OXFORD TEXTBOOK OF
MEDICINE

OXFORD MEDICAL PUBLICATIONS

OXFORD TEXTBOOK OF
MEDICINE

THIRD EDITION

VOLUME 3
Sections 18–33 and Index

Edited by

D. J. Weatherall

Regius Professor of Medicine, University of Oxford;
Honorary Director, Institute of Molecular Medicine, Oxford

J. G. G. Ledingham

Clinical Professor and May Reader in Medicine,
Nuffield Department of Clinical Medicine, University of Oxford

D. A. Warrell

Professor of Tropical Medicine and Infectious Diseases,
Nuffield Department of Clinical Medicine, University of Oxford

Oxford   New York   Tokyo
OXFORD UNIVERSITY PRESS
1996

Oxford University Press, Walton Street, Oxford OX2 6DP

Oxford   New York
Athens   Auckland   Bangkok   Bombay
Calcutta   Cape Town   Dar es Salaam   Delhi
Florence   Hong Kong   Istanbul   Karachi
Kuala Lumpur   Madras   Madrid   Melbourne
Mexico City   Nairobi   Paris   Singapore
Taipei   Tokyo   Toronto
and associated companies in
Berlin Ibadan

Oxford is a trade mark of Oxford University Press

Published in the United States
by Oxford University Press Inc., New York

A catalogue record for this book is available from the British Library

Library of Congress Cataloging in Publication Data
(Data Available)

ISBN 0 19 262140 8 (Three volume set)
ISBN 0 19 262706 6 (vol 1)
ISBN 0 19 262707 4 (vol 2)
ISBN 0 19 262708 2 (vol 3)
Available as a three volume set only

Typeset by University Graphics Inc, New Jersey, USA
Printed in the United States of America

Preface to the Third Edition

As the third edition of the *Oxford Textbook of Medicine* begins to see the light of day, medical textbooks are having a bad press in Great Britain. The stimulus to the recent resurgence of the age-old argument about the educational value, or lack of it, of textbooks was a presentation to a House of Lords Select Committee that suggested that many patients are losing their lives because doctors rely on information obtained from outdated texts and clinical teaching based on archaic practice.

In the preface to the first edition of the *Textbook* we discussed the late Professor Mitchell's similarly jaundiced views on the value of medical textbooks. He had suggested that they were likely to suffer the same fate as dinosaurs in that their very weight would preclude survival (it is not just the medical sciences that need constant revision; this view of the reason for the extinction of the dinosaurs may also have to be modified!). He went on to say that textbooks were already out of date before they were published, and hence, as well as being a health hazard due to their weight, were of limited educational value to their readers. However, having had a few more years to ponder further on Professor Mitchell's forecasts, we remain largely unrepentant.

A number of factors have combined greatly to increase the complexity of medical practice over the relatively short timespan since this *Textbook* was first published. There has been a major revolution in the basic biological sciences that has enormous implications for clinical practice in the future. In the richer countries the mean age of the population has risen dramatically and hence the pattern of disease has become much more complex and multifactorial. The populations of the developing countries continue to expand and, if anything, malnutrition and infectious disease present an even more frightening problem than they did fifteen years ago. And the remarkable achievements of the basic biomedical sciences combined with the inability of the richer countries to contain the costs of health care, and the poorer ones to provide it, are raising many new ethical problems for doctors.

Set against this complex and rapidly changing scene what should be the objective of a textbook of medicine? Clearly, no student or practitioner can own a library of monographs and journals that covers the whole of internal medicine. One important function is to provide a sound basic account of the many disorders that comprise internal medicine and thus give the background to more recent advances that are best sought in specialist journals. Furthermore, as well as the greater complexity of the diseases of the richer countries, the increasing ease of international travel and the movements of massive refugee populations round the world mean that internal medicine today is truly global; diseases that once were restricted to tropical climates or particular countries can turn up in hospitals or consulting rooms anywhere in the world. It is clear, therefore, that some basic textbooks that give students and doctors a 'way in' to the literature on the bulk of the diseases that they are likely to encounter, common or rare, are still required. With this background in mind we have added a number of new chapters and topics to this edition and have had many of the previous ones completely rewritten. We have expanded some of the background chapters on the basic sciences, particularly for students and doctors in countries in which access to current literature in these fields is limited. We have introduced new sections on medical ethics, clinical trials and evidence-based medicine, forensic medicine, and related topics that are an important part of the modern medical scene. As in previous editions, we have attempted to provide a global view of internal medicine rather than describe it as it is seen in day-to-day practice in the richer industrialized countries. And because of the increasing evidence of the clinical value of the management of cancer by specialists in the field we have included a new section on clinical oncology as a background to the descriptions of malignant disease in individual sections.

We are well aware that parts of this book will rapidly date and hence it is important that students and practitioners continue to augment their reading with up-to-date journals, and refresh themselves by regular visits to postgraduate meetings. Information systems and related technology are rapidly changing the face of communication in medicine and readers should avail themselves of every opportunity of learning the complexities and potentials of this rapidly evolving branch of practice.

As before we are particularly grateful to those of our colleagues who helped in the planning of particular sections: Dr J.A. Vale (poisoning by drugs and chemicals); Dr E. Hodgson and Professor J.M. Harrington (occupational and environmental health and safety); Dr R.W.E. Watts (metabolic disorders); Professor Alan McGregor (endocrine disorders); Professor C. Redman (medical disorders of pregnancy); Dr Derek Jewell, Dr Margaret Bassendine, and Professor Sir Leslie Turnberg (gastroenterology); Professor Stuart Cobbe (cardiovascular disorders); Drs Julian Hopkin and Donald Lane (respiratory medicine); Professor M.W. Adler (sexually-transmitted diseases and sexual health); Professor Paul Dieppe (rheumatology); Professors John Goldman and Sam Machin (disorders of the blood); Drs J. Strang, I. Glass, and M. Farrell (alcohol and drug-related problems); Professor J. Newsom-Davis (neurology and disorders of voluntary muscle). The section on Psychiatry was organized and edited by Professor Michael Gelder.

We wish to thank Dr Irene Butcher who has edited this edition of the *Textbook*; her forbearance with its editors, some of its more errant authors, and Oxford University Press has, at times, bordered on the saintly. We also thank Mrs Pam Herridge for invaluable editorial work. Finally, we are particularly grateful to our personal secretaries who have stayed the course with us through yet another phase of this saga, Mrs Janet Watt, Mrs Maureen Stacey, and Miss Eunice Berry.

Oxford
April 1995

D.J. WEATHERALL
J.G.G. LEDINGHAM
D.A. WARRELL

Summary of Contents

Volume 1

Volume 2

Volume 3

Contents

Volume 1

Volume 2

Volume 3

Contributors

P. AABY
Senior Researcher, Statens Seruminstitut, Copenhagen, Denmark
7.10.2 Measles

J.P. ACKERS
Senior Lecturer, Department of Medical Parasitology, London School of Hygiene and Tropical Medicine, London, UK
7.13.13 Trichomoniasis

A.A. ADISH
% McGill Community Health Project, Addis Ababa, Ethiopia
8.5.5(h) Podoconiosis (non-filarial endemic elephantiasis of the lower legs)

M.W. ADLER
Professor of Genito-Urinary Medicine, Academic Department of Genito-Urinary Medicine, University College London Medical School, UK
21.1 Sexually transmitted diseases and sexual health

D. ADU
Consultant Nephrologist, Queen Elizabeth Hospital, Birmingham, UK
20.4.2 Idiopathic glomerulonephritis
20.5.2 Infections and associated nephropathies

M.P. ALPERS
Director, Papua New Guinea Institute of Medical Research, Goroka, Papua New Guinea
24.7.5 Kuru

P.D. ANDERSON
Consultant, World Health Organization Regional Office for Europe, Copenhagen, Denmark
28.2.1 Alcohol and drug-related problems: screening and brief intervention

H. ANNETT
Head, Health Department, Secretariat de Son Altesse l'Aga Khan, Aiglemont, Gouvieux, France
3.4 Health care in developing countries

J.K. ARONSON
Clinical Reader in Clinical Pharmacology, University of Oxford; Honorary Consultant Physician, Anglia and Oxfordshire Health Authority, Oxford, UK
9 Principles of clinical pharmacology and drug therapy

A.W. ASSCHER
Principal, St George's Hospital Medical School, University of London, UK
20.9.4 Balkan (endemic) nephropathy and irradiation nephritis

TAR-CHING AW
Senior Lecturer in Occupational Medicine, Institute of Occupational Health, University of Birmingham, UK
8.3.6 Poisoning from metals
8.5.5(k) Environmental factors and disease: vibration

J.G. AYRES
Consultant Respiratory Physician, Heartlands Hospital, Birmingham, UK
8.5.5(l) Environmental factors and disease: air pollution

R.R. BAILEY
Nephrologist, Christchurch Hospital, New Zealand
20.8.1 Urinary tract infection
20.8.2 Vesicoureteric reflux and reflux nephropathy

M.J. BAINES
Consultant Physician, St Christopher's Hospice, London, UK
32 Terminal illness

E.L. BAKER
Centers for Disease Control and Prevention, Atlanta, Georgia, USA
8.5.3(d) The main occupational diseases: neurological disorders

L.R.I. BAKER
Consultant Physician and Nephrologist, St Bartholomew's Hospital, London, UK
20.10 Urinary-tract obstruction
20.15 Genitourinary tuberculosis

J.E. BANATVALA
Professor of Clinical Virology, United Medical and Dental Schools of Guy's and St Thomas's Hospital, St Thomas's Campus, London, UK
13.12.1 Viral infections in pregnancy

C.R.M. BANGHAM
Consultant Virologist, John Radcliffe Hospital, Oxford, UK
7.10.31 HTLV-I and -II associated diseases

SIR ROGER BANNISTER
Honorary Consultant Neurologist, The National Hospital for Neurology and Neurosurgery, London, and Oxford Regional and District Health Authority, UK
24.3.7 The autonomic nervous system

K.M. BANNISTER
Senior Consultant, Renal Unit and Department of Nuclear Medicine, Royal Adelaide Hospital, South Australia
20.1 Clinical physiology of the kidney: tests of renal function and structure

D. BARLOW
Consultant Physician, Department of Genitourinary Medicine, St Thomas's Hospital, London, UK
7.11.6 Neisseria gonorrhoeae

A.J. BARRETT
Chief, Bone Marrow Transplant Unit, National Heart, Lung, and Blood Institute, National Institutes of Health, Bethesda, Maryland, USA
22.3.3 Acute myeloblastic leukaemia

C. BASS

Consultant in Liaison Psychiatry, John Radcliffe Hospital, Oxford, UK
27.3.1 Psychological factors and the presentation and course of illness

M.F. BASSENDINE

Professor of Hepatology, Department of Medicine, The Medical School, University of Newcastle; Consultant Physician, Freeman Hospital, Newcastle upon Tyne, UK
14.27.2 Primary biliary cirrhosis

P.J. BAXTER

Consultant Occupational Physician, University of Cambridge and Addenbrooke's Hospital, Cambridge, UK
8.5.5(m) Environmental factors and disease: environmental disasters

M.A.H. BAYLES

Senior Specialist and Senior Lecturer, Department of Dermatology, King Edward VIII Hospital and Medical School, University of Natal, Durban, South Africa
7.12.3 Chromoblastomycosis

P.H. BAYLIS

Professor of Experimental Medicine, University of Newcastle upon Tyne; Consultant Physician, Royal Victoria Infirmary, Newcastle upon Tyne, UK
12.3 The posterior pituitary
20.2.1 Water and sodium homeostasis and their disorders

J.I. BELL

Nuffield Professor of Clinical Medicine, John Radcliffe Hospital, University of Oxford; Consultant Physician in General Medicine, Oxford Radcliffe NHS Trust, UK
5.2 Immune mechanisms of disease
11.11 Diabetes mellitus

E.J. BELL*

Regional Virus Laboratory, Ruchill Hospital, Glasgow, UK
7.10.13 Enteroviruses

M.K. BENSON

Consultant Chest Physician, Osler Chest Unit, The Churchill Hospital, Oxford, UK
17.11 Pleural disease
17.13.2 Pleural tumours
17.13.3 Mediastinal tumours and cysts

V. BERAL

Director, Imperial Cancer Research Fund's Cancer Epidemiology Unit, Oxford, UK
21.8 Cervical cancer and other cancers caused by sexually transmitted infections

R.J. BERRY

Director, Westlakes Research Institute, Moor Row, Cumbria, UK
8.5.5(i) Environmental factors and disease: radiation

* It is with regret that we report the deaths of those authors marked with an asterisk. Although their deaths occurred between the appearance of the second edition and preparation of the third edition, much of their contribution to the former has been incorporated into this edition, with appropriate updating from their coauthors.

P.C.L. BEVERLEY

Professor of Tumour Immunology and Staff Member of the Imperial Cancer Research Fund, University College London Medical School, UK
6.4 Tumour immunology

C.M. BLACK

Professor of Rheumatology, Royal Free Hospital and School of Medicine, University of London, UK
18.11.1 Connective tissue disorders and vasculitis—introduction
18.11.4 Systemic sclerosis

S.R. BLOOM

Professor of Endocrinology, Royal Postgraduate Medical School, Hammersmith Hospital, London, UK
12.10 Non-diabetic pancreatic endocrine disorders and multiple endocrine neoplasia
14.8 Hormones and the gastrointestinal tract

L.D. BLUMHARDT

Professor of Clinical Neurology, University of Nottingham; Consultant Neurologist, University Hospital, Queen's Medical Centre, Nottingham, UK
24.4.2 Syncope

N.A. BOON

Consultant Cardiologist, Royal Infirmary of Edinburgh, UK
15.14.2 HIV-related heart muscle disease
15.28.3 Coarctation of the aorta as a cause of secondary hypertension in the adult

R.T. BOOTH

Professor of Safety and Health, Health and Safety Unit, Aston University, Birmingham, UK
8.5.4 Occupational safety

I.C.G. BOWLER

Consultant Microbiologist, Oxford Regional Public Health Laboratory, John Radcliffe Hospital, Oxford, UK
7.9 Nosocomial infection

D. BRADLEY

Professor of Tropical Hygiene, London School of Hygiene and Tropical Medicine, University of London, UK
7.13.2 Malaria

R.D. BRADLEY

Emeritus Professor of Intensive Care Medicine, St Thomas's Hospital, London, UK
16 Intensive care

D.P. BRENTON

Reader in Inherited Metabolic Diseases, Department of Medicine, University of College London School of Medicine, UK
11.3 Inborn errors of amino acid and organic acid metabolism

R.P. BRETTLE

Consultant Physician and Part-time Senior Lecturer, Regional Infectious Disease Unit, City Hospital, Edinburgh, UK
28.3.1 Complications of drug use, particularly injecting drug use

V. BROADBENT
Consultant Paediatric Oncologist, Addenbrooke's Hospital, Cambridge, UK
22.5.6 The histiocytoses

M. BROWN
Professor of Clinical Pharmacology, University of Cambridge; Honorary Consultant Physician, Addenbrooke's Hospital, Cambridge, UK
15.28.2 Phaeochromocytoma

A.D.M. BRYCESON
Consultant Physician, Hospital for Tropical Diseases, London
7.13.12 Leishmaniasis

C. BUNCH
Medical Director, Oxford Radcliffe Hospital NHS Trust, John Radcliffe Hospital, Oxford, UK
22.5.2 Introduction to the lymphoproliferative disorders
22.5.3 The lymphomas
22.8.2 Marrow transplantation

DANAI BUNNAG
Professor Emeritus, Clinical Tropical Medicine, Mahidol University, Bangkok, Thailand
7.16.2 Liver fluke diseases of humans

W. BURGDORFER
Scientist Emeritus, Laboratory of Vectors and Pathogens, National Institutes of Health, Rocky Mountain Laboratories, Hamilton, Montana, USA
7.11.30 Lyme disease

A.K. BURROUGHS
Consultant Physician and Hepatologist, Liver Transplantation and Hepato-biliary Medicine, Royal Free Hospital, London, UK
14.29 Cirrhosis, portal hypertension, and ascites

T. BUTLER
Professor of Internal Medicine and of Microbiology and Immunology, Texas Technical University, Health Sciences Center; Attending Physician, University Medical Center, Lubbock, USA
7.11.6 Plague

A.E. BUTTERWORTH
Medical Research Council External Scientific Staff and Honorary Professor of Medical Parasitology, Department of Pathology, University of Cambridge, UK
7.16.1 Schistosomiasis

F.I. CAIRD
Formerly David Cargill Professor of Geriatric Medicine, University of Glasgow, UK
31 Medicine in old age

J.S. CAMERON
Professor of Renal Medicine, United Medical and Dental Schools, Guy's Campus, London, UK
20.3 Common presentations of renal disease
20.5.6 Rheumatological disorders and the kidney
20.9.2 Gout, purines, and interstitial nephritis

D.M. CAMPBELL
Senior Lecturer in Obstetrics and Gynaecology and Reproductive Physiology, University of Aberdeen, UK
13.11 Nutrition in pregnancy

M.J. CARDOSA
Lecturer, School of Pharmaceutical Sciences, Universiti Sains Malaysia, Penang, Malaysia
7.10.20 Dengue haemorrhagic fever

D.J.S. CARMICHAEL
Consultant Nephrologist, Southend Health Care NHS Trust, Essex, UK
20.14 Drugs and the kidney

J. CARMICHAEL
J.B. Cochrane Professor of Clinical Oncology, University of Nottingham, UK
6.8. New approaches to cancer therapy

C.C.J. CARPENTER
Professor of Medicine, Brown University, Providence, Rhode Island, USA
7.11.11 Cholera

R.W. CARRELL
Professor of Haematology, University of Cambridge, Addenbrooke's Hospital, Cambridge, UK
11.15 α_1-Antitrypsin deficiency

D.P. CASEMORE
Clinical Scientist, PHLS Cryptosporidium Reference Unit, Glan Clwyd District General Hospital, Bodelwyddan, Clwyd, UK
7.13.5 Cryptosporidium and cryptosporidiosis
7.13.6 Cyclospora

A. CASSELS
Independent Health Systems Development Consultant, Chilham, Canterbury, Kent, UK
3.4 Health care in developing countries

D. CATOVSKY
Professor of Haematology, Institute of Cancer Research and Royal Marsden Hospital, London, UK
22.3.2 The classification of leukaemia
22.3.6 Chronic lymphocytic leukaemia and other leukaemias of mature B and T cells
22.3.7 Myelodysplastic syndromes

D.A. CHAMBERLAIN
Consultant Cardiologist, Royal Sussex County Hospital, Brighton: Senior Visiting Research Fellow, University of Sussex, UK
15.6.2 Digitalis

H.M. CHAPEL
Consultant Immunologist and Senior Clinical Lecturer, John Radcliffe Hospital, Oxford, UK
5.4 Complement and disease

L.E. CHAPMAN

Supervising Medical Epidemiologist, Division of Viral and Rickettsial Diseases, National Center for Infectious Diseases, Center for Disease Control, Atlanta, Georgia, USA
7.10.5 Human infections caused by simian herpesviruses

R.W. CHAPMAN

Consultant Gastroenterologist, John Radcliffe Hospital, Oxford, UK
14.27.3 Primary sclerosing cholangitis

SEUNG-YULL CHO

Professor of Parasitology, College of Medicine, Chung-Ang University, Seoul, Korea
7.15.4 Diphyllobothriasis and sparganosis

A.B. CHRISTIE*

Honorary Consultant, Fazakerley Hospital, Liverpool, UK
7.10.11 Mumps: epidemic parotitis
7.11.1 Diphtheria
7.11.18 Anthrax

M.L. CLARK

Senior Lecturer, St Bartholomew's Hospital Medical College, London, UK
14.16 Tumours of the gastrointestinal tract

A.R. CLARKSON

Associate Professor of Medicine, University of Adelaide; Director, Renal Unit, Royal Adelaide Hospital, Australia
20.4.1 IgA nephropathy, Henoch-Schönlein purpura, and thin membrane nephropathy

SIR CECIL CLOTHIER

Formerly Parliamentary Commissioner for Administration and Health Service Commissioner for England and Wales, and Scotland
1 On being a patient

A.J.S. COATS

Senior Lecturer and Honorary Consultant Cardiologist, Royal Brompton Hospital, London, UK
15.5 The syndrome of heart failure

S.M. COBBE

Professor of Medical Cardiology, University of Glasgow, Glasgow Royal Infirmary, UK
15.8.1 Cardiac arrhythmias

J. COHEN

Professor of Infectious Diseases and Bacteriology, Royal Postgraduate Medical School, Hammersmith Hospital, London, UK
7.19.3 Infection in the immunocompromised host

R.D. COHEN

Professor of Medicine, The London Hospital Medical College, University of London, UK
11.14 Disturbances of acid-base homeostasis
20.19.1 The renal tubular acidoses

J. COLLINGE

Wellcome Senior Research Fellow in the Clinical Sciences and Honorary Consultant in Neurology and Molecular Genetics, St Mary's Hospital Medical School, Imperial College London, UK
24.7.4 Prion diseases

R. COLLINS

British Heart Foundation Research Fellow and Co-ordinator, Clinical Trial Service Unit, Nuffield Department of Clinical Medicine, University of Oxford, UK
2.4 Large-scale randomized evidence: trials and overviews

G. COLMAN

Formerly Consultant Microbiologist, Division of Hospital Infection, Central Public Health Laboratory, Colindale, London, UK
7.11.2 Pathogenic streptococci

D.A.S. COMPSTON

Professor of Neurology, University of Cambridge, UK
24.9 Demyelinating disorders of the central nervous system

C.P. CONLON

Consultant Physician, Infectious Diseases Unit, Nuffield Department of Medicine, John Radcliffe Hospital, Oxford, UK
7.8 Travel and expedition medicine
7.10.29 HIV infection and AIDS
14.18 Gastrointestinal infections

M. CONTRERAS

Chief Executive and Medical Director, North London Blood Transfusion Centre, London, UK
22.4.13 Acquired haemolytic anaemia

M.R. COOPER

Formerly Commonwealth Bureau of Animal Health, Central Veterinary Laboratory, Addlestone, Surrey, UK
8.4.2 Poisonous plants and fungi

J. COUVREUR

Associate Professor of Paediatrics, Hôpital Trousseau, Paris, France
7.13.4 Toxoplasmosis

P.J. COWEN

Medical Research Council Clinical Scientist, University Department of Psychiatry, Littlemore Hospital, Oxford, UK
27.4.1 Psychopharmacology in medical practice

T.M. COX

Professor of Medicine, University of Cambridge, and Honorary Consultant Physician, Addenbrooke's Hospital, Cambridge, UK
11.2.1 Glycogen storage diseases
11.2.2 Inborn errors of fructose metabolism
11.2.3 Disorders of galactose metabolism
14.9.5 Disaccharidase deficiency

W.I. CRANSTON

Emeritus Professor of Medicine, United Medical and Dental Schools, St Thomas's Hospital, London, UK
8.5.5(b) Environmental factors and disease: drug-induced increases of body temperature

D.H. CRAWFORD

Professor of Microbiology, London School of Hygiene and Tropical Medicine, UK
7.10.4 The Epstein-Barr virus

P. CREAMER
Senior Registrar in Rheumatology, Bristol Royal Infirmary, UK
18.3 Rheumatology: use and abuse of investigations

I.B. CROME
Consultant Psychiatrist, Keele, Staffordshire, UK
28.1.2 Assessing substance use and misuse
28.1.3 Diagnoses and classifications: substance problems and dependence—what is the difference?
28.3.2 The management of substance-related problems in a general ward

D.W.M. CROOK
Consultant Microbiologist, Public Health Laboratory, John Radcliffe Hospital, Oxford, UK
7.9 Nosocomial infection
15.17 Infective endocarditis
15.21 Cardiovascular syphilis
17.6.3 Microbiological methods in the diagnosis of respiratory infections
24.15.1 Bacterial meningitis

G.W. CSONKA
Consultant Physician in Genitourinary Medicine (retired), Charing Cross Hospital, London, UK
7.11.34 Syphilis

J. CUNNINGHAM
Consultant Physician and Honorary Senior Lecturer in Nephrology, Royal London Hospital and Medical College, London, UK
20.19 Renal tubular disorders

SIR JOHN DACIE
Emeritus Professor of Haematology, Royal Postgraduate Medical School, University of London, UK
22.3.12 Paroxysmal nocturnal haemoglobinuria

D.A.B. DANCE
Director/Consultant Microbiologist, Public Health Laboratory, Derriford Hospital, Plymouth, Devon, UK
7.11.15 Melioidosis and glanders

J.H. DARGIE
Consultant Cardiologist, Western Infirmary, Glasgow, UK
15.6.3 Vasodilators

J.H. DARK
Consultant Cardiothoracic Surgeon, Freeman Hospital, Newcastle upon Tyne, UK
15.7 Cardiac transplantation

P.G. DAVEY
Reader in Clinical Pharmacology and Infectious Diseases, Ninewells Hospital and Medical School, Dundee, UK
7.6 Antimicrobial chemotherapy

M.J. DAVIES
BHF Professor of Cardiovascular Pathology, St George's Hospital Medical School, University of London, UK
15.10.2 The pathology of ischaemic heart disease

S.W. DAVIES
Consultant Cardiologist, The Royal Brompton Hospital, London, UK
15.3.1 Breathlessness
15.3.4 Fatigue

P.D.O DAVIES
Consultant Respiratory Physician, Cardiothoracic Centre and Aintree Hospital NHS Trust, Liverpool, UK
7.11.22 Tuberculosis
7.11.24 Disease caused by environmental bacteria

A.M. DAVISON
Consultant Renal Physician, St James's University Hospital, Leeds, UK
20.5.4 Renal manifestations of malignant disease
20.5.5 Sarcoid and the kidney

P.T. DAWES
Consultant Rheumatologist, Staffordshire Rheumatology Centre; Senior Lecturer, University of Keele, Staffordshire, UK
18.2 Rheumatology: clinical presentation and diagnosis

K. DAWKINS
Consultant Cardiologist and Clinical Services Manager, Wessex Cardiothoracic Centre, Southampton General Hospital, UK
15.4.7 Exercise testing

D.P. DE BONO
British Heart Foundation Professor of Cardiology, University of Leicester Medical School, UK
15.10.5 Coronary angioplasty

M. DE SWIET
Consultant Physician, Queen Charlotte's Hospital for Women and University College Hospital, London and Northwick Park Hospital, Harrow, Middlesex, UK
13.5 Thromboembolism in pregnancy
13.6 Chest diseases in pregnancy

D.M. DENISON
Professor and Director, Lung Function Unit, Royal Bromptom Hospital, London, UK
8.5.5(e) Environmental factors and disease: aerospace medicine
8.5.5(f) Environmental factors and disease: diving medicine

J. DENT
Gastroenterology Unit, Royal Adelaide Hospital, South Australia
14.2.1 Dysphagia and other symptoms in oesophageal disease
14.6 Diseases of the oesophagus

R. DICK
Consultant Radiologist, Royal Free Hospital Trust, London, UK
14.20.1 Computed tomography and magnetic resonance imaging of the liver and pancreas

P. DIEPPE
ARC Professor of Rheumatology, Bristol University, UK
18.1 Rheumatology: introduction
18.3 Rheumatology: use and abuse of investigations

M. DOHERTY
Reader in Rheumatology, University of Nottingham Medical School, Rheumatology Unit, City Hospital, Nottingham, UK
18.7 Crystal-related arthropathies

SIR RICHARD DOLL
Honorary Consultant, Imperial Cancer Research Fund, Radcliffe Infirmary, Oxford, UK
6.2. Epidemiology of cancer

M. DONAGHY

Clinical Reader in Neurology, University of Oxford; Consultant Neurologist, Radcliffe Infirmary, Oxford, UK
24.1 Neurology: introduction
24.16 The motor neurone diseases

S. DOVER

Senior Registrar in Medicine and Gastroenterology, Fazakerley Hospital, Liverpool, UK
11.5 Porphyrin metabolism and the porphyrias

R.H. DOWLING

Professor of Gastroenterology, United Medical Schools of St Thomas's and Guy's Hospitals, Guy's Campus, London, UK
14.9.3 Small-bowel bacterial overgrowth

R.M. DU BOIS

Consultant Physician, Royal Brompton Hospital and Honorary Senior Lecturer, National Heart and Lung Institute, London, UK
17.10.1 Alveolar and interstitial disease: introduction
17.10.2 Cryptogenic fibrosing alveolitis

C.R.K. DUDLEY

Consultant Nephrologist, The Richard Bright Renal Unit, Southmead Hospital, Bristol, UK
15.12 Cholesterol embolism

B.O.L. DUKE

River Blindness Foundation, Lancaster, UK
7.14.1 General principles of filarial infections and diseases

M.S. DUNNILL

Fellow of Merton College, Sometime Consultant Histopathologist, John Radcliffe Hospital, Oxford, UK
17.6.5 Histopathology and cytology in diagnosis of lung disease

G.R. DUNSTAN

Professor Emeritus of Moral and Social Theology, University of London; Honorary Research Fellow, University of Exeter, UK
2.2. Medical ethics

D.T. DURACK

Consulting Professor of Medicine, Duke University Medical Center, Durham, North Carolina, USA
7.19.1 Fever of unknown origin

S.R. DURHAM

Senior Lecturer and Honorary Consultant Physician, Royal Brompton Hospital, London, UK
17.8.1 Allergic rhinitis ('hay fever')

B.G.M. DURIE

Division of Hematology/Oncology, Department of Medicine, Cedars-Sinai Medical Center, Los Angeles, California, USA
22.5.5 Myeloma and other paraproteinaemias

P.N. DURRINGTON

Reader in Medicine, University of Manchester Department of Medicine, Manchester Royal Infirmary, Chester, UK
11.6 Lipid and lipoprotein disorders

G.M. DUSHEIKO

Reader in Medicine, Royal Free Hospital and School of Medicine, London, UK
14.33 Hepatic granulomas

C.J. EASTMOND

Consultant Physician, Department of Rheumatology, Aberdeen Royal Infirmary, UK
18.5 Seronegative spondarthropathies

S. EBER

Professor of Paediatrics, Universitäts-Kinderklinik, Göttingen, Germany
22.4.10 Genetic disorders of the red cell membrane

A.L.W.F. EDDLESTON

Professor of Liver Immunology and Dean of Clinical Medicine, King's College School of Medicine and Dentistry, London, UK
14.27.1 Autoimmune hepatitis

C.R.W. EDWARDS

Professor of Clinical Medicine, University of Edinburgh, UK
12.7.1 Adrenocortical diseases

G. EDWARDS

Emeritus Professor of Addiction Behaviour, National Addiction Centre, University of London, UK
28.1.1 Drug problems as every doctor's business

A.M. EL NAHAS

Consultant Renal Physician, Sheffield Kidney Institute, Northern General Hospital, Shefffield, UK
20.17.1 Chronic renal failure

M. ELIA

Head of Clinical Nutrition Group, MRC, Dunn Clinical Nutrition Centre; Honorary Consultant Physician, Addenbrooke's Hospital, Cambridge, UK
10.6 Special nutritional problems and the use of enteral and parenteral nutrition

M. ELIAKIM

Professor of Internal Medicine; Chairman, Department of Medicine, Bikur Cholim Hospital, Jerusalem, Israel
11.13.2 Recurrent polyserositis (familial Mediterranean fever, periodic disease)

E. ELIAS

Consultant Physician, Liver Unit, Queen Elizabeth Hospital, Birmingham, UK
14.25 Jaundice

C.M. ELLIOTT

Dean of Trinity Hall, Cambridge, UK
3.1 The diseases of gods: some newer threats to health

B.T. EMMERSON

Professor of Medicine, University of Queensland and Consultant Physician, Princess Alexandra Hospital, Brisbane, Australia
20.13 Toxic nephropathy

SIR ANTHONY EPSTEIN

Professor Emeritus of Pathology, University of Bristol; Fellow of Wolfson College, Oxford, UK
7.10.4 The Epstein–Barr virus

S.J. EYKYN

Reader (Honorary Consultant) in Clinical Microbiology, United Medical and Dental Schools, St Thomas's Hospital, London, UK
7.11.4 Staphylococci
7.11.4 Anaerobic bacteria

E.A. FAGAN

Senior Lecturer in Medicine, Royal Free Hospital School of Medicine and University College London Medical School, London
13.13 Liver and gastrointestinal disease in pregnancy

C.G. FAIRBURN

Wellcome Trust Senior Lecturer, Department of Psychiatry, University of Oxford, UK
10.4 Eating disorders
27.2.7 Psychiatric disorders as they concern the physician: eating disorders

M. FARRELL

Senior Lecturer/Consultant Psychiatrist, National Addiction Centre, the Maudsley Hospital, London, UK
28.1.2 Assessing substance use and misuse
28.2.2 Harm reduction
28.3.2 The management of substance-related problems in a general ward
28.3.8 Caring for the HIV-positive drug user

M.J.G. FARTHING

Professor of Gastroenterology and Honorary Consultant Physician, St Bartholomew's Hospital, London, UK
14.9.9 Malabsorption in the tropics

M.F. FIELD

Associate Professor of Medicine, University of Sydney, Concord Hospital, New South Wales, Australia
20.1 Clinical physiology of the kidney: tests of renal function and structure

J.D. FIRTH

Wellcome Fellow, Honorary Consultant Physician, Oxford, UK
15.3.3 Oedema
20.16 Acute renal failure

S. FISHER-HOCH

Department of Pathology, Aga Khan Hospital Medical School, Karachi, Pakistan
7.10.22 Arenaviruses

R.A. FISHMAN

Professor of Neurology, University of California, San Francisco, USA
24.2.6 Lumbar puncture

E. FITZSIMONS

Consultant and Senior Lecturer in Haematology, Monklands Hospital, Airdrie and Western Infirmary, Glasgow, UK
11.5 Porphyrin metabolism and the porphyrias

A.F. FLEMING

Professor of Haematology at Baragwanath Hospital, Soweto School of Pathology of the South African Institute for Medical Research and the University of the Witwatersrand, Soweto, South Africa
22.4.3 Anaemia as a world health problem

E.W.L. FLETCHER

Consultant Radiologist, John Radcliffe Hospital, Oxford, UK
14.3.2 Methods for investigation of gastrointestinal diseases: radiology

D. FLISER

Physician, Department of Internal Medicine, Division of Nephrology, University of Heidelberg, Germany
20.5.1 Diabetic nephropathy

P. FOËX

Nuffield Professor of Anaesthetics, University of Oxford, Radcliffe Infirmary, Oxford, UK
17.10.20 Adult respiratory distress syndrome

J.C. FORFAR

Consultant Physician, John Radcliffe Hospital, Oxford, UK
13.4 Heart disease in pregnancy
15.6.4 Catecholamines and the sympathetic nervous system

I. FOULDS

Senior Lecturer, Occupational Dermatology, Institute of Occupational Health, University of Birmingham, UK
8.5.3(a) Occupational dermatology

G.H. FOWLER

Reader in General Practice, University of Oxford; Honorary Director, Imperial Cancer Research Fund General Practice Research Group, Oxford, UK
3.3 Primary care

A.J. FREW

Senior Lecturer in Medicine, University Medicine, University of Southampton, UK
17.9.1(a) Asthma: basic mechanisms and pathophysiology

P. FRITH

Consultant Medical Ophthalmologist, University College Hospitals, London, UK
26 The eye in general medicine

H.R. GAMSU

Professor of Neonatology, King's College Hospital School of Medicine and Dentistry, University of London, UK
13.12.2 Bacterial, fungal, and protozoal infections in pregnancy and the newborn

D. GARDNER-MEDWIN

Consultant Paediatric Neurologist, Newcastle General Hospital, Newcastle upon Tyne, UK
24.18 Developmental abnormalities of the nervous system

C. GARRARD

Consultant Physician in Intensive Care, John Radcliffe Hospital, Oxford, UK
17.10.20 Adult respiratory distress syndrome
17.14.3(a) Acute respiratory failure: intensive care

J.S. GARROW

Professor of Human Nutrition, St Bartholomew's Hospital Medical College, University of London, UK
10.5 Obesity

D.H. GATH

Clinical Reader in Psychiatry, University Department of Psychiatry, Warneford Hospital, Oxford, UK
27.2.8 Affective disorders

K.C. GATTER

University Lecturer in Pathology, Department of Cellular Science, John Radcliffe Hospital, Oxford, UK
22.5.2 Introduction to the lymphoproliferative disorders
22.5.3 The lymphomas

M.G. Gelder

Handley Professor of Psychiatry, University of Oxford, UK
27.1 Psychiatry in medicine: introduction
27.2.1 Reactions to stressful events
27.2.2 Anxiety and obsessional disorders
27.2.3 Psychiatric conditions with physical complaints
27.2.4 Dissociative disorder
27.2.5 Malingering and factitious disorders
27.2.6 Personality and its disorders
27.2.9 Schizophrenia
27.4.2 Psychological treatment in medical practice

C. GERADA

Principal in General Practice, Hurley Clinic, Kennington, London, UK
28.3.6 The pregnancy drug abuser

A.H. GHODSE

Professor of Psychiatry and Director, Centre for Addiction Studies, St George's Hospital Medical School, University of London, UK
28.3.5 Drug misusers and addicts in accident and emergency

C.J. GIBSON

Professor of Respiratory Medicine, University of Newcastle upon Tyne and Consultant Physician, Freeman Hospital, Newcastle upon Tyne, UK
17.10.19 Drug-induced lung disease

D.G. GIBSON

Consultant Cardiologist, Royal Brompton Hospital, London, UK
15.18 Valve disease
15.20 Pericardial disease

A.M. GILES

Medical Laboratory Scientific Officer, Department of Clinical Biochemistry, John Radcliffe Hospital, Oxford, UK
33 Reference intervals for biochemical data

F.J. GILES

Assistant Professor, University of California at Los Angeles; Director, Myeloma Research and Treatment Center, Bone Marrow Transplantation Unit, Cedars-Sinai Medical Center, Los Angeles, California, USA
22.5.5 Myeloma and other paraproteinaemias

C.F. GILKS

Senior Lecturer and Consultant Physician, Liverpool School of Tropical Medicine, Liverpool, UK
7.10.30 Human immunodeficiency virus in the developing world

M.D.G. GILLMER

Honorary Lecturer, Nuffield Department of Obstetrics and Gynaecology, University of Oxford and Consultant Obstetrician and Gynaecologist, John Radcliffe Hospital, Oxford, UK
13.8 Diabetes in pregnancy

D.J. GIRLING

Clinical Coordinator, MRC Cancer Trials Office, Cambridge, UK
7.11.22 Tuberculosis
7.11.24 Disease caused by environmental mycobacteria

R. GOKAL

Consultant Nephrologist and Honarary Lecturer, Manchester Royal Infirmary, UK
20.17.2 Replacement therapy by dialysis

M.J. GOLDACRE

Consultant in Public Health Medicine, Anglia and Oxford Regional Health Authority, and Honorary Senior Clinical Lecturer in Public Health, University of Oxford, UK
3.2 Health and sickness in the community

M.H.N GOLDEN

Professor of Medicine (Nutrition), University of Aberdeen, UK
10.3 Severe malnutrition

S.J. GOLDING

Lecturer in Radiology, University of Oxford, UK
6.5 Medical imaging in oncology

J. GOLDMAN

Professor of Leukaemia Biology, Royal Postgraduate Medical School, Hammersmith Hospital, London, UK
22.3.5 Chronic myeloid leukaemia

S. GORDON

Glaxo Professor of Cellular Pathology, Sir William Dunn School of Pathology, University of Oxford, UK
4.2.3 The mononuclear phagocyte system and tissue homeostasis

E.C. GORDON-SMITH

Professor of Haematology, St George's Hospital Medical School, University of London, UK
22.3.11 Aplastic anaemia and other causes of bone marrow failure
22.4.11 Haemolysis due to red-cell enzyme deficiencies
22.4.13 Acquired haemolytic anaemia

M. GOSSOP

Head of Research, Drug Dependence Unit, National Addiction Centre, The Maudsley Hospital, London, UK
28.3.7 Management of pain in the drug abuser

J.M. GRANGE

Reader in Clinical Microbiology, National Heart and Lung Institute, University of London, UK
7.11.22 Tuberculosis
7.11.24 Disease caused by environmental mycobacteria

R. GRAY

Senior Research Fellow, Clinical Trial Service Unit, Nuffield Department of Clinical Medicine, University of Oxford, UK
2.4 Large-scale randomized evidence: trials and overviews

D.W.R. GRAY

Reader in Transplantation and Consultant Surgeon, Nuffield Department of Surgery, University of Oxford, UK
20.17.3 Renal transplantation

J.R. GRAYBILL

Professor of Medicine, University of Texas Health Science Center, San Antonio, USA
7.12.2 Coccidioidomycosis

M.F. GREAVES

Professor of Cell Biology and Director, Leukaemia Research Fund Centre at the Institute for Cancer Research, London, UK
22.3.1 Cell and molecular biology of leukaemia

M. GREAVES

Reader in Haematology, Central Sheffield University Hospital, UK
22.6.7 Thrombotic disease

B.M. GREENWOOD

Director, MRC Laboratories, Fajara, The Gambia
7.3 The host's response to infection
7.11.3 Pneumococcal infection
7.11.5 Meningococcal infection

R.J. GREENWOOD

Consultant Neurologist, St Bartholomew's and The National Hospitals for Neurology and Neurosurgery, London, UK
24.15.5 Neurosyphilis

B. GRIBBIN

Consultant Cardiologist, The John Radcliffe Hospital, Oxford, UK
15.17 Infective endocarditis
15.21 Cardiovascular syphilis

J. GRIMLEY EVANS

Professor of Clinical Geratology, University of Oxford, UK
31 Medicine in old age

N.R. GRIST

Emeritus Professor of Infectious Diseases, University of Glasgow; formerly Consultant Virologist, Head of Regional Virus Laboratory, Ruchill, Glasgow, UK
7.10.13 Enteroviruses

D.I. GROVE

Director of Clinical Microbiology and Infectious Diseases, The Queen Elizabeth Hospital, Woodville, South Australia
7.14.5 Nematode infections of lesser importance

D.J. GRUNDY

Consultant in Spinal Injuries, The Duke of Cornwall Spinal Treatment Centre, Salisbury District Hospital, UK
24.3.10 Spinal cord injury and the management of paraplegia

J.-P. GRÜNFELD

Professor of Nephrology, Necker Medical School, University René Descartes, Necker Hospital, Paris, France
20.5.3 Amyloid, myeloma, light chain deposition disease, fibrillary glomerulonephritis and cryoglobulinaemia
20.7 Clinical aspects of inherited renal disorders

W.J. GULLICK

Principal Scientist, Imperial Cancer Research Fund, Hammersmith Hospital, London, UK
6.3 Growth factors and oncogenes

H.H. GUNSON

Medical Director, National Blood Authority, Manchester, UK
22.8.1 Blood transfusion

M.R. HAENEY

Consultant Immunologist, Salford General Hospitals Trust, Salford, UK
14.4 Immune disorders of the gastrointestinal tract

A.M. HALLIDAY

Formerly Consultant in Clinical Neurophysiology, National Hospital for Neurology and Neurosurgery, London; Member of the External Staff of the Medical Research Council, UK
24.2.3 Evoked potentials

P.J. HAMMOND

Senior Registrar, St James's University Hospital, Leeds, West Yorkshire, UK
12.10 Non-diabetic pancreatic endocrine disorders and multiple endocrine neoplasia
14.8 Hormones and the gastrointestinal tract

D.M. HANSELL

Consultant Radiologist, Royal Brompton Hospital, London, UK
17.6.1 Thoracic imaging

A.E. HARDING

Professor of Clinical Neurology, Institute of Neurology; Consultant Neurologist, National Hospital for Neurology and Neurosurgery, London, UK
25.9 Mitochondrial myopathies and encephalomyopathies

KHUNYING TRANAKCHIT HARINASUTA

Professor of Tropical Medicine and Consultant, Faculty of Tropical Medicine, Mahidol University, Bangkok, Thailand
7.16.4 Intestinal trematodiasis

J.M. HARRINGTON

Professor of Occupational Health, University of Birmingham, UK
8.5.1 Occupational and environmental health and safety: general introduction
8.5.2 The investigation of occupational disease
8.5.3 The main occupational diseases. (b) Occupational cancer. (e) Cardiovascular system. (f) Genitourinary system

A.L. HARRIS

Imperial Cancer Research Fund Professor of Clinical Oncology, University of Oxford, ICRF Clinical Oncology Unit, Churchill Hospital, Oxford, UK
6.8 New approaches to cancer therapy
13.15 Malignant disease in pregnancy

SIR HENRY HARRIS

Regius Professor of Medicine Emeritus, University of Oxford
6.1 General characteristics of neoplasia

M.J.G. HARRISON

Professor in Clinical Neurology, University College London Medical School; Consultant Neurologist, Middlesex Hospital and the National Hospital, London, UK
24.4.4 Coma
24.21 Neurological complications of systemic diseases

C. HASLETT

Professor of Respiratory Medicine, Edinburgh University and Honorary Consultant Physician, Royal Infirmary, Edinburgh, UK
17.3.1 Non-immune defence mechanisms of the lung
17.3.2 Inflammation and the lung

I. HASLOCK

Consultant Rheumatologist, South Tees Acute Hospitals Trust; Visiting Professor of Clinical Bio-engineering, University of Durham, UK
18.8 Back pain and periarticular disease

D.A. HAWKINS

Consultant Physician in Genitourinary Medicine, Chelsea and Westminster Hospital, London, UK
28.2.3(b) Physical complications of drug abuse

K.E. HAWTON

Consultant Psychiatrist, University Department of Psychiatry, Warneford Hospital, Oxford, UK
27.3.4 Sexual problems associated with physical illness

R.J. HAY

Mary Dunhill Professor of Cutaneous Medicine, United Medical and Dental Schools, Guy's Hospital, London, UK
7.11.28 Nocardiosis
7.12.1 Fungal infections

B. HAZLEMAN

Consultant Rheumatologist, Addenbrooke's Hospital, Cambridge, UK
18.10 Miscellaneous conditions

A.H. HENDERSON

Professor of Cardiology, University of Wales College of Medicine, Cardiff, UK
15.3.2 Chest pain

D.J. HENDRICK

Consultant Physician and Honorary Senior Lecturer, Newcastle General Hospital, University of Newcastle upon Tyne, UK
17.10.8 Lymphocytic infiltrations of the lung
17.10.9 Extrinsic allergic alveolitis
17.10.12 Pulmonary alveolar proteinosis
17.10.13 Pulmonary amyloidosis
17.10.14 Lipoid (lipid) pneumonia
17.10.15 Pulmonary alveolar microlithiasis
17.10.21 Lung disorders in genetic syndromes

M.F. HEYWORTH

Associate Professor of Medicine, University of California; Staff Physician, Veterans Affairs Medical Center, San Francisco, USA
7.13.8 Giardiasis, balantidiasis, isosporiasis, and microsporidiosis

TRAN TINH HIEN

Clinical Research Unit, Centre for Tropical Diseases (Cho Quan Hospital), Ho Chi Minh City, Vietnam
7.11.1 Diphtheria

T.W. HIGENBOTTAM

Consultant Physician and Respiratory Physiologist, Papworth and Addenbrooke's Hospitals, Cambridge, UK
17.14.4 Lung and heart-lung transplantation

S.L. HILLIER

Research Associate Professor of Obstetrics and Gynecology, University of Washington, Seattle, USA
21.4 Vaginal discharge

D. HILTON-JONES

Consultant Neurologist, Radcliffe Infirmary, Oxford, and Milton Keynes General Hospital, UK
25.8 Metabolic and endocrine myopathies

T.D.R. HOCKADAY

Honorary Consultant Physician, Radcliffe Infirmary, Oxford, UK
11.11 Diabetes mellitus

J.R. HODGES

University Lecturer and Consultant Neurologist, University of Cambridge Clinical School, Addenbrooke's Hospital, Cambridge, UK
24.7.1 Dementia: introduction
24.7.3 Pick's disease (focal lobar atrophy)

H.J.F. HODGSON

Professor of Gastroenterology, Royal Postgraduate Medical School, London, UK
14.9.6 Whipple's disease
14.9.7 Short gut syndrome

E.S. HODGSON

Occupational Health Physician and Lecturer in Occupational Health, University of Oxford: Honorary Consultant Occupational Physician, Radcliffe Hospital, Oxford, UK
8.5.1 Occupational and environmental health and safety: general introduction
8.5.2 The investigation of occupational medicine
8.5.3 The main occupational diseases: (g) Gastrointestinal tract; (h) The haematopoietic system; (i) Infections

A.V. HOFFBRAND

Professor of Haematology, Royal Free Hospital, London, UK
22.4.6 Megaloblastic anaemia and miscellaneous deficiency anaemias

S.T. HOLGATE

MRC Clinical Professor of Immunopharmacology, Southampton General Hospital, UK
17.9.1(a) Asthma: basic mechanisms and pathophysiology

P. HOLLOWAY

Clinical Lecturer and Senior Registrar, Department of Clinical Biochemistry, John Radcliffe Hospital, Oxford, UK
33 Reference intervals for biochemical data

J.M. HOPKIN

Consultant Physician, John Radcliffe Hospital, UK
7.12.5 Pneumocystis carinii
17.1 Respiratory medicine: introduction
17.7.1 Upper respiratory tract infection
17.7.3 Suppurative pulmonary and pleural infections
17.7.4 Chronic specific infections
17.7.5 Respiratory infection in the immunosuppressed
17.10.3 Bronchiolitis obliterans
17.10.5 Pulmonary vasculitis and granulomatosis
17.10.17 Toxic gases and fumes
17.10.18 Radiation pneumonitis

A.P. HOPKINS

Director of the Research Unit, Royal College of Physicians: Consultant Neurologist, Royal Hospital NHS Trust, London, UK
24.4.1 Epilepsy in later childhood and adult life

J.A.C. HOPKIRK

Consultant Physician, King Edward VII Hospital, Midhurst, West Sussex, UK
8.5.5(e) Environmental factors and disease: aerospace medicine

A. HORWICH

Professor of Radiotherapy, Institute of Cancer Research, London University; Consultant in Clinical Oncology, Royal Marsden Hospital, London, UK
6.7 Role of radiotherapy in the treatment of cancer

I.A. HUGHES

Professor of Paediatrics, University of Cambridge, UK
12.7.3 Congenital adrenal hyperplasia

B.J. HUNT

Consultant/Honorary Senior Lecturer in Haematology, St Thomas's Hospital; Honorary Senior Lecturer in Cardiothoracic Surgery at The National Heart and Lung Hospital, London, UK
22.6.6 Acquired coagulation disorders

C.W. HUTTON

Consultant Rheumatologist, Mount Gould Hospital, Plymouth, UK
18.6 Osteoarthritis

C.W. IMRIE

Honorary Senior Lecturer, University of Glasgow; Consultant Surgeon, Royal Infirmary, Glasgow, UK
14.23.1 Acute pancreatitis

M. IRVING

Professor of Surgery, Hope Hospital (University of Manchester School of Medicine), Salford, UK
14.19 The peritoneum, omentum, and appendix

D. ISAACS

Head of Department of Immunology and Infectious Diseases, Royal Alexandra Hospital for Children, Sydney: Associate Professor, University of Sydney, Australia
7.7 Immunization
7.10.1 Respiratory tract viruses

P.G. ISAACSON

Professor of Morbid Anatomy, University College London Medical School, London, UK
14.9.8 Enteropathy-associated T-cell lymphoma

D.A. ISENBERG

Professor of Rheumatology, Bloomsbury Rheumatology Unit, The Middlesex Hospital, London, UK
18.11.3 Systemic lupus erythematosus and related disorders

I. ISHERWOOD

Emeritus Professor of Diagnostic Radiology, University of Manchester, UK
24.2.1. Principles of neuroradiology

K. ISHIKAWA

Director, Department of Internal Medicine, Higashi Nagahara Hospital, Osaka, Japan
15.13 Takayasu's disease

C.A. ISON

Lecturer in Medical Microbiology, St Mary's Hospital Medical School, London, UK
7.11.6 Neisseria gonorrhoeae

A. JACKSON

Senior Lecturer in Neuroradiology, University of Manchester, UK
24.2.1 Principles of neuroradiology

H.S. JACOBS

Professor of Reproductive Endocrinology, University College London Medical School; Consultant Physician, The Middlesex Hospital, London, UK
12.8.1 The ovary
12.8.3 The breast

R.J. JACOBY

Clinical Reader in Old Age Psychiatry, University of Oxford, UK
27.2.11 Mental disorders of old age

O.F.W. JAMES

Professor of Geriatric Medicine, University of Newcastle upon Tyne, UK
14.28 Alcoholic liver disease

W.P.T. JAMES

Professor and Director, Rowett Research Institute, Aberdeen, UK
10.1 Nutrition: introduction

J.L. JAMESON

C.F. Kettering Professor of Medicine, Northwestern University School of Medicine, Chicago, Illinois, USA
12.1 Principles of hormone action

B. JENNETT

Emeritus Professor of Neurosurgery, Institute of Neurological Science, Glasgow, UK
24.4.5 Brain death and the vegetative state

D.P. JEWELL

Consultant Physician, John Radcliffe Hospital; Clinical Lecturer, University of Oxford, UK
14.1 Gastroenterology: introduction
14.2.2 Vomiting
14.2.3 Abdominal pain
14.2.6 Gastrointestinal bleeding
14.3.1 Endoscopy
14.9.4 Coeliac disease
14.10 Crohn's disease
14.11 Ulcerative colitis
14.36 Miscellaneous disorders of the gastrointestinal tract and liver

A.R. JOHNS

Senior Lecturer, Division of Psychiatry of Addictive Behaviour, St George's Hospital Medical School, University of London, UK
28.3.4 Management of withdrawal syndromes

A.M. JOHNSON

Reader in Epidemiology, Academic Department of Genito-urinary Medicine, University College London Medical School, UK
21.2 Sexual behavior

A.W. JOHNSON

Formerly Commonwealth Bureau of Animal Health, Central Veterinary Laboratory, Addlestone, Surrey, UK
8.4.2 Poisonous animals and plants

P.J. JOHNSON

Institute of Liver Studies, King's College School of Medicine and Dentistry, London, UK
14.27.1 Autoimmune hepatitis

E.A. JONES

Chief of Hepatology, Department of Gastrointestinal and Liver Diseases, Academic Medical Centre, Amsterdam, The Netherlands
14.30 Hepatocellular failure

M. JOY

Consultant Cardiologist, St Peter's District General Hospital, Chertsey, Surrey, UK
15.10.7 Vocational aspects of coronary artery disease

R.W. JUBB

Consultant Rheumatologist, Selly Oak Hospital, Birmingham, UK
8.5.3(c) The main occupational diseases: musculoskeletal disorders

B.E. JUEL-JENSEN

Honorary Consultant Physician, Nuffield Department of Clinical Medicine, John Radcliffe, Hospital, Oxford, UK
7.10.2 Herpes simplex virus infections
7.10.3 Varicella-zoster virus infections: chickenpox and zoster
7.10.9 Orf
7.10.10 Molluscum contagiosum

J.A. KANIS

Professor in Human Metabolism and Clinical Biochemistry, University of Sheffield Medical School, UK
12.6 Disorders of calcium metabolism
20.18 Renal bone disease

TOMISAKU KAWASAKI

Director, Japan Kawasaki Disease Research Center, Tokyo, Japan
18.11.10 Kawasaki disease

W.R. KEATINGE

Professor of Physiology, Queen Mary and Westfield College, University of London
8.5.5 Environmental factors and disease: (a) heat; (c) Cold, drowning, and seasonal mortality

P.G.E. KENNEDY

Burton Professor of Neurology, University of Glasgow, UK
24.15.2 Acute viral infections of the central nervous system
24.15.3 Neurological manifestations of infections with human immunodeficiency virus type 1

S. KESHAV

Research Fellow, Sir William Dunn School of Pathology, University of Oxford, UK
4.2.4 Cytokines

M. KETTLEWELL

Consultant Surgeon, Oxford Radcliffe Trust; Fellow, Green College, Oxford, UK
14.14 Colonic diverticular disease

M. KING

Honorary Research Fellow, University of Leeds, UK
3.1 The diseases of gods: some newer threats to health

M.M. KLIKS

President and Director of Research, CTS Foundation, Honolulu, Hawaii, USA
7.14.3 Guinea-worm disease: human dracunculiasis

B. KNIGHT

Professor of Forensic Pathology, University of Wales College of Medicine, Cardiff, Wales, UK
29 Forensic medicine

R. KNIGHT

Associate Professor of Parasitology, Department of Medical Microbiology, Faculty of Medicine, Unity of Nairobi, Kenya
7.13.1 Amoebiasis
7.14.4 Strongyloidiasis, hookworm, and other gut cestodes
7.15.1 Gut cestodes

J.B. KURTZ

Consultant Virologist, John Radcliffe Hospital, Oxford, UK
7.11.36 Legionellosis and legionnaires' disease

H.P. LAMBERT

Emeritus Professor of Microbial Diseases, St George's Hospital Medical School, London; Visiting Professor, London School of Hygiene and Tropical Medicine, UK
7.1 Clinical approach to the patient with suspected infection

D.J. LANE

Consultant Chest Physician, Oxford Radcliffe Hospital, The Churchill, Oxford
17.1 Respiratory medicine: introduction
17.5 The clinical presentation of chest diseases
17.9.2 Cystic fibrosis
17.9.1(b) Asthma: clinical features and management
17.10.5 Pulmonary vasculitis and granulomatosis
17.10.6 Pulmonary haemorrhagic disorders
17.10.7 Pulmonary eosinophilia

H.E. LARSON

Consultant in Infectious Disease and General Medicine, Southborough, Massachusetts, USA
7.11.21 Botulism, gas gangrene, and clostridial gastrointestinal infections

N.F. LAWTON

Consultant Neurologist, Wessex Neurological Centre, Southampton General Hospital; Honorary Senior Lecturer, University of Southampton, UK
24.13 Benign intracranial hypertension

J.G.G. LEDINGHAM

May Reader in Medicine and Honorary Consultant Physician, John Radcliffe Hospital, Oxford, UK
13.3 Renal disease in pregnancy
15.3.3 Oedema
15.6.1 Diuretics
15.26 Pulmonary embolism
15.28.1 Renal and renovascular hypertension
15.29 Lymphoedema
20.20.2 Idiopathic oedema of women
20.20.3 Disorders of potassium metabolism
24.17.1 The POEMS syndrome

J.W. LeDUC

Medical Officer, Division of Communicable Diseases, World Health Organization, Geneva, Switzerland
7.10.21 Bunyaviridae

T. LEHNER

Head of Division of Immunology, United Medical and Dental Schools of Guy's and St Thomas's Hospital, Guy's Hospital, London
14.5 The mouth and salivary glands
18.11.8 Behçet's disease

G.G. LENNOX

Senior Lecturer in Clinical Neurology, University of Nottingham Medical School, UK
13.10 Neurological disease in pregnancy

E.A. LETSKY

Consultant Haematologist, Queen Charlotte's and Chelsea Hospitals, London, UK
13.9 Blood disorders in pregnancy

S.M. LEWIS

Emeritus Reader in Haematology, University of London; Senior Research Fellow, Department of Haematology, Royal Postgraduate Medical School, London, UK
22.5.4 The spleen and its disorders

D.C. LINCH

Professor of Haematology, University College London, UK
22.2.2 Stem-cell disorders

C.C. LINNEMANN JR.

Professor, Departments of Medicine and Pathology and Laboratory Medicine, University of Cincinnati, Ohio, USA
7.11.14 Bordetella

D. LIPKIN

Consultant Cardiologist, The Royal Free Hospital, London, UK
15.3.1 Breathlessness
15.3.4 Fatigue

W.A. LISHMAN

Emeritus Professor of Neuropsychiatry, Institute of Psychiatry, London, UK
27.3.3 Specific conditions giving rise to mental disorder

A. LLANOS-CUENTAS

Professor of Medicine and Public Health, Universidad Peruana Cayetano Heredia; Senior Research Assistant at Instituto de Medicina Tropical 'Alexander von Humboldt', Lima, Peru
7.11.45 Bartonellosis

C.M. LOCKWOOD

Wellcome Reader in the School of Clinical Medicine, Addenbrooke's Hospital, Cambridge, UK
18.11.3 Small-vessel vasculitis

S. LOGAN

Senior Lecturer in Paediatric Epidemiology, Institute of Child Health, London, UK
7.10.18 Rubella

D.A. LOMAS

Lecturer in Medicine/Honorary Consultant Respiratory Physician, University of Cambridge, UK
11.5. α_1-Antitypsin deficiency

M.S. LOSOWSKY

Professor of Medicine and Dean of the Faculty of Medicine, University of Leeds, UK
14.9.2 Investigation and differential diagnosis of malabsorption

P.F. LUDMAN

Senior Registrar in Cardiology, Papworth Hospital NHS Trust, Papworth Everard, Cambridgeshire, UK
15.4.5 Magnetic resonance and computed X-ray tomography

S.E. LUX

Professor of Pediatrics, Harvard Medical School; Chief, Division of Hematology/Oncology, Children's Hospital, Boston, Massachusetts, USA
22.4.10 Genetic disorders of the red-cell membrane

L. LUZZATTO

Professor of Haematology, Royal Postgraduate Medical School, Hammersmith Hospital, London, UK
22.3.12 Paroxysmal nocturnal haemoglobinuria
22.4.12 Glucose 6-phosphate dehydrogenase (G6PD) deficiency

D.C.W. MABEY

Professor of Communicable Diseases, London School of Hygiene and Tropical Medicine, UK
7.11.42 Chlamydial infections

J.T. MacFARLANE

Consultant Physician in General and Respiratory Medicine, City Hospital, Nottingham; Clinical Teacher, University of Nottingham, UK
7.11.36 Legionellosis and legionnaires' disease
17.7.2 Acute lower respiratory tract infections

B.B. MacGILLIVRAY

Physician in charge, Department of Clinical Neurophysiology, Royal Free Hospital; Consultant in Clinical Neurophysiology, National Hospitals for Neurology and Neurosurgery, London, UK
24.2.2 Electroencephalography

S.J. MACHIN

Professor of Haematology, University College London, UK
22.6.2 Introduction to disorders of haemostasis and coagulation
22.6.3 Purpura

D.W.R. MacKENZIE

Visiting Professor of Medical Mycology, London School of Hygiene and Tropical Medicine, UK
7.12.1 Fungal infections (mycoses)

I.J. MACKIE

Non-Clinical Lecturer in Haematology, University College London, UK
22.6.1 The biology of haemostasis and thrombosis
22.6.2 Introduction to disorders of haemostasis and coagulation

C.R. MADELEY

Professor of Clinical Virology, University of Newcastle upon Tyne, UK
7.10.14 Viruses in diarrhoea and vomiting

A. MADEN

Senior Lecturer in Forensic Psychiatry, The Institute of Psychiatry, London, UK
28.3.9 The needs of the alcohol/drug user in custody

M.M. MADKOUR

Consultant Physician, Military Hospital, Riyadh, Saudi Arabia
7.11.19 Brucellosis

C. MAGUIÑA-VARGAS

Professor of Medicine, Cayetano Heredia Peruvian University; Physician, Instituto Nacional de Salud; President, Instituto de Medicina Tropical 'Alexander von Humboldt', Lima, Peru
7.11.45 Bartonellosis

J.I. MANN

Professor in Human Nutrition and Medicine, University of Otago, Dunedin, New Zealand
10.7 Diseases of overnourished societies and the need for dietary change
15.10.1 Ischaemic heart disease: epidemiology and prevention

M.G. MARMOT

Professor of Epidemiology and Public Health, University College London, UK
15.10.1 Ischaemic heart disease; epidemiology and prevention

T.J. MARRIE

Professor of Medicine and Associate Professor of Microbiology, Dalhousie University; Active Staff Physician, Victoria General Hospital, Halifax, Nova Scotia, Canada
7.11.39 Coxiella burnetti infections (Q fever)

T.C. MARRS

Senior Medical Officer, Department of Health, London, UK
8.3.7 Poisoning by conflict

P.D. MARSDEN

Professor of Medicine, University of Brasilia, Brazil
7.13.11 American trypanosomiasis

C.D. MARSDEN

Professor and Head of Neurology, Institute of Neurology and the National Hospital for Neurology and Neurosurgery, London, UK
24.4.3 Narcolepsy and related sleep disorders
24.10 Movement disorders
24.19 Metabolic and deficiency disorders of the nervous system
24.20 Neurological disorders due to physical agents

V.J. MARTLEW

Chief Executive and Medical Director, National Blood Service: Mersey and North Wales, Liverpool, UK
22.8.1 Blood transfusion

A.D. MASON

Chief, Laboratory Division, US Army Institute of Surgical Research, Fort Sam Houston, Texas, USA
8.5.5(g) Environmental factors and disease: lightning and electric shock

W.B. MATTHEWS

Professor Emeritus of Clinical Neurology, University of Oxford, UK
24.3.2 The motor and sensory systems, midbrain, and brain-stem
24.3.9 Spinal cord

R.S. MAURICE-WILLIAMS

Consultant Neurosurgeon, The Royal Free Hospital, London, UK
24.3.11 Disorders of the spinal nerve roots

R.L. MAYNARD

Senior Medical Officer, Department of Health, UK
8.3.7 Poisoning in conflict

R.T. MAYON-WHITE

Consultant in Communicable Disease Control, Oxfordshire Health Authority, Oxford, UK
7.4 Epidemiology and public health

R.A. MAYOU

Clinical Reader in Psychiatry and Honorary Consultant, Warneford Hospital, Oxford, UK
27.2.10 Organic (cognitive) mental disorders
27.3.2 Emotional reactions in the bereaved and dying
27.4.3 Psychiatric emergencies

E. McCLOY

Medical Adviser to the Civil Service; Director, Civil Service Occupational Health Service, Edinburgh, UK
8.5.3 The main occupational diseases: reproductive system

K.E.L. McCOLL

Professor of Gastroenterology, University Department of Medicine and Therapeutics, Western Infirmary, Glasgow, UK
11.5 Porphyrin metabolism and the porphyrias

J.B. McCORMICK

Center for Bacterial and Mycotic Diseases, Centers for Disease Control, Atlanta, Georgia, USA
7.10.22 Arenaviruses

A.M. McGREGOR

Professor of Medicine, King's College School of Medicine, London, UK
12.4 The thyroid gland and disorders of thyroid function
13.7 Endocrine disease in pregnancy

N. McINTYRE

Professor of Medicine, Royal Free Hospital School of Medicine, London, UK
14.29 Cirrhosis, portal hypertension, and ascites

W.J. McKENNA

Professor of Cardiac Medicine, St George's Hospital Medical School, London, UK
15.14.1 The cardiomyopathies, myocarditis, and specific heart muscle disorders

A.J. McMICHAEL

MRC Clinical Research Professor of Immunology, Nuffield Department of Medicine, Institute of Molecular Medicine, Oxford, UK
5.1. Principles of immunology

A. McMILLAN

Consultant Physician, Department of Genito-urinary Medicine, Edinburgh Royal Infirmary, UK
21.6 Infections and other medical problems in homosexual men

T.W. MEADE

Director of MRC Epidemiology and Medical Care Unit and Professor of Epidemiology, Medical College of St Bartholomew's Hospital, London, UK
15.9.3 Haemostatic variables in ischaemic heart disease

A. MEHEUS

Professor of Epidemiology and Community Medicine, University of Antwerp, Belgium
21.1 Sexually transmitted diseases and sexual health

T.J. MEREDITH

Professor of Medicine and Pathology, School of Medicine, Vanderbilt University and Director, Center for Clinical Toxicology, Vanderbilt University Medical Center, Nashville, Tennessee, USA
8.1.1 Poisoning: introduction and epidemiology
8.1.2 Poisoning: clinical and metabolic features and general principles of management
8.2.1 Poisoning caused by analgesic drugs
8.2.2 Poisoning from antidepressants, hypnotics, antihistamines, anticonvulsants, and antiparkinsonian drugs
8.2.3 Poisoning from cardiovascular drugs
8.2.4 Poisoning caused by respiratory drugs
8.2.5 Poisoning caused by drugs acting on the gastrointestinal system
8.2.6 Poisoning by haematinics and vitamins
8.2.7 Poisoning by endocrine drugs
8.2.8 Poisoning from antimicrobials
8.2.10 Poisoning from drugs of abuse
8.2.11 Poisoning due to miscellaneous drugs
8.3.1 Poisoning from household products
8.3.2 Poisoning by alcohols and glycols
8.3.3 Poisoning by hydrocarbons and chlorofluorocarbons
8.3.4 Poisoning by inhalational agents
8.3.5 Poisoning due to corrosive substances

K.R. MILLS

University Lecturer and Consultant in Clinical Neurophysiology, The Radcliffe Infirmary, Oxford, UK
24.2.4 Investigation of central motor pathways: magnetic brain stimulation

A. MINDEL

Professor of Sexual Health Medicine, Universities of Sydney and New South Wales, Sydney, Australia
21.3 Genital herpes

S.A. MISBAH

Consultant Immunologist, Leeds General Infirmary; Senior Clinical Lecturer in Immunology, University of Leeds, UK
18.11.10 Cryoglobulinaemia

J.J. MISIEWICZ

Consultant Physician and Joint Director, Department of Gastroenterology and Nutrition, Central Middlesex Hospital, London, UK
14.7 Peptic ulceration

T.P. MONATH

Chief, Virology Division, USAMRIDD, Fort Detrick, Frederick, Maryland, USA
7.10.19 Flaviviruses

M.R. MOORE

Professor of Medicine, National Research Centre for Environmental Toxicology, University of Queensland, Australia
11.5 Porphyrin metabolism and the porphyrias

H.G. MORGAN

Professor of Mental Health, University of Bristol, Avon, UK
27.2.12 The patient who has attempted suicide

P.J. MORRIS

Nuffield Professor of Surgery and Director of the Oxford Transplant Centre, University of Oxford, John Radcliffe Hospital, Oxford, UK
5.5 Principles of transplantation immunology
15.11 Peripheral arterial disease

W.L. MORRISON

Consultant Cardiologist, Cardiothoracic Centre, Liverpool, UK
15.3.6 Cardiac cachexia

N.J.McC. MORTENSEN

Consultant Surgeon and Clinical Reader in Colorectal Surgery, John Radcliffe Hospital, Oxford, UK
14.14 Colonic diverticular disease

A.G. MOWAT

Honorary Senior Clinical Lecturer in Rheumatology, Oxford University; Consultant Rheumatologist, Nuffield Orthopaedic Centre, Oxford, UK
18.11.7 Polymyalgia rheumatica and giant-cell arteritis

J. MOXHAM

Professor of Thoracic Medicine, King's College Hospital, London, UK
17.14.1 Respiratory failure: definition and causes
17.14.3(b) Chronic respiratory failure

E.R. MOXON

Action Research Professor of Paediatrics, University of Oxford, UK
7.7 Immunization
7.11.12 Haemophilus influenzae

M.F. MUERS

Consultant Physician, Respiratory Unit, Regional Cardiothoracic Centre, Killingbeck Hospital, Leeds, UK
17.6.4 Diagnostic bronchoscopy and tissue biopsy

P.A. MURPHY

Professor of Medicine, Johns Hopkins University School of Medicine, Baltimore, Maryland, USA
7.5 Physiological changes in infected patients
7.19.2 Septicaemia

I.M. MURRAY-LYON

Consultant Gastroenterologist, Charing Cross Hospital, London, UK
14.32 Liver tumours

D.G. NATHAN

Robert A. Stranahan Professor of Pediatrics, Harvard Medical School, Boston, Massachusetts, USA
22.2.1 Stem cells and haematopoiesis

G. NEALE

Consultant Physician, Addenbrooke's Hospital, Cambridge, UK
14.17 Vascular and collagen disorders

G.H. NEILD

Professor of Nephrology, Institute of Urology and Nephrology, University College London Medical School, UK
20.6 Haemolytic uraemic syndrome

J. NEUBERGER

Consultant Physician, Queen Elizabeth Hospital, Birmingham, UK
14.34 Drugs and liver damage
14.35 The liver in systemic disease

J.M. NEUTZE

Chairman, Department of Cardiology, Green Lane Hospital, Auckland, New Zealand
15.16 The cardiac aspects of rheumatic fever

C.I. NEWBOLD

University Lecturer, University of Oxford, UK
7.13.2 Malaria

A.J. NEWMAN TAYLOR

Professor of Occupational and Environmental Medicine, National Heart and Lung Institute and Consultant Physician, Royal Brompton Hospital, London, UK
17.9.13 Occupational asthma

J. NEWSOM-DAVIS

Professor of Clinical Neurology, University of Oxford, Radcliffe Infirmary, Oxford, UK
24.1 Neurology: introduction
24.3.8 Respiratory problems in neurological disease
25.7 Disorders of neuromuscular transmission

S. NIGHTINGALE

Consultant Neurologist, Midland Centre for Neurosurgery and Neurology, West Midlands, UK
7.10.31 HTLV-I and -II associated diseases

SUCHITRA NIMMANNITYA

Consultant Paediatrician, Children's Hospital, Bangkok, Thailand
7.10.20 Dengue haemorrhagic fever

D.J. NOLAN

Consultant Radiologist, John Radcliffe Hospital, Oxford, UK
14.3.2 Methods for investigation of gastrointestinal disease: radiology

G. NUKI

Professor of Rheumatology, Department of Medicine, University of Edinburgh; Consultant Rheumatologist, Western General Hospital and Royal Infirmary of Edinburgh, UK
11.5 Disorders of purine and pyrimidine metabolism

R.E. O'HEHIR

Academic Head of Allergy and Clinical Immunology, St Mary's Hospital Medical School, London, UK
5.2 Immune mechanisms of disease

J.D. ORIEL

Formerly Consultant Physician in Genito-Urinary Medicine, University College Hospital, London, UK
21.7 Genital warts

D. OVERBOSCH

Consultant Physician, Department of Internal Medicine and Imported Tropical Medicine, Red Cross Hospital, The Hague, The Netherlands
7.15.3 Cysticercosis

S.M. OXBURY

Consultant Clinical Neuropsychologist, Radcliffe Infirmary, Oxford, UK
24.3.1 Disturbances of higher cerebral function

J.M. OXBURY

Consultant Neurologist, Radcliffe Infirmary, Oxford, UK
24.3.1 Disturbances of higher cerebral function

S. PARISH

Senior Research Fellow, Clinical Trial Service Unit, Nuffield Department of Clinical Medicine, University of Oxford, UK
2.4 Large-scale randomized evidence: trials and overviews

J.R. PATTISON

Professor of Medical Microbiology, University College London Medical School, UK
7.10.25 Parvoviruses

J. PAUL

Senior Registrar, Public Health Laboratory, John Radcliffe Hospital, Oxford, UK
7.11.46 'Newer' and lesser known bacteria causing infection in humans
7.17 Non-venomous arthropods

J. PAYAN

Consultant in Clinical Neurophysiology to Guy's and King's College Hospitals and the Hospital for Sick Children, London, UK
24.2.5 Electrophysiological investigation of the peripheral nervous system

I. PEAKE

Professor of Molecular Medicine, University of Sheffield, UK
22.6.4 The pathogenesis of genetic disorders of coagulation

J.M.S. PEARCE

Honorary Consultant Neurologist, Hull Royal Infirmary, Hull, UK
24.11 Headache

A.D. PEARSON

Senior Lecturer in Microbiology and Public Health Medicine; Clinical Director, Infection Control Department, St Thomas's Hospital, London, UK
7.11.17(a) Tularaemia (b) Pasteurellosis. (c) Yersiniosis

P.E. PELLETT

Chief, Herpesvirus Section, Centers for Disease Control and Prevention, Atlanta, Georgia, USA
7.10.7 Human herpesvirus 6

M.E. PEMBREY

Professor of Paediatric Genetics, Institute of Child Health, University of London, UK
4.3 Genetic factors in disease

M.B. PEPYS

Professor of Immunological Medicine, Royal Postgraduate Medical School, Hammersmith Hospital, London, UK
11.13.1 Amyloidosis
11.13.3 The acute phase response and C-reactive protein

S. PEREIRA

Research Fellow in Gastroenterology, United Medical Schools of St Thomas's and Guy's Hospitals, Guy's Campus, London, UK
14.9.3 Small-bowel bacterial overgrowth

B.A. PERKINS

Medical Epidemiologist, Childhood and Respiratory Diseases Branch, Centers for Disease Control and Prevention, Atlanta, Georgia, USA
7.11.41 Cat scratch disease, bacillary angiomatosis, and trench fever

P.L. PERRINE

Professor of Epidemiology, School of Public and Community Medicine, University of Washington, Seattle, USA
7.11.33 Non-venereal treponemes: yaws, endemic syphilis, and pinta
7.11.43 Lymphogranuloma venereum

C.J. PETERS
Chief, Special Pathogens Branch, Centers for Disease Control and Prevention, Atlanta, Georgia, USA
7.10.5 Human infections caused by simian herpesviruses

T.J. PETERS
Professor of Clinical Biochemistry, King's College; Consultant Physician and Chemical Pathologist, King's College Hospital, London, UK
28.2.3(a) Physical complications of alcohol misuse

R. PETO
Professor of Medical Statistics and Epidemiology, ICRF Cancer Studies Unit, Radcliffe Infirmary, Oxford, UK
2.4 Large-scale randomized evidence: trials and overviews
6.2 Epidemiology of cancer

T.E.A. PETO
Consultant Physician, Infectious Diseases, John Radcliffe Hospital, Oxford, UK
7.10.2 Herpes simplex virus infections
7.10.3 Varicella-zoster infections: chickenpox and zoster
7.10.9 Orf
7.10.10 Molluscum contagiosum
7.10.29 HIV infection and AIDS
17.6.3 Microbiological methods in the diagnosis of respiratory infections

R.K.H. PETTY
Lecturer in Neurology and Neurovirology, Institute of Neurological Sciences, University of Glasgow, UK
24.15.3 Neurological manifestations of infection with human immunodeficiency virus type 1

P.A. PHILIP
Senior Registrar in Medical Oncology, ICRF Clinical Oncology Unit, Churchill Hospital, Oxford, UK
13.15 Malignant disease in pregnancy

PRIDA PHUAPRADIT
Professor of Neurology, Division of Neurology, Department of Medicine, Ramathibodi Hospital, Mahidol University, Bangkok, Thailand
24.15 Bacterial meningitis

M.J. PIPPARD
Professor of Haematology, Ninewells Hospital and Medical School, University of Dundee, UK
22.4.4 Iron metabolism and its disorders

J.M. POLAK
Professor of Endocrine Pathology, Royal Postgraduate Medical School, Hammersmith Hospital, London, UK
14.8 Hormones and the gastrointestinal tract

P.A. POOLE-WILSON
Professor of Cardiology, National Heart and Lung Institute; Honorary Physician, Royal Brompton Hospital, London, UK
15.1 Cardiovascular disease: physiological considerations: biochemistry and cellular physiology of heart muscle
15.5 The treatment of heart failure

J.S. PORTERFIELD
Formerly Reader in Bacteriology, Sir William Dunn School of Pathology, University of Oxford, UK
7.10.21 Bunyaviridae

R.E. POUNDER
Professor of Medicine, Royal Free Hospital School of Medicine, University of London, UK
14.7 Peptic ulceration

M.A. PREECE
Professor of Child Health and Growth, Institute of Child Health, University of London, UK
12.9.2 Normal growth and its disorders

E.W. PRICE*
Research Fellow, Department of Clinical and Tropical Medicine, London School of Hygiene and Tropical Medicine, London, UK
8.5.5(h) Podoconiosis (non-filarial endemic elephantiasis of the lower legs)

J.S. PRICHARD
Professor of Medicine, St James's Hospital, Dublin, Eire
15.22.7 The pulmonary circulation in health and disease
15.23 Pulmonary oedema
15.24 Pulmonary hypertension
15.25 Cor pulmonale

N.B. PRIDE
Professor of Respiratory Medicine, Royal Postgraduate Medical School, Hammersmith Hospital, London, UK
17.6.2 Tests of ventilatory mechanics
17.9.4 Chronic obstructive pulmonary disease

J. PRITCHARD
Senior Lecturer in Paediatric Oncology, Institute of Child Health and Consultant, Hospital for Sick Children, Great Ormond Street, London, UK
22.5.6 The histiocytoses

A.T. PROUDFOOT
Consultant Physician, Royal Infirmary of Edinburgh NHS Trust; Director, Scottish, Poisons Information Bureau, Edinburgh, UK
8.1 Poisoning: introduction and epidemiology
8.1.2 Poisoning: clinical and metabolic features and general principles of management
8.2.1 Poisoning caused by analgesic drugs
8.2.2 Poisoning from antidepressants, hypnotics, antihistamines, anticonvulsants, and antiparkinsonian drugs
8.2.3 Poisoning from cardiovascular drugs
8.2.4 Poisoning caused by respiratory drugs
8.2.5 Poisoning caused by drugs acting on the gastrointestinal system
8.2.6 Poisoning by haematinics and vitamins
8.2.7 Poisoning by endocrine drugs
8.2.8 Poisoning from antimicrobials
8.2.10 Poisoning from drugs of abuse
8.2.11 Poisoning due to miscellaneous drugs
8.3.1 Poisoning from household products
8.3.2 Poisoning by alcohols and glycols
8.3.3 Poisoning from hydrocarbons and chlorofluorocarbons
8.3.4 Poisoning by inhalational agents
8.3.5 Poisoning due to corrosive substances
8.3.8 Pesticides

* It is with regret that we report the deaths of those authors marked with an asterisk. Although their deaths occurred between the appearance of the second edition and preparation of the third edition, much of their contribution to the former has been incorporated into this edition, with appropriate updating from their coauthors.

B.A. PRUITT
Commander and Director, US Army Institute of Surgical Research, Fort Sam Houston, Texas, USA
8.5.5(g) Environmental factors and disease: lightning and electric shock

SWANGJAI PUNGPAK
Associate Professor of Clinical Tropical Medicine, Mahidol University, Bangkok, Thailand
7.16.2 Liver fluke diseases in man

SOMPONE PUNYAGUPTA
President and Chairman, Department of Medicine, Vichaiyut Hospital, Bangkok, Thailand
7.14.8 Angiostrongyliasis

C.D. PUSEY
Reader in Renal Medicine, Royal Postgraduate Medical School, Hammersmith Hospital, London, UK
20.4.3 Rapidly progressive glomerulonephritis and antiglomerular basement membrane disease

N.P. QUINN
Reader in Clinical Neurology, Institute of Neurology, London, UK
24.3.3 Subcortical structures—the cerebellum, thalamus, and basal ganglia

A.J. RADFORD
Professor of Primary Health Care, Flinders University of South Australia
7.15.1 Hydatid disease
7.17 Non-venomous arthropods

PRAYONG RADOMYOS
Associate Professor of Parasitology, Bangkok School of Tropical Medicine, Faculty of Tropical Medicine, Mahidol University, Bangkok, Thailand
7.16.4 Intestinal trematodiasis

A.E.G. RAINE
Professor of Renal Medicine, St Bartholomew's Hospital Medical College, London, UK
15.6.1 Diuretics
15.28.1 Renal and renovascular hypertension
20.11 Hypertension: its effects on the kidney

A.C. RANKIN
Senior Lecturer in Medical Cardiology, Glasgow Royal Infirmary, UK
15.8.1 Cardiac arrhythmias

P.J. RATCLIFFE
University Lecturer and Honorary Consultant Physician, Nuffield Department of Medicine, Oxford, UK
20.17.3 Renal transplantation

C.W.G. REDMAN
Professor of Obstetric Medicine, Nuffield Department of Obstetrics and Gynaecology, John Radcliffe Hospital, Oxford, UK
13.2 Hypertension in pregnancy
13.3 Renal disease in pregnancy

A.J. REES
Regius Professor of Medicine, University of Aberdeen; Honorary Consultant Physician, Aberdeen Royal Hospitals, UK
20.4.3 Rapidly progressive glomerulonephritis and antiglomerular basement membrane disease

D. RENNIE
Professor of Medicine, Institute for Health Policy Studies, University of California, San Francisco, USA
8.5.5(d) Environmental factors and disease: diseases of high terrestrial altitudes

J. RICHENS
Clinical Lecturer, University College London Medical School, UK
7.11.8 Typhoid and paratyphoid fevers
7.11.9 Rhinoscleroma
7.11.45 Donovanosis (granuloma inguinale)

B.K. RIMA
Professor of Molecular Biology, School of Biology and Biochemistry, The Queen's University of Belfast, UK
7.10.11 Mumps: epidemic parotitis

E. RITZ
Professor of Medicine and Head of the Division of Nephrology, Ruperto Carola University of Heidelberg, Germany
20.5.1 Diabetic nephropathy

I.A.G. ROBERTS
Senior Lecturer and Honorary Consultant in Haematology, Royal Postgraduate Medical School, Hammersmith Hospital, London, UK
22.3.4 Acute lymphoblastic leukaemia

A.R. RONALD
Associate Dean, Research University of Manitoba; Director of Infectious Diseases, St Boniface Hospital, Winnipeg, Canada
7.11.13 Haemophilus ducreyi and chancroid

R.J.M. ROSS
Senior Lecturer in Endocrinology, Northern General Hospital, Sheffield, UK
12.9.3 Puberty

R.W. ROSS RUSSELL
Consultant Physician, St Thomas's Hospital, National Hospital of Neurology and Neurosurgery, and Moorfields Eye Hospital, London, UK
24.3.4 Visual pathways

M.N. ROSSOR
Consultant Neurologist, National Hospital for Neurology and Neurosurgery and St Mary's Hospital, London, UK
24.7.2 Alzheimer's disease

D.J. ROWLANDS
Consultant Cardiologist, Royal Infirmary, Manchester, UK
15.4.2 The electrocardiogram
15.4.4 Nuclear techniques

M.B. RUBENS
Consultant Radiologist, Royal Brompton Hospital, London and Honorary Senior Lecturer, National Heart and Lung Institute, University of London, UK
15.4.1 Chest radiography in heart disease

P.C. RUBIN
Professor of Therapeutics, University of Nottingham; Consultant Physician, University Hospital, Birmingham, UK
13.16 Prescribing in pregnancy

P. RUDGE
Consultant Neurologist, National Hospital for Neurology and Neurosurgery, London, UK
24.3.5 The eighth cranial nerve

T.K. RUEBUSH
Chief, Malaria Section, Division of Parasitic Diseases, Centers for Disease Control and Prevention, Atlanta, Georgia, USA
7.13.3 Babesia

R.C.G. RUSSELL
Consultant Surgeon, The Middlesex Hospital, London, UK
14.23.3 Tumours of the pancreas

T.J. RYAN
Clinical Professor of Dermatology, Oxford Radcliffe Trust, UK
23 Diseases of the skin

D.L. SACKETT
Professor of Clinical Epidemiology and Director, Centre for Evidence-Based Medicine, University of Oxford, UK
2.3 Evaluation of clinical method

P.J. SANSONETTI
Professeur à l'Institut Pasteur, Chef de l'Unite de Pathogenie Microbienne Moleculaire and INSERM U389, Institut Pasteur, Paris, France
7.2.1 Introduction to the diversity of bacterial pathogens
7.2.2 Molecular taxonomy of bacterial pathogens

M.O. SAVAGE
Reader in Paediatric Endocrinology, St Bartholomew's Hospital, London, UK
12.9.1 Normal and abnormal sexual differentiation
12.9.3 Puberty

G.F. SAVIDGE
Director, Haemophilia Reference Centre, St Thomas's Hospital, London, UK
22.6.5 Clinical features and management of the hereditary disorders of haemostasis

J.W. SCADDING
Consultant Neurologist, The National Hospital for Neurology and Neurosurgery, London, UK
24.5 Pain: pathophysiology and treatment

K.P. SCHAAL
Professor and Director, Institutes of Medical Microbiology and Immunology, University of Bonn, Germany
7.11.27 Actinomycoses

R.B.H. SCHUTGENS
Associate Professor and Clinical Chemist, Department of Paediatrics, University of Amsterdam, The Netherlands
11.9 Peroxisomal disorders

T.G. SCHWAN
Acting Head, Arthropod-borne Diseases Section, Laboratory of Vectors and Pathogens, National Institutes of Health, Rocky Mountain Laboratories, Hamilton, Montana, USA
7.11.30 Lyme disease

J. SCHWEBKE
Assistant Professor of Medicine, University of Alabama at Birmingham, USA
21.4 Vaginal discharge

J. SCOTT
Professor of Medicine, Royal Postgraduate Medical School, Hammersmith Hospital, London, UK
15.9.1 The pathogenesis of atherosclerosis

D.G.I. SCOTT
Consultant Rheumatologist, Norfolk and Norwich Health Care Trust, UK
18.11.1 Connective tissue diseases: introduction

A. SEATON
Professor of Environmental and Occupational Medicine, University of Aberdeen Medical School, UK
17.10.16 Pneumoconioses

A.W. SEGAL
Charles Dent Professor of Medicine, The Rayne Institute, University College London Medical School, UK
22.5.1 Leucocytes in health and disease

M.H. SEIFERT
Consultant Rheumatologist and Honorary Clinical Senior Lecturer in Medicine, St Mary's Hospital Medical School, London, UK
18.9 Septic arthritis

G.R. SERJEANT
Director, MRC Laboratories (Jamaica), University of the West Indies, Kingston, Jamaica
20.5.7 Renal manifestations of systemic disease: sickle-cell disease

C.A. SEYMOUR
Professor of Clinical Biochemistry and Metabolism and Honorary Consultant Physician, St George's Hospital Medical School, University of London, UK
11.7 Trace metal disorders
14.22 Hereditary disease of the liver and pancreas

K.V. SHAH
Professor of Immunology and Infectious Diseases, Johns Hopkins University School of Hygiene and Public Health, Baltimore, Maryland, USA
7.10.24 Papovaviruses

M. SHARPE
Clinical Tutor in Psychiatry, Oxford University, UK
7.19.4 Chronic fatigue syndrome (postviral fatigue syndrome and myalgic encephalomyelitis)

R.J. SHAW
Senior Lecturer and Consultant Physician in Respiratory Medicine, St Mary's Hospital Medical School, London, UK
17.10.4 The lung in collagen–vascular diseases
17.10.11 Pulmonary histiocytosis X (eosinophilic granuloma of the lung) and lymphangiomatosis
17.10.21 Lung disorders in genetic syndromes

M.C. SHEPPARD
Professor of Medicine, University of Birmingham, UK
12.5 Thyroid cancer

J.M. SHNEERSON

Director, Respiratory Support and Sleep Centre, Papworth Hospital, Cambridge, UK
17.12 Disorders of the thoracic cage and diaphragm

M. SIEBELS

Department of Internal Medicine, Division of Nephrology, University of Heidelberg, Germany
20.5.1 Diabetic nephropathy

C.A. SIEFF

Associate Professor in Pediatrics, Harvard Medical School and Dana Farber Cancer Institute; Senior Associate in Medicine, Children's Hospital, Boston, Massachusetts, USA
22.2.1 Stem cells and haematopoiesis

H.A. SIMMONDS

Senior Lecturer, Purine Research Laboratory, United Medical Schools of Guy's and St Thomas's Hospitals, London Bridge, UK
20.9.2 Gout, purines, and interstitial nephritis

I.A. SIMPSON

Consultant Cardiologist, Southampton General Hospital, UK
15.4.3 Doppler echocardiography

D.I.H. SIMPSON

Professor of Microbiology, Department of Microbiology and Immunology, Queen's University of Belfast, UK
7.10.17 Alphaviruses
7.10.23 Filoviruses: Marburg and Ebola fevers

V. SITPRIJA

Professor and Chairman, Department of Medicine, Chulalongkorn University; Director of Queen Saovabha Memorial Institute, Thai Red Cross, Bangkok, Thailand
7.11.32 Leptospirosis

M.B. SKIRROW

Honorary Emeritus Consultant Microbiologist, Public Health Laboratory, Gloucester Royal Hospital, UK
7.11.7 Enterobacteria and miscellaneous enteropathogenic and food-poisoning bacteria

P. SLEIGHT

Field Marshal Alexander Professor Emeritus of Cardiovascular Medicine, John Radcliffe Hospital, Oxford, UK
15.10.4 Myocardial infarction

R. SMITH

Consultant Physician and Consultant in Metabolic Medicine, John Radcliffe Hospital and Nuffield Orthopaedic Centre, Oxford, UK
10.1 Nutrition: introduction
10.2 Nutrition: biochemical background
11.6 Metabolic effects of accidental injury and surgery
19 Disorders of the skeleton

G.L. SMITH

Reader in Bacteriology, Sir William Dunn School of Pathology, University of Oxford, UK
7.10.8 Poxviruses

D.H. SMITH

Senior Lecturer and Honorary Consultant Physician in Tropical Medicine; Head of Division of Tropical Medicine, Liverpool School of Tropical Medicine, UK
7.13.10 Human African trypanosomiasis

M.L. SNAITH

Senior Lecturer in Rheumatic Diseases, Section of Rheumatology, University of Sheffield Medical School, UK
18.11.3 Systemic lupus erythematosus and related disorders

J. SOMERVILLE

Consultant Physician for Congenital Diseases, Cardiology Directorate, Royal Brompton Hospital, London, UK
15.15 Congenital heart disease in adolescents and adults

R.L. SOUHAMI

Kathleen Ferrier Professor of Clinical Oncology, University College London Medical School, UK
6.6 Cancer: clinical features and management

B.A. SOUTHGATE

Senior Lecturer in Tropical Disease Epidemiology, London School of Hygiene and Tropical Medicine, University of London, UK
7.14.2 Lymphatic filariasis

S.G. SPIRO

Consultant Physician, University College Hospitals London Trust, UK
17.13.1(a) Lung cancer. (b) Pulmonary metastases

C.J.F. SPRY

B.H.F. Professor of Cardiovascular Immunology, St George's Hospital Medical School, University of London, UK
15.4.3 The hypereosinophilic syndrome and the heart
22.5.7 The white cells and lymphoproliferative disorders: the hypereosinophilic syndrome

A. SPURGEON

Lecturer in Occupational Health Psychology, Institute of Occupational Health, University of Birmingham, UK
8.5.3(k) The main occupational disorders: neuropsychological disorders

S. STAGNO

Katharine Reynolds Ireland Professor and Chairman, Department of Pediatrics, University of Alabama, Birmingham, USA
7.10.6 Cytomegalovirus

J.C. STEVENSON

Director, Wynn Institute for Metabolic Research; Honorary Senior Lecturer, National Heart and Lung Institute, University of London; Honorary Consultant Physician, Royal Brompton Hospital, London, UK
13.17 Benefits and risks of hormone therapy

J.A. STEWART

Chief, Clinical Virology Section, Centers for Disease Control and Prevention, Atlanta, Georgia, USA
7.10.7 Human herpesvirus 6

J.H. STEWART

Professor in Medicine and Associate Dean, Western Clinical School, University of Sydney, Australia
20.9.1 Kidney disease from analgesics and non-steroidal anti-inflammatory drugs

R.A. STOCKLEY

Reader in Respiratory Medicine, Queen Elizabeth Hospital, Edgbaston, Birmingham, UK
17.9.3 Bronchiectasis
17.9.4 Chronic obstructive pulmonary disease

J.R. STRADLING

Consultant Physician, Oxford Radcliffe Trust (Churchill), Oxford, UK

17.2.2 The upper respiratory tract
17.8.2 Upper airways obstruction
17.14.2 Sleep-related disorders of breathing

J. STRANG

Professor and Director, Addiction Research Unit, National Addiction Centre, The Maudsley/Institute of Psychiatry, London, UK

28 Alcohol and drug-related problems: introduction
28.1.2 Assessing substance use and misuse
28.2.2 Harm reduction
28.3.2 The management of substance-related problems in a general ward
28.3.3 Drugs and the law
28.3.8 Caring for the HIV-positive drug user

P.R. STUDDY

Consultant Physician, Harefield Hospital NHS Trust and Mount Vernon and Watford Hospitals Trust, Hertfordshire, UK

17.10.10 Sarcoidosis

P.H. SUGDEN

Reader in Biochemistry, Department of Cardiac Medicine, National Heart and Lung Institute, University of London, UK

15.1 Cardiovascular disease: physiological considerations: biochemistry and cellular physiology of heart muscle

J.A. SUMMERFIELD

Professor of Experimental Medicine, St Mary's Hospital Medical School, Imperial College London, UK

14.21 Congenital disorders of the biliary tract and pancreas
14.24 Diseases of the gallbladder and biliary tree

PRAVAN SUNTHARASAMAI

Associate Professor, Department of Clinical Tropical Medicine, Mahidol University, Bangkok, Thailand

7.14.9 Gnathostomiasis

R. SUTTON

Consultant Cardiologist and Director of Pacing and Electrophysiology, Royal Brompton Hospital, London, UK

15.3.5 Syncope and palpitation
15.8.2 Pacemakers

J.D. SWALES

Professor of Medicine, University of Leicester, UK

15.27 Essential hypertension

R.H. SWANTON

Consultant Cardiologist, University College London, UK

15.4.6 Cardiac catheterization
15.10.3 Angina and unstable angina

D.M. SWIRSKY

Senior Lecturer in Haematology, Royal Postgraduate Medical School; Honorary Consultant, Hospital, London, UK

22.5.4 The spleen and its disorders

D.A. TABERNER

Clinical Director, Thrombosis Reference Centre, University Hospital of South Manchester, UK

22.6.7 Thrombotic disease

I.C. TALBOT

Consultant Pathologist, St Mark's Hospital, London, UK

14.16 Tumours of the gastrointestinal tract

C.R. TAYLOR

Charles P. Lyman Professor of Biology, Harvard University, Cambridge, Massachusetts, USA

17.2.1 Functional anatomy of the human lung

D. TAYLOR-ROBINSON

Professor of Genitourinary Microbiology and Medicine, St Mary's Hospital Medical School, Paddington, London, UK

7.11.41 Chlamydial infections
7.11.43 Mycoplasmas

G.M. TEASDALE

Professor of Neurosurgery, Institute of Neurological Sciences, University of Glasgow, UK

24.14 Head injuries

P.J. TEDDY

Consultant Neurosurgeon, The Radcliffe Infirmary, Oxford, UK

24.12 Intracranial tumours
24.15.4 Intracranial abscess

H.J. TESTA

Consultant in Nuclear Medicine, Royal Infirmary, Manchester, UK

15.4.4 The clinical assessment of cardiovascular function: nuclear techniques

A.C. THOMAS

Senior Specialist and Consultant in Tissue Pathology, Institute of Medical and Veterinary Science, Adelaide, South Australia

20.4.1 IgA nephropathy, Henoch-Schönlein purpura, and thin membrane nephropathy

P.K. THOMAS

Emeritus Professor of Neurology, Royal Free Hospital School of Medicine and Institute of Neurology, London, UK

24.3.6 Neurology: organization and features of dysfunction; other cranial nerves
24.8 Neurology: inherited disorders
24.17 Peripheral neuropathy

H.C. THOMAS

Professor of Medicine, St Mary's Hospital Medical School, Imperial College of Science, Technology and Medicine; Consultant Physician and Hepatologist, St Mary's Hospital, London, UK

14.26 Clinical features of viral hepatitis

J.E.P. THOMAS

Formerly Professor of Medicine, University of Zimbabwe, Harare, Zimbabwe

7.16.1 Schistosomiasis

D.G. THOMPSON

Senior Lecturer in Medicine and Consultant Physician, Hope Hospital, Salford, UK

14.2.5 Constipation
14.13 Functional bowel disease and irritable bowel syndrome

M.O. THORNER

Kenneth R. Crispell Professor of Medicine; Chief, Division of Endocrinology and Metabolism, University of Virginia School of Medicine, Charlottesville, USA

12.2 Anterior pituitary disorders

A.J. THRASHER

Honorary Lecturer and Wellcome Training Fellow, University College London Medical School, UK
22.5.1 Leucocytes in health and disease

P. THULLIEZ

Head, Laboratoire de la Toxoplasmose, Institut de Puériculture de Paris, France
7.13.4 Toxoplasmosis

P. TOOKEY

Research Fellow, Department of Epidemiology and Biostatistics, Institute of Child Health, London, UK
7.10.18 Rubella

P.P. TOSKES

Professor and Associate Chairman for Clinical Affairs; Director, Division of Gastroenterology, Hepatology and Nutrition, Department of Medicine, University of Florida College of Medicine, Gainsville, USA
14.23.2 Chronic pancreatitis

T.A. TRAILL

Associate Professor of Medicine, Johns Hopkins University School of Medicine, Baltimore, Maryland, USA
15.19 Cardiac myxoma

D.F. TREACHER

Consultant Physician, Department of Intensive Care, St Thomas's Hospital, London, UK
16 Intensive care

T. TREASURE

Consultant Cardiothoracic Surgeon, St George's Hospital, London, UK
15.10.6 Coronary artery bypass grafting

G.S. TREGENZA

Associate Specialist, Division of Addictive Behavior, St George's Hospital Medical School, University of London, UK
28.3.5 Drug misusers and addicts in accident and emergency

J.D. TREHARNE

Reader in Virology, Institute of Ophthalmology, University of London, UK
7.11.41 Chlamydial infections

SIR LESLIE TURNBERG

Section of Gastroenterology, Hope Hospital, Salford, Lancashire, UK
14.2.4 Diarrhoea

P.C.B. TURNBULL

Head, Anthrax Section, Centre for Applied Microbiology and Research, Porton Down, Salisbury, Wiltshire, UK
7.11.18 Anthrax

R.C. TURNER

Clinical Reader, Nuffield Department of Clinical Medicine, Diabetes Research Laboratories, Radcliffe Infirmary, Oxford, UK
11.12 Hypoglycaemia

F.E. UDWADIA

Emeritus Professor of Medicine, Grant Medical College and J.J. Group of Hospitals; Consultant Physician, Breach Candy Hospital and Parsee General Hospital, Bombay, India
7.11.20 Tetanus

S.R. UNDERWOOD

Senior Lecturer in Cardiac Imaging, National Heart and Lung Institute; Honorary Consultant, Royal Brompton Hospital NHS Trust, London, UK
15.4.5 Magnetic resonance and computed X-ray tomography

C.G. URAGODA

Physician, Chest Hospital, Welisera; Course Director of Clinical Studies, Postgraduate Institute of Medicine, University of Colombo, Sri Lanka
7.11.23 Particular problems of tuberculosis in developing countries

J.A. VALE

Director, National Poisons Information Service (Birmingham Centre), West Midlands Poisons Unit, City Road Hospital, Birmingham; Senior Clinical Lecturer, University of Birmingham, UK
8.1.1 Poisoning: introduction and epidemiology
8.1.2 Poisoning: clinical and metabolic features and general principles of management
8.2.1 Poisoning caused by analgesic drugs
8.2.2 Poisoning from antidepressants, hypnotics, antihistamines, anticonvulsants, and antiparkinsonian drugs
8.2.3 Poisoning from cardiovascular drugs
8.2.4 Poisoning caused by respiratory drugs
8.2.5 Poisoning caused by drugs acting on the gastrointestinal system
8.2.6 Poisoning by haematinics and vitamins
8.2.7 Poisoning by endocrine drugs
8.2.8 Poisoning from antimicrobials
8.2.10 Poisoning from drugs of abuse
8.2.11 Poisoning due to miscellaneous drugs
8.3.1 Poisoning from household products
8.3.2 Poisoning from alcohols and glycols
8.3.3 Poisoning from hydrocarbons and chlorofluorocarbons, and volatile substance abuse
8.3.4 Poisoning by inhalational agents
8.3.5 Poisoning due to corrosive substances
8.3.6 Poisoning from metals
8.3.8 Pesticides

P. VALLANCE

Senior Lecturer and Honorary Consultant in Clinical Pharmacology, St George's Hospital Medical School, London, UK
15.9.2 Vascular endothelium, its physiology and pathophysiology

SIRIVAN VANIJANONTA

Associate Professor, Head, Department of Clinical Tropical Medicine, Faculty of Tropical Medicine, Mahidol University, Bangkok, Thailand
7.16.3 Lung flukes (paragonimiasis)

D.J.T. VAUX

Lecturer in Experimental Pathology, Sir William Dunn School of Pathology, University of Oxford, UK
4.2.2 Cell biology of organelles and the endomembrane system

P.J.W. VENABLES
Reader in Rheumatology, Charing Cross and Westminster Medical School; Consultant Rheumatologist; Charing Cross Hospital, London, UK
18.11.5 Sjögren's syndrome

M.P. VESSEY
Professor of Public Health, Department of Public Health and Primary Care, University of Oxford, UK
3.2 Health and sickness in the community
13.1 Benefits and risks of oral contraceptives

P.D. WAGNER
Professor of Medicine, University of California San Diego, La Jolla, California, USA
17.4 Pathophysiology of lung disease

D.H. WALKER
Professor and Chairman, Department of Pathology, University of Texas Medical Branch at Galveston, USA
7.11.37 Rickettsial diseases including the ehrlichioses

J.A. WALKER-SMITH
Professor of Paediatric Gastroenterology, Medical College of St Bartholomew's Hospital and Queen Elizabeth Hospital for Children, London, UK
14.15 Congenital abnormalities of the gastrointestinal tract

J.R.F WALTERS
Senior Lecturer, Gastroenterology Unit, Royal Postgraduate Medical School, Hammersmith Hospital, London, UK
14.9.1 Mechanisms of intestinal absorption

LORD WALTON OF DETCHANT
President, World Federation of Neurology; Former Professor of Neurology, University of Newcastle on Tyne; Honorary Consultant Neurologist, Oxford, UK
18.11.6 Polymyositis and dermatomyositis
25.1 Disorders of voluntary muscle: introduction
25.2 The muscular dystrophies
25.3 The floppy infant syndrome
25.4 Myotonic disorders
25.5 Inflammatory myopathies
25.6 Miscellaneous disorders (of voluntary muscle)

R.J.A. WANDERS
Senior Biochemist and Associate Professor, University Hospital Amsterdam, Academic Medical Centre, Amsterdam, The Netherlands
11.9 Peroxisomal disorders

C.P. WARLOW
Professor of Medical Neurology, University of Edinburgh, UK
24.6 Cerebrovascular disease

D.A. WARRELL
Professor of Tropical Medicine and Infectious Diseases, University of Oxford
7.8 Travel and expedition medicine
7.10.15 Rhabdoviruses: rabies and rabies-related viruses
7.10.16 Colorado tick fever and other arthropod-borne reoviruses
7.11.29 Rat bite fevers
7.11.31 Other Borrelia infections

7.11.44 Bartonellosis
7.13.2 Malaria
7.13.5 Cryptosporidium and cryptosporidiosis
7.18 Pentastomiasis (porocephalosis)
8.4.1 Injuries, envenoming, poisoning, and allergic reactions caused by animals
24.15.1 Bacterial meningitis
24.15.2 Acute viral infections of the central nervous system
25.10 Tropical pyomyositis (tropical myositis)

M.J. WARRELL
Clinical Virologist, Centre for Tropical Medicine and Infectious Diseases, John Radcliffe Hospital, Oxford, UK
7.10.15 Rhabdoviruses: rabies and rabies-related viruses
7.10.16 Colorado tick fever and other arthropod-borne reoviruses

J.A.H. WASS
Professor of Clinical Endocrinology, St Bartholomew's Hospital Medical College, London, UK
12.11 Endocrine manifestations of non-endocrine disease

M.F.R. WATERS
Consultant Leprologist, Hospital for Tropical Diseases, London; sometime Member of the Medical Research Council External Scientific Staff, Middlesex Hospital, London, UK
7.11.25 Leprosy (Hansen's disease, hanseniasis)
7.11.26 Mycobacterium ulcerans infection

G. WATT
Chief, Department of Medicine, AFRIMS, Bangkok, Thailand
7.11.38 Scrub typhus

R.W.E. WATTS
Royal Postgraduate Medical School Visting Professor and Honorary Consultant Physician, Hammersmith Hospital, London, UK
11.1 The inborn errors of metabolism: general aspects
11.8 Lysosomal storage diseases
11.10 Disorders of oxalate metabolism
20.9.3 Hypercalcaemic nephropathy
20.12.2 Urinary stone disease (urolithiasis)

SIR DAVID WEATHERALL
Regius Professor of Medicine and Honorary Director of the Institute of Molecular Medicine, University of Oxford, UK
2.1.2 Scientific method and the art of healing
4.1 Molecular biology and medicine
4.2.1 Medical applications of cell biology: introduction
15.26 Pulmonary embolism
22.1 Disorders of the blood: introduction
22.3.8 Polycythaemia vera
22.3.9 Myelosclerosis
22.3.10 Primary thrombocythaemia
22.4.1 Erythropoiesis and the normal red cell
22.4.2 Anaemia: pathophysiology, classification, and clinical features
22.4.5 Normochromic, normocytic anaemia
22.4.7 Disorders of the synthesis or function of haemoglobin
22.4.8 Other anaemias resulting from defective red cell maturation
22.4.9 Haemolytic anaemia: the mechanisms and consequences of a shortened red cell
22.4.11 Haemolysis due to red-cell enzyme deficiencies
22.4.14 The relative and secondary polycythaemias
22.7 The blood in systemic disease

A.D.B. WEBSTER
MRC Immunodeficiency Research Group, Royal Free Hospital Medical School, London, UK
5.3 Immunodeficiency

E.R. WEIBEL
Professor of Anatomy Emeritus, University of Bern, Switzerland
17.2.1 Functional anatomy of the lung

R.A. WEISS
Professor of Viral Oncology, Institute of Cancer Research, London, UK
7.10.27 Viruses and cancer
7.10.28 Human immunodeficiency viruses

I.V.D. WELLER
Professor and Head of the Academic Department of Genitourinary Medicine, University College London Medical School, UK
7.10.29 HIV infection and AIDS

L. WESTRÖM
Associate Professor of Obstetrics and Gynaecology, University of Lund, Sweden
21.5 Pelvic inflammatory disease

N.J. WHITE
Director, Wellcome-Mahidol University, Oxford Tropical Medicine Research Programme, Faculty of Tropical Medicine, Mahidol University, Bangkok, Thailand
9 Principles of clinical pharmacology and drug therapy

H.C. WHITTLE
Deputy Director, Medical Research Council Laboratories, The Gambia, West Africa
7.10.12 Measles

D.E.L. WILCKEN
Consultant Physician, The Prince Henry and Prince of Wales Hospitals, Sydney, Australia
15.2 Clinical physiology of the normal heart

P.J. WILKINSON
Consultant Medical Microbiologist and Director, Public Health Laboratory, University Hospital, Nottingham, UK
7.11.35 Listeria and listeriosis

D.G. WILLAMS
Professor of Medicine, United Medical and Dental Schools of Guy's and St Thomas's Hospitals, University of London, UK
20.5.2 Infections and associated nephropathies
20.5.6 Rheumatological disorders and the kidney

R.C. WILLIAMS
Chief Medical Officer, GKN plc, Redditch, Worcestershire, UK
8.5.5(j) Environmental factors and disease: noise

A.C. de C. WILLIAMS
Consultant Clinical Psychologist, INPUT Pain Management Unit, St Thomas's Hospital, London, UK
28.3.7 Management of pain in the drug abuser

R. WILLIAMS
Director, Institute of Liver Studies and Consultant Physician, King's College Hospital, London, UK
14.31 Liver transplantation

C.B. WILLIAMS
Consultant Physician in Gastrointestinal Endoscopy, St Mark's Hospital, Northwick Park, London, UK
14.16 Tumours of the gastrointestinal tract

D.H. WILLIAMSON
Medical Research Council, External Scientific Staff, Nuffield Department of Clinical Medicine, Oxford University, UK
10.2 Biochemical background

BRIGADIER GENERAL KYAW WIN
Director and Consultant Physician, Directorate of Medical Services, Ministry of Defence, Union of Myanmar
7.11.38 Scrub typhus

C.G. WINEARLS
Consultant Nephrologist, Churchill Hospital, Oxford, UK
20.16 Acute renal failure
20.17.1 Chronic renal failure

D.L. WINGATE
Professor of Gastrointestinal Science, London Hospital Medical College, University of London, UK
14.12 Disorders of motility

P.A. WINSTANLEY
Senior Lecturer in Clinical Pharmacology, Department of Pharmacology and Therapeutics, University of Liverpool, UK
8.2.9 Poisoning from cinchona alkaloids and other antimalarials

F. WOJNAROWSKA
Consultant Dermatologist and Senior Clinical Lecturer, Churchill Hospital, Oxford, UK
13.14 The skin in pregnancy

A.J. WOODROFFE
Renal Physician, Royal Adelaide Hospital, Australia
20.4.1 IgA nephropathy, Henoch-Schönlein purpura, and thin membrane nephropathy

H.F. WOODS
Sir George Franklin Professor of Medicine, University of Sheffield, UK
11.14 Disturbances of acid-base homeostasis

B.P. WORDSWORTH
Clinical Reader in Rheumatology, Nuffield Department of Clinical Medicine, University of Oxford, UK
18.4 Rheumatoid arthritis

V.M. WRIGHT
Consultant Paediatric Surgeon, Queen Elizabeth Hospital for Children and University College London Hospitals, London, UK
14.15 Congenital abnormalities of the gastrointestinal tract

D.J.M. WRIGHT
Reader in Medical Microbiology, Charing Cross and Westminster Medical School, London, UK
7.11.34 Syphilis

F.C.W. WU
Senior Lecturer, Department of Medicine, University of Manchester, UK
12.8.2 Disorders of male reproduction

M.A.S. YASUDA

Associate Professor, Department of Infectious and Parasitic Diseases, São Paulo University School of Medicine (USP), Brazil
7.12.4 Paracoccidioidomycosis

A. YOUNG

Professor of Geriatric Medicine, Royal Free Hospital School of Medicine, London, UK
30 Sports medicine

V. ZAMAN

Professor of Microbiology, Aga Khan University, Karachi, Pakistan
7.13.7 Sarcocystosis
7.13.9 Blastocystis hominis
7.14.6 Other gut nematodes
7.14.7 Toxocariasis and visceral larval migrans

A.J. ZUCKERMAN

Dean and Professor of Medical Microbiology and Director of the World Health Organization Collaborating Centre for Reference and Research on Viral Diseases, Royal Free Hospital School of Medicine, London, UK
7.10.26 Viral hepatitis

J.N. ZUCKERMAN

Clinical Research Fellow, Royal Free Hospital School of Medicine, London, UK
7.10.26 Viral hepatitis

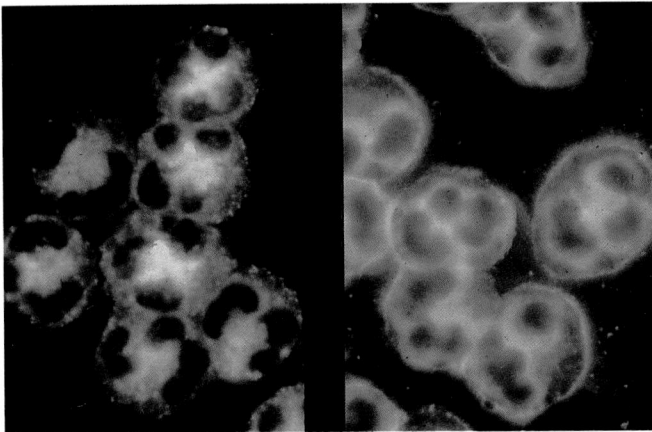

Plate 1 Indirect immunofluorescence tests for antineutrophil cytoplasm antibodies; left panel c-ANCA showing granular appearance with interlobular accentuation; right panel, p-ANCA producing perinuclear staining (note: with these two strong sera, there is punctate binding of the c-ANCA to the neutrophil cell membrane and additional, linear binding of the p-ANCA to the neutrophil cell membrane, also.) (Pathological section kindly provided by Dr D. Peat.)

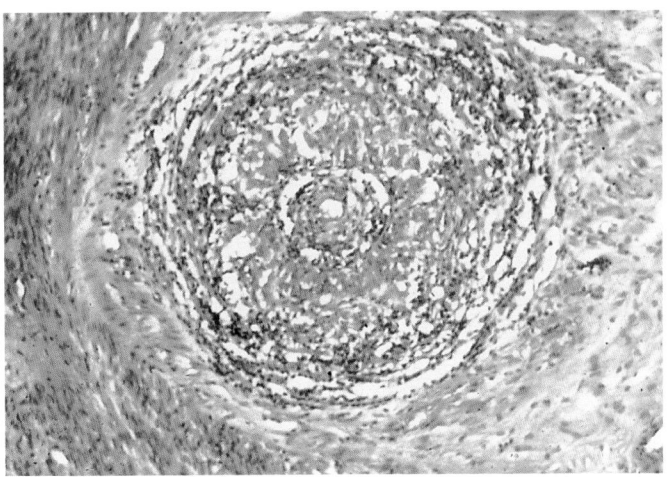

Plate 2 Small artery with granulomatous inflammation and central eosinophilic palisading histocytes, with occasional giant cells and peripheral rim of lymphocytes (multinucleate giant cells are present amongst the histocytes). (Pathological section kindly provided by Dr F. Wegener.)

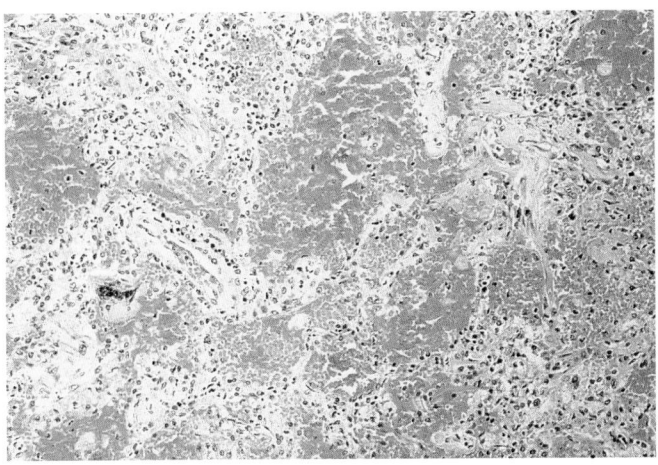

Plate 3 Transbronchial biopsy of lung showing severe haemorrhage into alveolar spaces. Note small blood vessel with multinucleate giant cell in the vicinity. There is a prominent infiltration of neutrophils and eosinophils within alveolar spaces and interstitium. (Pathological specimen kindly provided by Dr S. Thiru.)

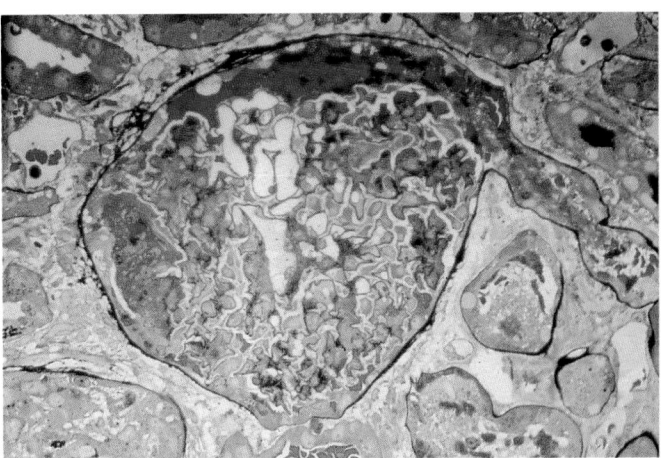

Plate 4 A single glomerulus showing segmental necrosis associated with fibrinoid necrosis and nuclear debris. Note red cells in Bowman's space and the tubular space, secondary to disruption of capillary wall. (Pathological specimen kindly provided by Dr D. J. Evans.)

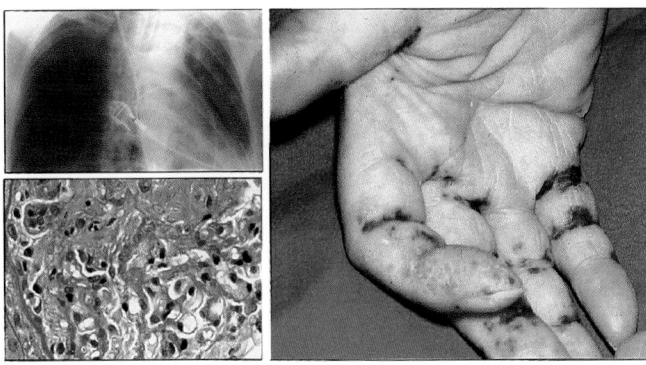

Plate 5 Microscopic polyangiitis in a 50-year-old woman, affecting predominantly left lung (radiograph), kidneys (biopsy showing a high power view of the glomerulus with segmental fibrinoid necrosis—staining orange with Martius Scarlet Blue) and skin (hand). (Pathology kindly provided by Dr D. Peat.)

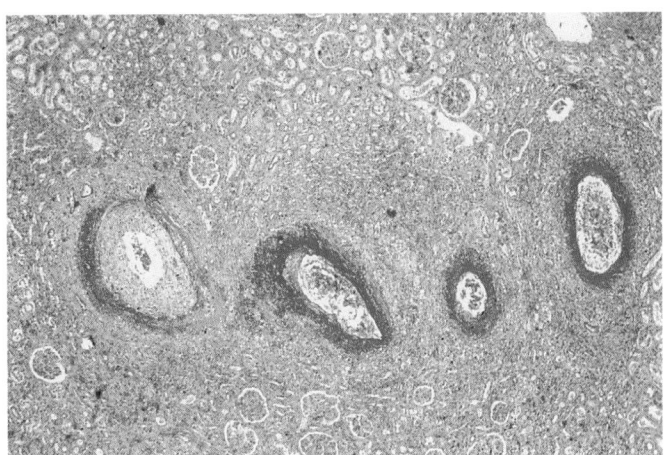

Plate 6 Renal cortex showing circumferential fibrinoid vasculitis in the medium size interlobular arteries of a patient with polyarteritis nodosa; the fibrinoid necrosis stains red with Martius Scarlet Blue. Note there is no evidence of glomerular (capillary) involvement. (Pathology kindly provided by Dr D. Peat.)

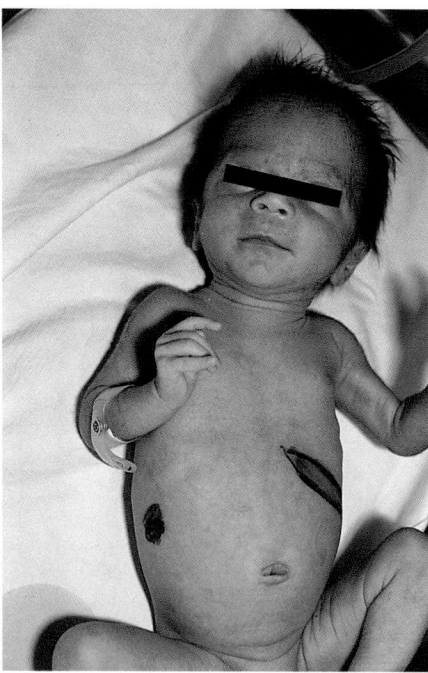

Plate 1 Neonatal lupus syndrome: a boy of 6 days of age, with rash, thrombocytopenia, splenomegaly, and hepatomegaly. His mother was clinically well, but had been known to carry anti-Ro and anti-La antibodies since she had given birth some years earlier to a child with congenital heart block.

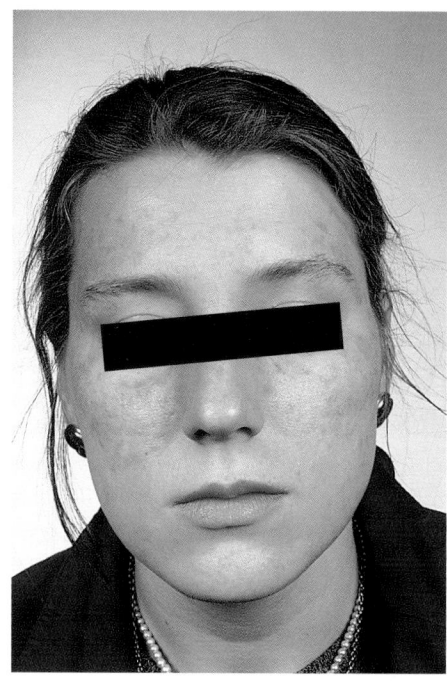

Plate 2 Butterfly (malar) rash: subacute malar rash, with erythema, vasculopathy, and early scarring.

Plate 3 Subacute cutaneous lupus erythematosus in a patient with anti-La antibodies.

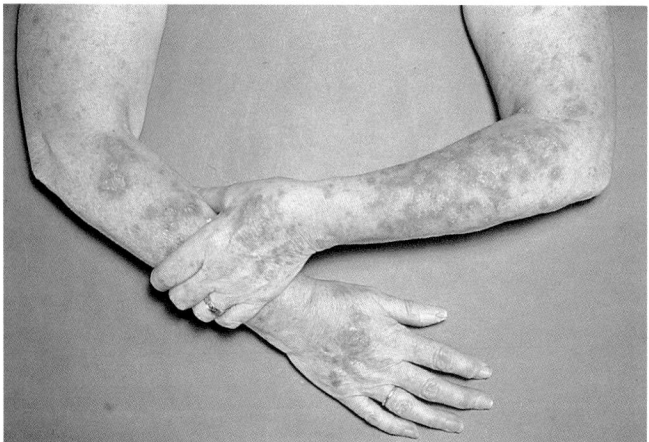

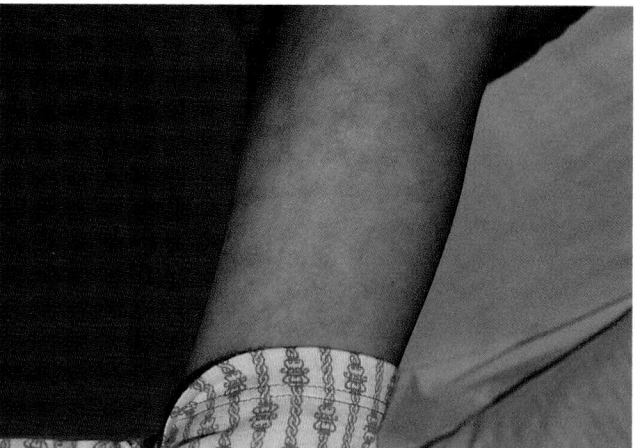

Plate 4 Livedo reticularis: mild livedo reticularis pattern in a patient without the antiphospholipid syndrome.

Plate 5 Lupus band test: deposition of IgG and complement at the dermoepidermal junction in the clinically normal skin of a lupus patient.

Plates for Section 20
CHAPTER 20.4.1

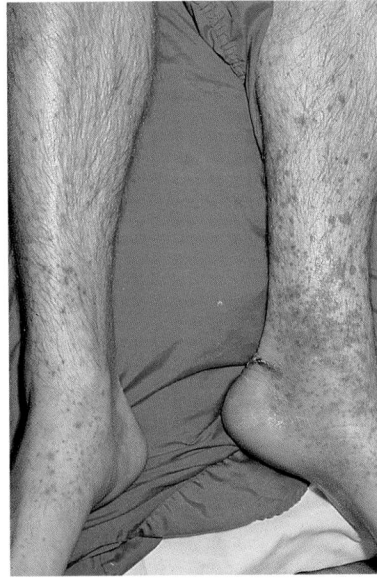

Plate 1 Characteristic purpuric rash affecting the lower limbs in Henoch-Schönlein purpura.

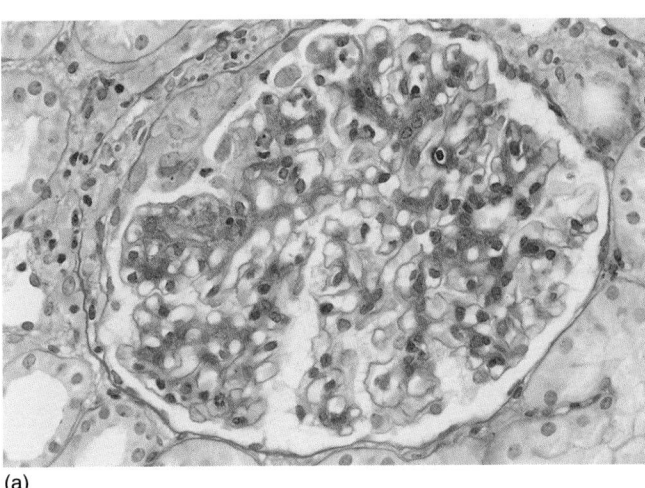

(a)

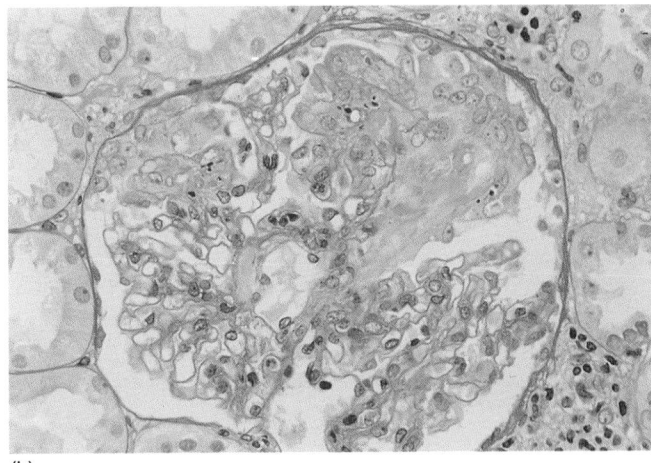

(b)

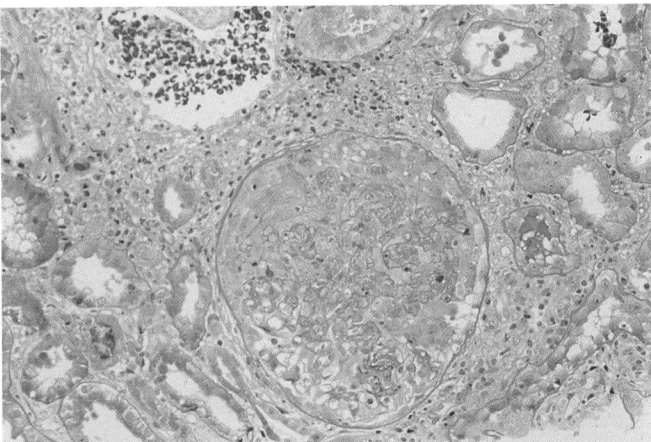

Plate 3 Light microscopic appearance of crescentic glomerulonephritis (arrows) in IgA nephropathy. The majority of the glomerular tufts appear collapsed and shrunken beneath the crescent. Note the surrounding interstitial scarring with tubular separation and atrophy, interstitial fibrosis, and chronic inflammatory cell infiltrate (Masson Trichrome stain, × 200).

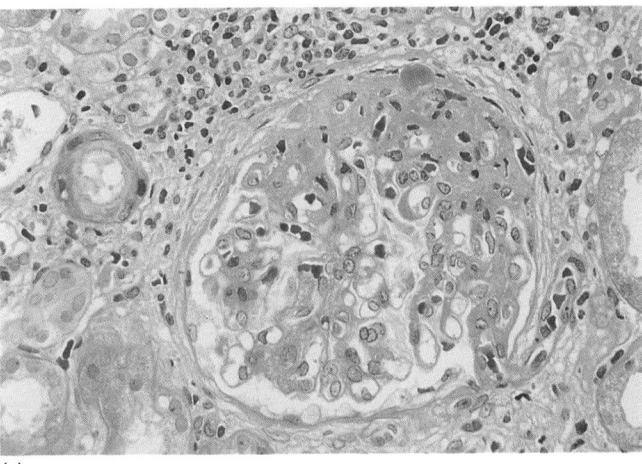

(c)

Plate 2 Light microscopic appearances of IgA nephropathy. (a) The glomerulus is enlarged and shows a segmental increase in both mesangial matrix and mesangial cellularity (small arrows). In addition, there is some early proliferation of the parietal epithelium of Bowman's capsule (large arrow) (Alcian Blue/PAS stain, × 375). (b) Glomerulus showing segmental increase in mesangial matrix and hypercellularity with fibrinoid necrosis and synechiae formation between the segmental lesion and parietal epithelium of Bowman's capsule (arrows) (Alcian Blue/PAS stain, × 375). (c) Glomerulus showing segmental increase in mesangial matrix, segmental sclerosis with synechia formation to overlying Bowman's capsule, and glomerular hyalinosis (arrow) (Masson Trichrome stain, × 375).

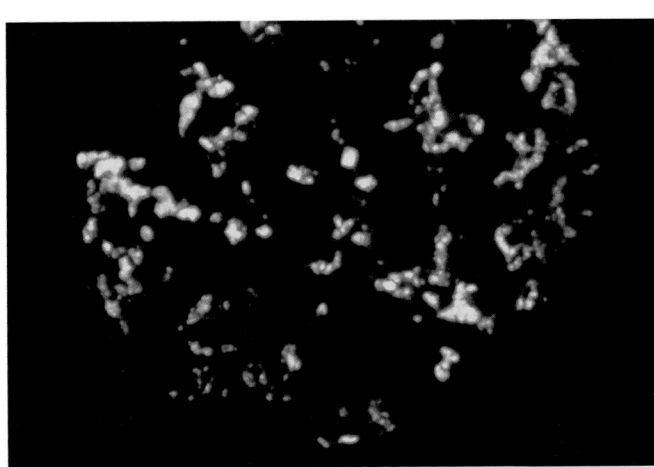

Plate 4 Immunofluorescence of a glomerulus in IgA nephropathy. Brightly fluorescent staining is seen within the mesangium with labelled antibodies to IgA. In some cases, some staining may also be observed along the capillary loops. A similar distribution of staining is normally seen with labelled antibodies to C3 (anti-human IgA, × 375).

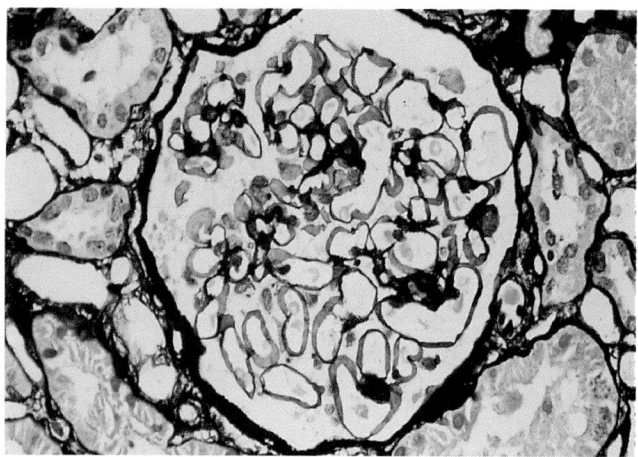

Plate 1 Minimal change nephropathy. Small glomerulus that looks normal on light microscopy (periodic acid–silver, magnification × 325). (By courtesy of Dr A.J. Howie.)

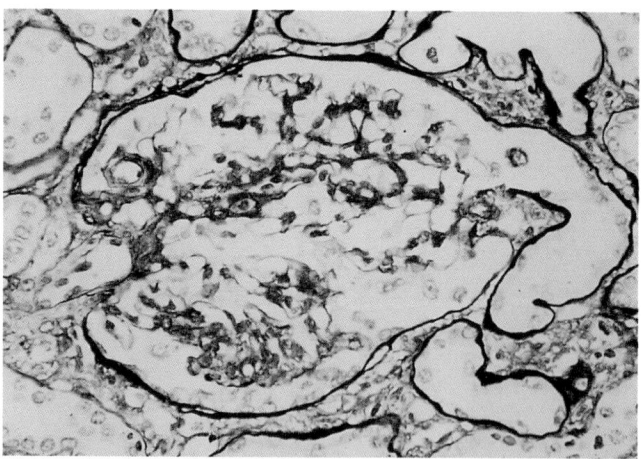

Plate 2 Late classical segmental glomerulosclerosis. Multiple erratic sclerosing lesions, including at origin of tubule (periodic acid–silver, magnification × 260). (By courtesy of Dr A.J. Howie.)

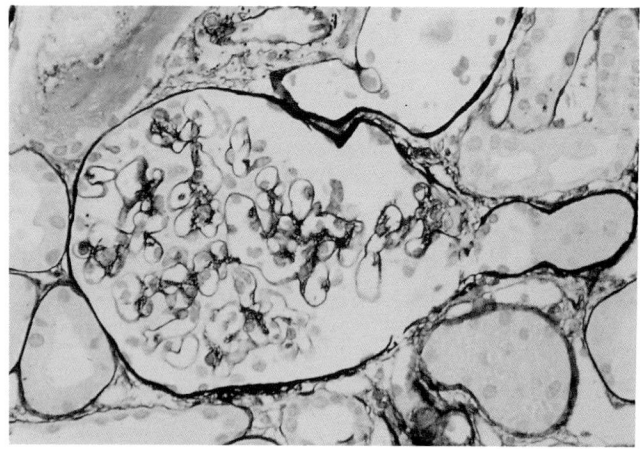

Plate 3 Glomerular tip lesion. Small glomerulus, adhesion of tuft to origin of tubule, otherwise normal (periodic acid–silver, magnification × 325). (By courtesy of Dr A.J. Howie.)

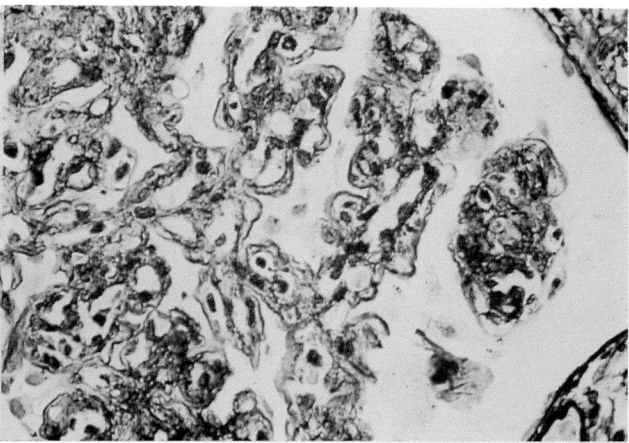

Plate 4 Subendothelial-type mesangiocapillary glomerulonephritis. Mesangial increase, doubled basement membranes (periodic acid–silver, magnification × 390). (By courtesy of Dr A.J. Howie.)

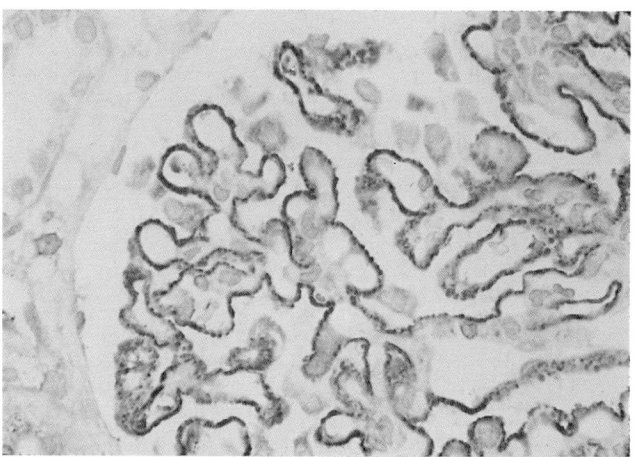

Plate 5 Membranous nephropathy. Regular granular deposits of IgG on outside of glomerular capillary loops (immunoperoxidase, magnification × 520). (By courtesy of Dr A.J. Howie.)

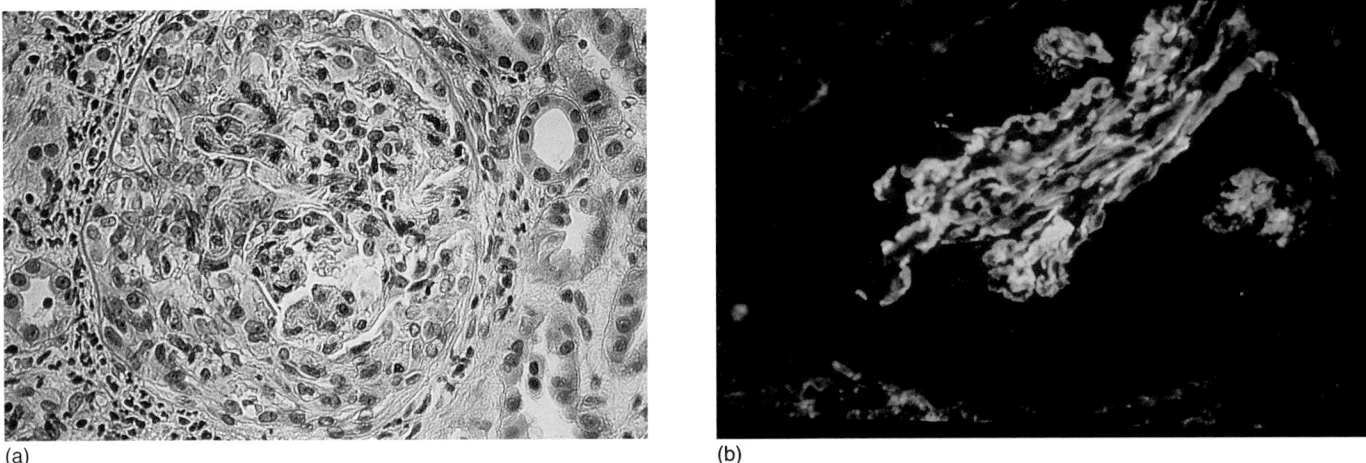

CHAPTER 20.4.3

(a)

(b)

Plate 1 Renal biopsy from a patient with antiglomerular basement membrane disease. (a) Light microscopy showing extracapillary proliferation with crescent formation. (b) Direct immunofluorescence showing linear deposits of IgG (note compression of glomerular tuft by a crescent). (By courtesy of Professor D. J. Evans.)

CHAPTER 20.16

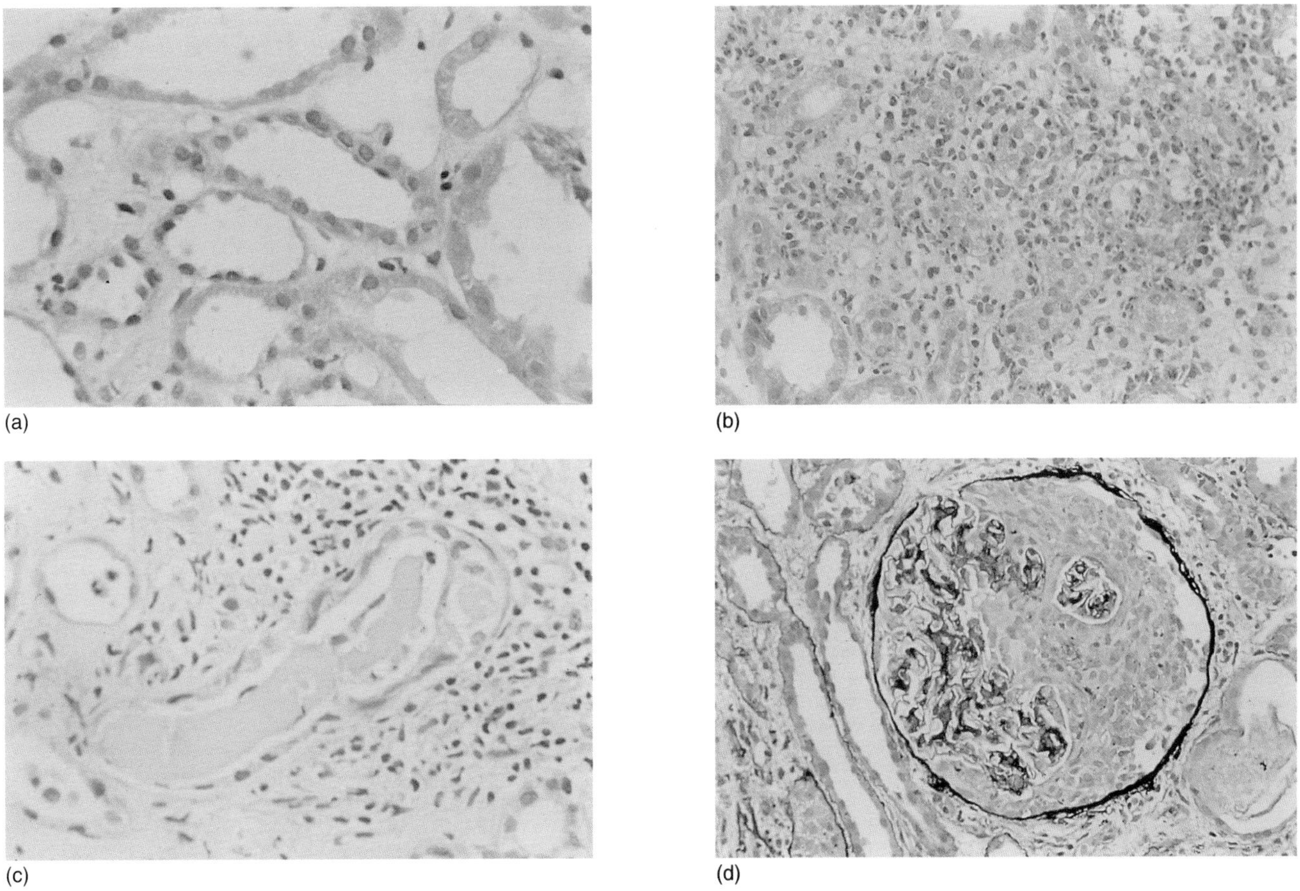

(a)

(b)

(c)

(d)

Plate 1 Renal biopsy appearances in acute renal failure. (a) Haematoxylin and eosin (H & E) stained section showing appearances of acute tubular necrosis, with dilated tubules, flattened tubular epithelium, and loss of cells over the tubular basement membrane. (b) H & E stained section of a case of drug induced interstitial nephritis, demonstrating separation of the tubules and a heavy infiltrate of cells in the interstitium. (c) H & E stained section from a patient whose myeloma presented with acute renal failure. A fractured cast is seen, together with reactive changes in the tubular epithelium and an inflammatory infiltrate in the interstitium. (d) Periodic acid-methenamine silver stained section from a case of rapidly progressive glomerulonephritis. Silver staining of the basement membrane of the glomerular tuft and Bowman's capsule highlights the filling of Bowman's space with proliferating cells forming a crescent. (Pictures by courtesy of Dr. D. Davies.)

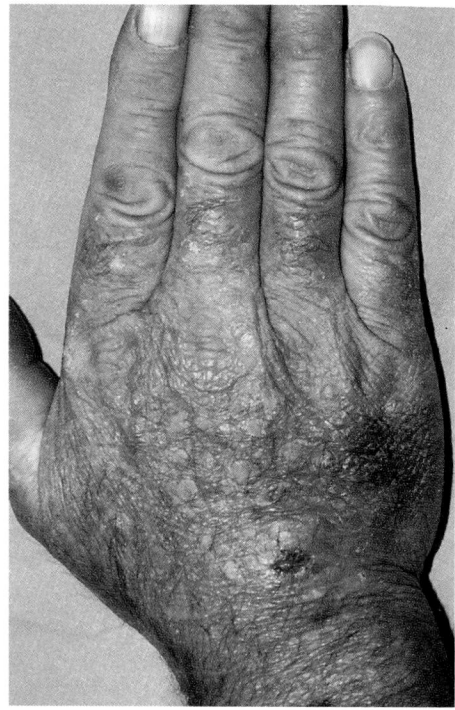

Plate 1 Sun damaged skin on the hand of a long-term renal transplant patient. There are widespread dysplastic changes and a squamous cell carcinoma of atypical appearance. (By courtesy of Dr Vanessa Venning.)

Plates for Section 22*

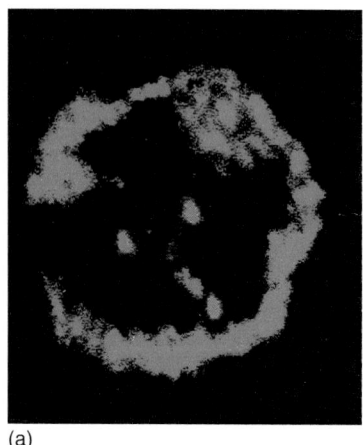
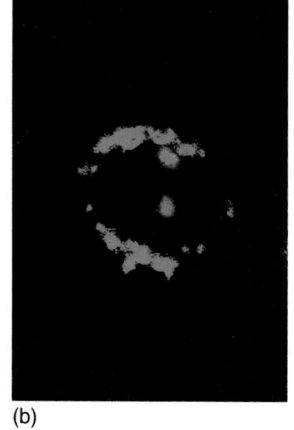

(a)   (b)

Plate 1 Combined detection of cell type (immunophenotype) and abnormal genotype in single interphase leukaemic cells. (a) Myeloid cell stained red in the cytoplasm with monoclonal antibody (CD11c) and green (three spots with a chromosome 8-specific probe revealing triploidy for chromosome 8. (b) Lymphoid cell (from same patient sample as (a)) stained red in the cytoplasm with a monoclonal antibody (CD3) and green (two spots) with a chromosome 8-specific probe revealing a normal (diploid) number for chromosome 8. Data such as these can reveal the cell type or lineage in which a particular chromosomal abnormality has arisen and this is a sensitive test as dividing cells are not required (see Price *et al.* in reference list, Chapter 22.3.1, for details).

*We are indebted to Drs D.M. Swirsky and S.M. Lewis for supplying the bulk of the Plates in this Section. Plate 1 was provided by Professor M.F. Greaves and Plates 13–15, 17–19, and 21–24 were provided by Professor D. Catovsky.

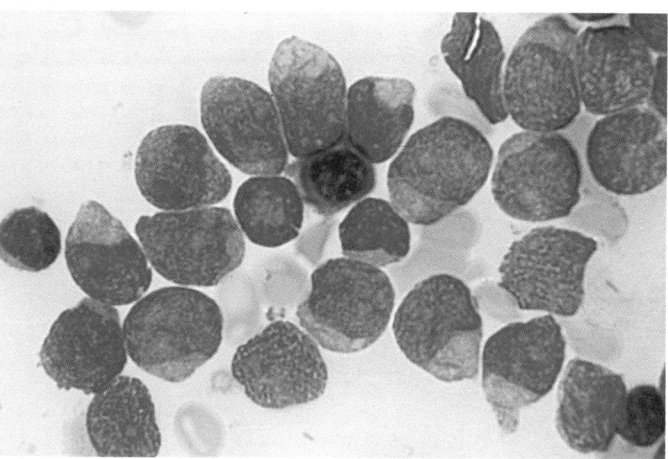

Plate 2 Acute myeloblastic leukaemia without maturation. Auer rods are present in the cytoplasm of several blasts.

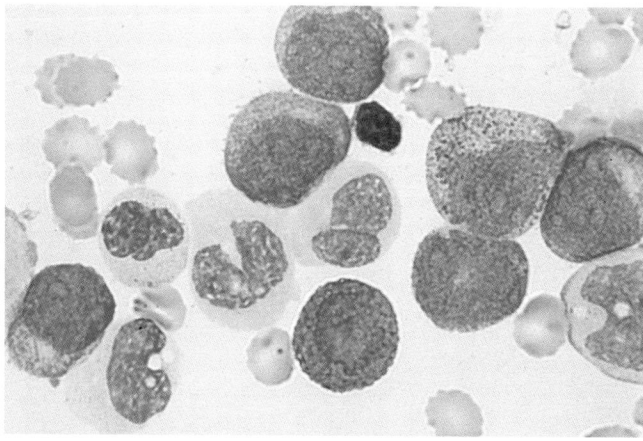

Plate 3 Acute myeloblastic leukaemia with maturation. In addition to the blast cells, one of which contains an Auer rod, there are two promyelocytes and three very dysplastic agranular neutrophils. These appearances are characteristic of the t(8;21).

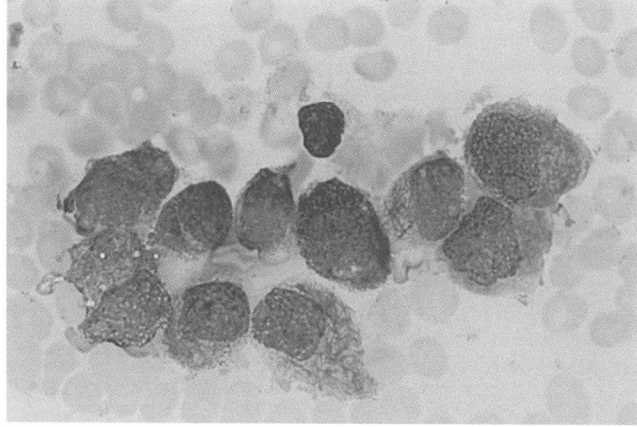

Plate 4 Acute promyelocytic leukaemia, hypergranular type. Bone marrow aspirate showing extensive deep purple cytoplasmic granules in the promyelocytes, and two cells with the pathognomonic sheaves of Auer rods.

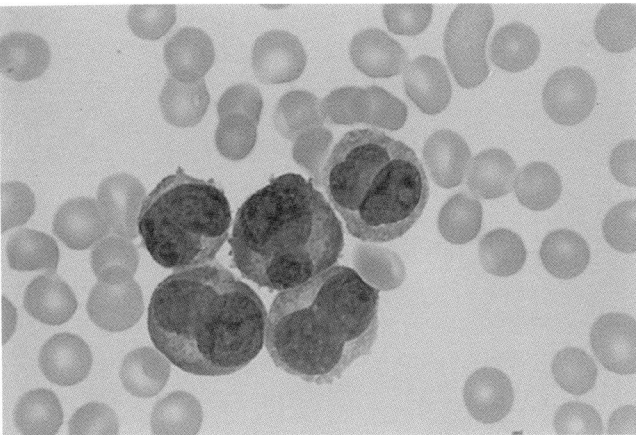

Plate 5 Acute promyelocytic leukaemia, hypogranular/microgranular variant. Peripheral blood smear, showing cells with deeply basophilic cytoplasm, and very striking bilobed or figure-of-eight nuclei. The cytoplasm is filled with granules too small to be resolved by the light microscope, but which are revealed by the electron microscope.

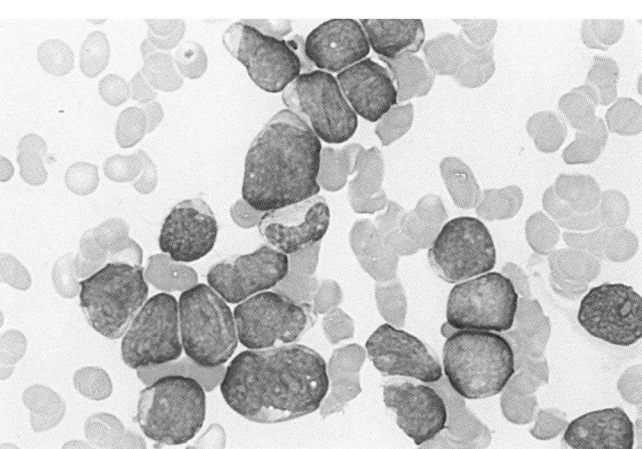

Plate 8 Acute lymphoblastic leukaemia. Bone marrow aspirate showing replacement by blasts. These have a high nuclear/cytoplasmic ratio, homogeneous chromatin, inconspicuous nucleoli, and clear weakly basophilic cytoplasm devoid of granules.

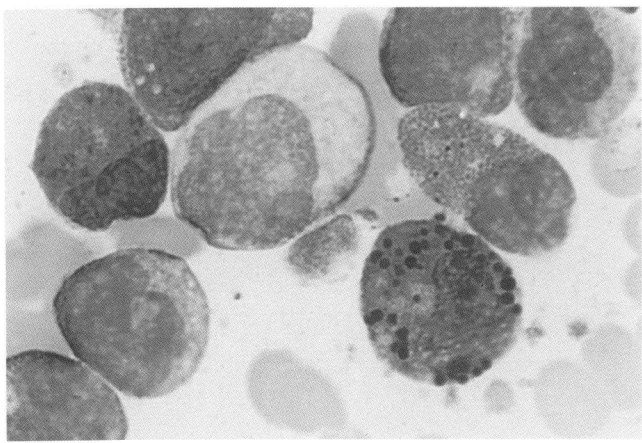

Plate 6 Acute myelomonocytic leukaemia with abnormal 'eosinobasophils' usually occurring when a pericentric inversion of chromosome 16 is present (M4Eo). Bone marrow aspirate shows several blasts, an abnormal nature eosinophil (right centre) a typical eosinobasophil (right bottom), and an earlier similar cell (left centre).

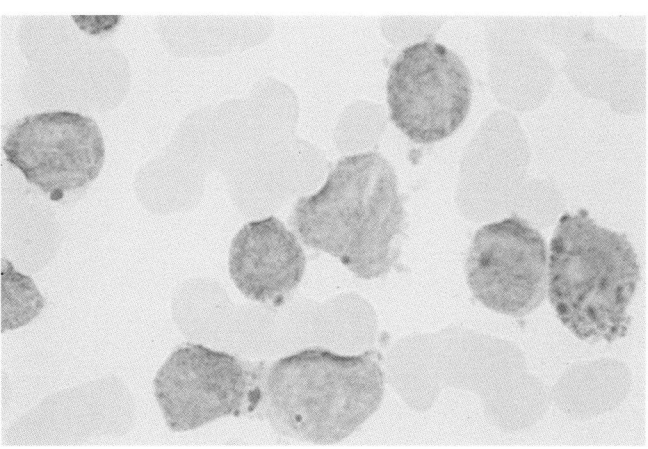

Plate 9 Acute lymphoblastic leukaemia, periodic acid–Schiff stain, showing the characteristic deep red discrete blocks and granules.

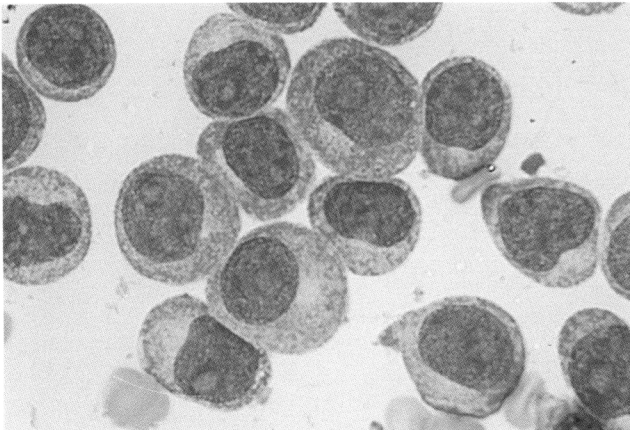

Plate 7 Acute monoblastic leukaemia. Bone marrow shows large monoblasts with round nuclei and a single prominent nucleolus. There is abundant basophilic cytoplasm surrounding the nucleus, and very fine azurophil granules in a few cells.

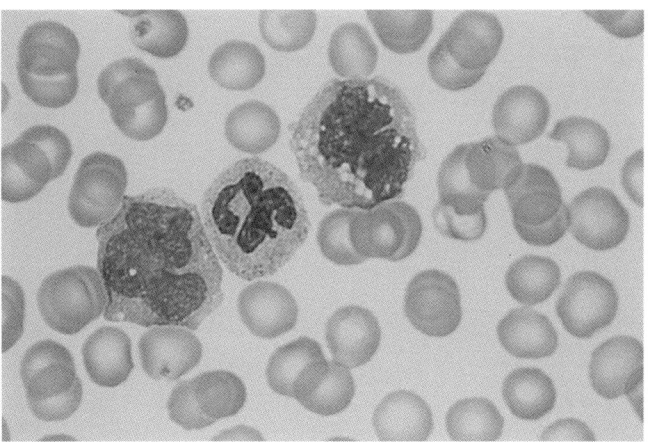

Plate 10 Chronic myelomonocytic leukaemia. Peripheral blood showing two abnormal monocytes and a dysplastic neutrophil with a poorly segmented nucleus.

Plates for Section 22 *(continued)*

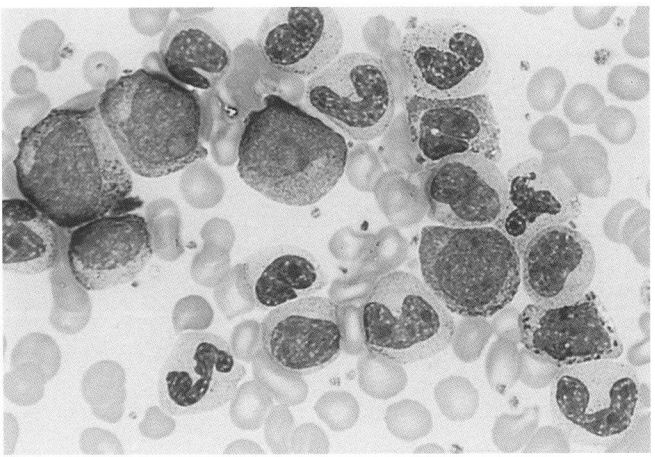

Plate 11 Chronic myeloid leukaemia. Peripheral blood, WCC 237 × 10⁹/l. All stages of granulocyte maturation from blast to neutrophil, with one basophil and one eosinophil.

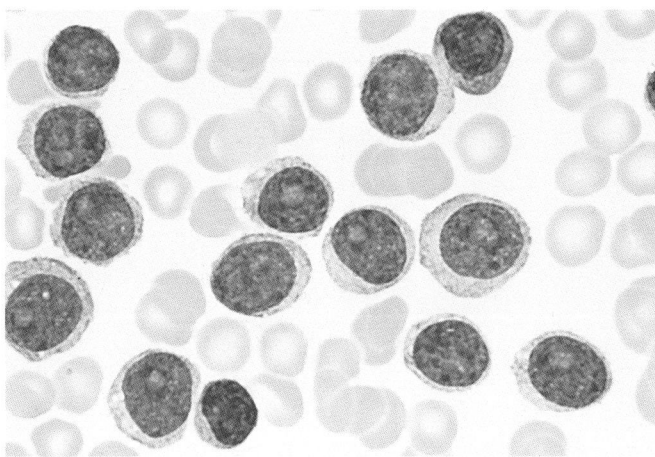

Plate 14 Peripheral blood film from a case of B-cell prolymphocytic leukaemia with characteristic nucleolated prolymphocytes.

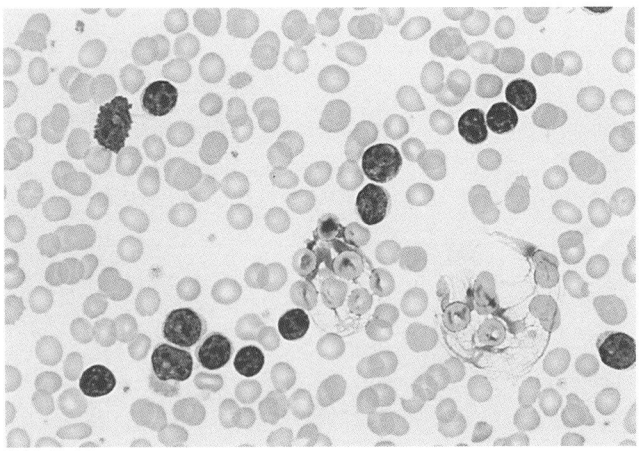

Plate 12 Chronic lymphatic leukaemia. Peripheral blood, WCC 116 × 10⁹/l, showing small lymphocytes and two smear cells (×63).

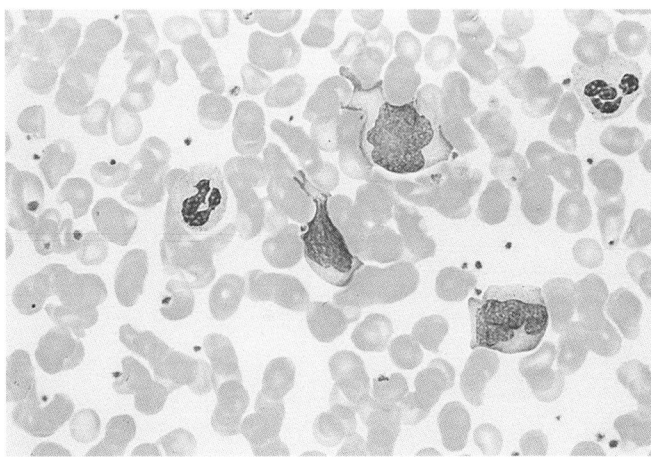

Plate 15 Circulating lymphocytes from a case of mantle-cell lymphoma.

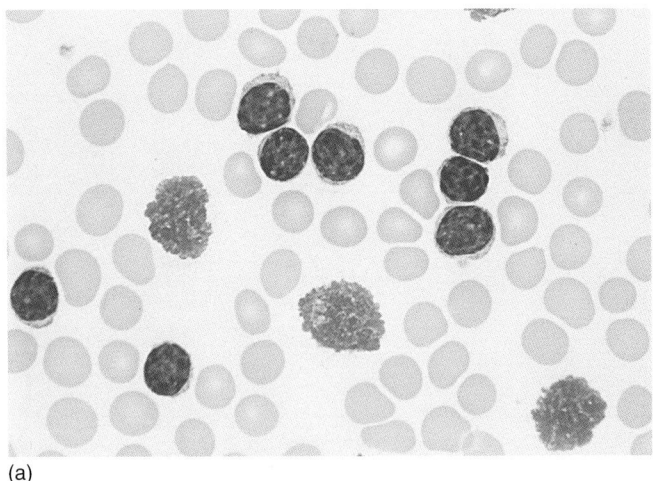

(a)

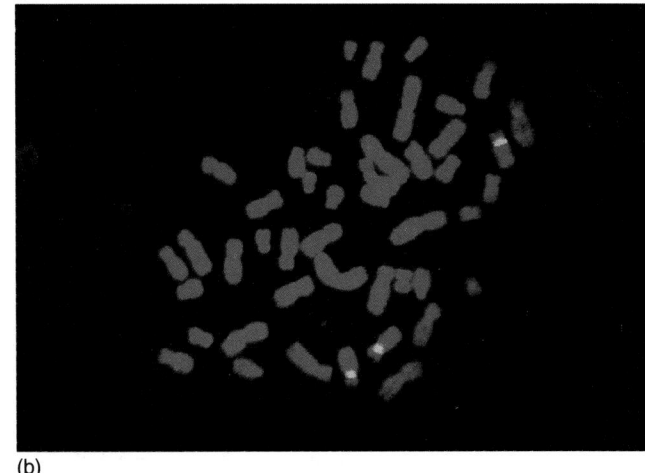

(b)

Plate 13 (a) Peripheral blood film from a case of chronic lymphocytic leukaemia showing small lymphocytes and smear cells. (b) Lymphocyte metaphase demonstrating trisomy 12 by *in situ* hybridization with a centromeric probe shown as single fluorescent dots in three chromosomes no. 12.

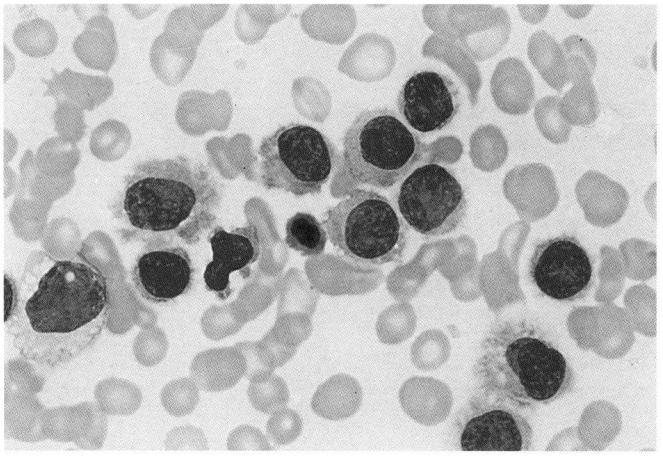

Plate 16 Hairy cell leukaemia, bone marrow aspirate. Many typical hairy cells with deep magenta nuclei, coarse chromatin and a tendency to nuclear folding. The abundant pale cytoplasm has the typical irregular spiked or indeterminate border. (This patient also has B-Thal trait with appropriate changes in the erythrocytes, although not very clear on the marrow smear.)

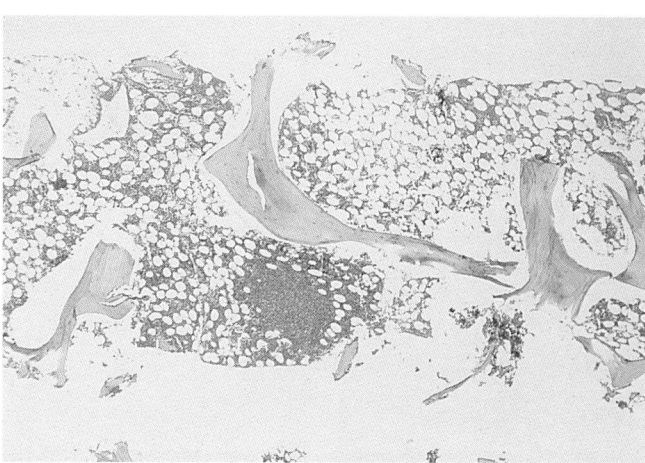

Plate 19 Nodular lymphocytic infiltration pattern in a bone marrow section from a case of mantle-cell lymphoma.

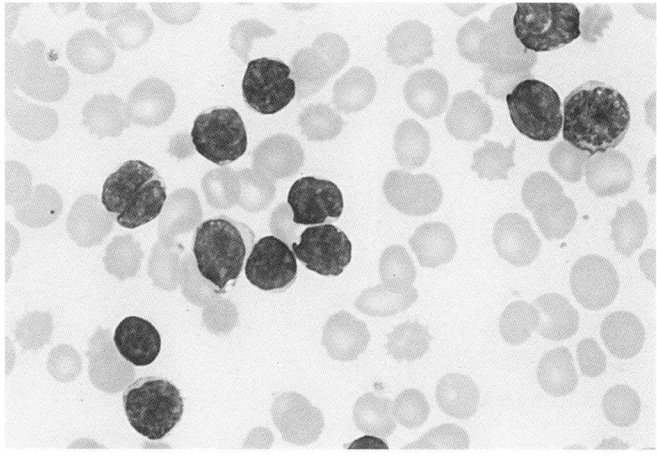

Plate 17 Peripheral blood cells from a case of follicular lymphoma presenting with leukaemia and a high leucocyte count.

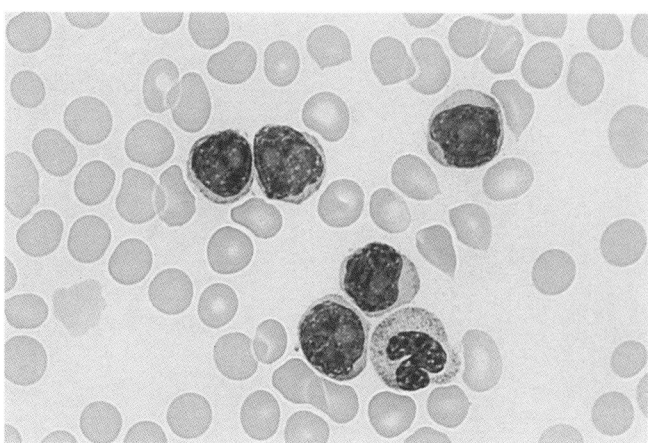

Plate 20 Prolymphocytic leukaemia. Peripheral blood showing five typical prolymphocytes with irregular nuclei, coarse clumped chromatin, a single prominent nucleolus, and moderate amounts of pale cytoplasm.

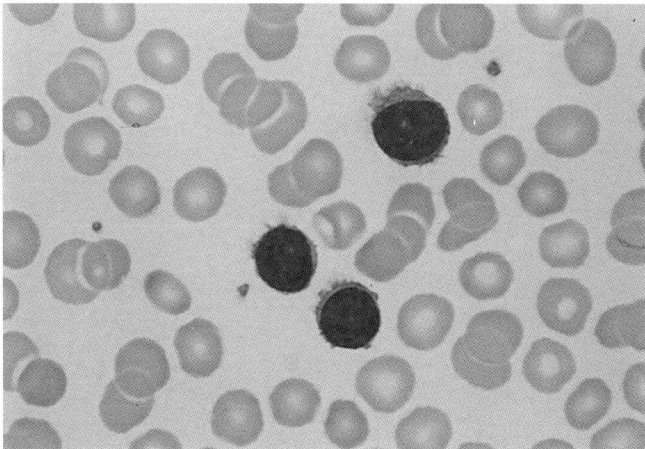

Plate 18 Peripheral blood lymphocytes with short villous projections from a case of splenic lymphoma with villous lymphocytes.

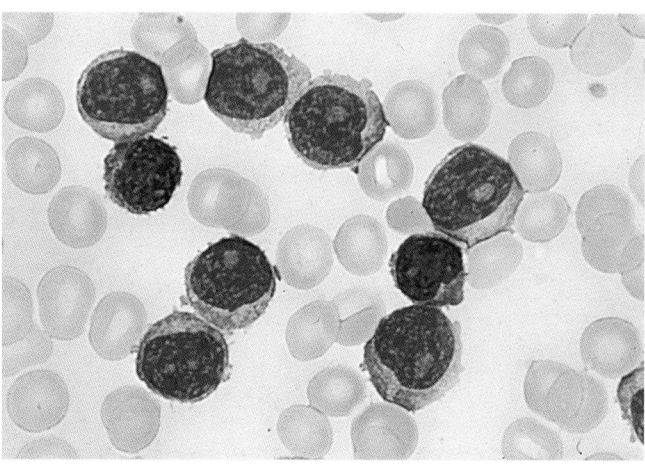

Plate 21 Peripheral blood from a case of T-cell prolymphocytic leukaemia.

Plates for Section 22 *(continued)*

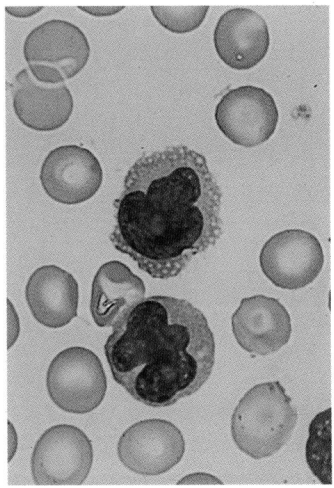

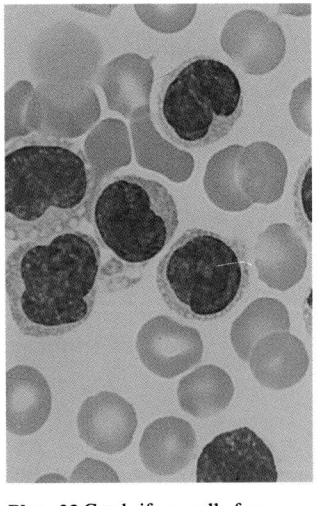

Plate 22 Circulating convoluted T cells from a Caribbean-born patient with adult T-cell leukaemia/lymphoma.

Plate 23 Cerebriform cells from a case of Sezary syndrome evolving with erythroderma and a high lymphocyte count.

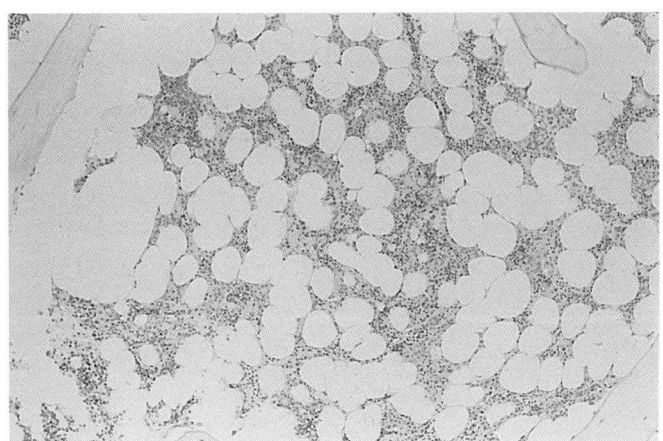

Plate 26 Bone marrow trephine. Normal cellularity (×25).

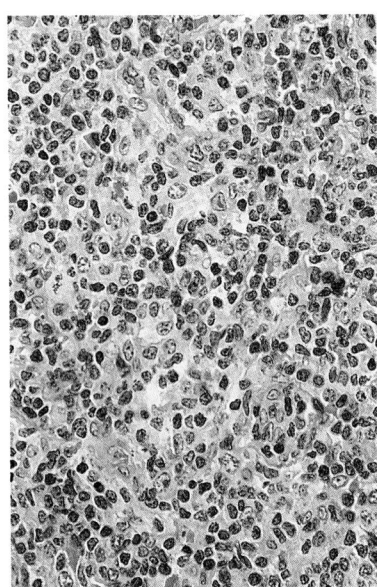

Plate 24 Lymph-node section from a case of adult T-cell leukaemia/lymphoma showing diffuse infiltration with pleomorphic small, medium, and large cells.

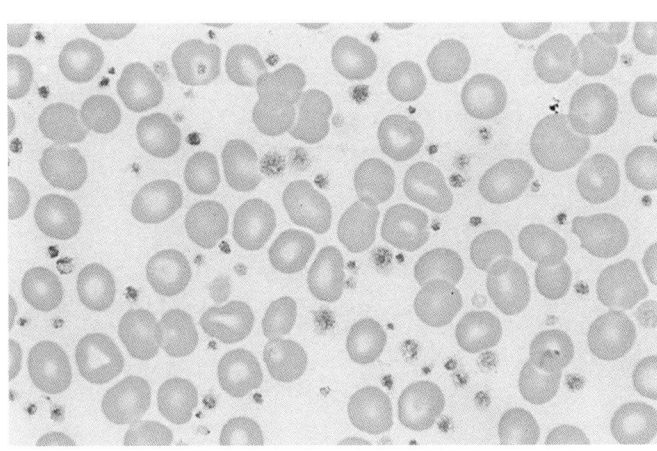

Plate 27 Essential thrombocythaemia, blood film from a patient with a machine platelet count of 2870 × 10⁹/l.

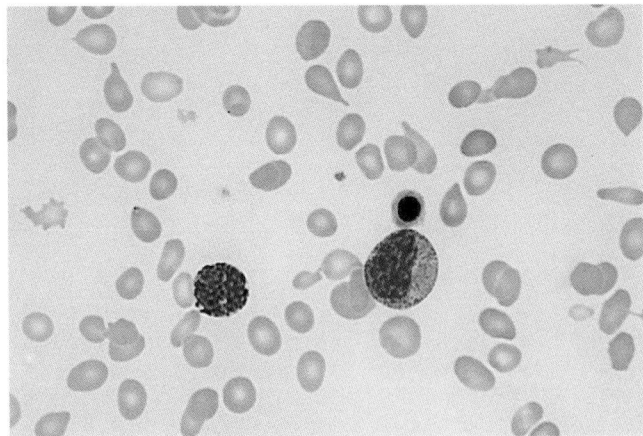

Plate 25 Myelofibrosis. Blood film showing anaemia, many characteristic tear-drop cells, a myelocyte, basophil, and nucleated red cell.

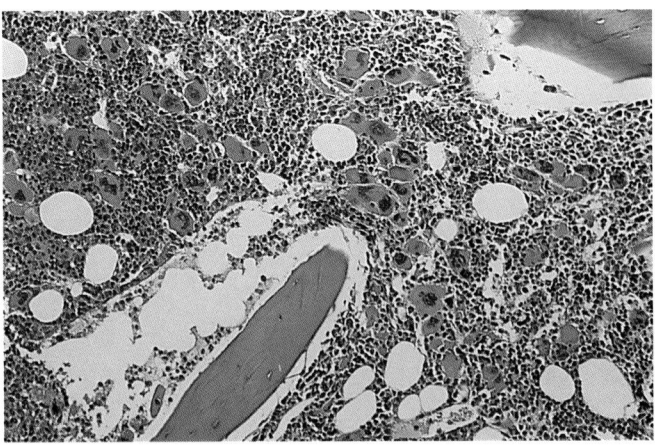

Plate 28 Bone marrow trephine. Essential thrombocythaemia, hypercellular (×25).

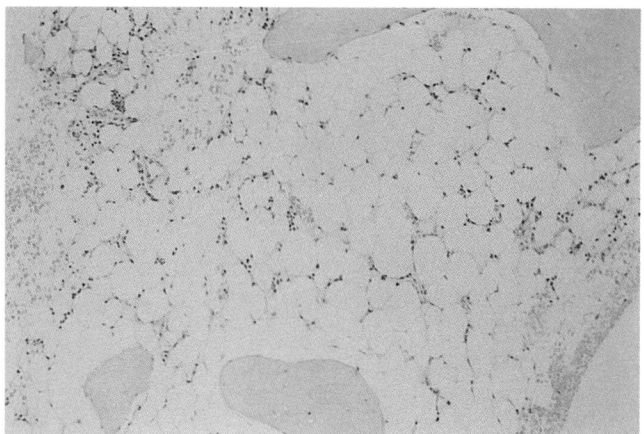

Plate 29 Bone marrow trephine. Aplastic anaemia (×25).

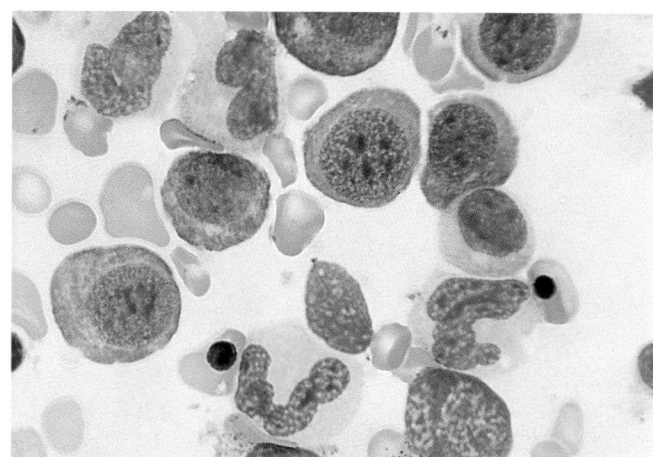

Plate 32 Megaloblastic anemia. Bone marrow aspirate showing mainly intermediate megaloblasts and four giant metamyelocytes.

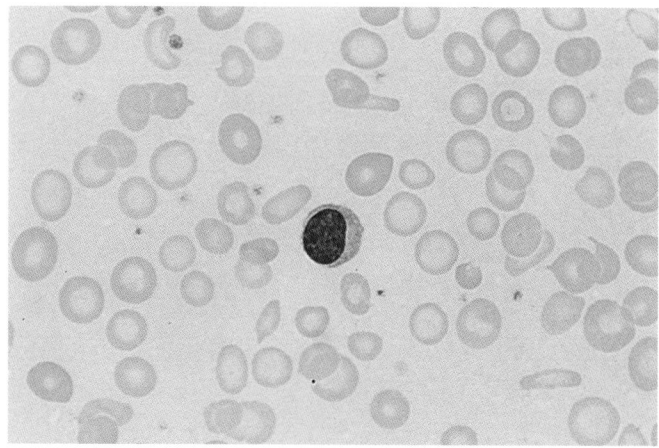

Plate 30 Iron deficiency. Hb 7.5 g/dl. Mainly pale cells with a thin rim of haemoglobin. Red cells are small in comparison to the nucleus of the small lymphocyte. Oblong 'pencil' cells present.

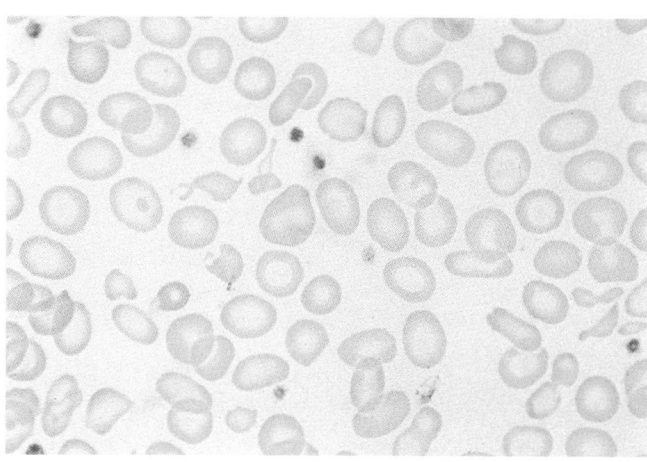

Plate 33 Haemoglobin H disease, showing poikilocytes, occasional target cells, marked anisocytosis, and red cell pallor.

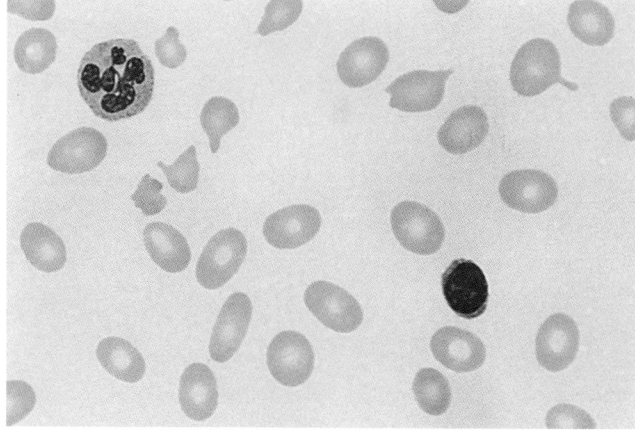

Plate 31 Megaloblastic anaemia. Hb 4.0 g/dl, MCV 120 fl. Hypersegmented neutrophil, oval macrocytes, and a small lymphocyte to show size of macrocytes. The fragmentation of advanced megaloblastosis is present. Thrombocytopenia is marked.

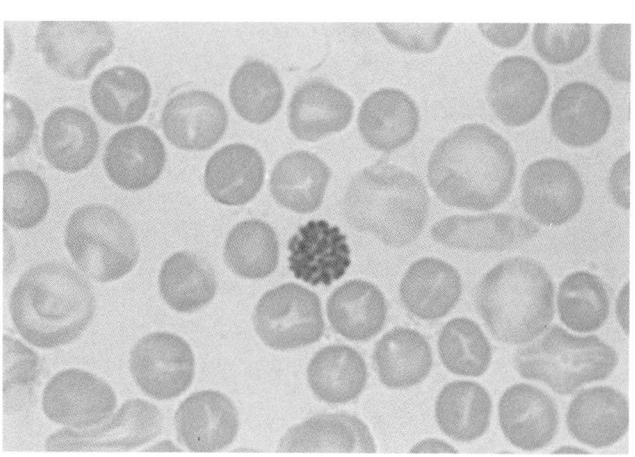

Plate 34 α-Thalassaemia trait. H-body preparation showing one 'golf-ball' cell in the centre.

Plates for Section 22 (continued)

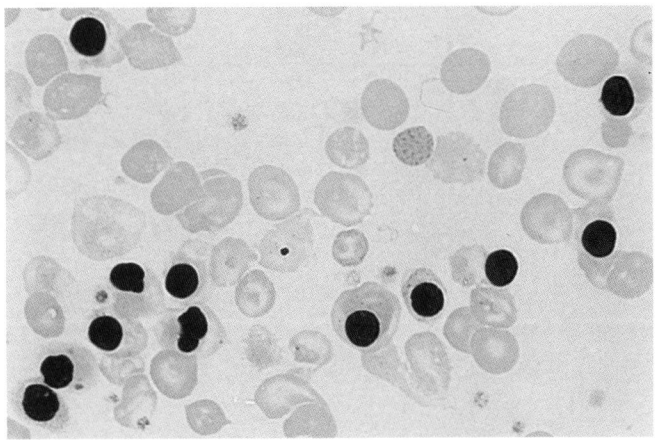

Plate 35 β-Thalassaemia intermedia/major. Peripheral blood film, previous splenectomy. Twelve nucleated red cells, hypochromia, marked anisocytosis, basophilic stippling, and target cells present. There are a few normochromic transfused erythrocytes.

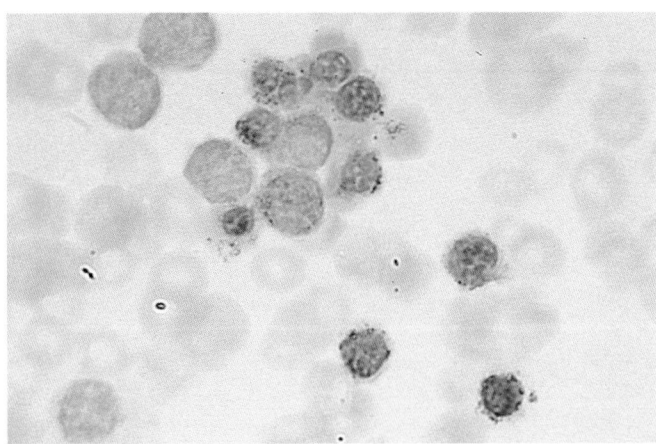

Plate 38 Sideroblastic anaemia (acquired). Bone marrow Perl's stain shows rings of siderotic granules around erythrocyte nuclei, and some mature red cells which still contain many granules.

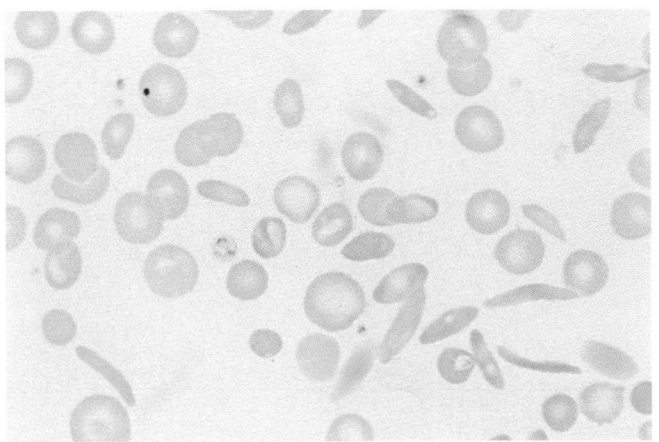

Plate 36 Sickle cell disease (SS), showing many ISC and a Howell-Jolly body.

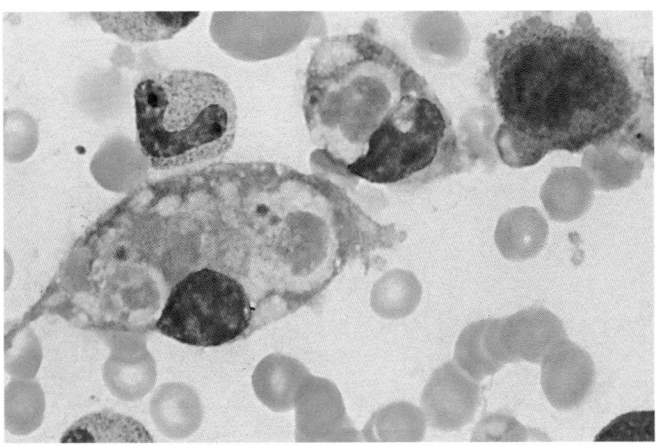

Plate 39 Haemophagocytic syndrome. Bone marrow showing macrophages ingesting red cells and platelets. In association with non-Hodgkin's lymphoma.

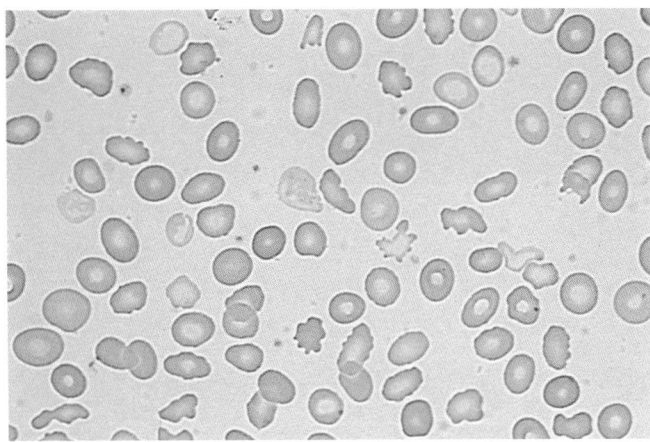

Plate 37 Sideroblastic anaemia (acquired). Blood film shows anisocytosis and some poikilocytes. Variable haemoglobin content of red cells, giving a dimorphic appearance.

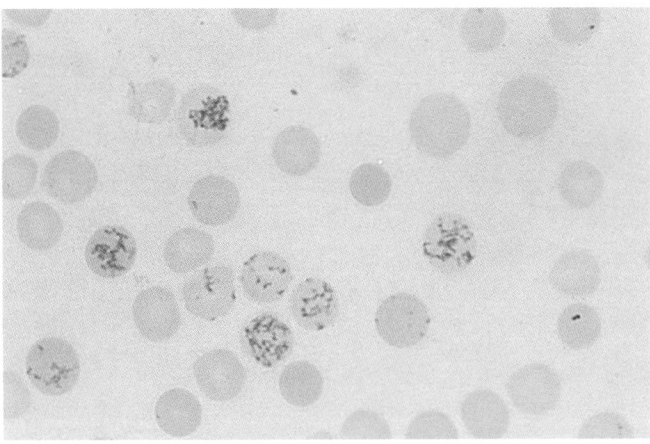

Plate 40 Reticulocyte preparation from same case as shown in Plate 39. Nine cells show reticular staining with brilliant cresyl blue.

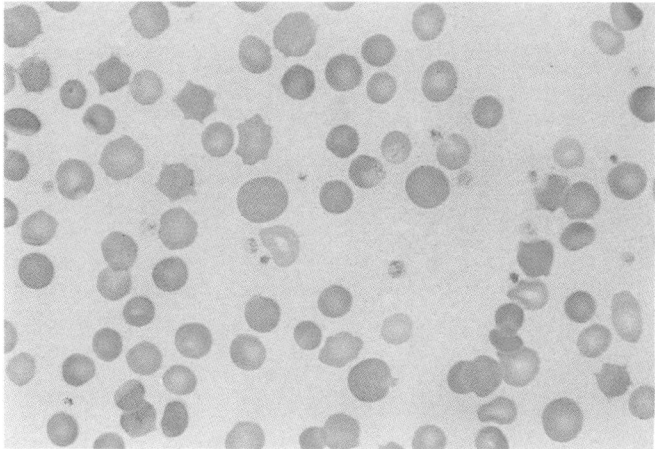

Plate 41 Hereditary spherocytosis. Severe chronic haemolysis, presplenectomy. Many dense spherocytes, marked polychromasia.

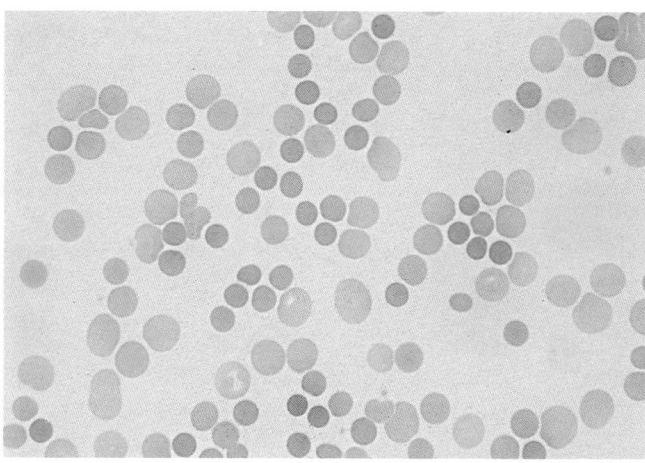

Plate 44 Autoimmune haemolytic anaemia. Strongly positive Coombs' test. The whole blood film consists of dense spherocytes and large polychromatic cells.

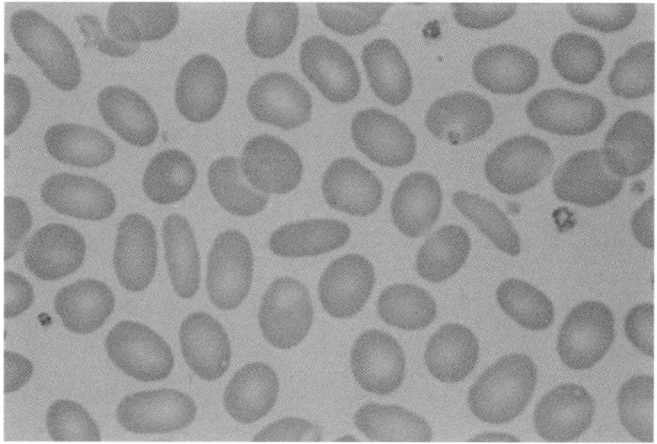

Plate 42 Hereditary elliptocytosis, blood film showing many ovoid red blood cells.

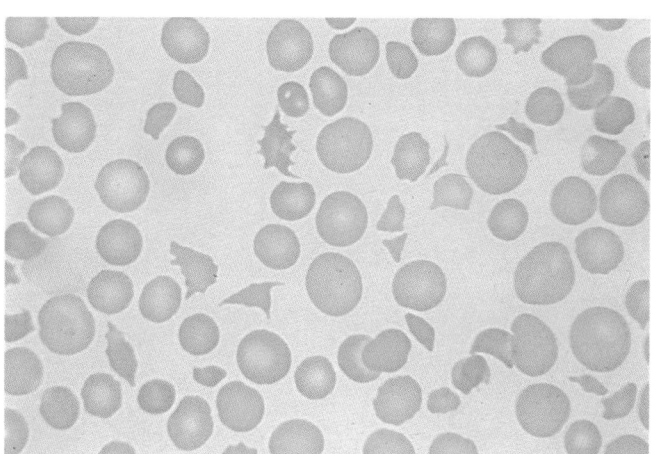

Plate 45 Microangiopathic red cell changes. Many poikilocytes—triangles, helmet cells, etc. There is also thrombocytopenia. Patient with extensive hepatoma.

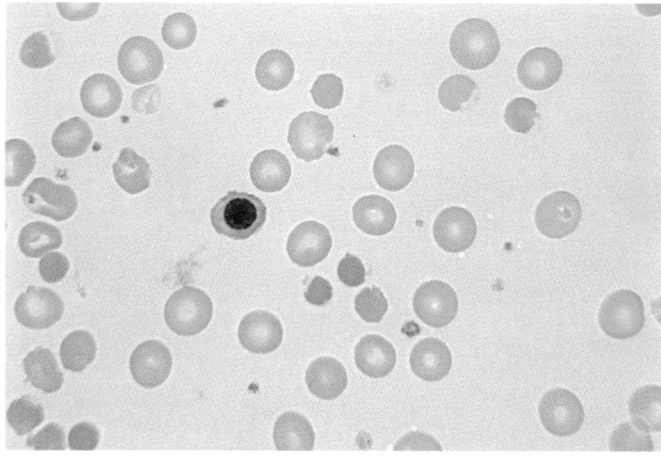

Plate 43 Favism. Acute phase showing many contracted cells, some with damaged membranes. One nucleated red cell and a few contracted cells.

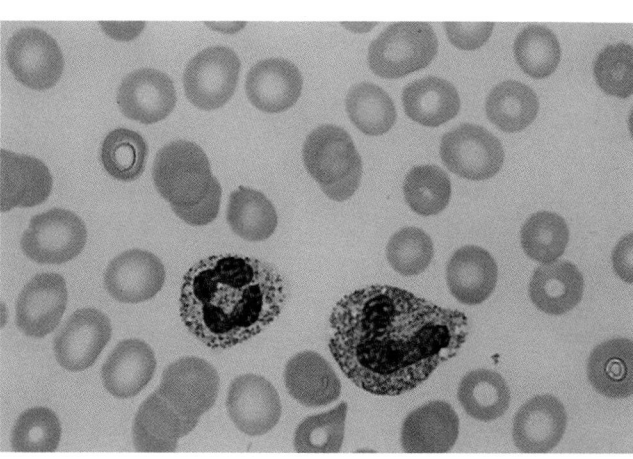

Plate 46 Toxic granulation of neutrophils in the peripheral blood.

Plates for Section 22 (continued)

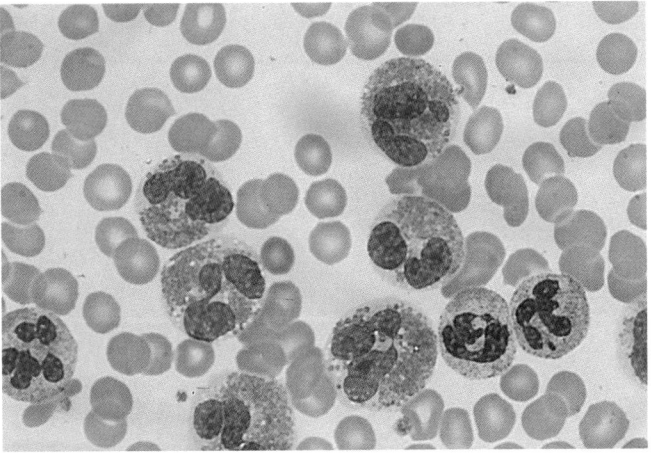

Plate 47 Hypereosinophilia, blood film showing six eosinophils, some partially degranulated, and three neutrophils. White cell count was 106 × 10⁹/l, in association with an underlying T-cell lymphoma.

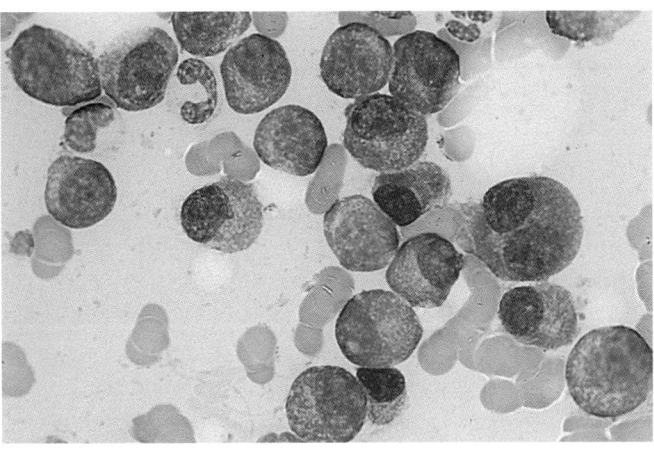

Plate 50 Multiple myeloma. Bone marrow aspirate showing almost complete replacement by large plasma cells. These have eccentric nuclei with coarse chromatin, a prominent perinuclear Golgi region, and deep blue cytoplasm. One binucleate cell is present.

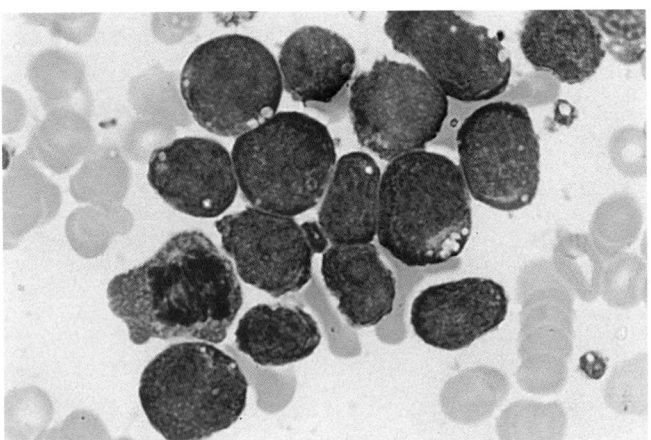

Plate 48 Burkitt type B-cell acute lymphoblastic leukaemia. The cells show coarse homogeneous chromatin, with deeply basophilic cytoplasm and frequent vacuoles.

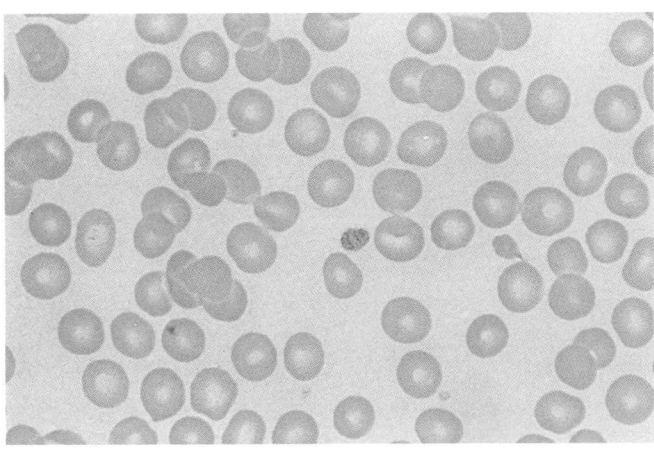

Plate 51 Chronic immune thrombocytopenia, showing one large platelet.

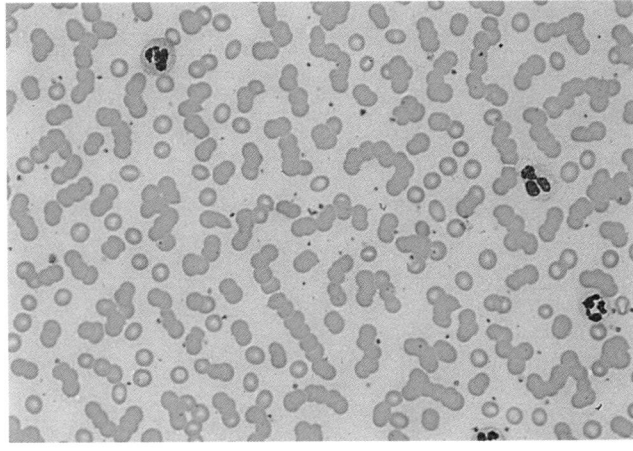

Plate 49 Rouleaux formation in peripheral blood. This example, from a case of myeloma, also shows a blue background tinge due to the raised protein.

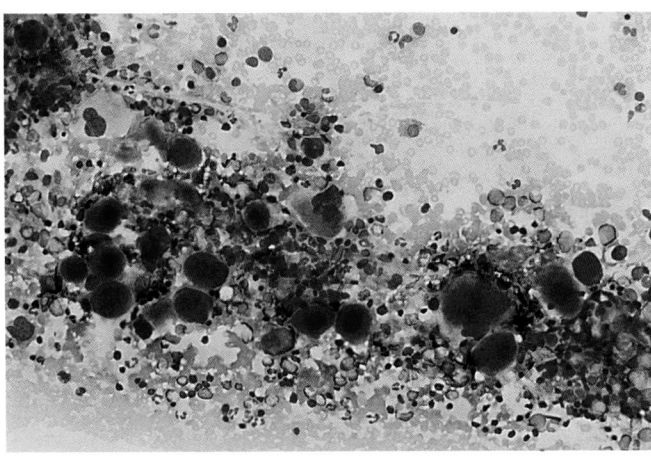

Plate 52 Bone marrow aspirate in idiopathic thrombocytopenic purpura, showing superabundant megakaryocytes.

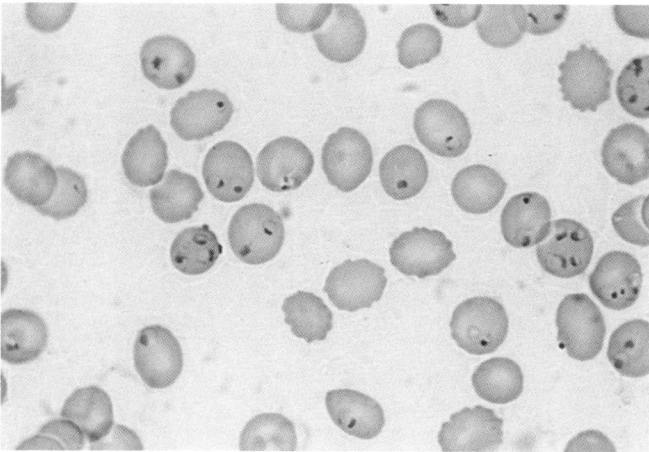

Plate 53 Malaria. Blood film showing fatal *Plasmodium falciparum* infection in a Gambian child.

Plates for Section 23

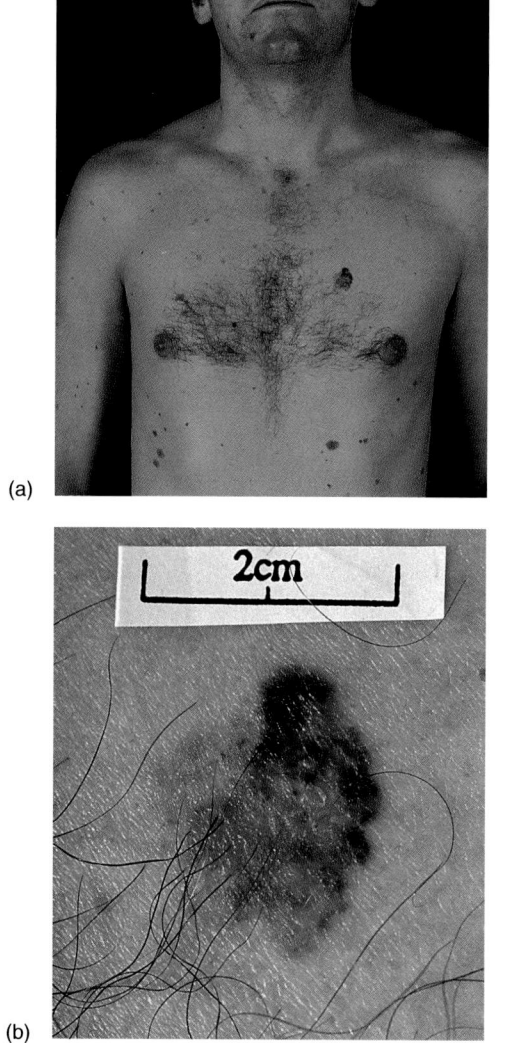

(a)

(b)

Plate 1 In a patient with multiple atypical naevii, one may stand out as different from the others (a) and on closer inspection (b) can be seen to be a melanoma. It has an irregular outline and contains numerous different shades of brown pigmentation.

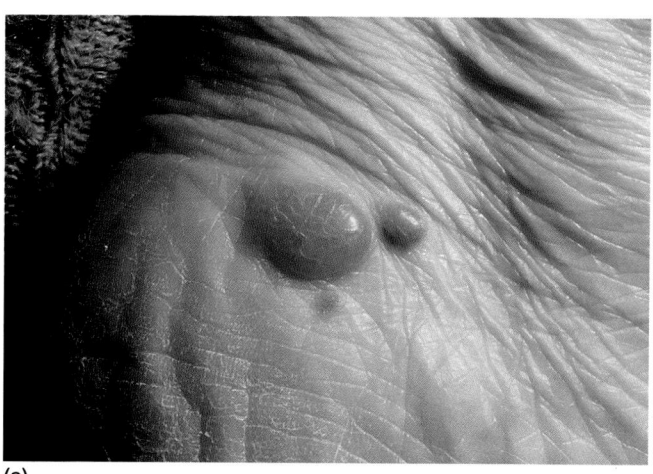

(a)

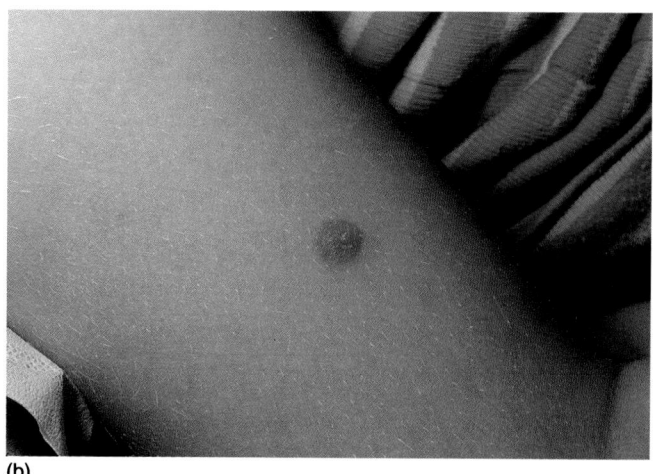

(b)

Plate 2 Most primary melanomas will have some pigmentation even so-called amelanotic melanoma (a). Spitz naevii (b) were formerly called juvenile melanoma because of their histological resemblance to melanoma, but their biological behavior is benign.

Plates for Section 23 *(continued)*

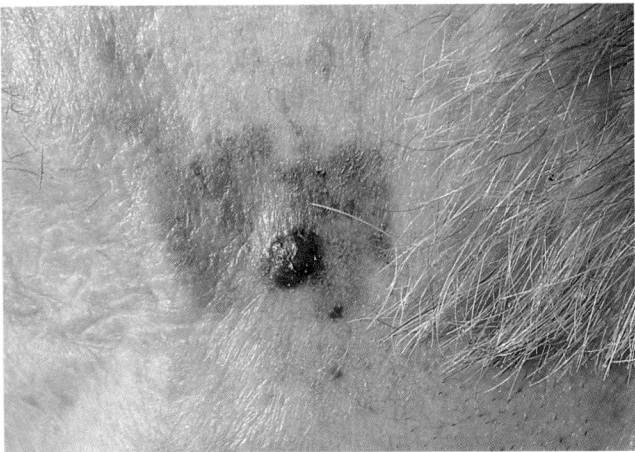

Plate 3 Nodular melanoma arising in a macular lentigo maligna (lentigo maligna melanoma).

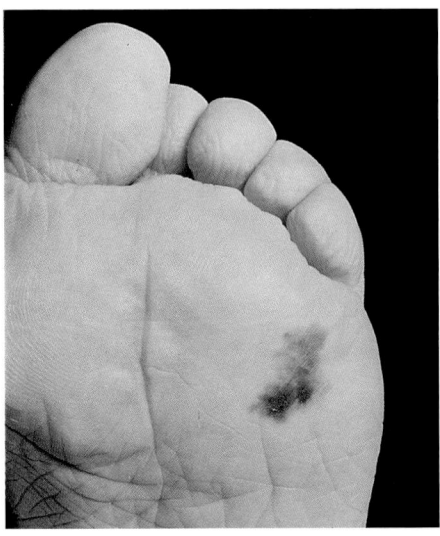

Plate 6 Acral lentigenous melanoma can be difficult to distinguish from benign junctional naevii on the palms and soles.

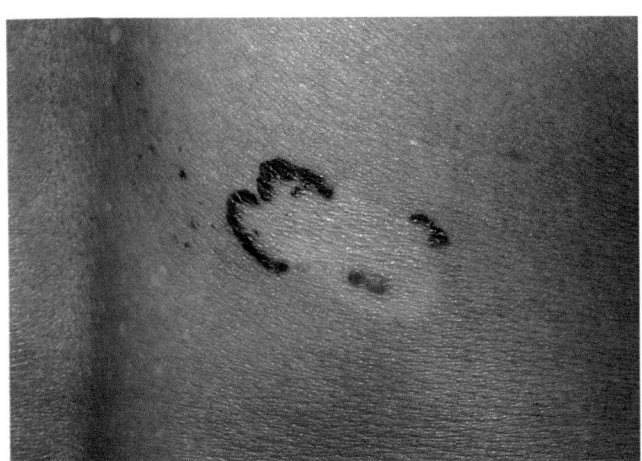

Plate 4 Regression in a melanoma making histological assessment of prognosis impossible.

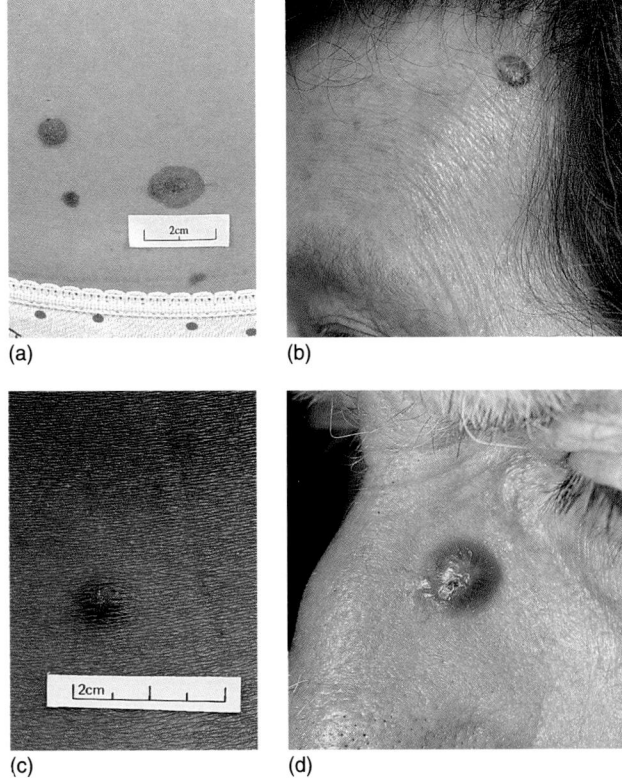

(a)   (b)

(c)   (d)

Plate 7 Lesions commonly confused with melanoma include (a) naevus *en cocarde,* which are central compound naevii with a surrounding macular junctional component, giving the appearance of a fried egg. Blue naevii (b) are often deeply pigmented, but the pigmentation is uniform and a blue tinge is discernible. Dermatofibromas (c) are sometimes easier to diagnose on palpation as they are hard and tethered to the skin. They may feel like a split pea. Pigmented basal cell epitheliomas (d) often have a rolled edge; however sometimes biopsy provides this unexpected diagnosis.

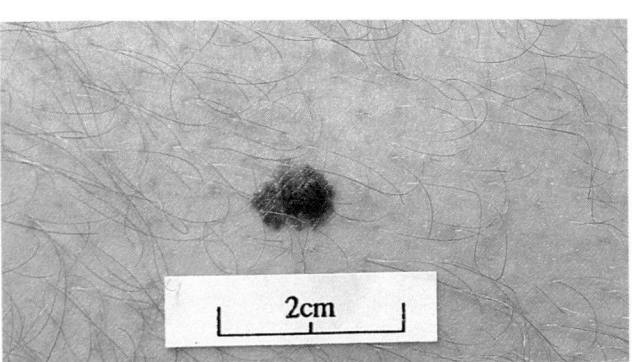

Plate 5 Melanoma most ofter arises *de novo* on normal skin and grows radially as well as vertically. Early detection requires identification of atypical morphology of smaller lesions.

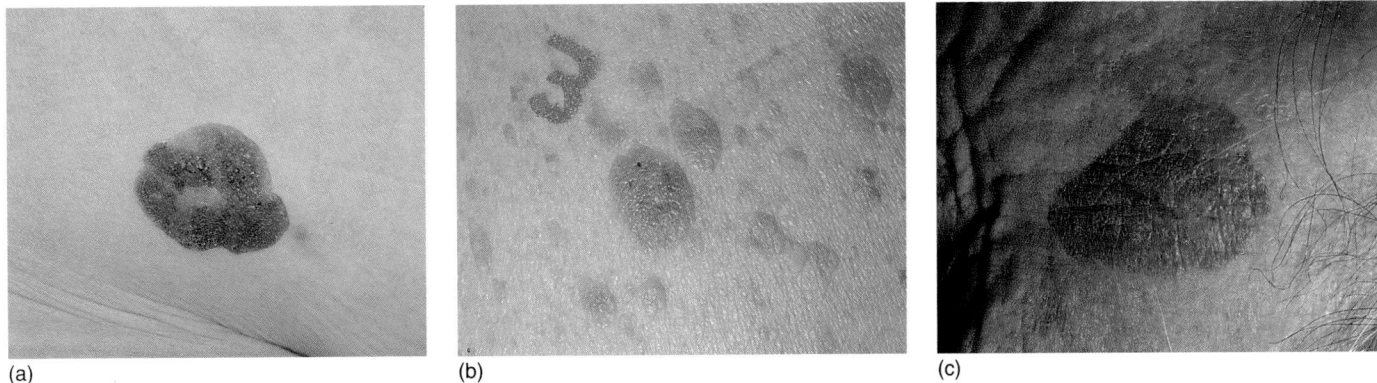

(a)   (b)   (c)

Plate 8 Seborrhoeic warts are often numerous and come in a variety of shapes and sizes. They may be deeply pigmented and elevated (a) or pale (b). They may also be macular (c). Characteristically they have a waxy surface and a 'stuck on' appearance.

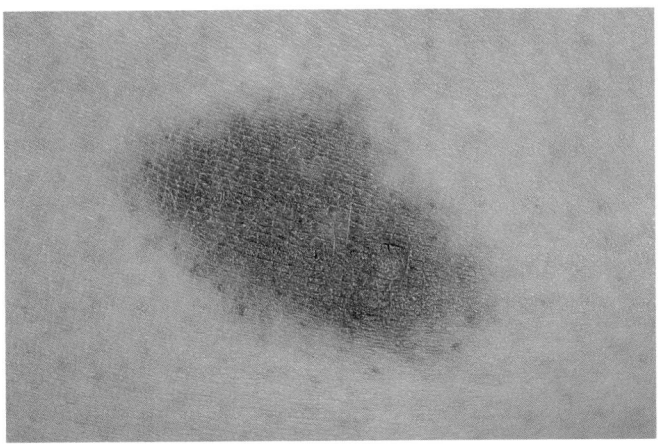

Plate 9 Congenital naevii are often larger than acquired naevii, but are usually evenly pigmented. They have a greater risk of malignant change.

Plates for Section 24
CHAPTER 24.15.1

(a)

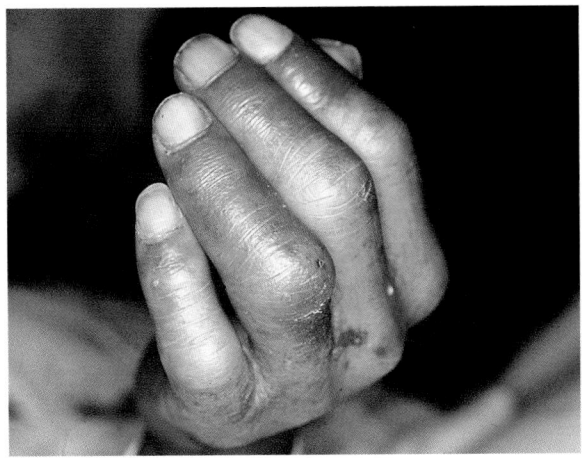

(b)

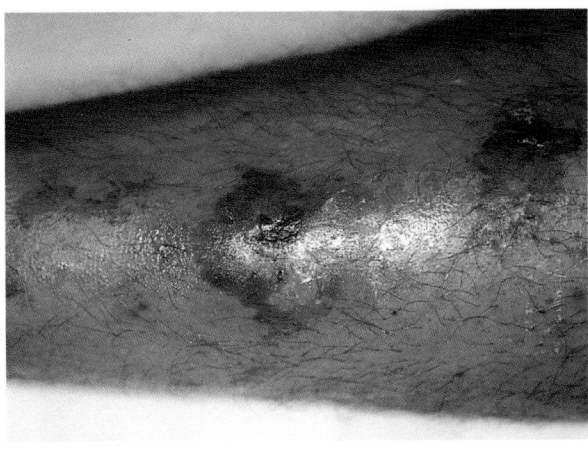

Plate 1 Septic arthritis of the interphalangeal joints in a 73-year-old Thai man with *Strep. suis* meningitis. (Copyright Prida Phuapradit.)

Plate 2 Haemaphagic lesions on the face (a) and shin (b) of a 63-year-old Thai man with *Strep. suis* meningitis. (Copyright Prida Phuapradit.)

Plates for Section 26

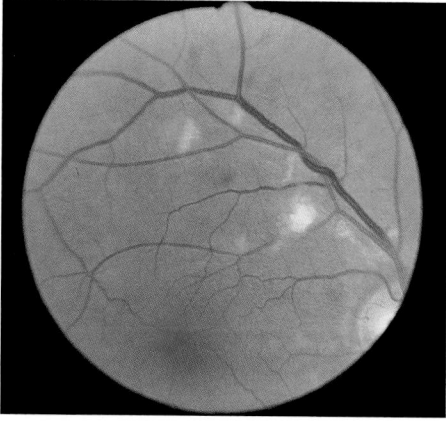

Plate 1 Cotton wool spots. Fluffy pale patches represent retinal microinfarcts, here following coronary artery bypass surgery.

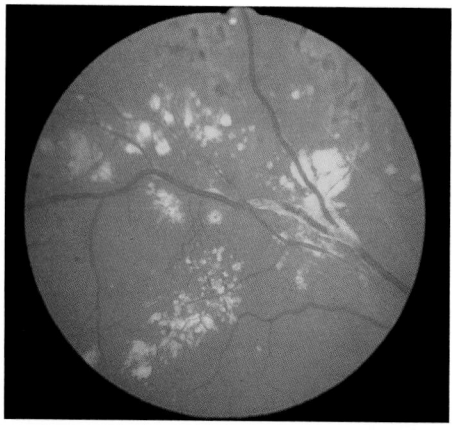

Plate 2 Hard exudates. Shiny pale hard exudates in a diabetic patient with type III hyperlipidaemia represent areas of lipid and protein leaked from plasma. The patient also had xanthomata.

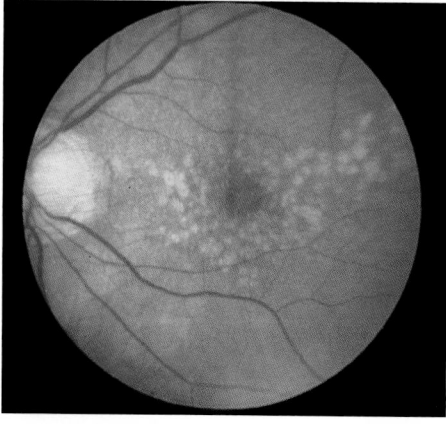

Plate 3 Retinal drusen. Pale lesions grouped round the fovea in an elderly patient are degenerative drusen which may precede disciform macular scarring.

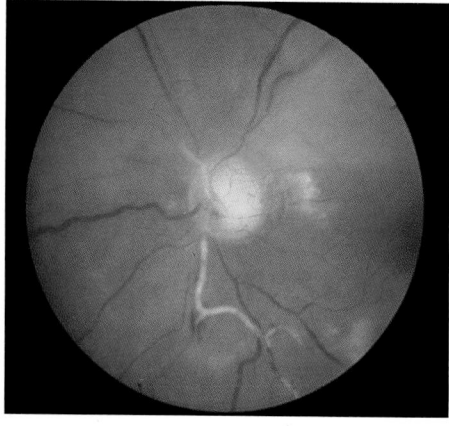

Plate 4 Retinal artery occlusion. Much of the retina is infarcted and hazy though the fovea is spared. The main retinal arterioles are sheathed. This patient had attacks of transient blindness before full occlusion.

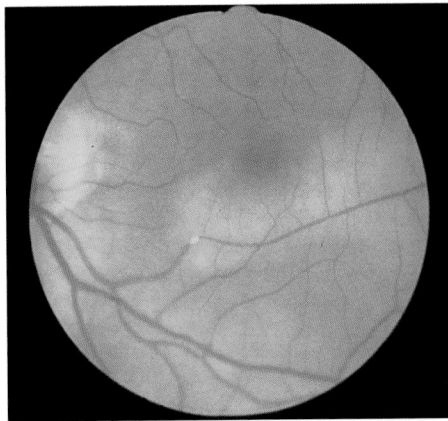

Plate 5 Retinal embolus. A small white embolus lodged in a branch retinal arteriole with surrounding area of pale retinal infarction. The embolus may be a fragment of atheromatous cholesterol or of cardiac valve.

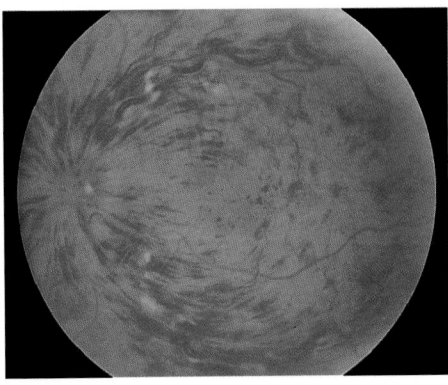

Plate 6 Retinal vein occlusion. Occlusion of the central retinal vein with a characteristic 'bloodstorm' appearance.

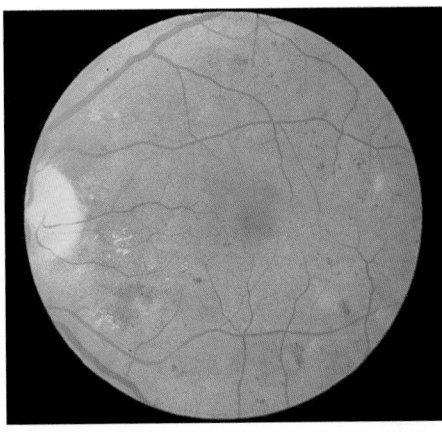

Plate 7 Diabetes, background retinopathy. There are scattered blot haemorrhages and sparse hard exudates but vision is normal.

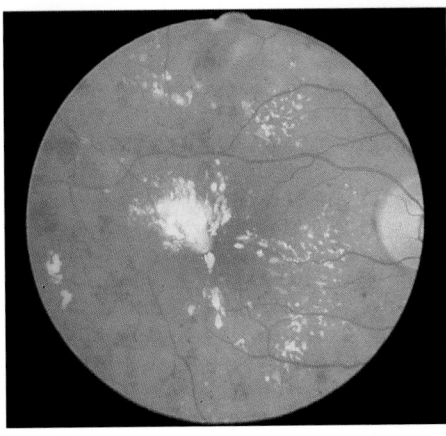

Plate 8 Diabetic maculopathy. Hard exudate at the fovea reduces vision irretrievably.

18.1 Introduction

P. DIEPPE

THE SCIENCE AND ART OF RHEUMATOLOGY

Rheumatology is concerned with the diagnosis and management of a wide group of disorders that affect particularly joints and periarticular tissues. They vary from problems of mild, regional pain, such as a tennis elbow, to severe multisystem, life-threatening disorders, such as systemic lupus erythematosus.

The basic pathological processes involved in diseases of the musculoskeletal system include genetic abnormalities of structural components of the body, inflammation, abnormalities of immune surveillance, crystal formation, ageing and degeneration, and alterations in the normal turnover of connective tissues such as bone and cartilage. Rheumatology therefore involves many of the most pertinent and exciting areas in the medical sciences.

People who aquire these common disorders often develop severe pain and physical disability as well as a variety of general medical problems. Many of the diseases are chronic and progressive, and result in a complex interaction between physical disease processes and psychosocial issues.

THE CLASSIFICATION OF RHEUMATIC DISEASES AND THEIR CONSEQUENCES

The World Health Organization classifies the rheumatic disorders into four main categories:

1. Back pain.
2. Periarticular disorders.
3. Osteoarthritis and related disorders.
4. The inflammatory arthropathies.

The main consequences of these disorders include musculoskeletal pain, stiffness, and physical disability. Pain in muscles and joints, particularly after excess or unusual physical activity, is normal. It can sometimes be difficult, therefore, to distinguish an abnormal response to normal pain, from disease-related pain.

The outcome of disorders of the system should be considered within the WHO framework for defining impairment, disability, and handicap (Table 1).

THE PREVALENCE OF THE RHEUMATIC DISORDERS

Rheumatic disorders are extremely common. Back pain occurs in a large proportion of the population, and severe attacks, sufficient to interrupt work or leisure activities, are frequent in developed countries, particularly in young adults. Furthermore, a large percentage of the population will suffer from some form of transient periarticular disorder (such as 'tennis elbow' or a 'frozen shoulder') at some stage in their life. Osteoarthritis causes problems in up to 10 per cent of the adult population, and inflammatory arthropathies are present in about 2 to 3 per cent.

These diseases cause major problems in the provision of health care; about 1 in 5 of all consultations with a general practitioner are caused by disorders of the locomotor system, and rheumatic diseases are responsible for 30 per cent of all physical disability, and about 60 per cent of the burden of severe disability in older people. The financial costs of lost work, medical and surgical interventions (including joint replacement surgery), and caring for those disabled by arthritis, are enormous.

Table 1 *Outcome of rheumatic disorders*

Rheumatic disease +/− pain
Impairment, e.g. reduced range of movement
Disability, e.g. inability to perform tasks
Handicap, e.g. social isolation and depression
(disadvantage)

Table 2 *Diagnosis of rheumatic diseases*

Pain in or around a joint:
history = pathological process
examination = anatomical localization
Differentiate pain as:

Periarticular	or	Articular
↓		↓
which anatomical structure		mechanical
(bursa, tendon,		or
ligament, etc.)		inflammatory

Consider the consequences (impairment, disability, handicap)

Most rheumatic diseases cause a degree of pain and disability, but have little or no effect on life expectancy. Many start in middle age or older adults. Thus, as the population becomes older, generally fitter, more health conscious, and more demanding of good quality of health in later life, the rheumatic diseases are likely to assume an increasingly important place in the priorities of the health care system.

SORTING OUT PATIENTS WITH RHEUMATIC DISEASES

Pain in or around a joint(s) is the most frequent presenting complaint. The history will help to define the type of pathological process that is involved; for example, trauma may have preceded the onset, sepsis will cause rapid worsening, whereas a degenerative process will result in a slow, variable evolution of symptoms. A working diagnosis can then be made by examining the patient, and following the algorithm outlined in Table 2. Rheumatology is largely a clinical discipline, in which accurate diagnoses, as well as a full assessment of the consequences of a condition, can usually be sorted out through a good history and physical examination alone.

THE MANAGEMENT OF RHEUMATIC DISORDERS

An holistic approach is needed to help patients with chronic, painful, disabling disorders. The major modalities of intervention available to the physician are shown in Table 3.

Family and others involved may need to participate in therapy given to the patient, and rheumatologists often act as the co-ordinators of a team of therapists, normally including physiotherapists, occupational therapists, specialist nurses, and community-based health-care workers. The wide variety of interventions available, as well as the heterogeneous expression and progression of rheumatic diseases, makes management

Table 3 *Treatment modalities for rheumatic disorders*

Patient education, including facilitating self-help
Physical treatments including hydrotherapy
Occupational therapy
Aids and appliances
Local or systemic drug therapy
Complementary techniques for pain relief
Surgery

a major challenge, involving much of the art of medicine, as well as the science.

LEARNING ABOUT RHEUMATIC DISEASES

Students need an adequate basis of factual knowledge, including an understanding of the epidemiology, clinical features, and principles of management of the most common forms of rheumatic disease. However, clinical skills are more important than theoretical knowledge; it is essential that the techniques required to achieve a full assessment of the musculoskeletal system are acquired at the bedside. Appropriate attitudes which will help patients to cope with chronic, painful disorders are also essential. Bedside teaching is more important than book learning.

18.2 Clinical presentation and diagnosis

P. T. DAWES

Introduction

Clinical rheumatology requires a practical understanding of the musculoskeletal system and its relationship to the other body systems. Patients may present with swollen, painful, stiff joints, or in more subtle ways with non-specific pains, arthralgias, or myalgias. Alternatively some rheumatic diseases may present when an associated organ becomes involved, for instance when acute uveitis unmasks a case of previously undiagnosed ankylosing spondylitis. The clinical history and examination should enable the clinician to make a working differential diagnosis, assess disability, and plan investigations and therapy.

Taking a history

PRESENTING COMPLAINT

Patients with rheumatic disease often present with a combination of joint swelling, pain, loss of function, deformity, and stiffness. There may also be systemic involvement with fever, sweating, malaise, fatigue, weight loss, and anorexia. All patients with an acute rheumatic disease must be asked about any prodromal event such as an upper respiratory tract infection, diarrhoeal illness, genitourinary infection, insect bite, or recent vaccination. It is also important to encourage patients to describe their problems in relation to their physical and functional disabilities, as well as to ask about specific keypoints in the functional enquiry.

  The full history should include the past medical history, drug usage, family history and ethnic origin, and dietary, social, and occupational factors. Some forms of rheumatic disease, systemic lupus erythematosus for example, can be precipitated by drugs (such as hydralazine), and many forms of arthritis have a genetic predisposition and racial preferences. Diet is particularly important in bone diseases and occupations are a frequent cause of periarticular disorders.

FUNCTIONAL HISTORY

Any patient with a chronic or potentially chronic rheumatic disorder it is essential to assess the effect of the disease on daily activities; can the patient climb stairs, get outside his or her home, or go shopping? Have they become socially isolated? How many different people have they been able to see in the last week? Can they independently transfer from bed, chairs, toilet, and cope with self-hygiene? Are they able indepen-

dently to cook, feed, and dress themselves? Who is at home and what support do they provide?. If working, is their job at risk, are there particular problems, and are they financially embarrassed? Depending on the answers to these enquiries, the help of an occupational therapist, medical social worker, or disablement resettlement officer may be required.

PSYCHOLOGICAL ASSESSMENT

Patients with chronic disease can have the ill effects of their disease compounded by associated anxiety or depression. An assessment of the mental attitude and motivation in patients with conditions like fibrositis and other chronic pain syndromes is always important. There may also be problems with sexual activity consequent on the disease or the patients perception of it. Correcting (when possible) these emotional and social problems can be just as important as pharmacological treatment of the patient with complex chronic disabling disease.

Key articular symptoms

Three specific screen questions should be asked of all patients (Table 1). It is important to establish in the history how a symptom started, whether the onset was sudden or gradual, and if episodic, self-limiting, or persistent and progressive. Precipitating or relieving factors such as overuse and exercise, rest, emotional stress, temperature, sunlight, and treatment should be identified as well as the pattern and extent of musculoskeletal involvement. Other important issues concern the first joint to be affected, how many are now affected, whether or not joint pains have migrated, and whether the joint involvement has been symmetrical or asymmetrical. It is also important to determine whether the major disability is due to pain; stiffness, or weakness.

PAIN

In osteoarthritis pain is often worse at the end of the day and after activity, and is relieved by rest; whereas in active inflammatory diseases it tends to be worse after rest, particularly in the morning, and may improve with exercise. Joint abnormalities often cause referred pain; for example, disease of the cervical spine can present with shoulder pain, shoulder disease with upper arm pain, lumbar spine lesions with hip or thigh pain, and hip disease with knee pain. Referred pain from internal

Table 1 *Key screen questions to detect rheumatological disease*

1. Have you any pain or stiffness in your muscles, joints, or back?
2. Can you dress yourself completely without any difficulty?
3. Can you walk up and down stairs without any difficulty?

organs is usually unrelated to activity, is often diffuse and may, for example, be altered by coughing, eating, defaecating, urinating, or menstruating. Psychogenic pain is also often diffuse, varies little in intensity with rest or activity, is often associated with other non-specific symptoms, and is unresponsive to analgesics.

STIFFNESS

A joint may be stiff either because of mechanical deformity or because of a local inflammatory process. In chronic arthritis stiffness is often due to a combination of both of these factors. Early morning stiffness is a feature of all inflammatory synovial diseases and its duration is often recorded (usefully) as a measurement of disease activity. Acute or subacute onset of severe bilateral shoulder and pelvic girdle stiffness in the early morning in an elderly patient should always arouse suspicion of polymyalgia rheumatica. Transient joint stiffness after rest occurs in osteoarthritis. With increasing age, joints often become stiffer and complaints of stiffness may be a particular feature of Parkinson's disease, not always clinically obvious.

SWELLING

Swelling of joints may be due to bony hypertrophy, synovitis, intra-articular fluid, or a swollen periarticular structure. Unlike tenderness, objective evidence of swelling indicates organic disease. Occasionally, patients complain of swelling which is not confirmed by examination and the clinician must then question the patient closely to establish or refute its presence. In general, synovial swelling is most pronounced on the extensor surface of joints where the capsule is more distensible.

LOSS OF FUNCTION

In chronic rheumatic disease, impaired function is often due to a combination of pain, stiffness, tendon and joint damage, neurological impairment, and muscle weakness. Patients with such chronic disability often under-report their problems and loss of function from a joint does not always relate to deformity. Some patients, for instance, complain of their joint 'giving way'. This occurs commonly with the knee and may indicate intra-articular pathology or muscle weakness. If the primary complaint is of weakness, observations of gait and ability or otherwise to sit up from a supine position with arms folded across the chest will help assessment of any primary muscle disease. Patients who describe a loss of function out of proportion to the physical findings often are found to have compounding psychological problems.

Key extra-articular symptoms

There are many extra-articular associations with rheumatic disease, some of which deserve specific consideration.

RAYNAUD'S PHENOMENON

Symptoms are usually bilateral, affect fingers more often than toes, and are provoked by cold, albeit sometimes by a very small change in temperature. Symptoms are of numbness, tingling, and burning, with three sequential colour phases of pallor, cyanosis, and, finally, erythema on recovery. Raynaud's phenomenon is often idiopathic, especially in

young women, but is associated with many of the connective tissue diseases, particularly systemic sclerosis in which it is the initial complaint in over 70 per cent of patients.

SKIN AND MUCOUS MEMBRANES

Rashes that often fluctuate with symptoms occur with rheumatic fever, erythema nodosum, adult and juvenile Still's disease, and connective tissue diseases, particularly systemic lupus erythematosus, when it may be photosensitive. Psoriasis may be present but missed when quiescent or hidden, for example in the natal cleft or scalp. Circinate balanitis in Reiter's disease may be asymptomatic, is not always admitted, and specific examination for it is important. Oral ulceration may be a feature of Reiter's and Behçet's disease as well as the connective tissue disorders; Sjögren's syndrome will cause a dry mouth (xerostomia), when oral hygiene may be poor.

EYES

Patients should be asked whether they have ever had red, gritty, or painful eyes. Conjunctivitis occurs in Reiter's disease, uveitis in the other spondyloarthropathies; episcleritis (painless), scleritis (painful), and keratoconjunctivitis sicca in rheumatoid and related diseases. Disturbance of vision and blindness can occur in giant cell arteritis. Rarely, tenosynovitis in rheumatoid disease can affect the occular muscles and cause diplopia.

GASTROINTESTINAL

A transient diarrhoea precipitating a reactive arthritis may have been relatively mild. Chronic bowel symptoms including diarrhoea, blood loss, and malabsorption should arouse suspicion of an enteropathic arthritis secondary to ulcerative colitis, Crohn's, Whipple's, or coeliac disease. Oesophageal reflux and dysphagia are common symptoms of systemic sclerosis; dysphagia may also be a prominent symptom in polymyositis and also occurs in Sjögren's syndrome secondary to a dry mouth or even an oesophageal web. Acute abdominal pain from mesenteric ischaemia or, on occasion, cholecystitis due to ischaemia occur in the vasculitic syndromes, particularly polyarteritis nodosa.

CARDIORESPIRATORY

Episodes of pericardial and/or pleuritic chest pain may indicate the presence of a connective tissue disease. Asthma may be a feature of Churg–Strauss syndrome or polyarteritis. Musculoskeletal chest pain is a common feature of the spondylarthropathies. Breathlessness may indicate associated pulmonary fibrosis or a cardiac defect such as aortic regurgitation in the spondylarthropathies. Chronic nasal, sinus, or middle-ear diseases are usual in Wegener's granulomatosis and may also complicate relapsing polychondritis.

GENITOURINARY

Symptomatic urethritis or an asymptomatic urethral discharge may point to a diagnosis of Reiter's disease. Testicular pain is sometimes a feature of polyarteritis. Dyspareunia occurs in Sjögren's syndrome. Miscarriages, particularly in the second trimester may be one important clue to the presence of the antiphospholipid antibody syndrome.

NEUROLOGICAL

Peripheral neuropathies, particularly an entrapment neuropathy (e.g carpal tunnel syndrome) may be early features of inflammatory synovitis. A history of migraine, depression, psychoses, dementia, or stroke may point to a diagnosis of systemic lupus erythematosus, vasculitis, or the antiphospholipid antibody syndrome. Headaches, scalp tenderness, and jaw claudication are well-recognized features of giant-cell arteritis.

Examination

A full and effective examination requires the patient to be in their under-clothes in a warm environment with easy access to an examination couch. In assessing the musculoskeletal system, of comparison between the two sides of the body, looking for asymmetry in colour, deformity, swelling, function, and muscle, wasting, can be helpful. Separate and careful examination of gait, arms, legs, and finally spine is a useful routine, perhaps best performed by the examiner undertaking the movements and then asking the patient to copy them.

GAIT

The patient should be observed while walking, turning, and walking back, looking for smoothness and symmetry of leg, pelvis, and arm movements, normal stride length and the ability to turn quickly.

ARMS

Inspection from the front allows assessments of shoulder girdle muscle bulk and symmetry. After placing both hands down by the side with elbows straight in full extension, the patient should attempt to place both hands behind the head and then push elbows back, to test the glenohumeral, acromioclavicular, and sternoclavicular joints. Hands should be examined palms down and fingers straight to detect swelling or deformity. It is important to assess movements of pronation/supination and grip, and placement of the tip of each finger on to the tip of the thumb in turn allows evaluation of normal dexterity. Discomfort in response to squeezing across the second to fifth metacarpals suggests synovitis.

LEGS

Observation of the standing patient reveals any gross knee, hindfoot, midfoot, or forefoot deformity. Later examination on the couch should include flexion of each hip and knee while holding the knee to test normal movement and help detect knee crepitus.

Each hip should be passively internally rotated in flexion, and the knee carefully examined for the presence of fluid in the joint. Synovitis in the feet is best detected by squeezing across the metatarsals. The soles of the feet may show callosities; keratoderma blennorrhagicum may be present in patients with Reiter's syndrome.

SPINE

This is best examined with the patient standing. A view from behind detects lateral spinal curvature, differences in the levels of iliac crests, and any asymmetry in paraspinal and girdle muscle bulk. Lateral flexion of the cervical spine can be assessed by asking the patient to place his or her ear on the tip of the shoulder on either side. Tenderness over the midpoint of the supraspinatus muscle suggests the presence of fibrositis.

Anteroposterior curvature of the spine is best observed from the side. Lumbar spine and hip flexion are easily assessed when patients bend to touch their toes with knees straight.

Clinical presentations

PERIPHERAL JOINTS

Peripheral arthritis may present as a monoarthritis or polyarthritis, which may either be acute (Tables 2 and 3) or chronic. Often there is overlap; monoarthritis may have an acute exacerbation and may, with time, become polyarticular. Many types of chronic polyarthritis may start with an acute onset.

Table 2 *Common causes of acute monoarticular arthritis*

Crystal arthritis—gout, pseudogout, calcific periarthritis
Septic arthritis
Haemarthrosis
Traumatic synovitis
Foreign-body synovitis—plant thorn

Table 3 *Common causes of acute polyarticular arthritis*

Rheumatoid arthritis
Palindromic arthritis
Reactive arthritis—Reiter's disease, rheumatic fever
Gonococcal arthritis
Post-viral arthropathies—rubella, parvovirus, hepatitis B
Adult and childhood Still's disease
Psoriatic arthritis and associated spondylarthropathies
Systemic lupus erythematosus
Paraneoplastic syndromes
Polymyalgia rheumatica

Table 4 *Detection of early synovitis in the absence of major joint deformity*

1. Evidence of vasospasm in the fingers can be detected by stroking the dorsum of the examiner's hand across the patient's palm and fingers to detect sweating and a distal temperature drop
2. Proximal interphalangeal joint skin discoloration and local joint tenderness suggest synovitis
3. The knuckles of a clenched fist should be white and stand out clearly with no infilling between them
4. Squeezing across all four metacarpophalangeal joints together may elicit tenderness
5. Pain elicited by forcibly stressing the inferior radio-ulnar joint at the extremes of pronation/supination often indicates early wrist involvement
6. When the elbow is held in full extension a bulge of synovium may be detected just above the radial head
7. Small effusions in the knee can be detected by pressure on the lateral side of the joint, when any fluid present is moved to produce a contralateral bulge
8. Pressure across the heads of the metatarsals may detect local tenderness, reflecting synovitis

Monoarthritis

Certain causes of acute monoarthritis show a preference for particular joints; for instance gout in the first metatarsophalangeal joint, pseudo-gout in the knee, calcific periarthritis in the shoulder, haemarthroses in the knees, foreign body synovitis in the feet (plant-thorn synovitis). Distribution is often in a lower limb in Reiter's disease and the spondylarthropathies, and in an upper limb in gonococcal arthritis. Palindromic rheumatism (self-limiting attacks lasting 1–2 days) often starts in the knees, shoulders, or small joints of the hand. Swelling and pain in a single joint arising on its own or as part of a generalized arthritic state should always raise the possibility of septic arthritis. The most critical test is the examination of the synovial fluid for the presence of infectious agents or crystals.

Polyarthritis

Detection of early synovitis (Table 4) is paramount in the management of certain disease, such as early rheumatoid disease, where there is mounting evidence that treatment is most efficacious if instituted early.

SPINE

Spinal disease can be broadly categorized into inflammatory and non-inflammatory types, although the differentiation is not always clear-cut.

Inflammatory spinal pain

Sleep disturbance due to back pain should arouse suspicion of ankylosing spondylitis, infection, Paget's disease, or malignancy. Vertebral collapse gives rise to acute unremmiting, progressive, and severe pain associated with localized tenderness. Spinal stiffness, worse in the morning and relieved by exercise, suggests ankylosing spondylitis; tenderness of the sacroiliac joints when pressure is applied downward and outward on the iliac crests of the supine patient, or discomfort elicited or by placing the flexed knee on to the opposite shoulder suggests an associated sacro-iliitis. Schobers test of flexibility of the spine, is performed on the erect patient; a mark is made on the middle of the back at the level of the posterior iliac crest (approximately L5) and a point 10 cm above. If the increase in the distance between these two points on maximum forward flexion is less than 3 cm, spondylarthritis is the likely cause of symptoms.

NON-INFLAMMATORY SPINAL PAIN

Pain due to degenerative spinal disease is worse with overuse and weight bearing, and improved by rest. The symptoms are often episodic with periods of acute exacerbation followed by improvement. Spinal movements are impaired, and during the acute episodes there may be scoliosis and associated paraspinal muscle spasm. Degenerative spinal disease is often associated with neurogenic symptoms. Pain, weakness, paraesthesiae, or numbness radiating into the arm or leg are caused by nerve compression, have a dermatome distribution, and are aggravated by movements which irritate the nerve root, such as straight-leg raising and sciatic and femoral nerve stretch tests. Wasting of muscles, loss of power, impaired reflexes and sensation may be present. Spinal cord claudication from a localized or diffuse spinal stenosis classically presents with weakness in the legs on walking with the patient having to sit down for relief of symptoms; this contrasts with the patient with peripheral vascular claudication, who gets relief at rest by standing. Patients with spinal claudication often walk with a flexed spine and adopt a 'simian' posture as this increases the spinal canal diameter.

SOFT TISSUE

Soft tissue symptoms may be due to a localized anatomical problem, with or without an associated systemic disease, or be the result of a condition such as fibrositis. Localized periarticular tenderness from epicondylitis, such as tennis elbow (lateral epicondyle) or golfer's elbow (medial epicondyle), can be confirmed by appropriate movements, such

as forced extension of the wrist which exacerbates tennis elbow pain. Enthesitis describes an area of pain arising from inflammation at a bony interface with a joint capsule, ligament, or tendon, and can be a feature of the spondylarthropathies, for example plantar fasciitis. Localized ligamentous problems around a joint can also be aggravated by an appropriate stress test; for example, tenderness around the medial aspect of the knee due to ligamentous strain will be aggravated by stressing the joint into a valgus position. A more diffuse tenderness around the joint line is more likely to occur with intra-articular disease. Tendons may become diffusely painful and swollen from repetitive trauma, chronic infection, or from synovial diseases such as rheumatoid disease and pigmented villonodular synovitis. Pain from inflamed tendons may be elicited by specific stress tests such as Finkelstein's test for De Quervain's tenosynovitis (extensor tendon of the thumb). Tendons should be palpated during movement to detect crepitus, nodules, and triggering. Tenderness around joints may be due to a superficial bursitis with obvious swelling, as in prepatellar bursitis, or be in the deeper tissues when less obvious, for example subtrochanteric bursitis of the hip. Diffuse swelling around a joint may be due to local oedema or be part of an inflammatory process such as leakage of synovial fluid from a ruptured popliteal cyst, causing symptoms and signs suggestive of venous thrombosis. Periarticular soft tissue hypertrophy may be due to a lipoma or a more diffuse fatty swelling, as seen in the tender medial fat pad syndrome of obese middle-aged ladies' knees, or the benign fibrofatty pads seen over the proximal interphalangeal joints of the fingers (Garrod's pads). Periarticular swellings also occur with arthritis and may be due to gouty tophi, or the nodules of rheumatoid disease and rheumatic fever, xanthomata, calcific deposits associated with systemic sclerosis, or rarities such as multicentric reticulohistiocytosis. If fibrositis is suspected, trigger points and specific sites of tenderness should be sought, particularly in the lateral neck strap muscles, the belly of the trapezius, the epicondylar area, the medial aspect of the knee, and over the greater trochanter of the femur. Hypermobility can cause arthralgia, and is detected by the ability to appose the thumb to the forearm, to hyperextend fingers, elbows, knees, by subluxation of patella, and the abilities of affected patients to place palms of hands on the floor with knees fully extended.

REFERENCES

Doherty, M., Dacre, J., Dieppe, P., and Snaith, M. (1992). The 'GALS' locomotor screen. *Annals of Rheumatic Diseases* **51**, 1165–9.
McCarty, D.J. (1989). Differential diagnosis of arthritis: analysis of signs and symptoms. In *Arthritis and allied conditions,* (ed. D.J. McCarty), pp. 55–68. Lea & Febiger, Philadelphia.
Michet, C.J. and Hunder, G.G. (1989). Examination of the joints. In *Textbook of rheumatology,* (ed. W.N. Kelley, E.D. Harris, S. Ruddy, and C.B. Sledge), pp. 425–41. W.B. Saunders, Philadelphia.

18.3 Use and abuse of investigations

P. Creamer and P. Dieppe

Introduction: The use and abuse of investigations in rheumatology

Most rheumatic disorders are easily diagnosed from the history and physical examination alone but, there are important roles for many types of investigation in rheumatology. They include:

1. To confirm or refute such diagnostic questions as the precise anatomical abnormality of an affected joint or the exact category of inflammatory disease.
2. To assist clinical monitoring of the activity and progression of chronic rheumatic diseases and their response to treatment.
3. To elucidate the nature of some complications of a rheumatic disease or its treatment.

Table 1 *Investigations in rheumatology*

Imaging
  Anatomical
    Plain radiograph[a]
    Tomographic radiographic images (CT)
    Arthrography
    Ultrasound
    Magnetic resonance imaging
    Arthroscopy
  Physiological
    Bone and joint scintigraphy[a]
    Thermography
    Magnetic resonance imaging

Synovial fluid analysis
  Cellular content[a]
  Bacteriology[a]
  Crystal identification[a]
  Biochemical tests
  Immunological tests

Assessment of systemic inflammation
  Erythrocyte sedimentation rate (or plasma viscosity)[a]
  C-reactive protein[a]
  Full blood count (haemoglobin, white cell/platelet count)[a]
  Other acute phase proteins
  Other biochemical/haematological tests

Immunological assays
  Rheumatoid factors[a]
  Antinuclear antibodies[a]
  Other autoantibodies
  Total immunoglobulins
  Assays of circulating immune complexes
  Assays of cellular immune function

Biochemical tests
  Uric acid[a]
  Others

Tissue biopsy
  Arterial biopsy[a]
  Muscle biopsy[a]
  Synovial biopsy
  Bone biopsy
  Lip-gland biopsy
  Others

Neurophysiological tests
  Electromyography
  Nerve conduction tests

[a]Tests of most value in routine clinical practice.

Investigations should be used only to answer well-formulated questions relevant to management of the patient. It is a good discipline to ask 'Will the result of this test alter my management?' before ordering a test. 'Screening' tests and 'baseline investigations' are rarely justified and are often used to conceal ignorance or sloppy thinking.

Investigations rarely have anything approaching 100 per cent sensitivity or specificity, and must be interpreted in the light of their intrinsic variation and error rate, which may vary in different centres. Furthermore, it is often the case that the overall pattern of clinical and investigation findings is more important than any single test result or clinical sign.

Types of available investigation

The spectrum of available tests will vary from centre to centre. However, tests can be subdivided into a small number of categories from which a limited number of key investigations can be picked, as indicated in Table 1.

In this chapter, each of the main categories of investigation will be considered, with an emphasis on their practical value in routine clinical practice.

Imaging

Imaging of bones and joints is one of the oldest and most valuable investigations in rheumatology. Normal and abnormal anatomy of the musculoskeletal system can be visualized in a number of ways; in addition, pathophysiological changes, such as alterations in blood flow or bone turnover can be imaged. The most important investigation in this category remains the plain radiograph.

THE PLAIN RADIOGRAPH

Plain radiographs provide excellent images of bones, with some ability to discern the surrounding soft tissues, such as the synovial cavity of

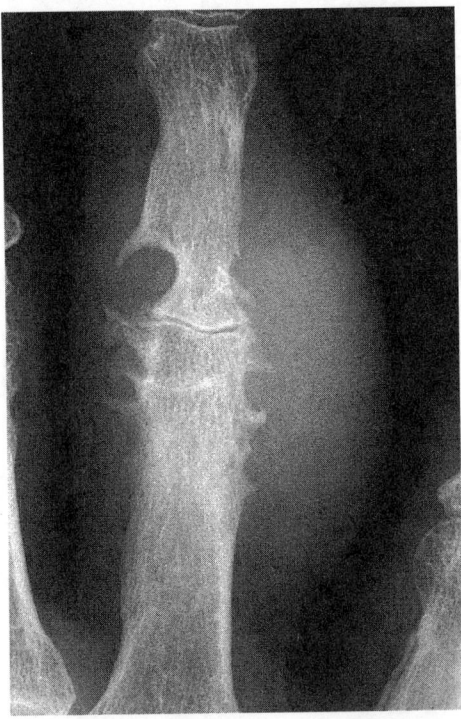

Fig. 1 Erosion of chronic tophaceous gout. The erosion is punched out and occurs along the shaft of the phalanx rather than on the articular surface. There is considerable soft-tissue swelling.

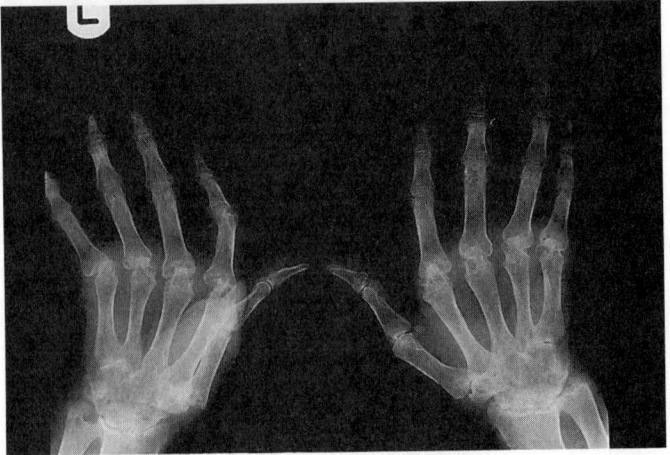

Fig. 2 Rheumatoid arthritis.

joints. Many bone and joint diseases result in characteristic changes in bony texture or contour, resulting in pathognomonic radiograph images (Figs. 1 and 2). However, there are several drawbacks, including the limitations of a two-dimensional image of three-dimensional structures, the variability introduced by small differences in patient position when radiographs are taken, and exposure to potentially dangerous radiation. For these reasons, radiography is best used when a limited number of views are obtained in order to answer a specific question.

The value of plain radiography lies in diagnosis, monitoring, and detection of disease and its complications.

Diagnostic examples include the detection of the characteristic erosions of gout, rheumatoid arthritis, or psoriatic arthropathy, or the features of osteoarthritis or chondrocalcinosis. A single anteroposterior view of the hands and feet is sufficient to demonstrate erosions and many other signs of joint disease; chondrocalcinosis is best detected on a single anteroposterior view of the knees. Sacroiliitis, a feature of seronegative arthropathy, is best seen on a plain anteroposterior view of the pelvis. If a single joint is abnormal, it may be useful to obtain identical views of both sides for comparison, but indiscriminate radiography of painful joints is of no value.

The plain radiograph is also important in monitoring disease progression. By the time a radiograph shows the characteristic features of either rheumatoid arthritis or osteoarthritis, the condition is well established and the diagnosis is likely to be easy without the aid of investigations. However, progression of disease over a period of years may be best monitored by radiography, provided that there is good reason to record this.

Several complications of rheumatic diseases, such as subluxations or dislocations, can be detected by plain radiography. An important example is subluxation of the cervical spine in rheumatoid arthritis, best seen by a single lateral view of the neck held in flexion.

The abuse of plain radiographs is a major problem. Doctors tend to order too many views of too many joints at unnecessarily frequent intervals. Symptoms and disability correlate poorly with the degree of radiographic change in radiographic appearance of a joint, and radiographic changes alone are rarely a reason for clinical action. Spinal radiographs for back pain are a special problem as changes of osteoarthritis are common in the elderly; they rarely provide information of any clinical value.

MODIFIED RADIOGRAPHIC TECHNIQUES

The views taken will determine what is seen on a radiograph, structures which are tangential to the X-ray beam being imaged best. Special views may be helpful. In the knee, for example, weight-bearing films are needed to optimize visualization of the interbone distance (or 'joint space', indicative of the thickness of the articular cartilage), long leg films or stress films may help measurement of angulation deformities and loading of the knee joint, and special views, such as the 'skyline view' are needed to image the patellofemoral joint.

Magnification techniques and digital imaging are being explored to help detection and measurment of subtle changes on plain radiographs of the limbs.

Radiographic imaging of the axial skeleton has been revolutionized by computerized tomography (CT). Multiple scan sections can be reconstructed to give a three-dimensional image, allowing facet joints, the spinal canal, and other structures to be visualized. CT is of great value in conditions such as spinal stenosis (Fig. 3), although it does require sophisticated equipment, specialized interpretation and exposure to a considerable radiation dosage. Arthrography, involving the injection of contrast medium into a joint or other tissue space, is another valuable way of increasing the amount of information that can be obtained from radiograph. Soft tissues are outlined, and the technique is useful in diagnosis of anatomical changes in the knee joint, as well as in spinal disease. In many centres, these modified radiography techniques are now being superseded by magnetic resonance imaging (MRI).

'PHYSIOLOGICAL' IMAGING TECHNIQUES

Radiography is limited by the fact that it can only provide a static historical record of previous anatomical changes that have occurred in a bone or joint. For example, septic arthritis will take several days or weeks to produce significant radiographic changes, and rheumatoid erosions rarely appear until the disease has been active for several months. Other types of imaging can visualize physiological as well as anatomical change. Such techniques include scintigraphy and MRI.

Scintigraphy

This involves the gamma-camera imaging of body tissues that have localized a radioisotope injected intravenously. The isotope most widely used is $^{99}Tc^m$-labelled diphosphonate. 'Early' images, obtained within minutes of injection, reflect blood flow, whereas 'late' images, taken a few hours after injection, indicate bone activity, due to localization of diphosphonate to areas of active bone turnover. Scintigraphy offers an extremely sensitive but non-specific way of detecting bone and joint disease. The particular value of bone scintigraphy results from its sensitivity in the detection of important lesions that may otherwise be missed; for example, bone metastases (Fig. 4), stress fractures, or occult infection such as septic discitis. The main problems in its use come from a lack of understanding that it has little or no specificity, so that a 'positive bone scan' means nothing unless it answers a highly specific clinical question.

Magnetic resonance imaging

MRI has enormous potential in the investigation of musculoskeletal diseases. Its ability to image soft tissue anatomy and biochemistry as well as bone means that it can provide superior information not only on anatomy but also on pathophysiology of bones and joints. A further advantage is the safe, non-invasive nature of the technique, without radiation exposure. The information obtained by the MRI of the cervical spine of a patient with rheumatoid arthritis, shown in Fig. 5, would otherwise have had to be obtained by cervical myelography, an unpleasant, time-consuming procedure involving considerable radiation. The main limitation of MRI is the cost of the procedure and time taken to obtain the information required to construct images. Its general value depends on availability of hardwear, money, software programs for bone and joint imaging and, availability of specialists who can operate his equipment and interpret the data. MRI can be abused because of the seduction afforded by beautiful but costly images, sometimes obtained more for 'oh my' value than to solve a clinical problem.

Fig. 3 CT scan of lumbar spine at L4/5 level. There is gross degenerative disease in the facet joints with a degenerative spondylolisthesis. The result is an acquired spinal stenosis.

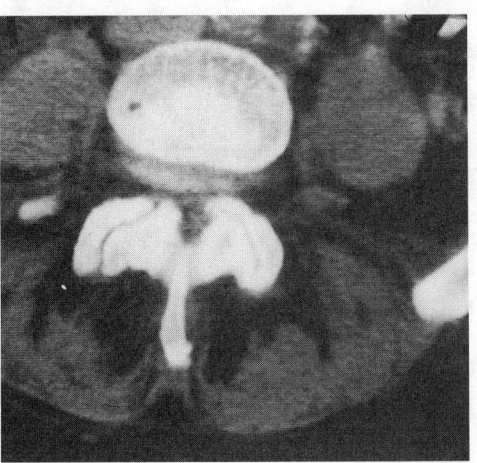

OTHER IMAGING TECHNIQUES

Arthroscopy is particularly useful in the investigation of a monoarthritis of uncertain aetiology. It can be used to obtain a sight-directed biopsy from a suspected pathological area: for example in tuberculous arthritis or pigmented villonodular synovitis. It is of great value in detecting internal derangements, such as cartilage or ligamentous injuries; moreover, treatment can often be undertaken via the arthroscope. In general, arthroscopy has little place in the management of arthritis where the diagnosis is known, although it can be useful as a means of giving a therapeutic lavage or washout. The knee is the joint most accessible to arthroscopy although instruments are now available which allow the shoulder, hip, and even smaller joints to be examined. Thermography detects the infrared radiation from the skin, and can be used to quantify changes in blood flow and inflammation in limbs and joints. Ultrasound imaging is a useful non-invasive way of detecting some soft tissue changes, including effusions in the hip joint and a Baker's cyst at the knee. Bone mineral density may be measured using dual-emission X-ray absorbitometry or DEXA scanning: this is helpful in some cases of osteoporosis.

Synovial fluid analysis

Synovial fluid analysis can provide answers to five types of question (Table 2). It is possible to obtain a small amount of synovial fluid from almost any joint and the contents of a needle are sufficient for many of

Table 2 *Synovial fluid analysis*

1. Intra-articular bleeding?
    Blood-staining of the synovial fluid
2. How much synovial inflammation?
    Fluid volume, viscosity, and opalescence
    Total and differential white cell count
    Biochemical assays, e.g., lactate dehydrogenase
3. Joint sepsis?
    Organisms visible on Gram stain
    Culture of organisms from synovial fluid
    Antigen detection, e.g. by molecular techniques
4. Crystal-associated arthropathy?
    Polarized light microscopy
    Stains for calcium crystals (e.g. alizarin red)
    Analytical electron microscopy
5. How much joint destruction?
    Number and size of cartilage fragments
    Biochemical assays, e.g. proteoglycan levels

Fig. 6 Synovial fluid: (a) non-inflammatory, e.g. osteoarthritis; (b) inflammatory, e.g. rheumatoid or psoriatic arthritis.

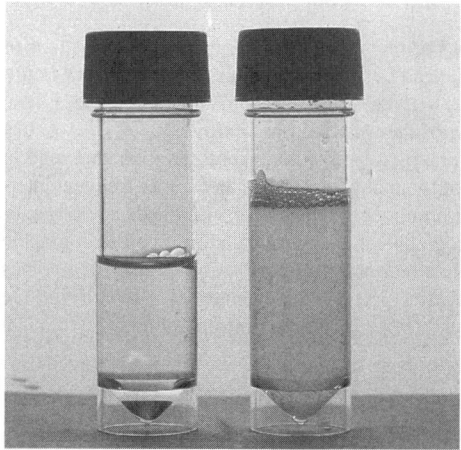

Fig. 4 Bone scan indicating multiple metastatic deposits.

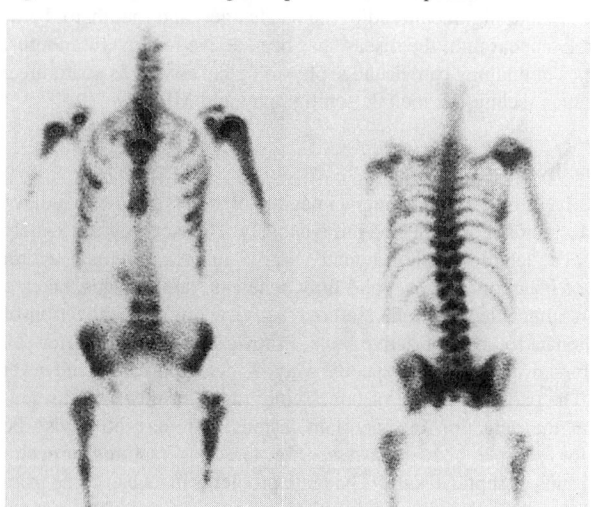

Fig. 5 MRI of the cervical spine in rheumatoid arthritis. There is atlantoaxial instability; the cervical cord is displaced by the protruding peg.

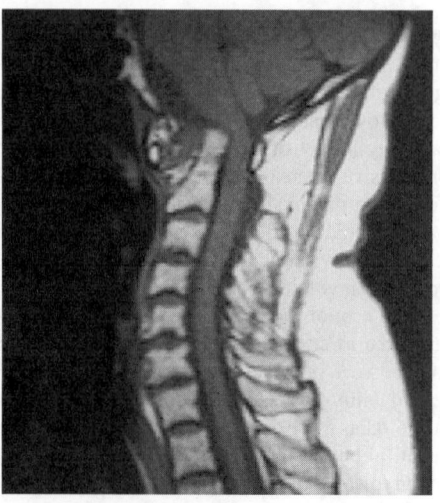

Fig. 7 Synovial fluid crystals, as seen under polarized light. (a) Monosodium urate, which is strongly negatively birefringent; (b) calcium pyrophosphate, which is weakly positively birefringent.

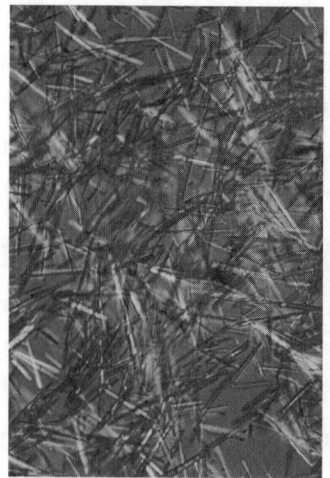
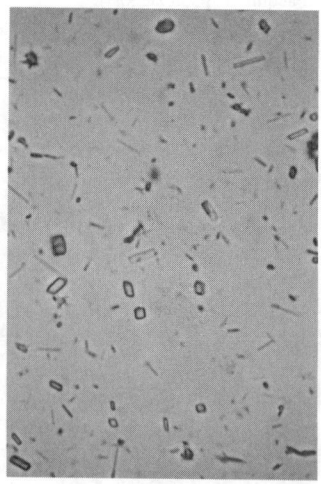

the most important assays. The fluid should always be examined by naked eye (blood-staining, viscosity, and opalescence; see Fig. 6) and a differential white cell count performed. This is the best index of synovial inflammation (proportional to the number of polymorphonuclear cells). The fluid should be examined for organisms and crystals and cultures set up.

The detection of crystals is a specialized technique, particularly dependent on the diligence and experience of the microscopist. Polarized light microscopy is the preferred technique for the identification of both monosodium urate monohydrate (the gout culprit) and calcium pyrophosphate dihydrate crystals (associated with pseudogout and chronic arthropathies) (Fig. 7). Hydroxyapatite and other crystals that may be associated with arthritis are much more difficult to detect and require specialized approaches, such as high-resolution analytical electron microscopy.

The main value of synovial fluid analysis is in the diagnosis of acute arthritis. Crystal arthropathies and septic arthritis can only be confirmed by detection of the crystals or organisms in the synovial fluid.

The main abuse of synovial fluid analysis includes mindless application of tests in chronic arthropathies, where it provides little or no information of clinical value, and from lack of sufficient care and training of technicians asked to examine the fluids. Arthrocentesis is a surprisingly safe procedure but there is a small risk of infection and, although mandatory in acute synovitis of unknown cause, there is no justification for diagnostic joint puncture in most other clinical settings.

Tests for systemic inflammatory disease

A variety of blood tests are indicative of a focus of inflammation somewhere in the body. They are very sensitive but non-specific; they provide semiquantitative information, giving some indication of the volume of inflammatory tissue as well as its presence or absence.

The background to these tests is shown in Fig. 8. Inflammation results in the release of soluble mediators (cytokines, including interleukin-1 and interleukin-6) from the mono- or polymorphonuclear cells involved. These cytokines have numerous local and systemic effects, including altering the rate of synthesis of proteins in the liver, and affecting blood cell release from the bone marrow. Liver synthesis of some 'acute-phase proteins', such as C-reative protein rises dramatically: other proteins, such as albumin, show a reduction in synthesis. Blood levels of white cells and platelets rise, at the expense of red cells. As a result, the measures of inflammation in the blood include those given in Table 3.

There are two main uses for these tests: the distinction of inflammatory from non-inflammatory disease and the monitoring of the progression of inflammatory arthropathies and their response to treatment.

Most inflammatory rheumatic diseases cause a significant rise in all acute-phase proteins. Measurement of the erythrocyte sedimentation rate and C-reactive protein is usually sufficient to detect the presence of inflammation, and this may be of great value in excluding inflammatory diseases that can be difficult to detect clinically, such as polymyalgia rheumatica. An exception is systemic lupus erythematosus, which may be active without causing a rise in C-reactive protein. In this condition, measuring the acute-phase response may help distinguish active systemic lupus erythematosus from a complication such as an infection (see Chapters 11.13.3 and 18.11.3).

Rheumatoid disease usually causes a persistent marked acute-phase response, and its degree and duration has some relationship to disease progression. These tests can be used to follow disease activity and are particularly useful in helping assess the value of slow-acting drug therapy. In an acute illness with day-to-day changes, the C-reactive protein

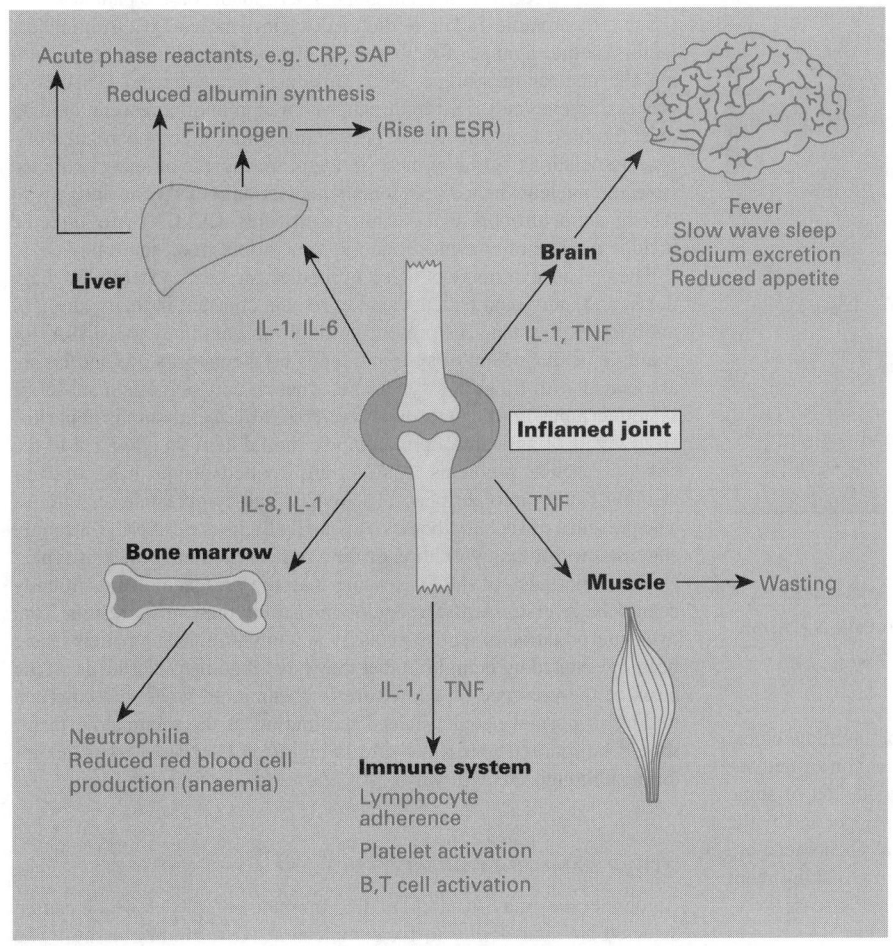

Fig. 8 Simplified diagram of the acute phase response of an inflammatory arthritis. Examples of relevant cytokines have been given.

Table 3 *The acute phase response*

Increased serum levels of proteins (the acute-phase proteins)
C-reactive protein
Some complement components (e.g. C3, C4)
Some antiproteases (e.g. α_1-antitrypsin)
Some transport proteins (e.g. ferritin)
Serum amyloid P protein
Decreased levels of serum proteins (negative acute phase reactants)
Albumin and prealbumin
Others
Raised erythrocyte sedimentation rate or plasma viscosity (Results from increases in fibrinogen and other acute-phase protein changes)
Blood cell changes:
Reduced red cells/low haemoglobin
Increased platelet count
(sometimes an increased white cell count)

The changes occur in the blood in response to inflammation anywhere in the body. Some changes occur quickly (e.g. an increase in C-reactive protein takes hours), others (such as a low haemoglobin) only appear with chronic inflammation. The degree of these changes can be a rough guide to the severity of the condition or volume of inflamed tissues.

Table 4 *Some antibody assays used in diagnosis and monitoring of the rheumatic diseases*

Antibody	Disease association
Rheumatoid factor	Rheumatoid arthritis
Antinuclear factors	Systemic lupus erythematosus, other connective tissue diseases
Extractable nuclear antigens	
Ro	Sjögren's syndrome, systemic lupus erythematosus
La	Sjögren's syndrome, systemic lupus erythematosus
Sm	Systemic lupus erythematosus
Scl 70	Systemic sclerosis
Jo-1	Polymyositis
U1 RNP	Mixed connective tissue disease
centromere	Limited scleroderma
Antineutrophil cytoplasmic antibody	Systemic vasculitis
Anticardiolipin antibody	Antiphospholipid antibody syndrome, systemic lupus erythematosus, other connective tissue disease

can be repeated usefully at quite short intervals (see Chapter 11.13.3) but other measurements are often repeated more often than is sensible.

Immunological tests

Many rheumatic diseases are associated with a lot of 'immunological noise', including lymphocyte activation and the production of autoantibodies. Many of these changes are non-specific. Production of some autoantibodies is a normal, age-related phenomenon, exaggerated by the presence of a rheumatic disease. Other immunological phenomena are clearly pathological; some have high disease specificity, making them valuable diagnostic aids, still others provide a reflection of disease activity and can be used to monitor progression of the disorder.

Table 5 *Some miscellaneous investigations used for the diagnosis of specific rheumatic conditions*

Disease	Investigations
Myositis	Electromyography
	Muscle biopsy
	Plasma creatine phosphokinase
	Jo-1 antibodies
Vasculitis	Arterial biopsy
	Factor 8 related antigen
	ANCA antibodies
Amyloidosis	Fat aspiration
	Rectal biopsy
	Renal biopsy
	Scintigraphy (see Chapter 11.13.3)
Villonodular synovitis	Synovial biopsy
Tuberculosis of joints	
Nerve entrapment syndromes	Nerve conduction studies
Gout	Uric acid metabolism
Paget's disease	24-h urinary hydroxyproline
Sjögren's syndrome	Lip gland biopsy

ANTIBODY TESTS

Close liason between clinician and pathologist is important if these tests are to be properly used and interpreted. Laboratory standards vary, and the normal values and test variability for antibody assays must be known for the local laboratory. Assays commonly used to diagnose and monitor rheumatic diseases include those listed in Table 4. All of these are autoantibodies, directed against antigenic determinants on the patient's own tissue. Rheumatoid factor is directed against native IgG. Antinuclear factors include a range of antibodies against nuclear components, including the nuclear membrane, DNA, histones, nucleoli, and DNA/RNA processing enzymes. Different patterns of immunofluorescent staining exist (homogeneous, nucleolar, peripheral) which suggest particular disease associations. Some of these antigens are capable of being extracted from the nucleus: hence 'extractable nuclear antigens'. The antigens to which antineutrophil cytoplasmic antibodies (ANCA) are directed include a range of enzymes found in the cytoplasm of neutrophils.

The presence of many of these antibodies can be very helpful in diagnosis, and individual patients tend to remain constant in their pattern of antibody expression. The presence of high-titre antibody to dsDNA, for example, is diagnostic of systemic lupus erythematosus. Ro and La are associated with Sjögren's syndrome, whereas Sm suggests a subset of systemic lupus erythematosus characterized by membranous nephritis. High levels of anticardiolipin antibody should alert the clinician to the risk of vascular problems. ANCAs are divided on the basis of their staining pattern into peripheral (p-ANCA) and cytoplasmic (c-ANCA). The presence of such antibodies, especially high-titre c-ANCA, strongly suggests necrotizing vasculitis of the Wegener's granulomatosis type.

The importance of the titre, rather than the presence of the antibody cannot be overstressed. The major misuse of these tests results from over interpretation of a positive assay at a low titre. Many patients have been devastated by being told that they have rheumatoid arthritis on the basis of the presence of a low titre of rheumatoid factor – a common finding in normal people: indeed the finding of the rheumatoid factor should be ignored unless the titre is high (over 1:128 in most laboratories, although this will vary).

OTHER IMMUNOLOGICAL TESTS

Autoantibodies may form circulating immune complexes which can be detected by their ability to fix complement (C1q binding assay). The total haemolytic complement activity remaining in serum can be assayed by measuring the ability of serum to lyse antibody-coated red blood cells (expressed as the 50 per cent lysis point or CH50). Such techniques are useful in monitoring the activity of connective tissue diseases and vasculitis. The detection of immune complexes fixed in tissues such as the kidney can also be of diagnostic value. Complement levels in the serum may be reduced by immune complexes, although in some disorders the tendency for inflammation to raise the level of production of some complement components can make the interpretation of serum levels difficult.

Such tests should always be viewed in the clinical context and abnormalities (frequently seen, for example, in rheumatoid disease) should not in themselves be regarded as an indication for treatment.

Other more sophisticated tests of immune cell function and antibody and complement production may be valuable in rare immune deficiency disorders—either primary or secondary.

The HLA class 1 allele B27 is found in over 90 per cent of subjects with ankylosing spondylitis. Although this finding may support a clinical diagnosis, it must be remembered that the great majority of HLA-B27 positive individuals are healthy. There is no place for routine assessment of HLA-B27 status in the evaluation of suspected seronegative spondylitis.

Other investigations

Several other investigations are important in the diagnosis or monitoring of specific rheumatic diseases or their complications. Some examples are shown in Table 5.

18.4 Rheumatoid arthritis

B. P. WORDSWORTH

The term rheumatoid arthritis was first used by Sir Archibald Garrod in 1876 to describe a chronic non-suppurative inflammatory arthropathy distinct from gout and osteoarthritis. It is generally regarded as an autoimmune disease but details of its pathogenesis remain unclear. Its prevalence is remarkably consistent worldwide (approximately 1 per cent) with a few important exceptions that have helped to highlight environmental influences and the role of the immune response genes. Inflammation of the synovial joints leading to destruction of joints and periarticular tissues is the most obvious clinical and pathological characteristic of the disease, but a wide variety of extra-articular features can also develop. In contrast to gout, osteoarthritis, ankylosing spondylitis, and many other forms of bone and joint disease, there is a remarkable dirth of evidence for the antiquity of rheumatoid arthritis raising speculations that it is a relatively 'new' disease. Another remarkable characteristic of this condition is that it is confined to humans, being virtually unknown in any other species.

Aetiology

Rheumatoid arthritis has a complex multifactorial aetiology. There is considerable evidence for an important genetic component. Twin studies indicate a concordance rate of around 20 per cent in monozygotic twins, although this figure is probably influenced by the severity of the disease in the proband. Thus, concordance rates may be lower when the index twin has mild, non-erosive disease but as high as 40 per cent if only index twins with erosive, rheumatoid factor-positive disease are considered. Confirmation of an important genetic contribution comes from comparing monozygotic and dizygotic twins, since disease concordance is approximately five times higher in the former despite their presumably similar exposure to environmental influences. However, susceptibility to rheumatoid arthritis must be determined predominantly by non-genetic factors since concordance rates are substantially lower than 50 per cent.

The pan-global distribution of rheumatoid arthritis could be explained by the involvement of a ubiquitous organism. However, strong supporting evidence for this concept is lacking. Although rheumatoid arthritis has many similarities to reactive arthritis, in which a wide range of different Gram-negative organisms are known to trigger the disease, infection at sites distant from the joints has not been identified, in spite of claims that infections of the urinary tract (*Proteus* sp.) may be more common in patients with rheumatoid arthritis than in healthy controls.

Likewise, no particular organism has ever been found reproducibly in the joints of patients with rheumatoid arthritis, although there have been sporadic reports of the isolation of viruses (rubella, parvovirus), atypical mycobacteria, and mycoplasma.

Some populations appear to be at unusually high or low risk of developing rheumatoid arthritis, and the study of these has yielded some clues to its aetiology. Such observations could be explained by genetic or environmental differences. For example, the prevalence of the disease is very low in much of Africa. In the case of South African negroes there is strong support for an environmental influence: in the rural areas this ethnic group has the same low prevalence of the disease as elsewhere in rural subSaharan Africa, but this is greatly increased in those who have migrated to the townships where the prevalence is similar to that in the population of European descent. In contrast, the high prevalence (5 per cent or more) in the Yakima and Chippewa Amerindians is more likely to be, at least in part, genetically determined. Both these tribes have a high frequency (c. 70 per cent) of HLA class II alleles associated with susceptibility to rheumatoid arthritis (DR4 in the Chippewa and DR6Dw16 in the Yakima).

The genetic component of rheumatoid arthritis has been clarified by studying families, and also from the definition of specific genetic markers associated with the disease. The risk to the first-degree relatives of probands with mild, non-erosive, seronegative disease (2–3 per cent) is little greater than in the risk in the general population. In contrast, the prevalence of rheumatoid arthritis among the first-degree relatives of probands with erosive, seropositive disease may be as high as 15 per cent, underlining the importance of genetic factors in determining disease severity. Estimates of the risk to the siblings of affected individuals range between 4 and 10 per cent, but there may be a delay, of decades even, before the development of the disease in the second sibling. Increasingly, interest in the genetic component of rheumatoid arthritis has focused on immunogenetic factors, particularly the immune response genes in the major histocompatibility complex on chromosome 6.

IMMUNOPATHOLOGY

In the early stages of rheumatoid arthritis the most obvious histological changes are confined to the synovial microvasculature, which shows evidence of endothelial damage, infiltration by polymorphonuclear leucocytes, and obliteration by thrombus. In the chronic phase, polymorphonuclear leucocytes are less obvious but the synovium is infiltrated by large numbers of inflammatory cells (macrophages, T and B lymphocytes, dendritic cells, and plasma cells). Among the lymphocyte population, B cells appear to be somewhat under-represented while T cells with the CD4+ (helper/inducer) phenotype are increased, particularly in the perivascular areas. The plasma cells in the subsynovium synthesize large quantities of immunoglobulin, much of which is IgM and IgG rheumatoid factor (i.e. immunoglobulin with reactivity to self-IgG). The precise role of these autoantibodies in the pathogenesis of the disease is not clear, but their ability to form immune complexes that can activate complement could be important in either initiating or prolonging local inflammation within the joint. Evidence for complement activation in the inflamed joints and serositis associated with rheumatoid arthritis is demonstrated by the presence of complement breakdown products such as C3a and C5a, both highly potent chemotactic agents for polymorphonuclear leucocytes and powerful mediators of inflammation. Rheumatoid factors are not specific for rheumatoid arthritis, being found in some 5 per cent of the normal population (usually in low titre) and in other diseases, particularly chronic infections such as tuberculosis, leprosy, and osteomyelitis. Their presence may precede the development of rheumatoid arthritis by months or even years, while in a minority of cases classical IgM rheumatoid factor may be persistently absent or only detectable long after the development of the disease.

Several observations suggest that the inflammatory reaction in rheumatoid arthritis is a T-cell mediated phenomenon. First, there is a clear physical association between CD4-positive T cells and dedicated antigen-presenting cells (dendritic cells and cells of the macrophage/monocyte lineage) in the perivascular areas of the synovium. Second, certain therapeutic measures including thoracic duct drainage, total body lymphoid irradiation, and, perhaps, the use of anti-CD4 monoclonal antibodies are associated with a decline in circulating T-cell numbers as well as clinical improvement. Third, cyclosporin, which is primarily

directed against CD4-positive T cells is effective in rheumatoid arthritis. Finally, a role for a selected population of T cells might be inferred from the limited array of HLA class II antigens (eg. DR4, DR1) that are strongly with associated with rheumatoid arthritis. Most of these cells are activated and have a mature (CD45Ro) phenotype but, somewhat surprisingly, it has been difficult to demonstrate increases in the levels of cytokines (interleukin-2, interleukin-4, and γ-interferon) that might have been expected in the synovium and synovial fluid. One explanation for these findings might be that there is an accumulation of an unusual lymphocyte subset in the synovium. In contrast, large quantities of macrophage-derived cytokines (interleukin-1, tumour necrosis factor-α) are present, perhaps indicating an important role for the macrophage in the synovial inflammation. Preliminary trials of the efficacy of chimeric antitumour necrosis factor antibodies have proved promising.

Unusual glycosylation patterns of immunoglobulins have been observed in patients with rheumatoid arthritis, similar to those which may be seen in mycobacterial infections and sarcoidosis. Curiously, these changes in glycosylation have also been noted in the unaffected spouses of those with the disease. It has been suggested that this may render self-immunoglobulins potentially immunogenic, leading to the development of rheumatoid factors, but this is speculative. A reduced capacity to oxidize certain sulphur-containing compounds has also been described in patients with rheumatoid arthritis. Whether either of these phenomena is of primary importance is not known, but both have been used successfully as predictors of progression to chronic rheumatoid arthritis in patients with signs of early inflammatory joint disease.

IMMUNOGENETICS

Susceptibility to rheumatoid arthritis is associated with the immune response (HLA) genes in the major histocompatibility complex. The products of these genes are cell-surface glycoproteins that play a fun-

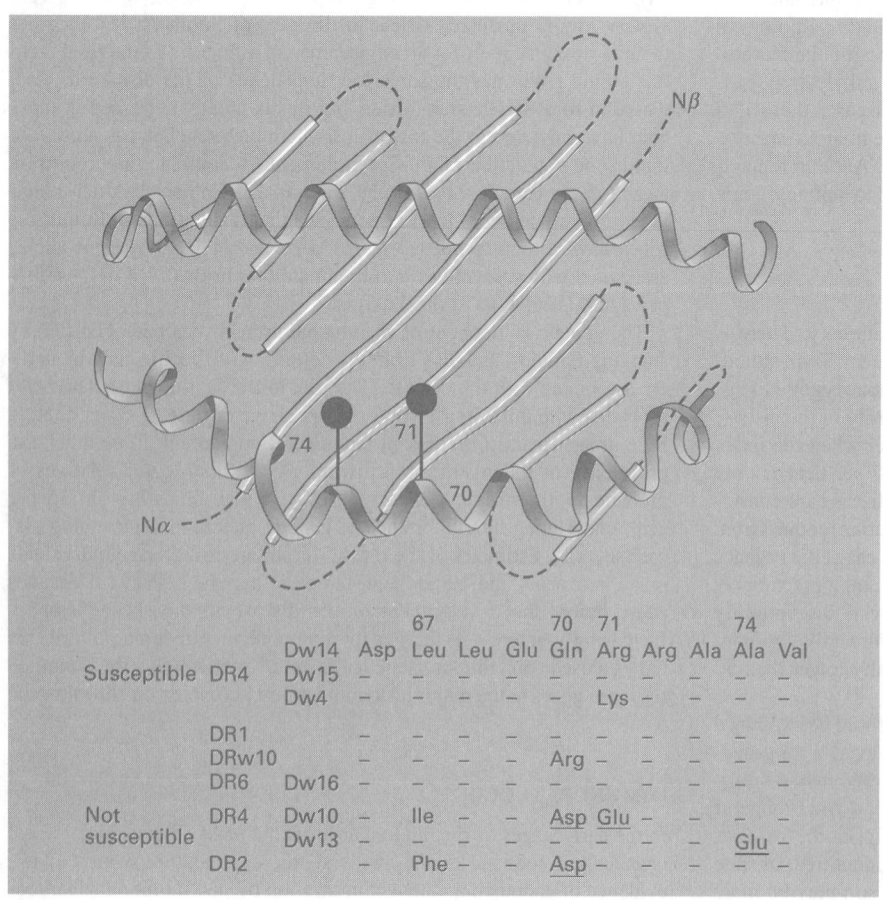

					67		70	71		74	
		Dw14	Asp	Leu	Leu	Glu	Gln	Arg	Arg	Ala	Ala	Val
Susceptible	DR4	Dw15	–	–	–	–	–	–	–	–	–	–
		Dw4	–	–	–	–	–	Lys	–	–	–	–
	DR1		–	–	–	–	–	–	–	–	–	–
	DRw10		–	–	–	–	Arg	–	–	–	–	–
	DR6	Dw16	–	–	–	–	–	–	–	–	–	–
Not susceptible	DR4	Dw10	–	Ile	–	–	<u>Asp</u>	<u>Glu</u>	–	–	–	–
		Dw13	–	–	–	–	–	–	–	–	<u>Glu</u>	–
	DR2		–	Phe	–	–	<u>Asp</u>	–	–	–	–	–

Fig. 1 Schematic representation of some HLA-DR molecules positively or negatively associated with rheumatoid arthritis. Charged amino-acid substitutions (underlined) at positions 71 and 74 in the antigen binding-site are crucial in influencing susceptibility among the DR4 subtypes.

damental role in the binding of peptide antigens and their presentation for recognition by T cells. The class I antigens (HLA-A, -B, and -C) are present on all nucleated cells and are particularly important in the immune surveillance of viral infections. The class II antigens (HLA-DR, -DQ, and -DP), in contrast, are found only on certain cells specialized in antigen presentation, such as dendritic cells, macrophages, and also B lymphocytes.

The observation from family studies that affected sibling pairs tend to inherit HLA haplotypes in common from their parents more frequently than would be expected by chance incriminates a gene (or genes) linked to HLA in susceptibility to rheumatoid arthritis. Furthermore, in most populations there are strong associations with specific alleles at the HLA-DRB1 locus which encodes the DRβ chain. Thus, the relative risk associated with alleles at this locus, defined serologically, ranges from nearly twofold for DR1 to over six-fold for DR4. The most likely explanation for this lies in the structure of the HLA molecule, in which polymorphic amino acid residues are concentrated around the antigen-binding site (Fig. 1). Those molecules which are associated with the disease share considerable homology in this region which is likely to have considerable influence on the range of peptide antigens that can be bound by particular HLA molecules. This is most clearly exemplified by the differential association of the various allelic subtypes of DR4 with rheumatoid arthritis where even one amino acid substitution in this region is sufficient to abrogate susceptibility to the disease (Table 1).

The association between DR4 and rheumatoid arthritis is strongest in the more severe variants of the disease. In community-based studies, which tend to include many milder cases, the association may be weak or even absent; in patients with erosive, seropositive disease 70 per cent of patients are likely to be DR4 positive, compared to about 25 per cent of the normal Caucasian population; in the Felty syndrome the frequency of DR4 is over 90 per cent. Furthermore, in the more severe forms of rheumatoid arthritis there is an increased frequency of the Dw4 subtype of DR4 (up to 90 per cent in the Felty syndrome) and also of DR4 homozygotes, the majority of whom have the Dw4/Dw14 genotype. It is likely that HLA accounts for no more than 30 per cent of the total genetic effect in rheumatoid arthritis, although no other genes contributing to susceptibility have yet been defined.

Clinical features

Rheumatoid arthritis is a systemic disorder characterized by a chronic inflammatory synovitis which typically affects the peripheral joints but may affect any synovial joint in the body. In addition to the articular features that are the hallmark of the disease, many other tissues may also be affected, although this, like the severity of the articular disease, is highly variable. It is a disease of exacerbations and remissions, the clinical variability of which suggests that it might represent the end result of a number of different disease pathways. Diagnosis is based on the aggregation of a series of common clinical features rather than any specific pathognomonic abnormality: until there is a fuller understanding of the aetiology of the disease the possibility that the single diagnosis 'rheumatoid arthritis' masks considerable heterogeneity cannot be excluded.

The development of various classification systems, based predominantly on clinical criteria, has been of substantial benefit in the study of the epidemiology and aetiology of the disease. The diagnostic criteria developed by the American Rheumatism Association in 1958 have been used widely. They allow the recognition of three grades of rheumatoid arthritis according to the number of diagnostic criteria present ('classical', seven or more criteria out of 11; 'definite', five criteria, 'probable', three criteria). However, the specificity of these criteria for rheumatoid arthritis is considerably increased if the milder variants are excluded. For this reason the 1987 American College of Rheumatology criteria, corresponding approximately to the 1958 'classical' and 'definite' groups, are now generally employed (Table 2). In individuals presenting with early inflammation of the joints, these criteria have proved good

predictors of those likely to progress to chronic destructive rheumatoid arthritis.

DISEASE PREVALENCE AND ONSET

Rheumatoid arthritis may occur at any age but has a peak incidence in the fifth decade. The lifetime incidence of the disease in women (1.8 per cent) is three times that in males (0.5 per cent) and the prevalence of the disease in women over 65 years old is more than 5 per cent. The sex difference is most pronounced (as high as 6:1) in those with early onset disease but is almost equal by the age of 65. The disease starts twice as commonly in winter, but whether this represents a non-specific effect, such as the increased sensitivity to joint symptoms, or a more specific process, such as the precipitation of vasculitis, is not clear. Several distinct patterns of onset are recognized which can be of some use in predicting the prognosis.

Palindromic onset

In about one-fifth of patients with rheumatoid arthritis, persistent joint disease may be antedated by repeated attacks of acute self-limiting synovitis, affecting a variable number of joints. Typically the inflammation develops over a few hours and is accompanied by erythema and swelling of the affected joints but resolves completely within 48 to 72 h, leaving no residual features. About 50 per cent of individuals who suffer from attacks of palindromic rheumatism ultimately develop chronic rheumatoid arthritis, and they can usually be identified by the presence of rheumatoid factor in the blood, although this may not be present at the outset. The number of joints involved is usually small but increases with time and with the onset of persistent joint disease. If joint symptoms are sufficiently frequent to be troublesome during the palindromic phase, they can often be controlled by intramuscular gold injections or D-penicillamine (often in low doses) as in the case of established rheumatoid arthritis.

Explosive onset

In about 10 per cent of cases the onset of the disease is very rapid, even overnight, with severe symmetrical polyarticular involvement. Many patients with this type of onset do surprisingly well in the long term.

Systemic onset

This is particularly common in middle-aged men in whom non-articular features may dominate the clinical picture. Fever, myalgia, weight loss, anaemia, pleural effusions, and vasculitic lesions may be severe, sometimes in the absence of marked joint pathology. Although rheumatoid factor is usually present in high titres, it is often be necessary to exclude other causes such as other connective tissue disorder, malignancy, or infection.

Insidious onset

The majority of cases of rheumatoid arthritis develop insidiously over weeks or months, with gradually increasing joint involvement. This pattern of onset, which is seen in up to 70 per cent of cases, is associated with a relatively poor prognosis. Progression from predominantly peripheral small-joint disease to the involvement of the more proximal joints, including the knees and hips, is the most common pattern. However, in a subset of patients the earliest joint involvement is in the knees and wrists, these patients are particularly likely to be positive for IgA rheumatoid factor.

Polymyalgic onset

Limb girdle muscle symptoms may precede the onset of an overt arthropathy, particularly in the elderly. Not all patients with this pattern are rheumatoid-factor positive and it may be difficult to distinguish with certainty from polymyalgia rheumatica. It is therefore of considerable

Table 1 *Differential association of rheumatoid arthritis with the various subtypes of HLA-DR4 in the United Kingdom. HLA-Dw4 and Dw14 are positively associated while Dw10 and Dw13 are negatively associated*

	n	Dw4	Dw14	Dw10	Dw13
DR4-positive controls	185	119 (64%)	53 (29%)	7 (4%)	15 (8%)
DR4 positive rheumatoid arthritis	178	133 (74%)	66 (37%)	0	2 (1%)
Probability		0.02	0.05	<0.01	0.01

Table 2 *American College of Rheumatology criteria for rheumatoid arthritis*

1. Morning stiffness of at least 1 h
2. Arthritis of three or more joint areas
3. Arthritis of hand joints
4. Symmetric arthritis
5. Rheumatoid nodules
6. Serum rheumatoid factor positive
7. Typical radiographic changes in the hand and wrist

Criteria 1–4 must have been for at least 6 weeks.

interest that both these conditions are associated with the HLA-DR4 antigen. The initial response to corticosteroid therapy in these cases is impressive but is less well maintained as progressive synovitis supervenes.

Mono- and pauci-articular onset

In young women there may initially be very limited joint involvement, particularly involving the knees. While there is no doubt that a proportion of these cases go on to develop full-blown rheumatoid arthritis, many do not. It is therefore important to exclude other potential causes of monoarthritis, such as low-grade infection or pigmented villonodular synovitis. Intermittent hydrarthrosis causes effusions which recur with remarkably consistent periodicity in the absence of pronounced systemic or joint inflammation. The sedimentation rate and C-reactive protein are normal and joint fluid white cell counts are typically less than 200/mm³. Patients with such limited joint disease who are persistently seronegative for rheumatoid factor usually pursue a benign course and probably represent an entirely different type of joint disease from classical rheumatoid arthritis.

JOINT FEATURES

Rheumatoid arthritis is typically a distal, symmetrical, small-joint polyarthritis involving the proximal interphalangeal and metacarpophalangeal joints of the hands, the wrists, metatarsophalangeal joints, ankles, knees, and cervical spine. The shoulders, elbows, and hips are less frequently involved, but can be a major source of morbidity. Any synovial joint in the body may be affected, including the cricoarytenoid and the temporomandibular joints. In addition, periarticular synovial structures, such as bursae and tendon sheaths, are commonly inflamed.

It may be difficult to distinguish between symptoms and signs of joint disease due to inflammation and those that result from secondary mechanical problems arising from joint destruction. This is an important distinction since it will often dictate the most appropriate form of treatment. Anti-inflammatory and disease-modifying drugs may be appropriate in the early inflammatory phase, but the use of analgesics and physical approaches, such as splints or corrective surgery, would be more likely to aid patients with severe joint damage.

The most common symptoms described by patients are pain and pronounced stiffness. The latter frequently exhibits a diurnal rhythm, worse on rising in the morning and then recurring towards the evening, perhaps reflecting the diurnal variation in plasma cortisol levels. Gentle activity may alleviate the symptoms but is followed by stiffening or 'gelling' with subsequent inactivity. The affected joints are frequently tender, swollen, and warm and there may be limitation of both active and passive movement. Muscle wasting serves to accentuate the local swelling of the joint, which is in part due to proliferation of the synovial tissue and in part to synovial effusion within the joint. Progressive destruction of the articular cartilage, subchondral bone, and periarticular soft tissues eventually combine to produce the characteristic deformities seen in long-standing rheumatoid arthritis.

In parallel with these clinical changes there are characteristic radiological appearances which may be helpful in the diagnosis of early rheumatoid arthritis and in monitoring its progress (Fig. 2). In the early stages of the disease it is common for the first evidence of erosions to be in the feet, and these should always be included in diagnostic views. Radiological changes include:

(1) soft-tissue swelling;
(2) juxta-articular osteoporosis;
(3) loss of joint space due to erosion of the articular cartilage;
(4) bone erosions at the points of attachment of the synovium; and
(5) joint deformities.

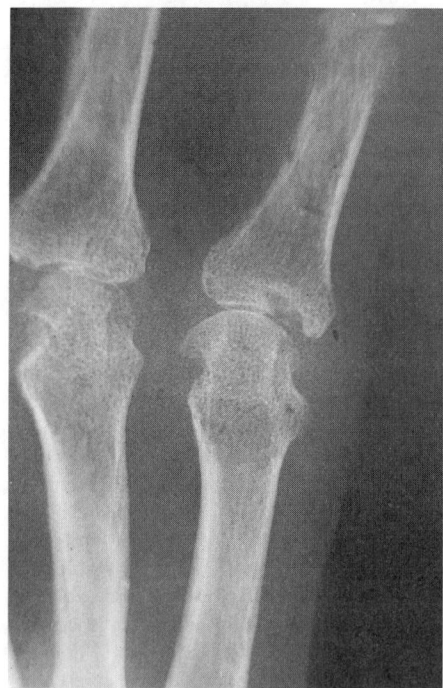

Fig. 2 Typical radiological features of rheumatoid arthritis in the metacarpophalangeal joints, showing osteoporosis, joint space narrowing, periarticular erosions, and angular deformity.

UPPER LIMBS

Hands and wrists

The appearance of the hands in rheumatoid arthritis is highly characteristic. However, there are numerous potential patterns of deformity, and distinction from other arthropathies is occasionally difficult. Early in the disease there may be soft-tissue swelling around the affected joints. Involvement of the proximal interphalangeal joints gives a spindle-shaped appearance to the fingers, and soft-tissue swelling can be observed over the ulnar styloid, and in the second and third metacarpophalangeal joints. Distal interphalangeal joint involvement is less common (about 15 per cent of cases) but rheumatoid arthritis may sometimes be superimposed on pre-existing osteoarthritis of these joints.

Tenosynovitis of the long flexor tendons in the palm of the hand may exacerbate stiffness of the fingers and cause 'trigger finger'. This may be associated with palpable crepitus over the tendon on active or passive movement of the corresponding finger. Similar synovitis at the wrist within the flexor retinaculum may cause compression of the median nerve with the typical features of carpal tunnel syndrome—paraesthesiae of the first three digits and the radial side of the ring finger, wasting and weakness of the thenar mucles, with night pain frequently extending proximally as far as the elbow; typically these symptoms can be relieved by shaking the hand or movement of the fingers. Tinel's sign is sometimes positive but relatively insensitive. Phalen's sign (pressure over the carpal tunnel with the wrist in flexion) may be more useful, not only because it is more frequently positive but also because it reproduces the symptoms accurately. The diagnosis can be confirmed if necessary by nerve conduction studies.

On the dorsal surface of the wrist, synovitis of the extensor tendons is common and may lead to rupture (Fig. 3). A 'dropped finger' affecting the little finger is an important indication for surgical exploration and synovectomy, since it may presage the progressive rupture of the rest of the extensor communis tendon. Similar rupture of the extensor pollicis longus and extensor indicis proprius may occur.

Persistent synovitis with erosion of the articular surfaces, weakening of the joint capsules, and muscle weakness, with or without tendon rupture, will inevitably lead to deformities. There are several commonly occurring variants:

Volar subluxation of the fingers at the metacarpophalangeal joints occurs as a result of destruction of the articular cartilage, and subsequent instability of these joints. Since the flexor tendons provide the strongest force acting across these joints progressive subluxation towards the palm may develop, leaving the metacarpal heads relatively prominent.

Ulnar deviation and subluxation of the fingers as a result of instability of the metacarpophalangeal joints. The fingers may tend to drift in an ulnar direction because of the ulnar vector of the action of both the flexor and extensor finger tendons. The process may be exacerbated by radial deviation of the carpus and also by ulnar subluxation of the extensor tendons if the supports which usually hold them in place over the centre of the metacarpophalangeal joints are weakened by synovitis (Fig. 4).

Swan neck deformities occur following volar subluxation of the proximal phalanges at the metacarpophalangeal joints, with subsequent contracture of the intrinsic muscles which become extensors rather than flexors of the proximal interphalangeal joints. Compensatory flexion of the distal interphalangeal joint occurs as a result of a tenodesis effect as the flexor digitorum profundus tendon is stretched over the hyperextended proximal interphalangeal joint.

Boutonnière (button-hole) deformity occurs when a chronic effusion within the proximal interphalangeal joint stretches or even ruptures the dorsal slip of the extensor hood, allowing dorsal migration of the joint through the discontinuity. A similar process at the carpometacarpal joint of the thumb may give rise to the Z-thumb deformity.

Piano-key sign can be detected when weakening of the distal radioulnar ligament by synovitis allows the distal ulna to migrate dorsally so that it overrides the radius (caput ulnae syndrome). The ulna can be depressed by pressure like a piano key (while the patient emits a note!). Progressive destruction of the carpal joints may be followed by volar subluxation and ultimately ankylosis.

Carpal collapse and fusion may occur late in the disease, particularly in those with an early onset rheumatoid arthritis, when instability of the wrist may lead to collapse of the carpal bones, causing foreshortening of the carpus and, ultimately, spontaneous fusion of the wrist.

Elbows and shoulders

Involvement of the elbows is less common than of the wrist but severe destruction may occur, leading to pronounced deformity and disability.

Fig. 3 'Bull's horn' deformity due to rupture of the extensor communis tendon from synovitis near the ulnar styloid. Selective sparing of the extensor indicis proprius and extensor digiti minimi tendons has in this instance preserved the ability to point the index and little fingers independently.

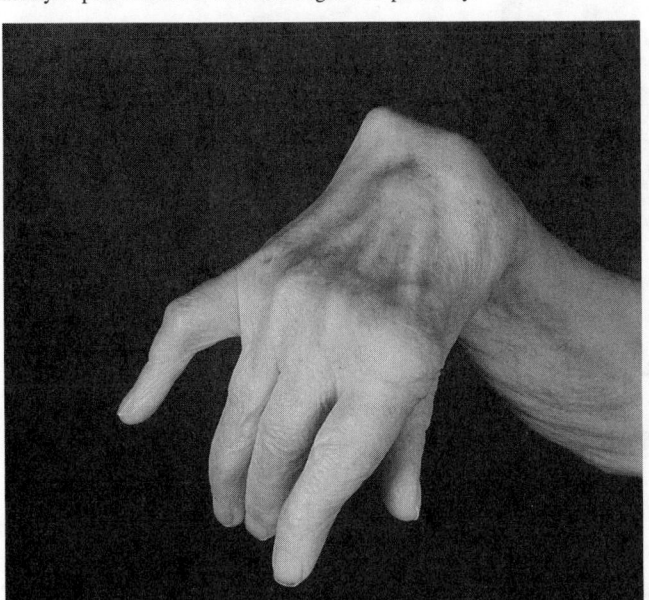

Fig. 4 Volar and ulnar subluxation of the fingers at metacarpophalangeal joints which results respectively from the relative strength of the long flexors and the ulnar direction of pull arising from both the long flexors and extensors. Cutaneous nodules are present on the fingers.

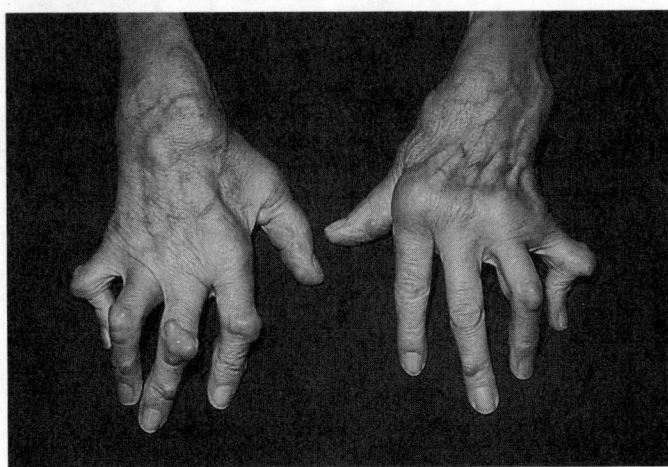

The radiohumeral joint is more commonly symptomatic than the humeroulnar joint and presents problems particularly with pronation/supination. Periarticular structures (olecranon bursa, ulnar nerve) may also be affected by synovitis and subcutaneous nodules are commonly found on the extensor surface of the forearm close to the elbow.

Pain around the shoulder may arise from the glenohumeral joint itself, periarticular structures (particularly the subacromial bursa), the acromioclavicular joint, or the cervical spine. Frequently more than one cause may coexist, necessitating careful evaluation of the anatomical cause of the pain if appropriate treatment is to be applied. There may be inflammation of the subacromial bursa or supraspinatus tendon in addition to glenohumeral joint synovitis, producing a typical painful arc syndrome. Involvement of the acromioclavicular joint can give rise to pain particularly with overhead activities, and is associated with localized tenderness. Referred pain from the neck or cervical radiculopathy may closely mimic shoulder pathology but tends to persist at rest. In late disease of older people, severe destruction of the shoulders can occur, with loss of the whole of the head of the humerus.

LOWER LIMBS

Feet and ankles

Involvement of the feet is common from an early stage of the disease. It frequently gives rise to problems which go unrecognized despite the fact that they can often be overcome relatively simply by the provision of appropriate footwear. Active synovitis of the metatarsophalangeal joints, with or without effusions, leads to spreading of the forefoot and a marked increase in width, necessitating a larger shoe fitting. Collapse of the transverse arch of the forefoot causes the weight to be taken predominantly on the second and third metatarsal heads rather than the first and fifth which is customary (Fig. 5). Patients frequently complain of pain arising in the ball of the foot (metatarsalgia) which can vary in intensity from 'walking on pebbles' to 'like walking on broken glass'. Dorsal subluxation of the toes leads to their progressive defunctioning for weight bearing and commonly causes pressure problems as they rub against the shoe uppers. In addition, the specialized weight-bearing skin and subcutaneous tissue lying under the metatarsal heads is drawn forward to be replaced by unprotected skin, which becomes hyperkeratotic in response to repeated loading. The resulting plantar callosities exacerbate the pain of metatarsalgia and may require regular chiropody. Hallux valgus almost invariably develops as a consequence of the spreading of the forefoot and the bowstring effect from the extensor hallucis longus.

Involvement of the ankle joint in isolation is rare but may occur in association with disease of the subtalar and midtarsal joints, which occurs in two-thirds of patients. Valgus deformity of the hindfoot is usual and may be exacerbated by rupture of the tibialis posterior tendon which buttresses the medial aspect of the ankle. Associated collapse of the medial longitudinal arch of the foot may add to the resulting mechanical problems, which include severe pain around the lateral aspect of the ankle from joint compression. Extensive synovitis, particularly of the long flexor tendons, may lead to compression of the medial plantar nerve in the tarsal tunnel.

Fig. 5 Forefoot deformity is common from an early stage of rheumatoid arthritis as a result of destruction of the normal transverse arch by synovitis of the metatarsophalangeal joints.

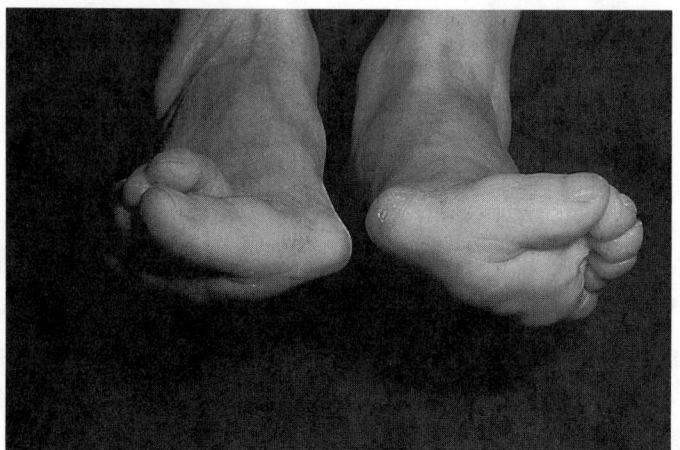

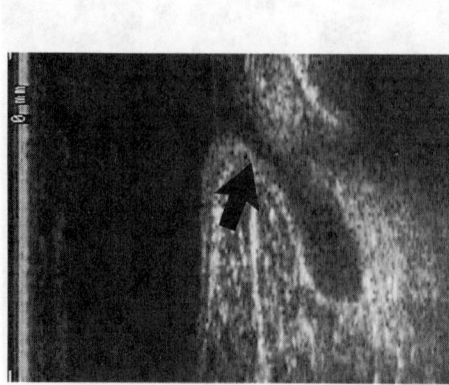

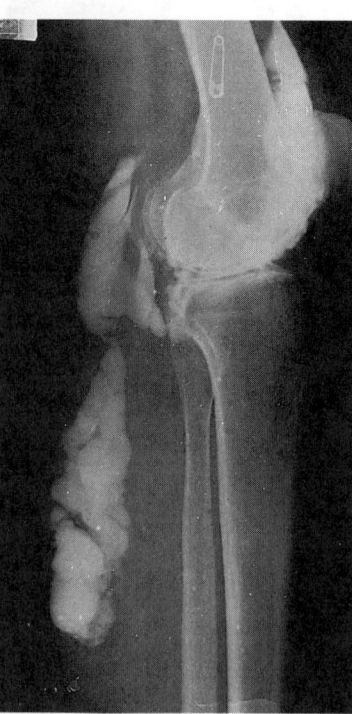

Fig. 6 Ultrasound of a large popliteal cyst communicating with the knee joint (left). This technique has superseded arthrography (right) and the neck of the cyst (arrowed) communicating with the joint is clearly seen.

Knees

Involvement of the knee is an important and relatively common cause of disability from an early stage in the disease because of its role in load bearing. Synovial proliferation is usually most obvious in the supra-patella pouch and there may be pronounced wasting of the quadriceps as a result of reflex muscle inhibition. Synovial effusion typically produces posterior knee pain in the early stages by stretching the posterior capsule of the joint. This may lead to the development of a popliteal cyst communicating with the joint via a valve-like opening which does not easily allow fluid back into the joint. Rupture of the joint or a popliteal cyst may cause extravasation of highly irritant synovial fluid into the calf where the inflammation and swelling may mimic a deep vein thrombosis. These two pathologies can sometimes coexist because there may be partial obstruction to the venous return by the presence of an extensive popliteal cyst (Fig. 6). It may be necessary to investigate both diagnoses by ultrasound and phlebography.

Tricompartmental damage to the articular surfaces of the knees is the usual outcome of late disease and may cause severe instability of the joint as the collateral and cruciate ligaments become lax. Valgus deformities of the knees are the usual consequence of loading such unstable joints, and are often combined with a degree of fixed flexion deformity. Pain may also arise from periarticular structures, such as the insertion of the collateral ligaments which are chronically under strain in the unstable knee joint. Even in the end stages of destruction of the knee joint it may be possible to afford the patient considerable relief by attention to specific anatomical sites of injury.

Hips

Involvement of the hips in rheumatoid arthritis is relatively uncommon overall (c. 25 per cent) but is a major source of morbidity in those patients with more severe diseases who tend to make up the hospital outpatient population. Pain is usually experienced in the groin and the buttock but may radiate to the knee, sometimes mimicking knee arthritis. Rotation and abduction of the hip are reduced before flexion, but ultimately fixed flexion deformity of the joint may occur. Even in patients with advanced hip arthritis a considerable contribution to the pain may come from periarticular tissues, in particular trochanteric bursitis. Typically, this is associated with tenderness over the greater trochanter (which may stop the patient lying on that side), and pain on adduction of the hip which may be referred to the lateral aspect of the knee. In late disease these may be relatively sudden collapse of the femoral head, with a severe increase in pain and disability, necessitating joint replacement.

AXIAL SKELETON

In contrast to the spondyloarthropathies, involvement of the sacroiliac joints is rare in rheumatoid arthritis. However, spinal arthritis is common, up to 80 per cent of patients demonstrating radiological evidence of the disease in the cervical spine. This may be asymptomatic but the most frequent result is painful limitation of movement, often in several planes. The most common radiological abnormalities consist of osteoporosis, erosion of the zygapophyseal joints, erosions of the vertebral end plates, and loss of disc space in the absence of florid osteophytosis.

There may be evidence of atlantoaxial subluxation in up to 25 per cent of patients attending hospital, but less than one in four of these will be symptomatic. In the normal joint the odontoid peg is closely opposed to the posterior aspect of the anterior arch of the atlas by a network of ligaments, including the cruciate, posterior longitudinal, and alar ligaments. Instability of the atlantoaxial joint results from erosion of the odontoid peg or rupture of the supporting ligaments and will be apparent on lateral radiographs of the cervical spine taken in flexion and extension. Lateral or vertical subluxation of the atlantoaxial joint may also occur. Separation of the odontoid peg from the arch of the atlas by 4

mm or more is abnormal. The risk of cord compression is greatest in males, in those with a subluxation exceeding 8 mm, and where there is also vertical subluxation of the atlantoaxial joint. Minor degrees of atlantoaxial subluxation can be relatively well tolerated because the cervical canal is relatively wide at this level. Subaxial subluxation presents a serious risk of cord compression because the cervical canal there is narrower.

Serious erosive change in the cervical spine is more likely in patients who have pronounced peripheral joint disease and in those on corticosteroids. Erosions, when present, usually develop within 2 years of the onset. Symptoms suggestive of atlantoaxial disease include high cervical pain radiating to the occiput and temporal regions, exacerbated by neck movements. There may be audible or palpable clunking on flexion, and inability to place the chin on the sternum is a useful screening test. At its worst, compression of the cervical cord or vertebral blood vessels may lead to quadriplegia or sudden death. More commonly it causes shooting pains in the arms or legs, weakness, and unsteadiness of gait or sphincter disturbance. A mild spastic weakness in the arms or legs may be difficult to detect in a patient whose limbs have already been rendered weak and stiff by arthritis, but pathologically brisk tendon jerks, a positive Hoffman sign, or upgoing plantar response are important signs. Loss of proprioception, vibration sense, and balance may indicate significant damage to the posterior columns, but can be difficult to distinguish from the peripheral neuropathy that is common in rheumatoid arthritis.

Acute subluxation of the cervical spine with neurological signs will initially require immobilization with skeletal traction. A proportion of cases will improve with such conservative measures but most will be left with marked residual neurological impairment and handicap. It has been estimated that atlantoaxial subluxation is responsible for as many as 5 per cent of all deaths in rheumatoid arthritis. However, although there may be pre-existing radiological evidence of atlantoaxial subluxation in a small proportion of these, it is rare for overt cervical myelopathy to have developed. The most common indication for fusion is intractable pain, and it is notoriously difficult to predict individuals at risk of catastrophic neurological damage on the basis of symptoms and physical examination alone. Patients with atlantoaxial slip of 8 mm or more should certainly be considered for posterior fusion, particularly if there is also evidence of vertical migration of the joint or if neurological signs suggestive of myelopathy are present. Magnetic resonance imaging provides an accurate, non-invasive method of assessing the degree of compromise to the spinal cord that can be particularly useful in patients with subaxial subluxation (Fig. 7).

Other joints

Hoarseness of the voice may occasionally be caused by effusion within the cricoarytenoid joints. Temporomandibular joint disease causes pain on chewing and may particularly restrict opening of the mouth. Discitis can occur in the lumbar as well as the cervical spine.

EXTRA-ARTICULAR FEATURES

The majority of patients with rheumatoid arthritis exhibit at least some extra-articular features and these tend to be more numerous and more severe in those with high titres of rheumatoid factor in the blood. However, these systemic features are highly variable, ranging from the fairly trivial (e.g. episcleritis, subcutaneous nodules) to the potentially life-threatening (e.g. systemic vasculitis, pleuropericarditis). Actuarial studies indicate that rheumatoid arthritis significantly reduces life expectancy. This is not explained by the effects of progressive immobility alone but by the systemic nature of the illness. Long-term studies suggest that rheumatoid arthritis itself is either responsible directly or contributes to death in about one-third of patients. This effect appears to be particularly pronounced in seropositive middle-aged men with pronounced extra-articular features.

The extra-articular disease may pursue a course quite dissociated from the joint disease. For example, systemic vasculitis may appear for the first time when joint synovitis has been suppressed by disease-modifying drugs.

The precise cause of many of the extra-articular features of rheumatoid arthritis remains to be elucidated. However, three major pathological phenomena dominate the disease: inflammation of membranes (pleura, pericardium, and others as well as the synovium), nodule formation, and vasculitis. Nodules correlate with titres of IgM rheumatoid factor, and vasculitis appears to depend more on the formation of IgG-containing immune complexes. Combinations of these phenomena explain most extra-articular events.

Rheumatoid nodules

Subcutaneous and intracutaneous nodules are a hallmark of the disease, occurring in about one-quarter of patients. They are discrete, firm, non-tender swellings varying from a few millimetres to several centimetres in size, and in rare instances, usually seropositive males, they may occur in the absence of typical articular disease (rheumatoid nodulosis). They occur most frequently on the extensor surface of the forearm and ole-cranon, sites where repeated minor trauma from leaning could initiate their formation. They also commonly occur around tendons, including the Achilles, the flexor and extensor tendons of the fingers, and over the sacrum. Sometimes superficial nodules may break down with ulceration of the surrounding skin.

Histological examination of these nodules reveals central fibrinoid necrosis surrounded by palisades of fibroblasts and chronic inflammatory cells, suggesting a combination of proliferative and destructive tissue responses.

Rheumatoid nodules may also develop in many other tissues including the eye (scleromalacia), pleura, pericardium, and parenchyma of the lungs and heart (where they may be found at autopsy in as many as 10 per cent of patients). They sometimes occur on the vocal cords and very occasionally they may cause dysfunction of the heart valves or conducting tissue. The Caplan syndrome, describing the combination of massive pulmonary fibrosis and pulmonary nodules, was first described in miners with rheumatoid arthritis but it may also develop, following occupational exposure to inorganic dusts (e.g. silica, asbestos), in seropositive individuals without arthritis. Such intrapulmonary nodules may be mistaken for other pathology, including tumours or abcesses, particularly if they break down and cavitate.

Fig. 7 Sub-ascial subluxation of the cervical spine (C 5/6) with compression of the spinal cord. The loss of disc height and subluxation in the absence of marked osteophytosis on the standard radiographs (left) is typical of rheumatoid arthritis. Magnetic resonance imaging (right) reveals the extent of the spinal cord compression.

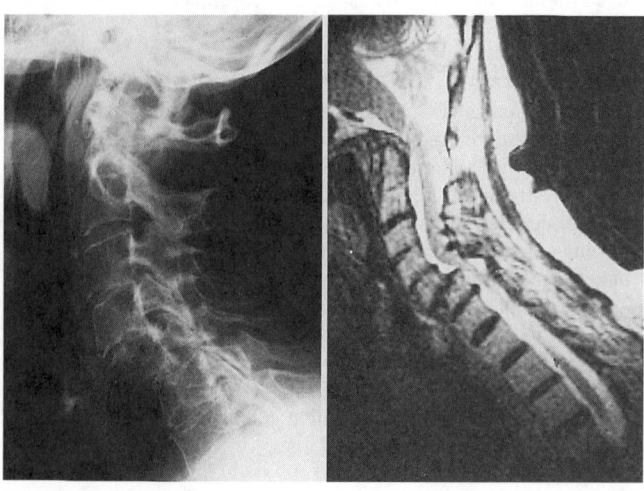

Anaemia

A moderate normochromic normocytic anaemia is an almost invariable finding in active rheumatoid arthritis and appears to be multifactorial in origin. A number of factors related to the inflammatory process probably contribute to this anaemia. Iron may be sequestered in an unusable form (haemosiderin) by the reticuloendothelial system; there may be ineffective erythropoiesis and red blood cell survival is reduced; haemodilution may occur as a result of increased blood volume. The potential influence of increased levels of cytokines (interleukin-1 and interleukin-6) and blunted erythropoietin responses are the foci of considerable research interest. The potential therapeutic role of recombinant erythropoietin has not yet been established.

The most important practical consideration is the differentiation of iron-deficiency anaemia secondary to gastrointestinal haemorrhage from the anaemia of chronic disease. This may be particularly difficult when the two coexist. As a general rule, a microcytic hypochromic blood picture indicates iron deficiency anaemia and should be treated and investigated as such. In the chronic anaemia of rheumatoid disease the blood picture is usually normocytic and normochromic or hypochromic (but rarely microcytic). Assessment of the bone marrow iron stores is the most reliable indicator of iron deficiency but is rarely necessary if the mean corpuscular volume, serum iron-binding capacity, and ferritin are used in combination. Iron-binding capacity is typically reduced in active rheumatoid arthritis: normal or slightly raised levels in the presence of a low serum iron are therefore highly indicative of iron deficiency. In contrast, as part of the acute phase response, ferritin levels are typically elevated in active rheumatoid arthritis unless there is iron deficiency. The typical anaemia of chronic disease seen in rheumatoid arthritis correlates closely with the sedimentation rate as a marker of disease activity and does not respond to iron, folic acid, or vitamin B_{12}. In contrast, suppression of the disease by corticosteroids appears to mobilize iron stores rapidly, resulting in increased haemopoiesis and a subsequent rise in haemoglobin concentration.

Platelets

The platelet count is commonly increased to levels greater than 5×10^5 in active disease and this may also occur when there is active bleeding from the intestine. In contrast, the platelet count may be low in the Felty syndrome or as a result of marrow toxicity from antirheumatic drugs.

Vasculitis

Vascular lesions are evident at autopsy in as many as 25 per cent of individuals with rheumatoid arthritis, with an equal sex-incidence. Many different sizes of blood vessels may be affected. The resulting clinical spectrum of disease is therefore highly variable. Intimal hyperplasia of the small terminal digital vessels causes very limited cutaneous lesions (nailfold infarcts, rashes, and splinter haemorrhages) and has a generally good prognosis in the absence of other signs suggestive of more severe systemic involvement. In contrast, severe life-threatening systemic tissue infarction (widespread cutaneous ulceration, infarction of the bowel, mononeuritis multiplex) may develop if there is involvement of the larger blood vessels by leucocytoclastic or necrotizing vasculitis. This may be indistinguishable from polyarteritis nodosa with fibrinoid necrosis of the intima and infiltration of the outer layers by lymphocytes and occasional polymorphonuclear leucocytes.

Vasculitis is more common in patients with high levels of IgM rheumatoid factor and severe joint disease, although the activity of the synovitis and extra-articular disease is often temporally dissociated. Its incidence increases with the duration of the disease, but occasionally it may be present from the outset, even, rarely, in the absence of joint disease. It is possible that the vasculitis may be initiated by IgG rheumatoid factor containing immune complexes deposited in the vessel walls, since these can activate complement. Vasculitis is increased somewhat in patients in whom antinuclear antibody can be detected and correlates more closely with raised circulating levels of IgG than IgM rheumatoid factor. In some patients with vasculitic features there may be detectable circulating cryoglobulins and low concentrations of complement in plasma.

Rheumatoid vasculitis is associated with significant mortality but this can be significantly reduced with appropriate therapy. Oral or intravenous pulses of corticosteroids alone are probably ineffective in the long term; indeed some observers have suggested that the reduction in the incidence of rheumatoid vasculitis since the 1960s can be attributed to the reduced use of steroids. However, regimens based on intermittent boluses of cyclophosphamide coupled with corticosteroids appear to induce effective and sustained suppression similar to that obtained in other forms of necrotizing vasculitis.

Lung involvement

Several patterns of lung disease may occur:

Pleurisy has an incidence of about 1 per cent overall, but pleural effusions due to rheumatoid arthritis may go undetected. Pleural involvement is five times more common in men than in women and often needs differentiation from other causes, particularly when other systemic features, such as weight loss and fever, are present. The fluid has raised protein, low glucose, and low complement levels and is typically positive for rheumatoid factor. The cell count is high due to the presence of lymphocytes, macrophages, and, to a lesser extent, multinucleate giant cells, including comet cells. Pleural biopsy may reveal rheumatoid granulomata, like an 'opened-out rheumatoid nodule', but typically there is the appearance of non-specific inflammation which does not allow differentiation from other causes of pleurisy.

Nodules are more common in the upper than the lower zones and may be single or multiple. Cavitation may occasionally lead to haemoptysis, and tissue diagnosis can usually be obtained by percutaneous or transbronchial needle biopsy without recourse to thoracotomy.

Pulmonary fibrosis is common in rheumatoid arthritis but is often subclinical. Ten per cent of patients have radiological evidence of fibrosis and many more have evidence of impaired vital capacity and gas transfer. Classical fibrosing alveolitis occurs in 2 per cent of patients with rheumatoid arthritis and causes progressive dyspnoea, clubbing of the fingers, fine late-inspiratory crepitations, and lower-zone reticulonodular shadowing on the chest radiograph. It carries a 5 year mortality of 50 per cent and responds poorly to treatment with corticosteroid, D-penicillamine, or cytotoxic agents.

Obliterative bronchiolitis is a rare but rapidly progressive and fatal process manifesting with an acute onset of breathlessness. Widespread small airways obstruction is present in the absence of alveolar fibrosis and there is little evidence of inflammation.

Many patients with rheumatoid arthritis have evidence of airways obstruction irrespective of their smoking habits. Bronchiectasis also appears to be more common in those with the disease and to predate its onset.

Cardiac involvement

This is more common in men and is frequently subclinical. Small pericardial effusions can be found by ultrasonography in up to half those patients with seropositive nodular disease admitted to hospital but this represents the severe end of the disease spectrum. The true overall prevalence is probably between 5 and 10 per cent. Clinically symptomatic pericarditis has an annual incidence of about 0.4 per cent and may occur at any stage of the disease. However, potentially life-threatening complications such as tamponade or constrictive pericarditis are very rare.

Valvulitis may be apparent at autopsy in 20 per cent of cases but is rarely symptomatic during life. Granulomatous thickening of the cusps of the aortic valve occurs more frequently than in the mitral valve but only rarely produces incompetence of the valve. Acute aortic regurgitation following perforation of one of the cusps is described and may need emergency valve replacement.

Autopsy studies reveal a patchy myocardial fibrosis in about one-sixth of patients and myocardial nodules can be found in some patients. Although evidence of a small-vessel vasculitis may be apparent at postmortem in 20 per cent of patients, the incidence of myocardial infarction resulting from necrotizing vasculitis during life seems to be very low. However, there is an excess cardiac mortality among patients with rheumatoid arthritis that appears to be caused through ischaemic heart disease, although the precise mechanisms involved are not clear.

Eye involvement (see Section 26)

This is common in rheumatoid arthritis and may be due to localized tissue involvement or as part of a more generalized disorder involving the exocrine glands—Sjögren's syndrome. Exceptionally there may be diplopia resulting from stenosing tenosynovitis of the superior oblique tendon (Brown's syndrome).

Sjögren's syndrome is characterized by diffuse infiltration of the exocrine glands and other tissues by lymphocytes, resulting in destruction and glandular insufficiency (see Chapter 18.11.5). The syndrome occurs in one-fifth of patients with rheumatoid arthritis (secondary Sjögren's syndrome).

Typical symptoms consist of pain, erythema and grittiness in the eyes, photosensitivity, and stickiness associated with adherent strands of mucus. Secondary bacterial infection is relatively common due to the loss of lysozymes, bacteriostatic agents normally present in tears. Corneal damage may occur.

Extraglandular involvement is less common in secondary Sjögren's syndrome than in the primary disease, but half of those with rheumatoid arthritis exhibit at least some degree of parotid gland enlargement. General malaise is common and cutaneous vasculitis, peripheral neuropathy, renal tubular acidosis, interstitial pulmonary fibrosis, and myositis may all coincide. Lymphoproliferation occurs in one-quarter of all patients (particularly those with primary disease), and there is a measurable excess of individuals who subsequently develop lymphoma.

In difficult cases the diagnosis may be aided by the following: lymphocytic infiltration of labial salivary glands on biopsy; the presence of anti-salivary gland antibodies; reduced secretion of saliva measured by cannulation of the parotid or submandibular ducts; abnormalities of the parotid ductular architecture at sialography. Rheumatoid factor is almost invariably positive and 70 per cent of patients are also positive for antinuclear factor.

Episcleritis usually appears as a raised lesion in the anterior sclera with hyperaemia of the deeper layers. The lesions are often transient but may be associated with vasculitis elsewhere. Low-grade discomfort is not uncommon and may require the use of topical corticosteroids.

Scleritis is less common but potentially more serious since it may lead to progressive thinning of the sclera (scleromalacia) and even perforation. Treatment with systemic corticosteroids is usually required. Keratolysis (corneal melting) and limbal guttering are rare complications of vasculitis of the circumcorneal vessels which can also cause perforation.

Peripheral nerve involvement

This is common in rheumatoid arthritis but is quite frequently masked by the severity of the joint disease. Entrapment neuropathies have already been considered and are amendable to treatment by corticosteroid injection and other measures to relieve local pressure.

A mild glove and stocking sensory neuropathy is relatively common in rheumatoid arthritis but is usually benign and does not imply inflammation of nervous tissue. However, there may be lymphocytic infiltrates of the dorsal root ganglia in Sjögren's syndrome. In contrast, the presence of a mixed sensorimotor neuropathy or mononeuritis multiplex is indicative of underlying vasculitis of the vasa nervorum and dictates the use of high-dose corticosteroid therapy with cyclophosphamide as outlined above.

Muscle involvement

In rheumatoid arthritis muscle involvement is usually attributed to the reflex inhibition and wasting resulting from severe joint pain. Focal lymphocytic infiltration may be present on muscle biopsy, but its relevance to symptoms is in doubt and there is no increase in muscle enzyme concentrations in the serum to suggest active myositis in all but a tiny minority of patients. It is important to remember that some drugs used in the treatment of the disease may cause a myopathy (e.g. corticofjsteroids, antimalarials) and that D-penicillamine is well documented to cause myasthenia gravis in some patients.

Liver involvement

This is evident in about 10 per cent of patients with active disease. There may be mild hepatosplenomegaly and asymptomatic elevation of the serum alkaline phosphatase but liver biopsy rarely shows specific changes. Minor degrees of fatty change, Kupffer cell hyperplasia, and lymphocytic infiltration of the portal tracts may be seen. The potential hepatotoxicity of many drugs used in the treatment of rheumatoid arthritis should be recalled, particularly high-dose salicylates, sulphasalazine, gold salts, and antimalarials.

Renal involvement

This is less of a problem in rheumatoid arthritis than might be expected from analogy with other disorders associated with vasculitis, such as systemic lupus erythematosus and polyarteritis nodosa. Renal biopsy studies have consistently failed to reveal evidence of renal vasculitis. Renal papillary necrosis and interstitial nephritis occasionally occur and are probably related, at least in part, to the use of non-steroidal analgesics (see Section 20). IgA nephropathy associated with elevated serum levels of IgM and IgA is described in rheumatoid arthritis but is probably no more common than in age-matched controls.

Gold salts and D-penicillamine can cause proteinuria due to membranous glomerulonephritis in about 10 per cent of patients. This may persist for up to 2 years after the drug has been stopped but rarely progresses to frank nephrotic syndrome.

Bone involvement

This occurs in the vicinity of the joints, where juxta-articular osteoporosis is an early feature. It also occurs as a more generalized phenomenon, partly as a result of the relative immobility of patients with severe arthritis but particularly in those receiving corticosteroids. Osteoporotic fractures are common and may occur at sites such as the pubic rami or ankle where they mimic exacerbations of the joint disease. Fractures of the long bones may develop with minimal trauma and are particularly common where there is pre-existing angular deformity of the limb (Fig. 8). A small proportion of patients may develop osteomalacia. However, its prevalence in patients with rheumatoid arthritis is probably no greater than in similarly handicapped, age-matched populations who also receive little exposure to direct sunlight and have diets poor in vitamin D.

The Felty syndrome

Lymphadenopathy is common in patients with rheumatoid arthritis, biopsies showing nodular hyperplasia. It is most obvious in patients with the Felty syndrome (rheumatoid arthritis, splenomegaly, and leucopenia). Other extra-articular features are frequently present and include anaemia, thrombocytopenia, persistent vasculitic leg ulceration, cutaneous pigmentation, weight loss, and recurrent infection. It is uncommon (less than 1 per cent of all cases) and rarely develops in patients who have had the disease for less than 10 years. It also seems to be particularly uncommon in certain ethnic groups, including Greeks and Chinese. This may reflect the weaker association of rheumatoid arthritis with the Dw4 antigen in these populations, since this marker is present

in about 85 per cent of individuals with the Felty syndrome in the United Kingdom.

Susceptibility to recurrent infection is closely related to the absolute neutrophil count, which may be less than $100/mm^3$. Antineutrophil antibodies may be detected in a proportion of cases, but the pathogenesis of the Felty syndrome is uncertain. Inadequate granulopoiesis, sequestration in the bone marrow, excessive margination of the circulating polymorphonuclear leucocytes, and destruction in the spleen have all been invoked. Splenectomy usually results in a temporary increase in the neutrophil count but does not provide reliable protection against recurrent infection. It is probably best reserved for those cases in which severe anaemia is due to hypersplenism. The potential role of recombinant granulocyte colony stimulating factors is interesting but remains to be evaluated.

CLINICAL COURSE OF THE DISEASE

The outcome of rheumatoid arthritis is unpredictable and observations in hospital populations are an unreliable guide to the clinical picture in the disease overall. Many patients with mild disease are never referred to hospital and may run a relatively benign, self-limiting course. Ten-year follow-up of patients admitted to hospital suggests that 25 per cent will remain fit for most activities, 40 per cent will exhibit moderate functional impairment, 25 per cent will be severely disabled, and 10 per cent will be wheelchair-bound.

An adverse outcome is suggested by an insidious, progressive onset of the symptoms, pronounced extra-articular disease (including nodules), the early development of erosions and failure to respond adequately to anti-inflammatory analgesics. Relatively severe disease also correlates with the presence of high titres of circulating rheumatoid factor and the presence of the HLA-DR4 antigen (particularly DR4 homozygosity). Although it is standard practice to begin treatment at an early stage in patients with more aggressive joint disease, evidence that this approach really does have a major influence and modifying effect on the long-term degree of disability and handicap is equivocal.

Fig. 8 Osteoporotic fracture of the tibia in a patient with severe arthritis of the knee joint and consequent angular deformity. The patient continued to walk on the leg for several weeks with increasing pain before seeking medical assistance.

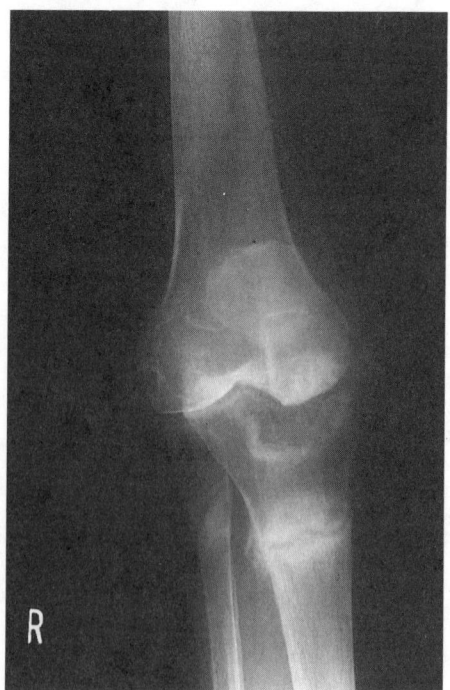

COMPLICATIONS

Septic arthritis (see Chapter 18.9) is a serious complication of rheumatoid arthritis, with a mortality rate of 25 per cent in some series. It is typically monoarticular but may be polyarticular in a quarter of cases. The expected clinical features (fever, rigors, neutrophil leucocytosis, and local inflammation of the joint) are frequently blunted or absent. Staphylococci account for three-quarters of all infections and may cause very rapid destruction of the articular surface if left untreated. In addition to systemic antibiotics, daily aspiration of the purulent synovial fluid at least is required. Open surgical drainage is sometimes necessary, particularly if the diagnosis has been delayed.

Rheumatoid arthritis is the commonest cause of AA amyloidosis in the United Kingdom (see Chapter 11.13.1). Its prevalence on rectal biopsy may be as high as 5 per cent, but rapidly progressive disease is very unusual. Suppression of disease activity with disease-modifying agents is probably as effective as the use of cytotoxic agents, although chlorambucil may be effective, particularly in juvenile rheumatoid arthritis and Still's disease.

DIFFERENTIAL DIAGNOSIS

When present in its mature, classical form the diagnosis of rheumatoid arthritis presents few problems. However, particularly during the early stages it may be difficult to distinguish from other, sometimes self-limiting, inflammatory arthropathies. For this reason it is probably best to be guarded about the diagnosis if there is any significant doubt. This is particularly true when rheumatoid factor is absent.

Viral infections are commonly associated with transient arthralgias and sometimes more prolonged attacks of synovitis. Numerous types of bacterial infection may also be followed by reactive arthropathies, and serological tests may confirm recent infection. These syndromes can usually, but not invariably, be distinguished from rheumatoid arthritis by the history, but a strongly positive test for rheumatoid factor is undoubtedly the most useful discriminatory laboratory test. In practice it is rare for there to be much difficulty distinguishing the seronegative spondarthropathies from rheumatoid arthritis, with the exception of psoriasis. This may be associated with an identical arthritis to seronegative rheumatoid arthritis and may sometimes develop before skin lesions (psoriatic arthritis without psoriasis) although there is usually a family history in such cases. Peripheral joint involvement in ankylosing spondylitis may be confusing, particularly in children, in whom it frequently antedates overt spinal disease. However, the asymmetrical pauciarticular lower limb distribution contrasts starkly with the polyarticular distribution typical of juvenile-onset rheumatoid arthritis.

Widespread synovitis commonly occurs in systemic lupus erythematosus but, although joint deformities may develop, bony erosion is very unusual. Rheumatoid factor is often present in low titre in addition to antinuclear antibodies, but evidence of renal disease, photosensitivity, mouth ulcers, pleuropericarditis and the presence of anti-DNA antibodies should clarify the diagnosis.

About 10 per cent of patients with gout have polyarticular disease from the outset but this tends to have an asymmetrical distribution and a predilection for the lower limbs, in particular the great toe. Negative tests for rheumatoid factor plus the demonstration of an elevated plasma urate level are suggestive, but the demonstration of urate crystals within the affected joints provides the definitive test. Gout may also preferentially affect joints involved by osteoarthritis, causing discrete episodes of inflammation. These, and osteoarthritis itself, can usually be distinguished without too much difficulty. However, rheumatoid arthritis superimposed on osteoarthritis can be difficult unless there are raised titres of rheumatoid factor.

The several forms of juvenile chronic arthritis can usually be distinguished from juvenile-onset rheumatoid arthritis by the absence of rheumatoid factor and the distinctive pattern of joint involvement. Still's disease has a systemic onset with fever, neutrophilia, rash, lymphadenopathy, and hepatosplenomegaly. Rheumatoid factor is absent and the sysemic features of the disease may predate the onset of joint symptoms by weeks or even months. It is uncommon in adults but may cause severe systemic upset requiring extensive investigation to exclude other connective tissue disorders, sepsis, or malignancy.

Management

Effective management of the patient with any but the mildest form of rheumatoid arthritis requires a multidisciplinary approach usually coordinated by a rheumatologist. Accurate diagnosis is essential for the early application of appropriate forms of therapy, the education of the patient in joint protection, and for counselling in adapting to disability and planning adequate social support.

In addition to standard pharmaceutical preparations, there are many other options for amelioration of symptoms, some orthodox and others not. Most patients seek relief from proprietary medicines and heterodox treatments such as copper bracelets, acupuncture, and various dietary regimes at some time in their illness. The value of many of these has undergone little rigorous testing but should not be discounted entirely.

The value of physical measures is well established. Acutely inflamed joints benefit from rest which may be accomplished either with bedrest or splintage of the affected joints, depending on the clinical context. Local application of heat or cold to affected joints and gentle massage are also frequently effective, and can be combined with stretching exercises to prevent the development of deformities consequent upon tendon and joint contractures. Regular exercise to strengthen muscles can help to stabilize damaged joints and should be initiated as early in the disease as practicable to prevent excessive muscle wasting. Many varieties of supporting splints are available to allow patients to continue to use joints that have been rendered painful or unstable by arthritis, and access to good orthoses may revolutionize the life of a patient, even with severe disease. In particular, careful attention to footwear with the provision of 'depth' shoes with soft uppers and adequately supporting insoles is important, both for immediate comfort and the prevention of future deformities.

Patients with more severe disabilities often benefit greatly from a careful assessment of the home environment, with advice on how to save labour and the provision of aids to give a mechanical advantage for specific tasks. Wheelchairs are often viewed negatively by patients and doctors alike but may greatly increase the range of activities and mobility open to the patient, thereby reducing the potential for social isolation.

DRUG TREATMENT

The dominant complaints of most patients from an early stage in the disease are pain and stiffness. These can arise as a mechanical phenomenon in damaged joints as well as from the primary inflammatory process. Analgesics ('first-line drugs') are therefore relevant at all stages of the disease. In contrast, the use of disease-modifying agents ('second-line drugs') is most logically restricted to those patients with potentially reversible soft-tissue inflammation and early erosive damage. 'Third-line drugs' include various cytotoxic agents and corticosteroids.

First-line drugs

These should include simple analgesics, such as paracetamol, codeine, and dextropropoxyphene. If these are effective, they should be used in preference to other non-steroidal anti-inflammatory drugs (NSAIDs) because of their relative safety. Many patients with mild or quiescent disease may require only intermittent analgesia.

A large number of NSAIDs are available with a broadly similar pattern of efficacy and side-effects, but there may be differences in response between individual patients. Many of the newer variants have prolonged half-lives which give a more sustained action, even allowing a single daily dosage regimen. Others may rely on sustained slow-delivery systems to achieve the same effect, despite the relatively short half-life of the drug being administered. It is logical to develop familiarity with a small selection of these drugs, including representatives from different chemical groups (Table 3). It is most appropriate to prescribe only one drug at a time and to use an adequate dose before abandoning it as ineffective. The use of nocturnal suppositories (indomethacin, diclofenac, naproxen) for the relief of morning stiffness is one particular exception to this general rule. Before embarking on long-term administration of these drugs it should be clear that there is a definite benefit to the patient, and the requirements for these drugs in the light of varying disease activity and symptoms should be critically reviewed periodically. The potential for serious adverse side-effects should not be underestimated. Gastrointestinal problems alone are very common, particularly as a result of superficial mucosal erosion, which may cause dyspepsia and haemorrhage. The relationship with chronic gastroduodenal ulceration is less clear-cut but it is important to remember that almost half of all patients admitted to hospital with acute gastrointestinal bleeding are taking non-steroidal anti-inflammatory drugs.

Second-line drugs

These are believed to exert an influence on the underlying pathological processes involved in rheumatoid arthritis. In contrast to the first-line drugs, they may retard the progression of erosive joint damage, but their effects are not usually apparent until they have been taken for at least 2 to 3 months. Commonly used second-line drugs include gold salts, D-penicillamine, antimalarials (hydroxychloroquine), and sulphasalazine. They are most appropriately used in patients who have evidence of widespread synovitis with inadequate control of symptoms by first-line drugs. Patients with advanced secondary degenerative changes and mechanical deformity are unlikely to respond to this form of therapy. Highly active disease limited to one or two joints may be best managed in the first instance by local measures, such as intra-articular corticosteroid injection, splintage, or synovectomy (surgical or radiochemical).

The effectiveness of these second-line agents can be monitored not only by the demonstration of improvement in such clinical parameters as pain, morning stiffness, and grip strength, but also by a fall in the sedimentation rate, platelet count, level of rheumatoid factor and acute-phase reactants. They should only be continued where a clear beneficial effect can be demonstrated after an adequately prolonged trial, because of the wide range of potential ill-effects. These include skin rashes, bone-marrow toxicity, and mouth ulcers (with gold, D-penicillamine, and sulphasalazine), nephrotic syndrome (gold and D-penicillamine), hepatitis ((gold and sulphasalazine), and retinopathy (antimalarials). Accordingly, careful monitoring (e.g. urinalysis, full blood count, and liver function) for side-effects is essential when these drugs are prescribed, an important responsibility of the clinician instigating the therapy even if not responsible for prescribing.

After 1 year, about two-thirds of patients started on second-line drugs will be doing well, while the remainder will have stopped the drug because of side-effects or lack of efficacy.

Third-line drugs

These include azathioprine, cyclophosphamide, chlorambucil, and methotrexate, all of which can modify the course of rheumatoid arthritis. Low-dose methotrexate (7.5–15 mg weekly), in particular, has found a firm place in treatment, and in many centres is used frequently as a second-line agent. In low dose it does not have the hepatotoxicity otherwise associated with its use; bone-marrow suppression is uncommon, but occasionally severe episodes of pneumonitis occur.

Corticosteroids are highly potent inhibitors of the inflammatory response that can have dramatic effects on the synovitis of rheumatoid arthritis. Unfortunately the plethora of unwanted side-effects (osteoporosis, fluid retention, atrophy of the dermis, increased susceptibility to infection) strictly limits their usefulness. Nevertheless about a quarter of hospital outpatients ultimately receive corticosteroids, usually in doses less than 10 mg daily, and such an approach may be highly effec-

Table 3 *Chemical groupings of the non-steroidal anti-inflammatory analgesics*

Phenylacetic acids (propionic acids)	Ibuprofen, fenoprofen, ketoprofen, flurbiprofen
Indoleacetic acids	Indomethacin, sulindac
Heterocarboxylic acids	Aspirin, salicylsalicylic acid, diflunisal
Naphthaleneacetic acids	Naproxen
Oxicams	Piroxicam, tenoxicam
Pyrazolidinediones	Phenylbutazone, oxyphenbutazone

tive in keeping patients mobile and independent when other drugs have failed.

A number of forms of experimental therapy have proved of some benefit in the treatment of rheumatoid arthritis, although their use is restricted to a few centres. These include total lymphoid irradiation, thoracic duct drainage, anti-CD4 monoclonal antibodies, and antibodies directed against the lymphocyte cell-surface determinant, CDw52.

SURGERY

Many aspects of the disease are amenable to surgical correction, and access to good orthopaedic services is critical to its management. The main indications for surgical intervention are to relieve pain, to correct deformity, to reduce instability, and to increase the effective range of movement and function.

Soft-tissue procedures

These include the repair of ruptured tendons, tendon transfers, decompression (carpal tunnel), or transfer of nerves (ulnar nerve at the elbow).

Synovectomy

This can be a useful procedure in joints with persistent active synovitis, particularly when the damage to the articular surface is relatively mild. It is also frequently performed in conjunction with excision arthroplasties (proximal radial head, lower end of ulna, forefoot arthroplasty).

Arthrodesis

This still plays a useful role in the surgical management of arthritis despite the loss of movement that it necessarily produces. It is particularly useful for the painful wrist or finger, and can correct pain and instability in the ankle and thumb. Fusion of the cervical spine may be essential to prevent catastrophic neurological damage to the cervical spinal cord.

Joint replacement arthroplasty

This has revolutionized the treatment of patients with severe arthritis of the large, weight-bearing lower limb joints. Total hip replacement is successful in 95 per cent of individuals, although ultimately revision due to loosening of the prosthesis and pain may be necessary. For this reason it is wise to consider using an uncemented prosthesis in individuals under the age of 60. Thromboembolism in the postoperative phase is rare in patients with rheumatoid arthritis compared to those with osteoarthritis. Sepsis occurs occasionally and can be a disastrous complication which may require removal of the prosthesis. The introduction of partially constrained total condylar prostheses for the knee has increased the success from replacement of this joint to rates similar to those of the hip although postoperative mobilization and recovery tends to be a little slower.

Replacement of other joints such as the elbow and shoulder may be highly successful in many patients but is less predictable. It should therefore be reserved for individuals with severe pain and limitation of movement. Prosthetic replacement of the wrist and ankle is not yet satisfactory and pain relief is better achieved in most cases by arthrodesis.

FURTHER READING

Arnett, F.C., Edworthy, S.M., Bloch, D.A., *et al.* (1988). The American Rheumatism Association 1987 revised criteria for the classification of rheumatoid arthritis. *Arthritis and Rheumatism,* **31,** 315–22.

Bacon, P.A. (1993). Extra-articular rheumatoid arthritis. In: *Arthritis and allied conditions* (eds. D.J. McCarty and W.J. Koopman). 12th edn. pp. 811–40. Lea and Febiger, Philadelphia.

Barrett, D.S., Brick, G.W., and Cobb, J.P. (1993). The surgery of rheumatic diseases in adults. In: *Oxford Textbook of Rheumatology* (eds. P.J. Maddison, D.A. Isenberg, P. Woo, and D.N. Glass) pp. 1099–114. Oxford University Press.

Campion, G., Maddison, P.J., Goulding, N., *et al.* (1990). The Felty syndrome: a case-matched study of clinical manifestations and outcome, serological features and immunogenetic associations. *Medicine,* **69,** 69–80.

Elliott, M.J., Mani, R.N., Feldman, M., *et al.* (1993). The treatment of rheumatoid arthritis with chimeric monoclonal antibodies to tumor necrosis factor α. *Arthritis and Rheumatism,* **36,** 1681–90.

Luukainen, R., Isoinaki, H., and Kajander, A. (1983). Prognostic value of the type of onset of rheumatoid arthritis. *Annals of the Rheumatic Diseases,* **42,** 274–5.

Panayi, G.S., Lanchbury, J.S. and Kingsley, G.H. (1992). The importance of the T cell in initiating and maintaining the chronic synovitis of rheumatoid arthritis. *Arthritis and Rheumatism,* **35,** 729–35.

Pinals, R.S. (1987). Survival in rheumatoid arthritis. *Arthritis and Rheumatism,* **13,** 903–6.

Porter, D.R., McInnes, I., Hunter, J., and Capell, H.A. (1994). Outcome of second line therapy in rheumatoid arthritis. *Annals of the Rheumatic Diseases,* **53,** 812–15.

Saway, P.A., Blackburn, W.D., Halla, J.T., and Alarcon, G.S. (1989). Clinical characteristics affecting survival in patients with rheumatoid arthritis undergoing cervical spine surgery; a controlled study. *Journal of Rheumatology,* **16,** 890–6.

Thomson, W., Pepper, L., Payton, A., *et al.* (1993). Absence of an association between HLA-DRBI*04 and rheumatoid arthritis in newly diagnosed cases from the community. *Annals of the Rheumatic Diseases,* **52,** 542–4.

Veale, D. and Pullar, J. (1994). Drug therapy of rheumatic diseases. *Hospital Update,* **20,** 93–101.

Waring, R.H. and Emery P. (1992). Genetic factors predicting persistent disease: the role of defective enzyme systems. *Baillière's Clinical Rheumatology,* **6,** 337–50.

Wollheim, F.A. (1993). Rheumatoid arthritis—the clinical picture. In: *Oxford Textbook of Rheumatology* (eds. P.J. Maddison, D.A. Isenberg, P. Woo, and D.N. Glass) pp. 639–60. Oxford University Press.

Wordsworth, P. and Bell, J.I. (1992) The immunogenetics of rheumatoid arthritis. *Springer Seminars in Immunopathology,* **14,** 59–78.

Young, A., Corbett, M., and Wingfield, J. (1988). A prognostic index for erosive changes in the hands, feet and cervical spine in early rheumatoid arthritis. *British Journal of Rheumatology,* **27,** 94–101.

18.5 Seronegative spondarthropathies

C.J. EASTMOND

INTRODUCTION AND HISTORICAL PERSPECTIVE

The diseases comprising the seronegative spondarthropathies and the associations between them are now well recognized. Some were accurately described more than a century ago but others have only been recognized within the past 20 years. The first detailed description of ankylosing spondylitis was probably made by Benjamin Brodie in 1888.

Reiter's syndrome acquired its eponymous title from a description in 1916, although Benjamin Brodie had provided a classical description of the syndrome in 1818.

Wright established psoriatic arthritis as a specific disease distinct from other inflammatory arthritides in 1959.

In 1973 Aho introduced the term 'reactive arthritis' to describe an inflammatory arthropathy following infection with *Yersinia* spp. The term has since been extended to describe other forms of postinfective arthritis due to gastrointestinal infection when the extra-articular features of Reiter's syndrome are absent. Reactive arthritis and Reiter's syndrome probably represent aspects of the same response to infection, the former being manifest by an arthropathy alone and the latter with the classical extra-articular features.

The association between ulcerative colitis and inflammatory joint disease was recognized by Bargen in 1930, although it was almost 30 years later that distinction of this arthropathy from rheumatoid arthritis was fully established.

The concept of the seronegative spondarthropathies was proposed in 1974 following detailed studies among individuals and families in Leeds of the rheumatological manifestations of inflammatory bowel disease and psoriatic arthritis. These established not only the associations between individual diseases and sacroiliitis but also the familial associations with sacroiliitis and ankylosing spondylitis. The concept of the seronegative spondarthropathies arose on the basis of a greater-than-expected frequency of both sacroiliitis and ankylosing spondylitis, dis-

tinctive patterns of peripheral arthropathy, associations with inflammatory eye disease, mucosal ulceration, absence of IgM rheumatoid factor, and familial associations. These observations coincided with the discovery of the association between ankylosing spondylitis and the histocompatibility antigen HLA-B27. Later work has demonstrated an association between HLA-B27 and the majority of the other diseases included in the seronegative spondarthropathies (Table 1).

Ankylosing spondylitis

DEFINITION AND DIAGNOSTIC CRITERIA

Criteria for the diagnosis of ankylosing spondylitis have been established, but they are more applicable to epidemiological studies than to the clinical diagnosis of an individual case. Diagnosis is usually made on the basis of inflammatory back pain with radiological evidence of sacroiliitis in the absence of evidence of microbial infection. Inflammatory back pain is commonly of insidious onset, with persistent low back or buttock pain for more than 3 months, together with early morning stiffness and improvement with exercise. In most cases symptoms arise before the age of 40 years.

PREVALENCE

Racial variation in the prevalence of ankylosing spondylitis closely matches that of HLA-B27. In white European and North American populations the prevalence lies between 1 in 250 and 1 in 100 males, but is less frequent in females, male : female ratio about 5 : 1.

AETIOLOGY AND PATHOGENESIS

Approximately 90 per cent of Caucasians with ankylosing spondylitis are HLA-B27 positive, contrasting with a general population frequency

Table 1 *Diseases included in seronegative spondarthropathies and their respective HLA-B27 frequencies*

	HLA − B27 + ve(%)
Ankylosing spondylitis	80–96
Psoriatic arthritis	4.5–27
with sacroiliitis	9–77
Reactive arthritis	80–90
Reiter's syndrome	65–96
Enteropathic synovitis	
Ulcerative colitis	C
Crohn's disease	C
Intestinal bypass	C
Chronic inflammatory bowel	28–72
disease with ankylosing	
spondylitis	
Uveitis	56
Whipple's disease	30
Behçet's syndrome	C
Undifferentiated	?

C, Control population frequency.

of about 8 per cent. It is possible that HLA-B27 is not itself important in the pathogenesis of the disease, but no evidence has been produced to support the alternative proposition that a linked gene is responsible. The association with HLA-B27 has given rise to a number of ideas regarding pathogenesis, although all at present remain hypotheses. The main suggestions are centred around molecular mimicry, receptor theories, and abnormal host defence mechanisms.

Molecular mimicry theories emphasize shared amino acid residues between HLA-B27 and *Klebsiella* species or other organisms, perhaps resulting in:

(1) this shared molecular structure leading to an impaired immune response and hence to disease;

(2) the shared structure leading to the production of antibodies directed against self, resulting in disease; or

(3) proteins encoded by the pathogen resulting in antibody formation against self structures in joints and entheses.

In the third model, HLA-B27 is required to bind peptide from the pathogen or self and present this to the immunocompetent cell with resultant disease.

In the original receptor theory, HLA-B27 was proposed as a receptor for Klebsiella and other bacterial cell products. An alternative possibility is that bacterial plasmids may transfect HLA-B27-positive cells to express new determimants specific for ankylosing spondylitis, resulting in HLA-B27 being a specific receptor rather than non-specific as in the original theory. Finally, there may be abnormal host defence mechanisms related to the presence of HLA-B27 (or products of closely linked genes) which in a more generalized way lead to a defective immune response.

CLINICAL FEATURES

The initial symptoms predominantly affect people under the age of 40 with a strong male predominance, and classically comprise pain and stiffness in the low back, buttocks, and the back of the upper thighs, more marked in the mornings, eased by moderate exercise and activity, tending to recur with rest or inactivity. Some patients experience disturbance of sleep because of these symptoms and many find lying in bed after waking uncomfortable. Radiation of the pain into the thighs is classically bilateral but may be unilateral and can mimic sciatica; it rarely goes much below the knee and virtually never into the foot. There are no associated paraesthesiae. Cough impulse pain may be present. Initially limitation of spinal movement may not be evident, particularly

in mild cases; but once it begins it involves movements in all planes, to include lateral flexion as well as forward flexion and extension. There is frequently a flattening of the lumbar lordosis or an inability to reverse this on forward flexion (Fig. 1). Scoliosis may or may not be present but is not usually a marked feature. With more advanced disease a thoracic kyphosis develops, with concomitant restriction of thoracic rotation and chest expansion due to involvement of the costovertebral and costotransverse joints. In advanced and severe cases movements of the cervical spine are also restricted in all planes, usually with dramatic limitation of lateral flexion. The combination of a thoracic kyphosis and cervical stiffness may lead to difficulties with forward vision or marked hyperextension of the cervical spine (Fig. 2).

There is peripheral joint involvement in some 30 to 40 per cent of patients during the course of disease and this is a presenting feature in 10 to 20 per cent of patients. This type of onset is more common in younger patients, particularly teenagers. Initial diagnosis is difficult if back symptoms are absent. The joints most commonly involved are

Fig. 1 Limitation of spinal forward flexion. Note the flat lumbar spine.

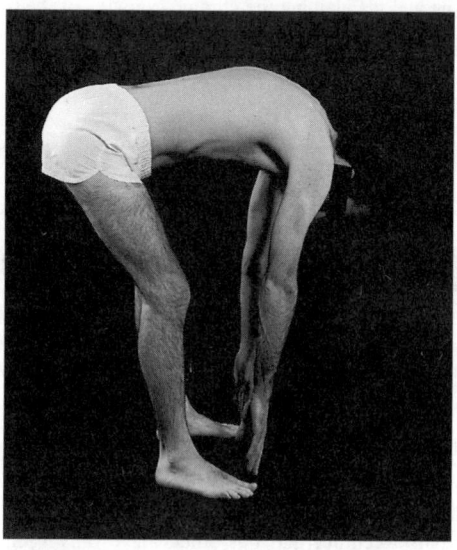

Fig. 2 Advanced ankylosing spondylitis with marked thoracic kyphosis and flexion deformity of the hip.

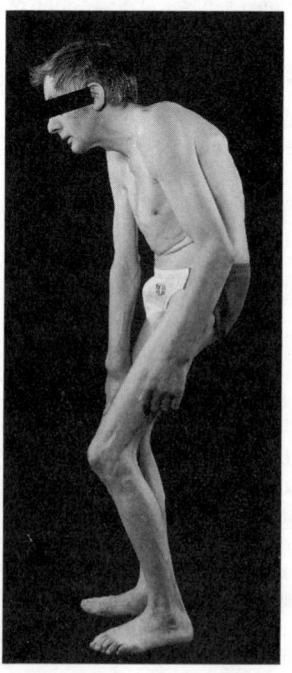

those of the lower limb, particularly the knees and ankles. There may be dactylitis of the toes and involvement of the hip. In the upper limb the shoulders and wrists are most commonly involved with comparative sparing of the small joints of the hands. The temporomandibular joints may be affected, as may the sternoclavicular and manubriosternal joints. Joint involvement is usually oligoarticular and asymmetrical. The junctional areas between ligament or tendon and bone (entheses) are characteristically involved, particularly at the heel at the insertions of the plantar fascia and the Achilles tendon to the calcaneum. This enthesopathy is associated with pain, tenderness, and sometimes swelling. Other sites include the iliac crests, ischial tuberosities, and greater trochanters. It tends to be an early feature of the disease but may occur at any time and is often associated with other peripheral joint involvement.

Acute anterior uveitis occurs at any time in the course of the disease and is seen in up to 20 per cent of patients. Recurrent attacks are common, occuring in 60 per cent of affected patients. Either eye may be affected in separate episodes but simultaneous bilateral involvement is uncommon.

Limitation of chest expansion results in a restrictive pulmonary defect, partially compensated for by diaphragmatic movement. It is often associated with a rather flat-looking chest and a pot-belly. Approximately 1 per cent of patients with advanced disease will develop apical pulmonary fibrosis and cavitation radiologically similar to the appearance of tuberculosis. Superinfection with Aspergillus may occur.

Aortic regurgitation secondary to aortitis has been found in approximately 1 per cent of patients, usually in those with advanced severe disease. Atrioventricular block is also a recognized association.

A cauda equina syndrome may complicate advanced disease with resultant disturbance of bladder and bowel function. In most cases myelographic examination reveals lumbar diverticulae.

Some patients have associated psoriasis or chronic inflammatory bowel disease. Ileocolonoscopy studies have recently revealed ileal ulceration in a high proportion of patients with ankylosing spondylitis and other seronegative spondarthritides. The significance of this finding has yet to be fully determined.

LABORATORY AND RADIOLOGICAL FEATURES

The radiological hallmark of ankylosing spondylitis is sclerosis and erosion of both sides of both sacroiliac joints over an extensive segment, most marked in the lower half (Fig. 3). When these changes are combined with classical clinical features the diagnosis is straightforward. Lesser degrees of radiological abnormality of the sacroiliac joints are more difficult to interpret, and in early and mild disease there may be no radiological abnormality for several years, making early diagnosis

Fig. 3 Radiological sacroiliitis. Note the sclerosis and erosions on both the ilial and sacral sides of the joint.

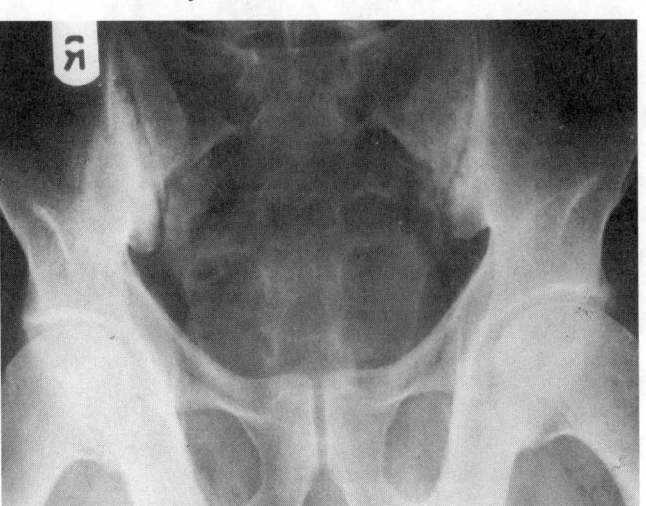

difficult. In established disease, bony bridging (syndesmophytes) occurs between the vertebrae (Fig. 4), usually first observed in the upper lumbar spine and increasing with progression of the disease. Preceding or coinciding with syndesmophyte formation, squaring of the lumbar vertebrae is often observed in lateral radiographs, with loss of the normal anterior concavity. This may be preceded by an eroded sclerotic (Romanus) lesion at the upper or lower border of the vertebrae best seen on lateral films. In advanced cases syndesmophyte formation will extend throughout the spine. Ligamentous calcification may occur, resulting in linear calcification joining the posterior spinus processes and laminae, best seen in the anteroposterior radiograph (Fig. 4).

The erythrocyte sedimentation rate and C-reactive protein are raised in only 25 to 30 per cent of patients. Less commonly there may be raised plasma concentrations of immunoglobulins, particular IgA. Mild degrees of normochromic normocytic anaemia are common but are not usually as profound as in rheumatoid arthritis. Abnormalities of the liver function tests, particularly the alkaline phosphatase and γ-glutamyl transferase, are also well recognized but are not usually severe.

TREATMENT

There is no cure for ankylosing spondylitis. Control of symptoms can usually be achieved by the use of one of the non-steroidal anti-inflammatory drugs combined with a daily programme of mobilizing, postural, and chest expansion exercises. These exercises may help to limit the degree of subsequent spinal stiffness and deformity. Intra-articular depot corticosteroids can be useful for short-term improvement of peripheral synovitis. Slow-acting antirheumatic drugs as used in peripheral chronic inflammatory joint disease are ineffective, although there is some evidence to suggest that sulphasalazine may be useful in patients responding inadequately to non-steroidal anti-inflammatory drugs. The response is probably better for peripheral arthropathy than for spinal disease. The recommended dose is sulphasalazine 1 to 1.5 g twice daily, and the response will be delayed by 2 to 4 months from initiation of therapy.

Regular daily exercises may need to be supplemented by specific physiotherapy for exacerbations or when there is increased spinal stiffness. Regular swimming is recommended as additional exercise. Contact sports are usually best avoided, particularly for those with more advanced disease.

Fig. 4 (a) Lumbar spinal syndesmophytes and (b) linear posterior ligamentous calcification, in ankylosing spondylitis.

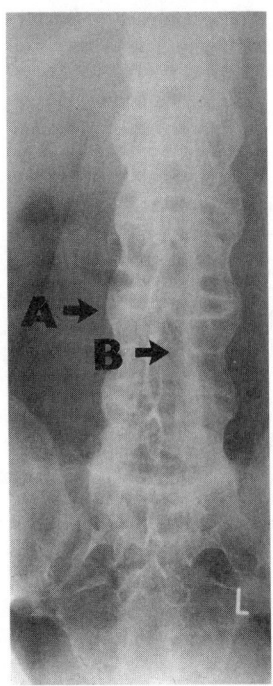

Braces and corsets should be avoided. They do not limit spinal deformity nor reverse it. For severe kyphosis, lumbar osteotomy may be valuable in some cases. Osteotomy at higher levels is particularly hazardous and requires assessment by a surgeon fully familiar with the procedure and its complications.

Combined restriction of spinal movements and involvement of hips is particularly disabling. When hip involvement is painful, a good outcome can be anticipated from hip joint replacement.

Persistent peripheral arthropathy involving single joints, such as a knee joint, may require synovectomy if painful and disabling.

PROGNOSIS

The few long-term follow-up studies performed have indicated that the majority of patients do well, with about 90 per cent either fully independent or minimally disabled. This is despite some 40 per cent of patients having severe spinal restriction. Early onset of peripheral arthritis or the presence of iritis is associated with more severe spinal restriction.

The longer-term prognosis can probably be determined after about 10 years of disease. Seventy-four per cent of those with mild restriction at 10 years do not progress further, and 80 per cent of those found to have severe spinal restriction after prolonged follow-up had marked spinal restriction after 10 years' duration. Those who do not develop hip involvement within the first 10 years appear to retain normal hips thereafter.

Long-term follow-up of manual workers with ankylosing spondylitis indicates that one-third are unable to continue working after 25 years. Of those still in employment, at least half are doing the same job, whereas a slightly smaller proportion have had to change to lighter work. For those with less physically demanding jobs a higher proportion are able to remain in work.

Mortality is not necessarily entirely relevant to a chronic disease, but a third to a half of deaths are due to cardiovascular causes. There is a 2.5–4 to threefold excess mortality due to respiratory causes. Radiotherapy is not currently used as a form of treatment, but studies of those who have previously received it demonstrate an overall two-thirds excess mortality, with a fivefold increase in death due to leukaemia and a 60 per cent excess of death due to carcinoma in the irradiated sites. The mortality is highest amongst those who have received radiotherapy late in the course of the disease.

The effect of pregnancy is less predictable than in rheumatoid arthritis, with the disease being unaffected in over one-half of patients, a quarter being worse, and a fifth improving during pregnancy. Slightly less than a half of patients suffer a mild postpartum flare. There is no evidence that pregnancy affects the overall course of the disease, or that the disease itself affects the course of pregnancy or the fetus.

Psoriatic arthritis

Psoriatic arthritis is characterized by a peripheral inflammatory polyarthritis associated with the presence of psoriasis and the absence of IgM rheumatoid factor. Psoriatic nail dystrophy is strongly associated and radiological sacroiliitis may be present.

PREVALENCE

Psoriasis affects about 1.6 per cent of the general population and seronegative arthritis occurs in some 6.8 per cent of these patients. These figures form part of the case for psoriatic arthritis being a distinct entity. No formal epidemiological studies have been conducted but its prevalence is estimated to be 0.1 per cent.

CLINICAL FEATURES

Psoriatic arthritis has been divided into five subgroups (Table 2). Their relative frequency tends to vary between series and may reflect different

Table 2 *Categories of psoriatic arthritis*

Distal interphalangeal
   (predominantly but not exclusively)
Asymmetrical
Symmetrical
Mutilans
Spinal

Table 3 *Characteristic features of psoriatic arthritis*

Asymmetry
Dactylitis
Distal interphalangeal joints
Oligoarticular
Radiological/clinical sacroiliitis

methods of ascertainment. In addition, patients may present with overlap between these subgroups during follow-up. It is probably more useful to identify those characteristics which distinguish psoriatic arthritis as a separate clinical entity from rheumatoid arthritis (Table 3 and Fig. 5). Additionally, many patients have relatively self-limiting episodes rather than persistent destructive synovitis, although the latter does occur.

There is a poor correlation between the presence or severity of arthritis and the severity and extent of psoriasis; or between the activity and time of onset of arthritis and psoriasis. There is a closer relationship between the onset of the nail dystrophy and the arthritis. In addition, nail dystrophy occurs in 85 per cent of patients with psoriatic arthritis, contrasting with only 20 per cent of patients with uncomplicated psoriasis. Nail dystrophy occurs more commonly in those patients with distal interphalangeal joint involvement than other patterns of joint disease. Several patients demonstrate a close association between involvement of individual finger distal interphalangeal joints and the corresponding nail (Fig. 6). Features of the nail dystrophy which are particularly helpful in diagnosis are onycholysis in the absence of infection or trauma and large numbers of nail pits. Horizontal ridging may also be helpful diagnosti-

Fig. 5 Dactylitis of the finger in psoriatic arthritis. Note the uniform swelling of the whole digit.

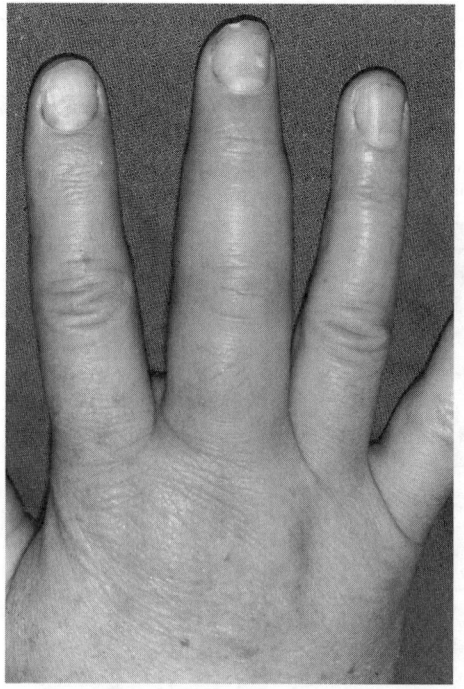

cally, but usually when associated with one of the other two features. Longitudinal ridging of the nail is not a specific associated feature.

Occular inflammation has been documented in 30 per cent of patients with psoriatic arthritis. Acute anterior uveitis is particularly prevalent in patients with radiological sacroiliitis (15 per cent) and those with ankylosing spondylitis (18 per cent). It does, however, occur in 6 per cent of patients with only peripheral arthritis. Non-suppurative conjunctivitis has been documented in 10 to 20 per cent of patients. Episcleritis and keratoconjunctivitis sicca are seen occasionally.

The differential diagnoses can include any other form of arthritis. Some patients have an acute onset involving only one joint, in which case, sepsis and crystal arthritis must be exclude by appropriate synovial fluid examination. The symmetrical form of psoriatic arthritis needs to be distinguished from rheumatoid arthritis on the basis of the presence or absence of other extra-articular features more characteristic of rheumatoid arthritis, in addition to the presence or absence of IgM rheumatoid factor.

LABORATORY AND RADIOLOGICAL FEATURES

In common with other inflammatory arthropathies, the acute-phase reactants (such as erythrocyte sedimentation rate and C-reactive protein) are often raised. This may not occur if only one or two small joints are involved. Anaemia is not as common or marked as in rheumatoid arthritis. By definition, IgM rheumatoid factor is absent. There may be mild elevations of the alkaline phosphatase and γ-glutamyl transferase, particularly in patients with widespread and active disease.

The distribution of radiological changes on the whole reflects the clinical distribution, with changes characteristically involving the distal interphalangeal joint of the fingers with asymmetrical involvement of these and other joints. The small joints of the hands and feet will generally show radiological changes before the larger joints. Periarticular osteoporosis is less severe than in rheumatoid arthritis. Erosion, joint-space narrowing, and, later, sclerosis occur. There may be periosteal elevation along the shafts of the phalanges. A characteristic pencil-in-cup deformity may occur with resorption of the distal end of a phalanx or metacarpal with deep uniform erosion of the proximal end of the next distal phalanx (Fig. 7). When widespread, these changes conform to the classical arthritis mutilans. Rarely, the severity of bone resorption may be such that individual finger or toe phalanxes seem to disappear. This would be clinically evident as a telescoping digit.

Sacroiliitis demonstrable by radiology occurs in 20 to 30 per cent of patients. Spinal changes with bony bridging (syndesmophytes) occurs in a lesser proportion of patients and also in those who have predominant spinal disease. Characteristically the syndesmophytes are more coarse than in classical ankylosing spondylitis and they may be asymmetrical.

Fig. 6 Psoriatic arthritis of a distal interphalangeal finger joint with onycholysis of the associated nail.

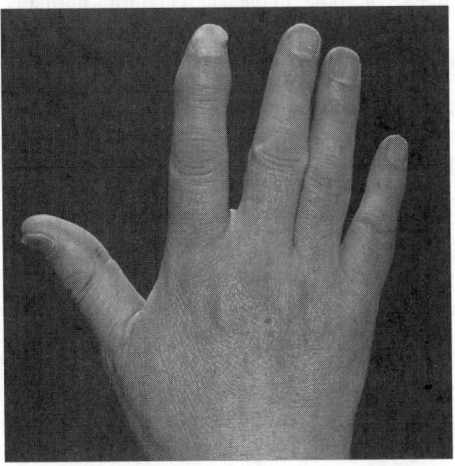

Coarse syndesmophyte formation has been described in the absence of sacroiliitis (Fig. 8).

TREATMENT

The majority of patients improve with the use of non-steroidal anti-inflammatory drugs given together with judicious use of intra-articular depot corticosteroid. The latter is most useful when only one or two larger joints are involved or there is localized flexor tenosynovitis in the hand.

In patients with more persistent or active disease not adequately responding to these measures, the use of selected slow-acting drugs is

Fig. 7 Radiological appearances of the pencil-in-cup changes at the interphalangeal joint of the right great toe in psoriatic arthritis.

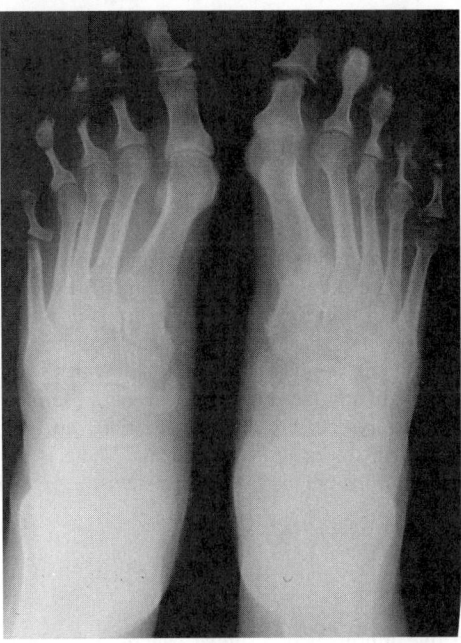

Fig. 8 Coarse syndesmophyte in psoriatic spondylitis.

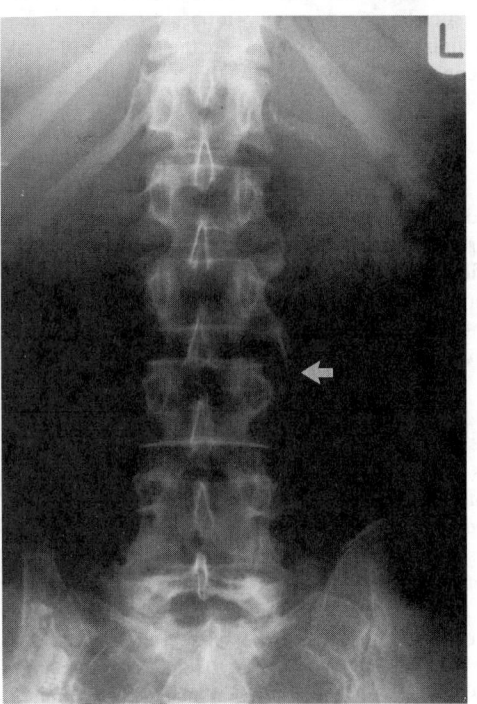

appropriate. The antimalarials should be avoided as they may exacerbate psoriasis. There is little or no evidence to suggest that penicillamine has any useful effects, but intramuscular gold can be helpful without any increased risk of mucocutaneous toxicity. Sulphasalazine is efficacious in some patients. In addition, cytotoxic agents such as methotrexate and azathioprine can be used with benefit, and may additionally improve psoriasis itself, unlike other slow-acting drugs.

Systemic corticosteroids are not used routinely as psoriasis may flare when they are withdrawn; they may, however, need to be used occasionally for persistently active disease which has not responded to other treatment.

Local treatment of the skin has no effect on the arthropathy. There is no conclusive evidence that PUVA therapy (psoralen with ultraviolet light) or etretinate have any predictable benefit on the arthropathy, although occasional patients have been found to improve coincident with these treatments.

Bedrest for short periods during episodes of active synovitis is appropriate, but joints should be mobilized early to reduce the risk of fibrous ankylosis and improve muscle tone and power. If there is spinal involvement, it is essential for patients to also carry out a similar programme of exercises to that used in ankylosing spondylitis.

PROGNOSIS

There have been few long-term follow-up studies of this disease. In general, the prognosis is better than in rheumatoid arthritis. One 8 year follow-up found 60 per cent of those with psoriatic arthritis in work, compared with only 36 per cent of those with rheumatoid arthritis; 23 per cent of the psoriatic arthritics were disabled, compared with 43 per cent of rheumatoid arthritics. In a further study, 11 per cent of psoriatic arthritics were severely or very severely disabled. Psoriatic arthritis improves during pregnancy in the majority of patients. There is no adverse effect on the course of the pregnancy or on the fetus.

Reactive arthritis

DEFINITION

The arthropathy of reactive arthritis is of a similar pattern to that seen in Reiter's syndrome, and it is sensible to consider these two disorders together. They both represent a sterile synovitis associated with recent infection at a distant site. There may or may not be extra-articular features. The features defining Reiter's syndrome are the presence of synovitis, urethritis, and conjunctivitis, occurring within a short time of each other.

PREVALENCE

Epidemiological studies of gastroenterological causes of reactive arthritis and Reiter's syndrome have shown that 1 to 2 per cent of a population exposed to a specific trigger infection may develop articular disease. Similar studies of large numbers of patients with non-specific urethritis attending departments of genitourinary medicine suggest a similar frequency for articular disease in this group.

AETIOLOGY AND PATHOGENESIS

The infective causes of reactive arthritis and Reiter's syndrome can be divided into those of gastrointestinal or of urogenital origin (Table 4). Epidemiological studies indicate that the delay between symptoms of the initial gastrointestinal infection and the arthropathy may vary from 3 to 30 days. The serum IgA levels are increased during active disease and antigen-specific IgA levels are increased for longer in those who develop arthropathy compared with those who do not. Bacterial cell wall fragments have been demonstrated within synovial fluid and membrane in the arthropathy associated with Chlamydia, Salmonella, and Yersinia.

Table 4 *Common precipitating infections of reactive arthritis and Reiter's syndrome*

Chlamydia
Salmonella spp. (not *S. typhi* or *S. paratyphi*)
Campylobacter jejuni
Shigella flexneri
Yersinia spp.

Table 5 *Characteristic features of the arthropathy of reactive arthritis and Reiter's syndrome*

Oligoarticular
Predominantly lower limb
Asymmetrical
Dactylitis
Enthesitis (especially heels)
Low back/buttock pain (inflammatory sacroiliitis)

Table 6 *Characteristic extra-articular features of reactive arthritis and Reiter's syndrome*

Arthritis[a]
Conjunctivitis[a]
Urethritis[a]
Circinate balanitis
Oral ulceration
Acute anterior uveitis
Keratoderma blennorrhagicum
Dystrophic nails
Fever

[a]Features defining Reiter's syndrome.

Whether these fragments are present in a free form or as immune complexes is not currently determined, although the latter seems likely.

There is enhanced synovial fluid T-cell responsiveness to causative bacterial antigens, suggesting a specific intra-articular immune response. However, synovial fluid lymphocytes are predominently CD4 rather than CD8 cells. The latter would normally be expected to be the responding T-cell subset in relation to class I antigens such as HLA-B27, which is strongly associated with reactive arthritis and Reiter's syndrome. As with ankylosing spondylitis, the precise role of HLA-B27 remains undetermined, nor is it clear whether or not the mechanism in these two disease is similar.

CLINICAL FEATURES

The arthropathy has certain characteristics (Table 5) common to both reactive arthritis and Reiter's syndrome. In the latter, urethritis normally predates other features. Conjunctivitis is either simultaneous with urethritis or follows very quickly thereafter, with arthropathy the third feature to develop, although this is not always the sequence. In sexually acquired Reiter's syndrome the urethritis is due to Chlamydia in 60 per cent of patients. Urethritis following gastrointestinal infection is sterile. Conjunctivitis is usually sterile, although secondary infection may occur. Some patients with so-called 'incomplete Reiter's' do not demonstrate all features of this classical triad. It may therefore be preferable to use the term reactive arthritis to encompass all patients and qualify this according to the presence of individual extra-articular features. Other extra-articular features that can occur are shown in Table 6. Oral ulceration may be due to multiple aphthae or a superficial erosive ulceration (Fig. 9) somewhat similar in appearance to balanitis (Fig. 10). This latter form of oral ulceration, as with balanitis, is usually symptomless. Symptoms alone may not differentiate between severe conjunctivitis and mild acute anterior uveitis. The latter occurs during the acute episode in some 10 per cent of patients and requires expert ophthalmic assessment and treatment. Acute anterior uveitis may also predate or succeed by several years an episode of Reiter's syndrome. Keratoderma blennorrhagicum (Fig. 11) affects less than 10 per cent of patients. It is usually seen in patients who are systemically unwell and is rare in patients without the full triad of Reiter's syndrome; it is most common in the soles of the feet, but may also affect the palms. In severe cases it may extend to other areas of skin. Nail dystrophy is usually more florid, often with onycholysis and hyperkeratosis, than that occurring in psoriasis. Fever may be present on its own or in association with other extra-articular features. Its presence requires the exclusion of coincidental infection, both systemic and articular.

LABORATORY AND RADIOLOGY

During the active phase the erythrocyte sedimentation rate and acute-phase reactants are raised. These may be anaemia broadly reflecting the overall severity and degree of systemic illness. Abnormalities of liver function tests, particularly alkaline phosphatase and γ-glutamyl transferase, are not uncommon in active disease.

By the time that arthropathy has developed there is often no continuing bacteriological evidence of active infection. This should, however, be sought by appropriate urethral and stool cultures. If sexually acquired disease is suspected, it is important to seek evidence for coincidental gonorrhoea and syphilis. In some circumstances it will be necessary to test for HIV infection after appropriate counselling.

Serum agglutinin tests are available for the currently known causes. They are not entirely reliable but may be an adjunct to diagnosis when titres are high, rise over the first 2 weeks, or fall over succeeding months.

Fig. 9 Ulceration of the tongue in Reiter's syndrome.

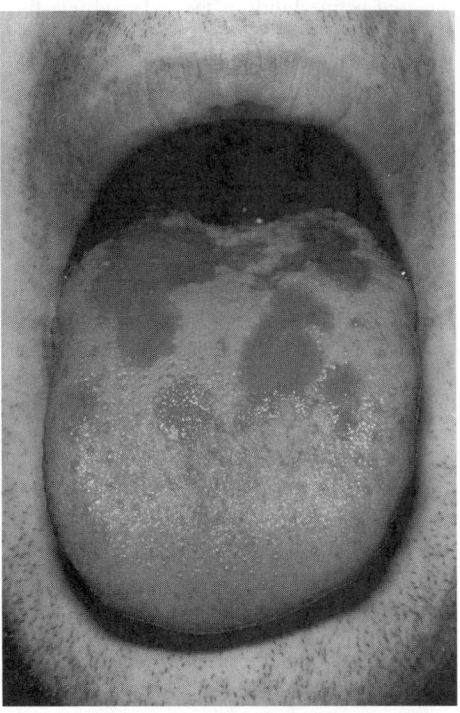

Fig. 10 Circinate balanitis in Reiter's syndrome.

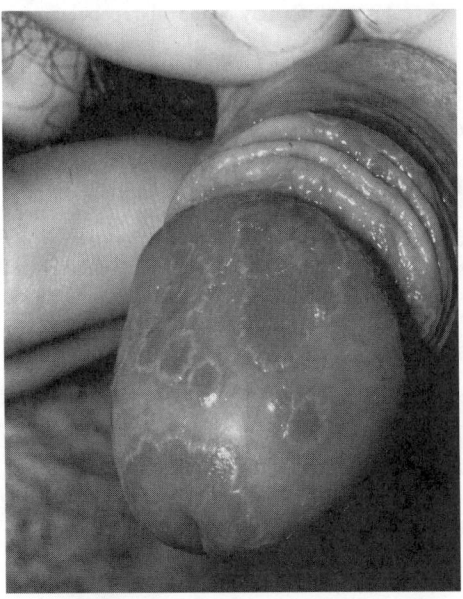

Fig. 11 Keratoderma blennorrhagicum in Reiter's syndrome.

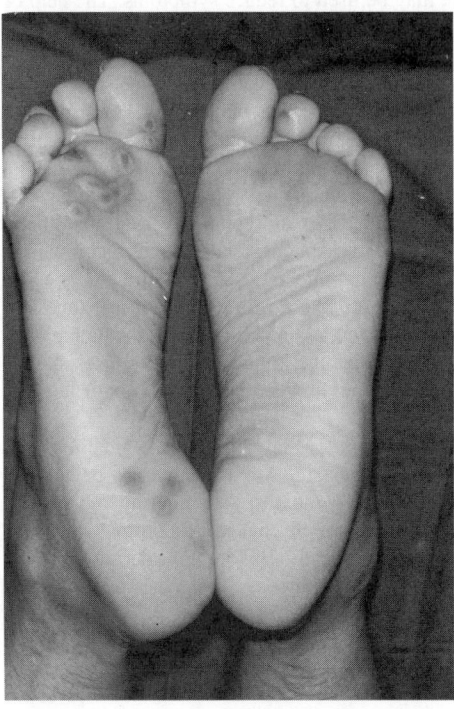

Fig. 12 Erosion at the insertions (entheses) of the Achilles tendon and plantar fascia in Reiter's syndrome.

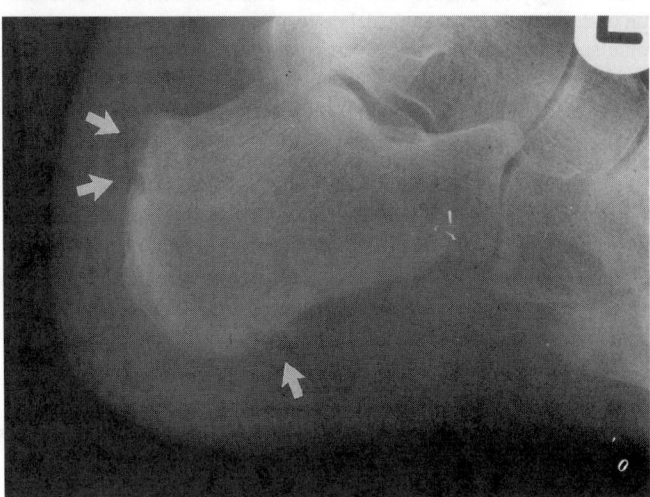

During the acute phase it is uncommon to find any radiological abnormality of the joints. In the small number of patients who have persisting disease, radiological erosions may occur, particularly in the metatarso-phalangeal joints and around the heel entheses (Fig. 12). Some patients develop radiological sacroiliitis, and a small proportion of these may acquire spinal disease. The syndesmophytes are then often coarse and asymmetrical, resembling the changes characteristic of psoriatic spondylitis rather than those of in classical ankylosing spondylitis.

TREATMENT

The joints should be rested during the acute phase. Effusions in the larger joints should be aspirated. Non-steroidal anti-inflammatory drugs help to reduce pain and stiffness. If effusions are recurrent, intra-articular depot corticosteroids can be useful if intra-articular infection has been excluded.

Secondarily infected conjunctivitis requires local antibiotic treatment; otherwise hypromellose may be used to reduce symptoms. The help of an ophthalmologist is required if acute anterior uveitis is present or suspected.

There is no current evidence that treatment of gastrointestinal infection or of infective urethritis alters the course of the arthropathy, although active urethritis, gonorrhoea, or syphilis require treatment in their own right. Local hygiene is required for balanitis, and, if it is, severe, 1 per cent hydrocortisone ointment can be applied with benefit.

Oral ulceration usually responds to antiseptic and local anaesthetic mouth washes; local cortiosteroid preparations may be needed if pain is persistent. Any coincidental fungal infection should be treated.

It is important during the acute phase to maintain muscle tone and power with isometric exercises and, as soon as the active inflammatory joint disease improves, to mobilize the joints. Spinal exercises similar to those used in ankylosing spondylitis can be useful in patients with symptomatic sacroiliitis.

A small proportion of patients develop chronic inflammatory joint disease; for these patients sulphasalazine 2 to 3 g daily may be helpful, but benefit may delayed for 2 to 4 months. Azathioprine and methotrexate have also been used with benefit, but it is important to ensure that there is no coincident HIV infection before considering these, in view of their adverse effects on the course and prognosis of HIV-associated disease.

PROGNOSIS

Some patients have a short, acute illness lasting only a few weeks, rarely leading to any residual disability. More commonly, the active phase of inflammatory joint disease lasts between 3 and 6 months. With resolution of the clinical features, the laboratory features also return to normal. Some such patients may, however, continue to have arthralgia, which can be sufficient to limit physical activity, but the symptoms are rarely sufficient to warrant the use of anti-inflammatory agents. Active disease can extend beyond 6 months in a few patients, who are then at risk of developing erosive disease. Classical psoriatic arthritis may also develop in some patients whose initial manifestations include severe systemic Reiter's syndrome and keratoderma blennorrhagicum. The prognosis in this situation is usually poor, and slow-acting or immunosuppressive drugs are commonly required.

Recurrences after full recovery do occur, and since it is not always possible to identify an infecting organism at the time, it is difficult to determine whether there has been reactivation of previous disease or reinfection with an unidentified organism.

There is evidence that Reiter's syndrome may be especially severe and associated with more severe extra-articular features in those who have coincident HIV infection and AIDS.

Enteropathic synovitis

DEFINITION

Enteropathic synovitis is a sterile synovitis occurring in association with chronic inflammatory bowel disease or after intestinal bypass surgery.

AETIOLOGY AND PATHOGENESIS

Enteropathic synovitis occurs in 10 per cent of patients with ulcerative colitis and in 10 to 20 per cent of patients with Crohn's disease. It has also been found in 8 to 30 per cent of those treated by intestinal bypass surgery for morbid obesity.

The arthropathy associated with chronic inflammatory bowel disease is more frequent in those with severe and extensive disease and during exacerbations of bowel disease. The precise mechanism is unknown, but it may be related to increased permeability of the inflamed intestinal mucosa to intraluminal antigens. Experimental models of intestinal bypass arthropathy have demonstrated IgA immune complexes associated with blind loops, and complexes of IgG and secretory IgA have been found in individuals with bypass arthropathy.

CLINICAL FEATURES

Chronic inflammatory bowel disease
The arthropathy has a predilection for lower limb joints, particularly knees and ankles, with a similar distribution in both ulcerative colitis and Crohn's disease, but upper limb joints can also be involved. Dactylitis of the toes is characteristic. Classically, the arthropathy relapses and remits in association with exacerbations and remissions of bowel disease. Joint destruction does not occur. Exceptionally, Crohn's granulomata have been observed in synovial membranes leading to a persistent arthropathy and joint destruction.

The arthropathy is frequently associated with other complications, in particular uveitis, episcleritis, and conjunctivitis, erythema nodosum, pyoderma grangrenosum, and oral ulceration (especially in Crohn's disease), and clubbing of the fingers.

Bypass surgery
This also tends to affect lower limb joints, particularly the knees and ankles, although fingers and shoulders may be involved. It usually occurs within 1 year of the bypass procedure. Males are more commonly affected than females. The pain is usually intense, with only slight swelling. Joint destruction does not occur, and there is no association with radiological sacroiliitis. Eighty per cent of patients with arthropathy have associated cutaneous features which may be macular, papular, pustular, urticarial, or erythema nodosum.

Sacroiliitis and ankylosing spondylitis
These occur with an increased frequency in patients with inflammatory bowel disease but not following bypass surgery. They also occur with an increased frequency in the relatives of patients with chronic inflammatory bowel disease. They are similar to classical ankylosing spondylitis, and are associated with HLA-B27 but in lower frequency (28–72 per cent). The course of the spinal disease is independent of the bowel disease. There is no association between the severity of chronic inflammatory bowel disease and the presence, absence, or severity of sacroiliitis and ankylosing spondylitis.

TREATMENT

Enteropathic synovitis associated with chronic inflammatory bowel disease
Control of synovitis is associated with successful medical treatment of the bowel disease. In ulcerative colitis removal of the affected colon

leads to complete remission of the arthropathy. Complete surgical exclusion of disease is not possible in Crohn's disease and the arthropathy may therefore continue despite surgical treatment if medical treatment cannot fully control the disease. The additional use of non-steroidal anti-inflammatory drugs may be useful, but some of these may aggravate the bowel disease. In large joints, aspiration of synovial fluid and local injection of depot corticosteroid may be helpful while other measures are undertaken to control the bowel disease. The presence of severe recurrent arthropathy may be an indication for colectomy in ulcerative colitis.

Intestinal bypass arthropathy

The use of antibiotics and non-steroidal anti-inflammatory drugs, respectively, may be useful in eliminating bacterial overgrowth and reducing synovitis. The syndrome can be fully reversed with corrective bowel surgery.

Ankylosing spondylitis and sacroiliitis

This should be treated in the same way as ankylosing spondylitis occurring independently of bowel disease (see above).

PROGNOSIS

The prognosis of enteropathic synovitis is largely dependent on that of the bowel disease. It is not usually destructive, with the rare exception of intra-articular granuloma formation in Crohn's disease, when systemic treatment with immunosuppressives and steroids may be helpful.

The prognosis for ankylosing spondylitis and sacroiliitis is similar to that for the spinal disease in the absence of bowel disease (see above).

Whipple's disease

(See also Section 14.9.6.)

Whipple described this rare disease of general wasting, diarrhoea inflammatory joint disease, widespread intestinal fat infiltration, and PAS-positive staining of the intestinal lesion in 1907. It predominantly affects middle-aged male Caucasians. HLA-B27 was present in 30 per cent of one reported series.

Arthropathy is a presenting feature in 60 per cent of patients and occurs in 90 per cent during the course of the disease, being either oligoarticular or polyarticular. Occasionally it may precede other manifestations by more than 10 years. It is rarely erosive and is frequently migratory. It tends to fluctuate independently of the gastrointestinal symptoms. Sacroiliitis has been found in 7 per cent of patients and ankylosing spondylitis in 4 per cent.

Diagnosis is confirmed by PAS-positive staining material in joint fluid and macrophages in the lamina propria of the intestine. Many other tissues may also have PAS-positive staining material. The finding of bacterial cell fragments on electron microscopy adds further confirmation.

Despite the electron microscopic features and a response to antibiotics, no precise causative organism has been found.

Treatment is with prolonged courses of penicillin, 500 mg 4 times per day; tetracycline, 500 mg 4 times per day; or erythromycin, 500 mg 4 times per day. Relapse may occur if treatment is stopped prematurely.

Behçet's syndrome

This chronic relapsing syndrome of oral ulceration, genital ulceration, and uveitis is more fully discussed in Chapter 18.11.8.

Synovitis occurs in some 40 per cent of patients (Table 7). The synovitis is subacute or chronic, involving large and small joints. It particularly affects the knees and ankles, and is usually oligoarticular or monoarticular. Erosive change is rare. Symptomatically it responds to corticosteroids. Sacroiliitis is a rare association.

Table 7 *The clinical features of Behçet's syndrome and their frequency*

	Percentage
Oral ulceration	100
Genital ulceration	74
Uveitis	52
Synovitis	40
Cutaneous vasculitis (similar to erythema nodosum)	54
Meningoencephalitis	30
Large artery aneurysms	
Phlebitis	
Discrete intestinal ulcers	

Table 8 *Characteristic features of seronegative spondarthritis*

Oligoarthritis
Lower limb predominance
Asymmetry
Enthesitis
Dactylitis
Back/buttock pain and stiffness
Family history of a seronegative spondarthritis or associated disease

Undifferentiated spondarthritides

Clinical observation has led to the necessity to define a group of undifferentiated seronegative spondarthritides. Ankylosing spondylitis may have a peripheral joint onset in 10 per cent of patients, especially in teenagers in whom radiology of the sacroiliac joints is unreliable; arthropathy may precede the onset of the dermal manifestations of psoriasis; Crohn's disease may be initially silent and present with arthropathy; and 50 per cent of patients with gastrointestinal infection may be asymptomatic, but a proportion still develop reactive arthritis. In addition, studies of patients with undifferentiated seronegative spondarthritis have found associations with HLA-B27 with a variable frequency.

The clinical features that should direct the clinician to consider a seronegative spondarthritis are shown in Table 8. In addition, the European Seronegative Spondarthritis Group has suggested criteria for the diagnosis of undifferentiated seronegative spondarthritis on the basis of analysis of a large number of patients from many centres (Table 9).

Repeated and careful search for additional diagnositic articular and extra-articular features is important as the evolution of the disease may allow more precise diagnosis with time; but long-term follow-up studies of such patients have not been undertaken.

Treatment and prognosis are largely dependent upon the most likely cause. Non-steroidal anti-inflammatories, joint aspiration, and injection with depot corticosteroid, periods of immobilization, and physiotherapy will be effective for most. Appropriate slow-acting or cytotoxic drugs may rarely be required.

Adult Still's disease

Adult Still's disease may not form one of the classical seronegative spondarthritides but has previously been included in the group. It is a rare disease of unknown prevalence, which is unlikely to be more than 1 per 100 000 population. It principally affects young adults aged between 16 and 35 years. It has the same characteristics as systemic juvenile chronic arthritis. Its cause is unknown, although in a small

Table 9 *European Seronegative Spondarthritis Group criteria for undifferentiated spondarthritis*

1. Inflammatory-type back pain:
   ≤40 years age at onset
   insidious onset
   improvement with exercise
   early morning stiffness
   ≥3 months' duration
   Or
2. Asymmetrical lower-limb synovitis
Plus two of:
(a) Positive family history:
    ankylosing spondylitis
    psoriasis
    acute anterior uveitis
    reactive arthritis
    chronic inflammatory bowel disease
(b) Psoriasis
(c) Chronic inflammatory bowel disease
(d) Urethritis preceding by ≤1 month
(e) Acute diarrhoea preceding by ≤1 month
(f) Alternating buttock pain
(g) Definite radiological sacroiliitis

Table 10 *Diagnostic criteria for adult Still's disease*

Each of:
1. Quotidian fever >39°C
2. Arthralgia/arthritis
3. Negative rheumatoid factor
4. Negative antinuclear factor
Plus two of:
(a) Leucocytosis >15 × 10⁹/l
(b) Evanescent macular/maculopapular rash
(c) Serositis (pleuritic/pericarditic)
(d) Hepatomegaly
(e) Splenomegaly
(f) Generalized lymphadenopathy

number of cases there has been evidence to suggest a preceding viral infection, principally of echovirus or rubella. There is no association with HLA-B27. Studies suggest associations with HLA-B14 and DR7, BW35 and CW4 and DR4. The principal criteria for diagnosis are given in Table 10. It is essential to exclude infection and primary haematological disease such as lymphoma and leukaemia. In some patients it is necessary to consider the differential diagnoses of sarcoidosis and endocarditis.

Initial treatment should be with high-dose non-steroidal anti-inflammatories, such as aspirin, indomethacin, or naproxen. If unsuccessful, or if there are severe systemic features, anaemia, pericarditis, or myocarditis, corticosteroids are usually required. High doses may be needed initially, but the aim should be to achieve a maintenance dose of less than 15 mg of prednisolone per day and finally to discontinue corticosteroid treatment within 6 months of its commencement. For patients failing to respond adequately to corticosteroids, or requiring more prolonged treatment, it may be necessary to consider slow-acting antirheumatic drugs or cytotoxic agents. No adequate trials of these have been performed in adult Still's disease but there are anecdotal reports of success with intramuscular sodium aurothiomalate, penicillamine, antimalarials and sulphasalazine. Cytotoxic agents have rarely been used, but there are anecdotal reports of improvement with azathioprine, chlorambucil, cyclophosphamide, or methotrexate.

Although initially considered to be a relatively benign disease, it is now recognized that 50 per cent of patients have progressive joint disease, particularly involving the wrists and hind feet leading to carpal and tarsal fusion, respectively. In addition, systemic complications including disseminated intravascular coagulation, acute hepatic failure, sometimes in combination with associated renal failure, cardiac tamponade, constrictive pericarditis, myocarditis, endocarditis, severe lung disease, peritonitis, and amyloidosis have all been reported. There have been single case reports of panophthalmitis, status epilepticus, and polymyositis with rhabdomyolysis.

REFERENCES

Archer, J.R., Winrow, V.R., and McLean, I.L. (1988). The role of HLA B27 in arthritis. *British Journal of Rheumatology* **27**, 306–9.
Archer, J.R. (1994). HLA-B27 and its role in arthritis. *Rheumatology in Europe,* **23**, 97–9.
Brewerton, D.A., Hart, F.D., Nicholls, A., Caffrey, M., James, D.C.O., and Sturrock, R.D. (1973). Ankylosing spondylitis and HL-A27. *Lancet* **i**, 904–7.
Carette, S., Graham, D., Little, H., Rubenstein, J., and Rosen, P. (1983). The natural disease course of ankylosing spondylitis. *Arthritis and Rheumatism* **26**, 186–90.
Dougados, M., et al. (1991). The European spondylarthropathy study group preliminary criteria for the classification of spondylarthropathy. *Arthritis and Rheumatism* **34**, 1218–27.
The International study group for Behçet's disease (1992). Evaluation of diagnostic ('classification') criteria in Behçet's disease—towards internationally agreed criteria. *British Journal of Rheumatology* **31**, 299–308.
Maki-Ikola, O. and Granfors, K. (1992). Salmonella-triggered reactive arthritis. *Lancet* **339**, 1096–8.
Mapstone, R. and Woodrow, J.D. (1975). HLA B27 and acute anterior uveitis *British Journal of Ophthalmology* **59**, 270–5.
Moll, J.M.H., Haslock, I., McCrae, I.F., and Wright, V. (1974). Association between ankylosing spondylitis, psoriatic arthritis, Reiter's disease, the intestinal arthropathies, and Behçet's syndrome. *Medicine (Baltimore)* **53**, 343–64.
Russell, A.S. (1988). Klebsiella and ankylosing spondylitis. *Clinical and Experimental Rheumatology* **6**, 1–2.
Schlosstein, L., Terasaki, P.I., Bluestone, R., and Pearson, C.M. (1973). High association of an HL-A antigen, W27, with ankylosing spondylitis. *New England Journal of Medicine* **288**, 704–6.
Seronegative spondarthropathies (1985). *Clinics in Rheumatic Diseases* **11**, (No.1).
A useful monograph containing good reviews.
Tertti, R. and Toivanen, P. (1991). Immune functions and inflammatory reactions in HLA B27 positive subjects. *Annals of the Rheumatic Diseases* **50**, 731–4.
van der Putte, L.B.A. and Wouters, J.M.G.W. (1991). Adult onset Still's Disease. In *Rheumatic manifestations of haematological disease. Clinical rheumatology, international practice and research,* (ed. R.D. Sturrock), Vol. 5, (No. 2), pp. 263–75. Ballière Tindall, London.
Wollheim, F.A. (1989). Enteropathic arthritis. In *Textbook of rheumatology,* (ed. W.N. Kelly, E.D. Harris, S. Ruddy, and C.B. Sledge), (3rd edn). W.B. Saunders, Philadelphia.
Wright, V. and Moll, J.M.H. (1976). *Seronegative polyarthritis.* North-Holland, Amsterdam.
A monograph marking an important milestone in the understanding of these diseases and containing a wealth of information.

18.6 Osteoarthritis

C. W. HUTTON

Osteoarthritis is an enigmatic condition. Fatalism about the process being simply due to 'wear and tear' and old age has delayed systematic study. However, present knowledge of osteoarthritis allows a more rational approach to its management, underlines its importance as a public health problem, and delineates the directions for future research.

The concept of osteoarthritis

As osteoarthritis is poorly understood, it is difficult to define. Some features are recognized as important in diagnosis but whether they are necessary or sufficient remains controversial. Historically, it was recognized from morbid anatomy and later radiographic changes. Some forms of arthritis were characterized by loss of articular cartilage associated with bone increase ('hypertrophic'), in contrast to that associated with bone loss ('atrophic'). With the recognition of the role of chronic infection and the evolution of the diagnosis of inflammatory arthritis the 'atrophic' group became well defined. A rump of 'disease' remained associated with bone proliferation that can loosely be described as osteoarthritis. The age association and premature development of osteoarthritis after trauma meant that it was seen as a degenerative process, resulting in the delineation of 'degenerative joint disease'.

Osteoarthritis is a chronic condition, and although it may develop acutely, its evolution usually takes years. Current knowledge is primarily based on observations made at a single time in the evolution of the disorder. In humans, short-term follow-up studies are few and long-term studies exceptional. Any understanding of the mechanism of osteoarthritis must take account of its key features, which include: age association, the pattern of joint involvement, the common homogeneous features, and the contrasting marked heterogeneity.

A current pathological definition of osteoarthritis is 'a disease process of synovial joints characterized by focal areas of loss of hyaline articular cartilage, associated with increased activity in marginal and subchondral bone'. These features, when severe, result in the characteristic radiographic changes of reduced interbone distance (joint space narrowing), osteophyte formation, and subchondral sclerosis and cysts. A proportion of people with these changes develop symptoms, including use-related pain in the affected joints, with stiffness after inactivity.

The sites most frequently affected include knees, hips, certain joints of the hands, and the spinal apophyseal joints. Various clinical subgroups have been proposed, both on the basis of joint site, and on presumed aetiology. Osteoarthritis is often described as 'secondary' if a clear abnormality is associated with it, and 'primary' if there is no obvious association. However, if osteoarthritis is a common pathway, produced by a variety of joint insults, multiple association may be apparent.

Osteoarthritis as a public health problem

Osteoarthritis is a common cause of pain and handicap and has a major economic impact on society. It may also be associated with decreased survival, from drug-related morbidity, immobility, and handicap. There are direct medical costs; for instance those of drugs, physiotherapy, and surgery. In the United States an estimated US $1 billion is spent annually on hip surgery alone. There are also ill-effects on productivity, the cost of people functioning below optimum. Those who look after incapacitated patients at home or in hospital add to the costs. Over 180 000 people in the United States are wheelchair-bound by osteoarthritis. There are legal compensation and pension costs. In Quebec in 1983 lumbar pain compensation alone exceeded $150 million.

Epidemiology

PREVALENCE: AGE, SEX, AND PATTERN OF JOINT INVOLVEMENT

Radiographic evidence of osteoarthritis increases with age (Fig. 1). Population-based studies show a low prevalence in all joint sites in young adults. In the commonly affected joints (hands, knees, hips, spine) prevalence rates rise steeply with age so that radiographic changes are almost universal in the elderly. Some joints, such as the ankle, are rarely affected. Radiographic osteoarthritis also depends on race and gender. In Caucasians, osteoarthritis of the hip has a roughly equal sex incidence, contrasting with the 2:1 excess in females of knee and hand osteoarthritis. Some of the less commonly affected sites, such as the elbow, are affected more commonly in males.

Fig. 1 The relationship of age to increasing prevalence of osteoarthritis at different joint groups. Radiographic prevalence of osteoarthritis in (a) the hand and (b) the knee.

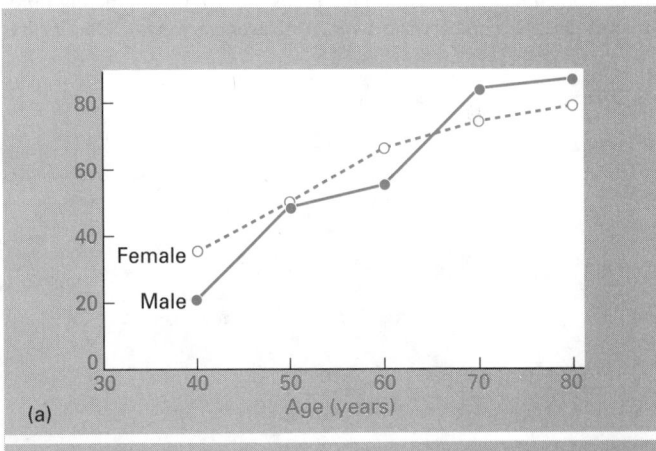

(a)

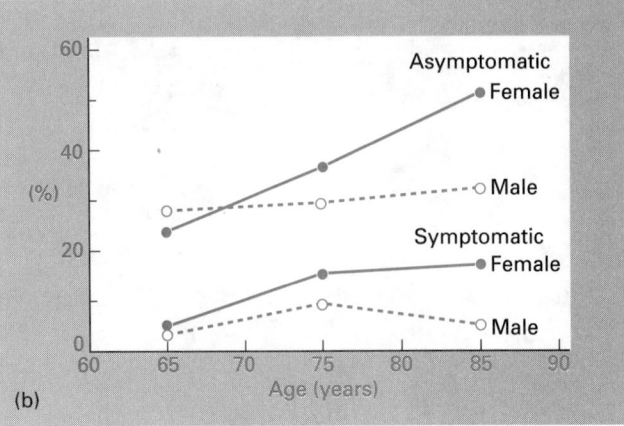

(b)

Symptomatic osteoarthritis is less common than radiographic change, many damaged joints remaining asymptomatic. It has been estimated that the overall adult prevalence of symptomatic osteoarthritis is 1 per cent, with some 10 per cent of the over-sixties affected. Common clinical patterns include lone hip osteoarthritis in younger males, knee and hand disease in middle-aged, obese females, and involvement of several joints in the elderly.

RISK FACTORS

If 'wear and tear' were to be the cause of osteoarthritis there should be a close correlation with joint trauma. Untreated fractures through a joint do result in a high frequency of subsequent osteoarthritis, but population studies have failed to show a clear relationship of osteoarthritis to previous trauma.

Studies of occupational groups such as footballers, parachutists, and ballet dancers give confusing results. This may partly be due to other confounding effects, such as hypermobility, which may determine why certain people have certain occupations, but it may also be evidence that the etiology of the condition is multivariate. Development of disease at unusual sites, for example at the ankle in footballers and ballet dancers, and 'miners elbow', suggest repetitive trauma is important. This is supported by studies of mill-workers, showing that the pattern of hand osteoarthritis reflects their repetitive occupation. Knee disease is increased by previous major knee injury and occupations involving frequent bending; and hip osteoarthritis is increased in farmers.

SYSTEMIC FACTORS

Osteoarthritis is now thought to be due to a combination of systemic influences leading to a predisposition to joint damage, and local biochemical influences, which dictate the distribution and severity of the condition (Table 1).

Obesity is an important risk factor for osteoarthritis of the knees, obese women having seven to nine times the risk of contracting tibiofemoral disease, compared to women of average weight. Obesity has

Table 1 *Factors associated with osteoarthritis: severity, symptoms and incidence*

Strong:
Age, sex, familial, geographical, major joint trauma
Weak:
Chondrocalcinosis, occupation, obesity
Uncertain:
Hypermobility, osteoporosis

weak associations with hip and hand disease, and it is unclear how much of its effect is systemic, and how much is biomechanical.

Hypermobility is another predisposing factor that may involve general as well as local factors. In contrast, osteoporosis has a negative association with hip osteoarthritis. Other evidence of systemic predisposition comes from the geographical and genetic data outlined below.

GEOGRAPHY

Osteoarthritis is present in all populations around the world, but there are hints that patterns vary in different populations (Fig. 2). For example, there is a low incidence of hip disease in the Near and Far East, in Chinese and Japanese populations. In contrast, there is a relatively higher incidence of knee disease but low levels of nodal hand disease in Black and sub-Saharan Africans. Sadly there are no population migration studies to help define whether this variation is from environmental rather than genetic factors, although anthropological studies suggest that the pattern of disease has been different in different cultures and at different times.

In addition, endemic forms of osteoarthritis are seen in certain parts of the world:

Kashin–Beck disease
In Manchuria and along the Amur River there is a very high prevalence of a severe disease developing in adolescence with interphalangeal joint, wrist, and metacarpophalangeal stiffness, swelling, and pain. There is

Fig. 2 The geography of osteoarthritis.

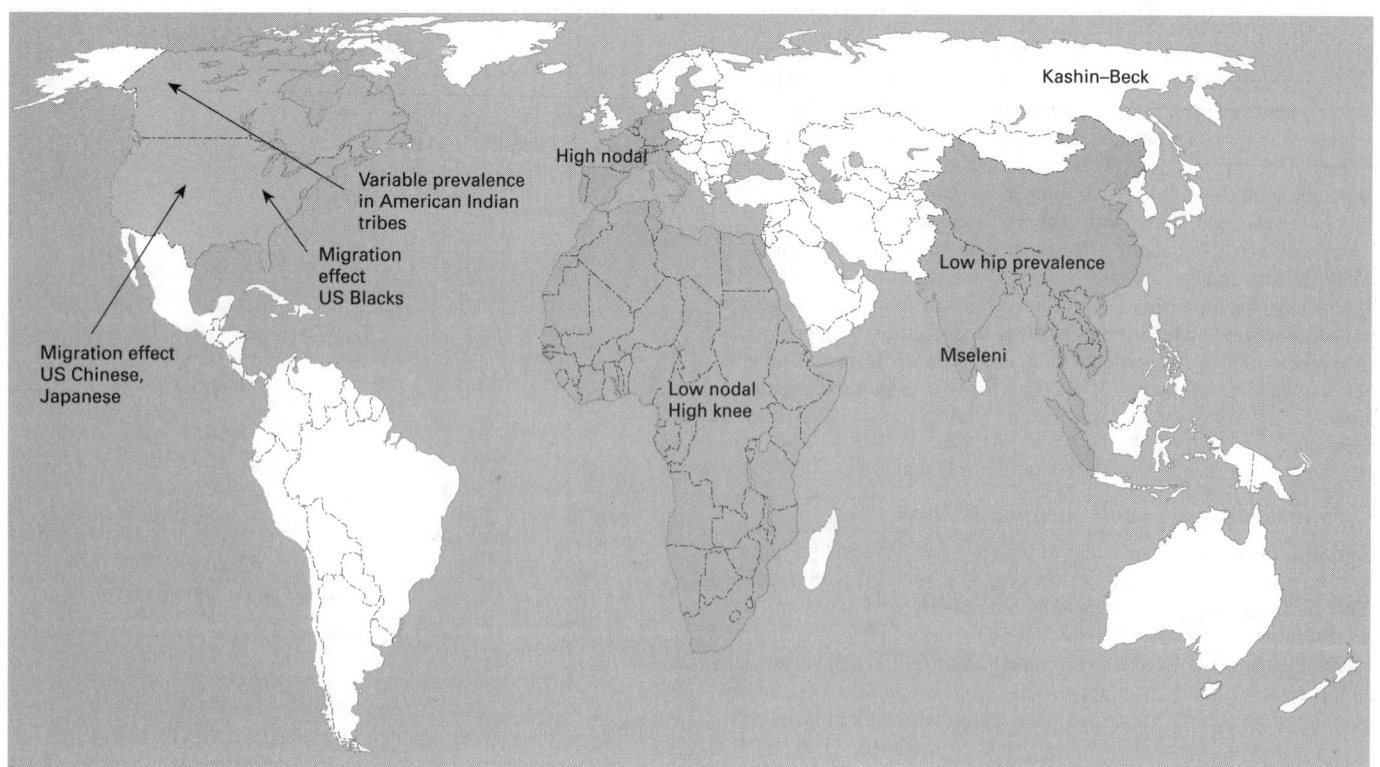

irregular epiphyseal growth and premature focal ossification. By early adult life a severe premature osteoarthritis develops with involvement of elbows, knees, and ankles. Hip involvement is uncommon. Histologically there is zonal necrosis of the growth plate. Environmental toxicity by trace metals or mycotoxins has been suggested as a cause.

Mseleni disease

In Natal there is a high prevalence of hip disease with protrusio acetabuli, associated with ankle, knee, shoulder, and elbow involvement; it appears to have a genetic basis.

Genetics

Genetic factors are important in the development of osteoarthritis (Table 2). This is apparent in that 'secondary' osteoarthritis can result from developmental and metabolic disorders like the chondrodysplasias, congenital dislocation of the hip, and ochronosis. Indications of the genetic basis of 'primary' osteoarthritis come from twin studies, family studies, and molecular genetics.

Specific and possible polygenetic effects are shown by a familial tendency, particularly for generalized nodal osteoarthritis, concordance in

Table 2 *Heredity disorders associated with premature osteoarthritis*

Mucopolysaccharidosis type I, aa; II, X; IV, aa
Familial chondrocalcinosis, Aa
Multiple epiphyseal dysplasia, Aa, aa
Spondyloepiphyseal dysplasia tarda, X
Ehlers-Danlos syndrome types I and III, osteo-onychodystrophy (nail-patella syndrome), Aa
Progressive hereditary arthro-ophthalmopathy (Sticker's syndrome), Aa

identical twins, and the identification of an abnormality in the type II collagen gene in a few families with premature osteoarthritis.

Animal models

Osteoarthritis occurs in most mammals studied, from rodents to chimpanzees. It is rare in the wild, perhaps reflecting a negative effect on survival. It can be induced in experimental animals, by ligament or meniscal removal in the dog, guinea-pig, and rabbit, for example. Some animals such as the SRT/ORT mouse strain have an increased sponta-

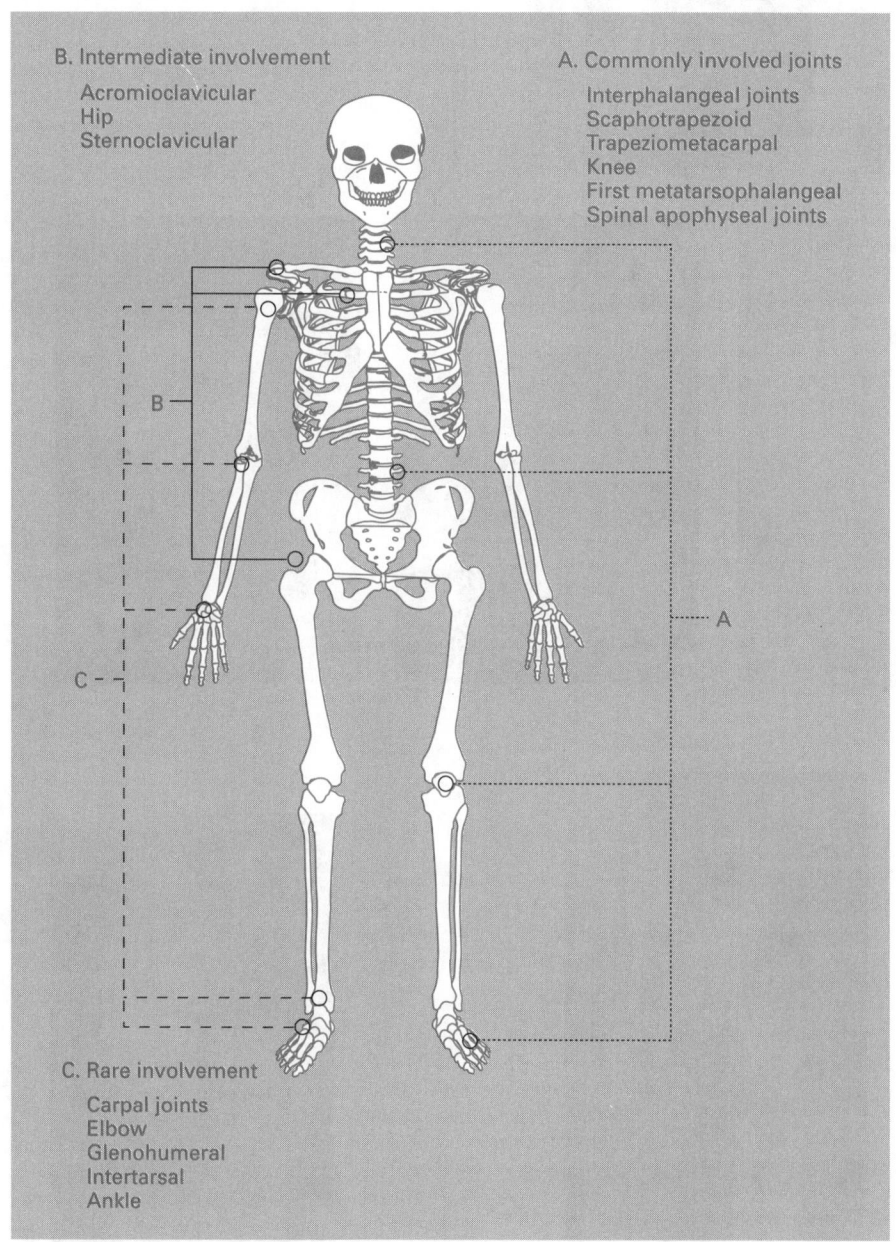

B. Intermediate involvement

Acromioclavicular
Hip
Sternoclavicular

A. Commonly involved joints

Interphalangeal joints
Scaphotrapezoid
Trapeziometacarpal
Knee
First metatarsophalangeal
Spinal apophyseal joints

C. Rare involvement

Carpal joints
Elbow
Glenohumeral
Intertarsal
Ankle

Fig. 3 The pattern of involvement at different joints.

neous incidence of a disease with features of osteoarthritis. These animals have marked variation in susceptibility and experiments have shown that the process can be manipulated by diet, drugs, and sex hormones.

Subgroups

Osteoarthritis is not a single diverse entity. The risk factors outlined above vary with joint site (Fig. 3); thus knee disease has strong asso-

Fig. 4 Examples of subgroups of osteoarthritis. (a) The Heberden's node. (b) Scaphotrapezoid, trapeziometacarpal, and metacarpal osteoarthritis in haemochromatosis. (c) Acromegalic hand osteoarthritis. Note joint space widening. (d) Interphalangeal erosive osteoarthritis. (e) Knee osteoarthritis. Anterior and lateral views. (f) Superior pole hip osteoarthritis. (g) Medial pole hip osteoarthritis. (h) Atrophic hip osteoarthritis. (i) Osteoarthritis in congenital dislocation of the hip. (j) Concentric osteoarthritis of the hip with protrusio acetabulae.

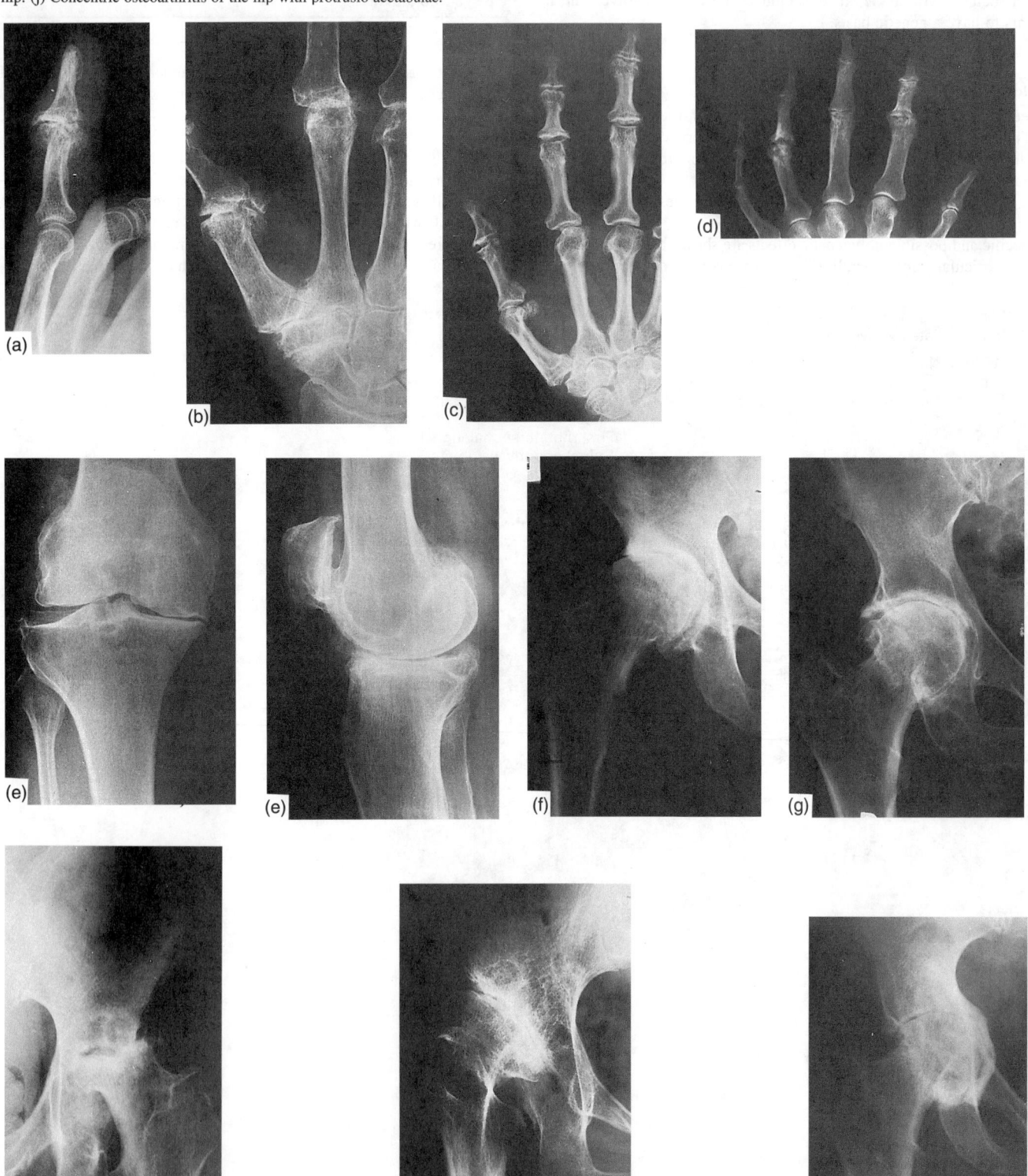

ciations with obesity and the female sex, whereas hip osteoarthritis has an equal sex incidence, little or no link to obesity, and a strong association with farming. This indicates that osteoarthritis of each of the major joint sites should be regarded as a different disorder. In addition, the implication of having developed osteoarthritis in different sites varies—in general, hip and knee osteoarthritis produce much more pain and disability than does upper limb disease. Subgroups of osteoarthritis can also be distinguished, independent of risk factors and site of joint involved:

Examples of subgroups of osteoarthritis are illustrated in Fig. 4.

GENERALIZED OSTEOARTHRITIS

A specific controversy concerns whether or not there is a 'generalized' form of osteoarthritis. This has been suggested from clinical and epidemiological studies, and it has been defined as involvement of three or more joint groups. If this is a true entity, a common predisposing factor should result in osteoarthritis developing in all joints; such a pattern should therefore be a feature of known generalized problems like collagen gene defects. However, there are marked differences in the frequency of individual joint involvement which remains unexplained. The alternative hypothesis is that joints in which it is common for osteoarthritis to develop will be involved, so as to give a generalized pattern purely by chance.

Generalized osteoarthritis is often diagnosed when osteoarthritis involves the distal interphalangeal joints, knees, apophyseal joints of the spine, and first metatarsophalangeal joints. Bony swellings in the distal interphalangeal joints (Heberden's nodes) may form insidiously or from a hyaluronate-filled cyst that may be painful and warm. Nodal disease appears more common in women, with a strong familial pattern. The joint involvement is strikingly asymmetrical, with individual finger joints going through different phases of evolution of the disease; some becoming quiescent and non-painful while others become inflamed and active. This type of nodal hand osteoarthritis is common in women around the menopause and has been termed 'menopausal' osteoarthritis. Polyarticular hand osteoarthritis may be associated with marked inflammation of the joints and the pattern of destruction may include erosive damage. This has led to some cases being classified as 'inflammatory' or 'erosive' osteoarthritis of the hand. Ankylosis of the interphalangeal joints can also occur.

ATROPHIC/HYPERTROPHIC OSTEOARTHRITIS

Classification of osteoarthritis according to the bone response seen on radiographs suggests two polar groups: atrophic and hypertrophic disease—atrophic being rapidly progressive, associated with apatite crystal deposition, and more common with age, while more subchondral sclerosis and osteophytosis (seen in the hypertrophic group) may be associated with a better prognosis.

DIFFUSE IDIOPATHIC SKELETAL HYPEROSTOSIS (FORESTIER'S DISEASE)

This is a spinal disease characterized by exuberant 'flowing candle wax' ossification bridging at least four vertebral disc spaces, with no loss of vertebral height or disc space. The changes are most marked in the lower thoracic spine. It is associated with calcification of anterior spinal ligament, without sacroiliitis, although there may be para-articular osteophytes. There may be ligamentous calcification around peripheral joints, with wiskering of muscle insertions. It is a common, age-related disorder with an estimated adult prevalence rate of 3.8 per cent in men and 2.6 per cent in women.

Although diffuse idiopathic skeletal hyperostosis is most often asymptomatic, backache, stiffness, and pain or tenderness at osseous spurs has been described. It is associated with obesity and diabetes. Spinal encroachment can cause myelopathy, and spinal stenosis, and large cervical osteophytes may causes dysphagia. There may be an association between diffuse idiopathic skeletal hyperostosis and the hypertropic type of peripheral joint osteoarthritis, but this remains controversial.

Table 3 *Conditions favouring later development of osteoarthritis*

Infection, inflammation
Trauma
Frostbite
With abnormal development
Congenital dislocation of the hip
Slipped upper femoral epiphysis
Perthe's disease
With bone disease
Paget's disease
Osteopetrosis
Avascular necrosis of bone
In metabolic and endocrine disease
Acromegaly
Ochronosis
Haemochromatosis
Wilson's disease

CHARCOT'S JOINTS

A destructive osteoarthritic disease associated with a proliferative bone response is sometimes seen in patients with diabetes mellitus, syringomyelia, meningomyelocele, and neurogenic syphilis. It is non-inflammatory, often with a haemorrhagic effusion. It is probably due to neurovascular, not neurotraumatic, change.

'SECONDARY' OSTEOARTHRITIS

Osteoarthritis may develop following any process damaging a joint (Table 3).

In Paget's disease and osteopetrosis the most common site of osteoarthritis is in the hip. Ochronosis, due to an abnormality of homogentisic acid oxidase results in the deposition of homogentisic acid in connective tissues such as cartilage, and degenerative changes are seen in the spine (with disc calcification), in the knee, shoulder, and hip. Haemochromatosis results in degenerative disease in the metacarpophalangeal, interphalangeal, and shoulder joints, often with pyrophosphate deposition. In Wilson's disease 50 per cent of adults show osteoarthritis changes in metacarpophalangeal joints, wrists, elbows, hips, and knees, and these are associated with periarticular osteopenia.

The localization of osteoarthritis—within and between joints

The commonly affected sites are the spine, hips, knees, hands, and feet. In the spine the atlantoaxial joint, apophyseal joints in the mid-cervical and low lumbar regions, and oncovertebral joints are most vulnerable, probably because these are the sites of greatest stress. Three different radiographic patterns have been identified on the hip joint: concentric, superior pole, and medial pole disease (Fig. 5; see also Fig. 4), stressing the fact that osteoarthritis localizes to specific sites within a joint, as well as to different joint sites. Similarly, at the knee osteoarthritis may affect the medial tibiofemoral or patellofemoral compartments, and in the hand the only sites to be affected commonly are the thumb base (trapezometacarpal and scaphotrapezial joints) and the distal interphalangeal joint. The base of the big toe (first metatarsophalangeal) is the major site involved in the foot.

Pathology

Changes occur throughout an affected joint and can be identified at macroscopic, microscopic, and biochemical levels (Fig. 6).

CARTILAGE

Cartilage becomes fibrillated, thins, and develops 'ulcers' or craters. These changes are usually focal within the joint, becoming more extensive with progression. Areas of new cartilage proliferation may be seen, particularly in association with osteophytes and fibroblast invasion from the marrow. There is invasion by blood vessels into the cartilage across the subchondral plate, and reduplication to the tide mark delineating change in the calcified cartilage layer. Chondrocytes may appear grouped in nests, and other areas have empty lacunae. Fibrocartilage menisci disintegrate.

Fig. 5 Classification of osteoarthritic hip. 1. Normal. 2. Superior pole. 3. Medial pole. 4. Concentric. 5. Dysplastic.

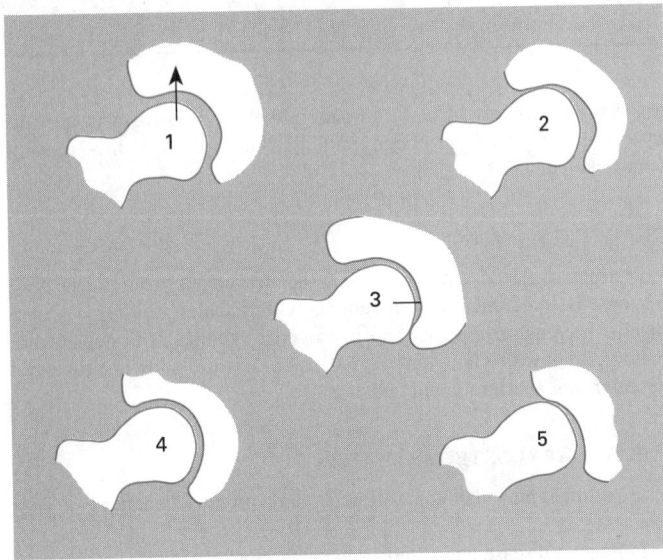

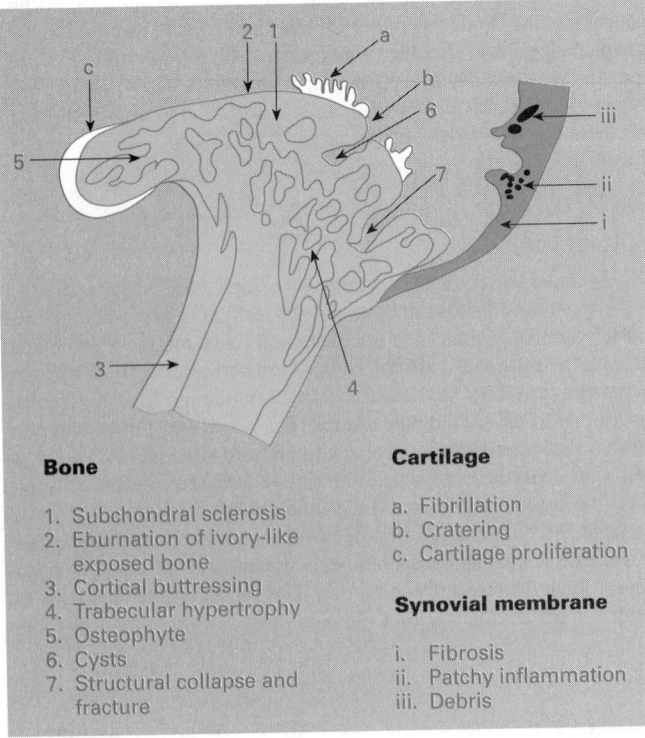

Fig. 6 Pathological features of osteoarthritis.

Bone

1. Subchondral sclerosis
2. Eburnation of ivory-like exposed bone
3. Cortical buttressing
4. Trabecular hypertrophy
5. Osteophyte
6. Cysts
7. Structural collapse and fracture

Cartilage

a. Fibrillation
b. Cratering
c. Cartilage proliferation

Synovial membrane

i. Fibrosis
ii. Patchy inflammation
iii. Debris

BONE

The hallmark of osteoarthritis is the change in bone; osteophyte formation, sclerosis, and cyst formation. The subchondral plate and trabecular network thicken. Cortical bone thickens, particularly in the hip to 'buttress' the femoral neck. The cartilage surface may be lost and the exposed bone becomes eburnated—thick and ivory-like. Bony outgrowths, osteophytes develop; there may be formation of subchondral cysts (Fig. 7). The marrow becomes hyperaemic and big sinusoids develop. Late stages of the disease are associated with collapse of the subchondral bone.

SYNOVIUM AND PERIARTICULAR STRUCTURES

The synovium is usually bland. It may contain bone debris, foci of mild, chronic inflammation, and proliferation of fibrous tissue. Tendons hypertrophy and there is wasting of muscle. The synovial fluid may increase in volume and become less viscous. It may contain cartilage and bone debris in addition to crystals, including pyrophosphate and apatite.

Aetiology

MECHANICAL CONSIDERATIONS

Joints are mechanical systems. Understanding how they malfunction and how to modify such malfunction must be considered in this mechanical context. Essentially, joints allow stable, controlled movement of a system of levers under load. The power for movement from muscle is transmitted through tendons to bone. Systems must be designed to

Fig. 7 The formation of bone cysts.

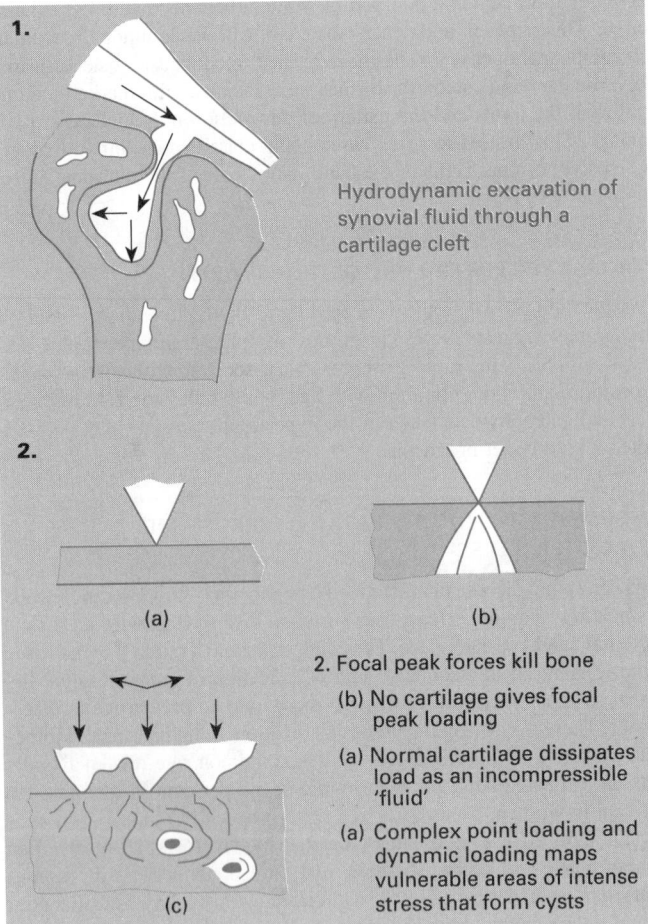

1.

Hydrodynamic excavation of synovial fluid through a cartilage cleft

2.

(a)   (b)

(c)

2. Focal peak forces kill bone

(b) No cartilage gives focal peak loading

(a) Normal cartilage dissipates load as an incompressible 'fluid'

(a) Complex point loading and dynamic loading maps vulnerable areas of intense stress that form cysts

reduce wear of moving surfaces and control fatigue of components during life. Movement with excessive load induces wear. The coeffiecient of friction in the joint surface is below 0.02, but once damage has started this may change. In gel and fluid phases there is also a possibility of cavitation damage. Considerable uncertainty exists whether wear is a problem in normal joints. One possibility is that cartilage continues to grow *pari passu* with wear.

If loading on a bone increases, the bone will hypertrophy, and the highest loads will produce a fracture: either a fatigue (stress) fracture or a catastrophic disintegration. The transmission of force across non-congruent surfaces results in non-uniform distribution of stress. This distribution will change with movement but results in localized intense foci of force that may prevent viable cell function with resultant development of focal cysts. Cartilage acts like a fluid and disperses load to counteract these forces. However, photoelastic models demonstrate that a change in the character of the cartilage may prevent this dispersion of stress. Cyst formation may result from hydrodynamic stress transmitted through cartilage fissures into bone.

The distribution of cartilage fibrillation in the hip, knee, and elbow in pathological studies shows a focal development in areas of relative disuse: the less loaded areas. For example, the hip areas covered by the acetabulum are less affected than a zone in the periphery and around the fovea. This runs counter to the concept that stressed areas should develop change first, and suggests the reverse: that inadequate loading may be a cause of damage.

The lack of data on stress distribution *in vivo* underlies the difficulty of identifying whether or not loading keeps the surface intact and inadequate loading induces damage. Immobilized dog cartilage will thin and, if then exercised, vigorously disintegrates with loads that have no effect on joints normally exercised.

The vulnerability of the system to develop these changes and capacity to tolerate damage is a function of the design or any joints. This includes biological factors determining the configuration of the joint and its material composition. Degenerative change will therefore be provoked by factors such as failure of remodelling, design limitation, defects in materials, and control of development.

A unifying hypothesis therefore emerges of osteoarthritis as a common pathway that can be triggered by any damage to a joint, and accelerated by a wide range of factors, although it is difficult to identify independent variables in each case.

Repair

Osteoarthritis may be considered as an ill result or the process of joint repair. The cartilage may not regenerate perfectly as the joint adapts to limit damage and maintain function. The anabolic processes in bone, particularly osteophyte growth, can be seen as part of this response. In progressive osteoarthritis the repair process is inadequate.

Biochemistry

In experimental osteoarthritis there is an initial increase in cartilage hydration and resultant swelling. There must be a change in the collagen network that restrains the proteoglycan matrix for this to occur. It is unclear how the network of collagen type II is damaged, but changes occur in proteoglycan turnover, altering the size and charge density of cartilage macromolecules, and thus the behaviour of matrix. The increase in chondroitin sulphate is suggestive of the proteoglycan composition of developmental cartilage. Antibodies recognizing epitopes on these 'juvenile' molecules may offer a method of monitoring the progress of osteoarthritis. Proteoglycans may also be important in determining the development of a joint. The limb bud is rich in dermatan sulphate, but with cartilage formation chondroitin sulphate synthesis is turned on. With maturation there is a decrease in chain length. In ageing, at least in bovine cartilage, this is associated with an increase in der-

matan sulphate formation. The collagen subtype profile also changes, with increased synthesis of type II cartilage.

These changes may be mediated by cytokines and hormones. Interleukin-1α and 1β act on the same chondrocyte receptor to increase release of enzymes. α-Tumour necrosis factor acts on a different receptor, to release collagenase and the protoglandin, PGE_2. The chondrocyte also has oestrogen, growth hormone, and somatomedin receptors. For the anabolic response, a switch on of genes controlling cell proliferation and synthesis, changes in the stability of mRNA, or decreased catabolic degradation must occur. Growth factors such as insulin-like growth factor, platelet-derived growth factor, and transforming growth factor β, may be involved in this control.

Clinical features

Osteoarthritis causes pain and joint malfunction. These combine to provide a varying handicap, dependent on a multitude of other factors.

PAIN

Pain must result from changes in the bone or periarticular structures, as hyaline cartilage contains no nerves. Ligamentous strain and inflamed bursae and synovial tissue may also contribute. Pain is characteristically worse on loading, and may be due to secondary effects on loaded tissue such as the bone marrow. In severe disease, night pain is a particular feature, possibly due to raised interosseous pressure.

MALFUNCTION

In joints involved with locomotion, malfunction gives limitation of mobility, instability, stiffness, secondary muscle weakness and pain. Lower limb disease, particularly hip and knee osteoarthritis, cause the greatest problems, resulting in major difficulties with steps, stairs, and walking. Upper limb involvement is uncommon, except around the thumb and interphalangeal joints, resulting in restricted manipulation. In the spine osteoarthritis contributes to postural deformity and causes pain. Osteoarthritis joints are stiff, particularly after resting.

Management

Osteoarthritis cannot be reversed and the aim must be to modify a problem that cannot be eliminated (Fig. 8). The principles of management may be summarized as:

(1) prevention;
(2) early diagnosis and the identification of its causes and complications;
(3) assessment of the main symptoms and dysfunction;
(4) assessment of handicap;
(5) assessment of the patient's emotional, cognitive, and psychological response to the disease.

There is a dearth of guidance from controlled trials, but inference from what is known about osteoarthritis allows a logical plan of treatment to be developed, directed at one or more of these areas.

Prevention is widely practised under different guises; for example, detection of congenital deformity of the hip, reducing trauma, and improving the management of fractures as well as an improved public health policy on exercise, obesity, and fitness; this despite the lack of data on effectiveness of such modifications of lifestyle on osteoarthritis.

Of particular importance in the clinician's approach to the patient is the need to assess the degree of handicap in relation to other problems. For example, if the patient has poor sight, is on inappropriate medication, is under family stress, or is isolated, the osteoarthritis may result in much greater handicap than would otherwise be the case. The psychological response to the disease, possible difficulties in sexual relationships, and the impact on work and leisure activities are important issues, not always properly addressed.

A joint that is unstable and painful may be made less painful and more stable by appropriate aids. In someone who is refusing, or is at too high a risk for surgery, wheelchairs, and adaptations such as bath rails and stair lifts, may make it possible to maintain independence. Walking sticks can be remarkably helpful, but only if used with appropriate attention to detail; for a painful hip or knee, holding the stick in the contralateral hand transfers the weight off the painful joint; for instability, use in the most reassuring hand is appropriate. Splinting to correct instability, correction of varus or valgus at knee and ankle, use of a rocker sole to ease hallux rigidus pain, or a heel raise for leg inequality, all allow reduction of symptoms at low risk. Many people with osteoarthritis find great relief from use of shoes with good shock absorbing insoles, which can reduce pain related to joint loading.

Also important is the correction of the secondary effects of a flexion deformity or muscle wasting. In the knee, quadriceps wasting produces a weak leg with a perception of instability and loss of confidence in movement. Getting up from a chair and using stairs become difficult. If there is a knee flexion, the gait is abnormal and the inequality of leg length tends to weight the painful knee. Exercise, including hydrotherapy, continuous passive motion, and splinting, may correct any deformity, as well as strengthening muscles. Quadriceps exercises have been shown to be an effective way of reducing pain and increasing mobility in people of all ages with osteoarthritis of the knee.

MODIFYING PAIN

In osteoarthritis, drug-related pain control is rarely good, either with simple analgesics, or with non-steroidal anti-inflammatory agents,

Fig. 8 Management of the patient with osteoarthritis.

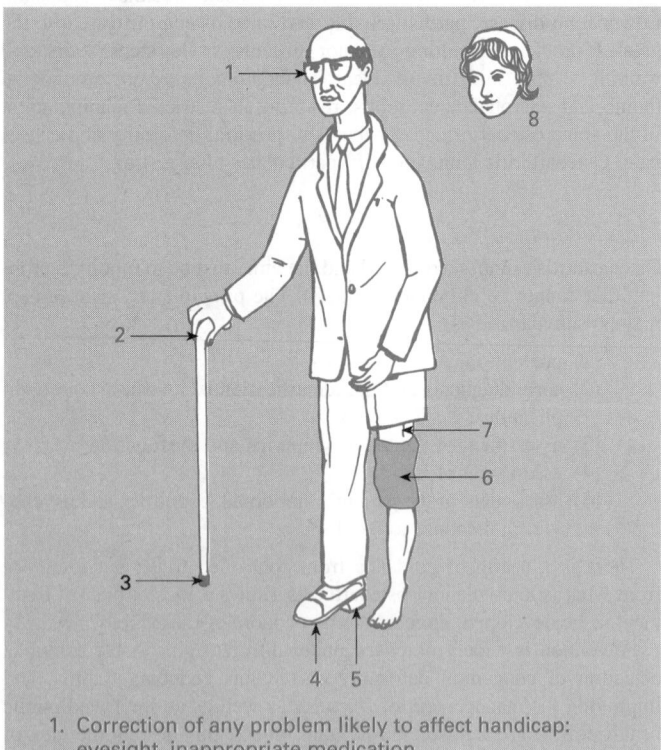

1. Correction of any problem likely to affect handicap: eyesight, inappropriate medication.
2. Correct stick length in contralateral hand to painful leg.
3. Ferrule with rubber grip.
4. Rocker sole for hallux rigidus, wide deep fitting shoe for hallux valgus.
5. Heel raise to correct leg length inequality.
6. Knee support splint.
7. Good quadriceps and corrected knee flexion deformity.
8. Happy, informed, and supported carer.

which carry a risk of gastropathy. It is important to appreciate that pain is multifactorial, with exacerbation from mood, fear, uncertainty, and other associated factors, which may be helped by education and support. Improved sleep, combined with physical treatment, may reduce the need for analgesics. Soft-tissue pain may be underdiagnosed, and may follow postural change induced by pain. This and joint pain and swelling may respond to local steroid injection. Postural pain may alter with changes in the work environment, or advice on posture, sitting, and lifting. However, uncontrolled pain remains the major indication for surgery.

SURGERY

Arthroplasty has transformed the outlook for people with severe osteoarthritis of the hip and knee, but for other joints is still experimental, partly because of the technical problem of surgery and partly from the lack of understanding of the natural history of the disease in most joint sites.

Other procedures, short of arthroplasty, may be appropriate, particularly in high-risk patients, to ease symptoms. In the hip, a Girdlestone's operation may control pain and allow some mobility. Osteotomy of the knee, and adductor muscle release at the hip, may allow treatment in younger people as well as correcting contributing deformity. Arthroscopy with lavage of debris and meniscal cartilage debridement may ease knee locking and reduce symptoms for a period. Joint fusion will give a pain-free joint albeit at the cost of immobility.

Investigation

The diagnosis is usually clear from history and examination, continued if necessary by imaging. Analysis of serology and crystallography of synovial fluid may be important in excluding other inflammatory disease, and biochemical investigation is occasionally necessary to exclude underlying metabolic causes.

Radiographs remain the major *in vivo* assessment of the bone response and delineation of osteoarthritis. Their limitation is poor definition of soft tissues and lack of information about cartilage unless contrast agents are used. Isotope bone scans show increased activity in osteoarthritic joints and can have some prognostic value, but do not contribute to diagnosis or management.

Cartilage can be imaged by magnetic resonance, and major advances in this technique, such as magnetization transfer, are likely to make this more and more valuable. Methods of following the osteoarthritic process by tracking biochemical markers of the different processes are also being developed.

Summary

Osteoarthritis is a poorly understood and complex disease process. This complexity and lack of understanding provide a stimulus to the investigator, and a challenge to the clinician. It is such a widespread problem that better management must make a substantial impact on the health of the ageing population.

REFERENCES

Bland, J.H. and Cooper, S.M. (1984). Osteoarthritis: a review of the cell biology involved and evidence for reversibility. Management rationally related to known genesis and pathophysiology. *Seminars in Arthritis and Rheumatism* **14**, (2), 106–33.
Bullough, P.G. (1981). The geometry of diarthrodial joints, its physiological maintenance, and the possible significance of age related changes in geometry to load distribution and the development of osteoarthritis. *Clinical Orthopaedics and Related Research* **156**, 61–6.
Danielsson, L.G. (1964). Incidence and prognosis of coxarthrosis *Acta Orthopaedica Scandinavica* **S66**, 8–114.
Felson, D.T. (1990). The epidemiology of knee osteoarthritis: results from

the Framlington Osteoarthritis Study. *Seminars in Arthritis and Rheumatism* **20**, 42–50.

Hadler, N.M., *et al.* (1978). Hand structure and function in an industrial setting. Influence of three patterns of stereotyped repetative usage. *Arthritis and Rheumatism* **21**, (2), 1019–25.

Hull, R. and Pope, F.M. (1989). Osteoarthritis and the collagen genes. *Lancet* **ii**, 1337–8.

Kellgren, J.H. and Moore, R. (1954). Generalised osteoarthritis and Heberden's nodes. *British Medical Journal* **1**, 181–4.

Peyron, J.G. (1979). Epidemiologic and etiologic approach of osteoarthritis. *Seminars in Arthritis and Rheumatism* **8**, 288–306.

Radin, E.L. and Burr, D.B. (1984). Hypothesis: joints can heal. *Seminars in Arthritis and Rheumatism* **13**, 293–302.

Resnick, D., Shaul, S.R., and Robins, J.M. (1975). Diffuse idiopathic skeletal hyperostosis (DISH) Forestier's disease with extraspinal manifestations. *Radiology* **115**, 513–20.

Sokoloff, L. (1968). *The biology of degenerative joint disease.* University of Chicago Press, Chicago.

18.7 Crystal-related arthropathies

M. DOHERTY

INTRODUCTION

Diversity and terminology

A large number of crystals have been associated with acute synovitis, chronic arthropathy, or periarticular syndromes (Table 1). In practice only monosodium urate monohydrate, calcium pyrophosphate dihydrate, and basic calcium phosphates (mainly hydroxyapatite) are commonly encountered.

The taxonomy of these conditions is not universally agreed. Difficulties arise from our poor understanding of pathogenesis, historical extrapolation from gout to other crystal-related conditions, and multiple terms for the same clinical syndrome. Possible relationships between crystals and disease are outlined in Fig. 1. A 'crystal-deposition disease' is defined as a pathological condition associated with mineral deposits which contribute directly to the pathology. This is probably the situation for all manifestations of gout, for acute syndromes associated with calcium pyrophosphate dihydrate, and for acute apatite periarthritis. The role of non-urate crystals in chronic arthropathy, however, is unclear and confounded by the following observations:

1. Most crystals lack disease specificity and occur in a variety of clinical settings, often unaccompanied by symptoms or other abnormality.
2. Crystal deposition may coexist with other rheumatic disease, most commonly osteoarthritis, and often follows rather than precedes articular damage.
3. Combined deposition of several crystal species is common ('mixed crystal deposition').

For descriptive purposes, confusion may be avoided by itemizing the crystal, the site of involvement, and the clinical syndrome (for example, chronic urate olecranon bursitis, acute pyrophosphate arthritis of thè knee).

Crystal deposition and clearance

Many factors determine crystal formation and dissolution (Fig. 2). High solute concentrations alone are often insufficient to initiate crystal formation, and the presence of nucleating factors that aid initial particle formation and the balance of growth-promoting and inhibitory factors are probably more important. Little is known of such tissue factors, although they may in part explain:

(1) the characteristic, limited distribution of different crystals;
(2) the frequency of mixed crystal deposition (via epitaxial nucleation and growth of one crystal on another); and
(3) non-specific predisposition to crystal formation in osteoarthritic tissues (via accompanying alterations in proteoglycan, collagen, and lipid).

Table 1 *Crystalline particles associated with joint disease*

Intrinsic
  Monosodium urate monohydrate
  Calcium pyrophosphate dihydrate (monoclinic, triclinic)
  Calcium phosphates
    basic: hydroxyapatite, octacalcium phosphate,
            tricalcium phosphate
    acidic: brushite, monetite
  Calcium oxalate
  Lipids
    cholesterol
    lipid liquid crystals
    Charcot-Leyden (phospholipase) crystals
  Cystine
  Xanthine, hypoxanthine
  Protein precipitates (e.g. cryoglobulins)
Extrinsic
  Synthetic corticosteroids
  Plant thorns (semicrystalloid cellulose), especially
    blackthorn, rose, dried palm fronds
  Sea-urchin spines (crystalline calcium carbonate)
  Methylmethacrylate

Formation of crystals *in vivo* is a dynamic, although usually slow, process. At any time the crystal load will depend on the rate of formation, the rate of dissolution, and trafficking of crystals away from their site of formation (via 'shedding' from preformed deposits with secondary uptake by synovial and other cells).

Crystal-induced inflammation and tissue damage

Crystals implicated in joint disease are stable, hard particles that exert biological effects via surface-active and mechanical properties. With respect to acute inflammation, they are all markedly phlogistic agents in a wide range of *in vitro* and *in vivo* systems. Surface-active interaction has been demonstrated with:

(1) humoral mediators, for example complement activation via classical and alternative pathways; activation of Hageman factor;
(2) cell-derived mediators, for example superoxide production and release of lysozymes, chemotactic factor, and lipoxygenase-derived products of arachidonic acid by neutrophils; release of interleukin-1, interleukin-6, and tumour necrosis factor by monocytes and synoviocytes,
(3) cell membranes, for example membranolysis of lysosomes,

erythrocytes, and neutrophils; non-lytic platelet and neutrophil secretory responses.

In general, monosodium urate monohydrate is the most inflammatory, followed by calcium pyrophosphate dihydrate, then apatite and the less common crystals. In general, smaller particle size, marked surface irregularity, and high negative surface charge correlate with inflammatory potential. Some surface effects result from direct crystal contact but others are mediated via adsorbed protein, particularly immunoglobulin. Although adsorbed IgG may enhance inflammation, most other protein binding is inhibitory.

Less is known of chronic crystal-induced tissue damage. Postulated effects include persistent synovial inflammation, altered cell metabolism, and deleterious mechanical effects from large deposits. Evidence for activation of inflammatory mediators in chronic crystal-associated synovitis is lacking, although a chronic 'granulomatous' reaction often occurs around large accretions. The physicochemical effects of hard, highly charged crystals embedded within cartilage, or occurring as wear particles at the surface, are largely unknown.

Gout (see also Chapter 11.4)

Monosodium urate monohydrate crystals are undoubted causal agents in gout, usually depositing in previously normal tissues and eliciting acute inflammation and eventual tissue damage. Their effective removal halts progression and results in 'cure'. In these respects gout is a true 'crystal deposition disease'.

The incidence of gout varies in populations from 0.2 to 0.35 per 1000,

Fig. 1 Possible relationships between crystals and joint disease.

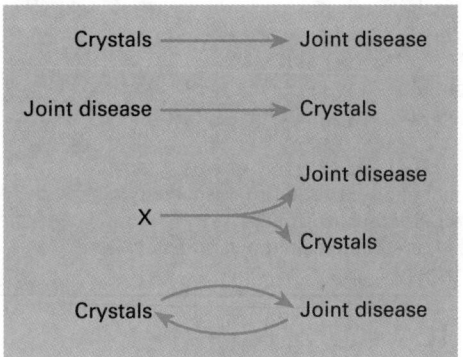

Fig. 2 Factors affecting crystal formation.

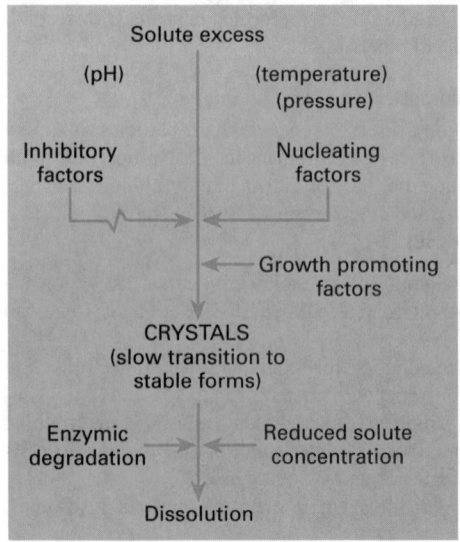

with an overall prevalence of 2.0 to 2.6 per 1000. Prevalence increases with age and increasing serum urate concentration. There is strong predominance in men (c. 10:1), particularly under 65 years of age. The natural history of untreated gout slowly evolves through four clinical phases: asymptomatic hyperuricaemia, acute gout, intercritical gout, and chronic tophaceous gout.

ASYMPTOMATIC HYPERURICAEMIA

Monosodium urate monohydrate crystals preferentially deposit in peripheral connective tissues in and around synovial joints, favouring lower rather than upper limbs. Deposits occur first in articular cartilage, most commonly the first metatarsophalangeal and small joints of feet and hands. Deposits later develop in synovium, capsule, and periarticular soft tissues, with progressive involvement of more proximal sites. Monosodium urate monohydrate crystals probably take months if not years to grow *in vivo* to detectable size, implying a long asymptomatic phase. Absence of inflammation during this period may relate to low crystal yield, positioning within hypovascular tissues, or inhibitory protein coating. Probably 95 per cent of hyperuricaemic subjects remain asymptomatic throughout life, although how many have occult monosodium urate monohydrate deposits is unknown. Of those who develop gout, one in five will have suffered renal colic due to uric acid urolithiasis, sometimes more than a decade earlier. The first presentation of gout is usually acute synovitis, although an insidious onset of chronic arthropathy or nodular deposits ('tophi') occasionally occurs without preceding attacks.

ACUTE ATTACKS

Classical attacks are highly characteristic but atypical presentations may cause diagnostic problems.

The classical attack

In almost all initial episodes a single peripheral joint is involved. This is the first metatarsophalangeal joint ('podagra') in 50 per cent of first attacks and 70 per cent of all attacks. Other common sites are the ankle, midtarsal joints, knees, small hand joints, wrist, and elbow. The axial skeleton and large central joints are rarely involved and never as the first site.

Attacks often wake the patient in the early morning with localized irritation and aching. Within a few hours the joint and surrounding tissues are swollen, hot, red, shiny, and extremely painful. The patient cannot bear even bedclothes to touch the joint and often describe it as 'the worst pain ever experienced'. Inflammation is maximal within 24 h and often associates with pyrexia and malaise. Examination reveals florid synovitis and swelling, extreme tenderness, and overlying erythema. If left untreated, the attack resolves spontaneously over 5 to 15 days, often with pruritus and desquamation of overlying skin.

Although many attacks occur spontaneously, certain situations encourage shedding of preformed monosodium urate monohydrate crystals and triggering of acute attacks. Suggested mechanisms include mechanical loosening (local trauma); partial dissolution and reduced crystal size (initiation of hypouricaemic treatment); and local increase in cytokines which encourage inflammatory responses to crystals and facilitate crystal escape via alterations in cartilage matrix (intercurrent illness, surgery). Although some triggers (alcohol, dietary excess, diuretics) increase local urate levels, acute crystallization is considered unlikely.

Atypical attacks

Acute attacks may manifest as tenosynovitis, bursitis, or cellulitis. Many patients describe mild episodes of discomfort without swelling lasting a day or so ('petite attacks'). Ten per cent of all typical attacks involve more than one joint; sometimes acute gout, by triggering the acute phase response, provokes migratory attacks in other joints over subsequent days ('cluster attacks'). Polyarticular attacks are rare, usually occurring after a long history of recurrent attacks; marked systemic upset, fever, and confusion may dominate the clinical picture.

INTERCRITICAL PERIODS

These are asymptomatic intervals between attacks. Some patients never have a second attack, in others the next episode occurs after many years; in most, however, a second attack occurs within 1 year. Subsequently the frequency of attacks and number of sites involved gradually increase with time. Later attacks are more often pauci- or polyarticular and more severe. Eventually recurrent attacks and continuing monosodium urate monohydrate deposition cause joint damage and chronic pain; the interval between the first attack and development of chronic symptoms is variable, but averages about 10 years. The principal determinant is the serum uric acid—the higher it is, the earlier and more extensive the development of joint damage and tophaceous deposit.

CHRONIC TOPHACEOUS GOUT

Large crystal deposits ('tophi') produce irregular firm nodules, principally around extensor surfaces of fingers, hands, ulnar surface of forearms, olecranon bursae, Achilles tendons, first metatarsophalangeal joints, and cartilaginous helix of the ear. Marked asymmetry, both locally and between sides, is particularly characteristic (Fig. 3); monosodium urate monohydrate crystals beneath the skin may give a 'chalky' appearance (Fig. 4). If untreated, tophi can enlarge into gross knobbly swellings that may ulcerate; discharging material is white and gritty and associates with local inflammation (erythema, pus) even in the absence of secondary infection. If extensive, tophi may rarely involve the eye, eyelids, tongue, larynx, or heart (causing conduction defects and valvular dysfunction).

Joints most commonly involved with signs of damage (restricted movement, crepitus, deformity) and varying degrees of synovitis are the first metatarsophalangeal joints, midfoot, small finger joints, and wrists. As with tophi, joint involvement is usually asymmetrical. Occasionally gross destruction may occur in feet and hands, and less commonly other sites. Acute attacks may become less of a feature as chronic symptoms become established. If untreated, the combination of extensive joint destruction and large tophi may cause grotesque deformities, particularly of hands and feet. Ankylosis is a rare late event. Although axial involvement is rare even in late stages, gouty involvement of hips, shoulders, spine and sacroiliac joints, and spinal cord compression by tophi, are all reported.

CLASSIFICATION

Traditional classification into primary or secondary gout depends on defined predisposing factors for hyperuricaemia.

Fig. 3 Chronic tophaceous gout affecting the hands. Note the eccentric nature of the tophi and the asymmetry between sides.

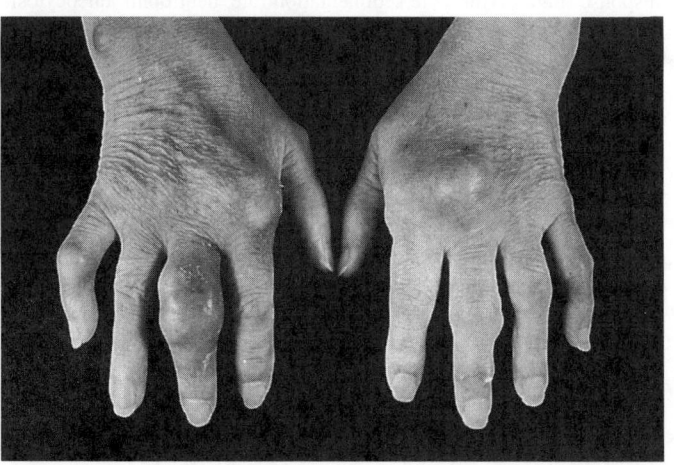

Most gout is primary, strongly predominating in men, with initial onset between 30 and 60 years of age (Table 2). Presentation is with acute attacks, and untreated disease progresses to chronic tophaceous gout. Such patients often give a family history of gout and are 'undersecretors' of uric acid; abnormal proteoglycan metabolism, indicated by high serum uronic acid levels, is also detectable, suggesting that an inherited tissue factor that promotes crystal formation is equally important.

Secondary gout usually results from chronic diuretic therapy and presents in older subjects (>65 years). This increasingly common form affects women and men and often associates with osteoarthritis; the distribution equally favours upper and lower limb joints. Acute attacks are less prominent and presentation is often with painful, sometimes discharging, tophaceous deposits in Heberden's and Bouchard's nodes (Fig. 4). In such 'impostumous' gout the combination of diuretic-induced hyperuricaemia and local alterations in tissue factors accompanying nodal osteoarthritis predispose to tophaceous deposition in osteoarthritic tissue.

ASSOCIATIONS

Hyperuricaemia

Mechanisms resulting in decreased excretion or increased production of uric acid are fully discussed in Chapter 11.4. Though hyperuricaemia and gout are strongly linked, they are not synonymous. Most hyperuricaemic subjects never develop gout (emphasizing the importance of local tissue factors in crystal nucleation/growth) and gouty patients may not be hyperuricaemic at presentation. Associations also differ; for example, impaired glucose tolerance, ischaemic heart disease, and hypertension are common in men with gout but do not associate with hyperuricaemia *per se*. The majority (75–90 per cent) of patients with primary gout are 'undersecretors' of uric acid, having inherited an isolated renal lesion that reduces fractional urate clearance; fewer than 10 per cent are 'overproducers' of uric acid; the cause usually remains unclear, although a very few have an inherited purine enzyme defect (see Chapter 11.4). Some patients are both undersecretors and overproducers.

Fig. 4 Diuretic-induced gout in an elderly women, showing tophaceous deposition on pre-existing nodal osteoarthritis; the white monosodium urate monohydrate crystals are clearly visible beneath the skin.

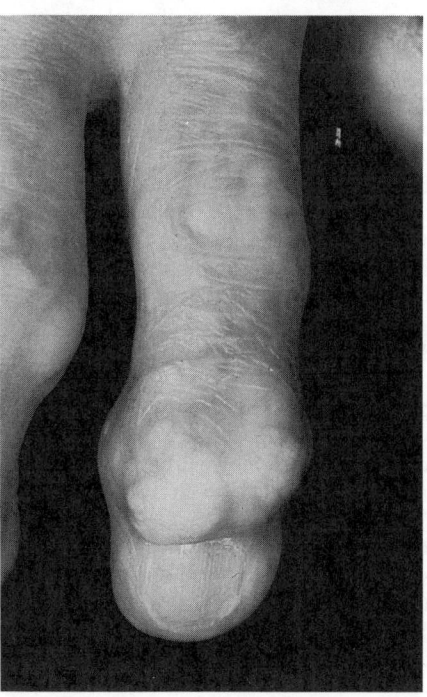

Table 2 *Comparison between primary and diuretic-induced gout*

	Primary	Diuretic-induced
Sex	Male >> female	Male = female
Age	Middle aged	Elderly
Acute attacks	Common	Uncommon
Tophi	Develop late	Develop early
Associations	Obesity, hypertension, hyperlipidaemia, high alcohol intake	Renal impairment, osteoarthritis

Clinical associations differ according to gender. In men important associations are obesity, excessive alcohol intake, type IV hyperlipoproteinaemia, impaired glucose tolerance, and ischaemic heart disease. Obesity and lifestyle, rather than hereditary factors, appear to be central factors linking these 'associations of plenty'. Excessive beer drinking, with its high calorie and alcohol intake, is a common form of alcohol abuse associating with gout. The nineteenth century association with port is partly explained by addition of lead to sweeten the port; lead inhibits uric acid excretion and also promotes nucleation of monosodium urate monohydrate, predisposing to 'the gout, the colic and the palsy' (all features of lead poisoning). However, 'saturnine' gout still occurs in individuals who drink alcohol distilled or stored in lead-contaminated containers ('moonshine'). Alcohol is a less common association in women, usually occurring in young to middle-aged, thin, spirit drinkers; in women the main associations are diuretic therapy, chronic renal impairment, and pre-existing osteoarthritis.

A strong negative association exists between gout and rheumatoid arthritis. This remains unexplained, but probably reflects impaired nucleation/growth of monosodium urate monohydrate crystals rather than masking of monosodium urate monohydrate crystal-induced inflammation (for example, by crystal coating with rheumatoid factors).

Renal disease (see also Section 20)
Urolithiasis
Uric acid stones account for 5 to 10 per cent of all stones in the United Kingdom and United States, and up to 40 per cent in Israel (Chapter 20.12). A history of renal colic is seen in 10 to 25 per cent of patients with gout (75 per cent in Israel), the most important aetiological factor being the urinary uric acid concentration. In particular, high urinary concentrations occur in overproducers of uric acid, if renal urate clearance is increased (uricosuric drugs, defects in tubular reabsorption), and in situations of dehydration with lowering of urinary pH (diarrhoea, ileostomy). Gouty subjects also have an increased incidence of calcium-containing stones, particularly calcium oxalate, with no detectable uric acid nidus. Rarely, xanthine, oxipurinol, or orotic acid stones may occur with allopurinol treatment.

Acute uric acid nephropathy describes rapid precipitation of uric acid crystals in renal collecting ducts with secondary acute obstructive renal failure. This event correlates with the amount of uric acid excreted rather than the level of hyperuricaemia; strongly acid urine, which reduces uric acid solubility, potentiates the problem. Acute obstructive uropathy is most likely in ill, dehydrated patients with lymphoma or malignancy subjected to aggressive chemotherapy without adequate prophylactic treatment with allopurinol, but also occurs in gouty patients with markedly accelerated purine synthesis, following excessive exercise, and after epileptic seizures. The condition is largely avoidable by appropriate hydration, urine alkalization, and allopurinol prophylaxis.

Chronic urate nephropathy
Progressive renal disease is an important complication of untreated chronic tophaceous gout, accounting for up to 25 per cent of deaths (Section 20). Albuminuria and inability to concentrate urine maximally are early manifestations. Widespread monosodium urate monohydrate deposition in the interstitium of the medulla and pyramids results in crystal-induced inflammation with surrounding giant-cell reaction and fibrosis, affecting particularly the tubular epithelium of the loop of Henle and juxtaposed interstitial tissues. Subsequent changes include glomerular hyalinization and hypertrophy of the intima and media of arterioles; hypertensive damage, tubular obstruction, and secondary pyelonephritis may all complicate this picture. In late renal disease of any cause, calcium oxalate or phosphate crystals may deposit in renal parenchyma but are predominantly cortical in location (cf. the medullary site of monosodium urate monohydrate).

The association between parenchymal disease and less severe gout remains controversial, being confounded in males by frequent accompanying obesity, hypertension, and drug therapy. The minor progression of renal insufficiency that occurs in most gouty patients, however, is probably largely age-related and life expectancy is not reduced.

INVESTIGATIONS AND DIAGNOSIS
Investigations are to confirm the diagnosis, identify associated conditions, and assess cartilage and bone damage.

The history and signs of classical acute or chronic tophaceous gout are highly characteristic, and with a raised serum uric acid a strong presumptive diagnosis is readily made. However, definitive confirmation requires demonstration of monosodium urate monohydrate crystals by compensated polarized light microscopy of fluid from a gouty joint, bursa, or tophus. Synovial fluid in acute attacks is typically turbid with diminished viscosity and greatly elevated cell count (>90 per cent neutrophils); chronic gouty fluid is more variable, but occasionally appears white due to the high crystal load. Only a few drops collected directly on to a slide are required for crystal identification (Chapter 18.3). Monosodium urate monohydrate crystals are seen readily as strongly birefringent (negative sign) needle-shaped crystals, 5 to 20 μm in length, within cells or occurring freely in fluid; in tophaceous material they occur as dense, tightly packed sheets. During intercritical periods, aspiration of an asymptomatic first metatarsophalangeal joint or knee still often permits monosodium urate monohydrate crystal confirmation.

Hyperuricaemia is confirmed if two or more fasting serum uric acid levels exceed the normal range for the patients age and sex. In primary gout of young onset, determination of undersecretion or overproduction of uric acid is best undertaken by measuring total urinary excretion on a low purine diet, but a quick guide is given by the creatinine/uric acid ratio estimated on a single urine sample (normally <0.5). In young overproducers, a purine enzyme defect becomes more likely and should be sought (Chapter 11.4). Assessment of renal function (creatinine, urea, electrolytes, urine testing) should always be undertaken. Measurement of fasting lipoprotein concentrations should be made in all patients with primary gout. An intercritical full blood count and measurement of erythrocyte sedimentation rate/viscosity should detect any underlying myeloproliferative disease. During acute attacks a marked acute phase response (high erythrocyte sedimentation rate, neutrophil leucocytosis, thrombocytosis, elevated C-reactive protein) is usual; modest elevations of erythrocyte sedimentation rate also accompany chronic gout.

Radiographs supplement the clinical assessment of structural damage but may also aid diagnosis; in early disease they are usually normal. During acute gout, non-specific soft-tissue swelling (rarely juxta-articular osteopenia) may be evident. After repeated attacks, and in chronic disease, joint space narrowing, sclerosis, cysts, and osteophyte (that is, the changes of osteoarthritis) become more frequent in feet and hands. Gouty 'erosions' are a less common but more specific abnormality, occuring as para-articular 'punched-out' bone defects with well-demarcated sclerotic margins, overhanging hooks of bone, and retained bone density (Fig. 5). They are typically asymmetric, eccentric lesions positioned away from the 'bare area' of the joint, contrasting with more symmetrical, ill-defined marginal erosions (with osteopenia) of rheumatoid. Tophi appear as eccentric soft-tissue swellings, occasionally with patchy calcification due to epitaxial growth of apatite. In late disease, severe destructive change with osteopenia may occur and distinction from rheumatoid or other conditions becomes more difficult.

DIFFERENTIAL DIAGNOSIS

Acute attacks

Sepsis and other crystal-associated synovitis are the main considerations. Furthermore, gout and sepsis may coexist, as may monosodium urate monohydrate and calcium pyrophosphate dihydrate deposition (particularly in elderly subjects). Examination of aspirated fluid for both crystals and sepsis (Gram stain, culture) is the only sure way of obtaining the correct diagnosis. In ill patients particularly, a wider search for sepsis may be indicated (for example blood and urine cultures). With less classic attacks, other conditions that may be considered include psoriatic and acute Reiter's arthropathy, acute sarcoid arthropathy, traumatic arthritis, palindromic rheumatism, and exacerbation of osteoarthritis.

Chronic tophaceous gout

Other causes of arthritis and periarticular swellings/nodules that may require differentiation are rheumatoid arthritis, generalized nodal osteoarthritis, xanthomatosis with arthropathy, and multicentric reticulohisticytosis. Gout is usually less symmetrical in distribution than these conditions and, except for hyperlipidaemia, acute attacks are not a feature. Nodal osteoarthritis, of course, may coexist with gout. Aspiration (joint fluid, nodules) and plain radiographs readily facilitate correct diagnosis.

TREATMENT

Acute gout

The treatment aim is pain relief by reducing inflammation and intra-articular hypertension. Alteration of uric acid levels is avoided until the attack has resolved; initiation of hypouricaemic drugs may only prolong the attack.

Rapid symptom relief may be obtained with a quick-acting non-

Fig. 5 Characteristic radiographic changes of established gout in a finger: joint space loss and cystic change at the distal interphalangeal joint, 'pressure erosions' with overhanging bony 'hooks' at both interphalangeal joints, and eccentric soft-tissue swelling at the proximal joint.

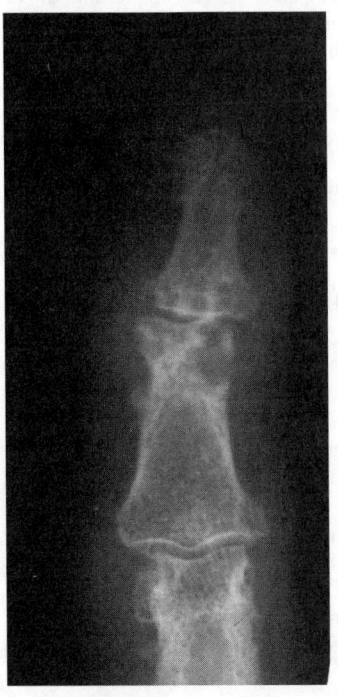

steroidal anti-inflammatory drug (NSAID), given in full dosage. Although indomethacin has a long tradition in this context, it is preferably avoided in the elderly due to its frequent renal, gut, and nervous system side-effects.

Oral colchicine is rapidly effective within a few hours (1 mg immediately, followed by 0.5 mg every 6 h until symptoms abate). Unfortunately, at effective doses diarrhoea, nausea, and abdominal cramps are common, causing the patient 'to run before he can walk'. Colchicine, however, is a useful alternative if NSAIDs are contraindicated. Intravenous colchicine is particularly toxic and should never be used. Although previously used as a 'diagnostic test' the efficacy of colchicine is not specific to gout (it also ameliorates other crystal-associated syndromes).

Joint aspiration often provides immediate relief by reducing intra-articular hypertension. Intra-articular steroid is useful for large joints such as the knee, or when NSAIDs or colchine are contraindicated or unsuccessful. In difficult cases, joint lavage may terminate an attack, and for troublesome polyarticular attacks there is anecdotal support for the use of parenteral steroid.

Long-term management

Once any acute attack has resolved, long-term strategies need consideration. Gout is potentially curable. Treatment may involve:

(1) considering and eliminating modifiable factors that cause hyperuricaemia; and
(2) utilizing hypouricaemic drugs.

Management of gout may require alteration in lifestyle and chronic medication; patient compliance and motivation, which depend on appropriate education and counselling, are essential for success.

Modification of provoking factors

In early primary gout, gradual weight loss, reduction in alcohol consumption, and avoidance of toxins (low-dose aspirin, lead) may alone be sufficient. Similarly, in diuretic-induced gout stopping the diuretic (± substitution of alternative therapies) may prove possible and be all that is required.

Hypouricaemic drug therapy

Indications for drug therapy are:

(1) recurrent, troublesome acute attacks;
(2) presence of tophi;
(3) bone or cartilage damage;
(4) coexistent renal disease, uric acid urolithiasis;
(5) very high uric acid levels (particularly with overproduction and hyperexcretion).

The logical approach would be allopurinol for overproducers and uricosurics for undersecretors. In practice, however, allopurinol is the usual drug of choice, permitting flexible tailoring of dose to reduce urate levels below the solubility limit. Allopurinol inhibits xanthine oxidase and often also depresses *de novo* purine synthesis. The starting dose is 100 to 300 mg daily, which is then adjusted within the range 100 to 900 mg daily according to the serum uric acid level (initially checked monthly). In patients with renal insufficiency, particularly the elderly, excretion of the active metabolite oxypurinol is delayed; the starting dose should therefore be 100 mg daily and adjustments made cautiously. The uricosurics probenecid (0.5–1.0 g twice a day) and sulphinpyrazone (100 mg 3–4 times daily), which prevent proximal tubular reabsorption of urate, are rarely used, but have partly been replaced by uricosuric NSAIDs (for example azapropazone 600 mg twice a day). Because of their symptomatic benefit, compliance with NSAID uricosurics is good; a drawback is the usual spectrum of NSAID side-effects. Uricosurics are alternatives to allopurinol in patients with normal renal function but are contraindicated in those with renal impairment, urolithiasis, or gross overproduction of uric acid. The therapeutic aim of hypouricaemic therapy is to maintain the serum uric acid well within the normal range (preferably the lower half).

Acute attacks may be provoked during the first few months of hypouricaemic treatment. Prophylactic colchicine (0.5 mg twice a day) or a standard dose of NSAID given for the first 2 to 3 months of treatment largely avoids 'breakthrough' attacks. Uricosuric NSAIDs do not require such cover. With any uricosuric, high fluid intake and urine alkalinization in the early weeks of treatment are recommended to avoid uric acid deposition within the kidney. Serious side-effects are unusual with any hypouricaemic drugs. Rare problems include toxic epidermal necrolysis and vasculitis (allopurinol), nephrotic syndrome (probenecid), and hepatitis and marrow suppression (both drugs). Important interactions with allopurinol occur with coumarin anticoagulants (due to hepatic microsomal enzyme inhibition) and purine analogues (such as azathioprine) which are inactivated by xanthine oxidase. Associated hypertension should be treated, but preferably not with diuretics which elevate serum urate and may provoke acute attacks during initial therapy.

Pyrophosphate arthropathy

Deposition of calcium pyrophosphate dihydrate crystals ($Ca_2P_2O_7 \cdot 2H_2O$) in articular cartilage is a common age-related phenomenon. Calcium pyrophosphate dihydrate crystals preferentially deposit within fibrocartilage and are the most common cause of cartilage calcification (chondrocalcinosis).

Calcium pyrophosphate dihydrate deposition may occur in otherwise normal cartilage or associate with structural change and clinical arthropathy—'pyrophosphate arthropathy'. A causal role for calcium pyrophosphate dihydrate crystals in acute inflammation is accepted but their role in chronic arthropathy is unclear. The strong association/overlap with osteoarthritis has led some to consider pyrophosphate arthropathy not as a crystal deposition disease but as a 'subset' of osteoarthritis, with calcium pyrophosphate dihydrate a 'process' marker associating with a hypertrophic articular response.

The prevalence of radiographic chondrocalcinosis is rare under 50 years of age, but rises from 10 to 15 per cent in those aged 65 to 75, to 30 to 60 per cent in those over 85, showing female preponderance (relative risk 1.33) and association with osteoarthritis (relative risk 1.52 at the knee). No epidemiological data exist for pyrophosphate arthropathy, but in patient series the mean age of presentation is c. 65 to 75 with female preponderance (c. 2–3:1), particularly in older patients.

Clinical features

Common presentations are acute synovitis, chronic arthritis, or incidental finding. Other presentations are rare.

ACUTE SYNOVITIS ('PSEUDOGOUT')

This is the most common cause of acute monoarthritis in the elderly. Attacks may occur as isolated events or be superimposed upon a background of chronic symptomatic arthropathy. Most attacks occur spontaneously but provoking factors include intercurrent illness, surgery, and local trauma. Although any joint may be involved, the knee is by far the most common site, followed by the wrist, shoulder, and ankle. Concurrent attacks in several joints are uncommon (<10 per cent of cases) and polyarticular attacks rare.

The typical attack develops rapidly with severe pain, stiffness, and swelling, becoming maximal within 6 to 24 h of onset. Examination reveals a very tender joint with signs of florid synovitis (increased warmth, tense effusion, restricted movement with stress pain) and often overlying erythema. Fever is common and elderly patients may appear unwell or mildly confused. Attacks are self-limiting, usually resolving within 1 to 3 weeks.

CHRONIC PYROPHOSPHATE ARTHROPATHY

This common condition affects mainly elderly women and targets the same large and medium-sized joints as pseudogout. Knees are the usual and most severely affected joint. Presentation is with chronic pain, stiffness, and functional impairment ($\pm$ superimposed acute attacks). Symptoms usually relate to just a few joints, although examination often reveals more widespread abnormalities. Affected joints show signs of osteoarthritis (crepitus, bony swelling, restricted movement) with varying degrees of synovitis (often most marked at the knee, radiocarpal, or glenohumeral joint). Knees typically show abnormality of two or three compartments; valgus or varus deformity may occur.

Although symptoms and signs are those of osteoarthritis, chronic pyrophosphate arthropathy may often be distinguished from uncomplicated osteoarthritis by:

(1) the joint distribution: in osteoarthritis wrist, glenohumeral, ankle, elbow, and midtarsal involvement are uncommon;
(2) the often marked inflammatory component; and
(3) superimposition of acute attacks.

The outcome for chronic pyrophosphate arthropathy is generally good, most patients running a relatively benign course, particularly with respect to small and medium-sized joints. Most progression that occurs is slow and related to knees, hips, or shoulders. Occasionally severe, rapidly progressive destructive arthropathy develops at these sites; this is virtually confined to very elderly women and associates with severe pain, recurrent haemarthrosis (shoulder, knee), and occasional joint leakage.

INCIDENTAL FINDING

As with osteoarthritis, clinical or radiographic evidence of pyrophosphate arthropathy and chondrocalcinosis are not uncommon incidental findings in the elderly, and may confound the cause of regional pain if a through history and examination are not undertaken.

UNCOMMON PRESENTATIONS

Acute tendinitis (triceps, Achilles), tenosynovitis (hand flexors, extensors), and bursitis (olecranon, infrapatellar, retrocalcaneal) occur uncommonly, usually in patients with widespread calcium pyrophosphate dihydrate crystals. Median and ulnar nerve compression at the wrist may accompany flexor tenosynovitis. Rare tophaceous deposits of calcium pyrophosphate dihydrate usually present as solitary lesions in areas of chondroid metaplasia.

CLASSIFICATION AND ASSOCIATIONS

Calcium pyrophosphate dihydrate deposition is traditionally classified as:

(1) hereditary;
(2) associated with metabolic disease; or
(3) sporadic/idiopathic (by far the commonest, associated with osteoarthritis).

Familial predisposition

This is reported from many countries and different ethnic groups. Two clinical phenotypes occur: early onset (third to fourth decade) florid polyarticular chondrocalcinosis with variable severity of accompanying arthropathy; and late-onset (sixth to seventh decade) oligoarticular chondrocalcinosis (mainly knee) with arthritis resembling sporadic disease. The pattern of inheritance varies, although autosomal dominance is usual. The mechanism of familial predisposition remains unclear and may differ between families: a primary cartilage abnormality that promotes calcium pyrophosphate dihydrate crystal nucleation and growth

(Swedish and Japanese families), and a generalized abnormality of pyrophosphate metabolism resulting in a local increase in cartilage levels (French and American kindreds) have both been reported.

Metabolic disease associations

Inorganic pyrophosphate (PPi) is a byproduct of many biosynthetic reactions, with a turnover of several kilograms per day. Much extracellular PPi derives from ATP via the action of NTP pyrophosphatase, and is rapidly converted to orthophosphate by pyrophosphatases (particularly alkaline phosphatase) (Fig. 6). A number of metabolic diseases associate with calcium pyrophosphate dihydrate deposition (Table 3), their association being rationalized through putative effects on PPi metabolism. Suggested mechanisms include:

(1) reduced PPi breakdown by alkaline phosphatase, due to:
    (a) reduced levels,
    (b) inhibitory ions (calcium, iron, copper), or
    (c) impaired complexing with magnesium;

(2) enhanced nucleation by iron or copper;
(3) increased calcium concentration; and
(4) increased production of pyrophosphate through stimulation of adenylate cyclase by parathyroid hormone.

Osteoarthritis and joint insult

Several observations support a relationship between osteoarthritis and calcium pyrophosphate dihydrate deposition, the latter often following rather than preceding joint damage. However, a negative association exists between calcium pyrophosphate dihydrate deposition and rheumatoid arthritis, with atypical radiographic features in coexistent disease (retained bone density, marked osteophyte, cyst, and bone remodelling) suggesting that the primary association of calcium pyrophosphate dihydrate is with hypertrophic tissue response/osteoarthritis and not joint damage *per se*. The explanation for this association is unknown. Synovial fluid PPi levels are increased in pyrophosphate arthropathy and osteoarthritis, and low in rheumatoid arthritis, but the order of change is unlikely to influence calcium pyrophosphate dihydrate formation, significantly. These crystals form in pericellular sites and associate with lipid, proteoglycan depletion, and adjacent hypertrophic chondrocytes containing lipid granules; it is therefore possible that reduction of inhibitors (such as proteoglycan) and increase in promotors (such as lipid)

may combine to co-promote calcium pyrophosphate dihydrate formation in metabolically active osteoarthritic tissue.

INVESTIGATIONS AND DIAGNOSIS

Critical investigations are synovial fluid analysis and plain radiographs. In pseudogout aspirated fluid is often turbid or bloodstained with elevated cell count (>90 per cent neutrophils); fluid from chronic pyrophosphate arthropathy shows variable characteristics. Compensated polarized microscopy reveals calcium pyrophosphate dihydrate crystals as weakly birefringent (positive sign) rhomboids or rods, c. 2 to 10 μm long. Calcium pyrophosphate dihydrate crystals are less readily identified and often less numerous than those of monosodium urate monohydrate; examination of a spun deposit may increase detection.

Radiographic aspects relate both to calcification and arthropathy. Chondrocalcinosis signifies extensive deposition and is not always evident; it mainly affects fibrocartilage (particularly knee menisci, wrist triangular cartilage, symphysis pubis), less commonly hyaline cartilage (Fig. 7). Although occasionally monoarticular, it usually affects several sites. Calcification of capsule, synovium, and tendons is less common. Chondrocalcinosis and calcification may increase or decrease with time, diminishing chondrocalcinosis often accompanying crystal 'shedding' or cartilage loss.

Changes of arthropathy are those of osteoarthritis: cartilage loss, sclerosis, cysts, and osteophyte. However, characteristics which suggest pyrophosphate include:

(1) distribution between and within joints that is atypical of osteoarthritis (for example glenohumeral disease; isolated or predominant patellofemoral or radiocarpal involvement);
(2) prominence of osteophytes and cysts; and
(3) prominent osteochondral bodies.

Such combined features may present a distinctive 'hypertrophic' appearance even in the absence of chondrocalcinosis (Fig. 8). In destructive arthropathy, marked cartilage and bone attrition with fragmentation and loose osseous bodies may resemble a Charcot joint.

Metabolic predisposition is rare and routine screening of all patients is unrewarding. Nevertheless, arthritis associated with calcium pyrophosphate dihydrate crystals may be the presenting feature of metabolic disease, and a search is warranted in the following circumstances:

(1) early onset arthritis (<55 years);
(2) florid polyarticular chondrocalcinosis; or
(3) presence of additional clinical or radiographic clues.

A reasonable screen would include serum calcium, alkaline phosphatase, magnesium, ferritin, and liver function.

DIFFERENTIAL DIAGNOSIS

The principal differential diagnosis for pseudogout is sepsis or gout (both of which may coexist with calcium pyrophosphate dihydrate deposition). Gram stain and culture of joint fluid should be undertaken even when calcium pyrophosphate dihydrate (± monosodium urate monohydrate) crystals are identified. Marked bloodstaining may lead to consideration of other causes of haemarthrosis (especially a bleeding disorder or subchondral fracture).

Chronic pyrophosphate arthropathy is usually readily distinguished from rheumatoid by the synovial fluid and radiographic findings, the infrequency of severe systemic upset, absence of extra-articular features, and only modest acute-phase response. Proximal stiffness due to glenohumeral involvement may suggest polymyalgia rheumatica, although clinical examination and near normal erythrocyte sedimentation rate should exclude the diagnosis. Destructive pyrophosphate arthropathy may simulate a neuropathic joint, although such joints are severely symptomatic and neurological abnormality is absent.

Fig. 6 Simplified scheme of extracellular pyrophosphate metabolism, showing putative sites of interaction by metabolic diseases. Hyperparathyroidism, 1, 2, 3; haemochromatosis, 2, 4; hypophosphatasia, 2; Wilson's disease, 2, 4; and hypomagnesaemia, 2.

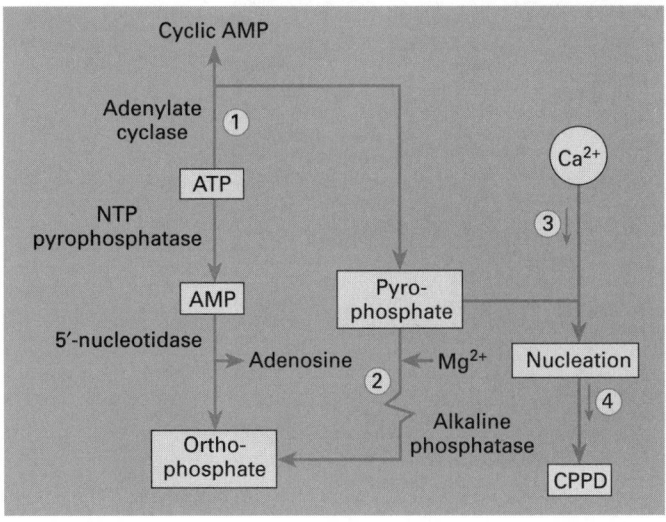

Table 3 *Metabolic diseases associated with calcium pyrophosphase dihydrate (CPPD) crystal deposition*

	Chondrocalcinosis	Pseudogout	Chronic CPPD arthropathy
Definite associations			
Hyperparathyroidism	+	+	−
Haemochromatosis	+	+	+
Hypophosphatasia	+	+	−
Hypomagnesaemia	+	+	−
Possible associations			
Hypothyroidism	+	−	−
Gout	+	+	−
X-linked hypophosphataemic rickets	+	+	+
Familial hypocalciuric hypercalcaemia	+	−	−
Wilson's disease	+	−	−
Ochronosis	+	−	−
Acromegaly	+	−	−

TREATMENT

Pseudogout

Since pseudogout usually affects only one or a few joints in elderly patients, local therapy is preferred. Aspiration alone often relieves symptoms, but may be combined with intra-articular steroid in florid cases. Simple analgesics and NSAIDs give additional benefit but should be used cautiously in the elderly. Joint lavage is reserved for troublesome steroid-resistant cases. Colchicine is effective but rarely warranted. Triggering illness (for example chest infection) will require appropriate treatment. Rapid mobilization should be instituted once the synovitis is settling.

Chronic pyrophosphate arthropathy

Unlike gout there is no specific therapy, and treatment of any underlying metabolic disease does not influence outcome. Aims are to reduce symptoms and maintain or improve function. This may include education of the patient in appropriate use of the affected joints, reduction in obesity, improvement of muscle strength, use of stick or other walking aid, and surgery for severe disease. Chronic synovitis may be improved by intermittant steroid injection or intra-articular radiocolloid (yttrium-90). As with pseudogout, symptomatic drugs are to be used with caution in older patients; simple analgesics are generally preferable to NSAIDs.

Fig. 7 Radiographic chondrocalcinosis of the knee, affecting meniscal fibrocartilage (central, triangular) and hyaline cartilage (linear, parallel to bone).

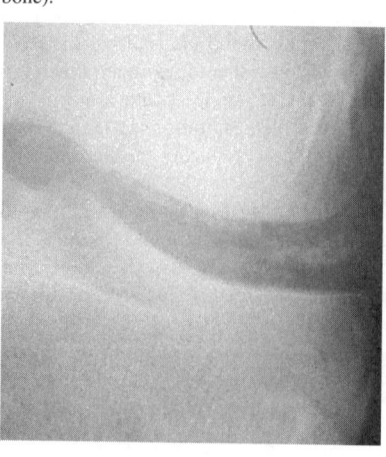

Other crystal-related disorders

Apatite-associated syndromes

Hydroxyapatite is the principal bone mineral. Apatites or basic calcium phosphates (partially carbonate-substituted hydroxyapatite, octacalcium phosphate, rarely tricalcium phosphate) are also the usual mineral to deposit in extraskeletal tissues (for example tuberculous lesions, arteries).

The [calcium × phosphate] product must be kept high to maintain skeletal integrity. Specific cellular mechanisms activate calcification where appropriate (for example matrix vesicles in growing cartilage) while other mechanisms (such as pyrophosphate and aggregated proteoglycan) inhibit calcification elsewhere. In general, abnormal calcification results from:

Fig. 8 Lateral knee radiograph showing predominant patellofemoral involvement by 'hypertrophic' osteoarthritis characteristic of pyrophosphate arthropathy.

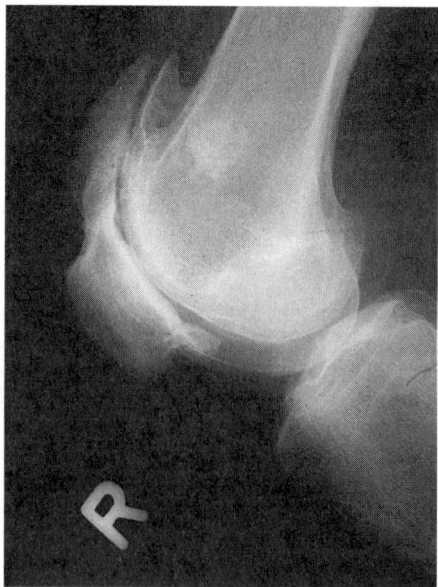

(1) elevation of the calcium phosphate product, causing widespread 'metastatic' calcification, or

(2) alteration in the balance between inhibitory and promoting tissue factors, resulting in local 'dystrophic' calcification.

In rheumatic diseases abnormal deposition of basic calcium phosphates may occur in:

(1) periarticular tissues (particularly tendon);

(2) hyaline cartilage, in association with osteoarthritis; or

(3) subcutaneous tissues and muscle, principally in connective tissue diseases.

Apatite crystals are too small (5–500 nm) to be seen by light microscopy. Particles may aggregate, however, to form spherulites visible by light microscopy. Confirmation of basic calcium phosphates requires sophisticated analytical techniques and most clinical diagnoses are presumptive, based on radiographic calcification or non-specific staining of joint fluid or histological material.

ACUTE CALCIFIC PERIARTHRITIS

Apatite deposition in the supraspinatus tendon (Fig. 9) is a relatively common incidental finding (c.7 per cent of adults). It occasionally results in severe acute inflammation of the subacromial bursa, periarticular tissues, or joint itself. Periarticular sites around the greater hip trochanter, the foot, or the hand are less commonly affected.

Acute episodes may follow local trauma or occur spontaneously. Within a few hours pain and tenderness are often extreme and the area appears swollen, hot, and red. Modest systemic upset and fever are common. Sepsis is usually considered first but the diagnosis is made following demonstration of radiographic calcification. If the lesion is aspirated, thick white fluid containing many apatite aggregates may be obtained. The condition usually resolves spontaneously over 1 to 3 weeks, often accompanied by radiographic dispersal of modest-sized calcifications (crystal 'shedding'). NSAIDs ameliorate symptoms and the attack can be abbreviated by aspiration and injection of steroid. Large deposits may require surgical removal. Calcific periarthritis rarely results from metabolic abnormality (renal failure, hyperparathyroidism, hypophosphatasia) and measurements of serum calcium, alkaline phosphatase, and creatinine are usually normal. Rare families are predisposed to calcific periarthritis at multiple sites with no evidence of altered calcium phosphate product.

OSTEOARTHRITIS AND APATITE-ASSOCIATED DESTRUCTIVE ARTHRITIS

Modest amounts of basic calcium phosphates are commonly found in synovial fluid from osteoarthritic joints, in isolation or with calcium pyrophosphate dihydrate ('mixed crystal deposition'). Whether apatite plays any part in inflammatory exacerbations, or associates with severity or progression of osteoarthritis remains uncertain.

The uncommon condition 'apatite-associated destructive arthritis' is often considered a 'subset' of osteoarthritis. It is virtually confined to elderly women and affects the hip, shoulder ('Milwaukee shoulder') or knee. It has the general appearance of severe large joint osteoarthritis but is particularly characterized by:

(1) rapid progression, often leading to severe pain and disability within a few months of onset;

(2) development of marked instability;

(3) large, cool effusions;

(4) an atrophic radiographic appearance with marked cartilage and bone attrition and little osteophyte or bone remodelling.

Aspirated fluid has normal viscosity and a low cell count but contains large amounts of apatite aggregates, seen readily on light microscopy

following non-specific calcium staining (alizarin red, acidic pH). The differential diagnosis may include sepsis (excuded by synovial fluid culture), late avascular necrosis, or neuropathic joint. The pathogenesis of this condition remains unclear. Although apatite particles could contribute to tissue damage by stimulating release of collagenase and other proteolytic enzymes from synovial cells, it is most likely that the apatite is non-contributory and principally reflects the severity of subchondral bone attrition. The outcome is poor and inevitably requires surgical intervention.

Other apatite syndromes

Tophaceous periarticular apatite deposition may occur in patients with chronic renal failure managed by dialysis. Apatite has also been incriminated in the occasional erosive interphalangeal arthropathy seen in such patients.

Other crystals

Cholesterol

Cholesterol crystals may induce acute synovitis, acute tenosynovitis, and chronic xanthomatous tendinitis in hypercholesterolaemic subjects. Cholesterol and other lipid crystals may also occur as a non-specific finding in chronic synovitis, most commonly due to rheumatoid; in this situation the lipid probably derives from cellular debris and its pathogenic significance is uncertain.

Oxalate

Oxalate crystals have been incriminated in acute and chronic articular and periarticular syndromes occurring in association with either primary familial oxalosis (types I and II) or secondary oxalosis (Chapter 11.10). Chronic renal failure managed with dialysis is the commonest cause of secondary oxalosis, particularly if ascorbic acid supplementation has been given. Acute symmetrical interphalangeal and metacarpophalangeal arthritis, with or without tenosynovitis, and digital calcific deposits are the usual manifestation; large joint involvement, chondrocalcinosis, and tophaceous periarticular masses are less common. Calcium oxalate crystals may also induce life-threatening organ involvement, with peripheral vascular insufficiency and digital necrosis, myocardiopathy, peripheral neuropathy, and aplastic anaemia. There is no effective treatment.

Extrinsic crystals

These are a rare cause of locomotor problems. Acute flares following intra-articular injection of corticosteroids are uncommon but may represent iatrogenic crystal-induced inflammation. Penetrating injuries involving plant thorns and sea-urchin spines may cause acute and chronic inflammatory synovitis, periostitis, or periarticular lesions

Fig. 9 Shoulder radiograph showing florid supraspinatus tendon calcification (calcific periarthritis).

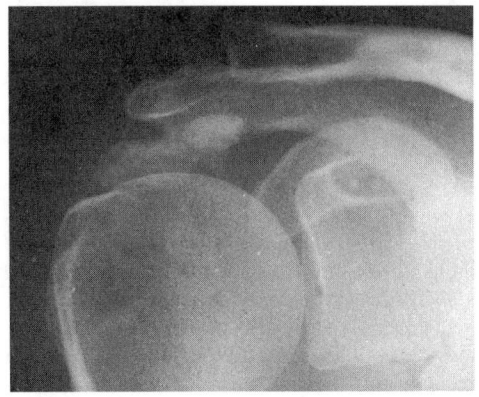

which only resolve following surgical removal of the crystalline material.

REFERENCES

Dieppe, P.A. and Calvert, P. (1983). *Crystals and joint disease.* Chapman & Hall, London.

Doherty, M. and Dieppe, P.A. (1986). Crystal deposition disease in the elderly. *Clinics in Rheumatic Diseases* **12**, 97–116.

McCarty, D.J. (ed.) (1988). Crystalline deposition diseases. *Rheumatic Disease Clinics of North America* **14**, 2.

Reginato, A. and Kurnik, B. (1989). Calcium oxalate and other crystals associated with kidney diseases and arthritis. *Seminars in Arthritis and Rheumatism* **18**, (3), 198–224.

18.8 Back pain and periarticular disease

I. HASLOCK

Aches and pains in the musculoskeletal system are common features of everyday life. Each year about 40 per cent of the population develop some symptoms relating to their locomotor system. Despite the fact that 60 per cent of these symptoms do not lead to medical consultation, about 8 million people consult their general practitioner each year. The commonest locomotor symptom is pain in the back, with 15 per cent of the adult population reporting at least 3 days' back pain annually. The epidemiology of back pain has been reviewed recently by the Clinical Standards Advisory Group (United Kingdom).

APPROACH TO THE PATIENT WITH BACK PAIN

Traditional medical diagnosis aims to attribute a pathological cause to the patient's symptoms through a deductive process based on history taking, physical examination, and appropriate investigations. These three diagnostic processes are equally important in elucidating the cause of back pain, but several complicating features interfere with the simplicity of the deductive process. For example, comparisons of patients with acute back pain who consult a doctor with those who manage their own symptoms reveals no significant difference in clinical findings between the two groups. There is no agreed pathological cause for the patients symptoms in 85 per cent of cases, but there are large numbers of medical and non-medical specialists in the care of back pain who offer precise and superficially convincing detailed explanations and consequential therapies, which have rarely been exposed to scientific evaluation. Outcome appears to relate more to factors such as educational level and perception of illness than to diagnostic categories or treatment methods. Further complexity is added when, as is often the case, ideas about the pain being caused by an incident, accident, or occupation are present, with attendant interference from legal or compensatory processes. Attempts to dissociate these 'non-medical' factors has led to the development of an examination system which encompasses the distinction of a series of non-appropriate clinical signs as well as organically understandable ones. In particular, dramatic and nonanatomical descriptions of unvarying pain accompanied by widespread superficial tenderness, lumbar pain on axial loading or simulated rotation, and jerky giving-way on motion assessment all alert the examiner to the contribution of 'illness behaviour' to the patient's symptoms.

PATHOLOGY

In its totality, the behaviour of the spine is that of a flexible rod. Its function is to absorb loads and permit movement while protecting the spinal cord and emerging nerve roots. The vertebrae are separated from each other by intervertebral discs, designed to allow absorption of loads, and synovial apophyseal joints which are angled so that the appropriate movement is facilitated—flexion/extension, side flexion, and rotation in the cervical spine; predominantly rotation in the dorsal spine, and predominantly flexion/extension and side flexion in the lumbar region. The

normal spinal posture is vertical, with cervical and lumbar lordoses and a mild thoracic kyphosis, this alignment facilitating absorption of impact loads during walking and running.

The intervertebral disc comprises an outer annulus fibrosus comprising tough, obliquely arranged collagenous fibres surrounding a thick gelatinous nucleus pulposus. This provides a good shock-absorbing mechanism, which becomes less efficient with age as the nucleus becomes more fibrotic.

The apophyseal joints may be involved as a part of any inflammatory polyarthritis, and are particularly important in ankylosing spondylitis (see Chapter 18.5). They are particularly prone to osteoarthritis, especially when loading is abnormal as a result of degeneration and narrowing of the adjacent disc, or in a more widespread fashion from alignment abnormalities such as scoliosis.

Spondylosis is the association of the degeneration and narrowing of the disc space with the development of osteophytic lipping at the adjacent vertebral margin. There is often secondary osteoarthritis in the associated apophyseal joints.

Prolapse of the intervertebral disc occurs when the nucleus pulposus is no longer contained within the annulus but bulges through it. Because of the increased curvature of the posterolateral border of the vertebra, prolapse takes place preferentially at this site, which is adjacent to the emerging spinal nerve roots. The force distribution throughout the spine is such that the L5–S1, then the L4–L5, discs are by far the most commonly affected, although prolapse can occur at any level. Root pressure at these sites gives rise to pain and neurological signs in the ipsilateral leg, usually referred to as sciatica. The second commonest site of prolapse is at the posterior margin of the disc where the extruded nucleus presses on the tightly bound posterior spinal ligament. This causes pain without lateralizing signs, and, if large, may result in cord or, more usually, cauda equina compression, leading to interference with bladder function and anal sphincter competence. More chronic disc protrusion associated with degeneration can lead to the condition of spinal stenosis. This causes symptoms of 'cord claudication' with pain in the legs on exertion. The canal diameter is increased by flexion, which produces the characteristic symptom that cycling is easier than walking, or that the patient bends forward in order to hurry, for example across the road.

The integrity of the bony spinal cord may be interrupted at the pars interarticularis, either because of a congenital defect or trauma. The resultant forward slippage of the vertebra is called spondylolisthesis.

The bony spine and its attendant articulation is surrounded by powerful muscles and ligaments, with a particularly complex ligamentous array at the junction with the pelvis. Both local and referred pain may arise from irritation of these structures, and the work of Kellgren (1939) illustrated the range of responses produced by irritation of these structures using local injection of hypertonic saline. It is assumed that a great deal of back pain arises from these structures, but the nature of the nociceptive insult, the precise attribution of symptoms to sites, and the appropriate treatment for these putative insults are all obscure.

In addition to the mechanical causes of back pain described above, the spine may be the site of infection or tumour. The classical spinal infection was tuberculosis, which started from haematogenous spread to a disc and spread through the vertebral end plates into the two adjacent vertebrae. This led to vertebral body collapse with preservation of the posterior spinal elements, leading to severe angulation—the gibbus—now seen almost exclusively in the elderly. Infection is now most commonly with staphylococci, with streptococci becoming increasingly important, and more exotic infections occurring in the iatrogenically immunocompromised and those with AIDs. Primary malignancy may occur, but is less common than secondaries, particularly from breast, bowel, and prostate. Myeloma may present with back pain. Pain from infection and malignancy is often both severe and unvarying. Pain which lacks periodicity and association with activity, especially unremitting night pain, raises the suspicion of a sinister cause.

Acute low back pain

The majority of the estimated 23 million episodes of back pain occurring in Britain annually are acute. The sudden onset may be associated with an incident such as bending, lifting, or turning. Pain is usually in the lumbar area and often radiates to one or both legs.

In evaluating treatment, it is important to know the natural history of acute back pain. Only a minority come to medical attention, and of those severe enough to warrant consultation with a general practitioner, 40 per cent recover each week. Thus by 3 weeks 80 per cent of acute episodes have settled, irrespective of the intervention used. A short period of rest—2 or 3 days is as effective as 2 weeks—followed by progressive resumption of activity is the treatment of choice. Analgesia should be adequate, with paracetamol or co-dydramol being sufficient for most patients. Severe pain may require an intramuscular analgesic. Non-steroidals given intramuscularly are as effective as narcotics, and avoid the risk of constipation. Where muscle spasm is severe, intramuscular diazepam is valuable.

Extensive evaluation is only needed in the acute phase where there is disturbance of bladder or bowel function which might indicate a massive central disc protrusion. Examination under these circumstances should include reflexes, power, and sensation in the lower limbs, including the saddle area particularly. The motor and sensory signs shown in Table 1 may be seen, often involving both legs.

Persistence of acute back pain

If the pain fails to settle with simple measures, or the symptoms become more severe, a full physical evaluation is needed. The pain may present in the back, in the affected leg alone, or in both. Persistence of sciatica with resolution of the back pain deserves just as much attention as when the back pain persists. The presence of a cough impulse—dysaesthesiae in the leg produced by raising the intrathecal pressure by coughing or sneezing—demands further investigation.

CLINICAL EXAMINATION

The patient must stand undressed and the spinal posture is noted. Flexion, extension, and side flexion are observed for range and symmetry. Finger-floor distance, often suggested as a measure of spinal flexion, is an inconsistent blend of spinal and hip movement and should never be used. The patient then lies down to allow neurological examination of the legs. The most important sign to seek is restriction of straight leg raising (Lasague's sign). Although straight leg raising to 90 degrees is usually quoted as normal, not everyone can achieve this. Comparison with the contralateral side is valuable, but restriction to less than 75 degrees is almost always significant, and below 45 degrees strongly suggestive of disc prolapse. Increasing the pressure on the irritated sciatic nerve by sharply dorsiflexing the foot at the limit of straight leg raising (the sciatic stretch test) produces extra pain.

Finally, there should be a general examination to look for signs suggesting infection or malignancy. This should include stigmata of weight loss, presence of pyrexia and lymphadenopathy, and examination of the breasts in women and the prostate in men. Non-mechanical disease may be accompanied by severe, local spinal tenderness.

INVESTIGATION

Investigations will be guided by the physical signs. Plain radiographs are usually the first investigation undertaken. They are rarely of value in mechanical back pain, as some degree of disc degeneration is almost universal with increasing age, and the severity of the radiological signs bears almost no relationship to symptoms. The major value of radiography is to show them to the patient, usually to demonstrate the absence of serious disease; without this educational use the majority are worthless. Plain radiographs are capable of showing major anatomical abnormalities, spondylolisthesis, vertebral collapse, or malignancies producing isolated or multiple lesions, usually destructive but occasionally sclerotic. If the history and neurological signs indicate the possibility of nerve root compression or central disc protrusion, a computed tomography (CT) scan is the most generally available next investigation (Fig. 1). Disc protrusion or other anatomical abnormalities are well shown, but nervous tissue is better shown by magnetic resonance imaging (MRI) (Fig. 2). Myelography should now be reserved for clearer delineation of a lesion pre-operatively, if the surgeon desires it. Where non-mechanical disease is considered, plain radiography is essential in revealing infection or tumours. A raised erythrocyte sedimentation rate or plasma viscosity, a raised white cell count, raised alkaline or acid phosphatase, and a monoclonal band on electrophoresis of plasma are all indications of serious disease, and form part of the diagnostic work-up. Isotope bone scanning is the most useful way of identifying infective or malignant lesions, with CT and MRI scanning providing complementary methods of delineating them, and CT-guided percutaneous biopsy providing histological material.

Chronic back pain

The proportion of patients developing chronic back pain is small, but their symptoms may last for many years, producing significant disability regarding work and social activities. They consume large amounts of medical time, and are often referred to specialists in many disciplines, undergoing frequent fruitless investigations. Chronicity is as much caused by social and psychological factors as by underlying pathology. Re-referral to hospital is often precipitated by events such as refusal or downgrading of benefits. The major obligation is to take a careful history to ensure no new features suggesting a new cause of pain are present, and to undertake and document a careful clinical examination. Without new guiding symptoms, reinvestigation of patients with chronic back pain is almost invariably fruitless.

TREATMENT

A valuable protocol for the evaluation and management of back pain has been produced by the Clinical Standards Advisory Group (United Kingdom). Patients found to have non-mechanical causes for back pain, such as infection or malignancy, require treatment guided by the underlying diagnosis.

Persistent acute pain

Patients with persistent mechanical back pain first require an explanation of their symptoms. Phrases such as 'spinal arthritis' should be avoided, as they imply chronicity and inevitable incapacity, and inhibit recovery. A progressive re-educative exercise regime should be accompanied by postural correction and advice, and advice regarding lifting and work. 'Back schools' designed to convey this advice are found in a lot of physiotherapy departments, but many people fail to respond to group activities such as these. Patients should be encouraged to lose weight if obese, and take regular exercise, swimming being ideal. Although cor-

Table 1 *Neurological signs in the legs*

Nerve root	Pain and distribution	Weakness	Sensory loss	Reflexes
S1	Buttock Back of thigh Back of calf	Eversion and plantar flexion of foot	Lateral foot	Ankle jerk diminished
L5	Buttock Back and side of thigh Lateral calf	Dorsiflexion of hallux Eversion of foot	Dorsum of foot	
L4	Lateral thigh Medial calf	Inversion of foot	Medial calf	Knee jerk diminished

sets may be helpful in the short term, their long-term use should be discouraged as it tends to cause paraspinous muscle weakness. Analgesia should be simple, non-costive, and given for the shortest possible duration. Non-steroidal anti-inflammatory drugs are often prescribed. Their use is illogical in absence of demonstrated inflammation, but pragmatically they are sometimes helpful. Manipulation often helps mobilize the patient in the early stages of treatment. Various 'schools' of manipulation appear to offer no differential advantage. Many patients have some intermittent residual back pain. Whether this is considered tolerable will depend on their personality and occupation.

Patients with distinct neurological symptoms and signs often show spontaneous recovery. Manipulation, epidural injection, and out- or in-patient traction may all be useful in settling symptoms. Surgery should only be considered where conservative treatment has failed. Modern surgical techniques are designed to be minimally invasive and hence reduce unnecessary damage to the spine.

Fig. 1 (a) CT scan at L4/5 showing unilateral osteoarthritis in the right facet joint. (b) CT scan of L2/3 showing a combination of an isolated osteophyte associated with the right facet joint in association with a right-sided bulge of the disc causing nerve root compression.

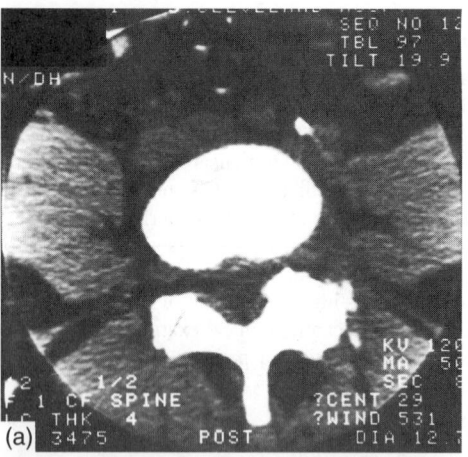

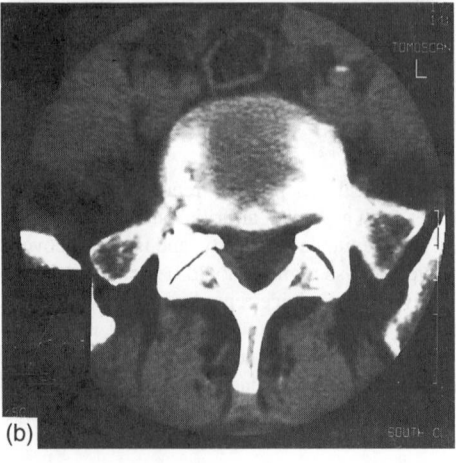

Chronic pain

The treatment of chronic back pain follows the same principles, but is unsatisfactory. Approaches such as the 'school of bravery' attempt to persuade patients to 'push through' their pain and increase their physical capability. Skilled psychological input helps with these approaches, and also with pain control programmes and teaching patients coping skills. Very rarely surgery, usually in the form of spinal fusion, may be helpful, especially where degenerative disease has led to spinal instability. Unfortunately, many patients continue to be regular attenders to their family doctor, chronic consumers of analgesics and frequent visitors to physiotherapy departments and pain clinics.

Pain in the dorsal spine

Mechanical dorsal spine pain is less common than lumbar pain, but does occur. Pain may radiate around the chest wall.

Examination of the dorsal spine is best done with the patient seated. A dorsal kyphosis is common, especially in those such as seamstresses who bend forward at work. Fixed kyphosis accompanies osteoporosis. The 'gibbus' caused by spinal tuberculosis may be seen in some older patients, and in some patients who have had osteoporotic crush fractures.

Severe local tenderness may be caused by fracture, sepsis, or malignancy, usually secondary. Referred pain from penetrating peptic ulcer, pancreatitis, and occasionally gallbladder disease may be felt in the dorsal region, so the history must be appropriate for these conditions, and the examination should include the abdomen.

INVESTIGATIONS

The radiological appearances of spondylosis and of diffuse idiopathic skeletal hyperostosis (DISH) are too ubiquitous to be discriminating in dorsal pain. Osteoporotic wedging or crush fracture, sepsis, or malignancy may be seen on radiography and confirmed by scintigraphy, CT,

Fig. 2 MRI scan showing a degenerate L5/S1 disc.

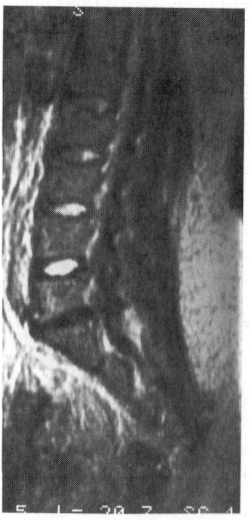

or MRI in case of doubt. Measurement of erythrocyte sedimentation rate, white cell count, and plasma alkaline phosphatase concentration also aids these diagnoses. Myeloma may produce single or multiple lesions, and protein electrophoresis and Bence Jones proteins should be included in the diagnostic work-up of the ill patient with dorsal pain.

TREATMENT

Mechanical dorsal pain is treated by postural correction, which is difficult, and active exercises. These may be enabled by mild simple analgesia. Osteoporosis with or without fracture requires appropriate treatment (Section 19), as do malignancy and sepsis. Acute dorsal disc protrusion requiring surgery is extremely rare.

Pain in the cervical spine

Radiological changes of spondylosis are almost universal in those over 35 years, but correlate as poorly with symptoms as do similar changes in the lumbar region. Cervical pain is often associated with spasm in the trapezius, paraspinous muscles, and the muscles of the scalp. These in turn are frequently caused by poor posture, especially at work, and emotional trauma. However, osteophytic lipping may occasionally impinge on surrounding structures such as the oesophagus (Fig. 3 or the vertebral vessels. Radiating symptoms to the arms are very common in patients with neck pain, the dysaesthesiae often following a non-anatomical pattern. Distinct radiculopathy raises the suspicion of nerve compression by disc protrusion or impinging osteophytes. MRI is the investigation of choice under these circumstances.

TREATMENT

This involves reassurance, especially when head pain occurs, and an exploration of physical and emotional lifestyle causes for muscle spasm. Local and general methods to induce relaxation are valuable, and the temporary use of a soft collar at night only is helpful in diminishing pain—a daytime collar is often used as a badge of disability and encourages perpetuation of symptoms. Simple analgesics or short courses of non-steroidal anti-inflammatories may be helpful. Physiotherapy may help alleviate immediate pain, but should be supplemented by a home exercise and postural correction regime continued on a long-term basis. Despite these measures, chronic neck pain is a frequent cause of persistent misery.

Periarticular disorders

Rheumatism has been defined as 'pain within a mile of a joint', drawing attention to the fact that much musculoskeletal pathology is non-articular. These syndromes are best considered regionally.

Fig. 3 Osteophytic lipping impingeing on the oesophagus.

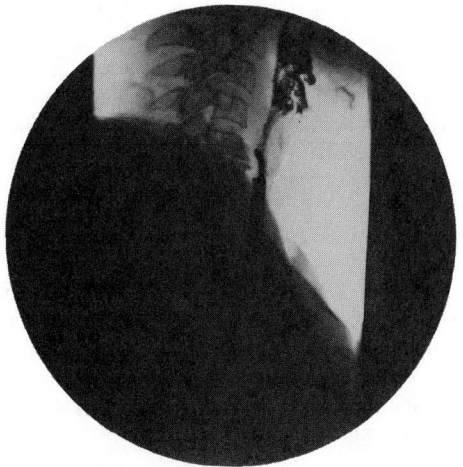

THE SHOULDER

The complex interrelationships of the muscles, tendons, and bursae related to the shoulder joint, together with its wide range of movement, appear to make it particularly vulnerable to the development of pain and restriction. Unfortunately, there is considerable confusion in the nomenclature of shoulder disease, with different authorities referring to the painful restricted shoulder syndrome as capsulitis of the shoulder, periarthritis, adhesive capsulitis, frozen shoulder, rotator cuff lesion, and subacromial or subdeltoid bursitis. Subtle differences among these 'different' entities are often described but appear to be of little practical importance.

Examination of the painful shoulder usually reveals diminished abduction and rotation, both active and passive, with reversal of the normal scapulohumeral rhythm of movement. Tenderness may be related to the anterior part of the shoulder joint, the subacromial region or the posterior aspect of the shoulder. There is often muscle spasm, particularly of the upper fibres of the trapezius, leading to pain in the neck, and pain may also be referred to the deltoid muscle or the medial condyle of the elbow as well as being felt diffusely around the whole of the shoulder girdle.

Pathologically the primary lesion appears to be tearing of fibres at the insertion of the rotator cuff with secondary inflammation, both in relation to the healing fibres and in the subacromial bursa. As movement may exacerbate the pain, the limb tends to be held to the patient's side with consequent adhesion formation both within the joint and between the surrounding soft tissue structures.

Treatment is by reduction of pain, muscle spasm, and inflammation using non-steroidal anti-inflammatory agents and physical methods such as infrared radiation or ice. Thereafter the shoulder is remobilized, the accent being on teaching the patient an active home exercise regime which gradually but progressively increases the range of pain-free movement. Full relief of symptoms takes up to 2 years to accomplish and the range of movement is rarely normal after an episode of capsulitis, although an adequate functional range is usually achieved. Resolution of symptoms may be accelerated by local corticosteroid injection into the rotator cuff, the joint itself, or into the subacromial bursa. Occasionally, manipulation, either under the influence of intravenous diazepam or general anaesthesia, is used to regain movement in a recalcitrant joint.

More localized lesions occasionally form part or all of the painful stiff shoulder syndrome. A painful arc of abduction between about 45 degrees and 90 degrees can be associated with calcification in the supraspinatus tendon, the pain being related to the position in which the calcified portion is squeezed between the humeral head and the acromion. Patients with this condition can hold their arm fully elevated if it is passively moved to that position, but are inhibited from achieving elevation by the painful arc, and tend to drop the arm suddenly as the pain strikes rather than achieving smooth depression from an elevated position. Treatment is by local corticosteroid injection, ultrasound application to disrupt the calcium deposit, or, occasionally, surgical removal of the deposit.

Bicipital tendinitis is differentiated by the finding of local tenderness over the insertion of the long head of the biceps and pain on resisted flexion of the pronated forearm. Local corticosteroid infiltration into the paratenon is usually effective, but care must be exercised not to inject into the body of the tendon as this may lead to tendon rupture.

THE ELBOW

Pain related to the common extensor origin on the lateral epicondyle is called tennis elbow, and the less common syndrome of pain related to the common flexor origin on the medial epicondyle is called golfer's elbow. Both these are overuse phenomena, usually relating to easily identifiable, often sporting, activities, as their names imply. Tearing of muscle fibres near the bony insertions, or pulling up of the periosteum in that area, sets off a low-grade inflammatory reaction. There is local tenderness, and pain occurs when the muscles are brought into action. Ideally the precipitating movement should be avoided and the elbow rested, but this is usually advice the patient will not, or cannot, follow. It is very important in relation to all overuse injuries in sportsmen to examine the player's technique in conjunction with an experienced coach. Many such overuse injuries are the result of bad technique, and coaching to correct the technique is as important as medical treatment, for if faulty style is not eliminated recurrence is inevitable. Local corticosteroid injection is often helpful in reducing the pain, although several injections may be necessary. Both manual frictions, applied by a physiotherapist, and ultrasound have also been used effectively in these conditions. Rarely, surgery is required to achieve full symptom relief, especially where lifting of the periosteum has led to formation of a spicule of new bone which is often both palpable and visible on radiographs.

THE WRIST AND HAND

Tenosynovitis of the wrist and hand occurs as part of inflammatory disease such as rheumatoid arthritis, but may occur as a discrete entity as the result of overuse. The extreme example of this is cane-cutter's disease, a severe form of tenosynovitis of the wrist extensors suffered by sugar-cane cutters in the harvesting season. Lesser degrees of the same condition are associated with racquet sports and unaccustomed house-painting. As the thumb is, functionally, half the hand, the extensors of the thumb are particularly prone to develop overuse inflammation. Clinically the affected tendon sheath becomes painful, especially on use, tender and swollen, and exhibits soft crepitus on movement. The overlying skin is often red and warm. The thickening induced by swelling of the tendon sheath may become sufficient, especially as it becomes more chronic, to prevent smooth running of the tendon. This condition is known as stenosing tenovaginitis or, in relation to the thumb extensors and abductors, de Quervain's disease. Treatment of simple tenosynovitis is by rest, either in a splint or a plaster cast. Resolution may be aided by injection of corticosteroid into the tendon sheath, but significant obstruction requires surgical release of the stenotic sheath.

Tenosynovitis is recognized as an occupational disease, and patients with non-specific pain in their forearms, felt during their work, often describe it as 'teno' in the knowledge that this diagnosis implies compensation. Non-specific use-related pain and fatigue in the forearms associated with non-specific physical signs such as diffuse tenderness has been called 'repetitive strain syndrome' or sometimes 'repetitive strain injury', this latter term confirming the patients' feelings about the causation. These symptoms are common in workers making repetitive movements, especially keyboard operators. The complexity of the disease was demonstrated by the epidemic that occurred in Australia when it became recognized as an industrial disease. Many repetitive workers suffer similar symptoms, which the majority simply tolerate, and which can be relieved by minor changes in working posture or practice, including short periods of rest, in well-motivated people.

THE THIGH AND KNEE

Subtrochanteric bursitis produces symptoms that are often diagnosed as hip pain. The pain is felt in the lateral side of the thigh and is exacerbated by hip movement. Examination reveals local tenderness just distal to the greater trochanter, and the symptoms are relieved by local corticosteroid injection, which may need to be repeated two or three times to achieve complete resolution. This syndrome is often related to abnormalities of gait, and these need to be eliminated to ensure persistent resolution of the symptoms. The prepatellar bursa becomes inflamed when subjected to repeated trauma—beat knee of miners, housemaids' knee, or clergyman's knee—producing painful swelling distal to the lower pole of the patella. This area becomes red and oedematous and secondary infection may occur. Local injection is less effective in this site and excision is frequently required.

Ligamentous injuries to the knee are common accompaniments of sport and recreation. Pain may be accurately located at the medial or lateral side, but more diffuse pain and swelling may make differentiation from an internal derangement difficult. Local tenderness and swelling occurs, usually related to the tibial attachments of the medial or lateral ligaments, and pain may be produced on stressing the appropriate ligament by flexing the knee to about 20 degrees and then forcibly abducting or adducting the leg with the thigh fixed. Local corticosteroid injection, frictions, ultrasound, and muscle strengthening may all be effective, but severe strains require a period of immobilization in a Robert-Jones bandage, or plaster of Paris. Muscle wasting, in the quadriceps especially, takes place with extreme rapidity when the knee is immobilized. To some extent this can be prevented by isometric exercises in the plaster, but it is of great importance not to allow vigorous use of the leg, either in sport of at work, until muscle strength and bulk have been progressively restored by graded exercise, or further sprains around the knee will almost inevitably occur.

Fat pads related to the knee, especially the medial side, may be painful either in isolation or as part of Durcum's disease. Local treatment with pain-relieving physiotherapy methods or infiltration with local anaesthetics such as bupivacaine, sometimes mixed with Hyalase® is often ineffective. Intravenous infusions of lignocaine may help intractable or widespread symptoms.

THE LEG AND ANKLE

In contrast to the partial tears seen elsewhere, the calf is the site of sudden rupture of tendons, usually the plantaris, or of parts of the gastrocnemius muscle belly. The patient feels sudden pain in the calf, with local tenderness and swelling. Plantaris rupture is of no significance and requires only an antalgesic heel-raise until the pain subsides. Achilles tendon or gastrocnemius rupture requires surgical repair. The ankle is prone to sporting ligamentous injuries and also those arising from accidents such as stepping awkwardly off kerbs. The stability of the ankle joint is almost entirely dependent on the integrity of the surrounding ligaments, and minor tears in them may produce serious problems, resulting in a chronically 'weak' or unstable ankle. The ankle is also particularly prone to swelling after injury, as the hydrostatic pressure here is very high, and ligaments may be stretched or disrupted as a result of this. Strains or partial tears of the ankle ligaments should, therefore, be treated by immobilization in a tight bandage or plaster of Paris for a short period (2 or 3 days) followed by assessment of the severity of the damage and subsequent therapy aimed to reduce oedema and improve muscle tone. Post-traumatic rehabilitation with especial attention to fine balancing movements, most easily stimulated by use of a wobble-board, is essential if recurrent strains are to be avoided.

THE FOOT

Bursal lesions in the foot are common. The great toe is subject to valgus deviation, especially when ill-fitting shoes are worn which force the great toe into valgus and cause rubbing on the lateral surface of the metatarsophalangeal joint. Inflammation of the bursa at this position produces a bunion. Treatment is by prophylaxis—avoiding ill-fitting shoes—local pressure relief by padding, or surgical correction of the hallux valgus. The calcaneal bursa, between the Achilles tendon and the calcaneum, may become inflamed, often in conjunction with Achilles tendinitis. This latter condition produces heel pain and the swollen Achilles tendon sheath is easily visible and palpable and is often red. This condition usually arises as a result of overuse, and may be exacerbated or caused by local pressure. Unfortunately the heel-tabs on running shoes which are often claimed to protect against this problem appear to be a prime cause of it. Rest and infiltration of corticosteroid into the paratenon are effective forms of treatment but, especially in sportsmen, it is important to modify the footwear to prevent recurrence. A rarer overuse condition is central core degeneration of the Achilles tendon. Here the tendon itself is swollen, and at operation is found to contain a degenerate central core which requires excision. The longitudinal arch of the foot is maintained by the long plantar (spring) ligament. Laxity of this ligament produces a flat foot. Pain felt at the insertion of the ligament into the calcaneum occurs as part of the enthesopathy of seronegative spondarthritis but also as an isolated, idiopathic condition. Plantar spurs may be seen on radiographs of these patients, but well-defined spurs are of no pathological significance, occurring as often in normal subjects as in patients with heel pain; in contrast, fluffy spurs are indicative of the presence of an inflammatory process. Initially, treatment is by removing impact trauma by use of sorbo heel pads. If this fails, local corticosteroid injection may be effective, although this procedure is painful. Surgery may be necessary.

Metatarsalgia, or pain felt under the metatarsal heads, is a common accompaniment of rheumatoid arthritis, but also occurs as an isolated, idiopathic complaint. Overuse and inappropriate footwear are the usual precipitating causes. Treatment is by use of a metatarsal bar attached to the sole of the shoe or appropriately padded insoles. Morton's metatarsalgia is a variant of this condition caused by neuroma formation in the digital nerve at the level of the metatarsal heads. Careful examination reveals the tenderness to be located in the web space between the toes rather than under the metatarsal heads. Treatment is by local anaesthetic and corticosteroid injection or, more usually, surgical excision of the neuroma.

Generalized musculoskeletal pain

Increasing numbers of patients present with 'pain all over'. A careful history and detailed clinical examination is required to sort such patients into different categories.

SORTING OUT GENERALIZED MUSCULOSKELETAL PAIN

Inflammatory joint disease may present as diffuse pain rather than localized articular symptoms. Examination reveals signs of rheumatoid arthritis, ankylosing spondylitis, or other arthritides. The symptoms of the diffuse connective tissue diseases are often rather non-specific, reflecting the generalized nature of these disorders. A careful history must be coupled with examination for features such as Raynaud's phenomenon, rashes, or vasculitis. Polymyalgia rheumatica is particularly prone to present as a rather non-specific illness with diffuse pain in older people (Chapter 18.11.7).

Rheumatic complaints associated with general medical disorders are often characterized by diffuse aching or pain. Thyroid disorders, both hyper- and hypothyroidism, and diabetes are particularly prone to present in this way. Metabolic bone disease may cause diffuse pain, although it should be noted that osteoporosis, even when severe, is not intrinsically painful, and should not be blamed for pain in absence of fractures.

Although many patients assume all their musculoskeletal symptoms have a simple common cause, this is often not the case. Soft-tissue rheumatic disorders are very common, and they coincide commonly. They also coincide with common articular disease such as osteoarthritis or spondylosis. A careful history and examination might, for example, reveal that a patient with pain 'from head to toe' has got cervical spondylosis to explain his neck and shoulder pain, tennis elbow causing

symptoms in one arm and carpal tunnel syndrome symptoms in the other, trochanteric bursitis causing thigh pain, and flat feet producing chronic aching in the feet and ankles. Such combinations are not rare, and the individual components, which are only found by meticulous, skilled physical examination, should be treated individually rather than by the blanket diagnosis 'rheumatism'—or even worse, 'arthritis'—being followed by the unthinking prescription of a non-steroidal anti-inflammatory drug.

Increasingly, 'pain all over' is attributed to the group of syndromes variously called postviral fatigue syndrome, fibromyalgia, or myofascial pain syndrome, which in some aspects blends into myalgic encephalomyelitis (ME). This group of syndromes is characterized by severe diffuse pain, morning stiffness, subjective swelling, especially in the hands, incapacitating fatigue, and often severe resultant disability. They are occasionally preceded by a viral infection. The only significant physical finding is multiple tender spots in muscles and ligaments. There is an association with irritable bowel syndrome and tension headaches, and many patients have psychological disturbance, particularly depression. Despite many theories of causation, the aetiology of this condition, which in the United States is more common than rheumatoid arthritis, remains obscure. Treatment is unsatisfactory, the only helpful therapies appearing to be antidepressants coupled with a progressive exercise programme aimed at improving aerobic fitness and improving function. This group of diseases is unique in that membership of the relevant patients' association appears to produce a worse prognosis.

REFERENCES

Badley, E.M. and Tennant, A. (1992). Changing profile of joint disorders with age: findings from a postal survey of the population of Calderdale, West Yorkshire, United Kingdom. *Annals of the Rheumatic Diseases* **51**, 366–71.

Clinical Standards Advisory Group. (1994). *Back pain.* HMSO, London.

Clinical Standards Advisory Group. (1994). *Epidemiology review: the epidemiology and cost of back pain.* HMSO, London.

Deyo, R.D. and Diehl, A.K. (1988). Psychosocial predictors of disability in patients with low back pain. *Journal of Rheumatology* **15**, 1557–63.

Dixon, A. St. J. and Graber, J. (1989). *Local injection therapy in rheumatic diseases* (3rd edn.). EULAR publishers, Basle. A comprehensive pocket-sized guide, with useful diagnostic tips as well.

Doherty, M., Hazleman, B.L., Hutton, C.W., Maddison, P.J., and Perry, J.D. (1992). *Rheumatology examination and injection techniques.* W.B. Saunders, London.

Hadler, N.M. (1987). *Clinical concepts in regional musculoskeletal illness.* Grune and Stratton, Orlando. A broad view of the medical and non-medical influences on common locomotor disorders.

Hazleman, B.L. and Dieppe, P.A. (ed.) (1989). The shoulder joint. *Baillière's Clinical Rheumatology* **3**, (3).

Jayson, M.I.V. (ed.) (1992). *The lumbar spine and back pain,* (4th edn). Churchill Livingstone, London.

Kellgren, J.H. (1939). On the distribution of pain arising from deep somatic structures with charts of segmental pain. *Clinical Science* **4**, 35–46.

Waddell, G. (1987). Clinical assessment of lumbar impairment. *Clinical Orthopaedics and Related Research* **221**, 110–20.

Yunus, M.B., Masi, A.T., and Aldag, J.C. (1989). A controlled study of primary fibromyalgia syndrome: clinical features and association with other functional syndromes. *The Journal of Rheumatology* **16**, (Suppl. 19), 62–71.

18.9 Septic arthritis

M. H. SEIFERT

INTRODUCTION

This chapter is concerned with those rheumatic diseases that have been associated with a proven infectious agent, but excluding the conditions broadly termed reactive arthritis. Many different organisms can cause septic arthritic, including bacteria, fungi, viruses, and spirochaetes.

Bacterial arthritis

PATHOGENESIS

Joints become directly infected most often by haematogenous spread of micro-organisms from a remote site or less commonly, as a result of direct penetration by instrumentation or trauma. Once in the joint the organism multiplies in the synovium and can usually be recovered from the synovial fluid or synovium itself. The resultant pathophysiological sequence is the same for all bacterial infections in joints. The synovial membrane is extremely vascular and the micro-organisms soon migrate from the vascular compartment into the interstitial space where the reaction to the infection varies markedly, depending on the amount and type of organism present, its virulence, and the host's defence mechanisms. The bacteria multiply and set off a cascade of inflammation in the synovium and synovial fluid. Proteolytic enzymes are released by activated polymorphonuclear leucocytes and these destroy the articular cartilage first by altering the proteoglycan matrix and then destroying the collagen superstructure, with resultant deformation of cartilage. With the increase in synovial fluid the intra-articular pressure rises. Other synovial tissues, such as bursae and tendon sheaths, also suffer from this inflammatory damage, but it is the destruction of articular cartilage that causes the most serious sequelae to septic arthritis, and dictates the urgency of treatment (Table 1). The septic stage must be halted urgently prior to collagen loss and chondrocyte death to prevent cartilage destruction and joint damage.

PREDISPOSING CAUSES

Although previously more common in young children, joint sepsis is now found increasingly in the elderly and in those with chronic illness such as malignancy, diabetes, alcoholism, or anaemia. Intravenous drug abusers and immunosuppressed patients are also predisposed to septic arthritis. Chronic joint disease due to rheumatoid arthritis, crystal synovitis, trauma, or surgery also increases the risk of infection (Table 2).

INFECTING ORGANISMS

A wide variety of bacteria can cause septic arthritis, but some particular organisms have varying predilection for different age groups and predisposing causes. For example Staphylococcus aureus is more likely to be found in the septic joints of children aged between 2 and 15 years and the elderly, than Haemophilus influenzae, which is more likely to be encountered in children under 2 years of age. In rheumatoid arthritis Staphylococcus aureus is the likely cause, while in acute leukaemia a Gram-negative bacillus is most common. In the years of sexual activity Neisseria gonorrhoeae is the likely cause, and infections of joints due

Table 1 Sequence of joint destruction in bacterial arthritis

1. Synovial membrane hypertrophy
   (a) Infiltration by polymorphonuclear cells (PMNs)
   (b) Release from PMNs of proteolytic enzymes
   (c) Activation of lining cells
   (d) Cartilage erosions by membrane proliferation
2. Synovial fluid accumulates
   Pressure necrosis of cartilage
3. Articular cartilage destruction (enzymatic and bacterial)
   (a) Proteoglycan depletion
   (b) Collagen degradation
4. Bone involvement

Table 2 Predisposing causes of non-gonococcal bacterial arthritis

Systemic disease
  Chronic liver disease
  Diabetes mellitus
  Cancer
  Chronic renal disease
  Sickle-cell anaemia
  Systemic lupus erythematosus
Chronic arthritis, joint trauma
  Rheumatoid arthritis
  Trauma, arthroscopy, joint replacement
  Gout
Systemic immunosuppressive medications
Intravenous drug abuse
Infection with the human immunodeficiency virus

to streptococci and Gram-negative organisms, such as enterobacteria and Pseudomonas aeruginosa, can occur at any age. Specific clinical pictures are recognized to be associated with particular organisms, including brucella, gonococci, and meningococci and are considered in Section 7.

CLINICAL FEATURES

The onset is generally abrupt with the development of severe pain and inflammation over a few days. Weight-bearing joints, particularly the knee, are most commonly involved in adults. Less common joints to be infected include the small joints of the hands and feet. Although usually monoarticular, polyarticular involvement is well recognized, particularly with streptococcal infections. Most patients have a fever, although it can be low grade or absent; rigors are not common unless there is bacteraemia reflected by a positive blood culture. Movement of the involved joint is painful and restricted and examination reveals swelling, heat, and joint tenderness, sometimes, but not always, with erythema of the overlying skin.

DIFFERENTIAL DIAGNOSIS

Acute arthritic disorders such as gout, pseudogout, palindromic rheumatism, rheumatic fever, or trauma with haemarthrosis may be confused with infectious arthritis. Systemic symptoms such as fever or chills and marked leucocytosis are however, uncommon or less marked in these conditions. Pre-existing joint disease such as rheumatoid arthritis may cause difficulty in recognizing the development of a septic joint. Any patient with rheumatoid arthritis who has a joint that is inappropriately swollen and hot should be suspected of having developed sepsis in that joint, and whenever there is this possibility the joint must be aspirated promptly to exclude bacterial infection.

BACTERIAL AND JOINT FLUID EXAMINATION

After a complete medical and physical examination, paying particular attention to potential portals of entry of infection, such as the skin, nasal passages, middle ear, lungs, rectum, urethra, and pelvis, it is essential for the joint to be aspirated. This is of vital diagnostic value but also removes debris and destructive enzymes and relieves pain by reducing the joint pressure. The laboratory should be warned that the aspiration is to be performed in order that the fluid may be inoculated into appropriate culture media while still warm. Samples of fluid should be placed in sterile tubes for culture and into heparinized containers for cell counting. The fluid should also be examined for the crystals of gout or pseudogout. Infected synovial fluid usually appears purulent and thick with a high white cell count of predominantly polymorphonuclear leucocytes, but occasionally the fluid is not obviously purulent and there may be only modest increases in the cell count. The fluid should be Gram stained and inoculated into appropriate media.

Other potential sites of infection should be sought, and culture from skin, nasopharynx, sputum, urine, and stool obtained routinely. At least two blood cultures for aerobic and anaerobic organisms should be obtained. These may yield positive results when culture of synovial fluid is negative. Cerebrospinal fluid should be cultured when clinically indicated. Occasionally, all these cultures are negative despite joint sepsis, especially if antimicrobial treatment has been initiated prior to joint aspiration.

RADIOLOGICAL EXAMINATION

Early in the course of infection radiographs of the affected joint are normal or show only the changes of soft tissue swelling and the presence of effusions. Films at this stage are useful, however, to compare with later ones which characteristically reveal juxta-articular osteoporosis, followed by joint space narrowing resulting from destruction of articular cartilage. Vertebral bone and disc destruction can occur within weeks of infection. Sacroiliac joint infection is predominately unilateral. Radioisotope scanning using either gallium or technetium is particularly useful in detecting sepsis in deep joints such as the hip, shoulder, and spine, as are CT or MRI, especially where there is suspicion of osteomyelitis. MRI has been shown to detect the early changes in infected joints, especially in cartilage.

TREATMENT

General

A septic joint is extremely painful and the natural reluctance of the patient to move it should be respected. A splint helps to reduce pain and, by immobilization, to control inflammation. This should be only a temporary measure and physiotherapy must be started early to prevent stiffness, contractures, and muscle wasting. Pain is relieved by aspirating as much synovial fluid as possible, daily or more frequently if the fluid reaccumulates rapidly. When this is a persistent problem, it is helpful to wash out the joint with physiological saline. It is sometimes difficult in shoulder and hip joints to eliminate sepsis, particularly when there are loculated pockets of fluid; then it may be necessary to establish open surgical drainage, a procedure which should always be considered in the absence of clinical or laboratory signs of improvement despite 4 to 7 days of adequate antimicrobial therapy. Consultation from the outset

with an infectious disease specialist and an orthopaedic surgeon is invaluable in planning treatment.

Antimicrobial treatment

This should be initiated as soon as the diagnosis of septic arthritis is made, and even before the infecting organism has been identified. A preliminary estimate of the type of micro-organism can be made on the result of the initial Gram stain smear of the synovial fluid. Parenteral antimicrobials should be continued for at least 7 to 14 days, and because some Gram negative and staphylococcal infections are slow to respond, it is often necessary to continue for 4 to 6 weeks. Parenteral administration of antimicrobials provides maximal serum and synovial fluid concentrations, and there is no indication for intra-articular injections, which can cause a chemical synovitis and may even introduce further infection. Improvement is indicated by a decrease in the frequency of the need for joint aspiration and the return to normal of the joint fluid. A progress chart recording temperature, the volume and content of aspirated fluid, the results of repeated Gram stains, and the antimicrobial prescribed is helpful in assessing the response to therapy.

Suppurative arthritis, sometimes monoarticular, is a rare feature of brucellosis and of infection with *Neisseria gonorrhoeae* or *Neisseria meningitidis* (see Chapters 7.11.19, 7.11.5, and 7.11.6).

Arthritis due to mycobacteria and fungi

Mycobacterial and fungal arthritis are characterized by a slowly progressive evolution of symptoms and signs. Constitutional symptoms may be few, and extra-articular involvement absent. It is therefore not surprising to find a long delay between the onset of symptoms such as pain and the final diagnosis. Patients with unexplained chronic monoarthritis or with spondylitis and chronic tendonitis with erythema nodosum should be considered as potentially infected.

Tuberculous arthritis

Although there has been a steady decline until recently in the prevalence of tuberculosis in advanced countries, there is a huge morbidity and mortality in the developing world, and the disease is being seen more frequently in accultured societies. The age incidence has changed from being a disease of children and young adults to one that affects all ages, including the elderly. In the United Kingdom tuberculosis is particularly common among Asian immigrants, often with atypical presentation (see Chapters 7.11.22, 7.11.23). Rheumatological presentations include tendon sheath involvement and dactylitis, but half the cases of skeletal tuberculosis occur in the spine, while the rest involve the hip, knee, ankle, and wrist. There is often an absence of active pulmonary disease, although in 40 per cent there is radiological evidence of previous infection. The most frequent symptom is pain on movement, and gross synovial proliferation with effusion is a common sign. Predisposing trauma may have been noticed, and there is an association with debilitating diseases, alcoholism, drug addiction, and acquired immune deficiency syndrome (AIDS). The tuberculin skin test is usually positive and this should be included in the investigation of any unexplained monoarthropathy. Radiographical features of skeletal tuberculosis are not pathognomonic. Soft-tissue swelling and diffuse osteoporosis of bone appear early. Later cystic lesions develop initially adjacent to joints with little periosteal reaction. The joint space tends to be preserved until gross adjacent cortical bone destruction has developed. There is no osteophyte formation.

Spinal tuberculosis (Pott's disease)

Fifty per cent of skeletal tuberculosis occurs in the spine, often in the absence of pulmonary or extrapulmonary disease. The lower thoracolumbar area is most often involved. Infection typically starts at the margin of adjacent vertebral bodies and invades the disc spaces early. These spaces narrow with vertebral collapse and consequential kyphosis or gibbus formation. Cold paraspinous abscesses may develop and dissect along the spine, causing multiple sites of destruction with skip areas in the vertebral column and ribs, and pointing in the neck, groin, or chest wall. There is overlying muscle spasm, nerve root irritation, and spinal cord involvement in 10 to 25 per cent of patients.

Peripheral tuberculous arthritis

This is usually monoarticular, and the hip is a common site. In children the initial complaints are of pain in the groin with a limp and the hip held in flexion and abduction when at rest. Later, destruction of the femoral neck and acetabulum occurs with the appearance of a cold abscess pointing to the outer thigh. In the knee and other peripheral joints pain is the prominent symptom, with synovial swelling and warmth. The majority of patients have both bone and synovial infection. Non-specific symptoms of low-grade fever and weight loss frequently occur, but florid reactions such as high fever, night sweats, malaise, and anorexia are limited to patients with concomitant pulmonary or miliary tuberculosis.

Synovial fluid findings include elevated protein and, in 50 per cent, a low sugar content. There is a polymorphonuclear leucocytosis in the blood and the white cell count varies widely. In 80 per cent of cases synovial fluid cultures are positive but a higher yield is obtained by culturing synovial biopsy tissue. In 90 per cent of cases caseating granulomata and acid-fast bacilli are found on microscopic examination.

TREATMENT

There is debate about the number and choice of drugs to use and the duration of treatment, although all would agree the need for at least two drugs. One favoured regimen is the combination of isoniazid, ethambutol, and rifampicin, at least for the first 6 to 8 weeks. Overall, treatment should continue for 18 to 24 months and should be adjusted in the light of the sensitivity of the organism. Surgical intervention has been recommended to clean infected synovium and to deal with a spinal abscess, to secure an unstable spine, or to provide material for culture and sensitivity testing.

Atypical mycobacterial arthritis

A heterogeneous group of organisms usually having a low pathogenicity for man, shares some of the characteristics of infection with *Mycobacterium tuberculosis*. Pulmonary and joint disease is indistinguishable from that produced by the tubercle bacillus. The pathological lesions are also similar and diagnosis depends on the isolation of the organism and analysis of growth characteristics and biochemical and serological properties.

Previous joint disease and compromise of immune defences predispose to these infections. Treatment may prove difficult and resistance to antituberculous drugs results in more recourse to surgical intervention than with *Mycobacterium tuberculosis* infection. The problem of drug resistance by these organisms dictates that a number of drugs must be used in combination before sensitivity data are available.

Fungal arthritis

Fungi invade bone locally to cause septic arthritis and only rarely is fungal arthritis the result of haematogenous spread. Diagnosis usually requires synovial biopsy, because culture from synovial fluid is difficult and serological tests are disappointing. Synovial fluid changes are non-specific. A chronic joint destruction occurs. Radiologically the lesions resemble other forms of granulomatous infection, such as tuberculosis.

Coccidioidomycosis (see also Section 7)

Coccidioides immitis infection is endemic in the south-western United States and Mexico. Following inhalation, in one-third of previously fit patients there is transient arthralgia with erythema nodosum, fever and malaise. Within a month all symptoms resolve without residual arthritis. Dissemination occurs in a small percentage of patients, and of these, 20 per cent have bone and joint involvement. The affected joints are ankles, knees, and, less commonly, the feet and wrists. The chronically infected joint has a thick, grey synovial membrane with serous or purulent fluid and often a discharging sinus. Diagnosis, often delayed, is made by identification of the organisms in the synovium or by culture from these tissues. Treatment is by surgical synovectomy and intravenous amphotericin B. Intra-articular amphotericin B has also been used.

Blastomycosis

Blastomyces dermatitidis is endemic in the Mississippi and Ohio River basins. The fungus gains entry through the lungs, causing a mild flu-like illness, but in some cases more florid pulmonary and cutaneous lesions develop. Up to 50 per cent of patients systemically infected also develop bone and joint lesions. Most of the joint infection is from osteomyelitic spread, although primary arthritis without bone disease also occurs. Joints commonly involved are the ribs, vertebrae, long bones, and skull. Because the organisms are so numerous, synovial fluid examination frequently reveals the yeast-like organisms. Treatment is with amphotericin B.

Sporotrichosis ('rose grower's arthritis')

Penetration of the skin by a thorn or other plant material carrying *Sporothrix schenckii* may result in the development of cutaneous sporotrichosis. Rarely, there is a systemic infection secondary to the cutaneous lesions, and in 8 per cent of these an arthritis develops. Large joints are most frequently involved although other joints and tendon sheaths can also be infected. Delay in diagnosis averages 2 years and can result in irreversible joint damage. Cultures of synovial fluid and tissue yield Sporothrix. Serological tests may be suggestive but not diagnostic. Treatment is with intravenous or intra-articular amphotericin B.

Candidiasis

This is now perhaps the most common fungal arthritis in the United Kingdom, due to an increased incidence of systemic candidiasis in the compromised host. Nevertheless, bone and joint infection is rare. The knee is the most frequently involved joint and usually the adjacent bone is infected. Treatment is with amphotericin B, accompanied by appropriate measures to improve immunological defences whenever possible.

Viral arthritis

Characteristic symptoms of any viral infection include malaise, fatigue, chills, fever, headache, and arthralgia, together with sore throat, regional lymphadenopathy, and a mild pyrexia; arthritis is unusual at this stage. On close questioning though, these prodromal features will be found to have preceded arthritis when it occurs. There is no characteristic pattern of joint involvement, although there is a tendency towards a polyarticular pattern. A papular or macular rash is frequently present. The risk of chronicity and tissue necrosis is slight and it is rare for any persisting arthritis to develop. Investigations are not often helpful, although an elevated sedimentation rate is the rule and there may be abnormal circulating lymphocytes. Synovial fluid analysis and synovial biopsies show only non-specific inflammation. Only rarely, as in rubella, have viruses been cultured from these specimens. A number of viral infections are most commonly associated with later development of arthritis; these include hepatitis B, rubella, parvovirus, group A arboviruses, mumps, varicella zoster, and vaccinia. Diagnosis depends largely on a good clinical history, for example the detection of intravenous drug abuse in patients with hepatitis B infection, or recent immunization for rubella.

Hepatitis B (see also Chapter 7.10.26)

Arthritis occurs in approximately 50 per cent of people infected with hepatitis B, often together with a skin rash and the prodromal features of the infection. There is a sudden onset of arthritis which is usually polyarticular and symmetrical with involvement characteristically of the small joints of the hands. These joint symptoms last for a few weeks and are often associated with tendonitis. Fifty per cent of patients with arthritis also develop a pruritic urticarial rash on the legs. These features have disappeared by the time jaundice develops. During the prodrome, surface antigen (HBS Ag) is present in the blood in excess over antibody (anti-HB), and immune complexes containing both these are present, together with depressed C4 and CH50 serum complement levels. With resolution of the arthritis there is disappearance of HBS Ag, normalization of complement, and increase of anti-HB. Tests for HBS Ag are positive in both blood and synovial fluid during the arthritic phase, but become negative as the arthritis resolves and the tests for anti-HB become positive. There are few other significant haematological abnormalities and synovial fluid analysis is also unrewarding. The arthritis is helped by salicylates and varies in duration from a few days to several weeks.

Rubella (see also Chapter 7.10.18)

In naturally acquired rubella infection, arthritis is extremely common. Ninety per cent of women infected with the virus develop a symmetrical polyarthritis affecting the small joints of the hands, wrists, and knees in a distribution similar to that of rheumatoid arthritis. The arthritis is self-limiting and rarely lasts more than 3 weeks. As well as the characteristic morbilliform rash and lymphadenopathy, a carpal tunnel syndrome may develop. Tests for rheumatoid factor may be positive and the virus has been isolated from synovial fluid. Rubella virus has also been isolated from the synovial fluid of some patients with an inflammatory polyarthritis in the absence of clinical evidence of rubella and it has been suggested that some form of rubella infection may be the primary pathogenic event in the aetiology of the chronic arthritis in these patients.

Parvovirus (see also Chapter 7.10.25)

The parvovirus (PV) demonstrated to cause disease in humans is PV B-19 and at least 30 per cent of adults in Great Britain have antibodies to it by the age of 16. B-19 is associated with a mild illness of fatigue, leukopenia, and rash and is the aetiological agent of erythema infectiosum, slapped cheek disease, and fifth disease, mainly found in children and producing very red cheeks. Other symptoms are of mild upper respiratory tract infection, mild gastroenteritis, and arthropathy. More serious problems resulting from infection with PV B-19 are acute aplastic crises in patients with haemoglobinopathies and intrauterine infection leading to spontaneous abortion (see Chapter 13.12.1). PV B-19 is also associated with an acute and chronic arthropathy in adults with either clinical or inapparent infections. Common features of this complication in adults include a symmetrical polyarthropathy involving small joints of hands, wrists, and knees. Prodromal symptoms are reported in under half the cases, when an 1gM and IgG response to B-19 can be measured. Adult females are more frequently affected in a ratio of 4:1. Within 2 to 8 weeks joint symptoms resolve, but occasionally persistent disease develops.

Arboviruses (see also Chapter 7.10.16)

Arboviruses are transmitted via arthropods to vertebrates. The vector is usually a mosquito and the host a mammal. The most common manifestations of arboviral diseases are fever, arthritis or arthralgia, and rash. The three main arbovirus infections causing arthritis are epidemic polyarthritis of Australia, chikungunya and O'nyong-nyong.

Epidemic polyarthritis of Australia

This is caused by the Ross River virus and transmission to man is via the mosquito. Outbreaks have been reported in New South Wales, and the north and south of eastern Australia. An incubation period of 10 days is followed by fever, malaise, myalgia, and 2 days later an urticarial rash which is associated with lymphadenopathy and arthritis. Young adult women are more frequently affected and the small joints of the hands, ankles, and wrists are involved. A maculopapular rash often develops on the trunk, fading after a week. There are no specific investigations and the Ross River virus has only been isolated once from the blood of a patient. The arthritis clears after 2 or 3 weeks, sometimes longer, and aspirin gives partial relief of symptoms.

Chikungunya (Swahili for 'he who walks doubled up')

This is also an epidemic infectious arthritis and occurs in wide areas of Africa, southern India, and southern Asia. There is acute onset of fever, chills, and arthritis involving the knees, wrists, fingers, and lumbar spine. The arthritis lasts from 5 to 7 days and sometimes recurs for months. A maculopapular rash develops on the trunk or extremities and follows the arthritis by 4 or 5 days. The chikungunya virus can be recovered from blood within 3 days of the onset of symptoms, but its recovery from synovial fluid has never been reported. Aspirin and non-steroidal anti-inflammatory drugs help the symptoms.

O'nyong-nyong ('joint breaker')

This virus is transmitted by mosquitoes and results in a disease characterized by the acute onset of fever with severe joint pains, headaches, rash, and lymphadenopathy. Epidemics occur in East Africa and have the added complication of conjunctivitis and eye pain. The virus is similar to that of chikungunya and has been isolated from the blood of only a few patients.

Arthritis associated with miscellaneous viruses
MUMPS

Arthritis in young adult males is well recognized and occurs 10 days after the onset of parotitis. The arthritis is migratory and lasts for 2 weeks, leaving no residual joint damage.

CHICKENPOX

Characteristic swelling and heat in the knees occurs very rarely a few days after the typical vesicular rash. The arthritis resolves after a few weeks. The virus has never been recovered from the synovial fluid.

SMALLPOX

Variola and, rarely, vaccinia have been associated with arthritis, especially in children. The elbows were involved most often, then the wrists, hands, and knees in a symmetrical fashion. Unlike other viral infections causing arthritis, the synovitis originated from adjacent bone, and residual joint disease and deformity occurred in those continuing to grow.

INFECTIOUS MONONUCLEOSIS

Arthritis rarely occurs in patients with infectious mononucleosis. Large joints are involved and the arthritis settles within a week.

RETROVIRUSES

The arthritis encephalitis syndrome in goats is caused by the lentevirus, caprine arthritis encephalitis virus (CAEV). Adult goats develop slowly progressive arthritis, occasionally interstitial pneumonia, and leucoencephalomyelitis. The virus is grown from the synovial fluid and synovial biopsies. Some patients infected with human immunodeficiency virus (HIV), another retrovirus, have been shown to have a polyarthritis. Although this is likely to be a reactive arthritis, the virus has been isolated from synovial fluid in infected patients.

Arthritis due to spirochaetal infections

Syphilitic arthritis

Bone and adjacent joints can be affected in both congenital and acquired treponemal infection, but this is rare. Congenital syphilis can present in the first weeks of life as osteochondritis or epiphysitis with pseudoparalysis of a limb and para-articular swelling. Eventual complete fracture of the epiphysis may occur. From the age of 8 to 16 painless effusions of the knees can develop (Clutton's joints). These may be confused with an inflammatory polyarthritis, although there is little pain or loss of function. Mild stigmata of congenital syphilis, such as interstitial keratitis, Hutchinson's teeth, or nerve deafness may be present, and synovial biopsy shows lesions suggestive of microgummata. Acquired syphilis presents in its secondary stage with arthralgia and arthritis. As well as back pain, large joints are involved and painful effusions occur in the knees. Tenosynovitis and periostitis are common, and the latter can be identified on bone scan. Other stigmata of secondary syphilis such as rash, mucous plaques, alopecia, and lymphadenopathy should also be sought. In tertiary syphilis it is common to find periostitis of the tibia and the clavicle. The ossification that follows produces a characteristic lacy pattern of the bone. Joint disease results from the spread of gummatous infiltration from the bone. Charcot (neuropathic) joints associated with tabetic lesions usually present as a monoarthropathy. There is progressive enlargement, effusion, and instability of the painless joint with marked crepitus. The knee is the most frequent site, followed by the hip and the ankle. Serological tests for syphilis are strongly positive in all patients in these latter two stages of the disease.

Lyme disease (see also Chapter 7.11.30)

Lyme disease is a tick-borne, immune-mediated inflammatory disease caused by the spirochaete *Borrelia burgdorferi*. In 1975 an unusually high incidence of arthritis was reported from Old Lyme and Lyme in Connecticut. Cases were more common in summer and autumn, particularly among children and young adults. A characteristic rash, erythema chronicum migrans, had been reported in about 25 per cent of patients prior to the development of the arthritis. The disease is now known to occur worldwide, wherever Ixodes ticks are found. In Europe the vector is *Ixodes ricinus*. Ixodes ticks are widespread throughout the United Kingdom but are found in greater numbers in forests and woodland areas where deer are farmed. The skin eruption appears over the trunk or proximal extremities, is hot to touch, and is associated with systemic symptoms of malaise, fatigue, headache, and stiff neck. Fever and lymphadenopathy are common and the skin lesions fade after 3 weeks. Joint manifestations occur in approximately half the patients, mostly affecting the knees. This initially lasts for 1 week but recurrent attacks

may follow. In a small minority chronic arthritis develops years after the initial manifestations of Lyme disease. Immune complexes and cryoglobulins have been detected in both serum and synovial fluid. The erythrocyte sedimentation rate is frequently elevated.

Penicillin clears the skin disease and shortens the duration of arthritis. Non-steroidal anti-inflammatory drugs and intra-articular steroids also help. Other manifestations of the disease and their management are discussed in Chapter 7.11.30.

REFERENCES

Bacterial arthritis

Esterhai, J.L. and Gelb, I. (1991). Adult septic arthritis. *Orthopedic Clinics of North America* **22**, 503–14.

Gardner, G.C. and Weisman, M.H. (1990). Pyarthrosis in patients with rheumatoid arthritis: a report of 13 cases and a review of the literature from the past 40 years. *American Journal of Medicine* **88**, 503–11.

Petty, R.E. (1990). Septic arthritis and osteomyelitis in children. *Current Opinion in Rheumatology* **2**, 616–21.

***Brucella* arthritis**

Gotuzzo, E., *et al.* (1982). Articular involvement in human brucellosis: a retrospective analysis of 304 cases. *Seminars in Arthritis and Rheumatism* **12**, 245–55.

Gonococcal arthritis

Masi, A.T. and Eisenstein, B.I. (1981). Disseminated gonococcal infection and gonococcal arthritis. *Seminars in Arthritis and Rheumatism* **10**, 173–98.

Meningococcal arthritis

Kidd, B.L., Hart, H.H., and Grigor, R.R. (1985). Clinical features of meningococcal arthritis: a report of four cases. *Annals of the Rheumatic Diseases* **44**, 790–2.

Arthritis due to mycobacteria and fungi

Dall, L., Long, L., and Stanford, J. (1989). Poncet's disease: tuberculous rheumatism. *Review of Infectious Disease* **11**, 105–7.

Evanchick, C.C., Davis, D.E., and Harrington, T.M. (1986). Tuberculosis of peripheral joints: an often missed diagnosis. *Journal of Rheumatology* **13**, 187–9.

Fungal arthritis

Bayer, A.S. and Guze, L.B. (1979). Fungal arthritis II. Coccidiodal synovitis: clinical, diagnostic, therapeutic, prognostic considerations. *Seminars in Arthritis and Rheumatism* **8**, 200–11.

Bayer, A.S., Scott, V.G., and Guze, L.B. (1979). Fungal arthritis IV. Blastomycotic arthritis. *Seminars in Arthritis and Rheumatism* **9**, 145–51.

Bayer, A.S., Scott, V.J., and Guze, L.B. (1979). Fungal arthritis III. Sporotrichal arthritis. *Seminars in Arthritis and Rheumatism* **9**, 66–74.

Campen, D.H., Daufman, R.L., and Beardmore, T.D. (1990). *Candida* septic arthritis in rheumatoid arthritis. *Journal of Rheumatology* **17**, 86–8.

Viral arthritis

Calabrese, L.H., Kelley, D.M., Myers, A., O'Connell, M., and Easley, K. (1991). Rheumatic symptoms and human immunodeficiency virus infection. *Arthritis and Rheumatism* **34**, 257–63.

Inman, R.D. (1982). Rheumatic manifestations of hepatitis B infection. *Seminars in Arthritis and Rheumatism* **11**, 406–20.

Gordon, S.C. and Lauter, C.B. (1984). Mumps arthritis: a review of the literature. *Review of Infectious Diseases* **6**, 338–44.

Rotbart, H.A. (1990). Human parvovirus infections. *Annual Review of Medicine* **41**, 25–34.

Smith, C.A., Petty, R.E., and Tingle, A.J. (1987). Rubella virus and arthritis. *Rheumatic Disease Clinics of North America* **13**, 265–74.

Tesh, R.B. (1982). Arthritides caused by mosquito-borne viruses. *Annual Review of Medicine* **33**, 31–40.

Arthritis due to spirochaetal infections
Cooper, J.D. and Schoen, R.T. (1992). Epidemiology, clinical features and diagnosis of Lyme disease. *Current Opinion in Rheumatology* **4**, 520–8.

Reginato, A.J. and Falasca, G. (1988). Immunologic and musculoskeletal manifestations of syphilis. In *Infections in the rheumatic diseases*, (ed. L. Espinoza, D. Goldenberg, F. Arnett, and G. Alarcon), pp. 215–28, Grune and Stratton, Orlando.

18.10 Miscellaneous conditions

B. Hazleman

Joint symptoms may be either the presenting feature, or major component of many conditions. These include metabolic disorders, blood dyscrasias, sarcoidosis, neoplasia, and amyloidosis. The pattern of joint involvement and the accompanying systemic features help in this differentiation but diagnosis requires a careful assessment of the history and physical signs and an accurate interpretation of laboratory tests.

Dermatological disorders

ACNE ARTHRALGIA AND ARTHRITIS

Severe acne may be associated with myalgias, arthralgia, and non-septic joint effusions. Large joints are usually involved. Most reported cases have been in young males. There is a tendency for improvement with resolution of the acne.

An arthritis can be present which resembles psoriatic arthritis or rheumatoid arthritis. These patients have severe acne, palmar and plantar pustules, hyperostotic reactions (particularly in the clavicles and sternum), sacroiliitis, and peripheral inflammatory arthritis.

ERYTHEMA NODOSUM

Joint manifestations occur in about 75 per cent of patients with erythema nodosum. Arthralgia is more common than a synovitis and can precede the appearance of skin lesions. A symmetrical synovitis occurs in one-third of patients, usually involving the knees and ankles, but it can involve wrists, elbows, small joints of the hands, and shoulders. The affected joints are painful, tender, and stiff, with synovial thickening and effusion. The presence of erythema nodosum around the ankles may be confused with involvement of these joints, because of the redness and swelling with pain and stiffness on movement which arise from the skin and subcutaneous lesions.

Erythema nodosum is considered to be an allergic cutaneous vasculitis or a hypersensitivity response to a number of agents, including streptococcal infection, sarcoidosis, tuberculosis, meningococcal and fungal infections, Crohn's disease, and ulcerative colitis and drug therapy, particularly sulphonamides.

The synovitis is self-limiting and non-erosive. Anti-inflammatory drugs usually provide effective relief, but corticosteroid therapy may be necessary.

HAEMANGIOMA OF SYNOVIUM

True haemangiomas of the synovium or joint capsule are rare and most are associated with soft-tissue vascular abnormalities, particularly arteriovenous malformations or skin vascular lesions. The most common symptoms include unilateral intermittent joint pain and enlargement with subsequent limitation of movement.

Therapy for a localized haemangioma of the joint is excision of the tumour. However, those lesions associated with soft-tissue vascular mal-formations may have recurrences due to the extensive vascular abnormalities. Radiation therapy has been advocated in such cases, with mixed results.

PYODERMA GANGRENOSUM

This painful, non-infective, ulcerating skin lesion of unknown aetiology may be associated with ulcerative colitis, rheumatoid arthritis, a paraproteinaemia, or occur without an identifiable underlying disorder. A seronegative, progressive, symmetrical erosive polyarthritis has been described, and about 30 per cent of patients have arthralgia or arthritis. The arthritis may develop before and is unrelated to the activity of the skin lesion. It is unlike rheumatoid arthritis in that the joints involved include the first carpometacarpal and terminal interphalangeal joints, in addition to the elbows, temporomandibular joints, and cervical spine. Depressed complement levels in synovial fluid suggest immune complex deposition, but skin histology does not reveal arteritis or immune complex deposition.

SWEET'S SYNDROME

The characteristic tender, red or purple, discrete skin plaques are associated with myalgias, arthralgias, or non-inflammatory joint effusions, manifestations which usually resolve over 2 to 3 months. Sjögren's syndrome and a facial rash have been reported to coincide in some cases, causing confusion with systemic lupus erythematosus.

Endocrine and metabolic disorders

AMYLOID ARTHROPATHY (SEE ALSO SECTION 11)

Articular involvement has been described most frequently in cases of myeloma associated amyloidosis, and is also present in primary generalized amyloidosis. In most instances, the associated monoclonal protein is either a κ Bence Jones protein or an intact immunoglobulin with a κ light chain. Arthropathy is not a significant feature of secondary amyloidosis nor of familial amyloidosis.

Amyloid arthritis can mimic a number of rheumatic diseases, presenting as it does with a symmetrical peripheral arthritis associated with nodules, morning stiffness, and fatigue. Small and large joint involvement can occur. The initial symptoms of pain and stiffness are associated later with soft-tissue flexion contractures of the hands. The joints are often swollen, firm, and occasionally mildly tender, but without redness or severe tenderness. The shoulder may be prominently involved, giving the appearance of a 'padded shoulder'. Subcutaneous nodules are present in 70 per cent of patients. An associated carpal tunnel syndrome is often present; amyloidosis should always be excluded in cases of apparently idiopathic carpal tunnel syndrome occurring in middle-aged and elderly men, by histopathological examination of tissue removed at operation.

Synovial fluid analysis usually reveals a non-inflammatory fluid but staining of sediment by Congo red and examination under polarized light may reveal amyloid deposits in fragments of synovial villi. Radiographs show osteoporosis or lytic lesions, but erosions are rare. Large deposits in bone stimulate neoplasms and can lead to pathological features.

HYPERLIPOPROTEINAEMIA AND JOINT SYMPTOMS

Articular symptoms may occur with type II and type IV hyperlipoproteinaemia. Type II hyperlipoproteinaemia (high total cholesterol and low density lipoprotein) may cause a migratory polyarthritis affecting small and large peripheral joints which resembles rheumatic fever. Xanthomata may produce tendon nodules and involve bone with the formation of peri-articular bone cysts.

In type IV hyperlipoproteinaemia (characterized by an increase in plasma triglyceride and very low density lipoprotein levels) the onset of musculoskeletal symptoms occurs later than those in type II, most usually in the early forties. The most frequent joint complaints are of morning stiffness, pain on movement, or joint tenderness. There is little evidence of joint inflammation, despite the intensity of joint pain.

HYPERPARATHYROIDISM (SEE ALSO SECTION 12)

This may present with musculoskeletal complaints. Arthralgia then usually affects hands, wrists, and, when persistent, is an indication for parathyroidectomy. Muscle weakness and pain may also be a prominent feature, affecting over 50 per cent of patients; improvement can follow parathyroidectomy.

Three types of arthropathy are reported:

(1) subchondrial bone lesions due to bone disease with loss of the integrity of the subchondral plate;
(2) hyperuricaemia and gout;
(3) articular chondrocalcinosis and pseudogout.

The mechanism by which chondrocalcinosis occurs in primary hyperparathyroidism is still not understood.

Osteitis fibrosa cystica, the pathognomonic form of skeletal disease, usually manifests as bone pain, but is declining in frequency with earlier diagnosis.

OCHRONOSIS

In ochronosis or alkaptonuria, homogentisic acid accumulates in cartilage, causing it to become leathery and rigid, and thus prone to rapid degeneration. This affects the spinal joints in particular, the disc spaces becoming thin and ragged. Any peripheral joint may also be affected and severe disability may result.

The diagnosis is usually obvious, homogentisic acid appearing in the urine causing it to go black on exposure to the light or on alkalinization. The deposits in the cartilage of the ear or in the sclera also become blackened when exposed to light.

The treatment is that of osteoarthrosis, but in the absence of the capacity to correct the underlying metabolic abnormality it is largely ineffective.

WILSON'S DISEASE (SEE ALSO SECTION 11)

Wilson's disease not infrequently presents in childhood and this may be a reason why joint damage is less obvious than in haemochromatosis, where the mean age of onset is much later, and where age changes in cartilage may be contributory factors. Chondrocalcinosis occurs, as does bone fragmentation at the joint margins, with irregularity and sclerosis of the underlying bone. Osteochondritis and chondromalacia patellae have also been described.

The pathogenesis of the arthropathy is not understood, although copper inhibits pyrophosphatase. Joint manifestations do not correlate with other features of the disease. A lupus-like syndrome with an inflammatory polyarthritis is a known but rare accompaniment of penicillamine therapy, which is the mainstay of treatment in Wilson's disease.

Gastroenterological disorders

COELIAC DISEASE

Well-recognized musculoskeletal manifestations of coeliac disease include metabolic bone disease, muscle weakness, and a seronegative arthritis which improves on a gluten-free diet. The varied pattern of arthritis affecting hip, knee, and shoulder most frequently makes identification difficult, particularly as 50 per cent of patients have no bowel symptoms. Malaise, weight loss, and a low serum folate are useful clinical pointers.

HEPATIC DISORDERS AND ARTHRITIS

The association of hepatic disorders and arthritis is well described. Polyarthritis or arthralgia occurs in 25 per cent of patients with chronic active hepatitis. An acute self-limiting arthritis affecting large joints is described with viral hepatitis, and about 4 per cent of patients with alcoholic cirrhosis suffer from arthropathy during their illness. An erosive inflammatory arthritis commonly accompanies primary biliary cirrhosis. The arthritis is non-deforming and usually asymptomatic. The erosions are symmetrical and involve the distal small joints of the hands. Bone lesions similar to those seen in hyperlipoproteinaemia have been described and tend to be periarticular rather than true joint lesions.

Haematological disorders

ANAPHYLACTOID (HENOCH–SCHÖNLEIN) PURPURA (SEE ALSO SECTION 20)

This syndrome, due to a widespread vasculitis involving arterioles and small capillaries, can present predominantly with arthritis, particularly in children. In general the joint involvement is mild, consisting of transient, non-migratory synovitis with synovial swelling, pain, and stiffness, usually affecting more than one joint. The ankles, knees, hips, wrists, and elbows are usually affected, with a tendency to lower limb involvement. The synovial fluid is inflammatory in character. Joint destruction does not occur. The disease usually settles in 4 to 6 weeks without sequelae, but may recur.

COAGULATION DEFECTS (SEE ALSO SECTION 22)

Acute haemarthrosis is the most constant feature of severe haemophilia and, in the majority, preceding trauma does not occur. The incidence and severity of haemarthrosis are closely related to the severity of the coagulation defect in this disease and in Christmas disease. Joint bleeding usually begins before the age of 5 years but is rare before the child begins to walk and tends to recur repeatedly during childhood, after which it becomes less frequent. The preponderance of knee, elbow, and ankle bleeds over those into other joints is pronounced, and is presumably because these are hinge articulations, subject to angulatory and rotatory strain. Patients often comment that haemarthroses occur in cycles, perhaps because of associated hypertrophy and vascularity of the synovial membrane. If haemarthrosis is not treated early or adequately with factor VIII replacement, it will progress with synovial proliferation and atrophy of surrounding muscles.

In acute haemarthrosis the joint becomes hot, painful, swollen, and very tender, often with preceding sensations of prickling, increased warmth, and stiffness in the joint. Pain is the most disabling complaint and is due to a local irritant effect of blood and also to joint distension. The joint is usually held in flexion and the degree assumed is that in which the volume of the joints are maximal and the intrascapular pressure minimal.

Immediate treatment is indicated at the earliest suggestive symptom and before the development of obvious physical findings. There are four aims of treatment: to stop bleeding, to relieve pain, to maintain and restore joint function, and to prevent chronic joint changes. These aims are achieved by some or all of the following measures: clotting factor replacement, immobilization, local measures such as ice packs and elevation of the limb, aspiration, and rehabilitation. Many of these procedures can be avoided by prompt replacement therapy and, in the majority, this alone is sufficient. Pain is relieved by splinting and analgesics when necessary. Joint aspiration may be required if the haemarthrosis is under tension.

Permanent joint damage depends upon the frequency of bleeding into a joint and the length of time that blood remains in a joint. The end-stages of haemophilic arthropathy have features in common with both degenerative joint disease and long-standing rheumatoid arthritis. Joint function is lost and motion is severely restricted. There is often an associated flexion deformity, and subluxation, joint laxity, and alignment abnormalities are not uncommon. Hyperaemia of epiphyseal plates with resultant irregular overgrowth and periarticular fibrosis, both contribute to the deformity and loss of function. Once chronic joint changes have developed, treatment depends on physiotherapy, orthotic appliances, corrective plasters/traction, and reconstructive surgery.

HAEMOCHROMATOSIS

The patient with haemochromatosis who develops arthritis is nearly always a man over the age of 50. Although other clinical features of the disease is usually antedate the onset of arthritis, it can occasionally be the presenting complaint, when the first symptoms are usually in the second and third metacarpophalangeal joints, becoming more severe in the dominant hand. Early, there is minor pain on flexion of the fingers, with bony swelling of the involved joints, as in degenerative arthritis. Later, other small joints in both hands may be involved, with bony swelling and deformity, but ulnar deviation does not occur. The arthritis causes little in the way of symptoms. In a few patients more severe progressive changes take place, especially in the hip joints. Superimposed on this slowly progressive degenerative joint disease there may be attacks of acute synovitis due to pyrophosphate arthropathy; this usually involves the knees, but can involve several joints at the same time, leading to a mistaken diagnosis of rheumatoid arthritis.

The earliest radiological change is the appearance of small cysts in the metacarpal heads; prominent cystic changes can be seen in the carpal bones. In the shoulder, subchondral sclerosis occurs, and in the hips cystic changes with loss of cartilage. The most striking change is that of chondrocalcinosis affecting the knee most commonly; extra-articular sites of calcification include the tendo Achilles, the ligamentum flavum, and intervertebral discs.

The development of arthritis is not related to the length of time the patient has had evidence of haemochromatosis, but the age at which the first symptom occurs is an important determining factor, those with a later onset developing arthritis.

The calcification that occurs in articular cartilage in the intervertebral disc is due to deposition of calcium pyrophosphate dihydrate. Iron and haemosiderin can be found in the chondrocytes and synovium of untreated cases. The mechanism by which the arthritis occurs is unknown. A direct relationship with iron overload is supported by reports of identical joint lesions in secondary haemochromatosis. Pyrophosphatase inhibition by metal ions has been cited as a possible mechanism, but does not explain the distribution of the joint changes in haemochromatosis, with the predilection for the metacarpophalangeal joints, which differs from that seen in other types of idiopathic chondrocalcinosis. Venesection therapy is disappointingly ineffective in influencing the arthritis.

HAEMOGLOBINOPATHIES (SEE ALSO SECTION 22)

Sickle-cell disease is by far the most common haemoglobinopathy to produce rheumatic symptoms, but they are seen also in patients with sickle-C haemoglobin, sickle-thalassaemia, and sickle-F haemoglobin.

Expansion of the bone marrow occurs in all haemoglobinopathies associated with haemolysis but except when secondary mechanical problems have developed these changes seem to be asymptomatic. Gout and hyperuricaemia occur in about 40 per cent of adults with sickle-cell disease. Sickle-cell dactylitis may be seen in children from 6 months to 2 years of age. This consists of diffuse, symmetrical, tender, warm swelling of hands and/or feet. Infarction of marrow, cortical bone, periosteum, and periarticular tissues appear most likely to be the underlying mechanism. Patients with sickle-cell disease are susceptible to bacterial infections or osteomyelitis or, less frequently, septic arthritis.

Bone infarction and avascular necrosis is a prominent feature of sickle-cell disease and can occur in thalassaemia. The bone pains in sickle-cell crises are felt to be due largely to infarction. Aseptic necrosis of the head of the femur is the most disabling complication. Similar aseptic necrosis occurs at the humeral head, tibial condyles, and occasionally other sites.

Joint effusions involving the knee usually occur during crises and are far more common than either gout or septic arthritis. Synovial effusions are usually non-inflammatory and result from infarction of the synovium. Haemarthrosis is not uncommon.

HYPOGAMMAGLOBULINAEMIA (SEE ALSO SECTION 22)

Primary hypogammaglobulinaemia is associated with a non-erosive inflammatory synovitis in 10 to 30 per cent of patients. It resembles rheumatoid arthritis with symmetrical pain, stiffness, tenderness, and synovial swelling occurring in the small and medium-sized peripheral joints.

The natural history is variable in that the synovitis can be transient or persist for many years with continuing tenderness and effusion. Little evidence of permanent joint damage is seen. Subcutaneous nodules are occasionally found. The histology of synovium and subcutaneous nodules differs from that of rheumatoid arthritis, in that plasma cells are absent. Tests for rheumatoid factor are negative. Patients with hypogammaglobulinaemia are also prone to develop septic arthritis.

LEUKAEMIA

Joint symptoms include symmetrical or occasionally migratory polyarthritis, arthralgias, and bone pain and tenderness. Sixty per cent of patients with lymphocytic leukaemia have joint symptoms, usually involving large peripheral joints.

Acute lymphoblastic leukaemia in young children can mimic Still's disease, with fever, lymphadenopathy, and splenomegaly. An acute suppurative arthritis or haemarthrosis can occur; but aching in the limbs is more common due to sub-periosteal infiltration. Joint symptoms with a leukaemoid reaction in young children with infections, lymphoma, or neuroblastoma, may cause diagnostic confusion.

LYMPHOMA

Bone pain is a common symptom. Synovial reaction is rarely caused by direct invasion; but is most often associated with adjacent bone disease. Articular symptoms are less frequent than one might expect in view of the frequency of skeletal invasion.

SERUM SICKNESS

A generalized polyarthritis may be associated with serum sickness, usually following the therapeutic injection of foreign serum. After some 2 to 16 days an acute reaction develops consisting of fever, rash, and headache. Arthritis and arthralgia, usually of the larger joints, occurs in 50 per cent of patients. There may be transient proteinuria. These patients should be treated with antihistamines or corticosteroids.

Neoplastic disorders

THE POLYARTHRITIS OF CARCINOMA

A polyarthritis resembling rheumatoid arthritis may be the presenting manifestation of malignancy, particularly in elderly men. This is a distinct entity separate from hypertrophic osteoarthropathy and from symmetrical metastases. Although most often confused with rheumatoid disease, it has been mistaken for adult Still's disease when associated with unexplained fever. There is a close temporal relationship between the onset of a low-grade, seronegative polyarthritis and discovery of the malignancy; improvement of the joint symptoms parallels the successful treatment of the underlying tumour, and recurrence of the joint symptoms is associated with re-appearance of the tumor. Arthritis is most common in patients with carcinoma of the bronchus, prostate, or breast.

Other rheumatic disorders that may be complications of malignancy include polymyositis, secondary gout, necrotizing vasculitis, systemic sclerosis, and a syndrome resembling polymyalgia rheumatica.

HYPERTROPHIC OSTEOARTHROPATHY

This syndrome consists of chronic proliferative periostitis of the long bones, clubbing of the fingers or toes, or both, and oligo- or polyarticular synovitis. It can be primary or secondary. Diseases associated with it are usually neoplastic, inflammatory, or infectious, involving the pulmonary, cardiovascular, gastrointestinal, or hepatobiliary systems. Most cases relate to intrathoracic disease, particularly lung neoplasia. The reported incidence in primary lung tumours varies from less than 1 per cent to 10 per cent, and is seen less in small-cell carcinomas.

The cause is uncertain. A number of mechanisms have been suggested: reflex disturbance of the autonomic nervous system, toxic materials, and hormones secreted by neoplasms. Many theories involve a circulating vasodilator normally inactivated by the lungs. Relief of symptoms as well as signs may be achieved by vagotomy.

Neurological disorders

ALGODYSTROPHY (REFLEX SYMPATHETIC DYSTROPHY)— SUDEK'S ATROPHY

Algodystrophy is a term used in the European literature to describe a condition characterized by pain, vasomotor disturbance, and trophic changes usually affecting part, or the whole, of a limb. There are many synonyms, including some that refer to the autonomic features, such as reflex neurovascular atrophy. In other synonyms, for instance Sudeck's atrophy and regional migratory osteolysis, the radiological changes are highlighted. The common association with trauma is emphasized by the term postraumatic dystrophy. Involvement in particular locations has led to the use of terms such as shoulder–hand syndrome and transient osteoporosis of the hip. This confusing army of terminologies represents an attempt to describe a disorder that is poorly understood and that represents a spectrum of acute, subacute, and chronic clinical manifestations, some of which may be atypical and of varying severity.

Typical clinical features include burning pain, hyperaesthesiae, vasomotor changes, hyperhidrosis, and trophic changes. It can occur at all ages, in females more than males, and its incidence probably increases with age until late middle-age. The condition frequently follows an injury, but in up to 50 per cent of cases there may be no identified precipitating cause. Metabolic changes, such as occur in pregnancy, diabetes, and hyperlipidaemia, may contribute to the disorder. Essentially the diagnosis is a clinical one. Severity of pain out of proportion to the preceding injury and its persistence is characteristic.

Physiotherapy aimed at restoring movement and function, and hence desensitizing abnormal reflex changes, remains the main treatment. When identifiable, the underlying disorder should be treated. Physical therapy alone may be effective, but pain can make patient co-operation difficult. Analgesics may help but further measures are frequently required. Sympathetic blockade is logically the best way of suppressing the sympathetic hyperactivity, but is invasive and requires specialist techniques; multiple blocks are often required and the effect may be short-lived. Stellate ganglion or lumbar sympathetic chain blockade is achieved by infiltration with a long-acting anaesthetic such as bupivacaine hydrochloride. Guanethidine can be incorporated into an intravenous regional Bier block. These techniques are likely to be most effective given early and combined with an active intensive rehabilitation programme. Early treatment is most successful, before reflex patterns, tissue changes, and any (common) psychological response to chronic pain become relatively fixed. Algodystrophy was originally described as a self-limiting condition but in many cases it persists for years, sometimes with major disability.

NEUROPATHIC JOINTS: SYNONYM, CHARCOT'S JOINTS

Any loss of joint sensation renders that joint liable to develop a gross osteoarthrosis with prolific new bone formation and marked instability. In practice, Charcot's joints are seen in association with tabes dorsalis, syringomyelia, and diabetes mellitus. They may also occur in association with paraplegia, Charcot–Marie–Tooth disease, myelomeningocele, and leprosy. An associated pyrophosphate arthropathy leads to inflammation. The joints are usually painless, although the diabetic tarsal neuropathic joint may be painful and present a clinical and radiological appearance suggestive of sepsis.

Renal disorders

RENAL TRANSPLANTATION AND HAEMODIALYSIS

Joint disorders occurring in patients given renal replacement therapy include septic arthritis, acute episodic synovitis, and acute calcific periarthritis. In those receiving renal transplants, a transient synovitis may develop in the early postoperative period. Avascular necrosis affecting the head of the femur or lower femoral condyle is a later complication.

Disorders of uncertain aetiology

FAMILIAL MEDITERRANEAN FEVER (SEE ALSO SECTION 11)

The joint symptoms consist of episodic, recurrent attacks of synovitis marked by pain and swelling of the joint. Although less frequent than the attacks of peritonitis, they are experienced by 75 per cent of the patients and, in one-third, are the presenting feature. In some patients they may be the only feature for years, in others they dominate the clinical picture because of their severity and resulting incapacity. Protracted attacks persisting for months sometimes occur. The joints most commonly affected are the knees, ankles, and hips; occasionally more than one joint is involved and recurrent attacks usually involve the site affected originally. Fluid from the affected joint shows a high polymorphonuclear cell count and is sterile.

One of the typical features of the disease is the propensity for recovery of the joints after what appears to have been a potentially damaging arthritis. There is no treatment available to abort an attack once it has started and complete bedrest and anti-inflammatory drugs, including corticosteroids, provide no demonstrable effect. Colchicine therapy prevents attacks and secondary amyloidosis is a rare complication now that prophylactic colchicine is used routinely.

MULTICENTRIC RETICULOHISTIOCYTOSIS

This is a rare systemic disease of unknown aetiology, with a large number of synonyms. It is characterized by an infiltration of lipid-laden histiocytes and multinucleated giant cells into various tissues. The onset of the disease is usually insidious, with almost two-thirds presenting with a polyarthritis. Skin nodules may precede the arthritis or appear concurrently. Middle-aged females are most commonly affected. Rapid development of a severe incapacitating, deforming arthritis is well recognized. The interphalangeal joints are most frequently involved but other joints, including the spine, may be affected. In contrast to rheumatoid arthritis, the distal interphalangeal joints are commonly involved. Radiographs show 'punched out' bone lesions in the early stages, followed later by severe destructive changes.

Nodules appear most frequently on the face and hands, but can occur in any part of the body. They can range in number from a few to hundreds, and are light copper to reddish-brown in colour. Mucosal surfaces are also frequently involved. Associated malignant disease has been reported in 20 to 30 per cent of patients. There is no satisfactory treatment for this condition.

PALINDROMIC RHEUMATISM

Described in 1941 and derived from the Greek work meaning to recur, this episodic synovitis consists of episodes of joint pain, swelling, redness, tenderness, and stiffness, developing spontaneously and lasting from 3 to 7 days. Joints most commonly involved are the wrists and hands, knees, ankles, and elbows, with only one or two joints being involved at any one time. During the interval between attacks the joints appear normal. Up to one-third progress to develop a more typical pattern of rheumatoid arthritis. Treatment consists of anti-inflammatory drugs and, in those with frequent attacks, treatment with gold salts or penicillamine is often effective.

PIGMENTED VILLONODULAR SYNOVITIS

This is a hyperplastic overproduction of the synovial tissue of the joints, tendon sheaths, bursae, or the fibrous tissue adjacent to the tendons. It may present in the diffuse villous or villonodular form or in the localized nodular form. The localized nodular form is found almost exclusively in the tendon sheaths and peritendinous tissue. The diffuse villous and the localized nodular form are found with equal frequency in the joints. Paratendinous localized nodular synovitis (usually in the hand) is frequent, whereas diffuse villonodular synovitis is rare. It is usually found in adults with a maximum incidence between 20 and 40 years of age.

In localized nodular tenosynovitis the patient complains of a nodule in relation to a tendon sheath, it is generally not painful and is never greater than 3 cm in diameter. It causes pain only when it becomes enlarged and compresses surrounding structures, or after trauma. Impairment of tendon function is usually mild and late in its course. The histological findings of crowded and confluent nodules of yellow to brown colour are unmistakable.

The symptoms of diffuse villonodular synovitis are initially mild but long in duration. Often the diagnosis is made years after the onset of symptoms. The principal symptoms are diffuse synovial thickening, mostly confined to the knee, with recurrent effusions. The synovial fluid is often brown in colour, and the synovium itself is also brown, a feature which distinguishes it from all other conditions. The synovial membrane is greatly thickened, with long villi and numerous nodules. Macrophages from affected joints contain haemosiderin pigment.

Surgical excision of the localized nodular form is not associated with recurrence, but in the diffuse villonodular forms complete surgical excision is difficult or impossible. An yttrium synovectomy is often the first line of therapy, and radiotherapy is sometimes used to complement surgery. It is not clear whether these treatments reduce the incidence of relapse.

SARCOIDOSIS

Arthritis is the most frequent rheumatological manifestation of sarcoidosis, occurring in up to 37 per cent of patients. It is three times more common in females. Two distinct clinical patterns, acute and chronic, have been recognized in adults. An acute onset is most common. Frequently associated with erythema nodosum and hilar lymphadenopathy (Löfgren's syndrome), the synovitis is symmetrical, migratory, and most frequently affects the knees and ankles, proximal interphalangeal joints, wrists, and elbows; monoarthritis is unusual. The arthritis reaches maximal intensity within 3 days and may last from 2 weeks to 4 months. Joint deformity and destruction does not occur.

Chronic sarcoid arthritis may occur at any time in the course of the disease and may occur with acute exacerbations over a period of years. This is more common in those of African ancestry and is usually accompanied by other signs of sarcoidosis. Biopsy of synovial membrane may reveal granulomata. Radiological changes appear late, and therefore are of limited diagnostic value. The joint space may become narrowed, and mottled rarefactions and multiple 'punched out' cystic lesions can be seen in the metacarpals and phalanges.

Acute synovitis responds to salicylates or, if necessary, corticosteroids. The response to corticosteroid therapy in the chronic group is poor.

TIETZE'S SYNDROME AND COSTOCHONDRITIS

Both these disorders are characterized by inflammation of one or more costal cartilages at the costochondral junction, but the less common Tietze's syndrome is associated with local swelling while costochondritis is not. The cause is unknown; violent coughing an direct trauma are suspected of playing a role, although there is often no history of trauma. Patients of all ages can be affected, including children. In Tietze's syndrome one or more tender lumps of the upper costal cartilages gradually develop. A single costal cartilage is involved in 80 per cent of patients, the second and third being most affected. Deep breathing and coughing may produce local pain. The lumps are firm and somewhat tender, but not warm. The onset of pain may be acute or insidious. Investigations show no evidence of a generalized disorder, and only nonspecific minor inflammatory changes are found on biopsy. The course is variable; there may be spontaneous remission, or painless lumps may persist for years. If the pain is troublesome, local injections of lignocaine and/or corticosteroid preparations may give relief. The diffuse nature of costochondritis and its occurrence in an older age group make it more likely that it will be confused with visceral pain.

Costochondritis is too diffuse to inject but anti-inflammatory drugs are often effective. These syndromes should not be confused with sepsis or rheumatoid arthritis involving the manubriosternal joint.

REFERENCES

Barrow, M.V. and Holubar, K. (1969). Multicentre reticulohisticytosis. *Medicine* **48**, 287.

Bourne, J.T., Kumar, P., Huskisson, E.C., Mageed, R., Unsworth, D.S., and Wojtulewski, J. (1985). Athletes and coeliac disease. *Annals of the Rheumatic Diseases* **44**, 592–8.

Bywaters, E.G.L. (1950). The relation between heart and joint disease including 'rheumatoid heart disease' and chronic post-rheumatic arthritis (type Jaccoud). *British Heart Journal* **12**, 101.

Chamot, A.M., Benhamon, C.L., Kahn, M.F., Beraneck, L., Kaplan, G., and Prost, A. (1987). Le syndrome acne pustulose hyperostose osteite (SAPHO) – 85 observations. *Revue du Rhumatisme et des Maladies Ostea-articularies*, **54**, 187.

Cohen, A.S. and Canoso, J.J. (1975). Rheumatological aspects of amyloid disease. *Clinics in Rheumatic Diseases* **1**, 149.

Cream, J.J., Gumpel, J.M., and Peachey, R.D.G. (1970). Schönlein–Henoch purpura in the adult: a study of 77 adults with anaphylactoid or Schönlein–Henoch purpura. *Quarterly Journal of Medicine* **39**, 461.

Doury, P. (1988). Algodystrophy: reflex sympathetic dystrophy syndromes – review. *Clinical Rheumatology* **7**, 173–80.

Dumonde, D.C., Steward, M.W. and Brown, K. A. (1979). Role of microbial infection in rheumatic disease. In *Textbook of the rheumatic diseases*, (ed. J.T. Scott), p. 411. Churchill Livingstone, Edinburgh.

Duthie, R.B., Matthews, J.M., Rizza, C.R., and Steel, W.M. (1972). *The management of musculoskeletal problems in the haemophilias.* Blackwell Scientific Publications, Oxford.

Golding, D.N. and Walshe, J.M. (1977). Arthropathy of Wilson's disease. *Annals of the Rheumatic Diseases* **36**, 99.

Hamilton, E., Williams, R., Brlow, K.A., and Smith, P.M. (1968). The arthropathy of idiopathic haemochromatosis. *Quarterly Journal of Medicine* **37**, 171.

Hazleman, B. and Adebajo, A.O. (1993). Alcaptonuria. In *Connective tissue and its heritable disorders,* (ed. P. Royce and B. Steinmann). Wiley-Liss, New York.

Hench, P.S. and Rosenberg, E.F. (1941). Palindromic rheumatism. *Proceedings of the Mayo Clinic* **16**, 808.

Holt, P., Davies, M.G., and Nuki, G. (1977). Polyarthritis in association with pyoderma gangrenosum. *Annals of the Rheumatic Diseases* **36**, 285.

Khachadurion, A.K. (1968). Migratory polyarthritis in familial hypercholesterolemia (Type II hyperlipoproteinemia). *Arthritis and Rheumatism* **11**, 385.

Lansbury, J.C. (1953). Collagen disease complicating malignancy. *Annals of the Rheumatic Diseases* **12**, 301.

Loewi, G., Webster, A.D.B., and Asherson, G.L. (1975). Arthritis in immune deficiency. *Scandinavian Journal of Rheumatology* **4**, (Suppl. 8), 11.

Marx, W. and O'Connell, D. (1979). Arthritis of primary biliary cirrhosis. *Archives of Internal Medicine* **139**, 213.

Rooney, P., Ballantyne, D., and Watson Buchanan, W. (1975). Disorders of the locomotor system associated with abnormalities of lipid metabolism and the lipoidoses. *Clinics in Rheumatic Diseases* **1**, 163.

Rosenthal, R.E., Spickard, W.A., Markham, R.D., and Rhamy, R.K. (1982). Osteomyelitis of the symphysis pubis: a separate disease from osteitis pubis. Report of 3 cases and a review of the literature. *Journal of Bone and Joint Surgery* **64A**, 123–8.

Schumacher, H.R. (1975). Rheumatological manifestations of sickle-cell disease and other hereditary haemoglobinopathies. *Clinics in Rheumatic Diseases* **1**, 37.

Sohar, E., Pras, M., and Gafric, J. (1975). Familial Mediterranean fever and its articular manifestations. *Clinics in Rheumatic Diseases* **1**, 195.

Spilberg, I., Silzbach, L.E., and McEwen, C.E. (1969). The arthritis of sacroidosis. *Arthritis and Rheumatism* **12**, 126.

Truelove, C.H. (1960) Articular manifestations of erythema nodosum. *Annals of the Rheumatic Diseases* **19**, 174.

18.11 Connective tissue disorders and vasculitis

18.11.1 Introduction

C. M. BLACK AND D.C.I. SCOTT

THE SPECTRUM OF DISEASES

The connective tissue diseases comprise a group of syndromes of unknown aetiology affecting as many as 1 person in 40, often with a predilection for the female sex. Included are systemic lupus erythematosus, polymyositis and dermatomyositis, Sjögren's syndrome, scleroderma, overlap syndromes, and the vasculitides (polyarteritis nodosa, Wegener's, giant cell arteritis, etc.) (Table 1).

Although many of these illnesses in their mild forms are unlikely to have life-threatening consequences, they may be extremely debilitating and distressing, significantly reducing quality of life for the patient and his or her family. In their severe form they are life-threatening. The socioeconomic effects of these disorders are also considerable.

The connective tissue disorders have in common evidence for an autoimmune pathogenesis, which in most instances is linked to the major histocompatibility locus HLA-DR. Several can be precipitated or mimicked by exposure to drugs or chemicals in the environment, as in drug-induced lupus or scleroderma-like illnesses. A high level of clinical suspicion may be necessary in order to recognize these diseases, particularly in their evolutionary stages. The symptoms and signs are often diffuse and involve several systems, for example arthralgias, myalgias, breathlessness, chest pains, headaches, malaise, weight loss, dry eyes and mouth, nasal discharge, fever, skin rashes, and hair loss. This is particularly true of the vasculitides, systemic lupus erythematosus, and Sjögren's syndrome. Organ-specific features may be more noticeable with conditions such as myositis/dermatomyositis or the cutaneous changes found in scleroderma. The autoantibody profile may add considerable weight to the clinical features, but it must be remembered that a low titre of antinuclear antibody is found in a small percentage of the normal population (1–2 per cent) and is found more frequently in older people; that some antibodies, such as U$_1$-RNP, are found in more than one connective tissue disease and p-ANCA (antineutrophil cytoplasmic antibody) is found in more than one form of vasculitis. Because of such shared clinical features, differentiation must rest on the combination of history, physical examination, and laboratory investigations. Indeed, many patients (perhaps some 20 per cent of cases) do not fit easily into one disease entity: these patients may have true overlap syndromes fulfilling the diagnostic criteria for more than one of these diseases—the most common amongst these are scleroderma/systemic lupus erythematosus, scleroderma/polymyositis, and systemic lupus erythematosus/rheumatoid overlaps; or they have insufficient features for an established diagnosis, in which case the term undifferentiated connective tissue syndrome (UDCTS) is a more accurate description of the clinical state (Figs. 1 and 2). Attempts to classify these diseases are also complicated by the fact that many of them are heterogeneous and contain several subsets.

IMMUNOPATHOGENESIS

The pathogenic mechanisms operating in these diseases are complex and not necessarily the same in each patient. The organs that bear the brunt of the damage vary, as does the extent of injury that they sustain. For example, in systemic lupus erythematosus immune complex deposition results in widespread vasculitis. In polymyositis the pathogenic T cells make an organ-specific attack. In scleroderma the initial damage may lead to vascular compromise and increased extracellular matrix, but there is no evidence of a necrotizing vasculitis and minimal evidence of immune complex deposition.

Recent findings in immunogenetics and the identification of disease-specific antibodies show promise for identifying specific biochemical and biological markers which are strongly linked to a disease, part of a disease or a process within the disease.

The products of several major histocompatibility complex (MHC) genes appear to play an important role in connective tissue diseases and some are associated with multiple HLA antigens. Systemic lupus erythematosus is associated with a null allele at C4A (poor prevention of amino-rich immune complex formation and dissolution) and with MHC class II antigens (often on the same A1, B8, C4Q0, DR3, DR52, DQ2 haplotype). Mixed connective tissue disease, in contrast, has a strong single antibody type association (to the message and/or protein for RNP) and a strong single MHC class II association with an HLA-DR4 subgroup epitope (also shared with HLA-DR2).

Table 1 *The spectrum of the connective tissue diseases*

Disease	Major organ/system involvement	Principal immunological abnormalities
Systemic lupus erythematosus	Skin, joints, kidneys, brain, heart, lungs	AB to polynucleotides, histones, ENA phospholipids, abnormalities in T and B lymphocytes and accessory cells
Poly-/dermatomyositis	Muscle, skin, blood vessels, lungs	Disease-specific AB (e.g. anti-Jo-1) and infiltrates of T lymphocytes in muscle
Scleroderma	Skin, gut, lungs, kidneys, heart, muscle	Disease-specific AB (e.g. anti-Scl-70, anti-centromere); T-cell and cytokine abnormalities
Sjögren's syndrome	Exocrine glands, notably lacrimal and parotid	AB to ENA, SSA/Ro, SSB/La; major infiltrate of T lymphocytes in glands
Vasculitides (PAN, Wegener's, giant cell arteritis)	Skin, joints, muscles, lungs, CNS, kidneys, blood vessels of all sizes	Cellular infiltration of blood vessel walls; disease-related antibodies, c-ANCA, p-ANCA

AB, antibody; ANCA, antineutrophil cytoplasmic antibody; ENA, extractable nuclear antigen; PAN, polyarteritis nodosa; SS, Sjögren's syndrome.

All these diseases have associations with genetic polymorphisms in the MHC region. In general there are MHC class II associations with the production of IgG autoantibodies. It is not known how these antibodies relate to the pathogenesis of the primary disease, but in clinical practice they do help in subset definition. The presence of IgG antibodies and the known role of MHC class II in peptide presentation to CD4 T-cells support an important role for helper T cells in these diseases. Several of the strategies for immune intervention in connective tissue disorders utilize reagents that affect the proportion of CD4-cells.

The triggers that initiate the connective tissue diseases are still poorly understood but may represent a genetically determined host response to external factors. Depending on the disease in question, genetic factors (gender being the strongest influence), viral, environmental, and hormonal factors may all play a part. Scleroderma, for instance, is associated with the use of solvents and other chemicals, whereas drugs of various kinds can induce both systemic lupus erythematosus and scleroderma.

The mechanisms by which autoimmune processes cause damage are numerous, ranging from antibody and immune-complex mediated injury, to damage orchestrated by activated T cells, monocytes, macrophages, or mast cells, either directly or through their products, such as cytokines. The response of the tissues and the site of ultimate damage determine the diversity of the diseases we classify as connective tissue disorders.

Fig. 1 Venn diagram illustrating the overlap between systemic lupus erythematosus (SLE), polymyositis/dermatomyositis (PM/DM), and scleroderma, showing the usual overlap associated with mixed connective tissue disease (MCTD).

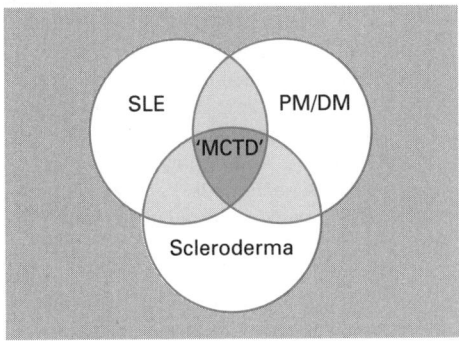

GENERAL CLINICAL CONSIDERATIONS

Connective tissue diseases present to a variety of clinicians, most commonly rheumatologists, nephrologists, or dermatologists, but not uncommonly to neurologists, infectious disease physicians, haematologists, chest physicians, or cardiologists; sometimes the major clinical features determine a surgical referral. Increasing specialization in medicine may, on occasion, hinder early diagnosis, sometimes with serious or fatal consequences.

Urgent problems

When faced with a patient with possible connective tissue disease, it may be more important to assess the severity of the disorder and the specific organ dysfunction involved than to try to find a diagnostic label. This is particularly so when delay in treatment leads to serious and irreversible morbidity or death. Among the protean manifestations of the connective tissue disorders, some constitute a medical emergency. Chief among these for the nephrologist is rapidly progressive glomerulonephritis (systemic lupus erythematosus; polyarteritis; Wegener's granulomatosis) associated or not with lung haemorrhage; or the scleroderma renal crisis, when severe hypertension needs urgent treatment. For the neurologist, presentations requiring most urgent recognition and management include fits, disturbed consciousness level, focal neurological signs, and occasionally acute tranverse myelitis. Myocardial infarction can be the result of vasculitic illnesses; pericarditis can, on occasion,

Fig. 2 Venn diagram illustrating the overlap between Fig. 1 connective tissue diseases, Sjögren's syndrome, rheumatoid arthritis, and primary vasculitis (polyarteritis nodosa, Wegener's granulomatosis, etc.).

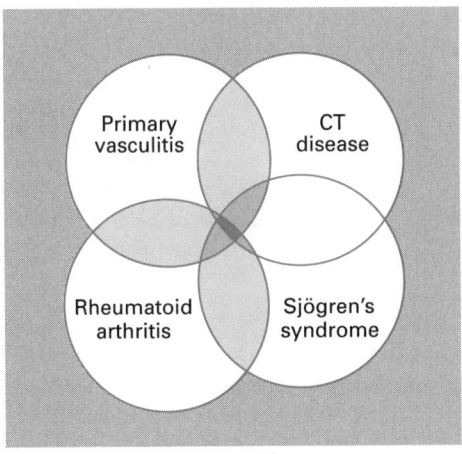

Table 2 *Antinuclear antibodies*

Staining pattern	Clinical association
Homogeneous	SLE
Rim	SLE
Speckled	Overlap syndromes, Sjögren's
Nucleolar	Scleroderma

SLE, systemic lupus erythematosus.

Table 3 *Common antibodies seen in connective tissue diseases*

Antibody	Disease
Anti-dsDNA	SLE
Anti-Sm	SLE
Anti-U$_1$RNP	SLE, overlap syndrome (MCTD)
Anti-Ro	SLE, Sjögren's
Anti-La	SLE, Sjögren's
Anticentromere	Limited cutaneous scleroderma (CREST)
Anti-Scl-70	Diffuse cutaneous scleroderma
Anti-Jo-1	Polymyositis, lung involvement
c-ANCA	Wegener's granulomatosis
p-ANCA	Microscopic PAN, other vasculitides
Anticardiolipin	SLE with thrombosis, miscarriages, etc.

ANCA, antineutrophil cytoplasmic antibody; MCTD, mixed connective tissue disease; PAN, polyarteritis nodosa; SLE, systemic lupus erythematosus.

produce tamponade; and acute myocarditis may induce complex arrhythmias or severe heart failure. Pneumonitis due to systemic lupus erythematosus, or associated with a myositic syndrome, can be life-threatening if unrecognized and treated only with antimicrobials. Acute venous or arterial thrombosis complicating the antiphospholipid antibody syndrome can affect any organ, whereas polyarteritis affecting gut vasculature can result in a surgical 'acute abdomen'.

In all these conditions prompt diagnosis is essential; too often physicians hesitate to treat because of a lack of certainty in diagnosis, which is a common problem.

DIAGNOSIS

In 'classical' cases there is no difficulty, but clinical features are not always characteristic, and may change with time as the disease evolves.

An understanding of the epidemiology of these diseases is helpful in suggesting the likely diagnosis. For example, polyarthritis in young men is more likely to be due to seronegative spondylarthritis or connective tissue disease than rheumatoid arthritis. Systemic vasculitis most commonly affects middle-aged men, but the use of newer laboratory tests (e.g. antineutrophil cytoplasmic antibody) has increased our awareness of Wegener's granulomatosis, especially in elderly women. The incidence of many other connective tissue diseases also appears to be increasing in the elderly.

Laboratory investigations sometimes conflict with clinical features, and vice versa. When a connective tissue disorder is suspected, it is common to use the presence or absence of an antinuclear antibody or extractable nuclear antigen as a screening test. Although this is a satisfactory approach in most cases, the result must not be assessed without close consideration of all the other clinical and laboratory findings. The type of staining of antinuclear antibodies, although not specific, often gives a clue to the diagnosis (Table 2). Extractable nuclear antibodies also have some common associations with specific diseases (Table 3). Anti-Scl-70 is one of the most specific of these in its association with diffuse cutaneous scleroderma, and anticentromere antibodies correlate best with benign limited scleroderma or the CREST syndrome.

One variety of the antineutrophil cytoplasmic antibody (c-ANCA) is relatively closely associated with Wegener's granuloma, but the p-ANCA is much less specific and has been found in microscopic polyarteritis, idiopathic crescentic glomerulonephritis, and a variety of other vasculitic syndromes, including Churg–Strauss syndrome, adult Henoch–Schönlein purpura, and the vasculitis of rheumatoid arthritis.

18.11.2 Small-vessel vasculitis

C. M. LOCKWOOD

INTRODUCTION

The primary systemic vasculitides are characterized by the presence of inflammation and necrosis of the blood vessels themselves, with disease outside the vasculature being subordinate to this. As such they are distinct from the secondary forms of vasculitis, which arise in the context of other pathology, for example close to a necrotic tumour or downstream from an abscess cavity. According to the site and size of vessel involved, a number of eponymously defined primary vasculitic syndromes have been recognized. However, their classification has been difficult, because so little was known about either their aetiology or pathogenesis, and much confusion has arisen. The simple classification used here, reached by recent consensus, is largely a morphological one, based on the size of vessel involved and the presence or absence of granulomata near the vasculitic lesions (Table 1). It is worth reviewing briefly the way in which difficulties with classification have arisen, since these have led to different terminologies being used for the same vasculitides in Europe and the United States; these are unfortunately still widely used in literature on both sides of the Atlantic.

The first vasculitic syndrome to be identified was in a case report by Kussmaul and Maier in 1866 which contained a classical description of a patient with polyarteritis nodosa. The autopsy revealed widespread nodular inflammation in muscular arteries which had the calibre of coronary and hepatic vessels. In 1948 Davson drew attention to two types of polyarteritis which could coexist, especially in the kidney. The first was the typical arteritis of large vessels found in polyarteritis nodosa, the second was a necrotizing glomerulonephritis or microscopic polyarteritis. How frequently polyarteritis nodosa is accompanied by microscopic polyarteritis is still debated, but the latter became recognized as a separate entity, also affecting extrarenal sites; as such it was given the term 'hypersensitivity angiitis' in the 1950s, on the basis that it might be caused by an abnormal response to drugs or infections. This approach was understandable, given that systemic vasculitis frequently presents with a fever for which antibiotic treatment is ineffective, therefore leading to the suggestion, as the vasculitis developed clinically, that the antibiotic treatment was causal. Subsequently the term 'hypersensitivity vasculitis' was used to describe idiopathic small-vessel vasculitis of the microscopic polyarteritis variety. More recently the same term was also used to describe a cutaneous leucocytoclastic vasculitis in which visceral involvement was absent or occurred only rarely: present-day assessment would probably consider the latter as an example of microscopic polyarteritis with predominantly skin involvement. To try to provide a more accurate description, consensus has now been reached that the term 'microscopic polyangiitis' should be used to indicate that a venulitis and capillaritis may be present, as well as inflammation of small arteries, in those conditions previously described as microscopic polyarteritis or hypersensitivity angiitis.

As well as the identification of polyarteritis nodosa and microscopic polyangiitis as separate syndromes, other small vessel vasculitides have emerged as entities, based largely on the pattern of organ involvement and, to a varying extent, distinctive associated pathology. Thus Henoch–Schönlein purpura is characterized by its gastrointestinal, kidney, joint, and skin symptomatology, with distinctive IgA deposition in kidney,

Table 1 *Classification of the systemic vasculitides*

	With granulomata	Without granulomata
Large vessel	Takayasu's disease Giant cell arteritis	
Medium vessel		Polyarteritis nodosa Kawasaki disease
Small vessel	Wegener's granulomatosis Churg-Strauss syndrome	Microscopic polyangitis Henoch-Schönlein purpura

gut, and skin; Wegener's granulomatosis by the granulomatous involvement of the upper respiratory tract, lungs, and kidneys; and Churg–Strauss syndrome by its asthma and peripheral eosinophilia. Most recently, Kawasaki disease has been recognized as a childhood vasculitis in which aneurysmal dilation of affected medium-sized arteries, particularly the coronary vessels, can have substantial clinical and pathological consequences.

The vasculitides considered in this chapter are restricted to those involving the small vessels; large-vessel vasculitides are considered elsewhere. The reasons for this segregation are twofold: first, there is growing evidence that autoimmune mechanisms may play an important role in the pathogenesis of small-vessel vasculitis, and, second, that similar therapeutic strategies may be useful in their management. Thus these small-vessel vasculitides will be grouped for discussion of their pathogenesis and treatment, and discussed individually as clinical syndromes.

It is important to note that, with the recent availability of the first diagnostic tests, the prevalence of small vessel vasculitis can now be appreciated. Based on clinical criteria, together with the serological identification of their associated specific circulating autoantibodies, an overall incidence rate of small vessel vasculitis of 40 per million has been derived from general population studies. This is almost certainly an underestimate, firstly, because patients with biopsy proven vasculitis do not necessarily completely fulfil all the clinical criteria and, secondly, because patients with their wide ranging manifestations of vasculitis, may present to any medical discipline, not just that performing the study. An annual incidence of 100 per million seems more likely, of which Wegener's granulomatosis forms the largest diagnostic category.

AETIOLOGY AND PATHOGENESIS

The aetiology of the small-vessel vasculitides is poorly understood. A genetic predisposition, viral or bacterial infectious agents, as well as abnormal responses to drugs, have been suggested as important factors. A weak genetic linkage of systemic vasculitis with DQw7 has been reported but not yet confirmed by other studies. Hepatitis B infection has been associated with polyarteritis nodosa and the virus identified in both circulating immune complexes and vasculitic lesions, although whether, because of the infectious load, the virus is deposited ubiquitously in any immune complex has yet to be determined. That environmental factors, such as microbial pathogens, may be important is suggested by the seasonal incidence of vasculitis, with a peak in winter in the North American population. However, whether these environmental factors are initiators or amplifiers of injury is uncertain since, for example, there is a well-documented association of vasculitis relapse after episodes of intercurrent infection. Better evidence supports the role of drugs in producing vasculitis. Both hydralazine and propylthiouracil have been reported to cause a clinical vasculitis characterized by the associated development of autoantibodies to neutrophil cytoplasmic antigens. Withdrawal of the drugs was accompanied by disappearance of the vasculitic lesions. Experimental models to study the aetiology of vasculitis have been difficult to develop, but in both the Kinjoh mouse and the Brown Norway rat the role of genetic factors in predisposing to vasculitic injury is now emerging, and in the latter the role of infection

in exacerbating the vasculitis has been found to be closely analogous to the situation in man.

Humoral autoimmunity in systemic vasculitis

A major advance in our understanding of the small-vessel vasculitides has come with the identification of circulating autoantibodies, antineutrophil cytoplasmic antibodies (ANCAs) in a variety of the syndromes that make up the spectrum of vasculitis. They can be found in the majority of untreated patients with Wegener's granulomatosis, microscopic polyangiitis, and Kawasaki disease, as well as to a variable extent in Churg–Strauss syndrome and polyarteritis nodosa. Their immunochemical properties and pathophysiological effects have led to the belief that they are important in pathogenesis.

Initially these autoantibodies were characterized by the pattern of indirect immunofluorescence which was produced when sera from patients were overlaid on to immobilized normal human polymorphonuclear leucocytes. Two binding specificities were recognized: the first a cytoplasmic granular immunofluorescence with an interlobular accentuation (c-ANCA) and the second a perinuclear (p-ANCA) pattern (Plate 1). Subsequently, the molecular nature of the ligands was identified, the target of c-ANCA being one molecule, a neutral serine proteinase, proteinase 3, those giving p-ANCA comprising a number of different molecules, including myeloperoxidase, the most frequent, as well as elastase, lysozyme, lactoferrin, and cathepsin G. Careful clinical correlation has shown that antiproteinase 3 antibodies are closely associated with the development of Wegener's granulomatosis. However, although antimyeloperoxidase antibodies are associated with the development of microscopic polyangiitis, the association is not as close as that for antiproteinase 3 antibodies and Wegener's granulomatosis: antimyeloperoxidase antibodies have been described in a number of conditions, particularly chronic inflammatory gastrointestinal lesions, such as sclerosing cholangitis, chronic active hepatitis, ulcerative colitis, and Crohn's disease. In none of these is a primary vasculitis a dominant component. Furthermore, conditions indistinguishable from microscopic polyangiitis have been described in association with ANCA with specificity for elastase, cathepsin G, and lactoferrin.

ANCA in diagnosis and management

Approximately 85 per cent of patients with untreated Wegener's granulomatosis will have antiproteinase 3 antibodies. It appears that those with limited disease are less likely to have positive serology. The presence of antiproteinase 3 antibodies in conditions other than vasculitis is exceptionally rare, and thus the presence of antiproteinase 3 antibodies has come to be recognized as highly specific for Wegener's granulomatosis. Approximately 70 per cent of patients with microscopic polyangiitis have circulating antimyeloperoxidase antibodies; as mentioned above, other antigenic specificities have been identified, notably to elastase, cathepsin G, and lactoferrin. Thus the presence of antimyeloperoxidase antibodies is a less valuable aid to diagnosis in conditions suggestive of vasculitis than is the case for antiproteinase 3 antibodies, particularly since the presence of antimyeloperoxidase antibodies is increasingly being noted in a variety of inflammatory gastrointestinal conditions. Antimyeloperoxidase antibodies have also been recorded in a number of patients with other forms of vasculitis, such as the Churg–

Strauss syndrome and polyarteritis nodosa, perhaps reflecting a component of microscopic polyangiitis in these conditions. When indirect immunfluorescence was the only diagnostic test available, false-positive ANCA tests were recorded rarely in acquired immunodeficiency syndrome (AIDS) and other chronic infections, such as infective endocarditis. However, such false-positive results have not been substantiated in studies using molecularly defined antigens.

Levels of ANCA have been shown to correlate with disease activity, and in many centres their value as a guide to management has been established. Hence, in individual patients, rising titres have often been found to be reliable predictors of relapse. Thus, in management, many physicians use ANCA as a better guide to disease activity than measurements of the acute-phase response, such as erythrocyte sedimentation rate and C-reactive protein, which were hitherto the only indices available but which are relatively non-discriminatory, varying with other intercurrent events, such as infection. Nevertheless, there are certain patients in whom high ANCA levels persist, despite little evidence of disease activity being apparent clinically, and there are others in whom vasculitis activity seemingly continues in the absence of detectable ANCA. Thus rising titres of ANCA should be viewed with caution and alert the physician to extra vigilance and readiness to treat early, rather than dictate treatment escalation.

ANCA in pathogenesis

Several studies have suggested that ANCA can stimulate polymorphonuclear leucocytes directly, by binding to membrane-expressed proteinase 3 and myeloperoxidase. As a consequence, neutrophil adhesion is increased through upregulation of the expression of the adhesion molecule CD18 and eventual activation brings about the release of injurious oxygen free radicals. Thus at inappropriate sites, for example within the microvasculature, the neutrophil may mediate endothelial cell injury and so initiate vasculitis. *In vitro* studies have confirmed the toxic effects of purified ANCA and polymorphonuclear leucocytes on cultured endothelial cells, suggesting that this is indeed a route by which vasculitic damage may occur. Other work has focused on the ability of cytokines, particularly tumour necrosis factor, to orchestrate the expression of proteinase 3 on the surface of the endothelial cell. This ligand is then the target for ANCA-mediated cytolysis. Finally, another school of thought has suggested that ANCA may inhibit the complexation of neutrophil enzymes with their physiological inactivators, such as α_1-antitrypsin. Thus tissue destruction may take place wherever inactivation of these enzymes is impeded by the autoantibodies.

Wegener's granulomatosis

Wegener's granulomatosis is a necrotizing granulomatous vasculitis which involves both the upper and lower respiratory tracts. Typically this is accompanied by a small-vessel vasculitis affecting the kidney, and to a variable extent by a vasculitis in other organs. Circulating autoantibodies to neutrophil cytoplasmic antigens, usually to proteinase 3, can be found in most untreated patients at presentation.

CLINICAL PRESENTATION

Many patients develop clinical evidence of their vasculitis against a background of non-specific symptoms such as malaise, weight loss, fever, and night sweats, reflecting a constitutional disturbance, together with evidence of multisystem disease, reflecting the pattern of vasculitic involvement. The disease has an equal sex incidence and no ethnic group is exempt. The course is variable: some patients have indolent disease which takes months or years to declare itself, during which long periods occur when the patient is relatively symptom-free; others develop fulminating life-threatening organ failure within weeks. Because any organ system may be involved, the patient may be seen first by a wide range of specialists, so that a varying spectrum of clinical involvement may be reported. However, with the predilection of the vasculitis to affect the airways, usually respiratory-tract symptoms and signs predominate.

Upper respiratory tract

Bloody, foul-smelling nasal discharge, paranasal sinus pain, nasal ulceration and septal perforation, as well as eventually a saddle nose deformity, may be present. Here involvement includes the development of chronic suppurative otitis media, due to eustachian tube blockage and occasionally painless deafness, due to eighth nerve involvement. Hoarseness or stridor may also be a feature due to granulomata developing on the vocal chords or vasculitis in the trachea producing tracheal stenosis, respectively. Granulomatous space-occupying lesions in the sinuses may erode locally, leading to fistula formation, and bacterial superinfection may be a significant clinical problem wherever the mucosal epithelium is breached (see below).

Lower respiratory tract and lungs

Chronic non-productive cough, dyspnoea, pleurisy, and haemoptysis may all reflect vasculitic injury and or development of granulomata in the airways or lung parenchyma. Occasionally, formation of exuberant endobronchial granulomatous tissue can occlude the airway and lead to segmental collapse, or more rarely an obliterative bronchiolitis may spread, sleeve-like along the bronchi or bronchioles. The extension of this into the alveolar spaces, either as a capillaritis or as a necrotizing granulomatous pneumonic process, may bring about a rapid deterioration in pulmonary function and is an ominous development when it is accompanied by lung haemorrhage, this being particularly resistant to treatment. Although on radiographs characteristically there are pulmonary nodules which may cavitate, transient pulmonary infiltrates or more permanent changes of pulmonary fibrosis may also be found.

Renal involvement

This is dealt with in detail elsewhere and has particular importance because before renal replacement therapy became widely available the prognosis of the disease was determined by the nature of the renal injury and its response to treatment. Even in the presence of normal renal function, early renal involvement may be suspected from the findings of asymptomatic proteinuria and haematuria. Renal biopsy at this stage may only show a minor focal proliferative glomerulonephritis. The tempo of the renal disease is unpredictable and the sudden deterioration in renal function, in the presence of red cell casts in the urine, may indicate the development of an acute focal necrotizing glomerular capillaritis with crescent formation, the histological hallmark of rapidly progressive nephritis. Although the glomerulus usually bears the brunt of the vasculitic injury, capillaritis may be found elsewhere in kidney, for example in the peritubular vessels, so that occasionally the histological picture may be that of a granulomatous tubulointerstitial nephritis.

The eye

Conjunctivitis, uveitis, and scleritis may all occur in Wegener's disease, but the finding of proptosis, due to retro-orbital development of granulomatous vasculitis forming a pseudotumour, is particularly important. First, in the context of respiratory-tract disease or nephritis it is strongly suggestive of Wegener's disease; second, in approximately 50 per cent of patients it causes loss of vision because of optic nerve ischaemia; and, third, due to involvement of the extraocular muscles, it may be responsible for the loss of conjugate gaze and diplopia.

Other manifestations

Most patients experience generalized myalgias and arthralgias at some stage in the disease; less frequently a symmetrical polyarthritis may develop. Occasionally the arthritis may be restricted to one or few joints. However, joint deformity is not a feature of arthritis in Wegener's granulomatosis. A variety of lesions can be found in the skin. These may vary from nailfold infarcts and purpuric rashes to isolated ulcers, vesicles, and papules. Biopsy occasionally discloses granulomata typical of Wegener's disease. Nervous system involvement is unusual but can be severely debilitating. Mononeuritis multiplex is the commonest neurological lesion; occasionally, central nervous system abnormalities are found, including isolated lesions of the cranial nerves, meningeal involvement, and stroke.

Wegener's granulomatosis affecting the heart is rare, but pericarditis and coronary arteritis have been reported, as well as arrhythmias attributed to granulomata in the conducting bundles of His. Very rarely, biopsy-proven Wegener's granulomatosis has been described in the breast, ureter, vagina, cervix, and parotid gland.

'Limited' Wegener's granulomatosis is the term given to the condition where there is only restricted involvement evident clinically, and in most patients it describes disease limited to the upper respiratory tract. Sometimes this situation may persist for many years before progression to other organ involvement occurs; occasionally subclinical disease is only discovered at autopsy. There was an impression that limited Wegener's disease ran a more benign course and was easier to treat, but with the advent of serological tests to diagnose the condition more readily it has become evident that milder forms of the generalized disease also exist and so the prognostic and therapeutic distinction is no longer evident.

DIAGNOSIS

The diagnosis may be suspected clinically from the combination of upper or lower airways disease together with renal involvement. Usually there is evidence of constitutional disturbance producing malaise, fever, night sweats, and weight loss. Biopsy confirmation may prove to be frustrating since histological evidence of a typical granulomatous vasculitis (Plate 2) is often hard to obtain in life. Usually the kidney provides the most suitable tissue, although transbronchial biopsies are also useful (Plate 3). In the kidney the diagnostic requirement is the demonstration of focal necrosis of the glomerular capillary wall in the absence of any other primary glomerular pathology. The differential diagnosis then lies between other small-vessel vasculitides, such as microscopic polyangiitis and Henoch–Schönlein purpura, systemic lupus erythematosus, or Goodpasture's syndrome associated with antiglomerular basement membrane antibodies. Immunofluorescence of the renal biopsy may be helpful in this differential since mesangial deposits of IgA are characteristic of Henoch–Schönlein disease, glomerular and extraglomerular capillary immunoglobulin deposits of any, and sometimes each, isotype, as well as complement, are found in lupus nephritis, and linear deposits of IgG along the glomerular basement membrane are the hallmark of antiglomerular basement membrane nephritis. Glomerular immunoglobulin deposits, if found at all, are typically scanty in Wegener's granulomatosis or microscopic polyarteritis, accounting for the term 'pauci-immune nephritis' often used to describe the renal lesion in both disease. Because granulomata are rarely found in the kidney, further distinction between these two disorders has to depend on the clinical context and ANCA specificity.

Until recently there was no diagnostic laboratory test for Wegener's granulomatosis. However, growing evidence now suggests that ANCAs with specificity for proteinase 3 are closely associated with the development of the disease; rarely have autoantibodies with this specificity, validated by accepted criteria (immunoblotting, immunoprecipitation, and competitive inhibition studies using pure molecular species), been reported in other conditions, and in none consistently. Thus antiproteinase 3 antibodies are proving to be valuable for the diagnosis of Wegener's granulomatosis, frequently alerting the physician to the need for careful evaluation of multisystem symptomatology and close supervision during follow-up of a suspected case. As mentioned above, these antibodies can be found in 85 per cent of untreated patients with generalized disease and in approximately 60 per cent of those with limited Wegener's granulomatosis. Other abnormal laboratory findings, char-

acteristic of any small-vessel vasculitis in the untreated acute phase, include, almost invariably, normochromic normocytic anaemia, neutrophil leucocytosis, thrombocytosis, and evidence of an acute-phase response (raised erythrocyte sedimentation rate and C-reactive protein), as well as, in 80 per cent of patients, a polyclonal increase in immunoglobulins and, in 50 per cent, a positive rheumatoid factor.

DIFFERENTIAL DIAGNOSIS

The clinical presentation, with pulmonary and renal involvement together with distinctive serology, has made the differential diagnosis of the patient with Wegener's granulomatosis relatively straightforward. Atypical forms, either with limited disease expression or negative serology, may still cause problems. In such circumstances lung tumours or other causes of granulomatous change, such as tuberculosis or sarcoid may be suspected. Differentiation from other vasculitides or connective tissue diseases may be troublesome, and distinction from the pulmonary renal presentation of Goodpasture's syndrome may be difficult because the two can coexist; it, however, is important because the implications for treatment are different. The presence of circulating antiglomerular basement membrane antibodies in patients with Goodpasture's syndrome is usually helpful here.

Idiopathic 'lethal' midline granuloma may present with features suggestive of Wegener's disease limited to the head and neck. This condition is now thought to be a variant of a T-cell lymphoma which is locally invasive and not found elsewhere other than the head and neck. Unlike Wegener's disease, it may produce destructive ulceration of facial tissues, although both can erode through upper airways. In idiopathic midline granuloma, laboratory tests reflect the absence of inflammatory vasculitis with near normal erythrocyte sedimentation rate or C-reactive protein and absence of neutrophilia or thrombocytosis.

Lymphomatoid granulomatosis is extremely rare but closely resembles Wegener's granulomatosis in the multisystem distribution of tissue involvement, where it can affect lungs, kidney, upper respiratory tract, and central nervous system. It differs from Wegener's disease in the nature of the blood vessel involvement, with an absence of an inflammatory infiltrate: instead the vessel destruction appears to be mediated by infiltrates of lymphocytes of either T- or B-cell lineage. In approximately half the patients lymphomatous transformation eventually occurs. In keeping with absence of the inflammatory component, a raised C-reactive protein, erythrocyte sedimentation rate, and neutrophilia are usually not found.

Microscopic polyangiitis

Microscopic polyangiitis is a small-vessel vasculitis which may affect any organ in the body, either individually or in multisystem fashion. However, disease limited to a single organ is not uncommon, being well described for kidney, gut, and skin, although evolution to a multisystem disease may occur up to several years after presentation. Circulating autoantibodies to a variety of neutrophil cytoplasm antigens, predominantly myeloperoxidase, can be found in many patients.

CLINICAL PRESENTATION

The disease has an equal sex incidence and is not restricted by age or race. Constitutional disturbance manifested by fever, night sweats, weight loss, and profound malaise is common and it may not be for some weeks before organ-specific symptoms arise. In one-third of the patients an influenza-like prodromal illness may occur prior to presentation.

Renal involvement

The kidney is almost always involved in microscopic polyangiitis, and up to 100 per cent of patients in some series have proteinuria and haematuria during their illness. Although occasionally mild at first, more frequently there is a glomerulonephritis of moderate severity, which may run a rapidly progressive course. However, it is not possible to predict the outcome, based on the level of plasma creatinine at referral. Renal biopsy usually, but not always, reflects the severity of the vasculitis (Plate 4), the presence of focal necrosis of glomerular capillary walls supporting the diagnosis. For some time nephrologists have recognized idiopathic rapidly progressive nephritis as a *forme fruste* of microscopic polyangiitis limited to the kidney, which should be treated in the same way as generalized polyangiitis.

Lung involvement

This may present with cough, pleurisy, dyspnoea, or haemoptysis. Radiologically there may be transient infiltrates or segmental atelectasis. The most serious complication is lung haemorrhage which can be profuse and occasionally fatal.

Other manifestations

Purpuric rashes (Plate 5) are common and splinter haemorrhages may be found. Arthralgias are a frequent complaint, the joint involvement usually being symmetrical; however, arthritis is less usual and joint deformation is not a feature of this vasculitis. Mononeuritis multiplex is a particularly debilitating complication of microscopic polyangiitis. Gastrointestinal symptomatology may include non-specific abdominal pains, diarrhoea, or gastrointestinal haemorrhage. Although sometimes present, patients with microscopic polyarteritis do not frequently have nasopharyngeal or ocular symptoms, in contrast to patients with Wegener's granulomatosis; nor do they have asthma and flitting pulmonary infiltrates, in contrast to those with the Churg–Strauss syndrome; nor do they present with severe hypertension and large viscus perforation or organ infarction, as may occur in polyarteritis nodosa.

DIAGNOSIS

This may be suspected clinically in a patient in whom constitutional symptoms of malaise, fever, weight loss, and night sweats have failed to be accounted for by an infective or neoplastic aetiology and in whom there is evidence of multiple organ dysfunction. Confirmation of the diagnosis may come from biopsy of the affected organ, of which the best is usually the kidney, although segmental vascular necrosis with an inflammatory cell infiltrate at any site may provide a useful clue to the diagnosis. However, it must be remembered that these pathological changes may be seen near epithelial surfaces which have been breached due to a variety of causes, infective, traumatic, or neoplastic, or in association with other pathologies such as tumour, abscess cavity formation, or in other connective tissue diseases such as rheumatoid arthritis and systemic lupus erythematosus. The finding of focal segmental necrosis of glomerular capillary walls does, however, restrict the diagnosis to microscopic polyangiitis or to other small-vessel pathologies, such as found in Wegener's granulomatosis, systemic lupus, Goodpasture's syndrome, cryoglobulinaemia, or Henoch–Schönlein purpura. The first four of these have distinctive circulating immunoglobulins: autoantibodies to proteinase 3, DNA, glomerular basement membrane, or cryoglobulins, respectively. All have characteristic deposits of immunoglobulin in the renal biopsy except microscopic polyangiitis and Wegener's granulomatosis, where such deposits are not found.

The detection of circulating antibodies to neutrophil cytoplasmic antigens has contributed greatly to the laboratory diagnosis of microscopic polyangiitis. Usually these have specificity for myeloperoxidase, but occasionally identical clinical syndromes present with autoantibodies to other neutrophil cytoplasmic antigens, such as lactoferrin, elastase, and cathepsin G. In the right clinical context, the detection of these antibodies is very helpful, but it must be remembered that autoantibodies with similar specificities may be found in a number of other conditions which are not primary vasculitides, for example, inflammatory gastrointestinal diseases, such as chronic active hepatitis, sclerosing cholangitis, Crohn's disease, and ulcerative colitis. Other laboratory investigations which are almost invariably abnormal, as in other vasculitides, include a normochromic normocytic anaemia, raised erythrocyte sedimentation rate or C-reactive protein and a neutrophilia. Frequently there is thrombocythaemia as well as hyperglobulinaemia, and occasionally positive rheumatoid factors may be found.

DIFFERENTIAL DIAGNOSIS

This usually has to be considered amongst three categories of patients, those presenting with pyrexia of unknown origin, with malignancies, and with covert infection. The differential diagnosis may be particularly difficult since vasculitis may be evident as a rash in patients from any of those, for example associated with sarcoid or endocarditis in those with pyrexia of unknown origin, with carcinoma or leukaemia in those with malignancy, or with tuberculosis or syphilis in those with infection. All of these disorders may also show additional multisystem involvement due to the underlying disease. Hence, such diagnostic problems underscore the importance of ANCA detection, since in none of the preceding conditions have ANCAs consistently been found.

Polyarteritis nodosa

Polyarteritis nodosa is a vasculitis of medium-sized arteries in which aneurysm formation is a frequent occurrence. The clinical manifestations reflect the size of vessel involved: major organ infarction may affect the gut, renal, or cerebral vasculature. Moderate to severe hypertension is common. In many patients an overlap with microscopic polyangiitis is apparent clinically and at biopsy. Circulating ANCAs are rarely found, and when present may indicate the coincident development of the smaller-vessel vasculitis. An association with hepatitis B antigenaemia is evident in certain patient populations.

CLINICAL PRESENTATION

The disease may present at any age and is more common in men (male to female ratio 2:1). Constitutional disturbance with tachycardia, fever, and weight loss is frequent and may be accompanied by striking clinical signs such as an acute abdomen, myocardial infarction, juvenile stroke, or severe hypertension.

Renal involvement

Extraglomerular arteritis rarely occurs alone (Plate 6) and often a glomerular capillaritis similar to microscopic polyarteritis is found. Thus proteinuria, haematuria, and urinary casts are evidence of renal involvement; additional clinical findings such as malignant hypertension or frank haematuria may reflect the contribution of arterial ischaemia or infarction due to larger-vessel vasculitis. Progressive renal failure was an important cause of death before renal replacement therapy was available.

Cardiac involvement

Coronary arteritis is an important cause of intractable heart failure or death due to myocardial infarction in polyarteritis. The cardiac involvement may be compounded by renovascular hypertension, and other cardiac complications include the development of an acute vasculitic pericarditis.

Gastrointestinal tract

Typically the presentation may be with severe abdominal pain or gastrointestinal haemorrhage due to mucosal ulceration or perforation. Polyarteritis may also affect single organs, mimicking acute cholecystitis, pancreatitis, or appendicitis. Liver involvement may produce a hepatitic presentation or even hepatic necrosis. However, there is no distinctive clinical entity associated with hepatitis B polyarteritis.

Skin

Cutaneous involvement may vary from vasculitic purpura or urticaria to subcutaneous haemorrhage with gangrene. The presence of palpable nodules, which may occur near to the course of superficial arteries, is a distinctive feature of polyarteritis nodosa. These may reach the size of a large pea, and can persist from days to months. Rarely these small 'nodosed' aneurysms may cause the surrounding skin to ulcerate.

Other manifestations

Arthralgias and myalgias are frequently present in polyarteritis nodosa. Neurological manifestations are rare, with stroke due to cerebral vasculitis or visual disturbance due to retinal aneurysms and haemorrhage (visible fundoscopically) being the most striking. Mononeuritis multiplex secondary to arteritis of the vasa nervorum may also produce peripheral neurological signs. Rarely, polyarteritis nodosa may be found to affect ovaries, testes, epididymis, and bladder.

DIAGNOSIS

It is unusual for the disease to present without clinical features to suggest a microscopic polyarteritis but a superimposition of substantial dysfunction of any of the major organs, together with hypertension, are useful pointers to a diagnosis of polyarteritis nodosa. The diagnosis may be confirmed by angiography or by histology of affected tissue.

There are no specific laboratory tests for polyarteritis nodosa. However, almost all patients have a normochromic normocytic anaemia, raised erythrocyte sedimentation rate or C-reactive protein, and neutrophilia.

DIFFERENTIAL DIAGNOSIS

As well as the differential diagnosis for microscopic polyarteritis, the size of vessel involved in polyarteritis nodosa makes it worth excluding two other multisystem vascular occlusive diseases. The first, thrombotic thrombocytopenic purpura is readily identified by the presence of thrombocytopenia and intravascular haemolysis; the second, Degos disease, which is an occlusive arterial disease affecting skin, gastrointestinal tract, and brain, is distinguished by its skin lesions, which are distributed centrifugally towards the extremities and undergo a typical course starting as pink-grey papules which then develop a depressed scaly centre surrounded by an elevated red margin.

Henoch–Schönlein purpura

This condition is described in Chapter 20.6. Its characteristic features generally allow confident diagnosis, but on occasion its features may overlap with, or more closely mimic, the conditions described in this chapter.

Churg–Strauss syndrome

This is probably a variant of polyarteritis in which there is a granulomatous necrotizing vasculitis predominantly affecting the lungs and to a lesser extent other organs. Typically, patients present with asthma and eosinophilia with clinical evidence of multisystem vasculitis.

CLINICAL PRESENTATION

As with other vasculitides, marked constitutional disturbance is frequently found at presentation.

The lungs

Asthma is the clinical feature which distinguishes the patient with Churg–Strauss syndrome from the other vasculitides; it is often severe and usually predates the development of the systemic vasculitis. Transient pulmonary infiltrates may be seen radiologically.

Gastrointestinal tract

There may be disturbance of bowel habit and abdominal pain due to gut vasculitis. Biopsy usually shows an eosinophilic infiltrate which may be present extensively throughout the gastrointestinal tract.

Other manifestations

Occasionally involvement of other organs similar to that seen with microscopic polyarteritis occurs. When present, mononeuritis multiplex and coronary vasculitis may prove particularly refractory to treatment.

DIAGNOSIS

This may be suspected on clinical grounds in a patient with asthma and evidence of multisystem vasculitis. Confirmation comes from demonstration of vasculitis on biopsy in which frequently the affected tissues show eosinophilic infiltrates. Moderate ($<20 \times 10^9$/l) peripheral eosinophilia is common. In occasional patients ANCAs, with specificity for myeloperoxidase, are to be found.

DIFFERENTIAL DIAGNOSIS

The main disorder to consider in the differential diagnosis is the hypereosinophilic syndrome (Chapter 15.14.3) that accompanies endomyocardial fibrosis (Löffler's endocarditis). In this condition hypereosinophilia may be intense (usually $>20 \times 10^9$/l) and the eosinophils are morphologically abnormal, displaying loss of granules and vacuole formation. Asthma is rare in the hypereosinophilic syndrome, and although involvement of other organs with eosinophilic infiltrates may occur, rarely is there evidence of overt vasculitis.

Relapsing polychondritis

This is a very rare condition in which a small-vessel vasculitis appears predominantly to affect cartilaginous structures such as the pinna of the ear, nasal cartilage, larynx, and trachea.

CLINICAL PRESENTATION

Males and females are equally affected and the onset is most frequent in the seventh decade; untreated it carries a poor prognosis. Fever, weight loss, and malaise are common at the onset.

Cartilage

Tenderness, inflammatory swelling, and eventual destruction of the cartilage, often in cyclical fashion, are the main features of relapsing polychondritis. Thus there may be gross deformation of the pinna of the ear, a saddle nose, and stridor due to collapse of the larynx or trachea. Involvement of the heart valves or aorta may produce heart failure or aneurysm, respectively.

Other manifestations

There may be episcleritis and monoarticular arthropathy as well as, infrequently, evidence of small-vessel vasculitis in other organs.

DIAGNOSIS

The diagnosis is usually made on clinical grounds, with biopsy showing necrotizing vasculitis and cartilage destruction in affected tissue. There is no specific laboratory test, but normochromic anaemia, a marked acute-phase response, and leucocytosis are frequently found.

Table 2 *Direct complications of conventional immunosuppression in Wegener's granulomatosis (n = 158)*

Cyclophosphamide		Prednisolone	
Female infertility	57%	Cushingoid features	100%
Cyclophosphamide cystitis	43%	Cataracts	21%
Hair loss	17%	Fractures	11%
Bladder cancer	3%	(aseptic necrosis 3%)	
Myelodysplasia	2%	Diabetes mellitus	8%
		(requiring insulin 3%)	
Development of malignancy*	↑ ×2.4		
Development of bladder cancer*	↑ ×33		

*Related to age and sex matched population (after Hoffman *et al.* 1992).

Kawasaki disease

This childhood form of systemic vasculitis is described in Chapter 18.11.9.

Treatment of systemic vasculitis

Cytotoxic drugs and steroids are the mainstays of treatment for the small-vessel vasculitides. Usually these are combined, at high dose, in an induction regimen to gain effective control of the disease activity at presentation, which is followed after 2 months by a lower-dose, maintenance regimen for the longer term, in which other immunosuppressive agents may substitute for the cyclophosphamide. Prophylaxis against opportunistic infection should be considered for all patients receiving cytotoxic drugs and steroids long term.

It should be noted that often these treatment regimens need to be followed long term, since particularly in Wegener's granulomatosis remissions are slow to achieve and relapses are frequent. There is thus substantial morbidity due not only to the vasculitis itself but also to the direct cumulative toxicity of the drugs themselves. (Table 2).

INDUCTION THERAPY

Empirically it has been determined that doses of cyclophosphamide at 3 mg/kg body weight (rounded down to the nearest 50 mg) are suitable for the induction regimen to control the disease at the outset. This dosage should be lowered or discontinued temporarily if the total white cell count falls to less than 4.0×10^9/l, or the neutrophil leucocyte count falls to less than 2.0×10^9/l. Cytotoxic therapy should also be modified if severe infection occurs. In the older patients, aged 55 years or over, a lower induction dose of 2 mg/kg is often given because of the greater susceptibility of the elderly to bone marrow immunosuppression and infection. Steroids are given at high dose, initially prednisolone 60 mg/day, tapering at weekly intervals until at 2 months (when possible) the patient is receiving 10 mg/day.

MAINTENANCE THERAPY

Usually cyclophosphamide can be substituted by the same dose of azathioprine at 2 months and at the same time steroid treatment may be converted to an alternate-day regimen. Both drugs may then be withdrawn gradually at 12 months.

MONITORING DISEASE ACTIVITY

Standard tests of organ function should be used to monitor the effect of treatment on disease activity. Serial measurements of the erythrocyte sedimentation rate and C-reactive protein are a useful guide as to whether the vasculitis has been brought under control, but are relatively non-specific, being elevated during intercurrent infection or by other causes of inflammation as well as by vasculitic injury. Many centres now use serial ANCA measurements to help monitor treatment, with an aim to reduce levels to background during induction therapy, withdrawing treatment at an earlier stage if control of the autoimmune response can be demonstrated in this manner. However, it must be noted that certain patients have persistently raised ANCA levels despite no evident disease activity, and also that, vice versa, a very small number of patients apparently have undetectable ANCA but continuing vasculitis.

Objective, non-invasive whole body monitoring of vasculitis inflammation is also possible using autologous, polymorphonuclear leucocytes which after isotope labelling and reinjection can be imaged using gamma-camera scanning. Sequential studies can be helpful in monitoring the effect of drug treatment or warning of relapse.

OTHER THERAPEUTIC STRATEGIES

Use of pulse dose (0.75–1 g intravenously) cyclophosphamide or prednisolone has been advocated by some. However, recent evidence suggests that pulse cyclophosphamide is less effective at maintaining remission than oral cyclophosphamide. Furthermore, since the active metabolites of cyclophosphamide are in part renally excreted, then, in patients with nephritis, lower-dose oral therapy should allow more accurate titration of dose effect. It remains to be demonstrated whether pulse dosage of prednisolone is superior for the management of systemic vasculitis.

For patients who are intolerant of cyclophosphamide, perhaps the most useful drug is azathioprine. Where disease activity is not controllable by either drug, then other immunomodulatory agents, such as methotrexate or cyclosporin A, have been tried. Although some patients benefit, as yet there is no substantial evidence to warrant their use as first-line agents in management.

The use of trimethoprim-sulphamethoxazole has enjoyed a vogue for the management of systemic vasculitis, particularly Wegener's granulomatosis. However, with the advent of better diagnostic criteria, careful exclusion of intercurrent infections (particularly a problem in Wegener's affecting the upper respiratory tract), and study of controls given trimethoprim-sulphamethoxazole alone, doubts have been cast over the efficacy of this agent.

In patients who have fulminating vasculitis, threatening vital organ function, intensive plasma exchange may be beneficial. There is now evidence from several studies that such an approach may benefit patients with severe renal vasculitis (requiring dialysis support), lung haemorrhage due to pulmonary vasculitis, or in coma due to cerebral vasculitis.

Finally, for patients with intractable vasculitis, resistant to conventional immunosuppression, a few reports now point to the value of more specific forms of immunotherapy, such as pooled high-dose intravenous immunoglobulin, 0.4 g/kg/day for 5 days, believed to exert one of its immunomodulatory effects through anti-idiotypic control of B-cell function, or humanized monoclonal antibody therapy which targets T cells.

RESPONSE TO TREATMENT
Wegener's granulomatosis and microscopic polyangiitis

Approximately 75 per cent of patients with Wegener's granulomatosis and microscopic polyangiitis treated with cytotoxic drugs and steroids will achieve complete remission. However, the rate by which patients enter remission varies, in that 60 per cent of patients with microscopic polyangiitis may gain complete remission within 2 months compared with patients with Wegener's granulomatosis, of whom only 50 per cent may have achieved remission by 12 months. Although the data are difficult to compare from different series of patients, the rate of relapse does not appear to differ between the two disorders. These occurred in approximately 50 per cent of patients, although in patients followed for long periods the remission interval could amount to several years before relapse was identified.

Henoch–Schönlein purpura

Most cases of childhood Henoch–Schönlein purpura resolve spontaneously within 2 to 3 weeks; although relapses do occur within the first 2 years, these are usually also self-limiting and permanent sequelae are rare. For patients with progressive disease, induction of remission may be effected by short courses of steroids alone, or, for resistant cases, similar regimens used for the other small-vessel vasculitides may be employed.

Polyarteritis nodosa and Churg–Strauss syndrome

The pathogenesis of these large-vessel vasculitides is not understood, although the accompaniment of a small-vessel vasculitis and occasional ANCA reactivity suggest that a similar autoimmune diathesis underlies their development. Consequently, treatment for both polyarteritis nodosa and Churg–Strauss syndrome generally follows a similar pattern to that for small-vessel vasculitis, with the minor variation that high-dose steroids (prednisolone 40–60 mg/day) may be effective when given alone initially. These are then tapered according to disease activity. Cyclophosphamide should be added if there is a slow response, or in any case where small-vessel vasculitis may also play a prominent part.

REFERENCES

Hoffman, G.S., Kerr, G.S., Leavitt, R. Y., *et al.* (1992). Wegener's granulomatosis: an analysis of 158 patients. *Annals of Internal Medicine,* **116,** 488–98.

Savage, C.O.S. and Lockwood, C.M. (1993). Systemic vasculitides. In: *Clinical aspects of immunology* (ed. D.K. Peters and P.J. Lachmann). pp. 1205–16. Blackwell, Oxford.

Savage, C.O.S., Winearls, C.G., Evans, D.J., Rees, A.J., and Lockwood, C.M. (1985). Microscopic polyarteritis: presentation, pathology and prognosis. *Quarterly Journal of Medicine,* **220,** 467–83.

18.11.3 Systemic lupus erythematosus and related disorders

M. L. SNAITH and D. A. ISENBERG

Introduction

Systemic lupus erythematosus (SLE) is variously classified as a non organ-specific autoimmune disease, as an inflammatory multisystem rheumatic disorder, or, formerly, as one of the 'collagen vascular' diseases. These classifications indicate some unease as to whether the patients with this condition should be identified by their clinical expression (multisystem, rheumatic), by the nature of the presumed aetiology (autoimmune), or their pathophysiology (collagen vascular [*sic*]).

The disease may have been recognized for centuries, but the term is ascribed to Cazenave in 1851. There is a broad spectrum of clinical features (Table 1). Patients with minor forms of the condition may continue with near normal health for many years, but eventually most present to one of various subspecialists, such as a dermatologist, rheumatologist, or nephrologist. Treatment with corticosteroids, immunosuppressives, and supportive measures such as antibiotics and antihypertensive agents has improved life expectancy somewhat in recent years; nevertheless SLE should be regarded as a serious and potentially fatal disorder, affecting as it does an otherwise predominantly healthy age group.

Epidemiology

The disease is encountered worldwide and can affect any race but is most commonly found amongst women of childbearing years. The highest frequencies are in women of Afro-Caribbean, Chinese, Asian, and South American Indian ancestry, with northern European patients on average affected to a less frequent and less severe degree. Large-scale epidemiological surveys have been sparse in some of the populations apparently most frequently affected, but reported incidences of new cases range from 4.8 cases per 100 000 population in Sweden to 7.6 in San Francisco. Prevalence ranges from 39 to 65 per 100 000 in the same studies. If age as well as ethnicity is taken into account, the prevalence and incidence in the at risk population may be even higher in certain Black female groups in the United States and in the Caribbean. Intriguingly, indigenous West Africans appear to be less affected than descendants of West Africans in North American or the Caribbean.

In population studies, the acquisition of cases will depend upon the criteria for selection. In the absence of a single screening test with a high specificity and sensitivity, the application of classification criteria has clarified the frequency of the disease. The American Rheumatism Association (ARA) (now the American College of Rheumatology) developed initial criteria, later modified to exclude Raynaud's phenomenon and to include certain specific or immunological tests (Table 2). The convention of using four ARA criteria, whether present simultaneously or sequentially, to classify patients as having definite SLE has been helpful, but patients with fewer than four criteria may still have lupus. However, with the inclusion of immunological tests the practicability of using these criteria may be different in the context of different health-care systems. It is also apparent from series emanating from different centres across the world, that there are some differences in presentation between different races, for example with regard to the expected frequency of skin disease or fever.

INFLUENCE OF HORMONES AND AGE

The majority of patients with SLE are female: most series indicate an overall ratio of 9:1 F:M; however, this ratio is less in older patients and possibly in certain racial groups. In male, and probably also female, patients there is an abnormal degree of 16-hydroxylation of oestriol. There is a relatively high frequency of SLE in Klinefelter's syndrome (XXY males), and in lupus-prone mice the disease can be manipulated very considerably by alteration in the androgen/oestrogen status of the animals (see below). Previously it was thought that pregnancy in patients with SLE was accompanied by a greater risk of flare in the puerperium, but this is now considered to have been due to a selection bias. Pregnancy is an important issue in these patients and is discussed below. SLE may develop in women long past the menopause, so that female susceptibility cannot be attributed only to the higher levels of oestrogen found in women in the reproductive phase of life.

The pattern of disease at onset in patients over the age of 50 differs from that in younger patients. There is a lower ratio of females to males and the disease seems to be less aggressive in those past middle age. The age of onset is, on average, higher in Caucasians than in those of African descent. There is a relative lack of long-term data on patients

Table 1 *The common clinical features in systemic lupus erythematosus, by system*

System	Clinical features
Musculoskeletal	Arthralgia, arthritis, myositis, tendinitis
Cardiorespiratory	Pleurisy, pericarditis, endocarditis, myocarditis, atelectasis, 'shrinking lungs'
Nervous system	Polyneuritis, cranial nerve lesions, migraine, spinal cord lesions, cerebritis, epilepsy, stroke, chorea
Urogenital	Cystitis, primary ovarian failure, miscarriages
Renal	Glomerulonephritis, tubular syndromes
Vascular	Raynaud's, vasculitis, arterial and venous thromboses
Constitutional	Fever, fatigue, anorexia, nausea
Haemopoietic	Anaemia (haemolytic or normochronic–normocytic), thrombocytopenia, lymphopenia, leucopenia, splenomegaly, lymphadenopathy
Mucocutaneous	Mucositis/ulcers, rashes, photosensitivity, alopecia
Ocular	Uveitis, retinal lesions

Table 2 *A summary of the 1982 American Rheumatism Association revised criteria for the classification of systemic lupus erythematosus*

Criterion	Definition
Malar rash	Fixed erythema, flat or raised
Discoid rash	Erythematous raised patches with adherent keratotic scaling and follicular plugging
Photosensitivity	By history or observation
Oral ulcers	Observed by a physician, usually painless
Arthritis	Non-erosive; two or more joints
Serositis	Pleuritis or pericarditis
Renal disorder	Proteinuria >0.5g/24 h or casts
Neurological disorder	Seizures (not otherwise explained) *or* psychosis
Haematological disorder	Haemolytic anaemia *or* leucopenia *or* lymphopenia *or* thrombocytopenia
Immunological disorder	Lupus erythematosus cells *or* anti-native DNA *or* anti-Sm *or* biological false positive test for syphilis
Antinuclear antibody (ANA)	ANA positive, in the absence of possible drug induction

followed through the menopause to ascertain in individuals whether the disease changes its characteristics with age and the associated change in hormonal environment.

Children can be affected in several rather distinct ways. Neonatal lupus may appear in the newborn of patients with lupus, or in babies of mothers with the autoantibody profile characteristic of lupus or a related condition. For example (Plate 1) a florid rash, splenomegaly, and thrombocytopenia were present at birth in the infant of a clinically well woman but in whom anti-Ro and anti-La antibodies were found. Another manifestation is of neonatal heartblock (see later). Finally, a small number of children, born healthy, develop juvenile lupus, which is broadly similar to the spontaneous adult disease, although often rather severe.

Clinical course

The pattern of disease is episodic. Depending upon the clinical expression, flares of disease may be superimposed upon an increasing burden of disability. Examples of this are increasing hand deformity, cutaneous scarring, intellectual blunting, or renal failure. In addition to this disease-related disability, problems may develop from treatment of the disease. For example, osteonecrosis and coronary vascular disease are both related to high-dose or a long duration of steroid treatment (Fig. 1); the effects of this are probably on vascular endothelium and also, in the case of the latter, disturbance of lipid metabolism. This makes it difficult to interpret some of the mortality data. However, if the patient survives the more active phases of the disease, there is an impression that amelioration may come with advancing years. Spontaneous remission is

more likely to occur in younger patients presenting acutely. In patients with advanced renal disease, the non-renal features may regress or remit completely, perhaps because of a degree of immune suppression caused by uraemia. The same is true after successful renal transplantation, in this case perhaps because of the associated immunosuppressive therapy.

Fig. 1 Radiograph of the femoral condyle: steroid-induced avascular necrosis (osteonecrosis).

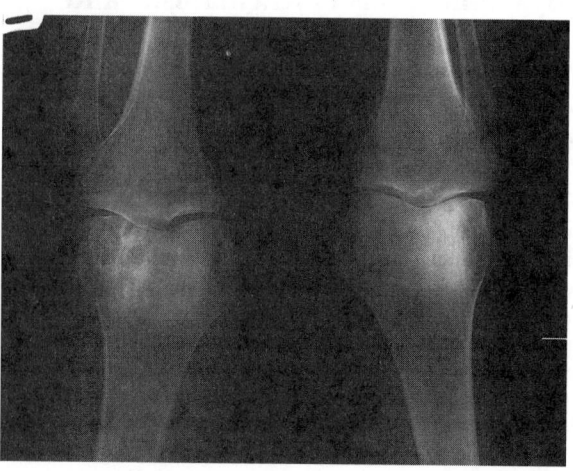

Clinical features

CONSTITUTIONAL

Probably the most common symptom is undue fatiguability. This can often be marked without evidence of involvement of any particular organ, a matter which gives rise to considerable misery. Unstable disease may also be characterized by unexplained weight change, (gain or loss) and low-grade fever. Fever should always alert the physician to the possibility of infection, but it is also a characteristic of disease flare. Lymphadenopathy, which can be gross enough to mimic lymphoma, can be regarded as a non-specific feature, which may precede disease flare by years, but is of course an illustration of the florid immunological changes of the disease.

CUTANEOUS AND MUCOSAL (SEE ALSO SECTION 24)

The skin is a target organ in over 70 per cent of cases: rashes range from erythematous lesions resembling a drug reaction to severe ulceration and scarring. Unusually rapid hair loss often heralds a flare, can proceed to alopecia and, ultimately, scarring. The classical 'butterfly rash' (Plate 2) is far from universal but is characteristic when seen. It involves the 'blush' area, perhaps because of the particular vascular reactivity in this part of the face, because of local susceptibility to vasculitis, or as a consequence of particular exposure to the sun in the area. Additional cutaneous features include non-specific rashes, apparently allergic or hypersensitive drug-induced rashes (particularly to sulphur-containing compounds and antibiotics), urticaria, and bullous lesions. About 50 per cent of patients with SLE are photosensitive and a fairly well-demarcated subgroup Subacute Cutaneous Lupus Erythematosus (Plate 3) can be identified, which is associated with the presence of anti-Ro/La antibodies. Oral ulceration is a common feature of active disease, but may be relatively painless.

VASCULAR INVOLVEMENT

The vascular theme runs throughout the disease; 20 to 30 per cent of patients have Raynaud's phenomenon (compared with up to 15 per cent of the general population), and nail-fold capillaritis, dermal infarcts, and other minor forms of vasculitis can extend to ulceration, and major vessel thrombosis, especially in the context of a coagulopathy (see below).

MUSCULOSKELETAL SYSTEM

Over 90 per cent of patients experience arthralgia, arthritis, or tendinitis. Although bone or cartilage erosions are not characteristic of SLE, as they are of rheumatoid arthritis, deformity resulting from joint capsule and/or tendon contracture may mimic the latter. The Z-deformity or 'hitch-hiker's thumb' is especially characteristic (Fig. 2). Tendinitis may be quite acute and painful and joint effusion may be painfully tense. Avascular (aseptic) osteonecrosis (Fig. 1) most frequently affects the subchondral cancellous bone of the femoral head, but other sites include the shoulder, knee, or other joints. This condition is associated with a combination of long-standing severe disease and high-dose steroid treatment. With lower long-term steroid dosage osteonecrosis is less commonly seen, but minor degrees may now be detected with isotope bone scans or magnetic resonance imaging.

RENAL INVOLVEMENT (SEE ALSO SECTION 20)

Nephritis is still probably the most likely manifestation of SLE to be associated with mortality, although with good treatment for hypertension and effective dialysis the final cause of death is usually a complication such as infection rather than uraemia itself. The presentation of nephritis may be acute, with rapid onset of an acute nephritic and/or nephrotic syndrome, or with asymptomatic haematuria or proteinuria. Urinalysis is crucial in the diagnosis, assessment, and management of

patients with lupus (Fig. 3): simple stick testing for protein and blood should be accompanied, in positive cases, by direct microscopy of a fresh uncentrifuged specimen of urine. The subject is addressed more fully in Chapter 20.5.6. It is important to recognize that a small group of patients experiences insidious loss of glomerular function as part of the antiphospholipid syndrome (see below) without haematuria or proteinuria. In this instance the major histopathological finding is of multiple, small glomerular thrombi rather than glomerulonephritis. Such patients may be better treated by anticoagulants than by immunosuppressive agents.

NEUROLOGICAL INVOLVEMENT (SEE ALSO SECTION 24)

The central nervous system is reported to be involved in about 20 per cent of patients in most series, but a much larger proportion is affected in a more subtle way: for example patients will say that they feel 'distant', a form of depersonalization. There is also the difficulty of deciding whether a patient with, for example, severe headache, can be said to have cerebral involvement. Patients may have classical or atypical migraine, and visual phenomena (teichopsia or scotomata) may feature without headache. However, less doubt arises in patients with strokes, cranial nerve palsies, fits, chorea, long-tract signs, or organic confusional states, all of which may occur as single manifestations or as part of a multifaceted clinical syndrome. There is evidence for increasing loss of intellectual function with cerebral atrophy in some patients with long-term cerebral lupus.

Fig. 2 Tendon contractures of the hand: including 'hitch-hiker's thumb' or 'Z-deformity'.

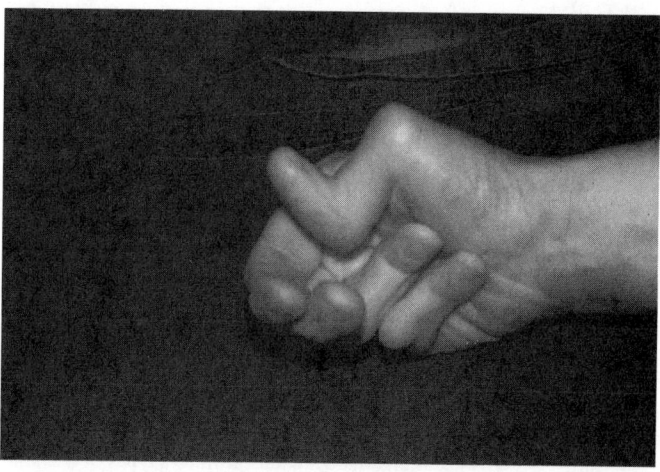

Fig. 3 An active urine sediment in lupus nephritis, with casts.

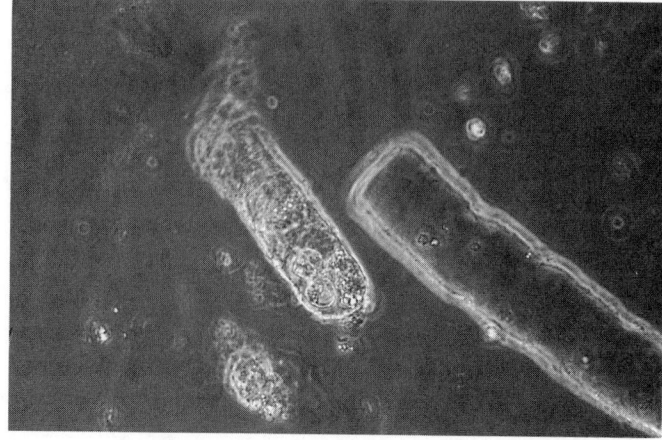

The peripheral nervous system is less commonly involved, but spinal infarction can give rise to devastating paraplegia. Cranial nerve lesions, particularly trigeminal, are curiously associated with use of non-steroidal anti-inflammatory drugs, particularly ibuprofen.

CARDIORESPIRATORY SYSTEM

The most common manifestation is serositis. A patient with lupus can give a history of an unexplained episode of pleurisy some years prior to multisystem disease. Acute chest pain with shortness of breath may be due to basal atelectasis, which over time manifests itself as 'shrinking lungs'. The pain can be confused with infective pleurisy, pulmonary infarction, or, in patients with steroid-induced osteoporosis, dorsal vertebral collapse. Primary pulmonary hypertension is a rare manifestation; pulmonary hypertension secondary to lung involvement is probably more common. Pericarditis may be acute and symptomatic, or identified only on cardiac ultrasound. Valvular involvement and Libman–Sachs endocarditis are less common clinical features, but recent Doppler ultrasound techniques suggest a greater prevalence than previously recognized, particularly among patients with severe disease.

GASTROINTESTINAL INVOLVEMENT

Sterile peritonitis is a further, rarer, example of serositis. Vasculitis may present acutely as mesenteric infarction, but usually does so in the presence of skin vasculitis. Pancreatitis is uncommon but can be severe. Elevated concentrations of transaminase enzymes are commonly found, but it is unusual for this to reflect inflammatory hepatitis and the possibility that such changes are drug induced must always be suspected. The term 'lupoid hepatitis' is confusing and should be abandoned. An episode of diarrhoea often seems to precede a flare of disease, but it is not clear if this represents a subtle manifestation of the disease process or an incidental infection which may trigger a flare.

ANAEMIA AND CYTOPENIAS

Haematological involvement is manifested commonly as a mild (but sometimes severe) normocytic, normochromic or hypochromic anaemia of chronic disease. Cytopenias are almost universal in active disease: lymphopenia and neutropenia are manifestations of the disease process itself, with lymphopenia in particular being an indicator of propensity to disease, leucopenia being more often associated with active disease. Haematological involvement may on occasion extend to pancytopenia.

Immune thrombocytopenia is a well-recognized feature, which may be the mode of presentation of SLE. It is also an important contributor to mortality. Broadly speaking, there are three different types of immune thrombocytopenia in lupus.

1. Rapid onset, with counts falling to below $10 \times 10^9/l$, usually responsive to steroid treatment;
2. Progressive severe, resistant to steroids alone and requiring considerable support with pooled immunoglobulin infusions, cytotoxic treatment, and possibly splenectomy (see below); and
3. Chronic low-grade thrombocytopenia with counts ranging from about 30 000 to 100 000, without need for aggressive management.

THE LUPUS ANTICOAGULANT AND THE ANTIPHOSPHOLIPID SYNDROME

Some patients with lupus have long been known to show positive tests for syphilis (i.e. positive Wassermann reactions or VDRL tests) without evidence of this disease pre-existing or current. An increased frequency of early miscarriage with retention of normal fertility has also long been recognized as part of the lupus syndrome. Sneddon's syndrome (livedo reticularis with cerebral thrombosis; Plate 4), in patients not otherwise identified as having lupus was described in 1965. A connection between these and other features, including thrombocytopenia, has now been recognized and appears to depend, if not directly, on the presence of antibodies to negatively charged phospholipids. These may coincide with other antibodies and clinical findings suggestive of SLE, or may be found in isolation with the associated clinical features attributed to the 'primary antiphospholipid syndrome'. The presence of these antibodies may be detected by a variety of tests, particularly for the 'lupus anticoagulant' or for anticardiolipin antibodies. The phospholipids with which these antibodies react include cardiolipin, phosphatidyl serine, phosphatidyl inositol, phosphatidic acid, and phosphatidyl glycol. Clinical manifestations of the syndrome (part of lupus or independent) include particularly venous and arterial thrombosis and recurrent miscarriage. Deep vein thrombosis without obvious precipitating cause may be complicated by thromboembolism; Budd–Chiari syndromes and renal vein thrombosis have also been described. Less common is arterial thrombosis, but this may affect any artery. An association with stroke in young people is particularly well-recognized, but events in the retinal, coronary, renal, brachial, femoral, and more distal arteries or arterioles can also occur and are not always diagnosed promptly, particularly if other features (laboratory or clinical) of SLE are absent. In the appropriate clinical context, the presence of these antibodies may be considered causative or closely related markers of the causative antibody, and should lead to treatment by long-term anticoagulation. A caveat is that such antibodies have also been described in such chronic disorders as syphilis or leprosy, and antiphospholipid antibodies (usually IgM) may appear transiently after acute infections (e.g. viral pneumonia, Epstein–Barr virus, viral hepatitis, measles, chickenpox, Lyme disease, and many others). These infection-associated antibodies are not associated with clinical manifestations and do not require treatment by anticoagulation.

CLINICAL SUBGROUPS

There is an apparent panoply of heterogeneous presentations of lupus. Nevertheless, various subgroups can be discerned within the spectrum. Not only do these patients tend to run to type but there are reasonably clearly defined autoantibody associations with the clinical syndromes. These groups are summarized in Table 3.

Investigations

Investigations will be discussed as measures of illness or inflammatory activity, as measures of disease activity, or as measures of organ structure and function.

ILLNESS OR INFLAMMATORY MEASURES

The erythrocyte sedimentation rate is a very non-specific test. Some patients may have severe cerebral disease with a normal rate, whereas others may feel and be quite well with a very raised rate, which, in such a case, probably reflects involvement of the coagulation cascade, or of hyperglobulinaemia. The C-reactive protein level, commonly raised in other inflammatory rheumatic disorders such as rheumatoid arthritis or seronegative arthropathies, tends to be normal in most patients with active SLE. It has recently been suggested that patients with active heart/lung involvement may have a raised level of C-reactive protein but in the main (although not always) a raised level in SLE implies concurrent infection. For this reason, a C-reactive protein estimation is a very useful laboratory test in the evaluation of the lupus patient with fever. In such patients culture of blood, urine and sputum are essential investigations.

Table 3 *Autoantibody associations with clinical syndromes in systemic lupus erythematosus*

Clinical syndrome	Typical autoantibody profile
Nephritis, photosensitivity, serositis	Anti-dsDNA
Photosensitivity (subacute cutaneous lupus erythematosus)	Anti-Ro/La
Neonatal lupus syndromes	Anti-Ro/La
Coagulopathy, thrombocytopenia, miscarriages, CNS syndromes	Lupus anticoagulant, antiphospholipid
Overlap features such as Raynaud's, myositis, and cardiopulmonary lesions	Anti-RNP (certain epitopes)
Drug-induced lupus (serositis, rashes, fever)	Antihistone

This table is presented in order to indicate that, contrary to the sometimes apparently random profusion of autoantibodies and clinical features, there is some consistency. These clinical syndromes are not necessarily found in their entirety in any individual patient, nor are the antibodies always found with the syndromes. Therefore it is still appropriate to recognize the overall complex as SLE, within which are several recognizable subgroups.

Leucocytosis is not necessarily observed in an infected lupus patient. Leucopenia or lymphopenia may be related to the disease, or sometimes to immunosuppressive medication.

MEASURES OF DISEASE ACTIVITY

Complement deficiency may be inherited or acquired. Inherited complement deficiency (of one of the complement proteins such as C2 or C4) carries an increased risk of developing SLE, but not necessarily of having severe disease. A low serum level of complement components (CH50, C4, or C3, measured by immunodiffusion or nephelometry) is found in most patients with active renal disease, but is less predictably helpful in other presentations. This finding is evidence of increased complement consumption, but there may also be disease-related reduced synthesis. In turn, because of the beneficial effects of complement components in solubilizing immune complexes, this may have an exacerbating effect on disease. Levels of breakdown products (e.g. C3d) fluctuate with disease flare, but the tests are not widely available and perhaps too sensitive for routine use.

Antibodies to DNA are commonly raised in patients with active lupus nephritis, less frequently when other systems are the major site of disease. It is important to test the urine regularly in lupus patients with raised anti-DNA antibodies, as renal disease may develop several years after the onset of other clinical features. Disease flare may be predicted by a rise (and in some cases, subsequent falls) in the level of anti-DNA antibodies, which should also be measured for diagnostic purposes in any patient suspected of having lupus. Enzymatic assays (enzyme-linked immunosorbent assays, ELISA) are now readily available, but users should be aware of the rather different affinity and avidity of antibodies detected with these methods compared with those using radioactively labelled DNA in immunoprecipitation (Farr) assays. The micro-organism *Crithidium lucilliae* has contributed usefully to diagnosis: its tightly coiled DNA is used as the substrate in a simple but elegant and highly specific immunofluorescent assay for double-stranded DNA. Its value lies in confirming that antibodies detected using one of the methods involving the isolation of DNA as an antigen have bound to true double-stranded DNA, especially since these antibodies are closely associated with nephritis. Antibodies to single-stranded DNA are not specific for SLE.

Most patients with active systemic lupus will demonstrate a significantly raised titre of antinuclear antibodies associated with hypocomplementaemia (low C3, C4) and raised DNA-binding antibodies. There is, however, an important entity of antinuclear antibody-negative systemic lupus erythematosus, characterized clinically by prominent cutaneous disease (in over 80 per cent of such patients) and variable joint, kidney, and neurological involvement. Despite the absence of conventional antinuclear antibodies, the presence of antibodies to Ro and La antigens in many of these patients is a useful diagnostic aid. The precise frequency of antinuclear antibody-negative lupus is unclear, but estimates of around 5 per cent have been made. It is important always therefore to consider clinical features as well as detailed immunological laboratory profiles in cases of doubt.

The titre of antibodies to phospholipid (see below) bears some relationship to thrombotic disease severity. Tests of coagulation (PKTT and Russell's viper venom test) are important for diagnosis of the lupus-associated coagulopathies.

ORGAN STRUCTURE AND FUNCTION MEASURES

These will include such investigations as renal function (e.g. proteinuria and creatinine clearance, or, preferably, glomerular filtration rate by a more accurate method); respiratory function tests; or psychological tests for cognitive dysfunction. Magnetic resonance imaging will sometimes reveal focal lesions in cerebral white matter in patients with neurological manifestations of lupus when CT scanning has been unhelpful.

Renal biopsy must be considered in a patient with clinical evidence of renal disease, but there is rarely a good reason to biopsy the kidney of a lupus patient with no evidence of nephritis. If nephritis is suspected but renal function is normal, it is justified to begin treatment without knowledge of the histological picture, which may be one of several different types. If the initial response is poor, it is helpful to know the nature of the nephritis, to determine whether to proceed to immunosuppression sooner rather than later when there is evidence of active disease, which is unlikely to respond to steroids alone. In more chronic renal disease, it is also useful to know if there is evidence of persisting, potentially reversible glomerulonephritis; whereas if there is widespread scarring and little active inflammation, it may not be helpful to persist with potentially toxic immunosuppression.

Skin biopsy is helpful not only in the assessment of a rash in a patient with known lupus, but in diagnosing a patient with suspected lupus, with or without a rash. Clinically normal skin should be biopsied in such a patient: the presence of immune complexes (C3 and immunoglobulin) in a linear band at the dermo-epidermal junction (Plate 5) is very suggestive of SLE. Lymph node biopsy may reveal the unusual but characteristic pattern of lymphorrhexis.

MONITORING

The frequency of outpatient visits will depend upon the need, the circumstances, and the facilities available. However, it cannot be stressed too strongly that sophisticated immunopathological tests are no substitute for regular careful clinical assessment.

Management and treatment

MANAGEMENT AND PASTORAL CARE

Patients with lupus tend to be female and relatively young. The social implications of this are important. The young working woman with SLE has to cope with her disease while sustaining and developing her own occupation. She is probably hopeful of eventually becoming pregnant. If she is married, her husband is likely to be of a similar age and coping with the problems of a career himself or perhaps struggling to maintain employment in a difficult economic climate. If the woman concerned has already completed her family, her children are still likely to be young and dependent upon her, or certainly unable to provide much support themselves. Whatever her situation, the questions of family planning, contraception, primary or secondary infertility, and lack of social support are all considerations with which the doctor must be sympathetic and helpful.

CONTRACEPTION AND FAMILY PLANNING

As indicated above, the probable oestrogen dependency of at least some patients with lupus raises doubt over whether oestrogen contraception should be advised. Ideally it should be avoided, certainly in the context of a thrombotic tendency. Barrier methods should be used where possible. Intrauterine contraceptive devices are usually contraindicated in a patient with any form of bleeding tendency such as thrombocytopenia or when on oral anticoagulation. Progesterone contraception is an alternative, slightly less certain strategy which can cause breakthrough bleeding.

PREGNANCY IN SLE

Whether or not pregnancy affects the severity of the disease depends largely on disease activity at the time of conception. The risk of flare caused by pregnancy or during the puerperium has been exaggerated as a result of observations on a selected series of patients. Exacerbations of SLE are less frequent in those who are in remission at the start of pregnancy. Maternal deaths, though rare, are most often recorded in patients with active renal disease at the onset of pregnancy. The timing of pregnancy therefore requires careful consideration. A patient in the early stages of SLE cannot be confident that her disease is likely to go into long-term remission in the near future; therefore one cannot usually recommend deferment of pregnancy into the late thirties with the additional inherent age-related risks over and above those of a younger primipara. This aspect of care of a patient with lupus requires time for full discussion between physician, obstetrician, the patient, and her partner.

A common concern is the fear of adverse effects on future children of medication taken to control current disease. Against this is the risk of delaying pregnancy whilst being treated with inadequate medication. The antimalarials are relatively contraindicated during pregnancy because of fetal ototoxicity. Warfarin, used for the treatment of recurrent thromboses in a patient with the phospholipid syndrome, is contraindicated because of teratogenesis. Yet to confine the treatment of the patient to corticosteroids (relatively safe during pregnancy) and ignore the possible advantages of additional treatment with antimalarials or immunosuppressive drugs, is to expose her to higher doses of prednisolone than would otherwise be required, whilst probably decreasing the chance of adequate control of the disease. Ideally one would advise choosing a time of relative clinical quiescence of the disease for pregnancy but this may be impracticable. Close collaboration between obstetrician and physician is crucial to good outcome.

There is no evidence for reduced fertility in SLE patients, but spontaneous abortions, premature labour, and perinatal deaths all occur more commonly than expected. Impairment of renal function (plasma creatinine >150 μmol/l) correlates with a poor outcome, and increased fetal loss is particularly associated with the antiphospholipid syndrome. Low dose aspirin may be a useful treatment for some women with the syndrome, but suppression of the antibody by immunosuppressive regimens is often difficult to achieve, although it may result in successful pregnancy in women with a past history of repeated fetal loss.

A particular problem of SLE during pregnancy is the development of hypertension and proteinuria which may be difficult to distinguish from pre-eclampsia. Furthermore, during the third trimester pre-eclampsia can be superimposed on SLE, increasing the difficulty of precise diagnosis. Pre-eclampsia does not cause joint, skin, or pleuritic problems, and is not associated with signs of active glomerular disease such as the presence of red cell casts in the urinary sediment. Monitoring of complement components and of anti-DNA antibodies is especially helpful in this situation.

Neonatal SLE is a rare complication of maternal SLE arising from the transfer of maternal antibodies. Features may include cardiac problems, particularly congenital heart block, classical discoid skin lesions, and more rarely haematological complications such as haemolytic anaemia or thrombocytopenia (see Plate 1 and above). The skin and haematological problems are transient and do not usually present a major difficulty. Heart block, however, may lead to heart failure *in utero* and fetal hydrops; a pacemaker may be required early after delivery. Up to 80 per cent of mothers who deliver a child with congenital heart block have antibodies to a cytoplasmic antigen designated Ro or SSA. The neonatal heart block syndrome is found in babies of about 1 in 20 mothers with Ro/La antibodies, who may have no clinical symptoms and perhaps features more suggestive of Sjögren's syndrome than of SLE. Anti-Ro antibody has also been detected in affected babies up to 3 months of age. Occasionally, neonatal disorders of this kind are the first indication of a previously unsuspected disorder in the mother.

PRECIPITATION OF FLARE

Fatigue requires sympathetic assurance from a physician; there is no specific treatment, although the antimalarials do tend to improve the relatively minor symptoms of arthralgia, skin rashes, and intermittent low-grade fever. There is anecdotal evidence that physical, mental, or emotional stress can precipitate flare. There is also some anecdotal evidence that intercurrent viral infections may be associated with a precipitation of flare. Interferon levels are raised in active SLE as part of the disease process, and therefore it is difficult to be sure whether influenza-like symptoms are due to the disease or a viral infection. Sympathetic consideration of these various factors may include, for example, advising the patient to work part time or to give up work altogether; to avoid obvious stresses such as moving house if there is an option; and to adhere to available immunization schedules. There is no evidence that any form of immunization is contraindicated in lupus. Smallpox vaccination, to be avoided in patients on steroids, is no longer required worldwide. Live polio vaccination appears to be safe.

PROGNOSIS

Patients wish to know their future. The physician is not able to foresee this with certainty, and although lupus tends to improve with age, this can by no means be guaranteed. At the same time a depressing pessimistic outlook is unhelpful to a patient having difficulty in coping with the present. A 90 per cent 10-year survival rate sounds encouraging when viewed in the context of a malignant disease such as leukaemia, but to be given a 10 per cent chance of dying in the subsequent 10 years is of no great assurance to a patient aged 20. The prognosis has improved in the past generation; this is partly due to more frequent diagnosis of milder disease but management has also got better and has greatly improved the care of renal disease, hypertension, and infection which used to be common causes of death. The late complications of atherosclerosis, manifested by premature coronary thrombosis are a cause for concern. Where opportunities exist, specialist advice from a physician experienced in managing patients with lupus is likely to provide a greater degree of confidence in patients than from one who rarely sees

Table 4 *Problem-directed treatment in systemic lupus erythematosus*

	Analgesics	NSAID	Local steroid	Physical therapy	Vascular modifiers	Antimalarials	Cortico-steroids	Immuno-suppression	Adjunctives[a]
Arthralgia	(+)	+				+	(+)		
Synovitis	(+)	+	+	+		+	(+)	(+)	(+)
Tendinitis		+	+	(+)					
Vasospasm					+				
Photosensitivity			(+)			+			+
Vasculitis					(+)	(+)	+	(+)	
Thrombosis					(+)		(+)		+
Serositis	(+)	(+)				+	(+)	(+)	
Pneumonitis							(+)	(+)	
Myositis				+			+	(+)	
Neuropathies				(+)			+	(+)	(+)
Cerebritis							(+)	(+)	(+)
Convulsions							(+)	(+)	+
Nephritis							+	+	(+)
Cytopenias							(+)	(+)	(+)
Sicca syndrome						(+)	(+)	(+)	(+)

[a]Adjunctives include (for example) local treatments for rashes or sicca symptoms, transfusions, intravenous globulin for cytopenias, etc.

+, Of clear therapeutic value; (+), of less certain effectiveness, or under specific circumstances.

This table illustrates the range of treatments which may be appropriate for patients with SLE. It is **not** prescriptive. In one individual, for example, tendonitis may be treated effectively with just a local intralesional injection of corticosteroid, and an accompanying skin rash may respond to hydroxychloroquine. In another patient active nephritis may necessitate systemic steroids and immunosuppression, rendering an antimalarial superfluous. The importance of physical therapy as part of a programme of rehabilitation in patients with locomotor or neurological disability must not be overlooked.

such patients. In large series of patients, the most important correlates with mortality have been the levels of haemoglobin and creatinine.

Treatment

PROBLEM-DIRECTED MANAGEMENT

Before considering treatment with corticosteroids, it is important to remember that there are other therapies available for individual problems. Table 4 illustrates these, with approximate indications. Antimalarial medication with hydroxychloroquine (200–400 mg/day) or chloroquine (200–250 mg/day) is useful in managing many forms of inflammatory rash, photosensitivity, fever, arthralgia, and serositis. This dose may be temporarily exceeded for hydroxychloroquine, as the risk of macular damage and blindness is much less than with chloroquine; but should be reduced in patients of body weight less than 50 kg. Regular (at least 6 monthly) ophthalmic monitoring is mandatory for patients on long-term therapy. Retinopathy due to chloroquine is more likely if the total accumulative dose exceeds 300 g. Ultraviolet barrier cream with a protection factor in excess of 15 is essential for patients with photosensitivity and is advisable in any patient with a fair skin likely to be exposed to the sun.

Anti-inflammatory medication ranging from aspirin to one of the more newly developed non-steroidal anti-inflammatory drugs may be adequate to contain minor arthralgia or provide a helpful addition to corticosteroids. The degree of risk of cranial nerve lesions with ibuprofen is not clear. Isolated convulsions may be treated appropriately with anticonvulsants. There seems to be no risk or of exacerbating established disease by the addition of a drug (e.g. procainamide or phenytoin) known to be capable of producing a drug-induced SLE syndrome.

In patients with recurrent thromboses, long-term anticoagulation is necessary. Antidepressants, antimigraine medication, and oral or depot phenothiazines are all examples where adjunctive management of particular clinical problems may be successful without necessarily requiring an increase in steroid medication. Splenectomy for immune thrombocytopenia is controversial. It seems to be most successful when combined with immunosuppression; supportive treatment with danazol or

intravenous stabilized gammaglobulin is a common requirement in persisting thrombocytopenia; the morbidity and mortality of severe (type 2, as defined above) immune thrombocytopenia are high. Raynaud's syndrome is occasionally helped by calcium-channel blockers such as nifedipine, but severe ischaemia necessitates more powerful vasodilators with antithrombotic potential, of which prostacyclin given intravenously is currently the most effective. Nifedipine, often supported by angiotensin-converting enzyme inhibitors, is also valuable in controlling the hypertension that frequently accompanies renal disease.

CORTICOSTEROIDS

Corticosteroids (principally prednisone or prednisolone) remain the mainstay for long-term management of patients with SLE. Doses for acute flare need to be of the order of 0.75 to 2.0 mg/kg body weight/day. The dose should be tapered slowly with clinical resolution but not discontinued. Most patients with SLE are best managed, even when in clinical remission, with maintenance of a low dose of prednisolone (e.g. 2.5–5.0 mg/day) perhaps for many years, with a temporary increase in dose to control any recrudescences of disease.

MANAGEMENT OF THE ACUTE FLARE

Large doses of oral prednisolone (2–3 mg/kg) can be used and are relatively well tolerated in the short term. Intravenous methylprednisolone 'pulse' infusions of 0.5 to 1.0 g, repeated daily or on alternate days three to five times, have become standard practice in managing patients with acute active lupus. Trial data indicate the efficacy of this treatment for patients with acute severe glomerulonephritis and vasculitis, but chronic progressive nephritis is better managed with a combination of immunosuppression and steroids (see below). The treatment is usually well tolerated and to offset its cost relative to oral pulses, one can be reassured that the medication has actually been taken. The infusions, given slowly over half an hour or longer, can be managed without admission to hospital, but the patient should rest under supervision for 2 or 3 h afterwards. Dose-finding studies have been rare and it may be that much smaller doses of intravenous or intramuscular prednisolone (e.g. 100–200 mg) may be just as effective as 0.5 or 1.0 g for symptomatic flare, other than active renal disease. Similarly, it is quite likely that oral prednisolone pulses are actually as effective and much cheaper than intravenous boluses for many patients and are well worth considering if inpatient facilities are limited.

Plasma exchange is usually reserved for severe unremitting multisystem disease. Large-scale trial data are lacking, but the consensus is that it is unhelpful used without simultaneous immunosuppression and that it is probably more effective if the replacement fluid includes plasma containing complement, probably aiding immune complex removal. It is not clear whether removal of antibody is crucial to its effect. It is very expensive: although mere removal of whole blood and replacement with blood transfusion is feasible and simple, to perform large-volume replacement requires sophisticated haemapheresis technology and blood products.

CYTOTOXIC OR IMMUNOSUPPRESSIVE TREATMENT

Azathioprine (1.0–2.5 mg/kg) is relatively ineffective alone, but in combination with prednisolone enables disease control with a lower dose of steroid. Cyclophosphamide is best reserved for acute flare resistant to high-dose oral prednisolone. It is probably more effective in combination with prednisolone than is azathioprine for nephritis, where monthly pulses of cyclophosphamide for at least 6 months following initial pulse treatment are recommended in order to maintain remission. There is less good evidence that it is effective in cerebral disease. Methotrexate is less well tested in lupus, but is often used in inflammatory myositis and in severe synovitis of rheumatoid arthritis and so may be an alternative treatment for patients intolerant of cyclophosphamide or azathioprine.

Precautions: A single intravenous pulse of 0.75 to 1.0 g of methylprednisolone preceding 0.5 to 1.0 g of cyclophosphamide reduces, but does not usually eliminate, the need for antiemetics such as metoclopramide; a high fluid intake during infusion of cyclophosphamide combined with mesna (sodium mercoptoethanesulphonate) reduces urothelial toxicity. Whether immunosuppressive medication in SLE operates by cytotoxic destruction of polygenic B-cell clones or by less specific effects on inflammatory cascades is uncertain. Whichever the mechanism, suppression of host defences is an inevitable consequence, with an increase in the risk of sepsis. The nadir (lowest level) of leucocytes following intravenous cyclophosphamide is at about 10 days, hence the advisability of leaving a gap of 2 weeks between infusions. Hair loss is occasionally encountered but is rarely severe. Azathioprine side-effects include raised liver enzyme levels, and methotrexate can cause hepatic fibrosis after long-term use and, rarely, pulmonary toxicity. Both may cause marrow suppression.

The biology of lupus

ANIMAL MODELS

Models of lupus have been described in dogs and in several strains of mice. The economic advantages of working with the murine strains are such that most animal model research in lupus has been done in this species. Amongst these strains, the best known are the New Zealand Black/White (NZB/W) F_1 and the MRL/lpr/lpr strain. A more recently described model, the SWR/NZB, appears to be particularly useful for studying renal disease. None of the lupus mouse strains reflects the totality of the clinical and serological features of human lupus. Rather, each model reflects particular features reminiscent of the human disease.

The NZB/NZW F_1 murine disease is clearly influenced by sex hormones. Females develop the disease by the age of 6 months, males 6 months later. The animals develop oedema, severe immune complex nephritis, haemolytic anaemia, and some degree of lymphocytic infiltration of the lacrimal and parotid glands. Thus they have features of Sjögren's syndrome as well as SLE. The animals have antibodies to erythrocytes, DNA, and RNA. The class of antibody appears to be

important in the development of the disease. Up to the age of 6 months, female NZB/W mice produce anti-DNA antibodies, primarily of the IgM class. Thereafter, and simultaneously with the onset of clinical symptoms, a class switch occurs and IgG becomes the dominant anti-DNA isotype. Many T-cell abnormalities have also been detected in this model, and there is a notable involution of the thymus at an early age, with concomitant loss of production of thymic hormones.

The female MRL/lpr mouse also suffers a more severe disease than the male. The lifespan of the female is approximately 6 to 8 months. The most notable clinical feature in these animals is the development of massive lymphoproliferation (hence the term lpr). Intriguingly, some colonies develop a deforming arthritis, with synovitis, pannus formation, and joint effusions reminiscent of rheumatoid arthritis. These mice develop a severe immune complex nephritis accompanied by antinuclear antibodies, including anti-DNA and anti-Sm antibodies.

In a recent development, it has been shown that mice carrying the lpr mutation have defects in a gene encoding the 'Fas' antigen. This antigen is a cell-surface protein that mediates the process of apoptosis (programmed cell death) and it seems likely that it has an important role in the negative selection of autoreactive T cells in the thymus. Furthermore, because the Fas antigen can be expressed in activated B lymphocytes, B-cell producing autoantibodies may survive longer in lpr mice than in normal mice and this may, at least partly, explain the excessive numbers of autoantibodies seen in this strain. Further support for a primary defect in the B lymphocyte comes from studies of a transgenic model in which a single disregulated gene, Bcl-2, capable of enhancing B-cell lifespan was shown to induce hypergammaglobulinaemia and widespread systemic autoimmunity.

AUTOANTIBODIES IN SLE

The serological hallmark of lupus is the presence of circulating autoantibodies directed against a range of plasma membrane, cytoplasmic, and, especially, nuclear antigens (Table 5). In a recent study, 98 per cent of patients had antinuclear antibodies, and 56 per cent had raised levels of antibodies to double-stranded DNA. The antibodies to double-stranded DNA thought to be associated with immunopathology are of the IgG isotype. Renal biopsies from lupus patients show the deposition of IgG and complement components, indicating a localized immune response and subsequent inflammation. Eluates from affected kidneys show that the IgG has specificity for double-stranded DNA. It is generally thought that such antibodies are cationic in charge, clonally restricted, and of relatively high affinity. The deposition of these antibodies in the kidney may be due to the trapping in the glomerulus of circulating immune complexes consisting of DNA and anti-DNA antibodies. More recently it has been suggested that anti-DNA antibodies may cross react with heparan sulphate, the glycosaminoglycan sidechain of heparan sulphate proteoglycan, which is a major constituent of the glomerular basement membrane. This binding has been reported to be mediated via bound complexes containing both DNA and histones. Histones have a very high affinity for heparan sulphate and antihistone antibodies are also a feature of systemic lupus.

Whereas anti-DNA antibodies have been identified in roughly equal proportions across the range of ethnic groups in which lupus has been studied, antibodies to Sm have shown an interesting restriction. In European Caucasian patients, the prevalence of anti-Sm antibodies is generally less than 10 per cent, whereas amongst the Afro-Caribbean population of the United States, the prevalence of anti-Sm antibodies is approximately three times higher. Antibodies to the closely associated U1 ribonucleoprotein lack this ethnic distinction and seem to be associated with relatively mild lupus, a lower incidence of renal involvement, and the major histocompatibility complex HLA-DR4 (DRβ 10401 in the new nomenclature).

Antibodies to Ro and La are more frequently associated with Sjögren's syndrome where this complicates SLE.

Recently, conflicting claims have been made about the importance of

Table 5 *Prevalence of autoantibodies in systemic lupus erythematosus*

Autoantigen	Prevalence (%)	Autoantigen	Prevalence (%)
dsDNA	40–90	Cardiolipin	20–50
ssDNA	50–70	Lupus anticoagulant	15–20
Histones	50–70	IgG Fc	20–30
Sm	5–30	Thyroglobulin	10–30
RNP	25–35	Thyroid microsomes	10–30
Ro/SSA	25–35	Red cell membrane	5–10
La/SSB	10–15	(Coombs' test)	
poly(ADP-ribose)	50–70		

The wide ranges may be accounted for by differences in laboratory technology and also in the populations of patients studied in the various reported series. For example, anti-Sm antibodies are found predominantly in black populations and only rarely in white Europeans.

Table 6 *Major cellular and cytokine abnormalities in systemic lupus erythematosus*

B lymphocytes	$\uparrow$ nos activated B cells
	Hypergammaglobulinaemia
	$\uparrow$ IgG (and some IgM) autoantibodies reacting with self-antigens (see Table 5)
	$\uparrow$ IL-2R; $\downarrow$ CR1 expression
	$\uparrow$ surface expression of hsp90 (or some component of it) but not hsp 70 or 65
T lymphocytes	$\downarrow$ CD4$^+$CD45R$^+$ subset
	$\uparrow\uparrow$ CD4$^-$8$^-$TCR$\alpha\beta^+$T helper (probably escape thymic deletion)
	In vivo studies show activated T cells are HLA class II$^+$ (DP, DR); defective suppression and impaired cytotoxicity
Cytokines	
IL-1	Either insufficient production by accessory cells or defective T-cell
IL-2	IL-1 receptor
IL-4	Normal or $\downarrow$ production by CD4$^+$ and CD8$^+$ T cells
IL-6	Increased
IL-10	Increased
TNFα	Increased especially in those with serositis
	MHC-linked production, thus:
	$\downarrow$ in DR2, DQw1 + nephritis
	$\uparrow$ in DR3, DR4, − nephritis
γ-IFN	Normal levels produced; NK cells refractory

This table reviews the abnormalities which have been most consistently described in the literature. There are some variations between reports, especially where there is a question of comparable degrees of disease activity.

Adapted from Isenberg and Horsfall (1993).

antibodies to ribosomal P-protein in lupus patients. There appear to be roughly equal numbers of reports claiming that these antibodies are, or are not, associated with cerebral involvement, in particular with psychosis.

During the past decade the development of assays to measure cardiolipin (and other phospholipids) has enabled the identification of the subgroup of lupus patients with the phospholipid syndrome discussed previously. It has become clear that the antibodies in lupus patients require an additional cofactor (β2 glycoprotein I, molecular weight 55 kDa). The combination of phospholipid and cofactor appears to bring about the formation of a new, or neo-antigen. The precise relationship between the levels of this antibody and clinical features remains obscure.

Lupus may be regarded as a disorder of intolerance of immune complexes: deposition or formation *in situ* is an important component of the immunopathology. Solubilization is probably impaired and complement deficiencies, both inherited and secondary to disease activity, are associated with the disorder (see below). Reticuloendothelial clearance of complexes is impaired in active disease. Yet the assay of immune complexes is no longer regarded as a useful measure, either as a diagnostic test or as a measure of disease activity: there is too much true variation in response to such physiological factors as sleep, rest, and food diges-

tion, and too little agreement between methods for the measurement of complexes.

In patients with drug-induced lupus syndromes, such as those due to hydralazine or procainamide, antibodies to histones H2A/B are found. The syndrome includes rashes, fever, and serositis, but rarely nephritis or cerebritis. Clinical illness only develops in a minority of the patients who become antinuclear antibody positive, which in turn is only a proportion of those treated with the relevant drug. The HLA-DR3 genotype, slow acetylation, and complement deficiencies are powerful genetic risk factors, which then require the combination of hypertension and the relevant drug for development of the disease. This interaction of genetic and environmental factors has obvious implications for the development of spontaneous SLE. Once the drug is withdrawn, the illness remits but antinuclear antibody remains positive for many months, confirming that autoantibody expression is not synonymous with clinical disease.

CELLULAR IMMUNOLOGY

Many cellular abnormalities have been identified in patients with lupus, of which the more important and consistent are shown in Table 6. The increase in activated B lymphocytes contributes to the hypergammaglobulinaemia associated with the disease. Receptors for the cytokine IL-2 are increased on circulating B cells, while the expression of CR1 (the receptor for C3b) is decreased.

Among the two major T-cell populations, there is a marked reduction of a subset bearing the CD4 and CD45Ro phenotypes. Since this population helps to induce suppression by providing a positive signal for the CD8 population, the reduction in their numbers may well contribute to the failure of T cells to suppress hyperactive B lymphocytes. There has been a recent suggestion that $CD8^+$ lymphocytes in lupus patients act to enhance, instead of suppress, IgG production by antibody-secreting B cells.

It has been postulated that a biochemical defect of T cells underlines the impairment of their responses in patients with SLE. Abnormalities in the levels of adenylate cyclase and of cAMP-dependent protein kinase have been found. The cAMP pathway mediates the mobility of certain transmembrane and glycolipid-anchored surface molecules, resulting in ligands bound to T-cell membrane molecules being selectively internalized, cleared from the cell surface by capping and endocytosis or by shedding. T lymphocytes from lupus patients have shown a markedly abnormal level of capping of T-cell surface proteins (in CD3, 4, and 8 cells). These cells have also shown decreased cAMP production in response to adenosine, associated with an inability to switch phenotype or to express suppressor activity.

CYTOKINES

A number of abnormalities in cytokine production have been identified in lupus, but the importance of their role in the aetiopathogenesis of the disease has not been determined as clearly as in rheumatoid arthritis. However, it seems that accessory cells in lupus patients produce impaired amounts of interleukin 1, which provides the necessary activation signals for T cells. Both CD4 and CD8 T lymphocytes may, according to some reports, produce decreasing amounts of IL-2 in response to a variety of exogenous antigens and autoantigens. There appears to be altered expression of IL-2 receptors on $CD4^+$ T cells. The $CD8^+$ T-cell subset (suppressor cytotoxic) has IL-2 receptors but fails to respond in SLE patients as there is no IL-2 signal from $CD4^+$ T cells. In addition both IL-6 and IL-10 levels are often raised.

Both macrophage- and natural killer cell-mediated cytotoxicity are often impaired in lupus patients. γ-Interferon-induced enhancement of both types of cytotoxicity is also reduced in spite of relatively normal levels of production of α-interferon by lupus cells. Natural killer cells from patients with lupus seem unable to release the soluble factors necessary for killing. Intriguingly, recombinant γ-interferon has been used to induce remission in patients with rheumatoid arthritis but was found to exacerbate disease in lupus patients and in lupus-prone strains of mice.

GENETIC COMPONENTS

An analysis of the genetic component in the aetiopathogenesis of lupus includes studies of both populations and individuals. The different prevalence of lupus in different ethnic populations has already been referred to. The lower prevalence in West Africans than in Americans of African descent raises the likelihood of an environmental contribution to the pronounced inherited risk. Amongst monozygotic twins a concordance rate for lupus was thought to be around 70 per cent but more recent studies indicate that 30 per cent is a more accurate figure. This compares with 5 per cent for dizygotic twins.

Lupus is strongly associated with deficiencies of the early classical pathway of complement components, notably C1, C4, and C2. Two alleles are inherited for each complement component, so deficiencies may be partial or complete (homozygous). Congenital deficiencies of C2 and C4 are often in linkage disequilibrium with HLA-DR3 and -DR2 markers, known to be associated with lupus. C4 is composed of

two distinct but homologous proteins, C4A and C4B. A single null C4A allele increases the relative risk for lupus by a factor of three, and two null alleles by a factor of 17. It has been shown that deficiencies of C4A can arise by two mechanisms. In the first, a 30 kb deletion of DNA encoding all C4A along with the small portion of C4B occurs, while the other mechanism does not involve a deletion but may be the result of the regular gene linked to the MHC complex causing reduced synthesis of C4A.

The complement receptor CR1 is the only receptor to have been studied in detail in systemic lupus. The receptor is present on peripheral B lymphocytes, erythrocytes, monocytes, and tissue macrophages. The expression of CR1 on these cells has been described as reduced in patients with systemic lupus and their healthy family members. Although this was originally interpreted as an inherited defect, it is now thought to be an acquired phenomenon. The extent of the CR1 deficiency appears to correlate with disease activity.

Many studies have analysed the relationship between the MHC genes and both lupus as a whole and the presence of certain autoantibodies in particular. Amongst Caucasians those expressing the HLA-A1, B8, DR3 haplotype are approximately 10 times more likely to develop lupus. The haplotype also appears to be in linkage disequilibrium with a null allele of C4A. In Japanese lupus patients, however, the disease is more strongly associated with DR2. Other weaker associations with tumour necrosis factor α and certain T-cell receptor polymorphisms are also evident. Intriguingly, the major autoantibody specificities appear to have distinct genetic associations. There has been much interest recently in trying to determine whether there is any bias in the usage of certain V_H and V_L genes in the production of autoantibodies. It has now been established that germline genes may encode for autoantibodies, but in the main IgG antibodies are found to utilize a variety of somatic mutations. There are at least seven V_H families in man and of these the V_H1 and V_H3 families are easily the largest. Although the number of human anti-DNA antibodies sequenced to date remains relatively small, there appears to be some bias to the usage of the smaller V_H families 4, 5, and 6 amongst panels of hybridoma-derived monoclonal autoantibodies. In particular V_H4-21 seems to be particularly predisposed to the development of autoantibodies, notably cold agglutinins and, as identified recently, anti-DNA antibodies.

Over 20 different DNA antibody idiotypes have been identified in the past decade. Since sharing of an idiotype strongly suggests that there may be sharing of genes which encode the amino acids that constitute the idiotype, there has been much interest in determining the frequency with which certain anti-DNA antibody idiotypes are found in lupus patients. Some idiotypes, including the 16/6 Id, and Id GN2, are found frequently (in more than 40 per cent of patients) on the immunoglobulins in the serum of lupus patients or deposited in their kidneys. These observations suggest that such idiotypes may be involved in the immunopathology of lupus. The identification of these and other idiotypes in the healthy relatives of lupus patients, albeit at much lower frequencies, also suggests that their expression is inherited. However, it is also clear that idiotypes first identified on antibodies binding to DNA are not confined to antibodies with this antigen-binding specificity. Indeed, the expression of, for example, the 16/6 idiotype on anti-Klebsiella antibodies and the 3I idiotype on antipneumococcal antibodies points strongly to the links between autoimmunity and infectious disease. Perhaps those individuals expressing idiotypes on autoantibodies which are usually present on antibacterial antibodies are predestined to developing SLE and other related conditions.

REFERENCES

Ainsun Rahman, M.A. and Isenberg, D.A. (1994). Autoantibodies in systemic lupus erythematosus. *Current Opinion in Rheumatology*, **6**, 468–73.

Arnett, F.C. (1992). Genetic aspects of human lupus. *Clinical Immunology and Immunopathology* **63**, 4–6. A useful overview of the genetic association of SLE and its autoantibodies.

Beynon, H.L.C., Walport, M.J. (1992). Antiphospholipid antibodies and cardiovascular disease. *British Heart Journal* **67**, 281–4.

Brinkman, K., Termaat, R.M., Berden, J.H.M., and Smeenk, R.T.J. (1990). Anti-DNA antibodies and lupus nephritis: the complexity of cross-reactivity. *Immunology Today* **11**, 232–4.

Fessel, W.J. (1988). Epidemiology of systemic lupus erythematosus. *Rheumatic Disease Clinics of North America* **14**, 15–24.

Hay, E. and Isenberg, D.A. (1992). Autoantibodies in central nervous system lupus. *British Journal of Rheumatology*, in press.

Hay, E.M. and Isenberg, D.A. (1993). Autoantibodies in central nervous system lupus. *British Journal of Rheumatology*, **32**, 329–32.

Hughes, G.R.V. (1993). The antiphospholipid syndrome: ten years on. *Lancet* **342**, 341–4.

Isenberg, D.A. and Horsfall, A. (1993). Systemic lupus erythematosus. In *Oxford Textbook of Rheumatology* (ed. P. Maddison, D. Isenberg, D. Glass, and P. Woo). pp. 733–55. Oxford University Press.

Kammer, G.M. and Stein, R.L. (1990). T lymphocyte dysfunctions in systemic lupus erythematosus. *Journal of Laboratory and Clinical Medicine* **1156**, 273–82.

Lahita, R.G. (ed.) (1987). *Systemic lupus erythematosus*. Churchill Livingstone, Edinburgh.

Morgan, B.P. and Walport, M.J. (1991). Complement deficiency and disease. *Immunology Today* **12**, 301–6.

Nived, O., Sturfelt G., and Wollheim, F. (1985). Systemic lupus erythematosus in an adult population in Southern Sweden: incidence, prevalence and validity of ARA revised classification criteria. *British Journal of Rheumatology* **24**, 147–54.

Pascual, V. and Capra, J.D. (1991). Human immunoglobulin heavy chain variable region genes: organisation, polymorphism and expression. *Advances in Immunology* **49**, 1–74.

Strasser, A., *et al.* (1991). Enforced BCL2 expression in B-lymphoid cells prolongs antibody responses and elicits autoimmune disease. *Proceedings of the National Academy of Sciences, USA* **88**, 8661–5.

Symmons, D.P. (1991). Review of UK data on the rheumatic diseases – 8:SLE; *British Journal of Rheumatology*, **30**, 288–90.

Takahashi, T., Dixon Gray, J., and Horwitz, D.A. (1991). Human CD8$^+$ lymphocytes stimulated in the absence of CD4$^+$ cells enhance IgG production by antibody-secreting B cells. *Clinical Immunology and Immunopathology* **58**, 352–65.

Triplett, D.A. (1993). Antiphospholipid antibodies and thrombosis: a consequence, coincidence or cause. *Archives of Pathology and Laboratory Medicine* **117**, 78–88.

Vaarala, O., Palosuo, T., Kleemola, M., and Aho, K. (1986). Anticardiolipin response in acute infections. *Clinical Immunology and Immunopathology* **41**, 8–15.

Watanabe-Fukunaga, T., Brannan, C.I., Copeland, N., Jenkins, N.A., and Nagata, S. (1992). Lymphoproliferation disorder in mice explained by defects in Fas antigen that mediates apoptosis. *Nature* **356**, 314–17.

Worrall, J.G., Snaith, M.L., Batchelor, R., and Isenberg, D.A. (1990). SLE – a rheumatological view. *Quarterly Journal of Medicine* **275**, 319–30. An overview of the clinical, serological, and immunogenetic links of SLE.

18.11.4 Systemic sclerosis

C. M. BLACK

Systemic sclerosis is a connective tissue disease which results in widespread damage to small blood vessels and fibrosis in both the cutaneous tissue and the internal organs. Consequent disability may be minimal or it may be life-threatening. Skin thickening is the hallmark of the disease. Historically, the term 'scleroderma' has encompassed both the skin lesions of Systemic sclerosis (Table 1) and the heterogeneous group of dermal fibrotic conditions known as localized scleroderma in which vascular and internal organ involvement are absent (Table 2). A transition from localized scleroderma to systemic sclerosis is excessively rare, as is the coexistence of the two diseases. Environmental and chemical agents have been implicated in the development of Systemic sclerosis (Table 3) and, in addition, many conditions have scleroderma-like fea-

Table 1 *Spectrum of systemic sclerosis*

1. **'Pre-scleroderma'**
   Raynaud's phenomenon plus nailfold capillary changes and circulating antinuclear antibodies (topoisomerase I, anticentromere, nucleolar).

2. **Diffuse cutaneous systemic sclerosis**
   Onset of skin changes (puffy or hidebound) within 1 year of onset of Raynaud's phenomenon
   Truncal and acral skin involvement
   Presence of tendon friction rubs
   Early and significant incidence of interstitial lung disease, oliguric renal failure, diffuse gastrointestinal disease, and myocardial involvement
   Nailfold capillary dilatation and capillary drop out
   Antitopoisomerase I (Scl-70) antibodies (30% of patients)

3. **Limited cutaneous systemic sclerosis**
   Raynaud's phenomenon for years (occasionally decades)
   Skin involvement limited to hands, face, feet, and forearms (acral) or absent
   A significant (10–15 years) late incidence of pulmonary hypertension, with or without interstitial lung disease, skin calcifications, telangiectasia, and gastrointestinal involvement
   A high incidence of anticentromere antibody (ACA) (70–80%)
   Dilated nailfold capillary loops, usually without capillary dropout

4. **Scleroderma sine scleroderma**
   Raynaud's phenomenon +/−
   No skin involvement
   Presentation with pulmonary fibrosis, scleroderma renal crisis, cardiac disease, gastrointestinal disease
   Antinuclear antibodies may be present (Scl-70, ACA, nucleolar)

Table 2 *Localized scleroderma*

Morphea types:	plaque
	guttate
	bullous
	morphea profunda (subcutaneous)
	nodular (keloid)
	generalized
Linear types:	*en coup de sabre*
	facial hemiatrophy
Morphea ⟷	eosinophilic fasciitis

Table 3 *Chemical agents implicated in the development of scleroderma*

Organic chemicals
   aliphatic hydrocarbons, e.g. vinyl chloride, trichlorethylene
   aromatic hydrocarbons, e.g. benzene, toluene
Epoxy resins
Toxic oil (aniline-treated rape-seed oil)
Silica, in stone masons, coal miners, gold miners
Foam insulation (urea-formaldehyde)
Drugs, e.g. L-tryptophan, bleomycin, cocaine, pentazocine, and appetite suppressants
Augmentation mammoplasty, silicone, paraffin

Table 4 *Scleroderma-like syndromes*

Immunological/ Inflammatory	Chronic graft-versus-host disease, eosinophilic fasciitis, overlap syndromes (with rheumatoid arthritis, systemic lupus erythematosus syndrome, for example) undifferentiated connective tissue disease
Metabolic	Sclerodema of Buschke ⎫ with or without Scleromyxoedema ⎬ paraproteinaemia Insulin-dependent diabetes mellitus (digital sclerosis) Carcinoid syndrome Acromegaly Lichen sclerosis et atrophicus Acrodermatitis chronica atrophicans Amyloidosis
Inherited	Phenylketonuria Porphyrias Premature ageing syndromes—progeria, Werner's syndrome
Localized systemic sclerosis and visceral diseases	Idiopathic pulmonary fibrosis Amyloidosis Sarcoidosis Infiltrating carcinomas Infiltrating cardiomyopathy Oesophageal and intestinal hypomotility syndromes

tures, e.g. amyloid, carcinoid, and scleromyxoedema (Table 4). In some patients the disease is not clearly defined, there being in addition features of other connective tissue diseases.

The disease is global in distribution and appears to affect all races. It strikes 18 people per million in the United Kingdom every year, and 20 per million in the United States. Age, sex, race, and genetic factors all influence the development of the disease. Systemic sclerosis is the only connective tissue disease in which several environmental factors have been implicated as initiating factors, and the finding of antinuclear antibodies in the serum of the spouses of patients with the disease adds weight to the supposition of environmental influences.

The disease usually begins between the ages of 30 and 60, although it is also found in children and may strike the elderly. It affects women approximately four times as often as men, and this ratio increases during the child-bearing years. It is slightly more common in the Afro-American than the Caucasian, and more severe in the non-Caucasian patient. Scleroderma usually occurs in a sporadic fashion, and familial occurrence is unusual but it, or other connective tissue disorders, has been reported in the families of patients with systemic sclerosis; this, and the increased incidence of antinuclear antibodies in blood relatives (particularly females), suggests a genetic susceptibility to developing these disorders. Current evidence would suggest that this to the susceptibility is related to the HLA system.

The typical patient presents with Raynaud's phenomenon, often with other complaints such as swollen hands, tight skin, and painful joints and muscles. Swallowing difficulties may be an early symptom too, and the challenge is then to defect those patients destined to have a progressive and complicated course as opposed to those whose disease will remain mild. The duration, both of Raynaud's phenomenon and of other symptoms and signs, helps place the patient in one of the two major subsets (Table 1), the relatively benign and at worst slowly progressive limited cutaneous systemic sclerosis or the aggressive diffuse cutaneous form. Patients with the rarer scleroderma *sine* scleroderma often have Raynaud's phenomenon and express the appropriate antibodies; they lack changes in the skin but not in other tissues susceptible to the changes of sclerosis. Within the spectrum overall should be included patients who appear to have primary Raynaud's phenomenon, but with positive autoantibodies and abnormal nailfold capillaries; these patients may be developing more classical systemic sclerosis.

Raynaud's phenomenon

Raynaud's phenomenon, is an episodic event characterized by pallor, cyanosis, suffusion and/or pain of the fingers, toes, ears, nose or jaw in response to cold or stress. It affects 3 to 10 per cent of the adult population worldwide and has a predilection for females. About 1 per cent of those showing the phenomenon develop a connective tissue disease, the most common of which is scleroderma. Other conditions associated with Raynaud's include cervical rib, vibration white finger, hypothyroidism, and uraemia. It is important to make an accurate diagnosis; Raynaud's is intermittent and is commonly not the cause of cold extremities, chilblains, or digital ulceration. Associated symptoms such as rash, ulcers, changes in skin texture, calcium deposits in skin, painful swollen joints, myalgia, muscle weakness, difficulty in swallowing, or breathlessness would indicate that the primary condition has developed into one of the connective tissue disorders, if not systemic sclerosis itself.

Limited cutaneous scleroderma

This was formerly described as the CREST type of the disease (Calcinosis circumscripta, Raynaud's, Esophagus, Sclerodactyly, and Telangiectasia) and is the most common form of the disease, accounting for some 60 per cent of cases overall. The patient destined to develop it is usually female, between 30 and 50 years old. Raynaud's phenomenonon will already be long-standing in such a patient, often of up to 20 years' duration. Skin changes are noticed, but at first disturbing only from a cosmetic point of view. She will often complain of swelling of her hands with some thickening of the skin or the fingers, with local pain which may extend to the wrist with some of the features of a carpal tunnel syndrome—a not infrequent misdiagnosis. However, the bilateral nature of the problem, with furrowing and puckering around the mouth as well as telangiectases on the face and anterior chest and painful crusting lesions on the fingertips, should lead to the correct diagnosis Fig. 1. The patient may also complain of dyspepsia from reflux desophagitis.

Diffuse cutaneous scleroderma

The patient who develops this form of systemic sclerosis often has a very short history of Raynaud's phenomenon, which may indeed have arisen concurrently with other symptoms and signs and sometimes even follows the skin changes. These patients (less than 40 per cent of the total) are often in their fourth decade, although the range extends from the first to the eighth. In contrast to those with the limited cutaneous disease, they are more likely to be male. The onset of the disease is often abrupt and may present as diffuse, bilateral, and sometimes itchy and painful swelling of the fingers, arms, feet, legs, and face. Rapid weight loss and fatigue are common and the muscles may be weak. Oesophageal symptoms are frequent and the patient may complain of a substernal discomfort on eating. Exertional dyspnoea may also be a problem. If the patient presents at a later stage, i.e. 2 to 3 years after onset, widespread skin thickening with painful joint contractures, muscle wasting, and digital ulcers are usually the major complaints, along with those related to disease of the internal organs. Should a patient with early disease present with headaches, blurring of vision, and significant hypertension, this is a medical emergency, as it portends hypertensive renal crisis, and requires immediate action.

Scleroderma sine *scleroderma*

These patients are the most difficult group to recognize. They may or may not have Raynaud's phenomenon, but never have the skin changes of scleroderma: common presenting problems include oesophagitis, malabsorption, pseudo-obstruction, renal failure, cardiac arrhythmias, and interstitial lung disease.

Physical examination

RAYNAUD'S PHENOMENON

Most patients with Raynaud's destined to develop systemic sclerosis will have done so within the first 2 years of the onset of the phenomenon. After this time, fewer than 5 per cent will develop it. The clinical examination must include the nailfold capillaries, looking for the typical changes that are highly predictive of the subsequent development of sclerosis. There are several ways to do this:

Fig. 1 This patient shows the typical facial features of scleroderma—microstomia, thickened shiny skin, and beaking of the nose, with telangiectasia on lips and forehead, and alopecia.

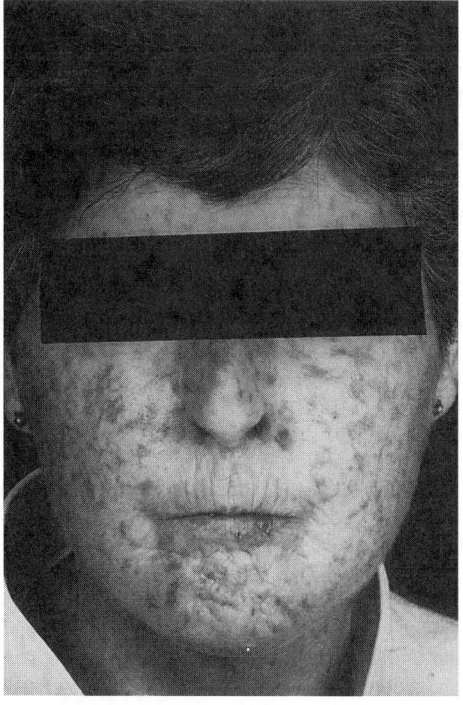

(1) with the naked eye—only occasionally rewarding;
(2) with an ophthalmoscope or other form of magnification (some workers regard this method as having a sensitivity equal to that of microscopy); and
(3) capillary microscopy, which is highly sensitive and also allows for a permanent photographic recording of a row of horizontal capillary loops at the nailfold, just proximal to the cuticle.

On microscopy two morphological patterns may be seen, either dilatation of many loops, or 'giant' loops associated with avascular areas without visible capillaries. The latter pattern is associated with diffuse disease. The capillary patterns appear early and are remarkably constant over time. Taken together with the presence of specific autoantibodies, they can detect more than 95 per cent of patients in a stage transitional to the full-blown disease.

LIMITED CUTANEOUS SYSTEMIC SCLEROSIS

The physical examination of these patients is often rewarding. Early in the disease there is non-pitting oedema of the fingers (sausage-shaped fingers) which after several weeks or months is gradually replaced by skin thickening. The thickening occurs in the dermis and is accompanied by epidermal thinning, leading to loss of skin creases, hair, and secretions. The skin involvement in this subset is minimal. Although the skin may thicken and become shiny, it is not usually so closely adherent to the underlying structures that mobility of tendons, joints, and muscle is severely impaired—this is in sharp contrast to findings in the diffuse disease. The skin involvement does not spread proximally on to the trunk, but the face should be examined carefully for thin, tightly pursed lips and microstomia. The most striking cutaneous finding is digital and facial telangiectasiae, representing dilated capillary loops and venules. Other evidence of structural vascular change is to be seen in the fingertips, where small areas of ischaemic necrosis or ulceration are common, often leaving pitting scars and pulp atrophy. The reabsorption of the tufts of the terminal phalanges, suspected clinically and confirmed on radiography, is also presumed to be due to ischaemia. Patients with limited cutaneous disease often develop intracutaneous and subcutaneous calcification. These deposits frequently occur in the fingers, particularly in the digital pads, and periarticular tissues such as the pre-patellae area and olecranon bursa. Such calcinotic masses vary in size from tiny lumps, not clinically apparent, to large masses in the forearms and legs. They are often complicated by ulceration of overlying skin, extrusion of calcium, and secondary bacterial infection.

In an early case the rest of the clinical examination may be entirely normal. If the patient has had the disease for more than 10 to 15 years, two major complications may be clinically apparent: small bowel involvement and pulmonary hypertension. There may be evidence of malabsorption, with anaemia and a history of marked weight loss, oily, bulky, offensive stools, and abdominal distension. This complication, except for those few patients who have a functional ileus (pseudo-obstruction), has a slower clinical evolution than that of pulmonary hypertension. Severe pulmonary arterial hypertension is found in up to 10 per cent of patients in the limited cutaneous subset, and is not secondary to pulmonary interstitial fibrosis, which in such patients is either absent or mild. In addition to marked dyspnoea, these patients develop right ventricular hypertrophy, an accentuated pulmonary component of the second heart sound, and eventually signs of right heart failure. The prognosis is extremely poor and mean duration of survival from detection is only 2 years.

DIFFUSE CUTANEOUS SCLERODERMA

The clinical findings in diffuse scleroderma depend entirely on the stage of the disease. If the patient is examined at the onset, which is often

Table 5 *Gut involvement in scleroderma*

Region	Disorder	Symptom	Investigation	Treatment
Mouth	Sicca syndrome	Dry mouth	Salivary gland biopsy	Artificial saliva
Oesophagus	↓ Motility	Dysphagia	Oesophageal scintiscan	Domperidone Metoclopramide Cisapride
	↓ Lower oesophageal sphincter pressure → Reflux	Retrosternal discomfort/pain	Endoscopy Barium swallow	Omeprozole
	Stricture	Dysphagia	Endoscopy	Dilatation and omeprazole
Stomach	Ulceration secondary to NSAIDs	Dyspepsia	Endoscopy	H_2 blockers then misoprostol
	Gastric paresis	Anorexia, nausea/ vomiting, early satiety	Scintigram	Metoclopramide
Small bowel	Hypomotility, stasis/bacterial overgrowth, adynamic ileus, pseudo-obstruction	Weight loss, abdominal distension, steatorrhoea, episodes of abdominal pain and distension	Ba follow-through, hydrogen breath test or [14] [C] glycocholate breath test jejunal aspiration, 3-day faecal fat, plain abdominal radiograph	Antibiotics (anti-anaerobes) Metoclopramide/cisapride Pancreatic supplements Total parenteral nutrition
	Small bowel ulcers secondary to NSAIDs	Chronic anaemia, abdominal pain	Small bowel enema	Misoprostol
	Pneumatosis intestinalis	Diarrhoea and blood, benign pneumoperitoneum	Plain abdominal radiograph	Oxygen
Large bowel	Sigmoid/rectal hypomotility	Alternating constipation/ diarrhoea	Barium enema	Dietary manipulation + stool expanders (e.g. ispaghula)
	Colonic wide-mouthed pseudodiverticulae	Rare perforation	Barium enema	(Resection)
	Anal sphincter involvement	Anal incontinence	Rectal manometry	??Stimulation

abrupt, examination of the cutaneous tissue will usually reveal cold, painful, swollen hands, with the swelling and stiffness already extending into the arms, the feet, the lower legs, the face, and the trunk. The oedematous phase is usually replaced within a few months by the indurative phase, when the skin becomes tight and shiny, and bound to underlying structures. Pigmentation (hyperpigmentation or hypopigmentation) accompanies the skin thickening in many patients.

The natural history of skin involvement in this subset is quite different from that in the limited form of the disease, and can be mapped semi-quantitatively, by the measurement of the degree and extent of cutaneous thickening in multiple sites, from which is derived a skin score. In diffuse scleroderma, the skin score increases rapidly at first and often peaks after 1 to 3 years. This rapid progression is accompanied by impaired mobility in tendons, joints, and muscles, which is clinically all too apparent. The contractures and stretching of the skin over the bony points often lead to painful ulcers which are slow to heal. The most frequent site for the ulcers are the proximal interphalangeal joints; the elbows and malleoli of the ankles are other favoured sites.

In its earliest stages diffuse scleroderma may be confused with an acute inflammatory arthropathy, particularly if Raynaud's phenomenon is absent. The oedematous puffy skin is often accompanied by symmetrically stiff, painful joints (hands, feet, knees, ankles, and wrists) but the classic synovitis of rheumatoid arthritis is usually absent. A clinical sign which must be carefully sought in this group of patients is a tendon friction rub. These rubs have a distinctive leathery crepitus: they are elicited over elbows, knees, fingers, wrists, and ankles, during joint movement. They are rather ominous signs, frequently antedating a rapid increase in cutaneous involvement, or the onset of visceral disease. Signs of a carpal tunnel syndrome may be present and are due to a flexor tenosynovitis at the wrist. Mild muscle disease is common, and can be detected on examination. This is not usually accompanied by an increase in plasma creatine phosphokinase or inflammatory changes on muscle biopsy. It is also non-progressive. A few patients have florid changes of polymyositis, and are usually classified to have an overlap syndrome. As with limited disease, evidence of structural vascular damage may be found in the nailfold capillaries and the digital pads, and can be extensive.

It is the timing of the onset of visceral disease that distinguishes the patient with diffuse from the one with limited scleroderma; the signs of, for example, gastrointestinal involvement are similar in both subsets (Table 5), but occur earlier in the diffuse form of the disease. Lung involvement (Table 6) occurs in 70 per cent of patients, and is the most common cause of death directly related to scleroderma. It has two components, interstitial lung disease and pulmonary hypertension. The hypertension is either secondary to lung fibrosis and then mild; or severe and associated with limited cutaneous scleroderma. Unfortunately, patients with interstitial lung disease often have few clinical signs, although careful auscultation may reveal fine bilateral basal crepitations. Primary heart disease in scleroderma consists of pericarditis with or without effusion, heart failure (left or bi-ventricular), or arrhythmias

Table 6 *Pulmonary disease in scleroderma*

Disorder	Symptoms	Signs	Investigations	Therapeutic possibilities
Pulmonary fibrosis	Dry cough	↓ Chest expansion	Chest radiography Lung function tests	Steroids +/−
	Dyspnoea	Basal crepitations	High-resolution CT scan DTPA scan Bronchoalveolar lavage Lung biopsy	cyclophosphamide, azathioprine, D-penicillamine, cyclosporin, α-interferon Intravenous or intra-arterial prostacyclin
Pulmonary hypertension	Dyspnoea Ankle oedema	Loud P$_2$ right ventricular heave	Chest radiography Doppler-echocardiography cardiac catheter	Nifedipine ?ACE inhibitor

Rare complications
  Bronchiectasis
  Spontaneous pneumothorax
  Lung carcinoma (squamous, adenocarcinoma, small cell)
				Antibiotic treatment if necessary
				Try to avoid a tube
				Use drugs and radiotherapy; most cases unsuitable for surgery

Table 7 *Cardiac involvement in scleroderma*

Disorder	Effect	Frequency	Symptom	Investigation	Treatment
Pericardial involvement	Pericardial effusion	10–15% clinically 35% at autopsy More common in localized than diffuse scleroderma	Chest pain Dyspnoea	Chest radiography Electrocardiography Echocardiography	NSAIDS Steroids Rarely drainage
Myocardial fibrosis	Congestive cardiac failure Arrhythmias	30–50% More common in diffuse than localized	Dyspnoea Oedema Atypical chest pain Palpitation	Thallium scan MUGA scan Holter monitor	Diuretics Calcium channel blockers Antiarrhythmics
Myocarditis	Congestive cardiac failure	Rare	Dyspnoea Ankle oedema	Electrocardiography Echocardiography	Corticosteroids

MUGA = multiple uptake gated acquisition scan.

(Table 7) Again, clinical signs are not common. Acute symptomatic pericarditis is unusual, congestive cardiac failure occurs in less than 5 per cent of patients, and arrhythmias are often asymptomatic.

The regular recording of the blood pressure is particularly important in early diffuse disease (less than 5 years' duration). Between 15 and 20 per cent of these patients develop a scleroderma renal crisis, with the abrupt onset of malignant arterial hypertension. Clinical features which accompany the hypertension include visual difficulties with severe retinopathy, severe headaches, seizures, or left heart failure. Normotensive renal failure has been reported in this group of patients and is often accompanied by severe microangiopathic haemolytic anaemia. Renal crisis may also be precipitated by sudden severe volume depletion in a susceptible patient who has had clinically undetected reduced renal blood flow.

Major organ involvement, suitable investigations, and treatment suggestions are given in Tables 5, 6, and 7.

Disease course

Patients with limited disease have an 'early phase' that lasts about 10 years, when the picture is usually dominated by vascular problems such as Raynaud's phenomenon, pitting scars, digital ulcers, and telangiectasiae. Later there may be worsening of the vascular disease, both cutaneously and in the pulmonary circulation. Pulmonary interstitial disease, usually more indolent than that seen in the diffuse form, can also occur as a late complication. Gut involvement may worsen with time, and oesophageal strictures, malabsorption, pseudo-obstruction, and anal incontinence are all potential late and troublesome events in this subset.

During the early phase of diffuse disease (the first 5 years), the patient is fatigued and loses weight. Hypertensive renal crisis is a real risk and rapid progression of pulmonary and cardiac disease may occur. Arthritis, myositis, and tendon involvement can be most marked at this time. After 5 years, considered to be the late stage of diffuse disease, the constitutional symptoms settle down, the skin and musculoskeletal problems have usually reached a plateau, and there is progression of existing visceral disease but reduced risk of new organ involvement. These differences in pattern and natural history influence evaluation and therapy.

Pathogenesis

The pathophysiology of systemic sclerosis includes immunological, vascular, and connective tissue abnormalities. The concept of an initial immune attack on the endothelial cell and fibroblast or other component of the extracellular matrix is an attractive one. Currently, the precise relationship between these components is unknown. They may represent separate processes, different target responses to a common process, or a sequential event with the initial target being the endothelial cell and the resultant factors acting on the fibroblast to cause fibrosis (Fig 2).

The use of the laboratory

Any patient with Raynaud's phenomenon may develop scleroderma; the identification of one of the scleroderma-specific autoantibodies has been shown to be a useful predictor. Studies using an immunoblotting technique, more sensitive than immunofluorescence and the gold standard for future work, have demonstrated that the anticentromere antibody (the antigen actually resides in the kinetochore region of the chromosome) has a predictive value for the development of the limited cutaneous disease (sensitivity 60 per cent, specificity 98 per cent) and Scl-70 (an antibody known to recognize the nuclear enzyme DNA topoisomerase I) for the diffuse subset (sensitivity 38 per cent, specificity 100 per cent). Other serum autoantibodies, notably those to nucleolar antigens, are also relatively specific for scleroderma, and the proportion of patients having one or more antibody is over 80 per cent of the total. Some of these antibodies have been shown to have correlations with class II MHC polymorphisms. A summary of the clinical and laboratory characteristics of patients according to serum autoantibody type is shown in Table 8. Although these antibodies are good markers of individual subsets, a pathogenic role for them has yet to be assigned: there is evidence for either molecular mimicry or an antigen-driven process.

Other less specific serological abnormalities are found in scleroderma and include hypergammaglobulinaemia, the presence of immune complexes, low concentrations of complement components, and a weakly positive rheumatoid factor. Antibodies to SSA/Ro and SSB/La are found

in 50 per cent of the scleroderma patients who also have Sjögren's syndrome, and are nearly always found in patients with glandular lymphocyte infiltration rather than fibrosis.

Once the patient has developed full-blown disease, other investigations will be needed. Assessment of the function of internal organs susceptible to involvement should be done early in relation to the recognition of disease evolution. The extent and frequency of the investigations will depend on the subset of the disease, its stage and local facilities.

In a patient with limited cutaneous disease, only a few of these tests need be repeated regularly; however, the longer the disease has been present, the greater the need for careful monitoring for pulmonary hypertension and for small bowel disease. Thus, Doppler echocardiography and pulmonary function tests may be repeated every year and the investigation of malabsorption instigated if clinically indicated.

The monitoring of the diffuse syndrome is quite different. In the first 3 to 4 critical years of the disease, patients need closely spaced assessments of renal function (monthly serum creatinine and urinary micros-

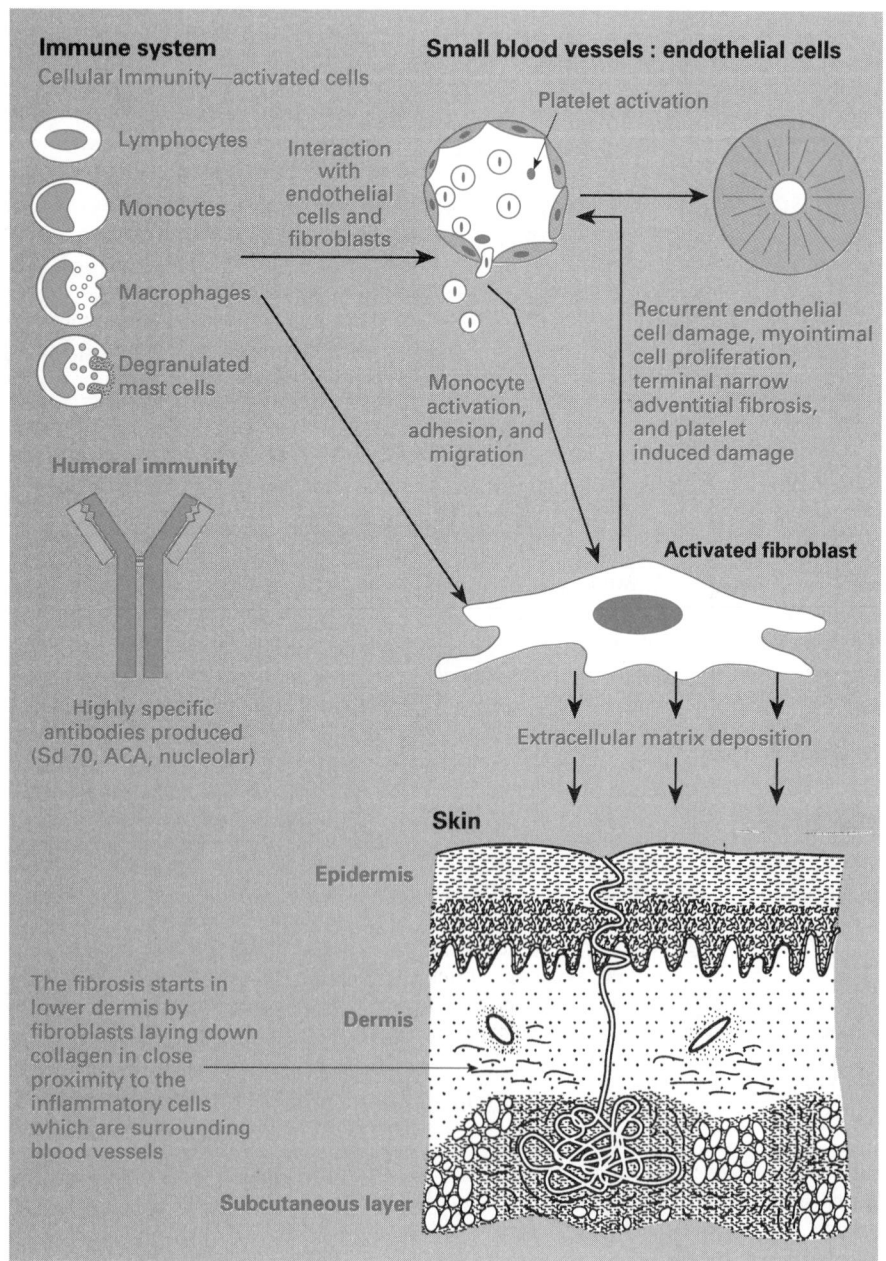

Fig. 2 Pathophysiology of systemic sclerosis.

Table 8 *Serum autoantibodies with clinical and laboratory correlates*

Antigen	Antinuclear antibody staining pattern	HLA associations	Frequency in all patients (%)	Clinical associations	Organ involvement
Scl-70 Topoisomerase 1	Speckled	DR5 (DR11) DR3/DR52a DQ7 DQB1	15–20	Diffuse	Lung fibrosis
ACA centromere	Centromere (kinetochore)	DR1 (DQ5) DQB1 DR4 (D13 subtypes)	25–30	Limited	Pulmonary hypertension
RNA I and III	Speckled/nucleolar	?	20	Diffuse	Renal Skin
U₃RNP	Nucleolar	?	5	Overlap Mixed	Pulmonary hypertension Muscle
U₁RNP	Speckled	?	10	Limited overlap Afro-Caribbeans	Muscle
Th (To)	Nucleolar	?	5	Limited	Pulmonary hypertension Small bowel
PM-Scl	Nucleolar	DR3 DR52	3–5	Overlap Mixed	Muscle

copy and measurements every 3 months creatinine clearance), and monitoring of cardiac and lung function every 6 months.

Reliable laboratory tools for the assessment of activity in systemic sclerosis have yet to be developed, but several markers are under review. Immune activation is reflected by the serum levels of interleukin-2 (IL-2) and soluble IL-2 receptors, microvascular damage by plasma factor VIII/von Willebrand factor antigen, and fibroblast activity by serum procollagen III peptide concentrations.

Lung disease is the current major therapeutic challenge. Technical developments have made early detection of interstitial lung disease possible. Chest radiography is not sufficiently sensitive to identify early organ involvement. Pulmonary function tests, particularly exercise ones, are more sensitive, but neither they nor chest radiography provide a guide to the course of the disease in the lung. The combined use of thin-section (3 mm) high-resolution computed tomography, bronchoalveolar lavage, and diethylenetriaminepentaacetic acid (DTPA) scans is beginning to provide much earlier diagnosis and indices of progression. The earliest detectable abnormality in high-resolution CT is usually a narrow, often ill-defined, subpleural crescent of increased attenuation in the posterior segment of the lower lobe. Other early CT changes are of an amorphous ground-glass pattern of parenchymal opacification, or, alternatively, a more reticular appearance (Fig. 3). The relative extent of each pattern is important because there is good correlation between these appearances and histological findings at open-lung biopsy; an inflammatory biopsy equating to an amorphous pattern and fibrosis to a reticular one. Such information may reduce the need for an invasive biopsy. Bronchoalveolar lavage identifies patients with an alveolitis often before the onset of symptoms or abnormalities on chest radiography or in pulmonary function tests. DTPA scans, particularly serial ones, may become useful predictors of progression or improvement: a persistently abnormal DTPA scan is associated with a higher rate of decline in pulmonary function tests subsequently, whereas a reversion to normal clearance is associated with a sustained improvement in pulmonary function. These tests have obvious value in the assessment of progress of the disease and are critically important in evaluation of new treatments.

Other organ involvement

Neurological involvement is uncommon, but in the late stages of limited cutaneous disease a small but significant proportion of patients develops unilateral or bilateral trigeminal neuralgia.

Impotence is also a major problem for males with the diffuse syndrome. It usually occurs 1 to 2 years after the onset and is thought to have an neurovascular cause which is refractory to treatment. Dryness

Fig. 3 Thin section CT scan images illustrating: (a) the ground glass appearance of early pulmonary involvement posteriorly, associated with a normal chest radiograph. (b) Extensive honeycomb shadowing and cystic air spaces involving both lower lobes, with the corresponding chest radiographic appearances of advanced interstitial lung disease (bibasilar reticulonodular shadowing). (With grateful acknowledgement to Drs A. Wells, R. du Bois, and Dr B. Strickland, Departments of Respiratory Medicine and Radiology, Royal Brompton National Heart and Lung Hospitals (Chelsea).)

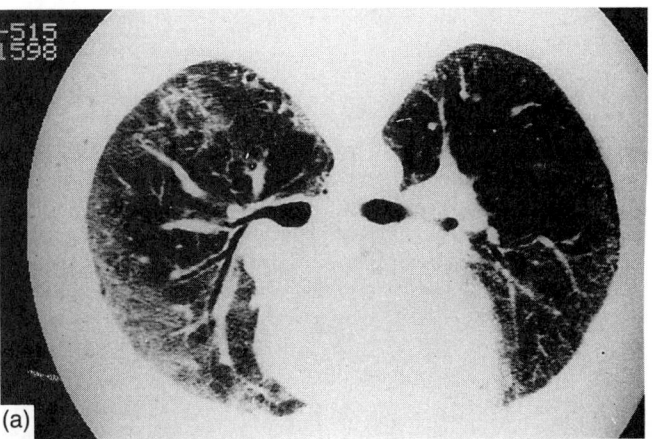
(a)

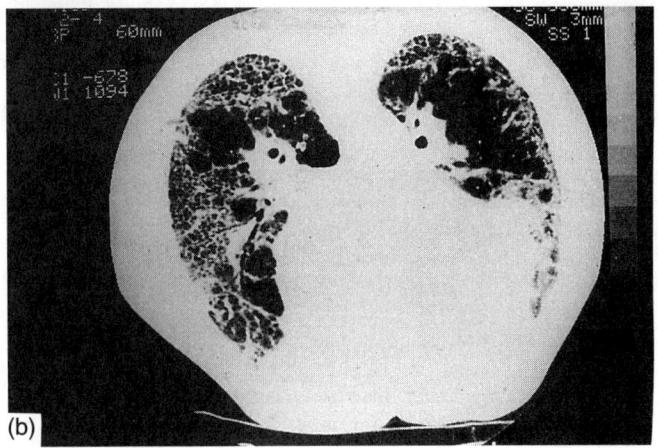
(b)

Table 9 *Treatment of Raynaud's phenomenon*

Stages of Raynaud's phenomenon	Recommended treatment
Simple short attacks	Warmth, heating appliances No smoking or β-blockers Fish oil and evening primrose oil
Frequent prolonged attacks interfering with daily living often accompanied by digital infarcts	Calcium-channel blockers, e.g. nifedipine, diltiazem, felodipine, isradipine, norcardipine Transdermal glyceryl trinitrate Ketanserin—selective 5HT$_2$ receptor antagonist reducing 5-hydroxytryptomine (5HT)-induced vasospasm and platelet aggregation AcE inhibitor, e.g. captopril
Severe prolonged attacks with ulceration and incipient gangrene	Prostacyclin infusion
Secondary infection	Antibiotics, surgery (e.g. debridement, nail removal, nail bed removal)
Gangrene	Amputation—auto, surgical
Surgical measures	Cervical sympathectomy—should be avoided Lumbar sympathectomy—still has a place for Raynaud's phenomenon of the lower limb Digital sympathectomy for severe pain and ulceration of fingers or toes: may be used in conjunction with intravenous prostacyclin

of the mucous membranes is common and dyspareunia frequent. Hypothyroidism occurs in as many as 50 per cent of patients with systemic sclerosis and is frequently missed. Some patients have antithyroid antibodies but lymphocytic infiltration in the gland is uncommon, fibrosis being the more typical finding.

Survival

There have been a number of studies of survival in the past 50 years, and the 5-year cumulative survival rate ranges from 34 to 73 per cent. Even prolonged survival does not protect against an increased mortality risk, which continues over time for at least 15 years. Factors which adversely affect outcome are increasing age, being male, extent of skin involvement, and heart, lung, and renal disease. Survival has altered but little in the past 50 years, reflecting the lack of any truly effective therapy.

Treatment

Scleroderma is a chronic disease, difficult to manage, and patients are often unduly pessimistic at the onset. The first responsibility of the physician is therefore to discuss with the patient and his or her relatives the particular form of his or her disease. Such discussions help the patient understand future risks and likely outcome. An adjunct to such discussion is provided by the excellent publications available through patient support groups, and these should be recommended. Current treatments include general management measures to improve Raynaud's phenomenon, treatments aimed to modify the immune system and encroaching fibrosis, and treatment of specific organ problems.

The patient must protect hands and feet against both trauma and cold; thermal clothing, hand warmers, and heated gloves and socks may all be helpful. There must be abstinence from tobacco and the avoidance of drugs known to precipitate Raynaud's phenomenon, such as β-blocking agents.

Skin care is critical and many patients find lanolin and other oils, creams, and bath oils helpful for protecting and moisturizing the skin. Unsightly telangiectasiae can be covered with an appropriate cosmetic preparation. Infection of ulcerated fingers must be treated promptly, and troublesome calcinotic deposits may be removed surgically. Treatment with low-dose warfarin and colchicine has not been successful in treating calcinosis. The role of physiotherapy, exercises, and splinting is controversial—if these therapies are to be of any use they must be started at the onset and performed regularly.

The treatment of primary Raynaud's phenomenon is less complicated than that of Raynaud's phenomenon associated with scleroderma, in which there is additional structural damage underlying the vasospasm. A graded scheme for the management of Raynaud's phenomenon with some of the drugs in current usage and the appropriate surgical procedures is found in Table 9. Unfortunately, none of the treatments used so far to control the vasoactive features of scleroderma can stop the continuing vascular damage in the viscera or prevent continuing fibrosis.

The variable prevention of renal failure is possible by the use of angiotensin-converting enzyme inhibitors to control the accelerated hypertension of scleroderma renal crisis, but there is no effective treatment for vascular insufficiency and fibrosis in the lung, heart, and gastrointestinal tract. Many drugs seem promising in pilot studies but none has proved able to halt the progression of systemic sclerosis in a controlled prospective trial. The difficulties of evaluating a therapy in this disease are well-recognized. Scleroderma is variable in its severity and rate of progression. Spontaneous improvement occurs after several years, particularly in the skin, and objectives and points for ascertaining improvement (or deterioration) in the condition have been difficult to establish.

Current concepts of the pathogenesis of systemic sterosis are helpful when considering treatment. Therapy would be designed logically to:

(1) contain and repair endothelial damage;
(2) prevent the mononuclear cells and their products from activating fibroblasts or interacting with each other;
(3) stop mast cell degranulation;
(4) down-regulate collagen synthesis; and
(5) increase the degradation of extracellular matrix molecules.

There are drugs that do many of these things. Some have been tried in scleroderma and found wanting, e.g. 5-fluouracil, chlorambucil, total lymphoid irradiation, ketotifen and colchicine; others have unacceptable side-effects (e.g. retinoids) and some are under review (see Table 10). Any new therapies must be tested in controlled trials with sufficient numbers of patients of defined subsets and stage of disease.

Overlap syndromes

There are patients who are not easily defined, having features overlapping with those of other connective tissue diseases. A variety of terms

Table 10 *Drugs currently used in treatment of scleroderma*

Drug	Mechanism of action	Efficacy in trials	
		Uncontrolled	Controlled (double blind)
D-Penicillamine	Forms a complex with hydroxylysine aldehyde and lysine groups needed for formation of stable collagen cross-links, so reducing collagen production	Yes: lung, skin, renal	?
Interferon α and γ	Specific inhibitory effect on collagen production by fibroblasts, possibly by elimination of a subpopulation of high-collagen-producing fibroblasts, or by inhibiting procollagen mRNA synthesis	Yes	?
Cyclosporin A	Alters early immune response by reducing IL-2 production ? via reduced m-RNA transcription; also reduction in IL-1 from monocytes	Yes	?
Methotrexate	Folic acid antagonist	Yes	?
Azathioprine	Purine antagonist—thus reducing DNA synthesis	?	?
Cyclophosphamide	Alkylating agent	+	?
+ prednisolone	Immunosuppressant	Yes for arthralgia, myositis	
Plasmapheresis + prednisolone and cyclosporin	Removes immune complexes and vasoactive substances	Alone no good ? in combination	
Pentoxifylline	Reduces fibroblast proliferation and synthesis of collagen glycosaminoglycans and fibronectin	Yes	?
Antithymocyte globulin	Disruption of T-cell activity early in disease, may reduce cytokine production and hence fibroblast activation	Yes	?
Photopheresis	Extracorporeal exposure of blood to photoactivated 8-methoxypsoralen to reduce activity of aberrant T cells	Yes	?
Factor XIII	Inhibits collagen synthesis	Yes	?

such as mixed connective tissue disease, undifferentiated connective tissue syndrome, and overlap syndromes have emerged to describe such patients.

Whether or not mixed connective tissue disease is a true entity as first suggested by Sharp and colleagues in the 1970s is controversial. The term described patients with some of the features of polymyositis, lupus, and scleroderma who ran a benign course with no pulmonary, cerebral, or renal involvement, and no vasculitis. They supposedly responded well to low-dose steroids, and could be identified by the presence of an antibody with a specificity for a nuclear U_1 ribonucleoprotein (RNP) antigen. However, neither the clinical features, the laboratory tests, nor the response to therapy have proven to be specific, and these patients do not fulfil the definition of and diagnostic criteria for a single disease. Neither do they fall within the 'overlap syndromes', assuming the definition for this subset to be the coexistence of two separate diseases. These patients do not 'conform'. Many with long-term follow-up develop major internal organ involvement and evolve into a defined connective tissue disease. It has also become apparent that ribonucleoprotein antibodies can be found in patients with scleroderma or systemic lupus erythematosus. The typical patient with this syndrome presents with Raynaud's phenomenon, puffy hands, arthralgia, myositis, abnormal oesophageal motility, and lymphadenopathy. Over a period of a few years, the skin may become thickened, telangiectasiae and calcinosis may appear, and signs and symptoms of interstitial lung disease emerge; such a patient has developed scleroderma. Another patient with similar initial findings may develop alopecia, photosensitivity, mouth ulcers, renal disease, antibodies to dsDNA and has developed systemic lupus erythematosus. Patients who remain undifferentiated (about 50 per cent at 5 years) are almost invariably a subset carrying HLA-DR4, the exceptions carrying HLA-DR2. Whether these observations imply the presence of a single disease entity remains unclear.

REFERENCES

Black, C.M. (1989). Raynaud's phenomenon, scleroderma, overlap syndromes, and other fibrosing syndromes. *Current Opinion in Rheumatology* **1**, (4), 473–523.

Black, C.M. (1990). Raynaud's phenomenon, scleroderma, overlap syndromes, and other fibrosing syndromes. *Current Opinion in Rheumatology* **2**, (6), 917–67.

Black, C.M. (1991). Raynaud's phenomenon, scleroderma, overlap syndromes, and other fibrosing syndromes. *Current Opinion in Rheumatology* **3**, (6), 941–95.

Black, C.M. (ed.) (1991). Systemic sclerosis (scleroderma). *Annals of the Rheumatic Diseases, Heberden Papers* **50**, (Suppl, 4).

Jablonska, S. (1975). *Scleroderma and pseudo-scleroderma.* Polish Medical Publishers, Warsaw.

Jayson, M.I.V. and Black, C.M. (ed.) (1988). *Systemic sclerosis: scleroderma.* John Wiley and Sons, New York.

LeRoy, E.C. (ed.) (1990). Scleroderma. *Rheumatic Disease Clinics of North America* **16**, 1.

LeRoy, E.C. (1992). Raynaud's phenomenon, scleroderma, overlap syndromes, and other fibrosing syndromes: editorial overview. *Current Opinion in Rheumatology* **4**, (6), 821–78.

Maddison, P.J. (1991). Mixed connective tissue disease, overlap syndromes, and eosinophilic fasciitis. *Annals of the Rheumatic Diseases* **50**, 887–93.

Medsger, T.A. Jr (1989). Systemic sclerosis (scleroderma), eosinophilic fasciitis, and calcinosis. In *Arthritis and allied conditions*, (11th edn. (ed. D.J. McCarty), pp. 1118–1165. Lea & Febiger, Philadelphia.

Medsger, T.A. Jr (1991). Treatment of systemic sclerosis. *Annals of the Rheumatic Diseases* **50**, 887–86.

18.11.5 Sjögren's syndrome

P. J. W. VENABLES

Introduction

Sjögren's syndrome, originally described in 1933 as the triad of dry eyes, dry mouth, and rheumatoid arthritis, is characterized by inflammation and destruction of exocrine glands, principally the lachrymal and salivary glands. The syndrome is now classified as primary when it exists on its own, or secondary when associated with other diseases. Well-recognized secondary associations are with rheumatoid arthritis, systemic lupus erythematosus, systemic sclerosis, polymyositis, and primary biliary cirrhosis. More recently, the syndrome has been described in chronic graft-versus-host disease after bone marrow transplantation and in infection with HTLV-1 and HIV-1, in the latter case with infiltration by CD8 T cells, not only in the salivary and lachrymal glands, but also in the gastrointestinal tract, kidneys, and liver—so-called diffuse infiltrative lymphocytic syndrome (DILS).

Aetiology and pathology

The aetiology of Sjögren's syndrome is not known, but is often considered to be related to an interaction between genetic and environmental factors, leading to autoimmunity. Primary Sjögren's syndrome is strongly associated with HLA-DR3 and the linked genes B8 and DQ2 and the C4A null gene. The syndrome occurring with HIV infection, on the other hand, is associated with alleles of HLA-DR5 and DR6, with a decreased frequency of HLA-B35.

Obvious aetiological candidates for triggering autoimmunity in Sjögren's syndrome are viruses which infect the salivary glands; Epstein–Barr virus and cytomegalovirus have been the main subjects of investigation, with conflicting results. Using DNA hybridization techniques, Epstein–Barr virus has been detected in biopsies of parotid and labial glands, but it remains controversial whether or not the virus has truly triggered the lymphocytic infiltration and inflammation in Sjögren's syndrome.

The cardinal pathological features of the syndrome are inflammation and destruction of salivary gland tissue. In primary and connective-tissue-associated Sjögren's syndrome the infiltrating cells are mainly CD4-positive T cells, found largely around ducts and acini. In cases associated with HIV-1 infection, the infiltrating lymphocytes are CD8-positive T cells, but the simple microscopic appearances are very similar. Scattered interstitial plasma cells are common, but are also seen in the glands of normal people. The destructive changes are predominantly of duct dilatation, acinal atrophy, and interstitial fibrosis. These latter findings can also be seen in biopsies of glands in patients without Sjögren's syndrome, particularly in the elderly, and cannot be regarded as specific in diagnosis.

Clinical features

Sjögren's syndrome is nine times more common in women than men and its onset is at any age from 15 to 65. Patients rarely complain of dry eyes, but rather a gritty sensation, soreness, photosensitivity, or intolerance of contact lenses. In early disease excessive watering or deposits of dried mucus in the corner of the eye and recurrent attacks of conjunctivitis may occur. The dry mouth is often manifest as the 'cream cracker' sign, inability to swallow dry food without fluid, or the need to wake up in the night to take sips of water. About half of the patients complain of intermittent parotid swelling, sometimes misdiagnosed as recurrent mumps. When the swelling is excessively painful it is often due to secondary bacterial infection. On examination, xerosto-

mia can be detected as a diminished salivary pool, a dried fissured tongue, often complicated by angular stomatitis and chronic oral candidiasis. The eyes may be reddened and roughened due to shallow erosions in the conjunctiva. Occasionally the front of the eye is eroded to reveal strands of underlying, collagen leading to the appearance of filamentary keratitis.

Other exocrine glands may be affected. Dry nasal passages and upper airways may lead to recurrent bouts of sinusitis, a dry cough, and, possibly, a higher than expected frequency of chest infections. Dry skin and dry hair are symptoms frequently elicited on direct questioning. About 30 per cent of patients have diminished vaginal secretions and may present with dyspareunia. Involvement of the gastrointestinal tract leads to reflux oesophagitis or gastritis due to lack of protective mucus secretion, and some patients complain of constipation which may be attributed to defective mucus in the colon and rectum. Pancreatic failure, leading to malabsorption syndromes, occurs rarely. Endocrine disease in the form of a higher than expected frequency of thyroid autoimmunity also occurs. Whether this is part of the same pathological process is debatable. Nevertheless, it underlines the importance of checking thyroid function from time to time in patients with Sjögren's syndrome.

The secondary Sjögren's syndrome associated with HIV infection has somewhat different clinical and laboratory features, as shown in Table 1.

Systemic manifestations

True Sjögren's syndrome is a systemic disease. Two-thirds of patients complain of fatigue and depression. Occasionally weight loss and fever mimicking an occult malignancy may be the presenting symptoms, particularly in the elderly. Other features include an arthritis which resembles the Jaccoud-like arthritis of systemic lupus erythematosus (Fig. 1). There have been intermittent reports of a higher frequency of osteoarthritis in Sjögren's syndrome, which has been termed 'SOX', but whether this is a true association is still debated. Raynaud's phenomenon occurs in about 50 per cent of patients, although a true vasculitis is less common. Waldenström's benign hypergammaglobulinaemic purpura affecting the lower legs is found in patients with very high IgG levels. Patients may present with polymyalgia rheumatica or, much less frequently, polymyositis. Pleurisy occurs in about 40 per cent, and a high prevalence of pulmonary function abnormalities has been described, although these are rarely clinically significant. A wide range of neurological diseases, including central nervous system disorders resembling multiple sclerosis, have been described, although these appear to be rare in unselected populations. Peripheral neuropathies are relatively common, particularly mononeuritis multiplex mediated by vasculitis. Interstitial nephritis leading to renal tubular acidosis or nephrogenic diabetes insipidus occurs in about 30 per cent of patients; the manifestations are usually subclinical but may lead to hypokalaemia causing muscular weakness or, occasionally, nephrocalcinosis. Lymphomas, almost always of B-cell lineage, are a characteristic but unusual feature. They occur in about 5 per cent of patients in referral units and are particularly found in patients with high levels of immunoglobulins, autoantibodies, and cryoglobulins. As the lymphoma develops, the immunoglobulin levels often fall and the autoantibodies become undetectable. Women of child-bearing age are at increased risk of giving birth to babies with congenital heart block. Although rare (about 1 in 20 000 births), this complication is of great immunopathogenic interest as it is thought to be mediated by transplacental transfer of anti-Ro and La antibodies.

In secondary Sjögren's syndrome the sicca symptoms are often said to be less severe than in primary disease. In rheumatoid arthritis with Sjögren's syndrome, the patients tend to have more frequent extra-articular manifestations, such as digital infarcts and subcutaneous ulcers. In systemic lupus erythematosus, those with Sjögren's syndrome have a lower frequency of renal disease and a relatively good prognosis.

Table 1 *Contrasting features of 'true' Sjögren's syndrome and that complicating HIV infection (diffuse infiltrative lymphocytosis syndrome; DILS) (reproduced from Itescu and Winchester 1992, with permission)*

	Sjögren's syndrome	DILS
Glandular changes	Moderate parotid swelling Frequent xerostomia Frequent xerophthalmia	Massive parotid swelling Frequent xerostomia Occasional xerophthalmia
Extraglandular features	Infrequent, but may have pulmonary, gastrointestinal, renal, and neurological involvement	Prominent pulmonary gastrointestinal, renal, and neurological involvement
Infiltrative lymphocyte phenotype	CD4 positive	CD8 positive
Autoantibodies	Common Rheumatoid factor ANA, anti-Ro (SSA), anti-La (SSB)	Rare Rheumatoid factor ANA, anti-Ro, and anti-La
HLA association	B8 DR2 DR3 DR4 (in rheumatoid)	DR5 DR6

ANA, antinuclear antibody.

Diagnostic tests

Keratoconjunctivitis sicca can be detected by Schirmer's test, tear break-up time, and Rose Bengal staining, and xerostomia by a reduced parotid salivary flow rate and by reduced uptake and clearance on isotope scans. It is important to remember that both salivary and lachrymal function decline with age and may be impaired in conditions other than Sjögren's syndrome. One cause of diagnostic confusion arises from treatment with drugs with anticholinergic side-effects, the most frequent being the tricyclic antidepressants.

Biopsy and histology of the labial glands from behind the lower lip provides the most definitive diagnostic test. The area is anaesthetized with lignocaine containing adrenaline and an incision 1.5 cm long allows access to five to ten glands, 2 to 4 mm in diameter, which are removed by simple blunt dissection. A diagnosis of Sjögren's syndrome depends on finding foci of periductular infiltrates of at least 50 lymphocytes and/or plasma cells at a density of more than one focus/4 mm^2 (Fig. 2).

The majority of patients have a raised erythrocyte sedimentation rate, and a mild normocytic anaemia with leucopenia in about 50 per cent. One of the most remarkable features of primary Sjögren's syndrome is the high level of IgG, which can be up to 50 g/l. Complement levels are usually normal, although those of C4 can sometimes be reduced, because of the link between Sjögren's syndrome and the C4A null gene. Anti-La antibodies occur in about 50 per cent of patients with primary Sjögren's syndrome. Although of relatively low sensitivity, they are of great diagnostic help when present. Rheumatoid factors, as measured by routine assays, occur in all forms of Sjögren's syndrome and their detection in primary disease is a common reason for misdiagnosing rheumatoid arthritis in such patients. Similarly, antinuclear antibodies can occur. Both rheumatoid factors and antinuclear antibodies, although not diagnostically specific, can help in distinguishing true Sjögren's syndrome from non-autoimmune causes of sicca symptoms. Anti-salivary gland antibodies have been described in patients with Sjögren's syndrome and rheumatoid arthritis, but this assay is not widely available and has not established itself as a useful diagnostic test.

Diagnostic criteria

Precise diagnostic criteria, although not important in clinical practice, are essential for the standardization of any research involving patients, particularly in the case of a disease, or group of diseases, as heterogeneous as Sjögren's syndrome. Currently used criteria depend on the demonstration of keratoconjunctivitis sicca, xerostomia, and a positive

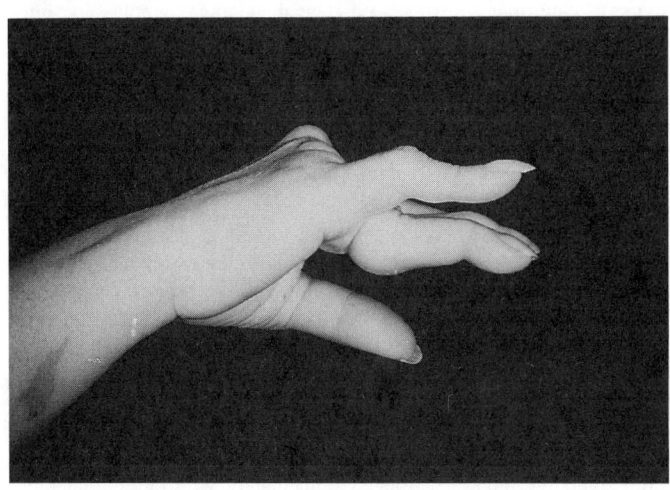

Fig. 1 Hands of a patient with long-standing primary Sjögren's syndrome, showing correctable swan-necking deformities similar to the Jaccoud-like arthritis seen in systemic lupus erythematosus.

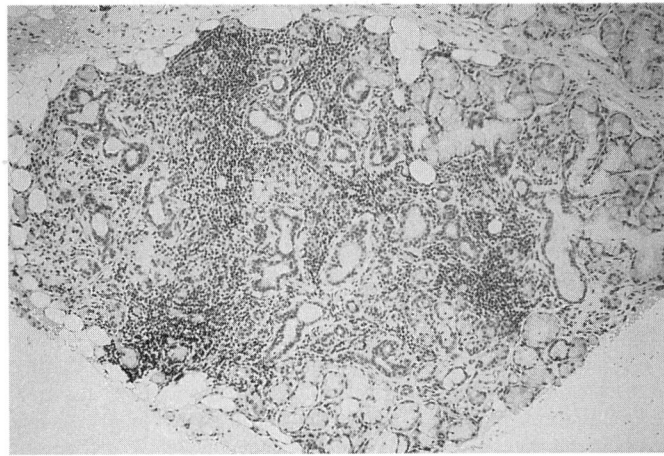

Fig. 2 Biopsy showing a lobule of minor salivary gland from a patient with Sjögren's syndrome. There are focal inflammatory infiltrates surrounding blood vessels and ducts, with the acini being relatively spared.

Table 2 *Questionnaire for eliciting the main ocular and oral symptoms of Sjögren's syndrome (from Vitali et al. 1992, with permission)*

Ocular symptoms: a positive response to at least one of the three selected questions:

1. Have you had daily, persistent, troublesome dry eyes for more than 3 months?
2. Do you have a recurrent sensation of sand or gravel in the eyes?
3. Do you use tear substitutes more than three times a day?

Oral symptoms: a positive response to at least one of the three selected questions:

1. Have you had a daily feeling of dry mouth for more than 3 months?
2. Have you had recurrently or persistently swollen salivary glands as an adult?
3. Do you frequently drink liquids to aid in swallowing dry food?

labial gland biopsy. Recently proposed criteria, based on the results of a multicentre European study, are probably the most thoroughly evaluated and simplest to apply. They are based on a short questionnaire (Table 2) of ocular and oral symptoms. Other essential criteria are ocular signs (by Schirmer's test or Rose Bengal staining), lymphocytic infiltrates on lip biopsy, salivary gland involvement (scintigraphy, sialography, or decreased salivary flow rate); and demonstration of serum autoantibodies (rheumatoid factors, antinuclear antibodies, and/or Ro or La antibodies).

Treatment

Most treatment in Sjögren's syndrome is topical and symptomatic. Simple measures can help preserve the integrity of the cornea as well as the gums and teeth, and are worth pursuing with enthusiasm rather than with the negative attitude which some patients find in their physicians. Tear substitutes, such as hypromellose eye drops, are the mainstay of treatment of the dry eye and it is generally worth trying several different types before settling on the most suitable preparation. Where thick mucus strands are a particular problem, topical acetylcysteine may help. Eye ointments, particularly at night, can help lubricate sticky eyes. Bacterial infection should be treated immediately with chloramphenicol ointment or drops. Some benefit can be achieved by preventing evaporation of tears by fitting side panels to spectacles. Temporary or permanent occlusion of the canaliculi or, rarely, tarsorraphy may help to retain tears within the conjunctival sac.

Dry mouth may be treated by saliva substitutes which are now available as convenient sprays. Candidal infections are extremely common in Sjögren's syndrome and are often missed. They are best treated with prolonged courses of anticandidal drugs, such as fluconazole, 50 mg daily for 10 days. Attention to dental hygiene may help to prevent the premature caries which is a common problem in Sjögren's syndrome.

Attempts to treat the underlying disease with steroids or cytotoxic drugs is generally thought ill-advised unless there are systemic complications. Fever and weight loss often respond well to a low dose of steroids. Serious systemic complications such as polymyositis, mononeuritis multiplex, or fibrosing alveolitis are treated with steroids and cytotoxic drugs as in other connective tissue diseases. The arthritis of primary Sjögren's syndrome may be treated with anti-inflammatory drugs, although it has been reported to respond to hydroxychloroquine. It is generally agreed that other second-line agents for rheumatoid arthritis, such as gold or sulphasalazine, are associated with a high frequency of side-effects. This is one of the most important reasons for distinguishing between the arthritis of primary Sjögren's syndrome and that of rheumatoid arthritis.

REFERENCES

Alexander, E.L., Malinow, K., Lijewski, J.E., Jerdan, M.S., Provost, T.T., and Alexander, G.E. (1986). Primary Sjögren's syndrome with central nervous system dysfunction mimicking multiple sclerosis. *Annals of Internal Medicine* **104**, 323–30.

Dwyer, E., Itescu, S., and Winchester, R. (1993). Characterization of the primary structure of T-cell receptor beta genes in cells infiltrating the salivary gland in the Sicca syndrome of HIV-1 infection. *Journal of Clinical Investigation* **92**, 495–502.

Flescher, E. and Talal, N. (1991). Do viruses contribute to the development of Sjögren's syndrome? *American Journal of Medicine* **90**, 283–5.

Fox, R.I., Robinson, C., Kozin, F., and Howell, F.V. (1986). Sjögren's syndrome: proposed criteria for classification. *Arthritis and Rheumatism* **29**, 577–85.

Itescu, S. and Winchester, R. (1992). Diffuse infiltrative lymphocytosis syndrome: a disorder occurring in human immunodeficiency virus-1 infection that may present as a Sicca Syndrome. *Rheumatic Disease Clinics of North America* **18**, 683–97.

Itescu, S., Brancato, L.J., and Winchester, R. (1989). A Sicca syndrome in HIV infection; association with HLA-DR5 and CD8 lymphocytosis. *Lancet* **2**, 466–8.

Manthorpe, R., Frost-Larsen, K., Isager, H., and Prause, J.U. (1981). Sjögren's syndrome: a review with emphasis on immunological features. *Allergy* **36**, 139–53.

Morrow, J. and Isenberg, D. (eds.) (1987). Sjögren's syndrome. In *Autoimmune rheumatic diseases*, pp. 203–33, Blackwell Scientific Publications, London.

Pease, C.T., Shattles, W., Charles, P.J., Venables, P.J.W., and Maini, R.N. (1989). Clinical, serological and HLA phenotypes subsets in Sjögren's syndrome. *Clinical and Experimental Rheumatology* **7**, 185–90.

Venables, P.J.W. (1992). Sjögren's syndrome and overlap syndromes. In *Oxford textbook of clinical nephrology* (ed. J.S. Cameron *et al.*), pp. 693–9. Oxford University Press.

Venables, P.J.W. and Brookes, S. (1992). Retroviruses: potential agents in autoimmune rheumatic disease? *British Journal of Rheumatology,* **31**, 321–5.

Vitali, C., Bombardieri, S., Montsopoulos, H. M., *et al.* (1993). Preliminary criteria for the classification of Sjögren's syndrome: results of a prospective concerted action supported by the European community. *Arthritis and Rheumatism,* **36**, 340–8.

18.11.6 Polymyositis and dermatomyositis

J. WALTON

DEFINITION

These names have been given to clinical syndromes produced by combined degenerative and inflammatory changes in skeletal muscle. They do not include suppurative, infective, and parasitic varieties of myositis, which are dealt with in Section 25.5. In some instances skin and mucous membranes are also involved, when the condition is called dermatomyositis, but often the main brunt of the disease process falls upon the skeletal muscles.

AETIOLOGY

Although the syndrome may embrace several diseases of varying aetiology, in most cases the pathological process is clearly autoimmune. Until recently it was customary to group together polymyositis and dermatomyositis, but it is now known that in several respects the two conditions are different. Thus polymyositis is due to a lymphocyte-mediated autoimmune process in which sensitized T4 and T8 cells invade and destroy skeletal muscle; the typical histological picture is one of muscle fibre necrosis and regeneration with interstitial and perivascular infiltration with such cells, which can be identified in histological preparations with monoclonal antibodies. In dermatomyositis, the intramuscular blood vessels may be damaged by circulating immune complexes and the autoimmune process is humoral rather than cell-mediated. Histologically, vasculitis is common and so is perifascicular atrophy of muscle fibres.

CLINICAL FEATURES

These syndromes are seen in patients of all ages and in both sexes. The peak incidence is in middle life. Acute polymyositis in adults is uncommon but dermatomyositis is much more so; it sometimes occurs in childhood. It is characterized by generalized muscular pains and weakness of comparatively rapid progression, associated often with a widespread erythematous rash on the face, limbs, and trunk. The proximal limb muscles are more severely affected than the distal. The affected muscles are tender and the patients are often ill and febrile; the respiratory muscles may be involved and the illness may end fatally within a few weeks or months. Subacute polymyositis is much more common. In such cases muscular pain and tenderness and symptoms of constitutional upset are often absent, and the presenting features are those of progressive weakness and moderate atrophy of the muscles of the shoulder and pelvic girdles. This clinical picture can resemble closely that of muscular dystrophy, save for the fact that in polymyositis all the proximal limb muscles are usually weakened, and the deltoid, for instance, is not spared; furthermore the neck muscles are often weak, dysphagia and a Raynaud phenomenon in the hands are common (although these two features occur more often in dermatomyositis), and the muscular weakness is often greater than the degree of atrophy would suggest. This form of subacute polymyositis is particularly common in middle and late life.

When dermatomyositis occurs in childhood or adolescence there are often minor skin changes on the face and the hands and fingers, resembling those of early systemic sclerosis or acrosclerosis. In some cases, the skin lesions resemble those of lupus erythematosus, while in others there may be associated evidence of another connective tissue disease such as rheumatoid arthritis. Subcutaneous and intramuscular calcification (calcinosis universalis) is common in childhood dermatomyositis. Many cases of dermatomyositis in middle and late life develop in association with malignant disease in the lung or in some other organ. The relationship between adult polymyositis and malignant disease is much less striking and may not, indeed, be significant.

DIAGNOSIS

In diagnosis, a raised erythrocyte sedimentation rate may be helpful but this test is normal in more than a third of all cases. The serum creatine kinase activity and immunoglobulins are also often raised, but in most cases final diagnosis depends upon a combination of the clinical findings on the one hand, with the results of electromyography and muscle biopsy on the other.

PROGNOSIS AND TREATMENT

The prognosis of polymyositis and dermatomyositis is variable. Some acute cases are eventually fatal, despite modern methods of treatment. A few subacute cases in childhood have been known to remit spontaneously and even to recover incompletely; others enter a chronic stage with the development of fibrous contractures in the muscles and severe deformity (chronic myositis fibrosa). Most subacute cases occurring in adult life are progressive; very few arrest if untreated. Many cases remit completely or partially when treated with prednisone and immunosuppressive drugs (for example azathioprine, cyclophosphamide, or methotrexate), but maintenance therapy may have to be continued for many years. Plasma exchange can be useful as a temporary measure in acute dermatomyositis; and in some intractable cases of polymyositis wholebody irradiation has been successful. Treatment is considered further in Section 25.5.

Related conditions

Several rare forms of inflammatory myopathy resembling polymyositis have been identified. Eosinophilic myositis is clinically similar and is steroid-responsive, as are granulomatous myositis (resembling sarcoidosis of muscle) and localized nodular myositis, a focal form of polymyositis which causes painful swellings in one or more muscles. An eosinophilic fasciitis giving a scleroderma-like syndrome has been described in patients receiving L-tryptophan for the treatment of depression. Inclusion-body myositis, which is more common in the older age groups, often affects distal limb muscles predominantly and is insidiously progressive in most cases, usually being uninfluenced by steroids and immunosuppressive agents. Histologically, ringed vacuoles and intranuclear filamentous inclusions are characteristic of the latter condition.

Polymyalgia rheumatica (see also Chapter 18.11.7)

This is a disorder of middle-aged and elderly patients, of whom some prove to be suffering from temporal or cranial arteritis. Typically it presents with diffuse muscle pain and aching which may restrict movement (getting out of the bath is often particularly difficult) but there is no muscular weakness or wasting. The erythrocyte sedimentation rate is invariably raised and the response to prednisone is dramatic. Maintenance treatment is often required for several months or years.

REFERENCES

Cumming, W.J.K., Weiser, R., Teoh, R., Hudgson, P., and Walton, J.N. (1977). Localised nodular myositis: a clinical and pathological variant of polymyositis. *Quarterly Journal of Medicine* 46, 531–46.
Emslie-Smith, A.M. and Engel, A.G. (1990). Microvascular changes in early and advanced dermatomyositis: a quantitative study. *Annals of Neurology* 27, 343–56.
Engel, A.G. (1990). Immune effector mechanisms in the idiopathic inflammatory myopathies. *Journal of the Neurological Sciences* 98, (Suppl.), 6.
Engel, A.G. and Emslie-Smith, A.M. (1989). Inflammatory myopathies. *Current Opinion in Neurology and Neurosurgery* 2, 695–9.
Mastaglia, F.L. and Walton, J.N. (1991). Inflammatory myopathies. In *Skeletal muscle pathology,* (ed. F.L. Mastaglia and J.N. Walton), (2nd edn), pp. 453–91. Churchill Livingstone, Edinburgh.
Whitaker, J.N. and Engel, W.K. (1972). Vascular deposits of immunoglobulin and complement in idiopathic inflammatory myopathy. *New England Journal of Medicine* 286, 333–8.

18.11.7 Polymyalgia rheumatica and giant-cell arteritis

A. G. MOWAT

Polymyalgia rheumatica and giant-cell arteritis are common debilitating conditions that may represent opposite ends of a disease spectrum, but since they appear to present with different clinical symptoms and signs and demand rather different treatment, it is convenient to describe them separately.

Polymyalgia rheumatica

Polymyalgia rheumatica is a clinical condition occurring predominantly in patients over the age of 60 years in which there is marked pain and stiffness in shoulder and pelvic girdles associated with variable systemic symptoms and elevated c-reactive protein and erythrocyte sedimentation rate. The incidence has been difficult to establish, partly because firm diagnostic criteria do not exist and partly because, with wide-ranging symptoms, patients present to several hospital departments. While an incidence of some 50 per 100 000 of the population aged 50 years and over has been accepted for hospital referrals on both sides of the Atlantic, careful study of defined elderly populations has shown an incidence of 1.5 per cent which exceeds that of any other inflammatory rheumatic disease in the elderly.

DISEASE CHARACTERISTICS

Although the most common age group involved is that between 60 and 70 years, a third of patients are under 60 years old. Initial symptoms are seldom seen before 45 years or after 80 years. The male-to-female ratio is 1:2.

The onset is often dramatic, with some patients giving the precise date of their first symptoms, and in most cases it is fully developed within a month. The source of pain and stiffness is usually localized to the muscles, although tenderness is not as severe as in myositis. There may be additional tenderness involving periarticular structures such as bursae, tendons, and joint capsules. The onset is most common in the shoulder girdle, spreading to involve both shoulders, the pelvic girdle, and proximal muscles with striking symmetry. Although a range of variants is possible, involvement of distal muscles is unusual. Immobility is most severe on waking; a characteristic complaint is a need to roll out of bed, often with the aid of the spouse. Such morning stiffness may persist for hours, making the patient totally dependent. Most patients look unwell and complain of general malaise, fatigue, and depression. Anorexia and weight loss (mean 6 kg) can be striking, often suggesting neoplasia, while night sweats and fever are frequent and occasionally are the presenting feature.

The extent of joint involvement is disputed: an incidence of mild inflammatory polyarthritis varying from 0 to 100 per cent has been recorded. Almost any joint may be affected, particularly knee and finger joints, but because the arthritis is mild and non-deforming some argue that central joint involvement, which may be the basis for the referred pain patterns, is underdiagnosed. Distinctive radiographic erosion is claimed in some central joints (e.g. sternoclavicular), while isotopic and arthroscopic studies of the shoulder support this contention, which was originally claimed by Bruk in 1967. Carpal-tunnel syndrome is an occasional accompaniment. Despite the prominent muscle symptoms, EMG studies and serum muscle enzyme values are normal while changes on sequential muscle biopsy are non-specific and largely due to disuse.

LABORATORY FINDINGS

An acute phase response (raised erythrocyte sedimentation rate, C-reactive protein, and plasma viscosity) is typical. The elevation in erythrocyte sedimentation rate, often to more than 100 mm/h, should not be overinterpreted since polymyalgia rheumatica accounts for only 2 per cent of such high values. Although untreated patients with a normal erythrocyte sedimentation rate do exist in whom C-reactive protein values will be helpful, an ESR of 40 mm/h has good diagnostic value. A mild hypochromic normocytic anaemia (mean 12.2 g/dl, range 8.0–14.5 g/dl) is common, with normal marrow and low plasma iron values. Iron therapy is ineffective; the haemoglobin rises with disease control. Other cell counts are normal. There are no consistent changes in protein electrophoresis, immunoglobulins, or complement values, and rheumatoid factor shows a low incidence of positivity consistent with the patient's age. Several studies have demonstrated a profound and selective decrease in the CD8+ suppressor–cytotoxic T cells that persists for a year or more after apparent disease control. Serum values of liver enzymes, alkaline phosphatase, and γ-glutamyl transferase are elevated in most patients, and can be correlated with the erythrocyte sedimentation rate and disease severity. Liver biopsy shows only a mild cellular infiltrate and minor changes in the bile canaliculi.

Apart from the changes in CD8+ cells, all other clinical and laboratory features clear rapidly with corticosteroid therapy.

DIFFERENTIAL DIAGNOSIS

In the absence of a unique feature or confirmatory laboratory test polymyalgia rheumatica remains a clinical diagnosis; thus it is axiomatic that a careful history is taken and a full examination carried out. Diagnostic criteria have been validated and the seven best discriminatory features are shown in Table 1. A patient should be considered to have polymyalgia rheumatica if three or more criteria are fulfilled. Until recently there was a mean delay in diagnosis of 6 months, with the striking features being ascribed to osteoarthritis or psychological illness. Now, greater awareness and fear of the link with giant-cell arteritis and possible blindness has led to overdiagnosis and overtreatment, with the frequency of muscle aching in middle age being forgotten. This has been compounded by an over-reliance on the specificity of the corticosteroid response. Many elderly patients feel better on taking corticosteroids, and most rheumatic diseases including osteoarthritis respond dramatically to these drugs.

Differential diagnosis will include a wide range of conditions (Table 2). Infection may be viral or bacterial, with miliary tuberculosis and infective endocarditis causing confusion. Bone diseases may be difficult to separate as they are common incidental findings in this elderly group and the alkaline phosphatase is raised in polymyalgia rheumatica. This is also the case with neoplastic disease, which may be associated with myalgia even in the absence of secondary spread to bone. Primary muscle disease can be distinguished by EMG, biopsy, and enzyme values, but inflammatory joint disease, particularly osteoarthritis, rheumatoid arthritis, and other connective tissue diseases, all of which may start with a polymyalgic pattern lasting for some months in older patients, cause confusion although appropriate serological tests should help.

AETIOLOGY AND PATHOGENESIS

While the arteritis in giant-cell arteritis ensures a homogeneous group, it is possible that polymyalgia rheumatica includes several different conditions, one of which is due to arteritis occurring in 15 per cent of cases. A distinct prodromal malaise noted by many patients and a possible summer/winter peak incidence has promoted an unrewarding search for infective causes. The evidence for a central arthritis affecting clavicular, shoulder, and sacroiliac joints could explain the pain patterns in polymyalgia rheumatica; one elegant study reproduced these patterns by injecting hypertonic saline into these joints. In those with proven arteritis, which need not be confined to the temporal and other central vessels but, rather, is found in larger arteries all over the body and is associated with bruits and tenderness, a similar pattern of referred pain can be implicated. An immune destruction of the internal elastic lamina is proposed and supported by finding circulating immune complexes, together with immunoglobulins, complement deposition, and mononuclear cell infiltrate adjacent to the lamina (Fig. 1).

Although polymyalgia rheumatica is found worldwide, it is more common in Caucasians, particularly those of Scandinavian extraction. The infrequency of the disease in spouses argues against environmental factors, while familial aggregation and association with HLA DR4 suggests both genetic and immunological mechanisms.

TREATMENT

Once the diagnosis is secure there is no justification for treating polymyalgia rheumatica with non-steroidal anti-inflammatory drugs; all patients should receive prednisolone. The dose should be just sufficient to abolish symptoms (e.g. 10–20 mg/day in two divided doses), and it is rarely necessary to use an arteritic suppressing dose (60–100 mg) since those patients at risk of visual and neurological complications can be separated by symptoms and signs (see below). The initial erythrocyte sedimentation rate or C-reactive protein values are no guide to disease type or steroid dose, and are not even of much value in deciding upon dose reduction. It is usually possible to reduce the dose to 10 mg/day

Table 1 *Validation of diagnostic criteria for polymyalgia rheumatica*

Discriminatory feature	Sensitivity* (%)	Relative value†
Shoulder pain and/or stiffness bilaterally	86	155
Onset duration 2 weeks or less	88	151
Initial ESR > 40 mm/h	74	149
Stiffness duration > 1 h	80	141
Age 65 + years	70	139
Depression and/or weight loss	58	130
Upper-arm tenderness bilaterally	36	132

$$*\text{Sensitivity} (\%) = \frac{\text{individuals with disease with positive test}}{\text{all individuals with disease}}$$

$$\text{Specificity} (\%) = \frac{\text{individuals with disease with positive test}}{\text{all individuals without disease}}$$

†Relative value = sensitivity + specificity (range 0–200)

After H. A. Bird *et al.* (1979). *Annals of the Rheumatic Diseases,* **38,** 434–9.

Table 2 *Differential diagnosis of polymyalgia rheumatica*

Infection
  Viral
  Brucellosis
  Tuberculosis
  Endocarditis

Bone disease
  Osteoporosis
  Osteomalacia
  Paget's disease
  Senile hyperostotic spinal ankylosis

Joint disease
  Osteoarthritis
  Rheumatoid arthritis
  Connective tissue diseases

Others
  Neoplasia
  Muscle disease
  Fibromyalgia syndrome
  Chronic fatigue syndrome
  Parkinsonism
  Hypothyroidism

within 2 to 3 months, but thereafter the rate must be slow. Alternate-day therapy is ineffective, while withdrawal at any time may be followed by a relapse perhaps months later. Azathioprine has a modest steroid-sparing effect.

As the average duration of symptoms is 2 to 3 years, with some persisting for 7 or more years corticosteroid side-effects are common. Up to 50 per cent of patients subjected to this treatment experience some side-effects, usually weight gain and fluid retention. Serious side-effects, including osteoporotic fractures, avascular necrosis of bone particularly at the hip, diabetes, and hypertension, are related to high initial and maintenance dosage, and prolonged therapy with high cumulative doses. The difficulties in diagnosis and the risk of corticosteroid therapy argue for management to be shared with a specialist, certainly in younger or unusual cases.

Relationship of polymyalgia rheumatica to giant-cell arteritis

William Bruce, a physician practising in Strathpeffer Spa, Scotland, described polymyalgia rheumatica in 1888 using the term senile rheumatic gout, and Jonathan Hutchison described giant-cell arteritis in 1890. The current names were applied much later. For more than 20 years a common cause has been suggested, emphasized by the term polymyalgia arteritica, based upon the following observations:

(1) the age and sex distribution is the same, and Caucasians (Scandinavians) are mostly affected;

(2) the similarity of the myalgia and associated systemic features;

(3) the similarity of the laboratory features (both are associated with a reduction in CD8+ T cells and HLA DR4);

(4) the positive biopsy findings show an identical pattern of giant-cell arteritis (Fig. 1);

(5) the similarity in the corticosteroid response;

(6) the failure to demonstrate differences in disease cause between positive and negative biopsy patients with polymyalgia rheumatica (Table 3).

The last finding may be explained by the patchy involvement that can be missed even in long specimens from temporal or occipital arteries. Angiography at the time of biopsy has not increased the sensitivity. The importance of positive biopsy to a clinician is less as a guide to initial steroid dosage, which reflects clinical and not laboratory features, but rather as reassurance about later questioning over the diagnosis and true need for steroid therapy.

Giant-cell arteritis

Giant-cell (cranial, senile, or temporal) arteritis, which is rare before the age of 50 years, chiefly affects those between 65 and 75 years with a male-to-female ratio of 1:2. An annual incidence of biopsy-proven disease amongst those in the population aged 50 years or more of 18 per 100 000 (25 per 100 000 for women and 10 per 100 000 for men) has been recorded in the United States and Scandinavia, with the rate for women appearing to rise.

DISEASE CHARACTERISTICS

The features of giant-cell arteritis are protean, being variable in presentation and on examination, but typical series are shown (Table 4). The diagnosis depends upon a high degree of clinical suspicion in less typical cases. As with polymyalgia rheumatica, the onset may be dramatic and

Fig. 1 Photomicrograph of a temporal artery biopsy showing giant cells, a monocellular infiltrate, and disruption of the internal elastic lamina.

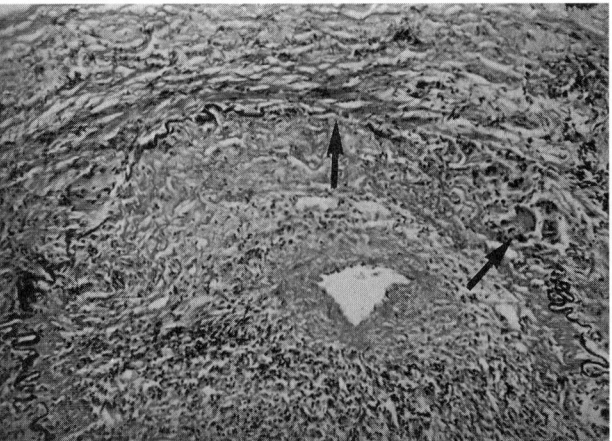

Table 3 *Biopsy findings in 148 patients with polymyalgia rheumatica or giant-cell arteritis*

Symptoms	Biopsy findings		No biopsy	Total
	Positive	Negative		
Local symptoms of TA without myalgia	27	1	0	28
Local symptoms of TA with myalgia	42	4	1	47
Myalgia without local symptoms of TA	29	39	5	73

TA, temporal arteritis.

Table 4 *Clinical presentation and features of giant-cell arteritis (percentage of cases affected)*

Chief presentation		Clinical features	
Symptoms of temporal arteritis	30%	Signs of temporal arteritis	90%
Polymyalgia rheumatica	27%	Polymyalgia rheumatica	55%
Weight loss, malaise	14%	Weight loss, malaise	50%
Fever	13%	Visual disturbance	40%
Visual disturbance	6%	Fever	32%
Headache	4%	Cranial features	24%
Anaemia	4%	Peripheral neuropathy	12%
Claudication (leg)	2%	Claudication (leg)	7%

the condition always becomes fully developed over a few weeks although the delay in diagnosis may be months. The malaise, fever, and anaemia are similar to those in polymyalgia rheumatica; the differences are in the vascular symptoms. The majority have temporal features with headache, scalp sensitivity, and tender thickened arteries; the classical nodular red streaks are unusual. Overwhelming generalized headache and the feared complication of irreversible loss of vision are more readily recognized. The clinical features listed emphasize developing arteritis. A wide range of cranial manifestations reflects the involvement of larger arteries with an internal elastic lamina in the face, neck, and brain base but not in the cerebral vessels. They include headache, scalp tenderness, skin necrosis, jaw claudication while talking or chewing, tongue pain and claudication, and face and neck pain with nerve damage. The visual manifestations, which include blurred vision, amaurosis fujax, transient and permanent blindness, diplopia, and visual hallucinations, are due to ischaemic changes in the ciliary arteries causing optic neuritis or infarction, with a smaller number of cases being due to central retinal artery thrombosis. A few patients may have evidence of arteritis elsewhere, with intermittent claudication, peripheral neuropathy, widespread vessel tenderness with bruits, myocardial ischaemia and damage, and occasionally an aortic arch syndrome with valve disease. Stroke due to brain-stem vascular disease is uncommon, accounting for only 1 to 2 per cent of such cases. In contradistinction to other vasculitides, renal involvement is rare.

LABORATORY FEATURES

Laboratory features are exactly the same as in polymyalgia rheumatica. Temporal artery biopsy is the definitive diagnostic test. A 2 cm segment of a tender artery obtained after local anaesthetic infiltration will provide positive histology in 70 per cent of cases. The rate may be enhanced by taking longer segments or by the biopsy of other tender scalp vessels. While biopsy confirmation of the diagnosis is important, it should not be a reason for withholding steroids since characteristic pathological features persist for 2 weeks after treatment has begun.

DIFFERENTIAL DIAGNOSIS

Since the diagnosis of giant-cell arteritis depends upon a positive biopsy, the differential diagnosis does not include other causes of headache,

neck pain, anaemia, and weight loss. The vasculitis of rheumatoid arthritis or systemic lupus erythematosus affects arterioles and is associated with other disease features, particularly arthritis and characteristic immunological tests. Polyarteritis, although not always nodular, affects small arteries with cutaneous, abdominal, and renal rather than cranial features and the histology is distinctive. Although cranial and central nervous system features occur in Wegener's granulomatosis, involvement of many systems includes characteristic lesions of the respiratory tract with diagnostic histological features. Takayasu's arteritis, in which the pathological lesions mimic those of giant-cell arteritis, is confined to the aortic arch and its major branches and occurs chiefly in young oriental women.

TREATMENT

The only treatment is corticosteroids; immunosuppressive therapy has no direct effect and the modest steroid sparing rarely warrants the additional hazard. With clear arteritic features 60 to 100 mg of prednisolone in two to four divided doses per day is required. Ophthalmologists, who are likely to see patients with established visual effects or threatening features in the second eye, may use higher doses or methylprednisolone infusions. Dosage reduction must be gradual and be judged solely on clinical features as acute phase responses (erythrocyte sedimentation rate or C-reactive protein) are no guide. Most should have achieved a maintenance dose of 10 mg/day after 1 year. Subsequently the known persistence of disease in a significant proportion for 4 years or more and the possible recurrence of symptoms, including blindness, even a year after corticosteroid withdrawal argues for very gradual dosage reduction and careful monitoring even after withdrawal. Unfortunately there are no predictors of these risks. Accordingly, the hazards of therapy are even greater than in polymyalgia rheumatica. Despite all the problems, giant-cell arteritis does not reduce life expectancy.

REFERENCES

Achkar, A.A., Lie, J.T., Hunder, G.G., O'Fallon, M., and Gabriel, S.E. (1994). How does previous corticosteroid therapy affect the biopsy findings in giant cell arteritis? *Annals of Internal Medicine,* **120,** 987–92.

Allison, M.C. and Gallagher, P.J. (1984). Temporal artery biopsy and corticosteroid treatment. *Annals of the Rheumatic Diseases,* Disease, **43,** 416–17.

Bird, H.A., Esselinckx, W., Dixon, A.St. J., Mowat, A.G., and Wood, P.H.N. (1979). An evaluation of criteria for polymyalgia rheumatica. *Annals of the Rheumatic Diseases*, **38**, 434–9.

Bruk, M.I. (1967). Articular and vascular manifestations of polymyalgia rheumatica. *Annals of the Rheumatic Diseases*, **26**, 103–13.

Hazleman, B. and Bengtsson, B.A. (1991). Giant-cell arteritis. *Clinical Rheumatology*, **5** (3).

Kyle, V. and Hazleman, B.L. (1989). Treatment of polymyalgia rheumatica and giant cell arteritis. Relation between steroid dose and steroid associated side-effects. *Annals of the Rheumatic Diseases*, **48**, 662–6.

Mason, J.C. and Walport, M.J. (1992). Giant cell arteritis. Probably under-diagnosed and overtreated. *British Medical Journal*, **305**, 68–9.

Sandercock, P.A.G., Warlow, C.P., Jones, L.N., and Starkey, I.R. (1989). Predisposing factors for cerebral infarction: the Oxfordshire Community Stroke Project. *British Medical Journal*, **298**, 75–80.

18.11.8 Behçet's disease

T. LEHNER

Introduction

Behçet's disease is a recurrent, multifocal disorder which usually persists over many years. It was first described by Hippocrates in ancient Greece and later by Behçet, a Turkish dermatologist. Initial description of the disease comprised oral and genital ulcers and uveitis, but later a number of other clinical features were added, notably skin, joint, neurological, and vascular manifestations. This creates considerable difficulty in diagnosis and a multidisciplinary approach is often required.

An international study group has recently proposed a set of diagnostic criteria based on data from 914 patients with the disease from 12 centres and seven countries, requiring the presence of oral ulcers plus any two of the following; genital ulcers, defined eye lesions, defined skin lesions, or a positive skin pathergy test. These criteria (Table 1) show better discrimination in sensitivity, specificity, and relative value than did their predecessors. A large number of important clinical manifestations of Behçet's disease have not been included (Table 2) because their lower frequency does not contribute to the accuracy of diagnosis. The same group have proposed that the term 'Behçet's syndrome' be replaced by 'Behçet's disease'.

Epidemiology

The striking feature of the disease is the relatively high prevalence in Japan (1 in 10000). Indeed, in 1977 there was an estimated total of 11000 patients with Behçet's disease in Japan. The prevalence is also high in countries bordering the Mediterranean: Italy, Greece, Turkey, Israel, Egypt, Lebanon, Syria, Jordan, Saudi Arabia, as well as Algeria and Tunisia. An epidemiological study in the United Kingdom has shown a prevalence of 1 in 170 000 which compares with 1 in 800 000 in a study in the United States.

Although the disease may develop at any age, the most common onset is in the third decade. However, it can start in childhood with orogenital ulcers, followed by the other manifestations years or decades later. Male predominance is found in most reported series, but this may vary from 2:1 in Japan to 9:1 in the Middle East. Increased familial prevalence of the syndrome has been recorded frequently, and there is an immunogenetic basis for the disease.

Aetiology

The cause of Behçet's disease is unknown but an immunogenetic basis has now been established. HLA-B51 is significantly associated and HLA-B51, B12, DR7, and DR2 might in some way be associated with tissue localization of the disease. As with other HLA disease associations, there are at least two interpretations of these findings:

Table 1 *International study group criteria for diagnosis of Behçet's disease: recurrent oral ulcers plus any two of the four other manifestations*

Recurrent oral ulcers	Minor aphthous, major aphthous, or herpetiform ulcers which recurred at least three times a year
Recurrent genital ulcers	Ulcers or scarring
Eye lesions	Anterior uveitis, posterior uveitis, or cells in the vitreous on slit-lamp examination; or retinal vasculitis
Skin lesions	Erythema nodosum, pseudofolliculitis, papulopustular lesions, or acneiform nodules in postadolescent patients not on corticosteroid treatment
Positive pathergy test	Read by physician at 24–48 h

Table 2 *Clinical manifestations of Behçet's syndrome*

Mucocutaneous
    Recurrent oral ulcers: aphthous or herpetiform
    Recurrent genital ulcers: vulval, vaginal, penile, or scrotal
    Skin lesions: pustules, erythema nodosum, perianal ulceration, erythema multiforme
Arthritic
    Polyarthritis of predominantly large joints
    Polyarthralgia of large joints
Neurological
    Brain-stem syndrome, resembling minor strokes
    Meningomyelitis or meningoencephalitis
    Organic confusional syndromes
    Multiple sclerosis-like disorder
Ocular
    Uveitis with or without hypopyon
    Iridocyclitis
    Retinal vascular lesions
    Optic atrophy
Vascular
    Venous thrombosis
    Aneurysms
Gastrointestinal
    Abdominal pain, diarrhoea, distension, nausea, and anorexia
Others
    Pulmonary: haemoptysis
    Renal: asymptomatic proteinuria and haematuria

(1) the HLA antigen might function as a specific receptor for viruses (or pathogens); or

(2) the antigenic determinants of some pathogens might mimic the HLA antigens.

A viral aetiology for Behçet's disease has often been claimed, but attempts to isolate viruses from patients have failed. An indirect approach to the study of a viral aetiology in autoimmune diseases has been the finding that herpes simplex virus failed to replicate in inactivated cultures of mononuclear cells from patients with Behçet's disease. The interference with the growth of virus was considered to be consistent with a viral aetiology of the disease. However, a direct approach, using herpes simplex virus DNA probes and *in situ* hybridization with the complementary RNA mononuclear cells, revealed a significant increase in hybridization in those with Behçet's disease. These results suggest that at least part of the herpes simplex virus genome is transcribed in the circulating mononuclear cells of these patients. The role of the virus in the immunopathogenesis of Behçet's disease, however, has not been elucidated; it may induce some defect in immunoregulation or invoke an autoimmune response.

A variety of streptococci (*Streptococcus sanguis*, *Strep. pyogenes*, *Strep. faecalis*, and *Strep. salivarius*) have been implicated in the aetiology of Behçet's disease, leading to the hypothesis that heat-shock protein might be a common and perhaps causative agent among these bacteria. Indeed, a significant increase in serum IgA antibodies to the mycobacterial 65 kDa heat-shock protein has been found in patients with Behçet's disease. Earlier reports of autoimmune responses to oral epithelial antigens have also been re-investigated, and a 65 kDa band has been identified with polyclonal and monoclonal anti-65 kDa heat-shock protein antibodies and mucosal homogenate, as well as streptococci. This evidence, that the 65 kDa heat-shock protein might be involved in the disease, is consistent with the finding of a significant increase in circulating T cells with the γδ T-cell receptor. Furthermore, four peptides derived from the sequence of the mycobacterial 65 kDa heat-shock protein and the corresponding four homologous human heat-shock protein peptides specifically stimulate T cells from patients with Behçet's disease. The potential pathogenicity of some of these peptides has now been established in rats that developed anterior uveitis when the peptides were injected with adjuvant by the subcutaneous route. Overall, the evidence is growing that Behçet's disease may be closely associated with heat-shock protein peptides of microbial and cross-reactive human origin.

Immunopathology

An early lymphomonocytic infiltration is usually found at the onset of ulceration in the lamina propria, the adjacent epithelium, and around small blood vessels. The latter may show endothelial cell proliferation and some obliteration of the lumen. Although the early stages are suggestive of the type IV cell-mediated immune reaction, this is followed by a polymorphonuclear infiltration and fibrinoid necrosis in the blood vessels, consistent with a type III Arthus reaction. The keratinocytes of oral epithelial cells adjacent to an ulcer express HLA class II antigen.

Cell-mediated immune responses can be induced *in vitro* by homogenates of oral mucosa; these elicit lymphoproliferative responses, leucocyte migration inhibition, and cytotoxicity. The proportion of CD4 cells may be decreased, but that of CD8 cells remains within the normal range.

Circulating immune complexes have been detected in 40 to 60 per cent of patients with Behçet's disease and are associated with disease activity. Although the concentrations of serum C3 and C4 are normal, careful sequential studies revealed that C3, C4, and C2 were significantly reduced before an attack of uveitis, suggesting complement consumption by the classical pathway. Electron microscopical examination of centrifuged pellets of serum revealed the presence of small membrane fragments, some of which showed complement-dependent holes. These findings suggest that the soluble immune complex may generate C5b-9 complexes which may bind to the surface of cells and result in cell lysis.

Acute-phase proteins are increased in Behçet's disease, especially serum C-reactive protein and C9. However, α_1-acid glycoprotein is significantly increased in the ocular type and factor B in the neurological type of Behçet's disease. Serum C9 is a good marker of disease activity and can be useful in monitoring treatment.

An increased serum chemotactic activity is found with normal polymorphonuclear leucocytes and this might be due to IgG complexes releasing chemotactic factors. However, leucocytes from patients with Behçet's disease may show a depressed response to chemotactic stimuli and this might be ascribed to IgA complexes. It should be noted that serum IgA is often increased but IgG and IgM are variable in Behçet's disease.

Unlike most autoimmune diseases, nuclear, thyroid, and gastric autoantibodies are not found in greater proportion in Behçet's disease than in the normal population. Rheumatoid factor is also negative, even in patients with joint involvement.

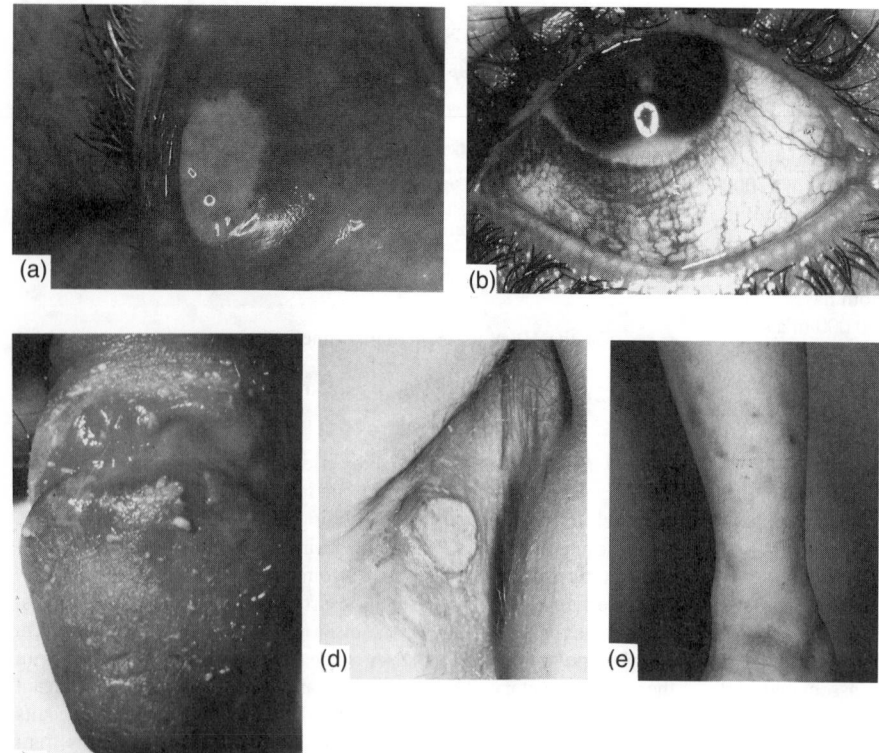

Fig. 1 Behçet's disease: (a) oral ulcer, (b) hypopyon in the eye, (c) ulceration of the head of the penis, (d) vulval ulcers, (e) multiple erythema nodosum lesions of the leg.

Clinical features

The patients often appear to be generally well and complain only of the localized lesions. However, occasionally they may present with acute exacerbation of malaise, fever, dysphagia, and loss of weight. Other manifestations are listed in Table 2.

RECURRENT ORAL ULCERS

Oral ulcers are the presenting feature in most but not all patients with Behçet's disease. The ulcers can be of the minor or major aphthous or herpetiform type (see Section 7). However, since these ulcers are rather common in the general population and usually give rise only to local discomfort, they may be missed in the patient's history. Indeed, the least severe minor aphthous ulcers are found in 67 per cent of the neurological and 76 per cent of the ocular types of Behçet's disease, whereas the most severe type of major aphthous ulcers are found in 40 and 64 per cent, respectively, of the mucocutaneous and arthritic types. Herpetiform ulcers are found mostly in the mucocutaneous type (45 per cent). An essential feature in relation to the diagnosis of Behçet's disease is that the ulcers recur frequently, at intervals of weeks or months, but this varies from one patient to another. The long-cherished view that oral ulcers in Behçet's disease are rather severe and associated with scarring is no longer tenable. The clinical manifestations can be readily recognized and differentiated from those of similar disorders. The pharynx can also be the site of aphthous ulcers which tend to be rather large, shallow, and covered with a fibrinopurulent exudate (Fig. 1).

GENITAL ULCERS

These are found in most, but not all, patients and can be of the three types described for oral ulcers. They affect females more commonly than males, and scars may follow healing in either sex. Females develop recurrent ulcers on their labia or vagina and they suffer from dysuria and dyspareunia which can ruin their marriage. Males develop recurrent ulcers on the penis or scrotum, again with dysuria and pain on sexual intercourse; some patients develop epididymo-orchitis.

SKIN LESIONS

These vary, but diffuse pustular lesions on the face and particularly the back are most common. Erythema nodosum may affect the limbs or other parts of the body. Occasionally, erythema multiforme is found. Both females and males may develop perianal ulcers and, curiously, these may present in the young, well before genital ulcers have appeared.

OCULAR LESIONS

These are the most serious developments in Behçet's disease. Relapsing uveitis, with or without hypopyon, iridocyclitis, retinal vascular lesions, and optic atrophy are common findings. Relapsing conjunctivitis, keratitis, and choroiditis are also features. Gross retinal vascular changes affect both arteries and veins, and fluorescein angiography is particularly helpful in such cases. Both eyes tend to be involved in 90 per cent of patients, within a period of 2 years of onset of symptoms in one eye. Visual prognosis is then poor, as useful vision (less than 6/60) is lost in about half the patients within 4 years of onset of the ocular symptoms.

NEUROLOGICAL FEATURES

These are found in 10 to 25 per cent of patients with Behçet's disease (see also Section 24). The patients develop transient or persistent brain-stem syndromes resembling minor strokes. Transient focal cerebral syndromes and spinal cord involvement are also found. Others may present with meningomyelitis or meningoencephalitis and some with organic confusional syndromes. Multiple sclerosis-like features have also been described. The cerebrospinal fluid sometimes shows pleocytosis and raised protein concentrations but more often is normal. Computed tomography (CT) scanning does not often reveal abnormalities but the electroencephalogram (EEG) can show slowing of basic rhythm. Magnetic resonance imaging (MRI) is the most sensitive and reliable examination, since most patients with neurological involvement may manifest:

(1) atrophy of the cerebral cortex, cerebellum, or brain-stem;
(2) the sinuses may be enlarged;
(3) high-intensity signals may be recorded in the pons, brainstem, or the midbrain; and
(4) demyelinating processes may be found in the pons and medulla.

MRI can help to differentiate Behçet's disease from multiple sclerosis and other neurological diseases, as well as in assessing the response to treatment.

The prognosis of Behçet's disease with neurological features used to be poor, with mortality of about 40 per cent in the literature before 1970. However, the prognosis has recently been improved with reduced mortality, although whether this can be attributed to steroid and/or cytotoxic agents remains uncertain.

ARTHRITIS OR ARTHRALGIA

The joints are involved in about half the patients with Behçet's disease, at irregular intervals and usually in more than one joint. The knees, ankles, and elbows are most commonly involved, and less frequently the joints of the hands, feet, shoulders, and hips. Effusions, especially in the knees, cause considerable disability. Radiography of the joints does not usually demonstrate erosive or destructive changes, but a number of exceptions have now been recorded with erosive change in the hips, wrists, and elbows. The test for rheumatoid factor is negative.

VASCULAR LESIONS

Recurrent thrombophlebitis of leg veins is a significant feature of Behçet's disease. This has been ascribed to decreased plasma fibrinolytic activity. Less frequently, superior or inferior vena cava thrombosis may develop. Arterial aneurisms have also been reported.

GASTROINTESTINAL MANIFESTATIONS

These are ill-defined. The Japanese literature records diarrhoea, distension, nausea, and anorexia in more than half the patients. Radiological examination has revealed abnormalities affecting predominantly the small intestine; dilatation, gas and fluid retention, segmentation and thickening of intestinal folds. However, a British series failed to identify consistent gastrointestinal manifestations, although various transient symptoms were noted in 13 of 70 patients; two of these had rectal ulcers and one each an anal ulcer, a small intestinal ulcer, perianal fistula, and coeliac disease. It should be noted that patients with inflammatory bowel disease are excluded from the diagnosis of Behçet's disease by the Mayo Clinic, although they may fulfil current criteria for that diagnosis.

RENAL INVOLVEMENT

This has not been established in Behçet's disease. A small number of patients have been reported with Behçet's disease and amyloidosis affecting the kidneys, and a few also with glomerulonephritis. It is doubtful if these renal changes can be considered as primary manifestations of the disease, and they may well be coincidental. Asymptomatic proteinuria and haematuria without evidence either of amyloidosis or nephritis have also been reported in a small number of patients. In a prospective British study, two out of 38 patients with Behçet's disease showed evidence of renal disease. One of these, with biopsy-proven focal proliferative glomerulonephritis, has had no clinical symptoms, and in a 5-year follow-up period the glomerular filtration rate has remained normal.

PULMONARY MANIFESTATIONS

These have been reported occasionally, usually with haemoptysis. In some of these patients, pulmonary tuberculosis has been suspected.

Diagnosis

There are no definitive criteria for the diagnosis of Behçet's disease and the various schemes suggested rely on the association between two, three, or four clinical features (Table 1). Accordingly, the terms incomplete and complete Behçet's disease are often used. The spectrum of the disorder can be divided into four types, which appear to have an immunogenetic basis.

(1) Mucocutaneous disease which involves oral and genital ulcers with or without skin manifestations; in these, HLA-B12 and/or DR2 is significantly raised.

(2) Arthritic type, in which joint involvement is combined with some or all of the muco-cutaneous manifestations; again HLA-B12 and/or DR2 is raised.

(3) Neurological type, which involves the central nervous system and some or all of the features in (1) and (2); here, HLA-DR7 or DRw52 (MT2) is raised.

(4) Ocular type, which affects the eyes with some or all the features described in (1), (2), and (3); HLA-B51 and/or DR7 is raised.

Thrombosis of blood vessels can be found in any one of the four types of Behçet's disease, as can some of the other inconsistent features.

HLA-B51 is significantly associated but is not diagnostic of the disease.

The pathergy test, whereby a sterile subcutaneous puncture (without injection of any material) elicits a pustular reaction within 24 to 48 h, has been used as a diagnostic test in the Middle Eastern countries and in Japan. The presence of immune complexes is consistent with Behçet's disease and so are the raised levels of acute-phase-reacting proteins; C9 is particularly useful in monitoring the course of the disorder.

Patients with rheumatoid arthritis, osteoarthritis, or Reiter's syndrome are excluded from the diagnosis of Behçet's disease, as are patients with a firm diagnosis of ulcerative colitis or Crohn's disease. Stevens–Johnson syndrome may mimic Behçet's disease but the recurrences are less frequent and tend to be seasonal, the ulcers are large and shallow, the lips are often covered with haemorrhagic crusts, and the skin may show typical lesions of erythema multiforme.

Treatment

The management of patients with Behçet's disease can be difficult, as it requires close liaison between different specialties. Whenever possible, topical treatment of local lesions should be attempted before embarking on systemic anti-inflammatory or immunosuppressive therapy. Oral and genital ulcers often respond to topical application of steroids or tetracycline or both, as described elsewhere. Uveitis is also initially treated with local steroids. However, at some stage systemic prednisolone is usually administered, with a starting dose of 30 to 60 mg/day which is rapidly brought down to a minimum effective maintenance dose of about 10 mg. There is usually a prompt response, although a small core of patients are resistant to steroid therapy. Aza-

thioprine is often used with prednisolone (2–3 mg/kg body weight daily) and, quite a[ ] from its steroid-sparing function, it may have additional beneficial effects. Colchicine has been particularly advocated by Japanese and Turkish physicians for the treatment of the disease and a recommended dose of 0.5 mg twice a day. The rationale is that this drug inhibits the motility of polymorphonuclear leucocytes, which is increased in Behçet's disease. Colchicine can be helpful, although it is not certain whether the drug may not have a selective beneficial effect on some lesions. There is a general consensus that cyclosporin (2.5–5 mg/kg body weight) should be used in patients with unresponsive uveitis in spite of possible serious side-effects. Chlorambucil has also been applied successfully in the treatment of uveitis, but side-effects have limited its application. Thalidomide has recently been found to be effective in the treatment of orogenital ulcers, but the teratogenic effect of this drug may severely restrict its use.

REFERENCES

Barnes, C.G. (1979). Behçet's syndrome–Joint manifestations and synovial pathology. In *Behçet's syndrome. Clinical and immunology features. Proceedings of a conference sponsored by the Royal Society of Medicine, February 1979,* (ed. T. Lehner and C.G. Barnes), pp. 199–212. Academic Press, London.

BenEzra, D. and Nussenblatt, R. (1978). Ocular manifestations of Behçet's disease. *Journal of Oral Pathology* **7**, 431–5.

Chajek, T. and Fainaru, M. (1975). Behçet's disease. Report of 41 cases and a review of the literature. *Medicine* **54**, 179–96.

Chamberlain, M.A. (1977). Behçet's syndrome in 32 patients in Yorkshire. *Annals of the Rheumatic Diseases* **36**, 491–9.

Fukuda, Y., Hayashi, H., and Kuwabara, N. (1982). Pathological studies on neuro-Nehcet's disease. In *Behçet's disease. Pathogenitic mechanism and clinical future. Proceedings of the International Conference on Behçet's disease, 23–24 October 1981, Tokyo,* (ed. G. Inaba) pp. 127–43. University of Tokyo Press, Tokyo.

Hughes, R.A.C. and Lehner, T. (1979). Neurological aspects of Behçet's syndrome. In *Behçet's syndrome. Clinical and immunological features. Proceedings of a conference sponsored by the Royal Society of Medicine, February 1979,* (ed. T. Lehner and C.G. Barnes), pp. 241–58. Academic Press, London.

International Study Group for Behçet's Disease (1990). Criteria for diagnosis of Behçet's disease. *Lancet* **335**, 1078.

Jorizzo, J.L., *et al.* (1986). Thalidomide effects in Behçet's syndrome and pustular vasculitis. *Archives of Internal Medicine* **146**, 878–81.

Lehner, T., *et al.* (1993). T and B cell epitope mapping with heat shock protein in peptides in Behçet's disease and induction of uveitis in rats. In *Excerpta Medica International Congress. 6th International Conference on Behçet's Disease, Paris, 30 June–1 July, 1993.* Elsevier Science, Holland.

Masuda, K., Nakajima, A., Urayama, A., Nakae, K., Kogure, M., and Inaba, G. (1989). Double-masked trial of cyclosporin versus colchicine and long-term open study of cyclosporin in Behçet's disease. *Lancet* **1**, 1093–5.

Mizushima, Y., *et al.* (1977). Colchicine in Behçet's disease (letter). *Lancet* **2**, 1037.

Nussenblatt, R.B., Palestine, A.G., Chan, C.-C., Mochizuki, M., and Yancey, K. (1985). Effectiveness of cyclosporine therapy for Behçet's disease. *Arthritis and Rheumatism* **28**, 671–9.

O'Duffy, J.D., Lehner, T., and Barnes, C.G. (1983). Summary of the third international conference on Behçet's disease, Tokyo, Japan, October 23–24, 1981. *Journal of Rheumatology* **10**, 154–8.

O'Duffy, J.D., Robertson, D.M., and Goldstein, N.P. (1984). Chlorambucil in the treatment of uveitis and meningoencephalitis of Behçet's disease. *American Journal of Medicine* **76**, 75–84.

Ohno, S. (1982). Clinical and immunological studies on ocular lesions in Behçet's disease. In *Behçet's disease. Pathogenetic mechanism and clinical future. Proceedings of the International Conference on Behçet's Disease, Tokyo, 23–24 October 1987,* (ed. G. Inaba), pp. 127–36. University of Tokyo Press, Tokyo.

Pervin, K., *et al.* (1993). T cell epitope expression of mycobacterial and homologous human 65-kilodalton heat shock protein peptides in short term cell lines from patients with Behçet's disease. *Journal of Immunology* **151**, 2273–82.

Plotkin, G.R., Calabro, J.J., and O'Duffy, J.D. (1988). *Behçet's disease: a contemporary synopsis.* Futura Publishing, Mount Kisco, New York.

Stanford, M.R., Kasp, E., Whiston, R., *et al.* (1994). Heat shock protein peptides reactive in patients with Behçet's disease are uveitogenic in Lewis rats. *Clinical and Experimental Immunology,* **97,** 226–31.

Yazici, H., *et al.* (1981). A controlled trial of azathioprine in Behçet's syndrome. *New England Journal of Medicine* **322,** 281–5.

18.11.9 Kawasaki disease

TOMISAKU KAWASAKI

SYNONYMS

MCLS: Infantile acute febrile mucocutaneous lymph-node syndrome.

Introduction

Kawasaki disease is an acute febrile eruptive disease commonly occurring in infants and young children under 5 years of age. It was first described by Kawasaki in 1967. Originally, the prognosis was believed to be favourable. However, as more studies were carried out, the fatality rate was found to be 0.3 to 0.5 per cent, and autopsy findings revealed unique pathological features, such as coronary artery aneurysms with thrombosis in many cases. Since this disease cannot be differentiated histopathologically from infantile periarteritis nodosa, which has rarely been reported in American and European literature, it is still unclear whether it is a new entity or a disease which had previously been overlooked. This problem will remain unsolved until the pathogenesis is determined.

The disease has attracted much attention recently because asymptomatic coronary artery lesions (mainly aneurysms) have remained as sequelae in 5 to 10 per cent of the patients. These lesions are considered to cause sudden death, myocardial infarction, or mitral insufficiency, probably due to the papillary muscle dysfunction syndrome.

Kawasaki disease is a clear-cut clinical entity which can be diagnosed after recognition and analysis of six principal symptoms.

Clinical manifestations

The clinical features of Kawasaki disease can be classified into two categories: principal and subsidiary. At least five of the six principal features should be present for the diagnosis of this disease. However, patients with four features can also be diagnosed as having the condition provided that coronary aneurysms are identified by echocardiography or coronary angiography.

PRINCIPAL FEATURES

Fever of unknown aetiology lasting 5 days or more

In general, the onset of Kawasaki disease is usually with abrupt high fever but without prodromal symptoms such as coughing, sneezing, or rhinorrhoea. Sometimes, however, lymphadenopathy is felt, particularly if the patient complains of neck pain. At times, these symptoms precede the abrupt high fever by a day. Usually there is remittent or continuous fever ranging from 38 to 40 °C for 1 to 2 weeks. High fever lasting more than 2 weeks is seen in 14 to 20 per cent of cases. Fever lasting 30 days is rarely seen, while high fever lasting any longer suggests another disease. There is no response to antibiotics. The mean temperature reached is between 39.0 and 39.9 °C. It is believed that the longer the fever continues, the greater the possibility of coronary artery aneurysm.

Bilateral congestion of ocular conjunctiva

Two to 4 days after the onset, conjunctival injection occurs. On close examination each capillary vessel is dilated. There is no purulent discharge so the term 'conjunctivitis' is not appropriate. In most cases redness of the eyes is obvious, but in some cases it can be seen only upon very close examination. Pseudomembrane formation, iris adhesion, or visual disturbance has not been reported. With careful slit-lamp examination early in the course of the disease, anterior uveitis can be observed in some cases. Conjunctival injection usually subsides within 1 week and rarely continues for more than several weeks. It is seen in nearly 90 per cent of confirmed cases.

Changes of lips and oral cavity

Three to 5 days after the onset, dryness, redness, and fissuring of lips is present. In some cases there is bleeding and crust formation; it seems as if there is lipstick on the lips. The membranes of the oral cavity and pharyngeal mucosa are diffusely red. There is no vesicle, aphtha, or pseudomembrane formation. Frequently there is prominence of the tongue papillae, referred to as a strawberry tongue and similar to that seen in scarlet fever. These changes subside 2 weeks after the onset, but often the reddening of the lips continues for 3 to 4 weeks.

Acute non-purulent swelling of cervical lymph-nodes

From the day before the onset of fever, or together with fever, there is swelling of the cervical lymph-nodes. The patient complains of pain and often suffers a wryneck. In some cases the swelling occurs several days after the onset of fever. The nodes range from 1.5 to 5 cm and form a firm, non-fluctuant mass. Sometimes there is bilateral swelling leading to misdiagnosis of mumps. Cervical lymphadenopathy is seen in about two-thirds of cases in Japan. Significant lymph-node enlargement is the least important of the criteria for diagnosis. Usually it disappears with defervescence.

Polymorphous exanthema

From the first to the fifth day after the onset of fever, a polymorphic rash appears on the trunk or extremeties. It is variously morbilliform, scarlatiniform, urticariform, or erythema multiforme-like. In each case the rash is a different combination of these forms. The individual lesions measure 5 to 30 mm in diameter and spread over the trunk and extremeties within 2 days. Each lesion becomes increasingly large, and they often coalesce. They are not accompanied by vesicles or crusts but sometimes there are small aseptic pustules on the knees, buttocks, or other sites. The eruptions usually disappear in less than a week. There may also be localized redness at the sites of BCG inoculations in the acute stage.

Changes of the extremeties

Approximately 2 to 5 days after the onset of the disease, when the rash on the trunk has appeared, there is reddening of the palms and soles. Simultaneously, there is an indurative oedema. Sometimes the degree of swelling is considerable and the skin is shiny and appears to be about to burst (Fig. 1). When the fever goes down the swelling usually disappears. From 10 to 15 days after the onset of the illness, desquamation begins from the tip of the fingers, and membranous desquamation spreads over the palms up to the wrist. From a month and a half to 2 months after onset, transverse furrows frequently appear in the nails of both fingers and toes.

OTHER CLINICAL MANIFESTATIONS AND COMPLICATIONS

Cardiovascular changes

The most important complications of Kawasaki disease are changes in the cardiovascular system. In the acute stage, pancarditis and coronary arteritis frequently occur. Auscultation reveals gallop rhythms and distant heart sounds, and in some cases the ECG shows variable PQ and QT prolongation, low-voltage, ST- and T-wave changes, and arrythmias.

Two-dimensional echocardiography or selective angiography (Fig. 2) reveals that coronary artery aneurysms or dilation occur in about 40 per cent of cases, 10 to 20 days from the onset of the illness. However, about 30 days after the onset, the incidence decreases to about 20 per cent of all cases; by 60 days, the incidence is reduced to about 10 per cent of cases.

Kato (1974) first reported regression of aneurysms, and it has been confirmed subsequently that aneurysms in Kawasaki disease regress with time. In general, stenosis and obstruction do not occur in aneurysms which quickly regress; regression depends upon the shape (saccular, cylindrical, or fusiform) and diameter of the aneurysm.

If the diameter is more than 8 mm, there is little possibility of regression and often stenosis or occlusion occur. If the diameter is less than 4 mm, almost all cases show regression. In cases in which the diameter is between 4 and 8 mm, the prognosis is usually favourable. In general, stenosis or occlusion is liable to occur in large saccular and cylindrical aneurysms. Consequently, cases with aneurysms or dilation larger than 4 mm should have selective angiography carried out from 1 to 3 months after onset to determine accurately the shape and diameter of the aneurysm. According to recent Japanese literature, stenosis or occlusion occurs in 3 to 5 per cent of all cases studied with coronary artery angiography.

Gastrointestinal tract

Diarrhoea occurs in about 35 per cent of patients. Patients with gallbladder involvement often suffer severe abdominal pain, especially in

Fig. 1 Indurative oedema of the hands in Kawasaki disease.

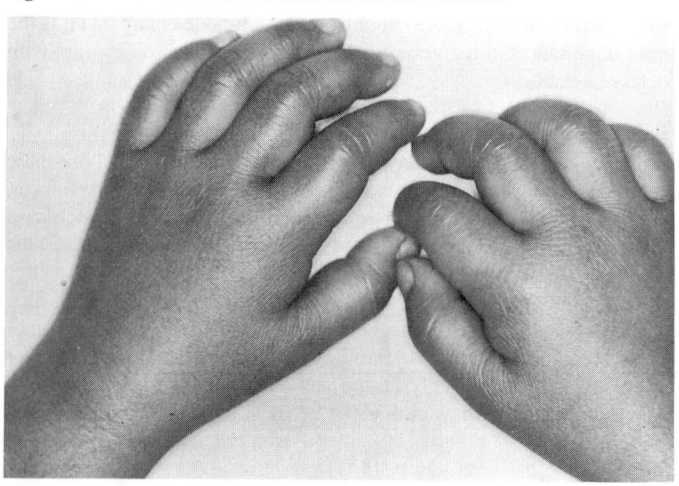

Fig. 2 Multiple aneurysms of the coronary artery in Kawasaki disease.

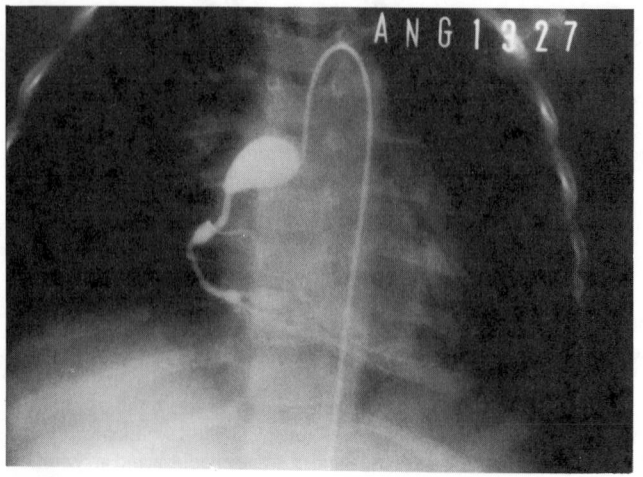

the upper right quadrant. Ultrasound examination is useful in the diagnosis. Mild jaundice occurs in about 5 per cent of cases. The total serum bilirubin level is almost always lower than 10 mg/dl. In the acute phase, serum transaminase levels are often increased. Serum GOT and GPT increase from 60 to 200 IU and LDH increases from 600 to 900 IU. Paralytic ileus has been reported.

Blood

In almost all cases there is a leucocytosis with a shift to the left, an increased erythrocyte sedimentation rate, positive C-reactive protein, and an increased α_2-globulin level. The platelet count increases from the second week and may reach 1000 to 1500 $\times$ 10^9 per litre. Hypoalbuminaemia and slight anaemia frequently occur.

Urinary tract

Albuminuria is frequently seen in the acute phase with aseptic microscopic pyuria. These findings disappear in the convalescent phase.

Respiratory system

Cough and rhinorrhoea may be present at the onset. Abnormal infiltrates are occasionally seen on the chest radiograph.

Joints

Arthralgia or arthritis are seen in about 25 per cent of cases. These symptoms disappear within 30 days after onset in most cases.

Nervous system

Aseptic meningitis occurs in 20 to 50 per cent of cases. Aseptic meningitis in Kawasaki disease, compared to mumps meningitis, shows higher numbers of macrophages, ependymal cells and pia-arachnoid cells. Other neurological complications such as facial palsy, hemiplegia, and encephalopathy have been reported.

Pathological findings

Kawasaki disease is an acute inflammatory disease with systemic angiitis which is distinguishable from classic periarteritis nodosa of Kussmaul–Maier type. Coronary aneurysms are usually present at autopsy (Fig. 3). The angiitis is characterized by acute inflammation with no or mild fibrinoid necrosis. The course of the angiitis can be classified into four stages according to the duration of the illness:

Stage 1 (1–2 weeks from onset) shows perivasculitis and vasculitis of microvessels, small arteries, and veins. There is inflammation of the intima, externa, and perivascular areas in the medium- and large-sized

Fig. 3 Postmortem findings in Kawasaki disease. This 9-month-old boy died suddenly at 49 days after the onset of the illness. A large aneurysm of the coronary vessels is shown.

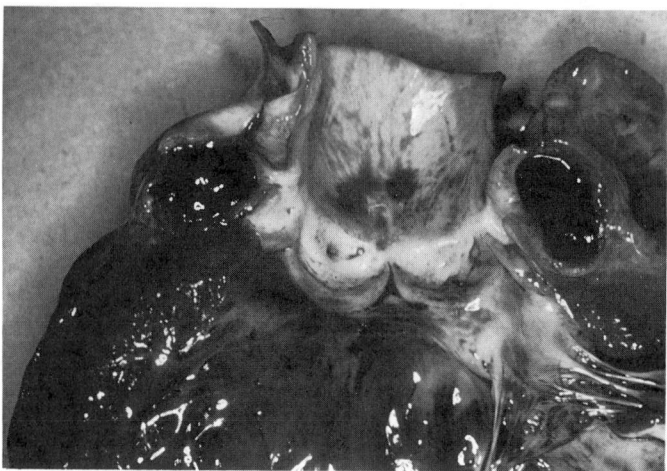

arteries. Oedema and infiltration with leucocytes and lymphocytes is also present.

Stage 2 (2–4 weeks from onset) shows less inflammation in the vessels than in stage 1. Aneurysms with thrombus and stenosis in the middle-sized arteries, especially in the coronary arteries, are present.

Stage 3 (4–7 weeks from onset) shows subsidence of inflammation in the vessels. Granulation may occur in the medium-sized arteries.

Stage 4 (more than 7 weeks from onset) reveals scar formation and intimal thickening with aneurysms, thrombus, and stenosis in the medium-sized arteries.

Other lesions include myocarditis involving conduction systems, pericarditis, endocarditis, and inflammation of almost all organs. All these lesions are frequently seen in Stages 1 and 2, but rarely in Stage 4.

Ischaemic heart disease usually occurs in Stages 2 to 4. The major cause of death in Stage 1 is myocarditis, including inflammation of conduction systems. In Stages 2 and 3, the causes are ischaemic heart disease, rupture of an aneurysm (rare), and myocarditis. In Stage 4, there may be ischaemic heart disease and, in rare cases, heart failure due to mitral insufficiency.

Epidemiology

In 1970 the first nationwide survey was conducted by the Japanese Kawasaki Disease Research Committee. Since then, 12 surveys have been carried out at 2-year intervals up to December 1992. A total of 116 848 cases (67 815 males and 49 033 females, M/F = 1.4) have been reported, including 392 (0.3 per cent) deaths. The number of cases reported has been steadily increasing since 1971. A high incidence of the disease was recognized in the early winter to late spring of 1979, 1982, and 1985 to 1986 throughout Japan. A shift of the epidemic wave from warm to cool geographical areas was observed in 1979, but not in 1982 or 1985 to 1986. The male:female ratio was 1.3 to 1.5:1. The age distribution of the cases showed monomodal curves reaching a peak at 8 to 11 months. Eighty-five per cent of cases were less than 5 years of age. The sex ratio (M/F) tended to be lower and the age of incidence to be younger in epidemic years.

Since 1974, outside Japan, a number of cases have been reported from Korea, China, the United States, Canada, Germany, France, the United Kingdom, and other countries. However, reports from the developing countries are still few.

Aetiology

Many agents such as rickettsia, viruses, bacteria (streptococcus, staphylococcus, propionibacterium, etc.), chemical substances (detergents, mercury, drugs, etc.), and mite antigens have been suggested as the cause of Kawasaki disease. Other possible factors, such as an abnormal host reaction to a variety of agents and circulating immune complexes, have been reported. HLA typing specific to Kawasaki disease and other genetic factors have not been confirmed. Another hypothesis is that Kawasaki disease may be triggered or initiated in a susceptible child by an infection with a variety of common viruses prevalent among children in the community. This disease, therefore, may be a unique clinical reaction pattern to several agents, just as a variety of agents may trigger such disorders as Reye's, Guillain–Barré, or Stevens-Johnson syndromes.

Recently it has been shown that scarlet fever's causative bacterial exotoxin is SPE-ABC and toxic shock syndrome's causative bacterial exotoxin is TSST1. These bacterial exotoxins act as superantigens. Kawasaki disease, scarlet fever, and toxic shock syndrome possess clinical similarities. Therefore, it has been suggested that Kawasaki disease may be caused by a superantigen (for example a bacterial toxin that stimulates T cells expressing a particular T-cell receptor B-chain variable gene segment).

Treatment

High-dose gammaglobulin treatment for the acute phase is now accepted as the best way to prevent coronary artery abnormalities. Furusho and colleagues first recommended the dosage of 400 mg/kg/day for 5 days plus 30 to 50 mg aspirin/day, but in the United States Newburger and colleagues have found that 400 mg/kg/day for 4 days plus 100 mg aspirin/day was as effective. In addition, a new regimen of 2 g/kg in one infusion has been reported by Newburger to be as effective and as safe as the 4 day regimen. A comparison of various regimens by Furusho has shown that high-dose gammaglobulin prevents coronary artery abnormalities, depending on the dosage. The minimum effective total dosage was 1000 mg/kg. The recommended regimen was 200 mg/kg/day plus 50 mg/kg aspirin/day for 5 days.

High-dose gammaglobulin is expensive; when costs are affordable, the American regimen is recommended, but if not, the Japanese one is perfectly adequate. A regimen of a single dose of 1 g/kg of intravenous gammaglobulin has also been reported, repeated if there has been relapse. Hypoalbuminaemia should be corrected before or with high-dose gammaglobulin treatment. However, sometimes, gammaglobulin in high dosages of 2 g/kg or more, administered within 7 days after onset, has been ineffective.

Caution should be used during infusion; too fast a rate leads to shivering, nausea, and shock-like effects. There have also been reports of congestive heart failure with oedema. However, these are transient adverse side-effects.

After the acute phase, aspirin in a dose of 3 to 5 mg/kg/day for 2 months is recommended. If coronary artery complications remain, aspirin should be continued until two-dimensional echo- or angiography show normal vessels.

In cases in which gammaglobulin is not available during the acute phase, a good regimen is with aspirin, 30 to 50 mg/kg/day, plus prednisolone 2 mg/kg/day for 1 to 2 weeks. Attention should be paid to possible bacterial infection during prednisolone treatment. After clinical signs have subsided, 3 to 5 mg/kg/day of aspirin should be continued for 2 months, but prednisolone should not be continued beyond 2 weeks.

Management

Patients with Kawasaki disease should be admitted to hospital and closly monitored for coronary artery changes by two-dimensional echocardiography. If there are no changes, drug treatment can be discontinued. For those patients with persistent coronary artery aneurysms, low-dose aspirin, 3 to 5 mg/kg/day, should be administered until the aneurysms disappear. As mentioned earlier, patients with large aneurysms should have selective coronary angiography performed from 1 to 3 months after the onset; this should be repeated after 1 or 2 years.

If myocardial infarction or myocardial insufficiency due to mitral regurgitation occurs, bypass surgery should be considered; this complication is more likely in younger patients.

REFERENCES

Abe, J., *et al.* (1992). Selective expansion of T cells expressing T-cell receptor variable regions VB2 and VB8 in Kawasaki disease. *Proceedings of the National Academy of Sciences, USA* **89**, 4966–5070.

Cremer, H.J. and Rieger, C. (1988). Considerations on treatment in Kawasaki-Syndrome (KS). *Proceedings of the 3rd International Kawasaki Disease Symposium, Japan Heart Foundation, Tokyo, Japan*, pp. 297–300.

Fujiwara, H. and Hamashima, Y. (1978). Pathology of the heart in Kawasaki disease. *Pediatrics* **61**, 100–7.

Furusho, K., Ohta, T., Soeda, T., Kimoto, K., Okabe, T., and Hirota, T. (1981). Possible role for mite antigen in Kawasaki disease. *Lancet* **ii**, 194–5.

Furusho, K., *et al.* (1984). High-dose intravenous gammaglobulin for Kawasaki disease. *Lancet* **ii,** 1055–8.

Furusho, K., *et al.* (1988). Gammaglobulin treatment for Kawasaki disease – long-term follow up of coronary arterial lesion and changes of WBC counts in acute phase. *Proceedings of the 3rd International Kawasaki Disease Symposium, Japan Heart Foundation, Tokyo, Japan,* pp. 311–13.

Kato, H., Koike, S., and Yokoyama, T. (1979). Kawasaki disease: effect of treatment on coronary artery involvement. *Pediatrics* **63,** 175–9.

Kato, H., *et al.* (1982). Fate of coronary aneurysms in Kawasaki disease: serial coronary angiography and long-term follow-up study. *American Journal of Cardiology* **49,** 1758–66.

Kawasaki, T., Kosaki, F., Okawa, S., Shigematsu, I., and Yanagawa, H. (1974). A new infantile acute febrile mucocutaneous lymph node syndrome prevailing in Japan. *Pediatrics* **54,** 273–6.

Landing, B.H. and Larson E.J. (1977). Are infantile periarteritis nodosa with coronary artery involvement and fatal mucocutaneous lymph node syndrome the same? Comparison of 20 patients from North American with patients from Hawaii and Japan. *Pediatrics* **59,** 651–62.

Melish, M.E., Hicks, R.V., and Larson, E.J. (1976). Mucocutaneous lymph node syndrome in the United States. *American Journal of Diseases in Childhood* **130,** 599–607.

Newburger, J.W., *et al.* (1991). A single intravenous infusion of gamma globulin as compared with four infusions in the treatment of acute Kawasaki syndrome. *New England Journal of Medicine* **324,** 1633–9.

Shigematsu, I., Tamashiro, H., Shibata, S., Kawasaki, T., and Kusakawa, S. (1980). World wide survey on Kawasaki disease. *Lancet* **i,** 976.

Tanaka, N., Sekimoto, K., and Naoe, S. (1976). Kawasaki disease: relationship with infantile periarteritis nodosa. *Archives of Pathology and Laboratory Medicine* **100,** 81–6.

Yanagawa, H., Kawasaki, T., and Shigematsu, I. (1987). Nationwide survey on Kawasaki disease in Japan. *Pediatrics* **80,** 58–62.

Yanagawa, H., *et al.* (1988). A nationwide incidence survey of Kawasaki disease in 1985–1986 in Japan. *Journal of Infectious Diseases* **158,** 1296–301.

Yanagawa, H. and Kato, H. (1993). *Report of the 12th Nationwide survey of Kawasaki disease in Japan,* (ed. Kawasaki Disease Research Committee; Chairman, Hirohisa Kato) (in Japanese).

Yoshikawa, J., *et al.* (1979). Cross-sectional echo-cardiographic diagnosis of coronary artery aneurysms in patients with the mucocutaneous lymph node syndrome. *Circulation* **59,** 133–9.

18.11.10 Cryoglobulinaemia

S.A. MISBAH

DEFINITION AND CLASSIFICATION

The term cryoglobulinaemia refers to the presence in blood of immunoglobulins that reversibly precipitate in the cold (4 °C; Fig. 1), redissolving at higher temperatures (37 °C). Although the phenomenon was first described by Wintrobe in 1933, the term cryoglobulin was introduced only in 1947. Since then three distinct types of cryoglobulins have been recognized on the basis of their immunoglobulin composition and associated diseases (Table 1). Type I cryoglobulins are composed entirely of monoclonal immunoglobulin (usually IgM or IgG) and account for approximately 25 per cent of all cryoglobulins. Type II, which are made up of a mixture of monoclonal IgM exhibiting rheumatoid factor activity and polyclonal IgG, constitute up to 25 per cent of all cryoglobulins, whereas the remaining 50 per cent are made up from type III cryoglobulins, which are composed entirely of polyclonal immunoglobulins (IgM rheumatoid factor and polyclonal IgG).

Usually cryoprecipitation only occurs below a temperature of 10 °C, although a thermolabile type I cryoglobulin may sometimes precipitate out in the syringe soon after venepuncture if the syringe has not been prewarmed to 37 °C. The precise reason(s) for the cryoprecipitation of immunoglobulins is not known. It is plausible to suggest that tempera-

ture-dependent conformational changes in paraproteins might account for the cryoprecipitation of type I cryoglobulins, but the evidence for this is conflicting. Analysis of immunoglobulin light chains of mixed (types II and III) cryoglobulins suggests a correlation between the presence of certain subgroups of κ variable-region chains and cryoprecipitability. Biochemical abnormalities noted include instability of disulphide bonds linking heavy chains and sialic acid deficient side-chains, but no single structural abnormality has provided a unifying explanation for cryoprecipitability. This is not surprising in view of the heterogeneity of cryoglobulins.

AETIOLOGY

In the majority of patients with cryoglobulinaemia an underlying condition in the form of malignant paraproteinaemia, lymphoma, autoimmune disease, or infection is evident. Type I cryoglobulinaemia is typically associated with plasma cell dyscrasias, with only a small minority of patients failing to show evidence of underlying lymphoproliferative disease. In mixed cryoglobulinaemia (types II and III) detailed clinical investigation fails to uncover associated disease in up to one-third of patients. These patients were originally classified as having idiopathic or mixed essential cryoglobulinaemia.

The immunopathogenesis of cryoglobulinaemia is poorly understood. A wide range of primary antigen–antibody complexes has been detected in the cryoprecipitates of type II and III cryoglobulins, in addition to the complex of rheumatoid factor and IgG. This has led to the view that the formation of mixed cryoglobulins is the end result of a sequence of events driven by an antibody response to either infective agents or endogenous antigens, as in systemic lupus erythematosus. It is hypothesized that prolonged antigenic stimulation leads to production of IgG antibodies and soluble IgG–antigen complexes. This is followed by the formation of IgM rheumatoid factor directed against IgG with enhanced affinity at lower temperatures, leading to the formation of insoluble cryoimmune complexes. Features of lymphoproliferative disease such as monoclonal B-cell populations in bone marrow, clonal immunoglobulin gene rearrangement in peripheral blood lymphocytes, and idiotypic

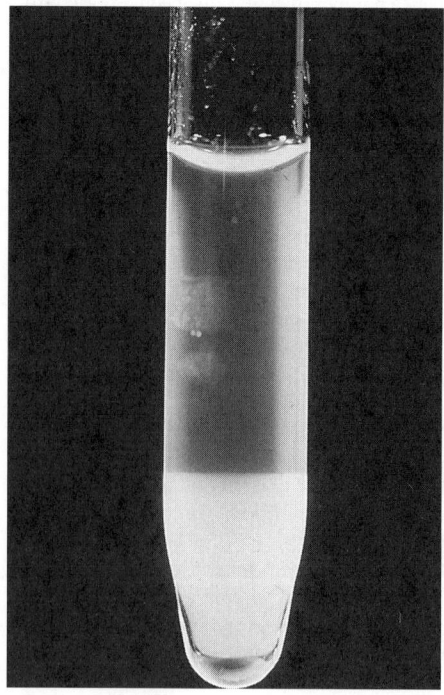

Fig 1. Serum of patient with type II cryoglobulinaemia, showing cryoprecipitate after 24 h at 4 °C.

Table 1 *Classification of cryoglobulins*

	Levels of cryoglobulin	Composition	Disease associations
Type I	>5 mg/ml Cryocrit >1–30%	Monoclonal immunoglobulin, usually IgM or IgG	Waldenström's macroglobulinaemia Myeloma, lymphoproliferative disease
Type II	1–5 mg/ml Cryocrit <1–10%	Monoclonal IgM rheumatoid factor plus polyclonal IgG	Infections Bacterial endocarditis Viral hepatitis C, hepatitis B, Epstein–Barr, cytomegalovirus
Type III	<1 mg/ml Cryocrit <1%	Polyclonal IgM rheumatoid factor plus polyclonal IgG	Spirochaetal Lyme disease, syphilis Fungal Coccidioidomycosis Parasitic Malaria Autoimmune disease Systemic lupus erythematosus, rheumatoid arthritis, Sjögren's, scleroderma Idiopathic Mixed essential cryoglobulinaemia

cross-reactivity between the monoclonal IgM rheumatoid factors characteristic of the disease, may also occur in type II cryoglobulinaemia. However, overt lymphoma develops only in a minority of such patients on long-term follow-up. Recent studies from the United States, Italy, France, and Switzerland suggest that many patients with type II cryoglobulinaemia have underlying hepatitis C virus infection, as evidenced by the presence of hepatitis C virus RNA and antibody in the cryoprecipitate and serum.

CLINICAL FEATURES

The clinical signs of cryoglobulinaemia are due to a combination of vascular obstruction and the inflammatory nature of these immune complexes. Type I cryoglobulins may occur in either sex and are characterized by features of hyperviscosity and vasculitis. These include Raynaud's phenomenon, arterial thrombosis, gangrene, and retinal haemorrhage. Mixed cryoglobulins, in contrast, affect females in particular and present with diverse clinical features due to deposition of cryoprecipitable immune complexes in blood vessels causing systemic vasculitis (Table 2). The triad of skin, renal, and joint disease is of particular importance. Cutaneous vasculitis is seen in virtually all patients with prominent lower limb purpura, often progressing to frank ulceration. Skin biopsies of affected areas show leucocytoclastic vasculitis with deposition of immunoglobulins and complement. Renal disease due to membranoproliferative glomerulonephritis with immunoglobulin and complement deposition occurs in up to 50 per cent of all patients with mixed cryoglobulinaemia. Distinctive histological features of cryoglobulinaemic glomerulonephritis include marked glomerular monocytic infiltration, amorphous Congo-red-negative eosinophilic deposits in capillaries, and a double-contoured glomerular basement membrane due to interposition of monocytes. The presence of these features on renal biopsy in a patient with so-called idiopathic glomerulonephritis should prompt a search for cryoglobulins. Nephrotic syndrome and hypertension are common sequelae.

Although arthralgia is seen in three-quarters of all patients with mixed cryoglobulinaemia, frank arthritis with deformity is uncommon. Impaired liver function with a wide spectrum of histological abnormality, ranging from chronic persistent hepatitis to cirrhosis, occurs in up to 70 per cent of patients and is of interest in view of the strong association with hepatitis C virus infection in type II cryoglobulinaemia.

Table 2 *Frequency of clinical features in 50 patients with mixed cryoglobulinaemia*

	Number	(%)
Female	33	(66)
Purpura	50	(100)
Arthralgia	35	(70)
Leg ulcers	15	(30)
Raynaud's phenomenon	11	(22)
Abdominal pain	9	(18)
Sjögren's syndrome	7	(14)
Sensorimotor peripheral neuropathy	10	(20)
Liver disease	35	(70)
Renal disease	26	(54)
Hypertension	17	
Oedema	20	
Azotaemia	13	
Nephrotic syndrome	6	
Haematuria	24	
Proteinuria		
>4 g/day	5	
1–4 g/day	17	
>0.5–<1 g/day	3	

Adapted from Samter *et al.* 1988,. Table 69–9, with permission.

INVESTIGATION OF SUSPECTED CRYOGLOBULINAEMIA

Close liaison between clinician and the clinical immunology laboratory is essential for the proper investigation of suspected cryogloblinaemia. Meticulous attention to the collection of blood samples is vital. Blood should be collected into a plain tube without anticoagulant and immersed into a flask containing water at 37 °C, followed by immediate transfer to the laboratory. Failure to collect samples at 37 °C enables the cryoglobulin to precipitate out with the blood clot and hence escape detection. Blood samples are centrifuged at 37 °C and serum stored at 4 °C for 5 to 7 days, with daily inspection for the presence of a cryoprecipitate. Most significant cryoglobulins are evident within 24 to 72 h.

Once a cryoglobulin has been found, quantification of the cryoprecipitate (cryocrit) and typing by immunoelectrophoresis at 37 °C follows. In patients with type I cryoglobulin, appropriate investigations for plasma cell dyscrasias and lymphoproliferative disorders should be carried out. The presence of type II or type III cryoglobulin should instigate a search for underlying autoimmune disease or infective agents stimulating an immune response, in particular hepatitis C.

OTHER LABORATORY FEATURES

The presence of IgM rheumatoid factor with marked depletion of early serum complement components (C4, C1q) due to activation of the classical pathway by immune complexes is highly suggestive of mixed cryoglobulinaemia and occurs in over 90 per cent of patients. It is an useful rule of thumb that patients with an unexplained low serum C4 and renal or skin disease should be investigated for cryoglobulinaemia. Cryoglobulins interfere with the routine immunochemical measurements of serum immunoglobulins, leading to artefactually low levels; they may also interfere with routine full blood count analysis by automated Coulter counters leading to spurious apparent leucocytosis and thrombocytosis. Collection and analysis of samples at 37 °C would prevent such errors.

MANAGEMENT

The aims of treatment are twofold: to treat the underlying disease process and to reduce the concentration of cryoglobulin. In type I cryoglobulinaemia treatment of the associated plasma cell dyscrasia or lymphoma is often combined with regular plasmapheresis to remove cryoglobulins.

In patients with mixed essential cryoglobulinaemia, symptomatic treatment alone may suffice for those with mild disease limited to the skin. Although no controlled trials of immunosuppressive therapy in mixed essential cryoglobulinaemia have been carried out, the presence of progressive renal, hepatic, or neurological disease warrants immunosuppressive therapy in the form of corticosteroids and cytotoxic agents to attempt to halt disease progression. Plasmapheresis is an useful adjunct and is particularly useful as a short-term measure in the management of acute exacerbations of disease. Rigorous control of hypertension is of utmost importance if further renal damage is to be avoided. Not surprisingly, the long-term outcome of patients with mixed cryoglobulinaemia is largely determined by the extent of renal disease. The demonstration of a high prevalence of hepatitis C virus infection in type II cryoglobulinaemia suggests that a completely different approach to treatment should now be considered, with the emphasis shifting away from immunosuppression to specific antiviral treatment. Recent controlled trials from Italy in patients with mixed cryoglobulinaemia associated with hepatitis C suggest that α-interferon may be an effective therapeutic agent, leading to significant improvement of skin, renal, and hepatic disease, and stabilization of steroid dosage. It is unclear whether treatment with α-interferon alone will suffice in these patients, and further controlled trials are required to answer this question. At present the use of α-interferon should be considered in all patients with mixed cryoglobulinaemia and clear evidence of hepatitis C virus infection.

REFERENCES

Cacoub, P. *et al.* (1994). Mixed cryoglobulinaemia and hepatitis C virus. *American Journal of Medicine,* **96,** 124–32.

Gorevic, P.D. (1988). Cryopathies: cryoglobulins and cryofibrinogenaemia. In *Immunological diseases,* (4th edn), (ed. M. Samter, D.W. Talmage, M.M. Frank, K.F. Austen, and H.N. Claman), Vol. II, pp. 1687–713. Little, Brown and Company, Boston. A comprehensive, well-referenced account of cryoglobulins covering both basic and clinical aspects.

Misiani, R., *et al.* (1994). Interferon alpha-2a therapy in cryoglobulinaemia associated with hepatitis C virus. *New England Journal of Medicine* **330,** 751–6.

Section 19 *Disorders of the skeleton*

19 Disorders of the skeleton

R. SMITH

Introduction

Bone is the only tissue, apart from teeth, that is normally mineralized to allow it to perform its structural role. The presence of mineral should not encourage the view that bone is inert or neglect of the metabolic activity that occurs within it. Many disorders affect the skeleton and only some can be considered here. Fractures, infections, and tumours, more often dealt with by orthopaedic surgeons, are excluded. The descriptions that follow may be divided into:

(1) those disorders generally considered to be metabolic, such as osteoporosis, osteomalacia, Paget's disease of bone, and parathyroid bone disease;

(2) those arising primarily from synthetic defects in the major components of the organic bone matrix and connective tissue, including osteogenesis imperfecta and Marfan's syndrome;

(3) skeletal disorders that are clearly the result of enzyme defects, such as hypophosphatasia, homocystinuria, and the storage diseases;

(4) the skeletal chondrodysplasias;

(5) those that appear to be disorders of bone cell biology, such as osteopetrosis, fibrous dysplasia, and inherited ectopic ossification; and

(6) various bone disorders due to the effects of excessive minerals, vitamins, and metallic poisons.

To understand how these disorders arise and how to recognize them, a brief account of relevant aspects of bone physiology and clinical features is given here. More detail can be found in specialized texts (see references).

Physiology of bone

In the past few years our understanding of bone physiology has widened considerably. There is an increasing interest in the cells of bone, their control, activities, and communications, and in the non-collagen as well as the collagen components of the organic bone matrix. Advances in bone diseases such as osteoporosis, osteopetrosis, osteogenesis imperfecta, and Paget's disease reflect this. The causes of many rare skeletal disorders have been discovered. Examples are Marfan's syndrome (mutations in the fibrillin gene); vitamin D-dependent rickets type II (mutations in the 1,25-dihydroxycholecalciferol receptor); pseudohypoparathyroidism and polyostotic fibrous dysplasia (abnormalities in the G-protein signalling system); osteogenesis imperfecta (mutations in the type I collagen gene) and some skeletal dysplasias (similar mutations in the type II collagen gene). Other outstanding advances in bone physiology include the identification of the parathyroid hormone like peptide (PTHrP) and the bone morphogenetic proteins, known as BMPs. These advances, mostly in the field of molecular genetics, have, as yet, done little to reduce our ignorance of bone cell biology, and many mysteries remain.

The mammalian skeleton serves two main functions, the demands of which often conflict. The first is to provide a rigid structure, the second is to act as an accessible mineral store.

Both depend on the activities of specialized bone cells, controlled by genetic, mechanical, nutritional, and hormonal influences, and by a host of short-acting messengers produced by cells, collectively known as cytokines.

Structure

Bone tissue consists of cells and an extracellular mineralized matrix (35 per cent organic and 65 per cent inorganic). Ninety per cent of the organic component is type I collagen. The remainder includes many non-collagen products of the osteoblast, such as osteocalcin, osteonectin, and proteoglycans. The mineral is present mainly as a complex mixture of calcium and phosphate in the form of hydroxyapatite.

Two anatomical types of bone may be defined, trabecular (cancellous) and cortical. The proportion of these differs from one bone to another; for example, vertebral bodies are predominantly trabecular, and the shafts of the long bones cortical. Such a distribution is related both to the functions of the bones and to the development of disorders with them, such as osteoporosis. Trabecular bone contains more metabolically active surfaces in a given volume than cortical bone. Cellular activities take place on the surfaces of trabecular bone and through resorbing channels (cutting cones) in cortical bone. The finer structure of bone is dealt with in anatomical texts.

Bone is often thought to be inert, because of its structural rigidity and persistence after death, and also to be composed entirely of chalk because it contains 99 per cent of the body's calcium. Both assumptions are superficially reasonable; neither is correct.

Bone cells

Conventional histological sections of bone demonstrate three types of bone cells which are clearly different (Fig. 1): osteoblasts, which may be plump and apparently active, or flat and apparently inactive—otherwise called bone-lining cells; multinuclear osteoclasts, which most

Fig. 1 A diagram showing the structure of bone and the relationship of the different cell types (from *Oxford textbook of rheumatology,* with permission).

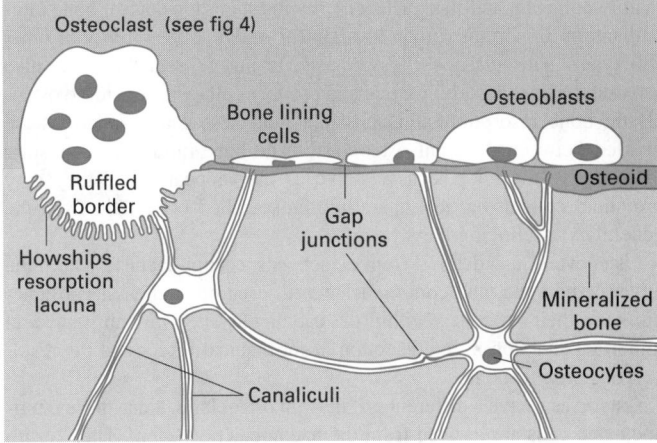

often occupy areas of resorption; and osteocytes within their lacunae in the mineralized bone, apparently in contact with other osteocytes and bone cells through their extensions in the canaliculi. All these cells are in close contact with the bone marrow, which contains their precursors and brings them into close relationship with the immune system.

Bone cells are at the centre of an information system of astonishing complexity; and it is this complexity of bone that provides both the challenge and the fascination for those interested in its disorders. Histological techniques have now been developed to study sequential cellular events in bone tissue; and the techniques of cell biology are used to study the origin and functions of different types of cells and the communications between them. All bone cells communicate with each other to control bone modelling during growth and remodelling throughout life. The constant processes of osteoclastic bone resorption and osteoblastic bone formation which achieve this are closely linked and take place in multicellular units, BMUs. The cellular cycle of such a unit begins with activation of multinucleate osteoclasts from their macrophage-like mononuclear precursors, which produce resorption (Howship's) lacunae on the surface of trabecular bone, or cutting cones in cortical bone. These are identical processes; in cancellous (trabecular) bone the BMU may be looked upon as a sagittal section of a cortical BMU. Resorption is followed by a reversal phase, during which a cement line is deposited, and the formation by osteoblasts of new bone matrix which is subsequently mineralized. In the young adult, when the bone mass is constant and there may be several million resorbing sites in the skeleton at any one time, the amount of newly formed bone equals that resorbed. In childhood more bone is formed than resorbed; and in later years there is an imbalance between the two processes in favour of resorption, leading to osteoporosis. The estimated time scale of the remodelling cycle is approximate. In the adult the replacement of old bone with new occurs at an annual turnover rate of 25 per cent in cancellous bone, and 2 to 3 per cent in cortical. In the BMU resorption takes 1 to 2 weeks and new bone formation about 7 weeks. A complete BMU cycle, including reversal and mineralization, takes several months.

The turnover of bone at a given site is determined by the frequency with which BMUs are activated and the rates of function of individual cells. Bone loss and gain depend on both factors; and the mechanism of bone loss is different in different disorders. For example, in thyrotoxicosis the activation frequency is increased, there is increased activity of the forming and resorbing cells and the period of both activities are shortened, with an imbalance at each BMU in favour of resorption.

Although the existence of the BMU system is widely accepted, it is far from understood. For instance, what factors lead to activation of the osteoclasts to initiate the resorbing cycle; how do cells talk to each other; and what links osteoblast and osteoclast activity?

It is clear that osteoblasts occupy a central position in bone physiology (Fig. 2). They are derived from the mesenchymal stromal cell system. They respond to hormonal factors, both systemic and local (cytokines), and to mechanical stress. They synthesize the organic bone matrix, mainly collagen, and non-collagen proteins, and they control bone mineralization. Importantly, they also appear to direct the activity of other cell types, particularly the osteoclasts. In this respect they may also activate the bone resorbing cycle and produce collagenase prior to osteoclastic bone resorption. It is possible that these many functions are divided between different osteoblasts. The bone-lining cells—resting osteoblasts—may not be as inactive as they appear, since they may provide a cellular barrier separating the so-called bone fluid from the general extracellular compartment.

Osteocytes, also derived from osteoblasts, occupy lacunae within the mineralized bone, and communicate with each other though gap junctions via their processes within the canaliculi. They probably have an important function in the detection of mechanical forces and the resultant response of bone.

Osteoclasts have a different origin from osteoblasts, since these multinucleated cells are derived from the haemopoietic system. They resorb bone by attaching themselves to its surface and forming a seal to isolate their area of activity. Within this sealed zone they produce a very acid environment, with the aid of a proton pump linked to the enzyme carbonic anhydrase II, to enable digestion of whole bone by lysosomal enzymes. Interestingly, the absence of carbonic anhydrase II is linked to a rare form of osteopetrosis (see below). Osteoclasts have receptors to calcitonin which, when occupied, directly suppress their activity; the existence of any other hormone receptors is controversial. However, they are activated by prostaglandins. The resorptive effects of parathyroid hormone and of 1,25-dihydroxycholecalciferol are probably mediated through the osteoblast.

Bone formation

The factors that control bone formation are complex and not fully understood, but must work largely through the osteoblast. The precursors of osteoblasts are found in the periosteum and the endosteal surfaces close to the bone marrow. The local remodelling stimulus for new bone formation appears to come from some product, or products, of bone resorption, which could, for instance, be a group of polypeptide growth factors or morphogenic proteins liberated from resorbed bone. Such substances are included in the category of cytokines. A cytokine may be defined as a peptide produced by a cell which acts as an autocrine, paracrine, or endocrine mediator. This definition includes a large number of substances with effects on metabolism of bone and cartilage. Such effects have largely been shown in experimental (and artificial) situations and their physiological role is unknown. Many cytokines have alternative names and multiple actions, featuring both synergism and antagonism. They include interleukins (1 and 6), tumour necrosis factor, γ-interferon, platelet-derived growth factor, fibroblast growth factors, insulin-like growth factors, transforming growth factor β, and bone morphogenic proteins.

Since bone cells contain, synthesize, and respond to many cytokines, the situation is complex. As an example, transforming growth factor β (TGFβ) appears to belong to a family of multifunctional regulatory peptides, and bone is probably its most abundant source. Not only do osteoblasts synthesize TGFβ, but they also have high-affinity receptors for it, and are mitogenically stimulated by it. In addition, most of the bone morphogenic proteins belong to the TGFβ family.

Fig. 2 To show the central position of the osteoblast in bone physiology (from *Oxford textbook of rheumatology,* with permission).

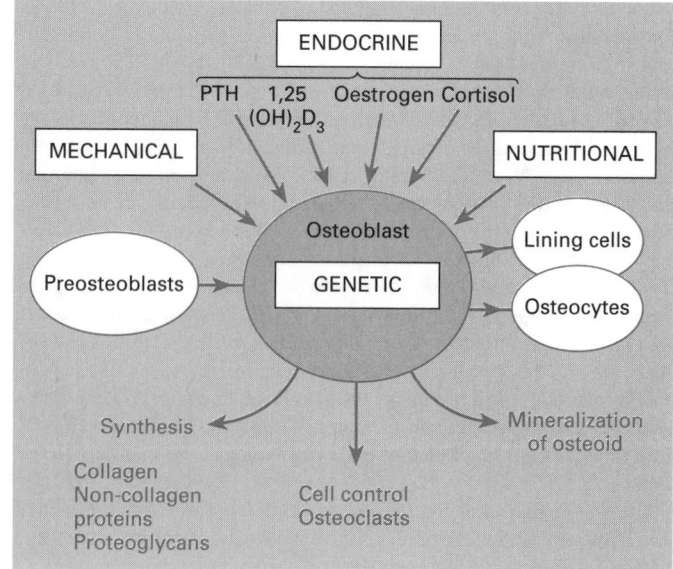

Table 1 *The major fibrillar collagens*

Collagen types	Subunits	Gene locus	Chromosome assignment	Molecular configuration	Major tissue distribution
I	$a1(I)$	COL 1A1	17q21–22	$(a1(1))_2 a2(1)$	All tissues except cartilage and vitreous; abundant
	$a2(I)$	COL 1A2	7q22	$(a1(1))_3$	in stress-bearing structure—tendon, bone dentine, skin, blood vessels
II	$a1(II)$	COL 2A1	12q13	$(a1(II))_3$	Cartilage, vitreous of the eye
III	$a1(III)$	COL 3A1	2q23	$(a1(III))_3$	Most tissues, except bone and dentine; high concentration in skin, gut, blood vessels

Bone resorption

Osteoclasts are controlled by systemic and local hormones, but there is no direct evidence that they are influenced by mechanical stress. Calcitonin directly inhibits the osteoclast, temporarily abolishes the active ruffled border, and suppresses the generation of new osteoclasts. Bone resorption is increased by parathyroid hormone and 1,25-dihydroxycholecalciferol. Since the osteoclast contains no receptors to either of these hormones it is proposed that their resorbing effect is mediated via the osteoblast. Again the messages that the osteoblasts use to turn on the resorbing activity of the osteoblasts are unknown, but amongst these are the prostaglandins (PGs). The number and activity of the osteoclasts are also increased by a variety of cytokines produced by lymphocytes or monocytes (lymphokines and monokines, respectively), and by peptide growth factors such as epidermal growth factor. In myeloma the malignant plasma cells release interleukin-1 and -6 and tumour necrosis factor, all of which stimulate osteoclastic destruction of bone.

Bone mass (see also osteoporosis)

The development of the skeleton and its eventual size and density are influenced by important genetic factors modified by mechanical stress, nutrition, the systemic effects of endocrines, and by local factors produced by the bone cells themselves. These determine the balance between resorption and formation, and their relative contribution varies with age.

Recent work re-emphasizes the importance of the genetic contribution to bone mass. Apart from the difference in bone mass between races, this work has confirmed the hereditability of bone mass at all sites, which is greater in monozygotic than dizygotic twins, and has demonstrated that the bone density of daughters of osteoporotic women is less than that of daughters of non-osteoporotic women. Clearly, mutations in the structural collagen genes will have a considerable effect on bone mass.

The main function of the skeleton is mechanical, and it has long been known that bone is laid down along its lines of stress. Although the way in which this occurs is obscure, *in vitro* experiments show that osteoblasts in culture respond to mechanical stress by an increase in levels of cyclic adenosine monophosphate (cAMP) and phosphinositol, partly mediated by prostaglandins. It also seems common sense that the size and density of the skeleton should be related to nutrition, particularly concerning calcium, protein, and energy. This has been difficult to prove, but recent co-twin studies in growing children have demonstrated a significantly greater density of bone in those on calcium supplements; and the starvation associated with anorexia nervosa reduces bone mineral content. This may also be due to oestrogen deficiency and emphasizes the important effect of systemic hormones on the skeleton. Sex hormones, testosterone and oestrogen, encourage new bone formation. Growth hormone is an important anabolic skeletal agent during the early years of life, partly through the local production of somatomedins (insulin-like growth factors). A number of hormones primarily thought of as resorptive may also have anabolic actions on the osteoblasts. One is parathyroid hormone, which increases proliferation of osteoblast precursors.

Collagen

Collagen is the major extracellular protein in the body, more than half of which is within the skeleton, and the major synthetic product of the osteoblast. There are many different molecular types, with different functions, each with their own genes (Table 1). Collagen in bone is of type I. This is a heteropolymer composed of two $\alpha1$-chains and one $\alpha2$-chain. The general structure of the $\alpha1$-chain is $(Gly-X-Y)_{338}$. The α-chains are synthesized as precursors within the osteoblasts and undergo a number of synthetic steps, including post-translational hydroxylation of proline and lysine residues; certain hydroxylysine residues are further modified into aldehydes and also glycosylated (Fig. 3).

After removal of their extensions the triple helical molecules form an exact structure with a quarter stagger overlap which is subsequently cross-linked. The so-called hole zones within this structure provide a template for early mineralization. Mutations in the collagen genes and defects in post-translational modification cause inherited disorders of connective tissue, of which osteogenesis imperfecta (type I collagen) and Ehlers–Danlos syndromes (type III collagen) are examples. Excretion of hydroxyproline peptides is an indicator of bone collagen turnover, and excretion of pyridinium compounds is a measure of bone resorption (see below).

Non-collagen proteins

Many such proteins may be extracted from bone and their abundance differs according to the starting material and the methods used. They include osteocalcin (Gla protein), sialoproteins, various phosphoproteins, such as osteonectin and osteopontin, the bone morphogenetic proteins, and bone-specific proteoglycans.

The nature of non-collagen substances sequestered in bone matrix is complex and most are synthesized by the osteoblasts. Few, if any, are unique to bone, since they can be expressed transiently in other tissues, and to date no unambiguous function has been determined for any of these proteins. Osteonectin is the most abundant non-collagen protein produced by human osteoblasts. It binds strongly to calcium ions, hydroxyapatite, and native collagen, but is not limited to mineralizing tissue, being also found in human platelets. Although osteonectin mRNA is widely distributed in developing tissues, osteonectin is most abundant in bone. Two bone sialoproteins are now recognized (BSP1 and 2). Their relative abundance varies with species studied. Thus BSP1 is a minor component of human bone, but a major contributor to total sialoprotein in rat bone. The protein contains an RGD (Arg–Gly–Asp) cell attachment sequence and is therefore called osteopontin. The major human sialoprotein is BSP2.

There are two bone Gla-containing proteins; osteocalcin—bone Gla protein (BGP)—and matrix Gla protein (MGP). The term Gla refers to the γ-carboxylated glutamic acid residues, formed by vitamin K modulated post-translational carboxylation of peptide-bound glutamic acid. These proteins have some sequence homology but are products of different genes. MGP is also a cartilage protein, and is found at an earlier developmental stage than BGP. The function of BGP is unknown. Warfarin-treated animals do not show abnormal mineralization. BGP biosynthesis is regulated by 1,25-dihydroxycholecalciferol $(1,25(OH)_2D_3)$ (and no other hormone), which enhances its nuclear transcription and eventual secretion from bone cells. Plasma BGP has been linked to the rate of bone formation or, less specifically, bone turnover.

Proteoglycans are proteins with one or more attached glycosaminoglycan chains. They vary widely in form and function. Those of bone, which include decorin and biglycan, have been studied less extensively than those from cartilage, and differ from them in their small overall size and relatively larger amounts of protein. Such small proteoglycans are thought to interact with growing collagen fibrils in a precise manner and to regulate their growth, maturation, and interactions. Type IX collagen, closely associated with type II collagen, bridges the gap between the collagens and proteoglycans since it contains a chondroitin sulphate glycosaminoglycan chain. It has been known for many years that demineralized bone matrix contains substances capable of inducing ectopic bone formation. Because they are present in such small amounts their extraction and isolation have presented great difficulties, but these bone morphogenic proteins have now been isolated and their genes localized and cloned. Interestingly most belong to the TGFβ supergene family included amongst the cytokines.

Bone mineral and mineralization

Mineralization occurs on the background of bone matrix collagen. The way in which it occurs has been long debated, but there is now good evidence that in most mineralized tissues calcifying vesicles derived from chondrocytes or osteoblasts provide a focus for mineralization. These vesicles are easily demonstrable in cartilage, but their function in the organized matrix of bone is controversial. The precipitation of calcium within these vesicles may be controlled by the action of a pyrophosphatase which locally destroys pyrophosphate, itself an inhibitor of mineralization. Alkaline phosphatase is one such pyrophosphatase which is readily demonstrable both in osteoblasts and in mineralizing vesicles. It is possible, for the purpose of clarity, to consider two types of mineralization; namely, homogeneous nucleation, which occurs in the lumen of the matrix vesicles, from amorphous calcium phosphate to form crystalline hydroxyapatite; and heterogeneous nucleation, which is collagen-mediated and may partly rely on absorbed non-collagen proteins as nucleators. After this first phase (mediated either by vesicles or collagen) there is a second phase of rapid spread of mineralization initially in the hole zones and later the overlap regions of the collagen matrix.

Calcium and phosphorus balance (see also Section 12)

Much has been written about calcium balance and the main hormones that control it. Phosphate balance is less well understood. The circulating level of plasma calcium is determined by the amount of calcium that is absorbed by the intestine, the amount that is excreted by the kidney, and the exchange of mineral with the skeleton. The relative importance of these exchanges differs during growth and in different disorders. Total plasma calcium is closely maintained between 2.25 and 2.60 mmol/l, of which nearly half is in the ionized form (47 per cent ionized, 46 per cent protein bound, and the remainder complexed). The skeleton contains approximately 1 kg (25 000 mmol) of calcium. The main fluxes of calcium in the young adult are shown in Fig. 4.

Parathyroid hormone (see also Chapter 12.6)

The gene for parathyroid hormone (PTH) is on chromosome 11. PTH is synthesized as a large precursor, in the way of proteins packaged for

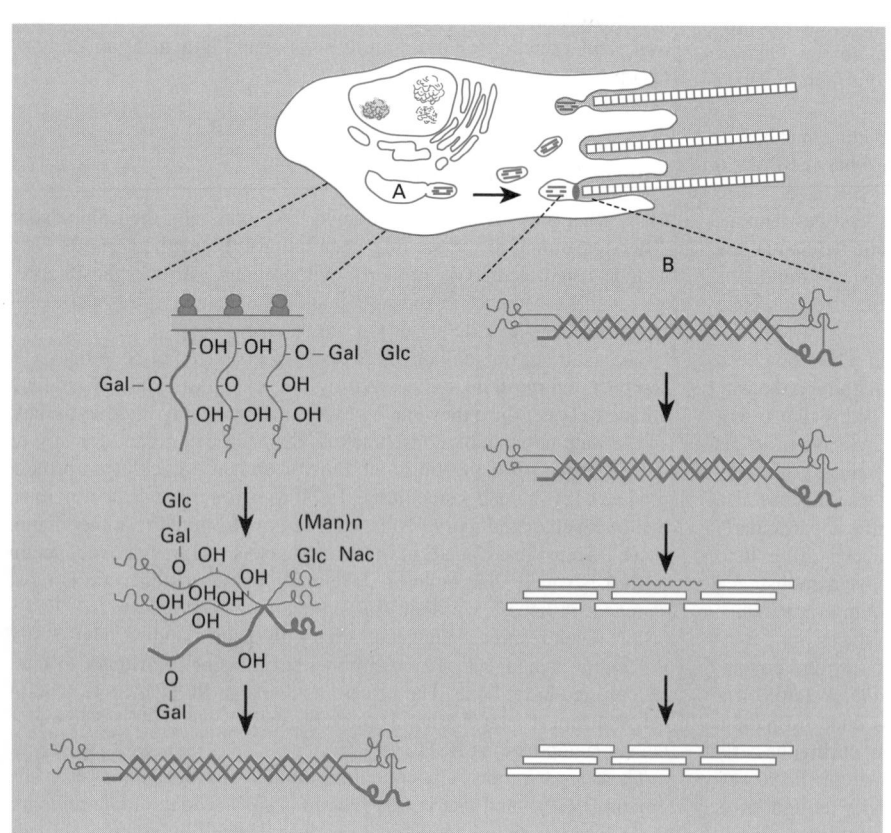

Fig. 3 The synthesis and assembly of collagen molecules. Within the fibroblast (A) the individual pro-α-chains are modified, assembled, and folded into the triple helix. In (B) these chains are exported, shortened, and self-assemble. (From Prockop and Kivirikko (1984) by permission of the *New England Journal of Medicine* and the authors.)

export, and its secretion is stimulated by a reduction in plasma ionized calcium concentration. This leads to an increase in calcium absorption through the gut, an increase in calcium reabsorption through the kidney, and an increase in bone resorption. Intestinal calcium absorption is mediated by 1,25-dihydroxycholecalciferol, and the 1α-hydroxylation of 25-hydroxycholecalciferol is stimulated by parathyroid hormone, so that the effect of parathyroid hormone in increasing intestinal calcium absorption is indirect. In contrast, the renal effect of parathyroid hormone on calcium reabsorption is direct. The cellular effects of parathyroid hormone on kidney and bone appear to involve two cellular systems, namely cAMP and phosphoinositol. Parathyroid hormone encourages osteoclastic bone resorption by its effects on the osteoblast (as previously described). Peripheral resistance to the effect of PTH due to an inherited defect in the G-protein signalling system occurs in pseudohypoparathyroidism (see below and Chapter 12.6).

Vitamin D

Vitamin D is synthesized either as vitamin D_3 (cholecalciferol) within the skin from its precursor 7-dehydrocholesterol under the influence of ultraviolet light (usually as sunlight), or taken in with food, either as vitamin D_3 or D_2 (ergocalciferol) (Fig. 5). It is transported to the liver by a binding protein where it undergoes 25-hydroxylation. 25-hydroxyvitamin D is then hydroxylated in the 1α-position by the renal 1α-hydroxylase. $1,25(OH)_2D$ is the active metabolite of vitamin D, which has widespread effects, the extent of which is only just being appreciated. These are mediated through a widely distributed vitamin D receptor which has DNA- and hormone-binding components. In addition to its classic effect on intestinal calcium transport, vitamin D is linked with the immune system and the growth and differentiation of a wide variety of cells. Measurement of plasma 25-hydroxy-vitamin D concentration has proved to be a useful indicator of vitamin D status, and work on $1,25(OH)_2D$ and its receptors has illuminated the cause of the rarer forms of inherited rickets (see below). The kidney is the main source of $1,25(OH)_2D$ but it is now clear that this metabolite can be synthesized by a variety of granulomata, providing an explanation for the hypercalcaemia of sarcoidosis and (occasionally) lymphomas.

Calcitonin

The main effect of administered calcitonin is to reduce bone resorption by direct and reversible suppression of osteoclasts and by inhibition of their production from precursors. The role of calcitonin is uncertain, although it is thought to protect the skeleton during physiological stresses such as growth and pregnancy. It is produced by alternative splicing of the primary gene transcript also responsible for the production of calcitonin gene-related peptide. Recent work has shown that its receptor is widely distributed.

Parathyroid hormone-related protein (PTHrP)

This hormone was recently discovered by studies on patients with nonmetastatic hypercalcaemia of malignancy. PTHrP has close sequence homology to PTH at the amino terminal end of the molecule and has very similar effects. Its gene is located on the short arm of chromosome 12, which is thought to have arisen by a duplication of chromosome 11, which carries the human PTH gene. It has been detected in a number of tumours, particularly of the lung. There is also evidence that it may have a role in fetal physiology, controlling the calcium gradient across the placenta to maintain the relatively higher concentrations in the fetal circulation.

Other hormones

Apart from the recognized calciotrophic hormones, the skeleton is influenced by corticosteroids, the sex hormones, thyroxine, and growth hormone. The main effect of excess corticosteroids (either therapeutic or in Cushing's syndrome) is to suppress osteoblastic new bone formation, although there is also an element of secondary hyperparathyroidism. In the appropriate gender, androgens and oestrogens promote and maintain skeletal mass. Osteoblasts have receptors for oestrogens, although they are not abundant. Thyroxine increases bone turnover and increases resorption in excess of formation; thyrotoxicosis thus leads to bone loss. Excess growth hormone leads to gigantism and acromegaly (according to the age of onset) with enlargement of the bones. Absence of growth

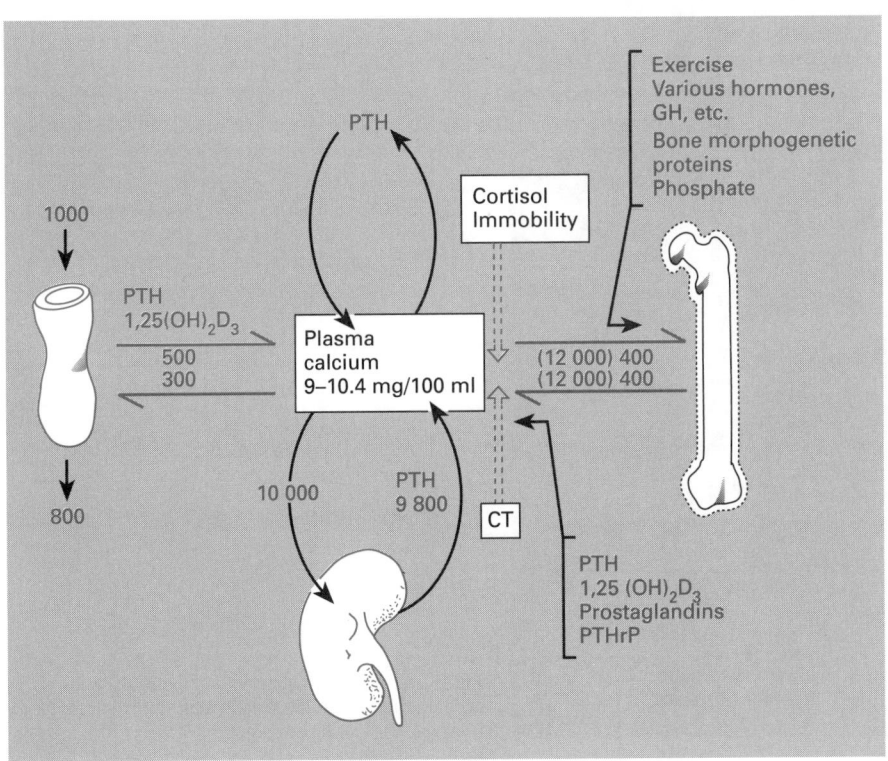

Fig. 4 Factors that control calcium balance. Units are in mg/day (to convert to mmol divide by 40) and refer to an adult. The figures in parentheses are an estimate of exchange through the cellular barrier of bone. CT, calcitonin; GH, growth hormone; PTH, parathyroid hormone; PTHrP, parathyroid hormone related peptide. (From *Oxford textbook of rheumatology*, with permission.)

hormone will lead to proportional short stature; where there is wider pituitary failure the reduction in gonadotrophins will cause bone loss.

Biochemical measures of bone turnover

Knowledge of bone physiology allows one to interpret biochemical measures of bone turnover. These include plasma bone-derived alkaline phosphatase and osteocalcin (BGP), and the urinary total hydroxyproline and cross-linked collagen-derived peptides. The first two are produced by osteoblasts and indicate bone formation, the second two bone resorption. Since formation and resorption are closely coupled, such measurements are usually closely related to each other, and to overall bone turnover.

Plasma alkaline phosphatase (largely derived from osteoblasts) provides a crude but readily accessible index of bone formation, being increased during periods of rapid growth and particularly when bone turnover is greatly increased, as in Paget's disease. Early measurements of serum BGP gave widely variable results and depended on the origin, sensitivity, and stability of the antibodies used. Total urinary hydroxyproline excretion is influenced by dietary collagen (gelatin) and reflects both resorption and new collagen synthesis. The recent development of methods for the measurement of urinary collagen-derived pyridinium cross-links promises to give a reliable indication of bone resorption rate, unrelated to new collagen formation, and uninfluenced by diet. There are two forms of cross-linked peptide—pyridinium and deoxypyridinoline, depending on their origin from oxidized hydroxylysine or lysine residues. Initial measurements were on acid-hydrolysed samples by high-pressure liquid chromatography (HPLC). Specific immunoassays are now being developed.

REFERENCES

Avioli, L.V. and Krane, S.M. (1990). *Metabolic bone disease,* (2nd edn). W.B. Saunders, Philadelphia.

Byers, P.H. (1989). Disorders of collagen biosynthesis and structure. In *The metabolic basis of inherited disease,* (ed. C.R. Scriver, A.L. Beaudet, W.S. Sly, and D. Valle D.), (6th ed), pp. 2805–42. McGraw Hill, New York.

Coe, F.L. and Favus, M.J. (1993). *Disorders of bone and mineral metabolism.* Raven Press, New York.

Evered, D. and Harnett, S. (1988). *Cell and molecular biology of vertebrate hard tissues,* p. 136. Ciba Foundation Symposium.

Hardingham, T.E. and Fosang, A.J. (1992). Proteoglycans: many forms and many functions. *FASEB Journal* **6**, 861–70.

Nordin, B.E.C., Need, A.G., and Morris, H.A. (1993). *Metabolic bone and stone disease,* (3rd edn). Churchill Livingstone. Edinburgh.

Prockop, D.J. and Kivirikko, K.I. (1984). Heritable diseases of collagen. *New England Journal of Medicine* **311,** 376–86.

Royce, P.M. and Steinmann, B. (1992). *Connective tissue and its heritable disorders. Molecular, genetic and medical aspects,* (1st edn). Wiley-Liss, New York.

Seibel, M.J., Robins, S.D., and Bilezikian, J.P. (1992). Urinary pyridinium crosslinks of collagen. *Trends in Endocrinology and Metabolism* **3**, 263–70.

Smith, R. (1993). Bone in health and disease. In *Oxford textbook of rheumatology,* (ed. P.J. Maddison, D.A. Isenberg, P. Woo, and D.N. Glass), pp. 242–56. Oxford University Press.

The diagnosis of bone disease

The diagnosis of bone disorders increasingly depends on investigation, with the result that important clinical points tend to be forgotten.

HISTORY

Deformity, pain, and fracture are common features. To these may be added proximal myopathy (in osteomalacia and rickets) and the symptoms of any underlying disease. The family history is always important.

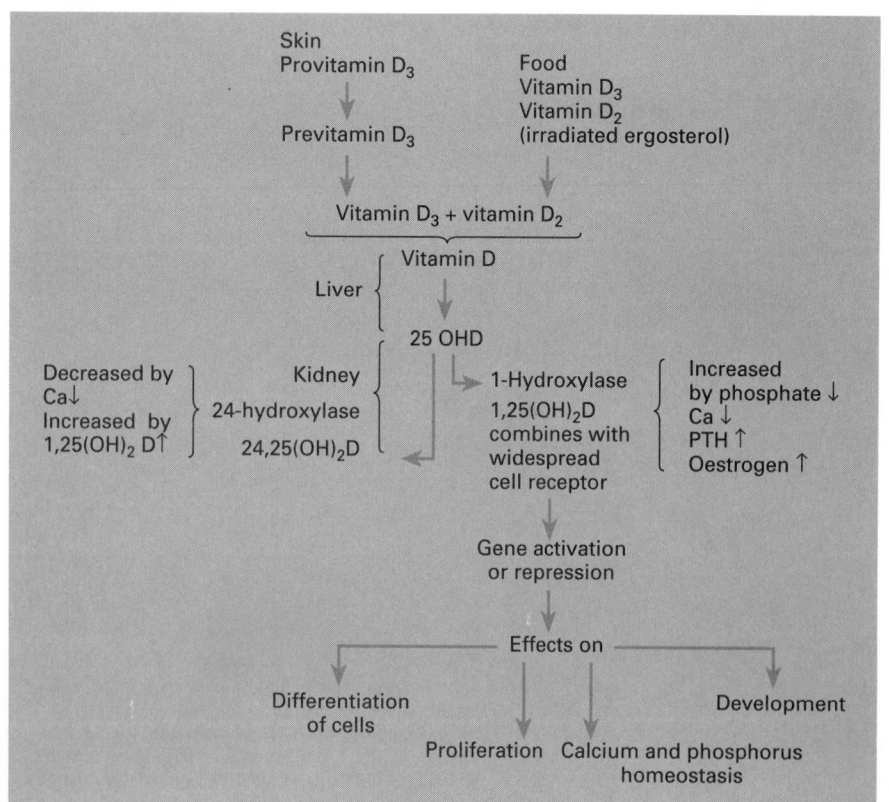

Fig. 5 The synthetic pathways and molecular and cellular effects of 1,25(OH)$_2$D (from *Oxford textbook of rheumatology,* with permission)

DEFORMITY

Deformity suggests previous skeletal disorder, especially if there is a disturbance of growth. Short stature and disproportion are more frequent than excessive height. In children a knowledge of growth is essential; in the normal adult height and span are approximately equal and the crown to pubis measurement is equal to the pubis to heel. Those with short stature can be divided into proportionate and disproportionate, of which the most frequent cause is short limbs. Proportionate short stature may occur in children who appear to be otherwise normal, whereas subjects with disproportionate short stature usually appear abnormal from birth. Some causes of short stature are given in Table 2. Skeletal chondrodysplasias are dealt with further below.

Kyphosis, with loss of trunk height, as in osteoporosis and osteomalacia, is the commonest acquired deformity of adult life. It is often noticed because clothes no longer fit. In childhood vertebral collapse will slow growth rate. Other deformities are characteristic of the underlying disease; for instance active childhood rickets produces knock knees, bowed legs, enlarged epiphyses, and bossing of the skull; Paget's disease produces thick limb bones and an enlarged skull vault; and severe osteogenesis imperfecta, very short limbs.

BONE PAIN AND FRACTURE

The cause of bone pain is not well understood. In osteomalacia it may be generalized and associated with tenderness on pressure. It may be due to excessive vascularity, with stretching of the periosteum; certainly it can be rapidly relieved by appropriate treatment, such as calcitonin for Paget's disease, or parathyroidectomy for parathyroid bone disease. Fractures of different sorts occur, examples are the partial, multiple, and painful microfractures ('fissure' fractures) on the convexity of Pagetic bone; the Looser's zones on medial borders of osteomalacic bones; and the repetitive vertebral compression fractures of osteoporosis.

MYOPATHY

The cause of the proximal muscle weakness in osteomalacia and rickets remains unknown. The symptoms include a waddling gait, and inability to rise from a chair, to lift objects off high shelves, or to climb stairs. Limbs may be described as stiff rather than weak. Myopathy does not occur in inherited hypophosphataemia.

UNDERLYING DISEASE

It is necessary to be alert for the symptoms of the underlying disease, such as renal failure, steatorrhoea, or myeloma, and to enquire particularly about previous abdominal operations, including hysterectomy and oophorectomy.

PHYSICAL SIGNS

It is important to see the patient out of bed so that, for instance, an abnormal gait or stature is not missed. The appearance may give vital clues; for instance, the large vault of Paget's disease; the coarse features, large nose, big lower jaw, and the widely spaced teeth of acromegaly; and the round face, simplicity, and cataracts of pseudohypoparathyroidism. Endocrine disorders affecting the skeleton, such as hypogonadism and hypopituitarism, are readily recognizable. Special facial features should receive attention; these include the eyes for such signs as corneal calcification, arcus juvenilis, and lens dislocation shown by the shimmering of the unsupported iris, iridodinesis. Further examples are corneal clouding, (some mucopolysaccharidoses) and cystine crystals (cystinosis). In dentinogenesis imperfecta, often found with osteogenesis imperfecta, the teeth are abnormal in shape, tend to be transparent and vary in colour from yellow to grey. Enamel defects occur in hypopara-

Table 2 *Some examples of short stature*

Proportionate	
Genetic	Familial
Endocrine	Growth hormone lack
	Hypothyroidism
Metabolic	Lysosomal storage diseases
	Renal glomerular failure
	Cystic fibrosis
Nutritional	Coeliac disease
	Starvation
Chronic disease	Cyanotic heart disease
Intrauterine	Low birth weight dwarfism
Chromosomal	Turner's syndrome
Social	Emotional deprivation
Disproportionate[a]	
Short limbs	
Lethal	Type II osteogenesis imperfecta
	Thanatophoric dwarfism
	Achondrogenesis
Non-lethal	Achondroplasia
	Inherited hypophosphataemia
	Metaphyseal dysostosis
Short spine	Spondyloepiphyseal dysplasia

[a]For further details see skeletal dysplasias and osteogenesis imperfecta.

thyroidism, teeth are lost early in hypophosphatasia; and dental abscesses are common in hypophosphataemic rickets.

Hands and feet need particular attention. The fingers may be abnormally long and thin, as in Marfan's syndrome, or excessively short and mobile, as in pseudoachondroplasia; alternatively they may be short, wide, and stiff in some mucopolysaccharidoses; or the hands may have short metacarpals, as in pseudohypoparathyrodism, or additional digits, as in the Ellis–van Creveld syndrome. The monophalangic big toe (and less often short thumbs) is characteristic of fibrodysplasia ossificans progressiva. Abnormal body proportions are common; the limbs are relatively long after vertebral collapse. Scoliosis often dates from adolescence; occasionally it may be a clue to an inherited connective tissue disorder. A thoracolumbar gibbus is a particular (though not exclusive) feature of the mucopolysaccharidoses. Spinal deformity produces secondary changes; thus a young patient with severe osteoporosis will develop a prominent sternum with ribs that touch the iliac crest and a transverse crease across the front of the abdomen. Spontaneous tetany is a rare symptom, but there are two recognized tests for latent tetany; of these Chvostek's sign is more convenient but that of Trousseau more reliable. The first involves tapping the branches of the facial nerves as they spread out from within the parotid gland; a positive sign is twitching of the appropriate facial muscle. In the second the forearm is made ischaemic with a sphygmomanometer cuff for up to 3 min; if positive, carpal spasm will occur.

BIOCHEMICAL INVESTIGATIONS

Many generalized disorders of the skeleton, such as postmenopausal osteoporosis, achondroplasia, osteogenesis imperfecta, and the epiphyseal dysplasias, have normal routine biochemical values; in others changes are diagnostic (Table 3). In normal persons the fasting plasma calcium concentration remains virtually constant through life, the plasma phosphate declines in adolescence, and the plasma alkaline phosphatase increases during rapid adolescent growth. Since total plasma calcium includes a protein-bound fraction, it is usual to relate it to the plasma albumin and, if necessary, correct it to a plasma albumin of 4 g per 100 ml. Acceptable corrections include: corrected calcium (mg per 100 ml) = measured calcium − albumin (g per 100 ml) + 4; or for SI

Table 3 *Biochemical and other features in disorders of the skeleton*

Disorder	Most common symptoms	Plasma Ca	P	Alkaline phosphatase	Urine Ca	THP[a]	Other biochemical features	Comments
Osteoporosis	Fracture	N	N	N	N	N	None	Hypercalcuria if immobilized
Osteomalacia (and rickets)	Bone pain; proximal weakness	N or L	L	N or H	L	N or H	Depends on cause	Plasma P increased in renal glomerular failure
Paget's disease	Pain; deformity	N	N	H	N	H	None	Hypercalcaemia if immobilized
Hyperparathyroidism (with bone disease)	Bone pain; hypercalcaemic symptoms	H	L	H	H	H	Aminoaciduria	P'ase and THP normal if clinical bone disease absent
Pseudohypoparathyroidism	Simple; short metacarpals; cataracts	L	H	N	N	N		Mutation in G-protein
Osteogenesis imperfecta	Brittle bones	N	N	N	N	N	None	Many collagen gene mutations
Marfan's syndrome	Tall with scoliosis; dislocated lenses; aortic dissection	N	N	N	N	$\pm$H	None	Dominant inheritance; clinically heterogeneous
Homocystinuria	Mentally subnormal; look like Marfan's syndrome	N	N	N	N	N	Homocystine in urine	
Alkaptonuria	Back pain; early arthritis; dark urine	N	N	N	N	N	Homogentisic acid in the urine	Calcified intervertebral discs
Mucopolysaccharidoses	Short stature; thoracolumbar gibbus; mentally subnormal (depends on type)	N	N	N	N	N	Characteristic mucopolysaccharide in urine	See text
Osteopetrosis (marble bones disease)	Anaemia; blindness; deafness (severe form)	$\pm$H	N	N	Low	N	Increase in acid phosphatase in some	Mild form fractures only; rarely carbonic anhydrase lack
Hypophosphatasia	Lethal short-limbed dwarfism; bone disease like rickets	N	N	Low	N	N	Phosphoethanolamine in urine increased	Fractures in adult
Hyperphosphatasia	Large head, bowing of long bones; occurs in childhood	N	N	Very high	N	Very high	None	Similar to Paget's disease
Fibrous dysplasia	Fracture; sexual precocity in girls; pigmentation	N	N	Slight increase	N	Slight increase	Biochemical changes in polyostotic form only. Mutation in G-protein	Occasional hypophosphataemic osteomalacia
Myositis ossificans progressiva	Pain and swelling in muscles; fixation of joints	N	N	? Increased during myositis	N	N	None	Monophalangic big toe

[a]THP = total hydroxyproline. The same changes occur in pyridinium cross-link collagen-derived peptides.

units: 0.02 mmol/l for every 1 g/l change of albumin from 40 g/l. The fasting plasma calcium is normal in osteoporosis and also in Paget's disease unless the patient is immobilized. It is increased in primary hyperparathyroidism, various neoplasms (including humoral hypercalcaemia of malignancy), in sarcoidosis, in vitamin D overdosage, and in a number of other states, such as acromegaly and thyrotoxicosis (Table 3). It is often low in osteomalacia but may be restored towards normal by secondary hyperparathyroidism, and is low in parathyroid insufficiency. Normal values are to be expected in inherited hypophosphataemia and in other forms of renal tubular rickets.

Since the main determinant of the fasting plasma phosphate concentration is its renal tubular reabsorption, hypophosphataemia occurs in primary hyperparathyroidism, in the humoral hypercalcaemia of malignancy, and it is also low in inherited hypophosphataemic rickets. Oral aluminium hydroxide and prolonged intravenous nutrition also both lower plasma phosphate. Hyperphosphataemia occurs in hypoparathyroidism, in renal glomerular failure, and in the rare recessively inherited form of tumoral calcinosis. It is also a transient finding after surgery in patients given intravenous fluids for 24 to 48 h or longer.

The plasma alkaline phosphatase is normally increased in adolescence and in osteomalacia, particularly in the young, but it may be near normal in renal tubular osteomalacia. Increases occur in primary hyperparathyroidism, but only where there is coexistent bone disease. The highest values for plasma alkaline phosphatase are found in young patients with active Paget's disease, and in idiopathic hyperphosphatasia; and the lowest in hypophosphatasia.

Sugar detected in the urine in a patient with inherited rickets suggests multiple renal tubular defects, and proteinuria is an important clue to myeloma.

The amount of calcium excreted in the urine is related both to the plasma levels and to the percentage of the filtered load reabsorbed through the renal tubules, itself altered by parathyroid hormone. Hypocalcaemia therefore causes hypocalciuria, particularly in osteomalacia and rickets; and hypercalcaemia leads to hypercalciuria, especially when this is due to rapid bone loss as in neoplastic disease of the skeleton, leukaemia, myeloma, and immobilization. Since parathyroid hormone increases the renal tubular reabsorption of calcium, the normal relationship between plasma and urine calcium is disturbed in parathyroid disease; however, most hypercalcaemic hyperparathyroid patients excrete more calcium than normal. Total hydroxyproline in the urine (after acid hydrolysis of the peptides) is a good indicator of breakdown and collagen turnover in bone, provided the patient is on a low-gelatin diet. The physiological changes in hydroxyproline excretion are striking, with a particularly sharp peak in adolescence coinciding with the maximum height velocity. The highest values are seen in active Paget's disease, where the excretion may be up to fiftyfold the normal value. Hydroxyproline excretion correlates well with plasma alkaline phosphatase, and is therefore increased in some forms of osteomalacia and in hyperparathyroidism with bone disease. Since thyroxine increases collagen turnover, urinary hydroxyproline is also abnormally high in thyrotoxicosis and abnormally low in myxoedema (either primary or secondary).

Hydroxyproline excretion can be most usefully expressed as the amount in a 24 h urine sample in a patient on a gelatin-free diet, or in a fasting urine sample in relation to creatinine. However, hydroxyproline peptide excretion is related both to newly formed and mature collagen, and is not, therefore, a direct measure of bone resorption. The urinary excretion of pyridinium compounds (see above) from the lysyl- and hydroxylysyl-derived cross-links of mature collagen is a direct measure of bone resorption, irrespective of dietary collagen.

RADIOLOGY

The diagnosis of bone disease often depends on the radiographic appearances, especially where there are no demonstrable biochemical changes. A particular example is in the differential diagnosis of lethal dwarfism. Conventional radiographs demonstrate well structural changes such as fractures, deformity, areas of resorption, and alteration size, but are unreliable for the assessment of bone density. As radiographic techniques develop, increasing use is made of isotope bone scans and CT scans. Diphosphonate-labelled scanning agents are selectively taken up in areas of increased vascularity or turnover. They are very useful in demonstrating the skeletal extent of Paget's disease of bone, the presence of bony metastases, the pathological fractures of osteoporosis, and Looser's zones in osteomalacia. An isotope scan is preferable to multiple radiographs to assess the distribution (but not the structure) of abnormal bone.

CT scanning can also be very useful in bone disease. Examples include the delineation of ectopic ossification, of spinal cord compression, and of bone tumours. Although magnetic resonance scanning (MRI) finds its most important application in soft tissue pathology, it is also useful in giving an idea of the composition as well as the structure of bone.

Methods for measuring bone mass are considered under osteoporosis (see below).

BONE BIOPSY

Direct examination of bone is a valuable but under-used investigation. Bone can be taken by a transiliac trephine (using a local anaesthetic) and sections should be examined with and without decalcification. In the various metabolic bone diseases the appearances are characteristic, with the excess osteoid of osteomalacia; the disorganized mosaic pattern, excessive cellular activity, and fibrosis of Paget's disease; and osteitis fibrosa cystica in hyperparathyroid bone disease. In mild osteogenesis imperfecta there is typically an increase in the number of osteocytes, and, in the more severe form, a considerable increase in the amount of woven bone. A normal biopsy will exclude these diseases except where the pathological changes are patchy. Where possible, histological examination should now include transmission and scanning electron microscopy, and the report should include quantitative histomorphometry. More details are given in larger texts (see references).

FURTHER INVESTIGATIONS

The measurement of external calcium and phosphorus balance is a classic way of investigating generalized bone disease and the effects of treatment upon it, but it is also tedious. The use of isotopes to measure calcium absorption and apparent bone formation and resorption rates is less direct and also depends on a number of assumptions. This leaves a large number of measurements available for specific problems. Examples (in the plasma) are intact PTH assays (to investigate hyper- and hypocalcaemia), PTHrP (mainly in research), 25-hydroxyvitamin D, and 1,25-dihydroxyvitamin D (for investigation of rickets and osteomalacia), and osteocalcin (as an indicator of osteoblast activity). In inherited disorders analysis of DNA (from white cells), RNA from lymphocytes, and enzyme activity and collagen synthesized from fibroblast cultures are increasingly used.

DIAGNOSIS

The diagnosis of a skeletal disorder is not difficult where there are clear biochemical disturbances (Table 3) although, as in osteomalacia, the causes may be many. When the standard biochemical results are normal an exact diagnosis may be impossible, and this is particularly so in some of the rare heritable disorders. Guidance based on the age of the patient and frequency of the disorder is given in Table 4.

REFERENCES

Avioli, L.V. and Krane, S.M. (1990). *Metabolic bone disease,* (2nd edn). W.B. Saunders, Philadelphia.

Table 4 *Diagnosis of disorders of the skeleton*

Age	Main presenting symptom	Most likely diagnosis	Frequency	Exclude
Over 50 years	Pain in the back loss of height fracture	Osteoporosis, most common in women	Common	Myeloma (especially in men)
				Secondary deposits
	Deformity of long bones pain in hips and pelvis fracture	Paget's disease of bone, most common in men	Common	Coexistent osteomalacia
				Osteomalacia
				Hyperparathyroid bone disease
				Skeletal metastases
	Bone pain, and tenderness, difficulty in walking, unable to climb stairs, pathological fracture	Osteomalacia	Uncommon, especially in the adult	Carcinoma
				Polymyalgia rheumatica
	Bone pain and deformity, thirst, nocturia, depression vomiting, constipation	Osteitis fibrosa cystica, most common in women	Rare	Carcinoma with hypercalcaemia myeloma
20–50 years	loss of height	Probably secondary deposits, or myeloma	Rare	Osteomalacia
				Accelerated osteoporosis
	Muscle weakness, loss of height, bone pain	Osteomalacia	Rare	Late muscular dystrophy
				Neoplastic neuromyopathy
				Cushing's syndrome
0–20 years	Bowing of bones, deformity, weakness	'Nutritional' rickets	Most common in Asian immigrants in Northern cities	Other causes of rickets
				Hypophosphatasia
	Multiple fractures bruising	In infants, inflicted by parents, 'battered baby'	Not uncommon	Osteogenesis imperfecta
	Bone pain, ill-health	Leukaemia	Uncommon	Osteomyelitis
				Rickets
	Pain in back, difficulty in walking, pain in ankles, less rapid growth	Juvenile osteoporosis	Rare	Leukaemia
				Osteogenesis imperfecta
	Failure to grow (short stature)	Many causes (Table 2)	Common	Particularly hypothyroidism, Turner's syndrome, and coeliac disease
	Excessive or disproportionate growth	Several causes, often familial	Less common than short stature	Particularly pituitary tumour
				Marfan's syndrome
				Homocystinuria
				Hypogonadism and chromosomal abnormalities
	Fracture and deformity at birth (often lethal)	Severe osteogenesis imperfecta	Uncommon	Hypophosphatasia
				Achondrogenesis
				Thanatophoric dwarfism

Eyre, D. (1992). New biomarkers of bone resorption. *Journal of Clinical Endocrinology and Metabolism* **74**, 470A–470C.

Lancet (1992). Pyridinium cross links as markers of bone resorption. *Lancet* **340**, 278–9.

Nordin, B.E.C., Need, A.G., and Morris, H.A. (1993). *Metabolic bone and stone disease*, (3rd edn). Churchill Livingstone, Edinburgh.

Osteoporosis

Osteoporosis is the most common metabolic bone disease, and it is important because of its contribution to fractures, particularly in the elderly. In osteoporosis there is a reduction in the amount of bone per unit volume without a change in its composition. There are two additions to this definition, one of which is statistical and the other clinical; the first defines osteoporosis as a reduction in bone mass by more than 2 standard deviations (SD) below the mean for a young adult population; the second as a reduction in the amount of bone sufficient to predispose to fracture. The term osteopenia, that is, a reduction in the amount of bone, defines the stage of bone loss without clinical fracture. There are microarchitectural changes in bone before such fracture and these are seen particularly in trabecular bone. Such changes are mediated by bone cell activity. The trabeculae become thinner and non-weight-bearing bone is selectively removed. The exact mechanism by which bone is removed varies according to the cause of the osteoporosis.

Although osteoporosis is not a new disease, widespread interest in this disorder is comparatively recent. This is because of the recognized financial and medical burden that results from osteoporosis-related fractures, the ability to measure bone loss and to prevent it, and the medical, social, and financial benefit that would result from such prevention. Osteoporosis and osteoporosis-related fractures occur particularly in women after the menopause, but the disorder is not restricted to this group since it can occur in the young, in both sexes, and at all ages. It is important for the clinician to be able to recognize all the underlying causes of osteoporosis, since at least some of these are treatable.

BONE MASS AND FRACTURE

The amount of bone in the adult depends on the peak bone mass and the rate of its subsequent loss. Peak bone mass depends on the interaction between genetic and mechanical factors, modified by nutritional and endocrine influences, which together determine the balance between bone resorption (by osteoclasts) and bone formation (by osteoblasts) (Fig. 6).

Thus known genetic determinants of bone mass are race—the peak bone mass of Negroid adults is greater than that of Caucasian adults, a difference which appears in adolescence—family, and collagen gene mutations.

Bones that are used are denser than those that are not, and bone loss in later life is delayed, to a variable extent, by appropriate exercise. Additional calcium intake increases peak bone mass and reduces subsequent loss. The most important hormones determining peak bone mass are the sex hormones, and varying degrees of oestrogen lack in the growing skeleton produce osteopenia. The effects of the interaction of these nutritional, mechanical, and endocrine factors on bone mass is particularly seen in anorexia nervosa (nutrition and oestrogen lack) often associated with obsessional exercise. Interestingly, the vertebral bone density of some competitive female athletes can be low rather than high compared with age-matched normals, demonstrating that the beneficial effects of mechanical stress on the skeleton are at least blunted by hormone lack.

Bone mass reaches a peak at about 30 years of age, and is higher in men than in women; when lean body mass is taken into account the difference in axial bone mineral density lessens or disappears (not unexpectedly, bone mass and body size are related). From young adult life bone is progressively lost in men at a steady rate, and in women rapidly after the menopause for some 10 years and then at the same rate as men. Endosteal resorption of bone dominates over new periosteal bone formation and the increase in external diameter is less than the internal expansion. At a certain bone density fracture becomes likely (theoretical fracture threshold). Fractures are more frequent in women than men because they reach the fracture threshold earlier and live longer. There are certain life-style features which increase the rate of bone loss—such as excess smoking, alcohol, thinness, and immobility, together with medical events such as hysterectomy, early natural or surgically induced menopause, and episodes of amenorrhoea in early life.

Fig. 6 A diagram to demonstrate the main known determinants of peak bone mass and examples of disorders that affect it (from Smith (1993), with permission)

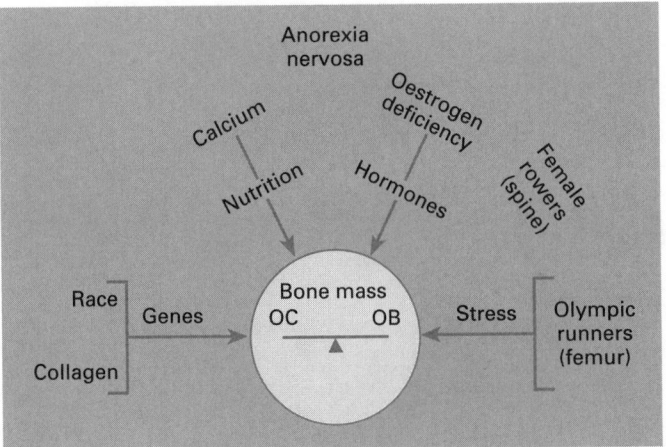

Assessment of the likelihood of fracture should take into account the presence or absence of such risk factors, together with the measurement of prevailing bone density.

Research has shown that the likelihood of subsequent fracture is directly and linearly related to bone density. However, there is an overlap in the bone densities of those who fracture and those who do not, so that fracture may occur in persons with normal bone density and not all persons with low bone density break bones. Thus in groups of subjects the mean bone density in those who sustain a femoral neck fracture is not more than 1 SD lower than those who do not. This means that the measurement of bone density within a population susceptible to osteoporosis (postmenopausal women) will not detect a significant proportion who are liable to fracture and, therefore, makes osteoporosis 'screening' of populations not medically or economically worthwhile. The problem is very similar to that of the measurement of cholesterol within populations as a predictor of cardiovascular events (Chapters 15.10.1 and 11.6). This does not mean that in the individual patient measurement of bone density is useless. In contrast, low bone density is an important risk factor for fracture.

The reason why bone density and fracture are not more closely related is that fracture depends on more than bone mass. An important cause of fracture, especially in the elderly, is falling. This may be increased by the physical and mental frailty of later years, by hypothermia, drugs and alcoholism, and by environmental factors. Whether or not a fall results in a fracture depends on the strength of the bone, related to its density, and the effect of the impact; for instance, protective pads over the upper hips may reduce femoral neck fracture rate. Some investigations suggest that falling is more important than osteoporosis in causing fracture in the elderly.

Fractures at three main sites—vertebrae, femoral neck, and forearm—are those most often considered to be related to osteoporosis. (Clearly, fractures at other sites such as the pelvis and other limb bones may also occur in osteoporotic bones.) The composition of the bone differs at these sites, with vertebral bone being predominantly trabecular and hip predominantly cortical. Vertebral fractures occur in younger people than hip fracture, probably because bone loss occurs more rapidly from the vertebral site. The frequency of both fractures increases with age, but they may have different causes. Thus in the immediate perimenopausal years bone loss is largely due to excess bone resorption and vertebral fractures predominate; later, reduced osteoblast activity reduces new bone formation and femoral neck fractures become important. The difference between the two groups (type I and II) and the proposed causes are outlined in Table 5.

Fractures of the forearm in mixed trabecular and cortical bone do not show an increase with incidence with ageing. This may be because this type of fracture often results from putting out the arm to prevent a fall, and in the elderly person the reflex to do so is diminished.

Both vertebral and femoral neck fractures produce disability—pain in the back with loss of height and inability to walk, respectively. The medical and economic effects of femoral neck fracture are considerable; for instance it has been estimated that 20 per cent of all orthopaedic beds in the United Kingdom are occupied by elderly women with hip fractures, and that after a femoral neck fracture up to 25 per cent of patients are dead 6 months later and the majority are disabled. The annual cost of such fractures in the United States approaches $16 billion. Recent reviews have shown that the immediate treatment of hip fractures is often unsatisfactory.

MEASUREMENT OF BONE MASS

Methods that measure the amount of bone present in different parts of the skeleton all depend on the assumption that the bone is normally mineralized, since they measure the amount of calcium and do not detect changes in the organic bone matrix. Apart from radiological methods of measuring cortical thickness and density compared with standards such

Table 5 *The different causes of bone loss and fracture after the menopause*

	Type I	Type II
Age (years)	51–75	70
Sex ratio (F:M)	6:1	2:1
Type of bone loss	Mainly trabecular	Trabecular and cortical
Rate of bone loss	Accelerated	Not accelerated
Fracture sites	Vertebrae (crush) and distal radius	Vertebrae (multiple wedge) and hip
Parathyroid function	Decreased	Increased
Calcium absorption	Decreased	Decreased
Metabolism of 25-OH-D to 1,25-(OH)$_2$D$_3$	Secondary decrease	Primary decrease
Main causes	Factors related to menopause	Factors relating to ageing

as aluminium wedges, current methods are single and dual photon densitometry, quantitative CT scanning, and dual X-ray absorptiometry.

Single photon densitometry relies on the absorption of photons from a single isotope source and is applied to the forearm; dual photon absorptiometry enables measurement of hip and spine bone density; quantitative CT scanning allows one to select a particular area for measurement; dual X-ray absorptiometry scanning utilizes two X-ray sources and is the method used most often. Much has been written on the measurement of bone density or mass. Bone mineral density (BMD) is expressed as the amount of mineral within a given area and the result is expressed as an area density.

Single photon forearm bone density is relatively inexpensive and reproducible; dual photon methods are more expensive. CT methods result in a high dosage of radiation, while dual X-ray absorptiometry methods are rapid and do not require a replaceable isotope source.

Although various differences have been recorded in accuracy and reproducibility, other factors influence the choice of method. It is clear that if one is concerned with density (and fractures) at a particular site, it is important to measure the density at that site. However, if one is making sequential measurements in individuals, forearm bone density measurements continue to be useful; and there is some evidence that the forearm bone density provides a good indication of overall fracture risk. However, since spinal bone density reflects the changes in trabecular bone, which is metabolically more active than other sites, it will, in general, be a more sensitive indicator of bone loss (and gain) than other sites. It is important to recognize that in the care of a patient undue importance should not be given to bone density alone. Fig. 7 shows the way in which a dual X-ray absorptiometry bone density result is commonly expressed.

Causes of osteoporosis

Many patients have more than one cause for their osteoporosis. The main recognized causes are shown in Table 6. Osteoporosis occurs most commonly in postmenopausal and elderly women, and is classified as age-related bone loss. At this age it is due to a triad of causes—menopause, increasing age, and reduced mobility. A significant number of elderly men also develop osteoporosis. Osteoporosis not clearly related to age is often associated with accelerated bone loss. Rarely, this occurs in childhood, in adolescence, and also in young adults, sometimes associated with pregnancy in women. Accelerated bone loss may also occur as the result of immobility, endocrine disease, chromosomal disturbances, and a number of other conditions. In some of these there is also a reduction in peak bone mass. Bone loss is increased by a number of medical and life-style factors, grouped as osteoporosis risk factors. These include excessive smoking and alcohol consumption, lack of exercise, early menopause, excessive thinness, and possibly nulliparity. The relative importance of these factors in regard to bone density is not clear. It is possible to make a very long list of the causes of osteoporosis but this is often done more for the sake of completeness than for any prac-

tical reason. To include other bone diseases, such as those due to secondary malignant deposits or to parathyroid overactivity, where loss of bone is merely one feature of the bone disorder, is confusing. However, it is important to remember these disorders in the differential diagnosis of osteoporosis (Table 7).

SYMPTOMS AND SIGNS

Osteoporosis produces symptoms by predisposing to fracture. The features differ according to the fracture site. The most common is deformity and loss of height due to vertebral collapse. The loss of height may be noticed more by others than by the patient, who rarely knows her original height. However, this may be determined by measurement of the span (since in the young adult, height and span are approximately equal). In the younger person vertebral collapse is accompanied by deformity of the chest and protrusion of the manubrium sterni. Vertebral collapse is at first clearly related to a recognized stress, for instance, moving heavy furniture; usually it produces severe and localized pain, and the vertebrae are tender to percussion. However, there is evidence that vertebral collapse frequently occurs without symptoms. Examination of the patient will confirm the loss of trunk height, the thoracic kyphosis, the proximity of the ribs to the iliac crest, and transverse abdominal crease, and may give some clue about the cause of the structural collapse. Thus

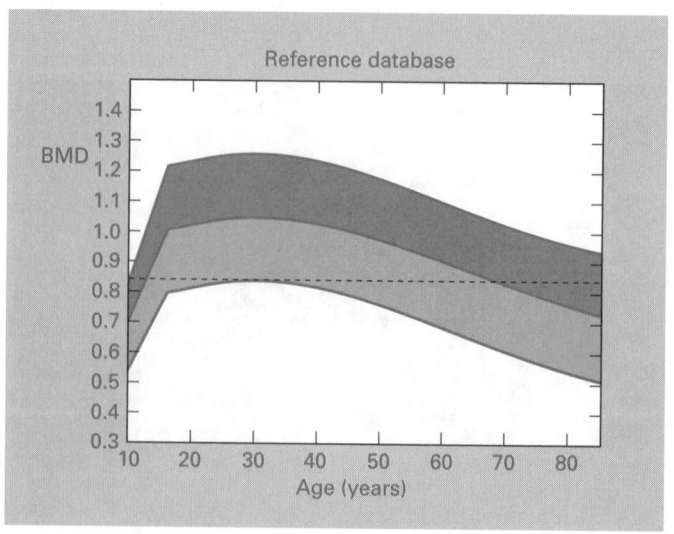

Fig. 7 The measurement of bone mineral density (BMD) by dual X-ray absorptiometry. The shaded area represents the changes of BMD with age, expressed as mean ± 2 SD (95 per cent confidence limits). 2 SD below the peak bone mass, i.e. below the shaded area for young adults, is a statistical definition of osteoporosis, and the horizontal dotted line extended from this represents the theoretical fracture 'threshold'.

Table 6 *The main causes and types of osteoporosis*

Age-related
  Postmenopausal
  Elderly
Not age-related
  Immobility
    General
      prolonged bed rest, neurological injury, space flight
    Local
      rheumatoid arthritis
  Endocrine
    Oestrogen lack
      Oophorectomy
      Hysterectomy
      Obsessional athletes
      Early menopause
    Testosterone lack in young men
    Cushing's syndrome, spontaneous or iatrogenic
    Thyrotoxicosis
    Hypopituitarism
  Nutritional
    Anorexia nervosa
    Starvation
    Coeliac disease
  Genetic
    Osteogenesis imperfecta
    Familial and racial (Oriental, Caucasian)
  Lifestyle (risk factors)
    Smoking
    Alcohol
  Idiopathic
    Pregnancy-related osteoporosis
    Juvenile osteoporosis
    Osteoporosis in young adults
  Other
    Mastocytosis
    Heparin administration
    Cytotoxic agents

Table 7 *The main differential diagnosis of osteoporosis*

Multiple myeloma: especially in men; high erythrocyte sedimentation rate, monoclonal gammopathy, light chains in the urine, plasma cells in the marrow, sometimes hypercalcaemia
Metastatic carcinoma: breast, bronchus, prostate, kidney, thyroid
Osteomalacia: may coexist with osteoporosis, especially in the elderly; identify by biochemistry and bone biopsy
Hyperparathyroidism: occasionally associated with generalized osteoporosis; biochemistry diagnostic
Osteogenesis imperfecta: distinguish by family history, blue sclerae, wormian bones

in middle age bone tenderness, anaemia, and general ill-health should suggest multiple myeloma or secondary carcinoma, and in children leukaemia may mimic juvenile osteoporosis. Clues to the various endocrine causes of osteoporosis should always be sought. Clearly, fractures at other sites (forearm, femoral neck) will have their own features.

RADIOLOGY

Plain films of the skeleton do not detect osteoporosis until there is a considerable loss of bone, and they are mainly useful in detecting the major complication of osteoporosis, that is, structural collapse. In the vertebrae, fractures due to osteoporosis appear as irregular anterior wedging affecting some vertebrae and not others. The end plates may be biconcave but this change does not have the uniformity of distribution seen in osteomalacia, except where it occurs in juvenile osteoporosis or in osteogenesis imperfecta. Different grades of vertebral fracture are defined, from a moderate loss of anterior height through conspicuous anterior wedging to complete flattening of the whole vertebra. Various changes are also described in osteoporotic bones before fracture. These include loss of the less important (horizontal) trabeculae in the vertebrae with apparent accentuation of those in the vertical direction; reduction of cortical thickness in the long bones; and progressive loss of trabeculae also in these bones, particularly at the upper end of the femur. In the vertebrae, herniation of the disc through the end plate causes a 'Schmorl's node'; it is said by some that this is unrelated to osteoporosis. In the peripheral bones the cortex is thinned and, especially in severe or acute osteoporosis (as with immobilization), the endosteal surface may appear scalloped, and the mineral loss has a 'spotty' or 'rain-drop' appearance. Osteoporosis is said not to affect the skull except where it is due to an excess of adrenal cortical steroids.

BIOCHEMISTRY

Biochemical measurements in osteoporosis are usually normal; however, recent immobility in a young person considerably increases the urine calcium, and after the menopause the ratios of calcium and of hydroxyproline to creatinine measured in the urine after an overnight fast may both be increased, which implies increased bone resorption. Likewise the urinary excretion of the collagen-derived pyridinium compounds may be increased. Measurements of plasma osteocalcin have given variable results.

Recent long-bone fracture may slightly increase plasma alkaline phosphatase. Where the osteoporosis is due to some underlying disorder, the biochemical changes reflect this; for example in thyrotoxic bone disease the plasma calcium, phosphate, and alkaline phosphatase, and the urinary hydroxyproline excretion may all be increased. Patients with active osteoporosis may be in negative calcium balance with a high urine calcium excretion and/or reduced intestinal absorption of calcium.

OTHER INVESTIGATIONS

Bone biopsy is not a useful or necessary way of confirming osteoporosis. However, it helps to identify its underlying cause, to exclude coexisting metabolic bone disease such as osteomalacia, and also to exclude disorders with a similar presentation. It should also probably be combined with bone marrow aspiration to exclude haematological disorders, especially in the young. In osteoporosis the reduction in trabecular volume may be associated with a reduction in mean wall thickness, a measure of bone formation rate. Isotope scanning may be useful to show the presence of fresh fractures, and to exclude such obvious features as multiple secondary deposits. The role of bone density measurements is not yet established. The most frequently used instrument is a dual X-ray source. Recommended specific indications are to confirm (or not) a radiological suggestion of osteoporosis, to provide a baseline measurement for treatment, to aid with decisions about hormone replacement therapy, and in clinical research. Densitometry should be considered in specific forms of osteoporosis, such as corticosteroid osteoporosis. Since bone density is an important indicator of future fracture it may be used to identify those at particular risk. The difficulty of applying this to populations has been mentioned.

DIAGNOSIS

In the diagnosis of osteoporosis there are two steps; first to establish that osteoporosis is present and that other significant bone diseases are absent, and secondly to try to establish its cause—since amongst these are some which can be improved by treatment. Osteoporosis itself will be readily excluded from other forms of metabolic bone disease because of its usually normal biochemistry, and from other causes of loss of trunk height and vertebral collapse by examination of the patient, the peripheral blood, the bone marrow, and the bone itself (Table 7). To establish the exact reason for osteoporosis can be difficult, since the causes are often multiple.

Types of osteoporosis

Age-related bone loss

The most common type of osteoporosis is that which occurs in women after the menopause. For clinical purposes we may separate bone loss occurring in the first decade after the menopause from 'senile' or 'elderly' osteoporosis, since the causes are probably different (Table 5). In the early postmenopausal years the main cellular abnormality is excess bone resorption, whereas later defective new bone formation becomes relatively more important. The rapid loss of bone in women immediately after the menopause is well documented, and likely to be due to oestrogen deficiency. Osteoporosis is generally considered to be the main cause of fractures in postmenopausal women and as such is an enormous (and potentially preventable) health problem.

MANAGEMENT OF AGE-RELATED OSTEOPOROSIS

Once the diagnosis has been made the management should be easy, but many controversies have arisen.

Since in later adult years the amount of bone depends on the peak bone mass and its subsequent loss, it is clearly important to build up an optimum bone mass in early years by exercise, adequate nutrition (especially calcium), and the avoidance of risk factors. In practice the opportunities to do this have usually disappeared, so that the main steps are to prevent any further bone loss and, where possible, to stimulate effective new bone formation. Further bone loss may be slowed by general measures such as increased exercise, additional calcium, appropriate hormone replacement therapy, and cyclical etidronate (Didronel®). Calcitonin has a tenuous position in the prevention of bone loss. New bone formation can also be stimulated by exercise and, most specifically, by sodium fluoride.

Whichever of these approaches is taken, it is important that each osteoporotic patient is regarded as an individual. Patients often have unnecessary worries about osteoporosis, especially because of the widespread publicity about it, and reassurance and explanation is important.

Dealing with each of these in turn, moderate weight-bearing exercise (and the avoidance of immobility) encourages new bone formation and osteoblastic activity and reduces osteoclastic bone resorption. This has been well demonstrated in animals and by densitometric measurements at the appropriate site in patients.

There is a continuing controversy about the role of additional calcium in the prevention of bone loss, but increasing evidence of its usefulness. It does not provide an alternative to hormone replacement therapy in the early postmenopausal years, but it may reduce bone loss (and fracture rate) in later years in women, and also in men.

It is in the use of hormone replacement therapy that the most advance has been made and the most controversy has arisen.

There seems little doubt that hormone replacement therapy prevents further bone loss at whatever postmenopausal age it is given. However, because bone loss is most rapid in the first 10 postmenopausal years, hormone replacement therapy is most effective if given during that time. It also reduces femoral neck fracture rate. Oestrogen given on its own increases the risk of endometrial cancer, and this risk is abolished by giving cyclical progestogen. Long-term oestrogen appears to increase the incidence of breast carcinoma, with a slightly increased mortality after 10 years. The relative risk is small and debated (values of 1.3–1.7 have been given). A number of epidemiological studies have shown that oestrogen alone significantly reduces cardiovascular deaths. If this is so, the cardiovascular benefits would be far greater than any benefit on the skeleton since cardiovascular disease is the most frequent causes of death in postmenopausal women. For opposed hormone replacement therapy, that is oestrogen plus progestogen, the situation is not clear; the majority of studies have been made on patients taking oestrogen alone, and it is not known whether adding progestogen to abolish uterine carcinoma will also abolish the apparent cardiovascular benefit of oestrogen alone. It is also possible that patients who take hormone replacement therapy and continue with it are self-selected in the sense that they also have a lifestyle which could prevent bone loss (exercise, sufficient oral calcium, and few or no risk factors). At present, therefore, hormone replacement therapy is widely recommended to prevent bone loss, both before and after fracture; but it is not widely accepted since oestrogen plus progestogen will induce cyclical bleeding. Progestogen is, of course, not necessary in a patient who has had a hysterectomy. The development of more acceptable forms of hormone replacement therapy and confirmation of their cardiovascular benefit when progestogen is added will be important.

A recent American consensus emphasizes the advantages of oestrogen in hysterectomized women, but is less positive about the advantages of oestrogen plus progestogen in women with an intact uterus.

Within the past few years the bisphosphonate, disodium etidronate, has been given in a cyclical manner (together with oral calcium) to prevent bone loss by suppression of osteoclastic bone resorption. This treatment is licensed for treatment of established vertebral osteoporosis with vertebral collapse.

Calcitonin reduces bone resorption when given by injection (which has side-effects) and also by nasal inhalation.

Antiresorptive agents produce their effects by modification of the BMU cycle. The activities of osteoclasts and osteoblasts are closely linked, so the effect on bone mass of reducing resorption is only temporary. This means that within the first year or so treatment with any antiresorptive will give an increase in bone mass which will only be temporary. This does not seem to be so for hormone replacement therapy or cyclical etidronate treatment.

Exercise probably has a dual effect, increasing new bone formation as well as decreasing resorption. Sodium fluoride stimulates the osteoblasts to form new bone and increases bone density. However, the newly formed bone is woven and mechanically unsound. In osteoporotic patients given sodium fluoride, vertebral bone density increases, but fractures do not decrease. There is, however, a controversy about the effect of different doses of fluoride on the skeleton. Other agents have also been used in the treatment of osteoporosis; thiazides reduce urine calcium excretion and femoral neck fracture rate; and vitamin D or its metabolites may also reduce the fracture rate (particularly in those with malabsorption of calcium). Detailed work has yet to establish the usefulness of the 1–34 amino acid fragment of parathyroid hormone.

In practice, the prevention of bone loss and its subsequent treatment depend on a triad of recommendations—exercise, adequate calcium intake, and hormone replacement therapy where appropriate—together with the avoidance of known risk factors, particularly (according to some) smoking. Since fractures are not due to osteoporosis alone, it is also important not to forget the importance of preventing falls.

Osteoporosis not related to age

Immobility contributes to many forms of osteoporosis, particularly with increasing age. In such instances it is difficult to exactly define its importance relative to other factors. There are other situations, especially in the young, where the contribution of immobilization to bone loss is clearly very significant. This immobility may be local, around inflamed joints or fractured limbs, or it may be general. Thus rapidly progressive osteoporosis follows severe injury in the young associated with enforced immobilization. This is due to a sudden 'uncoupling' of bone resorption and formation. It may produce hypercalcaemia or hypercalciuria; radiographically there is a spotty 'rain-drop' form of rarefaction. Similar events probably occur in space travel.

Treatment is difficult, but the osteoporosis will improve when mobility is resumed. Two localized forms of osteoporosis whose cause is unknown in which immobility may be important are a self-limiting transient osteoporosis which tends to affect the bones adjacent to larger joints, and that associated with Sudeck's atrophy.

Osteoporosis and pregnancy

Women occasionally develop vertebral fractures during pregnancy. Pain in the back and kyphosis are noticed near term or shortly after delivery. The pain generally improves after 2 or 3 months and the loss of height may cease; however, the bones remain osteoporotic. Further vertebral collapse in subsequent pregnancies does not necessarily occur.

It is possible that this very rare form of osteoporosis is associated with failure of the normal changes in calciotrophic hormones which appear to protect the maternal skeleton during pregnancy. The relationship to transient regional osteoporosis, which particularly affects the femoral necks in pregnancy, is obscure.

Osteoporosis in the young

Occasionally osteoporosis with structural collapse occurs during growth. The particular form that occurs around puberty (idiopathic juvenile osteoporosis) is usually self-limiting. Growth rate is reduced and shortness of the trunk with kyphosis due to vertebral fracture may develop. There is pain in the back which may follow injury. In this condition there may be metaphyseal fractures at the ends of the long bones which can be confused with Looser's zones. Such fractures are associated with pain in the ankles and difficulty in walking. Excessive bone resorption has been reported but decreased bone formation also occurs. The cause of the condition is unknown. Although it is generally associated with the rapid growth of adolescence, similar conditions occur in childhood. Except in rare cases, it is not progressive and the bones may return to a nearly normal structure within a few years, especially in the spine, although spinal deformity often persists (Fig. 8). The real incidence of this condition may be underestimated; it could account for a number of cases of idiopathic kyphosis. The condition most difficult to distinguish from it is mild osteogenesis imperfecta (see below) and the rare osteoporosis-glioma syndrome, especially where the characteristic family history and blue sclerae are absent.

Osteoporosis and endocrine disease

The skeleton is affected by many hormones. In some conditions, for instance thyrotoxicosis, the clinical effects are minor, but in others, such as Cushing's syndrome and hypogonadism, osteoporotic collapse of the skeleton is a significant feature.

Fig. 8 Changes in the vertebrae with age in a boy with idiopathic juvenile osteoporosis.

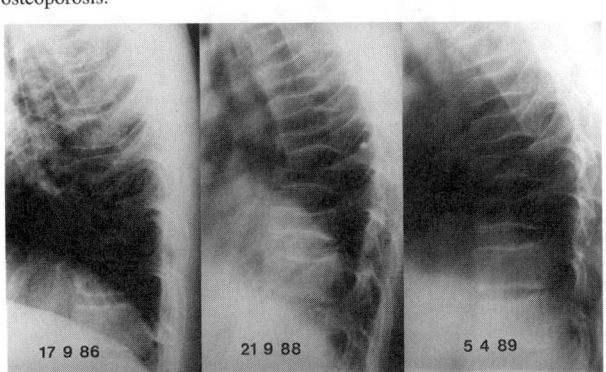

17 9 86   21 9 88   5 4 89

THYROID BONE DISEASE

In thyrotoxicosis bone turnover is excessive, bone resorption is more increased than bone formation, and after many years of thyroid overactivity significant osteoporosis may occur. Biochemically there may be hypercalcaemia, hyperphosphataemia, and an increase in plasma alkaline phosphatase; hypercalciuria and increased urinary hydroxyproline also occur. Since thyrotoxicosis is often recognized early, significant bone disease is uncommon; rarely it may be seen in patients who are thyroid addicts. It should be considered in all cases of obscure osteoporosis. Histologically there is an increase in the amount of bone surfaces covered by osteoid, in fibrous tissue, osteoclasts, and osteoblasts; mineralization is normal.

CORTICOSTEROIDS AND OSTEOPOROSIS

The most frequent endocrine bone disease after postmenopausal osteoporosis is osteoporosis due to prolonged administration of corticosteroids. Osteoporosis also occurs in Cushing's syndrome. In patients treated with corticosteroids there is not a close association between corticosteroid dose and osteoporosis, although the duration of treatment and reduction in bone mass are significantly related. However, there is wide individual variation, and in some subjects vertebral collapse may occur within a month or so of starting corticosteroid therapy.

The main effect of excess corticosteroids on the skeleton is to reduce osteoblast activity and bone formation. This appears to be direct; indirect suppression of bone formation also results from the inhibitory action of corticosteroids on the pituitary, affecting the production of oestrogen and testosterone. Early in corticosteroid treatment there is also an increase in osteoclast resorption secondary to intestinal malabsorption of calcium and hypercalciuria.

In children excess glucorticoids delay growth. Osteoporosis particularly affects the vertebrae and, in contrast to other forms, the skull. There is also excessive callus formation around fractures. Such fractures may occur in the same regions as Looser's zones (pubic rami, ribs), and be relatively painless. Another skeletal feature of excess corticosteroids is necrosis of the femoral heads.

THE PITUITARY AND OSTEOPOROSIS

Hypopituitarism in childhood produces infantilism. The epiphyses fuse very late and the rarefied bones tend to collapse in adult life. Acromegaly, due to excessive growth hormone secretion after growth has ceased, is often said to be a cause of osteoporosis because of the radiographic appearance of the skeleton, but there is little other evidence of this. Reactivation of endochondral growth at certain cartilage–bone junctions, and stimulation of periosteal bone formation, increases the size of the bones, particularly the vertebrae. An increase in plasma phosphate and urine calcium occurs; when the plasma calcium is increased this may be part of a multiple endocrine adenoma syndrome (Chapter 12.10).

HYPOGONADISM

Bilateral oophorectomy in young women is a well-recognized cause of severe osteoporosis. There is also some evidence that in a significant proportion of women oestrogen deficiency follows a year or so after hysterectomy, despite leaving the ovaries in situ.

Bone mass is similarly reduced in young women with anorexia nervosa, and in others in whom illness results in temporary amenorrhoea.

In men, hypogonadism is a potentially reversible cause of osteoporosis and should always be considered in a young patient. Clues are provided by the relatively long extremities, low hair line, smooth skin, high-pitched voice, and absence of secondary sexual characteristics. There may also be a past history of surgical attempts to correct cryptorchidism. Treatment with testosterone derivatives is important.

Osteoporosis and chromosomal abnormalities

The most common chromosomal cause of osteoporosis is probably Turner's syndrome, the chromosomal XO anomaly. Classically, patients are girls with growth retardation, webbing of the neck, cubitus valgus, cardiac lesions, and lack of sexual development; but many patients with Turner's syndrome may be chromosomal mosaics with no symptoms apart from growth failure and apparently delayed puberty. In Down's syndrome osteopenia is described in childhood which does not persist after adolescence.

Other possible causes of osteoporosis

Osteoporosis may occur in association with alcoholism, liver disease, diabetes, heparin administration, and rheumatoid arthritis. It is said to occur more frequently in cigarette smokers and in thin people. The evidence for these statements varies. There are many reasons why alcoholics should have osteoporosis and some evidence that alcohol has a direct effect on osteoblasts. Recent studies demonstrate that diabetics do not have clinically significant osteoporosis. The relation to heparin administration is of interest since systemic mastocytosis is a rare cause of osteoporosis. In rheumatoid arthritis, osteoporosis may be mainly due to local immobilization, but bone resorbing cytokines are also important. Osteoporosis in osteogenesis imperfecta, homocystinuria, and scurvy are dealt with separately.

REFERENCES

Cooper, C. and Melton, L.J. (1992). Epidemiology of osteoporosis. *Trends in Endocrinology and Metabolism* **3**, 224–9.

Dempster, D.W. and Lindsay, R. (1993). Pathogenesis of osteoporosis. *Lancet* **341**, 797–801.

Grady, D., *et al.* (1992). Hormone therapy to prevent disease and prolong life in postmenopausal women. *Annals of Internal Medicine* **117**, 1017–37.

Lindsay, R. (1993). Prevention and treatment of osteoporosis. *Lancet* **341**, 801–5.

Riggs, B.L. and Melton, L.J. (1988). *Osteoporosis, etiology, diagnosis and management.* Raven Press, New York.

Smith, R. (1993). Osteoporosis: advances and controversies. In *Horizons in Medicine 4,* (ed. C.A. Seymour and A.M. Heagerty), pp. 263–71. McGraw-Hill, New York.

Smith, R., Stevenson, J.C., Winearls, C.G., Woods, C.G., and Wordsworth, B.P. (1985). Osteoporosis of pregnancy. *Lancet* **i**, 1178–80.

Osteomalacia and rickets

Osteomalacia is the condition that results from a lack of vitamin D or a disturbance of its metabolism; in the growing skeleton it is referred to as rickets, and the terms are often used interchangeably. Very rarely, severe calcium deficiency can lead to rickets. Inherited hypophosphataemia and a number of other renal tubular disorders may also cause rickets without clear evidence of abnormal vitamin D metabolism.

The main histological feature of osteomalacia is defective mineralization of bone matrix (Fig. 9). Our present understanding of osteomalacia relies on advances in knowledge of vitamin D metabolism (Fig. 10). For clinical purposes two aspects of the physiology of vitamin D require emphasis. The first is the quantitative importance of vitamin D synthesis in the skin in comparison with that in the diet, and the second concerns the relative role of different vitamin D metabolites. The measurement of circulating concentrations of 25-hydroxy vitamin D (25(OH)D) as an index of vitamin D status has identified those groups (Asian immigrants and the elderly) most at risk from vitamin D deficiency; importantly it has also shown the large amounts of vitamin D

which can be synthesized in the human skin when exposed to ultraviolet light. The causes of osteomalacia can now be partly understood in terms of its metabolites, and the major importance of $1,25(OH)_2D$ (1,25-dihydroxy vitamin D) is established. However, the effects of giving vitamin D cannot be ascribed to the actions of $1,25(OH)_2D$ alone, and probably include other biologically active derivatives, such as 25-hydroxy vitamin D (25(OH)D) and possibly 24,25-dihydroxy vitamin D $(24,25(OH)_2D)$.

PATHOPHYSIOLOGY

The features of osteomalacia can be predicted largely from the known calciotropic effects of vitamin D. Examination of undecalcified bone shows wide osteoid seams with many birefringent lamellae of collagen (Fig. 9) covering more of the bone surface than normal, and absence of the 'calcification front'. The absence of this front is important since excessive osteoid may also be found in conditions other than osteoma-

Fig. 9 Bone from a patient with osteomalacia. The birefringent osteoid is abnormally thick (up to 12 lamellae, arrows) and covers all bone surfaces. The bone preparation is undecalcified and viewed under polarized light (stain von Kossa; magnification ×300).

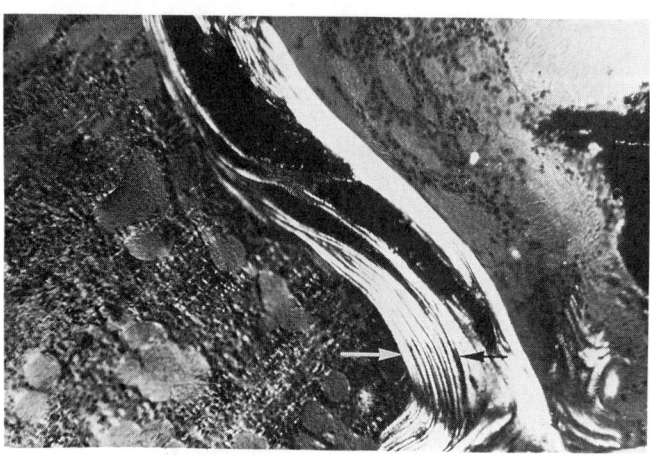

Fig. 10 The causes of rickets and osteomalacia related to the sources and metabolism of vitamin D (from *Oxford textbook of rheumatology,* with permission).

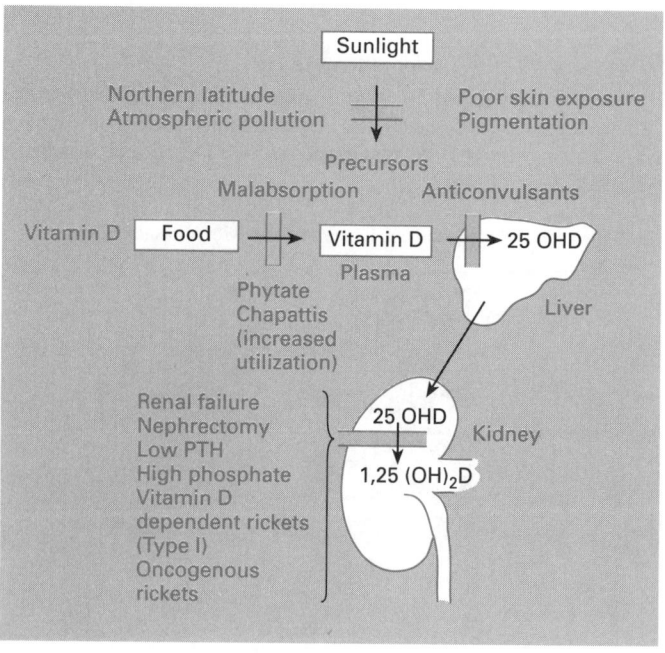

lacia, such as hypophosphatasia, Paget's disease of bone, and thyrotoxicosis, where the calcification front is normal; in these disorders the increase tends to be in the amount of bone surface covered rather than in the thickness of osteoid. Excess osteoid also occurs when bisphosphonates, such as etidronate, or aluminium accumulate in the skeleton. In rickets the main change is disorganization of the growth plate.

Since there is intestinal malabsorption of calcium in vitamin D deficiency, both the plasma and urine calcium are lower than normal; absorption of phosphorus is also defective, with resultant hypophosphataemia. Since hypocalcaemia stimulates the secretion of parathyroid hormone, this will correct the low plasma calcium and exaggerate hypophosphataemia. In osteomalacia, osteoblastic activity is increased and the plasma alkaline phosphatase is therefore also increased. There appears to be no difficulty in laying down bone matrix collagen, but it cannot be properly mineralized. One should recall that the effects of vitamin D are not confined to the skeleton, although they are clinically most obvious in this tissue; thus vitamin D has important effects on cellular differentiation and on the immune system.

CAUSES

There are many causes of osteomalacia (and rickets), some of which are very rare. They may conveniently be divided into three main groups: nutritional, malabsorptive, and renal (Table 8). Most can be understood in terms of vitamin D metabolism (Fig. 10). In the elderly and immigrant the intake of vitamin D in the food is often deficient and the requirements may be increased; the absorption of vitamin D is poor in coeliac disease, after partial gastrectomy, intestinal resection or bypass, and in biliary disease. The intestinal absorption of calcium is reduced by phytate and chapattis which may also increase vitamin D requirements (see below). Endogenous synthesis of vitamin D in the skin is poor in towns and northern cities, and is reduced by pigmentation of the skin. The 25-hydroxylation of calciferol may be impaired in some chronic liver diseases, and anticonvulsants may induce hepatic enzymes which degrade vitamin D. The 1α-hydroxylation of 25(OH)D is reduced or absent in renal failure, after nephrectomy, in hyperphosphataemia, parathyroid insufficiency, in type I vitamin D-dependent rickets and probably in some bone tumours. Many patients have more than one cause for their osteomalacia; in the elderly person vitamin D intake is poor, exposure to sunlight is limited, and renal glomerular failure progressive. Reduced exposure to sunlight is a frequent consequence of physical immobility and may contribute to osteomalacia in rheumatoid arthritis.

The effects of renal glomerular failure on the skeleton are complex (Chapter 20.18). Two main events occur: one is an increase in plasma phosphate which leads to a fall in plasma calcium and to secondary hyperparathyroidism with excessive bone resorption; the other is reduced formation of 1,25(OH)$_2$D with defective intestinal absorption of calcium and defective mineralization of bone. The combination of these events rapidly produces severe deformity, especially in the growing skeleton. In patients on dialysis they are sometimes complicated by aluminium intoxication (see Chapter 20.18).

CLINICAL FEATURES

The main symptoms of osteomalacia are bone pain and tenderness, skeletal deformity, and proximal muscle weakness, often accompanied by the features of the underlying disorder and by those of hypocalcaemia. In severe osteomalacia all the bones are painful and tender, often sufficiently so to disturb sleep. The tenderness can be particularly marked in the lower ribs and may also be accentuated over Looser's zones. Deformity is most often seen in rickets when the effects of vitamin D deficiency are superimposed on a growing skeleton. The linear growth rate is reduced, there is bowing of the long bones, enlargement of the costochondral junctions (rickety rosary), and bossing of the frontal and parietal bones. Later osteomalacia may produce a triradiate pelvis, a gross kyphosis, and corresponding deformities of the chest.

Table 8 *The main causes of rickets and osteomalacia*

Lack of vitamin D
  Deficient synthesis in the skin
  Low intake in the diet
  Probably increased requirement
Malabsorption
  Gluten-sensitive enteropathy (coeliac disease)
  Gastric surgery
  Bowel resection
  Intestinal bypass surgery
  Biliary cirrhosis
Renal disease
  Renal-tubular disorders
    inherited hypophosphataemia (vitamin D-resistant rickets)
    others[a]
  Renal glomerular failure
    renal osteodystrophy
    dialysis bone disease
Others
  Anticonvulsant osteomalacia
  Tumour rickets
  Vitamin D-dependent rickets
  Phosphate-deficiency rickets

[a]See Table 9.

Proximal muscle weakness is an important symptom. Its cause is unknown (although cultured myoblasts respond to 1,25(OH)$_2$D) and it is more marked in some forms of osteomalacia than in others. Most commonly there is a waddling gait, a difficulty in getting up and down stairs, out of low chairs, and in and out of small cars. In the elderly, weakness may make walking impossible and suggest paraplegia. In younger subjects muscular dystrophy may be simulated.

Features of the underlying disorder include anaemia; tiredness and steatorrhoea in coeliac disease; pigmentation, thirst, and nocturia in renal failure. Occasionally hypocalcaemia may cause spontaneous tetany; in children the manifestations of carpopedal spasm, stridor, and fits are more dramatic than in the adult.

Examination of the patient with osteomalacia or rickets confirms the main symptoms. Measurement of the body proportions is useful. Thus patients with inherited hypophosphataemia and rickets have relatively short limbs, whereas those with late-onset osteomalacia will have a relatively short trunk. It is important to look for clues of the cause of the osteomalacia, particularly the scars of previous gastric or intestinal surgery.

BIOCHEMISTRY

Since there are many causes of osteomalacia, the detailed biochemical changes differ from one to another. In vitamin D deficiency or malabsorption there is a low plasma calcium and phosphate, a low urine calcium, and an increase in the plasma alkaline phosphatase level. However, these may vary with the stage of the disease. Initially hypocalcaemia may be the only abnormality. Later, with secondary hyperparathyroidism, the plasma calcium returns towards normal, the plasma phosphate falls, and the alkaline phosphatase increases. In inherited hypophosphataemia (vitamin D-resistant rickets) plasma phosphate is low, but the plasma calcium is normal and the alkaline phosphatase may also be normal. Renal glomerular failure causes an increase in the plasma phosphate, urea, and creatinine, and hypocalcaemia, and in the rare renal tubular syndromes there may be a marked systemic acidosis. In patients with osteomalacia the urine should always be examined for the presence of glucose and protein. If these are present, it is important to check for the aminoaciduria characteristic of renal tubular disorders.

The measurement of vitamin D metabolites is not routine, but a low plasma 25(OH)D is a good indication of vitamin D deficiency. The more complicated estimation of plasma 1,25(OH)$_2$D is important to elucidate the very rare causes of rickets, and particularly to distinguish between type I (low 1,25(OH)$_2$D) and type II (high 1,25(OH)$_2$D) vitamin D-dependent rickets.

RADIOLOGY

The radiological appearances differ according to whether growth has ceased or not. In rickets the main abnormalities are at the ends of the long bones, where the width of the growth plate is increased, and the metaphysis is widened, cupped, and ragged (Fig. 11). Osteomalacia may show the deformities previously described, but the radiological hallmark of active osteomalacia is the Looser's zone (Fig. 12). This is a ribbon-like area of defective mineralization, which may be found in almost any bone but is seen particularly in the long bones, the pelvis, and the ribs, and also around the scapulae. Looser's zones may be bilateral and symmetrical; in bones such as the femur they occur on the medial border of the shaft or neck and are usually single, in contrast to the multiple fissure fractures on the lateral convexity of the bone in Paget's disease. In osteomalacia the vertebral bodies are often uniformly biconcave, to pro-

Fig. 11 The radiological appearance of rickets in a child with inherited hypophosphataemia. The growth plates are widened and the metaphyses cupped and ragged.

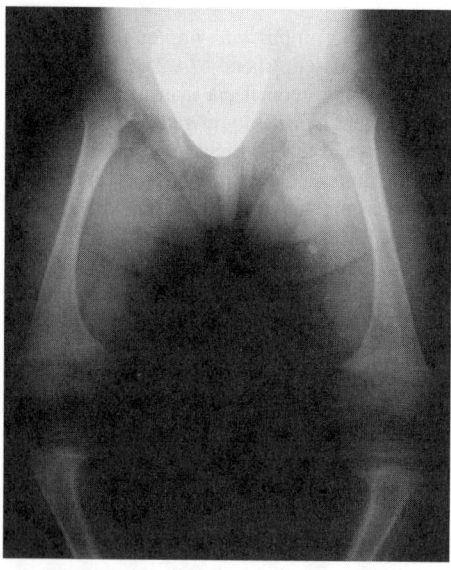

Fig. 12 To demonstrate the bilateral Looser's zones on the medial border of the femora in a woman with osteomalacia due to adult Fanconi's syndrome.

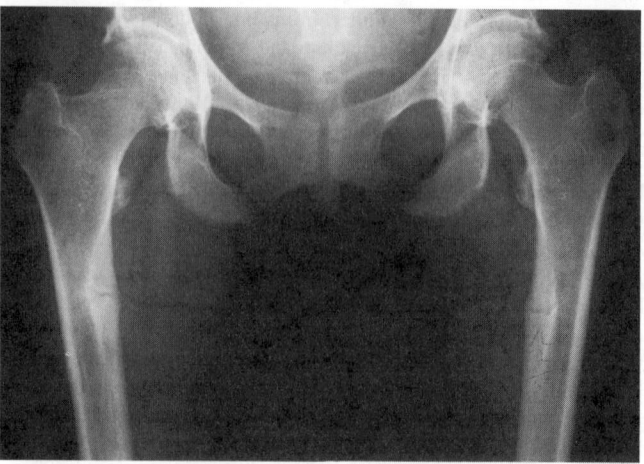

duce an appearance likened to a fish spine. Additionally, in renal glomerular osteodystrophy, the end plates may become relatively more dense than the rest of the vertebral body, to produce the so-called 'rugger jersey' spine. In the adult with inherited hypophosphataemia the bones may also become deformed, buttressed, and dense; in this disorder calcification of the tendons and ligaments at their insertions (enthesiopathy) and of the vertebral ligaments can produce an appearance similar to that of ankylosing spondylitis. Ossification of the ligamenta flava narrows the spinal canal and compresses the spinal cord and its roots. This is well shown on CT scans. In patients with osteomalacia and hypocalcaemia the radiological features of secondary hyperparathyroidism appear with subperiosteal bone resorption which affects the phalanges, the pubic symphysis, and the outer ends of the clavicles. In rickets, periostitis of the distal ends of the long bones, such as the radius and ulna, often occur.

The most extreme effects of parathyroid overactivity are seen in the skeleton of the child with renal osteodystrophy, where the region of the growth plate and metaphyses may fracture (an appearance likened to a 'rotting stump'). An isotope scan may be very useful in osteomalacia, demonstrating multiple pathological fractures often not seen on the plain films. The appearance is similar to that of bony metastases.

BONE BIOPSY

The diagnosis of osteomalacia is often clear without examining the bone. Where doubt exists, a transiliac biopsy examined before and after decalcification will demonstrate the failure of mineralization and the wide osteoid seams. It is important to take all surgical opportunities to examine bone, particularly during operations on fractured femurs in the elderly.

OTHER INVESTIGATIONS

Further investigation is not usually needed to diagnose osteomalacia, but may be necessary to identify its cause. Thus patients with vitamin D-deficient rickets and osteomalacia will have a low plasma 25(OH)D, but not all subjects with such low levels have osteomalacia. In the very rare condition of vitamin D-dependent rickets, measurement of circulating 1,25(OH)$_2$D will be necessary to sort out absence of the 1α-hydroxylase from resistance to 1,25(OH)$_2$D. Further, CT scanning may help to identify the presence of a mesenchymal tumour causing hypophosphataemic osteomalacia.

DIAGNOSIS

Osteomalacia is not difficult to diagnose once it is thought of. It should be distinguished from other forms of metabolic bone disease (Table 4), from other causes of proximal muscle weakness, and from other disorders causing bone pain. In patients with proximal muscle weakness, polymyalgia rheumatica, thyrotoxic myopathy, muscular dystrophy, neoplastic neuropathy, dermatomyositis, and polymyositis all need to be considered. Multiple myeloma and leukaemia may need to be excluded as causes of pain. Provided that the plasma calcium, phosphorus, and alkaline phosphatase are always measured in patients with these symptoms, those with osteomalacia should be easily identified. Patients with psychological illness may have an abnormal gait and complain of pain and weakness in their limbs, but in such patients the biochemistry will be normal. In practice, symptoms of pain and stiffness often first lead the patient with osteomalacia to a rheumatologist.

TREATMENT

Rickets and osteomalacia should respond rapidly to vitamin D (or to its metabolites) in an appropriate dose, which is a useful way confirming the diagnosis. Increased mobility with increase in muscle strength may be the first clinical response, despite a temporary increase in bone pain.

Biochemically, plasma phosphate and urine hydroxyproline are the first to increase. The alkaline phosphatase level may show a temporary rise and then falls slowly to normal levels. As the plasma calcium and 25(OH)D concentrations increase towards normal, the parathyroid hormone concentration falls.

The effective dose and preparation of vitamin D depends on the cause of the osteomalacia. That due to vitamin D deficiency will respond to microgram doses, but it is often useful to give considerably more than this, such as calciferol 1.25 mg daily for 1 to 2 weeks only. Where there is doubt about compliance, vitamin D may be injected intramuscularly in one large dose (up to 15 mg = 600 000 units). Lack of response to microgram doses suggest that the osteomalacia is not due to simple vitamin D deficiency but, for instance, to malabsorption or renal failure. It is particularly in the last group that the 1α-hydroxylated metabolites of vitamin D are effective (see Chapter 20.18). Clearly, underlying disorders must be treated at the same time. For example patients with coeliac disease will need a gluten-free diet.

Particular forms of osteomalacia and rickets

Nutritional osteomalacia

In the United Kingdom so-called nutritional osteomalacia occurs particularly amongst the elderly and in Asian immigrants of all ages. In the elderly the high incidence of osteomalacia is mainly due to poor exposure to sunlight and to a low intake of vitamin D; and may be contributed to by the effects of drugs such as anticonvulsants and by increasing renal glomerular failure. Since the elderly are often housebound, they may develop osteomalacia despite a sunny climate. Certainly, the prevalence of osteomalacia in the elderly population is significant. The frequency of osteomalacia in patients with fractures of the femoral neck is also higher than previously suspected, but figures of up to 30 per cent, which continue to be reported (according to the histological definitions used), are probably overestimates. Osteomalacia should always be excluded in elderly people with bone disease, and particularly in those with femoral neck fractures. Where possible this should be done by histological examination of bone taken at operation or by biopsy. When this is not appropriate, a therapeutic trial with vitamin D is often useful. Since it is often difficult to define osteomalacia accurately in elderly people it is important to consider the use of such empirical treatment. In the geriatric population the mean concentration of 25(OH)D is much lower than in non-elderly patients; it shows the usual seasonal variation, with lowest values in the winter and early spring and highest in late summer.

Asian immigrants to the United Kingdom develop osteomalacia and rickets more often than the indigenous population. There are probably several reasons for this. They tend to live in northern cities away from sunlight and, especially in women, do not expose their skin to the limited ultraviolet light. Where dermal synthesis of vitamin D is limited, dietary factors become more important, and it is particularly those on a meat-free diet containing chapattis who develop osteomalacia. The role of chapattis and the phytate they contain is not yet fully understood. Phytates bind to calcium, preventing its absorption, and it can be shown, at least experimentally, that reduced calcium absorption increases vitamin D requirement by increasing its parathyroid-mediated breakdown. It has been suggested that such a mechanism of reduced calcium absorption may also contribute to the osteomalacia of malabsorptive syndromes, such as that following partial gastrectomy.

Pigmentation of the skin can be shown experimentally to reduce vitamin D synthesis by a standardized dose of ultraviolet light, but in practice this is of little significance. Since those of Afro-Caribbean descent have a lower incidence of rickets than Asians in the same environment, it is clear that factors other than skin colour are important.

As in the elderly, 25(OH)D levels can be very low in Asian immigrants. They increase in the summertime, when there may be sponta-

Table 9 *Renal tubular disorders, rickets, and osteomalacia*

Inherited hypophosphataemia
Adult-onset hypophosphataemic osteomalacia
Renal tubular acidosis
Inherited
Proximal (bicarbonate wastage)
Distal (H$^+$ gradient defect)
Acquired
Ureterocolic anastomosis
Multiple renal tubular defects (Fanconi's syndrome)
Inherited
Cystinosis
Oculocerebrorenal syndrome (Lowe's syndrome)
Wilson's disease
Galactosaemia
Acquired
Cadmium poisoning
Multiple myeloma
Ifosfamide toxicity

neous healing of rickets. Important work in Glasgow has shown that Asian rickets can be prevented by fortifying food such as chapatti flour with vitamin D, although the incidence of osteomalacia in Asian adults remains unaffected. Other Western lifestyle changes will also influence the diet of children.

Osteomalacia and malabsorption

Coeliac disease (gluten-sensitive enteropathy) is a relatively common cause of osteomalacia. It should be suspected at any age and confirmed by a small intestinal biopsy showing an atrophic mucosa. Other causes of malabsorption vary in their frequency according to surgical practice. Thus it is well established that osteomalacia follows classic partial gastrectomy, but the actual incidence is debated and its cause is probably multifactorial. Post-gastrectomy subjects tend to take little vitamin D in their diet and there is defective calcium absorption. Available evidence suggests that clinical osteomalacia is rare after vagotomy and pyloroplasty. Osteomalacia can also follow removal of long segments of small intestine for conditions such as Crohn's disease, and complicates some intestinal bypass operations used for extreme obesity.

Osteomalacia and liver disease

In liver disease osteomalacia is uncommon; in theory it may be due to a number of factors such as malabsorption of vitamin D and its defective 25 hydroxylation. Most research has concerned the osteomalacia of biliary cirrhosis, and osteomalacia in chronic liver disease appears to be a complication related to prolonged cholestasis.

Osteomalacia and renal disease

It is important to distinguish the osteomalacia and rickets of renal glomerular failure from that attributable to renal tubular disorders. Bone disease in renal glomerular failure (renal osteodystrophy) is dealt with elsewhere (see Chapter 20.18); this includes bone disease in the dialysed patient and the effects of aluminium. Renal glomerular osteodystyrophy is a complex disease with excessive bone resorption, defective bone mineralization, and in some cases osteoporosis. Previously it was treated with large doses of native vitamin D; current therapy now includes 1α-hydroxycholecalciferol or 1,25(OH)$_2$D.

Many renal tubular disorders lead to osteomalacia (Chapter 20.19) (Table 9). Of these, the most common is inherited hypophosphataemia, so-called vitamin D-resistant rickets, which is normally inherited as an X-linked dominant characteristic, and in which the main abnormality is hypophosphataemia due to a reduction in the maximum renal tubular reabsorption rate of phosphate. Some patients in a family will have hypophosphataemia alone, whereas others will have hypophosphataemia with accompanying bone disease. The cause of the renal abnormality has not been fully established. It is not due to overactivity of the parathyroids. Measurements of $1,25(OH)_2D$ concentrations show that these are within the normal range; since hypophosphataemia would normally increase 1α-hydroxylation this suggests a reduced sensitivity of the 1α-hydroxylase in inherited hypophosphataemia. Children with hypophosphataemic rickets or osteomalacia are unlike patients with other forms of rickets. They present with deformity but are otherwise well, without muscle weakness; however, growth is defective and eventual height is usually less than 150 cm. Apart from hypophosphataemia there may be no other abnormality in biochemical values routinely available, and the plasma alkaline phosphatase can be normal for age. Radiographs show severe rickets, and later the bones are often dense with buttressing and exostoses. The enthesiopathy with ossification of the ligamenta flava can lead to paraplegia. Ligamentous calcification may also contribute to deafness. Finally, abnormal teeth in this disorder cause periapical translucencies and may lead to abscesses.

Treatment of inherited hypophosphataemia is controversial. For many years its mainstay was large doses of vitamin D; this posed a continuous danger of vitamin D poisoning and did not correct the eventual short stature. When oral phosphate is given in addition to vitamin D, there is an improvement in growth rate, but the condition does not appear to respond to phosphate alone. More recently it has been shown that combined oral phosphate and $1,25(OH)_2D$ produces healing of both epiphyseal and trabecular bone, and this is now the recommended treatment. This combination produces bone healing and increases eventual stature. However, it is still unusual for affected patients to have an eventual height of more than 1.5 m (5 ft). Accounts of the effects of medical treatment on deformity and height differ; the necessity for corrective osteotomy on the lower limbs is less than previously, but discussion with an orthopaedic surgeon is important.

It is also important that the parents should know the genetics of this condition. Because the defect in phosphate transport is inherited as a dominant on the X chromosome, an affected mother transmits the condition to 50 per cent of her children regardless of their gender. All the daughters of an affected father will have the disease, but none of his sons. In general, affected sons have a more severe disease and some affected daughters may be asymptomatic. Diagnosis can be made from birth, but demands accurate knowledge of the normal plasma phosphate at that age. Now that more is known about the exact gene location, prenatal diagnosis may be possible in future. Recently cloned human X-chromosome sequences which reveal restriction fragment length polymorphisms have been used in linkage studies of affected families to map the hypophosphataemic rickets gene. Flanking markers are potentially useful in the identification of mutant gene carriers and in presymptomatic diagnosis, but the distance between these markers and the hypophosphataemic gene is still large, at approximately 10 million base pairs. Hypophosphataemic animal models continue to help in understanding this disorder. A recently described *gy* mutation in, which hypophosphataemia is associated with gyratory activity, has no clear human equivalent. Rare human variants include an autosomal form of hypophosphataemia.

Other renal tubular osteomalacic syndromes include hypophosphataemic osteomalacia presenting in adult life, which may be due to a tumour (see below), inherited and acquired forms of renal tubular acidosis, and rickets associated with multiple renal tubular defects and generalized aminoaciduria (Fanconi's syndrome; see also Chapter 20.19). Renal tubular acidosis may be proximal or distal, with inability to reabsorb bicarbonate or to acidify the urine. The osteomalacia may be cured by giving bicarbonate alone or with vitamin D. A persistent acidosis with resultant osteomalacia may also result from ureterosigmoid anastomosis. The commonest cause of Fanconi's syndrome in childhood is nephropathic cystinosis or cystine-storage disease (see

Chapter 20.19), where there is a widespread deposition of cystine crystals throughout the tissues, and in which thirst, polyuria, dehydration, photophobia, and loss of weight begin at about the age of 1 year. The rickets will heal with the correction of the acidosis, and the administration of phosphate and 1α-(OH)D; renal transplantation corrects the renal failure and prolongs survival, but does not prevent non-renal complications.

Other rare causes of renal tubular rickets and osteomalacia with generalized aminoaciduria are inherited, such as Wilson's disease and the X-linked oculocerebral renal syndrome, or acquired, such as multiple myeloma, cadmium poisoning, and the toxic effects of ifosfamide, used in the treatment of childhood malignant disease.

Anticonvulsant osteomalacia

In patients treated with anticonvulsants the incidence of rickets and osteomalacia is higher than normal. This has been attributed to the induction by the anticonvulsants of hepatic enzymes which metabolize vitamin D to biologically inactive derivatives. However, epileptic patients in institutions are often deficient of vitamin D because they are deprived of sunlight, and osteomalacia in such patients probably has several causes.

Tumour rickets

An interesting but rare form of hypophosphataemic rickets or osteomalacia occurs in patients who have mesenchymal tumours, often of a particular pathological type, namely sclerosing haemangiopericytomata or non-ossifying fibromas. In any adult who develops hypophosphataemic osteomalacia, particularly with prominent myopathy, a tumour should be considered. The disorder is improved by oral phosphate and cured by removal of the tumour. The way in which the tumour induces hypophosphataemia and subsequent osteomalacia is unknown, but current evidence suggests that it interferes with renal 1α-hydroxylation of $25(OH)D$, since the circulating levels of $1,25(OH)_2D$ are abnormally low and rapidly return to normal when the tumour is removed. Rarely, hypophosphataemic osteomalacia may become apparent in adults with neurofibromatosis and polyostotic fibrous dysplasia.

Osteogenic osteomalacia has also been described in prostatic and oat-cell carcinoma.

Vitamin D-dependent rickets

Patients with these rare, recessively inherited forms of rickets show the features of severe rickets without vitamin D deficiency. There are at least two types of vitamin D-dependent rickets. In type I the activity of the renal 1α-hydroxylase is reduced so that the concentration of $1,25(OH)_2D$ is abnormally low. However, it can be increased by large doses of the native vitamin, which shows that the enzyme block is not complete; in type II there is an end-organ resistance to $1,25(OH)_2D$, which is present in high concentrations. In both forms there is severe rickets and myopathy from infancy; in type II, lifelong total alopecia is a striking feature. Vitamin D-dependent rickets type I responds to very large doses of vitamin D or physiological doses of $1,25(OH)_2D$; type II may also respond to large doses of vitamin D or its metabolites, or to prolonged intravenous calcium, but some recorded cases suggest that recovery occurs spontaneously with age.

Recent work on type II vitamin D-dependent rickets (otherwise known as hereditary $1,25(OH)_2D$ resistant) shows that the $1,25(OH)_2D$ receptor defects which are responsible for the end-organ resistance in this disease are due to a variety of point mutations in the gene for the 1,25 receptor, either at its steroid- or DNA-binding domains.

Phosphate deficiency rickets

If patients take a large amount of phosphate-binding drugs, such as aluminium hydroxide, a form of hypophosphataemic osteomalacia may develop. This differs clinically from inherited hypophosphataemic osteomalacia by the presence of severe muscle weakness. Other biochemical features include increased calcium absorption with hypercalcuria, associated with an increase above normal in the concentration of $1,25(OH)_2D$.

REFERENCES

Balsan, S., et al. (1986). Long term nocturnal calcium infusions can cure rickets and promote normal mineralisation in hereditary resistance to 1,25 dihydroxy vitamin D. Journal of Clinical Investigation 77, 1661–7.

Eisman, J.A. (1988). Osteomalacia. Baillière's Clinical Endocrinology and Metabolism 2, 125–55.

Parfitt, A.M. (1990). Osteomalacia and related disorders. In Metabolic bone disease, (ed. L.V. Avioli and S.M. Krane), (2nd edn), pp. 329–96. W.B. Saunders, Philadelphia.

Petersen, D.J., Boniface, A.M., and Schranck, F.W. (1992). X-linked hypophosphataemic rickets: a study of linear growth response to calcitriol and phosphate therapy. Journal of Bone and Mineral Research 7, 583–97.

Smith, R. (1990). Asian rickets and osteomalacia. Quarterly Journal of Medicine 76, 899–901.

Stanbury, S.W., and Mawer, E.B. (1990). Metabolic disturbances in acquired osteomalacia. In The metabolic basis of acquired disease, (ed. R.D. Cohen, B., Lewis, K.G.M.M. Alberti, and A.M. Denman,), pp. 1717–82. Ballière Tindall, London.

Thakker, R.V. and O'Riordan, J.L.H. (1988). Inherited forms of rickets and osteomalacia. Baillière's Clinical Endocrinology and Metabolism 2, 157–91.

Weidner, N. (1991). Oncogenic osteomalacia-rickets. Ultrastructural Pathology 15, 317–33.

Paget's disease of bone

Paget's disease of bone, osteitis deformans, was first described a century ago, but existed for many years before. Next to osteoporosis it is the most common of the so-called metabolic bone diseases. Its hallmark is excessive and disorganized resorption and formation of bone. Its cause is unknown, but recent studies on pagetic bone cells, particularly osteoclasts, have provided clues. The new generation of bisphosphonates now provide effective treatment.

PATHOPHYSIOLOGY

The natural history of Paget's disease is similar to that of a multicentric neoplasm or a slow virus disease which begins in young adult life. Electron microscopy shows virus-like inclusion bodies in the osteoclasts of patients with Paget's disease. Immunofluorescence studies suggest that these could represent the measles or respiratory syncytial virus. Another candidate is the canine distemper virus. The results of polymerase chain reaction amplification of reverse transcribed DNA from Paget's tissue to identify the putative virus are controversial.

Histology shows multinucleate osteoclasts which appear to be resorbing bone, and busy osteoblasts which appear to be replacing it; these activities are closely linked. There is also excess fibrosis in the marrow. The bone matrix is laid down in all directions and partially loses its birefringence and strength. Mineralization may be defective, probably because of the excessive rate at which the organic bone matrix is laid down. The cement lines and the mosaic appearances of the bone result from the tidemarks of resorption followed by formation. Osteosarcoma which occurs in Paget's disease is presumably the result of the excessive and prolonged activity of the bone cells. Pagetic bone is large, vascular, and deformed. Its physical characteristics depend on the stage of the disorder, and it may be hard or soft. In any case, it fractures more readily than normal.

Table 10 *The radiological prevalence of Paget's disease*

	Prevalence (%) of Paget's disease	
	Men	Women
Preston	8.6	6.3
Bolton	7.7	6.4
Blackburn	8.8	3.8
Bradford	7.9	3.6
Hull	7.6	3.1
Southampton	6.6	3.6
Bath	5.3	4.7
Stoke	4.7	4.2
York	5.8	2.5

These data are based on more than 500 patients in each town. The age standardized incidence is always higher in men than in women. The high incidence in Lancashire towns is not explained. Modified from Barker et al. (1977).

INCIDENCE

Paget's disease occurs in about 3 to 4 per cent of subjects over 40, is more common in men, and in women its frequency increases with age. It is not unknown in younger people. In Britain about 750 000 people may have Paget's disease, of whom fewer than 5 per cent have symptoms. It seems to be an Anglo-Saxon affliction, being very rare in countries such as Scandinavia and Japan. Within England early radiological surveys showed that it occurs most often in Lancashire towns and in northern industrial regions (Table 10). It is also more frequent in recent British immigrants to Western Australia than in the Western Australian population, but less frequent than in those relatives who remained in Britain. Such studies do not distinguish between the effect of environment and heredity. In a disorder as common as Paget's disease many striking examples of 'familial' Paget's disease occur by chance.

CLINICAL FEATURES
Pain, deformity, fracture

In Paget's disease the bone itself may be painful, or pain may be due to arthritis of a nearby joint, to an associated fracture, or to the development of sarcoma. It has been suggested that there is a specific type of hip joint disorder associated with Paget's disease. Bone pain could be due to stretching of the periosteum, since this part of the bone (and the vessels within bone) contain nerves sensitive to pain. Clinically, the affected bones are enlarged, deformed, and warm. The enlargement is well seen in bones such as the tibia and the skull; in the former the bone is typically bowed forwards; the latter shows a characteristic enlargement of the vault which is said to look like a soft beret, or 'tam-o'-shanter', which appears to descend over the ears. Other long bones may become bent and a kyphosis may develop. Although any of the bones can be affected, including the maxilla and the phalanges, the most common sites for Paget's disease are the pelvis and the spine. Fracture may be the first symptom of undiagnosed Paget's disease, for instance at the junction of a resorbing front with normal bone (Fig. 13), or across a fissure fracture (see Fig. 14).

Deafness and nerve compression

Deafness in Paget's disease is one of its most disabling symptoms and responds little to treatment. It has many causes, of which nerve compression is only one.

Most nerves can be compressed by enlarging pagetic bone. The spinal cord is particularly at risk, due to the combined effects of increased bone mass, vertebral collapse, and excessive vascularity. Paraplegia or cauda equina lesions may occur. Alterations in the shape of the skull may produce multiple cranial nerve palsies and brain-stem lesions, with dysphagia, dysarthria, and ataxia. Basilar invagination with obstruction of cerebrospinal fluid drainage can lead to internal hydrocephalus, raised intracranial pressure, and confusion.

Heart failure

In severe Paget's disease cardiac output is considerably increased, due to the excessive vascularity of the affected bones, but there is no convincing evidence of large arteriovenous shunts within the skeleton. The heart failure which results may be of the high-output variety, but this is rare. Since heart failure and Paget's disease of bone are common in the elderly, their occurrence together is usually coincidental.

Sarcoma

In the past the incidence of sarcoma in Paget's disease has sometimes been overestimated; it probably occurs in 1 per cent or less of those with symptoms. Paget's sarcoma often occurs in the humerus, although Paget's disease itself is most common in the pelvis and spine. Sarcoma should be considered in a patient known to have Paget's disease if pain has developed for the first time, or worsened, or if deformity has altered. Radiologically, the appearance of the pagetic bone alters, with evidence of bone destruction (Fig. 15); the tumours occur most often in the medulla. A recent review of 85 bone sarcomas associated with Paget's disease confirmed the humerus as a high-risk site. Rapidly worsening pain was the main symptom; lytic lesions were more common than sclerotic; periosteal reaction was uncommon; and radionuclide diphosphonate scans often showed areas of decreased uptake (contrasting with the underlying pagetic bone).

Fig. 13 A fracture in the region of a resorbing front in a pagetic bone (arrowed). Proximal to the area of bone resorption the cortex is thickened and the bone widened by disorganized formation of new bone.

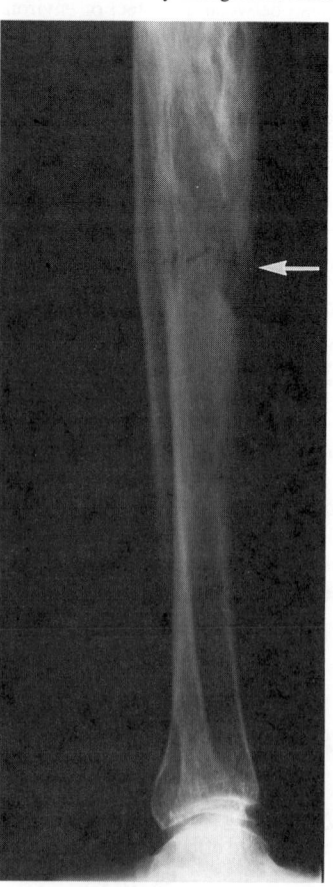

Associated disorders

Paget's disease is said to be associated with other disorders such as osteoarthritis, gout, vascular calcification, and articular chondrocalcinosis. Since all these occur more often in the elderly the associations have little significance.

BIOCHEMISTRY

There is a marked increase in the level of plasma alkaline phosphatase, derived from the overactive osteoblasts, which is roughly related to the extent of clinical and radiological involvement with Paget's disease. In contrast, the acid phosphatase (derived partly from osteoclasts) is only slightly increased. The rapid turnover of bone matrix collagen increases the urinary hydroxyproline (and hydroxylysine), in proportion to the increase in alkaline phosphatase and also the urinary excretion of cross-linked collagen-derived peptides. The plasma calcium and phosphate are normal; hypercalcaemia suggests coexistent hyperparathyroidism, malignant disease, or immobility.

RADIOLOGY

The radiological appearances of Paget's disease are legion. The most characteristic is an increase in size of the affected bone. Resorption predominates early in the disease and in the young patient. A resorbing front may be seen in a long bone (as a flame-shaped area) (Fig. 13) or in the skull (as 'osteoporosis circumscripta'). Excessive resorption is inevitably followed by disordered formation, and at this stage the bone becomes thick and deformed. In elderly subjects the affected bone may be very osteoporotic and liable to fracture. Multiple partial fractures (microfractures, fissure fractures) are common on the deformed convex surface of long bones (Fig. 14), particularly the femur and tibia.

Fig. 14 Multiple microfractures ('fissure fractures' arrowed) on the convex surface of a pagetic femur.

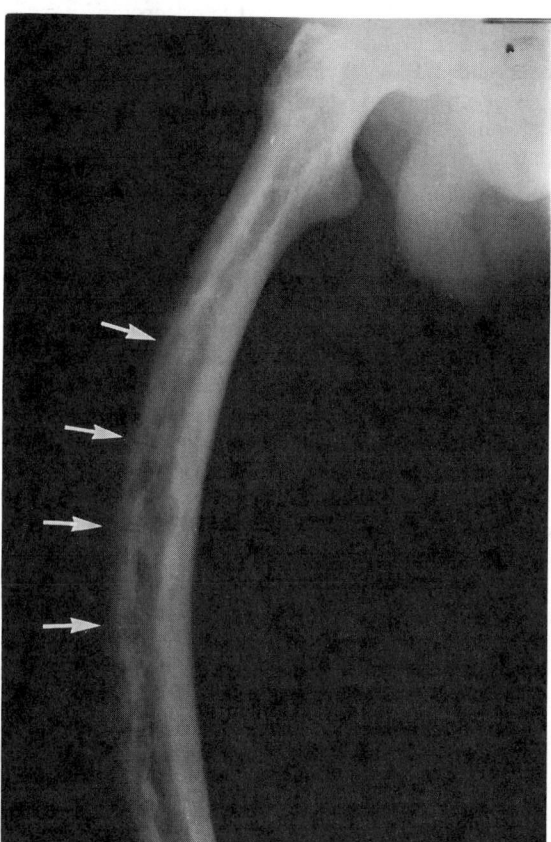

The use of bone-scanning agents (such as $^{99}Tc^m$-labelled disodium etidronate (EHDP) has been particularly informative in Paget's disease. Affected bones take up the isotope avidly, which demonstrates both the extent of the bone lesions and the effects of treatment. In one study, 180 patients with Paget's disease had whole-body scintigraphy and 826 lesions were identified. One-third of the patients had only one lesion, and only 10 patients had no symptoms. The increase in plasma alkaline phosphatase and urinary total hydroxyproline was proportional to scintigraphic involvement, and patients with skull involvement had the highest values. Apart from the number of sites involved, any distinction between monostotic and polyostotic disease appeared to be artificial.

DIAGNOSIS

The diagnosis of Paget's disease is usually obvious. Bone biopsy is useful to exclude other generalized bone diseases, such as osteomalacia, as well as to confirm Paget's disease. Paget's disease may initially be confused with osteomalacia because of the high plasma alkaline phosphatase; rarely an elevated plasma calcium should suggest additional hyperparathyroidism or malignant disease. In prostatic carcinoma with osteoblastic bone secondaries the dense bones are not enlarged (as they are in Paget's disease) and the acid phosphatase is considerably and disproportionately increased in relation to the alkaline phosphatase. Of many other conditions with similar radiological appearance, fibrous dysplasia (see below), in which the alkaline phosphatase may also be slightly increased, may be difficult to distinguish; in the generalised form the unilateral bone lesions, pigmentation, and sexual precocity (in the female) are characteristic. Another rare disorder usually mistaken for Paget's disease is fibrogenesis imperfecta ossium (see below), where the bone trabeculae are thickened without bony enlargement and there are multiple abnormal fractures.

Fig. 15 A sarcoma in the upper end of the left humerus in a man of 70 with Paget's disease. The destructive lesion in the proximal humerus has been treated with radiotherapy; there are secondary deposits around the distal end of the bone.

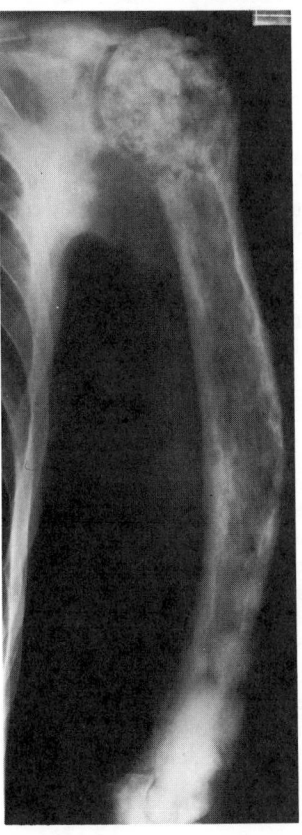

TREATMENT

Many patients with Paget's disease require no treatment, but it may be required for symptoms, to suppress the activity of the disease, and to prevent its further progress. Indications include bone pain, nerve compression, and the suppression of vascularity before elective orthopaedic surgery. Since medical treatment is now so effective these indications may be widened, especially in young people.

Medical treatment

Patients with pain associated with Paget's disease should first be treated with a simple analgesic. Where possible it should be determined whether the pain is directly due to the bone disease or to associated arthritis. In those who have pain due to bone disease despite analgesia, or have the complications of deformity, nerve compression, deafness, or heart failure, specific treatment aimed at the pagetic bone should be considered. This should also be considered in the young person with Paget's disease to prevent further progress. There is no evidence that the rapid course of pagetic sarcoma is altered by any treatment. Of the many agents previously tried in Paget's disease, such as aspirin, fluoride, and corticosteroids, only three are currently in use, mithramycin, phosphonates, and calcitonin. Mithramycin is now rarely used. It is an antimitotic agent given intravenously which is hepatotoxic in high doses. It may rapidly abolish pain in Paget's disease, and rapidly reduce the plasma alkaline phosphatase, but the effect is usually temporary. Mithramycin has been used on its own or in combination with bisphosphonates or calcitonin.

The bisphosphonates (once diphosphonates) are a series of compounds with a P–C–P structure resistant to the naturally occurring phosphonates and pyrophosphatases. They are effective orally or parenterally and reduce excessive bone turnover in Paget's disease. The first bisphosphonate used (and still the only one licensed for Paget's disease), ethane-l-hydroxy-l,l-bisphosphonate (disodium etidronate, EHDP, Didronel®), also interferes with mineralization if given in high doses (20 mg/kg body weight); subsequent derivatives, dichloromethylene diphosphonate (Cl_2 MDP) and 3-amino-hydroxypropylidine-l,l-bisphosphonate (APD, pamidronate) do not appear to do this. According to their dose, the bisphosphonates may take up to 6 months to produce their effect on symptoms, histology, and biochemistry. The recommended dose for EHDP is 5 mg/kg/day for up to 6 months. It also has been used in combination with calcitonin, and together these agents suppress Paget's disease more effectively than when given alone. The biochemical effects of EHDP appear to last for a long time (possibly several years) after the drug is stopped. Recent work shows that both Cl_2 MDP and APD effectively suppress resorption in Paget's disease without disturbing mineralization.

The calcitonins are widely used for the treatment of Paget's disease, and salmon calcitonin is the most effective commercially available form. Various dose regimens are used, for which 100 IU 3 times a week is average. Injected calcitonin may produce nausea and vomiting; if side-effects are troublesome, it is best given in the evening with an antiemetic. Its main effects are in the first 3 months of treatment, and continued treatment is ineffective, especially when the alkaline phosphatase level has ceased to decline.

Antibodies to calcitonin do develop but are not necessarily related to calcitonin 'resistance'. Indications for the bisphosphonates and calcitonins are different. Calcitonin is preferred to treat bone pain, for osteolytic Paget's disease, and for preoperative treatment (below). Some evidence suggests that calcitonin may halt the progression of deafness. Spinal cord compression is also alleviated. Thus treatment of eight patients with paraparesis due to pagetic vertebrae with either calcitonin or bisphosphonate produced marked clinical improvement, at least comparable to the results of surgical decompression.

Finally, calcitonin can also be given preoperatively to reduce excessive bleeding when operations such as total hip replacement have to be done on pagetic bone.

Within the past few years the bisphosphonates have become more

Table 11 *The main causes of hypercalcaemia*

Diagnosis	Features	Comments
Neoplastic disease[a] (usually hydrocortisone sensitive)	Common. With or without secondary deposits. Biochemistry often like hyperparathyroidism	Including tumours of lung, breast, and others. Plasma PTHrP increased; PTH decreased
Multiple myeloma	Bone pain, fractures	High ESR, Bence Jones (light chain) proteinuria
Hyperparathyroidism	Multiple; does not respond to corticosteroids	Plasma whole-molecule PTH increased
Vitamin D overdosage	May give acute hypercalcaemic symptoms; thirst, vomiting, sore eyes	Most often in patients treated with vitamin D
Sarcoidosis (and other granulomata)	Nephrocalcinosis, splenomegaly, hilar lymphadenopathy. Precipitated by sunlight or physiological amounts of vitamin D	May be due to inappropriate formation of $1,25(OH)_2D$
Immobility	Especially in young people or in Paget's disease	
Thyrotoxicosis	Increased bone turnover. Plasma phosphate increased	Alkaline phosphatase and hydroxyproline increased
Milk alkali syndrome	Associated with milk and alkali ingestion for peptic ulceration; more commonly due to 'indigestion' tablets	Very uncommon in acute forms
Thiazide diuretics Hypoadrenalism Acute renal failure		

[a]The relative frequency of neoplastic disease and hyperparathyroidism as a cause for hypercalcaemia varies with the population. In screening of healthy outpatients more than 85 per cent of patients with hypercalcaemia have primary hyperparathyroidism; with symptomatic inpatients neoplastic disease is the most common cause.

widely used than calcitonin, partly because of their more prolonged effectiveness and partly because of their lack of side-effects. However the most widely used second-generation bisphosphonate (APD) must be given intravenously and is restricted to research centres; and calcitonin is more acceptable and effective given by the nasal route.

Surgical treatment

Fractures through pagetic bone require the usual surgical treatment, although union may be delayed. Where fracture occurs through a deformed bone, this deformity should be corrected. In addition, elective osteotomy and intramedullary nailing may be considered for severe long bone deformity. Spinal cord compression not responding to medical treatment requires surgery. Rarely, hydrocephalus may require a ventriculojugular shunt. Whatever form of surgery is undertaken, it is important that the period of immobility is as short as possible, to avoid hypercalciuria and hypercalcaemia.

REFERENCES

Barker, D.J.P., Clough, P.W.L., Guyer, P.B., and Gardner, M.J. (1977). Paget's disease of bone in 14 British towns. *British Medical Journal* **1**, 1181–3.

Basle, M.F., Rebel, A., and Audran, M. (1990). Paget's disease of bone. In *The metabolic basis of acquired disease*, (ed. R.D. Cohen, B. Lewis, K.G.M.M. Alberti, and A.M. Denman), pp. 1783–1802. Ballière Tindall, London.

Douglas, D.L., Duckworth, T., Kanis, J.A., Jefferson, R.A., Martin, T.J., and Russell, R.G.G. (1981). Spinal cord dysfunction in Paget's disease of bone. *Journal of Bone and Joint Surgery* **63B**, 495–503.

Harinck, H.I.J., Bijvoet, O.L.M., Vellanga, C.J.L.R., Blanskma, H.J., Frijlink, W.B., and Tevelde, J. (1986). The relation between signs and symptoms of Paget's disease of bone. *Quarterly Journal of Medicine* **58**, 133–51.

Kahn, A.J. (1990). The viral aetiology of Paget's disease of bone; a new perspective. *Calcified Tissue International* **47**, 127–9.

Kanis, J.A. (1991). *Pathophysiology and treatment of Paget's disease of bone* Martin Dunitz, London.

Smith, J., Botet, J.F., and Yeh, S.D.J. (1984). Bone sarcomas in Paget's disease: a study of 85 patients *Radiology* **152**, 583–90.

Smith, R. (1992). Paget's disease of bone. Advance and controversy. *British Medical Journal* **305**, 1379–80.

Parathyroids and bone disease

Knowledge of the physiology of parathyroid hormone has expanded so rapidly that it now occupies a large and deserved part of any clinical description of parathyroid disorders (see Chapter 12.6). With increasing recognition of the many alternative ways in which parathyroid disorders may present, the close relationship between these endocrine glands and the skeleton becomes less obvious. However, primary hyperparathyroidism was first identified because of its effects on bone, and only later was it realized that it might more often present with renal stones, with pancreatitis, and with the signs and symptoms of hypercalcaemia, or be discovered by multichannel biochemical screening. Pseudohypoparathyroidism also has characteristic skeletal effects.

The subject is discussed further in Chapter 12.6.

Hypercalcaemia

Of the known causes of hypercalcaemia in hospital inpatients, neoplasm is the most important (Table 11). It should always be considered and excluded clinically. The relative frequency of the causes of hypercalcaemia varies according to the population studied. In healthy subjects primary hyperparathyroidism is the most frequent cause. In those patients with primary hyperparathyroidism, with hypercalcaemia, hypophosphataemia, hyperphosphatasia, and radiological evidence of osteitis fibrosa, and without clinical evidence of neoplasm, no further investigation is needed. Since only a few patients with hyperparathyroidism have clinical bone disease, further differentiation from other causes of hypercalcaemia is usually necessary. In practice this means the exclusion of neoplasm, sarcoidosis, thyrotoxicosis, vitamin D overdosage, treatment with thiazide diuretics or the 'milk alkali' syndrome. The subject is addressed further in Chapters 20.9.3 and 20.18.

Familial benign hypercalcaemia

This rare condition is dominantly inherited. Mild hypercalcaemia occurs without hypercalciuria (the alternative name is familial hypocalciuric hypercalcaemia) and is not improved by parathyroid surgery. The PTH level may be normal or slightly increased. Symptoms are few and include mild fatigue, sleepiness, and amnesia, but pancreatitis and chondrocalcinosis occur in heterozygotes.

Multiple endocrine adenoma syndromes (see also Chapter 12.10)

Familial isolated overactivity of the parathyroid is rare, and more often it is associated with overactivity of other endocrine organs. Two particular associated syndromes are recognized. Type 1 multiple endocrine neoplasia (MEN1) syndrome includes hyperparathyroidism, pituitary adenomata, insulin- and gastrin-secreting tumours of the pancreas, and gastric hyperacidity (Zollinger–Ellison syndrome). Type 2 multiple endocrine neoplasia (MEN2) syndrome, also known as Sipple's syndrome, includes hyperparathyroidism, medullary carcinoma of the thyroid, and phaeochromocytoma. It has been proposed that these associations occur because the cells have a common origin from the neural crest, and form part of a general endocrine system. Recently it has been shown that there is allelic loss from chromosome 11.

Secondary (and tertiary) hyperparathyroidism

Where hypocalcaemia is prolonged, as in renal glomerular failure or gluten-sensitive enteropathy, the parathyroid glands increase both their size and activity in an attempt to restore the plasma calcium to normal. This increases bone resorption and is a particular feature of renal glomerular osteodystrophy. Occasionally in such patients hypercalcaemia develops and persists. It has been proposed that one of the hyperplastic parathyroid glands becomes autonomous, and the label 'tertiary hyperparathyroidism' has been given to this. Hypercalcaemia may also occur after renal transplantation (see Chapter 20.18).

Hypoparathyroidism (see also Chapter 20.18)

Parathyroid insufficiency may occur after surgical removal of the parathyroids, in idiopathic hypoparathyroidism, and in a familial form of hypoparathyroidism which is often associated with manifestations of autoimmune disease, including moniliasis, malabsorption, thyroid and adrenal failure, and pernicious anaemia. In such patients the levels of immunoreactive parathyroid hormone are undetectably low but the cAMP response to exogenous PTH is maintained. This distinguishes parathyroid insufficiency from pseudohypoparathyroidism, in which the biochemical features of hypoparathyroidism are associated with characteristic skeletal abnormalities. Pseudohypoparathyroidism is inherited and in the most common form, as an autosomal dominant, the cAMP response to exogenous PTH is defective, and the circulating level of immunoreactive PTH is high. Variations of pseudohypoparathyroidism appear to exist, and disorders are described in which the cAMP response is present but there is still end-organ resistance, and also where the cAMP response is restored by giving vitamin D. Patients who have the skeletal manifestations of pseudohypoparathyroidism but with normal biochemistry may be found in families with pseudohypoparathyroidism, and to them the term pseudopseudohypoparathyroidism is applied. Investigation has shown that end-organ resistance is due to point mutations in the genes controlling one component of the G-protein signalling system.

So far as the skeleton is concerned, the most striking changes are found in pseudohypoparathyroidism. Clinical features include mental simplicity, short stature, round face, short neck, and abnormal metacarpals (or metatarsals), of which the most common change is shortness of the fourth and fifth. The bones may be excessively dense, and widespread ectopic calcification and ossification may also occur, particularly in the basal ganglia and the subcutaneous tissues. Treatment of the hypocalcaemia is the same as for idiopathic hypoparathyroidism, with 1α-hydroxycholecalciferol.

REFERENCES

Consensus Development Conference Panel (1991). Diagnosis and management of symptomatic primary hyperparathyroidism. Consensus development statement. *Annals of Internal Medicine* **114**, 593–7.

Paterson, C.R., Burns, J., and Mowat, E. (1984). Long term follow up of untreated hyperparathyroidism. *British Medical Journal* **289**, 1261–3.

Potts, J.T. (1992). Management of asymptomatic hyperparathyroidism. *Trends in Endocrinology and Metabolism* **3**, 376–9.

Woodhead, J.S., Silver, A.C., Aston, J.P., and Brown, R.C. (1989). Measurement of circulating parathyroid hormone. *Hormone Research* **32**, 97–100.

Wynne, A.G., van Heerden, J., Carney, J.A., and Fitzpatrick, L.A. (1992). Parathyroid carcinoma: clinical and pathological features in 43 patients. *Medicine* **71**, 197–205.

Osteogenesis imperfecta: the brittle bone syndrome

This disorder, which has emerged from the status of an obscure osteopathy to a metabolic bone disease, provides remarkable lessons concerning the effects of mutations in the collagen genes. The correlation between genotype and phenotype is by no means exact and leaves interesting problems.

Osteogenesis imperfecta is said to occur in about 1 in 20 000 births; since the milder forms may never be diagnosed, this could be an underestimate. It is a leading cause of lethal short-limbed dwarfism and crippling skeletal dysplasia. There is no convincing evidence of different racial frequency. Many patients with osteogenesis imperfecta do not fit easily into the Sillence classification (Table 12), and in some hypermobility and features of the Ehlers–Danlos syndrome (see below) are dominant.

PATHOPHYSIOLOGY

Osteogenesis imperfecta involves those tissues that contain the major fibrillar collagen, type I. These include particularly bone and dentine, but also the sclerae, joints, tendons, heart valves, and skin. The pathology in bone varies with the type and severity of the disease, with age, previous fracture, and surgery. The skeletal effects of osteogenesis imperfecta are most severe in the lethal forms (type II) and at the region of the growth plate. There is faulty conversion of apparently normal mineralized cartilage to defective bone matrix. The collagen fibres are thin but show the normal striated pattern. The endoplastic reticulum of the osteoblasts is dilated by retained mutant collagen. In type III osteogenesis imperfecta, which is less severe, there are variable amounts of woven immature bone, with disorganized trabeculae and an apparent excess of osteocytes—as in other forms of the disorder. At the growth plate there are multiple islands of cartilage in the epiphyses and metaphyses. Accounts of the bone pathology in type IV are sparse.

In mild, type I osteogenesis imperfecta there is a reduction in the amount of bone (and hence in measured bone mineral density) and defective bone formation at the cellular level, such that the osteoblasts each make approximately half as much bone collagen as normal. The result is an osteoporotic bone with an apparent excess of osteoblasts and osteocytes. This appearance of 'hyperosteocytosis' suggests (to some) an increase in bone turnover rate. The overall bone structure is otherwise normal, apart from occasional woven bone. In affected dentine, the

Table 12 *Current clinical classification of osteogenesis imperfecta*

Type	Clinical features	Inheritance
I	Few fractures Little or no deformity Normal stature Prominent extraskeletal features	Autosomal dominant
II	Multiple fractures Perinatal lethal, short limbs	New dominant mutations
III	Bones deform with age Extreme short stature Dentinogenesis imperfecta common Sclerae less blue with age	Some new mutations Some recessive
IV	Moderate bone deformity and short stature Sclerae normal colour	Autosomal dominant

odontoblasts produce short, branched dentinal tubules and fill in the dental pulp. In the ear, the auditory ossicles may be imperfect or fractured.

The reduction in collagen is repeated in non-skeletal tissues. Thus, the sclerae are thin (leading to their blueness since the pigmented coat of the choroid becomes visible), the tendons are gracile and weak, the thin heart valves may become incompetent, and the aortic root dilated.

CLINICAL FEATURES

Type I is the most frequent and least serious form, and accounts for 60 per cent of all patients with the disorder. Fractures can occur in the perinatal period or even be delayed until the early perimenopause. After the menopause the overall fracture rate has been recorded at seven times more than in the normal population, and the vertebral bone mineral content in adults with type I osteogenesis imperfecta has been found to be 70 per cent of normal.

Childhood fractures in type I osteogenesis imperfecta may be numerous, but rarely lead to deformity unless treated inappropriately. Any type of fracture can occur; they become less frequent with age. Overall, fractures are more frequent in the lower limbs. Significant scoliosis is rare. The skull shows interesting changes; in addition to multiple wormian bones (Fig. 16) (which can occur in other disorders, such as pyknodystosis, cleidocranial dysostosis, Menkes' syndrome, Prader–Willi syndrome, progeria, and, rarely, in normal subjects), the vault may overhang the base, leading to basilar impression requiring surgical correction.

Clinical dentinogenesis imperfecta occurs in only some patients; the appearance varies widely and affects some teeth more than others; the teeth are discoloured and the enamel (which is normal) fractures easily from the dentine, leading to rapid erosion of both the first and second dentition. Blueness of the sclerae is a particularly important physical sign of osteogenesis imperfecta. The cause of the frequently early (juvenile) arcus is unknown: limited investigation excludes hypercholesterolaemia. The cardiac manifestations of osteogenesis imperfecta are also important, not only because of their effects but because tissue fragility makes surgery dangerous. Aortic incompetence, aortic root widening, and mitral valve prolapse all occur. Patients with osteogenesis imperfecta often show hypermobility of joints, with resultant flat feet, hyperextensible large joints, and dislocation.

Type II is nearly always lethal but the severity does differ: some children may be born dismembered whereas others may (rarely) survive the perinatal period to later merge into the type III form. Not all infants with multiple fractures at birth succumb immediately. It is possible to give a prognosis from the extent of ossification of the skull, the shape of the long bones and ribs, and the number of fractures. In the most frequent form of lethal osteogenesis imperfecta (IIA) the infant is short with disproportionately short and deformed limbs, the skull is deformed and soft, the sclerae are often deep grey-blue. Whole-body radiographs which distinguish osteogenesis imperfecta from other forms of lethal short-limbed dwarfism show grossly defective mineralization of the skull, short broad limbs with multiple fractures, and broad ribs with innumerable fractures (Fig. 17). In type IIB, the ribs have some structure; in IIC, the long bones are narrow and beaded at the site of fractures and show some evidence of modelling. Perinatal death results from the mechanical uselessness of the skeleton, which leads to respiratory failure or intracranial haemorrhage.

Type III osteogenesis imperfecta causes most clinical difficulty, since its cause and forms of inheritance are obscure and its disability is severe and progressive. During the early years of life, progressive deformity affects the skull, the long bones, the spine, chest, and pelvis; the deformity is associated with fractures but can probably occur without them. The radiological appearance of the bones changes rapidly with age. The face appears triangular, with a large vault, prominent eyes, and small jaw. The sclerae may be blue in infancy but take on a normal colour in childhood. Eventual disability and deformity is considerable. Such patients rarely walk, even after multiple operations, and have a very short stature (-4 to -6 standard deviations (SD) below the mean). The changes in the long bones are often bizarre, with long, thin diaphyses and comparatively wide metaphyses. Cartilaginous islands often develop at the end of the long bones in the epiphyses and the metaphyses, spreading into the diaphysis, giving the appearance of 'popcorn' bone. Early death may occur from respiratory infections superimposed on the restrictive reduction in vital capacity associated with severe kyphoscoliosis (Fig. 18). Progressive deformity requires specialized orthopaedic care.

Fig. 16 The innumerable centres of ossification in the occipital region, wormian bones, in an infant with severe (type III) osteogenesis imperfecta.

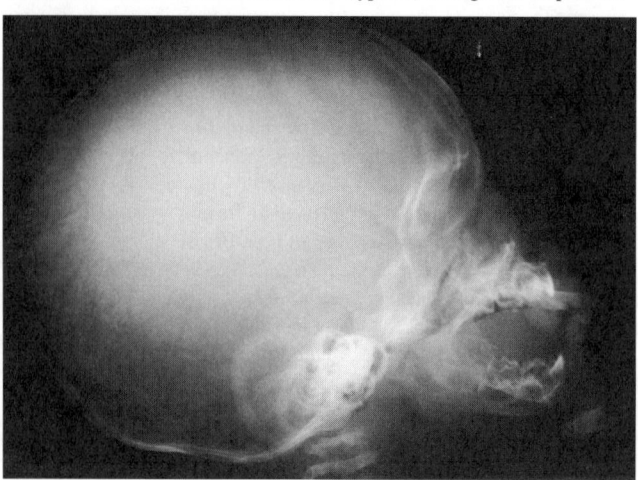

Type IV osteogenesis imperfecta is clinically intermediate between type I and type III and is inherited as a dominant trait. The sclerae are of normal colour after infancy. Overall stature is reduced and disability is variable. The rare complication of hyperplastic callus occurs most often in this form (Fig. 19). This begins with a swollen, painful, and vascular swelling, most often over the long bones, an increase in plasma alkaline phosphatase, and sometimes a systemic illness.

DIAGNOSIS

In the perinatal period, the concern is with alternative causes of lethal short-limbed dwarfism. These include severe hypophosphatasia (see below); achondrogenesis (see below), thanatophoric dwarfism, and the asphyxiating thoracic dystrophies. A perinatal whole-body radiograph is essential.

In the first few years of life non-accidental injury, 'the battered baby syndrome', is the main differential diagnosis. This is suggested by multiple fractures at different sites and of different ages, especially if associated with clinical signs of neglect. Some fractures, such as metaphyseal 'corner' fractures and posterior rib fractures are more often seen in non-accidental injury, but any type of fracture can occur in osteogenesis imperfecta. The distinction between osteogenesis imperfecta and non-accidental injury is legally important and can be difficult.

In late childhood and adolescence idiopathic juvenile osteoporosis needs to be distinguished (see above). This begins during growth with fractures of the long bones, reduction in growth rate (due to vertebral collapse), and metaphyseal compression fractures. In adult life, mild osteogenesis imperfecta may go unrecognized.

BIOCHEMISTRY

It is impossible to generalize about the clinical effect of a collagen gene mutation, but some patterns are emerging. In type I osteogenesis imperfecta there appears to be a null allele for collagen I, so that only 50 per cent of collagen is produced but this is of normal composition. Lethal osteogenesis imperfecta (type II) may result from large gene deletions, but more commonly from single base changes in COL1A1 or COL1A2. Such changes convert a glycine codon to one for another amino acid with a side chain. The effect on the triple helix of incorporating such a mutant chain appears to be most marked when the substitution occurs near the carboxy-terminal end of the chain (the helix winds up from this end), when the substituting amino acid is large; and when it occurs in the α1- rather than the α2-chain. Such mutations delay helix formation and render collagen mechanically and thermally unsound, and also lead to overhydroxylation and overmodification of the lysine residues, detectable by slowing and widening of the α-chains run on conventional polyacrylamide gels. Such abnormalities are common in type II osteogenesis imperfecta and less well defined in type III, which may rarely result

Fig. 18 Severe kyphoscoliosis in type III osteogenesis imperfecta.

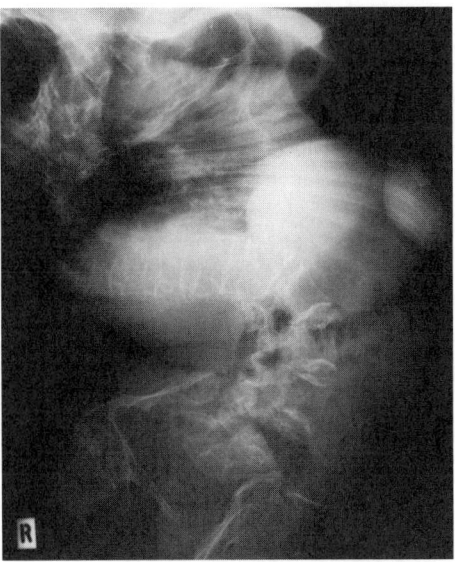

Fig. 17 Whole-body perinatal radiograph (babygram) of lethal (type II) osteogenesis imperfecta. The vault of the skull is not calcified, the ribs and long bones show multiple fractures. There was no family history.

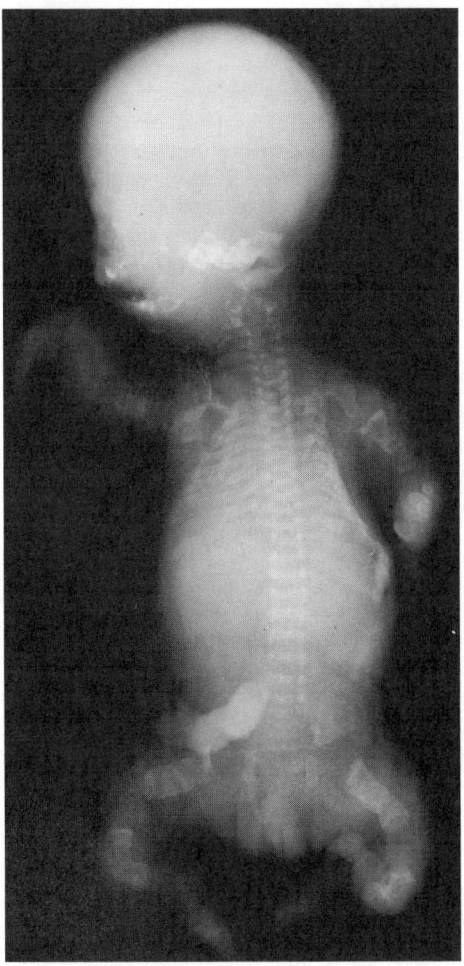

Fig. 19 The appearance of hyperplastic callus in a patient with osteogenesis imperfecta.

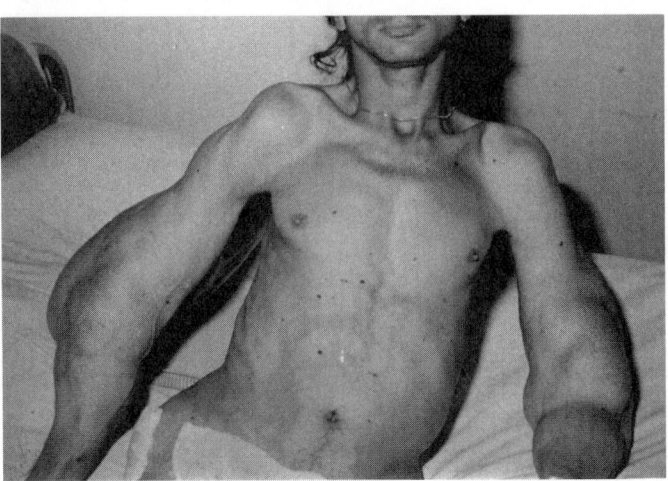

from failure to synthesize α2-chains. Type IV osteogenesis imperfecta is most often due to changes in the α2-chain.

Since the genes for α1- and α2-collagen have now been mapped and polymorphic sites identified, the mutant locus for osteogenesis imperfecta can be followed through large, dominantly inherited families. Such information can provide the basis for accurate prenatal diagnosis using fetal DNA derived from a chorionic villus biopsy. Methods are also now becoming available which make it possible to identify the mutation directly in the fetal DNA.

GENETIC ADVICE

Parents who have already had an infant with osteogenesis imperfecta need accurate advice about further pregnancies. This can be difficult, because the facts are not clear. Where the mutant gene is dominant (type I and IV) and where one parent is affected, the likelihood of affected children is 50 per cent. Difficulties arise where neither parent is clinically affected and in the lethal and progressive deforming varieties of the brittle bone syndrome. It is impossible to give a statistically accurate prediction of the likelihood of another affected child, particularly since the strict application of mendelian principles may be inappropriate because of germ-line and somatic cell mosaicism. However, there are some guidelines. Where one offspring of clinically unaffected parents has a form of osteogenesis imperfecta which fits into type I or type IV, this is likely to be a new dominant mutation (50 per cent of whose offspring will be affected) and risk of a further affected sibling is probably no more than normal. It used to be considered that infants with the severe lethal form of osteogenesis imperfect (type II) had inherited a mutant gene from both clinically normal parents and were, therefore, homozygous recessives, so that the risk of a further affected infant was 25 per cent. The evidence is now that the great majority (if not all) result from a new dominant (and lethal) mutation. To allow for the possibility of some recessives, the likelihood of phenotypically normal parents having a second baby with lethal osteogenesis imperfecta is put at approximately 7 per cent (more than normal but significantly less than 25 per cent).

The recurrence risk in progressively deforming osteogenesis imperfecta (type III) is unknown. If recessive inheritance is included in the definition, it is 25 per cent; if not, it is considerably less.

It is now recognized that germ-line and somatic cell mosaicism are important factors in the inheritance and expression of osteogenesis imperfecta, and probably in many other disorders. In brief, germ-line mosaicism means that the sperm (or ova) of an apparently normal person may contain a proportion of mutant genes for lethal (or other forms) of osteogenesis imperfecta. This accounts for those pedigrees where a phenotypically normal man has two babies with lethal osteogenesis imperfecta by separate partners. Somatic mosaicism, with variable proportions of mutant cells in different tissues, likewise provides one (but not the only) explanation for phenotypic variability and differing tissue expression. The many factors that control the regulated expression of the vertebrate collage genes in different tissues are only partly understood.

PRENATAL DIAGNOSIS

This may be done from the second trimester by ultrasound and appropriate radiographs, and in the first trimester by analysis of fetal DNA from a chorionic villus biopsy. The appropriateness of such an investigation depends on the information previously available. In a dominantly inherited form of osteogenesis imperfecta, analysis of DNA from affected and unaffected family members can establish linkage to a particular collagen gene polymorphism. In such a situation, analysis of chorionic villus DNA is the most direct approach. Alternatively the cells from such a biopsy may be cultured and the synthesized collagen examined for abnormalities. Where the collagen mutation is known in a previously affected family member, this method may directly confirm the presence of the mutation in the fetus. Except in well-organized laboratories, culture of cells and analysis of collagen will introduce unacceptable delays. Further, it is usually not possible to exclude an affected fetus merely on the grounds of apparently normal collagen. The rapid direct detection of the mutation in DNA from the chorionic villus is an eventual aim.

Amniocentesis also provides amniocytes for DNA linkage analysis and mutation detection. Amniotic fluid cells tend to produce an α1(I) homotrimer and are not, therefore, appropriate for collagen analysis.

Diagnosis by ultrasound is possible only in the more severe forms of osteogenesis imperfecta (types II and III). Since the severe forms of osteogenesis imperfecta are sporadic and therefore unsuspected, it is important to be able to detect them by routine scanning. Ultrasound features which suggest osteogenesis imperfecta are shortness and deformity of the limbs, abnormal skull shape with lack of mineralization, which makes the intracranial structures abnormally visible, and deformity of the ribs leading to a 'champagne cork' appearance on the A–P projection.

PROGNOSIS AND MANAGEMENT

For an infant born with manifest osteogenesis imperfecta, important questions are asked: how long will he or she survive; what will be the likelihood of further offspring being affected? The immediate prognosis may already be answered by perinatal death, so that it remains to deal with the prognosis of survivors. Not all born with multiple fractures succumb immediately and radiographic appearances can give a good guide to outcome.

It is in those severely affected survivors classified as type III that management will be a lifelong and specialized problem. Such individuals are of normal intelligence and prolonged admission to hospital, either for repeated surgery or for investigation, should not necessarily take precedence over education. Intramedullary rodding and osteoclasis to correct deformity and improve mobility should be very selective since the bones are often so abnormal as to take no advantage from such procedures. An organized programme of rehabilitation is important. There is no convincing evidence that medical treatments such as fluoride (to increase bone formation) or calcitonin (to decrease bone resorption) have any beneficial effect in this disorder. Intermittent bisphosphonate (in the form of 3-amino-hydroxypropylidine-1,1-bisphosphonate (APD) may produce intermittent increases in bone density, but without evidence that the fracture rate, which normally declines with age, is significantly reduced. The management of non-skeletal features of osteogenesis imperfecta, such as dentinogenesis imperfecta, aortic incompetence, and deafness, is important.

REFERENCES

Byers, P.H. (1989). Disorders of collagen biosynthesis and structure. In *The metabolic basis of inherited disease,* (6th edn), (ed. C.B. Scriver, A.L. Beaudet, W.S. Sly, and D. Valle), pp. 2805–42. McGraw–Hill, New York.

Byers, P.H. (1993). Osteogenesis imperfecta. In *Connective tissue and its heritable disorders,* (ed. P.M. Royce and B. Steinmann), pp. 317–50. Wiley-Liss, New York.

Cole, W.G. (1988). Osteogenesis imperfecta. *Baillière's Clinical Endocrinology and Metabolism* 2, 243–65.

Rowe, D.W. and Shapiro, J.R. (1990). Osteogenesis imperfecta. In *Metabolic bone disease,* (ed. L.V. Avioli and S.M. Krane), (2nd edn), pp. 659–701. W.B. Saunders, New York.

Smith, R. (1986). Osteogenesis imperfecta. *Clinics in Rheumatic Diseases* 12, 655–87.

Smith, R. (1993). Heritable metabolic bone diseases, chondrodysplasias and skeletal poisons. In *Metabolic bone and stone disease,* (ed. B.E.C. Nordin, A.G. Need, and H.A. Morris), (3rd edn), pp. 213–48. Churchill Livingstone, Edinburgh.

Sykes, B. (1990). Bone disease cracks genetics. *Nature* 348, 18–20.

The Marfan syndrome

The Marfan syndrome (Marfan's syndrome) is most often regarded as an inherited disorder of connective tissue rather than as a metabolic bone disease. Where connective tissue disorders significantly affect the skeleton, this distinction is blurred. For many years, it was thought that the defect underlying the Marfan syndrome involved collagen, but recent work excludes this.

PATHOPHYSIOLOGY

It is now recognized that Marfan's syndrome is caused by mutations in the epidermal growth factor-like regions of the fibrillin gene on chromosome 15. Fibrillin is the major constituent of the microfibrillar system and of the suspensory ligament of the lens; and it is also associated with elastin-containing tissues such as the aorta. This explains the association between dislocation of the lens and dissection of the aorta. The aorta dilates at its proximal part at the sinuses of valsalva, and returns to normal diameter below the innominate artery, unless a dissection is present. The cusps of the aortic valve do not close efficiently. Dissection is most often above the aortic valves in the area of greatest dilatation. The dissection may progress forwards or backwards. Retrograde dissection may tear the attachment of the coronary arteries and rupture into the pericardial sac. Histopathology shows a reduction in elastic fibres which are swollen and fragmented. The valve cusps are usually diaphanous and redundant. In the eye the suspensory ligament of the lens is disorganized.

CLINICAL FEATURES

The Marfan syndrome is dominantly inherited. Its major effects are on the skeleton, cardiovascular, and ocular systems. There is considerable phenotypic variation. In the typical patient with the Marfan syndrome, the overall height is increased (relative to unaffected siblings or a matched population) and the limbs are long relative to the trunk (so that the crown to pubis measurement is less than pubis to heel). Long, thin fingers (arachnodactyly) are common. Together with hypermobility, this disproportion forms the basis of clinical signs of variable utility. However, not all patients with Marfan's syndrome are long and thin. The skeletal phenotype differs from one family to another and within families. Asymmetric anterior chest deformity is associated with either depression or prominence of the sternum. Scoliosis is common, may be severe and worsens during preadolescent growth as in the idiopathic form. The hard palate is often narrow and high-arched (gothic).

Dislocation of the lens is the main ocular feature of Marfan's syndrome. Typically, this occurs upwards or sideways (in contrast to the downward dislocation in homocystinuria), and this may be present at birth or occur later. Dislocation causes the unsupported iris to wobble on movement (iridodinesis). Less important ocular features are myopia and retinal detachment. The axial length of the globe is increased and the cornea tends to be flattened.

The most severe complication of the Marfan syndrome is dilatation of the ascending aorta leading to aortic incompetence and dissection. Progressive widening of the aorta can be readily measured by serial echocardiography. Less well known manifestations of the Marfan syndrome include cutaneous striae, herniae, spontaneous pneumothorax, and dural ectasia. The mean life expectancy in Marfan's syndrome is reduced by nearly 50 per cent, predominantly due to cardiovascular catastrophe.

DIAGNOSIS

At present, there is no certain biochemical way of excluding or confirming Marfan's syndrome, although this is likely to change, and in those with few clinical features and no family history, the diagnosis of Marfan's syndrome can be difficult.

In the absence of an unequivocally affected first-degree relative, evidence of involvement of the skeleton, together with at least two other systems, and one major manifestation is necessary; when one first-degree relative is affected, involvement of at least two systems, with one major manifestation preferred, confirms the diagnosis. Homocystinuria (see below), which has a recessive mode of inheritance, should be excluded. Other important alternative diagnoses include congenital contractural arachnodactyly, familial tall stature, isolated mitral valve prolapse, familial or isolated annulo-aortic ectasia, and Stickler's syndrome. The latter is a dominantly inherited connective tissue disorder that affects the eyes, ears, and skeleton with severe myopia in childhood, sensorineural hearing loss from adolescence, and degenerative arthritis from early adult life. The diagnosis can be made at birth if cleft palate and micrognathia are present. There is considerable phenotypic variation. In some families the disorder is linked to the type II collagen gene.

Contractures can occur in Marfan's syndrome but are of a late onset. In congenital contractural arachnodactyly, which is inherited as an autosomal dominant trait, contractures involving the hands, feet, and larger joints are present from birth and tend to improve. Abnormal ears are described. Limited studies suggest that this disorder involves mutations of an additional fibrillin gene on chromosome 5.

TREATMENT

There is no specific treatment for the underlying defect, but major clinical manifestations require attention. Scoliosis may be progressive and severe, particularly in adolescence. Bracing is largely ineffective and operative stabilization may be necessary. Excessive height in girls may be prevented by giving oestrogen together with progestogen in the prepubertal years. Marked sternal deformity may need correction for cosmetic or cardiopulmonary reasons, but opinions on the value of surgery vary widely. In the eyes, it is rarely necessary to remove dislocated lenses unless they prolapse into the anterior chamber, but myopia should be corrected. The main decisions concern the management of the cardiovascular problems; when and if to operate on the dilated ascending aorta or to replace incompetent valves, and whether aortic dilatation can be prevented by reducing the intermittent force on its walls due to left ventricular systole. As far as the second point is concerned, it has not yet been proved convincingly that giving a β-blocker such as propranolol has any significant beneficial effect on aortic dilatation, but it is common practice to do so. As regards surgery on the aorta, it is clear that progressive aortic widening (measured regularly by echocardiography), together with progressive aortic incompetence and left ventricular strain provide strong indications for replacement of the proximal aorta by a prosthesis. Mitral valve replacement may also be necessary.

Since both aortic and mitral valves are susceptible to endocarditis, prophylactic antimicrobials must be given at the time of dentistry.

GENETIC ADVICE

Genetic advice is at present based on clinical observations and the knowledge that inheritance is of the autosomal dominant pattern. Advances in understanding of the biochemical and molecular biological factors underlying the disease are likely to contribute further before long.

REFERENCES

Dietz, H.C., *et al.* (1991). Marfan syndrome caused by a recurrent *de novo* missense mutation in the fibrillin gene. *Nature* **352,** 337–9.
Hewett, D.R., Lynch, J.R., Smith, R., and Sykes, B.C. (1993). A novel fibrillin mutation in the Marfan's syndrome which could disrupt calcium binding of the epidermal growth factor-like module. *Human Molecular Genetics* **2,** 475–7.

Table 13 *Classification and clinical features of the Ehlers-Danlos syndrome*

	Type	Inheritance	Skin extensibility and fragility	Bruising	Joint mobility	Other significant features	Biochemical defects
I	Gravis	Dominant	Gross	Severe	Generalized gross	Prematurity Molluscoid pseudotumours Musculoskeletal deformity	?Abnormal collagen fibrils and fibre packing
II	Mitis	Dominant	Mild	Mild	Moderate, often limited to hands and feet	None	Not known
III	Benign hypermobile	Dominant	Variable, usually minimal	Mild	Generalized gross	Recurrent joint dislocations Osteoarthritis Skilled contortionists	Not known
IV	Ecchymotic (arterial or Sack-Barabas type; includes acrogeria)	Dominant or recessive	Thin pale skin with prominent veins	Gross	Minimal limited to digits	Rupture of great vessels and bowel Elastosis perforans serpiginosa	In synthesis, secretion, and structure of type III collagen
V	X-linked	X-linked	Moderate with variable fragility	Variable	Mild	Floppy value syndrome	Lysyl oxidase deficiency (unconfirmed in other patients)
VI	Ocularscoliotic (hydroxylysine deficient disease)	Recessive	Moderate	Moderate	Generalized gross	Scoliosis Microcornea Ocular fragility	Procollagen lysyl hydroxylase deficiency
VII	Arthrochalasis multiplex congenita	Recessive	Moderate	Moderate	Severe	Short stature Congenital dislocations	N-terminal cleavage sites for procollagen peptidase mutated
VIII	Periodontitis	Dominant	Minimal with marked fragility	Mild	Moderate limited to digits	Advanced generalized periodontitis	Not known
IX	X-linked skeletal	X-linked recessive	Moderate		Moderate	Moderate	Occipital exostoses Deformed clavicles Bowed long bones	Abnormal copper metabolism

McKusick, V.A. (1991). The defect in Marfan syndrome. *Nature* **352**, 279–81.

Pyeritz, R.E. (1993). The Marfan syndrome. In *Connective tissue and its heritable disorders*, (ed. P.M. Royce and B. Steinmann), pp. 437–68. Wiley-Liss, New York.

Ehlers–Danlos syndrome

This syndrome initially included only those conditions with the common clinical features of abnormal velvety hyperelastic skin which healed poorly, hyperextensible joints, and lax ligaments. However, the disorders included in this syndrome have now been increased and have brought with them additional specific features, amongst which is vascular rupture, especially in type IV Ehlers–Danlos syndrome, associated with various mutations in type III collagen. In the currently expanded Ehlers–Danlos syndrome the skeleton is particularly affected in types VI and VII (Table 13).

In type VI (ocular scoliotic Ehlers–Danlos syndrome), the first disorder in which an inborn error of collagen metabolism was identified, the clinical features are due to lysyl hydroxylysase deficiency. Since hydroxylation of peptide-bound lysine is an essential posttranslational step in collagen synthesis and a necessary precursor to cross-link formation, this defect weakens collagen structure. The main clinical features are severe scoliosis, microcornea, and ocular fragility.

In type VII (arthrochalasia) there is excessive mobility, perinatal joint dislocations (especially of the hips) and short stature. There is persistence in the tissues of collagen molecules with a retained amino-terminal propeptide which leads to defective fibrillogenesis.

REFERENCES

Steinmann, B., Royce, P.M., and Superti-Furga, A. (1993). The Ehlers–Danlos syndrome. In *Connective tissue and its heritable disorders*, (ed. P.M. Royce and B. Steinmann), pp. 351–401. Wiley-Liss, New York.

Homocystinuria (see also Chapter 11.3)

Homocystinuria is phenotypically similar to Marfan's syndrome but with a different cause and additional important complications. It is due to a deficiency of cystathionine β-synthase, an enzyme whose gene is located on chromosome 21, and which contains firmly bound pyridoxal phosphate (vitamin B_6). Homocystinuria is inherited as an autosomal recessive condition. The amount of residual cystathionine synthase varies from 0 to 10 per cent in patients, and in obligate heterozygotes it is less than 50 per cent of normal.

PATHOPHYSIOLOGY

Homocysteine lies at the crossroads of two metabolic pathways and is converted to cystathionine by the addition of serine. This reaction is controlled by cystathionine β-synthase. The alternative fate of homocysteine is methylation to methionine. Cystathionine β-synthase activity is controlled by pyridoxine, but not all patients with cystathionine deficient homocystinuria are pyrodoxine sensitive, although this sensitivity or dependency is constant in sibships. In homocystinuria, there is an increase in both homocysteine and homocystine, which accumulate proximal to the metabolic block. Cystathionine, normally present in the brain, is no longer detectable and cysteine (normally made from methionine) becomes an essential amino acid.

The pathological findings include fraying and disruption of the zonular fibres of the lens, defective bone formation, and multiple central nervous system infarcts. It is not known how the biochemical changes lead to the clinical features. The increased thrombotic tendency is not fully explained by changes in platelet function, cellular endothelium, or soluble factors, although abnormalities have been described in all of them. The neurological abnormalities and mental backwardness have not been proven to be due to the biochemical consequences of cystathionine β-synthase deficiency or to repeated vascular thromboses. There is evidence that homocyst(e)ine increases the solubility of collagen and interferes with its synthesis; for some this explains the dislocation of the lens due to failure of the ciliary zonule. Since it is now known that this structure is composed largely of fibrillin, a further explanation is required. There is current interest in the possibility that young adults with premature vascular disease may be heterozygotes for the mutant cystathionine synthase gene.

CLINICAL FEATURES

The clinical features of cystathionine β-synthase deficiency involve four systems and develop some time after birth; they are ocular, skeletal, central nervous, and vascular. The main ocular manifestation is downward dislocation of the lens. Myopia, glaucoma, retinal degeneration, and detachment also occur, and cataracts, optic atrophy, and corneal abnormalities are described. Some skeletal features suggest Marfan's syndrome. They include a long, thin habitus, pectus excavatum, scoliosis, and genu valgum. There is often radiological osteoporosis and abnormal modelling of the long bones with epimetaphyseal widening. Many subjects with homocystinuria are mentally backward and may also have seizures and strokes. It is unknown how closely these follow the increased tendency to thrombosis or the biochemical changes, especially lack of cystathionine. Thromboembolism may occur in any vessel and at any age.

Any patient who has the phenotypic features of Marfan's syndrome associated with thrombosis, mental simplicity, and affected siblings should have a cyanide-nitroprusside test performed on the urine.

The outlook for patients whose biochemical abnormalities are corrected by large amounts of pyridoxine (i.e. have pyridoxine-sensitive homocystinuria) is usually better than those who are pyridoxine resistant. The main cause of death is thromboembolism.

The management of patients with homocystinuria differs according to the time of diagnosis and whether or not the patient responds to pyridoxine. In pyridoxine-responsive patients diagnosed after the newborn period, giving pyridoxine, in doses that vary from 250 to 1200 mg a day, appears to prevent thromboembolism.

When homocystinuria is detected in the newborn infant (most are discovered by screening and are pyridoxine non-responsive), a diet low in methionine appears to reduce the incidence of low intelligence. After the new-born period, in those who are not responsive to pyridoxine, methionine restriction and the administration of betaine (as a methyl donor) are also possibly useful lines of approach.

REFERENCES

Mudd, S.H., Levy, H.L., and Skovby, F. (19xx). Disorders of transulfuration. In *The metabolic basis of inherited disease,* (ed. C.R. Scriver, A.L. Beaudet, W.S. Sly, and D. Valle), (6th edn), pp. 693–734. McGraw-Hill, New York.
Skovby, F. (1993). The homocystinurias. In *Connective tissue and its heritable disorders,* (ed. P.M. Royce and D. Steinmann), pp. 469–86. Wiley-Liss, New York.

Alkaptonuria (see also Chapter 11.3)

In this rare autosomal recessive disorder, decreased activity of homogentisate oxidase leads to accumulation of homogentistic acid in the urine and increased pigmentation (ochronosis) in cartilage and connective tissues. Darkening of the urine, alkaptonuria, is due to the presence of 2,5-dehydroxyphenylacetic acid derived from the oxidation and polymerization of homogentisic acid. Polymerization increases in alkaline urine and is slowed down by antioxidants such as vitamin C. The structure of the pigment which causes ochronosis is not known. It is granular or homogeneous and may occur within or outside the cell. It is said to be associated with a reduction in lysyl hydroxylase in the tissue concerned, and impairment of the cross-links of collagen.

Alkaptonuria is more frequent in the former Czechoslovakia and Germany than elsewhere and occurs equally in the sexes. It is recessively inherited. Abnormal pigmentation is found in the cartilage of the ear (which may be calcified), the nasal cartilage and the sclerae. The most important effects of this disease are on the spine (Fig. 20) and later on the larger joints. The intervertebral discs lose height and later calcify;

Fig. 20 The appearance of the spine in a man of with alkaptonuria. There is universal calcification of the intervertebral discs.

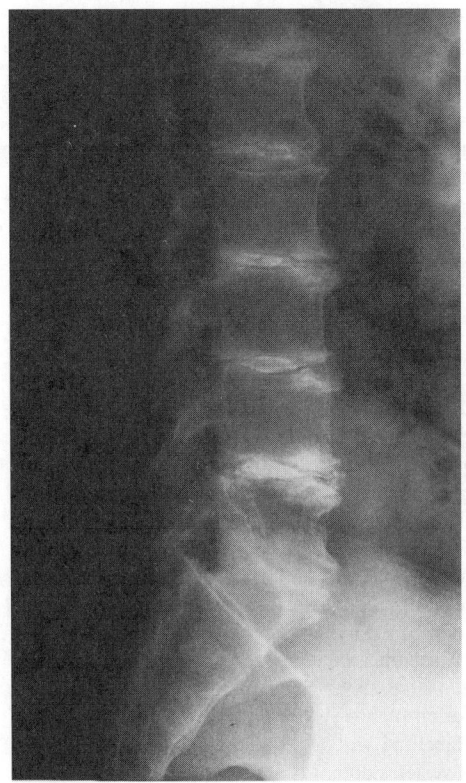

they may also herniate acutely. The spine becomes rigid and short and the lumbar lordosis is lost. In the large joints, such as the knees, shoulders, and hips, there are effusions and loose bodies. The symphysis pubis may be affected but not the sacroiliac joints. Ochronotic 'arthritis' is described with episodes of acute inflammation which resemble those of rheumatoid arthritis. Calcification of the aorta is an additional feature.

The diagnosis of alkaptonuria—often made late—should be suspected where there is a premature disc degeneration, even if there is no excessive darkening of the urine. Early degenerative arthritis suggests the disease, confirmed by finding deeply pigmented articular cartilage at the time of operation. In those patients with life-long discoloration of the urine, the differential diagnosis is from other rare causes of urinary pigmentation. The urine of a patient with alkaptonuria contains reducing substances and will therefore give a positive result suggesting glycosuria except where glucose oxidase is used. An increase in homogentisic acid in the urine and plasma confirms the diagnosis.

In theory, it should be possible to reduce the amount of homogentisic acid, and presumably the side-effects, by cutting down the protein intake to 30 or 40 g/day, thereby reducing tyrosine intake. There is no evidence that such a procedure alleviates the symptoms of alkaptonuria. For the moment, it is not possible to detect the heterozygotes for this disease and the chromosomal location of the defective gene has not been identified.

REFERENCES

Ladu, B.N. (1989). Alkaptonuria. In *The metabolic basis of inherited disease,* (ed. C.R. Scriver, A.L. Beaudet, W.S. Sly, and D. Valle), (6th edn), pp. 775–9. McGraw Hill, New York.
Hazleman, B.L. and Adebajo, A.O. (1993). Alcaptonuria. In *Connective tissue and its heritable disorders,* (ed. P.M. Royce and B. Steinmann), pp. 591–602. Wiley-Liss, New York.

Hypophosphatasia (see also Chapter 12.6)

This rare disorder has similarities to rickets and osteomalacia. It is due to a reduction in the tissue non-specific alkaline phosphatase (TNSAP) which leads to defective mineralization and a triad of biochemical disturbances; increased urinary phosphoethanolamine, plasma pyrophosphate, and plasma pyridoxal phosphate.

Studies on Manitoba Mennonites, where the incidence of hypophosphatasia is high, have linked the defective gene to chromosome 1 and provide knowledge on which to base prenatal diagnosis. Although TNASP is widely distributed, its absence leads to lesions only in the bone and teeth.

PATHOPHYSIOLOGY

The characteristic biochemical changes result directly from the alkaline phosphatase deficiency. Various mutations have been described in the alkaline phosphatase gene. Increased urinary pyrophosphate excretion is more reliable than urinary phosphoethanolamine as a marker for carriers of the hypophosphatasia gene. There is often also hypercalcaemia and hypercalciuria in childhood; and up to half affected children and adults have an increase in plasma phosphate levels. Hyperphosphataemia is described in carriers of the hypophosphatasia gene. The recorded plasma alkaline phosphatase must be compared with age-matched control values.

Histological examination of bone shows an excess of osteoid with abnormal tetracycline labelling without evidence of secondary hyperparathyroidism. Matrix vesicles do not contain alkaline phosphatase or hydroxyapatite crystals. The primary dental defect is in the cementum;

additionally, the predentine is widened and the dentinal tubules are enlarged and few.

CLINICAL FEATURES

Hypophosphatasia occurs in all races. Since the severe forms are inherited as autosomal recessive traits they are more frequent where there is consanguinity. It has been estimated that hypophosphatasia occurs in 1 in 100 000 live births in Toronto. Four clinical types provide a continuous spectrum from a lethal perinatal disorder to an asymptomatic disease in adults.

The first is an important cause of lethal short-limbed dwarfism (see above). Some newborn infants survive for a few days but fever, failure to thrive, anaemia, seizures, and intracranial haemorrhages occur. Radiographs show grossly defective mineralization, especially in the skull, where only the base may be mineralized, and in diaphyses of the long bones which, rarely, may have bony spurs.

In the infantile form (within the first 6 months) hypotonia, failure to thrive, hypercalcaemia, and hypercalciuria occur. Clinical rickets is noticed and the fontanelle appears wide but there is a functional synostosis. Craniostenosis can produce optic atrophy, exophthalmos, and raised intracranial pressure requiring surgery.

The most variable expression occurs in childhood. Early loss of deciduous teeth, due to defective cementum, may be the only feature (ondontohypophosphatasia). The pulp chambers are enlarged, the root canals short (shell teeth). If bone disease is present, walking is delayed and deformities occur; for instance bow legs, knock knees, short stature, and enlargement of the epiphyses at the wrist, knees, and ankles.

In the adult progressive stiffness, pain in the bones, and apparent 'stress' fractures can occur. Approximately 50 per cent of such patients have a history of bone disease resembling rickets, or premature loss of deciduous teeth, or both in childhood. There may also be premature shedding of adult teeth, short stature, and abnormal skull shape. Recurrent poorly healing metatarsal fractures occur. Partial fractures of the long bones characteristically occur on the convex outer surface (in contrast to the concave inner position of the Looser's zones in osteomalacia), most often in the upper one-third of the femoral shaft, and are often bilateral; other sites include ribs, tibia, and ulna. They may be unaltered for years or increase in size and eventually fracture. Secondary hyperparathyroidism is not seen. Chondrocalcinosis is common and in a proportion is associated with clinical pyrophosphate gout (pseudogout).

MANAGEMENT

In the management of hypophosphatasia, premature synostosis leading to raised intracranial pressure requires surgical relief. Hypercalcaemia may be dealt with by reducing dietary calcium and by giving prednisone. Replacing the defective enzyme by the transfusion of alkaline phosphatase-rich plasma does not produce consistent results. Intramedullary rods may prevent and treat fractures of the long bones. Dental abnormalities, which can occur in biochemically normal members of hypophosphatasia families, require treatment.

Prenatal diagnosis of a severely affected child can be made by ultrasound. There is also reduced alkaline phosphatase activity in the amniotic fluid cells.

REFERENCES

Henthorn, P.S. and Whyte, M.P. (1992). Missense mutations of the tissue non-specific alkaline phosphatase gene in hypophosphatasia. *Clinical Chemistry* **38**, 2501–5.
Whyte, M.P. (1993). Osteopetrosis and the heritable forms of rickets. In *Connective tissue and its heritable disorders,* (ed. P.M. Royce and D. Steinmann), pp. 563–9. Wiley-Liss, New York.

Lysosomal storage diseases (see also Section 11)

This large group of diseases is due to various inborn errors which affect the function of specific lysosomal enzymes normally responsible for the breakdown of a variety of complex molecules. As a result, these molecules or their partially degraded derivatives accumulate in the lysosomes and the tissues that contain them. The effect of this accumulation varies from one tissue to another according to the particular disorder, and the skeleton is significantly involved in only a proportion of them. They include some mucopolysaccharidoses and Gaucher's disease.

Mucopolysaccharidoses

Failure of the normal lysosomal breakdown of complex carbohydrates leads to their accumulation in the tissues, and produces many clinical abnormalities. The disorders may be divided into two main groups, according to the chemistry of the accumulated substance, namely the mucopolysaccharidoses and the mucolipidoses. Specific biochemical defects are described elsewhere in this book (see Section 11). Since some of these disorders have a prominent effect on the skeleton, they should also be briefly mentioned here; they are the Hurler syndrome (MPS IH), the Hunter syndrome (MPS II), and the Morquio syndrome (MPS IV). With certain exceptions the bone changes themselves do not permit precise diagnosis of the type of dysplasia present, or distinction from the mucolipidoses.

The Hurler syndrome (MPS IH)

This is the most severe type of mucopolysaccharidosis and causes death at an early age. The enzyme defect is recessively inherited and all patients have the same appearance, to which the term gargoylism was previously applied. Affected infants appear to develop normally in the first few months of life, but then deteriorate mentally and physically. Death often occurs in late childhood, commonly due to pneumonia or to coronary artery disease associated with mucopolysaccharide deposits.

The physical features include proportionate short stature (Table 3), a typical facial appearance, a short neck with a lumbar gibbus and chest deformity, and a protuberant abdomen. The facial features are coarse and ugly, with flattening of the nasal bridge, with large open mouth and tongue, and often with hypertrophied gums over enlarged alveolar ridges. The eyes are prominent with corneal clouding. There is noisy breathing and variable deafness. The vault of the skull may show scaphocephaly or acrocephaly. Other striking features include the stiff, broad trident hands and the large abdomen with hepatosplenomegaly. Radiographs show the abnormal shape of the skull, the slipper-shaped sella turcica, the beaking of the vertebrae with the thoracolumbar kyphosis, and the bullet-shaped phalanges. Similar but less severe features are seen in the Hunter syndrome, inherited as an X-linked recessive.

The Morquio syndrome (MPS IV)

In this disorder the orthopaedic manifestations are striking, and intelligence is normal. Although the disorder is probably heterogeneous and only a proportion of cases excrete an excess of keratan sulphate in the urine, the skeletal changes are uniform. In the first years of life the child becomes progressively more deformed and dwarfed. Characteristically the neck is short, the sternum is protuberant, and there may be a flexed stance with knock knees. There is a striking loss of muscle tone in comparison to the stiffness of MPS IH; hypermobility and a loose skin are features. Radiographs in infancy show a spine similar to that of Hurler syndrome, but later flattening of the vertebrae with anterior beaking lead to relative shortening of the trunk. The small bones of the hands are very different from those of MPS IH and the metacarpals show diaphyseal constriction (Fig. 21).

Importantly the odontoid may be hypoplastic, leading to atlantoaxial instability, compression of the long spinal tracts, and paraplegia.

Gaucher's disease (see also Section 11)

This is a very rare lysosomal storage disorder in which glucocerebroside-containing reticuloendothelial histiocytes accumulate within the bone marrow. It is recessively inherited and largely restricted to Ashkenazi Jews, where the incidence of the adult form (type I) is about 1 in 2500 births. The skeletal manifestations are often severe and disabling. They vary from a characteristic symmetrical failure of remodelling in the lower femora (Erlenmeyer-flask appearance) to diffuse and localized bone loss and osteosclerotic and osteonecrotic lesions, which cause pain and pathological fracture.

REFERENCES

Leroy, J.G., and Weismann, U. (1993). Disorders of lysosomal enzymes. In *Connective tissue and its heritable disorders,* (ed. P.M. Royce and B. Steinmann), pp. 613–39. Wiley-Liss, New York.
Mankin, H.J., Doppelt, S.H., Rosenberg, A.E., and Barranger, J.A. (1990). Metabolic bone disease in patients with Gaucher's disease. In *Metabolic bone disease,* (ed. L.V. Avioli and S.M. Krane), (2nd edn), pp. 730–52. W.B. Saunders, Philadelphia.

Skeletal dysplasias

The term skeletal dysplasia has been used traditionally to cover a wide range of generalized disorders of the skeleton, often of unknown cause, affecting both cartilage and bone. With increasing knowledge it is now

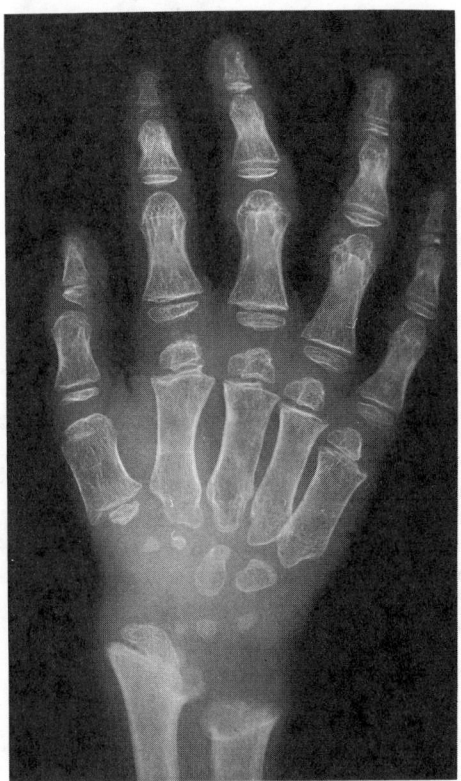

Fig. 21 The appearance of the hands in MPS IV (Morquio syndrome).

correct to distinguish the chondrodysplasias, which primarily affect cartilage (and in which biochemical changes in cartilage are being described) from such disorders as diaphyseal hyperostosis and assorted dense bone diseases, where the cause is unknown. Since osteopetrosis is a well-defined disorder of osteoclast function, it should be dealt with separately.

Most skeletal dysplasias are familial, and many are rare. They are more fully described in atlases and orthopaedic texts. It seems probable that the defects in some of the chondrodysplasias will mirror those in osteogenesis imperfecta, with the mutant collagen being type II (cartilage collagen) rather than type I. Type II collagen is synthesized in the same way as other fibrillar collagens (see above) but is a homopolymer of three α1(II) chains rather than heteropolymeric type I. It is the major, but not the only, collagen of cartilage, and is also found in other tissues such as the eye. Linkage studies have excluded the type II collagen gene as the mutant locus in many of the dysplasias, but type II collagen gene mutations have been identified and linkage established in achondrogenesis type II, spondyloepiphyseal dysplasia, and in Stickler's syndrome (hereditary arthro-ophthalmopathy).

CLINICAL FEATURES

The physician confronted by a patient with a skeletal dysplasia is unlikely to make the correct diagnosis without much additional help unless it is clearly one of the most frequent, for instance achondroplasia. However, accurate classification of the dysplasias is important and will make clinical and biochemical advance possible. The most convenient classification is a clinical one (Table 14). Most patients with skeletal dysplasias have restricted growth, and most are short limbed. The bodily proportions of skeletal dysplasias will provide a clue about whether the limbs are mainly affected, or the spine, or both. In the short-limbed group, achondroplasia and achondroplasia-like dwarfs are the most typical. Those without conspicuous dwarfing include various inherited epiphyseal dysplasias, diaphyseal dysplasias, and some metaphyseal dysplasias. An alternative classification, not based on height, groups the dysplasias according to whether they are predominantly epiphyseal or metaphyseal, whether the spine is predominantly involved, and whether single limbs or segments are involved. Radiographs, taken as soon as possible and, where possible, consecutively, are essential to determine whether the metaphyses of the long bones or the epiphyses are primarily affected.

For the purpose of this section, osteopetrosis (marble bones disease) is dealt with separately as a disorder of bone cell biology. Other sclerosing disorders of bone, in some of which biochemical abnormalities have been described (Engelmann's disease, van Buchem's disease), receive brief mention.

Achondroplasia

This is the prototype of short limbed, short stature. It is inherited as an autosomal dominant, with a high mutation rate and the incidence increases with paternal age. The cause remains unknown. Until recently any undiagnosed patient with excessively short limbs had the label of achondroplasia. This explains the apparent frequency of achondroplasia and its apparently high mortality, since different forms of lethal short-limbed dwarfism were then included.

As the clinical definition of achondroplasia has not always been exact, its true incidence and natural history are not well defined. There is a failure of the epiphyseal growth cartilage, and bulbous masses of cartilage appear at the ends of the long bones. In contrast, periosteal and membrane bone formation and bone repair are normal. This selective effect on growth cartilage accounts for the skeletal deformity.

Achondroplasia can be diagnosed at birth or within the first year of life, when the disparity between the large skull and short limbs becomes obvious. There is a striking disproportion between the trunk of normal

Table 14 *Clinical classification of the main chondrodysplasias with short stature*

Disproportionate
  Short limbs
    Lethal
      Type II osteogenesis imperfecta
      Hypophosphatasia
      Achondrogenesis
      Thanatophoric dwarfism
    Not lethal
      Achondroplasia
  Short limbs and trunk
    Pseudoachondroplasia
    Diastrophic dwarfism
    Kneist disease
  Short trunk
    Spondyloepiphyseal dysplasia
Proportionate
  Mucopolysaccharidoses
Without obvious short stature
  Multiple epiphyseal dysplasia
  Diaphyseal dysplasias
  Some metaphyseal dysostoses
With increased limb length
  Marfan syndrome
  Homocystinuria
  Some diaphyseal dysplasias
Sclerosing bone dysplasias
Others[a]
  Fibrodysplasia ossificans progressiva
  Polyostotic fibrous dysplasia

[a]Many obscure disorders can be added to this list.

length and the short arms and legs. Thus the finger tips may only come down to the iliac crest. The shortness of the limbs particularly affects the proximal segment. The limbs themselves look very broad, with abnormally deep creases, and the hands are trident-like. In contrast to the short limbs is the enlarged bulging vault of the skull, the small face, and flat nasal bridge or 'scooped out' glabella. There is a marked lumbar lordosis and also sometimes some wedging of the upper lumbar vertebrae, which may later lead to a thoracolumbar kyphosis. Radiological features include metaphyseal irregularity and flaring in the long bones, irregular and late-appearing epiphyses, a pelvis which is narrow in its antero-posterior diameter, with short iliac wings and deep sacroiliac notches, and a spine which shows progressive narrowing of the interpeduncular distance from above downwards, which is the reverse of normal.

Children with achondroplasia are of normal intelligence, and the complications of this disease arise particularly from the skeletal disproportion. This may lead to early osteoarthritis, to obstetric difficulties and the need for caesarian section, to hydrocephalus, and to paraplegia. Eventual height can vary from between about 80 to 150 cm. Recent reviews emphasize how often narrowing of the spinal canal produces symptoms of spinal stenosis.

Homozygous achondroplasia (the offspring of two affected parents) is severe and lethal. In contrast, the condition of hypochondroplasia is probably inherited independently from achondroplasia; the skeletal disproportion and the spinal abnormalities are less and the skull is unaffected.

Achondroplasia-like dwarfs

For the details of these and other causes of short-limbed dwarfism the reader should consult more specialized texts (see also Table 14). Those which most closely resemble achondroplasia at birth are thanatophoric dwarfism, achondrogenesis, severe hypophosphatasia and type II osteogenesis imperfecta. All can be distinguished radiologically.

Spondyloepiphyseal dysplasias

This is a heterogeneous group of disorders in which the spine is predominantly affected and the short stature is due to shortness of the trunk. The most severe type is spondyloepiphyseal dysplasia (SED) congenita; milder forms are referred to as SED tarda. There are various forms of inheritance.

SED tarda often has an X-linked mode of inheritance, so that males only are affected and females are carriers. In affected males the disproportionately short trunk becomes obvious at adolescence. Failure of ossification in the anterior part of the so-called ring epiphyses leads to central and posterior humps on the upper and lower parts of the flattened bodies. The condition needs to be distinguished from multiple epiphyseal dysplasia, which involves other major joints more than the spine.

SED congenita can be diagnosed at birth because of the short stature associated with a short trunk. There may be a close resemblance to Morquio's disease (MPS IV). The severe form may be distinguished from the age of about 4 years. The appearance of the capital femoral epiphyses is delayed (in some patients it may never be seen, except by arthrography). Marked lumbar lordosis waddling gait, back pain, and progressive disproportion may occur. The otontoid is hypoplastic, kyphoscoliosis may develop and the interpeduncular distances of the vertebrae do not increase in the lumbar region. Because of all these changes paraplegia may occur. In this disorder there is often myopia and retinal detachment.

There is a form of SED, pseudoachondroplasia, which resembles achondroplasia because of the short limbs but the facial appearances are normal. The short stature becomes obvious from about 2 years of age. Lumbar lordosis and scoliosis may develop. The tubular bones are short with irregular metaphyses and small, deformed epiphyses. Hypermobility is marked and early osteoarthritis occurs.

Proportionate dwarfism

Although it is important to classify short stature into proportionate and disproportionate (Table 14), there are many conditions in which this distinction is difficult to make. Hypophosphataemic rickets, mucopolysaccharidoses, vitamin D-dependent rickets, and osteogenesis imperfecta may come into both categories.

Bone dysplasias without conspicuous short stature

The height of patients with multiple epiphyseal dysplasia may only be slightly reduced. Although many epiphyses are affected, the spine is virtually normal. There are also variable forms of inheritance.

In patients with multiple hereditary exostoses (often referred to as diaphyseal aclasis) there is a juxtaepiphyseal disorder of bone growth, limited to bones developed in cartilage, which gives rise to cartilage-capped exostoses which point away from the joint. Inheritance is autosomal dominant and stature is normal.

The metaphyseal disorders are rare; some, such as the Jansen type of metaphyseal dysostosis do cause severe dwarfing. In others with less severe growth disturbance, such as Type Schmid, rickets is simulated, and confusion with inherited hypophosphataemia is possible. In progressive diaphyseal dysplasia (see below) the limbs are disproportionately long.

Sclerosing disorders of bone

Apart from marble bones disease (see below) the experience of most physicians of the osteoscleroses is limited by their extreme rarity.

Engelmann's disease (progressive diaphyseal dysplasia: Camurati–Engelmann disease)

This rare condition is autosomal dominantly inherited. It affects endocrine and muscular systems in addition to the skeleton, where the main feature is a variable but progressive endosteal and periosteal thickening of the diaphyses of the long bones. In severely affected subjects the spine, skull, and axial skeleton are all affected. The cause is unknown.

There is a waddling broad-based gait, muscle wasting and weakness, loss of subcutaneous tissues, and pain in the legs during childhood. The appearance is characteristic; the head is large with a prominent forehead and proptosis, the muscle mass is reduced, and the bones are palpably thickened. Cranial nerve palsies, deafness, and blindness with raised intracranial pressure can occur. Puberty is delayed. Bone pain resistant to analgesia is often a presenting and troublesome feature.

Radiographic appearances vary, from limited thickening of the diaphyses (often in the lower extremities) to widespread new bone formation, affecting all bones, including the skull, demonstrated by scintigraphy.

The increased bone turnover causes a moderate increase in plasma alkaline phosphatase and urinary hydroxyproline levels. There may be a markedly positive calcium balance, associated with hypocalcaemia and hypocalciuria. Hyperphosphataemia has been recorded.

Pathological examination confirms gross thickening of the bone with disorganization of internal structure and external shape. The peripheral subperiosteal new bone is woven. The muscles show non-specific type II fibre atrophy.

In the differential diagnosis the proximal myopathy and abnormal gait simulate muscular dystrophy. The radiographic appearances are diagnostic, although idiopathic hyperphosphatasia may present some difficulties.

The course of this disorder is unpredictable and remission of symptoms may occur during adolescence or adult life, so it is difficult to assess treatment. Bone pain may repond to corticosteroids in small, alternate-day doses. Etidronate (20 mg/kg daily) has produced hypocalcaemic tetany but intermittent administration is reported to reduce pain. Limb pain may be relieved by surgical removal of a cortical window in the diaphysis.

Pyknodystosis

In contrast to Engelmann's disease, pyknodystosis has an autosomal recessive inheritance, with parental consanguinity in some 30 per cent of subjects. It has some similarities to osteopetrosis. Marked reduction in stature with short limbs is a particular feature.

The vault of the skull is large, the face and chin small, the palate high-arched, and the teeth crowded, with retained deciduous teeth. The anterior fontanelle (and other cranial sutures) are typically open. The fingers may appear to be clubbed because of associated acro-osteolysis. The chest is deformed with kyphoscoliosis and pectus excavatum. Recurrent fractures of long bones occur, and occasionally rickets. Radiologically, there are similarities to osteopetrosis with generalized osteosclerosis and fractures. However, the osteosclerosis is uniform; there are no defects of modelling and no endobones. In addition to delayed closure of the cranial sutures there are also wormian bones; the bony fragility, wormian bones, and blue sclerae simulate osteogenesis imperfecta.

Idiopathic hyperphosphatasia

This very rare condition is also labelled juvenile Paget's disease. It has autosomal recessive inheritance. The long bones are abnormal, thickened, and bowed from the first year of life, and the skull may be enlarged. Muscular weakness is common and the plasma alkaline phosphatase level is continuously very high.

Sclerosteosis

This condition is due to an autosomal recessive trait. There is progressive overgrowth and sclerosis of the skeleton, including the skull and

20.1 Clinical physiology of the kidney: tests of renal function and structure

K. M. BANNISTER AND M. F. FIELD

Assessment of the function of the kidneys and the urinary tract

The investigation of the patient with suspected renal disease usually requires assessments of both structure and function of the kidneys. Structural evaluation includes macroscopic imaging and microscopic examination of tissue samples acquired by biopsy. Function is assessed by microscopic and biochemical examination of the urine, biochemical determinations on plasma samples, and, more rarely, by procedures involving administration of test substances.

Examination of the urine

Urine volume

In health there is a diurnal variation in renal function, with relative retention of both water and solute by night. Normal adults excrete between 1 and 2 litres of urine in 24 h, of which 60 to 80 per cent is passed by day. This diurnal rhythm may be abolished or even reversed in oedematous states, in chronic renal disease, malabsorption, adrenal insufficiency, and in some cases after head injury or renal transplantation. It is therefore sometimes useful to record day and night urine volumes separately.

Polyuria, arbitrarily defined as a regular urine volume in excess of 3 l/24 h, is most commonly caused by a high fluid intake, but is also a feature of the glycosuria of diabetes mellitus and renal failure. Less common causes include diabetes insipidus of cranial or nephrogenic origin and hypokalaemia and hypercalcaemia. Patients suffering from frequency of micturition may complain of passing excessive amounts of urine, and it is thus important to distinguish true polyuria from frequency in such cases.

Nocturia may be defined as the passing of more than one-third of the total 24-h urine volume by night. This symptom must also be distinguished from nocturnal frequency, with which it is often confused.

Oliguria is traditionally defined as the production by an adult of less than 400 ml of urine/24 h.

Urinalysis and urine microscopy

These simple procedures often give the first clue to the presence of renal disease and their value, too often neglected, cannot be overemphasized.

SAMPLE COLLECTION

A reliable midstream urine sample can be collected from males after retraction of the foreskin, and from females with the labia separated by their fingers. Ideally the genitalia should be swabbed with sterile saline but this is often impracticable. Antiseptics should be avoided if a sample is required for culture. The patient should have a full bladder and should collect the midstream specimen by moving the container in and out of a free-flowing stream.

Suprapubic bladder puncture, a well-accepted and safe procedure in infants and young children, is perhaps under utilized in the investigation of adult patients when it is difficult to obtain uncontaminated midstream specimens. The bladder should be sufficiently full to be palpable in the slim adult and dull to percussion well above the pubes in the obese. If there is any doubt, a potent diuretic should be given to fill the bladder before aspiration. No local anaesthetic is needed; the urine is aspirated through a thin, preferably all-metal, needle. Such bladder samples are free of vulval contamination and therefore allow more precise interpretation of findings on microscopy and culture.

Diagnostic catheterization should be reserved for the infirm from whom midstream or bladder puncture specimens cannot be obtained. The risk of introducing infection is reduced by instilling 120 ml of 0.2 per cent neomycin after taking the diagnostic sample of urine, before withdrawing the catheter.

The urine sample must be sent promptly to the laboratory to avoid growth of contaminant organisms and the dissolution of cellular elements and casts. It should be cooled in a refrigerator at 4 °C if the delay is likely to be greater than 2 h.

Urinalysis

The versatile dipstick is the only method in common use today. We refer to one widely used variety (Ames' Labstix®, Multistix®, etc.) for which there are several commercial alternatives available.

PROTEIN

The detector square contains the indicators methyl red and bromophenol blue, with buffering salts. When the latter dissolve on contact with urine they stabilize the pH of the paper at a level which keeps the colour of the indicators a pale yellow-green. Protein in the urine lowers the pH at which the indicators change colour, so the detector becomes progressively more deeply green in response to increasing protein concentrations. The test is particularly sensitive to albumin, which is the main constituent of most pathological proteinurias, but is insensitive to low molecular weight proteins (for example, Bence Jones proteins). The protein content of the urine of normal individuals can rise to about 150 mg/l when the urine is concentrated, a figure sufficient to give a trace positive result with the dipstick.

False positive results can occur with very alkaline urine, for example during infection with urea-splitting organisms. There is considerable observer error when poorly trained hospital staff use the dipstick as a semiquantitative test of proteinuria, but patients taught to test their own urine (for relapsing nephrotic syndrome) become adept at detecting the onset of proteinuria. Doubtful positive tests, and those in alkaline urine, should be checked with 25 per cent sulphosalicylic acid, which is a little less sensitive.

In view of the influence of diurnal variations in urinary concentration and the effects of posture (see below) on the detection of proteinuria by urinalysis, it is of great importance that any suspected abnormality be further investigated by measuring the total protein excretion in a carefully timed 24-h urine collection. The upper limit of normal on this test is generally taken to be 150 mg, of which up to half is Tamm–Horsfall mucoprotein and less than 30 mg is albumin, the remainder being mainly unidentified low molecular weight proteins. Levels of proteinuria above this amount nearly always indicate significant renal parenchymal disease and require further investigation.

Benign proteinuria
Postural

Three to five per cent of young adults, males more commonly than females, are found to have abnormal proteinuria when up and about, but not after a period of horizontal rest. Standing in a position of exaggerated lordosis can induce significant proteinuria in a substantial proportion of people who do not otherwise show it. These findings do not imply the presence of renal disease and do not require further investigation.

Functional

Abnormal proteinuria can also be observed in subjects without renal disease after severe exercise, in fever, or on exposure to extremes of heat or cold. Patients with cardiac failure may also have proteinuria without renal disease. After prolonged severe exercise, proteinuria, cystinuria, and microscopic haematuria may persist for as long as 24 h.

Microalbuminuria

Interest has recently been focused on the significance of minimally elevated rates of urinary albumin excretion that fall below the level at which a convincing positive reaction is obtained by dipstick. This so-called 'microalbuminuria', which is quantitated by a sensitive radioimmunoassay, corresponds to albumin excretion rates in the range 20 to 200 μg/min (approximately 30 to 300 mg/day), and has been found to be a useful early marker of the development of diabetic glomerular disease and carries potential prognostic and therapeutic significance (Chapter 11.11). A qualitative test kit for detection of these low levels of urinary albumin is now available (Ames' Micro-Bumintest®).

BLOOD

The detector in the stick turns green in the presence of very low concentrations of haem pigments, either haemoglobin or myoglobin. Haematuria is usually accompanied by lysis of some red cells and therefore commonly produces uniform colour change, reflecting positive haemoglobin. Scanty intact red cells produce small green spots by lysis on contact with the detector. The chemical test should always be complemented by microscopy to detect minimal haematuria, and its absence when the stick test is clearly positive should raise the possibility of myoglobinuria.

DEXTROSE

The test square contains glucose oxidase and is specific for dextrose. Although the colour depth is semiquantitative, it is not sufficiently accurate for assessment of the degree of glycosuria. Renal glycosuria may occur during pregnancy, in association with heavy proteinuria, and in renal tubular disorders such as the Fanconi syndrome. Glycosuria due to hyperglycaemia may rarely reflect rapid gastrointestinal absorption of large glucose heads, and transient glycosuria and hyperglycaemia may be associated with cerebrovascular events involving the floor of the fourth ventricle.

URINE pH

Random urine pH readings are of little diagnostic value. The pH detector square is useful in detecting infection with urea-splitting organisms, which raise urine pH to 8 or above, in alerting the observer to false positive tests for proteinuria, and in ensuring that the urine is being kept alkaline in patients with salicylate poisoning, uric acid calculi, cystinuria, and urinary infection during treatment with aminoglycosides.

NITRATE

An extended dipstick (N-multistix®, Ames) or a separate commercial stick can be used to detect nitrates. Most Gram-negative organisms reduce nitrates to nitrites and produce a red colour in the reagent square. False negative tests are common (about 30 per cent), partly because some patients do not excrete sufficient nitrate and partly because of non-nitrate-reducing bacteria. However, the test has some use in giving immediate confirmation of urinary infection and in screening large populations. Its low cost compensates for a detection rate well below 100 per cent.

LEUCOCYTES

Dipsticks that detect significant pyuria depend on the release of esterases. They give results in close accord with quantitative microscopy but it is important to observe the required 2-min wait before the result can be read; all other detectors can be read within 1 min.

Urine microscopy

Together with detection of protein and blood in the urine, the careful examination of the urine sediment is of the utmost importance in deciding whether the patient has renal disease, either primary or associated with a systemic illness. The urine sample should be fresh. If this is not possible, a trace of formalin will preserve cells and casts while boric acid (0.5 g/30 ml of urine) will also inhibit bacterial growth while maintaining viability of cellular components, allowing both microscopy and culture after a delay of some hours.

The commonest indication for urine microscopy is in the diagnosis of acute urinary infection. It can be performed by the doctor in the clinic or from the bedside when time is at a premium. A drop of urine under a coverslip can be examined under high power ($\times$40 objective) within about 1 minute, since the answer is usually obvious (Fig. 1). The heavy pyuria, often accompanied by some haematuria and visible bacilluria, is readily distinguishable from normal urine without quantitative tests. When the answer is not so clear-cut, the unspun urine may be examined in a counting chamber and the findings expressed quantitatively.

If renal disease is suspected, a centrifuged urine should be examined. The Kova® system (Boehringer, Mannheim) facilitates recognition of formed elements and gives quantitative results if the urine is a timed specimen. Urine, 12 ml, is spun for 2 to 5 min at 2000 to 3000 r.p.m. in a disposable tube. A bulbous pipette is pushed down the tube to isolate the lowest 1 ml, and the supernatant is poured off. One drop of stain is mixed with the remaining 1 ml. A drop is placed in a disposable plastic

Fig. 1 Pus cells, red cells, and bacteria in an unspun urine sample from a patient with an acute urinary infection. (High power.)

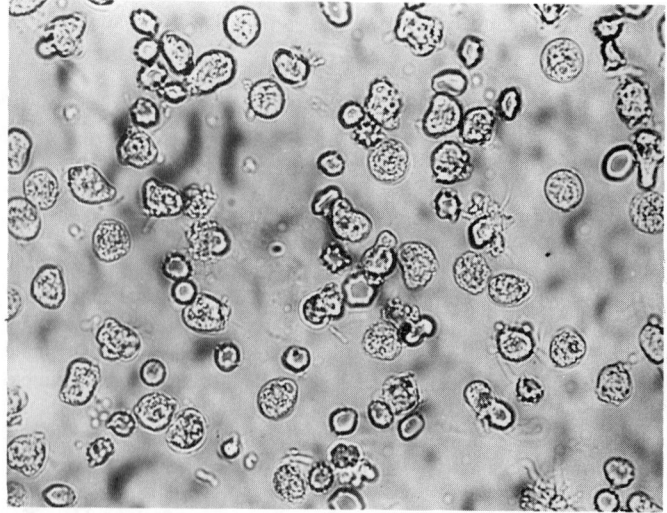

slide with built-in coverslip and counting chamber. Experienced microscopists can obtain much the same information from a qualitative examination of an unstained sediment. A thick, uncovered drop is scanned for casts then a coverslip is added and the high power used to distinguish cells, bacilli, yeasts, and trichomonads. Illumination is kept down by lowering the condenser and closing the diaphragm. Phase contrast is necessary for the study of red cell morphology (see below). Polarized light for urinary lipids and crystals is rarely of diagnostic importance.

WHITE CELLS

In the uncentrifuged urine, less than 3 leucocytes/ml is normal; 3 to 10, of doubtful significance; and greater than 10, abnormal. However, these figures only apply to well-taken midstream samples, free of gross vulval contamination, which can be judged by the absence, or scanty presence, of squamous epithelial cells. When squames are numerous, one can only make a guess, from experience, whether the leucocytes are out of proportion to the squames; there is little point in expressing this guess quantitatively; the best solution is to obtain a cleaner sample. It is abnormal to find any leucocytes in a bladder-puncture sample.

Not all pyuria is due to infection, nor is bacteriuria always accompanied by pyuria; the causes of a dissociation between the two are summarized in Table 1.

RED CELLS

Although there are a few red cells in normal urine, if there are enough to produce any count in unspun urine they are almost certainly pathological. There is considerable observer error in detecting slight haematuria; scanty red cells are often confused with small oxalate crystals, yeasts, and small air bubbles. Their presence should always be confirmed under high power, when a count of greater than 2000 red cells/ml is probably abnormal.

There has been considerable interest over the past decade in using the morphology of red cells excreted into the urine as a guide to the origin of abnormal bleeding within the urinary tract. Using phase-contrast microscopy, several authors have reported that the presence of significant numbers of 'dysmorphic' red cells, that is, those showing irregularities of size or shape, membrane spiculation, or crenation, shows good correlation with a glomerular source of bleeding, while red cells that are predominantly normal in morphology are more likely to be of lower urinary tract origin (from the bladder, for example). While the criteria for making predictions on this basis have varied quite widely in reported studies, in general it appears that a cut-off of 80 per cent or more of cells being dysmorphic correlates quite closely with a glomerular source of blood loss, while less than 20 per cent of dysmorphic cells is usually associated with a non-glomerular source.

Several limitations have emerged over recent years in the general utility of this method of diagnosis. It is clear that the technique is observer dependent, making comparison of results between different individuals or centres difficult. Furthermore, when haematuria is heavy the cells tend to be of normal morphology whether the bleeding is of glomerular or lower-tract origin. Finally, it appears that red cell dysmorphism may more precisely reflect a renal rather than a glomerular source of blood loss, since bleeding caused by renal biopsy was found to be of dysmorphic pattern in one study. None the less, in experienced hands this non-invasive technique may provide a useful guide to the next step in evaluation of a patient with haematuria of indeterminate cause.

Casts

These are cylindrical bodies formed in the lumen of the distal tubule, particularly the collecting tubule, where flow and pH are low and osmolality high. Their matrix is formed from Tamm–Horsfall mucoprotein, a viscous glycoprotein with a molecular weight of about 23 000 kDa, which is secreted by the cells lining the distal convoluted tubule. Cells,

Table 1 *Dissociation between bacteriuria and pyuria?*

Bacteriuria without pyuria
　Asymptomatic bacteriuria (covert-bacteruria)
　Contamination
True heavy pyuria without bacteriuria
　Culture inhibited by
　　antibacterial agent
　　specimen contaminated by antiseptic
　　wrong growth conditions for fastidious organisms
　Urinary tuberculosis
　Renal or bladder calculi
　Analgesic nephropathy
　Chemical cystitis, e.g. cyclophosphamide
　Acute glomerulonephritis
　Non-bacterial (e.g. chlamydial) infections of the urethra
True minor pyuria without bacteriuria
　Many chronic renal diseases (e.g. glomerulonephritis,
　　polycystic disease, interstitial nephritis)
False pyuria (not confirmed on bladder puncture)
　Vaginal discharge

cell debris, and other proteins in the tubular lumen may be agglomerated and caught up in the gel to form the different varieties of cast discussed below.

HYALINE CASTS

These consist entirely of Tamm–Horsfall protein. They are the clear, colourless cylinders, close to the refractive index of urine, which are occasionally seen in the urine of normal people, particularly when it is concentrated, or after exercise. Showers of hyaline casts appear in the urine during any febrile illness and after the administration of loop diuretics.

GRANULAR CASTS

The granules in these casts are formed from disintegrated cells or from aggregated serum proteins; immunofluorescence studies have identified albumin, lipoproteins, and immunoglobulins in the granules. It is therefore surprising that they are not seen more often with the heavy proteinuria of nephrotic syndrome due to minimal change nephropathy.

Finely granulated casts (Fig. 2) occur in much the same situations as hyaline casts and have similar significance. They are found with hyaline casts in the urine of normal subjects after exercise. Densely granular

Fig. 2 A finely granular cast surrounded by red cells. (High power.)

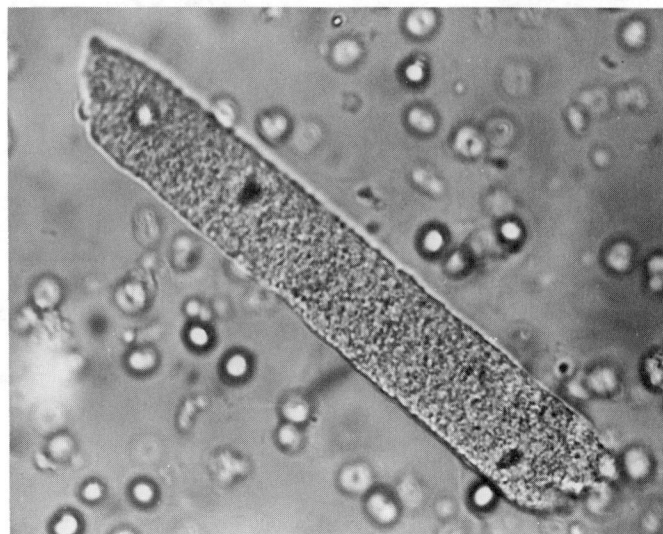

casts (Fig. 3) are always pathological. When the granules are very coarse they are often misidentified as red cell casts. They are found in many types of renal disease but are particularly characteristic of chronic proliferative or membranous glomerulonephritis, diabetic nephropathy, and amyloidosis.

FATTY CASTS

These are composed of highly refractile fat globules of varying size, some of which may be mistaken for red cells. They are often accompanied by oval fat bodies which are epithelial cells stuffed full of fat granules, and by the presence of free fat globules in the urine; they are most commonly seen when there is moderate to heavy proteinuria. Such a sediment when viewed with polarized light reveals the classical 'Maltese crosses' that are thought to be due to cholesterol esters.

RED CELL CASTS

These are pathognomonic of glomerular bleeding. The cells may be densely packed (Fig. 4) and appear red but more commonly a few cells are trapped in a hyaline or granular cast (Fig. 5); when the cells degenerate, a rusty coloured granular cast is formed, called a haemoglobin cast. Commonly seen in large numbers at the height of an attack of acute nephritis, they may be found in any condition in which there is a continuing glomerulonephritis or vasculitis. They may be found in malignant hypertension, in company with red cells and granular casts.

Scanty red cell casts and granular casts are found in association with microscopic haematuria in several forms of focal proliferative glomerulonephritis. The discovery of even one red cell cast is of great diagnostic value, indicating a renal cause for the haematuria. A thorough search of the deposit from several concentrated urine samples is well worth undertaking and may be supplemented by the examination of a urine filtrate, which is stained and examined on the filter paper.

WHITE CELL CASTS

White cell casts are relatively rare but may appear in considerable numbers during an episode of acute pyelonephritis. A few may be found in the urine in chronic pyelonephritis, and their numbers may increase if the patient develops a pyrexia for any cause. Sheets of leucocytes, or leucocytes clumped around other objects in the urine, may be mistaken for white cell casts.

Fig. 3 A densely granular cast. (High power.)

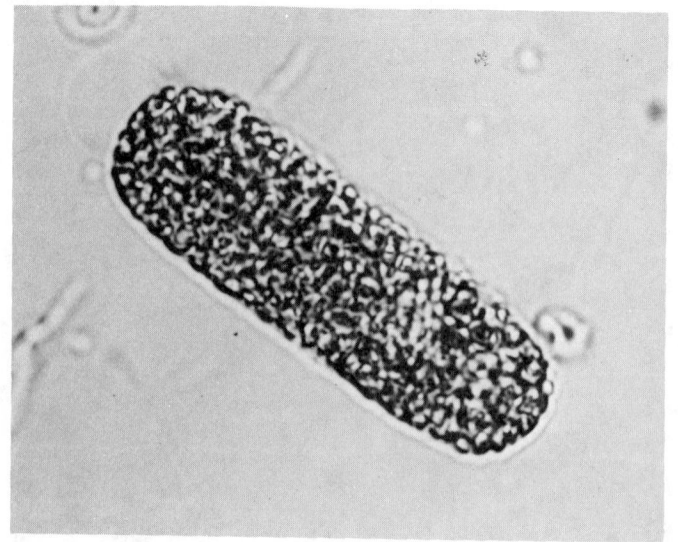

Fig. 4 A red cell cast from the urinary deposit of a patient with acute glomerulonephritis. (High power.)

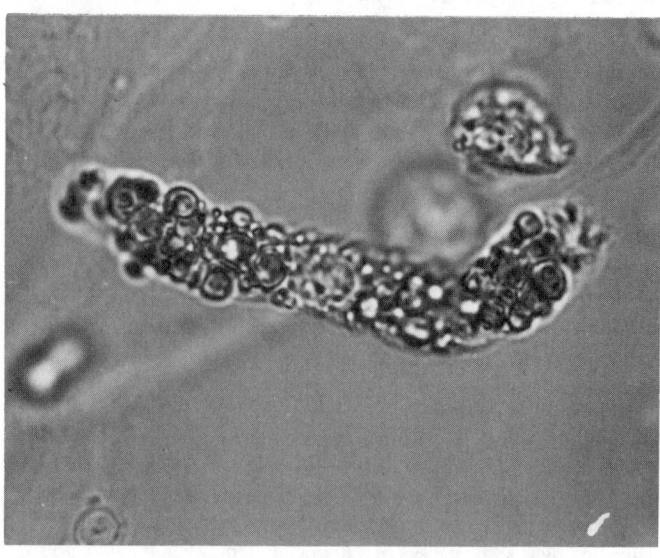

Fig. 5 One end of a cast predominantly hyaline but with a few red cells enmeshed in it. (High power.) Diagnostically this ranks as a red cell cast.

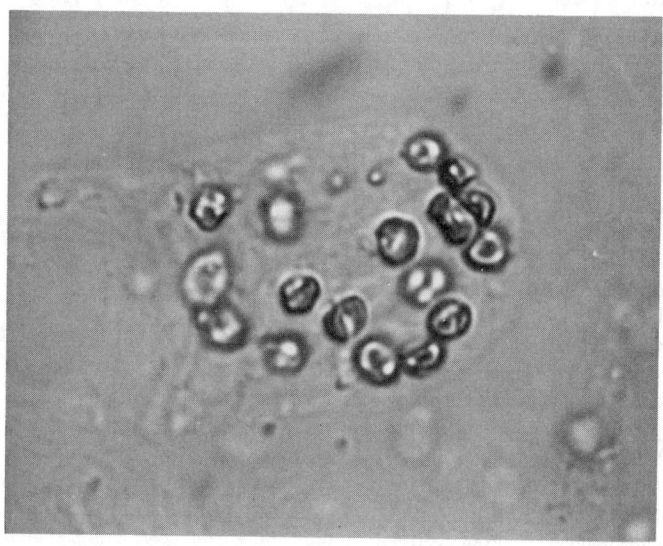

Fig. 6 Crystals of cystine in the urinary deposit of a patient with cystinuria and calculi. (High power.)

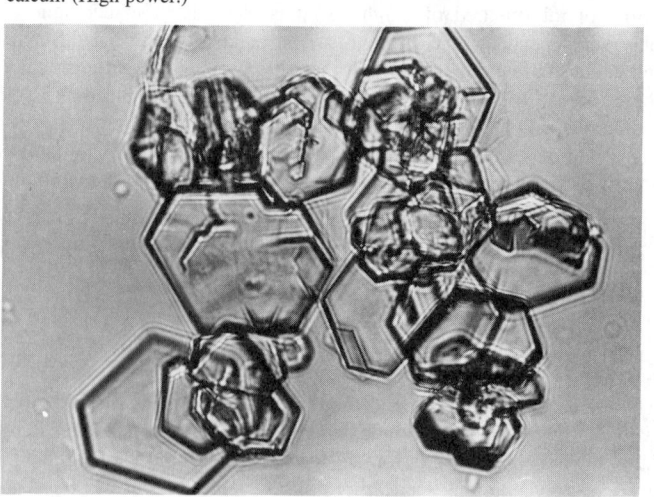

EPITHELIAL CELL CASTS

Casts with a regular arrangement of epithelial cells, suggesting that the epithelium has been shed in one piece, are found in the urine of patients with acute tubular necrosis or the more acute forms of glomerulonephritis. A commoner phenomenon is a hyaline or finely granular cast with one or two epithelial cells attached; these are seen in many forms of chronic renal disease.

TRANSITIONAL EPITHELIAL CELLS

These are smaller than vulvar squames and of a more uniform, oval shape. They are seen in small numbers in normal urine and are sometimes plentiful in the presence of urinary infection. Clumps of transitional cells, often with bizarre nuclei, are found in the urine of patients with bladder cancer or papilloma; they give a clue to this diagnosis but their absence does not exclude it. When there is reason to suspect cancer of the urinary tract, formal cytology and other appropriate investigations are required.

CRYSTALS

Cystine crystals (Fig. 6) may be found in freshly passed urine but are found more consistently if a concentrated sample is acidified and cooled in a refrigerator; their presence is diagnostic of cystinuria. Oxalate crystals (Fig. 7) are common in urine from normal individuals when it has stood for an hour or two. When present in freshly passed urine, in large numbers or in aggregates, they may indicate an increased liability to form oxalate stones, but firm conclusions can only be drawn if the urine is kept at 37 °C until examined on a warm-stage microscope.

It must be emphasized that although urinalysis and urine microscopy yield valuable information, it is possible for significant renal disease to be present without anything abnormal being detected in the urine.

REFERENCES

Damsgard, E.M., Frolaud, A., Jorgensen, O.D., and Mogensen, C.E. (1990). Microalbuminuria as a predictor of increased mortality in elderly people. *British Medical Journal* **300**, 297–300.

Fairley, K.F. and Birch, D.F. (1982). Haematuria: A simple method for identifying glomerular bleeding. *Kidney International* **71**, 105–8.

Mogensen, C.E. and Christensen, C.K. (1984). Predicting diabetic nephropathy in insulin-dependent diabetic patients. *New England Journal of Medicine* **311**, 89–93.

Pollock, C., *et al.* Dysmorphism of urinary red blood cells – Value in diagnosis. *Kidney International* **36**, 1045–9.

Fig. 7 Oxalate crystals, sketched from a urinary deposit.

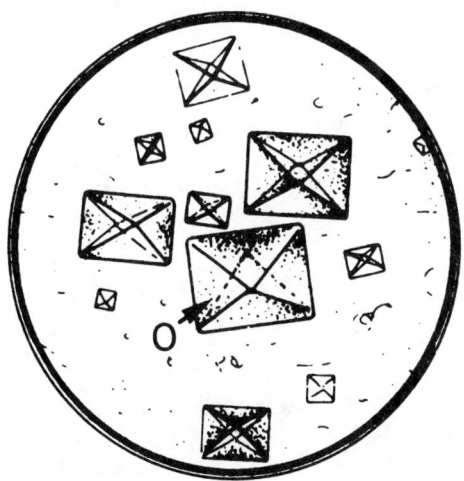

Estimation of glomerular filtration rate

Inulin clearance

The glomerular filtration rate can be measured accurately using a substance that is completely filtered at the glomerulus, not secreted or reabsorbed in the renal tubule, stable in urine, and readily measured. The traditional choice has been inulin, a polymer of fructose with a molecular weight of about 5200 Da. A wealth of investigation has confirmed its physiological suitability, but it has several disadvantages. It is poorly soluble and so must be dissolved by heating, which may partly hydrolyse it to fructose; it activates complement when injected, though no harm to patients has yet been reported; the chemical estimation is tedious and poorly reproducible in inexpert hands. Consequently, it is the gold standard against which all other methods are measured but it is seldom employed in clinical practice. A more soluble and homogenous analogue, polyfructosan-S (molecular weight about 2700 Da), and ^{14}C-labelled inulin are available and offer advantages over the parent compound but have never become popular.

The glomerular filtration rate is measured by infusing inulin intravenously at a constant rate until it is evenly distributed in the extracellular space and the plasma concentration is almost steady, typically after 90 to 120 min. The glomerular filtration rate is then equal to the renal clearance of inulin, defined as:

$$\text{Clearance} = \text{Urinary excretion rate/Plasma concentration} = UV/P$$

where U and P are the inulin concentrations in urine and plasma and V is the urinary flow rate. To measure this flow rate it is necessary to induce a moderate diuresis by regular administration of fluid before and during the test. The patient is asked to void several timed urine samples and blood is taken at the beginning and end of each. Catheterization is necessary if there is doubt about the patient's ability to empty the bladder completely, and is one of the unattractive features of the test.

Since the extrarenal clearance of inulin is very low (about 2 ml/min) urinary excretion is virtually equal to infusion rate once a steady state has been achieved. Consequently, the glomerular filtration rate can be calculated from the infusion rate and the plasma concentration. This method is preferred in children and others who have difficulty with complete bladder emptying. However, the infusion period must be prolonged to ensure complete stability of the plasma level; unlike the classical method it cannot be corrected for a slowly changing plasma level. A infusion lasting 3 h is sufficient in most patients.

Clearance of DTPA and other radiopharmaceuticals

The problem of measuring inulin can be circumvented by substituting a radioactive substance with similar properties. The two agents most extensively studied are the radiolabelled metal chelates, [^{51}Cr]EDTA (ethylenediaminetetraacetic acid) and [[99]Tc[m]]DTPA (diethylenetriaminepentaacetic acid). Several comparisons have shown that both agents correlate closely with inulin clearance, although both EDTA and DTPA clearance slightly underestimate the glomerular filtration rate using single-injection or continuous-infusion techniques. Currently the simplicity and ready availability of DTPA-labelling kits, in combination with the physical properties of [99]Tc[m], which also allow imaging of the kidneys, makes [[99]Tc[m]]DTPA the radiopharmaceutical of choice when accurate measurement of glomerular filtration rate is required.

These radiopharmaceuticals can be substituted for inulin in the standard infusion test, with timed urine samples, with the added advantage that an external count over the bladder confirms complete voiding. They can also be used in the constant-infusion technique without urine collection, or can be given by a single injection followed by timed plasma and urine samples over the exponential phase of the plasma activity curve. However, these techniques are seldom used outside research laboratories.

The usual method provided for routine hospital use is single intravenous injection followed by timed plasma samples. Plasma radioactivity falls steeply initially, reflecting diffusion into the extracellular space. An exponential fall follows from about 2 h postinjection. The slope of this part of the line is determined by the glomerular filtration rate plus extrarenal clearance. The latter term is usually ignored since it is small and fairly constant. The glomerular filtration rate is calculated by multiplying the slope of the exponential part of the curve by the volume of distribution, which is calculated by dividing the injected dose by the plasma activity at zero time.

Three blood samples are drawn at intervals determined by the expected result, judged from plasma creatinine. If renal function is close to normal, samples are drawn at 2, 3, and 4 h; if it is thought to be between 30 and 60 per cent of normal, at 2, 4, and 6 h; if renal function is below 30 per cent of normal, at 3, 6, 9, and 12 h. The test becomes unreliable, if the patient is oedematous.

Clearance of DTPA and other radiopharmaceuticals is most reliably measured when renal function is normal or moderately reduced. It then has a reproducibility of about ±5 per cent, which is adequate for clinical purposes since the glomerular filtration rate has a circadian rhythm, varying by about 10 per cent between its peak in mid-afternoon and its trough during the night, and is disturbed by emotion or exercise. DTPA clearance is therefore used to confirm the normality of renal function in patients with isolated proteinuria or haematuria, or other minor abnormalities which interfere in employment, superannuation, and insurance, and in the selection of kidney donors. It is measured repeatedly to assess the results of such procedures as surgery for obstruction or drug therapy for glomerulonephritis, and to plot the progress of renal diseases to provide prognosis, or when treatment with undesirable side-effects is to be given only in the presence of declining function.

In late renal failure the test is inaccurate and is decreasingly reliable as the glomerular filtration rate declines because the extrarenal clearance assumes greater importance and the error in calculating the slope increases as it approaches the horizontal. At this stage in renal disease clinicians are forced to rely on measurement of plasma creatinine, despite the limitations discussed below.

Endogenous creatinine clearance

Creatinine is a breakdown product of skeletal muscle metabolism, and maintains a nearly constant plasma concentration, proportional to the total body muscle mass, throughout 24 hours. Since under normal conditions it undergoes minimal transport along the renal tubular system, its excretion is largely determined by glomerular filtration, and thus the glomerular filtration rate can be estimated by determining the endogenous creatinine clearance rate. This approach has the advantage over the more precise methods listed above that no intravenous infusion of a test substance is required. However, it is important to recognize that the accuracy of creatinine clearance as a measure of the glomerular filtration rate is limited in situations of renal impairment, since tubular secretion of creatinine becomes more significant under these conditions, leading to systematic overestimation of the glomerular filtration rate.

In practical terms, the procedure involves collection of a precisely timed specimen of urine, with the drawing of a blood sample at some time during this period. While collection periods as short as 1 hour may be employed, greater accuracy is obtained using a 12- or 24-h interval. Regrettably, even with good supervision in hospital, there is a high rate of error in the completeness of urine collection, leading to poor reproducibility (around ± 20 per cent) of the resulting clearance calculation. For this reason, the popularity of the clearance protocol has declined over recent years, especially since it has been shown that it gives no better an estimate of the glomerular filtration rate than calculation from the plasma creatinine (see below), except where this calculation itself is prone to error (states of muscle atrophy and wasting, oedema, obesity, and pregnancy).

Interpretation of plasma creatinine

Since the production of endogenous creatinine remains constant (in the absence of rapid changes in body muscle mass), the daily excretion rate of creatinine, given by the product UV in the clearance formula, is also a constant for a given individual with stable renal function. It follows that the relationship between the creatinine clearance, as an estimate of the glomerular filtration rate, and the plasma creatinine concentration will be a rectangular hyperbola, of the form shown in Fig. 8.

Two important consequences arise from consideration of this relationship. First, it is evident that very small changes in plasma creatinine concentration in the low (normal) range where the hyperbolic curve is steepest, imply, for a given individual, very significant changes in glomerular filtration rate. This makes the test very powerful as a sensitive indicator of early renal impairment, although the impact of laboratory error in this range is also proportionally greater. Secondly, it is clear that individuals with differing muscle mass will fall along different hyperbolic curves (see Fig. 8). This means that the interpretation of a given plasma creatinine result must be made in relation to a particular patient; for example, a value of 0.1 mmol/l might reflect a normal glomerular filtration rate in a well-built young man, but would indicate significant renal impairment in a frail elderly woman.

Since age and sex are the principal factors known to determine the relative proportion of body weight attributable to muscle (in the absence of gross obesity, oedema, or wasting), it has been possible to devise empirical formulae that relate creatinine clearance to plasma creatinine and body weight, taking into account the age and sex of the subject. Several refinements of the relations originally published by Cockcroft and Gault (1976) have been reported, and a well-validated set is given in Table 2. Such formulae are in widespread use, and are most reliable when the glomerular filtration rate is moderately reduced, when they provide a quick guide to modification of dosing with nephrotoxic or renally excreted drugs. However, it must be remembered that the calculation assumes constant renal function and the result can be misleading if the patient has suffered a recent depression of glomerular filtration rate from acute illness.

The best-established use for the plasma creatinine is in following the course of renal failure in individual patients in whom a reliable baseline assessment of renal function has previously been made. The production of creatinine remains fairly constant as renal disease advances, until the terminal stage when anorexia, nausea, and vomiting lead to

Fig. 8 Compound graph showing theoretical relationship between plasma creatinine concentration and creatinine clearance for three subjects of differing muscle mass, with creatinine excretion rates (UV) of 14, 10, and 6 mmol/day.

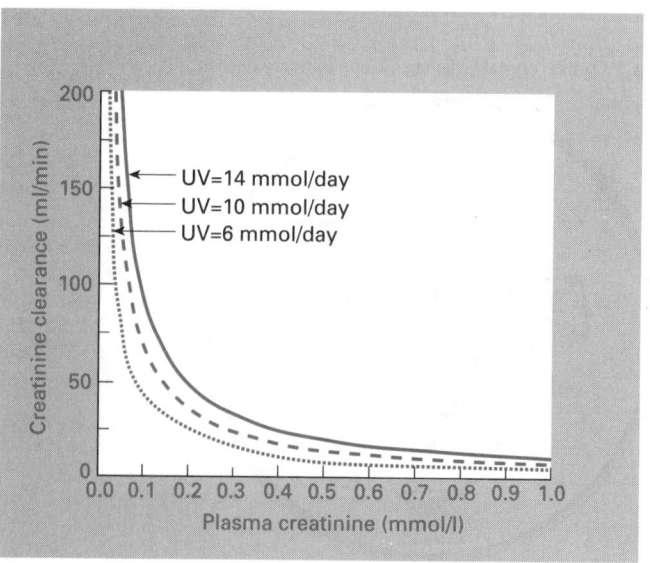

Table 2 *Formulae for calculating creatinine clearance from serum or plasma creatinine*

Males
Creatinine clearance in ml/min per 70 kg

$$= \frac{(145 - \text{age in years})}{(\text{serum creatinine in mg/dl})} - 3$$

$$= \frac{(88(145 - \text{age in years}))}{(\text{serum creatinine in } \mu\text{mol/l})} - 3.$$

Females
Creatinine clearance in ml/min per 70 kg

$$= \frac{(0.85(145 - \text{age in years}))}{(\text{serum creatinine in mg/dl})} - 3$$

$$= \frac{(75(145 - \text{age in years}))}{(\text{serum creatinine in } \mu\text{mol/l})} - 3$$

Note: These formulae and all others studied by Hull *et al.* (1981) are inaccurate in the presence of liver disease.

(Source: Hull, J.H. *et al.* (1981).)

loss of muscle mass. Consequently, a plot of the plasma creatinine against time gives a good indication of changing glomerular filtration rate in most patients, although in some individuals the expected rise in creatinine does not occur, presumably because of unusually rapid secretion by the tubules. Since the fall in glomerular filtration rate is frequently linear over time in the absence of intercurrent illness, it is sometimes valuable to plot the reciprocal of a patient's plasma creatinine versus time, which yields a declining straight-line relation. In selected cases, it may be possible, by extrapolating this plot, to obtain a rough forecast of when end-stage renal failure requiring haemodialysis will supervene.

REFERENCES

Cockcroft, D.W. and Gault, M.H. (1976). Prediction of creatinine clearance from serum creatinine. *Nephron* **16**, 31.

Hull, J.H., Hak, L.J., Koch, G.G., Wargin, W.A., Chi, S.L., and Mattocks, A.M. (1981). Influence of range of renal function and liver disease on predictability of creatinine clearance. *Clinical Pharmacology and Therapeutics* **29**, 516.

Interpretation of plasma urea

Prior to the widespread availability of reliable assays of creatinine, the plasma urea concentration was frequently used as the principal biochemical indicator of reduced glomerular filtration rate. This was based on the understanding that plasma urea varied reciprocally with the glomerular filtration rate, since the renal clearance of urea could be considered a relatively fixed fraction (approximately one-half) of the simultaneously determined inulin clearance.

There are two basic reasons why urea, when used alone, is an unsatisfactory marker of the filtration rate. First, its clearance is not in fact a constant fraction of the glomerular filtration rate, but varies with the urine flow rate, from less than 40 per cent of the glomerular filtration rate at low flows to 60 per cent or more during diuresis induced by vigorous hydration. Secondly, a number of other (non-renal) factors, relating to the prevailing metabolic state, affect urea production rate within the liver, and these must be taken into account in interpreting the plasma urea concentration. Thus, catabolic states such as infection, trauma or burns, or therapy with corticosteroids or tetracyclines will elevate the plasma urea, as will a high dietary intake of protein, or bleeding into the gut. Conversely, when urea synthesis is low, such as during periods of low dietary protein intake, or in advanced liver disease, plasma urea will be low without necessarily implying good renal function.

Current practice in most centres is to take advantage of the simultaneous knowledge of plasma concentrations of both urea and creatinine,

Table 3 *Diagnostic significance of differential changes in plasma urea and creatinine*

Plasma urea raised out of proportion to plasma creatinine
  Sodium and water depletion
  Heart failure
  Gastrointestinal haemorrhage
  High protein intake (oral or intravenous) in the presence of renal disease
  Protein catabolism
    corticosteroid therapy
    tetracycline in overdose or in presence of renal disease
  Following trauma
  Pure water depletion (modest effect)
Plasma creatinine raised out of proportion to plasma urea
  Some cases of rhabdomyolysis
  Drugs that block creatinine secretion (aspirin, cotrimoxazole) or increase creatinine production (penacemide): (modest effect)
Plasma urea depressed out of proportion to plasma creatinine
  Pregnancy
  Liver failure
  High fluid intake
  Low protein diet
Plasma urea and creatinine raised in parallel
  Chronic renal failure
  Established acute renal failure

thereby gaining diagnostic clues as to the possible contributing factors involved in any apparent disturbance of glomerular filtration rate. Some illustrations of the interpretation of differential changes of these two markers are given in Table 3.

Estimation of the glomerular filtration rate from plasma β_2-microglobulin

β_2-Microglobulin is a low molecular weight protein of about 11 800 Da which is a surface constituent of most cells, representing the constant zone of HLA antigens. It is filtered at the glomerulus, reabsorbed almost completely in the renal tubule but catabolized in the process. It is produced at a nearly constant rate, unaffected by diet, so that its plasma concentration reflects the glomerular filtration rate; its plasma concentration rises with age as the glomerular filtration rate declines, since its production rate does not fall, like that of creatinine, with declining muscle mass. Plasma β_2-microglobulin is raised, probably as a result of overproduction, in some malignant, immunological, and hepatic diseases; in the absence of these it is probably a better guide to changes in the glomerular filtration rate than is plasma creatinine, but is unlikely to replace the latter in clinical practice since its radioimmunoassay is far more tedious and expensive than is the automated chemical test for creatinine.

There are perhaps two situations in which the extra expense of measuring plasma β_2-microglobulin is justified, where it is available. It is a more sensitive indicator of a slight fall in glomerular filtration rate than is plasma creatinine, for example in monitoring nephrotoxic drug therapy, or detecting the onset of transplant rejection or diabetic nephropathy. It can also be used as an index of the glomerular filtration rate in terminal renal failure, when measured serially, superior perhaps to measurement of plasma creatinine, which is seriously affected by variable tubular secretion in this situation.

Estimation of renal plasma flow

Renal plasma flow is more subject to variation with physical or emotional stress than is the glomerular filtration rate but it has a similar and parallel circadian rhythm. Its measurement is an important research investigation but it is seldom requested in clinical medicine.

Estimation of renal plasma flow from clearance of p-aminohippurate

Renal plasma flow can be measured using an agent that is completely removed from plasma in one passage through the kidney by a combination of glomerular filtration and tubular secretion. *p*-Aminohippurate (**PAH**) approaches this ideal since about 92 per cent of plasma PAH is removed by the time it reaches the renal vein, in healthy subjects. It diffuses rapidly through its volume of distribution and a steady plasma level can be achieved more quickly than with inulin. PAH clearance is therefore a convenient and reliable test of renal plasma flow for physiological studies. The result is corrected by assuming that the test subject has the usual 92 per cent extraction rate and is converted to renal blood flow on the assumption that the haematocrit in the kidney is the same as that in the peripheral blood (an approximation to the truth).

In renal disease the extraction of PAH during one passage through the kidney falls substantially and unpredictably so it is necessary to measure renal vein PAH concentration by cannulating the renal vein with a Seldinger catheter, rendering the test unsuitable for routine use.

Estimation of renal plasma flow by radiohippurate clearance

Hippurate (hippuran) has a slightly lower extraction rate on single passage through the kidney than PAH and has the same limitation that its extraction rate falls in the presence of renal disease. In other respects it is a suitable agent for measuring renal plasma flow and can be labelled with any of the radioisotopes of iodine. It can then be used by the single shot technique on the same principles as in measuring glomerular filtration rate by DTPA clearance. Simultaneous administration of the two agents, labelled with different isotopes, permits simultaneous measurement of glomerular filtration rate and renal blood flow, and therefore the calculation of filtration fraction (the proportion of blood perfusing the kidney which passes into the glomerular filtrate). The crude ratio 'clearance of DTPA or iothalamate/hippurate clearance is often referred to as the filtration fraction, no account being taken of the unknown extraction rate for hippurate in the patient. This misnomer should be avoided, but the crude ratio may have some diagnostic value, for example in the detection of transplant rejection, which causes a high ratio (high 'filtration fraction').

CORRECTION FOR BODY SIZE

Both the 'glomerular filtration' rate and the renal plasma flow are determined by body size, and in the adult they correlate better with surface area than with other measures of body size such as height or weight. Consequently they are often expressed per 1.73 m², calculated as: actual clearance × 1.73/surface area in m². Surface area is estimated from height and weight by the nomogram in *Documenta Geigy*. Since 1.73 m² is an out-of-date mean size in a population that is growing larger, it would be more logical to express the results per m², and this practice is gaining ground.

Measurement of tubular functions (see also Section 20.19)

Overview of tubular dysfunction

A number of renal diseases involve, initially or predominantly, the tubulo-interstitial structures rather than the glomeruli, and these may present with, or be complicated by, physiological disturbances in function of the various tubular epithelia within the nephron. Furthermore, a number of inherited disorders of metabolism or transport may manifest with quite specific abnormalities in tubular function some time before overall filtration function is impaired. In what follows, an approach will be given to the evaluation of representative disorders affecting both the proximal and the distal segments of the tubular system.

It is often useful in pathophysiological conditions to have a means of assessing the overall state of renal tubular handling of a filtered solute whose normal pattern of tubular transport is known. A useful concept in this context is the fractional excretion (FE) of the substance, defined as the fraction of the filtered load of the solute which is excreted in the urine, expressed as a percentage. In mathematical terms, this can be expressed for freely filtered solutes as follows:

$$\text{FE of substance x} = (\text{excreted x})/(\text{filtered x}) \times 100\%$$
$$= (U_x V)/P_{P_x}\text{GFR} \times 100\%,$$

where U_x and P_x are the urine and plasma concentrations of x, respectively, GFR is the glomerular filtration rate, and V is the urine flow rate. Since, however, GFR can be estimated as the clearance of endogenous creatinine (cr), this relation can be simplified thus:

$$\text{FE of x} = (U_x V)/(P_x((U_{cr}V)/P_{cr})) \times 100\%$$
$$= (U_x/P_x)/(U_{cr}/P_{cr}) \times 100\%.$$

Expressed in this form, it can be seen that this valuable descriptor of net tubular handling of the substance in question can be calculated simply from the analysis of the concentrations of both x and creatinine in a single sample of urine and plasma obtained at the same time. The term is clearly equivalent to the ratio of the clearance of the substance in question to that of creatinine.

Application of this analysis to the handling of sodium, phosphate, and urate will be referred to where relevant, elsewhere in this section.

Assessment of glycosuria

The approach to the investigation of glycosuria provides a model for the clinical evaluation of overexcretion of a solute that undergoes rate-limited reabsorption in the renal proximal tubule. Similar considerations apply in principle to the handling of phosphate and amino acids, which will not be described further here.

Glucose is freely filtered by the glomerulus and reabsorbed actively by the proximal tubule. Under normal circumstances, reabsorption is complete but if the blood glucose rises sufficiently, a plasma level is reached (the threshold) at which the transport mechanism is saturated (the maximum tubular reabsorption rate, or T_m), and glucose starts to spill into the urine (see Fig. 9). In practice, the moment of saturation is not a sharp end-point, possibly because nephrons vary in length and transporter activity; the gradual slowing in the rate of increase as tubular absorption approaches its maximum is called splay.

With this background, it can be seen that glycosuria could arise in principle in two different ways. First, if the plasma glucose concentration rises above the threshold level (around 10 mmol/l in man) the unreabsorbed glucose will appear in the urine, and this occurs in uncontrolled diabetes mellitus, the commonest clinical cause of glycosuria. Alternatively, if the tubular mechanism for reabsorption is defective (low T_m and hence low threshold), glucose will appear in the urine even when the plasma glucose is within the normal range. This can occur as the result of an inherited abnormality in the protein(s) mediating glucose transport across the proximal tubular cells, or as a consequence of a disease process interfering with the function of this epithelium, as in cystinosis or tubular damage by heavy metals and other toxins.

Finally, it should be noted that the appearance of more than one proximally reabsorbed solute in the urine in significant amounts can generally be taken as a clue to a non-specific cause of proximal tubular damage, while spillover of any one species (or closely related molecules such as the various classes of amino acids) is more likely to reflect a specific defect of a particular transport carrier, and this is more likely to be inherited.

Measurements of urinary concentrating ability

In the course of any chronic renal disease, the tubules of surviving nephrons are exposed to an increased osmotic load, partly because the glomerular filtration rate per nephron is increased and partly because the plasma concentration of solutes such as urea, sulphate, and phosphate is elevated. Consequently, the patient's ability to concentrate the urine declines, even if tubular function is preserved in the remaining nephrons. It is possible to relate urinary concentrating ability to the patient's glomerular filtration rate and to deduce whether the concentrating ability is disproportionately reduced, indicating tubular disease. This test has been advocated for the differentiation of advanced chronic glomerulonephritis from chronic pyelonephritis or analgesic nephropathy (concentrating ability being best preserved in glomerulonephritis and worst affected in analgesic nephropathy). However, the typical ranges for these groups of diseases at each level of renal function have not been defined well enough to make the test of much practical value.

Special precautions are needed if fluid is to be withheld from patients in renal failure. Consequently, concentrating ability is only tested in those patients with normal or nearly normal glomerular filtration rate. The indications for its use are now restricted to a few specific circumstances where isolated distal tubular damage is suspected, for example in monitoring chronic lithium therapy or detecting early analgesic nephropathy.

Maximum concentration is achieved only after all fluids have been withheld for more than 24 h, an uncomfortable test which requires hospital admission to ensure compliance. Consequently it is usual to accept evidence of a submaximal concentrating ability above the lower limit of normal for the patient's age, tested for by three simpler manoeuvres. A few random early morning urine samples are collected and their osmolality tested. If none of these achieves the required level (for example 550 mosmol/kg) the patient is tested by fluid withdrawal or vasopressin (Chapter 12.3).

Fig. 9 Relationship between plasma glucose concentration and glucose transfer rates (filtration, reabsorption, and secretion) during 'titration' of the renal tubules with glucose in man. T_{mG} is the tubular maximal reabsorptive capacity for glucose. Threshold and splay are explained in the text. (Modified from Pitts 1963.)

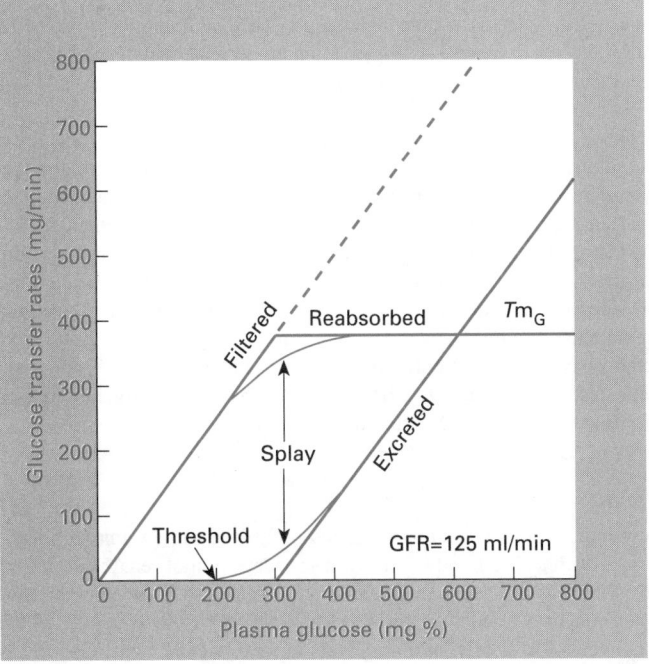

Fluid withdrawal is imposed by ensuring that the patient avoids drinks after 4 p.m., takes a dry supper, and and has no bedtime or morning drinks. The first two urine samples passed after rising are tested. This is a test of both the pituitary's ability to secrete antidiuretic hormone and the kidney's ability to respond.

The vasopressin tests investigate only the response of the kidney. In most countries, desmopressin is given intranasally; 20 μg are instilled into each nostril at 5 p.m. and the last evening and first morning urine samples are tested. The traditional stimulus was 5 units of Pitressin® in oil given intramuscularly at 8 a.m. The ampoule needed to be warmed and shaken before the contents were withdrawn. All urine samples passed over the next 8 h were tested. However, Pitressin® is no longer available in many countries. Fluid intake should be kept low during these tests but total abstention from drinks is not necessary. Normal adults should achieve a urine osmolality of 750 mosmol/kg in one of the samples in these tests. The lower limit of normal falls with age, to reach about 600 in those patients in their 60s. Subjects on a high-fluid intake (for example those with compulsive water drinking) require a more prolonged stimulus before reaching maximum urinary concentration.

Measurement of urinary acidification

This subject is addressed in Chapter 20.19.1.

Urinary enzyme excretion

Enzymuria is usually measured as an early indication of tubular damage during clinical trials of new drugs; during treatment with drugs of known nephrotoxicity (such as aminoglycoside antibiotics, antitumour agents such as cis-platinum); and as an early warning of overexposure to chromates, cadmium, and other industrial toxins. The enzyme chosen should be present in tubular cells and readily released by minor injury. The most popular is N-acetyl-β-glucosaminidase. It is measured on a spot urine taken at a constant time of day, to allow for diurnal fluctuation, and expressed per gram (or millimole) of creatinine, to correct for urinary concentration.

Other causes of enzymuria include: increased glomerular permeability alone (Goodpasture's syndrome) or with raised blood level (pancreatitis); pyuria; and urinary neoplasm. Diagnostic accuracy is increased if isoenzymes are identified by ion-exchange chromatography.

Excretion of small proteins and cellular antigens

An alternative to measuring urinary enzymes is the detection of low molecular weight proteins which are normally filtered by the glomerulus and reabsorbed almost completely by the tubules. Their appearance in urine, if plasma level is not increased, indicates proximal tubular damage. The best studied is urinary β2-microglobulin which is more sensitive than plasma creatinine but less sensitive than urinary N-acetyl-glucosaminidase in detecting early aminoglycoside toxicity.

Assessment of individual renal function, regional function, and renal structure: renal imaging

Plain radiography of the urinary tract

A plain radiograph of the kidneys, ureters, and bladder is an essential preliminary to urography. On this film it is often possible to trace the renal outlines and measure the renal size. If the outlines are obscured by bowel gas, they are often clarified by tomography. The left kidney is normally about 1 cm longer than the right. The length should be recorded in centimetres for comparison with subsequent films, but the normal range is wide (11–16 cm in the adult) so substantial reduction in renal mass must take place before it is possible to say with confidence using this technique that the kidneys are small. In children, the renal length is approximately equal to that of the first four lumbar vertebrae and their intervening discs. The other main function of a plain abdominal film is to detect calcification in the kidneys or radiopaque calculi in the ureters or bladder, which may be obscured in the subsequent pyelogram. Oblique views and films taken in inspiration and expiration may be necessary to confirm that suspected calculi are in kidneys. The film may yield other diagnostic information; gallstones are often detected and renal osteodystrophy or myelomatosis may be recognized in the skeleton.

Excretion urography

SYNONYMS: INTRAVENOUS PYELOGRAPHY; IVP; IVU

The older hyperosmolar contrast media, such as diatrizoate and metrizoate, are now being replaced in many centres by low osmolar, non-ionic compounds such as iopamidol and iohexol. Although the cost is higher, patient comfort is much improved, with elimination of flushing, nausea, vomiting, and headache that often accompanied bolus injection of the older agents. Occasional reactions include hypotension, asthma, urticaria or angioedema, convulsions, and cardiac arrythmia. There appears to be a lower risk from the new molecules, with a fatality rate of 1:75 000 to 1:100 000. Contrast-associated nephropathy is a risk in patients with pre-existing renal failure, diabetes mellitus, and multiple myeloma and is characterized by oliguria and a rise in serum creatinine within 2 days of contrast injection. High-risk patients should be identified if any contrast procedure (including arteriography or computed tomography (CT) scanning) is definitely indicated. Volume depletion should be avoided and adequate hydration ensured. There appears to be a similar incidence of nephrotoxicity with ionic and non-ionic contrast media.

The contrast medium is excreted almost entirely by glomerular filtration. A film at 1 min after injection gives the best view of renal outlines, with contrast concentrated in the tubules (the nephrogram). Later images, from 2.5 to 30 min, often with tomography, will show excretion of contrast into the collecting system (the pyelogram). If calyceal detail is not adequately visible the pelvis and calyces may be distended by applying compression over the lower ureters with an abdominal belt. A film immediately after release of compression will provide detail of ureteric filling. Pre- and postmicturition films of the bladder will provide information on prostatic indentation, space-occupying lesions, and the presence of bladder diverticula and will assess bladder emptying. However, in many centres ultrasound has replaced the IVU for assessment of prostatic volume, bladder capacity, and residual urine volume. Impaired renal function will cause a delayed pyelogram and extra films will need to be taken as late as 12 to 24 h in this situation or in the presence of severe obstruction.

The IVU is clearly the best choice for anatomical detail and filling defects of the collecting system, but it has been largely replaced by ultrasound and CT scanning for the investigation of abnormalities of renal anatomy, and by nuclear renal scanning or angiography for the investigation of renovascular hypertension.

Retrograde pyelography/ureterography

This technique is very useful for determining the site of complete obstruction to a ureter and for visualizing the ureter distal to the obstruction. It is particularly useful in cases of poor renal function where the kidneys and ureter show poor opacification on the IVU. A cystoscopy and anaesthetic is required and contrast is injected through a ureteric catheter. If an obstruction, such as sloughed papillae or epithelial tumour, is shown, then the catheter may be left in situ as a temporary drain pending surgery. Complications of the procedure include renal

colic, temporary ureteric obstruction from mucosal oedema, infection, and intrarenal or extrapelvic extravasation of contrast.

Antegrade ureteropyelography

This procedure is performed by percutaneous puncture of the renal pelvis under ultrasound guidance to locate the dilated pelvis. Urine is aspirated and contrast injected. A nephrostomy tube may be left in situ temporarily as a drainage procedure or to allow measurement of pressure change (Whittaker test for severity of an obstruction). The procedure will allow visualization of the ureter proximal to a stenosis and is increasingly used in the assessment of renal transplant obstruction. The other indication is in any case of renal obstruction where retrograde ureteric catheterization is likely to be difficult. Complications include haematuria, extravasation of urine, and infection of the urinary tract.

Renal arteriography

The renal arteries may be opacified either by intra-arterial injection or by peripheral intravenous injection of contrast medium. The latter requires larger doses of contrast and, in our experience, the quality of images obtained is often not sufficient to allow accurate evaluation of renal artery branches and intrarenal vessels. Intra-arterial injection is therefore the preferred method, but is an invasive procedure with a greater risk, including contrast nephrotoxicity, than urography, ultrasound, or nuclear renal scanning. It is performed by retrograde femoral catheterization under local anaesthesia. The narrow catheters now used have reduced the local complication rates substantially, often enabling patients to be discharged from hospital on the same day.

Contrast medium is injected rapidly into the aorta at the level of the renal arteries. Selective catheterization of the renal arteries is often required to evaluate the intrarenal vasculature, particularly in renal tumours and in assessment of living renal transplant donors. Digital techniques have now largely replaced standard angiographic imaging, allowing subtraction of superimposed tissue and contrast enhancement. Digital angiography also allows the use of 50 per cent lower doses of contrast medium, lower flow rates, and smaller catheters.

Current indications for renal arteriography are limited, as refinements of less invasive procedures such as CT scanning and ultrasound may provide appropriate information. The chief use is in the evaluation of renovascular disease where the diagnosis has been suggested by a nuclear renal scan, often after captopril challenge (see below). If the renal artery stenosis is amenable to transluminal angioplasty, the dilatation (or renal artery stenting) can be performed at the same time as the arteriogram, thus saving the patient the cost and inconvenience of a repeat arteriogram and hospital admission.

Other indications include suspected renal artery occlusion from thrombus, embolus, dissection or trauma, screening for arterial aneurysms in the diagnosis of classical polyarteritis nodosa, and when an intrarenal vascular lesion is suspected, as in persistent haematuria following a renal biopsy. In the latter situation arteriography can confirm an arteriovenous fistula or false aneurysm, and renal embolization via an endovascular catheter at the same time will prevent further bleeding. Renal angiography is always required in the surgical evaluation of the renal vasculature of potential live donors of kidney grafts. CT and magnetic resonance imaging (MRI) scanning have now largely replaced arteriography in the evaluation of renal tumours.

Renal venography

Few indications now remain for this procedure as new imaging techniques such as MRI and CT allow easier detection of renal vein thrombosis. However, an iliocavagram may be necessary to document caval extension of a renal vein thrombosis. Selective catheterization of the renal veins for renal vein renin levels in renovascular hypertension has now largely been replaced by the more reliable and quicker technique of nuclear renal scanning following captopril challenge (see below).

Micturating cystourethrography

The usual purpose of a micturating cystourethrogram is the demonstration of vesicoureteric reflux, but it can also be used to display abnormalities of the bladder neck and urethra. Contrast is injected into the bladder via a urethral catheter. The patient voids while sitting on a commode in front of the radiographic screen. The reflux is recorded on spot film or cineradiography. The risk of subsequent urinary infection is substantial and it is sensible practice to administer an antibacterial for 2 or 3 days after the procedure.

Computed tomography (CT scanning)

CT scanning of the trunk displays the kidneys particularly well in contrast to the surrounding perinephric and peripelvic fat. It can reveal abnormalities of the retroperitoneal and perirenal spaces that cannot be shown with conventional techniques. Contrast media used in CT scanning are the same as those used for intravenous urography. The prime indications for CT scanning of the kidneys are to detect renal mass lesions and suspected renal trauma.

Generally, simple renal cysts and polycystic renal disease can be equally well diagnosed with the cheaper technique of ultrasound. However, CT is the method of choice for the diagnosis of renal tumours, since it can confirm the solid nature of the tumour and allow determination of its local extension. Central calcification is very suggestive of a malignancy, as is contrast enhancement due to hypervascularity of the tumour. Extension of renal cell carcinoma has implications for prognosis and surgical intervention. CT is the best technique for documenting tumour thrombus in the renal veins (Fig 10). Lymph node involvement by tumour can be detected if the nodes are greater than about 1 cm in diameter.

In renal trauma, CT scanning is clearly the best technique for demonstrating parenchymal damage, subcapsular haematoma, and perirenal urinary collections, as well as assessing damage to other organs such as the liver and spleen.

Finally, CT scanning is useful in the investigation of retroperitoneal fibrosis, which may be idiopathic or secondary to the use of drugs. The appearance of the fibrous plaque, which starts below the level of the aortic bifurcation and extends upwards, often enveloping the ureters, can usually be distinguished from lymphoma or sarcoma involving this region.

Magnetic resonance imaging (MRI)

MRI is a digital tomographic imaging system where tissue contrast depends on the manipulation of intrinsic magnetic fields. The technique employs a strong uniform magnetic field combined with transient oscillating magnetic fields to create images without the use of ionizing radiation.

MRI offers very superior soft-tissue contrast and the ability to distinguish easily simple renal cysts, complex cysts, and solid renal masses. Like CT scanning, it is particularly useful in detecting tumour extension into veins. MRI angiography of the renal circulation is yet to be assessed but may have a future role in renovascular disease. Presently, MRI is mainly indicated to clarify equivocal CT findings in renal tumours.

Ultrasonography

This is now the initial investigation for the majority of patients in renal failure and has displaced conventional radiology as the first structural investigation of the urinary tract. High-resolution real-time (moving picture) scans are standard equipment.

Tissue density is the major determinant of acoustic impedance and when sound waves are passed into tissues of widely different acoustic impedances most of the waves are reflected, for example tissue/gas 99 per cent echo, tissue/bone 70 per cent echo. Fat is highly reflective and thick subcutaneous tissues lengthen the distance from the probe to the kidney, making ultrasonography difficult and occasionally impossible in obese patients.

Ultrasound findings are independent of renal function. They can therefore be used to study patients with renal failure, measuring with considerable accuracy the shape, depth from the surface, and internal architecture of the kidney and upper urinary tract (Fig. 11). Ultrasound generally detects the dilated calyces, pelvis, and ureter of the obstructed kidney, although in the presence of very recent obstruction the calyceal system may not have dilated sufficiently to make a firm diagnosis on ultrasound, and other investigations such as retrograde ureterography may be necessary. In unexplained renal failure, ultrasound is very useful to assess renal size and cortical thickness, with the presence of small kidneys suggesting chronic renal disease and enabling the renal physician to make appropriate decisions about whether or not renal biopsy is indicated.

Ultrasound is often helpful in identifying the cause of abnormalities detected on the IVU. It may show whether an enlarged kidney is the site of hydronephrosis, an infiltrative process, or a space-occupying lesion. It is particularly useful in deciding whether a localized swelling detected on IVU is cystic (and probably benign) or solid (and probably malignant). However, solid lesions may undergo some cystic change and therefore if a cystic lesion is not absolutely classical (unilocular, uniformly thin walls) then further investigation is indicated. This may be by CT scanning, MRI, invasive cyst puncture, or biopsy.

Ultrasonography has replaced excretion urography as the screening

Fig. 10 CT scan of the kidneys, showing (a) a large renal cell carcinoma arising from the left kidney; (b) extension of tumour into left renal vein (arrow) and a metastic deposit in the vertebral body.

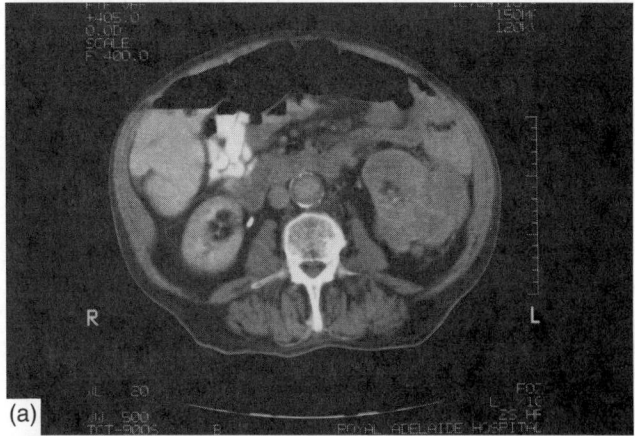

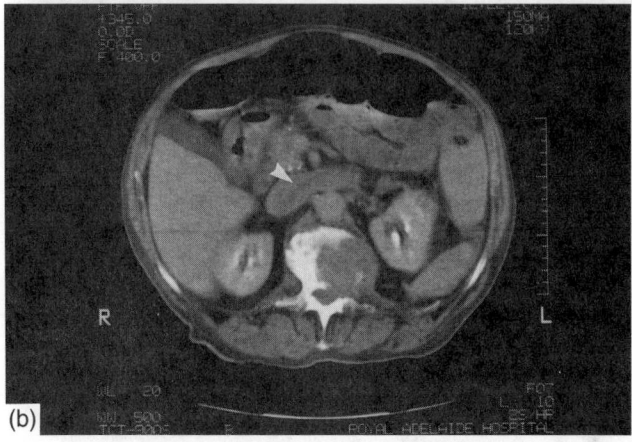

test for polycystic disease; the two techniques are comparable in accuracy but ultrasonography is faster, cheaper, and devoid of the risk of contrast injection and irradiation. However, cysts and tumours below 5 mm in diameter are not detected reliably by either ultrasound or excretion urography so polycystic disease cannot be excluded with certainty below the age of about 30 years.

Perinephric lesions are readily displayed by ultrasound; it is used to detect extravasation of blood after trauma or renal biopsy, although CT scanning may provide more accurate information in this regard. Ultrasonography is the first test for radiolucent calculi; it is also used for detecting radio-opaque calculi, but straight radiography remains the first investigation.

Finally, ultrasound is very useful in the assessment of complications of renal transplantation, particularly the surgical complications of extrarenal collections of blood, pus, and lymph, and in the identification of an obstructed transplant kidney (Fig. 12). An ultrasound-guided percutaneous nephrostomy can then allow temporary decompression of the obstruction. Doppler ultrasound may have a limited role in the diagnosis of vascular rejection of the transplanted kidney, but at this stage cannot reliably distinguish acute tubular necrosis and cyclosporin nephrotoxicity from acute rejection.

Nuclear renal imaging

The value of radiolabelled tracers in the investigation of renal disease lies in the ability to obtain important information about organ function as opposed to the predominantly structural information obtained from the previously described imaging procedures. In particular, nuclear imaging of the kidneys provides the only non-invasive quantitative assessment of individual kidney function.

Renal radiopharmaceuticals

Radionuclides (such as ^{123}I, ^{99}Tc^m) are linked to compounds that depend on either glomerular filtration alone, tubular excretion, or a combination of both for excretion from the body. These compounds can therefore provide quantitative information on these functions of the kidney, in addition to dynamic images.

The most widely used currently available renal radiopharmaceuticals include:

[^{99}Tc^m]diethylenetriaminepentaacetic acid (DTPA)

DTPA is a chelating agent which is filtered by the glomerulus and can bind to reduced ^{99}Tc^m, a radionuclide with excellent imaging properties with a Γ-ray energy of 144 keV and a short half-life (6 h). [^{99}Tc^m]DTPA is cheap, readily available, and is the most commonly used radiopharmaceutical in most countries for routine renal imaging. It has the additional advantage that the glomerular filtration rate can be easily assessed as part of the renal study, using plasma sampling. However, in patients with poor renal function the low extraction efficiency of DTPA will result in inferior images compared to agents dependent on tubular excretion.

[^{131}I]- and [^{123}I] iodohippurate

Iodohippurate, on the other hand, has a high renal extraction efficiency due to its tubular secretion, and can provide high-quality images even when renal function is poor. However, ^{131}I is an unsatisfactory radiolabel as a result of its γ-radiation energy (364 keV), β-emission, and long half-life, and can no longer be justified for routine renal imaging. ^{123}I is more suitable for imaging, with a γ-ray energy of 159 keV and a shorter half-life (13 hours), but it is expensive and not readily available.

[^{99}Tc^m]mercaptoacetyltriglycine (MAG3)

This new radiopharmaceutical combines the advantages of technetium as an imaging radionuclide with the extraction efficiency of a tubular-secreted compound. However, there is a small component of glomerular filtration and biliary excretion, making MAG3 unsuitable for the quantitative assessment of effective renal plasma flow. Nevertheless, in patients with poor renal function and in the renal transplant recipient it is the radiopharmaceutical of choice.

[^{99}Tc^m]dimercaptosuccinic acid (DMSA)

This agent is filtered by the glomerulus and then retained in proximal tubular cells with no significant urinary excretion. Static images with tomography at 3 h after injection therefore provide excellent images of the renal cortex and are particularly useful for defining renal scarring in reflux nephropathy.

Methodology

Modern gamma-camera renography has now replaced external probes for studies of individual and regional renal function. The gamma-camera

Fig. 11 Normal kidney displayed by ultrasonography, in longitudinal section. The small curved upper edge of the wedge represents the skin of the back, to which the probe is applied. The high-echo areas in the kidney are the calyces.

Fig. 12 Ultrasonogram of transplanted kidney showing dilation of renal pelvis and widening of ureter due to obstruction.

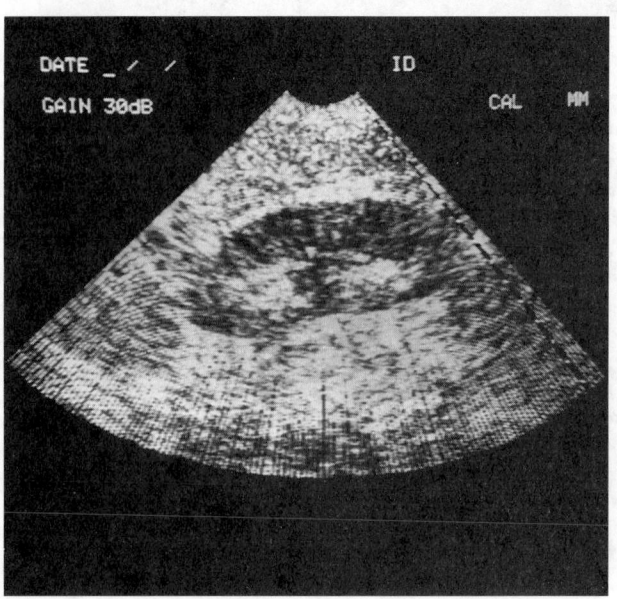

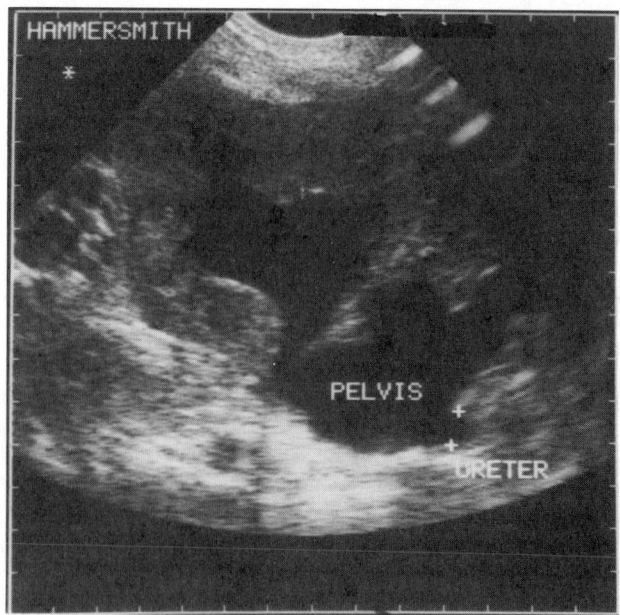

Table 4 *Clinical features suggesting a higher risk of renovascular hypertension*

Malignant or accelerated hypertension
Worsening of previously controlled hypertension
Hypertension and unexplained renal impairment
Hypertension and vascular disease
Hypertension and an abdominal bruit
Hypertension in a young female or any patient aged less than 40 years without a family history of hypertension
Rise in serum creatinine after angiotensin-converting enzyme inhibitor therapy for hypertension

is interfaced with a computer, with the latest generation of digital cameras having the computer as an integral component with resultant improvement in image resolution and tomographic cross-sectional image reconstruction.

The basic technique of imaging is similar for all of the radiopharmaceuticals. The patient should be well hydrated prior to the study and empties the bladder immediately before the procedure. The subject is placed in either a supine or sitting position with the gamma-camera positioned posteriorly. After rapid bolus injection of the radiopharmaceutical, imaging with computer acquisition is carried out for at least 30 min. Early images (for example, every 2 s for the first 30 s) reflect arterial perfusion of the kidney; later images at 2 to 4 min reflect the glomerular filtration rate if [^{99}Tc^m]DTPA is being used. Remaining images, to 30 min, will demonstrate excretion into the collecting system and pelvis. Delayed views and postdiuretic imaging will be required if renal obstruction is suspected.

Regions of interest are selected from the computer-acquired data and time–activity curves (corrected for background activity) are generated for the whole kidney (renogram), renal cortex, and renal pelvis. The renogram curve peaks normally at 150 to 180 s, after which time the tracer will be excreted from the kidney. Between the initial upstroke of the curve, reflecting the radionuclide entering the renal circulation, and the start of excretion into the collecting system, a reasonable assumption is made that virtually all activity is in the cortex of the kidney and therefore quantitative differences of activity between the two kidneys will reflect relative renal function. When corrected for attenuation due to depth differences of individual kidneys, and allowing for biological variation, the normal range for individual relative renal function is 50 ± 8 per cent.

Computed mathematical analysis of the renal time–activity curve, using deconvolution, simulates direct injection of the radiopharmaceutical into the renal artery and enables the calculation of transit times of tracer across the whole kidney, cortex, and pelvis. Normal ranges for these times have been established, and abnormalities in such times have been reported to be of value in the diagnosis of renovascular disease and obstructive nephropathy.

Indications for nuclear renal imaging

INVESTIGATION OF RENOVASCULAR HYPERTENSION (SEE ALSO CHAPTER 15.28.1)

This is now the prime indication for nuclear renal scanning in most departments of nuclear medicine. The aim is to identify functionally significant renal artery stenosis in 'at risk' patients with hypertension (see Table 4). The nuclear renal scan performed after challenge with the angiotensin-converting enzyme inhibitor, captopril, has been shown to have a higher sensitivity and specificity than non-invasive screening investigations, such as stimulated peripheral renin estimation, IVP, or intravenous digital subtraction angiography.

The basis of the test relates to the dependence of the glomerular filtration rate on angiotensin II-mediated efferent arteriolar vasoconstric-

Fig. 13 (a) [^{99}Tc^m]DTPA renal scan, showing a dramatic fall in uptake in the left kidney following captopril administration. (b) This is reflected in the computed differential function of this kidney. (c) The renal arteriogram confirms a high-grade stenosis in the left renal artery, which is amenable to angioplasty.

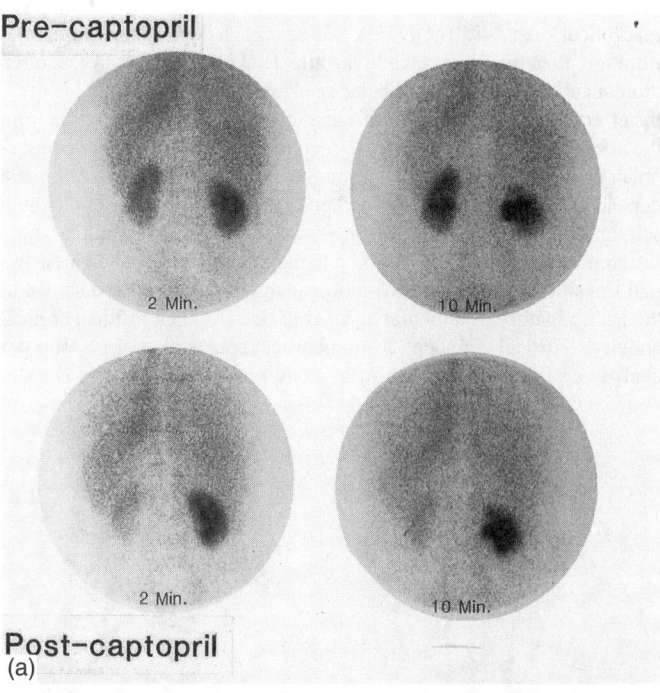

Pre-captopril

Post-captopril
(a)

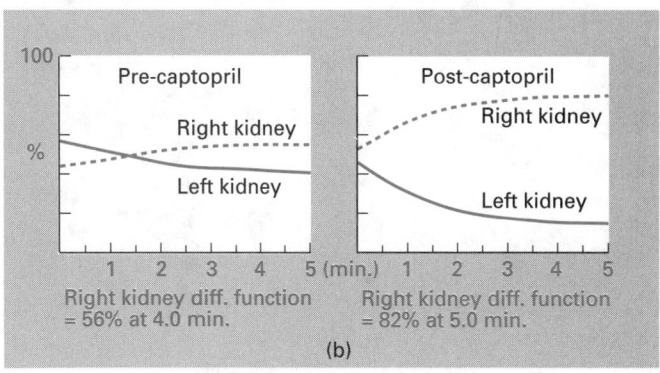

(b)

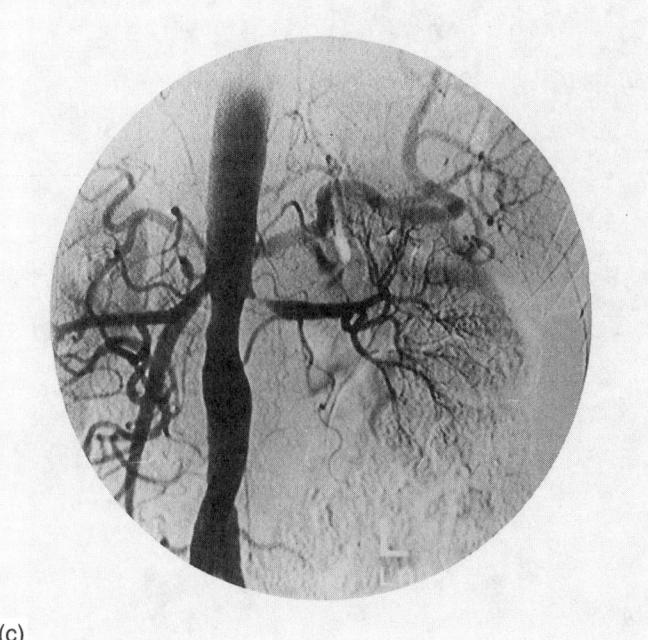

(c)

tion in the presence of significant renal artery stenosis. The addition of a short-acting angiotensin-converting enzyme inhibitor, such as captopril (25 mg orally), will result in dilatation of the efferent arteriole of the glomerulus, with a consequent fall in glomerular filtration rate as the glomerular transcapillary hydraulic pressure falls. If a radiopharmaceutical such as [^{99}Tc^m]DTPA is used, which depends on glomerular filtration, then relative uptake in the affected kidney will decrease, often dramatically (Fig. 13). If a tubular agent such as [^{99}Tc^m]MAG3 is used, the effect of captopril is to cause a marked delay in tracer excretion from the affected kidney, presumably reflecting decreased urine flow rate secondary to reduced glomerular filtration rate. Interpretation of the test depends on comparison of pre- and postcaptopril studies, assessing both scintigraphic images and renal time–activity curves. Most important is differential renal function, but time to maximum activity and parenchymal transit times from deconvolution analysis have also been shown to be discriminatory. If a tubular agent is to be used, then residual cortical activity ((cortical counts at 20 min/cortical counts at peak) × 100 per cent) is useful. The detection of bilateral renal artery stenosis is more difficult, and we would recommend the concurrent measurement of global glomerular filtration rate pre- and postcaptopril, using at least two plasma samples. Although scintigraphic appearances may not change significantly, the presence of bilateral renal artery stenosis will usually result in a significant fall in global glomerular filtration rate after captopril. In our experience and that of others, a positive captopril scan is predictive of a good response of hypertension to balloon angioplasty or surgery.

The danger of a single dose of captopril appears to be small but the potential exists for significant hypotension, and blood pressure should be closely monitored during the test. In addition, patients should be well hydrated and avoid diuretics on the day of the procedure.

ASSESSMENT OF INDIVIDUAL KIDNEY FUNCTION

Nuclear renal scanning is the only non-invasive way of quantitatively assessing the contribution of each kidney to total renal function. The measurement of split renal function is often critically important in con-

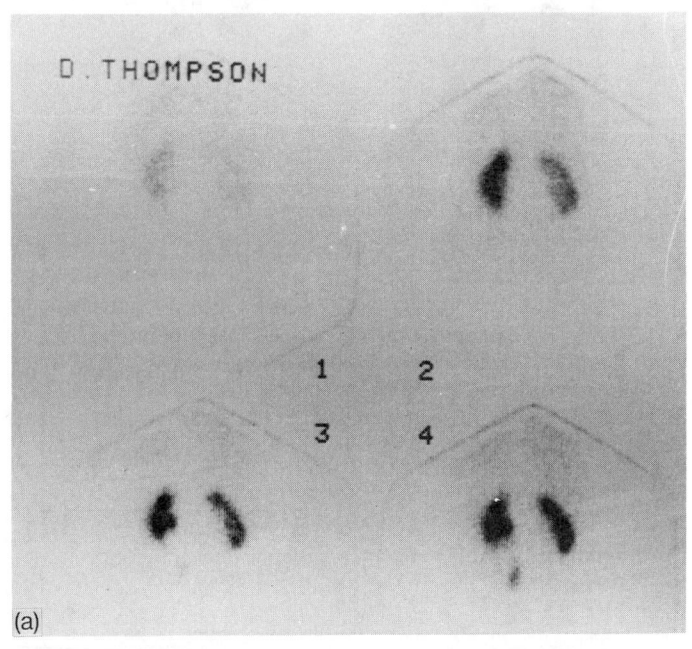

(a)

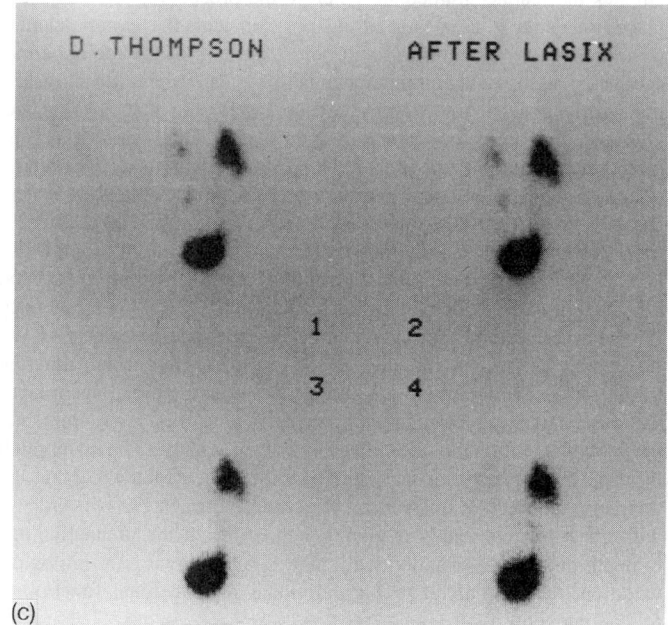

(c)

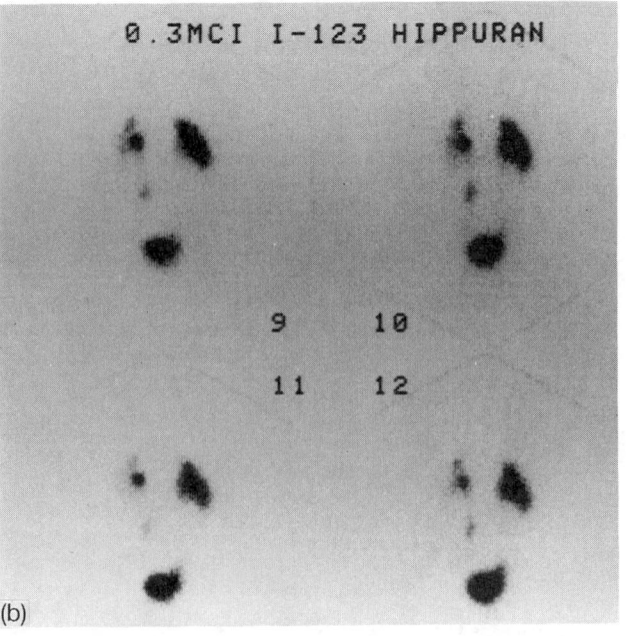

(b)

Fig. 14 (a) Gamma-camera scan of a patient with right pelviureteric obstruction. The right renal tract is on the right of the picture (mirror image of an IVU). Images at 1 to 4 min show slow appearance of radioactivity in parenchyma and pelvis of obstructed side. (b) Later images of scan shown in (a). Poor display of right ureter and persistence of radioactivity in right renal pelvis. (c) Frusemide test at the end of the scan shown in (a) and (b). Rapid clearing of radioactivity from the normal left side and persistence on the obstructed right side.

ditions that can affect renal function unilaterally, such as reflux nephropathy, nephrolithiasis, and obstruction. Decisions about surgical intervention in such cases should depend on measurements of global glomerular filtration rate, individual kidney function, and sometimes function within an individual kidney (for example, upper and lower moieties of a duplex collecting system). In the absence of knowledge of such data, surgical removal of a kidney contributing, for example, 40 per cent of a global glomerular filtration rate of 30 ml/min may well result in a patient becoming unnecessarily dialysis dependent.

RENAL OBSTRUCTION

Although ultrasound or IVU will usually be used to determine dilatation of the renal collecting system, in cases of suspected renal obstruction diuretic renography remains the best choice to answer the question of true obstruction versus a dilated but non-obstructed collecting system. The gamma-camera protocol involves normal acquisition of images for 20 minutes after injection of tracer. Frusemide (0.3 mg/kg intravenously) is administered and images collected for a further 15 min (Fig. 14). Background corrected time–activity curves are generated for the renal pelvis and the slope of the curve and the pattern of reponse to frusemide can be analysed qualitatively and quantitatively. Radiopharmaceuticals dependent on tubular function (such as [^{99}Tc^m]MAG3) may be the best choice in this situation as a higher target/background ratio can be obtained than with a glomerular agent, particularly if renal function is impaired.

Three major patterns emerge:

(1) Normal, in which frusemide accentuates the normal rate of washout of tracer with a very steep rate of fall.
(2) Dilated and obstructed collecting system, in which frusemide fails to cause wash out of activity.
(3) Dilated but non-obstructed system, in which frusemide causes a fall in counts in a system that was slowly accumulating activity prior to the diuretic.

Results are generally expressed in terms of half-clearance times (normal < 10 min; obstructed > 20 min) and percentage washout in 15 min (normal > 50 per cent).

The test needs to be interpreted with caution in cases of poor renal function where the tracer is not adequately taken up by the kidney which is unable to respond adequately to the diuretic.

RENAL TRANSPLANT ASSESSMENT (SEE ALSO SECTION 20.17.3.)

Nuclear renal scanning can provide information on graft perfusion and function earlier than changes in blood chemistry. However, such scans need to be performed in a reproducible way, commencing shortly after graft insertion and repeated regularly in the post-transplant period. The patient is scanned in the supine position with the gamma camera over the anterior pelvis. Early dynamic images will reflect perfusion of the graft and later images to 20 minutes will assess excretion of tracer into the collecting system. Quantitative measurements from time–activity curves of kidney and iliac artery (for example, Hilsons's perfusion index) may be useful in comparing subtle changes in perfusion from day to day. Choice of radiopharmaceutical depends on graft function. In the presence of primary non-function, a tubular agent such as [^{99}Tc^m]MAG3 will provide useful images (tracer will be retained in tubules) whereas a glomerular agent such as [^{99}Tc^m]DTPA may fail even to visualize the graft.

Infarction of the kidney following renal artery thrombosis is readily recognized from the scan, as a non-perfused kidney will appear as a photon-deficient region against the background radiation. In uncomplicated acute tubular necrosis, renal perfusion gradually improves, but if transplant rejection or cyclosporin nephrotoxicity is superimposed, perfusion will deteriorate. Unfortunately the nuclear renal scan is currently unable to differentiate between acute rejection and cyclosporin nephrotoxicity. Nevertheless, the scan is useful in recognizing other complications, such as leaks, obstruction, and renal arterial problems, and when assessed in conjunction with other clinical parameters can be very helpful in arriving at decisions regarding the need for graft biopsy or surgical intervention.

ACUTE RENAL FAILURE

Nuclear renal scanning has only a limited role in the assessment of acute renal failure in native kidneys. The main indication is the differentiation of acute tubular necrosis from cortical necrosis. In the former, [^{99}Tc^m]DTPA scan will show mild to moderate reduction of perfusion and no excretion, whereas in the presence of cortical necrosis the scan will fail to show perfusion or excretion.

REFERENCES

Blaufox, M.D. (1989). *Evaluation of renal function and disease with radionuclides: the upper urinary tract*, (2nd edn). Karger, Basel.

Cameron, J.S, Davison, A.M., Grunfeld, J.-P. Kerr, D., and Ritz, E. (1992). *Oxford textbook of clinical nephrology*, Vol. I, Sections 1.2 (urinalysis and microscopy), 1.3 (renal function testing), and 1.6 (visualizing the kidney). Oxford University Press, Oxford.

Pitts, R.F. (1963). *Physiology of the kidney and body fluids*. Year Book Medical Publishers, Chicago.

Schumann, G.B. (1980). *Urine sediment examination*. Williams and Wilkins, Baltimore

20.2 Water and electrolyte metabolism

20.2.1 Water and sodium homeostasis and their disorders

P. H. BAYLIS

Introduction

Total body water accounts for about 60 per cent of body weight of a healthy adult, of which two-thirds is intracellular and one-third extracellular. The extracellular fluid compartment is divided into the vascular, or blood, volume and the interstitial fluid compartment, in the ratio 1:2. Thus, for a 75-kg adult, the total body water volume is approximately 45 litres, with intracellular and extracellular volumes of 30 and 15 litres, respectively; the latter comprising the blood (5 litres) and interstitial (10 litres) compartments. Sodium is the main extracellular cation, which with its anion, chloride, contributes 95 per cent of the extracellular solute. In contrast, the major intracellular cation is potassium. Cell membranes are freely permeable to water but not to most electrolytes, which results in the same total solute but very different electrolyte concentrations in the extracellular and intracellular compartments (Fig. 1).

The maintenance of stable volume and solute concentrations is essen-

Fig. 1 Composition of body compartments. Body water is distributed uniformly throughout all compartments. Major and some minor (in parentheses) anions and cations are indicated. Osmolality remains the same inside and outside the cell.

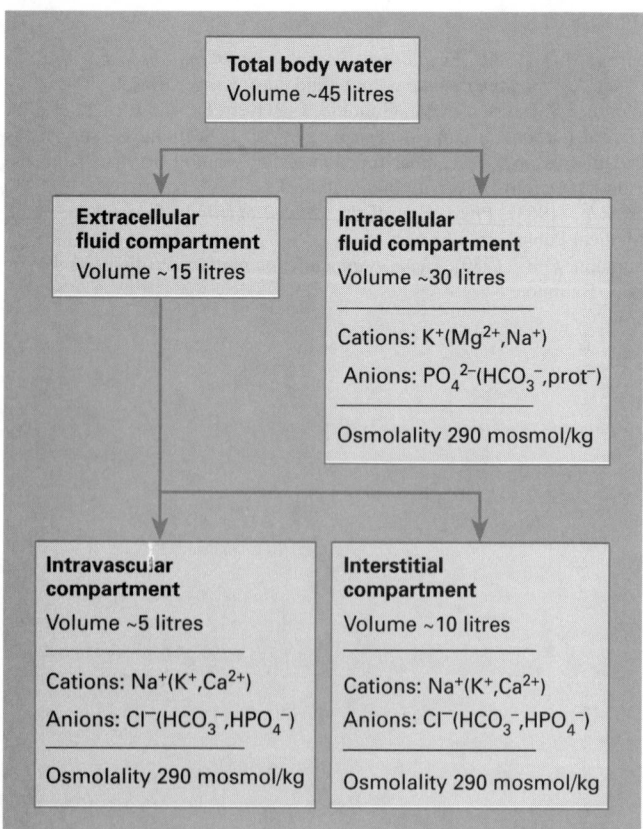

tial to all complex animals, including man. In the extracellular fluid compartment, particularly the vascular component, the control of water and sodium balance are inextricably linked. Water is distributed uniformly throughout all compartments, and clearly is a determinant of volume, but also is essential in establishing the concentration of sodium (and other solutes). Sodium, however, not only contributes to its own concentration, but its total quantity in the excellular compartment is the major factor determining the compartment's volume. There are a variety of integrated mechanisms that ensure that minimal fluctuations, probably less than 1 per cent, in blood volume and in sodium concentration occur in healthy adults. Body water, and therefore solute concentration, is regulated mainly by altering renal water excretion mediated by vasopressin (antidiuretic hormone), but also to some extent by thirst, which will motivate drinking. The secretion of vasopressin and thirst are influenced principally by changes in circulating concentrations of sodium, but also in part by considerable falls in blood volume or pressure. The volume of the extracellular compartment is determined by its total sodium content, which is regulated by numerous mechanisms. Sodium intake is poorly controlled in man, although some animals do demonstrate a specific sodium appetite. The kidney is the major effector organ influencing sodium homeostasis. Complex intrarenal mechanisms contribute to the maintenance of sodium homeostasis, in addition to endocrine factors that conserve renal sodium excretion (for example the renin–angiotensin–aldosterone system) or that produce a natriuresis (for example atrial natriuretic peptide, oubain-like substances). Furthermore, blood volume and pressure are influenced by a variety of vasoactive substances acting locally or systemically (such as catecholamines, prostaglandins, nitric oxide, endothelins), as well as changes in sympathetic nerve outflow. Changes in blood volume and/or pressure will, in turn, have an effect on vasopressin secretion. It can therefore be appreciated that there is an intricate network of homeostatic mechanisms controlling both sodium and water balance.

In clinical practice, the precise measurement of circulating concentrations of electrolytes, specific non-electrolytic solutes (such as glucose), and total solute is relatively simple, and approximates closely to their concentrations in interstitial fluid. Sodium is measured in molar terms (mmol/l) using flame-photometry or an ion-selective electrode. Total solute concentration is assessed by determining the depression of freezing point of the sample plasma with an osmometer, and is expressed as the number of osmoles of solute per kilogram (osmolality). Thus, a solution of glucose at 1 mmol/l will provide an osmolality of 1 mosmol/kg but 1 mmol/l solution of a salt (for example NaCl) which dissociates completely in the solvent into its sodium and chloride ions will have an osmolality of 2 mosmol/kg. The assessment of volume, whether it be intravascular, interstitial, or extracellular, is extremely difficult and inaccurate, and therefore estimations of the total quantity of electrolytes, particularly sodium, in these compartments is almost impossible.

The physiology of water homeostasis

The maintenance of normal water balance is achieved by the inter-relationship of three major factors, vasopressin, the kidney, and thirst. There must be secretion of adequate quantities of osmotically stimulated vasopressin, which binds to the renal tubule to modulate the flow of solute-free water across the cells, thus causing an antidiuresis. The kidney is capable of wide variations of urine output, ranging from 0.5 to 20 l/24 h, but most healthy adults excrete 1 to 2 l/24 h. The third determinant is osmotically stimulated thirst, which promotes drinking and is particularly important when the kidney is concentrating urine maximally but there is still persistent water loss from, for example, excessive sweating in hot climates or from copious watery diarrhoea. Under these circumstances it is essential that there is adequate fluid intake to maintain water homeostasis.

Fine control of water balance ensures that the concentration of solutes, particularly extracellular sodium, remains stable. The extraordinary sensitivity of the function of these three factors allows plasma osmolality to be maintained within the narrow range, 285 to 295 mosmol/kg (equivalent to serum sodium, 137–142 mmol/l) in healthy adults.

Thirst and water intake

Drinking behaviour of humans can be divided into two types. The first, called primary drinking, occurs as a result of physiological stimulation of thirst. As the body loses water, blood osmolality starts to rise, which is sensed by putative osmotically sensitive cells, the osmoreceptors, in the brain. This initiates drinking behaviour to allow ingestion of sufficient fluid to lower blood osmolality. Secondary drinking, which is far more common in our culture, occurs for social reasons (the endless cups of coffee throughout the day or the ritual visit to the 'pub'), habit, or the need to drink with food. For the majority of adults living in temperate climates, secondary drinking ensures that they remain in a state of mild water excess, and water balance is maintained by regulating renal water excretion.

Progressive water loss or dehydration stimulates the thirst osmoreceptors. Studies in animals indicate that they are situated in the anterior hypothalamic structures, probably in the organum vasculosum of the lamina terminalis (OVLT) or the subfornical organ (SFO) where a defect in the blood–brain barrier exists (see Fig. 1, Chapter 12.3). In humans, isolated lesions in this area following haemorrhage from an anterior communicating artery aneurysm, have resulted in loss of thirst appreciation, suggesting that human thirst osmoreceptors are located in an area similar to that of animals. The precise mechanism by which blood hyperosmolality stimulates thirst is not known, but it is believed that the increase in extracellular osmolality draws water from within the osmoreceptor cells of the OVLT and SFO, resulting in cellular hypovolaemia. The latter is translated into neuronal impulses which migrate to the cortex to allow conscious appreciation of thirst.

With the use of visual analogue scales it is possible to obtain an estimate of the degree of thirst sensation. There is a clear simple relationship between increasing blood osmolality and the intensity of thirst (Fig. 2(b)). Furthermore, there is also a direct relationship between thirst intensity and the amount of fluid drunk to quench thirst. The act of drinking quickly reduces thirst, usually within a few minutes and certainly before there are substantial falls in blood osmolality, which is probably mediated by an oropharyngeal reflex. It therefore appears that drinking is able to override or inhibit osmotically stimulated thirst.

Thirst is not only stimulated by increases in blood osmolality, but also by substantial acute falls in blood volume and/or pressure. A sudden decrease in volume in excess of 15 per cent is required before thirst is influenced. Low-pressure baroreceptors located in the atria and great veins of the chest mediate the response. In addition, significant extracellular hypovolaemia is a potent stimulus to the release of renin from the juxtaglomerular area of the nephron to generate increasing concentrations of circulating angiotensin II, known to be a profound dipsogen in animals. It is, therefore, possible that systemic angiotensin II augments the baroregulatory influence on thirst in acute hypovolaemia. Animal studies have also revealed that intrahypothalamic angiotensin II is the most potent neurotransmitter involved in the development of thirst sensation.

As humans age so their thirst appreciation appears to become blunted and primary drinking is reduced, so that individuals tend to become mildly hyperosmolar and hypernatraemic. Fortunately, most elderly people continue secondary drinking, rely on mechanisms to control renal water excretion, and are therefore protected against severe hypernatraemia.

During human pregnancy there is a fall in plasma osmolality of the order of 10 mosmol/kg with an appropriate fall in serum sodium, which is due to alteration in the osmoregulatory systems for both thirst and vasopressin secretion. The thirst osmoregulatory line (Fig. 2) is displaced to the left of the normal, non-pregnant position, which runs parallel, but the abscissal intercept, known as the osmotic threshold for thirst, is reset to about 275 mosmol/kg. Similar changes occur with the osmoregulatory line for vasopressin secretion (see below). The precise mechanisms for this 'resetting of the osmostat' are unknown, but it is believed that the hormonal environment (for example, human chorionic gonadotrophin) is responsible, at least in part.

Vasopressin and renal water excretion

The antidiuretic hormone of man is arginine vasopressin, a nonapeptide, the gene of which is located on chromosome 20 (see Fig. 2, Chapter 12.3). In brief, arginine vasopressin is synthesized from a large precursor molecule in the supraoptic and paraventricular nuclei of the hypothal-

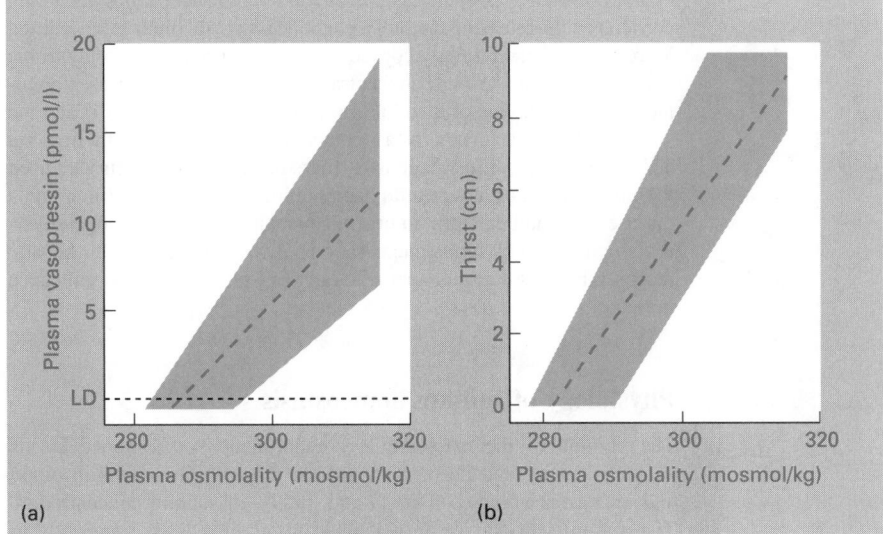

Fig. 2 (a) The relationship between plasma osmolality and plasma vasopressin during infusion of hypertonic (850 mmol/l) saline in healthy adults. There is a linear relationship between the two variables, represented by the dashed line, termed the mean osmoregulatory line for vasopressin secretion. The abscissal intercept of the line represents the threshold for vasopressin secretion, approximately 283 mosmol/kg. LD is the limit of detection of the assay, and the shaded area is the extent of the normal response. (b) The relationship between plasma osmolality and thirst intensity assessed by a visual analogue scale during the same hypertonic infusion. The dashed line is the mean osmoregulatory line for thirst, which has an abscissal intercept (thirst threshold) of 281 mosmol/kg. (Adapted from Thompson et al. 1986, Clinical Science 71, 651–656, with permission.)

amus, transported in neurosecretory granules to the posterior pituitary, median eminence of the hypothalamus, and to a lesser extent to other areas of the brain and brain-stem. It is secreted into the systemic circulation from the posterior pituitary to influence renal function; and into the hypothalamo-pituitary portal circulation to enhance pituitary adrenocorticotropic hormone secretion.

Control of vasopressin release

Secretion of vasopressin from the posterior pituitary is regulated mainly by changes in blood osmolality, but can be influenced by non-osmotic factors. The vasopressin osmoreceptors, although probably distinct from the thirst osmoreceptors, are located in the same anterior hypothalamic structures—the circumventricular structures, OVLT, and possibly the SFO. Rising blood osmolality causes water to flow out of the osmoreceptor cells and the cellular hypovolaemia is believed to initiate a neuronal signal which passes principally to the supraoptic nucleus to stimulate the process of vasopressin secretion. There exists an exquisitely sensitive linear relationship between blood osmolality and vasopressin secretion (Fig. 2(a)). The slope of the vasopressin osmoregulatory line is a measure of the sensitivity of the system and the abscissal intercept represents the threshold for vasopressin release. At plasma osmolality values less than 285 mosmol/kg, on average, vasopressin secretion is inhibited to allow a maximum water diuresis (15–20 l/24 h) with urine osmolality of 50 to 70 mosmol/kg (Fig. 3). Increases in blood osmolality above this threshold induce progressive vasopressin release, thus increasing urine concentration, so that at plasma vasopressin values of 2 to 4 pmol/l, maximum antidiuresis occurs. Drinking inhibits osmoregulated vasopressin secretion.

Each individual has a unique threshold and sensitivity for both thirst and vasopressin release. Circulating solutes have varying abilities to stimulate the osmoregulatory system, with sodium chloride being the most potent but glucose having little or no effect. In contrast to osmoregulated thirst, there is no blunting of the vasopressin response to osmotic stimulation with ageing. Pregnancy is associated with a lowering of the vasopressin threshold similar to the thirst threshold, which allows osmoregulation to occur about a lower set-point of 275 rather than 285 mosmol/kg.

Non-osmotic release of vasopressin may be influenced by large acute reductions in blood volume or pressure, of the order of 10 to 15 per cent or more, nausea and/or emesis, hypoglycaemia, and a variety of circulating substances (for example angiotensin II). Low-pressure receptors in the great veins of the chest and cardiac atria mediate the effect of hypovolaemia, while receptors in the arch of the aorta and carotid vessels sense reductions in arterial pressure. The information is carried via the vagus and glossopharyngeal nerves to the brain-stem vasomotor centres and is then transmitted to the hypothalamus, principally the paraventricular nucleus. There is an exponential relationship between the fall in blood volume/pressure and vasopressin release, such that large reductions ('40 per cent of normal) raise plasma vasopressin to huge values (100–500 pmol/l), concentrations that have vasoconstrictor effects. Similarly, high vasopressin concentrations can be achieved with nausea/emesis.

Actions of vasopressin

The major physiological action of vasopressin is to induce urinary concentration and, therefore, antidiuresis (Fig. 3). Circulating arginine vasopressin binds to a specific renal tubular receptor, designated the V_2 receptor, of the collecting ducts. Adenyl cyclase is stimulated to produce cyclic 5'-AMP, which activates intracellular protein kinases to organize microtubules and microfilaments that open water channels in the luminal cell membrane. Since there exists an osmotic gradient across the collecting tubular cell in healthy kidneys, with very high osmolality within the renal medullary interstitium, opening the water channels allows solute-free water to flow from the hypo-osmolal intraluminal fluid into the renal medulla, thus concentrating the urine.

Animal studies have indicated that vasopressin also stimulates the transport of urea across the collecting tubule and of sodium chloride across the medullary thick ascending limb of Henle's loop, thus both enhancing the osmotic gradient. As renal prostaglandins reduce cyclic 5'-AMP generation, they blunt the effect of vasopressin, and therefore prostaglandin synthetase inhibitors augment the antidiuretic action of arginine vasopressin.

The original action attributed to vasopressin was its ability to increase systemic blood pressure by peripheral vasoconstriction. Arginine vasopressin binds to vascular smooth muscle receptors (V_1 receptors) that increase intracellular calcium concentrations by activation of phosphatidylinositol pathways, to cause vascular muscle contraction. High circulating concentrations of vasopressin are necessary to achieve its pressor effect, and at physiological values it probably plays little, if any, role in maintaining blood pressure. Vasopressin, however, is involved in the pressor response to hypovolaemia/hypotension. There is no evidence that vasopressin is responsible for hypertension in man, although circulating concentrations may be elevated in malignant hypertension.

Vasopressin released from the hypothalamic median eminence acts as a physiological co-secretagogue of adrenocorticotropic hormone with corticotrophin-releasing factor. Arginine vasopressin binds to a modified V_1 receptor on the pituitary corticotroph to enhance adrenocorticotropic hormone release. At high concentrations, vasopressin increases circulating concentrations of the clotting factors, plasma factor VIII and the von Willebrand factor, by releasing them from vascular endothelium via a V_2 receptor. Specific V_2 agonists (for example desmopressin) are used to improve haemostasis in mild haemophilia A and in von Willebrand's disease, and can be helpful in uraemic bleeding. Hepatic glycogenolysis is also promoted by high concentrations of vasopressin via a V_1 hepatic receptor, but this does not appear to have any physiological significance in man.

Physiology of sodium homeostasis

The volume of the extracellular compartment is determined by its sodium content, and changes in sodium result in alterations in blood and interstitial volumes (Fig. 1) and, rarely, in sodium concentration. The reason is that a rise in sodium concentration leads transiently to

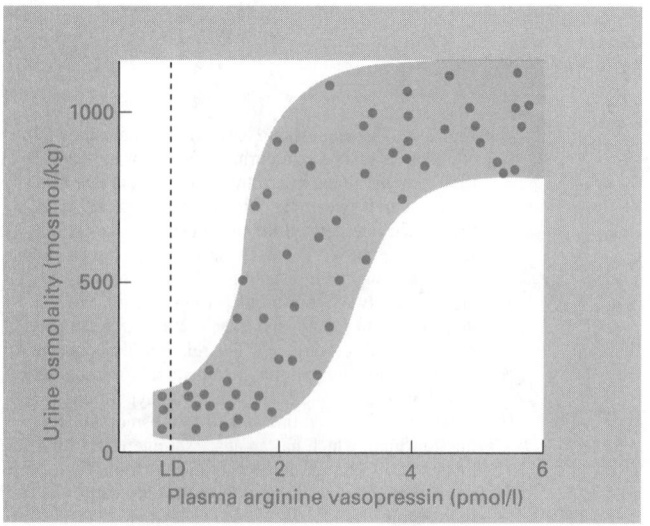

Fig. 3 The effect of vasopressin on urinary concentration during varying states of hydration in man. Each closed circle represents a single value, and the stippled area the normal range. Values of plasma vasopressin greater than 4 pmol/l fail to increase urinary concentration further. LD is the limit of the assay.

thirst stimulation and increased water intake and to vasopressin secretion to reduce renal water excretion, leading to an increase in body water and a return to normal concentrations of extracellular sodium. It appears that extracellular osmolality is conserved at the expense of volume in healthy adults. This integration indicates the close links between sodium and water homeostatic mechanisms.

Sodium intake

Control of sodium balance is maintained largely by the healthy kidney, which is capable of excreting a very wide range of sodium, 1 to 500 mmol/24 h. There is little regulation of sodium intake in man, although some animals do demonstrate a specific sodium appetite, with sodium receptors in the hypothalamus. In Western countries, including Britain, sodium intake is in gross excess for body needs, being about 100 to 200 mmol/24 h. There is little sodium loss from the healthy bowel and in temperate climates sweating is minimal (sweat sodium concentration is 40–50 mmol/l). Thus, the majority of people are in a state of potential sodium excess, which is prevented by the normal kidney but which leads commonly to salt retention in renal failure.

Control of renal sodium excretion

The glomerular filtration rate of normal kidneys is 170 l/24 h, the filtrate containing 140 mmol of sodium/l. Most of the filtered sodium is reabsorbed iso-osmotically by the proximal tubule (60–75 per cent), the remainder being reabsorbed in the medullary thick ascending limb of Henle's loop and the distal nephron, where the fine adjustment of sodium balance is largely regulated. Also, a glomerulotubular feedback mechanism operates at the single nephron level to maintain a balance between the reabsorptive function of each nephron and the amount of sodium and fluid filtered by the glomerulus. The mechanisms responsible for glomerulotubular feedback are not known precisely, but prob-

Fig. 4 The renin–angiotensin–aldosterone system. The enzyme, renin, secreted by juxtaglomerular cells of the renal afferent arterioles, acts to produce angiotensin I (inactive). The active peptides, angiotensin II and III are potent vasoconstrictors and stimulate aldosterone secretion from the adrenal cortex to expand blood volume and raise blood pressure.

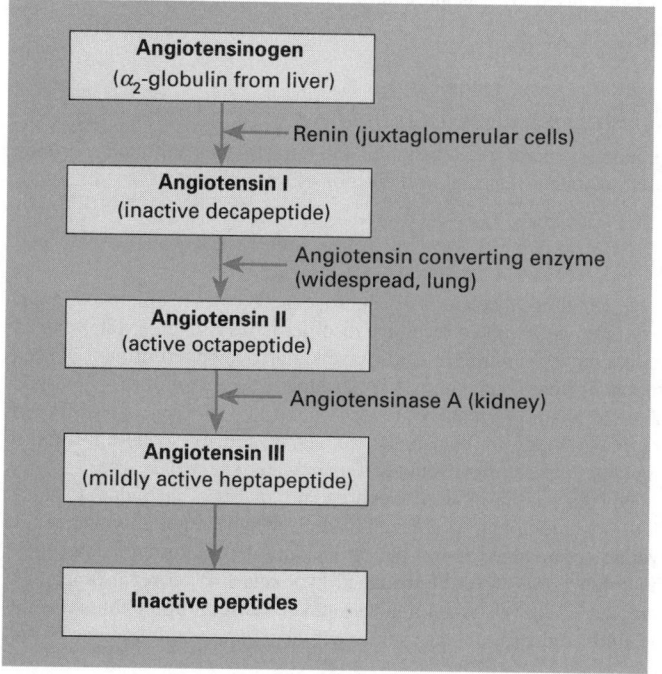

ably the macula densa cells of the thick ascending limb detect changes in composition of tubular fluid entering the terminal portion of this limb and transmit signals (possibly intrarenal angiotensin II) to modulate glomerular vascular resistance and glomerular pressure. Thus, acute changes in glomerular filtration will determine appropriate changes in sodium reabsorption in the proximal tubule. Most regulation of sodium balance, however, occurs in the distal nephron, which is under the control of a variety of mechanisms.

Renin–angiotensin–aldosterone system

Not only do the macula densa cells of the thick ascending limb detect decreases in sodium load within this portion of the nephron, but they also influence the juxtaglomerular cells of the renal afferent arterioles to synthesize and secrete renin into the systemic circulation as well as locally. In addition, reductions of renal perfusion pressure appear directly to increase renin secretion, while baroreceptors within the great veins of the chest influence renin secretion via the sympathetic nerves. Renin catalyses the conversion of angiotensinogen to angiotensin I (Fig. 4), which, in turn, is converted into the highly active octapeptide angiotensin II. The activity of angiotensin III is about 30 per cent that of angiotensin II. These peptides influence extracellular sodium content and volume in a number of ways. Angiotensin II, which acts both locally and systemically, is a potent vasoconstrictor which readily increases systemic blood pressure, stimulates the secretion of aldosterone from the zona glomerulosa of the adrenal cortex to enhance sodium reabsorption in the distal nephron, stimulates thirst, and is involved in the glomerulotubular feedback mechanism.

Atrial natriuretic peptide

Following the observation that blood volume expansion caused a large rise in renal sodium excretion which could not be accounted for by inhibition of the renin–angiotensin–aldosterone system, specific humoral natriuretic factors were proposed. One that has been well characterized is human α-atrial natriuretic peptide, which is synthesized and secreted primarily by cardiac atrial myocytes. Moderate increases in blood volume and postural changes influence α-atrial natriuretic peptide release, probably mediated by direct distension of the atrial muscle. Its most important actions are on the kidney. At physiological concentrations, α-atrial natriuretic peptide appears not to alter glomerular filtration rate, but causes a modest natriuresis, minimal diuresis, and reduces plasma renin activity and plasma aldosterone concentration. In addition, it acts as a vasodilator, reduces systolic blood pressure and cardiac contractility, and is a potent inhibitor of aldosterone synthesis and release. Indeed, many of the effects of α-atrial natriuretic peptide could be explained by antagonism of the renin–angiotensin–aldosterone system. Specific receptors for this peptide have been identified in the kidney, on cortical glomeruli, the inner medulla, the vasa recta in the outer medulla, and the collecting duct.

Thus, it appears that α-atrial natriuretic peptide plays a minor role in regulating extracellular sodium content and volume, but does counterbalance to some extent the actions of the renin–angiotensin–aldosterone system. It is likely that other natriuretic factors exist. For example ouabain-like substances that inhibit renal sodium–potassium ATPase activity have been described, but have yet to be characterized fully and their physiological significance in sodium homeostasis has yet to be determined. Furthermore, there are numerous other intrarenal factors that may influence renal sodium excretion. Local production of dopamine appears to augment natriuresis following increased dietary sodium intake. Prostaglandins within the kidney, particularly PGE_2, inhibit sodium transport in the medullary thick ascending limb. The role of the renal kallikrein–kinin system is even less clear, although there is evidence that the natriuretic effect of bradykinin is due to inhibition of sodium reabsorption in the distal nephron. It is therefore apparent that control of renal sodium

Table 1 *Causes of the polyuria–polydipsia syndromes*

Cranial diabetes insipidus	Nephrogenic diabetes insipidus	Primary polydipsia

Familial
  Dominant (rarely recessive) inheritance
  *DIDMOAD or Wolfram syndrome
    (autosomal recessive)
Acquired
  Idiopathic
  Trauma (neurosurgery, head injury)
  Neoplasia (craniopharyngioma,
    dysgerminoma, pinealoma,
    hypothalamic metastasis, large
    pituitary tumour)
  Infection (meningitis, encephalitis)
  Vascular (sickle-cell anaemia,
    aneurysms of anterior
    communicating artery, Sheehan's
    syndrome)
  Granuloma (sarcoid)
	Familial
	  X-linked recessive inheritance
	Acquired
	  Idiopathic
	  Metabolic (hypercalcaemia, hypokalaemia)
	  Vascular (sickle-cell disease)
	  Osmotic diuresis (glycosuria, post-
	    obstructive uropathy)
	  Chronic renal disease (renal failure,
	    amyloid, sarcoidosis, pyelonephritis)
	  Drugs (lithium, demeclocycline,
	    amphotericin, glibenclamide,
	    methoxyfluorane)
		Familial
		  Psychogenic (compulsive water drinking)
		  Psychotic (schizophrenia, mania)
		  Idiopathic
		Secondary
		  Granuloma (sarcoid)
		  Vasculitis
		  Multiple sclerosis
		  Drugs (phenothiazines, tricyclic
		    antidepressants)

*DIDMOAD: diabetes insipidus, diabetes mellitus, optic atrophy, deafness.

excretion and extracellular volume is multifactual, complex, and has yet to be elucidated fully.

Disorders of water and salt homeostasis

The polyuric states

Polyuria is a state of excessive hypotonic urine excretion, normal urine volume output being less than 2.5 to 3.0 l/24 h. Three basic pathogenetic mechanisms account for polyuria. The first is a lack of osmoregulated vasopressin secretion, termed cranial, central, hypothalamic, or neurogenic diabetes insipidus. The second mechanism is a reduction in renal tubular responsiveness to adequate vasopressin, called nephrogenic or vasopressin-resistant diabetes insipidus. Thirdly, persistent excessive intake of fluid due to inappropriate thirst or drinking behaviour, known as primary polydipsia or dipsogenic diabetes insipidus, causes polyuria.

Cranial diabetes insipidus

Cranial diabetes insipidus is a disorder of urinary concentration which is due to decreased secretion of vasopressin. At least 80 per cent of vasopressin-synthesizing neurones must be destroyed before overt clinical features become manifest.

AETIOLOGY

The causes of cranial diabetes insipidus are given in Table 1. Familial varieties of this disorder are very rare, and, in some incidences, are due to point mutations or deletions in the vasopressin gene. Recent studies suggest that about 30 per cent of causes are idiopathic, of which a third of patients have circulating antibodies to the hypothalamic neurones that produce vasopressin, indicating a possible autoimmune aetiology. Trauma to the hypothalamus or pituitary stalk is a frequent cause of cranial diabetes insipidus, but the trans-sphenoidal approach to the pituitary is less traumatic than transfrontal surgery, and rarely causes cranial diabetes insipidus. Head injury may cause this disorder, but some patients follow a triple-phase response to trauma, characterized by initial polyuria for a few hours or days, followed by antidiuresis for a variable period, which progresses to permanent polyuria. Primary pituitary tumours rarely cause cranial diabetes insipidus.

CLINICAL FEATURES

The major clinical manifestations of cranial diabetes insipidus are polyuria, nocturia, excessive thirst, and drinking. Children may present with enuresis. Most patients have partial deficiency of vasopressin. Urine volumes range between 3 and 20 l/24 h with random urine osmolalities less than 300 mosmol/kg. Patients with cranial diabetes insipidus maintain plasma osmolality and serum sodium usually within the normal reference ranges because they have an intact osmoregulated thirst mechanism. Defective thirst, hypodipsia, leads to hypernatraemia and hyperosmolality. With severe polyuria the slightest urinary tract outflow obstruction can lead to hydronephrosis and hydroureter. Cranial diabetes insipidus may be masked by glucocorticoid hormone deficiency due either to hypopituitarism or primary adrenal failure, because cortisol is necessary for the maximal diluting function of the distal nephron.

The symptoms of partial cranial diabetes insipidus often worsen in pregnancy due to the increase in metabolic clearance of arginine vasopressin caused by vasopressinase, a circulating enzyme of placental origin.

Nephrogenic diabetes insipidus

In nephrogenic diabetes insipidus the renal tubules are totally, or more often, partially, resistant to the action of vasopressin.

AETIOLOGY

Table 1 outlines the causes of nephrogenic diabetes insipidus. Although very rare, the X-linked recessive disorder is very severe. Males express these symptoms while females have slightly impaired urinary concentration. Different gene mutations, occurring across families, are responsible for abnormal renal V_2 receptors and loss of cyclic 5'-AMP generation. A subgroup of patients can activate adenyl cyclase but fail to stimulate intracellular events that open water channels.

Hypercalcaemia-induced nephrogenic diabetes insipidus (Chapter 20.9.3) is due in part to reduced medullary hyperosmolality and adenyl cyclase stimulation, and in part to calcium deposition with scarring of the kidney. The effect of sustained hypokalaemia on renal function is complex. It inhibits sodium–potassium cotransport in the thick ascending limb; reduces adenyl cyclase activity; increases intrarenal prostaglandin synthesis, which blunts vasopressin's antidiuretic effect; and may reduce intracellular protein kinase function. Reversal of these metabolic derangements often, but not always, returns renal function to normal.

A third of patients taking long-term lithium carbonate develop nephrogenic diabetes insipidus. Lithium blunts the generation and action of cyclic 5'-AMP in the distal nephron and may reduce osmoregulated vasopressin secretion and/or stimulate thirst. Demeclocycline also inhibits cyclic 5'-AMP generation and function.

CLINICAL FEATURES

Nephrogenic diabetes insipidus in adults is usually partial, with mild symptoms. As is the case in patients with cranial diabetes insipidus, these individuals usually have serum sodium and plasma osmolality within the normal range, but low urine osmolality (< 300 mosmol/kg). The X-linked disorder presents soon after birth with profound polyuria, dehydration, fever, vomiting, and failure to thrive.

Primary polydipsia

There is a group of patients that, for reasons that are ill-understood, drink copious quantities of fluid in excess of body requirements, a disorder termed primary polydipsia.

AETIOLOGY

Many patients have a psychological disturbance leading to compulsive drinking, some of whom have a lowered osmotic thirst threshold but a normal threshold for vasopressin release. Very rarely a structural hypothalamic lesion (such as sarcoidosis) is believed to be the cause of primary polydipsia (Table 1). Some drugs stimulate thirst, by causing a dry mouth.

CLINICAL FEATURES

Although the clinical manifestations of primary polydipsia are similar to those of cranial and nephrogenic diabetes insipidus, nocturia is less of a feature perhaps because intact renal function and their pattern of drinking allows them to sleep through the night. Individuals with primary polydipsia may drink at a rate faster than their kidneys can excrete free water, despite suppression of vasopressin, and therefore their serum sodium tends to be lower than that of patients with cranial and nephrogenic diabetes insipidus, but usually remains within the reference range. Indeed, many primary polydipsia patients can drink up to 20 l/24 h and still remain normonatraemic.

Diagnostic evaluation of polyuric patients

Before embarking on expensive and time-consuming tests, it is always wise to establish that the urine volume is in excess of 3 l/24 h. Urine output less than this with a normal serum sodium and plasma osmolality excludes significant disturbance of water balance. Routine biochemical investigations of glucose, calcium, and potassium will focus on the cause of polyuria (Table 1). Three types of diagnostic tests are available: dehydration tests, measurement of plasma vasopressin after dehydration or osmotic stimulation, and a therapeutic trial of desmopressin.

DEHYDRATION TESTS

These are useful in the diagnosis of severe forms of cranial and nephrogenic diabetes insipidus. Although many protocols have been described, they are all based on observing the urine and blood responses to a period of fluid deprivation followed by noting the urine concentrating ability of exogenous vasopressin (for example, desmopressin). A typical, commonly used test is described in Table 2 of Chapter 12.3. Patients should be encouraged to drink adequately during the night prior

Table 2 *Interpretation of results from the water deprivation–desmopressin test*

Urine osmolality (mosmol/kg)		
After dehydration	After desmopressin	Diagnosis
> 750	> 750	Normal*
< 300	> 750	CDI
< 300	< 300	NDI
300–750	< 750	Partial CDI or Partial NDI or PP

* Assumes that plasma osmolality remains in the normal reference range, 285–295 mosmol/kg.

CDI, cranial diabetes insipidus; NDI, nephrogenic diabetes insipidus; PP, primary polydipsia.

to the test starting in the morning. Basal urine, to measure volume and osmolality, and blood for plasma osmolality is taken and the patient is weighed. All fluid is then withheld for 8 h with regular 1 to 2 hourly urine and blood samples and weighing of the patient. Thereafter, 2 μg of desmopressin is injected intramuscularly the patient, being allowed to drink cautiously and eat. Urine samples are collected over the subsequent 16 h. This test should be stopped if there is a weight loss in excess of 5 per cent.

A guide to interpretation of the results of the water deprivation test is given in Table 2. A major difficulty arises with the interpretation of results in the differentiation of the partial diabetes insipidus disorders from each other and from primary polydipsia. The reason for the poor differentiation is that prolonged polyuria, irrespective of its cause, leads to a reduction in maximal renal concentrating ability by removing renal medullary interstitial solute. Therefore, vasopressin cannot elicit its maximal renal effect. Direct measurement of plasma vasopressin aids diagnosis in these circumstances.

PLASMA VASOPRESSIN RESPONSE TO OSMOTIC STIMULATION AND DEHYDRATION

Measurement of plasma vasopressin and osmolality during a 2-h hypertonic (850 mmol/l) saline infusion at a rate of 0.04 ml/kg/min will diagnose precisely partial and compete cranial diabetes insipidus, as the vasopressin response to osmotic stimulation is subnormal (Fig. 5(a)). Patients with nephrogenic diabetes insipidus or primary polydipsia have results that fall within the normal range. After a period of water deprivation, the measurement of urine osmolality and plasma vasopressin will define nephrogenic diabetes insipidus (Fig. 5(b)), as vasopressin will be inappropriately elevated with respect to the low urine osmolality.

THERAPEUTIC TRIAL OF DESMOPRESSIN

If the water deprivation–desmopressin test gives equivocal results and facilities to measure vasopressin are not available, then a formal therapeutic trial of desmopressin should be instituted to differentiate the cause of polyuria. Because of the potential hazard of severe water intoxication in primary polydipsia patients, the trial must be supervised closely, preferably in hospital. After a basal period of 3 to 4 days, desmopressin (1–2 μg, intramuscularly) is administered to patients who are weighed and have urine and plasma osmolalities or serum sodium and urine volume measured daily. Patients with cranial diabetes insipidus will be identified by a reduction of thirst, little or no weight gain, a reduction in urine flow, and normal plasma osmolality. Nephrogenic diabetes insipidus is characterized by lack of response, although a tenfold increase in desmopressin dose might alleviate some symptoms. Primary polydipsia patients remain thirsty, continue to drink, gain weight, and become progressively hyponatraemic.

Having established the pathogenetic mechanism causing polyuria, it is important to search for a specific underlying cause (Table 1).

Treatment

CRANIAL DIABETES INSIPIDUS

Mild forms of cranial diabetes insipidus (urine output less than 4 l/24 h) may not require any specific therapy other than advice to drink sufficient quantities to quench thirst. In more severe forms, the drug of choice is desmopressin, a synthetic vasopressin V_2 receptor agonist analogue, possessing potent antidiuretic but no pressor activity, with a prolonged duration of action. Desmopressin is administered intranasally by spray or tube, parenterally or orally. There are wide individual variations in the intranasal dose required to control symptoms, ranging between 5 and 80 μg daily. Patients require 100 to 600 μg of oral desmopressin. Dilutional hyponatraemia is a potential hazard if desmopressin is given in excess for a prolonged period. This can be avoided by instructing the patient to forgo the drug 1 day each week. Desmopressin is a safe drug with which to treat cranial diabetes insipidus in pregnancy, and is resistant to the circulating placental enzyme, vasopressinase.

Lysine vasopressin, also given intranasally, is a shorter-acting alternative, but as it possesses pressor activity it may cause intestinal and/or renal colic, increase blood pressure, and induce coronary artery vasospasm.

Chlorpropamide, clofibrate, carbamazepine, and thiazide diuretics have been used, either singly or in combination, to reduce urine volume by up to 50 per cent, but are prescribed rarely these days because of their side-effects and the efficacy of desmopressin.

NEPHROGENIC DIABETES INSIPIDUS

Correction of the underlying cause of acquired nephrogenic diabetes insipidus (for example, removal of drug or correction of hypercalcaemia) may allow recovery of renal concentrating ability, but it may take a number of weeks to resolve. Polyuria of the severe familial form of nephrogenic diabetes insipidus can be reduced by about 50 per cent using the combination of thiazide and/or amiloride diuretics with a prostaglandin synthetase inhibitor (for example, indomethacin, 100 mg daily).

PRIMARY POLYDIPSIA

There is no efficacious drug treatment available for primary polydipsia although propranolol in doses up to 120 mg daily has been recommended to reduce thirst. Therapy directed towards underlying psychiatric problems may prove helpful.

Hyponatraemic states

Hyponatraemia, defined as a serum sodium less than 130 mmol/l, is a common electrolyte disturbance, affecting up to 5 per cent of hospital patients. Severe hyponatraemia (serum sodium < 115 mmol/l) is rare.

PSEUDOHYPONATRAEMIA

Spuriously low measurements of sodium can occur in serum from patients who have very high circulating concentrations of lipids or proteins because the volume of these substances contributes substantially to serum volume. The concentration of sodium, however, in the water of phase of blood remains normal; as plasma osmolality is normal its measurement provides an easy diagnostic test. A similar situation arises with severe hyperglycaemia, although the mechanism is different. High blood glucose concentrations draw intracellular water into the extracellular space, resulting in spurious hyponatraemia. Plasma osmolality, however, will be elevated due to the hyperglycaemia.

CLASSIFICATION AND CAUSES OF HYPONATRAEMIA

In all hyponatraemic states there is an excess of extracellular water relative to the total sodium content of the extracellular compartment. The sodium content, however, can vary markedly, and may be divided into three groups, thus forming the basis of the classification of hyponatraemia. Total extracellular sodium quantity can be:

(1) lower than normal, resulting in extracellular hypovolaemia;
(2) normal, with approximately normal or slightly expanded extracellular volume; and
(3) higher than normal, causing extracellular hypervolaemia.

Gross extracellular volume changes can be detected clinically: hypovolaemia leading to thirst, tachycardia, reduced skin turgor, and hypotension; and massive hypervolaemia to dependent oedema, possibly elevation of jugular venous pressure, and ascites. Minor volume changes are very difficult to assess clinically and there are no simple quick diagnostic tests to aid classification.

Table 3 presents the pathogenesis, provides some examples of causes, and emphasizes the importance of measuring urinary sodium in the three types of hyponatraemia. It should be appreciated that the majority of hyponatraemic patients have urine osmolalities in excess of 300 mosmol/kg and, of course, plasma is hypo-osmolar (< 280 mosmol/kg).

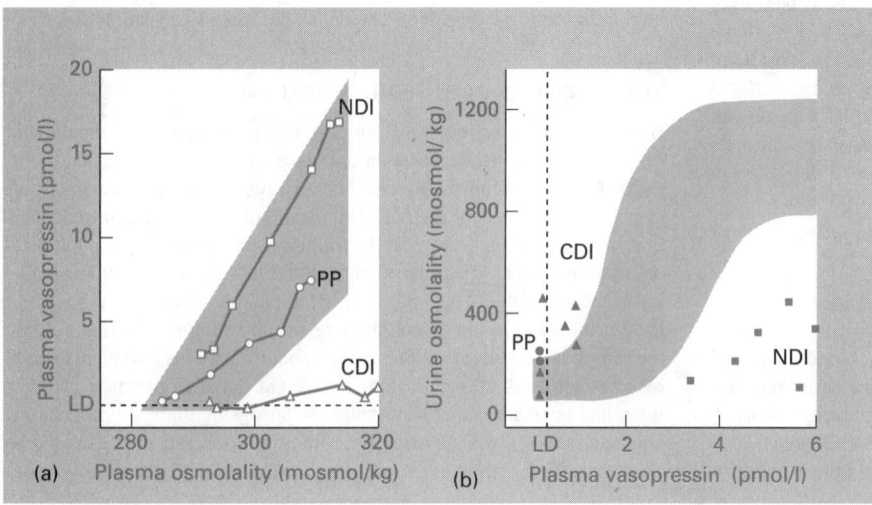

Fig. 5 (a) Relationship between plasma vasopressin and plasma osmolality during hypertonic saline infusion in typical patients with (i) cranial diabetes insipidus (CDI), (ii) nephrogenic diabetes insipidus (NDI), and (iii) primary polydipsia (PP). The shaded area represents the normal response. (b) Relationship between urine osmolality and plasma vasopressin in patients with CDI (▲), NDI (■), and PP (●) after a period of dehydration. The shaded area is the normal relationship under various degrees of hydration. LD represents the limit of detection of the plasma vasopressin assay.

Table 3 *Classification of hyponatraemia*

	Hypovolaemia: deficit of *TBW; larger deficit of *ExNa		Normovolaemia; normal or slight excess of TBW	Hypervolaemia: excess of ExNa; larger excess of TBW	
	Renal loss	Non-renal loss		Renal loss	Non-renal loss
Aetiology (examples)	Mineralocorticoid deficiency	Vomiting	Syndrome of inappropriate antidiuresis	Acute and chronic renal failure	Cardiac failure
	Sodium-losing renal disorders	Diarrhoea	Glucocorticoid deficiency		Cirrhosis
	Diuretic excess	Burns Excessive sweating	Hypothyroidism Inappropriate IV therapy (5% glucose)		Nephrotic syndrome Inappropriate IV therapy (normal saline)
			'Sick-cell' concept		
Urinary sodium concentration (mmol/l)	> 20	< 10	> 20	> 20	< 10

* TBW, total body water; ExNa, extracellular sodium; IV, intravenous.

Large sodium losses can occur commonly from persistent vomiting and/or diarrhoea, extensive skin burns, and excessive prolonged sweating. The healthy kidney will conserve sodium, urinary concentrations will be less than 10 mmol/l, and can be as low as 0.5 to 1 mmol/l. Renal sodium loss leading to hyponatraemia can be due to renal diseases (analgesic nephropathy, chronic pyelonephritis, polycystic kidneys, recovery from acute tubular necrosis or after bilateral ureteric obstruction), mineralocorticoid deficiency (Addison's disease, hyporeninaemic hypoaldosteronism), or diuretic excess.

Normovolaemic hyponatraemia is usually due to the syndrome of inappropriate antidiuresis (see below) or inappropriate administration of intravenous fluid (for example, 5 per cent dextrose solutions) in the postoperative period, and rarely to isolated glucocorticoid deficiency (for example partial hypopituitarism) or severe prolonged hypothyroidism. Beer drinker's potomania occurs in some individuals who drink excessive volumes of beer over short periods, for example 10 litres in 6 h, which overwhelms the kidney's capacity to excrete water.

Hypervolaemic hyponatraemia is observed commonly in severe heart failure, decompensated cirrhosis, and nephrotic syndrome. In these disorders glomerular filtration is reduced and proximal tubular sodium reabsorption increased. Renal afferent arteriole perfusion falls, leading to increased circulating angiotensin II concentrations, contributing to thirst stimulation. Furthermore, non-osmotic release of vasopressin also contributes to water retention (see Chapter 15.28.1).

CLINICAL FEATURES

In addition to the features associated with extracellular (and therefore blood) volume reductions described above, there are clinical manifestations due to hyponatraemia *per se* (Table 4). The severity of hyponatraemic features depend upon partly the absolute serum sodium concentration and partly its rate of fall. Chronic mild hyponatraemia (serum sodium 120–130 mmol/l) is often totally asymptomatic; but a fall to only 125 mmol/l from normal values over a few hours (usually iatrogenic) can cause convulsions.

GENERAL PRINCIPLES OF MANAGEMENT

Specific therapy for mild hyponatraemia is often not necessary and is reserved for symptomatic or severe life-threatening hyponatraemia. Treatment of the underlying cause is obviously essential and frequently corrects the serum sodium concentration.

For hypovolaemic hyponatraemia, volume replacement is mandatory. Infusion of isotonic saline is usually sufficient, but occasionally intra-

Table 4 *Clinical features of hyponatraemia*

Mild	Moderate	Severe
Anorexia	Personality change	Drowsiness
Headache	Muscle cramps	Diminished reflexes
Nausea	Muscle weakness	Convulsions
Vomiting	Confusion	Coma
Lethargy	Ataxia	Death

*Features depend upon the absolute serum sodium concentration or its rate of fall.

vascular volume expanders are required to maintain blood pressure, particularly in an acute situation. Immediate hydrocortisone as well as intravenous saline and subsequently fludrocortisone are essential to treat Addison's disease. Details of the treatment of normovolaemic hyponatraemia are given below.

The approach to hyponatraemia associated with hypervolaemic disorders is to give single or combined therapy with potent diuretic drugs to remove extracellular sodium, and to restrict water to less than 1 l/24 h. In cardiac failure, but not in cirrhosis, there may be benefit from angiotensin-converting enzyme inhibitors.

There is a high morbidity and mortality in patients in whom the plasma sodium concentration has fallen below 110 mmol/l, particularly when it has done so acutely. Although the underlying cause of such a change may be water intoxication from primary polydipsia in psychotic patients, or a combination of water excess and the use of amiloride-containing diuretics, the most common and always avoidable cause is probably iatrogenic ill-advised postoperative fluid administration. Modest hyponatraemia is common postoperatively and there are now more than 50 reports of symptomatic hyponatraemia after elective surgery in previously healthy women, all of whom died from the neurological sequelae. In the state of water intoxication, early symptoms include headache, nausea, vomiting, and later drowsiness proceeding to confusion, stupor, fits, respiratory arrest, and death.

CENTRAL PONTINE MYELINOLYSIS

When faced with a hyponatraemic patient with neurological features, urgent treatment is required to prevent this course of events; but over-rapid correction of the sodium concentration by whatever means can result in a different, but equally severe, neurological syndrome due to local areas of demyelination, called central pontine myelinolysis or the

Table 5 *Criteria for the diagnosis of the syndrome of inappropriate antidiuresis*

Dilutional hyponatraemia, i.e. plasma hypo-osmolality
  proportional to hyponatraemia
Urine osmolality greater than plasma osmolality (usually)
Persistent renal sodium excretion (> 50 mmol/l)
Absence of hypotension, hypovolaemia, and oedema-forming
  states
Normal renal and adrenal function

Table 6 *Classification and causes of hypernatraemia*

Hypervolaemic (excess extracellular sodium)
  Accidental (salt emetics, infant feeds)
  Iatrogenic (e.g. infusion of hypertonic bicarbonate or saline)
Hypovolaemic (insufficient total body-water)
  Decreased water intake
    Hypo- or adipsia
      Neoplasia of the hypothalamo-pituitary region
      Vascular (anterior communicating artery aneurysm)
      Granuloma (sarcoidosis, Langerhans cell histiocytosis)
      Miscellaneous (trauma, hydrocephalus, ventricular cyst)
    Reduced access to water
      Travel in desert
      Limitation of movement (stroke)
      Coma
  Acute excessive fluid loss
    Gastrointestinal
    Burns

osmotic demyelination syndrome. Features of this include quadriparesis, respiratory arrest, pseudobulbar palsy, mutism, and, rarely, fits. The distribution of the areas of demyelination include most often the pons, but also, in some cases, the basal ganglia, internal capsule, lateral geniculate body, and even the cerebral cortex.

This condition usually arises 24 to 48 h after over-rapid correction of profound hyponatraemia, and probably results from large shifts of intracellular water consequent on rapid changes in osmotic gradient between cells and extracellular fluid. Because of adaptations to chronic hyponatraemia resulting in reduced osmolality in brain cells, myelinolysis is particularly a risk when treatment of severe hyponatraemia is delayed for more than 24 h. A number of guidelines to the management of this dangerous clinical state have been proposed. All depend on a more or less rapid rate of infusion of physiological or hypertonic saline with the following caveats.

(1) The plasma sodium concentration should not rise by more than 10 to 12 mmol/l/24 h or 25 mmol/l in the first 48 h.

(2) When the fall is known to have occurred within 12 to 24 h it is safe to correct more quickly than if the hyponatraemia is more chronic.

Syndrome of inappropriate antidiuresis (siad)

This syndrome, due to inappropriate secretion of vasopressin, is the most common cause of normovolaemic hyponatraemia, and accounts for

Fig. 6 Types of osmoregulated vasopressin secretion patterns in SIAD. A, erratic vasopressin secretion; B, reset lowered, vasopressin threshold; C, failure to suppress vasopressin secretion; D, normal. The shaded area represents the normal range and LD, the limit of the assay. (Adapted from Zerbe *et al.* 1980, *Annual Reviews of Medicine.* 31, 315–327, with permission.)

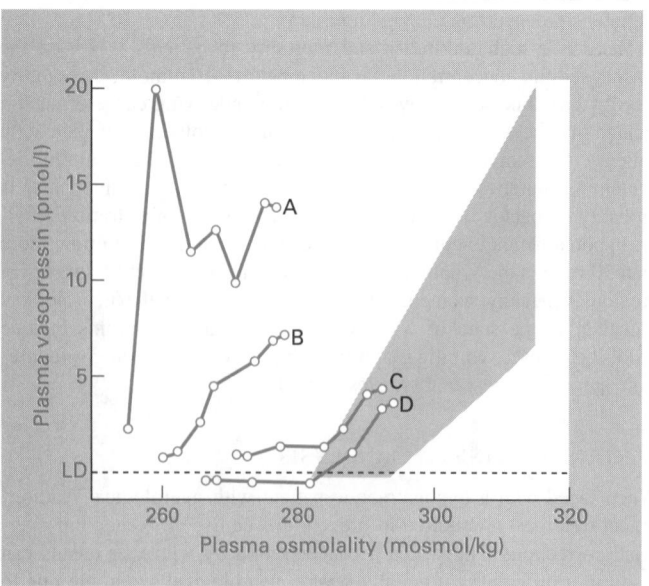

about 50 per cent of all hyponatraemia. The diagnosis of SIAD is established by ensuring that all the syndrome's criteria are fulfilled (Table 5). Only too often the first two criteria are met, leading to incorrect diagnoses. Measurement of urinary sodium is essential, which is persistently elevated (50–70 mmol/l). The final two criteria help to exclude hypo-and hypervolaemic states. Plasma vasopressin estimations are unhelpful in differentiating SIAD from other causes of hyponatraemia, because the majority of all hyponatraemic states (> 90 per cent) have detectable or elevated values, due to non-osmotic release of the hormone. It is in fact the persistent circulating vasopressin that largely causes the relative water excess in all types of hyponatraemia.

PATHOPHYSIOLOGY AND CAUSES OF SIAD

A very large number of disorders has been associated with SIAD, some of which are listed in Table 4 of Chapter 12.3. In brief, they include a variety of neoplasic conditions, the most common being small-cell carcinoma of bronchus; non-malignant chest diseases including infections; neurological disorders (infective and vascular); drugs (cytotoxic agents, chlorpropamide, carbamazepine, antidepressants, oxytocin, and thiazide diuretics); and a miscellaneous group (porphyria, cortisol deficiency, idiopathic).

Although measurement of plasma vasopressin plays no part in the diagnosis of SIAD, interesting insights into the pathophysiology of the syndrome are gained by studying osmoregulated vasopressin secretion. Four patterns of vasopressin secretion have been defined (Fig. 6); the most common (Type A) demonstrates erratic secretion of vasopressin. About 30 per cent of patients have an osmoregulated vasopressin release with a lowered threshold (type B), while some patients fail to suppress vasopressin secretion at low plasma osmolality (type C). A very small proportion have normal osmoregulated vasopressin (type D). The cause of SIAD does not correlate with the pattern of secretion. For example, patients with small-cell bronchial carcinoma may not only demonstrate type A (presumably ectopic vasopressin secretion by the tumour) but can have types B or C (likely to be due to abnormal neurological or neurotransmitter signals).

The persistent natriuresis, central to the diagnosis of SIAD, can be explained, in part, by the expanded total body-water producing a reduction in aldosterone production, an increase in circulating natriuretic factors, and a decrease in proximal sodium reabsorption.

TREATMENT OF SIAD

Identification and successful treatment of the underlying cause of SIAD will usually correct the hyponatraemia. If chronic symptomatic or life-threatening hyponatraemia remains, specific measures to remove the excess of total body-water are required.

Fluid restriction to 500 ml/24 h to increase serum sodium to about 130 mmol/l remains the fundamental therapy. If this approach is unsatisfactory, additional methods to remove water are justified, the most successful of which is the induction of partial nephrogenic diabetes insipidus with demeclocycline (600–1200 mg daily in divided doses) but maximal effect may take 2 weeks to achieve. It is preferable to lithium carbonate which, although inducing nephrogenic diabetes insipidus, is more toxic. An alternative approach is the administration of frusemide (40–80 mg daily) in combination with oral sodium chloride supplementation (3 g daily). Phenytoin has occasionally proved helpful by suppressing inappropriate neurohypophysial vasopressin secretion. Treatment of SIAD will be enhanced once specific V_2 receptor antagonists are developed. Infusion of isotonic or hypertonic solutions of saline are not advised because of the real danger of rapid serum sodium increases causing osmotic demyelination syndrome (see above).

SICK-CELL CONCEPT

This concept was formulated following the observation that hyponatraemia developed quickly in severe trauma or overwhelming infection in man or animals, but also in malnourished, very ill patients. It is a normovolaemic hyponatraemia that resembles type B SIAD (Fig. 6). It has been suggested that there is a shift of intracellular water into the extracellular compartment due to reduction of intracellular solute by either leakage across a damaged cell membrane or enhanced intracellular catabolism, or possibly due to movement of sodium into the cell. There is no specific therapy other than treatment of the underlying cause.

Hypernatraemic states and thirst deficiency

Hypernatraemia is less common than hyponatraemia and may be defined by a serum sodium greater than 150 mmol/l.

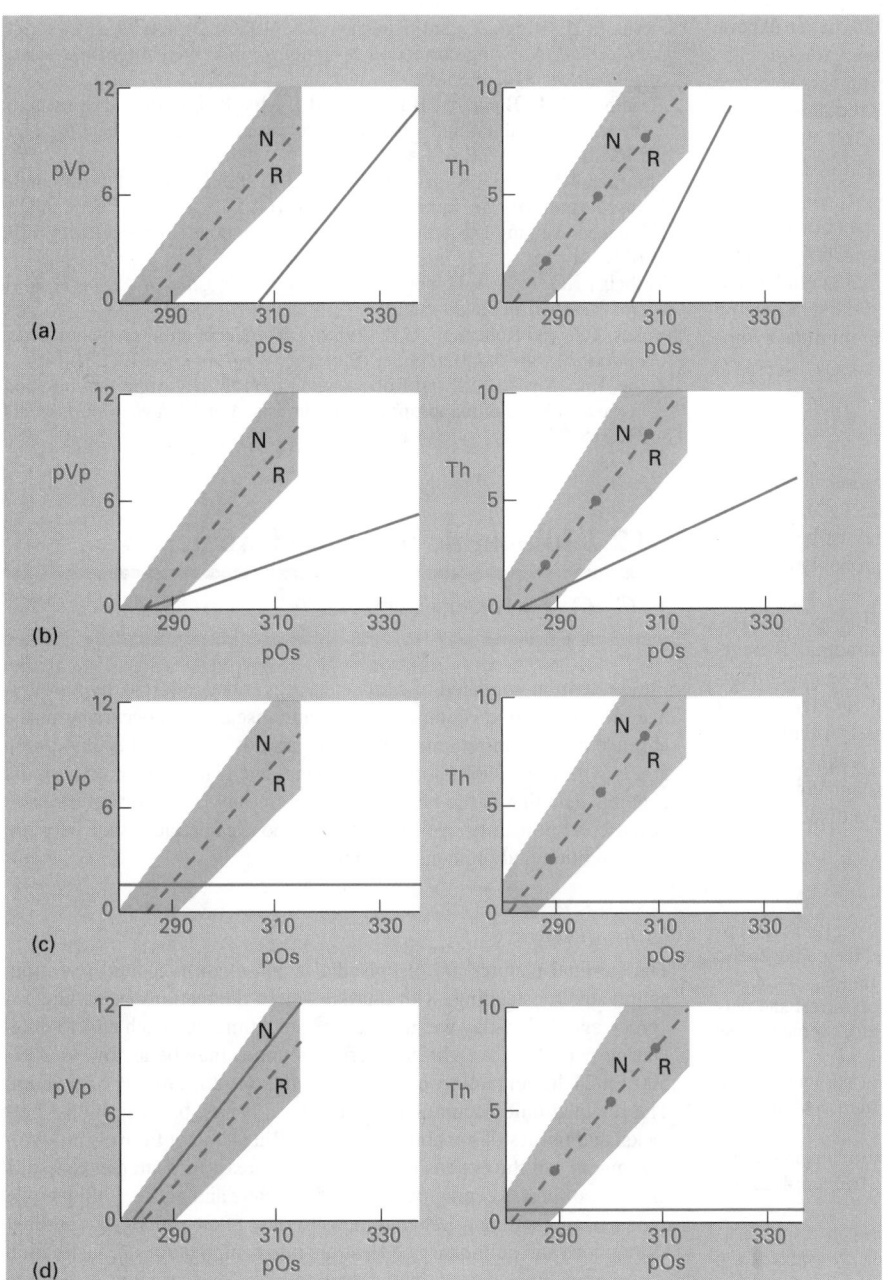

Fig. 7 Types of osmoregulated thirst (Th) and vasopressin secretion (Vp) in hypodipsic hypovolaemic hypernatraemia. Stippled areas are the normal responses to increases in plasma osmolality (pOs) and the dashed lines represent mean osmoregulatory lines. (a) Reset, raised, thirst and vasopressin thresholds or 'essential' hypernatraemia; (b) decreased sensitivity of thirst and vasopressin release; (c) complete destruction of both osmoreceptors; (d) absent thirst osmoregulation with normal osmoregulated vasopressin release. (Reproduced from Baylis, P.H., and Thompson, C.J. (1988). *Clinical Endocrinology*, **29**, 549–76, with permission.)

AETIOLOGY AND PATHOPHYSIOLOGY

Hypernatraemia is classified into two categories, dependent on extracellular volume states (Table 6). Hypervolaemic hypernatraemia is caused by extracellular sodium excess, usually as a result of accidental iatrogenic overdoses of sodium-containing preparations. Acute hypovolaemic hypernatraemia occurs when patients lose large quantities of hypotonic fluid (for example, gastrointestinal).

Chronic hypovolaemic hypernatraemia is the result of prolonged water deficit, usually the result of impaired or absent thirst, hypo- or adipsia, which implies a lesion of the thirst osmoreceptor. It is sometimes associated with abnormal osmoregulated vasopressin secretion. Four patterns of osmoregulatory dysfunction have been described (Fig. 7). The first, type A, shows elevation of osmotic thresholds for both thirst and vasopressin. It has been termed 'essential' hypernatraemia; patients continue to dilute and concentrate urine normally, but do so around a higher serum sodium. Type B is characterized by decreased sensitivity (slope) of the vasopressin and thirst osmoregulatory lines. The most serious defect, termed adipsic hypernatraemia (type C), is due to complete destruction of both osmoreceptors. Patients never experience the desire to drink even when serum sodium reaches values as high as 190 mmol/l. In the very rare fourth pattern (type D), there is selective complete loss of thirst but vasopressin osmoregulation remains normal.

CLINICAL FEATURES

Hypervolaemic hypernatraemia causes severe thirst, irritability, hypotonia, and may lead to convulsions, seizures, and death. Clinical manifestations of hypovolaemic hypernatraemia relate to extracellular and intracellular fluid loss, and the striking feature is lack of thirst. The slow development of hypernatraemia is often associated with minimal symptoms of confusion or drowsiness.

TREATMENT OF HYPERNATRAEMIA

Patients require water to lower serum sodium concentration slowly. The safest route of administration is oral, but unconscious patients will require infusion of 5 per cent dextrose solutions. Care must be taken to avoid rapid falls in serum sodium, with the rate of fall probably no faster than 10 mmol/24 h.

'Essential' hypernatraemia (Fig. 7, type A) requires little specific therapy as patients are protected from extremes of hypernatraemia. Patients with total loss of thirst and vasopressin osmoregulation pose major management problems. They should be instructed to drink a daily volume of about 2 litres which is adjusted according to changes in daily body weight. Desmopressin may be required. Regular checks of serum sodium are essential to avoid wide fluctuations. Constant vigilance is necessary to maintain water balance in chronic hypo- or adipsic patients.

REFERENCES

Anderson, R.J., Chung, H.-M., Kluge, R., and Schrier, R.W. (1985). Hyponatremia: a prospective analysis of its epidemiology and the pathogenetic role of vasopressin. *Annals of Internal Medicine* 102, 164–8.

Arieff, A.I. (1986). Hyponatraemia, convulsions, respiratory arrest and permanent brain damage after effective surgery in healthy women. *New England Journal of Medicine* 314, 1529–35.

Arieff, A.I. and Guisado, R. (1976). Effects on the central nervous system of hypernatremic and hyponatremic states. *Kidney International* 10, 104–16.

Bartter, F.C. and Schwartz, W.B. (1967). The syndrome of inappropriate secretion of antidiuretic hormone. *American Journal of Medicine* 42, 790–806.

Baylis, P.H. and Robertson, G.L. (1980). Plasma vasopressin response to hypertonic saline to assess posterior pituitary function. *Journal of the Royal Society of Medicine* 73, 255–60.

Baylis, P.H. and Thompson, C.J. (1988). Osmoregulation of vasopressin secretion and thirst in health and disease. *Clinical Endocrinology* 29, 549–76.

Berl, T. (1988). Psychosis and water balance. *New England Journal of Medicine* 318, 441–2.

Berl, T. (1990). Treating hyponatraemia; damned if we do and damned if we don't. *Kidney International* 37, 1006–18.

Berl, T., Anderson, R.J., McDonald, K.M., and Schrier, R.W. (1976). Clinical disorders of water metabolism. *Kidney International* 10, 117–32.

Davison, J.M., Shiells, E.A., Philips, P.R., and Lindheimer, M.D., (1988). Serial evaluation of vasopressin release and thirst in human pregnancy. *Journal of Clinical Investigation* 81, 798–806.

de Zeeuw, D., Janssen, W.M.T., and de Jong, P.E. (1992). Atrial natriuretic factor: Its (patho)physiological significance in humans. *Kidney International* 41, 1115–33.

Kenyon, C.J. and Jardine, A.G. (1989). Atrial natriuretic peptide: water and electrolyte homeostasis. Baillière's Clin Endocrinol. Metab. 3, 431–450.

Mitchell, K.D. and Navar L.G. (1989). The renin-angiotensin-aldosterone system in volume control. *Baillière's Clinical Endocrinology and Metabolism* 3, 393–430.

Robertson, G.L. (1989). Syndrome of inappropriate antidiuresis. *New England Journal of Medicine* 321, 538–9.

Sterns, R.H., Riggo, J., and Schochet, S.S. (1986). Osmotic demyelination syndrome following correction of hyponatremia. *New England Journal of Medicine* 314, 1535–42.

Thompson C.J., Bland, J., Burd, J., and Baylis, P.H. (1986). The osmotic thresholds for thirst and vasopressin release are similar in healthy man. *Clinical Science*, 71, 651–6.

Thrasher, T.N., Keil, L.C., and Ramsay, D.J. (1982). Lesions of the organum vasculosum of the lamina terminalis (OVLT) attenuate osmotically induced drinking and vasopressin secretion in dogs. *Endocrinology* 110, 1837–41.

Verbalis, J.G. (1989). Hyponatraemia. *Baillière's Clinical Endocrinology and Metabolism* 3, 499–530.

Vokes, T.J., and Robertson, G.L. (1988). Disorders of antidiuretic hormone. *Endocrinology and Metabolic, Clinics of North America* 17, 281–99.

Zerbe, R.L., Stropes, L., and Robertson, G.L. (1980). Vasopressin function in the syndrome of inappropriate antidiuresis. *Annual Review of Medicine* 31, 315–27.

20.2.2 Idiopathic oedema of women

J. G. G. LEDINGHAM

Fluid retention unrelated to cardiac, hepatic, renal, allergic, hypoproteinaemic, obstructive venous, or lymphatic disease, and occurring in the absence of sodium-retaining drugs occurs not uncommonly in women and has been labelled idiopathic oedema, cyclical oedema, or periodic oedema. The first is the best name, since in only a proportion of cases is the condition truly cyclical. There is no clear relationship between this condition and premenstrual tension.

Clinical features

The cardinal features are of episodic or more constant fluid retention, aggravated by standing, with diurnal weight fluctuations exceeding 1.4 kg/day and day-to-day weight changes sometimes as much as 4 to 5 kg. During periods of weight gain, urine volumes may be as low as 300–500 ml/24 h, containing minimal amounts (1–20 mmol/l) of sodium. The retained fluid accumulates in the face, hands, breasts, thighs, buttocks, and tissues of the abdominal wall. Rings do not fit over the swollen fingers and the expansion in waist and breast measurements results in some sufferers keeping two sizes of brassiere and girdle. Pitting ankle oedema is uncommon but may be observed after prolonged standing. Orthopnoea and pulmonary oedema are rare complications. Constipation is common. Episodes of fluid retention or of exacerbation of a more chronic state may occur unpredictably, but emotional stress, obesity, food high in carbohydrate, as well as prolonged standing, are recognized triggers.

The condition occurs only after menarche, is seen more often in the third and fourth decade but may persist with amenorrhoea, after oophorectomy, and may continue after the menopause. Sufferers are characteristically emotionally labile and are prone to neurosis and depression. Extreme physical and mental lethargy is usual and the patient's misery during periods of retention is aggravated by the sense of bloated ugliness and distortion of appearance that she feels. Most, but not all, patients have found access to diuretics when first seen in hospital practice. Hypokalaemic hypochloraemic alkalosis with hyperuricaemia may reflect diuretic abuse, and rare patients abuse purgatives as well.

Pathophysiology

There is no strong consensus of opinion about pathophysiology. It may be that this is a heterogeneous condition. Certainly there is a subset of women in whom overconcern with weight and appearance leads to diuretic abuse and rebound oedema when diuretics are stopped, as described by de Wardener. Some of this group have features in common with anorexia nervosa. Whilst diuretic abuse may be an aggravating factor in some women and the primary factor in others, it cannot be the whole story since cases were described before potent diuretics became available and because withdrawal of diuretics in hospital over 2 to 3 weeks reverses the condition in only a few patients.

No good evidence exists of primary abnormalities in the renin–angiotensin–aldosterone system, nor in the metabolism of oestrogens or progestogens. Hyperprolactinaemia, dopamine deficiency, and high plasma adenosine monophosphate have been described in a few cases, but it is unlikely that these changes are of aetiological significance in many patients. There is evidence of an orthostatic leak of plasma volume and plasma proteins into the tissue fluids in women subject to idiopathic oedema. The increase in venous blood haematocrit on standing is greater than normal, and reflects a fall in plasma volume which initiates renal salt and water retention, probably through enhanced proximal tubular reabsorption since there is a fall in fractional free water clearance and osmolar clearance. The renal response is then entirely appropriate to changes in plasma volume. Diurnal weight gains amounting to 4–5 kg must reflect an abnormally high fluid intake during periods of fluid retention, perhaps because of thirst stimulated by volume receptors. The mechanism of the presumed increase in capillary permeability is unknown, but could relate to abnormal arteriolar regulation of capillary hydrostatic pressures.

The distribution of oedema is an odd feature of this disorder, if it is indeed due to an abnormality of capillary permeability however caused. Such an abnormality would explain the aggravation of fluid retention on standing and its relief by lying flat, but does not explain why fluid is so predominantly distributed in face, breasts, fingers, abdomen, and thighs, while ankle oedema of the kind seen in nephrotic states, for instance, is remarkably rare.

Management

Sympathetic explanation of the nature of the problem helps management. Patients should be advised to avoid long periods of standing and to use supine rest to relieve oedema instead of diuretics whenever possible. Elastic stockings, put on before getting up, help to reduce the orthostatic loss of plasma volume. Clothes fitting tightly around the waist may aggravate the condition by increasing venous pressure in the legs and should be avoided. Obesity increases the tendency to fluid retention and some women associate exacerbation with an increase in dietary carbohydrate. Diuretics, by further decreasing an already reduced plasma volume, are an illogical treatment and should be used as sparingly as possible; but most patients' symptoms are unacceptable without some diuretic treatment. Resistance develops quickly and many patients are very difficult to wean from massive doses of loop agents, often combined with amiloride or spironolactone. Psychotherapy may help the neurotic and depressive traits but is of no proven benefit in reducing the frequency or severity of episodes of oedema.

Drugs have little to offer in this condition. Among those that have been tried occasional success has been reported with L-dopa, combined with carbidopa, bromocriptine, and most recently the tricyclic drug nomifensine but all must be considered of unproven value.

REFERENCES

de Wardener, H.E. (1981). Idiopathic edema: role of diuretic abuse. *Kid. Int.* **19**, 881–892.

Dunnigan, M.G. and Pelosi, A.J. (1993). Familial idiopathic oedema in prepubital children; a new syndrome. *Quarterly Journal of Medicine*, **86**, 301–13.

Edwards, O.M. and Bayliss, R.I.S. (1976). Idiopathic oedema of women. *Q. J. Med.* **45**, 125–144.

Gill, J.R. (1983). Idiopathic edema. *Sem. Nephol.* **3**, 205–210.

20.2.3 Disorders of potassium metabolism

J. G. G. LEDINGHAM

Hypokalaemia and hyperkalaemia

Physiological considerations

Potassium, the chief intracellular cation, is present in cells in a concentration between 150 and 160 mmol/l. Total body potassium ranges between 37 and 52 mmol/kg body-weight depending very largely on muscle mass, so that amounts are greater in the young than the old and in men than in women. Ninety-eight per cent of potassium is intracellular, the ratio of the intracellular to the extracellular components being a critical determinant of the membrane potential of excitable tissues. The movement of potassium into cells and the maintenance of the consequently large concentration gradient is chiefly dependent on the Na–K ATPase enzyme, which extrudes sodium and takes in potassium in a ratio of three sodium to two potassium molecules. This active transport of potassium into cells is normally balanced by passive losses, largely through ion-selective potassium channels present in all cell membranes.

Dietary potassium intake in Western society normally varies between 50 and 150 mmol/day, but homeostasis can be maintained with intakes as high as 500 mmol/day in health. In normal circumstances, the kidney is the only important route of excretion, with only some 5 to 15 mmol appearing daily in the stools.

The plasma potassium concentration (normally 3.5–4.5 mmol/l) is regulated by homeostatic mechanisms controlling internal as well as external balance. External balance, which determines total body potassium, is largely controlled by the kidney but with a small and sometimes important contribution by the gut. Internal balance determines the proportions of intracellular and extracellular potassium under the influence of pH, bicarbonate, aldosterone, insulin, adrenergic stimuli, glucagon, and osmolality.

INTERNAL BALANCE

PH and bicarbonate

The ratio of intracellular to extracellular potassium appears to be influenced by pH and plasma bicarbonate concentrations separately, with a rise in either increasing intracellular at the expense of extracellular potassium. The hyperkalaemia of acidosis has long been attributed to an exchange of hydrogen for potassium in cells, but inhibition of the Na–K ATPase by acidosis, although countered by an associated reduction in the conductance of potassium to cell membranes, must also contribute. The degree of change in plasma potassium depends on the cause of the associated change in pH. An hyperchloraemic acidosis may increase plasma potassium by some 0.7 mmol/l for each 0.1 unit fall in pH, whereas the change associated with respiratory acidosis is considerably less, around 0.1 mmol/l per 0.1 unit change of pH. In most clinical states of acidosis there is hyperkalaemia or at least a high plasma potassium concentration in relation to external balance; but hyperkalaemia is not a feature of post-ictal lactic acidosis, nor does infusion of organic acids (as opposed to mineral acids) in dogs induce hyperkalaemia. The reasons for these observations are not clear, but it may be that potassium shifts are not induced in organic acidaemic states when the origin of the excess acid is intracellular. There is also some evidence that organic acids may stimulate the release of insulin, which would tend to blunt the effect of acidosis *per se*.

Aldosterone

A rise in plasma potassium stimulates aldosterone secretion and a fall retards it. Although the major contribution of aldosterone in protecting against hyperkalaemia is to increase renal and, to a much lesser extent, colonic potassium excretion, it is possible that aldosterone also affects internal potassium balance. The adrenal gland is known to be essential for the phenomenon whereby acute potassium loads are taken up by cells in animals accustomed to a high potassium diet (potassium adaptation), but more direct evidence for an increased cellular uptake of potassium under the influence of aldosterone is lacking. One mechanism of potassium adaptation is by an increase in the activity of cell-membrane Na–K ATPase in response to major increases in dietary intake.

Insulin

An increase in plasma potassium stimulates insulin release which might be expected to induce a net uptake of potassium into cells. High concentrations of insulin given intravenously certainly lower plasma potassium by promoting uptake into the liver and muscle by a mechanism involving stimulation of the sodium–potassium pump, and independent of that promoting transport of glucose. The much lower concentrations of endogenous insulin have not yet been proven to influence internal potassium balance significantly, but it may be that the larger amounts present in portal vein blood influence potassium uptake by the liver substantially. Tolerance of potassium loads is impaired in insulin-deficient diabetics and in normal subjects infused with somatostatin, suggesting at least a permissive role for insulin in the regulation of cellular uptake of potassium.

Glucagon has been shown to increase plasma potassium concentrations independently of its effects on glucose and insulin, and, conversely, hyperkalaemia may be associated with the release of glucagon.

Adrenergic stimuli

The rise in plasma potassium concentrations resulting from an infusion of potassium chloride is increased in the presence of non-selective β-adrenergic blocking drugs, such as propranolol, or of the α-agonist phenylephrine. Adrenaline infusions induce hypokalaemia by increasing potassium flux into skeletal muscle by β_2-activation of membrane-bound adenylate cyclase and subsequent stimulation of Na–K ATPase. Sympathetic nervous discharge may also promote a shift of potassium from extra- to intracellular fluid, since the tolerance of intravenous potassium is reduced in animals which have been chemically sympathectomized.

Heavy muscular exercise results in a loss of potassium from muscle to extracellular fluid, and plasma concentrations can rise as much as 50 per cent after 10 to 15 min, falling precipitously in the postexercise period. β-Blocking drugs exaggerate the hyperkalaemia of exercise, while phentolamine reduces it. α-Agonists increase net loss of potassium from cells into the extracellular fluid while β-adrenergic stimuli are well recognized to promote hypokalaemia, particularly the β_2-selective agents such as salbutamol and terbutaline. Theophylline preparations also induce the entry of potassium into cells and it has been suggested that one reason for sudden death in asthmatics may be a hypokalaemia-

associated arrhythmia induced by high endogenous adrenaline, the use of salbutamol, and of theophylline derivatives all at the same time.

Plasma concentrations of adrenaline may rise to levels known to promote hypokalaemia after the pain and anxiety of myocardial infarction, and it is not surprising that there are increasing reports of hypokalaemia in patients in coronary care units who have not yet been treated with potassium-losing diuretics. The hypokalaemia which may complicate delirium tremens after alcohol withdrawal is also likely to be β-adrenergically mediated.

Non-selective β-blocking drugs may increase plasma potassium significantly in some patients with chronic renal failure or with insulin-deficient diabetes mellitus.

Osmolality

Hyperosmolar states caused by hyperglycaemia or, for instance, by mannitol infusion tend to increase plasma potassium by some 0.6 mmol/l per increase in osmolality of 10 milliosmoles/kg.

EXTERNAL BALANCE

External balance is regulated mainly by the kidney, with a small contribution by the gastrointestinal tract in health. The colon can be an important route of potassium excretion in renal failure.

Renal control of external potassium balance

Renal tubular handling of potassium is complex, but ultimate control of urinary potassium excretion is still believed to lie in the mechanisms of potassium secretion in the distal nephron.

Proximal tubular reabsorption is at least in part an active process and appears complete by the end of the proximal segment. Potassium then re-enters tubular fluid in the pars recta and the descending limb of Henle's loop to be reabsorbed in the thick ascending limb by sodium–potassium cotransport. Potassium present in the descending limb may come from reabsorption in the collecting ducts via the medullary tissue, thereby contributing to medullary hypertonicity by a recycling process which takes place largely in the juxtamedullary nephrons. The system may contribute to the regulation of potassium excretion in several ways. Reduced potassium absorption by the thick ascending limb of Henle's loop can contribute to kaliuresis. Further, a high medullary concentration of potassium tends to decrease sodium reabsorption in the thick ascending limb; the resultant increase of delivery to sodium to the distal nephron also favours kaliuresis.

In the early distal tubule there are mechanisms of active transport of potassium into cells on both the peritubular and luminal surfaces. Movement of potassium into tubular urine at this site is dependent on electrical and chemical gradients, and is therefore passive. The luminal concentration of sodium and the nature of its accompanying anion are important factors in controlling these gradients.

Further down the nephron in the cortical collecting ducts, potassium transport into tubular fluid is active, not strictly linked to sodium reabsorption but in some way dependent on intraluminal sodium concentration and the rate of flow of tubular fluid. Further secretion of potassium may occur in the medullary collecting ducts under conditions of metabolic alkalosis, solute diuresis, potassium loading, and facilitated by antidiuretic hormone (ADH).

A number of factors influence distal nephron potassium secretion and determine the rate of potassium excretion in the urine.

Potassium adaptation

A chronic high potassium intake enhances distal tubular potassium secretion by a number of mechanisms, which result in a kidney able to excrete as much as 10 or 20 times more than it does in normal circumstances. In this situation, there is an increased content of Na–K ATPase and of surface area in the basolateral membranes of the cortical collecting tubules, and the colon also increases its capacity to secrete potassium, again by an increase in Na–K pumps. These changes can occur independently of an increase in plasma aldosterone concentration, but hyperaldosteronism stimulated by hyperkalaemia is required for full adaptation by the kidney to chronic, very high potassium intakes.

Sodium delivery to the distal nephron

Any condition which increases sodium delivery to the distal nephron (for example loop diuretics, osmotic diuretics, or salt loading) enhances urinary potassium excretion. The precise mechanisms by which this phenomenon occurs are not clear but relate to sodium concentrations and tubular flow rates in the distal tubules.

Aldosterone

Mineralocorticoids enhance sodium reabsorption and potassium secretion in the cortical collecting ducts by increasing Na–K ATPase activity in the basolateral membranes and by increasing the conductance of potassium in the luminal membrane of the principal cells of the collecting duct.

pH changes

Alkalosis, by increasing the uptake of potassium in the basolateral membranes and the conductance of the luminal membranes of the distal nephron, promotes kaliuresis so that alkalotic states are associated with enhanced potassium excretion by the kidney. The reverse is the case in chronic acidosis. In addition, the mechanism whereby potassium and hydrogen may exchange for one another favours renal potassium wasting in alkalosis and retention in acidosis.

Flow rates of tubular fluid

There is good evidence from micropuncture studies that increased flow rates in distal tubular fluid enhance potassium excretion in potassium replete, but not in potassium deplete, animals.

ADH

A significant stimulation of distal tubular potassium secretion by ADH suggests that this hormone may help to prevent potassium retention and hyperkalaemia in oliguria secondary to dehydration. The effect appears to be mediated by activation of sodium and potassium channels in the luminal membrane, together with an increase in Na–K ATPase activity in the basolateral membrane; the effects of ADH and aldosterone in this context are additive.

Anions

An increased delivery of poorly reabsorbable anions in the glomerular filtrate (for example sulphate) also enhances distal tubular potassium secretion by a combination of increased fluid and sodium delivery and by the enhanced transepithelial electrical potential gradient.

Hypokalaemia

Severe hypokalaemia (plasma potassium less than 2.4 mmol/l) occurred in one per cent of patients admitted to hospital in one large series. Malignant disease, especially acute myeloid leukaemia, was a surprisingly frequent association, attributed in some cases to the sodium load given with massive doses of carbenicillin or penicillin. These and other causes of hypokalaemia are listed in Table 1. Dietary deficiency alone is an uncommon cause but a high intake may prevent, or a low one exacerbate, changes in internal or external balance.

PATHOPHYSIOLOGICAL EFFECTS OF HYPOKALAEMIA

Whether hypokalaemia is the consequence of overall potassium depletion or because of a shift of potassium into cells, there will be an increase in the ratio of intracellular to extracellular potassium. This change causes hyperpolarization across excitable membranes, an effect which underlies the most serious clinical consequences of hypokalaemia. The resultant

Table 1 *Causes of hyperkalaemia*

Intracellular shifts	
Alkalosis	Theophylline overdose
High-dose insulin	Periodic paralysis
β$_2$-adrenergic stimulation	? Aldosterone
	Poisoning by barium salts
	Toluene intoxication (glue-sniffing)
Renal wasting	
Alkalosis (metabolic and respiratory)	Cushing's syndrome
Diuretics	Adrenogenital syndromes
Solute diuresis	Bartter's syndrome
Glucose	Liddle's disease
Urea	Magnesium depletion
Mannitol	Carbenoxolone sodium
Saline	Liquorice addiction
Carbenicillin	Renal tubular acidosis
Penicillin	Ureterosigmoidostomy
Aldosteronism	Gentamicin
Primary	Amikacin
Secondary	Acute leukaemia
Renin-secreting tumours	Renal tubular acidosis
Renal tubular disorders	
Gastrointestinal	
Pyloric stenosis	Chloride-diarrhoea
Bulimia nervosa	Villous adenoma of the rectum
Ileostomy	Purgative abuse

increase in myocardial excitability can precipitate a variety of cardiac dysrhythmias ranging from unifocal extrasystoles to ventricular tachycardia or fibrillation. The toxicity of digitalis preparations is also enhanced and may be associated particularly with atrial tachycardia with block and with atrioventricular dissociation. Changes in the electrocardiogram, (**ECG**), which may be evident when plasma potassium concentrations fall below 3 mmol/l, include depression of the ST segment, flattening of the T-waves, and prominent U-waves. These changes, however, correlate poorly with the development of serious dysrhythmias. The force of myocardial contraction is increased *in vitro* when the bath fluid potassium concentration is low, but *in vivo* function is well maintained despite hypokalaemia.

Marked potassium depletion impairs striated muscle function, with weakness and absent reflexes sometimes progressing to paralysis which can affect the respiratory muscles causing a life-threatening emergency. Frank rhabdomyolysis occurs particularly after exercise when depletion is profound, but an increase in plasma levels of creatine phosphokinase without obvious myalgia is more common and may occur when plasma concentrations fall below 3 mmol/l. The smooth muscle of the gut is also affected, with reduced motility or frank ileus frequently complicating hypokalaemia.

The effects of low plasma potassium concentrations on the kidney include nephrogenic diabetes insipidus, a fall in glomerular filtration rate, a tendency towards sodium retention, and increased renal acid excretion resulting in metabolic alkalosis. Failure to concentrate urine appears to be due to a reduction in medullary solute concentration, perhaps related to altered local blood flow as well as resistance to ADH because of increased production of prostaglandins. The mechanism whereby very low potassium diets result in sodium retention and sometimes to oedema are not understood.

Chronic hypokalaemia is associated with morphological changes in the kidney with the appearance of prominent vacuoles in the cytoplasm of both proximal and distal cortical tubular cells. Although it is often claimed that severe and prolonged potassium deficiency causes irreversible and progressive interstitial nephritis with consequent renal failure, the evidence for this is not conclusive.

Potassium deficiency *per se* has long been reported to cause a metabolic alkalosis. The association is probably a true one linked to retention of sodium and bicarbonate and is most likely to be seen with coincident volume depletion. Deficits of 200 mmol of potassium alone, however, do not induce alkalosis in normal subjects under experimental conditions, and in most clinical states of hypokalaemic alkalosis there are other participating factors.

Potassium deficiency with hypokalaemia also impairs renal tubular absorption of phosphate and resultant hypophosphataemia is an occasional associated finding.

There are commonly no symptoms or serious adverse effects from hypokalaemia in otherwise healthy subjects. Even mild degrees of hypokalaemia may, however, lead to cardiac arrhythmias in the presence of established cardiac disease, and the link between hypokalaemia and ventricular tachycardia or fibrillation in acute myocardial infarction is well established. Muscle weakness or paralysis are features of extreme depletion. In surgical wards the commonest manifestation is paralytic ileus. Polyuria and polydipsia are again rare and late features. Paraesthesiae and, in very rare cases, tetany have also been described.

Specific syndromes of hypokalaemia

GASTROINTESTINAL

Vomiting

The concentration of potassium in gastric and upper intestinal secretions varies between 5 and 10 mmol/l, so that direct losses in vomitus contribute only partially to potassium deficiency. Major losses of chloride and gastric acid result in hypochloraemic alkalosis, which induces a renal potassium leak. This, together with a shift of potassium from the extracellular to the intracellular fluid spaces, is largely responsible for the hypokalaemia. Patients with pyloric stenosis may present with deficits of sodium and potassium exceeding 500 mmol, of chloride rather more, and of water in excess of 5 litres. In such extreme cases, with massive chloride depletion, the urine may be 'paradoxically' acid despite profound metabolic alkalosis. The excretion of an alkaline urine is not possible, then, until the chloride deficit has been reduced by rapid intravenous infusion of sodium chloride with added supplements of potassium chloride.

Covert vomiting is a cardinal feature of bulimia nervosa, which in many respects resembles Bartter's syndrome (see below).

Diarrhoea

There is more potassium (50–100 mmol/l) in liquid stools than in vomitus, so that potassium deficiency from diarrhoea does not require an additional renal leak. Any condition in which stool volumes are high may cause hypokalaemia (for example cholera or enteritis caused by *Escherichia coli*). Most usually, potassium loss in diarrhoeal states is paralleled by loss of bicarbonate, with a resultant metabolic acidosis, so that plasma potassium concentrations do not accurately reflect the true deficit. In some cases the opposite is the case, when potassium and chloride are jointly lost with resultant metabolic alkalosis. A villous adenoma of the colon or rectum may result in profound hypokalaemia, believed to be due to disturbances of ion transport in the colonic mucosa mediated by the tumour. Similar disturbances underlie the hypokalaemia of patients with non-insulin-secreting islet-cell tumours (Verner–Morrison syndrome, see Chapter 12.10). More common than these rarities is laxative abuse, in which hypokalaemia may be profound without a change in the acid–base balance. Ureterosigmoidostomy leads to profound hypokalaemia hyperchloraemic acidosis if urine is allowed to remain stagnant in the colon and is not evacuated regularly.

RENAL

Diuretics (see Chapter 15.28.1.)

All diuretics other than those acting directly on the distal tubules (amiloride, triamterene, and spironolactone) tend to increase urinary potassium excretion in an amount dependent on the dose, the natriuretic response, and the degree of prevailing secondary hyperaldosteronism. Hypokalaemia may or may not occur. It is most commonly observed early in treatment but potassium concentrations rarely fall below 3 mmol/l. The loop agents are chloruretic and may cause an hypochloraemic hypokalaemic alkalosis with renal potassium wasting, correctable by supplements of potassium chloride but not of potassium bicarbonate.

In an analysis of published data, the average fall after treatment with benzothiadiazines or chlorthalidone was 0.69 mol/l. Levels below 3.5 mmol/l have been described in some 48 per cent of treated patients. The tendency to hypokalaemia can be reduced by using minimal effective doses, avoiding the longer-acting agents (such as chlorthalidone), reducing sodium intake, and using potassium-retaining diuretic-thiazide combinations. The need to prescribe potassium supplements routinely or not has been much debated. The risks of hypokalaemia are of cardiac arrhythmias and an enhancement of digitalis toxicity. In the longer term, impairment of carbohydrate tolerance is a recognized problem, related to an impaired insulin secretory response to hyperglycaemia rather than to insulin resistance. An excellent correlation between total body potassium and impairment of insulin secretion has been described. On the other hand, most patients with modest hypokalaemia come to no particular harm and potassium supplements are variably absorbed, are a nuisance to take, and can, on very rare occasions, cause jejunal ulceration and stricture formation. Most physicians would prescribe supplements of the chloride in patients who are prone to cardiac arrhythmias and in patients with severe liver disease in whom electrolyte imbalance may precipitate encephalopathy.

BARTTER'S SYNDROME

The first description of the syndrome which now bears his name was made by Bartter in 1962. Two Negro patients aged 5 and 25 years were reported, in whom there was profound hypokalaemic alkalosis, Pitressin®-resistant diabetes insipidus, secondary hyperaldosteronism without hypertension, resistance to the pressor effects of angiotensin II, and hypertrophy and hyperplasia of the juxtaglomerular apparatus of the kidneys. Since then, many further cases have been described, more in children than in adults, but presenting at any age from the neonatal period to the opposite extreme of life. Reports of the disorder in siblings and in the first generation of children of consanguineous parents have been taken to suggest an occasional autosomal recessive inheritance, but most cases are not familial. Disorders of red cell cation transport have been described in patients with Bartter's syndrome and in otherwise unaffected relatives (see below). The sexes are probably equally susceptible, and evidence that the syndrome may be more common in Afro-Caribbeans than in other races is inconclusive.

Clinical findings

There is considerable heterogeneity in clinical and biochemical features which reflect the heterogeneity of causative mechanisms. In some patients the condition may be asymptomatic, with biochemical abnormalities detected by chance. At the other extreme, there are marked features of hypokalaemia, including muscle weakness, polydipsia, polyuria, tetany, fits, vomiting, and, in young children, marked stunting of growth. While the cardinal features of the disorder are hypokalaemic alkalosis with urinary potassium and chloride wasting and a normal, or marginally low, arterial pressure, a proportion of cases show additional abnormalities, including hyponatraemia, hypophosphataemia (with or without rickets), hypercalciuria, hypercalcaemia, nephrocalcinosis, hypomagnesaemia, and hyperuricaemia. Blood urea and plasma creatinine concentrations are usually normal. Urinary potassium wasting is a constant feature, and losses may exceed the filtered load, reaching amounts as high as 400 to 600 mmol over 24 h in rare patients. Plasma renin activity and angiotensin II levels are high, as is aldosterone secretion, unless retarded by profound hypokalaemia. Other abnormalities that have been described include increased urinary prostaglandin E (**PGE**) and kallikrein, high plasma levels of bradykinin, and abnormalities of platelet aggregation.

Renal histology

A variety of abnormalities of renal histology have been described, including, apart from juxtaglomerular cell hyperplasia, some examples of hypercellularity of glomeruli, periglomerular fibrosis, arteriolar sclerosis, and chronic interstitial nephritis. Primary renal damage may, in some cases, coincide with Bartter's syndrome if not be its underlying cause. Medullary interstitial hyperplasia is not now considered a feature confined to patients with true Bartter's syndrome.

Theories of pathogenesis

Theories continue to abound, and none has yet found general acceptance. Bartter's original hypothesis was of a primary lack of response to angiotensin II by arteriolar smooth muscle; but pressor insensitivity to angiotensin II is now known to be a feature of any patient with persistently high plasma renin activity, because of a reduced number or avidity of vascular receptors for angiotensin II. Pressor insensitivity to noradrenaline is also a non-specific feature. Profound falls of arterial pressure in patients with Bartter's syndrome given saralasin (an angiotensin II antagonist) or captopril indicate the inaccuracy of the original idea and the important contribution made by angiotensin to the maintenance of blood pressure in these patients. Strong support has been given to the concept of disordered chloride transport in the ascending limb of Henle's loop, or of a primary abnormality provoking distal tubular potassium secretion. A difficulty in distinguishing these is that not only does chronic severe potassium deficiency result in reduced chloride reabsorption, but also chloride deficiency results in increased urinary potassium loss. A primary defect in sodium reabsorption in the distal nephron has also been suggested on the basis of attempts to assess tubular function using free water clearance under conditions of water loads, but sodium can be conserved normally in most patients with Bartter's syndrome, and these studies cannot be considered conclusive.

A variety of different abnormalities in cation transport have been described in the red cells of such patients and their otherwise unaffected first-degree relatives, resulting in increased sodium and decreased potassium concentration in their erythrocytes. But the inconsistencies in the abnormalities described and reports of similar phenomena in disorders as disparate as essential hypertension and thyrotoxicosis make these findings difficult to interpret. A report that changes in erythrocyte sodium transport can be reversed by correction of hypokalaemia adds to uncertainty in this area.

A number of different observations indicate overproduction of prostaglandins (**PGs**) as one of the major if not primary features of the syndrome. Plasma PGA concentrations and urinary PGE_2, 6-keto $PGF_{1\alpha}$, kallikrein, and bradykinin are increased. Renal interstitial cells, a site of PG synthesis in the medulla, are hyperplastic. Abnormalities of platelet aggregation appear to be caused by a circulating PG or a PG metabolite. Clinical and biochemical abnormalities are improved by treatment with prostaglandin-synthetase inhibitors and platelet function can be restored to normal. But overproduction of PGs is now recognized to be a secondary phenomenon which occurs in any condition of profound and prolonged potassium depletion.

If the postulated defect in sodium chloride transport in the ascending limb of Henle's loop is not proven, it is the most widely quoted hypothesis, and its acceptance is implicit in recommended methods of differential diagnosis.

Differential diagnosis

Primary renal tubular disorders such as cystinosis can closely mimic Bartter's syndrome. Laxative and diuretic abuse, together with vomiting, produce all the features, including urinary potassium wasting, if alkalosis or potassium depletion are extreme. Urinary chloride estimations will detect covert vomiting as occurs in bulimia nervosa. In that condition, in purgative abuse, and in the 'rebound' chloride retaining state after diuretic abuse, urinary chloride on a high chloride intake is as low as 1 to 3 mmol/24 h. Indexing of urinary chloride loss by glomerular filtration rate (**GFR**) and free water clearance has been shown in Bartter's syndrome to indicate an *increase* in fractional chloride excretion together with a reduction in maximal free water clearance.

Diuretic abuse mimics Bartter's syndrome precisely, but can be detected by urinary assays for benzothiadiazines or loop agents. Villous adenoma of the rectum, renal tubular acidosis, chronic pyloric stenosis, and the effects of liquorice or carbenoxolone sodium are more easily detected, but the diagnosis of a proximal tubulopathy of familial origin presents more difficulty. In this syndrome, described in four siblings in 1983, all the classical features of Bartter's syndrome were present, but fractional delivery of solute and ascending limb reabsorption of chloride was normal. Paradoxically, although histological changes were prominent in proximal tubules (without change in juxtaglomerular cells), physiological changes were thought to be distal tubular.

Treatment

In some asymptomatic patients with mild biochemical disturbance, an increase in dietary potassium and supplements of potassium chloride (150–200 mmol/day) may suffice. Others can be improved by the addition of spironolactone, amiloride, or triamterene. Propranolol has been advocated to reduce the activity of the renin–angiotensin–aldosterone system, but in severe cases, particularly in children with stunted growth, prostaglandin synthetase inhibitors should be prescribed. Most experience has been gained in the use of indomethacin, which should be given in a dose up to 2 mg/kg.day. Secondary aldosteronism is always improved, but some degree of hypokalaemia usually persists. Remarkable improvement in clinical features can be expected.

Other causes of renal potassium wasting

In primary aldosteronism, hypokalaemia is more severe in adenoma than in hyperplasia (see Chapter 12.7.1). Secondary hyperaldosteronism with hypokalaemia may complicate malignant hypertension, renal artery stenosis and the fluid retention of heart failure, cirrhosis of the liver, and nephrotic syndrome treated by diuretic agents. Cushing's syndrome may be associated with renal potassium wasting, especially if caused by carcinoma of the adrenal cortex or by a non-endocrine tumour. Adrenogenital syndromes due to 11β-hydroxylase or 17α-hydroxylase deficiency result in hypokalaemia due to overproduction of deoxycorticosterone. Renin-secreting tumours increase urinary potassium loss by stimulating hyperaldosteronism. Liquorice consumed in large amounts or chronic use of carbenoxolone sodium for the treatment of peptic ulcer produce renal potassium wasting and hypokalaemia, not by a direct mineralocorticoid-like effect on the distal tubule as was once thought, but by inhibition of renal 11β-hydroxysteroid dehydrogenase (see Chapter 12.7.1). A congenital deficiency of that enzyme, critical in the renal metabolism of cortisol, appears to be responsible also for Ulick's 'mineralocorticoid excess syndrome', now described in one adult as well as in children. The syndromes of renal tubular acidosis may also be associated with hypokalaemia and are described in Chapter 20.19.

LIDDLE'S SYNDROME

Hypokalaemia in this rare familial syndrome is accompanied by hypertension, but with a low aldosterone secretion. The condition may be caused by increased sodium–potassium exchange in the distal renal tubules, and both hypertension and hypokalaemia respond to treatment with triamterene or amiloride, but there is no response to spironolactone.

11β-HYDROXYSTEROID DEHYDROGENASE DEFICIENCY (SEE CHAPTER 12.7.1)

A number of children and one adult have now been described with a congenital absence of this enzyme, which is normally concerned with the renal metabolism of cortisol. In its absence, unaltered cortisol activates the mineralocorticoid receptors in the distal nephron, with resulting hypertension, hypokalaemia, and suppression of both renin and aldosterone. Spironolactone improves both hypertension and hypokalaemia in these patients.

ACUTE LEUKAEMIAS

Renal potassium wasting and hypokalaemia may complicate acute myeloid, monocytic, and myelomonocytic leukaemias. Increased urinary lysozyme excretion, either causing or reflecting renal tubular damage, is found in many, but not all, cases.

In some patients renal tubular damage by aminoglycosides may be the cause (see below), and in others avid transmembrane transport of potassium by leukaemic cells may continue to remove potassium from plasma after venesection.

ANTIMICROBIALS

Amphotericin B, gentamicin, and amikacin may cause renal tubular damage, leading on occasion to urinary potassium wasting and hypokalaemia.

MAGNESIUM DEFICIENCY

Any cause of profound and chronic magnesium deficiency can enable the kidneys to conserve potassium. Hypokalaemia is then difficult to correct unless supplements of potassium are combined with those of magnesium also.

Hypokalaemic periodic paralysis

In this rare condition, episodes of muscle weakness or paralysis lasting up to 24 or even 72 h occur sporadically or at more regular intervals. In most cases there is a family history reflecting a mendelian autosomal dominant inheritance. Symptoms first appear late in the first or in the second decade. Attacks appear to be caused by a shift in potassium from the extracellular to the intracellular fluid with profound hypokalaemia, although on occasion the plasma potassium can be normal. Precipitating factors may include rest after severe exercise, large carbohydrate meals, tension, anxiety, and an habitual high-salt diet. Attacks may also occur during sleep with the patient awaking weak or paralysed. Histological changes in affected muscles include vacuolation and sometimes evidence of damage to myofibrils.

The mechanism of the disease is not known, but attacks can be provoked by administration of glucose and insulin or adrenaline, and prevented by diazoxide, which blocks insulin release. Long-term treatment by diazoxide is considered to be too toxic for use in this condition.

A number of other treatments have been recommended, including potassium supplements, spironolactone, amiloride, and propranolol or other non-selective β-adrenergic blocking drugs. Acetazolamide or ammonium chloride may also prevent attacks by inducing extracellular fluid acidosis, but their long-term use may be associated with nephrocalcinosis.

A very similar hypokalaemic syndrome may complicate thyrotoxicosis, especially in Oriental races. Excess of thyroid hormone increases markedly the number of sodium–potassium pumps in skeletal muscle

cell membranes and this, together with an associated increase in plasma catecholamines, must favour movement of potassium into cells. There is some evidence of higher than normal fasting and post-glucose insulin concentrations in thyrotoxic hypokalaemic periodic paralysis too, but the reason for the particular susceptibility of Oriental subjects for this complication of thyrotoxicosis is not known. This variant of the condition is always corrected by reversal of the hyperthyroidism, and responds acutely to the use of β-adrenergic blocking agents.

HYPOKALAEMIA AND SUDDEN DEATH IN NORTH-EAST THAILAND

Poor socio-economic status, nutritional deficiency, and possible loss of electrolytes in sweat may underlie a metabolic syndrome described in young people in north-east Thailand, which includes renal stone disease, distal renal tubular acidosis, diabetes mellitus, and a hypokalaemia with low dietary and urinary potassium. The possible importance of the hypokalaemia relates to recent reports of sudden unexplained deaths at night, usually afflicting young, muscular men, some of whom are known to have been hypokalaemic. In some cases there has been evidence of ventricular fibrillation. The suggestion has been made, but not proven, that vanadium toxicity could be an important factor mediating some of the metabolic changes by inhibition of Na–K ATPase and H–K ATPase.

TREATMENT OF HYPOKALAEMIA

Potassium replacement in hypokalaemia caused by shifts from extracellular to the intracellular fluid is rarely necessary. In those cases in which it is probable that there is a true deficit, the need to provide supplements or to retard urinary losses with amiloride or triamterene varies according to clinical circumstances. In patients with myocardial disease, there is a good case for treating all levels of hypokalaemia. In otherwise healthy subjects, most physicians will treat those in whom potassium concentrations are consistently below 3 mmol/l. The case when concentrations lie between 3.0 and 3.5 mmol/l is much less clear.

In most conditions in which oral supplements are required, there is an associated metabolic alkalosis provoking renal potassium losses which are not then corrected by the bicarbonate or citrate salts of potassium. In this situation the chloride salt is essential and can be given as an elixir but is better accepted embedded in a wax medium (Slow-K®). Enteric-coated potassium chloride preparations cause occasional ulceration and stricture formation in the jejunum and should be avoided. The bicarbonate preparations are particularly indicated when hypokalaemia is associated with acidosis, for instance in renal tubular acidosis.

Indications for rapid elevation of plasma potassium by parental infusion are few, but include hypokalaemic cardiac arrhythmias, paralysis, and hypokalaemic diabetic ketoacidosis. In every case care should be taken to assess the adequacy of renal function. No rule is absolute, but it is rarely wise to infuse potassium in a concentration exceeding 40 mmol/l, at a rate exceeding 40 mmol/h or 200 mmol/day. Care must be taken to monitor plasma levels closely, particularly in patients treated at these or faster rates.

Hyperkalaemia

Hyperkalaemia is less common than hypokalaemia but more dangerous. Very rarely, hyperkalaemic patients may develop muscle weakness, but cardiac arrest is the major complication and most commonly occurs without premonitory symptoms. Diagnosis therefore depends on clinical suspicion, on measurement of potassium in plasma, and on the characteristic changes in the electrocardiogram.

Some causes of hyperkalaemia are listed in Table 2. Although renal failure, acute or chronic, underlies most cases of hyperkalaemia, all too commonly there has been an iatrogenic contribution from unwise use of

Table 2 *Causes of hyperkalaemia*

Excessive intake

Impaired renal excretion
  Renal diseases
    Acute renal failure
    Chronic renal failure
    Renal tubular disorders (including
      pseudohypoaldosteronism)
  Endocrine effects on the kidney
    Addison's disease
    Isolated hypoaldosteronism
    C-21 hydroxylase deficiency
    3β-hydroxydehydrogenase deficiency
    Corticosterone methyloxidase deficiency
  Pharmaceutical effects on the kidney
    Potassium-retaining diuretics
    Angiotensin-converting enzyme inhibitors
    Non-steroidal anti-inflammatory agents
    Cyclosporin

Changes in internal balance
  Acidosis
  Rhabdomyolysis
  Burns
  Massive death of tumour cells
  Hyperkalaemic periodic paralysis
  Succinyl choline
  Digitalis poisoning
  Malignant hyperthermia
  Familial hyperkalaemic acidosis

Pseudohyperkalaemia
  Haemolysed blood samples
  Leukaemia with very high white cell counts
  Familial pseudohyperkalaemia

potassium supplements, potassium-retaining diuretics, angiotensin-converting enzyme inhibitors, and non-steroidal anti-inflammatory drugs (**NSAIDS**).

EXCESSIVE INTAKE

An individual's ability to handle an excessive intake of potassium depends mainly on renal function, but also on the phenomenon of adaptation, whereby a chronic high intake increases potassium tolerance because of enhanced uptake in the distal tubular cells and, perhaps, also in striated muscle as a consequence of increased numbers of Na–K pumps. This adaptive mechanism can increase maximal renal excretion of potassium in health by some ten- to twenty-fold. Examples of hyperkalaemia due solely to excessive intake of potassium by mouth in healthy people are therefore rare, but have been described after overdosage with slow-release potassium preparations (Navidrex-K®, Neo-NaClex-K®, and Slow-K®). Hyperkalaemia of dietary origin is a commonenough problem in the presence of renal failure, and may complicate mineralocorticoid deficiency or the inappropriate prescription of potassium-retaining diuretics. Parental infusion of potassium may cause dangerous hyperkalaemia if rates of infusion exceed 40 mmol/h or concentrations of potassium exceed 40 mmol/l or less in the presence of renal insufficiency. There is a particular risk of hyperkalaemia if patients with impaired renal function are transfused with stored blood, or treated with large doses of the potassium salts of penicillin.

ACUTE RENAL FAILURE

Hyperkalaemia is to be expected in any case of acute renal failure (see Chapter 20.16), especially when the condition is associated with muscle

injury tissue necrosis, gastrointestinal bleeding, or severe infection. The excess potassium is derived only partly from the diet, sometimes from unwise infusion of crystalloid or stored blood, from catabolism and necrosis of cells, and from intracellular stores in the presence of acidosis.

CHRONIC RENAL FAILURE

Hyperkalaemia is rarely a problem in chronic renal failure (see Chapter 20.17.1) until the glomerular filtration rate falls below 15 to 20 ml/min. At lower levels of function, plasma potassium can usually be maintained at normal or near normal concentration by restriction of dietary intake, treatment of acidosis, and avoidance of potassium-retaining diuretics. The adaptive changes, identical to those that occur in healthy individuals on a high potassium diet, increase the capacity of surviving nephrons to excrete potassium, and similar changes in the Na–K pump numbers and potassium conductance probably also occur in colonic mucosa. Animal studies suggest an increased capacity of the intracellular space to take up potassium by a mechanism that requires the presence of the adrenal cortex but does not depend on increased secretion rates of glucocorticoid or mineralocorticoid.

PSEUDOHYPERKALAEMIA

Samples in which plasma or serum have not been promptly separated from red cells will contain excessive amounts of potassium derived from leakage out of red cells after venesection. Pseudohyperkalaemia usually appears in blood samples that have been taken some distance away from the laboratory, in which case the red cells and plasma have not been separated for many hours. This problem is well known and easily circumvented. Haemolysed samples, of course, also show hyperkalaemia without long storage. Less common and less known is the pseudohyperkalaemia associated with leukaemias when the total white cell count is so high that leakage from white and red cells together induce pseudohyperkalaemia in unseparated blood samples within a few minutes after venesection.

    Another cause of pseudohyperkalaemia is so-called 'familial pseudohyperkalaemia', a condition which may be familial with an autosomal dominant inheritance of abnormal cation transport across red cell membranes. The prime feature of this condition is that there is an abnormal net efflux of potassium from red cells stored over 2 to 6 h at room temperature. The leak can be prevented by storing the cells at 37 °C rather than at room temperature. Radioisotope cation studies *in vitro* show a decreased temperature sensitivity by the 'passive leak' transport mechanism for potassium, accounting for the potassium leak at low temperatures. The blood film of these patients may show a few target cells and there is evidence of a mild compensated haemolytic state.

POTASSIUM-RETAINING DIURETICS

Large doses of amiloride or triamterene (and to a lesser degree of spironolactone) may cause severe hyperkalaemia, even in healthy people with normal renal function. These drugs are particularly to be avoided in renal failure.

ADRENAL INSUFFICIENCY

Addison's disease (see Chapter 12.7.1) is commonly associated with modest hyperkalaemia (plasma potassium 5.0–6.5 mmol/l), hyponatraemia, and a rise in blood urea. Other clinical features are likely to suggest the diagnosis, which is commonly further investigated by measurements of cortisol and its response to stimulation of the cortex by synthetic adrenocorticotropic hormone (**ACTH**) (see Chapter 12.7.1). This approach is satisfactory enough in most cases but will miss the diagnosis of isolated hypoaldosteronism, a condition that may occur more frequently than is currently recognized (see below).

ISOLATED HYPOALDOSTERONISM

The commonest cause of chronic hyperkalaemia without severe renal failure is probably hyporeninaemic hypoaldosteronism. The condition is caused by a relative or absolute deficiency of aldosterone. In many cases, plasma renin activity is low and unresponsive to the erect posture and sodium depletion. The associated hyperchloraemic metabolic acidosis (type 4 renal tubular acidosis—see Chapters 11.14 and 20.19) is largely the consequence of suppression of renal ammonia synthesis by hyperkalaemia. In most cases, there is also evidence of an acquired enzymatic defect in aldosterone biosynthesis with a reduced response to infusions of either angiotensin II or ACTH. A chronic low concentration of angiotensin II may contribute, and in this context increased aldosterone secretion, normally stimulated by potassium infusion, is blunted when angiotensin-converting enzyme inhibitors are given at the same time.

The plasma aldosterone concentrations may be 'normal' or low, but can be considered reduced in every case when indexed by the plasma potassium concentration (hyperkalaemia being normally a very potent stimulus to aldosterone secretion). Glucocorticoid metabolism is normal in these patients.

Clinical features

Patients are usually over the age of 60 years, although younger cases have been described. Vascular and ischaemic heart disease are common. Some 50 per cent of patients have been diabetic and 70 per cent have evidence of renal disease, most commonly some form of chronic interstitial nephritis, with modest impairment of glomerular filtration rate. Symptoms may include muscle weakness, but in most cases hyperkalaemia with hyperchloraemic acidosis is detected during laboratory investigation, or the disorder declares itself more dramatically with episodes of hyperkalaemic heart block, or cardiac arrest, often precipitated by vomiting or diarrhoea which tends to reduce sodium delivery and flow in the distal tubules and thus reduces renal potassium excretion. A similar course of events may follow discontinuation of potent diuretics previously overgenerously prescribed. Blood pressure is normal or even high.

The associations of this disorder with old age, diabetes, and renal disease may reflect the decreasing activity of the renin–angiotensin system with age, reduced sensitivity of the renal stretch receptors with increasing rigidity of arteriolar walls, insulin deficiency, and autonomic neuropathy.

The condition should be suspected in any patient with hyperkalaemia without other obvious explanation. Investigation is complex and requires measurements of renin activity and plasma aldosterone in response to sodium deprivation, with assessment in addition of the aldosterone response to infusions of angiotensin and ACTH.

Cyclosporin treatment

In some patients treated by cyclosporin after renal transplantation, hyperkalaemia (serum potassium 6.0–7.1 mmol/l) and acidosis may occur that are quite disproportionate to glomerular filtration rate and dietary intake. This condition is probably another variant of hyporeninaemic hypoaldosteronism and responds to treatment by fludrocortisone (see below).

Treatment

Most patients with hypoaldosteronism respond well to replacement therapy of 0.1 to 0.2 mg daily of fludrocortisone, but doses as high as 0.4 or even 1.0 mg may be needed to reduce the potassium concentration to normal, often at the cost of inducing oedema, hypertension, or cardiac failure. The failure of normal replacement doses to correct hyperkalaemia indicates a renal tubular component to the disease in some patients. In those in whom mineralocorticoids alone do not suffice, the combination of 9α-fluorohydrocortisone with a benzothiadiazine diuretic may be successful. Supplements of sodium bicarbonate may correct acidosis and facilitate renal potassium excretion.

CONGENITAL ADRENAL SYNDROMES

Adrenogenital syndromes due to C-21 hydroxylase deficiency or to 3β-hydroxydehydrogenase deficiency are associated with renal salt wasting and hyperkalaemia due to impaired synthesis of aldosterone, which is also a feature of the autosomal recessive condition of deficiency of methyloxidase I and II, enzymes normally responsible for the conversion of corticosterone to aldosterone. Most such cases present in infancy.

ANGIOTENSIN-CONVERTING ENZYME INHIBITORS

These agents are used increasingly in the treatment of hypertension in cardiac failure and now after myocardial infarction. The fall in angiotensin II concentrations induced by the drugs results acutely in much reduced aldosterone secretion, and, initially at least, in low plasma and urinary aldosterone. Some elevation of plasma potassium occurs, but severe hyperkalaemia (potassium more than 6.0 mmol/l) is only likely when the inhibitors are given to patients with creatinine clearances of less than 20 ml/min.

NON-STEROIDAL ANTI-INFLAMMATORY SUBSTANCES

These drugs are amongst the most commonly prescribed and will inevitably be given from time to time to patients with renal dysfunction. Inhibition of prostaglandin synthetase reduces glomerular filtration rate and delivery of sodium to the distal tubular exchange sites, and may interfere with renal renin secretion. These effects together are the reason for some 25 per cent of patients with chronic renal failure becoming hyperkalaemic when given indomethacin or similar agents.

RENAL TUBULAR DISORDERS

Hyperkalaemia with impaired renal excretion of potassium may be a feature of any cause of renal tubular acidosis (see Chapters 11.4 and 20.19). Hyperkalaemia and acidosis disproportionate to the degree of loss of glomerular filtration rate are also occasionally seen in chronic obstructive nephropathy, in sickle-cell disease with renal involvement (see Chapter 20.5.7), in systemic lupus erythematosus, and in renal amyloidosis.

More rare still are the conditions of type I and type II pseudohypoaldosteronism. In type I disease, an autosomal recessive disorder, hyperkalaemia of renal origin is associated with salt wasting and hypotension, features which are absent from type II disease. In neither condition is there evidence of aldosterone deficiency and in neither does mineralocorticoid in high dosage correct the hyperkalaemia (in contrast to true hypoaldosteronism). Type I disease is probably caused by a deficiency of mineralocorticoid receptors in the distal nephron, and responds well to treatment with salt supplements. In type II disease (Gordon's syndrome), hyperkalaemia is accompanied by hyperchloraemic acidosis, hypertension, and suppression of renin activity. The primary abnormality may then lie in increased chloride and thereby sodium reabsorption in the ascending limb of Henle's loop. This, by limiting sodium delivery to the distal tubules, impairs secretion of both potassium and hydrogen ions. Potassium clearance in type II disease is not increased by mineralocorticoid nor by sodium loading, but can be corrected by the infusion of non-reabsorbable anions in the form of sodium sulphate. Thiazide diuretics and loop agents are useful in correcting hyperkalaemia and reducing the arterial pressure.

HYPERKALAEMIC PERIODIC PARALYSIS

Even more rare than hypokalaemic periodic paralysis, this disease is familial with an autosomal dominant mode of inheritance. Attacks of paralysis begin in the first decade of life, usually precipitated by rest after exercise, when pronounced hyperkalaemia is associated with a flaccid paralysis lasting from a few minutes to several hours. Bulbar muscles may be involved. Myotonia may be a striking feature and can be demonstrated by McArdle's sign. Established attacks can be reversed by salbutamol inhalation, but treatment is best given prophylactically by use of benzothiadiazine diuretics of fludrocortisone. Both are effective.

SUCCINYL CHOLINE

Agents that depolarize muscle membranes increase plasma potassium by some 0.5 mmol/l in healthy subjects. In patients already at risk of hyperkalaemia because of renal failure, complicating burns, crush injuries, or other hypercatabolic states, the rise after muscle relaxants may be much greater and should be considered when such patients need general anaesthesia.

DIGITALIS

Severe hyperkalaemia may occur in patients who have taken an overdose of digitalis, presumably secondary to loss of intracellular potassium, following massive inhibition of Na–K ATPase.

MALIGNANT HYPERTHERMIA

This syndrome, which occurs in patients with a genetically determined increase in calcium concentration in skeletal muscle, is precipitated by inhaled anaesthetics. Hyperthermia and rhabdomyolysis are accompanied by hyperkalaemia which may reach dangerous levels in subjects with impaired renal function.

TREATMENT OF HYPERKALAEMIA

The need to treat hyperkalaemia, how urgently and how aggressively, depends on its degree, whether it is stable or increasing, its cause, and most importantly on the presence or not of associated changes in the electrocardiogram. Stable concentrations under 6.0 mmol/l may not need specific therapy. Concentrations over 6.5 mmol/l with ECG changes and levels exceeding 7.0 mmol/l constitute a medical emergency. ECG abnormalities, in order of severity, include tenting of T-waves, diminution or absence of P-waves, widening of the QRS complex, slurring of the ST segment into the T-waves, and a sine-wave pattern immediately preceding cardiac arrest (see Chapter 20.16).

If ECG changes are absent or involve only changes in P- and T-waves, intravenous glucose (50 g) and insulin (10–20) units soluble or Actrapid® will lower plasma potassium by approximately 1.0 mmol/l within 30 minutes, the effect persisting some 1 to 2 h; 50 to 100 ml 4.2 per cent sodium bicarbonate increases intracellular at the expense of extracellular potassium and is particularly effective when hyperkalaemia and acidosis are combined.

When the ECG changes are more advanced, with widening of the QRS complexes, intravenous 10 per cent calcium gluconate should be given over 2 to 5 min in whatever dose (usually 10–30 ml) is required to correct the ECG. The beneficial effects of calcium salts are evident within 2 min of infusion but are short lived.

A combination of calcium gluconate, glucose and insulin, and hypertonic bicarbonate provides control of hyperkalaemia for 2 to 3 h and can be supplemented, when necessary, by haemodialysis, peritoneal dialysis, or by cation exchange resins in the calcium or sodium phase. These agents in a dose of 15 to 20 g three or four times daily can be given by mouth or as a retention enema. Constipation, or worse, faecal impaction, may be avoided by adding 10 to 30 ml of a 70 per cent solution of sorbitol with each dose. Exchange resins begin to exert an effect on external potassium balance in some 1 or 2 h.

There is evidence that a variety of β₂- adrenergic agonists can be used to treat hyperkalaemia by virtue of their action in transferring potassium from the extracellular fluid into cells. There may be occasions in which this approach has advantages, but in general the established methods, which are thoroughly effective, are to be preferred.

REFERENCES

Adu, D., Michael, J., Turney, J., and McMaster, P. (1983). hyperkalaemia in cyclosporin-treated renal allograft recipients. *Lancet* ii, 370–2.

Carmine, Z., Ettore, B., Giuseppe, C., and Quirino, M. (1982). The renal tubular defect of Bartter's syndrome. *Nephron* 32, 140–8.

Dawson, D.C. (1987). Cellular mechanisms for K transport across epithelial cell layers. *Seminars in Nephrology* 7, 185–92.

DeFronzo, R.A. (1980). Hyperkalaemia and hyporeninaemic hypoaldosteronism. *Kidney International* 17, 118–34.

Delaney, V.B., Oliver, J.F., Simms, M., Costello, J., and Bourke, E. (1981). Bartter's syndrome: physiological and pharmacological studies. *Quarterly Journal of Medicine* 50, 213–32.

Epstein, F.H. And Rosa, R.M. (1983). Adrenergic control of serum potassium. *New England Journal of Medicine* 309, 1450–1.

Glassock, R.J., Goldstone, D.A., Goldstone, R., and Hsuch, W.A. (1983). Diabetes mellitus, moderate renal insufficiency and hyperkalaemia. *American Journal of Nephrology* 3, 233–40.

Hamill, R.J., Robinson, L.M., Wexler, H.R., and Moote, C. (1991). Efficacy and safety of potassium infusion therapy on hyperkalaemic critically ill patients. *Critical Care Medicine* 19, 694–9.

Hayslett, J.P. And Binder, H.V. (1982). Mechanism of potassium adaptation. *American Journal of Physiology* 243, F103–12.

Jamison, R.L. (1987). Potassium recycling. *Kidney International* 31, 695.

Kaji, D. and Kahn, T. (1987). Na⁺–K⁺ pump in chronic renal failure. *American Journal of Physiology* 252, F785.

Kaplan, N.M. (1984). Our appropriate concern about hyperkalaemia. *American Journal of Medicine* 77, 1–3.

Kokko, J.P. (1985). Primary acquired hypoaldosteronism. *Kidney International* 27, 690–702.

Korff, J.M., Siebens, A.W., and Gill, J.R. (1984). Correction of hypokalaemia corrects the abnormalities in erythrocyte sodium transport in Bartter's syndrome. *Journal of Clinical Investigation* 74, 1724–9.

Lancet (1981). Hypokalaemic periodic paralysis. *Lancet* i, 1140–1.

Layzer, R.B.I. (1982). Periodic paralysis and the sodium potassium pump. *Annals of Neurology* II, 547–52.

Licht, J.H., Amundson, D., Hsuch, W.A., and Lombardo, J.V. (1985). Familial hyperkalaemic acidosis. *Quarterly Journal of Medicine* 54, 161–76.

Medbø, J.T. and Sejevsted, O.M. (1990). Plasma potassium changes with high intensity exercise. *Journal of Physiology (London)* 421, 105–22.

Montolin, J., Lens, X.M., and Revert, L. (1987). Potassium lowering effects of albuterol for hyperkalaemia in renal failure. *Archives of Internal Medicine* 147, 713–17.

Nørgaard, K. and Kjeldsen, K. (1991). Interrelation of hyperkalaemia potassium depletion and its implications: a re-evaluation based on studies of the skeletal muscle sodium–potassium pump. *Clinical Science* 81, 449–55.

Ornt, D.B., Scandling, J.D., and Tannen, R.L. (1987). Adaptation for potassium conservation during dietary potassium deprivation. *Seminars in Nephrology* 7, 193.

Schamberlan, M., Sebastian, A., and Rector, F.C. (1981). Mineralocorticoid-resistant renal hyperkalaemia without salt wasting (type II pseudohypoaldosteronism). Role of increased renal chloride reabsorption. *Kidney International* 19, 716–27.

Sitprija, V., *et al.* (1991). Metabolic syndromes caused by decreased activity of ATPases. *Seminars in Nephrology* 11, 249–52.

Solomon, R. (1987). The relationship between disorders of K⁺ and Mg⁺ homeostasis. *Seminars in Nephrology* 7, 253.

Spital, A. and Sterns, R.H. (1989). Extrarenal potassium adaptation: the role of aldosterone. *Clinical Science* 76, 213–19.

Stein, J.H. (1985). The pathogenetic spectrum of Bartter's syndrome. *Kidney International* 28, 85.

Stewart, G.W., Corrall, R.F.M., Fyffe, J.W., Stockdill, G., and Strong, J.A. (1979). Familial pseudohyperkalaemia. *Lancet* ii, 175–7.

Tannen, R.L. (1985). Diuretic-induced hypokalaemia. *Kidney International* 28, 998.

Veldhuis, J.D. (1983). The many faces of hyperkalaemia. *Archives of Internal Medicine* 143, 1521–2.

Whang, R., Flink, E.B., Dyckner, T., Wester, P.O., and Ryan, M.P. (1985). Magnesium depletion as a cause of refractory potassium repletion. *Archives of Internal Medicine* 145, 1686–9.

Williams, F.A., Schambelan, M., Biglieri, E.G., and Case, R.M. (1983). Acquired primary hypoaldosteronism due to isolated zone glomerulosa defect. *New England Journal of Medicine* 309, 1623–7.

Ypersele de Strihou, C. van (1977). Potassium homeostasis in renal failure. *Kidney International* 11, 491–504.

20.3 Common clinical presentations and symptoms in renal disorders

J. S. Cameron

Renal disease presents with rather few syndromes. The complex state of uraemia is dealt with elsewhere in this section (Chapter 20.17.1), and the purpose of this chapter is to review other outward signs of renal disease and their clinical consequences. Here we discuss the patient showing haematuria and/or proteinuria, and discuss renal pain and variations in urinary output and in passing urine.

The patient with proteinuria

The nature and quantity of protein in the urine are of importance in many areas of medicine, and urine has been routinely tested for protein as part of the clinical examination of any patient for nearly 200 years. The patient will not notice any outward signs of protein in the urine unless a large amount is excreted—more than several grams per 24 h: in that case the urine may become frothy, because the protein lowers the surface tension of the urine and permits a relatively stable foam to form. Some patients will volunteer this information spontaneously, others in response to direct questioning, and it may be a valuable way of dating when profuse proteinuria began. The other cardinal symptom of profuse proteinuria is oedema as part of the nephrotic syndrome.

The physiological and pathological basis of proteinuria

The basis for the virtual exclusion of protein from glomerular filtrate is only partially understood. The complex glomerular filter, made up of modified vascular endothelial cells, a unique basement membrane, and a unique pericyte (the epithelial cell) permits a high flux of solvent (water) and does not retard the passage of molecules of up to an Einstein–Stokes radius of about 1.5 nm. Above this value, however, there is a gradual cut-off with increasing molecular size (Fig. 1). Thus in health, the urinary clearance of albumin is less than 0.01 per cent, while the clearance of proteins of lower molecular weight, such as Ig light chains, approaches that of the glomerular filtration rate. These findings can be modelled by the supposition of the presence of water-filled cylindrical pores of about 4.7 nm diameter occupying about 10 per cent of the glomerular filtration area; but it must be emphasized that the physical existence of these 'pores' is in doubt.

Figure 1 also shows that the human glomerulus permits greater penetration of uncharged molecules, such polyvinylpyrrolidone (PVP) or dextran, suggesting an effect of charge on transit through the glomerular capillary wall. This effect almost certainly relates to the high density of negative charges present on the structures of the glomerular capillary wall. In the rat, experimental glomerular disease facilitates penetration of anionic molecules through the membrane, while neutral or cationic molecules are somewhat retarded. In humans, data are available only for the urinary clearances of various proteins in proteinuric states, but the effect of tubular reabsorption cannot be assessed (see below). In general, some degree of size discrimination ('selectivity') is preserved in all clinical proteinurias resulting from glomerular damage, and remains highest in nephrotic patients with minimal change lesions. The clearances approximate to that expected for molecular weight, so that

the effects of charge seem to be subordinate for most proteinurias, despite the fact that plasma proteins, although all anionic at physiological pH, have different isoelectric points.

Studies in diabetic nephropathy have shown that as glomerular filtration rate falls, proteinuria reflects a gradual loss of glomerular discrimination for proteins of molecular size within the range 60 to 1000 kDa (Einstein–Stokes radius 3.5–20 nm). In minimal change disease, the clearance of smaller molecules of dextran (less than 4.8 nm) is actually decreased compared with normal clearance, while that of larger dextrans is normal or increased. A similar pattern has been found in nephrotic syndromes of varying types, including diabetes, lupus, and membranous nephropathy. Again, these data have been interpreted in terms of a heteroporous model, which supposes the enlargement of existing pores or the appearance of larger pores in the membrane which permit the abnormal proteinuria.

A practical consequence of this selectivity of the glomerular filter, even in disease, is that glomerular proteinuria consists largely of albumin, even in the most poorly selective and severely damaged glomeruli; the fact that the concentration of albumin in the plasma is normally higher than that of any other protein must also contribute.

Fig. 1 The selectivity of the normal human and mammalian glomerulus to proteins, which carry a negative charge (shaded area) and uncharged polydisperse macromolecules (PVP or dextran) which are uncharged (dotted line). The glomerulus shows both size- and charge-selective properties. Urinary clearances (vertical axis) for infused proteins of various molecular weights (dots) are progressively reduced below the GFR as molecular weight and size (horizontal axis) increases. At any molecular size, the clearance of a neutral dextran or PVP is much greater than that of negatively-charged proteins. Albumin has an Einstein-Stokes radius of 37 Å and a molecular weight of 67 kDA. (10 Å = 1 nm).

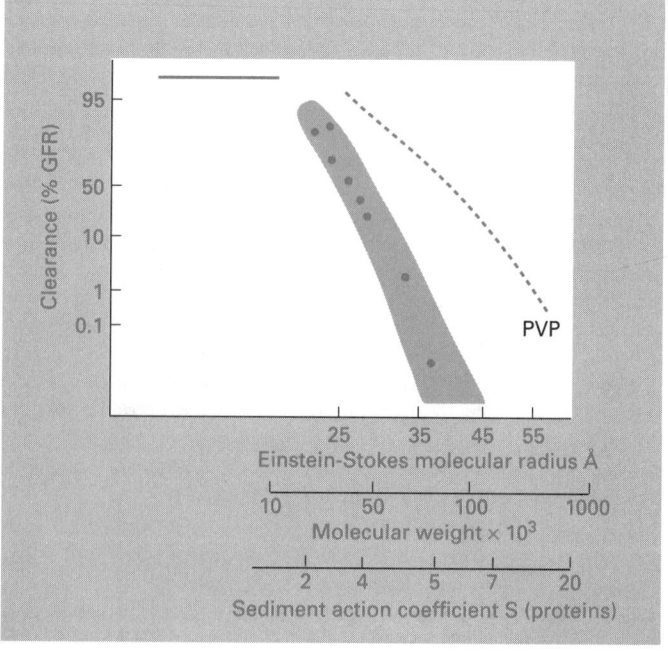

In humans, direct measurement of the tubular reabsorption of larger molecular weight protein (>60 kDa) is impossible, and there is dispute about how much albumin is normally filtered but reabsorbed in the proximal tubule by endocytosis and catabolized, either in health or in disease, and thus is not reflected by the amount in the urine. There is no evidence of competition between large anionic molecules for reabsorption, but this is not true for cationic or smaller molecules. In the rabbit the uptake of albumin is a low affinity–high capacity process, which accounts for the fact that some albumin normally escapes into the urine, even though the amount filtered is very small.

Proteins of lower molecular weight (10–45 kDa; 1.5–3.0 nm) are filtered at rates of 1 to 80 per cent of the glomerular filtration rate, the latter figure being reached for lysozyme and β_2-microglobulin, as well as fragments of IgG light chains. There is extensive reabsorption of low molecular weight protein in the proximal tubule, so that only about 100 mg/24 h are normally excreted, along with some 30 to 100 mg of albumin. Thus in proximal tubular damage of any kind, low molecular weight protein will predominate in the urine. Because of their ready filtration and extensive reabsorption, the plasma concentrations of low molecular weight proteins are in health very low (although they accumulate in uraemia) and their turnover by renal catabolism is very rapid. Thus the kidney is a major site of disposal for small molecular weight or peptide hormones such as insulin.

Clinical proteinuria

NORMAL PROTEINURIA

The amount of protein excreted in the urine per 24 h is 80 ± 24 mg (mean ± SD), so that 128 mg /24 h represents the upper limit of normal (+ 2 SD). As noted above, more than half of this amount consists of small molecular weight proteins or protein fragments, although albumin is the largest single component.

PATHOLOGICAL PROTEINURIA

Proteinuria in excess of this modest limit can come about in three ways:

1. The glomerular filter becomes more permeable to proteins of large molecular size, as well as permitting those of small molecular weight to pass ('glomerular' proteinuria). This is by far the commonest cause of proteinuria in clinical practice.
2. There is a marked rise in the plasma concentration of protein in the circulation, so that the amount filtered exceeds the reabsorptive capacity of the proximal tubule ('overflow' proteinuria). Apart from deliberate infusions of albumin, the only clinical circumstances in which this occurs is the excretion of IgG light chains and light chain fragments in myeloma, and of lysozyme in monomyelocytic leukemia.
3. The proximal tubule is damaged so that normally reabsorbed proteins, principally of low molecular weight, pass into the urine ('tubular' proteinuria).

'Glomerular' proteinuria

The earliest clinical test for albumin, of producing a visible cloudiness or even a solid coagulum by heat, is rarely used today, having been all but replaced by various 'stick' tests. The principle of their operation is that the titration curve of certain dyes is shifted in the presence of protein, especially albumin; it must be remembered that light chains or some low molecular weight proteins are not detected by stick tests. The sticks are buffered to keep the pH constant, which is important; leaving the stick in the urine will wash out the buffer and give a false reading; they should therefore be read immediately. Observer variation in reading the sticks must be remembered; those with colour blindness may have difficulties.

Commercial sticks such as Albustix® are very sensitive, giving a trace or positive reading with many normal urines containing only about 100 mg protein/l. There is only a crude relationship between the true concentration of protein and the stick reading. An alternative test is sulphosalicylic acid precipitation (0.5 ml of 3 per cent solution to 0.5 ml urine), which will give a rough quantitative reading when measured in a densitometer. The reference methods are the Kjeldahl measurement of precipitated nitrogen or the biuret method, which measures peptide bonds and is used for some automated methods of clinical protein measurement.

The concentration of protein in the urine will vary with the urine flow rate, and thus throughout the 24 hours. Also, protein excretion varies throughout the day, being least at night; therefore overnight collections, although easier, may not represent the 24 h output of protein. However, the difficulties of obtaining accurate 24 h urine collections in clinical practice apply to 24 h urine protein measurements. Given the relative constancy of creatinine excretion, the urine creatinine can be used to correct the protein concentration in 'spot', untimed samples of urine. In normal children, the urinary albumin/creatinine ratio is less than 10 mg albumin/mmol creatinine, 100 mg/mmol being moderate proteinuria, representing about 1.4 g /24 h in a 70 kg adult. In adults, an upper limit of 0.2 mg/mg creatinine has been suggested, that is 21 mg/mmol. More than 3.5 mg protein/mg creatinine (360 mg/mmol) represents nephrotic-range proteinuria.

'Tubular' proteinuria

All except the most specific chemical tests will miss some low molecular weight proteins, which are not only poorly precipitated in the sulphosalicylic acid test, but are also not denatured reliably on heating and do not react with sticks that are principally sensitive to albumin. This applies particularly to immunoglobulin light chains. Cellulose acetate electrophoresis is the easiest way of assessing the pattern of proteinuria, and is particularly valuable in the diagnosis and assessment of tubular proteinuria. An important pointer to the presence or absence of tubular proteinuria in tubular damage is the quantity of protein in the urine; in tubular proteinuria, there is almost never more than 1.5 to 2 g/24 h at most in the urine, whereas in glomerular proteinuria more than 100 g/24 h may be found on occasion. In myeloma, however, there may be concomitant glomerular damage, and thus albuminuria as well.

Specific radioimmunoassays and enzyme-linked immunosorbent assays (ELISAs) are available for β_2-microglobulin, one of the many microglobulins forming the majority of tubular proteinuria. Unfortunately this protein, although a very sensitive indicator of tubular damage, is unstable in urine of normal pH (5–6.5) and even alkalinization of the urine to pH 7 or above immediately on voiding may not stop loss of protein in the bladder. Normally, less that 0.4 μ/l of β_2-microglobulin is present in urine, but many times more is found in the presence of tubular damage, or in glomerular disease with a prominent tubulointerstitial component. Lysozyme can also be used to assess proximal tubular damage: normally the excretion is less than 1 mg/mmol creatinine (10 μ/mg), and α_1-microglobulin and retinol-binding protein have also been studied. Any of the causes of proximal tubular damage discussed in Section 20.19 will produce tubular patterns of proteinuria, proximal tubular damage from metabolic disorders such as cystinosis, heavy metal poisoning, and autoimmune disorders.

Assays for κ and λ chains by immunoelectrophoresis are an essential part of the diagnosis of myeloma, and may also be found in the urine of patients with primary amyloidosis and light chain nephropathy. The most accurate and sensitive method for their detection is immunofixation using specific antisera to probe blots of electrophoresed urines. The problem at the clinical level is to remember to test for them—in the presence of good renal function their concentrations in the plasma may often be negligible, compared to their abundance in the urine.

Secreted proteins, urinary casts

Some 20 to 30 mg/24 h of non-plasma protein is contributed by the renal tubules and the lower urinary tract. Much of this is Tamm–Horsfall protein, an easily polymerized, 200 kDa glycoprotein which appears to be identical with the previously described urinary immunosuppressant factor, uromodulin. Tamm–Horsfall protein is secreted only by the ascending thick limb of Henle's loop and early distal convoluted tubule into the tubular fluid. It is a major constituent of renal tubular casts, along with albumin and traces of many plasma proteins, including immunoglobulins. In myeloma, casts contain paraprotein polymerized with Tamm–Horsfall protein, and may show a microfibrillar structure that will stain positively with Congo red, even though no amyloid is present in the renal tissue.

Some secretory IgA is added by the lower urinary tract including the urethral glands, along with trace quantities of proteins of prostatic or seminal vesicular origin. Some of the secretory IgA found in the urine may have its origin from the renal tubules in renal disease as well as in health, together with some IgM.

Postural proteinuria (orthostatic proteinuria) and persistent symptomless proteinuria

Many healthy individuals have their urine tested for screening or insurance purposes. In a proportion, usually adults and especially males, proteinuria is found in excess of the normal limits outlined above, but which returns to normal during recumbency; the most usual way of testing this is to take the first urine passed on rising in the morning. This postural or orthostatic proteinuria has been recognized for more than a century, but its exact pathogenesis still eludes us; almost certainly it represents a response to haemodynamic change with posture. What is clear, however, is that its long-term prognosis is benign in virtually all cases.

Isolated modest proteinuria (0.5–1.5 g/24 h), even when present in all samples tested but in the absence of haematuria, is likewise almost always benign. The first thing is to ascertain that it is not postural and is persistent by repeated testing and perhaps quantitation. The mild proteinuria of uncontrolled hypertension, recent exercise (which can induce several g/l of protein) and cardiac failure should be excluded. If renal function is normal, blood pressure is normal, and no haematuria is present, then renal biopsy is not necessary, at least in the first instance. However, unlike the situation with postural proteinuria, biopsy will not always show an entirely normal glomerulus: as well as minimal change lesions, mild mesangial nephritis, membranous nephropathy, or, occasionally, sclerosing lesions may be found. As many as 5 per cent of schoolchildren may show isolated proteinuria persisting for months or even years, which is benign in the great majority.

However, proteinuria together with persistent microscopic haematuria should alert the clinician to the possibility of structurally damaged kidneys. In some cases this will be benign glomerular disease, such as resolving acute nephritis or IgA-associated nephropathy, but focal segmental glomerulosclerosis, crescentic nephritis, membranous nephropathy, or mesangiocapillary glomerulonephritis may be present. In the middle-aged or older patient amyloid or even diabetes may be found. Thus a renal biopsy will usually be necessary, especially if reduced renal function, hypertension, or both are present. In addition, some form of renal imaging will be needed, not just for the biopsy, because reflux nephropathy, polycystic kidneys, and renal tuberculosis may present as haematuria with proteinuria. Finally, serology for lupus and hepatitis B should be performed, and on estimation of at least the C3 component of complement.

An algorithm for the investigation of proteinuria is given in Fig. 2.

Selectivity of proteinuria

Tests of relative glomerular permeability are of limited value, except to distinguish minimal change nephrotic syndromes from other forms of nephritis or glomerular disease. Even here, they are more useful in children, in whom steroid therapy is often tried without a renal biopsy in younger patients with proteinuria but no haematuria, and because the distinction in terms of the selectivity profile between the two groups is clearer than in adults; moreover, a renal biopsy is almost always performed in older patients, at least in those with nephrotic-range proteinuria.

A common test or selectivity is to compare the clearance of IgG with that of a protein of lower molecular weight abundant in the urine, either albumin, or transferrin. This requires only a roughly simultaneous sample of plasma and a 'spot' untimed urine, since the urine volume cancels out in the relationship $C_{IgG} / C_{transferrin}$. A clearance of IgG greater than 20 per cent of transferrin or albumin represents 'non-selective' proteinuria; less than 10 per cent indicates a 'highly selective' proteinuria, suggesting that a minimal change lesion may be present, whereas the range between 10 and 20 per cent is of little discriminatory value. The proteins are measured conveniently in urine and plasma by radial immunodiffusion or laser nephelometry.

Microalbuminuria

There has been much interest in the increased excretion of albumin by apparently healthy diabetics, which exceeds normal but is less than that detected by Albustix® or similar tests. As noted above, normal individuals excrete less than 30 μg of albumin/min (43 mg/24 h), whereas the sensitivity of Albustix® is at best about 100 mg/l (150 mg/24 h). Diabetics who show proteinuria greater than 30 μg/h, but less than that detected by Albustix® (that is, 50–200 mg/24 h), are said to have 'microalbuminuria'. These individuals have been demonstrated to develop clinically evident proteinuria and diabetic nephropathy later in their course. Significant microalbuminuria by this definition may also be found in patients with poorly controlled or severe untreated hypertension.

In patients with systemic lupus erythematosus, but without evident nephritis, microalbuminuria is present in the majority, some of whom go on to develop obvious clinical proteinuria and nephritis. In minimal change nephrotic patients after remission, however, normal albumin excretion rates are present. Kits (for example Microalbutest®, Ames) are now available to test for microalbuminuria.

Enzymuria and brush border antigens in the urine

Urinary excretion of small amounts of enzymes from the cells of the renal tubules, and in particular in the brush border of the proximal tubules, occurs in normal individuals. Increased excretion of these enzymes has been shown to be a sensitive index of renal damage. Determination of these enzymes in the urine is easy and very sensitive, but unfortunately is non-specific so far as disease processes are concerned. Thus, these measurements are not very useful for diagnostic purposes, and their main value lies in screening populations at risk for renal damage, and for examining the fine nephrotoxicity of agents used clinically or commercially; or for examining consecutively the activity of processes already identified. Most urinary enzyme excretion measurements indicate tubular damage with some specificity, since many of these molecules are too large to pass through the glomerular filter under normal circumstances. Various enzymes have been studied, especially *N*-acetylglucosaminidase.

The consequences of proteinuria: the nephrotic syndrome

When proteinuria is prolonged and severe, a set of symptoms appear, the cardinal one being oedema. By convention, this combination of profuse proteinuria, oedema, and hypoalbuminaemia is called the nephrotic syndrome. Usually proteinuria of more than 3 to 4 g/24h for more than a few weeks is necessary to induce oedema with a serum albumin below 30 g/l, but it must be remembered that there is no firm and absolute boundary between persisting heavy proteinuria without oedema and a nephrotic syndrome; many patients will cross the boundary in either direction, sometimes because of a change in salt intake or activity rather than a change in proteinuria.

In the history, particular attention needs to be paid to medicines ingested, prior acute or chronic infections, allergies, or any features suggestive of a systemic disorder such as lupus. A history of macroscopic haematuria may be obtained, but this is unusual except in postinfectious or mesangiocapillary nephritis. The possibility of an associated tumour needs to be kept in mind in older patients. Finally, the family history may be revealing, as in Alport's syndrome or the Finnish form of congenital nephrotic syndrome.

The signs of the nephrotic syndrome centre on the oedema, which is soft, pitting, and dependent, often with facial swelling in the morning and ankle oedema at night. The arms may show oedema about the elbows and forearms, with wasting of the muscle in the upper arm— 'Popeye' arms. Genital oedema may be massive and a major source of distress. The puffy appearance leads to an apparent pallor, even when the haemoglobin is normal. If massive, the oedema may lead to spontaneous rupture of the protein-depleted skin, even in the absence of corticosteroids, with formation of striae and weeping wounds. Needle punctures may also leak for prolonged periods; this was formerly used to achieve drainage. The skin may show also xanthomata in patients with the most severe forms of an associated hyperlipidaemia, around the eyes or on the elbows. The oedema may extend to the pleurae, with bilateral hydrothorax, and ascites is common. The jugular venous pressure is usually normal, and if raised gives a suspicion in older patients that amyloidosis with cardiac amyloid may be present. In the case of progressive disorders, features of hypertension and uraemia may be

present. The liver will often be enlarged, especially in younger patients, presumably because of its increased synthetic work.

The microscopic appearance of the urine largely depends upon the underlying cause of the proteinuria: from a bland sediment with no red cells and only fatty casts in the case of minimal changes, to an 'angry' sediment with abundant red cells, and red cell and granular casts in a case of mesangiocapillary or crescentic nephritis.

Investigation of nephrotic patients follows closely that of patients with persistent proteinuria and haematuria, discussed above. The majority opinion is that all adult nephrotics and all nephrotic children over 10 years of age should be biopsied, even if their urine shows no casts or red cells (Fig. 3). Renal imaging will be needed, and renal function, assessed by measurement of glomerular filtration rate using an isotopic method, is desirable in addition to the obligatory measurement of plasma creatinine; in some very oedematous patients it may be better to wait until oedema has subsided under treatment because of problems with equilibration of the isotope. The proteinuria should be quantitated on several 24 h urines. Serological measurements should include a DNA antibody test, hepatitis B serology, complement concentrations, and, in older patients, chest radiograph and protein electrophoresis searching for paraproteins, as discussed above. Antineutrophil cytoplasmic antigen

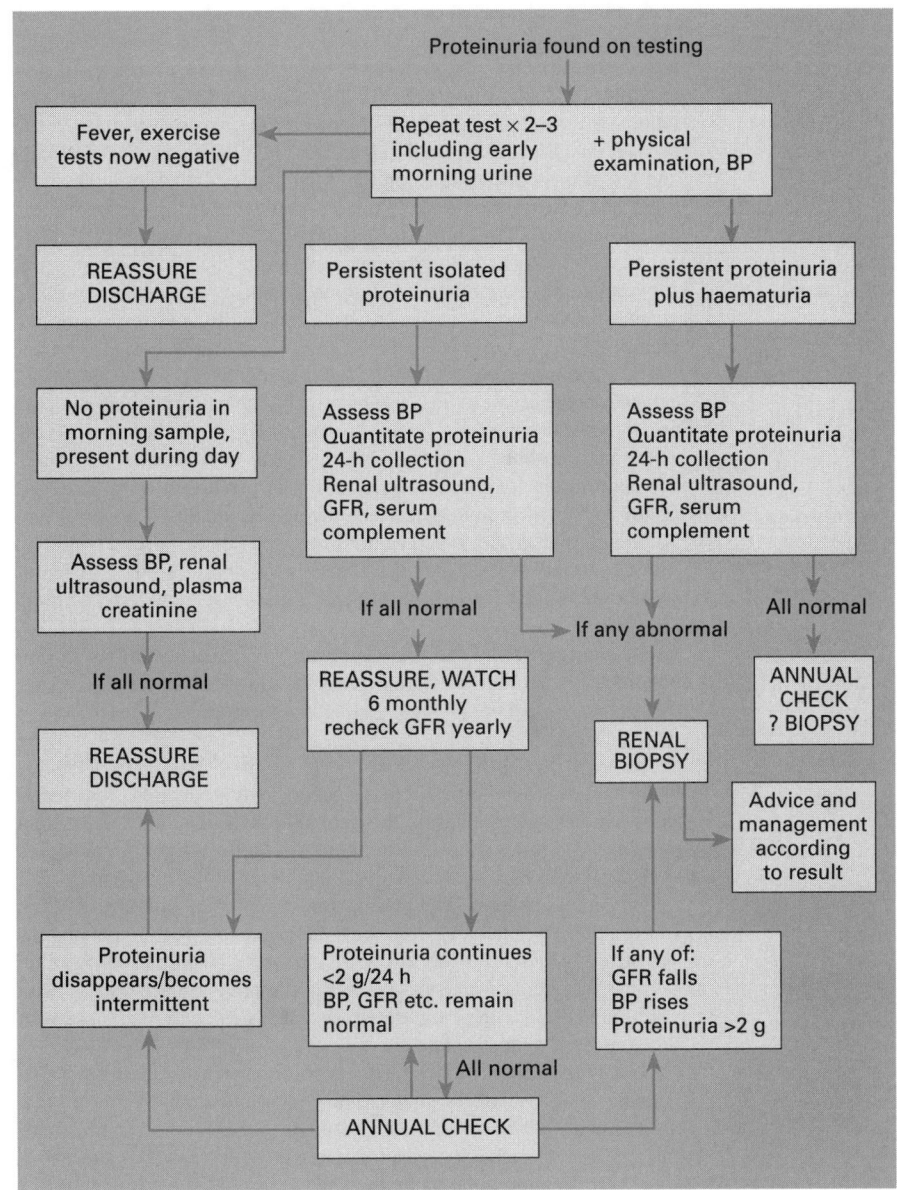

Fig. 2 An algorithm for the investigation of a patient found to have proteinuria on stick testing.

(ANCA) tests will rarely be needed since vasculitic patients very rarely develop a nephrotic state, unless they have recovered function after severe renal damage.

The genesis of nephrotic oedema

Until recently the 'classical' description of the genesis of nephrotic oedema was widely accepted: this pictured renal protein loss leading to a diminished plasma oncotic pressure because of a low serum albumin, which in turn led to hypovolaemia and triggering of salt-retaining humoral stimuli to which the kidney responded by avid salt retention, with consequent increased water absorption and oedema formation.

Clinical observation of patients accumulating or losing oedema showed that this story could only be partially true, and the finding that most stable adult nephrotics had normal or even increased plasma volumes struck the hypothesis a severe blow. Furthermore, studies, first on unilateral proteinuric disease in rats and then on isolated perfused kidneys, showed that the level of serum albumin is not an important stimulus to salt retention, and suggested that proteinuria per se leads to salt retention. Proteinuria probably influences salt retention through inducing resistance to atrial natriuretic factors (ANP), but at the moment we have no satisfying hypothesis as to the genesis of proteinuric oedema.

One or two ideas survive from older concepts: the difference between nephrotic and nephritic oedema is that although there is retention of salt and water in both conditions, the nephrotic syndrome occurs in a setting of a low plasma albumin, and the nephritic syndrome in one of a normal plasma albumin. Thus in the former peripheral oedema forms as interstitial water expands, and in the latter pulmonary oedema is more likely as intravascular volume expands as well.

Management of the nephrotic syndrome

The nephrotic syndrome is often chronic, and the psychological effects of a condition which (together with its treatment) distorts the patient's body must never be forgotten. Prolonged hospital admissions and fear of renal failure take their toll of morale. The main physical problem is to diminish or abolish the oedema. In the case of some disorders discussed in the next section this can achieved by specific treatment; here we will consider only general measures applicable to all nephrotics, whatever their underlying disease may be.

Salt intake should be modestly limited (to, say, 60 mmol/24 h) because stricter regimes are never followed. Water intake may also need to be watched because nephrotics excrete water loads poorly and excessive intake may precipitate hyponatraemia. Diuretics are the mainstay of oedema removal. In practice, loop diuretics are often the only effective agents, although both metolazone and spironolactone may be useful as adjuncts. Sometimes very big doses will be required, as much as 500 mg twice a day of frusemide or an equivalent drug. If this proves ineffective, or if oedema is massive, then the patients can be admitted to hospital and a daily regime of intravenous salt-poor albumin and intravenous diuretics (frusemide, 250 mg) used. Alone, the former carries the risk of pulmonary oedema and the latter the risk of hypovolaemic shock, but the two together are safe. This may need to be continued daily for a week or two, and 20, 30, or even 40 litres of oedema removed. It is interesting to note that, without any change in serum albumin or proteinuria, the patient is often able to sustain the new steady state with a much reduced burden of oedema.

A number of agents can reduce proteinuria, in every case at the expense of some reduction in glomerular filtration rate. The angiotensin-converting enzyme inhibitors have the best ratio of reduction in proteinuria to reduction in glomerular filtration rate; usually a 50 per cent reduction in proteinuria can be obtained at the expense of only 25 per cent off the glomerular filtration rate. Doses should be watched carefully and the plasma potassium monitored. Non-steroidal anti-inflammatory drugs and cyclosporin present a poorer profile, the change in proteinuria and glomerular filtration rate usually being identical, and a risk of acute or irreversible renal failure being much larger than with angiotensin-converting enzyme inhibitors. All these agents to be effective should be given after volume depletion has been induced by salt restriction and diuretics.

The recommended protein intake in nephrotics has been much debated. There seems to be little doubt that protein restriction diminishes proteinuria and a high protein diet augments it. On the other hand, giving a low protein diet in a protein-wasting state runs the risk of protein depletion in the long term. Some confusion has arisen from the terms 'high' and 'low' protein diet: in the United Kingdom 70 g/24 h represents a normal intake, whereas in North America it represents protein restriction, and in India luxury. After reviewing all the data, it seems about right to feed 1 g/kg/24 h of mainly first-class protein to nephrotic patients.

The management of specific complications such as infections, thrombosis, and hyperlipidaemia are dealt with below.

Complications and consequences of the nephrotic state

In the nephrotic syndrome, there is a general overproduction of all hepatically synthesized proteins, with selective loss of low molecular weight protein in the urine (Fig. 1). Thus low molecular weight proteins tend to be depleted in the plasma, with accumulation of the higher molecular weight protein species. The plasma concentration of proteins of about 180 to 200 kDa tends to be approximately normal; for proteins below this size, levels tend to be lowered, above this limit, raised. Another factor is the rate at which the protein is normally replaced, those with fast turnover in health being more resistant to depletion than those with slower normal synthetic rates.

Most of the complications of the nephrotic syndrome listed in Table 1 result from the effects of these profound alterations in the protein environment, either directly as a result of altered concentrations (for example in the coagulation system) or as a secondary result of alterations in cellular function induced by the change in protein environment (for

Fig. 3 The underlying histological appearances found in renal biopsies done in nephrotic patients in the developed world. During childhood, by far the most common appearance is that of minimal glomerular changes, and this appearance may be found even in the elderly. In young adults, the proportion of minimal change patients falls, and proliferative glomerulonephritis and lupus in young women form a significant proportion. In the elderly, membranous nephropathy becomes the dominant appearance together with diabetes and primary amyloidosis. The proportion of diabetics among older nephrotics is probably a considerable under estimate because many nephrotic diabetics do not have a renal biopsy. HSP, Henoch-Schönlein purpura; MCGN, mesangiocapillary glomerulonephritis; FSGS, focal segmental glomerulosclerosis.

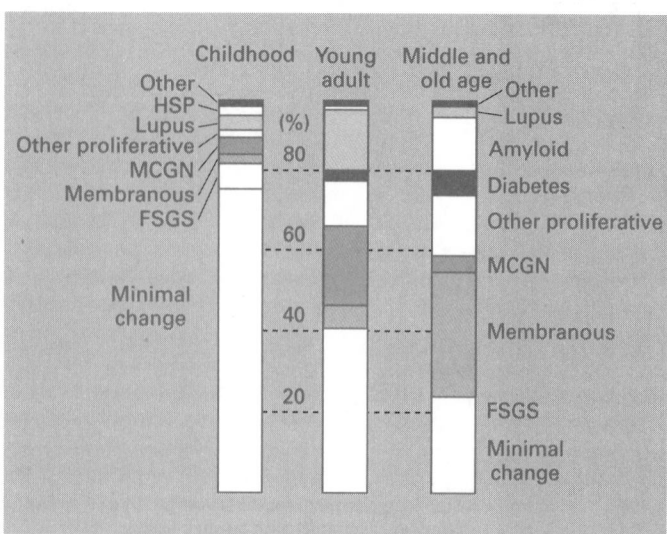

Table 1 *Complications of the nephrotic syndrome*

Susceptibility to infection
Thromboses
Hyperlipidaemia
Acute renal failure
Loss of binding proteins in urine
Protein malnutrition

example binding of increased quantities of low-density lipoprotein to cells or enhanced platelet activity).

INFECTIONS

Early reports from the pre-antibiotic era emphasized the high incidence and considerable mortality of bacterial infections in patients with a nephrotic syndrome, especially children. In the latter, peritonitis remains a threat even today. In the developing world, sepsis is still a major problem in nephrotics.

Primary peritonitis is particularly characteristic of nephrotic children. The onset may be insidious but is usually sudden, and should be suspected in any nephrotic child who develops abdominal pain. Unfortunately this is a common symptom associated with hypovolaemia, and the diagnosis must be confirmed by direct microscopic examination of a Gram stain, or an immunochemical search for bacterial antigens, on ascitic fluid removed by needle. Signs of attendant systemic infection make the diagnosis easier. Blood cultures are usually positive also, but take much longer to perform. Hypotension, shock, and even acute renal failure may follow rapidly, sometimes with disseminated intravascular coagulation (see below). In the past the organism was almost always *Streptococcus pneumoniae,* but other organisms, such as β-haemolytic streptococci, Haemophilus, and Gram-negative organisms may be found

Cellulitis is equally characteristic, especially in severely oedematous nephrotics. Many such infections arise from skin punctures, either spontaneous or as a result of venepuncture, or (in the past) attempts at mechanical drainage by puncture or scarification. Organisms responsible include β-haemolytic streptococci and a variety of Gram-negative bacteria. Usually the clinical diagnosis is clear, with obvious demarcation of the infected area, which may spread rapidly within hours to include most of the limb; the patient may be very toxic, febrile, or even become hypotensive. Other patients run a more indolent course with a well-demarcated area of infection which remains localized. It is difficult to stain or culture organisms from fluid aspirated from the area, but, as in primary peritonitis, blood cultures are usually positive.

It has been suggested that urinary tract infections are commoner in nephrotic children, and that they might inhibit the response to corticosteroids, but this has not held up under further examination. Both varicella and measles do, however, present a major danger to children receiving either corticosteroid or cytotoxic agents.

Causes of susceptibility to infection in nephrotic patients

Infections are commonest in children, reports of severe infections in adults being rare. Also, the predominance of pneumococcal infections is striking and organisms are nearly always encapsulated; some others, such as staphylococci, are notable for their almost complete absence. Large fluid collections are present in the abdomen and pleural cavity, providing a good site for the growth of bacteria, as in liver disease. Nephrotic skin is fragile, and may even rupture spontaneously under the pressure of oedema. Local humoral defences may be diluted by oedema. However, it seems likely that immunological factors play the major role in the susceptibility to infection of nephrotic patients.

Immunoglobulin G provides the main defence against infection in tissues, and low serum IgG concentrations are characteristic of nephrotic patients. The reasons for these low IgG concentrations are complex and may relate to a primary defect of T-lymphocyte function as well as to

urinary losses and tubular catabolism. However, in patients with inherited common hypogammaglobulinaemia, levels of IgG below 2 g/l are required before serious infections are seen, and such levels are rarely reached in nephrotic patients.

Pneumococcal infections are a particular problem in patients with some congenital deficiencies of the complement system, and alternative pathway activation is crucial in the phagocytosis of encapsulated organisms. Factor B, a major factor in this pathway, has a molecular weight of only 55 kDa and is lost in nephrotic urine. By 20 years of age, most adults have acquired antibodies against a variety of pneumococcal capsular antigens. Thus it is only during childhood that there is this peculiar vulnerability to *Strep. pneumoniae* from poor alternative pathway activity. Transferrin is essential for normal lymphocyte function, and acts as a carrier for a number of metals, including zinc. Added transferrin can restore normal lymphocyte function in nephrotics.

Treatment and prophylaxis

Prompt induction of remission of oedema and proteinuria are the most important goals in prevention, together with skin care and asepsis. In children there is a good case for using prophylactic penicillin to avoid pneumococcal infections, at least while the child is oedematous. Antipneumococcal vaccines against capsular antigens induce an adequate response when given in remission, but are not always protective when given during steroid therapy and are frankly defective when given shortly after cytotoxic therapy.

Treatment of established sepsis in nephrotics requires rapid action, which in turn depends on anticipation, suspicion, and rapid diagnosis. The erythrocyte sedimentation rate is a useless measurement in nephrotic children, and the white cell count may be misleading, especially in those taking corticosteroids. C-reactive protein may be useful in the diagnosis of serious sepsis, but the results may not be known rapidly enough. Parenteral antibiotics should always be used, even when the infection appears to be localized, because septicaemia is often already present. They should be begun as soon as cultures have been taken and should not await the return of sensitivities. In children benzylpenicillin should always be a component of the antibiotic therapy, and when pneumococcus is observed, back-up broad-spectrum therapy is needed, because it may not be the only organism present. A broad-spectrum cephalosporin, together with an aminoglycoside, may be used as initial 'blind' treatment in adults. Blood pressure, peripheral temperature, and venous pressure need careful watching and colloid may be necessary. The risk of secondary thrombosis suggests the need for anticoagulation. Supplementary corticosteroid is essential in those taking these drugs, or who have just stopped them.

THROMBOEMBOLIC COMPLICATIONS

Thrombosis in both the arterial and the venous circulations is a relatively frequent and serious complication of the nephrotic syndrome. Both corticosteroids and diuretics may contribute to thrombosis, the former from effects on coagulation proteins, and the latter through effects on blood viscosity, but the underlying reasons depend upon the nephrotic state itself.

Peripheral venous thrombosis and pulmonary embolism are common in nephrotic patients: overt deep venous thrombosis is evident in about 6 per cent of nephrotic adults and can be detected 25 per cent if Doppler ultrasonography is used. It is much less common in childhood (0.6 per cent). Clinically diagnosed pulmonary emboli are present in 6 per cent of adult nephrotics and, if ventilation-perfusion scanning is used, as many as 12 per cent are affected. However, only a single patient in our own series up to 1982 (followed for 2100 patient-years) actually died of pulmonary embolism. Other venous thrombi are much less common; however, subclavian or axillary, jugular, iliac, portal, splenic, hepatic, sagittal sinus, and mesenteric vein thrombosis have all been described, along with renal vein thrombosis.

In adults arterial thrombosis is much less common than venous thrombosis. In contrast, children show about an equal incidence of arterial and venous thrombosis. Even so, the incidence of arterial thrombosis in adults is still twice that in children, because of the rarity of deep venous thrombosis in children. Almost every artery has been involved: aorta, femoral, coronary, pulmonary, mesenteric, cerebral, renal, ophthalmic, and carotid arteries, together with major intracardiac thrombi.

Controversy exists about the incidence and significance of renal venous thrombosis. All agree, however, that it is commonly found in association with membranous nephropathy (usually idiopathic but also in lupus membranous nephropathy), after gold therapy or transplantation, as well as in the Heymann model of membranous nephropathy in rats. The reason for this predilection for patients with membranous nephropathy eludes explanation so far.

The prevalence of renal vein thrombosis at a clinical level is about 6 to 8 per cent in nephrotics with membranous nephropathy and only 1 to 3 per cent in other forms of glomerulopathy. However, if venograms are performed, the prevalence is seen to be 10 to 45 per cent in membranous patients and around 10 per cent in others.

Clinically evident renal venous thrombosis may present acutely, with loin pain, haematuria, renal enlargement, and deterioration in renal function; or as a slower fall-off in renal function without dramatic signs or symptoms. Otherwise, the thrombosis may be quite silent clinically, being found incidentally by venography or other evaluation. Leg oedema increases if the vena cava is involved, although caval thrombosis can be surprisingly silent. Thrombosis of renal veins is frequently bilateral, but may be unilateral. Men are more commonly affected than women. About 35 per cent of patients with renal venous thrombosis will have pulmonary emboli which are clinically evident or show up on scanning.

Nevertheless, few (if any) nephrologists have adopted a policy of doing renal venous venography in all nephrotic patients, or even in all those with membranous nephropathy. In general, those worth investigating are those with clinical signs suggestive of renal venous thrombosis (flank pain, otherwise unexplained deterioration in renal function, sudden onset of haematuria) and those with pulmonary emboli. It has yet to be established that seeking symptomless renal venous thrombosis is useful, since its prognosis appears to be benign; and how frequently or at what intervals re-screening must be undertaken is not established. If Doppler ultrasound, CT, or MRI scanning can be established as reliable, much of this will change. Functional renal impairment is an adverse prognostic sign but in most instances there is recovery of renal function and recanalization of the veins.

Abnormalities of coagulation in nephrotics

Nephrotic patients are relatively immobile and may have haemoconcentrated blood from hypovolaemia, especially in childhood. Whole-blood viscosity is increased by both the increase in haematocrit and as a result of increased plasma viscosity, in turn related to high fibrinogen concentrations. Many proteins involved in the initiation or regulation of clotting show altered concentrations in nephrotic patients. In general, zymogens of the intrinsic pathway are reduced in nephrotics, and occasional patients with a bleeding tendency from this have been reported. All other zymogens or cofactors are either present in normal amounts, or raised, particularly von Willebrand factor, fibrinogen, and factors V, X, and VII. In general, concentrations of prothrombin (factor II) are normal. Alterations in fibrinolytic and regulator proteins are complex because some are concerned both with inhibiting fibrinolysis and thombin generation. Thus even though levels of antithrombin III are very low, total antithrombin activity is normal in the nephrotic syndrome because of the rise in α_1-macroglobulin concentration. Plasminogen concentrations have been found consistently to be low in nephrotics, but the role of plasmin inhibitors is not clear. Protein C remains normal or raised, but free protein S activity is low. Recent studies suggest a major role for raised fibrinogen in flowing blood. In addition, there are indications that platelet hyperaggregability may play a significant role in the thrombotic state of nephrotic patients, even though there is as yet no firm evidence that the many phenomena described *in vitro* operate *in vivo*. A lowered serum albumin affects platelet protaglandin metabolism, hyperlipidaemia alters platelet membrane lipids, and von Willebrand factor concentrations are high. The platelet count in nephrotic patients has variously been reported as either normal or raised, but the elevation, if present, is usually mild.

Treatment and prophylaxis of thrombosis in nephrotics

Patients should be mobilized, sepsis avoided or treated promptly, dehydration from incidental causes (for example diarrhoea) treated, diuretics used with care, and haemoconcentration minimized. Anticoagulation carries the usual risks and presents additional difficulties in nephrotic patients. Heparin acts mainly through the activation of antithrombin III, the concentration of which is usually greatly diminished in nephrotics. Warfarin is albumin bound and the levels of albumin may change therapeutically or spontaneously. However, warfarin also raises antithrombin III levels. However, whether some or all nephrotics should receive anticoagulation remains a problem. Clearly, those with symptomatic thromboses, including renal vein thrombosis, should be anticoagulated for at least 3 to 6 months. At this point their serum albumin should be assessed, and if under 25 g/l, or especially if 20 g/l, then anticoagulation should probably be continued until it exceeds this level, because of the risks of re-thrombosis.

Whether nephrotic patients with symptomless deep venous thrombosis should be anticoagulated has never been studied; if these patients also have symptomless pulmonary emboli most physicians would anticoagulate. If the physician does decide to anticoagulate all nephrotics with symptomless deep vein thromboses, then one patient in four will be so treated. Many physicians give anticoagulants to patients with symptomless renal venous thrombosis, but there is no proven basis for doing this. A minority of nephrologists use prophylactic warfarin in all nephrotic patients; some, however, only treat those with very low albumin concentrations (<20 g/l). Others concerned about this at-risk subgroup use low-dose aspirin (75 mg daily, which is safe with steroids) and dipyridamole (100–200 mg three times a day).

ALTERATIONS IN LIPID METABOLISM

Much of the recent interest in the alterations in lipid metabolism occurring in the nephrotic syndrome has centred on possible effects on the induction of atheromatous vascular disease, and what might be learnt from this secondary phenomenon about risks of primary hyperlipidaemia, and vice versa. Early descriptions reported atheroma even in nephrotic children, and several small series of nephrotic patients with myocardial infarction were published, suggesting that the incidence in nephrotics was much higher than in controls. However, two careful case-control studies, one in the United Kingdom and one in California came to discordant conclusions: the question remains open. Nephrotic patients with a particularly severe or prolonged course are almost certainly at extra risk; the majority of these patients will have membranous nephropathy or focal segmental glomerulosclerosis.

It has also become received dogma that the (only possibly) increased incidence of ischaemic vascular disease in nephrotics is the result, in the main, of alterations in circulating lipids. Again, this proposition ignores the influence of other powerful risk factors, such as hypertension and smoking.

Concentrations of cholesterol triglycerides and lipoproteins

Total cholesterol (both free cholesterol and cholesterol esters) is raised in almost all nephrotics, with a strong negative correlation with the serum albumin. Increases in fasting triglyceride levels are less common, and are found largely in the more severe nephrotic syndromes, again correlating with depression of serum albumin. Free fatty acid levels are reduced, probably because of their binding to albumin, although the concomitant increase in lipids results in normal total fatty acid concentrations. Susceptibility to hyperlipidaemia is not in dependent on the underlying glomerular lesion: in particular, diabetics and those with lupus are, perhaps surprisingly, no different from those with glomerulonephritis of various other types. Diminished renal function does affect

Table 2 *Treatment of nephrotic hyperlipidaemia*

Agent	Effect on cholesterol	Effect on triglycerides	Deleterious side-effects
Bile-acid-binding resins	Reduction	Increase	Gastrointestinal side-effects
Fibric acid derivatives	Reduction	Strong reduction	Myonecrosis; gallstones
Probucol	Reduction	No effect	Reduces high density lipoprotein
Nicotinic acid	Reduction	Reduction	Flushing
HMG CoA reductase inhibitors	Strong reduction	Reduction	?Myonecrosis; no long-term studies

Fibric acid derivatives = clofibrate, benzafibrate, gemfibrozil.

Bile-acid-binding resins = cholestyramine, colestipol.

Nicotinic acid derivatives = nicotinamide, Bradilan®, Acipimax®.

HMG CoA reductase inhibitors = lovastatin, simvastatin, pravastatin, etc.

triglyceride levels profoundly. Also, there is some evidence that, at least in nephrotic children, the lipid abnormalities may persist into remission, or between relapses.

Very low density lipoproteins (VLDLs) and low density lipoproteins (LDLs) are increased in the more severe nephrotic states, but may be normal in mild cases. The lipoprotein fraction contains much of the excess triglyceride, and the cholesterol: phospholipid ratio is increased. Reduced apolipoprotein C2 is present in VLDL from nephrotics. Like cholesterol and triglyceride concentrations, VLDL and LDL concentrations vary inversely with the serum albumin concentration. Apolipoprotein (a) concentrations are usually raised.

Data on high density lipoprotein (HDL) concentrations in nephrotics are conflicting: low concentrations, normal levels, and high concentrations of HDL have all been reported. In most of these studies, the reduced HDL concentrations have been noted only in the most severe nephrotic syndromes. However, these differences probably arise from the heterogeneity of nephrotic patients of various ages, renal function, treatments, duration, and severity included in the studies. In parallel normal, low, or high apolipoprotein A1 concentrations were found. HDL2 concentrations are reduced, and those of HDL3 are normal or increased, except in the most severe cases.

Lipiduria

Lipiduria is well recognized in the nephrotic syndrome, and fatty urinary casts are a characteristic feature (see Chapter 20.1). Cholesterol, phospholipid, free fatty acids, and triglyceride are all present in nephrotic urine. HDL is also present, which is not surprising when one considers that it is only a little larger than albumin, whereas LDL is much larger. It seems that little catabolism of lipoproteins occurs in the kidney in the nephrotic syndrome: although apolipoproteins E and C1 may be dissociated from lipoprotein molecules, apolipoproteins B and A1 remain relatively unaffected. Thus it seems that only easily degradable or surface proteins are catabolized during their passage through the kidney.

Causes of lipid alterations in the nephrotic syndrome

The causes of the raised plasma lipids in the nephrotic syndrome are still not understood in full, but both a major increase in production of all types of lipid and a minor decrease in receptor-mediated removal of lipoproteins and decrease in lipoprotein lipase seem to be present, and abnormalities at almost every step in the production and removal of lipids have been described.

Hypoalbuminaemia was thought for some time to be the non-specific stimulus inducing increased liver apoprotein (and thus lipoprotein and lipid) synthesis. However, there is evidence that this is not so in the long term, since alterations in albumin synthesis by changing diet were not accompanied by alterations in lipids, and there is evidence that inert molecules such as dextrans also influence lipoprotein synthesis in hepatocytes.

Reduced activity of lecithin cholesterol acyltransferase (LCAT),

which could reduce HDL production, has been noted in nephrotics. Again, the reasons for this deficiency, which would reduce the ability to mobilize lipid from endothelium or other peripheral tissues, are obscure.

Treatment of lipid alterations in nephrotics

Because of the possibility that nephrotic hyperlipidaemia is a risk factor for accelerated vascular disease, as outlined above, attempts have been made to correct the abnormalities in the hope that there might be a consequent reduction in vascular disease, as has been shown in primary hyperlipidaemias. It seems reasonable to give dietary advice to nephrotic as to any other hyperlipidaemic patients, but surprisingly few studies have been done on compliance or effects of such advice on circulating lipids in nephrotics. There seems to be no justification in treating all nephrotic patients with hypolipidaemic agents. Most nephrotics remit spontaneously, are treated, or go on to develop chronic renal failure within 3 to 5 years of onset. The decision to treat hyperlipidaemia or not in a patient with a nephrotic syndrome can therefore be postponed until a year or so has passed, or until the decision can be made in the light of the probable duration of this syndrome in relation to biopsy appearances and response, or lack of it, to treatment.

Several possible modes of treatment are available (Table 2). There are no reports of studies on attempted dietary modification of plasma lipids, nor of the administration of ω-3 unsaturated fish oils, which might affect platelet function favourably. Neither is there any indication as to which of the various hypolipidaemic drugs may be the most useful in treating nephrotics, since no long-term studies have addressed this question. Now that more effective agents for treating hyperlipidaemia are available, interest has revived in this aspect of the nephrotic syndrome, but because there is as yet no way of knowing whether or not, in any individual, reduction of the lipids towards normal has achieved any good; the risks and side-effects of any drugs must be considered particularly carefully. The efficacy of the various agents in nephrotic patients is noted in Table 2. The statins are effective in lowering lipids in nephrotics and seem the preferable drugs at present.

LOSSES OF BINDING TRANSPORT PROTEINS IN THE URINE

A number of plasma proteins important in the transport of metals, hormones, and drugs are of relatively small molecular weight and thus are lost easily into the urine of nephrotic patients. However, such losses appear to be of little clinical significance.

Low concentrations of iron in nephrotic plasma are well known with losses of transferrin (molecular weight 87 kDa) and iron into the urine. Transferrin turnover studies in nephrotics show both increased synthesis and degradation; however, iron deficiency is rare, although cases of anaemia attributed to this cause have been described. Since losses of iron are at most 0.5 to 1.0 mg/24 h, even with the heaviest proteinuria, other factors must operate to produce iron deficiency. In addition, the transferrin–iron complex binds to many proliferating cells, and the effects of transferrin depletion on immunity may not depend entirely upon a lowered zinc-albumin complex.

The copper-binding protein, caeruloplasmin, has a molecular weight of 151 kDa and although low red cell and plasma copper concentrations in nephrotic patients have been described, most authors have reported normal levels of the metal, even though the binding protein is lost in the urine, and its plasma concentration is low. No clinical consequences of copper losses have been reported.

Zinc circulates bound mainly to albumin and also to transferrin, and thus the reported reduction in plasma, hair, and white cell zinc concentrations in nephrotics is not surprising. Hypogeusia has also been reported, and the possible reduction of cell-mediated immunity has been mentioned above.

Vitamin D binding protein (molecular weight 59 kDa) and its associated vitamin are lost in nephrotic urine. Clinically, both osteomalacia and hyperparathyroidism have been described in nephrotic children more often than in adults, but bone biopsies are commonly normal and bone disease or clinical significance is very rare. There is evidence, however, that patients with renal failure accompanied by nephrotic rates of proteinuria may be particularly prone to develop osteodystrophy, when early treatment with vitamin D preparations may have a place. The biochemical abnormalities described have varied but include hypocalcaemia, both total (protein-bound) and ionized; hypocalciuria, reduced intestinal absorption of calcium and negative calcium balance in both adults and children; reduced plasma 25-hydroxycholecalciferol and 24,25-dihydroxycholecalciferol and, surprisingly, also 1,25-dihydroxycholecalciferol; a blunted response to administration of parathyroid hormone (PTH); and raised PTH concentrations. Clinical consequences of any of these changes are remarkably rare.

The puffy face and low metabolic rate when uncorrected for the weight of retained fluid led many early observers to suppose that all nephrotic patients were hypothyroid. In fact, despite losses of thyroid-binding globulin (molecular weight 85 kDa) in the urine, proportional to total proteinuria and accompanied by bound T3 and T4, plasma concentrations of T3, T4, and thyroid stimulating hormone are usually normal in nephrotic patients; although the T3 may be rather low and the T4 somewhat elevated, with increased reverse T3 perhaps because of the loss of T3 in the urine. These findings, although potentially confusing, are not of clinical significance except when pursuing a diagnosis of incidental hypothyroidism in a nephrotic patient, when the plasma level of thyroid stimulating hormone is the important investigation.

Cortisol binding protein (molecular weight 52 kDa) is lost in nephrotic urine and the plasma concentration may be reduced.

Despite the large number of drugs normally bound in part to albumin, the gross reductions in serum albumin in nephrotics give rise to remarkably few problems. Those concerning warfarin and fibrates have been mentioned above. Prednisolone is frequently given to nephrotics, especially those with minimal glomerular changes, and is normally bound to albumin. Despite this fact, even severe hypoalbuminaemia does not render dose modification necessary, since the levels of free drug equilibrate rapidly to nearly normal concentrations; although in the Boston drug surveillance programme, there was a direct relationship between the side-effects of steroid treatment and serum albumin concentrations.

HYPOVOLAEMIA AND ACUTE RENAL FAILURE IN THE NEPHROTIC SYNDROME

Although acute renal failure is exceptionally rare in children with nephrotic syndromes, hypovolaemia is probably more common in children than in adults, even in the absence of diuretic therapy. Thus a nephrotic child in the initial attack or relapse may have a cold periphery, collapsed peripheral veins, and a low central venous pressure, a high haematocrit, a variable but sometimes very low blood pressure, and oliguria with urine almost devoid of sodium; all of which reverse on infusion of albumin. The frequency of hypovolaemia in children and the rarity of an associated acute renal failure suggests strongly that the acute renal failure described in older nephrotics does not result from hypovolaemia: when acute renal failure does occur in nephrotic children it is almost always associated with either sepsis or thrombosis.

Renal tubular dysfunction in nephrotics

Renal tubular dysfunction has been described in a rather small number of nephrotic patients, usually with multiple proximal tubular deficiencies in reabsorption, to give a complete or partial Fanconi syndrome. Although undoubtedly some of these cases have had reversible tubular defects dependent upon their nephrotic syndrome (presumably associated in some way with heavy proteinuria), in many others the defect has arisen from tubular damage as part of the underlying disease, often focal segmental glomerulosclerosis. Indeed, in children the presence of glycosuria or β_2-microglobulinuria can help to differentiate those children with focal segmental glomerulosclerosis from those with minimal change lesions only.

Proteinuria as factor in the progression of renal failure

There is a well-recognized correlation between the amount of proteinuria, its persistence, and the decline of renal function into renal failure. Until recently it had been assumed that this reflected intrinsically more severe disease, which in turn gave rise to a poorer prognosis. However, evidence has mounted that proteinuria is of itself deleterious to the kidney.

Three consequences of profuse proteinuria may contribute to progression of renal failure. Hypercoagulability has been implicated in the progression of remnant kidney renal failure in rats. Hypercoagulability in the nephrotic state results principally from platelet hyperaggregability, as discussed above. If a persistent nephrotic syndrome is present, this could contribute through intraglomerular thrombosis and sclerosis induced by release of platelet-derived factors. Treatment with antiplatelet agents might therefore be expected to slow progression of renal failure in persistent nephrotic syndromes, and there is evidence from animal models that this is so.

The second factor is hyperlipidaemia, which has a complex relationship with glomerulosclerosis. The analogy has been drawn between the macrophage infiltration and foam cell formation of atheroma, and events in the glomerulus in progressive glomerulosclerosis. Certainly, mesangial cells bear LDL receptors, and there is growing evidence from in vitro studies that binding of excess LDL can damage these cells. The renal disease seen in inherited LCAT deficiency is well recognized. Thus control of hyperlipidaemia in persistent nephrotic syndromes (see above) could have the aim not only of preventing generalized atheroma, but also of preventing progressive renal failure, or at least slowing its progression.

The third factor is the recent description that the proteinuria of intravenous protein overload will cause renal damage associated with an interstitial infiltrate. Renal tubular reabsorption of lipid-bearing albumin leads to the generation of a lipid chemotactic factor active on macrophages, which leads in turn to the infiltrate. Although this describes a potential mechanism for direct toxicity of filtered albumin, it does not account for the absence of renal failure in many patients with chronic minimal change disease unresponsive to steroids.

The patient with haematuria

Visible blood in the urine, blood detected on microscopy, or the finding of haemoglobin in the urine, is one of the cardinal ways by which renal disease is detected. The urine may be bright red, but more often, after

Table 3 *Causes of haematuria*

Disorders of coagulation	Anticoagulants Bleeding disorders (haemophilia, etc.)
Glomerular diseases	IgA nephropathy Endocapillary nephritis Alport's syndrome Thin membrane nephropathy Mesangiocapillary glomerulonephritis Crescentic glomerulonephritis Fabry's disease Vasculitis/lupus, etc.
Interstitial diseases	Interstitial nephritis Polycystic disease

Medullary diseases	Papillary necrosis from:
	  analgesic nephropathy
	  sickle-cell disease
	  diabetes mellitus
	Sponge kidney
	Tuberculosis

Renal and urinary tract tumours	Wilms' Renal cell carcinoma Transitional cell lesions Carcinoma of prostate Carcinoma of urethra
Infections	Acute pyelonephritis/cystitis Schistosomiasis Urethritis Prostatitis
Stones	Anywhere in urinary tract Calcium oxalate crystalluria Urate crystalluria
Obstruction	NB release of obstruction
Trauma Miscellaneous	To kidney, bladder, ureter Hypertension Loin pain haematuria syndrome Familial telanglectasia Arteriovenous malformations Endometriosis Chemical cystitis Meatal ulcers Urethral caruncle Foreign body Factitious (added blood)

a dwell time in the bladder, is brownish, likened to tea or Coca Cola, especially in acid urine. Usually the amounts of blood lost are trivial, but the presence of clots, with or without colic, suggests bleeding from the renal pelvis, ureters of bladder, although major bleeding may also complicate polycystic kidney disease as well as renal tumours. Haematuria may arise from anywhere in the urinary tract. The list of conditions capable of causing it is long (Table 3). The likelihood of finding any one of these conditions in a patient presenting with haematuria varies with age: the causes in an infant, a child or young adult, and a middle-aged or elderly subject are quite different.

Testing for blood in the urine

Only 5 ml of blood containing 25×10^9 red cells are needed to give visible haematuria in a litre of urine at a concentration of 25 000 cells/μl; twice this amount will give visible haematuria throughout the day in every specimen. In health, fewer than 10^7 red blood cells are excreted per day, at least some of which originate from the lower urinary tract; this represents the loss of less than 1 μl of blood per 24 h into the urine. The upper limit of the number of red cells in normal urine is less clearly defined than for protein excretion, perhaps because of the existence of normal individuals with thin glomerular capillary basement membranes: 90 per cent of normal individuals will have 1 red cell or less per μl of urine, that is an excretion rate of about 10^5 cells/h, but a few will have up to 10 times this figure. Even if all these came though the kidney, given that there are 2 million nephrons, probably only one, and at most 10, red cells pass through each nephron in 24 h. Thus it is not surprising that histopathological detection of red cells crossing the glomerular basement membrane is unusual, even in haematuric illnesses. Nevertheless this is how glomerular haematuria is supposed to originate, although why some forms of nephritis affecting the mesangium, such as IgA nephropathy, may cause macroscopic haematuria is obscure.

A number of drugs and foods that give a pink-red colour to the urine (phenindione, phenolphthalein, beetroot, rifampicin, and others) may be confused with haematuria. Haemoglobin and myoglobin may be excreted as free compounds when intravascular haemolysis or rhabdomyolysis occur, and will need to be differentiated from haematuria. Porphyrins may also discolour urine and be mistaken for haematuria.

Dipstick tests tests detect the haemoglobin from lysed red cells, which break up more quickly in dilute alkaline urine. The reaction is between the haemoglobin and *o*-toluidine, and the sensitivity of dipsticks is close to the normal range, about 1 to 5 cells/μl, so that some normal individuals will show positives from time to time, for example after vigorous exercise ('jogger's nephritis'). Microscopy of unspun urine usually shows about one cell per μl and is best done in fresh concentrated acidic urine to avoid breakup of the cells. Haemoglobinuria can only be excluded by doing both tests. Counts of red cells should be done in a Fuchs–Rosenthal counting chamber on unspun unstained urine; the use of phase-contrast rather than bright field illumination improves precision of the count. Concentration of the urine by centrifugation is useful for qualitative analysis, but counts are hopelessly unreliable in spun urines. In any case, microscopy is necessary to look for casts and for white cells.

Haematuria in patients taking anticoagulants presents special problems. Most will have underlying disease and require investigation.

Given the long list of causes of haematuria in Table 3, it is obviously valuable to be able to distinguish the site of origin of the red cells if possible. Some clues include the presence of concomitant proteinuria, which almost always indicates a renal (usually, but not always, glomerular) origin of the haematuria. This is because except in major bleeding (more than 50 ml/24 h), there is simply not enough protein lost in the blood to give a positive result on stick tests for albumin. Similarly, the presence of red cell casts indicates glomerular haematuria. Since Birch and Fairley reintroduced the idea in 1979, there has been much interest in distinguishing urinary tract bleeding from glomerular haematuria by red cell morphology. Both phase-contrast microscopy of unspun urine, which is strongly observer dependent, and red cell analysers have been used to make the distinction. However, these do not provide accurate information at low red cell excretion rates. Basically, glomerular haematuria usually contains a high proportion of bizarre-shaped acanthocytes with considerable anisocytosis; whereas the red cells of bleeding are usually smooth discs (Fig. 4).

Persistent symptomless isolated haematuria

The significance of this finding varies greatly with age. In young individuals in whom malignant disease of the urinary tract is very uncommon, significant disease in as few as 2 per cent of a haematuric population has been reported. Red cell casts and dysmorphic red cells imply glomerular haematuria, and in such cases renal biopsy often shows minor patterns of glomerular change, but may show thin membrane nephropathy or mesangial IgA deposition. Alport's syndrome will often present as isolated haematuria before any deafness or associated proteinuria is present.

Figure 5 gives an algorithm for the investigation of a patient with haematuria. If no red cell casts or dysmorphic cells are present and a clotting screen is normal, an intravenous urogram followed by a cystoscopy are usual practice, but in many young cases no abnormalities are detected. In patients of African origin the possibility of sickle-cell heterozygosity as a cause of minor papillary necrosis must not be forgotten. Infections of the urinary tract, including the prostate in males and the urethra in both sexes, are common causes of haematuria. Factitious haematuria may be induced by adding blood obtained by finger-prick to the urine. Rarely, parents will even add blood to their child's urine. Schistosomiasis may occur in individuals exposed in endemic areas.

In older patients the position is quite different. From 2 to 20 per cent of middle-aged and elderly males show microscopic symptomless haematuria, most commonly as manifestation of stones or renal tract malignancy, so that the percentage with significant findings is high and investigation is mandatory.

Persistent microscopic haematuria with associated proteinuria

This has been discussed above. Non-glomerular causes such as renal tuberculosis, polycystic kidneys, papillary necrosis, interstitial nephritis, and reflux nephropathy may cause confusion, but in general, glomerular disease will be present, commonly thin membrane nephropathy or IgA or other mesangial nephropathy, but other proliferative patterns and membranous nephropathy may be the cause. Patients with Alport's syndrome develop added haematuria as their glomerulopathy evolves, but usually show some high tone deafness by this stage. Therefore, especially if red cell casts, hypertension, or reduced renal function are present, renal biopsy will be the critical investigation.

Acute macroscopic haematuria with proteinuria: the acute nephritic syndrome

This has also been called 'acute glomerulonephritis', but because this term carries implications of histology, pathogenesis, and outcome which apply to only some patients, the term acute nephritic syndrome is preferable. Usually there is associated oliguria; circulatory overload and pulmonary oedema; hypertension, usually with normal fundi; and variable, often non-pitting oedema. If severe overload and malignant hypertension are present, convulsions may result. There is often a prodrome of an infection, either cutaneous or anginal, arising from *Streptococcus haemolyticus;* but many other infections can precipitate this syndrome.

Most frequently some form of proliferative/infiltrative nephritis is present, particularly endocapillary nephritis or mesiangiocapillary nephritis (MCGN), with or without some crescent formation. However, sometimes there is no tuft proliferation only a necrotizing glomerulitis with severe crescent formation; in many such cases, the underlying diagnosis is a vasculitis, when purpura, arthritis, or uveitis help to make a clinical diagnosis, but quite often the renal disease is, at least for a time, the only manifestation. Rarely, antiglomerular basement membrane disease with linear deposition of IgG along the glomerular capillary basement membrane is found. In neither vasculitic nor antiglomerular basement membrane disease is hypertension as common a problem as it is in those forms of glomerulonephritis in which glomeruli are infiltrated by monocytes.

Recurrent macroscopic haematuria, with or without proteinuria

This may result from glomerulonephritis, usually IgA nephropathy, but also from recurrent bleeding from urinary tract lesions; again the difference between younger and older patients needs emphasis. In some patients the volume overload and hypertension are absent, and the syndrome is called 'recurrent haematuria'. In these patients, the haematuria may be accompanied by loin pain, fever, and adenopathy, or precipitated by exercise. Usually, renal biopsy in such patients will show IgA nephropathy. Some patients' urine may be reddish almost all the time, and this and the haematuria of sickle-cell disease are almost the only states in which glomerular bleeding can be so profuse as to cause anaemia.

Disorders of micturition: oliguria, polyuria

The volume of urine passed varies greatly from day to day in normal individuals, under very precise regulatory stimuli, to maintain an essentially constant body fluid volume. Response to increased or decreased fluid intake, and greater or lesser extrarenal losses, are all smoothly regulated. Individuals are remarkably insensitive to the volume of urine they pass—only being aware of the frequency with which voiding occurs.

Oliguria is normal in hot climates or where intake has been restricted. Depending on the size and degree of catabolism of the individual, it is impossible to excrete the nitrogenous end-products of normal metabolism (mainly urea and amounting to about 800 mosmol/24 h) in less than about 500 to 600 ml of urine, even if it is maximally concentrated. Oliguria is abnormal when the kidney is damaged and unable to excrete water—as in obstruction, acute renal parenchymal disease, or failure of renal perfusion. In any oliguric patient the first steps in diagnosis are to establish whether the patient has had an adequate intake, has had excess extrarenal losses, is already overloaded because of failure to excrete a normal amount of intake, or has urinary tract obstruction at some level with an enlarged bladder or dilated upper tract. The composition of the urine, the state of the circulation and renal perfusion, as well as the

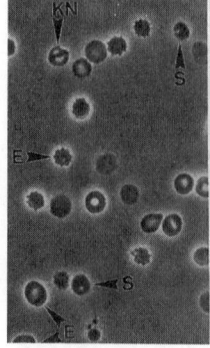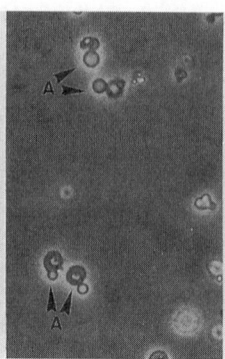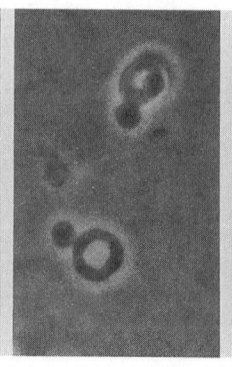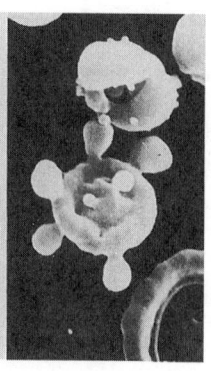

Fig. 4 Normal and dysmorphic red cells in the urine. On the left, dysmorphic red cells shown by phase-contrast microscopy at 400 diameters, with echincocytes (E) showing their crenellated edges. This appearance can be induced by changes in the composition of the urine, but is also common in renal bleeding, both glomerular and non-glomerular. In contrast, acanthocytes (A) with their knob-like protrusions (centre panels, phase contrast × 400 and × 1000, right scanning electron microscopy × 5000) appear to be relatively specific for glomerular bleeding (reproduced from Köhler, H. and Wandel, E., (1993). *Nephrology, Dialysis, Transplantation,* **8,** 879 with permission.)

history if available, will help in differentiating the different possibilities. These topics are discussed further in Chapter 20.16 including the clinical approach to diagnosis of oliguric states.

Polyuria describes the excretion of larger than normal volumes of urine. Often polyuric patients will continue to pass large volumes during the night, in contrast with the normal relative oliguria, thus giving rise to nocturia. It should be noted, however, that normal elderly subjects tend to pass almost the same amounts of urine during the night and the day.

The commonest cause of polyuria is a habitual high fluid intake. There may be no difficulty in obtaining a history of high fluid intake, but a few individuals with compulsive drinking may conceal this and cause diagnostic difficulty. The ability to pass normal volumes of urine depends upon several regulatory circuits. There may be defective secre-

tion of arginine vasopressin (pituitary diabetes insipidus) or a failure of the renal tubules to respond normally to arginine vasopressin (nephrogenic diabetes insipidus).

The increased solute load of glycosuria in diabetes mellitus or of hypercalcaemia commonly presents with polyuria and thirst, and urine volumes are increased by the same mechanism during infusion of saline, mannitol, or urea. Occasional patients take diuretics to achieve weight loss and may create puzzlement until this is discovered.

Polyuria and nocturia are to be expected in any case of chronic renal failure. A major cause in this context is the increased solute load per surviving nephron, with a contribution in addition from pathological changes in the distal nephron where arginine vasopressin has its major site of action. In disorders affecting the medulla more than the cortex (nephronophthisis, sickle cell disease, urinary tract obstruction, hypo-

Fig. 5 An algorithm for the investigation of a patient found to have haematuria. Note the different strategies in those aged less than or more than 45 years of age.

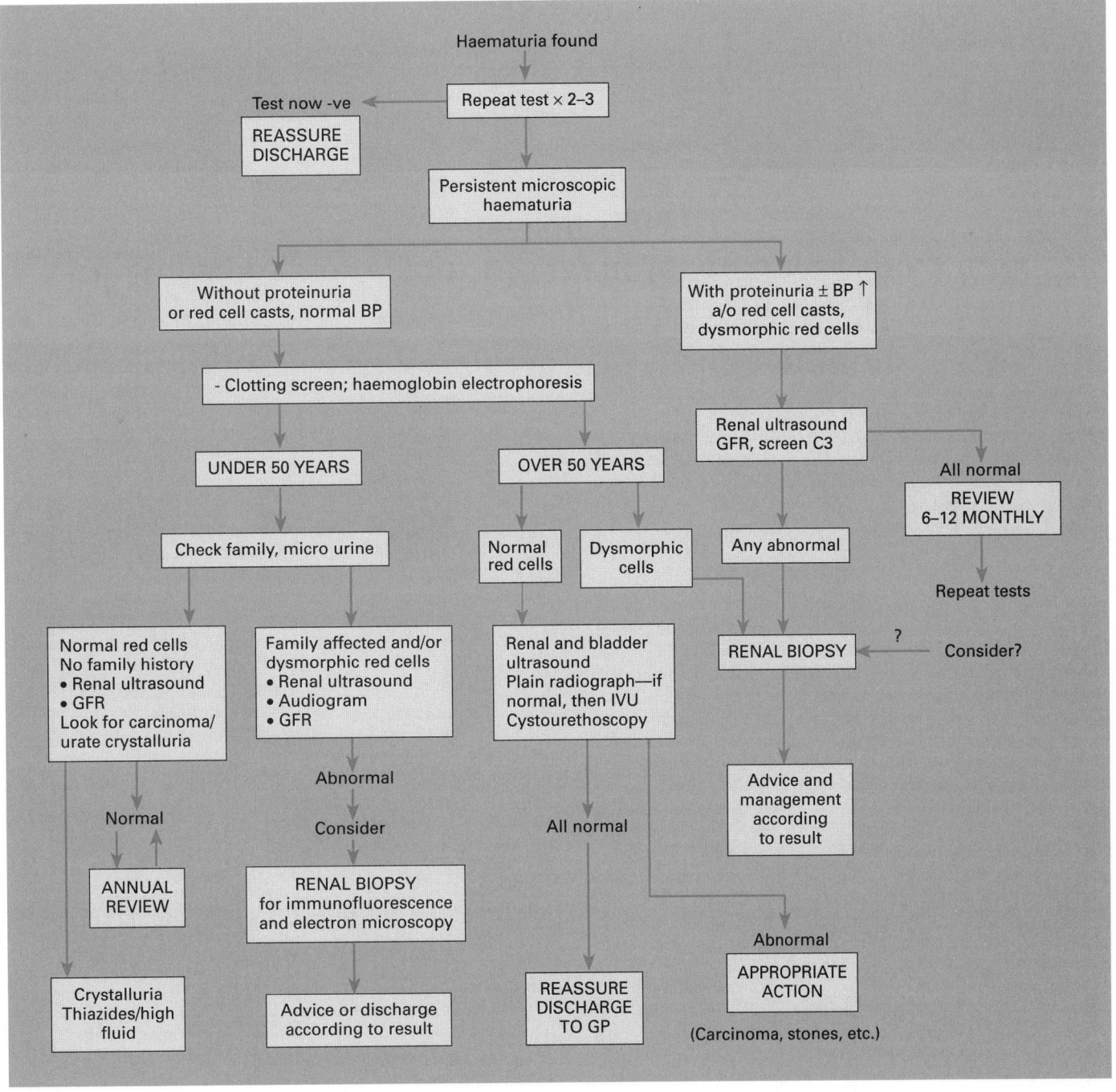

kalaemia) polyuria is particularly prominent. The polyuria associated with supraventricular tachycardia may be striking, and possibly relates to an associated increased rate of secretion of atrial natriuretic peptide.

Polyuric states require investigation by measuring the osmolarity of plasma and urine at the same time. In a water diuresis, the urine will be hypotonic compared to plasma, that is U_{osm}/P_{osm} will be less than unity, with a normal solute excretion. In a solute diuresis, U_{osm}/P_{osm} is 1.0 or greater with a raised solute excretion, and in mixed states usually the ratio will be 0.9 or below, accompanied by an increased solute diuresis. The other crucial observation is the response to overnight thirst, reinforced if necessary by injection or inhalation of dDAVP. Assay of plasma AVP concentrations is occasionally necessary, particularly in patients with compulsive water drinking whose medullary gradient of urea has been 'washed out' and who are therefore incapable of concentrating their urine maximally. If a solute diuresis is present, then the nature of the solute must be determined: electrolytes must be distinguished from non-electrolytes, by measuring urinary sodium and potassium, and testing for glucose.

Renal pain and dysuria

Ureteric colic

Loin pain was described by Hippocrates and remains an important symptom. The classic form is ureteric colic, often misnamed 'renal colic'. This is acute, usually severe, often indescribably so, and waxes and wanes in a typical colicky pattern; the sufferer thrashes about, unable to find comfort, sweats with the agony, and is often pale. Pain radiates from the loin into the abdomen, and down into the testicle, labium, or upper thigh. Vomiting may appear and mislead diagnostic enquiry. Sudden relief may occur if the stone, blood clot, sloughed papilla, or whatever is causing the obstruction moves on, only to recur when it impacts again. At the end of all this agony a surprisingly tiny, innocent looking stone may be passed. Once it has reached the bladder signs of irritation in the trigone may appear instead. The obvious differential diagnoses are appendicitis and biliary colic, if the pain is on the right side of the abdomen. Other differential diagnoses include colonic pain, especially left-sided. Ultrasound usually reveals the problem, although neither this technique nor straight radiographs of the abdomen is good at revealing small stones in the middle third of the ureter. An intravenous urogram is then the definitive investigation.

Renal pain

Renal pain, as opposed to ureteric colic, is usually static, dull, constant, and felt in the loin. Sometimes there is obvious renal swelling, with or without tenderness, and heat if infection is present. The commonest cause of this pain is obstruction to the urinary outflow, especially at the pelviureteric junction, and may be made worse by diuretics or consumption of large amounts of fluid, or alcohol, which acts as a diuretic. Acute pyelonephritis will also give rise to similar pain, and a rare differential diagnosis is of renal infarction by *in situ* thrombosis or embolism in the renal arterial tree. Less severe (and uncommon) renal pain may be a symptom of acute nephritic conditions and IgA nephropathy, presumably caused by distension of the renal capsule. Renal abcesses may be acutely tender, but it is surprising how symptomless indolent abcesses forming around large staghorn calculi can be. Renal venous thrombosis, if acute, also leads to acute renal pain. The main differential diagnosis is musculoskeletal pain, usually derived from pain referred around segments D10 to D12 from the back.

A special type of renal pain, which may be intractable and require cyst puncture or nephrectomy, is pain from bleeding or infection within cysts of polycystic kidneys. For some patients this is the main or only problem, and can be very difficult to manage. Renal colic may also occur from torrential bleeding from polycystic kidneys, which again may lead to nephrectomy in a few cases.

Loin pain in parenchymal renal disease; the loin pain–haematuria syndrome

An unusual group of patients, who cause great diagnostic difficulty present with recurrent or persistent extremely severe loin pain, often with intermittent or persistent microscopic haematuria but sometimes without (the 'loin pain–haematuria syndrome'). They are predominantly young women, and often have some connection with the practice of medicine. Many require opiates, and have disturbed personalities by the time they are seen. At this point it is impossible to know if this is the result of chronic pain, or preceded or perhaps is provoked by the illness. The pain is often unilateral to begin with and nephrectomy is often requested and sometimes performed. Usually the pain then recurs at another site, usually in the opposite kidney. In some, angiography reveals tortuous, middle-sized arteries, and renal biopsy may show onion-skinning of the vessels, but this is not common.

These patients present many problems of management: loin pain is quite a common symptom and it is difficult to sort out patients within this group. Around cases of what could be described as a 'typical' loin pain–haematuria syndrome cluster a more varied group of patients with unexplained severe loin pain who behave similarly. Some have had experience of renal colic from stones; many seek opiates for relief. Nephrectomy rarely solves the problem, and nor do attempts to denervate of the kidney by injection, surgical stripping of nerves, or autotransplantation. Although successful on occasion, the pain often recurs, perhaps because the kidney is re-innervated within 6 to 12 months. Both corticosteroids and antiplatelet drugs have been used in view of the arterial changes, but usually without effect. Management finally settles round establishing a regime for pain relief. Transcutaneous nerve stimulation, carbamazepine, and amitriptyline are usually ineffective, and establishing a stable analgesic regime, usually employing narcotics, is often required. It is usual for a stable dosage to be effective and most patients will give up the drugs without difficulty. Few patients have been followed long term, but the impression is that it remits when the patients are in their 40s and 50s, which perhaps supports hypotheses suggesting an important role for oestrogens, since the vascular changes have been linked with the use of oral contraceptives.

Frequency and dysuria

These are amongst the commonest symptoms in medicine, accounting for 20/1000 patient attendances in general practice. Dysuria describes pain or scalding on the passage of urine, and a sensation of incomplete voiding which often follows the slight relief after passing urine and leads to frequent painful passage of small amounts of urine. Microscopic haematuria is usually present, and bleeding from the inflamed mucosa may be sufficient to produce macroscopic haematuria. The complaint is much more frequent in women than in men, and is frequently attributed to cystitis. Dysuria can also occur in acute pyelonephitis, but is often absent; loin pain, headache, vomiting, and high fever are the cardinal features of this condition. The commonest cause is inflammation of the urethra, trigone, and bladder, most commonly with Gram-negative bacteria of gut origin. The full differential diagnosis and approaches to management are discussed in Section 20.8.

REFERENCES
General

Davison, A.M. and Grünfeld, J.-P. (1992). History and clinical examination of the patient with renal disease. In *Oxford textbook of clinical nephrology,* (ed. J.S. Cameron *et al.*), Vol. 1, pp. 3–24. Oxford University Press, Oxford.

Mallick, N.P. and Short, C.D. (1992). The clinical approach to haematuria and proteinuria. In *Oxford textbook of clinical nephrology,* (ed. J.S. Cameron *et al.*), Vol. 1, pp. 227–40. Oxford University Press, Oxford.

Proteinuria and nephrotic syndrome

Abuelo, J.G. (1983). Proteinuria: diagnostic principles and procedures. *Annals of Internal Medicine* **98**, 186–91.

Albright, P., Brensilver, J., and Cortell, S. (1993). Proteinuria in congestive heart failure. *American Journal of Medicine* 3, 272–5.

Anon (1988). Is routine urinalysis worthwhile? *Lancet* i, 747.

Cameron, J.S. (1992). The clinical consequences of the nephrotic syndrome. *Oxford textbook of clinical nephrology,* (ed. J.S. Cameron *et al.*), pp. 276–97. Oxford University Press, Oxford.

Cameron, J.S. and Glassock, R.J. (1988). *The nephrotic syndrome.* Marcel Dekker, New York.

Garella, S. (1990). Pathophysiology and clinical implications of proteinuria. *Nephrology Dialysis Transplantation* 3, (Suppl. 1), 10–15.

Pesce, A. and Roy First, M. (1979). *Proteinuria. An integrated review.* Marcel Dekker, New York.

Springberg, P.D. *et al.* (1982). Fixed and reproducible orthostatic proteinuria: results of a 20 year follow-up study. *Annals of Internal Medicine* 97, 516–19.

Sumpio, B.E. and Hayslett, J.P.H. (1985). Renal handling of proteins in normal and diseased states. *Quarterly Journal of Medicine* 57, 611–35.

Haematuria

Birch, D.F. and Fairley, K.F. (1979). Haematuria: glomerular or non-glomerular? *Lancet* ii, 845–6.

Briner, V.A. and Reinhart, W.H. (1990). *In vitro* production of glomerular red cells: role of pH and osmolality. *Nephron* 56, 13–18.

Britton, J.P., Dowell, A.C., and Whelan, P.O. (1989). Dipstick haematuria and bladder cancer in men over 60: results of a community study. *British Medical Journal* 299, 1010–12.

Culclasure, T.F., Brady, V.J., and Hasbargen, J.A. (1994). The significance of haematuria in the anticoagulated patient. *Archives of Internal Medicine* 154, 649–52.

Froom, P., Ribak, J., and Banbassat, J. (1984). Significance of microhaematuria in young adults. *British Medical Journal* 288, 20–1.

Kincaid-Smith, P. (1982). Haematuria and exercise-related haematuria. *British Medical Journal* 285, 1595–7.

Köhler, H., Wandel, E., and Brunsk, B. (1991). Acanthocyturia – a characteristic marker for glomerular bleeding. *Kidney International* 40, 115–20.

Schröder, F.M. (1994). Microscopic haematuria requires investigation. *British Medical Journal,* 309, 70–2.

Shichiri, M., *et al.* (1988). Red cell volume distribution curves in diagnosis of glomerular and non-glomerular haematuria. *Lancet* 1, 908–10.

Spencer, J., Lindsell, D., and Matorakou I. (1990). Ultrasonography compared with intravenous urography in the investigation of adults with haematuria. *British Medical Journal* 301, 1074–6. (But see also discussion of this paper: Stenlake, P.S., Wallace, D.M.A. *and* Cattell, W.R., Webb, J.A.W., and Whitfield, H.G. Investigation of adults with haematuria. *British Medical Journal* 301, 1396–7, and the authors' reply.)

Topham, P.S., Harper, S.J., Furness, P.N., Harris, K.P.G., Walls, J., and Feehally, J. (1994). Glomerular disease as a cause of isolated haematuria. *Quarterly Journal of Medicine,* 87, 329–35.

Loin pain

Fox, M. and Saunders, N.R. (1978). Significance of loin pain in women. A study of 100 cases referred to a urological clinic. *Lancet* i, 115–17.

Leaker, B.R., Gordge, M.P., Patel, A., and Neild G.H. (1989). Haemostatic changes in the loin-pain haematuria syndrome; secondary to renal vasospasm? *Quarterly Journal of Medicine* 79, 969–79.

Macdonald, I.M., Fairley, K.R., Hobbs, J.B., and Kincaid-Smith, P. (1975). Loin pain as a presenting symptom of idiopathic glomerulonephritis. *Clinical Nephrology* 3, 129–33.

Dysuria

Komaroff, A.I. (1986). Urinalysis and urine culture in women with dysuria. *Annals of Internal Medicine* 104, 212–18. (See also Section 9.)

Polyuria

Kirkland, J.L., Lye, M., Levy, D.W., and Banerjee, A.K. (1983). Patterns of urine flow and electrolyte excretion in healthy elderly people. *British Medical Journal* 287, 1665–7.

Zerbe, R.L. and Robertson G.L. (1983). A comparison of plasma vasopressin measurements with a standard indirect test in the differential diagnosis of polyuria. *New England Journal of Medicine* 305, 1539–46.

20.4 Primary renal glomerular diseases

20.4.1 IgA nephropathy, Henoch–Schönlein purpura, and thin membrane nephropathy

A. R. CLARKSON, A. J. WOODROFFE, AND A. C. THOMAS

Introduction

In this chapter major nephrological causes of symptomatic macroscopic haematuria and asymptomatic microscopic haematuria are discussed. While they are linked by the common symptom of haematuria, the clinical, pathological, pathogenetic and prognostic features are quite variable. A careful history can often provide valuable clues towards the correct diagnosis. For example, in thin membrane nephropathy there is often a positive family history. Recurring episodes of 'synpharyngitic' macroscopic haematuria are characteristic of IgA nephropathy, and in Henoch–Schönlein purpura, arthritis, cutaneous vasculitis, and gut symptoms occur to varying degrees. Renal biopsy confirms the diagnosis in each.

Central to the recognition of haematuria as glomerular in origin is the finding of dysmorphic red cells and casts in the urinary sediment (see

Chapter 20.1). Such findings demand nephrological rather than urological investigation to obtain appropriate information regarding diagnosis, prognosis, and treatment.

IgA nephropathy and Henoch–Schönlein purpura

Iga nephropathy

Only known as an entity since the initial description by Berger and Hinglais 25 years ago, IgA nephropathy is now recognized as the commonest form of glomerulonephritis in the world. There are racial differences in prevalence and in certain geographical areas the disease seems less common, but in most developed countries where the use of diagnostic renal biopsy is accepted and widespread, IgA nephropathy is found in approximately 30 per cent of all biopsies for primary glomerular disorders. Population studies indicate an occurrence rate of 1 in 10 000, but some autopsy studies suggest that the incidence of IgA mesangial deposits is between 1 in 100 and 1 in 1000.

CLINICAL FEATURES

IgA nephropathy is characteristically found in young males in the second or third decades of life (male to female ratio 3:1) who have recurring episodes of 'synpharyngitic' macroscopic haematuria. The onset of hae-maturia usually occurs within 12 to 24 h of the pharyngitis and fre-quently is accompanied by diffuse muscle pains, loin pain, high fever, and lethargy out of proportion to the severity of the sore throat. On occasion, infections involving other mucosal (or IgA secreting) surfaces may initiate the haematuria. These include bronchial, gastrointestinal, bladder, female genital tract, and breast infections. Unlike the smoky, grey-coloured urine seen 10 to 14 days after the throat infection in post-streptococcal glomerulonephritis, urine in IgA nephropathy is frankly bloody for between 1 and 5 days. Most commonly, blood pressure is normal during these episodes, there is no periorbital or ankle oedema, and recovery is rapid. However an acute decrease in renal function (sometimes to the extent that dialysis is needed) may accompany a hae-maturic episode in IgA nephropathy and delay recovery. In our expe-rience about one-third of patients with IgA nephropathy present initially with an episode of macroscopic haematuria, and a further 10 to 15 per cent will suffer such an episode after the diagnosis is made. These epi-sodes are frequently recurrent.

In a further one-third of patients diagnosis is made following the discovery of proteinuria and/or microscopic haematuria. The urinary sediment contains numerous dysmorphic erythrocytes and granular and red cell casts. Other features, such as hypertension, nephrotic syndrome, acute or chronic renal failure, and, rarely, the acute nephritic syndrome, may be the presenting problem in the remainder. In summary, the renal disease of IgA nephropathy may present anywhere in the spectrum of minor urinary abnormalities to rapidly progressive glomerulonephritis.

DIAGNOSIS

Unfortunately there is, as yet, no serological 'marker' for IgA nephrop-athy and renal biopsy is the only definitive diagnostic investigation. Positive mesangial immunofluorescence for IgA and C3 is the diagnostic hallmark. Variable findings include high circulating concentrations of IgA and IgA-containing immune complexes. There are no characteristic abnormalities in serum complement components.

CLINICAL COURSE

In children IgA nephropathy has a good prognosis for at least a decade, but it should be remembered that the disease evolves slowly. Complete clinical remission occurs in 30 per cent of these children after 10 years, and in the remainder, varying degrees of proteinuria, hypertension, and renal impairment may be found. Very few (1–3 per cent) develop end-stage renal failure in childhood.

In adults the outlook is worse, but development of the disease is usually slow. A small group of patients has a rapid downhill course into renal failure over 3 to 5 years ('malignant' IgA nephropathy) but more commonly renal failure develops after 15 to 25 years of indolent and often asymptomatic progress. Numerous reports from worldwide sources suggest strongly that 25 to 50 per cent of adult patients with IgA nephropathy will eventually develop endstage renal failure. Very few data exist on the proportion of patients entering complete clinical remission, but estimates of 10 per cent are not unusual.

Henoch–Schönlein purpura

Henoch–Schönlein purpura has been recognized as an entity for over 100 years. Easily diagnosed by the association of arthritis, palpable pur-pura, gut symptoms, and glomerulonephritis it can be viewed as the systemic manifestation of IgA nephropathy. The skin disease begins with urticarial spots on the extensor surfaces of arms and legs, especially around the ankles, buttocks, and elbows. The face and trunk are spared. Development to purpura which is often palpable occurs quickly, with some lesions coalescing to become necrotic (Plate 1). Resolution occurs over 2 to 4 weeks, but fresh crops frequently appear. Polyarthritis, often flitting, occurs in about two-thirds of patients, characteristically involv-ing large joints (knees and ankles) and is manifest by varying degrees of pain and periarticular swelling. Resolution is usually within 10 days, but recurrence is common.

Abdominal symptoms, when present, include colicky pain, melaena, haematemesis, and obstruction due to intramural haematomas and intus-susception. The most frequently observed clinical sequence is the devel-opment of one or more of the joint, gut, and skin manifestations soon after an intercurrent infection. As with IgA nephropathy, upper respi-ratory tract infections are the most frequent precipitants.

When there is renal involvement (reported frequency 20–100 per cent depending on the criteria used to define it), glomerulonephritis is usually noticed later, although careful examination may detect microhaematuria from the onset. Rarely, but significantly, extrarenal manifestations occur a considerable time after the initial diagnosis of IgA nephropathy. Recurrence may be frequent. Overt acute nephritis, nephrotic syndrome, and macroscopic haematuria are recognized more frequently in adults than in children, in whom serious or progressive glomerulonephritis occurs at an incidence of about 5 per cent of cases. Urinary abnormalities occur in about 50 per cent of the remainder of childhood cases. Prog-nosis in children and adults generally depends on the severity of the initial renal disease, but progressive renal failure may develop in patients whose initial renal disease is mild.

DIAGNOSIS

Diagnosis is usually made by noting the association of gut, joint, abdom-inal, and renal symptoms and signs, and can be confirmed by finding positive immunofluorescence for IgA and C3 within the 'vasculitic' skin lesions and the glomerular mesangia. Approximately 50 per cent of patients have elevated serum IgA concentrations, and IgA-containing immune complexes are found during the active phase of the disease.

CLINICAL COURSE

Apart from the occasional catastrophe associated with intussusception, the major cause of morbidity and mortality in Henoch–Schönlein pur-pura is glomerulonephritis. Fifty per cent of children with Henoch–Schönlein purpura glomerulonephritis are in complete clinical remission after 2 years. About 30 per cent have persisting urinary abnormalities with normal renal function, while a minority (3–5 per cent) progress quickly to renal failure. Proteinuria and decreased renal function persist in the remaining 15 to 20 per cent, and a significant proportion of these patients will have developed endstage renal failure after 10 years. Sim-ilar observations have been made in adults with Henoch–Schönlein pur-pura glomerulonephritis. It is noteworthy, however, that glomerulo-nephritis occurs more frequently in Henoch–Schönlein purpura of adults than children, so that the overall prognosis is much better in children.

Pathology of IgA nephropathy and Henoch–Schönlein purpura

Glomerular pathology is similar in IgA nephropathy and Henoch–Schönlein purpura although widely variable in both. The basic lesion is a mesangial proliferative glomerulonephritis. In their mildest form the mesangial changes are focal, and much of the glomerular tuft may appear normal. More frequently there is diffuse disease, the mesangial expansion and cellular proliferation appearing like a tree trunk (Plate 2 (a)). Sometimes mesangial expansion occurs to the extent that mesan-giocapillary changes are apparent. Added to the basic mesangial prolif-erative lesion, three distinct types of focal-segmental lesion may be seen.

The first is seen in 'active' disease and consists of areas of tuft necro-sis manifest by fibrin exudates and leucocyte infiltration (Fig. 2(b)). Small crescents are frequently associated with these lesions and, on occasion, circumferential crescents may be seen, but these are uncom-mon (Plate 3). The second probably represents healed areas of tuft necrosis, and consists of segmental glomerular scars with associated synechiae joining the tuft to Bowman's capsule (Plate 2(c)). In long-standing disease, areas of tuft collapse and sclerosis with hyalinosis occur (Plate 2(c)). These are most frequently seen in progressive disease, in which there is progressive glomerular obsolescence.

Mononuclear cells and neutrophils surround glomeruli with 'active' areas of tuft necrosis and crescents. Interstitial scarring, tubular atrophy, and hypertensive vascular changes complicate long-standing disease.

The diagnostic hallmark of both conditions is the occurrence of IgA and C3, found by immunofluorescence or immunoperoxidase techniques, within the glomerular mesangia (Plate 4). IgG and IgM are found variably, as is fibrinogen. IgA, which always predominates, is of subclass IgA$_i$.

Electron microscopy reveals electron-dense deposits in paramesangial areas (Fig. 1), with an associated expansion of mesangial areas, an increase in mesangial matrix, and, in long-standing cases, mesangial fibrosis. Occasionally, electron-dense deposits are seen in the glomerular capillary basement membranes.

Extrarenal pathology is more obvious in Henoch–Schönlein purpura, most features being a consequence of a leucocytoclastic vasculitis. Deposits of IgA and C3 are found in blood vessel walls, and serve to distinguish this form of vasculitis from that seen in polyarteritis nodosa and cryoglobulinaemia. Electron-dense deposits have been demonstrated in early lesions.

Although no clinically obvious changes are seen in the skin of patients with IgA nephropathy, in most cases deposits of IgA and C3 can be found in dermal blood vessels.

Pathogenesis of IgA nephropathy and Henoch–Schönlein purpura

Recognition of secondary forms of these diseases has cast some light on pathogenesis. While idiopathic forms of IgA nephropathy and Henoch–Schönlein purpura predominate, these diseases may occur in association with disease of the liver (cirrhosis) and gut (coeliac disease, Crohn's disease), and mucin-secreting carcinomas, wherein disorders of antigen processing may occur, leading to overproduction of IgA. For example, increased absorption of antigen from the gut in coeliac and Crohn's disease, and defective antigen handling in cirrhosis and portal

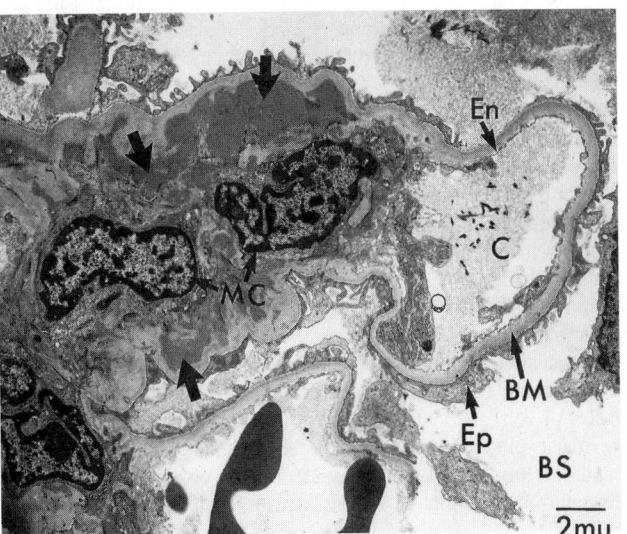

Fig. 1 Electron micrograph of glomerular capillary loop in IgA nephropathy. Numerous electron-dense deposits representing deposits of IgA can be seen within the expanded mesangium (arrows) (×5200). BM, basement membrane; C, capillary lumen; Ep, visceral epithelium; En, fenestrated endothelium; MC, mesangial cell nucleus; BS, Bowman's space.

systemic shunts, may occur. Additionally, IgA nephropathy has been described in other diseases where there is a clearly demonstrable immunoglobulin response of the IgA class, for example dermatitis herpetiformis, ankylosing spondylitis, and IgA monoclonal gammopathy.

In primary or idiopathic IgA nephropathy and Henoch–Schönlein purpura 50 per cent of patients have elevated serum concentrations of IgA and, at times of disease activity, have increased circulating concentrations of IgA immune complexes. Therefore it is postulated that increased uptake of antigen (in many cases probably related to upper respiratory or gastrointestinal infections) and decreased hepatic sequestration (possibly related to saturation of receptors) may give rise, together with the high concentrations of preformed antibody, to circulating IgA containing immune complexes. These complexes contain subclass IgA$_i$, as do the mesangial deposits. On the basis of this evidence, the mesangial proliferative glomerulonephritis is probably a response to the local deposition of circulating immune complexes. But why the high circulating levels of preformed IgA?

GENETIC FACTORS

A genetic susceptibility to IgA nephropathy and Henoch–Schönlein purpura is likely. Racial differences in prevalence are reported, and many instances have been described of first-degree relatives with the diseases and even more relatives without disease who have similar abnormalities of IgA production *in vitro*. In addition, disease associations with HLA-DR4-DQW4, and complement genes have been described. However, associations are not highly discriminatory, and other factors probably determine the final disease expression.

Immune profiles in IgA nephropathy and Henoch–Schönlein purpura

ABNORMAL IgA PRODUCTION

Increased serum IgA concentrations are found in 50 per cent of patients. The production of IgA by peripheral blood lymphocytes is increased *in vitro*, with both increases in IgA-specific T-helper-cell and B-cell activities being described. If studies with tonsillar cells can be extrapolated to other IgA-producing mucosal areas, mucosal production of IgA is also increased.

Conceptually, genetic determinants make the susceptible individual over-respond with IgA antibodies to a plethora of mucosally presented antigens, whether they be viral, bacterial, or dietary. Many clinical observations suggest that antigens such as influenza, Epstein–Barr virus *E. coli*, Campylobacter, gluten, soyabean, and alcohol (probably by increasing gut permeability to a multiplicity of macromolecules) can exacerbate disease, presumably by an increased immune complex load and subsequent glomerular deposition.

PRODUCTION OF ABNORMAL IgA

In the glomerular deposits, the IgA$_i$ subclass predominates, as does, in some but not all studies, the λ light chain. Furthermore, there is evidence that the glomerular IgA is abnormally anionic. Increased lectin-binding properties, perhaps attributable to abnormal glycosylation near the hinge region of the IgA molecule, may render the IgA more likely to deposit in mesangial sites. Autoantibody reactivities are also identified. These include rheumatoid factors, mesangial antibodies (these are IgA class), IgA–ANCA (antineutrophil cytoplasmic antigen), and fibronectin–IgA aggregates.

DEFECTIVE IMMUNE CLEARANCE

Impaired *in vivo* hepatic clearance of IgA aggregates has been shown. This might reflect saturation of receptors, resulting from the original IgA immune complex load. Further support for this premise comes from the observed occurrence of mesangial IgA deposits in cirrhotic patients and in animal models of cirrhosis.

Mediation of glomerular injury

It is still not known how the mesangial IgA deposits lead to glomerular injury. Acute exacerbations of disease such as 'synpharyngitic' haematuria and acute Henoch–Schönlein purpura are presumably mediated by the classical pathways of inflammation, but mediation of the indolent mesangial proliferative glomerular sclerotic lesions seems to be more complex. In the acute episode associated with heavy haematuria, necrotizing lesions are common and involve the glomerulus in a segmental or global manner. Crescent formation is frequent. These lesions presumably are initiated by immune complex deposition in glomerular capillary walls, which are damaged because of complement activation and leucocyte infiltration with subsequent platelet aggregation and fibrin formation. Crescents, which may be small or circumferential, are initiated by this process and potentiated by periglomerular and intraglomerular monocyte infiltration. Varying degrees of tubular injury, interstitial cellular infiltration, and tubular luminal red cell inspissation may account for reversible decreases in the glomerular filtration rate observed during these episodes, and probably occur secondary to glomerular injury.

Explanation of the chronic sclerotic glomerular changes is speculative, and several mediating influences may be involved. The most widely studied is the renin–angiotensin system. Mesangial cells have receptors for angiotensin II and contract in its presence, thereby reducing the glomerular filtration area.

Mesangial 'overload' caused by immune complex deposition and the consequent cellular matrix and fibrous tissue reaction, may stimulate local angiotensin II production and down-regulate glomerular filtration rate. Glomerular hypertension would then follow, with associated haemodynamic alterations contributing to the process of glomerular sclerosis and permanent renal function impairment.

Other factors potentiate this process. Platelets, platelet factor IV, platelet-derived growth factor, and platelet activating factor have all been incriminated, while interleukins, especially interleukin-1 and interleukin-6, and a large number of other cytokines may act as mitogens for mesangial cells. Transforming growth factor-β may play a role in the integration of these inflammatory events. Finally, hyperlipidaemia, by stimulating lipid accumulation in damaged glomeruli, may hasten the sclerotic process.

Transplantation

Host factors in the development of IgA nephropathy and Henoch–Schönlein purpura are highlighted by the repeated observations that IgA nephropathy recurs in kidneys transplanted into recipients whose primary disease is IgA nephropathy. Kidneys already with IgA nephropathy, inadvertently transplanted into recipients not suffering from IgA nephropathy are free of disease within a few weeks of transplantation. Prevention, or cure, of these diseases therefore rests with further understanding of those pathogenetic factors leading to immune complex deposition within the glomeruli, as the kidney itself does not seem to be at fault. Disease modification, on the other hand, may involve understanding the intrarenal events more precisely.

Treatment of IgA nephropathy and Henoch–Schönlein purpura

There is no known effective treatment for these diseases. However, examination of a simple schema of pathogenetic processes thought to be important in the genesis of the renal disease (Table 1) suggests several areas where therapeutic intervention may be helpful. Crude attempts to alter environmental factors with prophylactic antibiotics and tonsillec-

Table 1 *Simple schema of proposed pathogenetic mechanisms in IgA nephropathy and Henoch–Schönlein purpura.*

Genetic determinants
↓ Environmental agents
Abnormal IgA production
↓ Defective immune clearance
Mesangial IgA deposits
↓ Mediators
Glomerular injury

tomy, avoidance of certain dietary antigens, such as gluten and soyabeans, and desisting from alcohol have proved unsuccessful. Likewise, interference with IgA production by therapeutic use of phenytoin, a drug known to reduce serum IgA levels, has had no influence on disease progression in controlled trials. Collective experience with anti-inflammatory and immunosuppressive drugs is disappointing, although some reports of favourable responses to long-term corticosteroid therapy have prompted extensive controlled trials. Intuitively, however, the recurrence of disease in transplanted patients treated with corticosteroids, cyclosporin A, and azathioprine predicates against their use in the primary diseases.

Recently considerable attention has been placed on slowing the progression of established disease. Angiotensin-converting enzyme inhibitors and calcium-channel blocking drugs have been advocated on the basis of animal studies of renal ablation, where progressive renal failure and focal glomerulosclerosis are largely prevented by these drugs, which alter the deranged intraglomerular haemodynamics. While they are widely used to treat hypertension in these conditions, such treatments have not been subjected to controlled trials.

Low-protein diets; the treatment of hyperlipidaemia with HMG-CoA reductase inhibitors, fibric acids, and other lipid-lowering agents; and antiplatelet drugs are also used frequently in an attempt to retard the progression of many renal diseases.

Thin membrane nephropathy

The clinical entity of 'benign familial haematuria' was first described in 1966, but the association of haematuria with thin glomerular basement membranes was recognized later. It is a common condition (11 per cent of non-transplant renal biopsies in our series), which is diagnosed as a result of investigations performed to determine the cause of persistent, usually asymptomatic, microscopic, or 'dipstick' discovered haematuria. Microscopy of urine reveals a significant number of dysmorphic red blood cells. Minor proteinuria may be present, but blood pressure and renal function typically are normal. Episodes of macroscopic haematuria occasionally occur and raise the possibility of a more sinister diagnosis, such as Alport's syndrome.

Family studies support an autosomal dominant inheritance. In many cases a dilemma exists when the patient is first seen, in deciding how far to investigate these otherwise well individuals. As there is no genetic marker for this condition it remains our policy to make a firm diagnosis by renal biopsy in at least one member of a family, informing others that further investigations are not necessary unless the nature of the haematuria changes.

There is no point in performing renal biopsy unless electron microscopy is routinely available; the light microscopic features of mild mesangial expansion and hypertrophy of the juxtaglomerular apparatus are non-specific, and immunofluorescence is negative apart from C3 in the arterioles of some patients. The key finding is decreased width of the glomerular capillary basement membrane (Fig. 2)—normally between 340 and 450 nm. Values as low as 250 nm are observed in thin membrane nephropathy. Direct visual assessment by an experienced electron microscopist using standard magnifications is generally sufficient. In some patients there is marked global thinning of the basement membrane associated with patchy lamellation, electron-lucent flocculation, and subendothelial nodularities. In others, these membrane changes occur intermittently between lengths of near-normal membrane. Immunogold studies suggest a reduction in the subepithelial portion of the basement membrane. Unlike some patients with Alport's syndrome, however, Goodpasture's antigen is readily identified within these thin glomerular basement membranes.

PROGNOSIS

Long-term follow-up suggests that the condition is benign. Accurate diagnosis is therefore important in preventing repeated intravenous urography and cystoscopy. In addition, the diagnosis of thin membrane nephropathy should not compromise life insurance, which may not be offered without accurate diagnosis.

Fig. 2 Electron micrographs of glomerular basement membranes, contrasting membranes of normal thickness (a) with those of patients with thin membrane nephropathy (b). The normal basement membrane thickness is in the order of 350 to 430 nm, whereas in the example of thin membrane nephropathy illustrated it is around 200 to 270 nm (×5200). BM, basement membrane; C, capillary lumen; Ep, visceral epithelium, En, fenestrated endothelium; BS, Bowman's space.

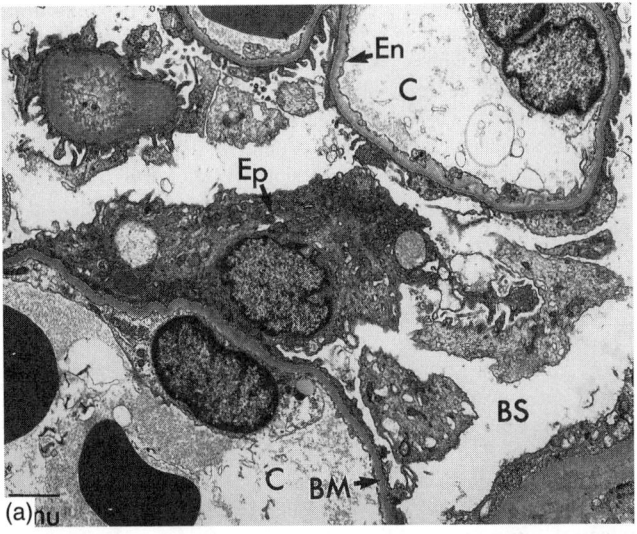

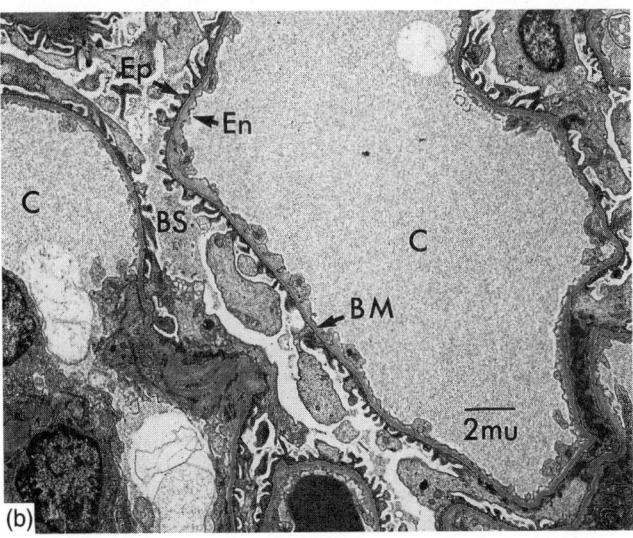

REFERENCES

Aarons, I., Smith, P.S, Davies, R.A., Woodroffe, A.J., and Clarkson, A.R. (1989). Thin membrane nephropathy: a clinico-pathological study. *Clinical Nephrology* **32**, 151–8.

Clarkson, A.R., Woodroffe, A.J., Bannister, K.M., Lomax-Smith, J.D., and Aarons, I. (1984). The syndrome of IgA nephropathy. *Clinical Nephrology* **21**, 7–14.

D'Amico, G. (1987). The commonest glomerulonephritis in the world: IgA nephropathy. *Quarterly Journal of Medicine* **64**, 709–27.

Feehally, J. (1988). Immune mechanisms in glomerular IgA deposition. *Nephrology, Dialysis, Transplantation* **3**, 361–78.

Meadow, S.R., Glascow, E.F., White, R.H.R, Moncrieff, M.W., Cameron, J.S., and Ogg, C.S. (1972). Schönlein–Henoch nephritis. *Quarterley Journal of Medicine* **41**, 241–58.

20.4.2 Idiopathic glomerulonephritis

D. ADU

The majority of patients with a glomerulonephritis in temperate regions of the world have an idiopathic glomerulonephritis. The aetiology and patterns of glomerulonephritis in tropical countries differ considerably and have been reviewed elsewhere. The understanding of glomerulonephritis is often hampered by the different levels of description used in classification. Classification has been based at the level of clinical expression, for example rapidly progressive glomerulonephritis; at the level of aetiology, for example post-streptococcal glomerulonephritis; at the level of pathogenesis, for example immune-complex glomerulonephritis; and at the level of histology, for example membranous nephropathy. Any good classification should guide diagnosis, clinical features, responsiveness to treatment, and prognosis.

Classification

The most helpful classification of glomerulonephritis is one based on histology. Careful clinicopathological studies in the 1960s and 1970s established the histological patterns of glomerulonephritis in patients with a nephrotic syndrome (Table 1). In children, idiopathic glomerulonephritis accounts for 90 per cent of all cases of the nephrotic syndrome, and in adults for approximately 80 per cent of patients with this syndrome. Although these histological changes are usually of unknown aetiology, they may also be secondary to well-defined aetiological factors.

Clinical presentation

The ways in which glomerulonephritis may present are fairly limited and are summarized in Table 2. Patients with glomerulonephritis can present with asymptomatic proteinuria and/or haematuria, with proteinuria that is heavy enough to cause a nephrotic syndrome, with an acute nephritic syndrome which may be severe enough to cause acute renal failure, or with chronic renal failure.

Diagnosis

Definitive diagnosis of most forms of glomerulonephritis is dependent on a renal biopsy, with careful interpretation of the renal histology in the light of clinical, biochemical, and immunological features of this disorder.

CHILDREN

In the original studies of the International Study of Kidney Diseases in Children (**ISKDC**) the diagnosis of minimal change nephropathy was

Table 1 *Histology of the nephrotic syndrome*

Histology	Children (%)	Adults (%)
Minimal change nephrotic syndrome	76	25
Mesangiocapillary glomerulonephritis	8	14
Focal segmental glomerulosclerosis	7	9
Proliferative (including diffuse mesangial proliferation)	2	13
Membranous	2	21
Other	5	–
Systemic lupus erythematosus	–	8
Amyloid	–	7
Diabetes	–	3

Children: ISKDC study (1978) (excludes secondary causes of nephrotic syndrome, such as systemic lupus erythematosus, Henoch–Schönlein purpura—about 10 per cent).

Adults: Cameron (1979).

Table 2 *Clinical presentation of glomerulonephritis*

Persistent microscopic haematuria
Persistent proteinuria
Nephrotic syndrome
Acute nephritic syndrome
Acute renal failure

Table 3 *Idiopathic nephrotic syndrome in childhood: histology and response to steroids*

Histology	Percentage of all cases	Remission with steroids (%)
Minimal change nephrotic syndrome	76	93
Mesangiocapillary glomerulonephritis	8	7
Focal segmental glomerulosclerosis	7	30
Proliferative glomerulonephritis	2	25
Diffuse mesangial proliferative glomerulonephritis	2	56
Focal and global glomerulosclerosis	1.7	75
Membranous nephropathy	1.5	0
Chronic glomerulonephritis	0.8	75
Unclassified	0.8	75

ISKDC (1978, 1981).

based on renal biopsies. From these and other studies it was established that in a child aged between 1 and 6 years with a nephrotic syndrome and highly selective proteinuria, and who did not have microscopic haematuria, hypertension, or renal impairment, the likely diagnosis was minimal change nephropathy. Such children had a greater than 90 per cent chance of going into remission with steroids within 4 weeks (Table 3). Based on these observations, children aged between 1 and 8 years with a nephrotic syndrome and the features summarized above are no longer subjected to renal biopsy and are instead treated with a trial of steroids. This leads to the term 'steroid-responsive nephrotic syndrome of childhood' and most, but not all, of such children will have minimal change nephropathy. In children characterized in this way, if there is no response of the proteinuria to steroids after a month, then a renal biopsy should be considered to establish the diagnosis. Children aged over 8

years are more likely to have a steroid non-responsive lesion and probably need a renal biopsy. In neonates and in children aged less than 1 year there is a high probability of the congenital nephrotic syndrome or diffuse mesangial sclerosis, and therefore renal biopsy should be considered. Neither of these lesions respond to steroids.

ADULTS

Only 25 per cent of adults with a nephrotic syndrome have minimal change nephropathy, and for that reason a renal biopsy is necessary to establish the type of glomerulonephritis. There have been suggestions that renal biopsy is not essential in the investigation of adults with a nephrotic syndrome, and that all such individuals should be treated with steroids. However, that approach means unnecessary treatment of a large proportion of patients with a potentially toxic drug. It also means that no assessment would be available of the type of glomerulonephritis nor an estimate of the likelihood of a response to treatment nor of the prognosis for long-term renal function. In skilled hands the dangers of renal biopsy are small and outweighed by those of steroid treatment.

Minimal change nephropathy, focal segmental glomerulosclerosis, mesangial proliferative glomerulonephritis: one disorder or many?

The majority of children in temperate countries with a nephrotic syndrome have minimal change nephropathy, focal segmental glomerulosclerosis (**FSGS**), or a mesangial proliferative glomerulonephritis. One school of thought argues that these are all variants of the same disease, termed the 'idiopathic nephrotic syndrome'. In favour of this view is the observation that in a proportion of patients with a steroid-responsive nephrotic syndrome, the histological lesion may evolve with time, usually from minimal change nephropathy or mesangial proliferative glomerulonephritis to focal segmental glomerulonephritis. The repeat renal biopsies were performed because affected patients were, or became, frequent relapsers, steroid dependent, or steroid resistant. One study suggested that patients with presumed minimal change nephropathy whose renal biopsies showed large glomeruli were more likely to develop FSGS. In general those patients with minimal change nephropathy who develop FSGS but remain steroid responsive have a good prognosis for renal function, whereas those who are steroid resistant develop progressive renal failure. The prognosis for renal function is therefore determined by the responsiveness to steroids and not by the histological lesion. Others have, however, argued that these are separate clinico-pathological entities with a different rate of response to steroids and differences in their progression to renal failure. The arguments for and against both views are complex, and further complicated by whether the studies were performed in children or in adults. In children these arguments cannot now be resolved as most children with an uncomplicated nephrotic syndrome no longer have a renal biopsy.

Minimal change nephropathy

AETIOLOGY

There is a well-recognized association between Hodgkin's lymphoma and minimal change nephropathy. Minimal change nephropathy has rarely been reported in patients with a carcinoma. There are also case reports of minimal change nephropathy in individuals exposed to bee stings, poison oak, grass pollen, and cow's milk. Some of these individuals had other atopic symptoms, leading to suggestions that in some patients minimal change nephropathy might be caused by reaginic antibodies. The evidence for this is not convincing. Non-steroidal anti-inflammatory drugs can cause an interstitial nephritis, which in some cases is accompanied by a nephrotic syndrome with renal histology showing the changes of minimal change nephropathy.

PATHOGENESIS

The responsiveness of the nephrotic syndrome of minimal change nephropathy to steroids, cyclophosphamide, chlorambucil, and cyclosporin is strong evidence that this disorder is immune mediated. However, the pathogenetic mechanisms remain obscure. Impairment of lymphocyte proliferation in response to mitogens has been described in minimal change nephropathy and appears to be due to inhibitory serum factors. These abnormalities are, however, also found in patients with other causes of the nephrotic syndrome. The low serum IgG and high IgM in these patients appear to be a consequence of the nephrotic syndrome *per se*, and sheds no light on pathogenesis. The hypothesis that the proteinuria in this disorder was caused by a lymphokine produced by an abnormal clone of T lymphocytes has been studied extensively. As yet it has neither been proved nor disproved. In Europe an increased incidence of HLA-DR7 is found in patients with minimal change nephropathy and in Japan the association is with HLA-DR8, suggesting a genetic predisposition to this disorder.

PATHOLOGY

The histological features are similar in both children and adults. On light microscopy the glomeruli appear normal and small (Plate 1) and on electron microscopy there is effacement of epithelial-cell foot processes over the outer surface of the glomerular basement membrane. Some authors accept a minor degree of mesangial IgM deposits and mesangial proliferation as being consistent with this disorder.

MINIMAL CHANGE NEPHROPATHY IN CHILDREN

Minimal change nephropathy is found in 70 to 80 per cent of children with an idiopathic nephrotic syndrome. Most affected children are aged less than 6 years (80 per cent), with a peak age of onset of 2 to 4 years. The incidence falls to some 60 per cent of those aged 6 to 15 years, and in adults it accounts for approximately 25 per cent of patients with the nephrotic syndrome. In children it is more common in boys than in girls, with a male to female ratio of 2:1.

Clinical presentation

The clinical presentation is with a nephrotic syndrome that is characterized by severe hypoalbuminaemia, with a serum albumin of less than 10 g/l in some 38 per cent of cases. Microscopic haematuria is infrequent (22 per cent) as is hypertension (9 per cent). Renal impairment is infrequent at diagnosis and is found in about 10 per cent of cases, and a presentation in acute renal failure is rare. These children are prone to infections, in particular cellulitis and pneumococcal peritonitis.

Diagnosis

This has already been discussed. In 75 per cent of children with minimal change nephropathy the proteinuria is highly selective or moderately selective. The concept of selectivity of protein clearances was based on the hypothesis that the glomerular basement membrane provided a size-selective barrier to the loss of protein molecules. Although it is now clear that glomerular permselectivity is also based on the charge on molecules, the selectivity test remains useful. A simple version of the test is derived by dividing the ratio of the urine and protein concentrations of a large protein (for example, IgG or α_2-macroglobulin) by the ratio of the urine and protein concentrations of a small molecule (such as albumin or transferrin).

Treatment of minimal change nephropathy in children

The first line of treatment of minimal change nephropathy is prednisolone at an initial dose of 60 mg/m² (maximum dose 80 mg) daily, reducing at 4 weeks to 40 mg/m² (maximum dose 60 mg) on alternate days for a further 4 weeks. With this treatment more than 90 per cent of children respond with complete loss of proteinuria within 8 weeks. This duration of treatment is more effective in maintaining a remission than a shorter course of steroids.

Relapses

Once remission is induced, however, 66 per cent of children develop at least one relapse. The major problem is that 40 to 55 per cent of children who initially respond to steroids develop multiple relapses when steroids are discontinued, or become steroid dependent and relapse when steroid dosage is reduced. Early frequent relapses (three or more) in the 6 months following the initial response to steroids predicts a frequently relapsing course.

Treatment of relapses

A standard regimen is prednisolone 60 mg/m² until the urine is free of protein for 3 days (maximum 4 weeks) and then prednisolone 40 mg/m² on alternate days for 4 weeks. During repeated steroid treatment of relapses, growth should be carefully monitored with growth curves.

Cyclophosphamide/chlorambucil

Treatment with an immunosuppressant drug should be considered in the following groups of patients: children who are frequent relapsers (two relapses within 6 months of the initial response or four relapses within any 1 year); children who are steroid dependent (two consecutive relapses occurring during alternate-day treatment for an earlier relapse) or who relapse within 14 days of treatment of an earlier relapse (fast relapse); children in whom two out of four relapses within 6 months were fast relapses; children who have developed serious side-effects from steroids. There is good evidence that short-term treatment with cyclophosphamide can induce sustained or even, on occasion, permanent remission in such children. Cyclophosphamide is given in a dose of 2 mg/kg/day (ideal height for weight) for 8 weeks. Approximately 50 per cent of treated children are in remission at 2 years and 40 per cent at 5 years. One study suggested that the duration of remission was longer with a 12 week course as compared with an 8 week course of cyclophosphamide, but this was not subsequently confirmed. Chlorambucil has also been used to treat these patients, but there is no evidence that it is better than cyclophosphamide and it is probably more toxic. Permanent gonadal toxicity occurs with chlorambucil at a cumulative dose of 8 mg/kg. Cyclophosphamide has been evaluated carefully in these children and is the drug of choice. The gonadal toxicity of cyclophosphamide and its oncogenic potential are well recognized. The borderline dose for permanent gonadal toxicity with cyclophosphamide is a cumulative dose of 200 mg/kg. Other toxic side-effects of cyclophosphamide include leucopenia, haemorrhagic cystitis, and alopecia. At the doses and duration of treatment outlined above it is relatively safe.

MINIMAL CHANGE NEPHROPATHY IN ADULTS

About 25 per cent of adults with a nephrotic syndrome have minimal change nephropathy. The mean age of onset is 40 years and the condition is found in individuals up to the age of 60 and over. The histology is identical to that found in children, with the exception of a higher incidence of globally sclerosed glomeruli, which are a feature of ageing.

Clinical presentation

As in children, the clinical presentation is with a nephrotic syndrome, although this is not as severe as in children. Profound hypoalbuminaemia (serum albumin < 10 g/l) is rare in adults and is found in only 6 per cent of cases. The disease is slightly more common in men than in women with a male to female ratio of 1.3:1. More adults than children are hypertensive (30 per cent), have microscopic haematuria (28 per cent), and have renal impairment at diagnosis (60 per cent). These abnormalities are more severe in patients aged over 60 years who are also at particular risk of developing acute renal failure albeit due to haemodynamic factors and reversible.

Diagnosis

Only 50 per cent of adults with minimal change nephropathy have highly selective proteinuria and this, together with the high incidence of microscopic haematuria and renal impairment, makes it impossible to differentiate minimal change nephropathy from other forms of glomerulonephritis on clinical grounds. In adults with a nephrotic syndrome, a renal biopsy is essential to make the diagnosis.

Treatment of minimal change nephropathy in adults

Treatment is with prednisolone at an initial dose of 60 mg/day. The nephrotic syndrome in adults with minimal change nephropathy responds to steroids slightly less often than in children, and also more slowly. Eighty per cent of adults with minimal change nephropathy respond to steroids but remission can take up to 16 weeks to occur. The number of relapses in adults is less frequent, at 1.7/patient, than in children, and only 21 per cent of adults develop multiple relapses or are steroid dependent. In adults, as in children, cyclophosphamide is effective in inducing a long-lasting remission. In one study, 62.5 per cent of patients treated with cyclophosphamide were in remission at 10 years.

Long-term outcome of minimal change nephropathy

In children, 5.5 per cent of patients continue to relapse into adult life. All such cases that have been published presented with a nephrotic syndrome before the age of 6 years. The long-term mortality rate in children ranges from 2.6 to 7.2 per cent. In adults, 6 per cent of patients are still nephrotic after a mean follow-up of 7.5 years. The survival in patients aged over 60 was 50 per cent at 10 years and in those aged 15 to 59 was 90 per cent. The progression of steroid-responsive biopsy-proven minimal change nephropathy to endstage renal failure is rare in both adults and children, and occurs in 1 per cent of cases. Progression to endstage renal failure is probably due to the subsequent development of focal segmental glomerulosclerosis.

Cyclosporin A in minimal change nephropathy

There is now good evidence that cyclosporin A is effective in the treatment of minimal change nephropathy in both adults and children. Patients who are steroid responsive or multiple relapsers are more likely to respond with complete or partial remissions (70–80 per cent) than patients who are resistant to steroids (40–50 per cent). Several guidelines can be drawn from the studies of cyclosporin A in minimal change nephropathy. The drug is effective in steroid-responsive minimal change nephropathy and its use could be considered in patients who develop steroid toxicity because they have multiple relapses or are steroid dependent. Cyclosporin A appears to be effective at blood levels of 100 to 200 ng/ml, and at these levels significant short-term nephrotoxicity and hypertension are uncommon. Relapses appear to recur with the same frequency after cyclosporin A has been discontinued as before. For that reason it is still advisable to use cyclophosphamide as the first choice of treatment in patients with a multiple relapsing or steroid-dependent minimal change nephropathy, in the hope of inducing a sustained remission. In essence, cyclosporin can best be viewed as a steroid-sparing agent in patients with minimal change nephropathy.

FOCAL SEGMENTAL GLOMERULOSCLEROSIS

This was first described by Rich (1957) at autopsy in children who died from a nephrotic syndrome. Fewer terms have generated more disagreement amongst pathologists and nephrologists than focal segmental glomerulosclerosis (**FSGS**). FSGS is not a disease entity but a histological lesion that is often of unknown aetiology.

Pathogenesis

In experimental models focal segmental sclerosis can develop from different pathogenic mechanisms. These include toxic injury (puromycin nephropathy), immunological injury (antiglomerular basement membrane nephritis), the nephritis of NZB/NZW F[1] lupus, and hyperfiltration

injury from five-sixths nephrectomy). Some of these models have clinical counterparts and the diversity of pathogenic mechanisms may explain the variability in the clinical presentation of FSGS as well as responses to therapy. As with minimal change nephropathy, there are suggestions that the glomerular injury in FSGS is caused by a lymphokine. The rapid development of heavy proteinuria following renal transplantation in some patients with FSGS suggests that the glomerular injury is caused by a circulating factor.

Pathology

Renal histology shows focal segmental sclerosing glomerular lesions affecting predominantly juxtamedullary glomeruli. The histological lesions of FSGS comprise segmental areas of glomerular sclerosis with hyalinization of glomerular capillaries. These segmental areas are usually adherent to Bowman's capsule. In childhood FSGS these lesions affect predominantly juxtamedullary glomeruli. Typically, the areas of segmental sclerosis are randomly distributed within the glomerular tuft, with a predilection for the hilar regions, and these patients may be regarded as having classical FSGS (Plate 2). In some biopsies the glomerular lesions are located peripherally at the glomerulotubular junction, the so-called glomerular tip lesion (Plate 3). Focal areas of tubular atrophy and interstitial nephritis are prominent. On immunofluorescent microscopy deposits of IgM and C3 may be seen in the sclerotic areas. Electron microscopy shows diffuse foot process effacement in apparently unaffected glomeruli.

Primary focal segmental glomerulosclerosis

Focal segmental glomerulosclerosis may be apparently idiopathic and found early on in the course of patients with a nephrotic syndrome. Even when FSGS is found early in the course of a nephrotic syndrome, there is no evidence to suggest that it represents a homogeneous disease.

Secondary focal segmental glomerulosclerosis

FSGS has also been found late on in the clinical course of patients with a nephrotic syndrome whose initial renal biopsy had shown minimal change nephropathy. FSGS may also be a sequel of glomerular scarring in patients with previous proliferative glomerulonephritis, and is seen in the biopsies of patients with Alport's syndrome (Table 4). It has also been found in the biopsies of patients with reflux nephropathy and other conditions leading to a reduced renal mass. It is a reasonable hypothesis that the segmental sclerosing lesions in these circumstances are a consequence of glomerular hypertension and hyperfiltration.

Clinical presentation of focal segmental glomerulosclerosis in children

Approximately 7 per cent of children presenting with an idiopathic nephrotic syndrome have FSGS. Males and females are equally affected and the peak age at onset is between 6 and 8 years. The majority of patients (75 per cent) present with a nephrotic syndrome, 20 per cent have persistent proteinuria, and 5 per cent haematuria as well as proteinuria. Clinically these patients differ from children with minimal change nephropathy in that two-thirds have microscopic haematuria, one-half have impaired renal function at diagnosis, and one-third are hypertensive. The proteinuria is usually poorly selective.

Clinical presentation of focal segmental glomerulosclerosis in adults

Approximately 10 per cent of adults with a nephrotic syndrome have FSGS. The clinical presentation in adults does not differ in any significant respects from that in children. The mean age at onset is between 20 and 30 years, but FSGS has been found in patients aged 70.

Treatment and prognosis of classical focal segmental glomerulosclerosis

In most studies, patients with classical FSGS and a nephrotic syndrome have been treated with steroids. The response to treatment is poor. Only

Table 4 *Secondary focal segmental glomerulosclerosis*

Alport's syndrome
Reduced renal mass
Reflux nephropathy
Remnant kidney
Healed glomerulonephritis
IgA nephropathy
Vasculitis
Diffuse proliferative glomerulonephritis
Sickle-cell disease
AIDS
Intravenous drug abuse (heroin)

Table 5 *Conditions associated with mesangiocapillary glomerulonephritis*

	MCGN
Autoimmune	
Systemic lupus erythematosus	Type I
Infection	
Post-streptococcal	Type I
Infective endocarditis	Type I
Visceral abscess	Type I
Shunt nephritis	Type I
Schistosomiasis	Type I
Leprosy	Type I
Filariasis	Type I
Hepatitis B	Type I
Hepatitis C	Type I
Mixed cryoglobinaemia	Type I
Candidiasis	Type II
Partial lipodystrophy	Type II
Miscellaneous	
Sickle-cell disease	Type I
Inherited complement deficiency	Types I and II
Carcinoma	Type I
α_1-Antitrypsin deficiency	Type I

10 to 30 per cent of patients respond by going into remission. These patients have a good prognosis and do not develop progressive renal failure. However, the prognosis in patients who do not respond to steroids is poor. Between 30 and 50 per cent of these patients develop endstage renal failure over 5 to 10 years. There is no difference in prognosis between adults and children. Patients with a nephrotic syndrome are more likely to develop endstage renal failure than those with more modest proteinuria. Cyclophosphamide at the same doses and duration as used in minimal change nephropathy has been given to some patients with FSGS who are resistant to steroids. A useful remission was induced in 25 per cent of cases and this approach may be tried in patients with a severe nephrotic syndrome.

Treatment of glomerular tip lesion

Some studies suggest that the site of the segmental sclerosing lesions predict steroid responsiveness. Adult patients with a peripheral segmental sclerosing lesion at the tubular origin, the glomerular tip lesion, have been reported to be responsive to steroids or immunosuppression and not to progress to endstage renal failure. Similar observations have been reported in children, although in neither children nor adults have these observations been confirmed beyond doubt.

Cyclosporin A in focal segmental glomerulosclerosis

Several studies have examined the effects of cyclosporin A in patients with FSGS and a nephrotic syndrome. In general, the responsiveness to cyclosporin A has been poor and has paralleled steroid responsiveness. Those patients who were steroid resistant achieved little or no benefit from cyclosporin A.

MESANGIOCAPILLARY GLOMERULONEPHRITIS

Mesangiocapillary, or membranoproliferative, glomerulonephritis (**MCGN**) is a disorder that is defined by its histological appearance. It is found in approximately 8 per cent of children and 14 per cent of adults with the nephrotic syndrome.

Aetiology

In most cases the disorder is idiopathic, but a similar histological appearance may be seen in infectious endocarditis, hepatitis B and C infections, systemic lupus erythematosus, Henoch–Schönlein purpura, mixed cryoglobulinaemia Candida infections, and other conditions (Table 5). Two major types of idiopathic MCGN are recognized on histology: Type I with subendothelial deposits and type II with electron dense deposits replacing the lamina densa of the glomerular basement membrane.

Pathogenesis

The pathogenesis of MCGN is uncertain. It has been known for some time that complement and immunoglobulin can be detected in deposits in glomeruli. More recently, in hepatitis B-associated nephritis evidence of virus (HBV) antigen has been found in serum, in immune complexes, in cryoprecipitates, and in glomerular deposits. In cases associated with hepatitis C, virus (HCV) RNA and antibodies have been found in plasma. These findings and the occurrence of complement abnormalities strongly favour a critical note for immune complexes, circulating or formed *in situ*. This case is strengthened by the frequent observation of subendothelial type I MCGN associated with infections.

Serum complement abnormalities

A low serum C3 is found in 60 to 100 per cent of patients with type II MCGN, and 36 per cent of patients with type I MCGN. Less commonly, C4 levels are low; 15 per cent in type II and 9 per cent in type I. These complement abnormalities indicate predominant activation of the alternative pathway of complement. A C3 nephritic factor (C3Nef) is found in 60 per cent of patients with type II and 27 per cent of patients with type I MCGN. The C3Nef factor is an IgG autoantibody directed at determinants on C3bBb, the alternative pathway convertase. Binding of C3Nef factor to C3bBb prevents its inactivation and this leads to continuous activation of the alternative pathway, with the generation of C3b and ticking over of this pathway. A small proportion of patients with both types of MCGN have been reported to have inherited deficiencies of the complement proteins C2, factor B, C6, C7, and C8.

Partial lipodystrophy and mesangiocapillary glomerulonephritis

A proportion of patients with partial lipodystrophy have C3Nef and develop type II MCGN and, rarely, type I MCGN. Partial lipodystrophy is a disorder in which there is asymmetrical loss of subcutaneous fat from the face, trunk and arms, leading characteristically to a gaunt face with sunken cheeks. Often the legs appear fatter than normal. The disorder at times follows childhood infectious illnesses, especially measles. About 80 per cent of patients with partial lipodystrophy have a low serum C3 and 66 per cent have C3Nef. Approximately one-third of patients develop MCGN between 5 and 20 years after the onset of partial lipodystrophy, with the complement abnormalities preceding the development of nephritis. It has been suggested that the hypocomplementaemia predisposes these individuals to infection, which in turn leads to the development of nephritis, but this has not been demonstrated to be so.

Pathology

Type I MCGN (subendothelial)

The glomeruli are increased in size and there is increased lobularity of the glomerular tuft. There is an increase in both mesangial cells and matrix, with extension of the latter between the glomerular basement membrane and the endothelium. This mesangial extension together with the basement membrane gives a 'double contour' appearance to the basement membrane (Plate 4). In a proportion of biopsies there is extra-capillary proliferation (crescent formation), although this is rarely exten-sive. On electron microscopy there are subendothelial, deposits of elec-tron-dense material (Fig. 1) and these deposits may also be found in the mesangium. Rarely, subepithelial electron-dense deposits or 'humps' are seen. On immunofluorescent microscopy subendothelial deposits of IgG and C3, and less commonly Ciq, C4, IgM, and IgA, are seen.

Type II (dense deposit disease)

Light microscopy shows enlarged glomeruli, which are hypercellular with an increase in mesangial cells and matrix, and subendothelial exten-sion leading to a double contour of the basement membrane. Glomerular lobularity may also be seen and, in about one-third of biopsies, crescents are seen. Occasionally an abnormal number of neutrophils are seen in glomeruli. The thickening of the glomerular capillary walls is due to replacement of the lamina densa of the glomerular basement membrane by a ribbon-like electron-dense material, that may in places be focal in extent (Fig. 2). This electron-dense material is often also present in the basement membrane of Bowman's capsule and the tubular basement membrane. In about one-third of biopsies there are subepithelial elec-tron-dense deposits or 'humps'. On immunofluorescent microscopy bright deposits of C3 are seen in the mesangium. Continuous linear deposits of C3 are also seen on the basement membrane, with rare depos-its of IgG, IgM, and IgA.

Fig. 1 Subendothelial-type mesangiocapillary glomerulonephritis. Electron-dense deposits on endothelial side of basement membrane (electron micrograph, magnification ×10 000). (By courtesy of Dr A.J. Howie.)

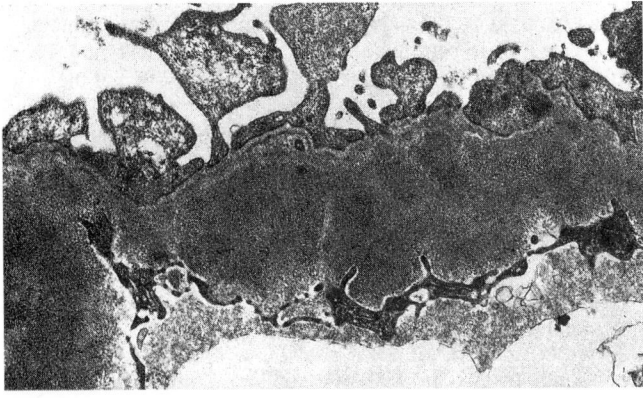

Fig. 2 Dense deposit disease. Electron-dense intramembranous material (electron micrograph, magnification ×2000). (By courtesy of Dr A.J. Howie.)

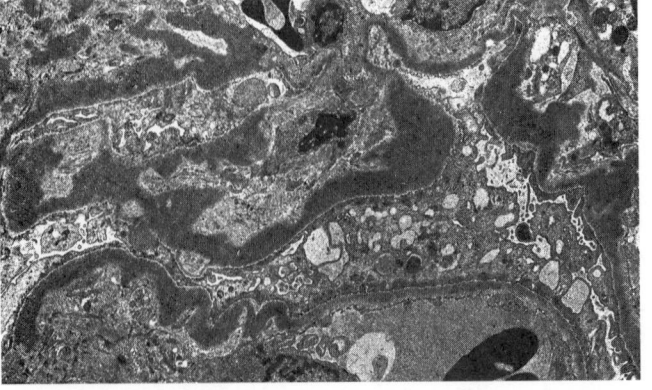

Type III MCGN

Some authors recognize a third type of MCGN in which there are con-tiguous subepithelial and subendothelial deposits, with formation of basement-like material on the surface of these deposits leading to a duplicated appearance of the glomerular basement membrane. As with the other types there is mesangial proliferation and an increase in mes-angial matrix with a variable increase in lobularity. On immunofluores-cent microscopy, C3 is found on capillary loops and in the mesangium, and rarely IgM, IgG, and IgA deposits are seen. It seems likely that type III MCGN is a variant of type I.

Clinical presentation

Type II MCGN is uncommon in infants and in old age. It is commoner in children aged over 8 years than in adults and has a median age of onset of 11 to 12 years. By contrast, the median age of onset in type I MCGN is in the twenties. Equal numbers of males and females are affected. The clinical presentations differ little between types I and II. Most frequent are a nephrotic syndrome (30–50 per cent), acute nephritis (20 per cent), or both, and less frequently the initial features are with macroscopic haematuria or asymptomatic proteinuria and/or haematuria. Approximately 30 per cent of patients are hypertensive and 40 to 60 per cent have renal impairment at diagnosis. Macroscopic haematuria, either on its own or as part of an acute nephritic illness, is more common in children than in adults, whereas adults are more likely to have renal impairment and hypertension at the onset of their disease.

Treatment

There is no treatment of proven benefit in MCGN. West's group have consistently supported the value of long-term alternate-day prednisolone in children with this disorder. In their hands this regimen was associated with a 74 per cent survival after 11 years and this improved to 90 per cent in patients starting treatment early. Although their results are impressive, they were uncontrolled and the potential toxicity of long-term prednisolone treatment is likely to be substantial. The only con-trolled trial of the use of steroids in MCGN was inconclusive, due to the large number of withdrawals because of steroid-induced hyperten-sion and encephalopathy. Suggestions that cyclophosphamide, warfarin, and dipyridamole are beneficial have been disproved by one controlled study, but another has suggested a benefit from warfarin and dipyridam-ole. The benefit was marginal and the complication rate from bleeding was high. One other controlled study showed early benefit from dipyr-idamole and aspirin, but this was not borne out on longer follow-up. At the present time there is no treatment of proven benefit to offer to patients with MCGN, but the use of α-interferon suggests that antiviral agents may ultimately prove to have a role in patients with viral induced glomerulonephritis.

Prognosis

The prognosis of MCGN is that of a slowly progressive disease, with the development of endstage renal failure in some 50 per cent of patients, 10 years after onset of disease. Patients with a nephrotic syndrome either at diagnosis or subsequently are more likely to develop endstage renal failure than patients with lesser degrees of proteinuria only. The pres-ence of sclerosed glomeruli or of crescents is often accompanied by more rapid development of renal failure. Although children have a better initial prognosis in terms of endstage renal failure than adults, this dif-ference disappears after 10 years. In adults, males with type I MCGN do worse than females. Serum complement levels, C3Nef, and the pres-ence or absence of hypertension do not correlate with the renal outcome.

MEMBRANOUS NEPHROPATHY

Membranous nephropathy accounts for between 20 and 30 per cent of cases of the nephrotic syndrome in adults, and about 2 to 5 per cent of cases of the nephrotic syndrome in childhood. Histologically it is defined by the presence of subepithelial immune deposits on the outer surface of the glomerular basement membrane. In most patients in temperate countries no cause for this histological lesion is found, and it is therefore termed idiopathic membranous nephropathy. It is unlikely that membranous glomerulonephritis is a homogeneous disorder. Its aetiology (where identifiable), genetic basis, frequency as a cause of the nephrotic syndrome, and clinical evolution with or without treatment differ substantially between studies from different countries.

Aetiology

In about 20 to 25 per cent of adults and 35 per cent of children with membranous nephropathy there is an identifiable associated condition (Table 6). The frequency of this varies in different parts of the world. Malignancy, usually a carcinoma and rarely Hodgkin's lymphoma or non-Hodgkin's lymphoma, is found in between 3 and 7 per cent of all patients with membranous nephropathy, and this rises to 16 per cent in patients aged over 60 years. The most common tumours are carcinoma of the bronchus, colon, kidney, breast, stomach, and prostate. Gold and penicillamine therapy are prominent causes of membranous nephropathy, and this complication is more common in individuals who carry the HLA-DR3 gene. There is also some evidence that membranous nephropathy can develop in patients with rheumatoid arthritis who are not on these drugs. Approximately 3 per cent of all patients with membranous nephropathy have systemic lupus erythematosus and a further 2 per cent of patients have serological features or histological changes that are suggestive of this disorder. These serological or histological features may predate the clinical evidence of systemic lupus erythematosus by many years. In northern Europe about 1 per cent of patients with membranous nephropathy have positive hepatitis B serology, although this probably causative association is much more common in South-East Asia and in Africa.

Pathogenesis

The immune mechanisms that lead to the development of membranous nephropathy are unknown. In rats, administration of antibodies to renal tubular epithelial antigen leads to a membranous nephropathy that histologically resembles human membranous nephropathy. The antibody responsible for this Heymann nephritis in rats binds to epitopes on glomerular epithelial cells and leads to the development of subepithelial deposits. There is no evidence that a similar mechanism plays a role in human membranous nephropathy. In Europe there is a strong association between membranous nephropathy and the major histocompatibility complex haplotype HLA-A1 B8 DR3; in Japan the association is with HLA-DR2. By contrast no such association is seen in the United States.

Pathology

Idiopathic membranous nephropathy is characterized histologically by diffuse thickening of the glomerular basement on light microscopy, usually with argyrophyllic subepithelial spikes. On immunofluorescent or immunoperoxidase microscopy this thickening is shown to be due to the presence of immune deposits consisting of usually IgG and C3 on the subepithelial surface of the glomerular basement membrane (Plate 5). The presence of mesangial proliferation, mesangial immune deposits, and IgA and C1q on immunofluorescent microscopy raises the possibility that the membranous nephropathy is secondary to systemic lupus erythematosus. In membranous nephropathy the size and extent of incorporation of immune deposits into the glomerular basement membrane on electron microscopy forms the basis of histological classification: Stage 1, subepithelial deposits without spikes; Stage 2, large subepithelial deposits separated by spikes of basement membrane; Stage 3, deposits incorporated into a thickened basement membrane with many spikes; Stage 4, a very thick irregular basement membrane with no spikes and resorbed deposits.

Table 6 *Conditions associated with membranous nephropathy*

Autoimmune diseases
Systemic lupus erythematosus
Rheumatoid arthritis
Drugs
Gold
Penicillamine
Captopril
Malignancy
Carcinoma (bronchus, colon, stomach, prostate, breast)
Infections
Hepatitis B
Syphilis
Filariasis
Leprosy
Miscellaneous
Autoimmune thyroid disease
Diabetes mellitus

Clinical presentation

In children, boys are affected three times as often as girls. In adults, the majority of patients are aged between 30 and 50, although membranous nephropathy has been described in patients aged up to 80 years. In most, but not all, studies there has been a preponderance of males, with a male to female ratio of 2:1 to 3:1. The clinical presentation is usually (some 70 per cent) with a nephrotic syndrome or with asymptomatic proteinuria. Microscopic haematuria is found in 50 per cent of adults and 90 per cent of children. Macroscopic haematuria occurs in about 10 to 20 per cent of children but is rare in adults. About 25 to 40 per cent of adults and 6 per cent of children are hypertensive at diagnosis, and between 10 and 30 per cent of patients have a raised serum creatinine at diagnosis.

Renal vein thrombosis

Patients with membranous nephropathy appear to be at particular risk of developing a renal vein thrombosis, although the prevalence is probably not as high as originally suggested. Approximately 5 to 10 per cent of these patients have clinical evidence of renal vein thrombosis, and a higher proportion will be detected by venography. In practice a renal vein thrombosis should always be looked for if there is sudden deterioration of renal function. It is now known that renal vein thrombosis is a consequence of the hypercoagulable state of the nephrotic syndrome and not a primary cause of membranous nephropathy.

Clinical evolution of untreated membranous nephropathy

In the long term, untreated membranous nephropathy evolves either to remission or to the development of chronic renal failure. The rate at which either outcome occurs varies in different studies. After a mean follow-up of 4.5 to 6 years, between 9.5 and 22 per cent of patients are in endstage renal failure, 9.5 to 19 per cent have significant impairment of renal function, and 23 to 50 per cent are in remission. Actuarial survival shows that about 75 per cent of patients are alive at 10 years and 60 per cent have functioning kidneys. Examination of the untreated patients in recent treatment trials shows that of 205 patients followed for between 2 and 5 years, 15 per cent were in complete remission and 9 per cent in endstage renal failure. Any study of treatment in membranous nephropathy must therefore address the difficulty of treating with toxic drugs large numbers of patients who have little risk of developing endstage renal failure.

Treatment

The twin aims of treating membranous nephropathy are, first, to induce a remission of the nephrotic syndrome and, secondly, to prevent the development of endstage renal failure. Despite several careful studies using steroids and immunosuppressants, there is still no agreement that these aims can be achieved.

Steroid treatment

In the Collaborative Study in the United States (1979), 72 adults with membranous nephropathy were randomized to treatment with either prednisolone (125 mg on alternate days) or placebo for 8 weeks. The steroid dose was then tapered and stopped over several weeks. Deterioration of renal function, as measured by the glomerular filtration rate, was significantly more rapid in untreated than in treated patients. Further, a significantly lower proportion of treated patients than untreated patients developed renal failure (serum creatinine > 440 μmol/l). In the MRC study in the United Kingdom (1990), 107 adult patients with membranous nephropathy were randomized to treatment with either prednisolone (125 mg on alternate days for 8 weeks) or placebo. At 36 months there were no significant differences in plasma creatinine, creatinine clearance, and 24-h urine protein between treated and untreated patients. In a Canadian study, 158 patients were treated with either prednisolone (45 mg/m²/day for 6 months) or no specific treatment. No benefits were seen in renal function or proteinuria after a mean follow-up of 48 months. These data indicate that short-term steroids are of no benefit in the treatment of membranous nephropathy.

Steroid and chlorambucil treatment

The study of Lagrue *et al.* (1975) suggested that chlorambucil was more effective than azathioprine or placebo in the treatment of membranous nephropathy. This provided the rationale for the Italian multicentre study (Ponticelli *et al.* 1989) in which patients were randomized to symptomatic treatment only or treatment with a regimen alternating (monthly for 6 months) high-dose methylprednisolone with chlorambucil. After a follow-up period of 31 to 37 months, significantly more treated than untreated patients were in remission. In addition, there had been a more than 50 per cent rise in serum creatinine in 8 of 30 untreated patients, but no such change in any treated patient.

A further study (1992) by the Italian group compared the effect of methylprednisolone alone to that of methylprednisolone plus chlorambucil. Those treated with the combination were more likely to have an early remission of the nephrotic state, but this advantage was no longer evident after 4 years, and there was no difference in the rates of decline of renal function between the two therapies.

Most nephrologists are hesitant to use the alternating regimen because of the gonadal toxicity and oncogenic risks of chlorambucil given to patients who might do well on no treatment. However, there may be a subgroup of patients with membranous nephropathy in whom renal function deteriorates more rapidly than is the norm. It is perhaps reasonable to consider some form of immunosuppressive regimen for these patients. It is important in this context, however, to first consider the possibility of a complicating drug-induced interstitial nephritis or a renal vein thrombosis. Several uncontrolled studies have suggested that intravenous methylprednisolone or prednisolone, combined with chlorambucil or cyclophosphamide, might reverse the rate of loss of renal function. Pending answers from controlled observations in this rare subgroup of patients, a trial of treatment is probably justifiable.

Prognostic factors

Identification of those patients who at onset of membranous nephropathy are most likely to do a badly would be helpful in deciding whom to treat. Most studies show that deterioration of renal function is more common in patients with a nephrotic syndrome, in those with tubulo-interstitial fibrosis or with initial poor renal function and whose renal function has deteriorated in the first 2.5 years after diagnosis. Some studies have shown that men do worse than women, but this has not been consistent. Children appear to do better than adults, and in one study 42 per cent of children went into complete remission and only 10

Table 7 *Proliferative glomerulonephritis*

Focal proliferative
  Systemic lupus erythematosus
Acute endocapillary proliferative
  Post-streptococcal
  Infective endocarditis
  Leprosy
Extracapillary proliferative (crescent formation)
  Idiopathic
  Microscopic polyarteritis/Wegener's
  Antiglomerular basement membrane antibody disease
  Systemic lupus erythematosus
  Henoch–Schönlein purpura
Mesangial proliferative
  Idiopathic
  IgA disease
  Henoch–Schönlein purpura
  Mesangial IgM
  Systemic lupus erythematosus
Diffuse proliferative
  Systemic lupus erythematosus

per cent developed endstage renal failure after a mean follow-up of 4 years.

PROLIFERATIVE GLOMERULONEPHRITIS

Modern renal histological techniques have led to a clear classification of proliferative glomerulonephritis into clinicopathological entities on the basis of the light, immunofluorescent, and ultrastructural appearances on renal biopsy. The histological appearances are diverse, as are the clinical associations, the clinical presentation, and the evolution of this disorder (Table 7). Most of the types of proliferative glomerulonephritis are described elsewhere (Chapter 20.5.2). Mesangial IgM proliferative glomerulonephritis is not, and so is discussed here.

MESANGIAL IgM PROLIFERATIVE GLOMERULONEPHRITIS

There is a great deal of disagreement on the significance of mesangial proliferation in patients with a nephrotic syndrome whose renal biopsies are otherwise normal. These changes have been reported in the renal biopsies of about 3 per cent of children with a nephrotic syndrome. In those early studies immunofluorescent microscopy was not performed or the details given were not such as to allow analysis. Although 95.3 per cent of children with pure minimal change nephropathy went into remission with steroid treatment within 8 weeks, only 55.5 per cent of children with biopsies showing a diffuse mesangial proliferation did so. Subsequent reports showed that some of these nephrotic patients, both children and adults, could be shown to have IgM glomerular deposits on immunofluorescence. One view is that mesangial proliferation with IgM deposits defines a subset of patients with a nephrotic syndrome who respond poorly to steroids and tend to develop progressive renal failure. The opposite view is that patients with this histological appearance cannot be differentiated by their clinical behaviour or responsiveness to steroids from patients with true minimal change glomerulonephritis. It is possible that patients with mild mesangial proliferation and minor deposits of IgM are a variant of minimal change glomerulonephritis.

Clinical presentation

Undoubtedly some patients usually presenting with a nephrotic syndrome, (but at times only with proteinuria or haematuria and proteinuria) have significant mesangial proliferation and mesangial IgM deposits on

Table 8 *Recurrence of glomerulonephritis after renal transplantation*

	FSGS	MCGN Type II	MCGN Type I	Membranous nephropathy
Histological recurrence	?	88 ⎫		
Clinical recurrence (%)	23	24 ⎬ 15–35 ⎫		rare
Graft loss (%)	11	10 ⎭ 5–10 ⎭		

biopsy—and this finding is commoner in adolescents and adults than in children.

Pathology

Renal biopsy shows mesangial proliferation with diffuse mesangial deposits of IgM and in some cases deposits of C3 also. Ultrastructural studies have shown electron-dense deposits in 20 to 70 per cent of cases, suggesting that the IgM is part of an immune complex lesion. Some IgM deposits may represent, alternatively, only trapping of a large molecule in the mesangium.

Treatment and prognosis

In those who present with a nephrotic syndrome, between 25 and 55 per cent go into remission with steroids and, of these, 25 to 50 per cent become dependent on steroids to maintain remission. In most studies, the majority of patients who do not respond to steroids also fail to respond to cyclophosphamide or chlorambucil. In a variable proportion of patients who have had a repeat renal biopsy, evolution into focal segmental glomerulosclerosis has been seen. Between 3 and 20 per cent overall develop progressive renal failure, and in one study the 10-year survival of renal function was 64 per cent. The prognosis for those who present with microscopic haematuria alone has not been analysed.

At present it is difficult to provide a unifying view of the place of mesangial IgM glomerulonephritis in a classification of idiopathic glomerulonephritis. In practice, patients with this lesion and a nephrotic syndrome could reasonably be given an 8 week course of steroids in an attempt to induce a remission.

RECURRENT IDIOPATHIC GLOMERULONEPHRITIS FOLLOWING RENAL TRANSPLANTATION (SEE ALSO CHAPTER 20.17.3)

Several types of idiopathic glomerulonephritis may recur after renal transplantation. These recurrences must be differentiated from glomerular disease that is a consequence of rejection or allograft glomerulopathy, which can lead to *de novo* histological lesions indistinguishable from FSGS, membranous nephropathy, and MCGN type I, and hence to an overestimate of rate of recurrence. The frequency of recurrences and their clinical significance are summarized in Table 8. Recurrence of FSGS is commoner in patients whose original disease led to renal failure within 3 years of onset. Proteinuria is often detected within days or weeks of transplantation. Although type II MCGN is often found on biopsy, clinical recurrence and graft losses from this are infrequent. The incidence of recurrent membranous nephropathy is difficult to estimate as this lesion often develops *de novo* in patients whose original disease was not membranous nephropathy. The possibility of recurrent glomerulonephritis is not a contraindication to renal transplantation.

REFERENCES

Appel, G.B. (1993). Immune complex glumerulonephritis-deposits plus interest. *New England Journal of Medicine* **328**, 505–6.

Cameron, J.S. (1979). The natural history of glomerulonephritis. In *Progress in glomerulonephritis*, (ed. P. Kincaid-Smith, S.J. D'Apice, and R.W. Atkins), pp. 1–25. John Wiley & Sons, New York.

Cameron, J.S. (1982). Glomerulonephritis in renal transplants. *Transplantation* **34**, 237–45.

Cameron, J.S. and Glassock, R.J. (ed.) (1988). *The nephrotic syndrome*. Marcel Dekker, New York.

Cameron, J.S., et al. (1983). Idiopathic mesangiocapillary glomerulonephritis: Comparison of types 1 and 11 in children and adults and long-term progression. *American Journal of Medicine.* **74**, 175–92.

Cameron, J.S., Healy, M.J.R., and Adu, D. (1990). The Medical Research Council Trial of short-term high-dose alternate day prednisolone in idiopathic membranous nephropathy with nephrotic syndrome in adults. *Quarterly Journal of Medicine*, **274**, 133–56.

Cameron, J.S., Davison, A.M., Grunfeld, J.P., Kerr, D., and Ritz, E. (ed.) (1992). *Oxford textbook of clinical nephrology*. Oxford University Press, Oxford.

Collaborative Study of the adult idiopathic nephrotic syndrome (1979). A controlled study of short-term treatment in adults with membranous nephropathy. *New England Journal of Medicine.* **301**, 1301–6.

International Study of Kidney Disease in Children (1974). Prospective controlled trial of cyclophosphamide treatment in children with the nephrotic syndrome. *Lancet* **ii**, 423–7.

International Study of Kidney Disease in Children (1978). Prediction of histopathology form clinical and laboratory characteristics at time of diagnosis. *Kidney International*, **13**, 159–65.

International Study of Kidney Disease in Children (1981). The primary nephrotic syndrome in children. Identification of patients with minimal change nephrotic syndrome from initial response to prednisolone. *Journal of Pediatrics* **98**, 561–4.

Lagrue, G., Bernard, J., Bariety, P., Druet, P., and Gunuel, J. (1975). Traitement par la chlorambucil et l'azathioprine dans les glomerulonephrites primitives. Résultats d'une étude controlée'. *Journal d'Urologie Nephrologie* **9**, 655–72.

Meyrier, A., and Collaborative Group of the Societé de Néphrologie (1989). Ciclosporin in the treatment of nephrosis. *American Journal of Nephrology* **9**, (Suppl.1), 65–71.

Nolasco, F., Cameron, J.S., Heywood, E.F., Hicks, J., Ogg, C., and Williams, D.G. (1986). Adult-onset minimal change nephrotic syndrome. A long-term follow-up. *Kidney International* **29**, 1215–33.

Ponticelli, C., et al. (1989). A randomized trial of methylprednisolone and chlorambucil in idiopathic membranous nephropathy. *New England Journal of Medicine* **320**, 8–13.

Ponticelli, C., Zucchelli, P., Paserini, P., and Cesana, B., and the Italian idiopathic membranous nephropathy treatment study group, (1992). Methylprednisolone plus chlorambucil as compared with methylprednisolone alone for the treatment of idiopathic membranous nephropathy. *New England Journal of Medicine.* **327**, 599–603.

Rich, A.R. (1957). A hitherto undescribed vulnerability of the juxtamedullary glomeruli in the lipoid nephrosis. *Bulletin of Johns Hopkins Hospital* **100**, 173–86.

Sissons, J.G.P., et al. (1976). The complement abnormalities of lipodystrophy. *New England Journal of Medicine*, **294**, 461–45.

Trompeter, R.S., Lloyd, B.W., Hicks, J., White, R.H.R., and Cameron, J.S. (1985). Long term outcome for children with minimal change nephrotic syndrome. *Lancet* **1**, 368–70.

West, C.D. (1986). Childhood membranoproliferative glomerulonephritis: an approach to management. *Kidney International* **29**, 1077–83.

20.4.3 Rapidly progressive glomerulonephritis and antiglomerular basement membrane disease

C. D. PUSEY and A. J. REES

DEFINITION

The term rapidly progressive glomerulonephritis is used to describe those cases of glomerulonephritis which progress from onset to endstage renal failure within weeks or months. The characteristic histological appearance is of a focal necrotizing glomerulonephritis with crescent formation, and the term crescentic nephritis has been used almost synonymously with rapidly progressive glomerulonephritis. Attempts have been made to define crescentic nephritis in terms of the percentage of glomeruli involved and extent of the crescents. However, there is no consensus, and a rigid definition seems inappropriate because of the sampling error implicit in renal biopsy material and the fact that the biopsy represents only one stage in the evolution of the disease.

DIAGNOSIS

The two principal causes of rapidly progressive glomerulonephritis are antiglomerular basement membrane disease and primary systemic vasculitis. So-called idiopathic rapidly progressive glomerulonephritis may be regarded as a renal-limited form of systemic vasculitis (see below). However, rapidly progressive glomerulonephritis may also occur in other systemic diseases, such as systemic lupus erythematosus, and may complicate most types of primary glomerulonephritis (Table 1). The diagnosis of rapidly progressive glomerulonephritis should be suspected when rapid deterioration in renal function occurs in the context of a particular clinical syndrome. However, since it can occur without systemic features, it should also be included in the differential diagnosis of unexplained acute renal failure.

In the absence of associated systemic disease, presentation may be delayed until renal failure leads to oliguria, peripheral oedema, shortness of breath, or symptoms of uraemia. However, some patients complain of non-specific symptoms such as malaise, fever, myalgia, and weight loss. Macroscopic haematuria and loin pain are sometimes reported. Examination may reveal features of renal failure, although hypertension is uncommon in the absence of fluid overload. An essential part of the clinical assessment of such patients is microscopy of a fresh sample of urine. This will generally reveal many dysmorphic red cells, together with red cell and granular casts. Proteinuria is usually modest, but occasionally reaches nephrotic levels. Renal ultrasound will confirm the presence of normal-sized non-obstructed kidneys. Once rapidly progressive glomerulonephritis is suspected, renal biopsy should be performed urgently, together with appropriate serological tests (Table 2) to confirm the diagnosis and detect any underlying cause.

MANAGEMENT

The specific management of antiglomerular basement membrane disease is considered below, and that of systemic vasculitis in Chapter 18.11.2. However, taken overall, the prognosis of rapidly progressive glomerulonephritis has been greatly improved by immunosuppressive therapy. The natural history of the untreated patient was death within a year, and even after the introduction of dialysis and corticosteroids irreversible renal failure occurred in around 75 per cent of patients. The review by Heaf et al. in 1983 showed that renal mortality at 2 years had improved with the progressive introduction of different forms of treatment: it was 87 per cent in untreated patients; 69 per cent in those receiving oral steroids ± immunosuppressive drugs; 36 per cent following high-dose intravenous steroids; and 42 per cent following plasma exchange. Although of historical interest, this analysis does not accurately reflect

Table 1 *Causes of rapidly progressive glomerulonephritis*

Antiglomerular basement membrane disease
  Goodpasture's disease [a,b]
  Isolated antiglomerular basement membrane nephritis[a]
Primary systemic vasculitis
  Wegener's granulomatosis[a,b]
  Microscopic polyarteritis[a,b]
  Idiopathic rapidly progressive glomerulonephritis[a]
  Churg–Strauss syndrome [b]
  Polyarteritis nodosa
  Giant-cell arteritis
  Takayasu's arteritis
Systemic disorders
  Systemic lupus erythematosus[a,b]
  Essential mixed cryoglobulinaemia[b]
  Henoch–Schönlein purpura[b]
  Relapsing polychondritis
  Behçet's syndrome[b]
  Rheumatoid disease
Primary glomerulonephritis
  Mesangiocapillary glomerulonephritis[a]
  Mesangial IgA nephropathy[a]
  Membranous nephropathy
Infection-related glomerulonephritis
  Post-streptococcal (and other causes of acute proliferative) glomerulonephritis[a]
  Infective endocarditis
  Ventriculoatrial shunt infection
  Visceral abscess
Neoplastic disease
  Carcinoma
  Lymphoma (Hodgkin's and non-Hodgkin's)
Drug reactions
  Penicillamine[b]
  Hydralazine
  Rifampicin

[a]Relatively common cause of rapidly progressive glomerulonephritis in adults.

[b]Association with pulmonary haemorrhage.

Postinfectious glomerulonephritis is common worldwide but now rare in Europe.

the current situation, in which attempts are made to tailor treatment to individual causes of rapidly progressive glomerulonephritis.

Since many patients will be treated with pulse doses of methylprednisolone or plasma exchange, in addition to oral immunosuppressive drugs, the adverse effects of each of these approaches should be recognized (Table 3). The risk of infection is particularly related to the steroid dosage, and there should be an aggressive policy in the diagnosis and treatment of suspected infection. Regular cultures of available material (blood, urine, sputum, peritoneal dialysis fluid, wound swabs) should be performed. There should be a low threshold for performing invasive investigations such as bronchoscopy or needle aspiration. Opportunistic infections are relatively common, particularly with nosocomial bacteria, fungi, Pneumocystis, and cytomegalovirus. When infection is suspected, treatment may need to be started on the basis of the likely diagnosis, pending microbiological results. There is no convincing evidence for the use of prophylactic antimicrobial drugs, although oral antifungal agents are widely used. It is important to ensure adequate nutrition, which may involve enteral or parenteral feeding, and to reduce the risk of upper gastrointestinal haemorrhage, by use of prophylactic H_2-antagonists.

The principles of management of 'medical' cases of acute renal failure apply. Indications for dialysis are conventional, but early treatment is preferred in order to avoid complications of renal failure—this is particularly important when rigorous immunosuppressive therapy is being

Table 2 *Selected blood tests in rapidly progressive glomerulonephritis*

Specific	
Antiglomerular basement membrane antibodies	Goodpasture's disease
Antineutrophil cytoplasmic antibodies	Systemic vasculitis
Anti-dsDNA antibodies, anti-Sm antibodies	Systemic lupus erythematosus
Cryoglobulins	Essential mixed cryoglobulinaemia type II
C3 nephritic factor	Mesangiocapillary glomerulonephritis type II
Raised ASOT	Post-streptococcal glomerulonephritis
Non-specific	
Complement	
low C4, normal C3	Essential mixed cryoglobulinaemia type II
low C4 ± C3	Systemic lupus erythematosus
low C3, normal C4	Mesangiocapillary glomerulonephritis type II
low C3 ± C4	Postinfectious glomerulonephritis, mesangiocapillary glomerulonephritis type I
raised C3, C4	Systemic vasculitis
Immunoglobulins	
raised IgG, IgM	Systemic lupus erythematosus, systemic vasculitis, postinfectious glomerulonephritis
raised IgE	Churg–Strauss syndrome
raised IgA	IgA nephropathy, Henoch–Schönlein purpura
paraprotein (usually IgM)	Essential mixed cryoglobulinaemia type II
Acute phase response	
raised C-reactive protein + ESR	Systemic vasculitis
raised ESR ± C-reactive protein	Systemic lupus erythematosus
raised alkaline phosphatase, low albumin	Systemic vasculitis
Haematology	
neutrophilia, thrombocytosis	Systemic vasculitis
eosinophilia	Churg–Strauss syndrome
leucopenia, thrombocytopenia	Systemic lupus erythematosus
severe anaemia	Goodpasture's disease
moderate anaemia	Systemic vasculitis, systemic lupus erythematosus, essential mixed cryoglobulinaemia
Microbiology	
blood cultures positive	Infective endocarditis
	Ventriculoatrial shunt nephritis

Some of the non-specific tests are abnormal only in a proportion of patients.

ASOT, anti-streptolysin O titre; ESR, erythrocyte sedimentation rate.

given. Peritoneal dialysis, intermittent haemodialysis, and continuous haemofiltration/haemodialysis have all been used successfully, and each has particular advantages and drawbacks. Peritoneal dialysis provides good control of fluid balance, but may be contraindicated if breathing is compromised or if there is gastrointestinal disease, and may not adequately treat the catabolic patient. Haemodialysis is more effective, but may need to be performed daily for adequate fluid management, and involves the risks of heparin therapy in those with lung haemorrhage. Continuous haemodialysis techniques can only be performed on intensive care or high dependency units. Since some patients will not recover renal function, care is needed with vascular and peritoneal access, and early consideration should be given to suitability for long-term dialysis.

Antiglomerular basement membrane disease

DEFINITION

The association of crescentic nephritis and lung haemorrhage was first described by Ernest Goodpasture, an American pathologist, in 1919. This combination of clinical features was designated Goodpasture's syndrome by Stanton and Tange, almost 40 years later. The development of immunofluorescence microscopy led to the identification of immunoglobulin deposits on the glomerular basement membrane in renal biopsies of similar cases. These deposits were later shown to be due to autoantibodies directed against a specific antigen in the membrane, sometimes referred to as the Goodpasture antigen.

However, it is clear that 'Goodpasture's syndrome', the combination of rapidly progressive glomerulonephritis and lung haemorrhage, may

be due to a variety of immunopathological processes, including systemic vasculitis (Table 1). Thus, the term antiglomerular basement membrane disease (or Goodpasture's disease) is preferred for those cases associated with antiglomerular basement membrane antibodies. An identical form of glomerulonephritis may occur without lung haemorrhage, and is included in the definition of antiglomerular basement membrane disease.

AETIOLOGY

Antiglomerular basement membrane disease is rare, with an estimated annual incidence of 0.5 to 1 cases per million population. It accounts for up to 5 per cent of cases of glomerulonephritis, and 2 per cent of the endstage renal failure population. It is reported mainly in Caucasians, and appears to be even rarer in other races. The disease can occur at any age, but is most frequent in the third and again in the sixth/seventh decades. In recent series, males are affected about twice as often as females.

Environmental factors

Geographical clustering of cases, and peaks of incidence in spring and early summer, have been described, suggesting a role for environmental factors. Both viral infections and hydrocarbon exposure have been reported in association with antiglomerular basement membrane disease, although the evidence for a causative role is not strong. Isolated cases have followed lithotripsy and obstructive nephropathy. There is a strong association between cigarette smoking and lung haemorrhage. However, the contribution of environmental factors to the development of antiglo-

Table 3 *Adverse effects of plasma exchange and pulse methylprednisolone*

Plasma exchange
  Vascular access complications
  Technical mishaps
  Fluid and electrolyte imbalance
  Citrate reactions (if used as anticoagulant)
  Reactions to fresh, frozen plasma (FFP), very rarely to
    albumin
  Risk of transfer of infection (FFP)
  Bleeding tendency

Methylprednisolone
  Susceptibility to infection
  Fluid retention
  Hypertension (especially in systemic lupus erythematosus)
  Arrhythmias
  Acute hyperglycaemia
  General effects of corticosteroids (diabetes, myopathy,
    cataracts, peptic ulceration)

merular basement membrane disease is unclear. They could induce the autoimmune process by revealing or altering self-antigens, or, in the case of micro-organisms, by bearing cross-reactive epitopes. However, they may act only to precipitate the clinical features of a pre-existing autoimmune process, since infection can upregulate inflammation non-specifically, and smoking may increase pulmonary capillary permeability, allowing access of antibodies to the alveolar basement membrane.

Genetic factors

There are several reports of sibling pairs, including monozygotic twins, who have developed antiglomerular basement membrane disease, sometimes following a common environmental stimulus. As in other autoimmune disorders, there are associations with particular class II HLA genes. The strongest association is with HLA-DR2(DRw15), which was found in over 80 per cent of Caucasian patients in the original Hammersmith series, and which has been confirmed by other authors. More recently, the use of molecular typing techniques has revealed an additional association with HLA-DR4, and negative associations with DR1 and DR7. In patients with HLA-DR2, the possession of the class I gene HLA-B7 is associated with more severe glomerulonephritis. Antiglomerular basement membrane disease is also associated with a particular immunoglobulin Gm haplotype. In one series of Caucasians, Gm 1, 2, 21 (axg) was present in 54 per cent of patients, compared with 17 per cent of controls. Antiglomerular basement membrane disease has also been described in association with other autoimmune diseases, including systemic vasculitis, and with primary glomerulonephritis, malignancy, and drug therapy.

PATHOGENESIS

Autoantibodies

There is good evidence for the pathogenicity of antiglomerular basement membrane autoantibodies. This was established by the classic transfer experiments of Lerner *et al.* in 1967, who showed that antibodies eluted from the kidneys of patients with antiglomerular basement membrane disease were capable of inducing glomerulonephritis in monkeys. Clinical studies support this observation: there is an extremely close association between the presence of antiglomerular basement membrane antibodies and the disease; antibody levels generally correlate with severity of disease; nephritis recurs in renal transplant recipients with detectable circulating antibodies; and treatment designed to lower antibody levels is often effective.

The distribution of the Goodpasture antigen has been studied by indirect immunohistology. Human antiglomerular basement membrane anti-

bodies, and a mouse monoclonal antibody (P1) raised to human glomerular basement membrane, bind only to glomerular basement membrane, distal tubular basement membrane, and Bowman's capsule, but not to other renal basement membranes. They also bind to alveolar basement membrane in the lung, and to a few other sites, including basement membranes of the choroid plexus, lens, choroid and retina of the eye, and the cochlea. This pattern of distribution explains the principal clinical features of rapidly progressive glomerulonephritis and lung haemorrhage, and rarely patients with choroid plexus or retinal involvement have been described.

The antigenic target of antiglomerular basement membrane antibodies has been localized to type IV collagen, a major structural component of the glomerular basement membrane. Type IV collagen molecules are linked to form a three-dimensional network common to all basement membranes. Each collagen molecule comprises a triple helix of α-chains, typically two $\alpha1(IV)$- and one $\alpha2(IV)$-chains. However, it has been found that glomerular basement membrane possesses an additional network of 'novel' $\alpha(IV)$-chains, which so far includes $\alpha3$, $\alpha4$, and $\alpha5$. There is evidence, from studies of biochemically separated glomerular basement membrane, that autoantibodies bind principally to the non-collagenous (NC1) domain of the $\alpha3(IV)$-chain. The gene encoding this protein (COL4A3) has recently been cloned and sequenced, and localized to chromosome 2.

Cell-mediated immunity

Although there is good evidence that antiglomerular basement membrane antibodies are pathogenic, it is also clear that cell-mediated immunity plays a role in pathogenesis. First, the restricted specificity of the antibody response, and the strong HLA class II associations, make it highly likely that autoantibody production is T-cell dependent. Thus, the induction of the disease presumably involves antigen-specific T-helper cells. Secondly, infiltration of the glomeruli and interstitium by T-cells and macrophages is observed on renal biopsy, suggesting a direct role for cell-mediated immunity in tissue injury. Several attempts have been made to identify T-cell responses to glomerular basement membrane antigens in patients with antiglomerular basement membrane disease, but this has proved difficult, largely due to lack of sufficiently pure antigen preparations.

CLINICAL FEATURES

Most presenting symptoms can be related directly to rapidly progressive glomerulonephritis or lung haemorrhage, although a proportion of patients complain of minor non-specific features of malaise. Tiredness and dyspnoea may be due to anaemia, which can be severe even in the absence of haemoptysis and is probably caused by subclinical lung haemorrhage.

The renal manifestations of antiglomerular basement membrane disease are similar to those of other causes of rapidly progressive glomerulonephritis (see above), except that renal function may be lost even more rapidly—sometimes within days. There are no clinical features specific for antiglomerular basement membrane nephritis, but the absence of signs of systemic vasculitis is of help in the differential diagnosis. The diagnosis can be confirmed by the detection of circulating antiglomerular basement membrane antibodies by various solid-phase immunoassays, most of which are rapid, sensitive, and specific.

Although treatment may be started on the basis of the immunoassay result, renal biopsy remains the definitive investigation. Early changes are of a focal and segmental proliferative glomerulonephritis, progressing to a more diffuse nephritis with focal necrosis and extensive crescent formation. There is usually accompanying interstitial inflammation. Direct immunofluorescence shows linear deposits of IgG along the glomerular basement membrane and sometimes distal tubular basement membrane (Plate 1). IgA and/or IgM are present in addition to IgG in up to a third of cases, and rarely IgA or IgM are deposited alone. Complement component C3 is detected in about two-thirds of cases. On electron microscopy there is usually irregular thickening and mottling of the glomerular basement membrane, with intermittent breaks in its continuity.

About two-thirds of patients are reported to have pulmonary haemorrhage in recent series based on detection of antiglomerular basement membrane antibodies. There is sometimes a history of intermittent haemoptysis and dyspnoea over months or years, but others may present with massive haemoptysis or with dyspnoea alone. Smoking history is important, since almost all current smokers have lung haemorrhage whereas it is rare in non-smokers. Findings on clinical examination depend upon the severity of lung haemorrhage, and can be normal or reveal tachypnoea, cyanosis, or inspiratory crackles throughout the lung fields.

The radiological appearances are non-specific, and comprise alveolar shadowing, generally in the central and lower lung fields. These changes are usually symmetrical, and often transgress the fissures. They can clear rapidly, usually within days, and no long-term sequelae are apparent radiologically. Since similar appearances can result from fluid overload or infection, and since haemoptysis is not invariable, additional information is required to diagnose lung haemorrhage. The corrected carbon monoxide uptake, or KCO, is a sensitive test for lung haemorrhage, since free haemoglobin in the alveoli leads to an increased value. The KCO is often below normal in patients with renal failure, but a change of greater than 30 per cent from base-line usually indicates haemorrhage. Changes in KCO occur rapidly, and usually precede radiographic changes. Bronchoscopy may reveal haemorrhage, and transbronchial biopsies sometimes, but not always, yield diagnostic material. Histology reveals intra-alveolar haemorrhage accompanied by haemosiderin-laden macrophages and alveolar-cell hyperplasia. The alveolar walls may be thickened with oedema, fibrosis, and an inflammatory infiltrate. Direct immunofluorescence usually shows intermittent linear binding of IgG in areas of lung haemorrhage, but may be negative. Electron microscopy may show thickening and irregularity of the alveolar basement membrane.

TREATMENT AND OUTCOME

The outcome of untreated patients was extremely poor, most dying within 6 months from lung haemorrhage or renal failure. There were early reports that lung haemorrhage improved following bilateral nephrectomy, but these are hard to interpret since haemorrhage tends to be intermittent. Following the introduction of dialysis, patients without severe lung haemorrhage could survive with renal support. On the basis of anecdotal reports it was suggested that steroids and/or other immunosuppressive drugs were of benefit in preserving renal function. However, only those with mild renal disease showed improvement, and the majority continued to do badly.

The introduction of plasma exchange to remove circulating antibodies proved to be the most effective approach. The treatment regimen introduced in the mid-1970s comprised prednisolone, cyclophosphamide, azathioprine, and intensive plasma exchange. This generally led to resolution of pulmonary haemorrhage within a few days, and recovery of renal function in all but the most severely affected cases. The benefit of plasma exchange was soon confirmed, and a similar treatment regimen is now widely used (Table 4). The effects of plasma exchange are not fully understood, but it clearly leads to a rapid disappearance of circulating antibodies when used in conjunction with immunosuppressive drugs. Plasma exchange alone has only a temporary effect on antibody levels, while drug therapy alone acts too slowly to be of immediate benefit. Once antibody levels have been reduced to near background they do not usually rise again, suggesting that the autoreactive lymphocytes have in some way been inactivated. It should be remembered that removal by plasma exchange of other potentially proinflammatory plasma components, such as complement and clotting factors, could also be important.

Because of the rarity and severity of the disease, and the convincing improvement in outcome following the introduction of plasma exchange, there has only been one attempt at a controlled trial. The group receiving drugs and plasma exchange (in a less intensive regimen

Table 4 *Initial treatment of antiglomerular basement membrane (anti-GBM) disease*

Prednisolone 60 mg daily, reducing to 20 mg daily by 4 weeks
Cyclophosphamide 2–3 mg/kg daily (lower dose if > 55 years); discontinued if white cell count < 4.0×10^9/l or in presence of life-threatening infection
Plasma exchange 4 l daily for 5% albumin; continued for 14 days or until anti-GBM antibody levels controlled; fresh, frozen plasma 400 ml given at end of exchange in presence of lung haemorrhage or within 3 days of invasive procedure

After 2–3 months, depending on response, cyclophosphamide is discontinued and prednisolone tapered.

than most) had a better outcome than those receiving drugs alone, but the results were confounded by more severe renal disease in the drug-treated group. Many authors have observed that patients treated with serum creatinine 1 of less than 600 μmol/l frequently recover, whereas those treated later (especially if oliguric) have little chance of regaining renal function. Results of recent series are summarized in Table 5. The decision as to whether dialysis-dependent patients should be treated aggressively must be considered in each individual case, and lung haemorrhage provides a separate indication for treatment. The use of bolus doses of methylprednisolone has been proposed as an alternative to plasma exchange for lung haemorrhage or rapidly declining renal function, but this approach has not been compared with plasma exchange, and several reports suggest that it is ineffective.

Duration of treatment in antiglomerular basement membrane disease depends upon the immunological and clinical response. In general, plasma exchange is continued until antibody levels are close to background and the patient has improved, which usually takes at least 2 weeks. Regular monitoring of renal disease (serum creatinine, urine microscopy) and lung haemorrhage (KCO, radiography, haemoglobin) is required. Cyclophosphamide is continued for 2 to 3 months, and prednisolone tailed off by 6 months. Relapses of clinical disease during the initial treatment period may be provoked by the recurrence of antiglomerular basement membrane antibody, or by non-specific factors such as infection, and in the case of lung haemorrhage by fluid overload or smoking. Such episodes are treated by re-introduction of plasma exchange and by aggressive management of any precipitating factor. Late recurrence of the disease months or years later is rare and should be treated as for the initial episode. As with any other renal disorder, some patients left with significant renal impairment after treatment of the acute episode may show a progressive decline in renal function, despite absence of immunological abnormality or other obvious cause of renal damage.

Renal transplantation

Patients with antiglomerular basement membrane disease can be transplanted successfully, provided they do not have circulating antiglomerular basement membrane antibodies. There are several reports of recurrent antiglomerular basement membrane disease in grafts, with graft loss, when circulating antibodies were present at the time of operation. Rarely, immunological recurrence has followed transplantation and antiglomerular basement membrane antibody levels should therefore be monitored postoperatively. It is reasonable to wait for 6 months after antibody has become undetectable before transplantation.

The development of antiglomerular basement membrane disease after renal transplantation in Alport's syndrome is well recognized. Antiglomerular basement membrane antibodies fail to bind to the glomerular basement membrane of many cases of Alport's syndrome, suggesting an absence or alteration of the Goodpasture antigen in that disorder. This is consistent with an abnormality of the network of 'novel' α-chains in the glomerular basement membrane (see earlier), since the genetic defect in Alport's has been localized to the gene (COL4A5) encoding

Table 5 *Outcome of patients with antiglomerular basement membrane disease treated with immunosupressive drugs and plasma exchange*

| Series | Percentage with independent renal function at 1 year according to initial serum creatinine level (number of cases shown in parentheses) | | Notes on regimen used |
	≤ 600 μmol/l	> 600 μmol/l	
Briggs *et al.* 1979 (*n* = 15)	36(11)	0(4)	Only 4/15 received plasma exchange
Simpson *et al.* 1982 (*n* = 12)	70(10)	0(2)	8/12 received plasma exchange
Johnson *et al.* 1985 (*n* =17)	69(13)	0(4)	Less cyclophosphamide than in Table 4 Half received plasma exchange, but only every third day and using fresh, frozen plasma
Walker *et al.* 1985 (*n* = 22)	82(11)	18(11)	Slightly less cyclophosphamide and plasma exchange than in Table 4
Hammersmith 1976–88 (*n* = 56)	90(21)	11(35)	As Table 4, except some also received azathioprine 1 mg/kg/day

the α5(IV)-chain. Patients with Alport's syndrome may not have developed tolerance to the Goodpasture antigen, and so develop an immune response to antigen in the grafted kidney. Although linear deposits of IgG on the glomerular basement membrane of the graft are often noted, crescentic nephritis is rare and lung haemorrhage has not been reported.

Idiopathic rapidly progressive glomerulonephritis

Crescentic nephritis without significant immune deposits or concomitant systemic disease has been termed idiopathic rapidly progressive glomerulonephritis, to differentiate it from those cases with a proposed cause or association, such as antiglomerular basement membrane disease or systemic lupus erythematosus. Idiopathic rapidly progressive glomerulonephritis has also been referred to as 'pauci-immune' crescentic nephritis, because of the general lack of immune deposits on immunofluorescence. A major re-evaluation of idiopathic rapidly progressive glomerulonephritis has occurred in the past few years, because of the observation of Falk and Jennette in 1988 that patients with this condition frequently have circulating antineutrophil cytoplasmic antibodies. These autoantibodies had previously been described in association with Wegener's granulomatosis and microscopic polyarteritis, which are both small-vessel vasculitides within the spectrum of primary systemic vasculitis.

The renal lesions occurring in systemic vasculitis have many characteristics in common with those of idiopathic rapidly progressive glomerulonephritis, including a similar histological and immunohistological appearance, natural history, and response to treatment. Furthermore, some patients with idiopathic rapidly progressive glomerulonephritis have subsequently been observed to develop features of systemic vasculitis. With the recognition of a similar autoantibody response in these patients, it is now becoming accepted that idiopathic rapidly progressive glomerulonephritis most often represents a renal-limited variant of small-vessel vasculitis. There are occasional patients in whom antineutrophil cytoplasmic antibodies are not detectable, and some authors maintain that there is a subgroup of idiopathic rapidly progressive glomerulonephritis unrelated to vasculitis. The aetiology, clinical features, and management of idiopathic rapidly progressive glomerulonephritis are essentially the same as those of rapidly progressive glomerulonephritis in systemic vasculitis, which is considered in Chapter 18.11.2.

The response to treatment of the renal lesion in idiopathic rapidly progressive glomerulonephritis is similar to that in systemic vasculitis, provided that comparison is made between patients with a similar degree of renal impairment. Reports that idiopathic rapidly progressive glomerulonephritis responds less well to treatment are probably due to the fact that it presents at a later stage because the clinical features are less apparent. The outcome in these patients is difficult to analyse, because different authors have included various diagnostic groups and used a variety of treatment regimens. However, in recent series using a combination of corticosteroids and cytotoxic drugs, the 1-year survival was generally over 70 per cent. The addition of either pulse methylprednisolone or plasma exchange appears to be of benefit in advanced cases, and dialysis-dependent patients frequently regain independent renal function. In one controlled trial, including patients with systemic vasculitis and idiopathic rapidly progressive glomerulonephritis, those receiving plasma exchange in addition to drug therapy were more likely to come off dialysis than those receiving drugs alone. This outcome differs from that observed in patients with antiglomerular basement membrane disease, who rarely recover renal function once oliguric. It is therefore reasonable to treat all patients with idiopathic rapidly progressive glomerulonephritis with an aggressive immunosuppressive regimen. As in systemic vasculitis, relapses of idiopathic rapidly progressive glomerulonephritis may occur, and maintenance therapy is usually necessary.

Rapidly progressive glomerulonephritis in other disorders

Other causes of rapidly progressive glomerulonephritis are summarized in Table 1, and only aspects of management peculiar to rapidly progressive glomerulonephritis will be considered. Proliferative lupus nephritis generally responds well to high-dose oral steroids together with oral or intravenous pulses of cyclophosphamide. The addition of pulse doses of methylprednisolone or of plasma exchange has been proposed in severe crescentic nephritis, although neither approach has been subjected to adequate trials. Methylprednisolone in this situation may exacerbate hypertension or hypervolaemia, and is associated with a high risk of infection. A recent controlled trial of plasma exchange in proliferative lupus nephritis did not show an overall benefit, but its use in patients with rapidly progressive glomerulonephritis or severe systemic vasculitis should be considered. In essential mixed cryoglobulinaemia with rapidly progressive glomerulonephritis, the addition of plasma exchange to immunosuppressive drugs is logical, since this will reduce the concentration of the potentially pathogenic cryoglobulin. Although there is little convincing evidence in favour of specific treatment in Henoch–Schönlein purpura associated with rapidly progressive glomerulonephritis, recovery has been reported after the use of an immunosuppressive regimen similar to that used in primary systemic vasculitis. Occasional patients with crescentic changes superimposed on IgA nephropathy have responded to similar manoeuvres, but treatment of other forms of primary glomerulonephritis complicated by rapidly progressive glomerulonephritis is generally unsuccessful.

FURTHER READING

Bolton, W.K. and Sturgill, B.C. (1989). Methyl prednisolone therapy for acute crescentic rapidly progressive glomerulonephritis. *American Journal of Nephrology.* **9**, 368–75.

Briggs, W.A., Johnson, J.P., Teichman, S., Yeager, H.C., and Wilson, C.B. (1979). Antiglomerular basement membrane antibody-mediated glomerulonephritis and Goodpasture's syndrome. *Medicine (Baltimore)* **58**, 348–61.

Couser, W.G. (1988). Rapidly progressive glomerulonephritis: classification, pathogenetic mechanisms, and therapy. *American Journal of Kidney Diseases* **11**, 449–64.

Falk, R. and Jennette, J.C. (1988). Antineutrophil cytoplasmic antibodies with specificity for myeloperoxidase in patients with systemic vasculitis and idiopathic necrotising and crescentic glomerulonephritis. *New England Journal of Medicine* **318**, 1651–57.

Goodpasture, E.W. (1919). The significance of certain pulmonary lesions in relation to the etiology of influenza. *American Journal of Medical Science* **158**, 863–70.

Heaf, J.G., Jorgensen, F., and Neilsen, L.P. (1983). Treatment and prognosis of extracapillary glomerulonephritis. *Nephron* **35**, 211–14.

Johnson, J.P., Moore, J., Austin, H.A., Balow, J.E., Antonovych, T.T., and Wilson, C.B. (1985). Therapy of anti-glomerular basement membrane antibody disease: analysis of prognostic significance of clinical, pathologic and treatment factors. *Medicine (Baltimore)* **64**, 219–27.

Lerner, R.A., Glassock, R.J., and Dixon, F.J. (1967). The role of anti-glomerular basement membrane antibody in the pathogenesis of human glomerulonephritis. *Journal of Experimental Medicine* **126**, 989–1004.

Pusey, C.D., Rees, A.J., Evans, D.J., Peters, D.K., and Lockwood, C.M. (1991). A randomised controlled trial of plasma exchange in focal necrotising glomerulonephritis without anti-GBM antibodies. *Kidney International* **40**, 757–63.

Pusey, C.D., and Rees, A.J. (1992). Acute renal failure due to vasculitis and glomerulonephritis. In *Oxford textbook of clinical nephrology*, (ed. J.S. Cameron, A.M. Davison, J.-P. Grunfeld, D.N.S. Kerr, and E. Ritz), pp. 1060–76. Oxford University Press, Oxford.

Simpson, I.J., *et al.* (1982). Plasma exchange in Goodpasture's syndrome. *American Journal of Nephrology* **2**, 301–11.

Turner, N., *et al.* (1992). Molecular cloning of the human Goodpasture antigen demonstrates it to be the α3 chain of type IV collagen. *Journal of Clinical Investigation* **89**, 592–601.

Turner, A.N. and Rees, A.J. (1992). Antiglomerular basement membrane disease. In *Oxford textbook of clinical nephrology*, (ed. J.S. Cameron, A.M. Davison, J.-P. Grunfeld, D.N.S. Kerr, and E. Ritz), pp. 438–56. Oxford University Press, Oxford.

Walker, R.G., Scheinkestel, C., Becker, G.J., Owen, J.E., Dowling, J.P., and Kincaid Smith, P. (1985). Clinical and morphological aspects of the management of crescentic anti-glomerular basement membrane antibody (anti-GBM) nephritis/Goodpasture's syndrome. *Quarterly Journal of Medicine* **54**, 75–89.

Wilkowski, M.J., *et al.* (1989). Risk factors in idiopathic renal vasculitis and glomerulonephritis. *Kidney International* **36**, 1133–41.

20.5 Renal manifestations of systemic disease

20.5.1 Diabetic nephropathy

E. RITZ, D. FLISER, and M. SIEBELS

Definition

Diabetic nephropathy is one particular facet of diabetic microangiopathy. The hallmark of the renal lesion is a particular form of glomerulosclerosis (Fig. 1) which is associated with arteriolar hyalinosis and interstitial fibrosis. Increased urinary albumin excretion is the first clinical manifestation. Once overt albuminuria is present, diabetic nephropathy will inexorably progress to endstage renal failure, although this course may be modified by therapeutic intervention. The development of diabetic nephropathy is of paramount importance for the survival of the diabetic patient, not only because of its consequences for renal prognosis, but also because it is strongly correlated to the risk of coronary disease and of cardiovascular death.

History

The occurrence of renal problems in the diabetic patient has been recognized for centuries, but the specificity of the renal lesion was documented relatively recently and proof for the efficacy of therapeutic interventions (optimal metabolic control, antihypertensive treatment, protein-restricted diets) has been provided only in the past decade.

Cotugno, in 1764, was the first to describe proteinuria in diabetics, and the frequent occurrence of renal failure was commented upon by Rayer (1840) and Griesinger (1859). In 1936, Kimmelstiel and Wilson recognized the specificity of the nodular glomerular intercapillary lesion for diabetes and its link to a clinical syndrome of proteinuria, hypertension, and progressive renal failure. It took another decade before Lund-

baek recognized that the renal changes are a part of a generalized syndrome of diabetic microangiopathy.

Epidemiology

Up to 30 per cent of patients with type 1 diabetes develop albuminuria. Renal involvement is more frequent in the male and is particularly frequent in patients who develop diabetes in the second decade of life.

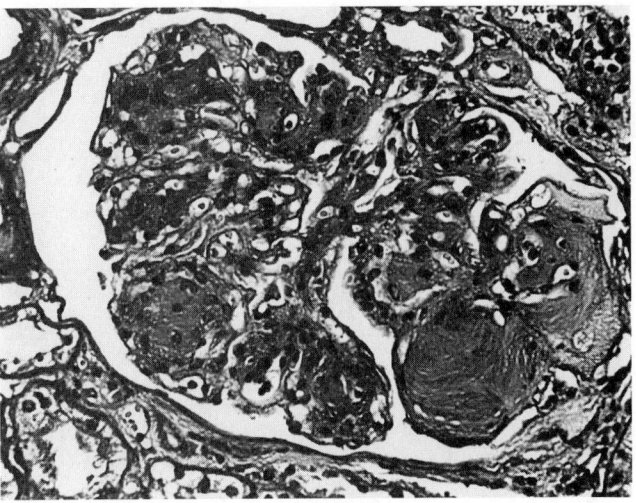

Fig. 1 Glomerulus from a patient with nodular diabetic glomerulosclerosis. Note the presence of two well developed acellular nodules in peripheral lobules (Masson trichrome stain, × 440). (By courtesy of Professor R. Waldherr, Department of Pathology, Heidelberg.)

Recently a trend has been noted towards a decrease in the frequency of nephropathy and a slower rate of progression in those affected, perhaps related to better metabolic control and blood pressure control, respectively.

Diabetic nephropathy was once thought an uncommon complication of type 2 diabetes because only 5 per cent of patients reached endstage renal failure. As shown in Fig. 2, however, the prevalence of proteinuria for any given duration of the disease is comparable in type 1 and type 2 diabetics, and so is the prevalence of renal failure. It appears that with current improvements in overall management, more of the elderly type 2 diabetics survive to experience renal failure. Even so, at the time of diagnosis of type 2 diabetes up to 40 per cent of patients already have albuminuria and 30 to 40 per cent of patients currently admitted for renal replacement therapy suffer from diabetic nephropathy.

In the past, once albuminuria was demonstrable, median survival was only 7 years and median time to the onset of endstage renal failure was around 10 years. Death usually occurred from cardiovascular causes and not from renal failure. Recently, both renal and overall prognosis have improved so that the 10-year survival of albuminuric diabetic patients is currently approximately 80 per cent.

Albuminuria is closely linked to the presence of risk factors for coronary artery disease, particularly dyslipidaemia and elevated lipoprotein a, but the excess cardiovascular risk is not explained by known risk factors alone. As shown in Fig. 3, the relative mortality (mortality relative to that of the matched general population) is strikingly higher in insulin-dependent diabetics with proteinuria, but only marginally higher in the diabetic patient without proteinuria. Although definite evidence is not yet available, it appears possible that albuminuria is a marker of a more generalized endothelial cell dysfunction. This may be present in

the microcirculation not only of the glomerulus, but also in that of the coronary arteries. A 'leaky endothelium' might then permit filtration of albumin into Bowman's space, and, in parallel, insudation of lipoproteins into the vascular wall of coronary arteries, thus promoting atherogenesis.

Evolution of diabetic nephropathy

Diabetic nephropathy has a rather predictable course. It can conveniently be categorized into different stages which differ with respect to renal haemodynamics, systemic blood pressure, urinary findings, and susceptibility to therapeutic interventions (Table 1). Early on there is renal overperfusion, accompanied by renal and glomerular hypertrophy. These changes are only partially reversible with insulin treatment. The first evidence of nephropathy demonstrable by clinical methods is a modestly elevated rate of urinary excretion of albumin (microalbuminuria; see below). Once microalbuminuria is established, blood pressure rises first within the range of normotension (according to WHO definition, that is < 140/90 mmHg), and only later reaches the range of established hypertension. Renal failure ensues after a median interval of approximately 10 to 20 years.

Pathophysiology of diabetic nephropathy

Since only some patients develop diabetic nephropathy, hyperglycaemia on its own is not a sufficient condition for the development of the nephropathy of patients with either type 1 or type 2 diabetes. Diabetic siblings of propositi who suffer from diabetic nephropathy have an 83 per cent risk of developing diabetic nephropathy, whereas the risk is only 17 per cent for diabetic siblings of propositi without nephropathy. A similar role of genetic predisposition to diabetic nephropathy has also been documented in type 2 diabetes. It is currently under investigation whether such predisposition is related to the genetic trait of primary (essential) hypertension, and, more specifically, to increased Na^+/Li^+ countertransport activity (as a surrogate marker for Na^+/proton exchange). The risk of developing diabetic nephropathy is particularly

Fig. 2 Similar risk of nephropathy in type I and type II diabetes. Cumulative prevalence of persistent proteinuria in type II and type I patients (a) and cumulative prevalence of renal failure, i.e. serum creatinine 1.4 mg/dl, in proteinuric type I and type II patients (b). (After E. Ritz *et al.* (1990). *Hypertension Pathophysiology Diagnosis and Management* (eds. J.H. Laragh and B.M. Brenner) pp. 1703–15. Raven Press, New York.)

Fig. 3 Cardiovascular mortality in insulin-dependent diabetics depends on proteinuria. Relative mortality from cardiovascular disease in insulin-dependent diabetics with persistent proteinuria (----) and without proteinuria (----). (After K. Borch-Johnsen and S. Kreiner. (1987). *British Medical Journal*, **294**, 1651–54.)

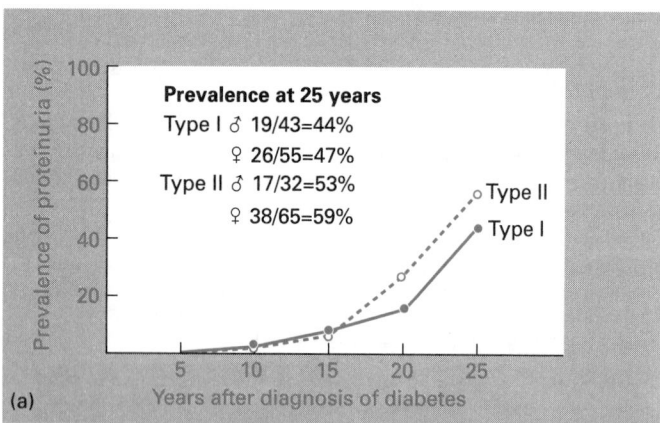

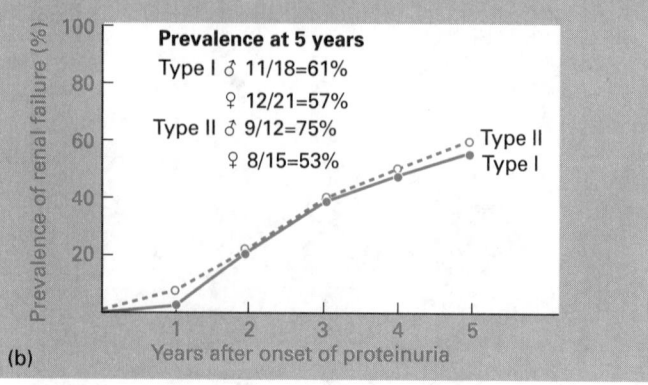

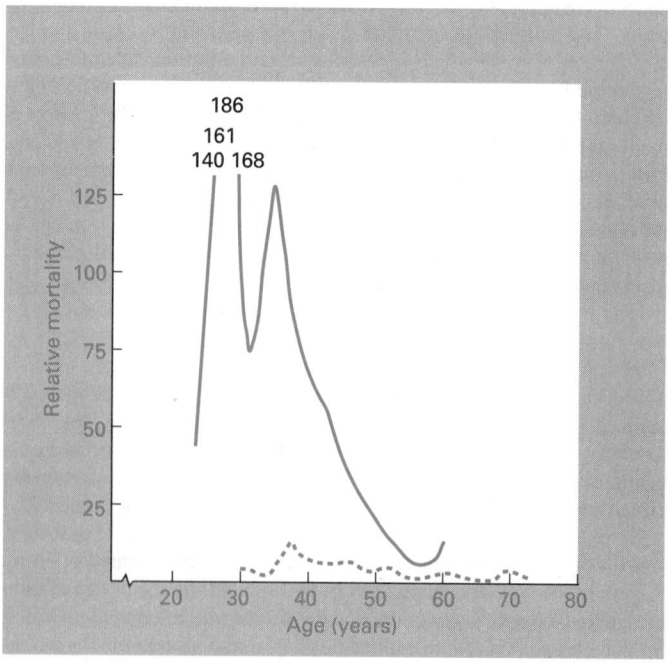

Table 1 *The stages of diabetic nephropathy—typical findings*

Stage	Glomerular filtration	Albuminuria	Blood pressure	Time course (years after diagnosis)
Renal hyperfunction	Elevated	Absent	Normal	At diagnosis
Clinical latency	High normal	Absent	Normal	
Microalbuminuria (= incipient nephropathy)	Within the normal range	20–200 µg/min (~ 30–300 mg/day)	Rising within or above normal range	5–15
Macroalbuminuria or persisting proteinuria (= clinically manifest nephropathy)	Decreasing	> 200 µg/min (> 300 mg/day)	increased	10–15
Renal failure	Diminished	Massive	Increased	15–30

great in genetically predisposed individuals (with high Na^+/Li^+ countertransport) who have poor metabolic control.

The mechanisms by which hyperglycaemia might be injurious have not been completely clarified. It appears possible, that glycation reactions (non-enzymatic reactions between glucose and amino groups of polypeptides) are involved. Glycation of protein ultimately leads to cross-linking of proteins and formation of advanced glycosylation end products. Glycation of the glomerular basement membrane may interfere with its breakdown and reduce its turnover, thus promoting its thickening. It may similarly predispose to accumulation of mesangial matrix. Aminoguanidine interferes with glycation reactions, but whether it has a beneficial effect on nephropathy in experimental or clinical diabetes is still controversial.

Another potential pathway is accumulation of sorbitol as a consequence of increased availability of glucose for reduction by aldose reductase in tissues with insulin-independent glucose uptake, such as mesangial cells. Excess sorbitol is thought to lead to osmotic damage to glomerular cells. Again, the beneficial effect of specific inhibitors of aldose reductase, the rate-limiting enzyme in the synthesis of sorbitol, on the development of glomerular pathology is controversial.

Of particular interest are recent findings of a reduced glycosaminoglycan, and particularly heparan sulphate, content of glomerular basement membranes. These observations are of note because polyanionic substances are responsible, at least in part, for the fixed negative charges of the glomerular basement membrane. They account for charge selectivity of the glomerular basement membrane which is responsible for restricted filtration of polyanionic macromolecules (such as albumin).

Alterations of glomerular haemodynamics may also be involved in the genesis of diabetic nephropathy. In experimental diabetes, renal perfusion, glomerular filtration, and glomerular capillary pressures are elevated, and this is associated with dilatation of both the afferent and efferent arterioles. Similarly, in those with untreated diabetes, the glomerular filtration rate and renal plasma flow are increased (unless hyperglycaemia is very severe). These abnormalities are partially reversed by institution of insulin treatment. Manoeuvres which reverse the elevation of glomerular filtration in experimental animals, for example antihypertensive treatment (particularly angiotensin-converting enzyme inhibitors) or a low-protein diet, will also reduce albuminuria and glomerular lesions, but extrapolation from rats (that do not develop Kimmelstiel–Wilson's glomerulosclerosis) to humans is problematical. An alternative, or complementary, pathogenetic pathway appears to be glomerular and renal hypertrophy, a common feature of diabetes in animals and humans. In several rodent models of renal damage the effects of glomerular hypertension and glomerular hypertrophy on the development of glomerulosclerosis can be dissociated, despite the presence of glomerular hypertension glomerulosclerosis developed only when glomeruli had undergone hypertrophy. It is therefore of note that renal hypertrophy of diabetic patients is not completely reversed even by closely controlled insulin treatment.

Albuminuria and proteinuria

Although there is some evidence of impaired tubular function in diabetics, particularly in those with poor metabolic control, it is commonly assumed that the presence of albumin in the urine points to disturbed glomerular permselectivity. Glomerular filtration of proteins depends on the size and the charge of the circulating molecule, as well as on the transcapillary pressure gradient. In diabetics, the presumed concentration of albumin in Bowman's space rises out of proportion to the concentration of other serum proteins; this is though to result from a selective loss of negative charges of the glomerular capillaries, favouring transcapillary passage of the polyanionic albumin molecule. Such loss of charge is apparently the consequence of depletion of heparan sulphate (see above). Only when glomerular damage is advanced do other serum proteins (IgG, lipoproteins, and others) permeate. With the use of dextran marker molecules it has been shown that such non-selective proteinuria is due to abnormal sieving characteristics leading to the appearance of pathways not dependent on molecular size, so-called shunt pathways. Dysfunction of endothelial cells is a well-known feature of diabetes, but the extent to which this might contribute to abnormal glomerular permselectivity, or to disturbed glomerular haemodynamics and mesangial cell dysfunction, is currently under investigation.

Blood pressure in diabetic nephropathy

Patients with type 1 diabetes are usually normotensive until albuminuria has supervened. Once microalbuminuria (see below) has appeared, blood pressure starts to rise; concomitantly, an abnormal circadian blood pressure profile is noted with a diminished nocturnal fall and excessive increments during exercise. The close relationship between elevated blood pressure and evidence of renal damage in type 1 diabetes suggests that the hypertension is the consequence of renal parenchymal changes. Renal sodium retention and increased responsiveness to pressor agents appear likely contributors to the raised pressure. Sodium retention is demonstrable even in non-hypertensive diabetics.

The relationship between nephropathy and hypertension is more complex in type 2 diabetics. Such patients have usually been hypertensive for years and decades prior to the onset of overt diabetes. At the time of diagnosis of type 2 diabetes, hypertension is found in approximately 70 to 80 per cent of the patients. Still, blood pressure rises further in those patients who subsequently develop diabetic nephropathy. An increased pulse pressure secondary to diminished aortic elasticity is also a feature, particularly of elderly type 2 diabetic patients. As a consequence, isolated systolic hypertension may be present (elevated systolic pressure without elevation of diastolic pressure) and this is linked to higher cardiovascular mortality even when the mean arterial pressure is normal.

A causal role for hypertension in the progression of nephropathy is suggested by studies documenting that lowering of blood pressure by antihypertensive agents reduces the rate of decrease of glomerular filtration.

Management of the patient with diabetic nephropathy

CLINICAL EVALUATION

Diagnostic strategies will depend on clinical circumstances. The asymptomatic diabetic patient must be monitored regularly for the presence of albuminuria and elevated blood pressure as early indicators of nephropathy.

Albuminuria

Albuminuria is the earliest and most sensitive indicator of diabetic nephropathy. The upper normal range of urinary protein excretion is 150 mg/24 h, but the greater part of the protein content of normal urine is of tubular or postrenal origin, so that total urinary protein excretion is not a sensitive index of glomerular damage. Direct determination of urinary albumin greatly improves sensitivity. The upper limit of albumin excretion is 30 mg/24 h, equivalent to approximately 20 μg/min.

Rates of albumin excretion below approximately 200 μg/min (or 300 mg/day) are not readily detected by conventional 'stix' routine methods of assessing proteinuria. More sensitive methods, such as enzyme-linked immunosorbent assays (ELISA), radioimmunoassay, and, more recently, dipsticks, have been developed to recognize incipient elevation of albumin excretion, so-called microalbuminuria. Albumin excretion is quite variable from day to day. It also increases during physical exercise, upright position (orthostasis), and when metabolic control or diabetes is poor, and it cannot be properly evaluated in the presence of urinary tract infection or other renal pathology. To minimize these confounding effects, it is best to examine early morning urine samples on at least three occasions. The diagnosis of microalbuminuria should be made only when, during a period of 6 months, three independent measurements confirm albumin excretion between 20 and 200 μg/min in morning urine specimens (approximately equivalent to 30–300 mg/24 h). The amount of albumin excreted is clearly related to blood pressure (Fig. 4) and is effectively reduced by antihypertensive treatment.

Fig. 4 Progression of microalbuminuria and loss of glomerular filtration depend on blood pressure. The graph gives the theoretical threshold of mean arterial blood pressure (MAP) for progression in microalbuminuria (95 mmHg) and the rate of decrease of GFR (105 mmHg) in insulin-dependent diabetic patients. (After C.E. Mogensen. (1992). In V.E. Andreucci, and L.G. Fine (eds.) *International Yearbook of Nephrology*, p. 141. Springer, London.)

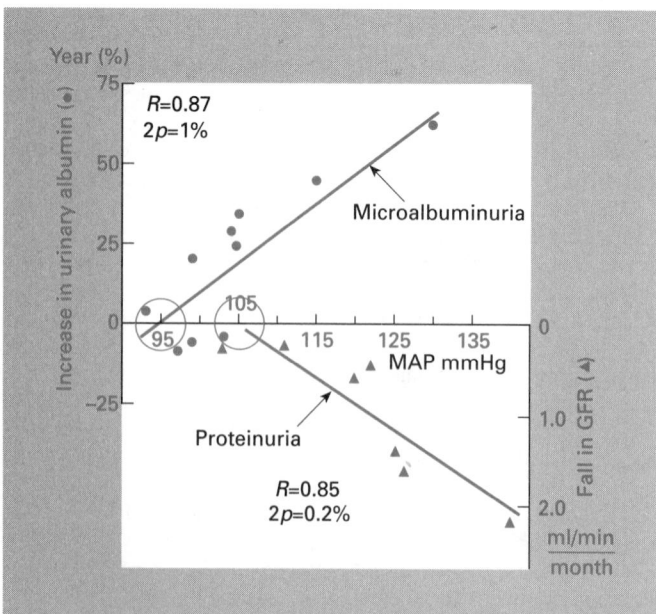

With progression of nephropathy, albumin excretion exceeds the arbitrary level of 300 mg/24 h, first intermittently and later permanently (so-called macroalbuminuria). Protein excretion can then be detected reliably even when using only the insensitive conventional methods, such as sulphosalicyclic acid and the biuret test. In the later stages, proteinuria may be in the nephrotic range of 3.5 g/24 h/1.73 m². Oedema, a common problem in the diabetic with renal failure, is poorly related to the amount of albumin lost in the urine. Nevertheless, the presence of heavy proteinuria is indicative of a particularly adverse renal prognosis.

Hypertension

In view of evidence that lowering raised blood pressure reduces albuminuria and attenuates progression of diabetic nephropathy, it is particularly important to detect hypertension accurately and early in order to institute prompt antihypertensive intervention.

Because of the variability of blood pressure, and the difficulty in taking casual pressures in excluding an 'alarm reaction' (white-coat hypertension), it is best to educate the patient to measure pressures at home or to use well-validated ambulatory devices. Echocardiography can be used to assess left ventricular hypertrophy. Because of the possibility of autonomic polyneuropathy and resultant susceptibility to an orthostatic fall in pressure, blood pressure should be checked on standing at regular intervals.

Renal function

Serum creatinine is commonly used as an index of the glomerular filtration rate, but there are particular problems with this method in diabetes; it does not adequately reflect the initial fall in glomerular filtration rate when it decreases from hyperfiltration through 'pseudonormal' filtration to frankly reduced rates. It also seriously underestimates the magnitude of loss of glomerular filtration rate in wasted diabetic patients with reduced muscular mass. In addition, methods to measure creatinine give spuriously elevated values in the presence of ketone bodies. On the other hand, endogenous creatinine clearance usually overestimates glomerular filtration rate. In patients with diabetic nephropathy, who are not on antihypertensive medication, the glomerular filtration rate decreases at an average rate of 10 ml/min each year, but the rate varies markedly between individuals. It is important to detect causes other than diabetic nephropathy when there is an unexpected increase in serum creatinine; these might include the effects of radiological contrast media, urinary tract infection with papillary necrosis, urinary tract obstruction, uncontrolled hypertension, congestive heart failure, untoward reactions to drugs, particularly non-steroidal anti-inflammatory agents and angiotensin-converting enzyme inhibitors, or hypovolaemia.

Differential diagnosis

Diabetic nephropathy is rare before the tenth year of diabetes, at least in type 1 disease, and is almost always associated with diabetic retinopathy. A cause of renal dysfunction other than diabetic nephropathy should be sought therefore when the onset is unexpectedly early and when there is no evidence of any diabetic retinopathy. If renal ultrasonography and excretory urography do not give an answer, a renal biopsy may be indicated, particularly when red cell casts are present. In the elderly diabetic, atherosclerotic renal artery stenosis is common and has been found at autopsy in approximately 20 per cent of such patients. This diagnosis may be suggested by finding asymmetry in length and width of the kidneys on ultrasound, particularly when there is clinical or radiological evidence of severe atheroma of the abdominal aorta. A rise in plasma creatinine concentration after therapy with angiotensin-converting enzyme inhibitors is another important clue. Bacteriuria is not strikingly more common in diabetic patients, at least in males, but urinary tract infection is more severe when it happens. Renal papillary necrosis, as well as intrarenal or perinephric abscess formation, must be carefully looked for in the febrile diabetic patient with pyuria and renal dysfunction.

PREVENTION AND TREATMENT

In the past 2 decades, clear evidence has been presented that the evolution of diabetic nephropathy may be influenced by preventive measures.

Metabolic control

There is reasonable evidence that consistently good control of glycaemia will delay the onset of albuminuria and reduce its prevalence. In prospective studies strict metabolic control by continuous subcutaneous insulin infusion or multiple injections of insulin has been shown to reduce albumin excretion in microalbuminuric patients and to prevent the otherwise inexorable increase of albuminuria. Results are less consistent once patients have progressed to the stage of macroalbuminuria. Meticulous correction of hyperglycaemia by continuous subcutaneous insulin infusion failed to alter the rate of decrease in glomerular filtration rate in one study. Others, in contrast, have shown a relationship between HbA1$_c$ levels and the rate of decline of glomerular filtrate rate, even in patients with renal failure.

Control of arterial pressure

A number of controlled prospective trials have shown that reduction in blood pressure has attenuated or even prevented the loss of glomerular filtration rate and reduced albuminuria in patients with diabetic nephropathy. In this context, a hypothesis based on animal studies has been advanced that angiotensin-converting enzyme inhibitors have a specific renoprotective action which may, in part, be related to relief of glomerular hypertension but may also involve non-haemodynamic mechanisms. At any given level of blood pressure, angiotensin-converting enzyme inhibitors reduce albuminuria more markedly than do cardioselective β-blockers. Furthermore, angiotensin-converting enzyme inhibitors may attenuate the decrease in glomerular filtration rate more effectively than do β-blockers (Fig. 5). Angiotensin-converting enzyme inhibitors have also been given to non-hypertensive insulin-dependent patients, and have successfully reduced the rate of microalbuminuria, but whether this will ultimately result in a lower incidence of progressive renal failure will have to be demonstrated by prospective studies. Despite the absence of definite proof, it appears to be acceptable practice to give angiotensin-converting enzyme inhibitors to microalbuminuric

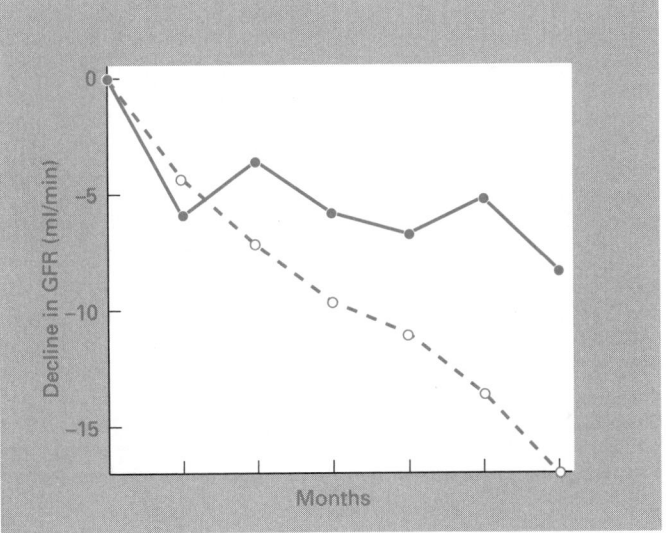

Fig. 5 Angiotensin converting enzyme inhibitors are superior to cardioselective β-blockers in attenuating the rate of decrease of glomerular filtration in 40 insulin-dependent diabetic patients with nephropathy observed over 36 months. Note that GFR declines less and urinary albumin rises less in patients treated with enalapril (●) than with metoprolol (○). (Reproduced from Björck, S.T., Mulec, H. Johnsen, S.A., Norden, G., and Aurell, M. (1992). *British Medical Journal* **304**, 339–43, with permission.)

patients in whom blood pressure starts to rise within the normotensive range.

Low-protein diet

Two studies of diabetic patients with moderately advanced nephropathy have shown a significant reduction of the rate of loss of glomerular filtration rate when dietary protein was restricted to approximately 0.6 to 0.8 g/kg body weight/day. Whether dietary protein is the only component involved in any efficacy of dietary intervention remains unproven; the intake of phosphate and sodium might also be important. It has been suggested that it is dietary restriction of animal protein, particularly red meat, which underlies any beneficial effect of protein-restricted diets. Renal functional changes similar to those produced by a low-protein diet are also seen on a vegetarian diet. Malnutrition and wasting are definite risks of a low-protein diet in diabetics with more advanced renal failure, and it is inadvisable when plasma creatinine levels exceed 500 µmol/l. Such patients rapidly develop profound catabolism during intercurrent illness or deficient intake of energy. Consequently, the diabetic patient on reduced intake of dietary protein requires close monitoring to detect malnutrition, for example regular measurements of serum albumin and anthropometric measurements such as midarm circumference.

The diabetic patient with renal failure

The case for meticulous metabolic control, careful treatment of hypertension, and perhaps some restriction of dietary intake of protein, fats, and salt has been made above, but diabetic patients continue to develop renal failure, ultimately culminating in the need for dialysis or transplantation. As renal failure progresses, the requirement for insulin or oral hypoglycaemic agents tends to fall, but in a way and to a degree that is difficult to predict. Renal catabolism and excretion of insulin is reduced, prolonging its half-life, but there is a coincident trend towards insulin resistance, insulin-dependent glucose uptake being reduced by up to 50 per cent. Consequently, frequent monitoring of blood glucose concentrations and reassessment of insulin requirements are recommended. With the exception of gliquidone, sulphonylurea compounds (or their active metabolites) are eliminated, at least in part, via the kidney. Because of the combined risks of hypoglycaemia from drug accumulation and from increased insulin half-life, there is need for particular care in the use of oral hypoglycaemic agents in uraemic diabetics. Metformin should never be used in the presence of renal failure because of the risk of lactic acidosis.

Values of HbA1$_c$ may be spuriously elevated in uraemia because of carbamylation of haemoglobin; but measurements by high-pressure liquid chromatography are less susceptible to this artefact.

There may be particular difficulty in controlling arterial pressure in diabetics with nephropathy, who are often particularly susceptible to salt and volume loads; and may require massive diuretic therapy. When control of arterial pressure is particularly difficult and renal failure advanced, it is often wise to start dialysis early to allow better correction of hypervolaemia and the associated hypertension. A particular problem is the combination of orthostatic hypotension with supine hypertension in nephropathic diabetic patients suffering from autonomic nephropathy. In these patients orthostatic hypotension may be further aggravated by hypovolaemia resulting from intense diuretic treatment. More than one antihypertensive agent is almost always required in the diabetic patient with advanced renal failure; a combination of diuretics (loop agents and thiazides), angiotensin-converting enzyme inhibitors, and calcium antagonists is often best. There is a reluctance by some to use β-blockers because of their untoward metabolic effect, but they should surely be given to the diabetic with ischaemic heart disease, albeit with consideration of the tendency for some cardioselective β-blockers to accumulate in renal failure. When angiotensin-converting enzyme inhibitors are administered there may be an abrupt increase of plasma creatinine, particularly, but not exclusively, in the presence of renal artery stenosis and when the glomerular filtration rate is less than 20 to 30 ml/min. There can be a significant rise in plasma potassium, to dangerous levels in the elderly diabetic with hyporeninaemic hypoaldosteronism (see Chapter 20.2.3). Evidence that insulin sensitivity is reduced by β-blockers, somewhat increased by angiotensin-converting enzyme inhibitors, and unchanged by calcium-channel blockers appears of little clinical importance in the patient taking insulin.

CARDIAC DISEASE

This is extremely common in the diabetic with nephropathy and is the single most common cause of death. Ischaemic heart disease is particularly common but may remain asymptomatic because of afferent denervation as a result of polyneuropathy. An abrupt onset of pulmonary oedema or congestive heart failure in such patients may be the first indication of severe ischaemic heart disease, particularly in the presence of renal dysfunction. Because silent disease of the coronary arteries is so common in diabetic endstage renal failure, some units undertake routine coronary angiograms in diabetics considered for renal transplantation.

DYSLIPIDAEMIA

This is also common in the nephropathic diabetic and is more severe, at any given level of glomerular filtration, than in the non-diabetic uraemic patient. The most common feature is hypertriglyceridaemia, resulting from accumulation of triglyceride-rich very low density lipoprotein (VLDL), associated with low high-density lipoprotein and inconstant elevation of cholesterol. Lp(a) is also high. Serum cholesterol is a strong predictor of cardiac death in the dialysed diabetic. Although no definite proof for the efficacy of the treatment is available, it appears sensible to advise reduced intake of saturated fat and to administer lipid-lowering agents, fibrates, or statins as indicated.

MANAGEMENT

At one time, most diabetics were severely cachectic by the time they were admitted to renal replacement therapy. Cachexia was the result of a combination of anorexia with poor intake of nutrients, poor glycaemic control, superimposed illness, particularly infection, and superimposition of catabolism related to uraemia. It is therefore important to supervise calorie and nutrient intake. If wasting develops, it may be wise to start dialysis early.

Diabetics, particularly elderly diabetic women, often have poor vessels with which to create vascular access. It is therefore good practice to create vascular access early, for example when serum creatinine has exceeded 500 μmol/l.

When the diabetic patient requires renal replacement therapy, three options are available, haemodialysis, continuous ambulatory peritoneal dialysis, or renal transplantation (isolated or combined with pancreatic or islet cell transplantation). There is no doubt that transplantation restores quality of life and rehabilitation best, and is certainly the treatment of choice in the younger patient. Despite past claims that continuous ambulatory peritoneal dialysis is superior to haemodialysis in the older diabetic, the two procedures give very similar results.

When the patient is on dialysis, insulin requirements usually decrease. It is wise to use glucose-containing dialysates, which allow continuation of the usual schedule of insulin administration on and off dialysis. Diabetic patients on dialysis tend to have higher blood pressures and require more antihypertensive agents than non-diabetic patients. Volume control is also more difficult in the diabetic than in the non-diabetic dialysis patient, and removal of excess fluid may require controlled ultrafiltration to avoid hypotensive episodes.

Renal transplantation is usually restricted to younger type 1 diabetics; this is not completely justified since, in selected series, good results have been achieved in type 2 diabetics, if high-risk patients with macrovascular disease have been excluded. Successful transplantation of diabetics has been helped by cyclosporin, which has allowed the use of a lower cumulative dose of steroids. The major causes of death after transplan-

tation are cardiac, specifically coronary, events, but whether clinically latent coronary disease should be dealt with by bypass surgery prior to transplantation is still controversial.

Transplantation of the pancreas from the same donor still presents a number of technical problems, and is not yet a routine procedure. To deal with the exocrine secretions of the pancreas, one strategy is to occlude the pancreatic duct by plastic material, the other (currently more in vogue) is drainage of pancreatic sections into the bladder. Islet transplantation, which eliminates these technical problems, is another approach with obvious potential.

FURTHER READING

Anderson, S. and Brenner, B.M. (1988). Pathogenesis of diabetic glomerulopathy: the role of glomerular hyperfiltration. In *The kidney and hypertension in diabetes mellitus*, (ed. C.E. Mogensen), pp. 139–46. Martinus Nijhoff, Boston.

De Chatel, R. *et al.* (1977). Sodium, renin, aldosterone, catecholamines and blood pressure in diabetes mellitus. *Kidney International*, **12**, 412–21.

DeFronzo, R.A. (1981). The effect of insulin on renal sodium metabolism. *Diabetologia* **21**, 165–71.

Drury, P.L., Smith, G.M., and Ferris, J.B. (1984). Increased vascular responsiveness to angiotensin II in type I (insulin-dependent) diabetic patients without complications. *Diabetologia* **27**, 174–9.

Earle, K., Walker, J., Hill, C., and Viberti, G. (1992). Familial clustering of cardiovascular disease in patients with insulin-dependent diabetes and nephropathy. *New England Journal of Medicine*, **326**, 673–7.

Feldt-Rasmussen, B., Mathiesen, E., and Deckert, T. (1986). Effect of two years of strict metabolic control on the progression of incipient nephropathy in insulin-dependent diabetes. *Lancet* **II**, 1300–4.

Feldt-Rasmussen, B., Mathiesen, E.R., and Deckert, T. (1987). Central role for sodium in the pathogenesis of blood pressure changes independent of angiotensin, aldosterone and catecholamines in type I (insulin-dependent) diabetes mellitus. *Diabetologia* **30**, 610–17.

Ferriss, J.B., *et al.* (1985). Diabetic control and the renin-angiotensin system, catecholamines, and blood pressure. *Hypertension* **7**, (Suppl. II), II-58-II-63.

Friedman, E.A. and L'Esperance, F.A. (1986). *Diabetic renal-retinal syndrome*, Vol. 3, *Therapy*. Grune & Stratton. Orlando, Florida, USA.

Hasslacher, C., Stech, W., Wahl, P., and Ritz, E. (1985). Blood pressure and metabolic control as risk factors for nephropathy in type I diabetics. *Diabetologia* **28**, 6–11.

Jarrett, R.J., Viberti, G.C., and Argyropoulos, A. (1984). Microalbuminuria predicts mortality in non-insulin-dependent diabetes. *Diabetic Medicine* **1**, 17–19.

Mogensen, C.E. (1982). Long-term antihypertensive treatment inhibiting progression of diabetic nephropathy. *British Medical Journal* **285**, 685–8.

Mogensen, C.E. (1984). Microalbuminuria predicts clinical proteinuria and early mortality in maturity onset diabetes. *New England Journal of Medicine* **310**, 356–60.

Mogensen, C.E. (1988). *The kidney and hypertension in diabetes mellitus*. Martinus Nijhoff, Boston.

O'Donnell, M.P., Kasiske, B.L., Daniels, F.X., and Keane, W.F. (1986). Effect of nephron loss on glomerular hemodynamics and morphology in diabetic rats. *Diabetes* **35**, 1011–15.

Parving, H.H., Smidt, U.M., Andersen, A.R., and Svendsen, P.A. (1983). Early aggressive antihypertensive treatment reduces rate of decline in kidney function in diabetic nephropathy. *Lancet* **i**, 1175–9.

Seaquist, E.R., Goetz, F.C., Rich, S.T., and Barbosa, J. (1989). Familial clustering of diabetic kidney disease. Evidence for genetic susceptibility to diabetic nephropathy. *New England Journal of Medicine* **320**, 1161–5.

Viberti, G.C., Keen, H., and Wiseman, M.J. (1987). Raised arterial pressure in parents of proteinuric insulin dependent diabetics. *British Medical Journal* **295**, 515–17.

Walker, J.D., *et al.* (1989). Restriction of dietary protein and progression of renal failure in diabetic nephropathy. *Lancet* **ii**, 1411–15.

Zeller, K., Whittaker, E., Sullivan, L., Raskin, P., and Jacobson, H.R. (1991). Effect of restricting dietary protein on the progression of renal failure in patients with insulin-dependent diabetes mellitus. *New England Journal of Medicine* **324**, 78–84.

20.5.2 Infections and associated nephropathies

D. C. WILLIAMS AND D. ADU

INTRODUCTION

Infections of many kinds can be associated with, or be the specific cause of, all clinical syndromes of renal diseases, for example acute tubular necrosis, acute interstitial nephritis, and glomerulonephritis resulting in proteinuria, the nephrotic syndrome, or the nephritic syndrome; obstructive uropathy; and chronic renal failure. The association between infection and the nephropathy may be overt, as in septicaemia with acute renal failure, or covert, for example when membranous glomerulonephritis is ascribed to infection with hepatitis B.

Globally, infection-associated nephropathies are common causes of renal disease, because of the high incidence, of postinfectious and parasite-associated glomerulonephritis in developing countries where the increased prevalence of infections is associated with poor hygiene and nutrition. Conversely, in developed countries the incidence of infection-associated nephropathies has fallen, mainly due to a marked decline in the occurrence of post-streptococcal glomerulonephritis. On the other hand, new infections affecting the kidney are appearing, either *de novo* such as AIDS-associated nephropathy, or due to geographical spread, for example Hantavirus nephropathy which is slowly progressing westward across Europe from Russia and the Far East. In many instances treatment of the infection will reverse, or at least halt progression of renal damage; notable exceptions are the glomerulonephridites due to malaria or schistosomiasis.

The association between infections and nephritis is of considerable interest because the elucidation of pathogenetic mechanisms, important in itself, may also help to define the pathogenesis of apparently idiopathic forms of nephritis. Classical experiments have established that glomerulonephritis can be induced by immunization with antigen, the development of the nephritis then coinciding with the production of specific antibody and the development of circulating antigen–antibody complexes. Many infections lead to the development of a nephritis that appears to be due to antigen–antibody complexes, the antigens being derived from infectious organisms.

The infection-associated nephropathies may be classified in different ways, according to pathogenetic mechanisms, the renal histology, or the nature of the infections themselves. The approach used here is to describe the renal manifestations, which in many instances will also have been defined histologically following a renal biopsy, or structurally following imaging of the renal tract, linked to discussion of the associated infections. Renal amyloidosis secondary to chronic infection, and antibiotic-associated nephropathies arising during the treatment of infections are not included, being described elsewhere (Chapters 20.5.3 and 20.9.1).

Glomerulonephritis

Although data are not firm, glomerulonephritis and its attendant syndromes of acute nephritic syndrome, proteinuria with or without a nephrotic syndrome, and acute or chronic renal failure, probably account for the majority of infection-associated nephropathies.

PATHOGENESIS

Although the precise mechanisms of most of the human nephritides ascribed to infection have not yet been demonstrated conclusively, analogies with experimental disease or circumstantial evidence in man suggest that the following mechanisms may be critically implicated.

Immune complex deposition/formation

Infectious organisms provide the largest number and widest range of exogenous antigens to which the human host makes an immune response, a major part of which (with few exceptions) is antibody formation. Circulating immune complexes can be detected in many infections without a complicating nephritis but in those in which nephritis does develop, hypocomplementaemia and deposition of immunoglobulins, complement, and, in some instances, antigen in glomeruli suggest that antigen–antibody complexes have become localized in the kidney. A variant of this mechanism is the renal deposition of antigen alone, with subsequent formation of antigen–antibody complexes *in situ*. Physical characteristics of the antigens and antibody, and their complexes, such as size, antibody class and subclass, and charge, are important determinants of renal deposition.

Cross-reactive antibodies or molecular mimicry

Among the wide range of antigens presented by infectious organisms, it is likely that there will be some that are sufficiently similar to endogenous antigens to evoke an antibody response cross-reacting with renal tissues with resultant nephropathy.

Polyclonal B-cell activation

Infections usually induce a specific antibody response alone (an oligoclonal B-cell response), when only those few B cells programmed to make the antibodies specific for the antigens of the infective organism will produce antibodies. Some infections, in addition, can stimulate a wide range of B cells whose immunoglobulins are less specific – polyclonal B-cell activation. Some of these latter antibodies may react with antigenic determinants in the host's own tissues. These are usually of lower affinity than antibodies produced in the oligoclonal-specific response and are therefore less likely to cause disease by direct fixation to tissue, but can cause renal damage by deposition of immune complexes in glomeruli.

Cell-mediated immunity

There is histological evidence to suggest that some infection-associated nephritides are caused by lymphocytes which are specifically targeting renal structures. This is particularly so in the case of infection-associated interstitial nephritis.

Post-infectious/acute endocapillary proliferative glomerulonephritis

The most common cause of acute proliferative glomerulonephritis is an infection with group A streptococci, but a similar type of glomerulonephritis has been reported in patients with other bacterial infections, for instance staphylococci, meningococci, *Streptococcus pneumoniae,* and Shigella. Post-streptococcal glomerulonephritis provides the typical model.

CLINICAL FEATURES

The distinctive feature is its development 1 to 2 weeks after a streptococcal pharyngitis or 3 to 6 weeks after skin infection (impetigo). With either site of infection the risk of an ensuing glomerulonephritis is higher in children aged between 2 and 12 years. The disease has become uncommon in Western countries but epidemic outbreaks following skin infections with streptococci still occur in tropical countries, where secondary streptococcal infection of scabies or insect bites is a common cause.

The clinical presentation ranges from asymptomatic haematuria and proteinuria, through an acute nephritic syndrome at times accompanied by nephrotic features, to, rarely, a rapidly progressive glomerulonephritis. The typical patient with an acute nephritic syndrome presents with oliguria, reddish-brown urine due to haematuria, proteinuria, a puffy face, and ankle oedema, often accompanied by hypertension and sometimes left ventricular failure. Headache, vomiting, and fits may also complicate the rise in blood pressure. There is some degree of impairment of glomerular filtration in the majority, usually only slight to moderate, and resolving within 1 to 2 weeks. A nephrotic syndrome is much less common and acute renal failure from extracapillary glomerulonephritis is rare, being found in less than 2 per cent of affected children.

AETIOLOGY AND PATHOGENESIS

Only certain M types (cell wall protein antigens) of Lancefield group A/β haemolytic streptococcal infections are followed by glomerulonephritis, but group C streptococci have also been associated with acute proliferative glomerulonephritis.

The frequent occurrence of hypocomplementaemia supports antigen–antibody-mediated nephritis. Some studies have indicated that the candidate antigen may be a water-soluble extractable antigen termed endostreptosin. Others have suggested that M proteins or M-associated proteins may be the pathogenic antigens, and in yet others, a cationic streptococcal proteinase has been implicated. An alternative mechanism is by way of the production of rheumatoid factor, when anti-IgG autoantibody is made to the host's IgG which has been rendered autoantigenic by removal of its sialic acid by neuraminidase, an enzyme produced by streptococci, as well as by other bacteria and viruses. As well as rheumatoid factors, the sera of some patients with poststreptococcal glomerulonephritis contain antinuclear antibodies, and antistreptococcal antibodies which cross-react with glomerular cell wall components.

Renal biopsies show the typical changes of an acute immune complex nephritis with deposits of C3, IgG, and sometimes IgM in the glomerular mesangium and in large subepithelial deposits (humps) detected by immunofluorescence studies and electron microscopy.

PATHOLOGY

There is increased hypercellularity of glomeruli from mesangial proliferation and an influx of polymorphonuclear leucocytes, monocytes, and T lymphocytes. Extracapillary proliferation (crescents) is infrequent. Rarely, the biopsy of patients with postinfectious glomerulonephritis shows typical mesangiocapillary glomerulonephritis which, in contrast with the idiopathic form of that disorder, usually carries a better prognosis.

SEROLOGY

Antibodies to various streptococcal antigens form the basis of diagnosis where culture techniques have not identified the organism. After streptococcal pharyngitis 95 per cent of children will have an antibody response to streptolysin O, deoxyribonuclease, deoxyribonuclease B, hyaluronidase, and streptokinase. After pyoderma antibody responses to deoxyribonuclease B are found but those to streptolysin O are infrequent. The rate of positive cultures from the site of suspected infection is low, so that failure to grow streptococci does not negate the diagnosis. Low serum concentrations of C3 occur in 80 to 90 per cent of cases and of C4 in a smaller proportion and, where present, they last for 4 to 6 weeks.

MANAGEMENT

All patients should be given a 10 day course of penicillin or erythromycin to eradicate infection and prevent secondary spread, but such treatment has no effect on the outcome of the renal illness. The management of the acute nephritic illness is based on meticulous attention to fluid balance together with diuretics and antihypertensive therapy as necessary. Very few patients will require dialysis.

OUTCOME

The acute illness usually resolves within 1 or 2 weeks, with return of normal renal function, although slight proteinuria and microscopic haematuria may persist for years in 20 per cent of patients. The long-term prognosis of post-streptococcal glomerulonephritis is good and there are few reports of resultant endstage chronic renal failure although in one American study of sporadic post-pharyngitic glomerulonephritis up to 50 per cent of patients ultimately developed some evidence of chronic renal damage, but this work has been criticized on several grounds and does not equate with the experience of most authorities.

Nephritis associated with current infection

Many forms of nephritis complicate infectious disease while the latter is still active. In such cases renal histological changes are much more variable, there is a poorer prognosis for renal function, and there is potential for improving the nephritis by successful eradication of the infection.

Infective endocarditis (see also Chapter 15.17.)

A variety of renal lesions are found in patients with infective endocarditis. These range from focal renal infarcts, glomerulonephritis, which may be of diffuse or focal segmental proliferative types, to acute tubular damage. The most common of these is glomerulonephritis. The incidence of this complication is not clear from recent studies but is probably of the order of 1 per cent. Glomerulonephritis has been reported in patients with acute as well as subacute endocarditis, and has been described with all types of infecting organism.

CLINICAL FEATURES

The presentation is often with an acute nephritic syndrome but some patients have only minimal urinary abnormalities. A small proportion have coincident cutaneous vasculitis and arthralgia.

LABORATORY INVESTIGATIONS

Low serum levels of the complement proteins C3 and C4 are found in approximately 50 per cent of patients and in some patients C3 nephritic factor can also be detected in serum. Circulating immune complexes and cryoglobulins are found in some 50 per cent of patients.

PATHOLOGY

The types of glomerulonephritis described include a focal segmental necrotizing glomerulonephritis, a mesangial proliferative glomerulonephritis, mesangiocapillary glomerulonephritis, and an endocapillary proliferative glomerulonephritis which may be accompanied by extracapillary proliferation (crescent formation). There is no clear association between the infecting organism and the type of glomerulonephritis. Immunohistology shows granular deposits of complement, IgG, IgA, and IgM in the glomerular basement membrane and mesangium. Electron microscopy shows subepithelial, subendothelial, and mesangial electron-dense deposits.

TREATMENT

Successful treatment of infective endocarditis leads to resolution of the glomerulonephritis in most cases. However, patients with extensive extracapillary proliferation (crescent formation) may develop chronic renal failure. Deaths are usually due to the infective endocarditis and not to the renal lesion.

Shunt nephritis

Infection of ventriculoatrial shunts for hydrocephalus is well recognized as a cause of nephritis.

CLINICAL PRESENTATION

The renal presentation is with haematuria which may be gross, and proteinuria which is often heavy enough to cause a nephrotic syndrome. Significant renal impairment is rarely present at diagnosis, but may develop in the absence of successful treatment. Fever is common, and anaemia, arthralgia, and a rash may develop.

AETIOLOGY AND PATHOGENESIS

The most common infective organism is *Staphylococcus epidermidis*, but a wide variety of other organisms has also been implicated in the development of shunt nephritis, including *Staph. aureus, Pseudomonas aeroginosa*, and diphtheroids. Glomerular deposits of IgM and C3, and in some cases of bacterial antigen with low serum complement levels and serum cryoglobulins, point to the glomerulonephritis being mediated by antigen–antibody complexes.

PATHOLOGY

Typically the renal lesion is a subendothelial mesangiocapillary glomerulonephritis with granular deposits of IgM and C3 in the glomerular mesangium and capillary walls, but other histological types of nephritis, for instance focal sclerosing glomerulonephritis, occur.

TREATMENT

Antibiotics alone are usually ineffective in eradicating infection. The shunt catheter should be removed as well; this usually leads to resolution of the nephritis.

Visceral abscesses

Chronic sepsis in the form of visceral abscesses, such as pulmonary, subphrenic, and pelvic abscesses, may be complicated by the development of a glomerulonephritis. The clinical presentation of renal disease, the types of glomerulonephritis, and the outcome with treatment resemble those seen in infective endocarditis.

Septicaemia

Staphylococcal septicaemia can cause a proliferative glomerulonephritis, particularly in intravenous drug abusers.

Typhoid fever

Salmonella typhi infection can be complicated by glomerulonephritis, which may be mesangial proliferative, diffuse proliferative, or IgA nephropathy. The presence of glomerulonephritis increases the mortality of typhoid fever from 5 to 10 per cent to 20 to 30 per cent.

Legionnaire's disease

CLINICAL FEATURES

Proteinuria, microscopic haematuria, and casts are found in 20 to 30 per cent of patients with legionnaire's disease. These features may be accompanied by mild impairment of renal function. Acute renal failure, which may be due to shock, rhabdomyolysis, endotoxaemia, and disseminated intravascular coagulation, develops in 7 to 14 per cent of patients. Renal biopsy typically shows an acute interstitial nephritis or acute tubular necrosis. The mortality in patients with legionnaire's disease who develop acute renal failure is high and ranges from 30 to 50 per cent.

Tuberculosis

Glomerulonephritis of different histological types, with or without detectable granulomata in the kidney, can complicate infection with *Mycobacterium tuberculosis*, most commonly in the presence of pulmonary lesions.

Hepatitis B infection

The renal complications of hepatitis B infection are found mainly in individuals with chronic disease and serological evidence of continued hepatitis B infection. The detection by immunological techniques of hepatitis B antigen or its antibody in affected tissues strongly suggests that the renal injury is immune mediated, although the precise mechanisms are unknown. The major renal lesions of hepatitis B infection are membranous nephropathy and vasculitis.

Hepatitis B-associated membranous nephropathy

CLINICAL FEATURES

This is seen particularly in children who are chronic carriers of hepatitis B virus. The frequency of hepatitis B as a cause of membranous nephropathy parallels the general carrier rate of this virus in the local population. Between 60 and 100 per cent of children with membranous nephropathy in Japan, Hong Kong, South Africa, and Zimbabwe have hepatitis B surface antigenaemia, contrasting with a rate of about 20 per cent in the United States. The rates in adults are less and range from 0 to 4 per cent in the United Kingdom to 30 to 40 per cent in Hong Kong. In children the age of onset is between 2 and 12 years, and over 80 per cent of affected children are male. The clinical presentation is usually with a nephrotic syndrome. Most affected children have no clinical evidence of liver disease, which is more common in adults.

AETIOLOGY AND PATHOGENESIS

The virus is thought to be the antigen in an antigen–antibody complex disease.

SEROLOGY

Sera from almost all patients with hepatitis B-associated membranous nephropathy show evidence of infection in the form of hepatitis B surface antigenaemia, hepatitis Bc antibodies, Be antigenaemia, and Be antibodies.

PATHOLOGY

The histological lesion of hepatitis B-associated membranous nephropathy differs from the idiopathic variety in that, in addition to subepithelial deposits, there are often subendothelial and mesangial deposits.

TREATMENT AND OUTCOME

There is no treatment of proven benefit in hepatitis B-associated membranous nephropathy. There is no evidence that steroids are beneficial and, indeed, their use and withdrawal may lead to rebound hepatitis. α-Interferon and adenosine arabinoside have been used in some patients but with no conclusive evidence of benefit. The prognosis in children is good, with reported spontaneous remissions of the nephrotic syndrome in up to two-thirds of cases.

Hepatitis C associated nephropathy

CLINICAL FEATURES

Hepatitis C virus infection is found in less than 0.6 per cent of the population of North America and Northern Europe but is more common in southern Europe and Africa and has a high prevalence in haemophiliacs and intravenous drug abusers. Hepatitis C infection may lead to chronic active hepatitis and cirrhosis. Hepatitis C infection is the main cause of mixed essential cryoglobulinaemia (Chapter 20.5.3). The renal presentation is with proteinuria or a nephrotic syndrome often accompanied by mild to moderate renal impairment.

PATHOLOGY

The renal lesion in mixed essential cryoglobulinaemia is a membranoproliferative glomerulonephritis Type 1 but other types of glomerulonephritis, e.g., focal and mesangioproliferative glomerulonephritis have been reported and rarely there is a granulomatous renal arteritis. Immunofluorescent microscopy shows subendothelial as well as mesangial and capillary wall deposits of IgM, IgG, and C3. On electron microscopy these deposits may show the characteristics of cryoglobulins. A membranoproliferative glomerulonephritis may also develop in patients without a cryoglobulinaemia.

SEROLOGY

Diagnosis is by serology for antibodies to hepatitis C and this is confirmed by the detection of hepatitis C RNA. Cryoglobulinaemia is often found and typically serum complement levels are low and there is a positive rheumatoid factor.

TREATMENT

Treatment with α-interferon improves liver function and proteinuria and possibly renal function but relapses occur once treatment is discontinued. Anecdotal reports suggest a possible benefit from prednisolone, plasma exchange, and cyclophosphamide but this may be complicated by infections and increasing viraemia with worsening liver function.

Other forms of glomerulonephritis

There are also reports of increased rates of hepatitis B surface antigenaemia in patients with a mesangiocapillary glomerulonephritis and mesangial proliferative glomerulonephritis.

HIV-associated glomerulonephritis

The evidence for a specific glomerulonephritis associated with HIV infection is strong, although it is argued that factors such as intravenous drug abuse or opportunistic infections may be important in the development of the renal lesions.

CLINICAL FEATURES

HIV-associated glomerulonephritis may be seen early in HIV infection as well as in patients with AIDS. The major clinical manifestations are proteinuria, a nephrotic syndrome, and renal impairment. This complication appears to be more common in the United States than in Europe; it is more common in intravenous drug abusers and black homosexuals than in white homosexuals. The clinical course in patients with HIV-associated focal segmental glomerulonephritis, once a nephrotic syndrome has developed, is of evolution to endstage renal failure within a few months.

AETIOLOGY AND PATHOGENESIS

It is suspected that direct viral invasion of the kidney is the basic cause; viral genome has been found in tubular and glomerular epithelia. Secondary infections, for instance with hepatitis B virus, may also play a role in pathogenesis.

PATHOLOGY

The characteristic histological lesion is of a focal segmental glomerulosclerosis that resembles the idiopathic variety. There is often a marked interstitial infiltrate of lymphocytes and plasma cells. Other histological types of glomerulonephritis which have been described include IgA nephropathy, mesangiocapillary, membranous, and minimal change nephropathy. Typically, on immunohistology mesangial deposits of IgM and C3 are seen.

MANAGEMENT AND OUTCOME

There is no evidence of benefit from treatment with azidothymidine or ddI, although this has not been systematically studied. Patients with HIV infection and endstage renal failure have been treated with chronic haemodialysis, but survival is poor.

Schistosomiasis

Significant glomerular disease has been reported only in patients with *Schistosoma mansoni* infections and hepatosplenic disease.

CLINICAL FEATURES

Overall, just under 5 per cent of patients with *S. mansoni* infection have hepatosplenic disease, and of these about 10 to 15 per cent develop glomerular lesions over a period of up to 10 years. The clinical presentation is with proteinuria or a nephrotic syndrome. In Egypt there is evidence that schistosomal glomerulonephritis is more common in individuals with concomitant chronic infections with salmonella.

PATHOLOGY

A mesangial proliferative glomerulonephritis is seen in mild or early cases, and the most common histological change in advanced cases, seen in 50 per cent, is a mesangiocapillary glomerulonephritis. The next most frequent histological lesion is a focal segmental glomerulosclerosis. There are also infrequent reports of membranous nephropathy and proliferative glomerulonephritis. Immunohistology shows granular deposits, predominantly of IgM, but also of IgG, IgA, IgE, and C3, in the mesangium and the subepithelial and subendothelial sites. Renal amyloidosis has been described in Sudanese patients with *S. mansoni* infection.

TREATMENT AND OUTCOME

Treatment of schistosomal glomerulonephritis with antischistosomal drugs, or prednisolone and cyclophosphamide, has been of no benefit. Progression to renal failure is usual.

Leprosy

The major renal lesions found in leprosy are amyloidosis and glomerulonephritis, although chronic interstitial nephritis has also been described.

CLINICAL FEATURES

Glomerulonephritis is found in up to 10 per cent of patients with leprosy at autopsy. It tends to be more common in patients with lepromatous than with tuberculoid leprosy and the onset of glomerulonephritis may coincide with an episode of erythema nodosum leprosum.

PATHOLOGY

The most common glomerular lesions are a mesangial proliferative glomerulonephritis and a focal or diffuse proliferative glomerulonephritis. Rarely, a membranous nephropathy is seen. Immunohistology shows granular glomerular deposits of IgG, IgM, and C3 in the mesangium or on capillary walls.

Filariasis

There are several reports from India and Cameroon of an association between filariasis and glomerulonephritis.

CLINICAL FEATURES

The clinical presentation is usually with a nephrotic syndrome and rarely with an acute nephritic syndrome.

PATHOLOGY

Patients with *Wuchereria bancrofti* infection may develop a mesangial proliferative or a diffuse proliferative glomerulonephritis. In patients with loa-loa infections both membranous and mesangiocapillary glomerulonephritis have been reported. Onchocerciasis infections have been reported to be associated with a nephrotic syndrome due to minimal change nephropathy, mesangial proliferative glomerulonephritis, and a mesangiocapillary glomerulonephritis.

On immunohistology glomerular deposits of IgG, IgM, and C3 are seen in the mesangium and capillary walls, and in one study onchocercal antigens were identified in glomerular capillaries.

TREATMENT

Treatment with diethylcarbamazine probably hastens recovery in those patients with an acute nephritic presentation but has no effect in patients presenting with a nephrotic syndrome.

Malaria

CLINICAL FEATURES

The majority of affected individuals are children and, to a lesser extent, young adults. In children the peak age of onset is between 5 and 8 years, and the sexes are equally affected. The clinical presentation is of a nephrotic syndrome, often with profound hypoalbuminaemia with ascites that is disproportionate to the degree of peripheral oedema. Microscopic haematuria is common and the proteinuria is usually poorly selective.

AETIOLOGY AND PATHOGENESIS

In the 1930s, in British Guiana, Giglioli established a long-suspected association between *Plasmodium malariae* infection and a nephrotic syndrome. Proteinuria, nephritis, and deaths from nephritis were then common in that country, and patients with a nephrotic syndrome had a higher incidence of *P. malariae* parasitaemia than did unaffected individuals, who more often had *P. vivax* or *P. falciparum* infection. Years later it was shown that following eradication of malaria from British Guiana there was a reduction in the incidence of proteinuria and nephritis and renal failure. The association between *P. malariae* infection and glomerulonephritis has also been confirmed by studies from Nigeria and Uganda in children with a nephrotic syndrome among whom the incidence of *P. malariae* parasitaemia (88 per cent) was significantly higher than that of healthy controls (20 per cent).

Immunohistology shows granular deposits of IgG and IgM. *Plasmodium malariae* antigen and antibody have been identified in the glomeruli of some children with a nephrotic syndrome in Nigeria and Uganda. Patients with malaria develop autoantibodies to single-stranded DNA and to IgG (rheumatoid factor), but their role in the pathogenesis of the nephritis is unclear.

Although *P. malariae* infection is widespread in many parts of the world, quartan malarial nephropathy has been described in only a few areas; it is uncommon in Ghana, Senegal, and Papua New Guinea. Glomerulonephritis, histologically similar to that associated with quartan malarial nephropathy, has been described in Senegalese children who, however, lacked evidence of *P. malariae* infection. There are several possible explanations for these observations. It is possible that only some strains of *P. malariae* are nephritogenic. It is also evident that only some individuals with *P. malariae* infection develop a glomerulonephritis, maybe because of the way that their immune system reacts to this infection or to environmental factors such as malnutrition or concomitant infections with other organisms. Finally, it is possible that whatever abnormality leads to quartan malarial nephropathy also leads to an increased susceptibility to *P. malariae* infection.

PATHOLOGY

The glomerular lesion comprises a segmental glomerular capillary wall thickening with expansion of the subendothelial area. In advanced cases there is segmental and mesangial sclerosis and global glomerulosclerosis. Mesangial hypercellularity and small fibroepithelial crescents are seen infrequently. Immunohistology shows coarse granular or fine diffuse deposits of IgG, IgM, and C3 in the glomerular capillary walls. Electron microscopy shows that the glomerular capillary wall thickening is due to increased amounts of basement membrane material in the subendothelial area.

MANAGEMENT AND OUTCOME

Antimalarial treatment of quartan malarial nephropathy does not produce remission of the nephrotic syndrome. Only a minority of children with minor glomerular lesions responded to steroids. In most children steroids were ineffective and had a substantial toxicity. Azathioprine and cyclophosphamide have not been shown to be effective, and in the case of azathioprine may actually worsen the prognosis. Most children with quartan malarial nephropathy develop progressive renal failure.

Syphilis

Although glomerulonephritis is an infrequent complication of syphilis, the rising incidence of this disease may make for an increasing problem. Secondary syphilis may rarely be complicated by a nephrotic syndrome caused by a mesangial proliferative glomerulonephritis or a histological appearance resembling membranous nephropathy. Immunofluorescent microscopy shows subepithelial deposits of IgG and complement. Treatment with penicillin leads to resolution of the nephritis.

Congenital syphilis may rarely be complicated by a membranous nephropathy with mesangial proliferation and at times crescent formation and a tubulointerstitial nephritis. The clinical presentation is with an acute nephritis or with a nephrotic syndrome. The renal lesion resolves following treatment with penicillin.

Other infections

Many other infections are rarely associated with glomerulonephritis—in some instances the association resting on a single case report. It is not surprising, in view of the probable pathogenetic mechanisms, that any infection might cause glomerulonephritis; of interest, and as yet not explained, are the marked differences in frequency with which different infections are associated with nephritis. Some of the infections that have rarely been associated with glomerulonephritis are shown in Table 1.

Table 1 *Some infections rarely associated with glomerulonephritis*

Bacteria	*Escherichia coli, Yersinia enterocolitica, Mycoplasma pneumoniae, Klebsiella pneumoniae*
Rickettsia	Rocky Mountain spotted fever
Viruses	Epstein–Barr virus, influenza (which has a particular association with antiglomerular basement membrane disease), cytomegalovirus, measles, varicella
Fungi	*Candida albicans, Histoplasma capsulatum*
Parasites	Toxoplasma, *Leishmania donovani*

Vasculitis

A number of infections have been associated with a systemic vasculitis involving the kidney and similar to the idiopathic form.

Hepatitis B-associated vasculitis

CLINICAL FEATURES

Hepatitis B surface antigenaemia has been reported in 10 to 40 per cent of patients in the United States, 18 to 50 per cent of patients in France, and 4 to 8 per cent of patients in the United Kingdom who have typical vasculitis. This may follow an episode of clinically apparent acute hepatitis, but in many patients there is no evidence of hepatitis. The renal involvement occurs mainly in adults and causes haematuria, proteinuria, and renal impairment.

PATHOLOGY

The renal histological lesions of an arteritis and arteriolitis and angiographic evidence of arterial aneurysms are indistinguishable from those of typical vasculitis.

SEROLOGY

The distinctive feature is the presence of antineutrophil cytoplasmic antibody.

TREATMENT AND OUTCOME

Most studies report that the prognosis of hepatitis B-associated vasculitis is improved by treatment with cyclophosphamide and prednisolone. Antiviral agents such as α-interferon and adenosine arabinoside have been used in small numbers of patients but with no compelling evidence of benefit. Unlike typical vasculitis, which tends to relapse in up to 40 per cent of cases, hepatitis B-associated vasculitis is more often a self-limiting disease.

Post-streptococcal vasculitis

A well-described but uncommon sequel of streptococcal infection is a systemic vasculitis occurring, like post-streptococcal glomerulonephritis, several days after the onset of skin or upper respiratory-tract infection.

Other infections

Vasculitis can occur in association with septicaemia caused by any organism, particularly staphylococci and streptococci. Heroin-associated vasculitis in intravenous drug abusers may be due to infection and septicaemia, or substances other than heroin in the mixture.

Interstitial nephritis

Interstitial nephritis, associated with infections, usually causes acute renal impairment, and can arise in two ways.

Direct infection

Invasion of the renal parenchyma by the micro-organisms produces a polymorphonuclear infiltration and microabscesses. This cause of renal failure is now uncommon in developed countries, owing to easy access to antibiotics for infections of the urinary tract that could lead to acute pyelonephritis. The usual organisms responsible are *Escherichia coli, staphylococcus aureus,* and *Proteus* species. The management is swift and effective treatment of the infection, and appropriate measures for renal failure. Scarring and chronic damage may occur, although in most cases that are treated promptly and effectively a full renal recovery is expected.

Leptospirosis

CLINICAL FEATURES

There is renal involvement in most cases of leptospirosis. Acute renal failure develops in about 50 per cent, and is usually accompanied by jaundice (Weil's syndrome). Characteristically, the acute renal failure is hypercatabolic, so hyperuricaemia, hyperkalaemia, and the rise in blood urea are disproportionate to the rise in serum creatinine.

PATHOLOGY

The major histological lesions are an acute interstitial nephritis with acute tubular necrosis. Minor glomerular mesangial proliferation may be seen.

MANAGEMENT AND OUTCOME

Treatment is with penicillin and erythromycin (see Chapter 7.11.25). Renal failure is treated by conventional methods. Most patients make a full recovery.

Haemorrhagic fever (hantavirus disease)

This disease is apparently increasing in frequency in Europe, spreading westwards.

CLINICAL FEATURES

In the severe form, haemorrhage into the skin and mucous membranes is the cardinal symptom, together with myalgia, fever, and loin pain. Oliguria with microscopic haematuria and proteinuria develop 7 to 10 days after the onset.

AETIOLOGY AND PATHOGENESIS

The Hantaviruses are carried by rodents; infection has occurred in laboratory workers exposed to rats.

PATHOLOGY

Acute tubular necrosis and medullary haemorrhage with mononuclear cell infiltrates are typical.

MANAGEMENT AND OUTCOME

There is no specific treatment; the outlook for renal function is good, recovery being the rule.

Immune-mediated interstitial nephritis

A whole range of infections has been associated with an acute interstitial nephritis which is characterized by a lymphocytic infiltration, without evidence of direct invasion by the micro-organisms. As with glomerulonephritis, many infections have been reported to cause this renal lesion. The clinical picture is similar, with tubular proteinuria, microscopic haematuria, and varying degrees of renal dysfunction.

AETIOLOGY AND PATHOGENESIS

The numerous organisms are thought to share a common mechanism, of an immune-mediated cellular (type IV) reaction against foreign antigens in the infecting agents.

PATHOLOGY

Focal or diffuse infiltration of the interstitium is typical; in some patients glomerulonephritis may coexist.

MANAGEMENT AND OUTCOME

Most patients recover on treatment of the underlying infection.

Haemolytic uraemic syndrome (see also Chapter 20.6.)

This is a syndrome of thrombocytopenia, microangiopathic haemolytic anaemia with fragmented red blood cells, and acute renal failure. The main cause of diarrhoea-associated epidemic haemolytic uraemic syndrome is verocytotoxin-producing *E. coli*. In the Indian subcontinent this syndrome may complicate *Shigella dysenteriae* type I infection. Rare infective causes of haemolytic uraemic syndrome include neuraminidase-producing pneumococci and *Salmonella typhi* infection.

Acute renal failure (see also Chapter 20.16.)

Acute renal failure may result from any of the acute proliferative glomerulonephritides and the acute forms of interstitial nephritis described above. Severe sepsis, without nephritis, may lead to acute renal failure. Typically this is accompanied by disseminated intravascular coagulation, most commonly from septicaemia with endotoxin-producing Gram-negative bacteria. A similar outcome may result from infections with Gram-positive cocci such as *Staphylococcus aureus* and meningococci. Acute renal failure from gynaecological sepsis is still common in some parts of the tropics. *Plasmodium falciparum* and *Salmonella typhi* infections can lead to massive intravascular haemolysis and acute renal failure, more commonly in individuals who are glucose 6-phosphate dehydrogenase deficient.

The main renal lesion in septicaemia is acute tubular necrosis. If disseminated intravascular coagulation occurs, then thrombosis of the vessels develops, which, if extensive, can lead to infarction. In cases of acute tubular necrosis alone, the outcome depends on the underlying infection, the renal prognosis being good.

Obstructive uropathy (see also Chapter 20.10.)

Obstruction due to infections can be caused by two mechanisms. Scarring and fibrosis of the ureters and/or bladder is caused by the chronic infections schistosomiasis and tuberculosis. The lesions can be extensive and multiple, resulting in narrowing of long segments of the ureters and a contracted non-expansile bladder. The bladder may calcify. In this more severe form, the ureteric lesions cannot be treated by operation.

In males acute gonococcal infection can cause urethral strictures and obstruction.

A second mechanism is seen in fungal infections of the urinary tract when a mycetoma may form and, acting as a space-occupying lesion in the pelvis of the kidney, the ureter, or the bladder, causes obstruction. Apart from antifungal treatment, removal of the mycetoma by an appropriate intervention is necessary.

REFERENCES

Andrade, Z.A., Rocha, H. (1979). Schistosomal glomerulopathy. *Kidney International,* **16**, 23–9.

Arze, R.S., Rashid, H., Morley, R., Ward, M.K., and Kerr, D.N.S. (1983). Shunt nephritis: report of two cases and review of the literature. *Clinical Nephrology,* **19**, 48–53.

Beaufils, M., Gibert, C., Morel-Maroger, L., *et al.* (1978). Glomerulonephritis in severe bacterial infections with and without endocarditis. *Advances in Nephrology,* **7**, 217–34.

Bhorade, M.S., Carag, H.B., Lee, H.J., Potter, E.V., and Dunea, G. (1971). Nephropathy of Secondary Syphilis. *Journal of the American Medical Association,* **216**, 1159–66.

Boonpucknavig, V. and Sitprija, V. (1979). Renal disease in acute Plasmodium falciparum infection in man. *Kidney International,* **16**, 44–52.

Bourgoignie, J.J. (1990). Renal complications of human immunodeficiency virus type 1. *Kidney International,* **37**, 1571–84.

England, A.C., Fraser, D.W., Plikaytis, B.D., Tsai, T.F., Storch, G., and Broome, C.V. (1981). Sporadic Legionellosis in the United States: the first thousand cases. *Annals of Internal Medicine,* **94**, 164–70.

Feinstein, E.I., Eknoyan, G., Lister, B.J., Kim, H-S., and Greenberg, S.D. (1985). Renal complications of bacterial endocarditis. *American Journal of Nephrology,* **5**, 457–69.

Giglioli, G. (1962). Malaria and renal disease with special reference to British Guiana II. The effect of malaria eradication on the incidence of renal disease in British Guiana. *Annals of Tropical Medicine and Parasitology,* **56**, 225–41.

Hendrickse, R.G., Adeniyi, A., Edington, G.M., Glasgow, E.F., White, R.H.R., and Houba, V. (1972). Quartan malarial nephrotic syndrome: collaborative clinicopathological study in Nigerian children. *Lancet,* **i**, 1143–9.

Johnson, R.J. and Couser, W.G. (1990). Hepatitis B infection and renal disease: clinical, immunopathogenetic and therapeutic considerations. *Kidney International,* **37**, 663–76.

Johnson, R.J., Wilson, R., Yamabe, H., *et al.* (1994). Renal manifestations of hepatitis C virus infection. *Kidney International,* **46**, 1255–63.

Lee, H.W. and van der Groen, G. (1989). Hemorrhagic fever with renal syndrome. *Progress in Medical Virology,* **36**, 62–102.

Poon-King, T., Potter, E.V., Svartman, *et al.* (1973). Epidemic acute nephritis with reappearance of M-type 55 streptococci in Trinidad. *Lancet,* **i**, 475–9.

Rao, T.K.S., Filippone, E.J., Nicastri, A.D., *et al.* (1984). Associated focal and segmental glomerulosclerosis in the acquired immunodeficiency syndrome. *New England Journal of Medicine,* **310**, 669–73.

Sitprija, V., Pipatanagul, V., Mertowidjojo, K., Boonpucknavig, V., and Boonpucknavig, S. (1980). Pathogenesis of renal disease in leptospirosis: clinical and experimental studies. *Kidney International,* **17**, 827–36.

20.5.3 Amyloid, myeloma, light chain deposition disease, fibrillary glomerulonephritis, cryoglobulinaemia

J. P. GRÜNFELD

These diseases, which are clinically heterogeneous, are characterized, however, by the presence of peculiar, often organized deposits within the kidneys. The main features of these deposits are summarized in Table 1.

Table 1 *Overall presentation of the renal histopathological changes found in the diseases discussed here*

Diagnosis	Myeloma	AL amyloidosis	Fibrillar glomerulonephritis	LCDD[a]	Mixed cryoglobulinaemia
Renal pathology	Cast nephropathy	Congo-red-positive fibrillar deposits in glomeruli and vessels	Non-amyloid fibrillar deposits in glomeruli	Granular peritubular deposits and mesangial nodules (in some cases), containing a monoclonal light chain (mostly κ)	Glomerular intracapillary cell proliferation Monocyte infiltration Subendothelial deposits, forming 'thrombi' Acute small vessel vasculitis (in some cases)
Pathogenesis	Renal toxicity of certain light chains	Certain fragments of certain light chains (mostly λ) prone to amyloid formation	Unknown; crystallization of immune aggregates?	Light chains, often abnormally glycosylated or polymerized	Mixed cryoglobulin deposits (usually IgG–IgM) which localize in glomeruli and trigger glomerular inflammation

[a]LCDD, Light-chain deposition disease.

Amyloid nephropathy

Clinical renal involvement is found in at least 50 per cent of the patients with AL amyloidosis (which is derived from fragments of light chains, mostly λ, of immunoglobulins) and almost all patients with AA amyloidosis (which is derived from amyloid protein A). Renal amyloid deposits can also be detected in some neuropathic hereditary forms of amyloidosis (see Chapter 11.13.1). β_2-microglobulin-derived amyloidosis is seen specifically in patients undergoing long-term dialysis for chronic renal failure, and is deposited in joints, tendons, the carpal tunnel, and bones.

Definition

Amyloidosis is characterized by intercellular accumulation of a protein substance forming non-branching fibrils with a diameter of 7 to 10 nm, in a β-pleated sheet conformation (the term 'β-fibrilloses' has been suggested as a common denominator of all types of amyloidosis). This tertiary configuration of amyloid is critical to its ability to bind the Congo red stain, and also produces green birefringence when viewed under polarized light. The chemical type of amyloid deposits may be identified by immunofluorescence. In the kidney, deposits are located in glomeruli (with a nodular-like appearance), in vessels, and, later in the course, in tubules and interstitium.

Symptoms

Proteinuria is the most usual presenting symptom of renal amyloidosis. It often progresses to a severe nephrotic syndrome. Renal vein thrombosis may complicate the nephrotic stage. Progressively, there is a decline in renal function, leading finally to endstage renal failure. In some rare patients in whom renal tubulointerstitial deposits predominate, renal failure may progress without a nephrotic stage. In some of these cases renal tubular dysfunction, e.g. Fanconi syndrome, renal tubular acidosis or even nephrogenic diabetes insipidus may have been the presenting problem. The kidneys are generally of normal size or large, even when renal function is impaired. Long-standing amyloidosis is often accompanied by postural hypotension which can be a disabling symptom. This is usually ascribed to amyloid autonomic neuropathy and/or adrenal insufficiency. Hypertension is relatively uncommon but it may develop concomitantly with renal failure.

Diagnosis

The diagnosis of amyloidosis is based on tissue specimen analysis. Rectal biopsy is a relatively simple procedure, often leading to diagnosis,

provided that the specimen includes submucosal tissue with vessels in it. Aspiration biopsy of abdominal fat is also safe and can give rapid diagnosis (but with a higher rate of false negative results). Bone marrow biopsy is of value in AL amyloidosis but renal biopsy may be necessary to prove the diagnosis in doubtful cases.

The associated clinical features may also contribute to diagnosis. AL amyloidosis is usually seen in patients over 50 years of age. It can complicate overt multiple myeloma but often lacks the classical features of that disease. The tongue (with macroglossia), skeletal muscle, skin (with ecchymoses, particularly in the upper part of the body), gastrointestinal tract, and heart are frequently involved. In most cases, a monoclonal component (frequently λ light chains) is detected in the serum or urine by immunofixation electrophoresis. The prognosis is more severe than in AA amyloidosis, mainly because of involvement of the heart which, when symptomatic, leads to death within a few months, unless prevented by cardiac transplantation.

AA amyloidosis frequently involves the liver, spleen, and adrenals, in addition to the kidneys. It is seen with chronic infections, inflammatory diseases, or malignant tumours, such as tuberculosis, empyema, osteomyelitis (the incidence of these three causes has dropped dramatically in recent decades), cystic fibrosis, bronchiectasias, leprosy, rheumatoid arthritis, Crohn's disease, Hodgkin's disease, and renal cell carcinoma. It can also complicate familial Mediterranean fever, an autosomal recessive disorder which affects Mediterranean populations (such as Sephardic Jews, Armenians, Turks, and Arabs). The mutant gene for this last disorder has been located on the short arm of chromosome 16. The disease is characterized by recurrent attacks of fever, abdominal pain, and arthritis, lasting 2 to 3 days and remitting spontaneously. The incidence of complicating amyloidosis is variable among different ethnic groups. It is high, approximately 25 to 30 per cent, in Sephardic Jews.

Prominent renal involvement is seen in two other forms of heredofamilial amyloidosis. In Muckle–Wells syndrome, AA amyloidosis is associated with nerve deafness and urticaria. In Ostertag amyloid nephropathy, the amyloid substance derives from a variant of apolipoprotein AI, from lysozyme or from the α-chain of fibrinogen.

Treatment

Prevention or suppression of chronic suppuration or inflammation is the best means for preventing or reversing secondary AA amyloidosis. In AL amyloidosis, chemotherapy similar to that used in myeloma may be beneficial. Continuous administration of colchicine is of great importance in familial Mediterranean fever:

(1) for preventing attacks; and
(2) most probably, for preventing the development of amyloidosis,

Colchicine, used since 1972, has dramatically changed the prognosis of this rare disease. It may also decrease the rate of progression of associated established renal amyloidosis, but convincing evidence for complete regression is still lacking. Colchicine has been advocated in other forms of amyloidosis but its efficacy in that context has not been established. Cytotoxic therapy with cyclophosphamide or chlorambucil are helpful in rheumatoid arthritis or Still's disease complicated by AA amyloidosis.

Amyloid nephropathy requires symptomatic management of the nephrotic syndrome and of renal failure. Patients in endstage renal disease are candidates for regular dialysis and/or kidney transplantation. The prognosis is compromised by the risks of extension of extrarenal deposition, and, after transplantation, of recurrence of amyloidosis in the graft. When the underlying disease before transplantation has been familial Mediterranean fever, colchicine therapy must be pursued to prevent renal recurrence and progression elsewhere.

REFERENCES

Gertz, M.A. and Kyle, R.A. (1991). Secondary systemic amyloidosis: Response and survival in 64 patients. *Medicine* **70**, 246–56.
Glenner, G.G. (1980). Amyloid deposits and amyloidosis. The β-fibrilloses. *New England Journal of Medicine* **302**, 1283–92, 1333–43.
Kyle, R.A. and Greipp, P.R. (1983). Amyloidosis (AL). Clinical and laboratory features in 229 cases. *Mayo Clinic Proceedings* **58**, 665–83.
Vigushin, D.M., *et al.* (1994). Familial nephropathic systemic amyloidosis, caused by antipoprotein AI variant Arg 26. *Quarterly Journal of Medicine*, **87**, 149–54.

Renal involvement in multiple myeloma

Multiple myeloma is characterized by the presence of a malignant clone of B lymphocytes (plasma cells) that produce excess intact monoclonal immunoglobulins or light chains or both. Renal impairment is found at presentation in 20 per cent of patients with myeloma and in half of them during the course of the disease. It is particularly common in patients with light-chain myeloma.

Monoclonal light-chain proteinuria (also called Bence Jones proteinuria) is a common abnormal finding in myeloma and may be the clue which leads to diagnosis when the light chain has been correctly identified. Light chains are not detected by dipstick analysis, but the conventional sulphosalicylic acid test is generally reliable for screening. The effects of heating on solubility, which were the basis of Henry Bence Jones' original observations, are now of historical interest only. Accurate identification of monoclonal light-chain (κ or λ) protein requires immunoelectrophoresis or, better, immunofixation electrophoresis of the concentrated urine. Due to high renal clearance (see below), the monoclonal light chain may not be detected in the serum and may be present in only small amounts in urine. Myeloma kidney only occurs when there are monoclonal light chains in the urine, but many patients similarly excreting monoclonal light-chains, sometimes large amounts, do not suffer from renal disease.

Free light chains of immunoglobulins are filtered through glomeruli, are totally or partially reabsorbed, and degraded in proximal tubular cells. They appear eventually in the urine when the catabolizing capacity of these cells has been exceeded. Certain light chains (critical characteristics undefined, but probably because of their physicochemical properties), exert tubular cell toxicity and/or precipitate within the tubular lumen; others appear harmless to the kidney. The precise mechanism of the nephrotoxicity is still unresolved. These deleterious effects can be amplified by additional factors, such as low urine flow rate and low pH, or hypercalcaemia, and can lead to the renal consequences listed below.

Other physicochemical properties most probably explain why other light chains form AL amyloidosis or granular light-chain deposits (Table 1).

Tubular dysfunction is rarely a presenting symptom. Fanconi syndrome (due to proximal tubular dysfunction) may result from intratubular crystalline inclusions of altered κ light chains. It may lead to osteomalacia and precede the development of overt myeloma by several years.

Bence Jones cast (or myeloma) nephropathy is the most common form of renal involvement. Myeloma kidney is characterized by the presence of typical polychromatophil protein casts, often lamellated, sometimes containing crystals, surrounded by multinucleated giant cells, located in the distal nephron, and associated with interstitial fibrosis and tubular atrophy. Casts occur in part because light chains co-aggregate with Tamm–Horsfall glycoprotein. This glycoprotein is synthesized exclusively by cells of the thick ascending limb of the loop of Henle. This explains the localization of the casts in the distal nephron. Clinically the patients present with either acute or chronic renal failure. Acute renal failure can be triggered by dehydration in conjunction with hypercalcaemia, infection, or injection of radiological contrast media, or by administration of nephrotoxic drugs, including non-steroidal anti-inflammatory drugs—all factors which precipitate intratubular cast formation. Chronic renal failure with insidious onset is secondary to the extent of tubular atrophy and interstitial fibrosis.

AL amyloidosis develops in approximately 10 per cent of myeloma patients. λ light chains are more amyloidogenic than κ, and in these cases the variable regions of certain λ chains favour the deposition of amyloid. The nephrotic syndrome is frequently found in these patients. Progressive heart failure, owing to restriction of ventricular filling due to amyloid infiltration, and arrhythmias are the leading causes of death in this subgroup of patients.

Light-chain deposition disease (see below) occurs in approximately 2 to 4 per cent of patients with myeloma. It may be the first manifestation or may develop in patients who have previously received chemotherapy, probably by selection of a clone of plasma cells which produce light chains of a particular abnormal structure. Renal and extrarenal features are described below. Not all myeloma patients with the nephrotic syndrome suffer from AL amyloidosis—some will be found to have light-chain deposition disease.

Renal impairment in myeloma may also be related to other factors—including atherosclerosis-induced kidney lesions in elderly patients. Hypercalcaemia is frequently found and results from increased osteoclastic bone resorption and decreased urinary calcium excretion, when glomerular filtration rate is reduced. The manifestation and management of hypercalcaemic nephropathy are more fully discussed in Chapter 20.9.3.

Treatment

The first aim of treatment is to prevent or retard renal impairment in all patients with myeloma, most particularly those with light-chain myeloma by prevention of dehydration, maintenance of a high urinary output and urine alkalinization, avoidance of nephrotoxic drugs, and control of any hypercalcaemia.

Renal failure of recent onset should be promptly and vigorously managed. Adequate salt and water administration and forced alkaline diuresis (which may help to prevent intratubular light-chain precipitation) are required when urine output persists. Chemotherapy (alkylating agents plus prednisone) may be given in the hope of decreasing production of light chains. Plasma exchange has been advocated to remove light chains more rapidly, but its value is unproven. In patients with oliguria, dialysis should be provided early. Hypercalcaemia requires correction of salt and water deficit, steroids, and/or diphosphonates, which are potent inhibitors of osteoclast activity.

Partial or total improvement of renal function is frequently obtained by such management. However, the progression to endstage renal disease is observed in about 30 per cent of the patients with renal failure.

Regular dialysis may be indicated if the clinical condition and bone lesions allow it. Recombinant human erythropoietin may be helpful to correct anaemia.

The survival rate of treated patients with myeloma is poor (median survival time, 30 to 40 months approximately); it is poorer in myeloma patients with renal failure (approximately 20 months), with a high mortality rate in the first 3 months after presentation. Prognosis depends on the tumor mass and response to chemotherapy. The modalities of chemotherapy, the place of other treatments, such as bone marrow transplantation, and the overall prognosis of myeloma independent of renal involvement, are beyond the scope of this chapter.

REFERENCES

Ganeval, D., Rabian, C., Guérin, Y., Pertuiset, N., Landais, P., and Jungers, P. (1992). Treatment of multiple myeloma with renal involvement. *Advances in Nephrology* **21**, 347–70.
Kyle, R.A. (1975). Multiple myeloma. Review of 869 cases. *Mayo Clinic Proceedings* **50**, 29–40.

Light-chain deposition disease

Light-chain deposition disease is characterized by the deposition of monoclonal light chains (mainly κ) in various tissues because of proliferation of an abnormal and small clone of B lymphocytes (plasma cells) in the bone marrow, which produces light chains, often with an abnormal structure (abnormally polymerized or glycosylated). The light-chain deposits are often widespread but the kidney is the most frequently involved organ and renal manifestations predominate.

Most patients are adults over 50 years of age. Most of them have an underlying malignant lymphoplasmacytic disorder, usually multiple myeloma. However, 20 to 30 per cent of them have no such overt disorder at presentation and do not develop it later in the course.

Symptoms

Proteinuria, either moderate or in the nephrotic range, is often the presenting symptom, associated with rapidly or slowly progressive renal failure. Extrarenal deposits may produce symptoms during the course of the disease, but cardiac lesions rarely result in heart failure or arrhythmias, and liver deposits are often asymptomatic, even when associated with marked capillary dilatations with the appearance of peliosis hepatis. In patients with myeloma and light-chain deposition disease, the prognosis is determined by the severity of multiple myeloma. In 'idiopathic' light-chain deposition disease, some rare patients have a fulminant course with multiorgan involvement. Most patients progress more slowly to endstage renal disease and some patients do not develop extrarenal manifestations even after years on dialytic therapy.

Diagnosis

The diagnosis is based on an immunofluorescence study of the renal biopsy specimen, using anti-light-chain antibodies. The most constant and prominent finding is the peritubular fixation of the monoclonal light-chain antibody, most often anti-κ, along the tubular basement membrane. By light microscopy, this membrane has a thickened and refractile appearance and appears outlined on its external aspect by ribbon-like, continuous deposits; by electron microscopy, the peritubular deposits have a granular structure. Fixation is also found in the glomerular mesangium, forming mesangial nodules in approximately 60 per cent of the patients. Of interest, in the absence of an immunofluorescence study, these lesions may be misdiagnosed as nodular diabetic (Kimmelstiel–Wilson) glomerulopathy.

In 'idiopathic' light-chain deposition disease, the monoclonal light chain can be detected in serum and/or in concentrated urine. However,

in some patients, it cannot be found with commonly available laboratory techniques. This is probably explained by a low level of synthesis, rapid tissue deposition, and/or accelerated rate of degradation.

Treatment

In patients with multiple myeloma, chemotherapy is indicated. In 'idiopathic' light-chain deposition disease, it is not established whether chemotherapy (alkylating agents plus prednisone) is beneficial. It has been advocated to prevent progression of renal changes and development of extrarenal deposits. Recurrence of light-chain deposition disease after renal transplantation has been reported.

REFERENCE

Ganeval, D., *et al.* (1982). Visceral deposition of monoclonal light chains and immunoglobulins: A study of renal and immunopathologic abnormalities. *Advances in Nephrology* **11**, 25–63.

Fibrillary glomerulonephritis

Fibrillary glomerulonephritis is a very rare disease, characterized by the deposition of randomly arranged fibrils in the glomerular capillary wall and mesangium. These fibrils do not bind the Congo red stain, and by electron microscopy are wider (18 to 22 nm) than are amyloid fibrils. By immunofluorescence, IgG4 and the C3 fraction of complement are predominantly found in fibrils.

The clinical presentation includes proteinuria of varying degrees, concomitant haematuria, hypertension, and renal failure in half the patients. No monoclonal protein is found in serum or urine. In one patient, haemoptysis due to intra-alveolar haemorrhage was ascribed to lung deposition of fibrillar deposits similar to those found in the kidneys. The evolution has generally been unfavourable, with progression of renal failure in the majority within 5 to 10 years.

The treatment is limited so far to symptomatic management. The disease may recur after renal transplantation.

Immunotactoid glomerulopathy has been considered as either belonging to the same spectrum or as a separate entity. It is characterized by the crystallization of immune aggregates into tactoids resulting in the deposition of fibrils or microtubules. These structures are arranged in parallel; their diameter ranges from 30 to 40 nm. Monoclonal immunoglobulin deposition is more common in immunotactoid glomerulopathy. In addition, these patients appear to be at risk for a concomitant dysproteinaemia and/or lymphoproliferative disorder.

REFERENCES

Iskandar, S.S., Falk, R.J., and Jennette, J.C. (1992). Clinical and pathological features of fibrillary glomerulonephritis. *Kidney International*, **42**, 1401–7.
Korbet, S.M., Schwartz, M.M., and Lewis, E.J. (1991). Immunotactoid glomerulopathy. *American Journal of Kidney Diseases* **17**, 247–57.

Renal involvement in cryoglobulinaemia

'Cryoglobulin' is a generic word used for any immunoglobulin that precipitates on cooling (at 4°C) and resolubilizes on warming (at 37°C). This stresses the need for proper methods of collecting and processing blood samples: the blood is taken from a fasting patient (lipids may interfere with the test by precipitating in the cold); it is placed in tubes in warm water and transported promptly to the laboratory, where it is allowed to clot at 37°C and is then separated in a warm centrifuge; the clear serum supernatant is removed, stored at 4°C and examined daily for cryoprecipitate.

Renal involvement is observed mainly in patients with mixed type II cryoglobulinaemia which usually consists of IgM rheumatoid factor, representing a monoclonal response against a polyclonal IgG. Both components form immune complexes which localize to the glomeruli, fix complement, serve as chemoattractants for macrophages, and trigger glomerular inflammation and cell proliferation. The typical glomerular lesions encompass intracapillary cell proliferation, infiltration of leucocytes, mainly monocytes-macrophages, and subendothelial deposits whose composition is identical to that of circulating cryoglobulin. The deposits may be massive, filling the capillary lumen and forming so-called 'thrombi'. By electron microscopy, the deposits often have a fibrillar or crystalline structure, similar to that of the cryoprecipitate. These glomerular changes may be associated with acute small vessel vasculitis of the kidney.

Aetiology

Mixed type II cryoglobulinaemia may be associated with lymphoproliferative disorders or chronic liver injury, but in many cases no underlying or associated disease is found and the cryoglobulinaemia is referred to as mixed essential cryoglobulinaemia.

Viral infections may trigger cryoglobulin formation. Whereas hepatitis B and Epstein–Barr virus infections have been implicated in the past, the role of hepatitis C virus infection is now recognized to be an unimportant factor in the pathogenesis of mixed type II cryoglobulinaemia. Hepatitis C virus antibodies and hepatitis C virus RNA are frequently found in the sera of patients with mixed type II cryoglobulinaemia. This might explain in part the uneven geographical distribution of mixed cryoglobulinaemia, which predominates in southern Europe where hepatitis C infection is more prevalent.

Symptoms

The symptoms and signs of mixed cryoglobulinaemia include palpable purpura, arthralgias, fatigue, Raynaud's phenomenon, peripheral neuropathy, hepatic involvement, and, frequently, glomerular disease. This syndrome occurs in adults in the fourth to fifth decades of life, and predominates slightly in females. In addition to cryoglobulin and IgM rheumatoid factor, laboratory testing shows very low serum C4 fraction and total haemolytic activity of complement.

The renal disease may present as an acute nephritic syndrome (in 20 to 30 per cent of the cases) with gross haematuria, heavy proteinuria, hypertension, and sudden-onset renal failure, sometimes with oliguria. The renal pathological counterpart in these patients is proliferative and exudative glomerulonephritis, with numerous intraluminal thrombi. Remission may occur spontaneously or during therapy. Clinical exacerbations may recur in up to 20 per cent of the patients.

Most patients with mixed cryoglobulinaemia have an indolent and protracted renal course. They present with proteinuria, haematuria, and hypertension, often several years after the onset of extrarenal symptoms. The pattern of kidney lesions in these patients is that of membranoproliferative glomerulonephritis, with some of the peculiarities described above. Endstage uraemia develops in fewer than 10 per cent of patients.

Treatment

The best way to treat this syndrome is not well established because the disease is rare, its course is unpredictable, and acute exacerbations may remit spontaneously. These episodes require symptomatic management, including antihypertensive therapy. High-dose steroids, cyclophosphamide, and plasmapheresis are usually restricted to the most severe cases, particularly those with signs of systemic vasculitis. The place of anti-hepatitis C virus therapy (such as α-interferon) has still to be evaluated in cases of mixed cryoglobulinaemia due to hepatitis C virus infection.

REFERENCES

Agnello, V., Chung, R.T., and Kaplan, L.M. (1992). A role for hepatitis C virus infection in type II cryoglobulinemia. *New England Journal of Medicine* **327**, 1490–5.
Appel G.B. (1993). Immune complex glomerulonephritis – deposits plus interest. *New England Journal of Medicine* **328**, 505–6.
D'Amico, G., Colasanti, G., and Ferrariof Sinico, R.A. (1989). Renal involvement in essential mixed cryoglobulinemia. *Kidney International* **35**, 1004–14.
Johnson, R.J., *et al.* (1993). Membrane-proliferative glomerulonephritis associated with hepatitis C virus infection. *New England Journal of Medicine* **328**, 465–70.
Misiani, R., *et al.* (1994). Interferon alfa-2a therapy in cryoglobulinemia associated with hepatitis C virus. *New England Journal of Medicine*, **330**, 751–6.

20.5.4 Renal manifestations of malignant disease

A. M. Davison

Introduction

Associated renal disease can occur in patients with benign and malignant tumours and with lymphoproliferative and myeloproliferative disorders. The renal manifestations may arise either as a direct effect of the tumour on the kidney, or as an indirect effect due to the systemic consequences of the tumour, the secretion of tumour products, or as a consequence of tumour therapy (Table 1).

Direct renal involvement

Metastatic spread of malignant solid tumours to the kidney is relatively uncommon in spite of the high renal blood flow relative to the renal mass. When present, metastases are usually multiple and often bilateral, presenting as either loin pain or haematuria; rarely do they cause significant impairment of renal function. On the contrary, renal infiltration is present in approximately 50 per cent of patients with leukaemia and 30 per cent of patients with lymphoma. The infiltration is most commonly nodular in patients with Hodgkin's lymphoma, but more diffuse in non-Hodgkin's lymphoma. The most common leukaemia to infiltrate the kidney is lymphoblastic leukaemia, which usually affects both kidneys diffusely throughout the cortex. As with metastatic disease, renal infiltration with lymphoma or leukaemia leads only uncommonly to significant renal functional impairment; and only very rarely is the initial manifestation of lymphoma or leukaemia due to renal infiltration.

Benign and malignant tumours, may, depending on their position, affect the renal blood supply, ureteric drainage, and bladder outflow. Tumours at the hilum of the kidney may compress the renal artery, resulting in diminished renal blood flow, increased secretion of renin, and subsequent hypertension. Only very rarely is the renal vein involved. Ureteric obstruction may arise from external compression of the ureters by retroperitoneal or pelvic tumours, for instance carcinoma of the cervix may extend laterally to the pelvic wall and occlude the pelvic ureters. Less commonly, adenocarcinoma of the sigmoid colon may produce a similar effect. Ureteric obstruction may also arise from lymphoma involving para-aortic nodes. Obstructive uropathy is most commonly produced by prostatic hypertrophy, which is benign in the

Table 1 *Renal manifestations of malignancy*

Direct effects
    Metastases
    Infiltration
    Obstruction
Indirect effects
    Electrolyte disorders
        Hypercalcaemia, hypokalaemia, hyponatraemia
    Acute renal failure
    Nephropathy
    Disseminated intravascular coagulation
    Renal vein thrombosis
    Hyperviscosity syndrome
    Fanconi syndrome
    Amyloidosis
Treatment associated
    Drug nephrotoxicity
    Tumour lysis syndrome
    Radiation

Table 2 *Evidence required to demonstrate a causal relationship between malignancy and nephropathy*

A close temporal relationship between the clinical presentation of the tumour and the nephropathy
Remission of nephropathy after cure or removal of tumour
Recurrence of nephropathy with recurrence of tumour
Demonstration of tumour antigen and associated antibody in glomerular deposits

majority of patients. Bladder cancer rarely causes obstruction unless it involves the trigone.

Indirect renal manifestation

ELECTROLYTE DISORDERS

Hypercalcaemia

This is a relatively common complication of many malignant disorders, arising from a variety of mechanisms. Hypercalcaemic nephropathy is a considerable problem in such patients. The subject is addressed fully in Chapter 20.9.3.

Hypokalaemia (see also Chapter 20.2.3)

This may arise from potassium loss as a consequence of prolonged diarrhoea or in patients with villous adenoma of the rectum. It can also develop as a consequence of prolonged vomiting and the accompanying metabolic alkalosis. Hypokalaemia has also been described in patients with multiple myeloma who develop a renal tubular acidosis due to degenerative changes, particularly in the proximal tubular cells. Rarely, hypokalaemia may arise in patients with acute leukaemia. Correction of hypokalaemia should be by oral supplementation wherever possible, and only rarely will intravenous therapy be required.

Hyponatraemia (see also Chapter 20.2.1)

This may arise from prolonged diarrhoea and vomiting, the secretion of antidiuretic hormone (ADH) or ADH-like peptides from oat-cell carcinomas (particularly of the lung), or from adrenal insufficiency due to metastatic disease. The hyponatraemia is rarely symptomatic, but if persistently less than 120 mmol/l, it may be life-threatening. Slow correction is most appropriate and should be undertaken by correcting fluid volume, restricting fluid intake, and stopping any diuretic therapy that may have been prescribed. The danger of rapid correction is that central pontine myelinolysis may develop.

NEPHROPATHY

The association between malignancy and glomerular disease was first described by Galloway in 1922, who described a patient with Hodgkin's disease who subsequently developed a nephrotic syndrome. There was a further report in 1931, but surprisingly, no further reports until 1966 when Lee *et al.* reported carcinoma in 11 of 101 adult patients presenting with nephrotic syndrome. Since then there have been many further series and anecdotal reports suggesting an association between malignancy and

nephropathy. The incidence of malignancy in adults presenting with a nephrotic syndrome is less than that suggested from the report of Lee *et al.* in 1966, and accounts for probably less than 1 per cent of such patients. A 1976 review of 14 published series with a total of 1643 patients with nephrotic syndrome revealed six (0.4 per cent) with associated malignancy. In children, glomerular involvement has only rarely been described in association with malignancy, although the triad of nephropathy, pseudohermaphroditism, and Wilms' tumour (Drash syndrome) is well recognized. Such patients present in the first 2 years of life with proteinuria, which may be sufficient to cause nephrotic syndrome, hypertension, and impaired renal function. The nephropathy is due to a diffuse mesangial sclerosis, which is usually progressive, leading to terminal renal failure.

The true incidence of glomerular involvement in malignancy is uncertain. Immune deposits have been detected at autopsy in from 2 to 30 per cent of patients with malignancy, but it is known that immunoglobulins may be detected in glomeruli at autopsy after sudden death in previously healthy adults, so that the causal relations of the immune deposits to the malignancy must be questionable. In one study of urinary abnormalities in patients with carcinoma, positive results were found in 58 per cent of 504 patients. However, again caution is required as such patients may have had renal metastases, nephrocalcinosis, analgesic effects, and would have been exposed to a wide variety of nephrotoxic drugs.

Demonstration of a causal relationship between malignancy and nephropathy requires that a number of conditions should be satisfied (Table 2). A literature review of 93 patients with carcinoma and nephropathy showed that the nephropathy had been described within 6 months of the detection of the tumour, in 63 per cent of cases; in most diagnoses were made simultaneously, but in 23 patients the nephrotic syndrome developed more than 12 months before or 12 months after tumour diagnosis. There can therefore be a prolonged time interval between the two presentations.

There are a number of reports indicating a prompt response between remission of the nephropathy and tumour removal. However, there have been few studies involving follow-up renal biopsies, and some patients fail to improve after remission or removal of the tumour. Recurrence of the tumour is usually associated with the recurrence of the nephropathy, but this is not invariable. The demonstration of tumour antigen and antitumour antibodies has been possible in a number of studies. Prostatic-specific antigen and melanoma antigen have been described, and in a number of patients eluates from the kidney have reacted with tumour cells. While these studies do not prove conclusively that the tumour antigen was primarily responsible for an immune-mediated inflammation they are, at least, suggestive. Overall, therefore, it seems that the criteria for establishing a causal relationship between the tumour and the nephropathy has been satisfied in a significant number of patients.

The pathogenesis of the nephropathy in the majority of patients is immunologically mediated, although in a number it may result from disseminated intravascular coagulation or amyloidosis. The immunopathological features of the nephropathy are similar to those found in immune-complex disease and possibly result from tumour-associated antigens, re-expressed fetal antigens, viral antigens, or the development of autoimmunity to autologous non-tumour antigens. Circulating immune complexes have been described in up to 80 per cent of patients with malignancy, but it is uncertain whether these are the cause of the nephropathy as it is most likely that the glomerular immune deposits are formed *in situ* from antigen and antibody deposited separately. Re-expressed fetal antigens, such as carcinoembryonic antigen have been demonstrated in glomerular deposits. In a number of malignancies, particularly in lymphoproliferative diseases, viral antigens may be the causal agent, but although glomerular deposition of viral antigen and antibody has been demonstrated in virus-induced mammary tumours in mice, no such association has yet been demonstrated with human solid tumours. However, antibodies to Epstein–Barr virus have been demonstrated in glomeruli in Burkitt's lymphoma. Glomerular deposition of autologous non-tumour antigens has been described, and this may be due to the fact that patients with malignancy have an increased incidence of autoimmunity.

The most common clinical presentation is with nephrotic syndrome, which, in about 40 per cent of patients becomes manifest before there are any signs or symptoms of malignancy. The true incidence of nephropathy in malignancy is unknown, as many patients have only minor degrees of proteinuria. Microscopic haematuria is common, but may not be directly related to nephropathy as urinary infection and high analgesic intake may be present. Renal functional impairment is uncommon in patients with solid tumours and the overall prognosis relates to that of the tumour rather than the nephropathy. In patients with multiple myeloma, renal involvement may present as a slowly progressive chronic renal failure, although in a number of patients the presentation is with acute renal failure, particularly if the patient has become dehydrated.

The tumours most commonly associated with nephropathy are adenocarcinomata of the lung and gastrointestinal tract (stomach, colon, and rectum), but there are reports of many other associated tumours, frequently in single-case reports. It is interesting that there are few reports of nephropathy in association with carcinoma of the breast, in spite of the common occurrence of this tumour. Nephropathy occurring in the presence of benign tumours is rare. Nephropathy complicating lymphoma or leukaemia, although recognized, is uncommon.

A wide variety of histological appearances have been described, although membranous nephropathy is the most common, occurring in approximately 70 per cent of patients with associated carcinoma. Mesangiocapillary glomerulonephritis has been described in a few reports in association with carcinoma of the breast, bronchogenic carcinoma, and adenocarcinoma of the stomach, and lymphocytic leukaemia. The very rare association of IgA nephropathy and malignancy is most likely to be fortuitous, although, mycosis fungoides has been reported in two patients with IgA nephropathy. In patients with Hodgkin's lymphoma the most common histological finding is that of minimal change nephropathy, although membranous nephropathy and mesangiocapillary glomerulonephritis have also been described. In all malignancies a wide range of glomerular appearances are described and in no instance does the glomerular appearance appear to be specific for a particular tumour type. In addition, there is no association between tumour load, as assessed by tumour size, or the presence of metastases and the development and severity of nephropathy.

Management consists of correcting any associated electrolyte disorder and diuretic therapy to control oedema. The overall prognosis is determined more by the malignancy than the glomerular findings. In general, complete resection or remission of the malignancy is associated with remission of the nephropathy. There may also be an improvement in the nephropathy with a reduction in tumour mass in patients in whom it is impossible to completely resect the tumour.

ACUTE RENAL FAILURE

Acute renal failure may occur as a consequence of hypovolaemia from prolonged diarrhoea and vomiting. In addition, it may arise as a complication of septicaemia occurring as part of the generalized immuno-suppression of advanced malignancy. In a number of patients, hepato-renal failure may develop as a result of metastatic disease in the liver. A few patients have been described who have developed disseminated intravascular coagulation in association with carcinoma of the pancreas or lung. It is generally recognized that patients with malignant disease have a hypercoagulable state, and renal vein thrombosis may develop. Acute renal failure is also seen in the tumour lysis syndrome (see below). In a few patients bilateral ureteric obstruction producing acute renal failure may be the first manifestation of malignancy.

AMYLOIDOSIS

Renal amyloidosis commonly complicates multiple myeloma, and in such patients the deposited amyloid is composed of immoglobulin light chains and has been termed AL amyloidosis. These AL proteins have also been described in Waldenström's macroglobulinaemia and benign monoclonal gammopathy. In patients in whom AL amyloidosis complicates myeloma, the AL proteins extracted from amyloid deposits are of the same composition as urinary Bence Jones protein, if present, suggesting a causal link between the excessive plasma cell production of the light chains and amyloid deposition. In general, the amyloid deposits are more likely to form in patients with excess λ light chains.

Amyloidosis of the AA type has most commonly been described in association with renal cell carcinoma, although other tumours have also been causally related.

Renal manifestations due to therapy

In patients with malignancy, nephrotoxicity may develop as a consequence of analgesic therapy, antibiotic therapy, or the use of cytotoxic drugs. A severe uric acid nephropathy (tumour lysis syndrome) may follow chemotherapy in patients with lymphoproliferative or myeloproliferative disorders, particularly acute lymphocytic leukaemia, where the rapid breakdown of cells is associated with increased nucleic acid catabolism increasing uric acid synthesis. This most commonly occurs in tumours which are very sensitive to chemotherapy, particularly if dehydration is present or if the patient has been given certain radiographic contrast agents, iopanoic acid or calcium ipodate, which are known to be uricosuric. Prevention of this complication of therapy is best achieved by pretreatment with allopurinol (300 mg daily), maintenance of a high urine flow rate, and avoidance of any drug known to be uricosuric.

Radiation nephritis is now uncommon as during such treatment care is taken to shield the kidneys. However, in a few instances it is impossible to protect the kidney completely, and acute radiation effects may become manifest within 6 to 12 months of radiation, whereas chronic effects develop over the years, becoming manifest by the development of proteinuria, hypertension, and impaired renal function.

REFERENCES

Beaufils, H., Jouanneau, C., and Chomette, G. (1985). Kidney and cancer: results of immunofluorescence microscopy. *Nephron* **40**, 303–8.

Beauvais, P., Vaudour, G., Boccon Gibod, L., and Levy M. (1989). Membranous nephropathy associated with ovarian tumour in a young girl: recovery after removal. *European Journal of Paediatrics* **148**, 624–5.

Cairns, S.A., Mallick, N.P., Lawler, W., and Williams, G. (1978). Squamous cell carcinoma of bronchus presenting with Henoch–Schönlein purpura. *British Medical Journal* **2**, 174–5.

Da Costa, C.R., Dupont, E., Hamers, R., Hooghe, R., Dupuis, F., and Potvliege, R. (1974). Nephrotic syndrome in bronchogenic carcinoma: report of two cases with immunochemical studies. *Clinical Nephrology* **2**, 245–50.

Drash, A., Sherman, F., Hartman, W., and Blizzard, R.M. (1970). A syndrome of pseudohermaphroditism, Wilm's tumour hypertension and degenerative renal diseases. *Journal of Pediatrics* **76**, 585–93.

Galloway, J. (1922). Remarks on Hodgkin's disease. *British Medical Journal* **2**, 1201.

Glenner, G.G. (1980). Amyloid deposits and amyloidosis. *New England Journal of Medicine* **302**, 1283–92.

Glenner, G.G., Terry, W.D., Harada, M., Isersky, C., and Page, D.L. (1971). Amyloid fibril proteins: proof of homology with immunoglobulin light chains by sequence analysis. *Science* **172**, 1150–1.

Haskell, L.P., Fusco, M.J., Wadler, S., Sablay, L.B., and Mennemeyer, R.P. (1990). Crescentic glomerulonephritis associated with prostatic carcinoma: evidence of immune-mediated glomerular injury. *American Journal of Medicine* **88**, 189–92.

Kaplan, B.S., Klassen, J., and Gault, M.H. (1976). Glomerular injury in patients with neoplasia. *Annual Review of Medicine* **27**, 117–25.

Keur, I., Krediet, R.T., and Arisz, L. (1989). Glomerulopathy as a paraneoplastic phenomenon. *Netherlands Journal of Medicine* **34**, 270–84.

Lee, J.C., Yamauchi, H., and Hopper, J. (1966). The association of cancer and the nephrotic syndrome. *Annals of Internal Medicine* **64**, 41–51.

Lewis, M.G., Loughbridge, L., and Phillips, T.M. (1971). Immunological studies in nephrotic syndrome associated with extra-renal malignant disease. *Lancet* **ii**, 134–5.

Olson, J.L., Philips, T.M., Lewis, M.G., and Solez, K. (1979). Malignant melanoma with renal dense deposits containing tumour antigens. *Clinical Nephrology* **12**, 74–82.

Pascal, R.R. (1980). Renal manifestations of extra-renal neoplasms. *Human Pathology* **11**, 7–17.

Pascal, R.R. and Slovin, S.G. (1980). Tumour directed antibody and carcinoembryonic antigen in the glomeruli of a patient with gastric carcinoma. *Human Pathology* **11**, 679–82.

Pascal, R.R., *et al.* (1975). Glomerular immune complex deposits associated with mouse mammary tumour. *Cancer Research* **35**, 302–4.

Pascal, R.R., Innaccone, P.M., and Rollwagen, F.M. (1976). Electron microscopy and immunofluorescence of glomerular immune complex deposits in cancer patients. *Cancer Research* **36**, 43–7.

Rossen, R.D., Reisberg, R.A., Hersh, E.M., and Gutterman, J.U. (1976). Measurement of soluble immune complexes: a guide to prognosis in cancer patients. *Clinical Research* **24**, 462A.

Row, P.G., *et al.* (1975). Membranous nephropathy, long term follow up and association with neoplasia. *Quarterly Journal of Medicine* **44**, 207–39.

Sawyer, N., Wadsworth, J., Winnen, M., and Gabriel, R. (1988). Prevalence, concentration and prognostic importances of proteinuria in patients with malignancies. *British Medical Journal* **296**, 1295–8.

Sutherland, J.C., Markham, R.V., and Mardiney, M.R. (1974). Subclinical immune complexes in the glomeruli of kidneys postmortem. *American Journal of Medicine* **57**, 536–41.

Vanatta, P.R., Silva, F.G., Taylor, W.E., and Costa, J.C. (1983). Renal cell carcinoma and systemic amyloidosis. *Human Pathology* **14**, 195–201.

Volhard, F. (1931). Cited by Revol, L., *et al.* (1964). Protéinuria associé à des manifestations paranéoplastiques au course d'un cancer bronchogenique. *Lyon Médecine* **212**, 907–16.

Wakashin, M., Wakashin, Y., and Iesato, K. (1980). Association of gastric cancer and nephrotic syndrome. An immunologic study in three patients. *Gastroenterology* **78**, 749–56.

Young, R.H., Scully, R.E., and McCluskey, R.T. (1985). A distinctive glomerular lesion complicating placental site trophoblastic tumour: report of two cases. *Human Pathology*, **16**, 35–42.

20.5.5 Sarcoidosis and the kidney

A. M. DAVISON

Sarcoidosis is a multisystem granulomatous disorder of unknown aetiology which may directly or indirectly involve the kidney (Table 1). Most commonly, renal involvement is a consequence of the associated disordered calcium metabolism, but in addition, acute or chronic interstitial nephritis, glomerulopathy, and a number of miscellaneous conditions may also arise (Kenouch and Méry 1992). In the majority of patients, renal complications develop in those known to have sarcoidosis, and only rarely are they a presenting feature.

Table 1 *Renal consequences of sarcoidosis*

Disordered calcium metabolism
  Nephrocalcinosis
  Nephrolithiasis
Interstitial nephritis
  Chronic renal failure
  Acute renal failure
Glomerulopathy
  Membranous nephropathy
  Rarely, other glomerulopathies
  Amyloidosis
Miscellaneous
  Obstructive uropathy
  Hypertension

Abnormal calcium metabolism

Hypercalciuria occurs in up to 65 per cent of patients with sarcoidosis, hypercalcaemia is much less common (Coburn and Barbour 1984). The disordered calcium metabolism arises due to the presence of 1α-hydroxylase in the macrophages of sarcoid granulomas, resulting in an uncontrolled production of 1,25-dihydroxycholecalciferol, particularly following exposure to sunlight or vitamin D ingestion.

The increased production of calcitriol results in an increased intestinal absorption of calcium and possibly also an increased reabsorption of calcium from bone. In the presence of normal renal function the plasma calcium remains normal, as does the serum phosphate. There is, as expected, a reduction in plasma parathyroid hormone and this, associated with the increased filtered load of calcium, results in hypercalciuria. Nephrocalcinosis may occur, but is rarely radiologically evident, although in some patients it is visible, particularly in the medulla as calcinosis in the papillae. Nephrolithiasis is less common, but may present as recurrent stone disease, in which small stones consisting of calcium oxalate and phosphate may be passed spontaneously.

In up to 20 per cent of patients, many with impaired renal function, the increased synthesis of calcitriol will result in hypercalcaemia. The effect of this is to reduce glomerular filtration rate and to impair urinary concentrating ability.

Corticosteroids have a rapid effect in reducing the activity of the macrophage 1α-hydroxylase. There is doubt as to the most appropriate dosage régime, but many will respond to prednisolone (10 mg on alternate days). The duration of treatment is dependent upon the response of the serum and urinary calcium.

Granulomatous interstitial nephritis

Granulomatous interstitial nephritis is usually associated with extrarenal manifestations of sarcoidosis and most commonly presents clinically as impaired renal function. This is usually chronic and slowly progressive, but some patients may present with acute renal failure. In only very rare cases has the granulomatous interstitial nephritis been the presenting feature of sarcoidosis. The impaired renal function is associated with mild proteinuria, which is predominately tubular in origin. Other tubular abnormalities include glycosuria, the Fanconi syndrome, proximal and distal tubular acidosis, and nephrogenic diabetes insipidus. The pathogenesis of the tubular disorders are most likely to be related to the accompanying hypergammaglobulinaemia, although hypercalcaemia may also play a part, particularly with respect to disorders of concentration, due to associated peritubular microcalcification.

The prevalence of granulomatous interstitial nephritis is difficult to determine, as infiltration may be clinically silent and small lesions may be missed on renal biopsy. However, it is likely to be in the region of 15 to 40 per cent of patients with sarcoidosis (Muther *et al.* 1981). The granuloma involve both the cortex and medulla and are similar to sarcoid granuloma found elsewhere. The lesions may progress to fibrosis with consequent tubular atrophy and resulting impaired renal function.

At diagnosis, many patients have severely impaired renal function, but this may respond dramatically to corticosteroid therapy. The dosage régime most commonly employed is 1 to 1.5 mg/kg.day with a gradual reduction in dose after 2 months of treatment. It is likely that prolonged therapy, up to and perhaps even exceeding a year, will be required. In patients requiring a high dose of corticosteroids, alternate-day therapy should be considered. The overall prognosis as far as renal function is concerned is determined by the extent of involvement and the subsequent fibrosis.

Glomerular involvement

Sarcoidosis-associated glomerulopathy is uncommon, but when present is usually manifest as a nephrotic syndrome associated with minor haematuria and mild impairment of renal function. It occurs most commonly as a late manifestation in patients with overt sarcoidosis. In approximately 50 per cent of patients the histological appearances are those of a membranous nephropathy, although focal and segmental glomerulosclerosis, diffuse endocapillary proliferative glomerulonephritis, and crescentic nephritis have also been described. In a few patients the glomerular abnormality is that of amyloidosis. There is considerable debate at present as to whether idiopathic membranous nephropathy responds to corticosteroid therapy, and it is as yet unclear whether sarcoidosis-associated membranous nephropathy is steroid responsive.

Miscellaneous

Other rare causes of renal involvement with sarcoidosis include obstructive uropathy due to retroperitoneal granuloma, producing ureteral compression. Hypertension has been described in one patient in whom there was stenosis of the renal artery due to peri-aortic fibrosis.

REFERENCES

Adams, J.S. and Gacad, M.A., (1985). Characterization of 1-α-hydroxylation of vitamin D_3 steroids by cultured alveolar macrophages from patients with sarcoidosis. *Journal of Experimental Medicine* **161**, 755–65.

Coburn, J.W. and Barbour, G.L. (1984). Vitamin D intoxication and sarcoidosis. In *Hypercalciuria states. Pathogenesis and treatment*, (ed. F.L. Coe), pp. 379–433. Grune and Stratton, Orlando.

Kenouch, S. and Méry, J.P., (1992). Sarcoidosis. In *Oxford Textbook of Clinical Nephrology*, (ed. S. Cameron, A.M. Davison, J.P. Grünfeld, D. Kerr, and E. Ritz), pp. 576–82. Oxford University Press, Oxford.

Muther, R.S., McCarron, D.A., and Bennett, W.M. (1981). Renal manifestations of sarcoidosis. *Archives of Internal Medicine* **141**, 643–5.

Taylor, R.G., Fisher, C., and Hoffbrand, B.I. (1982). Sarcoidosis and membranous glomerulonephritis: a significant association. *British Medical Journal* **284**, 1297–8.

20.5.6 Rheumatological disorders and the kidney: systemic lupus erythematosus, mixed connective tissue disease, scleroderma, Sjögren's syndrome, and rheumatoid arthritis

J. S. CAMERON and D. G. WILLIAMS

Systemic lupus erythematosus

This protean disease can affect almost any tissue or organ in the body, but the kidney is involved in a high proportion of patients. The pathogenesis of systemic lupus erythematosus and its general manifestations are dealt with in Chapter 18.11.3, and here we deal only with its effects on the kidney.

EPIDEMIOLOGY AND PRESENTATION

The proportion of patients with lupus who have renal involvement depends upon how assiduously the nephritis is sought. Thus in most unselected series of systemic lupus erythematosus 40 to 60 per cent of adults and up to 80 per cent of children show clinical evidence of renal involvement. However, if renal biopsies are performed in patients with normal renal function and normal urine, the proportion approaches 100 per cent. The histological appearances in these patients with clinically inapparent lupus nephritis are usually mild (see below). The proportion of males to females among those with renal involvement is the same as that for lupus as a whole, i.e. a predominance of females of around 8 to 12:1, which is lower in the few prepubertal children (5:1) and in the minority presenting later in life. Nor does the age at presentation differ: it peaks at 15 to 25 years in females, whilst in males most of those affected are less than 15 or over 45 years old at onset.

Clinical renal involvement is present in only about 20 per cent of adults at the time of presentation; the proportion with abnormal urine and/or renal function increases over the next 1 to 10 years, after which new involvement of the kidney is rare. Usually, patients in whom the renal condition becomes prominent later first present with fever, rashes, arthritis, or pleuropericarditis, and even if the urine is carefully tested it is found to be quite normal.

An important although unusual group of patients with lupus nephritis are those in whom the nephritis is initially the sole manifestation of the disease. This particularly applies to patients with membranous nephropathy. After a period, usually months or several years, other manifestations of lupus appear, and only then can the diagnosis be made. However, from the beginning these patients usually show positive antinuclear factor tests or the presence of anti-dsDNA antibodies, so that these should be sought in the evaluation of patients who appear to have primary nephritis, particularly young women and girls.

Renal involvement usually becomes evident in the form of proteinuria, amounting to a full nephrotic syndrome in 50 to 60 per cent of patients. Although this proteinuria is usually accompanied by microscopic haematuria, visible blood in the urine is rare and lupus nephritis almost never presents with isolated haematuria. At renal presentation, 40 per cent of patients have hypertension, 50 per cent have reduced renal function, and the occasional patient presents with acute renal failure. Many patients with lupus have, in association with the interstitial component of their nephritis, modest defects of distal tubular function of which renal tubular acidosis is the most important and is often associated with hyperkalaemia.

LABORATORY TESTS

As in lupus patients as a whole, abnormalities in laboratory tests (apart from those depending upon renal function) are usually haematological and immunological. Sixty per cent are anaemic, a similar number are leucopenic, 25 per cent have thrombocytopenia, and in 30 to 40 per cent phospholipid-dependent coagulation studies such as the APTT or reptilase tests are prolonged because of the presence of antiphospholipid antibody. By definition, almost 100 per cent have positive antinuclear factor tests and/or anti-dsDNA antibodies, and complement levels, particularly C4, are low in 75 per cent. The erythrocyte sedimentation rate is almost always increased, although in general levels of C-reactive proteins remain normal—an important point in differential diagnosis.

RENAL HISTOLOGY IN LUPUS NEPHRITIS

Although arguments have been advanced to the contrary, there is a good case for performing a renal biopsy in all patients with lupus who develop any clinical manifestation of renal disease, to provide information which

Table 1 *Summary of World Health Organization (WHO) classification of lupus nephritis*

Class	Optical microscopy	Immunohistology*
I (normal) (0–5%)	Virtually normal glomerulus	Scanty mesangial immune aggregates
II (mesangial) (15–20%)	Mesangial prominence and hypercellularity	Diffuse mesangial aggregates only
III (a) (focal) (20–30%)	Focal/segmental proliferative necrotic lesions usually on a background of diffuse mesangial hypercellularity	Diffuse mesangial aggregates
III(b)	As III(a) but much more diffuse with major disturbance of glomerular architecture focally in capillary wall	Diffuse mesangial aggregates plus segmental crescents in some glomeruli
IV (diffuse) (45–60%)	Diffuse proliferative/infiltrative glomerulonephritis plus irregular capillary wall thickening and frequent small and occasional large, crescents round glomeruli	Diffuse mesangial aggregates; diffuse capillary wall aggregates both inside and outside capillary wall
V (membranous) (10–15%)	Diffuse peripheral capillary wall thickening with little or no proliferation/infiltration	Predominant diffuse subepithelial capillary aggregates plus some mesangial aggregates in most cases

*In all forms of lupus nephritis, it is common to find IgG, IgA, IgM, C1q, C3, and C4 in the immune aggregates ('full-house' pattern), but this is by no means invariable; nevertheless this finding carries a high suspicion of lupus nephritis. IgG and C3 are almost always present, and lupus is very unlikely if they are absent

is diagnostically and therapeutically useful. Two approaches are useful in describing the histology of lupus nephritis: the first describes the pattern of involvement of the glomerulus, and the second assesses the activity and/or chronicity of the process.

The patterns of nephritis in lupus are bewildering in their variety. First a variety of appearances of the glomeruli have been described which are outlined in Table 1. These broad categories provide at best a general guide to analysis of the glomerular changes; in particular, class III (focal nephritis) covers a very wide range of appearances from occasional segmental lesions in a few glomeruli to segmental involvement of almost all gomeruli with other features more suggestive of a diffuse nephritis. Thus this category is often divided into mild (class IIIa) and severe (class IIIb) focal lupus nephritis. In addition, some patients may show varying patterns in different glomeruli, and even within a single glomerulus, so that the WHO classification is at best a simplification. Some patients are difficult or impossible to classify into a specific category.

The appearances seen on conventional optical microscopy are associated with the presence within the glomeruli of material which contains immune reactants, such as immunoglobulins and complement components, and therefore represents immune aggregates, although the putative antigens have not been identified. Although DNA and anti-DNA antibodies are present in immune aggregates within the glomeruli, they form only a very small proportion of this material, and the pathogenetic significance of DNA–anti-DNA complexes remains in doubt. The distribution of the immune material parallels the distribution of the lesions on optical microscopy (Fig. 1).

In the interstitium there is almost always an infiltrate of monocytes and T lymphocytes, together with a minority of plasma cells, natural killer cells, and a few eosinophils. This is associated with immune aggregates in the tubular basement membranes, which are more common in severe forms of nephritis. On occasion interstitial nephritis may be a dominant feature, with associated severe renal dysfunction or even acute renal failure. Varying degrees of tubular atrophy and interstitial fibrosis may be observed.

A variety of changes may be seen, in the intrarenal vessels including immune aggregates, rarely necrotizing angiitis, and premature vascular sclerosis. Sometimes, particularly in association with antiphospholipid antibodies, thrombi may be seen in glomerular capillaries or renal arterioles, and rarely this is accompanied by a clinical picture of a haemolytic-uraemic syndrome which is one cause of acute renal failure in lupus.

In parallel with this description of histological patterns, attempts have been made to assess how active the lesions are on the one hand and how

Fig. 1 The appearances of the glomeruli in the nephritis of systemic lupus erythematosus as classified by the WHO.
(a) Glomerulus normal to optical microscopy (class I) but with aggregates of immune reactants within the mesangium (arrows), in this case revealed by antibody directed against C1q labelled with peroxidase. The patient had fever, arthralgia, and glandular enlargement but only trivial proteinuria. (b) Obvious mesangial deposits associated with expansion of the mesangium on optical microscopy, together with a mild increase in mesangial cellularity, not visible in this preparation (WHO class II); (c) a more obvious mesangial hypercellularity, again associated with mesangial immune aggregates revealed by immunoperoxidase staining against C3. However, the peripheral capillary walls, however, show no aggregates (WHO class II). (d) WHO class III lesion with not only mesangial involvement but also a focal, predominantly necrotic, lesion containing nuclear debris (arrows). In some patients this may be associated with an overlying area of epithelial proliferation amounting to a segmental crescent. WHO class III includes a wide range of appearances, mild as here (WHO class III(a)) and also severe widespread lessions (but still predominantly focal and segmental) (class III(b)). (e) WHO class IV lesion with diffuse proliferative and infiltrative nephritis. There is a segmental crescent overlying part of the glomerulus. The capillary walls are thickened irregularly. The patient had a full nephrotic syndrome with reduced renal function and hypertension. (f) Appearance of such a glomerulus on immunohistological staining, in this case for IgG. There is mesangial deposition of the immune aggregates and also irregular deposition along the capillary walls, massively in some areas ('wire loops'). (g) A capillary loop from a class IV lesion at high power, stained with silver to show glomerular basement membranes. One of the thickened capillary loops is shown, and demonstrates the black silver-stained glomerular basement membrane, and at a subendothelial site massive clear aggregates of immune material (arrows) are present, with endothelial cells and mesangial cells completing the gross thickening of the capillary wall. (h) WHO class V membranous lesion. Although the mesangium contains immune aggregates, the most prominent lesion is a diffuse scattering of irregular-sized aggregates along the capillary walls which are on the subepithelial side of the membrane and protrude under the epitheial cells and Bowman's space. The patient was nephrotic but normotensive, with normal renal function. (See Table 1 for further identification.)

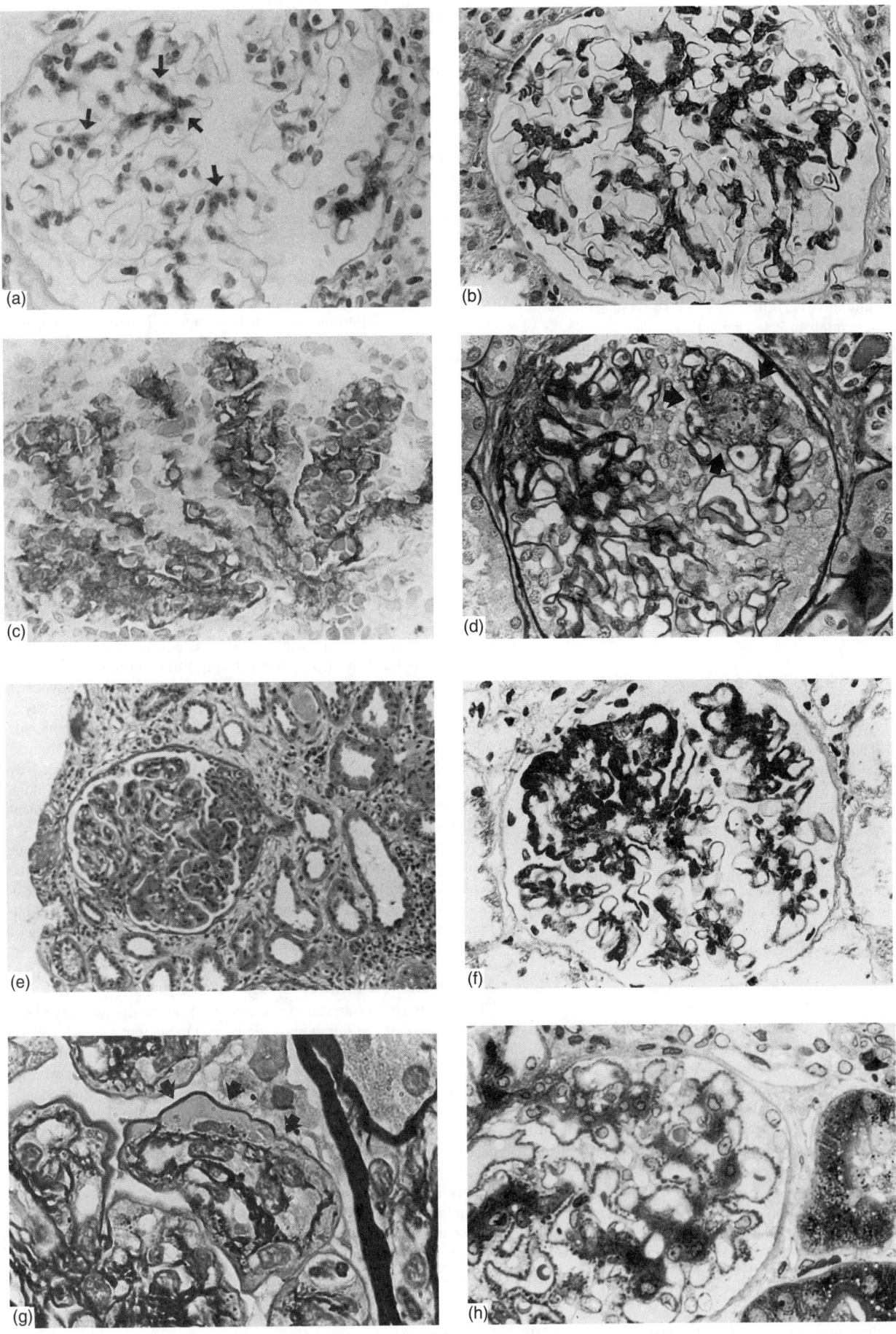

chronic on the other. The former assessment is based on features such as necrosis, nuclear dusting from fragmented cells, glomerular thrombi, and intensity of cellular infiltrate. The last depends essentially on an assessment of the amount of collagen (sclerosis) deposited within the glomeruli and within the interstitium. The former changes are judged to be susceptible to treatment, whilst sclerosis is assumed to be irreversible, although in chronic liver disease fibrotic changes can be reversible.

Clinicopathological correlations

Many apparent relationships between the clinical picture and the histological appearances of lupus nephritis have been modified or eliminated by the success of immunosuppressive treatment (see below). Thus in past years patients with WHO class I, II, and V lesions on biopsy did much better than those with severe focal glomerular lesions (class IIIb) or severe diffuse proliferative nephritis (class IV). Today under the prognosis for these more severely affected individuals under treatment is as good as for those with less severe histological appearances. This observation illustrates the value of renal biopsy, since when this is used as a guide more aggressive treatment can be given appropriately in patients with more severe clinical and histological disease. The additional information available in the renal biopsy probably allows prognosis to be made more accurately and treatment to be better focused. The interstitial infiltrate and interstitial fibrosis have been shown to be good predictors of outcome for renal function. Some controversy exists as to how valuable assessments of activity and chronicity are in predicting outcome in the presence of treatment: in some series predictive capacity has been good, but in others it has been poor.

In general there is no correlation between renal manifestations and levels of anti-dsDNA antibodies or complement, but patients with severe WHO class III and IV appearances in the glomeruli are more likely to be nephrotic, have reduced renal function, or be hypertensive.

TREATMENT OF LUPUS NEPHRITIS

Treatment remains a subject of controversy, with unresolved arguments on a number of points. None the less, an analysis of data from the past 40 years shows that the prognosis for severe forms of lupus nephritis has been transformed. In the 1950s almost no patient with WHO class IV nephritis survived for 5 years. Now, 80 per cent or more of such patients survive with useful renal function at 10 years. Today the problems are principally how to achieve and maintain this success with the minimum cost in side-effects and toxicity.

There are two phases of management in the treatment of lupus nephritis, as in any immune disorder: an initial induction phase during which the principal risk to the patient is the disease process and its effects, and a subsequent maintenance phase during which, although the risk of relapse persists, the main problem is the side-effects of the maintenance treatment.

Induction treatment of acute lupus nephritis

Induction treatment is often guided by the severity of the clinical and histological picture, although this approach has never been examined by a controlled trial. It is generally agreed that all patients with lupus nephritis should begin corticosteroid treatment, although some would dispute this for WHO class V patients with membranous nephropathy which tends to run an indolent course. Most nephrologists would use corticosteroids alone in the initial phase for WHO class I and II patients, and perhaps for mild class III patients with only a few segmental glomerular lesions.

The ideal regime for administration of corticosteroids has never been examined by controlled comparison. A regime comprising a high initial oral dose (e.g. 60 mg/daily) to control the disease, followed by tapering doses to a maintenance treatment of 10–15 mg/daily over 8 to 12 weeks depending on the clinical and immunological response, has been much used, but usually results in a cushingoid patient and can cause a high incidence of infections, some of which may be fatal. For the past 20 years large intravenous doses of methylprednisolone 'pulses' have been used as initial therapy, and there is little doubt that this approach coupled with a low maintenance dose by mouth from the start is less obviously toxic. With this regimen the number of intravenous pulses depends upon the response of the disease; three doses of 1 g on three consecutive days is a conventional but arbitrary programme, with a further similar course or courses if the condition appears resistant.

In more severe nephritis (severe class III and class IV nephritis with evidence of clinical activity), it is usual to use a cytotoxic agent in addition to corticosteroids. The evidence is strong that renal function can be preserved and renal scarring avoided if a cytotoxic agent is used in both the acute and maintenance phases of treatment, when compared with patients treated by corticosteroids alone. The problem is to know which cytotoxic agent to use, and by which route it should be given.

In the induction phase of treatment of acute lupus nephritis the choice lies between cyclophosphamide and azathioprine. No trial has compared these two drugs in this phase, and both seem effective. However, because of its powerful B-cell-suppressant action, cyclophosphamide quickly inhibits autoantibody formation and many nephrologists now feel that it should be used in the acute phase. Despite the popularity of intravenous administration of this drug in this phase of treatment (750–1000 mg as an infusion over several hours with hydration and an antiemetic), oral dosing for 8 to 12 weeks at 1–3 mg/kg/daily adjusted for renal function and white-cell count is as effective. Longer courses of oral daily cyclophosphamide should not be given because of bladder toxicity (which is avoided by the intravenous route), gonadal damage, and oncogenicity. The marrow toxicity of the intravenous regimen is greater than that of the oral route, and leucopenia is rarely a problem with the oral regime provided that renal function is taken into account. It does not seem to matter which route is used in terms of disease control.

There has been much debate as to whether the addition of plasma exchange to this acute induction regime has advantages, and two controlled trials have been performed. Neither trial showed any definite benefit, but neither used plasma exchange as aggressively as advocates of this treatment have suggested (daily 4 exchanges for 7 to 10 days). Others have suggested that pulsed intravenous cyclophosphamide administered 1 to 2 days after the exchanges has the advantage of attacking the B cells just as they are reacting to the removal of antibody by the exchange, and this synchronized approach is undergoing trials at the moment. Outside clinical trials, plasma exchange cannot at the moment be advocated in the induction treatment of severe lupus nephritis.

Another treatment still under evaluation is the use of intravenous pooled gammaglobulin. This has had some success in resistant patients, but there are difficulties in selecting a dose, and diversity of preparations and even between batches of the same preparation. In one study striking improvement was seen in nine resistant patients receiving 400 mg/kg of IgG daily on five consecutive days.

Maintenance treatment

The objective of maintenance treatment is to keep the disease suppressed as far as possible, at minimum toxicity, and to attempt to reach a stage where treatment can be stopped completely. The disease may run a course over 20 to 30 years or more, so that plans must be made in the light of the possible need for very prolonged treatment. Maintenance treatment is usually feasible some 12 weeks after the acute inductive phase when the disease will have come under clinical control in most cases.

Corticosteroids form the mainstay of maintenance treatment. They are given at the lowest effective dose, aiming at prednisolone between 7.5 and 15 mg daily according to clinical response. This alone will often suffice in mild forms of nephritis (WHO classes I, II, and V). In those with more severe or resistant disease, some back-up with cytotoxic agents is needed. Here there is less consensus than for the treatment of the acute phase. The options available are as follows.

1. Change oral or intravenous cyclophosphamide to oral azathioprine (2–2.5 mg/kg/daily) after 12 weeks. This is our usual practice, and has

the advantages of low toxicity in the long term, no increase in the incidence of infections over those treated with corticosteroids alone, no gonadal toxicity, and no adverse effects on pregnancy. The combination of steroid and azathioprine has never been demonstrated to improve results over corticosteroids alone, although most would concur that at the least it permits the use of prednisolone in lower doses. Complete remission, allowing withdrawal of all drugs, is rarely attained, at least for a decade or more.

2. Administration of intravenous cyclophosphamide (750–1000 mg) every month, and then every 2 months, for 1 to 2 years or more, again backed by low-dose maintenance corticosteroids in severe cases. This approach has been strongly advocated by the National Institutes of Health in the United States, and in their studies was clearly superior to corticosteroids alone in two controlled trials. However, their data showed no significant difference from those treated with corticosteroids and azathioprine, and only now is a trial comparing these two maintenance treatments being performed. The advantages of the intravenous cyclophosphamide regimen are that it is clear that the treatment has been received (non-compliance is a major problem in girls and young women with lupus), and it may be possible that a higher proportion of patients will go on to achieve an actual relapse-free cure and can cease all treatment. However, this important point has never been properly tested against the alternatives. The disadvantages of intravenous cyclophosphamide are that the patient must be treated in hospital as either an outpatient or an inpatient (although admission is not always necessary with modern antiemetic drugs such as ondansetron), quite severe chronic marrow depression may appear, there is considerable gonadal toxicity and teratogenicity, with inability to conceive whilst receiving treatment and premature menopause and infertility in more than 50 per cent of patients. There is also evidence of oncogenicity particularly with a risk of the later development of leukaemia much greater than that of azathioprine. Therefore it is reasonable practice to reserve treatment with intravenous cyclophosphamide for patients who require toxic doses of corticosteroids despite addition of azathioprine or for those with particular problems of compliance.

3. Administration of methotrexate 5–15 mg orally each week. The striking success of this drug in modifying the long-term course of rheumatoid arthritis has led to re-evaluation of its possible role in the long-term treatment of lupus. Certainly some patients resistant to other approaches may respond to the addition of this drug. The main limitation has been hepatotoxicity, but this is not usually a major problem in the low doses appropriate here.

4. Cyclosporine has been used in a number of patients with lupus at a dose of 4–5 mg/kg/daily or less, monitored by blood levels. It appears to have relatively little effect in acute lupus, but may have a role in its chronic management, particularly in allowing lower doses of corticosteroids to be used. It will also reduce proteinuria in patients (often with membranous nephropathy) who have particularly profuse proteinuria and severe nephrotic syndromes.

STOPPING TREATMENT

Some patients with lupus have disease which appears to 'burn out' or be driven into remission after about 5 years. However, it is more common for the condition to require indefinite treatment, and it is difficult to know whether, when, and how to stop if a patient is well but still receiving treatment.

It is reasonable practice to treat all patients with lupus nephritis for about 5 years. Then it may be possible to stop treatment in patients whose disease is clinically inactive, whose renal function is stable (although not necessarily normal), whose anti-dsDNA binding levels and complement levels are normal, and (if a biopsy is performed) whose biopsies do not show features of activity. The continued presence of proteinuria may indicate scarring only, and not activity, and need not be a contraindication. Nevertheless, even though some such patients can stop treatment without relapse, this may be as long as 25 years or more

from onset in occasional cases. The usual precautions with corticosteroid withdrawal need to be taken, and it is useful to put the patient on to a period of double doses on alternate days before tapering the dose out, since this allows the hypothalamic–pituitary–adrenal axis to recover more rapidly.

LONG-TERM OUTCOME AND COMPLICATIONS

Survival of renal function and of the patient can now be achieved in 80 per cent of patients with severe nephritis for as long as 10 years. However, it is not yet clear what the long-term outcome of patients given modern treatment regimes over several decades may be. Even if renal failure occurs, both dialysis and renal transplantation can be performed, and surprisingly the disease very rarely recurs in the transplanted kidney even in patients with continued active lupus requiring treatment.

Complications of lupus, and of its treatment, begin to assume increasing importance as time goes by, and some are important causes of morbidity and mortality. Particularly worrying are those complications which arise from lupus itself and are made worse by one or other of its treatments. These include infections of all types, but particularly opportunistic infections, thromboses, osteonecrosis, hypertension, and neoplasia, all of which are more common in untreated lupus patients than in a control population. In addition, an alarming incidence of accelerated atheroma is present in long-term survivors of lupus, the pathogenesis of which is not yet clear. All or any of the many complications of corticosteroids may be seen; diabetes mellitus and cataracts are particularly common, although the latter are rarely clinically significant. Growth failure can be major problem in children and adolescents.

Pregnancy in lupus was formerly discouraged, but it is now clear that relapses during pregnancy are no more common than in women who are not pregnant, although it is wise to escalate the prednisolone treatment for a few days immediately postpartum. Obviously it is wise to await until the lupus is well controlled before considering pregnancy, and in those women who present for the first time whilst pregnant the outlook remains disastrous for the baby, and poor for the mother. Surprisingly, there is no evidence that the combination of corticosteroids and azathioprine is teratogenic in humans (although it is strongly so in rodents). Fetal losses remain higher than in normal women (about 25 per cent compared with 8–10 per cent); a number occur in mid-pregnancy in association with the presence of antiphospholipid antibodies and/or a lupus 'anticoagulant' phenomenon, but in others they occur for unknown, probably immunological reasons. In particular, in women with anti-Ro antibody the fetus may be affected by complete heart block, which carries a high mortality.

Thus, although the recent story of the management of lupus nephritis shows outstanding success, this very success has led in turn to new problems of very-long-term survival of patients still receiving treatment with major potential or actual toxicity.

Mixed connective tissue disease

This rare disorder (Section 18.11) has features which overlap between systemic lupus erythematosus, systemic sclerosis, and polymyositis. It is characterized immunologically by a positive antinuclear factor dependent upon antiribonucleoprotein antibodies (U1 RNP), but serum complement concentrations are usually normal. Glomerular disease was once thought to be rare in mixed connective tissue disease, but it is now recognized to be present in 10 to 40 per cent of patients.

The presenting features of the renal disease are symptomless proteinuria and haematuria in most cases; a nephrotic syndrome is uncommon and renal failure is very rare. The histological appearances are varied; the most common are membranous nephropathy, mesangial proliferative, or proliferative glomerulonephritis. Nephritis in mixed connective tissue disease is usually mild and non-progressive, but if it is considered that it requires treatment, a good response to corticosteroid treatment is usual.

Sjögren's syndrome

Sjögren's syndrome is relatively common in elderly patients with rheumatological disorders. Unlike lupus, with which it shares some features, renal disease is uncommon, affecting only about 10 per cent of patients. Typical symptoms include a sicca syndrome, with dry eyes and mouth, and less commonly weight loss, arthritis, and Raynaud's phenomenon. Autoantibodies against nuclear antigens are present, with high concentrations of immunoglobulin in the plasma; the principal nuclear target antigens are the ribonucleoprotein antigens Ro (SS-A) and La (SS-B).

The commonest form of renal involvement is a tubulointerstitial nephritis which presents with renal tubular functional defects, particularly renal tubular acidosis. This is more commonly distal tubular (type I) rather than proximal tubular (type II) renal acidosis, and Sjögren's syndrome should be considered as a possible cause in any patient with tubular acidosis (Chapter 18.11.5). There may be polyuria and hypokalaemia from renal potassium wasting, which may lead to complaints of muscle weakness. Otherwise the renal involvement is usually symptomless. On histological examination, the kidney is infiltrated with plasma cells and CD5-positive T and B lymphocytes, and extensive tubular atrophy may be present. Peritubular immune aggregates of IgG and complement may be present, but severe disease can be seen in their absence. The condition is responsive to both corticosteroids and cyclophosphamide, but it is rarely justified to use these for the nephropathy alone. Otherwise, potassium supplements and sodium bicarbonate may be used. Rarely, nephrocalcinosis may appear together with renal failure.

Glomerular disease is very rare in Sjögren's syndrome. It usually takes the form of a membranous nephropathy, occasionally a focal proliferative nephritis associated in some cases with cryoglobulinaemia and low serum complement concentrations. Otherwise, serum complement concentrations are usually normal.

Systemic sclerosis (scleroderma) (see Chapter 18.11.4)

Systemic sclerosis (scleroderma) results from uncontrolled and irreversible proliferation of connective tissue, together with striking vascular changes. Renal involvement in systemic sclerosis was first described adequately by Osler, and primarily arises from the vascular changes which are central to this disease. Renal disorder is present in about one-third of patients, almost all with the diffuse form of the disease, and ranges from proteinuria, usually of modest degree, and haematuria, to slowly progressive renal failure with hypertension, to acute renal failure with accelerated hypertension. This last syndrome has been called the 'scleroderma crisis' and comprises rapid progression to acute renal failure, often accompanied by left ventricular failure against a background of accelerated hypertension. This form of renal disease is more common in black patients than in Caucasians. The renal manifestations of systemic sclerosis, and particularly of the scleroderma crisis, are associated with a raised plasma renin activity, but are not predictable by the level of plasma renin, by hypertension, or by the degree of renal failure. The diagnosis should be suspected in all patients presenting with severe hypertension and acute renal failure, but even careful examination of the digits and face may fail to reveal any changes in the skin. Raynaud's phenomenon is a valuable clue, and immunological testing shows a positive antinuclear factor resulting from antibodies against the centromere nuclear antigen topoisomerase I (also called scl 70) in a high proportion of those with renal involvement.

Histologically, the most important lesion in scleroderma affects the blood vessels, in which there is excess collagen production believed to be due to a circulating factor which has yet to be identified. Detailed examination shows proliferation of endothelial cells, with deposition of glycoproteins and mucopolysaccharides within the vessel wall (Fig. 2) together with fibrinoid necrosis and reduplication of the internal elastic lamina, giving rise to the so-called 'onion skin' appearance in histological preparations which is particularly common in interlobular and arcuate arteries of diameter 150–500 μm. These vascular changes can precede hypertension, as can functional changes in renal blood flow. The glomeruli usually only show changes due to ischaemia, but occasionally renal arteriolar thrombosis may be seen and the patients may have clinical features of thrombotic microangiopathy, such as thrombocytopenia and red-cell fragmentation. No specific immune aggregates are detected within the vessel wall by immunohistology, although IgM, C3, and fibrinogen may be present on occasion.

Management of renal disease has been much improved by the use of angiotensin-converting enzyme inhibitors in addition to other antihypertensive drugs. However, diuretics should not generally be used because they increase the plasma renin concentrations even further as a result of plasma volume contraction. Effective control of arterial pressure, particularly by angiotensin-converting enzyme inhibitors, has reduced the mortality of scleroderma renal crisis from 100 per cent to much lower levels, depending upon how early treatment is begun. It is now agreed that there is no role for corticosteroids or anticoagulants in the treatment of the condition.

If endstage renal failure supervenes, dialysis, on rare occasions with bilateral nephrectomy for hypertension, can be effective treatment. Interestingly, a small proportion of patients may recover some degree of renal function after several months of dialysis. Transplantation has also been an effective treatment, but recurrence of disease in the allograft has been reported in a few patients. The ultimate outcome of patients with systemic sclerosis and renal involvement may depend not only upon the severity of their renal disease but also upon involvement of other organs, particularly the lungs or oesophagus.

Pregnancy in systemic sclerosis is usually uncomplicated, except for the need to maintain control of hypertension and rarely, by a haemolyticuraemic syndrome of varying severity, sometimes complicated by digital or even limb ischaemia, during or immediately following the pregnancy.

Rheumatoid arthritis (see Chapter 18.4)

Glomerulonephritis

Glomerulonephritis, previously considered to be almost non-existent as a part of rheumatoid arthritis itself, does occur but is unusual, and is less important than the other two manifestations. Several forms of glomerulonephritis have been described as uncommon manifestations of rheumatoid arthritis.

Fig. 2 Lesions in medium-sized renal arterioles in a patient with systemic sclerosis. The intima shows swelling and proliferation, so that the lumen of the vessel is completely occluded. in addition the internal elastic lamina is reduplicated, the beginnings of an 'onion skin' appearance can be seen, and the media is vacuolated and swollen. A smaller vessel to the left of the picture shows similar changes.

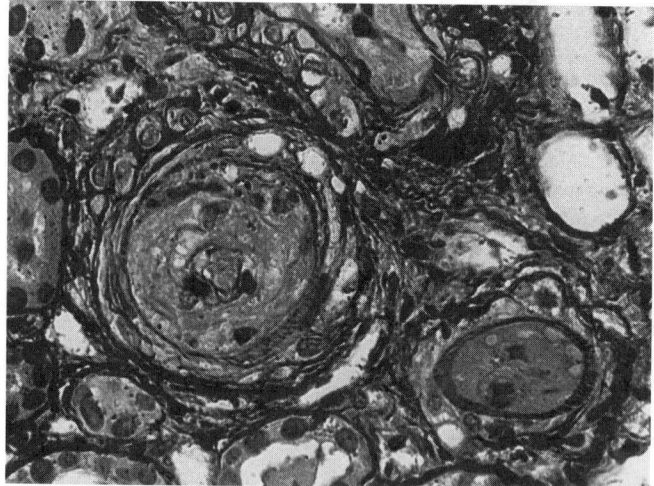

Mesangial proliferation may occur with or without visible deposits of IgA. In a proportion of patients with rheumatoid arthritis the serum IgA concentration is elevated, as it often is in idiopathic IgA-associated nephropathy. Whether or not these patients represent more than the coincidence of two relatively common conditions is unclear.

Membranous nephropathy can be found in occasional patients with rheumatoid arthritis who have never received gold or penicillamine. Again the possibility of coincidence arises, but seems unlikely.

Vasculitis in rheumatoid arthritis is common, but rarely affects the kidney. When it does the appearances are similar to those of microscopic polyangiitis, and it also responds well to treatment with corticosteroids or cyclophosphamide. The glomerular lesions may be segmental necrotizing lesions or full crescentic nephritis, as in the idiopathic forms.

Amyloidosis (Chapters 11.13.1, 20.5.3)

In developed countries, rheumatoid arthritis is now the most common underlying cause of amyloid affecting the kidneys. Amyloidosis affects about 15 per cent of all patients with rheumatoid arthritis in post-mortem studies and is a major cause of death (about 40 per cent), particularly in those with juvenile onset (Still's disease). Amyloidosis is particularly common in Finland, where it is a major cause of renal failure. Presentation is usually with proteinuria, either without symptoms or accompanied by a nephrotic syndrome. Microscopic haematuria is usually present also. Diagnosis is made by biopsy of the kidney, or inferred from biopsy of gum, abdominal fat, or rectal mucosa. There is some evidence of a decreased incidence of amyloid complicating rheumatoid arthritis in recent years, which may be the result of a more efficient therapeutic depression of the immune response during the course of the disease.

Management is similar to that of any form of secondary amyloid affecting the kidney. There is no specific agent which halts or diminishes the deposition of amyloid, and treatment is aimed at decreasing the inflammation of the arthritis itself. Claims have been made that early treatment with chlorambucil, particularly in juvenile rheumatoid arthritis, reduces the deposition of amyloid, but these results are uncontrolled and controversial. Likewise dimethylsulphoxide (DMSO) has been used to solubilize the amyloid, but the dreadful odour it confers on the patient makes it unusable. If renal failure finally supervenes, opportunities for self-dialysis by either continuous ambulatory peritoneal dialysis or haemodialysis may be limited because of severe joint involvement of the hands.

Drug-induced nephropathy

The sulphydryl-containing drugs penicillamine and sodium aurothiomalate, and less commonly auranofin (triethylphosphine gold), can induce a membranous nephropathy which may lead to proteinuria with or without a nephrotic syndrome depending on its severity. Risk factors for the appearance of proteinuria are the presence of HLA DR3 and low sulphoxidation capacity. The proteinuria is reversible on stopping the drug in almost all cases, but its disappearance may take as long as year or two. Indications for stopping are proteinuria above 2 g in 24 h, hypoalbuminaemia, or a diminution in the glomerular filtration rate. Rarely, penicillamine can induce pulmonary haemorrhage accompanied by crescentic nephritis, and in some of these patients antiglomerular basement membrane (anti-GBM) antibody is detectable in the plasma. Finally, non-steroidal anti-inflammatory agents may cause a reversible depression in glomerular filtration rate or an interstitial nephritis, occasionally complicated by papillary necrosis (Chapter 20.14).

REFERENCES
Systemic lupus erythematosus

Alexopoulos, E., Seron, D., Hartley, R.B., and Cameron, J.S. (1990). Lupus nephritis: correlation of interstitial cells with glomerular function. Kidney International, 37, 100–9.

Cameron, J.S. (1994). Lupus nephritis in childhood and adolescence. Pediatric Nephrology, 8, 230–49.

Cameron, J.S. (1993). What is the role of long-term cytotoxic agents in the treatment of lupus nephritis? Journal of Nephrology, 6, 172–6.

Donadio, J.V. and Glassock, R.J. (1993). Immunosuppressive drug therapy in lupus nephritis. American Journal of Kidney Diseases, 21, 239–50.

Esdaile, J.M., Federgrren, W., Quintal, H., Suissa, S., Hayslett, J.P., and Kashgarian, M. (1991). Predictors of one year outcome in lupus nephritis: the importance of renal biopsy. Quarterly Journal of Medicine, 81, 907–18.

Gruppo Intaliano per lo Studio della Nefrite Lupica (GISNEL) (1992). Lupus nephritis: prognostic factors and probability of maintaining life-supporting renal function 10 years after the diagnosis. American Journal of Kidney Diseases, 19, 473–9.

Hashimoto, M. et al. (1994) Methotrexate for steroid-resistant systemic lupus erythematosus. Clinical Rheumatology, 13, 280–3.

Kashgarian, M. (1994). Lupus nephritis: lessons from the path lab (Nephrology Forum). Kidney International, 45, 928–38.

Kozeny, G.A. et al. (1987). Occurrence of renal tubular dysfunction in lupus nephritis. Archives of Internal Medicine, 147, 891–5.

Lewis, E.J., Hunsicker, L.G., Lan, S.-P., Rohde, R.D., and Lachin, J.M. (1992). A controlled trial of plasmapheresis therapy in severe lupus nephritis. New England Journal of Medicine, 326, 1373–9.

Lin, C.-Y., Hsu, H.-C., and Chiang, H. (1989). Improvement of histological and immunological change in steroid and immunosuppressive drug-resistant lupus nephritis by high-dose intravenous gamma globulin. Nephron, 53, 303–10.

Nossent, H.C., Henzen-Logmans, S.C., Vroom, T.M., Berden, J.H.M., and Swaak, T.J.G. (1990). Contribution of renal biopsy data in predicting outcome of lupus nephritis. Arthritis and Rheumatism, 33, 970–7.

Pasquali, S., Banfi, G., Zucchelli, A., Moroni, G., Ponticelli, C., and Zucchelli, P. (1992). Lupus membranous nephropathy: long term outcome. Clinical Nephrology, 39, 175–82.

Ponticelli, C. and Banfi, G. (1992) Systemic lupus erythematosus (clinical). In Oxford textbook of clinical nephrology (ed. J.S. Cameron, A.M. Davison, J.-P. Grünfeld, D.N.S Kerr, and E. Ritz), pp. 646–67. Oxford University Press.

Mixed connective tissue disease

Kitridou, R.C., Akmal, M., Turkel, S.B., Ehresmann, G.R., Quismorio, F.P., and Massry S.G. (1986). Renal involvement in mixed connective tissue disease: a longitudinal clinicopathologic study. Seminars in Arthritis and Rheumatism, 16, 135–45.

Nimelstein, S.H., Brody, S., McShane, D., and Holman, H.R. (1980). Mixed connective tissue disease: a subsequent evaluation of the original 25 patients. Medicine, Baltimore, 59, 239–48.

Sjögren's syndrome

Kassan, S.S., and Talal, N. (1987). Renal disease in Sjögren's syndrome. In Sjögren's syndrome. Clinical and immunological aspects (ed. N. Talal, H.M. Moutsopoulos, and S.S. Kassan), pp. 96–101. Springer Verlag, Berlin.

Matsumura, R. et al. (1988). Immunohistochemical identification of infiltrating mononuclear cells in tubulointerstitial nephritis associated with Sjögren's syndrome. Clinical Nephrology, 30, 335–40.

Shiozawa, S., Shiozawa, K., Shinizu, S., Nakada, M., Isobe, T., and Fugita, T. (1987). Clinical studies of renal disease in Sjögren's syndrome. Annals of the Rheumatic Diseases, 46, 768–72.

Talal, N. and Moutsopoulos, H.M. (1987). Treatment of Sjögren's syndrome. In Sjögren's syndrome. Clinical and immunological aspects (ed. N. Talal, H.M. Moutsopoulos, and S.S. Kassan), pp. 291–5. Springer Verlag, Berlin.

Vitali, C., Tavoni, A., Sciuto, M., Maccheroni, M., Moriconi, L., and Bombardieri, S. (1991). Renal involvement in primary Sjögren's syndrome: a retrospective–prospective study. Scandinavian Journal of Rheumatology, 20, 132–6.

Systemic sclerosis

Altieri, P. and Cameron, J.S. (1989). Scleroderma renal crisis in a pregnant woman with late partial recovery of renal function. Nephrology Dialysis Transplantation, 3, 677–80.

Table 1 *Clinical presentations of urinary-tract infections*

Symptomatic
    Frequency–dysuria syndrome
        bacterial cystitis
        abacterial cystitis (urethral syndrome)
Acute pyelonephritis
Acute prostatitis
Asymptomatic (covert)

Table 2 *Classification of urinary-tract infections*

Uncomplicated
    Normal urinary tract
    Normal renal function
Complicated
    Abnormal urinary tract (e.g. calculi, vesico ureteric reflux,
        reflux nephropathy, analgesic nephropathy, obstruction,
        paraplegia, ileal conduit, atonic bladder, indwelling
        catheter)
    Impaired host defences (e.g. neutropenia,
        immunosuppressive therapy, organ transplant recipient,
        diabetes mellitus)
    Impaired renal function
    Virulent organism (e.g. urease-producing *Proteus* sp.
        metastatic staphylococcal infection)
All males

discomfort. If bacteriuria is demonstrated, this syndrome is referred to as bacterial cystitis. Up to one-third of women suffering from frequency and dysuria, however, do not have bacteriuria. This condition has been termed the urethral syndrome or abacterial cystitis.

Acute pyelonephritis is a much more serious illness. High fever (38–40 °C), rigors, and loin pain are cardinal features, commonly associated with vomiting and prostration. There is usually tenderness in one or both loins. Lower urinary-tract symptoms are often absent. When both kidneys are severely affected, oedema of the epithelium or the renal pelvis result in oliguric acute renal failure. The complication of papillary necrosis is discussed below. Nephro-urological conditions that may simulate acute pyelonephritis include urinary-tract obstruction, urinary colic, acute glomerulonephritis, renal infarction, renal vein thrombosis, and haemorrhage into a renal tumour or cyst, while the differential diagnosis should also include acute appendicitis, cholecystitis or pancreatitis, pelvic inflammatory disease, and a basal pneumonia.

Males with acute bacterial prostatitis, present with 'flu-like' symptoms, low backache, often few urinary tract symptoms and have a swollen, tender prostate gland.

A detailed physical examination is rarely very helpful, but a distended bladder should be excluded. In males it is important to do a rectal examination and to examine the genitalia, and in women to do a pelvic examination and view the cervix. Some women with urinary-tract infection may also have a vaginitis or cervicitis, often with enterobacterial organisms. These problems should be treated specifically, as they may be a focus for further ascending urinary-tract infection.

More unusual variations of complicated urinary-tract infections include pyonephrosis, where an obstructed hydronephrotic kidney has become infected. A variant of this is xanthogranulomatous pyelonephritis, which predominantly affects elderly women, and is commonly associated with calculous obstruction and infection with an organism such as *Proteus mirabilis*. In addition to loin pain and fever, these patients may have weight loss, constitutional symptoms, and a palpable renal mass. A renal carbuncle or cortical abscess is probably the result of a haematogenous infection with *Staphylococcus aureus*. The presentation is usually similar to that of acute pyelonephritis, and may also be mimicked by an infected renal cyst or a perinephric abscess. The latter is most likely to result from extension or rupture of an intrarenal abscess into the perirenal space. These generally present more insidiously than either acute pyelonephritis or a renal carbuncle, with the patient often having a prolonged period of progressive ill health and intermittent fever, often with loin pain.

ASYMPTOMATIC (COVERT) URINARY-TRACT INFECTION

Patients with bacteriuria are rarely completely asymptomatic. Those with truly covert bacteriuria come to attention only when the urine is cultured for some other reason.

Many different populations of healthy individuals have been screened for asymptomatic bacteriuria, but with the exception of pregnancy, there is no convincing evidence to suggest that routine screening or treatment is valuable. The prevalence of this condition is between 1 and 2 per cent in schoolgirls and 3 to 5 per cent in adult women. It is much rarer in the male (0.05 per cent of schoolboys and 0.5 per cent of male adults). In most studies, 5 to 6 per cent of pregnant women have been found to have bacteriuria. The reported rates have varied from 2 per cent in a private clinic in the United States to 18.5 per cent in urban New Zealand Maori women.

The importance of asymptomatic bacteriuria in pregnant women lies in a reported incidence of acute pyelonephritis developing late in the pregnancy or puerperium in the range 15 to 40 per cent (usually 15–20 per cent) (see Chapter 13.3). In some early studies of women with bacteriuria in pregnancy there appeared to be an increased risk of pre-eclampsia, lowered fetal birth weight, shortened gestation interval, more congenital fetal defects, increased perinatal mortality, infected amniotic fluid, and transference of the infection to the infant. Later reports indicate that these risks are not as high as was thought initially. Treatment of the bacteriuria when still asymptomatic effectively reduces the incidence of later acute pyelonephritis. About 20 per cent of women with asymptomatic bacteriuria in pregnancy have a radiological abnormality of the urinary tract (such as reflux nephropathy, stones, pelviureteric obstruction).

Otherwise healthy elderly women and men have a steeply increasing prevalence of bacteriuria with age, with the highest prevalence being in institutionalized women.

Classification of urinary-tract infections

From a clinical and management point of view it is useful to classify urinary-tract infections as uncomplicated or complicated (Table 2). All urinary-tract infections in males should probably be considered as complicated.

Diagnosis

The diagnosis of a urinary-tract infection can only be proven by culturing the urine. An accurate bacteriological diagnosis is the ideal, and must be made in all cases affecting infants, children, and males. A case can be made, however, to withhold a urine culture when it is difficult to obtain in women who have an isolated episode of cystitis. It may be more cost-effective to treat these women with a single dose or a 3 day course, and only culture the urine if the symptoms do not resolve or recur shortly after completing treatment.

MIDSTREAM SPECIMEN

The most widely used method of obtaining urine for culture is the clean-catch midstream (**MSU**) technique. However, it suffers from the disadvantage that some contamination of the specimen is inevitable in the female, making it necessary to quantitate the bacterial content. Kass provided systematic statistical analyses of urine bacterial counts in order to establish reliable criteria for separating contamination from true infection with Gram-negative bacilli. No data were produced for infections with Gram-positive cocci. These findings have been misinterpreted by many, even though it was stressed that it was necessary to accept several constraints when interpreting the results.

A single MSU specimen with a bacterial colony count of greater than 100 000/ml ($> 100 \times 10^6/l$) represents only an 80 per cent confidence level in diagnosing a urinary-tract infection in a female who is asymptomatic or has only mild lower urinary-tract symptoms. In this clinical context, therefore, 20 per cent of positive cultures may reflect only heavy contamination of the specimen. Such an error rate has been demonstrated under ideal conditions from populations of co-operative young women attending special clinics. To ensure more accuracy in diagnosis, multiple cultures of MSU specimens are necessary in those without symptoms. On the other hand, a bacterial count of more than 100 000 colonies/ml ($> 100 \times 10^6/l$) in an MSU from a patient with acute pyelonephritis has a confidence limit exceeding 95 per cent.

For women with marked frequency of micturition, or those infected with *Staphylococcus saprophyticus*, the bacterial count may be low. Stamm and colleagues have demonstrated that if a woman has urinary-tract symptoms and an MSU specimen has been collected particularly carefully, a single pathogen present in a count as low as 100/ml may indicate a urinary-tract infection. A recent international working party has suggested the use of a bacterial count of greater than 1000/ml ($> 10^6/l$) of a potential pathogen in a symptomatic female as a diagnostic criterion, although there was strong support for a more practical figure of greater than 10 000/ml ($> 10 \times 10^6/l$).

In most males, where there is a much reduced risk of contaminating a voided MSU specimen, a bacterial count of greater than 1000/ml ($> 10^6/l$) of a pathogen may be taken to indicate true infection with a high degree of confidence.

In most clinical situations there is usually little preparation or supervision of patients before or during the collection of MSU samples, and often an unacceptable delay in culturing the specimens. Special problems also exist in the collection of samples from infants and children, the elderly, bedridden or paraplegic patients, from women who are menstruating or who have a vaginal discharge, and from patients in the postsurgical or postpartum period. In infants and children the confidence limit for a single positive culture from an MSU, or from a specimen collected in an adhesive bag, is less than 40 per cent. For women in the puerperium, even with extremely careful urine collection, 30 per cent of MSU cultures have been demonstrated to give false positive results.

Colony counting of MSU is laborious, but this has been simplified by the introduction of the quantitative loop, the filter-paper method, and the many variations of the dip-inoculum method, which are now commercially available. Chemical screening tests have proved unsatisfactory and many are too crude for clinical use. Some dipstick reagent strips now include the nitrite test and/or a test to detect leucocytes. If a patient has acute symptoms, a positive nitrite test, and pyuria then it is extremely likely that the urine is infected.

Uncentrifuged fresh urine from patients with symptomatic urinary-tract infections invariably contains more than 10 leucocytes/mm³ ($> 10 \times 10^6/l$). If contamination of the specimen can be excluded, this is evidence of an inflammatory process. Of women with asymptomatic bacteriuria, only about one-half will have pyuria, so tests to detect pyuria are of no value in screening for bacteriuria in pregnancy, nor is the presence of proteinuria of specific value in this context.

Localizing the site of the infection by urological techniques is useful as a research tool, but is of little clinical value. The response to single-dose treatment (see below) may be a simple practical clue to the site of infection, in that most patients with bladder infections respond, whereas those with upper-tract infections often do not.

SUPRAPUBIC ASPIRATE

Suprapubic aspiration of the distended bladder has made the diagnosis of urinary-tract infection more rapid, efficient, and accurate. Contamination of the specimen is avoided and this eliminates the inconvenience of doing multiple MSUs and the need for quantitative bacterial counts, as any bacteria obtained by suprapubic aspiration can be regarded as significant. In most infected suprapubic aspiration specimens bacteria can be seen microscopically in a drop of unspun urine, and prompt treatment instituted. This simple technique is safe for all groups of patients, simpler than a venepuncture, quicker than obtaining a carefully collected MSU, readily acceptable to patients, and easily performed by trained nurses. Suprapubic aspiration must be used in order to appreciate its simplicity and obvious advantages, but it is important to ensure that there is a full bladder, when it is performed.

CATHETER SPECIMEN

There is little justification, except in unusual circumstances, for catheterizing the bladder specifically to obtain urine for culture. Although such a specimen rarely leads to false positive results, it may introduce bacteria into the bladder, and is uncomfortable and also time-consuming.

In elderly women, particularly those who are incapacitated, it is often difficult to obtain uncontaminated urine using the MSU technique and they may not be able to hold an adequate volume of urine in their bladder for suprapubic aspiration. In these circumstances the Alexa bag catheter or a straight plastic catheter is recommended.

PROSTATIC SPECIMENS

When prostatic infection is suspected it may be valuable to culture specimens derived from the urethra, the bladder, and the prostate separately, as described by Stanley. After cleaning the glans penis, the first few millilitres of urine are not discarded as in collecting a midstream specimen, but are collected for culture of organisms likely to have been present in the urethra. The midstream specimen is deemed to refect bladder urine. The prostate gland is then massaged and any secretion yielded collected with 5 to 10 ml or urine passed immediately after massage. Culture of the three specimens so obtained then gives some clue about localization of the infection. In the case of prostatitis the bacterial count in the third specimen exceeds that in the first.

Treatment

Although it is controversial, and may be inconvenient for both doctor and patient, to withhold antimicrobial therapy until the results of the urine culture and antibacterial sensitivity tests are known, this remains the best clinical practice particularly in the complicated case. Only in a very ill patient should it be essential to start treatment before this information is available. Many general practitioners, however, feel under pressure to start antimicrobial therapy at the initial visit.

Untreated patients may lose their symptoms, but in this event bacteriuria usually persists. The prescribing of an alkalinizing agent (for example, Citravescent or Ural) alone does not eradicate the infection, although it may temporarily alleviate lower urinary tract symptoms. The traditional advice to 'drink plenty' is a useful adjunct to antibacterial therapy, principally because it results in more frequent bladder emptying. Although the administered drug will have its urinary concentration reduced in the presence of a diuresis, this is of little practical importance.

Antimicrobial treatment regimens for urinary-tract infection can be classified as:

(1) curative;
(2) prophylactic or preventive; and
(3) suppressive.

Curative treatment

BACTERIAL CYSTITIS

A major error in the treatment of bacterial cystitis has been that most doctors have given too much drug for too long. The aim of treatment should be to use the shortest course of the simplest, safest, and cheapest drug that will eradicate the infecting organism. The possible side-effects of the chosen drug should be weighed against the severity of the illness. There is now considerable evidence that a single oral dose of an antimicrobial agent is as effective as a conventional short course for the treatment of uncomplicated cystitis. Algorithms of management are shown in Figs. 1 and 2.

Single-dose treatment

There is considerable enthusiasm for using single-dose antimicrobial therapy for treating uncomplicated urinary-tract infections. The first drug promoted in this way was amoxycillin, given in a single 3 g oral dose. This proved comparable to a standard course of amoxycillin. A single oral dose of 1.92 g co-trimoxazole or 600 mg trimethoprim is more effective than amoxycillin, and is equivalent to a 3 to 5 day course of either preparation. Amoxycillin and the cephalosporins are no longer recommended in single-dose regimens (Table 3).

Although single doses of many drugs have been shown to be efficacious, they are all less effective than trimethoprim or co-trimoxazole. Recently a single dose of some of the new 4-quinolones (e.g. norfloxacin, fleroxacin) have proven very effective, despite some doubt over their activity against *Staphylococcus saprophyticus*. A novel compound, fosfomycin trometamol has proved highly effective and has been marketed specifically for single-dose treatment of cystitis.

It is recommended that single-dose therapy be considered as the initial treatment for cystitis or asymptomatic bacteriuria in sexually active women, and also for girls who are known to have a normal urinary tract. The many advantages of single-dose therapy have now been well documented.

Short (3 day) course

An alternative to single-dose therapy for women with bacterial cystitis is a short course of treatment. Recent studies have demonstrated that 3 days is sufficient (Table 4).

One of the most popular antibiotics for this treatment has been amoxycillin, but in many areas up to 30 per cent of *E. coli* isolated in the community and 50 per cent in hospitals are now resistant to this drug. It is therefore a poor choice as a first-line drug before the antibacterial sensitivity profile is known. However, amoxycillin remains the drug of choice for treating *Streptococcus faecalis*. The problem of resistance to amoxycillin has been addressed by combining it with clavulanic acid or sulbactam, β-lactamase inhibitors, which are resistant to some bacterial β-lactamases. A clavulanic acid-potentiated form of amoxycillin (Augmentin®) has proved disappointing in some clinical studies, with a slow clinical response, a high proportion of bacteriological relapses, and a troublesome side-effect profile.

Co-trimoxazole is an effective agent for oral administration. This antibacterial combination, however, is a common cause of adverse drug reactions, most of which are related to the sulphamethoxazole component. In many countries trimethoprim alone has replaced co-trimoxazole for the treatment of urinary-tract infections. Many studies have shown trimethoprim to be just as effective as co-trimoxazole. It is also rational to use trimethoprim alone as, in the urinary tract, the antibacterial efficacy of the co-trimoxazole drug combination is almost entirely due to the trimethoprim component. In all countries, however, there is an increasing resistance of *E. coli* to trimethoprim.

Nitrofurantoin remains a valuable drug, although it is ineffective against *Proteus mirabilis*. Unfortunately, many doctors continue to prescribe a dose of 100 mg every 6 h, which often causes nausea or vomiting. Studies have shown comparable effectiveness with 50 mg every 8 h with minimal side-effects. A macrocrystalline formulation of nitrofurantoin is associated with fewer gastrointestinal side-effects.

The use of nalidixic acid and oxolinic acid has been superseded by a new generation of quinolones, including norfloxacin, enoxacin, ofloxacin, pefloxacin, ciprofloxacin, fleroxacin, and lomefloxacin. These orally absorbed, broad-spectrum, synthetic 4-quinolones are highly effective against a wide range of pathogens, including hospital-acquired organisms.

Cephalosporins, such as cephalexin, cephradine, and cefaclor remain

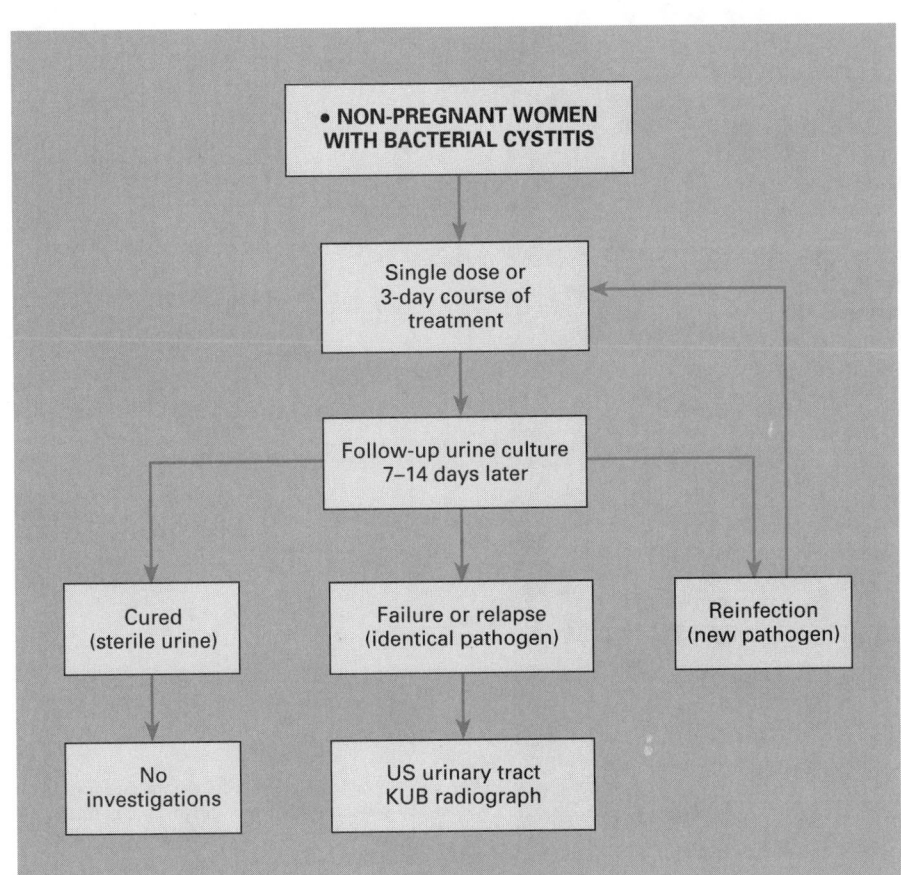

Fig. 1 A suggested algorithm for the management of non-pregnant women with bacterial cystitis (US, ultrasonography; KUB, plain abdominal radiograph, including kidney, ureter, and bladder areas).

useful drugs. The sulphonamides such as sulphamethizole have become unfashionable for the treatment of urinary-tract infections, although they remain efficacious.

The above recommendations apply only to patients with normal renal function. When renal function is impaired the renal handling of the drug must be known. Cephalexin is of well-proven value in patients with renal insufficiency.

URETHRAL SYNDROME

The management of women with the urethral syndrome is unsatisfactory, mainly because of ignorance regarding its aetiology. The symptoms usually settle, however, over a few days and may be improved by a high fluid intake. Alkalinization of the urine is rarely of much benefit. Antibacterial therapy appears to influence recovery in some women, particularly those with pyuria, but there have been no controlled studies comparing the effects of antimicrobial treatment with placebo in women with the urethral syndrome.

COURSE OF TREATMENT FOR SEVERE OR COMPLICATED URINARY-TRACT INFECTIONS

Acute pyelonephritis

Patients with uncomplicated acute pyelonephritis should receive a 5 day course of treatment, preferably with at least one dose of a parenterally administered drug if vomiting is a problem (Table 5). Many of these patients need to be in hospital for rehydration, analgesia, and administration of parenteral antibiotics. Blood cultures should be taken before antimicrobial treatment is started. Some clinicians still treat acute pyelo-

Table 3 *Suggested drugs for single-dose oral treatment of bacterial cystitis or asymptomatic bacteriuria*

Trimethoprim, 600 mg
Co-trimoxazole, 1.92 g
Norfloxacin, 800 mg
Ciprofloxacin, 500 mg
Fleroxacin, 400 mg
Fosfomycin trometamol, 3 g

nephritis for at least 2 weeks, but comparative studies have shown that this is unnecessary.

For patients who are particularly ill, the choice of drug now lies between an aminoglycoside, a 4-quinolone, or a β-lactam antibiotic. Many clinicians still prefer the aminoglycosides until the sensitivity profile is known. Tobramycin may be preferable to gentamicin, because of the reduced risk of nephrotoxicity. Netilmicin also has a reduced risk of nephrotoxicity and ototoxicity, but its use has been limited because of price. Amikacin is valuable for the treatment of resistant pathogens.

All patients, irrespective of their renal function, require a full loading dose of an aminoglycoside (for example, 2.5–3.0 mg/kg). The normal maintenance dose of 1.0 to 1.5 mg/kg should be adjusted according to the measured or assessed creatinine clearance, and given at an appropriately increased interval. This method is preferred to that of giving a smaller dose every 8 hours. However, the formula is no substitute for monitoring the peak and trough (predose) serum drug concentrations every second or third day, and even daily if treatment is extending

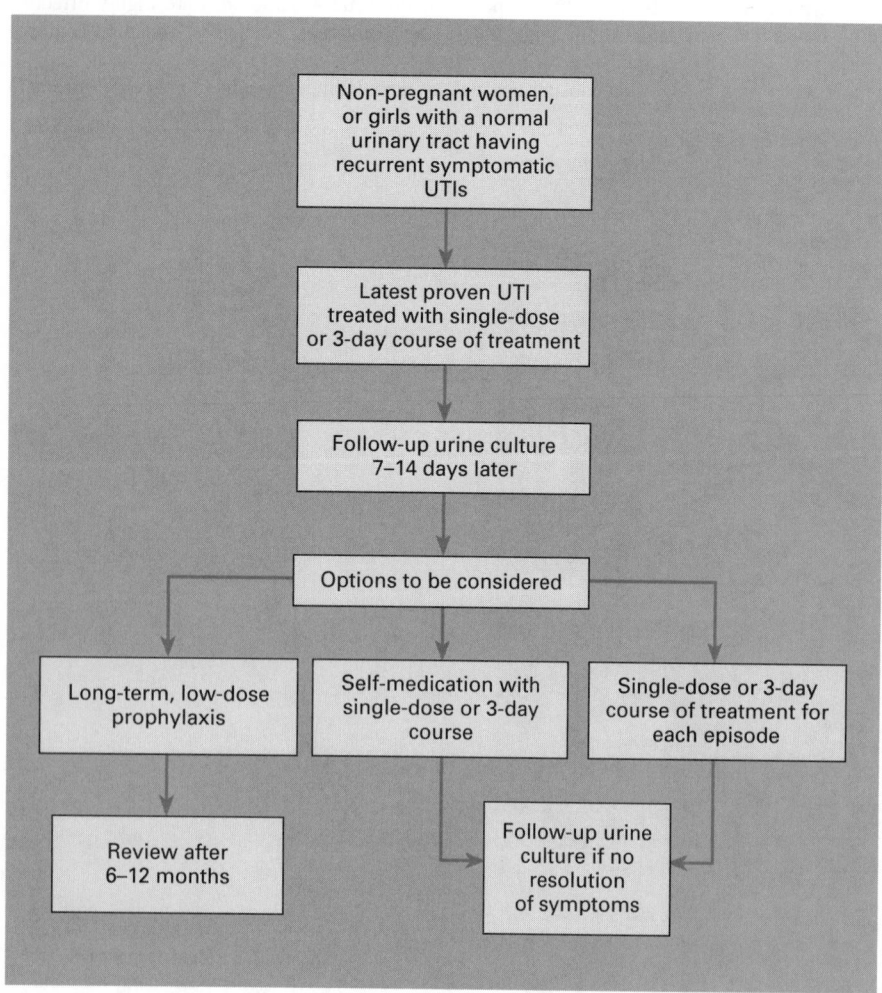

Fig. 2 A suggested algorithm for the management of either non-pregnant women or girls with a normal urinary tract who are having recurrent symptomatic urinary tract infections.

Table 4 *Drug regimens for an oral 3 day course of treatment for bacterial cystitis*

Drug	Dose	Comment
Trimethoprim	300 mg q24h	A useful agent
Co-trimoxazole	960 mg q12h	Should be replaced by trimethoprim alone
Nitrofurantoin	50 mg q8h	Not effective against *Proteus* sp.
Nalidixic acid	500 mg q8h	Not effective against *Staphylococcus saprophyticus*; superseded
Norfloxacin	400 mg q12h	
Ciprofloxacin	250 mg q12h	
Lomefloxacin	400 mg q24h	
Fleroxacin	400 mg q24h	
Cephalexin	250 mg q8h	Useful if renal insufficiency present
Cephradine	250 mg q8h	
Cefaclor	250 mg q8h	
Sulphamethizole	1 g q8h	Unfashionable
Pivmecillinam	200 mg q8h	
Amoxycillin	250 mg q8h	High incidence of resistance; useful for *Streptococcus faecalis*
Augmentin®	500 mg amox/125 mg clavulanic acid q12h	Proving disappointing

q24h, etc., every 24 h, etc.

Table 5 *Drug regimens for a parenteral 5 day course of treatment*

Drug	Dose
Gentamicin	Loading dose 3 mg/kg body weight; maintenance dose 1 mg/kg q8h*
Tobramycin	As for gentamicin*
Netilmicin	Loading dose 2 mg/kg body weight; maintenance dose 2 mg/kg q12h*
Amikacin	Loading dose 15 mg/kg body weight; maintenance dose 7.5 mg/kg q12h*
Ciprofloxacin	100 mg q12h } Can be switched
Lomefloxacin	400 mg q24h } to oral formulation
Cefazolin	1 g q8h
Cephradine	1 g q8h
Ceftriaxone	2 g q24h
Aztreonam	1 g q12h
Ipipenem/cilastin	500 mg/500 mg q8h
Amoxycillin	1 g q8h
Clavulanic acid/amoxycillin	200 mg/lg q8h

*Computer-derived individualized maintenance doses can be determined–drug concentrations should be monitored; single large daily doses are now being recommended rather than divided doses.

beyond 5 days. Some clinicians prefer to individualize aminoglycoside dosage based on measured pharmacokinetic parameters and computer predictions. Recently the aminoglycosides when given to subjects with normal renal function have been shown to be just as efficacious, easier to use, and safer if the maintenance dose is given as a single daily dose rather than in divided doses.

The 4-quinolones, such as norfloxacin, ciprofloxacin, and lomefloxacin, are highly effective for the treatment of acute pyelonephritis and rival the aminoglycosides as the drugs of choice. These compounds are highly effective against a wide range of pathogens, including hospital-acquired organisms. In addition, they are extremely efficacious for the treatment of prostatitis. Some of these quinolones are available in an intravenous formulation and after a few doses can be switched to tablets. This has enabled patients to be discharged from hospital earlier and thus greatly reduces the costs of treating acute pyelonephritis.

There is an extensive list of β-lactam antibiotics, including the new-generation cephalosporins, the semisynthetic- or ureido-penicillins, the monobactams, penems, and the β-lactamase inhibitors. These antibiotics have not replaced the aminoglycosides, are being superseded by the 4-quinolones, and have their own range of side-effects. Ceftriaxone has proved to be the most effective of the β-lactam drugs and is comparable to the aminoglycosides.

SPECIAL TREATMENT PROBLEMS

Men: bacterial prostatitis

This condition invariably responds well to standard therapy as described above, but chronic prostatitis presents a more difficult problem. Men with recurrent bacteriuria frequently carry the infecting organism in their prostatic fluid. Segmental cultures are needed to detect the organism and confirm the diagnosis. Until recently there were few antimicrobial agents that could effectively cross non-inflamed prostatic epithelium from plasma into prostatic fluid, but long-term (for example, 4–12 weeks) low-dose therapy (with, for example, nitrofurantoin, trimethoprim, norfloxacin) could prevent prostatic bacteria from initiating bacteriuria or even bacteraemia. However, the new quinolones penetrate prostatic tissue and are becoming established as the drugs of choice for bacterial prostatitis both acute and chronic.

Asymptomatic (covert) bacteriuria in pregnancy

The initial treatment should be with a single dose or a 3 day course of an appropriate drug. Studies have shown that either a single 1.92 g dose of co-trimoxazole or a single 600 mg dose of trimethoprim is highly effective in treating women with covert bacteriuria between 16 and 30 weeks' gestation. If bacteriuria returns, this treatment should be repeated and followed by prophylaxis in the form of 50 mg of nitrofurantoin each night until the puerperium (Fig. 3).

Women who have a recurrence of bacteriuria after treatment during pregnancy are those most likely to have a urinary-tract abnormality, which is best assessed by careful ultrasonography of the urinary tract and a plain abdominal radiograph after delivery.

Elderly women

The prevalence of bacteriuria rises with increasing age in women, with the lowest rate in those living independently and the highest in the residents of long-stay geriatric wards. Community studies have shown that about one-fifth of elderly women have bacteriuria. In the presence of a debilitating illness and in those cared for in institutions the rate of bacteriuria rises to frequencies between 25 and 50 per cent. Bacteriuria in these patients has been associated with mortality, but it seems improbable that this is the main cause of death in such cases; most often the bacteriuria is simply a complication of the primary cause(s).

If elderly women with bacteriuria are without symptoms, they are best left untreated because of the risk of inducing bacterial resistance. Symptoms may be atypical in the elderly, however, and bacteriuria in those who have become acutely confused, confined to bed, or in other ways have deteriorated should be treated. Improvement in such cases is not uncommon. Symptomatic urinary-tract infections (and not just smelly urine) should be treated in elderly patients of any age, and the approach to treatment should be no different to that for younger women.

The treatment of atrophic vaginitis should be given early consideration in elderly women with recurrent symptomatic urinary-tract infections. It can be corrected with the use of oral or topical oestrogen therapy. This promotes accumulation of glycogen by vaginal epithelial cells, thus allowing the growth of *Lactobacillus* species and the production of lactic acid, which causes a marked acidification of vaginal secretions with suppression of the growth of potential pathogens.

Asymptomatic bacteriuria in elderly women in whom there is also an underlying abnormality of the urinary tract that cannot be corrected is best left untreated, since antimicrobial therapy is likely in this situation to lead to the development of increasingly drug-resistant organisms—the more difficult to treat when symptoms do arise.

Urinary catheters

Long-term indwelling urinary catheters should be avoided if at all possible. All patients so treated will have bacteriuria. The responsible pathogen(s) will be resident in the biofilm lining the catheter. The latter is impermeable to antimicrobial agents. Catheters that are blocking up should be replaced, but the regular changing of catheters is no longer good practice provided that the patient is asymptomatic and urine is draining freely. A high fluid intake and consequent high urine flow is important.

Bacteriuria acquired after short-term catheter use in women often becomes symptomatic. For those with lower urinary-tract symptoms single-dose treatment is just as effective as a course of treatment.

In patients managed outside hospital or similar institutions, clean intermittent urethral catheterization constitutes a minimal risk since the introduction of bacteria rarely produces a serious infection. Such intermittent catheterization has revolutionized the care of patients with spinal cord disorders and neurogenic bladders. The risk of infection is greatly reduced by the absence of an indwelling catheter and the periodic elimination of residual urine. With each catheterization, bacteria may be introduced, but with good technique the risk is very low.

Acute papillary necrosis complicating acute pyelonephritis

Some patients, usually elderly, with severe acute pyelonephritis may develop acute papillary necrosis with complicating acute renal failure. This unusual complication may occur particularly in diabetics, alcohol-

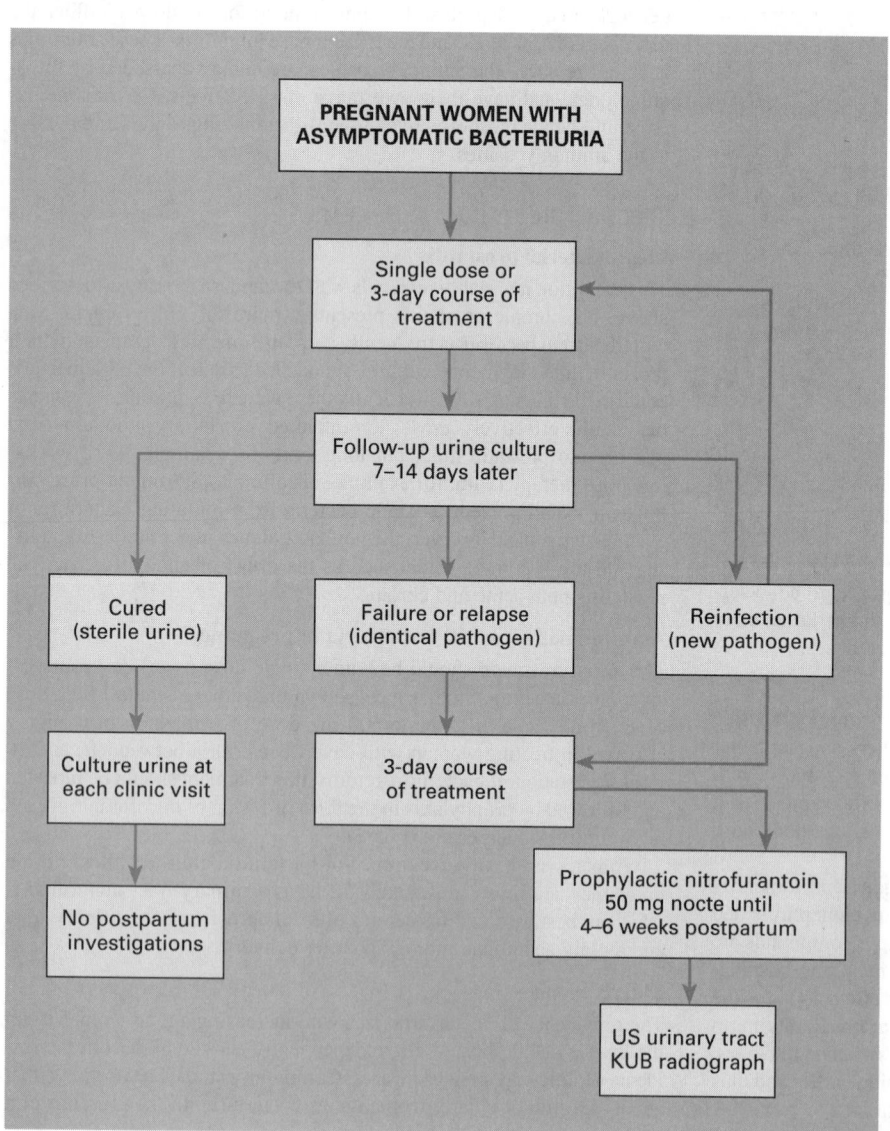

Fig. 3 A suggested algorithm for the management of pregnant women with asymptomatic bacteriuria (US, ultrasonography; KUB, radiograph—kidney, ureter and bladder areas).

ics, and those consuming non-steroidal anti-inflammatory drugs; the latter should always be discontinued at least temporarily in the presence of acute pyelonephritis.

PROPHYLACTIC OR PREVENTIVE TREATMENT

Many women have recurrent or closely spaced symptomatic urinary-tract infections, which cause much morbidity and considerable anxiety. They may benefit from advice always to empty the bladder completely, to avoid tight clothes round the perineum and to maintain a high fluid intake, especially at night. Others are helped by applying an antiseptic cream (for example 0.5 per cent cetrimide w/w) to the periurethral area before intercourse. If these simple techniques fail, the pattern of recurrences can be interrupted by instituting prophylactic therapy after the urine has been sterilized. Nitrofurantoin (50 mg taken last thing at night after the patient has emptied her bladder) is highly effective, as is trimethoprim (100 mg), co-trimoxazole (0.24 g), and norfloxacin (200 mg). There have also been satisfactory results with 1 g of hexamine hippurate and, in patients with renal insufficiency, 125 mg of cephalexin. Recent trials have shown that it is just as effective to give a dose on alternate nights, 3 nights a week, or in some women simply after intercourse (Table 6).

The excellent results with nitrofurantoin reflect the fact that the drug causes no alteration to the faecal flora. The development of resistant bacterial strains during the administration of nitrofurantoin is unknown. Trimethoprim and norfloxacin may have advantages as prophylactic agents as they are excreted partly through the vagina and thus eliminate a possible source of infecting pathogens.

SUPPRESSIVE TREATMENT

Some patients have urological abnormalities (for example calculi, ileal conduit, meningomyelocele, or neurogenic bladder) which make it impossible to sterilize the urinary tract. In some such patients, recurrent episodes of bacteraemia may occur, best managed by long-term suppressive treatment with an antimicrobial appropriate to the organism. If, however, there have been no such episodes and local symptoms are not a serious problem, suppressive treatment is best avoided because of the risk of bacteria or other serious events being caused by a more resistant organism.

Follow-up

Ideally all patients in whom a urinary-tract infection has been diagnosed and treated should be reviewed about 10 to 14 days after treatment, and a further urine specimen should be cultured. It was suggested earlier that 7 days was an ideal time to assess cure, but some of the new agents (such as the long-acting quinolones) may be excreted in the urine for up to a week.

The early reappearance of the same bacterial species or same serotype of *E.coli* suggests that the original pathogen was not eradicated and that the patient requires a longer period of treatment and further investigation. A genuine relapse will rarely occur if the urine is sterile 10 to 14 days after treatment. In practice, most recurrences are reinfections with a different bacterial species merely reflecting the recurrent nature of this problem.

Investigation

Any urinary-tract infection raises the question as to whether it is a marker of underlying urinary tract abnormality. This applies to all men but particularly to infants and young children, in whom there is a strong likelihood of a potentially damaging urinary-tract abnormality, the most important of which is primary vesicoureteric reflux (Chapter 20.8.2).

Every infant child and male must have their urinary tract investigated

Table 6 *Drug regimens for prophylactic therapy*

Drug	Dose each night, alternate nights, 3 nights a week, or after intercourse
Nitrofurantoin	50 mg
Trimethoprim	100 mg
Co-trimoxazole	0.24 g
Norfloxacin	200 mg
Cephalexin	125 mg; useful if renal insufficiency
Hexamine hippurate	1 g

following their first urinary-tract infection. In children under the age of 2 years a micturating (voiding) cystourethrogram should be undertaken to exclude vesicoureteric reflux, but this need not be done in older children if high-quality organ imaging (for example ultrasonography, intravenous urogram, or dimercaptosuccinic acid (**DMSA**) scan) has demonstrated a normal upper urinary tract. It is also important to assess renal function by measurement of plasma creatinine and, when feasible, creatinine clearance.

It is not cost-effective to undertake invasive investigations on sexually active women with occasional bacterial cystitis. When there is no evidence of urinary tract problems as a child, and occasional urinary-tract infections respond rapidly to a single dose of an oral antimicrobial agent, and when follow-up urine specimens show no microscopic haematuria and are sterile on culture, it is unnecessary to investigate further. In contrast, after an attack of acute pyelonephritis, or if there are unusual findings, such as persistent microscopic haematuria, pyuria, or recurrence of the same organism, imaging of the urinary tract (urinary-tract ultrasonography and a plain abdominal radiograph) should be undertaken, and prompt corrective treatment established when possible.

Cystoscopy in young women has been overused. In this large patient group cystoscopy rarely influences management. It should be considered, however, in most males, some older women, or when the clinical picture indicates the likelihood of abnormality in the lower urinary tract.

There are still many women who are concerned that recurrent urinary-tract infections may progressively damage their kidneys. There is ample evidence that infection in the presence of a normal urinary tract is a benign condition and patients should always be reassured of this.

REFERENCES

Bailey, R.R. (1992). Quinolones in the treatment of uncomplicated urinary tract infections. *International Journal of Antimicrobial Agents*, **2**, 19–28.

Bailey, R.R. (1987). Urinary tract infection. In *Textbook of renal disease*, (ed. J.A. Whitworth and J.R. Lawrence), pp. 196–207, Churchill Livingstone, Melbourne.

Cattell, W.R. (1992). Lower and upper urinary tract infection in the adult. In *Oxford textbook of clinical nephrology*, (ed. J.S. Cameron, A.M. Davison, J.-P. Grünfeld, D. Kerr, and E. Ritz), pp. 1676–1799. Oxford University Press.

Harding, G.K.M., *et al.* (1991). How long should catheter-acquired urinary tract infection in women be treated? A randomized controlled study. *Annals of Internal Medicine* **114**, 713–19.

Hooton, T.M., Hillier, S., Johnson, C., Roberts, P.L., and Stamm, W.E. (1991). *Escherichia coli* bacteriuria and contraceptive method. *Journal of the American Medical Association* **265**, 64–9.

Johnson, C. (1991). Definitions, classification, and clinical presentation of urinary tract infections. *Medical Clinics of North America*, **75**, 241–52.

Johnson, J.R. and Stamm, W.E. (1989). Urinary tract infections in women: diagnosis and treatment. *Annals of Internal Medicine* **111**, 906–17.

Kass, E.H. and Svanborg Eden, C. (1989). *Host–parasite interactions in urinary tract infections*. University of Chicago Press, Chicago.

Kaye, D. (1991). Urinary tract infection. *Medical Clinics of North America* **75**, 241–520.

Lipsky, B.A. (1989). Urinary tract infections in men: epidemiology, pathophysiology, diagnosis, and treatment. *Annals of Internal Medicine* **110**, 138–50.

Nicolle, L.E., Mayhew, W.J., and Bryan, L. (1987). Prospective randomized comparison of therapy and no therapy for asymptomatic bacteriuria in elderly, institutionalized women. *American Journal of Medicine* **83**, 27–33.

Ohkoshi, M. and Naber, K.G. (1992). International consensus discussion on clinical evaluation of drug efficacy in urinary tract infection. *Infection*, **20** (Suppl. 3), S135–S242.

Parker, S.E. and Davey, P.G. (1993). Antimicrobial therapy: once-daily aminoglycoside dosing (editorial). *Lancet*, **341**, 346–7.

Prins, J.M., Büller, H.R., Kuipjer, E.J., Tange, R.A., and Speelman, P. (1993). Once versus thrice daily gentamicin in patients with serious infections. *Lancet*, **341**, 335–9.

Privette, M., Cade, R., Peterson, J., and Mars, D. (1988). Prevention of recurrent urinary tract infections in postmenopausal women. *Nephron* **50**, 24–7.

Ronald, A.R. and Nicolle, L.E. (1993). Infections of the upper urinary tract. In *Diseases of the kidney* (eds. R.W. Schrier and C.W. Gottschalk), 5th edn. pp. 973–1006. Little Brown and Co. Boston.

Rubin, R.H., Beam, T.R. Jr, and Stamm, W.E. (1992). An approach to evaluating antibacterial agents in the treatment of urinary tract infection. *Clinical Infectious Diseases* **14**, (Suppl. 2), S246–S251.

Rubin, R.H., Shapiro, E.D., Andriole, V.T., Davis, R.J., and Stamm, W.E. (1992). Evaluation of new anti-infective drugs for the treatment of urinary tract infection. *Clinical Infectious Diseases*, **15** (Suppl. 1), S216–27.

Stamm, W.E., Counts, G.W., Running, K.R., Fihn, S., Turck, M., and Holmes, K.K. (1982). Diagnosis of coliform infection in acutely dysuric women. *New England Journal of Medicine* **307**, 463–8.

Stapleton, A., Latham, R.H., Johnson, C., and Stamm, W.E. (1990). Postcoital antimicrobial prophylaxis for recurrent urinary tract infection: a randomized, double-blind, placebo-controlled trial. *Journal of the American Medical Association* **264**, 703–6.

20.8.2 Vesicoureteric reflux and reflux nephropathy

R. R. BAILEY

Introduction

The term primary vesicoureteric reflux (**VUR**) describes the regurgitation of urine through a vesicoureteric junction rendered incompetent by a congenital defect of either the length, diameter, muscle, or innervation of the submucosal segment of ureter. The latter holds the key to ureteric continence. The defect is one of shortness of the submucosal segment due to congenital lateral ectopia of the ureteric orifice. As a child grows, the intravesical ureter lengthens. Hence the tendency for reflux to diminish or disappear with increasing age. The position and configuration of the ureteric orifice can be correlated with the presence and degree of VUR.

In infants and children the most frequent clinical presentation of VUR is with a complicating urinary-tract infection. The end-result of severe VUR is reflux nephropathy, which may present with urinary-tract infections, hypertension, proteinuria, or renal failure. The term 'reflux nephropathy' has replaced 'chronic (non-obstructive, atrophic) pyelonephritis', to describe the small, contracted, irregularly scarred kidney. The newer term emphasizes the fact that VUR is the essential component in the pathogenesis of this disorder.

The presence of intrarenal reflux determines the site of renal damage associated with the dilating degrees of VUR. Intrarenal reflux is associated with extensively fused or compound papillae, which occur almost exclusively at the renal poles. Simple or cone-shaped papillae are much less likely to permit intrarenal reflux. There is still some debate as to whether these papillary changes are congenital, or acquired as a direct result of continuing high-pressure reflux.

Organ imaging techniques for demonstrating vesicoureteric reflux (see also Chapter 20.1)

MICTURATING (VOIDING) CYSTOURETHROGRAPHY

The micturating cystourethrogram is the most precise method available for demonstrating VUR and will remain the reference against which new techniques will be evaluated. It also allows an assessment of bladder function and is best combined with measurements of bladder pressure and urine flow rate. The procedure, however, is invasive and unpleasant and has the potential for infecting the urinary tract. If repeated studies are required, the cumulative radiation dose should be considered.

When VUR is demonstrated, it is classified according to the extent of ureteric filling and the degree of dilatation of the collecting system, in particular, the minor calyces. There has not yet been agreement on a uniform radiological classification of VUR. There is still strong support for the simple and practical Rolleston classification which is as follows:

Slight (Grade I)	Incomplete filling of the upper urinary tract without dilatation.
Moderate (Grade II)	Complete filling of the upper urinary tract with slight dilatation but no ballooning of the minor calyces.
Gross (Grade III)	Complete filling of the urinary tract with marked dilatation and obvious ballooning of the minor calyces.

The most widely favoured classification at present is that agreed upon for the International Reflux Study in Children (Fig. 1). The essential difference between this and the Rolleston classification is that gross reflux using the latter classification is divided into three grades, and the former into five:

Grade I	Ureter only.
Grade II	Ureter, pelvis, and calyces with no dilatation and normal calyceal fornices.
Grade III	Mild or moderate dilatation and/or tortuosity of the ureter, and mild or moderate dilatation of the pelvis. No, or only slight, blunting of the fornices.
Grade IV	Moderate dilatation and/or tortuosity of the ureter, and moderate dilatation of the pelvis and calyces. Complete obliteration of the sharp angles of the fornices but maintenance of papillary impressions in the majority of calyces.
Grade V	Gross dilatation and tortuosity of the ureter, pelvis, and calyces. The papillary impressions are no longer visible in the majority of calyces (Fig. 2).

The grade of VUR is determined by the most severe reflux detected, and pressure which usually coincides with the peak of voiding. The

Fig. 1 Classification of grades of vesicoureteric reflux used by the International Reflux Study Committee (reproduced from International Reflux Study Committee Report (1981) with permission).

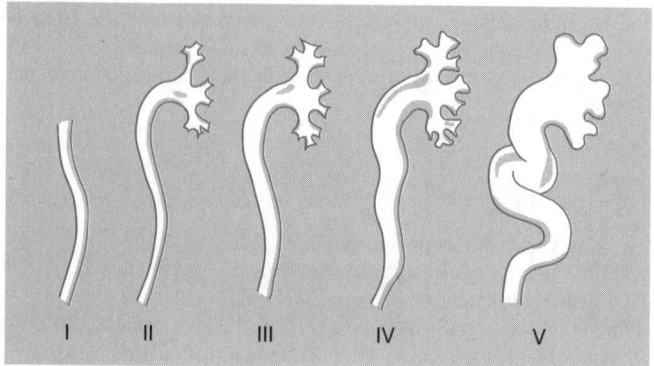

bladder volume and pressure at which reflux is first seen, as well as any intrarenal reflux, should also be noted, although these features are not part of the current grading systems. Intrarenal reflux may occur in association with either grade IV or V on the International classification (Fig. 3).

RADIONUCLIDE MICTURATING CYSTOGRAPHY

The development of radionuclides for investigating patients with VUR has been discussed elsewhere (Chapter 20.1). Radionuclide micturating cystography has become established for assessing and managing patients with VUR, and is ideal for the follow-up of those whose reflux has been treated surgically or managed conservatively (Fig. 4).

Fig. 2 Micturating cystourethrogram on a 9-week-old male infant, showing bilateral grade V (International classification) vesicoureteric reflux (reproduced from Bailey (1993), with permission.)

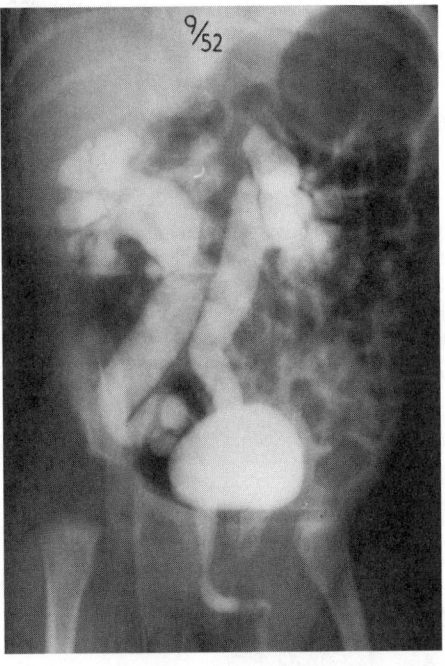

Fig. 3 Micturating cystourethrogram in a 10-month-old girl, showing bilateral grade IV (International classification) vesicoureteric reflux together with widespread intrarenal reflux. Some of the more obvious areas of opacification of the renal parenchyma are arrowed. (Reproduced from Bailey (1993) with permission.)

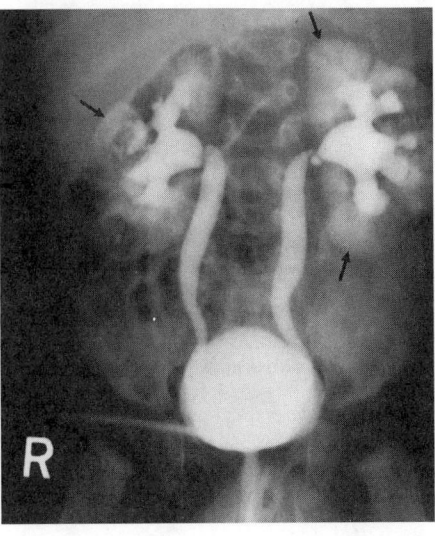

ULTRASONOGRAPHY

There has been interest in the use of dynamic ultrasonography for demonstrating VUR. The findings are essentially limited to the anatomical abnormalities of dilatation of the pelvicalyceal system and ureter, and dynamic information on ureteric function. Examination of the distal ureter may reveal a widely patent ureteric orifice, while the dynamic aspects of real-time ultrasonography allow an assessment of ureteric peristalsis. A limitation of this technique is its non-voiding nature and the inability to differentiate between urine passing up or down the ureter.

Recently, colour Doppler ultrasonography has been used to localize the ureteric orifices on the posterior bladder wall and assess their displacement from the midline.

Organ-imaging techniques for demonstrating reflux nephropathy

INTRAVENOUS UROGRAPHY

Intravenous urography with nephrotomography has been the traditional imaging technique for demonstrating reflux nephropathy. It should clearly delineate the renal outlines, so that their lengths and cortical thicknesses can be measured and compared. The morphology of the papillae can be assessed from the calyceal appearances. The irregularly scarred surface of the kidney should be demonstrated, along with clubbing of the underlying calyx. Clubbing indicates damage to the papilla and is evidence of full-thickness scarring on a lobar basis, which is the radiological hallmark of reflux nephropathy. Depending on the extent and severity of the scarring, two quite distinct types of radiographic damage emerge:

1. Full-thickness focal scars with calyceal clubbing and atrophy and retraction of the overlying cortex involving one or more renal lobes (Fig. 5). It is found most frequently in the polar regions and is pathognomonic of reflux nephropathy. There is always preservation of at least one normal renal lobe. This is the most common form of reflux nephropathy. The number of renal lobes involved determines the severity of the scarring process.

Fig. 4 Radionuclide micturating cystogram, showing vesicoureteric reflux into the left kidney. (Reproduced from Bailey (1993) with permission.)

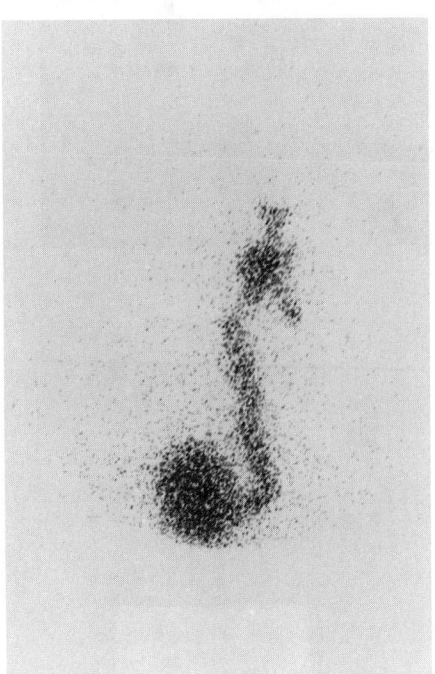

2. Occasionally, and associated with the most severe degrees of VUR, the renal damage is diffuse, resulting in a generalized reduction in parenchymal thickening with uniform papillary change. This type of reflux nephropathy resembles the changes seen in obstructive atrophy.

A classification (Fig. 6) of renal scarring is in use, but it leaves gaps that fail to account for many radiographic appearances.

RADIONUCLIDE SCANNING

Although the intravenous urogram has been the main imaging modality for detecting renal parenchymal injury, at times it fails to demonstrate focal scarring, particularly at the upper pole, and is of no value for determining renal function. This has resulted in the widespread use of radionuclides for the renal imaging of patients with reflux nephropathy. The most widely used radionuclides are those labelled with $^{99}Tc^m$ because of their excellent physical properties. The compound that has proved most successful is dimercaptosuccinic acid (**DMSA**). A focal defect on a DMSA scan reflects underperfusion, either because the proximal tubules in the damaged area extract a smaller amount of the radionuclide than the normal areas, or because they are damaged by ischaemia and are incapable of taking up the DMSA (Fig. 7).

Most clinicians currently consider the DMSA scan and the intravenous urogram to be complementary investigations in the diagnosis of renal scarring.

ULTRASONOGRAPHY

Reflux nephropathy can be detected using ultrasonography, but this requires a skilled operator using sophisticated equipment. A variety of features may be detected, including an assessment of renal size, focal cortical scarring (multiple views in coronal, parasagittal and transverse planes are necessary to detect small focal scars), calyceal dilatation and distortion, altered echogenicity of the renal parenchyma representing fibrosis, and the pattern of scarring such as would be seen in a duplex kidney with lower-pole scarring.

Natural history of vesicoureteric reflux

Some kidneys subjected to VUR become progressively damaged, while others remain unaffected. The observations by Rolleston and colleagues that the severity of the reflux was the single most important determining factor as to whether renal parenchymal damage would occur, was a major breakthrough in the understanding of this disorder. Support for renal parenchymal damage occurring in association with continuing reflux of a gross degree has come from studies of the function of individual kidneys. The critical period in the natural history of the renal scarring associated with VUR is during infancy and early childhood. The extent of the damage occurring during this period is directly related to the severity of the reflux and may occur in the absence of urinary-tract infection.

Clinical presentations of vesicoureteric reflux and reflux nephropathy

VUR may present in many ways. The most frequent, particularly in infants and children, is a complicating urinary-tract infection. The other clinical presentations are included in Table 1. Like VUR, reflux nephropathy may also present in many ways (Table 1), several of which overlap. The clinical presentations of VUR and reflux nephropathy will be discussed individually.

Fig. 5 Intravenous urogram in a 35-year-old woman, showing bilateral reflux nephropathy, more marked on the right side. Several focal scars (arrowed) involving the full thickness of the renal parenchyma and associated with calyceal clubbing are most obvious in the polar regions (reproduced from Bailey (1993) with permission.)

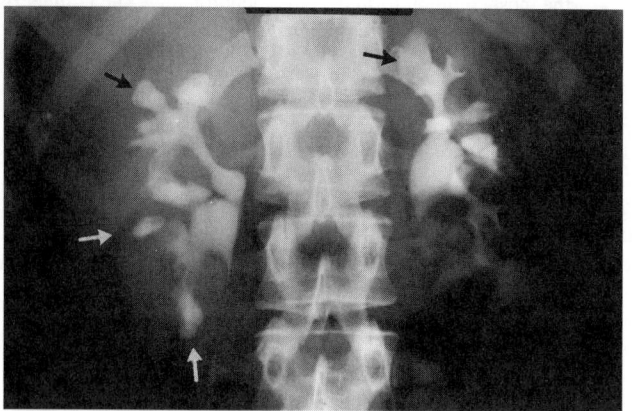

Fig. 7 DMSA scan showing focal scars (arrowed) in both kidneys.

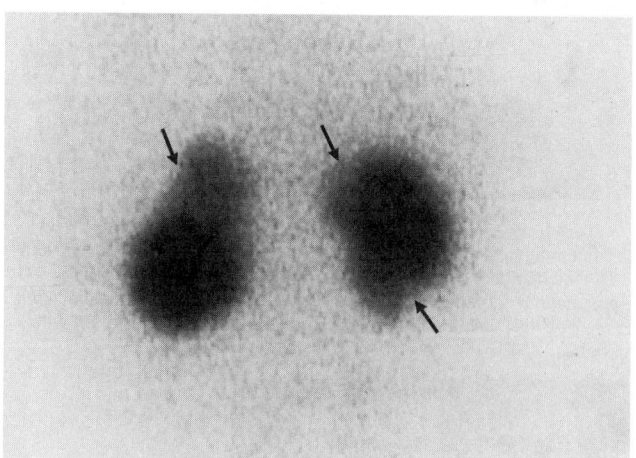

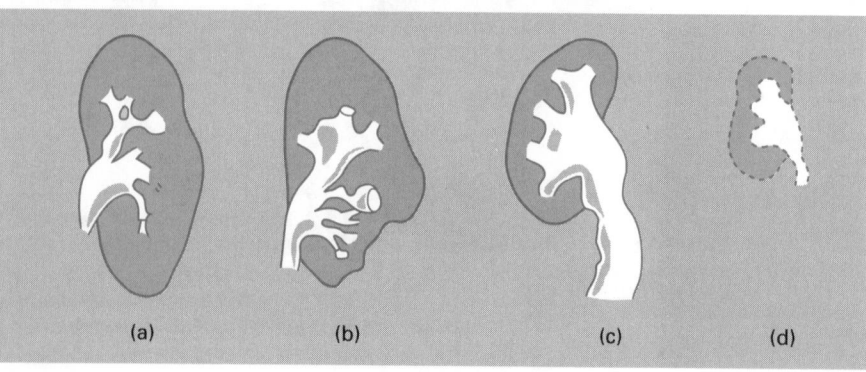

Fig. 6 Grading of parenchymal scarring in reflux nephropathy. (a) Mild scarring with not more than two scarred areas; (b) more than two scarred areas but some areas of normal tissue persist; (c) diffuse thinning of parenchyma with generalized calyceal clubbing—'back pressure' type; (d). shrunken kidney with insignificant parenchymal thickness (reproduced from Smellie, *et al.* (1975), with permission).

Table 1 *Clinical presentations*

Vesicoureteric reflux
Fetal ultrasonography
Urinary-tract infections
Family studies
Nocturnal enuresis or other urological complications
Associated with other congenital abnormalities
Loin pain
Coincidental
Reflux nephropathy
Fetal ultrasonography
Urinary-tract infections
Hypertension—benign or accelerated
During pregnancy—syndrome mimicking pre-eclampsia
Proteinuria
Renal failure
Urinary calculi
Family studies
Nocturnal enuresis or other urological complications
Associated with other congenital abnormalities
Coincidental

URINARY-TRACT INFECTIONS

Complicating urinary-tract infections are the commonest manifestation of VUR with or without nephropathy in infants and children. There are many reasons for susceptibility to infection, but these will not be addressed here. Depending on the age at which the initial investigations are undertaken, 15 to 60 per cent of infants and children with urinary-tract infection will be found to have some degree of reflux, and 8 to 13 per cent of the total will have radiological evidence of reflux nephropathy.

Any infant or child should undergo urinary tract investigation following a first bacteriologically proven urinary-tract infection. For the infant and child under the age of 2 years, the most appropriate initial investigation is a micturating cystourethrogram and ultrasonography of the urinary tract. If a competent ultrasonographer is not available, or either study is abnormal, a DMSA scan and/or an intravenous urogram should be done. Between the ages of 2 and 5 years a DMSA scan, and either ultrasonography or intravenous urography, are appropriate. A micturating cystourethrogram need only be done if an abnormality is seen on one of the initial examinations, or if recurrent urinary-tract infections occur. Over the age of 5 years ultrasonography and a plain abdominal radiograph are appropriate. If there is any abnormality, further imaging should be done as appropriate. The reasoning for omitting a micturating cystourethrogram in children over 2 years of age is that if dilating reflux had been present since birth it would already have caused renal parenchymal damage, which would be apparent on renal imaging.

With increasing age, other clinical presentations of VUR or reflux nephropathy become relatively more common, although some young women developing urinary-tract infections after the beginning of sexual activity can be shown to have underlying reflux nephropathy which had not presented in infancy or early childhood. About 5 per cent of sexually active women with symptomatic urinary-tract infections will have reflux nephropathy. These patients may present with either bacterial cystitis or acute pyelonephritis. The disorder may also come to attention because of the detection of asymptomatic bacteriuria in situations such as pregnancy.

FETAL ULTRASONOGRAPHY

Improved sophistication of high-resolution ultrasonographic equipment has permitted visualization of fetal anatomy capable of identifying up to 90 per cent of fetal kidneys by 17 to 20 weeks of intrauterine life.

After 20 weeks' gestation the rate of urine production can be measured by serial estimation of bladder volume. This knowledge has stimulated great interest. The commonest ultrasound findings are those of hydronephrosis or hydroureter. About 20 per cent of these neonates have been shown to have VUR.

Several recent reviews have recommended that any discernible degree of antenatal upper-tract dilatation should lead to postnatal investigation. The initial postnatal ultrasound examination should not be performed earlier than 5 days of age, and if normal, should be repeated at 2 months. Micturating cystourethrography is recommended for all neonates with postnatal upper-tract dilatation. Some investigators believe that all neonates with antenatal hydronephrosis require a micturating cystourethrogram and not just those with dilatation still present on postnatal ultrasonography.

Reflux diagnosed following the detection of antenatal hydronephrosis is characterized in most studies by a male preponderance, a relatively high grade of severity of reflux (over 60 per cent grades IV and V) and a resolution rate of reflux of about 40 per cent by the age of 2 years. In addition, approximately 20 per cent of refluxing kidneys which have been diagnosed following the detection of antenatal hydronephrosis, and which have not been affected by urinary-tract infection, have decreased function on DMSA scintigraphy. These kidneys are usually smooth, small, and may not demonstrate the focal defects that are characteristic of reflux nephropathy in later childhood. These findings, developing *in utero*, call into question the role of urinary-tract infections in the pathogenesis of the renal damage. Fetal ultrasonography promises to be a useful method of screening for the early detection of VUR in high-risk families.

FAMILIAL ASSOCIATION

There is convincing evidence of a familial occurrence of primary VUR. Until recently the mode of inheritance was uncertain. In a large study, 88 affected families were subjected to segregation analysis using a mixed model and a computer program. The model best fitting the data was that of a single dominant gene acting together with random environmental effects, suggesting a gene frequency around 1 in 600 and that mutation was uncommon. No definite or reliable genetic marker has yet been identified.

NOCTURNAL ENURESIS OR OTHER UROLOGICAL COMPLICATIONS

Infants and children with VUR have a high incidence of nocturnal enuresis or evidence of lower urinary-tract dysfunction, such as detrusor instability or detrusor-sphincter dyssynergia. Hypospadias, undescended testicles, bifid pelvicalyceal collecting systems, ureteric duplication, pelviureteric junction obstruction, and other urological conditions may be associated with primary VUR.

ASSOCIATED WITH OTHER CONGENITAL ABNORMALITIES

VUR has been reported in association with other congenital disorders such as Hirschsprung's disease, anorectal abnormalities (for example, short colon syndrome), and the prune-belly syndrome.

LOIN PAIN

Loin pain is probably the only urinary-tract symptom that can be attributed specifically to VUR. Although infants and young children rarely complain of loin pain, older patients may give a history of loin pain when their bladder is full, with worsening at the start of micturition followed by rapid relief after voiding. This is arguably the only indication for antireflux surgery in an older child or adult.

Table 2 *Total number of patients entering renal replacement programmes in Australia and New Zealand and the number with end-stage reflux nephropathy, 1971 to 1991 inclusive (ANZDATA Registry, A.P.S. Disney, personal communication)*

	Australia		New Zealand	
	Male	Female	Male	Female
Total number of patients	6752	5577	1283	940
Number with reflux nephropathy	405 (6.0%)	485 (8.7%)	83 (6.5%)	109 (11.6%)
Total number of patients aged < 16 years	286	219	56	57
Number aged < 16 years with reflux nephropathy	64 (22.4%)	55 (25.1%)	9 (16.1%)	15 (26.3%)

HYPERTENSION

Hypertension is a frequent late complication of reflux nephropathy. It may occasionally follow an accelerated course with deteriorating renal function. Reflux nephropathy is the commonest cause of severe hypertension in childhood.

The risk of patients developing hypertension increases progressively with the extent of the renal scarring. Approximately 15 per cent of patients with reflux nephropathy who reach adulthood will present with hypertension or its complications without a history of urinary-tract infections.

There has been considerable interest as to what role the renin–angiotensin system may have in the mechanism of the hypertension associated with unilateral reflux nephropathy. The balance of the published data would suggest that the renin–angiotensin system is not consistently involved unless the hypertension is in an accelerated phase.

There have been several reports of patients in whom unilateral reflux nephropathy was thought to be responsible for the hypertension, but in fact the contralateral renal artery was stenosed due to fibromuscular hyperplasia. This unusual clinical scenario should be considered in any hypertensive patient with a unilateral small kidney.

PRESENTATION DURING PREGNANCY (SEE ALSO SECTION 13)

If a female with reflux nephropathy does not come to clinical attention early in life with a complicating urinary-tract infection or hypertension, she may do so if she becomes pregnant. Apart from a urinary-tract infection, symptomatic or asymptomatic, the commonest presentation of reflux nephropathy in pregnancy is with a syndrome mimicking pre-eclampsia, often in the first or second trimester. Of women found to have bacteriuria during pregnancy, up to a third may have a urinary-tract abnormality, the commonest of which is reflux nephropathy.

In a large study of women who presented with severe pre-eclampsia or pre-eclampsia in a second or subsequent pregnancy, 4 per cent were found to have reflux nephropathy. Pregnancy in a patient with reflux nephropathy and moderately severe renal failure may have a deleterious effect on renal function.

If any woman develops hypertension during early pregnancy, or severe or atypical pre-eclampsia in a second or subsequent pregnancy, then reflux nephropathy should be considered.

URINARY CALCULI

Patients with reflux nephropathy have an increased frequency of urinary calculi. Some of these are staghorn calculi in patients (invariably women) with uncontrolled urinary-tract infections, usually with *Proteus mirabilis* or another urea-splitting organism. More frequently, however, the stones are found in scarred sections of the kidney, often in medullary cavities or clubbed calyces, or associated with papillary tips. The location of some of these stones suggests that urinary stasis may promote their formation.

PROTEINURIA

Persistent proteinuria is a bad prognostic feature. It indicates a complicating glomerulopathy, the histological hallmark of which is focal and segmental glomerulosclerosis with hyalinosis involving the unscarred segments of kidney, or the structurally normal contralateral kidney in patients with unilateral reflux nephropathy.

Proteinuria may not appear for many years after severe scarring has occurred, but it tends to increase as renal function declines. Hypertension then becomes an associated complication.

RENAL FAILURE

Reflux nephropathy is an important cause of chronic renal failure. In some centres it is clearly underdiagnosed as a cause of end-stage renal failure.

In Christchurch, New Zealand, 42 of 371 (11.3 per cent) consecutive patients entering the dialysis-transplant programme had reflux nephropathy. The majority presented with renal failure, hypertension, and proteinuria. Documented urinary-tract infections had occurred in 11 of the 24 females and in only 4 of the 18 male patients. Eight of the 24 women presented during a pregnancy, usually with features resembling pre-eclampsia. Six of the 42 patients started dialysis under 16 years of age and represented one-half of all children entering the programme. Between 1963 and 1982, 533 patients presented to a Melbourne renal unit with end-stage renal failure, and in 82 of these (15.3 per cent) the cause was reflux nephropathy. The mean age at which the 30 men developed renal failure was 22 years, and for the 52 women, 33 years.

In the Australia and New Zealand Dialysis and Transplant Registry from 1971 to 1991, 6.1 per cent of males and 9.1 per cent of females had reflux nephropathy, while among those under the age of 16 years this was the diagnosis in 21.3 per cent of boys and 25.4 per cent of girls (Table 2). As of 31 December 1989, 627 patients in Australia (37 per million population) and 119 patients in New Zealand (35 per million) with reflux nephropathy were dialysis-dependent or had a functioning transplant. This represented 11 and 12 per cent, respectively, of patients on renal replacement programmes in the two countries.

Although several recent editorials or reviews have drawn attention to reflux nephropathy being an important cause of end-stage renal failure, it continues to be regarded by many as a minor or insignificant problem. The diagnosis should be considered in any patient presenting with renal insufficiency and proteinuria, with or without hypertension or urinary-tract infections.

COINCIDENTAL FINDING

As more patients are having upper abdominal ultrasonography to evaluate abdominal symptoms, so is reflux nephropathy being detected coincidentally with greater frequency. The commonest situation is to find in a previously healthy individual an irregularly scarred kidney on one side with a hypertrophied contralateral kidney. Rarely, however, does the chance finding of a small kidney explain the abdominal symptoms, unless the patient has a urinary-tract infection or a urinary calculus.

Pathology of reflux nephropathy

A major step in elucidating the pathology of chronic pyelonephritis has been the recognition of the entity of reflux nephropathy (Fig. 8). Heptinstall has reviewed in detail the phases in the pathological diagnosis of chronic pyelonephritis. The role of urinary-tract obstruction in establishing and maintaining bacterial infection in the kidney has long been appreciated by pathologists, but the entity of 'chronic non-obstructive pyelonephritis' has been a puzzling exception. It is now clear that the pattern of renal injury resulting from VUR corresponds well with descriptions of both chronic non-obstructive pyelonephritis and the Ask–Upmark kidney.

Observations on the pig experimental model have contributed enormously to the understanding of the pathology of reflux nephropathy in humans. The latter has largely been inferred from descriptions of chronic pyelonephritis. The pathological changes have been based predominantly on the examination of kidneys removed because of uncontrollable urinary-tract infections or hypertension, or prior to renal transplantation. The pattern of evolving reflux nephropathy can be inferred from the appearances in the kidneys of some paraplegic patients.

Management

VESICOURETERIC REFLUX

There is still disagreement concerning the treatment of VUR. At one extreme are those clinicians who do not recommend surgical correction of any degree of reflux regardless of age, but choose to use long-term, low-dose antimicrobial prophylaxis; while at the other extreme are those who operate on any patient with any degree of reflux. In the past, many urologists have recommended antireflux surgery in an attempt to control complicating urinary-tract infections. The balance of evidence suggests, however, that surgical correction has no effect on the overall incidence of these infections. The latter are invariably easy to manage if attention is paid to careful bacteriological diagnosis, appropriate curative and prophylactic drug regimens, compliance with therapy, and regular follow-up.

Fig. 8 A small kidney showing all of the macroscopic features of severe reflux nephropathy, including an arrest of renal growth, focal cortical scarring, and adjacent calyceal clubbing. A preserved normal renal lobe is arrowed (reproduced from Bailey (1993), with permission).

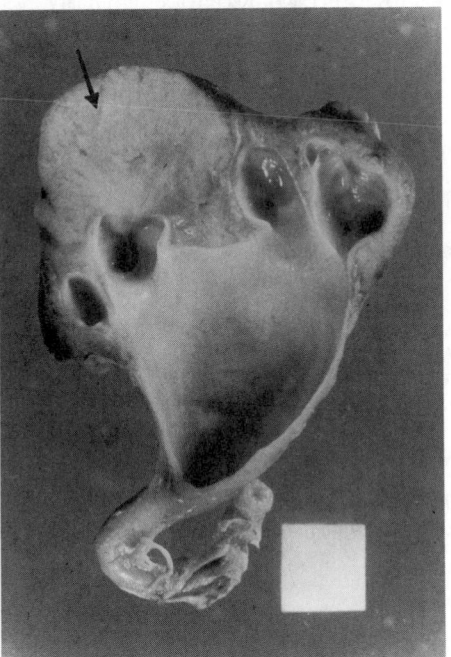

Recently there has been a more scientific approach to antireflux surgery. This has resulted directly from studies of the natural history of the different degrees of reflux in infants and children. The intentions of surgery must be to either prevent renal parenchymal damage developing in normal kidneys subjected to continuing reflux, or to reduce the risk of further damage to those kidneys that are already scarred. The important questions that have been addressed concern which kidneys are at risk of scarring, the age at which surgery should be done, and whether surgery prevents scarring, lessens further damage, or even allows the kidney to regain normal growth.

There have been many uncontrolled reports of surgery having little or no benefit, but the procedure has invariably been performed long after renal damage has developed, or has been undertaken on patients with a degree of reflux that does not result in parenchymal scarring. Surgery is of no benefit if the patient has developed proteinuria, renal insufficiency, or hypertension. The last persists, while renal function continues to deteriorate.

Several prospective controlled trials have been undertaken to assess the benefits of antireflux surgery compared with medical management (basically long-term, low-dose antimicrobial prophylaxis) of the more severe grades of VUR. The Birmingham Reflux Study Group concluded that neither treatment could claim superiority, nor could they fully protect the kidneys from further damage, and stressed that efforts must continue to be directed towards identifying those infants at risk before scarring develops. An important finding from the International Reflux Study in Children (grades III and IV) was that those patients treated surgically had fewer episodes of acute pyelonephritis, although the overall number of patients with recurrent urinary-tract infections (asymptomatic bacteriuria, cystitis, acute pyelonephritis), were the same in both treatment groups. Episodes of acute pyelonephritis frequently followed urinary-tract instrumentation. After 5 years the number of children with new renal scars and new renal parenchymal thinning were similar in both treatment groups. Following surgery new scars developed earlier than in the medical group. The younger the child at entry, the greater the risk of a new scar developing, while, irrespective of age, more boys than girls developed new scars. Children with grade IV reflux were much more likely to develop new lesions than those with grade III reflux. A full report on this study has been published. The most significant observation to date in the Auckland Reflux Study (grades III and IV) is that in children aged 2 to 10 years at entry, those treated surgically had a significant increase in glomerular filtration rate, but those in the medical group did not.

These three prospective studies had as their prime aim the study of the natural history of sterile VUR of a severe (usually only grades III and IV but not V) degree. However, as far as the long-term outcome of patients with VUR and reflux nephropathy is concerned it is probably more important to assess the effect of surgery on the natural history of reflux nephropathy and its complications.

In experienced surgical hands antireflux surgery is very successful and associated with a low morbidity rate. Cohen's transtrigonal advancement to lengthen the submucosal ureteric tunnel is the most popular technique because of its simplicity. A new procedure that has created great interest is the endoscopic injection of Teflon® behind the intravesical ureter. This simple technique can be undertaken in the outpatient department, but although it has been refined it clearly requires further evaluation. Because of concerns with migration of the injected Teflon®, granulomatous formation, and possible carcinogenic properties, this product has been withdrawn recently from use in some countries. Glutaraldehyde cross-linked to collagen is the best alternative substance tried to date. The specific indications for this simple approach to the correction of reflux have not yet been formulated.

The information available suggests that if antireflux surgery is beneficial it must be undertaken early in life in those with grade III to V reflux, as renal damage associated with reflux invariably develops within the first 2 or 3 years of life and usually within the first few months. The only specific indication for antireflux surgery in an adult is the very occasional patient who is troubled by loin pain when the bladder is full or after micturition.

REFLUX NEPHROPATHY

The management of reflux nephropathy and its complications such as urinary-tract infections, calculi, and renal failure is no different than for patients with other renal diseases and will not be discussed further. Pregnant women with reflux nephropathy require careful antenatal and postnatal supervision.

Treatment of the complicating hypertension is an essential part of the management of patients with reflux nephropathy and invariably responds well to the angiotensin-converting enzyme inhibitors or calcium-channel blockers.

Since 1929 when Ask–Upmark suggested a possible relationship between hypertension and unilateral renal disease and Butler reported that the removal of a small, scarred kidney cured severe hypertension in a 10-year-old girl with a urinary-tract infection, there has been interest in the question as to whether hypertensive patients with unilateral reflux nephropathy may benefit from nephrectomy. A review of the literature from 1956 to 1961 collated 326 patients with unilateral renal disease and hypertension who underwent unilateral nephrectomy. Fifty-seven of these had reflux nephropathy; 23 of them were normotensive after 1 year and 33 showed a substantial benefit. There has been an enormous published literature on this subject, but none of it was controlled and most of it was anecdotal. A long-term, prospective trial was undertaken in this institution to study the benefit of nephrectomy on the hypertension of patients with unilateral reflux nephropathy. This study has confirmed that normotensive patients are at risk of developing hypertension, but there was no evidence to show that this could be prevented by prophylactic nephrectomy. There was evidence, however, that some hypertensive patients benefited from nephrectomy.

Conclusion

Primary VUR is an important congenital abnormality, which may be familial, and is an essential component in the pathogenesis of reflux nephropathy. Early childhood is the critical period in the natural history of the renal scarring associated with reflux. In some infants renal damage occurs *in utero*. The extent of the renal damage is directly related to the severity of the reflux and the presence of intrarenal reflux. The precise role of complicating bacterial infections in the pathogenesis of reflux nephropathy remains uncertain, but renal damage may occur in the continued absence of urinary-tract infection. However, the most important clinical presentation of VUR is with a complicating urinary-tract infection in early childhood.

More investigation is required into the pathogenesis of this important cause of serious renal disease. A reliable way of detecting this abnormality at birth, or even *in utero*, is required so as to prevent, or at least reduce, the risk of renal damage, and to enable urinary-tract infections to be avoided. The search must continue for genetic markers, as well as a simple and reliable way of screening new-born infants for the presence of dilating degrees of VUR. Meanwhile, there is strong evidence to investigate those infants at birth who have parents or siblings with either VUR or reflux nephropathy. Antireflux surgery should be considered for young children with dilating forms of VUR.

REFERENCES

Bailey, R.R. (1973). The relationship of vesico-ureteric reflux to urinary tract infection and chronic pyelonephritis–reflux nephropathy. *Clinical Nephrology* **1**, 132–41.

Bailey, R.R. (1991). *Proceedings of the second C.J. Hodson symposium on reflux nephropathy*, pp. 1–79. Design Printing Services, Christchurch.

Bailey, R.R. (1992). Vesicoureteric reflux and reflux nephropathy. In *Oxford textbook of clinical nephrology*, (ed. S. Cameron, A.M. Davison, J.-P. Grünfeld, D. Kerr, and E. Ritz), pp. 1983–2002. Oxford Medical Publications, Oxford.

Bailey, R.R. (1993). Vesicoureteric reflux and reflux nephropathy. In *Diseases of the kidney*, (5th edn), (ed. R.W. Schrier and C.W. Gottschalk), pp. 689–727. Little, Brown, Boston/Toronto.

Birmingham Reflux Study Group (1983). Prospective trial of operative versus non-operative treatment of severe vesicoureteric reflux: two years' observation in 96 children. *British Medical Journal* **287**, 171–4.

Birmingham Reflux Study Group (1987). Prospective trial of operative versus non-operative treatment of severe vesicoureteric reflux in children: five years' observation. *British Medical Journal* **295**, 237–41.

Chapman, C.J., Bailey, R.R., Janus, E.D., Abbott, G.D., and Lynn, K.L. (1985). Vesicoureteric reflux: segregation analysis. *American Journal of Medical Genetics* **20**, 577–84.

Cotran, R.S. (1982). Glomerulosclerosis in reflux nephropathy. *Kidney International* **21**, 528–34.

Goldraich, N.P., Ramos, O.L., and Goldraich, I.H. (1989). Urography versus DMSA scan in children with vesicoureteric reflux. *Pediatric Nephrology* **3**, 1–5.

Heptinstall, R.H. (1983). *Pathology of the kidney*, (3rd edn), pp. 1323–96. Little, Brown, Boston.

Hodson, C.J., Maling, T.M.J., McManamon, P.J., and Lewis, M.G. (1975). The pathogenesis of reflux nephropathy (chronic atrophic pyelonephritis). *British Journal of Radiology* **48**, (Suppl 13), 1–26.

Hodson, C.J., Heptinstall, R.H., and Winberg, J. (1984). *Reflux nephropathy update: 1983*, pp. 1–388. Karger, Basel.

Hodson, J. and Kincaid-Smith, P. (1979). *Reflux nephropathy*, pp. 1–352. Masson, New York.

International Reflux Study Committee Report (1981). Medical versus surgical treatment of primary vesicoureteral reflux. *Pediatrics* **67**, 392–400.

International Reflux Study in Children. (1992). International Workshop on Reflux and Pyelonephritis. New Orleans, Louisiana, October 23–25, 1991. *Journal of Urology*, **148**, 1643–79.

Kincaid-Smith, P. (1975). Glomerular lesions in atrophic pyelonephritis and reflux nephropathy. *Kidney International* **8**, S81-S83.

Maling, T.M.J., Turner, J.G., and Bailey, R.R. (1987). Organ imaging. In *Textbook of renal disease*, (ed. J.A. Whitworth and J.R. Lawrence), pp. 64–77. Churchill Livingstone, Melbourne.

O'Donnell, B. and Puri, P. (1988). Technical refinements in endoscopic correction of vesicoureteral reflux. *Journal of Urology* **140**, 1101–2.

Olbing, H., Tamminen-Möbius, T., and Hirche, H. (for the International Reflux Study in Children (IRSC)) (1989). Recurrences of urinary tract infections in children with vesicoureteral reflux after surgical management in the International Reflux Study in children. *In Host–parasite interactions in urinary tract infection*, (ed. E.H. Kass and C. Svanborg Eden), pp. 292–6. University of Chicago Press, Chicago.

Roberts, J.A. (1987). The monkey as a model of urinary tract infection and reflux nephropathy in man. In *Nephrology, Vol. II*, (ed. A.M. Davison), pp. 844–53. Ballière Tindall, London.

Roberts, J.A. (1991). *International workshop on reflux and pyelonephritis*, pp. 1–58, Tulane Regional Primate Research Center, Covington.

Rolleston, G.L., Shannon, F.T., and Utley, W.L.F. (1970). Relationship of infantile vesicoureteric reflux to renal damage. *British Medical Journal* **1**, 460–3.

Rolleston, G.L., Maling, T.M.J., and Hodson, C.J. (1974). Intrarenal reflux and the scarred kidney. *Archives of Diseases in Childhood* **49**, 531–9.

Rolleston, G.L., Shannon, F.T., and Utley, W.L.F. (1975). Follow-up of vesico-ureteric reflux in the newborn.*Kidney International* **8**, S59–S64.

Smellie, J.M., Edwards, D., Hunter, N., Normand, I.C.S., and Prescod, N. (1975). Vesico-ureteric reflux and renal scarring. *Kidney International* **8**, S65–S72.

Walker, R.G. and Kincaid-Smith, P. (1987). *Proceedings of the first C.J. Hodson symposium*, pp. 1–125, Broughton, Melbourne.

20.9 Other interstitial nephritides

20.9.1 Kidney disease from analgesics and non-steroidal anti-inflammatory drugs

J. H. STEWART

Analgesic nephropathy

'Classical' analgesic nephropathy, identified in 1953, was for 20 to 30 years the commonest cause of both acute and chronic renal failure in parts of Europe and Australia, as well as occurring in nearly all developed and some developing countries. The disease is on the wane in most societies as a result of banning the sale of phenacetin or of compound analgesic preparations, but rather different syndromes caused by non-steroidal anti-inflammatory drugs have appeared.

The renal lesion

Papillary necrosis

The primary pathology is in the renal papilla. Initially the naked-eye appearance is virtually normal; microscopically the lesion is confined to the central part of the inner medulla and affects only the interstitial cells, the thin ascending limb of Henle's loop, and the peritubular capillaries (cellular necrosis; basement-membrane thickening; increased ground substance). In advanced disease there is full-blown necrosis of all medullary elements, commonly with partial or total papillary separation. Pigmentation and calcification are frequent and, while there is no granulocytic infiltration, lymphocytes and macrophages invade the outer medulla (Fig. 1).

Chronic interstitial nephritis

There is some atrophy of cortex overlying papillae, and hypertrophy of columns of Bertin between, which result from the location of the primary lesion. When papillary separation does not occur or is incomplete, there is progressive cortical atrophy with fibrosis and mononuclear infiltra-

Fig. 1 Analgesic-induced papillary necrosis showing loss of the papillary tip, calcification in the retained sclerotic tissue, and chronic inflammatory changes in the outer medulla.

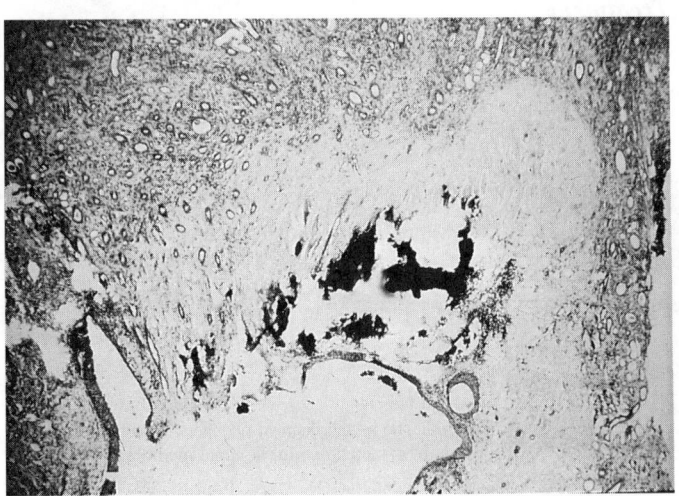

tion, attributed to intrarenal urinary obstruction. Glomerulosclerosis and arterial intimal thickening appear later, associated with chronic renal failure.

Capillary sclerosis

This is seen immediately under the urothelium, maximally at the pelviureteric junction but evident even in the bladder. It is due to repeated toxic lysis (by phenacetin metabolites) of endothelium, resulting in concentric deposition of layers of basement membrane on the inside of the damaged capillary wall.

Aetiology

Analgesic nephropathy has been common only in societies where the habit of taking compound antipyretic-analgesic preparations was widespread. Nearly always the amounts have exceeded 1 kg (represented by about two powders or tablets per day for 2 years), usually by many times. The preparations have contained at least three ingredients, each contributing to pathogenesis: phenacetin; caffeine and/or codeine; and either aspirin (in English-speaking countries and some of Europe) or phenazone or another pyrazolone (in much of Europe). Only rarely has phenacetin been taken without either aspirin or a pyrazolone, and other antipyretic-analgesics have not been consumed in the huge quantities characteristic of phenacetin abuse. Nevertheless, the potential of all analgesics and non-steroidal anti-inflammatory drugs to cause papillary necrosis is evident from testing in rodents; and some clinical studies tend to implicate paracetamol (acetaminophen in America), the major metabolic derivative of phenacetin. Aspirin taken by itself is not a cause of kidney disease in man although it has produced papillary necrosis in animals.

Habituation to analgesics

In societies where the taking of analgesics is common, the *habitué* is not readily distinguished by personality, social circumstances, or psychiatric abnormality, but all these play a part where the habit is unusual. There is evidence that phenacetin, alone or with another antipyretic-analgesic, is habituating, but more likely codeine or caffeine is responsible, the latter by causing withdrawal headache which then prompts taking further analgesics. Caffeine-containing preparations also are taken for their mildly stimulating effect.

Mechanism of disease

Glutathione normally protects tissues against the toxic metabolites of phenacetin and paracetamol (Fig. 2). However, high-dose salicylate consumption depletes glutathione reserves, possibly accounting for the nephrotoxicity of compound analgesics.

Clinical presentations

Renal papillary necrosis (Table 1)

This may be silent and discovered by organ imaging or histopathology. Proteinuria appears only with the onset of renal failure. The urine may be clear; more frequently there are casts, erythrocytes (especially if aspirin or non-steroidal anti-inflammatory drugs are being taken), or leucocytes (persistent asymptomatic sterile pyuria is characteristic).

Infection in or around necrotic papillae, not uncommon, may manifest as acute pyelonephritis or indolent urinary infection.

Separation of papillae may cause visible haematuria or colic, and the necrotic or calcified papillae may be voided. More seriously, pelvic ureteric or ureteric obstruction may occur, giving rise to hydronephrosis which frequently is infected (pyonephrosis). The last often results in Gram-negative septicaemia and acute renal failure, a life-threatening illness.

Chronic interstitial nephritis

In contrast to the sometimes florid manifestations of papillary necrosis, chronic interstitial nephritis almost always is covert, presenting with declining renal function or hypertension.

Chronic renal failure

Because of the primarily medullary pathology, impaired urinary concentration is the earliest abnormality, and distal renal tubular acidosis, salt-wasting, and hypocitraturia (possibly accounting for calcium deposition) are relatively common. Hypertension may appear late (when it may be volume-dependent), or early and severe (renin-dependent) due to secondary renal artery stenosis or intrarenal pathology. Acidosis and, possibly as a consequence, renal osteodystrophy occur more frequently during the stage of moderate renal failure than in other kidney diseases.

Urothelial cancer

Phenacetin is weakly carcinogenic in the kidney and urinary tract, perhaps in relation to 2-hydroxy and N-hydroxy metabolites, while renal papillary necrosis is a common precursor of the occurrence some years later of transitional cell carcinomas, often multiple, in the renal pelvis or bladder or both. These usually present with visible haematuria, but may be discovered by urinary cytology or imaging.

Extrarenal disease

Since analgesic nephropathy occurs only after prolonged and heavy consumption of compound analgesic preparations, the patient also will be at risk of the non-renal toxic effects of the components of the mixture consumed (Table 2).

Diagnosis

The diagnosis is certain only if both analgesic abuse and a characteristic renal lesion can be demonstrated.

The detection of analgesic abuse

The regular taking of analgesics may be denied; in such cases the detection in the urine of salicylate (by Phenistix®) or N-acetyl-p-aminophenol (by colorimetry) indicates surreptitious consumption, which is almost always excessive. In histopathology specimens, capillary sclerosis is pathognomonic of heavy phenacetin ingestion.

Organ imaging

On contrast pyelography, papillary necrosis gives a characteristic appearance of cortical scarring and calyceal irregularity (Fig. 3). The 'wavy' renal outline and random distribution of affected calyces often will discriminate from reflux nephropathy even when papillary necrosis

Table 1 *Differential diagnosis of renal papillary necrosis*

Aetiology	Pathology
Toxic:	
classical analgesic nephropathy	Non-inflammatory; calcification
Ischaemic:	
diabetes	Acute inflammation; infection
urinary obstruction	Acute inflammation; infection
acute pyelonephritis	Acute inflammation; infection
sickle-cell disease	Non-inflammatory; scarring
NSAID-induced	Non-inflammatory; scarring
profound shock (especially newborn)	Acute infarction

NSAID, non-steroidal anti-inflammatory drug.

Table 2 *The 'analgesic syndrome' (non-renal manifestations of analgesic abuse)*

Drug responsible	Clinical sequelae
Codeine	Constipation, laxative abuse
Caffeine	Recurrent headache; restlessness
Phenacetin	Methaemoglobinaemia; splenomegaly; pigmentation
Aspirin	Peptic ulcer, milk-alkali syndrome; iron deficiency; bleeding tendency; perinatal morbidity; salicylism
Uncertain aetiology	Accelerated atherogenesis; premature ageing; encephalopathy

is not evident. Medullary sponge kidney, tuberculosis, or simple calculi must be distinguished. The pyelogram may be normal, or nearly so, in early disease or when no papillae have separated.

Sonography or computed tomography will demonstrate calcified papillae, cortical scarring (which is not specific) and, rarely, medullary cavitation.

Histopathology

Chronic interstitial nephritis can be diagnosed only with certainty by biopsy, but the appearances do not identify the aetiology unless papillary necrosis is seen. Voided fragments of tissue or calculi may be identified as necrotic papillae by histology.

Treatment

Complete cessation of analgesic consumption is the only specific measure. Clinical evidence suggests that even normal doses of non-steroidal anti-inflammatory drugs, or of antipyretic-analgesics taken regularly,

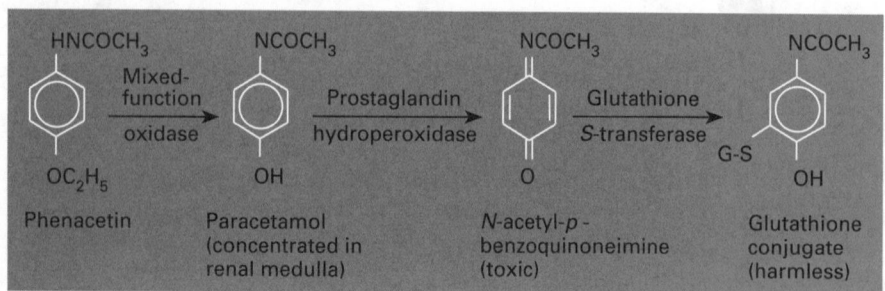

Fig. 2 The metabolism of phenacetin via paracetamol to a toxic metabolite in the renal medulla.

may cause progression of established renal damage whatever the original aetiology.

Infection

Acute pyelonephritis demands active antibacterial treatment. Pyonephrosis is a medical emergency, requiring both control of sepsis and relief of obstruction by percutaneous nephrostomy or ureteric catheterization. Dialysis may be necessary for the septicaemia-related acute renal failure or if obstruction is bilateral.

Indolent urinary infection should be eradicated by prolonged antimicrobial therapy to reduce the likelihood of acute pyelonephritis, but its role in causing progression of renal failure is debatable. Unlike in reflux nephropathy, where infection clears easily but recurs frequently, a prolonged course of rotating antibacterial agents may be required but long-term cure is usual unless a staghorn calculus is present.

Surgery

Normal surgical indications apply to the treatment of separated papillae, whether calcified or not, and of transitional-cell carcinoma.

Chronic renal failure

Patients with analgesic nephropathy generally are satisfactory candidates for maintenance dialysis and transplantation but have an increased likelihood of atheroma (particularly coronary) and urothelial cancer. In the latter context, since carcinomas may develop even when analgesics are no longer taken, it is important to perform regular cytological examination of the urine in those with stable chronic renal failure or after transplantation.

Prognosis

Autonomous progression despite cessation of abuse occurs less in analgesic nephropathy than in chronic renal failure of other causation. The major risk factor is hypertension, which all too often proves difficult to control. Rapid worsening of renal function or hypertension may be due to renal artery occlusion (atheroma) or ureteric obstruction; gradual deterioration is seen with focal glomerulosclerosis (indicated by proteinuria), diffuse accumulation of calcium salts in the kidneys or, more usually, continuing consumption of non-steroidal anti-inflammatory drugs, overt or occult.

Prevention

Education of doctors and the public has little impact, the dual effects of astute advertising and chronic habituation being more potent than rea-

soned persuasion. Either removing phenacetin from proprietary medications without its replacement by paracetamol, or prohibition from direct sale of any analgesic containing more than one ingredient, has proved effective in Scandinavia, Canada, Britain, and Australia (Fig. 4). Surprisingly, once denied access to their favourite analgesic, most *habitués* have little difficulty adjusting, and few have withdrawal symptoms or turn to other psychotropic agents.

Syndromes due to non-steroidal anti-inflammatory drugs (NSAIDs)

NSAIDs, all of which act by inhibiting the cyclo-oxygenase component of prostaglandin synthetase, may cause functional renal failure, or acute or chronic intrinsic renal disease. Virtually every NSAID has been implicated in each of the renal syndromes, but not aspirin nor paracetamol when taken alone. The latter, however, may cause toxic tubular necrosis.

Functional renal failure

Mechanism of disease

Each type of cell in the kidney elaborates one or more of the prostaglandins or thromboxane. These eicosanoids are paracrine agents, which modulate the effects of locally or distantly produced hormones or of autonomic nerves on renal function, particularly by regulating blood flow and pressure. They become important when renal function is already under haemodynamic stress (for example, from hypotension, diuretic administration, or effective plasma volume depletion as in nephrotic syndrome or cirrhosis) or chronically reduced (as in old age or chronic kidney disease). In such circumstances, when renal blood flow or its distribution is already compromised, the addition of NSAIDs may precipitate an acute fall in glomerular filtration unrelated to structural damage, a syndrome described as 'functional' renal failure.

Clinical presentation

Mild cases are manifest only as elevation of serum creatinine or salt and water retention, causing hypertension. When more severe, oliguria or frank acute renal failure occurs. Generally this syndrome is reversible and there are no residual defects, but occasionally the circulatory insult is severe and prolonged enough to cause tubular, or in isolated cases cortical, necrosis.

Fig. 3 A schematic drawing of the pyelographic appearances of analgesic nephropathy. From above down, the pyramids show: (i) central and (ii) total papillary calcification; (iii) central papillary cavitation; (iv) partial and (v) total papillary separation ('ring sign'); (vi) a 'clubbed' calyx from which the papilla has been passed. Note the areas of cortical atrophy over papillae, interspersed with hypertrophied columns of Bertin.

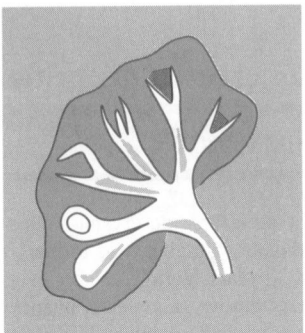

Fig. 4 The declining age-specific incidence of young and middle-aged women entering Australian endstage renal failure programmes as a result of analgesic nephropathy. Phenacetin was withdrawn in 1975, and all compound analgesic preparations in 1979. The decline occurred earlier, and was proportionately greater, in the younger age groups; much of the rise in the 55 to 64 year age group was due to increasing acceptance of older patients into renal failure treatment programmes.

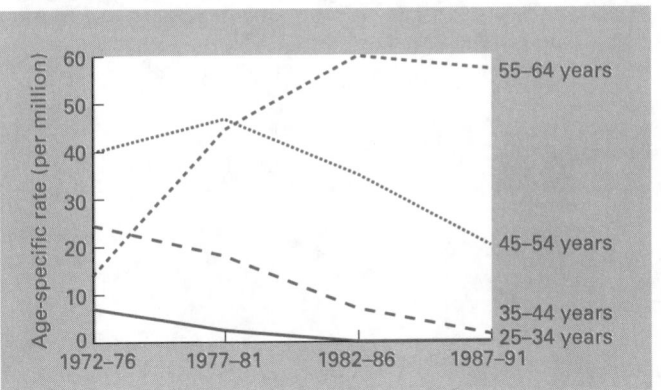

NSAID-induced kidney disease

Acute interstitial nephritis—minimal change nephrotic syndrome

In this condition, which is seen only with NSAIDs, the histological and clinical picture may be exclusively of either acute interstitial nephritis or minimal-change nephrotic syndrome, but usually both are present.

Mechanisms of disease

As there rarely is evidence of an immune reaction against the drug (onset is late, antibody is not detectable; neither eosinophilia nor systemic vasculitis), it seems likely that this syndrome is caused by disturbance of prostaglandin-modulated production of lymphokines, or the diversion of eicosanoid metabolism towards proinflammatory leukotrienes. The resulting T-lymphocyte abnormality is manifest at two sites in the kidney. In the interstitial tissue, there is mononuclear infiltration sometimes involving tubules, with formation of granulomata occasionally. The second target is the glomerular filtration barrier (perhaps specifically the epithelial foot processes)—hence the minimal-change nephrotic syndrome with its characteristic electron microscopic appearance.

Diagnosis

The insidious onset of worsening renal function, together with moderate proteinuria or the nephrotic syndrome several months after starting an NSAID is characteristic. Renal biopsy will confirm the diagnosis (Fig. 5), but often is unnecessary.

Treatment and prognosis

Not only should the offending NSAID be stopped, but all drugs of this class avoided, as the disorder appears to be a toxic rather than an allergic reaction. There is little evidence that corticosteroids help, except when granulomata are present. Nephrotic syndrome resolves spontaneously and completely within 1 month of withdrawing the drug, but recovery from acute interstitial nephritis is slow and incomplete.

Chronic interstitial nephritis

This may be a slowly evolving form of the acute disease described above, or analogous to classical analgesic nephropathy. However, papillary necrosis is relatively uncommon—when present, the cause may be medullary ischaemia rather than cytotoxicity (Table 1).

Diagnosis

Only recognition that NSAIDs may be nephrotoxic even at prescribed dosage, and the performance of a biopsy to show chronic interstitial

nephritis, will give the diagnosis with certainty. The majority of cases are overlooked because of the insidious nature of the chronic renal failure and the lack of urinary abnormalities.

Treatment and prognosis

Avoidance of all NSAIDs, and also of antipyretic-analgesics taken regularly, may protect against slow progression of chronic renal failure. On the whole, the severity of renal dysfunction seems to be less than in classical analgesic nephropathy, probably because papillary necrosis occurs rarely, and end-stage renal failure recognizably and primarily due to this cause is infrequent. However, this is an important and often unrecognized secondary cause of worsening chronic renal failure.

Toxic renal tubular necrosis

Two analgesic drugs, paracetamol and glafenine (an NSAID introduced in France but not used widely elsewhere) can cause nephrotoxic tubular necrosis. In the case of paracetamol, the mechanism of toxicity probably is the same as in hepatocellular necrosis (Chapter 8.2.1); in these cases, why the kidney rather than the liver should be the main target organ, is unknown.

REFERENCES

Burry, A.F. (1967). The evolution of analgesic nephropathy. *Nephron* **5**, 185–201.

Dubach, U.C., Rosner, B., and Stürmer, T. (1991). An epidemiologic study of abuse of analgesic drugs. Effects of phenacetin and salicylate on mortality and cardiovascular morbidity (1968–87). *New England Journal of Medicine* **324**, 155–60.

McCredie, M., Stewart, J.H., and Day, N.E. (1993). Different roles for phenacetin and paracetamol in cancer of the kidney and renal pelvis. *International Journal of Cancer*, **53**, 245–9.

Mohandas, J., Marshall, J.J., Duggin, G.G., Horvath, J.S., and Tiller, D.J. (1984). Differential distribution of glutathione and glutathione-related enzymes in rabbit kidney. Possible implications in analgesic nephropathy. *Biochemical Pharmacology* **33**, 1801–7.

Murray, M.D. and Brater, D.C. (1993). Renal toxicity of the nonsteroidal antiinflammatory drugs. *Annual Review of Pharmacology and Toxicology*, **33**, 435–65.

Murray, R.M. (1973). Dependence on analgesics in analgesic nephropathy. *British Journal of Addiction* **68**, 265–72.

Nanra, R.S. (1993). Analgesic nephropathy in the 1990s—an Australian perspective. *Kidney International*, **42**, S86–92.

Prescott, L.F. (1982). Analgesic nephropathy: a reassessment of the role of phenacetin and other analgesics. *Drugs* **23**, 75–149.

Sandler, D.P., Burr, F.R., and Weinberg, C.R. (1991). Nonsteroidal anti-inflammatory drugs and the risk for chronic renal disease. *Annals of Internal Medicine* **115**, 165–72.

Schwarz, A., Kunzendorf, U., Keller, F., and Offermann, G. (1989). Progression of renal failure in analgesic-associated nephropathy. *Nephron* **53**, 244–9.

Stewart, J.H. (ed.) (1993). *Analgesic- and NSAID-induced kidney disease.* Oxford University Press.

20.9.2 Gout, purines, and interstitial nephritis

J. S. CAMERON and H. A. SIMMONDS

Uric acid nephropathy of the classical type, a chronic crystal-related interstitial nephropathy in a middle-aged male with gout, was formerly common but has become rare in the past 30 years. Various factors may have contributed: a lower intake of dietary purines, a lower frequency of chronic lead intoxication, and early treatment of the majority of severely affected gouty subjects with allopurinol. Thus the relative

Fig. 5 Acute interstitial nephritis caused by naproxen. (By courtesy of Associate Professor R.S. Nanra, Newcastle.)

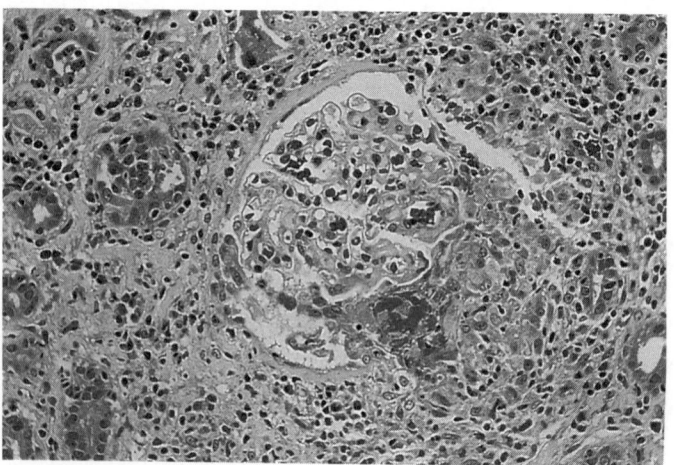

importance of rarer forms of metabolically induced or inherited gouty nephropathy has increased, and the average age of diagnosis of gout-associated or hyperuricaemic nephropathy has decreased.

Relevant aspects of purine metabolism and the genesis of uric acid are reviewed in Chapter 11.4.

CONTRIBUTION OF DIET TO URIC ACID EXCRETION; SOLUBILITY

Man has no requirement for dietary purines, and the intestine serves as an effective barrier capable of rapidly degrading dietary purine to uric acid, which can add to the endogenous load in subjects addicted to purine-rich diets. Clinical problems and pathological changes associated with uric acid arise entirely from its insolubility, and the ability of the resultant crystals to initiate inflammation. The solubility of urate at 37°C is about 1 mmol/l at pH 5, 12 mmol/l at pH 8. The precursor xanthine is even less soluble (about 1 mmol/l at either pH) and an analogue, 2,8-dihydroxyadenine (2,8-DHA), almost indistinguishable from uric acid in conventional laboratory testing, is the most insoluble of all (0.03 mmol/l at either pH).

URATE HANDLING BY THE KIDNEY: THE PATHOGENESIS OF GOUT

The exact nature of the renal handling of urate is not yet clear, since earlier pharmacological studies must be re-evaluated in the light of recent reports demonstrating that urate is transported across the brush border by a urate/anion exchanger which has affinity for a wide variety of inorganic and organic anions, such as Cl^- and HCO_3^-. However, there is no doubt that the transport of uric acid occurs predominantly in the proximal tubule, is bidirectional, and has both a secretory and reabsorptive component. Many factors acutely or chronically affect the amount of filtered urate reaching the urine, including circulating blood volume (which accounts for the low plasma urate of pregnancy and in part the rise with diuretic treatment) and competing metabolites or drugs.

If the role of relative excess of intake is assessed by putting the subject on a purine-free diet and measuring urinary urate, less than 1 per cent of gouty subjects are overproducers, in that they then continue to excrete abnormally large amounts of urate (> 3.0 mmol/day, or > 0.35 mmol/mmol creatinine). In these rare cases an underlying genetic metabolic defect can generally be demonstrated in which the normal feedback controls on *de novo* purine synthesis are overridden, resulting in gross uric acid overproduction. Two such enzyme defects have been identified: hypoxanthine guanine phosphoribosyltransferase (**HPRT**) deficiency and phosphoribosyl pyrophosphate synthetase (**PRPS**) superactivity (see below).

Primates display two peculiarities in their metabolism and renal handling of purines. First, they lack expression of the gene for the hepatic enzyme uricase, which degrades insoluble uric acid to the soluble allantoin in other mammals. Secondly, their renal tubules reabsorb around 90 per cent of the filtered urate, the fractional excretion ($FE_{ur} = C_{ur}/GFR$, where C_{ur} is the clearance rate of urate and GFR the glomerular filtration rate) being only about 10 per cent. Net reabsorption is slightly higher in males (92 per cent; FE_{ur}, 8 per cent) than in females (88 per cent; FE_{ur}, 12 per cent) and is lower in children of either sex (70–85 per cent; FE_{ur}, 15–30 per cent). This explains the higher plasma uric acid in men and the rarity of classical gout in women and children.

Current opinion suggests that the great majority of typical gouty patients underexcrete urate because of a defect in tubular secretion. Thus a combination of events is needed to produce hyperuricaemia and the clinical syndrome of gout: a large intake of readily absorbed purines, coupled with a defect in the renal handing of urate at the level of the renal tubule, which cannot respond to a purine load without an abnormal rise in plasma urate concentration. The ingestion of food rich in purines has been noted for millennia to be high in subjects with 'primary' gout. This is a disorder of affluent societies, and during times of food shortage this type of gout almost vanishes.

In addition, normal ranges for plasma and urine differ greatly in the healthy population from country to country. The majority of adults in the United Kingdom today ingest a diet relatively low in purines and a urinary uric acid excretion above 3.5 mmol/day would be considered abnormal. By contrast, the upper limit of normal for adults in Australia is about 7.0 mmol/day, values for the United States and France falling somewhere between.

In renal failure, in parallel with tubular rejection of sodium and an a number of other solutes, FE_{ur} progressively increases from the normal adult values of around 10 per cent of filtered urate in the urine up to as high as 85 per cent (Fig. 1) in advanced renal failure. The reasons for this are not understood, although retention of uricosuric metabolites, such as hippurates, has been suggested. Thus in patients with an initially subnormal FE_{ur} who develop renal failure, just at the point when their retention of urea and creatinine is barely evident their FE_{ur} becomes normal, at least for a time, and diagnosis becomes more difficult.

INHERITED DISORDERS OF URIC ACID AND PURINE METABOLISM

As noted above, 'classical' gout is probably a condition arising from purine overload in a patient with a kidney whose capacity to eliminate uric acid is lower than normal; thus classical gout can be considered to be an inherited renal disorder. However, a number of other rare conditions may present as gout, and in these renal involvement is common.

Fig. 1 The relationship between fractional excretion of urate (FE_{ur} vertical axis) and glomerular filtration rate (horizontal axis) in health and disease. In normal individuals, the FE_{ur} varies according to age and sex as discussed in the text, being greater in children and in women (10–14 per cent) than in men (8–12 per cent) and postmenopausal women. With decline in renal function, the FE_{ur} increases to reach as high as 85 per cent of filtered urate in terminal uraemia with a glomerular filtration rate of less than 5 ml/min. In some inherited uricosurias (stippled area, top right), both as isolated tubular defects or as part of a Fanconi syndrome, fractional excretion is usually 30 to 60 per cent, although in a few cases it can reach or even exceed the glomerular filtration rate, which is almost always normal. Again, in 'classical' male gouty patients (bottom right) renal function is usually normal when age is allowed for, but FE_{ur} is reduced below the normal male figures of 8 to 12 per cent. In lead nephropathy renal function (glomerular filtration rate) is frequently reduced and FE_{ur} is reduced, especially when the reduced renal function is taken into account. The same is true in familial juvenile hyperuricaemic nephropathy (FJHN), in which there is a very low FE_{ur} averaging only 4 to 5 per cent (both shown by hatched area).

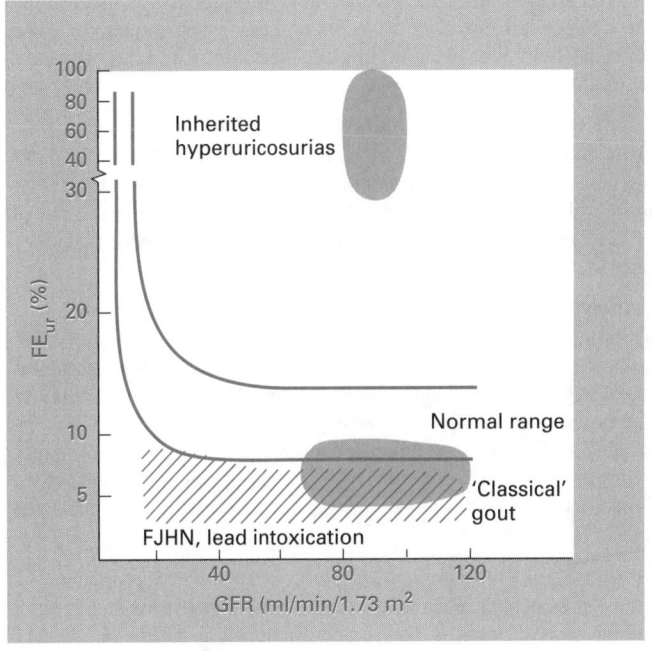

Glycogen storage disease type I

This results from a deficiency of the enzyme glucose 6-phosphatase. Purine overproduction arises from a combination of accelerated adenosine triphosphate breakdown and increased synthesis. The resulting hyperuricaemia is then amplified by a reduction in renal excretion related to the associated lactic acidosis.

Familial juvenile gout

Hyperuricaemia is also the presenting finding in a subset of patients who may develop a juvenile onset of gout affecting males and (unusually) females equally. This disorder, termed familial juvenile hyperuricaemic nephropathy, has been poorly characterized until recently. It is an autosomal dominant condition with high penetrance, and shows two major hallmarks: hyperuricaemia disproportionate to the degree of renal dysfunction and an extremely low FE_{ur}; clinical gout and hypertension are inconsistent features, and the condition may be misdiagnosed as 'familial nephritis'. The reason for the renal damage is obscure since there is no evidence of urate deposition within the kidney. However, the absence of detectable crystals does not necessarily preclude their original presence as the cause of the non-specific renal lesion frequently reported. It is most likely that there is a defect in a gene coding for one of the anion transporters in the proximal tubular epithelium, either in the basolateral or the brush border membranes. This would suggest that familial juvenile hyperuricaemic nephropathy may be the human analogue of the gouty chicken, in which a defect in a basolateral urate transporter has been described.

Deficiency of hypoxanthine guanine phosphoribosyltransferase (HPRT)

This X-linked disorder may present as the complete enzyme defect, the Lesch–Nyhan syndrome of severe neurological deficits, or as a partial defect associated only with uric acid overproduction and its consequences, presenting as gout or urolithiasis in adolescence or early adulthood. There is considerable variation in neurological abnormalities, enzyme activity, and genetic lesions, the majority being the result of point mutations or small deletions. All degrees of deficiency, however, result in gross uric acid overproduction and excretion. Patients may present with acute renal failure in childhood or infancy, uric acid stones, or chronic urate nephropathy, and are often misdiagnosed as 'cerebral palsy' in childhood. In acute renal failure, renal ultrasound may show the bright ultrasonogram of crystal nephropathy. Uric acid stones may be the sole manifestation in some cases.

The long-term prognosis is good in children and adolescents with partial HPRT deficiency and precocious gout, but patients with the complete deficiency mostly die of aspiration-associated infections, some with renal failure; there is no specific treatment for the neurological abnormalities.

Phosphoribosyl pyrophosphate synthetase (PRPS) superactivity

This is another rare X-linked disorder, of which only 24 families have been described. There is considerable heterogeneity of genetic defects and neurological manifestations, but there is gross overproduction of uric acid in all, and the majority present with severe gout or kidney stones in adolescence or early adulthood.

Adenine phosphoribosyltransferase deficiency

This is inherited as an autosomal recessive lesion of a gene on chromosome 16. The chief clinical manifestation is 2,8-dihydroxyadenine (2,8-DHA) urolithiasis and crystal nephropathy, sometime leading to acute or chronic renal failure. The nephrotoxicity relates to the extreme insolubility of 2,8-DHA at any pH, coupled with its high renal clearance as a result of tubular secretion. The condition is very rare in the United Kingdom, the majority of cases having been reported from Iceland and Japan.

Hereditary xanthinuria

This has previously been considered rare, generally affecting adults with xanthine stones, but it is now evident that this is not so. Hereditary xanthinuria arises from one of two recessively inherited deficiencies of

the enzyme xanthine dehydrogenase, coded on chromosome 2. As a result, there is an inability to degrade hypoxanthine and xanthine to uric acid, with accumulation of xanthine. Thus the potential for precipitation of this insoluble purine in the kidney or urinary tract is high, particularly in an infant with a history of vomiting, diarrhoea, or recurrent infection, and eventually can lead to tubular blockage or chronic renal failure.

ACUTE AND CHRONIC RENAL DISEASE ASSOCIATED WITH DISORDERS OF PURINE METABOLISM AND URATE HANDLING

Acute crystal nephropathy

Acute crystal nephropathy with acute renal failure may occur when insoluble purines (uric acid, 2,8-DHA, or xanthine) precipitate within the kidney, mainly within the tubular lumen; the increasing concentration and acidity of the distal tubular urine favours precipitation of uric acid crystals at that site. Intratubular uric acid crystals are usually easily visible in biopsy material in acute uric acid nephropathy, provided aqueous solutions do not wash them out during processing; alcohol-fixed or frozen biopsy material is best. These crystals induce inflammation as well as causing direct blockage of tubules, and are often detected by ultrasonography as a 'bright' appearance of the parenchyma; the urine also is loaded with the typical birefringent crystals. This syndrome is seen in settings of gross uric acid overproduction, and thus is found most commonly in the treatment of myeloid tumours, in which massive DNA breakdown occurs. Occasionally this may happen when such tumours go into spontaneous remissions, or in association with treatment of solid tumours, but this is rare. Finally it may occur in the gross overproduction of uric acid in the Lesch–Nyhan syndrome. In all these states, renal handling of uric acid is normal.

Treatment

This centres on prophylaxis: a good fluid intake with or without alkalinization of the urine is the central point of management, plus pretreatment with allopurinol. These measures lower urate retention by volume expansion, increase solubility in the urine, and distribute the purine load over three purine bases rather than just uric acid. If renal dysfunction or failure is already present, the dose of allopurinol may need to be reduced to doses as low as 100 mg thrice weekly in those on dialysis. Treatment with allopurinol of those overproducing uric acid increases the danger of xanthine nephropathy.

Hyperuricosuria–hypouricaemia

Some inherited tubular disorders, either as part of the Fanconi syndrome or as one of the heterogeneous isolated tubular defects (e.g., hereditary renal hypouricaemia) have uricosuria as a component. FE_{ur} is usually 30 to 50 per cent, but in occasional cases may equal, or even exceed, the glomerular filtration rate. Nevertheless, almost all of these hyperuricosuric patients are symptomless. Crystalluria or stones with colic have been noted in a minority, and acute renal failure has been reported after severe exercise in such patients.

Chronic urate nephropathy

In 'classical' gout, chronic urate nephropathy is more complicated and its pathogenesis more contentious than acute uric acid nephropathy. Certainly today, in most middle-aged male gouty patients, the main association of renal impairment is with renal vascular disease rather than in the urate crystal deposition, and glomerular function is often normal when corrected for age. A bland interstitial fibrosis with associated vascular changes are the usual histological findings; it is rare to find urate crystals, even though all insoluble purine crystals are known to be capable of inducing this type of tubulointerstitial injury in animal experiments. Even so, chronic interstitial deposits of sodium urate may occur in a few untreated gouty subjects, and may be associated with interstitial inflammation. Whether such crystals get there by erosion of initially intratubular deposits of uric acid, or form *in situ*, remains a matter of controversy. Crystals, when present, are most common in the medulla, and are surrounded by an inflammatory infiltrate of varying age. Crystals of 2,8-DHA or xanthine may appear similarly in the interstitium in adenine phosphoribosyltransferase and xanthine oxidase deficiencies, respectively, and present as chronic renal insufficiency.

One particular cause of gout-associated renal failure is chronic lead intoxication. Hyperuricaemia results from reduced tubular secretion of uric acid by unknown mechanisms, but it seems most likely that the renal damage relates more to the lead itself than the uric acid, since an interstitial nephritis without crystal deposits is usually seen, as is also the case in familial juvenile hyperuricaemic nephropathy, in which a disproportionate hyperuricaemic with low FE_{ur} is found (Fig. 1). In renal failure from other causes, despite raised plasma urate concentrations, gout is rare; and in the minority who do suffer clinical gout, either an increased body burden of lead will be detected by measuring its excretion after calcium edetate infusion, or familial juvenile hyperuricaemic nephropathy is identified.

Treatment

At the present time, treatment of chronic gouty nephropathy will almost always involve the use of allopurinol, since uricosuric agents such as probenecid become ineffective as the glomerular filtration rate falls and FE_{ur} increases concomitantly. The dose of allopurinol must be modified from the standard 300 mg/24 h down through 200 and 100 mg/day as glomerular filtration rate falls, to the lowest dose in dialysed patients, who require only 100 mg thrice weekly. Increasing fluid intake will not be of much use in established renal insufficiency, but it is worth trying in those with relatively normal renal function. In familial juvenile hyperuricaemic nephropathy, it is not clear yet whether allopurinol may protect against renal failure but it must be given in any event in order to control the hyperuricaemia.

Uric acid stones

As with tophaceous nephropathy, uric acid stones are much less common today in subjects suffering 'classical' middle-aged male gout than in the past; uric acid stones are discussed in Chapter 20.12. Other rare purine stones, such as those of 2,8-DHA in adenine phosphoribosyltransferase deficiency and xanthine in xanthine oxidase deficiency may occasionally be identified; the former are often confused with uric acid stones, but are grey and friable, unlike the yellow and hard uric acid stones.

FURTHER READING

Behringer D., Craswell, E., Mohl, C., Stoeppler, M., and Ritz, E. (1986). Urinary lead excretion in uremic patients. *Nephron* **42**, 323–9.

Bennett, W.M. (1985). Lead nephropathy. *Kidney International* **28**, 212–20.

Berger, L. and Yü, T.-F. (1975). Renal function in gout IV. An analysis of 524 gouty subjects including long-term studies. *American Journal of Medicine* **59**, 605–15.

Boumendil-Podevin, E.F., Podevin R.A., and Richet G. (1974). Uricosuric agents in uremic sera. Identification of indoxyl sulfate and hippuric acid. *Journal of Clinical Investigation* **55**, 1142–52.

Calabrese, G., Simmonds, H.A., Cameron J.S., and Davies, P.M. (1990). Precocious familial gout with reduced fractional excretion of urate and normal purine enzymes. *Quarterly Journal of Medicine* **75**, 441–50.

Cameron, J.S. and Simmonds, H.A. (1981). Uric acid, gout and the kidney. *Journal of Clinical Pathology* **34**, 1245–54.

Cameron, J.S., Moro, F., and Simmonds, H.A. (1993). Purine disorders, hyperuricaemia and gout in pediatric nephrology. *Pediatric Nephrology* **7**, 105–18.

Danovich, G.M., Weinberger, J., and Berlyne, G.M. (1972). Uric acid in advanced renal failure. *Clinical Science* **43**, 331–41.

Diamond, H.S. (1989). Interpretation of pharmacologic manipulation of urate transport in man. *Nephron* **51**, 1–5.

Palella, T. and Fox, I.H. (1989). Hyperuricemia and gout. In *The metabolic basis of inherited disease* (ed. C. Scriver *et al.*), pp. 965–1007. McGraw-Hill, New York.

Roch-Ramel, F., Werner, D., and Guisan, B. (1994). Urate transport in brush-border membrane of the human kidney. *American Journal of Physiology*, **35**, F797-F805.

Simmonds, H.A., Sahota, A., and van Acker, K. (1989). APRT deficiency and 2, 8 dihydroxyadenine lithiasis. In *The metabolic basis of inherited disease* (ed. C. Scriver *et al.*), pp. 1029–45. McGraw-Hill, New York.

Stone, T.W. and Simmonds, H.A. (1991). *Purines: basic and clinical aspects.* Kluwer, London.

Zöllner, N. and Gresser, U. (ed.) (1991). *Urate deposition in man and its clinical consequences.* Springer-Verlag, Berlin.

20.9.3 Hypercalcaemic nephropathy

R. W. E. WATTS

Renal handling of calcium

Only ionized calcium (concentration about 1.3 mmol/l or 47 to 52 per cent of the serum total calcium) and complexed calcium (concentration about 0.1 mmol/l or 6 to 8 per cent of the serum total calcium) enter the glomerular filtrate. Increases in the total serum calcium concentration are accompanied by parallel increases in the filtered calcium load, up to about 3.7 mmol/l. Above this level, rising serum phosphate concentrations with the formation of calcium phosphate–protein complexes, and possibly an increasing calcium-binding capacity of the plasma proteins, tend to destroy this linear relationship.

At normal serum calcium concentrations, the filtered load of calcium is 200 to 250 mmol/24 h, about 2 per cent of which is excreted in the urine. Calcium is reabsorbed by the proximal convoluted tubule (about 65 per cent), the thick ascending limb of Henle's loop (about 20 per cent), the distal convoluted tubule (about 10 per cent), and the collecting ducts (about 5 per cent). Passive diffusion and movement along electrochemical gradients between the epithelial cells, and energy-mediated active transcellular transport mechanisms are both involved. The former mediates calcium reabsorption in the proximal convoluted tubule and in the thick ascending limb of Henle's loop. There is also evidence for active reabsorption in the proximal convoluted tubule, although its nature is uncertain. Parathyroid hormone has been reported to increase calcium reabsorption in the cortical part, but not in the medullary portion, of the thick segment of Henle's loop. The thin segment of Henle's loop does not appear to be involved in calcium transport. The epithelium of the distal convoluted tubule exercises the final control of calcium excretion, although active and passive transport of calcium across the collecting duct epithelium have also been reported.

The amount of calcium filtered at the glomerulus is a major determinant of the flux of calcium across the renal tubular epithelium and the interstitium. This explains the development of calcium-mediated damage to the epithelium, and interstitial calcification in hypercalcaemic states.

The extracellular fluid volume is another factor that modifies the tubular reabsorption of calcium. Thus, extracellular fluid expansion increases the glomerular filtration rate and hence the absolute amount of calcium filtered. Saline infusion produces calciuresis as well as natriuresis. This has therapeutic implications in relation to the treatment of hypercalcaemia (see Chapter 12.6), and a low sodium chloride intake is recommended for recurrent calcium-containing stone formers.

Although the parathyroid hormone directly enhances the renal tubular reabsorption of calcium, its main effects are to enhance calcium and phosphate absorption from the intestine and to promote bone resorption. These actions increase the plasma concentration and filtered load of calcium, and cause a net calciuresis, the effects on the gut and bones exceeding any tendency for it to increase the tubular reabsorption of calcium, either directly or by reducing the glomerular filtration rate. Hyperthyroidism also increases urinary calcium excretion by augmenting the filtered load and not by modifying the renal tubular transport of calcium.

Physiological studies of possible direct effects of 1,25-dihydroxycholecalciferol $(1,25(OH)_2D_3)$ on the kidney have given conflicting results. Large doses of vitamin D are calciuric in man, due to enhanced intestinal absorption and an increased filtered load of calcium, which overwhelm any postulated direct effect on tubular transport.

Prostaglandins are involved in the regulation of calcium movement across the renal tubular epithelium. The intrarenal infusion of prostanoids causes a dose-related increase in renal blood flow and excretion of sodium, potassium, calcium, and magnesium. Inhibition of prostaglandin synthesis reduces calcium reabsorption in the thick ascending limb of Henle's loop and prevents experimentally induced nephrocalcinosis in rats.

Diuretics that inhibit sodium transport in either the proximal tubules or the loop of Henle (for example, the loop agents) also inhibit calcium reabsorption. Conversely, diuretics acting mainly on the distal tubule such as thiazides reduce calcium excretion and are used in the treatment of idiopathic hypercalciuria. Amiloride also promotes calcium reabsorption in the distal tubule, where it exerts its natriuretic effect. It is less potent as an hypocalciuric agent when used alone, although it acts synergistically with thiazides. The loop diuretics, on the other hand, are useful in the treatment of hypercalcaemia and are contraindicated in idiopathic hypercalciuria. The carbonic anhydrase inhibitors, acetazolamide and dichlorphenamide, which block hydrogen ion secretion and bicarbonate reabsorption, primarily in the proximal convoluted tubule, produce a small calciuresis as well as natriuresis.

PATHOPHYSIOLOGY

Acute hypercalcaemia causes a high flux of calcium through the renal parenchyma and interstitium, epithelial cell degeneration, necrosis and calcification, and the tubules become obstructed. Calcium deposits may also be found in the glomeruli and blood vessels. There is marked impairment of urine-concentrating ability, with resistance to antidiuretic hormone (ADH), which is probably of multifactorial origin. High levels of calcium ions either impair the ability of the ADH receptor to bind ADH, or the ability of the hormone–receptor complex to activate adenylate cyclase. In addition, impaired sodium chloride reabsorption in the ascending limb of Henle's loop may contribute by interfering with the medullary accumulation of solutes, which is the primary step in the generation of the countercurrent gradient on which water reabsorption by the thin segment of Henle's loop depends.

Acutely, this state of nephrogenic diabetes insipidus causes underhydration, which is aggravated by associated nausea and vomiting, resulting in additional sodium and chloride depletion.

Chronic hypercalcaemia leads to interstitial calcification and fibrosis, which are most marked in the medulla. It is sometimes associated with renal tubular losses of potassium and bicarbonate, resulting in some cases in hypokalaemia and acidosis. Thus chronic hypercalcaemic states can cause chronic renal failure with interstitial scarring often complicated by associated hypertension.

Clinical aspects

Hypercalcaemic nephropathy is most often associated with malignancy. Other major causes are primary hyperparathyroidism, multiple myelomatosis, sarcoidosis, and vitamin D intoxication. The milk-alkali syndrome, immobilization (especially if the patient has Paget's disease), tertiary hyperparathyroidism, and hyperthyroidism are less often encountered as causes of a sufficient degree of hypercalcaemia to damage the kidneys (see Chapter 12.6).

The severity of the clinical manifestations of hypercalcaemic nephropathy is roughly parallel the degree of hypercalcaemia, and serum total calcium concentrations greater than 3.5 mmol/l indicate a grave risk of developing a hypercalcaemic crisis. Whenever hypercalcaemia is found in a patient with renal failure it should be assumed in the first instance, that hypercalcaemia is the major factor in causing the impaired renal function. Tertiary hyperparathyroidism is very rare in chronic renal disease, although it occurs more often after successful renal transplantation, when, on occasion, hypercalcaemia may damage the grafted kidney.

Transient hypercalcaemia occurs occasionally during recovery from acute renal failure (Chapter 20.16).

The manifestations of calcium nephropathy may be the presenting feature or may form only a small part of the overall clinical picture of the primary disease. A hypercalcaemic crisis may arise suddenly and be life-threatening in a patient with, for example, primary hyperparathyroidism or malignant disease, who was previously in an otherwise relatively stable clinical state.

Hypercalcaemia is sometimes only discovered incidentally. There may be an antecedent history of the systemic symptoms of hypercalcaemia and circumcorneal calcification indicates relatively long-standing antecedent hypercalcaemia. Impaired urinary concentrating ability, with polyuria and polydipsia, are usually the earliest clinical indications of renal damage. Dehydration, oliguria, and uraemia follow, and the systemic manifestations of hypercalcaemia, which vary between individuals (anorexia, nausea, vomiting, constipation, lethargy, muscle weakness, stupor, and coma), appear or worsen. Proteinuria, haematuria, and pyuria may be present, even in the absence of nephrolithiasis and pyelonephritis. Medullary nephrocalcinosis and stones may be visible radiologically if there has been long-standing hypercalcaemia and hypercalciuria. Acute pancreatitis is a well-recognized complication of hypercalcaemia (Chapter 12.6).

Treatment

If possible, the underlying disease should be treated promptly and vigorously. Unless this is done, it is likely to prove impossible to control hypercalcaemia in the long term. The decision to treat hypercalcaemia has to be taken in the context of the patient's overall clinical condition. Those in whom hypercalcaemia is only an incident in a terminal illness should not be subjected to heroic measures but treated symptomatically.

PARENTERAL REHYDRATION AND SALINE-INDUCED CALCIURESIS

In the absence of such contraindications, hypercalcaemia of 3.0 mmol/l or more in the presence of renal impairment, or 3.5 mmol or more regardless of symptoms, indicates an urgent need for immediate treatment. The first step is to correct the deficit of salt and water by rapid infusion of isotonic sodium chloride, and to continue intravenous saline at a rate dependent on the severity of the hypercalcaemia, the degree of renal failure, and cardiac function. Most patients will tolerate 3 to 6 litres of isotonic saline given intravenously per 24 h, and the resulting calciuresis may be greatly enhanced and protection from pulmonary oedema achieved by the coincident use of a loop diuretic (frusemide, bumetanide, or ethacrynic acid) and a central venous line with central venous pressure monitoring. Usual doses range from 40 mg frusemide twice daily by mouth to 40 mg intravenously 2 hourly in the most severe cases. Infusion of 6 l of saline per 24 h, with two-hourly intravenous loop agents can induce urinary calcium excretion to some 25 mmol, and reduce plasma calcium concentrations by 1 to 1.5 mmol/l.day. Such aggressive treatment is rarely necessary.

BISPHOSPHONATES

If correction of dehydration and sodium chloride deficiency, together with judicious use of saline and diuretic-induced calciuresis, does not result in reducing plasma calcium concentrations below 3.0 mmol/l, and in those whose initial concentrations exceeds 3.5 mmol/l, additional treatment is required. The hypocalcaemic agents of choice in the United Kingdom are sodium clodronate or disodium pamidronate; in the United States, where clodronate is not yet available, etidronate is most commonly used.

These bisphosphonates are given by slow intravenous infusion. The recommended dose of clodronate is of 300 mg in 500 ml of 0.9 per cent saline, given over 2 h daily for periods not exceeding 10 days. The dose of disodium pamidronate may be adjusted in relation to the prevailing plasma calcium concentration, as shown in Table 1. The total dose of

Table 1 *Recommended doses of pamidronate according to plasma calcium concentrations*

Plasma calcium (mmol/l)	Dose
Less than 3.0	15–30 mg in 125–250 ml saline in 2 h
3.0–3.5	30–60 mg in 25–500 ml saline in 4 h
3.5–4.0	60–90 mg in 500–1000 ml saline in 8–24 h
More than 4.0	90 mg in 1000 ml saline in 24 h

pamidronate may be given as a single infusion or individual doses, but should not exceed 90 mg in a single course of treatment. Etidronate is also given intravenously in saline in a dose of 7.5 mg/kg body-weight over a 4-h period daily, given for between 3 and 7 days. If these bisphosphonates are given until the plasma calcium concentration has fallen to normal, a degree of hypocalcaemia may result, and so a reasonable target is to lower the concentration to below 3.0 mmol/l.

Oral doses of these drugs can be used in chronic hypercalcaemia, and although long-term administration of etidronate can cause osteomalacia, this ill-effect appears less likely to complicate the use of clodronate or pamidronate.

The bisphosphonates lower the plasma calcium by coating hydroxyapatite crystals in bone and thus inhibit osteoclastic resorption. In general, their effect on plasma calcium begins after 2 to 3 days and reaches full effect in 5 to 7 days.

Prednisolone (20 mg, 8 hourly by mouth) or hydrocortisone (150 mg, 8 hourly intravenously) can be effective treatments for hypercalcaemia in patients in whom the cause is sarcoidosis, vitamin D intoxication, and in some with lymphoma or myeloma, but glucocorticoids are generally not effective when the cause is a non-haematological carcinoma or primary hyperparathyroidism.

PHOSPHATE

Oral phosphate preparations (for example, phosphate-Sandoz®, dose equivalent to 500–1500 mg (16–48 mmol) of elemental phosphorus) and oral fluids can be used if nausea and vomiting are not prominent or have been controlled (for example by parenteral metoclopramide), but this approach has only a small effect on plasma calcium and larger doses cause diarrhoea.

Intravenous sodium phosphate can lower calcium levels rapidly, but because of the serious risk of deposition of calcium phosphate in tissues, particularly of the kidney and blood vessels, and it has been superseded.

MITHRAMYCIN

This cytotoxic drug, given at 25 μg/kg body-weight by intravenous infusion over a 4- to 24-h period, inhibits bone resorption and lowers the serum calcium concentration in 1 to 2 days. This effect lasts for several days. The infusion can be repeated at intervals of 24 to 48 h, but this increases the risk of myelotoxicity, hepatotoxicity, and nephrotoxicity.

CALCITONIN

Calcitonin inhibits bone resorption and increases the renal clearance of calcium, and is therefore of some value as an adjunct to other methods of controlling hypercalcaemia. An advantage is its rapid onset of action, with effects demonstrable sometimes within a few hours and maximal at 12 to 24 h. The effects are, however, relatively weak and short lasting. Perhaps the major indication is to initiate a reduction in particularly severe and symptomatic hypercalcaemia. Synthetic salmon calcitonin (salcatonin) is less immunogenic than other forms, and a preparation (Miacalcic®) for slow intravenous infusion (5–10 units/kg body-weight

over at least 6 h) is available. Co-administration of glucocorticoids may prolong the effects of calcitonin, but this is controversial, as is the question of whether or not down-regulation of receptors underlies a lesser effect with time.

NEWER AGENTS

The somatostatin analogue, octreotide (50 μg subcutaneously/day) has been shown to reduce malignancy-associated hypercalcaemia, possibly by inhibiting PTHrP (parathyroid hormone related protein) release. Its value relative to the other available treatments remains to be assessed.

GENERAL MANAGEMENT AND PROGNOSIS

Close supervision and frequent biochemical monitoring of blood and urine are necessary during the management of a hypercalcaemic crisis. Most patients survive the acute episode, provided that an adequate rate of urine flow can be established and that the hypercalcaemia is corrected without overloading the circulation with salt and water. Haemo- or peritoneal dialysis, using low-calcium dialysates, is occasionally needed.

Calcium nephropathy of short duration may be completely reversible, although total recovery may take many months after removal of the cause. The extent of the structural renal damage cannot be assessed during the acute episode, and some cases continue to deteriorate in spite of successful control of plasma calcium. Others remain oliguric and hypercalcaemic, and require continued treatment by haemo- or peritoneal dialysis.

In general, the cases diagnosed early, with a short total period of hypercalaemia, have the best prognosis. Apparently complete recovery may be followed by a gradual deterioration in renal function, due to slowly progressive, irreversible renal fibrosis initiated by nephrocalcinosis during the hypercalaemic periods.

REFERENCES

Attie, M.F. (1989). Treatment of hypercalcaemia. *Endocrinology and Metabolism Clinics of North America* **18**, 807–28.

Bilezikian, J.P. (1992). Drug therapy: management of acute hypercalcaemia. *New England Journal of Medicine* **326**, 1196–203.

Buck, A.C. And Lote, C.J. (1990). The renal handling of calcium. In *Renal tract stone; metabolic basis and clinical practice*, (ed. J.E.A. Wickham and A.C. Buck), Ch. 12. Churchill Livingstone, Edinburgh.

Harinck, H.I.J., *et al.* (1987). Role of bone and kidney in tumour-induced hypercalcaemia and its treatment with biphosphonates and sodium chloride. *American Journal of Medicine* **82**, 1133–42.

Hosking, D.J., Cowley, A., and Bucknall, C.A. (1981). Rehydration in the treatment of severe hypercalcaemia. *Quarterly Journal of Medicine* **50**, 473–81.

Singer, F.R., *et al.* (1991). Treatment of hypercalcaemia of malignancy with intravenous etidronate: a controlled multicenter study. *Archives of Internal Medicine* **151**, 471–6.

20.9.4 Balkan (endemic) nephropathy and irradiation nephritis

A. W. ASSCHER

Balkan nephropathy

DESCRIPTION

Balkan nephropathy is a form of chronic interstitial renal disease, which leads to extreme shrinkage of the kidneys due to interstitial fibrosis and causes progressive renal impairment. It is endemic in the adult populations of villages in parts of Romania, Bulgaria, Bosnia, Croatia, and

Serbia. The affected areas are all along the tributaries of the River Danube. All of the affected regions are within a distance of 60 miles of a bend of the river (Fig. 1). The disease occurs amongst the inhabitants of the low-lying plains that are subjected to frequent flooding, where villagers' water supply comes from shallow wells. It does not occur in hillside villages where the water supply comes from surface water. Local farming communities are affected, and it is not uncommon for several members of the same family to develop the disease. Women are affected somewhat more often than men, and immigrants to the region do not usually develop the disease until about 20 years after arrival. All of these features point to a chronic intoxication as a factor in the pathogenesis of the disease, but the nature of the toxin has yet to be determined with certainty. A genetic factor in the pathogenesis is suggested by the familial occurrence of the disease.

Clinical features

The disease presents with symptoms and signs of progressive kidney failure. The only distinguishing features from other causes of end-stage kidney failure are the coppery-yellow pigmentation of palms and soles, the marked β_2-microglobulinuria, and the increase (up to 200-fold) in the development of renal pelvic and ureteral tumours. These urothelial tumours may precede or follow the development of the nephropathy, or they may occur in isolation in the relatives of patients with Balkan nephropathy. It is noteworthy that hypertension, oedema, cardiovascular disease, and retinopathy are unusual.

Aetiology

The disease was first thought to be due to chronic poisoning with trace-metal contaminants in the water supply. Lead, cadmium, and uranium were thought to be likely candidates, but chemical analysis of post-mortem material failed to confirm this. Viral particles have been detected in the tubular epithelium of renal biopsy specimens, but their signifi-

cance is uncertain. Genetic factors in the pathogenesis of the disease are suggested by familial aggregation, correlation with particular blood groups and HLA types, and chromosomal abnormalities found in affected subjects and their families. A possible environmental cause of the disease is chronic exposure to fungal toxins. The main support for this view comes from the resemblance of the human disease to the ochratoxin A- and citrinin-induced nephropathy in pigs. The fungal origin of the nephrotoxin fits the year-to-year fluctuations in the mortality from the disease, which correlates with the previous autumnal rainfall. When rainfall is great, harvested grain is stored in moist conditions in the lofts of the local farmhouses, and growth of various fungi on the grain is thus promoted. In particular, *Penicillium* species (for example, *Pencillium verrucosum* var. *cyclopium*) are known to produce ochratoxins and are found in abundance growing on the stored maize, which is subsequently consumed in the locality. Since its first description, the disease has not shown any change in its incidence (3 per 1000 inhabitants of the endemic areas per year) but a tendency for the older inhabitants in the endemic regions to be affected has emerged in recent years.

Diagnosis and treatment

The diagnosis of this condition depends on a history of long-term residence and employment in the farming industry of the endemic areas. The urinary sediment is usually normal and the finding of haematuria should always suggest the development of urothelial neoplasia. Screening for β_2-microglobulinuria in endemic areas enables presymptomatic diagnosis of the disease, and a timely move from the endemic area may prevent progression of the disease. In the later stages of the disease, the symptoms and signs are those of end-stage kidney failure together with the tell-tale yellow pigmentation of palms of the hands and soles of the feet, and bilateral small, shrunken kidneys. Clinical evidence of the disease usually manifests between the ages of 40 and 50, and before the days of renal replacement therapy survival after the onset of symptoms was of the order of 2 to 3 years. Treatment by dialysis and/or trans-

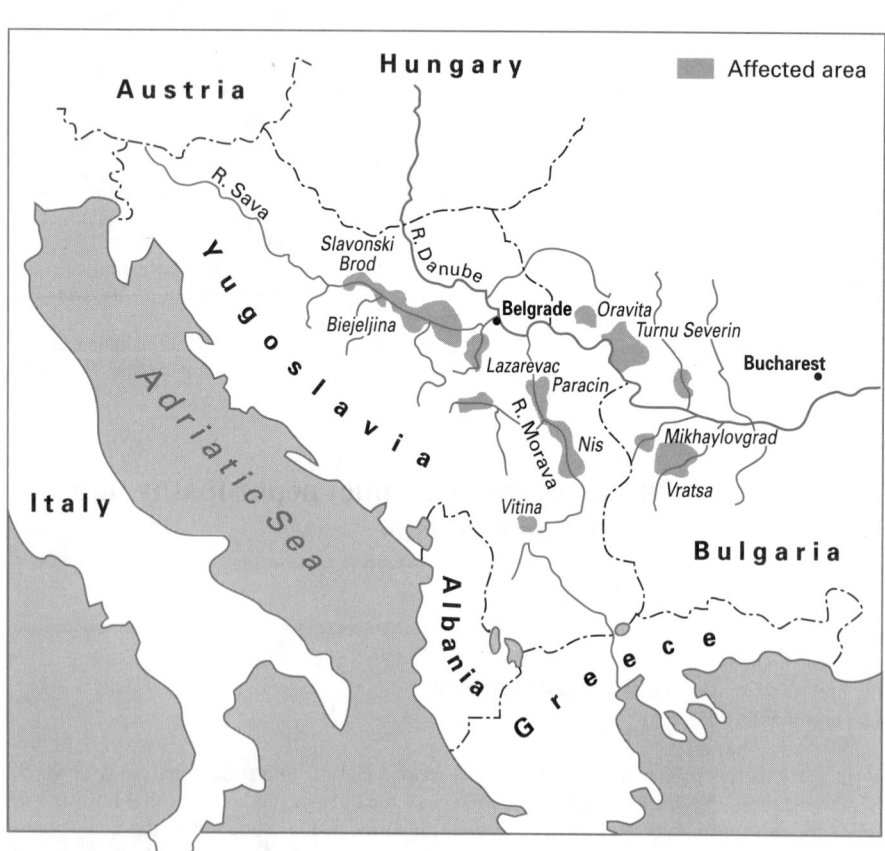

Fig. 1 Areas (shaded) along the bend of the River Danube with a high prevalence of Balkan nephropathy.

plantation is now effective in prolonging life, with the result that the neoplastic transformation of urothelium is becoming a more important cause of mortality. This may require both local treatment or more radical surgery. Recurrence of the nephropathy in transplanted kidneys has not been reported.

REFERENCES

Austwick, P.K.C., (1979). Endemic (Balkan) nephropathy. In *Renal Disease*, (4th edn.), (ed. Sir Douglas Black and N.F. Jones), pp. 879–83. Blackwell Scientific, Oxford.

Plestina, R., *et al.* (1990). Human exposure to ochratoxin A in areas of Yugoslavia with endemic nephropathy. *Journal of Environmental Pathology Toxicology and Oncology* **10**, 145–148.

Radovanovic, Z., Krajinovic, S., Petkovic, S., and Hall, P.W. (1981). Papillary transitional cell tumours, Balkan nephropathy and β-2-microglobulin. *Lancet*, **ii**, 689 (letter).

Stefanovic, V. and Polenakovic, M.H. (1991) Balkan nephropathy. Kidney disease beyond the Balkans? *American Journal of Nephrology* **11**, 1–11.

Irradiation nephritis

Damage to the kidney from inadvertent or unavoidable irradiation is now uncommon. The recognition of the damaging effects of ionizing radiations on the kidney, together with the introduction of more advanced radiotherapeutic techniques, have enabled shielding and/or exclusion of the kidney(s) from the irradiation field, with the result that the disease is now mostly of historical interest. Occasional reports of irradiation damage to kidneys continue to appear, in particular in patients undergoing total body irradiation in preparation for bone marrow transplantation.

Soon after the discovery of X-rays in 1895 there were several reports of experimental irradiation damage to the kidneys, but it was not until 1927 that Hartman, Bolliger, and Doub documented two cases of renal damage and hypertension following abdominal irradiation in man. An enquiry amongst 150 radiotherapists and 350 pathologists uncovered a further 16 similar cases. The largest and best-documented collection of cases was that of Luxton, originally reported in 1953 and subsequently followed up in 1961. From his studies five clinical patterns of the disease were defined (see Table 1).

Clinical features

ACUTE RADIATION NEPHRITIS

This condition develops some 6 to 12 months after irradiation of the renal areas with a dose of not less than 20 Gy, delivered over a period of 6 weeks. It manifests with symptoms of an acute nephritic illness, namely mild oedema, hypertension, and proteinuria with granular casts in the urine. Blood chemistry shows a rise of blood urea and a normochromic, normocytic anaemia. The hypertension is of the malignant variety in up to half the cases. Most of the patients with malignant hypertension progress to kidney failure and death within 3 to 12 months, but 25 per cent of them recover spontaneously, only to develop chronic nephritis at a later stage (see below).

CHRONIC RADIATION NEPHRITIS

Chronic radiation nephritis either develops 2 to 5 years after an acute episode of nephritis, or the condition may be discovered as a result of the development of proteinuria, benign hypertension, or symptoms of end-stage kidney failure some 2 to 5 years after exposure to irradiation. In most of the patients the condition slowly progresses to end-stage kidney failure and, in the few patients in whom malignant-phase hypertension develops, the decline to kidney failure is more rapid.

Table 1 *Clinical features of radiation nephritis*

Acute radiation nephritis
Onset 6–12 months after radiotherapy in adults
Shorter latent period in children
Hypertension/anaemia/proteinuria
Chronic radiation nephritis
May follow acute radiation nephritis or occur without prior acute radiation nephritis
Hypertension/anaemia/proteinuria/uraemia
Benign hypertension
Hypertension and variable proteinuria
Late malignant hypertension
Occurs 1–1.5 years after radiotherapy
Responds to nephrectomy of the atrophic kidney where one kidney is contracted
Asymptomatic proteinuria

Pathological findings

Little is known about the pathological findings in patients with acute radiation nephritis. In some, malignant hypertension appears to have occurred in the presence of minimal kidney damage. In others, glomerular endothelial swelling and fibrin deposition as well as basement membrane splitting are observed. In addition, in patients with malignant-phase hypertension, extensive fibrinoid necroses of small vessels, particularly afferent arterioles, are a feature.

In chronic radiation nephritis, the kidneys are shrunken and the renal capsule shows marked fibrosis. Histologically, the predominant feature is that of extensive interstitial fibrosis, tubular atrophy and dilatation, and glomerulosclerosis. Hypertensive vascular lesions usually abound in patients who develop high blood pressure. The prominence of hypertensive vascular lesions has been attributed to a sensitization of the irradiated blood vessels to the effects of raised intravascular pressure.

Treatment

The disease has now been largely eradicated by exclusion and/or shielding of the renal areas in patients in whom abdominal radiotherapy is administered. Where this is not possible, the minimum amount of renal tissue should be irradiated. Control of a rise of blood pressure is an important feature of the conservative management of patients with radiation nephritis, and will postpone the development of end-stage kidney failure. In patients in whom unilateral irradiation has led to shrinkage of one kidney and hypertension, removal of the shrunken kidney may lead to cure of the raised blood pressure. Once end-stage kidney failure has developed, renal replacement therapy must be instituted. In selecting patients for such treatment account must be taken of the prognosis of the underlying conditions for which the initial radiotherapy was given.

REFERENCES

Asscher, A.W., Wilson, C., and Anson, S.G. (1961). Sensitization of blood vessels to hypertensive damage by x-irradiation. *Lancet* **1**, 580–3.

Bergstein, J., Andrioli, S.P., Provisor, A.J., and Yum, M. (1986). Radiation nephritis following total body irradiation and cyclophosphamide in preparation for bone marrow transplantation. *Transplantation* **41**, 63–6.

Hartman, F.W., Bolliger, A., and Doub, H.P. (1926). Experimental nephritis produced by irradiation. *American Journal of Medical Science* **172**, 487–500.

Luxton, R.W. (1953). Radiation nephritis *Quarterly Journal of Medicine* **22**, 215–42.

Luxton, R.W. (1961). Radiation nephritis – a long term study of 54 patients. *Lancet* **2**, 1221.

Wilson, C., Ledingham, J.M., and Cohen, M. (1958). Hypertension following x-irradiation of the kidneys. *Lancet* **1**, 9–16.

20.10 Urinary-tract obstruction

L. R. I. BAKER

Introduction

If the flow of urine is impeded at any point in its course from renal calices to the exterior, urinary-tract obstruction is present. The terms 'obstructive uropathy', 'obstructive nephropathy', and 'hydronephrosis' are frequently used interchangeably and taken to have the same meaning as the term 'urinary-tract obstruction'. A more rigorous approach is preferable: 'obstructive uropathy' should be taken to mean pathological change occurring in the urinary-tract and kidney consequent upon urinary-tract obstruction. 'Obstructive nephropathy' is present when pathological change in the kidney resulting from urinary-tract obstruction is associated with prolongation of the transit time of glomerular filtrate down the nephron. The term 'hydronephrosis' should be taken to denote dilatation of the renal pelvis and calyceal system.

Intraluminal obstruction between the commencement of the proximal tubule and the distal end of the collecting duct, such as occurs in uric acid nephropathy, as a result of sulphonamide crystal deposition, and in multiple myelomatosis, falls outside the definition of urinary-tract obstruction employed here and will not be further considered.

Although dilatation of the outflow system proximal to the site of obstruction is a characteristic finding, widening of the ureter and/or pelvicalyceal system does not necessary indicate the presence of obstruction. Causes of such anatomical abnormality in the absence of obstruction are listed in Table 1.

Obstruction may be partial or complete, unilateral or bilateral. Bilateral obstruction, or obstruction of a single kidney, is a greater threat to the patient than unilateral obstruction. Obstruction associated with infection is a greater threat to kidney function and to life than obstruction in the absence of infection. Since it is common, and often reversible, obstruction of the urinary tract should be considered in every uraemic patient, whether acute or chronic.

Incidence

Urinary-tract obstruction occurs most frequently in the young and the old. Hydronephrosis is the most common cause of an abdominal mass in neonates, and obstruction, usually due to congenital abnormalities, is, also relatively common in children. Its incidence declines after the age of 10 and is at its lowest in middle age, but begins to rise again after age 60, particularly in males, in whom the cause is commonly prostatic enlargement. Although the overall frequency of urinary-tract obstruction is the same in both sexes, between 20 and 60 years of age it is more frequent in women, and over the age of 60 years the reverse is true.

Causes

Obstructing lesions may lie within the lumen or the wall of the urinary tract, or may cause obstruction by pressure from outside. The major causes in each group are listed in Table 2.

Calculi and neuromuscular dysfunction at the junction of renal pelvis and ureter are common causes of unilateral obstruction. Prostatic

Illustrations in this chapter have been reproduced from Baker, L.R.I and Whitfield H.N. (1992). The patient with urinary tract obstruction, *Oxford Textbook of Clinical Nephrology* (eds. S. Cameron, A.M. Davison, J.-P. Grünfeld, D. Kerr, and E. Ritz). pp. 2002–22. University Press, Oxford, with permission.

Table 1 *Causes of non-obstructive collecting system dilatation*

Anatomical variants
    Large major calyx
    Extrarenal pelvis
    Distensible system after relief of obstruction
    Pregnancy

Congenital anomalies
    Megacalyces

Vesicoureteric reflux
    Children
    Abnormality of ureteric insertion into bladder
    Adults
    Neuropathic bladder, after ileal loop diversion, following vesicoureteric surgery, after renal transplantation

Calyceal pathology
    Tuberculosis
    Caliceal cyst
    Papillary necrosis

obstruction, stone disease, and bladder tumours account for approximately 75 per cent of cases of bilateral obstruction in developed countries. Wide geographical variations occur in the relative incidence of some causes of obstruction, for example, schistosomiasis.

Urinary-tract obstruction has been found in 3.8 per cent of a large series of routine autopsies and 25 per cent of autopsies carried out upon uraemic patients. To the clinician, the most important questions are whether urinary-tract obstruction affects the upper or lower urinary tract, and whether it is of recent onset (acute obstruction) or is long-standing (chronic obstruction).

Pathophysiology

ACUTE UPPER-TRACT OBSTRUCTION

Urine flows from kidney to bladder as a result of ureteric and pelvic peristalsis, the effects of gravity, and the pressure of glomerular filtration. Peristalsis normally generates high pressures within the ureteric lumen, sufficient to propel urine down the ureter without the transmission of the increased pressure to the renal parenchyma. Initially, an upward movement occurs in the ureter: thereafter, proximal contraction of ureteric circular muscle, with eventual complete occlusion of the lumen, forms a bolus of urine. Contraction of longitudinal smooth muscle then propels the bolus along the ureter. Base-line ureteric pressure is similar to that in the renal pelvis, but during this process rises to values between 10 and 25 mmHg. These pressures are not transmitted to the renal pelvis, where pressure seldom rises above 4 mmHg.

In the normal dog, pressure within the ureter more than doubles when the ureteric lumen is occluded during peristalsis; similar changes occur in ureteric wall tension. Three minutes after acute ureteric obstruction, base-line and peak pressure and wall tensions are about twice as high as control values. Between 5 and 20 min after induction of obstruction, base-line pressure and wall tensions rise further and approximate to peak values. At 1 h there is a threefold increase in base-line and peak pressures and wall tensions compared with control values; base-line and peak values for pressure and tension do not then differ. At this point,

Table 2 *Some causes of urinary tract obstruction*

Within the lumen	Within the wall	Pressure from outside
Calculus	Pelviureteric neuromuscular dysfunction (congenital, 10 per cent bilateral)	Pelviureteric compression (bands, aberrant vessels)
Blood clot	Ureteric stricture (tuberculosis, especially after treatment; calculous; following surgery)	Tumours, e.g. retroperitoneal growths or glands, carcinoma of colon, diverticulitis, aortic aneurysm
Sloughed papilla (diabetes, analgesic abuse, sickle-cell disease)	Ureterovesical stricture (congenital, ureterocele, calculus, schistosomiasis)	Retroperitoneal fibrosis (peri-aortitis)
Tumour of renal pelvis or ureter	Congenital megaureter	Accidental ligation of ureter
Bladder tumour	Congenital bladder neck obstruction	Pancreatitis
	Neurogenic bladder	Retrocaval ureter (right-sided obstruction)
	Urethral stricture (calculous, gonococcal, after instrumentation)	Crohn's disease
	Congenital urethral valve	Chronic granulomatous disease
	Pin-hole meatus	Prostatic obstruction
		Tumours in pelvis, e.g. carcinoma of cervix
		Phimosis

occlusion of the ureter fails to occur and pressures generated by ureteric wall tension are transmitted to the renal pelvis and parenchyma. Any further increase in pressure results in dilatation of the ureter.

The effect of an increase in pressure within the ureter transmitted to the nephron depends upon the degree of obstruction (whether complete or incomplete), whether obstruction is unilateral or bilateral, and the duration of obstruction.

In the rat, pressure within the renal tubule shortly after occlusion of the ureter depends upon the state of hydration of the animal. In the hydropenic rat, intratubular pressure does not rise after occlusion of the ureter; if a solute diuresis is induced or if saline is administered intravenously, intratubular pressure rises, eventually approximating to glomerular filtration pressure. Intratubular pressure then declines progressively over the next 24 h. Whether pressures remain elevated thereafter depends upon the volume state of the animal and whether obstruction is bilateral or unilateral. Unilateral obstruction has a less marked effect upon intratubular pressure than does bilateral ureteric obstruction. In the former, intratubular pressure approximates to normal 24 h after induction of ureteric obstruction, but if obstruction is bilateral, intratubular pressures remain high at this time.

Any change in blood flow or glomerular filtration rate resulting from ureteric obstruction would have important effects on tubular pressures and flows. In man time of onset of obstruction is seldom known with any precision, and methods of measurement of renal blood flow or filtration rate using clearance techniques are indirect and depend upon tubular function, which is itself affected by urinary-tract obstruction, so that concepts must depend on animal experiments. In the dog, renal blood flow falls to 50 per cent of control values 3 or 4 days after induction of complete ureteric obstruction. At 4 weeks, blood flow is about one-third that to the contralateral unobstructed kidney. These phases are discernible in the relationship between changes in ureteral pressure and renal blood flow with time (Fig. 1). Phase I occurs during the first hour after induction of obstruction. Renal blood flow increases, presumably owing to a reduction in intrarenal vascular resistance, associated with a gradual increase in ureteric pressure. In phase II, which takes place over the next 2 to 5 h, ureteric pressure continues to rise and renal blood flow begins to fall. Thereafter, in phase III, renal blood flow continues to fall and ureteric pressure returns towards or to normal.

These changes are not completely understood. The rise in renal blood flow in phase I may be a direct effect of the increased ureteric pressure on inner medullary blood flow, which is known to decrease after induction of ureteric obstruction. A number of vasoactive hormones are produced in the renal medulla and an alteration in intrarenal hormone regulation may produce an abrupt change in overall vascular resistance, with resultant increased perfusion. The changes occurring in phase II

are thought to result from the direct effect of increased ureteric pressure on the renal interstitium, whereas in phase III, an increase in vascular resistance at the preglomerular level is thought to occur.

CHRONIC UPPER-TRACT OBSTRUCTION

Three months after production of experimental obstruction in dogs, base-line ureteric wall tension is increased and there is no difference between base-line and peak values of wall tension, the latter being measured during ureteric occlusion. By contrast, base-line and peak pressures within the ureteric lumen are not significantly different from control values. This is a consequence of the relationship between pressure and wall tension expressed in Laplace's law, which states that $P = K(T/$

Fig. 1 The relationship between ipsilateral renal blood flow and ureteric pressure during experimental ureteric occlusion in the dog. In phase I, renal blood flow and ureteric pressure rise. In phase II, blood flow declines while ureteric pressure continues to rise. In phase III, both renal blood flow and ureteric pressure decline. The arrow indicates the time of ureteric occlusion. Mean ± standard error; $n = 5$. (Reprinted with permission from Moody *et al.* 1975.)

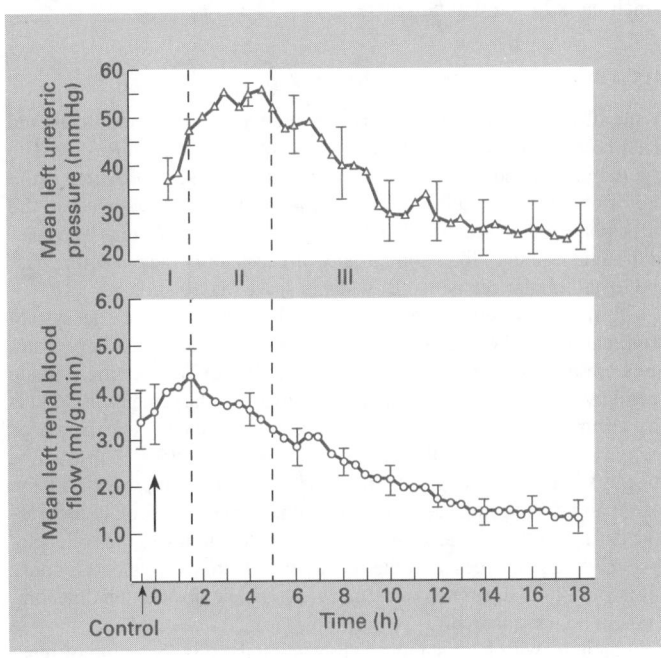

R), where *P* is the transluminal pressure, *K* is a constant, *T* is wall tension, and *R* is the radius of the ureter. In chronic obstruction, therefore, normal intraluminal pressures are maintained as a consequence of ureteric dilatation.

These experimental findings suggest that the major component of damage to the kidney due to obstruction occurs soon after its onset. Certainly, in man, the highest measured ureteric pressures have been found during acute obstruction (as high as 50 mmHg during passage of a stone) and there appears to be an inverse relationship between pressure within the renal pelvis measured in patients with complete obstruction and time. The notion that chronic obstruction with dilatation of the ureter may be relatively benign is supported by the observation that patients with incomplete urinary-tract obstruction due to congenital anomalies lose renal function only slowly.

ACUTE LOWER-TRACT OBSTRUCTION

The mechanical efficiency of smooth muscle fibres is reduced when they become overstretched,. As bladder outflow obstruction increases, a point is reached when acute urinary retention will result. Factors which may precipitate acute retention include a sudden diuresis, such as occurs after diuretic therapy (particularly loop agents) for heart failure, urinary infection, and drugs which have pharmacological effects upon the bladder, provoking retention, such as those with antimuscarinic and calcium-channel-blocking activity.

CHRONIC LOWER-TRACT OBSTRUCTION

In adults chronic outflow obstruction to the bladder is most commonly due to benign prostatic hypertrophy. Prostatic malignancy and urethral strictures may also be responsible. In children, posterior urethral valves and urethral strictures are most often the cause. Such organic causes are easy to understand, but functional obstruction may occur at the bladder neck and at the level of the distal sphincter owing to a failure of co-ordination between bladder contraction and sphincter relaxation. The bladder wall may become increasingly compliant or the opposite may occur: this is of significance to the urologist, since patients with poorly compliant bladders fare much better after removal of the obstruction than those with highly compliant bladders. The highly compliant bladder tends not to be associated with upper-tract dilatation, whereas the high pressure that exists within a bladder of low compliance may be transmitted to the upper tracts and may be the cause of renal impairment, which on occasion will be severe.

HISTOPATHOLOGICAL CHANGES

Acute obstruction results in increased ureteric pressure and decreased renal blood flow, and may be complicated by bacterial infection. The rise in intraluminal pressure and dilatation of the system proximal to the site of obstruction result in compression of the renal substance. In the early phase of obstruction the kidney becomes oedematous and haemorrhagic. Tubular dilatation initially affects mainly the collecting duct and distal tubular segments. Bowman's space may be dilated.

The ducts of Bellini are first affected by dilatation of the system proximal to the site of obstruction. Subsequently, other papillary structures are affected, and ultimately compression of renal cortical tissue occurs with thinning of the renal parenchyma. Enlargement of the kidney occurs in association with dilatation of the renal pelvis. Atrophy of the renal parenchyma with reduction in size of the kidney (obstructive atrophy) is believed to result from the effects of compression of the renal parenchyma and from prolonged renal ischaemia. Slowly progressive partial obstruction tends to result in gross dilatation of the collecting system, dilated calyces, and the renal pelvis being surrounded by only a thin rim of renal parenchyma. In acute complete obstruction dilatation tends to be less marked.

In patients with long-standing obstruction there is flattening of renal

tubular epithelium, periglomerular fibrosis, interstitial fibrosis, and mononuclear cell infiltration. These changes are thought to result in part from renal ischaemia and, in part, to reflect the effects of bacterial infection (Fig. 2).

EFFECTS OF OBSTRUCTION UPON RENAL FUNCTION

Little precise information is available about the effects of urinary-tract obstruction on glomerular filtration rate in man for reasons given earlier in relation to knowledge about ureteric pressures after the occurrence of obstruction in humans. It is clear, however, that ureteric obstruction results in a marked fall in glomerular filtration rate, and that bilateral incomplete obstruction causes progressive renal failure to develop. Glomerular filtration must continue to some extent even after development of complete acute obstruction since a nephrogram (albeit a delayed one) can be obtained after injection of intravenous contrast medium during urography.

The most common abnormalities in chronic partial ureteric obstruction are disturbances in renal function. As would be expected from the histopathological findings, distal tubular function is more strikingly disturbed than is that of the proximal tubule.

A characteristic feature of patients with chronic partial ureteric obstruction is an impaired ability to concentrate urine. The concentration defect is resistant to administration of antidiuretic hormone and is thus an example of nephrogenic diabetes insipidus. Such patients may present with polyuria, dehydration, and hypernatraemia secondary to a reduction in free water reabsorption. Animal experiments indicate that production of cAMP in response to vasopressin is reduced in chronic partial obstruction and this may, in part, explain the concentration defect. The extent to which the need to excrete an increased solute load in bilateral ureteric obstruction contributes to the concentration defect is unclear. Chronic partial bilateral obstruction in humans may be associated with a salt-losing state, although the frequency with which this occurs has not been defined.

Fig. 2 Histological appearances in long-standing obstruction. Note dilated tubules, interstitial fibrosis, vessel wall thickening, and global sclerosis of some glomeruli.

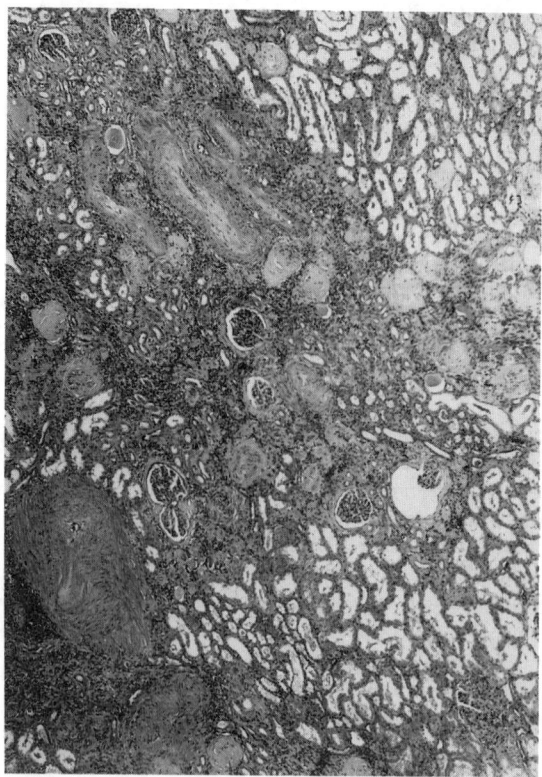

Most animal experiments which have examined the effects of ureteric obstruction upon renal tubular function have been performed after acute obstruction has been induced. In dogs, acute unilateral ureteric obstruction reduces urine flow and both absolute and fractional sodium and water reabsorption. Similar results have been obtained in the rat following 30 h of acute incomplete obstruction. More chronic ureteric obstruction in the dog also reduces the capacity to reabsorb sodium and water.

Since ureteric obstruction affects distal segments of the nephron more than proximal segments, an acidification defect is associated with chronic partial ureteric obstruction in man. In many patients with obstructive nephropathy, urinary pH is inappropriately high for any associated degree of metabolic acidosis. This distal renal tubular acidosis is present in both unilateral and bilateral ureteric obstruction, and may be associated with hyperkalaemia.

RENAL FUNCTION AFTER RELIEF OF OBSTRUCTION

In man the relationship between duration of obstruction and the extent of recovery of renal function after its reversal is unknown, and surprisingly few data have been published. Such studies as do exist indicate that renal blood flow increases after relief of obstruction, and glomerular filtration rate either remains the same or increases, but no large study has been performed in man in which duration of obstruction has been correlated with degree of recovery of glomerular filtration rate. There is no reason to doubt that the extent of recovery depends upon whether obstruction is partial or complete, the duration of obstruction, and whether or not obstruction is complicated by bacterial infection.

The relationship between duration of obstruction and recovery of function has been more clearly defined in experimental animals. Unilateral ureteric ligation has been performed in dogs. Glomerular filtration rate was measured before ligation and the glomerular filtration rate of each kidney was assumed to be 50 per cent of overall glomerular filtration rate. When the ligature was removed after 1 week of complete obstruction, the ipsilateral glomerular filtration rate was found to be 25 per cent of the ipsilateral control value and 16 per cent of that of the contralateral kidney measured at the same time. This discrepancy resulted from a compensatory increase in function of the non-obstructed kidney during the week of complete obstruction of its partner. Improvement in glomerular filtration rate of the previously obstructed kidney continued up to, but not beyond, 2 months after release of obstruction, but complete recovery never occurred, maximum improvement being only to 50 per cent of the glomerular filtration rate of the non-operated kidney.

HORMONAL CHANGES INDUCED BY OBSTRUCTION

Erythropoietin

Information regarding changes, if any, in serum erythropoietin in experimental acute and chronic obstruction is not available at present. Levels of erythropoietin are low in humans with renal failure due to obstructive uropathy, but neither the degree of anaemia nor the degree of depression of erythropoietin concentration is known to differ from that occurring in chronic renal failure of similar severity and different aetiology.

Erythraemia is a recognized association of chronic upper urinary-tract obstruction and correction after relief of obstruction has been recorded. Erythropoietin concentrations in such patients have rarely been documented.

Vitamin D metabolism

Anatomical considerations suggest that renal 1α-hydroxylase activity might be particularly severely affected in chronic obstruction. However, scant data are available in respect of vitamin D metabolite levels and vitamin D metabolism in renal failure associated with obstruction, compared with renal failure of similar degree but of different aetiologies.

An impression exists that osteomalacia may be more common in patients with chronic renal failure due to obstruction, but the fact that such renal failure is very slowly progressive may account for this. Among patients about to start dialysis, radiological evidence of hyperparathyroid bone disease is most common in those whose renal failure is a consequence of obstruction, even when a correction is applied for duration of renal failure and gender.

Hypertension and the renin-angiotensin system

Hypertension is more common in patients with bilateral urinary tract obstruction than in normal individuals matched for age and sex. The prevalence of hypertension resulting from unilateral obstruction is unknown.

An increase in total exchangeable sodium has been demonstrated in chronic bilateral upper-tract obstruction, and blood pressure frequently returns to normal with correction of obstruction. Patients of this sort appear to have a volume-dependent form of hypertension consequent upon salt and water retention. Concentrations of renin in renal and peripheral veins are normal.

Patients with chronic unilateral ureteric obstruction and hypertension have been described in whom renal vein renin concentrations were elevated on the side of obstruction and in whom both blood pressure and renal vein renin concentration returned to normal after relief of obstruction, but there are no clinical features or preoperative investigations which will predict outcome.

Atrial natriuretic peptide

Atrial natriuretic peptide release is augmented in patients with bilateral ureteric obstruction and uraemia, probably owing to salt and water overload, and this may contribute to the postobstructive diuresis and natriuresis which occurs after surgical correction of the problem.

Clinical features

ACUTE UPPER-TRACT OBSTRUCTION

Typically, this gives rise to pain in the flank which may radiate to the iliac fossa, inguinal region, testis, or labium. The pain may be dull or sharp, intermittent or persistent, though waxing and waning in intensity. It may be provoked by a high fluid intake, alcohol, or diuretics, measures which increase urinary volume and distend the collecting system: this is particularly noticeable when obstruction occurs at the pelviureteric junction. Loin tenderness may be detected and an enlarged kidney felt. Upper urinary-tract infection with malaise, fever, and symptoms and signs of septicaemia may dominate the clinical picture.

Complete anuria is strongly suggestive of complete bilateral obstruction or complete obstruction of a single kidney. The differential diagnosis includes bilateral total renal cortical necrosis, acute anuric glomerulonephritis, and bilateral renal arterial occlusion. Intermittent anuria indicates the presence of intermittent complete obstruction.

CHRONIC UPPER-TRACT OBSTRUCTION

Patients may present with flank or abdominal pain, renal failure, or both; the symptoms and signs of urinary-tract infection and septicaemia may be superimposed. Rarely, presentation is with erythraemia or hypertension and their complications. A proportion of patients are asymptomatic, obstruction being found during investigation of some other condition.

Polyuria often occurs in chronic partial obstruction owing to impairment of renal tubular concentrating capacity. Intermittent anuria and polyuria indicate intermittent complete and partial obstruction.

ACUTE LOWER-TRACT OBSTRUCTION

Acute urinary retention is often preceded by a history of symptoms of bladder outflow obstruction. Acute retention is typically associated with severe suprapubic pain, but this may be absent if acute retention is superimposed on chronic retention or if there is an underlying neuropathy.

A potential clinical pitfall is failure to recognize that patients who have had an epidural anaesthetic may develop painless acute retention of urine. Most modalities of bladder sensation are mediated via sacral parasympathetic nerves. The pain from bladder overdistension is sympathetically mediated and will be abolished by a high epidural reaching to D10. Obstetricians need to be particularly alert to this problem.

Pre-existing obstruction may have provoked changes in the bladder, such as muscle wall hypertrophy, sacculation, and diverticulum formation; these in turn predispose to persistence of lower urinary-tract infection once acquired and occasionally to bladder stones. Epididymo-orchitis may occur.

CHRONIC LOWER-TRACT OBSTRUCTION

Symptoms may be minimal or may be accepted by the patient as within normal limits. Hesitancy, narrowing, and diminished force of the urinary stream, terminal dribbling, and a sense of incomplete bladder emptying are typical features. If a large volume of residual urine remains in the bladder after urination, the frequency passage of small volumes of urine may be a prominent symptom even in the absence of infection. Incontinence of such small volumes of urine is termed overflow incontinence or retention with overflow.

There are no pathognomonic clinical features which differentiate high-pressure and low-pressure chronic retention. In each, if the residual urine volume is sufficient, the bladder may be palpably distended. The size and consistency of the prostate is variable.

Acute complete retention of urine, usually with severe suprapubic and perineal pain, may occur. In acute or chronic retention, the enlarged bladder can be felt or percussed after an attempt at voiding.

Lower urinary-tract infection occurs commonly in association with bladder outflow obstruction and may precipitate acute retention. Frequency, urgency, urge incontinence, dysuria, strangury, suprapubic pain, haematuria, and cloudy, smelly urine may be present. Asymptomatic bacteriuria is common.

Examination of the abdomen, genitalia, and rectal and vaginal examination are essential. It should be noted that the apparent size of the prostate is a poor guide to the presence of prostatic obstruction. Median-lobe enlargement of a palpably normal prostate may give rise to severe obstruction, whereas an apparently grossly enlarged gland may cause little or no obstruction.

Investigation

ACUTE UPPER-TRACT OBSTRUCTION

The investigation of acute obstruction must allow the site and cause to be identified rapidly, accurately, safely, and as economically as possible.

Intravenous urography

Emergency intravenous urography is the preferred method of investigating the patient with suspected acute upper-tract obstruction. It will confirm the diagnosis and will usually demonstrate the site, cause, and degree of obstruction, providing invaluable guidance for management. Ultrasonography, although demonstrating dilatation, cannot visualize the ureters adequately and may miss the site and cause of obstruction.

The initial sequence of radiographs must include full-length and coned renal plain films. The plain film must be examined carefully for opaque calculi along the line of the ureter—calculi overlying bone are easily missed (Figs 3, 4). Some obstructing calculi are very small and only faintly calcified or non-opaque. Ureteric calculi within the bony pelvis are often impossible to distinguish from calcified phleboliths on the plain film.

A large dose of contrast, preferably of low osmolality, should be given to compensate for the lack of preparation of the patient and the probability of a low glomerular filtration rate. After contrast injection, the recently obstructed kidney is typically enlarged and smooth in outline. The nephrogram is delayed owing to a reduction in glomerular filtration

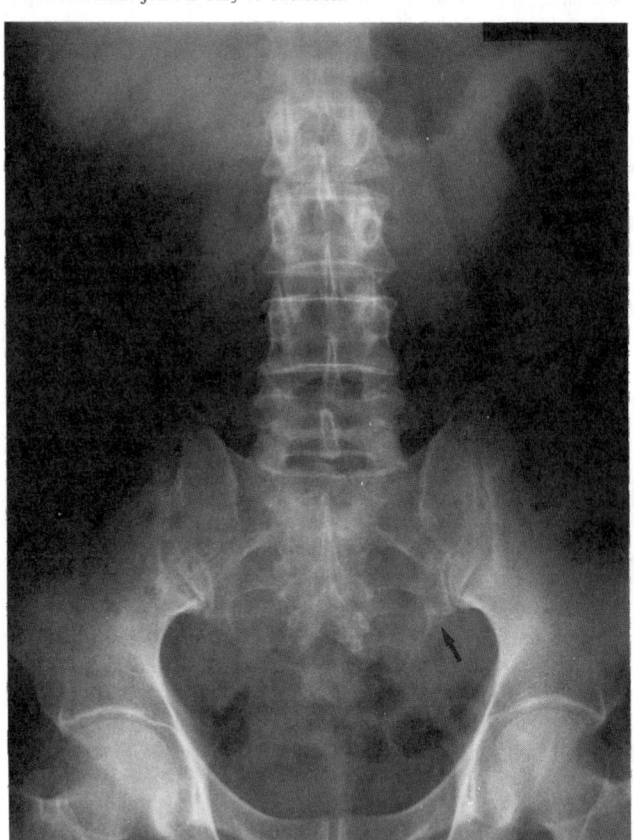

Fig. 3 Plain abdominal radiograph. Opaque calculus (arrowed) medial to left lower sacroiliac joint is easy to overlook.

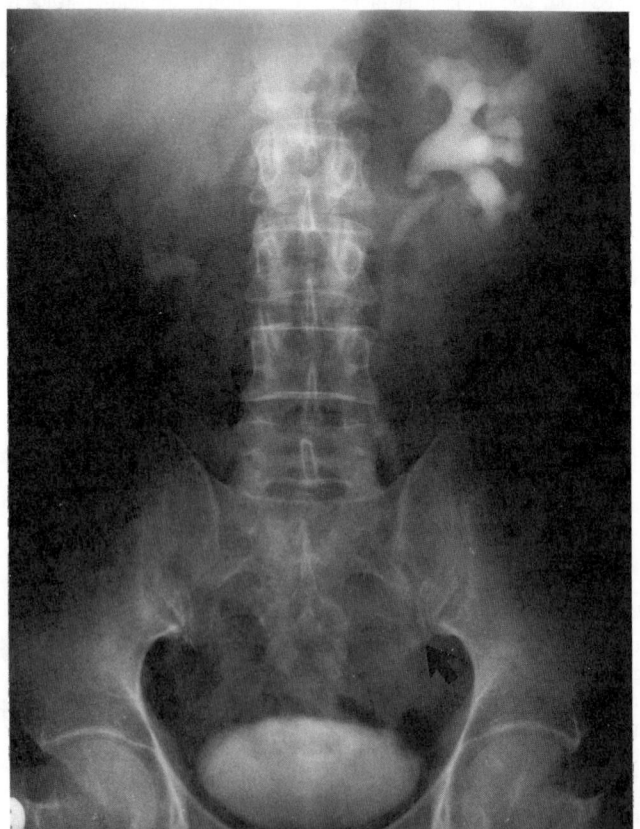

Fig. 4 Same patient as in Fig. 3, after-contrast radiograph. Note dilatation of collecting system and ureter to the level of the calculus.

rate and the calyces and pelvis fill with contrast later than normal. The nephrogram eventually becomes more dense than normal owing to the prolonged nephron transit time, which allows greater than normal concentration of contrast medium within the tubules. In time, the site of obstruction may become obvious owing to dilatation of the system to the level of the block (Figs 5, 6). A full-length film should be taken 20 min after contrast injection and after the patient has been asked to empty the bladder, since contrast in a full bladder may obscure the lower end

of the ureter and make it impossible to confirm that a ureter is dilated down to an opacity seen in the line of the ureter in the bony pelvis.

Since contrast medium enters the pelvicalyceal system and ureter slowly, opacification of the system and ureter may never be seen in severe acute obstruction. In most instances, filling of the pelvicalyceal system and ureter to the level of obstruction can be demonstrated on delayed films (Figs 7, 8). In acute ureteric obstruction the pelvicalyceal system and ureter may be only slightly dilated. Occasionally the only abnormality may be a ureter which remains full throughout its length to the level of the vesicoureteric junction, with this finding persisting on the full-length postmicturition film. Acute obstruction is characterized by increased excretion of contrast medium by the liver, leading to gall-bladder opacification on delayed films.

When typical obstructive changes are present, with a ureter dilated down to a calcified opacity, diagnosis is simple. If there is an obstructed nephrogram or dilatation of the pelvicalyceal system and/or ureter but no radiodense calculus is seen, diagnosis is more difficult. If the history is of recent-onset pain, the likely diagnostic possibilities are: recent passage of an opaque stone; uric acid stone; acute pelviureteric junction obstruction; blood clot; or sloughed papilla.

The presence of a uric acid stone may be suggested by a previous history of such stones, a personal or family history of gout, or clinical circumstances associated with uric acid stone formation, such as cytotoxic drug therapy or chronic small bowel disease. Urography shows uric acid stones as lucent filling defects (Fig. 9); similar filling defects may also occur with transitional cell tumours, sloughed papillae, or blood clots. Since most ureteric stones pass spontaneously, investigation of a possible transitional cell tumour or blood clot should be delayed. If a persistent lucency is present, CT scanning may be very helpful (Fig. 10).

Acute idiopathic pelviureteric junction obstruction should be suspected if there is a large, soft-tissue density inferomedial to the kidney

Fig. 5 Acute left ureteric obstruction. Note the increased density of the nephrogram and the absence of pyelogram on the left side 15 min after injection of contrast.

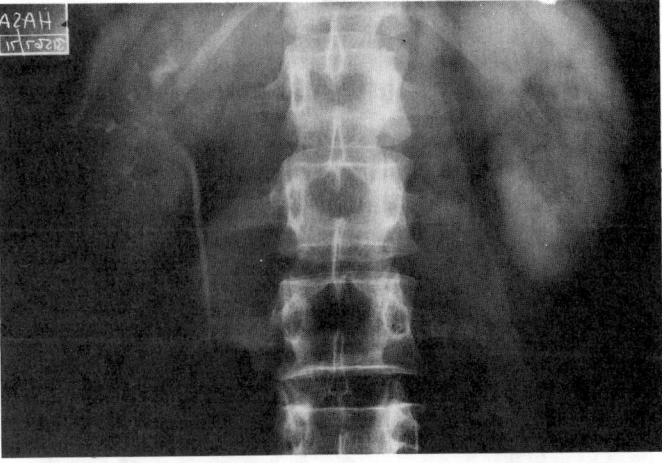

Fig. 6 Same patient as in Fig. 5. A later radiograph, showing a persistent dense nephrogram on the left. The pelivicalyceal system and ureter, which have now filled, are only slightly dilated due to the fact that obstruction is of very recent onset. The obstructing calculus at the left ureteric orifice is not visible.

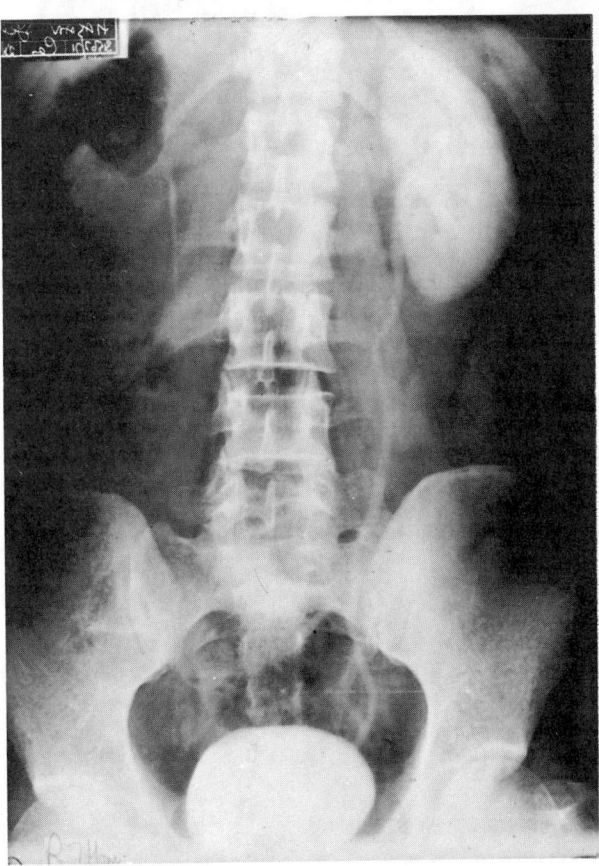

Fig. 7 Obstruction due to opaque calculus at the right vesicoureteric junction (arrowed). A nephrogram but no pyelogram is seen on the right, 10 min after contrast injection.

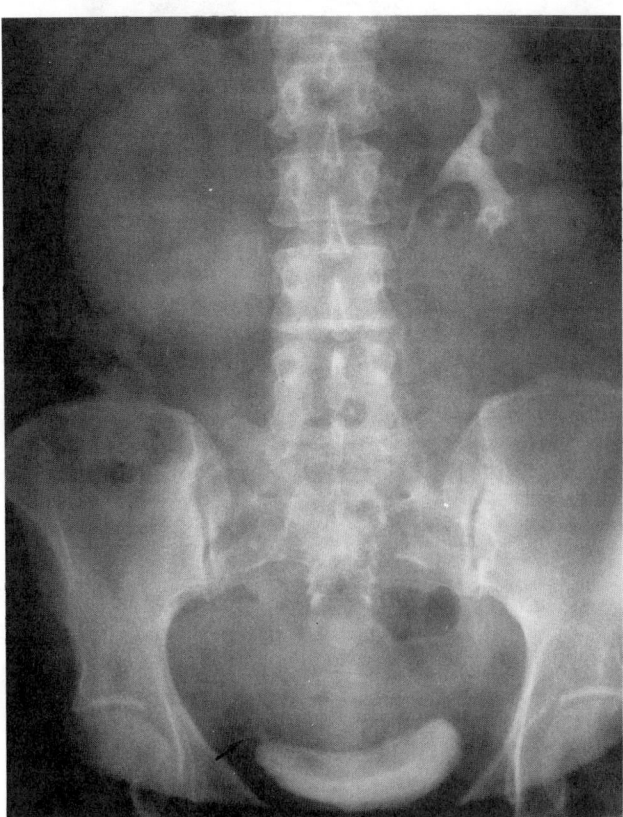

on the plain film produced by the distended pelvis. This usually fills on delayed films of the urogram, with no filling of the ureter.

Clot colic is always associated with macroscopic haematuria. When it is suspected, the urogram should be repeated after 2 weeks, by which time the clot should have lysed and any underlying lucent filling defect can be seen. Such patients require further investigation to define the cause of bleeding.

Sloughed papillae result from papillary necrosis. Typically, abnormal calyces are seen in both kidneys, but papillary necrosis may occasionally be unilateral, usually as a result of a previous episode of infection associated with unilateral obstruction, especially in diabetics. Occasionally, calcified papillae may mimic stones. (Fig. 11).

Ultrasonography

Ultrasound is less useful than urography in acute obstruction of the upper tract. It can define dilatation of the intrarenal collecting system in the upper third of the ureter, but dilatation of the middle and lower thirds of the ureter is not easily detectable ultrasonically, and the dilated ureter cannot usually be followed to the level of obstruction. Since dilatation is not synonymous with obstruction, and since acute obstruction can exist with only minimal dilatation, the value of ultrasonography in acute upper-tract obstruction is limited. The differentiation between collecting system dilatation due to obstruction and, for example, polycystic kidney disease, megacalycosis and non-obstructive hydrocalycosis cannot be made ultrasonically.

Ultrasound may be used to investigate patients with suspected acute urinary obstruction if they are pregnant or have a history of contrast allergy. It also has a role in the investigation of the patient in whom obstructive pyonephrosis is suspected—for example, with severe loin pain and fever plus significant bacteriuria—since the diuretic effect of contrast injection may cause severe pain in such a patient and the damage that has occurred may prevent contrast excretion. The risk of contrast nephrotoxicity in diabetics with moderate to severe renal impairment and in patients with myelomatosis is currently considered a relative contraindication to intravenous urography; ultrasonography therefore has a primary role in the investigation of such patients.

Fig. 8 Same patient as in Fig. 7. Film taken 1 h after contrast injection. Dilatation of the pelvicalyceal system and ureter to the level of the obstructing calculus is now seen. Delayed films may need to be taken as much as 24 or even 48 h after contrast injection to define the situation in some patients.

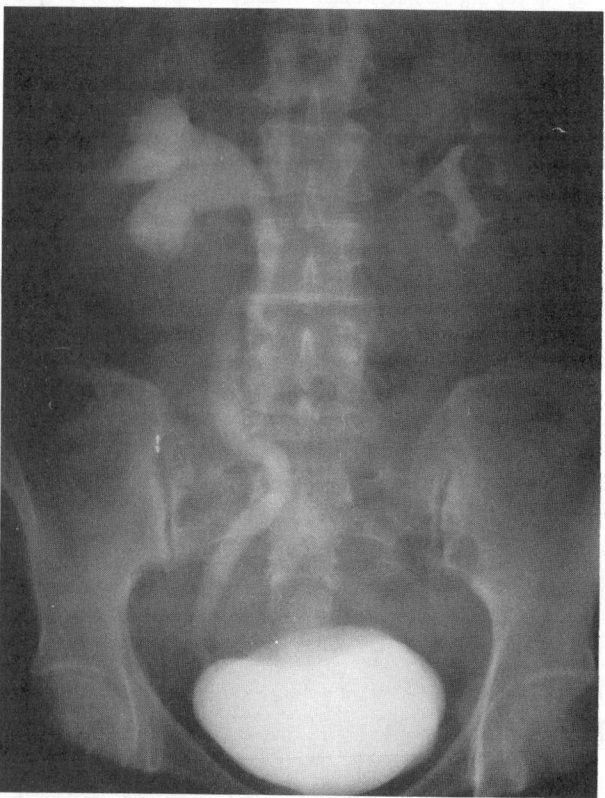

Fig. 10 Same patient as in Fig. 9. CT scan clearly shows uric acid stones as opacities within the collecting system.

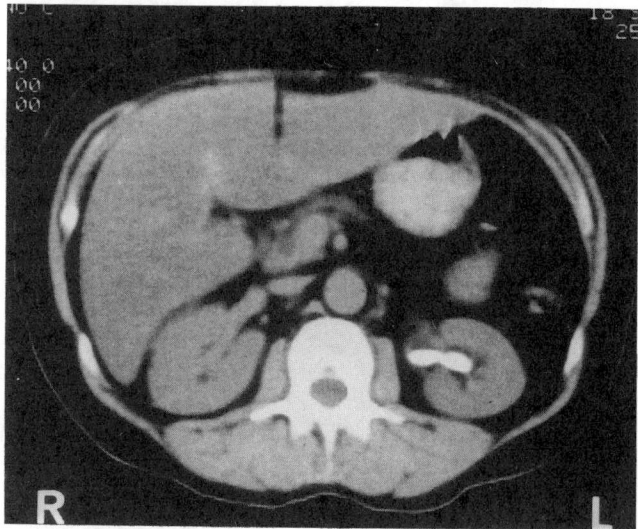

Fig. 9 Uric acid stones seen on intravenous urography as lucent filling defects in the collecting system on the left.

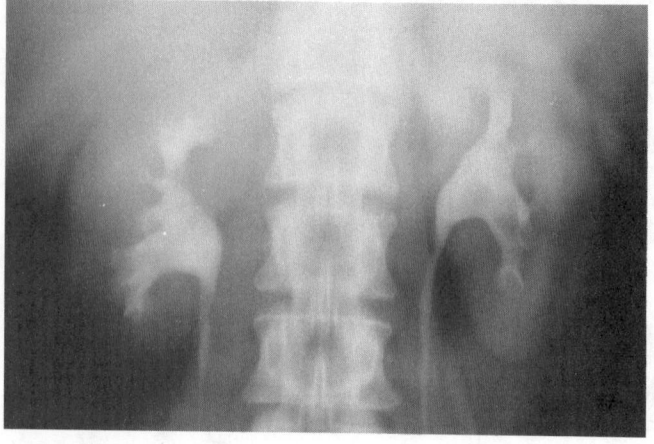

Fig. 11 Bilateral papillary necrosis with papillary calcification mimicking stones.

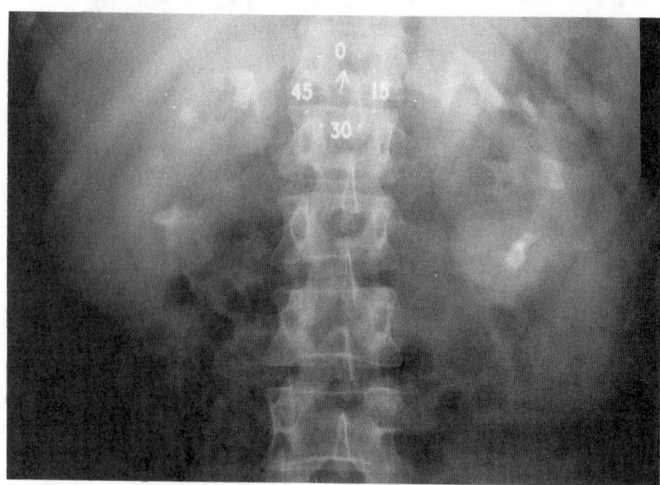

Antegrade and retrograde pyelography and ureterography

If the site of obstruction is not demonstrated by intravenous urography, antegrade or retrograde examination may be helpful. Both techniques can be initiated as a method of diagnosis and then extended to provide a therapeutic role by providing drainage.

CT scanning

Computerized tomography (CT) plays only a very minor role in the diagnosis of acute upper urinary-tract obstruction. The potential exists for demonstrating non-opaque stones, but since the first investigation performed is likely to be an intravenous urogram, the contrast given would probably negate the usefulness of a subsequent emergency CT scan. In any event, only non-opaque stones obstructing at the pelviureteric junction level could be diagnosed with certainty since ureteric stones are not reliably revealed by scanning.

Use of radionuclides

There is no role for the use of radionuclides in the investigation of acute urinary-tract obstruction.

CHRONIC UPPER URINARY-TRACT OBSTRUCTION

Obstruction must be excluded early in all patients with unexplained renal failure. In patients with known renal disease, rapid deterioration in renal function unexplained by the primary renal problem also demands investigation. Relapsing urinary-tract infections should also raise the possibility of an associated obstructing lesion. The diagnosis of partial obstruction should not be discounted simply because urine volume is normal or even increased.

The history should include questions relating to analgesic abuse (associated with papillary necrosis, transitional cell tumours, and periureteric fibrosis) and vitamin D consumption (associated with calculus formation). Ingestion of methysergide and other drugs may be associated with retroperitoneal fibrosis. Any history or family history of gout, diabetes, or renal stone formation should be sought.

The choice of imaging depends upon the mode of presentation. Intravenous urography is the method of choice in patients with loin pain since it best diagnoses the more common causes—calculous obstruction and idiopathic pelviureteric junction obstruction. Initial investigation of the patient with unexplained impairment of renal function should include ultrasonography, together with plain abdominal radiographs and renal tomography to screen for urinary-tract calculi. Tomography may be necessary to detect low-density calculi. Small unobstructed kidneys will be demonstrated in about 50 per cent of patients (Fig. 12) and other means of detecting upper-tract dilatation will be unnecessary. Since ultrasound cannot distinguish between an obstructed distended system and a baggy, low-pressure dilated system, an abnormality on ultrasound must prompt further definitive investigation. The cost and limited availability of CT mean that it is not the method of choice to detect obstruction. Scintigraphy is not recommended as the first investigation in suspected obstruction but is useful in defining whether dilatation shown by other methods is obstructive.

Intravenous urography

A high dose of contrast is required in patients with renal failure and tomograms and delayed films should be taken as necessary. In chronic obstruction, films taken immediately after contrast injection will show a dilated pelvicalyceal system as a lucent 'negative pyelogram' surrounded by opacified parenchyma. Later films usually show filling of the dilated pelvicalyceal system and ureter (Fig. 13). Tomography may be necessary to show the faint opacification of dilated calyces. Definition of the dilated ureter may be poor.

In very long-standing obstruction, generalized thinning of the renal parenchyma (obstructive atrophy) is seen. This is typically diffuse and symmetrical, and there is associated generalized calyceal dilatation.

When examining the intravenous urogram in known or suspected obstruction, the following questions should be asked:

1. Are calculi or nephrocalcinosis visible on the plain film taken before injection of contrast?
2. Are two kidneys present?
3. What is their size?
4. What is the pattern of development of the nephrogram?
5. Is the collecting system shown sufficiently well, whether filled with contrast or as a negative shadow, to allow a conclusion as to the presence or absence of dilatation?
6. Is there renal cortical thinning?
7. Is the ureter dilated and to what level? Is it displaced?

Fig. 12 (a) Ultrasound scan showing normal right kidney. (b) Ultrasound scan showing, for comparison, small unobstructed right kidney.

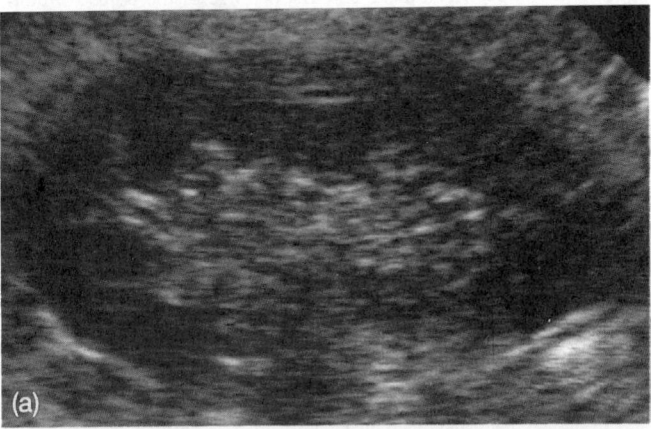

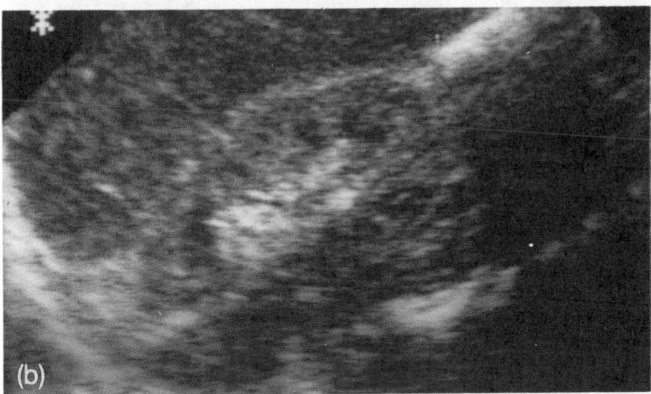

Fig. 13 High-dose intravenous urogram in chronic bilateral obstruction. Note dilated systems seen as lucent negative pyelograms.

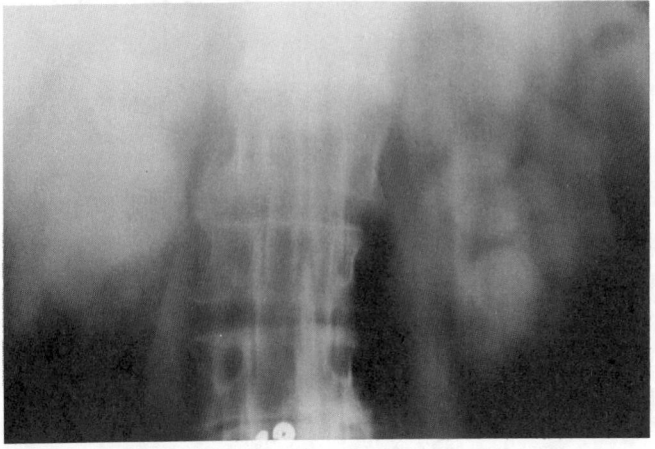

8. Does the bladder contain a filling defect?
9. Is bladder emptying complete on the after-voiding radiograph?

CT scanning

On CT the dilated collecting system appears as a multiloculate fluid collection of water density in the renal sinus. It is possible to distinguish the intrarenal collecting system from the extrarenal portion of the pelvis; this is important since obstruction can only be diagnosed on CT when there is dilatation of the intrarenal collecting system. A prominent extrarenal pelvis may be a normal variant. The whole dilated ureter is well shown on CT. The main value of CT in the investigation of chronic upper-tract obstruction is in defining the cause (Fig. 14).

Scintigraphy (see also Chapter 20.1)

Scintigraphy provides functional evidence of obstruction. A radioactive tracer is injected and its passage through the kidney is recorded by serial images and computerized data. The first passage of the bolus of radioactivity reflects renal perfusion; later images provide information on renal uptake, excretion, and drainage. [^{99}Tc^m]DTPA (diethylenetriaminepentaacetic acid) and [^{99}Tc^m] methylene diphosphonate (MDP) are frequently used and are excreted purely by glomerular filtration.

A rise in pressure in the collecting system, sufficient to result in impaired renal function, delays parenchymal clearance of tracer and emptying of the collecting system. On whole-kidney renograms, the time–activity curve fails to fall after the initial intake peak, or continues to rise (Fig. 15). This does not enable a distinction to be made between obstructive nephropathy, in which parenchymal transit time is prolonged, and retention of tracer within a large, baggy, low-pressure, unobstructed collecting system. Inspection of the analogue images may permit these two situations to be distinguished. Obstructive nephropathy

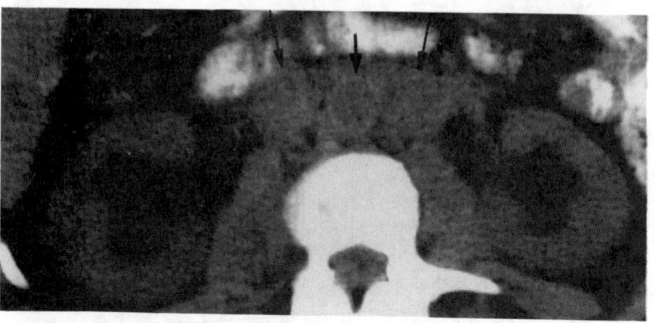

Fig. 14 CT scan in a patient with bilateral urinary tract obstruction due to prostatic cancer. Tumour tissue is clearly delineated on the scan (arrowed).

Fig. 15 Dynamic DTPA scintigram. Note the progressive rise of the right kidney curve to a plateau, in contrast to the normal left kidney curve.

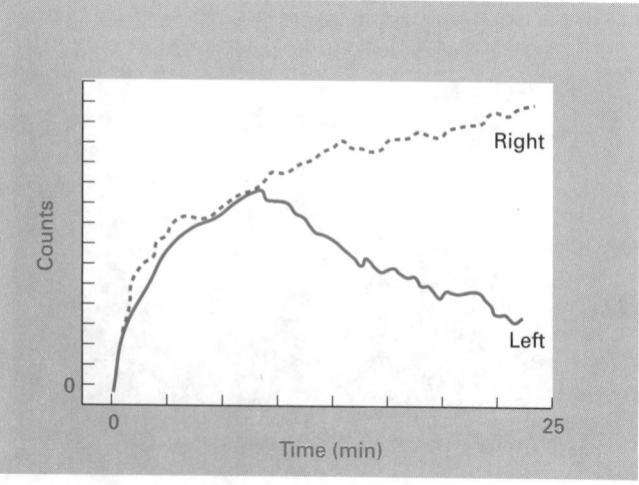

causes delayed clearance of tracer from the renal parenchyma and delayed outflow from the collecting system. A normal parenchymal clearance with delayed outflow suggests a non-obstructed, dilated collecting system.

A dynamic renal scintigram performed during diuresis may be of value in this situation. Frusemide (0.5 mg/kg) is given intravenously immediately after voiding, when a routing scintigram has raised the possibility of obstruction. Time–activity curves obtained over the renal pelvic area immediately after injection of frusemide show no significant change in the renogram. In normal subjects this is then followed by a rapid fall in activity. In the presence of obstruction the half-time is prolonged. A poor response may result from poor renal function or dehydration rather than from obstruction. In the presence of massive pelvic dilatation, washout may not be observed, and under these circumstances the test is uninterpretable.

Although scintigraphy has been used to screen for obstruction in patients with unexplained chronic impairment of renal function, ultrasonography is preferred in most centres. Radionuclide methods are of particular value in differentiating obstructive nephropathy from the prolongation of transit time associated with a baggy, dilated, but unobstructed system, and in defining the contribution of each kidney to overall uptake function. A decision as to whether conservative surgery or nephrectomy should be carried out in unilateral obstruction may be much facilitated by the latter assessment.

Intravenous urography and CT may both provide some limited information on renal function, whereas ultrasound provides none. An immediate nephrogram after intravenous injection of iodine-containing contrast medium, which increases in density with time is indicative of obstruction of recent onset.

Antegrade pyelography and ureterography

Percutaneous introduction of contrast medium directly into the renal pelvis or a calyx via a needle, with subsequent radiographic examination of the pelvicalyceal system and ureter (antegrade pyelography and ureterography), is used increasingly to define the site and cause of chronic upper-tract obstruction. Diagnostic antegrade examination can be combined with therapeutic drainage of an obstructed system.

Retrograde ureterography

Cystoscopy and catheterization of one or both of the ureters from below, followed by retrograde injection of contrast medium (retrograde ureterography) is indicated if antegrade examination cannot be carried out, or if there is a prospect of dealing with ureteric obstruction from below at the time of retrograde examination. The technique carries the risks of introducing infection into an obstructed urinary tract and of septicaemia, and should be performed only when absolutely necessary. In obstruction due to neuromuscular dysfunction at the pelviureteric junction and in retroperitoneal fibrosis, the collecting system may fill normally from below.

Pressure flow studies

This investigation provides a quantitative assessment of the effect of obstruction on the outflow tract. The technique involves the insertion of a needle transparenchymally into the upper collecting system. Local anaesthetic is sufficient in adults, but general anaesthesia is required in children. The bladder is catheterized and intravesical pressure measured. The pressure differential between the kidney and the bladder is monitored while the collecting system is perfused with dilute contrast at a rate of 10 ml/min. Perfusion must be maintained for long enough to ensure that the upper urinary tract is filled.

Normal systems can accommodate a flow rate of 10 ml/min without a pressure differential of more than 15 cm of water. If an obstruction is present, there will be a pressure differential of more than 22 cm of water. An equivocal range exists when the differential pressure is between 15 and 22 cm of water, but such a result occurs in only a small proportion of patients.

This diagnostic technique is relatively simple and can readily be extended into a therapeutic one by leaving a catheter *in situ*, to provide drainage of an obstructed system. The disadvantages are: first, that it is an invasive test with a risk (albeit small) of provoking infection; secondly, the technique investigates the collecting system and gives no information on parenchymal function; and thirdly, it is not readily repeatable.

With the advent of more sophisticated renography, pressure flow studies are performed less frequently, but still have a place in the investigation of obstruction in patients with very poor renal function, in whom radioisotope techniques are less reliable; in equivocal obstruction, particularly at the pelviureteric junction; and intraoperatively in patients with retroperitoneal fibrosis undergoing ureterolysis.

SIGNIFICANT INCOMPLETE CHRONIC UPPER URINARY-TRACT OBSTRUCTION

It may be very difficult to tell whether a given degree of partial or intermittent obstruction is impairing, or potentially impairing, renal function or causing symptoms. Symptoms may be present in the absence of deleterious effects upon renal function and the converse may also be true. Different methods of diagnosing obstruction define subtly different pathological features of the condition and a valid correlation between the results of different investigations cannot invariably be made. Incomplete obstruction is clinically important if it causes deterioration in kidney function which can be halted or corrected by intervention, or symptoms which are improved thereby. In patients with one kidney, or those with bilateral partial obstruction, a decline in serial measurements of glomerular filtration rate attributable to obstruction may define the situation. There may be a similar change in uptake of radionuclides in unilateral obstruction. Other proposed methods of detecting significant incomplete obstruction are given in Table 3. Strict validation of these methods would require them to be carried out in patients with supposed obstruction who would then be allocated randomly to intervention or no intervention. Deterioration in function predicted by each of the methods by comparison with matched controls would provide validation. This study is never likely to be done.

DIFFERENTIAL DIAGNOSIS OF NON-OBSTRUCTIVE COLLECTING SYSTEM DILATATION

A number of non-obstructive conditions may cause collecting system dilatation (Table 1). It is usually not possible for ultrasound to differentiate obstructive from non-obstructive dilatation because of its inability to show calyceal detail, differentiate an intrarenal from an extrarenal pelvis, and demonstrate the ureter. CT is also a poor indicator of whether dilatation is obstructive or non-obstructive, although it can identify cases of dilatation which are due to an extrarenal pelvis. Intravenous urography is of value in this connection.

Extrarenal pelves may mimic pelviureteric junctional obstruction. If frusemide is administered after the 20 min full-length contrast radiograph in this condition, contrast medium will have washed out of the affected side on a full-length film 15 min later. In the presence of pelviureteric junctional obstruction the contrast is retained and the pelvicalyceal system increases in size.

Megacalyces are readily identified on urography. The renal cortex is normal and calyceal infundibula, pelvis, and ureter are normal with no evidence of obstruction (Fig. 16).

Vesicoureteric reflux may be associated with dilatation of the ureters and in severe cases of the pelvicalyceal system too. The presence of reflux on urography is suggested by the degree of dilatation varying at different times during the examination, by dilatation which is greatest from the vesicoureteric junction upwards, and by a postmicturition film which shows a large volume of residual urine in the bladder composed of urine that has refluxed into the ureters during voiding and drained back thereafter.

Table 3 *Detection of significant incomplete obstruction*

Introduction of a needle into the renal pelvis with direct measurement of the pressure developing after infusion of fluid at a known flow rate (antegrade pressure flow measurement)

Urographic observation of the degree of distension of the renal pelvis induced by intravenous frusemide (frusemide urography)

Observation of the effect of intravenous frusemide upon the isotope renogram (frusemide renography)

Comparison of activity/time curves after injection of [^{99}Tc^{m}]-DTPA in whole kidney versus renal pelvis (retention function analysis)

Measurement of the nephron transit time of a non-reabsorbable tracer (outflow obstruction may increase the transit time)

A decision as to whether or not significant obstruction is present at the pelviureteric junction and whether operation is indicated may be facilitated by frusemide urography (Fig. 17) or frusemide scintigraphy. In some patients the urographic findings are unremarkable during asymptomatic periods, while emergency intravenous urography during an episode of pain may define the condition.

In women who have been pregnant, particularly those who have suffered pregnancy bacteriuria, one or both upper ureters (more often the right) may be dilated to the pelvic brim (Fig. 18). The system is seen to empty on a full-length postmicturition film (Fig. 19) and dilatation of pelvis and calyces is absent. Renographic examination carried out just before termination of pregnancy reveals abnormalities on the right side in almost 70 per cent of patients, and on the left in 50 per cent. Such studies do not define whether dilatation of the system is present in the

Fig. 16 Right-sided megacalyces—a normal variant. Note normal renal cortex, caliceal infundibula, pelvis, and ureter, with no evidence of obstruction.

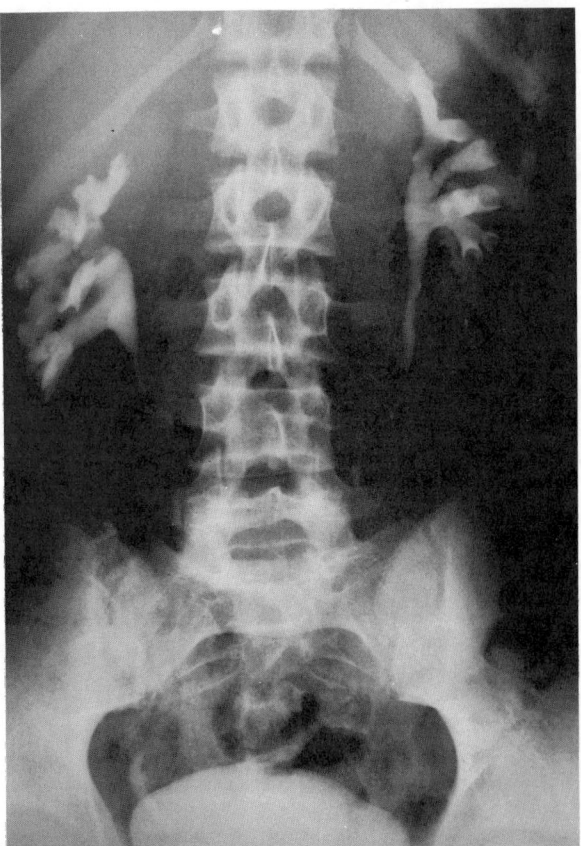

Fig. 17 (a) Right-sided pelviureteric obstruction. (b) Same urogram as in (a) 15 min after intravenous injection of frusemide. Note increase in size of pelvicalyceal system, indicating significant pelviureteric junction obstruction.

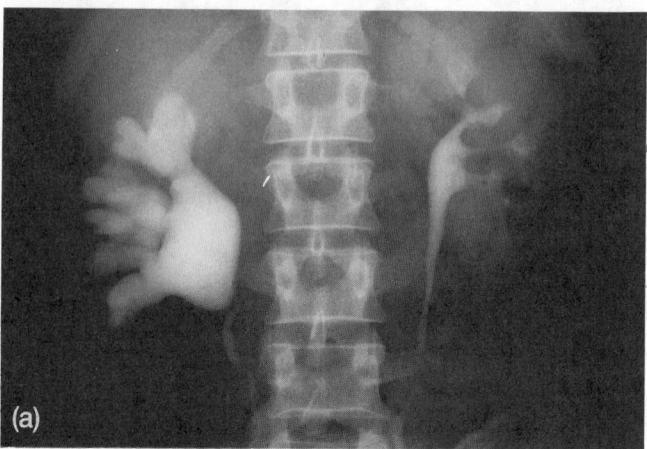

(a)

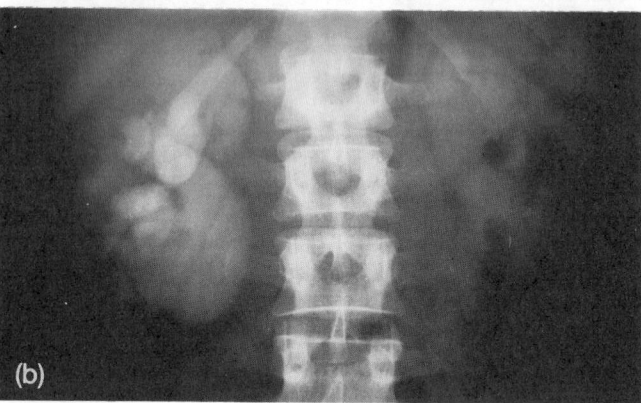

(b)

absence of prolongation of nephron transit times or whether true obstructive nephropathy is present. For obvious ethical reasons, the problem is difficult to study in normal pregnancy. Approximately one-third of women with asymptomatic bacteriuria in pregnancy develop acute pyelonephritis, compared with only 1 to 2 per cent of non-pregnant females. The relationship, if any, between this fact and the anatomical changes seen in pregnancy is unclear.

ACUTE LOWER URINARY-TRACT OBSTRUCTION

Most patients presenting with acute urinary retention require no investigation before treatment. Suprapubic pain coexisting with a bladder which is palpably or percussibly distended above the level of the symphysis pubis is sufficient evidence for immediate catheterization.

If doubt about the diagnosis exists, an ultrasound examination will confirm or refute the presence of a distended bladder. Transrectal ultrasound of the prostrate can demonstrate both the size of the gland and, to some extent, the benign or malignant nature of the enlargement. Such an investigation is not indicated in the acute situation but is of potential benefit after the relief of obstruction.

An ascending urethrogram may be indicated if an attempt at urethral catheterization proves unsuccessful. This is done as an elective procedure after bladder drainage has been achieved by suprapubic catheterization.

CHRONIC LOWER URINARY-TRACT OBSTRUCTION

In one series of patients presenting with acute retention of urine, approximately half had bladders of low and half of high compliance. Investigation is aimed at demonstrating associated pathology such as urinary-tract infection, upper-tract dilatation, stones, and renal impairment, and at defining the severity of bladder outflow obstruction.

Urine culture is essential. In most centres, ultrasonography of the upper and lower urinary tract, together with a plain abdominal radiograph and a urinary flow rate measurement have replaced the intravenous urogram. Full urodynamic investigations, with combined video-

Fig. 18 Right ureter dilated to level of pelvic brim after pregnancy. Note absence of dilatation of renal pelvis and calyces.

Fig. 19 Same patient as in Fig. 18, after voiding radiograph. Note good emptying of right ureter.

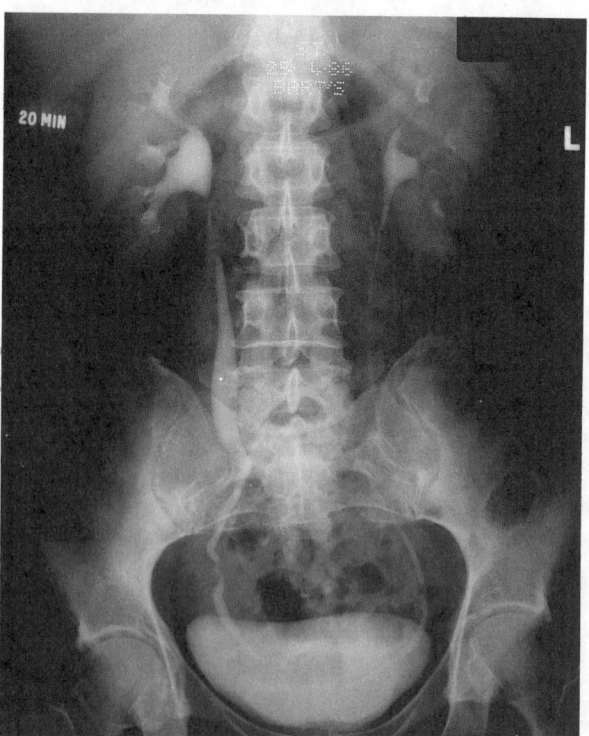

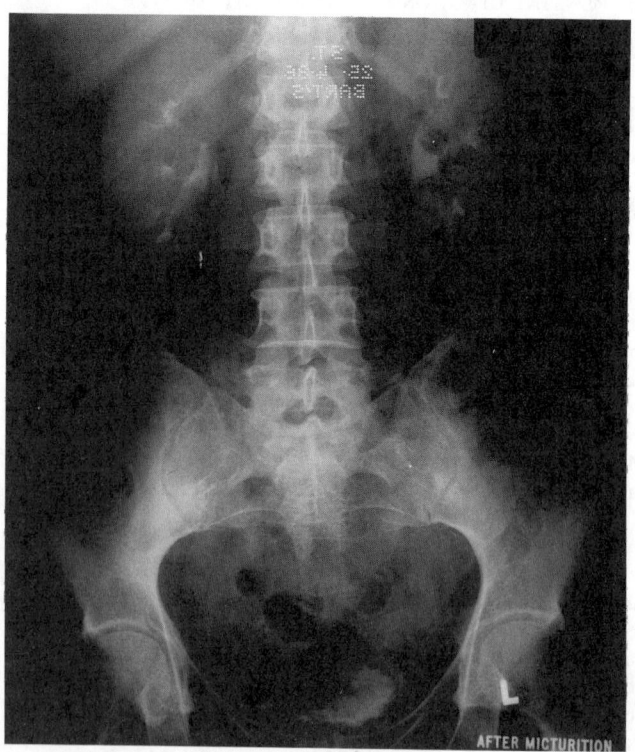

pressure cystourethrography may be necessary. Serum biochemistry and routine haematology are also required, as is measurement of prostatic-specific antigen level in males.

Management

ACUTE UPPER-TRACT OBSTRUCTION

Stones

The majority of patients presenting to an accident and emergency department with renal and ureteric colic will have a stone in the lower third of the ureter, often in that portion of the ureter lying within the bladder wall. Such patients can be managed conservatively, since the stone has already passed through two areas of relative ureteric narrowing: the pelviureteric junction, and the site at which the ureter crosses the bifurcation of the common iliac artery. A conservative policy is likely to prove successful if the stone is 5 mm or less in its maximum diameter. It is unusual for acute episodes of colic to persist for more than 72 h.

Patients with ureteric colic are usually admitted to hospital, although this is unnecessary in many cases since the only medical requirement is the provision of regular analgesia, which can be given parenterally, orally, or rectally. There is a time-honoured recommendation that patients with colic should be encouraged to maintain a very high fluid intake to induce a diuresis. An antimuscarinic drug such as propantheline is also often prescribed. There is no reason to think that these measures are of benefit, and they may even be harmful since both encourage ureteric dilatation and would be expected to reduce forward peristalsis of the ureter, which is the very effect needed to encourage spontaneous stone passage. A diuresis will also tend to increase intratubular pressure and may increase the risk of forniceal rupture. It might be argued that forniceal rupture may, by decompressing the system, encourage the return of peristalsis but few would regard this as an appropriate approach to management.

Although it has long been argued that morphine should be avoided as an analgesic as it may provoke ureteric spasm, there is no evidence that therapeutic doses of morphine have this adverse effect. Pethidine may provoke nausea and vomiting, particularly when administered parenterally, but since nausea and vomiting frequently accompany colic it is difficult to disentangle the effects of such treatment from the effects of colic alone. Very satisfactory pain relief can often be obtained using non-steroidal anti-inflammatory agents administered orally or rectally.

With the advent of new, less invasive methods of surgical management of ureteric stones there is a temptation to intervene earlier. With most lithotripters, whether imaging is by ultrasound or radiology, stones in the intramural ureter can be treated readily. Since most stones at that site will pass spontaneously, the extent to which lithotripsy will hasten the process is difficult to establish. Lithotripsy may be worthwhile for stones in the upper third of the ureter since, by disintegrating the stone into small fragments, spontaneous passage will be encouraged. The availability of lithotripsy for patients with acute colic varies very markedly between countries and the precise role and benefits of the technique have yet to be established.

Endoscopic manoeuvres, which are usually performed under general anaesthesia, are reserved for those patients with persistent colic.

Drainage of an obstructed system

If there is clinical evidence of infection above an obstruction, drainage must be established as a matter of urgency. The diagnosis is a clinical one. The patient will be pyrexial and the degree of loin tenderness will be greater than when obstruction is not associated with infection. Examination of bladder urine may be unhelpful since ureteric obstruction may prevent red and white blood cells and organisms from reaching the lower urinary tract. Leucocytosis may be present but this is not invariably the case, especially in the elderly.

The choice between antegrade and retrograde intervention will depend on the facilities and expertise available. In most specialist cen-

tres there is a clear preference for the insertion percutaneously of an antegrade needle to provide a nephrostomy under local anaesthesia. In a dilated high-pressure system the procedure is usually easy. Such a system may be used to provide drainage for weeks or even months if necessary. If excretion of intravenous contrast has outlined renal anatomy, renal puncture may be guided radiographically. If not, the initial puncture may be better directed under ultrasound control using a fine needle. The collecting system is then outlined with contrast and an accurate transparenchymal calyceal puncture can be placed, usually through a lower calyx.

A retrograde ureteric catheter, in contrast, can be relied on to provide drainage at best only for a matter of days. Occasionally, a retrograde catheter cannot be passed beyond the obstruction and the diagnostic role of retrograde ureterography cannot then be extended to a therapeutic one.

Other causes of acute obstruction

The two other most common causes are sloughed papillae and blood clots. The principles of management vary little from those already outlined for ureteric stones. However, greater attention must be paid in the acute phase to the underlying cause. In the patient with papillary necrosis, infection is a more common accompaniment of obstruction, and surgical intervention, usually with a percutaneous needle nephrostomy, is required more often. When colic results from blood clot, treatment of the underlying cause may be necessary at an early stage. Renal parenchymal tumours and transitional cell tumours of the collecting system may both cause persistent bleeding and colic, and ablative open surgery is usually required. More difficulty is encountered when bleeding occurs from a non-malignant cause. An arteriovenous fistula, whether spontaneous or traumatic, may be embolized with every prospect of success. The most difficult case of recurrent bleeding to manage is that associated with papillary necrosis in sickle-cell trait or disease. Antifibrinolytic agents may be of value, but administration of such treatment during active bleeding may produce hard, rubbery clots which fill the collecting system and require surgical removal.

CHRONIC UPPER-TRACT OBSTRUCTION

The aim of management is to relieve symptoms, improve or conserve renal function, and avoid complications such as septicaemia. Important surgical advances in the past decade include the increasing use of ureteric stents to provide short-term, or even long-term, relief of obstruction.

Obstruction is the most readily reversible cause of chronic renal failure. Acute obstruction caused by ureteric stones commonly resolves spontaneously; however, the longer a stone remains in the same position within the ureter the less likely it is that a conservative policy will be successful.

Probably the second most common cause of chronic obstruction in adults is pelviureteric junction obstruction. The Anderson–Hynes pyeloplasty gives very satisfactory results and provides the gold standard against which other open and endoscopic techniques (such as endopyelotomy) must be assessed.

Idiopathic obstruction at the pelviureteric junction may present in childhood. Obstructed megaureter and ureteric obstruction secondary to a ureterocele are also more common in children than in adults. Since all three congenital anomalies cause pelvicalyceal dilatation, it is becoming increasingly common for obstruction to be diagnosed *in utero*. Treatment of the obstruction *in utero* by the insertion of a nephrostomy tube has been reported: it is too early to know whether such early intervention will prove to have long-term benefits, but at the moment it seems, on balance, best to wait until immediately after delivery to investigate and relieve the problem.

Ureteric obstruction can occur in a transplanted kidney, most commonly at the site of the ureteroneocystostomy but sometimes more proximally in the ureter. Vesicoureteric stenosis is caused by ischaemia of the ureter, but it is never possible to define whether this ischaemia is associated with rejection or is a result of poor vascularization following donor dephrectomy. More proximal ureteric obstruction may be due to mechanical kinking of the ureter or, occasionally, to extrinsic compression by a lymphocele. Irrespective of the site and cause of the obstruction, the diagnosis presents special problems. The possibility of obstruction is raised either because of deteriorating renal function or because ultrasound during routine follow-up demonstrates increasing collecting system dilatation. The differential diagnosis includes rejection, cyclosporin nephrotoxicity, and arterial insufficiency. An obstruction may be demonstrated by intravenous urography and/or antegrade pyelography. Retrograde studies are usually difficult and not infrequency impossible, and since, in the case of stenosis at a ureteroneocystostomy, they involve passing a catheter across the segment of ureter under suspicion, the investigation is only indicated if intravenous urography and antegrade pyelography prove unsatisfactory.

Minimally invasive stone surgery

The past decade has seen a revolution in the management of urinary-tract stones, due to the adoption of minimally invasive techniques including percutaneous surgery and extracorporeal shock-wave lithotripsy.

Open operation for renal stones can now be avoided in many cases by creating a nephrostomy track to the calculus, dilating the track, and then either removing the calculus endoscopically via the track or causing it to disintegrate by direct application of an ultrasound probe. It is possible to extract ureteric stones endoscopically with the assistance of a ureteroscope, and bladder calculi may be disintegrated by the endoscopic application of electrohydraulically produced shock waves.

Externally delivered shock waves can be used to shatter calculi into many fragments which are then passed spontaneously. Extracorporeal shock-wave lithotripsy offers a solution to the problem of the presence of a calculus or calculi within the kidney without the need for a surgical operation, with the promise of a reduction in morbidity and perhaps mortality, a much shorter hospital stay for the patient, and a more rapid return to work. In addition, a number of patients who are unfit for conventional surgery may be suitable for shock-wave lithotripsy. The technique is unsuitable for hard uric acid and cystine stones, for very large stones (which must be 'de-bulked' percutaneously before lithotripsy), and for some ureteric stones (although a proportion of these can be manoeuvred into the upper collecting system endoscopically and then dealt with by this method. Other disadvantages include the high capital cost of the necessary equipment, its size and the need for further intervention in 10 to 15 per cent of patients in whom stone fragments do not pass. Such fragments can, in general, be removed endoscopically. Despite these problems, it seems likely that non-operative dissolution of calculi will be used increasingly in the developed world in future years, provided the stone recurrence rate in the long term proves to be no higher than after open surgery and no so-far-unforeseen long-term complication emerges. Large staghorn calculi are still usually removed by a cutting procedure. Surface cooling of the kidney at the time of operation allows time for more complete clearance of stones with the renal artery clamped, and protects against the development of ischaemic damage to the kidney.

Pelviureteric junction obstruction

Commonly, this appears to result from a functional disturbance in peristalsis of the collecting system in the absence of mechanical obstruction. A percutaneous procedure for managing pelviureteric junctional obstruction was first described in 1983. Subsequent experience has confirmed the usefulness of the technique, but there is no consensus on the indications. Currently, patients with secondary pelviureteric junction stenosis, in association with stones, infection, or previous surgery, are offered the operation, whereas those with primary idiopathic obstruction are better treated by open pyeloplasty. The percutaneous operation (endopyelotomy) involves a full thickness incision through the stenosed

region and a stent left *in situ*. Healing occurs by re-epithelialization from either side of the incision and very little new scar tissue is formed.

Malignant obstruction

A wide variety of tumours may cause ureteric obstruction, either by local spread (cervix, prostate, bladder), or secondary to para-aortic nodal enlargement (lymphoma, testicular tumours). The diagnosis rests upon the same investigations as for any other cause of chronic obstruction, but the treatment will vary widely, depending on the cause. An aggressive or radical approach is almost always indicated in a patient who has received no previous treatment for the underlying malignancy. Unilateral or bilateral percutaneous nephrostomies may be necessary to cover the period of time during which chemotherapy or radiotherapy are given with the expectation of controlling the tumour. More difficulty arises when ureteric obstruction is due to recurrent tumour, when the potential benefits of chemotherapy and radiotherapy are significantly less and patients may be facing debilitating treatment for an advancing malignant disease, the prognosis of which is poor. To be confined by nephrostomy drainage for what is left of life significantly diminishes its quality, but may be right in certain circumstances. A percutaneously placed pigtail nephrostomy, which can be inserted under local anaesthetic, has a tendency to fall out or to be pulled out. Open surgery can be avoided by the use of a ring nephrostomy inserted percutaneously under general anaesthesia: this provides secure long-term drainage, for years if necessary.

Obstruction in patients with urinary diversion

There are many reasons for diverting the urine into an isolated loop of ileum or colon. One of the recognized complications is stenosis at the site of anastomosis between the bowel and ureter(s).

The thin muscle wall of the ileum means that it is not possible to fashion an antireflux anastomosis between the bowel and the ureter when diverting the urine into an ileal conduit; a loopogram (a radiograph carried out after injection of contrast into an ideal loop) will normally therefore show bilateral ureteric reflux. The absence of reflux is strong evidence of a stenosis at the ureteroileal junction.

The operation of ureterosigmoidostomy, in which the ureters are anastomosed to sigmoid colon, has fallen into disfavour owing to the associated complications of infection, metabolic acidosis (caused by reabsorption of hydrogen ions from the gut), and osteomalacia.

Idiopathic retroperitoneal fibrosis (peri-aortitis)

In this condition the ureters become embedded in dense fibrous tissue, with resultant unilateral or bilateral obstruction, usually at the junction between the middle and lower thirds of the ureter. The condition is progressive: initially, the fibrous tissue is fairly cellular, later becoming relatively acellular. The mechanism by which obstruction occurs is unclear, not least because of the frequent observation that contrast medium injected into the lower ureter may pass freely up to the pelvicalyceal system despite the presence of clinical, radiological, and isotopic evidence of functional urinary-tract obstruction.

Pathogenesis

'Retroperitoneal fibrosis' is an unfortunate term, since there are many causes of fibrosis in the retroperitoneal area (including malignant disease of breast, colon, or prostate, for instance), and because it is anatomically misleading and says nothing about pathogenesis. Evidence has now accumulated to suggest that the condition is an autoimmune peri-aortitis. The peri-aortic nature of the condition has long been known to surgeons and pathologists, and this has been further emphasized by the advent of CT scanning (Fig. 20). In many ways the term 'peri-aortitis' is, therefore, preferable to retroperitoneal fibrosis.

Histologically, aortic atheroma, medial thinning, splits in the media, and an increase in the adventitia, which contains an inflammatory infiltrate, are seen. These findings are present to some extent in the aortae of some patients with advanced atherosclerosis who have not suffered a clinical illness and who may reasonably be classified as having 'subclinical peri-aortitis'. The fibrous tissue itself contains macrophages and plasma cells but not polymorphs.

It now seems likely that peri-aortic fibrosis is an autoimmune response to leakage of material derived from atheromatous plaques in the diseased aorta. The substance ceroid, an insoluble polymer of oxidized lipid and lipoprotein, which may be synthesized artificially by oxidizing low-density lipoprotein, may be involved in the reaction: it is found in atheromatous plaques and is identified by staining with oil-red-O. Sections of aorta containing such plaques incubated with mouse monoclonal antibody to human IgG localizes the antibody to the region of the plaque where ceroid has been identified by oil-red-O staining. Identical findings are obtained on incubation with polyclonal rabbit anti-human IgG. Moreover, IgG and some IgM, but not IgA or IgE, can be identified in plasma cells in the fibrotic tissue where there are splits in the adjacent media. Circulating antibodies to oxidized low-density lipoprotein and to ceroid extracted from human atheroma are detected in patients with peri-aortitis in much higher concentrations than in normal individuals and in those with ischaemic heart disease. Stored sera obtained from individuals subsequently shown at autopsy to have had subclinical peri-aortitis also show significantly increased antibody titres compared with controls. It seems likely then that chronic peri-aortitis has an autoimmune aetiology in which the allergen is a component of ceroid, probably oxidized low-density lipoprotein, produced in human atheroma, and that a specific immune response involves T cells and plasma cells, which secrete IgG. Oxidized low-density lipoprotein is known to be highly immunogenic.

This concept clarifies some issues which previously were difficult to explain. For example, the definite, although uncommon, association between mediastinal fibrosis and idiopathic retroperitoneal fibrosis has always been difficult to understand. If one regards at least some cases of mediastinal fibrosis (see below) as a peri-aortitis, occurring in this instance around the thoracic aorta, the association becomes comprehensible. Surgeons operating upon aortic aneurysms quite often see fibrosis around the aneurysm. Sometimes the surgeon encounters technical difficulties in adhesions between the aorta and duodenum, and a dense, fibrotic, chronic inflammatory infiltrate is present around the aorta: the term 'inflammatory aneurysm' is used to define this condition. The unifying hypothesis of an autoimmune peri-aortitis accounts for this finding. Certainly, so-called idiopathic retroperitoneal fibrosis, idiopathic mediastinal fibrosis, perianeurysmal fibrosis, and inflammatory aneurysm have much in common. The hypothesis also accounts for the well-known association between aortic disease, including aneurysm and aortic wall calcification, and retroperitoneal fibrosis. Finally, it may be no coincidence that carcinoid tumours and drugs such as methysergide and ergot derivatives which are sometimes responsible for the condition, all have well described effects on the vasculature.

Clinical features

The condition is three times as common in men as in women. Patients' ages range from the third to the ninth decade, but peak incidence occurs in the sixth and seventh decades; in one series of 60 patients the mean age of the group was 56 years. The early clinical manifestations are not distinctive. Most commonly there is pain in a girdle like distribution from the low back to the lower abdomen, occasionally spreading to buttocks or thighs. Examination is usually unremarkable apart from hypertension, which is found in over 50 per cent of patients. Oedema of the legs, a palpable kidney, and hydrocele, are found in less than 10 per cent of patients. There is usually a normochromic, normocytic anaemia and a raised erythrocyte sedimentation rate and plasma C-reactive protein, but a significant minority are normal in one or both of these respects. Proteinuria is uncommon and significant bacteriuria rare.

Diagnosis

Peri-aortic fibrosis is clearly more common than hitherto appreciated, if one takes into account subclinical forms of the condition. Even overt idiopathic retroperitoneal fibrosis is, in all probability, much more common than was generally thought. Diagnostic delay is the rule; in one series, 6 to 12 months, or even longer, elapsed from the onset of symptoms to diagnosis. Perhaps for this reason, bilateral rather than unilateral upper-tract obstruction was present in the majority of patients.

When taking the history, enquiry should be made regarding consumption of relevant drugs, including methysergide, β-blockers, methyldopa, and bromocriptine, another ergot-like drug.

Ultrasonography, isotopic methods, and the intravenous urogram will reveal findings typical of urinary-tract obstruction, and the last techniques may show medial deviation of the ureters. This last finding may also be present in normal subjects and is an unreliable guide to diagnosis. CT scanning will show the peri-aortic mass (Fig. 20). The differential diagnosis includes lymphoma (in which case splenomegaly and lymphadenopathy may be seen on CT scanning) and various forms of cancer, including particularly those of the bladder, bowel, and cervix.

A histological diagnosis should be obtained if at all possible, and laparotomy is required in order to obtain a sufficiently large sample to exclude lymphoma and cancer with certainty. Conversely, a CT-guided needle biopsy may be sufficient to make a definitive diagnosis of malignancy.

Management

Management of the idiopathic and probably autoimmune syndrome is empirical and controversial since controlled trials of treatment are lacking. Corticosteroid therapy, with or without temporary relief of obstruction by insertion of ureteric stents, ureterolysis alone, and ureterolysis followed by steroid therapy to shrink the peri-aortic mass and maintain remission have all been used. Corticosteroid therapy alone may correct obstruction, but is by no means invariably effective. Ureterolysis alone may also correct obstruction in the long term but is sometimes associated with recurrence or the development of a further obstruction in a previously unaffected kidney. Surgical relief of obstruction by ureterolysis followed by long-term corticosteroid therapy (prednisolone 20 mg daily begun when sutures are removed) has proved a reliable and successful strategy. When bilateral obstruction is present, bilateral ureterolysis followed by steroid therapy is preferable to unilateral ureterolysis with reliance upon corticosteroid therapy to free the contralateral side, since this is sometimes unsuccessful. Ureterolysis of kidneys shown to be nonfunctioning on high-dose excretion urography or by appropriate radionuclide techniques is usually unsuccessful in restoring useful renal function. A reasonable policy for management would seem to be to perform unilateral or bilateral ureterolysis, as appropriate, followed by corticosteroid therapy in patients fit for operation and able to take steroids safely. Surgery alone should be employed in those with a particular contraindication to corticosteroid treatment, such as the presence of a peptic ulcer or severe osteoporosis. Steroid therapy alone (methylprednisolone 500 mg intravenously daily for 3 days, followed by prednisolone 20 mg daily), with or without insertion of ureteric stents, should be reserved for patients unfit for ureterolysis. A dramatic response to

Fig. 20 CT scan in idiopathic retroperitoneal fibrosis (peri-aortitis) causing urinary-tract obstruction. Note the aortic calcification and peri-aortic nature of the mass.

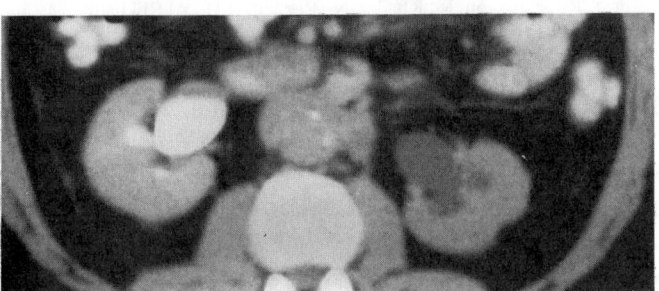

parenteral steroid treatment sometimes occurs, a marked diuresis being seen within 24 h of commencing treatment.

Prognosis

The older and the more uraemic the patient at the time of presentation, the worse is the prognosis. Nevertheless, if treated appropriately, most patients do well.

Follow-up

In some patients long-term remission is achieved by surgery alone. In those receiving maintenance prednisolone, the dose can be reduced progressively, and in some patients long-term remission occurs after complete withdrawal of corticosteroid therapy. In one series of 60 patients, 10 relapsed more than 5 years after the time of diagnosis when steroid therapy had been stopped, in that their erythrocyte sedimentation rates rose to an abnormal level, and obstruction and diminished renal function redeveloped. Five patients relapsed as late as 10 years after the onset of the disease. Lifelong follow-up is therefore mandatory. The best way to monitor such patients is not certain. Clinical assessment, serial measurement of erythrocyte sedimentation rate and C-reactive protein, and assessment of renal function, together with imaging to detect redevelopment of obstruction, are appropriate. Reduction in size of the periaortic mass can be detected on serial CT scanning, but residual periaortic tissue is seen frequently, even after steroid therapy, and the usefulness of CT in monitoring disease activity is limited.

Peri-aortitis in the absence of ureteric obstruction

The use of CT scanning in the investigation of abdominal pain has revealed an increasing number of patients to have peri-aortitis before the onset of urinary tract obstruction. Management of these cases is controversial. The development of bilateral ureteric obstruction with severe uraemia within 3 months of diagnosis (at which time renal function was normal and the ureters unobstructed) has occurred in at least one patient. Until more is known of the natural history of the disease in such patients, it would seem prudent to obtain a histological diagnosis at open operation and to consider corticosteroid therapy to shrink the mass. Whether an attempt to reduce the risk of ureteric obstruction by insertion of stents or displacement of the ureters from the mass at the time of the operation should be carried out is as yet unclear.

Chronic inflammatory bowel disease

Chronic inflammatory bowel disease is associated with chronic and unsuspected urinary-tract obstruction in 10 to 15 per cent of patients. The obstruction is nearly always right-sided in patients with Crohn's disease, and a valuable clue to its existence is pain radiating down from the right iliac fossa into the right leg. The ureter is usually involved in an inflammatory mass. In contrast, in patients with ulcerative colitis the problem may occur on either side and nearly always follows colectomy.

An ultrasound examination of the urinary tract to detect obstruction should be considered as part of the annual review in patients with chronic inflammatory bowel disease.

Mediastinal fibrosis

The pathological process described in connection with retroperitoneal fibrosis can also develop in the upper mediastinum. There, it tends to be located around the bronchi, the cardiac atria, the pulmonary arteries and veins, the superior cava, and the azygos vein; rarely, it also envelops the oesophagus. Symptoms vary according to the structures principally affected. There may be cardiopulmonary manifestations because of scar tissue about the atria, pulmonary vessels, or bronchi, and dysphagia can result from oesophageal constriction. One of the commonest clinical manifestations is due to obstruction of the superior vena cava, with distension of veins in the neck and upper extremities. When mediastinal fibrosis appears without discernible cause, it may be associated with retroperitoneal fibrosis and then probably has the autoimmune origin argued above. There are, however, other causes to consider. The con-

dition is encountered most commonly in people who reside in localities where histoplasmosis is endemic, notably in the central parts of the United States. Hence, most of the case reports have come from clinics located in the Mississippi River Valley. Studies of some of these patients have revealed the existence of large granulomata due to histoplasmosis, with eventual rupture into the superior mediastinum and subsequent growth of the dense masses of scar tissue characteristic of the fibrosing syndromes. A curious anomaly in this context is that tuberculosis rarely, if ever, causes the syndrome.

The diagnosis is suggested by radiographic demonstration of the fibrous tissue in the affected areas. CT scanning may be of great value in this context. Histological verification of the diagnosis can be made by needle biopsy or by employing the technique of mediastinoscopy.

Surgical treatment of mediastinal fibrosis is much more hazardous than of retroperitoneal fibrosis and is much less likely to be beneficial. There is a risk of injury to the vascular structures in the mediastinum during attempts to remove the fibrous tissue; furthermore, serious bleeding may be encountered because of the variable location of enlarged collateral veins. Despite this, some experienced thoracic surgeons recommend that attempts be made to remove large granulomatous masses of histoplasmosis when this is the diagnosis and it appears technically feasible. Also, attempts have been made to free the oesophagus from the constricting scar tissue when dysphagia is a special problem.

Chemotherapy for histoplasmosis has not been very effective. In view of the tendency of this fibrosing process to burn out eventually, it may be possible to ameliorate the manifestations by steroid therapy and thus gain time for a collateral circulation to develop.

Data about the effects of steroid treatment or other forms of immunosuppression as might be used for vasculitic syndromes have not been widely evaluated, but if the origin of the disorder is autoimmune, there is obvious potential for this approach.

Other rarer fibrosing syndromes

In association with retroperitoneal fibrosis and mediastinal fibrosis, other varieties of this process have been reported to involve the thyroid gland (Riedel's thyroiditis), the pancreas, the salivary glands, and orbital tissue. The last mentioned can cause severe proptosis and damage to the optic nerve leading to loss of vision. Some, at least, of these cases may be due to undiagnosed Wegener's granuloma with an atypical presentation.

Peyronie's disease is characterized by the deposition of fibrous plaques in the corpora cavernosa of the penis. These plaques, which can be detected by palpation, may cause discomfort and angulation during penile erection.

REFERENCES

Albarran, J. (1905). Retentionrenale par peri-ureterite. Liberation externe del'urétère. *Compte Rendu de l'Association Française d'Urologie* **9**, 511–17.

Arendshorst, W.J., Finn, W.F., and Gottschalk, C.W. (1974). Nephron stop-flow pressure response to obstruction for 24 hours in the rat kidney. *Journal of Clinical Investigation* **53**, 1497–500.

Baker, L.R.I., *et al.* (1988). Idiopathic retroperitoneal fibrosis. A retrospective analysis of 60 cases. *British Journal of Urology* **60**, 497–503.

Baker, L.R.I., Croxson, R., Khader, N., Reznek, R.H., Al Rukhaimi, M., and Wickham, J.E.A. (1992). Rate of development of ureteric obstruction in idiopathic retroperitoneal fibrosis (periaortitis). *British Journal of Urology* **69**, 102–5.

Better, O.S., Arieff, A.I., Massry, S.G., Kleeman, C.R., and Maxwell, M.H. (1973). Studies on renal function after relief of complete unilateral ureteral obstruction of three months' duration in man. *American Journal of Medicine* **54**, 234–40.

Brooks, A.P. (1990). Computed tomography of idiopathic retroperitoneal fibrosis ('periaortitis'): variants, variations, patterns and pitfalls. *Clinical Radiology* **42**, 75–9.

Brooks, A.P., Reznek, R.H., Webb, J.A.W., and Baker, L.R.I. (1987). Computed tomography in the follow-up of idiopathic retroperitoneal fibrosis. *Clinical Radiology* **38**, 597–601.

Buerkert, J., Martin, D., Head, M., Prasad, J., and Klahr, S. (1978). Deep nephron function after release of acute ureteral obstruction in the young rat. *Journal of Clinical Investigation* **62**, 1228–39.

Dines, D.E., Payne, W.S., Bernatz, P.E., and Pairolero, P.C. (1979). Mediastinal granuloma and fibrosing mediastinitis. *Chest* **75**, 320–4.

Früh, D., Jaeger, W., and Küfer, O. (1975). Orbital involvement in retroperitoneal fibrosis (morbus ormond). *Modern Problems in Ophthalmology* **14**, 651–6.

Ghose, R.R. (1990). Prolonged recovery of renal function after prostatectomy for prostatic outflow obstruction. *British Medical Journal* **300**, 1376–7.

Gillenwater, J.Y. (1986). The pathophysiology of urinary obstruction. In *Campbell's Urology*, (5th edn), (ed. P.C. Walsh, R.F. Gittes, A.D. Perlmutter, and T.A. Stamey), p. 554. WB Saunders, Philadelphia.

Graham, J.R., Suby, J.I., Le Compte, P.R., and Sandowsky, N.L. (1966). Fibrotic disorders associated with methysergide therapy for headache. *New England Journal of Medicine* **274**, 359–68.

Higgins, P.M., Bennett-Jones, D.N., Naish, P.F., and Aber, G.M. (1988). Non-operative management of retroperitoneal fibrosis. *British Journal of Surgery* **75**, 573–7.

Jaworski, Z.F. and Wolan, F.T. (1963). Hydronephrosis and polycythaemia, a case with erythrocytosis relieved by decompression of unilateral hydronephrosis and cured by nephrectomy. *American Journal of Medicine* **34**, 523.

Keuhnelian, J.G., Bartone, F., and Marshall, V.F. (1964). Practical considerations from autopsies in uraemic patients. *Journal of Urology* **91**, 467–73.

McDougal, W.S. and Wright, F.S. (1972). Defect in proximal and distal sodium transport in post-obstructive diuresis. *Kidney International* **2**, 304–17.

Mitchinson, M.J. (1970). The pathology of retroperitoneal fibrosis. *Journal of Clinical Pathology* **23**, 681–9.

Moody, T.E., Vaughn, E.D., and Gillenwater, J.Y. (1975). Relationship between renal blood flow and ureteral pressure during 18 hours of total unilateral occlusion. *Investigative Urology* **13**, 245–51.

Ormond, J.K. (1948). Bilateral ureteral obstruction due to envelopment and compression by an inflammatory process. *Journal of Urology* **59**, 1072–9.

Parums, D.V., Chadwick, D.R., and Mitchinson, M.J. (1986). The localisation of immunoglobulin in chronic periaortitis. *Atherosclerosis* **61**, 117–23.

Parums, D.V., Brown, D.L., and Mitchinson, M.J. (1990). Serum antibodies to oxidised LDL and ceroid in chronic periaortitis. *Archives of Pathology and Laboratory Medicine* **114**, 383–7.

Pryor, J.P., Castle, W.M., Dukes, D.C., Smith, J.C., Watson, M.E., and Williams, J.L. (1983). Do beta adrenoceptor blocking drugs cause retroperitoneal fibrosis? *British Medical Journal* **287**, 639–42.

Sacks, S.H., Aparicio, S.A.J.R., Bevan, A., Oliver, D.O., Will, E.J., and Davison, A.M. (1989). Late renal failure due to prostatic outflow obstruction: a preventable disease. *British Medical Journal* **298**, 156–9.

Schowengerdt, C.G., Suyemoto, R., and Main, F.B. (1969). Granulomatous and fibrous mediastinitis: a review and analysis of 180 cases. *Journal of Thoracic and Cardiovascular Surgery* **57**, 365–79.

Suki, W., Eknoyan, G., Rector, F.C., and Seldin D.W. (1966). Patterns of nephron perfusion in acute and chronic hydronephrosis. *Journal of Clinical Investigation* **45**, 122–31.

Webb, J.A.W., Reznek, R.H., White, F.E., Cattell, W.R., Kelsey Fry, I., and Baker, L.R.I. (1984). Can ultrasound and computed tomography replace high-dose urography in patients with impaired renal function? *Quarterly Journal of Medicine* **xx**, 411–25.

Whelan, J.S., Reznek, R.H., Daniell, S.J.N., Norton, A.J., Lister, T.A., and Rohatiner, A.S.Z. (1991). Computed tomography (CT) and ultrasound (US) guided core biopsy in the management of non-Hodgkin's lymphoma. *British Journal of Cancer* **63**, 460–2.

Whitaker, R.H. (1990). The diagnosis of upper urinary tract obstruction. *Postgraduate Medical Journal* **66**, (Suppl. 1), 25–30.

Whitfield, H.N., Britton, K.E., Hendry, W.F., and Wickham, J.E.A. (1979). Frusemide intravenous urography in the diagnosis of pelvi-ureteric junction obstruction. *British Journal of Urology* **51**, 445–8.

Whitfield, H.N., Britton, K.E., Nimmon, C.C., Hendry, W.F., Wallace, D.M.A., and Wickham, J.E.A. (1981). Renal transit time measurements in the diagnosis of ureteric obstruction. *British Journal of Urology* **53**, 500–3.

Whitfield, H.N., Mills, V., Miller, R.A., and Wickham, J.E.A. (1983). Percutaneous pyelolysis: An alternative to pyeloplasty. *British Journal of Urology* **55**, 93–6.

Wickham, J.E.A. and Buck, A.C. (ed.) (1990). *Renal tract stone*. Churchill Livingstone, London.

20.11 Hypertension: its effects on the kidney

A. E. G. RAINE

Introduction

Richard Bright observed in postmortem studies at Guy's Hospital over 150 years ago that left ventricular hypertrophy was common in patients with renal scarring and speculated that high blood pressure was a possible factor linking the changes in the heart and kidneys. Hypertension is indeed very common in patients with renal failure, and the reasons for this are discussed in more detail in Chapter 15.28.1. The aim here is to consider the effects of blood pressure on normal renal function, to review how the kidney adapts to systemic hypertension, and to ask in which circumstances hypertension may itself cause significant renal impairment. While there is no debate that accelerated-phase hypertension, characterized by grade III or IV hypertensive retinopathy, may cause severe and sometimes irreversible renal failure, whether or not mild and moderate essential hypertension lead to loss of renal function is much less certain.

Blood pressure and normal kidney function

Pressure natriuresis

The kidney is exquisitely sensitive to changes in systemic arterial pressure, and responds in a number of ways to achieve changes in fluid and electrolyte balance which will maintain circulatory homeostasis and normal blood pressure. First, an acute increase in renal perfusion pressure results in increased urine flow and sodium excretion, the phenomenon of 'pressure natriuresis'. The effect of this is to reduce intravascular volume and hence blood pressure. The increase in sodium excretion is not due to changes in renal blood flow or glomerular filtration rate, since the kidney displays a high degree of autoregulation of blood flow and glomerular filtration rate, which are relatively constant over a rather wide range of systolic blood pressure (80–180 mmHg). Rather, the increase in sodium excretion which occurs as blood pressure increases is due to reduced tubular sodium reabsorption. The mechanism of this is not fully established, but in part is due to increased interstitial hydrostatic pressure, especially in the renal cortex and papilla. In an analogous manner, acute reductions in renal perfusion pressure lead to a marked increase in tubular sodium reabsorption, which will counteract threatened volume depletion.

Renin–angiotensin system

The second means of response of the kidney to changes in blood pressure is through release of renin from the juxtaglomerular cells of the afferent arteriole which are sensitive to stretch and β-adrenergic stimuli and thus respond to rising or falling renal perfusion pressure by decreasing or increasing release of renin. Renin release is also stimulated by reduced delivery of filtered sodium to the macula densa. The sensing mechanism is located in the distal tubule, but adjacent to the juxtaglomerular apparatus.

Renin catalyses the formation of angiotensin I from renin substrate both locally and systemically. Angiotensin I is converted to angiotensin II by the action of angiotensin-converting enzyme, and systemic angiotensin II in turn stimulates release of aldosterone from the adrenal cortex. Local angiotensin II has intrarenal haemodynamic effects and effects on tubular function favouring sodium retention. The systemic renin-angiotensin cascade acts to restore blood pressure and renal perfusion in several ways. Both angiotensin II and aldosterone enhance renal tubular sodium reabsorption, thus increasing exchangeable sodium and intravascular volume. Angiotensin II is also itself a very potent vasoconstrictor. In addition to stimulating renin release, renal sympathetic nerves also directly enhance proximal tubular sodium reabsorption through activation of sodium–hydrogen exchange, an effect mediated by α_2-adrenoceptors.

Other factors

Neurohumoral systems which increase sodium excretion also exist. The best-characterized of these involves atrial natriuretic factor, a peptide hormone synthesized in the cardiac atria and released from them in response to volume expansion and atrial myocyte stretch. Atrial natriuretic factor acts to increase sodium excretion by the kidney through a

variety of actions, which include altered renal arteriolar tone, direct inhibition of papillary sodium reabsorption, and antagonism of the renin–angiotensin system. Other local intrarenal factors, such as vasodilator prostaglandins, endothelium-derived relaxing factor, and endothelin may also contribute to modulation of renal vascular tone and sodium excretion in response to changes in renal arterial pressure and in intravascular volume. Further, each of the above factors—angiotensin II, aldosterone, atrial natriuretic factor, catecholamines, and others—can modify the pressure natriuresis relationship.

These mechanisms normally interact very precisely to adjust renal sodium excretion in response to blood pressure changes, so that a normal set point arterial pressure is maintained, at which sodium balance is achieved. Guyton and colleagues (Fig. 1) were amongst the first to emphasize the fundamental importance of the pressure natriuresis mechanism in long-term blood pressure control, with the important corollary that resetting of pressure natriuresis must (and does) occur in established hypertension—otherwise a state of perpetual negative sodium balance and volume depletion would arise. Resetting of the renal pressure natriuresis mechanism has been confirmed in both human essential hypertension and in a number of experimental models. However, it has been more difficult to establish whether development of impaired pressure natriuresis is itself ever the primary event, initiating sustained hypertension.

Renal function in hypertension

As well as a rightward resetting of the pressure natriuresis relationship, a number of alterations in renal haemodynamics also take place in established uncomplicated essential hypertension. Renal blood flow is reduced and renal vascular resistance is increased. Glomerular filtration rate remains normal, and consequently filtration fraction (the ratio of glomerular filtration rate to renal plasma flow) is increased. Although increased vascular resistance in all tissue beds is a general finding in hypertension, in the case of the kidney it assumes particular significance. The glomerulus is unique in having a portal arterial circulation, and micropuncture studies in genetic models of hypertension, such as the spontaneously hypertensive rat, have shown that there is a balanced increase in resistance of both the afferent and efferent arterioles, so that glomerular capillary hydraulic pressure (P_{GC}), the major determinant of glomerular filtration rate, is maintained at a normal level (Fig. 2). The rarity of development of significant renal impairment in essential hypertension (see below) suggests that similar mechanisms operate in humans; an increase in afferent arteriolar resistance shields the kidney from the damaging effects of high systemic arterial pressure, while a simultaneous increase in efferent arteriolar resistance enables maintenance of normal glomerular filtration pressure.

Hypertension as a cause of renal failure

Despite the apparent protection conferred by renal vasoconstriction in the vast majority of hypertensive patients, there are clinical settings in which hypertension may result in severe or even endstage renal failure. The extent to which serious renal impairment develops in mild and moderate essential hypertension remains controversial. In contrast, there is no doubting the ability of accelerated hypertension to cause major renal dysfunction. The potential of coexisting hypertension to accelerate loss of renal function caused by underlying renal disease has now, too, become well established.

Essential hypertension

Essential hypertension in the so-called 'benign' phase appears to cause far less damage to the kidney than to other target organs such as the heart and brain. In contrast to left ventricular hypertrophy, for example,

Fig. 1 Renal function curves illustrating the normal pressure natriuresis relationship and resetting of the relationship in essential hypertension. A is the arterial pressure at which sodium balance is maintained in a normal subject. B is the corresponding arterial pressure in hypertension. (Reproduced from Guyton *et al.* 1972, with permission.)

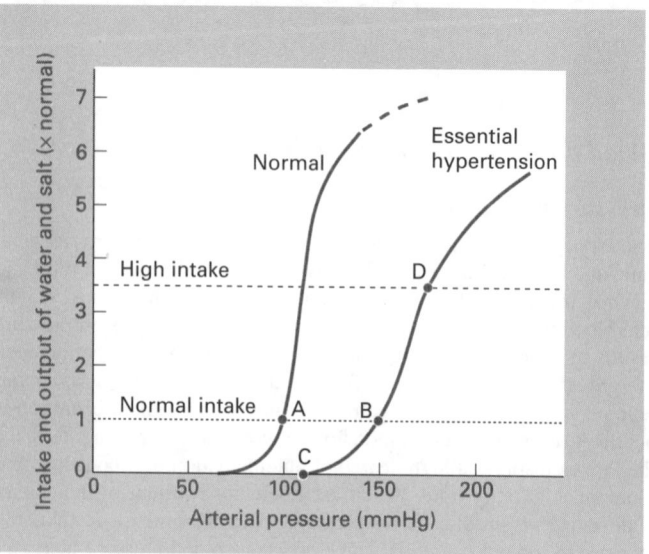

which occurs frequently even in mild hypertension, significant renal dysfunction is very rare in uncomplicated essential hypertension. Estimates in Caucasian populations have suggested that the relative risk of developing renal failure in primary hypertension is of the order of 1 in 6000 cases. The true incidence is probably even lower; many patients who present with severe renal failure and hypertension and are given a diagnosis of 'hypertensive nephrosclerosis' do not undergo histological examination by renal biopsy to exclude an underlying primary renal disease such as glomerulonephritis.

For reasons that remain unclear, hypertension appears to lead to progressive renal impairment much more frequently in patients of African or Afro-Caribbean origin, some American surveys suggesting that the relative risk of endstage renal failure due to hypertension in these patients is 18 times that of Caucasian patients. This racial difference in morbidity persists even when equal and adequate blood pressure control is achieved, implying the existence of genetic or environmental factors to account for it.

Fig. 2 Representation of glomerular haemodynamics: (a) normal; (b) essential hypertension, afferent and efferent arteriolar resistances are increased, P_{GC} (glomerular capillary hydraulic pressure) and GFR (glomerular filtration rate) remain normal; and (c) chronic renal failure (surviving nephron), systemic hypertension is transmitted to the glomerulus, P_{GC} and GFR are increased.

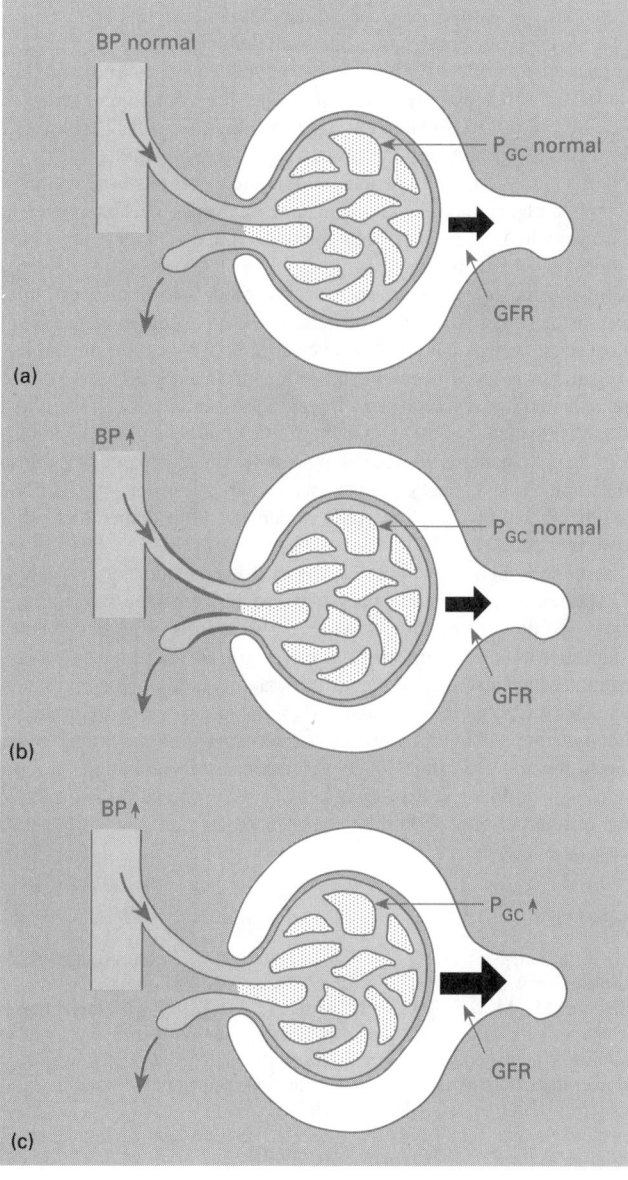

Both hypertension and a gradual and relatively modest decline in renal function due to glomerulosclerosis are common accompaniments of ageing. The renal microscopic appearances in the elderly are very similar to those of 'hypertensive' nephrosclerosis, with renal vascular changes including medial hypertrophy and reduplication of the internal elastic lamina. Hypertension, like hyperlipidaemia and smoking, is a major risk factor for both large-vessel and microvascular atherosclerotic disease. It appears likely that, in the elderly, essential hypertension sustained over many years results in significant atherosclerotic narrowing of intrarenal small vessels, and an ischaemic nephropathy with an increased rate of glomerulosclerosis. These changes need to be distinguished from renal dysfunction arising purely as a consequence of increased renal arterial pressure. This appears to be very rare indeed in mild and moderate primary hypertension, but in contrast, pressure-related damage to the kidney is characteristic of accelerated hypertension.

Accelerated hypertension

In accelerated phase (malignant) hypertension, caused by a rapid and severe increase in blood pressure and characterized by the presence of retinal haemorrhages and exudates and/or papilloedema in the optic fundi, renal involvement is very common. Kincaid-Smith and colleagues found that 73 of a series of 89 patients documented in the 1950s had impaired renal function at presentation, and uraemia was by far the commonest cause of death, at a time when maintenance dialysis was not available. Impairment of renal function at presentation, together with lack of adequate blood pressure control achieved during treatment, remain the most important adverse prognostic indicators in accelerated hypertension even today.

Animal studies have established that the changes in the optic fundi in accelerated hypertension are due to loss of retinal vessel autoregulation, and resultant overperfusion and increase in transmural pressure. Endothelial integrity is lost in dilated segments of arterioles, with leakage of plasma constituents and fibrin deposition in vessel walls, forming the characteristic 'fibrinoid necrosis'. Such changes result in ischaemic and hyperperfusion damage in the territory served by affected vessels. Similar changes are likely to occur in the renal vasculature, leading to the fibrinoid necrosis seen in afferent arterioles and the glomerular tuft in accelerated hypertension. The other characteristic pathological change

Fig. 3 Proliferative endarteritis of an interlobular artery in malignant hypertension. The arrow shows a severely narrowed arterial lumen: I, arterial intima with gross proliferative change and 'onion-skin' appearance; M, arterial media; T, tubulointerstitial fibrosis. (By courtesy of Dr A.J. d'Ardenne.)

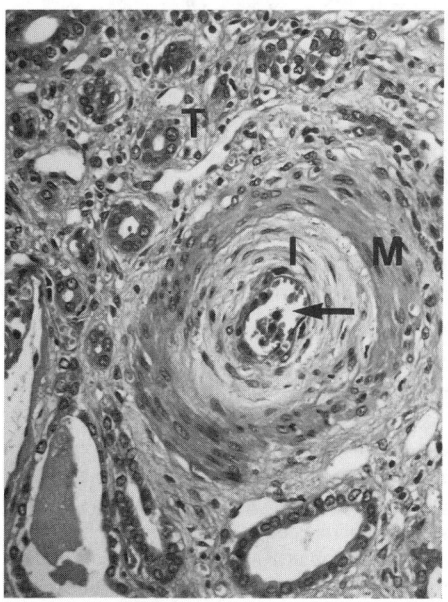

observed is a proliferative endarteritis of interlobular arteries (Fig. 3). It is likely that local release of mitogens, such as angiotensin II and endothelin, arising from endothelial injury promote this proliferation, although it is not yet known which are involved. The resulting narrowing or obliteration of the arterial lumen causes both glomerular and tubulointerstitial ischaemia and fibrosis (Fig. 3), with resulting loss of renal function.

Effective treatment of accelerated hypertension with potent antihypertensive therapy, combined with the availability of dialysis support if required, has transformed the previously bleak outlook for this condition. The goal is a gradual reduction in blood pressure to a level of 160 to 170/100 to 110 mmHg over a 24-h period, to avoid the risk of cerebral ischaemia. This is often best achieved with an intravenous infusion of sodium nitroprusside (0.5–3.0 μg/kg.min) or of labetalol (2 mg/min), although oral agents such as calcium-channel blockers have proved equally safe and effective. The long-term outlook for recovery of renal function is good if serum creatinine is 300 μmol/l or less at presentation, but patients with more marked initial renal impairment often progress to endstage renal failure, despite adequate blood pressure control.

Hypertension and progressive renal impairment

It is now generally accepted that when hypertension is present and uncontrolled in chronic renal failure it accelerates the rate of loss of renal function, and it is remarkable how greatly perceptions of this problem have altered. Until relatively recently, the consensus was that patients with chronic renal failure and hypertension who were free of serious complications required no treatment; indeed an elevated renal perfusion pressure was believed to help preserve the scarred and failing kidney. These beliefs were discarded in part because of experimental studies. These showed that when secondary hypertension, created for example by renal arterial clipping, was superimposed on kidney disease such as immune complex nephritis, the rate of loss of renal function was greatly increased. These observations led to suggestions that reduction in the number of functioning nephrons, by whatever disease process, would lead to adaptive alterations in renal vascular resistance, resulting in increased blood flow and transmission of systemic hypertension to the glomerulus in surviving nephrons (Fig. 2). The resulting glomerular capillary hypertension and hyperperfusion might then lead to increased proteinuria and ultimately to glomerular scarring. Micropuncture studies of glomerular haemodynamics in animal models of diabetic nephropathy and renal ablation nephropathy have shown that, here also, increases in systemic blood pressure are transmitted to the glomerulus and result in increased transcapillary hydraulic pressure and glomerular hyperfiltration. Brenner has argued that these latter haemodynamic changes may be a major factor in progressive renal impairment.

It appears likely now that other changes, such as glomerular hypertrophy and elaboration of growth factors within the glomerular mesangium, may play a role as important as glomerular hypertension, if not more so, in progressive glomerulosclerosis. However, further evidence for the direct or indirect influence of increased renal arterial pressure has been provided by a variety of experimental studies in models of chronic renal failure, in which blood pressure reduction resulted in preservation of renal structure and function, together with restoration of normal glomerular haemodynamics. Are these findings applicable to human disease?

Antihypertensive therapy and renal function

Most large-scale, controlled studies of mild and moderate hypertension have not been able to demonstrate any beneficial effect of treatment on renal function, since there is such a low incidence of renal dysfunction as a complication of essential hypertension in the malignant phase. Perhaps the most convincing clinical evidence has come from trials of antihypertensive therapy in patients with diabetic nephropathy. In patients with type 1 diabetes, the worsening of both incipient nephropathy with 'microalbuminuria' (urinary albumin excretion of 30–300 mg/24 h) and of established diabetic nephropathy with renal impairment appear to be retarded by effective antihypertensive therapy (see Chapter 20.5.1).

The benefit has, to date, been particularly apparent for converting enzyme inhibitors, and this is believed to relate to the ability of these agents to blunten angiotensin II-mediated efferent arteriolar constriction, thus reducing glomerular capillary pressure. The outcome of further trials of antihypertensive treatment, both in patients with diabetic nephropathy and in those with other forms of renal disease, is awaited. Nevertheless, there are already sufficient grounds for recommending that in all patients with progressive renal dysfunction, the aim should be to reduce arterial pressure to less than 140/90 mmHg whenever possible. Converting enzyme inhibitors may confer a particular benefit, although this is by no means proven, and caution with these agents is required in the presence of known or suspected renovascular disease (see Chapter 15.28.1).

The kidney and the pathogenesis of hypertension

The apparent normality of glomerular filtration rate and renal function in uncomplicated essential hypertension has, in some respects, diverted attention from the accumulation of evidence that the kidney is centrally involved in the pathogenesis of primary hypertension. For example, increased renal vasoconstriction has been demonstrated in young subjects who are normotensive but have two hypertensive parents, and thus are at risk of developing hypertension in later life. More direct evidence comes from cross-transplantation experiments in several different animal models of primary hypertension, which have shown that transplantation of a kidney from a hypertensive donor to a normotensive recipient confers hypertension on the recipient, and vice versa. This phenomenon still occurs when development of hypertension in the donor is prevented by antihypertensive therapy.

Although the relevance of such animal models to human essential hypertension remains a matter of debate, there is some evidence from clinical renal transplantation that reversal of both hypertension and target organ damage may occur when a kidney from a normotensive donor is transplanted into a recipient with previous essential hypertension. An increased prevalence of essential hypertension has been observed in parents of diabetic patients who develop nephropathy, compared with those who do not. Thus, a genetic predisposition to hypertension may increase the vulnerability of the glomerulus to damage from diabetes or other disease processes.

If an underlying renal abnormality is the fundamental cause of essential hypertension, its precise nature has so far remained tantalizingly elusive. We do not yet know whether certain forms of primary hypertension, such as occur in those of African origin, are conferred by genetic variations which also increase renal vulnerability to high blood pressure, or whether it is more the case that early renal disease leads to intrarenal haemodynamic adaptations which render surviving nephrons more prone to the adverse effects of hypertension in certain patient groups. What is not in doubt is that treatment of raised arterial pressure in all forms of renal disease should be commenced as early as possible, and it must be effective.

REFERENCES

Baldwin, S. and Neugarten, J. (1985). Treatment of hypertension in renal disease. *American Journal of Kidney Diseases* **5**, A57–A70.

Brenner, B.M., Meyer, T.W., and Hostetter, T.H. (1982). Dietary protein intake and the progressive nature of kidney disease: the role of hemodynamically mediated glomerular injury in the pathogenesis of progressive glomerular sclerosis in aging, renal ablation, and intrinsic renal disease. *New England Journal of Medicine* **307**, 652–60.

Brown, M.A. and Whitworth, J.A. (1992). Hypertension in human renal disease. *Journal of Hypertension* **10**, 701–12.

Cusi, D. and Bianchi, G. (1991). The kidney in the pathogenesis of hypertension. *Seminars in Nephrology* **11**, 523–37.

De Wardener, H.E. (1990). The primary role of the kidney and salt intake in the aetiology of essential hypertension. *Clinical Science* **79**, 193–200.

Guyton, A.C. (1992). Kidneys and fluids in pressure regulation. *Hypertension* **19**, (Suppl. 1), I-2–I-8.

Guyton, A.C., Coleman, T.G., Cowley, A.W., Scheel, K.W., Manning, R.D., and Norman, R.A. (1972). Arterial pressure regulation; over-riding dominance of the kidneys in long-term regulation and in hypertension. *American Journal of Medicine* **52**, 584–94.

Kincaid-Smith, P. (1991). Malignant hypertension. *Journal of Hypertension* **9**, 893–9.

Klahr, S. (1989). The kidney in hypertension—villain or victim? *New England Journal of Medicine* **320**, 731–3.

Lewis, E.J., Hunsickler, L.G., Bain, R.P., and Rohde, R.D. (1993). The effect of angiotensin-converting-enzyme inhibition on diabetic nephropathy. *New England Journal of Medicine*, **329**, 1456–62.

Rostand, S.G., Brown, G., Kirk, K.A., Rutsky, E.A., and Dustan, H.P. (1989). Renal insufficiency in treated essential hypertension. *New England Journal of Medicine* **320**, 684–8.

Van Hooft, I.M.S., Grobbee, D.E., Derkx, F.H.M., de Leeuw, P.W., Schalekamp, M.A.D.H., and Hofman, A.H. (1991). Renal haemodynamics and the renin–angiotensin–aldosterone system in normotensive subjects with hypertensive and normotensive parents. *New England Journal of Medicine* **324**, 1305–11.

20.12 Urinary stone disease (urolithiasis)

R. W. E. WATTS

INTRODUCTION

A urinary stone (calculus) consists of crystal aggregates with a small amount of associated protein and glycoprotein matrix material. Stones form in the urine outside the renal parenchyma and the smallest crystal aggregates probably begin within the collecting ducts. The term 'nephrocalcinosis' refers to the deposition of calcium salts in the renal parenchyma and this may be associated with urolithiasis.

EPIDEMIOLOGY

Urolithiasis is a common worldwide problem; Table 1 shows its high incidence in the United Kingdom. Many cases were previously regarded as being idiopathic when they were, in fact, due to the operation of multiple small but additive risk factors. The stone recurrence rate in such cases approaches 70 per cent after 10 years.

A view of the problem of urolithiasis in an international and historical context, suggests that overall socioeconomic development is associated with a decrease in childhood bladder stone disease and a progressive increase in renal stone disease in adults. The bladder stone disease in children which is hyperendemic in some countries resembles that seen in Europe in earlier times. X-ray crystallography has shown that in these cases calcium oxalate, ammonium urate, and uric acid were, and still are, the main stone components. Urate stones predominate in some parts of the Middle East, India, and North Africa. Calcium oxalate stones are most common in some parts of south-east Asia, although ammonium urate, calcium oxalate, and calcium phosphate stones occur in all areas. Calcium oxalate or mixed calcium oxalate and calcium phosphate renal stones in adults predominate in Europe, North America, Australasia, and South Africa.

Epidemiological studies suggest that urolithiasis is a hazard of both affluence and deprivation. The overall composition of the diet appears to be important in both groups: high protein, high carbohydrate diets appear to increase the risk of upper urinary tract calcium oxalate stones in the relatively affluent industrial societies; and protein deprivation, although not protein–calorie malnutrition (kwashiorkor), increases this risk in developing regions. 'Stone waves' (epidemics of urinary stone occurrence) in Europe during times of extreme deprivation after major wars have been well documented.

The cause of the extremely high incidence of pure calcium oxalate bladder stones in boys in Northern Thailand and adjacent areas is a special case. Here the practice of partly replacing breast milk with pre-

Table 1 *Incidence of urinary stones in the United Kingdom*

Patients discharged from hospital with diagnosis of stones	1.8 per 10 000
Incidence of stones in general practice	7 per 10 000
General practice incidence of stones in males aged 45–60 years	21 per 10 000

masticated glutinous rice (*Oryza glutinosa*) from the early neonatal period increases urinary oxalate excretion, partly because the rice contains a large amount of hydroxyproline, which is metabolized to glyoxylate and hence to oxalate. It also decreases fluid intake and urine volume and lowers urinary phosphate. The Thai villagers eat leafy vegetables which are a direct source of additional dietary oxalate. It has been shown that lowered urinary phosphate excretion favours calcium oxalate crystallization and microlith formation, and supplementing the infants' diet with orthophosphate reduces the incidence of stone formation in the very young children of this region. The mechanisms by which orthophosphate may reduce stone formation are discussed below. Inadequate milk-feeding in infancy was recognized as being associated with urinary stones in childhood in England during the early nineteenth century.

Except for occupations likely to cause underhydration and increased vitamin D biosynthesis due to prolonged exposure to sunlight, industrial exposure to beryllium and cadmium are the only well-recognized industrial hazards associated with an increased incidence of urinary stone. The potassium-sparing diuretic triamterine has been reported as either the sole constituent of urinary stones or mixed with calcium oxalate. Pure triamterine stones are radiotranslucent.

PATHOPHYSIOLOGY

Calcium-containing stones are the commonest type in the United Kingdom (Table 2). Even apparently pure calcium oxalate stones commonly contain a small central core of calcium phosphate or uric acid. This is due to the phenomenon of epitaxy, whereby a crystal can grow on a chemically different crystal because, in one or more particular orientations of the two crystals, there is a nearly geometrically accurate fit between the parts that are in contact.

Apart from stasis due to chronic urinary tract obstruction and infection, the main factors that predispose to stone formation are the urine

Table 2 *The composition of a series of approximately 1000 present-day renal calculi studied at the Institute of Urology, London (data kindly supplied by Dr G.A. Rose, Institute of Urology, London, England)*

Type of stone	Whole sample (%)	Adult	
		Males (%)	Females (%)
Pure calcium oxalate	39.4	47.9	22.2
Mixed calcium oxalate/phosphate	13.8	16.0	9.4
Magnesium ammonium phosphate	15.4	8.1	35.1
Stones which were virtually wholly composed of calcium and phosphate	13.2	11.3	17.8
Mixed stones containing: calcium, magnesium, ammonium, oxalate, phosphate, and uric acid	6.4	6.0	8.4
All or predominantly uric acid	8.0	8.9	1.0
Cystine	2.8	1.5	5.9
Total:	99.0	99.7	99.8

volume and overall composition of the urine in terms of potential stone-forming substances and the pH. The role of physiological inhibitors of crystallization is difficult to evaluate and attempts to measure the protective power of urine with respect to crystallization have not gained general application.

In normal urine, nephrocalcin is an acidic glycoprotein rich in γ-carboxyglutamic acid which inhibits calcium oxalate crystal growth. The nephrocalcin present in the organic matrix of calcium oxalate kidney stones resembles that present in the urine of the patient from whom the stone was removed but it differs from the nephrocalcin in normal urine. The stone-former's nephrocalcin lacks γ-carboxyglutamic acid residues and forms air–water interfacial films that are less stable than those formed by nephrocalcin from normal urine. The results of other studies suggesting a role for stone matrix in the genesis of urinary stones have been less clear cut. For instance, it has been proposed that the Tamm–Horsfall glycoprotein may aggregate and precipitate in the renal tubule, and is then made permanently insoluble by desialylation. The precipitated glycoprotein (uromucoid) might form microcalculi by enmeshing microcrystals of calcium oxalate and calcium phosphate. The microcalculi could then migrate to the pelvicalyceal system and grow into stones.

Differences in glycosaminoglycan (mucopolysaccharide) composition of the matrix in different stone types have been reported and correlated with the propensity of the glycosaminoglycans to promote or inhibit stone formation, hyaluronic acid and heparan sulphate favouring stone formation and chondroitin sulphate having a protective action. It has not yet been possible to extend this work into the clinical arena, either by means of chemical analysis to produce prognostic data based on glycosaminoglycan composition, or as a basis for modifying their concentrations therapeutically. Citrate and pyrophosphate ions are also physiological inhibitors of crystallization in urine.

The urine of those not forming stones is in such a physicochemical state that although crystallization of stone-forming salts will not begin spontaneously it is likely to progress once it has been initiated. This arises because the concentrations of the ions that contribute to calcium-containing stones are such that the activity products for octacalcium phosphate, hydroxyapatite, calcium oxalate, and magnesium ammonium phosphate are between their solubility products and their formation products, or at the most only a little below their formation products. In the case of urine, the calculation is complicated in order to allow for all the possible interacting ion species, some of which are not stone-constituents. Calcium oxalate is the salt which is most likely to precipitate from normal urine on the basis of physicochemical criteria, and this agrees with the clinical observation that calcium oxalate is the commonest constituent of urinary stones. Brushite ($CaHPO_4 2H_2O$) is the most likely salt to crystallize from persistently acidic urine.

Small postprandial and diurnal variations in the urinary calcium and oxalate excretions, as well as longer-term cyclic and seasonal variations occur. These can be quite small in absolute terms, but exert a marked effect on the degree of urine saturation.

The increased calcium and oxalate excretion in the summer months, with low values in the winter, are not associated with seasonal variations in the urine pH, volume, creatinine, phosphate, or magnesium excretion. These changes depend only on the seasonal variations in calcium and oxalate excretion. They are thought to reflect increased vitamin D synthesis in the skin during the summer months, which correlates with the 50 per cent higher rate of stone formation by recurrent stone-formers in the summer than in the winter. The diurnal variations in the degree of urine saturation due to changes in urine flow-rate, pH, and calcium and oxalate excretion, are superimposed on the seasonal variations. The diurnal and seasonal factors summate to increase the liability to crystallization at certain times in a 24-h cycle and emphasize that those forming calcium-containing stones, like other patients with urolithiasis, must maintain a water diuresis.

Decreasing the calcium intake only may actually increase the degree of urine saturation with respect to calcium oxalate by allowing more oxalate to be absorbed and therefore excreted. This arises because the oxalate ion has a greater effect than the calcium ion on the activity product that determines the degree of urine saturation (see below).

Most calcium-containing stones are of multifactorial origin. Epidemiological and urinary influences summate in different degrees and combinations in individual patients. The epidemiological risk factors include age, sex, occupation, overall nutritional status, diet, fluid intake, climate, and the presence of specific metabolic disorders. The urinary risk factors are high concentrations of calcium, oxalate, and uric acid in urine, lack of the normal diurnal rhythm of urinary pH, deficiency of crystallization-inhibiting glycosaminoglycans, and a low urine volume. Of these, the urine volume and the urinary oxalate excretion are the most important.

If genetic factors operate in the aetiology of the vast majority of idiopathic urinary stones, they do so in a multifactorial manner. However, there have been reports of families in which a rare syndrome comprising calcium containing urinary stones with renal tubular dysfunction beginning in childhood and progressing to nephrocalcinosis with renal failure in adult life has segregated in an X-linked recessive manner. Genetic linkage studies have shown linkage between the syndrome and a locus in the pericentric region of the short arm of the X-chromosome (Xq 11-22). Families in which an autosomal dominantly inherited factor may be operating, and in which the operation of a common environmental factor appears unlikely, are also very occasionally encountered.

CLINICAL DIAGNOSIS OF URINARY STONES

Urinary stones may be either clinically silent or they may present as summarized in Table 3. Pain due to urinary stones is either a dull ache in the renal angle due to pelvicalyceal distension, or colicky (ureteric colic) in the lateral part of the abdomen, classically radiating from the loin to the groin, perineum, scrotum, or penis. An attack of ureteric colic is often associated with retching and vomiting. Stones sometimes migrate down the ureter without pain and are occasionally passed *per urethram* with little or no discomfort. A history of recurrent urinary infections, which relapse after treatment, suggests the presence of a predisposing anatomical abnormality of the urinary tract, and this is commonly a stone. Occasional patients present with fever and rigors due to severe infection proximal to an obstructing calculus. Those with impacted bilateral ureteric stones present with acute oliguric renal failure and uraemia. Small stones that are voided spontaneously are generally composed of calcium oxalate, the larger calcium-containing stones which need removal usually contain appreciable amounts of phosphate. Predominantly phosphatic stones indicate past or present urinary tract infection.

Urolithiasis presents four diagnostic problems:

(1) the differentiation of the presenting symptoms from other types of renal disease and other causes of acute abdominal pain;

(2) the differential diagnosis of patients with calculus anuria or oliguria;

(3) the differentiation of the different types of urinary stone from one another;

(4) aetiology.

Renal colic has to be differentiated from other causes of acute abdominal pain: notably intestinal colic, appendicitis, biliary colic, torsion of an ovarian cyst, or ruptured ectopic pregnancy. Presentation with asymptomatic proteinuria may lead to initial confusion with chronic glomerulonephritis or chronic pyelonephritis. Painless haematuria with little proteinuria suggests a renal tract neoplasm rather than a stone, and haematuria with heavy proteinuria suggests glomerulonephritis. A history beginning with increased frequency of micturition, accompanied by sterile pyuria, and mild proteinuria (especially if the urine is acidic) will suggest renal tract tuberculosis as the provisional diagnosis, although such a picture can be produced by a stone, particularly if it is impacted in the intramural part of the ureter, causing bladder irritation. Anuria due to bilateral stone impaction (calculus anuria) may be preceded by remarkably little pain as the stones move down the ureter. The presence of a single, functionless kidney can sometimes be traced retrospectively to such a painless obstructive episode. Calculus anuria and oliguria have to be distinguished from the prerenal, renal, and other postrenal causes of acute renal failure.

Calcium oxalate stones are characteristically spiky and discoloured by altered blood, whereas phosphatic stones are generally larger, smoother, and more friable. Cystine stones are pale yellow and look crystalline. Xanthine stones are smooth, brownish yellow, and rather soft. The composition of urinary stones is markedly altered by complicating urinary infections. For example, a cystinuric patient may pass magnesium ammonium phosphate stones as well as cystine stones if there has been much infection. Similarly, the stone matrix which remains after a cystine stone has been dissolved medically may provide the basis on which a calcium oxalate stone develops subsequently.

IMAGING INVESTIGATIONS

The range of techniques available for the investigation of the kidneys and lower urinary tract are discussed in Chapter 20.1. Patients present-

Table 3 *Urinary stones: clinical presentations*

Pain
Ureteric colic
Lumbar ache
On micturition
Haematuria
Sterile pyuria
Asymptomatic proteinuria
Dysuria and increased urinary frequency
Urinary tract infections
Acute (single or recurrent attack)
Chronic
Pyonephrosis
Calculus anuria
Strangury and interruption of urine stream

ing with acute abdominal pain suggesting renal colic require immediate plain abdominal radiography with tomography and ultrasound examination, the latter to detect any degree of hydronephrosis or hydroureter. If these examinations leave the diagnosis in doubt, early intravenous urography may demonstrate lesser function on the side of the lesion and/or show evidence of a filling defect or spasm of the ureter around any very small calculus. If renal function is too poor to produce a pyelogram, and ultrasound shows evidence of hydronephrosis, the obstructive lesion is well shown by percutaneous antegrade pyelography, and this technique also allows nephrostomy when indicated by severe obstruction. Computed tomography (CT) and magnetic resonance imaging (MRI) scanning are also useful in those with renal failure in whom high-dose intravenous urography is inappropriate or ineffective. These last techniques are also particularly indicated when it is suspected that ureteric obstruction may be caused by enlarged retroperitoneal lymph nodes, retroperitoneal fibrosis, or other extraureteric obstructive lesions.

Intravenous urography and other imaging investigations after the acute episode show the overall state of the urinary tract and any persistent obstructive lesion, but they do not demonstrate the small stones which may have passed easily because the local spasm has relaxed.

Uric acid, xanthine, and dihydroxyadenine stones are characteristically radiolucent. The chemical nature and cause of the radio-opaque stones (that is, calcium-, cystine-, and silica-containing stones) cannot be established by their radiographic appearance. The presence of multiple stones detected simultaneously, especially if they are bilateral, is generally held to indicate that they are likely to arise from a metabolic cause. However, the presence of a single stone does not contraindicate investigation to identify a specific cause, although many patients repeatedly form stones for reasons which cannot be identified at present.

Table 4 summarizes the radiographic and other imaging results in patients presenting with renal colic. The causes of nephrocalcinosis are listed in Table 5.

BIOCHEMICAL INVESTIGATIONS

The minimum biochemical evaluation for a patient with urolithiasis is: (1) analysis, preferably quantitative, of the stone; (2) microbiological and microscopic examination of the urine; (3) measurement of serum calcium, phosphorus, creatinine, total protein, and albumin; (4) a qualitative test for urinary cystine; (5) measurement of the pH of the first morning urine, which should be in the pH range 5.3 to 6.8, as a screen for possible renal tubular acidosis (see Section 20.19); and (6) measurement of the 24-h excretion of oxalate, calcium, creatinine, and uric acid with the patient ambulant and taking a usual diet and fluid intake. A more comprehensive scheme of investigation is summarized in Table 6.

Although high dietary intake of vitamins C (an oxalate precursor) and D, animal protein, dairy products, oxalate, and calcium, and a low-fibre

Table 4 *Diagnostic imaging findings in patients presenting with renal colic*

Obstructive uropathy due to:
  Radio-opaque stone[a]
  Radiotranslucent obstructive lesion (stone[b], crystals, sloughed papillae, clots, carcinoma)
Generalized nephrocalcinosis[c]
Medullary sponge kidney
Adult polycystic kidney disease
Renal papillary necrosis (± sloughed papilla)
Cortical scars due to chronic pyelonephritis
Renal carcinoma (source of 'clot colic')
Coincidental calcific lesions (e.g. tuberculosis, Randall's plaques)

[a]Sites of calcific lesions which may be confused with radio-opaque calculi: gallstones, costal cartilages, mesenteric lymph nodes, adrenals, pancreas, renal and splenic arteries, pelvic veins.

[b]The radiotranslucent stones are: uric acid, xanthine 2,8-dihydroxyadenine, orotic acid, triamterin.

[c]Finely stippled nephrocalcinosis suggests long-standing hypercalaemia. Dense, coarse nephrocalcinosis suggests primary hyperoxaluria or renal tubular acidosis.

Table 5 *Causes of generalized nephrocalcinosis*

Mainly medullary (usual location)
  Primary hyperparathyroidism
  Idiopathic hypercalciuria
  Primary renal tubular acidosis
  Hypervitaminosis D
  Milk alkali syndrome
  Primary hyperoxaluria
  Sarcoidosis
  Chronic berylliosis
  Thyrotoxicosis
  Sulphonamide injury
Mainly cortical (very rare)
  Chronic glomerulonephritis
  Renal cortical necrosis ('tram-line' calcification)

diet have been suggested as causes or important contributors to recurrent stone formation. The evidence that they individually play a major role is difficult to establish in most cases. However, a dietary history is important in order to detect any gross excess. It is more important to assess customary fluid intake and urinary volume.

Table 7 summarizes the diagnostic experience of a large London-based stone clinic. The importance of chronic underhydration, even in a temperate climate, is apparent. When hypercalcaemia is detected with or without the symptoms listed in Table 8, slit-lamp examinations of the eye to detect circumcorneal calcification is an important part of the physical examination, giving some indication of the chronicity of the hypercalcaemia.

The many causes of sustained hypercalcaemia include primary hyperparathyroidism, sarcoidosis, multiple myelomatosis and other malignancies, hypervitaminosis D, and more rarely, thiazide diuretic therapy, familial hypocalciuric hypercalcaemia, thyrotoxicosis, lithium therapy, the milk alkali syndrome, Addison's disease, Cushing's syndrome, and chronic granulomatous diseases other than sarcoidosis. Hypercalcaemia in association with acromegaly raises the possibility of a pluriglandular syndrome with hyperthyroidism.

Table 6 *Detailed investigation of patients presenting with urinary stones*

Stone analysis:	Calcium, magnesium, ammonium, carbonate, oxalate, urate, cystine, xanthine, 2,8,-dihydroxyadenine[a], orotic acid[a]
Blood analysis:	(Collect fasting, recumbent, without venous occlusion)
	Calcium, phosphorus, total protein, albumin, plasma protein electrophoresis and quantitative immunoelectrophoresis, uric acid, alkaline phosphatase, urea, creatinine, sodium, potassium, bicarbonate, chloride
Urine analysis:	Calcium[b], urate, oxalate, creatinine (24-h excretion)
	pH[c] after NH_4Cl load (0.1 g/kg body-weight)
	Qualitative test for cystine
	Tests for xanthine if serum uric acid > 59 μmol/l (1 mg/100 ml)[a]
	Immunoelectrophoresis of any urinary protein
Others:	Chest radiograph, full blood count, erythrocyte sedimentation rate

[a]Only rarely needed.

[b]These measurements should be made with the patient taking his usual diet. They should be repeated on more than one occasion. The urinary creatinine assesses the consistency of the 24-h urine collections and allows the creatinine clearance to be calculated. Measuring the urine uric acid secretion after 5 days on a purine-free diet will identify uric acid overexcreters and therefore some of the patients with an excessive rate of uric acid synthesis.

[c]Measure urine pH hourly from 08.00 to 18.00 hours, give NH_4Cl at 10.00 hours. A urine pH of 5.2 should be achieved.

Table 7 *Final diagnosis in 708 patients with urolithiasis attending the Stone Clinic at the Institute of Urology, London (modified from Embon et al. 1990)*

Cause	No. of patients	%
Idiopathic hypercalciuria	230	32.5
Chronic dehydration	132	18.6
Medullary sponge kidney	95	13.4
Urinary tract infection	52	7.3
Primary hyperparathyroidism	41	5.8
Cystinuria	28	4.0
Uric acid stones	26	3.7
High dietary oxalate	26	3.7
Renal tubular acidosis	21	3.0
Secondary hyperoxaluria	13	1.8
Primary hyperoxaluria[a]	15	2.1
Miscellaneous (immobilization, gout, Paget's disease)	29	4.1
Total	708	100

[a] This figure includes the group of patients which Embon *et al.* (1990) refer to as having mild metabolic hyperoxaluria but which may be mild variants of primary hyperoxaluria type I (alanine–glyoxylate aminotransferase (AGT: EC 2.6.1.44) deficiency). Assay of AGT on liver tissue obtained by a percutaneous needle biopsy would be needed to establish this.

Table 8 *Systemic symptoms of hypercalcaemia*

Neuropsychiatric
    Depression
    Irritability
    Malaise
    Muscle weakness
    Confusion and coma
Gastrointestinal
    Anorexia
    Nausea and vomiting
    Abdominal pain (acute pancreatitis)
Renal
    Polyuria
    Polydipsia

PRIMARY HYPERPARATHYROIDISM AND URINARY STONES

Primary hyperparathyroidism is responsible for 5 to 10 per cent of cases of calcium-containing urinary stones and about 50 per cent of patients with primary hyperparathyroidism have urolithiasis. The diagnosis of primary hyperparathyroidism has been greatly simplified by the development of reliable two-site immunoradiometric assays for the parathyroid hormone (PTH), and in that context can be made biochemically by the demonstration of a level of circulating PTH which is inappropriately high for the prevailing plasma calcium concentration. This should be adjusted for the effect of the prevailing plasma albumin concentration. The adjusted calcium concentration should be altered up or down by 0.02 mmol/l (0.8 mg/100 ml) for each deviation of 1.0 g/l of plasma albumin from the mean normal value of 47 g/l. A mild degree of hyperchloraemic acidosis commonly occurs in primary hyperparathyroidism. Measurements of cAMP excretion, the tubular reabsorption of phosphate, and hydrocortisone suppression tests are now superflurous. Caution is needed in interpreting the results of some parathyroid hormone assays in the presence of renal failure. When a diagnosis of primary hyperparathyroidism has been made, the possibility that it might be either part of a multiple endocrine adenomatosis syndrome or one of the rare autosomal dominantly inherited forms should always be considered.

IDIOPATHIC HYPERCALCIURIA AND URINARY STONES

When renal stones are accompanied by high urinary calcium excretion rates and plasma calcium concentrations are normal, idiopathic hypercalciuria may be diagnosed. This is an important apparent cause of urinary calculi, but there are difficulties with this diagnosis as excretion rates vary across countries; healthy young men may excrete apparently excessive amounts of calcium without forming stones; and excessive excretion of oxalate may be more commonly associated with recurrent urolithiasis than calcium. A commonly accepted upper limit of the normal level of calcium excretion is 7.5 mmol per day.

Urinary calcium excretion much over 7.5 mmol in 24 h accompanied by urinary stones is commonly treated by thiazide diuretics, which increase renal tubular reabsorption of calcium and thus reduce hypercalciuria. Amiloride also reduces urinary calcium and can be used with thiazides to reduce the likelihood of hypokalaemia. There may then be a rise in plasma calcium, but this is rarely a problem. There is also a disputed case for the use of sodium cellulose phosphate, which, by binding calcium in the gut, reduces calcium absorption; but this manoeuvre may increase urinary oxalate and may cause diarrhoea and milky, offensive stools (see below). It is more important than either of these approaches to be sure of a sufficiently high fluid intake to reduce urinary calculi concentration.

Some cases of medullary sponge kidney have hypercalciuria and/or inability to acidify their urine normally. Hypercalciuria is also sometimes associated with type 1 (distal) renal tubular acidosis. These associations increase the likelihood of stone formation. The renal tubular dysfunction in chronic cadmium poisoning, berylliosis, and Wilson's disease may also cause normocalcaemic hypercalciuria. Although it classically causes hypercalcaemia, sarcoidosis can also be associated with normocalcaemic hypercalciuria. Hyperuricaemia, occasional aminoaciduria, and mild hypophosphataemia associated with idiopathic hypercalciuria may be attributable to renal tubular dysfunction caused by the hypercalciuria.

INTESTINAL DISEASE AND URINARY STONES

Two groups of patients with intestinal disease are predisposed to urolithiasis because of their primary disease. Continuous loss of alkaline intestinal secretions from an ileostomy and in chronic diarrhoea makes the urine concentrated and persistently acid. This predisposes to uric acid stone formation. Malabsorption due to diffuse small intestine disease or resection leaves increased concentrations of long-chain fatty acids in the bowel lumen. These bind calcium, leaving oxalate ions available for absorption and excretion in the urine. This predisposes to hyperoxaluria and to calcium oxalate urolithiasis.

TREATMENT

The treatment of urinary stones has been revolutionized by the development of non-invasive methods of stone disruption (extracorporeal shock-wave lithotripsy) and minimally invasive nephroscopic procedures. The latter comprise stone removal and stone fragmentation by either ultrasound, laser energy, or electrohydraulically derived shockwaves. When a complete range of extracorporeal and endoscopic techniques are available, only about 10 per cent of stone patients require open surgery for such problems as large infected and obstructing staghorn calculi.

Ureteric stones

A ureteric stone that is causing renal colic need only be removed immediately if infection is trapped above it. Otherwise, and provided it does not cause obstruction between attacks of colic, a ureteric stone can be treated conservatively. Stones less than 5 mm in diameter on a standard abdominal radiographic film usually either pass or migrate down the ureter and can be removed or fragmented endoscopically from below. Stones that are causing obstruction between attacks of colic should be removed without delay. If it is proposed to fragment a ureteric stone by extracorporeal lithotripsy, the stone is usually manipulated back into the renal pelvis for this procedure. Such manipulation is more difficult if the stone has been stationary in the ureter for more than a few weeks. Cases of ureteric stones that are being treated conservatively need regular supervision with serial abdominal radiographs, to assess the migration of the stone. In the absence of obstruction it is reasonable to wait 6 weeks after stone migration ceases before intervening. Recurrence of renal colic indicates further ultrasound and/or intravenous urography after the attack to determine whether obstruction has developed. A single kidney, impaired, and especially deteriorating, renal function, and bilateral ureteric stones indicate early surgical intervention. The spontaneous passage of stones is aided by maintaining a high fluid intake, if necessarily given intravenously, and the effect of this may be augmented by short bursts of vigorous diuretic therapy with, for example, intravenous frusemide.

Pelvicalyceal stones

Single pelvicalyceal stones of diameter less than 0.5 cm do not necessarily need treatment, unless they are obstructing a calyx or are associated with infection. They should, however, be kept under surveillance.

Small and moderate-sized stones (< 2 cm in diameter) which are associated with free drainage from the pelvicalyceal system are suitable for extracorporeal lithotripsy alone. Stones between 2 and 4 cm in diameter in a normal collecting system are also suitable for treatment by extracorporeal lithotripsy alone, provided that measures are taken to avoid obstructive complications. In these cases, a double-J ureteric stent is usually inserted preoperatively and the stone fragments then pass down the ureter around the stent. This may continue for several months. Larger calculi and those with multiple branching segments require preliminary percutaneous procedures to reduce their size ('debulking' operation). The contraindications to extracorporeal lithotripsy are: doubt about the location of the stone (intravenous urography and other imaging procedures are essential preliminary investigations), calyceal stenosis, large, peripherally located stone mass, distal obstruction, patient morphology (weight more than 135 kg, or height less than 100 cm, skeletal deformities), uncorrectable clotting disorders, and pregnancy. Very radiodense stones, cystine, uric acid, and rapidly growing soft stones associated with infection may all be difficult to break up with extracorporeal lithotripsy. However, in some of these cases extracorporeal lithotripsy can be a useful adjunct to other forms of treatment (for example, penicillamine in cystinuria). Fortunately, the common calcium oxalate stones and those of mixed composition usually fragment well.

The dissolution of pelvicalyceal stones by continuous irrigation, either from below or through a percutaneous nephrostomy, as a sole treatment modality has not gained wide acceptance, although it is used as an adjunct to extracorporeal lithotripsy and nephroscopic procedures.

Stone prevention

Identifiable biochemical causes of the stone, urinary infection, and anatomical abnormalities that obstruct the free flow of urine should be treated. The management of patients with urinary stones for which no cause has been found depends only partly on the composition of the stone. All patients who have had a stone should drink enough to maintain a urine volume of at least 3 litres/24 h, and should check this themselves. Some of the extra fluid should be taken late at night and larger volumes are needed in tropical climates and by those who work in hot environments. It is unnecessary to specify softened water, the final urine calcium concentrations achieved with hard tap water being only slightly higher than those with calcium-free water.

Those who form uric acid stones should have the diurnal change in their urine pH assessed by use of wide-range pH indicator papers. If they excrete persistently acid urine and do not have hyperuricaciduria, it is sufficient, in the first instance, to give enough alkali to keep the urine pH above 6. Allopurinol (100–300 mg/day) is recommended if there is proven hyperuricaciduria, or if an alkalinizing regime fails or is inappropriate for other reasons. Lack of a response to alkali indicates poor ability to inhibit crystal formation in the urine, undetected intermittently elevated uric acid excretion values, or non-compliance. The degree of dietary restriction of animal protein and other purine-containing foods necessary to lower uric acid excretion greatly is unacceptable to most European patients.

Patients who have had only one calcium-containing stone, for which no cause was found, need only be advised to maintain a high rate of urine flow, to avoid self-medication with vitamins D and C and calcium-containing antacids, and to avoid more than average intakes of dairy products and oxalate-rich beverages and fruits. The principles of the dietary management of patients with recurrent stones containing calcium salts are summarized in Table 9.

Urinary calcium excretion is modified by factors other than the dietary intake of calcium (Table 10). Responsiveness to dietary calcium restriction is variable, and decreasing the concentration of calcium in the intestinal lumen increases oxalate absorption and excretion. Dietary calcium restriction on the use of sodium cellulose phosphate therefore needs to be accompanied by dietary oxalate restriction and attention to other factors, such as the sodium and fibre contents of the diet (Table 10).

Table 9 *Dietary management of patients with recurrent calcium-containing stones*

Fluid intake	Sufficient to produce 3 litres of urine divided approximately uniformly over the 24-h period. Tap water is satisfactory. Increase fluid intake in hot environments. Check 24-h urine volume
Calcium	Reduce milk intake to 300 ml or less per day. This also reduces lactose intake. Omit cheese and yoghurt. Aim at an approximate 17.5 mmol (700 mg) per day calcium intake
Oxalate	Restrict intake because a low calcium diet increases oxalate absorption and excretion; urinary oxalate is a major risk factor for urolithiasis. Omit rhubarb, spinach, beans, beetroot, strawberries, nuts, chocolate, cocoa, and tea (or limit to 2 cups per day)
Fruits and fruit juices	Omit those that are rich in vitamin C (an oxalate precursor). These are oranges, lemons, grapefruit, limes, and blackcurrant syrup
Protein	Limit lean meat to 225 g (approximately 0.5 lb)/day.
Carbohydrate	Sufficient for estimated calorie needs
Fibre	Include high-fibre foods
Salt	Reduce dietary sodium chloride if urinary sodium > 250 mmol/24 h
Vitamin preparations	Omit vitamin D (promotes calcium absorption); omit vitamin C (oxalate precursor)
Pharmaceuticals	Omit any that are calcium salts, or which contain calcium salts, unless they are essential for the treatment of another disease. Examples are: calcium aspirin and many antacid preparations, including aluminium hydroxide preparations

A number of other treatments with probably marginal, if any, value include the use of allopurinol for the treatment of idiopathic calcium oxalate stone-formers, on the grounds that such stones may form on a nidus of uric acid and that uric acid removes inhibitors of calcium oxalate crystal nucleation. This is only recommended in exceptionally intractable cases unless there is associated hyperuric aciduria.

Orthophosphates and magnesium oxide (or hydroxide) have also been used as non-specific inhibitors of crystallization when stones recur in spite of apparently adequate treatment, or when no more specific treatment is available. Orthophosphates act by: (1) increasing the excretion of pyrophosphate; (2) binding some calcium in the gut; (3) increasing thirst; and (4) competing with oxalate ions for excreted calcium ions in the urine. A dose equivalent to between about 1 and 2 g of elemental phosphorus per day is given in effervescent tablets (Phosphate-Sandoz®). The dose of magnesium ions should be sufficient (for example, 200 mg magnesium oxide daily) materially to increase the urinary magnesium excretion. Hypocitraturia has been identified as an aetiological factor in some cases of urolithiasis. The administration of potassium citrate or mixed citrate preparations in large doses (for example, potassium citrate equivalent to 60 mmol) potassium/day) are sometimes helpful especially where alkalinization as well as the calcium complexing power of the citrate ion is desired.

Table 10 *Factors affecting the average urinary calcium excretion* (in general these effects are variable from one individual to another; individually they are usually small by comparison with the total daily calcium excretion, but their results are additive and cognizance of them may be helpful to patients with idiopathic hypercalciuria and to other patients with recurrent calcium-containing calculi)

Sex	Calcium excretion is lower in woman than in men
Age	Calcium excretion is lower in children and the geriatric age-group
Environmental	Exposure to sunlight increases calcium excretion in light-skinned subjects due to increased vitamin D synthesis. There are geographical differences which are independent of this effect, e.g. the higher urinary calcium excretion seen in the United States compared with Europe.
Associated diseases	Renal failure, nephrotic syndrome, and intestinal malabsorption syndrome reduce urinary calcium excretion
Diet	Calcium: high levels increase urinary calcium excretion
	Vitamin D: high levels increase urinary calcium excretion
	Inorganic phosphate: high levels reduce calcium absorption and excretion
	Fibre: high levels reduce calcium absorption and excretion
	Sodium content: high levels increase urinary sodium excretion; this is associated with an increase in urinary calcium
	Carbohydrate: high carbohydrate (glucose, sucrose, galactose) diets increase urinary calcium (and magnesium) in parallel with an increased hydrogen ion excretion
	Protein: high protein diets increase urinary calcium (and urate) excretion

COURSE AND PROGNOSIS

Urinary stones tend to recur even when a specific cause cannot be identified. Such recurrences may be separated by as much as 10 years, the total recurrence rate after this period being about 70 per cent. The treatability of a systemic or metabolic cause determines the immediate prognosis with respect to non-renal morbidity and mortality, and influences the prognosis for stone formation in the future. The amount of renal damage caused by the stones or nephrocalcinosis determine the prognosis with respect to renal function and hypertension. Urolithiasis does not cause hypertension unless it is accompanied by scarring of one or both kidneys. Nephrocalcinosis worsens the prognosis even if the underlying cause can be treated as, for instance, in primary hyperparathyroidism.

REFERENCES

Blacklock, N.J. (1990). Urolithiasis epidemiology. In *Scientific basis of urology*, (3rd edn), (ed. G.D. Chisholm and W.R. Fair), Ch. 2. Heinemann Medical Books, Oxford.

Buck, A.C. (1990). Risk factors in idiopathic stone disease. In *Scientific basis of urology*, (3rd edn), (ed. G.D. Chisholm and W.R. Fair), Ch. 22. Heinemann Medical Books, Oxford.

Embon, O.M., Rose, G.A., and Rosenbaum, T. (1990). Chronic dehydration stone disease. *British Journal of Urology*, **66**, 357–62.

Frymoyer, P.A., Scheinman, S.J., Dunham, P.B., Jones, D.B., Hueber, P., and Schroeder, E.T. (1991). X-linked recessive nephrolithiasis with renal failure. *New England Journal of Medicine*, **325**, 681–6.

Lancet (Editorial) (1987). Allopurinol for calcium oxalate stones. *Lancet* **1**, 258–9.

Lingerman, J.E., Smith, L.H., Woods, J.R., and Newman, D.M. (1989). *Urinary calculi. ESWL, endourology and medical therapy*. Lea and Febiger, Philadelphia. A comprehensive account of the management of urinary stones, with very good coverage of minimally invasive surgical techniques.

Mulloy, A.G. (1988). Management of nephrocalcinosis; new approaches to surgical kidney stones. *Annual Review of Medicine* **39**, 347–55. An account of the application of percutaneous nephrolithotomy, ultrasonic and electrohydraulic lithotripsy, and extracorporeal shock-wave lithotripsy.

Nakagowa, Y., Ahmed, M.A., Hall, S.L., Deganello, S., and Coe, S.L. (1987). Isolation from human calcium oxalate stones of nephrocalcin, a glycoprotein inhibitor of calcium oxalate crystal growth. Evidence that nephrocalcin from patients with calcium oxalate nephrolithiasis is deficient in gamma-carboxyglutamic acid. *Journal of Clinical Investigation* **79**, 1782–7.

Nordin, B.E.C., Need, A.G., and Morris, H.A. (1993). *Metabolic bone and stone disease*. Churchill Livingstone, Edinburgh. An authoritative and up-to-date multiauthor volume.

Pak, C.Y. (1991). Etiology and treatment of urolithiasis. *American Journal of Kidney Diseases* **18**, 624–37.

Polinsky, M.S., Kaiser, B.A., and Balmarte, H.J. (1987). Urolithiasis in childhood. *Paediatric Nephrology* **34**, 683–710. A generally useful review.

Robertson, W.G. (1990). Epidemiology for urinary stone disease. *Urological Research* **18**, 53–58.

Rose, G.A. (ed.) (1988). *Oxalate metabolism in relation to urinary stone disease*. Springer-Verlag, Berlin. Report of a workshop meeting, contains good sections on analytical problems and most aspects of the hyperoxalurias.

Scheinman, J.I. (1991). Primary hyperoxaluria: therapeutic strategies for the 90s. Editorial Review. *Kidney International* **40**, 389–99.

Scheinman, S.J., Pook, M.A., Wooding, C., Pang, J.T., Frymoyer, P.A., and Thacker, R.V. (1993). Mapping the gene causing X-linked recessive nephrolithasis to Xp11.22 by linkage studies. *Journal of Clinical Investigation*, **91**, 2351–7.

Shapiro, L.J. (1993). The genetic basis of X-linked nephrolithiasis: leaving no stone unturned. *Journal of Clinical Investigation*, **91**, 2339.

Smith, L.H. (1990). Idiopathic calcium oxalate urolithiasis. *Endocrinology and Metabolism Clinics of North America* **19**, 937–47.

Smith, L.H., *et al.* (1991). National blood pressure education programme (NHBPEP) review paper on complications of shock-wave lithotripsy for urinary calculi. *American Journal of Medicine* **91**, 635–41.

Watts, R.W.E. (1989). Factors governing urinary tract stone disease. *Pediatric Nephrology* **3**, 332–40.

Wickham, J.E.A. and Buck, A.C. (1990). *Renal tract stone; metabolic basis and clinical practice*. Churchill Livingstone, Edinburgh. An authoritative, comprehensive, and topical multiauthor work covering all aspects of the aetiology of urolithiasis, the pathophysiology of the condition, overviews of recent areas of research and well-balanced accounts of contemporary clinical practice.

Woolfson, R.G. and Mansell, M.A. (1991). Does triamterine cause renal calculi? *British Medical Journal* **303**, 1217–18.

Yendt, E.R. and Cohanim, M. (1989). Clinical and laboratory approaches for evaluation of nephrolithiasis. *Journal of Urology* **141**, 764–9.

20.13 Toxic nephropathy

B. T. EMMERSON

This term now refers to any adverse alteration in renal structure or function caused by an exogenous agent. In an acute toxic nephropathy, a cause and effect relationship is usually apparent between exposure to the toxin and the development of renal disease, the severity of the damage is usually related to the dose of the toxin, and the damage is potentially reversible. In those in whom the toxic renal damage has not reversed, follow-up of patients has established the entity of a chronic toxic nephropathy, although this might also develop as a sequel to prolonged low-grade exposure. More recently, immunologically mediated reactions to foreign substances have been recognized as another important mechanism for the production of toxic renal disease. Conventionally excluded from the concept are renal damage due to agents causing renal hypoperfusion or tubular obstruction, or due to renal involvement in systemic disease. None the less, the possibility that these might be contributing to an apparent toxic nephropathy needs always to be borne in mind. Thus, cyclosporin A may reduce renal blood flow, or high-dose treatment with acyclovir, methotrexate, or triamterene may cause intratubular obstruction.

Prevalence

The diagnosis of toxic nephropathy depends on both the recognition and the awareness of the causative agent as a nephrotoxin. Many cases of renal failure of unknown origin may have been caused by a drug or toxic agent. In addition, the detection of early cases is difficult because of the renal functional reserve and the lack of simple and reliable tests of early renal dysfunction. The prevalence will also vary in different parts of the world, in different races and in different climates. In developed countries, toxic renal damage may be seen in up to 3 per cent of hospital in-patients and up to 20 per cent of those undergoing intensive care.

Susceptibility of the kidney to toxins

Many factors increase the susceptibility of the kidney to toxic damage. Its normal concentrating function will increase the concentration of many potential toxins and this will occur in the intracellular as well as the intraluminal and interstitial compartments. This is of particular importance since the direct toxic effect of any agent depends upon the concentration achieved at the effector site. The vulnerability of each particular cell type to a particular toxin is dependent upon its transport function, its metabolic profile, and its detoxification mechanisms. The kidney's susceptibility is further increased by its function in excreting drugs and toxic substances. In addition, the kidneys receive 25 per cent of the cardiac output, and their large endothelial surface of reactive glomerular capillaries is especially susceptible to immune-mediated mechanisms. Glomerular structure and function may also be important in the localization of immune complexes. Host susceptibility is very variable, depending in part upon immunological reactivity, and in part upon modification of the toxic effect by the patient's age, blood pressure, pre-existing renal disease, concomitant drug therapy, and renal perfusion.

Pathogenetic mechanisms

CYTOTOXICITY

The commonest mechanism is a direct cytotoxic effect at the effector site, the effect being proportional to the concentration of the toxin and

the mechanism of its toxicity (Table 1). At low toxin concentrations, the effect is principally one of cell dysfunction, for example in the proximal tubule as the Fanconi syndrome of failure of reabsorption of glucose, phosphate, and amino acids, and in the distal tubule as a failure of concentrating capacity and/or of acid excretion. At higher concentrations of the toxin, cellular damage may occur and present with acute tubular necrosis and the syndrome of acute renal failure. If severe damage to distal tubular cells develops, either nephrogenic diabetes insipidus or renal tubular acidosis will result. Continued necrosis of cells and loss of nephrons may lead to chronic renal damage as an important mechanism of chronic renal failure due to prolonged exposure to a toxin.

The precise mechanisms of toxicity at the cellular level vary between the different cell types and the particular toxin involved. They range from impairment of calcium-messenger systems to free-radical generation with lipid peroxidation, and from covalent binding of sulphydryl groups with enzyme inactivation to interference with cell energy or damage to DNA.

IMMUNE-MEDIATED MECHANISMS

Immune mechanisms have been recognized only more recently as contributors to toxin-induced renal damage (Table 1). Characteristic of an immune-mediated process is the fact that the extent of the renal damage is not proportional to the severity of exposure (neither dose nor duration), and its development is less predictable, being found in only a small proportion of those exposed. In addition, when the adverse effect has subsided following removal of the cause, it will recur readily after further exposure, and other immunologically based systemic manifestations, such as fever, rash, arthralgia, and eosinophilia, may develop simultaneously.

Acute interstitial nephritis

One of the most important immunologically mediated manifestations presents as an acute interstitial nephritis, which usually develops as a reaction to a drug. Over 50 drugs have been recognized as provocative agents, including some of the penicillins, diuretics, antiepileptic agents, allopurinol, and some non-steroidal anti-inflammatory drugs. Almost any therapeutic agent can be regarded as having this potential, although it is particularly likely in some. Clinically, deterioration of renal function, usually with haematuria, is the dominant feature. Kidney size is usually increased. Involvement of other organs, particularly the skin and liver, is a common but not invariable feature. The characteristic lesion on biopsy shows oedema and infiltration of interstitial tissues by lymphocytes and plasma cells, together with eosinophils and occasional polymorphonuclear leucocytes. The glomeruli and vessels are usually normal, but interstitial oedema and dilatation of tubules may be seen with degeneration and necrosis of tubular epithelial cells. This is a most important pathogenetic mechanism with its own corresponding distinctive clinical syndrome.

Glomerulonephritis

The other immunologically mediated mechanism relates to the development of an autoimmune variety of glomerulopathy following exposure to a toxin or drug. This glomerulonephritis is usually of the so-called immune-complex type and presents as a membranous glomerulonephritis. In other cases, it is manifest as a nephrotic syndrome

Table 1 *Pathogenetic mechanisms of toxic renal damage*

	Syndrome	Example
Direct cytotoxin mediated		
Tubular dysfunction	Proximal:	
	Fanconi syndrome	Acute lead
	Distal:	
	Nephrogenic diabetes insipidus	Lithium
	Renal tubular acidosis	Amphotericin B
Acute tubular necrosis	Acute renal failure	Mercury
Chronic nephron damage	Chronic renal failure	Lead
Immunologically mediated		
Immunoallergic	Acute interstitial nephritis	Methicillin
Immune complex	Membranous glomerulopathy	Penicillamine
Cell-mediated	Minimal change nephropathy with nephrotic syndrome	Non-steroidal anti-inflammatory drugs
Hypersensitivity	Vasculitis	Sulphonamides

with minimal changes and this is probably cell mediated. In these situations, a cytotoxin, presumably by modifying a self-antigen, leads to glomerular disease with pathology similar to a membranous glomerulonephritis or minimal change nephrotic syndrome. Alternatively, the drug may modify immune regulation in the host. In the experimental animal, mercury can induce the production of autoantibodies to glomerular basement membrane and a membranous glomerulopathy. This occurs only with an appropriate dose and only with a susceptible strain of animal. The human parallel is the development of a membranous glomerulopathy in some patients with HLA-B8 or DR3 antigens after therapeutic exposure to gold or penicillamine. Penicillamine-induced glomerulopathy is also associated with abnormal sulphoxidation status. Study of the mechanism involved has great potential to expand our understanding of environmental or exogenous factors that may lead to the development of these types of glomerular disease. Certain other agents, particularly metals and some therapeutic agents, can also lead to chronic tubulointerstitial nephritis. However, at a later stage, the underlying mechanism is difficult to discern.

The various pathogenetic mechanisms mentioned are not mutually exclusive and various combinations can occur. However, it is important to stress that the immunologically based mechanisms, in particular, are complex and relatively poorly understood, and that one drug may act in different ways in different people. Although the various processes are not always as clearly separable as suggested, they are generally distinctive and are presented as such in order to provide workable concepts.

Clinical syndromes

This wide variety of pathogenetic mechanisms and their combinations result in a varied range of clinical presentations (Fig. 1). These depend upon the particular toxic agent and its mechanism of toxicity as well as the genetic make-up of the affected individual, which is currently poorly understood. None the less the following syndromes can often be defined.

Renal tubular dysfunction

This results from toxic damage mild enough only to impair function rather than cause tubular cell death. The effects include:

1. The Fanconi syndrome, showing as glycosuria, aminoaciduria, and phosphaturia, is a term used broadly to refer to renal damage in which proximal tubular dysfunction is disproportionately more severe than glomerular dysfunction. It is seen most frequently in some acute metal nephropathies.

2. Impairment of concentrating capacity leading in severe cases to nephrogenic diabetes insipidus with polyuria and polydipsia. Classically, this can result from toxicity from lithium, fluoride, and demethylchlortetracyline.

3. Impairment of acid excretion, which can lead to renal tubular acidosis. Typically, this can result from treatment with amphotericin B.

Acute renal failure

This may occur in varying degrees of severity. In its mildest form, only slight proteinuria with increased cell excretion in the urine may be found, associated with some degree of nitrogen retention and possibly oliguria. In its most severe form, the pattern will be that of acute tubular necrosis with the early development of oliguria and cessation of renal excretory function. Such tubular necrosis is potentially reversible after removal of the causative agent unless the damage has been extreme. A typical example is that seen with the aminoglycoside antibiotics.

Acute interstitial nephritis

This important syndrome presents with deterioration of renal function which develops some days or weeks after exposure to the causative agent. The renal failure is usually non-oliguric. Haematuria and proteinuria are usual, together with systemic manifestations, including fever, arthralgia, rash, eosinophilia, elevated IgE concentrations, and sometimes abnormal liver function. The diagnosis is supported by the demonstration of eosinophilic leucocytes in the urine, but a renal biopsy may be needed to establish the diagnosis. Mostly, the renal insufficiency is of moderate degree and remission occurs when the causative agent is withdrawn. However, continuing exposure can cause the acute insufficiency to develop into chronic renal impairment. If the renal insufficiency has not begun to reverse within a week of withdrawal of the cause, steroid therapy should be considered and has usually appeared to hasten remission.

Chronic renal failure

Chronic renal failure of toxic origin has few clinical features to distinguish it from other causes of renal damage. Lead is a model for this type of renal failure and, in this case, there is a slowly progressive deterioration of renal function over many years, even in the absence of continuing exposure to the underlying toxin. In other cases, hypertension with associated vascular disease may be an important contributor to progression.

Glomerulonephritis

An immune-mediated response to an exogenous toxin may be clinically indistinguishable from other varieties of glomerulonephritis, with insidious proteinuria, haematuria, and nitrogen retention. Sufficient proteinuria may lead to a nephrotic syndrome, usually due to a membranous or minimal-change nephropathy. Sometimes an autoimmune process is operating and in others a hypersensitivity vasculitis may be seen. Typical examples of this type of nephrotoxicity occur with some therapeutic agents, including penicillamine, gold, and trimethadione, and with certain exogenous poisons, including some snake venoms.

It is difficult to define consistent early clinical markers of nephrotoxicity. Nitrogen retention may be a relatively late manifestation of toxic renal damage, and abnormalities appearing on microscopy of urine deposits with haematuria and/or proteinuria are relatively non-specific. Thus, relatively few tests have been established as useful early diagnostic indicators, although increased urinary eosinophils may be found in at least 50 per cent of cases of acute interstitial nephritis. Determination of whether proteinuria is glomerular or tubular (low molecular weight) may prove useful in localizing the site of injury. Urinary excretion of N-acetylglucosaminidase as a marker of lysosomal enzyme loss from tubular epithelial cells shows potential as an indicator of tubular cell damage, but its clinical value as a predictor has yet to be established. Acutely affected kidneys are usually enlarged radiologically.

Prevention

In the prevention of toxic renal damage, one can only suggest constant vigilance and recognition of the potential for nephrotoxic reactions that exist with many therapeutic agents. When using a drug known to have dose-dependent cytotoxicity for the kidney, one can minimize the problem by using the lowest effective dose and by monitoring drug concentrations when possible. Potentially toxic combinations should be avoided, and appropriate monitoring for early signs of toxicity should be carried out. However, immune-mediated nephrotoxicity cannot be prevented, merely diagnosed and treated at an early stage. As a general principle, since hypovolaemia tends to aggravate nephrotoxicity, patients should be kept well hydrated, particularly when high doses of nephrotoxic drugs are given. However, acute renal failure in these situations is often non-oliguric.

REFERENCES

Bach, P.H. (1989). Detection of chemically induced renal injury: the cascade of degenerative morphological and functional changes that follow the primary nephrotoxic insult and evaluation of these changes by *in-vitro* methods. *Toxicology Letters* **46**, 237–49.

Druet, P. (1989). Contribution of immunological reactions to nephrotoxicity. *Toxicology Letters* **46**, 55–64.

International Programme on Chemical Safety (1991). Principles and methods for the assessment of nephrotoxicity associated with exposure to chemicals. *Environmental Health Criteria* 119. WHO, Geneva.

Kaloyanides, G.J. (1991). Metabolic interactions between drugs and renal tubulo-interstitial cells: role in nephrotoxicity. *Kidney International* **39**, 531–40.

Meyer, B.R., Fischbein, A., Rosenman, K., Lerman, Y., Drayer, D.E., and Reidenberg, M.M. (1984). Increased urinary enzyme excretion in workers exposed to nephrotoxic chemicals. *American Journal of Medicine* **76**, 989–98.

Porter, G.A. (1989). Risk factors for toxic nephropathies. *Toxicology Letters* **46**, 269–79.

Metal nephropathies

The spectrum of renal responses to metal intoxication depends upon the acuteness, severity, and duration of exposure, upon the mechanism of toxicity of the particular metal or its salt, and the responses of the host, particularly the immune mechanisms. Any of the clinical syndromes can

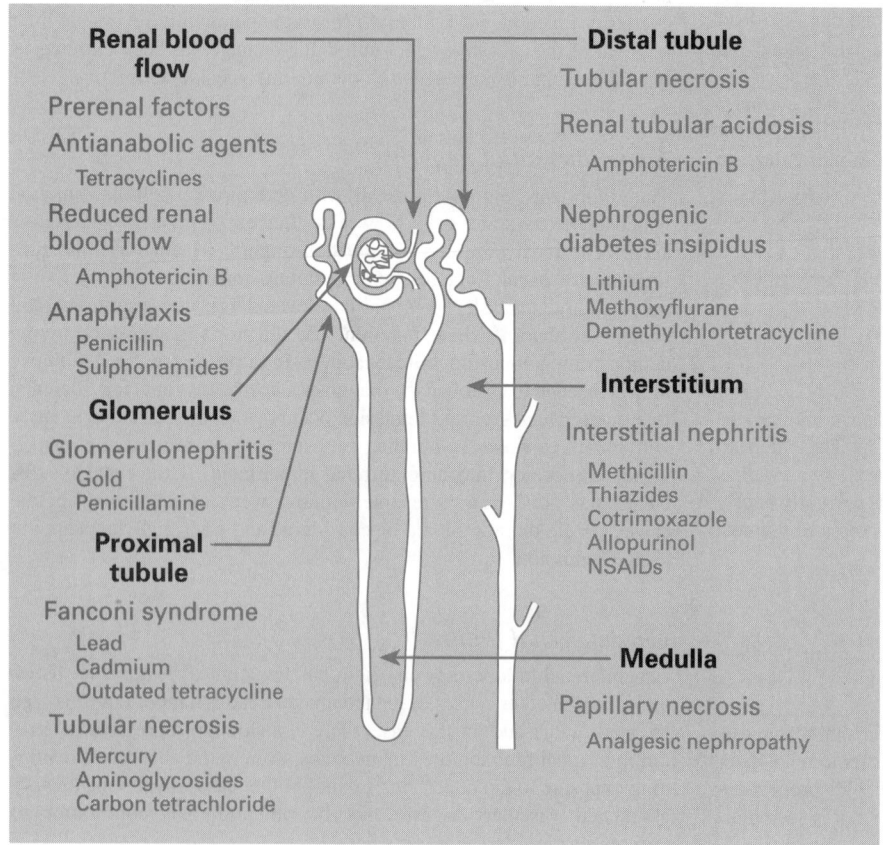

Fig. 1 Mechanisms of nephrotoxicity and representative factors involved in the pathogenesis of toxic renal damage affecting various parts of the nephron.

Table 2 *Features of metal nephrotoxicity*

| Metal | Acute nephropathy | | Chronic interstitial nephropathy | Glomerulonephritis/ nephrotic syndrome |
	Tubular necrosis	The Fanconi syndrome		
Lead	+	+	+	0
Cadmium	+	+	+	0
Mercury	+	0	?	+
Gold	0	0	+	+
Lithium	+	–	+	+
Platinum	+	+	+	–
Germanium	+	–	+	–
Uranium	+	+	+	0
Copper	+	+	+	0
Bismuth	+	+	+	0
Thallium	+	0	0	+

occur, although acute interstitial nephritis is less common (Table 2). Demonstrating an aetiolological association between the metal toxicity in man and the later development of chronic renal disease is particularly challenging and may require extensive epidemiological studies.

Lead

Lead poisoning is probably the commonest metal intoxication. Acute toxicity usually interferes principally with proximal tubular function, leading to glycosuria and amino aciduria as manifestations of a Fanconi syndrome. This probably reflects damage to brush-border membrane function and may be associated with enzyme loss in the urine. Nitrogen retention can occur but it is rarely severe enough to cause acute renal failure with oliguria. Intranuclear eosinophilic inclusion bodies (which consist of a lead–protein complex) are seen in proximal tubular cells and, if sought, these cells can often be demonstrated in the urine of an affected individual. Mitochondrial function is also affected. This nephrotoxicity is potentially reversible, either with removal from exposure or following treatment of the lead intoxication, usually with a chelating agent such as ethylene diaminetetraaecetic acid (**EDTA**). The symptoms of lead intoxication are often vague and may include intestinal colic, peripheral neuritis, and anaemia. When there is significant toxicity, prophyrin synthesis will usually be disordered and will result in coproporphyrinuria and an increased urinary excretion of δ-aminolaevulinic acid. Such acute lead poisoning is rapidly and effectively treated with calcium disodium-EDTA in a dose of 1 g/day in 5-day courses until the toxicity has remitted.

Chronic lead nephropathy can develop following prolonged low-grade lead intoxication. This leads to a reduced number of functioning nephrons and the pattern of a granular contracted kidney, principally with tubulointerstitial disease. This is best documented in three situations: in Queensland, Australia after childhood lead intoxication; in 'moonshine' drinkers from the southern states of the United States; and after long continued industrial lead intoxication.

In Queensland, acute childhood lead poisoning, from the ingestion of powdered and flaking paint, was common among children until lead paint was made illegal in 1930. Subsequent follow-up of patients affected with acute lead poisoning revealed a high prevalence of granular contracted kidneys. The distinctive entity of chronic lead nephropathy was established by detailed epidemiological follow-up and by correlation between the findings in the kidneys and the demonstration of increased concentrations of lead in bone. These patients demonstrated no continuing signs of lead intoxication and their kidneys demonstrated the effects of nephron loss, with hypertrophy of the remaining glomeruli and tubular atrophy. The criteria for diagnosis included the presence of uniform and equal contraction of both kidneys; long-standing chronic

renal disease of slow progression; exclusion of an alternative cause; and definite evidence of excessive past lead absorption, usually provided by demonstrating increased lead stores in bone or by the presence of an increased excretion of lead in urine after a standardized dose of calcium-EDTA. Affected patients showed disproportionate hyperuricaemia, and half developed gouty arthritis, an uncommon finding in other varieties of chronic renal failure. The hyperuricaemia was due to reduced renal excretion of urate, resulting from excessive reabsorption in the proximal tubule. Moderate hypertension was also a feature. It also seems that the kidney in early life is more susceptible to the adverse effects of lead.

A somewhat similar pattern was seen in 'moonshine' drinkers whose drink was produced in illicit stills with lead condensers. Their pattern of disease was similar to that seen in Queensland (where exposure occurred in childhood) and they shared a similar association with underexcretion of urate and gout. However, they demonstrated features of continuing lead intoxication with raised tissue lead concentrations and abnormal porphyrin metabolism. Prolonged industrial exposure to lead with resultant intoxication is now rarely seen in developed countries with good industrial hygiene. However, chronic lead intoxication is still seen in developing countries and occasionally in developed societies, and it seems likely that a number of such individuals with sufficiently prolonged and severe lead absorption can develop chronic renal damage. Clear proof of an aetiology for renal disease is more difficult in lead-exposed workers, because of the varying degrees of exposure and absorption, and of the variety of individual responses. However, on balance it seems likely that a sufficient degree of lead intoxication for a sufficient time can lead to chronic renal disease in man. Such exposure needs to be fairly heavy and to continue for years, and probably exceeds that which occurs in most industrial plants with good hygiene. The situation with lesser degrees of exposure to lead, usually without other features of lead intoxication or adverse effects on tissue function (so called subclinical lead exposure) is much more difficult to relate conclusively to the development of chronic renal disease, because adequate epidemiological studies have not been concluded.

The management of chronic lead nephropathy is that of chronic renal failure from whatever cause. However, the rate of progression is normally extremely slow and proteinuria is never severe. Unless there are signs of acute lead intoxication, no benefit to renal function can be obtained at this time from therapy with EDTA.

REFERENCES

Bernard, B.P. and Becker, C.E. (1988). Environmental lead exposure and the kidney. *Clinical Toxicology* **26**, 1–34.

Goyer, R.A. (1989). Mechanisms of lead and cadmium nephrotoxicity. *Toxicology Letters* **46**, 153–62.

Cadmium

Exposure to cadmium induces the production of a cysteine-rich protein, metallothionein, which binds the metal in a non-toxic form. Toxic effects are due to unbound cadmium, and the kidney may be affected by cadmium nephrotoxicity during its degradation of this cadmium–metallothionein complex. The toxic unbound cadmium initially affects cell membrane function and later intracellular organelles, resulting in cell necrosis.

Cadmium can be absorbed from either the respiratory or the alimentary tract. Although acute nephrotoxicity is rare because absorption is usually limited by the acute respiratory toxicity, renal tubular and cortical necrosis can occur. Chronic cadmium nephrotoxicity can result from prolonged low-grade exposure both in cadmium workers and in a population whose food and water has a high cadmium content because of environmental contamination. The early adverse effects on the kidney show principally as tubular dysfunction, with generalized aminoaciduria, glycosuria, and phosphaturia, as well as by a reduction in concentrating ability and acid excretion. A most distinctive feature is the excretion of 'tubular' proteins of low molecular weight ranging between 20 000 and 40 000. These consist principally of B_2-microglobulin and retinol-binding proteins but can also include mucoproteins and enzyme proteins. Albuminuria of glomerular origin may also be present at times. This type of renal damage appears to be progressive and not reversible. Even after removal from further exposure to cadmium, a progressive fall in the glomerular filtration rate occurs.

Another distinctive feature of chronic cadmium nephropathy is the association with hypercalciuria and hyperphosphaturia, which increase the risk of renal calculi and also of osteomalacia. This type of painful osteomalacia is the basis for 'itai-itai' or 'ouch-ouch' disease which occurs in Japanese populations who live in regions heavily contaminated with cadmium. The pathology is that of a chronic tubulointerstitial nephritis, somewhat similar to that due to lead. The difference from lead is the association with hypercalciuria and tubular proteinuria and the absence of disproportionate hyperuricaemia and gout.

Chelating agents have not been shown to be of value in this situation and removal from further exposure as soon as possible after toxicity is detected is the only course of action. The effects of the renal tubular acidosis and altered tubular functions can be corrected by appropriate specific supplements (for example, sodium bicarbonate).

REFERENCES

Thun, M.J., Osorio, A.M., Schober, S., Hannon, W.H., Lewis, B., and Halperin, W. (1989). Nephropathy in cadmium workers: assessment of risk from airborne occupational exposure to cadmium. *British Journal of Industrial Medicine* **46**, 689–97.

Mercury

Mercury is potentially the most nephrotoxic metal. Its toxicity may also affect the central nervous system. Its mechanism of toxicity involves an inhibition of membrane function, particularly of the brush-border membrane of the renal tubules, by interfering with reactive sulphhydryl groups. Thus high tissue concentrations of sulphhydryl-containing compounds such as glutathione and cysteine may be protective against its toxicity. Ultimately, mercury can interfere with the functions of the mitochondrial membrane and of sulphhydryl-containing enzyme systems.

Mercury can be absorbed by inhalation, via the mucous membrane, or skin. Mercurial compounds are no longer used in therapeutics, and most exposure is now either accidental or industrial. Acute mercurial poisoning usually causes acute oliguric renal failure. Early manifestations include proteinuria with cellular casts, but the damage is usually too intense to cause the proximal tubular dysfunction characteristic of the Fanconi syndrome. Regeneration of tubules may occur if damage is not too severe, but calcification of necrotic proximal tubules occurs more frequently with mercury than in other metal nephropathies. Although there are claims that mercury can produce a chronic interstitial nephropathy, most evidence suggests that this reflects residual damage after the acute tubular necrosis.

Acute mercury poisoning should be treated early with gastric lavage and charcoal, followed by full dosage of dimercaprol (BAL) given as soon as possible. Injections of 2.5 to 3.0 mg dimercaprol/kg bodyweight should be given every 4 h for up to six injections. Dimercaprol is readily dialysable so that its toxic effects (nausea, vomiting, diarrhoea, hypoglycaemia, and psychological change) as well as associated oliguria can be dealt with by dialysis after treatment.

There is increasing evidence that mercury can produce an immune-complex type of glomerulonephritis. This appears to develop as an autoimmune reaction to a self-antigen modified by the metal toxicity. A considerable component of individual and variable immunological reactivity is likely to be involved. The histological picture is usually consistent with a membranous glomerulonephritis. The level of proteinuria may vary widely and a full nephrotic syndrome may develop. Removal from exposure to mercury may cause a fall in mercury excretion and a lessening of this proteinuria. Some workers with chronic industrial exposure to mercury have developed proteinuria which has subsided after removal from exposure. The pathology of this type of proteinuria is not well documented but the lack of any dose–response effect suggests that it is more of the immune-complex glomerulonephritis pattern. Heavy environmental contamination with organic mercurials at Minimata Bay in Japan, although causing principally neurological features, was associated with a low molecular weight proteinuria and this was thought to reflect early renal damage.

REFERENCES

Tubbs, R.R., *et al.* (1982). Membranous glomerulonephritis associated with industrial mercury exposure. *American Journal of Clinical Pathology* **77**, 409–13.

Gold

Most toxic reactions to gold occur during the therapeutic administration of gold salts to patients with rheumatoid arthritis. Gold binds readily to proteins and accumulates in the kidneys, initially in the proximal tubular cells and later in the distal tubule and interstitial macrophages, where it may persist for up to 30 years. Toxic reactions to gold may involve the skin, the bone marrow, or the kidney in varying combinations, and the kidneys are not always involved. Acute tubular necrosis is rarely, if ever, seen with therapeutic doses and the first manifestation is usually mild proteinuria or microhaematuria, which may be seen in up to 30 per cent of treated patients and may be severe enough to induce the nephrotic syndrome in about 2 per cent. Proteinuria and glomerulopathy may develop at any stage of gold treatment, even as late as 2 years.

Within a few months of stopping gold therapy, the proteinuria begins to remit and has usually subsided completely within 2 to 3 years. Steroid therapy is indicated only rarely. After remission, there has usually been no further deterioration of renal glomerular function. Individual immune responsiveness is an important determinant and there is an increased association of renal damage in patients with HLA-B8 and DR3 antigens. Renal histopathology has usually shown a membranous glomerulonephritis with subepithelial deposits of immune complexes, sometimes containing IgG and complement. Gold is usually absent from the glomerular lesions. In a few cases the lesions may be of a minimal change, with mesangial-dense deposits, or without any morphological glomerular change. Gold nephrotoxicity, then, presents the pattern of a metal-induced glomerulonephritis of immune origin, rather than of direct nephrotoxic origin as is common with lead and cadmium.

REFERENCES

Hall, C.L., Fothergill, N.J., Blackwell, M.M., Harrison, P.R., MacKenzie, J.C., and MacIver, A.G. (1987). The natural course of gold nephropathy: long term study of 21 patients. *British Medical Journal* **295**, 745–8.

Wooley, P.H., Griffin, J., Panayi, G.S., Batchelor, J.R., Welsh, K.I., and Gibson, T.J. (1980). HLA-DR antigens and toxic reaction to sodium aurothiomalate and D-penicillamine in patients with rheumatoid arthritis. *New England Journal of Medicine* **303**, 300–2.

Lithium

Lithium is used extensively in the treatment of manic depressive psychoses. It is eliminated from the body almost entirely by the kidney, being filtered at the glomerulus and reabsorbed in the proximal tubule, resulting in a clearance of one-third of the creatinine clearance. It is known to move in and out of the intracellular compartment only slowly. Its principal toxicity relates to distal tubular function, which is probably related to its inhibition of adenylate cyclase and generation of cyclic AMP. This promotes the deposition of glycogen in distal tubular cells, which interferes with distal tubular function, leading to polyuria and, if sufficiently severe, to nephrogenic diabetes insipidus (see Chapter 20.2.1). Ultimately this can lead to tubular loss with scarring. Sufficiently severe acute toxicity can affect the proximal tubule to cause acute tubular necrosis.

Even during careful control of dosage and with the assistance of serum lithium concentrations, a number of patients may still show defective renal concentrating capacity with polyuria and polydipsia unresponsive to vasopressin. This effect is concentration dependent and reversible. Patients who develop polyuria should not be allowed to become salt depleted because this results in increased proximal tubular reabsorption of both sodium and lithium, which tends to increase the serum lithium and may lead to neurological disturbances and other signs of toxicity. In clinical practice, acute lithium toxicity is most commonly precipitated by diarrhoea or vomiting, or the unwise use of diuretic agents which should only be prescribed in those taking lithium with the greatest circumspection. The institution of indomethacin therapy, or the withdrawal of phenothiazines, in patients stabilized on lithium may also increase the serum lithium concentration. Occasional patients with serum lithium concentrations in the normal range may develop a nephrotic syndrome with minimal glomerular changes which remits on cessation of the lithium. Chronic low-grade intoxication appears to be associated with chronic renal impairment with focal atrophy of nephrons, tubular dilatation, and interstitial fibrosis. Haemodialysis is the most effective means of removing lithium during intoxication, particularly if there is associated oliguria.

REFERENCES

Hammersmith Staff Rounds (1991). Lithium intoxication. *British Medical Journal* **302**, 1267–9.

Platinum

Cisplatin, a platinum-containing compound widely used as an anticancer agent, causes a characteristic dose-related nephrotoxic reaction. The precise pathogenic mechanism of this toxicity is poorly understood. Doses of 20 mg/m^2.day for 5 days usually produce no nephrotoxicity, while high-dose therapy at twice this level usually causes depression of renal function, sometimes for up to 2 years. Minor renal dysfunction can show as aminoaciduria and proteinuria (principally of tubular origin during administration) with increased excretion of β_2-microglobulins and enzymes such as N-acetylglucosaminidase, which are preferentially localized to the proximal tubule. These can reverse rapidly and are not of value in monitoring therapy. The distal parts of the proximal tubule and the distal nephron are principally affected and can cause reversible

azotaemia in up to one-third of patients, and occasionally irreversible renal failure requiring dialysis. This interferes with sodium and water reabsorption in both proximal and distal tubules which may be depressed for up to 6 months after a course of treatment. Nephrotoxicity is associated with increased renal losses of potassium and magnesium, and monitoring of their serum concentrations and appropriate replacement is desirable. Chronic renal disease of the tubulointerstitial type can occur.

Partial protection against the nephrotoxic effect of cisplatin is provided by a mannitol and saline diuresis. This is attributed to a reduced duration of exposure of the renal tubule to toxic concentrations. There is some evidence that sodium thiosulphate and other SH-containing compounds may be protective. However, until the mechanism of nephrotoxicity is better understood, it will be difficult to design a rational preventative regimen. However, the newer platinum compounds, such as carboplatin, appear to be less nephrotoxic.

REFERENCE

Daugaard, G. and Abildgaard, U. (1989). Cisplatin nephrotoxicity. *Cancer Chemotherapy and Pharmacology* **25**, 1–9.

Germanium

Inorganic germanium, which usually occurs only as a trace metal, is increasingly being consumed in high doses as a tonic, particularly in Japan. Sufficient rapid accumulation can lead to acute renal failure, while prolonged low-grade intake can result in chronic impairment of renal function. This has no specific characteristics except that there is no proteinuria or haematuria. The histological pattern is of vacuolar degeneration, particularly affecting the distal tubules, with interstitial fibrosis and minor glomerular abnormalities. When consumption is stopped, there may be a gradual improvement in renal function. The excess absorption of germanium can be demonstrated by increased concentrations in hair and nails.

REFERENCE

Sanai, T., *et al.* (1990). Germanium dioxide-induced nephropathy: a new type of renal disease. *Nephron* **54**, 53–60.

Antimicrobial and chemotherapeutic agents

Aminoglycosides

Gentamicin is the most frequently used member of this group of antimicrobials especially active against Gram-negative organisms. It produces acute renal failure of the dose-related cytotoxic variety in a significant percentage (average 10 per cent) of all subjects to whom it is administered. The drug accumulates in proximal tubular cells where it is only slowly eliminated. Since nephrotoxicity is related in part to the serum concentration, the initial dosage regimen should be calculated from a consideration of body weight and renal function, with subsequent dosage adjustment according to trough-and-peak serum concentrations of the drug. One of the first clinical manifestations is the presence of non-oliguric renal failure with elevation of the serum creatinine concentration. Impaired urine concentrating ability will be present and enzymuria with N-acetylglucosaminidase, proteinuria with β_2-microglobulin, and lysozymuria may be observed. However, these do not invariably precede or predict the later development of renal failure. Renal function and antibiotic levels must be monitored during therapy. The associated renal failure is potentially reversible, depending upon the extent of the tubular damage and other complicating factors. In some cases, recovery may be slow and incomplete. The risk of renal damage may be increased by associated treatment with diuretics or cephalosporins, and any toxicity is potentiated by increasing age, pre-existing cardiac or renal failure or ischaemia, and the presence of endotoxinaemia.

The mechanism of aminoglycoside nephrotoxicity is being increasingly elucidated. Gentamicin, for instance, is cationic and hydrophilic and is first transported into and accumulated within the proximal tubular cells by crossing the apical membrane by a process involving endocytosis. Its toxicity is related to its potential to bind anionic phospholipids in the liposomal membrane. This can lead to necrosis of the proximal convoluted tubules. Experimentally, polyaspartic acid, a polyanionic compound, has been found to protect against this nephrotoxicity by an action within the lysosomes. However, these studies have not yet advanced to a clinical application.

Tobramycin has less potential for nephrotoxicity than gentamicin. None the less, careful calculation of dose and monitoring of serum concentrations are desirable. The other more toxic aminoglycosides, neomycin and kanamycin, are no longer used in therapeutics.

REFERENCES

Kacew, S. and Bergeron, M.G. (1990). Pathogenic factors in aminoglycoside-induced nephrotoxicity. *Toxicology Letters* **51**, 241–59.

Laurent, G., Kishore, B.K., and Tulkens, P.M. (1990). Aminoglycoside-induced renal phospholipidosis and nephrotoxicity. *Biochemical Pharmacology* **40**, 2383–92.

Penicillins

These agents rarely exhibit dose-related nephrotoxicity but almost all of the penicillin group have the potential to induce an acute interstitial nephritis. This occurred in up to 20 per cent of patients during methicillin therapy and was an important factor in the replacement of this drug with others of lesser toxic potential. It may still occasionally be seen after administration of any of the penicillin derivatives. Methicillin nephropathy usually presents with a steadily developing renal insufficiency, coming on some days after the beginning of treatment, usually associated with haematuria, and sometimes with fever, eosinophilia, and a rash. Eosinophils can often be found in the patient's urine and the histological picture is typical of an acute interstitial nephritis. The postulated mechanism is thought to involve an immune response to an antigen–protein complex, caused either by the coupling of the penicilloyl hapten to an intrinsic renal protein or by the development of antibodies to tubular basement membrane. Subsequent exposure to another penicillin derivative often results in a recurrence of the syndrome. With removal of the cause and conservative management of the associated renal insufficiency, the condition usually settles. If there is delay in resolution, however, or if the patient becomes severely ill, prednisone should be used since it seems to speed resolution significantly to a worthwhile degree.

Cephalosporins

The cephalosporins are rapidly excreted by secretory mechanisms within the proximal convoluted tubule. Accumulation in the cortex and any associated toxicity can be inhibited by probenecid and other inhibitors of tubular transport. The original cephalosporin, cephaloridine, demonstrated dose-dependent nephrotoxicity and should no longer be used. The newer cephalosporins are much less nephrotoxic but they accumulate in the cortex and may still have some nephrotoxic potential. The second- and third-generation cephalosporins have minimal nephrotoxicity, although there are a few reports of acute interstitial nephritis associated with their use. Nephrotoxicity is frequently reported during combined therapy with cephalosporins and the aminoglycosides. Seriously ill patients with pre-existing renal disease who are dehydrated with a contracted plasma volume are particularly susceptible, especially if exposed to high concentrations of antimicrobials for more than a few days.

Sulphonamides

During the early years of the use of sulphonamides, crystal nephropathy was not infrequent. With the newer agents, however, this is now rare and the main renal complications from these drugs are allergic. These usually manifest either as an acute interstitial nephritis, as an immune-complex glomerulonephritis, or as a necrotizing angiitis. Such reactions are particularly likely to be associated with the long-acting sulphonamides. Co-trimoxazole (trimethoprim–sulphamethoxazole) can also cause these reactions but they are uncommon in patients with normal renal function. The dose should be reduced in the presence of renal insufficiency. With this drug, it is wise not to rely on the serum creatinine concentration alone since trimethoprim interferes with the tubular secretion of creatinine.

Tetracyclines

The tetracycline tetracyclines increase urea production by inhibiting the utilization of amino acids for protein synthesis. This becomes a problem only in patients with pre-existing renal insufficiency in whom the excretion of the tetracycline is delayed and its protein catabolic effect intensified. Their use is also associated with an increase in salt and water excretion which, in patients with pre-existing renal insufficiency, can lead to weight loss, acidosis, and deterioration of renal function. However, doxycycline, which has only a slight antianabolic effect, does not have an adverse effect in patients with pre-existing renal disease because its excretion is unchanged.

Outdated or deteriorated tetracycline has caused toxic tubular damage with a reversible Fanconi syndrome and a marked renal tubular acidosis with hypocalcaemia and hypouricaemia. Proteinuria, glycosuria, phosphaturia, and aminoaciduria have also been reported. A degradation product of the tetracyclines, anhydrotetracycline, is thought to be responsible and to cause damage to both proximal and distal tubules. A change in the excipient used in the capsules has greatly reduced this risk but its potential should be borne in mind.

Demethylchlortetracycline (demeclocycline) can impair renal concentrating ability in normal subjects and induce a reversible nephrogenic diabetes insipidus. This tubular toxicity is reversible and dose related and is sometimes used in the treatment of the chronic syndrome of inappropriate secretion of antidiuretic hormone. Its use in patients with cirrhosis of the liver has been associated with the development of non-oliguric renal failure.

REFERENCE

Montoliu, J., Carrera, M., Darnell, A., and Revert, L. (1981). Lactic acidosis and Fanconi's syndrome due to degraded tetracycline. *British Medical Journal* **283**, 1576–7.

Antituberculous agents

Rifampicin (rifampin) may induce an immune-mediated variety of renal insufficiency, with associated influenza-like symptoms of chills, malaise, vomiting, and fever. This syndrome has often developed when recommencing therapy after a prior course of the drug. Anti-rifampicin antibodies have been found in the serum of many affected patients but not in all. However, similar antibodies have been demonstrated in the serum of patients receiving regular therapy with rifampicin who do not have such complications. It seems likely that a critical level of antigen–antibody complex is needed to induce the syndrome, and this tends particularly to occur when therapy is intermittent. Some of the patients have shown immunoglobulin deposits around the renal tubules, while some have had a positive Coombs test and others a positive macrophage migration inhibition reaction. The lesion is usually regarded as being an acute interstitial nephritis, though it has a number of unusual features.

The associated renal insufficiency is usually mild but may be sufficiently severe to require dialysis.

Ethambutol treatment may be associated with an episode of acute renal failure which subsides after withdrawal of the drug, only to leave persistent impairment of renal function in some patients. The pattern is that of an acute interstitial nephritis. This drug also causes hyperuricaemia by reducing the urate clearance but this does not seem to have an aetiological role in the renal disease. Rarely, p-aminosalicylate may be associated with an acute interstitial nephritis with allergic skin lesions.

Amphotericin B

This drug, which possesses major cytotoxic potential, still needs to be used for some of the serious systemic fungal infections. It is strongly protein bound, is not dialysable, and is only slowly eliminated from the body, largely by non-renal routes. It affects the permeability of cellular membranes, particularly the luminal membrane of the tubular epithelium, resulting in a failure of hydrogen ion excretion and an increased urinary loss of potassium. Proximal tubular damage may be reflected by the associated phosphaturia and uricosuria, and impairment of renal concentrating power may be sufficient to give a nephrogenic diabetes insipidus. The glomerular filtration rate falls, roughly in proportion to the dose of amphotericin B given, and some renal vasoconstriction has been postulated. The associated renal failure is potentially reversible at low dosage, and withdrawal of the drug will usually lead to a slow recovery of renal function. However, a sufficiently high dose can produce acute tubular necrosis with irreversible renal failure. Necrosis of the proximal and distal tubules may be sufficient to produce a characteristic nephrocalcinosis with calcium deposits in both tubules and interstitium.

Since it is used chiefly in life-endangering situations, the risk of nephrotoxicity must be weighed against the risk of the untreated disease. During therapy, the recognized potential adverse effects from the nephrotoxicity should be sought and diagnosed early and corrected where possible. This may involve the early administration of potassium and magnesium salts, alkali in the form of sodium citrate or bicarbonate, and adequate fluids to prevent any dehydration. A good urine volume should be maintained throughout, but there is no clear evidence that a mannitol diuresis reduces nephrotoxicity.

REFERENCE
Sabra, R. and Branch, R.A. (1990). Amphotericin B nephrotoxicity. *Drug Safety* **5**, 94–108.

Drugs and therapeutic agents

A significant degree of intrinsic nephrotoxicity would prevent the therapeutic use of a drug unless it possessed a unique action, particularly in a life-endangering situation. This has already been exemplified by the use of gentamicin for serious infections and cisplatin as an anticancer agent. For this reason, most drug-induced renal damage is immune mediated and presents either as an acute interstitial nephritis (Table 3) (often with involvement of other organs, such as skin or liver) or as a glomerulopathy with or without a nephrotic syndrome. In these types of reaction, the development of renal damage is unpredictable and the prevalence of renal damage is so low that routine monitoring of renal function is not indicated. Individual susceptibility is important but, apart from recognition of an association with certain tissue types and in slow drug metabolizers, no useful predictive indices have been developed. In addition, the lesion seen is not always specific, and several different pathological processes may be operating. Once the condition is recognized or suspected as being drug related, the drug should be withdrawn and the diagnosis established, usually by renal biopsy. If there is an acute interstitial nephritis which is not settling rapidly, steroids are indicated.

Table 3 *Some major drugs causing immune-mediated acute interstitial nephritis (This list is not comprehensive and a large number of drugs can infrequently cause this response)*

Antibacterial agents
  β-lactams
    methicillin
    ampicillin
    penicillin
    cephalothin
  Sulphonamides
    cotrimoxazole
  Rifampicin and ethambutol
Diuretics
  Thiazides
  Frusemide
Analgesics
  Non-steroidal anti-inflammatory agents (especially fenoprofen)
Others
  Allopurinol
  Sulphinpyrazone
  Phenindione
  Cimetidine
  Captopril
  Phenytoin
  Glafenine

REFERENCE
Pusey, C.D., Saltissi, D., Bloodworth, L., Rainford, D.J., and Christie, J.L. (1983). Drug associated acute interstitial nephritis: clinical and pathological features and the response to high dose steroid therapy. *Quarterly Journal of Medicine, New Series LII* **206**, 194–211.

Cyclosporin A

This potent immunosuppressive, used effectively to prevent transplant rejection or to treat some autoimmune diseases, is generally regarded as having some intrinsic nephrotoxicity. This has two components. The first is an unusual effect upon the renal vasculature which, in the acute situation, leads to renal vasoconstriction and is reversible by dopamine. This results in a 30 to 40 per cent reduction in renal blood flow and glomerular filtration, and an increase in the filtration fraction. There is also increased reabsorption of sodium and urate from the proximal convoluted tubule. The other component is a dose-dependent cytotoxicity affecting the proximal convoluted tubule. This is potentially reversible but may occasionally lead to necrosis of the proximal convoluted tubule, interstitial fibrosis, and chronic renal disease. This dose-dependent cytotoxicity can be minimized by the careful control of plasma cyclosporin concentrations and this is essential for safe clinical use. The drug itself is metabolized by the hepatic cytochrome P450 system, and drugs that inhibit this system, such as erythromycin, ketoconazole, and diltiazem, may increase blood cyclosporin concentrations and increase nephrotoxicity. The clinical pattern is associated with a gradual deterioration of renal function with increasing concentrations of creatinine, potassium, and urate. Usually, this will stabilize and not progress. A metabolic acidosis may develop together with fluid retention. Hyperuricaemia is found in over 70 per cent of patients. This appears to be due not only to the vascular effect upon the glomerular filtration rate, but probably also represents a combination of proximal tubular damage and excessive reabsorption of urate associated with the overabsorption of sodium in the proximal convoluted tubule. This hyperuricaemia is associated with an accelerated form of gout in up to 20 per cent of patients. Recent reports of the new immunosuppressive, FK506, originally said to be less toxic than cyclosporin A, suggest that nephrotoxicity may still be a problem.

REFERENCE

Kahan, B.D. (1990). Drug therapy: cyclosporin. *New England Journal of Medicine* **321**, 1725–38.

Phenindione

Rarely, patients treated with this drug may develop an acute interstitial nephritis with acute renal failure and multisystem involvement, including the skin and liver. The severity of the renal insufficiency varies considerably, but sometimes it may be prolonged and at times may be irreversible. Occasional patients may develop a nephrotic syndrome. A comparable risk does not exist with warfarin.

D-Penicillamine

This drug is used in the treatment of hepatolenticular degeneration, acute metal intoxications, and most commonly as a slow-acting antirheumatic agent in rheumatoid arthritis. Mild proteinuria occurs frequently, and initially may settle with dosage reduction. Less commonly, proteinuria may become severe. This usually occurs during the first 12 months of therapy and may be severe enough to cause a nephrotic syndrome. The condition usually settles on withdrawal of treatment and steroid treatment is not necessary. Although remission may be delayed, most have resolved completely within 2 years, although in some it may appear incomplete. There is minimal deterioration of renal function.

The mechanism is that of a drug-induced glomerulonephritis/nephrotic syndrome and the histology is usually that of a membranous glomerulonephritis. A few patients show mesangial-dense deposits or minimal glomerular changes. Patient susceptibility, as reflected by HLA-B8 and/or DR3 tissue antigens, and/or by an abnormal sulphoxidation status, is recognized as an important contributory factor. It is of particular interest that penicillamine inhibits the covalent binding of C4 and may thereby interfere with the handling of immune complexes. In addition, C4 levels may be low in DR3-positive individuals because DR3 is associated with an increased frequency of C4-null alleles.

REFERENCES

Hall, C.L., *et al.* (1988). Natural course of penicillamine nephropathy: a long term study of 33 patients. *British Medical Journal* **296**, 1083–86.
Sim, E., Dodds, A.W., and Goldin, A. (1989). Inhibition of the covalent binding reaction of complement component C4 by pencillamine, an antirheumatic agent. *Biochemistry Journal* **259**, 415–19.

Anticonvulsants

Phenytoin (diphenylhydantoin) may rarely cause a hypersensitivity reaction with multisystem involvement, including dermatitis, hepatitis, myositis, and fever, in which acute renal failure may occur. It should be managed as for an acute interstitial nephritis.

The oxazolidinediones, particularly trimethadione and paramethadione, occasionally cause proteinuria which may be severe enough to induce a nephrotic syndrome. The proteinuria usually settles on withdrawal of the drug, but the rate of recovery and the completeness of the remission vary. The pathology has varied widely, sometimes suggesting an acute interstitial nephritis and in others an immune-complex glomerulonephritis. It is difficult to advise on specific therapy because some patients have remitted, albeit slowly, on withdrawal of the drug, whereas others appear to have needed steroid and immunosuppressive drugs. None the less, remission following withdrawal of the cause and steroid therapy has not been invariable and chronic renal failure may develop.

Diuretics

Both frusemide and the thiazide diuretics have occasionally caused an acute interstitial nephritis. Some patients have shown the features of a hypersensitivity vasculitis. In other cases, diuretics appear to have augmented the nephrotoxicity of other agents.

Drugs altering urate concentrations

Allopurinol therapy is occasionally complicated by the development of an acute interstitial nephritis which can vary in severity up to the full syndrome with fever, exfoliative dermatitis, eosinophilia, eosinophiluria, and abnormal liver function. These reactions are more likely to occur in patients with pre-existing renal disease, especially if the dose of allopurinol has not been reduced in proportion to the glomerular filtration rate. The uricosuric agent sulphinpyrazone has also been implicated in a similar syndrome. Unless the syndrome clears rapidly and improvement is apparent within a week, steroid therapy is indicated and usually promotes rapid subsidence. High doses are usually used, either as intravenous methyl prednisolone (500 g daily for 4 days) or oral prednisolone (60 mg/day) until the creatinine begins to fall or a diuresis occurs. The dose is then reduced at a rate depending on the response, but usually over at least 2 weeks. If any relapse occurs following withdrawal of steroids, an increase in dose is needed and prolonged therapy may be justified. Occasionally, despite steroid treatment, the renal insufficiency has been severe, prolonged, and occasionally fatal.

Other drugs

A large number of other drugs, such as many of the extensively used non-steroidal anti-inflammatory agents, can induce one of the immune-mediated types of toxic renal disease, usually being categorized as either an acute interstitial nephritis or the glomerulonephritis/nephrotic syndrome pattern (Table 1). Captopril and some other sulphhydryl-containing compounds have also been incriminated. The number of drugs able to induce these rare immune-mediated reactions is very large and there are probably fewer drugs that cannot do so than there are drugs recognized as being occasionally associated with this type of nephrotoxicity.

Radiographic contrast media

This important cause of renal insufficiency usually shows initially as an increase in the serum creatinine concentration occurring within 24 h of a radiographic procedure using a contrast agent. Usually the elevated creatinine concentration reaches a maximum at 4 days and subsequently subsides to revert to normal within 7 to 10 days. The true incidence of this reaction is difficult to determine because of variation between patients in their response, and because it may pass unrecognized unless sought. The use of contrast media is relatively safe when used for most standard procedures in most patients, but there is a definable subgroup in whom there is a substantially increased risk of developing nephrotoxicity. Extensive analysis has shown that the most important risk factor is the presence of pre-existing renal disease and this seems to be particularly important when it is due to diabetes. Repeated administration of contrast in large doses also increases the risk, particularly soon after any previous administration. The pre-existing renal disease need not be severe to significantly increase the risk of nephrotoxicity, since mild elevations of the base-line serum creatinine to as little as > 140 μmol/l appear to contribute. The risk is also increased in those over 60 years of age, but this may merely be a reflection of declining renal function at this age. The higher the initial serum creatinine concentration, the longer does the reversible renal insufficiency take to subside. Sometimes the renal insufficiency may be prolonged, even to requiring dialysis, and in some cases, particularly those with significant prior nitrogen retention, the serum creatinine may never return to the previous level.

The mechanism of production of this nephrotoxic response has not been unequivocally elucidated. It is quite different from the acute anaphylactic reaction that can occur in some patients immediately after injection of contrast, and in most patients is asymptomatic. There appear to be two elements in its causation. The first is a reversible renal vasoconstriction leading to renal ischaemia, which is potentially damaging to residual nephrons in the presence of pre-existing renal disease. The other mechanism appears to be a direct tubule-cell cytotoxic response, which is largely dependent on the concentration of medium achieved within the cell. Both mechanisms are more likely in patients with pre-existing renal disease in whom residual nephrons are undergoing hyperfiltration and in whom there is likely to be associated vascular disease.

Prevention consists first in recognizing patients at risk and attempting to use an alternative radiographic procedure if possible. If the use of contrast is unavoidable, however, it is recommended that the dose be adjusted in accordance with the degree of nitrogen retention, and that repeated procedures be avoided—or at least that renal function be allowed to return to the base-line level before further medium is given. Patients should be well hydrated before the procedure and given a saline infusion of up to 500 ml/h throughout, provided the vascular system can tolerate this without overhydration. Since maintenance of a good urine volume is the goal, mannitol may be added for its diuretic effect, or frusemide if there is volume overload. The simultaneous use of prostaglandin synthetase inhibitors is particularly contraindicated. Use of the newer non-ionic contrast agents has not shown a reduction in nephrotoxicity in the higher risk patients and, in these patients, the same preventive programme should be adopted.

REFERENCE

Berns, A.S. (1989). Nephrotoxicity of contrast media. *Kidney International* **36**, 730–40.

Hydrocarbons and organic solvents

These comprise a large and varied group of compounds able to induce a variety of toxic responses in the kidney. Many, such as carbon tetrachloride and the halogenated hydrocarbons, are cytotoxic to renal tubular cells and can induce a range of damage to the tubule up to, and including, acute tubular necrosis. Functional tubular disorders, such as the Fanconi syndrome and renal tubular acidosis, have been reported following glue-sniffing. However, the largest group comprises those who develop an immune-complex type of glomerulonephritis following relatively low-grade exposure to a wide variety of hydrocarbons. Studies of hydrocarbon exposure in patients with glomerulonephritis, and of renal disease in persons with chronic industrial exposure to hydrocarbons, have suggested that such hydrocarbon exposure may be causal in the development of glomerular disease. Limitations of study design reduce the certainty with which causality can be established, but the accumulating data are increasingly supportive of such a relationship, particularly in Goodpasture's syndrome.

The clinical presentation is either as a membranous glomerulonephritis or as one arising as a response to toxic injury of mesangial cells. It is possible also that the hydrocarbons might modify the immune response. Certainly, in many of those exposed industrially to hydrocarbons, features of coexisting tubular damage, in the form of a tubular proteinuria and increased excretion of N-acetylglucosaminidase, may be found in those with features of glomerulonephritis. Glomerulonephritis, secondary to other nephrotoxins, has now become an established entity and an important feature of this type of nephrotoxicity is a component of individual susceptibility. To date this has been reflected only by an association with HLA tissue types. Future studies may well be informative in establishing the relationship further.

REFERENCES

Nelson, N.A., Robins, T.G., and Port, F.K. (1990). Solvent nephrotoxicity in humans and experimental animals. *American Journal of Nephrology* **10**, 10–20.

Yaqoob, M., Bell, G.M., Percy, D.F., and Finn, R. (1992). Primary glomerulonephritis and hydrocarbon exposure: a case-control study and literature review. *Quarterly Journal of Medicine, New Series* **82**, 409–18.

Ethylene glycol

Ethylene glycol is an aliphatic alcohol used as a freezing-point depressant. Nephrotoxicity is part of a more generalized toxic reaction often involving encephalitis, myocarditis, and myositis. The ethylene glycol is metabolized by alcohol dehydrogenase to oxalate and other toxic intermediates, and the brilliant birefringent crystals of calcium oxalate may be found in a wide variety of tissues. In the kidney, they can be seen within the lumina of the proximal tubules, many of which demonstrate necrosis. The clinical pattern is of acute oliguric renal failure which is potentially reversible, but which may pass into chronic renal failure if damage has been sufficiently severe.

The key points in the management of ethylene glycol nephrotoxicity are maintenance of a diuresis, early haemodialysis, correction of acidosis and the administration of alcohol. Since the ethylene glycol is metabolized by alcohol dehydrogenase, its metabolism to toxic compounds can be delayed considerably by the simultaneous administration of ethanol at a dose of 10 g/h. A vital aspect of management is the maintenance of a vigorous diuresis using both intravenous frusemide and mannitol. Early institution of these measures may prevent the development of acute renal failure and treatment may need to be continued for several days until the ethylene glycol has been slowly metabolized. Prevention depends upon the appreciation of the hazard of improper storage of this potentially toxic material.

REFERENCE

Jacobsen, D.A.G., Hewlett, T.P., Webb, R., Brown, S.T., Ordinario, A.T., and McMartin, K.E. (1988). Ethylene glycol intoxication: evaluation of kinetics and crystalluria. *American Journal of Medicine* **84**, 145–52.

20.14 Drugs and the kidney

D. J. S. CARMICHAEL

Introduction

The kidney is the major route of elimination of many drugs and their metabolites. This excretion may be by glomerular filtration, tubular secretion, or in some cases both. Patients on maintenance dialysis or following transplantation usually take large numbers of drugs as do those with acute or chronic renal failure. In practice, a minority of drugs need dose adjustment (dosage and/or interval) and it is those with a narrow therapeutic range or whose adverse effects are related to the drug or its metabolites which cause the major problems.

Excretion is affected most by renal impairment, but absorption, distribution (including protein binding), metabolism, and renal haemodynamics, as well as pharmacodynamics, may be altered. The major determinant of alteration in dosage is the change in drug clearance which can be broadly estimated by measurement of glomerular filtration rate. There are many handbooks that provide guidelines for the adjustment of dosage in renal impairment. The data in many of these are derived from measurement or estimation of changes in clearance, half-life ($t_{1/2}$) and volume of distribution (V_d). These measurements should be regarded only as approximations. In addition many of the adverse effects of drugs in kidney disease occur because there is often:

(1) ignorance of renal impairment before a drug is prescribed;
(2) ignorance of how a drug is cleared from the body; and
(3) failure to monitor therapeutic and adverse effects.

Pharmacokinetics

Gastrointestinal absorption

Renal impairment has minimal effects for most drugs, although increased gastric pH may reduce the absorption of acidic agents.

Distribution

Protein binding may be reduced by accumulation in the plasma of a number of acidic compounds that compete for binding sites on albumin and other plasma proteins. Phenytoin therapy is one of the few instances where these changes may be clinically significant. Binding of phenytoin to plasma protein is reduced in direct proportion to the fall in glomerular filtration rate and, consequently, the proportion of free (active) drug increases for a given total plasma concentration. The therapeutic range, estimated by total plasma concentration, has therefore to be adjusted to a lower level.

Digoxin is an example of a drug whose tissue binding (and consequently volume of distribution) falls in renal failure, and a smaller loading dose is needed.

Metabolism

The majority of drugs are excreted by the kidney either as the original compound or after metabolism in the liver to more polar (water-soluble) substances. There may be reduced clearance of metabolites which have therapeutic or adverse effects (see Table 1). Accumulation of inactive or relatively inactive metabolites may also confound interpretation of plasma concentration measurements of some drugs.

Renal failure may reduce drug metabolism and vitamin D is an important example of this phenomenon.

Renal excretion

Renal excretion of drugs depends upon filtration, active tubular secretion and reabsorption, and passive diffusion. Although renal clearance of drugs can be expressed as a function of glomerular filtration rate, this is often not a linear relationship because of the confounding effects of tubular reabsorption and secretion.

Compounds with a molecular weight below 60 000 Da are filtered to a variable extent depending on molecular size and on their degree of protein binding, since only the unbound portion is freely filtered. Non-polar (lipid-soluble) drugs diffuse readily across tubular cells, whereas polar (water-soluble) compounds do not. The latter generally remain in the tubular fluid and are excreted in the urine, while the former are reabsorbed by passive diffusion down their concentration gradient into plasma. Some polar drugs are eliminated in the urine as a result of active or facilitated transport mechanisms that transport organic acids or bases. Many drugs are metabolized, primarily in the liver, to produce more polar compounds, which cannot be passively reabsorbed and so are eliminated in the urine.

Examples of drugs that are actively secreted into the tubule are given in Table 2. In addition, some agents interact to inhibit tubular secretion of others (for example, probenecid with penicillin, with cephalosporins, and with frusemide). Elimination of organic acids (AH) or bases (B) is affected by the H^+ ion concentration of tubular fluid. In the non-ionized state these agents diffuse readily through the tubules, whereas ionization prevents such diffusion, changes in urinary pH which favour ionization therefore increase excretion rates:

$$H^+ + B \overset{pK_B}{\to} BH^+$$
$$AH \underset{pK_A}{\to} H^+ + A^-$$

The amount of ionized drug at any particular pH is determined by its pK. The pK is the pH at which 50 per cent of the drug is ionized. If an organic acid has a $pK_A < 7.5$, making the urine alkaline (that is, increasing its pH) increases the amount of ionized drug (A^-) and therefore its excretion. The converse is true for organic bases with a $pK_B > 7.5$, which are eliminated as the charged (BH^+) form favoured by acid pH. The excretions of salicylates (weak acids) and amphetamines (weak bases) exemplify these principles, which underlie the reason, for instance, of considering alkaline diuresis in the treatment of salicylate poisoning, to increase urinary clearance per unit glomerular filtration rate.

Drugs present in tubular fluid may affect the excretion of other compounds; for example, aspirin and paracetamol reduce methotrexate excretion. Although it is a simplification to disregard the tubular handling of drugs, in renal impairment both filtration and secretion of drugs appear to fall in parallel and in proportion to the glomerular filtration rate. It is paramount that, irrespective of what assumptions are made about the handling of drugs by the kidney, the most important aspect of prescribing in renal disease is awareness of the existence of renal impairment and of changes in renal function. Some measure of glomerular filtration rate is needed; serum creatinine measurement alone may be insufficient, particularly when renal function is changing (Chapter 20.1).

Table 1 *Parent drugs, metabolites, and possible adverse effects in renal failure*

Drug	Metabolite	Effect of metabolite
Allopurinol	Oxypurinol	? Cause of rashes
Clofibrate	Chlorophenoxyisobutyric acid	Muscle damage, neuropathy
Nitroprusside	Thiocyanate	Toxic symptoms
Primidone	Phenobarbitone	Active drug
Procainamide	N-Acetyl procainamide	Antiarrhythmic
Sulphonamides	Acetylsulphonamides	Rashes
Pethidine	Norpethidine	Causes seizures
Morphine	Morphine-6-glucuronide	Prolongs analgesia and respiratory depression
Codeine	Morphine	
Propoxyphene	Norpropoxyphene	Cardiotoxic
Acebutolol	N-Acetyl analogue	Confers selectivity
Nitrofurantoin	Metabolite	Peripheral neuropathy

Table 2 *Examples of drugs actively secreted into tubular fluid*

Organic acids	Organic bases
Penicillins	Amiloride
Cephalosporins	Procainamide
Sulphonamides	Quinidine
Frusemide	
Thiazides	
Salicylates	
Probenecid	

Drug kinetics

Most drugs that are eliminated by the kidney display first-order kinetics. This means that the rate of removal is proportional to the concentration of the drug. The elimination rate constant, k_e, is the proportion of total amount of drug removed per unit time. This produces a simple exponential decline (and therefore a straight line on a semilogarithmic plot) in concentration (Fig. 1). The half-life ($t_{1/2}$) of a drug is the time for its plasma concentration to fall by half after absorption and distribution are complete. It is useful in determining dosage interval, drug accumulation (both extent of accumulation and time taken to reach steady state), and persistence of drug after dosing is stopped. It is inversely related to k_e:

$$t_{1/2} = 0.693/k_e \qquad (0.693 = \ln 2)$$

The clearance of a drug depends upon $t_{1/2}$ (k_e) and volume of distribution (V_d). Volume of distribution does not usually correspond to a real volume, although for a drug confined exclusively to the plasma it would approximate the plasma volume. It represents an apparent volume that the drug would have distributed in to produce the measured plasma concentration. Volume of distribution itself may be affected by protein and tissue binding of drugs, changes in intravascular and extravascular fluid volumes, and lean body-mass.

Clearance can be used to calculate the steady-state concentration of a drug (C_{ss}) that can be anticipated in response to any particular dosage regimen. This concentration is proportional to the dose and $t_{1/2}$ of the drug and inversely proportional to the V_d and dosage interval. From these relationships it can be seen that C_{ss} will increase with a longer $t_{1/2}$ and a smaller V_d; the C_{ss} can be reduced either by lowering the dose or by increasing the dose interval.

The relationship between the elimination of a drug in the presence and absence of renal impairment can be estimated. This estimate, which has been calculated for a number of drugs, can be used to gauge the appropriate reduction in dose or increase in dose interval compared to a standard regimen. If non-renal clearance accounts for 50 per cent or more of total drug clearance, provided non-renal clearance is not affected by renal impairment no dose adjustment will be needed. Whether the dose, dose interval, or both is adjusted, the dose/unit time will be less than that in patients with normal renal function. In practice, however, the decision whether to reduce dose or prolong dose interval is not always equivalent. An example is the use of aminoglycoside antibiotics which must achieve a threshold peak concentration in order to kill bacteria effectively. In consequence, small but frequent doses may fail to achieve efficacy, whereas the same total dose delivered less frequently is more likely to achieve the desired therapeutic effect without leading to accumulation and toxicity.

Renal haemodynamics

Renal blood flow has little effect on the excretion of most drugs unless there is *pari passu*, a related fall in glomerular filtration rate. Non-steroidal anti-inflammatory agents may alter the glomerular filtration rate by inhibiting prostaglandin synthesis. Angiotensin-converting enzyme inhibitors may lower glomerular filtration rate by lowering glomerular efferent arteriolar tone under certain circumstances, such as dehydration or renovascular disease, when glomerular filtration rate is dependent upon the balance between afferent/efferent arteriolar tone.

Dialysis and haemofiltration

The clearance of drugs by haemodialysis and haemofiltration follows first-order kinetics. Estimates of clearance can be obtained by use of the sieving coefficient, which is the proportion of the drug (or solute) that will cross the membrane; it should be constant for a particular drug and membrane (Table 3).

The clearance of a drug depends on its molecular weight (and size) and protein binding. Haemofilter membranes have a pore size of 0.01 μm and those for haemodialysis 0.001 μm. In haemofiltration, drugs with a molecular weight below that of inulin (5200 Da) will pass through, whereas in haemodialysis most of those with a molecular weight below 500 Da (which includes many antibiotics) will be cleared,

Fig. 1 Plot of log concentration of a drug against time, to demonstrate the half-life of a drug.

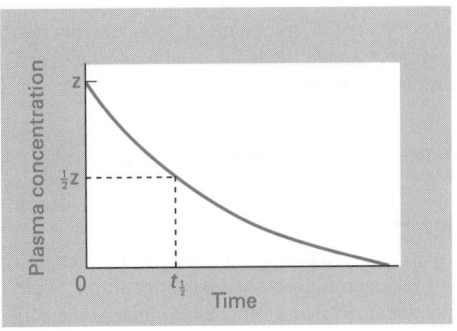

Table 3 *Factors influencing clearance of drugs by dialysis or filtration*

Properties of the drug	Molecular weight
	Protein binding
	Volume of distribution
Delivery of drug to the filter	Blood flow to filter
	Blood flow within filter
	Volume of distribution
Properties of the filter	Pore size
	Surface area

but drugs such as vancomycin (1800 Da), amphotericin (960 Da), and erythromycin (734 Da) behave differentially with respect to haemofiltration/haemodialysis. Heavily protein-bound agents, even with a lower molecular weight (for example, propranolol, 259 Da), will not be filtered, but drugs which are displaced from binding sites in the presence of renal impairment will become available for filtration. Water-soluble drugs pass through filters more readily than those that are fat soluble. A list of some commonly used drugs and their clearance by haemodialysis or peritoneal dialysis is shown in Table 4. Differences resulting from the use of the different techniques for haemodialysis, haemodiafiltration, and intermittent and continuous haemofiltration are dealt with in other texts.

Digoxin and antidepressants are examples of drugs with a large volume of distribution. They will have low plasma concentrations and therefore little will be available for filtration.

Peritoneal dialysis clears drugs very much less efficiently than do haemodialysis or haemofiltration. However, some drugs, particularly antibiotics, need readjustment in dosage regimens in the treatment of peritonitis complicating continuous ambulatory peritoneal dialysis (CAPD) (Chapter 20.17.2).

Drug prescribing

When a particular drug, known to be cleared largely by the kidney is to be given to a patient with impaired renal function, the dose can be adjusted in two main ways. Either the size of each dose or the frequency of administration can be reduced. Plasma drug concentrations can be used to confirm that the initial adjustment of dosage is correct for the particular individual. Steady-state concentrations of anticonvulsants, digoxin, and theophylline can be measured after the equivalent of five half-lives of the drug. For antibiotics such as gentamicin it is essential to measure the peak-and-trough level after the first day's administration and thereafter if renal function is impaired or changing.

A combination of reduction in dosage and less frequent administration is suitable for most drugs. Dosage reduction alone is more likely to lead to subtherapeutic plasma concentrations. Adjustments of doses must be kept simple and clear since unfamiliar dosages and administration at unusual times make for error. It is best to use a limited number of drugs so that those responsible develop familiarity with regimens used in renal failure or during renal replacement treatments.

Patients with multisystem failure

Many of the most complex prescribing problems arise in patients with multiple organ failure, commonly resulting in the need for artificial ventilation as well as renal replacement therapy.

VENTILATED PATIENTS AND THOSE IN INTENSIVE CARE UNITS

Neuromuscular blocking agents

Succinylcholine is rapidly hydrolysed by plasma cholinesterase; no dose adjustment is needed. For more prolonged paralysis atracurium, which is degraded by non-enzymatic Hofmann elimination independent of renal or hepatic function is preferable. It is removed by dialysis and haemofiltration and the dose is titrated to produce a therapeutic effect. Tubocurarine, gallamine, alcuronium, pancuronium, and vercuronium should be avoided.

Anaesthetic and sedating agents

Propofol, fentanyl, and alfentanil require no dose adjustment but the last two may have prolonged effects if there is concomitant hepatic dysfunction. Diazepam has metabolites that accumulate, and midazolam is preferable with dosage reduction if the glomerular filtration rate falls below 10 ml/min. Phenothiazines, butyrophenones, and Heminevrin® can be given in usual doses.

Narcotic analgesics

Opiates are affected by renal failure, and retention of metabolites can produce adverse effects. Reduced intermittent doses, epidural administration, or low-dose continuous infusions reduce the incidence of adverse effects. Diamorphine is metabolized into morphine and then to morphine-3-glucuronide and morphine-6-glucuronide, both of which accumulate to prolong both analgesia and respiratory depression. Pethidine (meperidine) is converted to norpethidine (normeperidine) which accumulates and can cause seizures. Papaveretum is a mixture of alkaloids of opium including morphine, codeine, noscapine, and papaverene: its use is not recommended.

Cardiac drugs

Adrenaline, dobutamine, or dopamine and noradrenaline should be used in the minimum possible doses in order to avoid renal vasoconstriction. Low-dose dopamine (2 μg/kg/min) is often used in conjunction with other agents to preserve renal blood flow. Intravenous nitrates can be given in normal dosage. Sodium nitroprusside is metabolized in the liver to sodium thiocyanate which is eliminated by the kidney, and so may accumulate in renal failure to cause toxicity. It is removed by haemodialysis or peritoneal dialysis.

Antiarrhythmics

In patients with abnormal renal function it is advisable to keep treatment simple. Most antiarrhythmic drugs are used without dose modification (for example, lignocaine, flecainide, mexiletine, and verapamil). Digoxin is a notable exception with a lower loading and much lower maintenance dose than usual. The maintenance dose of amiodarone should be reduced to 100 mg daily when the glomerular filtration rate falls below 20 ml/min.

ANTIMICROBIALS

Many antimicrobial agents are excreted by the kidney. With the exception of aminoglycosides and vancomycin, most have a wide therapeutic index and little or no dose adjustment is usually made until the glomerular filtration rate is less than 20 ml/min. Antimicrobials that are removed by dialysis should be administered after dialysis, or a supplemental dose should be given at that time. Adjustments are shown in Table 5.

Penicillins

All penicillins should be given in reduced dose. Carbenicillin and ticarcillin solutions contain approximately 5 mmol Na$^+$/g, and caution is needed in the presence of salt and water retention. Mezlocillin, unlike other penicillins, is not dialysed.

Intravenous cephalosporins and other β-lactams

Cephalosporins are excreted in similar fashion to penicillins and should be given in lower doses in renal impairment (Table 5). The combination of a loop diuretic and a first-generation cephalosporin, cephaloridine, caused nephrotoxicity; the later-generation drugs are safer but caution is still needed with cefuroxime. In the third-generation drugs, cefotax-

Table 4 *Effectiveness or otherwise of clearance of drugs by dialysis*

Dialysed	Slightly dialysed	Not dialysed
Haemodialysis		
Acyclovir	Amantadine	Acebutolol
Allopurinol	Cilastatin	Amphotericin B
Amikacin	Ciprofloxacin	Bretylium
Amoxycillin	Co-trimoxazole	Chloroquine
Ampicillin	Enalapril	Clonidine
Atenolol	Erythromycin	Cyclosporin
Aztreonam	Ethambutol	Diazoxide
Carbenicillin	Ethosuximide	Digoxin
Cefotaxime	Lorazepam	Disopyramide
Ceftazidime	Methylprednisolone	Flecamide
Cefuroxime	Nadolol	Glutethamide
Cephalexin	Procainamide	Heparin
Cephradine	Tetracyclines	Methicillin
Flucytosine	Vancomycin	Methotrexate
Gentamicin		Metoprolol
Isoniazid		Miconazole
Lithium		Oxazepam
Mecillinam		Pethidine
Metronidazole		Phenytoin
Moxolactam		Prednisone
Netilmicin		Procainamide
Penicillin		Propoxyphen
Ranitidine		Propranolol
Streptomycin		Valproic acid
Theophylline		Vancomycin
Ticarcillin		Warfarin
Tobramycin		
Trimethoprim		
Peritoneal dialysis		
Aztreonam	Aminoglycosides	Isoniazid
Ceftazidime	Aspirin	Phenobarbitone
Ethambutol	Cephalexin	Quinidine
Gallamine	Flucytosine	Theophylline
Ranitidine	Lithium	

ime and ceftazidime, cilastatin (an inhibitor of dipeptidase) confers protection against renal toxicity.

Aminoglycosides

Particular attention to dose adjustment is required for aminoglycosides, even in mild impairment of renal function. Furthermore, these agents are inherently nephrotoxic, and their use may worsen renal impairment and cause ototoxicity.

Several factors make nephrotoxicity more likely: prior or prolonged treatment, hypovolaemia, dehydration, concomitant administration of diuretics, hypokalaemia, and hypomagnesaemia. Obstructive jaundice also increases the risk. The only way to be sure of preventing aminoglycoside toxicity is to avoid the use of these drugs altogether in patients with any suspicion of renal impairment, but the risk of nephrotoxicity is often outweighed by the need for effective antimicrobial treatment in sick patients.

There are many nomograms and other guidelines for dose adjustment of aminoglycosides for patients with renal impairment, but each has drawbacks. Since the volume of distribution of aminoglycosides is not materially affected by renal impairment, an adequate loading dose of 1 to 1.5 mg/kg of gentamicin is required. Reduced doses given at the usual intervals may increase the likelihood of subtherapeutic peak plasma levels. If only the dose interval is prolonged, there is also the risk of subtherapeutic plasma concentrations when the drug is given over long periods. A combination of both methods with frequent peak measurements (taken 1 h after intravenous dosing) and trough measurements

(immediately before the next dose) is optimal. Such measurements should be made daily when alterations in renal function are anticipated and two to three times a week under other circumstances. The dose regimen is adjusted to produce peak plasma concentrations of gentamicin between 6 and 10 mg/l and trough concentrations not exceeding 2 mg/l. Doses and therapeutic concentrations are shown in Table 6.

Vancomycin and teicoplanin

Vancomycin is excreted by the kidney and is not dialysed. In patients with endstage renal failure on dialysis, therapeutic concentrations can be maintained for 5 days or more after a single intravenous dose; the target steady-state plasma concentration is approximately 15 mg/l. Following a loading dose of 15 mg/kg, further doses are given on the basis of plasma concentration. Vancomycin is not removed by haemodialysis or haemofiltration (except at extremely high flow rates in haemofiltration, by haemodiafiltration, or by haemodialysis with high flux dialysers). Teicoplanin, a glycopeptide related to vancomycin, behaves rather differently. The half-life is prolonged in renal failure (approximately three times) and after a loading dose of 400 mg the maintenance dose of 200 mg/day should be reduced after 3 days even in mild renal failure. It is not cleared by dialysis.

Ciprofloxacin

Renal excretion exceeds glomerular filtration rate, and in patients with normal renal function approximately 60 per cent is cleared by the kidneys. It is recommended that the dose should be reduced in renal impair-

Table 5 *Guidelines for adjustment of doses of antimicrobials in renal failure (GFR (ml/min))*

Drug	Renal function	Dose reduction	Comments
Ampicillin			Seldom needed
Flucloxacillin		Nil	
Amoxycillin + clavulanic acid	< 20	By 50%	Half dose postdialysis
Benzyl penicillin	< 20		Daily dose should not exceed 20 mU
Piperacillin	20–50	By 50%	Half dose postdialysis
	< 20	By 66%	
Cefotaxime ⎫	20–50	By 66%	
Ceftazidime ⎬	< 20	By 75%	Half dose postdialysis
Aztreonam	< 10	By 75%	
Imipenem/cilastatin	< 20	By 50%	Half dose postdialysis
Erythromycin		Nil	Half dose postdialysis
Trimethoprim	< 20	By half	
Ciprofloxacin	< 10		Half dose postdialysis
Rifampicin			500–750 mg per day maximum
Flucytosine	20–50	Nil	Avoid with cyclosporin
	< 20	By half	Half dose postdialysis
Fluconazole	< 50	By three-quarters	
Acyclovir		By half	After 2 days
	Stepwise reduction from 800 mg five times a day with GFR 50 ml/min to 10 ml/min		

GFR, glomerular filtration rate

Table 6 *Doses and therapeutic plasma concentrations of aminoglycosides*

Drug	Usual daily dose	Therapeutic concentration	
		Peak (mg/l)	Trough (mg/l)
Gentamicin	2–5 mg/kg	5–10	< 2.5
Tobramycin	2–5 mg/kg	5–10	< 2.5
Netilmicin	2–5 mg/kg	5–10	< 2.5
Amikacin	10–30 µg/kg	20–30	< 10
Kanamycin	10–30 µg/kg	20–30	< 10

Peak concentration is measured 1 h postinjection.

Trough concentration is measured immediately before next dose.

Usual daily dose is administered 8 hourly.

The netilmicin dose can be increased to 7.5 mg/kg/day in severe infections, but requires careful therapeutic monitoring.

ment but the proportion that is cleared by the liver and gut is increased in renal failure. Ciprofloxacin is not significantly removed by haemo-dialysis but may be removed by haemofiltration.

Tetracyclines

All the tetracyclines except minocycline and doxycycline are renally excreted. Plasma half-lives are markedly prolonged (up to 100 h) in renal impairment. Tetracyclines are antianabolic and increased plasma levels cause a concentration-related increasing uraemia, setting up a vicious cycle that leads to deterioration in renal function. Doxycycline or minocycline can be used cautiously in patients with renal impairment, but the other tetracyclines are always contraindicated.

Sulphonamides, co-trimoxazole, and trimethoprim

Sulphonamides are eliminated by acetylation followed by renal excretion, and acetylated metabolites (which have no antibacterial activity) are a cause of crystalluria and tubular damage. High doses of co-trimoxazole are needed in the treatment of *Pneumocystis carinii* infection, the risk of adverse effects being balanced against the seriousness of the condition in patients who often have impaired renal function. The initial dose of trimethoprim is 20 mg/kg body-weight/day and of sulphamethoxazole, 100 mg/kg/day divided in two or more doses. The plasma concentration should be maintained at approximately 5 to 8 µg/l mea-sured after five doses, and can sometimes be achieved by lower maintenance doses.

Pentamidine

The usual dose is 4 mg/kg, given by slow intravenous infusion over 90 min. There is considerable tissue binding and the drug is excreted in the urine over long periods. The dose should be reduced in patients with renal impairment and, since the drug is nephrotoxic, it should be reduce by 30 to 50 per cent if the serum creatinine increases by 80 to 100 µmol/l (around 1 mg/100 ml).

Antiviral agents

Acyclovir and gancyclovir are both eliminated by the kidney and are dialysed. Lower doses of both drugs are required in the presence of renal failure.

Antifungal agents

Amphotericin is nephrotoxic, and should only be used with great caution in patients who already have renal impairment. Toxicity may be ameliorated by sodium supplementation provided the kidney can excrete the extra load. Both flucytosine and fluconazole are excreted in the urine. Ketoconazole is less well absorbed in renal failure and interferes with cyclosporin metabolism (see Table 7).

Table 7 *Drugs affecting cytochrome P450 system*

Inhibitors	Inducers
Ketoconazole	Rifampicin
Erythromycin	Phenytoin
Oral contraceptives	Phenobarbitone
Methylprednisolone	Carbamazepine
Diltiazem	Sodium valproate
Nicardipine	
Verapamil	
Cimetidine	

Antiprotozoal agents and malaria

Quinine is given in usual doses unless acute renal failure develops, when the dose should be reduced after 2 to 3 days. The dose of chloroquine is reduced by half if the glomerular filtration rate is less than 50 ml/min, and to a quarter if the glomerular filtration rate is less than 10 ml/min; primaquine is given in usual doses. Prophylactic chloroquine can be given in the usual dose of 300 mg/week in patients with renal impairment. Proguanil (usual dose 200 mg daily) should be given in half the usual dose if the glomerular filtration rate is less than 10 ml/min.

Treatment of urinary tract infection

Only drugs that will attain satisfactory levels in the urine in the presence of renal impairment should be prescribed. Nalidixic acid and nitrofurantoin are of little use and the latter accumulates.

DRUGS ACTING ON THE CENTRAL NERVOUS SYSTEM

These may have a prolonged effect not only because of changes in pharmacokinetics but also because of increased sensitivity as a consequence of uraemia.

Antidepressants

Clinically significant effects of renal impairment on antidepressants have not been described and all can be given at the usual dosage.

Lithium

Lithium is used primarily in affective disorders. It is filtered and then reabsorbed, mainly in the proximal tubule. The dose should be reduced in renal impairment, with careful monitoring of plasma concentrations. In sodium depletion (for example with chronic thiazide diuretic use) tubular reabsorption of lithium is increased, leading to higher plasma concentrations and toxicity. The effect of non-steroidal anti-inflammatory drugs on renal haemodynamics may also increase toxicity when added to lithium therapy.

Major tranquillizers

No dose change is required when phenothiazines or butyrophenones are used in patients with renal impairment.

Minor tranquillizers

Benzodiazepines too can be prescribed in usual dosage, but diazepam and chlordiazepoxide have active metabolites that may accumulate. It is preferable, therefore, to use drugs without active metabolite, such as nitrazepam and temazepam, to avoid hangover the morning after use as night sedation.

Anticonvulsants

Phenytoin, carbamazepine, and valproic acid are given in usual dosages with the proviso concerning therapeutic concentrations of phenytoin.

Weaker analgesics

Codeine and dihydrocodeine, although relatively weak analgesics, still have the potential to cause severe respiratory depression in some patients, as does dextropropoxyphene (combined with paracetamol as co-proxamol). Its metabolite, norproxyphene, which accumulates in renal failure, sometimes causes cardiac toxicity.

Buprenorphine is metabolized in the liver and does not appear to have any important toxic metabolites that might accumulate in renal failure.

Non-narcotic analgesics

Paracetamol is excreted in small amounts by glomerular filtration with some passive tubular reabsorption. The major part of the drug is metabolized and the glucuronide and sulphide metabolites, which are subject to active tubular secretion, accumulate in renal impairment, and there is some regeneration of the parent compound. Despite this, paracetamol is used in normal doses. Aspirin has the disadvantage of causing gastric inflammation and increasing the bleeding diathesis of patients with renal failure. Renal elimination of its metabolite salicylate is enhanced in alkaline urine.

Antihistamines

Both terfenadine and prochlorperazine can be used at the usual dosage.

CARDIAC FAILURE AND OEDEMA

Diuretics

Spironolactone, triamterene, and amiloride, all potassium-sparing diuretics, should be avoided in renal impairment because of the danger of hyperkalaemia. The same applies for combination diuretics such as Moduretic® (amiloride and hydrochlorothiazide) or Dyazide® (triamterene and hydrochlorothiazide). Thiazides apart from metolazone (a quinolone) become less effective if the glomerular filtration rate is below 25 ml/min. Higher doses of loop diuretics are needed, but the synergistic effect with metolazone may overcome 'diuretic resistance' in refractory oedema.

Severe sodium and water depletion can result from poorly controlled diuretic therapy with secondary effects on renal function and concomitant drug therapy.

Angiotensin-converting enzyme

Whether angiotensin-converting enzyme inhibitors (ACE inhibitors) are being used to treat cardiac failure or hypertension, the same precautions apply. Starting doses should be low and increased slowly with careful monitoring of serum creatinine and potassium. Particular caution is necessary if these drugs are used in combination with diuretics or in other high-renin states (such as volume depletion), when marked hypotension (first-dose effect) may be anticipated. Caution is also necessary when there is (or may be) a possibility of renal artery stenosis, both because of the risk of hypotension and also because of reduced glomerular filtration rate in the affected kidney(s). They should generally not be used with potassium-sparing diuretics because of the added risk of hyperkalaemia. All are eliminated by the kidney, which accounts for the reduced dose often required in the elderly. Captopril has a shorter half-life than the others and dose adjustments can therefore be made more readily. They are all dialysed.

HYPERTENSION

Problems should be avoided by titration of a low starting dose of any drug to produce the required therapeutic effect. Thiazides are less effective as the glomerular filtration rate falls, and a loop diuretic is often necessary since many antihypertensive drugs tend to promote sodium retention.

β-Blockers

Atenolol, bisoprolol, pindolol, nadolol, and sotalol are all excreted by the kidney and reduced doses may be needed. The metabolites of acebutolol may accumulate. Other β-blockers can be prescribed unchanged.

Vasodilators, calcium-channel blockers, and α-blockers

No dose adjustment is needed for any of these drugs. Minoxidil therapy often requires concomitant use of a loop diuretic.

Centrally acting agents

α-Methyldopa and clonidine are given in usual doses.

DIABETES MELLITUS

Insulin

Insulin requirements fall with declining renal function, probably as a consequence of its reduced renal metabolism in both acute and chronic renal failure. In patients on haemodialysis it is often necessary to give supplemental insulin during treatment. The same situation applies in patients on haemofiltration in acute renal failure, particularly if they are being fed parenterally, and in continuous arteriovenous haemodialysis when the dialysate is a glucose-based solution. Non-diabetic patients may require insulin temporarily under these circumstances. Patients on CAPD may need a change in insulin preparation and adjustment in the frequency and route of administration. The intraperitoneal requirement is approximately 50 per cent of intravenous requirements.

Oral hypoglycaemic agents

Gliclazide and glipizide are the safest drugs to use in renal failure, although dose reduction may be needed if the glomerular filtration rate is below 10 ml/min. Other sulphonylureas, particularly chlorpropamide, have a prolonged half-life. The biguanides should not be used if the glomerular filtration rate is below 20 ml/min.

ASTHMA

Doses of β-agonists administered by inhalation, oral, or parenteral routes need no adjustment in patients with renal impairment. Aminophylline and theophylline can also be given in usual doses but metabolites may accumulate.

GASTROINTESTINAL DRUGS

H_2-antagonists and antiulcer drugs

Cimetidine is cleared by the liver but metabolites accumulate if the glomerular filtration rate is less than 20 ml/min. Ranitidine, which causes less cerebral confusion, is preferable in this situation; but it may interfere with creatinine secretion and raises plasma creatinine. It is partly cleared by the kidneys and the dose should be halved when the glomerular filtration rate is less than 10 ml/min. It is dialysed, and a supplemental dose is needed after dialysis but not after haemofiltration. Omeprazole and misoprostol are given in usual doses. Misoprostol may cause reductions in glomerular filtration rate through haemodynamic changes in the kidney.

Antacids

Alginates, magnesium trisilicate mixture (but not magnesium trisilicate powder), and sodium bicarbonate all have a high sodium content. The use of aluminium-containing compounds, such as aluminium hydroxide or sulcralfate in patients with severe renal impairment or those on dialysis is controversial because of the potential risks of aluminium retention with deleterious effects on bone, bone marrow, and the central nervous system. Calcium carbonate should not be used as an antacid but only as a phosphate binder.

HYPERURICAEMIA

Allopurinol

Allopurinol is metabolized to oxypurinol which is retained in renal impairment and may be responsible for some of the adverse effects, including rashes, bone marrow depression, and gastrointestinal upset.

The dose should be reduced to 100 mg/day when the glomerular filtration rate is less than 20 ml/min, and in haemodialysis patients this drug should be given at the end of treatment. Allopurinol interferes with the metabolism of 6-mercaptopurine, which is an active metabolite of azathioprine. When the two drugs are given together, therefore, it is often necessary to reduce the dose of azathioprine.

Probenecid

Probenecid inhibits secretion of acids in the proximal tubule and prevents reabsorption of urate from the tubular lumen. It prolongs the effect of penicillins, cephalosporins, naproxen, indomethacin, methotrexate, and sulphonylureas (all of which are weak acids), causing accumulation and the potential for toxicity. It also inhibits tubular secretion (and hence activity) of frusemide and bumetanide.

Colchicine

Colchicine has been largely replaced by non-steroidal anti-inflammatory drugs (**NSAIDs**) for the treatment of acute gout. However, it remains valuable in patients in whom NSAIDs are undesirable (for example, those with peptic ulcer disease, cardiac failure, or renal impairment) and can be given in the usual doses.

ANTI-INFLAMMATORY AGENTS

NSAIDs, including aspirin, inhibit prostaglandin synthesis by inhibition of cyclo-oxygenase. The principal renal prostaglandins in man are PGE_2 and PGI_2, each of which is a vasodilator and natriuretic. In addition to effects on renal blood flow, prostaglandins also influence tubular ion transport directly. In healthy individuals inhibition of cyclo-oxygenase has no detectable effect on renal function, but in patients with cardiac failure, nephrotic syndrome, liver disease, glomerulonephritis, and other renal disease cyclo-oxygenase inhibitors predictably cause a reversible fall in glomerular filtration rate, which can be severe. They also cause fluid retention, blunt the effects of antihypertensive drugs, and may also cause hyperkalaemia. There is some evidence that sulindac causes less inhibition of renal cyclo-oxygenase than a dose of ibuprofen that is equieffective on extrarenal tissues; it may therefore cause less renal impairment than other NSAIDs. Aspirin may also spare cyclo-oxygenase in the kidney to some extent. The clinical relevance of these observations remains uncertain and any of this class of drugs should only be given to patients with renal failure with circumspection.

Indomethacin, azapropazone, and diflunisal have important renal excretion, whereas most other NSAIDs are eliminated by metabolism. The NSAIDs are highly protein bound and are not removed by dialysis.

ANTICOAGULANTS

Warfarin is used in normal dosage and its effect monitored by measuring INR in the usual way. It is highly protein bound and there may be slight displacement and consequent reduction in the volume of distribution in renal failure. In nephrotic patients hypoalbuminaemia leads to increased sensitivity to warfarin. It is not dialysed. Heparin can be used in normal dosage.

Corticosteroids and immunosuppressive agents

Prednisone and prednisolone are not eliminated by the kidney. Methylprednisolone is cleared by haemodialysis, and should therefore be given after dialysis. Azathioprine accumulates in renal impairment and the dose should be reduced from a maximum of 3 mg/kg/day to 1 mg/kg/day if the glomerular filtration rate falls below 10 ml/min.

Cyclosporin is a highly lipid-soluble drug which is extensively bound to plasma proteins and has a large volume of distribution. It is metabolized by the liver via the cytochrome P-450 system by mono- and dihydroxylation as well as N-demethylation. Only minor amounts are excreted as parent drug or metabolites in the urine. Renal impairment does not affect the metabolism. However, since many other drugs may be prescribed to patients on cyclosporin therapy several important interactions may occur. These can increase plasma concentration and therefore increase the risk of nephrotoxicity or, in contrast, reduce plasma concentrations and increase the risk of transplant organ rejection. Aminoglycosides may have an additive effect upon the nephrotoxicity of cyclosporin. The common interactions are listed in Table 7.

MISCELLANEOUS DRUGS

Acetazolamide

Acetazolamide may produce systemic acidosis and hypokalaemia, particularly in renal impairment and in the elderly. Its use should be avoided or carefully monitored.

Lipid-lowering agents

The anion-exchange resins (for example, colestipol) and HMG-CoA reductase inhibitors (simvastatin, pravastatin) are given at their usual dose. The fibrates (gemfibrozil, bezafibrate) can be used with dose reduction at glomerular filtration rates of less than 20 ml/min. It is probably best to avoid clofibrate altogether as myopathy is more likely to occur in the presence of renal dysfunction.

Summary

Since the presence of impaired renal function affects the metabolism of so many drugs and their interaction with other agents, it is essential always to check the need for a modification of normal dosage in any patient in whom renal disease is known or suspected, and to watch carefully for adverse effects.

REFERENCES

Benet, L.Z., Mitchell, J.R., and Sheiner, L.B. (1990). Pharmacokinetics: The dynamics of drug, absorption, distribution, and elimination. In *Goodman and Gilman's The pharmacological basis of therapeutics*, (ed. A.G. Gilman, T.W. Rall, A.S. Nies, and P. Taylor), Section I, pp. 3–32. Pergamon Press, Oxford.

Bennett, W.M. (1990). Guide to drug dosage in renal failure. In *Clinical pharmacokinetics drug data handbook*, pp. 31–84. Adis Press, United Kingdom.

Carmichael, D.J.S. (1992). Handling of drugs in kidney disease. In *Oxford textbook of clinical nephrology*, (ed. S. Cameron, A.M. Davison, J.-P. Grunfeld, D. Kerr, and E. Ritz), pp. 175–96. Oxford University Press.

Drayer, D.E. (1983). Pharmacologically active drug metabolites: therapeutic and toxic activities, plasma and urine data in man, accumulation in renal failure. In *Handbook of clinical pharmacokinetics*, (ed. M. Gibaldi, and L. Prescott), pp. 114–32. Raven Press, New York.

Duchin, K.L. and Schrier, R.W. (1983). Inter-relationship between renal haemodynamics, drug kinetics and drug action. In *Handbook of clinical pharmacokinetics*, (ed. M. Gibaldi, and L. Prescott), Section I, pp. 183–97. ADIS Health Science Press, Balgowlah, Australia.

Fillastre, J.-P. and Singlas, E. (1991). Pharmacokinetics of newer drugs with renal impairment (Part I). *Clinical Pharmacokinetics* **20**, 293–310.

Golper, T.A. (1991). Drug removal during continuous hemofiltration or hemodialysis. *Contributions in Nephrology* **93**, 110–16.

Gugler, R. and Azarnoff, D.L. (1983). Drug protein binding and the nephrotic syndrome. In *Handbook of clinical pharmacokinetics*, (ed. M. Gibaldi, and L. Prescott), Section III, pp. 96–108. ADIS Health Science Press, Balgowlah, Australia.

Gulyassy, P.F. and Depner, T.A. (1983). Impaired binding of drugs and ligands in renal diseases. *American Journal of Kidney Diseases* **2**, 578–601.

Humes, H.D. (1988). Aminoglycoside nephrotoxicity. *Kidney International* **33**, 900–11.

Martindale. (1989). In *The extra pharmacopoeia*, (ed. J.E.F. Reynolds). The Pharmaceutical Press, London.

Park, G.D. (1987). Pharmacokinetics. In *The scientific basis of clinical pharmacology*, (ed. R. Spector), pp. 67–102. Little, Brown and Co., Boston.

Singlas, E. and Fillastre, J.-P. (1991). Pharmacokinetics of newer drugs in patients with renal impairment (Part II). *Clinical Pharmacokinetics* **20**, 389–410.

20.15 Genitourinary tuberculosis

L. R. I. BAKER

Social changes, public health measures, BCG vaccination, and effective chemotherapy have much reduced morbidity and mortality in tuberculosis, including genitourinary tuberculosis, in wealthy nations in recent decades. The disease remains a major public health problem in less fortunate parts of the world, immigrants from which (for example those from Asia) still have a high prevalence of the disease. The impact worldwide of acquired immunodeficiency syndrome upon the prevalence of active tuberculous infection amongst sufferers and their contacts may well be marked. The effect, if any, upon genitourinary tuberculosis incidence and prevalence rates is as yet unclear. In the United Kingdom, approximately 6000 new cases of tuberculosis are reported annually.

Genitourinary tuberculosis is typically a late manifestation of previous pulmonary infection. It probably develops in 4 to 5 per cent of cases of pulmonary tuberculosis.

Aetiology

Mycobacterium tuberculosis, the human tubercle bacillus, in common with all mycobacteria, is an obligate aerobe possessing the ability to take up certain aniline dyes and to resist decolorization by washing in acidified alcohol. Mycobacteria in general exist in soil, water, and various animal species, including reptiles, amphibia, birds, and mammals. Several mycobacteria are pathogenic to humans, for example *Mycobacterium bovis*, the bovine tubercle bacillus. This has almost completely disappeared as a human pathogen in developed countries, mainly owing to tuberculin testing of cattle and the pasteurization of dairy products. Other mycobacteria, such as *M. smegmatis*, are human saprophytes. *Mycobacterium smegmatis* is frequently identified in urine, giving rise to the potential for a mistaken diagnosis of true tuberculous infection.

Pathogenesis

Pulmonary tuberculosis is acquired by inhalation and a subsequent mismatch between the virulence of the organism and the host's immunological response. Spread via the bloodstream results in tuberculosis of the genitourinary tract. Rarely, the primary infection is derived from the gut rather than the lungs.

Bloodstream dissemination of mycobacteria most often affects the renal cortices. Small granulomas develop in the glomerular or adjacent capillaries, the high blood flow rate and oxygen tension in this region presumably favouring the organism. Subsequent rupture of capillaries spreads mycobacteria to the tubules, allowing the ultimate development of infection in the renal medulla. The immune response in the medullary region is weak, perhaps owing to increased hypertonicity, relatively slow blood flow, and increased ammonia concentration, amongst other factors, presumably explaining the usual location of renal tuberculous infection in the medulla. Medullary granulomas may enlarge and become closed lesions but more often rupture with consequent spread of tubercle bacilli. Infection of renal pelves, ureters, bladder, and the genital organs follows. Genital infection is more common in men. Direct seeding via the bloodstream and lymphatic spread to adjacent organs may also occur.

PATHOLOGY

The typical microscopic finding is of caseating granulomas. Tubercle bacilli may be identified by Ziehl–Neelsen staining. Granulomas in the renal cortex have little tendency to enlarge, in contrast to medullary and papillary granulomas which tend to increase, caseate, and cavitate with release of tubercle bacilli into the renal pelvis, ureters, and bladder. Subsequent healing of infection followed by fibrosis causes renal parenchymal atrophy, calyceal infundibular stenosis and fibrotic obstruction at the pelviureteric junction (uncommon), ureteric stenosis (most common at the vesicoureteral junction), and bladder fibrosis with marked bladder-wall thickening and loss of bladder capacity. Urinary tract obstruction resulting from stricture formation may lead to obstructive atrophy of the kidney, further compromising renal function already impaired by direct parenchymal infection. Calcification of diffuse parenchymal lesions may be localized or extensive. In the latter case renal destruction ('autonephrectomy') occurs. Occasionally, diffuse parenchymal infection may occur in the absence of cavitation, calcification, or distortion of the pelvicalyceal system, ureters, and bladder. A proportion of such patients develop endstage renal failure with the nonspecific finding of small, unobstructed kidneys on imaging.

Cystoscopic appearances vary from a region of inflammation or superficial granulation at one or other ureteric orifice to a generalized cystitis with oedema and widespread granulations. Healed bladder lesions have a stellate appearance caused by bands of fibrous tissue meeting at a central point, the main area of severe infection. Severe fibrotic change may cause the ureteric orifice to become withdrawn and widely patent ('golf-hole ureter').

PRESENTATION

Most patients are young men. The male : female ratio is 2 : 1 and the large majority of patients are aged between 20 and 40 years. The disease is rare before puberty. A previous personal or family history of tuberculosis is not uncommon.

Urinary tract tuberculosis often produces little in the way of symptoms until the bladder is involved. The most common presenting symptom is urinary frequency followed by dysuria. Macroscopic haematuria and renal pain, usually mild, are present in less than 30 per cent of patients. Ureteric colic is rare. Constitutional symptoms (malaise, tiredness, weight loss, night sweats, fever, and anorexia) are seen in less than one-fifth of patients. Much less commonly, patients present with polyuria, renal salt-wasting, hypertension, or chronic renal failure.

In many instances the suspicion of urinary tract tuberculosis is based on laboratory or imaging examinations carried out without the diagnosis in mind. A significant proportion of patients are diagnosed at operation or even at autopsy.

The patient may present with chronic epididymitis or other symptoms of infection of the genital tract.

Investigation

URINE EXAMINATION

On microscopy, pyuria may or may not be present. Pyuria in the absence of significant bacteriuria on conventional microbiological culture ('sterile pyuria') should raise the suspicion of urinary tract tuberculosis, although many other causes exist. Conversely, the finding of significant bacteriuria does not exclude the diagnosis of tuberculosis, since superimposed secondary infection may be present in advanced cases. The commonest causative organism is *Escherichia coli*.

The isolation of *Mycobacterium tuberculosis* by urine culture is the definitive diagnostic test for the confirmation of urinary tract tuberculosis. Sensitivity tests should be carried out on positive cultures to streptomycin, rifampicin, isoniazid, pyrazinamide, and ethambutol. Three to five early morning urine specimens should be provided and should reach the laboratory at the earliest opportunity, since the longer the urine remains in contact with the organism the less likely is the Mycobacterium to grow. *Mycobacterium tuberculosis* is present only intermittently in the urine and in low count, and grows poorly on culture media. Specimens should not be kept, pooled together, or brought up to the laboratory together, some of them being days old. Urine samples are exposed to acid and alkaline solutions and centrifuged, and a sample of the deposit inoculated on to either egg-based (Löwenstein–Jensen) or agar-based media, so constituted as to inhibit the growth of contaminant bacteria. Media with and without pyruvate may be employed, the latter to isolate the rare cases of bovine tuberculosis. It is important that drugs inhibiting mycobacterial growth, such as aminoglycosides and tetracyclines, be stopped for one week or more before urine is examined for Mycobacterium. Molecular biological techniques exploiting the polymerase chain reaction will, in all probability, come into use in future years, and these will permit the diagnosis of the presence of dead mycobacteria in the urine as well as living ones. The Ziehl–Neelsen stain (acid-fast stain) performed on concentrated urine sediment may reveal the presence of mycobacteria, although the yield of this approach is not high. Confusion may arise in the not infrequent presence of saprophytic *Mycobacterium smegmatis*. Guinea-pig inoculation is now seldom used in the diagnosis of urinary-tract tuberculosis.

The tuberculin test may be useful since almost all patients have a positive reaction to 5 IU of tuberculin, except for those immunosuppressed by medication, renal failure, or acquired immunodeficiency syndrome. Other methods of diagnosis of tuberculosis include culture of material aspirated from tuberculous abscesses, histological examination of biopsy specimens with Ziehl–Neelsen staining (the only method of diagnosis in some cases of diffuse interstitial tuberculosis with normal urinary tract anatomy and negative culture findings), and culture of such material. Conventional urine culture, full blood count, erythrocyte sedimentation rate, estimation of blood urea, electrolytes, and serum creatinine are also mandatory.

IMAGING

Plain radiographs of the chest and abdomen are essential to exclude an active pulmonary lesion and calcific deposits in the kidneys or elsewhere in the genitourinary tract.

Intravenous urography

A high-dose intravenous urogram is essential in all suspected cases of genitourinary tuberculosis to define the presence of extensive destructive renal lesions and urinary tract obstruction (Figs. 1–3). Tomograms may be required to define the presence of faint calcification. All cases of renal tuberculosis are initially bilateral, given that spread of the organism occurs via the bloodstream. On urography, however, unilateral lesions are commoner than bilateral ones.

If urinary tract obstruction is absent at the time of diagnosis, intravenous urography should be repeated 4 to 6 weeks after commencement of treatment, as healing by fibrosis may produce strictures in the urinary tract leading to obstruction. If obstruction is present at diagnosis, serial follow-up by ultrasonography or urography will be required.

The differential diagnosis of calyceal abnormality due to tuberculosis includes renal papillary necrosis from other causes, calyceal diverticulae, and medullary sponge kidney. Tuberculous granulomatous disease in renal parenchyma may be mimicked by lobar nephronia (the nephrological equivalent of lobar pneumonia), xanthogranulomatous pyelonephritis, and malignant renal tumours.

Retrograde ureterography and pyelography

This examination was formally helpful in the investigation of non-functioning or poorly functioning kidneys. It has now largely been replaced by computerized tomography (Fig. 4). It may be required in patients with a stricture at the lower end of the ureter, although, again, antegrade pyelography has largely replaced it.

Renal ultrasonography

Renal ultrasonography has a role in the follow-up of hydronephrosis secondary to obstructive lesion and in the differential diagnosis of a renal mass.

CYSTOSCOPY

Cystoscopy is not indicated as a routine investigation in suspected genitourinary tuberculosis. Not infrequently, it is carried out in the investigation of a patient with symptoms of 'cystitis' who does not have bacteriuria on conventional culture, and in those with haematuria. Biopsy of bladder mucosa may allow a rapid histological diagnosis of tuberculosis and may exclude (or confirm) the presence of a bladder neoplasm which may occasionally mimic tuberculosis. On the other hand, *Mycobacterium tuberculosis* is almost invariably grown when bladder biopsy shows active tuberculosis, and it has been claimed that tuberculosis meningitis may follow biopsy in acute tuberculous cystitis.

Indications for treatment

Treatment should usually be withheld until a positive culture of the organism has been obtained. However, when classical radiological appearances are accompanied by acid-fast bacilli on Ziehl–Neelsen staining, there has been a positive bladder biopsy, or the patient is ill, treatment may be begun immediately.

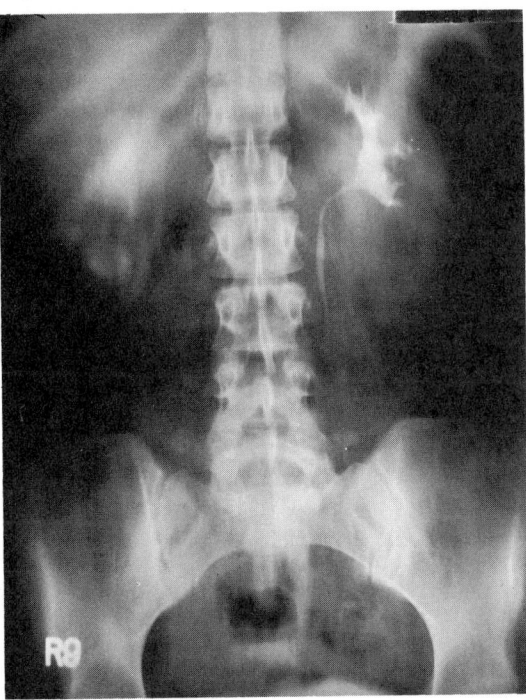

Fig. 1 Bilateral renal tuberculosis showing right hydronephrosis secondary to obstruction of the lower ureter and a closed cavity. Note the absence of normal calyces in the lower pole of the left kidney.

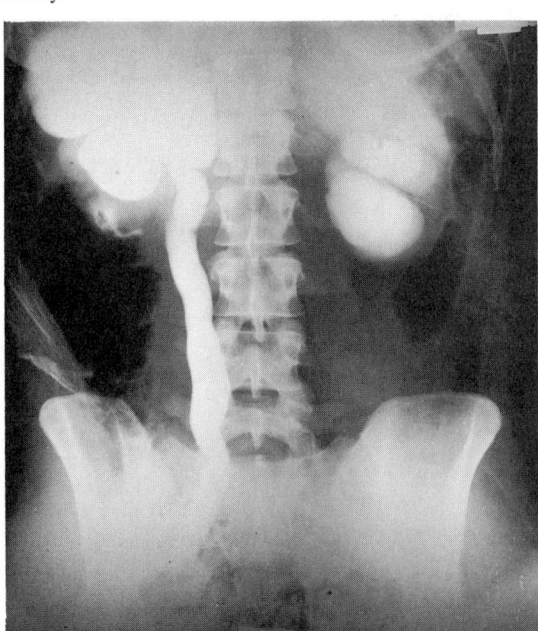

Fig. 2 Shows clearer detail outlined by right antegrade (percutaneous) pyelogram and left cyst puncture. Surgical treatment consisted of reimplantation of the right ureter and excision of the lower pole of the left kidney.

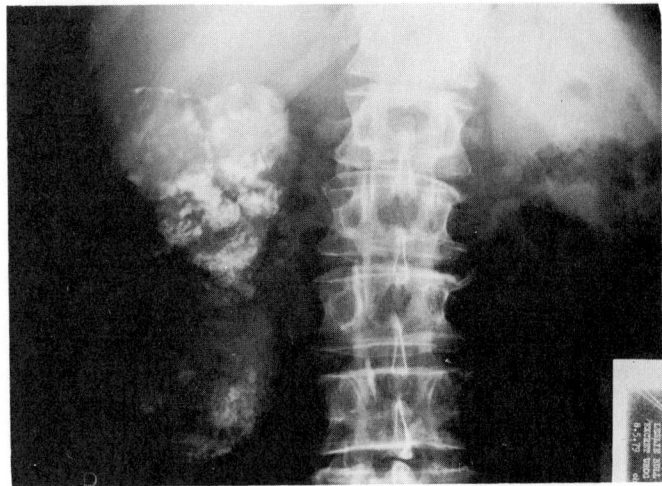

Fig. 3 Calcified tuberculous pyonephrosis. Nephrectomy is usually advisable in this condition as miliary spread may otherwise remain a threat for the future. The operation should be covered by a course of appropriate antituberculous chemotherapy.

MEDICAL TREATMENT

Several regimens have been advocated. The drug combination currently most often used includes isoniazid (300 mg daily as a single oral dose), rifampicin (600 mg daily before breakfast), and pyrazinamide (1 g daily). Drug doses need not be changed unless renal function is severely impaired. After 4 months the treatment regimen may be reduced to two drugs (rifampicin and isoniazid) unless the results of *in vitro* sensitivity tests dictate otherwise. Treatment is continued for a total of 9 months. Previously, medical treatment was continued for a total of 2 years, but trials indicating that pulmonary tuberculosis is controlled in the large majority of patients within 6 to 9 months have encouraged shorter treatment periods in tuberculosis of the urinary tract. Experience indicates that, in this way, excellent results can be obtained. Indeed, shorter treatment periods (2 months of three-drug therapy, 2 further months of two-drug therapy) have been advocated. The results of treatment of genitourinary tuberculosis should be at least as good, or better than, those of treating pulmonary tuberculosis with short-course regimens, for the following reasons.

1. Far fewer organisms are found in renal lesions than in the lung.
2. High concentrations of antituberculous drugs occur in urine.
3. Isoniazid and rifampicin penetrate tuberculous cavities at high concentration.
4. Rifampicin is known to penetrate the whole of the urinary tract.

Pyrazinamide, isoniazid, and rifampicin may be best tolerated if taken together at night. Many patients prefer to take them with milk.

In fulminating cases where the patient is very ill, streptomycin 1 g daily intramuscularly can be added to the three-drug regimen for the first 2 months of treatment. Blood levels should be measured regularly, particularly in patients with impaired renal function.

FOLLOW-UP

Three early morning urines are cultured on completion of the course of chemotherapy and at 6 and 12 months thereafter. If negative results are obtained and there is no other indication for follow-up, the patient may be discharged from supervision. Patients with renal calcification or impaired renal function need long-term follow-up.

CORTICOSTEROID ADMINISTRATION

In theory, the addition of corticosteroid administration to antituberculous chemotherapy might prevent or reduce healing by fibrosis and hence the development of urinary tract obstruction; it has been advocated for this reason. Unfortunately, controlled trials are lacking and the consensus is that such prophylaxis is not to be recommended.

In tuberculous interstitial nephritis with renal impairment, anecdotal evidence suggests a protective effect of concomitant corticosteroid administration upon renal function when antituberculous chemotherapy is administered, but again no controlled studies are available.

Corticosteroid treatment of obstruction

Many experienced clinicians believe that concomitant corticosteroid therapy is of benefit if urinary tract obstruction is present at the time of diagnosis. No adequately conducted prospective controlled trial data are available (some at least would find ethical difficulties in conducting a placebo-controlled trial) and unfortunately no definitive answer as to the benefits or otherwise of corticosteroid therapy in this context can be given.

SURGICAL TREATMENT

This falls into two categories, ablative and reconstructive surgery. Ablative surgery consists of nephrectomy, partial nephrectomy, cavernostomy, and epididymectomy. The indications for nephrectomy are:

1. Non-functioning kidney with or without calcification.
2. Extensive disease involving the whole kidney associated with superimposed secondary infection or haemorrhage.
3. Small, very poorly functioning kidney with extensive calcification and pelviureteric obstruction causing pain.
4. Coexisting renal cancer.
5. Very occasionally, severe hypertension poorly controlled by medical means.

Partial nephrectomy is now very seldom required. The two main indications are:

1. A localized, calcified lesion which has failed to respond to chemotherapy.
2. An area of calcification which is increasing in size and threatens to destroy the entire kidney.

Fig. 4 Computed tomography after administration of intravenous contrast. (a) The upper pole shows calcified parenchyma. (b) In the lower pole, low-density areas represent obstructed calyces with cortical thinning. (Reproduced from J.S. Cameron, *et al.* ed. (1992). *Oxford Textbook of Clinical Nephrology* p. 1724. University Press, Oxford, with permission.)

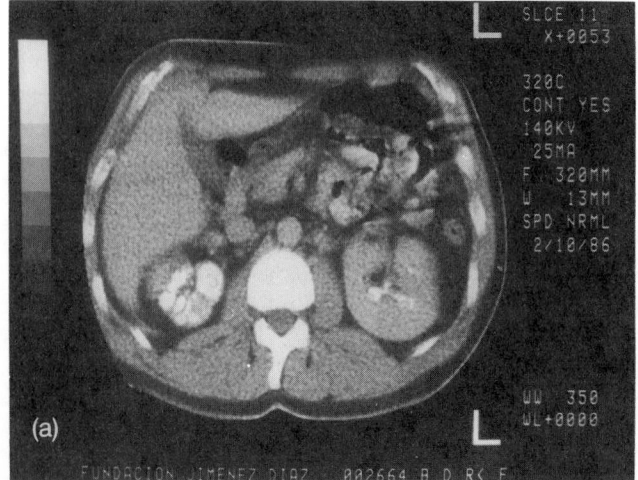
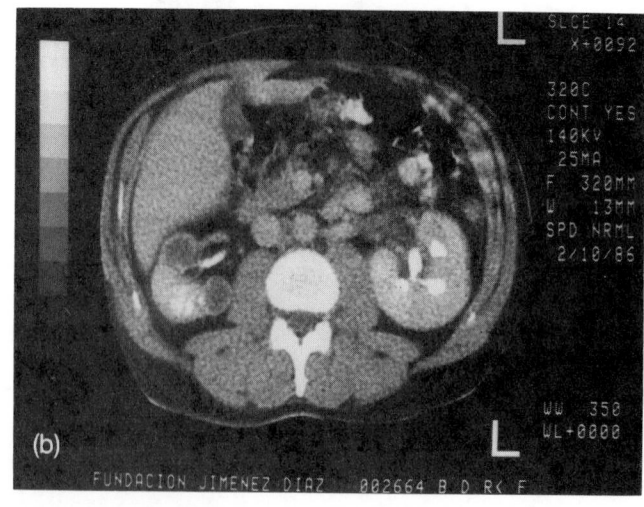

Cavernostomy still has a place in modern management of genitourinary tuberculosis, although modern imaging techniques allow the contents of a tuberculous abscess to be aspirated under imaging control and antituberculous drugs inoculated.

Epididymectomy is required rarely. The only indication is a caseating abscess which has failed to respond to chemotherapy. Involvement of the testes is common. Orchidectomy is required in only 5 per cent of cases.

Reconstructive surgery

This comprises correction of obstruction in the upper urinary tract and enlargement of the contracted bladder by enterocystoplasty.

If obstruction persists or increases despite antituberculous chemotherapy with or without corticosteroid treatment, surgery will be needed to correct pelviureteric junction obstruction (pyeloplasty) or ureterovesical junction obstruction (by reimplantation of the ureter using an antireflux technique). These operations should be carried out during the course of medical treatment, timing depending on the progress of the obstruction as judged by imaging and overall renal function.

Enlargement of the contracted bladder by ileo-, colo-, or caecocystoplasty is necessary where the healing process results in a contracted bladder with resultant severe daytime frequency and nocturia. It should

rarely be performed early in the course of treatment, for sometimes surprising improvement follows the use of antituberculous drugs. In most instances, the trigone can be preserved and the bowel simply used to increase the bladder capacity, leaving the ureterovesical valve *in situ*.

REFERENCES

Hernando, L. and Vela-Navarrete, R. (1992). Renal tuberculosis. In *Oxford textbook of clinical nephrology*, (ed. J.S. Cameron, A.M. Davison, J.-P. Grünfeld, D.N.S. Kerr, and E. Ritz), Vol. 3, pp. 1719–29. Oxford University Press, Oxford.

Howe, N.W. and Tulloch, W.J. (1975). Conservative management of renal tuberculosis. *British Journal of Urology* 47, 481–7.

Mallinson, W.J.W., Fuller, R.W., Levison, D.A., Baker, L.R.I., and Cattell, W.R. (1981). Diffuse interstitial renal tuberculosis – an unrecognised cause of renal failure. *Quarterly Journal of Medicine* 198, 137–48.

Mitchison, D.A. (1980). Treatment of tuberculosis. *Journal of the Royal College of Physicians (Lond.)* 14, 91–9.

Morgan, S.H., Eastwood, J.B., and Baker, L.R.I. (1990). Tuberculous interstitial nephritis – the tip of an iceberg? *Tubercle* 71, 5–6.

Prenkumar, A., Lattimer, J., and Newhouse, J.H. (1987). CT and sonography of advanced urinary tract tuberculosis. *American Journal of Roentgenology* 148, 65–9.

20.16 Acute renal failure

J. D. FIRTH and C. G. WINEARLS

Introduction

Acute renal failure is defined as a significant decline in renal excretory function occurring over hours or days. This is detected clinically by a rise in plasma concentrations of urea and creatinine. Oliguria, defined (arbitrarily) as a urinary volume of less than 400 ml/day, is usually present, but its absence is not infrequent. Acute renal failure may arise as an isolated problem, but much more commonly occurs in the setting of circulatory disturbance associated with severe illness, trauma, or surgery; transient renal dysfunction complicates some 5 per cent of medical and surgical admissions. There are many possible causes (Table 1), but in any given clinical context very few of these are likely to require consideration.

Diagnosis of the presence of acute renal failure

A high index of clinical suspicion is required to diagnose acute renal failure at an early stage of its development. This is because symptoms and signs attributable to the accumulation of uraemic wastes within the body are not apparent until the condition is far advanced. Unsuspected hyperkalaemia is the greatest danger, since this may produce no symptoms whatever before inducing cardiac arrest.

All patients admitted to hospital with acute illness should be considered at risk of developing acute renal failure. Those who have some pre-existing chronic impairment of renal function are particularly susceptible to acute exacerbations. This group includes all elderly patients, in whom a combination of low muscle mass and low dietary meat consumption may conspire to maintain an apparently 'normal' plasma creatinine, despite a reduction in glomerular filtration rate to as little as 25 per cent of that expected in a healthy young adult.

In order to recognize impairment of renal function early, basic care of all acutely ill patients should include careful monitoring of fluid input

Table 1 *Some causes of acute renal failure*

Prerenal uraemia
'Acute tubular necrosis'
    Following haemodynamic compromise, commonly with sepsis
    Following exposure to nephrotoxins: including drugs, chemicals, rhabdomyolysis, snake bite (see Tables 10 and 11)
Vascular causes
    Acute cortical necrosis
    Large vessel obstruction
    Small vessel obstruction: accelerated-phase hypertension and systemic sclerosis
Glomerulonephritis and vasculitis (see Table 12)
Interstitial nephritis (see Table 13)
'Haematological' causes
    Haemolytic uraemic syndrome/thrombotic thrombocytopenic purpura
    Myeloma
Hepatorenal syndrome
Urinary obstruction
    intrarenal: crystalluria
    postrenal; renal stones, papillary necrosis, retroperitoneal fibrosis, bladder/prostate/cervical lesions

and output, daily weighing (where practicable), lying and standing blood pressure, and regular estimation of plasma creatinine, urea, and electrolytes.

The estimation of urinary output and of gastrointestinal losses is usually not difficult. Precise determination of fluid input is often more problematic, excepting in those who are only receiving fluids parenterally. Cups of tea, often only partly drunk, seem to be recorded as an almost invariable '180 ml'; patients help themselves to extra jugs of water and have been known to use drinking water to revive the flowers; kindly domestic staff and relatives provide extra (uncharted) drinks. These considerations mean that the most likely explanation for fluid balance charts being difficult to interpret is that recording of intake is erroneous. Daily weighing on accurate scales provides a much more reliable picture of net overall fluid balance. Patients who are acutely ill invariably lose flesh weight, commonly at a rate of up to a few hundred grams per day. If weight appears to fall at a rate faster than this, then negative fluid balance is likely; the occurrence of greatly increased 'insensible' losses through the skin and lungs during fever being the commonest explanation. If weight rises at any time, then this must be due to positive fluid balance, whatever the input/output charts may suggest. It may not be obvious from clinical examination where the fluid has gone: the possibilities of sequestration in the peritoneal cavity or in the tissue interstitium should be recognized.

Plasma urea, creatinine, and electrolytes should be measured on admission in all acutely ill patients and repeated daily or on alternate days in those who remain so. Together with the keeping and regular inspection of proper fluid balance charts and daily weighing, these measurements will ensure that advanced acute renal failure does not seem to have occurred 'suddenly' in patients already in hospital. However, many patients will be found to have significant renal impairment on admission, and many more will develop some degree of renal impairment while on the ward. In all of these cases a diagnosis of the cause must be attempted.

Diagnosis of the cause of acute renal failure

In the initial assessment of a patient who appears to have acute renal failure three questions should be asked.

Question 1: is the renal failure really acute?

The only basis for excluding the possibility of pre-existing chronic renal impairment with absolute confidence is the knowledge of a previous normal measurement of renal function. In cases where there is uncertainty, a diligent search for previous notes and biochemical information may prevent a waste of time, effort, and money in unnecessary investigations. The finding of two small kidneys on ultrasound examination indicates the presence of chronic renal disease. Other clinical features are poor discriminators between acute and chronic renal impairment. A history of vague ill-health of some months' duration, of nocturia, of pruritus, or the findings of skin pigmentation or anaemia would all suggest chronicity (see Chapter 20.17.1). However, anaemia is not invariable in chronic renal failure (for example in polycystic kidney disease the haemoglobin concentration may be normal), and anaemia can develop over a few days in acute renal failure, as may hypocalcaemia and hyperphosphataemia. Radiological evidence of renal osteodystrophy is only found in patients with obviously long-standing renal failure and rarely, if ever, aids the clinical distinction between acute and chronic renal failure.

Question 2: is urinary obstruction a possibility?

One of the merits of the traditional division of the causes of acute renal failure into pre-renal, renal, and post-renal is that it encourages consideration of the possibility of urinary obstruction. This is not a common cause of acute or chronic renal impairment, but it is extremely important that the diagnosis should not be missed, since it is readily treatable and delay may cause permanent renal damage. Obstruction is particularly likely in those with a single functioning kidney, in those with a history of renal stones or of prostatism, and after pelvic or retroperitoneal surgery. It should be considered seriously in all cases where another positive diagnosis cannot be made. The presence of anuria, or of alternating

polyuria and oligoanuria are helpful clues; but it is not widely appreciated that a patient may pass normal or elevated volumes of urine despite significant obstruction. The mechanism is poorly understood, but three factors present in obstruction tend to impair urinary concentrating ability and thereby lead to preservation of urinary volume despite obstructive depression of filtration rate. These factors are structural damage to the inner medulla and papilla, functional changes in the distal nephron resulting from increased intraluminal or interstitial pressure, and loss of medullary hypertonicity at low filtration rates.

Ultrasound examination of the kidneys and bladder is the usual first method of investigation for the presence of obstruction. It should be remembered, however, that ultrasound detects calyceal dilatation, not obstruction, and cases of obstruction are not infrequently missed either because the calyces fail to dilate or do so minimally. Furthermore, the quality of the image obtained by renal ultrasonography is highly variable—depending on the patient, the equipment, and on the operator. If doubt as to the diagnosis persists in the clinician's mind, then the examination should be repeated, and if uncertainty still remains then diethylenetriaminepenta-acetic acid (DTPA) renography with frusemide injection and/or cystoscopy with retrograde ureteric catheterization should be undertaken. Obstruction, once diagnosed, must be relieved urgently by bladder catheterization, percutaneous nephrostomy, or cystoscopic insertion of ureteral stents, as a prelude to definitive treatment (where possible) of the underlying obstructive lesion. The most important causes of urinary obstruction are renal calculi, retroperitoneal fibrosis, and malignant diseases of the uterine cervix, prostate, bladder, and rectum (see Chapter 20.10).

Question 3: are glomerulonephritis, interstitial nephritis, vasculitis, or other rarities possible?

In order to help make these diagnoses, which, although rare, have critically important management implications, microscopy of the urinary sediment is an essential part of the assessment of any patient with unexplained acute renal failure. This should be done by spinning 10 to 15 ml of urine at 1500 r.p.m. for 5 min, carefully discarding all but 1 ml of the supernatant, and then resuspending the pellet. Examination should be made under high power, preferably after counterstaining. Red cell casts are present in acute glomerulonephritis, renal vasculitis, accelerated-phase hypertension, and (sometimes) in interstitial nephritis, but not in other conditions. Their presence indicates the need for urgent specialist renal referral. The conditions giving rise to them, and other rare causes of acute renal failure, are discussed later in this chapter.

Prerenal failure and acute tubular necrosis

The vast majority of cases of acute renal failure will fall into the categories of prerenal failure and acute tubular necrosis. The term 'prerenal failure' is used when renal dysfunction is entirely attributable to hypoperfusion, and restoration of renal perfusion leads to rapid recovery. The term 'acute tubular necrosis' is not a very good one, since it erroneously suggests that the pathological basis of the clinical syndrome is clearly understood. In fact necrosis of tubular cells can usually be found by diligent examination, but the lesion maybe inconspicuous and the pathophysiological implications of such necrosis may remain uncertain. The glomeruli and vessels are usually normal. In common usage (retained here) 'acute tubular necrosis' describes a clinical entity comprising acute renal failure with three main characteristics:

(1) it is seen in specific clinical contexts, frequently involving circulatory compromise and/or nephrotoxins;

(2) urinary abnormalities usually suggest tubular dysfunction; and

(3) essentially complete recovery of renal function is expected within days or weeks if the patient survives the precipitating

insult, with a period of polyuria commonly following oliguria.

The syndrome can be seen after virtually any episode of severe circulatory compromise, but it should be noted that not all causes of circulatory derangement are equally devastating to renal function. Primary impairment of cardiac performance, for example following myocardial infarction, may cause plasma creatinine to rise somewhat, but rarely causes renal failure of sufficient severity to require renal replacement therapy. By contrast an apparently similar haemodynamic upset caused by sepsis frequently does. Table 2 shows the causes of development of acute impairment of renal function (usually modest) in over 2000 consecutive medical and surgical admissions. Table 3 shows the causes of acute renal failure requiring renal replacement therapy in over 1000 cases treated at a single centre between 1956 and 1988. Circumstances associated with a particularly high risk of acute renal failure include repair of ruptured aortic aneurysm (20 per cent, as opposed to 3 per cent for elective repair), hepatobiliary surgery (10 per cent), pancreatitis (10 per cent), and burns.

Pathophysiology

When the circulation is compromised, the perfusion of the kidney is reduced before that of any other organ. In the face of modest underperfusion, the glomerular filtration rate is relatively preserved by a compensatory increase in filtration fraction. This increase has repercussions on tubular function which, along with other factors, leads to increased tubular reabsorption of sodium, water, and urea—a situation rapidly reversed by restoration of renal perfusion. However, following prolonged circulatory shock, renal function frequently deteriorates in a manner which is not immediately reversible, and it is not at all obvious why this should be so. Lack of a clear pathophysiological understanding has bedevilled all attempts at the development of rational therapy. Under normal conditions the kidney enjoys high blood flow, exceeded on a volume/weight basis only by the carotid body, and oxygen tension in the renal venous effluent is high, suggesting that oxygen supply greatly exceeds demand. Such a situation might be expected to confer protection from the effects of circulatory compromise, but no such benefit is observed: indeed the kidney appears more susceptible to damage than other organs. Acute renal failure resembling acute tubular necrosis can be produced in animal models by ischaemia. This, coupled with the setting of profound haemodynamic disturbance in which clinical acute renal failure is frequently seen, has led to the supposition that—despite apparently generous blood flow normally—renal ischaemia is the cause of renal failure in such circumstances. Two main hypotheses, not necessarily mutually exclusive, have been proposed to explain this. The first stresses that arteriovenous shunting of oxygen, resulting from the specialized anatomical relationships between intrarenal arteries and veins, leads to the presence of areas of profound hypoxia within the normal kidney. These areas might therefore be operating on the verge of anoxia in the normal organ and susceptible to ischaemic damage in response to modest compromise of whole-organ blood flow. The second hypothesis is based on clinical and experimental angiographic evidence of intense constriction of renal vessels during shock, and suggests that very severe reduction in renal blood flow (perhaps only transient) may be responsible for the initiation of ischaemic damage. The justification for many of the interventions proposed in the management of patients at risk of acute renal failure, or with established acute renal failure, is that they might preserve renal blood flow and/or reduce renal oxygen consumption, thus rendering the development of ischaemic injury less likely.

Once damage has been sustained, a variety of factors may be responsible for the persistence of excretory failure that is characteristic of the clinical syndrome of acute tubular necrosis. Renal blood flow remains reduced; hence continuing ischaemia may play some part, but in addition the glomerular ultrafiltration coefficient may be reduced, renal tubules may be obstructed, and backleakage of filtrate from damaged tubules

Table 2 *Causes of development of acute impairment of renal function in 2216 consecutive medical and surgical admissions*

Acute tubular necrosis	
Hypovolaemia	22
Congestive cardiac failure	10
Sepsis	10
Nephrotoxins	25
Postsurgical	23
Other	12
Hepatorenal syndrome	5
Obstruction	3
Vasculitis	2
Other/multifactorial/unknown	17
Total	129
	(5.8 per cent of admissions)

Acute impairment of renal function was diagnosed when serum creatinine rose by a predetermined amount (approximately one-third of the base-line) during the period of hospital admission.

During the period of study, 46 patients were excluded from analysis because they were either admitted specifically for treatment of acute renal failure or were recipients of long-term haemodialysis.

Dialysis was required in 10 cases. (Modified from Hou *et al.* 1983.)

may occur. It is impossible in clinical practice to determine which of these factors is most important at any given time. However, many of these abnormalities have a structural, rather than functional basis: hence rapid reversal cannot be expected.

Diagnosis

In prerenal failure the urinary biochemical composition reflects the response of normal tubules to impaired renal perfusion. There is avid retention of sodium and water, leading to low urinary sodium and high urinary urea and creatinine concentrations, together with a high urinary osmolarity. Restoration of renal perfusion leads to rapid improvement in renal function. By contrast, in the 'typical' clinical case of acute tubular necrosis the urinary sodium concentration is elevated and the urinary urea and creatinine concentrations and urinary osmolarity are relatively low (Table 4): indeed, it is these features that suggest tubular dysfunction. In such instances, whatever the treatment, renal function rarely improves rapidly. Consideration of cases such as these might lead to the view that biochemical analysis of the urine could provide useful prediction of the renal response to therapy. However, for reasons listed in Table 4 there are so many exceptions to the 'typical' findings described that such analysis is rarely of clinical value. From a practical point of view, treatment is begun on exactly the same lines whether the expected diagnosis is of prerenal failure or of acute tubular necrosis. The response to initial treatment retrospectively defines the diagnosis and determines further management.

Circumstances predisposing to prerenal failure are almost invariably associated with raised plasma levels of antidiuretic hormone (ADH). This acts on the collecting duct to increase tubular reabsorption of both water and urea; hence plasma levels of urea rise out of proportion to creatinine in prerenal failure. Plasma urea may also appear to be disproportionately raised with sepsis, steroids, tetracycline (catabolic effect), and gastrointestinal haemorrhage (protein meal).

Avoidance

One of the main aims of the basic care provided to all acutely ill patients is to minimize the chances of development of renal impairment. Of course, acute renal failure can arise despite exemplary treatment, but there is no doubt that poor care increases the likelihood. As described above, regular measurement of serum creatinine will permit early rec-

Table 3 *Causes of acute renal failure requiring renal replacement therapy at a single centre between 1956 and 1988*

	Number of patients (% total)	Diagnoses present (% patients)	
Surgical	638 (47.5%)	General surgery	445 (33.1%)
		Surgical sepsis	126 (9.4%)
		Urinary obstruction	116 (8.6%)
		Trauma	94 (7.0%)
		Cardiovascular surgery	81 (6.0%)
		Malignancy	52 (3.9%)
		Pancreatitis	24 (1.8%)
		Burns	17 (1.3%)
General medical	285 (21.2%)	Sepsis	112 (8.3%)
		Acute liver disease	44 (3.3%)
		Salt and water depletion	43 (3.2%)
		Ischaemic heart disease	36 (2.7%)
		Diabetes mellitus	30 (2.2%)
		Others	53 (3.9%)
Renal parenchymal disease	166 (12.4%)	Polyarteritis	31 (2.3%)
		Crescentic nephritis	25 (1.9%)
		Haemolytic uraemic syndrome	21 (1.6%)
		Proliferative glomerulonephritis	19 (1.4%)
		Histology unknown	19 (1.4%)
		Systemic lupus erythematosus	15 (1.1%)
		Others	36 (2.7%)
Obstetric	142 (10.6%)		
Poisoning	112 (8.3%)		
Total	1343 (100%)		

Modified from Turney *et al.* (1990)

Some patients fell into more than one diagnostic category.

During the period of study there were significant changes in case-mix. Between 1980 and 1988, the following categories were more frequent: general medical (33.2% of all cases) and cardiovascular surgery (15.1%); and the following categories were less frequent: general surgery (26.4%), trauma (2.8%), and obstetric (1.3%).

Table 4 *Urinary biochemical indices in prerenal failure and acute tubular necrosis*

Indices	'Typical' prerenal failure	'Typical' acute tubular necrosis
Urinary sodium (mmol/l)	< 20	>40
Urine osmolarity (mosmol/l)	>500	< 350
Urine/plasma urea	>8	< 3
Urine/plasma creatinine	>40	< 20
Fractional sodium excretion (%)	< 1	>2

Reasons why urinary biochemical indices are of very limited clinical use:

(1) Intermediate values are common.

(2) 'Typical' values do not reliably predict renal prognosis. It is increasingly recognized that cases which are otherwise indistinguishable from 'typical' acute tubular necrosis can have low urinary sodium.

(3) Diuretics and pre-existing tubular disease will impair tubules' ability to retain sodium in prerenal failure.

(4) In hepatorenal syndrome indices are prerenal.

(5) Treatment is not dictated by urinary indices.

ognition of declining renal function, but is not of itself therapeutic. The cornerstones of good management are: the maintenance of optimal intravascular volume, and the avoidance of, or reduction of, exposure to nephrotoxic agents.

MAINTENANCE OF OPTIMAL INTRAVASCULAR VOLUME

What is an optimal intravascular volume? From the point of view of the kidney it might be defined as the volume at which renal perfusion is optimal. However, as we have no method of measuring renal perfusion, a more practical target is to obtain improvement in the general state of the circulation and of the perfusion of those tissues about which a judgement can be made. The features listed in Table 5 are indicators of depletion or excess of intravascular volume, and the presence of any one of these should lead to consideration of whether the patient would benefit from increasing or decreasing that volume. Although a number of clinical signs are traditionally thought to be of use in the diagnosis of volume depletion, for example reduced skin turgor, reduced ocular tension, dry mouth and tongue, these are very poor guides and may be misleading, particularly in the elderly.

It is common practice in the management of ill patients for a central venous pressure line or pulmonary capillary wedge pressure line to be inserted to aid assessment of haemodynamic status. A central venous pressure line provides more precise measurement of right atrial pressure than can be gained from inspection of the jugular venous pulse, and the pulmonary capillary wedge pressure line provides information on left-sided filling pressure that cannot be obtained clinically with any degree of certainty at all (although in a patient with a normal heart and lungs the relationship between the left- and right-sided pressures are consistent). However, the advantages of inserting these lines must be seen in perspective. There are some patients, particularly those with 'bull-necks', in whom the jugular venous pulse cannot be seen at all. In such individuals a central venous pressure line is invaluable; indeed, it may not be possible to proceed safely without one. By contrast, in the majority of patients the jugular venous pulse can be seen, and the intravascular volume status is clinically obvious. In these cases the benefits of a cen-

Table 5 *Evaluation of intravascular volume*

Clinical signs of volume depletion
  Jugular venous pressure low[a]
  Hypotension, postural drop in blood pressure of >10 mmHg
    and rise in pulse rate of >10 b.p.m (lying and sitting, if
    lying and standing not possible)
  Collapsed peripheral veins and cool peripheries (nose,
    fingers, toes)
  Fast, thready pulse

Clinical signs of volume overload
  Jugular venous pressure high[a]
  Gallop rhythm
  Hypertension, peripheral oedema, liver congestion, basal
    crepitations

Directly measurable indices of intravascular volume
  Central venous pressure[a]
  Pulmonary capillary wedge pressure[a]

Therapeutic tests of volume depletion or excess
  Trial of fluid infusion[b]
  Trial of fluid removal (diuretic, haemofiltration/
    haemodialysis, venesection (exceptionally))

[a]Absolute values are deliberately not given: 'low' or 'high' relative to the estimated optimal value for that individual.

[b]Trials of fluid infusion should be undertaken with the patient under continuous medical observation, and should be terminated immediately in the event of deterioration in the patient's condition.

tral venous pressure line may not outweigh the risks of insertion, and the decision to use one is sometimes attributable to the bravado of junior medical staff, or to slavish adherence to rigid protocols, rather than to sensible analysis of the clinical situation. It is particularly dangerous to try and insert a central venous pressure line into someone whose intravascular volume is clearly low. The line itself is not therapeutic, and time spent on its insertion is time during which appropriate treatment is neglected. Furthermore, with constricted central veins the procedure is likely to be technically difficult, with greatly increased likelihood of complications. With the caveats stated in Table 5, in most patients central venous pressure should be maintained at a level of 5 to 8 cm of water (measured from the midaxillary line).

It must be stressed that, even with measurement of central venous pressure, it is not always easy to decide whether intravascular volume is optimal. Three brief examples should serve to illustrate this point:

1. Following a large myocardial infarction it is not at all uncommon to find a fast, thready pulse; postural hypotension; cool peripheries; a high jugular venous pressure, a gallop rhythm, and pulmonary crepitations.
2. Chronic cardiac or pulmonary disease may mean that an individual's habitual and optimal jugular venous pressure is greatly in excess of that which would generally be regarded as normal: ill-advised attempts to reduce the cardiac filling pressure can be catastrophic.
3. In many circumstances the presence of peripheral or pulmonary oedema is associated, not with excess, but with contraction of intravascular volume.

In each of these circumstances the relationship between left- and right-sided filling pressures may be abnormal, and measurement of pulmonary capillary wedge pressure can be very helpful. However, uncertainty as to whether intravascular volume is optimal may still persist, and the final strategy that can be employed is a trial of fluid infusion or removal (Table 5). If a decision to give a fluid challenge is made, then this should be done carefully, with the patient under continuous medical observation, paying particular attention to the possibility that pulmonary oedema might be induced. The administration of 250 ml of colloid or

0.9 per cent saline should be rapid, and the patient should then be observed closely for the next 5 min. If there is no perceptible deterioration, then the process can be repeated.

One common clinical situation worthy of specific note is the patient about to undergo a major elective surgical procedure such as repair of an abdominal aortic aneurysm. In the past the risk of acute renal failure following such an operation was substantial. It has been considerably lessened by recognition of the importance of careful attention to fluid management—with the aim of avoiding episodes of hypovolaemia—both before, during, and after the procedure. It is good practice to maintain a diuresis, which can often be accomplished simply by infusion of crystalloid solution at moderate rate, since this appears to render the kidney less susceptible to insult. Although the routine use of mannitol and other diuretic agents is advocated by some, they would appear to have no specific advantages over a simple saline diuresis in protecting the kidney. Moreover, the massive diuresis which may be provoked (urine output >500 ml/h) can lead to considerable difficulties in control of electrolytes (potassium particularly) postoperatively. For very high-risk cases the insertion of a central venous pressure line preoperatively is a sensible precaution: it should be remembered that the positioning of the patient for surgery and the presence of drapes may prevent the jugular venous pulse from being seen at all, and the risks of elective insertion of a central venous pressure line in the relative calm of the anaesthetic room are considerably less than those incurred if the attempt is made with the patient 'going off' on the operating table.

AVOIDANCE/REDUCTION OF EXPOSURE TO NEPHROTOXINS

Many drugs have been reported to cause alteration of renal function and hence might be described as nephrotoxins. Indeed, as virtually all acutely ill patients are receiving drugs of one form or another, and acute renal failure frequently develops on a background of multiple recognized risk factors, it is rarely possible to exclude the possibility that a drug may be an exacerbating factor. For the majority of drugs the evidence of frequent significant nephrotoxicity is unconvincing and, if prescribed for the correct indication, their likely benefit should far outweigh the renal risk. However, a few agents in common usage are either directly injurious to renal tissue or predictably induce detrimental renal haemodynamic changes: these are listed in Table 6. For these drugs the benefit/risk balance in the acutely ill patient is much more difficult to judge. They should only be prescribed when they can reasonably be said to offer significant advantage over less noxious alternatives.

Clinical findings in prerenal failure and acute tubular necrosis

In the early stages of acute renal failure there are few warning symptoms, and so unsuspected and potentially fatal hyperkalaemia is the greatest danger. The patient or nursing staff may notice a reduction in urinary volume, but non-oliguric renal failure comprises as many as 50 per cent of cases in some series. The clinical picture is likely to be dominated by the primary condition of which acute renal failure is a complication, and by the effects of intravascular volume depletion (see Table 5). In the later stages of acute renal failure there are manifestations of uraemia with anorexia, nausea, and vomiting (only occasionally diarrhoea); muscular cramps; and signs of encephalopathy—including a 'metabolic' flapping tremor (asterixis) progressing only rarely to depressed consciousness and grand mal convulsions. Skin bruising and gastrointestinal bleeding may occur. Uraemic haemorrhagic pericarditis occurs much less frequently in acute renal failure than in chronic renal failure, but when it does it is another potentially fatal complication.

If the patient does not die of acute renal failure, either because the degree of uraemia is modest or renal replacement therapy is provided, then renal recovery occurs in the vast majority of those who survive the precipitating insult. Only a few suffer acute cortical necrosis with little or no recovery of renal function. Recovery may begin at any time from

Table 6 *Drugs to be used with extreme caution in acutely ill patients*

Antimicrobials	
Aminoglycosides e.g. gentamicin	Strongly cationic agents which accumulate in the cells of the proximal tubule, probably as a result of electrostatic interaction with membrane phospholipids. Nephrotoxic and ototoxic
Amphotericin B	Membrane damage related to cumulative dose. Administration in/with lipid reduces toxicity
Tetracyclines (except doxycycline)	Retained in renal failure and exacerbate uraemia by catabolic effect
Cephaloridine (not other cephalosporins)	Toxicity dependent on cellular accumulation via organic anion transporter
Non-steroidal anti-inflammatory agents and angiotensin-converting enzyme inhibitors	
In the setting of circulatory compromise, renal blood flow and glomerular filtration are substantially supported by intrarenal generation of vasodilator prostaglandins and angiotensin II. Administration of these agents in such circumstances can lead to a dramatic reduction in renal perfusion and induce acute renal failure	

a few days to a few months (median 10–14 days) after the onset of acute renal failure, with a progressive increase in urinary volume typically preceding improvement in plasma levels of creatinine and urea. Due to a relatively persistent defect in renal tubular sodium reabsorption and concentrating ability, a period of polyuria may ensue, placing the patient at risk of sodium and water depletion. Young patients can be expected to recover clinically normal renal function; but in those over 70 years old recovery may be delayed, incomplete, and sometimes does not occur at all—leading to lifelong dependence on renal replacement therapy.

Biochemical changes

The clinical diagnosis of renal failure, acute or chronic, is made when plasma urea and creatinine concentrations rise. Other important biochemical changes include the development of hyperkalaemia, metabolic acidosis, hypocalcaemia, and hyperphosphataemia. Hyperkalaemia is due not only to reduced urinary excretion, but also to potassium release from cells—either as a consequence of cell death or as a result of metabolic acidosis. Particularly rapid rises are to be expected when there is extensive tissue damage or hypercatabolism, as in rhabdomyolysis, burns, and sepsis. Transfusion of stored blood is sometimes said to cause dangerous rises in plasma potassium concentration in oliguric patients. However, the transfused blood may not really be to blame, but the circumstances that demand transfusion. Loss of blood into the gastrointestinal tract or body tissues is followed by red cell lysis and the absorption of a considerable potassium load.

Protein catabolism produces sulphuric and phosphoric acids. These are normally buffered by bicarbonate and excreted by the kidney. In acute renal failure these systems fail, leading to the development of acidosis. This is usually modest in degree (plasma pH 7.2–7.35), but can be more severe, manifesting as sighing Kussmaul respiration and/or with circulatory compromise. Acidosis is sometimes the metabolic abnormality most obviously necessitating urgent institution of renal replacement therapy. Overzealous administration of bicarbonate should be avoided (see below).

Calcium malabsorption occurs early in acute renal failure and is probably secondary to disordered vitamin D metabolism. Hypocalcaemia can develop with surprising rapidity. It is usually asymptomatic, but tetany and fits may be provoked by injudicious over-rapid correction of acidosis with resultant depression of ionized calcium. Profound hypocalcaemia and marked hyperphosphataemia, together with hyperuricaemia, is to be expected in rhabdomyolysis. During the recovery phase of acute renal failure transient hypercalcaemia is frequently seen. This is also particularly common after rhabdomyolysis and probably caused by secondary hyperparathyroidism related to preceding hypocalcaemia. The hypercalcaemic phase may be prolonged and accompanied by metastatic calcification in patients in whom there has been extensive muscle injury.

In acute renal failure plasma sodium concentration is usually normal, since deficit of sodium is usually matched by that of water: hence the extracellular fluid volume is reduced, but the plasma sodium concentration remains unchanged. On occasion, however, intake of water—either driven by hypovolaemia or iatrogenic—may exceed the rate of excretion, and hyponatraemia results. The retention of uric acid, sulphate, and magnesium occurs in acute renal failure, but these biochemical abnormalities are rarely clinically significant. Levels of uric acid are likely to be particularly high in rhabdomyolysis and following tumour lysis.

Medical management

The immediate management of the patient with renal impairment is directed towards three goals. The first is treatment of any life-threatening complications of acute renal failure. The second is prompt diagnosis and treatment of hypovolaemia. The third is specific treatment of the underlying condition: if this persists untreated then renal function will not improve.

LIFE-THREATENING COMPLICATIONS

Hyperkalaemia (See also Chapter 20.2.3)

Hyperkalaemia is most commonly dangerous in the context of acute renal failure, and is important because it can cause cardiac arrest or ventricular fibrillation. Patients may occasionally notice muscle weakness or paralysis, but the significance of these symptoms is rarely appreciated, and usually there are no symptoms whatever. All doctors who work with acutely ill patients should be able to recognize the characteristic electrocardiogram (ECG) appearances, which are a better indicator of cardiac toxicity than the serum potassium level. As serum potassium rises, the following changes progressively occur (Fig. 1):

(1) 'tenting' of the T-wave;
(2) reduction in size of P-waves, increase in PR interval, widening of QRS complex;
(3) disappearance of P-wave, further widening of QRS complex;
(4) irregular 'sinusoidal' ECG;
(5) asystole.

Any change more severe than tenting of the T-waves demands immediate treatment, as described in Table 7.

Pulmonary oedema

The most serious complication of salt and water overload in acute renal failure (usually iatrogenic) is the development of pulmonary oedema. Severe cases are dramatic. The patient is terrified, restless, and confused. Examination reveals cyanosis, tachypnoea, tachycardia, widespread wheeze or crepitations in the chest, and a gallop rhythm (if the heart can be heard). Investigation demonstrates arterial hypoxaemia and widespread interstitial shadowing on the chest radiograph. The patient should be sat up and supported, and given oxygen by facemask in as high a concentration as possible. Frusemide is of little value in renal failure but morphine relieves symptoms rapidly, provided that it can be given safely. The definitive treatment is of removal of fluid by haemodialysis, haemofiltration, or, less satisfactorily, peritoneal dialysis, but the immediate beneficial effects of venesection of 100 to 200 ml blood from the patient *in extremis* should not be forgotten.

RECOGNITION AND TREATMENT OF VOLUME DEPLETION

If features suggestive of intravascular volume depletion (listed in Table 5) are present, the deficit should be corrected rapidly. Large-bore intravenous access should be established and fluid infused at maximum rate. The fluid should be of a type that remains substantially within the intravascular compartment (blood, colloid, saline) and which mimics as closely as possible the nature of the fluid lost. The patient should be continuously observed and the infusion stopped when features of volume depletion have disappeared, but before volume overload has been induced. There has been much debate about the best type of replacement fluid, but little evidence on which to base firm recommendations. It seems sensible to: (1) include blood in replacement when blood has obviously been lost, or the haemoglobin concentration is less than 10 g/dl, and (2) to include albumin when the serum albumin is very low (< 25 g/dl). Dextrose saline (containing 0.15 per cent saline) or 5 per cent dextrose infusions have no place in the correction of depleted intravascular volume, since these solutions partition throughout the total body water and only a small fraction remains within the vascular compartment. An all too common cause of gross oedema in patients referred to renal units with acute renal failure is previous inappropriate administration of dextrose-based solutions.

OTHER MEASURES ALLEGED TO IMPROVE RENAL FUNCTION

The importance of effective treatment of the underlying condition and of rapid correction of hypovolaemia are above clinical dispute, although neither has been subject to controlled trial as regards the outcome of acute renal failure. However, there is no really compelling clinical evidence in the literature of general benefit of any of the 'specific' remedies often prescribed in an endeavour to protect or to improve renal function. Recommendations (necessarily tentative) have to be made on the basis of frankly inadequate data. Modest doses of diuretics (frusemide 40–120 mg, mannitol 25 g) given intravenously to a volume-replete patient

undergoing a procedure that might compromise renal blood flow, for example bile duct surgery, resection of aortic aneurysm, cardiac bypass, will increase urinary volume and may afford protection from acute renal failure. This is not proven, but provided the patient is not volume depleted the treatment should do no harm. In established acute renal failure large doses of frusemide (0.5–2 g/day) may substantially increase urinary volume, and this can ease the management of fluid balance and reduce the degree of hyperkalaemia. They are most unlikely to lead to improvement in renal clearance of metabolic wastes, will probably not greatly alter the requirement for renal replacement therapy, and there is no evidence that they reduce mortality. The evidence in favour of 'renal dose' dopamine (1–3 μg/kg/min) is even weaker and, although dopamine receptors certainly exist in the renal vasculature and on the renal tubules, it may well be that the effects that are sometimes observed clinically relate to the diuretic effects of dopamine and to improvements in cardiac output rather than to any direct effect on renal vasculature. Practical recommendations are given in Table 8. All other medical treatments should be regarded as experimental and not given except in the context of controlled trials. The effect of calcium-channel blocking agents, perhaps administered by direct infusion into the renal artery, is an area of current interest.

FLUID AND ELECTROLYTE REQUIREMENTS IN ESTABLISHED ACUTE RENAL FAILURE

Many patients with acute renal failure will be volume depleted at the time of presentation. An urgent priority is to correct such depletion rapidly. Once this has been achieved, as judged by an improvement in peripheral perfusion, a fall in pulse rate, loss of postural drop in blood pressure, and rise in jugular venous pressure, the perspective changes. In the absence of normal renal function the greatest care must be taken to regulate the intake of fluids and electrolytes to match losses in the urine, from the gastrointestinal tract, and from other 'insensible' sources. As a working rule, fluid intake is limited to the volume of the previous day's urine output and gastrointestinal losses plus 500 ml; but this allocation may need to be substantially increased in the presence of fever or in hot environments, when insensible losses through the skin may be much increased. However, fluid balance charts are frequently inaccurate and unthinking adherence to the 'output plus 500 ml' rule can lead to grief. There is no substitute for careful, twice-daily clinical examination for signs of intravascular volume depletion or excess, supplemented by

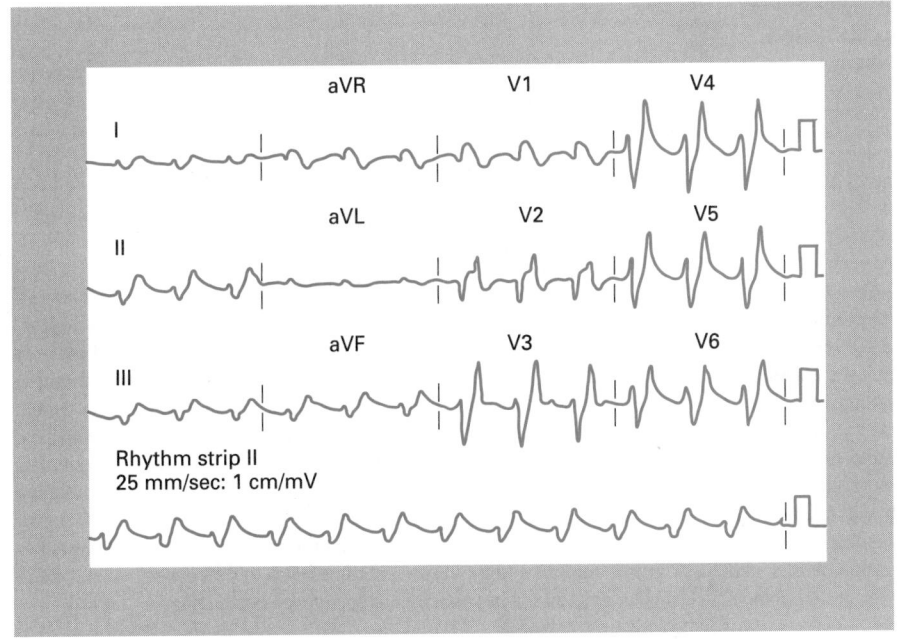

Fig. 1 An electrocardiogram showing severe hyperkalaemia changes in a patient with a serum potassium level of 8.6 mmol/l.

Table 7 *Treatment of hyperkalaemia*

Treatment	Comment
1. Intravenous calcium (10 ml of 10% calcium gluconate, over 60 s, repeated until ECG improves)	Acts instantly to 'stabilize' cardiac membranes (mechanism unknown). Does not alter serum potassium
2. Intravenous insulin and glucose (10 units rapidly acting insulin + 50 ml 50% glucose, over 10 min)	Insulin stimulates Na–K-ATPase in muscle and liver, thus driving potassium into cells. Serum potassium falls by 1–2 mmol/l over 30–60 min
3. Intravenous sodium bicarbonate (50–100 ml of 4.2% solution over 10 min)	Traditionally thought to increase blood pH, inducing exchange of intracellular protons for extracellular potassium. May not work in this manner since hypertonic saline has been shown to be effective
4. Cation exchange resins, e.g. sodium or calcium polystyrene sulphonate (15g by mouth 6 hourly or 15–30 g per rectum 6 hourly)	Exchanges sodium or calcium for potassium in the gut lumen and thus induces loss of potassium from body (unlike 1–3 above). Takes 4 h to produce an effect. Precautions against severe constipation are necessary
5. Haemodialysis/filtration	Except in those rare cases where renal function can rapidly be restored, e.g. relief of obstruction, it is likely that hyperkalaemia will recur and haemodialysis or high-volume haemofiltration will be required

Table 8 *Practical recommendations for medical treatment of prerenal failure or acute tubular necrosis*

1. Treat the precipitating condition vigorously (if possible) and stop drugs listed in Table 6 (if possible)
2. Correct intravascular volume depletion (see Table 5) rapidly by *infusion of blood/colloid/saline* until signs of volume depletion have disappeared **and then stop infusion** before volume overload is induced
3. If, despite measures described above, the urine output remains low, then it is reasonable to give a trial of frusemide and dopamine therapy. There is no evidence that these will generally be beneficial, but there are occasions when individual patients seem to respond:
   (a) give frusemide 80 mg intravenously. If no response:
   (b) infuse frusemide at 2–4 mg/min (to total dose of 0.5–1 g) together with dopamine 2.5 µg/kg/min. If no response, do not repeat. If apparent response, stop frusemide and observe, then stop dopamine and observe. Restart infusions if there is a clear-cut deterioration in urine output on cessation, but do not give more than 1 g of frusemide/day because of ototoxicity
4. After restoration of intravascular volume, fluid input should equal measured output plus 0.5–1 l/day (insensible losses). This fluid should probably have an average sodium concentration of 70–80 mmol/l

accurate daily weighing to gauge overall net fluid balance, and an intelligent flexible response to the findings.

In the undialysed patient, the intake of sodium must also be matched to output. In oliguric patients, requirements are usually very small, perhaps only 15 to 30 mmol/day. In polyuric patients, however, the requirements can be considerable, with a danger of volume depletion if these are not met. The urine will usually contain sodium at a concentration of 50 to 70 mmol/l: hence if urine output is 3 l/day then over 200 mmol of sodium may be required. On occasion, the urine output in polyuric acute renal failure can be even higher and, if the response is to administer an even greater quantity of fluid (output plus insensible losses), it is possible to contrive a vicious cycle whereby ever increasing urinary output is met by ever increasing fluid infusion. Such a danger should be recognized in the polyuric patient and arrangements made to avoid the situation, perhaps by limiting input to urinary output alone and allowing other fluid losses to establish a mild overall negative balance.

For reasons that are not known, excess of sodium and water in patients with tubular necrosis leads to peripheral or pulmonary oedema, whereas in those with glomerulonephritis it tends to produce hypertension.

Because hyperkalaemia is one of the most important problems in the management of acute renal function, it is essential to check plasma potassium levels at least daily; and in those with hypercatabolism or gastrointestinal bleeding, or who require surgery, more frequent estimations are advisable. In oliguric cases, dietary consumption should be limited to the minimum compatible with an adequate intake of protein and amino acids (20–30 mmol/day).

Distal tubular diuretics, such as spironolactone, amiloride, and triamterene, promote potassium retention and should never be used in renal failure. It is noteworthy that these agents are frequent constituents of tablets containing a combination of diuretic/antihypertensive compounds. Antimicrobial agents containing potassium should also be avoided whenever possible. In oliguric patients, excretion of potassium can sometimes be enhanced by the use of high doses of frusemide (0.5–1 g daily). By contrast, in polyuric acute renal failure substantial losses of potassium can occur and need to be replaced. Measurement of urine potassium concentration can be helpful in estimating how much potassium is required.

RENAL REPLACEMENT THERAPY

Mandatory indications for immediate instigation of renal replacement therapy are:

(1) overt uraemia manifesting as encephalopathy, pericarditis, or uraemic bleeding;
(2) refractory hyperkalaemia;
(3) intractable fluid overload; and
(4) acidosis producing circulatory compromise.

These indications will be present in some patients on admission to hospital. However, in a larger number of cases renal function will be seen to decline over a period of a few days, despite optimal medical therapy. In this situation there is no hard and fast rule as to when renal replacement therapy should be initiated. There is no level of nitrogenous waste at which the patient suddenly becomes susceptible to overt uraemic sequelae. Nevertheless, it is clearly not sensible to wait until an obvious uraemic complication (which might be fatal) arises. Modern practice is (whenever possible) to begin renal replacement therapy when the blood urea reaches 25 to 30 mmol/l and the serum creatinine 500 to 700 µmol/l, unless there is clear evidence that spontaneous recovery is occurring.

How should treatment be given? There are three basic options: haemodialysis, peritoneal dialysis, and haemofiltration. Because peritoneal dialysis is technically simple and is the least expensive, it is the method most commonly used worldwide. The principle is the same as that described for long-term treatment of patients with chronic renal failure (see Chapter 20.17.1), the major differences being: (1) that catheters are used that can be inserted percutaneously using a metal stylet; and (2) that smaller volume exchanges with shorter dwell-times are the norm. The technique requires an intact peritoneum; hence it is precluded in the many patients whose renal failure is associated with abdominal surgery. Other problems include difficulties in maintaining dialysate flow, leakage, peritoneal infection, protein losses, and restricted ability to clear fluid and uraemic wastes. These limitations mean that, particularly in the hypercatabolic patient, peritoneal dialysis is frequently unable to provide good dialysis as judged by modern standards. By contrast, traditional haemodialysis, performed daily or on alternate days, can provide much better control of uraemia. Major disadvantages (apart from cost) arise from the fact that it is an intermittent treatment. In each 4 hour treatment at least 2 to 3 litres of fluid must be removed to make 'space' either for infusion of drugs/parenteral fluids or for oral fluid intake in the 24- to 48-h period before the next dialysis. Such a procedure can impose substantial haemodynamic stress and so is frequently not tolerated by those with impaired cardiovascular function. This is the main reason why continuous haemofiltration techniques have largely replaced haemodialysis in intensive care units. Blood, driven either by the patient's own arterial pressure or by a mechanical pump, passes through a haemofilter of high hydraulic conductivity, such that roughly 1 litre of plasma ultrafiltrate is removed per hour. This is replaced, less the volume of other fluid inputs, using a lactate/acetate-based substitution fluid. The process is tolerated well, even by patients who are very ill, and the continuous nature of the technique permits continuous fine tuning of the intravascular volume (Fig. 2).

INDICATIONS FOR RENAL BIOPSY

Most cases of acute renal failure are due to prerenal failure or to the clinical syndrome of acute tubular necrosis. They occur in an appropriate clinical setting and follow a typical time course, with recovery of renal function over the course of a few weeks. In such instances renal biopsy should not be performed, since the information gained is exceedingly unlikely to influence management, and the risks of the procedure are therefore not warranted. There are, however, circumstances in which renal biopsy is essential to establish a correct diagnosis, with important implications for both management and prognosis. Biopsy should be considered:

(1) when the history, examination, or laboratory tests suggest a systemic disorder that could cause acute renal failure and could be diagnosed by renal biopsy;

(2) when the urine sediment contains red cell casts;

(3) when the case history is atypical; and

(4) when renal failure is unusually prolonged (say beyond 6 weeks).

In this context, cortial necrosis (see below) is better diagnosed by angiography.

NUTRITION

Patients with acute renal failure are invariably catabolic, and derive a larger fraction of their energy expenditure from protein breakdown than normal. Insulin resistance, metabolic acidosis, the release of proteinases into the circulation, and changes in the metabolism of branched-chain amino acids have all been suggested as possible reasons. If nutrition is neglected, patients with acute renal failure lose weight very rapidly, and those that lose most have the highest mortality. There is a consensus

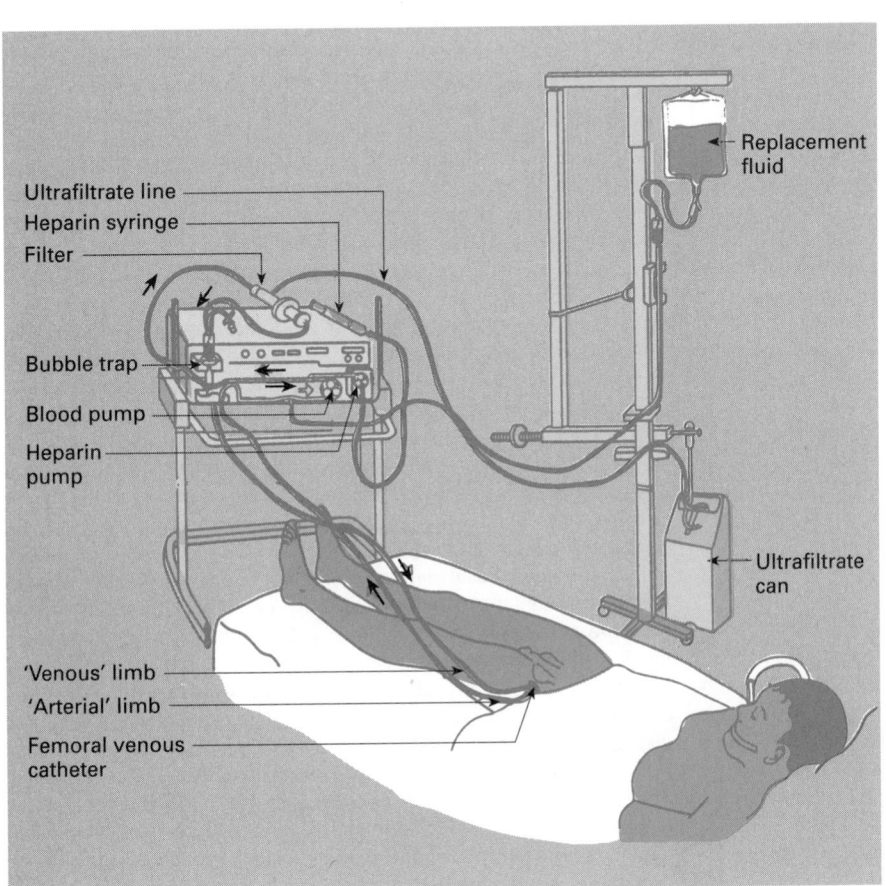

Fig. 2 Diagram of a patient undergoing pumped venovenous haemofiltration for acute renal failure using a gravity feed balance system for infusion of replacement fluid. (Reproduced from P.M. Morris and R.A. Malt. (1994). *Oxford Textbook of Surgery* p. 198. University Press, Oxford, with permission.)

that early institution of nutritional support probably improves prognosis, but despite this, action is frequently delayed or not taken at all—particularly if it is thought that the extra fluid load required will mandate the institution of dialysis or the need for additional dialysis sessions in an already busy unit. The diet for the undialysed patient with acute renal failure should provide all essential amino acids in a total protein intake of 0.3 to 0.5 g/kg bodyweight daily, with fat and carbohydrate to bring up the energy intake to at least 2000 calories, or 4000 calories in hypercatabolic cases. In patients too unwell to take adequate food by mouth, commonly those who need it most, tube feeding or parenteral nutrition should be started early. Protein restriction, aimed at moderating the rise of plasma urea, is no longer appropriate once a decision has been made to initiate dialysis.

BLEEDING

In uraemia the bleeding time is prolonged, and in acute renal failure this summates with any abnormality of haemostasis that might be simultaneously induced by the precipitating condition. Better control of uraemia and the routine use of H_2-receptor antagonists has been associated with a greatly reduced risk of upper gastrointestinal bleeding, a previously frequent and grave occurrence. In the majority of patients, impairment of haemostasis is not a cause of great clinical concern. There are, however, some patients who bleed—from anywhere and everywhere. Guidelines for the management of such cases are given in Table 9.

SEPSIS

Overwhelming septicaemia is a common cause of acute renal failure, and in such instances the diagnosis is often straightforward. However, in many more cases the role of sepsis is insidious and difficult to diagnose with certainty. There is often strong clinical feeling, but little in the way of hard proof, that sepsis underlies the slide towards worsening renal and multiorgan failure of patients who have been apparently successfully resuscitated from major trauma or surgery. Septicaemia is the commonest cause of death in those with acute renal failure. The index of clinical suspicion must therefore be very high: if a patient with acute renal failure appears to be deteriorating in any way, the question must be asked 'is this sepsis?'. Unused intravenous lines and urinary catheters should be removed, and those that are necessary but in any way 'suspicious' should be replaced. The patient should be examined regularly for signs of a septic focus. There should be a low threshold for repeated, thorough microbiological investigation. Proven infection should be treated promptly with modified doses of appropriate antimicrobials. In many cases, however, it will be necessary to start treatment 'blind', having taken specimens for culture and made an educated guess at the likely pathogen, with the possibility of Gram-negative septicaemia high on the list. In the patient who appears 'obviously septic', but in whom no cause can be found, attention should be directed towards the chest and abdomen since these are the most likely places of hidden mischief. Radiological investigations, including CT scanning, to search for abdominal sepsis should not be relied upon too faithfully, and surgical exploration should be undertaken if there is any doubt.

PRESCRIPTION OF DRUGS

Many drugs are excreted by glomerular filtration or tubular secretion and must be given in reduced dosage or at longer intervals than normal in patients with renal failure (see Chapter 20.14). Protein binding and extrarenal metabolism of drugs may be altered by the uraemic state. The changes in dosage recommended in renal failure should be regarded as a guide at best, and whenever possible plasma levels should be measured regularly to avoid toxicity. Agents to avoid include tetracyclines (increased protein catabolism) and cephaloridine (nephrotoxicity). Particular care should be taken with prescription of non-steroidal anti-

Table 9 *Practical strategies for the management of bleeding in acute renal failure*

1. Exclude the possibility of a heparin effect
2. Blood transfusion to obtain haematocrit >30% (occasionally erythropoietin is of value)
3. Cryoprecipitate (10 bags) has its maximal effect between 1 and 2 h after administration. Its effect disappears at 24–36 h
4. Desmopressin (0.3 μg/kg intravenously) acts by increasing factor VIII coagulant activity. Shown in acute renal failure to shorten prolonged bleeding time. Repeated doses have a lesser effect
5. Conjugated oestrogen: 0.6 mg/kg/day for 5 days. Shown to reduce bleeding time (for at least 14 days) in patients with chronic renal impairment and haemorrhagic tendency

inflammatory agents and converting enzyme inhibitors (potentially deleterious haemodynamic consequences), allopurinol (greatly reduced dosage in renal failure), and high-dose penicillin therapy for endocarditis (risk of encephalopathy). Despite its known nephrotoxicity, gentamicin is commonly used in patients with renal failure and Gram-negative septicaemia. Initial dosage should be estimated from nomograms that allow for the patient's age, weight, and plasma creatinine level. Thereafter dosage should be modified in the light of plasma levels checked before and 15 to 30 min after injection.

Other specific causes of acute renal failure

Nephrotoxic causes of acute renal failure
EXOGENOUS NEPHROTOXINS

A wide variety of exogenous agents, including therapeutically prescribed drugs, can cause acute renal failure. Some of these agents are listed in Table 10. The following are worthy of particular note.

Aminoglycosides

Gentamicin, amikacin, kanamycin, and streptomycin are all potentially nephrotoxic, as are tobramycin and netilmicin to a lesser degree. These drugs are usually prescribed for seriously ill patients suspected to be suffering from potentially fatal infections. Thus, in clinical practice it is frequently impossible to separate harmful effects of aminoglycosides from those of the underlying condition, or of other drugs used in treatment. However, evidence from animal models supports the view that these agents are genuinely nephrotoxic, rather than that their prescription is simply a marker for severe infection, which is itself a potent cause of acute renal failure. It has been stated that acute renal failure complicates up to 25 per cent of therapeutic courses of gentamicin, even when drug levels are optimally controlled by monitoring. Parenteral administration is not required for toxicity. Acute renal failure can occur as a result of systemic absorption when aminoglycosides are used in irrigating or bowel sterilizing solutions. The typical clinical picture is of relatively mild non-oliguric renal failure coming on 1 to 2 weeks after starting treatment. Tubular proteinuria and impaired ability to concentrate the urine precede loss of glomerular filtration rate. Proximal tubular damage involves the brush border, reflected by increased urinary excretion of γ-glutamyl transferase, alanine aminopeptidase, and of lysosomal enzymes. Recovery may be slow, delayed, or incomplete. It is known that gentamicin accumulates in the renal parenchyma, particularly in the cortex, but the exact mechanism of toxicity remains unknown. The risk of nephrotoxicity is increased by old age, pre-existing renal insufficiency, high dosage, prolonged treatment, combined treatment with other nephrotoxic drugs, renal ischaemia, and volume depletion.

Table 10 *Some nephrotoxins that can cause acute renal failure (excluding causes of interstitial nephritis—see Table 13)*

Exogenous	
Antibiotics	Aminoglycosides, tetracyclines, cephaloridine, amphotericin B, sulphonamides, polymyxin/colistin, bacitracin, pentamidine, vancomycin
Radiocontrast media	
Anaesthetic agents	Methoxyflurane[a], enflurane[a]
Chemotherapeutic/immunosuppressive agents	Cyclosporin A, *cis*-platinum, methotrexate
Organic solvents	Glycols (e.g. ethylene glycol[a]) Hydrocarbons (e.g. carbon tetrachloride, toluene)
Poisons	Insecticides/herbicides/rodenticides (including paraquat, copper sulphate, sodium chlorate); mushrooms (Amanita); venoms (snake bite, e.g. Russell's viper; stings); hemlock; carp bile; herbal medicines
Drugs of abuse	
Heavy metals	
Endogenous	
Pigments	Myoglobin, haemoglobin
Intrarenal crystal deposition	Urate, phosphate (tumour lysis syndrome)
Tumour-related	Immunoglobulin light chains

In many instances nephrotoxicity arises both from direct toxic action on renal tissue and from indirect systemic effects.

[a]May be associated with intratubular precipitation of oxalate crystals.

Radiographic contrast media

The incidence of acute renal failure associated with the use of radiographic contrast media has been reported to vary between 0 and 50 per cent. This extraordinary variability reflects differences in other risk factors in the populations under examination. Modern prospective studies, using non-ionic contrast media and in which careful attention has been paid to the maintenance of adequate hydration, have shown a very low incidence of significant renal impairment—even in groups reported to be at high risk (diabetes, myeloma). When renal impairment does occur it is usually mild.

ENDOGENOUS NEPHROTOXINS

Myoglobin

Myoglobinuric acute renal failure is associated with crush injury or other trauma to muscle, but the mechanism of renal failure remains unclear. It is not widely recognized, however, that there are a large number of causes of non-traumatic rhabdomyolysis (Table 11). Unless there is a high index of suspicion these will not be diagnosed, since muscular pain, swelling, and tenderness may not be prominent features, and may even be absent. The combination of dark-brown urine, positive for 'blood' on a reagent strip but without red cells on microscopy, indicates myoglobinuria and confirms the diagnosis. The findings of very high plasma urate (>750 μmol/l) and phosphate (>2.5 mmol/l) and of unusually low plasma calcium (< 1.5 mmol/l) in any patient with acute renal failure should lead to serious consideration of the condition. Gross elevation of plasma uric acid may conceivably contribute to the mechanism of renal damage. Extremely high levels of plasma myoglobin, aldolase, creatine phosphokinase, and lactic dehydrogenase—all released from damaged muscle—are to be expected.

If the diagnosis of rhabdomyolysis is made, then the question of whether to initiate an alkaline diuresis arises, since on theoretical grounds it would be anticipated that alkalinization of the urine would lead to enhanced excretion of the putative toxin and protect against acute renal failure. Victims of crush injury have been treated with infusion of very large volumes of fluid (12 l/day) and big doses of mannitol (160 g/day) and bicarbonate (240 mmol/day). In comparison with historical (volume-depleted) controls the incidence of renal failure was impressively reduced; but the difficulties of controlling potassium balance in the face of such a massive diuresis should not be underestimated. It may well be that avoidance of hypovolaemia using a less aggressive and more easily managed fluid regime would be equally efficacious.

Table 11 *Some causes of rhabdomyolysis*

Direct muscle injury

Ischaemic muscle injury
  Compression
  Vascular occlusion

Any cause of coma (e.g. opiate overdose, diabetes mellitus, cerebrovascular accident) or of prolonged immobility (e.g. following a fall in the elderly) can be associated with rhabdomyolysis due to a pressure effect.

Excessive muscular activity
  Seizures
  Sporting, e.g. marathon running

Inflammatory myositis
  Immunological, e.g. dermatomyositis, polymyositis
  Infection, e.g. viral (influenza, coxsackie)

Metabolic
  Hypokalaemia, hypophosphataemia
  Genetic abnormalities of carbohydrate metabolism, e.g. myophosphorylase deficiency (McArdle's syndrome), phosphofructokinase deficiency

Toxins/drugs
  Snake bite, carbon monoxide, alcohol, hemlock, paint/glue sniffing
  Clofibrate, aminocaproic acid, HMGCoA reductase inhibitors

Others
  Malignant hyperpyrexia
  Neuroleptic malignant syndrome
  Phaeochromocytoma 'storm'

Haemoglobin

In several situations, acute renal failure is seen in association with massive haemolysis: malaria, glucose 6-phosphate dehydrogenase deficiency, mismatched blood transfusion, arsine poisoning, copper sulphate poisoning, burns, and as a complication of bladder irrigation with hypotonic solutions. In each circumstance it is possible, but not proven, that the development of acute renal failure might be attributable to, or exacerbated by, the presence of large amounts of free haemoglobin within the circulation.

Urate

A rapid rise in plasma uric acid concentration complicating treatment of lymphoma, leukaemia, myeloma, or other 'high-turnover' tumours may result in the deposition of urate crystals in the distal tubule. These can both physically obstruct the tubule and initiate an inflammatory response, leading to acute renal failure in which freshly voided urine is found to be heavily laden with urate crystals. Hyperuricaemia and renal failure have been described on rare occasions after recurrent epileptic seizures.

In the context of the treatment of malignancy, hyperuricaemic acute renal failure is predictable, and an attempt should obviously be made to prevent it. Dehydration should be avoided at all costs. If possible, at least 24 h before the initiation of chemotherapy, a brisk saline or alkaline diuresis should be initiated, and allopurinol treatment started. In those with normal baseline renal function a dose of 900 mg/day may be preferred to the conventional dose of 300 mg/day. If hyperuricaemic acute renal failure does develop, then it is unlikely that these treatments, or diuretics, will reverse the condition. Indeed, administration of alkali may be contraindicated if plasma phosphate is raised concurrently (as it often is). Prompt improvement usually follows reduction in plasma uric acid levels, which can be accomplished much more effectively by haemodialysis than by peritoneal dialysis. On very rare occasions the ureters can become obstructed by urate crystals—indicated by colic, pelvicalyceal distension, or persistent oliguria—and ureteral catheterization and washout may be required.

Other endogenous nephrotoxins

More uncommon even than intratubular obstruction by urate crystals is similar obstruction by phosphate, also seen in the context of massive cell destruction in the treatment of malignant disease. Urinary alkalinization should be avoided because it may promote intratubular phosphate precipitation. The possible role of immunoglobulin light chains in causing acute renal failure related to myeloma is dealt with in Chapter 20.17.1 and Section 22.

Vascular causes of acute renal failure

ACUTE CORTICAL NECROSIS

Acute cortical necrosis is a rare cause of acute renal failure, accounting for perhaps less than 1 per cent of all cases of suspected acute tubular necrosis. Most cases used to be the result of obstetric disasters, particularly after postpartum haemorrhage, abruptio placentae, eclampsia, or septic abortion. With improved obstetric care such cases are now very rare. In the non-obstetric population, pancreatitis, endotoxaemia, and disseminated intravascular coagulation are risk factors. The pathological findings are of microvascular thrombosis, mainly affecting interlobular arteries, arterioles, and glomeruli, with complete infarction of affected areas of cortex. The medulla and a rim of juxtamedullary tissue are spared. The diagnosis is usually first suspected when renal function fails to recover as expected in a patient thought to be suffering from acute tubular necrosis. The investigation most likely to provide the diagnosis is renal angiography, which reveals attenuation of interlobular arteries, an increase in the subcapsular vessels, and a negative outer cortical nephrogram. Biopsy, which samples only a very small piece of tissue, may mislead because of the patchy nature of renal damage. Radiopharmaceutical investigations (DMSA scans) are sometimes advocated, but are frequently difficult to interpret in patients with poor renal function. Return of renal function in cases of acute cortical necrosis occurs very slowly, if at all, and is attributable to the survival of islands of intact cortical tissue. About 50 per cent of cases recover function sufficiently to get off dialysis, but the glomerular filtration rate rarely exceeds 10 to 20 ml/min; hypertension (including accelerated phase) may be a major problem, and a subsequent decline in renal function with the necessity for a return to dialysis/transplantation is not uncommon. The kidneys tend to contract, and cortical calcification, producing an eggshell or tramline appearance on the abdominal radiograph, is a characteristic sequela.

LARGE-VESSEL OBSTRUCTION

Occlusion of the main renal arteries—or of the artery of a solitary functioning kidney—by trauma, dissection, thrombosis, or embolism may rarely be the reason for acute renal failure. Loin pain sometimes occurs, and fever would be expected, but symptoms can be notable by their absence. Proteinuria and haematuria may occur. Diagnosis is important, because renovascular surgery can be surprisingly effective in restoring function, even when undertaken 24 h or more after onset. Symptoms may mimic acute pyelonephritis, and although suspicion should be aroused by complete, sudden anuria in the absence of urinary obstruction in an appropriate clinical setting, these suggestive features may be absent. DTPA renography and angiography are the appropriate diagnostic tests, but CT scanning can also reveal the characteristic wedge-shaped infarcts when occlusion is incomplete.

Renal vein thrombosis may cause acute renal failure, most commonly in adults as a complication of the nephrotic syndrome, but in infants and children as a result of abdominal sepsis or severe dehydration. Renal pain, increasing proteinuria and haematuria usually, but by no means always, herald this complication. Appropriate investigation includes ultrasound/Doppler examination of the renal veins and inferior vena cava, and renal angiography with late films taken specifically to look for filling of the renal veins. Treatment by anticoagulation is the usual practice.

SMALL VESSEL OBSTRUCTION

Accelerated-phase hypertension (See also Chapter 15.27)

'Accelerated-phase' hypertension (a term preferred to 'malignant' hypertension because it is less misleading and less terrifying for patients) is diagnosed when the blood pressure is elevated sufficiently to cause fibrinoid necrosis of blood vessels, leading to the development of haemorrhages and exudates in the ocular fundi. It may develop as a consequence of pre-existing renal disease, but does not always do so, and is itself a potent cause of renal damage. In those with previously normal renal function, renal impairment is a common complication, associated with proteinuria, haematuria, and the presence of urinary red cell casts. The higher the creatinine at presentation, the poorer the prognosis for both patient survival and renal outcome. In one study, only 9 per cent of patients with an initial plasma creatinine below 300 µmol/l progressed to endstage renal failure, compared with two-thirds of those with a plasma creatinine above this level. In the days before dialysis was available uraemia was the cause of two-thirds of deaths in these patients.

The main renal pathological findings consist of proliferative endarteritis of the intralobular arteries and fibrinoid necrosis of the afferent arterioles and glomerular capillary tuft. The ability of the kidney to autoregulate perfusion is disturbed; thus the lowering of arterial pressure may be associated with reduced renal perfusion and an abrupt decline in renal function. With control of blood pressure the fibrinoid lesions heal within days, but the proliferative lesions do not, eventually being converted to acellular fibrous and elastic tissue. Accelerated-phase hypertension is one of the conditions in which renal function sometimes recover after a lengthy period on dialysis.

Systemic sclerosis

This disease does not usually involve the kidney (see Chapter 18.11.4). However, a syndrome resembling accelerated-phase hypertension, the 'scleroderma renal crisis', is well recognized. It can occur at any time during the disease, often during the winter months. Rapid worsening of skin manifestations may precede the crisis, but frequently there is no warning. The patient may develop headaches, visual disturbance, and convulsions. Arterial pressure is usually grossly elevated, but the renal syndrome can occur without a rise in arterial pressure. Haemorrhages and exudates are often seen in the ocular fundi. Renal failure, with proteinuria and haematuria, develops rapidly. A microangiopathic haemolytic anaemia may complicate the situation. Plasma levels of renin are grossly elevated. There have been a number of case reports of arrest or reversal of the syndrome after treatment with angiotensin-converting enzyme inhibitors or nifedipine. These agents should be tried, but more in hope than expectation that they will prevent relentless progression to endstage renal failure.

Glomerulonephritic and vasculitic causes of acute renal failure

A large number of glomerulonephritic and vasculitic diseases can cause acute renal failure, sometimes in association with pulmonary haemorrhage. These are listed in Table 12, and they are discussed in detail elsewhere. Together they form only 5 to 10 per cent of cases of acute renal failure, but making the correct diagnosis is of extreme importance because of the management implications. Regrettably, most nephrologists have seen cases where the diagnosis has been much delayed because renal impairment has incorrectly been attributed to acute tubular necrosis, and infiltrates on the chest radiograph to oedema or infection. This error, which can be catastrophic, should be avoided in patients in whom the cause of acute renal failure is not obvious by:

1. A history and examination specifically directed towards determining whether one of the conditions listed in Table 12 might be present.
2. Microscopy of the urine to look for the presence of red cells and red cell casts.
3. The following blood tests:
   (a) measurement of antiglomerular basement membrane (anti-GBM) antibodies as a matter of urgency;
   (b) measurement of antineutrophil cytoplasmic antigen antibodies (ANCA)—positive in microscopic polyarteritis and Wegener's granulomatosis;
   (c) estimation of serum complement levels (C3 depressed in postinfectious glomerulonephritis, mesangiocapillary glomerulonephritis, systemic lupus erythematosus)
   (d) measurement of anti-streptolysin O titre (ASOT—elevated in post-streptococcal glomerulonephritis);
   (e) serological tests for systemic lupus erythematosus;
   (f) cryoglobulins.
4. Consideration of the possibility that pulmonary infiltrates in a patient with acute renal failure might be due to haemorrhage. The chances of this are increased if there is a history of haemoptysis (associated with several forms of rapidly progressive glomerulonephritis), nasal discharge or bleeding (associated with Wegener's granulomatosis), or if anaemia is unusually profound and otherwise unexplained. Lung function tests demonstrating an increase in carbon monoxide transfer factor can establish the diagnosis.
5. Performance of an urgent renal biopsy (Plate 1). In any patient with acute renal failure and an active urinary sediment, renal biopsy should be performed unless the diagnosis is clear, for example classical history of post-streptococcal nephritis, obvious infective endocarditis/shunt nephritis, or there is a strong contraindication, for example single kidney or serious bleeding disorder.

The possibility of the presence of a rapidly progressive glomerulonephritis/vasculitis constitutes a medical emergency. Anti-GBM disease responds well to immunosuppression with methylprednisolone/plasma exchange and cyclophosphamide, but only if treatment is begun before oliguria develops. Similar immunosuppressive treatment should be given as early as possible in the course of acute renal failure complicating microscopic polyarteritis/idiopathic rapidly progressive (crescen-

Table 12 *Glomerulonephritides and vasculitides causing acute renal failure*

Antiglomerular basement membrane (anti-GBM) disease
Primary glomerulonephritis
  Mesangial IgA nephropathy
  Mesangiocapillary glomerulonephritis
Primary systemic vasculitis
  Microscopic polyarteritis/idiopathic rapidly progressive (crescentic) glomerulonephritis
  Wegener's granulomatosis
  Churg–Strauss syndrome, polyarteritis nodosa, giant-cell arteritis, Takayasu's arteritis (all rarely cause renal failure)
Other causes
  Cryoglobulinaemia
  Systemic lupus erythematosus
  Infection—post-streptococcal, infective endocarditis, ventriculoatrial shunt, visceral abscess

tic) glomerulonephritis, Wegener's granulomatosis, and systemic lupus erythematosus. The urgency is such that it may well be appropriate to start these treatments while the results of blood tests and renal biopsy are awaited, and to stop them if the findings do not corroborate the initial clinical diagnosis. The management of these patients is complex and patients benefit from the judgement and expertise of specialists.

Interstitial nephritis as a cause of acute renal failure
DRUGS

Drugs are the commonest cause of acute interstitial nephritis. Those which are most frequently implicated are listed in Table 13, together with other (rarer) causes of the condition. The classical clinical picture aids prompt diagnosis; a few days or weeks after taking a drug the patient develops flank pain (sometimes), fever, a skin rash, arthralgias, haematuria, blood eosinophilia and elevated IgE, disturbed liver function (sometimes), interstitial pneumonia (rarely), and renal impairment. Often some or all of these features other than the renal manifestations are absent. The urine contains protein and blood, with white and red cell casts. Proteinuria may be in the nephrotic range, particularly in association with non-steroidal anti-inflammatory agents.

The diagnosis of acute interstitial nephritis can only be established by renal biopsy, since the associated clinical signs listed above may be absent or may also be found in conjunction with biopsy appearances deemed suggestive of acute tubular necrosis. The typical histological findings are of an interstitial infiltrate of lymphocytes and monocytes/macrophages, together with some eosinophils (see Plate 1). Epithelioid granulomata may be seen, and strongly support the diagnosis of a drug-induced interstitial nephritis, but they are not pathognomonic. When large numbers of cells are present in the renal interstitium the diagnosis is not contentious: more difficult are those cases (not too infrequent) in which the infiltrate is modest—how many cells turn 'acute tubular necrosis' into 'interstitial nephritis'? The importance of making the distinction lies in the belief that, apart from withdrawal of the offending drug, treatment of drug-induced interstitial nephritis with steroids is beneficial. There is some evidence that those given prednisolone have an earlier and more complete recovery of renal function than those left untreated.

LEPTOSPIROSIS (SEE ALSO CHAPTER 7.11.32)

Acute renal failure due to an interstitial nephritis may appear within a few days of the onset of disease, but more commonly occurs in the second week. It is frequently mild, but may be severe, with plasma urea rising rapidly due to hypercatabolism. The diagnosis of leptospirosis should be considered in any patient with unexplained acute renal failure

Table 13 *Some causes of interstitial nephritis causing acute renal failure*

Drugs	
β-Lactam antibiotics	Penicillin G, methicillin, ampicillin, cephalothin
Other antibiotics	Sulphonamides (co-trimoxazole), rifampicin
Anti-inflammatory agents	Fenoprofen, naproxen, ibuprofen, glafenin, mefenamic acid
Diuretics	Thiazides, frusemide, chlorthalidone, triamterene
Others	Cimetidine, phenindione, diphenylhydantoin, allopurinol
Note: Many other drugs have been incriminated on the basis of occasional association	
Infections	
Septicaemia	Direct invasion by Gram-negative organisms, Staphylococcus *Candida albicans*
Direct/indirect effects	Commonly in leptospirosis and Hantavirus disease. Less commonly in scarlet fever and diphtheria. Occasionally in infectious mononucleosis and HIV disease. Many other infections have been incriminated on the basis of occasional association
Infiltration	
Lymphoma, leukaemia, plasma cell dyscrasia (multiple pathogenic mechanisms)	
Other	
Sarcoidosis	
Idiopathic: no plausible cause found, diagnosed by exclusion. Occasionally associated with uveitis or iritis, chronic active hepatitis, primary biliary cirrhosis, ulcerative colitis	

who has myalgias/muscle tenderness, conjunctival infection, and/or haemorrhage or jaundice. Direct inquiry must be made as to whether any such patient has been exposed to rats. Thrombocytopenia is common, and mild changes of intravascular haemolysis/coagulation may be seen. The diagnosis is established by demonstration of elevated leptospiral antibody titres. Specific treatment is with benzylpenicillin.

HANTAVIRUS DISEASE

Several serotypes of Hantavirus produce a disease similar in many respects to leptospirosis. In both the European and Asian (more severe) forms, myalgias, conjunctival haemorrhage, and thrombocytopenia may be observed, but jaundice is rare. The diagnosis depends on serological evidence of infection. There is no specific treatment.

'Haematological' causes of acute renal failure

HAEMOLYTIC URAEMIC SYNDROME, THROMBOTIC
THROMBOCYTOPENIC PURPURA, AND IDIOPATHIC
POSTPARTUM RENAL FAILURE (SEE ALSO CHAPTER 20.6)

The haemolytic uraemic syndrome (HUS) is a condition, or group of conditions, in which acute renal failure, characterized on biopsy by thrombosis and necrosis of intrarenal vessels, occurs together with thrombocytopenia, haemolytic anaemia, and red cell fragmentation. It most frequently affects young children, in whom renal function usually recovers, but may (rarely) affect adults, in whom renal failure is often irreversible. The causes/associations can be divided on the basis of whether or not diarrhoea is a feature of the illness. Of infective diarrhoeal-associated HUS, that caused by infection with verocytotoxin-producing *E. coli* 0157 : H7 is the commonest and best described. The sporadic, non-infectious forms are less common. Familial cases have been described, as have associations with cyclosporin, mitomycin C, systemic lupus erythematosus, accelerated-phase hypertension, and scleroderma. Aside from standard supportive therapy, treatment with fresh frozen plasma may be of benefit. Steroids are of no value.

The haemolytic uraemic syndrome may develop within 24 h, or up to several weeks, after an entirely uneventful pregnancy and delivery ('idiopathic postpartum acute renal failure'), or complicate treatment by oral contraceptive drugs. In some reports cardiomyopathy has been noted in association. Two-thirds of women never recover renal function; in the remainder a variable degree of impairment occurs. In the very

rare cases of this condition, treatment with fresh frozen plasma is usually given, although there is no certainty of benefit.

The syndrome of thrombotic thrombocytopenic purpura (TTP) is closely related to HUS; indeed the two may represent the extremes of a continuum. Similar vascular injury occurs in both conditions, but in TTP it appears to be more widespread in its clinical impact, with fever and fluctuating central nervous system abnormalities added to those of HUS, and a lesser propensity for severe renal failure. In adults, usually women, the illness may run a chronic relapsing course. Treatment is as for US.

MYELOMA (SEE ALSO SECTION 22)

Acute renal failure complicates about 7 per cent of cases of myeloma, and is increasingly recognized as a presenting feature. A subacute form of progressive renal failure is much commoner (14–61 per cent of myeloma cases). Both are associated with the reversible factors of dehydration, infection, hypercalcaemia, and hyperuricaemia; with renal damage caused by free immunoglobulin light chains; and most commonly with a combination of these factors. The reason why only some patients with myeloma develop renal failure, and others do not, remains a mystery. There has been much speculation as to whether variation in the isoelectric point of light chains, and hence their capacity for reabsorption by the renal tubules, might be responsible. However, individual patients with light chains of very similar physicochemical properties can present totally different clinical pictures, varying from no perceptible renal involvement to irreversible renal failure.

In a patient with acute renal failure, a history of bone pain, the finding of clumping of erythrocytes on the blood film, or of gross and unexpected elevation of the erythrocyte sedimentation rate, are clues that myeloma might be the underlying diagnosis. Such clues may be absent when excess production of monoclonal light chains is the predominant problem. The best way to pursue the possibility is by bone marrow biopsy for immunochemical analysis of plasma cell population; and by careful examination of the urine for free κ or λ light chains ('myeloma kidney' only occurs with light chain proteinuria, but hypercalcaemic nephropathy can occur without). The renal biopsy appearances are of a tubulointerstitial nephritis, with fractured casts in the tubular lumina, tubular atrophy, interstitial oedema/fibrosis, and an interstitial infiltrate that may contain multinucleate giant cells (see Plate 1).

Apart from establishing the correct diagnosis, the first priority in management is to deal promptly with those factors that can be reversed—

dehydration, infection, hypercalcaemia, and hyperuricaemia. It has been suggested that alkalinization of the urine by use of intravenous sodium bicarbonate may be advantageous in promoting light chain excretion, but it is not clear that this is better than adequate rehydration with saline alone. If there is a clear precipitant for the decline in renal function, then the prospects for renal recovery are good; if not, then the renal outlook is less favourable. Although some report that aggressive treatment with cytotoxics and/or plasmapheresis can restore renal function in such cases, this is not everyone's experience, and renal recovery seems to be the exception rather than the rule.

The prognosis for patients with myeloma and established renal failure requiring dialysis is poor: 50 per cent 1-year survival, 30 per cent at 2 years. However, many patients will have few symptoms from their myeloma, excepting renal failure, and these should certainly be offered the opportunity of renal replacement therapy. In those with considerable extrarenal manifestations the situation is much more difficult, and it may not be appropriate or kind to offer aggressive haematological regimens, producing considerable side-effects, and/or dialysis, in such circumstances. The decisions to be made are rarely straightforward: they will substantially depend on an assessment of the overall burden to the patient of their disease and a realistic appraisal of what benefits treatment might produce.

Hepatorenal syndrome

The hepatorenal syndrome consists of the association of severe and usually progressive liver disease with acute renal failure. The renal failure is characterized by:

(1) no evidence of renal parenchymal damage—if the kidney is transplanted it functions normally in the recipient;
(2) characteristic 'prerenal' urine biochemistry (Table 4);
(3) no sustained response to volume expansion; and
(4) exclusion of other causes of acute renal failure.

The mechanism of renal failure is not known, but it is associated with markedly reduced renal perfusion. Recent suggestions of a contribution from endothelin require further evaluation.

One of the aims of general management of patients with liver disease is prevention of the hepatorenal syndrome, the most important consideration being avoidance of known precipitants (drugs, excessive diuresis, delay in treatment of sepsis). Nevertheless, the syndrome develops in up to 20 per cent of cirrhotics admitted to hospital. There is no specific treatment and the prognosis is extremely poor. In the presence of potentially reversible liver disease, or with the prospect of liver transplantation, intensive therapy and renal replacement therapy are justified. If these criteria are not met, then aggressive support is almost certainly inappropriate.

Tropical

Acute renal failure in the tropics, as elsewhere, is usually a consequence of acute tubular necrosis. However, the spectrum of diseases which causes it is substantially different from that encountered in the 'developed' world. Medical causes account for 65 per cent of cases, surgical causes 25 per cent, and obstetric causes 15 per cent (compared to 1–2 per cent in developed countries). Common tropical infections causing acute renal failure include falciparum malaria, leptospirosis, melioidosis, salmonellosis, and shigellosis. Snake bite is the cause of 2 to 3 per cent of cases, and a much higher proportion in some centres at some times of the year. Acute renal failure develops in two-thirds of those bitten by Russell's viper. Poisoning by deliberate (occasionally accidental) ingestion of paraquat (herbicide) or copper sulphate (leather industry) are not infrequent causes. Paraquat can lead to death due to inexorably progressive respiratory failure: treatment with corticosteroids and cyclophosphamide has been used in an attempt to prevent pulmonary fibrosis and may be of benefit. Heat stroke can cause acute renal failure. In infants, diarrhoea, various septicaemias, and the haemolytic uraemic syndrome account for most cases.

Prognosis and financial cost

Acute renal failure of sufficient severity to require renal replacement therapy has a high mortality. In a series of over 1300 cases the actuarial 1-year survival of all medical and surgical cases rose from 39 per cent to 58 per cent between 1956 and 1988, despite an increase in the median patient age from 41 to 61 years over this period. The prognosis varies according to the cause of acute renal failure: it is best in obstetric and poisoning cases (80–90 per cent survival) and worst in burns (15–20 per cent survival). Death is nowadays rarely attributable to a primary sequel of renal failure, for example uraemia or hyperkalaemia, and the incidence of life-threatening gastrointestinal haemorrhage is much reduced: sepsis is the major killer. The patients die *with* but not directly *of* renal failure. If they survive the precipitating insult, largely complete recovery of renal function can be anticipated, excepting in the elderly (over 70 years) in whom there is a substantial chance (10–20 per cent) that dependence on dialysis will be lifelong.

Treatment of acute renal failure is expensive, particularly in those patients with multiorgan failure needing to be managed in an intensive care unit, who account for 50 per cent of all cases requiring renal replacement therapy. At a time when, all over the world, there are pressures to reduce health care expenditure, it seems reasonable to ask what the financial costs of treating acute renal failure are. It is surprising that there are few good published data. However, the Oxford experience in 1990 of 41 patients, all requiring both mechanical ventilation and renal replacement therapy revealed the following. A total of 551 patient days of dual organ support were provided, at an estimated total cost of £715 000 (£1300/day). The 25 patients who died each received between 1 and 20 days of the combined treatments (median 6 days), and the group as a whole consumed 205 treatment days (£265 000). The 16 survivors (alive at 180 days) each received between 4 and 52 days of pulmonary/renal support (median 22 days), the group as a whole consuming 346 treatment days (£450 000). Nine of these survivors required a total of 140 days of further renal support before their kidneys recovered, and a tenth survivor remained dialysis-dependent 2 years later. From these figures it can be seen that the cost of intensive care treatment was approximately £48 000 for each patient with acute renal failure who was alive at 180 days. If subsequent renal unit and other ward expenditure were to be taken into consideration, then the cost per survivor would be higher.

REFERENCES

Anderson, R.J., *et al.* (1977). Non-oliguric acute renal failure. *New England Journal of Medicine* **296**, 1134–8.

Anon (1989). Hyperkalaemia – silent and deadly (Editorial). *Lancet* **i**, 1240.

Bennett, W.M. (1983). Aminoglycoside nephrotoxicity. *Nephron* **35**, 73–7.

Bennett, W.M., Aronoff, G.R., Golper, T.A., Morrison, G., Singer, I. and Brater, D.G. (1991). *Drug prescribing in renal failure*, (2nd edn). American College of Physicians, Philadelphia.

Better, O.S. and Stein, J.H. (1990). Early management of shock and prophylaxis of acute renal failure in traumatic rhabdomyolysis. *New England Journal of Medicine* **322**, 825–9.

Bonventre, J.V. (1993). Mechanisms of ischemic acute renal failure. *Kidney International* **43**, 1160–78.

Brosius, F.C. and Lau, K. (1986). Low fractional excretion of sodium in acute renal failure: role of timing of the test and ischaemia. *American Journal of Nephrology* **6**, 450–7.

Chugh, K.S., Sakhuja, V., Malhotra, H.S., and Pereira, B.J.G. (1989). Changing trends in acute renal failure in third-world countries – Chandigarh study. *Quarterly Journal of Medicine* **73**, 1117–23.

Cohen, D.J., Sherman, W.H., Osserman, E.F., and Appel, G.B. (1984). Acute renal failure in patients with multiple myeloma. *American Journal of Medicine* **76**, 247–56.

Couser, W.G. (1988). Rapidly progressive glomerulonephritis: classification, pathogenetic mechanisms and therapy. *American Journal of Kidney Diseases* **11**, 449–64.

Firth, J.D. (1993). Renal replacement therapy on the intensive care unit. *Quarterly Journal of Medicine,* **86,** 75–7.

Graziani, G., *et al.* (1984). Dopamine and frusemide in oliguric renal failure. *Nephron* **37**, 39–42.

Grunfeld, J.-P., Ganeval, D. and Bournerias, F. (1980). Acute renal failure in pregnancy. *Kidney International* **18**, 179–91.

Hayslett, J.P. (1985). Post-partum renal failure. *New England Journal of Medicine* **312**, 1556–9.

Hou, S.H., Bushinsky, D.A., Wish, J.B., Cohen, J.J., and Harrington, J.T. (1983). Hospital-acquired renal insufficiency: a prospective study. *American Journal of Medicine* **74**, 243–8.

Isles, C.G., Mclay, A., and Boulton-Jones, J.M. (1984). Recovery in malignant hypertension presenting as renal failure. *Quarterly Journal of Medicine* **53**, 439–52.

Kleinknecht, D., Grunfeld, J.-P., Gomez, P.C., Moreau, J.-F., and Garcia-Tores, R. (1973). Diagnostic procedure and long term prognosis in bilateral renal cortical necrosis. *Kidney International* **4**, 390–400.

Levy, M. (1993). Hepatorenal syndrome. *Kidney International* **43**, 737–53.

Milligan, S.L., Luft, F.C., McMurray, S.D., and Kleit, S.A. (1978). Intra-abdominal infection in acute renal failure. *Archives of Surgery* **113**, 467–72.

Myers, B.D. and Moran, S.M. (1986). Hemodynamically mediated acute renal failure. *New England Journal of Medicine* **314**, 97–105.

Parfrey, P.S., *et al.* (1989). Radiocontrast induced renal failure in diabetes mellitus and in patients with pre-existing renal failure: a prospective controlled study. *New England Journal of Medicine* **320**, 143–9.

Pusey, C.D., Saltissi, S., Bloodworth, L., Raniford, D.J., and Christie, J.L. (1983). Drug associated acute interstitial nephritis: Clinical and pathological features, and the response to high dose steroid therapy. *Quarterly Journal of Medicine* **52**, 194–211.

Remuzzi, G. (1987). Nephrology forum: HUS and TTP: variable expression of a single entity. *Kidney International* **32**, 292–308.

Remuzzi, G. (1988). Bleeding in renal failure. *Lancet* **i**, 1205–8.

Schlondorff, D. (1993). Renal complications of nonsteroidal anti-inflammatory drugs. *Kidney International* **44**, 643–53.

Solez, K. and Racusen, L.C. (ed.) (1991). *Acute renal failure: diagnosis, treatment and prevention.* Marcel Dekker, New York.

Solez, K., Morel-Maroger, L., and Sraer, J.D. (1979). The morphology of acute tubular necrosis in man: analysis of 57 renal biopsies and a comparison with the glycerol model. *Medicine,* **58**, 362–76.

Turney, J.H., Marshall, D.H., Brownjohn, A.M., Ellis, C.M., and Parsons, F.M. (1990). The evolution of acute renal failure, 1956–1988. *Quarterly Journal of Medicine* **74**, 83–104.

Winearls, C.G., Chau, L., Coghlan, J.D., Ledingham, J.G.G., and Oliver, D.O. (1984). Acute renal failure due to leptospirosis: clinical features and outcome in six cases. *Quarterly Journal of Medicine* **53**, 487–95.

van Ypersele de Strihou, C. and Mery, J.P. (1989). Hantavirus-related acute interstitial nephritis in Western Europe. Expansion of a world-wide zoonosis. *Quarterly Journal of Medicine* **73**, 941–50.

20.17 Chronic renal failure and its treatment

20.17.1 Chronic renal failure

A. M. EL NAHAS and C. G. WINEARLS

Introduction

Chronic renal failure affects every aspect of the lives of the patients who suffer it. Treatment must be provided over a lifetime and be directed against the cause, the progression, and the many consequences of the loss of renal excretory and endocrine function. Eventually, when all renal function is lost the patient embarks on a career of various renal replacement treatments (dialysis, in its various forms, and renal transplantation) in the hope of prolonging and maintaining the quality of life (see Chapters 20.17.2 and 20.17.3).

Compared to diseases such as cancer and ischaemic heart disease, renal failure is a small public health problem, but the expense of dialysis and transplantation, and the fact that chronic renal failure is particularly common in the elderly, mean that renal failure represents a substantial burden for the health services of even the wealthiest countries.

Definition

Chronic renal failure is defined as the irreversible, substantial, and usually long-standing loss of renal function causing ill-health, usually referred to as uraemia. Endstage renal failure is the degree of chronic renal failure that without renal replacement treatment would result in death. Diminished renal reserve precedes chronic renal failure; plasma biochemistry is then normal and there are no clinical consequences of the reduction in the glomerular filtration rate below the normal range.

The severity of chronic renal failure can be classified by clinical consequences and proportion of renal function lost, as mild, moderate, severe, and endstage (Table 1). All patients with renal failure should be assessed by a nephrologist but the care of those with mild loss of function can be shared with the general practitioner or the specialist in another discipline, for example the diabetologist. Despite the relationship between plasma creatinine concentration and glomerular filtration rate (Fig. 8 of Chapter 20.1), the severity of chronic renal failure cannot be accurately estimated from the plasma creatinine concentration (see Chapter 20.1), for it can remain within the normal range despite a significant loss of renal function. Plasma creatinine levels are also affected by the patient's age, gender, muscle mass, and diet. Changes in plasma creatinine must also be interpreted with caution. At low concentrations (< 200 μmol/l), small changes (such as 50 μmol/l) reflect large differences in glomerular filtration rate, whereas at higher concentrations (>500 μmol/l), they would indicate only slight changes in excretory function. Nevertheless, an estimate of glomerular filtration rate can be made from the plasma creatinine level, the patient's age, sex, and weight, using the formula:

$$GFR = \frac{(140 - \text{age in years}) \times \text{weight (kg)}}{\text{Plasma creatinine } (\mu\text{mol/l}) \times 0.82}$$
(For females, subtract 15% of calculated value)

It must be emphasized that there is a poor correlation between symptoms and signs of chronic renal failure and this classification of severity. Progression can be so insidious that patients become used to the effects of renal failure, attributing them to age or other illnesses so only presenting when they are close to needing dialysis.

Table 1 *Severity of renal failure*

	GFR (ml/min)	Symptoms and signs
Mild	30–50	None:± hypertension; early secondary hyperparathyroidism
Moderate	10–29	Few: anaemia, hypertension, early osteodystrophy, lassitude
Severe	< 10	Fluid retention, anorexia, vomiting, pruritus, poor intellectual performance
Endstage	< 5	Pulmonary oedema, fits and coma, pericarditis, hyperkalaemia, death

GFR, glomerular filtration rate.

Prevalance and incidence

The true prevalence of chronic renal failure (of all degrees of severity) is unknown because many patients are asymptomatic or its presence has not been recognized. A prospective study in the United Kingdom, which involved ascertainment through hospital biochemistry laboratories, revealed a point prevalence of abnormal plasma creatinine concentrations (>150 μmol/l) of 2058 adults per million population. This included patients with transient acute renal impairment. There were approximately 600 patients per million population (p.m.p.) with established renal failure not requiring renal replacement treatment, and an annual incidence of endstage renal failure needing dialysis of 78 p.m.p. Precise information has long been available for the incidence of endstage renal failure for which renal replacement has been provided, from national registers. Table 2 shows the incidence in the United States, various countries in Europe, and Australia. The difference between the estimated incidences and acceptance rates reflects the selection of patients for dialysis and transplant programmes. The prevalence of treated endstage renal failure (that is, the number of patients receiving dialysis or with a functioning transplant) will vary from country to country, and will depend on the incidence of particular diseases and the availability and capacity of dialysis and transplant programmes (Table 3).

The problems of ascertainment notwithstanding, there are real differences in the incidence of endstage renal failure according to age, gender, and race. In Western countries the incidence is lowest in children (10 p.m.p./year), and highest in the elderly (> 400 p.m.p./year in the population over 75 years of age). In Caucasians, 30 to 60 years of age, the incidence ranges between 50 and 150 p.m.p./year and is slightly higher in males than females. In the United States the annual incidence of endstage renal failure in those of African or native American descent is nearly four times higher (424 p.m.p.) than in Caucasian subjects (114 p.m.p.). This difference cannot be explained solely by the higher prevalence of diabetes mellitus and hypertension within these ethnic groups. It may reflect genetic and environmental predisposition to some forms of renal disease and socioeconomic factors including diet, and access to medical care, likely to influence the prevalence of some diseases and their rate of progression. Although the difference is less striking, the incidence of endstage renal failure in the United Kingdom is higher in Asian immigrants and their descendants than in the native British population. These factors may also explain the higher incidence of chronic renal failure in the developing countries (see below).

Causes

There are many causes of chronic renal failure, for most renal diseases can eventually lead to a significant reduction in function. Table 4 lists the major causes of endstage renal failure given in the European, American, and Australian registers. A list of rarer causes is given in Table 5.

Table 2 *Acceptance rates on to renal replacement programmes 1991: international comparisons*[a]

County	Patients (p.m.p./year)
USA (1990)[b]	169
Austria	110
France	77
Germany (West)	94
Sweden	99
United Kingdom	65
Australia[c]	61

[a]Geerlings, W. *et al.* (1994). Report on Management of renal failure in Europe XXIII. *Nephrology, Dialysis and Transplantation*, **Suppl. 1,** 6–25.

[b]United States Renal Data System 1993. (1993). Annual Data Report. Executive Summary. *American Journal of Kidney Diseases*, **22,** (Suppl. 2), 9–16.

[c]ANZDATA Report (1993). *Australia and New Zealand Dialysis and Transplant Registry*. (ed. A.P.S. Disney.) Adelaide, South Australia.

Table 3 *Prevalence of patients on renal replacement treatment: international comparisons*

Country	Patients (p.m.p.)
USA (1990)[a]	659
Japan (1990)[a]	836
Austria (1992)[b]	440
France (1992)[b]	409
Germany (West) (1992)[b]	387
Sweden (1992)[b]	509
United Kingdom (1992)[b]	382
Australia (1992)[c]	403

[a]United States Renal Data System 1993. (1993). Annual Data Report. X International Comparison of ESRD therapy. *American Journal of Kidney Diseases*, **22,** 85–8.

[b]Geerlings, W. *et al.* (1994). Report on management of renal failure in Europe XXIII. *Nephrology, Dialysis, Transplantation*, Suppl 1, 6–25.

[c]ANZDATA Report (1993). *Australia and New Zealand Dialysis and Transplant Registry* (ed. A.P.S. Disney). Adelaide, South Australia.

Conventional lists of causes of chronic renal failure were once compiled from the diagnoses of the selected cohorts of patients accepted on to renal replacement programmes. Such patients were young and did not suffer systemic diseases and so the lists were headed by glomerulonephritis. Now that dialysis programmes in most Western countries exclude very few patients, the spectrum of pathologies reflects the true pattern more accurately. One of the most important changes over the past decade is the increase in the referral of patients with diabetic nephropathy for renal replacement therapy (see Chapter 20.5.1). This diagnosis now accounts for approximately 30 per cent of patients on dialysis programmes in the United States. There is one caveat: hypertension is frequently given as the cause of renal failure when no specific pathological entity has been identified. Although some patients do indeed have pure primary hypertensive damage to the kidney, many others probably have an undiagnosed glomerulonephritis (see Chapter 20.11). Many patients present very late in their illness with small, shrunken kidneys from which no informative renal tissue can be obtained by biopsy and so they are classified as 'aetiology unknown'.

The influence of age on causes of chronic renal failure is illustrated by the higher prevalence of obstructive uropathy and reno-vascular dis-

Table 4 *Comparison of aetiology of endstage renal failure: estimates from the European and national registries*

	Percentage of cases		
	Europe[a] (1985–1987)	USA[b] (1987–1990)	Australia[c] (1992)
Glomerulonephritis	25	14	38
Diabetes	12	34	14
Cystic disease	8	3	8
Hypertension[d]	10	29	9
Analgesic nephropathy	2	1	9
Pyelonephritis/ interstitial nephritis	17	3	5
Unknown	15	7	5
Misc[e]	11	9	12

[a]EDTA Registry 1985–1987, from A.J. Wing (1992).

[b]United States Renal Data System (1993). Annual Data Report. III Incidence and causes of reported ESRD. *American Journal of Kidney Diseases*, **22**, (Suppl. 2), 30–7.

[c]ANZDATA Report (1992). *Australia and New Zealand Dialysis and Transplant Registry* (ed. A.P.S. Disney) Adelaide, South Australia.

[d] See text.

[e]Including: renal vascular disease, nephrolithiasis, and causes in Table 5.

Table 5 *Some rare causes of chronic renal failure (< 1% of cases)*

Medullary cystic disease
Hereditary nephritis with deafness (Alport's syndrome)
Cystinosis
Oxalosis
Systemic vasculitis (Wegener's granulomatosis and polyarteritis)
Systemic lupus erythematosus
Myeloma
Amyloid
Scleroderma
Haemolytic-uraemic syndrome
Kidney tumour
Nephrocalcinosis
Gouty nephropathy
Fabry's disease
Sickle-cell disease
Tuberculosis

ease (ischaemic renal disease) in the elderly. Obstruction of the lower urinary tract is common in elderly men, as up to 40 per cent of men over the age of 50 have symptoms of bladder outflow obstruction, although only a small proportion of these go on to develop hydronephrosis and serious loss of renal function. Amyloidosis and myeloma are also more common in the elderly.

There is a higher prevalence of reflux and analgesic nephropathies in women, and another effect of gender is that there is evidence of a faster rate of deterioration in male patients with polycystic disease and some forms of glomerulonephritis, which may explain the higher number of male patients treated by replacement therapy.

Apparent geographical variations in the causes of chronic renal disease within Europe have also been reported. More than 80 per cent of patients with endstage renal failure in Finland are thought to have chronic glomerulonephritis; the equivalent figure in the United Kingdom is less than 50 per cent, and in Greece only 5 per cent. It is unclear whether these reported differences are genuine or are accounted for by diagnostic approach or referral pattern. Diabetic nephropathy appears to

be commoner in Scandinavia and analgesic nephropathy more prevalent in Belgium, Switzerland, and Australia. Amyloidosis is very common in the Mediterranean basin and in Turkey, where it is the cause of 30 per cent of endstage renal failure. Balkan nephropathy is confined to the former Yugoslavia and Bulgaria. Overall, the incidence of glomerulonephritis appears higher in China, India, South-East Asia, Africa, and South America, when compared to Europe or the United States. This may reflect socioeconomic differences and the higher prevalence of glomerulonephritis caused or exacerbated by infections. In some parts of the Middle-East, schistosomiasis and its associated nephropathy are endemic.

In the United States, significant racial differences have been reported in the causes of chronic kidney disease. This may, in part, reflect underlying racial differences in the prevalence of diabetes mellitus and hypertension. Diabetes mellitus (particularly type II), is 1.35-fold more prevalent in Afro-Americans than Caucasians, and a higher prevalence amongst native and Hispanic-Americans is also well established. Likewise, there is a higher prevalence and incidence of renal failure due to hypertension in Afro- and Hispanic-Americans compared to Caucasians.

Pathophysiology of chronic renal failure

In chronic renal failure, compensatory and adaptive mechanisms maintain acceptable health until the glomerular filtration rate is about 10 to 15 ml/min, and life-sustaining renal excretory and homeostatic functions continue until the glomerular filtration rate is less than 5 ml/min. The popular explanation for continuing function in remaining nephrons is the 'intact nephron hypothesis': that is, most nephrons are non-functioning, while the remaining few function normally. These functioning nephrons produce an increased volume of filtrate and their tubules respond appropriately by excreting fluid and solutes in amounts which maintain external balance. For sodium and potassium, some balance exists at a glomerular filtration rate of 5 ml/min and plasma values are commonly normal. For phosphate and urate, adaptation is less precise and plasma concentrations are increased in many patients at a glomerular filtration rate of 20 ml/min and in almost all at 5 to 10 ml/min.

The 'trade off' hypothesis is to be considered together with the intact nephron hypothesis, that is the concept that adaptations arising in chronic renal failure may control one abnormality, but only in such a way as to produce other changes characteristic of the uraemic syndrome. Although the mechanisms involved are largely unknown, examples are the role of parathormone in phosphorus balance, of vasopressin in free water clearance, and of atrial natriuretic peptide in the control of sodium excretion. The best example of 'trade off' is increase of parathormone secretion essential for increased fractional excretion of phosphate; as the glomerular filtration rate falls, plasma phosphate rises, parathormone secretion increases, and plasma phosphate is lowered by decreased tubular reabsorption. The cost of normal plasma phosphate is then secondary hyperparathyroidism, and metastatic calcification (see Chapter 20.18). Other abnormalities have also been attributed to excess parathormone, including central and peripheral nervous disease, impotence, myopathy, carbohydrate intolerance, and lipid disorders. It is also suggested that there are 'trade offs' associated with the homeostasis of sodium, potassium, and other solutes.

Water

Inability to concentrate urine in the presence of dehydration is often the first symptom of chronic renal failure, resulting in polyuria, nocturia, and thirst when the glomerular filtration rate is about 30 ml/min or less. Diluting capacity is preserved until renal failure is advanced, the asymmetrical narrowing of the range of urinary osmolality eventually producing the fixed osmolality of chronic renal failure with its obligatory polyuria (Fig. 1). Diseases that affect predominantly the medulla, such as pyelonephritis, interstitial nephritis, and medullary cystic disease, may present with a concentration defect at an earlier stage of chronic renal failure. Defective urine concentration is due to increased solute load in surviving nephrons, with minor contributions from decreased tubular function and increased glomerular filtration rate per nephron. As a result, urine osmolality is fixed at 300 mosmol/kg. Thirst accompanies polyuria, and water balance is thereby maintained provided there is free access to fluid. As obligatory water loss is increased, there is need for careful attention to fluid balance in the presence of anorexia, fever, surgery, and other sources of extrarenal loss if dehydration, hypotension, and further impairment of renal function are to be avoided. Urinary dilution is maintained until late in chronic renal failure but large water loads are excreted more slowly than in normal subjects and excessive fluid results in hyponatraemia, mental disturbances, and convulsions (Chapter 20.2.1).

Sodium

As renal function decreases, hormonal mechanisms increase the fraction of filtered sodium excreted so that sodium balance and extracellular fluid volume are maintained until the glomerular filtration rate is less than 10 ml/min. The extent of this adaptation is such that the 1 per cent or less of filtered sodium excreted by normal subjects increases to 30 per cent in late chronic renal failure. Adaptive mechanisms are not unlimited; in late renal failure increased total body sodium, with water to maintain osmotic equilibrium, presents as fluid overload and hypertension. Initially excess extracellular fluid does not cause oedema, but maintains normal body contours and may mask tissue wasting. In late renal failure, there is often leg oedema, elevated jugular venous pressure, pulmonary congestion, and functional incompetence of mitral and aortic valves. The major consequence of sodium and fluid excess is hypertension, present in 80 per cent of patients in late chronic renal failure and often presenting in the accelerated phase. Precisely how sodium retention and increased extracellular fluid volume lead to hypertension is still quite uncertain, despite much research (see Chapter 20.11). In the presence of dietary sodium restriction or of loss of sodium by various routes, functioning nephrons cannot restrict sodium excretion promptly so that extracellular fluid, plasma volume, and glomerular filtration rate all decrease. Although this sodium and fluid loss has been attributed to an osmotic diuresis, other mechanisms are involved and may dominate; thus, if sodium restriction is induced slowly over months, patients can reduce urinary sodium to less than 10 mmol/l without a significant reduction in glomerular filtration rate. A small number of patients with early chronic renal failure, usually with disease affecting the renal medulla, present with a urinary sodium leak and sodium depletion on a normal sodium diet. In these patients blood pressure is normal or low, often with a postural drop of arterial pressure, and sodium supplements may be needed.

Fig. 1 Progressive loss of flexibility in water handling as renal failure worsens. Concentrating ability is impaired earlier than the ability to excrete a dilute urine.

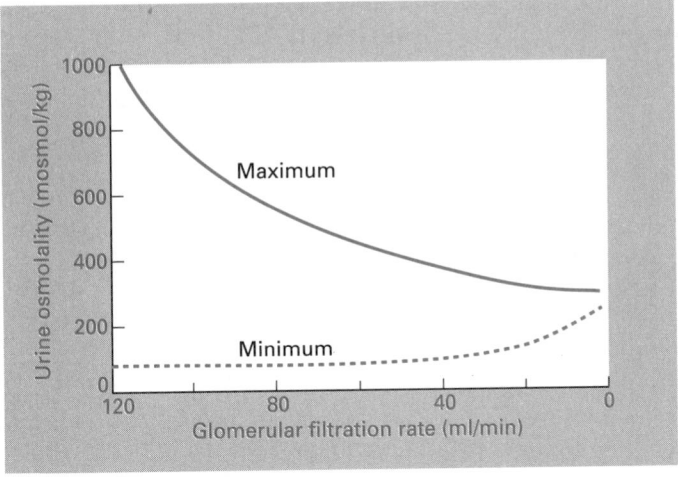

Potassium (see Chapter 20.2.3)

Most patients maintain normal external potassium balance until the glomerular filtration rate is less than 5 ml/min, but their capacity to excrete potassium is limited and severe hyperkalaemia may follow a sudden reduction in residual glomerular filtration rate, excess dietary potassium (chocolate, nuts, instant coffee, some fruits and their juices, wine), potassium-sparing diuretics (spironolactone, amiloride, triamterene), medication with high potassium content, surgery, and hypercatabolic states. Acidosis raises serum potassium by ion transfer out of cells and interference with renal excretion. Hypoxia causes hyperkalaemia by impaired uptake of potassium from extracellular fluid. In some patients, particularly those with diabetes mellitus and/or interstitial nephritis, and sometimes in early chronic renal failure, hyperkalaemia may be due to selective aldosterone deficiency (hyporeninaemic hypoaldosteronism) or the use of angiotensin-converting enzyme inhibitors, which responds at least partially to 9α-fluorohydrocortisone treatment. Tubular resistance to aldosterone is another rare cause of hyperkalaemia. Complications occur at plasma potassium concentrations greater than 7.0 mmol/l; weakness in pelvic and shoulder girdle muscles may be the presenting symptom, but in most patients serious electrocardiographic abnormalities and fatal cardiac arrhythmias are the first signs of hyperkalaemia (Chapter 20.2.3).

Acid–base

The kidney is the principal organ to maintain acid–base balance, by reabsorption of filtered bicarbonate, acidification of urinary buffers, and excretion of ammonia. As renal failure progresses, intact nephrons increase fractional reabsorption of filtered bicarbonate and excretion of hydrogen ion, which, with intracellular buffers and respiration, prevent acidosis, until the glomerular filtration rate is less than 20 ml/min. Increasing acidosis, variable between patients, occurs at a glomerular filtration rate of less than 10 ml/min: normal net acid production exceeds the excretory capacity of remaining nephrons and diminished tubule function impairs ammonia synthesis and bicarbonate regeneration. Renal diseases which principally affect tubules and interstitial tissues are associated with acidosis quite early in chronic renal failure. Acidosis seldom requires treatment unless bicarbonate is less than 15 mmol/l and pH less than 7.30, except in children in whom prevention of severe acidosis with bicarbonate supplements may have a beneficial effect on renal osteodystrophy and growth retardation. Delayed excretion of excess base is also a feature of late chronic renal failure, so that metabolic alkalosis may occur more easily and resolve more slowly after prolonged gastric aspiration, for instance.

Calcium and phosphate

The role of the kidney in regulating calcium and phosphate in body fluids and tissues is described in Chapter 20.18. Magnesium concentrations are usually high and care must be exercised with the use of magnesium-containing drugs.

Clinical presentation and assessment

The symptoms of uraemia develop insidiously and late, so it is unusual for the diagnosis to be reached because complaints have led to a specific request for a measurement of plasma urea or creatinine. Abnormalities are usually found in the course of assessment of patients with conditions known to lead to chronic renal failure, such as diabetes and adult polycystic kidney disease, glomerulonephritis, or with associated abnormalities such as hypertension, proteinuria, haematuria, or glycosuria. These are often picked up during pregnancy or at routine insurance or employment medical examinations. It is in this group that a specific diagnosis can be made, measures to preserve renal function put in hand, and complications prevented. The identification of such patients is one benefit of the wide availability of biochemical screens in hospital and general practice.

Eventually uraemic symptoms and signs do develop (Fig. 2) and these are used as part of the assessment to decide when dialysis should be started. The most common and dominant symptoms are fatigue, dyspnoea, ankle swelling, anorexia, vomiting, pruritus, and inability to concentrate. Regrettably a significant number of patients are referred to renal units when they have already reached endstage. They sometimes present as 'uraemic emergencies' requiring immediate dialysis or its institution within a month. Such patients may be comatose, may have fitted, and have asterixis. The skin shows excoriation from pruritus, purpura, and bruising on a sallow yellow-brown background. The blood pressure is raised and the fundi may show haemorrhages and exudates. The left ventricular impulse is displaced and there is often a pericardial friction rub. There are basal crepitations and oedema of the face, sacrum, and ankles. Blood investigations show a urea of greater than 50 mmol/l, a creatinine of greater than 1000 μmol/l, hypocalcaemia, hyperphosphataemia, hyperkalaemia, and a partially compensated metabolic acidosis. There is a normochromic normocytic anaemia, a normal white blood count, and a platelet count in the low normal range. History taking is difficult but the family report a general deterioration in health over the past 6 months, with dyspnoea, anorexia, pruritus, and nocturia. Such a patient is easy to diagnose, indeed the ammoniacal smell of the breath usually alerts the family practitioner. This medical emergency is now less frequently encountered than before, but the gradual deterioration in

Table 6 *Indications of chronicity of renal failure*

History	> 6 months ill-health, long-standing hypertension, proteinuria, nocturia for > 6 months; sexual dysfunction; abnormalities detected during routine medicals; pregnancies; recurrent illness during childhood
Examination	Pallor, pigmentation and pruritus, brown nails, evidence of long-standing hypertension. The patient often appears 'well' for their very abnormal biochemistry.
Investigations	Normochromic anaemia
Small kidneys on ultrasound (except: diabetes, amyloid, myeloma, adult polycystic kidney disease)
Renal osteodystrophy on radiography (this is rarely found but conclusive evidence if present)

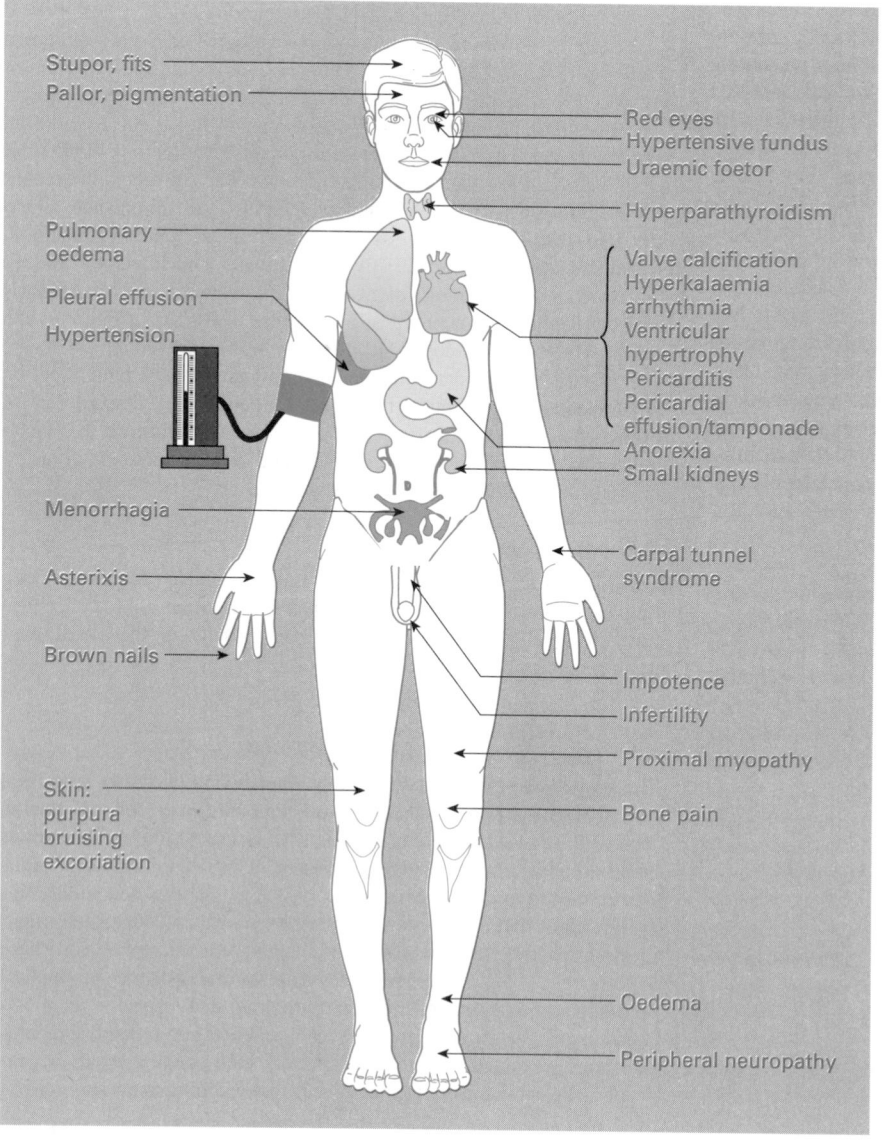

Fig. 2 Symptoms and signs of uraemia.

Table 7 *Causes of acute on chronic renal failure*

Renal hypoperfusion	Dehydration from diarrhoea, diuretics, surgery Cardiac failure Pericardial tamponade (rare) Renal vascular disease Drugs especially ACE inhibitors + NSAIDs Systemic infection
Obstruction and infection of the urinary tract	Papillary necrosis and sloughing Stones Bladder cancer Polycystic cysts Clot in the ureter
Metabolic and toxic	Hypercalcaemia Hyperuricaemia Contrast media (especially in diabetes) Drugs, especially aminoglycosides
Progression of underlying diseases	Relapse of nephritis
Development of accelerated phase hypertension	
Renal vein thrombosis	Usually in chronically nephrotic patients
Pregnancy	At the end or after delivery, e.g. in patients with reflux nephropathy

ACE, angiotensin-converting enzyme; NSAIDs, non-steroidal anti-inflammatory drugs.

the patient is such that it may take some final event like a fit to provoke referral. The morbidity in such patients is high and it is obvious that opportunities for halting the underlying pathology or slowing progression will have been lost. Most patients present with a much milder combination and are often irritated that their non-specific symptoms had not earlier been attributed to chronic renal failure. They need to be told that renal failure is rare and that, in the absence of obvious clues, no doctor should be criticized for missing the diagnosis in the early stages.

The approach to every new case of chronic renal failure should be systematic and resolve the following issues:

1. Is there any life-threatening complication of chronic renal failure that requires urgent treatment? These include pulmonary oedema, hyperkalaemia, metabolic acidosis, uraemic encephalopathy, or accelerated-phase hypertension. Urgent dialysis, peritoneal or haemo-, is required and where possible should be in a specialist unit (see management).
2. Does the patient really have chronic renal failure? Clues to aid in distinguishing acute from chronic renal failure are listed in Table 6.
3. Are there factors operating which have caused or are causing acute reduction in chronically impaired renal function? If so, can they be reversed? (Table 7). Examples include:
   (i) Hypoperfusion. Dehydration caused by diarrhoea, vomiting, iatrogenic deprivation of fluid, for example following surgery, or overzealous use of diuretics. An occult cause is the condition of renal loss of salt and water. Significant dehydration is associated with a reduction in weight and postural hypotension. Worsening renal arterial stenosis and cholesterol emboli are found in arteriopaths.
   (ii) Drugs. Many drugs, particularly non-steroidal anti-inflammatory drugs (NSAIDs), aminoglycosides, and antihypertensive agents, can cause a reduction in glomerular filtration rate and acute interstitial nephritis. Tetracyclines cause nausea and vomiting. Clofibrate causes rhabdomyolysis and myoglobinuria. Contrast media in the dehydrated patient are another cause.

(iii) Infection. Systemic infection such as pneumonia can reduce the glomerular filtration rate, and renal parenchymal infections in patients with diabetes, analgesic nephropathy, and adult polycystic kidney disease can damage the remaining functioning renal tissue.
(iv) Obstruction. The effect of obstructing one kidney in patients with chronic renal failure by calculi or papillary necrosis, for instance, will lead to a marked change in the severity of their renal failure. Sloughed papillae should be sought in those with analgesic nephropathy, diabetes, obstruction, and sickle-cell disease. Retroperitoneal fibrosis may be occult and is not always detected by ultrasound examination (see Chapter 20.10).
(v) Relapse of the underlying disease. Patients with diseases such as systemic lupus erythematosus, IgA nephropathy, or systemic vasculitic syndromes will deteriorate when the underlying disease relapses, causing further damage to glomeruli. Diagnosis can be difficult because the kidneys are too small to biopsy. Serology and examination of the urine deposit can be helpful. Occasionally membranous nephropathy and membranoproliferative glomerulonephritis can change in character with the development of extracapillary proliferation (crescent formation) and this is associated with a rapid decline in function. Renal vein thrombosis causes a deterioration in function and should be considered in those with chronic nephrotic syndrome, particularly with underlying membranous nephropathy or focal segmental glomerulosclerosis.
(vi) Hypertension. The development of accelerated-phase hypertension may cause a sharp and irreversible reduction in residual function.
(vii) Congestive heart failure itself, independent of salt and water retention of uraemia can lead to a reduction in glomerular filtration rate. This can be a result of hypertension, myocardial infarction, or arrhythmias.
(viii) Hypercalcaemia. The use of vitamin D analogues, such as alfacalcidol, to prevent hyperparathyroidism often

Table 8 *Causes of chronic renal failure in which specific treatment can halt progression*

Disease	Diagnostic method	Treatment
Obstruction	Ultrasound, CT scan	Surgical relief, retrograde or antegrade J-stenting
Analgesic nephropathy	History, urine testing for salicylates	Exhortation to stop consumption
Rapidly progressive nephritis	Renal biopsy, ANCA, urinalysis	Prednisolone, azathioprine, or cyclophosphamide
Membranous nephropathy	Renal biopsy	Prednisolone and alkylating agents
Systemic lupus erythematosus	Renal biopsy, anti-DNA antibodies	Prednisolone, azathioprine, or cyclophosphamide
Accelerated phase hypertension	Fundoscopy, renal biopsy	Drugs
Tuberculosis	Intravenous urogram, culture of early morning urine	Antituberculous drugs
Myeloma	Serum/urine protein electrophoresis, renal biopsy	Chemotherapy
Secondary amyloid	Rectal or renal biopsy	Eliminate source of sepsis or treat inflammation
Familial hyperuricaemia	History, urine, urate	Allopurinol
Ischaemic renal disease	Angiography	Angioplasty or surgical bypass

leads to hypercalcaemia. When marked (plasma $Ca^{2+}>3$ mmol/l), this causes a reduction in glomerular filtration rate, usually by causing dehydration (Chapter 20.9.3).

(ix) Pregnancy. Early in pregnancy the plasma creatinine concentration tends to fall but the course of diseases such as reflux nephropathy or glomerulonephritis may accelerate.

4. What is the cause of renal failure? A specific diagnosis is needed for several reasons:

(i) To consider specific measures to arrest the pathology. Opportunities to do so are infrequent but should not be missed. Examples include: obstructive uropathy, analgesic nephropathy, drug-related interstitial nephritis, rapidly progressive glomerulonephritis, systemic lupus erythematosus, vasculitic syndromes, accelerated phase hypertension, tuberculosis, myeloma, amyloid secondary to chronic infection or inflammation, ischaemic renal disease, and familial hyperuricaemic nephropathy (see Table 8).

(ii) To make the physician aware of potential complications and coincident disease, for example diabetes mellitus.

(iii) To advise the family in conditions such as polycystic kidney disease or other causes of familial renal disease.

(iv) To take into account when considering renal transplantation, for example focal glomerulosclerosis, antiglomerular basement membrane disease, mesangiocapillary glomerulonephritis (especially 'dense deposit disease').

5. What measures are needed to delay progression? See below.

6. Are there complications of chronic renal failure that require specific treatment?

The important examples are hypertension, renal osteodystrophy, and anaemia.

These issues are only resolved by application of routine clinical methods—a careful history and review of records, a comprehensive and focused physical examination, urinalysis including microscopy and investigations, both standard and specific.

HISTORY

A careful medical history may pin-point the onset of the first uraemic symptoms. Nocturia is a particularly useful and reliable indicator of chronicity. In women, an obstetric history may reveal pregnancy-related hypertension, oedema, or proteinuria, suggesting the presence of renal disease during or preceding the pregnancy. A history of urinary tract infections, enuresis, and failure to thrive will point to reflux nephropathy; a heavy intake of pain killers to analgesic nephropathy. Symptoms and signs of systemic diseases known to affect the kidney, such as diabetes mellitus, hypertension, and systemic vasculitis, should be sought. A careful family history of renal disease may raise the possibility of conditions such as adult polycystic kidney disease or Alport's syndrome. Careful enquiry about any drugs consumed regularly or irregularly is essential; some patients will not consider preparations which they can purchase without prescription a 'drug'. An occupational history may reveal exposure to lead, analgesics, or hydrocarbons. A full social history is needed to help in the choice of the most appropriate replacement therapy that may be needed in the future.

PHYSICAL SIGNS

Physical examination should focus on signs (Fig. 2) that point to a specific cause of renal failure, its degree of chronicity, and its likely complications. Signs of chronicity include pallor, yellow-brown skin discoloration, and nail dystrophy. Other manifestations of chronic uraemia include hypertension, cardiomegaly, congestive cardiac failure, and pericarditis. Retinal examination may reveal acute or chronic hypertensive changes, diabetic lesions, and, rarely, evidence of cholesterol emboli or retinitis pigmentosa. Associated physical signs may reveal evidence of diabetes mellitus, or systemic vasculitis. It is particularly important to try to detect any potentially reversible cause of renal insufficiency such as dehydration, overhydration, heart failure, and urinary tract obstruction, the latter perhaps resulting in bladder distension. In the elderly uraemic and hypertensive patient, the presence of bruits, particularly in the abdomen, suggest the possibility of underlying renal artery stenosis, the relief of which by angioplasty or vascular surgery may, in rare cases, restore sufficient renal function to delay or avoid dialysis.

INVESTIGATIONS

Laboratory

The chronicity of renal insufficiency can ultimately only be confirmed by laboratory and radiological investigations. A full blood count is likely to reveal a normocytic normochromic anaemia but this can occur quite quickly in acute renal failure. Severe hypocalcaemia and hyperphosphataemia are suggestive of chronicity, although they too can also be observed in acute renal failure, particularly after rhabdomyolysis. High levels of bone alkaline phosphatase reflecting osteodystrophy implies chronicity but this is a rare finding. Measurement of carbamylated haemoglobin may in the future be a helpful test. Urinalysis is of some value in establishing the chronicity of renal diseases, when large casts may reflect tubular dilatation, and white cell casts pyelonephritis or analgesic nephropathy. Sterile pyuria is a clue to analgesic nephropathy and renal tuberculosis. Urine osmolality when renal failure is chronic, closely approximates that of plasma (isosthenuria). Crenated red cells in profusion and red cells casts suggest acute glomerulonephritis, and eosinophiluria an acute drug-induced interstitial nephritis. In advanced uraemia, when the glomerular filtration rate is less than 15 ml/min and plasma creatinine in excess of 600 μmol/l, proteinuria seldom exceeds 1 g/24 h. Heavy proteinuria, despite such severe chronic renal failure, suggests the diagnosis of diabetic nephropathy or renal amyloidosis. It is usual to screen for immunological disease but the tests (for antinuclear antibody, ANCA, antiglomerular basement membrane antibodies, and complement) are rarely helpful in the absence of clinical clues. It is always worth looking for myeloma and other causes of hypercalcaemia. Hepatitis B surface antigen is sought to alert laboratories and those who will be exposed to the patient's blood during diagnostic manoeuvres and treatment.

Radiological

Radiological imaging of the kidneys and lower urinary tract, preferably by ultrasonography, is required to exclude obstruction and to determine kidney size. Chronicity is often, but not always, associated with shrunken kidneys; exceptions in which kidney size may be preserved in spite of advanced uraemia include diabetic nephropathy, polycystic disease, amyloidosis, myeloma, and systemic sclerosis. Dilatation of the calyces does not prove the presence of obstruction but indicates the need for it to be excluded either by a technetium-99-diethyltriaminepenta-acetic acid (DTPA) renogram with a diuretic challenge or retrograde pyelography (Chapter 20.10). Renal osteodystrophy may be revealed by radiography of the hands and clavicles (hyperparathyroidism), pelvis (osteomalacia), and spine (osteosclerosis). These changes will be found in fewer than 10 per cent of new cases of chronic renal failure. A chest radiograph is useful to measure cardiac diameter, and may, on occasion, raise the possibility of previously unsuspected pericardial effusion or pulmonary oedema. The presence of scars suggestive of tuberculosis should alert the clinician to possible reactivation.

Histological

Renal biopsy should not be undertaken in patients with small kidneys as its yield at this late stage is minimal and the procedure carries a high risk of complications. By contrast, in patients with normal-sized kidneys, a renal biopsy may be justified to rule out acute causes. Prognosis is difficult to equate with glomerular changes in chronic disease, but the presence of severe tubulointerstitial infiltrate or fibrosis usually indicates a poor outlook.

MEASUREMENT OF RENAL FUNCTION (CHAPTER 20.1.)

Serum creatinine and creatinine clearance measurements, together with a plot of the reciprocal of serum creatinine (1/Cr) against time, are used to determine the degree of renal failure and its rate of progression, respectively (Fig. 3).

More accurate assessments of glomerular filtration rely on the measurement of the clearance of substances eliminated exclusively by glomerular filtration. These include inulin, iodinated (^{125}I)-iothalamate, DTPA, or chromium-51-ethylenediaminetetra-acetic acid (EDTA), but these are rarely justified in routine clinical practice.

ELECTROCARDIOGRAM AND ECHOCARDIOGRAM

The electrocardiogram may reveal the presence of left ventricular hypertrophy and previous ischaemic events, and is a sensitive index of the cardiac effects of hyperkalaemia. More accurate assessment of left ventricular function and hypertrophy requires echocardiography.

Organ and metabolic dysfunction in chronic renal failure

The 'uraemic' syndrome is a consequence of a combination of the effects of the retention of toxic waste products on all organ systems (see Fig. 2) and the failure of both the endocrine and homeostatic functions of the kidney.

The potentially toxic substances that accumulate include purine metabolites, amines, indoles, phenols, myoinositol, and acid polyols. Retained 'middle molecules' of molecular weight 500 to 5000 Da are also suspected of contributing to uraemic toxicity. Recently β_2-microglobulin, a component of the HLA molecule, has been shown to cause a form of amyloid that occurs only in patients with chronic renal failure (Chapter 11.13.1).

The cardiovascular system

The single most important complication of chronic renal failure is raised arterial blood pressure, which contributes to accelerated atherosclerosis and left ventricular hypertrophy. Arterial pressure rises as renal function deteriorates and itself causes a further decline in renal function, maintaining a vicious cycle leading to hypertensive tissue damage and end-stage renal failure. There are many contributory causes to the rise in arterial blood pressure, but the major one, however mediated, is the retention of sodium and water. Overactivity of the systemic and local vascular renin angiotensin systems probably also contribute in most cases, and in some to a substantial degree.

Cardiac dysfunction in chronic renal failure may simply arise because of the combined effects of chronic hypertension with associated left ventricular hypertrophy together with chronic anaemia and coronary artery disease. Whether or not other factors, particularly disordered calcium metabolism and hyperparathyroidism, contribute to a specific 'uraemic cardiomyopathy' is debated. Certainly there is evidence of myocardial fibrosis and valvular calcification in uraemic patients. Whatever the cause(s), uraemic hypertensive patients are at much increased risk of heart failure, myocardial infarction, stroke, arrhythmia, and sudden death.

Uraemic pericarditis is a feature of advanced uraemia. The associated pericardial effusion can be either sero-fibrinous or haemorrhagic and can lead to cardiac tamponade.

It has been argued that accelerated atherosclerosis is a feature of chronic renal failure, probably due to the combined effects of chronic hypertension, hyperlipidaemia, and vascular calcification. Whether further exacerbation of atheromatous vascular lesions takes place in patients maintained on chronic dialysis is debatable.

Fig. 3 Plot of reciprocal plasma creatinine (μmol/l) against time, for a patient with adult polycystic disease: (a) work promotion, (b) arteriovenous fistula, (c) haemodialysis.

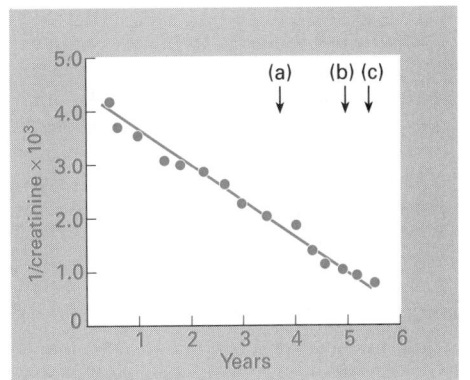

The skeleton

The important complications of chronic renal failure relating to calcium metabolism and related bone disease are described in Chapter 20.18.

Gastrointestinal system

Gastrointestinal symptoms such as anorexia, nausea, vomiting, and sometimes diarrhoea are symptoms usually observed in severe uraemia. Peptic ulcer disease as well as atrophic gastritis are known complications. Similarly, angiodysplasia of the gastrointestinal tract, in particular the colon, is relatively common and can cause severe and protracted bleeding. Gastrointestinal bleeding in renal failure is exacerbated by the underlying bleeding diathesis when uraemia is advanced.

The nervous system

The function of the central and peripheral nervous systems may be disturbed in chronic renal failure. Encephalopathy is a feature of severe uraemia and is characterized by a decline in higher mental functions, causing confusion, loss of memory, apathy, and irritability. These are often followed by motor disturbances causing myoclonic jerks, flapping tremor (asterixis), and seizures. Uraemic peripheral neuropathy is mixed motor and sensory in nature. Its presence is an indication to start dialysis. It causes paraesthesiae, including restless or burning feet. Autonomic nervous system dysfunction has also been described in uraemic patients.

Uraemic patients accumulate the metabolites of opioid drugs and their effects are easily mistaken for encephalopathy. Reversal with opioid antagonists reveals the diagnosis. The burden of illness frequently leads to severe depression which can be mistaken for dementia.

The skin

The cutaneous manifestations of chronic renal failure include pruritus, dry flaky skin, as well as darkening and yellow pigmentation of the skin, made more obvious by the pallor of anaemia. Bullous lesions in sun-exposed areas (pseudoporphyria cutanea) are occasionally seen in patients on dialysis. Proximal skin necrosis (thighs and trunk) is a consequence of ischaemia resulting from calcification and occlusion of arterioles. Trophic nail changes are frequent, including brown nail arcs ('half-and-half nails').

Endocrine system

Apart from the endocrine failure and derangement of the kidney itself (erythropoietin deficiency, failure to produce 1,25-dihydroxycholecalciferol, excess renin production), other disturbances are also commonplace in severe chronic renal failure. These result from the dysfunction of the hypothalamopituitary axis as well as the retention of many polypeptide hormones. End-organ resistance to the action of some hormones is observed in uraemia, explaining, in part, glucose intolerance (insulin resistance), anaemia (erythropoietin resistance), and stunting of growth in children (growth hormone resistance).

Sexual dysfunction in uraemia is a feature of the more generalized endocrine disturbance mentioned above. In males, low testosterone levels are associated with loss of libido and impotence, but vascular insufficiency, drugs, and neurogenic and psychological factors also contribute. Gynaecomastia is rare nowadays and its cause was never explained. In females, there is reduced libido, irregular menstruation, or amenorrhoea. Patients with severe renal failure are usually infertile and it is rare for those on dialysis to have successful pregnancies.

Haematological effects

A normochromic normocytic anaemia is an almost constant feature of uraemia. It is caused by a failure of the kidneys to produce sufficient erythropoietin to stimulate the erythroid marrow to a level of red cell production to compensate for the shorter than normal red cell survival associated with uraemia. The uraemic bone marrow is responsive to erythropoietin, but it remains a matter of debate whether this response is normal or blunted. Serum erythropoietin concentrations are usually above the normal range for non-anaemic subjects and yet ferrokinetic measurements suggest that the rate of erythropoiesis is subnormal. Nevertheless, exogenous erythropoietin in supraphysiological doses can reverse the anaemia completely. Other factors aggravate this anaemia—blood loss from the gastrointestinal tract or menstrual loss, which may be excessive, a consequence of the bleeding diathesis of uraemia. This blood loss eventually results in iron deficiency. Marrow fibrosis and hyperparathyroidism are thought to affect marrow function but these probably operate only in patients with severe renal failure and those on dialysis. Aluminium overload is similarly a problem of dialysis patients and not those with lesser degrees of renal failure.

The anaemia is relatively well tolerated until the haemoglobin falls below 10 g/dl. This tolerance may be explained by the shift in the haemoglobin-oxygen dissociation curve resulting from the increased red cell content of 2,3-diphosphoglycerate.

Platelet counts are usually normal in uraemia but function is not. Bleeding times, the comprehensive test of platelet endothelial cell interaction, are prolonged. Uraemic plasma affects platelet function adversely and their adherence to endothelium is then poor. Anaemia appears to contribute to this defect, for raising the haematocrit by transfusion shortens the bleeding time.

Polymorph function is depressed by mechanisms which remain unexplained and this may account for the poor response to bacterial infections. T-cell immunity is significantly impaired, which explains the higher risk of reactivation of tuberculosis and herpes zoster, the failure to respond to hepatitis B vaccine and to clear hepatitis B infection.

Metabolic effects

LIPIDS

Two-thirds of uraemic individuals have hypertriglyceridaemia and several lipoprotein abnormalities—increased very low-density lipoprotein (VLDL) with cholesterol enrichment; prevalence of VLDL subclass late pre-β lipoprotein; an increase in particle size and triglyceride content of low-density lipoprotein (LDL), and reduced concentration of high-density lipoprotein (HDL) cholesterol. Depressed lipoprotein lipase activity is also found in uraemia and suggests impaired peripheral metabolism as a likely cause for dyslipoproteinaemia. If an association between accelerated atherosclerosis and hyperlipidaemia is established, and at present this is not universally accepted, management of lipid abnormalities will become important in patients with chronic renal failure. Carnitine, which plays a part in the oxidation of fatty acids, may be deficient in patients with chronic renal failure, due to poor nutrition, diminished renal synthesis, and loss in the dialysate. Its administration as a dietary supplement may reduce cholesterol and triglyceride levels but is not yet routinely recommended because of unpredictable results and side-effects.

CARBOHYDRATE

Glucose intolerance is a feature of uraemia and is explained by a post-receptor block to the action of insulin in the peripheral tissues. It is partially reversed by dialysis. Insulin clearance is delayed in renal failure, so the development of renal failure can have contrasting effects on insulin requirements in diabetics.

PROTEIN

Uraemia favours protein breakdown and inhibits anabolism. The tendency to negative nitrogen balance is explained by the chronic metabolic acidosis, malnutrition, and the production of inflammatory mediators.

Protein synthesis is impaired partly because of resistance to the action of insulin. Patients with endstage renal failure frequently show the features of protein malnutrition. They are wasted, have reduced muscle bulk, and low concentrations of albumin, transferrin, and C_3. Dialysis will improve this and the aim is to achieve a protein catabolic rate of less than 1 g/kg/day, by encouraging an appropriate intake of high-class protein and covering the effects of this increased intake with adequate duration and frequency of dialysis treatment.

Natural history

The natural history of most nephropathies is characterized by a progressive decline in renal function. However, the rate of progression varies considerably between patients, with some displaying stable function over many years, perhaps most often when urinary-tract obstruction has been relieved or when nephrotoxic analgesics have been withdrawn.

It has been observed that the rate of progression of chronic glomerulonephritides is generally faster than that of tubulointerstitial nephritides. This may be the result of more severe proteinuria in the former. Proteinuria is the most reliable prognostic factor in chronic renal failure as its severity correlates with the rate of progression of the underlying nephropathy. In chronic glomerulonephritis, persistent heavy proteinuria (in the nephrotic range) predicts a poor outcome. Conversely, the absence of significant proteinuria, or its partial or complete remission, indicate a favourable prognosis. In patients with tubulointerstitial nephropathies, the onset of significant proteinuria (>1 g/24 h) is often associated with a steady decline in renal function. This is also true of patients with diabetes mellitus, where the onset of microalbuminuria and the severity of proteinuria predict progressive diabetic nephropathy. In these patients, the onset of proteinuria also indicates a higher morbidity and mortality from cardiovascular complications, perhaps because of associated hyperlipidaemia. The mechanism(s) by which heavy proteinuria might adversely affect the rate of loss of renal function is not known. It may of course be a marker rather than a directly causative factor.

The other important factor influencing the natural history is systemic hypertension, which appears early in the course of renal diseases and often precedes the onset of uraemia. It is associated with an accelerated decline in renal function and, although it is difficult to distinguish primary deterioration of renal function and secondary worsening of hypertension from vice versa, there is now sound evidence that uncontrolled hypertension can accelerate the loss of renal function (Chapter 20.11). Even when controlled, hypertensive patients with chronic nephropathies have a faster rate of deterioration of renal function when compared to their normotensive counterparts. The control of hypertension slows the rate of decline of renal function, certainly in patients with diabetic and probably also in non-diabetic nephropathies.

Other factors modulating progression
GENETIC RACIAL FACTORS

Certain antigens of the major histocompatibility complex have been associated with a poor outcome in some forms of glomerulonephritis. This is the case when Goodpasture syndrome occurs in patients with HLA, DR2, and B7. Associations have also been described in patients with IgA and membranous nephropathies. In the latter, carriers of the haplotype B8-DR3-BfF1 may be associated with a worse prognosis. In adult polycystic disease, it has been reported that patients carrying the PKD1 gene on the short arm of chromosome 16 have an earlier onset and a faster rate of decline compared to those whose abnormal gene is on chromosome 4 (Chapter 20.5.3). Genetic factors may also explain some race-related differences in susceptibility and outcome of nephropathies. Afro- and, to a lesser extent, Hispanic-Americans suffer a faster rate of progression when compared to Caucasians. Afro- and native Americans also have a faster rate of progression of diabetic nephropathy.

GENDER

In certain forms of chronic renal disease, function deteriorates faster in males than in females, for instance in adult polycystic kidney disease, Alport's syndrome, mesangial IgA, and membranous nephropathies. In Western societies, males also tend to have a higher blood pressure than age-matched females, and this may be one reason for a more rapid decline in renal function.

AGE

The age at onset of a nephropathy may affect its outcome. It has been suggested that an early onset of renal failure in polycystic disease may lead to faster progression. By contrast, elderly patients with idiopathic membranous and mesangial IgA nephropathies have a poorer prognosis.

Mechanisms of progression

Progressive loss of filtration rate in chronic renal disorders reflects the progression of the underlying scarring of the kidneys. The latter is characterized by progressive glomerulosclerosis, tubulointerstitial fibrosis, and vascular sclerosis. Over recent years, considerable progress has been made in the understanding of the pathophysiology of these changes.

GLOMERULOSCLEROSIS

It is currently thought that common mechanisms of scarring affect the kidneys regardless of the cause of the initial nephropathy and well after the initiating events have subsided. Glomerulosclerosis has been attributed to immunological (glomerulonephritis), haemodynamic (hypertension), or metabolic (diabetes mellitus) insults leading to glomerular endothelial injury. Glomerular capillary wall injury may also affect the glomeruli spared the initial insult. Much of the current view of the reasons for these findings depend on animal experiments. In these, glomeruli undergo adaptive morphological and functional changes, characterized by hypertrophy and hyperfunction (hyperperfusion and hyperfiltration). A compensatory increase in intraglomerular capillary pressure (glomerular hypertension) also takes place as the result of a disproportionate afferent arteriolar vasodilatation and the loss of autoregulation by remnant glomeruli exposing them to systemic hypertension. The unopposed transmission of systemic hypertension to the glomerular capillary bed leads to glomerular hypertension, which in turn is associated with endothelial damage. Injury to the glomerular endothelial lining favours platelet adhesion, aggregation, and the formation of glomerular microthrombi. It appears also to allow the transudation of macromolecules, including lipids and growth factors, into the glomerular mesangium. These may stimulate mesangial proliferation and increased synthesis of extracellular collagenous matrix. Both lipids and growth factors have been implicated in the progression of glomerulosclerosis in animal experiments.

Comparisons have been drawn between the process of glomerulosclerosis and that of atherosclerosis. In both processes platelets, monocytes/macrophages, and lipids infiltrate the vascular/glomerular wall. Interactions between infiltrating and resident cells through the release of autacoids and growth factors lead to mesangial proliferation and expansion of the glomerular extracellular matrix of collagen. Platelet-derived growth factor and transforming growth factor-β are likely candidates for the stimulation of the synthesis of glomerular collagen, and ultimately the development of fibrosis. The inability of scarred glomeruli to clear excessive collagen deposition may be due to loss of collagenase activity by scarred glomeruli and/or qualitative changes in glomerular collagen, making it resistant to degradation.

TUBULOINTERSTITIAL SCARRING

Good correlations have been observed between the severity of tubulointerstitial scarring and glomerular filtration rate. Tubulointerstitial inflammatory infiltrate as well as widespread interstitial fibrosis usually indicate a poor prognosis. The mechanism of tubulointerstitial fibrosis is an important area of current research. It bears some similarities to that described above for glomerulosclerosis. Like most forms of fibrotic processes, it is characterized by an inadequate healing process with excessive collagen deposition. It involves interactions between renal tubular cells, inflammatory cells, and resident fibroblasts through the release of cytokines and peptide growth-promoting factors, which ultimately leads to tubulointerstitial fibrosis.

VASCULAR SCLEROSIS

The extent and severity of renal vascular changes (arterial and arteriolar) can also affect the outcome of nephropathies. In elderly patients, atherosclerosis of renal arteries has been implicated, through renal ischaemia and cholesterol embolization, in the acceleration of renal scarring. Hyalinosis of smaller renal vessels is also common in patients of all ages with chronic renal disease. Severe arteriolar hyalinosis can often be seen in kidney biopsies of patients with chronic nephropathies even when systemic hypertension is mild. The severity of these vascular lesions often exceeds that observed in patients with essential hypertension. Arteriolar hyalinosis can further jeopardize glomerular and tubular blood supply and accelerate scarring.

Interactions between these various contributors to kidney scarring are likely to take place and ultimately lead to nephron destruction and loss of renal function.

Management

Once the full first assessment of the patient is complete (see above) and appropriate emergency measures applied (see Chapter 20.16), the plan of long-term management will be formulated and consist of three elements.

CONSERVATION OF RENAL FUNCTION

There are a few causes of renal failure the pathology of which can be arrested (see above and Table 8), but most forms of glomerulonephritis (apart from the rapidly progressive forms and membranous), diabetic nephropathy, and adult polycystic kidney disease are all 'unstoppable'. It is the progressive and often constant decline in renal function caused by the non-specific scarring of the remaining nephrons, which occurs irrespective of the underlying pathology, that attracts most experimental effort and therapeutic intervention. The purpose of follow-up is to monitor the progress of chronic renal failure, which for practical reasons is best assessed by measuring the plasma creatinine concentration and assessing the rate of decline by a 1/creatinine plot versus time (Fig. 4). Deviations from the established slope alert the clinician to the possibility of an additional insult or change in pathology (see Table 7).

Experimental data

Animal experimentation has suggested a wide range of dietary and pharmacological interventions aimed at slowing the progression of loss of renal function. These include dietary restrictions of protein, calories, phosphate, sodium, and sucrose, as well as lipids. Dietary supplementation with various polyunsaturated fatty acids, such as linoleic acid and eicosapentaenoic acid (fish oil), has also proved beneficial in experimental uraemia. Pharmacological interventions to reduce systemic as well as glomerular hypertension, hyperlipidaemia, or the prevention of platelet aggregation (causing glomerular microthrombosis) have also proved effective in slowing progression in experimental animals. Manipulation of fibrogenic cytokines and growth factors with neutralizing antibodies and/or antagonists has also proved beneficial.

Clinical data

The heterogeneity of renal diseases in humans makes the evaluation of the approaches suggested by animal data difficult. It should be empha-

sized that the evaluation of treatment requires accurate measurement of glomerular filtrate rate by isotope methods, for creatinine clearance is too inaccurate, especially at lower levels of renal function. With the exception of the control of systemic hypertension (a benefit which is most obvious in diabetic nephropathy, (see Chapter 20.5.1)), none of them has so far proved convincingly effective. This is also the case for dietary protein restriction, as careful review of most published literature shows its effects to be inconclusive. A reasonable approach in the light of current knowledge is to recommend the avoidance of a high-protein diet and the limitation of the intake of protein to 0.8 g/kg/day, since this could prove beneficial and is unlikely to be harmful. Dietary supplementation with eicosapentaenoic acid has so far shown conflicting results in the management of progressive glomerulonephritis. Other interventions, including immunosuppression, antiplatelet therapy, and anticoagulation, as well as lipid reduction, seem to have little impact on progression and are not without side-effects. Uraemic patients should be spared the potential side-effects of unproven therapies. The avoidance of potentially nephrotoxic drugs in patients with chronic renal diseases is especially important (Chapter 20.14).

COMPENSATION FOR THE EFFECTS OF CHRONIC RENAL INSUFFICIENCY

Control of blood pressure

The pathogenesis of hypertension of chronic renal failure is complex (see Chapter 20.11). The threshold for drug treatment should be lower than in essential hypertension and the aim is to keep diastolic blood pressure below 90 mmHg, not only to prevent the common complications of the raised pressure but also to break the cycle of accelerated glomerular scarring leading to worsening renal function and further hypertension. Before drugs are prescribed, simple measures should be instituted: modest dietary sodium restriction (60 mmol/day), reduction in body weight, exercise, and limiting alcohol consumption to less than 21 units/week. The first choice of monotherapy is open. β-Blockers, angiotensin-converting-enzyme inhibitors and calcium-entry blockers are all effective in early renal failure. A combination of angiotensin-converting-enzyme inhibitors and a loop diuretic is logical in more advanced renal failure, and is associated with a minimum of side-effects. If this is ineffective, a vasodilator (either an α-blocker or a calcium-channel blocker) should be added. In the most resistant cases, minoxidil (starting at 2.5 mg/day) and high doses of diuretics, including metolazone (2.5 mg/day), hardly ever fails. It is a moot point whether any particular agent is better in this respect, but the balance of opinion appears to favour the angiotensin-converting-enzyme inhibitors. It has been suggested that angiotensin-converting-enzyme inhibitors may have additional therapeutic advantages, contributing to their beneficial effect on the reduction of proteinuria and slowing the progression of chronic renal failure in diabetic and non-diabetic nephropathies. However, these agents should be prescribed with caution as they can accelerate the decline in renal function in the elderly, in advanced renal insufficiency, or underlying diffuse renovascular disease. It is worth remembering that 'difficult' blood pressures may be spurious, either because measurements are high in the alarming environment of an outpatient clinic or because the patient is not taking the drugs. Ambulatory blood pressure monitoring can be helpful in such cases.

Match dietary and fluid intake to the excretory capacity

It is possible to reduce the effects of uraemia by limiting protein intake without promoting breakdown of essential tissue protein such as muscle. An intake of 0.6 g/kg/day of high-quality protein will often reduce the blood urea (and presumably, therefore, uraemic toxins) significantly. More severe protein restrictions require special caloric supplements and do carry the risk of inducing malnutrition. Restriction should be started when symptom relief is needed. This is very variable in terms of blood urea. Symptoms may arise at levels as low as 25 mmol/l but can be absent at 40 mmol/l or more. Controlled trials have shown little advantage in the early introduction of a low-protein diet in chronic renal fail-

Table 9 *Drugs to be used with care in renal failure*

	Class	Comment
Antimicrobial	Aminoglycosides	Reduce dose, ototoxic
	Acyclovir	Reduce dose
	Cephalosporins	Reduce dose
	Co-trimoxazole	Reduce dose
	Ethambutol	Reduce dose, retinal toxicity
	Ganciclovir	Reduce dose
	Nitrofurantoin	Avoid, neuropathy
	Penicillins	Avoid high doses, fits
Anaesthetic drugs	Pancuronium	Avoid, prolonged paralysis
	Gallamine	Avoid, prolonged paralysis
	Opiates	Reduce dose, prolonged effect
Gastrointestinal	Metoclopramide	Be aware of extrapyramidal effects
	H_2 antagonists	Reduce dose
	Magnesium salts	Monitor magnesium concentration
Cardiac	Digoxin	Reduce dose and frequency
	β-Blockers	May need to reduce dose
	Spironolactone	Avoid, hyperkalaemia
	ACE inhibitors	Monitor creatinine and K^+
	Clofibrate	Avoid, muscle injury
Oral hypoglycaemics	Chlorpropamide	Avoid, hypoglycaemia
	Tolbutamide	Reduce dose
	Biguanides	Avoid, lactic acidosis

ACE, angiotension-converting enzyme.

ure. Phosphate restriction (1000 mg/day) will counter one of the stimuli to parathyroid hormone oversecretion and lower the calcium phosphate product, thus limiting vascular and other soft-tissue calcification. Modest sodium restriction to 60 mmol/day will contribute to control of arterial pressure and avoid oedema without making the diet unpalatable. Commonly, some patients are 'salt losers' and require supplements in the form of Slow Sodium® or sodium bicarbonate. This is most often needed in patients with interstitial nephropathy, such as medullary cystic disease. Potassium restriction is only needed when chronic renal failure is severe, unless bicarbonate loss leads to early acidosis; hyperkalaemia may then be corrected by bicarbonate supplements. The effects of potassium-sparing diuretics and angiotensin-converting-enzyme inhibitors on raising plasma potassium should be remembered before limiting the intake of enjoyable potassium-containing foods such as fruit and vegetables. Fluid restriction is not usually necessary until late in renal failure, the kidneys' ability to excrete free water being relatively well maintained. Dehydration is more common and results from a failure to match intake with output, visible and insensible.

A mild chronic compensated metabolic acidosis develops when the glomerular filtration rate falls below 30 ml/min. This usually causes few problems but may contribute to bone disease in children. Later, it is a contributory factor to the development of hyperkalaemia, and the symptom of breathlessness on effort. When plasma bicarbonate is less than 20 mmol/l, sodium bicarbonate 600 mg four times/day should be started if the sodium load can be tolerated. More severe acidosis is an indication to start dialysis.

Prevention and treatment of abnormalities of calcium homeostasis in renal bone disease

This is dealt with fully in Chapter 20.18.

Treatment of renal anaemia

Significant symptoms of anaemia start to appear when the haemoglobin falls below 10 g/dl and are disabling below 6 g/dl. Before instituting erythropoietin treatment the common aggravating causes should be sought and treated. These include blood loss from the gastrointestinal tract, iron deficiency, and chronic infection. These are screened for by faecal occult blood measurements, ferritin concentration, and C-reactive protein. Recombinant human erythropoietin (epoetin) is given at a dose of approximately 100 U/kg/week by subcutaneous injection as two or three injections. These cause a little local discomfort. The target haemoglobin should be 10 to 12 g/dl, or higher if symptoms such as angina persist. The haemoglobin response should be monitored monthly and the dose adjusted down if the rise in haemoglobin is more than 2 g/month. The dose can be adjusted up to more than 300 U/kg/week, but these high doses should prompt a search for confounding factors. Blood pressure tends to rise as anaemia is reversed. This requires treatment but it is prudent to stop the erythropoietin until blood pressure control is adequate.

Bleeding diathesis

This is usually only a problem when patients with renal failure undergo surgery. The first measure is to raise the haematocrit to improve platelet function. Vasopressin (DDAVP®) 0.3 microgram/kg in 100 ml NaCl in 30 min, administered before surgery, will reduce the risk of haemorrhage and can be given for bleeding, for example uncontrolled epistaxis. The next measure to try is administration of cryoprecipitate which shortens bleeding time for 24 to 36 h after infusion. A longer effect is obtained by a total dose infusion of 3 mg/kg conjugated oestrogen over 5 days. The onset of effect is delayed but lasts about 2 weeks.

Hyperlipidaemia

The treatment of hyperlipidaemia of renal failure is a daunting challenge, for the patients are usually oscillating between malnutrition and dietary restriction of foods containing phosphate, potassium, and sodium. A renal diet is not an appetizing one, and restriction of fat intake makes it even less so. There is a dual purpose in treating the hyperlipidaemia. First, it may contribute to progressive renal damage and, secondly, it underlies the probably greater risk of atherosclerosis that these patients run. A reasonable compromise is to advise patients to stay at their ideal weight, take regular exercise, and to avoid animal fats. If the cholesterol remains high, above 6.5 mmol/l, 3-hydroxy-3-methylglutaryl-CoA reductase inhibitor should be prescribed in preference to the fibrate drugs, which accumulate and can cause muscle damage.

Use of drugs

Because many drugs and their metabolites are excreted via the kidney, care must be taken with the selection of agent and dose in patients with renal failure. Table 9 lists the common drugs that should be used with caution.

Psychological

Patients with renal failure are understandably under unremitting emotional stress. Their general health affects their employment, social and sexual life, and recreation. Responses range from anger to depression and even suicide. It is unusual for these patients to require formal psychiatric assessment and it is left to their clinical carers, doctors, and nurses to counsel and console them. Sedatives should be used sparingly and antidepressants prescribed if an endogenous depression is diagnosed. Like a bereavement, most patients adjust to the loss of their kidney function and many limit its intrusion and live full and productive lives.

PREPARATION FOR DIALYSIS AND TRANSPLANTATION

Once endstage renal failure seems inevitable, the patient must be prepared physically and psychologically for renal replacement treatment. One can predict roughly when the endstage will be reached (Fig. 4). This information is useful for the patient and provides a guide for the timing for the creation of vascular access. One should avoid the temptation to delay starting dialysis for as long as possible, for the quality of life and health of a well-dialysed patient is superior to that of a non-dialysed, uraemic, malnourished one.

The absolute indications for dialysis are the development of complications that cannot be contained by conservative and pharmacological means. These are fluid overload, severe hypertension, pericarditis, hyperkalaemia, encephalopathy, and neuropathy. To wait for these is bad practice. Nephrologists generally wait until the patient has obvious uraemic symptoms such as anorexia, lassitude, and pruritus, if only because their relief reinforces the need to adjust to regular dialysis. Apart from potassium concentrations and the degree of acidosis, blood tests such as urea and creatinine do not provide a safe guide of when to start. Nevertheless it is advisable to start dialysis, in the absence of symptoms, in small-framed subjects, including women, when the urea is approximately 35 to 40 mmol/l and the creatinine 650 to 800 μmol/l; and in men when the blood urea is 45 to 50 mmol/l and creatinine greater than 1200 μmol/l. Initiation of dialysis at lower blood levels of urea and creatinine is also commonplace in diabetic patients.

The choice of modality—haemodialysis, continuous ambulatory peritoneal dialysis, or renal transplantation,—depends on many factors, not least their availability and the patient's preference. If transplantation (see Chapter 20.17.3) is appropriate, there is no reason not to perform it before dialysis is mandatory. If haemodialysis is chosen, vascular access should be created 2 to 3 months before the need for it. If continuous ambulatory peritoneal dialysis is to be used, the Tenckhoff catheter should be placed 2 to 3 weeks before dialysis needs to be started, to allow it to seal.

REFERENCES

Allon, M. (1993). Treatment and prevention of hyperkalaemia in end-stage renal disease. *Kidney International* **43**, 1197–209.
ANZDATA (1992). Report.
Appel, G. (1991). Lipid abnormalities in renal disease. *Kidney International* **39**, 169–83.
Cassidy, M.J.D. and Kerr, D.N.S. (1992). The assessment of the patient with chronic renal insufficiency. In *Oxford textbook of clinical nephrology*, (ed. J.S. Cameron, A.M. Davison, J.-P Grünfeld, D.N.S. Kerr, and E. Ritz), pp. 1149–73. Oxford University Press.
Chatenoud, L., Jungers, P., and Descamps-Latscha, B. (1994). Immunological considerations of the uremic and dialysed patient. *Kidney International* **44**, (Suppl. 44), S92–S96.
EDTA, Registry (1991).
El Nahas, A.M. and Wight, J.P. (1991). The management of chronic renal failure: ten unanswered questions. *Quarterly Journal of Medicine*, **81**, 799–809.
Eschbach, J.W. (1989). The anaemia of chronic renal failure: pathophysiology and the effect of recombinant erythropoietin. *Kidney International* **35**, 134–48.
Feest, T.G., Mistry, C.D., Grimes, D.S., and Mallick, N.P. (1990). Incidence of advanced chronic renal failure and the need for end-stage renal replacement treatment. *British Medical Journal* **301**, 897–900.
Klahr, S. (1991). Chronic renal failure management. *Lancet* **338**, 423–7.
Levinsky, N.G. (1993). The organisation of medical care. Lessons from the Medicare End-Stage Renal Disease Program. *New England Journal of Medicine* **329**, 1395–9.
May, R.C., Kelly, R.A., and Mitch, W.E. (1991). Pathophysiology of Uremia. In *The kidney*, (ed. B.M. Brenner and F.C. Rector), pp. 1997–2018. W.B. Saunders, Philadelphia.
Meyer, T.W., Scholey, J.W., and Brenner, B.M. (1991). Nephron adaptation to renal injury. In *The kidney*, (ed. B.M. Brenner and F.C. Rector), pp. 1871–908. W.B.Saunders, Philadelphia.
Mitch, W.E. (1991). Dietary protein restriction in patients with chronic renal failure. *Kidney International* **40**, 326–41.
Smith, S.R., Svetkey, L.P., and Dennis, V.W., (1991). Racial differences in the incidence and progression of renal disease. *Kidney International* **40**, 815–22.
US Renal Data System (1991). *Annual Report*.
Walser, M. (1990). Progression of chronic renal failure in man. *Kidney International* **37**, 1195–210.
Wing, A.J. (1992). Causes of end-stage renal failure. In *Oxford textbook of clinical nephrology*, (ed. J.S. Cameron, A.M. Davison, J.-P. Grünfeld, D.N.S. Kerr, and E. Ritz), pp. 1227–36. Oxford University Press.

20.17.2 Replacement therapy by dialysis

R. GOKAL

Introduction

Kidney function is replaced only in part by maintenance dialysis treatment, which, at best provides the equivalent of 5 to 10 per cent of excretory 'renal function'. In spite of this, survival and rehabilitation are good for up to 20 years, partly related to the ability of other organ systems to function in the face of continuing uraemia.

At the end of 1992 there were well over half a million people on dialysis worldwide, of which roughly 82 per cent were maintained on haemodialysis and the rest on peritoneal dialysis. The proportion of patients managed on the various modes of treatment in individual countries varies considerably (Fig. 1) and is dependent upon local factors such as financial constraints, physician bias, and limited haemodialysis facilities. Peritoneal dialysis as a proportion of the total dialysis population ranges from 5 per cent in Japan to over 90 per cent in Mexico, with the United Kingdom at 52 per cent. In most instances the treatments are used in an integrated sequence, with patients moving between different therapies dictated by medical and social factors.

Starting dialysis and patient selection

The decision of when to begin dialysis in a patient with chronic renal failure depends on clinical features of uraemia, biochemical abnormalities, and resources for treatment. Uraemic symptoms that do not respond to conservative measures are usually the indication for dialysis, which is rarely essential before the creatinine clearance has fallen below 5 ml/min. However, an earlier start (between 5 and 10 ml/min) may well be needed in the presence of cardiovascular problems and in patients with diabetes mellitus, who are less able to tolerate uraemia.

The selection of the appropriate treatment modalities for the individual patient is complex and requires consideration of a number of factors. If there is free choice, patient preference is an important consideration, but medical, social, and psychological factors need to be taken into

Table 1 *Factors influencing modality selection*

Haemodialysis preferred	Do well on either therapy	Peritoneal dialysis

Severe inflammatory bowel disease
Third trimester pregnancy
Severe active psychotic disorder
Market disability with no helper
Homeless
	In-centre haemodialysis oriented
	
	Dependent lifestyle
	Active diverticulitis
	Ischaemic renal disease
	Large polycystic kidneys
	Severe recurrent hernias
	Frequent and substantial therapy changes
	    CAPD oriented
	
	Independent lifestyle
	Severe pulmonary disease
	Transmissable disease
	APD oriented
	
	Same as CAPD plus
	Days free from exchanges
	More prescription flexibility
	Social support filled by helper at home
		Unstable cardiovascular disease
		Difficulty in vascular access
		Severe anaemia
		Age limitations (children under
		    5, elderly)
		Diabetes
		Strong need for independence,
		    autonomy, or control
		Distance from centre

Centre	Centre/home	Home

Fig. 1 Proportion of patients on various dialysis treatments in the United Kingdom (upper panel) compared to Europe as a whole (lower panel) over the years up to 1990. HD, haemodialysis; CPD, chronic peritoneal dialysis. The actual number of patients on various treatments in 1990 is displayed on the right-hand scale.

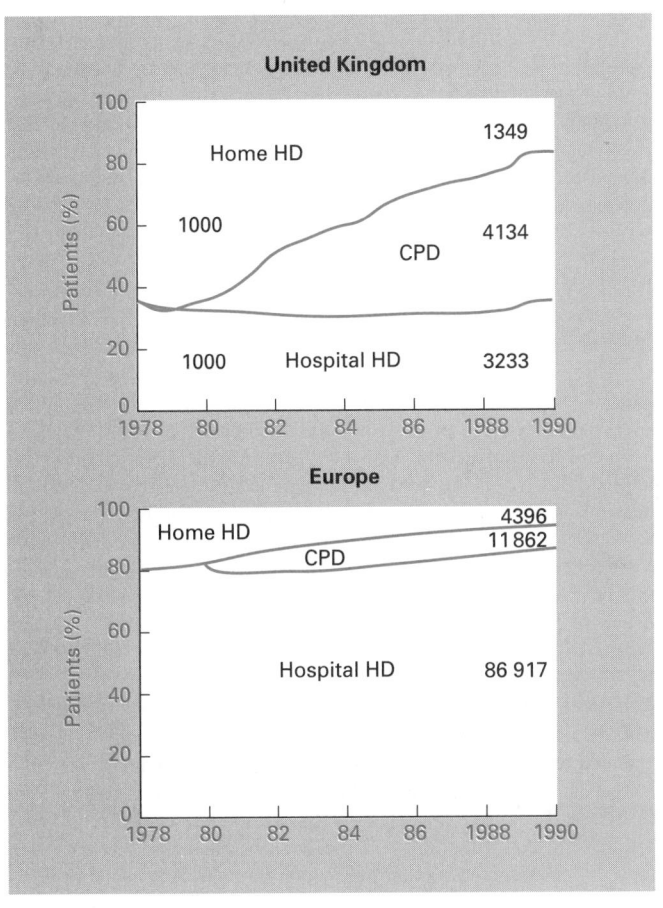

Table 2 *Techniques of peritoneal dialysis (home or hospital)*

	Number of exchanges (2l)	Duration of exchanges (hours)		Type/ duration
		Day	Night	
CAPD	3–5	4	8	Continuous
CCPD	3–5	16	1–2	Continuous
IPD	40	1/2–1	1/2–1	24 hours
NIPD	8–10	–	1/2–1	Nightly
TIPD	25–30	–	1/2	Nightly

CAPD, continuous ambulatory peritoneal dialysis; CCPD, continuous cyclic peritoneal dialysis; IPD, intermittent peritoneal dialysis; NIPD, night intermittent peritoneal dialysis; TIPD, tidal intermittent peritoneal dialysis.

All these peritoneal techniques (except CAPD) are automated, using a cycler to perform the exchanges.

account before a treatment modality is chosen (Table 1). The dialysis modalities that are available are shown in Tables 2 and 3.

Haemodialysis

PRINCIPLES OF HAEMODIALYSIS

The principle of haemodialysis is relatively simple. Blood flows on one side of a semipermeable membrane and dialysis fluid (an osmotically balanced solution of electrolytes, buffer, and glucose in water) flows countercurrent on the other side. Solute transfer across this membrane occurs mainly by diffusion and to some extent by convective transport. Removal of excess fluid (ultrafiltration) is achieved by creating a negative transmembrane pressure.

TECHNICAL ASPECTS OF HAEMODIALYSES

The extracoporeal blood and fluid circuits

Blood is pumped from the vascular access cannula of the patient through the dialyser and back to the patient. Within this circuit, venous and arterial pressure-measuring devices are incorporated to assess flow, as

Table 3 *Techniques using extracorporal circuits*

	Location	Blood flow (ml/min)	Dialysate flow (ml/min)	Duration	Comments
Haemodialysis	Home minimal/ care hospital	200–400	500	4–8 h 3 times per week	
Haemofiltration	In centre	400	–	3 times per week	40% of body weight exchanged
High-flux haemodialysis	In centre (home)	400	500	2–4 h 3 times per week	Requires: bicarbonate; volumetric control of ultrafiltration; synthetic membrane; monitoring of adequacy
Haemodiafiltration	In centre	400	Combination of haemodialysis and haemofiltration used mainly in acute renal failure		

are air detector systems to allow shutdown of the pump to prevent air embolus. Heparin is typically infused between the blood pump and the dialyser. Anticoagulation carries risks and newer products (low molecular weight heparin, bonded heparin-lined membranes) may make this safer.

Dialysis fluid, maintained at 37 °C, is continuously produced by proportioning devices, and flows countercurrent to the blood at a rate of 500 ml/min and then into the drain.

Dialysers

Two types of haemodialyser are most widely used: the parallel plate and hollow-fibre. The average membrane surface area is 1.1 m² (0.8–1.5). There are two types of dialyser membranes.

Cellulose-based membranes

Cuprophan is the most widely used dialyser membrane material, made of reconstituted cellulose.

Synthetic membranes

These include polysulfone, polycarbonate, polyamide, and polyacrylonitrate. They have a high solute and hydraulic permeability (high flux) and few membrane/blood interactions. They are regarded as being more 'biocompatible' but are also more expensive. These properties of synthetic polymers have been exploited for better haemodialysis when ultrafiltration is controlled (high-flux dialysis).

Dialysis fluid

The water used in dialysis must be treated and purified before use to remove bacteria, calcium and aluminium. Standard water-treatment devices utilize softeners to remove Ca^{2+} filters, and reverse osmosis. In the latter the water is forced through a highly semipermeable membrane under pressure, removing 90 to 100 per cent of inorganic and organic substances, pyrogens, bacteria, and particulate matter. Although acetate is still the commonly used buffer, it is thought to induce vasodilation and to have a cardiodepressant action. Bicarbonate buffer is now available and its use has reduced dialysis hypotension improving the treatment of those patients with cardiovascular instability and dialysis-related symptoms.

Ultrafiltration

Transmembrane pressure for ultrafiltration is determined by the mean hydrostatic pressure in the dialysate and blood compartment and the oncotic pressure in the blood compartment. Ultrafiltration control systems (the flow censor system and the volumetric balancing system), which measure and directly control the rate of ultrafiltration, have assured uniform, accurate, and predictable fluid removal. Dialysers with

high-flux synthetic membranes must be used in dialysis machines with reliable volume control of ultrafiltration to prevent excessive fluid loss.

Haemofiltration

Haemofiltration is an alternative form of renal replacement therapy, where solute removal is achieved only by convection, rather than by diffusion as in haemodialysis. Instead of a dialyser, a haemofilter (made of highly permeable synthetic membranes) is used, which produces ultrafiltration rates of between 120 and 180 ml/min under appropriate conditions of blood flow and transmembrane pressure. The ultrafiltrate, containing the waste products, is substituted with an equal volume of replacement fluid, usually bicarbonate based. Some of the requirements are shown in Table 3. The clinical advantages of haemofiltration over haemodialysis include better haemodynamic stability during treatment, less hypotension, and no exposure to dialysis fluid, which may contain pyrogen and other toxins. In spite of these advantages, only 3 per cent of all patients on dialysis in Europe are treated by this technique—the major reason being the higher cost.

VASCULAR ACCESS

The success of haemodialysis is very largely dependent on good vascular access, which usually takes the form of an arteriovenous fistula at the wrist. This primary access in not always possible, in which case use of vein grafts or synthetic materials is essential. Permanent internal jugular dialysis catheters can also provide adequate long-term access.

Problems associated with permanent access to the circulation to provide blood flows of 200 to 500 ml/min are the main reasons for hospital admissions, inadequate dialysis, and incomplete rehabilitation and anxiety. A strategy for vascular access is essential for all patients with chronic renal disease. Preparation for dialysis should begin with access provision well in advance of its need (glomerular filtration rate 10–15 ml/min).

Primary and secondary access

The important arm (cephalic and antecubital) and leg veins essential for haemodialysis are destroyed or damaged by infusions and repeated venepunctures. Use of these should be avoided in those at risk of renal failure or already in renal failure and undergoing dialysis therapy. Primary access for long-term dialysis is an arteriorvenous fistula between the radial and cephalic vein near the wrist of the non-dominant arm. After a period of maturation, during which time the vein becomes arterialized, the fistula can be needled and heparinized blood pumped around the extracorporeal circuit. Blood flows in excesss of 300 ml/min are needed for adequate, efficient dialysis. Secondary vascular access is constructed from vein grafts (saphenous, cephalic) between large proximal arteries and veins in the forearm, antecubital fossa, or thigh. In the absence of veins for grafting, use is made of vascular grafts made from various synthetic materials.

Temporary access

Temporary access uses the internal jugular, subclavian, and femoral veins and is achieved by introducing wide-bore double-or single-lumen catheters, using the Seldinger technique. This provides access for several weeks. A major advance is the use of polyurethane (which is softer and more pliable) catheters into the internal jugular vein; this avoids the complications of subclavian vein cannulation (that is, thrombosis and stenosis) and provides a more permanent access. The external part of the catheter is tunnelled and stabilized by Dacron® cuffs to minimize exit infection.

TREATMENT OF PATIENTS WITH ENDSTAGE RENAL DISEASE BY HAEMODIALYSIS

In most Western countries haemodialysis takes place in a specialized centre which may be integrated into a hospital or a private setting. The centre provides a full medical service and close monitoring during and between treatments. Such treatments are expensive, mainly due to a high staff to patient ratio and, because of the high cost, programmes have been developed to teach patients to haemodialyse themselves in minimal care units or at home, which nevertheless requires full medical, nursing, technical, and social support. Home haemodialysis therapy is on the decline (Fig. 1). Details of haemodialysis (both standard and high flux) are given in Table 3.

COMPLICATIONS OF HAEMODIALYSIS

These are shown in Table 4 and are related to those of the haemodialysis treatment itself and to vascular access. Technical failures are now rare and haemodialysis has become a safe therapy.

Symptomatic hypotension is very common during haemodialysis and may be accompanied by nausea, vomiting, and muscle cramps, and can proceed to circulatory collapse. Inappropriate volume removal by ultra-filtration is the usual cause of hypotension. However, other factors (auto-nomic neuropathy, the vasodilatory actions of acetate, and the bioin-compatibility/toxicity of cellulose membranes) may contribute. Current evidence also supports the role of inflammatory cytokines (such as inter-leukin-1 and tumour necrosis factor), and, because of activation of the alternative pathway of complement in this syndrome, C3a and C5a are released when membrane–blood interactions take place. The comple-ment activation leads to white cell sequestration in the lungs (hypoxia) and the cytokines induce hypotension, mediated by cytokine-induced nitric oxide production in vascular smooth muscle cells.

ADEQUACY OF HAEMODIALYSIS

The pathophysiology of the clinical syndrome of uraemia is not well defined, and so the complex question of how to assess adequacy of haemodialysis is unresolved. A clinical definition of adequate dialysis—that which permits the patients to be fully rehabilitated, in the widest sense of the word—does not provide a practical guideline for adequate prescription. A widely accepted definition was developed from the National Cooperative Dialysis Study in the United States. This pro-spective randomized study evaluated 'adequacy' of dialysis in four groups of patients treated by four different dialysis schedules, based on length of dialysis times and plasma urea concentrations. Morbidity and mortality were higher in the group with a high average serum concen-tration of urea (TAC). Urea clearance depends on the time on haemo-dialysis (T) and on the dialyser urea clearance (K). For practical dialysis prescription, the dialysis index of KT/V was arrived at, where the total

Table 4 *Complications of dialysis*

Haemodialysis
Acute
  Disequilibration syndrome
  Bleeding
  First use syndrome
  Technical faults
  Hypotension
  Haemorrhagic
    membrane
    bloodline
    vascular access
  Air embolus
  Hypohypernatraemia
  Cramps
  Complement and cytokine
    reactions
  Hardwater syndrome
  Haemolysis

Vascular access
  Inadequate flow
  Recirculation
  Infection
    cellulitis
    septicaemia
  Thrombosis
  Stenosis
  Haemorrhage
  Aneurysm
  Increased cardiac output
  Vascular steal syndrome
  Ischaemia
  Fistula thumb

Peritoneal dialysis
Infection
  peritonitis
  exit/tunnel infection
Catheter malfunction
  migration
  outflow/inflow
  obstruction
  fluid leakage
  biofilm
  formation
  cracking catheter material
Loss of ultrafiltration
Obesity
Hernias
Low back pain
Patient dislike and 'burn out'

Disorders common to all dialysis
Cerebrocardiovascular
  disease (cardiac failure,
  cerebrovascular accident)
Anaemia (erythropoietin
  therapy)
Abnormal bleeding
Hypertension
Hyperlipidaemia
Atherosclerosis
Renal bone disease
Infections
Malignancy
Malnutrition
Underdialysis
β_2-Microglobulin
  amyloidosis
Acquired renal cysts
Aluminium toxicity

urea clearance is normalized to the volume of distribution of the urea (V), corresponding to 65 per cent of the total body weight.

KT/V is calculated for a single treatment and a value of less than 1 is felt to be inadequate. A KT/V value of 1.2 to 1.3 and a TAC of less than 50 mg/dl with a protein intake of approximately 1 g/kg/day provides a reasonable guideline for adequate dialysis. Understanding and applying these concepts is particularly important in short dialysis when even minor deviations may result in undertreatment. It is thought that short dialysis without adequate monitoring has been responsible for the higher mortality in the dialysis population in the United States, and is a source of concern.

Peritoneal dialysis

PRINCIPLES OF PERITONEAL DIALYSIS

The principles of dialysis using the peritoneal membrane are essentially similar to those of haemodialysis. The peritoneum is used as a 'semi-permeable membrane', but the analogy is not exact since the peritoneum is a living membrane. In peritoneal dialysis, solutes in uraemic plasma diffuse across the peritoneal membrane towards the low concentration in the dialysis fluid; this gradient is maintained by replacing the used dialysis fluid with fresh solution at regular time intervals, depending upon the dialysis technique used (Table 2). Solute removal is also enhanced by convective loss related to ultrafiltration, which is achieved by the use of various osmotic agents, of which glucose is the most common.

PERITONEAL MEMBRANE

The normal peritoneum consists of three layers: the mesothelium, with elongated cells containing projecting microvilli; the interstitium, consisting of connective tissue; and the capillary endothelium in the microvessels. Introduction of peritoneal dialysis fluid into the peritoneal cavity has profound ultrastructural effects, which include interstitial oedema, diminished microvilli numbers, and submesothelial deposition of collagen fibres. Continuous exposure to unphysiological peritoneal dialysis solutions and repeated episodes of peritonitis appear to be responsible for these changes.

Recent studies show that there are minimal morphological alterations in the peritoneal membrane after 5 to 7 years on peritoneal dialysis in the absence of peritonitis. Duplication of basement membrane in the capillary endothelium and mesothelium, and increased collagen and fibrosis, appear to be seen only in patients who have experienced repeated peritonitis. These findings suggest that even transient breakdown of the mesothelial barrier during peritonitis may result in increased permeability of the peritoneum to glucose; glycosylation of the capillary membrane proteins may then result in basement membrane duplication and increased fibrosis.

The peritoneal membrane is also a secretory organ and releases surface-active material (phospholipids, mainly phosphatidylcholine) which act as lubricating agents and may well affect ultrafiltration.

PERITONEAL ACCESS

Despite the improvements in catheter survival over the past few years, catheter-related complications impart significant morbidity, resulting in a permanent change to haemodialysis treatment in 20 per cent of cases that fail continuous ambulatory peritoneal dialysis. A variety of catheters are available, all based on the one initially introduced by Tenckhoff. The straight intraperitoneal portion has been modified to the coil, double disc (Toronto Western), or column disc to prevent catheter migration and obstruction to flow. The extraperitoneal portion has been modified to create a permanent bend (Swan-Neck) such that the exit site points caudally. Infections and leaks around the catheter are avoided by ingrowth of fibrous tissue into two Dacron® cuffs.

Catheter implantation techniques vary considerably, but there appears to be general agreement on several fronts: the deep cuff needs to be placed in the musculature of the anterior abdominal wall, and the subcutaneous cuff near the skin surface within 2 to 3 cm of the exit, which is caudally directed. The insertion should be paramedian and implantation needs to be done by an experienced team of inserters, no matter which technique is used (blind, open surgical, or peritoneoscopic). Complications resulting from catheter malfunction are listed in Table 4.

PERITONEAL DIALYSIS SOLUTIONS

Current peritoneal dialysis solutions are unphysiological with pH 5 to 5.5 and high osmolality (350–500 mosmol/kg). Available solutions differ mainly in the amount of lactate, sodium, potassium, and calcium. The ideal buffer would be bicarbonate, but solutions containing mixes of bicarbonate, calcium, and glucose are difficult to prepare and sterilize, because of the formation of insoluble calcium salts. Two-chamber systems incorporating bicarbonate solutions are now being tried in clinical use.

Although glucose remains the safest osmotic agent for ultrafiltration, other agents have been tried in short-term dialysis; for example amino acids (predominantly as a protein supplement in malnourished patients) or glucose polymers, which provide isosmotic ultrafiltration based on colloid osmosis, appropriate for long-dwell peritoneal dialysis.

APPLICATION OF PERITONEAL DIALYSIS TO PATIENTS IN ENDSTAGE RENAL FAILURE

Peritoneal dialysis is simple and requires less complex equipment than does haemodialysis. Access to the peritoneum is not difficult. In addition, the slow correction of fluid and solute abnormalities makes it better suited for use in children, the elderly, and those with a cardiovascular disorder or diabetes mellitus. Treatment is easily undertaken at home. The disadvantages are chiefly related to the long duration of treatment, infective problems such as peritonitis, and the expense of hospital admissions.

TECHNIQUES OF PERITONEAL DIALYSIS

Various dialysis techniques have evolved to maximize the shortcomings of peritoneal dialysis, based on the need to deliver enough dialysis to keep the patient well, at the same time matching as far as possible the patient's psychosocial needs.

The peritoneal equilibration test This test, first devised by Twardowski, helps to determine whether the solute transport characteristics of the peritoneal membrane of individual patients are of high, average, or low transporters. This can then guide selection of treatment modality (Table 2) to formulate the dialysis prescription, and to identify patients with likely suboptimal dialysis performance.

Continous ambulatory peritoneal dialysis (CAPD)
Concept and technique

Conventional intermittent peritoneal dialysis techniques use large volumes with short dwell times to obtain adequate clearance of small molecular weight substances. In contrast, the concept of CAPD is to utilize the smallest daily volume of equilibrated dialysate, to prevent uraemia. Theoretical calculations have demonstrated that a patient will maintain a steady blood urea if 10 litres of peritoneal dialysis fluid are allowed to equilibrate daily with body fluids. This calculation underlies the CAPD technique of four daily exchanges of 2 litres to produce, with ultrafiltration, a total dialysate of 10 litres daily.

CAPD entails a closed system whereby fluid is initially instilled by gravity into the peritoneal cavity after the connection is made between the transfer set and a new bag, and fluid is then drained out into the same bag. A modification has been the use of the 'Y system', which entails drainage of the peritoneal effluent after the connection is made with a new bag, thereby enabling any resulting contamination to be flushed out. This 'flush before fill' concept has had a major impact on peritonitis and has considerably improved the outcome on CAPD.

Automated peritoneal dialysis

A cycler machine is used to enhance solute and fluid removal in patients in whom transport characteristics reveal a high transporter status or because there are psychosocial or medical factors which require short-dwell dialysis.

COMPLICATIONS OF PERITONEAL DIALYSIS (TABLE 4)

Peritonitis

Peritonitis has remained the most significant complication, accounting for considerable morbidity and when recurrent is a major cause of transfer to haemodialysis. With the newest techniques, episodes of peritonitis occur on average once in every 24 to 36 months. Peritonitis is diagnosed by the presence of a cloudy dialysate (WBC > 100/ml), with or without symptoms of abdominal pain or signs of peritonitis. The organisms responsible are Gram-positive (60 per cent, mainly *Staphylococcus epidermidis* and *S. aureus*), Gram-negative (20 per cent), and fungal (5 per cent) or no growth (culture-negative). Episodes related to *Staphylococcus aureus*, Pseudomonas, and fungal organisms have a poor outcome, need to be treated aggressively, and may need early catheter removal. The incidence of culture-negative peritonitis should be less than 10 per cent.

Treatment of peritonitis is dependent upon the isolation of the organism and treatment with appropriate antibiotics. A flow chart of management is shown in Fig. 2. Peritonitis remains a significant cause of hospitalization, accounting for about 4 days/patient year of therapy, but mortality from it is minimal.

Exit-site and tunnel infection

Exit infection is revealed by persistent seeping and/or erythema at the catheter epidermal interface. This is still a major problem. Better defined sites for insertion and exit, catheter immobilization, and the use of sterile dressings have reduced the incidence of this problem. Nasal carriage of *Staphylococcus aureus* may predispose to exit-site infections and peritonitis. Prophylactic use of nasal mupirocin or rifampicin appears useful.

Treatment of exit site infections is not satisfactory; but, since the main organism is *Staphylococcus aureus*, a combination of vancomycin and rifampicin has produced the best results.

Adequacy of dialysis and nutrition

As in haemodialysis (see above), there have been several attempts to define adequacy of dialysis by using various measures, including *KT/V*, total weekly creatinine clearance, and a derived dialysis index. Of these the *KT/V* index and creatinine clearance are gaining acceptance. Values of weekly *KT/V* of less than 1.5 are regarded as inadequate, as is the value of less than 40 l/week of total creatinine clearance. Clinical correlates with these indices appear to be reasonably good.

Another approach to prescription of CAPD involves tailoring dialysis according to the nitrogen balance. By determining daily nitrogen intake and non-urea nitrogen loss, the amount of urea and nitrogen to be removed and the corresponding drainage volume can be calculated. In stable patients nitrogen intake (dietary protein intake) should equal

Fig. 2 Flow chart of the management of peritonitis in continuous ambulatory peritoneal dialysis.

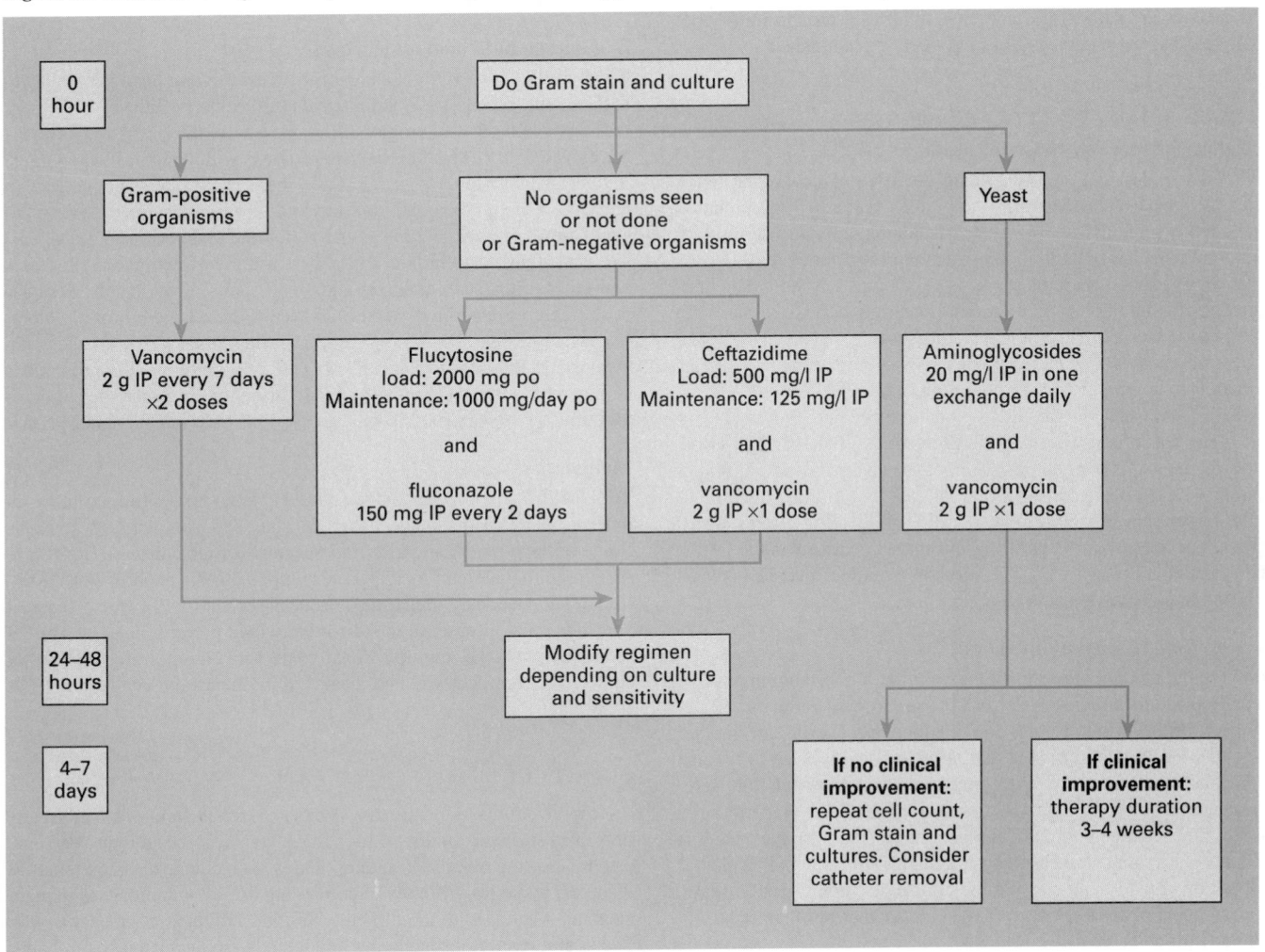

Table 5 *Daily dietary requirements in dialysis patients*

Calories	35–40 kcal/kg body-weight
Protein	1.0–1.2 g/kg body-weight
Carbohydrate	35% of ingested calories
Fat	remainder of ingested calories
P:S ratio	1.5:1
Vitamins	Supplements of B_6, C, folate, D
Calcium	1.0–1.5 g
Phosphorus	800–1000 mg
Bicarbonate	To maintain pH/serum bicarbonate within normal range
Sodium+ potassium	Limited to minimize fluid gain between dialysis of < 1 kg (HD); in CAPD based on residual renal function and ultrafiltration—by and large most need some restriction

CAPD, continuous ambulatory peritoneal dialysis; HD, haemodialysis.

nitrogen output (protein catabolic rate). This approach detects protein malnutrition or significant degrees of underdialysis, and several workers have shown a link between the amount of dialysis the patient receives and nutritional status reflected by serum albumin.

Appropriate protein intake is essential to make good the inherent losses in the peritoneal effluent. During an episode of peritonitis, protein losses are enhanced two- to threefold. Hence a dietary protein intake of at least 1 g/kg body-weight has been advocated, but levels of around 0.8 g/kg are normally achieved. The daily dietary requirements for CAPD patients are shown in Table 5. A significant proportion (40 per cent) of CAPD patients are mildly to severely malnourished.

Outcomes and complications of dialysis

Survival of patients and causes of death

Many reports of survival rates of patients on different renal replacement regimes have been published over the past 20 years, but interpretation of such reports remains very difficult. The demography of patients with renal failure has changed and therapy has improved. In the past decade the number of patients on renal replacement therapy has more than doubled, as has the number with additional, severe extrarenal diseases. In addition, more than 50 per cent of patients starting dialysis therapy are now over 60 years of age. Comparisons between replacement therapies must therefore be interpreted very carefully.

Overall, 5-year patient survival on renal replacement therapy begun in the 1980s was 85 per cent in patients aged less than 45 years at the start of treatment; 70 per cent in those between ages 45 and 54; 60 per cent in those aged between 55 and 64; 40 per cent in those aged 65 to 75; and 25 per cent in those above 75 years of age. These rates are 10 to 20 per cent better than for patients who started treatment in the 1970s. Diabetic patients do less well, but survival is similar overall between CAPD and haemodialysis patients.

Causes of death in patients on dialysis

Cardiovascular complications are a major cause of mortality in patients on renal replacement therapy. Cardiac causes account for about 40 per cent of all deaths, with vascular complications accounting for another 15 per cent. Death due to myocardial infarction and ischaemia is some 20 times more common than in a comparable general population; cerebrovascular accidents are 20 to 50 times more common. Hypertension, smoking, hyperlipidaemia (as in the general population), and uraemia itself have been established as being the major risk factors that should be addressed urgently and early in the course of chronic renal disease. Excessive gains of fluid between dialysis is another problem requiring regular attention (Table 4).

Technique survival and the need for admission to hospital

Problems that lead to a change in the method of renal replacement occur more commonly (by some 10–40 per cent) in CAPD than in haemodialysis. The major causes are peritonitis, catheter problems, loss of ultrafiltration, patient preference, and psychosocial causes. Elimination of peritonitis may well reduce the substantial differences in rates of failure between CAPD and haemodialysis. Hospital admissions are more frequent in CAPD than in haemodialysis patients (about 15 days/patient year of treatment on CAPD as opposed to 10 days/patient year of treatment on haemodialysis).

Chronic fluid overload and heart failure

Chronic overhydration is a long-term, and probably life-threatening complication leading to cardiovascular overload and increased mortality. The principal reasons for this are excess fluid intake and/or inadequate ultrafiltration. An increased cardiac output because of arteriovenous fistula, chronic anaemia, hypertension, or coronary artery disease also contribute to cardiac malfunction. Weight gain between haemodialysis sessions in excess of 3 kg is a predictor of poor survival, in addition to the immediate side-effects of rapid fluid removal, which can result in headaches, cramps, vomiting, and cardiovascular instability.

Hypertension

This persists in 25 to 30 per cent of patients treated by haemodialysis and to a lesser extent in patients treated by CAPD. Before resorting to long-term drug therapy, a trial of sodium and water removal is essential. The use of antihypertensive therapy in these patients is the same as in essential hypertension (Chapter 15.27).

β₂-Microglobulin and amyloidosis

β_2-Microglobulin is a light chain of the class 1 major histocompatibility antigen, composed of 100 amino acids (molecular weight 11 700). Less than 3 per cent of β_2-microglobulin is excreted extrarenally and its levels are elevated 20–40-fold in dialysis patients. Following prolonged intermittent dialysis (in excess of 5 years) there is a progressive increase in deposition of β_2-microglobulin amyloid at various sites, including the synovium, bone, carpal tunnel, and vertebrae. This results in carpal tunnel syndromes and chronic arthralgias, usually affecting the shoulders and other joints such as knees and small joints of the hands. Femoral neck fractures due to bone cysts can occur. There is no uniformly effective therapy although use of synthetic membranes can alleviate the symptoms. Renal transplantation is certainly helpful. This problem is similar in CAPD and haemodialysis, but better clearance of β_2-microglobulin can be achieved in the latter by use of synthetic membranes.

Malignant disease

The incidence of malignant disease is about three times higher in uraemic patients on dialysis then in age- and sex-matched controls. Some of the tumours are related to the cause of renal disease (for example, uroepithelial tumours in patients with analgesic nephropathy). Multiple renal adenocarcinomas also occur in the acquired cystic disease of endstage renal disease. In this disorder, which presents as renal or perirenal haemorrhage, multiple renal cysts and tumours are found after some years of dialysis, and death from metastatic malignancy has occurred.

QUALITY OF LIFE

As the techniques for treating endstage renal failure have greatly improved survival, quality of life issues have become an issue. Personal differences, the effects of ageing, and of coincident diseases (such as diabetes) make for difficulty in comparing different approaches to management—and it is all too difficult to define and measure quality of life. Successful renal transplantation undoubtedly achieves the best rehabilitation, which is complete in less than half the patients on dialysis, amongst which CAPD patients fare better than those on in-centre haemodialysis. Subjective measures of quality of life (as perceived by the patient) are not dissimilar to those of the general population, with little difference between dialysis modalities. Hitherto, employment and sexual activity in particular have been much reduced in dialysed patients, but the introduction of recombinant human erythropoietin (see Chapter 20.17.1) has improved the quality of life on dialysis quite remarkably.

REFERENCES

Ahlmen, J. and Kjellstrand, C. (ed.). (1990). Aspects of quality of life in renal replacement therapy and endstage renal disease. *Scandinavidan Journal of Urology and Nephrology* Supplement 131.

Diaz-Buxo, J.A. (1992). Is CAPD adequate longterm therapy for endstage renal disease? A critical assessment. *Journal of the American Society of Nephrology* **3**, 1039–48.

Dinarello, C.A. (1992). Cytokines: agents provocateurs in haemodialysis? *Kidney International* **41**, 683–94.

Dobbie, J. (1992). Pathogenesis of peritoneal fibrosing syndromes in peritoneal dialysis. *Peritoneal Dialysis International* **12**; 14–27. A review of peritoneal membrane changes based on a large international peritoneal biopsy registry.

Gokal, R. (1992). Peritoneal dialysis. In *Oxford Textbook of Clinical Nephrology,* (ed. S. Cameron, A. Davison, J.-P. Grunfeld, D.N.S. Kerr and E. Ritz), pp. 1466–505. Oxford University Press. A comprehensive review on peritoneal dialysis. This volume also has chapters on vascular access (pp. 1405–17); haemodialysis and complications (pp. 1417–36); and medical complications of long-term dialysis patients (pp. 1436–76).

Gokal, R. and Nolph, K.D. (1994) *Textbook of Peritoneal Dialysis.* Kluwer Academic Publishers, Amsterdam. A detailed, comprehensive book on peritoneal dialysis.

Gokal, R. *et al.* (1993). Peritoneal catheters and exit site practices: toward optimum peritoneal access. *Peritoneal Dialysis International* **13**, 29–39.

Henderson, L.W. and Jacobs, C. (ed.). (1992). Frontiers in renal disease. In *Kidney International* (Suppl. 38), **42**, S1–53 (Time, adequacy and mortality); S68–S100 (What's new in haemodialysis); S148–S171 (What's new in peritoneal dialysis). A special supplement issue of *Kidney International* covering the latest development and controversies in dialysis.

Keane, W.F. *et al.* (1993). Peritoneal dialysis related peritonitis treatment recommendations. *Peritoneal Dialysis International* **13**, 5–28.

Lindsay, R.M. *et al.* (1993). Contemporary management of renal failure. *Kidney International,* (Suppl. 41).

Mistry, C.D., Mallick, N.P., and Gokal, R. (1987). Ultrafiltration with an isosmotic solution during long peritoneal dialysis exchanges. *Lancet* **2**, 178–182. Landmark paper explaining the concept of colloid osmosis as applied to peritoneal dialysis.

Nelson, C.B., Port, F.K., Wolfe, R.A. and Guire, R. (1992). Comparison of CAPD and haemodialysis patient survival with evaluation of trends during the 1980s. *Journal of the American Society of Nephrology* **3**, 1147–55.

Steinman, T.I. (1992). Nutritional management of the chronic haemodialysis patient. **5**, 155–8.

United States Renal Data System, (1992). *Annual report*. Bethesda, National Institute of Health, National Institute of Diabetes and Digestive and Kidney Disease.

Van Holder, R.C. and Ringoir, S.M. (1992). Adequacy of dialysis: a critical analysis. *Kidney International* **42**, 540–58.

Winchester, J.F. *et al.* (1994). *Replacement of renal function by dialysis*, (4th edition). Kluwer Academic Publications, Amsterdam. A large multi-author book giving a comprehensive and detailed account of all aspects of dialytic therapies.

20.17.3 Renal transplantation

P. J. RATCLIFFE and D. W. R. GRAY

Assessment of patients prior to renal transplantation

Thirty years ago, renal transplantation was a risky and rather experimental treatment which was appropriate only for highly selected patients with chronic renal failure. With technical improvements and the availability of more effective immunosuppressive drugs, transplantation is now the treatment of choice for most patients with endstage renal failure. Patients from extremely disparate prognostic groups may benefit. For some, renal transplantation should be a relatively safe procedure; whereas for others it will be necessary to balance the chance of long-term improvement in quality of life against a significant risk of perioperative mortality. Such difficult decisions are compounded by the knowledge that the basic resource for transplantation, cadaver organs, is in limited supply. In contrast with cardiac or hepatic transplantation, the availability of dialysis means that renal transplantation is very rarely required as an emergency and time should be taken for careful medical assessment and for the advantages and disadvantages of dialysis or transplantation to be carefully considered. It is important for the patient to be aware of the possibility of failure, the side-effects of immunosuppressive drugs, and the need for very close monitoring in the first few months after transplantation.

Ideally, planning should begin as soon as irreversible renal failure is recognized so that renal transplantation can be performed before dialysis becomes necessary. Those suitable for transplantation should then enter a pool of waiting patients from which the most immunologically appropriate matches with cadaver grafts are determined and balanced against considerations of clinical urgency. Living, related donor transplantation is an alternative to that of cadaver, providing immunological advantages, and greater freedom in planning the exact time of transplantation.

GENERAL MEDICAL ASSESSMENT

Important considerations in preparing patients for renal transplantation are the assessment of medical fitness for major surgery and the anticipation of problems likely to arise from immunosuppression. Pre-existing diseases may interact with immunosuppressive treatment in several ways. Immune surveillance of malignant or infectious diseases is impaired. Metabolism of immunosuppressive drugs may be altered, and sensitivity to specific side-effects can be increased.

Cardiovascular disease

Chronic renal failure is associated with an increased incidence of vascular disease, which is particularly high in the elderly, in those presenting with renal failure from renovascular disease, and in patients with diabetic renal disease. Postoperative myocardial infarction is an important risk after renal transplantation and preoperative assessment must include a careful cardiovascular examination. However, coronary disease can be difficult to assess in chronic renal failure because coexisting hypertensive heart disease, anaemia, and mobility problems reduce the accuracy of exercise testing. Patients with symptoms of ischaemic heart disease will usually require coronary arteriography. It has also been argued that coronary angiography should be performed routinely on high-risk patients, such as those with diabetic renal disease, with a view to coronary revascularization prior to transplantation. Few centres possess the facilities for such a practice, and many perform renal transplantation without coronary arteriography in high-risk patients who are asymptomatic. Nevertheless, it is important to limit cardiovascular stress by use of perioperative blood transfusion or erythropoietin to avoid severe anaemia, by strict attention to accurate fluid balance, and by avoidance of hypoxaemia. Dependent on local facilities, an elective perioperative admission to the intensive care unit may be appropriate.

Vascular disease in the iliac vessels may also create difficulties with vascular anastomosis to the transplanted kidney. Calcification visible on a pelvic radiograph may alert the surgeon to potential difficulties; arteriography is required for definitive assessment.

Infectious disease

Active infection should always be treated before transplantation. Recurrent bacterial chest infections, such as occur in chronic bronchitis or bronchiectasis, are more difficult to treat when the patient is heavily immunosuppressed as early after transplantation; transplantation in the summer months may be appropriate in such cases. Recurrent urinary infections are more frequent after transplantation, but are usually easy to treat and rarely damage the graft. None of these conditions contraindicates transplantation, unless infection is active when the patient is called for surgery.

Certain viral infections require consideration. Cytomegalovirus infection (primary, reinfection or reactivation) is common after transplantation. Primary infection is generally more severe. Potential recipients should be tested for antibodies that indicate past infection. Those at risk of primary infection should be considered for vaccination and should, if possible, receive grafts and blood products from cytomegalovirus-negative donors. When heavy immunosuppression follows implantation of a cytomegalovirus-positive graft into a cytomegalovirus-negative recipient, the risk of serious disease is high and there should be a low threshold for treatment with ganciclovir.

Reactivation of herpes zoster in the form of shingles is common, and the patient's immune status should be determined prior to transplantation. Patients without antibodies should be immunized prior to transplantation, since primary infection (chicken pox) is dangerous in immunosuppressed patients.

Patients with past or present infection with hepatitis B virus require special consideration. Those with antibodies and without antigenaemia may lose immune status, develop antigenaemia, and become infectious. Liver disease almost certainly progresses more rapidly in infected individuals who are immunosuppressed. However, the rate of progression is rather variable, and liver biopsy is important assessing the likely outcome. Patients with more active and more advanced liver pathology do worst, and in these cases transplantation is inadvisable. Patients without such features may be transplanted and immunosuppressed although they have a high risk of chronic liver failure in the long term. Alcohol consumption compounds the injury and should be avoided. In units where the risk of infection is high, uninfected patients should be immunized prior to transplantation.

Patients being assessed for renal transplantation should be tested for human immunodeficiency virus (**HIV**) using appropriate guidelines. Since immunosuppression appears to hasten the progress of HIV infection, renal transplantation is rarely appropriate. Nevertheless, asymptomatic HIV-positive patients who have undergone renal transplantation, and others who have been infected by the graft, may remain asymptomatic for several years. In clinical acquired immunodeficiency syndrome (AIDS), immunosuppression arising from HIV infection does not prevent rejection. Immunosuppressive drugs accelerate disease, so transplantation is contraindicated.

Previous tuberculosis may be reactivated by immunosuppression. Many units give chemoprophylaxis with isoniazid during the first year of transplantation to those with a history of tuberculosis and those from countries where the incidence is high. The nematode worm *Strongyloides stercoralis* can cause potentially fatal disease due to hyperinfestation in immunosuppressed patients. In patients from endemic areas, such as the West Indies and the Far East, pretransplant assessment should include a search for infestation by examination of stool or duodenal aspiration. Treatment is with thiabendazole or mebendazole.

Some diseases make patients particularly susceptible to non-immu-

Table 1 *Drug interactions with cyclosporin A*

(a) Drugs which increase cyclosporin A levels
Major effects
Ketoconazole
Erythromycin
Diltiazem
Nicardipine
Verapamil
Minor or unproven interactions
Acetazolamide
Chloramphenicol
Ciprofloxacin
Colchicine
Fluconazole
Imipenem
Itraconazole
Methotrexate
Metoclopramide
Metronidazole
Omeprazole
Sex steroids
Methyltestosterone
Oxandrolone
Ethinyloestradiol
Danazol
Norethisterone
(b) Drugs which reduce cyclosporin A levels
Major effects
Rifampicin
Phenytoin
Phenobarbitone
Carbamazepine
Minor or unproven interactions
Cholestyramine
Ethambutol
Griseofulvin
Isoniazid
Sulphinpyrazone
(c) Drugs which may potentiate nephrotoxicity
Amphotericin B
Aminoglycosides
Non-steroidal anti-inflammatory agents
(d) Drugs whose metabolism is impaired by cyclosporin A
Lovastatin
Pravastatin
Simvastatin

nological side-effects from immunosuppressive drugs. Peptic ulcer was a common complication when patients were treated with high doses of steroids before the availability of H_2-antagonists. In patients with a history of ulcer disease, treatment and endoscopic demonstration of healing is required before transplantation. Prophylaxis with an H_2-antagonist is advisable for the first 6 months. Other patients in whom steroids may create particular difficulties are those with pre-existing osteoporosis or osteonecrosis, with psychiatric disease, diabetics, and children whose growth may be impaired. Since cyclosporin alone, or in combination with azathioprine, can provide effective immunosuppression, many units avoid the use of corticosteroids in such patients. Patients with pre-existing haematopoietic hypoplasias may be particularly susceptible to azathioprine. Cyclosporin metabolism is impaired in liver disease, and doses then need adjustment and monitoring with an assay specific for the parent compound. It is also important to note the possibility of interaction of cyclosporin or azathioprine with the patient's existing medications (Table 1).

Malignant disease

Transplantation of patients with a history of malignant disease raises the concern that immunosuppression will increase the risk of recurrence. Surveys have shown a much reduced incidence of tumour recurrence as the interval between cancer treatment and transplantation increases. These results form the basis of current practice, which is to wait 2 to 4 years after curative cancer therapy before transplantation.

RENAL ASSESSMENT

Few renal diseases constitute a contraindication to transplantation. Nevertheless, the underlying cause of renal failure should be determined as far as is possible. Implications for renal transplantation centre around the likelihood of associated extrarenal disease, urological problems, and the risk of recurrent disease in the graft.

Diseases with extrarenal manifestations

Diabetic renal disease is almost invariably associated with advanced extrarenal diabetic complications but life expectancy for patients with diabetic renal disease undergoing renal transplantation compares favourably with the results of maintenance dialysis. Nevertheless, renal transplantation does not halt the progression of diabetic complications. Limb amputation, myocardial infarction, and progressive retinopathy are common causes of serious morbidity and mortality. High doses of steroids are particularly poorly tolerated. These problems have led to attempts to replace pancreatic endocrine function using combined kidney and pancreas transplantation. Pancreatic graft survival rates are in the region of 70 per cent at 1 year, with most of the patients becoming independent of insulin. Even so, blood glucose control is not normal. Furthermore, it has not yet been possible to demonstrate an improvement in retinopathy or vascular disease, although some reduction in histological evidence of recurrent nephropathy and some improvement in neuropathy has been reported. The combined procedure is associated with increased operative morbidity and most units still manage diabetic patients with renal transplantation alone. Islet transplantation may offer a less risky alternative in the future.

Autoimmune renal diseases, such as antiglomerular basement membrane disease (Goodpasture's syndrome), polyarteritis, and Wegener's granulomatosis, all have important systemic manifestations. However, these diseases often remit and rarely cause important extrarenal problems after transplantation. This is also true of systemic lupus erythematosus; patients who have undergone prolonged relapsing and remitting courses often enter prolonged remission once endstage renal failure is reached and rarely present extrarenal problems after transplantation.

Other renal diseases which have specific implications for renal transplantation are renovascular disease, where generalized arterial disease may affect medical fitness and technical feasibility, and myeloma, where progressive disease may be hastened by immunosuppression. Extrarenal problems are also important in a number of relatively rare metabolic diseases. Anderson–Fabry disease (α-galactosidase A deficiency) results in glycosphingolipid deposition which affects endothelial cells, causing premature vascular disease. Enzyme replacement by the graft is inadequate to prevent progression. In primary hyperoxaluria, systemic oxalosis causes cardiac conduction defects, obliterative vasculitis, neuropathy, and osteosclerosis. These problems persist after transplantation and, in addition, oxalate deposition frequently damages the graft. The most frequent form of primary hyperoxaluria (type I) is due to alanine–glyoxylate aminotransferase deficiency; this enzyme is adequately replaced by liver transplantation and these patients should now be considered for combined hepatic and renal transplantation.

Recurrence of disease in the graft

Many types of primary glomerulonephritis, diabetic glomerulosclerosis, amyloidosis, and oxalosis recur in renal allografts, yet graft failure from recurrent disease is unusual. For instance, surveys of recurrent primary

glomerulonephritis have estimated the prevalence of recurrence at 6 to 27 per cent, but graft failure is very rarely reported. However, data are incomplete since proof of recurrent disease requires histological diagnosis of both primary renal disease and graft failure, and this is rarely achieved. The type of glomerulonephritis influences the risk of recurrence. In type II mesangiocapillary glomerulonephritis histological recurrence is almost universal but renal damage is only slowly progressive and the disease is compatible with good graft survival. Histological evidence of recurrence and haematuria is also common with IgA nephropathy although graft failure is again unusual. Nephrotic syndrome associated with focal segmental glomerulosclerosis may recur immediately and may lead to progressive renal failure. It is important, however, to distinguish this rather rare clinical syndrome from identical morphological lesions which commonly complicate other primary glomerular disease and other allograft pathologies.

Clinically important recurrence is most likely if primary glomerulonephritis has run an aggressive course immediately prior to transplantation, and it may then be wise to defer transplantation for 6 to 12 months after entry to a dialysis programme, particularly if living, related transplantation is planned. In the case of antiglomerular basement membrane disease, transplantation should be deferred until the antibody titre has declined. Native nephrectomy has not been shown to influence the development of recurrent disease.

Urological disease

This is rarely a contraindication to transplantation, although clearly an adequate urinary drainage system must be established. If necessary, implantation of the transplant ureter into a urinary diversion, such as an ileal or colonic conduit, is feasible but reconstructive surgery should be completed prior to transplantation. Dialysis patients with long-standing anuria have very small bladder capacity but normal bladder function returns rapidly with urine flow from a functioning transplant.

Pretransplant nephrectomy is occasionally required when large polycystic kidneys fill the entire abdominal cavity and hinder implantation of the graft. Nephrectomy is also indicated if the kidneys harbour a potential focus of sepsis. Kidneys containing staghorn calculi and grossly dilated systems will require removal, but asymptomatic recurrent urinary infection is not an indication for nephrectomy.

IMMUNOLOGICAL ASSESSMENT

Tissue typing

Both the ABO blood group antigens and the HLA system present potentially important barriers to transplantation. ABO incompatibility is associated with a high risk of hyperacute rejection but is easily avoided by blood grouping. The highly polymorphic HLA system presents much greater difficulty.

HLA antigens are cell-surface proteins which direct immune responses. In transplantation they provide the basis for allograft recognition and stimulation of the rejection response. There are two functionally and structurally distinct types of HLA molecule, termed class I and class II. The genes for both are situated on the short arm of chromosome 6, and for each there are several allelic systems, each of which is highly polymorphic. The class I systems are termed HLA A, B, and C, and those of class II, HLA DR, DQ, and DP. HLA molecules associate with endogenous and exogenous peptides; an immune response is stimulated by T-cell recognition of foreign peptide in association with HLA molecules. Normally, foreign peptide is generated from invading micro-organisms. In transplantation, either allo-HLA or other polymorphic molecules borne by the graft could act as a source of foreign peptide for presentation by host cells. However, the major allograft rejection response arises from direct recognition of allo-HLA molecules as foreign, whatever the associated peptide. Of particular importance is the direct recognition of graft class II HLA by helper T cells. Very large numbers of different host T-cells (1–2 per cent of the total repertoire) can recognize a particular foreign HLA molecule and the response is extremely powerful.

HLA matching and graft survival (Table 2)

HLA typing is performed using defined antisera in a lymphocyte cyto-toxicity test. Typing sera are incubated with the subject's lymphocytes and reactivity is detected by lysis following addition of complement. Unseparated peripheral blood lymphocytes or T lymphocytes are used as targets for class I typing, but because of restricted expression, B lymphocytes are required for class II typing. The procedure requires healthy lymphocytes, good-quality typing sera, and significant skill. Recently, methods have been developed to determine HLA polymorphisms by DNA analysis. Such methods may determine the DNA polymorphism directly or detect other polymorphisms which are commonly co-inherited with particular HLA genes. The optimum technique is still undecided, but DNA analysis is likely to offer improved reliability for some antigens. In addition, further subdivision is possible at the DNA level, but whether these subdivisions are important in allograft recognition remains to be determined.

In living, related transplantation a major effect of HLA matching on graft survival has long been clear. Across the HLA locus recombination is rare; consequently, within a family the whole HLA haplotype will almost always be inherited *en bloc*. Parents and offspring will share one haplotype; siblings will share both, one, or neither haplotype in a proportion 1 : 2 : 1. In patients receiving prednisolone and azathioprine, 1-year graft survival rates were greater than 90 per cent for HLA identical siblings, 70 to 80 per cent if one haplotype was shared, and approximately 60 per cent if neither was shared. These results have been substantially improved using cyclosporin, but although differences are less, they remain clear. More important perhaps, are graft 'half-life' estimates from audit of long-term survival. Estimated 'half-lives' are 25 years, 15 years, and 10 years for 'living, related' grafts sharing 2, 1, and 0 haplotypes. Even so, some HLA identical grafts are rejected despite immunosuppressive treatment, indicating that other antigens can elicit rejection. Equally, it is surprising that, in view of the powerful *in vitro* response to allo-HLA, graft survival can commonly be achieved even with complete mismatch of HLA antigens.

In the general population, particular sets of HLA genes at different loci often occur together, a phenomenon known as linkage disequilibrium. Despite this, recombination has been such that chromosomes which share alleles at one or more sites will most commonly differ at other sites within the HLA locus. Perhaps for this reason the advantage of matching at a particular locus has been more difficult to demonstrate in cadaver transplantation. Nevertheless, a consistent advantage is seen for matching at the DR locus. Improved graft survival at 1 year, reduced frequency of rejection crises, and more stable long-term graft function have all been reported, with increasing benefit for 2 versus 1 versus 0 DR matches. Large surveys have also provided evidence of apparently independent and additive effects for matching at HLA-B and HLA-A. Such matches are very uncommon in unrelated individuals. Tissue-typing laboratories therefore have to balance the expectations of improved results from HLA matching against the logistic difficulties presented by managing a large-enough pool of potential recipients to permit this approach.

Sensitization to HLA

Sensitization occurs from exposure to foreign HLA associated with blood transfusion, pregnancies, or previous allografts. An important feature is the production of circulating anti-HLA antibodies. Preformed complement-fixing antibodies against graft HLA can destroy the grafts in minutes or hours by hyperacute rejection. HLA antibodies also predict a high risk of graft loss from accelerated acute rejection involving cellular immune mechanisms. To monitor sensitization, sera are obtained from potential recipients and tested regularly for such antibodies using a panel of lymphocytes. Immediately prior to transplantation a cross-match test is performed against the donor's lymphocytes. A positive test

Table 2 *Some factors affecting long-term survival of transplanted kidneys*

		Predicted survival expressed as half-life in years
Source of graft		
Sibling (HLA identical)		32.9
Parent		11.2
Cadaver		10.3
Spouse/living unrelated		13.6
Recipient characteristics		
Original disease		
Polycystic kidneys		16.3
Glomerulonephritis		10.7
Juvenile diabetes		8.4
Gender		
Male → female		12.1
Male → male		10.4
Female → female		10.8
Female → male		8.1
Race		
Caucasian → Caucasian		10.3
Black → Caucasian		8.8
Caucasian → Black		4.7
Black → Black		4.6
HLA		
number of B, DR mismatches	0	18.0
(cadaver kidneys)	1	10.8
	2	9.7
	3	10.3
	4	8.8
Early function		
Dialysis at 1 week	Yes	7.7
	No	10.9

Data are from the United Network for Organ Sharing Kidney Transplant Registry, USA, by courtesy of Dr P. I. Terasaki. Half-life is calculated from the slope of the survival curve which is log-linear after the first year. Data are for first transplants in Caucasian recipients except when stated otherwise.

arising from IgG anti-HLA antibodies is a contraindication to transplantation. Highly sensitized patients react against most of the panel and will cross match positively against almost all potential donors. Unfortunately such patients, many of whom have had previous graft failures, are not infrequent and pose a major problem in transplantation. Several strategies have been applied to address the problem.

First, it has become clear that not all antibodies which react against donor lymphocytes reflect sensitization against HLA. For instance, autoantibodies reacting against non-HLA epitopes will generate a positive cross-match test but are quite benign. Characterization of the reactive antibody is therefore important in interpreting the cross match. Secondly, if a very large donor pool is used it may be possible to find a very closely matched graft which is cross-match negative. Thirdly, it is possible to remove antibodies prior to transplantation by plasmapheresis or immunoabsorption. This can permit more exact definition of the specificity of remaining antibodies, avoid hyperacute rejection, and enable successful transplantation in some cases.

Blood transfusion

Although blood transfusion can cause sensitization against allo-HLA antigens, it is also clear that it can reduce subsequent immune responses. In the 1970s it was observed that patients who had never received blood transfusions experienced substantially lower graft survival rates than did transfused patients. Following this demonstration, many units introduced a policy of deliberate blood transfusion in preparation for transplantation. More recent surveys have shown an overall improvement in graft survival and a smaller effect of transfusion, so that deliberate blood transfusion is now less frequently performed. The mechanism of improved graft survival is unknown. A few patients become sensitized and consequently will not receive grafts. However, the spurious effect created by removal of these few high-risk individuals from the pool cannot explain the large effect originally observed. In animal models, transfusion can lead to donor-specific unresponsiveness, but whether similar changes follow random transfusion of humans is not known.

Sources of kidneys

LIVING, RELATED KIDNEY DONATION

The ethical concerns regarding the practice of live donation of kidneys are complex, but the benefits to the recipient are clear. For related donations they include the immunological advantage of HLA haplotype matching and that of a planned surgical procedure conducted under optimal conditions.

Prospective donors must undergo thorough assessment, preferably by a physician who is not involved in the recipient's care. Assessment should confirm blood group compatibility, normal general health, and the presence of two kidneys with normal renal function, vascular supply, and urinary collecting systems. The donor should be free from vascular, malignant, or infectious diseases, including hepatitis B and C and HIV. Motivation should be carefully considered. Family pressures to donate a kidney are often very great and if there is a conflict it is appropriate to provide the donor with a medical 'opt out'.

The operation is performed via either a loin or midline incision and the potential donor should be aware that this is a major procedure in terms of the size of the incision, postoperative pain, and other surgical morbidity. Mortality has been carefully documented for western Europe and the USA, and is currently 1 : 3300. Apart from the remote risk of injury to the remaining single kidney, and occasional complications from adhesions, the long-term risk is very small, and kidney donors are accepted as normal risk by life insurance companies. Large follow-up surveys for as long as 20 years have not discerned evidence of functional sequelae such as hypertension or hyperfiltration renal injury following unilateral nephrectomy in this or other settings.

Improvements in immunosuppression could alter the indications for living, related transplantation. First, it has been argued that much improved results from cadaver renal transplantation should reduce the indication for living, related transplantation. On the other hand, long-term function is considerably better for living, related grafts. The advantage is large for HLA identical grafts, but very good long-term graft survival figures have been reported even for live donor HLA mismatched grafts. This has led some groups to perform transplants between genetically unrelated individuals such as spouses, with a high level of success.

CADAVERIC ORGAN DONATION

The medicolegal, ethical, and religious issues surrounding cadaveric organ donation vary from country to country and are beyond the scope of the present text. However, in western Europe and the United States cadaveric organ donation is actively sought from all patients declared dead due to brain-stem death.

The commonest cause of death leading to organ donation is head trauma, followed by primary cerebral haemorrhage. All age-groups are potentially suitable for organ donation and the only firm contraindications are serious infections (HIV, hepatitis B and C, severe bacterial infection) and past or present extracranial malignancy. Minor chest or urinary infections, benign tumours, and primary intracranial malignancies, are not absolute contraindications and should be discussed with the

transplant team. Even abnormal organ function, such as moderately impaired renal function, may not be a contraindication if the cause is likely to be reversible.

Brain-stem death

The concept of brain-stem death arose out of the need to define death in comatose patients receiving ventilatory support. Brain-stem death therefore defines death as a state in which there is irreversible loss of the capacity for consciousness, combined with irreversible loss of the capacity to breath. Clinical tests can reliably indicate brain-stem death but it is absolutely necessary to establish a set of preconditions. It is vital to realize that unless these preconditions have been fulfilled, and certain exclusions met, a diagnosis of brain-stem death cannot even be considered. The United Kingdom code of practice is summarized as follows:

1. Preconditions:
   (a) comatose patient on a ventilator,
   (b) establishment of an unequivocal diagnosis of the cause of coma.
2. Exclusions:
   (a) hypothermia,
   (b) all depressant drugs,
   (c) severe metabolic disturbances.
3. Tests of brain-stem function:
   (a) no pupillary response,
   (b) absent corneal reflex,
   (c) absent vestibulo-ocular reflexes,
   (d) no cranial nerve motor response to painful stimuli,
   (e) no gag reflex,
   (f) no respiratory movement with $PaCO_2$ above 6.65 kPa (50 mmHg).

Most countries specify that tests should be performed on two occasions to exclude the possibility of error. Once a diagnosis of brain-stem death has been made it is appropriate to issue a death certificate; if organs are to be donated then the operation should be conducted as soon as is practical.

Where legislation allows the organ donation procedure to be carried out while the donor's heart continues to beat, perfusion with oxygenated blood can be maintained while the organs are dissected and prepared for rapid cooling by the insertion of aortic and caval perfusion catheters. Particular care is required in the renal dissection to avoid damage to accessory vessels or to the ureteric blood supply.

The perfusion fluid used is a buffered, hypertonic electrolyte solution, usually containing an impermeant solute to reduced ischaemic cell swelling. The kidneys are removed when cool and stored cold (usually in an ice-cooled box, but sometimes on a special perfusion machine). The stored kidneys undergo slow deterioration during cold storage, but are usable for up to 3 to 4 days, although transplantation within 24 to 36 h is preferred. Transport of the kidney to other centres is possible and is frequently arranged by national co-ordinating organizations.

Operative management

Patients selected for a cadaveric transplant may wait for a time varying from a few days to many years before a suitable kidney becomes available, depending on factors such as blood group, HLA type and sensitization, and donor kidney supply. When there has been delay a thorough history and examination will be necessary, particularly to exclude adverse events that may have occurred during the waiting period, such as cardiac ischaemia or recent infection. Care should also be taken to ensure that there has been no unrecorded blood transfusion, since this may have induced sensitization against HLA.

Many patients require dialysis before surgery to reduce the likelihood of such treatment in the early postoperative period, when anticoagulation, hypotension, and fluid shifts could endanger a newly anastomosed transplant kidney. Excessive dehydration should be avoided during this procedure and the postdialysis weight should be recorded, to help in determination of postoperative fluid balance. Preoperative viral serology as well as routine haematological and biochemical investigations should be performed. Some immunosuppressive agents and prophylactic antibiotics will usually be given preoperatively. Diuretics and mannitol are commonly given just before revascularization, to promote diuresis.

During surgery the graft is anastomosed to the iliac vessels, using an incision in the iliac fossa that divides the abdominal muscles and allows an extraperitoneal approach, thus preserving the option of subsequent peritoneal dialysis. If possible, a patch of aorta, termed a Carrel patch, is left attached to the to the donor renal artery and used to anastomose the graft to the side of the external iliac artery. Multiple arteries may then be simply dealt with by using a larger patch. Otherwise the anastomosis is made to the recipient internal iliac artery end-to-end. The venous anastomosis is usually to an accessible portion of the external iliac vein. The ureter is anastomosed to the bladder using a tunnelling technique to prevent reflux. If there is insufficient length of viable ureter, anastomosis to the donor ureter is possible.

POSTOPERATIVE FLUID BALANCE AND MONITORING

Maintenance of accurate fluid balance is important. Generally, attempts are made to optimize graft perfusion and urine flow by maintenance of a high central venous pressure by infusion of colloid. Should unexpectedly large volumes be required, the possibility of haemorrhage should be considered. In patients with impaired cardiac function care is required to avoid pulmonary oedema. Urine output is measured hourly and replaced with crystalloid, generally given as isotonic saline and 5 per cent dextrose in a 2:1 ratio. When the urine output is very high it is helpful to measure its electrolyte content and match it in the crystalloid infusion. Dopamine infusion and frusemide may be given if urine output is low. Although they will usually increase urine flow, their protective action against acute tubular necrosis is uncertain. Acute tubular necrosis has little effect on eventual outcome but immediate function avoids the need for dialysis in the postoperative period and the presence of a urine output provides a useful means of monitoring for complications.

Careful monitoring of cardiorespiratory stability is required. Clearance of drugs and their metabolites by the transplanted kidney is variable and postoperative respiratory depression is a risk. For instance, if morphine is used, retention of the metabolite morphine-6-glucuronide may lead to severe respiratory depression. Hypotension should be avoided by appropriate volume replacement and dopamine infusion if necessary. Hypertension requires treatment only if severe; sublingual nifedipine is then usually effective.

TECHNICAL PROBLEMS

Haemorrhage

This usually occurs within 12 h postoperatively. Reduction in urine output and low central venous pressure which fails to respond promptly to colloid infusion should suggest this possibility. The diagnosis is rapidly confirmed by ultrasound showing a large perigraft haematoma. Early operation usually permits correction of the bleeding source.

Vascular thrombosis

This may be arterial or venous. Arterial thrombosis usually occurs early, either immediately after transplantation or in the first few postoperative days. There is abrupt loss of function; but other signs are often unremarkable. The diagnosis can be confirmed by ultrasound and isotopic scans, showing no pulsation and no perfusion. Fine-needle aspiration cytology or Trucut biopsy confirms necrosis. Venous thrombosis also occurs early but is sometimes observed in the first few weeks after transplantation, even in grafts with previously good function. The presentation is often dramatic with loss of function, pain, and swelling of the graft. The ipsilateral leg may be swollen, and bruising of the wound and flank may become apparent if the patient is left untreated: some cases

progress to graft rupture with life-threatening haemorrhage. Occasionally early venous thrombectomy is possible, but usually there is no alternative to graft nephrectomy. The aetiology of vascular thrombosis is not clear and it is of concern that venous thrombosis, in particular, appears to have become more frequent. Complex vascular anastomoses, postoperative haemodynamic instability, and cyclosporin may predispose, but cases occur in which none of these risk factors operate.

Postoperative infection

As with other surgery, there is the risk of infection of the wound, chest, urinary system, and sites of intravenous cannulation. Fortunately, these infections have become less common with reduced steroid dosage, good surgical technique, and prophylactic antibiotics.

Urinary leakage

Most commonly, urinary leakage arises from ischaemic necrosis of the lower end of the ureter, which is vulnerable because of its blood supply from the renal artery. Since the integrity of an ischaemic ureter is not lost immediately, presentation is usually delayed until after the first postoperative week. Symptoms include suprapubic or penile pain and swelling, although the signs are not always striking. A localized collection of urine can be visualized by ultrasound; biochemical analysis of aspirated fluid for urea and creatinine will prove urinary origin. Within the first postoperative week, urinary leak usually indicates a faulty ureteric implantation but can arise from blockage of the urinary catheter or placement of a drain injudiciously close to the ureterocystostomy. Catheter replacement or partial withdrawal of the drain may sometimes solve the problem.

Lymphocoele

Severed lymphatics may cause a lymphatic collection termed a lymphocele. A large collection causes swelling of the leg by pressure on the iliac vein or reduction in graft function by pressure on the ureter. Aspiration will relieve obstruction; definitive treatment is by surgical fenestration to drain the lymph into the peritoneal cavity.

DIAGNOSIS OF INITIAL NON-FUNCTION

Many grafts do not function immediately because of postischaemic acute tubular necrosis. Such kidneys will recover spontaneously and have a good long-term prognosis. Early failure of graft function may also arise from rejection, vascular thrombosis, ureteric obstruction, or cyclosporin nephotoxicity, and any of these conditions can supervene in a graft with pre-existing acute tubular necrosis. Isotope renography is used to measure vascular perfusion and to exclude major vessel occlusion; obstruction is demonstrated by retention of isotope in the pelvis. Good perfusion and lack of obstruction usually indicates acute tubular necrosis when immunosuppression with cyclosporin is generally reduced or substituted entirely by antithymocyte globulin or monoclonal antibodies, since cyclosporin can greatly delay recovery from acute tubular necrosis. Particular vigilance is required to detect and treat rejection. In unsensitized patients rejection is unusual in the first week, but many will have had contact with allo-HLA antigens through pregnancy, transfusion, or previous grafts; they are liable to early rejection and since graft function cannot be monitored, diagnosis is difficult. Fine-needle aspiration cytology of the graft can be performed within the first week, but biopsy is usually deferred until 7 days after transplantation. There should be low threshold for treatment for possible rejection and increased immunosuppression is often given prophylactically to recipients at high risk.

Immunosuppression and rejection
IMMUNOSUPPRESSIVE TREATMENT

With the exception of transplants between identical twins, rejection is a universal response and will almost always destroy the graft unless controlled by immunosuppression. Cyclosporin, a cyclic peptide of fungal origin, has made a major contribution to improved results over those previously achieved by the combination of prednisolone and azathioprine. A similar drug, FK506, has recently proved to be a very effective immunosuppressant, but whether or not it will provide a further advantage in renal transplantation is still to be determined. Most units currently use cyclosporin as the main agent, at least in the first 6 months, usually together with azathioprine, prednisolone, or both these drugs in a combination termed 'triple therapy'. Immunosuppressive drugs are commenced just prior to the operation. Antilymphocyte sera, antithymocyte sera, or anti-T-cell monoclonal antibodies may also be used to provide additional or alternative immunosuppression for limited periods. This approach is used to provide more powerful and immediate immunosuppression in sensitized patients or to avoid the effects of cyclosporin nephrotoxicity on the postischaemic grafted kidney.

During the course of the first year the risk of rejection declines, and doses of immunosuppressive drugs are gradually reduced. Maintenance doses are usually in the range, prednisolone 5–12.5 mg once daily, azathioprine 1 to 2.5 mg/kg, cyclosporin 3 to 5 mg/kg, the dose depending on the perceived risk of rejection and whether the drugs are used singly or in combination. The exact requirements for long-term immunosuppression are unclear. Withdrawal of cyclosporin with continued prednisolone and azathioprine has been associated with acute rejection in 10 to 30 per cent of patients. Withdrawal of prednisolone is less commonly associated with acute rejection but is not without risk. The need for long-term immunosuppression is currently the major drawback of renal transplantation. Since it was first demonstrated in animals by Medawar and colleagues 50 years ago, the induction of specific graft tolerance has been one of the main areas of research in transplantation biology, but the good results obtained in animal experiments are not yet applicable to man.

Cyclosporin nephrotoxicity

A central feature is vasoconstriction of the afferent arterioles of the glomeruli, leading to a persistent reduction in renal blood flow and glomerular filtration rate. Acute nephrotoxicity is due to an exacerbation of these changes, usually in association with high blood levels of the drug. The haemodynamic changes can be reversed by drug withdrawal even after a year or more of exposure. However, histological evidence of fibrosis indicates that the damage is not all reversible, and concern has been raised that progressive damage might seriously reduce allograft survival. Nevertheless, recent data suggest that improved immunosuppression obtained by the use of cyclosporin most likely outweighs this disadvantage. Hypertension is also commonly observed with therapeutic doses of the drug; sodium retention is an important component and vasoconstrictive effects outside the renal circulation may also contribute. Cyclosporin also causes a thrombotic tendency. It is quite probable that these effects all stem from a direct action of cyclosporin on vascular endothelium.

CLINICAL FEATURES OF REJECTION

Relatively distinct patterns of clinical presentation are observed.

Hyperacute rejection

This is now exceedingly rare. Loss of function occurs within minutes or hours of revascularization, due to the action of preformed complement-fixing antibodies against donor MHC (major histocompatibility complex). Graft loss is inevitable.

Acute rejection

Acute rejection was characterized classically by fever, painful swelling of the graft, and abruptly reduced function. In patients receiving cyclosporin this reaction is less dramatic and is often detected simply from a progressive rise in the plasma creatinine. Alternative diagnoses include urinary obstruction and cyclosporin nephrotoxicity, the latter favoured by high blood levels of cyclosporin. Lower levels, fever, and severe reduction in graft function all suggest rejection, but it is important to realize that rejection and cyclosporin nephrotoxicity may coexist. Aspiration cytology or graft biopsy demonstrating an immune cell infiltrate provides evidence of rejection and tubules may show regions of damage. Vascular abnormalities and interstitial haemorrhage are poor prognostic signs.

In the initial 3 to 6 months after transplantation acute rejection remains common, and more than 50 per cent of patients experience at least one episode. Thereafter the frequency declines, although episodes can occur even years later, then usually associated with withdrawal or reduction in immunosuppressive therapy. Most episodes of acute rejection respond well to treatment, and overall more than 90 per cent of episodes are reversed. In the first instance a short course of high-dose steroids is given. Resistant episodes may be treated with antithymocyte globulin or the monoclonal antibody OKT3.

Chronic rejection

This is a poorly understood entity which is clinically manifest by a gradual but progressive rise in serum creatinine associated with the development of proteinuria. Histological examination shows vascular changes, particularly intimal proliferation, together with fibrosis and tubular atrophy. Lymphocytic infiltration may be present but is not as striking as in acute rejection. This picture is most commonly seen in grafts which have already suffered early damage from acute rejection. It is not clear that progressive reduction in graft function is entirely due to immune rejection. Other possibilities include hyperfiltration injury, recurrent nephritis, and cyclosporin nephrotoxicity. The condition does not respond to increased immunosuppression.

Medical problems in transplanted patients

INFECTION (SEE ABOVE)

Changes in the use of immunosuppressive drugs have been associated with a shift in the spectrum of infectious complications. The incidence of wound infection and bacterial sepsis has decreased in line with reduction in corticosteroid dosage, whereas the introduction of cyclosporin A has been associated with an increased risk of specific infections with organisms which are normally controlled by T-cell immunity, such as cytomegalovirus and *Pneumocystis carinii*.

Infections which are common in the general population may present at any time after transplantation. Apart for the need for urgency in diagnosis and treatment, management is conducted along usual lines. Early infections most commonly arise from the surgical procedure. Opportunistic infections associated with immunosuppression usually present after the first month and they are most prevalent between 1 and 6 months postoperatively. The peak period of risk is offset with respect to the peak dose of immunosuppression, and particular vigilance is required in the weeks that follow a period of heavy immunosuppression. Important opportunistic infections are listed in Table 3, together with specific aspects of diagnosis and management. In the early period after renal transplantation patients should keep a daily record of temperature. The differential diagnosis of fever includes graft rejection, usually reflected by a rise in serum creatinine.

The diagnosis of many infections involving organisms which are difficult to culture is based on serum antibody responses. Antibody production can be delayed or reduced by immunosuppression. In general, positive responses are helpful but negative results provide insecure evidence against infection. The leucocytosis which is usually observed in bacterial infection may be blunted by azathioprine.

Fever with hypotension in an ill patient indicates probable bacterial septicaemia and requires immediate antibiotic treatment. The urinary tract is the commonest source. In contrast, certain viral infections will generate very high fever which is well tolerated. Striking remittant fever, leucopenia, and raised AST of hepatic origin are typical of cytomegalovirus infection.

The lungs, cranial sinuses, and the cerebrospinal fluid are important sites of opportunistic infections. Lumbar puncture and sinus radiographs should be performed in cases of diagnostic uncertainty.

Table 3 *Some opportunistic infections in renal transplant recipients*

Organisms	Common sites of infection	Treatment
Bacteria		
Mycobacterium tuberculosis	Lung/disseminated	Triple therapy (note drug interactions)
Nocardia	Lung/CNS/disseminated	Co-trimoxazole
Fungi		
Aspergillus	Lung/CNS	Amphotericin B
Candida	Disseminated/gastrointestinal tract/lung	± 5-h flucytosine
Cryptococcus	CNS/lung	
Parasites		
Pneumocystis	Lung	Co-trimoxazole
Strongyloides	Disseminated	Thiobendazole/albendazole
Toxoplasma	CNS	Sulphadiazine + pyrimethamine
Histoplasma	Lung	Amphotericin (itraconazole)
Viruses		
Cytomegalovirus	Lung/liver/disseminated	Gancyclovir
Herpes zoster	Skin/disseminated/lung	Acyclovir (high dose)

Early diagnosis of opportunistic pneumonia is a particular challenge. Dry cough and dyspnoea are important symptoms but are not always present; crepitations may be present but chest examination can be normal. Diffuse lung infiltrates can easily be overlooked on a chest radiograph unless careful comparison is made with previous films. Impairment of gas exchange detected by arterial gas analysis is an important pointer to pulmonary pathology. Since the differential diagnosis is wide and specific treatment is required for many pathogens, microbiological diagnosis is of paramount importance. Lavage specimens collected at fibreoptic bronchoscopy have a high diagnostic yield and should be obtained early in all cases of undiagnosed pulmonary infiltration.

Infection with *Pneumocystis carinii* is particularly frequent, and many units give prophylaxis with co-trimoxazole or nebulized pentamidine for the first 6 months after transplantation.

Urinary infections

These are common after transplantation, particularly in females. Although they are generally uncomplicated and often asymptomatic, septicaemia or graft pyelonephritis may occur. The risk is greater early after transplantation and with polycystic, calculus, or pyelonephritic disease of the native kidneys. In the first year after transplantation, urine should be cultured frequently and bacteriuria treated promptly. Recurrent symptomatic infections may require long-term suppressive antibiotic treatment, but recurrent asymptomatic infection is apparently benign and there is no established benefit from treatment.

Dermatological infections

Fungal infections occurring after transplantation include candidiasis, pityriasis versicolor, and dermatophyte infection of skin and nails. Treatment with topical antifungal agents is along conventional lines (see Section 23). Resistant cases sometimes require systemic treatment. It should be noted that ketoconazole blocks the metabolism of cyclosporin.

Warts, caused by the human papilloma virus, are extremely common and affect more than 50 per cent of long-term transplant patients. It is likely that they contribute to the risk of squamous cell carcinoma, and the two lesions may be difficult to distinguish. If atypical warts recur following treatment, histological examination is required.

Reactivation of herpes simplex and herpes zoster is common. Most herpes simplex reactivations are confined to labial and oral lesions, and will respond to topical acyclovir. Systemic treatment is indicated for inaccessible or disseminated disease. Reactivation of herpes zoster gives rise to the typical dermatomal rash of shingles. Since there is an increased risk of generalized disease, systemic acyclovir is indicated. Chickenpox is rare but dangerous; systemic antiviral treatment and immune globulin are indicated.

GASTROINTESTINAL PROBLEMS

Peptic ulceration

Peptic ulceration and its complications are now seen much less commonly than in the past, probably because of reduced corticosteroid usage. Never the less, patients with a history of peptic ulcer should receive prophylactic H_2-antagonists for the first 6 months after transplantation and persistent symptoms should be investigated by endoscopy.

Chronic liver disease

Persistent biochemical abnormalities of liver function are common in renal transplant recipients, but the aetiology and clinical significance is unclear. Some units have reported a substantial mortality from chronic liver disease in long-term renal transplant patients but this has been rare in others. Both azathioprine and cyclosporin A have the potential for hepatotoxicity, but the extent to which they contribute to the problem is not known. The incidence of chronic infection with hepatitis viruses B and C varies widely according to prevalence in the community. Although there is agreement that hepatitis B infection progresses more rapidly in immunosuppressed patients, very widely differing experiences of the prognosis in transplanted patients have been reported, and reasons for these differences are not understood.

BONE DISEASE (SEE CHAPTER 20.18)

In most cases, renal osteodystrophy improves rapidly following successful renal transplantation. The new kidney provides a source of 1α-hydroxylase and the excretory function to restore phosphate balance. Healing is manifest by a rise in serum alkaline phosphatase which gradually subsides over the months following transplantation. Quite commonly, however, parathyroid hormone levels remain modestly elevated, and 5 to 10 per cent of transplant patients have persistent, mild, asymptomatic hypercalcaemia. The benefits, or otherwise, of parathyroidectomy in these asymptomatic patients are unknown; in rare cases severe hypercalcaemia and its adverse effects dictate the need for parathyroidectomy.

The effect of transplantation on other components of renal bone diseases is less clear. Aluminium accumulation is cleared slowly over months or years. Symptoms from dialysis amyloid improve early after transplantation, but deposits remain and the natural history of this disease after transplantation is still unknown.

Corticosteroid medication causes osteonecrosis and osteoporosis. The risk of osteonecrosis is closely related to the dose of steroids. The weight-bearing joints (hips, knees, and the ankles), are most commonly affected.

ERYTHROCYTOSIS

Eythrocytosis develops in 10 to 20 per cent of patients. The peak incidence occurs around 1 year after transplantation. Many, but not all, cases remit over subsequent years. Usually the cause is dysregulated erythropoietin produced by the native kidneys, and the prevalence is highest in patients with polycystic native kidneys. The risks are not clear but most units venesect patients to maintain the packed cell volume below 0.55. Converting enzyme inhibitions and theophylline reduce the erythrocytosis by reducing erythopoietin production, but the benefits of these approaches are unknown.

MALIGNANT DISEASE

The increased risk of certain forms of cancer is most probably a consequence of immunosuppression *per se*. The pattern of tumour occurrence is well defined and similar to that observed in other states of immunodeficiency. Risk is correlated with the degree of immunosuppression, and sometimes tumours regress when immunosuppression is reduced. Particular cancers occur at a high frequency in transplanted patients. The incidence for some, such as lymphoma and squamous-cell carcinoma of the skin, is in the region of 20 to 50 times that observed in the general population, and contrasts strikingly with tumours of bronchus, breast, prostate, and colon which have been observed only slightly more commonly in transplant recipients. It is interesting that for many of the tumours that are more frequent after transplantation there is evidence of a viral component in the aetiology.

Lymphoma

In contrast with the pattern of disease observed in the general population, lymphoma in transplanted patients is most commonly a non-Hodgkin type, of B-cell origin. Extranodal disease, particularly affecting the central nervous system, is unusually common. The Epstein–Barr virus is strongly implicated in the aetiology; there is usually serological evidence of Epstein–Barr virus activity, and the viral DNA can be detected in the tumours. The risk is higher in Epstein–Barr virus-negative recipients of kidneys from Epstein–Barr virus-positive donors.

Although lymphoma may occur at any stage after transplantation, the peak incidence is in the first 6 months. The recent use of more powerful immunosuppressive agents has been associated with an increased incidence. High doses of cyclosporin A carry this risk, but the most striking association is with the use of large doses of anti-T-cell immunotherapy such as the monoclonal antibody OKT3. Lymphomas developing in this setting may be monoclonal or polyclonal. In addition to conventional treatment with radiotherapy and cytotoxic chemotherapy, reduction in immunosuppression is an important component of treatment and, in a few cases, has led to regression of the lymphoma without other specific treatment. The antiviral agent acyclovir may also contribute to therapy.

Skin malignancy

Squamous-cell carcinoma of the skin is the commonest malignancy in renal transplant patients (Plate 1). Related or premalignant conditions, such as solar keratoses, keratoacanthoma, and Bowen's disease, are also common. Malignant melanoma is also more common than in the general population. Not only is the frequency of squamous-cell carcinoma much increased, but the tumours may be unusually aggressive. Spread to local lymph nodes and more distant sites occurs in a significant minority of patients and death may result. Solar damage undoubtedly contributes to the aetiology and all transplanted patients should be advised to limit sun exposure and wear protective creams. There is a clear association with warts, but the exact role played by the papilloma virus is unknown. The incidence is strikingly related to ethnicity, being most frequent in Caucasians of fair complexion. Older patients are more susceptible and prevalence increases strikingly with the duration of immunosuppression. In the United Kingdom about 25 per cent of patients transplanted for more than 10 years will have suffered at least one squamous-cell carcinoma. It is too early to know precisely whether immunosuppression with cyclosporin A carries any less risk, but current data suggest that the risk is not dissimilar from that in patients receiving long-term azathioprine and corticosteroids.

Kaposi's sarcoma

This tumour accounts for about 6 per cent of reported post-transplant malignancies, a prevalence which is several hundred fold greater than that in the general Caucasian population. A viral aetiology has been suspected on epidemiological grounds, but has not been proven. Ethnic or geographical predisposition is striking, the majority of cases occurring in subjects of Arabic, Jewish, Mediterranean, or African origin, even though such groups form only a small proportion of the transplanted population. The tumour usually regresses if immunosuppression is reduced or withdrawn.

Anogenital carcinoma

Tumours in this region occur more frequently than in the general population and a younger age-group is affected. There is, however, a long latency following transplantation, with reported carcinoma of the perineum occurring a mean of 8 years following transplantation. The vagina, vulva, perianal skin, penis, and scrotum may be affected. Disease is more common in women.

Carcinoma of the cervix

Carcinoma *in situ* of the uterine cervix is commoner in transplanted patients and affects younger women than in the general population. The incidence of invasive carcinoma is also increased. It is recommended that adult female transplant recipients receive annual cervical smear tests.

VASCULAR DISEASE

Atheromatous disease is the leading cause of death in renal transplant patients. Coronary disease, peripheral vascular disease, and cerebrovascular disease all occur more frequently, and at a younger age, than in the general population. Vascular disease prior to transplantation is common and, as might be expected, this is a strong predictor of vascular complications after it. However, the high incidence of progressive disease many years after transplantation indicates that there must be additional contributory causes in the long-term post-transplantation period. Large epidemiological studies, such as those which established hypercholesterolaemia, hypertension, and smoking as factors for vascular disease in the general population, are not feasible in the much smaller and less homogeneous transplanted population. Nevertheless, there is every reason to suppose that these same risk factors do operate in renal transplant patients, and they are certainly common. Hypertension, hyperlipidaemia, obesity, insulin resistance, and hyperuricaemia are all more prevalent in transplanted patients than in the general population. Many of these changes are drug induced.

Hyperlipidaemia

This typically consists of a combination of raised total and low-density lipoprotein-associated cholesterol, together with raised triglyceride levels. Both corticosteroid and cyclosporin can cause these abnormalities, and in each case the effect is dose dependent. Hyperlipidaemia is most severe early after transplantation when doses of immunosuppressive drugs are high. Since blood cholesterol will interact with other risk factors over most of its range, there is a strong case that all patients with multiple risk factors should attempt dietary reduction of cholesterol, unless other life-threatening disease is present. Drug treatment for hyperlipidaemia must be determined for individual patients on the perceived balance of risks.

Hypertension

More than 50 per cent of renal transplant recipients are hypertensive. Aetiological factors are immunosuppressive drug therapy, the presence of diseased native kidneys, and dysfunction of the grafted kidney. Cyclosporin and corticosteroids both increase blood pressure in a dose-dependent manner, and the prevalence of hypertension is particularly high in patients receiving both drugs. The existence of a persisting pressor effect from the native kidneys is indicated by the lower prevalence of hypertension in patients who have undergone bilateral native nephrectomies prior to transplantation. In cases of severe post-transplant hypertension, native kidney nephrectomy or embolization can reduce blood pressure. Such treatment is not without risk and is reserved for resistant cases.

The function of the allograft is of great importance in determining blood pressure. Patients in whom rejection has resulted in chronically impaired graft function have a much greater prevalence of severe hypertension. Graft artery stenosis is a less common but important cause of post-transplant hypertension, since cure may follow angioplasty or surgical repair. When graft arteriography is performed on all patients, the incidence of radiographic abnormality may approach 25 per cent. However, in only a fraction of these patients is the stenosis haemodynamically significant. Impaired function in a graft which shows little histological damage will suggest that a coincident stenosis is haemodynamically significant. In other cases of transplant renal artery stenosis, glomerular capillary pressure, and hence glomerular filtration rate, is maintained by efferent arteriolar vasoconstriction. Administration of an angiotensin-converting enzyme inhibitor will block this compensation and promptly reduce the glomerular filtration rate. Such a response is a good predictor of improvement following surgical correction.

The medical management of hypertension in transplanted patients is similar to that of hypertension in the general population, but some aspects do differ. The common coexistence of multiple risk factors probably justifies a slightly lower threshold for treatment. However, as with the general population, it is important to distinguish sustained hypertension from spurious rises in the clinic. Home or ambulatory recordings are useful in cases of uncertainty. It should also be remembered that hypertension may ameliorate as immunosuppressive drugs are reduced towards the end of the first year after transplantation.

Sodium retention is an important component of hypertension induced by cyclosporin. Moderate dietary sodium restriction (60–80 mmol/day) can be useful in reducing the need for diuretics in such patients. It has been argued that calcium-channel-blocking drugs carry particular advantages in patients receiving cyclosporin, and in some studies their use has been associated with better graft function. No proof of advantage in the long term has yet been obtained. It should be noted that diltiazem and verapamil reduce the metabolic clearance of cyclosporin. Angiotensin-converting enzyme inhibitors are also very effective. Because of the risk of sudden reduction in the function of graft with arterial stenosis, careful monitoring of serum creatinine in the days following introduction of this medication is mandatory. However, most patients without graft arterial stenosis tolerate such drugs well.

Overall attention towards reducing the known risk factors for vascular disease is of particular importance in transplanted patients who must be strongly advised not to smoke, to take regular exercise, and to avoid obesity.

REFERENCES

Allen, R.D.M. and Chapman, J.R. (1994). *A manual of renal transplantation.* Edward Arnold, London.

Burdick, J.F., Racusen, L.C., Solez, K., and Williams, G.M. (1992). *Kidney transplant rejection: diagnosis and treatment,* (2nd edn) Marcel Dekker, New York.

Cameron, J.S., Davison, A.M., Grunfield, J.-P., Kerr, D., and Ritz, E., eds. (1992). *Oxford textbook of clinical nephrology.* Section 11 *The transplant patient.* Oxford University Press.

Curtis, J.J. (1993). Management of hypertension after transplantation. *Kidney International,* **43,** S45–49.

Frey, F. (1991). Pharmacokinetic determinants of cyclosporine and prednisolone in renal transplant patients. *Kidney International,* **39,** 1034–50.

Higgins, R.M. and Ratcliffe, P.J. (1991). Hypercholesterolaemia and vascular disease after transplantation. *Transplantation Reviews,* **5, 131–49.**

Mathew, T.H. (1991). Recurrent disease after renal transplantation. *Transplantation Reviews,* **5,** 31–45.

Morris, P.J., ed. (1994). *Kidney transplantation. Principles and practice* (4th edn) W.B. Saunders Co., Philadelphia.

Rubin, R.H. (1993). Infectious disease complications of renal transplantation. *Kidney International,* **44,** 221–36.

Schmahl, D. and Penn, I. eds. (1991). *Cancer in organ transplant recipients.* Springer-Verlag, Berlin.

Stephanian, E., Gruber, S.A. Dunn, D.L., and Matas, A.J. (1991). Posttransplant lymphoproliferative disorders. *Transplantation Reviews,* **5**(2), 120–9.

Terasaki, P.I., ed. (1994). *Clinical Transplants 1993.* UCLA Tissue Typing Laboratory, Los Angeles.

Thomson, A.W. and Cato, G.R.D., eds. (1993). *Immunology of renal transplantation.* Edward Arnold, London.

20.18 Renal bone disease

J. A. KANIS

Introduction

Of the disorders affecting survivors with chronic renal failure, much attention has been directed to the disturbances in mineral metabolism which give rise to bone disease, which develops in a high proportion of patients and is not favourably altered by dialysis treatment. Advances in the past few years have led to an understanding of some of the mechanisms by which such bone disease arises, so that the objectives of treatment and the way in which these objectives might be realized have become more accurately defined.

Features of renal bone disease

The skeletal disorders found in chronic renal failure (Table 1) are collectively termed renal osteodystrophy, and may occur singly or in various combinations. None of these is unique to renal failure nor to particular populations of patients, such as those managed conservatively, those on dialysis, or, indeed, transplanted patients. But there are differences in the incidence of the various abnormalities, not only within these populations but also between various renal units. The variable apparent prevalence of bone disease reflects in part the use of differing histolog-

Table 1 *Features of renal bone disease and some clinical manifestations of disturbed calcium and phosphate metabolism in chronic renal failure*

Feature	Clinical consequence
Hyperparathyroidism and osteitis fibrosa	Skeletal deformity, bone pain, pruritus, anaemia, impotence, neuropathy
Osteomalacia and decreased availability of vitamin D, calcium, and phosphate	Skeletal deformity, bone pain and tenderness, pathological fracture[a] Proximal myopathy, encephalopathy, microcytic anaemia,[a] haemolytic anaemia
Adynamic bone disease	Pain, pathological fracture, hypercalcaemia
Osteoporosis	Pathological fracture, skeletal deformity
Osteonecrosis	Joint pain
Osteosclerosis and periosteal new bone formation	None known
Extraskeletal calcification	Depends on site—skin ulcers, pruritus, vascular disease, cardiac failure, pseudogout

[a] More characteristic of aluminium toxicity

ical and radiographic criteria for diagnosis, but other important factors include age, the nature and duration of renal disease, and the treatment given.

By the time patients with progressive chronic renal failure start dialysis treatment, the majority have histological abnormalities of bone but skeletal symptoms are found in a minority (less than 10 per cent). However, the incidence of symptomatic bone disease increases thereafter as do the extraskeletal manifestations (Table 1).

BONE TURNOVER

Bone is continually remodelled by synthesis of bone matrix (osteoid formation), mineralization of this osteoid matrix, and its subsequent resorption. These processes are governed by the activity of bone cells, which include osteoblasts (the bone-forming cells), osteoclasts (the bone-resorbing cells), and osteocytes, which are probably osteoblasts buried in bone matrix (see Section 19).

Increased secretion of parathyroid hormone (**PTH**)—secondary hyperparathyroidism—is thought to be of major importance in renal bone disease by increasing the activity and the numbers of these bone cells and so increasing bone turnover. Rapid rates of bone turnover are associated with deposition of fibrous tissue in the marrow spaces (osteitis fibrosa) and the formation of new bone matrix which is not lamellar but disorganized in structure (woven bone). This impairs its strength and occasionally gives rise to serious mechanical consequences (Fig. 1), particularly in the young. If hyperparathyroid bone disease is severe, an imbalance between bone formation and bone resorption occurs and skeletal mass diminishes, particularly that of cortical bone. In adolescents, severe hyperparathyroid bone disease may resemble rickets on skeletal radiographs. Bone loss is not invariable and patchy osteosclerosis of trabecular bone (for example vertebral bodies) is also found. Biochemical indices of bone cell activity include serum measurements of PTH, alkaline phosphatase, and osteocalcin (both derived from bone-forming cells), and hydroxyproline (derived from the breakdown of collagen). Concentrations of all these are higher in patients with osteitis fibrosa than those without.

Osteomalacia is characterized by an increase in the amount of un-mineralized bone matrix. It is important to distinguish increased amounts of osteoid due to augmented bone turnover from that due to a defect in its mineralization. Osteomalacia arises because of an abnormal delay between the onset of bone matrix formation and its subsequent mineralization. Osteomalacia and hyperparathyroidism commonly coexist and are distinguished by histological measurements on bone biopsy which estimate the rate of mineralization. The most direct method is to administer two pulses of tetracycline before bone biopsy. The tetracycline is incorporated into bone at the site of mineralization and, since tetracyclines fluoresce under ultraviolet light, the rate and extent of bone mineralization can be measured.

In contrast to hyperparathyroid bone disease, in adynamic bone disease (low-turnover bone disease) all the elements of bone turnover are decreased—resorption, formation, and mineralization. This impairs the ability of the bone to self-repair fatigue damage and gives rise to pain and fractures.

Changes in bone mass are common in renal failure. There is commonly a redistribution of skeletal mass so that osteosclerosis and osteoporosis may coexist in the same patient. Severe osteoporosis is rarely found in patients not yet requiring dialysis treatment, but is common in the dialysis-treated population and after transplantation.

CLINICAL FEATURES

Disturbed mineral and skeletal metabolism in renal failure has many consequences other than those affecting bone (see Table 1). The skeletal manifestations of renal bone disease include bone pain, bone tenderness, fractures, retardation of growth, joint disease, and soft-tissue calcification.

Both osteomalacia and osteitis fibrosa may be associated with bone pain, tenderness, and muscle weakness. Pain in the lower limbs, pelvis, and back are particularly common and may be worse on exercise. Muscle weakness is frequently proximal. Symptoms are unusual in patients not yet requiring dialysis, except in children and in those in whom renal failure has been present for many years. In patients receiving dialysis treatment there is, however, great variability in the prevalence of symptoms between dialysis units, ranging from 10 per cent to nearly 100 per cent of those treated.

In patients attending dialysis centres which have a very high incidence

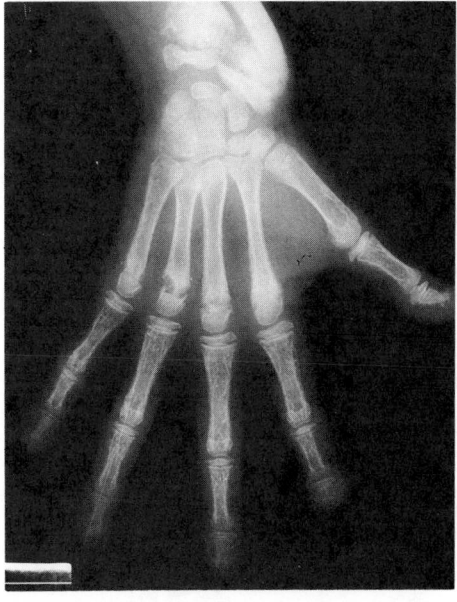

Fig. 1 Radiographic features of hyperparathyroid bone disease in an adolescent with chronic renal failure. Note the marked subperiosteal erosions of the phalanges. Erosion of the terminal, phalanges has resulted in the collapse of soft tissue, giving a drum-stick appearance of the fingers. Severe osteitis fibrosa at the wrist is indicated by the marked metaphyseal resorption, giving rise to skeletal deformity. Less marked hyperparathyroid bone disease may give rise to radiographic features resembling rickets.

of osteomalacia (reflecting a dialysis-induced cause, probably aluminium intoxication), indolent fractures occur, particularly of the ribs, spine, pelvis, and femoral neck. Multiple rib fractures may result in respiratory failure. The manifestations of adynamic bone disease are similar.

Osteosclerosis and periosteal new bone formation are not associated with symptoms and are therefore only incidental radiographic findings. Osteoporosis is asymptomatic unless fractures occur.

Extraskeletal calcification is characteristically found in the vascular tree and periarticular soft tissues (Fig. 2). A predisposing factor is an increase in the plasma calcium × phosphate product which induces precipitation when its solubility is exceeded. Calcification occurs commonly in the eye, as band keratopathy or in the conjunctiva. Acute conjunctival precipitation may cause a chemical conjunctivitis, the 'red-eye' of renal failure. Deposition of calcium in the skin may contribute to pruritus, frequently an unpleasant condition in patients with chronic renal failure. Ischaemic necrosis of the skin is unusual but disabling.

The abdominal aorta and the femoral and digital arteries are the most common sites of vascular calcification (usually medial) visible on radiographs.

Avascular necrosis occurs rarely in chronic renal failure but is a significant cause of morbidity in transplant recipients. The hip joint is the most commonly affected and presents with joint pain.

RADIOGRAPHIC FEATURES

Radiography is much used in the assessment of renal bone disease but is relatively insensitive since many patients with significant skeletal abnormalities may have normal radiographic appearances.

The characteristic radiographic feature of hyperparathyroid bone disease is subperiosteal erosion of bone (Fig. 3), most commonly found at the radial aspect of the middle phalanges of the hand, the tufts of the terminal phalanges, and the distal ends of the clavicles. Gross erosion may result in collapse of soft tissue normally supported by bone. In the terminal phalanges this may give rise to the appearance of pseudoclubbing (see Fig. 1).

Radiographic features are uncommon in osteomalacia, and a negative radiographic survey is therefore not helpful in excluding osteomalacia. There may be a generalized radiolucency of bone. Looser's zones (Fig. 3) are characteristic of osteomalacia and are most frequently seen in the

pelvis. The presence of coarse trabecular markings, osteosclerosis, and periosteal new bone formation (Fig. 3) has been attributed to hyperparathyroidism, but their appearance appears to be more consistently associated with osteomalacia. The radiographic features of osteosclerosis bear only a superficial resemblance to those of avascular necrosis.

Methods of assessing bone mass include measurement of cortical width, single photon absorptiometry, and dual-energy X-ray absorptiometry, which are becoming widely available and provide a useful adjunct in the diagnosis and management of osteoporosis. Bone biopsy is the only certain way to exclude the presence of osteomalacia and aluminium-related bone disease.

Children are particularly prone to renal bone disease and some may show radiographic features that resemble rickets. There are, however, important differences between uraemic 'rickets' and nutritional vitamin D deficiency, which are more evident on histological than radiographic examination: in uraemia there is often no widening of the metaphyseal zone, and the width of the growth plate is not as thick as in vitamin D deficiency (although it may appear so radiographically because of metaphyseal fibrosis and resorption below the growth plate).

The radiographic features of extraskeletal calcification (see Fig. 2) depend on its site. Clinically significant extraskeletal calcification may occur in the absence of radiographic abnormalities and occasionally can be detected by radionuclide scanning.

Fig. 3 Some of the radiographic features of renal bone disease: (a) subperiosteal bone resorption of the terminal phalanx due to secondary hyperparathyroidism; (b) changes in the lumbar spine manifest as alternate bands of increased and reduced radiodensity ('rugger jersey spine'); (c) periosteal new bone formation—the periosteal separation from the mineralized cortex of the femur is shown by the arrows; (d) radiographic characteristics of osteomalacia. A Looser's zone is present in the midshaft of the tibia. There is widening of both the epiphyseal plate and metaphysis.

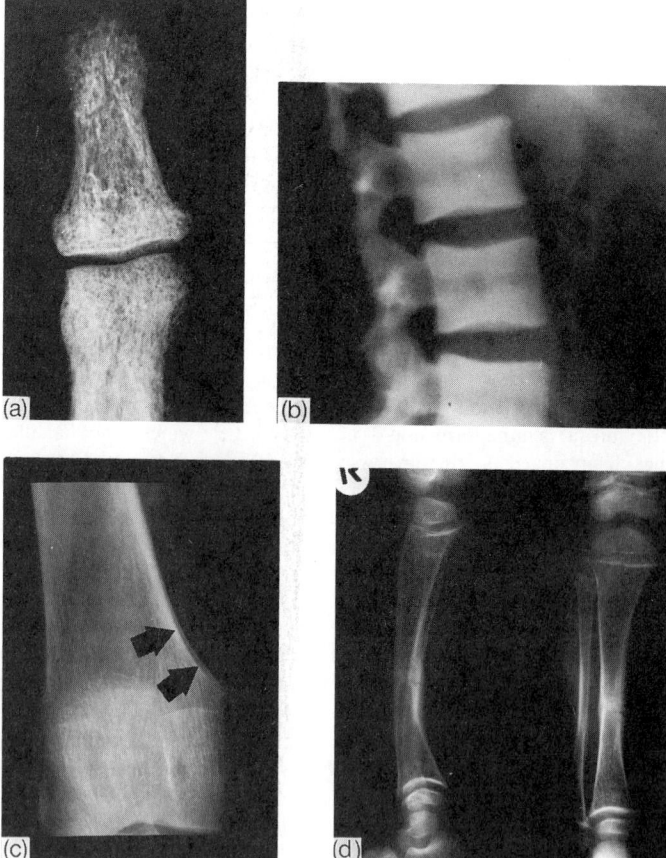

Fig. 2 Radiographic and clinical photographs of periarticular calcification due to hyperphosphataemia in a patient treated by intermittent haemodialysis.

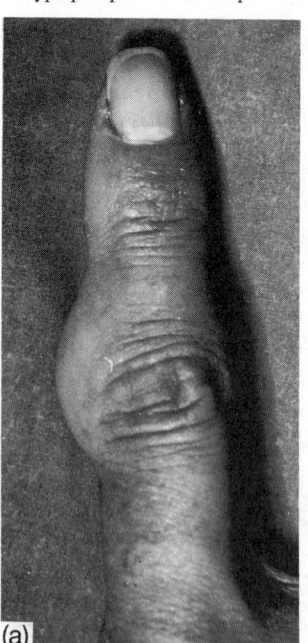
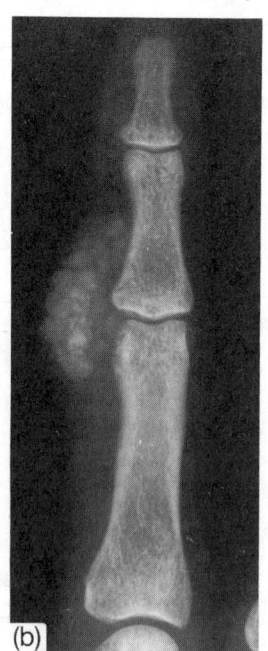

BIOCHEMICAL FEATURES

The classical biochemical findings related to disturbed skeletal metabolism in chronic renal failure include a low serum calcium, hyperphosphataemia, diminished intestinal absorption of calcium, raised plasma activity of alkaline phosphatase, and increased serum values of immunoassayable PTH. Plasma concentrations of calcium are lower in chronic renal failure than in health, particularly in children, and may be lower in patients with osteomalacia than those without. These differences persist in patients on intermittent haemodialysis, although they are less marked. Hypercalcaemia is less common but is found in dialysis-treated patients with severe hyperparathyroidism (so called tertiary or autonomous hyperparathyroidism), in vitamin D toxicity, and in some patients with aluminium retention or aplastic bone disease. The occurrence of mild or moderate renal failure and hypercalcaemia is sufficiently unusual that the diagnosis of primary hyperparathyroidism and secondary renal failure should always be considered. Transient hypercalcaemia occurs occasionally shortly after starting haemodialysis, and may be due to the resorption of pre-existing extraskeletal calcification.

Hyperphosphataemia occurs when the glomerular filtration rate falls below approximately 30 ml/min. The serum phosphate concentration is determined by the diet, the glomerular filtration rate, the tubular reabsorption of phosphate, the use of oral phosphate binding agents, and the dialysis regime. Patients with severe chronic renal failure also malabsorb phosphate, and hypophosphataemia may occasionally be noted despite the absence of renal function. As in the case of serum calcium, those patients with osteomalacia tend to have lower values of serum phosphate (Fig. 4), but neither the serum calcium nor phosphate is sufficiently different from patients without osteomalacia for clinical diagnosis.

Serum activity of alkaline phosphatase is commonly increased in chronic renal failure, but the increase is not always due to the bone-derived enzyme. Other sources in patients with renal failure are the gut and liver. The determination of hepatic enzymes such as 5′-nucleotidase activity may be helpful in excluding a hepatic source. In the absence of liver disease, hyperphosphatasia suggests increased bone-cell activity as seen in secondary hyperparathyroidism. In osteomalacia in the absence of hyperparathyroidism, serum activity of alkaline phosphatase is commonly normal.

Radioimmunoassays for PTH are becoming increasingly available, but there are several problems in interpreting immunoassayable PTH in chronic renal failure. The kidney is an important site of degradation of some of the biologically inactive fragments of PTH and, in some assay systems, values of immunoassayable PTH in serum may be twenty- or forty-fold higher than normal, even in the absence of significant secondary hyperparathyroidism. The development of assays which measure the intact hormone have partly resolved this difficulty. Irrespective of the assay used, serum values of immunoassayable PTH are higher in patients with hyperparathyroid bone disease and renal failure than those without. The finding of hypercalcaemia with inappropriately high values of PTH suggests the presence of aluminium bone disease.

Pathophysiology

The biochemical and endocrinological disturbances giving rise to renal bone disease include abnormalities in the excretory function of the kidney, alterations of its endocrine function, and the effects of drugs, diet, or differing dialysis regimens (Table 2).

METABOLISM OF VITAMIN D

Very large doses of vitamin D (calciferol) increase the intestinal absorption of calcium and may heal osteomalacia and osteitis fibrosa in some patients with renal failure. The bone disease is 'vitamin D resistant' in the sense that the doses of vitamin D required are greater than physiological. This resistance is due to defective renal metabolism of vitamin D, since the kidney is the major site of production of calcitriol (1,25-dihydroxyvitamin D_3 or $1,25(OH)_2D_3$) and secalciferol ($24,25(OH)_2D_3$). Defective production of calcitriol accounts for the vitamin D resistance but there are additional aspects of vitamin D metabolism important in renal bone disease.

The first step in the metabolism of vitamin D_3 is its hepatic conversion to calcidiol (25-hydroxyvitamin D or 25-OHD_3) (see Chapter 12.6). In most patients with chronic renal failure, serum calcidiol is normal. Low values, when present, are usually due to inadequate diet, reduced exposure to sunlight, or peritoneal losses during chronic peritoneal dialysis. Calcidiol may also be low in patients with the nephrotic syndrome due to urinary losses. Anticonvulsants, including barbiturates, induce hepatic microsomal enzymes, and might, therefore, increase the metabolism of calcidiol to inert products. A more important effect of anticonvulsants may be to block the action of vitamin D metabolites on gut and bone. Low values of calcidiol may contribute to osteomalacia, particularly when the degree of renal failure is modest.

Most of the actions of vitamin D_3 are mediated by the metabolism of calcidiol to calcitriol. Since the kidney is normally the sole site of synthesis of circulating calcitriol (apart from the placenta in pregnancy), the development of bone disease and its resistance to vitamin D and to calcidiol results from its impaired production due to loss of renal tissue and also to the inhibitory effects of hyperphosphataemia on the renal 1α-hydroxylase enzyme. Serum values of calcitriol decrease when the glomerular filtration rate is less than 40 ml/min and are very low in end-stage renal failure.

Deficiency of calcitriol in man retards skeletal growth and results in defective mineralization of matrix produced both by chondrocytes and osteoblasts. It also induces intestinal malabsorption of calcium and aggravates hypocalcaemia and secondary hyperparathyroidism. Calcitriol may also affect PTH secretion by a direct action on the parathyroid gland, so that deficiency exacerbates hyperparathyrodism. Reversal of many of these abnormalities by physiological doses of calcitriol provides convincing evidence for its importance in skeletal metabolism. However, it is not yet clear whether or not formation and mineralization of bone and cartilage are direct actions of the vitamin D metabolites (see Chapter 12.6).

Not all patients with osteomalacia respond to treatment with 1α-hydroxylated metabolites, and healing is commonly incomplete when histological indices of response are used. Also, the prevalence of osteomalacia has been low in some renal units despite the ubiquity of defective calcitiol production (Fig. 5). These observations suggest that factors other than defective production of calcitriol can contribute significantly to bone disease.

Fig. 4 Relationship between plasma phosphate (P_i) and a histological index of osteomalacia in patients with renal failure receiving dialysis treatment. Osteomalacia (five or more osteoid lamellae) is uncommon in patients with high plasma values of phosphate. Evidence of osteomalacia is often noted in patients whose plasma phosphate lies below the upper limit of the normal range (indicated by the dashed line).

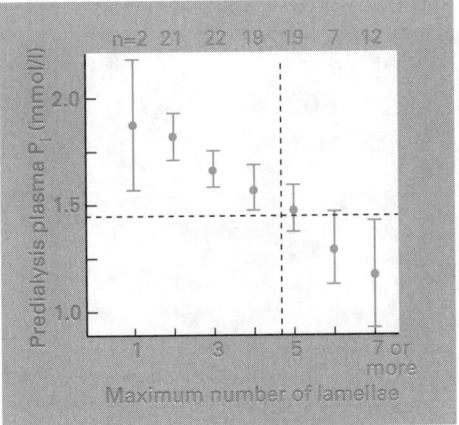

Table 2 *Factors of possible importance in the pathogenesis of renal bone disease*

Disturbances in endocrine function
   Defective production of dihydroxymetabolites of vitamin D_3
   Impaired metabolism, peritoneal or urinary losses of 25-hydroxyvitamin D_3 (CAPD, nephrotic syndrome)
   Secondary hyperparathyroidism
   PTH resistance
   Secretion, degradation, or action of other hormones, e.g. calcitonin, thyroxine, gonadal steroids, prolactin, and others
Accumulation of toxic products
   Aluminium, magnesium, and possibly other metals, e.g. iron cadmium, beryllium, manganese
   Products of metabolism such as hydrogen ions, middle molecules, etc.
Drugs
   Phosphate-binding agents
   Anticonvulsants and barbiturates
   Corticosteroids and cytotoxic agents
   Vitamins A, C, D
   Heparin
Deficiency states
   Phosphate
   Availability of calcium (diet, dialysis, malabsorption)
   Dietary protein
   Vitamin C, pyridoxine, vitamin D
Other
   Age (adolescence), female sex
   Duration and nature of renal disease

The production of secalciferol is also impaired in renal failure since the kidney converts calcidiol to this metabolite, but its administration alone does not heal bone disease. There is some evidence that both calcitriol and secalciferol are required for the actions of vitamin D on bone to be complete.

PHOSPHATE METABOLISM

Animal experiments suggests that the tendency for serum phosphate to rise as renal failure occurs stimulates the secretion of PTH by decreasing the ionized fraction of serum calcium. The increase in PTH so induced decreases tubular reabsorption of phosphate and hence lowers serum phosphate and increases serum calcium. Thus, during the course of progressive renal failure, serum values of calcium and phosphate may be kept relatively normal, but at the expense of an ever-increasing secretion rate of PTH and its resultant skeletal effect—osteitis fibrosa. When the decrement in glomerular filtration rate is too great, the number of residual nephrons is not sufficient to lower serum phosphate, and hyperphosphataemia and hypocalcaemia ensue (Fig. 6). Hyperphosphataemia may be one of the reasons for reduced synthesis of calcitriol.

In chronic renal failure, and renal tubular disorders, the concentration of plasma phosphate appears to be an important determinant of osteomalacia. Plasma phosphate concentrations in dialysis-treated patients correlate inversely with the degree of osteomalacia, such that those patients with normal amounts of osteoid have the higher values of phosphate. Plasma phosphate in such patients is considerably higher than the upper limit of normal in health, and a degree of hyperphosphataemia may therefore protect the patient from osteomalacia, despite defective vitamin D metabolism.

CALCIUM METABOLISM

It is probable that the skeletal effects of vitamin D are not solely dependent upon direct actions of the metabolites on bone itself but also due to consequent changes in extracellular concentrations of calcium, phosphate, and PTH. Severe dietary deficiency of calcium renders patients with chronic renal failure unresponsive to calcitriol, whereas healing of osteomalacia occurs when the diet is adequately supplemented.

The dialysis membrane provides a site for the loss or the incorporation of calcium into the body. The net transfer is dependent on shifts in extracellular pH and serum protein concentrations, and on the respective calcium concentrations of serum and dialysis fluid. The use of a low dialysate calcium (for example 1.25 mmol/l) induces osteoporosis, but calcium-rich dialysis fluids (for example 2.0 mmol/l) are not advised; extraskeletal calcification may be accentuated and, despite transient effects on the secretion of PTH, the long-term skeletal response is disappointing. The ideal calcium concentration of haemodialysis fluid lies somewhere between 1.63 and 1.75 mmol/l. In view of the uncertain effects of vitamin D on bone, it is unknown whether the combination

Fig. 5 The prevalence of osteomalacia in patients established on long-term intermittent haemodialysis as assessed by repeated bone biopsy. Note the large difference which once existed between Newcastle (a high aluminium area) and Oxford (low aluminium in the dialysate fluid) but a similar prevalence of osteomalacia at the time of starting dialysis. These observations antedate the use of methods to remove aluminium from dialysis fluid.

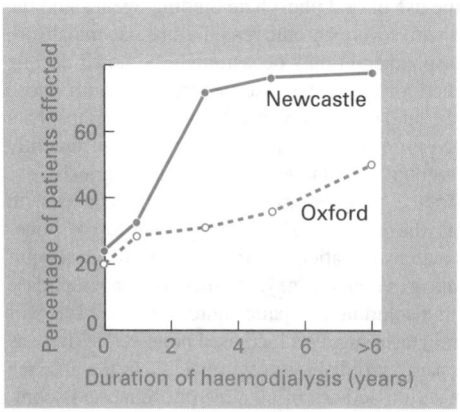

Fig. 6 The role of vitamin D, aluminium (Al), and parathyroid hormone (PTH) in the pathogenesis of renal bone disease. Progressive renal disease induces decrements in glomerular filtration rate (GFR) and synthetic capacity for calcitriol (1,25 $(OH)_2D_3$). An increase in serum phosphate (P_i) due to the fall in GFR stimulates the secretion of PTH indirectly by decreasing serum calcium concentrations (Ca). During progressive renal failure serum calcium and phosphate tend to remain normal (because of the renal and skeletal effects of PTH) at the expense of an increasing secretion rate of PTH and its skeletal consequence, osteitis fibrosa (OF). When the compensatory abilities of the kidney are compromised by renal failure, hyperphosphataemia and hypocalcaemia prevail. Hyperphosphataemia may further inhibit synthesis of calcitriol and cause osteomalacia (OM). Malabsorption of calcium may contribute to secondary hyperparathyroidism.

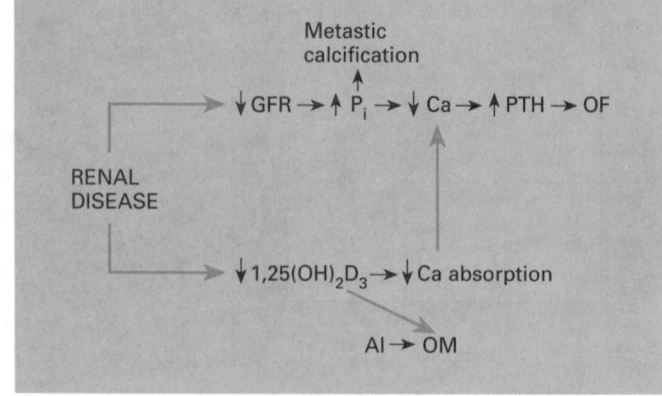

of a low-dialysate calcium and calcitriol would be advantageous, but such regimens are being increasingly used.

TRACE ELEMENTS AND WATER CONTAMINANTS

Many elements accumulate in skeletal tissues in patients with chronic renal failure due either to impaired excretory function or to their entry from the dialysate fluid during dialysis. These include iron, arsenic, strontium, molybdenum, magnesium, manganese, copper, aluminium, and fluoride, but, with the exception of aluminium and possibly iron, their role, if any, in the evolution of dialysis bone disease is not known.

Aluminium retention is an important factor in the pathogenesis of osteomalacia in some dialysis-treated patients. A form of osteomalacia associated with a high incidence of bone pain and fracture is common in certain geographical locations with a high aluminium content in the water (see Fig. 5), and its incidence decreases with deionization of the water. Skeletal retention of aluminium is not invariably associated with osteomalacia but also gives rise to adynamic bone disease and low rates of bone formation, which cause pathological fracture. A similar syndrome has been described due to iron retention. Both are refractory to treatment with vitamin D derivatives.

The question arises whether the phosphate- binding agents containing aluminium salts may themselves give rise to aluminium toxicity. Waterborne, rather than oral, aluminium was the major source of skeletal aluminium in the past, but oral aluminium is now a significant cause of aluminium retention.

Aluminium toxicity should be suspected in patients with bone pain and muscle weakness who have little radiographic or biochemical evidence for hyperparathyroid bone disease. The presence of hypercalcaemia or pathological fracture are additional features. The diagnosis can be confirmed by bone biopsy which shows focal aluminium accumulation by specific histochemical stains, and low rates of bone formation. Osteomalacia, when present, is characterized by a paucity of active-looking osteoblasts—aplastic osteomalacia.

ACIDOSIS

The role of acidosis in contributing to renal bone disease has been advocated for many years. The acute administration of acid loads to normal man results in a negative calcium balance and it has been noted that the rate of mineralization increases acutely when alkalis are administered to acidotic patients with osteomalacia. The correction of acidosis appears to influence uraemic bone disease in only a minority of patients.

PARATHYROID HORMONE METABOLISM

Not only is the kidney an important site of action for parathyroid hormone, it is also a major site for its degradation. Serum concentrations of immunoassayable PTH are increased in early renal impairment. Hypocalcaemia is a common finding in chronic renal failure, and this provides the major stimulus for the secretion of PTH. Some vitamin D metabolites exert direct effects on the parathyroid gland, and in chronic renal failure disturbed metabolism of vitamin D, and possibly of magnesium, may contribute to hypersecretion and hyperplasia of the parathyroids. Aluminium also directly affects the secretion of PTH and contributes to the suppression of bone turnover in adynamic bone disease.

There are several mechanisms by which hypocalcaemia arises in chronic renal failure. These include, hyperphosphataemia (see above), intestinal malabsorption of calcium, decreased renal tubular reabsorption of calcium, and 'skeletal resistance' to the action of PTH. Skeletal resistance to PTH is suggested by the finding of high concentrations of immunoassayable PTH irrespective of the prevailing concentration of serum calcium. Impairment of the acute calcaemic response to exogenous PTH is commonly found in chronic renal failure, but the relevance of such observations made in acute studies to long-term effects on bone are not clear.

PTH may also affect the mineralization of bone. Some patients develop osteomalacia after total parathyroidectomy when osteitis fibrosa has healed. The relative ease with which the woven osteoid (found in hyperparathyroidism) calcifies, compared to lamellar osteoid, may explain the appearance of osteomalacia, since lamellar bone is laid down after parathyroidectomy. A corollary is that a degree of hyperparathyroidism may protect against osteomalacia.

OTHER FACTORS

It has been known for many years that uraemic plasma contains factors that inhibit the calcification of cartilage. They include toxins such as guanidines, phenols, aliphatic amines, and other 'middle molecules' yet to be identified. Substances normally found in trace amounts, such as pyrophosphate, fluoride, aluminium, vitamin A, and cadmium, also accumulate and may contribute to disordered skeletal metabolism. Disturbances in the metabolism of hormones other than PTH and vitamins occur in chronic renal failure; affected hormones include calcitonin, growth hormone, insulin, gonadal steroids, prolactin, and thyroid hormone, all of which may variously influence skeletal tissue itself or the metabolism of its regulating hormones. In addition, protein-deficient diets tend to restrict the intake of vitamin C and pyridoxine, both of which are essential cofactors in the formation and maturation of collagen.

DRUGS AND DIET

The management of chronic renal failure, particularly before the advent of dialysis treatment, commonly included severe dietary restrictions. Deficiencies of Vitamin C, pyridoxine, and vitamin D occur commonly in chronic renal failure and may cause bone disease in patients with moderate renal impairment. Severe phosphate restriction may induce osteomalacia, and calcium-deficient diets will decrease the net intestinal absorption of calcium irrespective of the activity of the intestinal transport process.

Many drugs are known to affect skeletal metabolism. The effects of anticonvulsants and barbiturates on skeletal metabolism have been mentioned earlier. Heparin, which is commonly used during dialysis treatments, causes increased bone resorption when very high doses are used. The effect of low molecular weight heparins on bone are unknown. Avascular necrosis occurs most commonly when corticosteroids are used in the treatment of the underlying renal disorder and after transplantation. It is likely that the combination of corticosteroids and chronic renal failure are additive risk factors, since avascular necrosis is relatively uncommon in patients with chronic renal impairment not exposed to steroids, and in steroid-treated patients with normal renal function. The incidence of avascular necrosis appears to be lowest where very high doses of intravenous corticosteroids are avoided in the treatment of transplant rejection.

Treatment of renal bone disease

Treatment strategy should be based not only on the nature of the bone disease or associated symptoms but also on a careful assessment of the other non-skeletal effects of disturbed mineral metabolism (see Table 1) and the mechanisms responsible for the disorder (see Table 2). The proposed management of the chronic renal disease itself should also be considered since, for example, therapeutic approaches may depend on the probability of subsequent transplantation.

There are a number of preventative measures which should be considered in all patients with advanced renal impairment. It is probable that the severe restriction of dietary protein, as sometimes practised, is a greater factor in inducing morbidity than it is in achieving beneficial effects. Both vitamin C and B_6 should be given as dietary supplements, particularly in dialysis-treated patients. It is reasonable to ensure that the dietary intake of calcium and vitamin D is at least normal with the use of appropriate dietary supplements.

Plasma values of vitamin A are high in renal failure, due to increased binding by retinol-binding protein. Vitamin A increases bone resorption and may augment PTH secretion, so supplements containing this vitamin should be avoided.

PHOSPHATE METABOLISM

Serum phosphate is nearly always markedly increased in patients with severe renal impairment. Control of serum phosphate concentrations contributes to the prevention of hyperparathyroid bone disease and is also important in the management and prevention of extraskeletal calcification. It is impractical to limit the dietary intake of phosphate, but decreased availability of phosphate for absorption can be achieved with the use of phosphate-binding agents. The most commonly used agent is aluminium hydroxide, prescribed as a gel, in biscuits, or in capsule form. Calcium carbonate also binds phosphate in the gut and has potential advantages in correcting acidosis when present, increasing the dietary calcium load, and avoiding the ingestion of aluminium; but in practice the amounts of calcium carbonate required are large and they limit the use of vitamin D analogues. It is advisable to withdraw aluminium-containing drugs when aluminium toxicity is suspected.

Phosphate-binding agents should be given before meals and the dose regulated according to its effects on serum phosphate. Predialysis values of serum phosphate should be less than 2.2 mmol/l to avoid extraskeletal calcification. Factors which influence the dose required include the dietary intake of phosphate, concurrent treatment with vitamin D and its analogues or metabolites, and the dialysis treatment schedule prescribed. Profound hypophosphataemia should also be avoided since it is associated with osteomalacia (see Fig. 4). The values of serum phosphate which best balance the risks of extraskeletal calcification and osteomalacia lie between 1.4 and 2.2 mmol/l in dialysis-treated patients.

CALCIUM METABOLISM

Unlike the net intestinal absorption of phosphate which is largely dependent on the dietary load, the net absorption of calcium is more critically dependent on the presence of calcitriol. Nevertheless, net intestinal transport of calcium can be augmented by large amounts of calcium carbonate (5–20 g daily) and this may improve osteomalacia. It is often more practicable to give vitamin D or one of its metabolites (discussed later) but net intestinal absorption of calcium cannot be greatly augmented if the diet is severely deficient in calcium. Moreover, calcium deficiency impairs the response to vitamin D. It is important, therefore, to ensure at least a normal dietary intake of calcium (1 g daily) with the use of calcium supplements if necessary.

The dialysate calcium which best balances the risks of osteoporosis and extraskeletal calcification lies between 1.6 and 1.75 mmol/l/ in patients treated by haemodialysis.

VITAMIN D AND RELATED COMPOUNDS

A variety of vitamin D compounds are available for use in chronic renal failure. These include vitamin D_2 (calciferol), D_3 (cholecalciferol), dihydrotachysterol (DHT), calcitriol, and alfacalcidol (1α-hydroxyvitamin D_3). A great deal of clinical interest has focused on calcitriol and its synthetic analogue alfacalcidol since they bypass the metabolic block caused by uraemia: but dihydrotachysterol is also biologically active without the necessity for 1α-hydroxylation by the kidney. Dihydrotachysterol (DHT) and alfacalcidol undergo hepatic hydroxylation, and the 25-OHDHT or calcitriol so formed are the major circulating forms of these agents.

All the vitamin D-like compounds available for use are effective in augmenting calcium absorption, relieving symptoms of bone pain and muscle weakness, in increasing serum calcium, and in the majority of patients they suppress elevated serum values of alkaline phosphatase

and correct radiographic abnormalities (Fig. 7). Skeletal deformity in the young can probably be prevented and growth partly restored.

The histological response to treatment is often less marked than the clinical, biochemical, or radiographic responses, particularly in patients maintained on intermittent haemodialysis, where factors other than disturbed vitamin D metabolism presumably play a dominant role in the pathophysiology. Both osteitis fibrosa and osteomalacia appear to respond more readily when associated with each other. Once again, this may be related to the different pathogenic mechanisms.

Although most patients with end-stage chronic renal failure have histological evidence of bone disease, they are often symptomless. The treatment of asymptomatic patients with vitamin D metabolites should be considered, particularly in children in whom skeletal disease may progress rapidly.

Doses of the various agents required to maintain serum calcium within the normal range and to reverse bone disease are indicated in Table 3. In general, the dose tolerated in order to avoid hypercalcaemia decreases with time (Fig. 7). The greatest risks of hypercalcaemia occur at the start of treatment, in patients who ultimately respond poorly to treatment, particularly those with aluminium-related disorders; and, in others, later when biochemical responses are nearing completion. Serum calcium should be monitored frequently during these risk periods. It is also important to note that these agents increase the absorption of phosphate and the requirements for phosphate-binding agents may be increased.

There is no evidence that calcitriol, alfacalcidol, or DHT have any particular therapeutic actions not also possessed by other agents, such as calcidiol or vitamin D. The advantages of the 1α-hydroxylated derivatives of vitamin D and DHT lie in the ease with which doses are titrated according to requirements and the rapidity with which toxic effects are reversed on stopping treatment.

Treatment with vitamin D or its metabolites is not without risk. Prolonged increases in plasma calcium and phosphate give rise to extraskeletal calcification. Patients with pre-existing hypercalcaemia should be treated cautiously, if at all, since such patients often respond poorly to treatment. Prolonged hypercalcaemia may also impair renal function, sometimes irreversibly, and there has been concern that vitamin D com-

Fig. 7 Long-term treatment of renal bone disease with alfacalcidol (1α-HCC) in a dialysis-treated patient. Healing of osteomalacia and osteitis fibrosa (OM and OF) occurred within 15 months. Episodes of hypercalcaemia occurred suddenly and the dose of alfacalcidol tolerated decreased progressively once plasma alkaline phosphatase had fallen to normal values. Remission from bone disease was maintained using a dose of 1α-HCC of 1 μg thrice weekly.

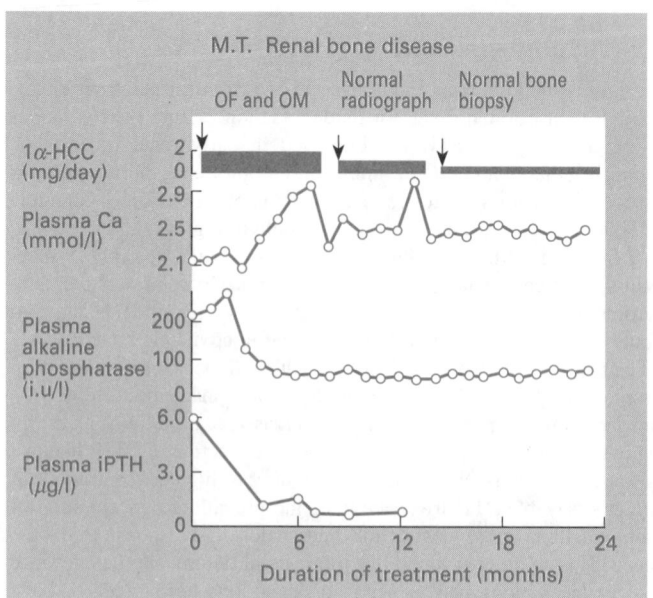

Table 3 *Usual dose requirements of vitamin D, dihydrotachysterol (DHT), alfacalcidol, and calcitriol in dietary deficiency rickets and in vitamin D resistance due to chronic renal failure*

	D_3	DHT	Alfacalcidol	Calcitriol
Approximate daily dose required to treat or prevent rickets (μg)	2.5–25	up to 200	up to 1.0	up to 0.5
Potency relative to vitamin D_3	100	10	250	500
Approximate daily dose required to treat renal bone disease (μg)	750–10 000	200–1000	0.5–2.0	0.25–2.0
Potency relative to vitamin D_3	100	1000	500 000	500 000

Potencies are shown relative to that of vitamin D (= 100 per cent). Note that although larger amounts of DHT than vitamin D are required to treat simple rickets, only slightly higher doses are required to treat renal bone disease with DHT (or with alfacalcidol or calcitriol—up to four times), whereas much larger doses of vitamin D (up to 400 times) are required to treat renal bone disease. Note 1 microgram D_3 or calcitriol is equivalent to approximately 40 IU.

pounds may themselves be nephrotoxic. A rise in serum creatinine associated with vitamin D is not always associated with a decrease in glomerular filtration. Close control of serum calcium and phosphate, and serial assessment of renal function in patients not yet established on dialysis treatment are particularly important when any form of vitamin D is prescribed.

ALUMINIUM TOXICITY

Neither osteomalacia nor adynamic bone disease resulting from aluminium retention respond to treatment with vitamin D or its metabolites. They may respond slowly to transplantation or adequate removal of aluminium from the dialysis fluid. This probably reflects the prolonged skeletal retention of aluminium and the difficulty with which it is removed by haemodialysis, and indicates the importance of prophylaxis. Thus, where aluminium levels in the dialysate exceed 20 μg/l, the water should be treated by reverse osmosis or by deionization.

Aluminium-containing antacids should not be prescribed except for the regulation of serum phosphate. They are most efficient when given immediately before meals, and requirements may be minimized by using in combination with calcium salts, such as calcium carbonate. The need for aluminium hydroxide can also be reduced by increasing the hours of dialysis treatment or the use of more efficient artificial kidneys.

The chelating agent desferrioxamine is used to decrease the body burden of aluminium. A typical regimen is to give desferrioxamine (15 mg/kg/h) by intravenous infusion during the first 2 h of each haemodialysis treatment, or to add a similar weekly dose (85 mg/kg) to the fluid used for peritoneal dialysis. In patients with significant aluminium retention, serum aluminium rises acutely due to its mobilization from tissues and chelation in the extracellular fluid. The rise in aluminium can be used as a diagnostic test and to judge the duration of treatment required. The amount of aluminium removed during each dialysis depends on the serum value and the type of dialyser used. Treatment is associated with clinical improvement (reduction in bone pain, muscle weakness) as well as improvements in the formation and mineralization of bone.

PARATHYROIDECTOMY

Surgical removal of parathyroid glands is an effective and rapid method of treating hyperparathyroid bone disease. It also improves extraskeletal calcification, but vascular calcification improves less readily than periarticular calcification. It should be considered in patients who fail to respond to medical treatment, particularly those with so-called tertiary or autonomous hyperparathyroidism—hyperparathyroid bone disease and a high serum calcium. Other indications include ischaemic necrosis of skin and intractable pruritus.

Recurrence of hyperparathyroidism is common following subtotal parathyroidectomy, and it has been suggested that total parathyroidec-

tomy should be considered in patients who are unlikely to receive renal transplants. The combination of vitamin D metabolites and subtotal parathyroidectomy does not avoid the risks of recurrence. The argument for total parathyroidectomy is that of avoiding recurrence, but the occurrence (or unmasking) of osteomalacia resistant to vitamin D treatment is one of the reasons why partial parathyroidectomy may be preferable.

The main management problem is the immediate postoperative control of serum calcium when severe bone disease is present. Large intravenous doses of calcium (up to 6 g daily) may be required to avoid postoperative tetany. Prior treatment of patients with 1α-hydroxylated derivatives of vitamin D appears to diminish the degree and duration of hypocalcaemia, and in some may even avoid the need for surgery.

RENAL TRANSPLANTATION

Theoretically, renal transplantation would be the treatment of choice for patients with bone disease. This rapidly restores the capacity to form calcitriol and, of course, reverses uraemia. Osteomalacia is often slow to reverse, particularly when associated with aluminium retention. Bone disease, including osteomalacia and avascular necrosis, may arise *de novo* in the transplanted population. There is a high incidence of hypercalcaemia and hypophosphataemia in the transplant population and this may be in part related to phosphate depletion by the use of antacids, the persistence of hyperparathyroidism, which is slow to regress after transplantation, and the effects of corticosteroids to decrease renal tubular reabsorption of phosphate.

EXPERIMENTAL APPROACHES

Several agents block or antagonize the effects of parathyroid hormone on bone, including calcitonin and the bisphosphonates. These might be of value in the management of renal osteodystrophy, either to prevent ectopic calcification in the case of bisphosphonates or to reduce the hyperparathyroid or osteopenic component. Calcitonin appears to be effective in the management of patients with hypercalcaemia which occasionally occurs spontaneously in patients just starting dialysis treatment, but has only transient effects on disturbed skeletal metabolism. There has been recent interest in the finding that high intravenous doses of calcitriol or alfacalcidol suppress the secretion of PTH without raising serum calcium concentrations. The long-term effects of intravenous regimens are not known. It is also possible other metabolites of vitamin D have effects either directly on the parathyroid gland to suppress its secretion, or on bone to increase bone formation. One such candidate is secalciferol, and its combination with calcitriol appears to have more complete effects on hyperparathyroid bone disease than the use of calcitriol alone.

Magnesium salts have been used to bind intestinal phosphate in combination with low dialysate magnesium concentrations, but may cause troublesome diarrhoea. Other aluminium-free phosphate-binding agents currently being evaluated are iron salts and synthetic polymers which deliver ionic calcium in the gastrointestinal tract.

REFERENCES

Kanis, J.A., Cundy, T.F., and Hamdy, N.A.T. (1988). Renal osteodystrophy. *Clinical Endocrinology and Metabolism.* **2**, 193–241.

Kanis, J.A., Hamdy, N.A.T., and McCloskey, E.V. (1992). Hypercalcaemia and hypocalcaemia. In *Oxford Textbook of Clinical Nephrology*, (ed. J.S. Cameron, A.M. Davison, J.-P. Grunfeld, D.N.A. Kerr, and E. Ritz), pp. 1753–82. Oxford University Press.

Ritz, E. and Slatopolsky, E. (1992). Renal osteodystrophy. In *Frontiers in renal disease*, (ed. L.W. Henderson and C. Jacobs). *Kidney International Supplement* **38**, S37–S67.

Slatopolsky, E. (1990). Update on Vitamin D. *Kidney International Supplement* **29**, S1–S68.

20.19 Renal tubular disorders

J. CUNNINGHAM

Introduction

Abnormalities of renal tubular function are common—most patients with renal disease of any type have demonstrable defects if studied in sufficient detail. Although in the majority of these the tubular disturbance is dominated by other clinical manifestations of the underlying renal disease, in some the abnormal tubular function is the major or sole cause of the clinical disease.

A reduced number of functioning nephrons implies an increase in the amount of water and solute to be processed by each residual nephron. This always leads to a reduction of the kidney's ability to operate at extremes of tubular water and solute conservation or excretion. Thus, a reduction in adaptive capacity is an extremely common finding in patients with renal disease.

The clinical significance of primary tubular defects depends principally on the nature of the renal defect (renal glycosuria has no clinical sequelae whereas renal phosphate wasting has many), and on the presence of associated transport or other defects elsewhere. For example, in Hartnup disease, a rare inherited disorder of neutral amino acid reabsorption in the proximal tubule, the renal lesion is of little or no consequence, but the associated abnormality of intestinal tryptophan absorption leads to a pellagra-like syndrome (see Chapter 11.3).

General physiology of tubular transport

The human kidney filters vast quantities of water and solute—the daily volume of the glomerular filtrate is about 180 l, containing large amounts of solute which must be reclaimed to prevent rapid and overwhelming depletion (see Table 1). Because water and solute reabsorption is so great, approaching 100 per cent in some instances, quite small changes in the percentage reabsorption leads to enormous changes of excretion rate.

The process of reclamation is energy dependent and to achieve the required metabolic support for solute transport on such a large scale, the kidney must hydrolyse substantial quantities of ATP. This is derived mainly from aerobic metabolism (95 per cent), except in the medulla where anaerobic metabolism contributes significantly to energy supply. The level of metabolic activity can be gauged roughly from consideration of renal O_2 consumption (Q_{O_2}), which is about 10 per cent of the whole body Q_{O_2} at rest, this being achieved by paired organs together comprising less than 1 per cent of body weight. Of the other major organs, only the heart is more active metabolically gram for gram.

Transepithelial movements may be intercellular or transcellular. Intercellular movement is by passive diffusion and occurs only down electrochemical gradients—'downhill'. Transcellular movement, on the

Table 1 *Quantitative aspects of tubular transport in health*

Substance	Filtered load (per 24 h)	Typical 24-h urinary output	Percentage reabsorbed (net)
Water	180 l	0.75–2.5 l	98.6–99.6
Sodium	25 000 mmol	100–250 mmol	99.0–99.6
Potassium	720 mmol	60–120 mmol	83–92
Bicarbonate	4300 mmol	5 mmol	99.9
Glucose	810 mmol	1 mmol	99.9
Calcium	234 mmol	5 mmol	98
Phosphate	200 mmol	6–40 mmol	80–97

other hand, is usually dependent on specific transporters located in the apical or basolateral membrane of the tubular epithelial cells. Many, although not all, of these transporters are energy linked, allowing active transport of solute against electrochemical gradients—'uphill'. Active transport may be classed in a general sense as primary, secondary, or tertiary (Fig. 1).

The major primary process in the kidney is the Na^+–K^+ ATPase, located on the basolateral membrane of all tubular epithelial cells. This pump is electrogenic (3 Na^+ out and 2 K^+ in) and both ions are moved 'uphill'.

Secondary active transport provides the means for reabsorption of sugars and amino acids against their electrochemical gradients. The uphill movement of, for example, a sugar across the brush border membrane of a proximal tubular cell is coupled to the parallel downhill movement of Na^+ into the cell, thereby establishing indirect linkage between the movement of the sugar and the hydrolysis of ATP by the Na^+–K^+ ATPase.

Tertiary linkage is more indirect still. In the example shown (Fig. 1) the object is to drive Cl^-–HCO_3^- exchange. To do this H^+ is moved uphill by a Na^+–H^+ antiporter (exchanger) which is driven by the movement of Na^+ down a gradient that is maintained by the ubiquitous basolateral Na^+–K^+ ATPase. The resulting electrochemical gradient for H^+ is then available for linkage to other transporters, for example a Cl^-–HCO_3^- antiporter.

In addition to those driving Na^+–K^+ exchange, ATP-powered pumps exist for the primary active transport of Ca^{2+}–H^+; H^+–K^+; H^+; and HCO_3^-. The location of these transporters along the nephron and their modulation is complex and the reader is referred elsewhere for more detailed discussion.

The movement of ions across transporting epithelia poses additional problems if the normal intracellular concentration of the ion is low and the mass transfer is high. For example, calcium must be moved in large quantities from apical to basolateral membrane, while still maintaining a low concentration of free calcium ions in the cytosol. This is achieved by means of calcium sequestration in or on intracellular organelles and the production of calcium-binding proteins, such that cellular integrity is not threatened by a rise of intracellular calcium concentration.

Defects of water handling—nephrogenic diabetes insipidus

DEFINITION AND AETIOLOGY

The pure form of this condition is a rare X-linked semirecessive disorder (affecting males more severely than females), resulting from a defective gene at the tip of the long arm of the X chromosome. The hallmark is failure of renal responsiveness to vasopressin. However, various acquired forms are much more common (Table 2), and many of these

Fig. 1 Examples of primary, secondary, and tertiary active transport. Primary active transport is driven directly by ATPases (e.g. Na^+–K^+ATPase) to move ions against an electrochemical gradient. Secondary active transport uses the electrochemical gradient created by primary transport to drive a secondary linked uphill movement. Tertiary active transport couples the transport of a solute to the electrochemical gradient created by a secondary transport process. (Redrawn from Hebert, S.C. and Gullans, S.R. (1991). Metabolic basis of ion transport. In: *The Kidney* (ed. Brenner and Rector), p. 77. W.B. Saunders, Philadelphia, with permission.)

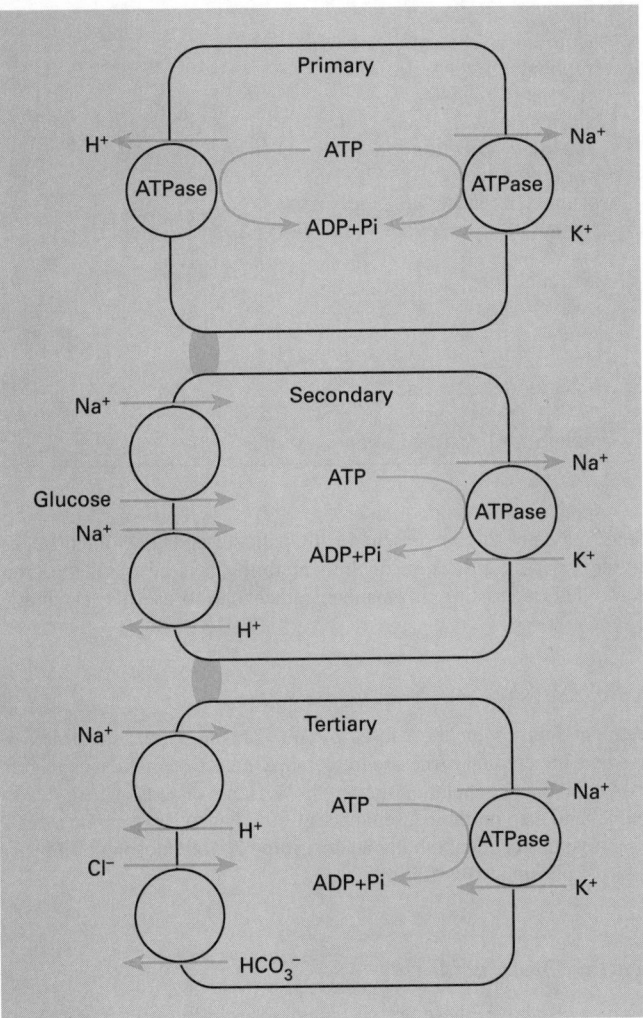

Table 2 *Causes of nephrogenic diabetes insipidus*

Primary
  Familial X-linked nephrogenic diabetes insipidus
Secondary and acquired
  Tubulointerstitial diseases
    obstruction (partial)
    pyelonephritis
    cystic diseases
    granulomatous diseases
    sickle-cell disease/trait
  Metabolic
    hypokalaemia
    hypercalaemia
  Chemical
    lithium
    demeclocycline
  Solute-driven
    glycosuria
    diuretic therapy

are associated with other tubular defects (salt wasting, acidification defects, etc.).

Many acquired forms of the syndrome are associated with structural damage of the medullary interstitium and the tubules contained therein, and, not surprisingly, it is those conditions that damage principally the interstitium that are most likely to cause nephrogenic diabetes insipidus (Table 2).

PATHOPHYSIOLOGY

Vasopressin has varied actions on the kidney, mediated by V_1 and V_2 receptors. The major actions are:

(1) glomerulus—mesangial cell contraction, increased prostaglandin synthesis (V_1);
(2) vasa recta and medullary interstitium—reduction of medullary blood flow and increased prostaglandin (PGE_2) synthesis (V_1);
(3) collecting tubule—increased sodium reabsorption and potassium secretion with increased permeability to water (V_2).

The last of these is the most important determinant of the kidney's antidiuretic response to vasopressin, and it is this system that is defective in X-linked nephrogenic diabetes insipidus. The precise nature of the defect is unclear, but the absence of a normal factor VIII increase after desmopressin infusions suggests that there is almost certainly a generalized failure of V_2-mediated vasopressin responses in these patients.

In both inherited and acquired forms, the renal insensitivity is more often partial than complete, so that adequate antidiuresis can sometimes be achieved, but only at the expense of high endogenous vasopressin secretion rates coupled with a high fluid intake. This, in turn, requires plasma osmolality to be at a level sufficient to stimulate thirst and vasopressin secretion, such that the new steady state is maintained. The incomplete nature of the defect also means that treatment with pharmacological doses of vasopressin analogues (for example desmopressin) is often effective.

PRESENTATION AND DIAGNOSIS

The polyuria imposes the need for a large water intake, which, if not met, leads rapidly to water depletion, hypernatraemia, prerenal uraemia, and ultimately death. Distinguishing nephrogenic causes of polyuria from others is usually easy and can often be made with reasonable certainty on the basis of associated conditions (Table 2) and a careful his-

Table 3 *Aminoacidurias*

Type	Diseases	Amino acid	Clinical
Neutral	Hartnup disease	Alanine, asparagine, glutamine, histidine, isoleucine, phenylalanine, serine, threonine, tryptophan, tyrosine, valine.	'Pellagra' rash, ataxia, mental retardation, diarrhoea (all resulting from defective gut tryptophan absorption)
Dibasic	Cystinuria	Cystine, lysine, arginine, ornithine	Cystine stones
Imino acids and glycine	Iminoglycinuria	Proline, hydroxyproline, glycine	No sequelae
Acidic	Acidic aminoaciduria	Glutamate, aspartate	No sequelae

tory. This needs to be backed up by assessment of the renal responsiveness to vasopressin.

Amino aciduria and Fanconi syndrome

General

Large amounts of amino acids appear in the glomerular filtrate and in health at least 95 per cent of these are reabsorbed by the proximal tubule. The appearance of excessive quantities of amino acids in the final urine is the result of defective proximal tubular transport.

Organic solute transport in the proximal tubule is a two-step process that is carrier mediated and sodium coupled; the amino acid must first enter the proximal tubule cell via the brush border membrane against an electrochemical gradient, and exit via another transporter across the basolateral membrane. Movement of amino acids is accomplished by secondary active mechanisms whereby coupling to Na^+ transport allows the movement of amino acids to be driven indirectly by the basolateral membrane Na^+–K^+ ATPase. This enzyme lowers the intracellular sodium to about 10 per cent of that in the extracellular fluid or proximal tubular fluid, so providing the energy source for any transport system linked to the downhill movement of sodium.

Although each amino acid has a unique structure, not all have specific carriers in the proximal nephron. Instead, based on loose structural similarities, the amino acids segregate into four groups, each with a group-specific carrier system (Table 3). Common to many defects of amino acid transport is a reduction of the electrochemical sodium gradient across the proximal tubular cells. This leads to impairment of linked transport of glucose, amino acids, phosphate, and a range of other solutes.

Because some of the tubular amino acid transporters are expressed in the intestine also, defects may be evident at both sites. In these the clinical disease can result from the intestinal defect, the renal defect, or both.

The Fanconi syndrome (see Chapter 20.7)

This term implies a disturbance of proximal tubular function with resulting generalized amino aciduria, phosphate wasting, metabolic bone disease (rickets in children and osteomalacia in adults), renal tubular acidosis type 2 (proximal RTA), and renal glycosuria.

Juvenile and adult Fanconi syndrome are expressions referring simply to the age of onset, and these terms serve no additional purpose. The causes are numerous and it is helpful to classify them on the basis of aetiology and pathogenesis as far as possible (Table 4).

The clinical presentation of the Fanconi syndrome usually depends more on the associated underlying abnormality than on the renal tubular defect *per se*. Nevertheless, the diagnosis ultimately depends on the demonstration of characteristic multiple proximal tubular defects. These

Table 4 *Classification of Fanconi syndrome*

Inherited
  Primary idiopathic
    sporadic
    familial
  Secondary to inborn error of metabolism
    cystinosis (intralysosomal cystine)
    tyrosinaemia (fumarylacetoacetate)
    Wilson's disease (copper)
    Lowe's syndrome
    galactosaemia (galactose 1-phosphate)
    hereditary fructose intolerance (fructose 1-phosphate)
Acquired
  Intrinsic renal disease
    acute tubular necrosis
    hypokalaemic nephropathy
    myeloma
    Sjögren's syndrome
    transplant rejection
  Hormonal
    primary hyperparathyroidism
    secondary hyperparathyroidism (vitamin D/calcium deficiency)
  Nutritional
    kwashiorkor
  Exogenous toxins
    heavy metals (mercury, lead, cadmium, uranium)
    outdated tetracycline
    6-mercaptopurine
    maleic acid (in experimental animals)

defects may not all be present in all patients and may fluctuate in individual patients. Because of this variability it is best to define the specific defects existing in a patient, rather than to use the 'catch all' eponym.

MANAGEMENT

Treatment focuses on the causes of the Fanconi syndrome (fructose avoidance in hereditary fructose intolerance, galactose avoidance in galactosaemia, copper chelation therapy in Wilson's disease) where this is feasible, and also on the consequences of the Fanconi syndrome (alkali and potassium for renal tubular acidosis type 2, oral phosphate and calcitriol for phosphate wasting).

Specific amino acidurias

As indicated above, these are classified according to the four group-specific carrier defects (Table 3).

Neutral aminoacidurias
HARTNUP DISEASE

Pathophysiology

This is a rare (1:16 000 births) autosomal recessive disorder comprising:

(1) intestinal tryptophan malabsorption;

(2) a pellegra-like syndrome with photosensitive skin lesions, ataxia, and neuropsychiatric disturbances;

(c) neutral aminoaciduria with increased renal clearance of alanine, asparagine, glutamine, histidine, isoleucine, leucine, phenylalanine, serine, threonine, tyrosine, valine, and tryptophan.

The clinical manifestations flow from the tryptophan malabsorption which leads to nutritional deficiency, exacerbated by the further loss of tryptophan in the urine.

Presentation and management

Presentation is much like that of pellagra, although usually is less severe and tends to fluctuate. Analysis of the urine distinguishes the two disorders and Hartnup disease responds well to oral nicotinamide (40–200 mg daily).

Basic aminoacidurias

These comprise cystinuria, lysinuric protein intolerance, and lysinuria.

CYSTINURIA

This is by far the most important, being quite common (1 in 7000 births) and having important clinical manifestations. Inheritance is autosomal recessive and three phenotypes have been recognized, the homozygous forms of which are characterized by cystine stone formation. Other basic amino acids (lysine, arginine, and ornithine) are also present in abnormal quantities, but only cystine, by virtue of its low solubility in urine, is of clinical importance.

Pathophysiology

The group-specific carrier protein for dibasic amino acids is located on the brush border membrane of proximal tubule cells and is thought to be the product of a single pair of allelic genes. Three potential mutant alleles appear capable of causing cystinuria when homozygous. Manifestation of cystinuria is dependent on homozygosity for any of the alleles, or heterozygosity for two of them. When expressed in the kidney, this transport defect is also found in intestinal epithelium.

Clinical features and management

Presentation is usually during childhood or young adult life, with symptoms and complications of stone formation, including pain, infection, and in some cases renal impairment and hypertension. The stones are radio-opaque (though less so than calcium-containing stones), are smooth, and sometimes staghorn. The diagnosis is confirmed by a positive nitroprusside test, the presence of typical hexagonal crystals in morning urine specimens, and measurement of urinary cystine output.

Treatment aims to reduce the cystine concentration in the urine and to increase its solubility, and entails a high fluid intake by night as well as by day, alkalinization of the urine to pH greater than 7.5, with large quantities of potassium citrate and sodium bicarbonate, often combined with penicillamine therapy. Solubility of cystine changes little across the acidic range of pH, but increases rapidly above pH 7. At 37 °C and pH 7, the solubility is only 1.66 mmol/l, but increases to about 3.3 to 3.5 mmol/l at pH 7.8. Pushing the pH to still more alkaline levels is often counterproductive owing to decreasing solubility of calcium phosphate and consequent deposition on the cystine stones. The regimen is arduous, and to be fully effective requires oral fluids on at least one occasion during the night. For obvious reasons compliance is often sub-optimal, but at least 50 per cent of patients respond to the above measures if they are rigorously applied and adhered to, and in some of these the stones regress significantly.

In the past, penicillamine has often been reserved for those who fail on the fluid/alkali regimen given alone. However, although potentially toxic (cutaneous reactions, marrow suppression, and glomerulopathy), serious reactions are rare and because it is so effective, penicillamine is now used much earlier and often forms part of initial therapy. Sulphhydryl-containing drugs, such as penicillamine, react with cystine to form penicillamine-cysteine which is much more soluble. Penicillamine is given at doses of 1 to 2 g daily and the aim is to reduce the cystine concentration to below 1.66 mmol/l. Stones already present can be dissolved and new ones prevented.

LYSINURIC PROTEIN INTOLERANCE

This rare autosomal recessive condition results from widespread defects of dibasic amino acid transport, involving particularly the intestine and proximal renal tubule, together with impaired hepatic uptake. Cystine transport is normal. Mental retardation, growth failure, and osteopenia are prominent and thought to result from reduced activity of the urea cycle with low plasma urea concentration and hyperammonaemia after food. The renal tubule defect plays no part in the development of the disease.

Treatment with citrulline has been effective, probably by regenerating the deficient urea cycle intermediates, arginine and ornithine.

Iminoacids and glycine
FAMILIAL IMMINOGLYCINURIA

This is a relatively common condition, arising in approximately 1 in 15 000 births. Inheritance is autosomal recessive, but it appears that there are multiple alleles and gene loci for the transport of imino acids and glycine. Transport of proline, hydroxyproline, and glycine in the proximal tubule is also impaired, and in some cases in the intestine as well, consistent with involvement of multiple alleles.

Originally iminoglycinuria was thought to be associated with mental retardation and seizures, but it now appears that this is almost certainly not the case and that in most, and possibly all, individuals the metabolic disturbance has no clinical sequelae.

Acidic aminoaciduria

These exceedingly rare disturbances of renal tubule transport of the dicarboxylic amino acids (aspartic acid and glutamic acid) are not fully understood. Renal clearance in excess of the glomerular filtration rate has been reported, possibly the result of excessive renal production and/or failure to transfer these amino acids into the circulation.

Renal glycosuria

Glucose reabsorption occurs in the proximal tubule and is a two-step process, coupling secondary active transport by carrier-mediated Na^+–glucose cotransport across the brush border (apical) membrane, with facilitated diffusion linked with active sodium extrusion across the basolateral membrane.

Patients with renal glycosuria exhibit glycosuria at normal blood glucose concentrations. The condition is seen most frequently in normal pregnant women, in whom an increased glomerular filtration rate is associated with a high filtered glucose load which may exceed the renal tubular maximum capacity for reabsorption. The isolated form is familial with a mixed inheritance pattern. This is consistent with the notion that the condition comprises any one of a number of mutations affecting the proximal tubular glucose transporter, in turn associated with subtle differences in the transport defect. The functional basis for these defects is either reduction of tubular maximum capacity for glucose reabsorption or reduction of the tubular threshold alone.

Abnormalities of glucose transport can also arise from defective linked mechanisms. For example, reduction of the electrochemical sodium gradient leads to a generalized proximal tubular transport defect with renal glycosuria, amino aciduria, bicarbonaturia, and phosphaturia (Fanconi syndrome—see above).

Renal glycosuria *per se* has no clinical sequelae, and is easily distinguished from diabetes mellitus by simultaneous documentation of a normal blood glucose concentration. The isolated form must be distinguished from more complex defects, including Fanconi syndrome, that are associated with tubulointerstitial damage in children with focal and segmental glomerulosclerosis, and finally a rare autosomal recessive form with associated intestinal malabsorption of glucose and galactose.

Disorders of renal phosphate handling

The renal handling of inorganic phosphate is the major determinant of extracellular phosphate concentration and, in health, shows an adaptive capacity capable of maintaining normal phosphate concentrations in the face of wide fluctuations of phosphate intake. Parathyroid hormone (PTH) and metabolic need in relation to dietary intake separately control the handling of phosphate at its major reabsorption site, the proximal tubule. About 20 per cent of tubular phosphate transport occurs in the distal convoluted tubule and collecting duct. PTH is phosphaturic and acts on the proximal nephron via an adenylate cyclase and cAMP, and possibly also by activation of protein kinase C. In addition, the renal tubules can respond to dietary phosphate intake, even when plasma phosphate changes little or not at all. The precise nature of the dietary phosphate signal is uncertain, and, like PTH, it operates on the proximal tubule. In parallel with the antiphosphaturic effect of reduced dietary phosphate, there is an increase in bone resorption leading to mobilization of phosphate (and calcium) from the skeleton. Both the renal and skeletal responses are unimpaired by parathyroidectomy and are therefore not mediated by PTH. A humoral message from gut to kidney and skeleton is possible, but its existence is unproven.

Tubular phosphate wasting

Phosphate transport defects are of several types and all cause hypophosphataemia, with inappropriate phosphaturia. The fractional excretion of phosphate (the percentage of filtered phosphate that appears in the final urine) is increased and the tubular transport maximum for phosphate (TmP/GFR) is decreased. The resulting clinical disturbances include rickets (in children) and osteomalacia (in adults), and depend on severity, chronicity, and associated non-renal abnormalities (Table 5).

X-linked hypophosphataemic rickets
AETIOLOGY AND PATHOGENESIS

This is the most important type and usually presents with poor growth and rickets in early childhood. Inheritance is X-linked dominant. Plasma calcium and PTH are usually normal but there is a subtle disturbance of vitamin D metabolism—plasma calcitriol concentration does not show the increase expected during hypophosphataemia and is normal in most cases. Females (heterozygotes) are less severely affected than males (hemizygotes). Studies in a murine model of X-linked hypophosphataemic rickets (the *hyp* mouse), have shown that the defect lies in the proximal tubular brush border membrane Na$^+$–P$_i$ transporter, and almost certainly the same holds for the human disease. Cross-circulation studies using affected and non-affected mice showed transfer of the defect from affected to non-affected mice, suggesting that a humoral factor mediates the tubular abnormality, although other studies demonstrating abnormal phosphate handling by cultured kidney cells from affected *hyp* mice favour an intrinsic cellular defect.

MANAGEMENT

Diagnosis is made on the basis of the characteristic clinical features coupled with persistent hypophosphataemia and a reduced TmP/GFR, indicating reduced tubular reabsorptive capacity for phosphate.

Treatment is aimed at increasing plasma phosphate to normal concentration—a difficult task. As phosphate rises towards normal levels during therapy, so also does the filtered load and total urinary loss of phosphate, necessitating large and frequent dosing with oral phosphate. This is usually combined with calcitriol to promote intestinal phosphorus absorption. The results are usually good, but the compliance of children with frequent dosing of oral phosphate therapy is often poor.

Oncogenous rickets

Rarely, a similar renal disturbance is acquired in association with certain mesenchymal tumours, especially giant-cell tumours of bone, neurofibromata, and cavernous haemangiomata. This condition is termed oncogenous rickets, and is almost certainly mediated by a humoral factor, as yet unidentified. The functional disturbance is indistinguishable from that of the X-linked form and successful removal of the tumour leads to complete recovery of renal phosphate handling.

Other phosphate-wasting disorders

In addition to X-linked inheritance, sporadic cases exist and present at any age, although most often in childhood. In addition, both autosomal recessive and autosomal dominant inheritance has been encountered. Although some heterogeneity of presentation and functional disturbance is found amongst these, common to all is impaired proximal tubular phosphate transport (low TmP/GFR), resulting in phosphate wasting and in most cases metabolic bone disease also (Table 5).

Tubular phosphate retention

Excessive tubular phosphate reabsorption (high TmP/GFR), with resulting hyperphosphataemia is seen in conditions of PTH lack or renal resistance to PTH (Table 5). All these patients have hypocalcaemia and hyperphosphataemia, the former largely the result of failure of calcitriol production by the PTH-deprived kidney and the latter the result of an inappropriately raised TmP/GFR.

Hypoparathyroidism

Here the renal tubular response to PTH is normal; the metabolic abnormalities merely reflect the PTH lack. Diagnosis depends on a low or absent PTH concentration in plasma, despite prevailing hypocalcaemia.

Pseudohypoparathyroidism

There are two main types, and renal resistance to PTH is common to both. In type I pseudohypoparathyroidism, a G-protein defect leads to failure of coupling between the PTH receptor and adenylate cyclase, and as a result PTH administration evokes neither urinary cAMP nor a phosphaturic response. In type II pseudohypoparathyroidism, G-protein activity is normal and PTH induces a cAMP response but no phosphaturia. This would be consistent with a defect of cAMP-dependent protein kinase C. In these disorders hypocalcaemia evokes an appropriate PTH

Table 5 *The kidney and phosphate metabolism*

Disturbance	Comments
Hypophosphataemia	
X-linked hypophosphataemic rickets	The most common
sporadic	Rare
acquired	
oncogenous rickets	
primary hyperparathyroidism	Increased PTH-dependent phosphaturia
secondary hyperparathyroidism due to vitamin D deficiency	
Hyperphosphataemia	
renal failure	Reduced filtered P_i load
hypoparathyroidism	Reduced PTH-dependent phosphaturia
pseudohypoparathyroidism	Renal PTH resistance
type I	Absent cAMP and phosphaturic responses to PTH (G-protein defect)
type II	Normal cAMP and absent phosphaturic response to PTH (cAMP-dependent protein kinase C defect)

response; plasma PTH is elevated but despite this TmP/GFR is high, with associated phosphate retention. The clinical features are characterized by manifestations of hypocalcaemia and hyperphosphataemia, and also by somatic features comprising short stature, short fourth and fifth metacarpals, and variable mental deficiency.

All types of hypoparathyroidism are treated using oral calcitriol or alfacalcidol at pharmacological doses to bring calcium into the normal range.

Disorders of the renal tubular handling of calcium and magnesium

Normal renal calcium handling (see also Chapter 20.18)

In health between 200 and 250 mmol of calcium are filtered at the glomeruli each day, assuming an ultrafilterable calcium of 1.3 mmol out of the total calcium present in blood at 2.5 mmol. About 70 per cent of this is reabsorbed proximally, and the rest in the thick ascending limb of Henle's loop (20 per cent), the distal convoluted tubule (5–10 per cent), and the collecting tubule (< 5 per cent), such that only about 5 mmol of calcium appears in the final urine each day. Assuming stable total body calcium, this urinary calcium loss is equal to the net intestinal calcium absorption.

Factors affecting renal tubule calcium handling are given in Table 6. Noteworthy is that both PTH and PTH-related peptide are anticalciuric. These effects contribute to the hypercalcaemia of primary hyperparathyroidism and humoral hypercalcaemia of malignancy, respectively.

Idiopathic hypercalciuria (see also Chapter 20.12)

This is an important metabolic disturbance because of an increased risk of calcium stone formation. The term implies hypercalciuria without hypercalcaemia, in the absence of factors known to accelerate bone resorption (for example acromegaly, hyperthyroidism, immobilization) or to reduce tubular calcium reabsorption (for example frusemide, metabolic acidosis). In some of these (a minority) a defect of tubular calcium reabsorption is the prime mover ('renal leak' hypercalciuria), with secondary increase of PTH, calcitriol, and intestinal calcium absorption. In the majority, however, calcium hyperabsorption by the intestine drives the hypercalciuria which is thus of 'overspill' type. In most of these there is a primary reduction of TmP/GFR (renal phosphate leak) stimulating calcitriol production.

Table 6 *Tubular calcium reabsorption*

Stimulus	Net effect on transport	Excretion
Hypercalcaemia	↓	↑
Volume expansion (sodium loading)	↓	↑
Hypomagnesaemia	↓	↑
Phosphate depletion	↓	↑
Metabolic acidosis	↓	↑
Metabolic alkalosis	↑	↓
PTH (parathyroid hormone)	↑	↓
PTH-related peptide	↑	↓
Loop diuretics (frusemide, bumetanide)	↓	↑
Thiazide diuretics	↑	↓

The assessment and management of stone-forming hypercalciuric patients has become increasingly sophisticated in order to identify the appropriate treatment for the particular underlying defect. For example 'renal leak' hypercalciuria requires enhancement of tubule calcium reabsorption by reducing protein intake (acid load) and sodium intake and also giving thiazide diuretics and amiloride. Conversely 'absorptive hypercalciuria' is more logically managed initially by reducing intestinal calcium absorption by means of moderate dietary calcium restriction, and, in those with evidence of calcitriol excess driven by hypophosphataemia, oral phosphate therapy as well. Thiazides and amiloride can be added if the above measures are inadequate. Further discussion of hypercalciuria in relation to stone formation appears in Chapter 20.12.

Hypocalciuria

Reduction of urinary calcium excretion is found in most patients with hypocalcaemia, in whom a reduced filtered load of calcium is sufficient to limit the calcium appearing in the final urine. This is particularly marked in patients with secondary hyperparathyroidism and underlying vitamin D and/or calcium deficiency, in whom a reduced filtered load of calcium is combined with avid tubular calcium absorption under the influence of increased PTH, resulting in very low urine calcium. The majority of patients with significant renal failure, and virtually all those with advanced renal failure, exhibit hypocalciuria.

Familial hypocalciuric hypercalcaemia (alternative designation: familial benign hypercalcaemia) is a rare dominantly inherited condition, in which an intrinsic acceleration of tubular calcium reabsorption coupled with an increase in the parathyroid 'set point' for calcium act synergistically to elevate blood calcium concentration. The condition is usually benign and the diagnosis depends on exclusion of other hypercalcaemic conditions and confirmation of the dominant inheritance by assessment of family members. Children of affected patients may suffer from neonatal hyperparathyroidism and severe hypercalcaemia.

Tubular magnesium handling: hypermagnesaemia and hypomagnesaemia

Tubular magnesium handling can be varied over a wide range and, although normally only about 3 per cent of the filtered magnesium appears in the urine (most of the remaining 97 per cent is reabsorbed in the proximal tubule and the thin limb of Henle's loop), this can rise dramatically in conditions of hypermagnesaemia and also as a result of tubular injury. Because of this high potential excretory capacity, hypermagnesaemia is rare in the presence of good renal function, unless inordinately large quantities of magnesium are given parenterally. In contrast, patients with renal failure are more prone to hypermagnesaemia, particularly when magnesium intake is high, as may be the case if magnesium containing antacids are used.

Hypomagnesaemia, on the other hand, is much more common and frequently results from renal magnesium wasting (Table 7). Iatrogenic causes are the most common, especially aminoglycoside and cisplatin toxicity. The diagnosis is easy—inappropriately high magnesium excretion (> 1.5 mmol/day in a hypomagnesaemic patient) is conclusive. Symptoms are rare, but when present are similar to those of hypokalaemia (see Chapter 20.2.3) and should be treated with parenteral magnesium chloride or sulphate (35–50 mmol given in 5 per cent dextrose or saline over 24 h). Smaller maintenance doses can be given by mouth but often provoke diarrhoea. In that case repeated intravenous replacement is required on rare occasions.

Disorders of tubular potassium handling

Renal potassium wasting (see Chapter 20.2.3)

Potassium depletion of renal origin always reflects abnormal tubular potassium handling with inappropriate kaliuresis despite progressive hypokalaemia. The tubular abnormality may reflect aberrant hormonal or neurogenic signals acting on a normal kidney, or there may be intrinsic disturbances of tubular function or abnormal tubular responsiveness to hormonal or other modulators. The causes are listed in Table 8.

Diuresis-associated potassium loss

By far the commonest loss of potassium is that resulting from diuretic therapy.

Mineralocorticoid and glucocorticoid excess

These syndromes are discussed in detail in Section 20.2. In all, there is increased potassium secretion in the distal nephron. The underlying mechanisms differ, however. Hyperaldosteronism (primary and secondary) and adrenogenital syndromes (deoxycorticosterone excess from 17α-hydroxylase or 17β-hydroxylase deficiency), together with exogenous mineralocorticoid (9α-fludrocortisone, hydrocortisone) all stimulate distal Na^+–K^+ exchange. The explanation for glucocorticoid hypokalaemia is less clear cut. Almost certainly, increased glomerular filtration rate and fluid delivery to the distal nephron account for the kaliuretic properties of glucocorticoids, with additional contribution

Table 7 *Renal magnesium wasting*

Diuretics
Tubular toxins
    aminoglycosides (gentamicin, tobramycin)
    cisplatin
    cyclosporin
Hypercalcaemia
Bartter's syndrome
Tubulointerstitial nephropathies
Obstruction

Table 8 *Renal causes of potassium depletion*

Mineralocorticoid excess
    hyperaldosteronism
    adrenogenital syndromes
    exogenous mineralocorticoids
    Liddle's syndrome
    liquorice ingestion (11β-hydroxysteroid dehydrogenase
        inhibition)
Diuretic states
    postobstructive
    post acute tubular necrosis
    diuretic therapy
Chloride depletion
    upper gastrointestinal losses (for example, pyloric stenosis)
    diuretic therapy
Magnesium depletion
Renal tubular acidosis
    RTA type 1
    RTA type 2
Non-renal metabolic acidosis
    diabetic ketoacidosis
    lactic acidosis
Bartter's syndrome
Drugs
    amphotericin B
    aminoglycosides
    cisplatin

from corticosterone and deoxycorticosterone in patients with Cushing's syndrome.

Ingestion of liquorice or therapy with carbenoxelone sodium can produce a state mimicking aldosterone excess. These compounds interfere with the inactivation of cortisol by blocking 11β-hydroxysteroid dehydrogenase, and the excess cortisol binds to mineralocorticoid receptors.

Bartter's syndrome

This eponymous syndrome, first described in 1962, is characterized by hypokalaemic alkalosis, renal potassium and chloride wasting, hypertrophy of the juxtaglomerular apparatus, hyperreninaemic hyperaldosteronism, and normotension. Associated with these abnormalities are resistance to the pressor effects of angiotensin II (controversial) and of noradrenaline, evidence of prostaglandin overproduction and elevated plasma bradykinin and urinary kallikrein.

Liddle's syndrome

This is a rare condition in which hypertension and hypokalaemic metabolic alkalosis of renal origin are found in combination with low plasma aldosterone levels. In many respects this resembles a state of mineralocorticoid excess, but no other mineralocorticoid has been identified, either directly or indirectly by means of abnormal salivary Na^+/K^+ ratio.

Hypomagnesaemic potassium wasting

Magnesium depletion of any cause leads to potassium wasting, in some cases with secondary aldosteronism as a likely mediator. However, cause and effect is not always easy to establish in coexistent magnesium and potassium depletion. For example, diuretic therapy is a common cause of both, and it is quite likely that the magnesium depletion helps to sustain the potassium wasting. Amiloride and triamterene are both antimagnesuric, an action that could account for some of their potassium sparing actions.

Renal magnesium wasting and secondary potassium wasting are often seen in aminoglycoside nephropathy, and even more consistently in cisplatin nephropathy, in which depletion of both cations is often severe.

Antibiotic therapy

Aminoglycosides (see above) and amphotericin B are both important causes of renal potassium wasting, often with associated (and possibly causal) magnesium depletion. So also are penicillins, but by a different mechanism. Here the penicillin anion is non-reabsorbable, and increases potassium excretion, although only to a significant extent when given at very high dose.

Renal hyperkalaemia

For general discussion of hyperkalaemia, see Chapter 20.2.3. Hyperkalaemia is most commonly seen in acute and chronic renal failure, but may be found when the GFR is normal or only moderately reduced. In these cases, the hyperkalaemia is the result of abnormal tubular potassium secretion.

Impaired tubular potassium secretion

Analogous with other cations, this may reflect intrinsic tubular malfunction or aberrant signalling to otherwise normal tubules.

ACQUIRED

Isolated hypoaldosteronism and hypoaldosteronism resulting from generalized adrenal insufficiency result in absent or reduced hormonal drive to the distal $Na^+–K^+$ exchange with resulting hyperkalaemia. Hypoaldosteronism secondary to hyporeninaemia (hyporeninaemic hypoaldosteronism) is discussed with other causes of renal tubular acidosis type 4 in Chapter 20.9.1.

Tubular resistance to mineralocorticoids is found in association with most types of tubulointerstitial nephropathy. The patients have reduced distal tubular potassium secretion and a low fractional excretion of potassium, but normal activity of the renal angiotensin system and normal plasma aldosterone (unlike those of with hyporeninaemic hypoaldosteronism) and cannot lower urine pH adequately. This implies tubular resistance (often partial) to aldosterone and is in many ways similar to the situation prevailing during spironolactone therapy. Such patients form an additional subtype of renal tubular acidosis type 4.

Treatment with pharmacological doses of fludrocortisone is effective in some, but not all, cases and is often combined with loop diuretics to increase the flow rate and potassium secretion in the distal nephron.

Three commonly used drugs, spironolactone, amiloride, and triamterene, have as their main therapeutic action a reduction of distal potassium excretion. Self-evidently, spironolactone reduces the aldosterone-dependent component of potassium secretion. Amiloride and triamterene act independently of aldosterone—the pharmacology of

Table 9 *Drugs causing renal potassium retention*

Potassium-sparing diuretics
amiloride
triamterene
spironolactone
Angiotensin converting enzyme inhibitors
Prostaglandin synthetase inhibitors
indomethacin, other non-steroidal anti-inflammatory drugs
Cyclosporin
Heparin

amiloride is best understood and involves the selective blockade of the apical sodium channel of the epithelial cells in the cortical collecting duct. The ensuing reduction of transtubular voltage impairs potassium and proton secretion, leading to hyperkalaemia and metabolic acidosis.

Several other drugs cause renal potassium retention—those to consider are listed in Table 9.

CONGENITAL

Pseudohypoaldosteronism type I is a rare autosomal recessive condition associated with mineralocorticoid resistance in all major target tissues. This results in renal salt wasting and potassium retention with metabolic acidosis, features identical to isolated hypoaldosteronism, from which the disorder is distinguished by the presence of elevated aldosterone. Mineralocorticoid receptors in the cytosol of lymphocytes are reduced in number, and quantitation of this is useful as a marker of the condition. Spontaneous regression is the rule, and by the age of 4 years most children are metabolically normal on no therapy. Treatment is with supplements of sodium chloride and sodium bicarbonate.

The type II variant (also designated Gordon's syndrome) has a completely different pathogenesis despite also manifesting hyperkalaemia and metabolic acidosis. Type II patients present in adolescence or as young adults and, in contrast to type I, these individuals are hypertensive, retain sodium, and are found to have suppressed aldosterone. The most likely primary defect is probably accelerated chloride reabsorption in the thick ascending limb of Henle's loop and the distal tubule, with resulting sodium chloride retention and volume expansion. This still does not explain the extreme suppression of aldosterone, which appears in excess of that attributable to volume expansion alone, and which also should be limited by the potent direct stimulus from hyperkalaemia. The pathogenesis may be more complex, with the possibility of an adrenal defect as well. Not surprisingly, fludrocortisone is ineffective but increased potassium excretion can often be achieved using a combination of sodium bicarbonate and thiazide or loop diuretics.

REFERENCES

Brenner, B.M. and Rector, F.C. (1991). *The kidney* (4th edn). Saunders, Philadelphia. A large comprehensive textbook of nephrology. Extensive sections on renal physiology and metabolism, ion and solute transport, and the scientific basis of disturbed tubular function. Comprehensive and scientifically orientated sections on clinical aspects of renal tubular disorders.

Giebisch, G. and Boulpaep, E. (ed.) (1989). Symposium on co-transport mechanisms in renal tubules. *Kidney International* **36**, 333–434.

Raine, A.E.G. (1992). *Advanced renal medicine*. Oxford University Press. A collection of review articles, including sections covering membrane transport in uraemia, and normal and abnormal regulation of salt and water metabolism.

Watts, R.D.E. (1982). Cystinuria and xanthinuria. In *Scientific foundation of urology*, (2nd edn) (ed. G.D. Chisholm and D.T. Williams), pp. 314–23. William Heinemann, London.

20.19.1 The renal tubular acidoses

R. D. COHEN

INTRODUCTION

Renal tubular acidosis (**RTA**) is the term used to describe metabolic acidoses whose cause is a disorder of the renal tubules. The designation distinguishes this type of acidosis from that accompanying generalized glomerulotubular failure (uraemic acidosis). It is, however, of considerable importance that glomerular failure may supervene in chronic renal tubular acidosis—an outcome which may in some instances be prevented by treatment. The pathogenesis of uraemic acidosis has been described in Chapter 20.17.1.

NORMAL ACID–BASE FUNCTION OF THE KIDNEY

Both the proximal and distal nephron actively secrete hydrogen ions (H^+) in normal acid–base functioning of the kidney (see Fig. 1(a)). A major function of H^+ secretion in the proximal tubule is the reabsorption of filtered bicarbonate. In the healthy adult about 4500 mmol of bicarbonate are filtered per day, and all but 10 to 15 per cent of this is titrated by secreted H^+ in the proximal tubule to form carbonic acid, which is rapidly dehydrated to carbon dioxide and water by brush-border carbonic anhydrase. The CO_2 diffuses into the proximal tubular cells; here it combines with hydroxyl ions (generated when the original H^+ was pumped out into the lumen) to form bicarbonate, which then passes into the peritubular capillaries. Thus for each H^+ secreted, a single HCO_3^- ion is effectively reabsorbed.

That HCO_3^-, which escapes reabsorption by the above mechanism in the proximal nephron, passes to the distal nephron, where, in the common situation where the final urine pH is less than 6.5, it is completely reabsorbed by further H^+ secretion. The events so far described have thus used H^+ secretion to reclaim filtered bicarbonate, and have done nothing to dispose of H^+ in response to any acid burden that requires correction. Nearly all authors describe how further H^+ secretion titrates phosphate buffer in the tubular lumen thus:

$$HPO_4^{2-} + H^+ \rightarrow H_2PO_4^-$$

and ammonia (NH_3), which has been formed in the tubular cells and has passed into the lumen by non-ionic diffusion, as follows:

$$NH_3 + H^+ \rightarrow NH_4^+.$$

The amount of H^+ 'locked up' in $H_2PO_4^-$ can be approximately determined by titrating the urine back to pH 7.4, and is known as 'titratable acidity'. The total amount of net acid excreted by the kidney is therefore conventionally regarded as the excretion of

$$(\text{titratable acid} + \text{ammonium} - \text{bicarbonate}).$$

The bicarbonate term has been included to cover the situation where an alkaline urine is passed and bicarbonate has not been completely reclaimed. The total net acid excretion in the urine calculated in this way amounts to 50 to 100 mmol/day, the contribution of ammonium being typically two to three times greater than that of titratable acidity, and that of bicarbonate is very small. During any tendency to acidosis, H^+ secretion is enhanced; the phosphate buffer is more completely titrated, resulting in an increase in titratable acidity and lowering of urine pH. Furthermore, ammonia synthesis and diffusion into the urine is increased by a variety of mechanisms, so more H^+ is excreted as NH_4^+. Bicarbonate excretion is reduced to zero and, given sufficient stimulus, the urine reaches its minimum possible pH, which varies between normal individuals in the range 4.4 to 5.3. The final acidification is achieved in the medullary collecting duct. The acidoses seen in different types of RTA are in conventional descriptions regarded as being ultimately due to various defects leading to inappropriately low excretion of H^+ buffered either as titratable acidity or NH_4^+, and/or to excessive excretion of bicarbonate.

However, a major interpretation of the role of the kidney in acid–base homeostasis has been proposed by Oliver and Bourke (1975) and by Atkinson and Camien (1982). They point out that, since ammonium is generated from glutamine virtually entirely as NH_4^+, there is no possibility of it acting as a significant buffer for H^+. This means that the ammonium term has to be deleted from the expression for net renal acid excretion, which now becomes:

$$(\text{titratable acid} - \text{bicarbonate}).$$

Nevertheless, renal excretion of NH_4^+ still remains of major importance for acid–base status, but indirectly in the following way. If one considers the total daily nitrogen load to be excreted, the majority of this excretion takes place by conversion to urea in the liver and subsequent urinary excretion, most of the remaining nitrogen being excreted as NH_4^+ in the urine. Now whenever a molecule of urea is synthesized, two H^+ ions are produced as byproducts. These H^+ ions are normally used to neutralize the large quantity of bicarbonate produced by metabolism of the non-amino portions of the amino acids constituting the proteins from which the urea was derived. If, however, there is a defect in the renal excretion of ammonium, the liver is forced to increase urea synthesis, with the consequent production of more H^+ ions than are needed to neutralize the amino acid-derived bicarbonate. Acidosis therefore results. Under this interpretation, therefore, that part of the acidosis in RTA which is due to underexcretion of NH_4^+ in the urine results from overproduction of urea, not from failure of excretion of H^+ buffered as NH_4^+. It is not known, however, how precisely the liver responds reciprocally by increasing urea synthesis when confronted with a decrease in urinary excretion of NH_4^+. The reader should bear this reinterpretation in mind when reading the extensive literature on RTA, which almost invariably regards the conventional calculation given above as a precise estimate of renal excretion of acid. The present author has yet to see a convincing argument against the above reinterpretation.

In the following description, RTA is broken down into three main categories, on the basis of clearly identifiable differences in pathogenesis.

Distal renal tubular acidosis ('classical' RTA, 'gradient RTA', RTA type 1)

This form of RTA (RTA-1) is characterized by an inability to generate a normal minimum urinary pH even in the presence of severe systemic acidosis. It may present in infancy, childhood, or adult life, most typically with acute acidosis and hyperventilation, often accompanied by muscular weakness due to hypokalaemia. In most patients the attacks of acute acidosis represent a worsening of a mild chronic hyperchloraemic metabolic acidosis which may have been fully compensated until presentation. About 70 per cent of patients are found to have either nephrocalcinosis or calcium-containing renal calculi. Rickets and growth stunting in childhood are frequent features, and osteomalacia may be seen in adults. Although the glomerular filtration rate is characteristically normal, or nearly so, at the outset, progressive nephrocalcinosis, obstructive uropathy related to calculi, and recurrent urinary tract infections may eventually result in glomerular failure.

The diagnosis in the acute state is usually simple and depends on the observation of a urinary pH greater than 5.5 (and usually greater than 6) in the presence of a normal anion gap metabolic acidosis (see Chapter 11.14), hyperchloraemia, and normal or nearly normal plasma urea and creatinine. Severe hypokalaemia, hypercalciuria, evidence of renal calcification, and the presence of clinical features related to one of the aetiologies discussed below may provide further evidence. The failure to acidify the urine maximally in the presence of severe acidosis (plasma bicarbonate < 12 mmol/l) serves to distinguish the condition from RTA types 2 and 4. Nephrocalcinosis is virtually confined to RTA-1. In the chronic non-acute state, which often presents with renal stones, incidental discovery of nephrocalcinosis, failure of growth, anorexia, or lethargy, the diagnosis may be confirmed by the short acid load test of

Table 1

	RTA-1	RTA-2	RTA-4
Urine pH when plasma HCO_3^- < 13 mmol/l	> 6	< 5.4	< 5.4
Plasma potassium	Low	Low	Raised
Nephrocalcinosis or renal lithiasis	+	−	−
Therapeutic requirement			
For bicarbonate	Modest	Large	Modest
For mineralocorticoid	−	−	+

Wrong and Davies, the critical finding being the failure to achieve normal minimum urinary pH after ingestion of a standard body-weight-related dose of ammonium chloride. Wrong and Davies also draw attention to a group of patients with nephrocalcinosis and failure to acidify the urine normally on ammonium chloride challenge, but did not have systemic acidosis ('incomplete syndrome of RTA'); these patients often show an unusually brisk excretion of NH_4^+ in response to the acid load. It is not safe to administer the acid load test if the plasma bicarbonate is below 19 mmol/l. Under such conditions, comparison of urinary pH with plasma bicarbonate is helpful (see Table 1).

PATHOPHYSIOLOGY

RTA-1 is due to a failure of the distal nephron and collecting duct, to generate the 800–900:1 H^+ gradient between tubular lumen and blood that a normal subject can achieve under acidifying conditions. Except in rare patients with mixed syndromes, proximal tubular function is normal in terms of H^+ secretion and bicarbonate reabsorption. In RTA-1, the distal nephron defect is variable in severity, but if the urine pH cannot be lowered below 6 to 6.5, increasingly large quantities of bicarbonate may appear in the urine. This bicarbonate represents that proportion of the 10 to 15 per cent of filtered bicarbonate which has reached the distal nephron, but has not been reabsorbed because of failure of distal H^+ secretion. The H^+ secretion defect also results in the failure of titration of phosphate buffer. Because NH_4^+ excretion is lessened in alkaline urine, it may be lower than appropriate for systemic pH; under the reinterpretation discussed above, failure of NH_4^+ excretion would encourage increased urea synthesis and H^+ generation. All these factors, which are direct consequences of the distal tubular defect, lead to acidosis (see Fig. 1(b)). In children in particular, loss of bicarbonate may be a major contributor.

The precise nature of the defect which results in failure to establish the normal H^+ gradient is, in most instances, unknown. Theoretically, it could result from a failure of active H^+ secretion in the distal nephron, or, alternatively, an abnormal permeability of the distal nephron to H^+, resulting in leak-back of H^+ after secretion. The latter mechanism is clearly seen in RTA-1 occurring during amphotericin B therapy. This antifungal agent acts as a protonophore—it inserts itself into the luminal cell membrane in the distal nephron and provides a channel for back leakage of H^+ into the cell, or, alternatively, of bicarbonate out of the cell into the lumen. Another possible mechanism is deficiency of distal cellular carbonic anhydrase; the isoenzyme present is carbonic anhydrase II, and hereditary deficiency has been described in association with osteopetrosis and RTA-1. However, carbonic anhydrase is normal in the vast majority of cases. Evidence that defects in distal tubular energy metabolism can result in RTA-1 has been provided by its occurrence in carnitine palmitoyltransferase (type I) deficiency.

A marked reduction in urinary citrate excretion is seen in RTA-1 and has been considered to be an indication of abnormal mitochondrial function in distal nephron cells, but there is no direct evidence to substantiate this view.

The hypokalaemia frequently present has two origins. First, lack of H^+ flux out of the tubular cell into the lumen encourages K^+ exchange for luminal Na^+ in the distal nephron; even so, overall distal Na^+ reabsorption is impaired, leading to secondary aldosteronism, which provides the second reason for renal K^+ wasting. Correction of the acidosis, which raises distal luminal pH and therefore permits more H^+ secretion, results in amelioration of Na^+ and K^+ wasting (in contrast to RTA-2, see below).

Renal lithiasis is generally attributed to the hypercalciuria and hypocitraturia. Citrate complexes with calcium ions to form the $CaCit^-$ ion, which is partly responsible for maintaining calcium ions in solution in the urine, and a situation in which there is both lack of citrate and increased calcium is likely to be lithogenic. The pathogenesis of the nephrocalcinosis is unclear. So is that of osteomalacia or rickets, which can be corrected by treatment of the chronic acidosis without vitamin D therapy. There is no evidence in humans for interference with vitamin D metabolism in acidosis, although transient depression of renal 1-hydroxylation of vitamin D by acidosis has been observed in animals.

CAUSES OF RTA-1

RTA-1 may occur as a primary disorder, or secondary to a whole range of conditions which, in one way or another, affect distal nephron function.

Fig. 1 Diagrams to indicate the site of the defects in different types of RTA. (a) Normal; (b) RTA-1, gradient defect in distal nephron; (c) RTA-2, proximal HCO_3^- reabsorption defect due to reduced H^+ secretion; (d) RTA-4, defects in NH_4^+ production and in capacity of H^+ pump in distal nephron due to hypoaldosteronism. The thickness of the arrows indicates semiquantitatively the magnitude of the ionic fluxes. See text for further explanation.

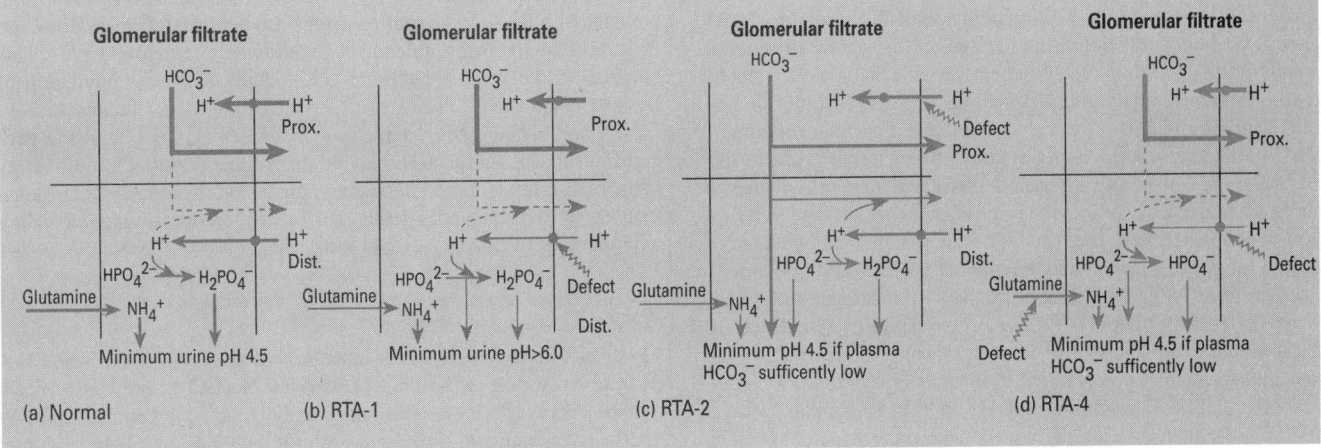

The primary disorder may be clearly hereditary, or may be sporadic. The hereditary form behaves as an autosomal dominant and may present in childhood or in adult life. There is, however, an infantile form of the condition which is transient and may occur in siblings without other family history. It is not clear whether this is a recessive disorder, or due to environmental factors. The rare hereditary carbonic anhydrase deficiency has been referred to earlier. RTA-1 has recently been reported in association with carnitine palmitoyltransferase (type I) deficiency.

In the acquired category, RTA-1 associated with presumptively autoimmune disorders accounts for a significant proportion of cases. Sjögren's syndrome is the most prominent association in this group, but other dysglobulinaemic or hypergammaglobulinaemic conditions also give rise to RTA-1. It does not appear, however, that the raised plasma globulin itself is the determining factor. RTA-1 is occasionally seen in primary biliary cirrhosis and, rarely, in fibrosing alveolitis. Although RTA-1 is a cause of nephrocalcinosis, it seems fairly clear that nephrocalcinosis itself can, by causing medullary damage, give rise to RTA-1. Thus, for instance, hyperparathyroidism and chronic vitamin D poisoning may cause RTA-1 because of nephrocalcinosis. Conditions directly damaging the renal medulla, such as pyelonephritis, papillary necrosis, chronic obstructive uropathy, medullary sponge kidney, and sickle-cell anaemia may also give rise to varying degrees of RTA-1. Amongst drug-related causes, analgesic nephropathy presumably acts through papillary damage; the RTA-1 associated with amphotericin B therapy has been explained above.

TREATMENT

The acutely acidotic patient will usually have moderate to very marked hypokalaemia. It is essential that the hypokalaemia be corrected before the acidosis. If, mistakenly, the acidosis is dealt with before the hypokalaemia, movement of K^+ into cells will further lower plasma K^+ and cardiac arrest may occur. Potassium, and then isotonic sodium bicarbonate, are administered intravenously, aiming to restore the abnormalities over a few hours.

In the chronic condition, therapy with oral sodium bicarbonate has markedly beneficial effects. Not only will it prevent recurrent exacerbations of acidosis, but renal potassium loss will be curtailed, hypercalciuria will be diminished, and hypocitraturia improved, osteomalacia or rickets healed, and growth restored in children. In addition, progression of nephrocalcinosis and nephrolithiasis and consequent renal damage may be halted. The daily bicarbonate requirement is usually in the range 1 to 3 mmol/kg body-weight, but often more in children. Not infrequently, potassium supplements are required in addition to sodium bicarbonate.

Proximal renal tubular acidosis (RTA type 2; bicarbonate wasting RTA)

This form of RTA (Fig. 1(c)) is superficially clinically similar to RTA-1, but there are notable distinguishing features. It is rare as an isolated defect and, in the great majority of patients, is associated with multiple abnormalities of proximal tubular functions, e.g. glycosuria, aminoaciduria, hyperphosphaturia, and uricosuria (the Fanconi syndrome). Provided the patient is sufficiently acidotic, the urine pH falls to the normal minimum. Nephrocalcinosis and renal calculi are virtually never present. Bicarbonate leakage into the urine is much greater than in RTA-1 and, in consequence, very large quantities of sodium bicarbonate may be required for therapy. There may be marked polyuria and polydipsia, especially in those patients in whom the acidosis has been fully controlled by bicarbonate therapy. Proximal myopathy, osteomalacia, or rickets are common associations of RTA-2, probably largely because of the frequent aetiological involvement of disorders of vitamin D supply or metabolism. RTA-2 resembles RTA-1 in that it presents with a chronic (or acute exacerbation of) normal anion gap hyperchloraemic acidosis, with a marked tendency to potassium deficiency due to renal potassium loss.

PATHOPHYSIOLOGY

The basic lesion in RTA-2 is a depression of the capacity of the proximal tubule to secrete H^+ and thus to reabsorb bicarbonate. In a normal individual or in a patient with RTA-1, the plasma bicarbonate above which bicarbonate appears in the urine is 25–28 mmol/l. In RTA-2 this bicarbonate 'threshold' is lowered, often markedly so, due to the proximal tubular defect. The result is that the distal nephron is flooded with bicarbonate which has escaped proximal reabsorption, and the low capacity (but high gradient) distal H^+ secreting mechanism cannot produce enough H^+ to reabsorb this bicarbonate, which therefore spills over into the urine. However, when, in consequence of the bicarbonate leak, plasma bicarbonate falls to a level which reduces the filtered bicarbonate load to one with which the defective proximal tubule can cope, then the distal nephron is fully capable of producing a normally minimal urinary pH of 4.5 to 5.3 (Fig. 1(c)). The acidosis in RTA-2 is predominantly due to the bicarbonate leak, but it is, to a lesser extent, related to failure of titration of phosphate and failure of appropriate NH_4^+ excretion due to the inappropriately high urine pH—at least while plasma bicarbonate remains above the renal threshold. The high distal load of sodium bicarbonate is also responsible for sodium wastage. This leads to secondary aldosteronism, which, together with the high demand created for Na^+/K^+ exchange in the distal nephron, results in potassium wastage and hypokalaemia. The polyuria is due both to the distal sodium bicarbonate load and to the effects of potassium deficiency on the renal concentrating mechanism. When osteomalacia/rickets is seen in RTA-2 it may be related both to the basic cause of the syndrome (see below) and possibly to the acidosis itself.

CAUSES OF RTA-2

Nearly always some factor which damages proximal tubular function can be identified. However, familial autosomal dominant RTA-2 has been reported as an isolated lesion. Isolated damage to the proximal tubular H^+ secretion mechanism occurs during treatment with the carbonic anhydrase inhibitor acetazolamide and in carbonic anhydrase II deficiency, in which there is also an element of RTA-1.

More usually, RTA-2 occurs as part of more generalized proximal tubular damage, with reabsorption defects for glucose, amino acids, and phosphate—the Fanconi syndrome. There are many causes of the Fanconi syndrome; in the genetic category are included cystinosis, Wilson's disease, and hereditary fructose intolerance, as well as the isolated hereditary variety. Amongst acquired causes of RTA-2/Fanconi syndrome may be listed vitamin D deficiency, lead poisoning, multiple myeloma, therapy with outdated tetracycline, hyperparathyroidism, and the nephrotic syndrome. A more comprehensive list has been compiled by Du Bose and Alpern (1989). The precise mechanisms of damage in patients with RTA-2/Fanconi syndrome are not usually clear. However, in hereditary fructose intolerance the absence of fructose-1-phosphate aldolase in the proximal tubular cells results in the accumulation of fructose-1-phosphate during fructose ingestion (see Chapter 11.2.2). Fructose phosphorylation depletes ATP stores markedly and the generalized tubular malfunction may be due to this perturbation of energy metabolism. In vitamin D deficiency, the lesion is probably contributed to both by the deficiency itself and by the accompanying secondary hyperparathyroidism.

THERAPY

The bicarbonate leak is much more severe in RTA-2 than in RTA-1, and the daily dose of sodium bicarbonate needed to prevent acidosis may be very large (3 to 20 mmol/kg body weight). In contrast to RTA-1, effective treatment of the acidosis in RTA-2 does not help, and may worsen the potassium deficiency and polyuria, by providing a greater sodium bicarbonate load to the distal tubule. If glomerular failure ensues, as for example in cystinosis, then the bicarbonate requirement may lessen. Potassium supplements in the form of oral bicarbonate will be required. If the amount of oral bicarbonate needed is intolerable, hydrochlorothiazide may be added. This agent appears to diminish the bicarbonate requirement by decreasing the filtered load of bicarbonate, but may necessitate an increase in potassium supplementation.

Hyperkalaemic renal tubular acidosis (RTA type 4)

RTA-4 is characterized by hyperkalaemia rather than hypokalaemia. As in RTA-1 and RTA-2, patients present with metabolic acidosis in which the anion gap is normal or nearly so and there is a similar tendency to hyperchloraemia. As in RTA-2, if the plasma bicarbonate falls sufficiently, then the distal tubule is able to mount a normal blood/urine pH gradient. These patients frequently have slight or moderate glomerular impairment, but the degree of hyperkalaemia is quite out of proportion to this (see Chapters 20.2.3, 20.17.1).

PATHOPHYSIOLOGY

The basic abnormality behind most aetiologies of RTA-4 is either hypoaldosteronism or failure of aldosterone action. Mineralocorticoid deficiency diminishes the capacity of the H^+ secreting mechanism in the distal nephron but not its power to sustain a pH gradient if bicarbonate delivery from the proximal tubule is small. There is no evidence of a proximal tubular defect in H^+ secretion and bicarbonate reabsorption. The hyperkalaemia is a direct consequence of the mineralocorticoid deficiency and has the additional effect of suppressing renal production of NH_4^+, the excretion of which is diminished in RTA-4. The nitrogen not thus excreted is converted to urea and H^+ in the liver. In this way the failure of NH_4^+ excretion in RTA-4 is largely responsible for the acidosis (Fig. 1(d)). A second mechanism of RTA-4 is illustrated by its induction by amiloride, which inhibits sodium reabsorption in the cortical collecting duct and thereby reduces the negative luminal potential required for K^+ and H^+ secretion.

CAUSES

Aldosterone deficiency leading to RTA-4 may be due to primary adrenal disease, as in Addison's disease and certain inborn errors of steroid synthesis. However, much more commonly it is related to deficient renin production, which may be seen in many chronic renal disorders, most notably in diabetes and chronic tubulointerstitial disease, including pyelonephritis. Renin production is, to some extent, dependent on prostaglandin synthesis and, increasingly commonly, RTA-4 is being seen in patients receiving prostaglandin synthetase inhibitors in the form of non-steroidal anti-inflammatory agents. It also may occur in association with the administration of angiotensin-converting enzyme inhibitors, β-blockers, and potassium sparing diuretics. Finally, RTA-4 is also seen in patients receiving aldosterone antagonists and in infants with pseudo-hypoaldosteronism; in both these circumstances there is a renal insensitivity to aldosterone action.

TREATMENT

Patients with RTA-4, in which acidosis is significant or hyperkalaemia is potentially dangerous, should be treated with a mineralocorticoid. Typically, 0.05 to 0.15 mg fludrocortisone daily improves NH_4^+ excretion, and restores hyperkalaemia and acidosis towards normal.

DIFFERENTIAL DIAGNOSIS OF THE DIFFERENT TYPES OF RENAL TUBULAR ACIDOSIS

For convenience, the principal points of distinction between the different types of RTA have been summarized in Table 1, the contents of which have been restricted to the simpler clinical considerations.

REFERENCES

Atkinson, D.E. and Camien, M.N. (1982). The role of urea synthesis in the removal of metabolic bicarbonate and the regulation of blood pH. *Current Topics in Cellular Regulation* **21**, 261–302.
Du Bose, T. and Alpern, R.J. (1989). Renal tubular acidosis. In *The metabolic basis of inherited disease* (6th edn), (ed. C.R. Scriver, A.L. Beaudet, W.S. Sly, and D. Valle). McGraw-Hill, New York.
Oliver, J. and Bourke, E. (1975). Adaptations in urea and ammonium excretion in metabolic acidosis in the rat. *Clinical Science and Molecular Medicine* **48**, 515–20.
Sebastian, A. and Morris, R.C. (1977). Renal tubular acidosis. *Clinical Nephrology* **7**, 216–30.
Wrong, O.M. and Davies, H.E.F. (1959). The excretion of acid in renal disease. *Quarterly Journal of Medicine* **28**, 259.

Section 21 *Sexually-transmitted diseases and sexual health*

The clinical features of non-gonococcal urethritis associated with infection with the oculogenital serovars (D–K) of *C. trachomatis* are described in Chapter 7.11.41. Pharyngeal infections are often symptomless but can be associated with pharyngitis lacking specific features. Most men with rectal infection are symptomless with normal proctoscopic findings but there may be features of a distal proctitis. Histologically, there is a non-specific proctitis consisting of a mild increase in the number of chronic inflammatory cells and polymorphonuclear leucocytes within the lamina propria.

Infection with lymphogranuloma venereum serovars is associated with a more severe proctitis with systemic features. The sigmoidoscopic findings are those of a severe proctitis but the inflammatory changes seldom extend more proximally than 12 cm from the dentate line. Occasionally, the inflammation is more localized, with the formation of an irregular ulcerated mass that may be polypoidal and extend circumferentially to produce stenosis. Inguinal lymph-node involvement may be a feature of lesions of the anal canal and distal rectum. Untreated, lymphogranuloma venereum can be complicated by perianal abscess formation, strictures, and fistulae in ano. Histologically, there is a dense infiltration of the lamina propria and submucosa by lymphocytes, plasma cells, hystiocytes, and sometimes eosinophils. Occasionally, granulomas with giant cells are found with focal areas of acute inflammation with crypt abscesses.

The treatment of non-gonococcal urethritis is detailed elsewhere. Although there are limited data on the treatment of rectal chlamydial infections, tetracyclines have proved useful. In the management of oculogenital chlamydial infection, oral oxytetracycline in a dosage of 500 mg six-hourly for 7 days is satisfactory, and doxycycline given in a dose of 100 mg twice daily by mouth for 14 to 21 days is effective against infection with lymphogranuloma venereum serovars.

Mycoplasma and ureaplasma infections

Although *Mycoplasma hominis* and *Ureaplasma urealyticum* can be cultured from rectal material from over one-third of homosexual men and probably can be transmitted to the rectum during anal intercourse, there is little evidence that either organism causes proctitis.

Chancroid

Chancroid, caused by the bacterium *Haemophilus ducreyi*, is common in tropical countries. Although there are few reports on the features of perianal chancroid, it is likely that the ulceration is similar to that occurring on the genitalia (Chapter 7.11.13).

Granuloma inguinale

Although usually regarded as a sexually transmitted disease, the mode of transmission of the causative organism *Calymmatobacterium granulomatis* is uncertain. Perianal granuloma inguinale most commonly occurs in homosexual men and presents as ulceration. Occasionally, extensive fibrosis may occur with anal stenosis and, in a few cases, extensive areas of skin and subcutaneous tissue undergo necrosis. Basalcell or squamous-cell carcinomas may result as a complication of the infection.

Shigellosis

The sexual transmission of *Shigella* spp. among homosexual men was first recognized in 1974 in San Francisco and subsequent reports have confirmed the spread of this organism through oroanal sexual contact.

Salmonellosis

Cases of typhoid fever that have been acquired from anilingus with symptomless carriers of *Salmonella typhi* have been described.

Campylobacter infections

In some areas of the United States, *Campylobacter* spp. (particularly *C. jejuni* but also to a lesser extent *C. fetus fetus*, *C. fennelliae*, and *C. cinaedi*) can be isolated from over 20 per cent of homosexual men with diarrhoea. The source of infection is often uncertain but symptomless carriers are known to exist.

Corynebacterium diphtheriae *infection*

In a recent study, non-toxigenic *C. diphtheriae* was isolated more commonly from the throats of homosexual men than heterosexual men who attended a clinic for sexually transmitted diseases in London. Although these organisms may be associated with pharyngitis, the significance of this finding is still uncertain.

Viral infections

Human papillomavirus (HPV) infection

The most common clinical presentation of HPV infection is the condyloma, a lesion that is almost always associated with HPV type 6/11, although occasionally other types may be detected concurrently. In homosexual men, condylomata are found most frequently in the perianal region and within the anal canal, where they may cause pruritus ani and bleeding during defaecation. Rarely, condylomata acuminata may be seen in the oropharynx. Although condylomata may be very extensive and persistent in immunocompetent individuals, this is particularly so in the immunocompromised patient, including those with HIV infection.

Treatment of perianal and anal warts can be difficult. Podophyllin can be used to treat perianal lesions but I prefer to avoid its use in the anal canal. Extensive lesions often require surgical treatment, for example, scissor excision or laser ablation.

Non-condylomatous HPV lesions of the anal canal have only recently been described by cytological screening and may be associated with intraepithelial neoplasia. The lesions, which can be identified by examination with an operating microscope or colposcope after the application of acetic acid (5 per cent v/v), are white, well-demarcated from the surrounding mucosa, and have a punctate appearance similar to that seen in HPV infection of the uterine cervix. Biopsy is required for the detection of associated anal intraepithelial neoplasia. The natural history of these lesions is still uncertain.

Herpes simplex virus (HSV) infection

Both types 1 and 2 of HSV can affect the anogenital region. In Edinburgh, between 1978 and 1991, primary or initial episodes of anogenital disease in homosexual men were associated with HSV-1 in 37 per cent of 66 cases and had probably been acquired during orogenital or oroanal sexual contact. Inapparent infection with either type is common and symptomless excretors of the virus may be important in the epidemiology of the infection.

In primary perianal herpes, there is anal pain, constipation, tenesmus, anal discharge, and bleeding on defaecation; in addition, systemic features are often prominent. Sacral nerve-root involvement may result in paraesthesiae in the distribution of the affected nerves, and urinary hesitancy or acute retention and impotence may be features. There are often multiple tender ulcers in the perianal region and within the anal canal. A distal proctitis is common; there may be no specific features but discrete vesicular or pustular lesions or ulcers may be seen. Herpetic proctitis can occur in the absence of perianal or anal ulceration. Rectal biopsies show a marked infiltration of the lamina propria with neutrophils (sometimes with the formation of crypt abscesses), perivascular infiltration of the submucosal vessels with lymphocytes, multinucleated cells, and, occasionally, intranuclear inclusions may be noted. HSV, however, is an uncommon cause of proctitis in homosexual men and in one study from London, the organism was isolated from only 6 per cent of 77 men with non-gonococcal proctitis.

Recurrences are more likely in HSV-2 than in HSV-1 infection but, generally, the symptoms and signs are much less severe and systemic features are not found.

Oral acyclovir given in a dosage of 400 mg five times per day for 10 days is effective in the treatment of primary or initial anorectal herpes. Recurrent disease can be treated with a lower dose of acyclovir, for example, 200 mg, five times per day for 5 days.

Cytomegalovirus (CMV)

Infection with CMV has been more prevalent among homosexual than heterosexual men and women. In a study from San Francisco in 1981, 94 per cent of sexually active, homosexual men were seropositive for CMV compared with only 54 per cent of heterosexuals. In addition, CMV was cultured from the urine of 14 per cent of 101 young (18–29 years of age) homosexual men but from none of 101 heterosexual men. In a subsequent study from the same group of workers, over 70 per cent of susceptible individuals became infected with CMV during a 9-month surveillance period. These findings suggested that CMV was transmissible amongst homosexual men. The virus is present in semen and receptive anal intercourse is the most likely means of acquisition. Restriction enzyme analysis of serial isolates from homosexuals has shown that infection with multiple strains of CMV is common and that multiple strains can be shed simultaneously.

Hepatitis A virus (HAV)

HAV is transmitted by the faecal–oral route and homosexual men are at increased risk of infection through oroanal and orogenital contact and occasionally from the ingestion of urine. In many areas of Western Europe and the United States, the prevalence of anti-HAV in the serum of homosexual men is higher than in that of heterosexual men. Epidemic outbreaks of homosexually acquired, acute hepatitis A are reported occasionally, and recently an increase in the number of acute cases has been noted in the United States, Canada, Australia, and London. In the prevention of spread of HAV, inactivated HAV vaccine may be indicated in sexually active homosexual men.

Hepatitis B virus (HBV)

The homosexual transmission of HBV was first recognized almost 20 years ago when it was shown that the prevalence of hepatitis B surface antigen (**HBsAg**) was significantly higher in the serum of Caucasian homosexuals than in that of Caucasian heterosexual men who attended a clinic for sexually transmitted diseases in London. In the United Kingdom at that time, about 5 per cent of homosexual men attending clinics for genitourinary medicine were hepatitis B surface antigenaemic, a rate that was some 20 times that of blood donors. Although the prevalence of serological markers for HBV in clinic attenders varies from city to city within a country and from country to country, in Europe and the United States it is significantly higher in the sera of homosexual men. Seropositivity for HBV has been related to the duration of regular homosexual activity and to the numbers of different sexual partners. Recently, in some areas there has been a decline in the prevalence of HBV infection, presumably as a result of the adoption of safer sexual practices to avoid HIV infection and to the more widespread use of hepatitis B vaccine. As HBsAg can be detected in saliva, seminal fluid, faeces, and the rectal mucosa, particularly when there is superficial ulceration following intercourse, anogenital and oral–anal sexual contact with an HBV carrier are significant risk factors for the homosexual transmission of the virus. As hepatitis B e antigenaemia is closely associated with infectivity and as the sera of some 70 per cent of homosexual men who

are persistent carriers of HBsAg contain e antigen, their sexual contacts are at particular risk of infection.

In the prevention of spread of HBV, active vaccination of sexually active homosexual and bisexual men who are antiHBs negative, is cost-effective. The antibody response to vaccination in HIV-infected homosexual men, however, is frequently impaired.

Hepatitis C virus (HCV)

Although the sexual transmission of HCV undoubtedly occurs, the risk of infection to homosexual men remains to be ascertained. In one recent study from a clinic for sexually transmitted diseases in London, however, 2.2 per cent of 275 serum samples from homosexual men but only 0.4 per cent of 763 samples from heterosexual men and women gave positive results for antiHCV in an enzyme immunoassay for antibodies to C100 protein.

Hepatitis D virus (HDV)

HDV is usually spread by parenteral exposure but in areas where vertical transmission of HBV occurs, HDV may be spread by close family contact (non-sexual). Epidemics of HDV hepatitis have occurred in susceptible populations (i.e. with a high HBsAg carrier rate) and homosexual men with their relatively high prevalence of HBV infection might therefore be considered to be a susceptible population for HDV. In a recent, large, multicentre study from the United States, sera from 7.7 per cent of 298 homosexual men who were HBsAg positive had anti-HDV. Analysis of the findings showed that there was an association between (i) the number of sexual partners and (ii) anorectal trauma in the 2 years before testing. These data and the finding of HDV markers in the serum and viral RNA in liver tissue from HBV-infected homosexuals who had never injected intravenous drugs suggests that sexual transmission of this virus occurs within this population group.

Human immunodeficiency virus

The epidemiology, pathogenesis, and manifestations of this viral infection are discussed in Chapter 7.10.29.

Human T-cell leukaemia viruses (HTLV) types 1 and 2

Although HTLV-1 can be transmitted sexually, the prevalence of infection among homosexual men is low. In one recent study from Los Angeles, the seroprevalence rate was 0.8 per 1000 men. HTLV-2 infection is rare in homosexuals, antibodies having been detected in the serum of only 1 of 883 homosexual men in the United States.

Other viral infections

Coronaviruses have been detected in the faeces of several homosexual men but their significance remains uncertain. Similar remarks pertain to the finding of echovirus 11 in the faeces of several symptomless men.

Protozoal infections

Amoebiasis

The existence of virulent and avirulent strains of *Entamoeba histolytica* has been postulated for many years but it has only been within the past 15 years that a relatively simple method for their differentiation has been described. Isoenzyme analysis of isolates of *E. histolytica* can be undertaken and it is now clear that only some isoenzyme patterns (zymodemes) are associated with pathogenicity. Amongst homosexual men in temperate climates, the prevalence of infection with *E. histolytica* varies between 10 and 35 per cent but it is now widely accepted that most of these men are infected with strains of the amoeba whose zymodemes are not associated with tissue invasion. Treatment is therefore not indicated. The situation is different, however, in tropical and subtropical areas where pathogenic zymodemes are more prevalent and can be transmitted sexually.

Giardiasis

The prevalence of *Giardia intestinalis* in homosexual men who attend clinics for sexually transmitted diseases in temperate climates has varied between 2 and 12 per cent and most of these men have become infected through oroanal sexual contacts. Although most infections were symptomless, a diarrhoeal illness may result.

Cryptosporidiosis

Infection with *Cryptosporidium parvum* can produce diarrhoeal illness. Usually transmitted by water, person-to-person spread of the organism has probably been responsible for the occurrence of infection in household contacts. Although the protozoan has been identified as a cause of diarrhoea in some homosexual men, the importance of sexual transmission in the epidemiology of cryptosporidium remains to be determined.

Nematode infection

Enterobius vermicularis

Although threadworms are most frequently transmitted by food or fomites contaminated by ova, sexual spread amongst homosexual men is common, oroanal contact being the most likely means of acquisition of the nematode.

Strongyloides stercoralis

In the case of *S. stercoralis*, non-infective rhabditaform larvae may develop into infective filariform larvae before leaving the colon. During oroanal contact, ingestion of faeces containing these larvae may enable transmission to occur. Penetration of the skin or mucous membrane of the penis by infective larvae may result in infestation following or during anal intercourse.

Other medical conditions in homosexual men

Urinary-tract infection and epididymitis

Although significant bacteriuria was found more commonly in homosexual than in heterosexual men who attended a clinic for sexually transmitted diseases in Seattle, this has not been the finding in other clinics, where the prevalence of urinary-tract infection was similar in both population groups. The Seattle workers also reported that acute epididymitis in homosexuals aged less than 35 years was more likely to be caused by enterobacteria than *N. gonorrhoeae* or *C. trachomatis*, the most common aetiological agent in young heterosexual men.

Anorectal trauma

Violent anal intercourse can cause anal fissures or the formation of a perianal haematoma. Profuse rectal haemorrhage may result from laceration of the mucosa during the insertion of a closed fist into the rectum, an activity that may also result in rupture of the colon, particularly at the rectosigmoid junction. Extraperitoneal microperforation of the rectum during fisting may result in pelvic cellulitis. Within a few days of such activity, lower abdominal, rectal pain develops and the temperature

rises. Abdominal examination is usually normal but there may be tenderness in the left iliac fossa. There is marked proctitis and induration of the pararectal tissues. Treatment is with broad-spectrum antimicrobial agents.

Anorectal sepsis

This may present as a chronic intersphincteric abscess with or without fistula formation, or as fistulae in ano.

Streptococcal infections

Streptococcal infection of the penis may result from fellatio. The lesions are erythematous, exude pus, and crusting may develop. Inguinal lymphadenitis associated with β-haemolytic streptococci may occur in immunocompromised individuals.

Rectal spirochaetosis

In this condition, spirochaetes lie parallel to the microvilli of the epithelial cells of the rectum and superficial portions of the crypts. The condition is indicated by the presence in a haematoxylin and eosin-stained section as a haematoxyphil zone, 3 μm wide, on the luminal surface of the cells. At least one species of spirochaete, *Brachyspira aalborgi*, has been associated with this condition.

Rectal spirochaetosis is found in at least one-third of homosexual men who attend clinics for sexually transmitted diseases but in between only 2 to 7 per cent of patients attending general medical and surgical departments. The source of these spirochaetes is uncertain but their increased prevalence in homosexual men suggests sexual transmission. Their pathogenicity is uncertain, although there have been occasional case reports on the occurrence of diarrhoea in individuals with rectal spirochaetosis and its resolution after treatment with penicillin.

Kaposi's sarcoma

In the early years of the epidemic of HIV infection, Kaposi's sarcoma accounted for some 50 per cent of AIDS cases in the United States; it was uncommon (less than 4 per cent) in other groups with AIDS. The percentage of people with an AIDS-defining illness reported to have Kaposi's sarcoma has declined over time, and, in 1989, just over 20 per cent of homosexual or bisexual men were affected. Although the aetiology of Kaposi's sarcoma is unknown, there is some indirect evidence that a sexually transmissible organism is causative. In the United States the condition is not related to age and race; it varies across the country but is greatest in the areas that were the initial foci of the epidemic. Women were more likely to have Kaposi's sarcoma if their partners were bisexual men than if they were intravenous drug users. A number of case reports on the development of Kaposi's sarcoma in HIV-seronegative homosexual men have also been published recently. Epidemiological data from London patients suggest that faecal–oral contact is the main route of transmission of the presumed agent of Kaposi's sarcoma. These findings, however, have not been confirmed in other areas.

Carcinoma of the anorectum

Over the past 20 years, several case reports on the occurrence of premalignant and malignant disease of the anorectum of homosexual men have been reported and epidemiological data appear to confirm that in men, receptive anal intercourse may be a risk factor for squamous- and transitional-cell carcinomas of the anal canal. Carcinomas of that area are relatively rare but in some cities of the United States such as New York, the incidence amongst homosexual men has been increasing. Parallels have been drawn between the aetiology of anal cancer in men and cervical cancer in women. HPV types 16 and 18 and to a lesser extent, types 31, 33 and 35, are usually found in high-grade cervical intraepithelial neoplasias (**CIN**) and invasive squamous-cell carcinomas. Recently, such types, particularly HPV-16, have also been detected in anal squamous-cell carcinomas.

As it is known that some women with higher grades of CIN will develop cervical carcinoma, a search has been made to detect premalignant lesions of the anal canal of homosexual men. Anal intraepithelial neoplasia (**AIN**) was first described in 1986 and is most commonly found at the transitional zone of the anal canal, that is, at the junction of the squamous epithelium of the anal canal and the columnar epithelium of the rectum. AIN has been found in tissue removed from the anal canal of homosexual men. With the operating microscope, after the application of acetic acid, severe AIN appears as irregular white areas with cobblestoning and mosaicism, and corkscrew vessels.

Minor degrees of AIN tend to be associated with HPV types 6 and 11 and more severe dysplasia with types 16 and 18. The natural history of AIN, particularly its progression to invasive cancer and whether treatment is necessary, is as yet unknown. The increasing incidence of anal cancers in homosexual men in the United States parallels that of HIV infection and indeed, there are case reports on the occurrence of squamous-cell carcinomas in HIV-infected individuals. Abnormal anal cytology is common in homosexual men with late-stage HIV disease (CDC group IV) and is significantly associated with HPV infection. HPV DNA often homologous with the DNA of multiple types of HPV but particularly types 16 and 18 is detectable in anal brushings from at least 50 per cent of these men. As the prevalence of HPV is inversely related to the number of CD4$^+$ cells in the peripheral blood, it has been postulated that the immune deficiency associated with HIV infection permits reactivation of latent HPV resulting in epithelial abnormalities. The situation may be analogous to development of cancers at other sites in iatrogenically immunosuppressed patients.

REFERENCES

Adler, M.W. (1988). *Diseases in the homosexual male*. Springer-Verlag, London.

Beral, V. *et al.* (1992). Risk of Kaposi's sarcoma and sexual practices associated with faecal contact in homosexual or bisexual men with AIDS. *Lancet*, **339**, 632–5.

Berger, R.E., Kessler, D., and Holmes, K.K. (1987). Etiology and manifestations of epididymitis in young men: correlations with sexual orientation. *Journal of Infectious Diseases*, **155**, 1341–3.

de Ruiter, A. and Mindel, A. (1991). Anal intraepithelial neoplasia. *European Journal of Cancer*, **27**, 1343–5.

Hunt, A.J., Davies, P.M., Weatherburn, P., Coxon, A.P.M., and McManus, T.J. (1991). Changes in sexual behaviour in a large cohort of homosexual men in England and Wales 1988–9. *British Medical Journal*, **302**, 505–6.

Kendall, P. *et al.* (1992). Hepatitis A among homosexual men—United States, Canada and Australia. *Mortality and Morbidity Weekly Report*, **41**, 155–64.

Meyer, R.D. *et al.* (1990). Prevalence of human T cell leukaemia viruses in selected populations of homosexual men. *Journal of Infectious Diseases*, **162**, 1370–2.

Quinn, T.C. and Stamm, W.E. (1990). Proctitis, proctocolitis, enteritis and esophagitis in homosexual men. In *Sexually transmitted diseases*, (ed. K.K. Holmes, P.A. Mardh, P.F Sparling, and P.J. Wiesner), pp. 663–83. McGraw-Hill, New York.

Solomon, R.D. *et al.* (1988). Human immunodeficiency virus and hepatitis delta virus in homosexual men. *Annals of Internal Medicine*, **108**, 51–4.

Tedder, R.S. *et al.* (1991). Hepatitis C virus: evidence for sexual transmission. *British Medical Journal*, **502**, 1299–302.

Weinstein, M.A., Sohn, N., and Robbins, R.D. (1981). Symptoms of pelvic cellulitis following rectal sexual trauma. *American Journal of Gastroenterology*, **75**, 380–1.

Wilson, A.P.R. *et al.* (1992). Unusual non-toxigenic *Corynebacterium diphtheriae* in homosexual men. *Lancet*, **339**, 998.

21.7 Genital warts

J. D. ORIEL

Genital warts are benign epithelial tumours caused by human papillomaviruses.

VIROLOGY

Human papillomaviruses (**HPV**) are a genus of the family Papovaviridae (see Chapter 7.10.24). HPV-6 and -11 are predominantly associated with genital warts, the lower grades of cervical intraepithelial neoplasia, and laryngeal papillomatosis in children.

PATHOGENESIS

HPV cause symptomatic tumours (genital warts) and subclinical lesions, but the viral genome may persist indefinitely in host cells as a latent infection. Genital warts may represent only 10 per cent, or less, of the whole range of genital HPV infections. Infection begins with the passage of viral material through the host epithelium, presumably via a breach in its surface, which enters the keratinocytes of the basal layer. Subsequent events are largely unknown, but the formation of viral proteins and the assembly of virions occur only in the nuclei of differentiated cells towards the surface of a lesion. Genital warts are characterized histologically by papillomatosis, an increased cellularity of the prickle-cell layer (acanthosis), and the appearance in the granular layer of koilocytes—large, vacuolated cells with pyknotic and often double nuclei; these nuclei contain basophilic inclusions composed of arrays of virions (Fig. 1).

Immune responses

Little is known about host defences to papillomaviruses, although both humoral and cell-mediated responses are known to occur. Patients with conditions that depress T-cell function, such as pregnancy, lymphoma, and immunosuppression for organ transplantation, have an increased risk of developing genital warts, which are often large and intractable.

EPIDEMIOLOGY

The incidence of genital warts is maximal between the ages of 16 and 24 years. The disease is usually transmitted by direct sexual contact, and 60 per cent of sexual partners of individuals with genital warts also develop them, after an incubation period of between 3 weeks and 9 months (mean 2.8 months). Other sexually transmitted diseases such as gonorrhoea, *Chlamydia trachomatis* infections, and trichomoniasis are often present, even in patients seen in dermatological practice. Occasionally, genital warts are secondary to common warts on non-genital areas. HPV can be transmitted vertically, and both anogenital warts and laryngeal papillomatosis may occur in children whose mothers had vulval warts at the time of delivery. Anogenital warts in children can also be due to close but non-sexual contact within a family, or be secondary to common skin warts, but in many cases sexual abuse by an infected adult is responsible. The existence of several modes of infection and the long incubation period of the disease may make the interpretation of anogenital warts in children difficult.

Genital strains of HPV can infect non-genital sites. Of these, the most common is the anus. Anal warts may be associated with penile or vulval warts; such multicentric HPV infection is not uncommon, and is also shown by the frequent coincidence of vulval and cervical lesions. Anal warts occurring alone, on the other hand, are strongly associated with anoreceptive intercourse and are therefore common in homosexual men. The age of onset of anal warts is similar to that of genital warts, and associated sexually transmitted diseases are common. The predominant viral types present in both anal and genital warts are HPV-6 and -11. Genital warts can also be transmitted sexually to a partner's lips or mouth.

CLINICAL FEATURES

The range of disease of genital epithelia caused by HPV infection is broad, and both clinical and subclinical lesions are recognized.

Lesions in men

Condylomata acuminata (exophytic condylomas) most often appear on areas exposed to coital trauma—the glans penis, coronal sulcus, prepuce, and terminal urethra. The soft, fleshy, vascular tumours are usually multiple and may coalesce into large masses (Fig. 2). Sessile or papular warts are more likely to occur on dry areas such as the shaft of the penis (Fig. 3). They are raised, pink or grey lesions, 0.5 to 3 mm in diameter, and may occur alone or in association with exophytic condylomas. Subclinical HPV lesions (flat condylomas) are identified by examining the genitals with magnification after the application of 5 per cent aqueous

Fig. 1 Human papillomavirus particle. Vulval wart extract, negative staining with phosphotungstic acid. ($\times$ 181 000)

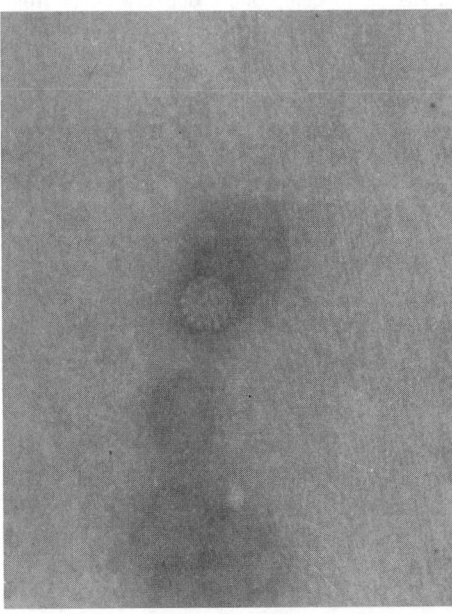

Fig. 3 Sessile (papular) warts of penis.

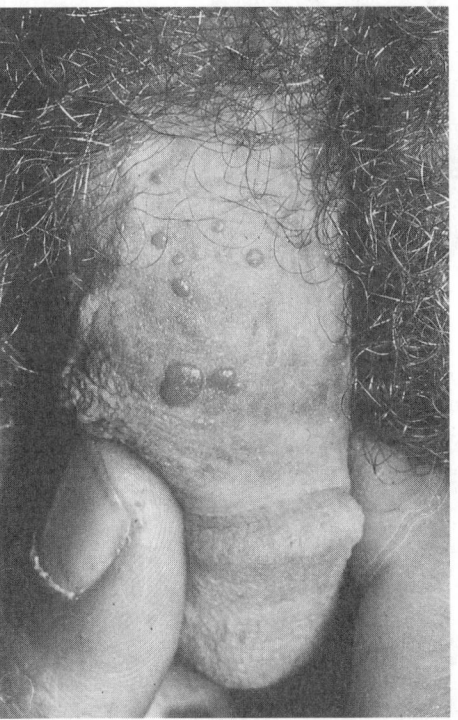

Fig. 2 Condylomata acuminata (exophytic condylomas) of penis.

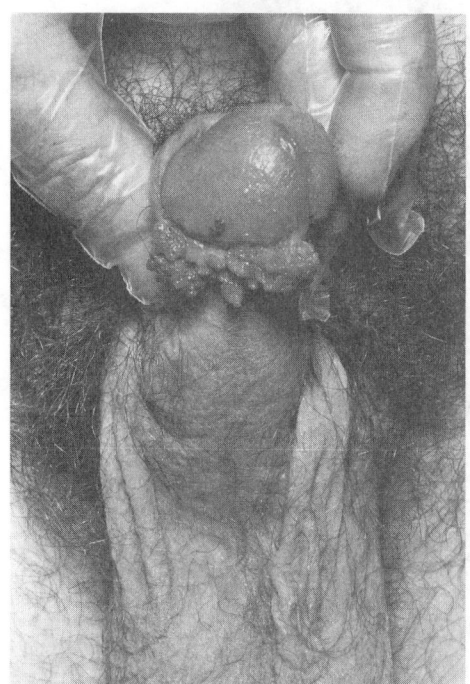

Fig. 4 Subclinical human papillomavirus lesions (flat condylomas) of penis after application of 5 per cent aqueous acetic acid.

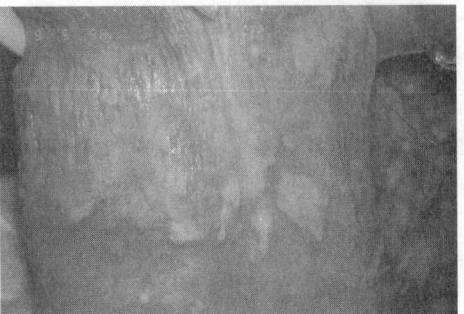

acetic acid solution. The affected areas are slightly raised, and shiny white (acetowhite), with a rough surface (Fig. 4). Flat condylomas affect the same areas as exophytic condylomas.

Perianal warts are usually exophytic, and in the moist conditions around the anus may reach a large size. In 50 per cent of cases, condylomas also appear in the anal canal (Fig. 5). Areas of acetowhite epithelium indicative of subclinical HPV infection may be associated with perianal warts, or occur alone.

Fig. 5 Condylomata acuminata of anal canal in an anoreceptive homosexual man.

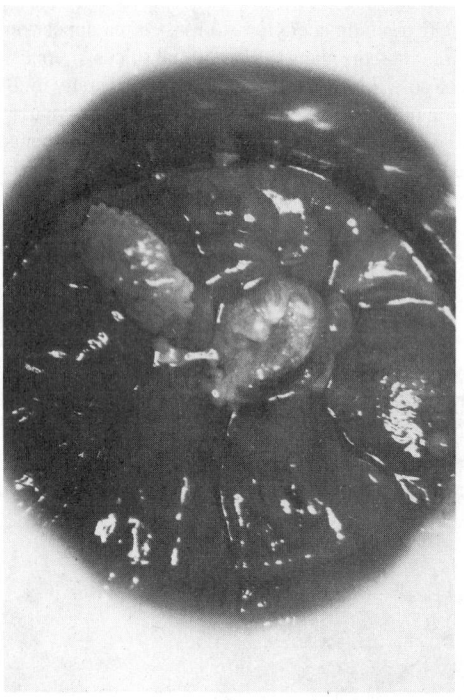

Fig. 6 Condylomata acuminata of vulva.

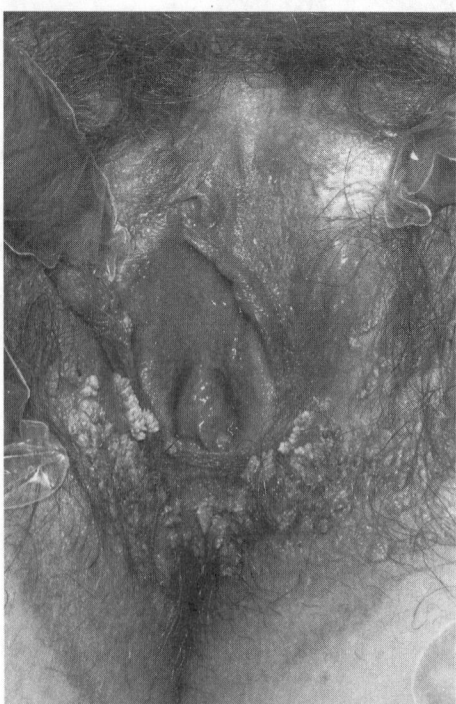

Lesions in women

Exophytic condylomas are the most common expression of HPV infection in women (Fig. 6). They appear at the fourchette and adjacent labia and may spread to the rest of the vulva, the perineum and anus, or the vagina and cervix. Multiple sessile warts may affect the labia majora and perineum. Subclinical HPV infection presents as slightly raised, acetowhite lesions; fissuring of these may cause dyspareunia.

About 15 per cent of women with vulval warts have exophytic condylomas on the cervix. Subclinical infection is more common, and acetowhite lesions, with punctation due to capillary loops, can be identified by colposcopy (Fig. 7). Altogether, one-half of women with vulval warts show evidence of clinical or subclinical HPV infection of the cervix. This is associated with characteristic koilocytotic cervical cytological appearances. Many women with cervical HPV infection also show evidence of cervical intraepithelial neoplasia.

Large, exophytic vulval condylomas may develop during pregnancy. They may reach such a size as to compromise delivery either from obstruction of the birth canal or because of the difficulty of suturing

Fig. 7 Subclinical human papillomavirus infection of cervix.

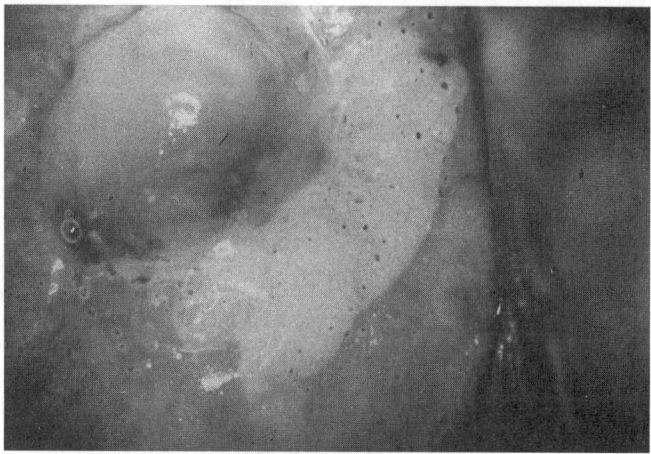

Fig. 8 Extensive anogenital condylomata acuminata in an infant.

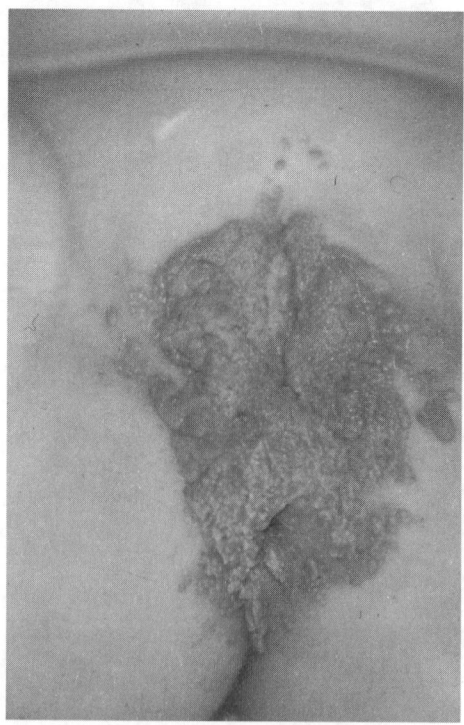

condylomatous tissue. Most of these large tumours regress, partly or completely, after delivery.

Lesions in children

Both exophytic condylomas and sessile warts may affect the anogenital region in children (Fig. 8). Laryngeal papillomatosis is an intractable disease that is often linked with maternal genital HPV infection. Its onset is usually in infancy, but older children may be affected.

COMPLICATIONS

Giant condyloma is a rare tumour that mostly occurs on the penis. An apparently harmless wart relentlessly enlarges and causes much tissue destruction. Although clinically it appears malignant, histologically it resembles condyloma acuminatum; transformation to squamous-cell carcinoma sometimes occurs.

Intraepithelial neoplasia comprises a group of papular lesions formerly known as Bowen's disease, Bowenoid papulosis, and carcinoma *in situ*. They may be associated with genital warts, but unlike these they contain sequences of HPV-16 or -18, and may progress to malignancy.

DIAGNOSIS

Genital warts must be distinguished from anatomical variants such as Fordyce's spots and fibroepithelial polyps, and from infective conditions like molluscum contagiosum or the papular lesions of secondary syphilis. The distinction from intraepithelial neoplasia may be difficult, and early biopsy of any lesions that appear atypical, or respond poorly to treatment, is essential. On the cervix, flat condylomas can be reliably distinguished from intraepithelial neoplasia only by biopsy.

MANAGEMENT

It is important to exclude associated sexually transmitted diseases by suitable laboratory tests, and to make arrangements for the examination of sexual partners. Next, the extent of the disease should be determined, and intraepithelial neoplasia excluded. Cervical cytological examination should always be done on women with vulval warts and on female partners of men with penile warts.

It is possible to type HPV extracted from genital warts; most contain HPV-6 or -11 but a few contain HPV-16, -18, and other types associated with genital epithelial cancer and regarded as 'high risk'. It has been suggested that typing the virus might be a useful way of indicating lesions requiring aggressive treatment and prolonged surveillance, but most investigators think that patients' treatment should depend on the history, clinical findings, and degree of histological abnormality rather than on the HPV type present.

No antiviral treatment for genital warts is available, and none of the local methods is entirely satisfactory. The oldest is the application of podophyllin preparations; although this is widely used, treatment failures are common. Other cytotoxic agents such as 5-fluorouracil and trichloracetic acid are even less effective. Initial treatment by destructive procedures is preferable. Those in use include cryotherapy by liquid nitrogen or a nitrous oxide cryoprobe, electrocautery, electrodesiccation, and scissor excision. Carbon dioxide laser therapy is often used for extensive or recalcitrant lesions. The treatment of cervical HPV infection, with or without associated intraepithelial neoplasia, is a matter for the gynaecologist.

Interferons α, β, and γ may be of value in the treatment of persistent anogenital warts. They have been given by local injection or systemically, either alone or to supplement destructive therapy.

REFERENCES

Bennett, R.S. and Powell, K.R. (1987). Human papillomaviruses: associations between laryngeal papillomas and genital warts. *Pediatric Infectious Disease Journal*, **6**, 229–32.

Brown, D.R. and Fife, K.H. (1990). Human papillomavirus infections of the genital tract. *Medical Clinics of North America*, **74**, 1455–85.

Chuang, T-Y. (1987). Condylomata acuminata (genital warts): an epidemiological view. *Journal of the American Academy of Dermatology*, **16**, 376–84.

Cohen, B.A., Honig, P., and Androphy, E. (1990). Anogenital warts in children. *Archives of Dermatology*, **126**, 1575–80.

Gross, G. (1990). Interferons in genital HPV disease. In *Genital papillomavirus infections*, (ed. G. Gross, S. Jablonska, H. Pfister, and H.E. Stegner), pp. 393–430. Springer-Verlag, Berlin.

Hatch, K.D. (1991). Vulvovaginal human papillomavirus infections in women—clinical implications and management. *American Journal of Obstetrics and Gynecology*, **165**, 1183–8.

Koutsky, L.A., Galloway, D.A., and Holmes, K.K. (1988). Epidemiology of genital human papillomavirus infection. *Epidemiological Review*, **10**, 122–63.

Roman, A. and Fife, K.H. (1989) Human papillomaviruses: are we ready to type? *Clinical and Microbiological Review*, **2**, 188–90.

Schlappner, O.L.A. and Shaffer, E.A. (1978). Anorectal condylomata acuminata: a missed part of the condyloma spectrum. *Canadian Medical Association Journal*, **118**, 172–3.

21.8 Cervical cancer and other cancers caused by sexually transmitted infections

V. BERAL

It is surprising how many cancers are caused by sexually transmitted infections. Cancer of the uterine cervix is the most common. A sexual cause was first suspected a century ago when clinicians noticed that the malignancy virtually never occurred in nuns. During the 1960s, epidemiological studies demonstrated that a woman's risk of developing cervical cancer increased with the number of sexual partners she had had, and this prompted the search for a sexually transmitted cause of the disease. Only in the last few years has it been established definitively that infection with certain types of the human papillomavirus is the main cause of cervical cancer. Cancers of the vulva, anus, and penis are now also known to be caused by the human papillomavirus. Kaposi's sarcoma is believed to be caused by an unidentified infection that can be transmitted sexually. Hepatocellular carcinoma is caused by hepatitis B or C viruses, which in Western countries can be transmitted sexually.

This chapter deals almost exclusively with cervical cancer because it is common, we know most about it, and because many of the findings and principles of management are likely to be applicable to the rarer and less-studied cancers that are also caused by certain types of human papillomaviruses.

Cervical cancer

OCCURRENCE

Worldwide, cervical cancer is the second most common cancer in women. Its incidence varies considerably from country to country and it is far more frequent in Third World countries than in the West (Fig. 1). About 1 per cent of women in Britain have invasive cervical cancer diagnosed during their lifetime and 0.4 per cent die from it. Mortality rates have been falling throughout the twentieth century, except among recent generations of women who became sexually active during the 1960s, a time when exposure to sexually transmitted diseases increased rapidly.

THE ROLE OF HUMAN PAPILLOMAVIRUSES AND OTHER FACTORS

There is now overwhelming evidence that the vast majority of cervical cancers are caused by specific types of the human papillomavirus (see Section 7) DNA from human papillomavirus types 16, 18, 31, 33 or 35 (mostly type 16) has been found in cervical cancers from as many as 90 percent of women with the malignancy. Fewer than 10 per cent of women without cervical cancer have these types of papillomavirus in their cervical cells, although as is shown in Fig. 2, the prevalence of infection is highest in women in their 20s and then tends to fall with age.

The risk of cervical cancer is increased in women who are poor, have little education, were young when they first had sexual intercourse, had many sexual partners and multiple sexually transmitted infections, had many children, especially when they were young, and who smoked cigarettes and used oral contraceptives. Until recently it was not clear whether these factors directly affected cervical cancer risk or whether they were merely markers of exposure to an infection that itself caused the cancer. The issue has not yet been resolved but recent evidence suggests that hormonal and reproductive factors may independently influence the development of cervical cancer in papillomavirus-infected women, whereas cigarette smoking and other sexually transmitted infections may be of no direct aetiological significance.

THE NATURAL HISTORY OF INFECTION WITH THE HUMAN PAPILLOMAVIRUS AND ASSOCIATED CHANGES IN THE CERVICAL EPITHELIUM

The natural history of cervical papillomavirus infection and the sequence of events leading to the development of cervical cancer are just beginning to be understood. An appreciation of the process is important for clinical practice because the human papillomavirus may cause a variety of changes in the cervical epithelium, most of which are not sinister; and the development of cervical cancer is comparatively rare, usually occurring decades after initial infection with the virus.

Because the cervix can be examined clinically, exfoliated cervical cells can be studied cytologically, biopsy specimens can be examined histologically, and much is known about the appearance of the cervix and cervical cells. The problem is that there is a plethora of terms describing these appearances, definitions keep changing, and there is little agreement between clinicians, cytologists, and pathologists about how to classify lesions. What is encouraging at the moment is that most of the macro- and microscopical changes regarded as premalignant seem to be manifestations of papillomavirus infection, and the systematic use of tests to detect papillomavirus infection could eventually help simplify and standardize the classification and nomenclature of clinical and pathological changes.

Some cervical papillomavirus infections cause no obvious epithelial changes—cervical colposcopy, cytology and biopsy are normal and the only way infection can be identified is by virological study. Other papillomavirus infections cause 'cervical warts', which are asymptomatic but can be seen as white patches at colposcopy after acetic acid has been applied to the cervix. Cervical smears from women with cervical warts

Fig. 1 Percentage of women who develop cervical cancer before age 75, by country.

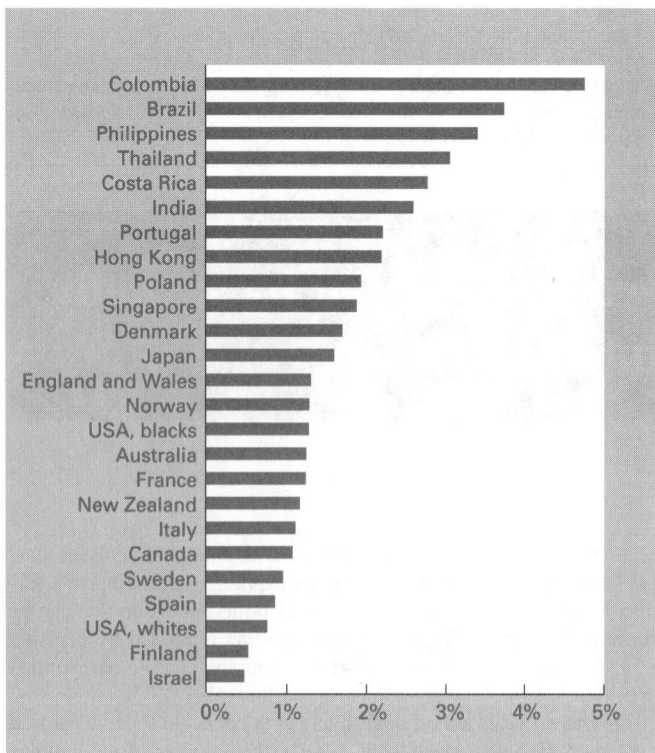

Fig. 2 Age-specific incidence of *in-situ* and invasive cervical cancer and of death from cervical cancer in England and Wales.

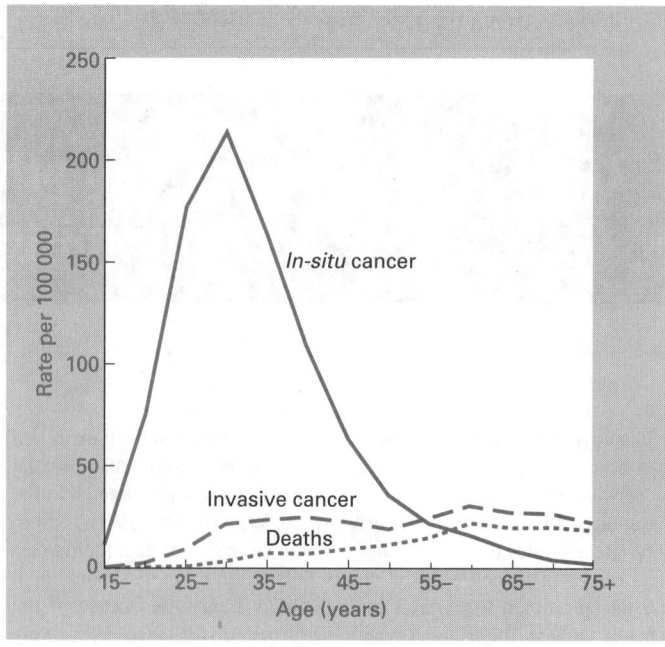

Table 1 *Estimated proportion of women in Britain likely to be infected by the papillomavirus and to develop abnormalities of the cervical epithelium, including cancer.*

Outcome	%*
Acquire cervical papillomavirus infection	10–20
Develop persistent infection with papillomavirus	5–10
Develop abnormalities of the cervical epithelium such as 'dyskaryosis' or 'cervical intraepithelial neoplasia' (CIN)	5–10
Have carcinoma *in situ* of the cervix diagnosed	2–5
Have invasive carcinoma of the cervix diagnosed	1.0–1.5
Die from cervical cancer	0.3–0.5

*Ranges are given because exposure to the papillomavirus and the risk of associated abnormalities of the cervical epithelium are not the same for different generations of women; definitions and diagnostic criteria for cervical lesions vary; and screening programmes are leading to a reduction in the incidence of invasive cervical cancer and mortality from it and the magnitude of this reduction cannot be estimated with precision.

may show various degrees of 'dysplasia' or 'dyskaryosis' and cervical biopsy may show various grades of 'cervical intraepithelial neoplasia' (CIN) (or 'squamous intraepithelial lesions' (SIL) according to a new classification known as the 'Bethesda system'). The most extreme change in the epithelium is the development of invasive cervical cancer, which seems to be associated with persistent viral infection and long-standing epithelial abnormalities.

Very little is known about what determines progression or regression of lesions. Most changes (up to the development of invasive cancer) seem to be reversible and lesions of different severity often coexist in the same woman. The more severe lesions tend to be rarer and found in older women: estimates of the proportion of women in Britain likely to develop various types of lesions are given in Table 1 and the age-specific prevalences of some of these lesions are shown in Figs. 2 and 3. Roughly one woman in 10, and possibly more, is likely to acquire a cervical infection with human papillomavirus types 16 or 18, but 1 in 20 women develops persistent infection or some abnormality of her cervical epithelium. One in 50 is diagnosed with *in situ* cervical cancer; and 1 in 100 develops invasive cervical cancer. Papillomavirus infection is most prevalent in women aged in their 20s, corresponding to the age when they acquire other sexually transmitted infections; the peak prevalence of *in situ* cancer tends to be about 10 years later (in women in their 30s) whereas invasive cancer is rare before 30 years of age.

CLINICAL IMPLICATIONS

If most cervical cancers are caused by certain human papillomavirus types, should all women be screened for those infections? How should infected women be treated? What should they be told? The important points to bear in mind are: most premalignant cervical changes are caused by papillomaviruses; most infections resolve spontaneously; cervical infection with papillomaviruses is especially common in young women but invasive cervical cancer is rare before the age of 30 years and seems to be associated with persistent infection and long-standing epithelial abnormalities.

We do not know why infection persists in some women and what determines who goes on to develop cervical cancer. Intensity of infection, age at exposure, immune response, genital hygiene, reproductive history, and the use of oral contraceptives could be relevant; future research should clarify which are. In the meantime it seems sensible not

to resort to active treatment in women in their 20s with papillomavirus infection and related mild cervical lesions, but to reassure them that most lesions will resolve spontaneously and encourage them to have regular cervical smears. Only in young women with severe lesions and older women with persistent epithelial abnormalities is there an appreciable risk of progression to invasive cervical cancer, and active treatment is required.

PREVENTION

Well-organized screening programmes, based on exfoliative cervical cytology, are known to be effective in reducing the incidence and mortality of cervical cancer. Testing for papillomaviruses should not replace cervical cytology as a first-line approach in screening, as this would result in unnecessary treatment in many young women and because not all cervical cancers are associated with papillomavirus infection. Testing for papillomaviruses may be useful, however, in deciding how to manage the large number of women who have equivocal cervical cytology. Its efficacy must be evaluated before it is adopted on a large scale.

The most important advance in cervical cancer is likely to come from the development of vaccines. Effective vaccines have already been produced for bovine tumours of the gastrointestinal tract caused by bovine papillomaviruses which are related to the human types. Bovine vaccines are effective not only in preventing infection with papillomaviruses but also in preventing tumour development in cattle already infected with the viruses. Similar types of vaccines against the human papillomaviruses would revolutionize the management and prevention of cervical cancer.

Other cancers

Cancer of the vulva, anus, and penis are also associated with infection with human papillomavirus types 16, 18, 31, 33, and 35. None of these cancers is common in Britain: 0.2 per cent develop vulval cancer, 0.2 per cent develop anal cancer, and 0.1 per cent develop penile cancer. Genital warts are common at these anatomical sites but are caused mostly by human papillomavirus types 6 and 11, which have extremely low malignant potential. Comments in the preceding section about the natural history of infection, clinical management, and prevention are also likely to apply to this group of cancers.

Kaposi's sarcoma was extremely rare in Western countries before the advent of AIDS. In Europe and the United States about 1 in 20 patients with AIDS have Kaposi's sarcoma and the disease is far more common

Fig. 3 Percentage of women whose cervical smears are positive for HPV 16/18, by age (from Meijer *et al.* in Munoz *et al.* (1992)).

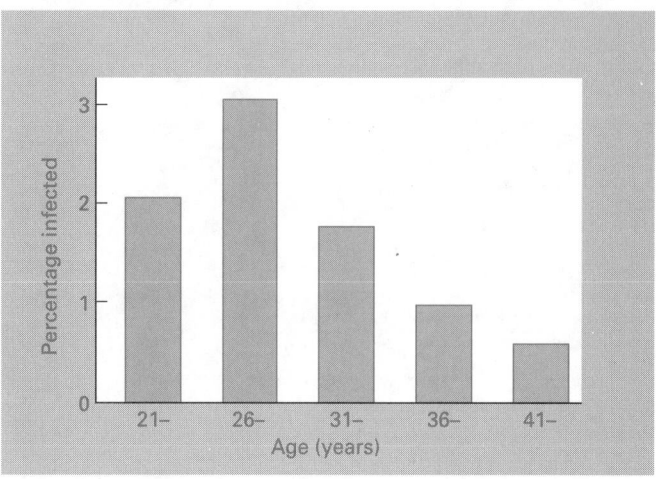

in homosexual men than in others with AIDS. Epidemiological evidence suggests that Kaposi's sarcoma is caused by a sexually transmitted infectious agent, in addition to the human immunodeficiency virus. The agent has not yet been identified but may be transmitted by contact with faeces.

REFERENCES

Beral, V. (1991). The epidemiology of cancer in AIDS patients. *AIDS*, 5 (suppl.), S99–S103.

Munoz, N., Bosch, F.X., Shah, K.V., and Meheus, A. (ed.) (1992). *The epidemiology of human papillomavirus and cervical cancer*, IARC Scientific Publication No. 119. International Agency for Research on Cancer, Lyon.

Schiffman, M.H. (1992). Recent progress in defining the epidemiology of human papillomavirus infection and cervical neoplasia. *Journal of the National Cancer Institute*, **84**, 394–8.

Section 22 *Disorders of the blood*

22.1 Introduction

D. J. WEATHERALL

The study of blood is one of the most fascinating branches of clinical medicine. There are very few diseases that do not produce changes in the blood at some time during the course of the illness. Furthermore, the primary disorders of the blood and blood-forming tissues can give rise to extremely diverse clinical manifestations, which may involve any of the organ systems. Textbooks often give their readers an unbalanced picture of haematology in the real world. Even in specialist haematological practice, primary disorders of the blood and blood-forming organs make up only a small fraction of the workload; most patients that are referred with haematological abnormalities have diseases in other systems. Anaemia is a good example. Most anaemias seen in medical wards are due to blood loss, infection, renal failure, malignant disease, and, in many parts of the world, malnutrition and parasitic infestation. Anaemia may be the first indication of a chronic urinary tract infection, hypothyroidism, pituitary failure, bacterial endocarditis, polymyalgia rheumatica, or even that endemic disease of 'medical grand rounds', atrial myxoma.

Thus, although this section concentrates heavily on the primary diseases of the blood and blood-forming organs, the reader should be aware that many of these conditions are relatively uncommon. Hopefully, the summary of the haematological manifestations of non-haematological diseases that appears later in the section will leave the reader with a more balanced view of the scope of this absorbing subject.

An approach to patients with haematological disorders

The diagnosis of blood diseases follows the same process as any other condition; expertise in the laboratory will never make up for an inadequate history and clinical examination. It should be remembered that many patients who are referred to hospital for a specialist opinion on their blood are worried about the possibility of leukaemia, although they will rarely say so. It is important to reassure them as soon as possible if this is not the diagnosis. Where leukaemia is suspected, no time should be lost in arriving at an accurate diagnosis and in developing a well-worked out plan of management. The situation can then be discussed frankly with the patient and their family; knowledge of what they are up against and precisely what form of treatment is to be instituted often engenders a great sense of relief after weeks or months of fearing the worst.

HISTORY

In taking a history from a patient who is suspected of having a haematological disorder, certain factors are of particular importance. The symptoms of anaemia are described in detail later in this section. However, it should be remembered that a slowly developing anaemia may be completely asymptomatic, even when the haemoglobin level is extremely low. Individuals who are otherwise healthy should be able to compensate for a relatively mild anaemia; a young woman with a haemoglobin level of 10.5 g/dl who complains of tiredness and inability to cope with life is more likely to be suffering from the effects of chronic anxiety due to marital problems than from mild anaemia. Other general symptoms are of great importance, particularly weight loss, night sweats, bone pain, and pruritis. While moderate nocturnal sweating is common in anxiety states, drenching sweats requiring several changes of nightclothes and sheets are a more ominous symptom, often associated with infection or lymphoproliferative disease. Pruritus occurs with many disorders of the blood. When associated with lymphoma it is non-specific, but when it accompanies the myeloproliferative disorders it is often precipitated by warmth such as getting into bed or a hot bath. A detailed drug history is also essential; there are very few drugs that do not produce haematological side-effects.

Although a complete systematic history must be taken, gastrointestinal and haemostatic functions are particularly relevant to diseases of the blood. When investigating anaemia a detailed dietetic history is essential and it is important to ask specifically about symptoms such as a sore tongue, bleeding gums, dysphagia, dyspepsia, disturbance of bowel habit suggestive of malabsorption, and rectal bleeding. Patients are often referred to haematological departments for investigation of easy bruising. Many people, particularly women, bruise easily and the key question is whether the bruising is unusual for them. Is it spontaneous or related to only mild trauma? It is also extremely helpful to enquire into certain key episodes in a patient's life that may provide a clue as to whether there is an inborn bleeding tendency. These include circumcision, dental extraction (was a return to the dentist for stitching or packing ever required?), menstruation, surgical procedures, and so on.

Assessment of menstrual blood loss is an important part of the history in women with iron deficiency, as well as for assessing haemostatic function. It is not enough to ask a woman whether she considers that her periods are normal. If she uses only internal tampons, she probably does not have menorrhagia. However, the use of one or more packets of the more absorbent brands of external pads, or having to get up at night to change pads or to stay at home during the menstrual period, suggests a heavy loss.

Family histories are particularly important for the diagnosis of blood diseases. It is not only essential to ask for a family history of anaemia or bleeding disorders; the racial origin of the patient's ancestors may also give valuable clues for the cause of anaemia. The long-forgotten Italian great-grandparent may have been the source of the thalassaemia gene that is responsible for a refractory hypochromic anaemia or the red-cell enzyme deficiency that leads to a haemolytic drug reaction. A detailed personal history is also essential. Cigarette or cigar smoking is probably the most common cause of mild polycythaemia, and alcohol can produce remarkably diverse haematological changes. A detailed occupational history may reveal exposure to industrial solvents or other agents responsible for bone marrow depression; unusual hobbies may also result in contact with toxic agents.

PHYSICAL EXAMINATION

The examination of a patient with a haematological disorder follows the same pattern as any physical examination but there are certain aspects of particular importance. On general inspection it is essential to examine the skin carefully for evidence of bruising, purpura, infiltration, or ulceration. The distribution and pattern of bruising or petechiae may be diagnostic, particularly in disorders such as Henoch–Schönlein purpura, senile purpura, scurvy, purpura due to venous obstruction, and the painful bruising syndrome. Thrombocytopenic purpura is often seen most easily over pressure areas; a few lesions in these regions are easily overlooked. Cutaneous lymphoma may mimic a variety of skin diseases. Chronic leg ulceration is a common finding in sickle-cell anaemia; it occurs occasionally with other genetic haemolytic anaemias. The perianal region and perineum should be carefully inspected. There may be perianal infiltration, particularly in the monocytic leukaemias, and it is very important to recognize perianal infection early in neutropenic patients. Rectal examination should be avoided in neutropenia for fear of disseminating infection. Potential sites of infection in compromised patients must be examined daily. They include the skin, intravenous infusion sites, the mouth and throat, and the perineum. The mucous membranes, nail beds, and palmar creases should be examined carefully for pallor, always remembering that the clinical assessment of anaemia is very inaccurate. Pigmentation of the face is sometimes a feature of folic acid deficiency. Mild jaundice may be a useful indicator of haemolysis, while a greyish pigmentation of the skin is common in patients with iron overload, both primary and secondary to repeated transfusion. There is an association between vitiligo and pernicious anaemia. In patients with polycythaemia there may be suffusion of the conjunctivae, a high colour, and prominence of the vessels over the face, neck and upper part of the chest. The nails should be examined for unusual fragility; flattened, spoon-shaped nails, koilonychia, which are supposed to be diagnostic of chronic iron deficiency, are now rarely seen.

An assessment of the size of the lymph nodes and an inspection of other lymphatic tissue are a major part of the examination of patients with haematological disorders. It is most important to develop a systematic approach to lymph-node examination. Each group of nodes in the head and neck, axillae and groins, together with the epitrochlear nodes, must be examined in detail. In the head and neck it is useful to start with the occipital nodes, then move to the preauricular and postauricular nodes, and, finally, to examine systematically the anterior and posterior triangles and supraclavicular regions. The scalp should be inspected for signs of infestation and secondary infection due to scratching in children with enlarged occipital or posterior cervical nodes. A simple way of describing enlarged lymph nodes should be used, without the use of too many adjectives. Nodes should be labelled as hard, firm or soft, and tender or non-tender. Ambiguous terms such as 'rubbery' should be avoided. Soft, tender nodes usually indicate infection. Large, firm nodes are characteristic of lymphoma. Hard nodes occur in secondary carcinoma, although calcified nodes, matted together and attached to skin, are still encountered in patients with tuberculous adenitis. The approximate size of the nodes should be recorded, together with whether they are mobile, attached deep or superficially, and discrete or matted together. It is also very important to examine the tonsils and adenoids, particularly in a patient suspected of having a lymphoproliferative disease.

A detailed examination of the mouth should include the state of the tongue, mucous membranes, gums, teeth, and fauces. Glossitis, as evidenced by a smooth, depapillated tongue, occurs in iron-deficiency and megaloblastic anaemia. Small, black bullae (blood blisters) on the tongue or mucous membranes, which burst and leave superficial ulcers, are characteristic of thrombocytopenic purpura. Gingival hypertrophy is sometimes found in patients with acute leukaemia, particularly the monocytic type, and in some individuals with megaloblastic anaemia due to phenytoin therapy. Ulcers of the mouth and fauces occur in all forms of acute leukaemia. Oral infection, often associated with ulceration, is very common in neutropenic patients. Candidosis may be seen on the fauces, tongue or mucous membranes. Candidal infection of the throat, associated with dysphagia, should raise the suspicion of oesophageal candidosis (-iasis). The teeth may be badly formed and the bite may be abnormal in patients with severe forms of thalassaemia. Dental abscesses are common in patients with neutropenia; suspect teeth should be gently percussed for evidence of apical infection. Telangiectases may be found on the lips and oral mucous membranes of patients with hereditary telangiectasia.

On abdominal examination the most important questions are the size of the liver, whether there is splenomegaly, and if there are any palpable para-aortic lymph nodes. It is not possible to learn how to examine the spleen from a textbook, but a few hints may be helpful. Large spleens can often be seen to move up and down on respiration if the abdomen is well illuminated and the observer stands at the end of the bed. Very large spleens tend to move downwards and medially towards the right iliac fossa and can be missed if the examiner does not start palpating from this region, moving upwards and medially towards the left subcostal region. A sure way to miss a moderately enlarged spleen is to go digging in with the fingers without eliciting the patient's help. With the left-hand hooked round the region above the left costal margin, and the right hand resting lightly on the abdomen, the patient should be asked to gently breathe in and out through the mouth. The secret of success is to persuade the patient to breathe just deeply enough to move the spleen down without contracting the abdominal muscles. The examiner should wait for the spleen tip to meet their fingers rather than to try to find it by deep palpation. Once defined, the position of the lower border of the spleen should be recorded in centimetres, vertically below the costal margin. Manoeuvres designed to facilitate the palpation of a slightly enlarged spleen, such as turning the patient on their right side, while useful for impressing clinical examiners, are rarely of much help in practice. Be gentle! The author has seen enlarged spleens ruptured by overenthusiastic medical students. If there is pain over the spleen or referred to the left shoulder, don't forget to listen for a rub. Finally, remember that spleens come in all sizes and shapes, and often lie more laterally than expected. Do not be disappointed not to feel the much publicized notch; it happens once or twice in a clinical lifetime! The differential diagnosis of palpable masses in the region of the spleen is considered later in this section.

The eyes are a mine of information in patients with haematological disorders. Periorbital oedema is sometimes seen in infectious mononucleosis. The conjunctivae may show mild icterus not obvious in the skin, and there may be haemorrhages in bleeding disorders. Pingueculae of the conjunctivae are seen in Gaucher's disease. Retinal haemorrhages are common in patients who have had a sudden fall in haemoglobin level. They are less frequent in severely thrombocytopenic patients with normal haemoglobin levels; the combination of anaemia and thrombocytopenia is particularly likely to lead to severe retinal bleeding. Papilloedema occurs commonly in patients with leukaemia involving the central nervous system. Proliferative abnormalities of the retinal vessels are often seen in patients with sickling disorders, particularly haemoglobin SC disease. The hyperviscosity syndrome associated with macroglobulinaemia and some forms of myeloma is characterized by fullness of the retinal veins, which are sometimes broken up into segments like a string of sausages. These changes are often associated with widespread retinal haemorrhages. Optic atrophy may occur in patients with severe vitamin B_{12} deficiency. Unilateral exophthalmos occurs occasionally in patients with myeloma deposits or lymphoma involving the orbit.

Examination of the musculoskeletal system may be particularly rewarding in patients suspected of having genetic disorders of blood. In patients with coagulation defects such as haemophilia or Christmas disease, recurrent bleeding into joints may produce a chronic deforming arthritis. Muscle haematomata are also common and are easily missed. For example, bleeding into the psoas sheath may produce a discrete swelling above the inguinal ligament, which may later be associated with nerve compression leading to weakness of the quadriceps and anaesthesia over the anterior aspect of the thigh. If muscle pain is the presenting symptom it is very important to palpate the muscle groups carefully for cystic swellings that may occur in haemophiliacs after bleeding into muscles. The joints have other important associations with blood disorders. A mild refractory anaemia is a very common accompaniment of rheumatoid arthritis. Painful arthritis of the large joints may be the presenting symptom of primary haemochromatosis. Gout is a common complication of all the myeloproliferative diseases; the ears should be examined carefully for tophi in addition to a full assessment of the joints. The value of bone tenderness in the diagnosis of acute leukaemia has been overemphasized. It is often absent. When present it is best elicited by carefully palpating the sternum or tibiae, or by rib compression. Be gentle, because sometimes the tenderness is quite exquisite. Bone tenderness or local swelling are also found in patients with myeloma or sickle-cell anaemia. In children with thalassaemia or other hereditary haemolytic anaemias there may be reduced growth, bossing of the skull, and facial deformities. A wide variety of skeletal changes may occur with congenital hypoplastic anaemia.

THE USE OF THE LABORATORY

Finally, the diagnosis and management of blood disease requires an examination of the blood and, if appropriate, the bone marrow. Clinicians will obtain the maximum information from their colleagues in the laboratory if they ask the right questions. Scribbling down 'full blood count' on a laboratory request form is useless. It is essential to ask for an examination of the blood film in any patient who is suspected of having a haematological disorder. More can be learnt from the help of an experienced morphologist than any other investigation in clinical haematology. Some haematological investigations are underused; others are requested far too often. For example, the often forgotten reticulocyte count is an invaluable guide to the response of the bone marrow to anaemia and for the recognition of bleeding or mild haemolysis. On the other hand, bone marrow examination, while invaluable in many cases, is an unpleasant investigation and should only be requested with very clear indications. For example, clinicians should stop and think why they are ordering a bone marrow examination in an elderly patient with a peripheral blood lymphocyte count of $80\,000\times10^9/l$. This can only be chronic lymphatic leukaemia; the bone marrow will be infiltrated with lymphocytes. Why put the patient through this traumatic investigation? The result is predictable and will not help in their management.

In the section that follows we shall describe briefly the normal blood count and what can be learnt from a peripheral blood film and bone marrow examination. It cannot be emphasized too strongly that the most useful information is obtained by very close liaison between the laboratory and the ward. Clinicians should visit the haematology laboratory regularly, review films and haematological data with their laboratory colleagues, and be very precise in setting out the reasons for the investigations they order. Much valuable information is lost because of lack of good liaison between the bedside and the laboratory.

Examination of the blood

Constituents of normal blood

Blood consists of several different types of cells suspended in plasma. The classification and morphological analysis of blood cells was made possible by the studies of Ehrlich, who, in 1877, described the use of

Fig. 1 A human erythrocyte as viewed through the scanning electron microscope. (By kind permission of Dr S.M. Lewis.)

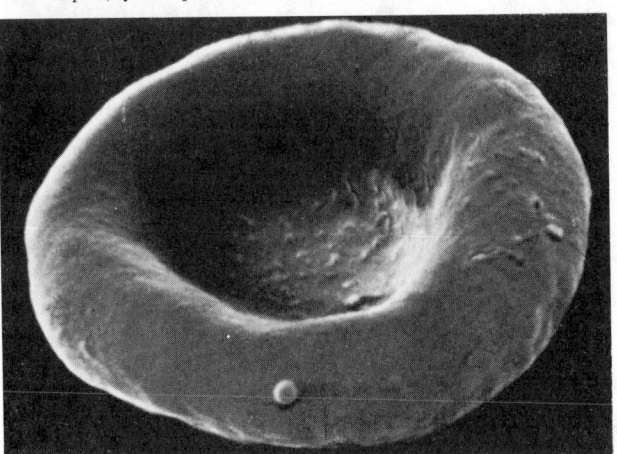

aniline dyes for staining dried blood films. This approach has been refined over the years with the gradual improvement of the microscope, and the fine structure of the blood cells has been analysed in greater detail with the electron microscope and, more recently, with the scanning electron microscope (Fig. 1).

The formed elements of the blood, or blood cells, consist of the red cells, white cells, and platelets. The red cells are biconcave discs approximately 7 to 8 μm in diameter (Fig. 1). They consist of a membrane that contains a concentrated solution of haemoglobin and a variety of other proteins, salts, and vitamins. Normally they are of a uniform shape and size, and contain similar amounts of haemoglobin. On supravital staining, approximately 1 per cent of the red cells show a reticular appearance. These are newly released cells and because of their staining characteristics are called reticulocytes.

The white cells are classified according to their morphological appearances into granulocytes (polymorphonuclear leucocytes), monocytes, and lymphocytes. The granulocytes and monocytes are phagocytic cells while the lymphocytes are involved in a variety of immune mechanisms. The granulocytes can be further classified according to their maturity. In the newly produced forms, band cells or juvenile polymorphonuclear leucocytes, the nucleus is horseshoe shaped but single. In a normal blood film the majority of the granulocytes have matured beyond this stage and their nuclei consist of two or more lobes separated by thin, filamentous chromatin strands. These cells are about 12 to 15 μm in diameter. The granulocyte series is further classified according to the staining characteristics of the granules into neutrophils, eosinophils, and basophils. The monocytes are of similar size to the granulocytes but have oval nuclei with a slate-coloured cytoplasm, which may contain some fine granules.

There are two morphologically distinct forms of lymphocyte: a large cell with a diameter of 8 to 16 μm and a smaller one measuring 7 to 9 μm. Both forms are round and have a light blue cytoplasm. In the large lymphocytes the nucleus fills about half of the cell whereas in the small lymphocytes it almost completely fills the cell.

The platelets are disc-shaped cells measuring approximately 2 to 3 μm in diameter. In normal blood they are relatively homogeneous in structure; their fine structure cannot be distinguished by conventional light microscopy.

A more detailed description of the structure and function of these different blood cells and their precursors appears later in this chapter.

Investigation of the blood—the normal blood count

A full blood count can be carried out on a 5-ml anticoagulated blood sample. A stained blood film is prepared for examination of the morphology of the different cells. Using either chemical and physical methods, or the more accurate electronic cell counters, the relative volume of packed red cells and white cells, the haemoglobin level, and the red-cell, white-cell, and platelet counts can be determined. From a series of calculations relating the volume of packed cells, haemoglobin level, and red-cell count, it is possible to derive a series of absolute indices that provide useful information about the size and degree of haemoglobinization of the red cells. Finally, the relative numbers of reticulocytes and the erythrocyte sedimentation rate can be determined.

THE STAINED BLOOD FILM

An examination of the stained blood film is the most important investigation in haematology. Each of the cell types is studied separately.

The red cells are examined to assess their degree of haemoglobinization and their shape; if both are normal, they are described as normochromic and normocytic. Disorders of the red cell are frequently associated with changes in their morphology or staining properties. These include variation in size or anisocytosis; an increase in size or macrocytosis; a reduction in size or microcytosis; variability in shape or poikilocytosis; pale staining or hypochromia, which suggests under-

Table 1 *Significance of morphological and staining variations of the red cells*

Change	Clinical significance
Hypochromia	Defective haemoglobinization; usually iron deficiency or defective haemoglobin synthesis
Microcytosis	As above
Macrocytosis	Dyserythropoiesis or premature release; may indicate megaloblastic erythropoiesis or haemolysis
Anisochromia	Variability of haemoglobinization or presence of young red-cell populations, e.g. in haemolysis
Spherocytosis	Usually indicates damage to membrane; may result from a genetic disorder of the membrane or an acquired defect often due to antibody or other damage to the cell
Target cells	Large 'floppy' cells that occur with deficient haemoglobinization or in liver disease; also occur in hypoplenism
Elliptocytes	May result from a genetic defect in the red-cell membrane but also occur in a variety of acquired conditions including iron deficiency
Poikilocytes: include burr cells, helmet cells, schistocytes, fragmented forms, etc.	Usually indicates trauma to red cells in microcirculation or severe oxidant damage
Sickle cells	Occur in the sickling disorders
Acanthocytes	Occur in genetic disorders of lipid metabolism
Inclusions: iron granules (siderocytes). Howell–Jolly bodies and Cabot's rings (nuclear remnants), basophilic stippling, and Heinz bodies	Iron granules and nuclear remnants are often seen after splenectomy Basophilic stippling indicates accelerated erythropoiesis or defective haemoglobin synthesis. Heinz bodies are precipitated haemoglobin or globin subunits

haemoglobinization; and variation in the degree of staining from cell to cell, which is called anisochromia. In addition to these changes there may be more specific alterations in the morphology of the red cells. Some of these, together with the different clinical disorders with which they are associated, are summarized in Table 1 and illustrated in Fig. 2.

The white cells may be abnormal in number or morphology. An increased white-cell count is called a leucocytosis. If this involves the polymorphonuclear series, it is called a polymorphonuclear leucocytosis or granulocytosis. An elevated eosinophil, basophil, monocyte, or lymphocyte count is called an eosinophilia, basophilia, monocytosis, or lymphocytosis, respectively. A reduced white count is called a neutropenia or lymphopenia, depending on the cell type involved. An absence of granulocytes in the blood is called agranulocytosis. As is the case for the red-cell series, much can be learned by morphological examination of the white cells. A blood film is said to show a 'shift to the left' if there are relatively more 'young' polymorphonuclear leucocytes present than normal. This is reflected by an increased proportion of band forms and, in more extreme cases, by a variable number of myelocytes or metamyelocytes. In acute bacterial infections, vacuoles may appear in the cytoplasm of polymorphonuclear leucocytes. In addition, the granules may become morphologically abnormal; heavy granulation of this type is called toxic granulation. This change is sometimes associated with the presence of small (1–2μ) oval bodies called Döhle bodies. A variety of genetic changes of nuclear configuration or of the granules of the polymorphonuclear leucocytes has been described; these are discussed later in this section.

THE PACKED-CELL VOLUME, HAEMOGLOBIN LEVEL, AND RED-CELL INDICES

A great deal can be learnt about the character of an anaemia from a few simple haematological tests. The volume of packed red cells (**PCV** or haematocrit) can be estimated either by centrifugation of a blood sample or by a conductivity method in which it is derived from measurement of the red-cell volume and the number of red cells using an electronic counting system. The haemoglobin concentration is usually determined spectrophotometrically by comparing a test sample with a stable standard, usually of the cyanmethaemoglobin derivative. Although for many years, red-cell counting fell into disrepute, it has now become part of a standard blood count because of the accuracy of electronic cell counters.

Normal values for the PCV, haemoglobin level, and red-cell count are shown in Table 2. It is important to become familiar with the variability of these figures at different stages of development and between

Fig. 2 Morphological changes of the red cells (×600–800). (a) Hypochromia and microcytosis. (b) Elliptocytosis. (c) Poikilocytosis (myelosclerosis). (d) Target cells and intracellular crystals (haemoglobin C disease). (e) Macrocytosis and anisocytosis (pernicious anaemia). (f) Dimorphic picture - normochromic and hypochromic (sideroblastic anaemia).

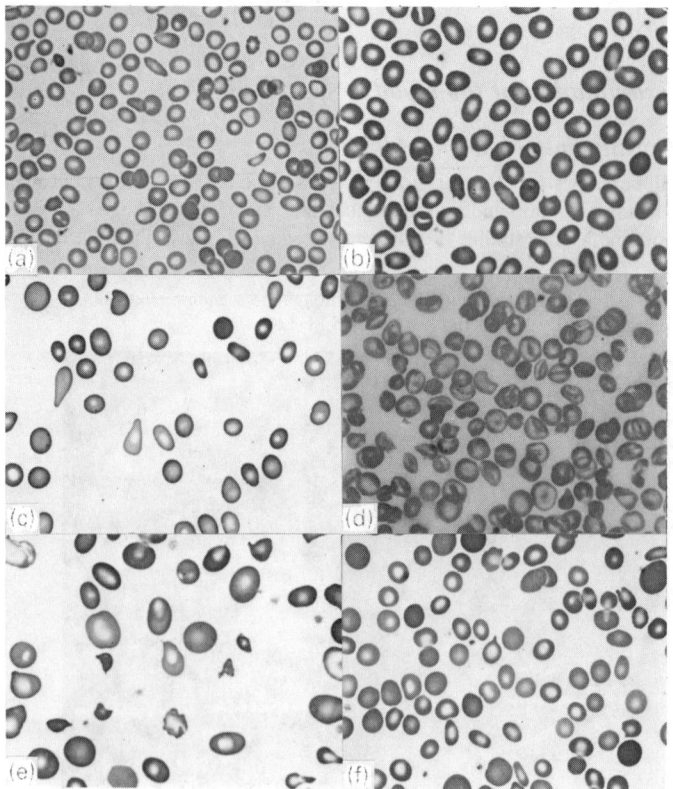

Table 2 *Haematological values for normal adults*

Red-cell count		*β-Thromboglobulin*	< 50 ng/ml
Men	$5.0 \pm 0.5 \times 10^{12}/l$	*Platelet factor 4*	< 10 ng/ml
Women	$4.3 \pm 0.5 \times 10^{12}/l$	*Protein C*	< 10ng/ml
Haemoglobin		Function	0.70–1.40 u/ml
Men	150 ± 20 g/l	Antigen	0.61–1.32 u/ml
Women	140 ± 20 g/l	*Protein S*	
Packed-cell volume (PCV;		Total	0.78–1.37 u/ml
haematocrit value)		Free	0.68–1.52 u/ml
Men	0.45 ± 0.05 (l/l)	*Heparin cofactor II*	55–145%
Women	0.41 ± 0.04 (l/l)	*Autohaemolysis* (37 °C)	
Mean cell volume (MCV)		48 h without added glucose	0.2–2.0
Men and women	92 ± 10 fl	48 h, with added glucose	0–0.9%
Mean cell haemoglobin (MCH)		*Cold agglutinin titre* (4 °C)	< 64
Men and women	29.5 ± 2.5 pg	*Serum iron*	13–32 μmol/l
Mean cell haemoglobin			(0.7–1.8 mg/l)
concentration (MCHC)		*Total iron-binding capacity*	45–70 μmol/l)
Men and women	330 ± 15 g/l		(2.5–4.0 mg/l)
Red-cell distribution width (RDW)		*Transferrin*	1.2–2.0 g/l
As CV	13.2 ± 1.6%	*Ferritin*	
As SD	42.5 ± 3.5 fl	Men	20–300 median 100 μg/l
Red-cell diameter (mean values)		Women	15–150 median 30 μg/l
Dry films	6.7–7.7 μm	*Serum vitamin B$_{12}$*	160–760 ng/l
Red-cell density	1092–1100 g/l	*Serum folate*	3–20 μg/l
Reticulocyte count	$0.5–2.0$% ($25–85 \times 10^9/l$	*Red-cell folate*	160–640 μg/l
Blood volume		*Plasma haemoglobin*	10–40 mg/l
Red-cell volume, men	30 ± 5 ml/kg	*Serum haptoglobin*	0.6–2.7 mg/l
women	25 ± 5 ml/kg	*HbA$_2$*	2.2–3.5%
Plasma volume	45 ± 5 ml/kg	*HbF*	< 1.0%
Total blood volume	70 ± 10 ml/kg	*Methaemoglobin*	< 2.0%
Real cell lifespan	120 ± 30 days	*Sedimentation rate*	
Leucocyte count	$7.0 \pm 3.0 \times 10^9/l$	(1 h at 20 ± 3 °C)	
Differential leucocyte count		(upper limits)	
Neutrophils	$2.0–7.0 \times 10^9/l$ (40–80%)	Men:	
Lymphocytes	$1.0–3.0 \times 10^9/l$ (20–40%)	17–50 years	10 mm
Monocytes	$0.2–1.0 \times 10^9/l$ (2–10%)	50–60 years	12 mm
Eosinophils	$0.04–0.4 \times 10^9/l$ (1–6%)	61–70 years	14 mm
Basophils	$0.02–0.1 \times 10^9/l$ (< 1–2%)	> 70 years	30 mm
Platelet count	$130–400 \times 10^9/l$	Women:	
Bleeding time		17–50 years	19 mm
(Ivy's method)	2–7 min	50–60 years	19 mm
(Template method)	2.5–9.5 min	61–70 years	20 mm
Prothrombin time	12–16 s	> 70 years	35 mm
Partial thromboplastin time (PTT)	30–46 s	*Plasma viscosity*	
Thrombin time	15–19 s	25 °C	1.50–1.72 mPa/s
Plasma fibrinogen	2.0–4.0 g/l	37 °C	1.16–1.33 mPa/s
Fibrinogen titre	≥ 128	*Heterophile* (anti-sheep red cell)	< 80
Plasminogen		agglutinin titre	
Function	0.75–1.35 u/ml	After absorption with guinea-pig	< 10
Antigen	0.76–1.36 u/ml	kidney	
Euglobulin lysis time	90–240 min		
Antithrombin III			
Function	0.86–13.2 u/ml		
Antigen	0.79–1.11 u/ml		

Expressed as mean ± SD (95% range).

After Dacie and Lewis (1994).

Table 3 *Haematological values for normal infants and children*

	At birth (full term)	Day 3	1 month	2–6 months	2–6 years	6–12 years
Red-cell count ($\times 10^{12}$/l)	6.0±1.0	5.3±1.3	4.2±1.2	3.8±0.8	4.6±0.7	4.6±0.6
Haemoglobin (g/l)	165±30	185±40	140±30	115±20	125±15	135±20
Packed-cell volume/haematocrit	0.54±0.10	0.56±0.11	0.43±0.12	0.35±0.07	0.37±0.03	0.40±0.05
Mean cell volume (MCV) (fl)	110±10	108±13	104±19	91±17	81±6	86±8
Mean cell haemoglobin (MCH) (pg)	34±3	34±3	34±6	30±5	27±3	29±4
Mean cell haemoglobin concentration (MCHC) (g/l)	330±30	330±40	330±40	330±30	340±30	340±30
Reticulocytes (%)	2–5	1–4.5	0.3–1	0.4–1	0.2–2	0.2–2
Leucocyte count ($\times 10^9$/l)	18±8	15±8	12±7	12±6	10±5	9±4
Neutrophils ($\times 10^9$/l)	5–13	3–5	3–9	1.5–9	1.5–8	2–8
Lymphocytes ($\times 10^9$/l)	3–10	2–8	3–16	4–10	6–9	1–5
Monocytes ($\times 10^9$/l)	0.7–1.5	0.5–1	0.3–1	0.1–1	0.1–1	0.1–1
Eosinophils ($\times 10^9$/l)	0.2–1	0.1–2.5	0.2–1	0.2–1	0.2–1	0.1–1

Expressed as mean ± 2 SD or 95% range.

After Dacie and Lewis (1994).

the sexes (Table 3). Furthermore, it should be emphasized that the accuracy of these measurements relies very much on the method used for their determination. For example, using an electronic cell counter, extremely reproducible results for all three measurements can be obtained, whereas a red-cell count made with a counting chamber is of little value. By combining information obtained from these measurements the red-cell indices can be estimated. The mean cell haemoglobin (MCH), which is derived from the haemoglobin value and the red-cell count and is expressed in picograms (pg), gives a reliable indication of the mount of haemoglobin per cell. The mean cell haemoglobin concentration (MCHC) represents the concentration of haemoglobin in g/dl (100 ml) of erythrocytes. The mean cell volume (MCV), calculated in femtolitres (fl), gives an indication of the size of the erythrocytes. Hence it is elevated in patients with macrocytic disorders and reduced in the presence of microcytic red cells. The normal values at different stages of development are summarized in Table 3.

It should be emphasized that the red-cell indices give an indication of the average size and degree of haemoglobinization of the red cells. Thus they are only of value if combined with an examination of a blood film to provide information about the relative uniformity of any changes in size or haemoglobin concentration.

THE TOTAL AND DIFFERENTIAL LEUCOCYTE COUNT

The leucocyte count can be determined either by using a counting chamber or electronically. The differential count is obtained from analysing the different types of white cells in a total of 200 to 300 cells, or more if the total white-cell count is unusually low. It should be remembered that the total white-cell count shows remarkable variability even in the same individual at different times. There are variations during the menstrual cycle and a marked diurnal rhythm with minimum counts in the morning with subjects at rest. Activity may increase the white-cell count slightly, as may emotional stress and eating. Furthermore, the differential white-cell count varies considerably during normal human development. There is a preponderance of lymphocytes during the first few years of life and of polymorphonuclear leucocytes during later development and in adult life. These normal variations are shown in Table 3.

THE PLATELET COUNT

This is most accurately determined with an electronic cell counter, although a rough approximation can be obtained by using a counting chamber. There is marked variation in the normal platelet count and the range in health is approximately 150 to 400×10^9/l. A slight drop in the

count occurs before menstruation but on the whole it varies less within an individual than the white-cell count.

BLOOD VOLUME, RED-CELL MASS, AND PLASMA VOLUME

Because the haemoglobin level or PCV may vary due to expansion or contraction of the plasma volume, it is sometimes necessary to measure the red-cell mass and plasma volume directly. This is usually done by radioisotope dilution. The red-cell volume (**RCV**) is measured by labelling the red cells with ^{51}Cr and the plasma volume (**PV**) by the use of isotope-labelled albumin. These measurements are fraught with difficulties because of the variation of vascularity and PCV between different organs, and because fat is a relatively avascular tissue. There is still considerable controversy about how best to express the results. A variety of correction factors has been derived, which attempt to relate the measured RCV or PV to an ideal body weight. In practice it is usual to simply calculate the RCV or PV in ml/kg. The wide range of normal values is summarized in Table 2.

THE ERYTHROCYTE SEDIMENTATION RATE (ESR)

The ESR is a measure of the suspension stability of red cells in blood. It is usually expressed in mm and is obtained by measuring the distance from the surface meniscus to the upper limit of the red cell layer in a column of blood after 60 min. The ESR depends on the difference in specific gravity between the red cells and plasma but is influenced by many other factors, particularly the rate at which the red cells clump or form rouleaux. The increased sedimentation rate of clusters of cells reflects reduced fluid friction resulting from a decreased surface:volume ratio. Rouleaux formation is related to the concentration of fibrinogen and, to a lesser extent, of α_2- and γ-globulins in the plasma. Unfortunately, the ESR is also subject to many technical difficulties including the dimensions of the tube, the nature of the anticoagulant used, and any degree of tilt of the tube from the horizontal.

The ESR is still widely used as a non-specific index of organic disease. It is elevated in many acute or chronic infections, neoplastic diseases, collagen diseases, renal insufficiency, and any disorder associated with a significant change in the plasma proteins. Anaemia may cause an increased rate of sedimentation, and although many attempts have been made to develop correction factors to allow for this variable, none is satisfactory. Like all haematological measurements, the ESR changes in certain physiological states, particularly in pregnancy and with increasing age. In men and women over the age of 60 a slightly elevated ESR is often found without an obvious cause (Table 2).

OTHER HAEMATOLOGICAL INVESTIGATIONS

The simple tests that have been outlined in this section form the general screening investigations for all haematological disorders. In later sections we will describe the more specialized investigations that are often required to diagnose specific disorders of the red cells, white cells, and platelets, or of haemostasis and coagulation. Normal values for some of these investigations are given in Table 2.

Examination of the marrow

Bone marrow can be examined by needle aspiration, closed needle biopsy, or open surgical biopsy. In adults the sites most easily available are the sternum and the anterior or posterior iliac crests, although the marrow at the iliac crests tends to become rather fatty in elderly subjects. In children of less than a year old the anterior surface of the tibia is the site of choice, but in older children the iliac crest or the lumbar vertebral spines are suitable. After aspiration of the marrow, films are made and stained with a Romanowsky stain. Needle or surgical biopsy samples are fixed and sectioned by standard methods.

The marrow films are examined initially under low power to assess the overall cellularity and for the presence of abnormal cells. It is sometimes useful to obtain a differential count and from this the myeloid/erythroid (**M/E**) ratio can be determined. This is approximately 3:1 in health, although, if there is increased erythroid activity, it may fall to unity or less. It should be remembered that differential counts may be quite inaccurate because the precursors may not be distributed homogeneously. This is a particular problem in disorders in which there are abnormal cells in the marrow. Having determined the overall cellularity, the morphology of the individual cells is examined. The degree of maturation of the red cells, white cells, and megakaryocyte series is assessed and the marrow is examined carefully for the presence of any abnormal cells.

A biopsy specimen is particularly useful for looking at overall cellularity and relating the amount of haemopoiesis to the amount of fatty tissue. It is of particular value if an aspiration yields a 'dry tap' when it may show replacement by fibrous or tumour tissue, which may not aspirate readily. Using appropriate stains it is possible to estimate the amount of iron and reticulin in the marrow.

ASSESSMENT OF BONE MARROW ACTIVITY AND DISTRIBUTION

Some indication of marrow function is obtained from its morphological appearances and from the M/E ratio. It is also possible to measure the rates of production and turnover of the red-cell series using radioactive iron (see Chapter 22.4.4). It is sometimes necessary to attempt to estimate the distribution of the haemopoietic marrow, and this is usually done by using isotopes to produce scintograms that show the distribution of erythropoietic or reticuloendothelial marrow throughout the body. Erythropoietic marrow can be visualized using the short-lived, positron-emitting isotope ^{52}Fe with a scintillation camera. In health this shows erythropoietic marrow in the ribs, spine, pelvis, scapula, and clavicle, with a variable amount in the skull. The reticuloendothelial portion of the marrow can be labelled with a radiocolloid with an appropriate particle size; the most effective and commonly used is ^{99}Tc^{m}-sulphurcolloid.

REFERENCES

Beutler, E., Lichtman, M.A., Coller, B.S., and Kipps, T.J. (ed.) (1994). *Williams hematology*, (5th edn). McGraw-Hill, New York (in press).

Dacie, J.V. and Lewis, S.M. (1994). *Practical haematology*, (8th edn). Churchill Livingstone, Edinburgh.

Nathan, D.G. and Oski, F.A. (1993). *Hematology of infancy and childhood*, (4th edn). Saunders, Philadelphia.

22.2 Haemopoietic stem cells

22.2.1 Stem cells and haemopoiesis

C. A. SIEFF AND D. G. NATHAN

INTRODUCTION

Normal haemopoiesis in the adult is sustained by the production of blood cells from their recognizable precursors in the bone marrow, their survival in the vasculature, and their demise in the reticuloendothelial system, predominantly in the spleen, the liver, the lung, and the marrow itself. Though the concentration of cells in the blood varies widely, it is notable that the values observed in normal individuals are, in fact, remarkably consistent, particularly considering the vast differences in the lifespans of these cells. For example, the mean lifespan of granulocytes in the peripheral blood may be measured in hours. In contrast, platelets survive for 7 to 10 days. Though platelets are removed from the blood in part by random forces, most of their lifespan is dictated by metabolic changes within them that lead to predetermined death in about 7 to 10 days. Normally, red cells are almost entirely lost by a process of metabolic decay that begins after the erythrocyte has attained an age

of approximately 100 days. Lymphocytes have very dramatic differences in lifespan. Some are removed from the circulation in 2 or 3 weeks by a process that is not at all understood. Others, particularly certain T lymphocytes, are thought to survive for the entire lifespan of the individual, carrying within them the programmes embossed upon them by the thymus.

Though steady-state concentrations of the blood cells vary from each other by three logs or more, the actual marrow production rates that maintain them are very similar. Approximately 5×10^4 red cells, 2×10^4 platelets, and 2×10^4 granulocytes must be produced per microlitre of blood per day to maintain a normal blood count. Lymphocyte production must be considerably lower because the bulk of lymphocytes in the peripheral blood are the long-lived T lymphocytes described above.

These relatively constant production rates of blood cells are regulated by a highly complex marrow tissue characterized morphologically by recognizable, differentiating precursor cells that are themselves partially renewed by a widely variable population of invisible progenitor cells, some of which have the characteristics of stem cells. These differentiating precursor cells and their progenitors are packed together into fronds surrounded by endothelial cells that separate the marrow cells from the venous sinuses. The completed blood cells find apertures through the endothelial cells and migrate between them to fall into the sinuses, the currents of which carry them into the peripheral blood.

In this chapter, we shall describe some of the important aspects of the physiology of haemopoiesis in the marrow. To understand this process, we must first review its ontogeny and comparative development.

PHYLOGENY AND ONTOGENY

John Hunter was a remarkable surgeon, but in our opinion he was wrong when he decided that the red cell is the least important element in the blood. Adaptation to terrestrial existence, accompanied by the development of a cardiorespiratory system, demanded that haemoglobin be encapsulated within erythrocytes rather than float free in the vasculature. This permits high oxygen delivery and acceptable blood viscosity. The renewal rate of red cells is a function of metabolic rate. Thus, turtles and crocodiles have remarkable low rates of red-cell production whereas pygmy shrews renew their red cells very rapidly. Marmots exhibit a marked reduction in red-cell renewal when they hibernate at cold temperatures. In the juvenile state, European eels lack erythrocytes but when they swim against the current of the rivers in northern Europe, nucleated erythrocytes appear. This is one of the most primitive demonstrations of the role of oxygen demand on erythropoiesis and is also observed in non-red cell-producing organisms such as Daphnia, the English water flea, that produces high molecular-weight haemoglobin in its ovaries when exposed to low oxygen tension in stagnant ponds.

In the developing human being, haemopoiesis moves through several overlapping anatomical and functional stages, beginning in the yolk sac, entering the hepatic phase at 6 weeks', and the marrow phase at 20 weeks' gestation. Transfer to the bone marrow phase is generally complete at birth. These anatomical shifts in sites of haemopoiesis are associated with marked alterations in functional properties, particularly with respect to the pattern of globin synthesis in the red cell. These changes are referred to as the 'fetal switch'. Clearly this transition is not a single event involving the γ-chains of fetal haemoglobin alone, but is instead polygenic involving a series of changes that are regulated in a programmed fashion. The mechanism of this coordinated series of changes of gene expression is as yet undetermined, but it appears to be mediated at the level of the progenitors of haemopoietic cells and is strongly influenced by site-specific regulatory factors.

MARROW ANATOMY

The relative red (active) marrow space of a child is much greater than that of an adult, presumably because the high requirements for red-cell production during neonatal life demand the resources of the entire production potential of the marrow. During postnatal life the demands for red-cell production ebb, and much of the marrow space is slowly and progressively filled with fat (Fig. 1). In certain diseases that are usually associated with anaemia, such as myeloid metaplasia, haemopoiesis may return to its former sites in the liver, spleen, and lymph nodes and may also be found in the adrenals, cartilage, adipose tissue, thoracic paravertebral gutters, and even in the kidneys.

The microenvironment of the marrow cavity is a vast network of endothelial cell-lined vascular channels or sinusoids that separate clumps of haemopoietic cells, including fat cells. The cells are found in the intrasinusoidal spaces. The vascular and haemopoietic compartments are separated by reticular cells (derived from fibroblasts) that form the adventitial surfaces of the vascular sinuses and extend cytoplasmic processes to create a lattice on which blood cells are found. The lattice is demonstrated by reticulin stains of marrow sections (Fig. 2). The conformation of the meshwork of fibroblast cytoplasmic extensions and the location of haemopoietic cells in the network of vascular sinuses are best illustrated by scanning electron microscopy (Fig. 3). The fibroblast–endothelial cell network provides two major functions: an adhesive framework on to which the developing cells are bound by fibronectin and other members of the integrin family, and the production by these cells of haemopoietic growth factors. These factors comprise a family of small glycoproteins that not only affect immature cells but also influence the survival and function of mature cells. They do so by binding to specific cell-surface receptors, and the genes for many of the growth

Fig. 1 A comparison of active red marrow-bearing areas in a child and adult. Note the almost identical amount of active red marrow in the child and adult despite a fivefold discrepancy in body weight. (Reproduced from MacFarlane, R.G. and Robb-Smith, A.H.T. (ed.) (1961). *Functions of the blood*, p. 357. Blackwell Scientific, Oxford, with permission.)

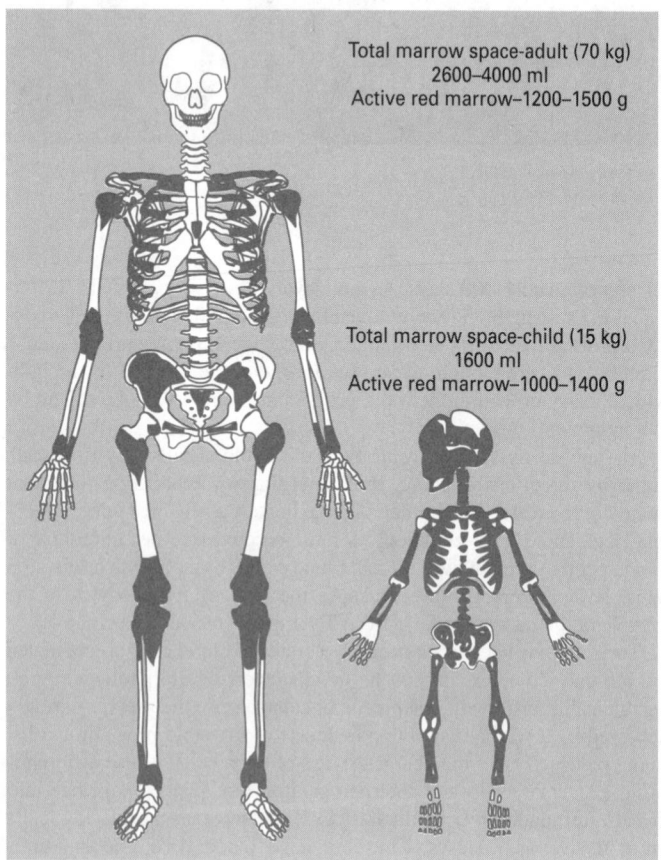

Total marrow space-adult (70 kg)
2600–4000 ml
Active red marrow–1200–1500 g

Total marrow space-child (15 kg)
1600 ml
Active red marrow–1000–1400 g

Fig. 2 Bone marrow biopsy of a patient with mild myelofibrosis. A slight increase in the number of reticulin fibres in a delicate discontinuous fibre network is present. (Gomori stain, ×350.) (Reproduced from Lennert, K. *et al.* (1975). *Clinical Haematology*, **4**, 335, with permission.)

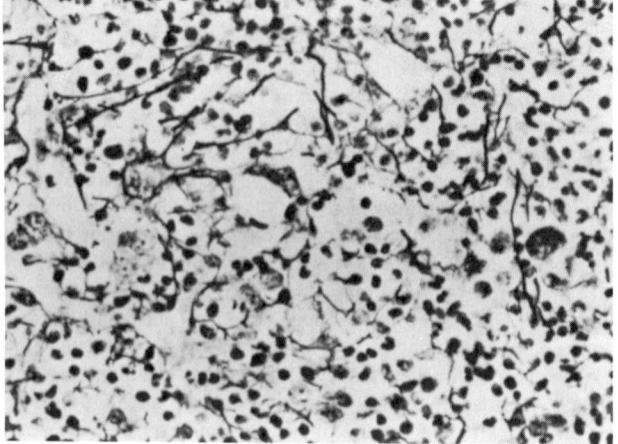

factors and their receptors have recently been isolated. The cellular origin and the major sites of action of important members of the haemopoietic growth-factor family are shown in Fig. 4. Two of the receptors, c-*kit*, the receptor for Steel factor, and c-*fms*, the monocyte colony-stimulating factor (**M-CSF**) receptor, are members of the transmembrane tyrosine kinase family. In contrast, the receptors for the other haemopoietic growth factors such as interleukin (**IL**) 3, granulocyte–macrophage colony-stimulating factor (**GM-CSF**), granulocyte-CSF (**G-CSF**), IL-5, IL-6, and erythropoietin are members of the haemopoietic growth-factor receptor family. They share several structural features but do not contain cytoplasmic tyrosine kinase domains, and they activate cells by an unknown mechanism likely to involve the association of the receptors with proteins that have kinase activity.

A schema of the marrow circulation is shown in Fig. 5. The central and radial arteries ramify in the cortical capillaries, which in turn join the marrow sinusoids and drain into the central sinus. Cells that egress from the marrow sinusoids then join the venous circulation through concomitant veins. The inner, or luminal, surface of the vascular sinusoids is lined with endothelial cells, the cytoplasmic extensions of which overlap, or interdigitate, with one another. The escape of developing haemopoietic cells into the sinus for transport to the circulation occurs through gaps that develop in this endothelial lining and even through endothelial-cell cytoplasmic pores (Fig. 6).

The location of the different haemopoietic cells is not random. Clumps of megakaryocytes are found adjacent to marrow sinuses. They shed platelets, the fragments of their cytoplasm, directly into the lumen. This reduces the requirement for movement of bulky mature megakaryocytes, a mobility characteristic of the granuloid- and erythroid-differentiated precursors as they approach the point at which they egress from the marrow. A schema that illustrates the transfer of haemopoietic cells into the sinuses is shown in Fig. 6.

As mentioned above, the formed elements of blood in vertebrates, including man, continuously undergo replacement to maintain a constant number of red cells, white cells, and platelets. The number of cells of each type is maintained in a very narrow range in normal adults—approximately 5000 granulocytes, 5×10^5 red blood cells, and 150 000 to 300 000 platelets per microlitre of whole blood. In the following section we shall examine the nature of the signals that affect the proliferation of the stem and progenitor cells, and the normal regulatory mech-

anisms that maintain a balanced production of new blood cells. They are still not completely understood, but present evidence strongly supports the following basic principles.

FUNCTION OF STEM CELLS AND PROGENITORS

The progenitors of the recognizable precursor cells are mononuclear 'blast' cells with large nuclei, prominent nuclei, and basophilic cytoplasm devoid of granules. These primitive progenitor cells are present at extremely low frequencies, approximately 1 in 10^4 to 10^5 marrow cells for the stem-cell population and 1 in 10^3 for their committed progenitor progeny. A single pluripotent stem cell is capable of giving rise, in a stochastic fashion, to increasingly committed progenitor cells according to the schema outlined in Fig. 4. These committed progenitors are destined to form differentiated recognizable precursors of the specific types of blood cells.

Pluripotent stem cells are defined as cells dually capable of self-renewal and differentiation under the influence of certain non-lineage-specific growth factors such as IL-1, IL-3, IL-6, IL-11, and Steel factor. Their differentiation programme is random and leads to a broad array of more mature lineage-committed progenitors that are themselves responsive to lineage-restricted growth factors, including erythropoietin, G-CSF, and M-CSF. Some of the lineage-restricted growth factors, particularly erythropoietin, are produced in response to the circulating levels of differentiated blood cells.

The lineage-committed progenitors are characterized by limited proliferative potential that depends upon the presence of specific growth factors. The latter interact with specific receptors on progenitor surfaces; therefore, they are not capable of indefinite self-renewal. In fact, they 'die by differentiation' to mature precursors of the blood cells. The maintenance of their numbers ultimately depends upon the presence of lineage-specific growth factor and on random influx into their pool from the pluripotent stem-cell pool.

Therefore, amplification of blood-cell production occurs at the level of the committed progenitor pool, while maintenance of the progenitors depends upon the capacity of members of the pluripotent stem-cell pool to differentiate into the committed progenitor pool.

Haemopoietic differentiation requires an appropriate microenvironment. In normal adult humans, this is confined to the bone marrow, whereas in the mouse it includes both the spleen and bone marrow. The existence of certain strains of mice that exhibit a deficiency in the haemopoietic microenvironment suggests that the interactions between haemopoietic cells and the bone marrow microenvironment involve very specific molecular mechanisms. Recent insight into the nature of one of these interactions has come from isolation of the genes that determine the White Spotting (**W**) and Steel (**S1**) mutations in mice. Animals affected by mutations at both of these loci have a severe macrocytic anaemia associated with defects in skin pigmentation and fertility. The mutations, however, map to different chromosome loci (W to chromosome 5, S1 to chromosome 10). This is consistent with the results of transplant experiments, which demonstrate that the W mutation is one of stem cells whereas the S1 defect is one of the bone marrow microenvironment. The W gene has now been shown to be allelic with the c-*kit* proto-oncogene, a member of the tyrosine kinase cell-surface receptor family; in contrast, the S1 mutation results in defective production of the ligand for this receptor (Steel factor, also known as kit ligand, stem-cell factor, or mast-cell growth factor). Interestingly, Steel factor is produced in both a secreted and membrane-bound form by fibroblasts and other cells, and the latter form may thus provide one molecular explanation for interactions between the stem cells and their microenvironment.

Progenitors can, however, exist outside the marrow. A number of early haemopoietic cells, including the pluripotent stem cells and certain committed progenitor cells, have been demonstrated in the circulation of normal individuals and experimental animals. The capacity of haemopoietic stem cells to negotiate the circulation is especially significant

Fig. 3 Scanning electron micrograph of rat femoral marrow. The haemopoietic cells are grouped between the interlacing network of vascular sinuses. Many cells are dislodged when the marrow is transected, and separate spaces are present where cells had been. (Reproduced from Lichtman, M.A. *et al.* (1978). Factors thought to contribute to the regulation of egress of cells from marrow. In *The year in hematology*, (ed. K. Silber *et al.*), pp. 243–79. Plenum Medical, New York, with permission.)

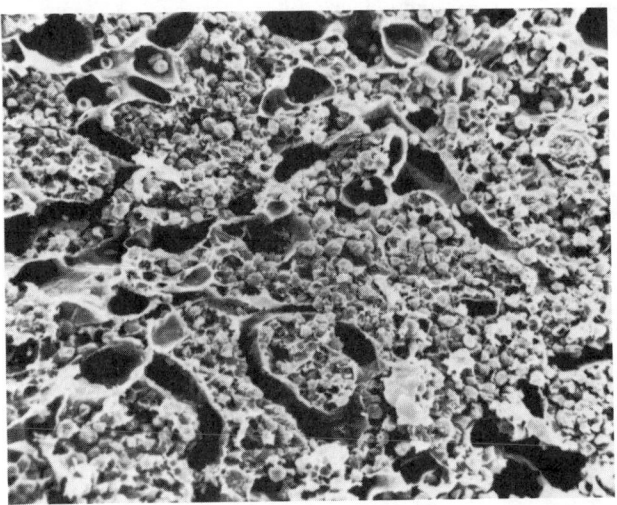

Fig. 4 Haemopoietic growth factors (HGFs). The predominant actions of several major HGFs are indicated diagrammatically. Interleukin-3 (IL-3), Steel factor (SF), IL-11, IL-6, and IL-1 act early during haemopoiesis on pluripotent stem cells (PSC), while GM-CSF probably acts slightly later, after commitment to myelopoiesis (myeloid stem cell (MSC)). The lineage-specific factors erythropoietic (epo), granulocyte-colony-stimulating factor (CSF) (G-CSF), monocyte-CSF (M-CSF), IL-5, and a putative thrombopoietin act on single lineage-committed progenitors and precursors. Monocytes and macrophages also produce IL-1 and tumour necrosis factor (TNF), potent inducers of HGF production by microenvironmental endothelial and reticular fibroblastoid cells. In addition, macrophages can produce these factors after induction with endotoxin (not shown) and T cells produce IL-3, GM-CSF, and IL-5 in response to IL-1 plus antigenic stimulation.

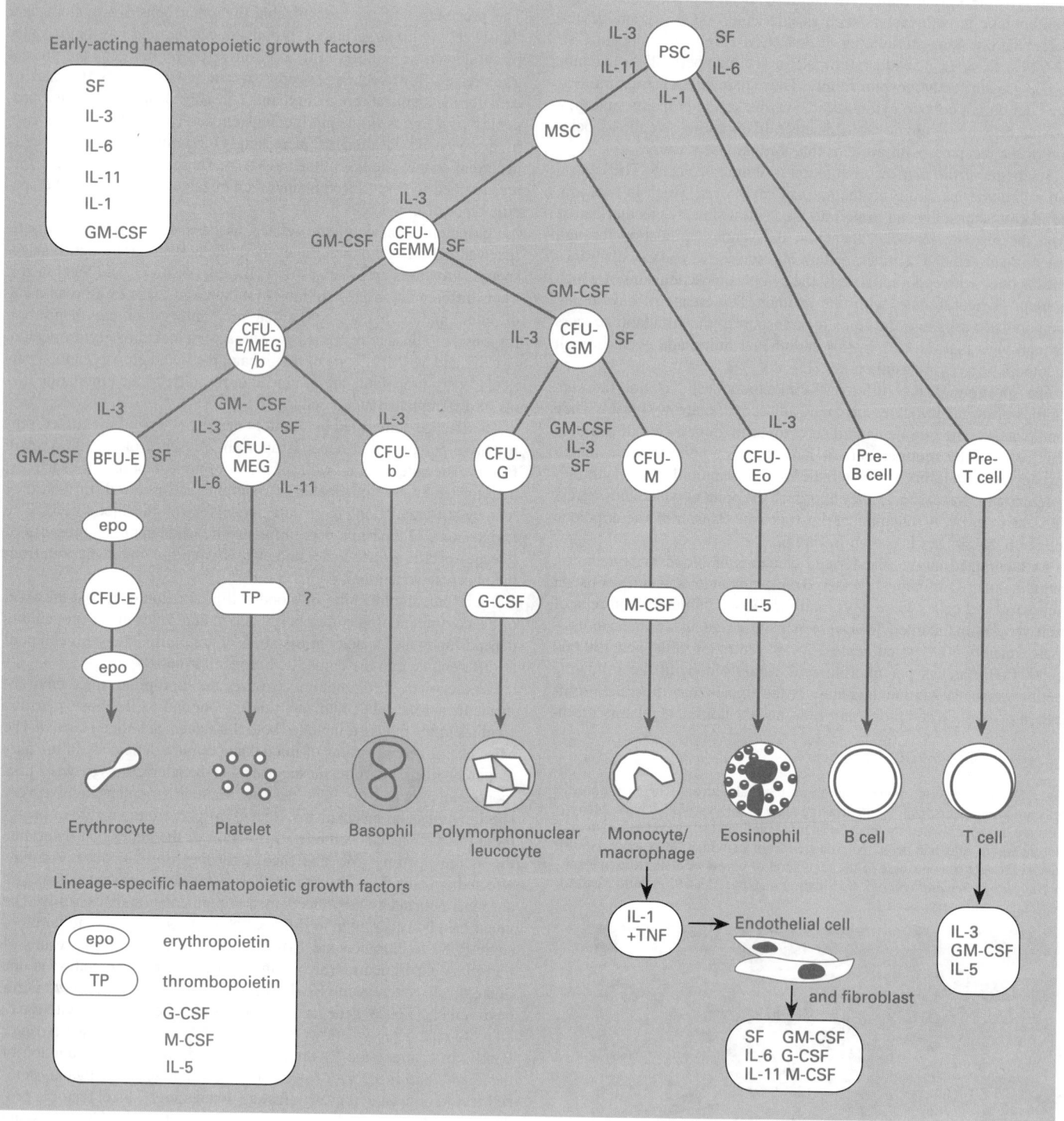

Fig. 5 A schematic representation of the circulation of the marrow. The nutrient artery, central arteries, and radial arteries feed the cortical capillaries. The cortical capillaries anastomose with the marrow sinuses, which drain into the large central sinus. The central sinus enters the comitant vein by which the marrow effluent enters the systemic venous circulation. An interesting feature of the circulation of marrow is the transit of nearly all arterial blood through cortical capillaries before entering the marrow sinuses. Not shown are the arterial communications from muscular arteries that feed the periosteum and penetrate the cortex to anastomose with intracortical vessels. (Reproduced from Lichtman, M.A. *et al.* (1978). Factors thought to contribute to the regulation of egress of cells from marrow. In *The year in hematology*, (ed. K. Silber *et al.*), pp. 243–79. Plenum Medical, New York, with permission.)

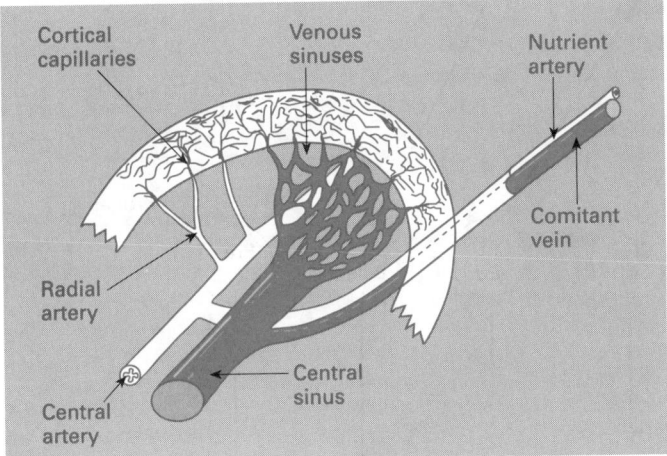

in relation to bone marrow transplantation, which is carried out by infusion of bone marrow cells from the donor into the circulation of the recipient. The relatively limited production of lymphocyte progenitors has made it difficult to demonstrate that the lymphocyte is derived from the same population of stem cells as the other cellular elements of blood. Present evidence indicates, however, that both T and B lymphocytes are in fact derived from a pluripotent stem cell that has the capacity to give rise to a myeloid stem cell that in turn matures to form the committed progenitors of red blood cells, phagocytes, and megakaryocytes.

THE PLURIPOTENT STEM CELL

Till and McCulloch demonstrated that colonies of haemopoietic cells could be observed in the spleen in bone-marrow transplanted, irradiated recipient mice within 10 days after the transplant. These spleen colony-forming units (**CFU-S**) produce colonies that contain precursors of erythrocytes, granulocytes, macrophages, and megakaryocytes. Subsequent experiments using karyotypically marked donor cells confirmed the clonal origin of the differentiated cells and recent experiments in which foreign genes have been inserted into spleen colony-forming cells have further substantiated this finding. It was also shown that each colony contains a variable number of stem cells that could again form spleen colonies of differentiated progeny in a second irradiated recipient, indicating the self-renewal property of stem cells. The demonstration of a stem cell that can differentiate to form progenitor cells for erythropoiesis, granulopoiesis, and megakaryopoiesis is completely consistent with subsequent observations in diseases such as chronic myeloid leukaemia and polycythaemia vera in which a clonal origin of abnormal erythroid, granulocytic, and megakaryocytic precursor cells can be demonstrated (see Chapter 22.3.5). In addition, these studies of chronic myeloid leukaemia have demonstrated a pluripotent stem cell that gives

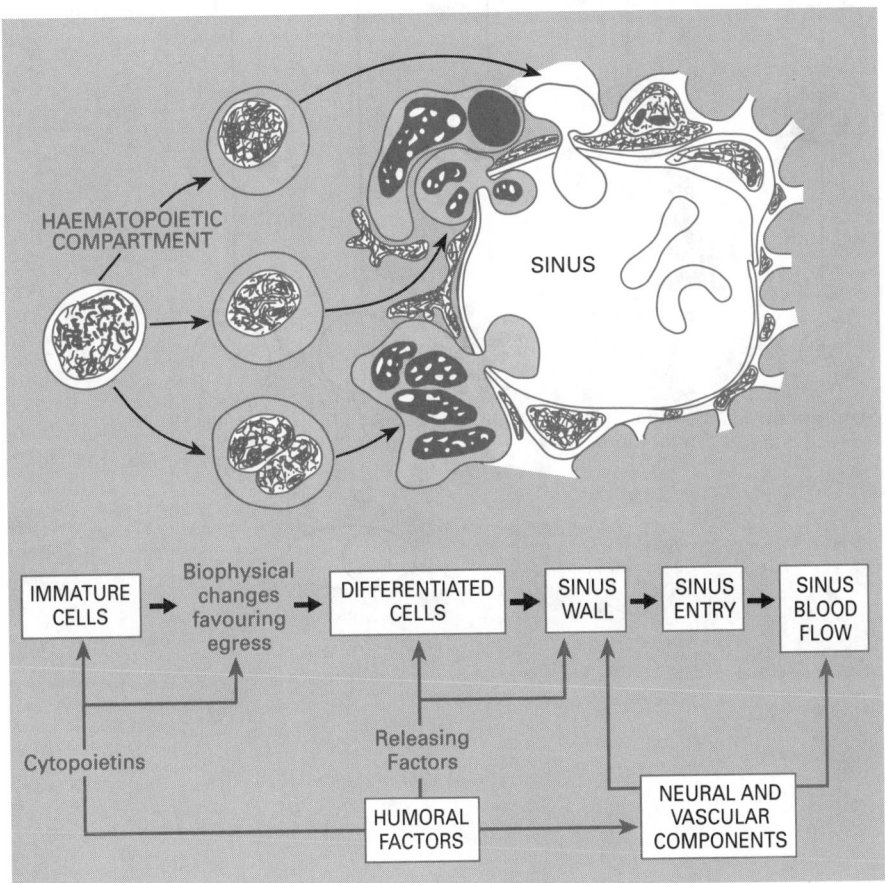

Fig. 6 A schematic diagram of the factors that may be involved in controlling the release of marrow cells. The central relation between the haemopoietic compartment and the marrow sinus is depicted. The drawing highlights the similarity of egress for the three major haemopoietic cells: reticulocytes in the top pathway, granulocytes and monocytes in the centre pathway, and platelets in the lower pathway. Immature cells undergo physical changes under the influence of cytopoietins that favour egress. In the case of the reticulocyte, enucleation precedes egress. This is shown by the solid black inclusion in the perisinal macrophage representing nucleophagocytosis antecedent to digestion of the erythroblast nucleus. The cytoplasmic protrusion of the megakaryocyte presumably detaches itself from the cell and will further fragment into platelets in the circulation. (Reproduced from Lichtman, M.A. *et al.* (1978). Factors thought to contribute to the regulation of egress of cells from marrow. In *The year in hematology*, (ed. K. Silber *et al.*), pp. 243–79. Plenum Medical, New York, with permission.)

Fig. 7 The maturation sequence of progenitor cells. The sequence is characterized by a progressive approach to single-lineage commitment. The term stem cell connotes high capacity for self-renewal, but all progenitors have some self-renewal capacity.

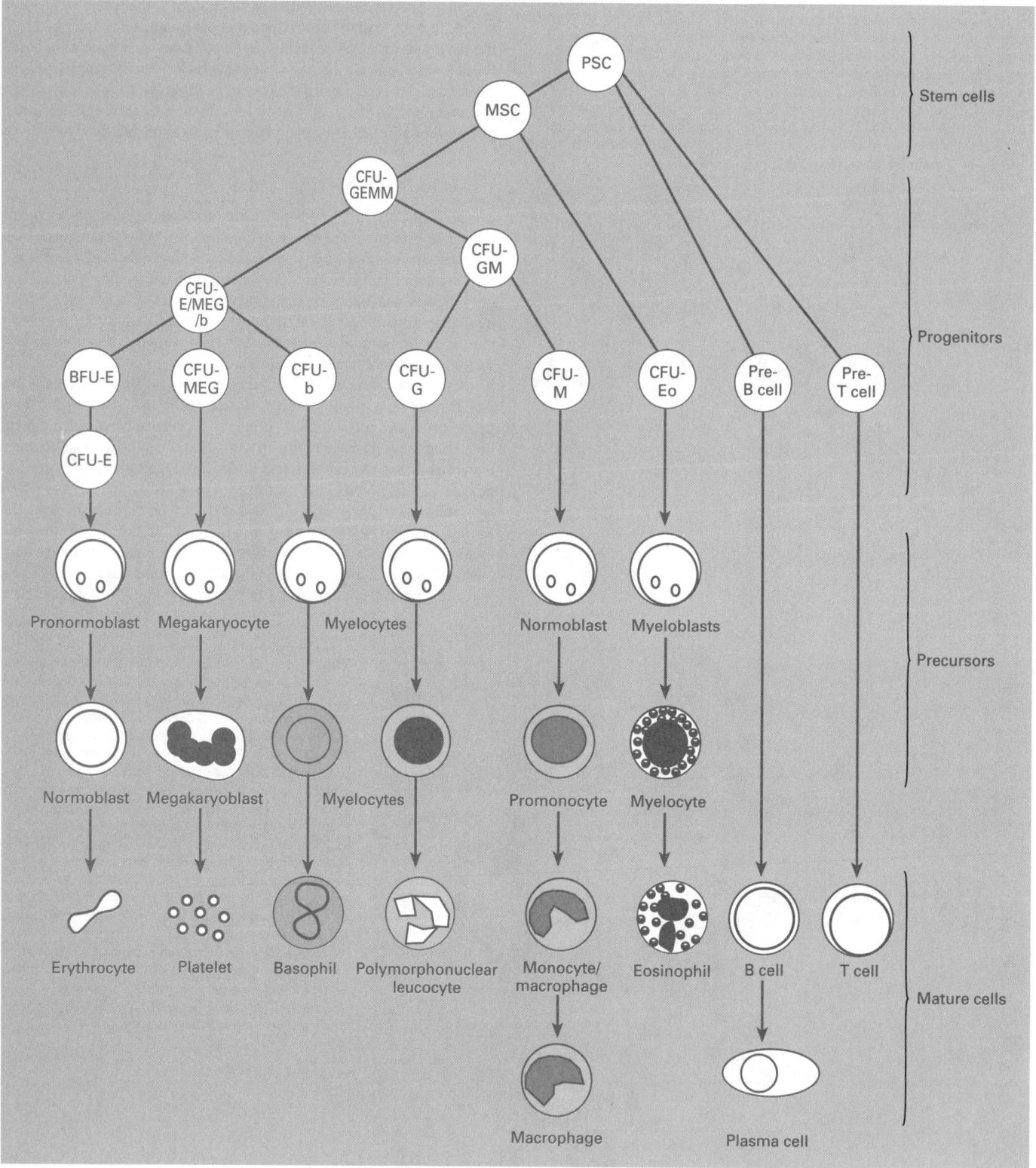

rise to B cells as well as to the aforementioned blood cells (Fig. 7). More recent studies provide a model of the stem-cell compartment in which the CFU-S is viewed as part of a continuum of cells with a decreasing capacity for self-renewal, increasing likelihood for differentiation, and increasing proliferative activity. The cells progress in a unidirectional fashion in this continuum. CFU-S can thus be distinguished from a more primitive precursor that has the capacity for long-term haemopoietic reconstitution after bone marrow transplantation. In the mouse, as few as 30 cells of a highly purified marrow population that lacks lineage-specific antigens but expresses Ly-6 (Sca-1) and low levels of Thy-1 (i.e. lin⁻ Sca-1⁺ Thy-1¹⁰) can reconstitute haemopoiesis in 50 per cent of lethally irradiated mice. Although this cell fraction appears to comprise virtually 100 per cent CFU-S, single-cell transfer experiments have shown that it is still heterogeneous in that only about 1 in 40 cells produces multi-lineage repopulating clones that persist for up to 2 to 3 months. Indeed, cell elutriation studies have shown that most of the CFU-S population is contained within a cell fraction that confers short-term radioprotective capacity, and can be separated from a cell fraction with the capacity for long-term haemopoietic reconstitution. Studies with purified populations of murine and human stem cells have shown that a combination of haemopoietic growth factors can act on at least some stem cells to induce cell cycling and proliferation. IL-3, produced by T and natural killer cells, or GM-CSF, a product of both stromal cells and T cells, appear to be factors essential for the survival in vitro of a class of stem cells that forms blast colonies in methylcellulose culture. These 'blast' colonies contain multilineage and unilineage progenitors and are probably at the myeloid stem-cell stage of differentiation (Fig. 4). When isolated from bone marrow, these stem cells are are mostly in a non-cycling, quiescent state. The addition to IL-3 or GM-CSF of Steel factor or other stromally produced haemopoietic growth factors such as IL-6, IL-11, or G-CSF shortens the G₀ phase in these cultures, thus hastening the onset of blast-colony formation. Interestingly, IL-3 and GM-CSF act on responsive cells by binding to a complex cell-surface receptor (R) that comprises α-chains specific for each ligand (IL-3Rα and GM-Rα) and a common β-polypeptide that does not bind ligand itself but that confers both high-affinity binding properties to each α-chain and also transduces the ligand-mediated signals to the interior of the cell. This common β-chain is also used by the eosinophil, lineage-specific, IL-5R α-chain.

The survival of a particular stem cell in the marrow requires a 'niche'; thus isogeneic marrow infusions are not successful unless the recipient is irradiated or treated with sufficient doses of cytotoxic drugs to create an adequate number of niches. Therefore, reports of failure of engraftment in aplastic anaemia using identical twin donors do not necessarily suggest an immunological basis for the disease but, equally as likely, imply persistence of non-functional pluripotent progenitors in the aplastic marrow niches. These abnormal cells must be destroyed in order to allow implantation of transfused normal progenitors.

ERYTHROPOIESIS

The rate of erythropoiesis is driven by anaemia or hypoxia, both of which stimulate a class of peritubular kidney cells through a haem-containing oxygen sensor to transcribe the erythropoietin gene and release the hormone into the blood. The hormone acts via the erythropoietin receptor found in erythroblasts and erythroid progenitors to stimulate their division and differentiation. The least mature committed erythroid progenitor is known as an erythroid burst-forming unit or **BFU-E** because when it differentiates in vitro it forms large colonies of erythroblasts and reticulocytes that may contain as many as 50 000 cells. The colonies, derived from single cells, have a burst-like appearance because they may be composed of multiple subcolonies. Thus one BFU-E may first divide in culture to form subcolony-forming cells, which then differentiate into colonies of erythroblasts and reticulocytes. BFU-Es progressively mature during their sojourn in the marrow and in doing so

lose their capacity to divide and migrate in vitro but gain in apparent sensitivity to erythropoietin until they reach the stage at which they are known as erythroid colony-forming units (**CFU-E**).

The regulation of the proliferation and maturation of erythroid progenitors depends on interaction with a number of growth factors. Erythropoietin is essential for the terminal maturation of erythroid cells. Its major effect appears to be at the level of the CFU-E during adult erythropoiesis, and recombinant preparations are as effective as the natural hormone. These very mature progenitors and proerythroblasts do not require 'burst-promoting activity' in the form of IL-3 or GM-CSF, and their dependence on erythropoietin is emphasized by the observation that they will not survive in vitro in its absence. As the majority of CFU-Es are in cycle, their survival in the presence of erythropoietin is probably tightly linked to their proliferation and differentiation to proerythroblasts and mature erythrocytes. Erythropoietin also acts on a subset of presumptive mature BFU-Es that require it for survival and terminal differentiation. A second subset of BFU-Es, presumably less mature, survive deprivation of erythropoietin if 'burst-promoting activity' is present, either as IL-3 or GM-CSF. Under serum-deprived culture conditions, the combination of erythropoietin and IL-3 or GM-CSF results in more BFU-E-derived colonies than when erythropoietin is added alone. Factors distinct from the classical colony-stimulating factors may positively regulate erythropoiesis, either directly or indirectly. Limiting dilution studies of highly purified CFU-Es in serum-free culture show that insulin and insulin-like growth factor I act directly on these cells. The presence of erythropoietin is also essential in these studies. Another factor that enhances both BFU-E and CFU-E colony formation is activin. This protein dimer, also known as follicle-stimulating hormone releasing protein, appears to have a lineage-specific effect on erythropoiesis that is indirect, as removal of monocytes and/or T lymphocytes abrogates its effect. It is interesting that activin has been identified as the factor produced by vegetal cells during blastogenesis which induces animal ectodermal cells to form primary mesoderm. Recently, Steel factor has also been shown to have marked synergistic effects on BFU-Es cultured in the presence of erythropoietin. Alone, it has no colony-forming ability.

CFU-Es and mature BFU-Es are highly responsive to the mitogenic effect of erythropoietin as well as to its differentiating role. Therefore, in haemorrhagic or haemolytic anaemias with elevated levels of erythropoietin, the numbers of CFU-Es and mature BFU-Es may rise remarkably in the marrow. Immature BFU-Es are less responsive to the mitogenic effect of erythropoietin, and therefore, the frequency of this subset of BFU-Es changes little in anaemia.

NEGATIVE REGULATION OF ERYTHROPOIESIS

Observations that subsets of lymphocytes with an immunological suppressor phenotype isolated from normal subjects can inhibit erythroid activity in vitro correlate with reports of patients with a variety of disorders in whom anaemia or granulocytopenia is associated with an expansion of certain T-lymphocyte populations. In the rare disorder T lymphocytosis with cytopenia, in vitro suppression of erythropoiesis (or granulocytopoiesis) has been correlated with the expansion of a T-lymphocyte population that may be the counterpart of the haemopoietic suppressor cells isolated from normal peripheral blood. The phenotype of these cells has been described in detail. The cell is a large, granular lymphocyte that is both E rosette-positive and CD8 (classic suppressor phenotype)-positive. Suppressor T cells may also be involved in some cases of aplastic anaemia or neutropenia without any underlying immunological disorder or an overt T-cell proliferation. Exactly how such suppressor T cells interact with haemopoietic progenitors, and what surface antigens are 'seen' by the suppressors, are currently under investigation. There is evidence to support the concept that suppression of erythroid colony expression in vitro can be regulated by T cells and may be genetically restricted. Cell–cell interactions in immunological systems have been well characterized with regard to surface determinants that allow for cellular recognition. That certain phenotypes of T cells 'recognize' distinct classes of histocompatibility antigens on immunological cell surfaces has been well described. Thus, the observation that haemopoietic progenitors have a unique distribution of class II histocompatibility antigens on their cell surface suggests a role for these antigens in the cell–cell interactions that regulate haemopoietic differentiation.

T cells may also inhibit erythropoiesis in a non-HLA restricted fashion by the production of inhibitory cytokines. Some lymphokines may inhibit erythropoiesis *in vitro* by a complex lymphokine cascade. Activation of T cells by the T-cell antigen receptor CD3 results in cell-surface expression of the IL-2 α-chain (p55) and the acquisition of IL-2 responsiveness. IL-2 inhibits BFU-Es in the presence of these IL-2R positive cells, possibly by inducing their release of interferon-γ (**IFN-γ**). CD2 can serve as an alternative pathway of T-cell activation, and may do so through binding to its ligand LFA-3 on antigen-presenting cells. Blockade of CD2 with monoclonal antibody leads to abrogation of IL-2/IFN-γ-mediated BFU-E suppression. These data are difficult to reconcile with the observation that IL-2 incubation of phorbol myristate acetate/calcium ionophore-activated, CD4+ T cells leads to marked expansion of IL-3 and GM-CSF mRNA-positive cells by *in situ* hybridization. Most, but not all, CD4+ T cells express CD28 as well, and there is evidence to suggest that IL-3 production is restricted to CD28+T cells. It thus appears paradoxical that potent stimulating and inhibitory lymphokines can be produced by activation of T cells through the same pathway.

Tumour necrosis factor also suppresses erythropoiesis *in vitro*. The injection of peritoneal macrophages into Friend murine leukemia virus-infected animals results in rapid but transient resolution of the massive erythroid hyperplasia associated with this disease. This may be due to elaboration by macrophages of IL-1α, which does not suppress erythropoiesis itself, but acts by the induction of tumour necrosis factor. This effect is reversed by erythropoietin.

Proerythroblasts represent the ultimate stage of differentiation of committed erythroid progenitors. In contrast to the progenitors, which compromise less than one-tenth of a per cent of the marrow cell population, proerythroblasts are present at 3 to 5 per cent, and their daughters, the recognizable erythroid precursors, comprise 30 per cent of the population.

Estimates of reticulocyte production and erythroblast content of marrows, together with measurements of the rate at which the proerythroblast compartment is renewed from the progenitor pool, suggest that approximately 10 per cent of the daily reticulocyte production is derived from the terminal differentiation of proerythroblasts newly developed from the progenitor department. During anaemic stress the rate at which progenitors differentiate to proerythroblasts may increase 10-fold or more. This increase in the rate of proerythroblast formation from progenitors is associated with an increase in the production of fetal haemoglobin in a large fraction of the erythroid cells derived from them. The basis of this reactivation of fetal haemoglobin synthesis in proerythroblast newly derived from progenitors is not understood, and the extent to which fetal haemoglobin may be increased in such settings could be genetically controlled. In any case, it is an important phenomenon because those with the capacity to develop large increases in fetal haemoglobin who are also homozygous for major β-chain haemoglobinopathies may have a remarkably mild course. Fetal haemoglobin elevation occurs in many forms of accelerated erythropoiesis and is indeed a marker of such a condition.

PHAGOCYTOPOIESIS

The development of a clonal assay for granulocyte and macrophage progenitors preceded the development of erythroid progenitor assays by nearly a decade, yet a clear understanding of the regulation of myeloid

differentiation remains elusive. Figure 4 describes the development and regulation of granulocyte, monocyte, and macrophage production from the pluripotent stem cell. The colony-forming unit–granulocyte-macrophage (**CFU-GM**) derived from the pluripotent progenitor gives rise to separate granulocyte and monocyte progenitors (CFU-G and CFU-M), which, under the influence of unique colony-stimulating factors, differentiate to mature granulocytes and/or monocytes, respectively. Both IL-3 and GM-CSF affect a similar broad spectrum of human myeloid progenitor cells. This includes colonies that contain granulocytes, erythrocytes, monocytes, and megakaryocytes (**CFU-GEMM**), CFU-GEMM, eosinophils (**CFU-Eo**) CFU-GM, CFU-G, and CFU-M. Data from serum-free cultures suggest that in the presence of IL-3 or GM-CSF alone, myeloid colony formation is much reduced, and the optimal CFU-G or CFU-M proliferation requires the addition of G-CSF or M-CSF, respectively, to the cultures. Even in serum-replete conditions, IL-3 acts additively or synergistically with G-CSF to induce more granulocyte colony formation than is observed with either factor alone. The serum-free studies may have important implications for the use of combinations of colony-stimulating factors *in vivo*, and it is apparent that the use of such culture conditions may provide further insight into the *in vitro* activities of the different factors.

In addition to their effects on progenitor differentiation, the colony-stimulating factors also induce a variety of functional changes in mature cells. GM-CSF inhibits polymorphonuclear neutrophil migration under agarose, induces antibody-dependent cellular cytotoxicity (**ADCC**) for human target cells, and increases neutrophil phagocytic activity. Some of these functional changes may be related to GM-CSF-induced increase in the cell-surface expression of a family of antigens that function as cell adhesion molecules. The increase in antigen expression is rapid and is associated with increased aggregation of neutrophils; both are maximal at the migration inhibitory concentration of 500 pM, and granulocyte–granulocyte adhesion can be inhibited by an antigen-specific monoclonal antibody. GM-CSF also acts as a potent stimulus of eosinophil ADCC, superoxide production, and phagocytosis.

G-CSF acts as a potent stimulus of neutrophil superoxide production, ADCC, and phagocytosis, while M-CSF activates mature macrophages and enhances macrophage cytotoxicity.

Monocytes leave the circulation and differentiate further to become fixed tissue macrophages. These tissue macrophages include alveolar macrophages and hepatic Kupffer cells, dermal Langerhans cells, osteoclasts, peritoneal macrophages, pleural macrophages, and possibly brain microglial cells though the origin of these is still uncertain. Thus, the wide variety of cells with diverse functions that must be supplied from the granulocyte–macrophage progenitor requires that this system be highly regulated at many levels of differentiation.

The granulocyte compartment itself is more complex than either the erythroid or megakaryocyte compartments. The circulating half-life of the newly rapidly deployed granulocyte is only 6.5 h. In order to meet sudden demands, an additional non-circulating granulocyte pool exists in the spleen, marginated around blood vessels, and in a readily releasable bone-marrow pool. The rate at which new myeloblasts or monoblasts are produced by progenitors *in vivo* is not known, but exhaustion of progenitors in infection, particularly in the neonatal period, is associated with a fatal outcome due to a failure of granulocyte production.

SUPPRESSION OF PHAGOCYTE PRODUCTION

An elaborate system of suppression of granulocyte and macrophage production involving T lymphocytes and their products, particularly IFN-γ, monocytes, and perhaps acidic isoferritins can be demonstrated *in vitro*; in some circumstances, clones of T cells that suppress granulocyte production *in vitro* and *in vivo* have caused profound granulocytopenia. Clearly, a twin regulatory system exists that contributes to the fine control of phagocyte production by close control between progenitors and adventitial cells that secrete inducer and suppressor molecules. It is well established that T lymphocytes capable of the suppression of phagocyte colony formation may be present in human marrow and induce neutropenia.

MEGAKARYOCYTOPOIESIS

The regulation of megakaryocyte progenitors, their development into acetylcholinesterase-positive cells or megakaryoblasts, and their subsequent progressive maturation into platelet-shedding, multinucleated cells are all influenced by growth factors. The fundamental system is very similar to that observed in erythropoiesis, in that at least two and perhaps as many as five factors interact synergistically for optimal function. Furthermore, there is strong evidence of positive feedback control.

For several years, it has been well established that megakaryocyte progenitor-derived colonies are best produced in short-term cultures that contain the plasma of patients rendered thrombogenic by aplasia. The activity is usually described as **meg-CSA** (colony-stimulating activity) and the search is on to define the factor(s) that contribute to the activity. The plasma of patients with aplasia due to chemotherapy or marrow transplant conditioning also supports the long-term culture of CFU-meg. While normal human plasma contains very little if any meg-CSA, the activity begins to rise immediately after ablative conditioning for marrow transplant and peaks 3 weeks after the transplant procedure. By day 30 after transplant, the activity has declined to baseline levels. Furthermore, the level of activity correlates with engraftment. Those with higher plasma activity have slower rates of engraftment, presumably because of persistent thrombocytopenia. Thus, there is little doubt that growth factors (some of which circulate) must play an important part in the regulation of thrombopoiesis, and much effort has been directed toward their molecular identity.

Just as is true of erythrocyte colony formation, the conditioned medium derived from T cells can contribute important growth-factor support to megakaryocyte colony formation. It is well established that T cells are excellent sources of both GM-CSF and IL-3 (see above). Furthermore, recombinant murine GM-CSF both promotes megakaryocyte colony formation, enhances the proliferation of megakaryocyte progenitors, and increases the size of megakaryocytes isolated from developing megakaryocyte colonies. In this last respect, GM-CSF has the functional characteristics of the so-called thrombopoiesis-stimulating factor. Yet GM-CSF itself has no effect on circulating platelets when it is given to mice *in vivo*. In addition to GM-CSF, IL-3 has also been shown to support megakaryocyte colony formation and human serum contains at least one other factor with meg-CSA.

THROMBOPOIETIN

Thrombopoietin has been a proposed factor for more than 30 years. Its biology, semipurification, and characterization have recently been reviewed and an assay of its activities developed. Recently, IL-6 and IL-11, haemopoietic growth factors derived from stromal cells, have been shown to have platelet-stimulating effects *in vitro*. Thrombopoietin enhances megakaryocyte ploidy *in vitro*, and thrombopoietin is released by stimulated epidermal cells, suggesting a mechanism by which inflammation causes thrombocytosis. Despite all of this work, the nature of thrombopoietin has remained elusive. Whether IL-6 or IL-11 contribute to its function are currently unclear.

CLINICAL STUDIES WITH HAEMOPOIETIC GROWTH FACTORS

Several recombinant haemopoietic growth factors are currently under evaluation in a variety of clinical settings. Largely because of availability, initial studies focused on erythropoietin in the anaemia of chronic renal failure, and GM-CSF and G-CSF in both transient and long-standing, bone marrow-failure syndromes; these three factors are now commercially available for clinical use. More recently, other haemopoietic growth factors such as M-CSF, IL-3, and SF are coming under scrutiny. Anaemia is a major complication of end-stage renal failure, and is due primarily to a reduction in erythropoietin production. Several phase I, II, and III studies have documented that recombinant human erythropoietin can induce a dose-dependent increase in effective erythropoiesis. The extension of this treatment to patients who do not yet require dialysis has met with similar success. Erythropoietin may also be useful in anaemia of chronic disease and in the anaemia that complicates azidothymidine treatment of patients with acquired immune deficiency disease (**AIDS**). G-CSF has proven to be useful for shortening the period of neutropenia following myelosuppressive anticancer chemotherapy, and has been approved in the United States and Europe for reduction of infection in patients with non-myeloid malignancies. GM-CSF and G-CSF can accelerate haemopoietic reconstitution after bone marrow transplantation, and GM-CSF has been approved for use in the United States in autologous transplantation. In the context of bone marrow failure, GM-CSF is a useful palliative treatment as it can increase the neutrophil count, particularly in the majority of children with acquired aplastic anaemia. GM-CSF can also increase the neutrophils, eosinophils, and monocytes in AIDS. Most patients with Kostmann's syndrome, a rare inherited severe failure of neutrophil production, respond dramatically to G-CSF treatment, and patients with other defects of neutrophil production such as cyclic neutropenia and chronic idiopathic neutropenia have also responded to this factor.

SUMMARY

Haemopoiesis is the process of terminal differentiation of recognizable immature precursors of the formed elements of the blood. Renewal of the precursor pool is accompanied by the differentiation of committed progenitor cells that are themselves renewed by a process of stochastic maturation of stem cells. A group of haematopoietins derived from T cells, monocytes, and fibroblasts governs the differentiation of committed progenitor cells by mechanisms yet to be defined.

The *mélange* of marrow cells described above exists in delicate fronds thrust into the venous sinuses. Cells are packed in close proximity within the fronds, held together by extensions of fibroblast cytoplasm and fibronectin. Such a delicate anatomy is subject to a myriad of abnormalities that can disturb the orderly progress of cell–cell interactions that govern the system. The multiple symptoms of bone marrow failure are the results of these disturbances.

REFERENCES

Cosman, D. *et al.* (1990). A new cytokine receptor superfamily. *Trends in Biochemical Science*, **15**, 265–70.
Hoffman, R. (1989). Regulation of megakaryocytopoiesis. *Blood*, **74**, 1196–212.
Lieschke, G.J. and Burgess, A.W. (1992). Granulocyte colony-stimulating factor and granulocyte-macrophage colony-stimulating factor. *New England Journal of Medicine*, **327**, 28–35; 99–106.
McDonald, T.P. (1989). The regulation of megakaryoctye and platelet production. *International Journal of Cell Cloning*, **7**, 139–55.
Metcalf, D. (1984). *The hemopoietic growth factors*. Elsevier, Amsterdam.
Metcalf, D. and Moore, M.A.S. (1971). Haematopoietic cells. In *Frontiers of biology*, (ed. A. Neuberger and E.L. Tatum). North-Holland, Amsterdam.
Miyajima, A., Kitamura, T., Harada, N., Yokota, T., and Arai, K-i. (1992). Cytokine receptors and signal transduction. *Annual Review of Immunology*, **10**, 295–331.
Moore, M.A.S., Muench, M.O., Warren, D.J., and Laver. J. (1990). Cytokine networks involved in the regulation of haemopoietic stem cell proliferation and differentiation. In *Molecular control of haemopoiesis*, CIBA Foundation Symposium 148, pp. 43–61. Wiley, Chichester.
Murphy, M.J. (1989). Megakaryocyte colony-stimulating factor and thrombopoiesis. *Hematologic/Oncologic Clinics of North America*, **3**, 465–78.

Nicola, N.A. (1989). Hemopoietic cell growth factors and their receptors. *Annual Review of Biochemistry*, **58**, 45–77.

Quesenberry, P. (1979). Hematopoietic stem cells. *New England Journal of Medicine*, **301**, 755–61.

Sieff, C.A. and Nathan, D.G. (1992). The anatomy and physiology of hematopoiesis. In *Hematology of infancy and childhood*, (4th edn) (ed. D.G. Nathan and F.A. Oski). Saunders, Philadelphia.

22.2.2 Stem-cell disorders

D. C. LINCH

Concept of stem-cell disorders

The notion of haemopoietic stem-cell disorders at first appears straightforward. There could be a quantitative or qualitative deficiency of stem cells with failure to proliferate and produce mature progeny, abnormal stem cells could produce normal numbers of abnormal end cells, or the stem cells could undergo malignant transformation. These possibilities are not mutually exclusive and transitional forms can be envisaged.

In practice, there are several reasons why classifying disease entities as stem-cell disorders (or not) is often extremely difficult. Although it is usually accepted that a stem cell has the ability to undergo self-renewal and exhibit multipotentiality, there is no clear-cut definition of a stem cell. Self-renewal cannot be considered in the context of malignant disorders, as any malignant clone, arising at any stage of differentiation, must have undergone immortalization and be capable of self-renewal. The term stem-cell disorder is thus used to imply that the target cell for the disease process has occurred in a cell with the potential to develop into cells of different lineages. Such a cell could be a relatively 'late' or lineage-restricted stem cell capable, for example, of giving rise to phagocytes and erythrocytes, or it could be a very primitive stem cell capable of giving rise to all myeloid and lymphoid lineages. A major difficulty arises, however, in that malignant change in a very primitive cell does not necessarily lead to the production of mature cells of multiple lineages. It is a feature of the acute leukaemias that there is a block in differentiation, and in some cases of acute myeloid leukaemia, no mature progeny is produced by the malignant clone. In other cases of acute myeloid leukaemia, neutrophils alone are produced, but it cannot be assumed that the target cell of the original oncogenic event was not a cell with potential to form all the myeloid elements including the red-cell series.

The concept of the stem-cell disorders is thus important, as it focuses attention on the early pathogenic events in the disease process and provides understanding of the natural history of these disorders, but it is of limited value in the practical classification of disease in individual patients.

DETECTION OF MULTILINEAGE INVOLVEMENT

In the bone-marrow hypoplastic states, stem-cell involvement is obvious because of the pancytopenia that occurs. In the myeloproliferative disorders, examination of the blood count and blood film also reveals involvement of multiple lineages; neutrophil leucocytosis may coexist with eosinophilia, basophilia, and thrombocytosis. A number of more sophisticated techniques have also been used to demonstrate that a particular cell lineage is involved in a clonal process (Table 1).

Analysis of non-random cytogenetic abnormalities represents one of the most longstanding techniques for examining cell-lineage involvement in the haematological malignancies. This approach was used in acute myeloid leukaemia to show that the large majority of T cells in the peripheral blood were not part of the malignant clone. Combination with immunophenotyping for lineage-specific markers provides a pow-

Table 1 *Assessment of clonality in haematological disorders*

1. *Chromosome analysis by microscopy*
   Conventional cytogenetic analysis
   Dual cytogenetic analysis with surface immunophenotyping
   Fluorescent *in situ* hybridization (FISH) for specific chromosome translocations, and changes in chromosome number, e.g. trisomy 8
   Dual FISH and immunophenotyping
2. *Detection of somatic mutations by non-microscopic means*
   Detection of chromosome loss ⎫
   Detection of translocations.   ⎬ RFLP analysis and
   Detection of point mutations. ⎭ PCR methodology
   DNA fingerprinting
3. *Lymphocyte gene rearrangements**
   Expression of surface light chains on B cells
   Rearrangement of immunoglobulin heavy- and light-chain genes
   Rearrangement of T-cell receptor genes, β, γ, δ
4. *X-chromosome inactivation*
   Protein expression, e.g. isoforms of G6PD
   DNA expression:
     PGK
     HPRT
     M27B
     HUMARA
   mRNA expression, e.g. G6PD polymorphisms

*Detection of lymphocyte gene rearrangements is not usually applicable to the stem-cell disorders, but a small proportion of cases of acute myeloid leukaemia do have rearrangements of the immunoglobulin heavy chains or T-cell receptor genes.

RFLP, restriction fragment length polymorphism (all other abbreviations in text).

erful addition to this approach. Conventional cytogenetic studies suffer the disadvantage that only cells in metaphase can be analysed, but techniques such as fluorescent *in situ* hybridization (with or without immunophenotyping) allow cells in interphase to be examined and will become widely used.

Somatic mutations, from major chromosomal alterations to point mutations, can also be detected using non-microscopic methods employing recombinant DNA technology. Point mutations in the *ras* oncogene family (see Section 6) are frequent in many malignancies and have been most studied. Such studies in essential thrombocythaemia have suggested that the disease arises in a cell with full myeloid and lymphoid potential. Methods that use the polymerase chain reaction (PCR) are particularly sensitive and make it possible to study small cell samples, but it is difficult to make the techniques fully quantitative and errors in interpretation can readily arise from minor contaminating cells in supposedly purified cell populations. Analysis of somatic mutations is subject to a further potential problem if the mutation is a secondary event in the disease process. Under these circumstances the mutation observed could have arisen in a subclone and not be present in all the malignant cells. In acute myeloid leukaemia, mutations in N-*ras* may be present in all or just a few cells and sometimes a mutation detected at presentation cannot be found in relapse, indicative of the process of clonal evolution.

Use of polymorphic X-linked markers has been a very useful tool for examining clonality in informative females and is not subject to the problems of clonal evolution. The original studies used the enzyme glucose 6-phosphate dehydrogenase (**G6PD**). There are many structural variants of this enzyme, the most common normally active variant being designated as B type. In populations of African Negro descent a common normal variant exists which is designated as A type. Although this variant only differs by one amino acid it can be readily separated from the B type on starch gel electrophoresis. Because the gene that codes for

G6PD is on the X chromosome, individual cells of a heterozygous female (AB) express only one enzyme type, with approximately half the cells expressing type A and half type B (i.e. the individual is a mosaic). This restricted pattern of gene expression arises because of the process of random X-inactivation, known as lyonization, which occurs in early embryonic life and is passed on to the progeny of those cells in a stable manner (Fig. 1). Malignant disorders nearly always arise in a single cell, and thus all the malignant cells in a particular patient will have the same X chromosome inactivated. In an informative G6PD female all the tumour cells will express either type A or type B enzyme. Analysis of the G6PD levels in blood cells of different lineages will help to determine whether they are involved in a haematological malignancy. This technique is limited by the low frequency of informative polymorphisms in populations other than those of African descent.

Clonality can also be investigated using X-linked DNA polymorphisms that do not result in different protein products, as the active and inactive genes are differentially methylated at specific cytosine residues. DNA samples are first digested with an appropriate restriction endonuclease to distinguish maternal and paternal copies of the gene, and subsequently with a restriction endonuclease sensitive to cytosine methylation in its recognition sequence to distinguish active from inactive copies of the gene. Useful genes to study include the hypoxanthine phosphoribosyl transferase (**HPRT**) gene and the phosphoglycerate kinase (**PGK**) gene (Fig. 2). The X-linked multiple tandem repeat recognized by the probe M27B is the most frequently informative methylation-sensitive sequence defined to date (approximately 90 per cent of females), but as this is not a gene, it is not really correct to talk about active and inactive copies. None the less, it acts as a useful marker of the inactivated X-chromosome, and results with this probe are concor-

dant with those obtained with HPRT or PGK. PCR-based assays have also been developed to examine the methylation status of the PGK gene, the 5' end of the monoamine oxidase A gene and the human androgen receptor gene (HUMARA), which require far fewer cells than for techniques based on Southern blotting. Recently, a sensitive technique for demonstrating X-inactivation patterns has been developed based on a common polymorphism (single-base change) in the G6PD gene. As only the active form of the gene can be expressed, determination of which copy of DNA is active can be done by the analysis of mRNA. This involves reverse transcription of the mRNA, with either PCR of the cDNA and hybridization with allele-specific probes, or use of the ligase detection reaction with specific primers, to distinguish between the two alleles.

Clonality studies based on X-chromosome inactivation patterns have two main drawbacks. Firstly, it must be appreciated that lyonization occurs early in embryogenesis when there are few stem cells destined to give rise to the different tissues. As a consequence of this and the random nature of X-inactivation, considerable skewing away from the expected 50:50 expression of maternal and paternal alleles occurs in some individuals. In approximately one-quarter of females more than 75 per cent of the expressed genes derive from the same allele, and it is therefore essential that X-chromosome inactivation patterns are interpreted with reference to normal tissue. This has frequently not been done and many of the reports in the literature are thus suspect. Furthermore, in the case of the haematological malignancies it is not always easy to obtain appropriate control samples. Non-haemopoietic tissues can be misleading controls, as X-inactivation patterns can vary between tissues. T cells are probably a good control in most myeloid malignancies as they derive from the same stem-cell pool as the myeloid cells and it is

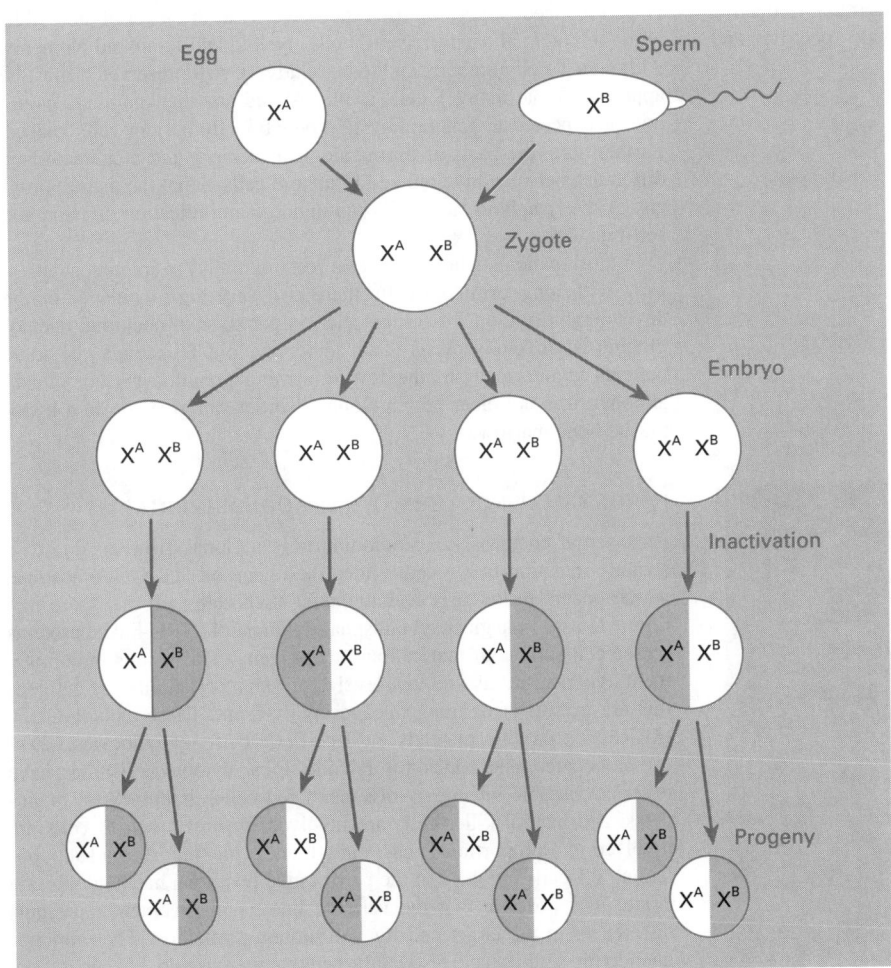

Fig. 1 X-chromosome inactivation.

unlikely that the majority of T lymphocytes will be involved in the malignant clone. This cannot, however, be assumed in all cases. The second problem with the study of X-inactivation patterns is that the technique cannot be used to detect a minor clone within a given population such as the T-cells where it is highly likely that the majority of cells will be long-lived normal polyclonal cells.

MYELOPROLIFERATIVE DISORDERS

The term myeloproliferative disorders was invented by Damshek and others in the 1950s in an attempt to explain the variability of the haematological findings in polycythaemia rubra vera, chronic myeloid leukaemia and myelofibrosis, and the existence of intermediate and transitional forms. The myeloproliferative disorders are characterized by the predominant cell type produced by the malignant clone, but they all arise from a primitive stem cell. (Fig. 3). Acute myeloid leukaemia should be considered as a myeloproliferative disorder and diseases such as chronic myeloid leukaemia and polycythaemia rubra vera not infrequently terminate in 'blastic transformation'. By convention, however, the term myeloproliferative disorders is usually reserved for the chronic malignancies where mature myeloid cells predominate.

Lineage involvement was first studied in chronic myeloid leukaemia because of the presence of the characteristic Philadelphia (Ph[1]) chromosome [t(9:22)(q34:q11)]. Not only were all cells of the phagocytic and red-cell series found to be involved, but Epstein–Barr virus-transformed B lymphocytes were also shown to contain the Ph[1] chromosome, thus indicating that the target cell for malignant transformation was a primitive stem cell with both myeloid and lymphoid potential. This is confirmed by the fact that about one-third of blastic transformations are due to the accumulation of primitive B cells. A similarly primitive stem cell is thought to be the cell of origin polycythaemia rubra vera, and essential thrombocythaemia. Damshek had considered that idiopathic myelofibrosis was part of the myeloproliferative disease spectrum, and

Fig. 2 Clonal analysis of PGK heterozygotes.

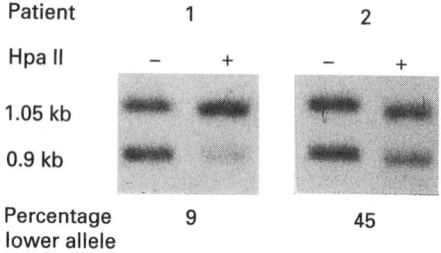

Fig. 3 The myeloproliferative disorders.

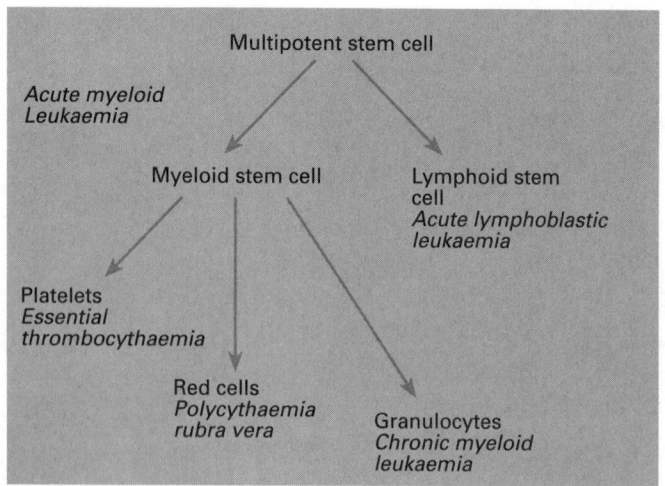

indeed this is the case. The fibroblasts are not part of the malignant clone, however, but are a reaction to an underlying myeloid malignancy. Fibrosis is particularly common when cells of the megakaryocytic series predominate, and may be due to the excessive local production of platelet-derived growth factors.

ACUTE LEUKAEMIAS

In children with acute myeloid leukaemia the red cells and platelets do not appear to be part of the malignant clone, whereas in adults, such trilineage involvement is frequent. There is no convincing evidence of lymphoid involvement. Considerable attention has been focused on the notion that remission in acute myeloid leukaemia frequently represents persistence of the malignant clone with full differentiation to give a normal blood count. This view was based on studies that did not pay adequate attention to the skewing of X-inactivation patterns that can occur in normal individuals, and true 'clonal remission' is rare.

Myelodysplasia, which frequently precedes acute myeloid leukaemia, often involves all myeloid lineages as is evident from examination of the blood and bone marrow films. There is considerable controversy within the literature, but the majority of studies do not demonstrate involvement of the lymphoid series.

Acute lymphoid leukaemia is usually restricted to the B-cell or T-cell lineage. An exception occurs in cases of Ph[1]-positive acute lymphoid leukaemia, where the myeloid lineages are often involved. This entity is akin to chronic myeloid leukaemic presenting in lymphoid blast crisis.

APLASTIC ANAEMIA

Aplastic anaemia by definition refers to involvement of multiple myeloid lineages (pancytopenia). In severe cases the lymphocyte count is also reduced, suggesting that the defect is at the level of stem cells with the potential to give rise to both myeloid and lymphoid elements. Although T-cell numbers tend to be relatively well preserved it must be appreciated that many T cells are long-lived and their numbers would not be expected to fall rapidly if production from stem cells ceased. Furthermore, the basis of immunological memory and a characteristic difference between myeloid and lymphoid cells is that the mature progeny of the lymphoid stem cells can undergo amplification division and self-renewal.

In those patients who respond (at least partially) to immunosuppression, with long-term follow-up there is a very high incidence of the development of clonal disorders such as paroxysmal nocturnal haemoglobinuria, myelodysplasia, and acute myeloid leukaemia. In some patients at presentation, the few remaining granulocytes are clonal, although it is not clear how a clonal disorder can give rise to a hypoplastic bone marrow.

PAROXYSMAL NOCTURNAL HAEMOGLOBINURIA

Paroxysmal nocturnal haemoglobinuria is a clonal disorder, due to a somatic mutation in a recently identified gene on the X chromosome, which occurs in an early haemopoietic stem cell such that there is a failure to assemble glucosyl phosphatidyl inositol (**GPI**)-linked proteins on the cell surface of that cell and its progeny. This results in complement hypersensitivity and low-level expression of a number of antigens that are useful for defining lineage involvement. These include CD59 (MIRL) for red cells, platelets and T cells, CD67 for granulocytes, CD14 for monocytes, and CD24 for B cells. Flow cytometric studies have revealed variable lineage involvement: red cells, granulocytes, monocytes, and natural killer cells are involved in most cases; B cells are involved in a proportion of cases and there is one report of a subpopulation of T cells involved in the paroxysmal nocturnal haemoglobinuria clone. It is possible that the variable lineage involvement represents differences in the target cell for the initiating mutation. The immunophenotypic studies have also confirmed that there is variable persistence of normal haemopoiesis, and some patients have more than one paroxysmal nocturnal haemoglobinuria clone with different levels of expression of GPI-linked molecules. One of the major unresolved questions in paroxysmal nocturnal haemoglobinuria is how does the clone, which is not usually considered to be a malignancy, acquire a growth advantage over the normal haemopoietic tissue.

REFERENCES

Abrahamson, G. *et al.* (1991). Clonality of cell populations in refractory anaemia using combined approach of gene loss and X-linked restriction fragment length polymorphism-methylation analyses. *British Journal of Haematology*, **79**, 550–5.

Allen, R.C., Zoghbi, H.Y. Moseley, A.B., Rosenblatt, H.M., and Belmont, J.W. (1992). Methylation of HpaII and HhaI sites near the polymorphic CAG repeat in the androgen receptor gene correlates with X-chromosome inactivation. *American Journal of Human Genetics*, **51**, 1229–39.

Beutler, E., Collins, Z., and Irwin, L.E. (1967). Value of genetic variants of glucose-6-phosphate dehydrogenase in tracing the origin of malignant tumours. *New England Journal of Medicine*, **276**, 389–91.

Boyd, Y. and Fraser, N.J. (1990). Methylation patterns at the hypervariable X-chromosome locus DXS255 (M27B): correlation with X-inactivation status. *Genomics*, **7**, 182–7.

Damashek, W. (1951). Some speculations on the myeloproliferative syndromes. *Blood*, **6**, 392–5.

Fialkow, P.J. (1972). Use of genetic markers to study cellular origin of development of tumours in human females. *Advances in Cancer Research*, **15**, 191–226.

Fialkow, P.J., Jacobson, R.J., and Papayanopoulou, T. (1977). Chronic myeloid leukaemia: clonal origin in a stem cell common to the granulocytic, erythrocyte, platelet and monocyte/macrophage. *American Journal of Medicine*, **63**, 125–31.

Fialkow, P.J. *et al.* (1987). Clonal development, stem cell differentiation and clinical remissions in acute non-lymphocytic leukaemia. *New England Journal of Medicine*, **317**, 468–73.

Gale, R.E. and Wainscoat, J.S. (1993) Clonal analysis using X-linked DNA polymorphisms. *British Journal of Haematology*, **85**, 2–8.

Gale, R.E., Wheadon, H., Goldstone, A.H., Burnett, A.K., and Linch, D.C. (1993). Frequency of clonal remission in acute myeloid leukaemia. *Lancet*, **341**, 138–42.

Kurzrock, R., Gutterman, J.U., and Talpaz, M. (1988). The molecular genetics of Philadelphia chromosome-positive leukaemias. *New England Journal of Medicine*, **319**, 990–8.

Lyon, M.F. (1961). Gene action in the X-chromosome of the mouse (*Mus musculus* L.). *Nature*, **190**, 372–3.

Nissen, C. *et al.* (1986). Acquired aplastic anaemia: a PNH-like disease? *British Journal of Haematology*, **64**, 355–62.

Rowley, J.D. (1973). A new consistent chromosomal abnormality in chronic myeloid leukaemia identified by quinacrine fluorescence and Giemsa staining. *Nature*, **243**, 290–3.

Rotoli, B., Bessler, M., Alfinito, F., and del Vecchio, L. (1993). Membrane proteins in paroxysmal nocturnal haemoglobinuria. *Blood Reviews*.

Turhan, A.G. *et al.* (1988). Molecular analysis of clonality and bcr rearrangements in Philadelphia chromosome positive acute lymphoblastic leukaemia. *Blood*, **71**, 1495–500.

van Kamp, H., Landegent, J.E., Jansen, R.P.M., Willemze, R., and Fibbe, W.E. (1991). Clonal haematopoiesis in patients with acquired aplastic anaemia. *Blood*, **78**, 3209–14.

Vogelstein, B. *et al.* (1987). Clonal analysis using recombinant DNA probes from the X-chromosome. *Cancer Research*, **47**, 4806–13.

22.3 The leukaemias and other disorders of haemopoietic stem cells

22.3.1 Cell and molecular biology of leukaemia

M. F. GREAVES

Our understanding of the biology of leukaemia has increased dramatically over the past 10 years, due in large measure to technological advances in molecular genetics. The picture that has emerged is remarkably rich in cellular and molecular detail but, more importantly, both novel insights and essential principles have been identified. These advances are now influencing patient management and offer considerable hope for the future in terms of highly selective or 'molecular' therapy. In these respects the biology of leukaemia provides an example for other cancers.

Leukaemia as a clonal disorder of haemopoiesis

At diagnosis, the acute and chronic leukaemias as well as the myelodysplastic or preleukaemic conditions are characterized by the presence of dominant, monoclonal cell populations. The evidence for this conclusion comes from the use of molecular markers (Table 1) and indicates that at some early stage in leukaemogenesis, a single cell with self-renewal or stem-cell properties has acquired a sustained net reproductive advantage over its neighbours. A Darwinian or evolutionary analogy is a useful way to think about this situation, which is similar to the origin, diversification, and selection of new species. A 'new' clone of leukaemic cells (or species) arises as a result of a mutation that endows the cell, via one of several possible routes, with an inheritable proliferative advantage (Fig. 1). The resultant clonal progeny will include both cells with self-renewing properties and others (the majority) that will differentiate and/or die. The former, as clonogenic cells, are subjected to continual selective pressure and, as a consequence, new mutant subclones will arise continuously and compete for dominance. Selective pressures will include both competition for space and response to positive or negative growth regulation and also the therapeutic intervention of physicians. The former is rather like the continual diversification of germ cells and selection of offspring in the evolution of sexually reproducing, eukaryotic organisms; the latter more akin to the development of antibiotic-resistant strains of bacteria. Either way, a dynamic, continuous process of mutation, diversification, and selection of clones lies at the heart of leukaemia and other cancers, and distinguishes these diseases from most others, including those with a genetic origin, the haemoglobinopathies and cystic fibrosis for example. Additionally, and crucially, the 'Darwinian' feature of continuous clonal diversification in leukaemia contributes very significantly to the often intractable nature of the disease clinically and the difficulty of complete eradication or cure.

Table 1 *Genetic markers of clonality in leukaemia*

1. X-linked glucose-6-phosphate dehydrogenase (G6PD) isoenzymes A/B
2. X-linked RFLPs (+ methylation status assay for transcribed allele)[1]
3. Unique or complex chromosome markers (e.g. translocations)
4. Oncogene rearrangements[2]
5. Immune recognition genes and their products:[3]

| Immunoglobulin | Ig_H, $I\kappa$, $Ig\lambda$ | Unique DNA rearrangements: κ or λ produced / Unique idiotypes |
| T-cell receptor (TCR) | γ, β, α | Unique DNA rearrangement / Unique idiotypes |

[1]RFPL: restriction fragment length polymorphism, e.g. in X-linked hypoxanthine phosphoribosyl transferase (HPRT), or phosphoglycerate kinase gene. This method has the advantage (cf. G6PD) that heterozygosity of HPRT (and other polymorphic genes) on the X chromosome is common.

[2]If rearrangements are in gene introns, then the precise position of the break will vary and provide a clone-specific marker (e.g. as restriction fragment size in Southern blot). See Ford *et al.* (1993). *Nature*, **363**, 358–60 for an example of the application of these different methods (used to demonstrate the common monoclonal origin of concordant acute lymphoblastic leukaemia in identical twin infants).

[3]Analysis of *Ig* or *TCR* gene rearrangements provides a unique identity tag for lymphoid clones and, in contrast to X-linked markers, can detect very small clonal populations. A limitation of using Ig_H and *TCR* gene rearrangements or idiotypes as clonal markers is that they are not entirely stable. For example, a single clone of leukaemic B-cell precursors may continue to rearrange its Ig_H gene segments (VDJ) resulting in an oligoclonal pattern.

Molecular diversity of leukaemia

Leukaemias, in common with most other cancers, are monoclonal because the mutations that drive the disease are sufficiently rare that only one cell is likely to incur an 'appropriate' hit. However, if we consider the enormous numbers of red and white cells produced per day and for most of our lifespan, the monoclonal nature of leukaemia and its relatively low incidence rate in the population are puzzling. This must, in part at least, be a testament to remarkably high-fidelity DNA copying with efficacious editing or repair of mistakes and damage. Other considerations and restraints also come into play. When mutations do arise in blood stem cells, as they will in all of us all the time, then of the 10^5 or so genes available in the genome, only a small fraction will be relevant to blood-cell production and only a minority of mutations in those genes will result in an altered function. Also, loss of function will usually be recessive and of no consequence unless and until the corresponding allele is also mutated.

These restrictions may still leave a rather large number of genes 'at risk' for leukaemogenesis and one of the striking discoveries of recent years has indeed been the remarkable diversity of genetic changes observed. It is difficult to gauge the total number of different mutations that can contribute to the development of leukaemia, either as initiating mutations or contributing to the progression of the disease, but somewhere between 200 and 500 may not be far off the mark. This extraordinary molecular diversity can be accommodated by considering both the cellular function of the genes involved and the diverse nature of the blood-cell types involved.

What matters for leukaemia (or new species!) development is net

reproductive advantage in the microenvironment of the bone marrow (or occasionally in thymus, lymph nodes or spleen). The number of cells at any given time is reflected in a 'balance sheet' of production and loss in which rates of proliferation, differentiation, and death are key variables (Fig. 2). Correspondingly, most oncogenes and other mutant genes contributing to the development of leukaemia can be expected to either promote proliferation or retard differentiation or death. In addition to these three 'sets' of genes, there can be an important contribution from genes influencing mutation frequency. These could, for example, be genes whose protein products (mostly enzymes) are involved directly in the recognition and repair of DNA damage, or alternatively a gene, such as *p53*, which is activated in response to some forms of DNA damage (ionizing radiation, some drugs) and brings about cell-cycle arrest in G_1 to provide the cell with time to repair DNA before replication. *p53* may be one of a number of genes whose functional absence through mutation or deletion in cancer and leukaemia may result in a mutation-prone phenotype, contributing very significantly to the risk or rate of accumulation of further mutations (see also Section 6).

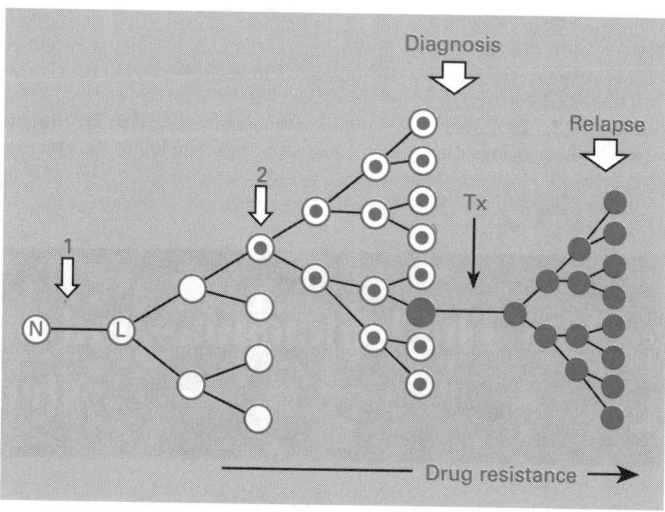

Fig. 1 Clonal evolution in leukaemia (1, 2, successive mutations; Tx, treatment; N, normal; L, leukaemic cell).

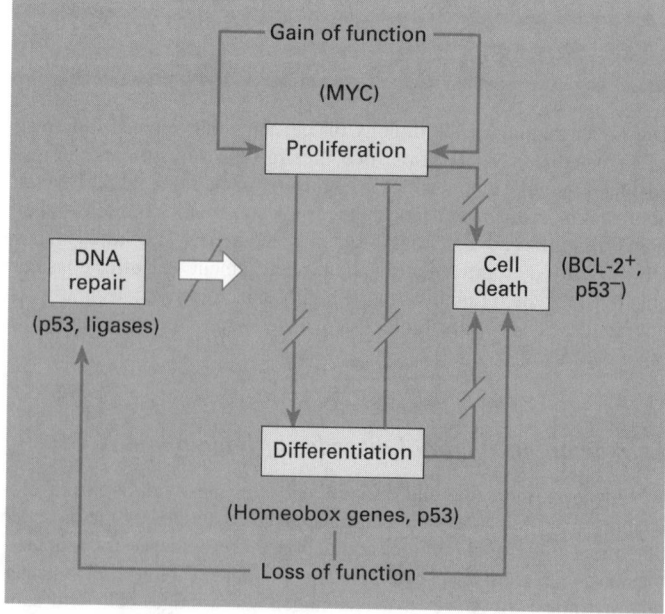

Fig. 2 Functional gene sets involved in leukaemia.

Table 2 *Diversity of genetic changes in leukaemia*

Type	Examples
Chromosomal breaks and rejoining→ illegitimate recombination/gene fusion:	
Reciprocal translocation (t)	t(9;22)(q34;q11) in Ph $^+$ CML and ALL
	t(15;17)(q22;q11) in AML (M3)
Inversion (inv)	inv(14)(q11;q32) in ATL and T-CLL
	inv(16)(p13;q22) in AML (M4)
Interstitial insertion (ins)	ABL(9q34) → BCR(22q11) in some Ph$^-$ CML
Chromosomal loss:	
Monosomy	Monosomy 7 in MDS, AML
Hypodiploidy/near haploid[1]	In ALL
Chromosomal gain/duplication (dup)	
Triploidy	Trisomy 8 in AML
	Trisomy 12 in B-CLL
Hyperdiploidy	In ALL
Partial chromosomal loss/deletion (del)	9p $^-$ in ALL
	5q $^-$ in MDS
Partial chromosomal gain: isochromosomes (i)[2]	i17q in CML-BC
Gene deletion	p53 in some AL
Gene base change	N-*ras* in AML
	p53 in CML-BC
Gene amplification	Rare in leukaemias, but common in some types of solid tumour
Gene activation by 'insertional mutagenesis'[3]	Common in some virus-induced animal leukaemias

[1]Near haploidy may, paradoxically, be associated with duplication of some chromosomes.

[2]Isochromosomes may involve loss of one arm of a chromosome and duplication of the other.

[3]Viral elements (viruses themselves or intercisternal particles) may insert into 'upstream' regulatory regions of cellular genes and by doing so disrupt the genes' normal pattern of regulated expression. Well described in several animal virus-associated leukaemias; anticipated, but not as yet demonstrated, for human leukaemia.

The catalogue of common, or relatively common, chromosome changes (as well as rare changes) is probably very nearly complete. For more subtle changes at the level of loci or individual genes, there are probably many more still to be discovered.

Abbreviations: AL, acute leukaemia; ALL acute lymphoblastic leukaemia; AML, acute myeloid leukaemia; ATL, adult T-cell leukaemia; CML, chronic myeloid leukaemia; CLL, chronic lymphocytic leukaemia; MDS, myelodysplastic syndrome.

These then are the gene 'sets' of major importance in the development of leukaemia. Other genetic elements that may indirectly influence disease development or clinical response include the major histocompatibility complex (HLA) loci for leukaemias in which viral infection may play a part, e.g. human T-cell lymphotropic virus-1-associated adult T-cell leukaemia and, possibly, childhood acute leukaemia, and genes encoding proteins that regulate metabolism or cellular response pathways of drugs.

In practice, in any single patient it is likely that several mutations are present in the leukaemic clone at the time of diagnosis (Fig. 1). In some cases, there is direct evidence for this from the microscopic detection of chromosomal changes (karyotype) and molecular analysis for mutant genes. Experimental studies with viral oncogenes and with mutant genes transfected into cells *in vitro* confirm that genes whose normal products have complementary functions (i.e. in different sets; Fig. 2) can co-operate as mutants to exacerbate the uncoupling of the normally integrated processes of cell proliferation, differentiation, and death.

This complex interplay of molecular mutants within a clone of cells is segregated in an interesting way with the diversity of cell type involved in leukaemia. More of this in a moment, but first a brief outline of the nature of the mutations in leukaemia. For a mutation to be effective, there has to be, in essence, gain or loss of function; this can be achieved by alterations in the level of expression of a gene or the time frame of its expression or the specificity of its end function. In practice, these changes are brought about by multiple alterations ranging from gross chromosomal structure to single base changes in DNA (Table 2).

The most intensively studied molecular alterations in the leukaemias are the reciprocal chromosomal translocations (Table 2). These were the first non-random chromosome abnormalities to be discovered—in the form of the Philadelphia (Ph) chromosome in 1961. With the more recent identification by cloning and sequencing of the genes that lie at the breakpoints and that are functionally altered as a consequence, some very striking insights have emerged. First, although most reciprocal translocations result in the illegitimate fusion of two genes that are normally independently regulated on separate chromosomes, in structural and functional detail, there appear to be two types of mechanism. In the first, exemplified by the association of the *myc* oncogene with the immunoglobulin heavy-chain (Ig$_H$) locus (in Burkitt's lymphoma and other mature B-cell leukaemias and lymphomas), an essentially intact *myc* gene is present and a normal *myc* protein produced, but the gene is constitutively expressed (i.e. fixed in the 'on' mode) as a result of sitting next door to the regulatory genetic elements of the (Ig$_H$) gene that are themselves fixed 'on' in B cells. Compulsive cell cycling is the consequence. In the second type of illegitimate union, exemplified by the Ph chromosome, two genes or parts of two genes are fused 'in frame' for transcription as a single chimeric unit and so produce a fused or chimeric protein with novel properties—in this case greatly enhanced or stable enzyme activity of the ABL kinase domain of the BCR/ABL chimeric protein (constitutively phosphorylating key substrates involved in growth control).

A second remarkable feature of the translocations in lymphoid leukaemias is the crucial involvement of immunoglobulin (Ig$_H$) and T-cell receptor (**TCR**) genes in rearrangements such as that described above for the *myc* gene. The explanation for the predominance of these rearrangements has to do with the 'availability' of (Ig$_H$) and TCR genes as natural sites in lymphoid cells for both recombination and constitutive expression, and therefore their potential selective advantage or 'hot spots' as recombination sites for oncogenes.

Table 3 *Involvement of transcriptional regulators in leukaemogenesis*

Type of regulator	Deregulated product	Fused product[1]
HLH proteins	MYC t(8;14)(*q24*;q34) B-cell leukaemias Lyl-1 t(7;19)(*q35*;p13)/T-ALL TAL-1 t(*1*;14)(*p34*;q11) or del/T-ALL TAL-2 t(7;9)(q35;*q34*)/T-ALL	Pbx-1—**E2a** t(1;*19*)(q23;*p13*) (B-lineage ALL)
Homeodomain	Hox 11 t(*10*;14)(*q24*;q11)/T-ALL	**Pbx-1**—E2a t(*1*;19)(*q23*;p13)
Cys-rich/Zn fingers	Rhom-1 (LIM) t(11;14)(*p15*;q11)/T-ALL Rhom-2 (LIM) t(*11*;14)(*p13*;q11)/T-ALL	**PML—RARα** t(*15*;17)(*q21*;q11–22)/APML
Others		DEK—CAN/AML t(6;9)(p23;q34) HRX (MLL)—11q23 with multiple partner chromosomes/infant AL AML1—MTG8 t(8;21)(q22;q22)/AML

[1]Relevant type of regulator in bold type.

APML, acute promyelocytic leukaemia; HLH, helix–loop–helix; CYS, cysteine residues (indicative of disulphide bonding); Zn fingers, finger-like projections of protein stabilized by zinc ions. (all other abbreviations as in Table 2).

The third extraordinary feature of chromosome rearrangements in leukaemias, only recently uncovered, is the extent to which genes encoding DNA-binding transcription factors are involved (some current examples in Table 3). Perhaps, in retrospect, it is not at all surprising that genes that play a crucial part as regulators of those other genes whose products perform the executive function in proliferation and differentiation should themselves be effective targets for mutation in leukaemia.

One additional and remarkable feature of genes involved in leukaemia (and other cancers) has come to light. Many of the altered genes that have been discovered are ancestrally very ancient and have been conserved in sequence, structure, and function over millions of years of evolution. The homologues of *ras*, *myc*, and the transcription-factor genes (Table 3), for example, are to be found in yeast and Drosophila. In the latter case, mutations in these genes result in bizarre developmental abnormalities. The explanation for this kinship probably lies in the fact that, although biological processes are extraordinarily diverse, as evolutionary solutions they also tend to be parsimonious. Once effective biochemical solutions to the key cellular functions of cell cycling, intracellular signalling (of external stimuli), and transcriptional regulation were 'invented', the key molecular players involved acquired permanent 'team status'.

Left largely blank in this story of molecular mishaps is the crucial issue of how and when these mutations arise or are induced. Inherited genetic changes appear to play only a very minor part in leukaemia and the majority of mutations are acquired somatically. Placing these mutations in the context of epidemiology, the aetiology, and natural history of leukaemia still poses a considerable challenge. We urgently need to discover if the different leukaemias have preventable causes. Recent advances in cell and molecular biology may help us to address these issues more effectively.

Genes, cells, and leukaemia subtypes

Although some of the genes discussed above will be expressed and have similar or identical functions in all proliferating cell types, for example, genes encoding aspects of DNA regulation or repair (*myc*, *p53*), others will be more restricted in their expression, including those encoding cell type-specific functions (e.g. erythropoietin receptors) or encoding regulatory switches for such functions (e.g. DNA binding, transcription

factors; Table 3). One consequence of this pattern of selective gene expression is that some mutant genes have a widespread distribution in different types of leukaemia and cancer, whereas others are more restricted. This is most clearly reflected in the many different chromosomal translocations that occur in leukaemia; some examples of these remarkable molecular gymnastics are listed in Table 2. In several cases, the 'logic' behind the cellular specificity is easy to discern. The first of these translocations to be understood was the t(8;14)(q24;q32) involving the transposition of most or all of the c-*myc* gene into the immunoglobulin locus, resulting in dysregulated but qualitatively normal function of Myc protein. The specificity of this particular translocation to the B-cell lineage (and functionally equivalent translocations involving TCR in the T-cell lineage) is determined by the selective, differentiation-linked activity of the (*Ig*_H) gene. This example suggests, and others endorse the view, that particular genes may be involved, as functional mutants, in subsets of leukaemia either because they become illegitimately coupled with other cell type-specific genes (or regulatory elements of the latter) and/or because of the functional relevance of the resultant protein product on the behaviour of that particular cell type. The fusion of retinoic acid-receptor (α) gene with other genes (*PML*, *PLZF*) in acute promyelocytic leukaemia provides an example of the latter case. It is a reasonable assumption, therefore, that genes of unknown function that are involved in subset-specific chromosomal rearrangements probably exercise an important function in equivalent normal cells of the same or related cell type.

The consistency with which some gene rearrangements, particularly translocations, are observed in leukaemia lends credence to the view that they are critical components of the causal pathway and not epiphenomena. The best evidence to support this view comes from experiments in which the same genes in their abnormal or 'mutated' format initiate leukaemia when transfected into fertilized eggs to generate transgenic mice. Interestingly, in almost all such examples, additional, independent mutations in other endogenous (mouse) genes are required for clinical leukaemia to develop which is then monoclonal.

The alignment of genetic abnormalities with haematological diagnostic subtypes (Table 2) carries obvious implications for the precise developmental level or actual cell type in which the mutation arises. Herein lies an unavoidable and important complication. The cell type dominating the leukaemic blood or bone marrow smear is not necessarily that cell type in which the initiating or all subsequent mutations arise, or the cell type with the stem-cell properties that sustains the disease. This situation arises because of the variable extent to which leukaemic mutations, singly or in combination, block differentiation. An example to illustrate this point would be with the Bcr/Abl p210 fusion protein product of the Ph chromosome in chronic myeloid leukaemia (see Chapter 22.3.5). Here, in the chronic phase of disease, immature granulocytes dominate the picture but the abnormal *BCR/ABL p210* gene has a subtle physiological effect (perhaps in apoptosis) that only marginally impedes differentiation, and clonal analysis indicates that this mutation arises in multipotential, lymphomyeloid stem cells. All that can be inferred from a particular cellular phenotype in leukaemia is that it evolved clonally from an equivalent cell type or antecedent cell type in the same developmental pathway. Clonal analyses of different cell lineages using the mutations themselves as markers are the only way to determine with confidence the likely developmental level at which particular mutations have arisen. In this respect, there are still some uncertainties concerning the precise cellular and lineage origins of the various leukaemias; Figure 3 represents a simplified and current consensus. The precise cell type in which mutations arise and the functional impact of the mutations with respect to self-renewal and differentiation will determine the clonogenic phenotype; that is, the cellular characteristics of the usually small (a few per cent) proportion of cells in a leukaemic clone that sustains the disease, providing the cellular venue for subsequent mutations and clonal progression, and the relevant cellular target for effective therapy. The precise nature of this cell is therefore of some considerable clinical importance.

Clinical implications of leukaemia cell and molecular biology

The biology of leukaemia is fascinating in its own right and, in concert with the biology of other cancers at the cell and molecular level, has provided unique insights into fundamental aspects of the regulation of proliferation, differentiation, and cell-death pathways in normal haemopoiesis. It would, however, be an enormous disappointment if this new knowledge could not be translated into clinical benefit. Fortunately, it is very likely that it will, although we are still at the beginning of this applied aspect of research. It is beyond the scope of this introductory chapter on the biology of leukaemia to go into many of the details of these potential developments but some major themes that are already emerging merit mention.

Monoclonal antibody-defined immunophenotype, chromosome karyotype, and abnormal genotype identified with DNA probes have already provided a new level of disease subclassification and diagnostic precision, with potential advantages for differential diagnosis in cases that are occult, difficult or ambiguous. The actual benefit of such laboratory-based analyses will depend upon the clinical correlates of particular cellular features identified and such associations, in turn, are at least in part dependent upon the therapeutic framework within which such associations are sought. Leukaemia research is replete with anecdotal examples of such diagnostic insights relevant to treatment outcome. One unambiguous example of the 'new biology' providing an important diagnostic guide to treatment strategy is in acute lymphoblastic leukae-

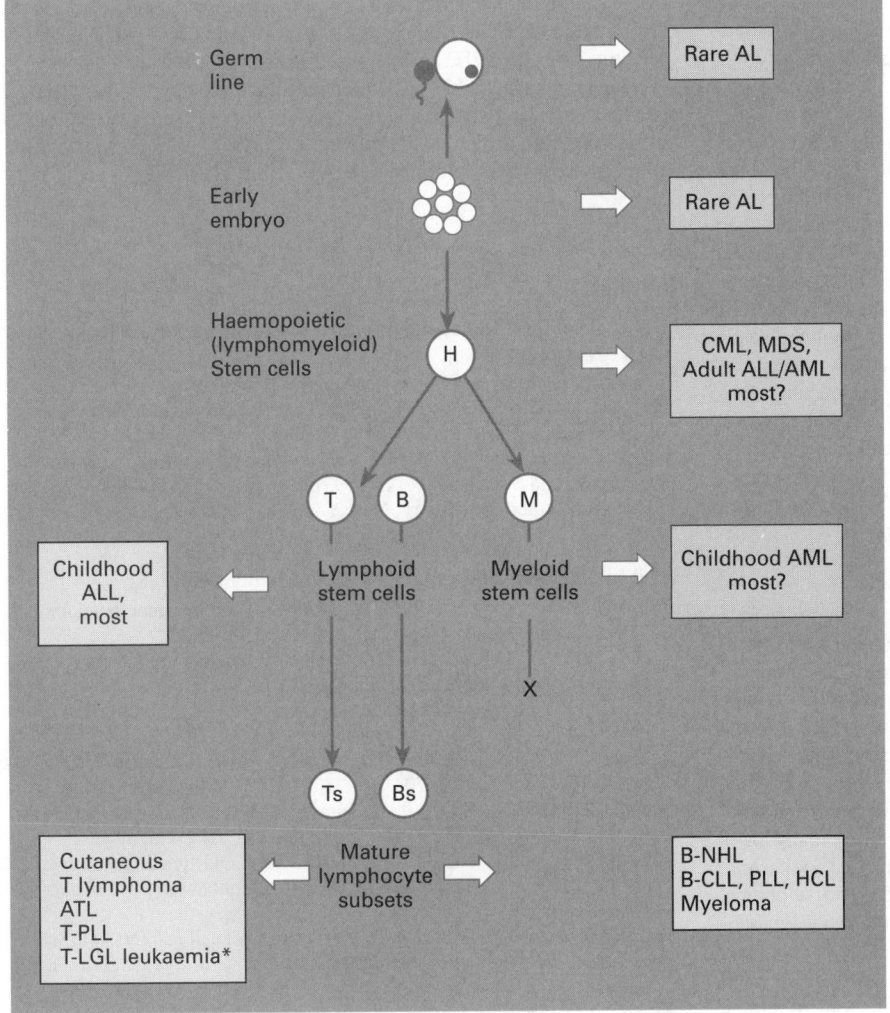

Fig. 3 Developmental and lineage origins of leukaemias and other haemopoietic malignancies. H, haemopoietic (stem cell); M, myeloid; Ts, Bs, subsets of mature T and B cells; x descendent progeny of myeloid stem cells are not relevant to leukaemogenesis, unlike mature lymphocytes, which are long-lived and have stem cell-like properties—one exception to this rule may, however, be APML (M3 AML), which involves promyelocytes with a specific gene rearrangement (see Tables 2 and 3).

mia, where the presence of a Ph chromosome, or the molecular event—the *BCR/ABL p210* or *p190* fusion gene—is a strong indicator of the likelihood that the leukaemia, whether in children or adults, is likely to be intractable to high-dose combination chemotherapy and radiation. In these circumstances, such patients, at diagnosis, are prime candidates for escalated therapy and stem-cell replacement via bone marrow transplantation.

Several of the new immunological and molecular diagnostic tools may find a unique and particularly informative application in the analysis of blood and marrow or tissue biopsies in patients in haematological remission but at risk of relapse. The sensitivity and specificity of the polymerase chain reaction (**PCR**) makes it a particularly suitable molecular method for detecting residual disease, accepting the need for very careful standardization and controls. This approach has already provided valuable new insights into the persistence of leukaemia or lymphoma clones in patients with chronic myeloid leukaemia and lymphoma post-transplantation and in those with acute lymphoblastic leukaemia. In all three situations, there is some correlation between presence or absence of PCR-based signal for residual disease and subsequent clinical course, suggesting that, in the future, PCR-based methods will contribute to the management of individual patients.

Chromosome karyotypes are too insensitive for disease monitoring but the rapidly evolving fluorescence *in situ* hybridization (FISH) technology, which combines chromosomal and molecular analysis at the single-cell level in non-dividing (interphase) cells, is a potentially powerful diagnostic indicator with broad applications in molecular medicine, including leukaemia. Multiple fluorescent tags used in combination and with appropriate detection devices (charged coupled device (CCD)) cameras allow all individual pairs of chromosomes to be simultaneously evaluated in interphase cells. With a judicious choice of reagents and sample preparation, it is also now possible to identify cell type and abnormal genotype in the same individual interphase cell (Plate 1).

The association between the presence of a molecular marker such as the *BCR/ABL* fusion gene in a leukaemic clone and clinical response begs the question of why this correlation exists, and of whether any other aspects of the cell and molecular biology of leukaemia can shed any light on the striking variation in clinical responses. To some extent, this smog of clinical heterogeneity was pierced some time ago with the demonstration that particular immunobiological subtypes of leukaemia, for example childhood common (B-cell precursor) acute lymphoblastic leukaemia, were more likely to be curable with available therapy. A more recent suggestion is that the clonogenic cell phenotype and genotype contribute critically to clinical response and outcome. For example, it is suggested that the remarkable success in treating childhood common acute lymphoblastic leukaemia owes much to the fact that, in most cases, the disease originates in a B-cell progenitor cell type that is programmed for apoptosis in the absence of an effective differentiation signal. Successful treatments, including ionizing radiation, steroids and methotrexate, somewhat fortuitously exploit this intrinsic feature of B-cell progenitors, the essential caveat being that leukaemogenic mutations (e.g. hyperdiploidy) do not subvert this cell-death pathway. Adult acute lymphoblastic leukaemia, even with a common B-cell precursor immunophenotype, is much less effectively treated. The reasons for this may be related to two observations. First, that the proportion of those with adult acute lymphoblastic leukaemia who carry the Ph chromosome abnormality increases substantially with age (to over 50 per cent), whilst the proportion with the more favourable chromosomal correlate—hyperdiploidy—decreases; and second, that the Ph chromosome in many cases of acute lymphoblastic leukaemia, as in chronic myeloid leukaemia, arises in a multipotential, lymphomyeloid stem cell. The lack of clinical response of poorly sustained remission in Ph-positive, acute lymphoblastic leukaemia may therefore be due: (a) to its origin in relatively drug-resistant, multipotential stem cells (in common with most adult acute leukaemias and myelodysplastic conditions; Fig. 3) in which the apoptotic response pathway is less accessible; and/or (b) to the expres-

sion of a mutated gene, such as *BCR/ABL*, whose function promotes cell proliferation and/or blocks apoptosis. This potential 'double burden' will lead to the rapid acquisition of clonal diversity via secondary alterations in DNA—as evidenced by karotypic studies on patients with Ph-positive, acute lymphoblastic leukaemia and experimental studies of transgenic mice developing acute lymphoblastic leukaemia driven by a human *BCR/ABL* transgene.

These ideas are at present speculative but they are in accord with current data and carry the implication that acute leukaemias of lymphomyeloid stem-cell origin and/or that have particular mutations such as *BCR/ABL* gene fusion (and perhaps others including *HRX*; Table 3) are unlikely to benefit from simple dose escalation alone and that more novel approaches, including stem-cell rescue or molecular therapy, are likely to be required.

This leads inexorably to the question of whether mutated genes or their products can themselves provide target molecules for therapeutic intervention. Much hope and even more venture capital has already been staked on a positive outcome to this question. It is a topic whose time may have come and is ripe for exploitation, but excitement over the real potential of this approach should be tempered with a realistic appraisal of some of the difficulties involved. For some strategies, there is already encouraging progress—anti-sense inhibition of mRNA, kinase inhibitors, 'toxic' monoclonal antibodies for example; others appear at present too far-fetched—*in vivo* replacement of defective genes (see also Section 4) for example. In principle, the presence of a mutant gene such as *BCR/ABL* provides a unique sequence and structure (at the DNA, mRNA, and protein level) that, for the first time, represents a leukaemia-specific target for therapy. It ought to be possible to design a therapeutic strategy that, in targeting such molecules, eliminates all clonogenic cells with the mutation whilst leaving normal stem cells untouched—that is, highly selective, non-toxic therapy. Leukaemias may be the ideal cancer type to pioneer this type of biology-based molecular therapy but the technical challenges in drug design and delivery are considerable. Attempting to overcome these difficulties is moving to the top of the agenda for the coming years, which promise to be every bit as exciting as the last 10 or so.

REFERENCES

General cell and molecular biology of cancer including leukaemia

Franks, L.M. and Teich, N.M. (1991). *Introduction to the cellular and molecular biology of cancer*, (2nd edn). Oxford University Press.

Furth, M. and Greaves, M. (1989). *Cancer cells 7. Molecular diagnostics of human cancer*. Cold Spring Harbor Laboratory Press.

Heim, S. and Mitelman, F (1987). *Cancer cytogenetics*. Liss, New York.

Varmus, H. and Weinberg, R.A. (1993). *Genes and the biology of cancer*. Scientific American Library, New York.

Cell biology and molecular genetics of leukaemia:

Adams, J.M. and Cory, S. (1991). Transgenic models of tumor development. *Science*, **254**, 1161–7.

Cleary, M.L. (1991). Oncogenic conversion of transcription factors by chromosomal translocations. *Cell*, **66**, 619–22.

Graf, T. (1988). Leukemia as a multistep process: studies with avian retroviruses containing two oncogenes. *Leukemia*, **2**, 127–31.

Greaves, M.F. (1986). Differentiation-linked leukemogenesis in lymphocytes. *Science*, **234**, 697–704.

Nichols, J. and Nimer, S.D. (1992). Transcription factors, translocations, and leukemia. *Blood*, **80**, 2953–63.

Rabbitts, T.H. and Boehm, T. (1991). Structural and functional chimerism results from chromosomal translocation in lymphoid tumors. *Advances in Immunology*, **50**, 119–46.

Raskind, W.H. and Fialkow, P.J. (1987). The use of cell markers in the study of human hematopoietic neoplasia. *Advances in Cancer Research*, **49**, 127–42.

Rowley, J.D. (1990). Recurring chromosome abnormalities in leukemia and lymphoma. *Seminars in Hematology*, **27**, 122–36.

Clinical applications of leukaemia biology

Greaves, M.F. (1993). Stem cell origins of leukaemia and curability. *British Journal of Cancer*, **67**, 413–23.

Potter, M.N. *et al.* (1993). Molecular evidence of minimal residual disease after treatment for leukaemia and lymphoma: an updated meeting report and review. *Leukemia*, **7**, 1302–14.

Price, C.M., Kanfer, E.J., Colman, S.M., Westwood, N., Barrett, A.J., and Greaves, M.F. (1992). Simultaneous genotypic and immunophenotypic analysis of interphase cells using dual-color fluorescence: a demonstration of lineage involvement in polycythemia vera. *Blood*, **80**, 1033–8.

Pui, C.-H., Behm, F.G., and Crist, W.M. (1993). Clinical and biologic relevance of immunologic marker studies in childhood acute lymphoblastic leukaemia. *Blood*, **82**, 343–62.

Pui, C.-H., Crist, W.M., and Look, A.T. (1990). Biology and clinical significance of cytogenetic abnormalities in childhood acute lymphoblastic leukemia. *Blood*, **76**, 1449–63.

Secker-Walker, L.M., Craig, J.M., Hawkins, J.M., and Hoffbrand, A.V. (1991). Philadelphia positive acute lymphoblastic leukemia in adults: age distribution, BCR breakpoint and prognostic significance. *Leukemia*, **5**, 196–9.

van Dongen, J.J.M., Breit, T.M., Adriaansen, H.J., Beishuizen, A., and Hooijkaas, H. (1992). Detection of minimal residual disease in acute leukemia by immunological marker analysis and polymerase chain reaction. *Leukemia*, **6**, 47–59.

22.3.2 The classification of leukaemia

D. CATOVSKY

INTRODUCTION

The classification of leukaemia has evolved over the years from a purely morphological approach, based on the appearances of the leukaemic cells in peripheral blood and bone marrow films, through cytochemical techniques and, lately, to a greater reliance on monoclonal antibodies against cellular antigens. The next decade will see a major input from cytogenetic and molecular methods. The object of any classification is to define disease entities with distinct biological and clinical features. The new methodologies are introducing greater precision and objectivity to the diagnostic criteria.

A broad classification includes two large groups historically designated acute and chronic (Table 1). Acute leukaemias are malignancies with little evidence of differentiation; the characteristic cells are immature blasts. It is in this group that techniques other than morphological are essential for classification. The chronic leukaemias show maturation, which is more easily recognized by morphology, although in the diseases of lymphocytes the various subtypes can only be accurately defined by means of monoclonal antibodies.

Acute leukaemias

There are two major groups of acute leukaemia, lymphoblastic (**ALL**) and myeloid (**AML**). Both affect children and adults but with different frequency: 80 per cent of patients with AML are adults (over the age of 15 years) and 20 per cent children, including infants; in contrast, 85 per cent of those with ALL are children (under 15 years) and 15 per cent adults. In AML there are few differences in most disease features between children and adults; conversely, the differences between childhood and adult ALL are significant.

For a diagnosis of acute leukaemia it is necessary to identify blasts as the main cellular component. With a few cytochemical reactions, namely myeloperoxidase, Sudan black B and α-naphthyl acetate (or butyrate) esterase (**ANAE**), it is possible to distinguish the two main forms, ALL and AML. However, because these cytochemical methods

Table 1 *The classification of leukaemia*

Acute leukaemias
Myeloid (AML):
  M0–M7 (see Table 3)
Lymphoblastic (ALL):
  B-lineage—common ALL etc. (see Table 5)
  T-lineage—T-ALL
Biphenotypic:
  Myeloid and lymphoid
Hypocellular

Chronic leukaemias
Myeloid:[1]
  Chronic granulocytic (CGL)[1]
  Atypical chronic myeloid (aCML)[1]
  Chronic neutrophilic
  Chronic myelomonocytic (CMML)[1]
  Juvenile CMML
  Chronic eosinophilic
Lymphoid:
  B-lineage—CLL and others[2]
  T-lineage—T-PLL and others[2]

[1]French, American, British (FAB) group classification (Bennett *et al.* 1994).

[2]See Chapter 22.3.6.

Table 2 *Immunological classification of acute leukaemia*

Marker	Lymphoblastic (ALL)[1] B-lineage	T-lineage	AML (MO–M7)
CD2	–	+	–
CD3(c)	–	+	–
CD7	–	+	–
CD10	+	–	–
CD19	+	–	–
CD22(c)	+	–	–
CD13	–	–	+
CD33	–	–	+
MPO(c)	–	–	+[2]

(c) Cytoplasmic expression.

[1]Classification of ALL subtypes, see Table 4.

[2]MPO (myeloperoxidase) is negative in erythroid precursors (M6) and megakaryoblasts (M7).

are largely negative in ALL, it is now customary to apply a battery of monoclonal antibodies, which can be used as markers for the two ALL cell lineages, B and T, and of AML blasts (Table 2). These monoclonals define the immunophenotype of the disease. In immature cells, some antigens are expressed first in the cytoplasm (c), then in the cell membrane. This must be taken into account when testing blasts in suspension by flow cytometry as this method needs to be adapted for the detection of cytoplasmic antigens. In fact, the three markers that are most specific for the T, B, and myeloid lineages, CD3, CD22 and myeloperoxidase, respectively (Table 2), are localized in the cytoplasm and not in the membrane. One alternative is to apply immunocytochemical methods on fixed cells for the demonstration of membrane and cytoplasmic antigens.

In addition to the monoclonal antibodies listed in Table 2, other markers can be used to distinguish ALL from AML. One is the DNA polymerase terminal deoxynucleotidyl transferase (**TdT**), which is demonstrated by a polyclonal antibody in all cases of ALL, both B and T. A proportion of AML (25–30 per cent) also expresses TdT, although not

Table 3 *The classification of acute myeloid leukaemia*

Myeloblastic leukaemia
M0: minimal differentiation
M1: poorly differentiated
M2: differentiated

Promyelocytic
M3: hypergraunlar
M3V: microgranular variant

Myelomonocytic
M4: granulocytic–monocytic
M4Eo: with bone marrow eosinophilia

Monocytic
M5a: monoblastic
M5b: monocytic
M6: Erythroleukaemia
M7: Megakaryoblastic

French, American, British (FAB) group classification:; Bennett *et al.* (1976, 1985*a*, 1985*b*, 1991).

in all cells and, if a quantitative procedure is applied, with less intensity. The routine use of monoclonals and TdT has also disclosed the existence of acute leukaemias that express antigens of more than one lineage, usually lymphoid and myeloid. These cases are designated mixed lineage or biphenotypic (see below).

Bone-marrow trephine biopsies are useful for the diagnosis of cases that yield a 'dry tap' or a hypocellular specimen in aspirates. This is the case in two forms of acute leukaemia: megakaryoblastic or AML-M7 (Table 3) and hypocellular acute leukaemia; the blasts in the latter are nearly always myeloid.

Acute myeloid leukaemia

The French, American, British (**FAB**) group aimed to standardize the diagnostic criteria for the different forms of AML (Table 3) that reflect all the lines of myeloid differentiation. Although most types can be recognized by morphology and cytochemistry, there are two types, M0 and M7, which require positive evidence by monoclonal antibodies. The significance of the FAB classification of AML was emphasized by the correlation of several of the defined subtypes with non-random chromosome translocations (Table 4).

AML-M0

This is the most immature form of myeloblastic leukaemia. The blasts are negative with myeloperoxidase and ANAE cytochemistry, negative with B- and T-lymphoid markers, as distinct from ALL, and positive with one or more of the AML markers (Table 2), including antimyeloperoxidase, which is more sensitive than the cytochemical method for myeloperoxidase. The incidence of M0 is around 5 per cent of all AML. There is evidence that this disease has poor prognosis with a lower remission rate and shorter survival than other forms of AML.

AML-M1

This form of AML is also poorly differentiated; it differs from M0 in the demonstration of myeloid features by the cytochemical reactions of myeloperoxidase and Sudan black B. The FAB criteria require at least 3 per cent of positive blasts with either myeloperoxidase or Sudan black B. The majority of cases have more than 25 per cent positive blasts and often show Auer rods. It is nowadays advisable, in cases with less than 10 per cent myeloperoxidase-positive blasts, to confirm the diagnosis of AML by positive myeloid markers (Table 2; Fig. 1).

Table 4 *Chromosome translocations in acute myeloid leukaemia (AML)*

AML type	Chromosome translocation	Genes involved[1]
M2	t(8;21)(q22;q22)	ETO-AML1
M3 & M3V	t(15;17)(q24;q21)	PML-RARa
M4Eo	inv(16)(p13;q32)	CBFB-MYH11
M5	t(11;19)(q23;p13)	MLL-ENL
AML with basophilia	t(6;9)(p23;q34)	DEK-CAN

[1]Detected by molecular methods: Southern blots, polymerase chain reaction or *in situ* hybridization.

AML-M2

This is AML with differentiation beyond promyelocytes. In 15 per cent of M2 cases the cells show the translocation t(8;21) (Table 4) and, in addition to myeloid antigens, express the B-cell antigen CD19.

AML-M3

This comprises 7 to 8 per cent of all AMLs. Typical cases can be recognized by morphology: the blasts are bilobed, heavily granular, and show bundles of Auer rods or 'faggots' (Fig. 2). Myeloperoxidase and Sudan black B are strongly positive, myeloid antigens are expressed but HLA-DR, which is a feature of myeloblasts, is negative. M3 affects young adults, who present with a low white blood-cell count and a bleeding tendency. M3 variant cases have a high white blood-cell count, the blasts are deceptively hypogranular and may resemble monocytes, but the nucleus is bilobed rather than reniform. Cytochemistry helps to exclude monocytic leukaemia by a strong myeloperoxidase and weak or negative ANAE. A unique feature of both typical and variant M3 is the translocation t(15;17) (Table 4) and the important role of all-*trans* retinoic acid in treatment.

AML-M4

These cases show evidence of granulocytic and monocytic differentiation. The latter is confirmed by the ANAE reaction in more than 20 per cent of the blasts, a raised serum and/or urine lysozyme, and peripheral blood monocytosis. M4Eo is a variant form defined by the presence of bone marrow eosinophilia, with these cells showing prominent basophilic granules in addition to the eosinophil granules. M4Eo cases have a high remission rate and overall good prognosis, and are associated with a unique chromosome abnormality (Table 4).

AML-M5

Two forms of monocytic leukaemia can be identified by morphology. M5a is immature, common in infants, and is recognized by a strong ANAE cytochemical reaction, sensitive to inhibition by sodium fluoride. In M5b the cells are more mature and lysozyme levels are raised. M5 is associated with a high white-cell count, lymphadenopathy, and gingival hypertrophy. A rare form of M5 has heavily granular blasts, prominent erythrophagocytosis and a bleeding diathesis, and is characterized by the translocation t(8;16) (p11;p13).

AML-M6

Because these cases always show features of trilineage myelodysplasia it is necessary to distinguish them from primary myelodysplasia. The FAB group recommended that the 30 per cent blasts required for the diagnosis of AML could be reached in M6 by excluding erythroblasts in the bone-marrow differential count. The blasts in M6 are nearly always myeloblasts; in rare cases they may be erythroid precursors and could be identified with monoclonal antibodies against glycophorin A.

AML-M7

This form of AML includes most cases with features of 'acute myelo-fibrosis', that is a fibrotic bone marrow with blasts, abnormal megakaryocytes, and circulating blasts shown to be megakaryoblasts by their reactivity with monoclonals against platelet glycoproteins, CD41/42/61 for example. Bone-marrow trephines are essential for diagnosis if there are insufficient blasts to examine with monoclonal antibodies. Both M6 and M7 are associated with poor prognosis.

Acute lymphoblastic leukaemia

ALL represents the clonal proliferation of immature lymphoid precursors. The characteristic cell is the lymphoblast, which has high nuclear : cytoplasmic ratio and lacks cytoplasmic granules. Myeloperoxidase, Sudan black B, and ANAE are negative. Because cases of AML-M0 or even M7 may resemble lymphoblasts, it is necessary to make a positive diagnosis of ALL by immunological markers (Table 2) and a positive TdT. In addition, the periodic acid–Schiff reaction may be positive in B-lineage ALL and the acid phosphatase reaction in T-lineage ALL.

The FAB group described three morphological types of ALL: L1, seen in 80 per cent of childhood cases, L2, seen in 20 per cent, and L3 or Burkitt type (Fig. 3), seen in 1 to 3 per cent. L2 is proportionally more common in adult-ALL (up to 40 per cent of cases). Both L2 and L3 are associated with poor prognosis. There is no correspondence between L1 and L2 and immunological subtypes of ALL, except for L3, which corresponds to membrane Ig-positive B-ALL and shares the same chromosome translocation, t(8;14), with Burkitt lymphoma.

The diagnosis and classification of ALL subtypes now relies on the immunophenotype (Table 2). Based on the sequential appearance of certain antigens during B- and T-cell differentiation, a subclassification of ALL can be delineated (Table 5). The most important marker of the B lineage is the common-ALL antigen, which is recognized by monoclonal antibodies of the CD10 cluster. CD10 is expressed in the blasts of 75 per cent of childhood ALL cases, hence the designation common ALL. Less mature lymphoblasts (early B-ALL) do not express CD10, and this is seen in 10 per cent of childhood cases and in 30 per cent of adult ALL. Pre-B-ALL blasts express cytoplasmic μ-chains (without light chains).

The various forms of ALL have distinct prognostic features that may be related to the associated chromosome abnormalities (Table 6). It could be argued that some types of ALL are best characterized by their chromosome rearrangements rather than morphology or phenotype. The best two examples are t(4;11) in infants and t(9;22), or Philadelphia (**Ph**) chromosome, in adults, which corresponds to 20 to 30 per cent of cases and increases in frequency with age. It may be justified to include in the classification of ALL the subtypes Ph-positive ALL and ALL with t(4;11).

The immunophenotype of ALL correlates at DNA level with the rearrangement of the Ig heavy-chain genes and T-cell receptor genes in the B and T lineages, respectively. This type of analysis is not necessary for diagnosis or classification but it is important for monitoring minimal residual disease. Molecular techniques, on the other hand, are becoming more informative for the detection of rearranged genes and chimeric mRNA involved in the specific chromosome abnormalities of ALL (Table 6) and AML (Table 4).

CLINICAL CLASSIFICATION

A practical classification of ALL is to divide the cases according to age into adult and childhood ALL. Adult ALL has many biological and clinical differences from childhood ALL: more cases of L2 morphology and with a Ph-positive karyotype and fewer with hyperdiploidy, which

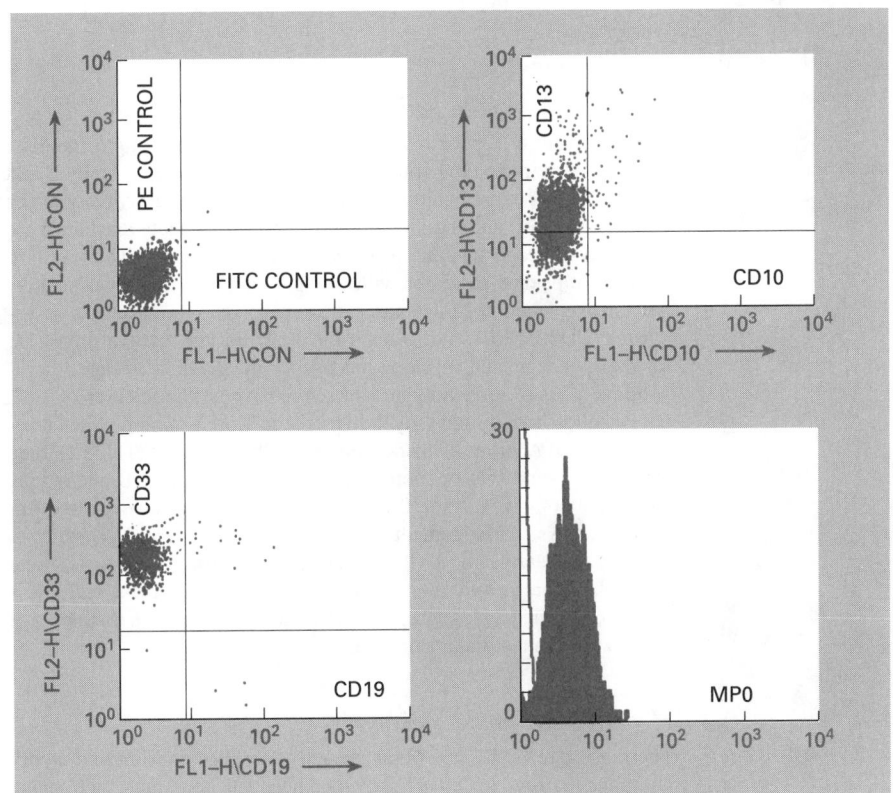

Fig. 1 Flow cytometric analysis of a case of acute myeloid leukaemia using double monoclonal antibodies conjugated with two different fluorescent dyes (PE (phycoerythrin) and FITC (fluorescein isothiocyanate)) shown in the control panel (top left). The blast cells are CD13+ and CD10− (top right), CD33+ and CD19− (bottom left) and anti-MPO+ (bottom right). See Table 3 and Farahat et al. (1994) for technical details.

is a good prognostic feature in children. The classification in Table 5 could be adapted to this division of childhood and adult cases.

Common ALL

This is the most frequent form of ALL in children and includes the cases with a better prognosis. The main diagnostic criterion is the demonstration of the common-ALL antigen (CD10+).

Early B-ALL

This was formerly described as null ALL and now redefined by the presence of early B-cell antigens CD19 and CD22 (cytoplasmic) and negative CD10.

Pre-B-ALL

Defined by the expression of μ-chain in the cytoplasm and persistence of CD10: a proportion of cases have the translocation t(1;19) (Table 6).

B-ALL

This is defined by evidence of membrane Ig (heavy and light chains) and is associated with L3 morphology (Fig. 3) and the translocation t(8;14) (Table 6). B-ALL probably represents the leukaemic presentation of non-endemic Burkitt lymphoma. In adults it may also represent the transformation of a pre-existing follicular lymphoma; in such cases t(8;14) coexists with t(14;18). The prognosis of B-ALL is very poor

Fig. 2 Bone marrow aspirate from a case of acute myeloid leukaemia M3 (hypergranular promyelocytic) showing a cell with multiple Auer rods ('faggots').

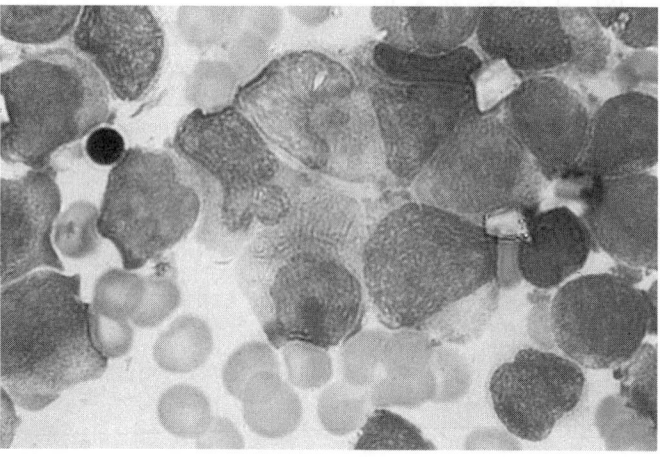

Fig. 3 Bone marrow film from a case of acute lymphoblastic leukaemia (ALL) L3 (Burkitt type) that corresponded immunologically to B-ALL (Table 4). The blasts have a deep basophilic cytoplasm with vacuoles.

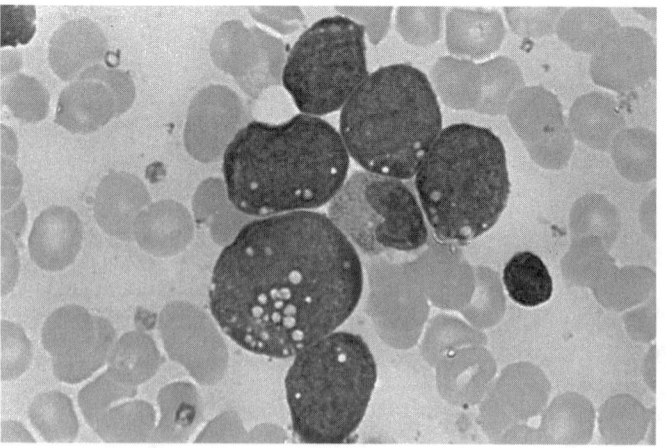

Table 5 *Immunological classification of acute lymphoblastic leukaemia (ALL)*

B-lineage
Early-B (CD10−)
Pre-B ALL (cyt. μ+)
B-ALL (membrane Ig)
T-lineage
Pre-T (CD2−)
T-ALL (CD2+)

Table 6 *Chromosome translocations in acute lymphoblastic leukaemia (ALL)*

ALL type	Chromosome translocation	Genes involved[1]
Early-B	t(4;11)(q21;q23)	*AFX-MLL*
Pre-B	(t(1;19)(q23;p13))	*PBX1-E2A*
Common	t(9;22)(q34;q11)	*ABL-BCR*
B-ALL	t(8;14)(q24;q32)	*MYC-IgH*
T-ALL	t(1;14)(p32;q11)	*TAL1-TCRd*
	t(10;14)(q24;q11)	*HOX11-TCRd*
	t(11;14)(p13;q11)	*RBTN-TCRd*

[1]Detected by molecular methods: Southern blots, polymerase chain reaction or *in situ* hybridization.

with conventional therapy, but has improved significantly with newer and more intensive regimens.

T-ALL

These cases, whether with an immature phenotype (CD2-) or more mature (CD2+), evolve with a thymic mass and high white-cell count. There is overlap with T-lymphoblastic lymphoma, a condition in which, by convention, the bone marrow contains less than 25 per cent lymphoblasts.

Biphenotypic acute leukaemia

The wider use of monoclonal antibodies has brought to light the existence of cases in which markers of different cell lineages (usually B and myeloid) are coexpressed on the same blast cells. Because many of the markers used for defining the immunophenotype of acute leukaemia are not always lineage specific, it is necessary to use restrictive criteria to define as biphenotypic cases with coexpression of at least two markers per lineage when specific markers are involved—for example, cytoplasmic CD22, Mb-1 and μ-chain for the B lineage, cytoplasmic CD3 for the T lineage, and myeloperoxidase for the myeloid lineage.

Some cases of biphenotypic leukaemia have all the features of ALL but coexpress two or more myeloid markers. More commonly they present as typical AML and, in addition to myeloid antigens (Table 2), they express TdT and two or more B (or rarely T) antigens. Biphenotypic leukaemia comprises 5 to 10 per cent of all acute leukaemias and frequently shows rearrangement of Ig and/or T-cell receptor genes, even in cases presenting as AML. Because of the distinct biological and molecular changes and poor prognosis associated with these cases, it is of clinical value to recognize biphenotypic leukaemia as a distinct type using well-defined diagnostic criteria.

Hypocellular acute leukaemia

These are rare AML cases that present with pancytopenia and a 'dry tap' bone marrow, which are shown on adequate bone-marrow trephine biopsies to be hypocellular (in contrast to the expected hypercellularity).

The biopsies may resemble aplastic anaemia but show distinct clusters of blasts as well as a number of these cells in the circulation. It is important when assessing the cellularity of bone marrow to take into account the patient's age, as the normal cellularity of marrow declines markedly with age and may be as low as 20 per cent in people aged between 65 and 85 years.

Chronic leukaemias

These are malignancies in which mature leucocytes are the predominant cell. As for the acute leukaemias, there are two main groups, myeloid and lymphoid, with two representative disorders, chronic granulocytic (CGL) and chronic lymphocytic (CLL). The latter, as well as the less common forms of leukaemias of mature B and T lymphocytes are described in Chapter 22.3.6. The myeloid leukaemias reflect granulocytic or monocytic differentiation or a combination of both, myelomonocytic. A pure monocytic leukaemia of chronic type without involvement of granulocytes is very rare.

Chronic granulocytic leukaemia

CGL is also known as chronic myeloid leukaemia (CML), although the former term describes more closely the haematological features of the disease. CML may be used as a generic term for the whole group. CGL has a distinct chromosome marker, the Ph chromosome, resulting from the reciprocal translocation t(9;22), which is found in 95 per cent of cases. Cases with similar haematological features but which are Ph negative often have the same molecular rearrangement as Ph-positive cases, which results from the juxtaposition of the *BCR* and *ABL* genes to form a hybrid *BCR-ABL* gene.

The diagnosis of CGL can be established by the morphological appearance of peripheral blood and bone marrow films, and is confirmed by cytogenetic and/or molecular analysis. The leucocyte differential count shows the full spectrum of granulocytic cells but with predominance of myelocytes (around 30 per cent) and mature neutrophils (around 50 per cent), almost invariably basophilia (around 5 per cent), and frequent eosinophilia; the percentage of monocytes is low, usually less than 3 per cent. Blasts comprise 1 or 2 per cent of the circulating cells unless the disease is in accelerated phase or in transformation; myelodysplastic changes are minimal. The bone-marrow aspirate is hypercellular, with granulocytic hyperplasia and numerous megakaryocytes, and is less useful than the peripheral blood for the differential diagnosis between CGL and the other chronic myeloid leukaemias. The myeloid : erythroid ratio is greater than 10 : 1 with few erythroblasts. The bone-marrow trephine is necessary to assess the degree of fibrosis and, occasionally, to distinguish from idiopathic myelofibrosis.

Atypical chronic myeloid leukaemia

Patients with high leucocyte counts who are Ph chromosome negative form an heterogeneous group. Some have morphological features of CGL and the molecular rearrangement *BCR-ABL*, and should be considered together with the Ph-positive cases as CGL because of their treatment response and natural history. Another group has atypical morphological features by comparison with CGL, namely, slight monocytosis (5–10 per cent), absence of or minor basophilia and eosinophilia, granulocytic dysplasia (Pelger and hypogranular neutrophils), and 2 to 3 per cent circulating blasts. Cases of atypical CML do not show *BCR-ABL* rearrangement, thus they are *Ph−/BCR−*, in contrast to CGL, which is *Ph+/BCR+* or *Ph−/BCR+*.

Chronic myelomonocytic leukaemia

Cases of CMML with high leucocyte counts (e.g. 20–40 per cent × $10^9/1$) could be considered together with other forms of CML rather than

with the myelodysplastic syndromes. The two main differences from atypical CML and CGL are the proportion of monocytes, which ranges from 25 to 50 per cent in CMML, and the lower percentage of immature granulocytes (5–10 per cent). The erythroid cells in the bone marrow are also more prominent in CMML, with a lower myeloid : erythroid ratio than in CGL and atypical CML. CMML cases are always *Ph−/BCR−*, show moderate to high levels of serum and urinary lysozyme, and have myelodysplastic changes in the bone marrow.

Rare forms of chronic myeloid leukaemia

Other types of chronic myeloid leukaemia that occur infrequently are chronic neutrophilic, juvenile CMML, and chronic eosinophilic leukaemia.

Chronic neutrophilic

This occurs in adults over 50 years, who have normal haemoglobin and platelet counts. The blood film shows predominantly neutrophils without immature forms. All cases are *Ph−/BCR−*. The neutrophil alkaline phosphatase score is high, in contrast with the very low levels in CGL.

Juvenile CMML

This comprises 2 per cent of childhood leukaemias. Patients are under 5 years of age and have systemic symptoms. In contrast to CGL, there is monocytosis without basophilia or eosinophilia. Characteristically, the levels of fetal haemoglobin are high. Cytogenetic analysis is important to distinguish this condition from Ph-positive CGL in childhood and from the myelodysplastic syndrome with monosomy 7 seen in young children.

Chronic eosinophilic leukaemia

It is difficult to distinguish this from the hypereosinophilic syndrome. In favour of the latter is the absence of chromosome abnormalities and immature forms, whilst their presence suggests eosinophilic leukaemia.

REFERENCES

Bartram, C.R. (1993). Application of molecular genetics to diagnosis in leukaemia. In *Haematology trends '93*, (ed. K. Lechner and H. Gadner), pp. 280–96. Schattauer, Stuttgart

Bennett, J.M. *et al.* (1976). Proposals for the classification of the acute leukaemias. *British Journal of Haematology*, **33**, 451–58.

Bennett, J.M. *et al.* (1980). A variant form of hypergranular promyelocytic leukaemia. *British Journal of Haematology*, **44**, 169–70.

Bennett, J.M. *et al.* (1981). The morphological classification of acute lymphoblastic leukaemia: concordance among observers and clinical correlations. *British Journal of Haematology*, **47**, 553–61.

Bennett, J.M. *et al.* (1985a). Criteria for the diagnosis of acute leukaemia of megakaryocyte lineage (M7). *Annals of Internal Medicine*, **103**, 460–2.

Bennett, J.M. *et al.* (1985b). Proposed revised criteria for the classification of acute myeloid leukaemia. *Annals of Internal Medicine*, **103**, 620–5.

Bennett, J.M., Catovsky, D., Daniel, M-T., *et al.* (1991). Proposal for the recognition of minimally differentiated acute myeloid leukaemia (AML-MO). *British Journal of Haematology*, **78**, 325–9.

Bennett, J.M., Catovsky, D., Daniel, M.-T., *et al.* (1994). The chronic myeloid leukaemias: guidelines for distinguishing chronic granulocytic, atypical chronic myeloid and chronic myelomonocytic leukaemia. *British Journal of Haematology*, **87**, 746–54.

Buccheri, V., Shetty, V., Yoshida, N., Morilla, R., Matutes, E., and Catovsky, D. (1992). The role of an anti-myeloperoxidase antibody in the diagnosis and classification of acute leukaemia: a comparison with light and electron microscopy cytochemistry. *British Journal of Haematology*, **80**, 62–8.

Buccheri, V., Matutes, E., Dyer, M.J.S., and Catovsky, D. (1993a). Lineage commitment in biphenotypic acute leukaemia. *Leukemia* 7, 919–27.

Buccheri, V., Mihaljevic, B., Matutes, E., Dyer, M.J.S., Mason, D.Y., and Catovsky, D. (1993b). mb-1: a new marker for B-lineage lymphoblastic leukaemia. *Blood*, **82**, 853–7.

Catovsky, D. and Matutes, E. (1992). The classification of acute leukaemia. *Leukemia*, **6**, (suppl. 2), 1–6.

Farahat, N., van der Plas, D., Praxedes, M., Morilla, R., Matutes, E., and Catovsky, D. (1994). Demonstration of cytoplasmic and nuclear antigens by flow cytometry in acute leukaemia. *Journal of Clinical Pathology* **47**, 843–9.

Galton, D.A.G. (1992). Haematological differences between chronic granulocytic leukaemia, atypical chronic myeloid leukaemia and chronic myelomonocytic leukaemia. *Leukemia and Lymphoma*, **7**, 343–50.

Janossy, G., Coustan-Smith, E., and Campana, D. (1989). The reliability of cytoplasmic CD3 and CD22 antigen expression in the immunodiagnosis of acute leukaemia: a study of 500 cases. *Leukemia*, **3**, 170–81.

Lilleyman, J.S. *et al.* (1992). Cytomorphology of childhood lymphoblastic leukaemia: a prospective study of 2000 patients. *British Journal of Haematology*, **81**, 52–7.

Martiat, P., Michaux, J.L., and Rodhain, J. (1991). Philadelphia-negative (Ph−) chronic myeloid leukemia (CML): Comparison with Ph+ CML and chronic myelomonocytic leukemia. *Blood*, **78**, 205–11.

Maruyama, F. *et al.* (1994). Detection of AML1/ETO fusion transcript as a tool for diagnosing t(8;21) positive acute myelogenous leukaemia. *Leukemia*, **8**, 40–5.

Soekarman, D. *et al.* (1992). *DEK-CAN* rearrangement in translocation t(6; 9) (p23;q34). *Leukemia*, **6**, 489–94.

Stasi, R. *et al.* (1994). Analysis of treatment failure in patients with minimally differentiated acute myeloid leukemia (AML-MO) *Blood*, **83**, 1619–25.

Warrell, R.P., de The, H., Wang, Z-Y., and Degos, L. (1993) Acute promyelocytic leukaemia. *New England Journal of Medicine*, **329**, 177–89.

Table 1 *Aetiology of acute myeloid leukaemia*

Primary (de novo)
Cause unknown
Secondary
Congenital disorders:
Fanconi anaemia
Trisomy 21
Chediak–Higashi disease
Wiskott–Aldrich syndrome
Acquired marrow disorders:
Myelodysplastic syndromes
Chronic myeloid leukaemia
Other myeloproliferative disorders (myelofibrosis, polycythaemia vera, essential thrombocythaemia)
Severe aplastic anaemia
Therapeutic agents:
Fractionated radiotherapy
Cytotoxics (alkylating agents, nitrosoureas, procarbazine, razoxane, others)
Environmental factors:
Accidental irradiation, nuclear weapons, benzene, toluene

22.3.3 Acute myeloblastic leukaemia

A. J. BARRETT

Introduction

Acute myeloid leukaemia (**AML**) affects adults and children but has an increased incidence with advancing age. Over 80 per cent of patients are over 60 years of age. This form of leukaemia, which has been recognized for at least 100 years, has a worldwide distribution. There is some evidence that the disease is becoming more common. AML has a reputation of being a poorly responding, incurable leukaemia. In comparison with acute lymphoblastic leukaemia of childhood, progress in treatment of AML has certainly lagged behind. However, the prospects for cure of younger adults and children with AML are now much better than they were even a decade ago. These improvements have arisen both from new treatment concepts derived from a better understanding of the disease process, and the development of intensive therapies such as bone marrow transplantation, facilitated by better supportive care.

The cause of AML is not known. In over half the affected individuals AML arises rapidly ('*de novo*') without any antecedent haematological changes. In other cases AML is secondary to an underlying bone marrow disorder, which may either be congenital (e.g. Fanconi aplastic anaemia) or acquired (e.g. myelodysplastic syndromes and myeloproliferative disorders). A variety of agents that damage bone marrow has been associated with an increased incidence of AML. These include anticancer drugs, toxic chemicals, and exposure to ionizing radiation. Some predisposing factors for AML are listed in Table 1.

Pathophysiology

In most, but not all, cases of AML the leukaemic process originates in a pluripotent stem cell. Leukaemic pluripotent cells give rise to committed progenitors of the granulocyte, erythroid, and megakaryocyte lineages. Leukaemic change in the stem-cell DNA causes a maturation arrest, usually at the myeloblast, monoblast, or promyelocyte stage. Occasionally the leukaemic maturation arrest can affect early erythroblasts or megakaryoblasts producing erythroleukaemia (AML M6), or megakaryocytic leukaemia (AML M7). The proliferation of leukaemic blast cells is not accompanied by the ordered process of differentiation that in normal myeloid cells switches off proliferation. The crowding of the bone marrow with this rapidly growing leukaemic blast population suppresses normal maturation of erythrocytes, granulocytes, and megakaryocytes derived from residual normal stem cells. The result is bone marrow failure. Patients become anaemic, thrombocytopenic, and neutropenic. The leukaemia cells spill into the blood and spread to the spleen, liver, and to a lesser extent the lymph nodes and other organs. Excessively high counts of leukaemic cells in the blood (usually over 500×10^9/l) can cause leucostasis in the lungs and brain. An important metabolic consequence of the rapidly proliferating mass of leukaemic blasts is the excess production of uric acid from nucleic acid turnover. Hyperuricaemia causing renal failure is a particular risk during the initial response to treatment. The extent to which normal stem cells persist is an important factor determining the response to treatment. In AML secondary to other diseases the residual normal stem-cell pool is very small or absent (Fig. 1) and full remissions are less common.

Presentation

In *de novo* AML the onset is typically abrupt, usually with a history of less than 6 weeks. The symptoms are often vague. Patients may complain of lassitude and headaches or may report that they have had influenza and never fully recovered. Many of these symptoms are related to the development of anaemia. Sometimes they may notice an increased tendency to bleed. Nosebleeds, menorrhagia, gum bleeding, bruising, or a petechial rash may prompt the patient to visit their doctor. Presentation with infection is less common: patients may develop bacterial infection causing mouth ulcers and septic skin lesions especially in the perianal area. Rarely, AML presents with acute appendicitis. Bone pain is less frequently a presenting feature than in childhood ALL. Sometimes the presence of extramedullary disease such as leukaemic skin deposits, gum hypertrophy, or neurological involvement may be the reason for presentation.

The clinical signs of AML are often subtle. Careful observation may reveal the presence of a poorly healing injury, petechial haemorrhage, modest hepatosplenomegaly, and lymphadenopathy. Patients may show the triad of features of bone marrow failure namely pallor from anaemia, petechial haemorrhage, bruising and bleeding as a consequence of thrombocytopenia, and evidence of bacterial and fungal infection as a result of neutropenia. Splenic enlargement may be detected by ultrasonography. Patients with secondary AML may show the features of the pre-existing disease—massive splenomegaly in AML following myeloproliferative disorders, abnormal facial appearance in Fanconi aplasia for example.

Particular features are associated with certain AML subtypes. Acute promyelocytic leukaemia (AML M3) is associated with a consumption coagulopathy and may present with catastrophic haemorrhage. Gum hypertrophy and skin deposits are a feature of AML M4 and M5. Children are more likely to present with central nervous leukaemia. Extramedullary (particularly extradural) deposits are a feature of M2. These conditions, and an explanation of their classification are considered in Chapter 22.3.7.

Diagnosis (Plates 2–7)

The diagnosis of AML may be suspected on clinical grounds but can only be confirmed by examination of the blood and bone marrow.

The blood count is variable. There is usually a mild to moderate anaemia. Severe anaemia below 7 g/dl suggests a secondary AML or significant bleeding. The platelet count is usually low—below 100×10^9/l. Higher counts suggest an AML arising from a transforming myeloproliferative syndrome. Almost any leucocyte count may be encountered, from below 1×10^9/l to over 200×10^9/l. In most cases, examination of the blood film reveals the presence of blast cells. These are scanty in pancytopenic presentations, but account for the majority of the circulating white cells in patients with leucocytosis. The blast population may show limited and aberrant maturation involving monocytoid cells, myelocytes, metamyelocytes, and neutrophils. The hallmark of AML is the presence of Auer rods in the cytoplasm of blast cells and abnormal granulocytes, often better seen in the blood film than in the bone marrow. This feature is diagnostic of AML but occurs in less than 25 per cent of patients. In differentiating AML from ALL it is useful to identify features of dysplasia in cells of the myeloid lineage such as neutrophil hypogranularity, abnormal monocytes, red-cell anisocytosis, and normoblasts with abnormal nuclei. These features strongly suggest a myeloid leukaemia.

Examination of a bone marrow aspirate is essential. The marrow is usually hypercellular, but in AML developing from a myelodysplastic disorder it may be hypocellular. Cellularity is best evaluated by examining a trephine biopsy. Typically the marrow is crowded with blast cells, which constitute over 90 per cent of the cells in the aspirate. Difficulties may arise in defining the precise point in time when a myelodysplastic syndrome of the refractory anaemia with excess of blasts (RAEB) variety has transformed into a frank acute leukaemia (Chapter 22.3.7). The accepted definition of transformation to AML is when the blast cells exceed 30 per cent of the marrow cells. These considerations are semantic. A functional definition that is used to decide when to apply AML therapy includes advanced bone-marrow failure to a stage where platelet transfusion support is required or neutropenia has become severe. Rapid progression of cytopenia is a further feature favouring introduction of AML treatment. It is not always possible on morphological grounds alone to determine whether the leukaemia is of myeloid or lymphoid origin. Furthermore, morphology can be deceptive. It is therefore sound practice to carry out routine cytochemical staining to differentiate AML from ALL. The presence in the blast population of lipid granules positive for Sudan black or myeloperoxidase confirms the

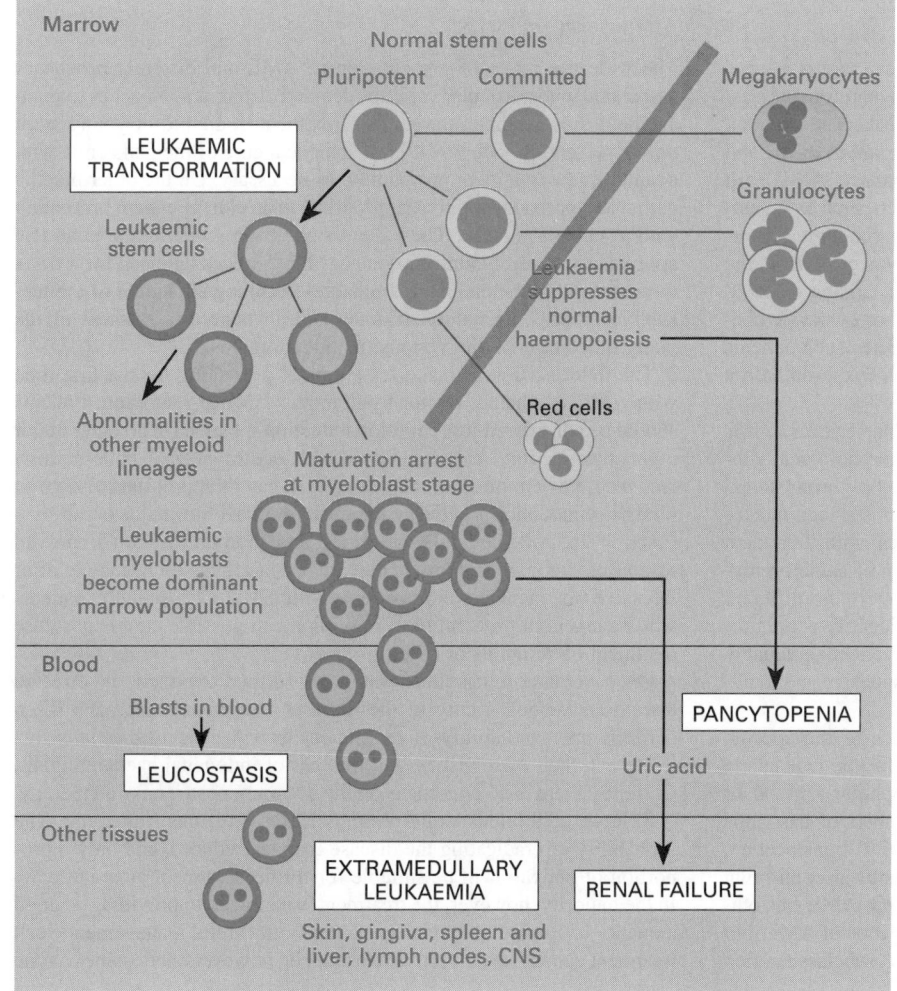

Fig. 1 Pathophysiology of acute myeloblastic leukaemia.

Table 2 *Prognostic classification of acute myeloid leukaemia*

Category	Unfavourable	More favourable
Presentation		
Aetiology	Secondary	*De novo*
Age	Older age, infants	Children > 1 year
Performance score	Low	100%
Extramedullary disease	Involvement of central nervous system	None
Morphological		
	MO Undifferentiated	M2 Myeloid with granulocytic differentiation
	M1 Undifferentiated myeloid	
	M4 Myelomonocytic	M3 Promyelocytic
	M5 Monocytic	
	M6 Erythroleukaemia	
	M7 Megakaryoblastic	
Karyotype		
	t (9;22) CML	t (15;17) promyelocytic
	del 5q)	t (8;21)
	del 7q) MDS	Inversion 16
	Chromosome breaks (Fanconi)	
	Deletion 11(q23)	

CML, chronic myeloid leukaemia; MDS, myelodysplastic syndrome.

diagnosis of AML. Some undifferentiated acute leukaemias remain untypable by cytochemical staining. It is usually possible to classify these cases as myeloid, lymphoid, or biphenotypic leukaemias using a panel of monoclonal antibodies as membrane markers.

SUBCLASSIFICATION OF AML

As our understanding of the disease process improves there is a trend towards diversifying the treatment approach used. It is therefore increasingly important to characterize the subtype of the AML. The first distinction that should be made is between primary (*de novo*) AML and secondary AML. Many patients developing secondary AML will already have been treated for defined myeloid disorders such as myeloproliferative diseases, myelodysplastic syndromes, or congenital disorders such as Fanconi aplasia. In some instances, however, AML is the first indication of another underlying disorder. AML arising even 20 years after significant exposure to ionizing radiation or cytotoxic chemotherapy should be considered a secondary event. Often such patients progress through a period of pancytopenia and myelodysplasia before developing overt acute leukaemia.

The morphological classification is described in Chapter 22.3.2. It is possible to characterize AML into at least seven morphological subtypes. In addition, some AML subtypes have specific chromosomal translocations. Morphology and karyotype have prognostic significance identifying favourable or less favourable outcomes with treatment (Table 2). Nevertheless (with the important exception of acute promyelocytic leukaemia described below) they do not determine different approaches to remission induction. It is essential to identify acute promyelocytic leukaemia (AML M3) because of the severe coagulopathy associated with this form of AML, and its specific responsiveness to all-*trans*-retinoic acid.

Morphology quite accurately predicts the presence of the specific chromosome translocations: t(15;17)—acute promyelocytic leukaemia; abnormalities of chromosome 16—M4 with eosinophilia; a blood or marrow appearance of blast cells and increased numbers of basophils strongly suggest an AML with the t(9;22) or the t(6;9) translocation. Monoclonal antibody membrane markers can be useful in confirming erythroid (M6), megakaryocytic (M7), or biphenotypic AML but otherwise have only minor importance in the subclassification of AML into prognostic subgroups at present. Other approaches to subclassification

of AML that measure proliferative behaviour and the degree of growth factor-independent proliferation are still being evaluated but may eventually prove useful.

Management

AIMS OF TREATMENT

The wide age range of presentation of AML and different prognoses associated with particular varieties demand different approaches to management. For example, the aim of treatment in a child or young adult newly presenting with AML is to achieve a cure of the leukaemia with as intensive a treatment programme as necessary. On the other hand, a palliative approach would be appropriate in an elderly patient presenting with a secondary AML. The patient's choice in selecting the treatment approach is of paramount importance. This implies the need for a frank discussion with the patient and relatives outlining the nature of the leukaemic process, its natural history, and an honest assessment of the likely outcome with the various treatment options.

The first decision to make for a patient presenting for the first time with AML is whether or not to attempt to induce remission. Patients should be considered for remission induction if they have no other major organ dysfunction, and if there is a chance of normal bone-marrow recovery. No definite rules can be made. It may be appropriate to attempt remission induction in elderly patients who have no major organ dysfunction and who are fully informed and motivated. With improved responses and good supportive care there is a growing tendency to offer intensive treatments to older patients with AML. Occasionally, patients who have a high probability of remission and possible cure may refuse treatment on religious or other grounds.

Once remission has been induced, further treatment is directed towards achieving a cure of the disease. The precise approach taken depends upon the ability of the patient to withstand further intensive treatment, their own wishes, and the bias of individual haematologists. Currently there is no consensus on the optimum post-remission therapy.

Relapse of the leukaemia presents a fresh treatment dilemma. The probability of eradicating the disease is much reduced, and only a proportion of patients will be suitable for further treatment aimed at cure. In the majority, however, the treatment is restricted to providing as good a quality of life for as long as possible. With careful management, such treatment can be very effective. Ultimately, however, there comes a time when it is necessary to abandon active leukaemia treatment and to use supportive care. Sadly, as more patients die with AML than are cured, it is important to emphasize the continuing responsibility the haematologist has beyond the stage of active treatment. Indeed, it is very important that the patient does not feel abandoned when the original treatment has to be modified. Particularly at this time, a good and honest rapport between the physician, the patient, and family provides the proper basis for instituting terminal care.

SUPPORTIVE CARE (TABLE 3)

Proper care of the cytopenic patient is a prerequisite to giving treatment of sufficient intensity to achieve remission and cure of AML. Patients undergoing treatment for AML experience prolonged periods of failure of normal bone-marrow function. They require almost constant venous access either for blood sampling, transfusion of blood products, or administration of chemotherapy and antibiotics. The installation of a semipermanent indwelling right atrial catheter greatly facilitates their management.

Thrombocytopenic bleeding is preventable by adopting a policy of checking platelet counts at least three times weekly, and transfusing 6 to 12 units of platelets whenever the count falls below $20 \times 10^9/l$. Sensitization to platelet and HLA antigens during the period of treatment is not usually a major problem and can be diminished by transfusion of leucocyte-poor blood products. Two situations merit special attention. Rapid platelet consumption occurs in patients who are infected, and those with acute promyelocytic leukaemia (AML M3). These patients may require twice-daily transfusions as well as coagulation-factor replacement.

Infections during the neutropenic period are derived from endogenous commensals, from bacteria and fungi present in the immediate environment, in food and drink, or acquired by direct human contact. Three approaches are employed to reduce the risk of infective death during treatment, as follows.

Prevention of autoinfection

Autoinfection is reduced by administration of non-absorbable oral antibiotics such as colistin or neomycin, and topical antiseptics. Alternatively, patients are given oral septrin, or ciprofloxacin. Candida infection can be prevented by use of an imidazole antifungal, and pulmonary aspergillosis may be reduced by regular application of an amphotericin aerosol.

Protective isolation

In the past this approach was taken to extremes, with patients cared for in environments supplied with filtered air under positive pressure, of operating-theatre level of sterility. Most AML treatment units now adopt a more relaxed approach to protective isolation, nursing the patient in a single room with restricted access to visitors and provision of 'clean' food. This approach has not been associated with any increase in infective problems. Such treatment is less expensive, better tolerated, and is practicable in most hospitals.

Prompt treatment of suspected infection

The practice of taking blood cultures and giving intravenous antibiotics to patients with fever is the key to successful management of neutropenia. A range of potent bactericidal broad-spectrum antibiotics is now available. Each hospital has its own particular treatment policy. In principle first-line agents should cover Gram-positive and Gram-negative organisms including *Pseudomonas* spp. This can be achieved with a combination of an aminoglycoside with a broad-spectrum penicillin. Failure to obtain a response of the fever requires a change to second-line treatment with a different antibiotic combination (e.g. vancomycin and ceftazidime). In patients not responding to antibacterial treatment an invasive fungal infection should be suspected and intravenous

Table 3 *Supportive care for acute myeloblastic leukaemia*

Monitoring
Daily or alternate daily: Blood count, electrolytes, liver function
Weekly: Bacteriological screen, chest radiograph
When indicated: Blood cultures, bone marrow aspirate

Anaemia
Transfusions of packed red cells to maintain haemoglobin above 10 g/dl

Haemorrhage
Transfusions of 3–12 donor units of platelets to maintain count above $10–20 \times 10/l$
Regular coagulation screens: replacement of coagulation factors with fresh frozen plasma, cryoprecipitate as required)

Infection prevention
Protective isolation: single room, reverse-barrier isolation, clean food
Oral antibiotics: septrin/ciprofloxacin/colistin/neomycin
Oral antifungals: amphotericin/nystatin/fluconazole
Pulmonary aspergillosis: amphotericin aerosol
Herpes simplex labialis: oral acyclovir

Infection treatment
Fever regimen: initiated if temperature rises above 38 °C
First line: aminoglycoside + broad-spectrum penicillin IV
Second line: (no response after 48 h, or deterioration) ceftazidime and vancomycin IV
Third line: (no response after 48 h, no organism isolated) amphotericin IV

Nutritional
Parenteral feeding if > 10% loss of body weight
Intravenous analgesia for painful stomatitis

Psychological
Frank discussions, optimistic attitude, regular daily visits and progress updates, family support, early discharge as soon as haematological recovery permits

amphotericin should be commenced even in the absence of any localizing features of infection.

Lastly, the importance of the psychological support of the patient by the care team cannot be overemphasized. Step-by-step explanation of treatment details and regular progress reports are essential aspects of the management of patients with life-threatening disorders who have to remain in hospital for considerable periods during their treatment.

REMISSION INDUCTION (FIG. 2)

The goal of remission induction treatment is to give chemotherapy to reduce the leukaemic load to a point at which the bone marrow becomes temporarily aplastic. This permits the recovery of normal haemopoiesis. It has become apparent that the more intensive the treatment given the more likely is remission to be achieved and the more rapidly it occurs. The shortening of remission induction time is associated with a shorter period of pancytopenia, and consequently a lower risk of infectious and haemorrhagic complications. To achieve these aims most remission induction schedules employ the combination of cystosine arabinoside and an anthracycline administered in a treatment block of 7 to 10 days. Many schedules also include a third agent such as thioguanine, etoposide, or a nitrosourea. Good results are also achieved with high-dose cytosine arabinoside alone. In responding patients the blood count falls, blasts disappear from the blood, and the bone marrow becomes hypocellular. At 2 to 3 weeks a marrow aspirate is done to assess progress.

There may be signs of haemopoietic recovery signalling early remission, the marrow may be aplastic, or there may be persisting leukaemia. Patients with persisting leukaemia 14 days after stopping treatment require further induction chemotherapy. The process of reassessment is repeated 2 weeks after stopping the second treatment course. Patients not aplastic or in remission at this time have a low probability of achieving remission. They may be suitable for salvage treatment with further chemotherapy or allogeneic bone-marrow transplantation. Alternatively, intensive treatment may be abandoned at this stage. Complete remission is defined as the presence of a normal blood count, and a cellular marrow containing fewer than 5 per cent blasts. Partial remission is defined as some degree of haematological recovery but with persisting leukaemia in the marrow, or persistence of gross dysplastic features.

Modern treatments achieve remission in up to 90 per cent of patients,

However, there are clear prognostic differences in the likelihood of achieving remission. Increasing age is a major negative prognostic factor. Secondary AML and the M4 and M5 subtypes of AML also have a lower probability of remission. Table 4 summarizes recent results of remission induction in the various AML categories.

POSTINDUCTION TREATMENT

The majority of patients achieving remission relapse unless further treatment is given. The choice is between treatment of lower intensity or greater intensity than that used in remission induction. The latter may be achieved using either intensive chemotherapy, or bone marrow transplantation from an autologous or allogeneic source. The precise choice of treatment remains an area of continuing controversy. There is, how-

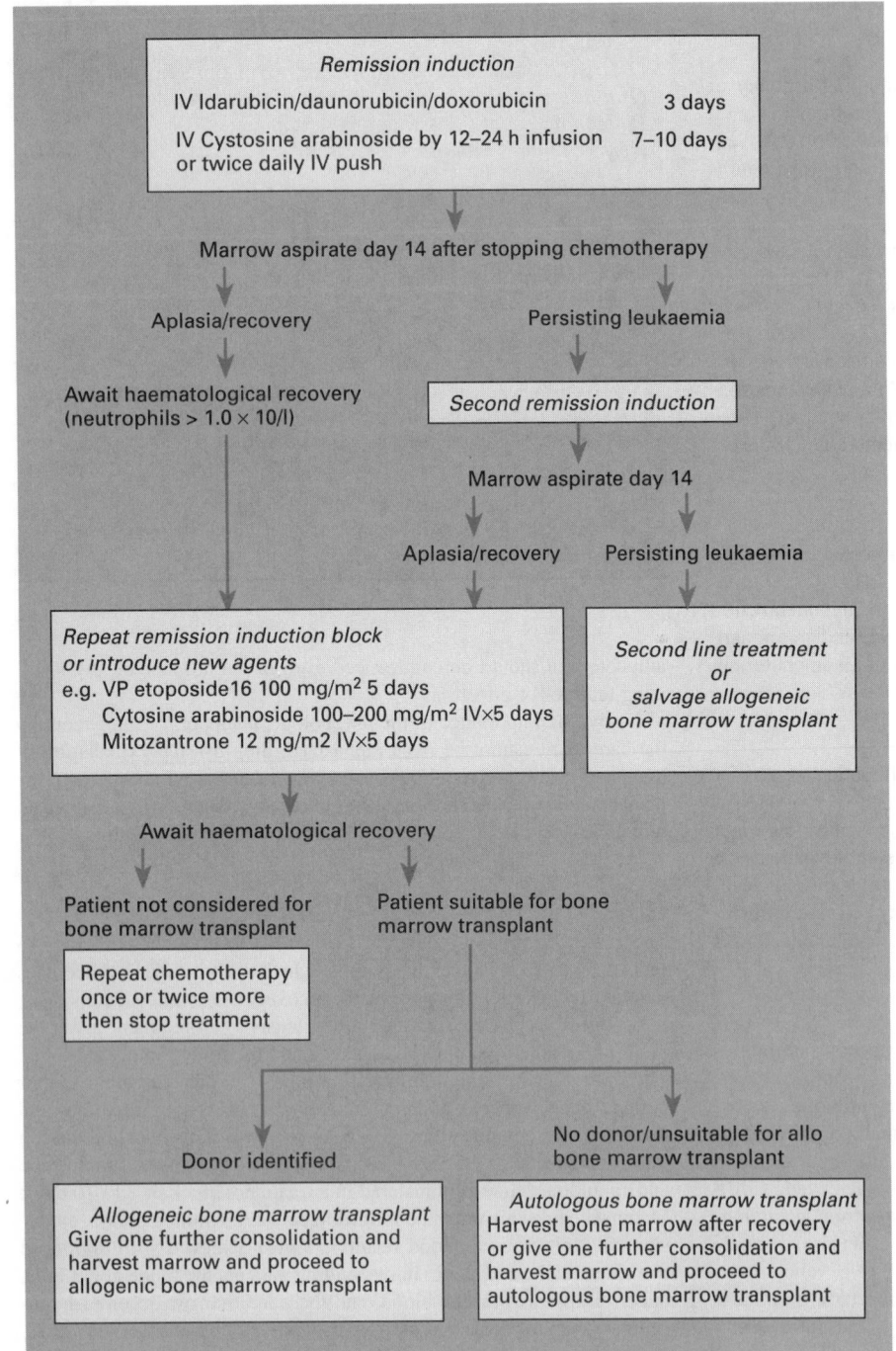

Fig. 2 Treatment of acute myeloblastic leukaemia.

Table 4 *Results of treatment for acute myeloblastic leukaemia (AML)*

Remission induction	
Children > 1 year	90%
15–65 years	60–85%
over 65 years	50–70%
De novo AML	60–85%
Secondary AML	30–70%
Postinduction 5-year disease-free survival	
Chemotherapy regimens	
De novo AML	20–50%
Secondary AML	0–20%
Autologous BMT	
First remission	40–60%
Second or subsequent remission	20–35%
Allogeneic BMT from a matched sibling donor	
First remission	45–70%
Second or subsequent remission	20–30%
subsequent relapse	5–15%
Primary induction failure	about 30%
Allogeneic BMT from partially matched donor or matched unrelated donor	
First remission	25–35%

BMT, bone marrow transplantation.

ever, a general consensus that neither maintenance treatment, so successful in the management of childhood ALL nor late intensification 1 year into remission have any important therapeutic potential in AML. In practice, most patients receive one to four postremission treatment cycles. The strategy is to use different combinations of agents than those employed in remission induction in order to protect against relapse from drug-resistant cells. Agents such as mitozantrone, 5-azacytidine, etoposide, and cytosine arabinoside are used in combination in treatment blocks of 5 to 10 days, with intervals of about a month between courses to allow for haematological recovery.

BONE MARROW TRANSPLANTATION (FIG. 3)

Only patients under the age of 60 are considered suitable for autologous bone-marrow transplantation, and under the age of 55 for allogeneic. The place of transplantation is still under evaluation. The high-intensity treatment approach provided by the pretransplant preparative regimen is considered to be more effective than chemotherapy alone for eradicating leukaemia, but differences in the outcome after chemotherapy alone and marrow transplantation in terms of disease-free survival are less clear-cut. This is because transplantation carries a significant treatment-related mortality, in the region of 25 per cent for allografts and 10 per cent for autografts. Furthermore, there is an as yet undefined risk that after autologous bone-marrow transplantation, residual leukaemia cells from the transplant inoculum may reseed in the recipient and cause relapse. Allogeneic transplantation is nevertheless considered the treatment of choice for younger patients with a fully HLA-matched sibling donor. Autologous transplantation is under evaluation in several trials where patients are randomized to receive marrow or chemotherapy as postremission treatment. Until the results of these studies are evaluated it is incorrect to hold dogmatic views in favour of one or other treatment.

Relapse rates for patients achieving remission vary widely according to the disease type. In general, *de novo* AML has a much greater chance of sustained remission than secondary AML. Younger patients and children especially have a lower chance of relapse. Even after consolidation chemotherapy alone some series report disease-free survivals for children in the region of 40 per cent. For adults this figure falls to around 25 per cent and decreases further in patients over the age of 65 years.

Allogeneic bone-marrow transplantation gives an overall 5-year disease-free survival of 65 per cent for patients transplanted in first remission. This is, however, in a selected group of patients under 50 years. Disease-free survival after autologous transplantation is similar, in the region of 50 to 60 per cent. Autologous marrow transplantation is done in a selected younger population of patients who are in a stable remission with a cellular marrow. With results of randomized trials still pending it is not possible to state categorically that bone marrow transplantation offers a better chance of survival than would be achieved with contemporary chemotherapy. Several national studies in Europe and the United States are in progress in an attempt to resolve the question of which treatment to use in patients in remission from AML.

TREATMENT OF ACUTE PROMYELOCYTIC LEUKAEMIA WITH ALL-*TRANS*-RETINOIC ACID

The t(15;17) chromosome translocation specific for acute promyelocytic leukaemia (**APML**) is believed to cause an alteration in the signalling properties of the retinoic acid receptor–ligand complex. The consequence is a block to granulocyte differentiation manifest as APML. Treatment with all-*trans*-retinoic acid (**ATRA**) appears to overcome this block allowing maturation of leukaemia cells to neutrophils, in the process exhausting the proliferative potential of the leukaemia, and inducing a remission. ATRA can be used alone to induce first and second remissions in APML by differentiating the leukaemic clone. In most patients treated with ATRA there is the rapid resolution of disseminated intravascular coagulation, followed by a progressive rise in the leucocyte count. At this stage the circulating leucocytes appear to represent the leukaemic clone with partially differentiated forms and some abnormal mature neutrophils. The leucocytosis persists for about 30 days. Following this there is a return to normal granulopoiesis and full haematological remission with normal marrow karyotype. The place of ATRA in the treatment of APML is still under evaluation. Its main value may lie in its ability to induce remission with or without additional chemotherapy. However, continued ATRA treatment does not maintain remission, and attempts to induce second remissions, in patients already treated with ATRA, are usually ineffective. To cure the leukaemia postremission treatment with chemotherapy or bone marrow transplantation appears to be necessary.

FUTURE DIRECTIONS

New antileukaemic drugs and other agents

The emergence of improved chemotherapeutic agents such as idarubicin (a new anthracycline), or new classes of drugs such as homoharringtonine are likely to produce only small improvements in remission induction and survival. The possibility of finding a chemotherapeutic agent

Fig. 3 Treatment response in acute myeloblastic leukaemia.

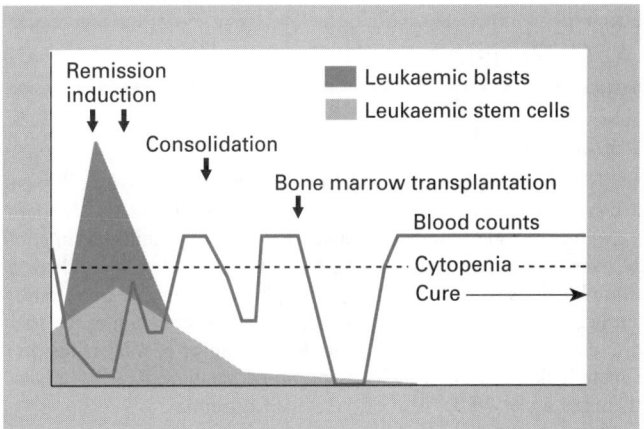

that possesses greater antileukaemic specificity remains more remote. Advances are more likely to be seen with the application of cytokines manufactured for clinical use by recombinant gene technology, probably in conjunction with chemotherapy. However, while agents such as the interferons, interleukins 2 and 6, and leukaemic inhibitory factor demonstrate therapeutic effects against leukaemia cells *in vitro*, much more has to be learned about their administration, interaction, and side-effects before they are likely to provide clinical benefit.

Immunotherapy

Initial attempts in the 1970s to stimulate the patient's own immune response to the leukaemia by immunization with BCG or irradiated leukaemia cells failed to demonstrate convincing benefit in AML. Antileukaemic activity can be induced in both autologous and alloreactive lymphocytes by culture with interleukin 2. Studies combining autologous bone-marrow transplantation with lymphokine-activated, killer-cell infusions are under way but this approach is at present experimental. In the future, more effective control of minimal residual disease could be achieved by combining cytoreductive chemotherapy with transfusions of lymphocytes with antileukaemic properties.

REFERENCES

Barrett, A.J. and Gordon, M.Y. (1990). Strategies in the treatment of acute myeloid leukaemia. In *Bone marrow disorders, the biological basis of treatment*, (ed. A.J. Barrett and M.Y. Gordon). Blackwell, Oxford (in press).

Bennett, J.M. *et al.* (1985). Proposed revised criteria for the classification of acute myeloid leukaemia: a report of the French-American-British cooperative group. *Annals of Internal Medicine*, **103**, 620–5.

Castaigne, S. *et al.* (1990). All *trans* retinoic acid as a differentiation therapy for acute promyelocytic leukaemia. *Blood*, **76**, 1704–9.

Devereux, S. (1991). Therapy associated leukaemia. *Blood Reviews*, **5**, 138–45.

Foon, K.A. and Gale, R.P. (1992). Therapy of acute myelogenous leukaemia. *Blood Reviews*, **6**, 15–25.

Swirsky, D.M., de Bastos, M., Parish, S.E., Rees, J.K.H., and Hayhoe, F.G.J. (1986). Features affecting outcome during remission of acute myeloid leukaemia of 619 patients. *British Journal of Haematology*, **64**, 435–53.

Swirsky, D. and Hoyle, C. (1989). Morphology and cytochemistry of species chromosome abnormalities in acute myeloid leukaemia. In *Leukaemia cytochemistry—principles and practice*, (ed. C.S. Scott), pp. 180–200. Ellis Horwood, Chichester.

Tiley, C. and Powles, R.A. (1992). The role of bone marrow transplantation in the management of acute myeloid leukaemia. In *Bone marrow transplantation in practice*, (ed. J.G. Treleaven and A.J. Barrett), pp. 11–19. Churchill Livingstone, Edinburgh.

22.3.4 Acute lymphoblastic leukaemia

I. A. G. ROBERTS

Introduction

Acute lymphoblastic leukaemia (**ALL**) is a biologically diverse disease that can affect any age group from neonates to the elderly. Modern therapeutic strategies can cure around 70 per cent of children. In contrast, over 70 per cent of adults with ALL ultimately die of their disease or complications of its treatment. Although malignant disease is infrequent in childhood, leukaemia constitutes the most common of the paediatric cancers. Approximately 30 to 40 per cent of paediatric cancers are acute leukaemias, of which around 80 per cent are ALL. In adults, ALL forms about 20 per cent of the acute leukaemias.

Incidence

Recent data from the United States show an age-adjusted incidence of ALL of around 1.0 to 1.3 cases per 100 000. This represents some 3000 cases diagnosed every year, approximately two-thirds of which are in children. The incidence of ALL in the United Kingdom and other Western European countries is similar and appears to have changed little since accurate records have been kept. It is difficult to look at trends before this time as earlier studies tended to group all types of leukaemia together; there have also been considerable changes in classification schemes and diagnostic capabilities. Another way of looking at the data is that there is a risk of around 1:2000 of a child developing ALL during the first 15 years of life.

The incidence of ALL varies with age, sex and, possibly, race. There is a well-recognized peak at the age of 2 to 5 years, then a drop which holds steady until the age of 60 years when the rate begins to increase again; this hints at the existence of two distinct diseases with independent risk factors. ALL in children is approximately 30 per cent more common in boys overall; this effect is more marked in T-ALL in which the ratio of affected boys:girls is 4:1. As for other childhood malignancies, the incidence of ALL appears to be lower in black children (only half that of white children). It is possible that this is due to a social class effect, although this observation remains true even in recent studies from the United States.

Aetiology

RISK FACTORS

A number of risk factors for the development of ALL have been identified. These broadly fall into two groups: those which are clearly hereditary and those which appear to be largely attributable to environmental influences (Table 1). Some single-gene defects associated with an increased risk of ALL are fairly well characterized. Patients with ataxia-telangiectasia, for example, who are homozygous for the A-T gene on the long arm of chromosome 11 (at 11q23), have an approximately 10 per cent risk of developing ALL, particularly T-cell ALL. Chromosomal disorders, which may involve several genes, such as Fanconi anaemia and Down's syndrome, are also important predisposing risk factors for the development of ALL, although in the former acute myeloid leukaemia (**AML**) is much more common than ALL. Recent reports show that around 2 per cent of all children with ALL have Down's syndrome. Familial cases of ALL are well described. There is an approximately four-fold risk that a sibling of a child with ALL will also develop the disease. The risk in monozygotic twins may be much higher, particularly in younger children, concordance rates in infancy approaching 100 per cent.

In the vast majority of cases of ALL, however, an underlying hereditary cause cannot be identified. A small proportion of these can be shown to be causally related to known leukaemogenic stimuli, such as radiation or retroviruses. Amongst children exposed to whole-body radiation from the atomic bombs in Japan, for example, there was an almost sixfold increase in the incidence of leukaemia, predominantly ALL. At least eight epidemiological studies since 1985 have addressed the issue of an increased risk of acute leukaemia (ALL and AML) in individuals living near power plants or nuclear reprocessing plants. Most studies have shown a small but not statistically significant increase in risk. In one recent review and meta-analysis, however, the crude summary measure of leukaemia risk among nuclear workers when age adjusted was about 1.5 and was statistically significant. Some important, but highly controversial, recent evidence suggests that childhood acute leukaemia, under special circumstances, may be initiated in the parental germ line. This conclusion was based on a very detailed case control study of young people born in Cumbria in the north of England and diagnosed with leukaemia or lymphoma while living there. A significantly high

Table 1 *Risk factors for acute lymphoblastic leukaemia*

Hereditary
Single-gene diseases:
  Bloom's syndrome
  Ataxia telangiectasia
  Schwachman's syndrome
  Achondroplasia
  Xeroderma pigmentosum
  Primary immunodeficiency diseases, e.g. congenital X-linked
    agammaglobulinaemia
Chromosomal disorders
  Fanconi anaemia
  Down's syndrome
Other familial associations
  Siblings, especially twins

Environmental
Radiation
  Diagnostic X-rays
  Radiotherapy
  Nuclear accidents/warfare
  ? Radiation from nuclear power installations
Viruses
  HTLV-1
Others*
  Smoking
  Electromagnetic fields
  Pesticides
  Chloramphenicol

* Causal association not proven.

relative risk was found for children whose fathers were employed at a nearby nuclear installation at the time of their conception and for those for whom dosimetry information was available the radiation doses in the period before conception were higher than the matched control fathers. This suggests that exposure of men to ionizing radiation may be leukaemogenic in their offspring. This fascinating observation remains to be confirmed in other and larger studies.

To date, human T-lymphotrophic virus 1 (**HTLV-1**) provides the only known example of retrovirus-induced leukaemia in humans. Infection with HTLV-1 is strongly associated with the development of adult T-cell leukaemia/lymphoma (**ATLL**). ATLL cells contain clonally integrated HTLV-1 genomic sequences, indicating the direct involvement of the virus in the oncogenic process. The genome of HTLV-1 encodes a 40-kDa protein, tax, which is able to transactivate a variety of viral and cellular promoters, including those involved in the regulation of T-cell growth (e.g. interleukin 2 and the α-chain of its receptor), and which may be responsible for the leukaemic transformation of infected T-cells.

PATHOPHYSIOLOGY

ALL results from clonal expansion of immature lymphoblastic cells. It is now clear that from the pathophysiological, as well as the clinical, point of view ALL is a heterogeneous disease; many subtypes can be identified by cytochemical, karyotypic, immunological, and molecular criteria. In most cases, however, the target cell which undergoes leukaemic transformation appears to be a lymphoid progenitor cell that is already committed to the B- or T-cell lineage and has therefore undergone immunoglobulin gene or T-cell receptor gene rearrangement, respectively. Equivalent normal cells are found in fetal tissues and in bone marrow and thymus after birth. Their leukaemic counterparts, however, may show asynchrony of gene expression resulting in an uncoupling of growth from differentiation. In addition, ALL cells tend to have diverse patterns of immunoglobulin and T-cell receptor gene rearrange-

ment, which may include incomplete or aberrant rearrangements and cross-lineage rearrangement of inappropriate genes. These patterns of gene rearrangement provide an indication of the clonality of ALL cells: each individual ALL cell clone is characterized by a unique junctional region of rearranged immunoglobulin and/or T-cell receptor genes.

The most frequently seen subtype of ALL, particularly in children, is common ALL, which has a pre-B-cell phenotype. One model proposes a two-stage pattern of leukaemogenesis specific for early pre-B-cell ALL that takes into account what is known about its epidemiology, the target cell, and its molecular basis. In this model the process of leukaemogenesis begins *in utero*. Spontaneous mutations, which are generated during the normal process of genetic recombination in lymphoid progenitor cells in the fetus, give rise *in utero* to a premalignant clone. After birth a second genetic event, determined by environmental influences, results in expansion of this clone into clinically overt ALL. The catalyst for this second event may simply be exposure of the child to a common childhood viral infection, which then results in immune stimulation. It is suggested that delayed exposure (i.e. in childhood rather than infancy) to a common infection may be the important factor that causes the proliferation of B-cell precursors to be abnormally regulated, leading to the development of ALL. This interesting hypothesis remains to be explored but it is certainly consistent with the higher frequency of ALL in the socially privileged classes and the many different characteristics of the disease in children compared to adults.

MOLECULAR BIOLOGY OF ACUTE LYMPHOBLASTIC LEUKAEMIA

Although it has been recognized for many years that specific karyotypic abnormalities are frequently associated with particular subtypes of ALL, it is only recently that the genes involved in these chromosomal rearrangements have begun to be identified. Some of the best characterized examples are shown in Table 2.

There is recent evidence that some of the translocations involve genes which code for transcriptional regulators. This can result in the activity of these genes becoming dysregulated or ectopically expressed, or a novel transcriptional regulator may be produced. For example, in the translocation t(1;19,q23,p13), which is the most common cytogenetic abnormality detected in childhood ALL, two such genes, *PBX1* and *E2A*, become fused to form a novel transcription factor gene. ALL carrying the t(9;22)(q34;q11) chromosomal abnormality is known as Philadelphia-positive ALL, the Philadelphia chromosome being the abnormal chromosome 22 bearing DNA translocated from chromosome 9. While the cytogenetic abnormalities appear identical to those seen in the majority of cases of chronic myeloid leukaemia, at the molecular level the *bcr–abl* fusion gene formed and the resultant fusion protein produced by the leukaemic cells, differ in ALL from that in most cases of chronic myeloid leukaemic. Philadelphia-positive ALL is now known to be a common form of adult ALL, although it is relatively uncommon in childhood. Most of the rearrangements in T-ALL involve the T-cell receptor-α, -β, or -δ loci; for example, in the translocation t(1;14)(p34; q11) the *tal-1* gene is transcribed as a result of rearrangement with the T-cell receptor-δ locus.

Clinical features

PRESENTATION

Patients may present acutely or insidiously with symptoms present for several weeks or even months. Many of the symptoms are non-specific. They reflect the uncontrolled growth of leukaemic cells in bone marrow and extramedullary sites, particularly the lymphoid system. The most common presentations and some of the more unusual ones are shown in Table 3. The differential diagnosis may include immune thrombocytopenia, neuroblastoma, rheumatoid or other forms of acute arthritis,

Table 2 *Cytogenetic and molecular genetic abnormalities in acute lymphoblastic leukaemia (ALL)*

Chromosomal abnormality	Genes involved	Subtype of ALL
t(9;22)(q34;q11)	*bcr, abl*	Often early or pre-B:
	bcr–abl fusion gene and mRNA are formed	3.5% of childhood ALL; 40% of adult ALL
t(1;19)(q23;p13)	*PBX1, E2A*	25% of childhood pre-B ALL
	PBX1–E2A fusion gene mRNA and protein are formed	Often pre-B:
t(8;14)(q24;q32)	*myc, IgH*	B-ALL:
	myc–IgH fusion gene	2% of childhood ALL
t(8;22)(q24;q11)	*myc, Igλ*	B-ALL
t(2;8)(p11;q24)	*myc, Igκ*	B-ALL
t(1;7)(p32–4;q34)	*tal*-1, *TCR*β	T-ALL
	tal–TCR-β fusion	
t(1;14)(p32-4; q11)	*tal*-1, *TCR*-δ	T-ALL
	tal–TCR-δ fusion	
t(7;9)(q34;q32)	*TCR*-β, *tal*-2	T-ALL
t(7;10)(q34-5;q24)	*TCR*-β, *HOX11*	T-ALL
t(7;19)(q35;p13)	*TCR*-β, *lyl*-1	T-ALL
t(11;14)(p15; q11)	Rhombotin-1/*TCR*-δ	T-ALL

TCR, T-cell receptor.

Table 3 *Clinical features of acute lymphoblastic leukaemia at presentation*

Common signs and symptoms
Lethargy and irritability
Pallor
Fever
Bone and joint pain
Bleeding, bruising, and petechiae
Hepatosplenomegaly
Lymphadenopathy: usually generalized and painless
Central nervous disease (5% of children, 15% of adults)
Mediastinal mass (especially in T-ALL)

Unusual presentations
Aplastic anaemia
Eosinophilia
Isolated renal failure
Pulmonary nodules
Pericardial effusion
Skin nodules

infectious mononucleosis and related viral infections, tuberculosis, aplastic anaemia, lymphoma and myeloproliferative disorders, including chronic myeloid leukaemia.

DISEASE OF THE CENTRAL NERVOUS SYSTEM

Central nervous system disease is uncommon at presentation, occurring in less than 5 per cent of children and around 15 per cent of adults. However, if prophylactic treatment is not given (see later), it has been shown to occur in the majority of patients. In most cases it is thought to result from seeding of the meninges by leukaemic cells, although direct spread from cranial bone marrow has been reported. The presenting symptoms and signs are due to raised intracranial pressure and include headache, nausea, vomiting, lethargy, irritability, papilloedema, and nuchal rigidity. Occasional. patients present with cranial nerve palsies, particularly of the IIIrd, IVth, VIIth, or facial nerves. The hypothalamic–obesity syndrome is a rare complication and is due to thalamic infiltration. The diagnosis of central nervous disease is made by examination of the cerebrospinal fluid; the pressure, protein, and leucocyte count are usually elevated, with a normal or reduced glucose. The peripheral blood count may be normal. However, relapse of ALL in the bone marrow is usually noted concurrently or within weeks.

OTHER SITES OF EXTRAMEDULLARY DISEASE

Although hepatosplenomegaly is common, liver function tests are usually normal or only mildly deranged. Renal enlargement may also occur due to leukaemic infiltration but this is also rarely associated with organ dysfunction. In boys the testis is a fairly common site of relapse of ALL, occurring in 10 to 15 per cent. It presents as painless, usually unilateral, testicular enlargement. Testicular relapse may be isolated but is often followed by relapse in the bone marrow. Routine testicular biopsies have now been abandoned due to difficulties in their interpretation and a high false-negative rate.

Diagnosis (Plates 8, 9)

In most cases the diagnosis is straightforward. The majority of patients are anaemic, neutropenic, and thrombocytopenic due to leukaemic infiltration of the bone marrow. The total leucocyte count is usually in the range of 5000 to 25 000×10⁹/l. However, leucocyte counts of in excess of 100 000×10⁹/l and under 5000×10⁹/l are not uncommon. All patients should have a bone marrow aspirate and trephine biopsy. This should allow an accurate diagnosis of the subtype of ALL to be made. This is based on the morphology of the leukaemic cells assessed by standard and special cytochemical stains, their immunophenotype and their karyotype. The diagnosis may be particularly difficult in patients who present with pancytopenia: in such patients it may be necessary to repeat the bone marrow aspirate and biopsy after a few weeks.

CLASSIFICATION OF THE SUBTYPES OF ALL

Morphology

The leukaemic blast cells in ALL can be quite heterogeneous in their appearance under the light microscope. As for AML, the French-American-British (**FAB**) Co-operative Working Group devised a classification scheme based on particular morphological characteristics. The FAB classification of ALL (Table 4) is widely used and appears to have some prognostic value although, with the exception of L3, it does not correlate with the immunophenotype or karyotype of the ALL cells.

Table 4 *The FAB classification of acute lymphoblastic leukaemia*

FAB class	Cytological appearance	Incidence (%)
L1	Small lymphoblasts with scanty cytoplasm and indistinct nucleoli	85
L2	Larger, more heterogeneous lymphoblasts with more cytoplasm, an irregular nuclear membrane and prominent nucleoli	10–15
L3	Large lymphoblasts with deeply basophilic vacuolated, cytoplasm and one or more nucleoli	1–3

Immunophenotyping

Classification of ALL cells by immunophenotyping has proved to be very helpful both for our understanding of the biology of the disease (see above) and, by providing useful prognostic information, for its management. Most haematology laboratories now use a panel of monoclonal antibodies that allow ALL cells to be classified into five main groups: **B cell;** early B, common, pre-B, and mature B; and **T cell**.

Useful monoclonal antibodies for identifying T cells are CD7, CD2 and CD3; antibodies for B cells include CD19 and CD22; common ALL cells are also positive with CD10, which is known as the CALLA or common ALL antigen.

Cytogenetics

Karyotypic abnormalities can be identified in leukaemic blast cells from 70 to 90 per cent of patients with ALL. These abnormalities are either numerical, that is chromosome loss (hypodiploidy) or gain (hyperdiploidy), or structural, usually translocations. Many of the structural karyotypic abnormalities can be related to specific immonophenotypes—t(8;14) with B-ALL, t(1;19) with pre-B ALL and t(1;7) with T-ALL for example; others (e.g. t(9;22)) have a variable immunophenotype. The most common structural cytogenetic abnormality in adults is t(9;22), that is, Philadelphia-positive ALL, and in children t(1;19).

Both numerical and structural cytogenetic abnormalities have been shown to have prognostic significance. The best prognosis is associated with hyperdiploidy with a modal number of chromosomes in excess of 50. The Philadelphia chromosome and certain other translocations such as t(8;14), t(4;11) and t(1;19) appear to be associated with a poor prognosis. In addition, the presence of residual cells with a normal karyotype appears to confer a better prognosis.

Management

Long-term survival in childhood ALL currently approaches 60 to 70 per cent and efforts are now directed towards minimizing the long-term side-effects of chemoradiotherapy by not overtreating children with a low probability of relapsing. In adults, however, long-term disease-free survival is 30 to 35 per cent at best and attempts to intensify treatment continue, including the optimum use of bone marrow transplantation. To address these issues, recent studies run by collaborative groups in Europe and the United States have stratified patients into different 'risk groups' based on factors found to have prognostic importance (see below) such as the presenting leucocyte count, age, and the immunophenotype and/or cytogenetics of the ALL cells.

CURRENT CONCEPTS OF TREATMENT

There are four main components to our current approach to treating ALL in any age group:

(1) remission induction;
(2) intensification chemotherapy;
(3) prophylaxis of central nervous involvement;
(4) maintenance treatment.

During all of these phases of treatment the importance of good supportive care cannot be overemphasized. The principles of supportive care for patients with ALL are identical to those for AML and are described in detail in the chapter on AML. They include the prevention and prompt treatment of viral, fungal, and bacterial infection, appropriate blood-product replacement for anaemia and thrombocytopenia, maintenance of good hydration and nutrition, and psychological support.

Remission induction

The aim of remission induction is to reduce the total number of leukaemic cells to levels undetectable by conventional means; that is, under 5 per cent leukaemic blast cells present on the marrow aspirate after this phase of treatment. The most useful drugs to achieve this have been shown to be oral prednisolone, intravenous vincristine, and intramuscular or subcutaneous L-asparaginase. These three drugs given in combination over 3 to 4 weeks are sufficient to induce complete remission in more than 95 per cent of children and around 80 per cent of adults. This approach is well established and supported by the results of national trials in thousands of patients in the United Kingdom, Germany, and the United States. Treatment is generally very well tolerated, without major immediate toxicity. Failure to induce remission is likely to be due to drug-resistant leukaemic cells present from the outset or to the early emergence of new drug-resistant clones. To try and prevent this, most patients now receive further intensive chemotherapy almost immediately after remission is induced.

Intensification chemotherapy

This aims to further reduce minimal residual leukaemia. The nature of the intensification used has been varied in different studies in order to try and target the patients at highest risk of relapse. The addition of drugs such as cytosine arabinoside and daunorubicin at this stage of treatment has been successful in improving survival. The role of allogeneic marrow transplantation as further intensification therapy in ALL once remission has been achieved is controversial and is discussed below.

Prophylaxis in the central nervous system

It was shown many years ago that one of the main reasons for ALL relapse was the presence of 'sanctuary' sites of disease where leukaemic cells were presumed to be exposed to non-lethal doses of chemotherapy. The most common of these sites is in the central nervous system; without prophylaxis up to 75 per cent of patients will relapse in the central nervous system. Most current treatment schedules recommend a combination of intrathecal chemotherapy (usually methotrexate) and cranial irradiation for the majority of patients. Cranial irradiation should not be given to infants under 1 year of age because of the risk of severe brain damage. It is possible that children estimated to be at low risk of relapse may also be satisfactorily managed with intrathecal therapy alone, but this remains controversial. Central nervous prophylaxis is started immediately after recovery from intensification chemotherapy.

Maintenance treatment

The addition of several years of maintenance treatment to the schedule of remission induction/intensification and central nervous prophylaxis has been shown to be of definite value in childhood ALL and probably also in adults; when it is omitted survival appears to be inferior. The aim of maintenance is to suppress the growth of any residual leukaemic cells. The drugs used are continuous oral 6-mercaptopurine and weekly methotrexate together with intermittent vincristine and prednisolone. The optimum duration of maintenance therapy has not been established, but trials suggest somewhere between 2 and 3 years. Recent studies show that the maintenance of adequate doses of 6-mercaptopurine on a continuous, rather than intermittent, basis is one of the most important factors influencing relapse: the dose used needs to be myelosuppressive and should usually only be reduced when the neutrophil count drops below 1000×10^9/l. During maintenance treatment all patients should be treated with continuous low-dose co-trimoxazole to prevent infection with *Pneumocystis carinii*.

TREATMENT OF CENTRAL NERVOUS LEUKAEMIA

A small proportion of patients present with disease in the central nervous system. This is treated by intrathecal chemotherapy, craniospinal irradiation and systemic chemotherapy as for marrow disease, including intensification and maintenance therapy. Some 10 per cent of patients without evidence of central nervous disease at diagnosis will experience a central nervous relapse despite appropriate prophylaxis. The choice of treatment is difficult, particularly for those who have previously received cranial irradiation, as the toxicity of further irradiation may be considerable. Nevertheless, reinduction with systemic chemotherapy and intrathecal therapy is successful in a proportion of patients and long-term cure is still possible.

TREATMENT OF RELAPSED ALL

The most common site of relapse of ALL, in patients who have received central nervous prophylaxis, is the bone marrow. In most children and in 50 to 60 per cent of adults a second remission can be induced. Patients who relapse while still on maintenance therapy tend to have a worse prognosis, fewer than 5 per cent having a disease-free long-term survival. The treatment for relapsed ALL usually consists of the same chemotherapy as employed to induce remission at the initial presentation, although in patients with early relapse alternative agents, such as high-dose cytosine arabinoside or methotrexate, may be used. Following this, most centres now offer allogeneic bone marrow transplantation to all suitable patients who achieve a second remission, who are under 50 to 55 years old and who have an HLA-compatible sibling.

THE ROLE OF BONE MARROW TRANSPLANTATION IN THE TREATMENT OF ACUTE LYMPHOBLASTIC LEUKAEMIA

The role of marrow transplantation in ALL is still controversial, although some consensus is beginning to emerge as a result of statistical analysis, by groups such as the International Bone Marrow Transplant Registry, of patient data contributed by transplant centres from all over the world. In summary, allogeneic transplantation is a valuable treatment option for those patients with a predictably poor treatment outcome ('high risk' ALL), for those that fail initial remission induction, and for relapsed patients who achieve a second remission. In all these patient groups, long-term disease-free survival appears to be significantly better; around 25 to 35 per cent compared to 5 per cent or less. The exception may be children with 'high risk' ALL in first remission for whom the results of chemotherapy seem to be equivalent to allogeneic bone-marrow transplantation.

For those patients without an HLA-compatible sibling, two other options have been explored: autologous bone-marrow transplantation and transplantation using marrow from an HLA-identical, unrelated donor. There are still insufficient data to evaluate the results of the latter. Similarly, although many thousands of patients have now been autografted, it remains to be proved that this approach is superior to conventional chemotherapy. Autologous bone-marrow transplantation in first remission appears to lead to long-term disease-free survival in 25 to 55 per cent of patients. Survival has been shown to be lower in patients autografted in second remission. The results are similar in children and adults.

LATE EFFECTS OF TREATMENT FOR ALL

The increasing number of patients surviving long-term after treatment for ALL, particularly childhood ALL, has highlighted the importance of lifelong follow-up of such patients to assess the late effects of high-dose chemoradiotherapy. The most common late effects are those due to structural damage in the central nervous system, endocrine abnormalities, and second malignancies.

The central nervous system changes include a reduction in head circumference and abnormalities of white matter detectable on computerized tomographic scan. Cognitive defects, though difficult to assess, appear to be mild but common and to be apparent even many years after treatment has been completed. These include reduction in Intelligence Quotient, impaired memory, and difficulty with mathematical problems and concentration. The degree of damage is greater in children treated when they are under 4 years old and those who need to have cranial irradiation repeated as a result of relapse in the central nervous system.

The most common endocrine abnormality is growth hormone deficiency, but this is rarely a clinical problem. Primary hypothyroidism occurs in around 3 per cent of children. Gonadotrophin levels are frequently low but are often unhelpful in predicting fertility and overall the long-term effects on fertility are unclear, owing to insufficient data. However, there are now many examples of successful parenthood after treatment for ALL in childhood and no excess of malignancies or congenital abnormalities has been reported in the offspring. Second malignancies occur in around 8 per cent of long-term survivors. The most common are intracranial tumours and haematological malignancies, including AML and non-Hodgkin's lymphomas.

Prognosis

PROGNOSTIC FACTORS AND RISK GROUPS

Over the years a large number of different groups have published lists of prognostic factors, some of which are common to all the studies while others are only significant in a minority. As more is learnt about the biology of ALL, more accurate classification of subtypes should help to identify much more accurately those patients with a better or worse prognosis. Currently, those factors that appear to be useful prognostically fall into two categories: pretreatment variables (e.g. age) and treatment-dependent variables.

The important pretreatment variables are age, the leucocyte count at diagnosis, the immunophenotype, and the karyotype of the ALL cells. For age, the poorest prognosis is in infants and in patients over 60 years. In general, the prognosis worsens progressively after the age of 10 years. For leucocyte count, different studies have established different ranges; however, it is clear that patients who present with a leucocyte count in excess of $100\,000 \times 10^9$/l fare worst. Patients with ALL with a T-cell or mature B-cell phenotype were thought to have a much worse prognosis. Recent results using more intensive chemotherapy have markedly improved the prospects for these patients, especially in childhood, but adults with T- and B-ALL still have a poorer prognosis than those with other ALL phenotypes. As mentioned above, the presence of the Philadelphia chromosome and other translocations such as t(8;14), t(4;11) and t(1;19), as well as hypodiploidy, appear to be associated with a poor prognosis.

The important treatment-dependent variables appear to be the initial response to a single cytostatic drug and the time taken to achieve complete remission. Patients with a good initial response and a short time to remission are twice as likely to achieve long-term disease-free survival.

The prognostic information from all of these studies has been used by several groups to stratify children, and more recently adults, into different risk groups. It has already led to improved survival in some subtypes of ALL, especially B-ALL in children. In the future it should result in more rational therapy for all patients with ALL and identify those who should be offered more intensive therapy, including BMT, new chemotherapy regimens, and perhaps more novel therapeutic approaches such as biological-response modifiers. In addition, the application of molecular techniques to the detection of minimal residual disease or early relapse may yield data critical for tailoring therapy to individual patients.

SURVIVAL

In childhood, 60 to 70 per cent of patients can now be cured using chemotherapy and central nervous prophylaxis. For those that relapse, allogeneic bone-marrow transplantation will cure around 25 to 35 per cent, chemotherapy possibly rather fewer. In adulthood, long-term disease-free survival with chemotherapy alone varies from 5 per cent in high-risk ALL to around 50 per cent in low-risk disease. Allogeneic transplantation in first remission probably cures around 40 per cent of patients and is therefore a good option for those with high risk ALL; in second remission, it still offers a 25 per cent chance of cure to adults who have relapsed. While these results offer grounds for more optimism than 20 years ago, it is salutary to note than more than half of the adults who develop ALL will die from their disease. Novel therapeutic strategies, perhaps based on the exciting new information becoming available from studying the molecular and biological basis of ALL, are an important goal for the future.

REFERENCES

Berger, R. (1992). The cytogenetics of haematological malignancies. *Clinical Haematology*, **5**, 791–814.
Champlin, R.E. and Gale, R.P. (1989). Acute lymphoblastic leukemia: recent advances in biology and therapy. *Blood*, **73**, 2051–66.
Eden, O.B. *et al.* (1991) Results of Medical Research Council Childhood Leukaemia Trial UKALL VIII (Report to the Medical Research Council on behalf of the Working Party on Leukaemia in Childhood). *British Journal of Haematology*, **78**, 187–96.
Gardner, M.J. *et al.* (1990). Results of a case control study of leukaemia and lymphoma among young people near Sellafield nuclear plant in West Cumbria. *British Medical Journal*, **300**, 423–9.
Godyn, J. (1988). Two different classification schemes of acute lymphoblastic leukemia. *British Journal of Haematology*, **69**, 100–2.
Greaves, M. (1992) Biological diversity of acute lymphoblastic leukaemia. *British Journal of Haematology*, **82**, 181–2.
Greaves, M. (1988). Speculations on the cause of childhood acute lymphoblastic leukaemia. *Leukaemia*, **2**, 120–5.
Hann, I.M. (1992). CNS-directed therapy in childhood acute lymphoblastic leukaemia. *British Journal of Haematology*, **82**, 2–5.
Horowitz, M.M. *et al.* (1991). Chemotherapy compared with bone marrow transplantation for adults with acute lymphoblastic leukaemia in first remission. *Annals of Internal Medicine*, **115**, 13–18.
Ochs, J. and Mulhearn, R.K. (1988). Late effects of anti-leukemic treatment. *Pediatric Clinics of North America*, **35**, 815–33.
Pui, C-H., Crist, W.M. and Look, A.T. (1990). Biology and clinical significance of cytogenetic abnormalities in childhood acute lymphoblastic leukaemia. *Blood*, **76**, 1449–63.
Rabbitts, T.H. (1991). Translocations, master genes and differences between the origins of acute and chronic leukaemias. *Cell*, **67**, 641–4.
Sachii, N. (1991). Leukemia in Down's syndrome. *Leukaemia*, **5**, 822–3.
Wheeler, K., Leiper, A.D., Jannoun, L., and Chessells, J.M. (1987). Medical cost of curing childhood acute lymphoblastic leukaemia. *British Medical Journal*, **296**, 162–6.
Yokota, S. *et al.* (1991). The use of polymerase chain reactions to monitor minimal residual disease in acute lymphoblastic leukemia patients. *Blood*, **77**, 331–9.

22.3.5 Chronic myeloid leukaemia

J. GOLDMAN

Chronic myeloid leukaemia, also known as chronic myelogenous or chronic granulocytic leukaemia, is a clonal disease of the pluripotential haemopoietic stem cell, whose progeny proliferates over months or more probably years and eventually usurps all normal marrow function. It was probably described originally in the 1840s but remained poorly characterized during most of the nineteenth century. It could be treated at the time with modest success with Fowler's solution (potassium arsenite). The disease was clearly recognized as a distinct form of leukaemia with the advent of panoptic stains for blood films at the end of the nineteenth century. One landmark in our understanding of the pathogenesis of chronic myeloid leukaemia was the discovery of the Philadelphia (**Ph**) chromosome in 1960; another was the characterization in the last decade of the *BCR-ABL* chimeric gene (see Sections 4 and 6). Until the 1980s, chronic myeloid leukaemia was assumed to be incurable and was treated palliatively, first with radiotherapy and more recently with alkylating agents, notably busulphan. It has become apparent in the last 10 years that it can be cured by bone marrow transplantation, but the proportion of patients eligible for this is still relatively small.

Classification

Most patients with chronic myeloid leukaemia have a relatively homogeneous disease characterized at diagnosis by splenomegaly, leucocytosis, and the presence of a Ph chromosome in marrow metaphases. A minority have a less typical disease that may be classified as atypical chronic myeloid leukaemia, chronic myelomonocytic leukaemia or chronic neutrophilic leukaemia. In none of these variants is there a Ph chromosome.

Epidemiology, aetiology, and natural history

The incidence of chronic myeloid leukaemia appears to be constant worldwide. It occurs in about 1/100 000 of the population in all countries where statistics are adequate. Chronic myeloid leukaemia is rare below the age of 20 years but occurs in all decades, with a median age of onset of 40 to 50 years. The risk is slightly greater in males than in females. The risk of developing chronic myeloid leukaemia is slightly but significantly increased by exposure to high doses of irradiation, as occurred in survivors of the atomic bombs exploded in Japan in 1945 and in patients irradiated for ankylosing spondylitis, but in general all cases are 'sporadic' and no predisposing factors are identifiable. In particular there is no familial predisposition and no known relevant infectious agent.

Chronic myeloid leukaemia is a biphasic or triphasic disease that is usually diagnosed in the initial 'chronic' or stable phase. The chronic phase lasts typically 2 to 6 years but it may on occasion last more than 10 or even 15 years. Unpredictably it transforms to a more aggressive phase that used to be referred to as blastic crisis and is now usually described as acute or blastic transformation. In the majority of cases the diseases evolves somewhat more gradually through an intermediate phase described as 'accelerated' disease, which may last for months or occasionally years, before frank transformation. Rare patients have a disease that progresses gradually to a myelofibrotic or myelosclerotic picture characterized by extensive marrow fibrosis with clinical problems due to failure of haemopoiesis rather than blast-cell proliferation. The duration of survival after onset of transformation is usually 2 to 6 months so the median survival from diagnosis is 4 to 5 years.

Many attempts have been made to subclassify or stage chronic myeloid leukaemia at diagnosis in a manner that would permit some prediction of the duration of the chronic phase in individual patients. The most commonly quoted classification, devised by Sokal in the 1980s, is based on a formula that takes account of the patient's age, blast-cell count, spleen size, and platelet count at diagnosis but it is still too inaccurate to be clinically useful. In practice the patient's response to initial treatment does give some information about duration of survival; those who have a low requirement for busulphan in the first year after diagnosis or who convert to Ph-negative haemopoiesis after treatment with interferon-α survive significantly longer than those who do not.

Cytogenetics and molecular biology

The Ph chromosome (see Sections 4 and 6) is an acquired cytogenetic abnormality that characterizes all leukaemic cells in chronic myeloid leukaemia. Reported originally in 1960 in metaphases from all dividing cells in the marrow of patients with chronic myeloid leukaemia, the Ph chromosome was the first example of a consistent chromosomal abnormality in malignant disease in man. It is formed as a result of a reciprocal translocation of genetic material between the long arms of one no. 22 chromosome and one no. 9 chromosome, an event described as t(9; 22)(q34;q11) (Fig. 1). The amount of material that moves from chromosome 22 to 9 is considerably greater than the amount that moves in the reverse direction, so the Ph chromosome appears in metaphase preparations of marrow cells as a 'stunted' 22 (formally 22q−). In patients with chronic myeloid leukaemia the Ph chromosome is present in all myeloid cell lineages, in some B cells, and in a very small proportion of T cells. It is found in no other cells of the body. This distribution is not altered by conventional treatment with busulphan or hydroxyurea. Though valuable as a marker of the leukaemic cells, its pathogenetic significance remained unclear for the next 24 years.

It was known since the early 1980s that the *ABL* proto-oncogene, the human homologue of the transforming sequence (v-*abl*) in the Abelson strain of the Moloney murine leukaemia virus, was situated normally on chromosome 9 and was translocated to chromosome 22 in patients with chronic myeloid leukaemia (see Sections 4 and 6). In 1984, Groffen and colleagues in Rotterdam showed that the precise position of the genomic breakpoint on chromosome 22 in a series of different patients with chronic myeloid leukaemia was clustered in a relatively small, 5.8-kb region to which he gave the name 'breakpoint cluster region' (bcr). Later it became clear that this region formed the central part of a relatively large gene now known as the *BCR* gene, whose normal function is unknown. The translocation results in juxtaposition of 5′ sequences from the *BCR* gene with 3′ *ABL* sequences derived from chromosome 9. Thus the Ph chromosome carries a chimeric gene, designated *BCR-*

ABL (Fig. 1), that encodes a protein of 210 kDa and has tyrosine kinase activity. The *BCR-ABL* gene is thought to play a pivotal part in the genesis of chronic-phase chronic myeloid leukaemia; the molecular basis of disease progression is still obscure, but evidence for involvement of the tumour suppressor gene p53 has been found in some cases.

Clinical features

Until recently the majority of patients presented with symptoms, usually attributable to splenomegaly or to anaemia. In recent years in 'developed' countries, chronic myeloid leukaemia has been diagnosed in almost 50 per cent of patients before the onset of symptoms as a result of 'routine' blood tests on healthy persons for pregnancy, before blood donation, or in the course of investigation for unrelated disorders. Symptoms when present may include lethargy, loss of energy, shortness of breath on exertion, or weight loss. Increased sweating is characteristic. Spontaneous bruising or unexplained bleeding from gums, intestinal or urinary tract are relatively common. Visual disturbances may occur. Fever and lymphadenopathy are rare in the chronic phase. The patient may have pain or discomfort in the splenic area or may have noticed a lump or mass in the right upper abdomen. Patients may present with features of gout or priapism, both of which are very rare.

Sixty to 80 per cent of patients have splenomegaly at diagnosis. The spleen varies from just palpable to being so large that it occupies all the left side of the abdomen and is palpable also in the right iliac fossa. The liver is frequently also enlarged but with a soft edge that is difficult to define. There may be no other abnormal findings. Ecchymoses of varying sizes and ages may be present, and some patients have asymptomatic retinal haemorrhages. Patients with very high leucocyte counts may have features of leucostasis with retinal-vein engorgement and pulmonary insufficiency.

Patients presenting with more advanced disease nearly always have some of the features described above. In addition they may have bone tenderness or signs of infection. In established transformation the spleen is frequently enlarged and may be painful. The liver may become very large. Patients may develop fever, lymphadenopathy, or, very rarely, lytic lesions of bone.

Haematology (Plates 10, 11)

Patients with splenomegaly are usually anaemic, while the haemoglobin concentration may be normal in those with 'early' disease. The leucocyte count at diagnosis is usually between 50 and 200 × 10⁹/l but the diag-

Fig. 1 A schematic representation of the Philadelphia chromosome showing the mechanism of formation of the chimeric *BCR-ABL* gene. Note that the positions of the normal ABL and BCR genes on chromosomes 9q34 and 22q11 respectively are shown to the left; to the right are the Ph (22q−) chromosome bearing the BCR-ABL fusion gene and the 9q+ (which bears the reciprocal chimeric gene designated ABL-BCR).

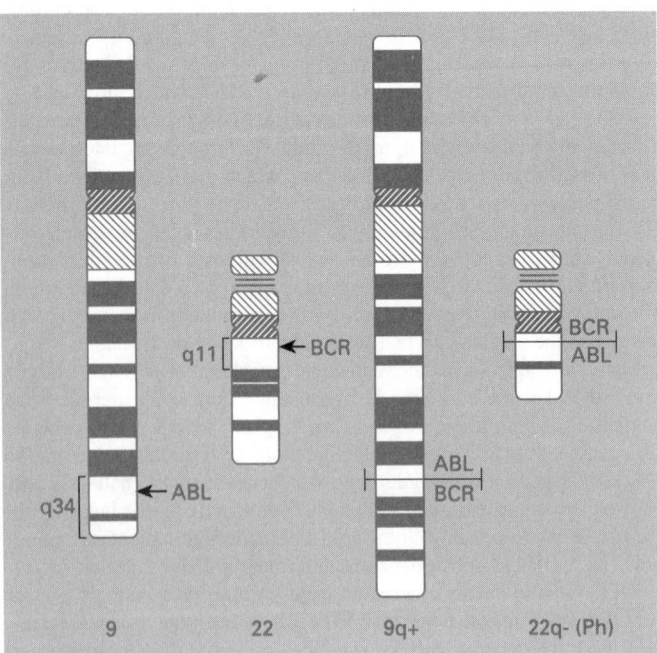

Fig. 2 Peripheral-blood appearances of a patient with chronic myeloid leukaemia at diagnosis. Note increased numbers of leucocytes including immature granulocytes and occasional blast cells.

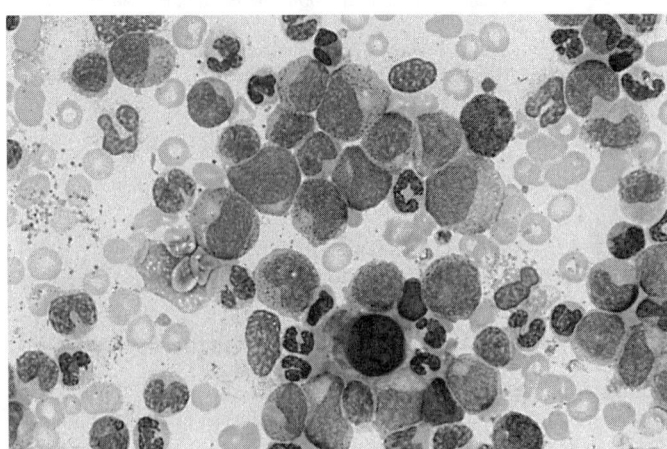

nosis of chronic myeloid leukaemia can be established in patients with persistent leucocytosis in the range 10 to 20 × 10⁹/l, and others may present with leucocyte numbers in the range 200 to 800 × 10⁹/l. The film shows a full spectrum of cells in the granulocyte series, ranging from blast forms to mature polymorphs (Fig. 2). The percentage of blast cells is loosely related to the absolute number of leucocytes but percentages higher than 12 suggest that the patient is already in acceleration or transformation. The percentage of eosinophils and basophils is increased. Absolute numbers of lymphocytes and monocytes are slightly increased but both are reduced as percentages in the differential count. Platelet numbers are usually increased in the range 300 to 600 × 10⁹/l, but may be normal or even reduced. Occasional nucleated red cells are present in the circulation in some patients. The alkaline phosphate content of the neutrophil cytoplasm is characteristically diminished or absent.

Examination of the bone marrow by aspiration or trephine biopsy is not necessary to confirm the diagnosis of chronic myeloid leukaemia but is usually done to assess the degree of marrow fibrosis, to make cytogenetic analyses, and to exclude transformation. The marrow aspirate shows multiple, small, hypercellular fragments and the trails show a cellular composition resembling that of the chronic myeloid leukaemic blood. Blast cells in chronic phase number 2 to 10 per cent. Eosinophils and basophils are usually prominent. Megakaryocytes are small, hypolobated but numerous. Occasionally, Gaucher-like cells are present. The marrow biopsy shows complete loss of fat spaces with dense hypercellularity. The reticulin content may be normal or modestly increased.

The haematological picture in acceleration is very variable. It may differ little from the chronic phase but the blast-cell number may be increased disproportionately. There may be anaemia in the presence of a normal leucocyte count. Platelet numbers may be greatly increased (over 1000 × 10⁹/10) or reduced (below 100 × 10⁹/l) in a manner not accounted for by treatment. The marrow also shows a picture no longer consistent with chronic-phase disease.

Blastic transformation is defined by the presence of more than 30 per cent blasts or blasts plus promyelocytes in the blood or marrow. Frequently this threshold is irrelevant because blast-cell numbers in both sites exceed 80 per cent. Their morphology is very variable. About 70 per cent of patients have blasts classifable generally as myeloid, which resemble to a degree the cells that characterize acute myeloid leukaemia (see Chapter 22.3.3). Such cells may be predominantly myeloblastic, monoblastic, erythroblastic, or megakaryoblastic, and mixtures of blast cells of different lineages frequently coexist. These cells are best defined by their cytochemical and immunophenotypic characteristics. About 20 per cent of patients have lymphoid blast cells; these may resemble the FAB-L1 cells that typify childhood acute lymphoblastic leukaemia (see Chapter 22.3.4) or more commonly have FAB−L2 appearances. Immunophenotyping shows the typical features of a B-cell acute lymphoblastic leukaemia, namely CD10 (CALLA) and CD13 positivity, and further studies show nuclear positivity for terminal deoxynucleotidyl transferase. Molecular studies usually show clonal rearrangement of Ig and sometimes also of T-cell receptor genes. The remaining 10 per cent of blast-cell transformations have mixed myeloid and lymphoid characteristics.

The biochemical changes in chronic myeloid leukaemia are non-specific. Patients diagnosed in chronic phase may have a slightly raised serum uric acid but the level is frequently normal. The serum alkaline phosphatase is usually normal or slightly raised. The lactic dehydogenase level is usually raised. Serum electrolytes are usually normal but the K⁺ may be spuriously raised due to leak of intracellular potassium from platelets, or less commonly from leucocytes, after the blood is drawn. In transformation the serum uric acid may be raised, sometimes substantially, and tests of liver function are usually moderately abnormal. Hypercalcaemia, when present, is usually due to bone destruction but may be attributable to a parathormone-like material ectopically produced by the blast cells.

Management

CHRONIC PHASE

The management of the newly diagnosed patient with chronic myeloid leukaemia has changed very greatly in the last 10 or so years. In the 1970s it was conventional for the physician to start treatment soon after diagnosis with busulphan and then to await further developments. When transformation occurred, hydroxyurea was administered until the patient died. The patient often was not informed that he or she had leukaemia. Today in most but not all countries the patient is informed of the diagnosis and given some information about prognosis at the time of diagnosis. The various options for treatment are discussed at this stage. For younger patients the question of bone marrow transplantation should be addressed as soon as possible after diagnosis. The patient, all siblings, and other family members should be HLA typed. The issue of gonadal function is important. Treatment with busulphan should not be initiated unless the patient is willing to accept permanent sterility. Conversely, a patient who might be a candidate for bone marrow transplantation should be offered the possibility of semen or embryo cryopreservation.

There is no immediate urgency to start treatment in asymptomatic patients with leucocyte counts below 100 × 10⁹/l. Most patients will, however, prefer to be treated once the diagnosis is confirmed. It the possibility of treatment by bone marrow transplantation is excluded or uncertain, treatment should be initiated with hydroxyurea or interferon-α. Hydroxyurea is a ribonucleotide reductase inhibitor whose precise mode of action in chronic myeloid leukaemia is not known. It seems to target a relatively mature myeloid progenitor because its pharmacological action is rapid and readily reversible. Treatment is usually started with 1.0 to 2.0 g daily by mouth and continued indefinitely. The leucocyte count starts to fall within days and the spleen gets smaller. It is usually possible to reverse all features of chronic myeloid leukaemia within 4 to 8 weeks of starting treatment with hydroxyurea. The dosage can then be titrated against the leucocyte count, the usual maintenance dose being between 1.0 and 1.5 daily. Any further reduction in the dose leads to a rapid increase in the leucocyte count, a phenomenon that disturbs the patient but has no ominous significance. The drug has relatively few side-effects. At high dosage it may cause nausea, diarrhoea, or other gastrointestinal disturbance. Some patients get ulcers of the buccal mucosa. Skin rashes are seen. Most patients develop megaloblastic changes in the marrow with macrocytosis in the blood.

Busulphan (1,4-dimethanesulphonyloxybutane) is a polyfunctional alkylating agent that was formerly used to treat all new patients but is now infrequently used. It seems to target a relatively primitive stem cell, as the effects of administration are prolonged for some weeks after stopping the drug. Treatment was conventionally started with 8 mg daily by mouth and the dosage was reduced as the leucocyte count began to fall. It was essential to reduce substantially or stop the drug before the leucocyte count fell below 20 × 10⁹/l because profound leucopenia might otherwise be produced. Busulphan could be administered in finite courses lasting up to 4 weeks or continuously at a maintenance dose between 0.5 and 2.0 mg/day. Occasional patients are 'hypersensitive' to the effects of busulphan and may develop severe, sometimes irreversible, pancytopenia with marrow hypoplasia on standard dosage. Overdosage can achieve the same effect in any patient. Gonadal failure (as mentioned above) invariably occurs within a year of starting treatment and is irreversible. Other toxic effects, which are related to cumulative dose over some years but have led to use of the drug only as second-line agent, include cutaneous pigmentation, pulmonary fibrosis, and a wasting syndrome resembling hypoadrenalism. These points notwithstanding, the drug is useful in older patients whose compliance is uncertain and forms a major component of some 'conditioning' regimens before bone marrow transplantation.

Interferon-α is a member of a large family of glycoproteins of biological origin with antiviral and antiproliferative properties. Studies in

22 DISORDERS OF THE BLOOD

the early 1980s using material purified from human cell lines showed that it was active in reducing the leucocyte count and reversing all features of chronic myeloid leukaemia in 70 to 80 per cent of patients. Of particular interest was the observation that 5 to 15 per cent of patients sustained a major reduction in the percentage of Ph-positive marrow metaphases, with restoration of Ph-negative (putatively normal) haemopoiesis. This effect was achieved only very rarely with standard cytotoxic drugs. It raised the important question of whether these 'cytogenetic responders' would have their life prolonged by treatment with interferon-α and prospectively randomized controlled studies were initiated in many European countries and in North America. It is too early to evaluate the results of these studies with certainty but it appears that treatment with interferon-α has two important effects: (i) it identifies, on the basis of speed of haematological response and degree of cytogenetic response, subgroups of patients who will survive longer than others; and (ii), it probably prolongs survival by perhaps 1 or 2 years in the majority of patients. For the present it seems reasonable to conclude that interferon-α should be offered to all newly diagnosed patients who are not candidates for allogeneic bone-marrow transplantation and that treatment should be continued for as long as the drug is tolerated.

Interferon-α is now available in various recombinant DNA preparations. It must be administered by subcutaneous injection. It may be started at low dosage, 3 mega units daily for example, with gradual increases, or at high dosage, for example 5 mega units/m² daily with dose reduction if necessary. There is some evidence that the greatest chance of cytogenetic response is achieved with the higher dose levels. However, the drug is not without side-effects. Almost all patients experience fevers, shivers, muscle aches, and general influenza-like features on starting the drug; these last 1 to 2 weeks but may be alleviated by paracetamol. They recur when dosage is increased. A significant minority of patients cannot tolerate the drug on account of lethargy, malaise, anorexia, weight loss, depression and other affective disorders, or alopecia. The drug is still very much more expensive than hydroxyurea.

Younger patients with HLA-identical sibling donors should be offered the opportunity of treatment by allogeneic bone-marrow transplantation (see Chapter 22.8.2). Most specialist centres exclude from consideration patients over the age of 50 or 55 years. In general, patients are 'conditioned' for transplant with cyclophosphamide at high dosage followed by total-body irradiation or with the combination of busulphan and cyclophosphamide at high dosage. Bone marrow collected from the donor is infused intravenously on day 0. If all goes well, reasonable marrow function is achieved in 3 to 4 weeks and the patient leaves the hospital. The possible major complications include graft-versus-host disease, reactivation of infection with cytomegalovirus or other viruses, idiopathic pneumonitis, and veno-occlusive disease of the liver. For patients with chronic myeloid leukaemia treated by transplantation with marrow from HLA-identical siblings, the overall leukaemia-free survival at 5 years is now 60 to 70 per cent. There is a 20 per cent chance of transplant-related death and a 15 per cent chance of relapse. Patients surviving without haematological evidence of disease can be monitored by serial cytogenetic studies and by use of the much more sensitive reverse-transcription polymerase chain reaction, which can detect very low numbers of *BCR-ABL* transcripts in the blood or marrow. These studies suggest (but do not prove) that the majority of long-term survivors have been cured of chronic myeloid leukaemia.

This qualified success with bone marrow transplants from matched siblings has led to increasing use of 'matched' unrelated donors for transplantation in patients with chronic myeloid leukaemia. At present, serologically matched unrelated donors can be identified for about 50 per cent of Caucasian patients and for lower percentages of patients of other ethnic origins. The results of transplants from unrelated donors are currently less good than results with HLA-identical siblings but some patients will probably prove to be cured.

The collated results of transplantation using matched sibling and unrelated donors are depicted in Fig. 3. Because only a minority of patients are eligible for allogeneic bone-marrow transplantation, much interest

has focused recently on the possibility that life may be prolonged and some cures effected by autografting patients with chronic myeloid leukaemia still in chronic phase. It is possible that the pool of leukaemic stem cells can be substantially reduced by an autograft procedure, and autografting may confer a short-term proliferative advantage on Ph-negative (presumably normal) stem cells. In practice, some patients have achieved temporary Ph-negative haemopoiesis after autografting. The

Fig. 3 A chart showing the availability of sibling donors and the probability of cure by bone marrow transplantation for a notional 100 patients with newly diagnosed chronic myeloid leukaemia.

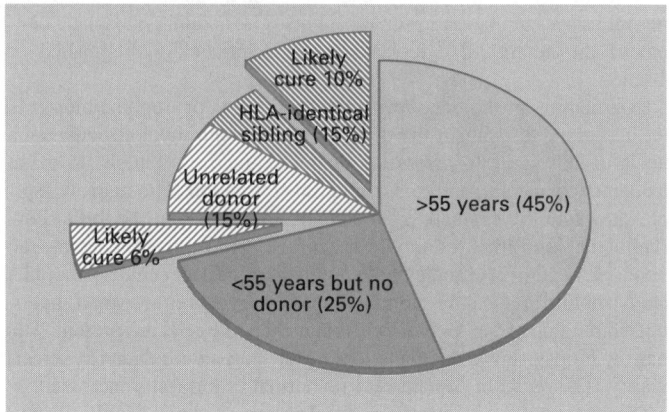

Fig. 4 An algorithm showing a possible approach to the management of a newly diagnosed patient aged 55 years or less. Blood- or marrow-derived stem cells can be cryopreserved at diagnosis. Patients with HLA-identical siblings may be allografted or treated first with interferon-α (IFN-α). In the latter case, those who achieve continuing cytogenetic responses (CCR) may have their bone marrow transplant (BMT) delayed. Patients without HLA-identical siblings may be treated initially with IFN-α. Non-responders may be treated with hydroxyurea (HU), by autografting (A/G) in chronic phase (CP), or by transplant with a 'matched' unrelated donor (MUD).

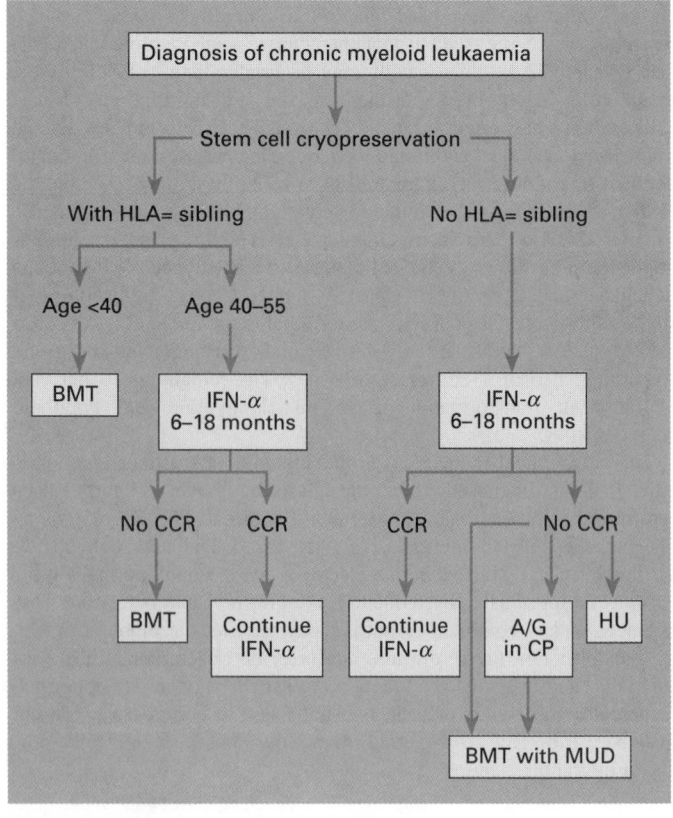

possibility that more durable Ph negativity may be achieved by auto-grafting with marrow or blood stem cells treated *in vitro* to reduce the proportion of Ph-positive stem cells is currently being studied in various centres. An integrated approach to the management of the 'younger' patient with chronic myeloid leukaemia is shown in Fig. 4.

ADVANCED-PHASE DISEASE

Patients in blastic transformation may be treated with combinations of cytotoxic drugs in the hope of prolonging life, but cure can no longer be a realistic objective. Conversely, it is reasonable to use a relatively innocuous drug such a hydroxyurea at higher dosage to restrain blast-cell numbers and maintain the patient at home for as long as possible. If the patient has a myeloid transformation, he or she can be treated with drugs appropriate to the induction of remission in acute myeloid leukaemia, namely daunorubicin, cytosine arabinoside with or without 6-thioguanine. The blast-cell numbers will be reduced substantially in most cases but their numbers usually increase again within 3 to 6 weeks. Perhaps 20 per cent of patients are restored to a condition resembling chronic-phase disease and this benefit may last for 3 to 6 months.

Patients in lymphoid transformation may be treated with a little more optimism. It is reasonable to initiate treatment with drugs applicable to the management of adult acute lymphoblastic leukaemia, namely prednisolone, vincristine, and daunorubicin with or without L-asparaginase. More than 50 per cent of patients will be restored to a 'second' chronic phase, at which point the status can be maintained with daily 6-mercaptopurine and weekly methotrexate. Patients who achieve a second chronic phase should have neuroprophylaxis with intrathecal methotrexate weekly for six consecutive weeks but the use of cranial irradiation is probably excessive. Some patients treated for lymphoid transformation of chronic myeloid leukaemia may sustain long periods of apparent 'remission'.

Allogeneic bone-marrow transplantation from HLA-matched sibling donors can be done in the accelerated phase; the probability of leukaemia-free survival at 5 years is 30 to 50 per cent. Bone marrow transplantation done in overt blastic transformation is nearly always unsuccessful. The mortality resulting from graft-versus-host disease is extremely high and the probability of relapse in those who survive the transplant is very considerable. The probability of survival at 5 years is consequently 5 to 10 per cent.

REFERENCES

Bergamaschi, G. and Rosti, V. (1994). Pathogenesis of chronic myelogenous leukaemia. *Haematologica*, **79**, 1–3.

Butturini, A., Keating, A., Goldman, J.M., and Gale, R.P. (1990). Autotransplants in chronic myelogenous leukaemia: strategies and results. *Lancet*, **i**, 1255–8.

Clift, R.A., Appelbaum, F.R., and Thomas, E.D. (1993). Editorial: treatment of chronic myeloid leukemia by marrow transplantation. *Blood*, **82**, 1954–6.

Gale, R.P., Goldman, J.M., Grosveld, G., and Goldman, J.M. (1993). Chronic myelogenous leukemia: biology and therapy. (Meeting Report.) *Leukemia*, **7**, 653–8.

Goldman, J.M. (1990). Options for the management of chronic myeloid leukemia—1990. *Leukemia and Lymphoma*, **3**, 159–64.

Goldman, J.M. (1994). Management of chronic myeloid leukemia. *Blood Reviews*, **8**, 21–9.

Kantarjian, H.M., Deisseroth, A., Kurzrock, R., Estrov, Z., and Talpaz, M. (1993). Review: chronic myelogenous leukemia: a concise update. *Blood*, **82**, 691–703.

Kurzrock, R., Gutterman, J.U., and Talpaz, M. (1988). The molecular genetics of Philadelphia chromosome-positive leukemias. *New England Journal of Medicine*, **319**, 990–8.

Lemoli, R.M. (1993). Characterization and selection of benign stem cells in chronic myeloid leukemia. *Haematologica*, **78**, 393–400.

Sokal, J.E. *et al.* (1984). Prognostic discrimination in 'good risk' chronic granulocytic leukaemia. *Blood*, **63**, 789–99.

Talpaz, M., Kantarjian, H., Kurzrock, R., Trujillo, J.M., and Gutterman, J.U. (1991). Interferon alpha produces sustained cytogenetic responses in chronic myelogenous leukemia Philadelphia chromosome-positive patients. *Annals of Internal Medicine*, **114**, 532–8.

The Italian Cooperative Study Group on Chronic Myeloid Leukemia (1994). Interferon alfa-2a as compared with conventional chemotherapy for the treatment of chronic myeloid leukemia. *New England Journal of Medicine*, **330**, 820–5.

Thomas, E.D., and Clift, R.A. (1989). Indications for marrow transplantation in chronic myelogenous leukemia. *Blood*, **73**, 861–4.

22.3.6 Chronic lymphocytic leukaemia and other leukaemias of mature B and T cells

D. CATOVSKY

Advances in diagnosis in the last decade have resulted in a greater recognition of the heterogeneity in leukaemias arising from immunologically mature B and T cells. These advances resulted mainly from the systematic use of monoclonal antibodies against lymphocyte differentiation antigens, greater attention to morphological detail, and a more consistent evaluation of the patterns of lymphocytic infiltration in the bone marrow, lymph nodes, and spleen. The need for a more precise diagnosis has been further stimulated by the availability of new treatments for these disorders and the related, low-grade non-Hodgkin's lymphomas (see Chapter 22.5.3).

The principal methods used for diagnosis and classification include peripheral blood and bone marrow films, bone-marrow trephine biopsies, a set of monoclonal antibodies and antibodies specific to immunoglobulin (Ig) heavy and light chains, and histological evaluation of involved organs. Other investigations that may provide useful information are protein electrophoresis, tests for free light chains in the urine, and imaging techniques. Physical examination should include palpation of lymph nodes, liver and spleen, and details of any skin infiltration. Results of cytogenetic and DNA analysis help to elucidate pathogenesis and may acquire a role in disease classification in the near future.

There are two broad disease categories to be considered: primary lymphoid leukaemias and leukaemia/lymphoma syndromes. Both can be subdivided, according to their cell derivation, into B- and T-cell types (Tables 1 and 2).

Chronic lymphocytic leukaemia

This is the most common form of lymphocytic leukaemia, accounting for 70 per cent of cases. In Western countries, chronic lymphocytic leukaemia accounts for 25 per cent of all cases of leukaemia. It is less common in the Far East, comprising 2 per cent of cases. Based on 1986/88 statistics, it is estimated that 1000 new cases are diagnosed in the United Kingdom each year.

Chronic lymphocytic leukaemia affects people over the age of 50 years, with only 5 per cent of patients aged between 30 and 50 years, and it is very rare below the age of 30. The peak incidence is between 60 and 80 years. The male to female ratio is 1.8:1. This ratio is greater in younger patients and lower in the elderly, as documented in the first Medical Research Council trial for the management of CLL.

Diagnostic criteria include a lymphocytosis of greater than $10 \times 10^9/l$ and more than 30 per cent lymphocytes in bone marrow aspirates. With the use of membrane markers it is possible to make a diagnosis with lower lymphocyte counts. The lymphocytes in chronic lymphocytic leukaemia have a distinct morphology: small size, round nucleus, clumped nuclear chromatin and scanty cytoplasm; smear cells are common (Plate 1(a)). A minority of cells are larger, with a prominent nucleolus, and have been designated prolymphocytes. Cases with more than

Table 1 *Primary lymphoid leukaemias*

B-cell type
Chronic lymphocytic leukaemia (CLL)
Prolymphocytic leukaemia (B-PLL)
Hairy-cell leukaemia (HCL)
HCL variant
T-cell type
Large granular lymphocyte leukaemia
Prolymphocytic leukaemia (T-PLL)
Sezary-cell leukaemia

Table 2 *Leukaemia/lymphoma syndromes**

B-cell type
Follicular lymphoma
Mantle-cell lymphoma
Splenic lymphoma with circulating villous lymphocytes (SLVL)
Lymphoplasmacytic lymphoma
Large-cell lymphoma (B)
T-cell type
Adult T-cell leukaemia/lymphoma (ATLL)
Sezary syndrome
Peripheral T-cell lymphoma
Large-cell lymphoma (T)

*Primary non-Hodgkin's lymphoma evolving with leukaemia.

10 per cent prolymphocytes have a progressive clinical course, a higher rate of proliferation than stable cases, and a correspondingly shorter lymphocyte doubling time. This variant form of chronic lymphocytic leukaemia has been designated **CLL/PL,** PL standing for prolymphocytes.

CLINICAL FEATURES (PLATE 12)

Almost one-third of patients are diagnosed by chance, with lymphocytosis and no specific symptoms or physical signs. Others present with lymphadenopathy or symptoms of anaemia. The lymphadenopathy is usually symmetrical and of moderate size, involving the neck, axillae, and inguinal regions. Other nodal areas can be ascertained by chest radiographs and abdominal computerized tomographic (**CT**) scan. Splenomegaly of variable size is found in 50 per cent of cases; hepatomegaly is less common and more difficult to document as being clinically relevant.

Systemic symptoms such as weight loss or night sweating are not common but, when present, correlate with bulky abdominal disease. Fever in chronic lymphocytic leukaemia usually indicates infection but if this is excluded it may suggest transformation (see below).

MEMBRANE MARKERS

Lymphocytes in chronic lymphocytic leukaemia are clonal B cells with weak κ or λ light-chain expression (SmIg) in the membrane. The immunophenotype of chronic lymphocytic leukaemia is unique within the B-cell disorders: CD5 and CD23 positive, FMC7 negative, and weak or negative CD22. These four markers and the weak SmIg expression represent the typical phenotype of chronic lymphocytic leukaemia. In the majority of cases (87 per cent), the lymphocytes show the expected findings with all five, or four, of the above reagents. The most consistent markers are CD5 and CD23, positive in 92 and 94 per cent of cases, respectively. This contrasts with observations in other B-cell leukaemias and non-Hodgkin's lymphomas in leukaemic phase (Table 3). CCL/PL has the same membrane markers as typical chronic lymphocytic leukaemia, although in 20 to 30 per cent of cases they depart slightly from

Table 3 *Membrane phenotype in leukaemias of mature B cells*

Marker	CLL	B-PLL	HCL	NHL[1]
SmIg	Weak	Strong	Strong	Strong
CD22	Weak	Strong	Strong	Strong
CD5	+	+/−	−	−/+
CD23	+	−	−	−/+
FMC7	−	+	+	+

[1]Non-Hodgkin's lymphoma (follicular, mantle-cell lymphoma, and SLVL); all other abbreviations as in Tables 1 and 2.

the usual phenotype by expressing strong SmIg or CD22 or FMC7. As CD5 is a marker of both B and T cells, it is important in the context of chronic lymphocytic leukaemia to establish by simultaneous double labelling, that another B-cell antigen, for example CD19, is co-expressed in the CD5-positive lymphocytes.

BONE MARROW FINDINGS

The patterns of bone marrow infiltration in chronic lymphocytic leukaemia are variable and correlate with clinical stages. Early chronic lymphocytic leukaemia shows minimal interstitial or nodular involvement; with disease progression the normal bone-marrow fat spaces are replaced by lymphocytes. There is a mixed interstitial and nodular pattern, and in advanced disease the involvement is diffuse or 'packed'. The latter correlates with the presence of anaemia and/or thrombocytopenia. A paratrabecular pattern, characteristic of non-Hodgkin's lymphoma and follicular lymphoma in particular, is not seen in chronic lymphocytic leukaemia. A nodular pattern, on the other hand, is common in lymphoplasmacytic, mantle-cell, and splenic lymphoma with villous lymphocytes (see below).

Examination of the bone marrow aspirate and trephine is important in chronic lymphocytic leukaemia for three reasons: (i) to assess the degree of infiltration, which is an independent prognostic factor; (ii) to establish the possible mechanism of anaemia or thrombocytopenia by assessing the normal haemopoietic reserves; and (iii), to distinguish chronic lymphocytic leukaemia from low-grade non-Hodgkin's lymphoma by the pattern of involvement in trephine biopsy sections. In patients with cytopenias and a large spleen, assessment of the bone marrow is critical in deciding whether splenectomy is indicated.

STAGING

The course of chronic lymphocytic leukaemia is very variable. Some patients may never require treatment and others have a progressive course with short survival. An important advance in management was the development of staging systems that can predict prognosis. The first system, widely used in the United States, was described by Rai and colleagues in 1975. A new, simplified proposal in 1981 by Binet and colleagues was subsequently adopted by the International Workshop on chronic lymphocytic leukaemia in 1981, while retaining some features of Rai's staging. Both systems use simple information: blood counts and physical signs, namely lymphadenopathy and hepatosplenomegaly. Findings by imaging techniques are not taken into account for staging but are useful for assessing accurately disease bulk and measuring response to treatment.

Binet's system is currently used in clinical trials in the United Kingdom. Stages A and B have no anaemia (Hb > 10g/dl) or thrombocytopenia (platelets > 100 × 10⁹/l), and have a different degree of organ enlargement. Stage A patients have either no palpable nodes (including liver and spleen as nodal areas) or have one or two involved areas. Stage B patients have three, four or all five nodal areas, which include nodes in cervical, axillary and inguinal regions, spleen, and liver. Stage C patients have anaemia (Hb < 10g/dl) and/or thrombocytopenia (platelets

$< 100 \times 10^9/l)$, and correspond to stages III and IV of the Rai system. The relative distribution of stages at presentation is as follows: stage A, 45 to 50 per cent; stage B, 25 to 30 per cent; stage C, 20 to 25 per cent. The proportion of patients in stages A, B, and C varies between the sexes; women are more likely to present with stage A, men with stages B and C. Stage A is also more common over the age of 70 years in both sexes. The stage of the disease is the most important prognostic factor (see below).

Attempts have been made to identify, within the stage A group, further prognostic substages. One is to retain Rai stage 0 (lymphocytosis with no physical signs) as stage A(0). The other, identified by the French Cooperative Group on chronic lymphocytic leukaemia, is to separate stage A into patients with Hb in excess of 12 g/dl and a lymphocyte count below $30 \times 10^9/l$, or Hb over 12 and lymphocytes over 30. The 5-year survival of the first group was 87 per cent and of the second 60 per cent.

COMPLICATIONS

Infections, particularly of the upper respiratory tract, are the chief cause of morbidity in chronic lymphocytic leukaemia. Pneumonia is the main cause of death in 30 per cent of cases, usually in patients with advanced disease. The main predisposing factor for the infections is hypogammaglobulinaemia.

Autoimmune phenomena, chiefly haemolytic anaemia with a positive direct antiglobulin test due to warm autoantibodies, are a feature in 5 per cent of cases. The proportion of cases with a positive Coombs' test is higher than the number with frank haemolysis. Not infrequently, the haemolytic anaemia is precipitated by the initiation of therapy with alkylating agents. Immune thrombocytopenia is seen in 2 per cent of cases.

Other malignancies are not uncommon in chronic lymphocytic leukaemia and it is not clear whether this relatively high incidence reflects age or a greater predisposition due to the disease itself or its associated immunodeficiency. Up to 30 per cent of patients may die of causes unrelated to the leukaemia and in half of them the cause is another cancer. In patients with early chronic lymphocytic leukaemia (stage A), half of the causes of death are not related to the leukaemia. In contrast, in advanced stages (stages B and C), 80 to 90 per cent of deaths are a direct consequence of it.

CHROMOSOME ABNORMALITIES

The most consistent chromosome abnormalities in chronic lymphocytic leukaemia are trisomy of chromosome 12, found in 15 to 20 per cent of cases, and deletions of the long arm of chromosome 13 (13q14) in 10 per cent. Trisomy 12 can be detected by in situ hybridization techniques in interphase nuclei as well as in metaphase spreads (Plate 13(b)) and is also a feature of some lymphoplasmacytic lymphomas.

PROGNOSTIC FACTORS

The main prognostic factors in chronic lymphocytic leukaemia are listed in Table 4. The most important for predicting survival is stage, assessed by either the Binet or Rai systems, followed by age, sex, and response to therapy. The median survival of stage A patients is over 10 years, of stage B 6 years, and stage C 4 years.

The lymphocyte doubling time is another important prognostic variable, in particular for stage A patients. A period of close observation, with blood counts every 2 or 3 months for the first year, is recommended in newly diagnosed stage A patients in order to assess the pace of the disease and calculate the doubling time. The degree of bone marrow infiltration is also an independent prognostic variable, particularly in stage B patients. A packed bone-marrow pattern is associated with worse prognosis. In contrast to the anaemia caused by bone marrow infiltration, autoimmune haemolytic anaemia is not considered to indicate poor

Table 4 *Prognostic factors in chronic lymphocytic leukaemia*

Clinical stage[1]
Age; sex
Response to therapy
Lymphocyte count
Lymphocyte doubling time
Bone marrow histology[2]
Percentage of prolymphocytes
Chromosome abnormalities

[1]Rai or Binet staging systems, adopted by the International Workshop on CLL (1981), take into account Hb, platelet levels, and number of lymph node sites.

[2]Diffuse or packed bone marrow worse than the other patterns (interstitial, nodular, and mixed).

prognosis. Because chronic lymphocytic leukaemia affects elderly people it is essential to investigate thoroughly the causes of anaemia and exclude, as unrelated to the leukaemia, those caused by iron, folate, or vitamin B_{12} deficiency, before deciding that the patient has stage C and requires chemotherapy.

TREATMENT

Because of the variable outlook, which relates to the stage of the disease and other features, it is important to consider treatment for those with early and stable disease and separately from those with progressive, symptomatic, and/or advanced disease. For this purpose, staging is the first criterion to take into account.

The majority of stage A patients have no symptoms and may be observed for a while to determine, by the lymphocyte doubling time, or other features, whether the disease has a stable pattern, before deciding whether treatment is necessary. Although this has been the conventional wisdom for many years, a number of trials have considered the question of early treatment for stage A patients with chlorambucil, with or without prednisolone (Table 5). This was based on two known premises: (i) that responses are better in early disease, and ii) that good responses correlate with improved survival (see Prognostic factors). To test this hypothesis the trials have randomized patients with stage A to early versus no therapy, or therapy deferred until disease progression. Several studies have shown conclusively that patients treated early did not fare better and, if anything, show a clear trend towards shorter survival. These data are now being analysed further as part of an international overview.

Treatment is indicated for patients with stages B and C or stage A with clear evidence of disease progression but short of the criteria for stage B or C. Disease progression is defined, in the context of chronic lymphocytic leukaemia, as a downward trend in Hb or platelets, rising lymphocyte counts, development of lymphadenopathy, and systemic symptoms. Most of the treatments listed in Table 5 have been, or still are, subject to clinical trials. It is accepted that the addition of prednisolone to an alkylating agent, chlorambucil or cyclophosphamide (as in COP; see Table 5), does not confer a survival advantage. There is good evidence, on the other hand, that the use of prednisolone alone for the first 4 weeks in patients who present at stage C facilitates the subsequent introduction of other drugs and corrects more rapidly the cytopenias.

The role of anthracyclines, as in the combination CHOP (see Table 5), was thought to be promising in an early trial but is currently still being tested in other trials and analysed in overviews. It is apparent that the response rates are slightly higher with anthracycline-containing combinations in previously untreated patients, 75 to 80 per cent for partial plus complete remissions, against 65 to 70 per cent with chlorambucil or COP for example.

A new generation of drugs, the nucleoside analogues (Table 5), has

Table 5 *Treatments used in chronic lymphocytic leukaemia*

Alkylating agents
Chlorambucil intermittently[1] (10 mg/m²/day × 6 days, monthly)
Chlorambucil continuously (4–5 mg/day)

Combinations
COP: cyclophosphamide, oncovin, prednisolone (5-day monthly courses)
Chlorambucil plus epirubicin (chlorambucil intermittently as above; epirubicin: 50 mg/m² IV day 1; both monthly)
Chlorambucil plus prednisolone intermittently (chlorambucil as above; prednisolone 40 mg/day × 5 or 7 days)
CHOP: COP plus doxorubicin (doxorubicin 50 mg/m² IV day 1, or 25 mg/m² 'mini' CHOP; monthly)
CAP: as CHOP without oncovin

Splenic irradiation
(1 Gy once or twice/week to 10 Gy)

Corticosteroids
Prednisolone 30 mg/m² for 3 weeks plus 1 week tailing off for stage C patients before other drugs
High-dose methylprednisolone IV (or oral) 1 g/m² (5-day monthly courses)

Nucleoside analogues
Fludarabine IV push 25 mg/m² daily (5-day monthly courses)
2'-Deoxycoformycin IV push 4 mg/m² (once a week or every 2 weeks)
2-Chlorodeoxyadenosine IV infusion (0.1 mg/kg per day × 7 days every 4–5 weeks)

[1]MRC CLL3 protocol.

shown promise for the treatment of chronic lymphocytic leukaemia and other low-grade lymphoid malignancies. The two with greater activity in chronic lymphocytic leukaemia are fludarabine and 2-chlorodeoxy-adenosine. The encouraging results with fludarabine result from higher remission rates, for example 33 per cent in previously untreated patients in one study, which compares favourably with the 15 per cent complete remissions that are observed with other agents. Furthermore, there is no evidence for cross-resistance between fludarabine and chlorambucil or anthracyclines. This makes fludarabine the agent of choice for second-line therapy in chronic lymphocytic leukaemia. It is not yet clear whether using it as first-line treatment provides any survival advantage as results of randomized trials are not yet available.

Splenectomy

There are three indications for splenectomy in chronic lymphocytic leukaemia: first, the most common, for therapy-resistant disease with significant residual splenomegaly; second, in patients with evidence of hypersplenism, that is cytopenia(s) and active bone-marrow haemopoiesis; and thirdly, for autoimmune complications, haemolytic anaemia or thrombocytopenia that do not respond to therapy with corticosteroids and immunosuppressive drugs. In my experience, splenectomy is always beneficial in any of the above indications. In patients in whom the spleen is the dominant organ affected, that is with little or no lymphadenopathy, splenectomy can revert the clinical staging from stage C to A, with corresponding improvement in survival.

Because of the poor humoral immunity in chronic lymphocytic leukaemia the prophylaxis after splenectomy should rely mainly on oral penicillin and less on antipneumococcal vaccines.

Supportive care

Recurrent infections in patients with chronic lymphocytic leukaemia, particularly those with advanced disease, makes supportive care an important component of management. This includes long-term antibiotic

prophylaxis and/or their availability for use as soon as signs or symptoms of infections appear, and intravenous immunoglobulin replacement therapy to prevent serious bacterial infections in selected patients. Other measures include blood transfusions and vitamin supplements to correct deficiencies. Anaemia in chronic lymphocytic leukaemia should always be thoroughly investigated and it should not be assumed that it is caused by bone marrow infiltration. The treatment of autoimmune complications includes corticosteroids, splenectomy, danazol, azathioprine, and cyclophosphamide.

TRANSFORMATION

There are two well-known forms of transformation in chronic lymphocytic leukaemia: a subtle one with an increased proportion of prolymphocytes, seen in some patients from presentation and known as CLL/PL, and a more dramatic change to a high-grade non-Hodgkin's lymphoma with diffuse large-cell/immunoblastic histology, known as Richter's syndrome. CLL/PL is seen in 10 per cent of patients, and Richter's syndrome in at least 5 per cent.

The large-cell transformation may be localized or generalized; rarely, it may resemble an acute leukaemia with circulating large blasts. The classical Richter's syndrome is associated with deteriorating clinical status and systemic symptoms: fever, weight loss, sweating, particularly when large para-aortic nodes are involved. It is possible that its true incidence is higher than hitherto reported as it is not common practice to biopsy suspicious large nodes in patients known to have chronic lymphocytic leukaemia. Systemic symptoms or rapidly enlarging, asymmetrical nodes should always raise the question of transformation and be properly investigated.

One question that has generated interest as well as conflicting results is whether Richter's transformation represents a new malignancy or a new change within the leukaemic B-cell clone. Studies with anti-light-chain antibodies and DNA analysis with probes for heavy- and light-chain genes seem to indicate that, although in two-thirds of cases the transformation occurs within the pre-existing leukaemia cells, in the rest—perhaps in up to 40 per cent of cases—it represents a new B-cell clone. Studies of many more cases will be required to document precisely which is the more common event.

Richter's syndrome has been associated with poor prognosis, with a median survival of less than 6 months from presentation. Alkylating agents are no longer effective at this stage, and probably neither is fludarabine, as we have observed the development of large-cell transformation on this therapy. Combinations of the type used in high-grade non-Hodgkin's lymphoma (e.g. CHOP; Table 5) may induce remissions in some patients. If complete remission is obtained, the outlook may be favourable. Patients with localized transformation seem to respond better than those with generalized lymph-node involvement. The survival in non-responders is very short.

Patients with CLL/PL have progressive disease that may respond to first-line therapy as for chronic lymphocytic leukaemia but the overall response rate is close to half that of patients with typical chronic lymphocytic leukaemia. Fludarabine may be effective too, but in a lower percentage of cases. There is no optimal approach for this group and, often, most forms of therapy listed in Table 5 achieve only moderate success.

B-cell prolymphocytic leukaemia

B-cell prolymphocytic leukaemia was originally described as a variant form of chronic lymphocytic leukaemia. Studies since the first description by Galton and colleagues in 1974 have shown that it is a distinct entity. The main features are splenomegaly without peripheral lymphadenopathy, anaemia and thrombocytopenia and high white-cell count, usually over 100 × 10⁹/l. The diagnosis is made by examination of peripheral blood films in which the predominant cells are prolymphocytes (Plate 14). Small lymphocytes, as in chronic lymphocytic leukaemia, are rarely seen.

The immunophenotype of B-cell prolymphocytic leukaemia (Table 3) is different from that of chronic lymphocytic leukaemia: most cases strongly express SmIg, FMC7, and CD22; two-thirds of cases are CD5 negative. The differential diagnosis should be with CLL/PL, mantle-cell non-Hodgkin's lymphoma, and the hairy-cell leukaemia variant. In CLL/PL there is splenomegaly with peripheral nodal involvement, the proportion of prolymphocytes is less than 50 per cent, there are many small lymphocytes in the blood films, and the immunophenotype is usually similar to that of chronic lymphocytic leukaemia. The circulating cells in the leukaemic phase of mantle-cell lymphoma have a pleomorphic appearance, the nucleolus is not prominent, and they often have an indented nuclear outline (Plate 15). The membrane phenotype may be similar to B-cell prolymphocytic leukaemia, except for CD5, which is positive in 70 per cent of cases of mantle-cell lymphoma. Lymph-node histology may help further in the differential diagnosis. The cells in the variant form of hairy-cell leukaemia have a prominent nucleolus resembling that of prolymphocytes but their cytoplasm is abundant and has distinct 'hairy' projections. Their immunological profile may be similar to that of B-cell prolymphocytic leukaemia.

TREATMENT AND PROGNOSIS

In contrast to chronic lymphocytic leukaemia, the evolution of B-cell prolymphocytic leukaemia is always progressive, with a median survival of 3 years. Several forms of treatment have been used in the past with moderate success: splenic irradiation, combination chemotherapy, and splenectomy. Recently, the nucleoside analogue fludarabine has been shown to induce partial plus complete remission in 50 per cent of patients. If this is confirmed, fludarabine could become the first line of therapy for B-cell prolymphocytic leukaemia, as chlorambucil and other alkylating agents are largely ineffective.

Hairy-cell leukaemia (Plate 16)

Hairy-cell leukaemia is characterized by cytopenia and splenomegaly in two-thirds of cases; monocytopenia is a consistent finding. Most patients have circulating hairy cells but leucocyte counts rarely exceed $10 \times 10^9/l$. Hairy cells are larger than lymphocytes, their nucleus has an homogeneous, loose chromatin pattern without a visible nucleolus (except in the hairy-cell leukaemia variant), and they have an abundant cytoplasm with broad-based projections or villi. The nuclear outline is often kidney shaped.

The bone-marrow trephine biopsy shows a unique pattern of infiltration with characteristic clear zones in between the cells. This infiltration is usually interstitial but may be also be focal. Bone marrow aspirates are, as a rule, unsuccessful (dry tap) due to the heavy deposition of reticulin fibres.

When hairy cells are tested with the five markers listed in Table 3, the immunophenotype is different from CLL but similar to other B-cell disorders. Four other monoclonal antibodies have shown specificity for hairy cells, B-ly-7, CD11c, CD25 and HC2, and are positive in most cases. Two of these, CD25 and HC2, are negative in the hairy-cell leukaemia variant.

A well-known cytochemical property of hairy cells is the presence of tartaric acid-resistant acid phosphatase, which is still useful for diagnostic purposes. In paraffin-embedded sections of bone marrow, hairy cells are positive with the monoclonal L26 (CD20) and DAB44. These reagents can help detect residual disease after treatment, as recognition of small clusters of hairy cells in histological sections is often difficult.

TREATMENT AND PROGNOSIS

The prognosis of patients with hairy-cell leukaemia has improved dramatically with the advent of three forms of treatment: interferon-α, 2'-deoxycoformycin (**DCF**), and 2-chlorodeoxyadenosine (**CdA**). Splenectomy, which was the mainstay of treatment in the past, is now reserved for patients presenting with very large spleens that are disproportionate to the degree of bone marrow involvement. Interferon-α improves the blood counts and the bone marrow but rarely induces prolonged complete remissions; treatment always needs to continue to maintain a response. DCF induces complete remissions in 75 per cent of patients with few (3 per cent) non-responders. Once treatment is discontinued the majority of responders remain in remission for more than 5 years. CdA is an equally effective agent, currently undergoing clinical trials in Europe and more widely used in the United States.

TRANSFORMATION

A subtle transformation takes place in patients with hairy-cell leukaemia (and hairy-cell leukaemia variant) in the form of massive abdominal lymphadenopathy with few systemic symptoms. The overall incidence of abdominal nodes in hairy-cell leukaemia is 28 per cent. This is assessed by routine CT scanning. The proportion with lymphadenopathy at presentation is only 17 per cent but is higher in patients who relapse after previously successful treatments and/or who have long-standing disease. Abdominal lymphadenopathy is associated with resistance to further therapy and with the presence of large hairy cells in both the bone marrow and the enlarged lymph nodes, supporting the concept of transformation as suggested by the clinical findings.

B-cell lymphomas in leukaemic phase

Several types of low- or intermediate-grade non-Hodgkin's lymphomas of B-cell type present or evolve with a leukaemic blood picture of more than $5 \times 10^9/l$ circulating lymphoid cells (Table 2). The two types of non-Hodgkin's lymphoma that most commonly develop a leukaemic phase are follicular lymphoma and splenic lymphoma with villous lymphocytes (**SLVL**). The main differential diagnosis is with chronic lymphocytic leukaemia, other non-Hodgkin's lymphomas and, in the case of SLVL, with hairy-cell leukaemia.

The circulating cells in follicular lymphoma are small, have no visible cytoplasm, the nuclear chromatin has a smooth pattern, and they show regularly deep nuclear clefts or indentations and an angular or irregularly shaped nucleus (Plate 17). Leukaemia in follicular lymphoma is associated with widespread disease, hepatosplenomegaly and lymphadenopathy for example. The membrane phenotype is different from that of chronic lymphocytic leukaemia (Table 3) and the cells often express CD10. Lymph-node biopsy is essential for a definitive tissue diagnosis. Cytogenetic analysis will show the translocation t(14;18) and molecular techniques the rearrangement of the *BCL-2* gene. Cases with leukaemia tend to run a more aggressive course and require more intensive treatment.

SLVL is a distinct, low-grade non-Hodgkin's lymphoma characterized by splenomegaly, moderate lymphocytosis ($10–30 \times 10^9/l$), a small monoclonal band, and/or free light chains in the urine in 50 per cent of cases. The circulating lymphocytes have a small nucleolus and a cytoplasm with conspicuous villous projections that are often seen polarized in one end of the cell (Plate 18). A minority of cells show plasma-cell differentiation. The bone marrow is minimally involved early in the disease and the biopsies show a nodular pattern. The immunophenotype of SLVL cells can be distinguished from that of chronic lymphocytic leukaemia (Table 3) and hairy-cell leukaemia, both diseases with which it can be confused. Splenectomy is a useful treatment for SLVL. The histological appearance of the spleen shows predominantly white-pulp involvement with a prominent marginal zone, which contrasts with the predominantly red-pulp infiltration pattern in hairy-cell leukaemia and its variant.

Leukaemia is uncommon in mantle-cell lymphoma. The circulating cells in mantle-cell lymphoma are of medium to large size with an irregular nuclear outline (Plate 15). The bone marrow biopsy shows nodular (Plate 19) or paratrabecular involvement. Mantle-cell lymphoma is also characterized by the translocation t(11;14) in 70 per cent of cases, involving the *BCL-1/PRAD-1* gene. This translocation is also seen in 20 per cent of cases of B-cell prolymphocytic leukaemia and SLVL.

Large granular lymphocytic leukaemia

Most cases with a persistent T-cell lymphocytosis of greater than 5 × 10⁹/l lasting for more than 6 months without an identifiable cause are likely to represent clonal proliferation of large granular lymphocytes. Clonality can be demonstrated by the rearrangement of T-cell receptor genes and, sometimes, also by chromosome translocations but these are not consistent in every case. Large granular lymphocytes have abundant cytoplasm with prominent azurophil granules and an eccentric nucleus without a visible nucleolus. Half of the patients have splenomegaly without lymphadenopathy and are neutropenic or, less frequently, suffer from other cytopenias. The membrane phenotype shows mature T cells that are CD4−, CD8+ and, characteristically, express one or more antigens associated with killer or natural killer cells, for example CD11b, CD16, CD56 or CD57. Bone marrow involvement is variable but is usually present in true, large granular lymphocyte leukaemia. The splenic involvement is in the red pulp, with reactive normal follicles (white pulp) and frequent granuloma formation. Although many patients do not require active treatment, a significant minority present a therapeutic problem. Treatments that have been effective in some patients are cyclosporin A, prednisolone plus an alkylating agent, and DCF.

T-cell prolymphocytic leukaemia (Plate 20)

This disease is characterized by splenomegaly, lymphadenopathy, and high leucocyte counts, usually rising rather rapidly above 100 × 10⁹/l. There is skin infiltration in the dermis around the blood vessels and appendages in 20 per cent of cases. The blood picture may resemble B-cell prolymphocytic leukaemia but typical T-prolymphocytes are smaller than B-prolymphocytes and have some distinct features: irregular nuclear outline and a deep basophilic cytoplasm with protrusions or blebs. The nucleolus is often prominent (Plate 21), although it may be hidden in some cases.

The membrane phenotype corresponds to that of mature (post-thymic) T lymphocytes with CD4+, CD8− markers. One-third of cases co-express CD4 and CD8 or are CD4−, CD8+. The diagnosis is made by examination of peripheral blood and bone marrow films and confirmed by the appropriate markers. Ultrastructural examination may be necessary to define the morphology in cases with small cells.

There are consistent chromosome abnormalities affecting chromosome 14, with breakpoints at 14q11 (locus for the T-cell receptor α and δ genes) and 14q32, the latter not involving the Ig heavy-chain gene. The abnormalities in chromosome 14 are manifested as inversion 14 or, less frequently, as the tandem translocation t(14;14). Another frequent chromosome change is trisomy 8q.

TREATMENT AND PROGNOSIS

The median survival of T-cell prolymphocytic leukaemia in our series has been 7 months. Complete and partial responses can be obtained in 50 per cent of cases with DCF. Complete responses have been obtained with the 'humanized' monoclonal antibody CAMPATH-1H in patients who were resistant and only partially responsive to DCF. It is too early to know whether these approaches will change the poor outlook for these patients.

T-cell lymphomas in leukaemic phase

T-cell non-Hodgkin's lymphomas develop leukaemia more frequently than do B-cell lymphomas. Two diseases in particular regularly evolve with circulating lymphoma cells in the peripheral blood: adult T-cell leukaemia/lymphoma (**ATLL**) and Sezary syndrome.

ATLL has a distinct geographic distribution affecting mainly the south-west islands of Japan, the Caribbean basin, and some parts of South America (Brazil and Chile). The demonstration of antibodies to human T-cell leukaemia lymphoma virus (**HTLV**)-I, the causative agent of ATLL, is one of the tests necessary for diagnosis. At the genomic level there is evidence of clonal integration of HTLV-I in the malignant T cells. Diagnosis is made by the demonstration of ATLL cells in peripheral blood films. These cells have an irregular nucleus with polylobed configuration and many atypical forms (Plate 22) including large transformed ones. These have been described as 'flower' cells. Patients with ATLL have generalized lymphadenopathy, splenomegaly, and skin rashes. Leucocyte counts are variable but often less than 50 × 10⁹/l. Hypercalcaemia is present in two-thirds of patients and tends to be difficult to control.

ATLL cells may resemble Sezary cells (Plate 23), which have more uniform features and a cerebriform rather than an hyperlobulated nucleus. Lymph-node histology shows diffuse infiltration with pleomorphic T cells of small, medium and large size (Plate 24). The median survival of ATLL is 6 months. Patients are treated as having high-grade non-Hodgkin's lymphoma but remissions are transient and opportunistic infections are common.

Sezary syndrome

This is a form of cutaneous T-cell lymphoma characterized by erythroderma and circulating Sezary cells, usually of small size. The skin infiltration is epidermotropic, with the formation of Pautrier microabcesses. Sezary cells, as well as ATLL cells, are mature T cells with a CD4+, CD8− immunophenotype. The main difference is the strong expression of the interleukin-2 receptor, demonstrated by the monoclonal CD25, in ATLL. Rare cases of T-cell leukaemia without skin involvement resemble Sezary cells morphologically but lack skin involvement and have been described as Sezary-cell leukaemia. The differential diagnosis with ATLL is sometimes difficult as some of these patients are HTLV-I positive. Treatment is as for high-grade non-Hodgkin's lymphoma (Chapter 22.5.3).

REFERENCES

Bennett, J.M. *et al.* (1989). Proposals for the classification of chronic (mature) B and T lymphoid leukaemias. *Journal of Clinical Pathology*, **42**, 567–84.

Binet, J.L. *et al.* (1981). A new prognostic classification of chronic lymphocytic leukemia derived from a multivariate survival analysis. *Cancer*, **48**, 198–6.

Catovsky, D. *et al.* (1994). Long term results with 2'deoxycoformycin in hairy cell leukaemia. *Leukemia and Lymphoma*, **14** (Suppl. 1), 109–13.

Catovsky, D. and Foa, R. (1990). *The lymphoid leukaemias*. Butterworths, London.

Catovsky, D., Fooks, J., and Richards, S. for the MRC Working Party on Leukaemia in Adults (1989). Prognostic factors in chronic lymphocytic leukaemia: the importance of age, sex and response to treatment in survival. *British Journal of Haematology*, **72**, 141–9.

Catovsky, D., Richards, S., Fooks, J., and Hamblin, T.J. (1991). CLL trials in the United Kingdom. The Medical Research Council trials 1, 2 and 3. *Leukemia and Lymphoma*, **5** (Suppl.), 105–12.

Coad, J.E., Matutes, E., and Catovsky, D. (1993). Splenectomy in chronic lymphoproliferative disorders: a report on 70 cases and review of the literature. *Leukemia and Lymphoma*, **10**, 245–64.

French Cooperative Group on Chronic Lymphocytic Leukaemia (1989). Long-term results of the CHOP regimen in stage C chronic lymphocytic leukaemia. *British Journal of Haematology*, **73**, 334–40.

French Cooperative Group on Chronic Lymphocytic Leukaemia (1990). Natural history of stage A chronic lymphocytic leukaemia. *British Journal of Haematology*, **76**, 45–57.

Galton, D.A.G., Goldman, J.M., Wiltshaw, E., Catovsky, D., Henry, K., and Goldenberg, G.J. (1974). Prolymphocytic leukaemia. *British Journal of Haematology*, **27**, 7–23.

International Workshop on CLL (1981). Chronic lymphocytic leukaemia: proposals for a revised prognostic staging system. *British Journal of Haematology*, **48**, 365–7.

Juliusson, G. *et al.* (1990). Prognostic subgroups in B-cell chronic lymphocytic leukemia defined by specific chromosomal abnormalities. *New England Journal of Medicine*, **323**, 720–4.

Keating, M.J. *et al.* (1989). Fludarabine: a new agent with major activity against chronic lymphocytic leukemia. *Blood*, **74**, 19–25.

Keating, M.J. *et al.* (1991). Fludarabine: a new agent with marked cytoreductive activity in untreated chronic lymphocytic leukemia. *Journal of Clinical Oncology*, **9**, 44–9.

Matutes, E. *et al.* (1991). Clinical and laboratory features of 78 cases of T-prolymphocytic leukemia. *Blood*, **78**, 3269–74.

Matutes, E., Morilla, R., Owusu-Ankomah, K., Houlihan, A., and Catovsky, D. (1994). The immunophenotype of splenic lymphoma with villous lymphocytes and its relevance to the differential diagnosis with other B-cell disorders. *Blood*, **83**, 1558–62.

Matutes, E., Morilla, R., Owusu-Ankomah, K., Houlihan, A., Meeus, P., and Catovsky, D. (1994). The immunophenotype of hairy cell leukemia (HCL). Proposal for a scoring system to distinguish HCL from B-cell disorders with hairy or villous lymphocytes. *Leukemia and Lymphoma*, **14** (Suppl. 1), 57–61.

Melo, J.V., Catovsky, D., and Galton, D.A.G. (1986). The relationship between chronic lymphocytic leukaemia and prolymphocytic leukaemia. I. Clinical and laboratory features of 300 patients and characterisation of an intermediate group. *British Journal of Haematology*, **63**, 377–87.

Melo, J.V., Hegde, U., Parreira, A., Thompson, I., Lampert, I.A., and Catovsky, D. (1987). Splenic B cell lymphoma with circulating villous lymphocytes: differential diagnosis of B cell leukaemias with large spleens. *Journal of Clinical Pathology*, **40**, 642–51.

Melo, J.V. *et al.* (1988). Morphology and immunology of circulating cells in the leukaemic phase of follicular lymphoma. *Journal of Clinical Pathology*, **41**, 951–9.

Mercieca, J. *et al.* (1992). Massive abdominal lymphadenopathy in hairy cell leukaemia: a report of 12 cases. *British Journal of Haematology*, **82**, 547–54.

Mulligan, S.P., Matutes, E., Dearden, C., and Catovsky, D. (1991). Splenic lymphoma with villous lymphocytes: natural history and response to therapy in 50 cases. *British Journal of Haematology*, **78**, 206–9.

Montserrat, E., Sanchez-Bisono, J., Vinolas, N., and Rozman, C. (1986). Lymphocyte doubling time in chronic lymphocytic leukaemia: analysis of its prognostic significance. *British Journal of Haematology*, **62**, 567–75.

Piro, L.D., Carrera, C.J., Beutler, E., and Carson, D.A. (1988). 2-chlorodeoxyadenosine: an effective new agent for the treatment of chronic lymphocytic leukemia. *Blood*, **72**, 1069–73.

Pombo de Oliveira, M.S., Jaffe, E.S., and Catovsky, D. (1989). Leukaemic phase of mantle zone (intermediate) lymphoma: its characterisation in 11 cases. *Journal of Clinical Pathology*, **42**, 962–72.

Que, T.H., Garcia Marco, J., Ellis, J., Brito-Babapulle, V., Boyle, S., and Catovsky, D. (1993). Trisomy 12 in chronic lymphocytic leukemia detected by fluorescence in situ hybridization: analysis by stage, immunophenotype and morphology. *Blood*, **82**, 571–5.

Rai, K.R., Sawitsky, A., Cronkite, E., Chanana, A.D., Levy, R.N., and Pasternack, B.S. (1975). Clinical staging of chronic lymphocytic leukemia. *Blood*, **46**, 219–34.

Rozman, C. *et al.* (1984). Bone marrow histologic pattern. The best single prognostic parameter in chronic lymphocytic leukemia: a multivariate survival analysis of 329 cases. *Blood*, **64**, 642–8.

Sivakumaran, M. *et al.* (1991). Patterns of CD16 and CD56 expression in persistent expansions of CD3+NKa+ lymphocytes are predictive for clonal T-cell receptor gene rearrangements. *British Journal of Haematology*, **78**, 368–77.

22.3.7 Myelodysplastic syndromes

D. Catovsky

Definition

Myelodysplastic syndromes are acquired, clonal, and progressive cytopenias associated with a hypercellular bone marrow and ineffective haemopoiesis. This pathogenesis should distinguish these disorders from cytopenias caused by peripheral destruction or resulting from aplastic bone marrows. As a rule, two or three of the bone marrow-cell lineages are involved in myelodysplastic syndromes but, rarely, only one may be affected. Because anaemia is the most common manifestation, these disorders have been designated as refractory anaemias of various types, although the term refractory cytopenia may be more accurate.

Two major types of myelodysplastic syndrome can be recognized, both carrying an increased risk of transformation to acute myeloid leukaemia: (i) primary myelodysplastic syndrome, the most common, has no known cause, and (ii) secondary myelodysplastic syndrome, which results from the use of chemotherapeutic agents, with or without radiotherapy, for the treatment of lymphomas, multiple myeloma, or solid tumours. Secondary or treatment-related myelodysplastic syndrome often precedes the development of overt acute myeloid leukaemia and occurs with a frequency that is in direct relation to the duration and intensity of the cytotoxic therapy, often 1 to 10 years after diagnosis of the original cancer.

Myelodysplastic syndromes have been described under other names in the past. Two terms, preleukaemic syndrome and smouldering acute leukaemia, have been widely used in the United States. The term preleukaemia was used mainly to define refractory cytopenias involving two cell lineages but without an increase in blast cells in the bone marrow. Smouldering leukaemia was used to describe cases with an increase in blast cells but short of the values frequently found in established acute myeloid leukaemia. The French, American, and British (**FAB**) cooperative group has proposed a classification of these heterogeneous conditions in order to learn more about their pathogenesis and clinical course, and to guide their management. The terms used by the FAB classification take into account the blood and bone marrow findings to define the various types of myelodysplastic syndrome and do not assume the development of acute myeloid leukaemia as inevitable, recognizing that a high proportion of patients die as a consequence of the cytopenias without features of acute leukaemia. In contrast to acute myeloid leukaemia, myelodysplasia is characterized by functional and morphological abnormalities resulting from defective haemopoiesis and is not, in its early stages, associated with the monomorphic cell proliferation characteristic of leukaemic processes. On the other hand, 10 to 15 per cent of acute myeloid leukaemias show features of trilineage myelodysplasia and it is likely that in these patients a subclinical phase of myelodysplastic syndrome preceded the development of acute myeloid leukaemia.

Clinical and laboratory features

Myelodysplastic syndromes almost always affect adults over the age of 50 years. The median age of patients with primary myelodysplastic syndrome is between 60 and 70 years, with slightly more males than females. Secondary myelodysplastic syndrome affects, as a rule, younger patients. The disease is rare but well documented in children.

Anaemia, fever or bleeding manifestations are the most common presenting symptoms. There are usually few, if any, significant physical signs. Splenomegaly is found in 20 per cent of cases, more often associated with one of the forms of myelodysplastic syndrome, chronic myelomonocytic leukaemia.

The key elements for diagnosis, in the presence of persistent anaemia or pancytopenia, are the examination of peripheral blood and bone marrow films.

HAEMATOLOGICAL FINDINGS

Anaemia (haemoglobin less than 12 g/dl) is the most constant feature; it is usually normocytic and normochromic, or moderately macrocytic (MCV greater than 104 fl). The red cells may show anisopoikylocytosis, polychromasia, punctate basophilia, and, commonly, nucleated forms with dyserythropoietic features. Reticulocyte counts are usually low (less than 0.5 per cent).

The white-cell count is variable, often low (less than $4 \times 10^9/l$) and, less commonly, normal. Leucocytosis with a monocytosis is only a feature of chronic myelomonocytic leukaemia. Neutropenia (less than $1 \times 10^9/l$) is seen in one-third of cases, depending on the type of myelodysplastic syndrome; it is almost always severe in cases transforming to acute myeloid leukaemia and it is rare in sideroblastic anaemia. A common finding in the blood films of patients with myelodysplastic syndrome is the presence of abnormal neutrophils (Fig. 1): (a) hypogranular or agranular forms, with absence or marked reduction of azurophil granules and/or specific secondary granules; (b) cells with a round or bilobed nucleus (acquired Pelger anomaly); (c) abnormal chromatin clumping; and (d) hypersegmented neutrophils. A proportion of myelocytes and blasts may be present, depending on the type of myelodysplastic syndrome. Cytochemical reactions for myeloperoxidase or Sudan Black B can highlight the neutrophil abnormalities by demonstrating two populations of neutrophils, positive, as normal cells, and negative, due to the absence of primary granules.

Thrombocytopenia (platelets less than $100 \times 10^9/l$) is less frequent than anaemia and neutropenia, again depending on the type of syndrome. It is seen with higher frequency in chronic myelomonocytic leukaemia (two-thirds of cases) and in cases with increased bone-marrow blasts or in transformation to acute myeloid leukaemia. The blood film may show large or even giant platelets and, rarely, megakaryocyte fragments.

BONE MARROW

The marrow aspirate is always normocellular or hypercellular, displaying quantitative and qualitative changes with maturation defects in two or three of the cell lineages. These features are summarized in Table 1. The presence of ringed sideroblasts (detected by the Prussian blue stain) is a feature of acquired idiopathic sideroblastic anaemia, in which over 15 per cent of the erythroblasts display the typical ring perinuclear arrangement of siderotic granules. Ringed sideroblasts may also be seen in the other types of myelodysplastic syndrome. Ultrastructural studies have shown that these granules result from the deposition of iron in the mitochondria and from aggregates of ferritin particles in the cytoplasm. Nuclear abnormalities in the erythroblasts, including cells with single, double, or more indentations and abnormal cytoplasmic features of various types are characteristic of dyserythropoiesis, and are seen in the majority of patients with myelodysplastic syndromes (Fig. 2). Dysgranulopoiesis is more marked in cases with excess marrow blasts. In addition to the abnormalities seen in the neutrophils, promyelocytes and myelocytes may show sparse granularity or coarse azurophil granules.

The presence of blast cells in the marrow is one of the main features considered for the classification of myelodysplastic syndrome. Two types of blasts have been recognized as significant: type I, with absent cytoplasmic granules and type II with few azurophil granules. Promyelo-

Table 1 *Features of myelodysplasia in the bone marrow-cell lineages*

> *Dyserythropoiesis*: ringed sideroblasts; nuclear fragments; multinuclearity; abnormal nuclear shape; karyorrhexis; cytoplasmic vacuolation; megaloblastic changes (Fig. 2)
> *Dysgranulopoiesis*: agranular or hypogranular neutrophils and myelocytes; hyposegmented nucleus (Pelger anomaly); abnormal chromatin clumping; hypersegmented neutrophils, occasionally with bizarre shapes; blasts with few or no granules; irregular distribution of cytoplasmic basophilia
> *Dysmegakaryopoiesis*: micromegakaryocytes; large or small mononuclear forms; megakaryocytes with multiple, small, round nuclei; small cells with bilobed nuclei (Fig. 3)

cytes are distinguished from myeloblasts by their eccentric nucleus with a clear zone in its vicinity (which corresponds to the Golgi zone seen at ultrastructural level), the presence of numerous azurophil granules, a low nuclear/cytoplasmic ratio, and a more condensed nuclear chromatin pattern.

Megakaryocytes may be decreased in number or show the qualitative abnormalities listed in Table 1 (Fig. 3). The degree of dysmyelopoiesis, in particular dysgranulopoiesis and dymegakaryopoiesis, has been shown to correlate with progression to acute myeloid leukaemia.

BONE-MARROW TREPHINE BIOPSY

In the presence of cytopenia and a leucoerythroblastic blood picture a marrow biopsy is necessary to exclude hypoplastic anaemia, rare cases of hypoplastic acute myeloid leukaemia, idiopathic myelofibrosis, and infiltration by neoplastic cells. Even though it is always possible to obtain a bone marrow aspirate in myelodysplastic syndrome, a trephine biopsy adds diagnostic and prognostic information. The features of dysmyelopoiesis are best seen in plastic-embedded marrow biopsy specimens and semithin sections (3 μm), which should include stains for reticulin fibres. Myelofibrosis is not a feature of primary myelodysplastic syndrome but it is not rare in secondary myelodysplastic syndrome. The megakaryocytic abnormalities can be appreciated in biopsy sections as well as films obtained from aspirates. The trephine biopsy is, as a rule, hypercellular, with few remaining fat spaces. The abnormal localization of immature precursors (**ALIP**), that is, clusters of blasts in the central spaces of the marrow and not along the endosteal spaces where they are normally found, has been considered a distinct feature of myelodysplastic syndromes. The presence of ALIP correlates well with the proportion of blasts seen in aspirates in cases with more than 5 per cent blasts. In addition, cases in which the aspirates do not show an excess of blasts may show ALIP clusters recognized only in trephine biopsies. This is important because the presence of ALIP is associated with worse prognosis and with a higher probability of developing acute myeloid leukaemia.

Classification

The FAB classification (Table 2) has been found to be reproducible and a basis for comparisons between different series. The main features considered for the classification, in the presence of dysmyelopoiesis, are (a) the proportion of marrow blasts (fewer than 5 per cent, 5–20 per cent, and between 21 and 30 per cent), (b) the presence of ringed sideroblasts, (c) blood monocytosis, and (d) the presence of blasts in blood films and/ or Auer rods.

The five categories of myelodysplastic syndrome should not be considered as rigid entities. Progression from one to another, usually from refractory anaemia to refractory anaemia with excess of blasts (**RAEB**), and from RAEB to RAEB in transformation (**RAEB-t**) (see Table 2) is frequently seen. In addition, all of them can progress to acute myeloid leukaemia, although with different frequency.

Fig. 1 Peripheral blood cells of myelodysplastic syndrome: (a) neutrophils with the Pelger anomaly; (b) monocytes and a neutrophil from a case of chronic myelomonocytic leukaemia. × 900.

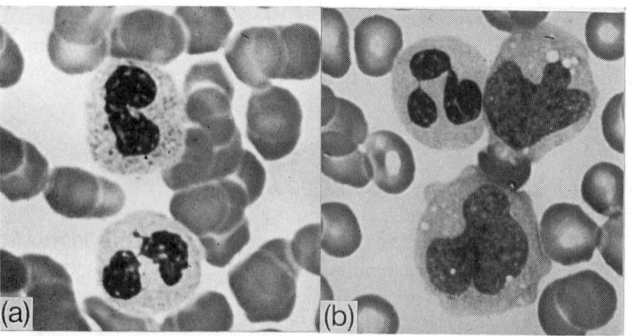

Fig. 2 Bone marrow appearances in myelodysplastic syndrome. (a) Erythroblasts from a case of refractory anaemia; one of them shows nuclear fragments. (b) Cells from a case of refractory anaemia with excess of blasts. Note a blast cell (arrow), hypogranular neutrophils and a late erythroblast with megaloblastic features. × 900.

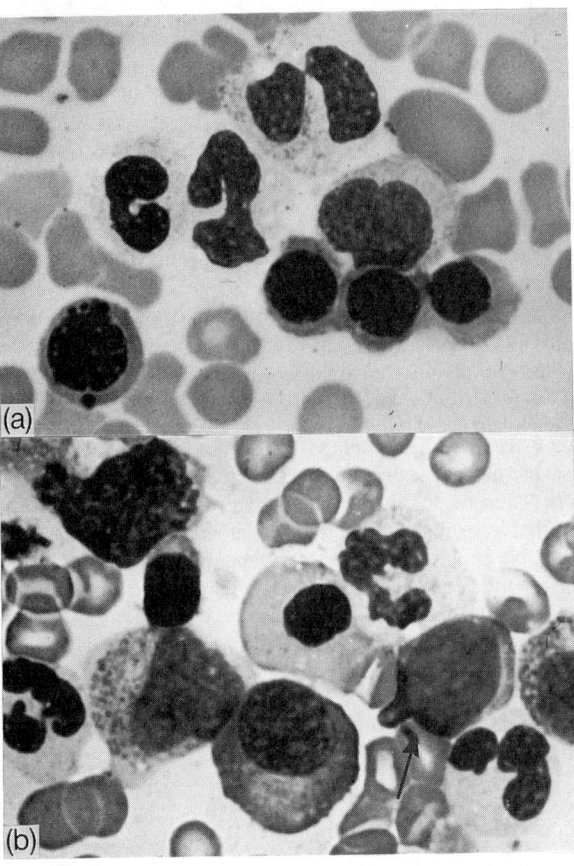

Fig. 3 Qualitative abnormalities of megakaryocytes: (a,b,d) binucleated or trinucleated micromegakaryocytes; (c) large mononuclear form. × 900.

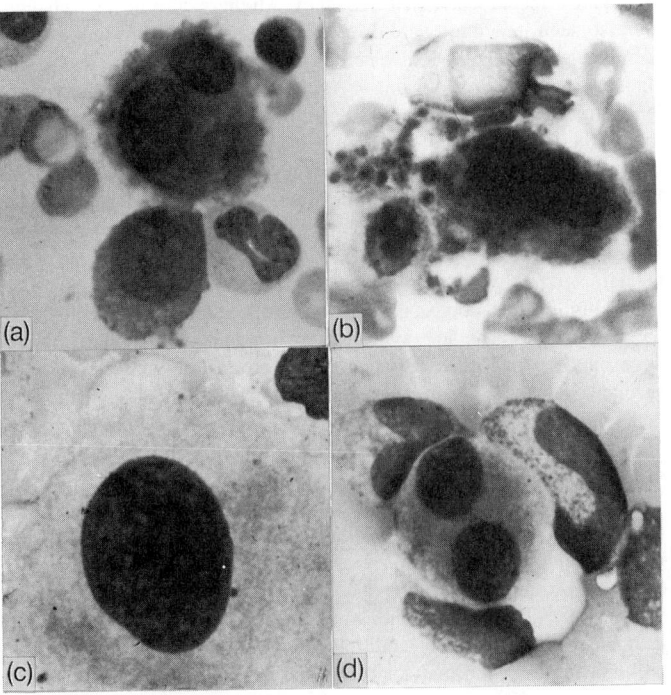

Table 2 *FAB classification of myelodysplastic syndromes*

Disease (abbreviation)	Percentage of blasts	
	BM	PB
Refractory anaemia (RA) / RA with ringed sideroblasts (RAS)	< 5	< 5
RA with excess of blasts (RAEB) / Chronic myelomonocytic leukaemia (CMML)*	5–20**	< 5
RAEB in transformation (RAEB-t)	21–30**	> 5

After Bennett *et al.* (1982).

BM, bone marrow; PB, peripheral blood.

*Absolute monocytosis ($> 1 \times 10^9/l$; frequently $>5 \times 10^9/l$).

**This percentage takes into account all BM cells; in cases with > 50% erythroblasts the percentage of blasts is calculated by excluding the erythroid cells. If this percentage is >30% in any of the assessments the diagnosis is acute myeloid leukaemia.

REFRACTORY ANAEMIA

Patients with refractory anaemia often have a macrocytic anaemia with erythroid hyperplasia in the marrow but with ineffective erythropoiesis, also shown by ferrokinetic studies. Neutropenia and/or thrombocytopenia are frequently associated features, although very rarely they can be seen without anaemia. Blast cells are not seen in blood films and are not prominent in the marrow (less than 5 per cent). Ringed sideroblasts are absent or seen in less than 15 per cent of the nucleated red cells. The diagnosis of refractory anaemia may be difficult in cases with minimal dysplasia. Infections and bleeding are the main clinical problems, and these depend on the severity of the cytopenia. Evolution to acute myeloid leukaemia is not uncommon, particularly in patients who showed clusters of blasts in trephine biopsies, defined as ALIP. The relative incidence of refractory anaemia within cases of myelodysplastic syndrome is between 20 and 30 per cent.

REFRACTORY ANAEMIA WITH RINGED SIDEROBLASTS

This condition is characterized by anaemia with erythroid hyperplasia and the presence of ringed sideroblasts in the marrow. Deficient haemoglobinization of some of the red-cell precursors results in a dimorphic blood picture; platelet and white-cell counts are often normal. It has a chronic course with a significantly lower risk of evolution to acute myeloid leukaemia than other types of myelodysplastic syndrome. The risk may be greater in cases with abnormalities of platelets and/or granulocytes; it is low in cases involving only the erythroid series. The frequency of this disease within the group of myelodysplastic syndromes has varied in different series according to whether pure erythroid cases (also described as acquired idiopathic sideroblastic anaemic) or those with involvement of other cell lineages were included; the incidence in recent studies was 10 to 15 per cent.

REFRACTORY ANAEMIA WITH EXCESS OF BLASTS

The characteristic of this group is the presence of between 5 and 20 per cent of type I or II blasts in the bone marrow. Cytopenias involving the three cell lineages are common and are associated with marked dysplastic changes, particularly dysgranulopoiesis and dysmegakaryopoiesis (see Table 1). Ringed sideroblasts are present in one-third of cases. The frequency of RAEB has varied from 20 to 30 per cent in different series. This condition has a higher incidence of bleeding complications, infections due to neutropenia, and evolution to acute myeloid leukaemia than refractory anaemia and refractory anaemia with ringed sideroblasts. Patients with RAEB have an equal chance of dying as a result of marrow failure or leukaemic transformation. In a proportion of patients without severe cytopenia the condition may remain stable for many months or even years. It is this group that has influenced the need to distinguish RAEB from *de novo* acute myeloid leukaemia (>30 per cent blasts in the marrow) and RAEB-t (>20 per cent and up to 30 per cent blasts) because of their different prognoses. This is a contentious issue because the differences in survival (ranging between 6 and 15 months) and the rate of evolution to acute myeloid leukaemia (c.50 per cent) can be similar between RAEB and RAEB-t.

RAEB IN TRANSFORMATION

This group differs from RAEB in that there are over 20 per cent (up to 30 per cent) of blasts in the marrow and/or 5 per cent or more blasts in the blood. Rarely, the presence of Auer rods in the granulocyte precursors is a feature of the disease. RAEB-t defines a group of cases with intermediate features between myelodysplastic syndrome and acute myeloid leukaemia. The incidence is of the order of 10 to 15 per cent and the poor prognosis of these patients (median survival of 4 to 6 months in most series) suggests that the clinical behaviour of RAEB-t, if untreated, is not very different from that of *de novo* acute myeloid leukaemia, in to which it evolves in at least 50 per cent of cases.

CHRONIC MYELOMONOCYTIC LEUKAEMIA

It is not generally agreed whether chronic myelomonocytic leukaemia should be considered a myelodysplastic syndrome or a myeloproliferative disorder. The appearances of the marrow are similar to RAEB, but with prominence of promonocytes, which morphologically may resemble promyelocytes. The peripheral blood, on the other hand, is characterized by neutrophilia and monocytosis (in excess of $1 \times 10^9/l$) and the only consistent cytopenia is thrombocytopenia, which is often responsible for bleeding manifestations. In contrast to other types of myelodysplastic syndrome, 30 per cent of patients with chronic myelomonocytic leukaemia have moderate splenomegaly. Gingival hypertrophy and lymphadenopathy, a feature of acute monocytic leukaemia, is not seen in chronic myelomonocytic leukaemia. The incidence of this leukaemia within the various series describing myelodysplastic syndromes is between 5 and 15 per cent. Some patients with chronic myelomonocytic leukaemia are diagnosed as atypical (Ph-negative) chronic myeloid leukaemia, although in that condition a higher proportion of immature granulocytes is present in the blood and the clinical course is shorter than in chronic myelomonocytic leukaemia. Patients with chronic myelomonocytic leukaemia are often elderly and in some the disease runs a chronic course. However, overall median survivals are short (1–2 years), with one-third of cases evolving to acute myeloid leukaemia.

Differential diagnosis

Myelodysplastic syndromes should be distinguished from other types of anaemia and from overt leukaemias. Other causes of aregenerative chronic anaemia, renal or liver disease for example, should always be excluded by appropriate investigations. In cases of refractory anaemia it is important to exclude nutritional anaemias by measuring iron, vitamin B_{12}, and folic acid levels. Even if this has been done it is customary to initiate a trial of treatment with vitamin B_{12}, folic acid, and/or pyridoxine. As a rule, patients with myelodysplastic syndrome will not respond. The guidelines of the percentage of blasts in RAEB and RAEB-t are useful to distinguish these two conditions from established acute myeloid leukaemia. One type of acute myeloid leukaemia, erythroleukaemia or FAB-M6, characterized by bizarre erythroid hyperplasia and increased numbers of blasts, may still present problems in the differential diagnosis with these two forms of myelodysplastic syndrome. This difficulty often arises from the variability in the overall percentage of erythroblasts in erythroleukaemia. To overcome this

Table 3 *Chromosome abnormalities in myelodysplastic syndromes (MDS)*

Monosomy or deletion of chromosome 5 [−5; del(5q)]*
Monosomy or deletion of chromosome 7 [−7; del(7q)]*
Translocation t(1;7)
Trisomy 8 (+ 8)
Abnormal 11q23**
Deletion 12p [del(12p)]
Isochromosome 17q
Trisomy 19 or 21 (+ 19,+ 21)
Deletion 20q [del(20q)]
Abnormal 21q22**

*These are seen in 30 to 40% of primary and secondary MDS; del(7q) is illustrated in Fig. 4.

**Seen in MDS/acute myeloid leukaemia secondary to treatment with drugs targeted against DNA-topoisomerase II, usually as balanced translocations with other chromosomes (Pedersen-Bjergaard *et al.* 1993).

problem the FAB group has proposed that if more than 50 per cent of erythroblasts are present in the bone marrow, the diagnosis of erythroleukaemia may still be possible if 30 per cent or more of the non-erythroid cells (that is, excluding erythroblasts) are blasts, even if the total percentage of blasts is less than 30 per cent. Bone-marrow trephine biopsies are useful to exclude aplastic anaemia and hypoplastic acute myeloid leukaemia (foci of blasts in a hypocellular bone marrow). Cases of secondary myelodysplastic syndrome may have atypical features including fibrosis, which is rare in primary myelodysplastic syndromes. Chromosome analysis may be useful in cases of refractory anaemia if one of the typical clonal abnormalities of a myelodysplastic syndrome is demonstrated (Table 3).

Chromosome and cellular abnormalities

Clonal karyotypic abnormalities can be demonstrated in the marrows of 50 to 70 per cent of patients with myelodysplastic syndromes. The incidence of chromosome abnormalities in secondary myelodysplastic syndrome is between 90 and 100 per cent. The most frequent abnormalities in myelodysplastic syndromes are listed in Table 3. These involve numerical or structural changes of chromosomes 5, 7 (Fig. 4), and 8, which are affected with equal frequency. All these chromosome changes are also seen in acute myeloid leukaemia. On the other hand, none of the changes associated with specific types of acute myeloid leukaemia, such as t(8;21) in myeloblastic (FAB-M2) or t(15;17) in promyelocytic leukaemia (FAB-M3), is found in myelodysplastic syndromes, and neither is the Philadelphia chromosome, t(9;22).

Some abnormalities have been described in association with particular types of myelodysplastic syndrome. For example, 5q−, when found in refractory anaemia or, less frequently, in RAEB, constitutes a distinct syndrome, 'the 5q− syndrome'. This is found more often in women and is characterized by macrocytic anaemia, normal white-cell counts, normal or high platelet counts, dyserythropoiesis, and hypolobulated micromegakaryocytes. The 5q− syndrome is associated with a relatively better prognosis than other types of myelodysplastic syndrome (median survival 5–6 years) and a lower incidence of evolution to acute myeloid leukaemia (10–15 per cent). Monosomy 7 (−7), on the other hand, has been associated with abnormal neutrophil function and childhood cases of myelodysplastic syndrome.

The frequency of chromosome abnormalities is greater in cases with more than 5 per cent marrow blasts, that is RAEB and RAEB-t. Similarly, the evolution to acute myeloid leukaemia is high (75 per cent) in cases with complex karyotype abnormalities, and twice as high in cases of myelodysplastic syndrome with chromosome abnormalities than in those without them. In addition to its prognostic significance, the presence of an abnormal karyotype is important in the differential diagnosis between myelodysplastic syndromes and non-preleukaemic anaemias.

Changes observed in therapy-related myelodysplastic syndromes seem to bear a relationship to the type of agent(s) used to treat the primary malignancy. In cases treated with alkylating agents the most common abnormalities are of chromosomes 5 and 7. In patients treated with agents that target DNA-topoisomerase II, such as the podophyllotoxin derivatives etoposide and teniposide, or anthracyclines combined with cisplatin or other drugs, there is a more rapid evolution to acute myeloid leukaemia and the most common abnormalities involve balanced translocations of chromosomes 11 and 21 with breakpoints at 11q23 and 21q22 (Table 3). The latter abnormalities have also been observed in secondary acute myeloid leukaemia, with or without a phase of myelodysplastic syndrome, and in 3.8 per cent of children in one study who developed acute myeloid leukaemia after treatment for acute lymphoblastic leukaemia with protocols that included epipodophyllotoxins. The deletion of chromosome 5, del(5q), has provided some clues about the pathogenesis of myelodysplastic syndrome because several genes encoding for growth and differentiation factors have been mapped to the long arm of chromosome 5, such as for the interleukins 3, 4, and 5, colony-stimulating factor (**CSF**) 1, granulocyte–monocyte CFS, and c-FMS (see below).

CHANGES IN ONCOGENES

Two abnormalities at the molecular level have been noted in myelodysplastic syndrome with slightly greater frequency than in acute myeloid leukaemia. These involve point mutations of the *ras* (40 per cent of cases) and c-*fms* (10 per cent of cases) genes, which result in activation of those genes. The *ras* mutations have been more extensively studied and affect codons 12/13 and 61, which involves, in 50 per cent of point mutations, the substitution of aspartate for glycine in the normal p21 RAS protein. Following mutational activation, the *ras* family of genes, h-*ras*, k-*ras*, and n-*ras*, functions as oncogenes. It is still not clear whether these changes are primary or secondary events in the development of myelodysplastic syndromes, or if they correlate with a greater frequency of evolution to acute myeloid leukaemia as suggested by some studies. The highest proportion of *ras* and c-*fms* mutations has been found in chronic myelomonocytic leukaemia.

BONE MARROW CULTURE

In vitro cultures in semisolid media that support the growth of haemopoietic precursor cells, cells forming granulocyte/macrophage colonies (**CFU-GM**), for example, have been used to predict the progression of myelodysplastic syndrome to acute myeloid leukaemia. This is often associated with an increase in cluster formation and/or a decrease in the number of colonies formed. The abnormalities in *in vitro* growth observed in myelodysplastic syndrome are similar to those in acute myeloid leukaemia.

Prognosis

Despite the chronic course of some cases, most series have shown that the median survival of patients with myelodysplastic syndrome ranges between 12 and 28 months. The main causes of death are complications resulting from the cytopenias, that is bleeding and infections, and evolution to acute leukaemia, almost always acute myeloid leukaemia.

A number of prognostic factors have been identified by several studies (Table 4). Most of them are closely interrelated so that it is difficult to identify which is the more important. The FAB classification (Table 2) has been shown to correlate with prognosis, the worst groups being RAEB and RAEB-t, both of which have the highest rate of evolution to acute myeloid leukaemia as well as the more severe neutropenias. The severity of the neutropenia and thrombocytopenia will have a direct bearing on some of the complications. An increase in blast cells, which is one of the determinants of the FAB classification, is one of the bad prognostic features. Patients with fewer than 5 per cent of marrow blasts, for example in refractory anaemia and refractory anaemia with ringed sideroblasts, have median survivals of 3 to 5 years in some series. The longest survivals are found in the latter when features of dyshaemopoiesis, other than the presence of ringed sideroblasts, are absent. The presence of ALIP (see above) identified in marrow trephine biopsies is a poor prognostic finding in patients with refractory anaemia and refractory anaemia with ringed sideroblasts, even if the marrow aspirates show less than 5 per cent blasts; it is often associated with transformation to acute myeloid leukaemia.

A number of scoring systems have been proposed that take into account the degree of cytopenia (Table 4) and the percentage of marrow blasts (above or below 5 per cent) (Mufti, Sanz, Aul); some of them also include age (above or below 60 years) and lactate dehydrogenase levels (over 200 u/l). Patients with myelodysplastic syndromes with high scores have a statistically significant shorter survival than those with low scores. These systems appear to recognize good and bad prognostic subgroups among patients with refractory anaemia, refractory anaemia with ringed sideroblasts, and RAEB. One scoring system (Varela) is based on the levels of neutrophils and platelets (quantitative components), and of dysgranulopoiesis and dysmegakaryopoiesis. The latter was found to be predictive of the evolution to acute myeloid leukaemia, whilst the overall score was important in predicting survival.

Cytogenetic findings have independent prognostic value. Recent studies have shown that incorporating these into a scoring system can predict both overall survival and evolution to acute myeloid leukaemia. Cases with complex rearrangements (at least three chromosome abnormalities)

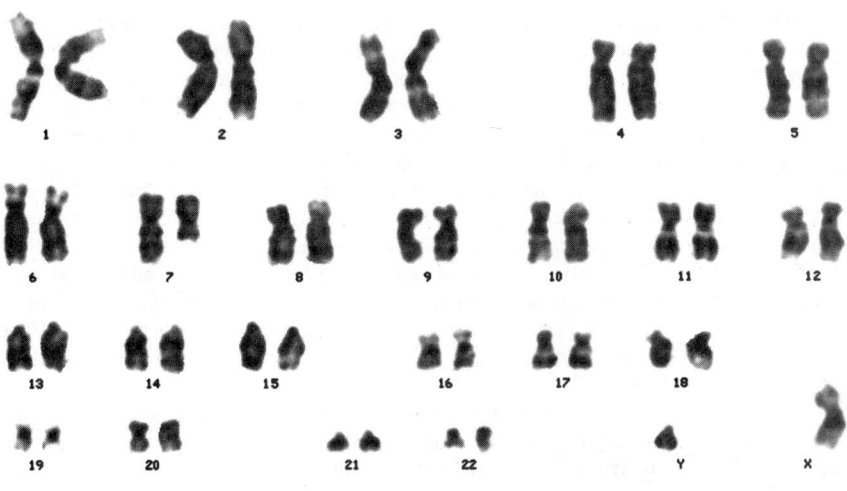

Fig. 4 Karyotype of a patient with myelodysplastic syndrome showing deletion on the long arm of chromosome 7, del(7q).

Table 4 *Prognostic factors in myelodysplastic syndromes*

Age > 60 years
Severity of the cytopenia*
Degree of myelodysplasia
Bone marrow blasts > 5%
FAB classification
ALIP** in bone marrow biopsies
Karyotypic abnormalities

*Hb < 10 g/dl, platelets < 100 × 10⁹/l and neutrophils < 2.5 × 10⁹/l in the Bournemouth score (Mufti *et al.* 1985); varying levels of neutrophils and platelets (Varela *et al.* 1985); Hb < 9 g/dl and platelets < 100 × 10⁹/l (Aul *et al.* 1992); platelet counts < 50 × 10⁹/l (Sanz *et al.* 1989).

**Abnormal localization of immature precursors, i.e. clusters of blast cells in the centre of the bone marrow spaces as opposed to their normal localization along the endosteal surface (Tricot *et al.* 1984).

have the worst prognosis. The myelodysplastic syndromes have been divided into low-, intermediate-, and high-risk groups based on blood counts, bone marrow blasts, ALIP, and cytogenetics. By combining karyotype (complex or not) and bone marrow blasts (above or below 10 per cent), rates of progression to acute myeloid leukaemia have been predicted by the combination in three groups of patients.

Although for clinical use, simple systems based only on blood counts and percentage of blasts are preferable, the more complex systems add important information that may be crucial in deciding on a treatment strategy, which could vary widely from supportive care only to radical attempts to cure. The prognostic as well as diagnostic information added to the clinical scores by chromosome analysis and bone marrow biopsies has implications for clinical management.

Complications

Infections due to neutropenia and bleeding due to thrombocytopenia are the main problems encountered in the management of myelodysplastic syndromes. Interestingly, these two factors are the most common causes of death in patients with refractory anaemia, with or without ringed sideroblasts. Neutrophil function (adhesion, chemotaxis, enzyme content, phagocytosis, microbicidal) is also depressed in myelodysplastic syndromes and, as a result, infections may be a feature in patients with normal neutrophil counts. Patients with RAEB have an equal chance of dying of these complications or of leukaemia.

PROGRESSION TO ACUTE MYELOID LEUKAEMIA

An evolution towards acute myeloid leukaemia is the inevitable outcome in 30 to 50 per cent of patients with RAEB and with chronic myelo-monocytic leukaemia, and in greater than 50 per cent of those with RAEB-t. This course is less common in refractory anaemia with or without ringed sideroblasts (5–15 per cent of cases); in these the finding of ALIP in marrow biopsy specimens may predict leukaemic evolution. Similarly, complex cytogenetic abnormalities and a high cluster to colony ratio in CFU-GM cultures, particularly if they progress, may precede the leukaemia. The group of myelodysplastic syndromes with the highest risk of progression to acute myeloid leukaemia has complex karyotypes and more than 10 per cent blasts in the bone marrow. The opposite, absence of a complex karyotype and less than 10 per cent blasts, defines the group with the lowest risk of leukaemic evolution.

Secondary myelodysplastic syndrome

This condition is seen now with increasing frequency in younger patients who have been treated intensively or for prolonged periods with cytotoxic drugs. Many cases of secondary acute myeloid leukaemia evolve through a phase of myelodysplastic syndrome. Therapy-related acute myeloid leukaemia/myelodysplastic syndrome is the most serious long-term complication of cancer chemotherapy. Several factors may help to distinguish secondary from primary myelodysplastic syndromes. Secondary myelodysplastic syndromes show early macrocytosis, a hypocellular marrow or an increase in reticulin fibres leading, sometimes, to myelofibrosis. The risk of secondary myelodysplastic syndrome and acute myeloid leukaemia increases with the duration of exposure, and may vary according to the type of cytotoxic agent used. In myelomatosis the use of melphalan for more than 3 years is associated with a 10 per cent risk of myelodysplastic syndrome and acute myeloid leukaemia in those surviving 5 years. As described above, there is a difference in patients treated primarily with alkylating agents and those treated with drugs, such as etoposide, that target topoisomerase II. The risk of leukaemia with the latter agents increases more steeply from the first year after treatment and is associated with chromosome translocations involving 11q23 and 21q22. The risk of leukaemia and myelodysplastic syndrome with alkylating agents increases by 1 per cent a year from the second year since starting therapy, and the most common cytogenetic changes are loss or deletion of chromosomes 5 or 7 (Table 3).

Treatment

Because of the life-threatening nature of myelodysplastic syndromes, the choice of active treatment to induce a remission or simple supportive care to protect the patient from the effects of the cytopenia must be made with extreme care. Anaemia without other evidence of marrow failure could always be supported by blood transfusions. Regular transfusions are indicated to keep haemoglobin levels above 8 g/dl. As stated earlier, a therapeutic trial of folic acid, pyridoxine, and/or vitamin B₁₂ should always be considered to identify responsive anaemias. For moderate neutropenias, antibiotics or antifungal agents should be given at the first sign of infection. For patients with more than 5 per cent blasts, or with marked cytopenia, supportive measures may not be enough to prolong survival. Anabolic steroids and glucocorticosteroids, although widely used in the past, are no longer indicated.

A number of agents that induce differentiation and maturation of leukaemic cells have been used to treat patients with myelodysplastic syndrome. One of them, *cis*-retinoic acid, can improve the anaemia in some patients with refractory anaemia or refractory anaemia with ringed sideroblasts but has little effect on other types of myelodysplastic syndrome. Another, cytosine arabinoside (**Ara-C**), is already known to be effective in acute myeloid leukaemia by its cytotoxic effect. Ara-C has been used at low doses, 10 mg/m² subcutaneously twice a day for 2 or 3 weeks, in order to induce haematological remissions. Although the exact mechanism of action of low-dose Ara-C in myelodysplastic syndrome is still not clear (whether inhibition of DNA synthesis and/or differentiation induction in myeloid cells), this agent has been shown to induce remissions (partial plus complete) in 30 to 40 per cent of cases. The median survival of patients treated with low-dose Ara-C is 9 months. Patients with thrombocytopenia and complex chromosome abnormalities respond less well to this form of treatment. Despite its differentiating effect, patients treated with low-dose Ara-C often undergo a transient deterioration of their cytopenia during the early stages of treatment and therefore require effective supportive care with blood products and antimicrobials until a full response is obtained. Significant myelotoxicity is observed in 80 per cent of patients and one-third may require hospital admission to treat the complications. High-dose Ara-C in combination with anthracyclines is indicated in RAEB-t where response rates can approach those obtained in acute myeloid leukaemia.

Oral etoposide and hydroxyurea may be beneficial in chronic myelo-monocytic leukaemia, particularly in cases with leucocytosis and involvement of such as spleen, lymph nodes, skin, and pleura. Two randomized trials are currently comparing these two agents, which can be given orally daily.

Intensive combination chemotherapy, as used in acute myeloid leukaemia, should be considered for younger patients with myelodysplastic syndrome. The finding of complete remissions with normal haemopoietic regeneration in patients treated with these regimens demonstrates that normal stem cells are still present in myelodysplastic bone marrows. The remissions with this approach are short (less than 1 year). Supralethal therapy with drugs and total-body irradiation, followed by a bone marrow transplantation from an HLA-identical sibling, have been tried with some success in younger patients with primary and secondary myelodysplastic syndromes. This is the only treatment that can achieve some cures but, because it can be used mainly in patients below 50 years of age, its overall benefits are limited. In contrast to acute myeloid leukaemia, allogeneic bone-marrow transplantation in myelodysplastic syndromes does not require prior induction of remission by combination chemotherapy. The best results have been gained in refractory anaemia with or without ringed sideroblasts and the worst in RAEB-t. There is little information at present on the use of autologous marrow transplants.

A new impetus for the treatment of myelodysplastic syndromes has resulted from the availability for clinical use of haemopoietic growth factors. These have been shown to correct cytopenias *in vivo* despite a defective response by bone marrows from myelodysplastic syndrome to these factors *in vitro*. Enhanced proliferative responses have been found in culture and this has caused concern about the possible stimulation towards acute leukaemia. The two most commonly used growth factors are GM-CSF and granulocyte (G)-CSF. Both increase significantly the levels of neutrophils in 60 to 70 per cent of patients and consequently decrease the risk of infections. Minor improvements in reticulocyte and platelet counts have been recorded with GM-CSF, although a drop in platelets has also been observed. The effect of both growth factors is seen only whilst they are being given and ceases once they are discontinued. At present it is not clear whether this therapy can have a significant impact on survival or whether long-term administration may accelerate transformation to acute myeloid leukaemia. The improvements in neutrophil counts will certainly enhance the quality of life in a proportion of patients. Results of long-term administration of G-CSF have been encouraging, with persistent improvement in neutrophil counts and their function, possibly as a result of a differentiating effect in the bone marrow. One area of possible application of GM- and G-CSF is in combination with low-dose Ara-C to facilitate prolonged courses of the latter without the risk of neutropenia.

Recombinant erythropoietin has been used in several studies to improve the anaemia of myelodysplastic syndrome on the basis of relative suboptimal serum levels of erythropoietin in some patients. Responses have been noted in 20 per cent of cases and combinations with G-CSF have been used, suggesting a synergistic effect in some of the studies.

The choice of treatment in a myelodysplastic syndrome depends on a number of factors, of which the patient's age and prognostic features are the most important. Even if a decision for active treatment is considered, it is not clear at present which are the best agents or drug combinations.

REFERENCES

Aul, C., Gattermann, N., Heyll, A., Germing, U., Derigs, G., and Schneider, W. (1992). Primary myelodysplastic syndromes: analysis of prognostic factors in 235 patients and proposals for an improved scoring system. *Leukemia*, 6, 52–9.
Bennett, J.M. *et al.* (1982). Proposals for the classification of the myelodysplastic syndromes. *British Journal of Haematology*, 51, 189–99.
Brito-Babapulle, F., Catovsky, D., and Galton, D.A.G. (1987). Clinical and laboratory features of *de novo* acute myeloid leukaemia with trilineage myelodysplasia. *British Journal of Haematology*, 66, 445–50.
Galton, D.A.G. (1984). The myelodysplastic syndromes. *Clinical and Laboratory Haematology*, 6, 99–112.

Hirst, W.J.R. and Mufti, G.J. (1993). Management of myelodysplastic syndromes. *British Journal of Haematology*, 84, 191–6.
Mathew, P. *et al.* (1993). The 5q− syndrome: a single-institution study of 43 consecutive patients. *Blood*, 81, 1040–5.
Morel, P. *et al.* (1993). Cytogenetic analysis has strong independent prognostic value in *de novo* myelodysplastic syndromes and can be incorporated in a new scoring system: a report on 408 cases. *Leukemia*, 7, 1315–23.
Mufti, G.J., Stevens, J.R., Oscier, D.G., Hamblin, T.J., and Machin, D. (1985). Myelodysplastic syndromes: a scoring system with prognostic significance. *British Journal of Haematology*, 59, 425–33.
Padua, R.A. *et al.* (1988). RAS mutations in myelodysplasia detected by amplification, oligonucleotide hybridization and transformation. *Leukemia*, 2, 503–10.
Pedersen-Bjergaard, J. *et al.* (1993). Therapy-related myelodysplasia and acute myeloid leukemia. Cytogenetic characteristics of 115 consecutive cases and risk in seven cohorts of patients treated intensively for malignant diseases in the Copenhagen series. *Leukemia*, 7, 1975–86.
Pierre, R.V. *et al.* (1989). Clinical-cytogenetic correlations in myelodysplasia (preleukemia). *Cancer Genetics and Cytogenetics*, 40, 149–61.
Pui, C-H. *et al.* (1991). Acute myeloid leukemia with epipodophyllotoxins for acute lymphoblastic leukemia. *New England Journal of Medicine*, 325, 1682–7.
Sanz, G.F. *et al.* (1989). Two regression models and a scoring system for predicting survival and planning treatment in myelodysplastic syndromes: a multivariate analysis of prognostic factors in 370 patients. *Blood*, 74, 395–408.
Sokal, G. *et al.* (1975). A new haematologic syndrome with a distinct karyotype: the 5q− chromosome. *Blood*, 46, 519–33.
Stephenson, J., Mufti, G.J., and Yoshida, Y. (1993). Myelodysplastic syndromes: from morphology to molecular biology. Part II. The molecular genetics of myelodysplasia. *International Journal of Hematology* 57, 99–112.
Tricot, G., De Wolf-Peeters, C., Hendrickx, B., and Verwilghen, R.L. (1984). Bone marrow biopsy in myelodysplastic syndromes and comparison with bone marrow smears. *British Journal of Haematology*, 57, 423–30.
Tricot, G. *et al.* (1985). Prognostic factors in the myelodysplastic syndromes: importance of initial data on peripheral blood counts, bone marrow cytology, trephine biopsy and chromosomal analysis. *British Journal of Haematology*, 60, 19–32.
Varela, B.L., Chuang, C., Woll, J.E., and Bennett, J.M. (1985). Modifications in the classification of primary myelodysplastic syndromes: the addition of a scoring system. *Journal of Hematologic Oncology*, 3, 55–63.

22.3.8 Polycythaemia vera

D. J. WEATHERALL

The term 'polycythaemia' is used to describe an increased red-cell count, packed-cell volume, or haemoglobin level. In his early descriptions of the disease William Osler realized that there are two main types of what he called 'polyglobulism': (i) relative, in which there is a reduction in plasma volume with a normal red-cell mass; and (ii) true, in which there is a genuine increase in the red-cell mass. It is now more usual to call these conditions relative and absolute polycythaemia. The absolute polycythaemias are divided into primary polycythaemia or polycythaemia rubra vera, usually shortened to polycythaemia vera, which is a myeloproliferative disorder of unknown aetiology, and the secondary polycythaemias, which result from a variety of different pathological mechanisms.

Here we shall consider polycythaemia vera because there is good evidence that this condition results from the neoplastic proliferation of a multipotent haemopoietic progenitor cell. The relative and secondary polycythaemias, and the differential diagnosis of an increased haemoglobin level, are considered in Chapter 22.4.14.

Aetiology

Polycythaemia vera results from abnormal proliferation of red-cell precursors derived from a single haemopoietic progenitor cell with the capacity for differentiation down red-cell, white-cell, and platelet lines. Evidence for this comes from studies of the red-cell enzymes of African females with the disorder who are also heterozygous for the A and B glucose 6-phosphate dehydrogenase (**G6PD**) variants. In excess of 90 per cent of their red blood cells carry only one G6PD-type, either A or B, whereas in other tissues a more or less equal number of cells containing A- or B-type enzymes are found. The lymphocytes do not appear to be involved in this abnormal proliferative process.

Thus the basic mechanism of polycythaemia vera is a change in the genetic constitution of a single multipotent haemopoietic progenitor so that its progeny proliferate independent of the normal control mechanisms involved in haemopoiesis. It has been suggested that some of the abnormalities of the bone marrow in this condition, particularly the tendency to myelosclerosis in the later stages of the illness, are the result of the production of growth factors, such as platelet-derived growth factor, by the abnormal megakaryocyte line.

Erythropoietin levels are normal or low in the blood and urine of patients with polycythaemia vera and there is an appropriate rise after venesection. On *in vitro* culture, the red-cell precursors from patients with this disorder show increased and prolonged unstimulated erythropoiesis and an unusual dose–response curve to erythropoietin. These studies suggest that polycythaemia vera is not due to a primary abnormality of erythropoietin metabolism, because as the red-cell mass increases the normal feedback reduction of erythropoietin output occurs. Thus it appears that the basic defect in polycythaemia vera is a proliferation of precursors that behave quite independently of the normal erythropoietin regulation system. Whether this is because they have an altered receptor state for the hormone remains to be determined. What is clear is that the abnormal clone of erythroid progenitors has the capacity to proliferate preferentially as compared with its normal counterparts.

There is a considerable incidence of acute leukaemic transformation in patients with polycythaemia vera. Many of them develop chromosomal abnormalities during the course of their illness, suggesting that the primary mutational event in the stem cell makes it more likely that unstable cell lines will develop with a tendency to leukaemic transformation. In this sense, polycythaemia vera can be looked upon as a pre-leukaemic condition. Indeed, the natural history of the disorder bears a strong resemblance to that of chronic myeloid leukaemia (see Chapter 22.3.5).

Haemodynamics and oxygen transport

When measured *in vitro*, the viscosity of blood increases exponentially with an increasing packed-cell volume (**PCV**). When the rate of flow is measured as a reciprocal of the viscosity at varying PCV levels, it decreases in a linear function with an increasing PCV. If the flow rate is multiplied by the oxygen content of the blood, the product provides a measure of the rate of oxygen transport at different PCVs. Optimum oxygen transport occurs at PCVs of between 40 and 50 per cent. If no compensatory mechanisms occurred, there would be a reduced rate of oxygen transport even with a moderate increase in the PCV. In fact, even at relatively high PCVs, oxygen transport is adequate because there is an increase in the total blood volume, particularly in the plasma volume, and an increased cardiac output together with an enlargement of the peripheral vascular bed leading to a fall in peripheral resistance. Indeed, at a PCV of 60 per cent there may be some increase in oxygen delivery. As pointed out many years ago by William Castle, hyervolaemia *per se* increases oxygen transport because the increased blood oxygen content and cardiac output more than compensate for the increased viscosity of the blood. Unfortunately, however, polycythaemia vera is a disease of middle and old age and is frequently associated with cardiovascular disorders such as hypertension and coronary artery and cere-

brovascular disease. Hence, these compensatory mechanisms tend to break down, and this is particularly likely to occur at PCVs in excess of 60 to 65 per cent, at which level there may be a marked increase in the workload on both left and right sides of the heart because of the high viscosity in the systemic and pulmonary circulations. In addition there may be a marked reduction in the cerebral blood flow at high PCV levels, and this, together with associated cerebrovascular disease and a high platelet count, makes the cerebral circulation particularly vulnerable to occlusive episodes.

While many of the complications of polycythaemia vera are related to the haemodynamic changes secondary to increased blood viscosity, there is the added factor of the abnormal function of the aberrant cell line. Thrombotic episodes probably result from reduced flow of thick, viscous blood together with the high platelet count that commonly accompanies the disorder. Damage to the intestinal mucosa following thrombotic episodes may account for the high incidence of mucosal ulceration. The abnormal platelets of polycythaemia vera and primary thrombocythaemia are able to produce microvascular changes that are distinct from the large-vessel thromboses characteristic of polycythaemia vera. There is also defective haemostasis, probably due to abnormal platelet function. The platelets do not aggregate in response to adrenaline or collagen, and show a reduced response to the aggregation inhibitor, prostaglandin D_2. Hence, polycythaemia vera is characterized by the bizarre association of both thrombotic and bleeding tendencies in the same individual, associated with cardiovascular complications consequent on increased cardiac work resulting from an increased blood viscosity. The effects of increased viscosity depend on a complicated series of factors that includes variability of shear rates in different vessels, the state of the vessel wall, the level of the PCV, and cardiovascular function.

Symptoms

The disorder sometimes starts insidiously. On the other hand, patients may first present with an acute, dramatic complication such as a cerebrovascular accident or major thrombotic episode.

Presenting symptoms may involve almost any organ system. Non-specific complaints, probably related to circulatory disturbances in the nervous system, are most common and include headache, dizziness, vertigo, tinnitus, and visual disturbances including blurring and diplopia. There may be a cardiovascular presentation with angina, intermittent claudication, or recurrent venous thrombosis or embolic disease. Other symptoms include an increased bruising tendency or more severe bleeding in the form of epistaxis or gastrointestinal haemorrhage, and abdominal pain due to a peptic ulceration or splenomegaly. The condition may be first recognized during the course of investigation for gout.

A particularly common symptom is severe and intractable pruritus. This has a very characteristic relation to warmth and frequently occurs after getting into bed at night or bathing. Some patients present with a burning sensation in the feet or toes. This may be associated with vascular lesions that cause small areas of gangrene on the tips of the toes, similar to those in primary thrombocythaemia (see Chapter 22.3.10).

Physical findings

Many patients with polycythaemia vera are plethoric and show a cyanotic tinge to the nose, ears, and lips. Typically there is injection of the conjunctivae and a flush over the neck and upper half of the trunk. At least 75 per cent of patients have splenomegaly sometime during their illness. The size of the spleen varies greatly and in some cases a straight abdominal radiograph, ultrasound, or a computed tomographic scan may be necessary to demonstrate that it is enlarged. A moderate degree of hepatomegaly is present in about one-third to one-half of patients. Although arterial hypertension has been thought to be a common accompaniment of polycythaemia vera, it is difficult to be sure about this because polycythaemia vera occurs at an age when hypertension is extremely common in the population and it is far from clear whether the association is real.

Neurological examination is normal unless there has been a cerebrovascular accident, although some patients have engorged retinal veins at presentation.

Haematological changes

Typically there is an increase in the haemoglobin and in the PCV, which may range from 50 to more than 70 per cent. These findings are associated with an absolute increase in the red-cell mass. In the majority of patients there is an elevation of either the white-cell or platelet count, or both. Bone marrow examination shows an active marrow, but erythropoiesis is normoblastic and there are no diagnostic features. A variety of abnormalities of platelet function have been demonstrated. The changes in splenic function in polycythaemia vera are considered in Chapter 22.3.8.

There are several other laboratory findings that help in making the diagnosis of polycythaemia vera. Many patients are hyperuricaemic, and secondary gout is quite common. The arterial oxygen saturation is usually normal, although, interestingly, mild degrees of unsaturation may occur occasionally in patients with otherwise well-documented polycythaemia vera. The leucocyte alkaline phosphatase is usually increased, which helps to distinguish cases with very high white-cell counts from chronic myeloid leukaemia, in which the level is reduced. The serum vitamin B_{12} content and the capacity of the serum to bind vitamin B_{12} are often markedly increased. There has been considerable interest in the last few years in the cytogenetic changes in polycythaemia vera. It is still not absolutely certain whether they are related to therapy, but there is increasing evidence that even patients who have not received radioactive phosphorus or cytotoxic drugs have an increased incidence of chromosomal abnormalities. These include aneuploidy and the presence of an extra C-group chromosome. The chromosomal changes are more marked in those patients who develop marrow failure or leukaemia; occasionally the Philadelphia chromosome may appear during an acute leukaemic transformation.

Differential diagnosis

Usually there is little difficulty in diagnosing polycythaemia vera. The finding of an increased haemoglobin level and PCV, an increased red-cell mass, splenomegaly, and an associated elevation in the white-cell and/or platelet count is diagnostic. Provided that an absolute polycythaemia has been demonstrated by red-cell mass estimation, the only difficulty is ruling out the various causes of secondary polycythaemia; this problem is considered in Chapter 22.4.14.

Occasionally, difficulty is encountered in patients with what is apparently polycythaemia vera but in whom the spleen is not enlarged and the white-cell and platelet counts are not elevated. Certainly, there is a small group of patients with persistently elevated red-cell masses in whom there is no other abnormality consistent with the diagnosis of polycythaemia vera and in whom no cause for secondary polycythaemia can be found. These individuals should be followed carefully and their polycythaemia managed by venesection. In the author's experience some of them have developed the typical features of polycythaemia vera after several months or years, while in others a cause of secondary polycythaemia such as a tumour has shown itself after an equally long period.

Course and prognosis

It is extremely difficult to give an accurate prognosis in this disorder. It appears that younger patients survive longer and that the prognosis for those who present with a major complication at the onset is considerably worse than those who present with minimal symptoms. There is still controversy about the relation between different forms of therapy and

prognosis (see below). Data collected from several large multicentre trials suggest that the median survival time varies from 9 to 14 years, with some variation depending on the form of therapy (see below).

During the course of the illness (Fig. 1) there may be vascular or thrombotic complications, particularly if the PCV is allowed to remain in excess of 55 per cent or more; a very high platelet count is also associated with an increased incidence of thrombotic and haemorrhagic complications. Any blood vessel may be involved, often the portal veins, fundal veins, cerebral circulation, and digital vessels of the hands and feet. In many of those patients who do not die of vascular complications, the polycythaemia gradually 'burns out' and is replaced by anaemia, massive splenomegaly, and progressive fibrosis of the bone marrow. At this stage the illness is indistinguishable from primary myelosclerosis (see Chapter 22.3.9).

The other form of termination of polycythaemia vera is acute leukaemia. It is now clear that the frequency of this complication is, at least in part, related to the form of treatment (see below). In some cases, leukaemic transformation is characterized by a sudden decline in general health, anaemia, thrombocytopenia, and the appearance of primitive white-cell precursors in the peripheral blood and bone marrow. The transformation may be much more subtle, with gradual enlargement of the spleen, slowly progressive thrombocytopenia, and the gradual accumulation of primitive precursors in the marrow and lymph nodes.

Management

Currently, polycythaemia vera is not curable and hence the objectives of management are to maintain well-being and to diminish the likelihood of complications for as long as possible. This is achieved by reducing a dangerously high PCV into a safer range by venesection and then by maintaining this level, either by regular venesection or the use of myelosuppressive agents, or both. At the same time an attempt is made to maintain the platelet count at a safe level and to control other complications such as hyperuricaemia and secondary folate deficiency with appropriate drugs.

Because patients with high PCVs are at great risk of thrombotic episodes it is important to initiate a venesection regimen as soon as the diagnosis is clear. It is usually possible to remove 350 to 500 ml of blood every other day until the PCV is reduced to the normal range. In older patients who find venesection distressing, smaller quantities of blood, in the 200 to 300 ml range, may be removed. In emergencies, preoperatively for example, more blood may be removed and replaced by an equal volume of plasma.

Once a normal PCV has been attained, maintenance therapy should be started. In young patients in whom the platelet count is not dangerously high, it is better to try to maintain the PCV at a normal level by

Fig. 1 Schematic representation of the natural history of polycythaemia vera.

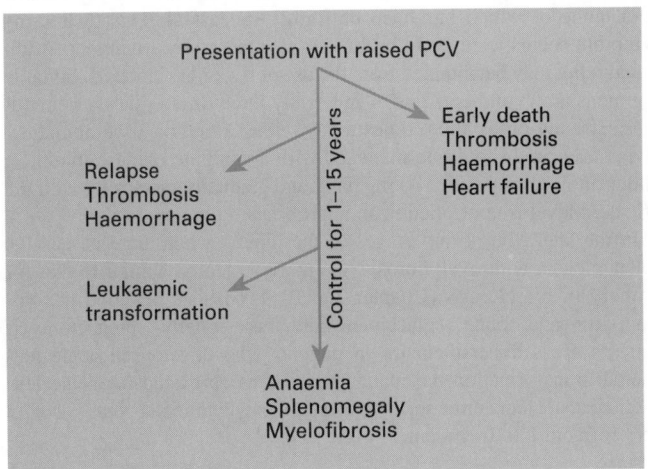

regular venesection. As mentioned earlier, it is important to keep the PCV below 50 per cent, and ideally below 45 per cent. After a while changes of iron deficiency will be observed. This does not matter, although some patients complain of glossitis, asthenia, and other symptoms that have been ascribed to iron deficiency. Thus it is customary to treat these patients with iron, although this probably increases the frequency with which venesection is required.

In older patients who cannot tolerate regular venesection, or in younger patients in whom there is a very high platelet count, myelosuppressive therapy is indicated. The type of myelosuppressive treatment has been a major controversy for many years, mainly because of the fear that use of these agents might provoke leukaemic transformation. This is the basis for several clinical trials to assess the best way of treating polycythaemia vera. Data from the Polycythaemia Vera Study Group suggest that the median survival for all ages is 8.9 years for those treated with chlorambucil, 11.8 years for ^{32}P, and 11.9 years for venesection alone. In a non-randomized study the survival for patients treated with venesection and intermittent, low-dose busulphan was approximately 11 years. It is quite clear from these studies that the use of chlorambucil is associated with a significantly higher frequency of leukaemic transformation. The use of ^{32}P also seems to increase the likelihood of the development of leukaemia, although because of the time interval involved this does not seem to preclude its use in older patients. Several studies have shown that it is possible to control high platelet counts and the other features of polycythaemia vera by the use of continuous hydroxyurea.

So which form of myelosuppressive therapy should be used in polycythaemia vera? In older patients it seems reasonable to use ^{32}P. Following venesection to a normal PCV, a dose of ^{32}P, 3 to 5 mCi (2.5 mCi/m^2), should be given intravenously. Sometimes a second, smaller dose, 2 to 3 mCi of ^{32}P, is required 3 to 4 months after the initial injection in order to bring the disease under complete control. The condition then often remains quiescent for months or even years. It is most unusual to produce severe marrow hypoplasia with this regimen. In younger patients, intermittent busulphan or hydroxyurea can be used. Busulphan should be given at a dose of 4 to 6 mg daily until the platelet count is approaching normal, at which time the dose should be reduced to 2 mg daily until a normal platelet count has been achieved. The drug should then be stopped and the patient carefully followed with regular blood counts. The count may remain under control for months or even years after a single course of busulphan, although usually intermittent courses with gaps of several months in between are required. Hydroxyurea is also useful as a myelosuppressive agent. It should be started at a dose of 500 mg to 1 g daily and the dose tapered down as control is achieved. It is a very valuable drug for achieving rapid control of the platelet count. Information from the Polycythemia Vera Study Group suggests that hydroxyurea is probably now the drug of choice for myelosuppression in this condition.

A variety of agents reportedly improve the pruritus of polycythaemia vera, none of which has been uniformly successful. This distressing symptom seems to respond best to myelosuppressive treatment. Additional relief may be obtained from the use of H$_1$- or H$_2$-blockers. Suitable regimens are cyproheptadine, 4 mg orally three times a day, or cimetidine, 300 mg orally three times a day, either alone or in combination. Hyperuricaemia should be managed with a xanthine oxidase inhibitor; allopurinol starting with 100 mg daily and gradually increasing until the uric acid level is controlled is an appropriate regimen.

In the later, 'burnt out' stages of the illness, when there is massive splenomegaly and myelofibrosis, the management is similar to that for primary myelosclerosis (Chapter 22.3.9). It consists of blood transfusion, iron and folate replacement and, occasionally, splenectomy if there is gross hypersplenism. In patients who develop an acute leukaemic transformation the management is as described for acute leukaemia; acute leukaemia superimposed on polycythaemia vera is usually very refractory to treatment.

REFERENCES

Adamson, J.W., Fialkow, P.J., Murphy, S., Prchal, J.F., and Steinmann, L. (1976). Polycythemia vera: stem-cell and probable clonal origin of the disease. *New England Journal of Medicine*, **295**, 913–16.

Berk, P.D. *et al.* (1986). Therapeutic recommendations in polycythemia vera based on Polycythemia Vera Study Group protocols. *Seminars in Hematology*, **23**, 132–43.

Beutler, E. (1994). Polycythemia vera. In *Williams hematology*, (ed. E. Beutler, M.A. Lichtman, B.S. Coller, and T.J. Kipps). McGraw-Hill, New York (in press).

Castle, W.B. and Jandl, J.H. (1966). Blood viscosity and blood volume: opposing influences upon oxygen transport. *Seminars in Hematology*, **3**, 193–8.

Ellis, J.T. and Peterson, P. (1979). The bone marrow in polycythemia vera. *Pathology Annual*, **14**, 383.

Ho, A.D. (1991). Chemotherapy of chronic haematological malignancies. *Baillière's Clinical Haematology*, **4**, 197–221.

Loeb, V. (1975). Treatment of polycythaemia vera. *Clinics in Haematology*, **4**, 441–8.

Messinezy, M., Pearson, T.C., Prochazka, A., and Wetherley-Mein, G. (1985). Treatment of primary proliferative polycythaemia by venesection and low dose busulphan: retrospective study from one centre. *British Journal of Haematology*, **61**, 657–66.

Pearson, T.C. (1987). Rheology of the absolute polycythaemias. *Baillière's Clinical Haematology*, **1**, 637–64.

Pearson, T.C. and Guthrie, D.L. (1984). The interpretation of measured red cell mass and plasma volumes in patients with elevated PC values. *Clinical and Laboratory Haematology*, **6**, 207–17.

Pearson, T.C. and Messinezy, M. (1987). Polycythaemia and thrombocythaemia in the elderly. *Baillière's Clinical Haematology*, **1**, 355–87.

Wetherley-Mein, G. and Pearson, T.C. (1982). Myeloproliferative disorders. In *Blood and its disorders*, (2nd edn). (ed. R.M. Hardisty and D.J. Weatherall), pp. 263–72. Blackwell Scientific, Oxford.

22.3.9 Myelosclerosis

D. J. WEATHERALL

The term 'myelosclerosis' is used to describe progressive fibrous replacement of the bone marrow; it is used synonymously with myelofibrosis. The condition may be part of the myeloproliferative syndrome or may be secondary to the effects of other neoplastic disorders of the bone marrow, metabolic changes involving vitamin D or its metabolites, and a variety of other conditions that provoke a fibrous reaction by an unknown mechanism.

Primary myelosclerosis

Primary myelosclerosis is a myeloproliferative disorder characterized by anaemia and abnormal proliferation of haemopoietic precursors associated with a variable degree of fibrosis of the bone marrow and myeloid metaplasia in the spleen, liver, and other organs. This last characteristic is the reason why the condition has many alternative names, including myeloid metaplasia, agnogenic myeloid metaplasia, and megakaryocytic splenomegaly. Furthermore, the curious pathological association of myeloid metaplasia and progressive fibrosis of the marrow explains the extremely bizarre and variable clinical and haematological pictures associated with this interesting disorder.

AETIOLOGY

The cause of myelosclerosis and myeloid metaplasia is unknown. It seems likely that the abnormal haemopoietic elements which constitute the myeloid metaplasia of the spleen, liver, and other organs result from the neoplastic proliferation of an abnormal stem-cell population. Recent evidence in support of this notion has come from enzyme studies similar to those used to demonstrate the clonal origin of polycythaemia. Fibroblasts grown from bone marrows of females with primary myelosclerosis who are heterozygous for glucose 6-phosphate dehydrogenase types A and B show both forms of the enzyme, while platelets and other blood cells contain only one form. These findings suggest that the fibroblast proliferation occurs secondarily to the effects of abnormal proliferation of a clone of haemopoietic progenitor cells. Similar results have been obtained from cytogenetic analyses. It is currently believed that the fibrotic reaction results from the release of platelet-derived growth factor for fibroblasts, or related factors from the abnormal line of megakaryocytes.

The fibrous tissue in the bone marrow of patients with myelosclerosis is demonstrated with the silver stain for reticulin. This staining reaction highlights many proteins, but in the bone marrow identifies mainly collagen and fibronectin. Platelet-derived growth factor, as well as stimulating fibroblasts to proliferate, induces collagen synthesis. Myelofibrosis is a dynamic process and there are several collagenases released from monocytes and macrophages that may degrade the fibrous tissue.

During the evolution of myelosclerosis the two major pathological processes, progressive fibrosis of the bone marrow and myeloid metaplasia of the liver, spleen, and lymph nodes, seem to occur simultaneously, although there is remarkable variability between patients in the rate and extent of these changes. The fibrosis of the marrow is extremely patchy and there may be areas of hyperplasia that can cause diagnostic difficulties. The hyperplasia involves all the precursor cells, particularly megakaryocytes. Indeed, megakaryocytic proliferation is a major feature of this disorder. Despite the existence of hyperplastic areas of the marrow, red-cell production is diminished, and, while in the early stages of the illness there may be a raised white-cell and platelet count, these tend to fall as fibrosis of the marrow progresses. Hence, a major factor in producing the clinical picture of myelosclerosis is progressive bone marrow failure. The second is hypersplenism due to increasing enlargement of the spleen. This process, and the associated hepatomegaly, seems to be largely due to myeloid metaplasia. It is now considered that this extramedullary haemopoiesis is part of a neoplastic proliferation which characterizes myelosclerosis, but that it may also play a role in compensating for bone marrow failure; while possible, there is no definite evidence that this is the case. The mechanism by which the massively enlarged spleen causes worsening of the anaemia, hypervolaemia, thrombocytopenia, and neutropenia is described in Chapter 22.5.4.

CLINICAL FEATURES

The presenting symptoms in myelosclerosis are extremely variable. The disorder may first be recognized because an enlarged spleen is discovered accidentally by the patient or physician. Sometimes it is large enough to cause abdominal distension or a dragging sensation in the left upper quadrant. On the other hand, the first symptoms may be progressive anaemia, weight loss or general ill health, bone pain, or acute abdominal pain due to a splenic infarct. Some patients are first referred to dermatologists with pruritus, which has the same distinctive relation to warmth as occurs in polycythaemia vera. Occasionally, the early clinical picture reflects abnormal platelet function and there may be increased bruising, unexplained gastrointestinal blood loss, or bleeding after minor trauma (Fig. 1).

The only physical finding that is almost invariably present is splenomegaly. The spleen ranges in size from just palpable to massive, and this is one of the few disorders in which the patient may present for the first time with a spleen in the pelvis. There is usually some degree of hepatomegaly.

Finally, since about a third of patients with myelosclerosis have a patchy osteosclerosis, the condition may first be recognized by the finding of an unusual bone radiograph in a patient who is having a radiological examination for another cause.

HAEMATOLOGICAL CHANGES (PLATES 25, 26)

Anaemia is present in over two-thirds of all patients when they are first seen. In the early stage of the illness it may be quite mild but usually becomes more severe as the disorder progresses. The red cells are characteristically misshapen, with many tear-drop-shaped forms, bizarre poikilocytes, and ovalocytes (Fig. 2). These changes are the real hallmark of myelosclerosis. Quite often there are nucleated red cells in the peripheral blood.

The white-cell count is often elevated. The white cells consist mainly of mature neutrophils but there are usually some immature forms, metamyelocytes, myelocytes, or even a few myeloblasts (Fig. 2). These changes, together with the presence of nucleated red cells, constitute a leucoerythroblastic reaction. The platelet count is variable. In the earlier stages of the illness there is often a moderate thrombocytosis. As the disease progresses and the spleen enlarges, the platelet count tends to fall and severe thrombocytopenia may be a troublesome feature in advanced myelosclerosis. The platelet morphology is abnormal; the changes are characterized by giant forms and occasional shreds of megakaryocyte cytoplasm in the peripheral blood (Fig. 2).

Bone marrow examination usually yields a 'dry' tap. However, it is always worthwhile looking carefully in the tail of such hypocellular preparations because there may be large platelet aggregates or scattered clumps of megakaryocytes, which will give a clue to the diagnosis. A needle or open biopsy shows extensive fibrosis with islands of haemopoietic cells, and megakaryocytic hyperplasia. Because of the patchiness of the myelofibrotic process, it is possible to aspirate fragments of hypercellular marrow. Even in these cases, however, silver staining for reticulin will show a marked increase in fibre formation (Fig. 3). Although many cytogenetic abnormalities have been reported in this disorder, there are no specific chromosomal changes that are of diagnostic help.

Fig. 1 A massive haematoma over the scapula region with tracking down in the tissue planes of the back in an 81-year-old patient with myelosclerosis and abnormal platelet function.

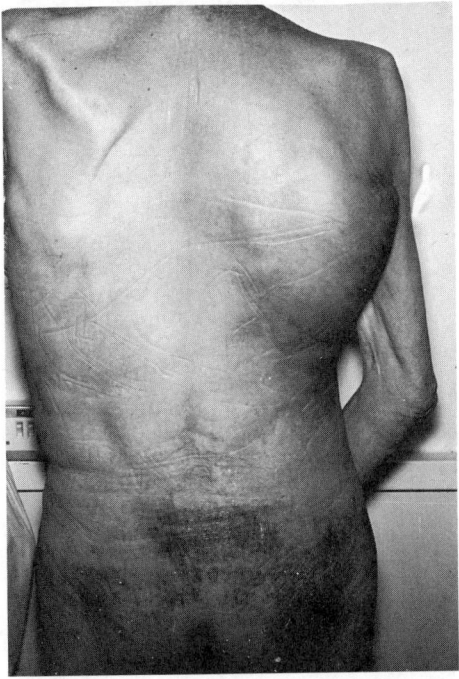

Fig. 2 Haematological changes in myelosclerosis. (a) A peripheral blood film showing tear-drop cells, a nucleated red cell, and a grossly distorted cell marked by the arrow. (From Liebold, P.F. and Weed, R.I. (1975). *Clinical Haematology*, **4**, 353, with permission.) (b) A scanning electron-microscope study showing characteristic poikilocytes. (From Liebold, P.F. and Weed, R.I. (1975). *Clinical Haematology*, **4**, 353, with permission.) (c) A leucoerythroblastic reaction in myelosclerosis showing young red-cell precursors. Note, in addition, the abnormal platelet morphology and platelet clumps.

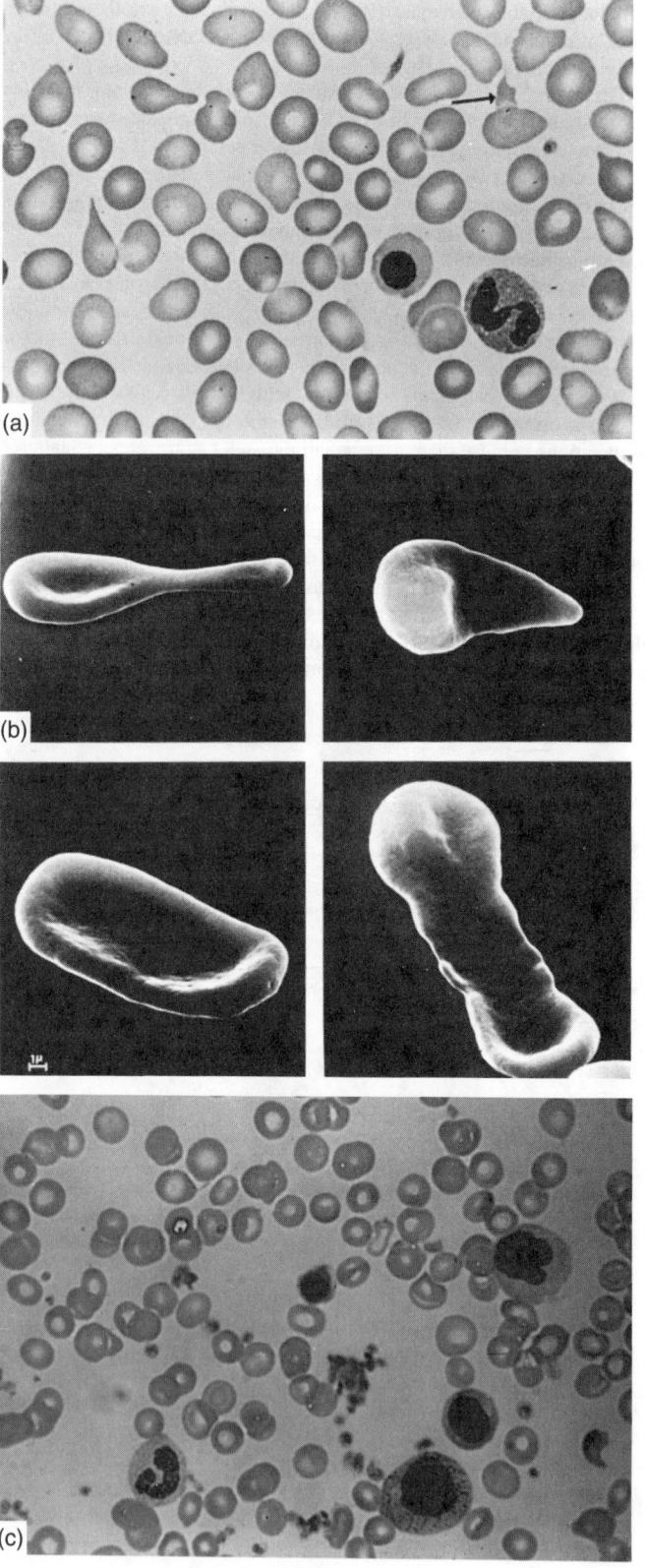

OTHER LABORATORY FINDINGS

There is usually an elevated uric acid level. The neutrophil alkaline phosphatase is variable, and normal, high, or low levels may be found.

Abnormalities of haemostasis and coagulation are common. In addition to thrombocytopenia many patients show abnormal platelet aggregation in response to collagen and adrenaline. The prothrombin time may be prolonged, often as the result of a deficiency of factor V. In some patients there may be features of disseminated intravascular coagulation although, curiously, they do not have the marked bleeding tendency usually associated with these findings.

Splenic or lymph-node aspiration almost invariably shows myeloid metaplasia. However, any form of biopsy except of the bone marrow should be avoided in myelosclerotic patients because of their bleeding tendency.

FERROKINETIC STUDIES

Although it is rarely necessary to use iron kinetic studies for diagnostic purposes, they may be useful for assessing the extent of the disease and the degree of effective splenic erythropoiesis, in cases in which splenectomy is being considered. This subject is considered in detail in Chapter 22.5.4.

DIFFERENTIAL DIAGNOSIS

The typical picture of myelosclerosis with a massive spleen and fibrosed bone marrow usually produces no diagnostic difficulty. However, in the

Fig. 3 Bone marrow appearances in myelosclerosis. (a) A biopsy showing a hyperplastic fragment with marked megakaryocytic hyperplasia; (b) silver stain showing the marked increase in reticulin.

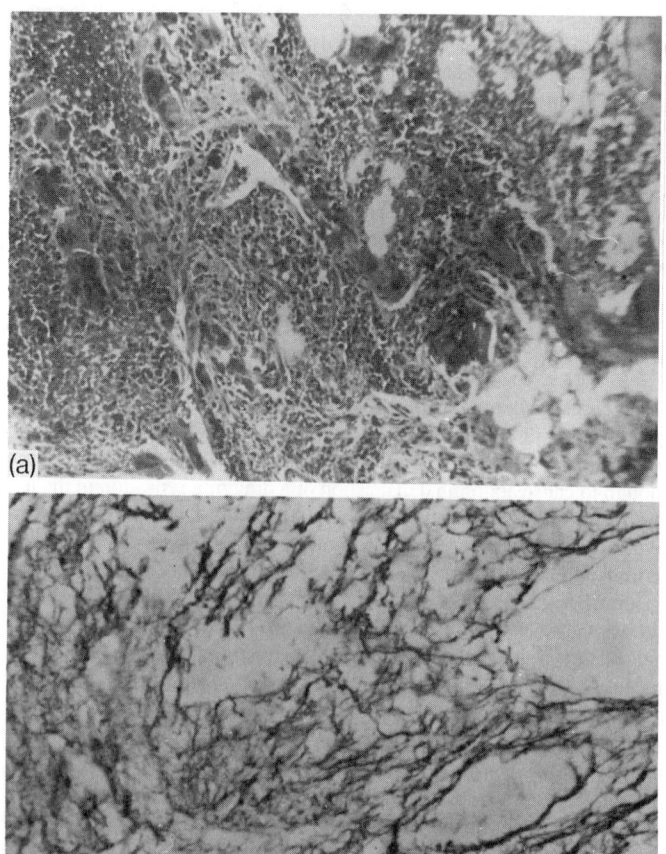

earlier phases of the illness when myeloid metaplasia predominates and the peripheral blood shows a leucocytosis and thrombocytosis, it is easy to confuse the condition with chronic myeloid leukaemia. However, the bone marrow in the latter disorder shows a predominance of myelocytes and promyelocytes, the leucocyte alkaline phosphatase is low, and a Philadelphia chromosome is present. In addition, the disorder must be distinguished from the causes of secondary marrow fibrosis mentioned later in this section and from other causes of a leucoerythroblastic anaemia, especially secondary carcinoma, other myeloproliferative disorders, and disseminated tuberculosis.

COMPLICATIONS

The major complications of myelosclerosis relate to the massive splenomegaly. The development of progressive hypersplenism has already been mentioned. Splenic infarction (Fig. 4) with associated pain over the spleen or in the left shoulder tip is relatively common. Trauma to the large spleen may cause it to rupture, either into the abdominal cavity or with the production of a perisplenic haematoma. Secondary gout is common. Because of the rapid turnover of the abnormal red-cell precursors, secondary folate deficiency is also common and may cause a sudden worsening of the anaemia with a marked macrocytosis and the appearance of megaloblasts in the blood. Presumably because of abnormal platelet function or peptic ulceration, chronic gastrointestinal blood loss occurs and the anaemia of myelosclerosis may be made worse by coexistent iron deficiency. Serious bruising and haematoma formation may result from mild trauma (see Fig. 1).

There appears to be a genuine association between myelosclerosis and portal hypertension, which may be accompanied by bleeding from oesophageal varices. The pathogenesis is not understood; presinusoidal obstruction due to infiltration of the hepatic sinusoids, portal or splenic vein thrombosis, and increased flow in the portal system have all been suggested.

COURSE AND PROGNOSIS

The course of myelosclerosis is variable. Some patients retain a relatively normal haemoglobin level and have a minimal splenomegaly for

Fig. 4 Autopsy showing massive splenomegaly together with a splenic infarct on the medial surface of the spleen in a patient with advanced myelosclerosis.

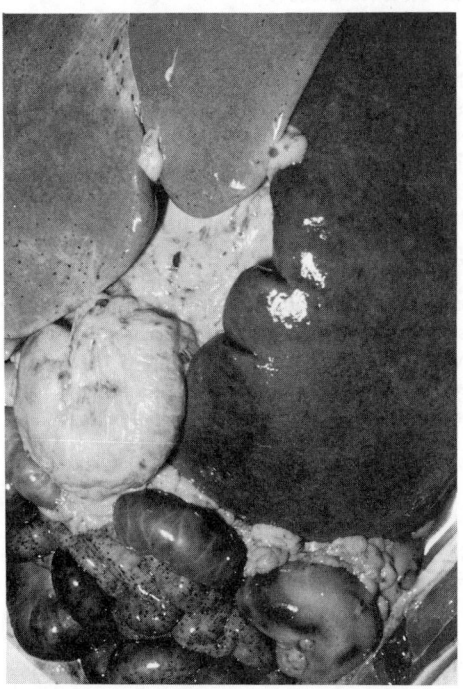

many years. More commonly there is a gradual decline in the patient's general condition with a progressive worsening of the anaemia, and increasing splenomegaly, which may reach enormous proportions. Although the median survival is usually given as approximately 5 years there is a very broad scatter and it is not at all uncommon for patients to live 10 to 20 years after myelosclerosis has been diagnosed. The usual cause of death is progressive anaemia, which becomes refractory to blood transfusion, due at least in part to haemodilution caused by the massive spleen. Approximately 20 per cent of cases terminate in acute myeloblastic leukaemia. There is a sudden worsening of the anaemia and a marked increase in the number of blast cells in the peripheral blood.

TREATMENT

There is no definitive treatment for patients with myelosclerosis. They should be followed carefully and complications such as iron or folate deficiency corrected. If they become symptomatic due to progressive anaemia, they should be started on a blood transfusion programme, although particular care is required when transfusing patients with this disorder. Because of the high blood volume associated with hypersplenism, it is very easy to overload them and to precipitate acute pulmonary oedema. Although splenic irradiation and chemotherapy have been used in an attempt to reduce the size of the spleen, the results are equivocal. Local irradiation is usually ineffective in reducing its size but some benefit may be obtained from a judicious use of busulphan or hydroxyurea. The author favours the latter drug because of its fewer side-effects and the fact that it is easier to titrate the white-cell and platelet counts than is the case with busulphan. It is wise to start with a low dose of hydroxyurea, 500 mg daily for example, and gradually to increase it keeping a careful watch on spleen size and white-cell and platelet counts. There have been a number of recent reports suggesting that interferon-α may have a part to play in the treatment of advanced myelosclerosis but, particularly in view of its severe side-effects, its true role remains to be established.

The place of splenectomy is controversial. It is argued that if the spleen is removed early on in the course of the illness, it may prevent the development of the problems of hypersplenism which occur as the disease progresses. Against this, however, is the fact that many patients with this disorder have many years of symptom-free life before the disease enters its terminal stage of massive splenomegaly. It is impossible to anticipate how long patients will take to develop symptoms referable to splenomegaly. Certainly when the spleen is large, surgery can be extremely hazardous. There are often multiple adhesions, which make the operation technically difficult, and postoperatively there may be a massive rise in the platelet count with subsequent thrombotic and bleeding complications. Although it is possible to control the platelet rise by the administration of busulphan or hydroxyurea, postoperative thrombocytosis can still be extremely difficult to manage. Furthermore, some patients develop progressive hepatomegaly after splenectomy. For these reasons it is better to manage myelosclerosis conservatively with careful iron and folate replacement therapy and the use of transfusion when required, and to reserve splenectomy for those rare cases in which splenic pain and severe hypersplenism become a major feature of the illness. The management of portal hypertension with bleeding oesophageal varices in patients with myelosclerosis is extremely difficult. Although there have been reports of successful shunt procedures, with or without splenectomy, surgery is so hazardous in these patients that it is better to try to manage the bleeding conservatively by sclerosing the varices (see Chapter 14.29).

Acute myelosclerosis and acute megakaryoblastic leukaemia

Although a very acute form of myelosclerosis has been recognized for a long time, it is only recently that evidence about its cellular origin has started to accumulate. Cytogenetic studies suggest that, as in chronic forms of myelosclerosis, the fibrotic reaction in the bone marrow is secondary to another pathological mechanism rather than the primary cause of the disease. Combined morphological and cytochemical analyses suggest that acute myelosclerosis is probably a myeloproliferative disorder that involves primarily the megakaryocyte or its precursor. For this reason it is preferable to call the condition acute megakaryoblastic leukaemia. It is currently believed that the myelofibrosis is mediated by growth factors released from the abnormal megakaryocytes, possibly platelet-derived growth factor. If this hypothesis is correct, acute myelofibrosis has the same basic pathophysiology as the more chronic form of the illness.

The condition has been seen in patients of all ages and is characterized by the rapid onset of symptoms of anaemia, low-grade fever, bleeding, increased disposition to infection, and, sometimes, generalized bone pain. On examination there is pallor and there may be a purpuric rash. The spleen is either impalpable or only slightly enlarged. There may be marked bone tenderness.

The blood picture is characterized by anaemia, neutropenia, and thrombocytopenia with a leucoerythroblastic reaction. Bone marrow aspiration almost invariably yields a 'dry tap' and a trephine biopsy shows increased reticulin, often accompanied by proliferation of bizarre cells that have the cytochemical characteristics of megakaryocytes.

The disease has an extremely poor prognosis and does not respond well to conventional leukaemia chemotherapy or radiotherapy. There has been one report of successful remissions following low-dose cytosine arabinoside (10 mg/m^2 per day in twice daily subcutaneous injections). It is not clear whether this drug is working as a cytotoxic agent or has a more subtle action in stimulating the resolution of myelofibrosis. Recently, several patients have been treated successfully by bone marrow transplantation following intensive chemotherapy and radiotherapy. Without transplantation the prognosis is extremely poor, with survival of greater than a year being uncommon. Apart from the use of cytosine arabinoside, treatment is largely supportive with blood transfusion, platelet infusions, and appropriate management of infection.

Secondary myelosclerosis

There is a wide variety of disorders that may be associated with increased reticulin formation in the bone marrow. Secondary myelosclerosis is frequently associated with a leucoerythroblastic anaemia. This is characterized by a variable degree of anaemia, changes in shape and size of the red cells, and the presence of nucleated red cells or myelocytes, or even an occasional myeloblast, in the peripheral blood. As in primary myelosclerosis, bone marrow aspiration results in a 'dry tap', and a trephine biopsy is required to establish the cause of the fibrotic reaction. Some of these conditions are summarized in Table 1.

NEOPLASTIC DISORDERS

All forms of leukaemia and chronic myeloproliferative disorders may give rise to some degree of myelofibrosis. It is quite common for polycythaemia vera or chronic myeloid leukaemia to enter a terminal myelosclerotic phase. Occasionally Hodgkin's disease or non-Hodgkin's lymphoma may also result in marrow fibrosis. Disseminated carcinoma invading the marrow can also give rise to a variable degree of fibrosis.

Systemic mast-cell disease

The mast-cell disorders are rare conditions that range from solitary benign mast-cell tumours to the bizarre syndrome of the malignant form of systemic mastocytosis. The syndrome of cutaneous mastocytosis with urticaria pigmentosa is described in Section 23.

The malignant form of systemic mastocytosis may develop *de novo* or superimposed on urticaria pigmentosa. It is a disease of the sixth and seventh decades and is more common in males. The symptoms are very varied and include general malaise, recurrent diarrhoea, paroxysmal

Table 1 *Disorders associated with myelofibrosis (full references are given by McCarthy (1985))*

Malignant
Idiopathic myelosclerosis
Acute myelosclerosis (acute megakaryoblastic leukaemia)
Chronic myeloid leukaemia
Acute lymphoblastic leukaemia
Hairy-cell leukaemia
Polycythaemia vera
Systemic mastocytosis
Hodgkin's disease
Myeloma
Secondary carcinoma

Non-malignant
Renal osteodystrophy
Vitamin D deficiency
Hypoparathyroidism
Hyperparathyroidism
Grey platelet syndrome
Systemic lupus erythematosus
Systemic sclerosis
Thorium dioxide administration

hypertension or hypotension, pruritus, the skin manifestations of urticaria pigmentosa, hepatosplenomegaly, dense sclerotic bone changes, and an increased number of mast cells in the skin, liver, lymph nodes, and bone marrow. Rarely, mast cells spill into the peripheral blood in large numbers giving rise to the picture of mast-cell leukaemia. The condition is diagnosed by demonstrating mast-cell infiltration of a lymph node or bone marrow using special staining techniques. Symptoms can sometimes be controlled by the use of H$_1$- or H$_2$-receptor antagonists. In some cases there appears to be overproduction of prostaglandin D$_2$ and symptoms may be reduced with aspirin. There have also been reports of successful control by blocking the uptake of calcium ions necessary for degranulation of mast cells with cromoglycate. Standard antileukaemia agents are not effective. The prognosis from the time of diagnosis is variable. Many patients run a long course, terminating, in some cases, in leukaemia.

Myelofibrosis and vitamin D deficiency

There have now been a number of reports of children with rickets, myelofibrosis, and myeloid metaplasia. There was associated splenomegaly and leucoerythroblastic blood changes. These changes reverted to normal after treatment with vitamin D or 1,25-dihydroxy vitamin D$_3$. Interestingly, it has been shown that the active metabolite of vitamin D$_3$ inhibits the proliferation of human megakaryocytes *in vitro* and also induces myeloid cells from normal individuals or patients with chronic myeloid leukaemia to mature into monocytes and macrophages.

Renal failure

Myelofibrosis occasionally occurs in patients with renal failure with or without other features of renal osteodystrophy. It has been suggested that complication may also be caused by a deficiency of vitamin D, although it has also been found that increased concentrations of parathyroid hormone, which occur in patients with renal failure, may also enhance the accumulation of collagen in the bone marrow.

Infection

It has been suggested that disseminated tuberculosis can produce a clinical picture very similar to myelosclerosis. However, it seems more likely that these are examples of tuberculous infection in patients with an underlying myeloproliferative disorder. There have been no really convincing cases of complete reversion to a normal blood picture after antituberculous therapy. This is a very confusing subject which requires further study. However, a sudden deterioration in a patient with a myelo-proliferative disorder, with no evidence of an acute leukaemic transformation, should raise the possibility of disseminated tuberculosis.

Other rare causes of marrow fibrosis are summarized in Table 1.

REFERENCES

Bain, B.J. *et al.* (1981). Megakaryoblastic leukaemia presenting as acute myelofibrosis—a study of four cases with platelet peroxidase reaction. *Blood*, **58**, 206–13.

Lichtman, M.A. (1994). Myeloid metaplasia. In *Williams hematology*, (ed. E. Beutler, M.A. Lichtman, B.S. Coller, and T.J. Kipps), McGraw-Hill, New York.

McCarthy, D.M. (1985). Fibrosis of the bone marrow: content and causes. *British Journal of Haematology*, **59**, 1–7.

Manoharan, A. (1988). Myelofibrosis: prognostic factors and treatment. *British Journal of Haematology*, **69**, 295–303.

Mulder, H., Steenburgen, J., and Hannen, C. (1977). Clinical course and survival after elective splenectomy in 19 patients with primary myelofibrosis. *British Journal of Haematology*, **35**, 419–26.

Sultan, C., Sigaux, F., Imbert, M., and Reyes, F. (1981). Acute myelodysplasia with myelofibrosis: a report of eight cases. *British Journal of Haematology*, **49**, 11–16.

Takácsi-Magy, L. and Graf, F. (1975). Definition, clinical features and diagnosis of myelofibrosis. *Clinics in Haematology*, **4**, 291–308.

Wetherley-Mein, G. and Pearson, T.C. (1982). Myeloproliferative disorders. In *Blood and its disorders*, (2nd edn) (ed. R.M. Hardisty and D.J. Weatherall), pp. 263–72. Blackwell Scientific, Oxford.

22.3.10 Primary thrombocythaemia

D. J. WEATHERALL

Primary thrombocythaemia is a myeloproliferative disorder characterized by hyperplasia of the megakaryocytes and a marked increase in the platelet count. There may be an associated increase in the white-cell count or even in the red-cell count, and the dividing line between this disorder and polycythaemia vera may be indistinct. Based on its varied clinical features this condition has collected a variety of names over the years including haemorrhagic thrombocythaemia, essential thrombocythaemia, and megakaryocytic leukaemia.

AETIOLOGY AND PATHOGENESIS

Recent evidence suggests that primary thrombocythaemia has a similar pathogenesis to the other myeloproliferative disorders and that it results from the abnormal proliferation of a stem-cell line, which, in this case, differentiates mainly towards the megakaryocyte/platelet compartments. It has been found that women with this disorder who are heterozygous for glucose 6-phosphate dehydrogenase types A and B have platelets that show predominantly the A or B types, indicating that they are all derived from a single abnormal progenitor.

The platelets are morphologically abnormal and the platelet count is usually higher than that observed in thrombocytosis, that is, an increased production of normal platelets. The clinical features of this disorder are the result of the high platelet count and the functional abnormalities of the platelets produced by the abnormal cell line. As expected, the very high platelet count is associated with a thrombotic tendency but, because of abnormal platelet function, bleeding is often a major feature of the disease. The platelets do not aggregate normally in response to adrenaline or collagen. On the other hand, they may aggregate spontaneously and they show a defective response to the inhibitory prostaglandin-D_2.

A few patients with primary thrombocythaemia have chromosome abnormalities, particularly a deletion of the long arm of chromosome 21.

CLINICAL FEATURES

The most common symptom is abnormal bleeding, usually spontaneous. The most usual site is the gastrointestinal tract but haematuria and spontaneous bruising occur commonly. Interestingly, the disorder is not associated with genuine purpuric lesions. Thromboembolic phenomena are less frequent than bleeding. Thrombosis of the splenic vein and the superficial or deep veins of the legs have been reported and may be followed by pulmonary emboli and infarction. Not infrequently the disorder presents to the vascular surgeon with curious thrombotic lesions of the vessels of fingers and toes, which cause small areas of gangrene not unlike those seen in the vasculitis of rheumatoid arthritis and collagen-vascular diseases (Fig. 1). Another common feature, which probably has the same underlying mechanism, is erythromelalgia. These bizarre peripheral vascular complications may be present for many years without a marked elevation in the platelet count.

The spleen is often enlarged, at least in the early stages of the illness. Splenic atrophy has also been reported and is thought to follow thrombosis of the splenic vessels. When this occurs, or when the spleen is mistakenly removed before the diagnosis is recognized, the platelet count may rise to a value almost approaching that of the red-cell count. Such patients are at particular risk of bleeding or thrombosis, or both.

LABORATORY FINDINGS (PLATES 27, 28)

The main finding is a greatly elevated platelet count, which is often in excess of 800 to 1000×10⁹/l. The platelet morphology is abnormal, with many large and bizarre forms, and aggregates in the peripheral blood. The bone marrow shows marked megakaryocytic hyperplasia. There is usually a mild polymorphonuclear leucocytosis and occasionally a slight elevation in the packed cell volume. Episodes of anaemia are quite common, almost certainly resulting from either acute or chronic blood loss. In patients whose spleens have atrophied typical changes of hyposplenism are found in the peripheral blood (Chapter 22.5.4).

Specialized tests of platelet function have shown a variety of abnormalities including reduced adhesiveness, reduced serotonin content and uptake, and reduced aggregation in response to ADP and adrenalin but not to collagen.

Fig. 1 A thrombotic lesion with infarction of the end of the toe in a patient with primary thrombocythaemia.

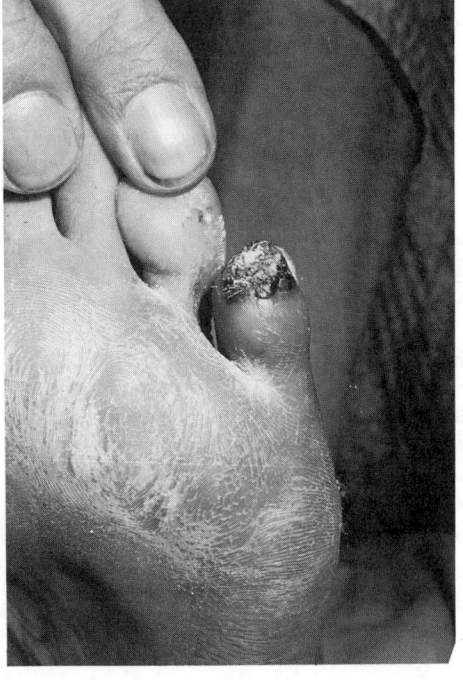

Table 1 *Causes of a raised platelet count*

Myeloproliferative disorders
Primary thrombocythaemia
Polycythaemia vera
Myelosclerosis
Chronic myeloid leukaemia

Secondary thrombocytosis
Bleeding
Inflammatory disorders
Rheumatoid arthritis
Malignant disease
Post-splenectomy
Splenic atrophy; sickle-cell disease, coeliac disease
Drugs: vincoids, adrenaline
Post-thrombocytopenia
Haemolytic anaemia

DIAGNOSIS

Thrombocythaemia must be distinguished from other causes of an elevated platelet count (Table 1). These include bleeding, malignant disease, rheumatoid arthritis, and infection. In these disorders it is very unusual to find platelet counts in excess of $800 \times 10^9/l$ and this, together with the remarkable morphological changes of the platelets, usually serves to distinguish primary thrombocythaemia from thrombocytosis.

COURSE AND PROGNOSIS

Because it is a relatively rare disease, very little is known about the natural history and prognosis of primary thrombocythaemia. Although many patients run a course punctuated by episodes of bleeding, thrombosis, embolism, and other complications, and the disease may be difficult to manage if the spleen has been mistakenly removed or if there is a thrombosis of the splenic vessels leading to splenic atrophy, the condition can also be surprisingly mild. Indeed, it is becoming apparent that young patients who present without symptoms may live for many years without suffering any ill effects. Furthermore, after a short course of alkylating agents or ^{32}P, many patients remain well for months or years before requiring another course of therapy when the platelet count finally rises again, as it always does.

For these reasons it is possible to give a reasonably good prognosis for patients with this condition. If it is found by chance there may be a long period of freedom from symptoms. Even if the disease presents with a complication it is usually possible to control the platelet count for many years. There have been occasional reports of acute leukaemic transformation.

TREATMENT

Because this condition is rare there have been few opportunities to study large numbers of patients to assess the best form of treatment. However, certain facts seem to be emerging. First, because young patients with this disorder, even with very high platelet counts, often remain asymptomatic for many years, it seems reasonable to leave them untreated under regular surveillance, and to initiate therapy only if symptoms occur or if the platelet count is progressively rising. In older patients there seems to be a genuine risk of vascular accidents and the platelet count should probably be reduced to below $500 \times 10^9/l$. Excellent control can usually be achieved using busulphan. Younger patients respond well

to a starting dose of busulphan 4 mg daily, which is reduced to 2 mg daily as the platelet count approaches normal. Once the count is normal the drug must be stopped; the count will often remain at a normal level for months or even years. It is very important to stop the drug when the platelet count has reached a normal level and not to persist with treatment, as a dangerous pancytopenia may result. In older patients, or in those who cannot be maintained under regular surveillance, ^{32}P therapy is the best approach. The dose regimen is similar to that described for the management of polycythaemia vera. If the platelet count needs reducing rapidly, hydroxyurea at a dose of 15 to 30 mg/kg per day is extremely effective. In emergencies the platelet count can be lowered rapidly by plateletpheresis.

Because of the relatively higher leukaemogenic risk, ^{32}P is now best restricted for older patients who may find it difficult to attend for the regular blood checks that are required during the administration of alkylating agents. It has been found recently that platelet counts can also be lowered by the administration of interferon-α. Satisfactory control can be achieved after 2 to 3 months at doses of 1 to 5 Mu daily in about 50 per cent of patients. However, side-effects may be quite severe and this is not an ideal form of treatment. Anagrelide, originally developed as an agent to prevent platelet aggregation, has recently been shown to cause a selective reduction in the platelet count. Induction doses of 1 to 1.5 mg given orally every 6 h produce a rapid decrease in the platelet count within 2 weeks with minimal side-effects. To date there is limited experience of the use of this drug, although several reports have suggested that it may be a valuable addition to the methods of treating thrombocythaemia. It is too early to advise an optimum regimen for the maintenance of a reduced platelet count using this agent.

In young patients who are being kept under surveillance without treatment it is important to monitor the platelet count carefully throughout pregnancy. It may rise, and if elective surgery is needed, or prior to childbirth, the platelet count can be reduced by plateletpheresis.

REFERENCES

Bellucci, S. *et al.* (1986). Essential thrombocythemia. Clinical, evolutionary and biological data. *Cancer*, **58**, 2440–7.

Fialkow, P.J., Faguet, G.B., Jacobson, R.J., Vnrdya, K., and Murphy, S. (1981). Evidence that essential thrombocythemia is a clonal disorder with origin in a multipotent stem cell. *Blood*, **58**, 916–19.

Ho, A.D. (1991). Chemotherapy of chronic haematological malignancies. *Baillière's Clinical Haematology*, **4**, 197–221.

Hussain, S., Schwartz, J.M., Friedman, S.A., and Chua, S.N. (1978). Aterial thrombosis in essential thrombocythaemia. *American Heart Journal*, **96**, 31–6.

Mitus, A.J. and Schafer, A.I. (1990). Thrombocytosis and thrombocythemia. *Hematology/Oncology Clinics of North America*, **4**, 157–78.

Pamlilio, A.L. and Reiss, R.F. (1979). Therapeutic plateletpheresis in thrombocythemia. *Transfusion*, **19**, 147–9.

Pearson, T.C. (1991). Primary thrombocythaemia: diagnosis and management. *British Journal of Haematology*, **78**, 145–8.

Pearson, T.C. and Messinezy, M. (1987). Polycythaemia and thrombocythaemia in the elderly. *Baillière's Clinical Haematology*, **1**, 355–87.

Schafer, A.I. (1994). Primary thrombocythemia. In *Williams hematology*, (ed. E. Beutler, M.A. Lichtman, B.S. Coller, and T.J. Kipps). McGraw-Hill, New York (in press).

Sedlacer, S.M., Curtis, J.L., Weintraub, J., and Levin, J. (1986). Essential thrombocythemia and leukemic infiltration. *Medicine*, **65**, 353–64.

Singh, A.L. and Wetherley-Mein, G. (1977). Microvascular occlusive lesions in primary thrombocythaemia. *British Journal of Haematology*, **36**, 553–64.

Van de Pette, J.E.W., Prochazka, A.V., Pearson, T.C., Singh, A.K., Dickson, E.R., and Wetherley-Mein, G. (1986). Primary thrombocythaemia. *British Journal of Haematology*, **62**, 229–37.

22.3.11 Aplastic anaemia and other causes of bone marrow failure

E. C. GORDON-SMITH

INTRODUCTION

The concept of bone marrow failure as a cause of peripheral blood cytopenias is imprecise but convenient. Broadly, it indicates that the cause of the peripheral blood disturbance lies within the dividing pool of cells in the marrow itself. Fundamental to the classification of disorders within this group of bone marrow failures is the idea that normal development of cells within the bone marrow and release of normal cells into the peripheral blood depend upon an interaction between haemopoietic cells and the environment in which they proliferate and differentiate. The pathogenesis of most of these disorders is unknown and their separation depends mainly upon morphological criteria. In most instances the conditions are metastable, that is, other changes may occur on the background of the damaged marrow usually, though not always, in the direction of malignant change. The classification shown in Table 1 attempts to group the syndromes where there is a failure of circulating cell production from the marrow according to the assumed mechanism of that failure and to give inherited or congenital syndromes that may mimic the acquired.

Acquired aplastic anaemia

DEFINITION

Acquired aplastic anaemia is a syndrome of haemopoietic stem-cell failure characterized by peripheral blood pancytopenia associated with hypoplasia of the bone marrow in which there is neither fibrosis nor infiltration by malignant cells. Vitamin B_{12} and folate levels are normal, and the disorder is not associated with other dietary deficiencies.

CLASSIFICATION

As defined above, the syndrome of aplastic anaemia may occur in a number of ways. There is no universally acceptable classification but a number of more or less well-defined entities may be identified. These are summarized in Table 2.

Inevitable aplastic anaemia

This occurs following exposure to cytotoxic drugs or irradiation. The severity and duration of aplasia is dose-related and recovery usually occurs 1 to 6 weeks after the cytotoxic agent is discontinued. With very high-dose radiation, stem-cell killing is complete and recovery does not occur. When high-dose radiation is used for a local lesion that includes an area of bone marrow, that area may later become fibrosed and, again, recovery does not occur.

Idiosyncratic acquired aplastic anaemia

This is the disease to which the term 'aplastic anaemia' is usually applied without further qualification. The disease arises spontaneously or may follow exposure to normal doses of a variety of drugs that do not usually cause haematological disturbances. The nature of these agents is discussed in greater detail below.

Immune aplastic anaemia

This is an uncommon disorder, which, again, may follow exposure to certain drugs or some virus infections, particularly infectious mononucleosis. It may also be associated with other autoimmune disorders. Unlike the idiosyncratic aplastic anaemias, recovery usually occurs 2 to 3 weeks after withdrawal of the offending agent, or spontaneously. In some instances it is possible to demonstrate inhibitors of granulopoiesis or erythropoiesis in vitro.

Inherited aplastic anaemia (Fanconi anaemia)

This is an autosomal recessive inherited disorder in which hypocellularity of the bone marrow and pancytopenia develop, usually during childhood. It is associated with skeleton and skin abnormalities, described in greater detail below.

'Malignant' aplastic anaemia

This occurs in association with acute leukaemia or myelodysplastic syndrome. The aplastic presentation of acute leukaemia is more common in childhood, particularly with acute lymphoblastic leukaemia.

Idiosyncratic acquired aplastic anaemia

AETIOLOGY

The term 'idiosyncratic' is used to indicate that only a small proportion of a population is susceptible to the disease and that the characteristics of the patient, derived from genetic and environmental factors, determine the peculiar sensitivity of that individual to the disease. Although the pathognomonic characteristic of aplastic anaemia is peripheral blood pancytopenia with a hypocellular marrow, there is some heterogeneity between cases and occasionally patients present with single or dual cytopenias that only slowly progress to full marrow failure.

In about two-thirds of cases of aplastic anaemia it is not possible to identify any likely cause. Amongst the rest, drugs, viruses, and environmental toxins may be identified as probable causes. As yet there is no test that can pinpoint with certainty the cause of the aplastic anaemia, and the implication of any particular agent depends upon temporal associations and previous reports. Drugs have been implicated in the aetiology of aplastic anaemia for 50 years or more and the list of such drugs is long. However, in many cases the association with the disease is weak and often confounded by the patient having received other drugs at the same time. The agents most commonly implicated are certain antimicrobials, of which chloramphenicol is the best known, and non-steroidal anti-inflammatory drugs, phenylbutazone and its derivatives being the most commonly involved. Table 3 lists the more frequently reported drugs. Aplastic anaemia is more likely to occur after a second or subsequent exposure to the drug than after the first exposure.

Viruses are also implicated in the aetiology of aplastic anaemia, particularly hepatitis viruses. Up to 10 per cent of patients in Western series of aplastic anaemia, particularly in the younger age group, give a history of jaundice and/or hepatitic symptoms some 6 weeks before the pancytopenia develops. In many instances, disturbances of hepatocellular function have been demonstrated. The hepatitis is usually hepatitis B surface-antigen negative, but the precise aetiology of the hepatitis is normally unidentified. Hepatitis A and C are not clearly associated with the disease. In one series of patients who received a liver transplant for fulminant non-A, non-B hepatitis, 9 out of 32 subsequently developed aplastic anaemia, whereas none of the patients transplanted for other causes of liver failure did so. Occasional reports of aplastic anaemia following Epstein–Barr virus infection have been published. In some instances the aplasia, though profound, is transient, suggesting that different mechanisms of marrow suppression may occur. Infection with human immunodeficiency virus (HIV) may be associated with profound marrow depression, sometimes compounded by treatment with azidothymidine, though it is not clear whether cases of genuine prolonged idiosyncratic aplastic anaemia occur with this virus.

Various domestic and recreational drugs and chemicals have been implicated in the cause of aplastic anaemia. 3,4-Methylenedioxymethamphetamine ('Ecstasy') has been associated with transient aplastic anaemia. DDT and other insecticides, particularly lindane and pentachlorophenol, have been linked to aplastic anaemia, although the evi-

Table 1 *Classification of bone marrow failure*

Pathogenesis	Diseases	
	Acquired	Congenital
Haemopoietic stem-cell failure	Acquired aplastic anaemia	Fanconi anaemia
		Dyskeratosis congenita
Haemopoietic failure during differentiation	Pure red-cell aplasia	Diamond–Blackfan anaemia
	Amegakaryocytic thrombocytopenia	Thrombocytopenia with absent radii (TAR)
	Chronic acquired neutropenia	Kostmann's syndrome
Proliferative dysplasias with abnormal differentiation	Myelodysplastic syndromes	Congenital dyserythropoietic anaemias
	Refractory anaemia (RA)	
	RA with ringed sideroblasts	
	RA with excess blasts	
	Chronic myelomonocytic leukaemia	
Abnormal environment	Proliferative dysplasias with fibrosis	Osteoporosis
	Myelofibrosis	
Infiltrations		
Leukaemias/lymphomas		
Lipid-storage disease (e.g. Gaucher's disease)		
Amyloid		
Infections	HIV	
	Dengue fever	
	Parvovirus B19	
Bone marrow necrosis		

Table 2 *Classification of aplastic anaemia (AA)*

Disease	Causes	Characterization
Inevitable AA	Cytotoxic drugs	Dose-dependent
	Radiation	Predictable recovery
Idiosyncratic AA	Drugs/chemicals	Not dose-dependent
	Viruses (e.g. hepatitis)	Prolonged course
	Idiopathic	Recovery unpredictable
Immune AA	Autoimmune disease	Usually short duration
	Viruses (e.g. Epstein–Barr)	Antibodies may be detectable
Inherited AA	Autosomal recessive disease	Fanconi anaemia
	Sex-linked (usually)	Dyskeratosis congenita
Malignant AA	Acute leukaemias (usually ALL*)	Transient: leukaemia develops later
	Myelodysplastic aplasia	Prolonged or preleukaemic
		Cytogenetic abnormalities common

*ALL, acute lymphoblastic leukaemia.

dence is not strong. Hair dyes have been incriminated in the past, but seem to be less commonly associated since aniline was discontinued as a constituent. The lack of suitable tests for possible aetiological agents, together with the delay between exposure and the development of pancytopenia, mean that the list of substances thought to cause aplastic anaemia is long and may be inaccurate.

INCIDENCE AND EPIDEMIOLOGY

Aplastic anaemia is a rare disease. In Europe and the United States the incidence is probably between 2 and 5 per million of the population per year. All age groups may be affected, possibly with peaks between 20 and 30 years, and again in older patients. There is a slight preponderance of males, possibly reflecting the greater risk amongst men of exposure to toxic substances at work. In the Far East the incidence of aplastic anaemia is much higher and the male preponderance much more obvious. This may be related to the greater use of chloramphenicol and the increased risk of hepatitis. The risk factors seem to be environmental rather than genetic, as people of the same ethnic groups in the West

have a lower incidence. The risk of developing aplastic anaemia following exposure to one of the drugs known to cause this disorder is equally uncertain. With chloramphenicol the incidence is probably somewhere in the region of 1 : 25 000 to 1 : 60 000 patients at risk. A realization that chloramphenicol could cause aplastic anaemia and the wide publicity given to this risk means that chloramphenicol is much less commonly prescribed in the West than before and it is no longer the single, most common cause of aplastic anaemia. Non-steroidal anti-inflammatory drugs now seem to be the most frequently associated with aplastic anaemia. Drugs suspected of being associated should be prescribed with caution and only for good reason.

PATHOGENESIS

The way in which the various agents bring about aplastic anaemia is unknown. The main defect is a failure of the pluripotent, haemopoietic stem cells in the bone marrow to proliferate and differentiate into mature blood cells. *In vitro* experiments with long-term bone marrow culture show that aplastic marrow stromal cells are able to support haemopoiesis

Table 3 *Drugs strongly associated with an increased risk of aplastic anaemia*

Class of drug	Specific drugs
Antibiotics	Chloramphenicol
	Sulphonamides:
	Salazopyrine
	Co-trimoxazole
Anti-inflammatory agents	Phenylbutazone
	Oxyphenbutazone
	Indomethacin
	Sulindac
	Diclofenac
	Piroxicam
	Penicillamine
	Gold salts
Thyrostatic	Carbimazole
	Thiouracils
	Potassium perchlorate
Anticonvulsant	Hydantoins:
	Phenytoin
	Mephenytoin
	Carbamazepine
	Phenacemide
	Ethosuximide
Psychotropic	Phenothiazines
	Remoxipride
Antimalarial	Quinacrine (Mepacrine)
	Maloprim
Antidiabetic	Chlorpropamide
	Carbutamide
	Tolbutamide

Note: Many of these drugs have also been associated with a variety of other blood dyscrasias, particularly neutropenia or agranulocytosis.

from normal stem cells but aplastic stem cells continue to grow abnormally on normal stroma. The abnormality might be initiated or prolonged by cellular immune pathways or there might be inhibitors circulating in the blood, though these have rarely been demonstrated.

DIAGNOSIS AND PATHOLOGY (PLATE 29)

The diagnosis of aplastic anaemia is made on the basis of findings in the peripheral blood and bone marrow. In the blood there is pancytopenia with no abnormal cells present. The anaemia is usually normocytic at presentation but may be macrocytic, even strikingly so, particularly in chronic cases. The reticulocyte count is low. Neutrophils are invariably reduced and the count may be very low. Circulating neutrophils may have rather heavy granulation, so-called 'toxic' granulation, and a high alkaline phosphatase content. The eosinophils and basophils are usually also depleted and monocytopenia is usual. The reduction in the lymphocyte count is more variable; in children particularly it may be relatively high so that the total white-cell count may be normal. It is only when the differential white-cell count is done that the severe neutropenia is recognized. The platelet count is reduced and the relatively uniform smallness of the platelets is an indication that production has failed.

Bone marrow aspiration is usually easy; fragments are obtained which are fatty, and there is a reduction of haemopoietic cells in the trails. The cellularity of the marrow may be judged to some extent from the marrow aspirate, but a so-called 'dry tap' (no material obtained from an aspirate) or 'blood tap' (no fragments obtained) do not allow an assessment of bone marrow activity. In aplastic anaemia there may be a patchy loss of cellularity throughout the marrow so that one aspirate may yield relatively normal-looking marrow. The diagnosis of aplastic anaemia

should therefore not be made on a bone marrow aspirate alone, and assessment of cellularity should be made on a trephine biopsy, which shows replacement of the normal cellular marrow by fatty marrow. The reticulin network of the marrow is reduced commensurately with the reduction in the overall cellularity. Focal areas of preserved cellularity may be seen in the trephine, and it is one of the mysteries of aplastic anaemia that these foci do not repopulate the remainder of the marrow (Fig. 1).

Dyserythropoiesis

In severe aplastic anaemia where normal haemopoiesis is almost completely abolished, there remain some cells within the marrow. These are normal lymphocytes, plasma cells, and macrophages. The cellular collection may be relatively uniform throughout the marrow or may occur in focal areas. Malignant cells are not seen. Where haemopoiesis has not been completely abolished, the remaining areas may demonstrate abnormalities of differentiation, particularly in the red-cell series (dyserythropoiesis). In the early stages of aplastic anaemia, erythrophagocytosis by macrophages may be quite prominent.

CLINICAL FEATURES

The clinical features of aplastic anaemia arise from the results of deficiencies of the cellular elements of the blood. Bleeding manifestations are often the first that take the patient to seek help from the doctor. The development of severe thrombocytopenia takes place over a matter of weeks or months so that catastrophic haemorrhage as a presenting feature is unusual; minor signs of the bleeding tendency present first. Excessive bruising or a petechial rash may be noticed. Commonly, there is bleeding from the gums or nose. Haemorrhages in the buccal mucosa may occur, and haemorrhages in the retinae may be a portent of serious bleeding. The anaemia also develops slowly and the patient may complain only of mild fatigue or shortness of breath on marked exertion. Infections, particularly of the oropharynx or upper respiratory pathways, may be a presenting feature. Infections anywhere aggravate the effect of thrombocytopenia, particularly in the mouth. Good oral hygiene may reduce the amount of bleeding as well as clearing up local sepsis. There are no specific physical findings in aplastic anaemia, as any abnormalities resulting from the pancytopenia would be the same whatever the cause. There is no lymphadenopathy except that associated with local infection. The liver and spleen are not enlarged. If the aplastic anaemia has followed an episode of apparent hepatitis, there may be some residual jaundice with enzyme abnormalities consistent with cholestasis.

The progression of the disease is variable and depends upon the severity and completeness of the marrow damage. In earlier series of patients with aplastic anaemia where only support in the form of transfusions and available antibiotics was given, about half the patients died within 3 to 6 months as a result of infection or haemorrhage. Patients alive at a year, however, had a better chance of surviving, at least for the next 2 or 3 years. This suggested that there was a group of patients with severe disease with a very poor chance of recovery and another group with a milder disorder. This led to the establishment of criteria for severe aplastic anaemia (Table 4), which have proved to be very useful in stratifying patients when different treatments have been compared.

The identification of the group with severe aplastic anaemia is important because, for these patients, early bone-marrow transplantation is the treatment of choice if a suitable donor is available. The subsequent course for patients who survive is variable. Spontaneous recovery, apparently to complete normality, may occur even after several years of pancytopenia. Other patients may remain stable for many years, and then gradually haemopoietic activity decreases further and they become anaemic and eventually die of infection or bleeding. Abnormal clones of cells may develop with a greater frequency in these patients than in a normal population. Paroxysmal nocturnal haemoglobinuria is the most frequent clonal abnormality to evolve in aplastic anaemia. It arises from a somatic mutation involving a gene that codes for one of the enzymes in the assembling pathway of the protein anchor—phosphatidyl inositol glycan (**PIG**). Two enzymes that inactivate comlement complexes, decay accelerating factor (DAF; CD59) and membrane inhibitor of reactive lysis (MIRL; CD55), are absent in red cells in paroxysmal nocturnal haemoglobinuria, which become sensitive to the action of complement. The condition may be recognized through the Ham's test or directly by using fluorescence-activated cell scanning to identify populations that lack the PIG-anchored proteins. Myelodysplastic syndromes and acute myeloid leukaemia may also develop following aplastic anaemia and the relation between these blood diseases is discussed below.

Before platelet transfusions became readily available, the usual cause of death in these patients was haemorrhage. Most now succumb to infection or a mixture of infection and haemorrhage, often after many months of treatment with antimicrobials. It is virtually impossible to eradicate infection in the severely neutropenic patient until such time as neutrophil production returns.

TREATMENT

The treatment of aplastic anaemia has two main components. The first is to protect and support the patient from the consequences of pancy-topenia and to keep him alive so that there may be a chance of spontaneous recovery. The second is to try to accelerate the recovery of the bone marrow by whatever means, without eradicating the chance of spontaneous recovery.

Support and protection

For the aplastic patient this depends upon reducing potential sources of infection to a minimum and replacing deficient cells by transfusion (see Chapter 7.19.3). Infections may arise from the environment or from sources of bacteria and other agents within the patient. As with all immunosuppressed patients, significant and lethal infections may arise from contamination with organisms that are not normally pathogenic. Exogenous infections are more likely in a hospital environment than at home, so any patient with aplastic anaemia admitted to hospital must be nursed in a clean and preferably sterile area. The two most important effective measures are for all medical and nursing staff to remove or cover outer garments that are likely to have been in contact with other infected patients, and for hands to be washed in bacteriocidal preparations before entering the patient's room and, again, before touching the patient. Other more stringent measures probably add little more in the way of protection. Virus infections are not in themselves especially likely in the neu-

Fig. 1 Trephine biopsies of adult posterior iliac crest. (a) Normal marrow. (b) Severe aplastic anaemia. (c) Cellular focus in severe aplastic anaemia. (d) Proliferative dysplasia with fibrosis.

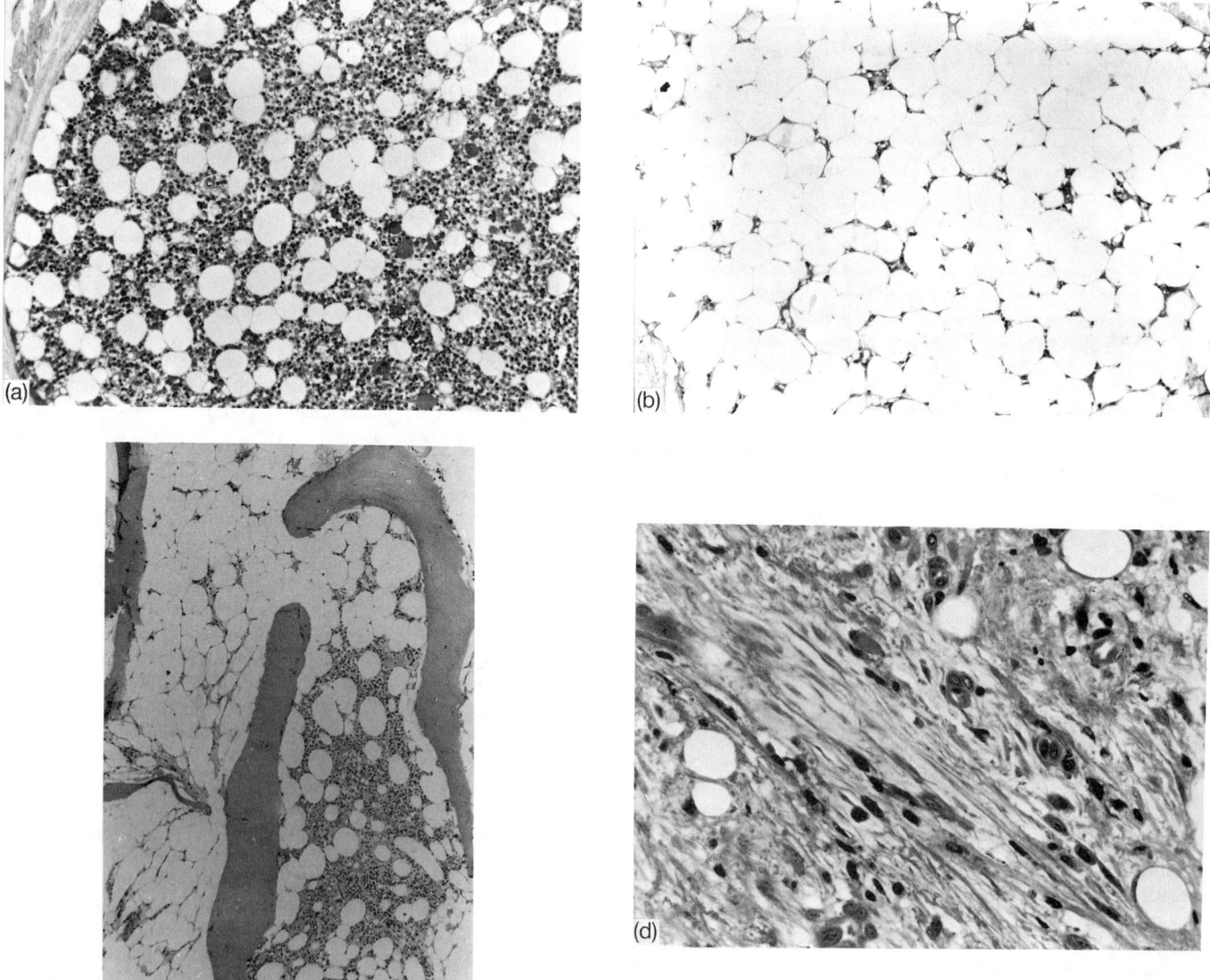

Table 4 *Criteria of severe aplastic anaemia**

Neutrophils	$< 0.4 \times 10^9/l$
Platelets	$< 10 \times 10^9/l$
Reticulocytes	$< 10 \times 10^9/l$
Bone marrow	>80 per cent of remaining cells are non-myeloid

*Any three of the above four present for at least 2 weeks.

tropenic host, but if they occur they produce an environment in which secondary bacterial infections may flourish. When the neutropenic patient is also immunosuppressed in other ways, virus infections assume a very important role in causing morbidity.

Endogenous infection arises from organisms carried within the patient, particularly in the upper respiratory passages and the gastrointestinal tract. Scrupulous skin and oral hygiene is essential. Repeated mouth washing with an antiseptic such as chlorhexidine or with hydrogen peroxide should be done regularly and after eating. The skin should be cleaned regularly with antiseptic. The extent to which potential pathogens should be removed from the gastrointestinal tract is debatable. Mostly these are aerobic organisms that are easily eliminated by antimicrobials. Some would argue that removal of the anaerobic bacteria may actually be harmful. So-called complete decontamination of the gut is achieved by giving a variety of non-absorbable antimicrobials together with antifungal agents such as nystatin or amphotericin. Co-trimoxazole together with an antifungal agent may be equally effective in eliminating most aerobic pathogens, although this has yet to be demonstrated conclusively. Recolonization of the bowel by potential pathogens can be avoided by using freshly cooked food and avoiding sources of hospital pathogens such as salads and fresh fruit. It must be remembered that patients with aplastic anaemia may require months of protective isolation and therefore measures must be practical as well as effective. Bowel decontamination is restricted to patients in hospital. In the outpatient department it is not possible to maintain a sterile gut, and patients are probably better protected by their own natural bowel flora than by non-absorbable antimicrobials. They should, however, be advised to avoid both food with high bacterial content and crowded places where they are liable to pick up infections.

Once an infection is established it is essential to treat it as soon as possible. Systemic antimicrobials must be given as soon as fever or signs of infection occur and appropriate samples have been sent to the laboratory. If an organism is isolated the antibiotics should be changed, according to the sensitivities of the organism. Because the most common exogenous infections arise from Pseudomonas or Klebsiella, and the endogenous ones from aerobic organisms of the gastrointestinal tract, the antimicrobials used in the first instance must be appropriate to those organisms. Most centres use a combination of aminoglycoside with a second antimicrobial likely to have activity against Pseudomonas or a third-generation cephalosporin (suitable regimens are described in Section 7). Localized skin infections carry a particularly grave prognosis because it is difficult to achieve adequate antimicrobial concentrations in the oedematous lesion. A major problem in aplastic anaemia is to decide when to discontinue the antimicrobials. The patient may become afebrile and apparently well, but when the antimicrobials are stopped, infection by the original organism is all too likely to return unless the neutropenia recovers. Granulocyte-stimulating cytokines, filgrastim or lenograstim or granulocyte-macrophage stimulating cytokine (rhGM-CSF) may sufficiently stimulate the remaining bone marrow to raise the neutrophil count enough to eradicate the infection. There is no place for granulocyte transfusions (see Section 7).

Transfusion of red cells and platelets is the other main standby in the management of aplasia. Red-cell transfusions usually present few problems, but it must be remembered that the platelet count will fall and catastrophic haemorrhage may occur during transfusion. Platelets should always be given before starting red-cell transfusion in the pancytopenic

patient and preferably also at the end in order to avoid this complication. Repeated platelet transfusions usually lead to the development of antibodies and resistance to platelet concentrates. The antibodies may be anti-HLA or antiplatelet-specific antigens. Resistance is indicated by an inability to raise the platelet count by platelet transfusion. It may become impossible to control bleeding manifestations. It is also possible that, with the development of antibodies, immune complexes will form, which leads to a fall in the granulocyte count as well as the platelet count as resistance increases. Conventionally, platelets are only given when there is a clinical indication for their use. These indications include the rapid development of purpura, extensive bleeding from the gums and in the buccal mucosa, retinal haemorrhages, and headache. Major haemorrhage from any site is also an indication for platelets. In aplastic anaemia, particularly when the individual is being managed as an outpatient, catastrophic and fatal haemorrhage may be the first indication of severe bleeding, particularly so if the patient develops an infection. For this reason, some centres manage their outpatients with regular platelet transfusions even though resistance may develop. This gives an opportunity for at least a weekly review of the patient and control of severe purpura. Sensitization to platelets may be avoided by using HLA-matched platelets or those that have been rendered free of white cells.

Further details of the management of patients with marrow failure are given in Section 7.

Specific measures

Androgens were the first drugs used in the treatment of aplastic anaemia that had any degree of success. High-dose anabolic (androgenic) steroids are given by mouth. Only those that are alkylated in the 17α position are absorbed from the gastrointestinal tract, and their usefulness is limited by hepatotoxicity, which includes the development of hepatocellular carcinoma and the formation of multiple venous lakes called peliosis hepatis. Other side-effects are associated with the virilizing action of androgenic steroids. Androgens may raise the responsiveness of the red-cell precursors to erythropoietin and also have a direct effect on stem-cell proliferation. In severe aplastic anaemia there has been no definite evidence that anabolic steroids improve survival, but when some marrow function remains they may produce a significant rise in all cell lines. In patients who do respond it takes about 3 months before effects are seen and recovery of the blood count is thereafter slow. Occasionally, patients become androgen dependent and stopping therapy leads to a relapse. For this reason, androgens should be tailed off slowly and the dose adjusted to response.

Bone marrow transplantation (see also Chapter 22.8.2)

Replacement of the aplastic bone marrow by normal marrow from a suitable donor has long been considered the most rational treatment for aplastic anaemia. Early attempts to establish allogenic grafts were universally unsuccessful but transient engraftment could be demonstrated in some immunosuppressed recipients. Immunosuppression together with unmatched bone marrow were occasionally followed by recovery of the patient's own marrow. These observations have led to two major forms of therapy for aplastic anaemia. In young patients (under 40 years or so) with severe aplastic anaemia who have a suitable HLA-matched donor, early transplantation is the recommended treatment. The transplant should be made as soon as possible after the diagnosis of severe aplastic anaemia has been established, to avoid sensitization of the patient to platelet antigens. Multiple transfusions increase the risk of graft failure. In bone marrow transplantation for severe aplastic anaemia, relatively mild immunosuppression is sufficient to permit engraftment without using whole-body irradiation. By using cyclophosphamide for pregraft immunosuppression, particularly when additional immunosuppression is given through antilymphocyte globulin, the risk of graft failure has been reduced to less than 10 per cent. Cyclosporin is given after bone marrow infusion to protect against rejection and to modify graft-versus-host disease. The success of HLA-matched, sibling transplants is now about 70 per cent, rising to better than 90 per cent for untransfused patients.

Immunosuppression

A somewhat serendipitous series of observations led to the introduction of immunosuppressive treatment using antilymphocyte globulin. The rate of recovery after such treatment is usually slow, with few patients showing a response before about 3 months, and in some instances much later. Many patients treated in this way still require some transfusion support even a year or more after treatment, and may indeed continue with neutropenia and/or thrombocytopenia for many years, though independent of transfusion or hospital care. It is worth achieving even a modest improvement in blood count because, with neutrophil counts above 0.5×10^9/l and platelets above 30×10^9/l, an independent and relatively safe existence is possible. If the patient fails to respond to the first course of antilymphocyte globulin (usually prepared in a horse), a second course using rabbit antihuman lymphocyte globulin may be given. Some 50 per cent of patients respond to the first course with partial or complete remission. About 40 per cent of non-responders to the horse protein will achieve some improvement with rabbit antilymphocyte globulin. The optimum timing of a second course still has to be determined but most groups wait about 4 months. There seems to be no advantage in giving more than a 5-day course of antilymphocyte globulin. Reactions during infusion of the globulin are common and serum sickness occurs in some 75 per cent of patients, requiring treatment with corticosteroids.

The addition of high-dose methylprednisone (5 mg/kg per day) has no obvious therapeutic advantage and produces a high incidence of avascular necrosis of the hip. Cyclosporin, 5 mg/kg per day, on the other hand, does appear to increase the rate of remission of aplastic anaemia when given after antilymphocyte globulin and may also be used alone as an alternative to that globulin. Recovery, as with antilymphocyte globulin, is slow and may be incomplete.

Anabolic steroids

Anabolic steroids may be useful in non-severe aplastic anaemia, though the virilizing side-effects make their use unpopular and hepatotoxicity is a problem. A trial of oxymethalone, 2.5 mg/kg per day may be warranted.

Congenital aplastic anaemia (Fanconi anaemia)

The most common of the inherited disorders which produce aplastic anaemia is that described by Fanconi in 1927. The disorder is inherited as an autosomal recessive and is associated with multiple developmental abnormalities, particularly of the skin and skeleton (Table 5).

HAEMATOLOGICAL FEATURES

Patients with Fanconi anaemia usually have a normal or nearly normal blood count at birth and during infancy. The disease presents with the effects of pancytopenia, usually about the age of 5 years or later. Bleeding due to thrombocytopenia is the most common presentation, with anaemia second. The neutrophil count is often relatively well preserved for some years after severe thrombocytopenia and anaemia develop. The bone marrow becomes progressively hypocellular over the years. In the initial stages, macrophages showing active phagocytosis and an infiltrate of lymphocytes are prominent. Granulopoiesis may be relatively well preserved. Dyserythropoiesis is common.

CYTOGENETIC FINDINGS

The characteristic finding in Fanconi anaemia is multiple, non-specific abnormalities in the chromosomes, particularly when cells are stressed by exposure to DNA cross-linking agents. These consist mainly of chromatid breaks and aberrations. It is suggested that these lesions arise as a result of failure of one of the DNA repair systems (Table 6). Although much work has been devoted to identifying such an enzyme defect, it

Table 5 *Abnormalities associated with Fanconi anaemia*

Condition	Patients affected (%)*
Hyperpigmentation of the skin	75
Malformation of the skeleton	
all patients	66
aplasia or hypoplasia of the thumb	50
aplasia or hypoplasia of the radii	17
syndactyly	15
reduced number of carpal bones	30
microsomy	60
microcephaly	40
malformation of kidneys	28
strabismus (in males)	30
crypogenitalism (in males)	20
Cryptorchidism	20
Mental retardation	17
Deafness	7
Short stature	80
Growth hormone deficiency†	Rare

*Percentages are approximate. Data derived mainly from Fanconi (1967).

†Most patients have normal levels despite short stature.

has so far eluded detection, but the gene that is abnormal in one of the several genetic variants of Fanconi anaemia has been identified.

CLINICAL FEATURES

The features of the full-blown Fanconi anaemia are characteristic (Table 5). In some cases, diagnosis may be difficult because of absence of the characteristic skeletal and skin features, and *formes frustes* probably exist. Infants are of low birth weight and remain small for age after birth. The skin is often mildly pigmented with areas of deeper pigmentation producing *café-au-lait* spots, sometimes with areas of depigmentation. Skeletal abnormalities involve particularly the bones of the forearm and thumbs. Abnormalities of the kidneys are also common. Mental development is only occasionally abnormal.

PROGNOSIS AND TREATMENT

The outlook in Fanconi anaemia is poor. Untreated, the disease is usually relentless. Despite support with transfusions over many years, most patients die of haemorrhage or infection. Treatment with anabolic steroids may bring about a remission of variable duration. Several years free from transfusion requirements may be obtained, but at the price of virilization and abnormalities of the liver. Hepatocellular carcinoma seems to be particularly common in children treated for years with 17α-alkylated anabolic agents (Fig. 2). The development of acute leukaemia is also common and may be the presenting feature. Fanconi anaemia should be suspected in all children presenting with acute myeloid leukaemia under the age of 10 years. Its detection would be important at least for identifying the familial nature of the disease for the purpose of genetic counselling.

There are well-documented reports of patients with Fanconi anaemia going into spontaneous remission at the time of puberty, and complete recovery of normal bone-marrow function has been described. Unfortunately, this does not happen often and there is no way of predicting who will recover. In general, the severity of the disease and the rapidity with which pancytopenia develops is predictable within one particular family but there is marked variation between different families. Leukaemia and other malignant disease is more common in the relatives of patients with Fanconi anaemia than in the population at large.

Table 6 *Disorders with possible defective DNA repair mechanisms associated with increased risk of leukaemia and other malignancies*

Disease	Clinical features	Evidence for DNA repair defect	Malignancy
Fanconi anaemia	Aplastic anaemia Skeletal disorders Skin disorders	Chromatid breaks	Acute leukaemia ?Hepatocellular carcinoma
Xeroderma pigmentosa	Keratosis of skin Neurological disease Mental deficiency Bone marrow failure	Excessive chromatid fragility to ultraviolet light Excision repair defect	Skin cancers
Bloom's syndrome	Growth disorder Sun-sensitive eruptions Disturbed immune function	Chromatid breaks Sister chromatid exchanges	Acute leukaemia
Ataxia telangiectasia	Cerebellar ataxis Oculocutaneous telangiectasia Combined immune deficiency	Defective excision	Acute leukaemia and other lympho-reticular malignancies

Bone marrow transplantation is the only curative form of treatment for these patients but unfortunately it carries special risks. The cells in Fanconi anaemia are very sensitive to the cyclophosphamide and irradiation used to immunosuppress patients before transplantation, and the doses given have to be greatly reduced to prevent severe skin and bowel toxicity. With these modifications the success of bone marrow transplants from HLA-matched donors is similar to that for acquired aplastic anaemia.

Aplastic presentation of malignant disease

Aplastic anaemia is one response to bone marrow damage and acute leukaemia is another. At presentation the distinction between the two may not always be clear, at least histologically and anatomically. There are a number of syndromes in which aplasia and acute leukaemia seem to be linked.

Acute lymphoblastic leukaemia of childhood

This may present in a form indistinguishable from aplastic anaemia. Blasts are not seen in the peripheral blood, and the bone marrow aspirate and trephine are hypocellular without any obvious infiltration by malignant cells. The aplasia in these children usually recovers rapidly, some-

Fig. 2 Hepatocellular carcinoma in the liver of a patient with Fanconi anaemia treated for 4 years with anabolic steroids; the liver also shows multiple venous lakes (peliosis hepatis), another side-effect of anabolic steroids.

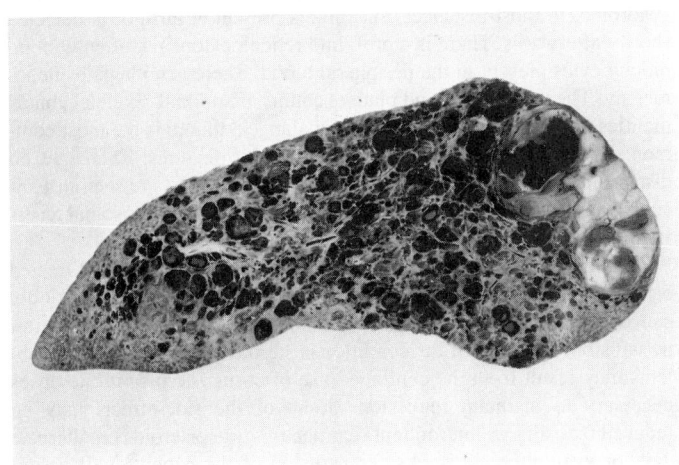

times in response to corticosteroids. Some 6 to 8 weeks later there is the emergence of leukaemic cells in the peripheral blood. It is suggested that the aplasia is an early result of the leukaemia or possibly part of the body's reaction against leukaemia. It has also been suggested that corticosteroids should be given to all young children with aplastic anaemia as a diagnostic test for acute leukaemia. Whilst acute lymphoblastic leukaemia in childhood is the most common association, aplasia preceding acute myeloid leukaemia in this way has been described and adults are occasionally affected.

Hypoplastic myelodysplasia (see also Chapter 22.3.7)

This is a term that has been applied to a disease characterized by a hypoplastic marrow in which a small proportion of blasts may be seen, usually with occasional blasts in the peripheral blood. The condition differs in a number of ways from aplastic anaemia, but the differences may be subtle. There is usually more reticulin present in the marrow and aspiration of the marrow may be difficult. The neutrophil alkaline phosphatase score may have low rather than high values as seen in aplastic anaemia. The condition may remain stable for months or years, during which the patient requires transfusions but is otherwise well. Slowly the proportion of blasts in the bone marrow and peripheral blood increases and eventually this condition becomes frankly leukaemic. Mostly, these patients do not respond to antileukaemic therapy, but remissions may occasionally be obtained so that it is probably worth trying chemotherapy when the frankly leukaemic phase emerges. If a suitable bone-marrow donor is available, transplantation is indicated, but under these circumstances additional chemotherapy and total-body irradiation must be given to eradicate the leukaemic clone.

Clonal disorders following aplastic anaemia

Some patients who survive for several years with aplastic anaemia may eventually develop acute leukaemia, though this is relatively rare (1–3 per cent). There may indeed be a period of apparent remission before the acute leukaemia develops, usually after a period of myelodysplasia. The emergence of clones associated with paroxysmal nocturnal haematuria has already been mentioned. Relapse or the emergence of an abnormal clone occurs in 25 to 40 per cent of patients with aplastic anaemia who have been treated with immunosuppression only.

The proliferative bone-marrow failures

There are a number of disorders characterized by peripheral blood pancytopenia in which the bone marrow is cellular but is ineffective in its

Table 7 *Bone marrow failure affecting single cell lines*

Disease	Cause	Example
Red cell aplasia	Inherited	Diamond-Blackfan syndrome
	Idiopathic, acquired (?autoimmune)	With or without thymoma
		With other autoimmune disorders
	Drug induced	Penicillamine
		Diphenylhydantoin
		Chlorpropamide
		Chloramphenicol
	Virus induced	Aplastic crisis in haemolytic anaemia (Parvovirus)
		Transient erythroblastopenia in childhood
	Riboflavin deficiency	Experimental
Neutropenia	Inherited	Infantile genetic agranulocytosis (Kostmann syndrome)
		With pancreatic insufficiency (Scwachman–Diamond syndrome)
		Others
	Idiopathic, acquired (?autoimmune)	?Cyclical
	Drug induced	Thiazides
		Semisynthetic penicillins
	Virus induced	Rubella
Amegakaryocytosis	Congenital	With total absence of radii
		Isolated
	Acquired	Variant of aplastic anaemia

production of normal peripheral blood cells (see also Chapter 22.4.8). Primitive cells are not usually present in the peripheral blood but there may be morphological, biochemical, or cytogenetic changes in the peripheral blood cells that are indicators of the disturbed haematopoiesis. These conditions have been given a number of names such as 'pre-leukaemia', 'smouldering leukaemia', and 'proliferative dysplasia'. It is particularly unsatisfactory to refer to this group as 'pre-leukaemia' because it suggests that these patients will inevitably develop leukaemia, whereas in certain circumstances the condition may be stable for many years and the problems that arise are not those of malignant change but of support for the patient. It is becoming apparent that there are various, reasonably well-circumscribed syndromes within this major group of proliferative bone-marrow failure. These are described in Chapter 22.3.7.

Proliferative dysplasia with fibrosis

Occasionally, fibrosis of the bone marrow appears without evident underlying cause and in the absence of hepatosplenomegaly or extramedullary haemopoiesis. The condition is characterized by increased pancytopenia, sometimes with the presence of red- and white-cell precursors in the peripheral blood—the so-called leucoerythroblastic picture. Bone marrow aspirate is usually unsuccessful, and a trephine biopsy shows a variable degree of reduction in haemopoietic cells, with the marrow replaced by reticulin and fibroblasts. Primitive cells are not seen at this stage of the illness. Ferrokinetic studies may indicate some remaining but ineffective erythropoiesis. Some of these patients probably have an unusual form of myelofibrosis.

Bone-marrow failure affecting single cell lines

There are a number of conditions in which anaemia, neutropenia or thrombocytopenia develop in isolation as a result of the failure to produce these cells by the bone marrow. The conditions may be inherited or acquired and the main disorders are listed in Table 7.

Pure red-cell aplasia (PRCA)

Pure red-cell aplasia is characterized by an anaemia with a marked reduction or absence of reticulocytes in which the neutrophils and platelet count are normal. The bone marrow is cellular, with normal granulopoiesis and megakaryocytes. There may be a complete absence of red-cell precursors or there may be precursors present up to a certain stage of development but not beyond, so-called 'maturation arrest'. Ferrokinetic studies show a grossly prolonged clearance time of ingested radioactive iron and no utilization. Apart from the changes in the red-cell series, there are no other abnormalities in the peripheral blood and there is no evidence of peripheral destruction of red cells. The patients are in other respects normal. Both congenital and acquired forms exist.

CONGENITAL PURE RED-CELL APLASIA (DIAMOND–BLACKFAN ANAEMIA)

This has also been called, rather confusingly, 'congenital hypoplastic anaemia', but is better known by its eponym, the Diamond–Blackfan syndrome. In most instances, anaemia is present at birth or is detected shortly afterwards. There is a profound reticulocytopenia, often with no reticulocytes present in the peripheral blood. There is no hepatosplenomegaly. The white count and platelet counts are normal. Skeletal abnormalities may be present, of which triphalangeal thumb is the most common, but many children have no dysmorphic features. There are no disturbances of growth, of the skin, or other organs as are seen in Fanconi anaemia. The disorder is mainly sporadic or has an autosomal recessive inheritance. There is no chromosomal instability.

Treatment presents many problems. Most of these children, if treated early enough with corticosteroids, will respond and the haemoglobin can be brought back to normal or maintained at normal levels after transfusion. However, if the condition is steroid dependent, major problems may result from the continued use of corticosteroids in the doses necessary to maintain remission. Some of the side-effects may be reduced by using an intermittent regimen of corticosteroids on alternate days or even alternate weeks. Transfusion of the patients will permit normal growth but will produce all the other problems of iron overload and chelation therapy is required from an early stage. Some patients fail to respond to corticosteroids, and this seems to be particularly true if the corticosteroids are instituted late in the illness. These patients rely on blood transfusions for survival.

During the course of the disease the spleen may enlarge and transfusion requirements increase. In these patients, splenectomy may reduce transfusion requirements and occasionally is associated with a marked increase in steroid responsiveness or even complete remission. This only seems to apply to those patients whose spleen is enlarged.

ACQUIRED PURE RED-CELL APLASIA

This may occur *de novo* or following the administration of various drugs. About 10 to 15 per cent of the idiopathic cases are associated with a thymoma. The red-cell aplasia may precede, accompany, or follow the development of the thymoma and excision of the tumour has variable effect with no guarantee of recovery of the anaemia. The haematological features of the disorder are similar to those seen in the congenital red-cell aplasia, with anaemia and reticulocytopenia associated with absence of red-cell precursors or maturation arrest of the red-cell series in the bone marrow. There is an unpredictable responsiveness to corticosteroids and there are reports of patients who are unresponsive to corticosteroids responding to immunosuppressive therapy with drugs such as cyclophosphamide. Autoantibodies have been thought to play a part in the genesis of this disease and occasionally immunoglobulins have been identified that inhibit haem synthesis or prevent the development of red-cell colonies *in vitro*. Very rarely, anti-erythropoietin antibodies have been found.

Apart from the association with thymoma, pure red-cell aplasia may be seen in other conditions where there is a high incidence of autoimmune disease. It may occur in association with acquired idiopathic hypogammaglobulinaemia and other autoimmune diseases. Occasionally, the direct antiglobulin test (Coombs' test) may be weakly positive, usually with complement on the surface of the red cell. There may be a severe thrombocytopenia in some cases. The presence of such autoimmune phenomena suggests that the patient has a better chance of responding to corticosteroids than in their absence. Pure red-cell aplasia may be associated with lymphomas, and evidence of an underlying lymphoma may be obtained by finding evidence of immunoglobulin or T-cell-receptor gene rearrangement in the marrow even when histological proof is lacking. Occasionally, splenectomy may increase responsiveness to corticosteroids or immunosuppression. An enlarging spleen that increases transfusion requirements is an indication for splenectomy.

Erythroblastopenic anaemia in childhood

'Aplastic crises' may occur in patients with haemolytic anaemia. The term is confusing because only the red-cell series is affected. Rapid anaemia develops as a consequence of failure of red-cell production in the presence of increased destruction. In many of these cases, infection with parvovirus seems to be the cause. Antibodies to the virus are absent at the time of crisis and the patient recovers as IgM antibodies appear, followed by the IgG response. Urgent transfusion may be required during the crisis. Transient erythroblastopenia of childhood may also have a viral aetiology, though this is not so clearly demonstrated. The anaemia, with reticulocytopenia, usually occurs in children from 18 to 26 months old (range 1–72 months). There is usually a history of preceding viral or bacterial illness. Recovery occurs within a few weeks of diagnosis though the patient may need transfusion in the mean time.

Isolated defects in white-cell or platelet production

These conditions are described in Chapter 22.5.1 and are summarized in Table 7.

REFERENCES

Brooks, B.J., Jr. Broxmeyer, H.E., Bryan C.F., and Leech S.H. (1984). Serum inhibitor in systemic lupus erythematosus associated with aplastic anaemia. *Archives of Internal Medicine*, **144**, 1474.

Camitta, B.M. *et al.* (1976). Severe aplastic anaemia: a prospective study of the effect of early bone marrow transplantation in acute mortality. *Blood*, **48**, 63–70.

Davis, L.R. (1983). Aplastic crises in haemolytic anaemia: the role of parvovirus-like agent. *British Journal of Haematology*, **55**, 391–3. Fanconi, G. (1967). Familial constitutional panmyelocytopathy: Fanconi's anaemia (FA). I. Clinical aspects. *Seminars in Hematology*, **4**, 233–40.

Gordon-Smith, E. (1992). Bone marrow transplantation for acquired aplastic anaemia. In *Bone marrow transplantation in practice*, (ed. J. Treleaven and J. Barrett), pp. 137–49. Churchill Livingstone, Edinburgh.

Gordon-Smith, E.C. and Issaragrisil, S. (1992). Epidemiology of aplastic anaemia. *Clinical Haematology*, **5**, 475–91.

Hagler, L., Pastore, R.A., Bergin, J.J., and Wrensch, M.R. (1975). Aplastic anemia following viral hepatitis: report of two fatal cases and literature review. *Medicine*, **54**, 139–64.

Kaufman, D.W., Kelly, J.P., Levy, M., and Shapiro, S. (1991). *The drug etiology of agranulocytosis and aplastic anemia*. Oxford University Press, New York.

Rosse, W.F. (1990). Phosphatidylinositol-linked proteins and paroxysmal nocturnal hemoglobinuria. *Blood*, **75**, 1595–601. Schroeder, R.M. and Kurth, R. (1971). Spontaneous chromosomal breakage and high incidence of leukemia in inherited disease. *Blood*, **37**, 96–112.

Schroeder-Kurth, T.M., Auerbach, A.D., and Obe, G. (1989). *Fanconi anemia. Clinical, cytogenetic and experimental aspects*. Springer-Verlag, Berlin.

Schwartz, R.S. (1994). PIG-A—the target gene in paroxysmal nocturnal hemoglobinuria. *New England Journal of Medicine*, **330**, 283–4. Storb, R. *et al.* (1983). Factors associated with graft rejection after HLVA-identical marrow transplantation for aplastic anaemia. *British Journal of Haematology*, **55**, 573–85.

Tzakis, A.G., Arditi, M., Whitington, P.F., Williams, D.M., Lynch, R.E., and Cartwright, G.E. (1973). Drug-induced aplastic anemia. *Seminars in Hematology*, **10**, 195–223.

Young, N.S. and Alter, B.P. (1994) *Aplastic anaemia, acquired and inherited*. Saunders, Philadelphia.

22.3.12 Paroxysmal nocturnal haemoglobinuria

J. V. DACIE AND L. LUZZATTO

Paroxysmal nocturnal haemoglobinuria (**PNH**) is an uncommon acquired disorder, bearing some relation to aplastic anaemia, and characterized by the production of an abnormal line of red cells that are unusually prone to lysis by complement. It affects both sexes and individuals of all racial groups. It is essentially a disease of adults, the majority of patients presenting between 20 and 40 years of age; it is rare, but not unknown, in childhood.

AETIOLOGY AND PATHOGENESIS

Paroxysmal nocturnal haemoglobinuria is an acquired disease originating in a haemopoietic stem cell. It is possible to demonstrate that not only the patient's red cells, but also the granulocytes, the platelets, and usually the lymphocytes are abnormal. There is evidence, from the use of X-linked markers subject to inactivation in females, and from the analysis of individual haemopoietic colonies, that PNH is a clonal disease, arising apparently as the result of somatic mutation. Although at one time in the evolution of the disease, the abnormal red-cell progenitors appear to have some advantage over normal red-cell progenitors and largely replace them—as happens in leukaemia—in PNH the abnormal clone gradually disappears in some patients, and if the patient has sufficient surviving normal stem cells he or she will eventually recover. The gradual elimination of the abnormal clone may result from ageing of the abnormal stem-cell population.

The relation between PNH and aplastic anaemia is intriguing and uncertain. There appears to be no connection with the cause of the aplasia. PNH has thus developed subsequent to marrow aplasia of idiopathic (unknown) origin, after marrow aplasia thought to be drug or chemically induced, and in at least one instance after aplasia of genetic origin (as in Fanconi anaemia). Possibly the marrow aplasia facilitates the growth of the abnormal clone by reducing competition by normal stem cells.

The abnormal red-cell line can be demonstrated by lysis in acidified serum, which reflects its increased sensitivity to complement. A characteristic phenomenon is that not all the patient's red cells undergo lysis under these conditions. The red cells thus vary considerably in their complement sensitivity. Two populations of abnormal red cells can be demonstrated in most patients: one abnormal and one normal. The abnormal population consists in some patients of cells that have a three- to fivefold increased complement sensitivity (these are called PNH type II cells); and in other patients of cells that have a 10- to 15-fold increased complement sensitivity PNH type III cells: the normal cells have been referred to as type I). In some patients both type II and type III cells may coexist with normal cells. The severity of a patient's illness correlates to some extent with the proportion of highly complement-sensitive type III red cells produced by the bone marrow.

Biochemical basis of paroxysmal nocturnal Haemoglobinuria

Apart from complement hypersensitivity, biochemical abnormalities of blood cells in PNH have been known for a long time: specifically, a deficiency of acetylcholinesterase in red cells and of alkaline phosphatase in granulocytes. Recently, it has become apparent that numerous surface proteins are either much reduced or completely lacking from PNH cells: these include, for example, CD59 (membrane inhibitor of reactive lysis) on red cells, on platelets, and on T lymphocytes, CD67 on granulocytes, CD14 on monocytes, and CD24 on B lymphocytes. At first sight, this multiplicity of deficiencies might have appeared difficult to reconcile with a single somatic mutation. However, a remarkable common feature shared by all of these proteins is attachment to the cell membrane through the same chemical structure: a glucosylphosphatidylinositol (**GPI**) anchor. This observation led to the notion that the most likely underlying lesion in PNH is a block in the biosynthesis of this anchor. Recent work on lymphoblastoid cell lines isolated from patients with PNH strongly favours this hypothesis, and has helped to localize the metabolic block at the transfer of *N*-acetylglucosamine to phosphatidylinositol. These findings provide a satisfactory explanation for hypersensitivity to complement of red cells in this condition, because three proteins involved in the interaction of complement within the membrane are GPI-linked: CD59, CD55 (decay accelerating factor, DAF) and the complement regulatory protein that binds C8 (C8bp: also referred to as homologous restriction factor). Recent evidence from a patient with isolated inherited deficiency of CD59, who clinically had a PNH-like syndrome, identifies this as the most critical molecule.

Mechanism of haemolysis

The increased haemolysis in PNH is primarily intravascular, hence the haemoglobinaemia, methaemalbuminaemia, ahaptoglobinaemia, haemoglobinuria, and the long-continuing haemosiderinuria. Lysis *in vivo* is thought to be determined by the continuous activation of the alternative complement pathway, which occurs normally. The PNH red cells pick up small amounts of activated C3, or C3b (normal red cells probably do this also to some extent), and these small amounts are sufficient to bring about the lysis of the sensitive PNH cells, although not causing lysis of normal red cells.

Why haemolysis should increase during sleep, thus explaining the nocturnal haemoglobinuria seen in seriously affected patients, is still not known: it has been attributed to the activation of the alternative pathway

during sleep, but the basis for this is unclear. The acute haemolysis that may complicate infections or follow inoculations, transfusions, or surgical interventions (e.g. splenectomy) also probably depends upon activation of the alternative pathway. Endotoxin derived from the gut seems likely to be an activating factor and to play a part in bringing about local haemolysis (and thrombosis) within the portal and hepatic venous systems.

CLINICAL FINDINGS

The onset of the disease is usually insidious, with gradually increasing weakness and dyspnoea on exertion, accompanied by pallor and perhaps slight jaundice, with or without the intermittent passage of dark urine (haemoglobinuria). In some cases, by contrast, an episode of massive haemoglobinuria may first bring the patient to the doctor. Haemoglobinuria is a striking sign, and as the title paroxysmal nocturnal haemoglobinuria signifies, it is in the urine formed at night and passed first thing in the morning that more haemoglobin tends to be found. Some patients may present simply with anaemia, or with attacks of abdominal pain, in which cases the diagnosis may be delayed considerably. In a minority of patients, rhythmic nocturnal haemoglobinuria persists for many days or weeks; in others, the haemoglobinuria is not obviously or regularly nocturnal. While the haemolysis generally occurs for no apparent cause, a number of factors can increase its severity and lead to intense and prolonged haemoglobinuria. Amongst such exacerbating factors are an infection, even a minor one such as the common cold, a blood transfusion, a surgical procedure, menstruation, exposure to cold, vaccine inoculations, and possibly 'stress'.

The physical signs are not distinctive. There is usually slight to moderate jaundice. The spleen is sometimes palpable a few centimetres below the costal margin and the liver may be slightly enlarged too; it becomes markedly so if intrahepatic venous thrombosis develops. Skin purpura or other evidence of a haemorrhagic tendency may be noticeable in the presence of marked thrombocytopenia.

The urine is red-brown to almost black in colour if it contains haemoglobin, methaemoglobin, or both. A constant finding, even in the absence of free haemoglobin, is haemosiderinuria—the presence in the urine deposit of numerous small granules giving a positive Prussian-blue reaction for free iron. The granules are derived from renal tubular cells that have taken in haemoglobin from the glomerular filtrate and, after the haemoglobin molecule has been broken down, retain the iron derived from haem in the form of haemosiderin. Despite the retention of iron, renal function is usually, although not invariably, well preserved.

Associated symptoms, signs, and complications

Many patients suffer from attacks of abdominal pain. This varies from a feeling of vague discomfort to severe colic or cramp and may be accompanied by vomiting, which may persist for hours. Sometimes the symptoms are experienced when haemolysis is particularly active, but this is not always the case. In a few patients the severity of the pain and doubt as to the diagnosis have led to laparotomy. The pain may result from thrombosis occurring within small veins in the portal system: however, even ultrasound and computerized tomographic scans may fail to document this.

Some patients have suffered from distressing headaches, but this symptom seems to be less common than that of abdominal pain. In a few instances, headache has presaged a cerebral vascular accident.

Venous thrombosis (in addition to causing abdominal pain when small vessels are affected) can lead to serious consequences. Thrombosis and thromboembolism are in fact the most frequent immediate cause of death in PNH. Veins almost anywhere in the body may be involved; particularly serious is major thrombosis within the portal system and intrahepatic venous thrombosis leading to the Budd–Chiari syndrome: in such cases there is sudden marked enlargement of the liver and ascites may develop. The tendency to thrombosis probably results from inappropriate activation of those platelets that are abnormally complement sensitive, although the precise mechanism has not yet been elucidated.

Some patients seem to be unusually susceptible to bacterial infections. This generally correlates with granulocytopenia and there is no clear evidence of defective neutrophil function.

Pigment gallstones may form in patients with PNH and may lead to cholecystitis or obstructive jaundice. This seems to be less common than in other types of haemolytic anaemia, probably because most of the haemoglobin is excreted through the urine.

Iron deficiency

As already mentioned, haemosiderinuria is a constant and persistent finding in PNH, even when the rate of haemolysis is insufficient to result in overt haemoglobinuria. As much as 10 mg of iron may be lost within 24 h in this way. Patients have presented as cases of iron-deficiency anaemia and the fact that there is, too, chronically increased haemolysis may be overlooked. At necropsy, it is characteristic of PNH that, while the kidney is heavily loaded with iron, in all other organs iron is conspicuous by its absence.

ASSOCIATION WITH HYPOPLASIA OF BONE MARROW

Many patients suffering from PNH have a history of pancytopenia and may have been diagnosed originally as suffering from aplastic anaemia. Thus of 80 personally observed patients, aplastic anaemia was the first diagnosis in 23, compared with haemolytic anaemia in 29. In 25 there was insufficient information to be certain as to the mode of onset and, in three patients, PNH had been preceded by myelosclerosis. The cause of the association between PNH and aplastic anaemia is not known for certain.

This association takes several forms:

1. Marrow hypoplasia is present at the onset and then a variable, but significant, degree of recovery of marrow function occurs and 'classical', haemolytic, PNH develops.
2. Marrow hypoplasia is present at the onset, there is no significant recovery of marrow function, tests for PNH become weakly positive, and the patient remains pancytopenic without increased haemolysis being obvious. A variant of this is the increasingly frequent appearance of a PNH clone in patients with aplastic anaemia treated with antilymphocyte globulin.
3. Haemolytic PNH is present at the onset, marrow hypoplasia subsequently develops, with a concomitant decrease in haemolysis: the patient develops frank aplastic anaemia.

In a small number of patients, PNH has been complicated by the development of leukaemia, which has been invariably acute myeloid leukaemia (**AML**). Although few such cases have been reported, PNH and AML are both sufficiently rare for us to suggest that their development in the same patient cannot be a coincidence. Indeed, in two cases it has been shown convincingly that AML has developed from within the PNH clone. Thus, PNH can be regarded as a preleukaemic condition. Fortunately, evolution to AML, which is the rule in chronic myeloid leukaemia, is the exception in PNH. In a few patients, too, PNH has been preceded by myelosclerosis (see above).

COURSE OF THE DISEASE AND CHANCES OF RECOVERY

PNH is a very chronic disorder. The median survival of 80 patients personally observed in London between 1946 and 1971 was 7.5 years. Fifty-five patients are now known to have died; six patients, however, recovered and became clinically well despite continuing weakly positive laboratory tests for PNH, while a further six also recovered both clinically and haematologically (although they tend to remain slightly macrocytic) and eventually gave completely negative laboratory tests for PNH. The longest follow-up, to the best of our knowledge, is a man who, having experienced a spontaneous recovery from PNH, eventually

died of bronchogenic carcinoma 48 years after the initial diagnosis of PNH. Thus an appreciable proportion of PNH patients (perhaps 10–15 per cent) recover completely: a remarkable and encouraging fact taking into account that PNH is a clonal disease of marrow stem cells.

BLOOD PICTURE

The characteristic finding is anaemia, neutropenia, and thrombocytopenia, accompanied by reticulocytosis. The severity of the changes depends upon the proportion of PNH red cells the patient is forming and the degree to which the bone marrow is hypoplastic. In some patients, anaemia is so severe that repeated blood transfusion is necessary; in others it is much less severe and transfusions are seldom if ever required. Reticulocyte counts vary widely from patient to patient and in individual patients from time to time. Thus counts range from less than 1 per cent to about 40 per cent depending upon the severity of haemolysis and the degree to which the marrow is able to respond to the consequent anaemia.

The neutrophil and platelet counts vary widely. Approximately 50 per cent of the patients may be expected to have fewer than $1.5 \times 10^9/l$ neutrophils and/or fewer than $50 \times 10^9/l$ platelets at one time or another. The neutrophils are unusual in that they lack alkaline phosphatase.

The appearance of the blood film is usually not remarkable. The red cells vary slightly to moderately in size and shape; polychromasia reflects the reticulocyte count. The MCV is normal or above normal (especially if the reticulocyte count is raised); the MCH is normal or less than normal when there is iron deficiency. The plasma contains free haemoglobin and is brownish in colour in cases in which haemolysis is active and methaemalbumin is present. Haptoglobins are typically absent. The haemoglobin pattern is typically normal on electrophoresis. However, raised levels of haemoglobin F have been recorded in a few patients.

DIAGNOSIS

A positive diagnosis of PNH depends on demonstrating that a proportion of the patient's red cells are unusually sensitive to lysis by human complement. The 'classic' test is the acidified serum test, often referred to as the Ham test. In this test the red cells to be tested for the abnormality are suspended in fresh normal ABO-compatible serum acidified to a pH of about 6.5. PNH red cells undergo lysis if the suspension is incubated at 37 °C for up to 30 to 60 min, while normal red cells do not. It is a characteristic of PNH that not all the patient's red cells undergo lysis under these circumstances and little or no lysis occurs in unacidified fresh serum at about pH 7.8. PNH red cells are not more sensitive than normal red cells to lysis by acid in the absence of fresh serum. The role of acidification is to activate the alternative complement pathway.

The acidified serum test, if carried out with proper controls, is a sensitive and reliable test for PNH. Subsequent to its introduction, a variety of other tests—the thrombin, sucrose low ionic strength (sugar-water), inulin, cobra venom, and cold antibody lysis tests for example—have been introduced, all similarly depending upon demonstrating the increased sensitivity of the red cells to lysis by complement via the alternative or classical pathway. None of these tests, however, seems to have a clear advantage over the simple acidified serum test. In the last few years, as flow cytometry has become popular, it has been used as a diagnostic aid in PNH, by demonstrating the presence of two cell populations when either red cells or white cells are stained with antibodies having specificity for one of the GPI-linked proteins characteristically lacking from the surface of the abnormal cells.

From the clinical point of view it is important not to forget that PNH is a possible diagnosis in any patient presenting with anaemia of obscure origin, particularly if accompanied by a slight to moderate reticulocytosis, neutropenia, and thrombocytopenia, even if the patient's chief (or only) complaint is of abdominal pain. It is wise to carry out the acidified serum test (or the sucrose test) and to look for haemosiderinuria at an early stage in such a patient's investigation.

TREATMENT

The only definitive treatment for PNH is bone marrow transplantation. In cases in which bone marrow failure has progressed to the stage of qualifying for severe aplastic anaemia, and if an HLA-identical sibling is available, transplantation must be regarded therefore as the treatment of choice. In haemolytic PNH without evidence of severe bone marrow failure, transplantation has been attempted only in a handful of cases in which an identical twin was available and it was carried out without myeloablative and immunosuppressive treatment: this type of marrow transplant has not been successful in these patients.

Therefore, for patients with haemolytic PNH, and for all those who do not have a potential donor, treatment must be supportive. Once the diagnosis is firmly established it is very important to explain to patients that they can live with it, perhaps for many years. Without raising hopes too high, it is fair to mention that adequate support may see them through to spontaneous recovery. Blood transfusion is imperative when exacerbation of haemolysis threatens life, but it should not be scheduled regularly. Rather, the (very variable) tolerance of the individual patient to anaemia should be assessed, as blood transfusion is indicated only when the haemoglobin level falls below the tolerated level.

As in other chronic anaemias, some patients can lead a virtually normal active life with a steady-state haemoglobin level as low as 70 g/l, and in our experience not infrequently patients are overtransfused. It is imperative to use on-line white-cell filters for all transfusions. This precaution has made it clear that the previously reported instances of haemoglobinuria triggered by blood transfusion resulted from white-cell reactions activating complement rather than from an increase in the haematocrit as such. A neglected cause of worsening anaemia is iron deficiency consequent to urinary iron loss. The mean corpuscular haemoglobin concentration (MCHC) and serum iron (rather than ferritin) should be monitored, and iron deficiency corrected with oral iron whenever necessary.

Any patient with PNH who has experienced venous thrombosis, whether peripheral or hepatic, should be placed on prophylactic warfarin for as long as he or she has evidence of the disease, because there is serious risk of recurrence, and venous thrombosis is one of the main causes of death. Although it may be regarded as perfectly rational to introduce warfarin in newly diagnosed patients even before they develop thrombosis, this has not been our policy thus far. For the treatment of hepatic venous thrombosis (Budd-Chiari), there is an immediate indication for thrombolytic therapy with tissue plasminogen activator. To our surprise, this has been effective in some patients even as late as 4 weeks after the onset of symptoms.

Although the haemolysis in PNH is complement mediated, there is no evidence that corticosteroids will decrease the rate of haemolysis, and there is no rationale for their use in PNH.

REFERENCES

Dacie, J.V. and Lewis, S.M. (1972). Paroxysmal nocturnal haemoglobinuria: clinical manifestations, haematology and nature of the disease. *Series Haematologica*, **5**, 3–23.

Hartmann, R.C. and Kolhouse, J.F. (1972). Viewpoints on the management of paroxysmal nocturnal hemoglobinuria (PNH). *Series Haematologica*, **5**, 42–60.

Hillmen, P., Hows, J.M., and Luzzatto, L. (1992). Two distinct patterns of glycosylphosphatidylinositol (GPI) linked protein deficiency in the red cells of patients with paroxysmal nocturnal haemoglobinuria. *British Journal of Haematology*, **80**, 399–405.

Kawahara, K., Witherspoon, R.P., and Storb, R. (1992). Marrow transplantation for paroxysmal nocturnal hemoglobinuria. *American Journal of Hematology*, **39**, 283–8.

Luther, A.B., Jenkins, D.E., Jnr., Tenorio, L.E., and Saba, H.I. (1980). Fulminant hepatic venous thrombosis (Budd-Chiari syndrome) in paroxysmal nocturnal hemoglobinuria: definition of a medical emergency. *Johns Hopkins Medical Journal*, **146**, 247–54.

Rosse, W.F. (1990). Phosphatidylinositol-linked proteins and paroxysmal nocturnal hemoglobinuria. *Blood*, **75**, 1595–601.

Rotoli, B. and Luzzatto, L. (1989). Paroxysmal nocturnal haemoglobinuria. *Baillière's Clinical Haematology*, **2**, 113–38.

22.4 The red cell

22.4.1 Erythropoiesis and the normal red cell

D. J. WEATHERALL

The circulating red cells and their nucleated precursors in the bone marrow comprise a functional unit called the erythron. As an introduction to the disorders of the red cells we shall consider the morphological and biochemical characteristics of erythropoiesis, i.e. the formation of red cells, and what is known about the regulation of the erythron.

Erythropoiesis

In order to appreciate the pathophysiology of anaemia and the complex compensatory mechanisms that are brought into play to maintain oxygenation of the tissues in patients with anaemia it is necessary to have a broad understanding of the way in which red cells are produced and how this is regulated.

THE EARLY STAGES OF ERYTHROPOIESIS

As described in the previous section, the red-cell precursors are derived from pluripotential stem cells by a differentiation step, the regulation and nature of which is still not understood. Recently, different populations of erythroid precursors have been defined which are probably part of the early committed erythroid population but which cannot be recognized as such under the microscope. Using either plasma clots or methyl cellulose as supporting media it has been possible to grow colonies of these erythroid precursors from mononuclear cells derived from human fetal or adult bone marrow or peripheral blood. The first colonies to appear are small and consist of about 8 to 16 cells; they are usually fully developed after a few days of incubation. After a longer period in culture larger colonies or 'bursts' appear that are made up of several thousand cells. The growth of these colonies depends on the presence of erythropoietin in the media. The cells that give rise to the small colonies are called **CFU-E** (colony-forming units, erythroid), and those that produce the 'bursts' are called erythropoietin-dependent burst-forming units, or **BFU-E**. It seems very likely that the CFU-E are the more differentiated of the two and are probably close to proerythroblasts in the differentiation pathway. On the other hand, the BFU-E are probably a much earlier population and are less sensitive to erythropoietin.

Nothing is known about the stimulus for the differentiation of early BFU-E from pluripotential stem cells. They require a factor (or factors) termed 'burst-promoting activity' for *in vitro* growth. Several of these burst-promoting factors have now been defined, including interleukin 3, granulocyte-monocyte colony-stimulating factor, and interleukin 4.

Current ideas about the function and regulation of BFU-E and CFU-E are shown in Fig. 1. It is believed that the BFU-E form an amplification compartment, which can respond to the requirements for erythropoiesis by rapid contraction or expansion. During maturation of the BFU-E their sensitivity to erythropoietin increases; by the time they reach the CFU-E stage they are highly responsive to this hormone. The CFU-E mature directly into pronormoblasts, which are the first cells in the erythroid maturation pathway that can be recognized morphologically.

MORPHOLOGICAL AND BIOCHEMICAL DEVELOPMENT OF THE RED CELL

The total maturation time of the identifiable red-cell precursors in the bone marrow is approximately 7 days. The first 4 days are spent in cell division; approximately 16 daughter cells are produced from each primitive red-cell precursor (Fig. 2). The remaining 3 days are devoted to maturation and haemoglobin synthesis, and during this period the nucleus is extruded. The red-cell precursor, which is now called a reticulocyte, remains in the marrow for a further 24 h and then moves into the peripheral circulation where it matures into a red-cell in approximately 1 day. As about 1 per cent of the total red-cell mass is destroyed every 24 h, in normal individuals there is a comparable number of reticulocytes delivered daily into the circulation.

The earliest recognizable red-cell precursor is the basophilic pronormoblast. This is a large cell with a diameter of about 24 μm. It has a deep-blue staining cytoplasm indicating that there is, as yet, no haemoglobin present. After several cell divisions there are well-marked maturation changes in the nucleus and in the cytoplasm. The next maturation stage is the polychromatophilic normoblast, which has a pink cytoplasm indicating that haemoglobin synthesis has commenced. The nucleus is smaller than that of the pronormoblast and the chromatin is starting to clump. By the fourth maturation division the cells reach the orthochromatic normoblast stage, in which the cytoplasm is uniformly pink and the nuclear chromatin is highly condensed. The nucleus is then lost from the cell, which becomes a reticulocyte, i.e. a cell containing some residual RNA and other organelles that, on supravital staining, clump and produce a characteristic appearance on light microscopy. It is estimated that between 5 and 10 per cent of the red-cell precursors are lost during their passage through the marrow. As we shall see later, in certain disorders of red-cell maturation this level of 'ineffective erythropoiesis' is considerably elevated above the normal baseline.

These morphological changes of red-cell maturation are accompanied by important alterations in the chemistry of the red-cell precursors. The early forms have a well-formed Golgi apparatus and mitochondria. They are capable of DNA, RNA, and protein synthesis, and oxidative metabolism. At the polychromatophilic normoblast phase of development, DNA and RNA synthesis cease. After further maturation the mitochondria and RNA are lost and the cell is then able to metabolize glucose only through the anaerobic Embden–Meyerhof pathway. In addition, the mature cell has a hexose monophosphate shunt that normally provides little energy but is of great importance in protecting the cell against oxidative damage. At first sight this seems to be a very simple and unsophisticated biochemical factory with which to go out into the turbulent world of the peripheral circulation. But as we shall see later it is beautifully suited to the needs of a cell that has to traverse a microcirculation and deal with the metabolically unfavourable environment of the circulation and, particularly, the spleen.

Regulation of erythropoiesis

It has been known for many years that the main stimulus to erythropoiesis is the degree of oxygenation of the tissues. It is now clear that information on the level of tissue oxygenation is transferred to the blood-forming organs by the action of a hormone called erythropoietin, which is capable of stimulating erythropoiesis. Thus, if the haemoglobin level falls or if the oxygen supply to the tissues is reduced in other ways, there is an increased production of erythropoietin, which stimulates the bone marrow to increase the output of red cells until oxygen delivery is restored to normal. This is an elegant example of a biological feedback loop (Fig. 3).

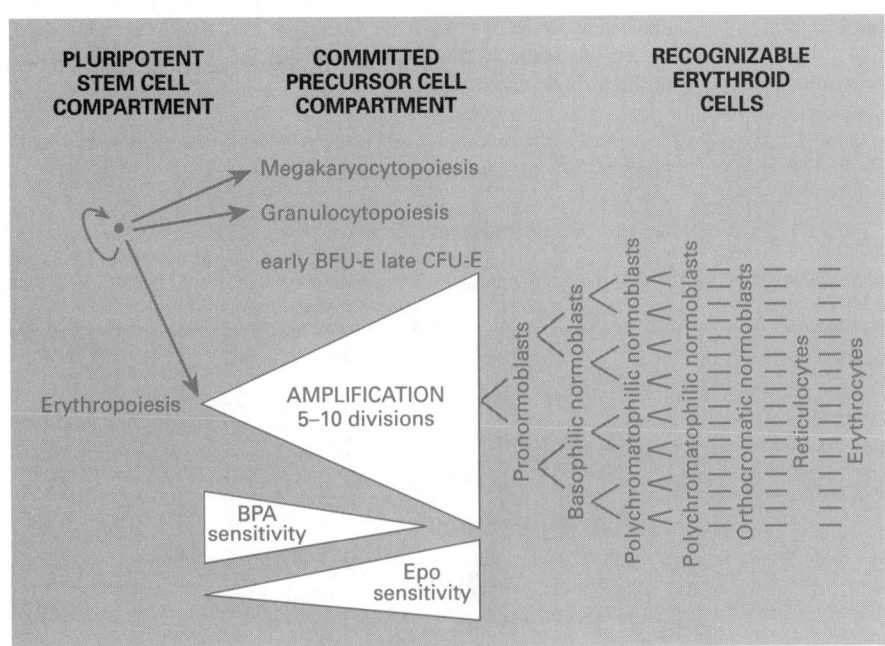

Fig. 1 Schematic representation of the various levels of erythropoiesis. (BPA = burst-promoting activity; Epo = erythropoietin). The details of the different compartments are described in the text.

Erythropoietin is a glycoprotein that is encoded by a gene on the long arm of chromosome 7. Its receptor is encoded by a gene that is on the short arm of chromosome 19. It is produced in response to hypoxia by fibroblasts that lie in the interstitium between the renal tubules. In fetal life it appears to be produced mainly in the liver. During the transition from BFU-E to CFU-E the red-cell progenitors become increasingly sensitive to erythropoietin and it is now considered to be the major physiological regulator of red-cell production. The sequences in the erythropoietin gene that are involved in oxygen sensing have been defined, although the precise mechanism whereby erythropoietin-producing cells respond to hypoxia remains to be determined, as does the way in which the hormone stimulates erythropoiesis. Although other hormones and mediators affect red-cell production, including corticosteroids, androgens, growth hormone, thyroxine, β-adrenergic agonists, cyclic AMP, and so on, these agents seem only to add some fine tuning to the rate of production.

The fact that erythropoiesis is regulated by a hormone produced by the kidney has important clinical implications. For example, the anaemia of renal disease is at least in part due to defective production of erythropoietin. Some renal tumours synthesize erythropoietin and cause polycythaemia. Severe hypoxia, as occurs in chronic lung disease or congenital heart disease, is associated with a marked drive to erythropoietin production and hence a variable increase in red-cell output. Further examples of the clinical importance of erythropoietin will be considered in later sections.

THE FACTORS REQUIRED FOR NORMAL ERYTHROPOIESIS

There are several factors that are essential for the normal function of the bone marrow. Iron is required for haemoglobin synthesis and also seems to have a direct effect on the regulation of erythroid proliferation. Vitamin B_{12} and folate are required for normal DNA synthesis and hence for nuclear maturation. A detailed account of the metabolism of iron, vitamin B_{12}, and folate is given later in this section. It has been suggested that certain other vitamins including pyridoxine, ascorbic acid, riboflavin, and vitamin E are essential for erythropoiesis in man, but it has been difficult to provide good evidence that this is the case. Similarly, certain trace elements such as copper, manganese, cobalt, and zinc may also be required; animals deprived of these metals show abnormalities of erythropoiesis. However, the relevance of these observations to human disease is not clear.

The red cell

The mature red cell is a biconcave disc, 7.5 μm in diameter, 2.5 μm thick at the periphery, and 1 μm thick at the centre. This shape provides an optimal surface area for respiratory exchange. The cell is composed of about 70 per cent water, the remainder consisting of haemoglobin and small amounts of lipid, sugar, and enzyme proteins.

The red cell has two main functions. First, it must maintain itself in the circulation for about 120 days. Second, it must maintain its haemoglobin in a state suitable for oxygen transport during this time. In describing the functions of the red cell we have to consider separately its three major components, membrane, haemoglobin, and metabolic pathways. However, it is important to appreciate that each of these is dependent on the others and can interact to modulate oxygen transport, protect haemoglobin from oxidant damage, and maintain the constancy of the osmotic environment of the cell.

Fig. 2 Erythropoiesis. (a) A schematic representation of the main steps involved in the maturation of red cells. (Reproduced by permission of Dr A. Erslev.) (b) The relationship between morphological differentiation and biochemical differentiation.

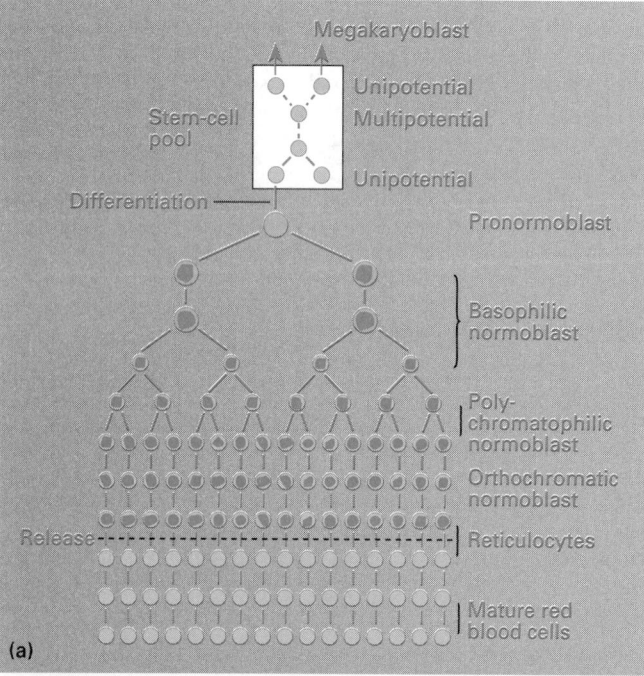

(a)

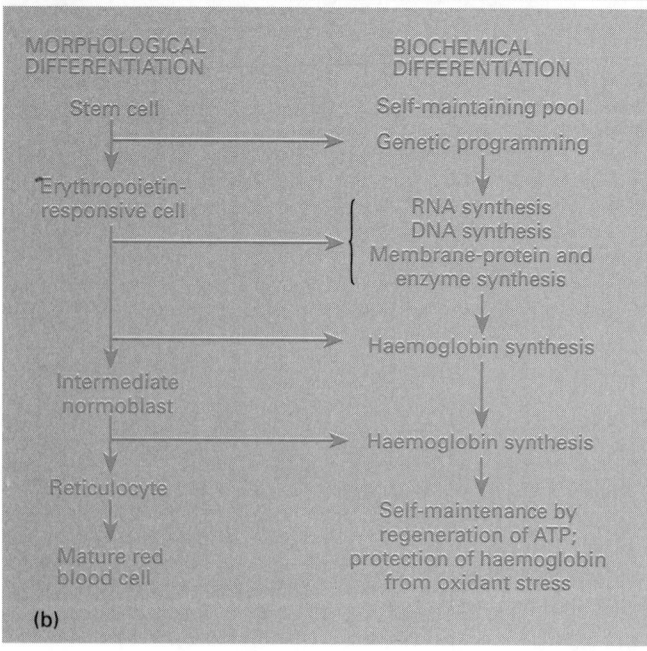

(b)

Fig. 3 The regulation of red cell production.

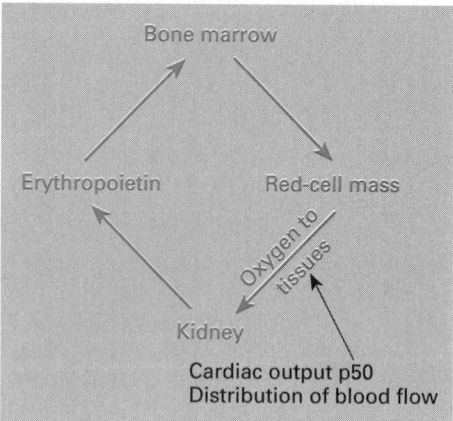

MEMBRANE (SEE ALSO CHAPTER 22.4.10)

A diagram of the structure of the red-cell membrane is shown in Fig. 4. It is composed of lipids, carbohydrates, and protein. Essentially, it consists of a lipid bilayer with intercollated proteins and glycoproteins. The carbohydrates are mainly glycolipids and glycoproteins. The mature red cell does not synthesize lipids *de novo*, and several lipid components, particularly cholesterol, exchange with lipids in the plasma. There are two main classes of membrane proteins, the peripheral proteins and the integral membrane proteins. The former make up an extensive submembranous reticulum called the red-cell cytoskeleton, which is responsible for the shape, integrity, and flexibility of the cell membrane. The basic building block of the cytoskeleton is the spectrin tetramer. The integral membrane proteins consist of an anion transport protein, a glucose transport protein and the sialoglycoproteins, glycophorins A, B, and C. The anion transport protein is the predominant integral protein and makes

Fig. 4 Diagram of the red-cell membrane showing the relation of integral and internal membrane proteins to the lipid bilayer. The numbers refer to individual membrane proteins. GPA and GPB are glycophorins A and B; PC, phosphatidylcholine; SM, sphingomyelin; PS, phosphatidylserine; PE, phosphatidylethanolamine. (Reproduced with permission from Brain, M.C. (1982). *Blood and its disorders*, (2nd edn) (ed. R.M. Hardisty and D.J. Weatherall), p. 45. Blackwell Scientific, Oxford.)

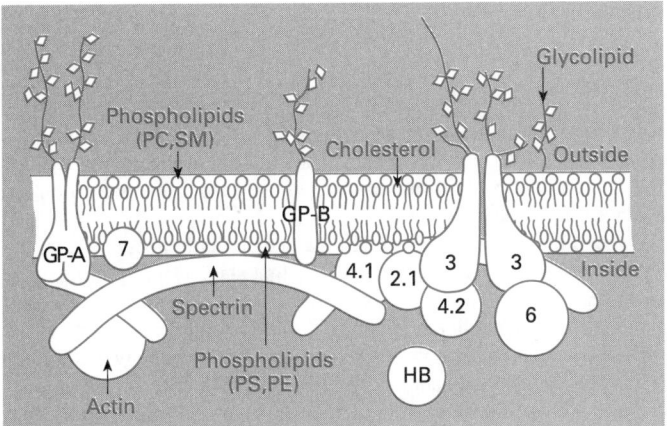

up 25 per cent of the membrane protein, which is equivalent to 1.2×10^6 copies per red cell. It is involved in the transport of HCO_3^- and Cl^-. The membrane also has a variety of transport systems, including Na^+, K^+-ATPase, which is involved in the transport of Na^+ out of and K^+ into the cell, Ca^{2+}, Mg^{2+}-ATPase, and acetyl cholinesterase. These membrane pumps are of critical importance for maintaining electrolyte homeostasis in the red cell. Sodium is actively pumped from the cell against a concentration gradient of 10 mEq/l inside the cell to 145 mEq/l in the plasma. Potassium, on the other hand, is pumped into the cell against a concentration gradient of about 4.5 mEq/l in the plasma to 100 mEq/l in the cell. The calcium/magnesium pump mediates calcium efflux against a 50- to 100-fold concentration gradient, converting one molecule of ATP to ADP for each two molecules of Ca^{2+} extruded. The membrane also has several protein kinases.

The critical functions of the red cell of maintaining its shape and deformability are mediated by these different components of its membrane. Considerable amounts of energy are required for the pumping activities needed to maintain the constancy of the electrolyte environment of the red cell. These functions can be modulated by hormones, cyclic nucleotides, calcium, and calmodulin. In later sections we shall see how primary or secondary abnormalities of the membrane lead to changes in function and hence to premature destruction of red cells.

HAEMOGLOBIN

The major haemoglobin of adult red cells, haemoglobin A, is a tetramer of two α- and two β-chains consisting of 141 and 146 amino acids, respectively. The heterogeneity and genetic control of haemoglobin is considered in Chapter 22.4.7. Each globin chain is attached to a haem molecule, a protoporphyrin ring that contains an iron atom and can reversibly bind oxygen. The oxygen binding of whole blood (Fig. 5) is ideally suited for oxygen transport. The sigmoid shape of the curve, which reflects the allosteric properties of haemoglobin, is beautifully adapted to oxygen transport. At relatively high oxygen tensions in the lungs, oxygen is rapidly taken up and it can be released readily at tensions encountered in the tissues. The curve is quite different from that of myoglobin, a molecule that consists of a single globin chain with haem attached to it, and which has a hyperbolic oxygen dissociation curve. It has been realized for many years that the transition from a

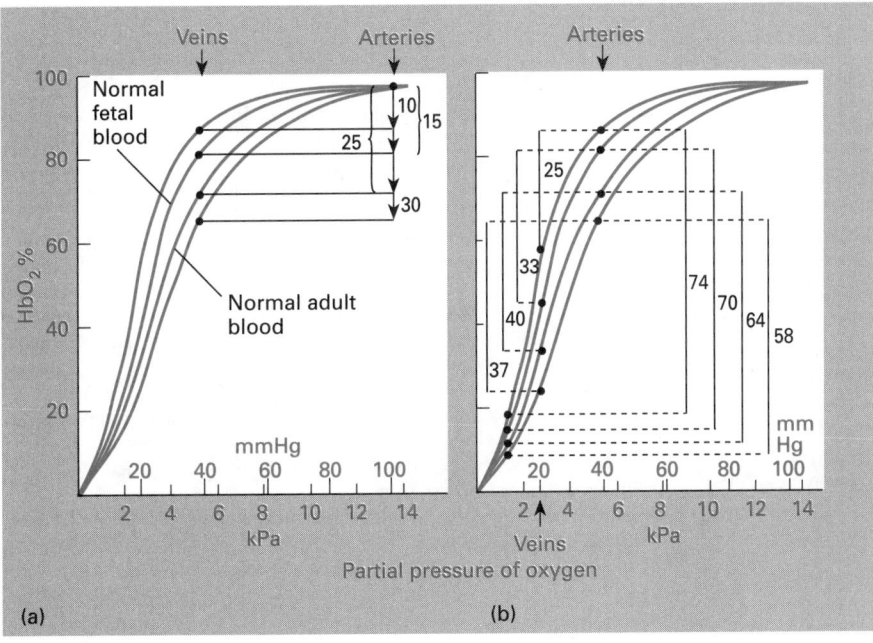

(a) (b)

Fig. 5 Oxygen dissociation curves of human blood. (a) The curves for normal adult and fetal blood and the effect of changing the oxygen affinity with normal partial pressures of oxygen in the arteries and veins, Pa_{O_2} and Pv_{O_2}. It is clear that lowering the oxygen affinity releases more oxygen to the tissues. (b) Effect of changing the oxygen affinity when there is a very low arterial P_{O_2} (40 mmHg). It is clear that if mean venous P_{O_2} is about 20 mmHg, lowering the oxygen affinity increases release. In contrast, with a low mean venous P_{O_2} less oxygen is released to the tissue as the curve shifts to the right. (Reproduced with permission from Huehns, E.R. (1982). *Blood and its disorders* (2nd edn) (ed. R. M. Hardisty and D. J. Weatherall), p. 333. Blackwell Scientific, Oxford.)

hyperbolic to a sigmoid curve must reflect cooperativity between the haem molecules. The molecular basis for this haem/haem interaction is now understood. When one haem molecule takes on oxygen the affinity for oxygen of the remaining haems of the tetramer increases markedly. This is because haemoglobin can exist in two configurations, deoxy (T) and oxy (R) (T and R stand for tight and relaxed states, respectively). The T form has a lower affinity than the R form for ligands such as oxygen. At some point during the sequential addition of oxygen to the four haems transition from the T to R configuration occurs; at this point the oxygen affinity of the partially liganded molecule increases dramatically. These allosteric changes involve a series of interactions between the iron of the haem groups and various bonds within the molecule that lead to subtle spatial alterations as oxygen is taken on and given up. We shall consider the clinical implications of haem/haem interaction later in this section.

The position of the oxygen dissociation curve can be modified in several ways. First, oxygen affinity is decreased with increasing CO_2 tensions. This phenomenon, which is largely pH dependent, is called the Bohr effect. It facilitates oxygen unloading at tissue levels, where a drop in pH due to CO_2 influx lowers oxygen affinity. In contrast, in the lungs efflux of CO_2 and increase in intracellular pH increases oxygen affinity, and hence uptake. Carbon dioxide influences haemoglobin in two ways. First, diffusion of CO_2 into the red cells, where carbonic anhydrase produces carbonic acid, decreases the pH, hence lowering the oxygen affinity by the Bohr effect. Second, by combining with the terminal amino-acid groups to form carbamino compounds, CO_2 further lowers oxygen affinity.

The position of the oxygen dissociation curve is modified by factors other than pH and CO_2. For example, another important constituent of the red cell that can modify oxygen transport is 2,3-diphosphoglycerate (**2,3-DPG**). Increasing concentrations of 2,3-DPG shift the oxygen dissociation curve to the right, that is, cause a state of reduced oxygen affinity, while diminishing concentrations have the opposite effect. 2,3-DPG fits into the gap between the two β-chains of haemoglobin when this becomes widened during deoxygenation, and interacts with several specific binding sites in the central cavity of the molecule. However, in the oxy configuration the gap between the two β-chains narrows and the molecule cannot be accommodated. It follows that, with increasing concentrations of 2,3-DPG, more haemoglobin molecules tend to be held in the deoxy configuration and the oxygen dissociation curve is therefore shifted to the right.

Thus it is apparent that the red cell has a remarkable facility for adaptation to different requirements for oxygen transport. In the next chapter we shall consider how these various adaptive mechanisms are utilized to facilitate oxygen transport in various disease states.

RED-CELL METABOLISM

The mature red cell has no nucleus or mitochondria and no tricarboxylic acid cycle. Hence the major source of energy is the glycolytic Embden–Meyerhof pathway. Glucose is metabolized via this pathway with the production of lactate, with a net gain of 2 mol of ATP and the reduction of 2 mol of NAD to NADH per mol of glucose. The other energy pathway is the hexose monophosphate shunt in which there is a reduction of 2 mol of NADP to NADPH per mol of glucose. In addition there is a 'metabolic siding' in the Embden–Meyerhof pathway that is regulated by diphosphoglycerate mutase and generates 2,3 DPG.

The metabolic functions of the red cell can be summarized as follows. First, it must maintain its osmotic stability through the activity of its membrane pumps. This critical transport function is driven by ATP. Second, it must maintain the iron of haemoglobin in the reduced state, by reducing Fe^{3+} to Fe^{2+}. The enzyme system involved, methaemo-

globin reductase, is driven by NADH. Third, 2,3-DPG must be generated to act as a modulator of haemoglobin function (see below). Fourth, the sulphydryl groups of haemoglobin and membrane proteins must be protected by maintaining adequate amounts of reduced glutathione. This system is dependent on NADPH generated from NADP via the pentose pathway. Finally, NAD must be synthesized from nicotinic acid, glutamine, glucose, and inorganic phosphate, and NADP formed by the reaction of NAD and ADP. As we shall see in a later section, a breakdown of any of these critical metabolic functions causes shortening of the red-cell survival and/or abnormal oxygen transport.

THE LIFESPAN OF RED CELLS

The lifespan of red cells, normally about 120 days, can be assessed by several methods. These include the use of antigenically recognizable cells by the Ashby technique, cohort labelling of newly produced red cells, or labelling of a sample of circulating cells with ^{51}Cr or $DF^{32}P$ (radiolabelled diisopropylfluorophosphate). In clinical practice, ^{51}Cr labelling of blood samples is the most convenient technique. Elution of label from red cells in the circulation causes an exponential decay of radioactivity. Correction for elution may be made, but the more usual method is to express the results in terms of half-life ($t_{1/2}$) of the label in circulation. The normal $t_{1/2}$ of ^{51}Cr-labelled cells is 25 to 36 days. By the use of suitable external counters it is possible to determine the sites of red-cell destruction.

RED-CELL DESTRUCTION AND THE FATE OF HAEMOGLOBIN

In health, erythrocytes are phagocytosed by the reticuloendothelial cells of the spleen, liver, and elsewhere. The changes of the ageing red cell that allow them to be identified and removed from the circulation are still not fully understood.

Once in reticuloendothelial cells, the haemoglobin liberated from the phagocytosed red cells is degraded. The first stage is the splitting up of haem and globin. The iron is split off from the haem molecule and reutilized for haemoglobin synthesis. Similarly, the globin fraction is broken down and the amino acids reutilized. Haem is converted to biliverdin by the enzyme haem oxygenase. One molecule of carbon monoxide is produced with each biliverdin molecule. The subsequent degradation of biliverdin via the action of biliverdin reductase, and the chemistry of the production and excretion of bilirubin is considered in detail in Section 14.

REFERENCES

Bull, B.S. (1994). Morphology of the erythron. In *Williams hematology* (ed. E. Beutler, M.A. Lichtman, B.S. Coller, and T.J. Kipps). McGraw-Hill, New York (in press).

Eaves, A.C. and Eaves, C.J. (1984). Erythropoiesis in culture. *Clinics in Haematology*, **13**, 371–91.

Erslev, A.J. (1994). Production and destruction of erythrocytes. In *Williams hematology*, (ed. E. Beutler, M.A. Lichtman, B.S. Coller, and T.J. Kipps). McGraw-Hill, New York (in press).

Krantz, S.B. (1991). Erythropoietin. *Blood*, **77**, 419–34.

Lajtha, L.G. (1979). Haemopoietic stem cells; concepts and definitions. *Blood Cells*, **5**, 477–91.

Metcalf, D. (1989). Haemopoietic growth factors 1. *Lancet*, **i**, 825–7.

Metcalf, D. (1989). Haemopoietic growth factors 2: clinical applications. *Lancet*, **i**, 885–7.

Testa, N.G. and Molineux, G. (1993). *Haemopoiesis: a practical approach*. IRL Press/Oxford University Press.

Wright, E.G. and Lord, B.I. (1992). Haemopoietic tissue. *Baillière's Clinical Haematology*, **5**, 499–507.

22.4.2 Anaemia: pathophysiology, classification, and clinical features

D. J. WEATHERALL

The main function of the red blood cells is oxygen transport. Hence a functional definition of anaemia is a state in which the circulating red-cell mass is insufficient to meet the oxygen requirements of the tissues. However, there are many compensatory mechanisms that can be brought into play to restore the oxygen supply to the vital centres, and therefore in clinical practice this definition is of limited value. For this reason anaemia is usually defined as a reduction of the haemoglobin concentration, red-cell count or packed cell volume (**PCV**) to below normal levels.

The definition of anaemia

It has been extremely difficult to establish a normal range of haematological values, and hence the definition of anaemia usually involves the adoption of rather arbitrary criteria. For example, the World Health Organization recommends that anaemia should be considered to exist in adults whose haemoglobin levels are lower than 13 g/dl (males) or 12 g/dl (females). Children aged 6 months to 6 years are considered anaemic at haemoglobin levels below 11 g/dl and those aged 6 to 14 years below 12 g/dl. The disadvantage of such arbitrary criteria for defining anaemia is that there may be many apparently normal individuals whose haemoglobin concentration is below their optimal level. Furthermore, the published 'normal values' for adults (see Chapter 22.1) indicate that there is such a large standard deviation that many adult females must be considered 'normal' even though they have haemoglobin levels below 12 g/dl.

Prevalence of anaemia

Anaemia is a major world health problem and its distribution and prevalence in the developing world are considered in detail in the next chapter.

The prevalence of anaemia has been studied in many populations but it is difficult to compare data from different sources because of variations in methodology and criteria. Certain patterns emerge, however. An early survey carried out in Great Britain established that haemoglobin levels were low in a significant proportion of the population, particularly susceptible groups being children under the age of 5 years, pregnant women, and those in social classes IV and V. A later random population study in the United Kingdom reported a prevalence of anaemia of 14 per cent for women aged 55 to 64 years and 3 per cent for men aged 35 to 64 years. These and similar studies have shown that anaemia is most common in women between the ages of 15 and 44 years and that it then becomes relatively less frequent, although the prevalence increases again in the 75-and-over age group. Interestingly, it is only in the latter group that the prevalence in males and females is almost the same. Where the cause of the anaemia has been analysed in these surveys, the majority of cases have been due to iron deficiency. No doubt these prevalence data vary considerably between the developed countries, but it is clear that nutritional anaemia is relatively common in most populations at certain periods during development and late in life.

Adaptation to anaemia

The function of the red cell is to carry oxygen between the lungs and the tissues. However, tissue oxygenation is the result of a complex series of interactions of different organ systems of which the red cell is only one (Table 1). Obviously the cardiac output, ventilatory function, and state of the capillaries are of great importance as well. Each of these

Table 1 *The steps involved in the transport of oxygen to the tissues*

Steps	Factors involved
Ambient O_2 tension	Altitude
Ventilation	Alveolar ventilation
	Gas to blood diffusion
	Ventilation/perfusion ratio
	Anatomical shunt
Circulation	Cardiac output
	Blood: haemoglobin concentration
	oxygen dissociation curve
Tissue diffusion	Intercapillary distance

oxygen supply systems is regulated differently. Ventilation responds to changes in pH, CO_2, and hypoxia. Cardiac output responds to the amount of blood entering the heart and this is regulated mainly by the effects of tissue metabolism as it modifies the resistance to blood flow in the microvasculature. The erythron itself responds to changes in haemoglobin concentration, arterial oxygen saturation, and to the oxygen affinity of the circulating haemoglobin. Thus a decreased capacity of any of these components may be compensated for by increased activity of the others in an attempt to maintain tissue oxygenation.

Oxygen diffuses across the alveolar membrane and into the blood, which equilibrates with the alveolar gas; the approximate oxygen tension is 100 mmHg, at which the blood is fully saturated with an oxygen content of 20 vols per cent. As blood is pumped through the tissue capillaries oxygen diffuses out. Although the venous oxygen tension varies between organs, the oxygen tension of the pooled venous blood in the pulmonary artery, the 'mixed venous oxygen tension', is remarkably constant at 40 mmHg. At this oxygen tension the oxygen content is 15 vols per cent. Hence, oxygen delivery as measured by the arteriovenous oxygen difference is normally 5 vols per cent. By reducing the oxygen-carrying capacity of blood, anaemia tends to reduce the arterial–venous oxygen difference and this may be compensated for by the following mechanisms: (a) modulation of oxygen affinity; (b) redistribution of flow between different organs; (c) increase in cardiac output; and (d) reduction of mixed venous oxygen tension to increase the arteriovenous oxygen difference.

INTRINSIC RED-CELL ADAPTATION

The consequences of anaemia on the normal oxygen-binding curve of blood are shown in Fig. 1. Anaemia, by lowering the haemoglobin concentration, reduces proportionately the oxygen-carrying capacity of the blood. As a response to this there is an increase in 2,3-diphosphoglycerate (**2,3-DPG**) concentration in the red cell, shifting the dissociation curve to the right, so significantly enhancing tissue oxygen delivery (Fig. 1).

With increasing severity of anaemia there is a progressive increase in 2,3-DPG, which may increase oxygen delivery by as much as 40 per cent for the same haemoglobin concentration. It should be noted, however, that a consequence of this adaptation is a lower venous oxygen content and hence a lower reserve of oxygen available for further increase in oxygen demand, as might occur on exercise for example. Hence the increase in 2,3-DPG in anaemia tends to ameliorate the effects of diminished oxygen carrying capacity of the blood, so reducing the adaptation required by other steps involved in tissue oxygen delivery (Fig. 2). 2,3-DPG levels vary in a variety of other clinical conditions; some of these are summarized in Table 2.

LOCAL CHANGES IN TISSUE PERFUSION

The total blood volume does not change greatly in anaemia and therefore increased tissue perfusion has to be achieved by shunting of blood from less to more vital organs. There is vasoconstriction of the vessels of the skin and kidney; this mechanism has little effect on renal function. The organs that gain from the redistribution seem to be mainly the myocardium, brain, and muscle.

CARDIOVASCULAR CHANGES

It seems likely that mild anaemia is compensated by shifts in the oxygen dissociation curve. Overall, oxygen consumption is unchanged in anaemia. However, when the haemoglobin level falls below 7 to 8 g/dl, there is an increase in cardiac output, both at rest and after exercise (Fig. 2). There is an increase in the stroke rate, and a hyperkinetic circulation develops characterized by tachycardia, arterial and capillary pulsation, a wide pulse pressure, and haemic murmurs. The circulation time is

Fig. 1 Enhancement of oxygen loading by decreased red-cell oxygen affinity in a patient with anaemia. An anaemic patient with 50 per cent reduction in haemoglobin concentration has only a 27 per cent reduction in oxygen unloading. (Based on Klocke, R.A. (1972). *Chest*, **69**, 795.)

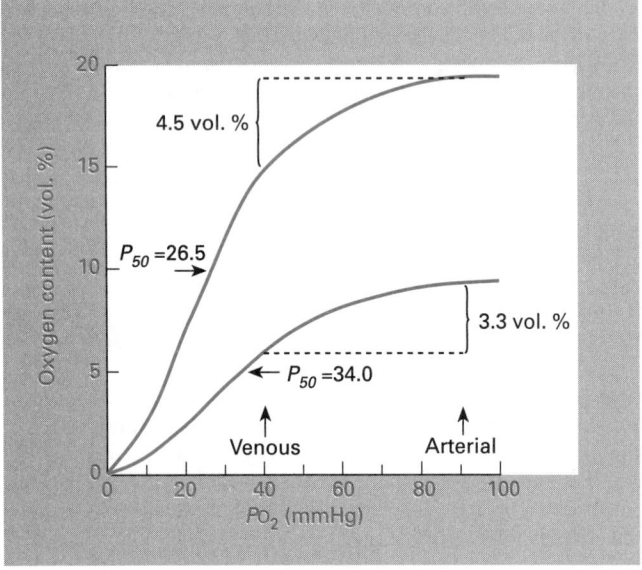

Fig. 2 The changes in factors involved in oxygen delivery with progressive anaemia. As anaemia becomes more severe, cardiac compensation becomes more significant ($p\text{v}O_2$, mixed venous oxygen tension). (From Bellingham (1974).)

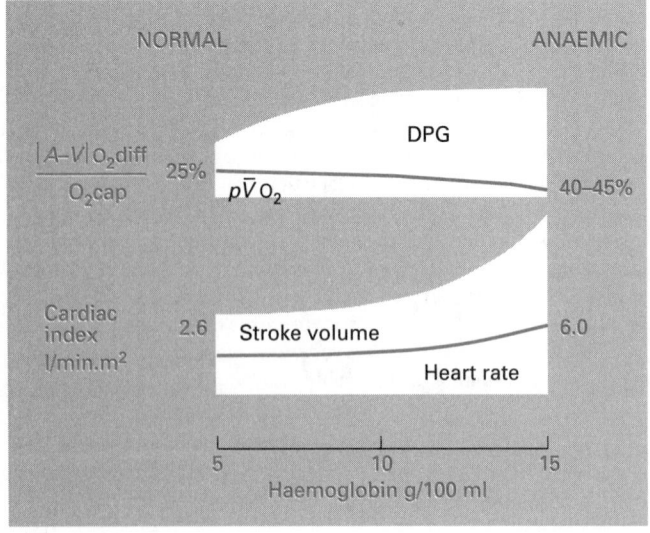

Table 2 *Some conditions in which there is a change in red-cell 2,3-diphosphoglycerate (DPG) levels leading to modification of oxygen transport*

Increased 2,3-DPG; increased P_{50}, reduced whole-blood oxygen affinity
Anaemia
Alkalosis
Hyperphosphataemia
Renal failure
Hypoxia
Pregnancy
Cyanotic congenital heart disease
Thyrotoxicosis
Some red-cell enzyme deficiencies
Decreased 2,3-DPG; decreased P_{50}, increased whole-blood oxygen affinity
Acidosis
Cardiogenic or septicaemic shock
Hypophosphataemia
Hypothyroidism
Hypopituitarism
Following replacement with stored blood

shortened, left ventricular stroke work is increased, and coronary flow increased in proportion to the increased cardiac output. It has been found that there is an acute reversal of the high-output state of chronic anaemia in response to orthostatic stress or pressor amines. This suggests that redistribution of blood volume and vasodilatation with reduced afterload play a dominant role in the hyperkinetic circulatory responses to chronic anaemia. The mechanism of the vasodilatation is not known; it may be a direct result of tissue hypoxia. An additional factor that may be of some importance in increasing cardiac output is the reduction in blood viscosity produced by a relatively low red-cell mass.

While the normal myocardium may tolerate sustained hyperactivity of this type indefinitely, patients with coronary artery disease or those with extreme anaemia may have impaired oxygenation of the myocardium. In such cases, cardiomegaly, pulmonary oedema, ascites, and peripheral oedema may occur, and a state of high-output cardiac failure is established. At this stage the plasma volume is almost always increased.

PULMONARY FUNCTION

As blood, regardless of its oxygen-carrying capacity, is almost completely oxygenated in the lungs, the oxygen pressure of arterial blood in an anaemic patient should be the same as that in a normal individual, and hence an increase in respiratory rate should not improve the oxygenation of the tissues. Curiously, however, severe anaemia is associated with dyspnoea. Although in some patients this may be related to incipient cardiac failure, in most cases it appears to be an inappropriate response to hypoxia which is centrally mediated.

Clinical manifestations and classification of anaemia

CLINICAL EFFECTS OF ANAEMIA

Because anaemia reduces tissue oxygenation it is not surprising that it is associated with widespread organ dysfunction and hence an extremely varied clinical picture. The picture depends, of course, on whether the anaemia is of rapid or more insidious onset.

After acute blood loss the red-cell mass and plasma volume are reduced proportionately and the symptoms are mainly of volume depletion. Depending on the amount of fluid replacement there may be a small fall in the PCV during the first 10 h; volume replacement by the influx of albumin from the extravascular compartment takes between 60 and

90 h. Hence the picture of rapid blood loss is characterized by the typical syndrome of shock, with collapse, dyspnoea, tachycardia, a poor volume pulse, reduced blood pressure, and marked peripheral vasoconstriction.

With anaemia of more insidious onset, the compensatory mechanisms outlined above have time to come into play. In mild anaemia there may be no symptoms or simply increased fatigue and slight pallor. As the anaemia becomes more marked the symptoms and signs gradually appear. Pallor is best discerned in the mucous membranes; the nail beds and palmar creases, although often said to be useful sites for detecting anaemia, are relatively insensitive for this purpose. Cardiorespiratory symptoms and signs include exertional dyspnoea, tachycardia, palpitations, angina or claudication, night cramps, increased arterial pulsation, capillary pulsation, a variety of cardiac bruits, reversible cardiac enlargement, and, if cardiac failure occurs, basal crepitations, peripheral oedema, and ascites. Neuromuscular involvement is reflected by headache, vertigo, lightheadedness, faintness, tinnitus, roaring in the ears, cramps, increased cold sensitivity, and haemorrhages in the retina. Acute anaemia may occasionally give rise to papilloedema. Gastrointestinal symptoms include loss of appetite, nausea, constipation and diarrhoea. Genitourinary involvement causes menstrual irregularities, urinary frequency, and loss of libido. There may be a low-grade fever.

In the elderly, in whom associated degenerative arterial disease is common, anaemia may present with the onset of cardiac failure. Alternatively, previously undiagnosed coronary narrowing may be unmasked by the onset of angina. Other symptoms of arterial degenerative disease may be also exacerbated or unmasked; intermittent claudication and a variety of neurological pictures associated with cerebral arteriosclerosis for example. It is important that anaemia is recognized as a contributing factor to the symptoms of these degenerative diseases as its correction may frequently bring about considerable symptomatic improvement.

CAUSES AND CLASSIFICATION OF ANAEMIA

A reduction in the red-cell mass can result from either defective production of red cells or an increased rate of loss of cells, either by premature destruction or bleeding. Decreased production of red cells may result from a reduced rate of proliferation of precursors in the bone marrow or from failure of maturation leading to their intramedullary destruction, i.e. ineffective erythropoiesis. Based on this approach we can derive a very simple pathophysiological classification of anaemia as shown in Table 3 in which the causes are divided into failure of red-cell proliferation, defective maturation, haemolysis, and blood loss.

Anaemia due to defective proliferation of red-cell precursors

The major causes of this group of anaemias are an inadequate supply of iron, primary diseases of the bone marrow that involve stem cells or later erythroid precursors, or a reduction in the amount of erythropoietin reaching the red-cell precursors (Table 4).

Iron deficiency results in defective erythroid proliferation and also in abnormal maturation of the red-cell precursors due to defective haemoglobin synthesis. Red-cell precursors require adequate iron supplies for normal proliferation, and the anaemia of iron deficiency tends to be hypoproliferative as well as dyserythropoietic. Chronic inflammatory disorders and related conditions also interfere with the iron supply to precursors, probably by blocking the release of catabolized red-cell iron from reticuloendothelial cells. The basic defect in iron-deficiency anaemia and that due to inflammation is similar, therefore, in that the supply of iron is inadequate to meet the requirements for erythropoiesis.

Defective proliferation of red-cell precursors can result from any of the causes of bone marrow failure including infiltration with leukaemic or other neoplastic cells, damage due to ionizing radiation, drugs, or infection, and various intrinsic lesions of the stem cells or red-cell precursors. The intrinsic disorders include the congenital hypoplastic anaemias, involving either all the formed elements or the red-cell precursors alone.

Finally, decreased proliferation of the red-cell precursors may result

Table 3 *The main groups of anaemias classified according to the underlying cause*

Reduced red-cell production:
Defective precursor proliferation
Defective precursor maturation
Defective proliferation and maturation
Increased rate of red-cell destruction:
Haemolysis
Loss of red cells from the circulation:
Bleeding

Table 4 *Main causes of anaemia due to defective production of red cells*

Reduced proliferation of precursors
Iron deficiency anaemia
Anaemia of chronic disorders:
Infections, malignancy, collagen disease, etc
Reduced erythropoietin production:
Renal disease
Reduced oxygen requirements:
Hypothyroidism
Hypopituitarism
Reduced O_2 affinity of haemoglobin
Primary disease of the bone marrow:
Aplastic anaemia:
primary
secondary to drugs, irradiation, chemicals, toxins, etc.
Pure red-cell hypoplasia
Infiltrative disorders:
leukaemia
lymphoma
secondary carcinoma
myelofibrosis
Defective maturation of precursors
Nuclear maturation:
Vitamin B_{12} deficiency
Folate deficiency
Erythroleukaemia
Cytoplasmic maturation:
Iron deficiency
Disorders of globin synthesis
Disorders of haem and/or iron metabolism
Disorders of porphyrin metabolism
Unknown mechanism:
Congenital dyserythropoietic anaemias
Myelodysplastic syndrome
Infection
Toxins and chemicals

from erythropoietin deficiency. The most common cause is chronic renal failure. A similar mechanism may be involved in conditions in which the tissue requirement for oxygen is reduced. These include various endocrine disorders such as hypothyroidism and hypopituitarism. It may also explain the mild anaemia associated with haemoglobin variants with decreased oxygen affinity.

As a group, the hypoproliferative anaemias are associated with a low reticulocyte count and defective proliferation of the bone marrow precursors. The red cells are usually normochromic and normocytic, although there may be a mild macrocytosis. If the anaemia is due to iron deficiency, the cells are hypochromic. If granulopoiesis is normal, the defect in red-cell proliferation is reflected by an increase in the myeloid:erythroid (**M/E**) ratio.

Defective red-cell maturation

Defects of red-cell maturation may involve primarily nuclear or cytoplasmic maturation (Table 4). Those involving nuclear maturation include vitamin B_{12} and folic acid deficiency and other causes of megaloblastic anaemia, and some of the primary marrow disorders including erythroleukaemia. The important causes of defective cytoplasmic maturation include the inherited disorders of globin synthesis, the thalassaemia syndromes, and the genetic and acquired defects of iron metabolism that characterize the sideroblastic anaemias. There are other genetic defects of red-cell maturation, the congenital dyserythropoietic anaemias, in which the aetiology is unknown. Furthermore, agents such as drugs, chemicals, and infections may interfere with erythroid maturation.

The main pathological mechanism common to all the anaemias that result from maturation abnormalities is ineffective erythropoiesis. In other words, there is marked erythroid proliferation but many of the precursors are destroyed in the bone marrow before they enter the circulation. Hence, the characteristic finding is marked erythroid hyperplasia with a reduction in the M/E ratio, associated with a low reticulocyte count. Because of the significant intramedullary destruction of precursors there is usually an elevated level of bilirubin and lactate dehydrogenase. Furthermore, there are nearly always morphological abnormalities of the red-cell precursors. The anaemias that are associated with abnormal nuclear maturation, such as those due to vitamin B_{12} and folic acid deficiency, are characterized by megaloblastic erythropoiesis and macrocytic red cells, while those caused by abnormal cytoplasmic maturation are characterized by normoblastic hyperplasia and hypochromic and microcytic red cells. However, even in the last conditions, there is marked anisocytosis and there may be a proportion of macrocytes in the peripheral circulation.

Blood loss

As mentioned earlier, the clinical picture associated with an acute loss of a large volume of blood is that of hypovolaemic shock.

Anaemias due to chronic blood loss may develop very insidiously and cause considerable diagnostic problems. Chronic blood loss from the gastrointestinal tract or uterus of more than 15 to 20 ml per day produces a state of negative iron balance. Assuming that the patient starts with a normal body store of iron, which is usually in the region of 1 g, the bone marrow will be able to maintain a normal haemoglobin level until the iron stores are totally depleted. At this stage there is no demonstrable iron in the bone marrow and the plasma iron level starts to fall but the patient is not anaemic. With a further fall in the plasma iron level, the haemoglobin level starts to fall, although at this stage the erythrocyte morphology may be relatively normal, as are the red-cell indices. It is only when iron-deficiency anaemia is well established that the typical morphological appearances of the red cells develop, and only after extreme periods of iron depletion that the tissue changes of iron deficiency become manifest.

From these considerations it is apparent that there may be prolonged blood loss before a patient presents with the symptoms and signs of anaemia. During the earlier stages the peripheral blood film may not be helpful in diagnosis, even though the serum iron level may be extremely low. Indeed, sometimes a dimorphic blood picture with normochromic and hypochromic cell populations may be seen. With chronic blood loss there is quite often a persistent thrombocytosis, and a hypochromic blood picture with thrombocytosis should always raise the possibility of chronic bleeding. In practice the most common sites of such bleeding are a hiatus hernia, peptic ulcer, and tumour of the large bowel or the uterus.

Haemolytic anaemia (Table 5)

When the lifespan of red cells is shortened there is a reduction in the circulating red-cell mass, which leads to relative tissue hypoxia. This causes an increased output of erythropoietin with stimulation of the bone marrow and an increased rate of red-cell production. This is reflected

Table 5 *General classification of haemolytic anaemia. A more detailed classification is shown in Chapter 22.4.9*

Genetically determined
Defects involving the structure and/or metabolism of the membrane
Haemoglobin disorders
Enzyme deficiencies involving the main metabolic pathways

Acquired
Immune (iso- or auto-)
Non-immune:
   Trauma
   Membrane defects
   Drugs, chemicals, toxins
   Bacteria, parasites
   Hypersplenism

by a raised reticulocyte count and a macrocytosis due to the presence of young cells in the peripheral circulation. Because of the increased rate of red-cell destruction, there is an increased production of bilirubin, which leads to mild icterus and the presence of increased amounts of urobilinogen in the urine and stool. Thus the haemolytic anaemias are characterized by a variable degree of anaemia, a reticulocytosis, and hyperbilirubinaemia. Their pathophysiology is considered in detail in Chapter 22.4.9.

Red cells are prematurely destroyed either because of an intrinsic lesion or as a result of the action of an extrinsic agent. The intrinsic abnormalities of the red cells that lead to their premature removal are nearly all genetic defects of either the membrane, haemoglobin, or metabolic pathways. The extrinsic agents that may cause premature destruction of the cells include a variety of antibodies, chemicals, drugs, and toxins, or bacteria and parasites. In addition, red cells may be damaged by direct trauma in the microcirculation or on body surfaces.

Premature destruction of red cells may take place either intravascularly or extravascularly, or, as occurs more commonly, in both sites. The site of destruction depends on the type and degree of damage to the red cell. For example, complement-damaged cells develop large holes in the membrane and are destroyed in the circulation, whereas IgG-coated cells are removed mainly in the reticuloendothelial system.

Clearly, there are numerous causes of premature destruction of red cells. These will be considered in detail later in this section. Usually it is easy to recognize that a particular anaemia has a haemolytic basis by virtue of the reticulocytosis and macrocytosis associated with erythroid hyperplasia of the bone marrow, hyperbilirubinaemia, and increased urinary urobilinogen. However, it should be remembered that many anaemias associated with abnormal proliferation or maturation of red cells have a haemolytic component. For example, there may be a slightly shortened red-cell survival in patients with pernicious anaemia or thalassaemia and yet there may be a very poor reticulocyte response. Similarly, there is a haemolytic component in the anaemia due to inflammation or malignancy but again the marrow response is poor. In such cases it may be necessary to measure the lifespan of the red cells directly in order to determine the magnitude of the haemolytic component as compared with defective proliferation or maturation.

General approach to the anaemic patient

CLINICAL ASSESSMENT

The clinical assessment of patients with anaemia has two main objectives. First, it is essential to determine the degree of disability caused by the anaemia and hence how quickly treatment must be started. Second, as much information as possible about the likely cause of the anaemia must be obtained from a detailed clinical history and physical examination. There is no place for the 'blind' treatment of anaemia without first establishing the cause.

In assessing the severity of the anaemia and how urgently treatment should be instituted, a detailed history of the patient's exercise tolerance must be obtained. This should include a specific enquiry of symptoms suggestive of cardiac complications including angina, dysrhythmias, positional dyspnoea, cough, or ankle swelling. The clinical examination should include a careful assessment of the degree of pallor, the position of the neck veins, whether there are warm extremities and a bounding pulse with a large pulse pressure, the presence of ankle or sacral oedema, and whether there are basal crepitations. The finding of profound anaemia with signs of cardiac failure indicates that urgent treatment is required. If the anaemia is associated with marked splenomegaly there will almost certainly be an increased blood volume and, particularly if there are already signs of cardiac failure, the patient may well go into acute left ventricular failure if transfused. Severely ill patients with profound anaemia require immediate treatment in an environment where they can be under constant observation, have regular measurements of the central venous pressure, and where they can be managed by experienced clinical and nursing staff.

An account of history taking and clinical examination in patients with haematological disorders was given earlier in this section (Chapter 22.1). It cannot be emphasized too strongly that in many cases the anaemia is a symptom of a non-haematological disorder. A detailed history and clinical examination will often provide a clue as to the likely cause of the anaemia and which laboratory investigations are likely to be most productive for confirming the diagnosis.

HAEMATOLOGICAL INVESTIGATION

A preliminary blood count and blood film examination should classify anaemia into hypochromic–microcytic, and macrocytic or normochromic, normocytic varieties (Table 6). In middle-aged women with a history of several pregnancies or heavy menstrual loss it is reasonable to assume that a hypochromic anaemia is due to iron deficiency and treat them with iron without further investigation. However, hypochromic anaemia in males or young or postmenopausal women always suggests blood loss and should be investigated accordingly. If there is any doubt about a hypochromic anaemia being due to iron deficiency, the serum iron level and total iron-binding capacity should be established. Hypochromic anaemia with a normal serum iron suggests a genetic or acquired defect in haemoglobin synthesis, common causes being thalassaemia and sideroblastic anaemia. The diagnosis of a macrocytic anaemia always requires further investigation and should be followed up with a bone marrow examination. A macrocytosis with a normoblastic bone marrow may result from alcohol abuse, haemolysis, or, occasionally, one of the refractory anaemias with hyperplastic bone marrow (see Chapter 22.4.8). Macrocytic anaemias with megaloblastic bone marrows are usually due to vitamin B_{12} or folate deficiency and should be investigated accordingly. If there is macrocytosis with a reticulocytosis, hyperbilirubinaemia, and a normoblastic marrow, a haemolytic anaemia is likely; an approach to the further investigation of haemolysis is described in Chapter 22.4.9.

The normochromic, normocytic anaemias often cause more diagnostic difficulty. Some help can be gained from a determination of whether the white-cell and platelet counts are normal. If there is associated neutropenia and thrombocytopenia, a primary disease of the bone marrow is likely and bone marrow examination should be made to determine whether there is hypoplasia of the various precursor forms, hypoplastic or aplastic anaemia, or whether the pancyptopenia results from infiltration of the bone marrow as occurs in the various forms of leukaemia. If there are nucleated red cells or young white cells on the peripheral film (i.e. a leucoerythroblastic picture), a bone marrow examination is essential as this type of reaction usually indicates infiltration of the bone marrow with abnormal cells, either as part of a primary marrow disease such as leukaemia, or metastatic carcinoma. In the normochromic–nor-

Table 6 *The main causes of anaemia classified according to the associated red-cell changes*

Hypochromic–microcytic (reduced MCV, MCH, and MCHC)
Genetic:
   Thalassaemia
   Sideroblastic anaemia
Acquired:
   Iron deficiency
   Sideroblastic anaemia
   Chronic disorders (mildly hypochromic, occasionally)

Normochromic–macrocytic (increased MCV)
With megaloblastic marrow:
   Vitamin B_{12} or folate deficiency
With normoblastic marrow:
   Alcohol, myelodysplasia

Polychromatophilic–macrocytic (increased MCV)
Haemolysis

Normochromic–normocytic (normal indices)
Chronic disorders:
   Infection, malignancy, collagen disease, rheumatoid arthritis
Renal failure
Hypothyroidism, hypopituitarism
Aplastic anaemia or primary red-cell hypoplasia
Primary disease of bone marrow, leukaemia, myelosclerosis,
   infiltration with other tumours

Leucoerythroblastic (indices usually normal)
Myelosclerosis
Leukaemia
Metastatic carcinoma

mocytic anaemias in which the white-cell count and platelet count are normal, it is also helpful to make a bone marrow analysis. The most common cause is anaemia of chronic disorders, the diagnosis of which is described in detail below. Another particularly common cause is chronic renal failure. After these conditions have been excluded, there remain the chronic anaemias associated with endocrine deficiencies (see Chapter 22.7) or the primary red cell hypoplasias (Chapter 22.3.11).

THE MANAGEMENT OF ANAEMIA

The management of specific forms of anaemia is described in detail in subsequent sections. However, a few principles can be outlined here. In general, a cause should always be sought before treatment is instituted. There is no place whatever for treating anaemia 'blind' with multi-haematinic preparations. As mentioned above, most cases of iron-deficiency anaemia require further investigation for a source of blood loss. If there is a clear-cut history of poor diet, multiple pregnancies, or obvious uterine bleeding, it is reasonable to start iron therapy and observe the haemoglobin level both during the period of treatment and for some months after iron therapy has been stopped. A rise in the haemoglobin level of approximately 1 g/dl per week indicates a full haematological response. In the megaloblastic anaemias it is quite reasonable to start treatment with vitamin B_{12} and folic acid once a diagnosis has been established and blood samples have been obtained for serum folate and B_{12} levels. The precise cause of the megaloblastic anaemia can be established at leisure once these samples have been obtained. A brisk reticulocyte response 5 to 7 days after initiating therapy suggests that there will be a full restoration of the haemoglobin level to normal. Failure of response of a hypochromic anaemia to adequate iron therapy should be managed by first finding out whether the iron is being taken and, if so, by determining the serum iron level. If it is normal, causes of hypochromic anaemia that are not associated with iron deficiency, thalassaemia and sideroblastic anaemia for example, should be sought. Similarly, refractory macrocytic anaemias require detailed analysis of the bone marrow morphology as there may be an underlying preleukaemic state.

Blood transfusion should always be avoided unless the haemoglobin level is dangerously low, when it is reasonable to transfuse the patient up to a safe level and then allow the haemoglobin to return to normal following appropriate treatment of the underlying cause. The decision whether to transfuse an anaemic patient depends mainly on the severity of the anaemia and its cause. For example, a young patient with a hae-moglobin of 5 g/dl who is shown to have an active duodenal ulcer should probably be transfused because they would be at severe risk from a further brisk bleed from the ulcer. On the other hand, a patient of similar age with a similar haemoglobin level due to chronic nutritional iron deficiency might well be allowed to restore their haemoglobin level on oral iron therapy.

Occasionally, patients present in gross congestive cardiac failure with profound anaemia. This picture is usually seen in elderly patients with long-standing pernicious anaemia or iron deficiency. This type of condition still carries a high mortality and requires urgent treatment. Such profoundly anaemic patients require transfusing up to a safe level, i.e. a haemoglobin value of 6 to 8 g/dl. This can usually be achieved by the slow transfusion of two or three units of red cells with the intravenous administration of a potent diuretic such as frusemide with each unit; the diuretic should never be mixed directly with the blood. A very careful check on the neck veins and lung bases should be made throughout the period of transfusion. Ideally, a central venous-pressure line should be inserted before the transfusion is started. Occasionally, patients are encountered in such gross heart failure that the administration of packed cells and diuretics worsens the failure. In this situation it is possible to raise the circulating red-cell mass by infusing packed cells or whole blood through one arm while removing an equal volume of blood from the other. By carrying out a two-to-three unit exchange transfusion of this type it may be possible to tide the patient over while treating the heart failure by conventional means.

REFERENCES

Adamson, J.W. and Finch, C.A. (1975). Haemoglobin function, oxygen affinity and erythropoietin. *Annual Review of Physiology*, **37**, 351–69.

Bellingham, A.J. (1974). The red cell in adaptation to anaemic hypoxia. *Clinics in Haematology*, **3**, 577–94.

Bunn, H.F. and Forget, B.G. (1986). *Hemoglobin: molecular, genetic and clinical aspects*. Saunders, Philadelphia.

Hjelm, M. and Wadman, B. (1974). Clinical symptoms, haemoglobin concentration and erythrocyte biochemistry. *Clinics in Haematology*, **3**, 689–704.

Oski, F.A. (1993). Differential diagnosis of anemia. In *Hematology of infancy and childhood*, (ed. D.G. Nathan and F.A. Oski), pp. 346–53. Saunders, Philadelphia.

Varat, M.A., Adolph, R.J., and Fowler, N.O. (1972). Cardiovascular effects of anemia. *American Heart Journal*, **83**, 415–26.

Viteri, F.E. and Torun, B. (1974). Anaemia and physical work capacity. *Clinics in Haematology*, **3**, 609–26.

Weatherall, D.J. and Bunch, C. (1985). The blood and blood forming organs. In *Pathophysiology*, (2nd edn) (ed. L.H. Smith, and S.O. Their), pp. 173–320. Saunders, Philadelphia.

Woodson, R.D. (1974). Red cell adaptation in cardiorespiratory disease. *Clinics in Haematology*, **3**, 627–48.

22.4.3 Anaemia as a world health problem

A. F. FLEMING

Introduction

Homo sapiens evolved over millions of years as a relatively rare species of hunter-gatherers. Their lack of specialization allowed them to adapt

Table 1 *Estimated prevalence of anaemia by region, age and sex, around 1980*

Region	Percentage anaemic				
	Children		Women 15–49 years		
	0–4 years[1]	5–12 years[2]	Pregnant[3]	All[4]	Men 15–59 years[5]
Developing	51	46	59	47	26
Developed	12	7	14	11	3
World	43	37	51	35	18

Definitions of anaemia: [1]Hb < 110 g/l; [2]Hb < 120 g/l; [3]Hb < 110 g/l; [4]Hb < 120 g/l; [5]Hb < 130 g/l.
Data from DeMaeyer and Adiels-Tegman (1985).

Table 2 *Causes of anaemia related to agriculture*

Infection	Genetic	Nutritional
Malaria	α^0-thalassaemia (hydrops fetalis)	Iron deficiency
Hookworm	Hb H disease	Folate deficiency
Schistosomiasis	β-thalassaemias	(Vitamin B$_{12}$ deficiency)
	Sickle-cell disease Hb E, Hb D	(Protein–energy malnutrition)
	G6PD deficiency	
	Ovalocytosis	

G6PD, glucose 6-phosphate dehydrogenase; Hb, haemoglobin.

to large variations of environment and diet, including the profound alterations introduced by the invention of agriculture and animal husbandry. Agriculture increased vastly the available energy-rich foods and permitted large leaps in the size of populations. Humans have adapted only partially to these self-imposed changes, which occurred recently in evolutionary terms, between about 300 generations ago in western Asia and 80 generations ago in the forests of Africa. The costs of agriculture follow from (a) increased density of population, (b) alterations of the natural distribution of water, soil and flora, and (c) changes in the food available. Anaemia is the most frequent manifestation of disease, especially in children and pregnant women, in the developing world (Table 1); the most common causes of anaemia are related directly or indirectly to agriculture (Table 2).

EFFECTS OF POPULATION DENSITY

Large populations carry the risk of famine, especially following natural disasters such as drought, or war. Secondly, density of population and inadequate disposal of waste intensify the transmission of infections. In terms of evolution it is probable that non-human primates, such as chimpanzees with population densities of about 4/km², were the principal hosts for malaria, and that humans were infected as zoonoses only when their populations were less than 1/10 km². As humans became numerous and replaced other primates, malarial species evolved and transferred to humans as their main host. *Plasmodium ovale* and *P. malariae* are probably the most ancient of malarial parasites infecting man. *P. malariae* remains a parasite common to chimpanzees and humans. *P. vivax* is likely to have evolved from *P. fragile* of Toque monkeys in South-East Asia. Surprisingly, *P. falciparum* is related closely to avian malarial species, and it may be speculated that it arose by lateral transfer following the domestication of poultry.

Table 3 *Annual number of births of homozygotes or compound heterozygotes for the major haemoglobinopathies (conservative estimates)*

	$\alpha^0\alpha^0$-thalassaemia (hydrops fetalis)	β-thalassaemia major	Hb E/β-thalassaemia	Hb S/β-thalassaemia	Hb SS and Hb SC	Total
Africa (subSaharan)		?		?	100 000	100 000
North Africa		850		300	100	1 250
Eastern Mediterranean		1 650		530	3 100	5 280
Asia	10 000	16 950	16 100	200	4 000	47 250
North America and Caribbean		100	?	200	2 300	2 600
South America		90		500	4 100	4 690
Oceania	?	?				?
TOTAL MINIMUM	10 000	21 990	16 100	1 830	113 700	163 620
POSSIBLE TOTAL	20 000	42 000	32 200	3 600	120 000	217 800

Numbers should be increased by about 40 per cent to allow for population growth by 1993.

From WHO Working Group (1983). The conditions are described in detail in Chapter 22.4.7.

CHANGES IN THE ENVIRONMENT CAUSED BY AGRICULTURE

Clearing of the forest and bush by slashing and burning creates open sunlit pools of water preferred for breeding sites by *Anopheles gambiae*. Irrigation dams and channels produce the swampy ground and vegetated shady water-edges favoured by *A. funestus*. These vectors of malaria can reach astonishing numbers: averages of over 250 bites per night and up to 145 sporozoite-positive bites per year per person have been recorded. Over 250 million clinical cases of malaria is certainly an underestimation. In the sudan savanna of Nigeria, the infant mortality rate was 245/1000 per year, and the death rate in the 1- to 4-year age group was 154/1000 per year: these figures were reduced by about two-thirds through antimalarial intervention. Severe malarial anaemia (haemoglobin < 50 g/l) (see Section 7) is seen often in young children and during first pregnancies. Recurrent malaria in the immune population causes more-or-less constant haemolysis and compensatory erythroid hyperplasia: control of malaria in areas of Africa and Papua New Guinea has been followed by an increase of mean haemoglobin values in both sexes and at all ages of about 20 g/l.

Hookworm and schistosomiasis are only two among the many other diseases whose transmission is favoured by agriculture, and both are major causes of anaemia. Hookworm is found throughout the tropical world and it is estimated that there are over 900 million infected people (see Section 7). About 200 million people are infected by *Schistosoma* spp., and transmission is increasing through ill-advised irrigation.

Evolutionary adaptations to malaria

The immensely heavy biological burden of malaria has led to the selection for inherited variants of red-cell haemoglobin, enzymes, and membrane, which confer partial protection against the worst effects of *P. falciparum* malaria. For several common variants, the advantage enjoyed by heterozygotes is balanced by hereditary anaemias, often severe in homozygotes or compound heterozygotes (Tables 2 and 3).

HAEMOGLOBINOPATHIES (SEE CHAPTER 22.4.7)

The genes for the α-thalassaemias, the β-thalassaemias and haemoglobins S, C, D-Punjab (or Los Angeles), and E, all achieve polymorphic frequencies in areas where *P. falciparum* malaria is or was endemic (Figs. 1–4). Migration and the slave trade have carried the haemoglobinopathies, especially haemoglobin S and β-thalassaemia, to the Americas, northern Europe, and Australasia. There are at least 240 million heterozygotes for the haemoglobinopathies in the world. More than 300 000 severely or lethally affected homozygotes and doubly heterozygotes are born each year, about equally divided between thalassaemias

and sickle-cell disease (Table 3). Unlike the anaemias from infectious diseases and malnutrition, the burden of the health services from haemoglobinopathies will increase with improved standards of living, as the life expectancies of the patients are prolonged, and the numbers born increase at about 3 per cent per annum.

α-Thalassaemia (see Chapter 22.4.7)

The total number of α⁰-thalassaemia heterozygotes in South-East Asia and southern China is about 42 million, with the highest frequencies in northern Thailand (Fig. 1). Homozygous inheritance occurs in between 14 000 and 28 000 infants per annum; it is lethal, resulting in a hydropic fetus who is stillborn or who dies soon after birth. Mothers bearing these infants suffer from toxaemia of pregnancy. The double heterozygous inheritance of α⁰-thalassaemia with either α⁺-thalassaemia or haemoglobin Constant Spring causes haemoglobin H disease, a thalassaemic condition of intermediate severity, most often presenting as acute haemolysis following infection. Haemoglobin H disease is seen commonly in South-East Asia: for example, about 70 000 infants are affected annually in Thailand.

β-Thalassaemia (see Chapter 22.4.7)

Thalassaemia major arises from the homozygous or compound heterozygous inheritance of various genes for β⁰-thalassaemia or β⁺-thalassaemia. Between 30 000 and 60 000 affected infants are born each year, the greatest number being in Asia (Table 3). The haemoglobin value is consistently less than 70 g/l: without treatment, death is usual before 6 years of age, usually from infection or heart failure. Treatment with repeated blood transfusions and deferoxamine to reduce iron overload controls the disease, and prolongs near-normal life, at least into the third decade of life and probably much longer. However, about 25 units of blood are needed per patient per year, and the total cost per patient of US $10 000 per year presents an impossible burden on the health resources of developing countries where the great majority of patients live.

Milder forms of β-thalassaemia, or combinations of β-thalassaemia and structural haemoglobin variants, are also extremely common. For example, haemoglobin E thalassaemia (Table 3; Figs 2 and 4) affects thousands of children throughout South-East Asia, Burma, and the eastern half of the Indian subcontinent.

There are approximately 94 million heterozygotes for β-thalassaemia in the world, including over 84 million in Asia (Fig. 2). The condition is essentially symptomless, but the haemoglobin level is about 20 g/l lower than normal. Anaemia is more pronounced in pregnancy, and is associated with placental hypertrophy, intrauterine growth retardation, and about 15 per cent of infants being born with Apgar scores of 3 or less.

Sickle-cell disease (see Chapter 22.4.7)

Sickle-cell trait is carried by about 84 million people in the world, of whom 70 million are in Africa (Fig. 3). The trait is almost harmless but over 160 000 infants are born each year with sickle-cell disease, the great majority in Africa (Table 3). Sickle-cell anaemia is by far the most common and most severe form of the disease, but haemoglobin SC disease is important locally in West Africa, especially Ghana and Burkina Faso where the frequency of the haemoglobin C gene is up to 0.15

(Fig. 4), and sickle-cell thalassaemia is not uncommon in Liberia, the Mediterranean basin, and in racially mixed populations of the Americas (Table 3).

Haemolysis, infarction, and infection result in death before the age of 4 years of the great majority of children with sickle-cell anaemia in rural tropical Africa. Those with the milder sickling disorders, SC disease and S β-thalassaemia are likely to survive childhood, and females present with complications during pregnancy. With improved social conditions

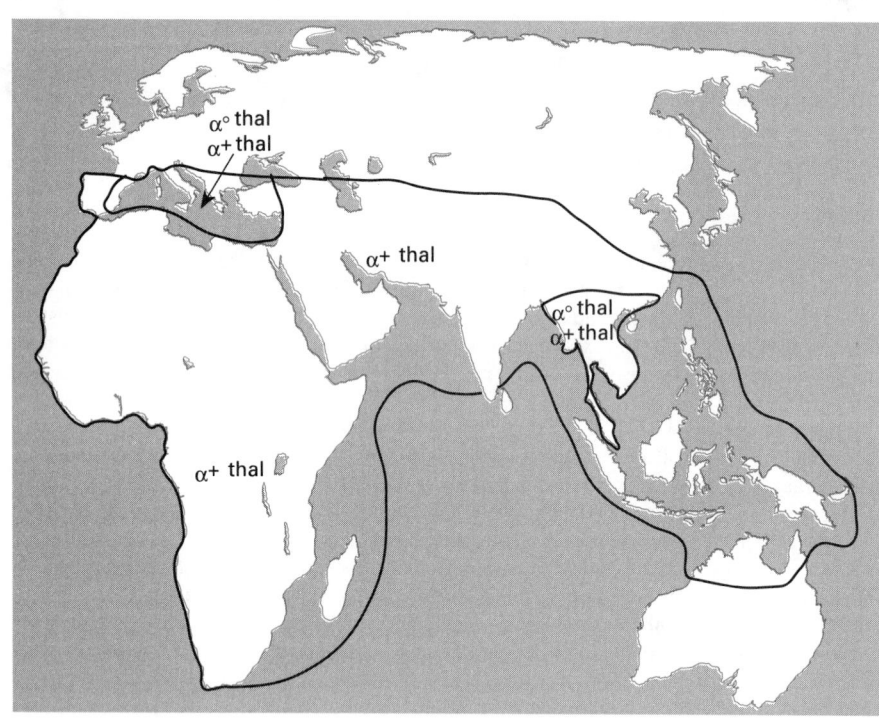

Fig. 1 Areas of the Old World where the α-thalassaemias occur commonly. The different types of α-thalassaemia are described in Chapter 22.4.7. (Reproduced from Fleming (1994) with permission.)

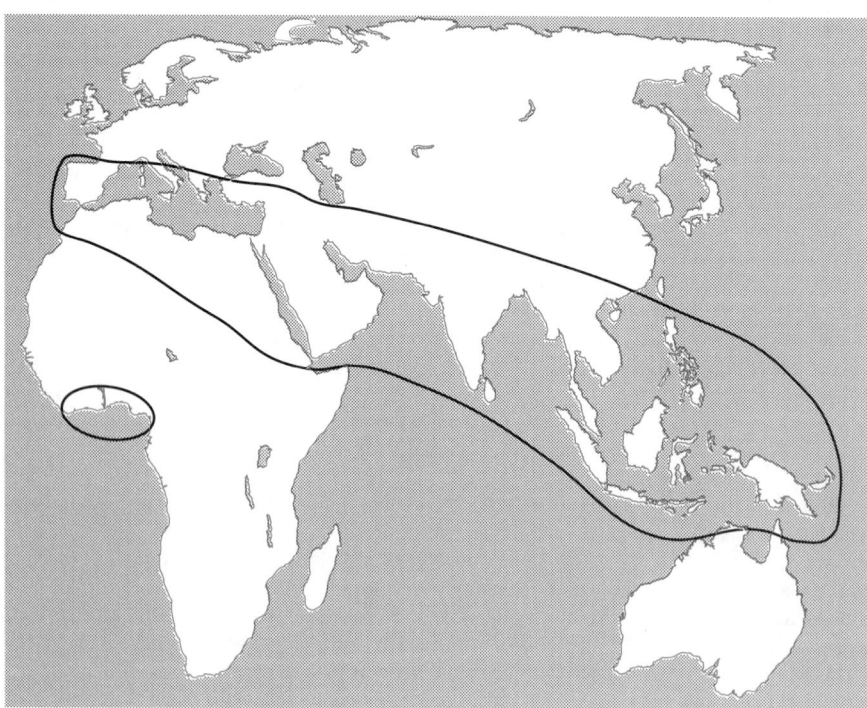

Fig. 2 Areas of the Old World where the β-thalassaemias occur commonly.

and the establishment of sickle-cell clinics, more children will lead near-normal lives, and sickle-cell disease will grow to be one of the greatest loads on the health services of tropical Africa.

ENZYMOPATHIES: GLUCOSE 6-PHOSPHATE DEHYDROGENASE DEFICIENCY (SEE CHAPTER 22.4.12)

There are numerous variants of the enzyme glucose-6-phosphate dehydrogenase (**G6PD**), but discussion is confined only to those that cause intermittent haemolysis and reach polymorphic frequency. There are three zones of the Old World where G6PD deficiency occurs commonly (Fig. 5).

The clinical and haematological manifestations of different G6PD deficiencies are discussed in Chapter 22.4.12. They present major health problems primarily through their contribution to neonatal jaundice, secondly by causing haemolysis and jaundice during acute infections, and finally, with the severe deficiencies only, through haemolysis triggered by certain oxidant drugs and foods (favism).

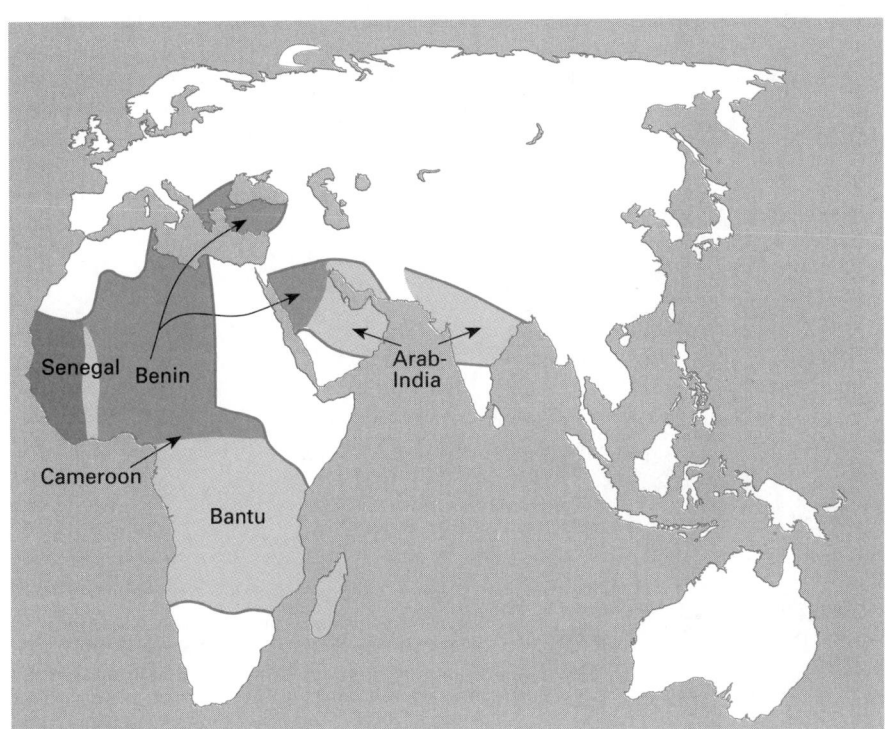

Fig. 3 Areas of the Old World where the haemoglobin S gene occurs at frequency greater than 0.02, and the distribution of β^s-haplotypes. Heavy arrows indicate probable spread of the Benin haplotype to the Mediterranean and western Asia. (Reproduced from Fleming (1994) with permission.)

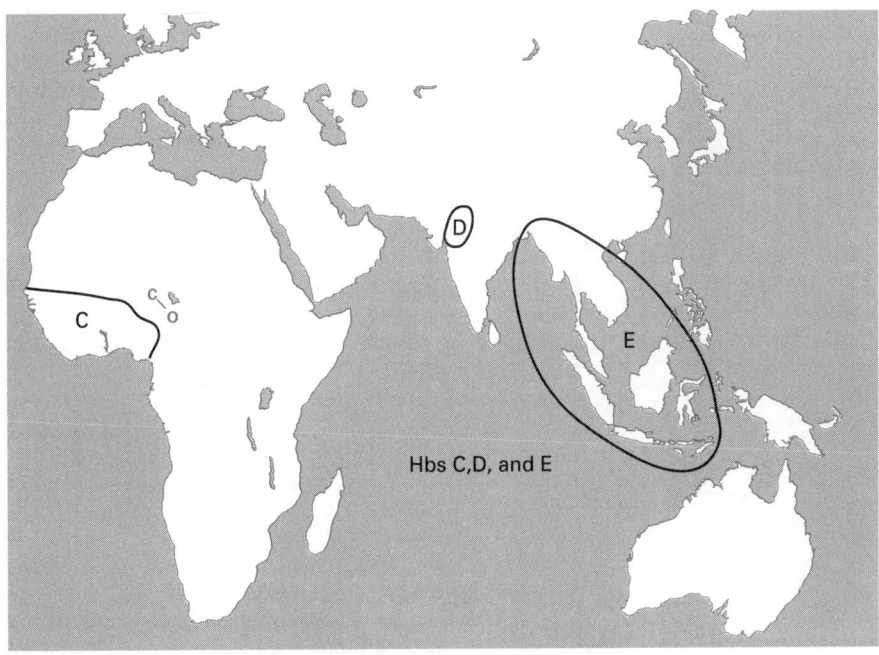

Fig. 4 Areas of the Old World where haemoglobins C, D-Punjab (or Los Angeles), and E occur commonly. (Reproduced from Fleming, (1982) with permission.)

HEREDITARY OVALOCYTOSIS AND ELLIPTOCYTOSIS

Ovalocytosis is widespread and common in Peninsular Malaysia, Borneo, Philippines, Indonesia, and Papua New Guinea (Fig. 6). It is present in more than 20 per cent of Melanesians in some areas of lowland Papua New Guinea, and their red cells have been shown to be highly resistant to invasion by *P. falciparum, in vitro*. About 80 per cent of subjects with South-East Asian ovalocytosis have otherwise normal red-cell indices. Others have a partially compensated haemolytic anaemia, with an average haemoglobin about 20 g/l lower than normal.

Congenital elliptocytosis is seen in up to 3 per cent of subjects in west and north Africa (Fig. 6). There is no agreement as to whether these red cells are resistant to invasion by malaria. In most, there is no or mild anaemia only, but the occasional child can have severe haemolytic anaemia, apparently triggered by successful invasion by *P. falciparum*.

Changes in the diet following agriculture

The domestication of plants by agriculture resulted in a reduction of the contribution of animal food in the diet from about 70 to 5 per cent or less. This affected profoundly the intake of biovailable iron, folate, and protein.

IRON DEFICIENCY

Humans are adapted to absorb haem efficiently as in intact metalloporphyrin, and to utilize the iron. As a consequence, iron deficiency and anaemia are uncommon amongst those groups who have persisted as hunter-gatherers, for example, the Hadza in Tanzania and the !Kung San in the Kalahari Desert, and amongst pastoralists who eat blood and meat, like the Masai in Kenya. In contrast, the absorption of non-haem iron (except from breast milk) is comparatively restricted, and iron deficiency and anaemia are common in communities whose food is predominantly

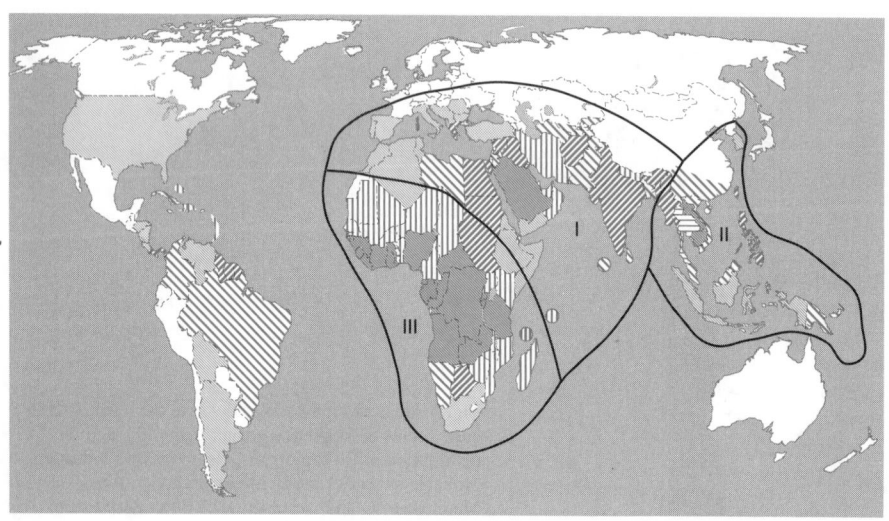

Expressed as percentage of the male population that is hemizygous

| <0.4% | 0.5–2.9% | 3–6.9% | 7–9.9% | 10–14.9% | 15–26% |

Fig. 5 World distribution of G6PD deficiency. (From WHO Working Group (1989) and Fleming (1993), with permission of the World Health Organization and W.B. Saunders.) Superimposed are three zones where different G6PD variants reach polymorphic frequencies. Zone I, Gd^{Mediterranean}; Zone II, Gd^{Mediterranean}, Gd^{Canton}, Gd^{Union}, Gd^{Mahidol}, Zone III, GdA$^-$.

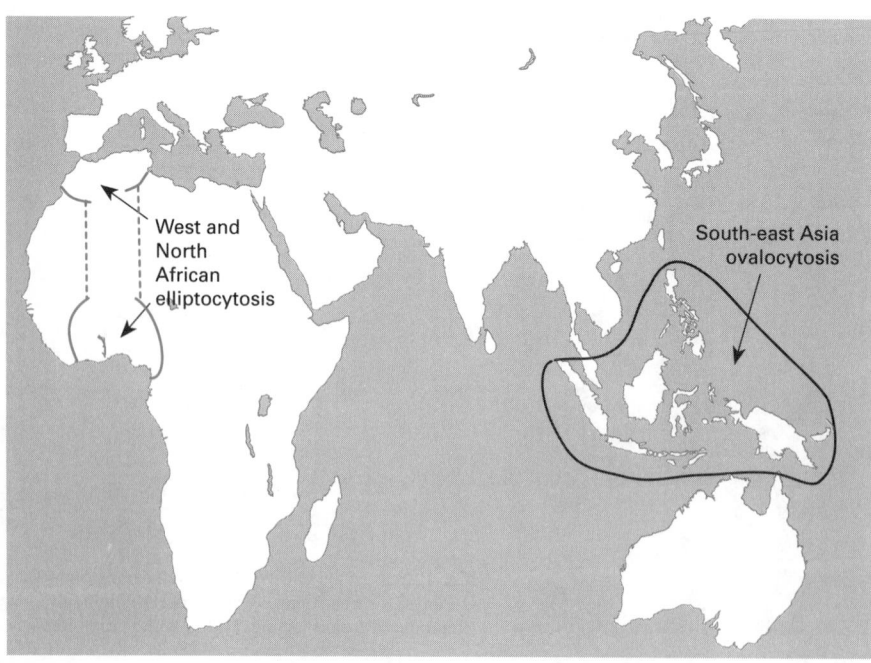

Fig. 6 Areas of the Old World where ovalocytosis and elliptocytosis achieve (or approach) polymorphic frequencies. (Reproduced from Fleming (1994) with permission.)

Table 4 *FAO/WHO recommended iron intakes (mg/day) to cover requirements of 97.5 per cent individuals in each age/sex group for diets with different bioavailabilities*

Age/sex group	Absorbed iron required	Bioavailability of dietary iron (percentage of iron absorbed)			
		Very low[1] (< 5%)	Low[2] (5–10%)	Intermediate[3] (11–18%)	High[4] (> 19%)
Children, both sexes					
0–4 months	0.5	*	*	*	*
4–12 months	0.96	24	13	6	4
13–24 months	0.61	15	8	4	3
2–5 years	0.70	17	9	5	3
6–11 years	1.17	29	16	8	5
Adolescents					
12–16 years (girls)	2.02	50	27	13	9
12–16 years (boys)	1.82	45	24	12	8
Adults					
Men	1.14	28	15	8	5
Women					
Menstruating	2.38	59	32	16	11
Pregnant:					
1st trimester	0.8				
3rd trimester	6.3	**	**	**	
Lactating	1.31	33	17	9	6
Postmenopausal	0.96	24	13	6	4

* Iron from breast milk is sufficient for about the first 6 months.

** Supplementation essential.

[1] *Very low bioavailability*: diet composed entirely of cereals (e.g. in India).

[2] *Low bioavailability*: monotonous diet based on cereals, roots, and tubers, with a preponderance of foods that inhibit iron absorption (maize, rice, beans, wheat, sorghum), and with negligible quantities of meat, fish, or ascorbic acid.

[3] *Intermediate bioavailability diet*: similar to above, but including some foods of animal origin and/or ascorbic acid.

[4] *High bioavailability*: a diversified diet containing generous quantities of meat, poultry, fish, or foods rich in ascorbic acid: typical of most populations in industrialized countries. The regular consumption with meals of inhibitors of absorption (e.g. tea or coffee) can reduce bioavailability to the intermediate level.

Modified from DeMaeyer *et al.* (1989), with permission of the World Health Organization.

of vegetable origin. The three great staples of humans are rice, wheat, and maize. Sorghum and millet are important in some dry areas of Africa and Asia. Soy and other legumes are essential sources of protein in many countries. Iron content is generally low, but more importantly, iron absorption is inhibited by fibre, phytates, phosphates, and polyphenols of these vegetable staples (Table 4). Ascorbic acid and amino acids (especially cysteine) from animal protein are the major enhancers of absorption of non-haem iron, but natural sources are expensive, and animal protein may be excluded from the food by religious beliefs, including Hinduism. Much of the world's population is restricted to a diet from which sufficient iron cannot be absorbed to meet physiological requirements, especially during infancy, early childhood, adolescence, menstruation, and pregnancy (Tables 1 and 4). Loss of iron from chronic haemorrhage due to hookworm or schistosomiasis contributes further to the high frequencies of iron deficiency and anaemia. About 1400 million persons or 36 per cent of 3800 million in developing countries (in 1989) have iron-deficiency anaemia. Iron-deficiency anaemia is an important, though lesser problem in the developed countries, where it is present in about 100 million or 8 per cent of 1200 million (Table 1).

MEGALOBLASTIC ANAEMIAS (SEE CHAPTER 22.4.6)

Deficiency of active folate coenzymes is common, resulting from low intake, malabsorption, high requirements or metabolic blocks. Deficiency of vitamin B_{12}, which figures prominently in medical textbooks, is comparatively less important from a global view.

Folate deficiency

There is scanty information about the folate content of foods eaten commonly in the tropics. Yams, sweet potatoes, other tubers, plantain, fresh peppers, locust beans (*Parkia fillicoidea*), and green vegetables are all rich sources, but rice, maize, cassava, sorghum, and millet are poor. Folates are heat labile so that prolonged cooking and repeated reheating are major factors contributing to the high prevalence of megaloblastic anaemia amongst Africans and Indians, as illustrated by the frequency in Indians in Singapore, compared to the Chinese, who cook vegetables lightly (Table 5). Low intake is not necessarily the result of a lack of folate in the food; the more or less continuous anorexia of recurrent infections such as malaria, or chronic infections like tuberculosis, is a most important cause of deficiency in the tropics.

Acute enteric infections, and also infections of other systems, for example pneumonia, are important causes of malabsorption in childhood. In southern India, over 70 per cent of patients with sprue for 3 months or more have megaloblastic marrows due to folate deficiency.

Children and pregnant women are particularly liable to depletion of folate because of high physiological requirements. Pathologically high demands result from erythroid hyperplasia secondary to haemolysis. The effects of recurrent malaria are seen most clearly during pregnancy: antenatal antimalarial prophylaxis alone in Nigeria was followed by higher serum folate levels, a reduction of the prevalence of megaloblastosis and the abolition of life-threatening anaemias (Table 5). Patients with sickle-cell anaemia and thalassaemia major are almost invariably folate depleted on first presentation in rural areas.

Table 5 *Prevalence of megaloblastic erythropoiesis in samples of all pregnant women and anaemic pregnant women*

	Country	Population sample	Percentage megaloblastic
All pregnant women	Nigeria	Primigravidae, Zaria	56
		Primigravidae, protected against malaria	25
	Southern India	Rural and urban	66
	Indonesia	Rural	25
	Western Australia	Urban	18
Anaemic pregnant women	Nigeria	Rural and urban, Ibadan	75
	Pakistan	Urban	25
	Malaysia	Urban	25
	Singapore	Urban Indian	45
		Urban Malay	30
		Urban Chinese	7

From various sources, including Luzzatto (1981), Fleming *et al.* (1986), and Fleming (1989).

Dihydrofolate reductase activity, and hence the conversion of folate to its active forms, is inhibited at 39 °C; pyrexia may lead to acute megaloblastic arrest of erythropoiesis, and may play a part in the megaloblastosis seen so often complicating infectious diseases.

Megaloblastic erythropoiesis is commonly a preanaemic state: 18 per cent of pregnant women in Western Australia showed frank megaloblastosis, but folate deficiency was associated only occasionally with anaemia. However, once the haemoglobin starts to fall, profound anaemia, often with neutropenia and thrombocytopenia is liable to develop rapidly.

Thirty-nine per cent of Indian and 34 per cent of Nigerian children with kwashiorkor have megaloblastic erythropoiesis. In northern Nigeria 40 per cent, and in Cameroon 79 per cent of anaemic preschool children have megaloblastosis. The highest prevalence recorded during pregnancy is in West Africa (Table 5).

Vitamin B₁₂ deficiency

The requirements for vitamin B_{12} are so low (rising to only 3 µg/day during pregnancy) that they are met by the smallest intake of animal products. Serum levels and liver stores are lowest in Hindu vegetarians, but even amongst the poorest in southern India, purely dietary deficiency is uncommon, probably because bacterial contamination of water and food provides sufficient vitamin. (Dietary deficiency can occur when Indians migrate to the United Kingdom, where clean food and piped water remove these sources of vitamin B_{12}.) Significant deficiency in the vegetarian adult is liable to develop if there is interference with absorption by the ileum following infection. Deficiency becomes progressively common with time of duration of tropical sprue. Infants of deficient Indian mothers are born with low stores and fed on breast milk containing insufficient vitamin B_{12}; after a few months they develop megaloblastic anaemia with locomotor complications, which may progress to coma and death.

Pernicious anaemia is rare in Asia and tropical Africa. As the condition is seen frequently in Africans in subtropical southern Africa, it is suggested that some environmental factors prevent the development of autoimmune parietal cell and intrinsic-factor antibodies.

Agriculture-related anaemias

There are three periods of life when anaemia is most prevalent and has the most serious consequences: (i) the neonatal period, (ii) childhood, and (iii) pregnancy. Maternal anaemia will be discussed first, as the frequency and severity of neonatal jaundice and anaemia in childhood are largely governed by intrauterine events. Although anaemia is less common in adult men and non-pregnant women, it reduces work capacity and hence has important economic consequences.

ANAEMIA IN PREGNANCY (SEE ALSO CHAPTER 13.9)

Women are liable to anaemia during pregnancy because they have higher requirements for iron and folate, and there is an increased susceptibility to infection, of which *P. falciparum* is by far the most important in endemic areas. Both frequency and density of parasitaemia increase progressively to reach a peak around mid-pregnancy, especially in first pregnancies. The major causes of anaemia in pregnancy in the world are iron deficiency and folate deficiency, malaria, and the haemoglobinopathies. The relative importance of these factors will vary around the world: for example, iron deficiency predominates in India, whereas malaria complicated by folate deficiency is the major cause of profound anaemia in West Africa (Table 5).

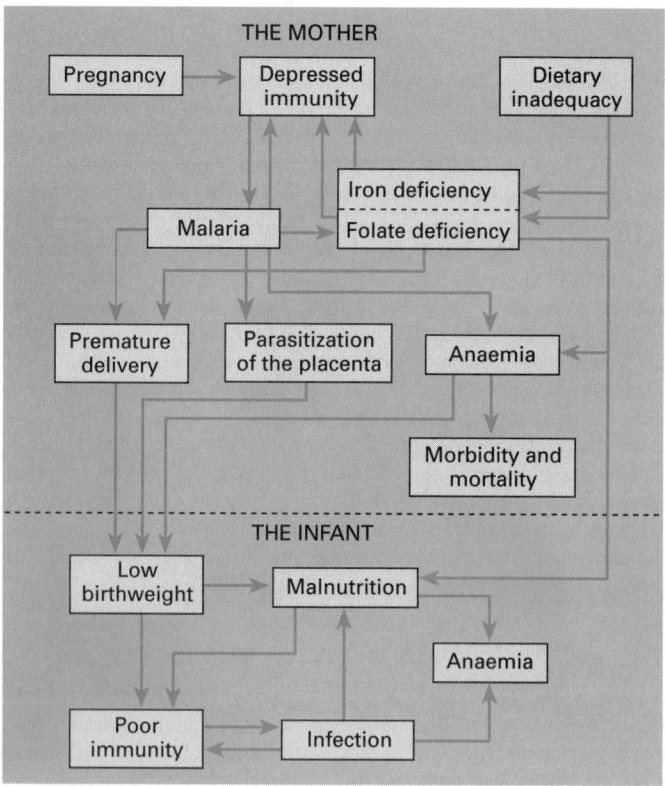

Fig. 7 The pathophysiology of malaria, iron deficiency, folate deficiency, and anaemia during pregnancy. (Reproduced from Fleming *et al.* (1986) with permission.)

The impact of anaemia, dietary deficiency, and malaria on the mother and the infant are shown schematically in Fig. 7. Deficiencies of iron and folate, and malaria lower further the immune responses, and the pregnant woman enters a vicious cycle of infection, nutritional deficiency, and depressed immunity. She is less able to withstand haemorrhage, and is breathless on exertion, or at rest when anaemia is severe. The full impact is seen if the haemoglobin level is less than about 30 g/l, when congestive cardiac failure may develop and, without treatment, mortality is around 50 per cent; appropriate transfusion of concentrated red cells with a rapidly acting diuretic and medication reduces mortality to about 2 per cent.

The consequences to the infant are more often disastrous. If anaemia persists throughout pregnancy, as with haemoglobinopathies or in the absence of treatment, fetal hypoxia results in compensatory placental hypertrophy and retarded intrauterine growth. Fetal distress is common and Apgar scores of 3 or less are observed in about 15 per cent if the mother's haemoglobin level is below 100 g/l. The prevalence of low birth weight is related directly to the severity of maternal anaemia; when Nigerian mothers' packed cell volumes were 0.23 or less at the time of delivery, 50 per cent of infants weighed less than 2.0 kg and perinatal mortality was more than 30 per cent. Successful treatment of maternal anaemia for about 6 weeks before delivery results in a dramatic improvement of birth weight and other measures and of infant health.

The causes of anaemia may themselves have directly adverse effects on the fetus. Malaria infects the placenta and causes low birth weight; pyrexia precipitates premature labour. Folate deficiency is itself a cause of premature delivery.

Infants of iron-deficient mothers have low iron stores; their folate status at birth reflects that of the mother, and the folate content of breast milk is diminished by maternal deficiency and maternal malaria. Low birth weight is strongly associated with poor immunity: neonatal infections lead to further depression of immunity and the infant has completed the same cycle of poor immunity, infection, and malnutrition as the mother, but in the infant the cycle is much more vicious as the immune system is undeveloped and nutrition is critical.

NEONATAL JAUNDICE

Jaundice (serum bilirubin above 250 μmol/l) during the first week of life is a common problem in hospitals in Asia and Africa, but estimates of its frequency are unreliable. Aetiology is nearly always multiple; four causes are most prevalent, sepsis, prematurity, G6PD deficiency, and ABO incompatibility. Rhesus incompatibility is unusual except among Caucasians, and intrauterine infections by toxoplasmosis, cytomegalovirus, herpes, and malaria present no problem where the mothers have high levels of acquired immunity.

Awareness by mothers and doctors, and early treatment by phototherapy and exchange transfusion, reduce mortality substantially, but despite treatment many infants show subsequent psychomotor retardation.

ANAEMIA IN CHILDHOOD

Preschool children in the underdeveloped countries are liable to be anaemic from 6 months of age onwards for several reasons. They have lost protection from maternally derived antibodies and have not yet acquired active immunity, breast feeding may be replaced by inappropriate or inadequate solid foods, they may be exposed to hookworm infection once they start crawling, and the β-globin haemoglobinopathies become manifest. The common causes of anaemia are malaria, viral and bacterial infections, iron and folate deficiency, protein–energy malnutrition (see Section 10), and haemoglobinopathies. Aetiology is almost always multiple; the children have been caught in a vicious cycle of infection, depressed immunity, and malnutrition, of which anaemia is only one major complication (as illustrated in the lower half of Fig. 7).

Infections suppress immunity

Many infections impair cell-mediated immunity especially, but also humoral immunity and phagocytic function. Measles and malaria in particular are commonly complicated by upper and lower respiratory tract and gastrointestinal infections frequently associated with anaemia in childhood.

Infections lead to anaemia and malnutrition

The anaemia of malaria has many mechanisms (Chapter 22.7). Viral and bacterial infections depress erythropoiesis, immobilize iron in the reticuloendothelial system, and cause toxic, microangiopathic, or immune haemolysis, but the strongest link from infection to anaemia in childhood is through malnutrition. Anorexia causes rapid depletion of folate stores and a negative iron balance, and jeopardizes energy and protein balance. Gastrointestinal and other infections cause malabsorption of folate and other nutrients. Measles is further complicated by protein-losing enteropathy. Demands for folate are increased by erythroid hyperplasia following haemolysis from infections. Dihydrofolate reductase is inactivated by pyrexia.

Malnutrition causes anaemia and suppresses immunity

Protein–energy malnutrition is associated with a mild normochromic, normocytic anaemia unless complicated by iron or folate deficiency and infection. The most important feature of protein–energy malnutrition in the aetiology of anaemia is impairment of resistance to infection. There are defects of the non-specific defences (skin, epithelial surfaces, secretions, complement, and function of the phagocytes), depletion of T lymphocytes, and some depression of humoral immunity. Iron deficiency results in depression of cell-mediated immunity and of the bacteriocidal activity of neutrophils, but there is no agreement as to whether iron deficiency leads to clinically significant liability to infection. Folate deficiency causes neutropenia and defective lymphocyte division, affecting cell-mediated more than humoral immunity.

Consequences of anaemia in childhood

The syndrome of infection, malnutrition, and anaemia in early life is commonly fatal, or leads to permanent defects of growth, development and intellectual function. Iron deficiency alone is associated with reduced weight gain and poor scholastic performance, both improving after the administration of iron supplements.

Anaemia and work capacity

Compensatory mechanisms (Chapter 22.4.2) ensure that oxygenation of the tissues is adequate at rest while haemoglobin levels are above about 70 g/l, but subjects will quickly become breathless on exertion. The performance of near-maximal work, as measured by the Harvard step test, shows a direct correlation to haemoglobin concentration, and the earning capacity of anaemic rural workers is reduced seriously. When the haemoglobin falls below 70 g/l the compensatory mechanisms fail, lactic acid accumulates, and subjects are breathless even at rest. Self-employed farmers often do not present for treatment until they have reached this stage, when any heavy manual work is impossible. Iron deficiency *per se* limits physical exertion as depletion of the iron-containing enzyme α-glycerophosophate dehydrogenase impairs glycolysis and results in excessive production of lactic acid.

Anaemia affects the whole family through inability to care for children, loss of earnings, or reduction of food production. The economy of the village suffers from a diminution of the area of ground under cultivation, and the national economy is affected by overall low productivity. The socioeconomic consequences of the high prevalence of anaemia in rural tropical communities are enormous.

Prevention of anaemia

The global control of anaemia is an immense and complex problem. The first step is research into the prevalence of anaemia in infants, children, pregnant women, non-pregnant women, and adult men, and into the relative importance of the common causes of anaemia. Recommendations can then be made as to the initial treatment required. Maternal child-health centres should be established, with objectives including the prevention of anaemia in pregnancy. Most of the causes of neonatal jaundice can be avoided by antenatal care, which reduces the frequency of low birth weight, birth trauma, and sepsis: oxidant drugs should not be prescribed without good reason, and ABO incompatibility can be anticipated. Antenatal care will go far to prevent anaemia in childhood by reducing prematurity, increasing average birth weight, and improving the nutritional status of the newborn. Anaemia will be controlled further by the encouragement of breast feeding, iron and folic acid supplementation for premature and other infants at risk, early detection and treatment of malnutrition and its prevention by education of mothers, prompt diagnosis and treatment of malaria, prevention by immunization and the early treatment of other infections, and the early diagnosis of haemoglobinopathies. The health of mothers and children will be enhanced by advice aimed at extending the intervals between births. Genetic counselling and prenatal diagnosis (see Chapter 22.4.7) will reduce the frequency of haemoglobinopathies.

On a national or international level, the eradication of malaria now seems to be beyond our present capabilities, but the impact of malaria can be minimized by mosquito avoidance and control near to homes. Transmission of many diseases associated with anaemia will be broken by clean water and adequate disposal of sewage. Hookworm may be eliminated by the use of pit latrines, abandoning the use of human faeces as fertilizer, the wearing of cheap plastic sandals when in the fields; hookworm has been virtually eradicated from South Korea by these simple methods.

Many countries are conducting trials of fortification with iron of commonly eaten foods: these include an acidified milk formula for infants and biscuits (with bovine haemoglobin) for children in Chile, sugar in Guatemala, salt in India, fish sauce in Thailand, and soy sauce in China. Results are promising and the global control of nutritional iron deficiency could be achieved in the foreseeable future.

Finally, there are many schemes, large and small, around the world aimed at boosting the production of food. Irrigation and agriculture will, however, increase the sum of human misery unless these plans include measures to avoid transmission of the diseases that in turn cause malnutrition and anaemia.

REFERENCES

DeMaeyer, E.M. and Adiels-Tegman, M. (1985). The prevalence of anaemia in the world. *World Health Statistics Quarterly*, **38**, 302–16.

DeMaeyer, E.M., Dallman, P., Gurney, J.M., Hallberg, L., Sood, S.K., and Srikantia, S.G. (1989). *Preventing and controlling iron deficiency anaemia through primary health care*. World Health Organization, Geneva.

Fleming, A.F. (1982). *Sickle-cell disease: a handbook for the general clinician*. Churchill Livingstone, Edinburgh.

Fleming, A.F. (1989). Tropical obstetrics and gynaecology. 1. Anaemia in pregnancy in tropical Africa. *Transactions of the Royal Society of Tropical Medicine and Hygiene*, **83**, 441–8.

Fleming, A.F. (1994). Haematological diseases in the tropics. In *Manson's tropical diseases*, (20th edn) (ed. G.C. Cook), Saunders, London, in press.

Fleming, A.F., Ghatoura, G.B.S., Harrison, K.A., Briggs, N.D., and Dunn, D.T. (1986). The prevention of anaemia in pregnancy in primigravidae in the guinea savanna of Nigeria. *Annals of tropical Medicine and Parasitology*, **80**, 211–33.

Flint, J., Harding, R.M., Clegg, J.B., and Boyce, A.J. (1993). Why are some genetic diseases common? *Human Genetics*, **91**, 91–117.

Foman, S.J. and Zlotkin, S. (eds.) (1992). *Nutritional anemias*. Raven Press, New York.

Hill, A.V.S. (1992). Molecular epidemiology of the thalassaemias (including haemoglobin E). *Baillière's Clinical Haematology*, **5**, 209–38.

Ho, N.K. (1992). Neonatal jaundice in Asia. *Baillière's Clinical Haematology*, **5**, 131–42.

Knox-Macaulay, H.H.M. (1992). Tuberculosis and the haemopoietic system. *Baillière's Clinical Haematology*, **5**, 101–29.

Luzzatto L. (ed.) (1981). Haematology in tropical areas. *Clinics in Haematology*, **10**, 697–1073.

Nagel, R.L. and Fleming, A.F. (1992). Genetic epidemiology of the β^s gene. *Baillière's Clinical Haematology*, **5**, 331–65.

Nurse, G.T., Coetzer, T.L., and Palek, J. (1992). The elliptocytoses, ovalocytosis and related disorders. *Baillière's Clinical Haematology*, **5**, 187–207.

Phillips, R.E. and Pasvol, G. (1992). Anaemia of *Plasmodium falciparum* malaria. *Baillière's Clinical Haematology*, **5**, 315–30.

Savage, D., Gangaidzo, I., Lindenbaum, J., *et al.* (1994). Vitamin B$_{12}$ deficiency is the primary cause of megaloblastic anaemia in Zimbabwe. *British Journal of Haematology*, **86**, 844–50.

Waters, A.P., Higgins, D.G., and McCutchan, T.F. (1991). *Plasmodium falciparum* appears to have arisen as a result of lateral transfer between avian and human hosts. *Proceedings of the National Academy of Sciences, USA*, **88**, 3140–44.

World Health Organization Working Group (1983). Community control of hereditary anaemias: memorandum from a WHO meeting. *Bulletin of the World Health Organization*, **61**, 63–80.

WHO Working Group (1989). Glucose-6-phosphate dehydrogenase deficiency. *Bulletin of the World Health Organization*, **67**, 601–11.

22.4.4 Iron metabolism and its disorders

M. J. PIPPARD

Iron is required by all cells, yet the chemical reactivity that underlies its requirement in many biological oxidation–reduction reactions carries with it the potential, when present in excess, for causing life-threatening tissue damage. It is thus not surprising that both iron deficiency and iron overload affect many body systems, with a wide range of clinical manifestations. Recognition of how the body utilizes, and is adapted to, the chemical peculiarities of iron is helpful in understanding disorders of iron metabolism and the laboratory tests used in their diagnosis.

Distribution of body iron

Iron-containing compounds may be separated into those in which iron has a vital functional role, and those that maintain body iron homeostasis through iron transport and iron storage. All three groups need to be considered when assessing disturbances of iron status.

FUNCTIONAL IRON-CONTAINING COMPOUNDS

Ferrous iron is an essential component of haem, allowing haemoglobin and myoglobin to bind oxygen reversibly as it is transported to, and stored in, the tissues. Of the 3 to 4 g of iron normally present in adults, 60 to 70 per cent is in the haemoglobin of circulating red cells and bone-marrow erythroid precursors, with another 10 per cent in the myoglobin of muscle cells. Other functional haem or iron–sulphur containing proteins account for less than 5 per cent of body iron. However, they are essential for the cellular utilization of oxygen, making use of the reversible electron-transfer reactions that allow iron to move between two oxidation states, ferrous (Fe^{2+}) and ferric (Fe^{3+}). They include mitochondrial cytochromes, which transfer electrons to oxygen with the parallel release of energy as ATP, various hydroxylating and oxidizing enzymes, including cytochrome P450 and xanthine oxidase, and ribonucleotide reductase, needed for DNA synthesis.

PROTEINS OF IRON TRANSPORT AND STORAGE

The redox activity of iron, upon which oxidative metabolism depends, is potentially toxic through its capacity to catalyse the production of damaging oxygen free radicals. In addition, at neutral pH and in the generally oxidizing conditions within the body, any 'free' iron risks conversion to highly insoluble, and biologically unavailable, ferric hydroxide. These chemical constraints have been met by the evolution of specialized proteins for plasma iron transport (transferrin), cellular uptake of transferrin-bound iron (transferrin receptors), and iron storage (ferritin). Transferrin and ferritin hold ferric iron in a soluble, relatively non-toxic, and available form. As iron stores accumulate, there is an increasing tendency for cytoplasmic ferritin to undergo partial lysosomal degradation to form insoluble haemosiderin. This second form of storage iron is responsible for the Prussian-blue staining of iron-rich tissues with Perls' reagent. Only a tiny fraction of the total body iron (less than 0.1 per cent) is bound to plasma transferrin. By contrast, storage iron may normally be up to 1 g, but the amount is variable and it may be much lower or absent. It is found mainly in macrophages and hepatocytes, as shown in Fig. 1, which also illustrates the principal pathways of iron exchange.

Iron exchange

Body iron is normally rigorously conserved and reutilized (Fig. 1) and there is no active iron-excretion mechanism. Iron absorption must therefore be regulated to balance small, unavoidable losses (approximately 1 mg each day in exfoliated mucosal and skin cells, and insensible blood losses from the gut), and increased physiological requirements associated with growth, menstruation, and pregnancy.

IRON ABSORPTION

Dietary iron is approximately 6 mg/1000 kcal. However, the overall bioavailability of the iron (about 15 per cent in 'Western' diets) is more critical than the absolute amount, and is dependent upon the dietary make-up and gut luminal factors (Table 1). Non-haem iron, which pre-

Table 1 *Factors influencing iron absorption*

Increase	Decrease
Dietary factors	
Increased haem iron	Decreased haem iron
Increased meat	Decreased meat
Luminal factors	
Acid pH (e.g. gastric HCl)	Alkalis (e.g. pancreatic secretions)
Soluble iron complexes with e.g.:	Insoluble iron complexes with e.g.:
Ascorbic acid	Phytates
Sugars	Phosphates
Amino acids	Tea (tannates)
'Meat' factor	Bran
Systemic factors	
Reduced iron stores	Increased iron stores
Increased erythropoiesis (especially in dyserythropoietic anaemias)	Decreased erythropoiesis
Hypoxia	Inflammatory disorders

dominates in vegetable foods, forms the majority in most diets. After solubilization by stomach acid, the amount that remains available to the absorptive surface of the mucosal cells after entering the alkaline medium of the duodenum depends upon the balance between promotional and inhibitory ligands derived from the diet. In vegetable foods, inhibitory ligands predominate. By contast, small amounts of dietary haem iron, derived from foods of animal origin, are relatively well absorbed by a separate pathway, the absorption being largely unaffected by other dietary constituents. Meat also contains a factor that enhances availability of non-haem iron in the gut lumen. Iron balance is thus more precarious, and iron deficiency more likely, in people eating a diet low in animal foods.

The mechanisms of mucosal iron uptake, transfer through the cell, and delivery to the plasma of the portal circulation are poorly understood. A number of internal factors influence these stages of absorption; reduced iron stores and hypoxia increase mucosal iron uptake, while changes in erythropoiesis are directly related to the amount of iron transferred to the plasma. Hypoxia and the erythroid expansion resulting from ineffective erythropoiesis are likely to be related to the excessive iron absorption seen in some iron-loading anaemias.

INTERNAL IRON EXCHANGE

Iron movements around the body are normally dominated by the need to supply adequate iron for haemoglobin synthesis in developing erythroblasts (Fig. 1). The uptake in iron-requiring tissues is determined by their expression of cell-surface transferrin receptors. These are normally mainly on erythroid precursors, which take up 80 to 90 per cent of the approximately 30 mg of iron passing through the plasma each day. Parenchymal cells throughout the body also express transferrin receptors, but those on hepatocytes predominate, accounting for a further 10 per cent of the plasma iron turnover. These two main alternative pathways for tissue iron uptake are seen by monitoring surface radioactive counts over particular organs after injection of trace amounts of radio-iron (^{59}Fe) bound to transferrin; in the absence of bone marrow erythroblasts (e.g. in aplastic anaemia), ^{59}Fe leaves the plasma more slowly than normal, and accumulates in the liver instead of the bone marrow. Such ferrokinetic studies are still occasionally useful in defining aberrant

Fig. 1 The principal metabolic pathways of iron. These are dominated by iron supply for erythropoiesis and turnover of iron from senescent red cells (heavy arrows). The normal minor component of ineffective marrow erythropoiesis is shown by the broken line.

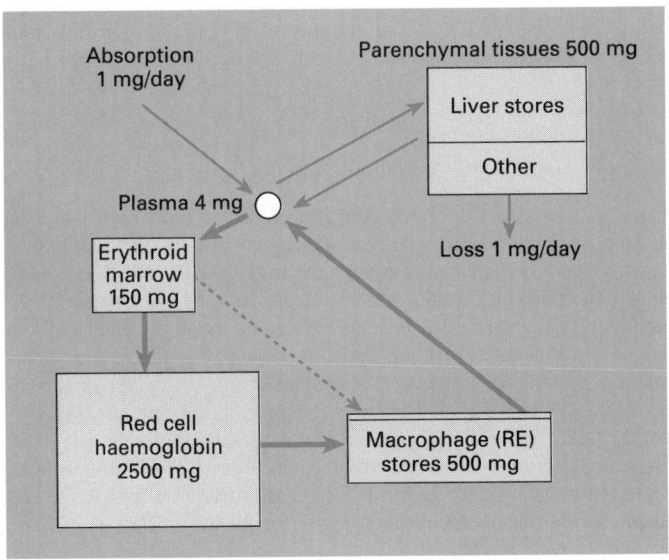

sites, and the effectiveness, of erythropoiesis (e.g. in primary myelo-fibrosis). Measurement of the plasma iron concentration and rate of iron clearance also allows calculation of the plasma iron turnover. Calculations based on this measure have been used to quantify erythropoiesis, and to validate alternative, less cumbersome measurements of erythropoiesis.

At the end of their life-span, red cells are broken down within macrophages, the iron being mobilized by microsomal haem oxygenase and either released back to circulating transferrin or stored as macrophage ferritin and haemosiderin. The control of iron release, normally closely matched to the iron requirements of the tissues, remains one of the most poorly understood aspects of iron metabolism; transferrin appears to act only as a passive acceptor of the iron released at the cell surface. The flow of iron through macrophages is unidirectional (Fig. 1), and there is no appreciable uptake of iron from transferrin. This contrasts with hepatocytes, which not only receive transferrin iron but also any haemoglobin (bound to plasma haptoglobin) released into circulation during red-cell breakdown. In addition, with iron overload the total iron-binding capacity (TIBC) of the plasma transferrin may be exceeded, and iron that continues to be released into the plasma from macrophages and intestinal mucosal cells may circulate as low molecular-weight, non-transferrin-bound iron; this too is cleared by hepatocytes, on first pass through the liver. The hepatocytes, with a two-way exchange of iron with plasma iron, thus act as a buffer, taking up and storing excess iron when the transferrin iron saturation is increased, and releasing it at times of increased iron need. As a result the liver is a principal target for iron accumulation in chronic iron overload.

IRON TRANSPORT AND CELLULAR IRON UPTAKE

Transferrin iron binds to transferrin receptors before being taken into cells by receptor-mediated endocytosis. The genes for both proteins are on chromosome 3. Transferrin is a single-chain glycoprotein (M_r 79 570) with two iron-binding sites, while transferrin receptor is a transmembrane glycoprotein dimer (M_r 185 000) with two transferrin-binding sites. As the iron loading of transferrin is largely random, transferrin circulates as diferric, one of two forms of monoferric, or apo-transferrin, the relative amounts being dependent on the iron saturation of the protein. This is important because the transferrin receptor has a much higher affinity for diferric transferrin than for monoferric, while at the neutral pH of the plasma apo-transferrin does not bind to the receptor at all. The long-established view that the per cent saturation of the serum transferrin is a better measure of the iron supply to the tissues than simply the serum iron concentration finds its support in this more recent observation of receptor preferences.

Transferrin synthesis occurs mainly in the liver and is transcriptionally regulated, the level of synthesis being inversely related to iron stores. Serum transferrin concentrations (measured by immunological assay or as a TIBC) are thus increased in iron deficiency and decreased in iron overload (Table 2).

Transferrin receptors are present in highest concentration on cells with a high iron requirement, including erythroid precursors, the placenta (with its role in satisfying fetal demands for iron), and on rapidly dividing cells. Their synthesis and expression are increased if cells are deprived of adequate iron, and reduced if they are iron replete. An immunoreactive, soluble, truncated form of the transferrin receptor is detectable in the serum, and is derived from the cells. In the absence of iron deficiency, serum transferrin concentrations reflect the level of erythropoiesis. Thus, the measurement is of potential value as a replacement for time-consuming ferrokinetic studies in quantitative studies of erythropoiesis. In the assessment of iron deficiency, increased concentrations of serum transferrin receptors provide an early indicator of impaired iron supply to the tissues. In this respect the measurement appears

more sensitive than the concentration of free red-cell protoporphyrin (Chapter 11.5).

Cellular iron metabolism

After cellular uptake the transferrin is separated from its iron in the acid environment of the endosome; at acidic pH, apo-transferrin remains bound to the transferrin receptor, is protected from degradation, and is recycled to the cell surface where, once more exposed to a neutral pH, it is released into the plasma to resume its role in iron transport. The separated iron enters an ill-defined cytosolic pool of low molecular-weight iron, metabolically available for incorporation within functional iron proteins or storage ferritin. Iron derived from other sources (e.g. from senescent red cells in macrophages, or haemoglobin–haptoglobin complexes in hepatocytes) also enters such a pool, as does iron released from existing cellular ferritin iron stores. In iron overload it is likely that the presence of excessive amounts of metabolically active iron in transit between iron proteins is responsible for tissue iron toxicity. In addition, within the liver it is a main source of the iron chelated by desferrioxamine, used in the treatment of secondary iron overload.

FERRITIN IRON

Ferritin is a spherical protein (M_r 440 000) made up of 24 subunits and capable of binding up to 4500 iron atoms in its core. The subunits are of two types, an H coded on chromosome 11, and L coded on chromosome 19; neither corresponds to the link with chromosome 6 seen in hereditary haemochromatosis see below, making a primary abnormality of the ferritin protein less likely in this disorder. Iron destined for storage enters the molecule through channels between the subunits and, after oxidation at a site on the H subunit, forms part of a polynuclear core of ferric hydroxide phosphate. Very little is known about the reverse process of iron mobilization; degradation of the ferritin after uptake by lysosomes is a likely mechanism for iron release, and it is possible that the formation of insoluble haemosiderin results when this process is overloaded and incomplete.

All cells possess the capacity to synthesize ferritin in response to iron excess. Early, basophilic erythroblasts normally take up more iron than they will subsequently require for haemoglobin synthesis. This is deposited as cytoplasmic ferritin aggregates, which are the siderotic granules visible on staining with Perls' reagent in normal marrow sideroblasts. Very small amounts of newly synthesized, iron-free apo-ferritin appear in the blood, being derived mainly from macrophages and hepatocytes. Immunological assay of serum ferritin concentration thus provides an indirect assessment of overall cellular iron status and body iron stores.

REGULATION OF CELLULAR IRON HOMEOSTASIS

Expression of several of the proteins of central importance in iron metabolism is controlled by an iron-dependent cytosolic protein known as iron-responsive element-binding protein (IRE-BP). The IRE-BP (M_r 98 000) is coded on chromosome 9, and is capable of binding to mRNAs containing a sequence that forms a regulatory structure called an iron-responsive element. Dependent upon the amount of available iron within the cell, the IRE-BP undergoes a reversible conversion between iron-poor and iron-rich forms. The latter contains an iron–sulphur (4Fe–4S) cluster, functions as a cytoplasmic aconitase and, unlike the iron-poor form, does not bind to the iron-responsive element. The 3' untranslated region of transferrin receptor mRNA contains five iron-responsive elements, while the 5' untranslated region of ferritin mRNA contains a

Table 2 *Factors influencing serum iron, total iron binding capacity (TIBC), and ferritin measurements*

Measurement	Increase	Decrease
Serum iron (normal 10– 30 μmol/1)	Iron overload Liver disease Decreased erythropoiesis (e.g. aplastic anaemia) Haemolysis/dyserythropoiesis (e.g. pernicious anaemia)	Iron deficiency Infection/inflammation
Serum TIBC (normal 45–70 μmol/1)	Iron deficiency Pregnancy Oral contraceptive	Iron overload Infection/inflammation Protein loss/malnutrition
Serum ferritin (normal 15–300 μg/l but age and sex dependent)	Iron overload Liver disease[1] Infection/inflammation Malignancy Haemolytic anaemia Hyperthyroidism Spleen or bone marrow infarction	Iron deficiency

[1]May be massive increase with severe hepatocellular damage.

single one. Binding of iron-poor IRE-BP retards cytoplasmic degradation of transferrin receptor mRNA, but represses translation of ferritin mRNA. By contrast, in the presence of increased amounts of intracellular iron, iron-rich IRE-BP no longer binds to the iron-responsive element, allowing ferritin production but reducing transferrin receptor synthesis. This coordinated regulation of the two iron proteins acts to maintain a constant intracellular iron content.

Measurement of iron status

Knowledge of the mechanisms of cellular iron homeostasis provides a rational basis for the hope that combined immunological assays for serum transferrin receptor and serum ferritin, in conjunction with haemoglobin concentrations, will provide epidemiological studies with a valid measure of body iron status over the complete range from iron deficiency to overload. However, in clinical practice there is no one test, or combination of tests, that is optimal for all circumstances. This is because abnormalities may affect only one iron compartment or may develop sequentially. In addition, factors other than iron status affect many of the measurements (Table 2). Investigations useful at different stages of the development of iron deficiency and in iron overload, together with normal values, are shown in Tables 3 and 8, respectively.

STORAGE IRON

Measurement of the serum ferritin concentration is reproducible and well correlated with iron stores in normal people. In the neonate, values increase as the high haemoglobin present at birth declines and its iron is moved into stores, and then falls to a nadir at 6 to 12 months of age as the growing infant exhausts the iron reserve. After puberty, the serum ferritin increases through adult life, except in premenopausal women, who have lower mean concentrations (approximately 30 μg/1) than men (approximately 100 μg/l). These values correspond to iron stores of around 300 and 1000 mg, respectively. Concentrations below 15 μg/l are specific for storage-iron depletion but values above 300 μg/l do not necessarily indicate iron overload. This is because ferritin synthesis is increased by factors other than iron, and because damage to ferritin-rich tissues can release large amounts into the circulation. Where doubt remains, it may be necessary to look for Prussian blue-stainable iron in

bone marrow macrophages (in the differential diagnosis of iron deficiency) or in a liver biopsy (in the diagnosis of parenchymal iron overload). Iron stores have also been assessed by measuring urinary iron excretion in the 6 h after a test dose of an iron-chelating agent (e.g. desferrioxamine, 500 mg intramuscularly). This is useful in assessing parenchymal iron overload but, like the serum ferritin, may give falsely high values in haemolytic and dyserythropoietic anaemias. Non-invasive approaches to determining tissue iron content include dual-energy computed tomography and magnetic resonance imaging. Both currently lack the sensitivity to detect early iron overload or to follow the response to treatment.

TRANSPORT IRON

Wide normal fluctuations, as well as a diurnal rhythm, in serum iron concentrations mean that it is unreliable as a measure of iron supply to the tissues. However, values tend to stabilize at low or high levels in iron deficiency and overload, respectively. For the reasons already discussed the percentage saturation of the TIBC is more closely related to iron supply. Alternatively, in iron deficiency, tissue iron needs may be assessed by the less labile measurement of free erythrocyte protoporphyrin concentration, or by determination of serum transferrin receptor concentration, if these tests are available. However, an increase in transferrin saturation is the first change in the development of parenchymal iron loading, and its measurement remains an essential part of screening for iron overload.

RED-CELL IRON

A reduction in the amount of haemoglobin iron may be part of an overall reduction of body iron in iron-deficiency anaemia or acute blood loss. Other anaemias result in the movement of iron from red cells into macrophage stores; a reciprocal increase in serum ferritin and bone marrow stainable iron should therefore be expected.

Disturbances in iron status

With much of the world's population eating a predominantly vegetarian diet containing poorly available iron, only slight increases in physiolog-

Pregnancy (see also Section 13)

This, associated with poor nutrition, is probably the most common cause of megaloblastic anaemia worldwide, if folic acid supplements are not taken. The frequency of the anaemia was about 0.5 per cent in most Western cities and up to 50 per cent in some areas of Asia and Africa until the introduction of prophylactic folic acid. The incidence increases with parity, is higher in twin pregnancies, and in some but not all series has been highest at the end of the winter. Folate requirements in a normal pregnancy are thought to be increased to about 300 to 400 μg daily, some 200 to 300 μg above normal. Serum and red-cell folate tend to fall as pregnancy progresses, with about 30 per cent subnormal red-cell folate levels in Britain in late pregnancy, and to rise spontaneously about 6 weeks after delivery. Lactation may prove an additional cause of folate deficiency, however, which may precipitate megaloblastic anaemia post partum.

The cause of the deficiency in pregnancy is increased degradation of folate due to hydrolysis at the C_9-N_{10} bond. Folate transfer to the fetus may play a minor part. Malabsorption of folate and increased urine folate excretion may be minor factors in some patients; in a few, megaloblastic anaemia of pregnancy is the first sign of adult coeliac disease. The statistical association of iron and folate deficiencies in pregnancy is probably due to a poor quality of the diet in certain women.

Prophylactic folic acid should now be given routinely in pregnancy; 400 μg daily is recommended (see earlier) and intake in women who may become pregnant should be at least this amount daily from food or supplements. Larger doses (4–5 mg daily) should be used if there has been a previous infant with a neural-tube defect. Conventional doses of 5 mg daily are satisfactory generally but have the theoretical drawback of being more likely to mask anaemia in the rare pregnant subject with untreated pernicious anaemia and thus might allow B_{12} neuropathy to develop.

Prematurity

Newborn infants have higher serum and red-cell folate concentrations than adults. These fall to a lowest value at about 6 weeks of age because utilization (and possibly excessive urinary loss) exceed intake. In premature infants, the fall in folate levels after birth is particularly steep and a number of such infants have developed megaloblastic anaemia, particularly if infections, feeding difficulties, or haemolytic disease with exchange transfusion have occurred. Prophylactic folic acid (e.g. 1 mg weekly for the first 3–4 weeks of life) may be given, particularly to those babies weighing less than 1.5 to 1.8 kg at birth.

Malignant diseases

Mild folate deficiency is frequent in patients with cancer (Table 5). In general, the severity correlates with the extent and degree of dissemination of the underlying disease. Patients with megaloblastic anaemia due to folate deficiency are unusual and folic acid might 'feed the tumour'; it should be withheld unless there is a real indication for its use, for example gross megaloblastosis causing severe anaemia, leucopenia, or thrombocytopenia.

Blood disorders

Chronic haemolytic anaemia

Requirements for folate are increased in patients with increased erythropoiesis, particularly when there is ineffective erythropoiesis with a high turnover of primitive cells. Occasional patients, presumably those with a poor folate intake, develop megaloblastic anaemia, particularly in sickle-cell anaemia, thalassaemia major, hereditary spherocytosis, and warm-type autoimmune haemolytic anaemia; prophylactic folic acid is usually given in these disorders.

Chronic myelofibrosis

Megaloblastic haemopoiesis was reported in as many as one-third of patients in a series in London (England) with this disease but a lower incidence occurred in a large series in the United States. Circulating megaloblasts, increased transfusion requirements, severe thrombocytopenia, or pancytopenia may be the first indication that folate deficiency has developed. Polycythaemia vera is not a cause of folate deficiency.

Sideroblastic anaemia

Folate deficiency, usually mild, may occur in about half of acquired cases. Megaloblastosis, refractory to folate or B_{12}, also occurs in the acquired form as in other myelodysplastic diseases.

Inflammatory diseases

Folate deficiency has been described in patients with tuberculosis, malaria, Crohn's disease, psoriasis, widespread eczema, and rheumatoid arthritis. The degree of deficiency is related to the extent and severity of the underlying disorder. Increased demand for folate probably is a factor but reduced appetite is also important in those who develop megaloblastic anaemia.

Metabolic

Homocystinuria (see Section 11)

Patients with the most common form of this disorder due to cystathionase deficiency may show folate deficiency, possibly due to excess conversion of homocysteine to methionine and thus excess utilization of the folate coenzyme concerned.

EXCESS URINARY LOSS OF FOLATE

Urine folate excretion of 100 μg a day or more occurs in some patients with congestive cardiac failure or active liver disease causing necrosis of liver cells. It is presumed that losses are due to release of folate from damaged liver cells. Haemodialysis and peritoneal dialysis remove folate from plasma. Folic acid (e.g. 5 mg weekly) is now usually given prophylactically to patients with renal failure who require long-term dialysis.

DRUGS

Dihydrofolate reductase (DHFR) inhibitors

Methotrexate, aminopterin, pyrimethamine, and trimethoprim all inhibit DHFR but have different relative activities against the human, malarial, and bacterial enzymes. Methotrexate is converted to polyglutamate forms, which increases its activity against DHFR and also increases its retention in cells. They cause varying degrees of impairment of folate metabolism in man. Trimethoprim, used as an antibacterial agent, may aggravate pre-existing folate or B_{12} deficiency but does not of itself cause megaloblastic anaemia.

Alcohol

Folate deficiency may occur in spirit-drinking alcoholics. The main factor is poor nutrition and it is likely that alcohol interrupts the enterohepatic circulation for folate. It also has a direct effect on haemopoiesis, causing vacuolation of normoblasts, impaired iron utilization, sideroblastic changes, macrocytosis, megaloblastosis, and thrombocytopenia, even in the absence of folate deficiency. Beer drinkers seem relatively immune to folate deficiency because of the high folate content of beer. The usual macrocytosis in less severe, non-anaemic alcoholics is not related to folate deficiency.

Anticonvulsants, barbiturates

Diphenylhydantoin, primidone, and barbiturate therapy may be associated with some degree of folate deficiency. The more severe deficiency is associated with poor dietary intake of folate and usually prolonged drug therapy at high doses.

The mechanism for the deficiency is undetermined. Malabsorption of folate, excess utilization due to induction of folate-requiring enzymes, displacement of folate from its binding protein, or competition for folate-requiring enzymes have all been suggested but not proven.

Other drugs

Nitrofurantoin, triamterene, proguanil, and pentamidine have been suggested to cause folate deficiency. Homofolates and carboxypeptidase G are two folate antagonists that have not been used in man.

Liver disease

Folate deficiency occurs most commonly in alcoholic cirrhosis where alcohol, poor nutrition, poor nutrition, poor storage, and excess urine losses may all be important. The deficiency is less frequent in other types of liver disease.

Laboratory investigation of megaloblastic anaemia

This consists of three stages: (i) recognition that megaloblastic anaemia is present; (ii) distinction between B_{12} or folate deficiency (or rarely some other factor) as the cause of the anaemia; (iii) diagnosis of the underlying disease causing the deficiency (Table 7).

Recognition of megaloblastic anaemia

THE PERIPHERAL BLOOD (PLATES 31, 32)

There is a raised mean corpuscle volume (**MCV**) to between 100 fl and 140 fl, and oval macrocytes are seen in the blood film. In mild cases, macrocytosis is present before anaemia has developed. Poikilocytosis and anisocytosis are also marked in severe cases, and Cabot rings (composed of arginine-rich histone and non-haemoglobin iron) and occasional Howell–Jolly bodies (DNA fragments) may occur due to extramedullary haemopoiesis in the liver and spleen. The MCV may be normal if there is associated iron deficiency, when the blood film appears dimorphic, or if the anaemia (usually due to folate deficiency or antimetabolite drug therapy) develops acutely over the course of a few weeks. The MCV is also normal in some severely anaemia cases due to excess red-cell fragmentation. The reticulocyte count is low for the degree of anaemia, usually of the order of 1 to 3 per cent.

The peripheral blood also shows hypersegmented neutrophils (which have nuclei with more than five lobes) and the leucocyte count is often moderately reduced in both neutrophils and lymphocytes, although the total leucocyte count rarely falls to less than $1.5 \times 10^9/l$. The lymphocyte CD4/CD8 ratio is reduced. The platelet count may be moderately reduced but rarely falls below $40 \times 10^9/l$.

BIOCHEMICAL CHANGES

These are confined to the anaemic patient and include a slight rise in serum bilirubin (up to 50 μmol/l), mainly unconjugated, a rise in serum lactic dehydrogenase of up to 10 000 i.u./l, with less marked rises in serum lysozyme and serum transaminases. The serum iron is also raised and falls within 12 to 24 h of effective treatment; the serum ferritin is mildly raised and falls over the first few days of therapy. The serum cholesterol is low and alkaline phosphatase mildly reduced. Absence of haptoglobins is usual. In severe cases, free haemoglobin may be present in plasma, Schumm's test for methaemalbumin in serum is positive, and haemosiderin and fibrin degradation products are present in urine. The direct Coombs' test is weakly positive in some patients, due to complement.

BONE MARROW

The bone marrow is hypercellular in moderate or severely anaemic cases and expanded along the lengths of the long bones. The myeloid–erythroid ratio is often reduced or reversed. The erythroblasts are larger than normal and show a number of morphological abnormalities; there

Table 7 *Laboratory diagnosis of megaloblastic anaemia*

1. *General tests*
   Peripheral blood film and count
   Bone marrow
   Serum bilirubin, iron, LDH
2. *Tests for B_{12} or folate deficiency*
   Serum B_{12} and folate; red-cell folate
   Serum homocysteine and methylmalonic acid levels
   Deoxyuridine suppression test
3. *Tests for cause of B_{12} or folate deficiency*
   B_{12} deficiency:
      Serum antibodies to parietal cell, intrinsic factor
      Serum immunoglobulins
      Gastric secretion; intrinsic factor, acid,
      Endoscopy, gastric biopsy
      Barium meal + follow-through
      Radioactive B_{12} absorption tests (alone, with intrinsic factor, after antibiotics, with food)
      Proteinuria, fish tapeworm ova, intestinal flora, etc.
   Folate deficiency:
      Small-intestinal function
      Xylose, glucose, vitamin A, fat, B_{12} absorption
      Duodenal or jejunal biopsy
      Barium follow-through
      Tests for many underlying conditions

is asynchronous maturation of nucleus and cytoplasm, nuclear chromatin remaining primitive with an open, lacy, fine granular pattern despite normal maturation and haemoglobinization of the cytoplasm. Fully haemoglobinized cells with incompletely condensed nuclei may be seen. Excessive numbers of dying cells, and nuclear remnants including Howell–Jolly bodies, mitoses, and multinucleate cells may be present. Because of death (by apoptosis) of later cells, there is a disproportionate accumulation of early cells. Giant and abnormally shaped metamyelocytes, and megakaryocytes with hypersegmented nuclear lobes are also usually present. Studies with labelled thymidine have shown an increase of cells in G_2 and mitosis, and of cells with intermediate amounts of DNA between 2C and 4C but not synthesizing DNA, and presumably destined to die.

The severity of these changes tend to parallel the degree of anaemia. In milder cases, changes, described as 'intermediate', 'transitional', or 'moderate', are principally in the size and nuclear chromatin pattern of the individual developing erythroid cells, with giant metamyelocytes present; hypercellularity and gross dyserythropoiesis may be absent. In very mild cases, megaloblastic changes are difficult to recognize. In patients with severe anaemia but only mild megaloblastic changes, some additional cause for the anaemia should be sought.

DEOXYURIDINE SUPPRESSION TEST

This is an *in vitro* biochemical test for B_{12} or folate deficiency based on the presence of a block in thymidylate synthesis (see Fig. 2). Deoxyuridine added to normoblastic cells reduces the incorporation of radioactive thymidine into DNA. The deoxyuridine is converted into deoxyuridine monophosphate (**dUMP**) and hence to mono-, di-, and trithymidine phosphates, which inhibit thymidine kinase and so uptake of the labelled thymidine. Uptake of labelled thymidine into DNA is not blocked as much by deoxyuridine in cells from patients with B_{12} or folate deficiency as in normoblastic cells because of the block in conversion of dUMP to dTMP (thymidine monophosphate) in megaloblasts. Correction of the test *in vitro* with B_{12} or methyl-THF can be used to differentiate the two deficiencies as B_{12} will correct in B_{12} deficiency whereas methyl-THF does not; the reverse occurs in folate deficiency. The test is normal in cells from patients with megaloblastosis due to a block in DNA synthesis other than at thymidylate synthetase.

CHROMOSOMES

Changes found in marrow and other proliferating cells include: (a) random chromatin breaks; (b) exaggeration of centromere constriction; and (c) thin, elongated, uncoiled chromosomes.

INEFFECTIVE HAEMOPOIESIS

The increased cellularity of the marrow with degenerate forms, and the low reticulocyte count account for the degree of anaemia and suggest that many developing cells are dying in the marrow. This occurs by apoptosis especially of late erythroblasts. Red-cell survival is moderately shortened, and radio-iron studies show rapid clearance, with increased plasma iron turnover but poor red-cell iron utilization. The raised unconjugated serum bilirubin, lactic dehydrogenase, and lysosyme are all due to infective haemopoiesis.

DIFFERENTIAL DIAGNOSIS

Other causes of macrocytosis include a high reticulocytosis (e.g. haemolytic anaemia or regeneration of blood after haemorrhage), aplastic anaemia, red-cell aplasia, liver disease, alcoholism and myxoedema, the myelodyplastic syndromes, myeloid leukaemias, cytotoxic drug therapy, chromic respiratory failure, myelomatosis, and other causes of a leucoerythroblastic anaemia. Once a bone marrow biopsy has been done, the principal differentiation is from other causes of megaloblastosis, particularly myelodysplasia. Other causes of megaloblastic anaemia not due to B_{12} or folate deficiency were listed in Table 6.

Some patients with rapidly developing megaloblastic anaemia, particularly due to folate deficiency, may develop almost complete aplasia of the red-cell series, and the peripheral blood and bone marrow may resemble that of acute myeloid leukaemia.

DIAGNOSIS FOR B_{12} OR FOLATE DEFICIENCY

The peripheral blood and bone marrow appearances are identical in folate or B_{12} deficiency. Special tests are, therefore, needed to distinguish between the two deficiencies. The deoxyuridine supression test has been described already (see above), and is used for reliable and rapid diagnosis in some laboratories.

Vitamin B_{12} deficiency

The assay of the B_{12} content of serum is now usually done by radioassays. The normal ranges have been reported to be higher with the radioassays (e.g. 200–1200 ng/l) than the previously used microbiological assays (e.g. 160–900 ng/l). Subnormal levels are found in cases of megaloblastic anaemia due to B_{12} deficiency, being extremely low in B_{12} neuropathy. Subnormal serum B_{12} concentrations in the absence of tissue B_{12} deficiency have been reported in pregnancy, in severe nutritional folate deficiency, in subjects taking large doses of vitamin C, and occasionally in iron. A false low result may also be found with the microbiological assays if the serum to be tested contains a drug (e.g. antibiotic or antimetabolite) that inhibits the growth of the assay organism.

Raised serum B_{12} levels, if not due to therapy or a contaminated serum, are most commonly caused by a raised B_{12}-binding capacity due to a rise in TC I as in a leucocytosis due to a myeloproliferative disease—chronic myeloid leukaemia, polycythaemia rubra vera, or in eosinophilic leukaemia for example. Raised levels of 'R' binder also occur in association with some tumours, especially hepatoma and fibrolamellar tumour of the liver. In benign leucocytosis, the rise is mainly of TC III and this is often not accompanied by a high serum B_{12}. Raised levels of TC II occur in conditions where macrophages are stimulated; for example, autoimmune diseases such as systemic lupus erythematosus, rheumatoid arthritis, in Gaucher's disease and in some monocytic or monoblastic leukaemias, in histiocytic lymphomas, and inflammatory

bowel disease. In active liver diseases, serum B_{12} leaks from the liver with saturation of the serum B_{12} binders.

A third and less widely used test for B_{12} deficiency is the measurement of the serum concentration of methylmalonic acid (**MMA**) or 24-h urine excretion of MMA. Serum MMA levels and excretion of MMA are raised in B_{12} deficiency but not in folate deficiency but may occur in renal failure. Rare cases of congenital methylmalonic aciduria have been described, owing to a variety of enzyme defects. The test is less sensitive than the serum B_{12} assay.

A sensitive method of measuring MMA in serum has been introduced and combined with serum homocysteine assay for the diagnosis of B_{12} or folate deficiency. In one study, 33 per cent of 196 serum samples with a serum B_{12} of less than 170 ng/l showed raised MMA and homocysteine levels, 22 per cent one or other variable raised, and 45 per cent both normal. Lindenbaum et al. (1988) and Stabler et al. (1990) have used the serum MMA concentration to diagnose B_{12} deficiency in the absence of macrocytes or anaemia in patients with neuropathy and serum B_{12} concentration of less than 200 ng/l. These reports are surprising and need to be confirmed; however, most find that patients with B_{12} neuropathy show haematological changes of B_{12} deficiency and there are not substantial numbers of patients with undiagnosed pernicious anaemia with normal haematological findings and borderline or even normal serum B_{12} levels, and clinical symptoms.

Folate deficiency

Direct tests include the serum and red-cell folate assay. In some laboratories, microbiological assays using *Lactobacillus casei* are still used but radioassays are now common. The serum folate is always low in folate deficiency (and is normal or raised in B_{12} deficiency unless folate deficiency is also present). The serum folate does not accurately measure the severity of folate deficiency. Raised levels occur after folate therapy and also in B_{12} deficiency and in the stagnant-loop syndrome. Red-cell folate is a better guide than the serum folate to tissue folate stores but is also low in a proportion of patients with megaloblastic anaemia solely due to B_{12} deficiency. Serum homocysteine levels are usually raised in folate deficiency.

DIAGNOSIS OF THE CAUSE OF B_{12} DEFICIENCY

Although the clinical and family history and the clinical findings may point to pernicious anaemia or some other cause of B_{12} deficiency, it is important to establish this for certain. A brief dietary history will rapidly establish whether or not the patient is a vegan or takes a very inadequate diet. Radioactive B_{12} absorption tests are valuable to demonstrate malabsorption of B_{12} and to differentiate gastric from small-intestinal lesions as the cause. The patient, after an overnight fast, is fed an oral radioactively labelled dose of cyanocobalamin, usually 1 μg cobalt-57 B_{12}. Absorption can be measured by whole-body counting, liver uptake, faecal excretion, by plasma radioactivity or by 24-h urinary excretion after a non-radioactive, parenteral flushing dose of 1 mg B_{12} (Schilling test). Hydroxocobalamin instead of cyanocobalamin as originally described can be used to flush absorbed, labelled B_{12} into urine.

Normal subjects absorb more than 30 per cent of the 1-μg dose. In patients with a gastric cause, malabsorption is corrected when the labelled B_{12} is given with IF, whereas if the lesion is small intestinal, the absorption does not improve with IF. Treatment with broad-spectrum antibiotics may improve the absorption in the stagnant-loop syndrome. In some patients with pernicious anaemia the absorption with IF only improves substantially after weeks of B_{12} therapy, possibly due to slow recovery of ileal function from the effects of B_{12} deficiency. A combined test 'Dicopac' has been devised in which B_{12} labelled with cobalt-57 is given simultaneously with [^{58}Co] B_{12} attached to IF. This is particularly convenient for the urinary excretion test if urine collection is likely to be incomplete but because of isotope exchange it is not as accurate as two separately performed tests. A double isotope test has also been developed in which [^{58}Co] B$_{12}$ is incorporated *in vitro* in egg yolk; [^{57}Co] B$_{12}$ is given in crystalline form. It is aimed to give a more accurate guide to food B$_{12}$ absorption. Some patients with atrophic gastritis, or after partial gastrectomy and low serum B$_{12}$ levels, may show normal absorption of crystalline B$_{12}$ but reduced absorption of food B$_{12}$. Patients with pernicious anaemia show malabsorption of both forms.

Gastric secretion studies after pentagastrin stimulation in pernicious anaemia reveal achlorhydria (resting pH 7.0 and not falling by more than 1.0 unit on stimulation) and grossly reduced or absent IF in gastric juice.

Endoscopy and gastric biopsy will show features of gastric atrophy and help to exclude gastric carcinoma. Follow-through radiographic examination of the small intestine will help to exclude a small-intestinal lesion, duodenal or jejunal diverticulosis for example.

The serum gastrin level is raised in most patients with gastric atrophy and the serum is tested for antibodies to IF, parietal cells, and thyroid; serum immunoglobulins are measured in view of the association with hypogammaglobulinaemia.

Diagnosis of the cause of folate deficiency

An inadequate diet is usually at least partly implicated, but an exact estimate of dietary intake from the clinical history is impossible because of variation in folate content of foods, losses in cooking, and size of portions. Often it is the general social circumstances that suggest a poor intake. Drug intake, particularly of barbiturates, is important. Many underlying inflammatory or malignant diseases may exaggerate the tendency to folate deficiency in patients with inadequate diets. The main cause of malabsorption of folate is gluten-induced enteropathy; in patients with severe folate deficiency, a jejunal biopsy is usually necessary. In certain tropical countries sprue may cause a generalized malabsorption syndrome in which folate deficiency commonly occurs. Tests of folate absorption have been devised, either by measuring the rise in serum folate after an oral dose of folic acid or of more natural folate derivatives (e.g. folate polyglutamates), or by measuring urinary or faecal excretion of radioactivity after feeding one or other labelled folate compound. None of these tests has achieved routine use.

TREATMENT OF MEGALOBLASTIC ANAEMIA

Therapy is aimed at correcting the anaemia, completely replenishing the body of which ever vitamin is deficient, treatment of the underlying disorder, and prevention of relapse. In most cases, it is possible to diagnose which deficiency is present before starting therapy.

Vitamin B$_{12}$ deficiency

Hydroxocobalamin 1000 μg intramuscularly given six times at several days' interval over the first few weeks will restore normal B$_{12}$ stores. There is no evidence that patients with B$_{12}$ neuropathy derive greater benefit from more frequent doses, although many physicians use these for 6 months or so.

Response to therapy

The patient feels better within 24 to 48 h, and the mild fever, if not due to infection, falls to normal. A painful tongue and uncooperative, disorientated state may also be improved in 48 h. The reticulocyte count begins to rise on the second day with a peak after 5 to 7 days. The white-cell count becomes normal by the third to seventh day and the platelet count rises and may reach levels of 500 to 1000 × 10^9/l before falling to normal at about 10 to 14 days. The bone marrow reverts to normoblastic by 36 to 48 h, although giant metamyelocytes persist for 10 to 12 days. The serum iron falls within 24 h, usually to subnormal levels, while the serum lactic dehydrogenase falls more generally during the first 14 days of therapy.

The neuropathy always improve with therapy but residual deficits remain in some patients, particularly those with the longest histories and the most severe manifestations.

Maintenance

Hydroxocobalamin, 1000 μg intramuscularly, is given once every 3 months for life in pernicious anaemia and most other causes of B$_{12}$ deficiency, to prevent relapse. The life expectancy in pernicious anaemia once treated, is as good as that in the general population in women, and slightly lower in men, probably due to the increased incidence of carcinoma of the stomach. In a few patients with B$_{12}$ deficiency, the underlying cause can be reversed; for example, expulsion of the fish tapeworm, improvement of vegan diet, surgical correction of an intestinal stagnant loop. A few micrograms of B$_{12}$ can be absorbed each day in pernicious anaemia from oral doses of 1000 μg or more by passive diffusion, but this maintenance therapy is reserved for those who cannot have injections—for example those with a bleeding disorder, or who refuse them—and for the extremely rare individual who is allergic to all injectable forms of B$_{12}$. Vegans may be maintained on much smaller oral doses of B$_{12}$ each day, such as 50 μg as a tablet or syrup.

Prophylactic maintenance

B$_{12}$ therapy should be given from the time of operation after total gastrectomy or after ileal resection if a B$_{12}$ absorption test postoperatively reveals malabsorption of the vitamin. Patients with pernicious anaemia tend to develop iron-deficiency anaemia and they may also develop thyroid disorders or carcinoma of the stomach. It is advisable that a regular blood count be made once a year. Routine regular endoscopy is not warranted but these diseases must be particularly borne in mind if relevant symptoms or signs develop.

Folate deficiency

This is corrected by giving 5 mg folic acid by mouth daily. It is essential to exclude B$_{12}$ deficiency so that precipitation of a neuropathy is avoided. It is usual to continue for at least 4 months until there is a completely new set of red cells, although body stores will theoretically be normal within a few days of therapy. In patients with severe malabsorption of folate, larger oral doses of folic acid (e.g. 5 mg three times daily) may be used but it is not necessary to give parenteral folate except for those unable to swallow tablets. The response to therapy is as described for B$_{12}$. The decision whether or not to continue folic acid beyond 4 months depends on whether or not the cause can be corrected. In practice, long-term folic acid is usually needed only in patients with severe haemolytic anaemias (e.g. sickle-cell anaemia and thalassaemia major), myelofibrosis, and in gluten-induced enteropathy when a gluten-free diet is either unsuccessful or not feasible. In patients on a gluten-free diet, assessment of folate status is one simple way of following the improvement in absorption.

Prophylactic folic acid

This should be given to all pregnant women (doses of 300 to 400 μg daily are used, often combined with an iron preparation) and, if the diet is poor, to all women likely to become pregnant. Larger doses are given if there has been a previous neural tube-deficit infant. Folic acid is given to patients undergoing regular haemodialysis or peritoneal dialysis, and to premature infants weighing less than 1.5 kg at birth, and to selected patients in intensive care units or receiving parenteral nutrition.

Folate therapy has been shown to improve chromosomal stability in the fragile X syndrome, even though these patients do not have folate deficiency or a demonstrable defect of folate metabolism.

Folinic acid (5-formyl-THF)

This reduced folate is used to prevent or treat toxicity due to methotrexate or other dihydrofolate reductase inhibitors.

Severely ill patients

Some patients, usually elderly, are admitted to hospital severely ill with megaloblastic anaemia, perhaps in congestive heart failure, or with pneumonia. In this case, it is necessary to commence therapy immediately after obtaining blood for B_{12} and folate assay and aspirating bone marrow, before it is known which deficiency is present. Both vitamins should be given stimultaneously in large doses. Heart failure and infection should be treated in conventional fashion but blood transfusion should be avoided, except in cases of extreme anaemia, when 1 to 2 units of packed cells may be given slowly, accompanied by removal of a similar volume of blood from the other arm, and diuretic therapy.

Other therapy

Hypokalaemia may occur during the response to therapy and oral potassium supplements should be given to those with initial heart failure or if severe hypokalaemia is demonstrated, but are not needed routinely. An attack of gout has been reported on the sixth to seventh day of therapy. Most patients develop hyperuricaemia at this stage but the clinical disease probably only occurs in those with a strong gouty tendency. Iron deficiency commonly develops in the first few weeks of therapy and this should be treated initially with oral ferrous sulphate in the usual way.

Megaloblastic anaemia due to inborn errors of folate or B_{12} metabolism

FOLATE

A number of babies have been described with congenital deficiency of one or other enzyme concerned in folate metabolism: 5-methyltetrahydrofolate, methylene THF-reductase, Figlu transferase, methenyl-THF cyclohydrolase. Some of the babies had multiple congenital defects including the heart and cerebral ventricles and nearly all showed impaired mental development. In the methylfolate transferase deficiency, megaloblastic anaemia was present.

VITAMIN B_{12}

Congenital deficiency of TC II was first reported in 1971 in two siblings who developed megaloblastic anaemia requiring therapy with large daily doses of B_{12} at 3 and 5 weeks of age. Similarly affected families have been described in which neuropathy developed in the absence of adequate therapy. A spectrum of loss of TC II occurs and functionally inactive TC II has been detected in some cases, often presenting later in life. The serum B_{12} level is usually normal, B_{12} being bound to TC I. Absorption of B_{12} is impaired. Treatment is with massive doses of B_{12} (e.g. 1000 μg intramuscularly three times each week). In contrast, in subjects with rare, inherited, low levels of TC I, low serum B_{12} levels occur, but haemopoiesis is normal.

Children with one form of congenital methylmalonic aciduria, which responds to B_{12} therapy in large doses, have been shown to have a defect in conversion of hydroxocobalamin to ado-B_{12}. They do not show megaloblastic anaemia. In a few, this defect has been associated with a defect of formation of methyl-B_{12} and with homocystinuria, but some of the children have also surprisingly not shown megaloblastic anaemia. Neurological abnormalities are usual. Homocystinuria and megaloblastic anaemia without methylmalonic aciduria have also been reported. In some cases the defect appears to be in maintaining B_{12} bound to methionine synthase in the reduced state.

Megaloblastic anaemia due to acquired disturbances of folate or B_{12} metabolism

FOLATE

Therapy with dihydrofolate reductase inhibitors may cause megaloblastic anaemia. This is usual with methotrexate and less likely with pyrimethamine unless high doses are used or the patient is already folate deficient. Trimethoprim and triamterene are very weak folate antagonists

in man, but may precipitate megaloblastic anaemia in patients already B_{12} or folate deficient (see earlier).

VITAMIN B_{12}

Nitrous oxide (N_2O)

This anaesthetic gas oxidizes B_{12} from the active fully reduce cob(I)alamin form to the inactive cob(II)alamin and cob(III)alamin forms, inactivating methyl B_{12} and hence methionine synthase. Megaloblastosis develops within several hours in man and a fault in thymidylate synthetase can be demonstrated by the deoxyuridine suppression test in human marrow exposed to N_2O. This recovers over several days when exposure to N_2O is discontinued. After many weeks exposure to N_2O, monkeys develop a neuropathy resembling B_{12} neuropathy in man; peripheral neuropathies have also been described in humans (e.g. dentists and anaesthetists) repeatedly exposed to the gas. When N_2O is used as anaesthetic for patients with low B_{12} stores, megaloblastic anaemia or neuropathy may be precipitated months later, due to failure to replenish B_{12} stores by absorption. Recovery from N_2O exposure needs new cobalamin and also synthesis of new apoenzyme (methionine synthase) because this protein is also damaged by active oxygen derived from the N_2O–cobalamin reaction. Methylmalonic aciduria has not been found in animals or humans exposed for short periods to N_2O, as methylmalonic CoA mutase does not have reduced B_{12}.

Megaloblastic anaemia not due to folate or B_{12} deficiency or metabolic defect

CONGENITAL

Orotic aciduria

This is a rare recessive disorder involving two consecutive enzymes (orotidylic pyrophosphatase and orotidylic decarboxylase) in pyrimidine synthetase and presents with megaloblastic anaemia in the first few months of life. The diagnosis is made if needle-shaped, colourless crystals of orotic acid are found in the urine, daily excretion ranging from 0.5 to 1.5 g. Heterozygotes excrete slightly raised amounts of orotic acid but show no haematological disorder. Treatment with uridine (1–1.5 g daily) leads to a haematological response, restoration of normal haemopoiesis and growth, and reduction in orotic acid excretion.

Lesch–Nyhan syndrome

A few patients with this rare disorder of purine synthesis have shown megaloblastic change but whether this was due to associated folate deficiency or a direct result of reduced purine synthesis is not certain (see Section 11).

Vitamin E deficiency

This has been reported to cause megaloblastosis in a group of children with kwashiorkor. However, many were also folate deficient.

Vitamin C deficiency

Megaloblastic appears to be due to associated folate deficiency.

Thiamine responsive

Seven cases have been well documented. They have also shown sideroblastic change and a fault in thiamine metabolism has been implicated.

Responding to large doses of vitamin B_{12} **and folate**

A single patient has been reported who needed both vitamins in large doses but the site of the defect was not elucidated.

Congenital dyserythropoietic anaemia

Some cases of congenital dyserythropoietic anaemia show megaloblastic changes not due to B_{12} or folate deficiency.

ACQUIRED

Megaloblastic changes are often marked in acute myeloid leukaemia/ (AML) M6 and less commonly in other forms of AML. They also occur in about 50 per cent of patients with primary acquired sideroblastic anaemia and in other myelodysplastic syndromes. The exact site of block in DNA synthesis in these syndromes is unknown.

Drugs that directly inhibit purine or pyrimidine synthesis (e.g. cytosine arabinoside, 5-fluorouracil, hydroxyurea, 6-mercaptopurine, or azathioprine) may cause megaloblastic anaemia. Alcohol has also been found to have a direct effect on the bone marrow, causing megaloblastosis in some cases even in the absence of B_{12} or folate deficiency. On the other hand, drugs that inhibit mitosis (e.g. colchicine or daunorubicin) or alkylate preformed DNA (e.g. cyclophosphamide, chlorambucil, or busulphan) do not cause megaloblastosis.

Other deficiency anaemias

VITAMIN C

Anaemia is usual in scurvy but the pathogenesis is complicated. It is likely that vitamin C has a direct effect on erythropoiesis but folate and iron deficiencies, haemorrhage, or haemolysis often complicate the picture.

Biochemical and nutritional aspects

Vitamin C is needed for collagen synthesis by its involvement in the hydroxylation of protein and for maintenance of intercellular substance of skin, cartilage, periosteum, and bone. It may also have a general role in oxidative–reduction systems, for example glutathione, cytochromes, pyridine, and flavin nucleotides. Although vitamin C is also thought to be needed for maintaining body folates in the reduced active state, the exact reactions involved are unclear. Vitamin C has a particular role in iron metabolism, iron excess causing increased utilization of vitamin C and in extreme cases clinical scurvy, whereas iron deficiency is associated with a raised leucocyte ascorbate concentration. Vitamin C is needed for incorporation of iron from transferrin into ferritin and for iron mobilization from ferritin. Vitamin C therapy increases iron excretion in patients receiving subcutaneous desferrioxamine infusions and also, at least in experimental animals, affects iron distribution by increasing parenchymal relative to reticuloendothelial iron. Minimum adult daily requirements for vitamin C are about 10 mg but 30 to 70 mg is recommended; utilization and therefore requirement are relatively higher in infants, children, and pregnant and lactating women. Vitamin C may be excreted as such but is also broken down to oxalate.

Vitamin C is present in food as its reduced (ascorbic acid) and oxidized (dehydroascorbic acid) forms, the highest concentrations occurring in greens, fruits, tomatoes, liver, and kidney. Potatoes are not a rich source but provide a substantial proportion of normal dietary intake. Cooking, particularly in alkaline conditions with large volumes of water, destroys the vitamin, which is also lost on storage with exposure to the air. Absorption occurs through the length of the small intestine and deficiency is never solely due to malabsorption.

The anaemia of scurvy is typically normochromic, normocytic with a slightly raised reticulocyte count to 5 to 10 per cent and a normoblastic marrow with erythroid hyperplasia. This suggests a direct role for vitamin C in erythropoiesis but not all patients with clinical scurvy are anaemic. Extravascular haemolysis with mild jaundice and increased urobilinogen excretion occurs in many of the patients. Moreover, in many the anaemia is complicated by folate deficiency (due to inadequate folate intake) with a megaloblastic marrow, or in a few by iron deficiency due to external haemorrhage, reduced diet intake, and possibly reduced iron absorption. In a few patients placed on a low folate diet, response of megaloblastic haemopoiesis to vitamin C alone has been described. In others, response of the megaloblastic anaemia to folic acid alone on a low vitamin C diet has occurred but in most such cases, both vitamin C and folic acid have been found necessary.

VITAMIN B_6

This, involved as its coenzyme, forms pyridoxal-5-phosphate in many reactions of the body, especially for transaminases and decarboxylases. It is also a cofactor in the important rate-limiting reaction in haem synthesis, δ-aminolaevulinic acid (**ALA**)-synthetase (see Section 11). It occurs in natural tissues in three major forms, pyridoxine, pyridoxamine and pyridoxal phosphate. Red cells are capable of interconverting them. Anaemia due purely to vitamin B_6 deficiency has been produced in animals. It is hypochromic and microcytic with a raised serum iron and increased iron in erythroblasts, with some partial or complete ring sideroblasts. A similar anaemia has occurred in humans with malabsorption, pregnancy, or haemolysis but has not been fully documented to respond to physiological doses of vitamin B_6 alone. Vitamin B_6-responsive anaemia is, however, well documented among patients with sideroblastic anaemia of all types. Pyridoxine responses occur particularly in the inherited form (when it is assumed that a fault in one or other enzyme of haemo synthesis, e.g. ALA-synthetase, increases the need for pyridoxal phosphate as cofactor) and when sideroblastic anaemia occurs in patients receiving pyridoxine antagonists, such as antituberculous drugs.

RIBOFLAVIN

On the basis of studies in experimental animals and humans fed a deficient diet together with a riboflavin antagonist, deficiency of this vitamin is known to cause a normochromic, normocytic anaemia associated with a low reticulocyte count and red-cell aplasia in the marrow, sometimes with vacuolated normoblasts. The exact biochemical basis is undecided. Clinically a similar anaemia may occur in pure form but is usually associated with the anaemia due to protein deficiency as in kwashiorkor or marasmus. Other clinical features of riboflavin deficiency—dermatitis, angular cheilosis and glossitis for example—may be present.

THIAMINE

For discussion, see under megaloblastic anaemia not due to folate or B_{12} deficiency or metabolic defect.

NICOTINIC ACID, PANTOTHENIC ACID, AND NIACIN

Deficiencies of these vitamins cause anaemia in experimental animals but anaemia purely due to one or other of these deficiencies has not been established to occur in man.

VITAMIN E

This vitamin is needed for preventing peroxidation of cell membranes. A haemolytic anaemia responding to vitamin E has been reported in premature infants. Less well documented is a macrocytic anaemia due to vitamin E deficiency in protein–calorie-deficient infants and aggravation of anaemia in patients with thalassaemia major because of vitamin E deficiency (see Chapter 22.4.7).

PROTEIN DEFICIENCY (SEE SECTION 10)

Anaemia is usual in both 'pure' protein deficiency, kwashiorkor, and in protein–calorie malnutrition (marasmus). It has been reported in many parts of the world where malnutrition, especially in children and pregnant women, is common. The anaemia also occurs in patients with gastrointestinal disease and severe malabsorption. The anaemia is typically normochromic, normocytic, and of the order of 8.0 to 9.0 g/dl. The reticulocyte count is usually reduced and the marrow may show a selective reduction in erythropoiesis. Experimental studies in animals suggest that the anaemia is largely due to reduced serum erythropoietin levels consequent on a lack of stimulus for erythropoietin secretion. Lack of amino acids for synthesis of erythropoietin or globin is not the cause. In many patients, the anaemia is complicated by infection, folate or iron deficiency and possibly other vitamin deficiencies (e.g. riboflavin, vitamin E) and then it may be more severe and show additional morphological abnormalities in the blood and marrow.

REFERENCES

General

Beck, W.S. (1991). Diagnosis of megaloblastic anaemia. *Annual Review of Medicine*, **42**, 311–22.

Chanarin, I. (1989). *The megaloblastic anaemias*, (3rd edn). Blackwell Scientific, Oxford.

Chanarin, I., Deacon, R., Lumb, M., and Perry, J. (1992). Cobalamin and folate: recent developments. *Journal of Clinical Pathology*, **45**, 277–83.

Hoffbrand, A.V. (ed.) (1976). Megaloblastic anaemia. *Clinical Haematology*, **5**,(3).

Hoffbrand, A.V. and Jackson, B.F.A. (1993). Correction of the deoxyuridine suppression test in vitamin B_{12} deficiency with tetrahydrofolate: evidence in favour of the methyl folate trap hypothesis. *British Journal of Haematology*, **83**, 643–7.

Hoffbrand, A.V. and Wickremasinghe, R.G. (1982). Megaloblastic anaemia. In *Recent Advances in Haematology*, Vol. 3 (ed. A.V. Hoffbrand), pp. 25–44. Churchill Livingstone, Edinburgh.

Metz, J. (1983). The deoxyuridine suppression test. *CRC Critical Reviews of Clinical and Laboratory Science* **20**, 205–41.

Savage, D.G. and Lindenbaum, J. (1994). Folate–cobalamin interactions. In *Folate in Health and Disease*. (Ed. L. Baily) pp. 237–85. Marcel Decker, New York.

Savage, D.G., Lindenbaum, J., Stabler, S.P. and Allen, R.H. (1994). Similarities of serum methylmalonic acid and total homocysteine determinations for diagnosing cobalamin and folate deficiencies. *American Journal of Medicine*, **96**, 239–46.

Scott, J.M. and Weir, D.G. (1980). Drug-induced megaloblastic change. *Clinical Haematology*, **9**, 587–606.

Shorvon, S.D., Carney, M.W.P., Chanarin, I., and Reynolds, E.H. (1980). The neuropsychiatry of megaloblastic anaemia. *British Medical Journal*, **281**, 1036.

Wickremasinghe, S.N. and Fida, S. (1993). Misincorporation of uracil into the DNA of folate and B_{12} deficient HL60 cells. *European Journal of Haematology*, **50**, 127–32.

Vitamin B_{12}

Carmel, R. (1988). Pepsinogens and other serum markers in pernicious anaemia. *American Journal of Clinical Pathology*, **90**, 442–5.

Carmel, R. (1992). Reassessment of the relative prevalences of antibodies to gastric parietal cell and to intrinsic factor in patients with pernicious anaemia: influence of patient age and race. *Clinical and Experimental Immunology*, **89**, 74–7.

Carmel, R. *et al.* (1988). Cobalamin and osteoblast-specific proteins. *New England Journal of Medicine*, **319**, 70–5.

Carmel, R., Sinow, R.M., Siegal, M.E., and Samtoff, I.M. (1988). Food cobalamin malabsorption occurs frequently in patients with unexplained low serum cobalamin levels. *Annals of Internal Medicine*, **148**, 1715–19.

Chanarin, I. (1982). The effects of nitrous oxide on cobalamins, folates and on related events. *CRC Critical Review of Toxicology*, **10**, 179–213.

de Aizpunia, H.J., Ungar, B., and Toh, B.H. (1985). Autoantibody to the gastrin receptor in pernicious anaemia. *New England Journal of Medicine*, **313**, 479–83.

Dieckgrafe, B.K. *et al.* (1988). Isolation and structural characterisation of a cDNA clone encoding rat gastric intrinsic factor. *Proceedings of the National Academy of Sciences (USA)*, **85**, 46–50.

Doscherholmen, A., Silvis, S., and McHahon, J. (1983). Dual isotope Schilling test for measuring absorption of food bound and free vitamin B_{12} simultaneously. *American Journal of Clinical Pathology*, **80**, 490–5.

Fish, D.T. and Dawson, D.W. (1983). Comparison of methods used in commercial kits for the assay of serum vitamin B_{12}. *Clinical and Laboratory Haematology*, **5**, 271–7.

Gleeson, P.A. and Toh, B.H. (1991). Molecular targets in pernicious anaemia. *Immunology Today*, **12**, 233–8.

Graham, S.M., Aruela, O.M., and Wise, G.A. (1992). Long-term neurologic consequences of nutritional vitamin B_{12} deficiency in infants. *Journal of Paediatrics*, **121**, 710–14.

Hall, C.A. (ed.) (1983). *The cobalamins: Methods in hematology*. Churchill Livinginstone, Edinburgh.

Healton, E.B., Savage, D.G., and Brust, J.C.M. (1991). Neurologic aspects of cobalamin deficiency. *Medicine*, **70**, 229–45.

Hoffbrand, A.V. (1983). Pernicious anaemia. *Scottish Medical Journal*, **28**, 218–27.

Kapadia, C.R. and Donaldson, R.M. (1985). Disorders of cobalamin (vitamin B_{12}) absorption and transport. *Annual Review of Medicine*, **36**, 93–110.

Karlsson, F.A., Burman, P., Loof, L., and Mardh, S. (1988). Major parietal cell antigen in autoimmune gastritis with pernicious anaemia is the acid producing H^+, K^+ adenosine triphosphatase of the stomach. *Journal of Clinical Investigation*, **81**, 475–9.

Kondo, H., Kolhouse, J.F., and Allen, R.H. (1980). Presence of cobalamin analogues in animal tissues. *Proceedings of the National Academy of Sciences (USA)*, **77**, 817–21.

Kuovonen, I. and Grasbeck, R. (1981). Topology of the hog intrinsic factor receptor in the intestine. *Journal of Biological Chemistry*, **256**, 154–8.

Lindenbaum, J.L. *et al.* (1988). Neuropsychiatric disorders caused by cobalamin deficiency in the absence of anaemia or macrocytes. *New England Journal of Medicine*, **319**, 1720–8.

Narayannan, M.N., Dawson, D.W., and Lewis, M.J. (1991). Dietary deficiency of vitamin B_{12} is associated with low serum cobalamin levels in non-vegetarians. *European Journal of Haematology*, **47**, 115–18.

Platica, O. *et al.* (1991). The cDNA sequence and the deduced amino acid sequence of human transcobalamin II show homology with rat intrinsic factor and human transcobalamin I. *Journal of Biological Chemistry*, **286**, 7860–3.

Remacha, A.F., Riera, A., Cadafalch, J., and Grimferrer, E. (1991). Vitamin B_{12} abnormalities in HIV-infected patients. *European Journal of Haematology*, **47**, 60–4.

Schilling, R.F. (1986). Is nitrous oxide a dangerous anaesthetic for vitamin B_{12} deficient subjects? *Journal of the American Medical Society*, **255**, 1605–6.

Stabler, S.P., Allen, R.H., Savage, D.G., and Lindenbaum, J. (1990). Clinical spectrum and diagnosis of cobalamin deficiency. *Blood*, **76**, 871–81.

Sweeney, B. *et al.* (1985). Toxicity of bone marrow in dentists exposed to nitrous oxide. *British Medical Journal*, **291**, 567–9.

Viera-Makings, E. *et al.* (1990). Cobalamin neuropathy: is 5-adenosylhomocysteine toxicity a factor? *Biochemical Journal*, **266**, 707–11.

Waters, H.M., Dawson, D.W., Howarth, J.E., and Geary, G.C. (1993). High incidence of type II antibodies in pernicious anaemia. *Journal of Clinical Pathology*, **46**, 45–7.

Weir, D.G. *et al.* (1988). Methylation deficiency causes vitamin B_{12}-associated neuropathy in the pig. *Journal of Neurochemistry*, **51**, 1949–52.

Wickremasinghe, S.N. and Mathews, J.H. (1988). Deoxyuridine suppression: biochemical basis and diagnostic applications. *Blood Reviews*, **2**, 168–77.

Folate

Antony, A.C. (1992). The biological chemistry of folate receptors. *Blood*, **79**, 2807–20.

Bailey, L. (ed) (1994). *Folate in Health and Disease*. Marcel Decker, New York.

Crellin, R., Bottiglieri, C.R., and Reynolds, E.A. (1993). Folates and psychiatric disorders: clinical potential. *Drugs*, **45**, 623–36.

Mills, J.L., *et al.* (1995). Homocysteine metabolism in pregnancies complicated by neural-tube defects. *Lancet*, **345**, 149.

MRC Vitamin Study Group (1991). Prevention of neural tube defects: results of Medical Research Council Vitamin Study. *Lancet*, **238**, 131–7.

Rosenblatt, D.S. (1989). Inherited disorders of folate transport and metabolism. In *The metabolic basis of inherited disease*, (6th edn) (ed. C.R. Scriver, A.L. Beaudet, W.S. Sly, and D. Valle) pp. 2049–64. McGraw Hill, New York.

Shane, B. (1989). Folypolyglutamate synthesis and role in the regulation of one-carbon metabolism. *Vitamins and Hormones*, **45**, 263–335.

Miscellaneous

Adams, E.B. (1970). Anemia associated with protein deficiency. *Seminars in Hematology*, **7**, 55–66.

Cox, E.V. (1968). The anaemia of scurvy. *Vitamins and Hormones*, **26**, 635–52.

Hillman, R.S. and Steinberg, S.E. (1982). The effects of alcohol on folate metabolism. *Annual Review of Medicine*, **33**, 345–54.

Rindi, G., *et al.* (1994). Further studies of erythrocyte thiamin transport and phosphorylation in seven patients with thiamin-responsive megaloblastic anaemia. *Journal of Inherited Metabolic Diseases*, **17**, 667.

22.4.7 Disorders of the synthesis or function of haemoglobin

D. J. WEATHERALL

Disorders of the synthesis or structure of haemoglobin may be either inherited or acquired. The inherited disorders of haemoglobin are the most common single-gene disorders in the world population. The World Health Organization has estimated that approximately 7 per cent of the world's population are carriers for important haemoglobin disorders. In many of the developing countries, where there is still a very high mortality from infection and malnutrition in the first year of life, these conditions are not yet recognized as an important public health problem. However, once economic conditions improve and infant death rates fall, the genetic disorders of haemoglobin start to place a major burden on the health services. This phenomenon has already been observed in parts of the Mediterranean region and South-East Asia.

As a result of mass migrations of populations from high incidence areas of the haemoglobin disorders these conditions are being seen with increasing frequency in parts of the world where they have not been recognized previously. Because some of them, particularly sickle-cell anaemia and the more severe forms of thalassaemia, can produce life-threatening medical emergencies, it is important for clinicians to have at least a working knowledge of their clinical features, management, and prevention.

The other reason why the haemoglobin disorders have become of particular interest in recent years is that they were the first group of diseases to be analysed by the new methods of recombinant DNA technology. More is known about their molecular pathology than any other genetic disorders and it is likely that their study has already given us a good idea of the overall repertoire of mutations that underlie human inherited diseases.

The World Health Organization has estimated that approximately 7 per cent of the world's population are carriers for important haemoglobin disorders.

The structure, genetic control, and synthesis of haemoglobin

STRUCTURE

Human haemoglobin is heterogeneous at all stages of development; different haemoglobins are synthesized in the embryo, fetus, and adult, each adapted to the particular oxygen requirements of these changing environments.

The human haemoglobins all have a tetrameric structure made up of two different pairs of globin chains, each attached to one haem molecule (Fig. 1). The reasons for this complex structure were considered earlier in this section (Chapter 22.4.1). Adult and fetal haemoglobins have α-chains combined with β-chains (Hb A, $\alpha_2\beta_2$), δ-chains (Hb A$_2$, $\alpha_2+\delta_2$)

or γ-chains (Hb F, $\alpha_2\gamma_2$). In embryos, α-like chains called ζ-chains combine with γ-chains to produce Hb Portland ($\zeta_2\gamma_2$), or with ϵ-chains to make Hb Gower 1 ($\zeta_2\epsilon_2$), and α- and ϵ-chains combine to form Hb Gower 2 ($\alpha_2\epsilon_2$). Fetal haemoglobin is itself heterogeneous; there are two kinds of γ-chains, which differ in their amino acid composition at position 136 where they have either a glycine or an alanine residue; those with glycine are called $^G\gamma$ chains, those with alanine $^A\gamma$. The $^G\gamma$ and $^A\gamma$ chains are the product of separate ($^G\gamma$ and $^A\gamma$) loci.

GENETIC CONTROL

The arrangement of the two main families of globin genes is illustrated in Fig. 2. The β-like globin genes form a linked cluster on chromosome 11, which is spread over approximately 60 kb (kb = kilobase or one thousand nucleotide bases); they are arranged in the order $5'—\epsilon—^G\gamma—^A\gamma—\psi\beta—\delta—\beta—3'$. The α-like globin genes also form a linked cluster, in this case on chromosome 16, in the order $5'\zeta2—\psi\zeta1—\psi\alpha2—\psi\alpha1—\alpha2—\alpha1—3'$. The $\psi\beta$, $\psi\zeta$, and $\psi\alpha$ genes are pseudogenes, that is, they have sequences which resemble the β, ζ or α genes but contain mutations that prevent them from functioning as structural genes. They may be 'burnt out' remnants of genes that were functional at an earlier stage of evolution.

Some of the important structural aspects of the globin genes and their flanking sequences are illustrated in Figs 2 and 3. Like most mammalian genes they have one or more non-coding inserts called intervening sequences (IVS) or introns at the same position along their length. The non-α globin genes contain two introns of 122 to 130 and 850 to 900 bp between codons 30 and 31 and 104 and 105, respectively. Similar though smaller introns are found in the α- and ζ-globin genes. At the $5'$ non-coding (flanking) regions of the globin genes there are several blocks of nucleotide homology that are found in analogous positions in

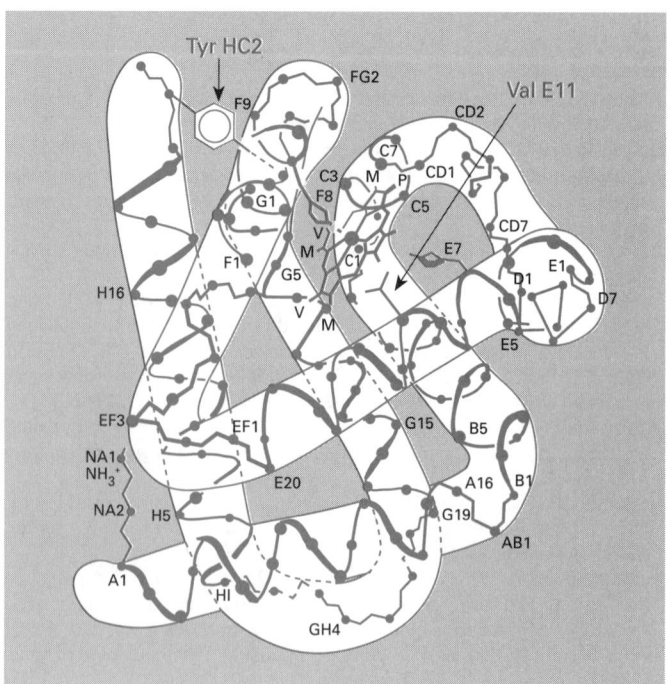

Fig. 1 The α-chain subunit of human haemoglobin showing the position of the haem molecule in a cleft formed by the globin chain. The helical parts of the chain are given letters of the alphabet and each amino acid residue in each helical region has a specific number, e.g. val E11 is the eleventh amino acid in the E helical region. The non-helical regions of the amino- and carboxyl-terminal ends of the chains are labelled NA and HC respectively. (Reproduced by permission of Dr M.F. Perutz and the Editors of the Cold Spring Harbor Symposia for Quantitative Biology.)

many species. One is AG-rich and is called the Hogness box. Another, called the CCAAT box, is found about 70 bp upstream (to the left) from the 5' end of the genes. These and other sequences are involved in the initiation of transcription and hence play an important part in the regulation of the structural genes. As we shall see later, mutations in these regions can reduce the output of the related genes. At the 3' non-coding regions of all the globin genes there is a sequence AATAAA (Fig. 3) which is believed to be the signal for polyA addition to RNA transcripts; we shall discuss the significance of this when we consider the disorders of globin-chain synthesis.

SYNTHESIS

The synthesis of a globin chain follows the same pattern as any protein (Fig. 3). There is a flow of information from the DNA of the structural gene through an intermediary, a form of RNA called messenger RNA (**mRNA**), to the cell cytoplasm where protein chains are assembled on a mRNA template, which is a mirror image of the gene from which it was transcribed. When a globin gene is to be transcribed a mRNA molecule is synthesized from one of its strands by the action of an enzyme called RNA polymerase. The primary transcript of the globin genes is a large mRNA precursor molecule, which contains both introns and coding regions (exons). While in the nucleus this molecule undergoes a number of modifications (Fig. 3). First, the introns are removed and the exons are spliced together. It should be noted that the exon/intron junctions always have the sequence GT at their 5' end, and AG at their 3' end. This appears to be essential for accurate splicing and, as we shall see later, if there is a mutation in these sites normal splicing cannot occur. The mRNAs are modified at their 5' end, by the addition of a CAP structure, and at their 3' end by the addition of a string of adenylic acid residues (polyA). The processed mRNA now moves into the cytoplasm to act as a template for globin-chain production. The mechanisms of globin chain synthesis in the cytoplasm are described in Section 5. Individual globin chains combine with haem, which is synthesized through a separate pathway, and with themselves to form definitive haemoglobin molecules. Very little is known about the way in which the globin genes are regulated or switched on and off during development. Control seems to be mediated mainly at the transcriptional level with some fine tuning during translation.

Classification of the disorders of haemoglobin

The main groups of disorders of haemoglobin are shown in Table 1. The genetic disorders are divided into those in which there is a reduced rate of production of one or more of the globin chains, the thalassaemias, and those in which there is a structural change in a globin chain leading to instability or abnormal oxygen transport. In addition, there is a harmless group of mutations that interfere with the normal switching of fetal to adult haemoglobin production; these conditions are known collec-

Table 1 *Disorders of haemoglobin*

Genetic
Thalassaemia
Structural variants
Hereditary persistence of fetal haemoglobin
Acquired
Methaemoglobin
Carbonmonoxyhaemoglobin
Sulphaemoglobin
Defective synthesis:
Haemoglobin H/leukaemia
Other neoplastic disorders

tively as hereditary persistence of fetal haemoglobin. Although of no clinical significance, they are important models for studying the regulation of gene switching during development. The acquired disorders of haemoglobin can also be subdivided into those characterized by defective synthesis of the globin chain and those in which the structure of the haem molecules is altered, leading to inefficient oxygen transport.

The thalassaemias

HISTORICAL INTRODUCTION

Thalassaemia was first recognized in 1925 by a Detroit paediatrician called Thomas B. Cooley who described a series of infants who became profoundly anaemic and developed splenomegaly over the first year of life. Subsequently, further cases were identified and the disorder was variously called von Jaksch's anaemia, splenic anaemia, erythroblastosis, Mediterranean anaemia, or Cooley's anaemia. However, in 1936 George Whipple and Lesley Bradford, in describing the pathological changes of the condition for the first time, recognized that many of their patients came from the Mediterranean region and hence they invented the word 'thalassaemia' from the Greek θαλασσα, meaning 'the sea'. Although more recently it has been realized that the disorder occurs throughout the world and is not localized to the Mediterranean region, the name has stuck.

During the last 10 years it has become clear that thalassaemia is extremely heterogeneous and that its clinical picture can result from the interaction of many different genetic defects.

DEFINITION AND CLASSIFICATION

The thalassaemias are a heterogeneous group of genetic disorders of haemoglobin synthesis, all of which result from a reduced rate of production of one or more of the globin chain(s) of haemoglobin. They are divided into the α-, β-, δβ- or γδβ-thalassaemias according to which

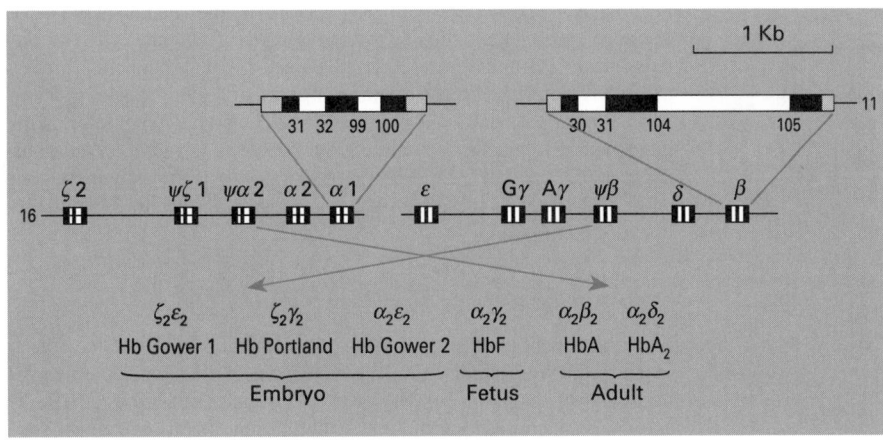

Fig. 2 The genetic control of human haemoglobin. Two of the genes are enlarged to show the introns (unshaded) and exons (dark staining). Kb = 1000 nucleotide bases.

globin chain(s) is produced in reduced amounts (Table 2). In some thalassaemias no globin chain is synthesized at all, and hence they are called α°- or β°-thalassaemias, whereas in others some globin chain is produced but at a reduced rate; the latter conditions are called α^+- or β^+-thalassaemias. The $\delta\beta$- and $\gamma\delta\beta$-thalassaemias are always characterized by an absence of chain synthesis; thus they are $(\delta\beta)^\circ$- and $(\gamma\delta\beta)^\circ$-thalassaemias. Because thalassaemia occurs in populations in which structural haemoglobin variants are common, it is not at all unusual for an individual to receive a thalassaemia gene from one parent and a gene for a structural haemoglobin variant from the other. Furthermore, both α- and β-thalassaemia occur commonly in some countries and hence individuals may receive genes for both types. These different interactions produce an extremely complex and clinically diverse series of genetic disorders, which range in severity from death *in utero* to extremely mild, symptomless, hypochromic anaemias.

The thalassaemias are inherited in a simple Mendelian codominant fashion. Heterozygotes are usually symptomless, although they can be easily recognized by simple haematological analysis. More severely affected patients are either homozygotes for α- or β-thalassaemia, compound heterozygotes for different molecular forms of α- or β-thalassaemia, or compound heterozygotes for one or other form of thalassaemia and a gene for a structural haemoglobin variant. Clinically, the thalassaemias are classified according to their severity into major, intermediate, and minor forms. Thalassaemia major is a severe transfusion dependent disorder. Thalassaemia intermedia is characterized by anaemia and splenomegaly though not of such severity as to require regular transfusion. Thalassaemia minor is the symptomless carrier state. While these descriptive terms do not have a precise genetic meaning, they remain useful in clinical practice.

The β-thalassaemias

The β-thalassaemias are the most important types of thalassaemia because they are so common and produce severe anaemia in their homozygous and compound heterozygous states (Table 3).

Fig. 3 Globin gene structure, mRNA processing, and globin synthesis. Each of the structures and steps illustrated is described in the text and in Section 5.

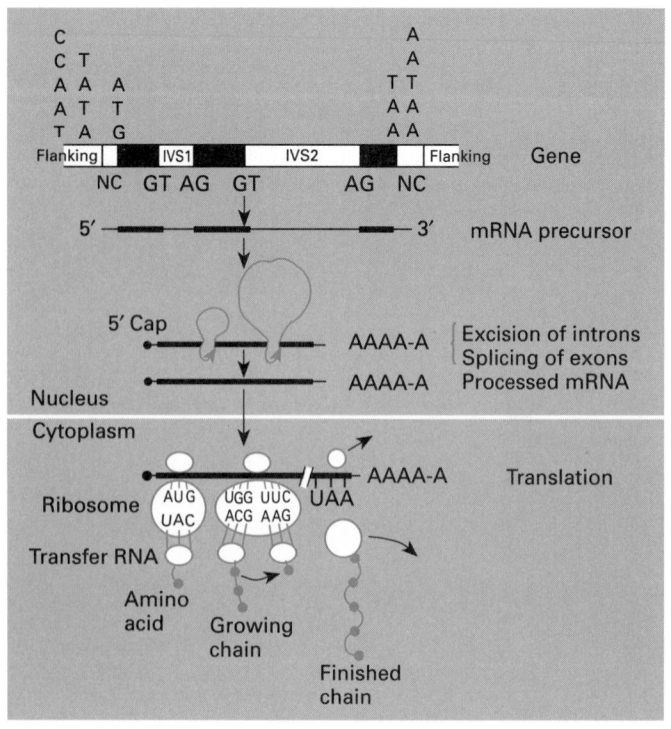

Table 2 *The thalassaemias*

α-Thalassaemia
  α°
  α^+
β-Thalassaemia
  β°
  β^+
$\delta\beta$-Thalassaemia
  $(\delta\beta)^\circ$
  Haemoglobin Lepore $(\delta\beta)^+$
$(\epsilon\gamma\delta\beta)^\circ$-Thalassaemia
δ-Thalassaemia

Table 3 *The β-, $\delta\beta$-, and $\gamma\delta\beta$-thalassaemias*

Type of thalassaemia	Findings in homozygote	Findings in heterozygote
β°	Thalassaemia major[1,2] Hbs F and A_2	Thalassaemia minor Raised Hb A_2
β^+	Thalassaemia major[1,2] Hbs F, A and A_2	Thalassaemia minor Raised Hb A_2
$\delta\beta$	Thalassaemia intermedia Hb F only	Thalassaemia minor Hb F 5–15 %; Hb A_2 normal
$(\delta\beta)^+$ (Lepore)	Thalassaemia major or intermedia Hbs F and Lepore	Thalassaemia minor Hb Lepore 5–15 %; Hb A_2 normal
$\epsilon\gamma\delta\beta$	Not viable	Neonatal haemolysis Thalassaemia minor in adults, with normal Hbs F and A_2

[1]Occasionally have thalassaemia intermedia phenotype.

[2]Many patients with thalassaemia are compound heterozygotes for different molecular forms of β° or β^+ thalassaemia.

DISTRIBUTION

The β-thalassaemias occur widely in a broad belt ranging from the Mediterranean and parts of north and west Africa through the Middle East and Indian subcontinent to South-East Asia. The high-incidence zone stretches north through Yugoslavia and Romania and the southern parts of Russia and includes the southern regions of the People's Republic of China. The disease is particularly common in South-East Asia where it occurs in a line starting in southern China and stretching down through Thailand and the Malay peninsula through Indonesia to some of the Pacific island populations. In these populations, and in some of the Mediterranean island and mainland countries, carrier frequencies for the various forms of β-thalassaemia range between 2 and 30 per cent. In many of these regions the β-thalassaemias cause a major public health problem and a drain on medical resources; this will become even greater as the incidence of infant or early childhood death due to infection and malnutrition declines. It should be remembered that β-thalassaemia is not entirely confined to these high incidence regions; it occurs sporadically in every racial group.

MOLECULAR PATHOLOGY

The β-globin genes from many patients with β-thalassaemia have been sequenced, and the molecular lesions responsible for the defective synthesis of the β-globin chains have been determined. The disease is extremely heterogeneous and over 100 different mutations can produce the clinical phenotype of β-thalassaemia. Some of these lesions completely inactivate the β-globin genes leading to the phenotype of β°-thalassaemia; others cause a reduced output from the genes and hence the picture of β⁺-thalassaemia.

The main classes of mutations that cause β-thalassaemia are summarized in Fig. 4. Long deletions are rare, and most of them are single-base changes or small deletions or insertions of one or two bases at various points in the genes. As shown in Fig. 4 they occur in both introns and exons, and also in the flanking regions. Some of the exon substitutions are nonsense mutations, i.e. a single-base change in a codon produces a stop codon in the middle of the coding part of the mRNA (Fig. 5a). This causes premature termination of globin-chain synthesis and hence leads to the production of a shortened and non-viable β-globin chain. Other exon mutations result in frameshifts; that is, one or more bases are lost or inserted and the 'reading frame' of the genetic code beyond the lesion is thrown out of phase (Fig. 5b). Several mutations have been described, either within introns or at intron/exon junctions, that interfere with the mechanism of splicing the exons together after the introns have been removed during the processing of the mRNA

precursor. Single-base substitutions at the intron/exon junctions prevent splicing altogether and result in the phenotype of β°-thalassaemia. Some intron mutations produce alternative splicing sites so that both normal and abnormal mRNA species are produced (Fig. 6). An incorrectly spliced mRNA is non-functional because it contains intron sequences; in some cases a nonsense mutation or frameshift is generated. Thus, the mRNA cannot act as a template for the synthesis of a normal globin chain.

Single-base substitutions have also been found in the flanking regions of the β-globin genes. Two are in the ATA box and others are further upstream, about 80–90 bases from the initiation codon. It seems likely that these mutations are in the regulatory regions involved in the initiation of transcription of the β-globin genes.

Because there are so many different β-thalassaemia mutations it follows that many patients who are apparently homozygous for β-thalassaemia are, in fact, compound heterozygotes for two different molecular lesions.

PATHOPHYSIOLOGY

The molecular defects in the β-thalassaemia result in absent or reduced β-chain production. α-chain synthesis proceeds at a normal rate and hence there is imbalanced globin-chain synthesis with the production of an excess of α-chains (Fig. 7). In the absence of their partner chains the α-chains are unstable and precipitate in the red-cell precursors, giving rise to large intracellular inclusions. These interfere with red-cell maturation, and hence there is a variable degree of intramedullary destruction of red-cell precursors, i.e. ineffective erythropoiesis. Those red cells that do mature and enter the circulation contain α-chain inclusions which interfere with their passage through the microcirculation, particularly in

Fig. 4 Some of the mutations that produce β-thalassaemia. The β-globin gene is divided into three exons (hatched) and two introns (IVS; unshaded). The different deletions are shown at the top of the figure while below the general position of the different point mutations is represented. PR, promoter; C, CAP site; I, initiation site; FS, frameshift; NS, nonsense; SPL, splice-site mutation; polyA, RNA cleavage and polyA addition site.

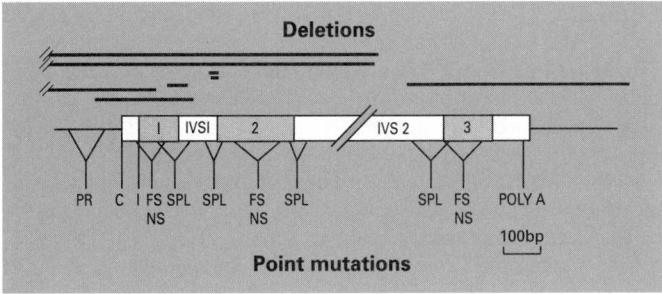

Fig. 6 A representation of the consequences of different splice-site mutations. In β°-thalassaemia two different mutations are shown, one that inactivates the normal splice site, and another that produces a new splice site. Two abnormal mRNA molecules are produced. In the β⁺-Thalassaemia case a new splice site is produced in the first intron. Both normal and abnormal mRNAs are produced, the latter in greater amounts.

Fig. 5 Point mutations that cause β°-thalassaemia: (a) premature stop codon (nonsense mutation); (b) frameshift mutation. See text for further details.

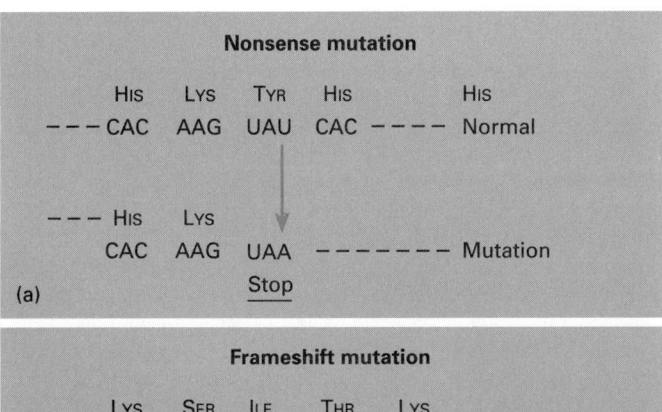

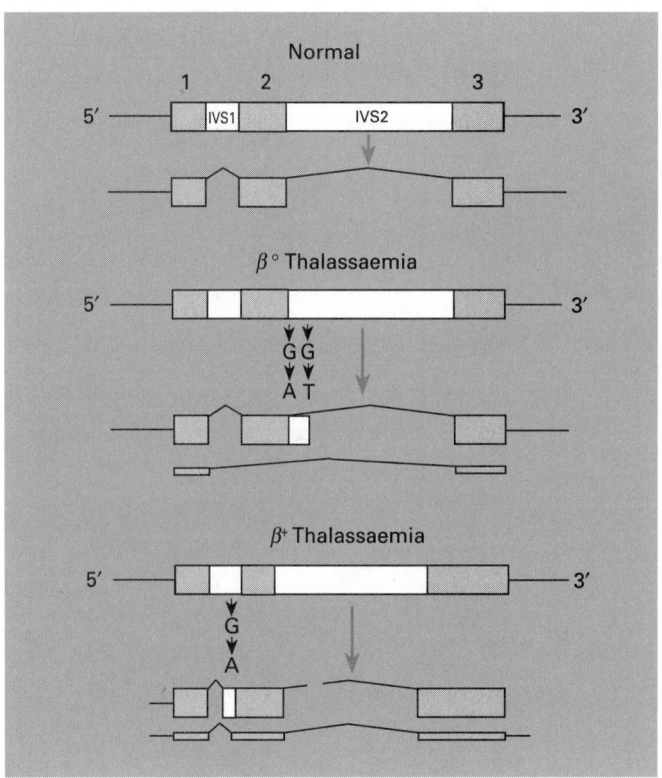

the spleen. These cells are prematurely destroyed and thus the anaemia of β-thalassaemia results from both ineffective erythropoiesis and a shortened red-cell survival. The anaemia is a stimulus to increased erythropoietin production from the kidneys and this causes massive expansion of the bone marrow, which may lead to serious deformities of the skull and long bones. Because the spleen is being constantly bombarded with abnormal red cells, it hypertrophies and the resulting splenomegaly causes an increase of the plasma volume, which contributes to the anaemia.

As mentioned previously, fetal haemoglobin production largely ceases after birth. However, some adult red-cell precursors (F cells) retain the ability to produce a small number of γ-chains. Because the latter can combine with excess α-chains to form haemoglobin F, cells that make relatively more γ-chains in the bone marrow of β-thalassaemics are partly protected against the deleterious effect of α-chain precipitation. Because these cells have a selective survival advantage they appear in the blood and hence a raised fetal haemoglobin level is characteristic of all the β-thalassaemias. Furthermore, because δ-chain synthesis is unaffected, the disorder is characterized by a relative or absolute increase in haemoglobin A_2 ($\alpha_2\delta_2$) production. These interactions are summarized in Fig. 7.

It follows that if the anaemia is corrected with blood transfusion the erythropoietic drive is shut off, growth and development are normal, and bone deformities do not occur. On the other hand, each unit of blood contains 200 mg of iron; with regular transfusion there is a steady accu-

Fig. 7 The pathophysiology of β-thalassaemia.

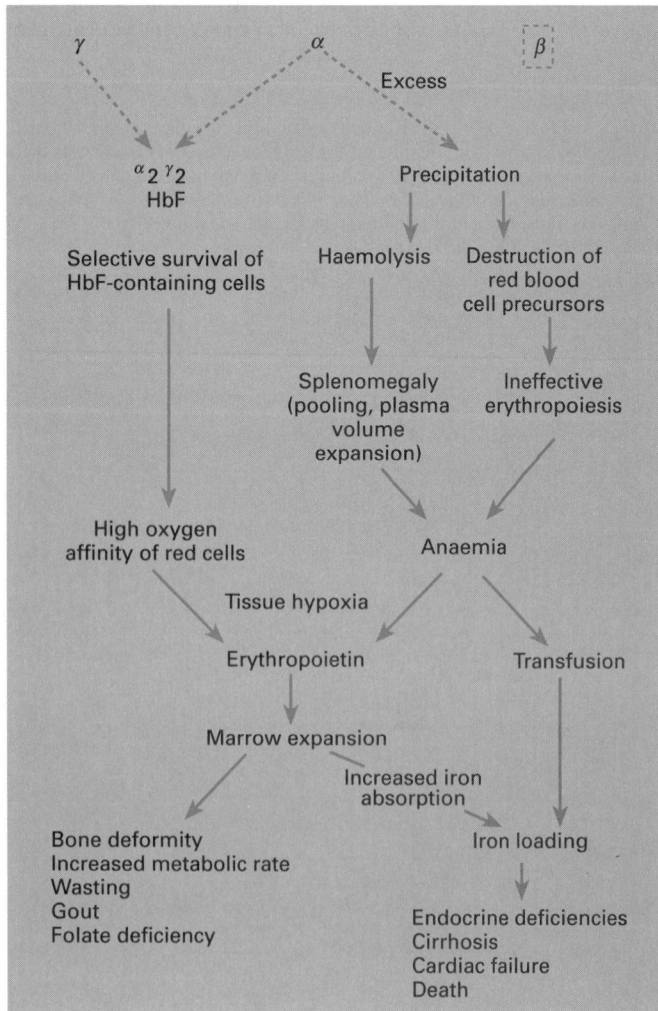

mulation of iron in the liver, endocrine glands, and myocardium. Thus, although well-transfused thalassaemic children grow and develop normally, they die of iron overload unless steps are taken to remove iron.

The severe homozygous or compound heterozygous forms of β-thalassaemia

These are the most common and most important forms of thalassaemia and give rise to a major public health problem in many parts of the world.

CLINICAL FEATURES

Most severe forms of β-thalassaemia present within the first year of life with failure to thrive, poor feeding, intermittent bouts of fever, or failure to improve after an intercurrent infection. At this stage the affected infant looks pale, and in many cases splenomegaly is already present. There are no other specific clinical signs and the diagnosis depends on the haematological changes outlined below. If the infant is put on a regular blood-transfusion regimen at this stage, early development is normal and further symptoms do not occur until puberty, when the effects of iron loading due to repeated blood transfusion start to appear. If, on the other hand, the infant is not adequately transfused, the typical clinical picture of homozygous β-thalassaemia develops. Thus the clinical manifestations of the severe forms of β-thalassaemia have to be described in two contexts, the well-transfused child, and the child with chronic anaemia throughout early life.

In the well-transfused thalassaemic child, early growth and development is normal and splenomegaly is minimal. However, there is a gradual accumulation of iron and the effects of tissue siderosis start to appear by the end of the first decade. The normal adolescent growth spurt fails to occur and hepatic, endocrine, and cardiac complications of iron overloading produce a variety of problems including diabetes, hypoparathyroidism, adrenal insufficiency, and liver failure. Secondary sexual development is delayed, or does not occur at all. The short stature and lack of sexual development may lead to serious psychological problems. By far the most common cause of death, which usually occurs toward the end of the second or early in the third decade, is progressive cardiac damage. Ultimately these patients die either with protracted cardiac failure or suddenly due to an acute arrhythmia. The use of intensive chelation therapy may prevent or delay this distressing termination.

The clinical picture in children who are inadequately transfused is quite different. Early childhood is interspersed with a series of distressing complications and the overall rates of growth and development are retarded. There is progressive splenomegaly, and hypersplenism may cause a worsening of the anaemia, sometimes associated with thrombocytopenia and a bleeding tendency. Because of the bone marrow expansion there may be hideous deformities of the skull, with marked bossing and overgrowth of the zygomata giving rise to the classical mongoloid facies of β-thalassaemia (Fig. 8a). These changes are reflected by striking radiological changes, which include a lacy, trabecular pattern of the long bones and phalanges and a typical 'hair on end' appearance of the skull (Fig. 9). These bone changes may be associated with recurrent fractures. There is an increased proneness to infection, which may cause a catastrophic drop in the haemoglobin level. Because of the massive marrow expansion resulting from the chronic anaemia, these children are hypermetabolic, run intermittent fevers, lose weight (Fig. 8b), have increased requirements for folic acid, and may become acutely folate depleted with worsening of their anaemia. Because of the increased turnover of red cell precursors, hyperuricaemia and secondary gout occur occasionally. There is a bleeding tendency, which, although partly due to thrombocytopenia secondary to hypersplenism, may also be exacerbated by liver damage associated with iron loading and extra-

Fig. 8 Homozygous β-thalassaemia: (a) skull and facial deformity due to bone marrow expansion; (b) gross wasting of the limbs and hepatomegaly in an undertransfused child.

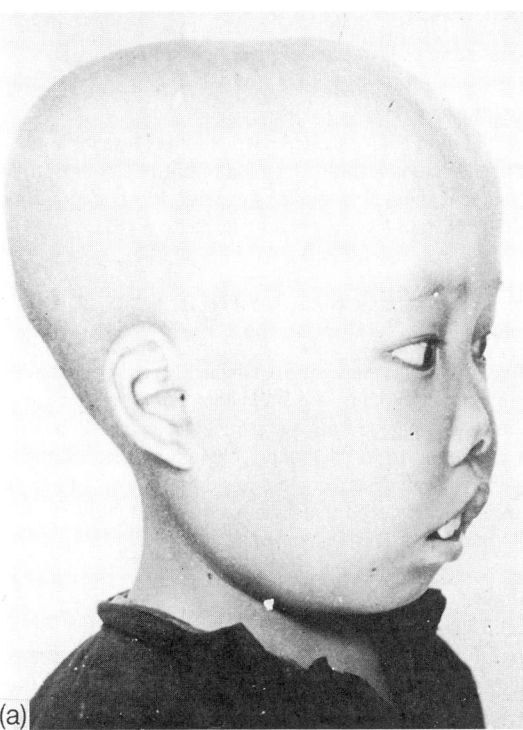

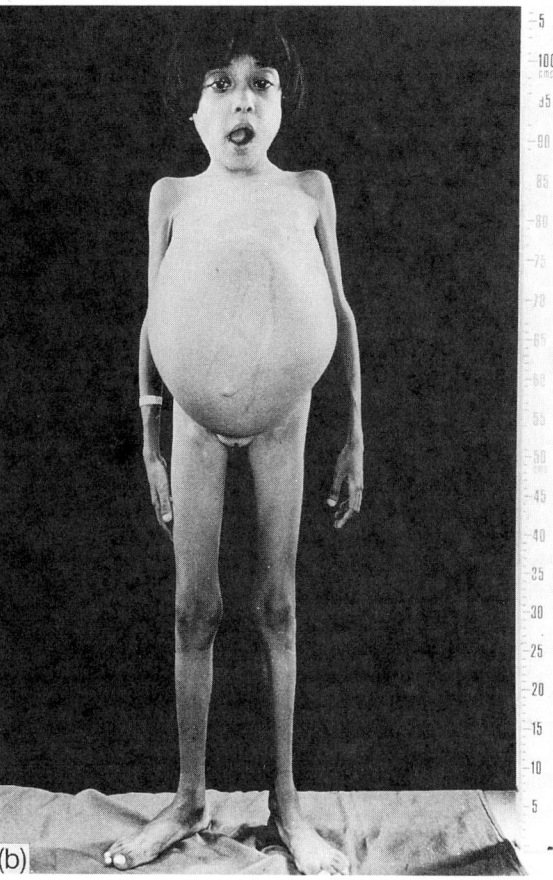

medullary haemopoiesis. Because of the bone deformities of the skull, there may be distressing dental complications, with poorly formed teeth and malocclusion, and inadequate drainage of the sinuses and middle ear may lead to chronic sinus infection and deafness. If these children survive to puberty, they develop the same complications of iron loading as the well-transfused patients. In this case some of the iron accumulation results from an increased rate of gastrointestinal absorption as well as that derived from the inadequate transfusion regimen.

The prognosis for poorly transfused thalassaemic children is bad. If they receive no transfusions at all they die within the first 2 years, and if kept at a low haemoglobin level throughout early childhood, they usually succumb to an overwhelming infection. As already mentioned, if they reach puberty, they die of the effects of iron accumulation with acute or chronic cardiac failure of the same type as occurs in the well-transfused child.

Haematological changes

There is severe anaemia and the haemoglobin values on presentation range from 2 to 8 g/dl. Although the red cells are hypochromic and microcytic, the red-cell indices, as derived from an electronic cell counter, may give surprisingly normal results, although usually the mean corpuscular haemoglobin and volume (**MCH, MCV**) are reduced. The appearance of the stained peripheral blood film is grossly abnormal (Fig. 10). The red cells show marked hypochromia and variation in shape and size. There are many hypochromic macrocytes and misshapen microcytes, some of which are mere fragments of cells. There is a moderate degree of anisochromia and basophilic stippling. There are always some nucleated red cells in the peripheral blood and, after splenectomy, these are found in large numbers. In the post-splenectomy film many of the nucleated cells and mature erythrocytes show ragged inclusions after incubation of the blood with methyl violet. There is usually a slight elevation in the reticulocyte count. The white-cell and platelet counts are normal unless there is hypersplenism when they are reduced. The bone marrow shows marked erythroid hyperplasia with a myeloid/erythroid (M/E) ratio of unity or less. Many of the red cell precursors show ragged inclusions after incubation of the marrow with methyl violet.

There are biochemical changes of increased haemolysis and progressive iron loading. The bilirubin level is usually elevated and haptoglobins are absent. The ^{51}Cr red-cell survival is shortened. The serum iron

Fig. 9 Radiological changes of the skull in homozygous β-thalassaemia.

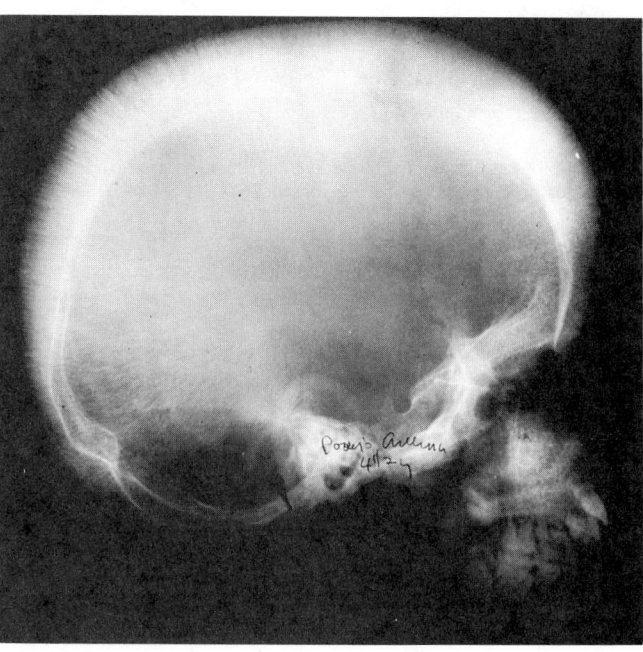

rises progressively and most transfusion-dependent children have a totally saturated iron-binding capacity. This change is mirrored by a high plasma ferritin level, and liver biopsies show a marked increase in iron both in the reticuloendothelial and parenchymal cells (Fig. 11).

Other biochemical changes

Many thalassaemic children are vitamin E and ascorbate depleted. Folic acid deficiency has already been mentioned. Frank diabetes may develop and endocrine function tests may reveal parathyroid or adrenal insufficiency, or inappropriate response by the pituitary to various release hormones; growth hormone levels are usually normal.

Haemoglobin changes (see Table 3)

The haemoglobin F level is always elevated. In β°-thalassaemia there is no haemoglobin A and the haemoglobin consists of F and A_2 only. In β^{+}-thalassaemia the level of haemoglobin F ranges from 30 to 90 per cent of the total haemoglobin. The haemoglobin A_2 level is usually normal and is of no diagnostic value.

HETEROZYGOUS B-THALASSAEMIA

Carriers for β-thalassaemia are usually symptom free except in periods of stress such as pregnancy when they may become anaemic. Splenomegaly is rarely present.

Fig. 10 Peripheral blood film in homozygous β-thalassaemia ($\times 630$, Leishman stain).

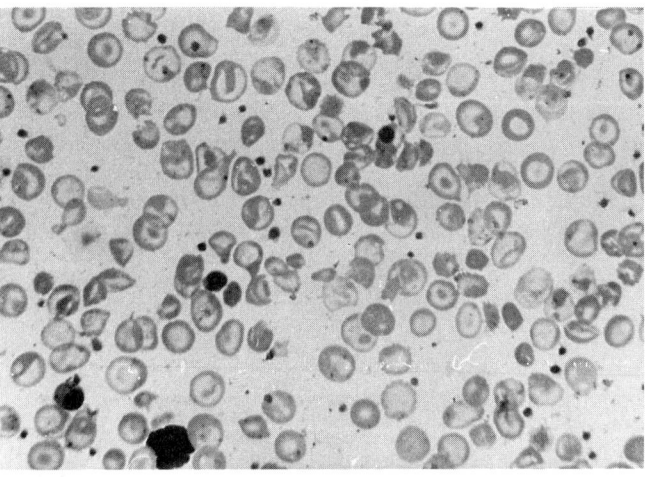

Fig. 11 Histological appearances of the liver in homozygous β-thalassaemia showing gross iron deposition ($\times 270$, iron stain).

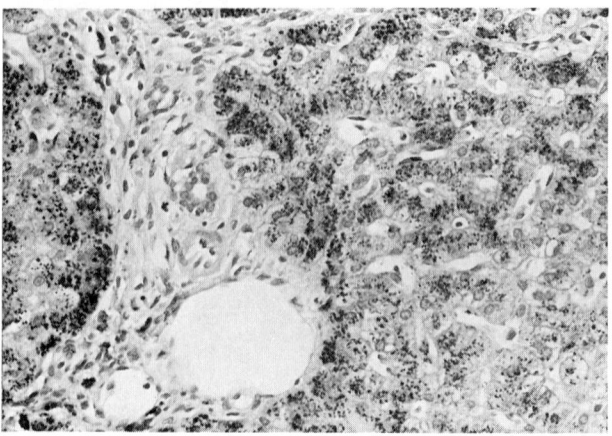

Haematological changes

There is mild anaemia with haemoglobin values in the 9 to 11 g/dl range. The red cells show hypochromia and microcytosis with characteristically low MCH and MCV values. The reticulocyte count is usually normal. The bone marrow shows moderate erythroid hyperplasia.

Haemoglobin changes

The characteristic finding is an elevated haemoglobin A_2 level in the 4 to 6 per cent range. There is a slight elevation of haemoglobin F in the 1 to 3 per cent range in about 50 per cent of cases. A less common form occurs in which the haemoglobin A_2 is not elevated.

β-THALASSAEMIA IN ASSOCIATION WITH HAEMOGLOBIN VARIANTS

In many populations, because there is a high incidence of β-thalassaemia and various haemoglobin variants, it is quite common for an individual to inherit a β-thalassaemia gene from one parent and a gene for a structural haemoglobin variant from the other. Although numerous interactions of this type have been described, in clinical practice only three are of real importance—sickle-cell β-thalassaemia, haemoglobin C β-thalassaemia, and haemoglobin E β-thalassaemia.

Sickle-cell β-thalassaemia

The clinical manifestations that result from the interaction of the β-thalassaemia and sickle-cell genes vary considerably from race to race. In African black populations there is an extremely mild form of β^{+}-thalassaemia, which, when it interacts with the sickle-cell gene, produces a condition characterized by mild anaemia and few sickling crises. This condition is compatible with normal survival and is often ascertained by chance haematological examination. On the other hand, in Mediterranean populations it is quite common for an individual to inherit a β°-thalassaemia determinant from one parent and a sickle-cell gene from the other. Sickle-cell β°-thalassaemia is often associated with a clinical picture indistinguishable from that of sickle-cell anaemia.

The diagnosis of sickle-cell thalassaemia rests on the clinical features of a sickling disorder found in association with a peripheral blood picture with typical thalassaemic red-cell changes, i.e. a low MCH and MCV. In the more severe forms of sickle-cell β°-thalassaemia there may be an elevated reticulocyte count, and sickled red cells are found on the peripheral blood film. The diagnosis can be confirmed by haemoglobin electrophoresis, which in sickle-cell β^{+}-thalassaemia shows haemoglobin S together with 10 to 30 per cent haemoglobin A and an elevated haemoglobin A_2 value. In sickle-cell β°-thalassaemia the haemoglobin consists mainly of haemoglobin S with an elevated level of haemoglobins F and A_2. To be absolutely certain about the diagnosis it is necessary to examine the parents; one should have the sickle-cell trait and the other the β-thalassaemia trait.

Haemoglobin C thalassaemia

This disorder is restricted to West Africans and some North African and southern Mediterranean populations. It is characterized by a mild haemolytic anaemia associated with splenomegaly. The peripheral blood film shows numerous target cells and thalassaemic red-cell changes with a moderately elevated reticulocyte count. Haemoglobin electrophoresis shows a preponderance of haemoglobin C. The diagnosis is confirmed by finding the haemoglobin C trait in one parent and the β-thalassaemia trait in the other.

Haemoglobin E β-thalassaemia

This is the most common severe form of thalassaemia in South-East Asia and throughout the Indian subcontinent. Recent work has shown that haemoglobin E is inefficiently synthesized, and hence, when a haemoglobin E gene is inherited together with a β°-thalassaemia determinant, which is the most common type of β-thalassaemia in South-East Asia, there is a marked deficiency of β-chain production, and the resulting clinical picture can closely resemble homozygous β°-thalassaemia.

The clinical and haematological changes in haemoglobin E thalassaemia are variable. There is usually a marked degree of anaemia and splenomegaly with typical thalassaemic bone changes (Fig. 12). Although not always transfusion dependent, patients with this disorder usually run low haemoglobin values in the 4 to 9 g/dl range with an average of 6 to 7 g/dl. The blood film shows typical thalassaemic red-cell changes and the bone marrow shows marked erythroid hyperplasia with α-chain inclusions in many of the red-cell precursors.

Although very little is known about the natural history of this disorder, it seems likely that in many parts of South-East Asia and India it causes a very high mortality in the early years of life. Complications include a marked proneness to infection, secondary hypersplenism, progressive iron loading leading to liver rather than cardiac damage, a variety of neurological lesions due to tumours caused by extramedullary erythropoiesis extending in from the inner tables of the skull or vertebrae, folate deficiency, and recurrent pathological fractures. On the other hand, some patients with haemoglobin E thalassaemia grow and develop normally with few complications and there are many recorded cases of pregnancy in women with this disorder.

The diagnosis of haemoglobin E thalassaemia is confirmed by finding only haemoglobins E and F on haemoglobin electrophoresis and by demonstrating the haemoglobin E trait in one parent and the β-thalassaemia trait in the other.

The δβ-thalassaemias (see Table 3)

MOLECULAR GENETICS AND CLASSIFICATION

Disorders due to reduced β- and δ-chain synthesis are much less common than those due to defective β-chain production alone. These conditions are remarkably heterogeneous at the molecular level. In some cases they result from deletions of the β- and δ-globin genes, while in others there appears to have been mispaired synapsis and unequal crossing over between the δ- and β-globin gene loci with the production of

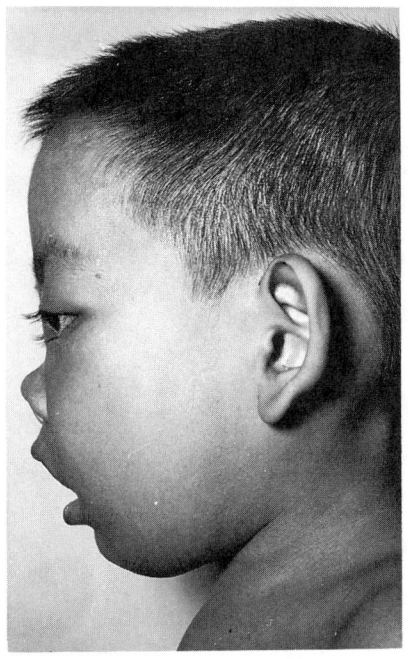

Fig. 12 Bossing of the skull in haemoglobin E thalassaemia.

δβ-fusion genes. These produce δβ-fusion chains, which combine with α-chains to form haemoglobin variants called the Lepore haemoglobins (Lepore was the family name of the first patient to be recognized with this disorder). Hence it is usual to classify this group of conditions into the δβ-thalassaemias and the haemoglobin Lepore thalassaemias.

CLINICAL AND HAEMATOLOGICAL CHANGES

In the homozygous state there is a mild degree of anaemia with haemoglobin values of 8 to 10 g/dl. There is often a moderate degree of splenomegaly but these patients are usually symptomless except during periods of stress such as infection or pregnancy. Haemoglobin analysis shows 100 per cent haemoglobin F. Carriers for this condition have thalassaemic blood pictures, elevated levels of haemoglobin F of 5 to 20 per cent, and normal levels of haemoglobin A_2.

The homozygous state for haemoglobin Lepore is similar to that of homozygous β-thalassaemia, although in some cases it may be milder and non-transfusion dependent. The clinical and haematological findings are similar to those of β-thalassaemia. The haemoglobin consists of F and Lepore only. Carriers have thalassaemic blood pictures associated with about 5 to 15 per cent haemoglobin Lepore.

There is a group of genetic disorders of haemoglobin production, encountered most commonly in African black populations, called collectively 'hereditary persistence of fetal haemoglobin'. Homozygotes have a mild thalassaemia-like blood picture but are not anaemic. They have 100 per cent haemoglobin F. Heterozygotes show no haematological abnormalities and carry 20 to 30 per cent haemoglobin F. These disorders are due to gene deletions involving the δ- and β-globin genes and therefore appear to be extremely mild forms of δβ-thalassaemia in which the lack of δ- and β-chain production is almost entirely compensated by the synthesis of the γ-chains of haemoglobin F.

The γδβ-thalassaemias

There are several rare forms of thalassaemia that result from long deletions of the β-globin gene cluster, which, as well as removing the β-genes, remove the δ, γ- and, in some cases, embryonic ε-genes. This means that there is no output of globin chains from this gene cluster at all. Clearly, the homozygous state for these disorders would not be compatible with survival. Heterozygotes have severe haemolytic disease of the newborn with anaemia and hyperbilirubinaemia. If they survive the neonatal period they grow and develop normally; in adult life they have the haematological picture of heterozygous β-thalassaemia with mild anaemia, hypochromic microcytic red cells, and a haemoglobin pattern consisting of haemoglobin A, no elevation of haemoglobin F, and a normal level of haemoglobin A_2.

Other β-thalassaemia variants

It is not uncommon to encounter patients with the clinical features of heterozygous β-thalassaemia who do not have an elevated haemoglobin A_2 level and yet who do not appear to have α-thalassaemia. This condition occurs in some Mediterranean populations. It is important to recognize it because if it is inherited together with a typical β-thalassaemia gene it can produce a severe transfusion-dependent disorder. Hence this variant is important in antenatal screening programmes. It can only be identified for certain by globin-chain synthesis analysis in a specialized laboratory.

Families are encountered occasionally in which there is a more severe form of heterozygous β-thalassaemia associated with anaemia, jaundice, and splenomegaly. In some of these families it is apparent that the affected individuals are in fact compound heterozygotes for β-thalassaemia and the so-called 'silent' β-thalassaemia gene, a determinant that cannot be identified haematologically in heterozygotes. In other families the severe form of β-thalassaemia behaves as a single-gene disorder with full expression in heterozygotes. The disorder results from the synthesis of a highly unstable β-globin chain variant.

The α-thalassaemias

Although the α-thalassaemias are more common than the β-thalassaemias they pose less of a public health problem. This is because the severe homozygous forms cause death *in utero* or in the neonatal period and the milder forms do not produce major disability.

DISTRIBUTION

The α-thalassaemias occur widely through the Mediterranean region, parts of West Africa, the Middle East, isolated parts of the Indian subcontinent, and throughout South-East Asia in a line stretching from southern China through Thailand, the Malay peninsula, and Indonesia to the Pacific island populations. For reasons that will become apparent when we consider the molecular pathology of these disorders the serious forms of α-thalassaemia are restricted to some of the Mediterranean island populations and South-East Asia (see Fig. 1, Chapter 22.4.3).

DEFINITION AND INHERITANCE

The genetics of α-thalassaemia is complicated, not least because the condition has collected such a confusing nomenclature over the years.

Because both haemoglobins A and F have α-chains, genetic disorders of α-chain synthesis result in defective fetal and adult haemoglobin production. In the fetus, deficiency of α-chains leads to the production of excess γ-chains, which form γ$_4$-tetramers, or haemoglobin Bart's (Fig. 13). In adults, a deficiency of α-chains leads to an excess of β-chains which form β$_4$-tetramers, or haemoglobin H, which is the adult counterpart of haemoglobin Bart's. Thus, the presence of haemoglobins Bart's or H in red cells is the hallmark of α-thalassaemia. If this was the whole story α-thalassaemia would pose no problems. However, for reasons that are not yet clear a critical level of globin-chain imbalance is required before detectable amounts of haemoglobins Bart's or H appear in the red cells. Unfortunately for clinicians, in persons heterozygous for different forms of α-thalassaemia this level is not reached; significant amounts of these variants only occur in the red cells of patients who have inherited two or more α-thalassaemia determinants

Table 4 *The α-thalassaemias*

Type	Homozygotes	Heterozygotes
α°	Hb Bart's hydrops	Thalassaemia minor
α$^+$ (deletion)	Thalassaemia minor	Normal blood picture[2]
α$^+$ (non-deletion)	Hb H disease[1]	Normal blood picture[2]

[1]Haemoglobin H disease more commonly results from the compound heterozygous inheritance of α° and either variety of α$^+$-thalassaemia.
[2]There may be very mild red-cell hypochromia.

and hence who have a severe degree of α-chain deficiency. This means that the carrier states for different forms of α-thalassaemia are difficult to diagnose.

The clinically important forms of α-thalassaemia (Table 4) result from the interaction of two main classes of α-thalassaemia determinants. It is still customary to define these conditions by the haematological changes in heterozygotes. First, there is a more severe form, which produces a mild but recognizable hypochromic anaemia in heterozygotes. Because we now know that this condition results from a genetic lesion that causes a complete absence of α-chain production from the affected chromosome, we call it α°-thalassaemia. The second type is almost completely silent in carriers; their red cells are normal or only slightly hypochromic. We call this α$^+$-thalassaemia because we know from molecular studies that the output of α-chains from the affected chromosome is only partially reduced. To put it another way, the terms α°- and α$^+$-thalassaemia describe haplotypes—the products of two linked α-chains on one of a pair of homologous chromosomes 16. Before we had all this information it was usual to call α°- and α$^+$-thalassaemia α-thalassaemia 1 and 2, respectively.

There are two symptomatic types of α-thalassaemia, the haemoglobin Bart's hydrops syndrome and haemoglobin H disease. The former

Fig. 13 The pathophysiology of α-thalassaemia.

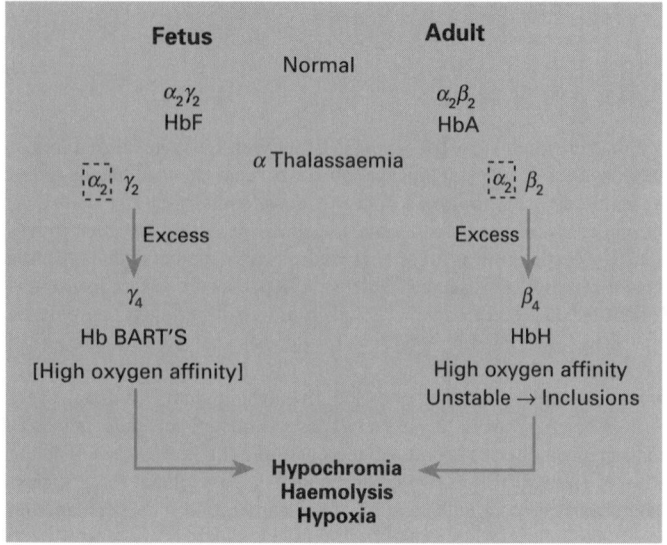

Fig. 14 The genetics of α-thalassaemia. The black α-genes represent gene deletions or otherwise inactivated genes. The open α-genes represent normal genes. α°-Thalassaemia and α$^+$-thalassaemia are defined in the text.

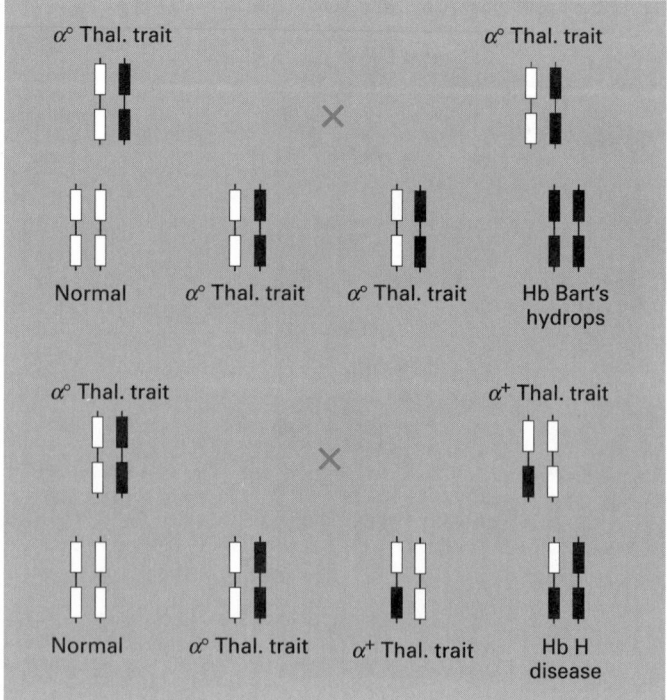

results from the homozygous inheritance of α°-thalassaemia. On the other hand, haemoglobin H disease usually results from the coinheritance of both α°- and α^+-thalassaemia. We now know that there are many different molecular types of both α°- and α^+-thalassaemia. These genetic interactions are summarized in Fig. 14.

MOLECULAR PATHOLOGY

The α°-thalassaemias result from the deletion (loss) of both linked α-globin genes. There are many different-sized deletions, one of which is particularly common in South-East Asia and another which occurs mainly in Mediterranean populations (Fig. 15). The molecular basis of the α^+-thalassaemias is more complicated. In some cases they result from deletions that remove one of the linked pairs of α-globin genes, leaving the other one intact. In others, both α-globin genes are intact but one of them has a mutation that either partially or completely inactivates it. These mutations are rather like those which cause β-thalassaemia. They may cause abnormal splicing or the production of a highly unstable α-chain incapable of producing a viable haemoglobin. One particularly common form of non-deletion α^+-thalassaemia occurs in South-East Asia and results from a single-base change in the chain termination codon UAA, which changes to CAA. The latter is the code-word for the amino acid glutamine. Hence, when the ribosomes reach this point, instead of the chain terminating, mRNA that is not normally translated is 'read through' until another stop codon is reached. Thus an elongated α-globin chain is produced, which is synthesized at a reduced rate. The resulting variant with an unusually long α-chain is called haemoglobin Constant Spring after the name of the town in Jamaica in which it was first discovered. It occurs in 2 to 5 per cent of the population of Thailand.

Another form of non-deletion α^+-thalassaemia is very common in the Middle East. It results from a single-base change in the highly conserved sequence at the 3' coding region of the α-globin gene, AATAAA, which is changed to AATAAG. As mentioned earlier, this sequence is the polyA signal site; the mutation probably interferes with polyadenylation of α-globin mRNA.

GENOTYPE/PHENOTYPE RELATIONS (SEE TABLE 5 AND FIG. 14)

These molecular studies explain much of the clinical variability of α-thalassaemia in different populations. Because the haemoglobin Bart's hydrops syndrome requires the homozygous inheritance of α°-thalassaemia, this condition will only occur in populations where α°-thalassaemia is common. Because it is largely confined to South-East Asia and the Mediterranean islands it is in these populations that the haemoglobin Bart's hydrops syndrome causes a public health problem. Similarly, because most forms of haemoglobin H disease are due to the inheritance of both α°- and α^+-thalassaemia, haemoglobin H disease is also restricted mainly to Mediterranean and Oriental populations. On the other hand, α^+-thalassaemia occurs very commonly throughout parts of West Africa, the Indian subcontinent and the Pacific island populations. However, because α°-thalassaemia does not occur in these regions the haemoglobin Bart's hydrops syndrome and haemoglobin H disease are not seen. The homozygous state for the deletion forms of α-thalassaemia is characterised by a mild hypochromic anaemia, very similar to the heterozygous state for α°-thalassaemias; the result of having only two out of the normal four α-genes seems to be the same whether the two genes are missing from the same chromosome or opposite pairs of homologous chromosomes. Curiously, the homozygous state for the non-deletion forms of α^+-thalassaemia is associated with a more severe defect in α-chain production and the clinical picture of haemoglobin H disease. In this case the remaining normal α-globin gene does not seem to be able to compensate for the lack of activity of its defective partner.

PATHOPHYSIOLOGY

The pathophysiology of α-thalassaemia is different to that of β-thalassaemia. A deficiency of α-chains leads to the production of excess γ-chains or β-chains, which form haemoglobins Bart's and H, respectively (Fig. 13). These soluble tetramers do not precipitate in the bone marrow and hence erythropoiesis is more effective than in β-thalassaemia, i.e. there is less intramedullary destruction of red cell precursors. However,

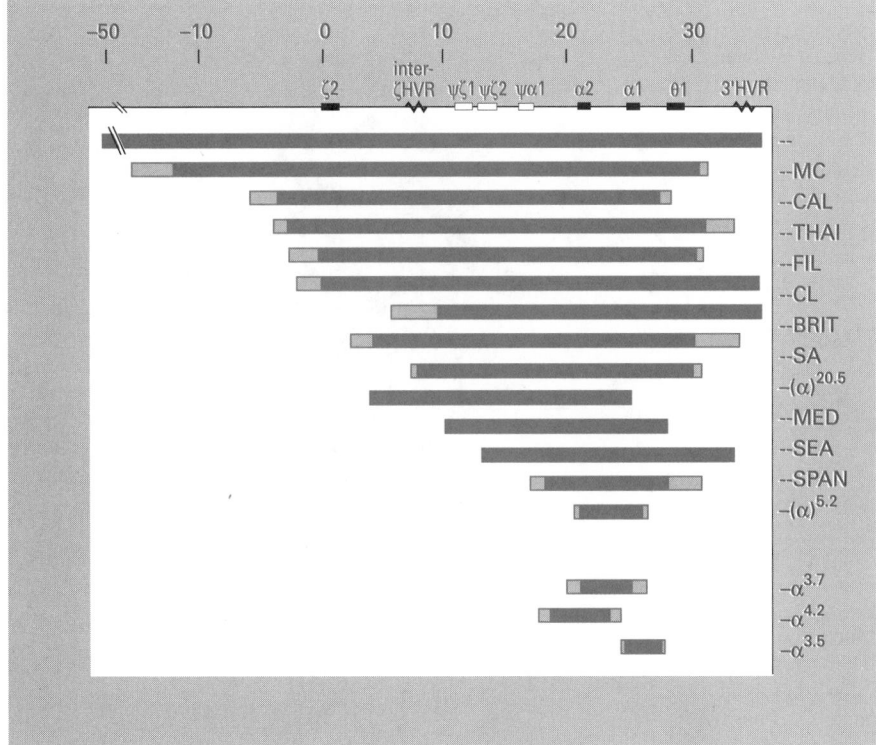

Fig. 15 The different-sized deletions responsible for some forms of α°- or α^+-thalassaemia. The α-globin gene cluster is shown at the top of the figure. Two highly variable regions (HVR) are shown. The abbreviations on the right-hand side indicate the source of origin of patients with the deletions, e.g.: MED, Mediterranean; SEA, South-East Asia. The three smaller deletions at the bottom of the figure show some of the main classes of α^+-thalassaemia. The superscripts 3.7, 4.2, and 3.5 indicate the size of the deletions.

haemoglobin H is unstable and precipitates in red cells as they age. The resulting inclusion bodies are trapped in the spleen and other parts of the microcirculation leading to a shortened red-cell survival. Furthermore, both haemoglobins Bart's and H have a very high oxygen affinity; because they have no α-chains there is no haem/haem interaction and their oxygen dissociation curves resemble myoglobin. Thus the pathophysiology of severe forms of α-thalassaemia is based on defective haemoglobin production, the synthesis of homotetramers, which are physiologically useless, and a haemolytic component due to their precipitation in older red cells.

The haemoglobin Bart's hydrops syndrome

This condition, which results from the homozygous state for α°-thalassaemia, is a common cause of fetal loss throughout South-East Asia and in Greece and Cyprus. Affected infants produce no α-chains at all and hence can make neither fetal nor adult haemoglobin.

The clinical picture is very characteristic (Fig. 16). These infants are usually stillborn between 28 and 40 weeks, or if they are live-born take a few gasping respirations and then expire within the first hour after birth. They show the typical picture of hydrops fetalis with gross pallor, generalized oedema, and massive hepatosplenomegaly. There is a very large, friable placenta. All these findings are due to severe intrauterine anaemia. The haemoglobin values are in the 6 to 8 g/dl range and there are gross thalassaemic changes of the peripheral blood film with many nucleated red cells. The haemoglobin consists of approximately 80 per cent haemoglobin Bart's and 20 per cent of the embryonic haemoglobin, Portland ($\zeta_2\gamma_2$). It is believed that these infants survive to term because they continue to produce embryonic haemoglobin at this level; haemoglobin Bart's has an oxygen dissociation curve like myoglobin and is therefore useless as an oxygen carrier.

Apart from fetal death this syndrome is characterized by a high incidence of toxaemia of pregnancy and considerable obstetric difficulties due to the presence of the large, friable placenta. Both parents have thalassaemic red cell changes with normal haemoglobin A_2 values, i.e. the characteristic finding of the heterozygous state for α°-thalassaemia.

Haemoglobin H disease

MOLECULAR GENETICS AND PATHOGENESIS

As mentioned earlier, haemoglobin H is a tetramer of normal β-chains with the formula β_4. It is produced when there is a marked reduction of α-chain synthesis. Haemoglobin H disease usually results from the inheritance of α°-thalassaemia from one parent and α+ from the other. It may also result from the homozygous state for non-deletion forms of α-thalassaemia. The latter form of inheritance is particularly common in the Middle East.

CLINICAL FEATURES

There is a variable degree of anaemia and splenomegaly but it is most unusual to see severe thalassaemic bone changes or the growth retardation characteristic of homozygous β-thalassaemia. Patients usually survive into adult life although the course may be interspersed with severe episodes of haemolysis associated with infection, or worsening of the anaemia due to progressive hypersplenism. In addition, oxidant drugs such as sulphonamides may increase the rate of precipitation of haemoglobin H and therefore exacerbate the anaemia.

HAEMATOLOGICAL CHANGES (PLATE 33)

Haemoglobin values range from 7 to 10 g/dl and the blood film shows typical thalassaemic changes. There is a moderate reticulocytosis, and on incubation of the red cells with brilliant cresyl blue, numerous inclusion bodies are generated by precipitation of the haemoglobin H under the redox action of the dye. After splenectomy large, preformed inclu-

sions can be demonstrated on incubation of blood with methyl violet. Haemoglobin analysis reveals from 5 to 40 per cent haemoglobin H together with haemoglobin A and a normal or reduced level of haemoglobin A_2.

FAMILY FINDINGS

One parent is heterozygous for α°-thalassaemia and the other for either deletion or non-deletion forms of α+-thalassaemia. In some cases both parents have extremely mild haematological changes characteristic of the carrier state for non-deletion forms of α-thalassaemia.

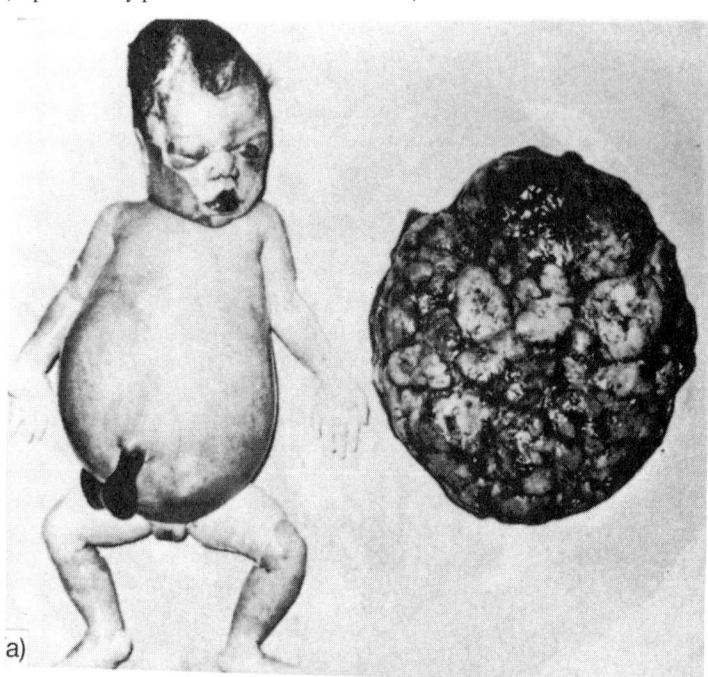

Fig. 16 The haemoglobin Bart's hydrops syndrome: (a) a hydropic infant with massively enlarged placenta; (b) autopsy findings with an enlarged liver. (Reproduced by permission of Professor P. Wasi.)

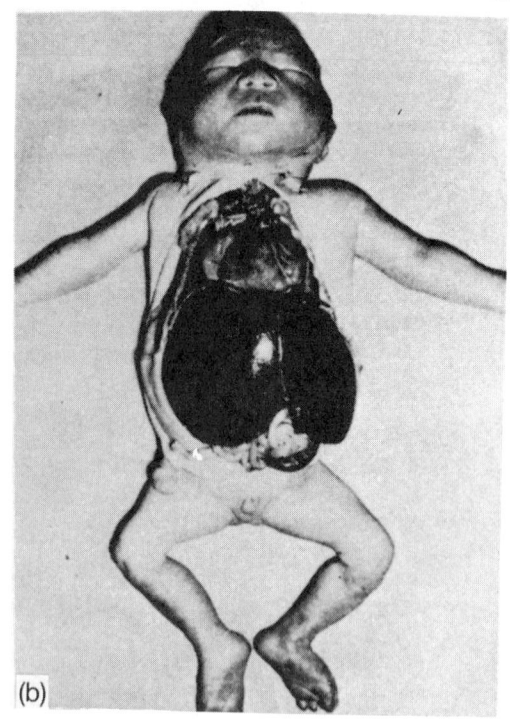

α-Thalassaemia traits (Plate 34)

The haematological findings in the different α°- and α^+-thalassaemia traits are summarized in Table 4.

Other forms of α-thalassaemia

α-Thalassaemia/mental retardation (ATR) syndromes

There are two clear-cut disorders in which acquired forms of α-thalassaemia are associated with mental retardation. The first, ATR 16, results from long deletions at the end of chromosome 16, which remove the α-globin genes and 1 to 2 megabases (million bases) of DNA. They may result from simple truncations of chromosome 16 or from more complex rearrangements such as balanced translocations. The mental retardation is associated with variable dysmorphic features and the disorder is thought to reflect the loss of a number of genes at the end of chromosome 16. The more common disorder, ATRX, is characterized by a more severe degree of mental retardation with a characteristic constellation of dysmorphic features. In these cases the α-globin genes are intact and appear to be defective both in *cis* and *trans* due to the action of a factor encoded by a locus on the long arm of the X chromosome. There may be multiply affected siblings and the pattern of inheritance is X-linked. The blood picture is that of a mild form of α-thalassaemia with occasional haemoglobin H inclusions in the red cells. Female carriers can be identified by the presence of a very small proportion of red cells that contain haemoglobin H inclusions. The defective gene on the X chromosome, *XH2* has now been identified.

Haemoglobin H and leukaemia

Elderly patients may develop a cell line containing haemoglobin H during the course of the evolution of a myeloproliferative disorder or acute leukaemia. The mechanism is unknown; the presence of haemoglobin H or haemoglobin H inclusions in an elderly patients should raise the suspicion of a preleukaemic disorder.

Thalassaemia intermedia

DEFINITION AND PATHOGENESIS

The term thalassaemia intermedia is used to describe patients with the clinical picture of thalassaemia, which, although not transfusion dependent, is associated with a much more severe degree of anaemia than that found in heterozygous carriers for α- or β-thalassaemia. Many of the conditions described earlier in this section follow this clinical course—haemoglobin C or E thalassaemia, the various δβ-thalassaemias and haemoglobin Lepore disorders, and the wide variety of conditions that can result from the interactions of the different β- and δβ-thalassaemia determinants for example. However, some children with this condition have parents with typical heterozygous β-thalassaemic blood pictures and elevated haemoglobin A_2 levels. These individuals appear to be homozygous for β-thalassaemia yet run a much milder course than is usually the case with this condition. There is increasing evidence that many of them have inherited an α-thalassaemia determinant as well as being homozygous for β-thalassaemia. This reduces the overall degree of globin-chain imbalance and consequently the severity of the dyserythropoiesis that usually accompanies homozygous β-thalassaemia; hence these children run a milder clinical course. In other cases, particularly in the African blacks, relatively mild forms of homozygous β-thalassaemia seem to reflect the action of less severe β-thalassaemia mutations.

CLINICAL AND HAEMATOLOGICAL CHANGES (PLATE 35)

The clinical features of the intermediate forms of thalassaemia are extremely variable. At one end of the spectrum are individuals who are virtually symptom-free, and except for moderate anaemia, are completely normal. At the other end there are patients who have haemoglobin values in the 5 to 7 g/dl range and who develop marked splenomegaly, severe skeletal deformities due to expansion of bone marrow, and, as they get older, become heavily iron-loaded because of increased intestinal absorption of iron. Recurrent leg ulceration, folate deficiency, symptoms due to extramedullary haemopoietic tumour masses in the chest and skull (Fig. 17), gallstones, and a marked proneness to infection are particularly characteristic of this group of thalassaemias.

Because of the heterogeneity of these disorders, it is only possible to determine the course that is likely to evolve in any individual patient by following the disorder very carefully from early childhood.

Differential diagnosis of the thalassaemias

There are few conditions likely to be confused with the more severe forms of homozygous β-thalassaemia or haemoglobin H disease. The racial background of the patient, the presence of anaemia from early in life, and the characteristic haematological changes make the diagnosis relatively easy. Once thalassaemia is suspected, the parents and near relatives should be examined for the carrier states for α- or β-thalassaemia. Both disorders can be distinguished from simple iron deficiency by the finding of a normal serum iron or ferritin level and by the associated changes in the haemoglobin pattern.

The laboratory diagnosis of thalassaemia

The thalassaemias should be suspected when a typical thalassaemic blood picture is found in an individual of an appropriate racial group. The homozygous states for the severe forms of β-thalassaemia are easily recognized by the typical haematological changes associated with very high levels of haemoglobin F; haemoglobin A_2 values vary so much that they are of no diagnostic help. The heterozygous states are recognized by microcytic hypochromic red cells and an elevated level of haemoglobin A_2. The δβ-thalassaemias are characterized by the finding of 100

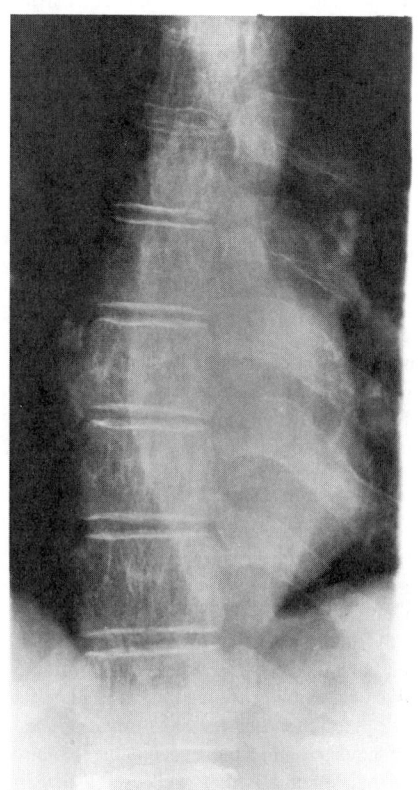

Fig. 17 An extramedullary haemopoietic mass in a patient with β-thalassaemia intermedia.

per cent haemoglobin F in homozygotes, and 5 to 15 per cent haemoglobin F together with a normal level of haemoglobin A₂ in heterozygotes (see Table 3).

When β-thalassaemia is diagnosed, a quantitative haemoglobin electrophoresis should be done to exclude the presence of an abnormal haemoglobin variant such as haemoglobin E or Lepore.

The haemoglobin Bart's hydrops syndrome is recognized by the finding of a hydropic infant with a severe anaemia, a thalassaemic blood
picture, and the presence of 80 per cent or more haemoglobin Bart's on
haemoglobin electrophoresis. Haemoglobin H disease is identified by
the finding of a typical thalassaemic blood picture with an elevated
reticulocyte count, generation of multiple inclusion bodies in the red
cells after incubation with brilliant cresyl blue, and the finding of variable amounts of haemoglobin H on haemoglobin electrophoresis. There
are no really useful diagnostic tests for the different α-thalassaemic carrier states although α°-thalassaemia heterozygotes usually have typical
thalassaemic red-cell changes with a normal haemoglobin A₂ value.

Prevention and treatment

Thalassaemia produces a severe public health problem and a serious
drain on medical resources in many populations. Because there is no
definitive treatment, most countries in which the disease is common are
putting a major effort into its prevention.

PREVENTION

There are two major approaches to the prevention of the thalassaemias.
As the carrier states for the β-thalassaemias can be easily recognized, it
is at least theoretically possible to screen populations and give genetic
counselling about the choice of marriage partners. If β-thalassaemia
heterozygotes marry other carriers, 1 in 4 of their children will have the
severe transfusion-dependent homozygous disorder. While large-scale
programmes of this type have been set up in Italy, the results are not
yet available, and in smaller pilot studies in Greece the outcome has not
been encouraging. Until more is known about the usefulness of this form
of prospective genetic counselling, most countries are developing
screening programmes at antenatal clinics. When heterozygous carrier
mothers are found, their husbands are tested and if they are also
carriers the couple are offered the possibility of prenatal diagnosis and
termination of pregnancies carrying fetuses with severe forms of
thalassaemia.

Prenatal diagnosis

Prenatal diagnosis may be offered to couples at risk for having children
with severe forms of β-thalassaemia. Because of the serious obstetric
complications and the trauma of carrying a hydropic fetus to term there
is also a good indication for prenatal diagnosis for the haemoglobin
Bart's hydrops syndrome. Termination of pregnancies at risk for milder
forms of thalassaemia is undertaken, but should only be considered after
very careful counselling of the parents. Some children with intermediate
forms of thalassaemia are symptom free and develop normally; others
have more severe anaemia and bone deformity.

Prenatal diagnosis of thalassaemia can be carried out in several ways.
The diagnosis can be made by globin-chain synthesis studies of fetal
blood samples obtained by fetoscopy at 18 to 20 weeks of gestation.
The diagnosis can also be made by fetal DNA analysis on amniotic fluid
cells obtained by amniocentesis earlier in the second trimester. More
recently it has been possible to carry out prenatal diagnosis of thalassaemia and sickle-cell anaemia by direct analysis of fetal DNA obtained
by chorion biopsy at about the tenth week of gestation. Because it
reduces the long period of uncertainty, during which the fetus is growing
and the mother and her relatives and friends are coming to accept she
is to have a child, and because late second-trimester terminations are
often difficult, first-trimester diagnosis is much more acceptable to many
women. Prenatal diagnosis of thalassaemia is now well established in

many countries, and in Sardinia, Greece, and Cyprus has already significantly reduced the number of new cases of thalassaemia in the
community.

Because prenatal diagnosis of thalassaemia is available it is very
important to discuss the genetic implications of the condition when carriers are detected by chance, regardless of the individual's racial background. They should also be given a letter explaining, in simple terms,
the pattern of inheritance and the dangers for their children. This
approach should always be followed, even for sporadic cases in low-
incidence regions such as northern Europe. Because of the increasing
movements of populations they might marry another carrier and have
severely affected children.

SYMPTOMATIC TREATMENT

The symptomatic management of severe β-thalassaemia hangs on regular blood transfusion, the judicious use of splenectomy if hyperaple-
nism develops, and the administration of chelating agents to attempt to
deal with the problem of iron overload from regular blood transfusion.
When the diagnosis of severe β-thalassaemia is suspected during the
first year of life, the infant should be followed for several weeks to make
sure that the haemoglobin level is falling to a level at which regular
transfusion will be necessary. It is difficult to be dogmatic about exactly
when transfusions should be started, but if the infant is severely anaemic
and it is feeding poorly or otherwise failing to thrive, it will almost
certainly need to be transfused. The object should be to maintain the
haemoglobin level between 9 and 14 g/dl and this usually requires transfusion every 6 to 8 weeks. Either washed or frozen red cells should be
used and whole blood should be avoided because of the danger of sensitization to serum or white-cell components. A careful check on the
pre- and post-transfusion haemoglobin level should be kept and the
transfusion requirements carefully plotted. If there is a marked increase
in blood requirement, hypersplenism should be suspected. A thalassaemic child with an easily palpable spleen probably has some degree
of hypersplenism. Splenectomy should be done as late as is feasible and,
if possible, not in the first 5 years because the incidence of post-splenectomy infection seems to be particularly high in early childhood.
Apart from increased transfusion requirements, the presence of neutropenia or thrombocytopenia is a useful guide to the presence of hypersplenism. After the operation children should be maintained on prophylactic penicillin indefinitely and the parents warned about the dangers
of infection. Advice on preoperative vaccination is given in Chapter
22.5.4.

The only useful chelating agent for the prevention or treatment of iron
overload in thalassaemia is desferrioxamine. The drug has to be given
systemically and there is convincing evidence that much better results
are obtained by a slow subcutaneous infusion using some form of
mechanical pump than by single bolus injections. Therapy should be
started as early as possible, but for practical purposes this usually means
somewhere between the second or third year or later. Desferrioxamine
is given at a dose of 30 to 40 mg/kg as an overnight infusion lasting 8
to 12 h using a butterfly needle placed subcutaneously in the anterior
abdominal wall. It is important to monitor progress by measuring the
urinary iron excretion in the 24-h period after the infusion. The most
common side-effects are local redness or small nodules at the site of the
infusion. When used over a long period there may be damage to the
auditory nerve and the development of high-frequency hearing loss. This
is not always reversible after stopping the drug. Visual failure with night
and colour blindness together with field loss has also been reported;
again this may be reversible after stopping the drug. Thus all patients
on long-term desferrioxamine treatment should undergo regular specialist assessment of hearing and vision.

There is considerable evidence that better levels of iron excretion are
achieved if patients are ascorbate replete and this can be achieved by
giving low doses of ascorbic acid at a dose of 3 mg/kg. There have been
a few reports of cardiac deterioration in heavily iron-loaded thalassaemic

children who have received high doses of vitamin C and this drug should be used with caution. It is customary to give folic acid supplements but if children are maintained on a good diet and adequately transfused they rarely become folate depleted. This complication is much more common in children with thalassaemia intermedia who live in impoverished conditions.

Current research is directed at developing oral chelating agents or methods for raising fetal haemoglobin production. The role of bone marrow transplantation is still controversial. Recent results suggest that if it is done early in life, with marrow donated from an HLA-compatible sibling, there is about an 80 per cent chance of curing the disease. These results need confirmation by larger series but at the time of writing there seems to be a genuine place for marrow transplantation, particularly in families who find regular transfusion and chelating agents difficult to manage.

The intermediate forms of β-thalassaemia and haemoglobin H disease require careful surveillance and splenectomy if hypersplenism develops. Haemoglobin H disease is usually fairly innocuous, although patients should be warned against the use of oxidant drugs, which tend to precipitate haemoglobin H and worsen the anaemia. Children with β-thalassaemia intermedia should be watched carefully in early childhood, and, if there are signs of growth retardation or increasing bone deformity, they should be placed on a transfusion regimen as outlined above.

Finally, it is most important that all thalassaemic children are under regular surveillance by an experienced paediatrician. Apart from the specific complications of the disorder, their proneness to infection and bony deformities lead to a series of general paediatric complications, particularly recurrent ear infection, deafness, sinus infection, emotional disturbances, and a variety of orthodontic problems. Hepatitis B or C, due to infected blood products, are common complications; their management is described in Section 14. In some parts of the world, AIDS, contracted in the same way, is becoming a major threat.

The families require constant encouragement and they should be told that the current form of chelation therapy is, in a sense, buying time until more active oral chelating agents become available or until a more definitive form of treatment is developed. If well looked after, these children can have a relatively normal childhood, and the recent advances in the use of chelating drugs may mean that some of the distressing side-effects of iron loading that occur at puberty may at least be delayed, and possibly prevented indefinitely.

Structural haemoglobin variants

Over 400 structural haemoglobin variants have been described, most of which result from single amino acid substitutions. Many of them are harmless and have been discovered during surveys of the electrophoretic patterns of human haemoglobin. Of course, this approach underestimates the number of variants because it only identifies those in which the amino acid substitution alters the charge of the haemoglobin molecule.

Single amino-acid substitutions cause clinical disorders only if they alter the stability or functional properties of haemoglobin. A classification of the diseases that result from structural abnormalities of haemoglobin is shown in Table 5. They include the sickling disorders, the unstable haemoglobins associated with congenital non-spherocytic haemolytic anaemia, the high oxygen-affinity variants, which lead to hereditary polycythaemia, and a group that produces methaemoglobinaemia. We shall consider the different varieties of genetic methaemoglobinaemias at the end of this chapter.

NOMENCLATURE

Originally, the structural haemoglobin variants were named by letters of the alphabet. By the late 1950s there were no letters of the alphabet left and it was decided to designate new haemoglobin variants by the

Table 5 *Clinical disorders due to structural haemoglobin variants*

Disorder	Variants
Haemolysis and tissue damage	Haemoglobin S
Drug-induced haemolysis	Haemoglobin Zürich and other unstable haemoglobins
Chronic haemolysis	Unstable haemoglobin variants
	Haemoglobin C
Congenital polycythaemia	High-affinity variants
Congenital cyanosis	Haemoglobin(s) M
	Low-affinity variants
Hypochromia: thalassaemic phenotype	Haemoglobin E
	Haemoglobin Constant Spring

Table 6 *The major sickling disorders*

Disorder	Genotype (normal = $\alpha\alpha/\alpha\alpha.\beta/\beta$)	
SS disease (sickle-cell anaemia)	$\alpha\alpha/\alpha\alpha$	β^S/β^S
SC disease	$\alpha\alpha/\alpha\alpha$	β^S/β^C
SD disease	$\alpha\alpha/\alpha\alpha$	β^S/β^D
S–β thalassaemia	$\alpha\alpha/\alpha\alpha$	$\beta^S\beta^0$ or β^S/β^+
S–hereditary persistence of fetal Hb	$\alpha\alpha/\alpha\alpha$	$\beta^S/-*$
S–α thalassaemia	$\alpha-/\alpha\alpha$ or $\alpha-/\alpha-\beta^S/\beta^S$	

* Indicates β-gene deletion.

place of origin of the first patient in whom they were characterized. It is customary to call the heterozygous (carrier) state the 'trait' and the homozygous condition the 'disease'. For example, haemoglobin S heterozygotes (genotype AS) are said to have the sickle-cell trait, while individuals homozygous for the sickle-cell mutation (genotype SS) are said to have sickle-cell disease. In practice it is very important to distinguish between the carrier state and the homozygous or compound heterozygous state for a sickle haemoglobin variant; carriers are always asymptomatic.

The sickling disorders

Sickling disorders (Table 6) consist of the heterozygous state for haemoglobin S, or the sickle-cell trait (AS), the homozygous state, or sickle-cell disease (SS), and the compound heterozygous state for haemoglobin S together with haemoglobins C, D, E, or other structural variants. In addition, there are several disorders that result from the inheritance of the sickle-cell gene, together with different forms of thalassaemia.

PATHOGENESIS

Haemoglobin S differs from haemoglobin A by the substitution of valine for glutamic acid at position 6 in the β-chain. Although this has been known since Vernon Ingram's work over a quarter of a century ago, it is still not absolutely clear how it gives rise to the sickling phenomenon. Sickling appears to be due to the unusual solubility characteristics of haemoglobin S, which undergoes liquid crystal (tactoid) formation as it becomes deoxygenated. In the deoxygenated state, aggregates of sickled haemoglobin molecules arrange themselves in parallel, rod-like structures with a diameter of about 11.6 nm. The molecules of these strands are in a helical configuration. It seems likely that there is a tendency for normal haemoglobin molecules to become lined up in a similar way when haemoglobin is in the deoxy configuration, and in sickle cells the β6 valine substitution somehow stabilizes these molecular stacks. There is considerable variation with which different haemoglobins are able to participate with haemoglobin S in the sickling process. This accounts for some of the clinical variability of the different sickling conditions. For example, haemoglobin F is almost completely excluded from the sickling process and therefore increasing concentrations in the red cell tends to reduce the rate of sickling.

During their passage through the circulation, red cells containing haemoglobin S at a high concentration go through a series of cycles of sickling and desickling and finally, owing to loss of membrane and changes in membrane permeability, the cells become irreversibly sickled (Fig. 18). Sickling has two main effects. First, sickled erythrocytes have an increased mechanical fragility and hence a significantly shortened survival. This leads to a chronic haemolytic anaemia. Secondly, because of the formation of aggregates of sickled erythrocytes, particularly in the microvasculature, the viscosity of the blood increases, which leads to vascular stasis, local hypoxia, further sickling and, in extreme cases, to complete blockage of small vessels and tissue infarction.

DISTRIBUTION

The sickling disorders occur very frequently in African Black populations and, sporadically, throughout the Mediterranean region and the Middle East. There are extensive pockets in India but the disease has not been seen in South-East Asia. It is thought that the high frequency of the sickle-cell gene occurs because carriers are more resistant than normal individuals to *Plasmodium falciparum* malaria.

CLINICAL FEATURES

Except in conditions of extreme anoxia such as flying in unpressurized aircraft, the sickle-cell trait causes no clinical disability. However, it is possible for individuals to suffer vaso-occlusive episodes if they become unusually hypoxic under anaesthesia and therefore all individuals of the appropriate racial background should have a sickling test (see below) before receiving an anaesthetic. If the test is positive, the anaesthetic should be given with adequate oxygenation and special care should be taken to avoid postoperative dehydration.

Sickle-cell anaemia (Plate 36)

This condition runs an extremely variable clinical course. At one end of the spectrum it is characterized by a crippling haemolytic anaemia interspersed with severe exacerbations or crises, while on the other hand it

Fig. 18 Irreversibly sickled cells in the peripheral blood (×1000, Leishman stain).

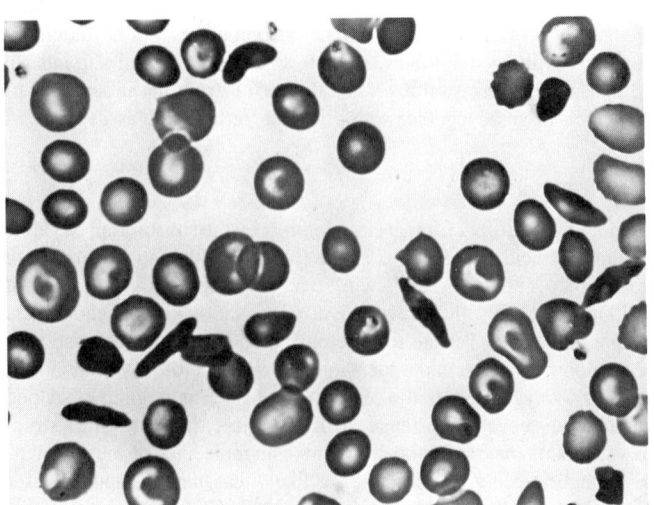

may be an extremely mild disorder, only found by chance on routine haematological examination. The reasons for these remarkable differences in phenotypic expression of what appears to be the same genetic defect, which are only partly understood, include the level of haemoglobin F, climate, and, probably most important, socioeconomic factors such as availability of early treatment of infection.

Typically, sickle-cell anaemia presents in infancy with a variable degree of anaemia and jaundice and most patients go through the rest of their life with a chronic haemolytic anaemia. A common presenting symptom is the so-called hand and foot syndrome, which occurs early in infancy and is characterized by a painful dactylitis with swelling of the fingers or feet. Epiphyseal damage during one of these episodes may lead to chronic shortening of a digit. Infants are anaemic from about the third month of life and during early development often have significant splenomegaly. In most cases this gradually resolves due to repeated infarction of the spleen, a condition called autosplenectomy. Indeed, it is most unusual to feel the spleen after the end of the first decade. Typically, these children have haemoglobin levels in the 6 to 8 g/dl range with a reticulocyte count of 10 to 20 per cent. There is chronic, mild icterus with an elevated bilirubin level. Examination of the peripheral blood film shows anisochromia and poikilocytosis with a variable number of sickled erythrocytes (Fig. 18). As the children grow older the haematological changes of hyposplenism develop with the appearance of pits on the surface of the red cells, Howell–Jolly bodies, and distorted red cells. The white-cell and platelet counts are usually normal or slightly elevated.

Apart from the signs mentioned above, growth and development are usually normal although there may be some skeletal deformities including frontal bossing of the skull due to expansion of the bone marrow. In some studies, children have tended to be short for their age, while postadolescents were usually tall. Inequalities between upper and lower segments, stressed in the early literature, are unusual. The only other physical sign that is frequently present is chronic leg ulceration; this is discussed in a later section.

COMPLICATIONS

The chronic haemolysis of sickle-cell disease is interspersed with acute exacerbations of the illness called sickling crises. Furthermore, a series of serious and life-threatening long-term complications develops in many patients with symptomatic sickle-cell anaemia.

The different forms of sickle-cell crises are summarized in Table 7. The most common is the painful crisis. This is sometimes precipitated by infection and dehydration or exposure to cold, although quite often no underlying cause can be found. The episode starts with vague pain, often in the back or bones of the limbs. The pain gradually worsens and its bizarre distribution may cause a major diagnostic puzzle. The pain is almost certainly due to blockage of small vessels with sickled erythrocytes, and marrow aspiration over areas of bone tenderness reveals infarction of the marrow tissue. Occasionally, abdominal pain is the major symptom and this may be associated with distension and rigidity, a picture very similar to an acute abdominal emergency. The diagnostic difficulties in distinguishing between an abdominal crisis and a surgical abdomen are compounded by the fact that the bowel sounds are often very quiet during abdominal crisis.

Two other serious forms of thrombotic crises occur, which are known as the 'lung' and 'brain' syndromes. The 'lung' syndrome is characterized by acute dyspnoea and pleuritic pain and is due to infarction of major pulmonary vessels. It is often preceded by a rapid fall in the packed cell volume, which may reflect sequestration of sickled cells in the pulmonary vessels. Neurological complications usually present in childhood, either as fits, transient neurological symptoms resembling ischaemic attacks, or with a fully developed stroke. There is a tendency for recurrent episodes. This crippling complication may reflect hypertrophic changes in the carotid vessels as well as abnormal blood rheology due to sickling. Recent evidence suggests that strokes may be

Table 7 *Acute exacerbations ('crises') in sickle-cell (SS) disease*

1. Thrombotic:
   Generalized or localized bone pain
   Abdominal
   Pulmonary
   Neurological
2. Aplastic
3. Haemolytic
4. Sequestration:
   Spleen
   Liver
   ?lung
5. Various combinations of above

predicted by regular transcranial Döppler ultrasonography to detect stenosis of cerebral vessels.

During painful crises there may be a marked increase in the rate of haemolysis with a fall in the haemoglobin level. Such haemolytic episodes are relatively uncommon. Much more serious are periods of transient bone marrow aplasia called aplastic crises. These seem to result from intercurrent infection, particularly due to parvoviruses, and frequently affect more than one sibling in the same family.

Finally, and most serious, are the sequestration crises. These occur mainly in babies and young children and are characterized by a rapid enlargement of the spleen or liver, which become engorged with sickled erythrocytes. As the crisis progresses a large proportion of the total red-cell mass may be trapped in the spleen or liver, and death may occur due to gross anaemia. These episodes show a tendency to recur in the same individual. Hepatic sequestration, which may occur in adults, is easily overlooked if the liver size is not monitored carefully (Fig. 19).

The most common cause of death in sickle-cell anaemia appears to be a sequestration crisis or acute infection, or both. It is not absolutely clear why patients with this disorder are so prone to infection, although splenic malfunction may play a part. Abnormalities of the alternate pathway of complement activation have also been described. A variety of organisms is involved, particularly the pneumococcus, and in some tropical countries typhoid infection of bone infarcts leads to typhoid osteomyelitis. Despite the relative resistance of heterozygotes to *P. falciparum* malaria, deaths due to malaria are extremely common in Africa.

Pregnancy may be uneventful, or associated with an increased incidence of painful crises. There is slightly increased incidence of maternal mortality and a definite increase in the rate of fetal loss.

Chronic complications

The chronic complications of sickle-cell anaemia result largely from repeated episodes of vascular occlusion. Almost any organ can be involved. Those of particular risk are areas that rely largely on small vessels for their blood supply. The bones are particularly prone to infarction. Aseptic necrosis of the humeral or femoral heads may lead to their destruction and to gross deformity of the shoulder and hip joints (Fig. 20). Bone infarcts may result in chronic sequestra, which may become secondarily infected to produce osteomyelitis. Infarction of the bone marrow does not seem to have any long-term sequelae, although occasionally pieces may break off and embolize to the lungs.

Progressive renal dysfunction and failure is of particular importance. In the renal medulla the low pH and oxygen tension and hypertonicity are conducive to sickling, and damage and disorganization of the system of vasa rectae have been demonstrated. There is progressive inability to concentrate the urine, leading to polyuria, nocturia, and the enuresis that is particularly common in children with the disease. But it is chronic glomerular damage that seems to lead to chronic renal failure, which is a major contributor to or cause of death, particularly in patients over the age of 40 years. The precise mechanism of glomerular damage is not known.

There may be a chronic pulmonary fibrosis, although cor pulmonale secondary to pulmonary hypertension seems to be uncommon. There is increasing evidence that chronic lung disease may be an important determinant of complications and death. Chronic leg ulceration is also an important problem and may run a relapsing course for 10 or 20 years. Recurrent attacks of priapism may lead to chronic deformity of the penis. Vaso-occlusion in the eye due to ischaemia of the retinal vasculature is reflected by proliferative retinopathy with progressive visual loss. This complication occurs more frequently in haemoglobin SC disease. Although there is cardiomegaly and a variety of flow murmurs, myocardial fibrosis seems to be extremely rare and, with the exception of cor pulmonale, there are no long-term cardiac complications.

Because of the chronic haemolysis, gallstones are very common and are seen in over 30 per cent of children by the age of 15 years. They

Fig. 19 Hepatic sequestration crisis in sickle-cell anaemia.

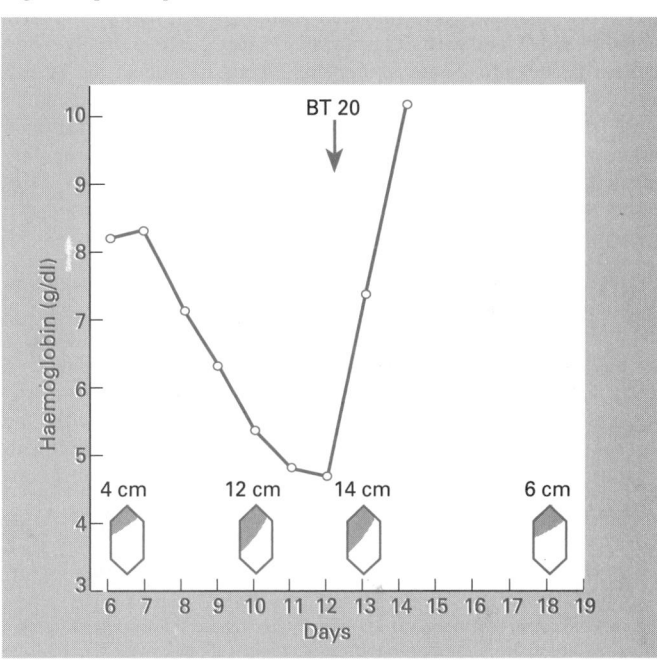

Fig. 20 Aseptic necrosis of the left femoral head in sickle-cell thalassaemia. (Reproduced by courtesy of Dr Graham Serjeant.)

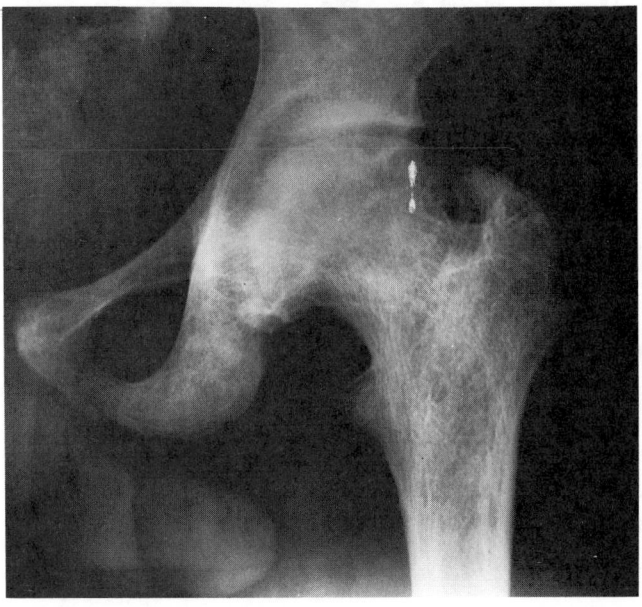

may cause acute or chronic cholecystitis or obstruction of the common bile duct.

COURSE AND PROGNOSIS

Some patients with sickle-cell anaemia go through life with few complications but there is a subset who undergo repeated crises, strokes, and incapacitating bone disease. Although factors such as the level of fetal haemoglobin, coexistent α-thalassaemia, and other genetic influences play a part in this heterogeneity, there is still a great deal to be learnt about the factors that modify the phenotype of the sickling disorders.

There is a marked difference in course and prognosis between populations. In Africa it seems likely that the disease still has a very high mortality early in life in rural populations. In Jamaica there appears to be about a 10 per cent mortality in the early years, although survival into adult life and old age is common. In the United States and Europe the use of prophylactic penicillin seems to have greatly reduced the early mortality and at least 80 to 90 per cent of patients seem to be surviving into early adult life. There are very little good data about the overall survival, although it seems likely that it is shortened. The most common cause of death at all ages is acute infection, while it appears that renal failure is becoming a more frequent cause of death in older sickling populations.

LABORATORY DIAGNOSIS

The sickle-cell trait causes no haematological changes and is diagnosed by the finding of a positive sickling test together with haemoglobins A and S on electrophoresis (Fig. 21). Sickle-cell anaemia is diagnosed by the finding of a variable degree of anaemia, an elevated reticulocyte count, sickled erythrocytes on the peripheral blood film, a positive sickling test, and a haemoglobin electrophoretic pattern characterized by the absence of haemoglobin A and a preponderance of haemoglobin S with a variable amount of haemoglobin F (Fig. 21). The diagnosis is confirmed by finding the sickle-cell trait in both parents.

There is a variety of simple sickling tests available, but for ward

Fig. 21 The haemoglobin pattern in the sickling disorders (starch gel electrophoresis, protein stain, pH 8.5). The following are shown (left to right): (1 and 2) the sickle-cell trait; (3) normal; (4) sickle-cell anaemia; (5) normal.

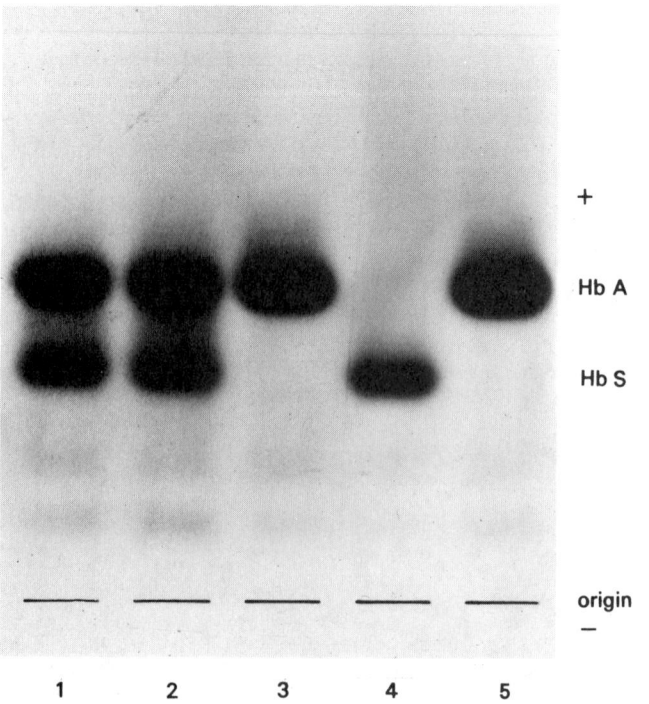

laboratories the simplest is to take a drop of blood and mix it with a drop of freshly prepared 2 per cent sodium metabisulphite, place a coverslip over the mixture, seal the edges with petroleum jelly and examine the slide for sickling after 1 h.

MANAGEMENT

Like all genetic diseases the first priority should be prevention. In the few places it has been tried, prospective genetic counselling and education of communities has not had much effect on the incidence of new cases. However, there are very effective methods for prenatal diagnosis and it is likely that programmes will be set up whereby women are screened at the antenatal clinic and at-risk couples advised about the possibility of therapeutic abortion of affected fetuses. However, before these programmes are fully developed, we need to know more about the natural history of sickle-cell anaemia and the burden that is placed on families and individual patients in high-incidence populations.

Apart from advice about anaesthesia and avoidance of unpressurized aircraft or deep-sea diving, individuals with the sickle trait require no treatment.

It is important to identify patients with sickle-cell anaemia as early as possible. In high-risk populations neonatal screening programmes should be established. As soon as the disease is identified babies should receive oral penicillin, daily; several trials have shown that prophylactive penicillin reduces morbidity in infancy and childhood. Patients should also receive a pneumococcal vaccine.

Most patients with sickle-cell anaemia manage well with relatively low haemoglobin levels, and regular blood transfusion is not ordinarily required. Adaptation to anaemia is particularly successful because of the low oxygen affinity of haemoglobin S. Episodes of infection should be treated early, and in populations in which the diet is low in folate, regular folate supplements should be added. Patients should be given access to a unit that is used to managing the disorder and advised to come early at the first sign of a painful crisis.

All but the mildest painful crises should be managed in hospital. The patient should be fully examined for evidence of underlying infection and then given adequate intravenous fluids, oxygen, antibiotics, and analgesia. It should be remembered that the pain may be excruciating. It may be necessary to administer strong analgesics, but because of the danger of respiratory depression, this should only be done in an environment in which patients are under close observation, with regular monitoring of blood gases. A recent report that the duration of painful crises can be reduced by a short course of high-dose corticosteroids requires confirmation.

The packed cell volume or haemoglobin level, and reticulocyte count should be estimated at least daily, and perhaps twice daily, but unless there is a fall in the haemoglobin level or evidence of an impending aplastic crisis as evidenced by a drop in the reticulocyte count, transfusion is not required. If the haemoglobin level falls due to increased haemolysis or bone marrow failure, a blood transfusion should be given to restore the haemoglobin level to normal or slightly higher. A sequestration crisis is an indication for urgent transfusion and very close surveillance because profound anaemia may develop over a period of hours. Hence, patients with a sickling crisis should have regular examination of the abdomen to assess spleen and liver size to try and anticipate impending episodes of sequestration. Complications such as the brain or lung syndrome should be treated by partial exchange transfusion. The level of sickle cells should be reduced to below 30 per cent. If the initial haemoglobin level is lower than 5 to 6g/dl, this can be achieved by transfusion up to 13/14g/dl followed by regular 'top-up' transfusions to reduce endogenous erythropoiesis. If the initial haemoglobin value is unusually high (e.g. in excess of 9 g/dl) it is better to carry out a partial exchange transfusion.

Hypertransfusion or exchange transfusion can be used to cover major surgical procedures or in patients who are having recurrent crises. Occasionally, the spleen may enlarge to such a degree that secondary hypersplenism occurs. This complication usually occurs in young children with sickle-cell disease, particularly in malarious areas. Splenectomy may be indicated in such cases. Similarly, because sequestration crises seem to recur in the same infant, this may also be an indication for splenectomy.

There is no special treatment required during pregnancy except for regular surveillance and folate supplementation. If the haemoglobin level drops significantly, or if there are recurrent crises, a regular transfusion regimen should be started to cover pregnancy and delivery. This should maintain a normal haemoglobin level and less than 30 per cent sickle cells (or haemoglobin S).

Occular complications, particularly proliferative retinopathy, require expert ophthalmological advice; early results of treatment of proliferative retinopathy with either zenon arc or argon laser indicate that the risk of vitreous haemorrhage is significantly reduced. Chronic hip pain and difficulty with walking due to aseptic necrosis of the femoral heads may require total hip replacement. It is frequently asked whether oral contraceptives are contraindicated in sickle-cell anaemia. There is no evidence that they increase the number of veno-occlusive episodes and should certainly not be withheld; it is probably wiser to use a low-oestrogen preparation. Any surgical procedure should be undertaken with great caution. It is critical to maintain high levels of oxygen and adequate hydration throughout the preoperative and postoperative period. Limb tourniquets should be avoided and any major procedures are probably best carried out after exchange transfusion. Haematuria is a worrying symptom and although drugs such as ϵ-aminocaproic acid have been advocated there is no evidence that they shorten the period of bleeding. Terminal renal failure should be managed as for any other form of renal insufficiency.

Priapism occurs quite frequently in patients with sickle-cell anaemia. It has been found that nearly two-thirds of major episodes are preceded by 'stuttering' attacks and therefore it has been suggested that effective therapy at this stage may reduce the risk of sustaining a major attack. Preliminary data suggest that stilboestrol 5 mg daily may be effective in preventing a major episode of priapism in patients who have had these spells in minor episodes. Fully developed priapism is a serious complication because if not relieved it frequently leads to permanent impotence. It has been suggested by the group in Jamaica, who have wide experience of this problem, that conservative treatment is restricted to 24 h at the most. During this time the patient should be hydrated, given adequate analgesia, and transfused up to a level at which the number of sickleable cells is below about 30 to 40 per cent. If there is no improvement by these simple measures, surgery should not be delayed. The most efficient procedure is a cavernosus–spongiosum shunt, which is a relatively minor procedure and produces a very good cosmetic result. Anticoagulants have no role in the treatment of priapism associated with sickle-cell anaemia; they have been advocated in cases of priapism associated with high platelet counts or hypercoagulable disorders; again, their role is uncertain. Whatever the cause of priapism the critical part of management seems to be to proceed to early surgery, rather than waiting in the hope of resolution, after 24 h. In patients who have become impotent after a severe episode of priapism it may be necessary to insert a penile prosthesis.

Although antisickling agents have been promoted, none has stood the test of a properly designed trial. Current research trying to prevent sickling with agents that inhibit polymerization of haemoglobin S decrease the intracellular concentration of deoxy haemoglobin S, or raise the level of fetal haemoglobin. A recent trial in the United States suggests that adults given daily hydroxyurea raise their HbF levels and have fewer crises.

OTHER SICKLING DISORDERS

The other sickling disorders include the interaction of haemoglobin S with haemoglobins C, D, and some of the rarer haemoglobin variants. The interactions with the different forms of β-thalassaemia were described earlier. In many of these conditions the clinical manifestations are little different from the sickle-cell trait, but haemoglobin SC disease and SD disease more closely resemble sickle-cell anaemia.

Haemoglobin SC disease

This disease is relatively common in West Africans. It is characterized by a milder anaemia than sickle-cell disease and many cases go unrecognized into adult life, when they may present with one of the complications of the disorder. These are the result of damage to the microvasculature, probably because of the relatively high haemoglobin level and the combined effects of sickling and red-cell rigidity caused by haemoglobin C (see below). Aseptic necrosis of the femoral or humeral heads or unexplained haematuria are common complications. Widespread thrombotic episodes, particularly involving the lungs, may occur during intercurrent infection or in pregnancy or the puerperium. The other serious complication is the damage that may follow repeated blockage of the retinal vessels, which leads to retinitis proliferans, retinal detachment, and permanent blindness. There is some evidence that patients with SC disease with an unusually high haemoglobin level are particularly at risk.

Haemoglobin SC disease is diagnosed by finding a mild anaemia with splenomegaly and characteristic morphological changes of the red cells including many target forms, intracellular crystals, and sickle cells. The sickling test is positive and haemoglobin electrophoresis shows haemoglobins S and C in about equal proportions. One parent shows the sickle-cell trait and the other the haemoglobin C trait.

In severe thrombotic episodes, patients with haemoglobin SC disease should be well hydrated and treated with anticoagulants. There is some evidence that regular venesection may help to delay the retinal changes in patients with unusually high haemoglobin levels, although this requires confirmation. Severe retinal disease is treated by coagulation therapy. In the life-threatening thrombotic episodes of pregnancy a partial exchange transfusion should be carried out.

Haemolysis due to other common haemoglobin variants

After haemoglobin S the second most common variant in West Africa is haemoglobin C. Haemoglobin C, because of its relatively low solubility, appears to exist in the precrystalline state in red cells and hence causes their rigidity and premature destruction in the microcirculation. The homozygous state for haemoglobin C, haemoglobin C disease, is characterized by a mild haemolytic anaemia with splenomegaly. The blood film shows 100 per cent target cells, and haemoglobin analysis shows C with small amounts of F. This is a mild disorder and no specific treatment is required.

The most common haemoglobin variant throughout South-East Asia and the Indian subcontinent is haemoglobin E. The homozygous state for this variant, haemoglobin E disease, is characterized by a very mild degree of anaemia with a slight reticulocytosis. The blood film shows mild morphological changes of the red cells, which are hypochromic and microcytic, resembling the changes seen in some forms of thalassaemia. Again, no treatment is required for this mild anaemia.

Haemoglobin variants that migrate in the position of haemoglobin S but do not sickle have been given the general title of haemoglobin D. There are several different molecular varieties of this variant. The homozygous state for some forms of haemoglobin D is associated with a moderately severe anaemia, splenomegaly, and a mild degree of haemolysis. The compound heterozygous state for haemoglobins S and D produces a disorder very similar to sickle-cell anaemia. It is diagnosed by finding one parent with the haemoglobin D trait and the other with the sickle-cell trait.

The unstable haemoglobin disorders

The unstable haemoglobin disorders are a rare group of inherited haemolytic anaemias that result from structural changes in the haemoglobin molecule, which cause its intracellular precipitation with the formation of Heinz bodies. Their true incidence is not known and there have been several families in which patients with one of these variants have had no affected relatives, suggesting that the condition has arisen by a new mutation.

AETIOLOGY AND PATHOGENESIS

Most of the unstable haemoglobins result from single amino-acid substitutions at critical areas of the molecule. For example, substitutions in or around the haem pocket can disrupt the normal anatomy and allow in water, with subsequent oxidative damage to haem, which leads to precipitation of the haemoglobin. Some substitutions, such as those involving proline residues, cause marked disturbance of the secondary structure of a globin chains. A few of these variants result from deletions of either single amino-acid residues or several residues. For example, in haemoglobin Gun Hill, five amino acids are missing including the haem-binding site. As the unstable haemoglobins precipitate in the red-cells or their precursors they produce intracellular inclusions or Heinz bodies, which make the cells more rigid and hence cause their premature destruction in the microcirculation (Fig. 22).

CLINICAL FEATURES

All these conditions are characterized by a haemolytic anaemia of varying severity and splenomegaly. There may be a history of the passage of dark urine, particularly during episodes of infection. Like all chronic haemolytic anaemias, there is an increased incidence of pigment gall-stones with their associated complications. The condition may become worse during periods of intercurrent infection and, in the more severe forms, such episodes are associated with life-threatening anaemia. Patients with unstable haemoglobins are at particular risk of haemolytic episodes following the administration of oxidant drugs such as sulphonamides.

Apart from intermittent icterus and splenomegaly there are no characteristic physical findings.

LABORATORY DIAGNOSIS

This condition should be thought of in any familial haemolytic anaemia, particularly if a red-cell enzyme deficiency cannot be demonstrated. The peripheral blood film shows the typical features of haemolysis but the red-cell morphology may be relatively normal. Occasionally there is a

Fig. 22 The peripheral blood film of a patient with an unstable haemoglobin disorder, haemoglobin Hammersmith. This is a postsplenectomy film, which shows small inclusions in many of the red cells (×1000, Leishman stain).

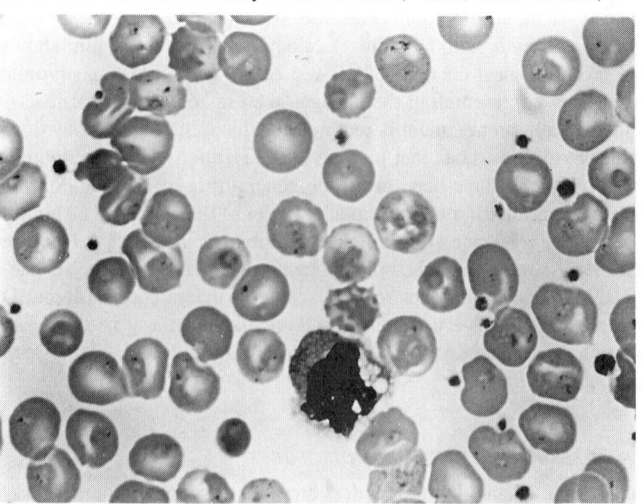

mild degree of hypochromia and microcytosis. Unless splenectomy has been carried out, Heinz bodies are not seen in the peripheral blood (Fig. 22).

The most characteristic feature of the unstable haemoglobins is their heat instability. If a dilute haemoglobin solution is heated at 50 °C for 15 min, most of the unstable haemoglobins precipitate as a dense cloud. A similar phenomenon can be induced by such agents as isopropanol. Some of these variants can be characterized by haemoglobins electrophoresis but others, because they result from the substitution of a neutral amino acid, produce no electrophoretic changes and can only be demonstrated by the heat precipitation test.

TREATMENT

Because these conditions are so rare there has been very little experience of the effects of splenectomy. From the little information that is available from the literature, and from the author's personal experience, it appears that if a child has had several life-threatening episodes of anaemia or is running a steady-state haemoglobins level that is impairing development or well-being, splenectomy should be done. Some of these haemoglobin variants produce a 'right shift' in the oxygen dissociation curve, and a measurement of the p_{50} as part of the presplenectomy assessment may help to decide whether to proceed to surgery; a marked right shift, i.e. an increased p_{50}, indicates that the anaemia should be more easily tolerated than if the oxygen dissociation curve is moved in the opposite direction with a low p_{50}. An accurate history from the child or its parents is probably more helpful, however.

Haemoglobin variants that cause abnormal oxygen binding

AETIOLOGY

The high oxygen-affinity haemoglobin variants result from single amino-acid substitutions at critical parts of the haemoglobin molecule which are involved in the configurational changes that underlie haem/haem interaction and the production of a sigmoid oxygen dissociation curve (see Chapter 22.4.1). Many of them occur at the junctions between the α- and β-subunits. Others involve the amino acids involved with the binding of 2, 3-diphosphoglycerate (**2, 3-DPG**) to haemoglobins. Increasing concentrations of 2, 3-DPG tend to push the oxygen dissociation curve to the right; fetal haemoglobin has a high oxygen affinity (left-shifted curve) because it cannot interact with 2, 3-DPG; mutations of the DPG-binding sites have a similar effect.

PATHOPHYSIOLOGY

All the high oxygen-affinity variants have a left-shifted oxygen dissociation curve with a reduced p_{50}. Thus the variant haemoglobin holds on to oxygen more avidly than normal haemoglobin and this leads to tissue hypoxia. This in turn causes an increased output of erythropoietin and an elevated red-cell mass.

CLINICAL FEATURES

Many patients with high oxygen-affinity variants are completely healthy and are only found to carry the variant when a routine haematological examination shows an unusually high haemoglobin level or packed cell volume. There have been one or two reports of arterial or venous thrombosis in these patients. However, this is uncommon and in most cases the patients are asymptomatic, there is no splenomegaly, and apart from the raised red-cell mass there are no associated haematological findings. Although it might be expected that a high oxygen-affinity haemoglobin would cause defective oxygenation of the fetus none of the reported families has had a history of frequent stillbirths.

DIAGNOSIS

The condition should be suspected in any patient with a pure red-cell polycythaemia associated with a left-shifted oxygen dissociation curve. The diagnosis can be confirmed by haemoglobin analysis.

TREATMENT

In asymptomatic patients with high oxygen-affinity haemoglobin variants no treatment is necessary. If the patient has associated vascular disease with symptoms of coronary or cerebral artery insufficiency the haematocrit should be reduced by regular venesection.

LOW OXYGEN-AFFINITY VARIANTS

At least six haemoglobin variants with reduced oxygen affinity have been reported. The first to be described, haemoglobin Kansas, was found in a mother and son with unexplained cyanosis. The subjects were asymptomatic and had normal haemoglobin levels without any evidence of haemolysis. Like many of the high-affinity variants the amino acid substitution in this variant was at the interface between the α- and β-globin chains. For reasons that are not clear, some substitutions in this region give rise to variants with a relatively low oxygen affinity. This condition should be thought of in any patient with an unexplained congenital cyanosis; the differential diagnosis is considered below.

Methaemoglobinaemia, carboxyhaemoglobinaemia, and sulphaemoglobinaemia

Methaemoglobinaemia

A condition characterized by increased quantities of haemoglobin in which the iron of haem is oxidized to the ferric (Fe^{3+}) form.

Carboxyhaemoglobinaemia (carbonmonoxyhaemoglobinaemia)

This results from the binding of carbon monoxide to the haem molecules.

Sulphaemoglobinaemia

A rare condition in which there is a mixture of haemoglobin derivatives whose structure is poorly characterized but which can be defined by their specific spectral characteristics.

PATHOGENESIS

As mentioned earlier in this section, each haemoglobin molecule has four haem molecules. At first sight it is not clear why the oxidation of a proportion of the iron atoms, or the fact that they are liganded to carbon monoxide, should cause such profound changes in oxygen transport. However, oxidation of 30 per cent of the haem molecules has a much more serious effect on tissue oxygenation than a reduction of the haemoglobin level by the same amount. This is because, if a single haem is oxidized, it so alters the conformation of the haemoglobin molecule that the oxygen affinity of the other three haems is increased. Thus methaemoglobin, carboxyhaemoglobin, and cyanmethaemoglobin all have very high oxygen affinities with 'left-shifted' oxygen dissociation curves, and hence are associated with impaired unloading of oxygen to the tissues.

Methaemoglobinaemia

Methaemoglobinaemia causes a variable degree of cyanosis and should be thought of in any patient with significant central cyanosis in whom there is no evidence of cardiorespiratory disease. The degree of cyanosis produced by 5 g/dl of deoxygenated haemoglobins can be produced by 1.5 g/dl methaemoglobin and 0.5 g/dl of sulphaemoglobin. Methaemoglobin concentrations of 10 to 20 per cent are tolerated quite well but, because it is useless as an oxygen carrier, levels above this are often associated with dyspnoea and headache. Much depends on the rapidity at which it is formed; many patients with lifelong methaemoglobinaemia are asymptomatic while individuals who have accumulated a similar level of methaemoglobin acutely after exposure to drugs or toxins may be acutely dyspnoeic. For reasons that are not clear it is unusual for patients with chronic methaemoglobinaemia to have an increased haemoglobin level or red-cell count.

Methaemoglobinaemia may arise as a result of a genetic defect in red-cell metabolism or haemoglobin structure, or may be acquired following the ingestion of various oxidant drugs and toxic agents.

GENETIC METHAEMOGLOBINAEMIA

There are two forms of inherited methaemoglobinaemia. The first results from a deficiency in red-cell NADH-diaphorase, the second from a structural alternation in either the α- or β-globin chains of haemoglobin.

NADH-diaphorase catalyses a step in the major pathway for methaemoglobin reduction. The enzyme reduces cytochrome b^5 using NADH as a hydrogen donor. The reduced cytochrome b^5 reduces, in turn, methaemoglobin to haemoglobin. Several different molecular forms of NADH-diaphorase deficiency have been identified by electrophoretic analysis of NADH-diaphorase in the red cells of affected patients. The condition is inherited as autosomal recessive. Homozygotes have elevated levels of methaemoglobin and are cyanosed from birth. Heterozygotes do not have elevated levels of methaemoglobin but seem to be unusually susceptible to the oxidant action of drugs. For example, severe cyanosis has been precipitated in heterozygotes for NADH-diaphorase deficiency by the use of antimalarial drugs.

There are several abnormal haemoglobin variants that are associated with genetic methaemoglobinaemia, all of which are designated haemoglobin M, and further identified by their place of discovery, e.g. haemoglobin M Boston, M Milwaukee, etc. These variants usually result from amino acid substitutions near the haem pocket. Normally, haem lies between two histidine residues, one called the proximal histidine, to which it is attached, and the other called the distal histidine. Oxygen is bound to haem at a site opposite to the distal histidine. If the distal histidine is substituted by tyrosine, as occurs in the α-chain variant haemoglobin M Boston and in the β-chain variant β-chain variant M Saskatoon, for example, a stable bond is formed between the haem iron and the phenolic ring of the tyrosine, and the iron atom is 'fixed' in the Fe^3 state. These haemoglobin variants are associated with cyanosis that is present from early life. In the case of the α-chain variants it is present from birth, while the β-chain haemoglobin variants only produce cyanosis after the first few months of life as adult haemoglobin synthesis becomes established. Unlike NADH-diaphorase deficiency, which is inherited as a recessive, the haemoglobins M have a dominant form of inheritance. Thus it is very simple to make the diagnosis of genetic methaemoglobinaemia and to determine the likely molecular basis by taking a good history; even the affected globin chain can be ascertained!

The diagnosis is confirmed by spectroscopic examination of the blood and by determination of methaemoglobin levels. The precise cause can be established by an assay of NADH-diaphorase or by haemoglobin analysis under appropriate conditions.

Genetic methaemoglobinaemia due to NADH-diaphorase deficiency is readily treated by the administration of ascorbic acid, 300 to 600 mg daily by mouth in divided doses, or by the administration of methylene blue, either intravenously (1 mg/kg body weight) or by mouth, 60 mg three to four times daily. On the other hand, the genetic methaemoglobinaemias due to structural haemoglobin variants do not respond to ascorbic acid, methylene blue, or any other treatment. In fact, most affected individuals go through life asymptomatic and require no treatment.

ACQUIRED METHAEMOGLOBINAEMIA

Acquired methaemoglobinaemia usually results from the administration of drugs or exposure to chemicals that cause oxidation of haemoglobin. There are many agents that are capable of exceeding the red cells' ability to reduce methaemoglobin. They include ferricyanide, bivalent copper, chromate, chlorate, quinones, and certain dyes with a high oxidation–reduction potential. Nitrite, often used as a preservative, is one of the most common methaemoglobin-forming agents; nitrates, after conversion to nitrites in the gut, may cause serious methaemoglobinaemia in infants. Other agents that commonly cause methaemoglobinaemia include phenacetin, primiquin, sulphonamides, and various aniline dye derivatives.

If any of the agents listed above is given in a low dose over a long period of time it may lead to chronic methaemoglobinaemia with or without a haemolytic anaemia. However, after exposure to a large amount of these agents, and the development of in excess of 50 to 60 per cent methaemoglobin, the symptoms of acute anaemia develop because methaemoglobin lacks the capacity to transport oxygen. Thus the clinical picture may be characterized by vascular collapse, coma, and death.

Methaemoglobinaemia with haemolytic anaemia

The haemolytic action of oxidant drugs is described later (Chapter 22.4.13). Chronic methaemoglobinaemia with haemolytic anaemia characterized by Heinz body formation and fragmented red cells occurs commonly in patients receiving dapsone, salazopyrine, or phenacetin. This condition is usually innocuous and can be modified by adjusting the dose of the drug.

Occasionally, acute intravascular haemolysis associated with methaemoglobinaemia and intravascular coagulation occurs and may lead to renal failure. It usually follows the ingestion or infusion of a strong oxidizing agent such as chlorate or arsine. There is gross intravascular haemolysis and methaemoglobinaemia together with evidence of disseminated intravascular coagulation. The haemoglobin level may fall very rapidly and the condition may be complicated by renal failure.

TREATMENT

In cases of chronic acquired methaemoglobinaemia, the drug or chemical agent should be removed where possible. If continued therapy is required, it should be at a lower dose.

Acute toxic methaemoglobinaemia may present a serious medical emergency. Methylene blue should be given in a dose of 1 to 2 mg/kg intravenously over a 5-min period. Repeated doses may be needed. Toxicity is uncommon although doses of over 15 mg/kg may cause haemolysis in young infants. The drug should not be used if the methaemoglobinaemia is due to chlorate poisoning as it may convert the chlorate to hypochlorite, which is an even more toxic compound.

In cases in which there is acute methaemoglobinaemia with intravascular haemolysis, haemodialysis with exchange transfusion is the treatment of choice.

Carboxyhaemoglobinaemia

Carbon monoxide has an affinity for haemoglobin approximately 210 times that of oxygen. Following acute exposure it is so tightly bound that it takes about 4 h for an individual with normal ventilation to expel half of it. At levels of 5 to 10 per cent there may be no symptoms, but above 20 per cent there is usually headache and weakness. Levels of 40 to 60 per cent or more lead to unconsciousness and death.

Carbon monoxide poisoning is discussed in Section 8 and secondary polycythaemia due to chronic exposure is considered in Chapter 22.4.14.

Sulphaemoglobinaemia

This poorly defined condition derives its name from the fact that it can be produced *in vitro* by the action of hydrogen sulphide on haemoglobin. It has not been reported as a genetic disorder and is usually associated with the administration of drugs, particularly sulphonamides or phenacetin. It has also been reported in patients with chronic constipation or malabsorption syndromes (enterogenous cyanosis), although its relation to these disorders is far from clear.

Other acquired abnormalities of the structure or synthesis of haemoglobin

GLYCOSYLATED HAEMOGLOBIN, HAEMOGLOBIN A₁C

Haemoglobin may undergo post-translational modification in patients with diabetes. The abnormal haemoglobin, haemoglobin A_1C, is formed by the non-enzymic combination of glucose with the N-terminus of the β-chain, forming first a Schiff base, which then undergoes a rearrangement to form a stable ketoamine. The level of haemoglobin A_1C is raised in diabetics and is related to the blood sugar level over the previous weeks. The value of the estimation of haemoglobin A_1C as an index of the control of diabetes is considered in Section 11.

REFERENCES

Beutler, E. (1995). Hemoglobinopathies associated with unstable haemoglobin. In *Williams hematology*, (ed. E. Beutler, M.A. Lichtman, B.S. Coller, and T.J. Kipps). McGraw-Hill, New York (in press).

Beutler, E. (1995). The sickle cell diseases and related disorders. In *Williams hematology*, (ed. E. Beutler, M.A. Lichtman, B.S. Coller, and T.J. Kipps). McGraw-Hill, New York (in press). McGraw-Hill Inc.

Bunn, H.F. and Forget, B.G. (1986). *Hemoglobin: molecular, genetic and clinical aspects*. Saunders, Philadelphia.

Cao, A. and Rosatelli, M.C. (1993). Screening and prenatal diagnosis of the hemoglobinopathies. *Baillière's Clinical Haematology*, **6**, 263–98.

Francis, R.B. and Johnson, C.S. (1991). Vascular occlusions in SS anemia. *Blood*, **77**,, 1405–14.

Gibbons, R.J., Suthers, G.K., Wilkie, A.O.M., Buckle, B.J., and Higgs, D.R. (1992). X-linked α-thalassemia/mental retardation (ATR-X) syndrome: localization to Xq12–21.31 by X- inactivation and linkage analysis. *American Journal of Human Genetics*, **51**, 1136–49.

Hebbel, R.P. (1991). Beyond polymerization. The red blood cell membrane and sickle cell disease pathophysiology. *Blood*, **77**, 214–17.

Higgs, D.R. (1993). α-thalassaemia. *Baillière's Clinical Haematology*, **6**, 117–50.

Higgs, D.R., Vickers, M.A., Wilkie, A.O.M., Pretorius, I-M, Jarman A.P., and Weatherall, D.J. (1989). A review of the molecular genetics of the human α globin gene cluster. *Blood*, **73**, 1081–104.

Kazazian, H.H. (1990). The thalasssemia syndromes: molecular basis and prenatal diagnosis in 1990. *Seminars in Hematology*, **27**, 209–28.

Mansouri, A. and Lurie, A.A. (1993). Concise review: methemoglobinemia. *American Journal of Hematology*, **42**, 7–12.

Nagel, R.L. and Lawrence, C. (1991). The distinct pathobiology of sickle cell-hemoglobin C disease. *Hematology/Oncology Clinics of North America*, **5**, 433.

Noguchi, C.T., Schechter, A.N., and Rodgers, G.P. (1993). Sickle cell disease pathophysiology. *Baillière's Clinical Haematology*, **6**, 57–92.

Serjeant, G.R. (1992). *Sickle cell disease*, (2nd edn). Oxford University Press.

Stamatoyannopoulos, G., Nienhuis, A.W., Majerus, P.W. and Varmus, H. (1994). *The molecular basis of blood diseases*, (2nd edn). Saunders, Philadelphia.

Thein, S.L. (1993). β-Thalassaemia. *Baillière's Clinical Haematology*, **6**, 151–76.

Weatherall, D.J. and Clegg, J.B. (1981). *The thalassaemia syndromes*, (3rd edn). Blackwell Scientific, Oxford.

Weatherall, D.J., Clegg, J.B., Higgs, D.R., and Wood, W.G. (1993). The hemoglobinopathies. In *The metabolic basis of inherited disease*, (7th edn) (ed. C.R. Scriver, A.L. Beaudet, W.S. Sly, and D. Valle). McGraw-Hill, New York (in press).

22.4.8 Other anaemias resulting from defective red-cell maturation

D. J. WEATHERALL

In the previous chapters we have considered anaemias that result from a reduced output of red cells due either to a lack of specific factors required for the nuclear or cytoplasmic maturation of their precursors, or from well-defined genetic defects of haemoglobin synthesis. However, in addition to these conditions there are other dyserythropoietic anaemias which are caused by either genetic or acquired disorders of red cell maturation but in which the precise defect is, as yet, unknown (Table 1).

Although the anaemias described in the following sections form a very diverse group, they have one major feature in common. In each case the marrow is able to respond to an increased output of erythropoietin by proliferation of its red-cell precursors. However, because maturation is defective many of these cells are destroyed before they reach the circulation. This process results in a haematological picture characterized by erythroid hyperplasia of the bone marrow associated with a low and inappropriate reticulocyte response in the blood, a combination of findings which is the hallmark of ineffective erythropoiesis.

The sideroblastic anaemias

The sideroblastic anaemias are a group of genetic or acquired disorders characterized by severe dyserythropoieses and marked iron loading of the red-cell precursors and, in some cases, widespread haemosiderosis (Table 2).

DEFINITION

The term sideroblastic anaemia is an unfortunate one. Normal red-cell precursors are sideroblasts in that they contain small aggregations of ferritin iron scattered throughout the cytoplasm. These remain in the cells until they reach the peripheral blood, after which they are removed in the spleen. Red cells that contain iron-staining granules, siderocytes, are only seen in the blood after splenectomy. In the sideroblastic anaemias there is an abnormal accumulation of iron in the erythroblasts. Much of the excess iron is situated in the mitochondria, which lie in a circle round the nucleus of the red-cell precursors, and hence on staining with Prussian blue or other iron stains, a ring or collar of heavy iron granules is seen in the perinuclear region (Fig. 1). Such red-cell precursors are called abnormal or 'ring' sideroblasts and are the characteristic feature of all the sideroblastic anaemias. The iron loading of the mitochondria can be easily seen on electron microscopy (Fig. 2).

AETIOLOGY AND PATHOGENESIS

The underlying aetiology of the sideroblastic anaemias has not been completely worked out. It is clear that there is a variable defect in erythroid maturation with intramedullary destruction of red-cell precursors and a considerable degree of ineffective erythropoiesis. It is believed that the marked accumulation of iron, and the resulting mitochondrial damage, plays an important part in this maturation defect. Whether this is the primary abnormality in sideroblastic anaemia is uncertain, however.

The sideroblastic anaemias are all characterized by the curious anomaly of hypochromic red cells together with iron loading of their precursors. This suggests that there is underlying abnormality of haemoglobin synthesis and it is currently believed that at least some forms of sideroblastic anaemia may result from defective haem production. There is some evidence that the rate of iron movement into red-cell precursors

Table 1 *Anaemias in which defective red-cell maturation and increased ineffective erythropoiesis is a major factor*

Abnormality of DNA synthesis
Vitamin B_{12} deficiency
Folate deficiency
Drugs (antipurines, antipyrimidines)

Defective cytoplasmic maturation
Disorders of globin synthesis:
    Thalassaemia
Disorders of haem and/or iron metabolism:
    Sideroblastic anaemia

Unknown mechanism
Congenital dyserythropoietic anaemias
Myelodysplastic syndrome (see Chapter 22.3.7)
Infection
Chemicals and toxins

Table 2 *The sideroblastic anaemias*

Congenital
X-linked
? others

Acquired
Primary or idiopathic (myelodysplastic syndrome)
Secondary:
    Drugs—INAH, chloramphenicol, etc.
    Alcohol
    Lead
    Malabsorption
    Secondary carcinoma
    Other systemic disorders

is regulated, at least to some degree, by the level of haem in the cells and, therefore, if there is a defect in haem synthesis, there may be increased movement of iron into the developing red cells.

The synthetic pathway for the production of haem is described in Section 11. Recent work on the genetic sideroblastic anaemias has shown that they are probably heterogeneous at the molecular level. In one family a mutation has been found in exon 9 of the δ-aminolevulinate synthase gene, which is located on the short arm of the X chromosome. The resulting asparagine for isoleucine substitution involves the pyridoxal 5-phosphate-binding site, thus accounting for the reduced ability of the cofactor to catalyse the formation of δ-aminolevulinic acid. There is increasing evidence that other mutations may be involved in the genetic form of sideroblastic anaemia and it has been suggested, though not yet proved, that some of them may involve mitochondrial DNA.

It is now clear that the primary, acquired form of sideroblastic anaemia is a neoplastic condition of the bone marrow that forms part of the myelodysplastic syndrome. So far no specific enzyme defects have been identified and there have been no consistent cytogenetic findings. The recent successes in finding the molecular pathology of genetic sideroblastic anaemia point the way for future research into the pathogenesis of the acquired forms, which may well result from somatic mutations. These might involve any of the genes in the haem synthesis pathway or mitochondrial DNA.

In some forms of sideroblastic anaemia, specific mitochondrial toxins can be implicated. These include chloramphenicol, phenacetin, and paracetamol. The sideroblastic anaemia of lead poisoning probably results from inhibition of δ-aminolaevulinic acid synthase and haem synthase by the action of lead. Agents such as alcohol and some of the antituberculous drugs may interfere with pyridoxine metabolism and hence with the early steps of haem synthesis.

The sideroblastic anaemias are a good example of what have been called 'iron-loading anaemias'. In most anaemias in which there is marked erythroid hyperplasia and ineffective erythropoiesis, there is an increased rate of gastrointestinal iron absorption. This occurs in the thalassaemias (see Chapter 22.4.7), sideroblastic anaemias, and in other dyserythropoietic disorders. The reason why patients with these conditions, who often have increased iron stores, continue to iron load is not clear. Ultimately they may develop generalized haemosiderosis with endocrine, liver, and cardiac damage (see Chapter 22.4.4).

THE GENETIC SIDEROBLASTIC ANAEMIAS

These are extremely rare conditions. In most cases they follow a sex-linked pattern of inheritance with males showing anaemia and female carriers only mild morphological changes of their red cells. More severely affected females have been encountered, however. This may reflect variability of X-chromosome inactivation or genetic heterogeneity of the disorder. The anaemia usually appears in early childhood, although presentation later in life has been well documented.

Fig. 1 Bone marrow treated with a stain specific for iron showing typical ring sideroblasts (×800).

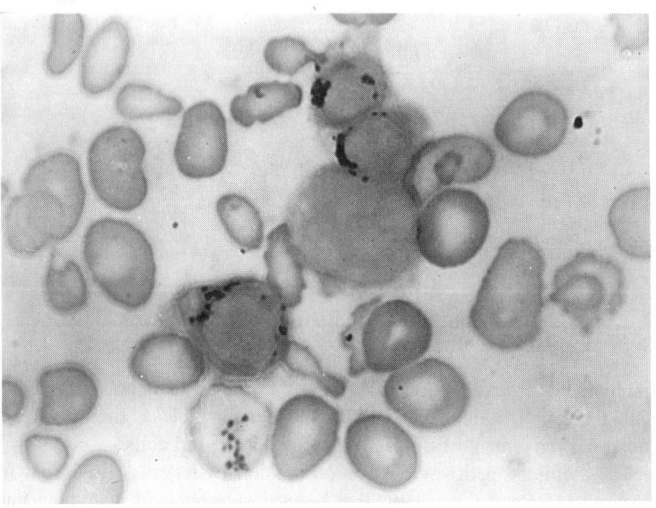

Fig. 2 Iron loading of the mitochondria in the perinuclear region in sideroblastic anaemia (electron microscopy, ×20 000). (Reproduced by permission of Professor S. Wickramasinghe.)

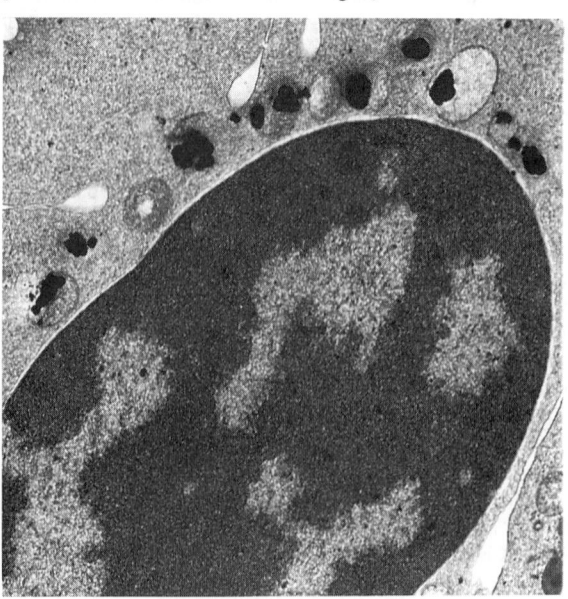

Table 3 *Clinical and haematological features of sideroblastic anaemia*

Congenital	Acquired
Mainly males	Both sexes
Mild splenomegaly	Splenomegaly unusual unless part of a myeloproliferative disorder
Dimorphic blood picture with an extremely hypochromic population	Dimorphic blood picture; usually a population of moderately hypochromic cells
Reduced MCH and MCV	MCV often normal or increased and MCH normal or slightly reduced
Marrow hyperplasia with large percentage of ring sideroblasts	Marrow hyperplasia, normal cellularity, or hypoplasia; variable numbers of ring sideroblasts
Platelets and white cells normal	White cells usually normal; platelets reduced in 30% of cases; occasionally increased
Red-cell protoporphyrin reduced	Red-cell protoporphyrin elevated
Hb A$_2$ reduced, Hb F normal	Hb A$_2$ reduced *or* normal. Hb F normal

The condition is characterized by a mild to moderate anaemia with haemoglobin values in the 6 to 9 g/dl range, and there is usually some degree of splenomegaly (Table 3). The peripheral blood film shows hypochromic cells interspersed with a normochromic population (Fig. 3). The bone marrow shows erythroid hyperplasia with abnormal nuclear and cytoplasmic maturation and the presence of a large proportion of ring sideroblasts (Plates 37, 38). The red-cell protoporphyrin level is usually reduced.

In the X-linked form the mother of affected sons shows small numbers of hypochromic cells mixed in a predominantly normochromic population and a few ring sideroblasts in the bone marrow. Some, but not all, patients with this disorder show progressive iron loading as they grow older with a steady increase in serum iron and ferritin values. Ultimately, they may develop generalized haemosiderosis, which may lead to diabetes, liver disease, and progressive cardiac failure.

ACQUIRED SIDEROBLASTIC ANAEMIA

Primary

By far the most common form of acquired sideroblastic anaemia is the primary idiopathic type, for which no underlying cause can be identified. This condition occurs equally in males and females and usually presents after the age of 50 years, although the author has seen several cases presenting in early childhood. There is usually a mild degree of anaemia, and splenomegaly occurs in only a small proportion of cases. The haematological changes are characterized by haemoglobin values in the 7 to 10 g/dl range and a 'dimorphic' blood film with both normochromic and hypochromic populations of red cells. The red-cell indices are often abnormal, with an increased MCV in the 100 to 120 fl range. The platelet count is usually normal, but both thrombocytosis and thrombocytopenia have been observed. The bone marrow shows marked erythroid hyperplasia and the presence of increased numbers of ring sideroblasts.

Many patients with this condition run a long course with chronic anaemia as the only abnormal finding. In some cases there is a steady increase in the serum iron and ferritin values, and occasionally generalized haemosiderosis may occur, with the development of diabetes, liver damage, and cardiac failure. A proportion of patients who present with sideroblastic anaemia develop leukaemia. The relation between this form of sideroblastic anaemia and the other disorders that comprise the myelodysplastic syndrome is considered in Chapter 22.3.7.

Secondary

In some individuals with acquired sideroblastic anaemia it is possible to demonstrate exposure to toxins or drugs. One of the most common causes of the condition, certainly in the United States although less frequently in the United Kingdom, is acute alcoholic intoxication. These patients are usually seen after a very high intake of alcohol and their blood films are dimorphic with marked macrocytosis; the bone marrow shows both dyserythropoietic and megaloblastic changes and variable numbers of ring sideroblasts. There is a high incidence of associated folic acid deficiency (see Chapter 22.4.6).

The antituberculous drugs, isoniazid, cycloserine, and pyrazinamide, given either alone or in combination, occasionally cause a secondary sideroblastic anaemia. The actual incidence of anaemia in patients receiving these drugs is low, although several studies have shown that a high proportion of them have ring sideroblasts in their bone marrows. Isoniazid therapy is frequently associated with sideroblastic changes in the marrow but severe anaemia is rare. In contrast, cycloserine and pyrazinamide quite often produce anaemia with sideroblastic changes. Chloramphenicol also causes sideroblastic anaemia in a small proportion of patients. A sideroblastic reaction is seen commonly in patients with lead poisoning, who are anaemic and who also have basophilic stippling of their red cells. There have been occasional reports of the association of sideroblastic anaemia with other drugs, phenacetin and paracetamol for example, but there has usually been evidence of associated haemolytic anaemia and folate deficiency.

Finally, sideroblastic changes are occasionally seen in a diverse series of systemic diseases. Among the non-haematological disorders in which a few ring sideroblasts occur are infections, hypothyroidism, rheumatoid arthritis, and collagen–vascular diseases. Among the haematological disorders in which ring sideroblasts are found are listed various haemolytic anaemias, pernicious anaemia, folic acid deficiency, different forms of leukaemia, myeloma, lymphoma, and the myeloproliferative diseases. In all these conditions the presence of ring sideroblasts is unexplained and the associated anaemia is clearly related to the underlying disorder rather than to the sideroblastic reaction.

There appears to be a distinct group of patients with sideroblastic anaemia who respond well to pyridoxine. Although, as mentioned earlier, many patients with acquired sideroblastic anaemia show some biochemical evidence of abnormal pyridoxine metabolism, the majority of them do not respond well to pyridoxyl phosphate. There are reports of individuals who did have a full haematological response, however, and whose haemoglobin values fell after withdrawal of pyridoxine. Whether this represents a separate and aetiologically distinct group of sideroblastic anaemias remains to be determined. True pyridoxine deficiency has been reported in a few patients with an underlying malabsorption syndrome. Both the sideroblastic changes and the steatorrhoea remitted on a gluten-free diet.

THE DIAGNOSIS OF SIDEROBLASTIC ANAEMIA (TABLE 3)

The sideroblastic anaemias are often missed because the morphological appearances of the red cells are not adequately examined. Most of these conditions are associated with a moderate degree of anaemia but the red-cell indices may be confusing. In the genetic group they usually show an overall hypochromic and microcytic picture with low MCH and MCV values, but in the acquired sideroblastic anaemias there may be a macrocytosis. In the genetic forms the blood picture is dimorphic (see Fig. 3), while the red-cell changes in the acquired variety are non-specific. The diagnosis depends on the marrow appearances. The diagnosis of primary or secondary sideroblastic anaemia rests on the determination of exposure to drugs, lead, or other toxins, and the presence or absence of another general systemic or haematological disorder.

TREATMENT

The genetic sideroblastic anaemias usually require no treatment. It is worth giving a trial of pyridoxine (see below), although in most cases there is no response. Secondary folate deficiency should be excluded and the patient should be followed up carefully with regular serum iron and ferritin estimations. If there is evidence of iron accumulation, it is worth starting on a programme of regular venesections or, if the patient cannot tolerate this approach, using a chelating agent such as desferrioxamine (see Chapter 22.4.4).

In the acquired sideroblastic anaemias a careful search for an underlying cause should be made. Particular care should be taken to obtain a good drug history and any evidence of exposure to toxins. Once an underlying disease has been excluded, these patients simply require regular surveillance. The haemoglobin level may remain constant for many years and no treatment is required. It is worth trying a course of pyridoxine, and high doses in the order of 25 to 100 mg or even larger thrice daily may be required to obtain a haematological response. In the majority of cases this type of therapy produces either no response or a short-lived reticulocytosis with no increase in the haemoglobin level. Trials of pyridoxal phosphate have been found to be equally unsuccessful. It is important to rule out secondary folate deficiency by measuring the serum folate level, and, if this is low, folic acid should be given. Splenectomy seems to have little place in the treatment of either genetic or acquired sideroblastic anaemia. Finally, if patients become symptomatic they should receive regular blood transfusions. In all cases of sideroblastic anaemia, it is important to monitor the serum iron and ferritin levels. If evidence of iron overload is obtained, these patients should be treated with desferrioxamine along the lines outlined in Chapter 22.4.4.

In the secondary sideroblastic anaemias due to drug therapy the drug should be stopped where possible. The management of lead poisoning is described in Section 8.

Other dyserythropoietic anaemias

To complete this review of anaemias due to defective erythropoiesis we must briefly describe some uncommon forms of congenital and acquired dyserythropoietic anaemia.

Fig. 3 Genetically determined sideroblastic anaemia. The peripheral blood film shows a dimorphic population with both normochromic and misshapen hypochromic microcytic red cells (×800. Leishman stain).

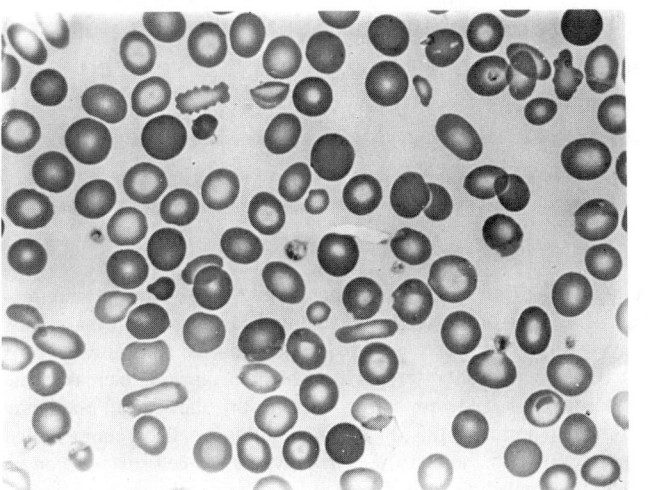

CONGENITAL DYSERYTHROPOIETIC ANAEMIAS

In recent years a group of disorders called congenital dyserythropoietic anaemias (CDA) has been defined by their bizarre red-cell precursor morphology and associated serological findings. These conditions usually, although not always, present early in life with anaemia and unusual red-cell changes characterized by anisopoikilocytosis and, sometimes, macrocytosis. Bone marrow examination shows marked erythroid hyperplasia, the most striking feature being multinuclearity of the red-cell precursors. The fact there is a very poor reticulocyte response indicates that these are primarily dyserythropoietic anaemias.

Several types of CDA are recognized. In type 1 there are megaloblastoid erythroblasts with internuclear chromatin-bridge formation, i.e. the cell nuclei are incompletely separated from each other. Type 2 is characterized by erythroblastic multinuclearity and a positive acid-serum lysis test using the sera of some but not all individuals, and not (in contrast to paroxysmal nocturnal haemoglobinuria, see Chapter 22.3.12) when using the patient's serum. This disorder has been called HEMPAS—*hereditary erythroblastic multinuclearity with positive acid serum lysis*. Type 3 CDA is characterized by erythroblast multinuclearity with large, abnormal erythroblasts which have been called gigantoblasts. At the time of writing the form of genetic transmission and underlying cellular defects in this group of disorders have not been determined and they can only be defined on morphological or serological grounds associated, in some cases, with a family history.

ACQUIRED REFRACTORY ANAEMIAS AND THE MYELODYSPLASTIC SYNDROME

Occasionally, patients are encountered with mild to moderate anaemia whose marrows show either erythroid hyperplasia or hypoplasia associated with marked dyserythropoiesis. Their bone marrow is characterized by marked abnormalities of red-cell maturation including asynchrony of nuclear and cytoplasmic maturation, mild megaloblastic change, mitotic abnormalities including nuclear fragmentation, karyorrhexis (abnormal lobulation of the nuclei), and binuclearity. It is now clear that disorders of this type, in which none of the identifiable causes of dyserythropoiesis can be found, are preleukaemic and therefore constitute part of the myelodysplastic syndrome (see Chapter 22.3.7). In a few cases, specific chromosomal abnormalities can be demonstrated. For example, in the 5q-syndrome there is a chronic macrocytic anaemia with normal or decreased erythroid precursors in the bone marrow, dyserythropoiesis, and an absence of ring sideroblasts or excessive iron accumulation. This condition seems to be part of the myelodysplastic syndrome and is associated with a relatively good prognosis. All patients who present with otherwise unexplained chronic dyserythropoietic anaemias should be maintained under regular surveillance because many of them develop other features of the myelodysplastic syndrome and may develop leukaemia, months or years after the onset of their anaemia.

DYSERYTHROPOIESIS AND INFECTION (PLATE 39)

The haematological manifestations of infection are considered later in this chapter. The bone marrow response to infection has been a neglected area of haematology for many years. However, there is increasing evidence that dyserythropoiesis may occur in association with a variety of infections, particularly viral and parasitic. There have been sporadic reports of acute dyserythropoietic changes in the bone marrows of patients with severe bacterial infections, although the incidence of this complication is uncertain. Similar changes may be found in patients with viral infections. The most extreme example of the association of viral infection and bone marrow damage is the recently described virus haemophagocytic syndrome. This disorder is usually seen in immunosuppressed patients and is characterized by a rapidly progressive anaemia together with marked erythroid hyperplasia, dyserythropoiesis, and erythrophagocytosis of red-cell precursors by bone marrow macro-

phages. Although little is known about the natural history of this disorder it seems to carry an extremely poor prognosis.

Dyserythropoiesis is also a feature of *Plasmodium falciparum* malaria infection. It is seen frequently in acute *P. falciparum* malaria infections in non-immune individuals and is also well documented in children with chronic malaria in West Africa. The bone marrows of these patients are often hyperplastic, with marked abnormalities of red-cell precursor maturation.

While, in general, very little is known about the bone marrow responses to infection it is becoming clear that in any severely ill patient with progressive anaemia in whom the marrow shows dyserythropoietic changes, an underlying infection should be suspected.

REFERENCES

Beutler, E. (1995). The hereditary dyserythropoietic anemias. In *Williams hematology*, (ed. E. Beutler, M.A. Lichtman, B.S. Coller, and T.J. Kipps). McGraw-Hill, New York (in press).

Bunn, H.F. (1986). 5q− and disordered haematopoiesis. *Clinics in Haematology*, **15**, 1023–35.

Cotter, P.D., Baumann, M., and Bishop, D.F. (1992). Enzymatic defect in 'X-linked' sideroblastic anemia: molecular evidence for erythroid δ-aminolevulinate synthase deficiency. *Proceedings of the National Academy of Sciences (USA)*, **89**, 4028–32.

Dewald, G.W., Pierre, R.V., and Phyliky, R.L. (1982). Three patients with structurally abnormal X chromosomes, each with Xq13 breakpoints and a history of idiopathic acquired sideroblastic anemia. *Blood*, **59**, 100–5.

Heimpel, H. (1976). Congenital dyserythropoietic anemia type I: clinical and experimental aspects. In *Congenital disorders of erythropoiesis*, (ed. R. Porter and D.W. Fitzsimons), Ciba Foundation Symposium 37, pp. 135–50. North-Holland, Amsterdam.

Jacobs, A. and Clark, R.E. (1986). Pathogenesis and clinical variations in the myelodysplastic syndromes. *Clinics in Haematology*, **15**, 925–51.

McKenna, R.W., Risdall, R.J., and Brunning, R.D. (1981). Virus associated hemophagocytic syndrome. *Human Pathology*, **12**, 395–8.

Mollin, D.L. (1965). A symposium on sideroblastic anaemia. Introduction: sideroblasts and sideroblastic anaemia. *British Journal of haematology*, **11**, 41–8.

Nusbaum, N.J. (1991). Concise review: genetic basis for sideroblastic anemia. *American Journal of Hematology*, **37**, 41–4.

Peto, T.E.A., Pippard, M.J., and Weatherall, D.J. (1983). Iron overload in mild sideroblastic anaemia. *Lancet*, **i**, 375–8.

Verwilghen, R.L. (1976). Congenital dyserythropoietic anaemia type II (HEMPAS). In *Congenital disorders of erythropoiesis*, (ed. R. Porter and D.W. Fitzsimons), Ciba Foundation Symposium 37, pp. 150–70. North-Holland, Amsterdam.

Weatherall, D.J. and Abdalla, S. (1982). The anaemia of *P. falciparum* malaria. *British Medical Bulletin*, **38**, 147–51.

22.4.9 Haemolytic anaemic: the mechanisms and consequences of a shortened red cell survival

D. J. WEATHERALL

INTRODUCTION

The normal red cell survives for approximately 120 days in the circulation. If its lifespan is significantly shortened, the red cell mass falls, relatively less oxygen is transported to the kidneys, and hence there is an increased output of erythropoietin which results in an increased rate of erythropoiesis. If the bone marrow is healthy, the red cell mass may be restored to normal in this way. This condition is called a compensated haemolytic state. If the marrow is healthy, the red cell survival can be reduced by as much as eight times without the development of significant anaemia. However, if the red cell survival time is less than 15 days

Table 1 *Mechanisms of haemolysis*

Mechanisms	Examples
Abnormalities of red cell membrane	
Genetic abnormality of membrane structure	Hereditary spherocytosis, elliptocytosis
Alteration in lipid constitution	Liver disease
Altered sulphydryl reactivity	Oxidant drugs
Altered properties resulting from interaction with complement or immunoglobulins	Immune haemolytic anaemia
Increased permeability, reduced plasticity	Glycolytic enzyme defects
Increased rigidity causing abnormal flow	
Aggregation of haemoglobin molecules	Sickle cell anaemia
Decreased solubility of haemoglobin	Haemoglobin C disease
Inclusion (Heinz) body formation	Thalassaemia, unstable haemoglobins, oxidant drugs
Direct physical trauma	
Direct external trauma	March and karate haemoglobinuria
Turbulent flow	Cardiac haemolytic anaemia
Cleavage by fibrin strands	Microangiopathic haemolytic anaemia

even a healthy marrow cannot compensate and a haemolytic anaemia results. If the bone marrow is abnormal or if there is inadequate supply of iron or other agents required for red cell production, anaemia may result even if the red cell survival is considerably greater than 15 days.

Before describing the different forms of haemolytic anaemia it is necessary to review briefly the mechanisms which cause a shortened red cell survival, the consequences of haemolysis, and the various compensatory mechanisms which are brought into action in order to attempt to restore the red cell mass to normal. The diagnosis of haemolytic anaemia depends on an understanding of these basic principles.

HAEMOLYTIC MECHANISMS

Premature destruction of red cells occurs either because the red cell membrane is abnormal in structure or function, the cells are subjected to excessive physical trauma in the circulation, or because they have become unusually rigid due to the precipitation or abnormal molecular configuration of haemoglobin (Table 1).

For a red cell to survive it must be capable of altering its shape to quite a remarkable degree as it passes through the microcirculation. This characteristic depends mainly on the surface-to-volume ratio of the red cell which is in turn related to the integrity of its membrane. Normal red cell membrane function requires the production of energy for active transport of Na^+ and K^+ ions in and out of the cells and for maintenance of the membrane protein SH groups in a reduced state. It also depends on the constant renewal of membrane lipids for the preservation of a normal lipid composition. If these functions fail, the red cell tends to become spherical, i.e. it develops a small surface area relative to volume, and hence is not so easily deformed. This in turn leads to its selective sequestration in the spleen and other parts of the reticuloendothelial system. This is the type of haemolytic mechanism which occurs in genetic disorders of the red cell membrane such as hereditary spherocytosis, or in which there is a defect in its energy pathways. The membrane may also be damaged by interaction of antibodies on its surface with macrophages of the reticuloendothelial system or by the direct action of trauma, chemicals, bacteria, or parasites.

Direct trauma to the red cells may occur in several ways including turbulence created by cardiac valve prostheses, rigid fibrin strands in the microcirculation, or excessive pressure on body surfaces.

Red cells which contain abnormally aggregated or precipitated haemoglobin molecules become less deformable and may be damaged in the spleen or other parts of the microcirculation. This is the basis for the shortened red cell survival in the sickling and thalassaemia disorders.

Precipitation of haemoglobin with the production of intracellular inclusions, or Heinz bodies, may result from the action of a variety of oxidant agents. Oxidative damage to the red cell may occur in several ways and the mechanisms are only partly understood. They include reduction in red cell glutathione levels, haemoglobin instability, generation of superoxides and other intermediates capable of causing peroxidation of the membrane lipids, deficiency of antioxidants such as vitamin E, and the accumulation of iron.

The site of red cell destruction depends on the type and degree of damage to the cells. For example, complement damaged cells develop large holes in their membrane and are destroyed in the circulation whereas IgG-coated cells are removed by interaction with macrophages in the reticuloendothelial elements of the spleen and liver. It should be remembered that the constant bombardment of the spleen by abnormal red cells results in splenomegaly, a phenomenon which is called 'work hypertrophy'. Thus many haemolytic anaemias are associated with progressive splenomegaly and secondary hypersplenism.

THE CONSEQUENCES OF HAEMOLYSIS

The haematological and biochemical changes which result from haemolysis reflect both compensatory mechanisms aimed at restoring the circulating red cell mass to normal, and the results of an increased rate of haemoglobin breakdown from the prematurely destroyed red cell population (Table 2).

COMPENSATORY MECHANISMS (PLATE 40)

If there is a significant reduction in the circulating red cell mass, there is a compensatory increase in erythropoietin production from the kidney. Within a few days of the onset of haemolysis the reticulocyte count increases and erythroid hyperplasia of the bone marrow becomes measurable by a decrease in the myeloid/erythroid (M/E) ratio. If the haemolysis is sustained there is expansion of the erythroid marrow and within 2 to 3 months the rate of erythropoiesis may rise to 10 to 15 times normal. The increased rate of red cell production is reflected in the peripheral blood by a reticulocytosis and the presence of deep-blue staining macrocytes on the blood film. The reticulocytes are larger than normal and hence are called 'shift' or 'stress' reticulocytes; they may have skipped a terminal maturation division.

The increased rate of red cell turnover has some important consequences. There is a greater-than-normal demand for iron and folate. The spread of erythroid marrow down the long bones may lead to bone

Table 2 *The main features of haemolytic anaemia*

1. Increased red cell production
   Polychromasia
   Macrocytosis
   Reticulocytosis
   Erythroid hyperplasia; M/E ↓
   Increased folate requirements
2. Increased red cell destruction
   Bilirubin level raised
   Increased faecal and urinary urobilinogen
   Haptoglobin and haemopexin levels reduced
   Evidence of intravascular destruction:
   　　Methaemoglobinaemia
   　　Raised plasma haemoglobin
   　　Haemoglobinuria
   　　Haemosiderinuria
3. Short red cell survival
   Reduced ^{51}Cr $t_{1/2}$
4. Secondary effects
   Splenomegaly
   Bone changes

Fig. 1 Pathways of haemoglobin catabolism in haemolytic anaemia.

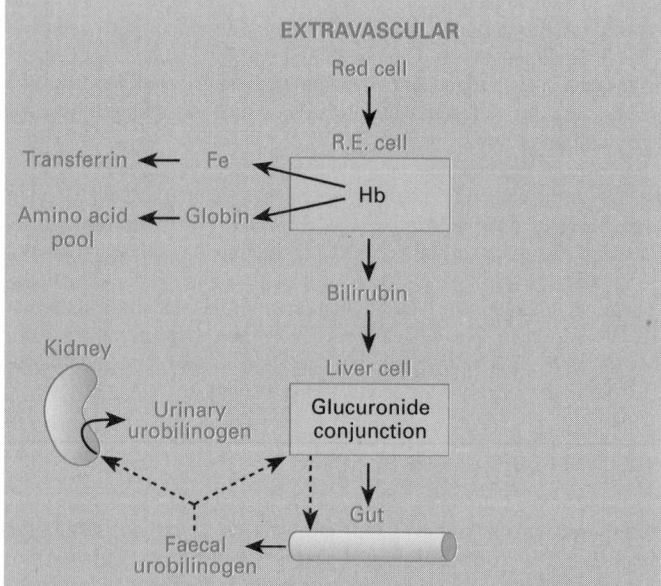

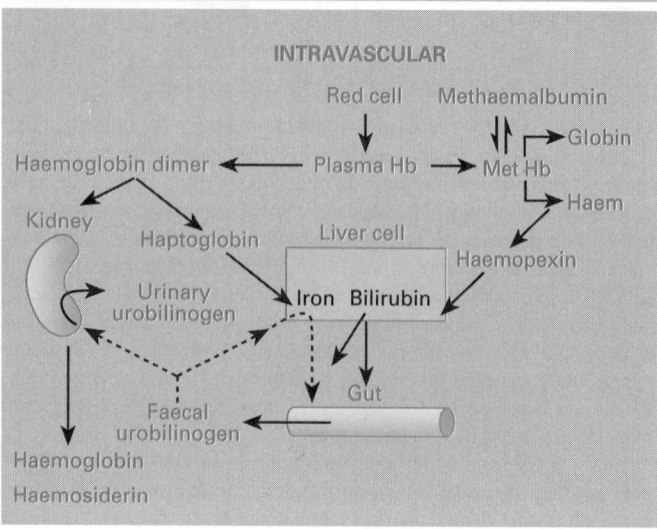

deformities similar to those observed in the severe dyserythropoietic anaemias. If the haemolysis has been present from early life, there is often extramedullary haemopoiesis in the spleen, liver, and lymph nodes.

HAEMOGLOBIN CATABOLISM

After haemoglobin is liberated into the circulation, it is bound to haptoglobin, and haptoglobin/haemoglobin complex is rapidly removed into the reticuloendothelial system (Fig. 1). Since this process may occur more rapidly than the liver's capacity to produce haptoglobin, a reduction in the serum haptoglobin level provides an extremely sensitive index of intravascular haemolysis. Even when the haemolysis is primarily extravascular, the haptoglobin level tends to fall, possibly because there is a small leak of free haemoglobin into the circulation. If the binding capacity of haptoglobin is exceeded, haemoglobin appears in the plasma where it is degraded and the haem which is liberated binds to a β-glycoprotein called haemopexin. Normally, sufficient haptoglobin is present to bind 100 to 140 mg of haemoglobin per 100 ml of plasma. The normal concentration of haemopexin is approximately 80 mg/100 ml of plasma.

When the haemoglobin binding capacity of haptoglobin and the haem binding capacity of haemopexin is saturated, free haemoglobin appears in the plasma where it is rapidly oxidized to methaemoglobin, dissociated, and the haem bound to albumin to form methaemalbumin. The latter produces a dirty brown discoloration of the plasma. If there is severe intravascular haemolysis, haemoglobin may be liberated into the plasma in sufficient amounts to saturate its haptoglobin, haemopexin, and albumin binding capacities and hence may appear in the urine. This happens because tetrameric haemoglobin dissociates into αβ dimers with a molecular weight of about 32 000. At a plasma haemoglobin level of 30 mg/dl or less no haemoglobin appears in the urine because it is reabsorbed in the proximal renal tubules. At levels in excess of this, free haemoglobin is found in the urine. Porphyrin and globin are rapidly catabolized in the renal tubular cells and much of the iron liberated is converted into haemosiderin. Cells containing the latter are cast off and appear in the urine; haemosiderinuria is the most reliable indication of chronic intravascular haemolysis.

There is increased production of bilirubin whenever the red cell survival is shortened. This is insoluble and is carried in the plasma bound to albumin. After conjugation in the liver cells it is excreted into the gut where it is converted by bacterial action to a group of compounds known collectively as faecal urobilinogen. Some is reabsorbed into the circulation and re-excreted via the enterohepatic circulation. However, being soluble these compounds pass through the glomeruli and appear in the urine as urinary urobilinogen where they can be demonstrated using Erlich's aldehyde reagent. Thus in all haemolytic anaemias there is an increased production of faecal and urinary urobilinogen. Because the formation of the former is dependent on the bacterial state of the gut, its level is not a reliable indicator of the degree of haemolysis. Furthermore, faecal urobilinogen may be derived from ineffective erythropoiesis, i.e. direct breakdown of developing erythroid precursors in the marrow, rather than from the peripheral destruction of mature erythrocytes. Thus its level may be elevated in dyserythropoietic anaemias as well as in haemolytic anaemias.

RECOGNITION OF HAEMOLYSIS

The clinical, haematological, and biochemical changes of haemolysis are easily understood if the principles outlined above have been followed. The degree of anaemia depends on the ability of the bone marrow to compensate by producing red cells at an increased rate, and the latter is recognized by the presence of deep-staining macrocytes on the blood film and by a variable reticulocytosis. The bone marrow shows variable erythroid hyperplasia with a decreased M/E ratio. There is an increased serum bilirubin level and serum haptoglobins are either reduced or

Table 3 *General approach to the diagnosis of haemolytic anaemia*

1. Is there evidence of an increased rate of red cell production?
   Blood film—polychromasia, macrocytosis
   Reticulocyte count—elevated
   Marrow–erythroid hyperplasia
2. Is there evidence of an increased rate of red cell destruction?
   Bilirubin level—elevated
   Faecal and urinary urobilinogen—elevated
   Plasma haptoglobin and haemopexin—reduced
   ^{51}Cr $t_{1/2}$—reduced
3. Is the haemolysis mainly intravascular?
   Plasma haemoglobin—elevated
   Methaemalbumin—present
   Haemoglobinuria—present
   Haemosiderin in urine—present (if chronic)
4. Where are the red cells being destroyed?
   ^{51}Cr labelling and external counting
5. Why are the red cells being destroyed?
   Genetically determined
     Morphology spherocytes, ovalocytes, etc.
     Haemoglobin analysis
     Enzyme assay
   Acquired
     Immune—Coombs' test
     Non-immune—red cell morphology
     Associated disease
     Ham's test, etc.

Table 4 *Main groups of haemolytic anaemias*

Genetic disorders of the red cell
  Membrane
    Hereditary spherocytosis
    Hereditary ovalocytosis
    Stomatocytosis
    Pyropoikilocytosis
    Other 'leaky' membrane disorders
    ?March haemoglobinuria
    Acanthocytosis
  Haemoglobin
    Sickling disorders
    Haemoglobins C, D, and E
    Unstable haemoglobins
    Thalassaemia syndromes
  Energy pathways
    Hexose-monophosphate shunt
    Embden—Meyerhof pathway
    Others
Acquired disorders of the red cell
  Immune
    Isoimmune; Rh or ABO incompatibility
    Autoimmune; warm or cold antibodies
  Non-immune
    Trauma
      Microangiopathy
      Valve prosthesis
      Body surface
    Membrane defects; PNH, liver disease
    Parasitic disorders
    Bacterial infection
    Physical agents, drugs, and chemicals
    Hypersplenism
    Defective red cell maturation

absent. In the presence of severe intravascular haemolysis there may be free haemoglobin in the plasma and urine, and in all states of chronic intravascular haemolysis there is a variable degree of haemosiderinuria which can be identified by staining a spun-down urinary deposit with the Prussian blue reagent. In addition to these findings, which are present in all forms of severe haemolysis, there are specific morphological, serological, and biochemical changes of the red cells which accompany the different types of haemolytic anaemia and which are described in detail in later sections.

In the majority of haemolytic anaemias there is some enlargement of the spleen. In some cases it is useful to measure the red cell survival directly and to try to determine the site of red cell destruction. This is usually done by labelling a peripheral blood sample with ^{51}Cr, reinjecting the cells, and measuring the rate of disappearance of the labelled population. In clinical practice it is unnecessary to correct for elution of label from the cells and it is usual to measure the time that it takes for 50 per cent of the label to disappear from the blood ($t_{1/2}$). The normal ^{51}Cr $t_{1/2}$ is 20 to 25 days. By using external counting and taking measurements over the heart as a background, it is possible to compare the rate of accumulation of radioactivity over the spleen and liver and to determine which site is most active in destruction of red cells. These data are usually converted to a simple spleen/liver radioactivity ratio. These procedures are usually carried out when splenectomy is contemplated, but otherwise are not often required for the recognition of haemolysis, which is based on the simple haematological and biochemical analyses outlined above.

An approach to the clinical and laboratory diagnosis of haemolysis is summarized in Table 3.

Classification of the haemolytic anaemias

The haemolytic anaemias are usually classified into two main groups: (a) genetically determined, and (b) acquired (Table 4). Like all biological classifications this is imperfect. For example, although certain

genetically determined red cell enzyme defects lead to haemolysis, they may require the action of an external agent such as a drug or toxin before a haemolytic episode occurs. Despite this difficulty it is convenient to describe the different clinical forms of haemolytic anaemia under these two main headings.

The commonest inherited haemolytic anaemias in the world population, the genetic disorders of haemoglobin structure and synthesis, are described in Chapter 22.4.7. In the chapters that follow the other common inherited and acquired forms of haemolytic anaemia are described.

REFERENCE

Williams, W.J., Beutler, E., Erslev, A.J., and Lichtman, M.A. (1994). *Hematology* (5th edn.). McGraw Hill, New York.

22.4.10 Genetic disorders of the red-cell membrane

S. W. EBER and S. E. LUX

Structure of the red-cell membrane

The red blood-cell membrane (or ghost) is composed of two parts, an external lipid bilayer (plasma membrane) and an inner, membrane-bound, proteinaceous network (membrane skeleton). A schematic illustration of the major components is shown in Fig. 1.

MEMBRANE LIPIDS

The lipid bilayer consists mainly of phospholipids, unesterified choles-terol, and glycolipids. The phospholipids are asymmetrically arranged: choline phospholipids (phosphatidyl choline and sphingomyelin) are found primarily in the outer half of the bilayer; aminophospholipids (phosphatidylethanolamine and phosphatidylserine) and phosphatidyl inositols are sequestered in the inner half. In the case of the amino-phospholipids this is accomplished by an ATP-dependent translocase of 'flippase', which transports phosphatidylethanolamine and phosphati-dylserine from the outer to the inner bilayer. It is probably important to sequester aminophospholipids, as their exposure in the outer bilayer triggers coagulation and causes red cells to adhere to phagocytes.

MEMBRANE PROTEINS

The red-cell membrane contains 10 to 15 major proteins and innumer-able minor ones (Fig. 1). The proteins fall into two classes, integral and peripheral. Integral membrane proteins include mainly band 3, the anion-exchange channel and the glycophorins, sialoglycoproteins that contribute most of the red cell's negative surface charge. Peripheral membrane proteins include a network of structural proteins, called the membrane skeleton, which line the inner surface of the bilayer, and some bound glycolytic enzymes.

Membrane skeleton

Spectrin

This, the major skeletal protein, is a long (100 nm) pliable molecule composed of two similar subunits called α- and β-spectrin. Each subunit is composed of tandem ≈106-amino acid repeats. The two subunits are aligned side-by-side to form spectrin heterodimers, but are oriented in opposite directions. The dimers bind to each other, head to head, at one end to form heterotetramers and some larger oligomers. This spectrin self-association is important because mutations that inhibit it cause most cases of hereditary elliptocytosis and pyropoikilocytosis (see below). It occurs because the head ends of the subunits contain complementary parts of a single, 106-amino acid repeat. These fit together to form a full repeat, attaching the two subunits.

Spectrin tetramers are cross-linked at their tail ends by short filaments of actin. On average, six spectrins bind to an actin filament, so the skeleton forms an hexagonal array. The spectrin–actin interaction is rather weak, but is greatly strengthened by protein 4.1, which binds to

the tail end of β-spectrin, next to the actin-binding site, and to actin. The spectrin–actin–4.1 junction also contains other proteins (dematin, adducin, tropomyosin, tropomodulin) that modify and regulate the inter-actions of the three core proteins.

The membrane skeleton is attached to integral proteins in the over-lying lipid bilayer by ankyrin and, to a lesser extent, by protein 4.1. Ankyrin binds to β-spectrin near the self-association site and links it to the cytoplasmic portion of band 3. Protein 4.2, which binds to both ankyrin and band 3, may strengthen the interaction. Protein 4.1 connects the skeleton to the bilayer via glycophorin C.

The structural importance of the membrane skeleton is best illustrated by the extraordinary haemolysis that occurs in mice whose red cells lack spectrin or ankyrin, and, to a lesser degree, by the membrane loss and fragmentation observed in human diseases of the membrane skeleton, such as hereditary spherocytosis and elliptocytosis (see below).

Congenital membrane defects

DIAGNOSTIC TESTS

Red blood-cell morphology and osmotic fragility are two of the most useful tests for detecting membrane defects. Almost all membrane dis-orders alter red-cell shape, and in many cases diagnostically useful shapes predominate on the blood smear, such as spherocytes, ellipto-cytes, membrane fragments, poikilocytes, stomatocytes, acanthocytes or target cells (Fig. 2). The osmotic fragility test measures the ability of red cells to swell in a graded series of hypotonic solutions. Spherocytes and stomatocytes have a reduced surface-to-volume ratio and can tol-erate less osmotic swelling than normal cells before they lyse. Xerocytes and other dehydrated red cells have an increased surface-to-volume ratio and are osmotically resistant.

Other tests are also useful in selected cases. Defects in membrane deformability or structural integrity can be readily detected in the ekta-cytometer, which uses laser diffraction to measure the deformation and disintegration of red-cell membranes exposed to shear stress. Sodium dodecyl sulphate (**SDS**)–polyacrylamide gel electrophoresis can detect missing membrane proteins or mutant proteins of altered molecular weight. The technique can be extended if it is combined with antibody staining (immunoblotting or Western blotting). SDS gels are often used to quantify membrane proteins, but the results can be rather inaccurate, especially for minor proteins or proteins like ankyrin that abut major

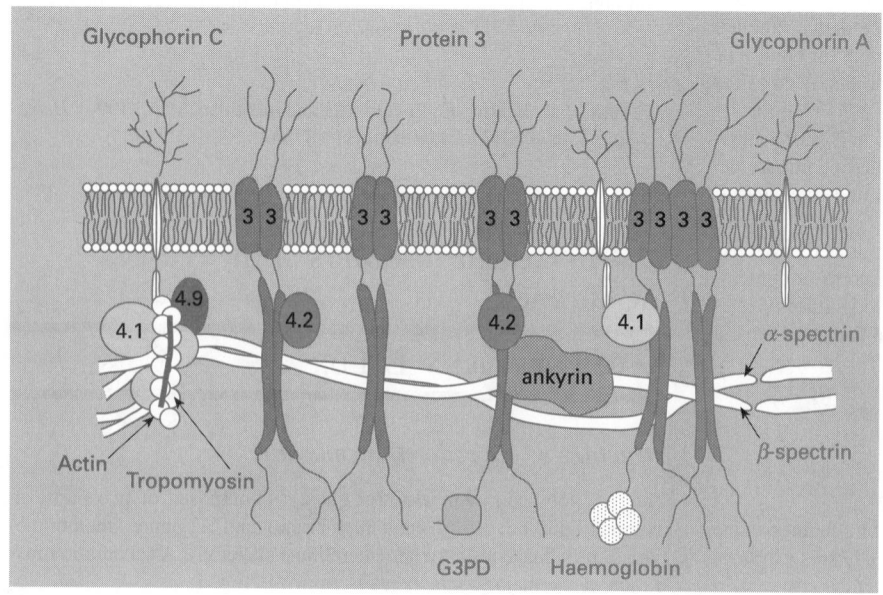

Fig. 1 Schematic illustration of the major components of the red-cell membrane and membrane skeleton. (Reproduced from Lux, S.E. (1989). Hereditary disorders of the red cell membrane skeleton. *Trends in Genetics*, **5**, 222–7, with permission.)

gel bands. Quantitation is best achieved with radioimmunoassays or enzyme immunoassays. Defects in spectrin self-association are common in hereditary elliptocytosis and pyropoikilocytosis, and can be detected by extracting spectrin at 0 to 4°C, where interconversion of spectrin dimers and tetramers is blocked, and separating the two species on non-denaturing polyacrylamide gels. Spectrin defects are also assessed by limited tryptic proteolysis. The sites of tryptic cleavage and, hence, the size of the resulting fragments are altered in many elliptocytic spectrins. Such spectrins are often heat sensitive and cause red cells to fragment at lower than normal (49°C) temperatures in the red-cell heat-stability test. Ultimately, membrane protein defects must be defined at the molecular level. This is complicated by the huge size of the proteins that are most often affected (i.e., spectrin and ankyrin), but has been done in selected cases.

Cation permeability defects, such as hereditary stomatocytosis and xerocytosis are ascertained by measuring steady-state red-cell Na$^+$ and K$^+$ concentrations, and cation fluxes.

Hereditary spherocytosis (Plate 41)

Hereditary spherocytosis is an inherited haemolytic anaemia, characterized by osmotically fragile, partially spherical cells that are selectively trapped by the spleen. The disease occurs in all races, but is particularly common in northern Europeans, in whom the prevalence is about 1:5000. There are at least two patterns of inheritance: 75 per cent of the families show a classic autosomal dominant pattern, most of the remainder have a non-dominant (probably autosomal recessive) form.

PATHOGENESIS

The molecular lesion in hereditary spherocytosis resides in spectrin or, more often, in the proteins that attach spectrin to the membrane: ankyrin, band 3, and protein 4.2. Preliminary studies suggest that at least 50 per cent of patients have mutations in ankyrin and 10 to 15 per cent have band-3 defects. Most red cells are spectrin and ankyrin deficient in this disease. The degree of deficiency correlates closely with the degree of spherocytosis, as measured by osmotic fragility, and with the severity of haemolysis and response to splenectomy. In general, patients with mild hereditary spherocytosis have only mild deficiency (spectrin and ankyrin content above 80 per cent of normal); patients with moderate hereditary spherocytosis have 50 to 80 per cent of the normal spectrin and ankyrin content; and some patients with severe hereditary spherocytosis have spectrin (and ankyrin?) values as low as 30 per cent of normal. Due to the reduced spectrin and ankyrin density, membrane stability and durability are decreased, leading to membrane vesiculation and marked spherocytosis. Rigid spherocytes are preferentially trapped in the splenic cords.

Fig. 2. Altered red-cell morphology: (a) spherocytes; (b) elliptocytes; (c) poikilocytes; (d) stomatocytes.

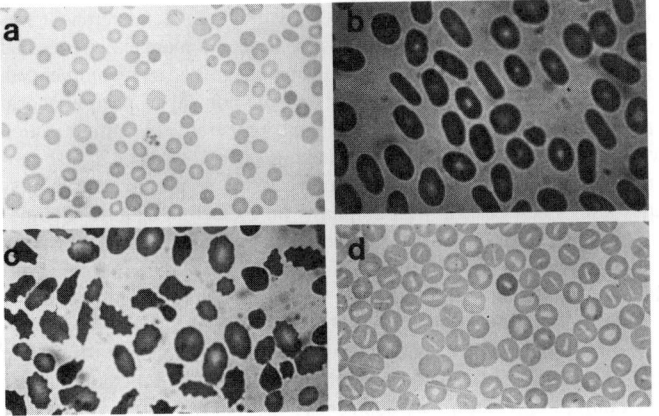

The molecular causes of hereditary spherocytosis have only been defined in a relatively small number of instances. Defects in ankyrin are common in dominant hereditary spherocytosis, particularly frameshift or nonsense mutations. These cause a variable decrease in ankyrin (and its attached spectrin), depending on the output of the normal ankyrin gene. Preliminary studies suggest that many mutations exist and that no single mutation is common. Mutations in band 3 are the second most common cause of dominant hereditary spherocytosis. The mutant molecules appear to be selectively lost as the defective red cells circulate, leading to band-3 deficiency. Rare families with dominant hereditary spherocytosis have a defect in β-spectrin that interferes with the stability of the molecule and with the binding of protein 4.1.

In recessive hereditary spherocytosis it appears that ankyrin-promoter mutations may be relatively common, perhaps in combination with structural defects. Less often, recessive hereditary spherocytosis is caused by the absence of protein 4.2, a protein that associates with both ankyrin and band 3, and probably strengthens their interaction. Finally, defects in α-spectrin appear to be responsible for rare cases of severe (transfusion-dependent) recessive hereditary spherocytosis.

The common theme in hereditary spherocytosis is that the responsible defects usually interfere with the 'vertical' interactions (spectrin–ankyrin–protein 4.2–band 3) that bind the membrane skeleton to the lipid bilayer rather than the 'horizontal' interactions (spectrin self-association and spectrin–actin–protein 4.1) that hold the skeleton together.

CLINICAL FEATURES

The clinical characteristics of hereditary spherocytosis are listed in Table 1. Mild, moderate and severe forms have been defined according to differences in the haemoglobin and bilirubin concentrations, and the reticulocyte count (Table 2). The semiquantitative evaluation of the osmotic fragility test in fresh and incubated blood as well as the determination of spectrin or ankyrin helps to further categorize hereditary spherocytosis. Patients with mild hereditary spherocytosis (about 40–50 per cent of cases) have 'compensated' haemolysis—that is a normal or near-normal haemoglobin concentration combined with an elevated reticulocyte count. The moderate form of hereditary spherocytosis accounts for roughly the other 50 per cent of cases. These patients have a chronic haemolytic anaemia. They may require exchange transfusions for hyperbilirubinaemia in the neonatal period, though in most cases this complication can be managed by phototherapy. Additional transfusions may be required during the first months of life, due to sluggish marrow erythropoiesis (i.e. a relatively low reticulocyte count for the degree of anaemia), but, by 1 year of age, patients with moderate hereditary spherocytosis reach a steady state, with haemoglobin values of 7 to 11 g/dl and reticulocyte counts of 5 to 15 per cent. On average, patients with recessive hereditary spherocytosis are more severely affected than those with dominant hereditary spherocytosis; however, there is considerable overlap.

About 3 per cent of patients have severe disease. They require regular transfusions in order to keep the haemoglobin level above 6 g/dl. The inheritance is nearly always autosomal recessive and both parents show minimal signs of increased haemolysis.

COMPLICATIONS

Crises

Most patients with moderate hereditary spherocytosis experience one or more haemolytic crises, usually with viral infections. These are characterized by increasing jaundice and haemolysis, and are probably due to transient splenomegaly or reticuloendothelial activation. Transfusions are rarely required. Severe, transfusion-dependent, aplastic crises occur, with few exceptions, only once in a patient's lifetime. They are mostly caused by parvovirus B19.

Table 1 *Characteristics of hereditary spherocytosis*

Clinical manifestations
Anaemia
Splenomegaly
Intermittent jaundice:
    From haemolysis
    From biliary obstruction
Aplastic crises
Inheritance:
    Dominant—75%
    Non-dominant—25%
Rare manifestations:
    Leg ulcers
    Extramedullary haemopoietic tumours
    Spinocerebellar degeneration
    Myocardiopathy
Excellent response to splenectomy

Laboratory features
Reticulocytosis
Spherocytosis
Elevated MCHC
Increased osmotic fragility (especially incubated osmotic
    fragility test)
Negative Coombs' test
Decreased red-cell spectrin, or spectrin and ankyrin, or protein
    3, or protein 4.2

Gallstones

Untreated older children and adults with hereditary spherocytosis often develop bilirubinate gallstones secondary to increased bilirubin production. Only 5 per cent of children under 10 years of age are affected, but the prevalence rises to 40 to 50 per cent in the second to fifth decades, and to 55 to 75 per cent thereafter. The frequency after the age of 30 parallels the frequency in the general population, which suggests that gallstones in patients with hereditary spherocytosis form primarily in the second and third decades. Ultrasonography is the most reliable method for detecting bilirubin stones.

Other complications

Occasional adult patients with hereditary spherocytosis develop gout, indolent ankle ulcers, or a chronic erythematous dermatitis on the legs. All of these complications disappear after splenectomy. A rare severe complication occurring mostly in elderly adults with otherwise mild hereditary spherocytosis is extramedullary haematopoietic tumours, often located in the thorax. Rare but potentially interesting associations of hereditary spherocytosis with spinocerebellar degeneration and familial myocardiopathy have also been described.

DIAGNOSIS

The hallmarks of hereditary spherocytosis are anaemia, jaundice, and splenomegaly. The diagnosis is made if osmotically fragile, partially spherical, red blood cells are found and if spherocytosis is the dominant morphology. Membrane analysis and detection of spectrin, ankyrin or band 3 deficiencies may help to ascertain the disease in unusual cases. It is fortunate that these are rare, as the membrane-protein analyses are only available in a few specialized centres.

There are only a few disorders that can be confused with hereditary spherocytosis. ABO incompatibility may be difficult to distinguish from hereditary spherocytosis in the neonatal period. In later life, autoimmune haemolytic anaemias must be excluded, particularly the warm-antibody type. This is best done with a Coombs' test. Spherocytes occur as a secondary phenomenon in some other diseases, but in these cases the diagnosis is either obvious (e.g. burns, snake bites, clostridial sepsis) or

spherocytes are not the dominant morphological abnormality (e.g. microangiopathic haemolytic anaemias, oxidant haemolysis, unstable haemoglobins, haemoglobin C disease).

TREATMENT

Splenectomy cures almost all patients with spherocytosis, eliminating anaemia and reducing the reticulocyte count to near normal levels (1–3 per cent). Patients with the most severe forms of the disease may not achieve a complete remission, but will still benefit greatly from splenectomy. However, the indications for splenectomy should be weighted carefully, as a small fraction of patients will die from overwhelming postsplenectomy infections or mesenteric/portal venous occlusion. The risk of postsplenectomy sepsis is very high in infancy and early childhood (see Chapter 22.5.4) and splenectomy should therefore be delayed until the age of 5 years or more if possible and to at least 2 to 3 years in all cases, even if chronic transfusions are required in the interim. It is difficult to estimate the risk later in life. The surveys of Schwartz and Green, the best available, are limited to adults and largely predate immunization for *Streptococcus pneumoniae* and other bacteria. They showed an incidence of fulminant sepsis of 0.2 to 0.5/100 person years of follow-up and a death rate of 0.1/100 person years; in addition, other serious bacterial infections (e.g. pneumonia, meningitis, peritonitis, bacteraemia) were much more common (4.5/100 person years) than normal, particularly in the first few years after the operation.

The incidence of ischaemic heart disease may also rise after splenectomy. In one careful study, Robinette and Fraumeni observed that death from ischaemic heart disease occurred 1.86 times as often in splenectomized men as matched controls, a significant difference. The cause is unknown, although the chronically higher platelet count after splenectomy would be a good candidate.

All patients with severe spherocytosis should be splenectomized, but lacking large clinical studies it is difficult to give a general rule for splenectomy for patients with mild to moderate hereditary spherocytosis. Patients with moderate spherocytosis should be splenectomized if they suffer from reduced vitality or physical stamina due to anaemia, or if, later in life, anaemia compromises vascular perfusion of vital organs or extramedullary haemopoietic tumours develop. We defer splenectomy in patients with mild, compensated haemolysis. Whether patients with moderate, asymptomatic anaemia should have a splenectomy remains controversial. The treatment of patients with mild-moderate hereditary spherocytosis and gallstones is also debatable, particularly as new treatments for gallstones (e.g. laparoscopic cholecystectomy, endoscopic sphincterotomy, and extracorporal choletripsy) lower the risk of this complication. In patients with distinct haemolysis and symptomatic gallstones a combined cholecystectomy and splenectomy may still be warranted, particularly if acute cholecystitis or biliary obstruction have occurred.

Recent studies suggest that partial splenectomy may be an effective compromise for many patients with hereditary spherocytosis, relieving haemolysis while maintaining some residual splenic phagocytic function. Complications were low and regrowth of the splenic remnant was not observed during a 4-year follow-up period, but more experience and longer follow-ups are needed before the procedure can be recommended.

All splenectomized patients must receive polyvalent pneumococcal vaccine, preferably given several weeks preoperatively. Immunization with *Haemophilus influenzae* and meningococcal vaccines is also recommended, particularly in children. We advocate prophylactic antibiotics after splenectomy, with emphasis on protection against pneumococcal sepsis (i.e. penicillin VK or equivalent, 125 mg orally twice daily in young children (under 7 years) and 250 mg twice daily in older children and adults), at least for the first 5 years after surgery and preferably for life.

Before splenectomy, patients with hereditary spherocytosis, like patients with other haemolytic disorders, should take folic acid (1 mg/day orally) to prevent folate deficiency.

Table 2 *Clinical classification of hereditary spherocytosis*

	Trait	Mild spherocytosis	Moderate spherocytosis	Severe[1] spherocytosis
Haemoglobin (g/dl)	Normal	11–15	8–12	6–8
Reticulocytes (%)	3	3.1–8	≥8	≥10
Bilirubin (mg/dl)	≤1	1–2	≥2	≥3
Spectrin content (% of normal)[2]	100	80–100	50–80	30–60[3]
Osmotic fragility				
Fresh blood	Normal	Normal or slightly increased	Distinctly increased	Distinctly increased
Incubated blood	Slightly increased	Distinctly increased	Distinctly increased	Distinctly increased

[1]Values before transfusion.

[2]Normal (± SD) = $245 \pm 27 \times 10^5$ spectrin dimers per erythrocyte. In most patients ankyrin content is decreased to a comparable degree. A minority of patients lack band 3 or protein 4.2 and have mild to moderate spherocytosis with normal or near normal amounts of spectrin and ankyrin.

[3]Some patients have severe hereditary spherocytosis despite normal concentrations of red-cell spectrin, ankyrin, band 3, and protein 4.2; their red-cell defect is unknown.

Hereditary elliptocytosis (Plate 42)

Although hereditary elliptocytosis is quite frequent (approx. 1 in 2500 in the Caucasian North European population), it is less important clinically than hereditary spherocytosis. Only about 10 per cent of patients have significant haemolysis; however, in some cases this can be life threatening. Four clinical phenotypes are distinguished: mild hereditary elliptocytosis, hereditary pyropoikilocytosis, spherocytic hereditary elliptocytosis, and South-East Asian ovalocytosis (see Table 3).

MILD HEREDITARY ELLIPTOCYTOSIS

As its name implies this form of hereditary elliptocytosis is usually very mild in heterozygous carriers; there is no anaemia and only mild haemolysis (reticulocyte counts of less than 4 per cent). However, moderate to severe haemolytic anaemia does occur in homozygous or combined heterozygous offspring.

Pathogenesis

In general, mild hereditary elliptocytosis and hereditary pyropoikilocytosis (see below) are caused by defects in the 'horizontal' interactions that hold the membrane skeleton together. The most common defects affect spectrin self-association and lead to an increased fraction of spectrin dimers in low-temperature spectrin extracts. These defects occur near the self-association sites: at the N-terminus of α-spectrin and the C-terminus of β-spectrin. α-Spectrin mutations are mostly single amino-acid substitutions that disrupt the structure of one of the 106 amino-acid repeats. β-Spectrin mutations typically truncate the C-terminal end of the β-chain. In general, particularly for α-spectrin mutations, the severity of the defect correlates directly with its effect on spectrin self-association and inversely with the distance of the mutation from the self-association site. However, this rule is complicated by the effect of the common α[LELY] mutation (see below).

The other common mutation in hereditary elliptocytosis involves protein 4.1. Heterozygous deficiency of 4.1 or loss of its ability to strengthen the spectrin–actin bond causes mild hereditary elliptocytosis. Homozygous defects result in severe poikilocytic anaemias.

Spectrin α[LELY]

This important polymorphism alters α-spectrin mRNA splicing so that half the α-spectrin molecules are defective (Sp α[LELY]) and cannot pair with β-spectrin. By itself the mutation is harmless, as α-spectrin is made in excess. However, when paired, in *trans*, with an α-spectrin mutation that causes hereditary elliptocytosis, the loss of normal α-chains results in an increased proportion of spectrin dimers bearing the hereditary elliptocytosis defect and greatly exacerbates the severity of the defect. The consequences are magnified because the α[LELY] defect is very common (20–30 per cent gene frequency in several populations).

HEREDITARY PYROPOIKILOCYTOSIS

Patients with this rare recessive disease have a moderately severe to life-threatening haemolytic anaemia characterized by remarkable red-cell fragmentation and microcytosis, bizarre poikilocytosis, and heat-sensitive red cells that fragment at 45 to 46°C instead of the normal 49°C. The more severe variants also feature spectrin deficiency (20–40 per cent) and spherocytosis. The haemolysis is diminished but not completely cured by splenectomy.

Hereditary pyropoikilocytosis typically results from homozygosity or compound heterozygosity for α-spectrin defects that produce mild hereditary elliptocytosis or from a combination of Sp α[LELY] with one of the more severe α-spectrin defects.

Transient infantile poikilocytosis

Interestingly, neonates with mild hereditary elliptocytosis and an inherited spectrin self-association defect may begin life with an hereditary pyropoikilocytosis-like syndrome, a severe poikilocytic, microcytic, haemolytic anaemia that sometimes requires transfusion. The condition converts to typical mild hereditary elliptocytosis during the first 6 to 12 months, in parallel with the loss of fetal erythrocytes. It appears that the high concentration of free 2,3-diphosphoglycerate in fetal cells weakens the spectrin–actin–4.1 interaction and aggravates the inherited defect in spectrin self-association.

SPHEROCYTIC HEREDITARY ELLIPTOCYTOSIS

Spherocytic elliptocytosis is a relatively rare autosomal dominant condition with features of both hereditary spherocytosis and hereditary elliptocytosis. Patients have a mild to moderate haemolytic anaemia characterized by rounded elliptocytes, occasional spherocytes, and a positive osmotic fragility test. The indications for splenectomy, which is curative, are the same as for hereditary spherocytosis. The molecular cause of the disease is unknown.

Table 3 *Clinical subtypes of hereditary elliptocytosis (HE)*

Clinical manifestations	Laboratory features

Mild HE
Asymptomatic
Dominant inheritance: one parent with HE
Variants:
   Some neonates with moderately severe
     haemolytic anaemia and HPP-like smear.
     Converts to typical mild HE by approx. 1
     year.
   Some patients with mild–moderate chronic
     haemolysis, due either to co-inheritance of
     low expression α-spectrin variant (α^{LELY}) or to
     coexistence of chronic disease producing
     splenomegaly
	Blood smear: elliptocytes, few or no poikilocytes
	No anaemia, little or no haemolysis (reticulocytes = 1–3%)
	Normal osmotic fragility
	Usually defect in spectrin self-association. Less often partial
	   deficiency or dysfunction of protein 4.1 or of glycophorin C (which
	   binds 4.1 to the membrane)

Hereditary pyropoikilocytosis (HPP) Moderate to severe haemolytic anaemia Splenomegaly Intermittent jaundice Aplastic crises Recessive inheritance: typically one parent with HE and one with α^{LELY} or both parents with HE Improvement following splenectomy	Blood smear: bizarre poikilocytes, fragments, spherocytes, elliptocytes Reticulocytosis Decreased MCV due to red-cell fragmentation Increased osmotic fragility Decreased red-cell heat stability Marked defect in spectrin self-association In most severe variants partial spectrin deficiency
Spherocytic HE Anaemia Splenomegaly Intermittent jaundice Aplastic crises Dominant inheritance pattern Excellent response to splenectomy	Blood smear: rounded elliptocytes, ± spherocytes Reticulocytes Increased osmotic fragility Primary defect unknown

South-East Asian ovalocytosis
Asymptomatic
Dominant inheritance
Lowland aboriginal tribes, especially in Melanesia
   and Malaysia
 	
No anaemia or haemolysis
Very rigid red cells that resist invasion by malarial
   parasites
	Blood smear: rounded elliptocytes, some with a transverse bar that
	   divides the central clear space
	Mutant band 3 that lacks anion exchange function and shows
	   increased aggregation and interactions with membrane skeleton →
	   rigid membrane.

SOUTH-EAST ASIAN OVALOCYTOSIS

This curious autosomal dominant polymorphism is very prevalent (up to 30 per cent) among Melanesian, Indonesian, and Malaysian aborigines, but is rarely seen in other populations. It is characterized by rounded elliptocytes, some with a unique morphology (a transverse bar that divides the central clear space), which are extraordinarily rigid and resist invasion by a variety of malarial parasites.

The primary defect is a deletion of eight amino acids in band 3 at the junction between the cytoplasmic and membrane domains. This either increases the binding of band 3 to ankyrin, causes band 3 to become entangled in the spectrin meshwork, or fosters band-3 aggregation, leading to the observed rigidity. Despite their stiffness, the red cells in this condition circulate freely and there is little or no associated haemolysis.

TREATMENT

Splenectomy is indicated only in severe cases of hereditary elliptocytosis or hereditary pyropoikilocytosis and, especially as spontaneous regression occurs in some infants, should be postponed to at least the third year of life and preferably the fifth year or later.

Hereditary defects in membrane cation permeability
HEREDITARY STOMATOCYTOSIS

In this rare autosomal dominant disease an inherited defect in membrane permeability causes massive Na^+ influx, which overwhelms the Na–K pump, and leads to an increase in total monovalent cation concentrations and cell water (Table 4). In some families this results in severe haemolysis. Patients with the severe form respond well to splenectomy, although mild to moderate haemolysis usually persists. The characteristic red blood-cell appearance shows a mouth-like band of pallor (i.e. 'stoma') across the centre of the red cell. Although the primary defect has not been identified, SDS gel electrophoresis of red-cell membrane proteins can be diagnostically helpful because stomatin, an integral protein within gel band 7, is absent or nearly absent in all patients.

HEREDITARY XEROCYTOSIS

In this rare autosomal dominant disorder, the permeability of K^+ is altered, due to an unknown membrane defect, so that the ratio of K^+ loss to Na^+ gain exceeds the normal ratio of 2:3. As a result, total monovalent cation concentrations and cell volume decrease (Table 4),

Table 4 *Characteristics of hereditary stomatocytosis and xerocytosis*

Characteristic	Stomatocytosis	Xerocytosis
Red blood-cell morphology	Stomatocytes	Targets, crenated cells, stomatocytes[1]
MCHC	Decreased	Increased
Osmotic fragility	Increased	Decreased
Total concentration of K^+ and Na^+	Increased	Decreased
Red blood-cell water content	Increased	Decreased
Active transport of Na^+	Increased (approx. 10-fold)	Increased (approx. 6-fold)
Active transport of K^+	Increased (approx. 10-fold)	Increased (approx. 2-fold)
Passive Na^+ flux	Increased (approx. 50-fold)	Increased (approx. 2-fold)
Passive K^+ flux	Increased (approx. 25-fold)	Increased (approx. 3-fold)

[1]Red blood-cell morphology is often normal or only shows a few target cells in patients with hereditary xerocytosis.

leading to dehydrated, viscous xerocytes that are cleared by the reticulocendothelial system. Patients have a mild to moderate haemolytic anaemia characterized by target cells, occasional stomatocytes and, in severe cases, irregular crenated cells. The osmotic fragility is decreased. Splenectomy is not beneficial, which suggests xerocytes are primarily destroyed in the liver.

SPECIAL SERIES OF REVIEWS

Palek, J. (ed.) (1992–1993). Cellular and molecular biology of the red blood cell membrane proteins in health and disease. Parts I–IV. *Seminars in Hematology*, **29**, 229–322 (Oct); **30**, 1–83 (Jan), 85–168 (Apr), 169–247 (Jul). This outstanding, up-to-date series of 18 reviews (340 pages, 2611 references) in four successive issues of *Seminars in Hematology* covers all aspects red cell membrane structure and function, normal and abnormal, except for membrane lipids.

REFERENCES

Agre, P., Casella, J.F., Zinkham, W.H., McMillan, C., and Bennett, V. (1985). Partial deficiency of erythrocyte spectrin in hereditary spherocytosis. *Nature*, **314**, 380–3.

Becker, P.S. and Lux, S.E. (1994). Disorders of the red cell membrane skeleton: hereditary spherocytosis and hereditary elliptocytosis. In *The metabolic basis of inherited disease*, (7th edn), (ed. C.S. Scriver, A.L. Beaudet, W.S. Sly, and D. Valle). McGraw-Hill, New York (in press).

Becker, P.S., Tse, W.T., Lux, S.E., and Forget, B. (1993). β Spectrin Kissimmee: a spectrin variant associated with autosomal dominant hereditary spherocytosis and defective binding to protein 4.1. *Journal of Clinical Investigation*, **92**, 612–16.

Conboy, G.J., *et al.* (1993). An isoform-specific mutation in the protein 4.1 gene results in hereditary elliptocytosis and complete deficiency of protein 4.1 in erythrocytes but not in nonerythroid cells. *Journal of Clinical Investigation*, **91**, 77–82.

Eber, S.W., Armbrust, R., and Schröter, W. (1990). Variable clinical severity of hereditary spherocytosis: relation to erythrocytic spectrin concentration, osmotic fragility and autohemolysis. *Journal of Pediatrics*, **177**, 409–16.

Eber, S.W., *et al.* (1993). Discovery of 8 ankyrin mutations in hereditary spherocytosis (HS) indicates that ankyrin defects are a major cause of dominant and recessive HS. *Blood*, **82(Suppl. 1)**, 308a. (abstract)

Green, J.B., Shackford, S.R., Sise, M.J., and Fridlund, P. (1986). Late septic complications in adults following splenectomy for trauma: a prospective analysis in 144 patients. *Journal of Trauma*, **26**, 999–1004.

Jarolim, P., *et al.* (1994). Duplication of 10 nucleotides in the erythroid band 3 (AE1) gene in a kindred with hereditary spherocytosis and band 3 protein deficiency (Band 3PRAGUE). *Journal of Clinical Investigation*, **93**, 121–30.

Liu, S-C., Palek, J., and Prchal, J. (1982). Defective spectrin dimer-dimer association in hereditary elliptocytosis. *Proceedings of the National Academy of Science (USA)*, **79**, 2072–6.

Liu, S-C. *et al.* (1990). Molecular defect of the band 3 protein in Southeast Asian ovalocytosis. *New England Journal of Medicine*, **323**, 1530–8.

Lux, S.E. and Palek, J. (1995). Disorders of the red cell membrane. In *Blood: principles and practice of hematology* (R.I. Handin, S.E. Lux, T.P. Stossel, eds), Chapter 54. J.B. Lippincott, Philadelphia, in press.

Lux, S.E. *et al.* (1990). Hereditary spherocytosis associated with deletion of the human erythrocyte ankyrin gene on chromosome 8. *Nature*, **345**, 736–9.

Mentzer, W.C., Jr., Iarocci, T.A., Mohandas, N., Lane, P.A., Smith, B., Lazerson, J., and Hayes, T. (1987). Modulation of erythrocyte membrane mechanical fragility by 2,3-diphosphoglycerate in the neonatal poikilocytosis/elliptocytosis syndrome. *Journal of Clinical Investigation*, **79**, 943–9.

Palek, J. and Jarolim, P. (1993). Clinical expression and laboratory detection of red cell membrane protein mutations. *Seminars in Hematology*, **30**, 249–83.

Robinette, C.D. and Fraumeni, J.F., Jr. (1977). Splenectomy and subsequent mortality in veterans of the 1939–45 war. *Lancet*, **ii**, 127–9.

Savvides, P., Shalev, O., John, K.M., and Lux, S.E. (1993). Combined spectrin and ankyrin deficiency is common in autosomal dominant hereditary spherocytosis. *Blood*, **82**, 2953–60.

Schwartz, P.E., Sterioff, S., Mucha, P., Melton, L.J., and Offord, K.P. (1982). Postsplenectomy sepsis and mortality in adults. *Journal of the American Medical Association*, **248**, 2279–83.

Tchernia, G. *et al.* (1993). Initial assessment of the beneficial effect of partial splenectomy in hereditary spherocytosis. *Blood*, **81**, 2014–20.

Tse, W.T. *et al.* (1990). Point mutation in the β-spectrin gene associated with $\alpha^{1/74}$ hereditary elliptocytosis. Implications for the mechanism of spectrin dimer self-association. *Journal of Clinical Investigation*, **86**, 909–16.

Whitfield, C.F., Follweiler, J.B., Lopresti-Morrow, L., and Miller, B.A. (1991). Deficiency of α-spectrin synthesis in burst-forming units-erythroid in lethal hereditary spherocytosis. *Blood*, **78**, 3043–51.

Wilmotte, R. *et al.* (1993). Low expression allele α^{LELY} of red cell spectrin is associated with mutations in exon 40 ($\alpha^{V/41}$ polymorphism) and intron 45 and with partial skipping of exon 46. *Journal of Clinical Investigation*, **91**, 2091–6.

Winkelmann, J.C. and Forget, B.G. (1993). Erythroid and nonerythroid spectrins. *Blood*, **81**, 3173–85.

22.4.11 Haemolysis due to red-cell enzyme deficiencies

E.G GORDON-SMITH AND D.J. WEATHERALL

Different inherited haemolytic anaemias that are the result of a deficiency of specific red-cell enzymes have been described. The resultant haemolytic anaemia is usually non-spherocytic, and may dominate the clinical picture or be part of a more generalized disorder, depending on whether or not the enzyme deficiency is expressed only in the red blood cells. Deficiencies of the enzymes of the glycolytic pathway produce a relatively constant degree of haemolysis; those of the hexose monophosphate shunt, which provides reducing power, produce haemolysis in the presence of oxidative stress.

Normal red-cell metabolism

During normal red-cell development the mitochondria are lost at about the time that the nucleus is extruded, and, therefore, mature red cells have no capacity for oxidative energy production. They are delivered into the circulation with a relatively simple, 'pay-as-you-go', energy-producing system that burns glucose as its main source of fuel.

Glucose is metabolized mainly through the anaerobic, glycolytic, Embden–Meyerhof pathway, with lactate as the end-product (Fig. 1). Energy required to maintain the shape and deformability of the cells, and for reduction of methaemoglobin, is provided by the net production of 2 mol of ATP and the reduction of 2 mol of NAD^+ to NADH per mol of glucose. About half of the ATP produced in this way is used for the red cell to maintain its volume and the integrity of its membrane by pumping sodium and water out, and potassium in. The role of the remainder of the ATP that is produced is unknown but loss of ATP leads to rigidity of the cell membrane. The production of NADH plays an important part in preventing the oxidation of the iron of haem. The other principal energy pathway is the hexose monophosphate shunt (Fig. 2) (also known as the pentose phosphate pathway), in which there is reduction of $NADP^+$ to NADPH. This pathway is stimulated by certain redox compounds and oxidants. One of the chief functions of the hexose monophosphate shunt is the maintenance of adequate levels of reduced glutathione in the red cell, which is essential for protection against oxidant damage. Under 'normal' conditions about 10 per cent of glucose is metabolized via the shunt but flux through the pathway can increase markedly in the face of oxidant stress.

There is a 'metabolic siding' in the Embden–Meyerhof pathway called the Rapoport–Luebering shunt, which is controlled by diphosphoglycerate mutase and which generates 2,3-diphosphoglycerate. The latter is the most abundant intracellular phosphate in human erythrocytes and plays an important part in controlling oxygen transport. Clearly, the

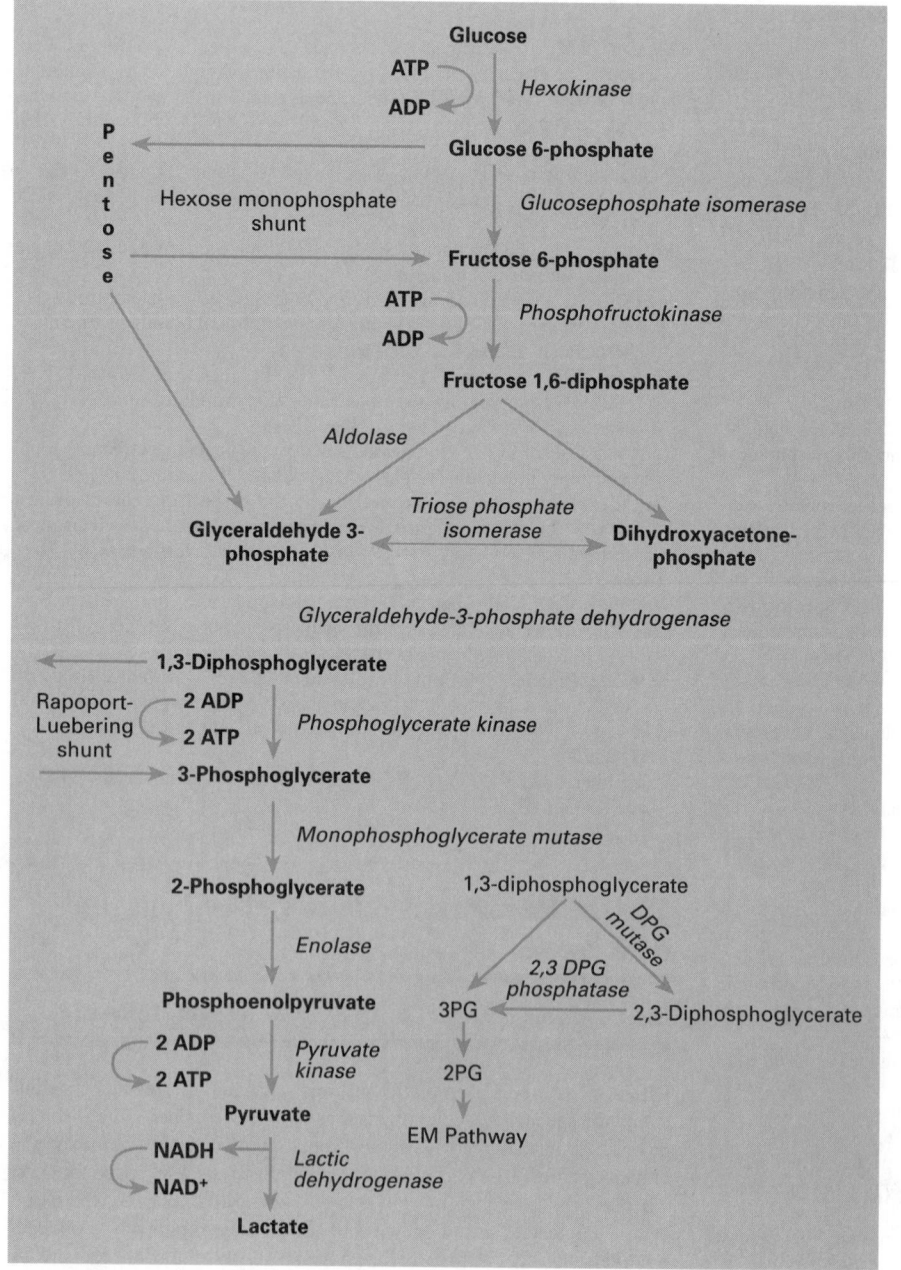

Fig 1. The relationship between the main red cell glycolytic pathway (Embden–Meyerhof) and the other metabolic pathways. The insert shows the production of 2,3-DPG in the Rapoport-Luebering shunt.

rate of production of 2,3-diphosphoglycerate is closely related to the rate of glycosis. Metabolic blocks early in the Embden–Meyerhof pathway reduce the production of 2,3-diphosphoglycerate, while blocks late in the pathway, pyruvate kinase deficiency for example, cause it to accumulate. Thus enzyme defects vary considerably in their effects on 2,3-diphosphoglycerate production, and hence on oxygen transport and the degree of compensation for anaemia.

The red cell contains enzyme systems for the utilization of substrates other than glucose under unusual conditions; these include adenosine, inosine, fructose, mannose, galactose, and lactate. Numerous other enzymes have been reported to be active in reticulocytes and mature red cells.

Inherited enzyme deficiencies

Deficiencies of many of the enzymes of the glycolytic and reducing pathways have been described but most are rare (Table 1). Two are relatively common, glucose-6-phosphate dehydrogenase (**G6PD**) deficiency in the reducing pathway and pyruvate kinase deficiency in the glycolytic. The various G6PD deficiency disorders are described in Chapter 22.4.12.

Pyruvate kinase deficiency

Pyruvate kinase catalyses the last step in the glycolytic pathway that produces the net gain in ATP from the metabolism of glucose (Fig. 1). Deficiency of pyruvate kinase is the most common of the inherited red-cell enzyme defects after G6PD deficiency. It has been reported in many different races, and the sexes are affected equally. The most commonly described form is inherited as an autosomal recessive. Homozygotes have haemolytic anaemia, mild to moderate splenomegaly, and a gross deficiency of red-cell pyruvate kinase activity, while heterozygotes are

Fig 2. The hexose-monophosphate pathway. Intermediates: G6P, glucose 6-phosphate; F6P, fructose 6-phosphate; Ga3P, glyceraldehyde 3-phosphate; 6PG, 6-phosphogluconate; Ru5P, ribulose 5-phosphate; R5P, ribose 5-phosphate; Xy5P, xylulose 5-phosphate; S7P, sedoheptulose 7-phosphate; E4P, erythrose 4-phosphate. Enzymes: G6PD, glucose 6-phosphate dehydrogenase; 6PGD, 6-phosphogluconate dehydrogenase; PKE, epimerase, PRI, phosphoribose isomerase. Cosubstrates: $NADP^+$ and $NADPH + H^+$, oxidized and reduced forms of nicotinamide-adenine dinucleotide phosphate.

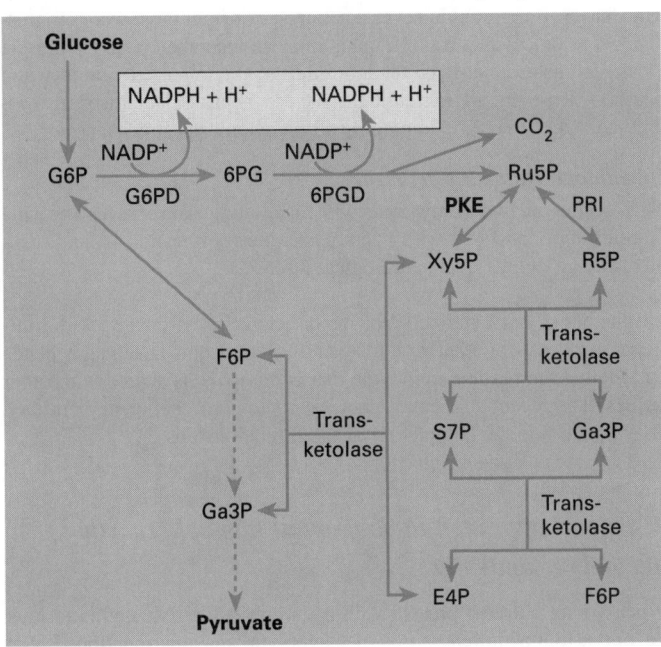

clinically and haematologically normal and have about half the usual amount of pyruvate kinase activity in their red cells.

AETIOLOGY AND PATHOGENESIS

Deficiency of pyruvate kinase results in a deficiency of ATP and the accumulation of glycolytic intermediates, particularly 2,3-diphosphoglycerate and phosphoenol pyruvate. In the absence of efficient glycolysis the red cell must obtain its energy requirements by other means. In the severe pyruvate kinase-deficient patient there is a marked reticulocytosis, and probably most of the red cells' energy is derived by oxidative pathways related to the residual mitochondria in the younger cell population. After splenectomy the reticulocyte count rises markedly, often up to 70 per cent or more of circulating cells. Removal of the spleen allows newly formed reticulocytes to remain in the circulation rather than being held in the spleen whilst mitochondria and DNA are removed.

Pyruvate kinase deficiency shows a remarkable degree of molecular heterogeneity. In some cases there is simply a quantitative defect in the enzyme but in others mutant enzymes with abnormal kinetic properties have been described. It appears that many apparent homozygotes are in fact compound heterozygotes with different genetic lesions at each of their pyruvate kinase loci.

CLINICAL FEATURES

Severe pyruvate kinase deficiency may present at birth with neonatal jaundice and haemolysis, sometimes requiring exchange transfusions. There is a variable degree of chronic haemolysis throughout life, with jaundice, anaemia, splenomegaly, and even bone changes similar to those seen in thalassaemia in the most severe cases. There is often a marked exacerbation of the anaemia during periods of stress such as infection or pregnancy. Interestingly, however, the anaemia is very well tolerated. This is probably because the high levels of red-cell 2,3-diphosphoglycerate cause a right shift in the oxygen dissociation curve and hence a more efficient oxygenation of the tissues. Aplastic crises due to human parvovirus infection have been reported.

LABORATORY DIAGNOSIS

The blood picture shows all the hallmarks of chronic haemolysis and the stained blood film shows polychromasia and macrocytosis with a varying number of irregularly contracted red cells. There is an increased rate of autohaemolysis, which is not corrected by glucose (type 2 autohaemolysis). The diagnosis is confirmed by an assay for pyruvate kinase.

THERAPY

There is no specific therapy but patients normally improve after splenectomy. Postsplenectomy the platelet count may be very much elevated ($600–1000 \times 10^9/1$) and patients may need long-term, low-dose aspirin to reduce the risk of deep-vein thrombosis. Pneumococcal vaccine should be given presplenectomy and penicillin V prophylaxis afterwards. As mentioned above, the reticulocyte count increases after the operation and may be extreme. Transfusion is required during periods of exacerbation of the haemolysis. Folic acid is required to prevent deficiency.

Pyrimidine 5'-nucleotidase deficiency

This condition, which is transmitted as an autosomal recessive trait, causes a variable haemolytic anaemia characterized by marked basophilic stippling of the red cells. It is of interest because it appears to be relatively common and, by 1980, 33 individuals from 24 separate kindreds had been reported. There appears to be a predisposition in Mediterranean, Jewish, and African populations. An acquired form of this

Table 1 *Some red-cell enzyme deficiencies*

Pathway	Enzyme	Clinical features
Embden–Meyerhof	Hexokinase	Rare; haemolytic anaemia (HA) mild to severe
	Glucose phosphate isomerase	HA mild to severe
	Phosphofructokinase	Mild HA ± myopathy (Tariu's disease)
	Aldolase	Rare; mild HA ± mental retardation
	Triosephosphate isomerase	Neuromuscular anomalies + moderate HA
	Phosphoglycerate kinase	Rare; HA ± mental and phagocytic deficiencies; X-linked
	Pyruvate kinase	Common; mild to severe HA
Hexose monophosphate shunt and glutathione (GSH) metabolism	Glucose-6-phosphate dehydrogenase	Very common, X-linked (see Chapter 22.4.12)
	GSH peroxidase or reductase	Rare; variable oxidant-sensitive HA
	GSH synthetase and α-glutamyl cysteine synthetase	
Nucleotide metabolism	Pyrimidine-5′-nucleotidase	Mild to moderate HA
		Basophilic stippling
	Adenylate kinase	Rare; mild HA
Methaemoglobin reduction	NADH: methaemoglobin reductase	10–35% methaemoglobin
		Heterozygotes cyanosed with oxidant drugs
	NADPH: methaemoglobin reductase	Methaemoglobinaemia only after oxidant stress
Nucleotide synthesis	Orotidine 5′-phosphate pyrophosphorylase	Megaloblastic anaemia
	Orotidine 5′-phosphate decarboxylase	± Mental retardation
	5′-phosphoribosyl 1-pyrophosphate synthetase	

enzyme deficiency occurs in severe lead poisoning and may be at least in part responsible for the haemolytic component of lead intoxication. Splenectomy does not appear to be effective in the genetic form of this condition.

Red-cell enzyme deficiencies associated with multisystem disease

The red-cell enzyme deficiencies that cause haemolytic anaemia are summarized in Table 1. Most of these conditions are rare and have only been encountered in a few families. Usually there is chronic haemolysis without involvement of other systems but there is an increasing number of examples of red-cell enzyme deficiencies that are associated with multisystem disease.

Triosephosphate isomerase deficiency

This combines a moderately severe haemolytic anaemia with a bizarre neurological disorder characterized by either progressive spasticity or flaccidity, diffuse muscle weakness, dysphasia, facial paresis, absent reflexes, fixed deformities of the hands, and tremor. Curiously, different neurological symptom complexes seem to occur in individuals with this disorder. Enzyme activity is greatly reduced in muscle, plasma, spinal fluid, skin fibroblasts, and white cells, suggesting that the deficiency involves most body tissues. Sudden death due to cardiac arrhythmias has been described and in some patients there is an unusual susceptibility to infection.

Phosphofructokinase deficiency

This produces a syndrome of myopathy and congenital, non-spherocytic, haemolytic anaemia. The condition is also known as Tarui's disease, after its discoverer, or glycogenosis type VII. The disorder shows marked clinical variability and is characterized by muscle weakness, exercise intolerance, intermittent myoglobinuria, and a variable degree of haemolysis. Hyperuricaemia and gout is a common complication.

Phosphoglycerate kinase deficiency

An X-linked disorder in which hemizygous males have a neurological syndrome characterized by seizures, variable mental retardation, emotional ability, speech impairment, and progressive extrapyramidal disease. There is severe, chronic haemolytic anaemia, which sometimes becomes transfusion dependent. There have been several reports of response to splenectomy. The haemolytic disorder is punctuated by severe exacerbations, often caused by infection, and characterized by worsening of the anaemia, jaundice, and a marked reticulocyte response.

γ-Glutamyl cysteine synthetase deficiency

This has been reported in several patients, in whom there were progressive neurological abnormalities including spinocerebellar ataxia, muscle weakness, absence of deep tendon reflexes, and impaired vibratory and position sense in all extremities. As the neurological disorder progressed, speech became impaired and myoclonic spasms occurred.

Glutathione synthetase deficiency

This occurs in two forms, one with haemolytic anaemia as the sole manifestation, and one with haemolysis, metabolic acidosis, and, usually, though not always, neurological disease.

Whether or not a red-cell enzyme deficiency is associated with multisystem disease, or whether it only causes haemolytic anaemia, depends on whether the particular enzyme that is defective is shared with other tissues. The recent studies on phosphofructokinase deficiency outlined above underline the complexity of these relationships.

A general approach to congenital non-spherocytic haemolytic anaemia

When young children present with haemolysis, the first step is to look for one of the acquired causes of haemolytic anaemia mentioned later in this section. Once these have been excluded, and abnormalities of the red-cell membrane and haemoglobin have been ruled out, the level of red-cell G6PD and pyruvate kinase should be determined. This will leave a number of patients in whom no diagnosis can be made, and they should then be referred to centres capable of analysing all the red-cell enzymes and glycolytic intermediates. In practice only a small proportion of cases of this type can be ascribed to a particular enzyme deficiency, and in the majority no specific abnormality can be found.

REFERENCES

Beutler, E. (1990). Hereditary nonspherocytic haemolytic anemia: pyruvate kinase and other abnormalities. In *Hematology*, (4th edn), (ed. W.J. Williams, E. Beutler, A.J. Erslev, and M.A. Lichtman), pp. 606–12. McGraw-Hill, New York.

Beutler, E. (1993). The molecular biology of enzymes of erythrocytic metabolism. In *The molecular basis of blood diseases*, (2nd edn), (ed. G. Stamatoyannopoulos, A.W. Nienhuis, P.W. Majerus, and H. Varmus), pp. 331–50. Saunders, Philadelphia.

Valentine, W.N., Tanaka, K.R., and Daglia, D.E. (1989). Pyruvate kinase and other enzyme deficiency disorders of the erythrocyte. In *The metabolic basis of inherited disease*, (6th edn), (ed. C.R. Scriver, A.L. Beaudet, W.S. Sly, and D. Valle), pp. 2341–66. McGraw-Hill, New York.

22.4.12 Glucose 6-phosphate dehydrogenase (G6PD) deficiency

L. LUZZATTO

Definition

Glucose 6-phosphate dehydrogenase (**G6PD**) is a key enzyme in redox metabolism. G6PD deficiency is an inherited condition in which red cells have a markedly decreased activity of G6PD, which predisposes to haemolytic anaemia.

Biochemistry

Red cells are very vulnerable to oxidative damage for two reasons. First, oxygen radicals are generated continuously from within the red cell in the course of methaemoglobin formation. Second, red cells are directly exposed to any oxidizing agent that may be present in the plasma and is able to penetrate the red cell. Oxygen radicals produced by such com-

pounds are converted by superoxide dismutase to hydrogen peroxide, which is itself highly toxic. The two enzymes able to detoxify hydrogen peroxide (by converting it to water) are glutathione peroxidase and catalase. G6PD, the first enzyme of the pentose phosphate pathway (see Fig. 1), catalyses the conversion of glucose 6-phosphate (G6P) and NADP to 6-phosphogluconolactone and NADPH. The most important product of the G6PD reaction, certainly in red cells, is NADPH, because it is crucial for the operation of both glutathione peroxidase (via glutathione reductase) and catalase (because it stabilizes this enzyme). Normally, G6PD activity in red cells is such that NADPH is maintained at a high level and there is practically no NADP: the NADPH/NADP ratio plays a large part in the intracellular regulation of G6PD activity.

The enzymatically active form of G6PD is either a dimer or a tetramer of a single protein subunit with a molecular mass of 59 096 Da. The sequence of the protein was deduced from the nucleotide sequence of the corresponding cDNA, and consists of 514 amino acids. Some regions of the molecule critical for its function have been identified because they are highly conserved in evolution. The G6P-binding site is located at or near lysine 205. Bound NADP is important for the stability of G6PD, but the location of the NADP-binding site and the overall three-dimensional structure of G6PD are not yet known.

Genetics

The inheritance of G6PD deficiency has long been known to have a mendelian X-linked pattern, and the gene encoding G6PD has been finely mapped to the telomeric region of the long arm of the X-chromosome (band Xq28), physically very close to the genes for haemophilia A and colour blindness. At the genomic level, the G6PD gene

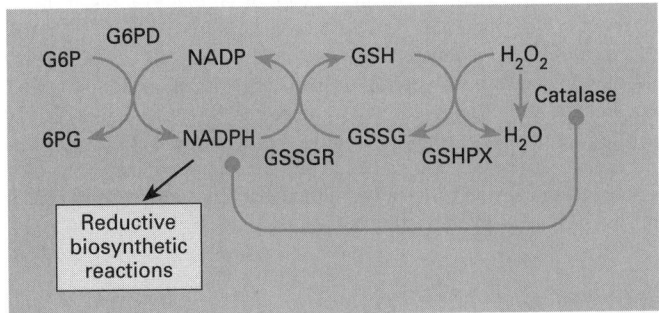

Fig. 1 The role of G6PD in red-cell metabolism: NADPH plays a dual role in (i) regeneration of glutathione (GSH) and (ii) stabilization of catalase (see also Chapter 22.4.11).

Fig. 2 Hetereogeneity of G6PD deficiency. The 13 exons of the *G6PD* gene are drawn approximately to scale; the introns (not drawn to scale) are shown by thin lines connecting the exons. The location of the mutations for the variants listed in Table 1 are shown; plus that of G6PD Sunderland, as example of an English sporadic variant associated with chronic non-spherocytic haemolytic anaemia and due to a deletion of a triplet of bases, corresponding to codon 35.

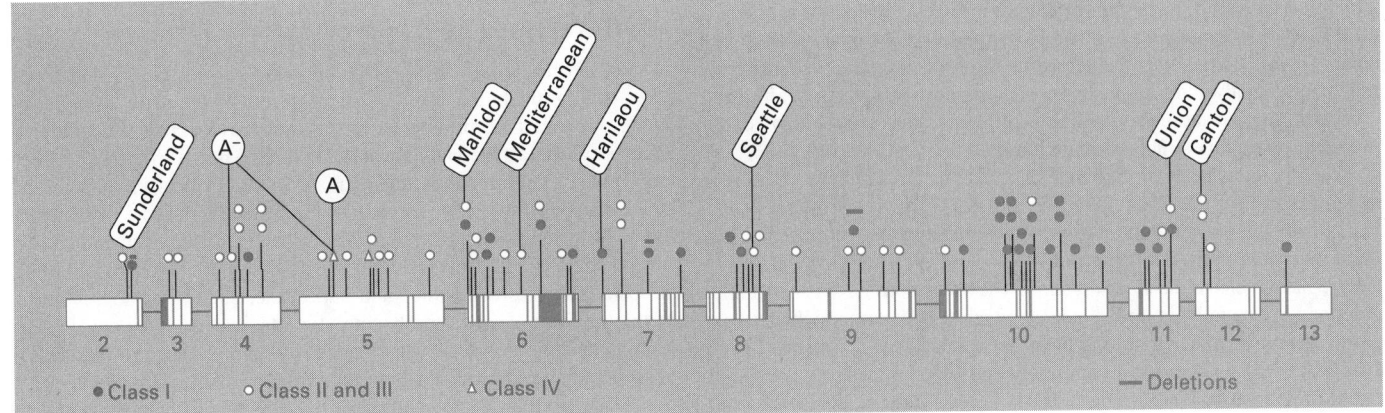

Table 1 *Genetic heterogeneity of G6PD deficiency*

Variant class	Clinical expression	Degree of enzyme deficiency	Examples	Amino acid replacements	Populations where prevalent	Mechanism of enzyme deficiency
I	Chronic non-spherocytic haemolytic anaemia	Usually less than 10% of normal	Harilaou Barcelona	216 Phe→Leu Not yet known	All class I variants are sporadic	Unstable Abnormal kinetics
II	Acute haemolytic anaemia triggered by fava beans, drugs or infection	Less than 10% of normal	Mediterranean Mahidol Canton Union	188 Ser→Phe 163 Gly→Ser 459 Arg→Leu 454 Arg→Cys	Mediterranean, Middle East, India South-East Asia China World-wide	Unstable Unstable Unstable ?
III	As for class II	10–50% of normal	A− ; Seattle	68 Val→Met 126 Asn→ASP 282 Asp→His	Africa; Southern Europe Europe	Unstable ?
IV	None	More than 60% of normal	A	126 Asn→Asp	Africa	None

consists of 13 exons and spans some 18.5 kb. Structural and functional studies have revealed features of a 'housekeeping gene'; this is in accord with the fact that G6PD is found in all cells.

X-linkage of the G6PD gene has important implications. First, as males have only one G6PD gene (i.e. they are hemizygous for this gene), they must be either normal or G6PD deficient. By contrast, females, having two G6PD genes, can be either normal or deficient (homozygous), or intermediate (heterozygous). Moreover, as a result of the phenomenon of X-chromosome inactivation, heterozygous females are genetic mosaics, and this in turn has clinical implications. Indeed, in most other cases, heterozygotes for enzyme deficiencies are asymptomatic because cells with an enzyme level close to 50 per cent of normal are biochemically normal. But in the case of G6PD, as a result of X-inactivation, the abnormal cells of a woman heterozygous for G6PD deficiency are just as deficient as those of a hemizygous deficient man, and therefore just as susceptible to pathology. Thus, although G6PD deficiency is still often referred to as an X-linked recessive trait, this is a misnomer because a recessive trait is, by definition, not expressed in a heterozygote: instead, G6PD deficiency is expressed in heterozygotes both biochemically and clinically—although it is true that heterozygotes are generally less severely affected.

Molecular basis of G6PD deficiency

Since the discovery of G6PD deficiency, one might have expected that some mutations would be located in regulatory regions of the gene, producing a reduction in the amount G6PD produced without changes in its structure (analogous to thalassaemias), whereas others would be located in the coding region of the gene, thus producing qualitative (or structural) as well as quantitative changes in G6PD (analogous to structural haemoglobinopathies). In fact, whenever G6PD from G6PD-deficient individuals has been subjected to careful biochemical characterization (by analysing, for instance, electrophoretic mobility, affinity constants, thermostability), qualitative differences have invariably been detected, predicting structural mutations.

Recently it has been verified that all mutations are structural (Fig. 2), as comparison of the DNA sequence of some 70 different mutant *Gd* genes with the normal gene has revealed, with few exceptions, single point mutations in the coding region of the gene, entailing single amino-acid replacements in the G6PD protein. The exceptions have been small deletions of one to eight amino acids, and a few instances in which two point mutations rather than one have been identified (for instance, in G6PD A−, the variant most commonly encountered in Africa). Regulatory mutations have not yet been discovered. Amino acid replacements can cause G6PD deficiency either by affecting its catalytic function or by decreasing the *in vivo* stability of the protein, or by both of these mechanisms. Enzyme instability is probably the most common mechanism (see Table 1).

Epidemiology

G6PD deficiency is distributed worldwide. Areas of high prevalence are found in Africa, Southern Europe, the Middle East, South-East Asia, and Oceania. In the Americas and in parts of Northern Europe, G6PD deficiency is also quite prevalent as a result of migrations that have taken place in relatively recent historical times.

Because the *Gd* gene is X-linked, frequencies of G6PD deficiency in males are identical to gene frequencies, and they are as high as 20 per cent or more in some of the areas just mentioned. The frequency of homozygous females is of course lower, but the frequency of heterozygous females is higher (according to the Hardy–Weinberg rule). Different G6PD variants underlie G6PD deficiency in different parts of the world: for instance G6PD Mediterranean on the shores of this sea, in the Middle East and in India; G6PD A− in Africa and in Southern Europe; G6PD Mahidol in South-East Asia; G6PD Canton in China; and G6PD Union worldwide. The overall geographical distribution of G6PD deficiency and its heterogeneity, together with findings from clinical field studies and *in vitro* experiments, strongly support the view that this common genetic trait has been selected by *Plasmodium falciparum* malaria, by virtue of the fact that it confers a relative resistance to heterozygotes against this highly lethal infection.

Clinical manifestations

ACUTE HAEMOLYTIC ANAEMIA

In view of the large number of people who carry a G6PD-deficiency gene, it is fortunate that the vast majority remain clinically asymptomatic throughout their lifetime. However, they are all at risk of developing acute haemolytic anaemia in response to three types of triggers: (i) drugs (see Table 2), (ii) infections, and (iii) fava beans. Typically, a haemolytic attack starts with malaise, sometimes associated with more or less profound weakness, and abdominal or lumbar pain. After an interval of several hours to 2 to 3 days (usually the onset is more abrupt in children), the patient develops jaundice and dark urine, due to haemoglobinuria. In the majority of cases the haemolytic attack, even if severe, is self-limiting and tends to resolve spontaneously. In the absence of additional or pre-existing pathology the bone marrow response is prompt and effective. Depending on the proportion of red cells that have been destroyed

Table 2 *Drugs and other agents that can cause haemolysis in G6PD-deficient people*

Drugs	Definite association	Possible of doubtful association[1]
Antimalarials	Primaquine	Chloroquine
	Pamaquine	Quinacrine
	Pentaquine	Quinine
Sulphonamides	Sulphanilamide	Sulphamethoxypyridazine
	Sulphacetamide	Sulphoxone
	Sulphapyridine	Sulphadimidine
	Sulphamethoxazole	Sulphadiazine
		Sulphamerizine
		Sulphisoxazole
Sulphones	Thiazolesulphone	
	Dapsone	
Nitrofurans	Nitrofurantoin	
Antipyretic/ analgesic	Acetanilide	Aspirin
		Aminopyrine
		Acetominophen
		Phenacetin
Other drugs	Nalidixic acid	Ciprofloxacin
		PAS
		Norfloxacin
		L-DOPA
	Niridazole	Chloramphenicol
		Doxorubicin
	Methylene blue	Vitamin K analogues
		Probenecid
	Phenazopyridine	Ascorbic acid
		Dimercaprol
Other chemicals	Naphthalene	
	Trinitrotoluene	
	Toluidine blue	

[1]These drugs can probably cause haemolysis only when given at high doses.

(reflected in the severity of the anaemia), the haemoglobin level may be back to normal in 3 to 6 weeks. The most serious threat in adults is the development of acute renal failure (this is exceedingly rare in children).

The anaemia is usually normocytic and normochromic, and it varies from moderate to extremely severe (haemoglobin of 4 g/dl or less has been recorded); it is due largely to intravascular haemolysis, and hence it is associated with haemoglobinaemia, haemoglobinuria and low or absent plasma haptoglobin The blood film shows anisocytosis, polychromasia, and other features associated with acute haemolysis, including spherocytes (Fig. 3); in severe cases the poikilocytosis is very marked, with bizarre forms, numerous red cells that appear to have unevenly distributed haemoglobin ('hemighosts'), and red cells that appear to have had parts of them bitten away ('bite cells' or 'blister cells'). Supravital staining with methyl violet, if done promptly, reveals the presence of 'Heinz bodies', consisting of precipitates of denatured haemoglobin (Fig. 3). The white blood-cell count may be elevated, with predominance of granulocytes. The platelet count may be normal, increased, or moderately decreased. The unconjugated bilirubin is elevated, but the 'liver enzymes' are usually normal.

FAVISM (PLATE 43)

This is one of the more spectacular forms of acute haemolytic anaemia associated with G6PD deficiency; it can occur at any age, but more commonly in children. Haemoglobinuria develops within 6 to 24 h and is associated with the child becoming first very fractious and then lethargic, and often with fever, abdominal pain, diarrhoea, and sometimes vomiting. Physical examination reveals pallor, tachycardia, jaundice,

and an enlarged spleen; in severe cases there may be evidence of hypovolaemic shock or, more rarely, of high-output heart failure. The cause of favism is the presence in fava beans (or broad beans *Vicia faba*) of vicine and convicine, two β-glycosides having as aglycones the substituted pyrimidines divicine and isouramil, which produce free radicals in the course of their autooxidation. Thus, haemolysis is highly specific for fava beans; other beans are safe. For reasons that are not yet clear, favism does not follow ingestion of fava beans in every case, especially in adults. On the other hand, the widespread notion that favism occurs only with some G6PD-deficient variants and not with others is incorrect.

Fig. 3 Blood film in a case of acute haemolytic anaemia in a G6PD-deficient patient (favism). (a) Romanovsky stain, showing marked poikilocytosis, polychromatic macrocytes, bite cells, nucleated red cells, and a shift to the left in the granulocytic series. (b) Supravital stain with methyl violet, showing the characteristic Heinz bodies.

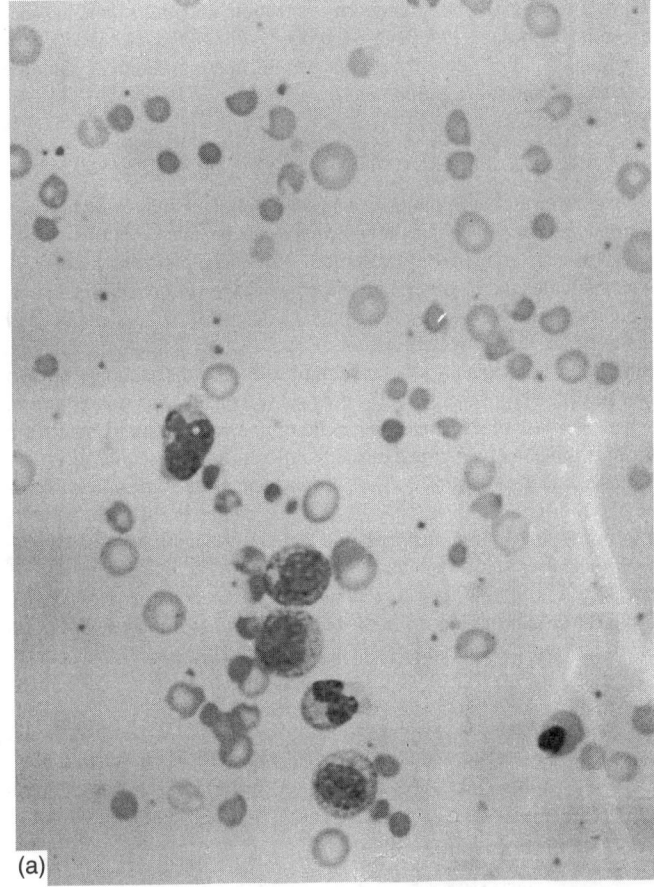

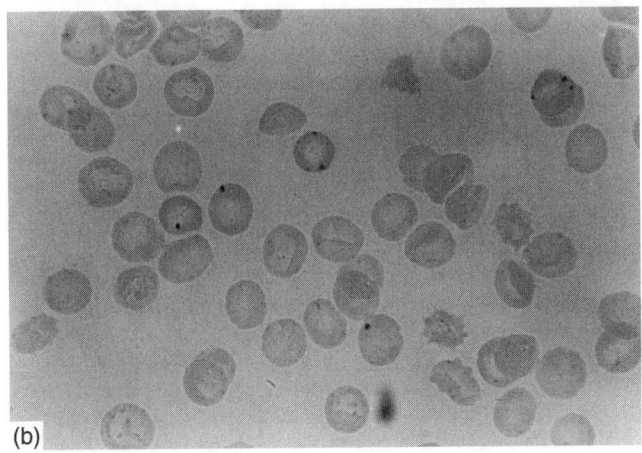

For instance, it has now been well documented with the A— variant, and even with the mildly deficient variant G6PD Seattle.

NEONATAL JAUNDICE

This is again commonly associated with all variants of G6PD deficiency, but it appears to be more common in some parts of the world than others. Not every G6PD-deficient baby becomes jaundiced after birth; however, the risk of developing neonatal jaundice is much greater in G6PD-deficient than in G6PD-normal newborns. The clinical picture of neonatal jaundice related to G6PD deficiency differs from the 'classical' Rhesus-related neonatal jaundice in two main respects: (i) it is very rarely present at birth, and the peak incidence of clinical onset is between day 2 and day 3; (ii) there is more jaundice than anaemia, and the anaemia is very rarely severe. The severity of G6PD-related neonatal jaundice varies enormously, from subclinical to overlapping with 'physiological jaundice' to imposing the threat of kernicterus if not treated. The reasons for this are not clear, but prematurity, infection, and environmental factors (for instance, naphthalene—camphor balls—used in babies' bedding and clothing) certainly play a part in making neonatal jaundice more severe and more dangerous.

CHRONIC NON-SPHEROCYTIC HAEMOLYTIC ANAEMIA

In contrast to the large majority of G6PD-deficient subjects who have minimal and subclinical haemolysis in the steady state, a small minority has chronic anaemia of very variable severity. The patient is practically always a male, and in general he presents because of unexplained jaundice. Frequently the onset is at birth, and a diagnosis is made of neonatal jaundice (see Fig. 4) which may be severe enough to require exchange transfusion. Subsequently the anaemia recurs and the jaundice fails to clear completely; or the patient is only reinvestigated much later in life, perhaps because of gallstones in a child or in a young adult. Usually the spleen is moderately enlarged in small children, and subsequently it may increase in size sufficiently to cause mechanical discomfort, or hypersplenism, or both. The severity of anaemia ranges in different patients from borderline to transfusion dependent. The anaemia is usually normochromic but somewhat macrocytic, because a large proportion of reticulocytes (up to 20 per cent or more) will cause an increased mean corpuscle volume and a shifted, wider than normal, size-distribution curve. The red-cell morphology is not characteristic, and for this reason

it is referred to in the negative as being 'non-spherocytic'. The bone marrow is normoblastic, unless the increased requirement of folic acid associated with the high red-cell turnover has caused it to become megaloblastic. There is chronic hyperbilirubinaemia, decreased haptoglobin, and increased lactate dehydrogenase. In this condition, unlike in the acute haemolytic anaemia described above, haemolysis is mainly extravascular. However, the red cells of these patients are naturally also vulnerable to acute oxidative damage, and therefore the same agents that can cause acute haemolytic anaemia in people with the ordinary type of G6PD deficiency will cause severe exacerbations with haemoglobinuria in people with the severe form of G6PD deficiency.

Chronic non-spherocytic haemolytic anaemia associated with G6PD deficiency is highly specific, in the sense that its molecular basis is always different from that of asymptomatic G6PD deficiency. Numerous point mutations in the G6PD gene causing this type of haemolytic anaemia have been identified, and there are several reasons why they cause a more severe clinical phenotype. In some cases the enzyme deficit is simply more extreme, because of severe instability of the enzyme. In other cases, alterations of the molecular properties of individual variants are important, particularly a decreased affinity for the substrate, glucose 6-phosphate. Molecular heterogeneity explains clinical variability, simply because in almost every case, chronic non-spherocytic haemolytic anaemia is due to a different G6PD mutation.

Laboratory diagnosis

Although the clinical picture of favism and of other forms of acute haemolytic anaemia associated with G6PD deficiency is quite characteristic, the final diagnosis must rely on the direct demonstration of decreased activity of this enzyme in red cells. With neonatal jaundice and chronic non-spherocytic haemolytic anaemia the differential diagnosis is much wider, and therefore this test is even more important. The most popular screening tests are the dye decolorization test, the methaemoglobin reduction test, and the fluorescence spot test. Any of these, provided it is properly standardized and subjected to quality control, is perfectly adequate for diagnostic purposes in patients who are in the steady state, but not those in the posthaemolytic period or with other complications; also, the tests cannot be expected to identify all heterozygotes. Ideally, every patient found to be G6PD deficient by screening should then be retested for confirmation by a quantitative assay. In normal red cells the range of G6PD activity, measured at 30 °, is 7 to 10

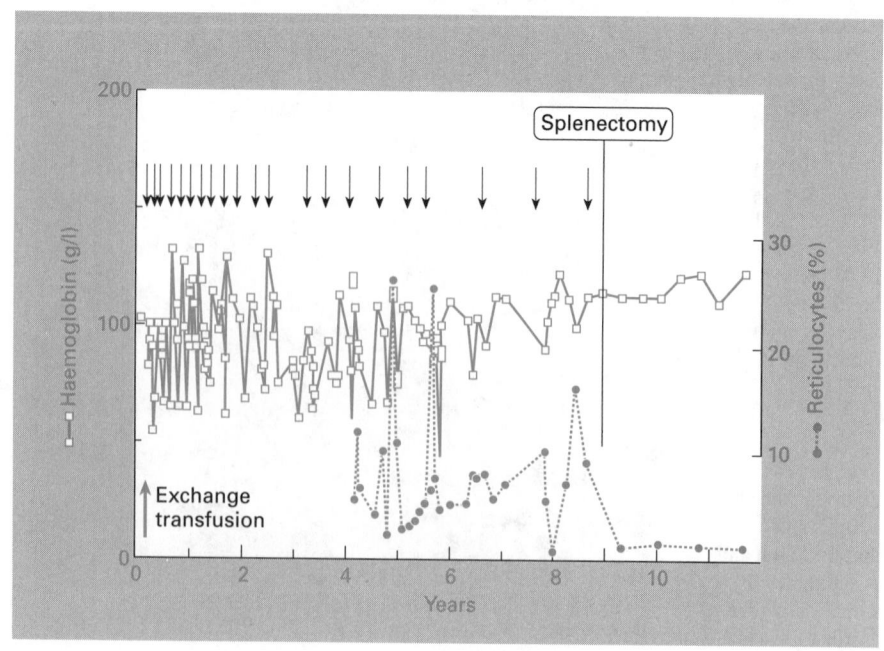

Fig. 4 Clinical course of a patient with chronic non-spherocytic haemolytic anaemia caused by severe G6PD deficiency, illustrating high transfusion requirement, which was alleviated after splenectomy.

iu/g Hb. In G6PD-deficient males (or homozygous females) the level of G6PD in the steady state is, by definition, less than 50 per cent of normal; but with most variants it is less than 20 per cent and with some it is practically undetectable. In heterozygous females the level is intermediate and extremely variable; in some cases the diagnosis may be therefore difficult without family studies or DNA analysis. However, for practical purposes it is most unlikely that a woman will have clinical manifestations if her G6PD level is more than 70 per cent of normal.

Pathophysiology

Acute haemolytic anaemia associated with G6PD deficiency clearly results from the action of an exogenous factor on intrinsically abnormal red cells. Although the sequence of events ending in haemolysis is not completely understood, we know that oxidative agents cause glutathione depletion in G6PD-deficient red cells. This is followed by oxidation of sulphydryl groups and consequent denaturation of haemoglobin (Heinz bodies) and probably of other proteins, which eventually causes irreversible damage to the membrane of red cells and hence their destruction, partly in the bloodstream and partly through phagocytosis by macrophages. An important feature of haemolysis in G6PD-deficient patients depends on the fact that G6PD decays gradually during red-cell ageing (for instance, in normal blood, reticulocytes have about five times more activity than the 10 per cent oldest red cells), and this process is accelerated with many G6PD variants. Thus, a haemolytic attack selectively destroys older red cells because they have a more severe shortage of G6PD. This phenomenon can be so marked with certain G6PD variants that patients in the posthaemolytic state are found to be relatively resistant to further challenge. By contrast, with some other variants the steady-state level of G6PD is so low, even in the absence of any oxidant challenge, that it becomes limiting for red-cell survival: this is the case in the patients with chronic non-spherocytic haemolytic anaemia, who may have a red-cell life-span of between 10 and 50 days.

Treatment

PREVENTION

The most common manifestations of G6PD deficiency, neonatal jaundice and acute haemolytic anaemia, are largely preventable or controllable by screening, surveillance, and avoidance of triggering factors. Of course, the practicability and cost-effectiveness of screening depends on the prevalence of G6PD deficiency in each individual community. Favism is entirely preventable by not eating fava beans. Prevention of drug-induced haemolysis is possible in most cases by choosing alternative drugs. A common practical problem is the need to give primaquine for the eradication of malaria due to *Plasmodium vivax* or *P. malariae;* in these cases the administration of a lower dosage for a longer time is the recommended approach, which will still cause haemolysis, but of an acceptably mild degree.

MANAGEMENT OF ACUTE HAEMOLYTIC ANAEMIA AND FAVISM

A patient with acute haemolytic anaemia may be a diagnostic problem, that once solved, does not require any specific treatment at all; or he or she may be a medical emergency requiring immediate action. With severe anaemia, immediate blood transfusion is definitely indicated. If there is acute renal failure, haemodialysis may be necessary. Recovery is the rule.

MANAGEMENT OF NEONATAL JAUNDICE

This does not differ from that of neonatal jaundice due to other causes than G6PD deficiency. In most cases, prompt phototherapy is highly effective and sufficient; but with bilirubin levels above 300 μmol/1 (or even less in babies who are premature, or who have acidosis or infection), exchange blood transfusion is imperative to prevent neurological damage.

MANAGEMENT OF CHRONIC NON-SPHEROCYTIC HAEMOLYTIC ANAEMIA

In general terms, this does not differ from that of chronic non-spherocytic haemolytic anaemia due to other causes, pyruvate kinase deficiency for example. If the anaemia is not severe, regular folic-acid supplements and regular haematological surveillance will suffice. It will be important to avoid exposure to potentially haemolytic drugs, and blood transfusion may be indicated when exacerbations occur, mostly in concomitance with intercurrent infection. In rare patients the anaemia is so severe that it must be regarded as transfusion dependent. In these cases, blood transfusion will be probably needed at approximately 2-month intervals, in order to keep the haemoglobin in the 8 to 10 g/dl range. A hypertransfusion regimen aiming to maintain a normal haemoglobin level is not indicated (as there is no ineffective erythropoiesis in the bone marrow). However, in patients requiring regular transfusions, appropriate iron chelation should be instituted by the age of 2 years, and must be continued as long as transfusion treatment is necessary; sometimes the transfusion requirement may decrease after puberty. Although there is no evidence of selective red-cell destruction in the spleen, as in heriditary spherocytosis, splenectomy has proven beneficial in severe cases. When a diagnosis of chronic non-spherocytic haemolytic anaemia is made, the family must be given genetic counselling, and an effort should be made to establish whether the mother is a heterozygote; if she is, the chance of recurrence is 1:2 for every subsequent male pregnancy. Prenatal diagnosis could be made by DNA analysis if the mutation is first identified in an affected relative.

REFERENCES

Beutler, E. (1978) Glucose 6-phosphate dehydrogenase deficiency. In *Hemolytic anemia in disorders of red cell metabolism,* (ed. E. Beutler), p.23. Plenum Medical, New York.

Beutler, E. (1991). Glucose 6-phosphate dehydrogenase deficiency. *New England Journal of Medicine,* **324,** 169–74.

Dacie, J.V. (1985). Hereditary enzyme deficiency haemolytic anaemias. Deficiency of glucose-6-phosphate dehydrogenase. In *Haemolytic anaemias,* III:*The hereditary haemolytic anaemias,* (ed. J.V. Dacie), p.364. Churchill Livingstone, London.

Luzzatto, L. (1993). Glucose 6-phosphate dehydrogenase deficiency and hemolytic anemia. In *Hematology of infancy and childhood,* (ed. D.G. Nathan and F.A. Oski), p.674. Saunders, Philadelphia.

Vulliamy, T., Mason, P., and Luzzatto, L. (1992). The molecular basis of glucose 6-phosphate dehydrogenase deficiency *Trends in Genetics,* **8,** 138–43.

Vulliamy, T.J., Beutler, E., and Luzzatto, L. (1993). Variants of glucose 6-phosphate dehydrogenase are due to missense mutations spread throughout the coding region of the gene. *Human Mutation,* **2,** 159–67.

22.4.13 Acquired haemolytic anaemia

E.G GORDON-SMITH AND M. CONTRERAS

The acquired haemolytic anaemias are caused by many different agents but the pathogenesis may be divided into three major groups: immune, physical and chemical changes in the environment, and damage to the membrane or contents of the cell by chemical agents (usually oxidant) or organisms.

Table 1 *Drug-induced immune haemolytic anaemia*

Mechanism	Drugs	Dosage of drug which produces haemolysis	Coombs' test	Reaction of eluate	Haemolysis
Hapten-membrane association	Penicillin, cephalosporins, insulin	High; exposure for some weeks	Mainly IgG	Reacts against drug-coated cells only	Extravascular
Immune complex	Stibophen, quinidine and quinine, p-aminosalicylic acid, isoniazid, phenacetin, anatzoline, sulphonamides, sulphonylureas, amidopyrine, dipyrone, rifampicin, insecticides	Low; second or subsequent exposure produces immediate haemolysis	Usually complement only	Reacts against drug-coated cells and sometimes against free drug	Intravascular acute
Autoimmune	α-Methyldopa, mefenamic acid, levodopa	Prolonged normal dosage	IgG	Reacts against normal red cells in the absence of the drug	Extravascular (usually slight)

The immune haemolytic anaemias (Plate 44)

PATHOGENESIS

Immune haemolysis may occur when antibody or complement are attached to the red-cell surface. Antibodies bound to the red-cell membrane cause binding to macrophages by the Fc receptors on the latter, with subsequent phagocytosis. The antibodies may be IgG, IgA, or IgM, depending upon the aetiology. When IgG is bound, there is competition between free IgG in plasma and the bound IgG for the Fc receptor sites. In the spleen, the plasma-skimming effect of the arteriolar network reduces the amount of free IgG so that destruction of IgG-coated red cells tends to be particularly active. IgM antibodies are bound most avidly at low temperatures and give rise to the cold autoimmune disorders (see below). IgM antibodies also fix complement to receptors on the red cell so that haemolysis occurs through complement activation (see Section 5). Macrophages have receptors for the activated component of C3, C3b, which does not exist in significant amounts in plasma, so that destruction of cells takes place throughout the macrophage system, not just in the spleen. If sufficient complement is bound and activated on the membrane, intravascular lysis occurs as a direct result of the action of the membrane-attack complex of the late complement components. In the acquired disorder paroxysmal nocturnal haemoglobinuria, the red-cell membrane is peculiarly susceptible to the action of activated complement, because the cells lack various surface inhibitors of the membrane attack complex.

Antibody directed against red-cell membrane may be provoked in a number of ways that will be discussed in more detail under the particular disorders. Briefly, antibodies may be directed against membrane components themselves, against components altered by binding of drugs, or against drug–plasma components, the antigen–antibody complex being passively bound to the membrane.

The presence of antibody or complement on the surface of the red cell is detected by the direct antiglobulin test, the Coombs' test. Antibody that reacts against normal red cells of similar blood group may be detected in the serum by the indirect antiglobulin test and eluates may be prepared from the antibody-coated cells to test the specificity of the antibody. The temperature at which the antibody is most active and the class of immunoglobulin involved are also required for reaching a diagnosis.

Drug-induced immune haemolytic anaemia

There are three principal ways in which drugs cause the development of antibodies that bind to the red cells' surface (Table 1).

Hapten–membrane association

Some drugs, of which penicillin is the best-understood example, are bound to red cell-membrane proteins by covalent bonds. The drug complex then acts as an antigenic determinant that binds specific antibody, which is mainly IgG in type. This type of haemolytic anaemia is produced by penicillin in high daily dosage (10–20 megaunits/day), as used in the management of bacterial endocarditis, but only occurs after prolonged exposure or a second course of treatment. Cephalosporins have a similar property and may cross-react with penicillin-induced antibodies.

The haemolysis is gradual in onset but may be profound in its effect, particularly if there is marrow depression due to chronic infection. The direct antiglobulin test is strongly positive but antibodies in the serum will not react with normal red cells of the same type unless penicillin is also present. When the drug is withdrawn, haemolysis ceases fairly promptly, though the direct antiglobulin test may remain positive for 60 to 80 days. The antibody reacts partially against breakdown products of penicillin but these patients rarely have the usual manifestations of penicillin sensitivity. There is no specificity of the antibody for normal blood-group substances.

Immune-complex formation

Many drugs have been incriminated in acute haemolytic anaemia (Table 1) but the number of case reports for each individual drug is small. The antibodies produced in most cases are IgM, which activates complement components and produces profound intravascular haemolysis with haemoglobinaemia and haemoglobinuria. Systemic symptoms are common and acute renal failure may ensue, though this is unlikely to be due to intravascular haemolysis alone but to a combination of haemoglobinuria with complement activation. The haemolysis follows a second or subsequent administration of a very small dose of the drug and is not seen after first exposure. The direct antiglobulin test is positive, owing to complement on the surface of the red cells, but antibody is rarely detected. Antibodies that are lytic for normal red cells only in the pres-

Table 2 *Autoimmune haemolytic anaemias (AHAs)*

	Warm	Cold

Primary	Idiopathic AHA
	  Evans' syndrome
	  (AHA and thrombocytopenia)
		Idiopathic, chronic cold
		  haemagglutinin disease (CHAD)

Secondary	Systemic lupus erythematosus,
	  other autoimmune disorders,
	Lymphomas (particularly
	  chronic lymphocytic
	  leukaemia and Hodgkin's
	  disease),
		Lymphomas (particularly histiocytic),
		  globinuria (PCH), paroxysmal cold
		  haemoglobinuria, infectious
		  mononucleosis

	Drugs, Ovarian teratoma, other cancers	Mycoplasma pneumonia Other virus infections (rare)

ence of the drug are found in the serum. Once the drug is withdrawn the haemolysis stops and the haemoglobin rapidly returns to normal.

'Autoimmune' drug-induced haemolytic anaemia

Three drugs, α-methyldopa, mefenamic acid, and levodopa have been found to provoke the development of autoantibodies directed against red cell-membrane constituents, occasionally producing haemolytic anaemia. The drugs have to be taken regularly for 3 to 6 months before the direct antiglobulin test becomes positive. If the drug is then discontinued the test becomes negative after a variable period, usually between 7 and 24 months. If the drug is then restarted, a further 3 to 6 months elapse before the test becomes positive again. The antibody is IgG in type; complement is not bound.

Haemolysis is extravascular and usually moderate. Spherocytes may be seen in the blood film but in general there are no specific features. Haemolysis stops fairly rapidly after withdrawal of the drug and steroid therapy is rarely indicated. One antidepressive drug, nomefensine, was withdrawn from the market because it produced both autoimmune and immune-complex haemolysis, often with acute renal failure.

Autoimmune haemolytic anaemia

Haemolytic anaemia due to antibodies directed against normal red cell-membrane constituents may arise as a 'primary' event in otherwise healthy individuals or may be associated with a number of other diseases. Table 2 shows that most secondary cases are associated with either malignancy of the lymphoid system or with more generalized autoimmune disorders. Autoimmune haemolytic anaemia may be further classified according to the temperature in which the antibodies are most active against normal red cells *in vitro*. In warm autoimmune haemolytic anaemia, the antibodies are most active at 37 °C, while in cold they are most active at low temperatures, 4 °C for example.

WARM AUTOIMMUNE HAEMOLYTIC ANAEMIA

This is an uncommon disorder that may arise at any age and affects females slightly more than males (about 3:2). It is more common in older age groups because of its association with lymphoid neoplasms.

Clinical features

The onset and severity are variable. Most patients present with a progressive anaemia or mild jaundice but rarely there is a fulminant illness with intravascular haemolysis. At the other extreme, the direct antiglobulin test may be positive but insufficient antibody is present to produce a shortening of the red-cell lifespan. Sometimes the symptoms and signs of the associated disorder dominate the clinical picture but the autoimmune haemolytic anaemia equally commonly precedes the discovery of the primary disease, sometimes by months or years. The spleen is usu-

ally palpable but rarely attains a great size, except in association with a lymphoma.

Haematological features

Anaemia and reticulocytosis are the most marked features of the blood count. There may be neutrophilia, often with a left shift, accompanying the massive erythropoietic drive that follows the onset of anaemia. Nucleated red cells may be seen in the peripheral blood. In uncomplicated autoimmune haemolytic anaemia the platelet count is normal or high, again a reflection of general marrow drive, but in some patients the platelets are also destroyed by antibody and the haemolysis is accompanied by thrombocytopenia (Evans' syndrome). Autoimmune haemolytic anaemia and immune thrombocytopenia may also occur at different times in the same person.

The peripheral blood film may suggest the diagnosis (Fig. 1). Spherocytosis occurs in many but not all cases, and the cells may show autoagglutination. This is not always easy to identify in warm autoimmune haemolytic anaemia, in contrast to the massive autoagglutination that occurs on slides made at room temperature from the blood of people with cold haemagglutinin disease (see below).

Red-cell antibodies

The direct antiglobulin test is positive in virtually all cases of warm autoimmune haemolytic anaemia. Specific antisera are used to detect immunoglobulin subtypes and/or complement components on the red-

Fig. 1 The peripheral blood changes in autoimmune haemolytic anaemia. There is marked anisocytosis and anisochromia with many macrocytes and microspherocytes. The macrocytes reflect the reticulocytosis (× 1000, Leishman stain).

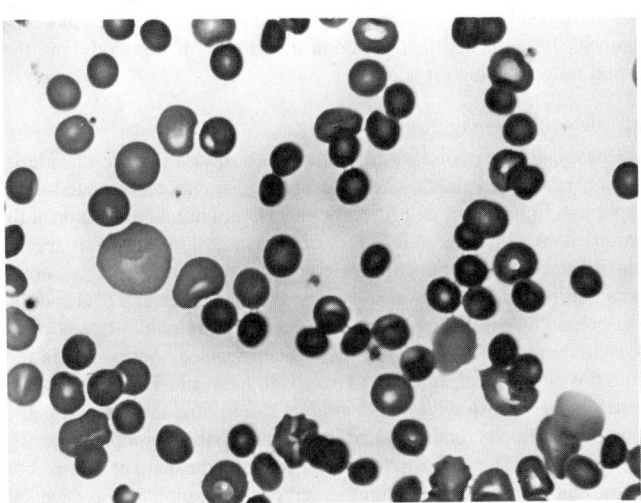

cell surface. Except in systemic lupus erythematosus there is no difference in the distribution or frequency of membrane-bound antibody between idiopathic and secondary autoimmune haemolytic anaemia. In systemic lupus, IgG and complement are both present during the phase of haemolysis but the IgG component may become very weak and finally disappear as the patient recovers.

Pathogenesis

The site of destruction of red cells depends upon whether sufficient complement is fixed to cause intravascular haemolysis or whether the antibody coating promotes phagocytosis by macrophages. When IgG only is bound to the red cell, destruction takes place mainly in the spleen. If complement only is detected, intravascular haemolysis or generalized destruction throughout the macrophage system is likely. When both IgG and complement are present the situation is unpredictable and radio-isotope studies with ^{51}Cr may be helpful in detecting the main site of red-cell destruction.

Treatment

The aim of treatment in autoimmune haemolytic anaemia is to keep the patient in the best possible health with the minimum of iatrogenic problems until the autoantibody disappears and haemolysis stops. In many patients with idiopathic autoimmune haemolytic anaemia the antibodies disappear or diminish to insignificant levels after a period varying from a few months to more than 10 years. Transfusion may be life saving in the acute phase and should not be delayed because of apparent incompatibility of cross-match; ABO matched blood that appears least incompatible should be used.

Corticosteroids are the first measure used to control haemolysis. Prednisolone, 80 mg daily, is effective in most patients and there is rarely any benefit in using higher doses. This dose may usually be reduced over a period of 2 to 3 weeks to 20 mg daily but thereafter a more cautious reduction should be used to find the minimum controlling dose. A maintenance dose of 10 mg prednisolone daily is acceptable in adults and side-effects may be reduced further if the drug is given on alternate days. Azathioprine may exert a steroid-sparing effect, allowing a reduction in steroid dose.

Splenectomy should done only when an adequate trial of corticosteroids has proved ineffective. The type of antibody present and the results of ^{51}Cr-survival studies with surface counting may sometimes provide some help in deciding whether to remove the spleen.

COLD AUTOANTIBODY SYNDROMES

Disorders due to autoantibodies that react most strongly at low temperatures may arise as primary (idiopathic) conditions or may be secondary to a variety of diseases (Table 2). The symptoms and signs of the diseases may result from agglutination of red cells or from haemolysis. Which of these occurs depends upon the titre of the antibody and the thermal range at which it is active.

Chronic cold haemagglutinin disease

Cold haemagglutinin disease in a chronic form is a disease of elderly patients, usually of unknown cause but occasionally associated with lymphoma. Episodes of painful acrocyanosis and numbness (Raynaud's phenomenon) with a variable degree of intravascular haemolysis are the main features. The blood film made at room temperature shows gross autoagglutination, which is absent if the blood is taken at 37 °C and the films prepared at this temperature. The direct antiglobulin test is positive, with complement bound to the red-cell surface. Antibodies in the serum are monoclonal, IgMκ, and nearly all have anti-I specificity. The disease progresses slowly, with a gradual rise in titre and thermal range of the cold antibody, and may end with a malignant lymphoma after 10 years or more. The main treatment is to keep the patient warm, but intermittent treatment with chlorambucil or fludarabine may reduce the antibody level and lead to temporary improvement. Steroids and sple-

nectomy are not of benefit. Blood transfusion should be avoided if possible; if absolutely necessary, it should be given slowly and via a warming coil.

Acute cold haemagglutinin disease

An acute intravascular haemolysis due to a rise in titre of anti-I antibodies may occur following *Mycoplasma pneumoniae* infection. The haemolysis appears about 10 to 14 days after the onset of respiratory symptoms and is usually transient, but occasionally patients require transfusion, which must be given through a warming coil. Rarely, the intravascular haemolysis is very severe and life threatening. The antibody is polyclonal IgM, usually with κ light chains.

A rise in anti-I IgM antibodies, usually with λ light chains, is found in infectious mononucleosis. Rarely, this may cause an acute haemolytic anaemia when the antibody reaches sufficient titre and thermal range. Serious consequences are rare.

Paroxysmal cold haemoglobinuria

Paroxysmal cold haemoglobinuria is a rare disorder caused by a complement-fixing antibody, the Donath–Landsteiner antibody, with anti-P activity. The condition used to arise most commonly in congenital syphilis but most cases are now associated with virus infections such as mumps, measles, or chickenpox. It may also arise without apparent antecedent infection and in this case, as well as in congenital syphilis, attacks may occur over many years. Acute intravascular haemolysis, accompanied by abdominal pain, peripheral cyanosis, and vascular symptoms of Raynaud type, occurs a few minutes after exposure to cold. In addition to the haemoglobinaemia and haemoglobinuria there may be a transient leucopenia. The diagnosis is confirmed by identification of the Donath–Landsteiner antibody, which fixes itself to the red cell in the cold and binds on complement; this causes lysis as the cells are warmed. Episodes are self-limiting and no specific treatment is required.

HAEMOLYTIC ANAEMIA OF THE FETUS AND THE NEWBORN

Haemolytic disease of the fetus and newborn (**HDN**) is a condition in which the lifespan of the infant's red cells is shortened by the action of specific IgG red-cell alloantibodies derived from the mother by active transfer across the placenta. The disease begins in intrauterine life and may result in death *in utero*. In liveborn infants, the haemolytic process is maximal at the time of birth; however, jaundice and anaemia become more severe after birth.

Most IgG red-cell antibodies have been shown to cause HDN, but in practice, and despite Rh prophylaxis, the most common cause of moderate and severe HDN in the Western world is anti-D, followed by anti-c, anti-K and anti-E. Although anti-A, and/or -B in group O women are the most common IgG antibodies, they only cause mild HDN in about 1 in 150 group A or B births and moderate-to-severe disease only very rarely, with very few affected infants needing exchange transfusion.

The binding of IgG antibodies to red cells leads in most, but not all, cases to red-cell destruction through interaction with the Fc receptors of the mononuclear phagocytic system; hence a positive direct antiglobulin or Coombs' test in a newborn infant is not synonymous with haemolytic disease. RhD-positive red cells may survive normally in a newborn infant with a positive direct antiglobulin test due to anti-D because the degree of IgG coating may be too weak; the IgG may have low avidity for Fc receptors, or blocking antibodies may have developed in the mother. It is often difficult to decide whether there is any increased red-cell destruction because, in almost all newborn infants, serum bilirubin concentration rises during the first 2 to 3 days of life and there is a fall in haemoglobin concentration, which continues for about 2 months.

Clinical manifestations of RhD haemolytic disease

Before prophylaxis, the incidence of RhD HDN was lower than expected, that is 1 in 100 second pregnancies. The disease due to anti-

RhD shows a wide spectrum of severity. Not all D-positive infants born to mothers with anti-D in their serum are affected by HDN. Some infants are only mildly affected, with jaundice and anaemia developing in the first week of life. More severely affected infants develop profound hyperbilirubinaemia that may impregnate a basal ganglion, causing kernicterus with signs of brain damage and leading to death within a week of birth in 70 per cent of cases; those who survive have permanent brain damage characterized by choreoathetosis and spasticity and, in milder cases, by high-frequency deafness. The most severe manifestation of HDN is profound anaemia, developing *in utero* as early as the eighteenth week of gestation and leading to hydrops fetalis with generalized oedema, ascites, hepatosplenomegaly, erythroblastosis, and a high mortality.

RhD immunization may occur in 10 per cent of pregnancies in RhD-negative Caucasian women who have a D-positive infant. Immunization is due mainly to transplacental haemorrhage from the fetus to the mother, which occurs at delivery in over 50 per cent of cases. Occasionally, immunization is due to the inadvertent transfusion of D-positive cells to a D-negative woman. About 1 to 3 per cent of women have significant, spontaneous transplacental haemorrhage in the third trimester and its volume can be quantitated by the acid-elution technique of Kleihauer. The chance of transplacental haemorrhage is increased in ectopic pregnancy and with interventions such as therapeutic abortion, chorionic villus sampling, amniocentesis, versions, fetal blood sampling, trauma, caesarean section, and manual removal of the placenta. The magnitude of detectable transplacental haemorrhage and the incidence of RhD immunization decrease when the fetus is ABO incompatible with its mother.

In approximately 1 per cent of D-negative women who deliver a first D-positive child, anti-D is detectable at the end of pregnancy; it is detectable 6 months postpartum in 7 to 9 per cent D-negative women with a D-positive child and in a further 9 per cent (17 per cent altogether) at delivery of the second D-positive infant.

Antenatal assessment of severity

All pregnant women should be grouped for ABO and D at least twice: at the first visit and at delivery. The serum should be tested for alloantibodies at the first visit and if found positive, followed-up monthly up to the twentieth week and at 2-weekly intervals thereafter. Unimmunized D-negative women should be retested at 20 weeks and, if negative, retested at 28 weeks, when antenatal prophylaxis should be considered. All women should have their serum retested at delivery and if D-negative, unimmunized, and carrying a D-positive child should be given RhD immunoglobulin (Ig) (see below). Amniocentesis can be done from the twenty-eight week of gestation onwards, if HDN is expected, to estimate the amount of bile pigment in the amniotic fluid. Ultrasonography also helps in the diagnosis of severe HDN from the eighteenth week onwards but measuring the haemoglobin and packed cell volume in a fetal blood sample is the best method to assess reliably the severity of haemolytic disease *in utero*.

Postnatal assessment of severity

If the direct antiglobulin test on cord red cells is positive, the cord haemoglobin level is the best indicator of severity in infants who may need exchange transfusion; 13.6 g/dl is the lower limit of normal in full-term infants. A cord plasma bilirubin concentration of 68 μmol/l (4 mg/dl) or more may also be an indication for exchange transfusion. If exchange transfusion is not indicated immediately, the plasma bilirubin concentration should be monitored every few hours; levels above 306 μmol/l (18 mg/dl) in mature infants may lead to brain damage. In premature infants the criteria of severity are stricter.

Treatment

In the antenatal period, severely affected fetuses can be transfused with D-negative blood intraperitoneally or, preferably, intravascularly by fetoscopy from the eighteenth to twentieth week of gestation onwards. High-dose IgG given intravenously to the mother has been reported to be beneficial. Premature delivery at 30 to 32 weeks also helps.

In the postnatal period, exchange transfusion with D-negative blood removes anti-D-coated cells, which have a short survival time, and also removes the bilirubin present in the plasma, thus preventing kernicterus. Phototherapy of the infants helps to convert bilirubin to biliverdin.

Prevention of RhD immunization

Some 20 μg of anti-D Ig are able to suppress maternal immunization by 1 ml of D-positive red cells (2 ml of blood). The standard dose of anti-D Ig varies in different countries between 100 to 300 μg given within 72 h of delivery of an RhD-positive child. Transplacental haemorrhages not covered by the standard dose should be quantitated and additional anti-D given as necessary. About 1 to 2 per cent of RhD-negative women are immunized earlier, during pregnancy. This can be prevented by giving anti-DIg antenatally, either by 100 μg anti-D at 28 and 34 weeks or by a single dose of 300 μg at 28 weeks.

Non-immune acquired haemolytic anaemias

Damage to the red-cell membrane leading to haemolysis may occur in certain infections, through oxidative damage brought about by various drugs and chemicals, or through physical damage to the red cell. Except in infection, where immune mechanisms probably play some part in the destruction of red cells, intravascular haemolysis is the usual result.

Infections causing haemolytic anaemia

Malaria
See Section 7 and Chapters 22.4.3 and 22.7.

Toxoplasmosis (see also Section 7)

Most infections with *Toxoplasma gondii* are symptomless or very mild. Infection of the fetus *in utero,* however, may give rise to a very severe disease resembling HDN. Stillbirth and premature delivery are common, and the infant may be hydropic and severely anaemic with erythroblasts in the peripheral blood. There are usually neurological symptoms due to the presence of cysts in the brain. Rarely, acquired toxoplasmosis produces a haemolytic anaemia in adults.

Bacterial infection

Depression of erythropoiesis is the common cause of the anaemia associated with bacterial infections but in some circumstances acute haemolysis is the dominant feature. Severe infections, particularly with Gram-negative organisms producing endotoxin, may lead to disseminated intravascular coagulation and a microangiopathic haemolytic anaemia (see below). *Clostridium perfringens* septicaemia is associated with an intense intravascular haemolysis, microspherocytosis, and fragmentation of the red cells. Renal failure usually occurs. Two mechanisms operate to produce the haemolysis—disseminated intravascular coagulation and direct destruction of red cells by lecithinase and proteolytic toxins produced by the organism. *Bartonella bacilliformis* causes Oroya fever, which is characterized by fever, chills, bone and muscle pain, and acute intravascular haemolysis. The organism occurs only in western South America and may be recognized on Romanowsky-stained blood films as red micrococci on or just inside the red-cell membrane (see Section 7).

Table 3 *Chemically induced haemolysis*

Drug or chemical	Probably haemolytic substance	Remarks
Phenacetin	2-Hydroxyphenetidin	Cyanosis and HB* haemolysis, renal papillary necrosis
Sulphonamides	Hydroxyamino derivatives	Acute haemolysis: hypersensitivity or G6PD deficiency: chronic haemolysis rare
Sulphones	4-Hydroxylamino derivatives	HB haemolysis, dose related
Salicylazosulphapyridine	Sulphapyridine	HB haemolysis, dose related
Phenothiazine	?	Overdose produces HB haemolysis
Phenazopyridine	?	Methaemoglobinaemia common, haemolytic HB anaemia may occur
p-Aminosalicylic acid	m-Aminophenol	Solutions of PAS stored in warm become brown: m-NH$_2$ phenol
Phenylhydrazine and acetyl phenylhydrazine	Phenylhydrazine	No longer used in treatment of polycythaemia vera; self administration may occur; used as experimental oxidizing agent
Water soluble vitamin K analogues	2-Methyl-14-naphthoquinone	Premature infants at risk
Sodium or potassium chlorate	CLO$_4^-$	Weed killer: DIC† as well as HB haemolysis and methaemoglobinaemia
Lead	—	The haemolytic component of lead poisoning is mild
Copper	—	Self poisoning or contaminated tubing
Naphthalene, naphthol	Naphthol	Moth balls, nappy sterilizer; may be absorbed through skin by infants
Wax crayons (red and orange)	p-Nitroaniline	Not permitted now in most countries: children and infants at risk
Well-water nitrates	Nitrite	Methaemoglobinaemia in infants; haemolysis may occur occasionally
Nitrobenzene derivates	Aromatic nitro groups	Industrial workers, especially in munitions, at risk
Nitrotoluene TNT arsine	Arsine	Metal smelters at risk
Insect and snake bites	?	Haemolysis occurs occasionally after bites by spiders and some snakes

*HB: Heinz body.

†DIC: Disseminated intravascular coagulation.

Chemically induced haemolysis

Haemolysis may be caused by a number of drugs and chemicals that are oxidative or produce oxidative metabolites (Table 3).

PATHOGENESIS

The principal pathways by which reducing power is generated in red cells were described earlier. Some drugs and chemicals are strong oxidants and may overcome these reduction mechanisms. There are several inherited conditions that make red cells more susceptible to oxidant damage. Glucose-6-phosphate dehydrogenase (G6PD) deficiency is described in Chapter 22.4.12, and there may be differences in the metabolism of drugs between individuals that alter the amount of oxidative metabolite produced. There is a relatively inefficient reduction system in the red cells of newborn infants and hence they are more prone than adults to develop haemolysis due to the administration of oxidants. Their susceptibility to the oxidative effects of nitrites may lead to a syndrome of methaemoglobinaemia and haemolysis if exposed to high levels of nitrites in drinking water. Variability in availability and absorption of oxidant substances may play a part in the development of the haemolytic anaemia. For example, partial gastrectomy may encourage overgrowth of bowel flora, which may in turn increase the level of oxidant metabolites. The use of dapsone and salazopyrine in inflammatory disorders of the bowel may change the pattern of their absorption and hence increase their toxicity at various times during the course of an illness.

There are several distinct syndromes that occur as a result of oxidant stress, as follows.

Intravascular haemolysis with renal failure

Some strongly oxidizing chemicals such as arsine or chlorate, which may be encountered in industry or used for self-poisoning, produce an intense haemolysis together with disseminated intravascular coagulation and acute renal failure. Constitutional symptoms occur and there may be cyanosis due to associated methaemoglobinaemia. The blood film is bizarre, with red-cell ghosts, fragments, and microspherocytes. The platelet count may fall. Treatment is urgent, the prime requirements being blood transfusion and the preservation of renal function. Haemodialysis and exchange transfusion have been used with success, though mortality is high. The management of acute methaemoglobinaemia is discussed elsewhere.

Acute intravascular haemolysis

Haemoglobinaemia by itself is not a cause of renal failure and acute intravascular haemolysis may follow drug ingestion without renal impairment. This may occur in apparently normal patients who have ingested drugs, such as phenylhydrazine, that have an oxidant action. In patients with G6PD deficiency, or in infants, this is the common result of exposure to oxidant drugs.

Chronic intravascular haemolysis

The usual result of normal individuals taking oxidant drugs such as dapsone or sulphasalazine for long periods is a chronic intravascular haemolysis. Cyanosis due to the presence of methaemoglobin and sulphaemoglobin may be prominent. Heinz bodies may be seen if there is a non-functioning spleen.

LABORATORY FINDINGS

There are features of intravascular haemolysis and the peripheral blood film shows red cells that are irregular and contracted, often with only a segment of the membrane apparently normal. Heinz bodies (precipitated haemoglobin) may be seen but are uncommon unless the spleen has been removed.

TREATMENT

Withdrawal of the drug will terminate the haemolysis but it is not always possible to stop treatment, particularly with dapsone or sulphasalazine. Provided the haemolysis is well compensated it is reasonable to continue the treatment together with iron and folate supplements. If anaemia is a problem, reduction of the dose of the drug may be necessary.

Mechanical haemolytic anaemias

Fragmentation of red cells by mechanical trauma occurs either when foreign material has been inserted into large blood vessels at surgery or where small blood vessels have been partially blocked by fibrin strands. The former has been called cardiac haemolysis and the latter micro-angiopathic haemolytic anaemia.

Cardiac haemolysis

The insertion of prosthetic valves or patches into the heart or aorta usually leads to some destruction of circulating red cells. Under certain circumstances this process can be sufficient to produce severe haemolytic anaemia. The first detailed description of such a case by Sayed et al. in 1961 contains most of the important clinical and laboratory findings.

PATHOGENESIS

Cardiac haemolysis is likely to develop where foreign material is present in a turbulent stream of blood. Homografts rarely produce marked haemolysis. Mitral-valve prostheses produce severe haemolysis less commonly than aortic but when they do the anaemia is often profound. The usual cause is a failure of the anchorage points of the mitral-graft ring so that blood leaks in a small jet around the side between the high-pressure left ventricle and low-pressure left atrium (paraprosthetic or paravalvular leak).

Cardiac haemolysis is aggravated by an increase in cardiac output so that exercise and anaemia itself may increase the rate of cell destruction.

CLINICAL FEATURES

The onset of significant haemolysis depends upon the development of suitable circumstances for mechanical destruction. This may occur at any time but there are certain periods where these conditions are most likely to be met and the acuteness of the haemolysis may give some indication as to its cause. Severe haemolysis occurring immediately postoperatively suggests a surgical cause, such as a defective stitch in the mitral-valve ring or incomplete occlusion of a foramen with a patch. Gradually increasing haemolysis after the patient has left hospital suggests that exercise is promoting turbulence or possibly that iron deficiency is aggravating the anaemia and increasing the turbulence. Delayed onset of haemolysis, particularly after some years in patients with ball-valve prostheses, suggests distortion of the ball or other abnormalities of the prosthesis and reoperation may be necessary.

LABORATORY FINDINGS

The peripheral blood film shows distorted and fragmented red cells with microspherocytes in most cases, but in very acute lesions fragmentation may be hard to find and does not correlate well with the severity of the mechanical haemolysis. The platelet count is usually normal or high, as is the white-cell count. Other features of intravascular haemolysis are present.

MANAGEMENT

Oral iron should be given so that iron deficiency does not develop as a result of haemosiderinuria. Intractable haemolysis may be an indication for surgical re-exploration.

CARDIAC HAEMOLYSIS AND BACTERIAL ENDOCARDITIS

Bacterial endocarditis may cause a severe and rapid anaemia that is difficult to distinguish from mechanical haemolysis due simply to foreign material. The anaemia is caused by marrow depression, usually associated with an increase in mechanical destruction of red cells. The mild hypochromia of infection may suggest iron deficiency but a low serum iron and raised ferritin suggest the anaemia of chronic disease and there is usually evidence of an acute-phase response. Serum complement components are normal in cardiac haemolysis but may be reduced in endocarditis. An enlarging spleen, and the presence of red cells as well as haemoglobin in the urine, point to bacterial endocarditis (Chapter 15.17).

Microangiopathic haemolytic anaemia (Plate 45)

Microangiopathic haemolytic anaemia is a term used to describe intravascular haemolysis due to mechanical destruction of red cells as a result of a variety of pathological changes in small blood vessels. The term was first used by Brain and his colleagues when they noted that fragmented red cells were associated with a wide range of conditions, all of which had in common damage to small blood vessels. The condition has been described in association with a variety of systemic disorders, some of which are summarized in Table 4.

PATHOGENESIS

Microangiopathic haemolytic anaemia develops in many different disorders associated with pathological changes in small vessels, of which microthrombi in capillaries and arterioles, fibrinoid necrosis, necrotizing arteritis, and invasion of capillary walls by malignant cells are the most common.

Some of the disorders that produce microangiopathic haemolytic anaemia are associated with disseminated intravascular coagulation and it has been suggested that microthrombi cause haemolysis because the red cells are fragmented during their passage through the fibrin clots in the small vessels. While this is certainly true in some cases, the relation between intravascular coagulation and microangiopathic haemolytic anaemia is far from clear-cut. Some patients show evidence of a severe form of disseminated intravascular coagulation and yet have virtually no fragmented red cells in their peripheral blood, while others may have a severe microangiopathic haemolytic anaemia and yet show no laboratory evidence of the coagulation. It is possible that these discrepancies reflect differences in the rate of fibrin deposition and the size of the vessels involved in the pathological process. However, there are still many gaps in our knowledge about the pathogenesis of this condition and its relationship to fibrin deposition is still uncertain.

CLINICAL FEATURES

Microangiopathic haemolytic anaemia is characterized by a haemolytic anaemia of varying severity. It is usually seen in a clinical setting of one of the disorders summarized in Table 4.

The haemolytic–uraemic syndrome and thrombotic thrombocytopenic purpura are considered separately later in this section. The presence

Table 4 *Causes of microangiopathic haemolytic anaemia*

Disease	Microangiopathy
Haemolytic-uraemic syndrome	Microthrombi in renal arteries and capillaries
Thrombotic thrombocytopenic purpura	Disseminated intravascular coagulation (DIC)
Renal cortical necrosis	Necrotizing arteritis
Acute glomerular nephritis	Necrotizing arteritis
Pre-eclampsia	Fibrinoid necrosis, DIC (?)
Malignant hypertension	Fibrinoid necrosis. Intimal proliferation in renal vessels
Disseminated carcinomatosis (especially mucinous types)	DIC, tumour emboli (?)
Polyarteritis nodosa	Arteritis
Wegener's granulomatosis	Arteritis
Systemic lupus erythematosus	Arteritis
Homograft rejection	Microthrombi in transplanted organ
Meningococcaemia and other septicaemias	DIC
Cavernous haemangioma	?Local vascular anomalies or thrombosis
Purpura fulminans	?Microthrombi in skin vessels
Polycarboxylate interferon induction	DIC

of renal disease, pre-eclampsia or septicaemia usually presents no diagnostic difficulty. If a patient presents with microangiopathic haemolytic anaemia with no obvious associated disease, it is important to rule out an underlying carcinoma or collagen–vascular disease. The most common tumours associated with this condition are mucus-secreting carcinoma of the stomach, lung, breast, or large bowel. These are nearly always widely disseminated and it is often possible to demonstrate tumour cells in the bone marrow. If disseminated carcinomatosis can be excluded, it is necessary to proceed to investigation for the various collagen–vascular disorders summarized in Table 4.

LABORATORY FEATURES

There is a variable degree of anaemia with a reticulocytosis and all the features characteristic of haemolytic anaemia. The diagnosis is made largely on the morphological appearances of the red cells, which show marked fragmentation and some microspherocytes (Fig. 2); the Coombs' test is negative. A reduced platelet count suggests that there may be an associated disseminated intravascular coagulation.

TREATMENT

The only really successful approach to the treatment of microangiopathic haemolytic anaemia is to find and eradicate the underlying cause. Severe anaemia requires blood transfusion. The use of heparin in the haemolytic uraemic syndrome and in thrombotic thrombocytopenic purpura is rarely of benefit (see later). The subject of heparin therapy for disseminated intravascular coagulation is considered further in Chapter 22.6.6.

Haemolytic–uraemic syndrome

In 1955, Gasser and his colleagues described five previously healthy children who developed acute renal failure and intravascular haemolysis. They gave the name haemolytic–uraemic syndrome to the association and since then many cases have been described. The renal aspects of the condition are considered in Chapter 20.6

PATHOGENESIS

Haemolytic–uraemic syndrome is a disease of infancy, although the peak incidence varies in different parts of the world, for example being about 13 months in Argentina and about 4 years in California. There is

also a seasonal variation and it is more common in the northern hemisphere in the late spring and early summer. There are several reports of more than one family member being affected. These observations, together with the acute febrile nature of the illness, suggest an infectious basis, and viruses, rickettsiae, and bacteria have been variously indicated.

The delay between the febrile illness and the onset of haemolysis and renal failure has cast doubt on whether there is a direct cause-and-effect relation between the infection and the haemolysis. Immune–complex deposition is rarely found in the microangiopathic lesions in this disorder. The lesions consist of widespread damage to the vascular endothelium with secondary fibrin deposition involving particularly renal arterioles and glomerular capillaries. These changes are also found widely throughout all the organ systems. It is presumed that the red-cell changes are secondary to damage during their passage through these small vessels. Laboratory evidence of a consumptive coagulopathy may be obtained, although the results are inconsistent.

Fig. 2 The peripheral blood changes in microangiopathic haemolytic anaemia. This patient had recurrent thrombotic thrombocytopenic purpura and the marked fragmentation of the red cells together with microspherocytosis is evident on the blood film (× 1000, Leishman stain).

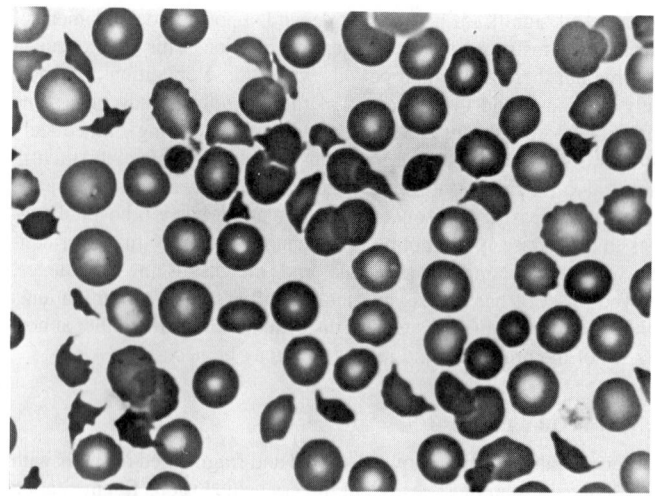

CLINICAL AND HAEMATOLOGICAL FEATURES

The syndrome usually develops after a febrile illness accompanied by diarrhoea, often bloody, and vomiting in a previously healthy child. There may be marked gastrointestinal symptoms, including bloody diarrhoea and abdominal pain. A virulent strain of verotoxin-producing *Escherichia coli*, 0157, has been responsible for a number of epidemics.

Evidence of acute intravascular haemolysis with rapidly developing anaemia develops during or shortly after the prodromal illness and may precede the onset of oliguria. Purpura and bleeding may also occur during the acute phase. Drowsiness, convulsions and coma may develop, and death may occur during the acute phase from uncontrollable anaemia, haemorrhage, or hypertension.

About a third of patients do not develop oliguria at all, about a third have oliguria for up to 10 days, and the remainder up to 4 weeks or longer. The majority of patients without oliguria recover completely without treatment. The longer the period of oliguria, the more likely it is that the condition will go on to a chronic renal failure.

The overall death rate from haemolytic–uraemic syndrome varies from about 2 to 10 per cent. Widespread differences in prognosis between southern and northern hemispheres may reflect differences in aetiology and supportive care in these areas.

The peripheral blood film shows fragmentation and distortion of the red cells with occasional spherocytes. In contrast to cardiac haemolytic anaemia, thrombocytopenia is common, although not invariable. There is often a moderate leucocytosis. Usually there is laboratory evidence of intravascular haemolysis with a raised plasma haemoglobin level, methaemalbumin, low or absent serum haptoglobins, and, sometimes haemoglobinuria. Coagulation studies give equivocal and often conflicting results, although in some cases there is evidence for a consumptive coagulopathy.

MANAGEMENT

The mainstay of treatment is supportive care, transfusion, hydration, control of hypertension, and, if necessary, dialysis. These measures are considered in greater detail in Chapter 20.6.

There have been many reports of the use of heparin therapy in this disorder. The results are, at the best, equivocal. More recently there have been anecdotal reports of the use of inhibitors of platelet aggregation and synthetic prostacyclins. The numbers treated so far are so small that no conclusions can be drawn about the value of this treatment. Corticosteroid therapy is ineffective.

Thrombotic thrombocytopenic purpura

Thrombotic thrombocytopenic purpura (Moschowitz syndrome) is a disorder that has some similarities to haemolytic–uraemic syndrome but occurs mainly in adults. The classical pentad of clinical features is thrombocytopenia, microangiopathic haemolytic anaemia, fluctuating neurological signs and symptoms, fever, and renal impairment. The renal aspects are considered in greater detail in Section 20.

AETIOLOGY AND PATHOGENESIS

The aetiology of thrombotic thrombocytopenic purpura is unknown although, because of the many similarities to haemolytic–uraemic syndrome, an infective basis has been suggested.

The pathological changes include the presence of hyaline material within the lumen of small vessels, endothelial proliferation, and aneurysmal dilation of the vessels. The first two changes may be the result of intravascular coagulation whereas the anatomical changes in the vessels have features in common with those seen in polyarteritis nodosa and systemic lupus erythematosus. Some patients with thrombotic thrombocytopenic purpura have other pathological changes more commonly associated with systemic lupus, including periarticular fibrosis of

the spleen, thickening of the glomerular basement membranes with the appearance of wire loops, atypical verrucous endocarditis, and occasionally positive LE-cell preparations. It is clear that at least at the tissue level there is a marked overlap between haemolytic–uraemic syndrome, thrombotic thrombocytopenic purpura, and the collagen–vascular disorder.

A principal pathogenetic pathway seems to be endothelial damage, which leads to the inappropriate or abnormal release of high molecular-weight von Willibrand multimers that enhance platelet aggregation and perhaps perpetuate endothelial-cell damage. In some cases there may be a plasma deficiency of factors that reduce the high molecular-weight multimers.

CLINICAL FEATURES

The disorder affects females more commonly than males (c. 2:1) and may occur at any age, with a peak incidence in young adults (c. 35 years). The onset is often sudden, with the development of fever and signs of neurological damage, which include convulsions, coma, transient or permanent paralyses, and bizarre psychiatric disturbances, sometimes with hallucinations; the neurological features often fluctuate widely. Purpura may accompany or follow the neurological signs and there may be severe bleeding, particularly from the gastrointestinal tract. Anaemia is not usually severe, although occasionally there may be dramatic intravascular haemolysis with haemoglobinuria.

The illness may run a fluctuating course of days or weeks and some patients may have a series of acute episodes with apparent recovery in between. The most common causes of death are sudden cardiac arrest, bleeding, cerebrovascular accident or renal failure.

HAEMATOLOGICAL AND BIOCHEMICAL CHANGES

There is a mild to severe haemolytic anaemia with fragmentation and contraction of the red cells. This is associated with a variable degree of thrombocytopenia; in some cases the platelets may almost disappear from the peripheral blood. The bone marrow is cellular and megakaryocytes are present in increased numbers but morphologically normal. There is usually a neutrophil leucocytosis. In some cases, coagulation studies show evidence of a consumption coagulopathy but this is not often marked. Examination of the plasma by gel electrophoresis and immunostaining may demonstrate the presence of high molecular-weight von Willebrand multimers, though these may disappear during the acute phase.

Proteinuria is usual, often with other evidence of renal damage in the form of casts and red cells, together with a raised blood urea and reduced creatinine clearance. In some cases there may be serological findings suggestive of systemic lupus erythematosus. Hypertension is common.

CHRONIC RELAPSING FORMS AND THROMBOTIC THROMBOCYTOPENIC PURPURA IN PREGNANCY (CHAPTER 13.9)

There appears to be a subgroup of patients with a thrombotic thrombocytopenic purpura-like illness who give a long history of relapses going back to childhood and often initiated by a disorder resembling the haemolytic uraemic syndrome.

Thrombotic thrombocytopenic purpura seems to be particularly prone to occur during pregnancy or in the postpartum period and this may account for the slight excess of young women affected by this disease. It is often associated with miscarriage. Removal of the fetus does not always lead to remission.

Plasma exchange is the most effective form of treatment. Up to 12 consecutive, daily exchanges may be required to produce a response and relapse is not uncommon. A proportion of patients may respond to infusion of fresh frozen plasma without exchange. Heparin and anti-platelet drugs are rarely of benefit but some patients improve with corticosteroids.

March haemoglobinuria

Haemoglobinuria following vigorous exercise in young men has been recognized for many years as a benign disorder but it was the studies of Davidson which showed that mechanical haemolysis was the cause. Haemoglobinuria follows walking or running on a hard surface and lasts for a few hours. Other sports such as karate may produce the same effect. There may be some systemic symptoms, such as nausea and abdominal pain, but usually the haemoglobinuria is symptomless. The haemolysis is produced by the interaction of a hard surface and red cells in the superficial vessels of the feet, but the blood film is normal in appearance and fragments are not seen. Treatment is not usually necessary but the insertion of a springy sole into running shoes will usually prevent haemolysis. As mentioned above, a structural change in the red-cell membrane may underlie the increased susceptibility to mechanisms of red-cell destruction in this condition; these observations await confirmation.

Haemolytic anaemia of burns

Extensive burns produce intravascular haemolysis with microspherocytosis and fragmentation in the peripheral blood. The direct action of heat is probably important in the pathogenesis but intravascular coagulation in the postinjury period may play some part.

Acquired disorders of the cell membrane

Paroxysmal nocturnal haemoglobinuria is the most common acquired disorder of the red-cell membrane. It arises from a somatic mutation that affects the production of phosphoinositol glycan anchor. The anchor attaches a number of membrane proteins on haemopoietic cells and its complete lack or deficiency leads to multiple abnormalities including susceptibility to complement attack and a thrombotic tendency. Paroxysmal nocturnal haemoglobinuria is considered in detail in Chapter 22.3.12.

Lipid disorders

Changes in the lipid content of plasma may induce red cell-membrane changes that lead to some shortening of the cell's survival. The cholesterol and part of the phospholipid content of the membrane are in equilibrium with plasma lipids. Changes in the latter influence the lipid content of the membrane and the shape and deformability of the red cell. Abnormalities of membrane lipid metabolism may contribute to the haemolysis of liver disease and disorders associated with hyperlipidaemia.

Liver disease

There is a shortening of the red-cell life-span in most patients with acute hepatitis, cirrhosis, and Gilbert's disease (see Section 14). In Gilbert's disease the decreased red-cell survival and slight reticulocysosis suggest that haemolysis may contribute to the increased unconjugated bilirubin, but it seems probable that it is only a minor factor and that deficiency of the enzyme UDP-glucoronyl transferase is mainly responsible. In biliary obstruction and mild liver disease, target cells are seen in the peripheral blood. In more severe disorders, acanthocytosis is prominent.

Zieve's syndrome

This is the association of haemolytic anaemia with abdominal pain, cirrhosis, hyperlipidaemia, and jaundice in chronic alcoholics. The peripheral blood contains spherocytes and the osmotic fragility is increased, unlike most liver disorders in which it is reduced.

Wilson's disease (see Chapter 11.7)

Acute haemolysis, usually intravascular, may be a presenting feature in Wilson's disease. It may be caused by the presence of free copper in the plasma.

Vitamin E deficiency

Vitamin E is necessary to prevent auto-oxidation of the unsaturated fatty acids in the red-cell membrane. Deficiency may occur in premature infants fed polyunsaturated fatty acids in artificial foods. A haemolytic anaemia with acanthocytosis occurs together with thrombocytosis. There is a prompt response to vitamin E administration.

Congenital pyknocytosis

This is a rare condition, seen in infants, characterized by haemolytic anaemia and the presence of bizarre, contracted red cells. The haemolysis may be marked but the disease is usually transient and the child recovers completely. The cause is unknown.

Hypersplenism

A significant enlargement of the spleen is frequently associated with a slightly shortened red-cell survival even though the red cells are intrinsically normal. The mechanism and methods for identifying this form of haemolysis are considered in Chapter 22.5.4.

Anaemia of chronic disorders and renal disease

The haemolytic component of the anaemia of chronic disorders is described in Chapter 22.4.5.

Physical agents

Haemolytic anaemia has been observed in astronauts exposed to 100 per cent oxygen. There have been occasional reports of acute haemolysis occurring in patients undergoing hyperbaric oxygen therapy. The mechanism for these changes is unknown. The shortened red-cell survival that occurs after total body irradiation has a complex basis which is ill understood; red cells are remarkably resistant to the direct effects of ionizing radiation.

REFERENCES

Byrnes, J.J. and Moake, J.L. (1986). Thrombotic thrombocytopenic purpura and haemolytic uraemic syndrome: evolving concepts of pathogenesis and therapy. *Clinical Haematology*, **15**, 413–42.

Brain, M.C., Dacie, J.V., and Hourhane, D. O'B. (1962). Microangiopathic haemolytic anaemia: the possible role of vascular lesions in pathogenesis. *British Journal of Haematology*, **8**, 358.

Clarke, C.A. and Whitfield, A.G.W. (1979). Deaths from rhesus haemolytic disease in England and Wales in 1977; accuracy of records and assessment of anti-D prophylaxis. *British Medical Journal*, **i**, 1665–9.

Davidson, R.J.L. (1969). March or exertional hemoglobinuria. *Seminars in Hematology*, **6**, 150.

Dacie, J.V. (1992). *The haemolytic anaemias*, Vol. 3, *The autoimmune haemolytic anaemias*, (3rd edn). Churchill Livingstone, Edinburgh.

Gordon-Smith, E.C. (1980). Drug induced oxidative haemolysis. *Clinical Haematology*, **9**, 557–86.

Gross, S. (1976). Hemolytic anemia in premature infants: relationship to vitamin E, selenium, glutathion peroxidase and erythrocyte lipids. *Seminars in Hematology*, **13**, 187.

Magilligan, D.J., Fisher, E., and Alam, M. (1980). Hemolytic anaemia with porcine xenograft aortic and mitral valves. *Journal of Thoracic and Cardiovascular Surgery*, **79**, 628–31.

Marsh, G.W. and Lewis, S.M. (1969). Cardiac hemolytic anemia. *Seminars in Hematology*, **6**, 133–45.

Moake, J.L. and McPherson, P.D. (1990). von Willebrand factor in thrombotic thrombocytopenic purpura and the hemolytic-uremic syndrome. *Transfusion Medicine Reviews*, **4**, 163.

Mollison, P.L., Engelfriet, C.P., and Contreras, (1993). *Blood transfusion in clinical medicine*, (9th edn), Ch. 3, 5, and 12. Blackwell Scientific, Oxford.

Rutkow, I.M. (1978). Thrombotic thrombocytopenic purpura (TTP) and splenectomy: a current appraisal. *Annals of Surgery*, **188**, 701–5.

Sayed, H.M., Dacie, J.V., Handley, D.A., Lewis, S.M., and Cleland, W.P. (1961). Haemolytic anaemia of mechanical origin after open heart surgery. *Thorax*, **16**, 356–60.

Shepherd, K.V. and Bukowski, R.M. (1987). The treatment of thrombotic thrombocytopenic purpura with exchange transfusions, plasma infusions, and plasma exchange. *Seminars in Hematology*, **24**, 178.

Walker, B.K., Ballas, S.K., and Martinez, J. (1980). Plasma infusion for thrombotic thrombocytopenic purpura during pregnancy. *Archives of Internal Medicine*, **140**, 981–3.

22.4.14 The relative and secondary polycythaemias

D. J. WEATHERALL

The word 'polycythaemia' means an increased red-cell count, packed cell volume, or haemoglobin level. In an earlier section we described the form of polycythaemia that is thought to be due to the neoplastic proliferation of a clone of haemopoietic red-cell progenitors, polycythaemia vera (Chapter 22.3.8). However, while it is quite common in clinical practice to encounter patients with a haemoglobin level above normal, this type of polycythaemia is quite rare. In this chapter we shall consider the more common causes of polycythaemia and how these are identified and managed.

Classification and pathogenesis

The mechanisms for the production of polycythaemia are summarized in Table 1. A high haemoglobin level can occur for two main reasons. First, there may be a reduction in the plasma volume with a normal red-cell mass. Second, there may be a genuine increase in the red-cell mass. Thus, it is usual to divide the polycythaemias into relative and absolute. The causes of a contracted plasma volume, which leads to a relative polycythaemia, are considered later.

The mechanisms for the production of an increased red-cell mass are best understood in terms of a breakdown of the normal regulation of erythropoiesis. The rate of red-cell production is controlled by the level of erythropoietin, the production of which is governed by the oxygen supply to the tissues. As well as the neoplastic proliferation of haemopoietic progenitors that occurs in polycythaemia vera there are several other ways in which the red cell mass can increase. First, there may be an appropriate response to an increased output of erythropoietin secondary to hypoxia. This is the mechanism of the polycythaemia of chronic obstructive airways disease, cyanotic congenital heart disease, altitude, hypoventilation, or defective release of oxygen by the red cells. Defective release may result from chronic carboxyhaemoglobinaemia due to cigarette smoking or, much less commonly, from intrinsic abnormalities of haemoglobin or red-cell enzymes. Second, there may be inappropriate secretion of high levels of erythropoietin. This usually results from an erythropoietin-secreting renal tumour or from ectopic production of erythropoietin from extrarenal lesions. It may also occur as a transient phenomenon after renal transplantation, or in families with a genetic defect in erythropoietin regulation. Finally, there are some endocrine disorders such as Cushing's disease in which there may be a genuine increase in the red-cell mass, the mechanism of which is not understood.

In clinical practice it is not uncommon to encounter patients with a genuine increase in the red-cell mass who do not appear to fit into any of these categories. They do not have splenomegaly or an elevated white-cell or platelet count characteristic of polycythaemia vera, and yet no other cause for polycythaemia can be found. They may have an elevated red-cell mass of approximately the same magnitude for many years. This condition has been called idiopathic or benign erythrocytosis. However, it is becoming clear that some of these patients, if observed for long enough, develop splenomegaly or an elevated platelet

Table 1 *Mechanisms for the production of polycythaemia*

Relative
Reduced plasma volume

Absolute
Normal or low erythropoietin levels; abnormal proliferation polycythaemia vera
Increased erythropoietin levels:
    Appropriate:
        lung disease, cyanotic heart disease, altitude, abnormal haemoglobin, hypoventilation, decreased 2,3-diphosphoglycerate production
    Inappropriate:
        renal tumour; other erythropoietin-secreting tumours; after renal transplant; genetic defect in erythropoietin regulation
    Mechanism unknown:
        endocrine disease; Cushing's disease; phaeochromocytoma

or white-cell count and other features which indicate that they have polycythaemia vera. However, this does not always happen and there appears to be a form of true polycythaemia which is not a myeloproliferative disorder and for which no cause can be found. It seems reasonable to retain the term benign erythrocytosis for this ill-defined condition.

An approach to the patient with polycythaemia

An usually high haemoglobin level or packed-cell volume (**PCV**) is one of the most common reasons for the referral of patients to haematology departments. If a great deal of unnecessary worry for the patient and expensive investigation is to be avoided it is very important to develop a logical approach to this problem (Fig. 1).

The first rule is that, unless the haemoglobin level is extremely high, it is wise never to diagnose polycythaemia on a single blood count. Care must be taken to ensure that a count is obtained when the patient is well hydrated, is not receiving large doses of diuretics, and has not had a heavy night's alcohol intake the day before the blood sample is taken. Heavy smokers who have a mild polycythaemia should be asked to stop smoking and their blood counts repeated several weeks later. Finally, it should be remembered that the haemoglobin level and PCV have a large standard deviation; many referrals for the investigation of polycythaemia stem from an ignorance of normal haematological values.

Having determined that the haemoglobin value or PCV is genuinely elevated the next step is to decide whether it is a true or relative polycythaemia. This requires a plasma volume and red-cell mass determination. We shall return to the problem of interpreting these data when we consider the diagnosis of relative polycythaemia.

If the red-cell mass determination shows that there is an absolute polycythaemia the next step is to decide whether this is a primary myeloproliferative disorder or a pure red-cell polycythaemia. The criteria for the diagnosis of polycythaemia vera are considered in Chapter 22.3.8. In the absence of a raised platelet and/or white cell count, or splenomegaly, another case for the elevated red cell mass must be sought.

The causes of secondary polycythaemia are summarized in Table 2. Hypoxia due to chronic obstructive airways disease is by far the most common. While this diagnosis can usually be made on clinical grounds, this is not always the case and it may sometimes be necessary to resort to blood-gas analysis, either at rest or after exercise, to rule out this diagnosis. Cyanotic heart disease usually presents no diagnostic problems but occasionally patients are encountered who have arteriovenous malformations that may not be obvious clinically. Again, analysis of the arterial oxygen saturation will provide a clue to the diagnosis. Before proceeding further it is very useful to carry out a P_{50} estimation. If the

P_{50} is reduced, indicating a left shift in the oxygen dissociation curve, the carboxyhaemoglobin level should be estimated; patients are often unreliable about their smoking habits! If this is normal and the P_{50} is low, there must be an intrinsic abnormality of the red cells, either of the haemoglobin or of the red-cell enzymes. If the P_{50} is normal, a source of inappropriate erythropoietin production should be looked for. The most likely site is the kidney, either a hypernephroma or a renal cyst. Thus a careful microscopic examination of the urine should be carried out followed by an ultrasound examination of the kidney, an intravenous urogram and, if indicated, a renal arteriogram. It may be necessary to do a computerized tomographic scan of the liver and posterior fossa to exclude a hepatoma or haemangioblastoma of the cerebellum. In women, a careful pelvic examination should be made to search for uterine fibroids, which are occasionally associated with polycythaemia. However, it should be emphasized that erythropoietin-secreting tumours are a very rare cause of polycythaemia and it is only necessary to go to these lengths in the minority of cases.

If in most cases these simple investigations will be sufficient to identify the cause of polycythaemia. However, where difficulty remains it is now possible to estimate the level of erythropoietin in the serum directly.

Finally, when all these investigations have been carried out there remains a number of patients who have an increased red-cell mass for which no cause can be found. It is worth assessing their close relatives to see if the condition falls into the rare group of hereditary polycythaemias due to abnormal erythropoietin control. Having excluded this

Fig. 1 Flow chart of investigations for polycythaemia.

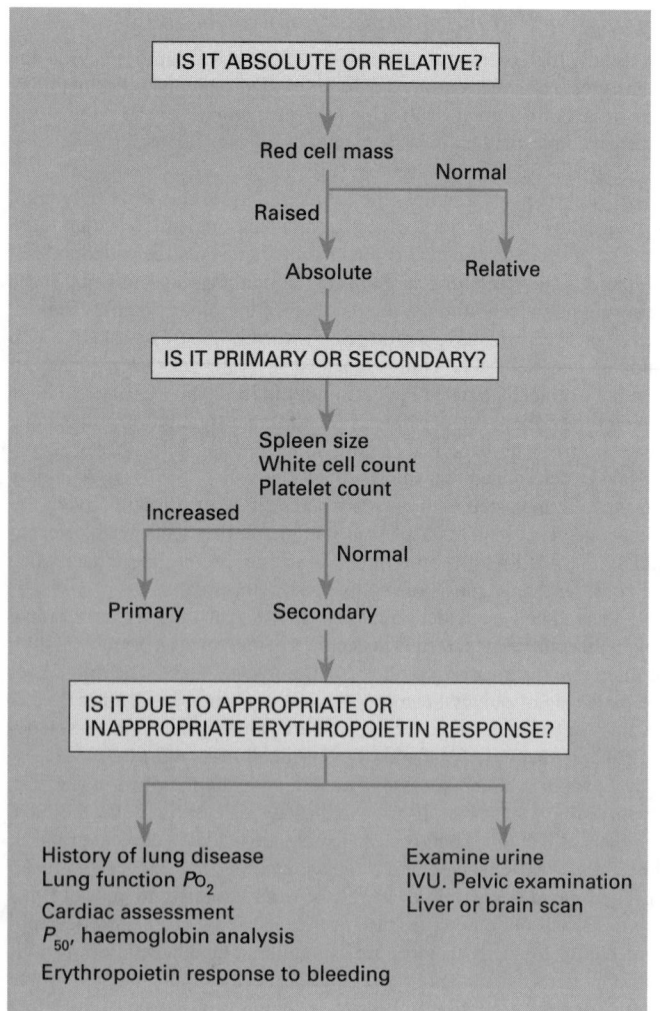

Table 2 *Clinical classification of polycythaemia*

Relative or *pseudopolycythaemia* ('stress' polycythaemia)

True polycythaemia
Primary
    Polycythaemia rubra vera
Secondary
    Altitude
    Chronic lung disease
    Cyanotic congenital heart disease
    Renal disease:
        tumours, cysts, hydronephrosis, post-transplant
    Non-renal tumours:
        hepatoma, cerebellar haemangioma, uterine fibromata
    Endocrine:
        Cushing's disease, phaeochromocytoma
    Genetic:
        abnormal haemoglobin
        abnormal erythropoietin response
        abnormal 2,3-diphosphoglycerate metabolism
    Obesity:
        Pickwickian syndrome
        other causes of hypoventilation

diagnosis these patients should be kept under regular surveillance because, as mentioned earlier, at least some of them develop features of polycythaemia vera, sometimes after many years.

Relative polycythaemia

Relative polycythaemia has collected several names over the years, including apparent, spurious, pseudo, stress, or benign polycythaemia, and Gaisböck's syndrome. The term describes an elevated haemoglobin level or PCV that results from a contraction of the plasma volume and is not associated with an absolute increase in red-cell mass. As will become apparent, the situation is not as simple as this definition might suggest.

CLASSIFICATION

There are two main groups of relative polycythaemias. The first is made up of patients who have a disturbance of fluid balance leading to a diminished plasma volume such as may occur in severe dehydration, following diuretic therapy, and in various endocrine disorders such as Addison's or Cushing's diseases. The second group is made up of patients who seem to have red-cell masses at the upper limit of normal and a slightly contracted plasma volume. We shall confine this discussion to the second group.

AETIOLOGY AND PATHOGENESIS

The relative polycythaemias in which there are no obvious fluid or electrolyte disturbances, although probably quite common, have been extremely difficult to define and virtually nothing is known about their pathogenesis. The real problem in this field is that it is extremely difficult to obtain accurate measurements of the red-cell mass, or for that matter the plasma volume. Where these have been done in a series of individuals labelled as having relative polycythaemia, the results have been inconsistent. In some cases the red-cell mass is at the upper limit of what is accepted as 'normal' and the plasma volume is at the lower limit of normal, while in others the red-cell mass may be normal and there may be a clear-cut reduction in the plasma volume. For technical reasons it is not possible to repeat these measurements very often in the same individual and hence to determine how constant the results are in the same person at different times. As a group these individuals tend to be obese, middle-aged males who are anxious and/or aggressive, overweight, and mildly hypertensive.

The mechanism for the plasma volume contraction is unknown. Recent studies have raised the possibility that it reflects an age-related defect in autonomic nervous function associated with changes in venous capacitance.

RELATION TO THROMBOTIC DISEASE

There is increasing interest in the relation between mildly elevated haemoglobin or PCV levels and cerebrovascular and coronary artery disease. There is some epidemiological data suggesting a relation between the haemoglobin level and the incidence of arterial thrombotic disease. Cerebral blood-flow studies suggest that there is a significant decrease in flow at PCV values ranging from 48 to 55 per cent, presumably due to increased blood viscosity. All these data indicate that a moderate elevation of the PCV may be an important risk factor in the pathogenesis of arterial disease, but more work is required before this is firmly established.

CLINICAL FEATURES

The typical clinical picture of relative polycythaemia is the overweight middle-aged male who is slightly hypertensive and has a haemoglobin value in the 18 to 20 g/dl range and a PCV of 49 to 55 per cent. There are no specific symptoms or signs that can be attributed to this 'disorder' and usually the presenting feature is an associated medical condition, most often cardiovascular disease or hypertension. An elevated haemoglobin level is found occasionally on routine investigation for a completely unassociated condition.

LABORATORY FINDINGS

With the exception of an elevated haemoglobin and PCV the rest of the haematological findings are completely normal. The red-cell mass is usually normal, and as mentioned above the plasma volume may be moderately contracted. Sometimes the red-cell mass is at the upper limit of normal and the plasma volume at the lower limit.

DIFFERENTIAL DIAGNOSIS

This type of relative polycythaemia should be diagnosed with caution. It should be remembered that a high haemoglobin level may be encountered in patients who are receiving diuretic therapy, who are dehydrated for any cause (including a heavy night's drinking) or who have one of the causes of a genuine increase in the red-cell mass. As emphasized earlier, tobacco smoking is one of the most common of the latter conditions. Hence extensive investigation should not be made until it has been demonstrated that the haemoglobin value or PCV are consistently elevated on two or three separate occasions. If this is the case, a red-cell mass should be estimated and the diagnosis confirmed by finding a normal value. The clinician should always bear in mind that normal male PCV is 47 per cent ± 6.2 per cent and therefore many normal men have PCVs of 50 to 52 per cent and should not, therefore, be classified as abnormal and subjected to extensive investigation.

MANAGEMENT

In the past it was thought sufficient, once the diagnosis of relative polycythaemia was made, to reassure the patient strongly and to stop examining his or her blood. Suitable advice was given about weight reduction, the control of hypertension, and stopping smoking. Although this is still the case, there is some evidence that the mild elevation of blood viscosity that occurs in patients with PCVs in the 50 to 55 per cent range may predispose towards coronary artery and cerebrovascular disease. At the time of writing this is a controversial subject and more data are required before the place of regular venesection of these patients is firmly established. At the present time it seems reasonable to venesect patients who have had episodes of coronary artery or cerebrovascular disease and who have persistently elevated PCVs, or those who have a particularly bad family history of cardiovascular disease. It is much more difficult to make a case for venesection in an asymptomatic middle-aged male with a slightly elevated PCV; if future studies show that these individuals are at considerable risk of developing vascular disease, a more aggressive approach will be required.

Secondary polycythaemia

Some of the causes of secondary polycythaemia are listed in Table 2.

ACUTE MOUNTAIN SICKNESS, MONGE'S DISEASE

These conditions, and a description of the secondary polycythaemia that results as part of adaptation to altitude, are discussed in Section 8.

RESPIRATORY DISEASE

This is probably the most common cause of secondary polycythaemia. The increased production of erythropoietin results from arterial hypoxia. There may be a right shift in the oxygen dissociation curve resulting from increased 2,3-disphosphoglycerate production secondary to hypoxia but this is probably of little functional significance. A curious feature of chronic pulmonary disease is that some patients do not show a compensatory polycythaemia, even if they are severely hypoxic. Although it has been suggested that this may be the result of bone marrow depression due to associated infection, this is not always the case and the lack of correlation between the PCV and degree of hypoxia in chronic chest disease remains unexplained. It should always be remembered that smoking may contribute to the polycythaemia of chronic lung disease.

The therapeutic value of venesection in patients with polycythaemia secondary to chronic obstructive airways disease remains controversial. There is some evidence for improvement in cardiac function and cerebral blood flow after venesection. Thus there may be a place for venesection in patients with PCV values of greater than 55 to 60 per cent, although this question requires further study.

ALVEOLAR HYPOVENTILATION

Central alveolar hypoventilation due to an impaired response of the respiratory centre has been reported in patients with cerebrovascular accidents or in association with Parkinson's disease, encephalitis, and barbiturate overdosage. Alveolar hypoventilation may also result from mechanical impairment of the chest in patients with muscular dystrophies, poliomyelitis, or ankylosing spondylitis (see Sections 17 and 18). The Pickwickian syndrome is characterized by gross obesity and somnolence; the associated polycythaemia seems to be caused by a combination of both central and peripheral hypoventilation. The precise aetiology is unknown but the mechanism appears to involve a vicious circle of somnolence, hypercapnia, and hypoventilation that leads to lack of respiratory response, which is further aggravated by mechanical impairment of ventilation due to extreme obesity.

There has been considerable recent interest in the problem of sleep apnoea. Intermittent alveolar hypoventilation is frequently observed in normal males, and in patients who are already hypoxic due to lung disease it may cause severe arterial hypoxaemia, hypercapnia, cyanosis, and marked secondary polycythaemia. This subject is considered in detail in Section 17.

CARDIOVASCULAR DISEASE

In any congenital heart disease with a right-to-left shunt there may be arterial oxygen unsaturation, severe cyanosis, finger clubbing, and extreme secondary polycythaemia. Some children with severe congenital heart disease of this type may have PCVs in excess of 80 per cent. There is a genuine risk of thrombotic episodes, particularly if these children become dehydrated due to an intercurrent illness. There may be an indication for venesection, particularly before surgery, although the precise value of reduction of the haematocrit is not clear.

Hypoxaemia and secondary polycythaemia occurs in association with other types of right-to-left vascular shunts. For example, it is well recognized as a complication of pulmonary arteriovenous aneurysms, and hereditary telangiectasia. Shunting of this kind may also be the mechanism for the mild secondary polycythaemia that is sometimes observed in patients with cirrhosis of the liver. For this reason it is important to carry out a blood gas analysis in any patient with unexplained polycythaemia.

DEFECTIVE OXYGEN TRANSPORT

Carboxyhaemoglobin due to smoking is one of the most common causes of secondary polycythaemia. Heavy smokers may have as much as 15 per cent of carboxyhaemoglobin, and because of the resulting increase in oxygen affinity there may be sufficient hypoxic drive to produce a moderate degree of polycythaemia. A mild degree of secondary polycythaemia is also seen in patients with genetic or acquired forms of methaemoglobinaemia.

A variable degree of polycythaemia is found in patients and their affected family members with high oxygen-affinity haemoglobin variants. These are described in detail in Chapter 22.4.7. They can be identified by haemoglobin analysis and are all associated with a left-shifted oxygen dissociation curve and a reduced P_{50}. Polycythaemia also occurs with red-cell enzyme deficiencies associated with low levels of 2,3-diphosphoglycerate.

TISSUE HYPOXIA

The only chemical that regularly produces secondary polycythaemia is cobalt. In the past this agent has been used to treat patients with refractory anaemias, although it is no longer in vogue because of its side-effects. It is thought to act by inhibiting oxidative metabolism.

INAPPROPRIATE ERYTHROPOIETIN PRODUCTION

There is a variety of disorders that cause inappropriate erythropoietin production and hence a variable degree of polycythaemia. The hormone is produced by renal tumours, or occasionally by tumours of the cerebellum or liver. It has been estimated that about 2 per cent of all patients with hypernephromas have erythrocytosis. It is possible to demonstrate an increased level of erythropoietin in the serum and urine in such patients. The precise mechanism for increased erythropoietin production in patients with renal tumours remains to be determined. Although it has been suggested that the tumour secretes the hormone the finding of increased erythropoietin production in some patients with Wilms' tumour, or even benign adenomas of the kidney, suggests that mechanically induced hypoxia due to the pressure of the tumour may stimulate normal renal parenchyma to increase erythropoietin production. Once these tumours are removed the red-cell mass returns to normal, although polycythaemia may recur in patients who develop metastatic tumours in the contralateral kidney.

There is a well-documented association between secondary polycythaemia and cerebellar haemangiomata. Cyst fluid has been shown to contain material with the properties of erythropoietin. Workers in Hong Kong, where hepatocellular carcinoma is common, have reported that up to 10 per cent of patients with these tumours have secondary polycythaemia. The mechanism is uncertain, as increased blood levels of erythropoietin have not been demonstrated.

There is also a well-documented association between mild polycythaemia and the presence of large uterine myomas. In some cases the polycythaemia regresses after removal of the tumour. The mechanism is not clear. It is possible that the large abdominal mass interferes with the vascular supply to the kidneys and so causes renal hypoxia. However, inappropriate erythropoietin secretion by the muscle cells of the tumour has been demonstrated in several patients and, interestingly, in a patient with cutaneous leiomyoma.

Mild polycythaemia has also been reported in patients with other forms of renal pathology including hydronephrosis, polycystic disease, renal artery stenosis, and Bartter's syndrome. Interestingly, it does not seem to be a common finding in patients with renal artery stenosis.

A transient polycythaemia occurs sometimes after renal transplantation. Although it was originally suggested that this might reflect a temporary overproduction of erythropoietin by the transplanted kidney there is recent evidence that the source of the erythropoietin is the patient's own kidney. The mechanism of this curious response to transplantation remains to be determined.

ENDOCRINE DISORDERS

Mild polycythaemia has been recorded in patients with phaeochromocytomas or aldosterone-producing adenomas. High levels of erythropoietin have been found in the serum of these patients and the polycythaemia regresses after removal of the tumour. The mechanism of increased erythropoietin production is unknown. A mild polycythaemia may occur in patients with Cushing's syndrome and is probably the result of non-specific stimulations of the marrow by steroid hormones.

GENETIC POLYCYTHAEMIAS

The most common form of hereditary polycythaemia is due to abnormal haemoglobins with a high oxygen affinity. When these have been excluded there remain families in which there is polycythaemia, affecting more than one generation, that appears to be inherited in either a recessive or dominant fashion. So far, the mechanism has not been determined. However, the availability of gene probes for erythropoietin and its receptor should clarify these issues. For example, at least one family has been described in which the polycythaemia segregates with the gene for the erythropoietin receptor.

AUTOTRANSFUSION

This recent addition to the list of causes of secondary polycythaemia is the result of athletes attempting to improve their performance. Athletes have also been observed to try to increase their PCVs by injecting themselves with erythropoietin. Autotransfusion can be recognized by observing a haemoglobin level in an appropriate setting associated with a low erythropoietin level.

REFERENCES

Adamson, J.W., Stamatoyannopoulos, G., Kontras, S., Lascari, A., and Detter, J. (1973). Recessive familial erythrocytosis: aspects of marrow regulation in two families. *Blood*, **41**, 641–52.

Erslev, A.J. (1994). Secondary polycythemia. In *Williams hematology*, (ed.) E. Beutler, M.A. Lichtman, B.S. Coller, and T.J. Kipps). McGraw-Hill, New York (in press).

Isbister, J.P. (1987). The contracted plasma volume syndromes (relative polycythaemias) and their haemorheological significance. *Baillière's Clinical Haematology*, **1**, 665–93.

Kazal, L.A. and Erslev, A.J. (1975). Erythropoietin production in renal tumors. *Annals of Clinical and Laboratory Science*, **5**, 98–109.

Murphy, G.P., Kenny, G.M., and Mirand, E.A. (1970). Erythropoetin levels in patients with renal tumors or cysts. *Cancer*, **26**, 191–4.

Pearson, T.C. and Guthrie, D.L. (1984). The interpretation of measured red cell mass and plasma volume in patients with elevated PCV values. *Clinical and Laboratory Haematology*, **6**, 207–17.

Russell, R.P. and Conley, C.L. (1964). Benign polycythemia: Gaisböck's syndrome. *Archives of Internal Medicine*, **114**, 734–40.

Smith, J.R. and Landaw, S.A. (1978). Smokers' polycythemia. *New England Journal of Medicine*, **298**, 6–10.

22.5 The white cells and lymphoproliferative disorders

22.5.1 Leucocytes in health and disease

A. J. Thrasher and A. W. Segal

Introduction

Leucocytes form the cellular basis of host defence against the numerous pathogens present in the environment. They can be divided into phagocytic cells, which include neutrophils, monocytes, and eosinophils, and non-phagocytic cells, the basophils and lymphocytes. Until quite recently, the phagocytic cells and basophils were regarded solely as primary effector cells in acute inflammation, but it is now clear that together with lymphocytes they fulfil an important role in the modulation of cellular and humoral immunity through the release of immunoregulatory cytokines. In addition, these cells are responsible for the ingestion and digestion of cellular and non-cellular debris that otherwise would accumulate during the normal processes of cell death and renewal. In this chapter we will concentrate on phagocytic cells, their role in host defence and inflammation, and specific defects of these cells in the context of their normal physiology. Lymphocytic cells are dealt with in more detail in an earlier chapter.

Morphology and composition

Granulocytes are classified into three main types, neutrophils, eosinophils, and basophils, on the basis of the staining characteristics of granules in their cytoplasm. They have irregularly shaped, lobed nuclei, and are sometimes referred to as polymorphonuclear leucocytes. Monocytes and lymphocytes have more regular nuclei, and are known as agranulocytes because of the absence of specifically staining granules in their cytoplasm.

NEUTROPHILS

A mature neutrophil contains about 5000 granules, of which one-third are known as primary (or azurophil) granules, because they are the first to be formed. These granules are heterogeneous in structure, density, and composition. They contain myeloperoxidase, lysozyme, and most of the antimicrobial molecules. The secondary (or specific) granules form at a later stage of cell maturation, and stain salmon pink with Romanowsky stains. These granules are smaller and contain membrane components that are stored and transferred to the plasma membrane when the cell is activated, in addition to lysozyme, lactoferrin, and vitamin B_{12}-binding protein. The stored components include chemoattractant receptors, adhesion receptors, and cytochrome b_{-245}, a major membrane component of the NADPH-oxidase (see later). The contents of the granules are activated by discharge into a phagosome or secretion to the exterior of the cell (Fig.1). The main function of these cells is in providing immunity against bacterial and fungal infections and in the removal of exogenous and endogenous debris.

EOSINOPHILS

Eosinophils are much less numerous than neutrophils, making up only 1 to 6 per cent of blood leucocytes. They are derived from a stem cell common to basophils and are characterized by the presence of elliptical crystalloid granules that stain yellow-pink with eosin (acidophilic granules), and that develop from large spherical primary granules. They contain high concentrations of basic proteins, such as major basic protein, eosinophilic cationic protein, and eosinophil protein X, as well as hydrolases and eosinophil peroxidase. Eosinophils are attracted to sites of inflammation by products released from T lymphocytes, mast cells and basophils, in particular eosinophil chemotactic factor of anaphylaxis. Functionally, they are capable of phagocytosis but they discharge granule contents primarily to the exterior of the cell. The eosinophil exerts its proinflammatory and cytotoxic action through the release of both preformed factors in the granules, and release of substances synthesized at the site of inflammation including prostaglandins E_2, D_2, $F_{2\alpha}$, thromboxane A_2, leukotriene C_4, platelet activating factor, and reduced oxygen species. The mode of action of the basic proteins is unclear but among other things they are strongly helminthotoxic, and play a primary part in host defence against metazoan parasitic infection. Major basic protein is also known to activate mast cells.

BASOPHILS

Basophils make up less than 0.2 per cent of blood leucocytes, and unlike other members of the granulocyte family, are non-phagocytic. The cytosol is filled with large heterogeneous granules that often obscure the nucleus, and that stain a deep violet colour with Romanowsky stains. Historically, because of common staining characteristics, it has been

Fig. 1 Electron micrograph of a neutrophil that has engulfed opsonized latex particles, which become enclosed in membrane bound phagocytic vacuoles. The dark staining primary granules fuse with the phagocytic vacuoles.

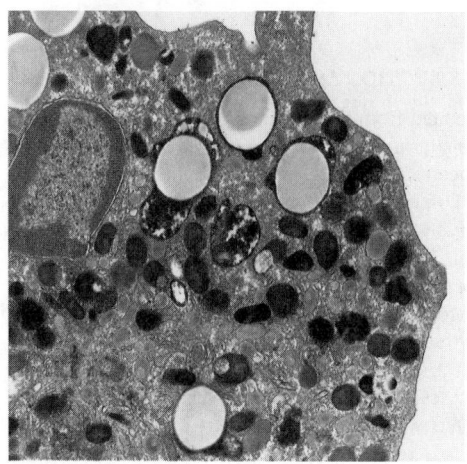

assumed that basophils and mast cells belong to the same lineage, but the true relationship between these cells remains undefined. Basophils release preformed mediators from granules including heparin, histamine, eosinophil chemotactic factor A, neutrophil chemotactic factor, tryptase, chymase, as well as newly formed mediators of inflammation—leukotrienes C_4, D_4, B_4, prostaglandins, and platelet-activating factor. Degranulation is initiated by antigens that cross-link specific IgE to the surface of the cell by high-affinity Fc receptors. These receptors are specific to basophils and mast cells. The ability of the basophil to release such a wide range of active compounds suggests not only a role in parasite elimination, and in type 1 hypersensitivity, but also in immunoregulation of other IgE-dependent and IgE-independent responses.

MONOCYTES/MACROPHAGES (SEE ALSO CHAPTER 4.2.3)

Many of the properties of the monocyte are similar to those of the neutrophil. They possess numerous cytoplasmic granules containing acid hydrolases and myeloperoxidase. The functional status of monocytes depends on their degree of activation, which itself is determined by macrophage-activating factors, such as interferon γ and colony-stimulating factors (see later), as well as by physical contact with tumour cells, micro-organisms, and many other molecules. Bacterial activating products include endotoxin (lipopolysaccharide), lipid A, and muramyl dipeptide. Phagocytosis of micro-organisms, and digestion of ingested cellular debris are the most prominent effector functions of monocytes/macrophages. In addition, activated cells produce many immunomodulatory molecules including interferon-β, interleukin 1 (**IL-1**), tumour necrosis factor-α, and IL-6, as well as reactive oxygen intermediates, reactive nitrogen intermediates, and arachidonic acid derivatives. Reactive oxygen and nitrogen intermediates may interact to form more toxic compounds, and seem to be particularly important in the killing of intracellular organisms such as mycobacteria and leishmania. Cytokines released from macrophages not only act locally, but exert hormonal effects throughout the body, resulting in fever, synthesis of acute-phase proteins, and tissue catabolism.

Apart from their role as effector cells, monocytes/macrophages and related specialized cells play an important part as antigen-presenting cells. Binding of T-cell receptors to the antigen–major histocompatibility complex (**MHC**) on the macrophage cell surface stimulates a complex series of cytokine- and cell contact-mediated interactions that regulate the immune response and direct proliferation and differentiation of B cells into mature plasma cells. MHC antigen expression is modulated by T cell-derived cytokines, but can be profoundly influenced by natural resistance genes such as the mouse macrophage-resistance gene *Bcg*. This single gene influences the functional status of the macrophage, and controls in an autosomal dominant fashion, innate resistance to growth of intracellular organisms such as mycobacteria, leishmania, and *Salmonella typhi*. The existence of an homologous human gene and its relevance to disease susceptibility remains to be determined, but is an intriguing prospect.

LYMPHOCYTES (SEE SECTION 5)

Lymphocytes are generated from pluripotential stem cells in the bone marrow, and undergo maturation in lymphoid tissues of the body. Normal lymphocytes are heterogeneous in size and staining characteristics. They constitute about 20 per cent of blood leucocytes, and can be separated into two main types, B cells and T cells, which are specialized for antigen recognition. B lymphocytes develop predominantly in the bone marrow while pre T lymphocytes migrate to the thymus where they are selected and processed before colonizing the lymphoid organs as mature T lymphocytes. A third population of lymphocytes contains large numbers of electron-dense granules, and account for up to 20 per cent of blood lymphocytes. These cells lack conventional surface antigens, and are associated with non-MHC-restricted natural killer-cell

activity, and antibody-dependent cellular cytotoxicity. Lymphocyte migration from blood to lymphoid tissues occurs through high endothelial venules and communication between cells is effected by direct cell contact, cytokine release, and antibody interaction. Further details on lymphocyte biology can be found in Chapter 5.1.

VARIATIONS OF LEUCOCYTE MORPHOLOGY

Variations in neutrophil morphology are frequently observed, and may involve the nucleus, the cytoplasm, or both. A drumstick appendage to the nucleus can be seen in a small number of neutrophils in normal females and represents the inactivated X chromosome. Hypersegmentation of the nucleus may be seen in megaloblastic anaemia due to vitamin B_{12} or folate deficiency, and rarely as an inherited condition. The Pelger–Huet anomaly is an inherited defect of nuclear segmentation, in which the nucleus may be rod-like, spherical, or dumb-bell shaped. A similar but acquired morphology may be seen in certain types of anaemia and leukaemia. Conditions that are accompanied by the premature release of cells from the bone marrow, such as sepsis, may result in primitive nuclear morphology, and an abnormal staining of primary granules that have not completed their normal maturational process, known as toxic granulation. Abnormalities in cytoplasmic morphology may also be seen in certain rare inherited disorders such as the May–Hegglin anomaly, which is characterized by the presence of large RNA-containing basophilic inclusions in most granulocytes and monocytes, and large poorly granulated platelets. Similar inclusions may be seen in septic states, pregnancy, malignancy, following cytotoxic drug therapy, and are known as Döhle bodies. Abnormalities of granule morphology are characteristic of certain rare inherited disorders of granule formation, and are discussed later.

Distribution and regulation of leucocytes

FUNCTIONAL DISTRIBUTION

Granulocytes and monocytes have short lifespans requiring constant production of new mature cells throughout adult life. All mature blood cells derive from pluripotential stem cells that arise during early embryonic development, and migrate from the yolk sac to the fetal liver. Subsequently, and throughout adult life, the bone marrow constitutes the major site of haemopoiesis.

Granulocytes occupy four functional compartments in the bone marrow through which the cells pass over a period of 10 to 14 days before release into the circulation. The stem-cell compartment contains the most primitive cells in the marrow and includes true pluripotential cells that have the capacity for extensive self-renewal and multilineage differentiation. The mitotic pool contains proliferating cells that are committed to the granulocyte lineage. Following a period of active cell division, the cells lose the ability to divide, and enter a non-mitotic pool in which the final stages of granulocyte maturation take place. The development of mature neutrophils with segmented nuclei takes about 7 days. Finally, before release from the bone marrow into the circulation, mature cells remain in a storage pool for a variable period of time. In normal states this contains 10 to 15 times the number of granulocytes found in peripheral blood, but these can be released prematurely from marrow should the need arise.

The myeloblast is the most immature recognizable cell in the bone marrow and gives rise to all three types of granulocyte. The most prominent event in maturation is the formation of characteristic storage granules, which lasts for about half of the cell maturation period. Primary granules are formed only at the promyelocyte stage, while the secondary granules increase in number throughout the myelocyte stage of development. In the final stages of maturation, the cell loses the ability to divide and passes through a metamyelocyte stage in which the nucleus becomes indented, and before assuming the lobed form typical of the mature cell, passes through a further intermediate stage in which the nucleus appears as a curved rod, the band form. At the same time the cell acquires properties essential to its function, such as the ability to respond to chemotactic stimuli, and to activate the respiratory burst (see later).

Once released from sites of haemopoiesis, neutrophils occupy three other functional compartments. In the circulation they are either in the circulating pool, or the marginating pool adherent to microvascular endothelium, each with roughly equal numbers of cells in dynamic equilibrium with each other. Mature neutrophils remain in the circulation for up to 12 h, and then migrate into the tissues where they perform their biological function and survive for 1 to 3 days.

Unlike granulocytes, which are terminally differentiated, monocytes can differentiate further into macrophages, and related specialized cells. After 24 to 48 h in the circulation, they enter tissues and differentiate into large macrophages that are widely spread throughout every tissue and organ of the body, particularly the spleen, lymph nodes, alveoli, liver, bone marrow and serous cavities, and may persist in these tissues for months or years.

REGULATION OF MYELOPOIESIS (SEE ALSO CHAPTER 22.2)

Adult haemopoiesis is regulated by stromal cells in the bone marrow, which by direct cell contact and release of local regulatory molecules, maintain multipotential stem-cell numbers, and direct the production of lineage-specific progenitors. These haemopoietic growth factors control the proliferation and maturation of progenitor cells by interacting with specific cell-surface receptors. The most important molecules controlling the production, maturation, and function of granulocytes and monocytes are the colony-stimulating factors. These are glycoproteins, and are produced by many cell types including bone-marrow stroma, lymphocytes, endothelial cells, and fibroblasts. Granulocyte–macrophage colony-stimulating factor (**GM-CSF**), granulocyte colony-stimulating factor (**G-CSF**), and multipotential colony-stimulating factor (multi-CSF or IL-3) consist of a single polypeptide chain, whereas macrophage colony-stimulating factor (**M-CSF**) is a dimer of two identical chains. Each factor induces mitosis and proliferation of particular responsive progenitors, and their immediate progeny, but is not alone able to stimulate progenitor formation from self-renewing stem cells. GM-CSF and IL-3 stimulate the production of both monocytes and granulocytes, while G-CSF and M-CSF seem to be more selective for their respective cell lineages. *In vivo*, the four colony-stimulating factors functionally interact with other regulators of haemopoiesis such as stem-cell factor, IL-5, and IL-6, to influence the behaviour of responding cells. When more cells of a particular lineage are required, for example during infection, the levels of the appropriate colony-stimulating factors are rapidly increased. As well as stimulating proliferation, the factors control differentiational commitment of granulocyte–monocyte progenitors, the initiation of maturation, and the functional activity of mature cells. Direct effects of these factors on mature effector cells include prolonged survival, expression of adhesion molecules, and enhanced synthesis of antimicrobial peptides. They also have indirect priming effects that may result in enhanced phagocytosis and oxidative killing, inhibition of chemotaxis, and enhanced biosynthetic function.

The most important haemopoietic factors regulating eosinophil proliferation, differentiation, and function are G-CSF, GM-CSF, IL-3, and IL-5, all of which augment cellular viability, cytotoxicity, and release of inflammatory mediators in mature cells. The cytokines known to be involved in basophil growth and differentiation are GM-CSF, IL-3, IL-4, IL-5, and stem-cell factor, the predominant factor being IL-3.

Molecular cloning of the genes coding for the colony-stimulating factors has resulted in the development of therapeutic strategies based on their biological properties. G-CSF and GM-CSF have been shown to accelerate myeloid recovery after high-dose chemotherapy and autologous marrow transplantation, and to enhance reconstitution in transplant patients with delayed engraftment or graft failure. They have also been used in the setting of aplastic anaemia, myelodysplastic syndrome, and drug-induced agranulocytosis. A further potential therapeutic benefit of these various factors is alleviation of dose-limiting neutropenia during chemotherapy, so permitting intensification of regimens. More recently, trials have been undertaken to facilitate haemopoietic reconstitution using G-CSF-primed peripheral blood progenitors.

Abnormalities of cell number

In white adults, 50 to 70 per cent of leucocytes circulating are granulocytes. During infancy there is a predominance of lymphocytes. In some areas of Africa, the adult neutrophil to lymphocyte ratio may be reversed.

Neutrophilia (Plate 46)

An increase in numbers of neutrophils in the circulating compartment is described as neutrophilia or neutrophil leucocytosis. The total leucocyte count is typically raised above 10×10^9 /l. Neutrophilia commonly accompanies bacterial infection and tissue injury, where there is increased production stimulated by colony-stimulating factors and early release of cells from the bone marrow. Consequently, immature band cells and metamyelocytes may be found in the circulation, giving rise to a blood picture described as left shifted. Intense muscular activity, the administration of adrenaline or corticosteroids, and other conditions such as acute haemorrhage that provoke an acute stress response, recruit cells from the marginating compartment and cause a transient neutrophilia without increasing production. Other causes of neutrophilia include hyposplenism and malignant disease. Extreme neutrophilia, often greater than 30×10^9/l, may occur in disseminated malignancy, disseminated tuberculosis and severe infection, particularly in splenectomized individuals, and needs to be differentiated from chronic granulocytic leukaemia and other myeloproliferative diseases. The neutrophil alkaline phosphatase score is characteristically low in leukaemic disorders, the hallmark of which is the uncontrolled clonal expansion of cells from a single transformed progenitor, and high in most other neutrophilic states.

Neutropenia

A circulating neutrophil count below 1.5×10^9/l is usually abnormal, although lower counts may be normal for certain non-white genetic groups, in particular blacks and Arabs. In these healthy individuals, there are relatively more cells in the marginating pool, and they are able to mount a normal response to infection. Patients with neutrophil counts less than 0.5×10^9/l for whatever reason are at increased risk of infection.

Inherited neutropenia

Congenital agranulocytosis (Kostmann's syndrome) This is characterized by persistent severe neutropenia, and bone marrow morphology suggestive of maturational arrest of neutrophil precursor cells at the promyelocyte stage. Other findings include varying degrees of monocytosis, eosinophilia, hypergammaglobulinaemia, and thrombocytosis. Children develop frequent and severe infections starting in infancy.

Cyclic neutropenia A rare condition characterized by cyclic fluctuations in numbers of neutrophils, monocytes, eosinophils, lymphoctes, platelets, and reticulocytes with a periodicity of 3 to 4 weeks. Patients suffer from fever, mouth ulceration, and serious infections at times when the neutrophil count is low. The defect appears to be at the level of the stem-cell regulation, but may improve spontaneously with time.

In both these conditions, regular G-CSF has been shown to augment neutrophil counts, and to decrease the frequency of serious infection.

Acquired neutropenia

The most common cause of acquired neutropenia is viral infection. It is particularly found in association with influenza, hepatitis, rubella, and infectious mononucleosis, but may also be caused by bacterial infections, particularly *S. typhi*, brucella, mycobacteria, and severe sepsis of any kind. Predictably, radiotherapy and cytotoxic drug therapy result in neutropenia, but many other drugs may produce idiosyncratic cytopenia due to decreased marrow production. Antithyroid drugs present a particularly high risk. Miscellaneous causes of neutropenia include hypersplenism, megaloblastic anaemia, autoimmune and isoimmune destruction, marrow infiltration by malignant cells, idiopathic aplasia, and drug-induced immune destruction. Felty's syndrome is a rare condition in which splenomegaly and neutropenia occur together with rheumatoid arthritis.

An increase in the marginating pool may result in apparent neutropenia, and has been observed during haemodialysis, in severe sepsis, and particularly in the adult respiratory distress syndrome, in which neutrophils rapidly accumulate in the pulmonary microcirculation, and contribute to tissue damage and hypoxaemia.

Eosinophilia (see also Chapter 22.5.7 and Plate 47)

An elevated eosinophil count above $0.5 \times 10^9/l$ is seen in a number of clinical conditions. It is most frequently associated with atopic disease, invasive parasitic infection, and drug hypersensitivity, but may also be a feature of malignancy, hypoadrenalism, and vasculitis.

Eosinopenia

This is most commonly encountered in conditions where endogenous cortisol levels are elevated, and during exogenous administration of corticosteroids.

Basophilia

The regulation of basophil and mast-cell lineages appears to be disordered in myeloproliferative disorders, and in systemic mastocytosis. Basophilia may herald terminal blast crisis in chronic granulocytic leukaemia, but the molecular basis of this relationship has yet to be identified. In systemic mastocytosis and the related cutaneous disorder urticaria pigmentosa, proliferation of mast cells within tissues is common, but systemic elevations of mast-cell numbers occur only rarely in mast-cell leukaemia. Increased turnover of mast cells in these conditions may be associated with increased numbers of mast-cell or basophil progenitors in the peripheral blood, and release of inflammatory mediators, leading to symptoms such as urticaria, anaphylaxis and asthma. The underlying cause for the induction of basophilia or mast-cell hyperplasia is currently unknown.

Monocytosis

Absolute monocytosis is an infrequent finding, but may occur in cases of chronic infection, such as tuberculosis, brucellosis, infective endocarditis, and protozoan disease, as well as in chronic neutropenia, Hodgkin's disease, and monocytic leukaemia.

Lymphocytosis

A lymphocytosis is most frequently associated with viral infection, in particular, infectious mononucleosis, acute human immunodeficiency virus (**HIV**) infection, rubella, cytomegalovirus, and infectious hepatitis. It may also occur during bacterial infection, particularly brucellosis and tuberculosis, and in toxoplasmosis.

Lymphopenia

Apart from lymphopenia associated with HIV, absolute lymphopenia is an uncommon finding, but may be associated with marrow failure, immunosuppressive therapy, corticosteroid therapy, autoimmune disease, and systemic lupus erythematosus in particular. Severe combined immunodeficiency and other inherited lymphopenias are described in Chapter 5.3.

Leucocyte biology

Human polymorphonuclear neutrophils are the primary effector cells in acute inflammation. They are rapidly recruited from the bloodstream to sites of infection or inflammation, initially by increase in local blood flow and vascular permeability, and then by the processes of adhesion to endothelial cells, transendothelial migration, and chemotaxis. Once at these sites they ingest and phagocytose foreign particles, and release a range of biological mediators (Fig. 2).

Leucocyte–endothelial cell recognition

Localization of leucocytes to areas of inflammation requires a complex series of leucocyte–endothelial cell interactions via adhesion molecules, which may be specific to the inflammatory stimulus, to the chronicity of the inflammation, and to the tissue site. Leucocyte–endothelial cell recognition may be regarded as an active process requiring at least three sequential events: primary adhesion, activation, and activation-dependent adhesion.

Primary adhesion

Within minutes of tissue injury, polymorphs begin to interact loosely with the walls of affected segments of venules at the site of inflammation. This initial interaction is mediated by selectin molecules both on the leucocyte and on the surface of endothelial cells. Neutrophil L-selectin is constitutively active, and mediates attachment of polymorphonuclear leucocytes to endothelial cells in the absence of neutrophil activation. E-selectin and P-selectin are transiently expressed on the surface of endothelial cells in response to products of the clotting cascade such as thrombin, and other inflammatory mediators. The counter-receptors that interact with selectin molecules have not been fully characterized, but both endothelial selectins recognize sialyl-Lewis X, a blood-group determinant, on the neutrophil surface. Primary adhesion is transient and

Fig. 2 Schematic representation of neutrophil transit from the circulation to areas of acute inflammation. The first interaction with the endothelium is mediated by selectin molecules, and is transient (1). The neutrophil must be activated before a more permanent adhesion, mediated by integrin molecules (2), and transendothelial migration (3) can take place. Directed by chemotactic gradients, the leucocyte interacts with the extracellular matrix, and migrates towards the inflammatory focus (4). Opsonized particles are recognized by receptors on the surface of the cell, and become enclosed in a phagocytic vacuole (5). The respiratory burst is then activated, and microbicidal molecules are discharged from cytoplasmic granules (6).

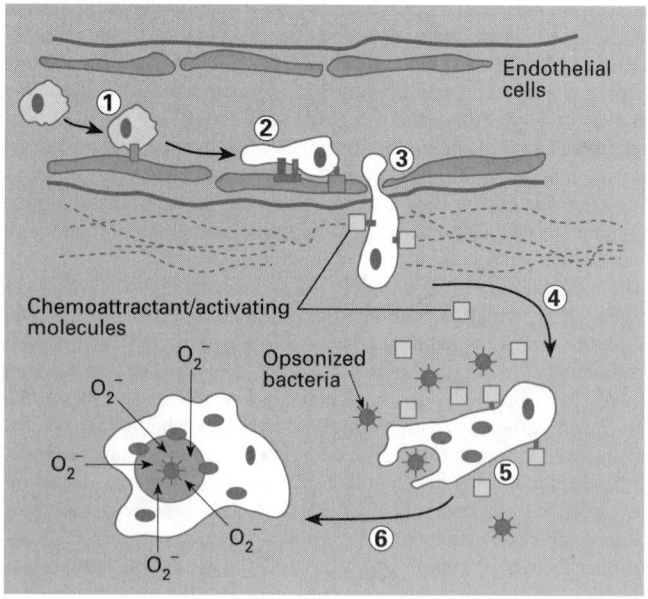

reversible and unless the polymorph is activated by specific chemoattractant or cell contact-mediated signals, transendothelial migration fails to take place, and the leucocytes detach.

Activation

The second step in the leucocyte–endothelial cell interaction is activation of the cell, which is accompanied by shedding of L-selectin from the cell surface, and up-regulation of leucocyte integrin adhesion molecules. These are responsible for more permanent interaction with the endothelium. The specific factors responsible for activation are unknown, but may include members of the intercrine family, platelet-activating factor leukotriene B$_4$, C5a, N-formyl peptides, and binding of E-selectin.

Activation-dependent adhesion

The third and final step is the interaction of activation-dependent adhesion molecules with their endothelial cell counter-receptors. Integrins are a large family of molecules involved in intercellular and cell–substratum adhesion. Each is a heterodimer of non-covalently linked α- and β-chains. The members of a particular family share a common β-chain, but each possesses a unique α-chain. The best known of the integrins are from the β$_2$-family, and expression of these is confined to leucocytes. This family consists of the molecules lymphocyte function-associated antigen (**LFA**)-1, CR3 (Mac-1,Mo-1) and CR4 (p150,95), which share a CD18 β-chain coupled to a CD11a,b,c α-chain. All three β$_2$-integrins are constitutively represented on the plasma membrane of the polymorphonuclear leucocyte, and are both quantitatively and functionally up-regulated by activation of the cell. The counter-receptors for leucocyte integrin molecules are members of the immunoglobulin gene superfamily, **ICAM**-1 and ICAM-2 (intercellular adhesion molecule), which are expressed on endothelial cells. Recent work has indicated that resting leucocytes themselves express a third ligand for LFA-1, ICAM-3, which is constitutively expressed particularly on B lymphocytes and cells of the monocyte/macrophage lineage, and which may play a part in interactions between leucocytes.

MIGRATION OF LEUCOCYTES INTO TISSUES

Movement of cells into sites of inflammation depends on leucocyte–endothelial cell interaction as described above. Following activation, the cell squeezes through gaps between endothelial cells, and directed by chemotactic molecules, interacts with the extracellular matrix and other cells at the site of inflammation via specialized adhesion molecules. Chemotactic molecules generated at sites of inflammation are short-range signalling molecules. C5a and LTB4 show no selectivity of action between neutrophils and monocytes, while members of the intercrine family are more cell specific. The α-intercrines IL-8 (NAP-1) and NAP-2 activate neutrophils but not monocytes whereas β-intercrines, monocyte chemotactic and activating factor (MCAF) and RANTES are predominantly chemotactic for monocytes. Platelet-activating factor is a potent chemotactic agent for human eosinophils.

DISORDERS OF LEUCOCYTE ADHESION AND MIGRATION

Leucocyte adhesion deficiency (LAD)

A rare inherited disease characterized in its severe form by delayed separation of the umbilical cord, recurrent life-threatening bacterial and fungal infections, gingivitis, impaired pus formation, and chronic leucocytosis. Lymphocytes, monocytes, and granulocytes show defects in adhesion to endothelial cells, cell migration, cell-mediated cytolysis, and antigen presentation. Patients with LAD are deficient in their cell-surface expression of the β$_2$-integrin family of molecules. At the molecular level, the defects have been found to be somewhat heterogeneous, and to occur in the gene coding for the common β$_2$-subunit. The degree of deficiency of these molecules correlates well with the severity of the clinical condition. Patients suffering from the severe form of the disease

usually die in childhood. Recently, two patients displaying a similar phenotype have been noted to be deficient in the ligand for the endothelial selectin molecules, sialyl-Lewis X.

A number of syndromes have been described in which depressed neutrophil mobility and a predisposition to pyogenic infection are associated with a cluster of physical signs. The causes are largely unknown. Schwachman's syndrome is characterized by the association of exocrine pancreatic insufficiency, abnormal neutrophil chemotaxis, metaphyseal chondrodysplasia, growth retardation and a predisposition to infection. Job's syndrome and other hyperimmunoglobulin E syndromes are characterized by grossly elevated IgE levels and recurrent staphylococcal 'cold abscesses', in which signs of inflammation are absent.

Neutrophil mobility is reduced in a number of acquired conditions, both idiopathic and in association with diabetes, viral infection, severe bacterial infection, malnutrition, severe burns and drug therapy. The clinical relevance of subtle abnormalities of mobility in isolation is questionable.

Phagocytosis and killing

Once localized to the area of inflammation, the phagocytic cells are in a position directly to combat invading micro-organisms. They do this by internalization of particles into phagocytic vacuoles, or phagosomes. On the cell surface, leucocytes express carbohydrate mannosyl-fucosyl receptors that can bind non-encapsulated microbes carrying these surface sugars in the absence of opsonization, in addition to high-affinity receptors for IgG and complement, FcR and CR1/CR3, respectively, which cooperate with each other to bind to their corresponding ligands. Opsonization of particles with IgG and fragments of complement, in particular C3 breakdown products such as C3bi, renders them much more susceptible to phagocytosis. Deficiency of these components results in susceptibility to infection by organisms whose main route of destruction is by phagocytosis, in particular pyogenic bacteria.

Polymorphonuclear leucocytes kill bacteria and fungi by a combination of oxidative and non-oxidative mechanisms. Although commonly regarded as two independent processes, they are interdependent, and efficient destruction of microbes requires both systems working in unison. For descriptive purposes, however, it is convenient to discuss them separately.

Oxidative killing

Activation of polymorphonuclear leucocytes and phagocytosis of opsonized particles is associated with a massive increase in oxygen consumption that cannot be accounted for by mitochondrial respiration. This is called the respiratory burst and is accomplished by an enzyme complex known as the NADPH-oxidase in the wall of the phagocytic vesicle. It consists minimally of a membrane-bound cytochrome b$_{-245}$ composed of two subunits α and β and three cytosolic factors that translocate to the membrane on activation of the cell, p47-*phox*, p67-*phox*, and p21rac, a small guanosine triphosphate-binding protein. This assembled complex, when activated, transfers electrons from the substrate NADPH across the membrane into the phagosome, where molecular oxygen is reduced to a free radical species superoxide anion O$_2^-$. In turn, two molecules of superoxide interact in a dismutation reaction to form hydrogen peroxide. Hydrogen peroxide in the presence of myeloperoxidase is able to oxidize halide ions to form hypohalous acids and chloramino compounds, which are more likely than superoxide and other free radical species alone to be directly toxic. Although these mechanisms play an important part in killing, one of the most important functions of the NADPH-oxidase is alkalinization of the phagosome during dismutation. This is a direct consequence of the consumption of protons that accompanies formation of hydrogen peroxide. Consequently, during activation of the respiratory burst, the pH in the vacuole rises to 8.0 before falling slowly to more acidic levels. This initial rise in pH optimizes activity of certain microbicidal enzymes released into the phagosome from the cytoplasmic granules.

Recently, considerable interest has been placed in a nitric oxide (NO) generating system, the NO-synthase, which is independent of the NADPH-oxidase. This system has been proposed to be a primary macrophage defence mechanism against intracellular micro-organisms, as well as against fungi and helminths that are too large to be phagocytosed. Whether it is dependent on products of the NADPH-oxidase for formation of toxic compounds, and whether it is important in neutrophil action remains to be determined.

Non-oxidative killing

Neutrophil cytoplasmic azurophil granules contain an abundance of antimicrobial proteins and peptides including defensins, lysozyme, bactericidal/permeability increasing factor, cathepsin G, and azurocidin. These are active against a wide range of bacterial, viral, and fungal organisms, even under anaerobic circumstances, although the efficiency of action may be suboptimal.

DISORDERS OF KILLING AND DIGESTION

Disorders of oxidative mechanisms

Chronic granulomatous disease

This is a heterogeneous group of inherited conditions characterized by failure of the NADPH-oxidase, and occurs with a frequency of about 1 in 500 000 births. Approximately two-thirds of cases are X-linked, and due to genetic lesions in the gene coding for the large β-subunit of the cytochrome, whilst one-third are recessively inherited and mostly due to defects in the gene encoding p47-*phox*. A few cases result from defects in the other components of the system. The clinical syndrome manifests as a marked susceptibility to pyogenic and fungal infection, and often considerable growth retardation. Onset of symptoms is usually in childhood, and appearance of symptoms at an early age predicts greater likelihood of complications and death. Common sites of infection include the skin, lymph nodes, lung, liver, and bone. The most prevalent organisms cultured from these sites are *Staphylococcus aureus*, Gram-negative bacteria, and *Aspergillus fumigatus*, although many other organisms may participate. A characteristic sterile granulomatous reaction develops in the tissues of many patients, and may represent an attempt to eliminate indigestible material.

Diagnosis is made on the basis of the clinical picture, and evidence of failure of superoxide production by neutrophils and monocytes, most simply demonstrated by their inability to reduce the yellow dye nitroblue tetrazolium to insoluble blue formazan in the nitroblue tetrazolium (NBT) slide test. Phagocytes from these patients show an impaired ability to kill *Staph. aureus in vitro*.

G6PD deficiency

In severe cases this may mimic certain aspects of chronic granulomatous disease due to greatly decreased production of the substrate NADPH by the pentose phosphate cycle.

Disorders of granule constituents

Myeloperoxidase deficiency

This is a relatively common autosomal recessive disorder that results in impaired killing of bacteria and fungi *in vitro*. Most patients remain asymptomatic and free of infection.

Chediak–Higashi syndrome

A rare autosomal recessive disorder characterized by partial oculocutaneous albinism, frequent pyogenic infection, and the presence of abnormally large cytoplasmic granules in neutrophils and other cells. These granules result from inappropriate fusion of granules to form large conglomerations in which the granule contents are sequestered. Death usually results in childhood or adolescence from infection or superimposed lymphoproliferative disease. Polymorphonuclear leucocytes of patients show normal or enhanced phagocytosis, and respiratory-burst activity, but defective killing of certain bacteria.

Specific granule deficiency

An infrequent congenital disorder characterized by recurrent pyogenic infection of skin, subcutaneous tissue, and respiratory tract. Abnormal composition of both primary and specific granules may be important in the pathogenesis of this syndrome, and may reflect arrest in the differentiation of these cells.

Tissue damage by leucocytes

In addition to their essential role in host defence, human leucocytes are being increasingly implicated as mediators of tissue damage in inflammatory disorders such as adult respiratory distress syndrome, inflammatory bowel disease, emphysema, and asthma. In a physiological inflammatory response, release of mediators by leucocytes is carefully regulated and directed towards foreign particles. However, persistent or innappropriate activation of these cells releases potent proinflammatory molecules that can inactivate tissue protease inhibitors such as α_1-protease inhibitor, α_2-macroglobulin, secretory leucoproteinase inhibitor, and plasminogen activator inhibitor 1, and activate latent proteinases such as elastase, gelatinase, and collagenase. In this setting, the tissue factors that normally protect against damage to cells and the extracellular matrix are overwhelmed, and tissue damage occurs. α_1-Antitrypsin (α_1-protease inhibitor) deficiency is an example of an inherited disease in which the balance is in favour of tissue damage because of deficiency of a protective factor.

Leucocyte function tests

Any patient who has suffered from recurrent episodes of infection or infection by unusual organisms should be investigated for defects in host defence. A careful history, family history, and clinical examination may suggest a specific diagnosis, and are important in focusing further investigation. As neutrophil functional defects are uncommon causes of increased susceptibility to infection, it is first necessary to exclude other more common conditions that involve complement, humoral, and cell-mediated mechanisms. Initial screening tests should include a full blood count and differential white-cell count, immunoglobulin levels with subsets, complement levels, and skin testing with purified protein derivative, and candida. HIV infection should be excluded in those individuals deemed to be at risk. If the patient is anergic, specific analysis of T-cell number, distribution, and function is indicated. Deficiency of one or more classes of immunoglobulin suggests a primary defect of B cells, or a secondary effect of T-cell dysfunction. Morphologic evaluation of the leucocytes may also be useful. If this initial evaluation fails to identify the cause, then more specific tests of white-cell function can be made.

The skin window technique examines the migration of cells through a dermal abrasion *in vivo*, and as such is an accurate though non-specific assessment of what is really happening at sites of inflammation. If this is normal then adhesion, migration and chemotaxis are intact. If abnormal, then specific assays can be done for these functions. Cell mobility can be assessed *in vitro* by a number of methods, the most common being with a variation of the Boyden chamber in which cells move through a porous membrane. The standard method for assessing activity of the respiratory burst is in the nitroblue tetrazolium slide test, in which the water-soluble yellow dye, nitroblue tetrazolium, is reduced to insoluble blue staining formazan by O_2^- when the cell is stimulated. A negative test is indicative of chronic granulomatous disease, and can be followed up by quantitation of superoxide production, and analysis of the various components of the NADPH-oxidase. The ability of a phagocyte to ingest and kill micro-organisms, in particular *Staph. aureus* and candida, forms the basis of an *in vitro* assay for phagocytosis and killing. Further tests of lymphocyte function, and of macrophage activation may be indicated in specific circumstances.

Treatment of patients with a leucocyte disorder

All defects in leucocyte function require correct identification of the cause of dysfunction, and treatment or removal of precipitating factors. Routine management is supportive and relies on avoidance of exposure to infectious material, prophylaxis with antibiotics such as co-trimoxazole and flucloxacillin, and where appropriate, immunization. Leucocyte numbers may be augmented with colony-stimulating factors, and other immunomodulatory cytokines such as interferon-γ may be used to augment functional activity of the immune system. A large trial recently conducted in the United States supports the use of interferon-γ as a prophylactic agent in chronic granulomatous disease, but suggestions that this partially restores the activity of the NADPH-oxidase seem in general to be unfounded. It is more likely that enhanced macrophage activity is responsible for the apparently beneficial action in these patients. Broad-spectrum intravenous antibiotics, and white-cell transfusions form the mainstay of treatment during intercurrent septic episodes. Inherited disorders of leucocytes with a poor prognosis may be considered for allogeneic bone marrow transplantation, if a suitable donor is available, although the morbidity and mortality associated with this procedure is considerable. In the future, genetic manipulation of autologous cells may become a curative procedure for some patients.

REFERENCES

Abramson, J.S. and Wheeler, J.G. (eds.). (1993). *The neutrophil.* IRL Press, Oxford.

Axtell, A.A. (1988). Evaluation of the patient with a possible phagocytic disorder. In *Haematology/oncology clinics of North America* (ed. J. Carnutte), pp. 1–12.

Butcher, E.C. (1991). Leukocyte–endothelial cell recognition: three (or more) steps to specificity and diversity. *Cell,* **67,** 1033–6.

Curnutte, J.T. (ed). (1988). Phagocytic defects 1: abnormalities outside of the respiratory burst. *Hematology/Oncology Clinics of North America,* **2,** No. 1. W.B. Saunders Co., Philadelphia.

Denburg, J.A. (1992). Basophil and mast cell lineages *in vitro* and *in vivo.* *Blood,* **79,** 846–60.

Finn, A., Hadzic, N., Morgan, G., Strobel, S., and Levinsky, R.J. (1990). Prognosis of chronic granulomatous disease. *Archives of Disease in Childhood,* **65,** 942–5.

Gordon, S. (1992). Monocytes/phagocytes. In *The Oxford textbook of pathology* (ed. J. O'D. McGele, P.G. Isaacson, and A.W. Wright), pp. 336–45. Oxford University Press.

Gordon, S. (1992). The mononuclear phagocyte system. In *The Oxford textbook of pathology* (ed. J. O'D. McGele, P.G. Isaacson, and A.W. Wright), pp. 236–57. Oxford University Press.

Hardisty, R.M. and Weatherall, D.J. (1982). *Blood and its disorders,* (2nd edn). Blackwell Scientific Publications, Oxford.

Lehrer, R.I. and Ganz, T. (1990). Antimicrobial polypeptides of human neutrophils. *Blood,* **76,** 2169–81.

Karlsson, S. (1991). Treatment of genetic defects in haematopoietic cell function by gene transfer. *Blood,* **78,** 2481–92.

Kroegel, C., Virchow, J.C., Kortsik, C., and Matthys, H. (1992). Cytokines, platelet activating factor and eosinophils in asthma. *Respiratory Medicine,* **86,** 375–89.

Long, M.W. (1992). Blood cell cytoadhesion molecules. *Experimental Haematology,* **20,** 288–301.

Metcalf, D. (1991). Control of granulocytes and macrophages: molecular, cellular, and clinical aspects. *Science,* **254,** 529–33.

Morel, F., Doussiere, J., and Vignais, P.V. (1991). The superoxide-generating oxidase of phagocytic cells: physiological, molecular and pathological aspects. *European Journal of Biochemistry,* **201,** 523–46.

Segal, A.W. and Walport, M.J. (1992). Neutrophil leukocytes. In *The Oxford Textbook of Pathology* (ed. J. O'D. McGele, P.G. Isaacson, and A.W. Wright), pp. 321–9. Oxford University Press.

Thrasher, A.J., Keep, N.H., Wientjcs, F., and Segal, A.W. (1994). Mini-review on molecular basis of disease: chronic granulomatous disease. *Biochemica et Biophysica Acta,* in press.

Weiss, S.J. (1989). Tissue destruction by neutrophils. *New England Journal of Medicine,* **320,** 365–76.

22.5.2 Introduction to the lymphoproliferative disorders

C. BUNCH AND K. C. GATTER

Proliferation of lymphocytes in response to antigenic stimuli is central to the immune response and commonly leads to enlargement of lymph glands and other participating lymphoid tissues. In most instances, the antigenic stimulus is an infecting organism, the lymphadenopathy is short lived, and the glands return to their normal size after successful control of the responsible infection. Occasionally, however, the proliferative response is more prolonged and may itself give rise to clinical problems.

Persistent lymphadenopathy may simply reflect repeated antigenic challenge—as commonly occurs in young children suffering upper respiratory infections during the winter months. Alternatively, it may be due to persistence of antigen, possibly because the immune response is inadequate for one reason or another or because an infecting organism (such as the tubercle bacillus) is relatively inaccessible and difficult to eliminate. In other instances, such as rheumatoid arthritis and other collagen–vascular disorders, lymphadenopathy is associated with an abnormal immune response directed against 'self' antigens. Finally, and much less commonly, autonomous proliferation of a neoplastic clone of lymphoid cells may occur—giving rise to one of the malignant lymphoproliferative disorders considered later in this section.

Organization of the immune system

Many of the clinical features of lymphoproliferative disorders can be explained by the fact that, structurally, the immune system is represented by lymphoid tissue strategically placed throughout the body, networked together by a system of lymphatic vessels and the bloodstream. In addition to 500–600 or so discrete lymph nodes, lymphoid tissue is found extensively in the oropharynx (Waldeyer's ring), bronchial tree, and gastrointestinal tract. Lymphocytes are also found in the bone marrow, where they tend to form small follicles, and of course in the spleen.

LYMPH-NODE STRUCTURE (FIG. 1)

The lymph nodes are loosely arranged into outer cortical and inner medullary areas within a connective tissue capsule. Lymph enters the node via afferent lymphatics and percolates through radial sinusoids to the hilum, where it leaves the node via efferent lymphatics. Blood enters and leaves the node through hilar vessels: an extensive vascular network extends throughout the node, and specialized postcapillary venules allow extensive traffic of lymphocytes between the blood and lymphatic vessels.

Cells in the cortical areas are arranged into a number of spherical nodules or follicles with a pale centre known as the germinal centre. These comprise mainly B cells with a smaller number of T cells and non-lymphoid cells. The cuff surrounding the germinal centre consists of mature small lymphocytes. Within the centre itself, the most characteristic cell is a slightly larger, small follicular lymphocyte known as a centrocyte or, because of its irregular nucleus, as a small cleaved cell. A number of larger cells can also be found, including macrophages (histiocytes), transformed lymphocytes or immunoblasts, and cells with a regular, centrally placed nucleus variously called centroblasts or non-cleaved follicle-centre cells. Also within the germinal centre are follicular dendritic cells, so called because of their network of interdigitating cytoplasmic processes that extend throughout the follicle. These cells are most likely of histiocytic origin but differ from tissue macrophages in having lost the ability to phagocytose. Their role is to handle antigen presented by other cells such as macrophages and Langerhan's cells via their surface receptors, particularly Fc and CD21.

Following antigenic challenge, intense proliferative activity takes place in the germinal centre as B cells recognizing foreign antigens undergo clonal expansion and differentiation. The associated morphological changes follow the appearance of different types of cell within the germinal centre, and the various stages of B-cell differentiation are also reflected in the expression of different antigens. This explains in part the diversity of lymphomas that can arise in the follicle centre, as malignantly transformed cells retain a limited but variable capacity for differentiation, which is reflected in their morphology, immunocytochemical phenotype, and behaviour.

The interfollicular and paracortical areas consist mainly of T cells. The medulla is comprised of cords of cells lining the sinusoids—the so-called medullary cords. These cells include fixed macrophages, plasma cells, lymphocytes, and connective tissue cells.

Lymphoid tissue in other sites is arranged in a broadly similar fashion. Gut-associated lymphoid tissue consists of a diffuse collection of lymphocytes throughout the submucosa, which coalesces patchily to form more discrete nodules (e.g. Peyer's patches). Bronchial lymphoid tissue is similarly arranged. The structure of the spleen is described in Chapter 22.5.4.

LYMPHOCYTE RECIRCULATION

Lymphocytes are not static, and there is extensive movement or recirculation of cells throughout the immune system. This is necessary because only a small number of lymphocytes are capable of responding to a given antigen, and it explains to some extent the clinical patterns of lymph-node involvement and spread of malignant lymphomas. Cells pass from the bloodstream to the lymphatic system through postcapillary venules within the lymph nodes, and return to the bloodstream by the thoracic duct. Part of the enlargement of lymph nodes that occurs following immune stimulation can be accounted for by a marked increase in lymphocyte traffic through the node.

Lymphadenopathy

Normal lymph nodes are impalpable, except in some very thin subjects. Palpable enlargement is commonly referred to as lymphadenopathy, even though the nodes may be simply reacting to antigenic stimulus in a normal fashion.

CAUSES

The main causes of lymphadenopathy are shown in Table 1. As indicated above, lymphadenopathy is most commonly due to infection, but

Table 1 *Principal causes of lymphadenopathy*

Inflammatory	*Granulomatous*
Suppurating	Infective
Pyogenic infection	Tuberculosis
Non-suppurating	Syphilis
Infection—local or systemic	Toxoplasmosis
Immunologically-based	Histoplasmosis etc.
Collagen disease	Non-infective
Rheumatoid arthritis	Sarcoidosis
Serum sickness	
Dermatopathic	*Malignant*
Drugs e.g. phenytoin	Primary
Addison's disease	Lymphoma
Thyrotoxicosis	Leukaemia
	Secondary
	Carcinoma
	Melanoma
	Sarcoma
	Congenital
	Lymphangiomas
	Cystic hygroma

other inflammatory disorders may be responsible. Lymphomas are relatively rare, and metastatic carcinoma is a more common cause of lymphadenopathy.

CLINICAL MANAGEMENT

In many instances the underlying cause will be apparent after taking a careful history and performing a thorough clinical examination. The history should encompass the patient's general health and past illnesses, possible exposure to infection, including contact with animals or birds, foreign travel, and constitutional upsets such as fever, weight loss, sweats or pruritus. Alcohol-induced pain at sites of affected nodes is characteristic if not pathognomonic of Hodgkin's disease.

Physical examination should take note of the location and extent of the lymphadenopathy, and the characteristics of the nodes themselves. Localized, tender lymphadenopathy should prompt a search for an infected lesion or portal of entry in the area drained by the node. Tender nodes are usually inflammatory or reactive, but rapid enlargement due to malignancy can stretch the capsule and produce pain and tenderness. Hard nodes, especially if fixed and matted together, suggest malignancy. When there is cervical lymphadenopathy, the throat and pharynx should be carefully examined. A full general examination should be performed, with particular attention to the size of the liver and spleen.

Investigations should include a full blood count, erythrocyte sedimentation rate, and examination of the blood film. These may be diagnostic in cases of leukaemia, or may point to a viral cause such as glandular fever. Additional investigations might include a chest radiograph, biochemical profile, and antibody screens for an infective cause, together with specific microbial cultures as appropriate.

LYMPH-NODE BIOPSY

The cause of lymphadenopathy can be determined in the majority of instances by history, clinical examination, and the simple investigations outlined above. If this fails to yield a diagnosis, a lymph-node biopsy may be necessary, but knowing just when to do this is often difficult and the usefulness of this investigation is reduced if it is done indiscriminately. If the clinical suspicion of lymphoma is strong, and there are good reasons why treatment should not be delayed—perhaps because the patient's condition is deteriorating—a biopsy should be undertaken as soon as possible. If the suspicion is less strong, then one should wait at least until the results of preliminary investigations are to hand: in this time a number of infective and inflammatory conditions will resolve spontaneously.

Fig. 1 Functional architecture of a normal lymph node. (Reproduced from Arno, 1980, with permission of the author and MTP Press.)

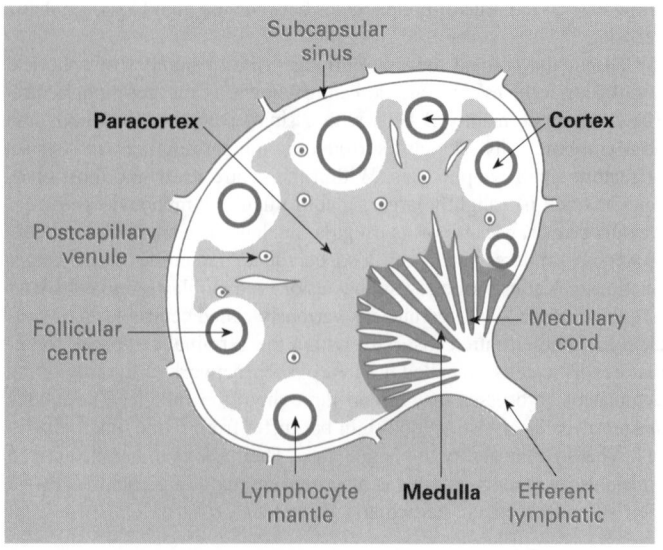

The diagnostic yield is improved by careful selection of the node to be biopsied. Supraclavicular nodes are preferred, as axillary or inguinal nodes may be involved in reaction to coincident local trauma or infection in hands or feet. Similarly, enlarged nodes close to a malignant node may show only a reactive pattern and it is better to remove the largest node, even if this is technically more difficult. Occasionally, lymph-node enlargement is confined to internal lymph nodes, such as those in mediastinum, para-aortic, or mesenteric areas, and is not readily accessible to routine surgical biopsy. In these circumstances, material may be obtained by needle-core biopsy or fine-needle aspiration under radiological guidance (see Fig. 2). The biopsied specimen should not be put automatically into formalin: many of the techniques described below require fresh, unfixed tissue, and close liaison with the histopathologist is essential.

Fine-needle aspiration biopsy

Fine-needle aspiration biopsy done in consultation with the cytologist is gradually becoming more widely available as a simple, safe, and cheap investigation that often reveals a definitive diagnosis without recourse to surgery. However, in the case of suspected lymphoma it is not always possible to provide full diagnostic information with this material and biopsy is still considered to be an essential part of management.

Methods for the study of lymphoproliferative disorders

Traditionally, the diagnosis of abnormal lymphoproliferative conditions, and especially the malignant lymphomas, has depended upon conventional histological evaluation of the tissues involved, the interpretation of which has been limited by the prevalent understanding of the structure and function of the lymphoid system. Less than 40 years ago the function of lymphocytes was largely unknown, but many of the techniques devised by basic scientists to unravel the complexities of the immune system have now been successfully applied to clinical problems and as a result have greatly refined our diagnostic ability and our understanding of these conditions.

HISTOPATHOLOGY

Conventional histological examination remains the cornerstone of diagnosis in a lymphoid biopsy. It is said that more errors are made in the diagnosis of lymph nodes than in any other organ and that the most common reason for this is poor preparation of the biopsied tissue. The clinician, by alerting the pathologist to an impending biopsy and providing fresh, unfixed tissue, will ensure that material is received in an optimal state. Needle-core biopsy, and more recently, fine-needle aspiration, have been advocated as a more convenient and rapid replacement for formal biopsy.

The histological evaluation of a lymph node depends on a systematic microscopic examination, taking into account the different compartments (capsule, follicles, paracortex, and sinuses) and cell types (lymphocytes, macrophages, plasma cells, etc.) of which it is composed. Although a few conditions can be diagnosed on the basis of a single abnormal feature, the major distinction between a benign and a malignant process can usually only be made after careful consideration of all the features mentioned above. Further details can be found in the discussion below on patterns of lymph-node reactivity and in Chapter 22.5.3.

The chief limitations of a purely morphological approach to lymph-node diagnosis are that it provides only a static view of a dynamic process and that the cellular composition and structure of a node is largely related to its immunological function, which can, at best, be perceived only indirectly in conventional histological preparations.

IMMUNOCYTOCHEMISTRY

The introduction of reliable immunoenzymatic staining techniques, coupled with the development of monoclonal antibodies, have added considerable refinement to the conventional histological examination of lymphoid tissue. The value of using an immunocytochemical technique such as the immunoperoxidase or immunoalkaline phosphatase method is that these provide permanent histological preparations that are similar

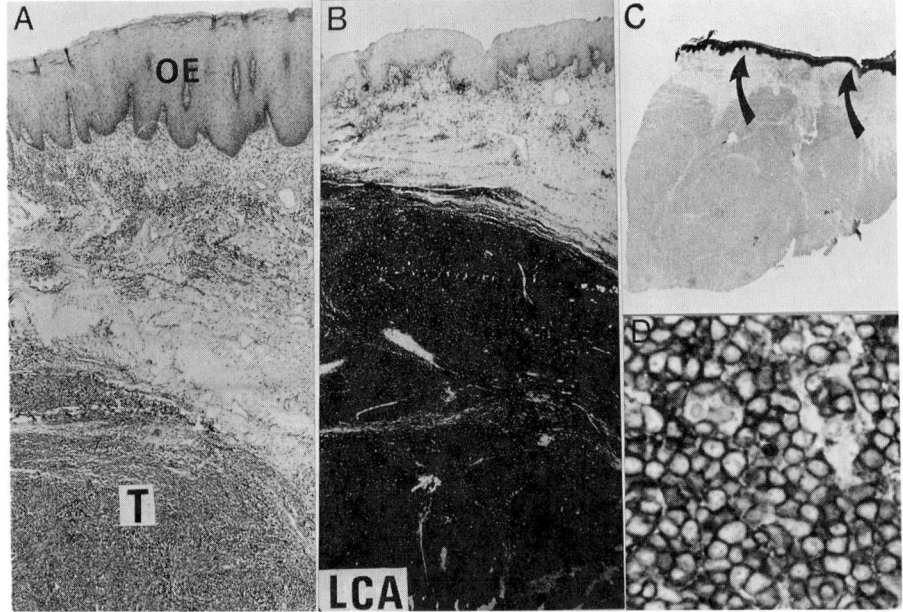

Fig. 2 This figure illustrates a typical problematical tumour biopsy. The patient, a middle-aged male, presented with a tumour in the oral cavity. A small biopsy was taken and, after considerable debate, reported as poorly differentiated squamous cell carcinoma. This led to an extensive resection involving hemimandibulectomy and deep neck dissection. However, it can be seen in (a) that the oral tumour (T) in the operation specimen lies deep to the epithelium (OE) and is not connected with it. A monoclonal antibody against the leucocyte common antigen (LCA) which stains leucocytes in conventionally-fixed paraffin sections shows (b) that the tumour is strongly positive. In contrast staining with antiepithelial antibodies (c) gave no reaction with this tumour. Note that the oral epithelium (arrowed in (c) gives a strong reaction with this antiepithelial antibody providing a built-in control. The strong surface membrane labelling for LCA (shown in detail in (d) in the absence of epithelial positivity is characteristic of lymphoma. On clinical reassessment this patient was found to have extensive mediastinal and abdominal lymphadenopathy. He was treated with systemic chemotherapy to which he made a good initial response although he died of his disease 2 years later. Undoubtedly the radical and mutilating operation was unnecessary. Subsequently other diagnostic errors of this type have been averted by similar immunocytochemical staining procedures performed in conjunction with routine histological examination of the biopsy specimen.

to, and can be easily compared with, routine histological specimens. Monoclonal antibodies are invaluable because of the wide range of antigens that can be detected, the purity of the preparations, the homogeneity of the antibodies, and their wide availability. Using these techniques and reagents the histologist can now readily identify the different cell types (B cells, T cells, dendritic reticulum cells, macrophages, etc.) within lymphoid tissue and can accurately classify the immunological origin of most lymphoproliferative disorders (Fig. 3).

The principal application of these techniques has been in the study of lymphomas, in the hope of improving their classification and ultimately their treatment. Although this has generated a great deal of information, it has as yet had little direct influence on patient management. This fact has unfortunately tended to obscure several genuine advances, one of which is the ability of a well-chosen panel of monoclonal antibodies to differentiate between anaplastic tumours such as carcinoma, lymphoma, melanoma, and various sarcomas (see Fig. 3). The final diagnosis in such conditions has considerable bearing on management, and it is of particular interest that using these methods most pathologists will have found cases of lymphoma that have been misdiagnosed as carcinoma or melanoma, with whose appearances they are more familiar.

MOLECULAR APPROACHES

One problem that puzzled immunologists for many years was how the body is able to respond to so many different antigens and yet produce a specific antibody for each new antigen encountered. It was clear that the total genome was not large enough to code for each possible antibody separately, and that there must be some mechanism to generate the necessary degree of antibody diversity. It is now known that this is achieved not by post-translational modification of a primitive antibody molecule, but by the assembly of a 'supergene' from smaller coding segments in a process of gene 'rearrangement' that occurs at a very early stage of a lymphocyte's differentiation into the B-cell lineage.

The process of rearrangement affects the immunoglobulin heavy- and light-chain genes sequentially, and precedes their expression and thus the synthesis of immunoglobulin. It is shown schematically for the κ light-chain gene in Fig. 4. A similar mechanism occurs for generating diversity in the T-cell antigen receptor. The state of the immunoglobulin genes within a given tissue can be analysed by hybridization of radioactive complementary DNA (cDNA) probes for segments of the rearranged genes to digests of DNA extracted from the tissue in question (Fig. 5).

Fig. 3 A scheme of lymphocyte differentiation based on surface markers, enzyme, and molecular studies. Each 'cell' illustrated represents a phenotypically discrete stage in a continuum of differentiation. The pathways of differentiation are indicated by a solid arrow → and the relationship of various developmental stages with lymphomas and leukaemias is indicated by a broken arrow (- - - →). The phenotypic characteristics are indicated beneath each cell. IGA indicates the arrangement of immunoglobulin genes as follows: G = germ line arrangement, H = heavy chain genes rearranged, L = light chain genes rearranged; T1, 3, 6, 8–11, and BA-1 represent reaction with monoclonal antibodies detecting various stages of T and B lymphocyte development, respectively; cALL = common acute lymphoblastic leukaemia antigen; TdT = terminal transferase; DR = HLA DR expression; E = sheep erythrocyte, rosetting; Cμ = cytoplasmic μ heavy chain; SmIg = surface membrane Ig; CIg = cytoplasmic Ig (heavy and light chain); CLL = chronic lymphatic leukaemia; PLL = prolymphocytic leukaemia; HCL = hairy cell leukaemia; HGL = non-Hodgkin's lymphoma (high grade); LGL = non-Hodgkin's lymphoma (low grade). (Modified from Foon, 1982.)

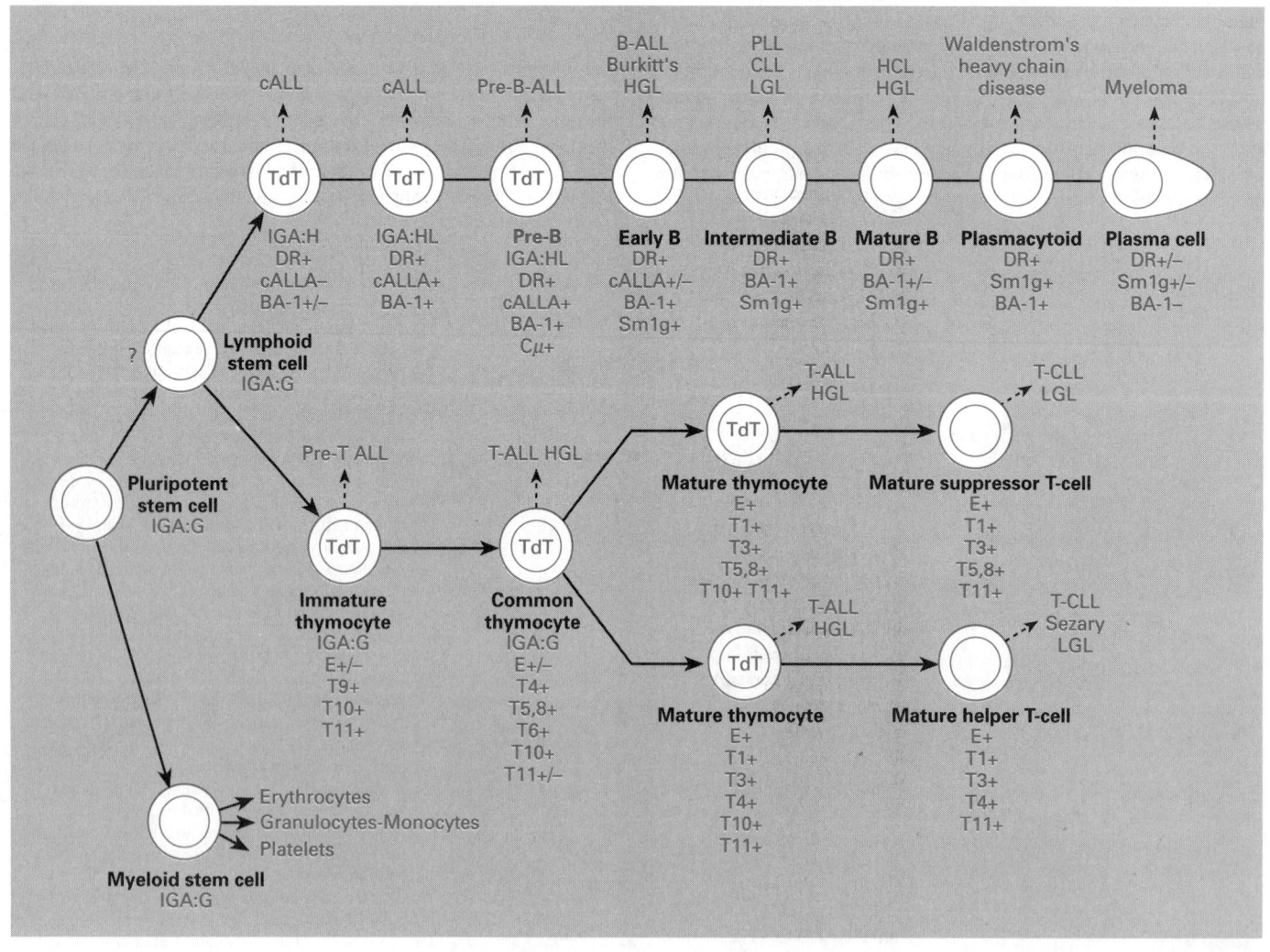

In non-lymphoid tissues, whether normal or neoplastic, the immunoglobulin genes remain in their germline configuration in all the cells and the cDNA probe hybridizes only with DNA fragments of a single size. If cells from a single clone (for example, from a malignant B-cell neoplasm) are analysed, the probe also hybridizes with large numbers of fragments containing the rearranged gene, but because the rearrangement effectively compresses the gene these fragments are of a different size and can readily be separated from those containing the germline genes. On the other hand, normal and reactive lymph nodes contain many clones of cells, each capable of producing a different antibody; in these circumstances the probe hybridizes with small numbers of many different-sized fragments, which cannot be readily distinguished from each other.

In addition to revealing how the immune system is able to respond to many different antigens, analyses of the immunoglobulin and T-cell antigen-receptor genes are proving to be a powerful tool in the investigation of lymphoproliferative disorders. For example, analysis of immunoglobulin genes has shown that the common (cALL) variety of acute lymphoblastic leukaemia, previously thought to lack markers of B- or T-cell lineage, is in fact of early B-cell origin. Similarly, hairy-cell leukaemia, the cellular origin of which was disputed for many years, is now known to be a B-cell neoplasm.

These techniques can also help in diagnosis. Whilst the majority of lymphoproliferative disorders can be confidently diagnosed with conventional light microscopy, establishing a malignant as opposed to the reactive nature of a lymph node is difficult in a small proportion—even with the immunocytochemical techniques outlined above. This is particularly true in T-cell malignancies, which lack any readily identifiable markers of monoclonality and in which analysis of the T-cell receptor gene can provide objective evidence of monoclonal expansion.

Patterns of lymph-node reactivity

Lymph nodes can be divided into three functional areas: the follicles, the paracortex, and the medullary sinuses. When lymph nodes respond to antigenic stimuli or invasion by infectious or neoplastic agents, changes often predominate in one of these areas, leading to one of three basic reactive patterns (Fig. 6).

Follicular hyperplasia

This occurs when either increases in the size or number of lymphoid follicles contribute to significant lymph-node enlargement. It is a common histological finding in enlarged lymph nodes during childhood and adolescence. The condition is self-limiting and an underlying cause is rarely discovered. Specific causes of marked follicular hyperplasia include rheumatoid arthritis, measles, and toxoplasmosis.

Paracortical expansion

Characteristically seen in many viral infections, presumably due to a greatly increased stimulation of T lymphocytes; florid persistent lymphadenopathy due to paracortical expansion is seen after vaccination for diseases such as smallpox, herpes zoster, whooping cough, or influenza. It also commonly occurs in adolescents with infectious mononucleosis. Another cause of exaggerated paracortical expansion occurs in granulomatous responses to tuberculosis, yersinia infections, or sarcoidosis. In these conditions the paracortex is filled with epithelioid histiocytes (cells of macrophage origin) rather than T lymphocytes. Finally, patients with chronic skin diseases, either benign (chronic dermatitis, psoriasis) or malignant (mycosis fungoides), show a massive expansion of the paracortex in regional draining lymph nodes. This reaction is due to an accumulation of interdigitating reticulum cells (which are closely related to the Langerhan's cells of the skin) rather than macrophages and is known as dermatopathic lymphadenopathy. There is also a neoplastic proliferation of Langerhan's cells, usually seen in children, known as histiocytosis X, which comprises three clinical syndromes: Letterer–Siwe disease, Hand–Schüller–Christian syndrome, and eosinophilic granuloma (Chapter 22.5.6).

Sinus hyperplasia

Commonly seen in nodes draining inflammatory or neoplastic conditions, this may overflow into the paracortex (leading to so-called passive paracortical expansion). Here the expansion and subsequent lymph-

Fig. 5 Autoradiographs of DNA digested with *Bam*H1, a restriction endonuclease which reproducibly cuts DNA at sites of specific sequences giving rise to DNA fragments which can be separated according to size. The fragment containing the constant (C) region of the κ gene is identified by hybridization with a probe consisting of a radioactively labelled complementary DNA sequence. Track 1 shows the pattern in normal DNA, in which the κ genes remain in the germ-line configuration. The probe has hybridized with a single 12 kilobase fragment. Track 2 shows DNA extracted from a B cell lymphoma expressing κ-chain synthesis. The single additional 9.0 kb band indicates not only that the κ genes have undergone rearrangement in this particular tumour, but also that a single rearrangement has occurred and that the tumour is monoclonal. Track 3 shows DNA extracted from a metastatic carcinoma: the κ genes have not rearranged. (Photograph by courtesy of Dr N.T.J. O'Connor.)

Fig. 4 The variable region of the κ light chain gene is assembled from separately encoded V and J segments that are brought together by genomic rearrangement during B-cell differentiation. The germ-line κ gene cluster contains in excess of 100 different V (variable region) segments and 5 J (joining) segments. In this example the rearranged DNA contains one V gene segment (V_{16}) and one J gene segment (J_5). The final messenger RNA containing the VJC sequence is produced by processing of the primary transcript from the rearranged gene segments.

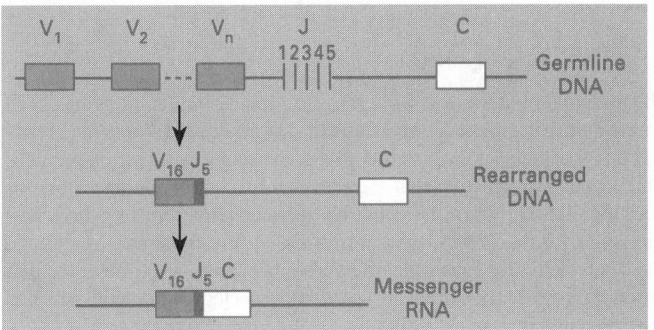

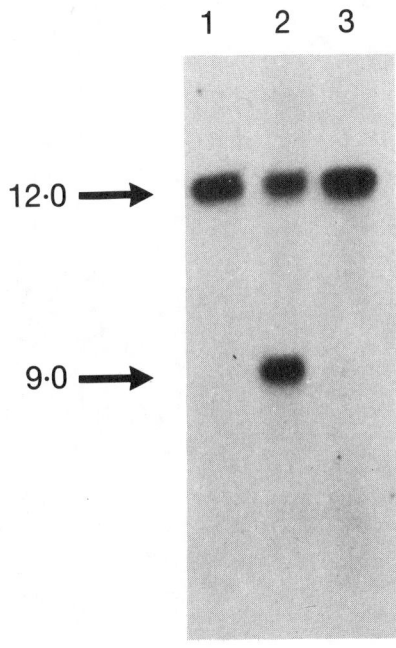

adenopathy is caused by a greatly increased drainage of macrophages into the sinuses from the periphery as well as their proliferation in the sinuses themselves. Specific conditions giving rise to sinus hyperplasia include the lipidoses and Whipple's disease, and it may also be seen after lymphangiography. There is also a rare entity of unknown cause termed sinus histiocytosis with massive lymphadenopathy or Rosai–Dorfman disease, in which lymph nodes, especially cervical, become extremely large due to the accumulation of giant macrophages in their sinuses. These macrophages are typically filled with engulfed small lymphocytes and are accompanied by a reactive plasmacytosis. The condition is more common in blacks than in any other race and usually resolves without any specific therapy, although fatalities have been recorded.

In conclusion, it should be emphasized that many conditions cause changes in each of the three areas of a lymph node, so that distinction between the three basic reactive patterns described above is not always clear.

Non-malignant lymphoproliferative disorders

Generalized lymphoproliferation is a feature of several infections, which may occasionally present in an unusual fashion, raising the possibility of something more sinister. The most obvious example is infectious mononucleosis (glandular fever), but cytomegalovirus infections and toxoplasmosis are other conditions in this category (see Section 7).

Several conditions that may be clinically confused with lymphoma are described in Chapter 22.5.3. Other lesions, such as angioimmunoblastic lymphadenopathy and lymphomatoid granulomatosis, are genuinely borderline and whilst not necessarily neoplastic (at least in their early stages) frequently progress to a true malignant lymphoma.

Infectious mononucleosis (see also Section 7)

Infectious mononucleosis is worthy of special mention as the virus responsible, the Epstein–Barr virus (**EBV**) preferentially infects B lymphocytes and most of the clinical features of the disease can be ascribed to an intense proliferation of T cells attempting to eliminate the infected

Fig. 6 Patterns of lymph-node reactivity. See text for description. (Reproduced from Arno, 1980, with permission of the author and MTP Press.)

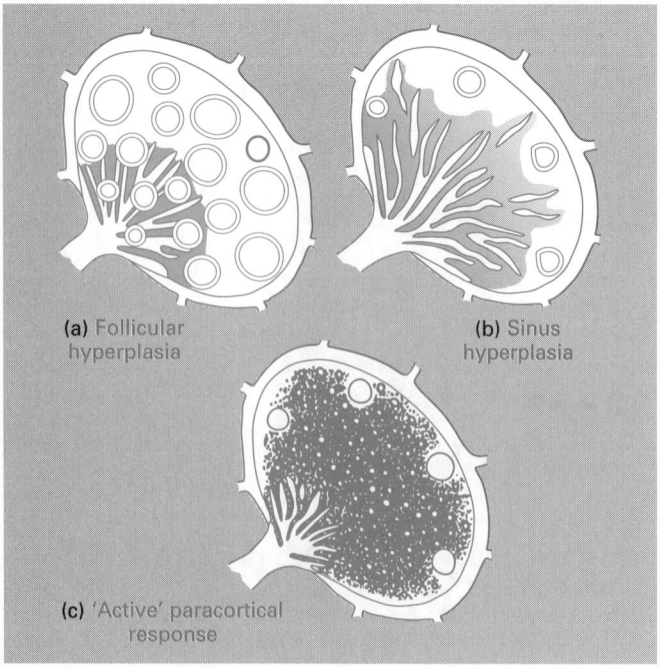

(a) Follicular hyperplasia

(b) Sinus hyperplasia

(c) 'Active' paracortical response

B cells. This is never fully achieved, and in common with other herpesviruses, the EBV lies dormant and may be reactivated at a later date in susceptible individuals. Whilst resolution of the clinical features of infectious mononucleosis normally occurs within a few weeks, in some patients the T-cell response is weak, and the condition may wax and wane, resolving eventually after several months.

One effect of EBV infection on B cells is to immortalize the cell, that is, to confer the potential for unlimited proliferation. This is most readily apparent *in vitro*: cells from individuals who have had infectious mononucleosis will proliferate quite easily in culture whilst it is generally impossible to encourage B-cell proliferation *in vitro* from previously uninfected individuals. Normally this tendency is kept in check by suppressor T cells *in vivo*, but in some highly immunodeficient individuals, such as transplant patients, uncontrolled B-cell proliferation may occur. At first this is polyclonal, but in some instances (and sometimes more than once in a given individual), a particular clone takes off, producing a condition indistinguishable from an immunoblastic lymphoma.

HIV infection and AIDS

A characteristic, generalized, painless lymphadenopathy may develop in human immunodeficiency virus (**HIV**) infection, often before the patient fulfils the criteria for having AIDS itself. This lymph-node enlargement, referred to as persistent generalized lymphadenopathy, develops independently of an identifiable infective cause other than HIV and is characterized by striking follicular hyperplasia with large irregular germinal centres. As AIDS supervenes, opportunistic infections with their own patterns of lymphadenopathy arise, leading usually to lymph-node atrophy—a type of burned-out syndrome—in the terminal stages.

Castleman's disease

This rare syndrome is a peculiar hyperplasia of lymph nodes that may be localized (particularly to the mediastinum) or generalized. It is characterized by the replacement of typical lymph-node follicles with nodules of small lymphocytes with a central, hyaline, vascular core replacing the germinal centre. In the plasma-cell variant these nodules are surrounded by a rich network of sinusoidal vessels with sheets of accompanying plasma cells, which are usually polyclonal. The generalized plasma-cell variant of this disease may accompany the so-called POEMS syndrome where patients demonstrate *p*olyneuropathy, *o*rganomegaly, *e*ndocrine abnormalities, *m*onoclonal gammopathy, and *s*kin rashes. Other vascular lesions such as Kaposi's sarcoma may also be associated.

Pathogenesis of malignant transformation

It is now widely accepted that the majority of malignant neoplastic disorders result from the transformation of a single progenitor cell to a cell with abnormal potential for growth and differentiation, rather than from a general breakdown of homeostatic mechanisms, although the latter could conceivably contribute to the survival of an abnormal clone in some instances. What is less certain is the nature of the transforming event, and how it arises in the first place.

EVIDENCE FOR CLONALITY

The malignant nature of a wide range of neoplastic disorders has been inferred either from the observation that any associated cytogenic abnormalities (see below) consistently affect the majority or all of the neoplastic cells—suggesting that they arise from a common ancestor—or from the fact that when the condition develops in a female patient heterozygous for the A and B variants of the X-linked enzyme glucose-6-phosphate dehydrogenase, the affected cells express only one of the two variants (A or B), not both as would be expected if the neoplasm had not originated in a single cell.

In the case of lymphoid neoplasms, additional evidence for clonality comes from the clonal nature of the immune response itself, although some care is required in its interpretation. The most easily demonstrated examples are the paraproteinaemias, in which a single clone of B cells produces a single type of immunoglobulin with either κ or λ light chains, but not both. Similar observations can be extended to the majority of B-cell neoplasms, and are carried to a greater degree of sophistication by the demonstration that each clone of B cells has a unique arrangement of its immunoglobulin genes, as described above. Similarly, although the clonal nature of T-cell neoplasms has been harder to demonstrate by other means, the recent discovery of analogous genetic rearrangements affecting the antigen-receptor genes has confirmed the clonal (and by inference the neoplastic) nature of many T-cell disorders.

CYTOGENETICS

It has been known for some time that some human malignancies are consistently associated with chromosomal abnormalities. With the advent of high-resolution banding techniques it has become apparent that cytogenetic abnormalities occur in the vast majority of tumours and that these are not necessarily random.

The most common defects are deletions of certain bands or in some circumstances of an entire chromosome, reciprocal translocations, or duplication of a chromosome (trisomy). Several examples are given in Section 22.3 and Chapter 22.5.3. Of particular interest is the observation that many of these defects involve the sites of cellular proto-oncogenes. For example, in Burkitt's lymphomas a consistent finding is a translocation between the long arms of chromosomes 8 and 14. One effect of this translocation is to move the c-*myc* gene from chromosome 8 and to juxtapose it to one of the immunoglobulin heavy-chain genes (which are actively transcribed in B cells) on chromosome 14.

AETIOLOGY (see also Section 6)

Although the precise nature of the alterations that occur within a cell to confer malignant properties remains unknown, a framework is beginning to emerge that helps us to understand in part the pathogenesis of malignant disorders. In many instances malignant transformation is associated with abnormal expression of one or more cellular proto-oncogenes. These are genes that show a great deal of homology with genes present in retroviruses associated with a number of animal and avian neoplasms. At first it was thought that the presence of these genes signified previous retroviral infection, but the converse is now thought to be true, that the genes have at some stage in evolution been 'captured' by the viruses from eukaryotic cells. The genes are, in fact, highly conserved, and in the majority of instances code for a protein (usually tyrosine) kinase that is thought to be intimately involved with the control of cell growth and proliferation.

It is thus not difficult to imagine how abnormal expression of such genes might play a part in the proliferation of malignant neoplasms. Evidence that oncogenes are directly related to malignant transformation has come from *in vitro* transfection experiments, in which certain (already abnormal) cell lines can be induced to proliferate uncontrollably by the introduction of genomic material from malignant tumours. As mentioned above, and elsewhere in this section, abnormal expression of an oncogene may result from its translocation to a site of high transcriptional activity and/or by mutation—resulting in an abnormal gene product. Alternatively, increased expression could result from gene duplication, as could occur in trisomy states.

Such events are unlikely to account entirely for the process of malignant transformation, and several discrete steps are probably required, with oncogene activation perhaps representing the last straw. The first step could involve an alteration in the kinetics or growth potential of a cell population that simply allows cells to go on growing indefinitely without altering their response to regulatory influences. An example is EBV infection of B cells, which, as we have seen, enables these cells to proliferate indefinitely *in vitro*. This behaviour is suppressed by T cells *in vivo*, but uncontrolled proliferation may result if T-cell activity is seriously impaired, as after tissue transplantation.

In areas of Africa where Burkitt's lymphoma is endemic, EBV infections are extremely common in infancy or early childhood, when they are often subclinical. It is of interest that the EBV was first isolated from cultures of Burkitt's lymphoma cells some years before its causative role in infectious mononucleosis was established. Although a direct aetiological association between the virus and this lymphoma has been postulated, it is most unlikely to be the sole factor. It has been suggested that persistent malarial infection, which has a similar geographical distribution to Burkitt's lymphoma, chronically stimulates the immune system, increasing its susceptibility to somatic mutation or to some other transforming event.

Recent advances in understanding control of cellular proliferation are beginning to shed light on some of the processes that occur during neoplastic transformation. Some of the best studied examples are the retinoblastoma and p53 proteins, which act as proliferation suppressants (their genes often being referred to as tumour-suppressor genes), and abnormalities of these proteins have been commonly described in many malignancies. A particularly important gene in lymphoma may be the recently described *bcl-2*, the protein product of which appears to be an important regulator of programmed cell death, a process known as apoptosis. Thus, overexpression of *bcl-2* protein, as seen for example in many follicular lymphomas, where the *bcl-2* gene on chromosome 14 is translocated next to the heavy-chain gene on chromosome 18, may be important in allowing unchecked proliferation of follicle centre cells.

REFERENCES

Adams, J.M. (1985). Oncogene activation by fusion of chromosomes in leukaemia. *Nature*, **315**, 542–3.

Arno, J. (1980). *Atlas of lymph node pathology.* MTP Press, Lancaster.

Desforges, J.F. (1985). T-cell receptors. *New England Journal of Medicine,* **313**, 470–577.

Foon, K.A., Schroff, R.W., and Gale, R.P. (1982). Surface markers on leukemia and lymphoma cells: recent advances. *Blood,* **60**, 1–19.

Gatter, K.C., Alcock, C., Heryet, A., and Mason, D.Y. (1985). Clinical importance of analysing malignant tumours of uncertain origin with immunohistological techniques. *Lancet,* **i**, 1302–5.

Greaves, M.F., Myers, C.D., Katz, F.E., Schneider, C., and Sutherland, D.R. (1984). Cell-surface structures involved in haemopoietic cell differentiation and proliferation. *British Medical Bulletin,* **40**, 224–8.

Klein, G. (1975). The Epstein–Barr virus and neoplasia. *New England Journal of Medicine,* **293**, 1353–7.

Klein, G. (1981). The role of gene dosage and genetic and genetic transpositions in carcinogenesis. *Nature,* **294**, 313–18.

Korsmeyer, S.J. *et al.* (1983). Immunoglobulin gene rearrangement and cell surface antigen expression in acute lymphocytic leukemias of T cell and B cell precursor origins. *Journal of Clinical Investigation,* **71**, 301–13.

Korsmeyer, S.J., Hieter, P.A., Ravetch, J.V., Poplack, D.G., Waldmann, T.A., and Leder, P. (1981). Developmental hierarchy of immunoglobulin gene rearrangements in human leukemic pre-B-cells. *Proceedings of the National Academy of Science* (USA), **78**, 7096–100.

Louie, S., Daoust, P.R., and Schwartz, R.S. (1980). Immunodeficiency and the pathogenesis of non-Hodgkin's lymphoma. *Seminars in Oncology,* **7**, 267–84.

O'Connor, N.T.J. *et al.* (1985). Rearrangement of the T-cell-receptor β-chain gene in the diagnosis of lymphoproliferative disorders. *Lancet,* **i**, 1295–7.

Purtilo, D.T. (1980). Epstein–Barr-virus-induced oncogenesis in immune deficient individuals. *Lancet,* **i**, 300–2.

Stansfeld, A.G. (1992). Non-neoplastic lymphoproliferative disorders. In *Oxford textbook of pathology,* (ed. J.O. McGee, P.G. Isaacson and N.A. Wright), Vol. 2b, pp. 1756–68. Oxford University Press.

Warnke, R.A. *et al.* (1983). Diagnosis of human lymphoma with monoclonal antileukocyte antibodies. *New England Journal of Medicine,* **309**, 1275–81.

Yunis, J.J. (1983). The chromosomal basis of human neoplasia. *Science,* **221**, 227–36.

Table 9 *A working formulation of non-Hodgkin lymphomas for clinical usage (equivalent or related terms in the Kiel classification are shown)*

Working formulation	Kiel equivalent or related terms
Low grade	
A. Malignant lymphoma	
Small lymphocytic	
consistent with CLL	ML lymphocytic, CLL
plasmacytoid	ML lymphoplasmacytic/lymphoplasmacytoid
B. Malignant lymphoma, follicular	
Predominantly small cleaved cell	
diffuse areas	
sclerosis	ML centroblastic-centrocytic (small),
C. Malignant lymphoma, follicular	follicular ± diffuse
Mixed, small cleaved and large	
cell diffuse areas	
sclerosis	
Intermediate grade	
D. Malignant lymphoma, follicular	
Predominantly large cell	
diffuse areas	
sclerosis	ML centroblastic-centrocytic (large),
	follicular ± diffuse
E. Malignant lymphoma, diffuse	
Small cleaved cell	
sclerosis	ML centrocytic (small)
F. Malignant lymphoma, diffuse	
Mixed, small and large cell	ML centroblastic-centrocytic (small), diffuse
sclerosis	ML lymphoplasmacytic/lymphoplasmacytoid,
epithelioid cell component	polymorphic
G. Malignant lymphoma, diffuse	
Large cell	ML centroblastic-centrocytic (large), diffuse
cleaved cell	ML centrocytic (large)
non-cleaved cell	ML centroblastic
sclerosis	
High grade	
H. Malignant lymphoma	
Large cell, immunoblastic	ML immunoblastic
plasmacytoid	
clear cell	
polymorphous	T zone lymphoma
epithelioid cell component	Lymphoepithelioid cell lymphoma
I. Malignant lymphoma	
Lymphoblastic	
convoluted cell	ML lymphoblastic, convoluted cell type
non-convoluted cell	ML lymphoblastic, unclassified
J. Malignant lymphoma	
Small non-cleaved cell	
Burkitt's	
follicular areas	ML lymphoblastic, Burkitt type and other B
	lymphoblastic
Miscellaneous	
Composite	—
Mycosis fungoides	Mycosis fungoides
Histiocytic	—
Extramedullary plasmacytoma	ML plasmacytic
Unclassifiable	—
Other	—

Reproduced with permission from the Non-Hodgkin's Lymphoma Pathologic Classification Project (1982).

with prognosis, but it was produced at a time when knowledge of the origin and functions of different cell types within normal and reactive lymph nodes was scanty, and its terminology is now frankly misleading.

In recent years our understanding of lymphoid differentiation has increased markedly, helped by immunological techniques that can pinpoint surface antigens on individual cells within suitable histological sections. This has led to a much clearer idea of the structure of normal lymph nodes, the traffic of cells through them, and the changes that occur after antigenic stimulation. More recent classifications of non-Hodgkin lymphomas have attempted to relate the nature of the malignant cell to its normal counterpart. Several such schemes have evolved, which vary mostly in their technical requirements and suitability for use with routine histopathological methods. All have prognostic significance, but it is unfortunately not possible to make direct translations between the various classifications, and this makes comparisons of therapeutic trials difficult to interpret.

Table 10 *Updated Kiel classification of non-Hodgkin's lymphoma*

Low-grade B	Low-grade T
Lymphocytic—chronic lymphocytic and prolymphocytic leukaemia; hairy-cell leukaemia	Lymphocytic—chronic lymphocytic and prolymphocytic leukaemia
Lymphoplasmacytic/cytoid (LP immunocytoma)	Small cerebriform cell—mycosis fungoides, Sézary's syndrome
Plasmacytic	Lymphoepithelioid (Lennert's lymphoma)
Centroblastic/centrocytic:	Angioimmunoblastic (AILD, LgX)
• follicular ± diffuse	T zone
• diffuse	Pleomorphic, small-cell (HTLV-1 ±)
Centrocytic	
High-grade B	*High-grade T*
Centroblastic	Pleomorphic, medium and large cell (HTLV-1 ±)
Immunoblastic	
Large-cell anaplastic (Ki-1+)	Immunoblastic (HTLV-1 ±)
Burkitt's lymphoma	Large cell anaplastic (Ki-1+)
Lymphoblastic	Lymphoblastic
Rare types	*Rare types*

From: Lancet (1988), **i,** 292–3.

Table 11 *The REAL classification of non-Hodgkin lymphomas (NHL)*

Morphology	% NHL	Immunotype
B-cell neoplasms		
Lymphocytic: small lymphocytes	7	Surface Ig CD5+ CD10− CD23+
Immunocytoma: lymphoplasmacytic	3	Cytoplasmic Ig CD5− CD10− CD23−
Follicular centre: centroblastic/centrocytic	25	Surface Ig CD5− CD10+ bcl-2+
Mantle cell: centrocytic	2	Surface Ig CD5+ CD10− CD23−
MALtoma: marginal zone (centrocyte-like)	3	Surface Ig CD5− CD10− CD23−
Large cell: centroblasts and immunoblasts	37	Surface Ig CD5− CD10−
Burkitt's: cohesive medium-sized blasts, 'starry sky' appearance	2	Surface Ig CD5− CD10+
Lymphoblastic: lymphoblasts	<1	Cytoplasmic Ig −/+ CD10+ Tdt+
T-cell neoplasms		
Lymphocytic: small lymphocytes	<1	CD4 or 8+
Cutaneous (mycosis fungoides/Sézary syndrome): small cerebriform cells	2	CD4+
Peripheral: extremely variable but usually includes medium and large pleomorphic cells with differing admixtures of reactive cells and blood vessels	8	May show marked heterogeneity of T-antigen expression CD4 or 8+
Lymphoblastic: lymphoblasts	‡	CD7+ may be CD4 or CD8+ Tdt+
Anaplastic large cell: Large pleomorphic blast cells with prominent nucleoli	5	CD15− CD30+ EMA+ may be, T, B or null phenotype

EMA, epithelial membrane antigen.

Note: Rare entities and primary bone-marrow neoplasms, e.g., myeloma and hairy-cell leukaemia, have been omitted. The percentages given reflect United States and European practice but may be considerably different elsewhere (especially in Asia). Full details of this classification are given in Harris *et al.* (1994). *Blood,* **84,** 1361–92.

In an attempt to circumvent this problem, in 1981 an expert international panel reviewed clinical and histological material from 1175 patients. All cases were classified by six systems: Rappaport, Kiel, British National Lymphoma Group, Lukes–Collins, World Health Organization, and Dorfman. The result was a *Working Formulation of Non-Hodgkin's Lymphoma for Clinical Use,* which can be readily translated into any one of the standard classifications. This scheme (Table 9) was not intended to supplant any of those already in use, but to be a common language through which, for example, comparison of results of clinical trials might be made. One point to note is the category of 'intermediate' malignancy, which does not appear in any of the original six classifications on which this formulation was based. This distinction has not achieved any practical value, with most pathologists and clinicians continuing to apportion non-Hodgkin lymphomas to either a low- or high-grade category. These grades are based on the morphological features of lymphoma types, which are believed to correlate well with the natural progression of untreated disease.

It should be noted that in spite of all the efforts put into the classification of non-Hodgkin lymphomas, accurate classification remains difficult or impossible in up to 10 per cent of cases with the material or techniques available.

The classification most widely used in Europe is that devised by Lennert's group in Kiel. This scheme was updated in 1988 (Table 10) to incorporate information gained from cell-marker studies, and when combined with a cytological/haematological approach enables a considerable consensus to be reached by non-specialist histopathologists working with routine biopsies. It has good prognostic correlations and, like other classifications, separates non-Hodgkin lymphomas into those with a relatively good prognosis (low-grade) and others with high-grade or poor prognostic features.

The Kiel classification has not received as much attention elsewhere, and in the United States a plethora of other classifications is used. Indeed, many centres now use the Working Formulation as a classification system, which is something it was specifically not designed to be. To overcome this lack of harmony and to incorporate new information into lymphoma classification a group of 19 haematopathologists from the United States, Europe, and Asia met in Berlin in 1993 to discuss existing schemes. The somewhat surprising result was that, despite their different origins, there was almost complete agreement between these pathologists on the entities that they were diagnosing. They have therefore put together a set of proposals as the REAL (Revised American European Lymphoma) classification in an attempt to simplify and coordinate diagnoses worldwide by emphasizing the recognition of disease entities (Table 11). In fact, the most radical aspect of this proposal is that for the first time it places emphasis on what pathologists do do rather than what a particular classification theory thinks they should do. If the concept of dealing with clinical and pathological entities is accepted, the artificial distinction of dividing lymphomas into low- and high-grade tumours can be eliminated.

Clinical and pathological features (see also Plates 14–19)

The non-Hodgkin lymphomas, with the exception of the lymphoblastic lymphomas, are relatively uncommon under the age of 40, and have a peak incidence in the 60- to 70-year-old age group (Fig. 6). The presenting features may be similar to Hodgkin's disease with local or general lymph-node enlargement, with or without systemic symptoms, and a biopsy is always required to establish the diagnosis. The spread of disease is, however, unlike Hodgkin's disease, with no clear anatomical spread from one area to a contiguous one and a much greater propensity to extranodal spread (Table 12).

There follows a brief description of some of the more important features of the main types of non-Hodgkin lymphoma.

Fig. 6 Age distribution of non-Hodgkin lymphomas expressed as new cases registered in England and Wales in 1973.

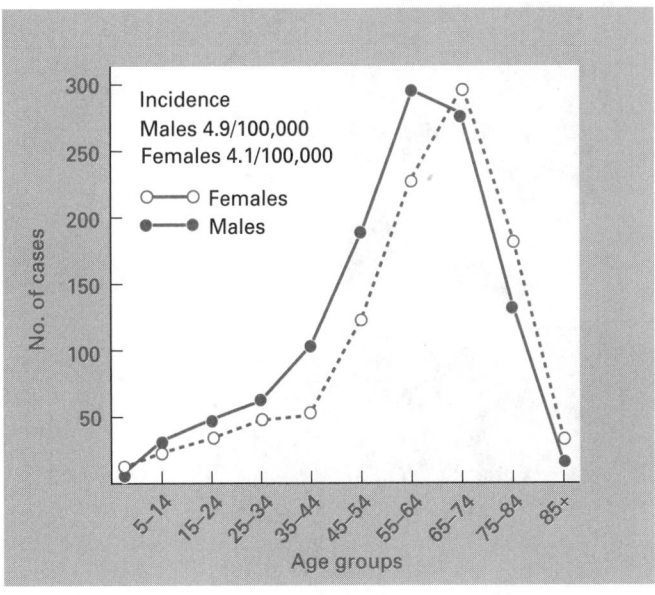

Table 12 *Some general clinical differences between Hodgkin's disease and non-Hodgkin lymphomas (NHL)*

Hodgkin's disease	Non-Hodgkin lymphomas
More often localized to one or more discrete groups or nodes	Commonly generalized (though not necessarily obvious clinically)
Waldeyer's ring and gut lymphatic tissue rarely affected	Waldeyer's ring and/or gut commonly involved
Extranodal involvement (marrow, skin etc.) uncommon	Extranodal involvement common
	Primary extramodal lymphomas are usually non-Hodgkin lymphoma

B-cell lymphomas

B-cell lymphomas are those that express at least one of the pan-B-cell antigens CD19, 20 and 22, and usually demonstrate surface or cytoplasmic immunoglobulin. Genotypically, all B-cell malignancies show clonal immunoglobulin-gene rearrangement.

LOW-GRADE B-CELL LYMPHOMAS

Lymphocytic lymphoma

The common B-cell type of lymphocytic lymphoma is often arbitrarily separated from chronic lymphocytic leukaemia (**CLL**) on the basis of the degree of involvement of the blood and/or marrow. The disease is confined to lymph nodes at presentation in a small number of cases, but the bone marrow usually becomes involved as the disease progresses. As with CLL, the pace of progression is variable and, in some patients, proliferation may reach a plateau and remain stable for many years. In general, the features are similar to those of CLL, described in detail in Chapter xxx, including impaired humoral immunity in a significant proportion and paraprotein production in a few.

Immunocytic lymphomas

In this group there is an accumulation of cells that appear intermediate in morphology between lymphocytes and plasma cells, and which contain monoclonal intracellular immunoglobulin. Lymph nodes, gut, or spleen may be involved singly or in combination, or plasmacytomas may develop—often in association with the respiratory tract.

The majority of these patients have an IgM paraprotein, when the condition is known as Waldenström's macroglobulinaemia. This may be associated with symptoms of hyperviscosity.

Myeloma is obviously related closely to this group of tumours but is traditionally considered separately as a primary haematological malignancy.

Follicular lymphoma

This is known as centroblastic/centrocytic lymphoma in the Kiel classification and is the most common type of non-Hodgkin lymphomas recognized in the West. It accounts for about 20 per cent of all non-Hodgkin lymphomas, and about one-third of all low-grade lymphomas It is characteristically a disorder of middle to old age, and most often presents with localized lymph-node enlargement. However, careful assessment will usually reveal more widespread involvement of other lymph nodes and the bone marrow.

Follicular lymphoma is believed to arise as a malignant transformation of germinal-centre cells and histologically comprises two cell types: the majority are small cleaved cells or centrocytes, together with scattered blast cells known as centroblasts. Most cases at presentation show a nodular pattern similar to reactive follicular hyperplasia, although mantle zones are poorly formed or absent and tingible-body macro-phages are scarce. The demonstration of light-chain restriction by immu-nocytochemistry is useful in confirming the histological diagnosis.

Although the clinical course of this type of lymphoma is often initially benign or indolent, treatment at best produces a temporary clinical regression or remission, and cure is usually impossible, even with aggressive treatment. Ultimately the disease progresses, often over many years, and may end in frank transformation to a high-grade, diffuse, large-cell lymphoma. Such high-grade transformations imply clonal evolutions, and in some cases aggressive treatment can eliminate the high-grade clone, although the original, low-grade disease eventually returns.

A frequent cytogenetic abnormality in follicular lymphoma is the translocation of part of chromosome 14 to chromosome 18, bringing the bcl-2 gene into apposition with immunoglobulin heavy-chain genes.

Mantle-cell lymphoma

This lymphoma was originally described by the Kiel group and named centrocytic lymphoma. This subtype is much less common than follic-ular lymphoma and constitutes a replacement of the lymph node by a pure proliferation of small, cleaved cells indistinguishable morpholog-ically from germinal-centre centrocytes. Initially it was believed to be a proliferation arising from the germinal centre, but immunophenotypic and genotypic studies have shown it to be quite distinct from germinal-centre cells. Currently, the evidence is much in favour of the tumour arising from cells in the mantle zone surrounding germinal centres, lead-ing to the suggestion it should be renamed mantle-cell lymphoma. Although generally grouped with the low-grade lymphomas, the clinical course is more aggressive, prompting the Working Formulation origi-nators to include this in their intermediate category.

HIGH-GRADE B-CELL LYMPHOMAS

Large-cell lymphoma

These tumours comprise about 20 per cent of non-Hodgkin lymphomas and include two separate tumour types in the Kiel classification, cen-troblastic and immunoblastic. Centroblastic lymphomas are believed to arise from germinal centres, either primarily or as a secondary transfor-mation from a low-grade lymphoma. In the case of immunoblastic lym-phoma, it is unclear whether it arises exclusively from a plasmacytic course of differentiation or as a further stage of germinal-centre cell differentiation. Both tumours are composed of diffuse, uniform infil-trates of large blast cells and may be primary (arising de novo) or sec-ondary (following transformation of a low-grade B-cell lymphoma).

There is debate amongst lymphoma pathologists as to whether or not these two categories can be separated reliably. Certainly, from a practical point of view, even the most ardent subclassifiers agree that the therapy should be identical for both tumours. The small survival advantage for centroblastic lymphoma claimed by some sources depends crucially on the grounds for recognizing the tumour.

Burkitt's lymphoma (Plate 48)

This very interesting lymphoma is the most common neoplasm in chil-dren in a wide equatorial belt of Africa and in New Guinea. This is known as endemic Burkitt's lymphoma to distinguish it from a small number of cases with a similar histological appearance seen in Europe and North America (so-called non-endemic Burkitt's lymphoma). The peak incidence is in the 4- to 7-year age group, and over 80 per cent of cases occur between the ages of 3 and 12 years.

Burkitt's lymphoma has a characteristic histological picture com-posed of a diffuse infiltrate of medium-sized blast cells. This tumour has a high proliferation rate, as evidenced by numerous mitotic figures, which is partially offset by the cell death demonstrated by the large number of apoptotic cells. This gives rise to large amounts of cellular debris, which is phagocytosed by macrophages giving the characteristic 'starry sky' pattern. Unlike lymphoblastic non-Hodgkin lymphoma, Burkitt's lymphoma has a tendency to grow in uneven clusters, giving

a pattern of apparent cohesion between the cells. To the experienced eye this can be the single most important feature in helping to distinguish Burkitt's lymphoma from either large-cell or lymphoblastic non-Hodg-kin lymphoma.

The clinical picture of endemic Burkitt's varies somewhat with the age of the subject, the typical jaw tumours (Fig. 7) being most common in the younger patients. These tumours usually arise in molar or pre-molar regions of the jaws, leading to loosening of the teeth. They may involve the mandible or maxilla, and in the maxilla may extend upward to involve the orbit.

Abdominal involvement is also present in the majority of cases, ret-roperitoneal masses, ovarian tumours, hepatic involvement, or gastro-intestinal tumours being common. Involvement of the testes and breast may also occur. The masses may extend into the cranium or involve the spinal cord to give paraplegia. There may also be involvement of bones with tumour. Lymph node involvement is relatively uncommon. A dif-ferent pattern of disease is seen in non-endemic cases, which predomi-nantly involve lymph node, bone marrow, and gastrointestinal tract.

One of the reasons that Burkitt's lymphoma has aroused such interest is the close association between the tumour and high titres of antibodies against EBV and the cellular antigens determined by it. Burkitt has drawn attention to the geographical distribution of the tumour and the importance of tumour-free gaps in tropical Africa, and has deduced that malarial infection may increase the tendency to neoplasia resulting from infection with a virus (the EBV) that usually produces a non-malignant lymphoid proliferation. The connection with the presence of EBV is not clear, although the viral genome is incorporated into the tumour-cell nuclei, a feature rarely seen in non-endemic Burkitt's or found in other conditions associated with the EBV such as nasopharyngeal carcinoma.

A translocation between chromosomes 8 and 14 (t[8;14][q24.13: q32.33]) is characteristic of Burkitt's lymphoma. The abnormalities involving chromosome 14 have been found in relation to a variety of other lymphomas, particularly of B-cell origin. Recent work describing the relation between the chromosomal changes in this condition and changes in cellular oncogenes is described in Section 6.

Burkitt's lymphoma is traditionally classified separately from other non-Hodgkin lymphomas, although for a time it was treated as a subtype

Fig. 7 Jaw tumour in a child with Burkitt's lymphoma (reproduced by courtesy of Professor D.H. Wright).

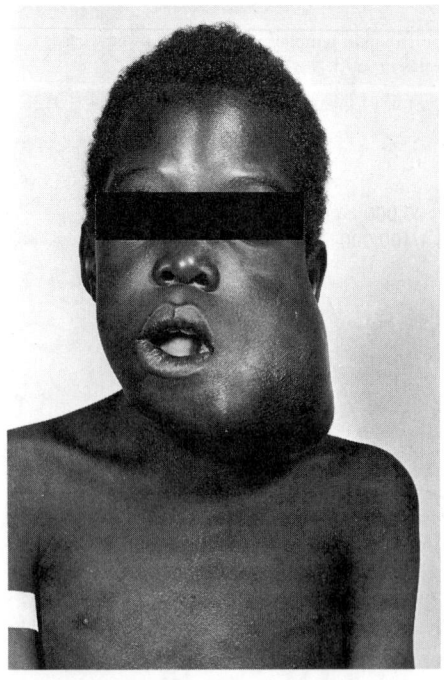

of lymphoblastic lymphoma in the Kiel classification. Although most research points to an origin from follicle-centre cells there are strong arguments for separating Burkitt's lymphoma from the common follicle-centre cell tumours. Burkitt's lymphoma shows no evidence of cytoplasmic immunoglobulin and no follicular pattern, and lymph node and spleen involvement, which is common in follicle-centre cell tumours, is relatively rare. Furthermore, the behaviour and response to therapy is quite different from that of centroblastic (large-cell) lymphoma in adults.

Lymphoblastic lymphoma

B-cell lymphoblastic lymphoma is an unusual condition occurring mostly in childhood, where it is almost always associated with acute lymphoblastic leukaemia. The tumour consists of a monotonous infiltrate of small to medium-sized blast cells with inconspicuous nuclear details. It can be difficult to distinguish morphologically from Burkitt's lymphoma, although the lack of nucleoli, phagocytic macrophages, and overcrowding and clumping of cells usually allows it to be recognized as a separate entity. Occasional adults with abdominal or mediastinal masses turn out to have B-cell lymphoblastic lymphoma that may not be associated with leukaemia.

T-cell lymphomas (see also Plates 22–24)

A T-cell lymphoma expresses, at least partially, one or more of the following pan-T-cell antigens: CD2, CD3, CD4, CD7, and CD8. Genotypically, all T-cell malignancies show T-cell-receptor rearrangement, usually of the β-chain but occasionally only of the γ/δ-chain.

T-cell non-Hodgkin lymphoma is less common than the B-cell variety, comprising no more than 20 per cent in most series of Western patients. However, it comprises a much higher proportion in those areas such as south Japan and the Caribbean where the human T-cell lymphotropic virus (**HTLV-1**) is endemic. Unlike most B-cell proliferations, T cells have a highly variable morphology, making the identity of neoplastic lesions and their classification extremely difficult. There are also no easily recognizable clonal markers, as both subtype antigens (CD4 or -8) may be absent or a reactive phenomenon. There is even debate over the reliability of T-cell-receptor gene rearrangements for this purpose. This places a considerable diagnostic burden on the pathologist, which can be eased, if not completely relieved, by close and sympathetic cooperation with clinicians.

LOW-GRADE T-CELL LYMPHOMAS

T-cell lymphocytic lymphoma

Morphologically these are similar to B-lymphocytic lymphomas and chronic lymphocytic leukaemias. A particular feature of the T-cell lymphocytic lymphomas is their predilection for the skin. This may be related to the known immunological functions of the skin and the fact that normal T cells interact dynamically with epidermal structures as part of the local immune response to invading antigen.

Primary cutaneous lymphoma

Primary lymphomas arising in the skin are almost always of T-cell origin and generally show a helper T-cell phenotype. Histologically, the epidermis is invaded by small cells with striking folded nuclei, often known as cerebriform or Lutzner cells. This infiltrate may form recognizable clusters in the epidermis known as Pautrier's microabscesses. As the lesion progresses, extension down into and beyond the dermis takes place.

Two forms of primary cutaneous T-cell lymphoma are recognized (mycosis fungoides and Sézary syndrome) and are distinguished by their clinical features.

Mycosis fungoides

A progressive disorder that presents initially with a non-specific, scaly eruption, progressing eventually to the formation of multiple skin plaques and tumours, some of which may ulcerate. The disease tends to affect middle-aged men, and may be present for 20 years or more before systemic spread follows, with lymphadenopathy and visceral involvement. Death is often from unrelated causes, although internal organs may be found to be involved at autopsy.

Sézary syndrome

This may be considered as a generalized though insidious leukaemic variant of mycosis fungoides. It starts with a non-specific, eczematous, or licheniform skin eruption, which progresses to an intensely pruritic, generalized, exfoliating erythroderma, with a particular predilection for the face, palms, and soles. At this stage the condition bears a striking resemblance to acute graft-versus-host disease. Patchy hyperpigmentation and also some degree of lymphadenopathy are common. Plaque formation resembling that of mycosis fungoides is often found, and the histology of the two conditions at this stage is similar. Spontaneous remissions and exacerbations do occur, but the disease is ultimately fatal, with an average life expectancy of 5 years.

In both mycosis fungoides and the Sézary syndrome the malignant cell usually has a helper T-cell phenotype. When chromosomal studies have been done these have generally been abnormal, with marked aneuploidy. Occasionally, marker chromosomes have been detected, confirming a clonal origin.

Peripheral T-cell lymphoma

There are four T-cell lymphomas classified as low grade in the Kiel classification that have a similar neoplastic component. They differ mainly in the reactive elements surrounding them, presumably elicited by the lymphoma cells. These four tumours are:

- Lennert's lymphoma,
- angioimmunoblastic lymphoma,
- T-zone lymphoma,
- small-cell pleomorphic lymphoma.

Their common feature is a proliferation of small to medium-sized T cells, often with an associated vascular response. Eosinophils are a common component of the reactive lymphocytic infiltrate. Individual features of these disorders are discussed separately below. There is still no clear consensus on their behaviour, with many authorities believing them all to be high grade regardless of their morphology. In the REAL classification the T-cell tumours are treated as entities so that the concept of low- and high-grade categories has less relevance.

Lymphoepithelioid (Lennert's) lymphoma

This was originally described by Lennert as a type of Hodgkin's disease but more detailed study has identified it as a T-cell lymphoma with a mixed population of malignant T cells interspersed with numerous small foci of epithelioid macrophages—that is, a granulomatous reaction. Its behaviour is that of a high-grade lymphoma.

Angioimmunoblastic lymphoma

This is a disease of older people, principally in their sixth or seventh decade, with only some 10 per cent being under 40 years of age. It presents with constitutional symptoms of fever, malaise, pruritis, polyarthralgia, anorexia, and weight loss. About half the patients have skin rashes, which may be maculopapular, purpuric or urticarial.

Lymphadenopathy is an almost invariable feature and it may involve both peripheral and internal lymph nodes. Hepatosplenomegaly is common, and lung involvement, arthritis, polyneuropathy, skin plaques and nodules, vasculitis, glomerulonephritis, oedema, and ascites have all been described in this condition. An autoimmune haemolytic anaemia is often found and a leucocytosis with eosinophilia is common. The erythrocyte sedimentation rate is usually raised, with a polyclonal hypergammaglobulinaemia.

The histological appearance of the glands is characterized by a proliferation of arborizing, postcapillary venules (the epithelioid venules) in the paracortex. In between the new vessels the interstitium is packed with a polymorphous selection of T cells with admixed polyclonal plasma cells. B-cell follicles are unrecognizable.

Initially, angioimmunoblastic lymphadenopathy with dysproteinaemia was believed to be non-neoplastic because, although virtually all patients died rapidly regardless of therapy, this seemed mostly to be due to the effects of immunodeficiency. However, the recognition that some developed obvious large-cell lymphomas, combined with careful molecular analysis, has identified the disease as a T-cell lymphoma.

Clinical behaviour and response to treatment is variable. Exposure to a known stimulus, for example, one which has produced an allergic drug reaction, should be avoided in future, and if the condition shows no tendency to regress spontaneously, treatment with prednisolone and possibly an immunosuppressive drug such as cyclophophamide is indicated. Once the condition has entered a clinically more obviously malignant phase, treatment appropriate to a high-grade lymphoma may be tried, but the prognosis is poor.

T-zone lymphoma

In this lymphoma the B-cell areas are usually intact but surrounded by a polymorphic T-cell infiltrate, very similar to that seen in angioimmunoblastic lymphoma.

Pleomorphic small-cell lymphoma

This lymphoma basically consists of the neoplastic infiltrate from the three tumours described above minus the granulomas, vascularity, or B-cell reaction. Like the high-grade pleomorphic T-cell lymphomas, with which it merges insidiously, it may be associated with HTLV-1 infection.

HIGH-GRADE T-CELL LYMPHOMA

Pleomorphic lymphoma

This is a lymphoma composed of a mixture of pleomorphic cells of medium to large size. It can be extremely difficult to distinguish from the low-grade small-cell variant, and indeed the REAL classification recognizes this by putting all these tumours together as a single entity. Many cases, particularly in endemic areas, are associated with HTLV-1 infection. These cases are usually associated with an accompanying leukaemia and thus are known as adult T-cell leukaemia/lymphoma syndrome.

Adult T-cell leukaemia/lymphoma syndrome (ATL)

As might be expected from the association with the type C retrovirus HTLV-1, ATL tends to occur in clusters. It was first described in patients from Japan and subsequently in the Caribbean, although it has now been detected in other populations. ATL is an aggressive systemic disorder characterized by widespread lymphadenopathy, bone lesions, refractory hypercalcaemia, bone marrow, peripheral blood, central nervous, and skin involvement.

Angiocentric lymphoma

These are T-cell neoplasms characterized by invasion of vascular walls. This pathological entity encompasses a number of clinical syndromes such as polymorphic reticulosis, midline granuloma, and lymphomatoid granulomatosis. It is a rare disorder, though more common in Asia than in the West. The clinical course appears to depend on the proportion of large atypical cells.

Other forms of non-Hodgkin lymphoma

Anaplastic large-cell lymphoma

This is a recently recognized entity composed of large cells with abundant cytoplasm and pleomorphic nuclei. This lymphoma has a characteristically cohesive growth pattern involving lymph nodes, often patchily, in the subcapsular sinuses and paracortex. Many cases were misdiagnosed as secondary cancer until antibodies against the activation

Table 13 *Primary gastrointestinal non-Hodgkin's lymphoma*

B-cell
Lymphomas of mucosa-associated lymphoid tissue (MALT):
   (a) low-grade B-cell lymphoma of MALT
   (b) high-grade B-cell lymphoma of MALT with or without a
       low-grade component
   (c) immunoproliferative small-intestinal disease (IPSID)
       low-grade, mixed or high-grade
Mantle-cell lymphoma (lymphomatous polyposis)
Burkitt's or Burkitt-like lymphoma
Other types of lymphoma corresponding to peripheral lymph-node equivalents

T-cell
Enteropathy-associated T-cell lymphoma (EATL)
Other types unassociated with enteropathy

antigen CD30 revealed the identity of this lesion as a malignancy of activated lymphocytes. Approximately 75 per cent of these lesions are T cell, 20 per cent B cell, and 5 per cent unidentifiable. Many have a characteristic t(2;5) chromosomal translocation.

This lymphoma occurs in two age peaks, one in older children and teenagers and one in elderly people. There is preliminary evidence in children that the tumour has a better prognosis than other high-grade large-cell lymphomas, whereas in adults there is no evidence yet that it is better or worse than other large-cell lesions.

Histiocytic lymphomas

Ever since the first description, in 1939, of a clinicopathological syndrome of hepatosplenomegaly, fever and anaemia termed histiocytic medullary reticulosis, the literature has been full of case reports of macrophage-based neoplasms. Like the Loch Ness monster they are frequently cited but never caught. Most cases have been shown to be tissue deposits of monocytic leukaemia or T-cell lymphoma. If histiocytic lymphoma does exist it is so rare that for practical purposes it can be dismissed or lumped in with the high-grade large-cell lymphomas.

PRIMARY EXTRANODAL LYMPHOMAS

As discussed earlier in this chapter, non-Hodgkin lymphomas have a tendency to involve structures other than lymph nodes, either by direct invasion (for example from mediastinal node into pleura, lung or pericardium) or more remotely. Extranodal spread occurs rarely in Hodgkin's disease. Primary extranodal presentations (without evidence of disease elsewhere) are less common and are almost exclusively confined to the non-Hodgkin group. A wide variety of tissues may be involved, most commonly the mucosa-associated lymphoid tissues (**MALT**) of gut, thyroid, lung, and salivary gland (the so-called MALTomas), the eye, and the skin.

MALTomas

These are a group of lymphomas showing common clinical and pathological features whose identity owes much to the painstaking studies of Isaacson and Wright. They most commonly involve the stomach but other affected tissues are colon, thyroid, lung, and salivary gland. Maltomas may be low or high grade and are the most common primary gastrointestinal non-Hodgkin lymphomas, a classification of which is given in Table 13.

MALTomas are believed to arise from small centrocyte-like cells surrounding gut lymphoid follicles. These cells give rise to a low-grade malignancy with a marked propensity for invading epithelial glands but remain localized to the organ site, be it stomach or thyroid, for many years. It is assumed that high-grade MALTomas arise as a transformation of these low-grade tumours into large-cell lymphomas. Strikingly, even these high-grade lesions may remain localized for relatively long periods. This results in the important feature that fully resected MAL-Tomas have a much better prognosis than their nodal counterparts, as shown by a detailed follow-up study of primary gastric lymphoma from the Kiel Lymphoma Group.

Recent studies suggest that early gastric MALTomas may be driven by antigenic stimulation from *Helicobacter pylori* infection. Appropriate antibiotic therapy can result in dramatic regression of these lesions. It may well be that other antigens are stimulating MALTomas in other sites and might similarly respond to appropriate therapy.

Immunoproliferative small-intestinal disease (IPSID) (see also Section 14)

This condition is virtually confined to countries bordering the Mediterranean. It presents with malabsorption and consists of infiltration of small bowel by lymphoplasmacytic and plasma cells synthesizing only the heavy chain of IgA. Hence it is also known as α-chain disease. In the early stages, prolonged remission may be obtained with broad-spectrum antibiotics, indicating that these lesions may be preneoplastic and thus reversible. As the lymphoma progresses, it becomes virtually indistinguishable from other MALTomas and has a similar clinical and pathological course.

Other primary gastrointestinal lymphomas (see Section 14)

There are two further primary gastrointestinal lymphomas, both of which are localized variations of nodal non-Hodgkin lymphomas (or at least are currently indistinguishable from them).

Lymphomatous polyposis

This presents with multiple small polyps in the small bowel infiltrated by a mantle-cell, non-Hodgkin lymphomas. These are true centrocytes and should be distinguished from the centrocyte-like cells of MAL-Toma. Like nodal mantle-cell lymphoma it has a worse prognosis than its bland cytology might lead one to expect, and unlike MALToma it tends to spread rapidly to other sites.

Enteropathy-associated T-cell lymphoma

This is similar or identical to nodal, high-grade, pleomorphic, T-cell non-Hodgkin lymphoma and usually arises as a complication of long-standing coeliac disease. There is some evidence that there are T cells that localize to the gastrointestinal tract and that enteropathy-associated T-cell lymphoma arises from these cells. This would make this lesion the T-cell equivalent of B-cell MALToma. Unlike the MALTomas, enteropathy-associated T-cell lymphoma has a grave prognosis.

OTHER EXTRANODAL NON-HODGKIN LYMPHOMAS

Nervous system

Secondary involvement of the nervous system is a fairly common late complication of a variety of non-Hodgkin lymphomas. It usually affects the meninges, producing radicular or cranial-nerve symptoms, but may involve the brain in a focal or diffuse manner with headache, altered conciousness, and/or focal neurological signs. The prognosis is poor, but a combination of intrathecal chemotherapy and radiotherapy may relieve symptoms sufficient for consideration of high-dose salvage therapy.

Primary brain lymphomas are rare cause of intracranial neoplasia but are occasionally found on biopsy of intracranial lesions. Treatment outcome is highly unsatisfactory. Initial symptoms may be relieved by radiotherapy but recurrence either intracranially or systemically is usual. Intensive systemic chemotherapy may be a better alternative, but the rarity of the condition means that there are no large studies to guide rational therapy.

Primary B-cell non-Hodgkin lymphomas also arise in the orbit and the skin. Cytologically these have many similarities to MALTomas, although there are important differences such as a tendency to systemic dissemination (orbit) or lack of epithelial invasion (skin). In the skin the most common lymphoma is of T-cell origin and presents as mycosis fungoides or Sézary syndrome, which have been dealt with above.

Management of non-Hodgkin lymphomas

The principles of management of patients with non-Hodgkin lymphoma are essentially the same as for Hodgkin's disease described above, and involve accurate diagnosis and the assessment of extent of disease and prognostic factors in order to determine optimal therapy.

The approach to staging is traditionally the same as for Hodgkin's disease, and the same Rye staging system is employed. It must be remembered, however, that non-Hodgkin lymphomas are frequently diseases of lymphocytes that may normally recirculate throughout the blood system and lymphatics. Non-Hodgkin lymphomas are thus more often widespread, and the pattern of spread is predominantly haematogenous rather than to contiguous lymph nodes via the lymphatics as in Hodgkin's disease. Extranodal involvement is thus also much more common, and special investigations such as endoscopy may be required in individual cases.

The most useful routine investigations are a full blood count and erythrocyte sedimentation rate, biochemical profiles (especially lactic dehydrogenase, which is elevated in some patients with high-grade tumours and may serve as a useful marker of disease activity), bone marrow examination, which should include aspirate and trephine, preferably from more than one site, chest radiograph (Fig. 8), and CT scan (Fig. 9).

TREATMENT

Over the years there has been less agreement about the optimal treatment for patients with non-Hodgkin lymphoma than with Hodgkin's disease, but recent improvements in classification, the introduction of less invasive investigations, and experience with different approaches to treatment have allowed a more rational approach to treatment to emerge, based on realistic, achievable goals. Many patients with non-Hodgkin lymphoma are elderly, their normal life expectancy may be limited, and attention to the quality of life is often at least as important as the duration of survival.

Low-grade tumours

It is now apparent that, despite their more indolent course, few patients with low-grade non-Hodgkin lymphoma can be cured, even with aggressive cytotoxic therapy (Fig. 10). Exceptions are those in the minority with disease localized to one or two nodes, who may be cured by surgical removal and/or radiotherapy. Even so, long-term follow-up of such patients over 10 years or more will reveal a proportion which relapses at other sites. The aim of treatment in most patients with a low-grade non-Hodgkin lymphoma is therefore the control of symptoms and prolongation of good-quality survival rather than cure.

Some patients may not require treatment at first and can be safely watched and treated only if symptoms occur, or can be anticipated from progression of the disease. Patients with stage I or II disease may be treated with radiotherapy to involved areas, particularly if node enlargement is producing local symptoms. Radiotherapy will generally produce good local control but the majority of patients will relapse in other sites sooner or later.

Various chemotherapeutic approaches for low-grade non-Hodgkin lymphoma have been suggested. Whilst the time required to achieve a remission is usually shorter with combination chemotherapy such as cyclophosphamide, vincristine and prednisolone, randomized trials have shown that single-agent therapy with chlorambucil or cyclophosphamide may achieve just as good results with less toxicity, although taking longer to do so. Newer agents such as fludarabine, deoxycoformycin, and chlorodeoxyadenosine are currently under evaluation. Preliminary studies indicate that they may induce more complete responses than chlorambucil, but they are more difficult to administer, more toxic, and considerably more expensive, and do not at the moment appear to confer any long-term survival advantage.

Splenectomy may sometimes be helpful, either in patients whose disease is largely confined to the spleen or where hypersplenism is a feature. It may also be useful in the occasional patient with an autoimmune

Fig. 9 The value of computed tomography in abdominal lymphoma. (a) A group of enlarged lymph nodes (arrowed) is seen surrounding the aorta (A); note the tip of an enlarged spleen (S), lying anteriorly. (L = liver; K = kidneys). (b) A few centimetres lower, a group of enlarged mesenteric nodes is seen (arrowed). (c) More inferiorly, there is a large soft-tissue mass (M) arising from the distal small bowel. Lymphangiography in this patient would have demonstrated the para-aortic lymphadenopathy, but not the disease in other areas (Reproduced by courtesy of Dr. S. Golding.)

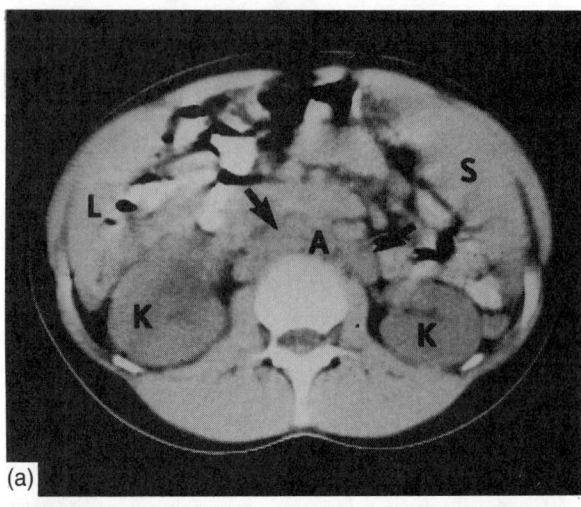

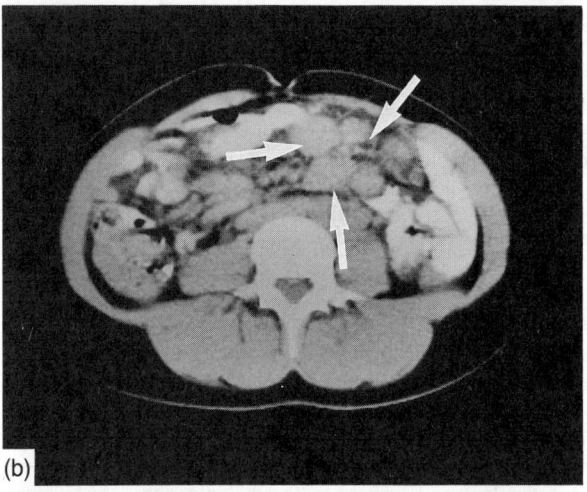

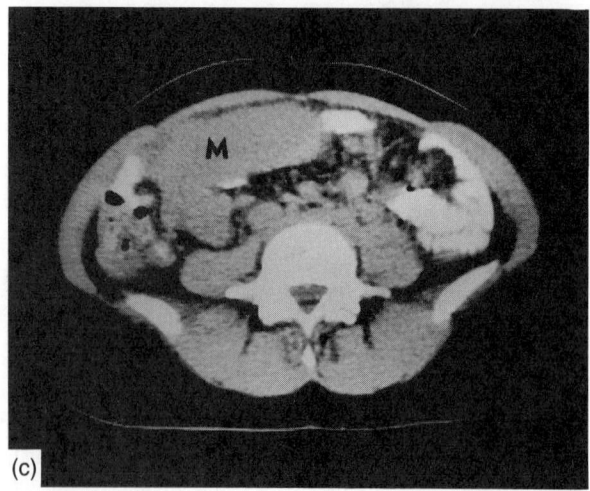

Fig. 8 JT, aged 31 at diagnosis, with malignant T-cell lymphoma associated with mediastinal obstruction, bilateral pleural effusions (which contained malignant T-cells) and involvement of the bone marrow but not of peripheral blood. Treated with aggressive chemotherapy on the lines of ALL, plus CNS prophylaxis with intrathecal methotrexate and 2 years maintenance chemotherapy. (a) chest radiograph at presentation; (b) 6 years later, when the patient remains well and in complete remission.

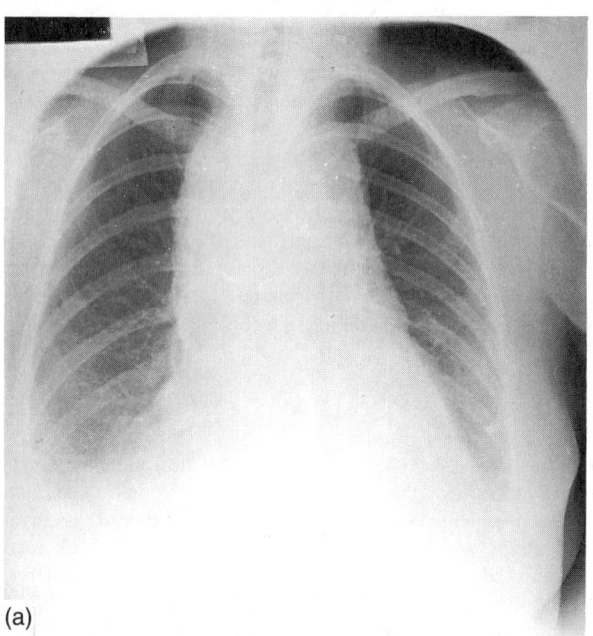

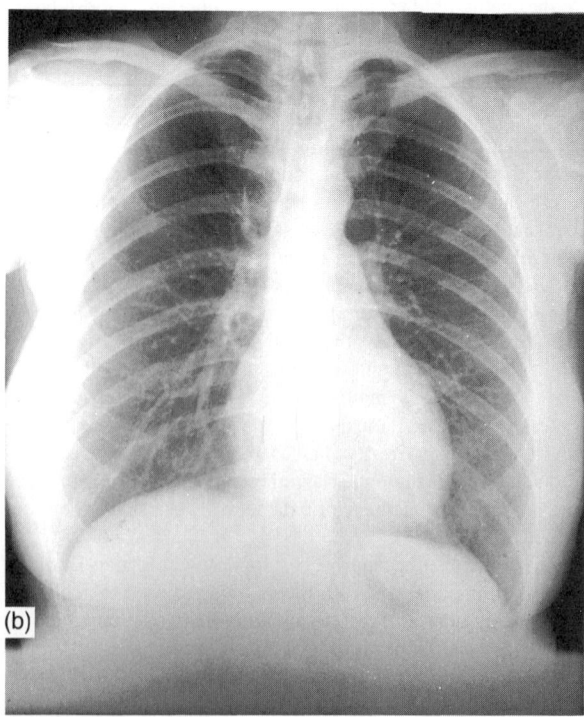

haemolytic anaemia where steroids or immunosuppressive treatment has failed or produced undesirable side-effects.

High-grade tumours

In high-grade non-Hodgkin lymphoma (lymphoblastic, large cell and anaplastic large cell) the prognosis without treatment is extremely poor and aggressive combination chemotherapy is generally used. In contrast to low-grade non-Hodgkin lymphoma, the early mortality of high-grade disease is high but, paradoxically, patients who do go into remission may have prolonged disease-free survival and about one-third may be cured (Fig. 10).

Lymphoblastic lymphomas are best treated in a similar fashion to acute lymphoblastic leukaemia, including prophylaxis for the central nervous system.

Large-cell (centroblastic and immunoblastic) lymphomas are best treated with combination chemotherapy containing doxorubicin, for example **CHOP**: cyclophosphamide, hydroxydaunorubicin (doxorubicin), vincristine (Oncovin), and prednisolone (Table 14). About one-half of all patients with large-cell lymphoma will have a complete response to CHOP, and about one-third overall will be cured. These somewhat disappointing results have led many to attempt more aggressive therapy with multiple (six, eight or more) drug combinations. Whilst initial small series in selected patients were highly encouraging, recent large-scale randomized studies in less highly selected patients have shown no overall advantage over CHOP.

Attention is now being focused on the role of high-dose chemo/radiotherapy with haemopoietic stem-cell (marrow or peripheral blood) support. This is worth considering in relapsed patients or in those who have responded to CHOP but have adverse prognostic features, and randomized studies of its use in initial therapy are under way. However, it is currently an experimental approach, which should be confined to formal trials in specialist centres.

Prognosis

The prognosis of non-Hodgkin lymphoma is generally less good than that of Hodgkin's disease, and until recently very few patients could

Table 14 *Chemotherapy regimens for the treatment of non-Hodgkin lymphomas*

Chlorambucil
   May be used continuously at a dose of 4–6 mg daily, or intermittently at a dose of 0.5 mg/kg daily for 3 days every 4 weeks

COP (CVP)
- Cyclophosphamide 400 mg/m² orally, days 1–5
- Vincristine (Oncovin) 1.4 mg/m² (max 2 mg) i.v., day 1
- Prednisolone 100 mg/m² orally, days 1 to 5

Course repeated every 3 weeks until remission or no further improvement

CHOP
- Cyclophosphamide 750 mg/m² i.v., day 1
- Vincristine (Oncovin) 1.4 mg/m² (max 2 mg) i.v., day 1
- Adriamycin (hydroxydaunorubicin) 50 mg/m² i.v., day 1
- Prednisolone 100 mg/m² orally, days 1 to 5

Course repeated every 3–4 weeks until remission + three further courses

expect to be cured. It must be remembered, however, that non-Hodgkin lymphoma represents a much more heterogeneous group of neoplasms, and this is reflected in the differing prognosis according to histological subtype, which is largely independent of the actual histological classification used.

Intuitively, one might expect patients with low-grade lymphomas to have a better prognosis than those with histologically more malignant forms. This generally holds true for patients followed up for up to 5 years after diagnosis (Fig. 10), but it is now becoming clear that, as in Hodgkin's disease, a proportion of patients with high-grade tumours histologically may be cured with more aggressive approaches to treatment.

On the other hand, with low-grade tumours, a cure is possible for only a very small minority of patients with very localized forms of disease, even with aggressive treatment. Indeed the failure of a variety of aggressive approaches to alter the ultimate outcome in low-grade disease suggests that a much more gentle approach is appropriate for these patients, especially as many are elderly. That antigenic stimulation by these tumours might be inhibited, as in gastric MALToma, is a valuable therapeutic possibility.

Other factors are important in determining prognosis. Age is clearly significant: the incidence of most forms of non-Hodgkin lymphoma increases with age and elderly patients tolerate aggressive treatment much less well.

In a group of unselected patients in Oxford the most powerful prognostic factors that emerged were the histological grade and the presence or absence of systemic symptoms. These two factors were largely independent. Clinical stage I disease (all groups) had a relatively good prognosis but stages beyond this were of no further prognostic value. The level of haemoglobin at presentation may be of some prognostic use, although the mechanism of anaemia is obscure and does not always appear to be related to marrow infiltration with tumour. In other series, overall bulk of disease at presentation has been shown to correlate inversely with prognosis.

The principal causes of death are advancing disease that is refractory to all forms of treatment, and infection.

Miscellaneous conditions resembling lymphoma

There are several uncommon conditions in which there is progressive, although often non-fatal, enlargement of lymph nodes. These conditions

Fig. 10 Actuarial survival of patients with non-Hodgkin lymphoma. The graph is divided into low-grade (grade 1) and high-grade (grade 2) forms of the disease. Patients with high-grade lymphoma have an initial high death rate but the survival curve forms a plateau at 5 years, indicating that a significant proportion of patients are cured of their disease. Low-grade lymphomas, although having an indolent initial course, show a continuing death rate after 5 years and appear to be incurable with current therapies. By 10 years the survival rates of low- and high-grade lymphoma are similar. (Data from the British National Lymphoma Investigation. (1988). *Lancet*, **i**, 292–3.)

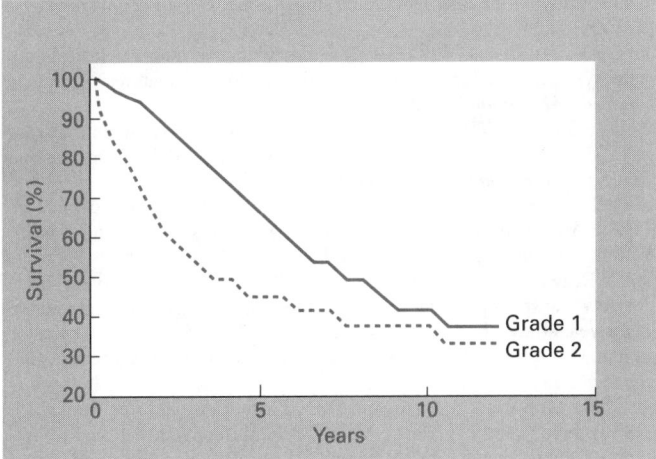

are not necessarily malignant, but some may subsequently progress to lymphoma, and may in time produce clues as to its aetiology. A common denominator appears to be an alteration of the vascular structure of nodes through which lymphoid cells have to pass.

Kaposi sarcoma

This condition shares a strikingly similar distribution in Africa to that of Burkitt's lymphoma and it accounts for approximately 16 per cent of all malignancies in some areas. It presents in children as a widespread lymphadenopathy. The lymph nodes are generally replaced by a sarcomatous proliferation of spindle cells that may be related to pericapillary fibroblasts, although the histogenesis is not known. They form slit-like clefts containing red cells. When the process involves an organ such as the gut, death may occur from massive haemorrhage.

In Europe, Kaposi sarcoma is diagnosed when a much more indolent, vascular spindle-cell proliferation involves the skin, particularly of the extremities. Nodal and visceral involvement may supervene. It is uncertain to what extent the African childhood lymph-node disease and the adult Western skin tumour are identical.

A striking association between Kaposi sarcoma and AIDS has been recognized. This is described in Chapter 7.10.29.

Castleman's disease

This is a rare condition, also known as angiofollicular lymph-node hyperplasia. The original description was of a mediastinal mass, detected on chest radiograph, which on biopsy showed 'pseudofollicles' with small lymphocytes surrounding capillaries, in the wall of which were concentric lamellae of plump, eosinophilic, endothelial cells, often resembling a Hassall's corpuscle in a normal thymus. Clinically, the condition may be asymptomatic, or associated with local symptoms such as cough and dyspnoea. Occasional patients may have constitutional symptoms such as fever and night sweats, and an associated anaemia and elevated erythrocyte sedimentation rate. In this form, the condition is generally benign, and asymptomatic patients may not require treatment, whilst surgical removal of the mass may relieve symptoms in those who are.

More recently, a histological form has been recognized, the 'plasma-cell variant', that is in contrast to the original description, which is now known as the 'hyaline vascular' variant. The plasma-cell variant is more often associated with systemic symptoms and a more generalized lymphadenopathy that may affect cervical, retroperitoneal or mesenteric lymph nodes. In some cases there may be one or more of *p*eripheral neuropathy, *o*rganomegaly (hepatomegaly and/or splenomegaly), *e*ndocrinopathy, a *m*onoclonal paraprotein, and *s*kin lesions—the so-called POEMS syndrome (Chapter 24.17.1). The aetiology of this condition is unknown, but high circulating levels of interleukin 6 have been observed. It is not thought to be neoplastic, but can be have in a clinically aggressive fashion and require treatment with corticosteroids, with or without cytotoxic chemotherapy. Occasional cases have been observed to progress to a frank non-Hodgkin lymphoma.

Lymphomatoid granulomatosis

This condition is characterized by a pleomorphic cellular infiltrate with atypical lymphocytoid and plasmacytoid cells, together with a granulomatous reaction. It affects adults between the third and sixth decades. The lungs are most commonly involved. Presenting features include cough, dyspnoea, pleuritic pain, fever, skin infiltrates, or neurological symptoms. A chest radiograph may show a nodular infiltrate. The diagnosis and distinction from Wegener's granulomatosis depends on biopsy.

The condition is now generally considered to be part of the angiocentric T-cell lymphomas and frequently progresses into an unequivocal florid lymphoma, often of a high-grade variety. The disorder is responsive to combined chemotherapy with cyclophosphamide and prednisone; long remissions can be obtained.

Histiocytic medullary reticulosis

This is a very rare disease of middle age, characterized by a fever, a rash, hepatosplenomegaly, and pancytopenia. Histiocytes in the splenic red pulp and hepatic sinusoidal cells show some erythrophagocytosis. As the disease progresses the architecture may be destroyed and tumour masses develop, especially in the skin and bones. Careful immunological review has shown that most of these cases are T-cell lymphomas.

Virus-induced haemophagocytic syndrome

This condition must be carefully distinguished from a purely reactive disorder that is seen occasionally in immunosuppressed patients. This has been termed the virus-induced haemophagocytic syndrome. There is often a history of a viral-like illness during the previous few weeks and laboratory investigation may reveal evidence of EBV or cytomegalovirus infection. Despite its reactive nature, this is a serious multisystem illness with a high mortality rate.

There is frequently an associated disseminated intravascular coagulation, and pancytopenia is invariable. The bone marrow shows increased numbers of histiocytes with prominent phagocytosis of red cells, platelets and nucleated cells. The histiocytes and cells are mature and morphologically normal.

Histiocytosis X

Proliferation of cells with histiocytic features is evident in the histiocytosis X group of tumours, but although some of these have a malignant clinical course there is no good evidence that they are neoplastic. They are described more fully in Chapter 22.5.6.

REFERENCES

Armitage, J.O. (1993). Drug therapy: treatment of non-Hodgkin's lymphoma. *New England Journal of Medicine*, **328**, 1023–30.
Armitage, J.O., Fyfe, M.A.E., and Lewis, J. (1984). Long-term remission durability and functional status of patients treated for diffuse histiocytic lymphoma with the CHOP regimen. *Journal of Clinical Oncology*, **2**, 898–902.
Bergsagel, D.E. *et al.* (1982). Results of treating Hodgkin's disease without a policy of laparotomy staging. *Cancer Treatment Reports*, **66**, 717–31.
Blayney, D.W. *et al.* (1983). The human T-cell leukemia/lymphoma virus associated with American adult T-cell leukemia/lymphoma. *Blood*, **62**, 401–5.
Brittinger, G. *et al.* (1984). Clinical and prognostic relevance of the Kiel classification of non-Hodgkin's lymphomas results of prospective multicenter study by the Kiel lymphoma study group. *Hematologic Oncology*, **2**, 269–306.
Burns, B.F. and Evans, W.K. (1982). Tumours of the mononuclear phagocyte system: a review of clinical and pathological features. *American Journal of Hematology*, **13**, 171–84.
Canellos, G.P. *et al.* (1992). Chemotherapy of advanced Hodgkin's disease with MOPP, ABVD, or MOPP alternating with ABVD. *New England Journal of Medicine*, **327**, 1478–84.
Carbone, P.B., Kaplan, H.S., Musshof, K., Smithers, D.W., and Tubiana, M. (1971). Report on the committee on Hodgkin's disease staging classification. *Cancer Research*, **31**, 1860–1.
Chopra, R. *et al.* (1993). The place of ?????? therapy and autologous bone marrow transplantation in poor-risk Hodgkin's disease. A single centre eight year study of 155 patients. *Blood*, **81**, 1137–45.
Coltman, C.A. (1980). Chemotherapy of advanced Hodgkin's disease. *Seminars in Oncology*, **7**, 155–73.
Dady, P.J., McElwain, T.J., Austin, D.E., Barrett, A., and Peckham, M.J. (1982). Five years' experience with ChlVPP: effective low-toxicity combination chemotherapy for Hodgkin's disease. *British Journal of Cancer*, **45**, 851–9.

DeVita, V.T. (1981). The consequences of the chemotherapy of Hodgkin's disease: the 10th David A. Karnofsky Memorial Lecture. *Cancer,* **47,** 1–13.

DeVita, V.T., Serpick, A.A., and Carbone, P.P. (1970). Combination chemotherapy in the treatment of advanced Hodgkin's disease. *Annals of Internal Medicine,* **73,** 881–95.

Fisher, R.I. *et al.* (1993). Comparisons of standard regimen (CHOP) with three intensive chemotherapy regimens for advanced diffuse non-Hodgkin's lymphoma. *New England Journal of Medicine,* **328,** 1002–6.

Goldie, J.A. and Coldman, A.J. (1982). The genetic origin of drug resistance in neoplasia: implications for systemic therapy. *Cancer Research,* **44,** 3643–53.

Gordon, L.I. *et al.* (1992). Comparison of second-generation combination chemotherapeutic regimen (m-BACOD) with a standard regimen (CHOP) for advanced diffuse non-Hodgkin's lymphoma. *New England Journal of Medicine,* **327,** 1342–69.

Gray, G.M., Rosenberg, S.A., Cooper, A.D., Gregory, P.B., Stein, D.T., and Herzenberg, H. (1982). Lymphomas involving the gastrointestinal tract. *Gastroenterology,* **82,** 143–52.

Haylittle, J.L. *et al.* (1985). Review of British National Lymphoma Investigation studies and development of a prognostic index. *Lancet,* **i,** 967–72.

Horning, S.J. (1994). Treatment approaches to the low-grade lymphomas. *Blood,* **83,** 881–4.

Kaplan, H.S. (1980). *Hodgkin's disease,* (2nd edn). Harvard University Press, Cambridge, MA.

Kaplan, H.S. (1981). Hodgkin's disease: biology, treatment, prognosis. *Blood,* **57,** 813–22.

Kinzie, J.J., Hanks, G.E., Maclean, C.J., and Kramer, S. (1983). Patterns of care study: Hodgkin's disease relapse rates and adequacy of portals. *Cancer,* **52,** 2223–6.

Lewin, K.J., Kahn, L.B., and Novis, B.H. (1976). Primary intestinal lymphoma of 'Western' and 'Mediterranean' type, alpha-chain disease and massive plasma cell infiltration: a comparative study of 37 cases. *Cancer,* **38,** 2511–28.

Linch, D.C. (1994). Management of histologically aggressive non-Hodgkin's lymphomas. *British Journal of Haematology,* **86,** 691–4.

Lukes, R.J. and Tindle, B.H. (1975). Immunoblastic lymphadenopathy: a hyperimmune entity resembling Hodgkin's disease. *New England Journal of Medicine,* **292,** 1–8.

Lungo, D.L. *et al.* (1991). The treatment of advanced stage massive mediastinal Hodgkin's disease: the case for combined modality therapy. *Journal of Clinical Oncology,* **9,** 227–35.

Lutzner, M., Edelson, R., Schein, P., Green, I., Kirkpatrick, C., and Ahmed. A. (1975). Cutaneous T-cell lymphomas: the Sézary syndrome, mycosis fungoides, and related disorders. *Annals of Internal Medicine,* **83,** 543–552.

McKenna, R.W., Risdall, R.J., and Brunning, R.D. (1981). Virus associated hemophagocytic syndrome. *Human Pathology,* **12,** 395–8.

Non-Hodgkin's Lymphoma Pathologic Classification Project (1982). National Cancer Institute sponsored study of classifications of non-Hodgkin's lymphomas. Summary and description of a working formulation for clinical usage. *Cancer,* **49,** 2112–35.

Parsonnet, J. *et al.* (1994). *Helicobacter pylori* infection and gastric lymphoma. *New England Journal of Medicine,* **330,** 1267–71.

Petersen, F.B. *et al.* (1990). Autologous transplantation for malignant lymphoma. A report of 101 cases from Seattle. *Journal of Clinical Oncology,* **8,** 638–47.

Portlock, C.S., Rosenberg, S.A., Glatstein, E., and Kaplan, H.S. (1978). Impact of salvage treatment on initial relapses in patients with Hodgkin disease, stages I–III. *Blood,* **51,** 825–33.

Porzig, K.J., Portlock, C.S., Robertson, A., and Rosenberg, S.A. (1978). Treatment of advanced Hodgkin's disease with B-CA Ve following MOPP failure. *Cancer,* **41,** 1670–5.

Prchal, J.T., Crago, S.S., Mestecky, J., Okos, A.J., and Flint, A. (1981). Immunoblastic lymphoma: an immunologic study. *Cancer,* **47,** 2312–18.

Robinson, B., Kingston, J., Costa, R.N., Malpas, J.S., Barrett, A., and McElwain, T.J. (1984). Chemotherapy and irradiation in childhood Hodgkin's disease. *Archives of Disease in Childhood,* **59,** 1162–7.

Rowley, J.D. and Fukuhara, S. (1980). Chromosome studies in non-Hodgkin's lymphomas. *Seminars in Oncology,* **7,** 255–66.

Safai, B. and Good, R.A. (1980). Lymphoproliferative disorders of the T-cell series. *Medicine (Baltimore),* **59,** 335–51.

Santoro, A., Bonfante, V. and Bonadonna, G. (1982). Salvage chemotherapy with ABVD in MOPP-resistant Hodgkin's disease. *Annals of Internal Medicine,* **96,** 139–143.

Scott, G.L., Myles, A.B. and Bacon, P.A. (1968). Autoimmune haemolytic anaemia and mefenamic acid therapy. *British Medical Journal,* **3,** 534–6.

Shipp, M.A. *et al.* (1993). A predictive model for aggressive non-Hodgkin's lymphoma. The International Non-Hodgkin's Lymphoma Prognostic Factors Project. *New England Journal of Medicine,* **329,** 987–94.

Smithers, D.W. (1967). *British Medical Journal,* **2,** 263.

Stuart, A.E., Stansfeld, A.G., and Lauder, I. (ed.) (1981). *Lymphomas other than Hodgkin's disease.* Oxford University Press.

Sutcliffe, S.B. *et al.* (1978). MVPP chemotherapy regimen for advanced Hodgkin's disease. *British Medical Journal,* **1,** 679–83.

Tester, W.J. *et al.* (1984). Second malignant neoplasms complicating Hodgkin's disease: the National Cancer Institute Experience. *Journal of Clinical Oncology,* **2,** 762–8.

Watanabe, S., Shimosato, Y., and Nakajima, T. (1983). Proliferative disorders of histiocytes. In *Malignant lymphomas,* (ed. S.C. Sommers and P.P. Rosen), pp. 65–108. Appleton-Century-Crofts, Norwalk, CT.

22.5.4. The spleen and its disorders

S. M. LEWIS AND D. SWIRSKY

Since Hippocratic times the role of the spleen has been controversial. Galen called it an organ of mystery; the elucidation of the mystery has been a long slow process! Its structure was described during the seventeenth and early eighteenth centuries by Harvey, Glisson, Wharton, Malpighi, and van Leeuwenhoek. In 1777, William Hewson recognized an association with the lymphatic system, and in 1846 Virchow demonstrated that the Malpighian follicles are concerned with the formation of white blood cells. In 1885, Ponfick showed that the spleen can remove particles from the blood and might be involved in its destruction. Two years later Spencer Wells performed a laparotomy on a 27-year-old woman with a lifelong history of the passage of dark urine with attacks of jaundice and who had an abdominal tumour thought to be a fibroid. This turned out to be a large spleen and its removal was followed by a complete remission. The retrospective diagnosis of hereditary spherocytosis was made by Lord Dawson of Penn some 40 years later, by which time splenectomy was being performed quite frequently for leukaemia, Hodgkin's disease, Banti's haemolytic jaundice, Gaucher's disease, polycythaemia, and thrombocytopenic purpura. The frequent success of the operation led Doan and Dameshek and their respective supporters to engage in a lively argument on the mechanisms whereby the spleen can destroy blood cells or suppress their formation, a process which Chauffard had earlier called 'hypersplenism'.

The past two decades have seen the resolution of many of these problems and there is now a much greater understanding of the functions of the spleen in health and its involvement in disease. Methods have been developed by which the various functions of the spleen can be defined and measured. Some of them have important clinical applications.

Structure of the spleen

At birth the spleen is about 4.5 cm in length, 2.5 cm wide, and 1.5 cm thick, and the mean weight is 11 g. By the age of 1 year the weight is 15 to 25 g; by 5 years it is 40 to 70 g, and by 10 years it is 80 to 100 g. It reaches its maximum weight of about 200 to 300 g soon after puberty, and is slightly lighter throughout adult life until the age of 65 years, when it decreases to 100 to 150 g or less. It is slightly heavier in the adult male than in the female. These figures have been derived from autopsy studies; they are probably underestimates. This is mainly due to the splenic red-cell pool, which will be described later. Ultrasound, computerized tomography, and scintigraphic radionuclide scans have shown that, *in vivo,* the normal adult spleen has a length of 8 to 13 cm, a width of 4.5 to 7 cm, a surface area of the order of 45 to 80 cm², and a volume less than 275 cm³. A spleen greater than 14 cm long is usually palpable. It should be noted, however, that the spleen is mobile and palpation does not always provide a reliable guide to its size.

The spleen has a complicated structure (Fig. 1). It consists of a connective tissue framework, vascular channels, lymphatic tissue, lymph drainage channels, and cellular components of the haemopoietic and reticuloendothelial systems. Histologically, there are two main components: (i) the red pulp; and (ii) the white pulp. The red pulp consists of sinuses and pulp cords. The sinuses, 20 to 40 μm in diameter, are lined by endothelial macrophages. The white pulp consists of periarteriolar lymphoid sheath and the adjoining follicles (Malpighian bodies), which contain a germinal centre and are structurally similar to lymphoid follicles. The outer capsule of the connective tissue framework consists of collagen tissue with elastic fibres covered by serous endothelium. From this come off a large number of lace-like trabeculae that extend into the pulp, carrying blood vessels, and autonomic nerve fibres. Within the spleen the trabeculae are in direct continuity with a mesh of reticular fibres that supports the pulp vessels and forms the basement membranes of arterial capillaries and the splenic sinuses. Along the reticular fibres lie adventitial reticular cells. These cells have an important role in regulating blood flow through the interendothelial slits of the vascular sinuses.

Blood is brought to the spleen via the splenic artery and thence, through the trabecular arteries, into the central arteries, which are sited in the white pulp. The central arteries run into the central axis of the peri-arteriolar lymphatic sheaths; they give off many arterioles and capillaries, some of which terminate in the white pulp whilst others go on to the red pulp. There they either connect directly with the sinuses and thence, via the collecting vein, to the trabecular vein (closed system), or they first pass into the cord spaces before joining up with the sinuses (open system).

Thus, as the blood flows through the spleen it will come into contact with the reticular fibres, and also with endothelial macrophages, which lie in the interstices of the reticular mesh.

BLOOD FLOW IN THE SPLEEN

Because the spleen has two vascular systems (closed and open) as described above, there are both rapid- and slow-transit components in the splenic circulation. The rapid transit (closed system) is of the order

Fig. 1 Diagramatic illustration of the circulation of the spleen. The blood passes either directly into a sinus (C, closed system) or first into the cord spaces in the red pulp (O, open system).

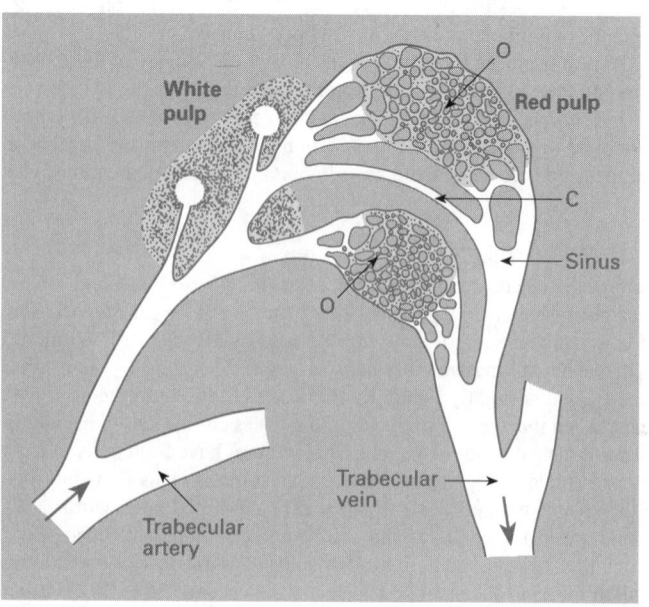

of 1 to 2 min and slow transit (open system) about 30 to 60 min. In normal subjects the open system has a minor role and the blood flows through the spleen as rapidly as through organs possessing a conventional vasculature, at a rate of 5 to 10 per cent of the blood volume per minute, so that each day the circulating blood has repeated passages through the spleen. In splenomegaly, the blood flow through the spleen increases up to 20 per cent or more of the blood volume per minute. At the same time, a certain proportion of the blood may be pooled in the cord spaces (see below). During the flow of the blood, the plasma and the leucocytes pass preferentially to the white pulp by a process of plasma skimming, and the plasma rapidly reaches the venous system, whilst blood with a relatively high packed-cell volume remains in the axial stream of the central artery. Some of this blood flows directly through the sinusoids to the venous system, while the remainder passes into the cords of the red pulp; the normally flexible red cells squeeze through endothelial slits into the sinuses, whilst cells with fixed membranes or with inclusions that render them relatively inflexible remain in the cords where they either become conditioned for later transit or are destroyed.

Functions of the spleen

In this section the physiological functions of the spleen will be described, together with the way in which these are changed in various pathological conditions.

HAEMOPOIESIS

In the fetus the spleen plays a relatively minor part in haemopoiesis in comparison with the liver. There is, however, some erythropoiesis and granulopoiesis in the spleen from the 12th week; this continues until birth, after which there is normally no demonstrable haemopoiesis. However, the potential remains, and under severe haematological stress, in thalassaemia and in chronic haemolytic anaemias for example, extramedullary erythropoiesis may occur together with intensive erythroid hyperplasia of the bone marrow, presumably as a compensatory mechanism. This must be distinguished from myeloid metaplasia occurring in myelofibrosis (Chapter 22.3.9) and occasionally in patients with leukaemia or secondary carcinoma. In these conditions, foci of haemopoietic tissue become established in the spleen and elsewhere outside the bone marrow. They represent an abnormal proliferation, which is distinct from compensatory erythropoiesis.

The spleen contains a large bulk of lymphoid tissue. It is not a major site of lymphopoiesis; most of the lymphocytes in the white pulp of the spleen migrate there from other sites of origin such as the bone marrow and thymus. However, the germinal centres of the spleen may respond to antigenic stimulus by proliferation of lymphocytes.

CELL SEQUESTRATION, PHAGOCYTOSIS, AND POOLING

The spleen has a remarkable ability to 'cleanse' or 'recondition' red cells for recirculation and also to remove from the circulation effete or damaged cells as well as foreign matter. Of particular importance is the trapping of encapsulated bacteria. Unfortunately, as is the case with so many physiological phenomena, these useful functions may become harmful under certain circumstances.

It is important to distinguish between the three mechanisms which are involved: sequestration is a temporary (reversible) process whereby cells are held in the spleen before returning to the circulation; phagocytosis represents the irreversible uptake of non-viable cells by macrophages or destruction of viable cells that have been damaged in some way, perhaps by prolonged sequestration or by deposition of antibody on the cell surface; pooling is the presence in the spleen of an increased amount of blood (or some of its component parts). In contrast to sequestration, pooled cells are in continuous exchange with the circulation.

As blood flows through the sinuses and cords, effete and damaged cells, and particulate foreign matter are promptly phagocytosed by the endothelial macrophages. Intact cells are held up temporarily, during which time siderotic granules, Howell–Jolly bodies, and Heinz bodies are removed by 'pitting'. In this process the particles are taken out with a small amount of cell membrane but without destroying the cell. After the inclusions have been removed the red cells return to the circulation. Sequestration of reticulocytes also occurs, and they are retained in the splenic cords for part of their last 2 or 3 days of maturation while they lose their intracellular inclusions, alter their surface membrane composition, and become smaller. The spleen normally sequesters 30 to 45 per cent of the total circulating platelet content of the blood. This platelet pool is rapidly mobilizable under conditions of stress, and normally there is a constant transit between spleen and vascular pools.

As the blood becomes more viscous in the spleen, red cells are subjected to a further hazard. Because they are packed together in the presence of metabolically active macrophages, they are deprived of oxygen and glucose. This increases their membrane rigidity and reduces their deformability. Cells may become inflexible if: (a) they are metabolically abnormal (as in certain congenital haemolytic anaemias) and thus unduly sensitive to the unfavourable environment of the spleen; (b) if they are held up in the spleen for a prolonged period and are thus rendered metabolically abnormal; and (c) if they are already spherical (as in hereditary spherocytosis), fragmented (as in microangiopathic haemolytic anaemia), or misshapen in some other way (see Chapter 22.1). This results in their being trapped in the cord spaces where they subsequently undergo phagocytosis. This is the process by which heat-damaged or chemically altered cells are taken up in the spleen. Cells that have been sequestered and damaged may also end their lives in this way. Identifying the role of the spleen or splenunculi in cell destruction is an important aspect of the management of patients with immune cytopenias.

IMMUNOLOGICAL FUNCTION

The spleen contains the largest single accumulation of lymphoid tissue in the body; about 25 per cent of the total T-lymphocyte pool and 10 to 15 per cent of the B-lymphocyte pool, with very marked exchange between circulating and splenic lymphocytes.

Micro-organisms or other antigens that find their way to the spleen are taken up by the cord macrophages and are delivered to immunocompetent cells in the lymphoid tissue. This stimulates antibody production and an increase in the size of lymphoid germinal centres of the spleen. Secondary stimulation with the antigen enhances antibody production, usually IgG. Red cells sensitized by IgG antibody do not, as a rule, agglutinate in the peripheral blood, but the environment in the spleen promotes local agglutination with consequent sequestration and destruction. At the same time the antibody-coated cells lose pieces of their membrane as they come in contact with Fc receptors on macrophages, and become spherical and less flexible each time they pass through the sinus vasculature, until finally they become too rigid to traverse the endothelial pores and thus are trapped, as described above. The rate of cell destruction in the spleen is influenced in opposite ways by two factors. On the one hand, increased cell destruction results in an expanding number of mononuclear macrophages in the splenic cords and hence in increased lysis. On the other hand, the damaged red-cell load tends to blockade the reticuloendothelial cells and thus reduce their phagocytic potential, at least temporarily.

BLOOD POOL

The normal red-cell content of the spleen is less than 80 ml of red cells, and always less than 5 per cent of the total red-cell mass; there is no significant red-cell pool. However, enlarged spleens are capable of developing remarkably large pools with a relatively slow exchange of red cells with the general circulation. In the myeloproliferative disorders, as much as 40 per cent of the blood volume, representing a litre of blood, may be present in the spleen. Increased pools also occur in lymphoproliferative disorders especially hairy-cell leukaemia and prolymphocytic leukaemia.

In health there is a good correlation between the amount of blood in the spleen and its size. In myeloproliferative disorders the pool is disproportionately large and is a major cause of splenomegaly. In lymphomas, however, the splenomegaly is sometimes greater than can be accounted for by the pool alone, possibly because in such cases the increase in spleen size is due primarily to an expansion of the lymphoid components with replacement of splenic sinuses by tumour. In myelofibrosis, on the other hand, there is an increase of the reticular element with expansion of the closed system in the red pulp. A similar effect occurs in hairy-cell leukaemia (see Chapter 22.3.6).

Not unexpectedly, the red-cell content of the spleen increases with increasing body haematocrit. There is a disproportionately increased pool in polycythaemia vera compared with secondary polycythaemia, where the pool remains small irrespective of the haematocrit level. This suggests that in polycythaemia vera there is a fundamental structural alteration in the spleen with an expansion of the closed system. Increased pools are also found in patients with hepatic cirrhosis. Here it is the increased portal pressure that leads to an increased splenic blood flow: the splenic arteries are dilated and the splenic pulp becomes expanded with prominent dilated sinuses. Conversely, it has been observed that portal hypertension is not uncommon as a secondary event in myeloproliferative disorders with splenomegaly (see Chapter 22.3.9).

In myeloproliferative disorders and some other conditions an enlarged splenic blood pool may contribute significantly to the anaemia. A low venous haematocrit can be present despite a normal red-cell mass (pseudoanaemia). Direct measurement of splenic red-cell volume makes it possible to predict the extent to which splenectomy will result in improvement in the anaemia and in reducing transfusion requirements.

Platelets also have a significant reservoir in the spleen, which is rapidly interchangeable with the circulation. In some cases of thrombocytopenia, destruction occurs mainly in the spleen and it is essential to distinguish this from pooling. As far as granulocytes are concerned, no pool is demonstrable in the normal spleen but an abnormally large marginal pool has been found in cases of splenomegaly associated with neutropenia.

PLASMA VOLUME CONTROL

The mechanism by which plasma volume is controlled is not clear. There is a complex neurohumoral mechanism that controls the fluid equilibrium between interstitial and intracellular compartments, ensuring that the water volume and electrolyte concentration in the circulating blood are both kept within normal limits. Under normal conditions, the red-cell volume is fairly constant while the plasma volume undergoes continual transient variations which trigger off the necessary adjustments which ensure that the total blood volume remains constant. There is no evidence that the spleen is involved in this mechanism. However, when the spleen is enlarged, it does play a role, and splenomegaly is frequently associated with an increased plasma volume, which may lead to an apparent anaemia (so-called pseudoanaemia or dilutional anaemia). Several possible mechanisms have been suggested to explain the expanded plasma volume in splenomegaly: (a) the enlarged organ requires an expansion of blood volume to fill the additional intravascular space; in conditions where marrow erythropoietic activity is reduced, as in myelosclerosis, it may not be possible to maintain the normal red-cell/plasma volume ratio and the additional volume is provided by plasma alone; (b) increased pressure in the portal vein and an increase in splanchnic blood volume resulting from obstructive or hyperkinetic portal hypertension; and (c) protein alterations, especially increased globulin levels with reduced albumin, resulting in an alteration in colloid oncotic pressure.

The last mechanism has been suggested as a factor in tropical splenomegalies and in cirrhosis. In blood dyscrasias, the increase in plasma volume is directly proportional to the size of the spleen; this is not so in cirrhosis.

Table 1 *Some characteristics of an enlarged spleen*

Moves downward and medially on inspiration
Dull to percussion
A notch may be palpable on medial margin
Does not push through from left loin (cf. left kidney)
Is difficult to insert fingers above mass under left costal margin (cf. left kidney)

Table 2 *Differential diagnosis of swellings in left upper quadrant of the abdomen*

Spleen
Left kidney
Tumours of splenic flexure of colon
Masses arising from the stomach
Retroperitoneal masses

Splenomegaly

A palpable spleen is usually enlarged. Occasionally a normal spleen is palpable if it is displaced downwards, by a pleural effusion for example. Useful information may be obtained from assessing the size of the spleen together with any related clinical and haematological findings, but a firm diagnosis often requires special investigations of splenic function and, occasionally, diagnostic laparotomy and splenectomy.

CLINICAL DETECTION OF SPLENOMEGALY (SEE ALSO CHAPTER 22.1)

As the spleen enlarges it moves forwards, downwards, and medially towards the right iliac fossa. The features which suggest that a left-sided mass is a spleen are summarized in Table 1.

The spleen has to be 1.5 to 2 times its normal size to be palpable; imaging procedures provide more reliable methods for measuring the actual spleen size. These include radionuclide scans, ultrasonic scans, computerized tomography (**CT**), and nuclear magnetic resonance imaging (**MRI**). In clinical practice the usual method for expressing the extent of splenomegaly is in centimetres below the left costal margin. The differential diagnosis of a mass in the left hypochondrium is summarized in Table 2.

CAUSES OF SPLENOMEGALY

So many conditions are associated with splenomegaly that it is impossible to give a comprehensive list. It is even more difficult to list the 'common' causes as these depend on geographical pathology. In western Europe and the United States viral infection and portal hypertension are the most common causes of splenomegaly and these together with leukaemias, malignant lymphomas, myeloproliferative disorders, haemolytic anaemias, and other infections account for most cases. Globally, however, the incidence of these haematological causes of splenomegaly is swamped by the great preponderance of splenic enlargement caused by parasitic infections, particularly malaria, leishmaniasis, and schistosomiasis. Human immunodeficiency virus (**HIV**) infection, particularly in the later stages of the disease, is an increasing cause of mild to moderate splenomegaly. In some countries haemoglobinopathies head the list. Portal hypertension is an important cause of splenomegaly in most tropical countries but it is especially prevalent in north-eastern India and southern China. The 'tropical splenomegaly syndrome' is seen commonly in New Guinea and Central Africa.

Some of the causes of splenomegaly are listed in Table 3, which also gives some indication of the relative size of the spleen in various conditions. The spleen sizes indicated are only a rough guide; clearly, where

Table 3 *Some causes of enlargement of the spleen*

Acute bacterial, viral, and other infections
Chronic bacterial infections: tuberculosis and brucellosis
Chronic parasitic infections: malaria, kala azar, schistosomiasis*
Idiopathic non-tropical splenomegaly*
Tropical splenomegaly*
'Congestive': portal and biliary cirrhosis; portal vein obstruction; splenic vein obstruction; Budd–Chiari syndrome; cardiac failure
Inherited haemolytic anaemia
Hereditary spherocytosis (HS)
Symptomatic elliptocytosis
Structural haemoglobinopathy
Thalassaemia
Red-cell enzyme defects
Acquired haemolytic anaemia
Warm-antibody haemolytic anaemia
Cold agglutinin disease
Primary blood disorders
Acute leukaemia
Chronic myeloid leukaemia*
Chronic lymphatic leukaemia
Hairy-cell leukaemia*
Polycythaemia vera
Myelofibrosis*
Megaloblastic anaemia
Malignant lymphoma
Hodgkin's disease
Non-Hodgkin's lymphoma
HIV infection
Acute seroconversion episode
Advancing disease, preAIDS
AIDS
AIDS-related lymphoma
AIDS-related opportunistic infection
Miscellaneous
Amyloid, sarcoidosis, tumour of the spleen
Connective tissue disorders
Systemic lupus erythromatosus
Felty's syndrome
Storage diseases
Gaucher's disease*
Niemann–Pick disease
Histiocytosis X*

* May be associated with massive splenomegaly.

the spleen is markedly enlarged, it will have been enlarging progressively at earlier stages and it may have been only just palpable at an earlier stage of the disease. Most of the conditions listed are described in other sections of the book. Those in which splenomegaly is the primary or an especially important feature are described below.

HYPERSPLENISM

Hypersplenism is a clinical syndrome of varied aetiology. It is characterized by:

1. Splenomegaly, although this may be only moderate.
2. Pancytopenia or a reduction in the number of one or more types of the blood cells: neutropenia is less common than anaemia and thrombocytopenia.

3. Normal production or hyperplasia of the precursor cells in the marrow or a so-called maturation arrest with paucity of the more mature cells but orderly maturation in the earlier stages. Some of the megakaryocytes show unusual features of sharply demarcated cytoplasmic borders and no granularity or signs of platelet formation.
4. Premature release of cells into peripheral blood, resulting in a mild reticulocytosis with nucleated red cells and occasional immature granulocytes.

Other features are:

5. Decreased red-cell survival.
6. Decreased platelet survival.
7. Hypervolaemia (i.e. increased plasma volume) if splenomegaly is marked.

The mechanisms which produce the various parts of the syndrome were considered earlier.

The haematological features may be obscured or dominated by the primary disease, especially if it involves the marrow. The diagnosis of hypersplenism is ultimately confirmed by response to splenectomy, although an immediate remission may be followed in the longer term by relapse with return of cytopenia.

TROPICAL SPLENOMEGALY SYNDROME (BIG SPLEEN DISEASE)

In areas where malaria is endemic, adults may present with moderate to massive splenomegaly, no obvious signs of active malaria, but all the features of hypersplenism including pancytopenia, expanded plasma volume, and haemolysis. It is apparently secondary to malaria, the evidence being its geographical incidence, the presence of raised titres of malaria antibody and the fact that, on continuous long-term antimalarial therapy, there is a marked and sustained reduction in spleen size, the pancytopenia remits, and the patient improves. The serum IgM level is usually high, and this decreases to normal concomitantly with response to antimalarial therapy. The spleen shows diffuse reticuloendothelial hyperplasia. These features suggest that the pathogenesis is an intense immunological response to circulating antigens with immune-complex formation and phagocytosis as a result of repeated exposure to the malarial parasite. It is not clear why this effect is only seen in a proportion of individuals in areas of the world where malaria is endemic (see above).

A similar degree of splenomegaly occurs in schistosomiasis (see Section 7) but in this condition there is the further complication that the eggs (especially *Schistosoma mansoni*) have a direct effect on the liver, resulting in hepatic fibrosis, and leading to portal hypertension.

NON-TROPICAL IDIOPATHIC SPLENOMEGALY

A number of patients present with marked splenomegaly and the haematological features of hypersplenism, but without exposure to malaria or other parasitic disorders. There may be a positive antiglobulin test and other evidence of autoantibody production. Some of these patients have a malignant lymphoma at the time of presentation but in others the essential feature is non-neoplastic lymphoid hyperplasia, which probably represents an immunological reaction to as yet unidentified stimuli. The chances of long-term cure after splenectomy appear to be good. However, a lymphoma may appear at periods ranging from months to years after splenectomy in this condition. The disorder is diagnosed by the finding of massive splenomegaly in the absence of any other cause and by the non-specific histological appearances of the spleen.

STORAGE DISEASE

The storage diseases are described in detail in Section 11. Some of them, notably Gaucher's disease and Niemann–Pick disease, may be compli-

cated by marked splenomegaly. Particularly in Gaucher's disease this may lead to hypersplenism and it is quite common for the question of splenectomy to arise. It has been suggested that this may lead to acclerated bone damage, and may render patients particularly prone to post-splenectomy sepsis. Although this view remains controversial, splenectomy should only be done in these conditions with great caution.

Niemann–Pick disease

The clinical picture of Niemann–Pick disease (see Section 11) is dominated by hepatosplenomegaly and mental retardation. The disorder presents in infancy, and death often occurs between the second and third years of age, but, as with Gaucher's disease, it may present later in life. In the older age groups hypersplenism becomes a feature, but in the childhood cases, anaemia and thrombocytopenia are uncommon and, if present, are mild. In contrast to Gaucher's disease, the serum acid phosphatase level is normal. The diagnosis depends on finding the characteristic Niemann–Pick cells in the bone marrow. These are 20 to 80 μm in size. The cytoplasm is engorged with globular droplets of sphingomyelin. The cells stain blue-green by Romanowsky stain and greenish yellow with haematoxylin and eosin. The PAS stain is variably positive, oil red O and Sudan black B are, as a rule, positive, and acid phosphatase is negative.

Other lipid storage diseases

Several other rare lipid storage diseases may cause hypersplenism. They include Tangier's disease, in which cholesterol esters fill the histiocytes, and Wolman's disease, which is associated with an accumulation of triglycerides and cholesterol esters. Sea-blue histiocytosis is characterized by splenomegaly, hepatomegaly, thrombocytopenia, and, occasionally, neurological damage. The bone marrow and spleen contain cells that have an accumulation of glycosphingolipids, phospholipids, and mucopolysaccharides. The cells stain blue-green by Romanowsky stain, but in contrast to those in Niemann–Pick disease they stain brownish yellow with haematoxylin and eosin. It is not clear whether this is a specific disorder. Similar cells occur in a wide variety of conditions in which there is excessive breakdown of leucocytes, platelets, and red cells. However, in these disorders there are usually only a few of the abnormal cells in the marrow.

Inborn errors of lipid mechanism give rise to a variety of disorders in which there may be secondary proliferation of histiocytic cells. These include Hand–Schüller–Christian disease, eosinophilic granuloma, and Letterer–Siewe disease, now usually referred to as histiocytosis X. The proliferation of histiocytes is especially active in the spleen, lymphnodes, and bone marrow. Splenomegaly is usually moderate, but occasionally it is more marked and may be associated with hypersplenism (see Chapter 22.3.6).

SPACE-OCCUPYING LESIONS AND INJURY OF THE SPLEEN

The most common causes of splenic masses are trauma leading to haematoma or rupture, abscesses, tumours, and cysts.

Splenic injury

The spleen is relatively unprotected and easily injured. Spontaneous rupture has been reported in a number of conditions in which the spleen is enlarged: these include typhoid, malaria Epstein–Barr virus infection, leukaemia, Gaucher's disease, and polycythaemia. This may be restricted to a subcapsular haematoma or there may be rupture into the peritoneal cavity.

The diagnosis is suggested by the symptoms of shock, left upper quadrant guarding and tenderness, pain referred to the left shoulder, and clinical and laboratory evidence of bleeding. Straight abdominal radiography is not, as a rule, helpful in diagnosis but CT scanning, splenic arteriography, ultrasound examination, or isotope scanning may be more useful.

22 DISORDERS OF THE BLOOD

3592 22 DISORDERS OF THE BLOOD

Abscess

Although the spleen is frequently enlarged in association with systemic infection, splenic abscesses are rare. They result from direct or haematogenous spread, or when a haematoma becomes infected. Conditions associated with splenic infarction, such as sickle-cell disease, are particularly likely to give rise to splenic abscesses. Almost any organism can be involved.

Metastatic tumour

Metastases in the spleen are uncommon by comparison to other organs; they occur late in the course of primary carcinoma and are not found in the absence of metastases elsewhere. Metastases in the spleen are most frequently derived from malignant lymphomas, especially Hodgkin's disease, and reticulum-cell sarcoma. Lung, breast, prostate, colon, and stomach are the organs from which carcinoma is most likely to disseminate to the spleen. Melanoma is also a relatively frequent primary source.

Cysts

Splenic cysts are rare. The most frequent is due to *Taenia echinococcus* (hydatid); other causes include haemangiomas, lymphangiomas, and dermoids. Cysts may also develop in area of haemorrhage or infarction. A splenic scan is a particularly useful method for identifying a cyst and recognizing it as the cause of apparent splenomegaly (Fig. 2)

Loss of spleen function and splenic infarction

SPLENIC HYPOPLASIA OR ATROPHY

Congenital hypoplasia is rare; in some cases it is associated with extensive developmental abnormalities of the heart and gut. Splenic atrophy may occur in a number of acquired conditions—sickle-cell disease, coeliac disease, dermatitis herpetiformis, ulcerative colitis, Crohn's disease, essential thrombocythaemia, and Fanconi anaemia. Steroid therapy and cytotoxic drugs cause atrophy of the white pulp, especially the germinal centres. The spleen shrinks in size in old age. Vascular blockade and infarction is the basis for splenic atrophy in sickle cell disease (see Chapter 22.4.7) and this may also be the case in thrombocythaemia (see Chapter 22.3.10). The peripheral blood changes of hyposplenism, when present, are proportional to disease activity in gut diseases. In coeliac disease, withdrawal of gluten from the diet reverses the changes unless splenic atrophy has occurred. The mechanism of splenic atrophy is unknown.

Splenic hypofunction and atrophy are characterized by changes in the blood film appearances; the main features are the presence of Howell–Jolly bodies and siderotic granules in some of the red cells. This is due to loss of the spleen's pitting function. Depression of sequestering activity, which usually occurs at the same time, can be identified by a scan after administration of isotope-labelled, damaged red cells, combined with the measurement of the rate of clearance of the cells from circulation (see below). Pitting and phagocytosis are, however, separate functions and there may be dissociation of these activities in an individual patient.

SPLENIC INFARCTION

Splenic infarction occurs quite frequently in patients who have very large spleens. It is particularly common in association with myelosclerosis and chronic myeloid leukaemia. It also occurs in the majority of patients with sickle-cell anaemia. In this disorder, splenic infarction occurs early in life and repeated episodes result in an autosplenectomy (see Chapter 22.4.7). Occasionally, when there is the rapid growth of the spleen in association with an aggressive form of non-Hodgkin's lymphoma, particularly histiocytic medullary reticulosis, there may be multiple infarctions and spontaneous rupture of the spleen with the signs mentioned in an earlier section.

Splenic infarction causes pain in the left upper quadrant. If the diaphragmatic surface of the spleen is involved, the pain may be referred to the left shoulder tip. The physical signs include tenderness over the spleen, and sometimes a loud splenic rub is heard. Treatment is by rest and analgesia. The occurrence of repeated splenic infarction may be an indication for splenectomy, although it should be remembered that the history of episodes of this type usually indicates that there will be multiple adhesions between the spleen and the overlying peritoneum.

Investigation of splenic function

Assessment of splenic function is often required in investigating a haematological disorder, particularly if splenectomy is contemplated. In many conditions it is sufficient to assess the spleen size, examine the peripheral blood for evidence of pancytopenia or a reduction in the number of neutrophils and platelets, and to examine the bone marrow to determine whether haemopoiesis is normal. Often this simple approach,

Fig. 2 Spleen scan (with radionuclide-labelled heat damaged cells) from a boy who presented with splenomegaly. (a) The scan showed uptake of the label predominantly in the area below the costal margin. (b) At laparotomy the upper two-thirds of the spleen was found to be occupied by a large splenic cyst. (Illustration by courtesy of Dr J. Pettit: reproduced by permission of *Clinics in Hematology* **6**, 640, 1977.)

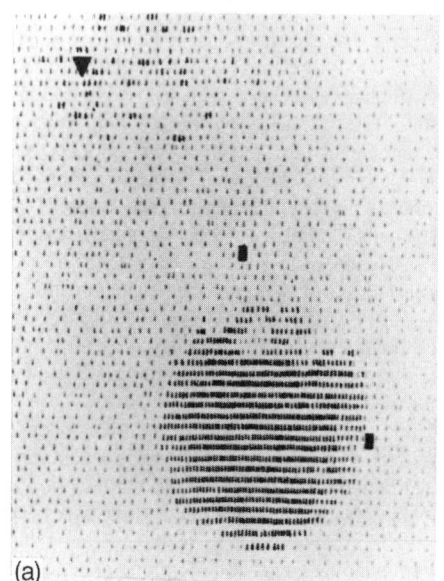

(a)

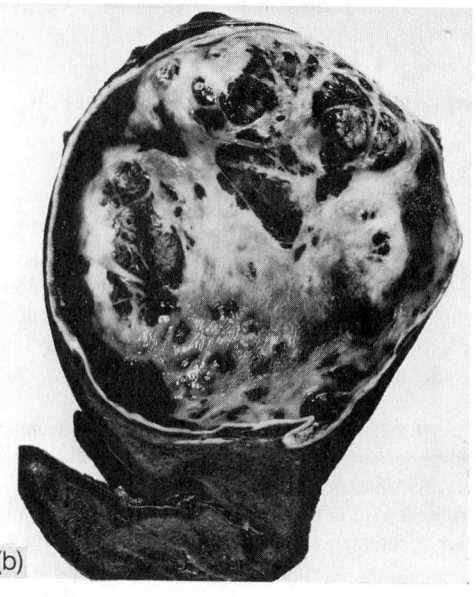

(b)

combined with a knowledge of the likely effects of splenectomy for a particular haematological disorder, will be all that is necessary to make a decision about whether to proceed to surgery. Sometimes, however, it is helpful to carry out more sophisticated studies to define more thoroughly the functions of the spleen. This approach is also useful occasionally for establishing an accurate haematological diagnosis.

Studies with radionuclides provide information about the extent of splenic involvement in a disease process, the role of the spleen in producing anaemia, and the likely benefits of splenectomy.

The following list summarizes the various *in vivo* tests that have been developed for investigating splenic function:

(1) delineation of functional splenic tissue;
(2) estimation of spleen size;
(3) measurement of splenic blood flow;
(4) measurement of splenic red-cell pool;
(5) measurement of phagocytic function (irreversible extraction);
(6) identification of sites of red-cell destruction ('surface counting');
(7) quantification of splenic red-cell destruction;
(8) plasma volume changes of splenomegaly;
(9) identification and quantification of splenic extramedullary erythropoiesis;
(10) role of spleen in platelet kinetics, especially in thrombocytopenia

Fig. 3 Images obtained by scintillation camera following administration of (a) ^{99}Tc-labelled red cells and (b) ^{111}In-labelled heat-damaged red cells.

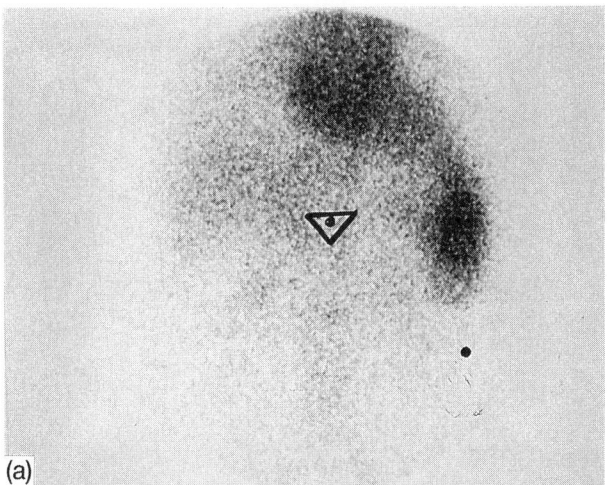
(a)

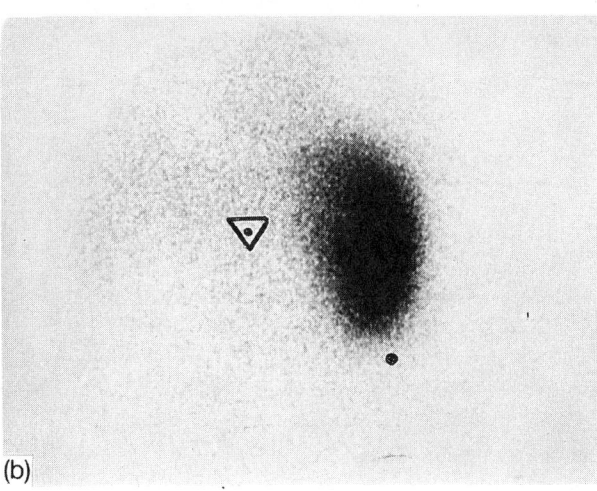
(b)

Details of the methods used and analysis of results obtained in various conditions are to be found in specialized textbooks (e.g. Dacie and Lewis, 1991). The combination of investigations used depends on the particular clinical problem. For example, spleen pool-size measurement may help to distinguish secondary polycythaemia from polycythaemia vera. In many conditions associated with splenomegaly, it is important to distinguish increased reticuloendothelial macrophage activity causing cell destruction from increased red-cell accumulation in a large pool, and to what extent enlargement of the spleen is due to tumour infiltration. Surface counting following injection of ^{51}Cr-labelled erythrocytes provides a qualitative indication of splenic red-cell destruction in various haemolytic anaemias; quantitative scanning provides a more accurate measurement of the actual proportion of the cells that are destroyed in the spleen and elsewhere. In myelofibrosis and hypersplenism, it may be helpful to determine the relative importance of the splenic red-cell pool, red-cell destruction, and extramedullary erythropoiesis (see below).

The most useful test is delineation of functional splenic tissue. The spleen can be visualized and its size estimated by scintillation scanning following injection of labelled red cells after they have been damaged artificially in a way which ensures that they will be removed from the circulation by the spleen, e.g. by heating to 50 °C. The picture obtained by a gamma-camera or rectilinear scanner (Fig. 3) demonstrates whether a mass in the left upper abdomen is a spleen. The technique is most useful for identifying accessory spleens (splenunculi) associated with post-splenectomy relapse of immune thrombocytopenia. It will help to diagnose space-occupying lesions of the spleen such as cysts (Fig. 2), haemangiomas, and haematomas. Infarcts and tumour deposits in the spleen are less easily demonstrated unless they are larger than 2 to 3 cm, in diameter. Conversely, functional asplenia, previous splenectomy, or splenic atrophy are readily detected. Hypofunction may occur when a tumour or cyst obliterates a large part of the splenic tissue.

Recording the spleen size is useful for monitoring response to therapy and for staging in myeloproliferative disorders. In polycythaemia vera, splenomegaly is an important diagnostic feature; in some cases in which the spleen is not palpable it is possible to show that it is none the less enlarged using this approach.

Fig. 4 Splenic enlargement and increased red cell pool in a patient with myelofibrosis. Demonstrated by scan after administration of ^{113}In^m-labelled red cells. The markings indicate the costal margin. The upper pole of the spleen merges with the image produced by labelled blood in the heart.

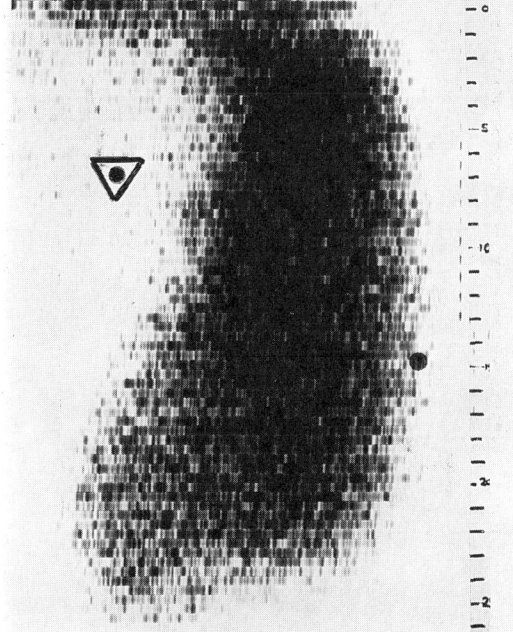

A similar procedure with undamaged, labelled red cells provides a measurement of the splenic red-cell pool. It is a relatively simple procedure that can be done with standard scanning equipment. (Figs 3 and 4).

The increased pool that occurs in the myeloproliferative and lymphoproliferative disorders has been described above. The extent of splenic red-cell pool should be taken into account when assessing the significance of associated anaemia. Measuring the pool is particularly useful for distinguishing polycythaemia vera from secondary polycythaemia.

The rate at which heat-damaged red cells are cleared from circulation provides a rough guide to the competence of splenic function. A slow clearance ($t_{1/2}$ greater than 15 min) is due to a combination of slow splenic blood flow and decreased phagocytic function. A slow clearance may identify splenic hypofunction before the blood film shows Howell–Jolly bodies and other morphological changes. Occasionally, there is the paradox of slow clearance and splenomegaly. This has been seen in children with sickle-cell disease, in malignant histiocytosis, and in amyloidosis.

EXTRAMEDULLARY ERYTHROPOIESIS

Normally, transferrin-bound iron passes to the bone marrow where the iron is released and enters erythroblasts for incorporation into the haemoglobin of developing erythrocytes. In the normal spleen, iron does not dissociate from transferrin. Hence uptake of iron, demonstrable by surface counts shortly after administration of ^{59}Fe, indicates that there is erythropoiesis in the spleen. The effectiveness of splenic erythropoi-esis can be assessed by the fall in surface counts on subsequent days coupled with the increase in blood radioactivity as a measure of red-cell production. Extramedullary erythropoiesis in the spleen occurs in the majority of patients with myelosclerosis. A different pattern of iron accumulation in the spleen is seen in patients with haemolytic anaemia with splenic destruction of red cells or in those with splenomegaly and red-cell pooling: initially, surface counting shows no evidence of uptake, but radioactivity increases during the first and second week of the study as the newly formed cells are destroyed or sequestered in the spleen (Fig 5).

A major limitation of surface counting as a means for measuring the extent of erythropoiesis at different sites is that, as only small segments of bone marrow and other organs are examined by a collimated counter, the results may be unrepresentative. Also, radioactivity in the ribs may be confused with splenic activity. Moreover, even if surface counting demonstrates the occurrence of extramedullary erythropoiesis in the spleen, it will fail to measure its extent and is thus of little value in deciding whether splenectomy may be disadvantageous. These limitations can be overcome by quantitative scanning, using cyclotron-produced ^{52}Fe, which has a half-life of only 8 h, and thus can be administered in relatively high doses and on repeated occasions for serial studies at conveniently short intervals. Thus, it is possible to assess the changes in erythropoiesis during the course of the disease, to define more accurately the fraction of an administered dose of labelled iron that is utilized in splenic erythropoiesis, and hence to distinguish splenomegaly due to myeloid metaplasia from that caused by red-cell pooling (Fig. 6). For example, in patients with polycythaemia vera and myelosclerosis, serial studies may be made at conveniently short intervals to assess changes

Fig. 5 ^{59}Fe ferrokinetic counting studies showing the patterns obtained in (a) a normal subject, (b) myelofibrosis with splenic extramedullary erythropoiesis, (c) hypersplenism with pronounced splenic red cell pooling, (d) dyserythropoiesis with splenic phagocytosis M = marrow, S = spleen, L = liver, H = heart (or blood) radioactivity, normalized to the count rate immediately after administration of the isotope.

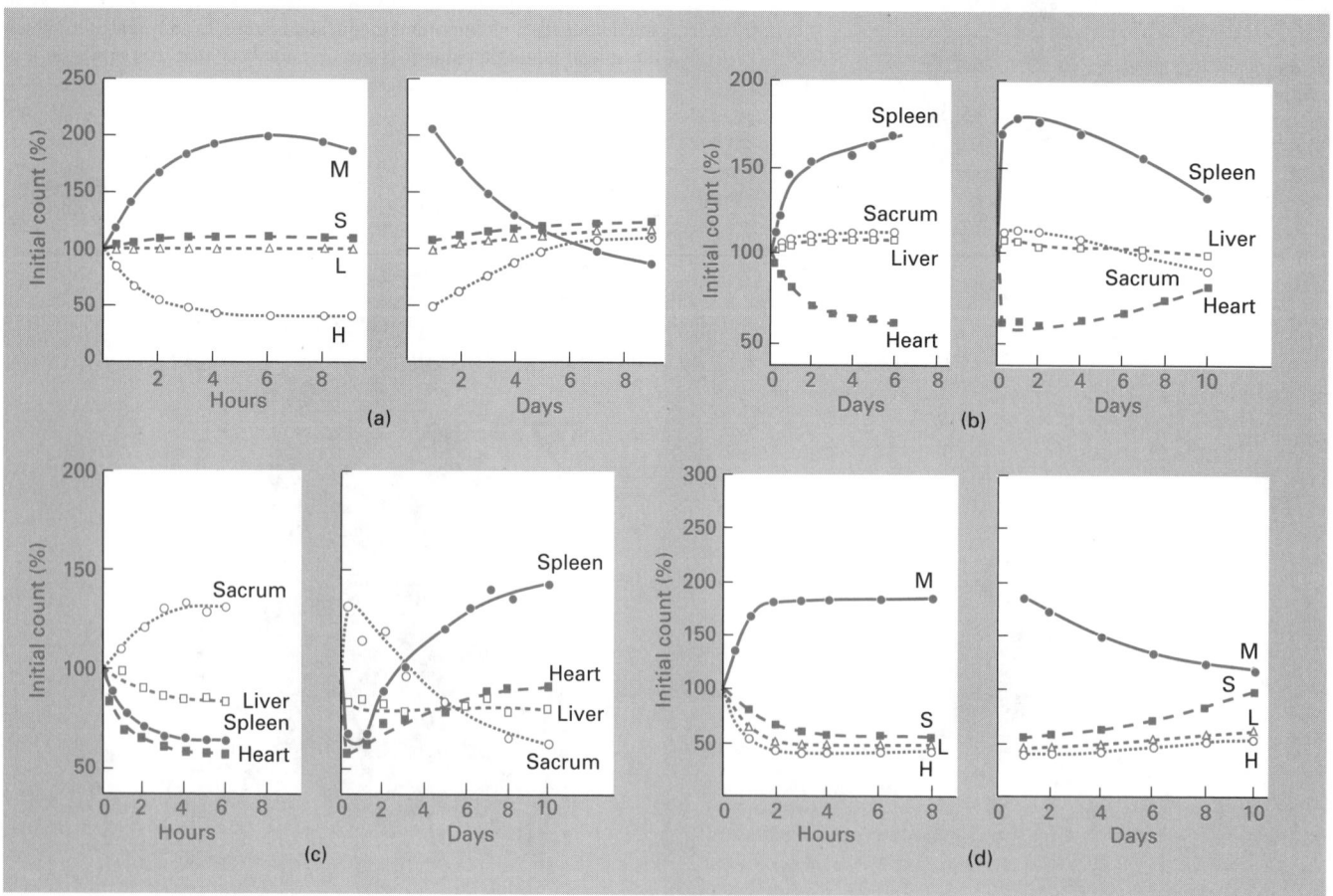

in erythropoiesis, and the effect of various forms of therapy on the clinical course in general and on the spleen in particular. ^{52}Fe studies are useful for detecting early stages of transition from polycythaemia vera to myelosclerosis and for diagnosing the syndrome of transitional myeloproliferative disorder (see Chapter 22.3.9).

PLATELET KINETICS

About one-third of an injection of ^{51}Cr-labelled platelets disappears from circulation during their lifespan, mainly in the spleen pool. Splenomegaly is associated with a marked increase in pooling: by contrast, in asplenia, nearly 100 per cent of the labelled platelets are recovered in the circulating blood. Surface counting has been used to identify the role of the spleen in thrombocytopenia. In some cases the spleen and in others the liver has appeared to be the main site of destruction. However, the clinical usefulness of such counting data in predicting the results of splenectomy is debatable. More reliable information can be derived from quantitative scanning following injection of platelets labelled with ^{111}In oxine. The spleen appears to deal with platelets by pooling and destruction in a manner similar to the way it handles red cells; normally platelets at the end of their lifespan are destroyed to an equal extent by the macrophages of the spleen and bone marrow. In thrombocytopenia there are three patterns of platelet distribution and destruction: (i) platelets have a normal lifespan but there is increased splenic pooling; (ii) there is accelerated destruction but this occurs to an equal degree in the spleen and marrow; (iii) platelet survival is markedly reduced and there is abnormal destruction in the bone marrow. Thus, quantitative platelet kinetic studies with ^{111}In can provide useful information in deciding whether to advise splenectomy for a patient with thrombocytopenia.

Indications for splenectomy

The main indications for splenectomy are summarized in Table 4. Splenectomy should never be undertaken lightly. Where traumatic damage, usually blunt injury, has occurred, every effort should be made to preserve the spleen. Ultrasound and CT imaging are vital in assessing the

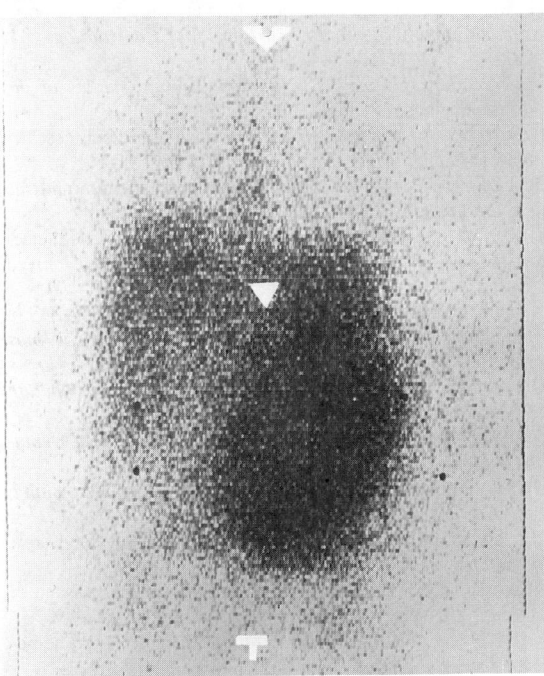

Fig. 6 ^{52}Fe scan in a patient with myelofibrosis showing the extent of splenic erythropoiesis. A small amount of erythropoiesis is demonstrable in the vertebral column.

Table 4 Indications for splenectomy

Definite
Irreparable trauma
Severe haemolytic hereditary spherocytosis
Refractory idiopathic thrombocytopenic purpura

Occasional
Disorders in which hypersplenism becomes a major feature of the clinical picture, e.g. hereditary or acquired haemolytic anaemia, myeloproliferative disease, some lymphomas, portal hypertension, Felty's syndrome, parasitic disease, etc.
Carcinoma of colon, pancreas, etc., involving spleen
Cases in which the cause of the splenomegaly cannot be determined by other methods

damage as rupture and haematoma can be confused clinically. Surgical techniques for repairing or partially preserving the spleen have improved and should be encouraged. The use of diagnostic laparotomy and splenectomy in Hodgkin's disease has fallen into disuse, partly as a result of improved imaging in the CT and MRI scans, and partly because of the absence of therapeutic advantage, combined with the long-term dangers of splenectomy. In primary haematological disorders, splenectomy is indicated to alleviate complications—repeated infarction, massive red-cell pooling, and hypersplenism for example. The decision is usually based on clinical assessment, but radioisotope studies to measure the splenic red-cell pool, splenic erythropoiesis, and red-cell survival may be helpful in difficult cases. Diagnostic splenectomy may still be required for splenic lymphomas where no other organ is affected. Increasingly diagnostic splenectomy may be required in HIV-related diseases, particularly for suspected lymphoma or opportunistic infection.

Clinical and haematological effects of splenectomy

Removal of the spleen is associated with certain immediate and delayed clinical complications, and by the presence of permanent changes in the peripheral blood picture.

CLINICAL COMPLICATIONS

Immediate

In some splenectomies, particularly when the spleen is bound down by adhesions following previous splenic infarction, there may be difficulty in achieving haemostasis. This is particularly so if the patient goes into surgery with a platelet count below 50×10^9/l. It is sometimes useful to administer platelets as soon as the splenic pedicle has been ligated to try to achieve a dry splenic bed. Postoperative collections of blood often become secondarily infected, with the production of a subphrenic abscess. Because the platelet count tends to rise immediately after the operation, there is an increased risk of thromboembolic disease in the first 2 or 3 weeks after splenectomy.

If the preoperative platelet count is 50×10^9/l or greater, subcutaneous heparin can be used. After wound healing, aspirin 75 mg daily should be given if the platelet count is elevated above 500×10^9/l, and continued until this normalizes. There is a small, long-term increase in myocardial infarction in splenectomized patients with persistently raised platelet counts, and in these patients aspirin should be continued indefinitely.

Long-term

All patients, whatever the reason for splenectomy, are at risk of overwhelming post-splenectomy infection (**OPSI**). Classically, OPSI presents with a vague general prodrome followed by prostration, bacteraemic shock, and, frequently, disseminated intravascular coagulation. Death may occur within 6 h of the first symptoms. The mortality rate in patients reaching hospital alive is in excess of 30 per cent. By far the most important causative organism is the pneumococcus (*Streptococcus pneumoniae*), but *Haemophilus influenzae*, *Neisseria meningitidis*, *Escherichia coli*, and Pseudomonas have all been implicated. In endemic areas, Plasmodium and Babesia infections are of increased severity. Special warnings should be given to splenectomized patients travelling to malarial areas. Viral illnesses may also be of increased severity post-splenectomy.

The risk of OPSI does not decline significantly in the years after splenectomy. Children are at greatest risk, followed by adults splenectomized for an underlying disorder that itself is immunosuppressive, or requires immunosuppressive treatment. Adults splenectomized for trauma are least at risk, but still carry a lifelong susceptibility. OPSI has been recorded more than 40 years after splenectomy. The relative risk of severe infection compared to the non-splenectomized population is about 10-fold for traumatic splenectomy and as much as 100-fold for small children and patients with Hodgkin's disease.

Strategies for preventing OPSI

All patients undergoing splenectomy should be immunized with pneumovax, which currently gives variable protection against 23 strains of *S. pneumoniae*. For elective splenectomies it should be given 1 month preoperatively to allow IgG antibody production. In patients with immunosuppressive diseases or treatment, or when it is given perioperatively in an emergency, antibody responses may be suboptimal. Children should also be immunized against *H. influenzae* type b and *N. meningitidis*. Pneumovax is not fully protective, and there are reports of OPSI occurring with strains of *S. pneumoniae* covered by the type of pneumovax given.

Prophylactic penicillin V, 250 mg twice daily, should be started postoperatively. Erythromycin can be substituted in penicillin-sensitive patients. The life-saving value of prophylactic penicillin V in children with sickle-cell disease (i.e. functional asplenia) has been proven beyond doubt, and there are only rare reports of OPSI in splenectomized patients taking regular penicillin. While the penicillin does not prevent infection, it prevents the rapid onset of the OPSI syndrome.

Following spleen rupture, splenic tissue may seed into the peritoneum, giving rise to nodules of recognizable splenic tissue (splenosis). These nodules have been shown to have some reticuloendothelial function. This has led to the deliberate autotransplantation of splenic tissue at the time of splenectomy where partial splenic preservation has not been possible. Although such nodules of splenic tissue can phagocytose damaged red cells and reduce hyposplenic changes on the blood film, their protective capacity from infection is not established. The presence of demonstrable splenosis should not be relied upon to replace vaccination and penicillin prophylaxis.

The safest course is to immunize all patients at the appropriate time, counsel them carefully about the dangers of infection, and impress upon them the need for lifelong penicillin prophylaxis. This should be reinforced at outpatient follow-up visits, and every effort made to maintain good compliance.

Other approaches to reducing the size of the spleen

Reduction of splenic size and function can also be achieved by ligation of the splenic artery or arterial embolization, and by irradiation. In the procedure for embolization, gel foam, silastic microspheres, or metallic coils are introduced by catheter into the splenic artery. It is an effective means of reducing the size and functions of the spleen. However, it carries the risk of infection of disseminated coagulopathy, while inaccurate delivery of the emboli may result in hepatic infarction. Because of the high risk of abscess formation and other complications, this procedure should be limited to patients needing splenectomy but unable to tolerate surgery, for example because of severe thrombocytopenia. Furthermore, it should be followed by surgical removal of the spleen as soon as the patient's clinical condition allows.

REFERENCES

Bateman S., Lewis S.M., Nicholas A., and Zaafran A. (1978). Splenic red cell pooling: a diagnostic feature in polycythaemia. *British Journal of Haematology*, **40**, 389–96.

Bowdler, A.J. (ed.) (1990). *The spleen. Structure, function and clinical significance.* Chapman and Hall Medical, London.

Bowring, C.S. (1977). Quantitative radioisotope scanning and its use in haematology. *Clinics in Haemat* **6**, 625–37.

Brubaker, L.H. and Johnson, C.A. (1978). Correlation of splenomegaly and abnormal neutrophil pooling (margination). *Journal of Laboratory and Clinical Medicine*, **92**, 508–15.

Castanada-Zungia, W.R., Hammerschmidt, D.E., Sanchez R., and Amplatz K. (1977). Nonsurgical splenectomy. *American Journal of Roentgenology*, **129**, 805–11

Christensen, B.E. (1973). Erythrocyte pooling and sequestration in enlarged spleens. Estimations of splenic erythrocyte and plasma volume in splenomegalic patients. *Scandinavian Journal of Haematology*, **10**, 106–19.

Crane, C.G. (1981). Tropical splenomegaly. Part 2: Oceanian. *Clinics in Haematology*, **10**, 976–82.

Crosby, W.H. (1980). The spleen. In *Blood, pure and eloquent*, (ed. M.M. Wintrobe). McGraw-Hill, New York.

Dacie, J.V. and Lewis, S.M. (1991). *Practical haematology*, (7th edn). Churchill Livingstone, Edinburgh.

Fakunle, Y.M. (1981). Tropical splenomegaly. Part 1: Tropical Africa. *Clinics in Haematology*, **10**, 963–75.

Ferrant, A.E., Glass, H.I., Lewis, S.M., and Szur, L. (1975). Quantitatve measurement of splenic and hepatic red-cell destruction. *British Journal of Haematology*, **31**, 467–77.

Ferrant, A., Cauwe, F., Michaux, J.L., Beckers, C., Verwilghen, R.L., and Sokal, G. (1982). Assessment of the sites of red cell destruction using quantitative measurements of splenic and hepatic destruction. *British Journal of Haematology*, **50**, 591–8.

Gaston, M. *et al.* (1986). Prophylaxis with oral penicillin in children with sickle cell anemia. *New England Journal of Medicine*, **314**, 1593–9.

Hocking, W.G., Machlede, H.I., and Golde, D.W. (1980). Splenic artery embolization prior to splenectomy in end stage polycythemia vera. *American Journal of Hematology*, **8**, 123–7.

Klonizakis, I., Peters, A.M., Fitzpatrick, M.L., Kensett, M.J., Lewis, S.M., and Lavender, J.P. (1981). Spleen function and platelet kinetics. *Journal of Clinical Pathology*, **34**, 377–80.

Lucas, C.E. (1990). Splenic trauma. Choice of management. *Annals of Surgery*, **213**, 98–112.

Pettit, J.E., Lewis, S.M., Williams, E.D., Grafton, C.A., Bowring, C.S., and Glass, H.I. (1986). Quantitative studies of splenic erythropoiesis in polycythaemia vera and myelofibrosis. *British Journal of Haematology*, **34**, 465–75.

Spencer, R.P. and Pearson, H.A. (1975). *Radionucleotide studies of the spleen.* CRC Press, Cleveland, Ohio.

Szur, L. (1970). Surface counting in assessment of sites of red cell destruction (annotation). *British Journal of Haematology*, **118**, 591–6.

Timens, W. and Leemans, R. (1992). Splenic autotransplantation and the immune system. *Annals of Surgery*, **215**, 256–60.

Traub, A. *et al.* (1987). Splenic reticuloendothelial function after splenectomy; spleen repair and spleen autotransplantation. *New England Journal of Medicine*, **317**, 1559–64.

Trindall, B., Swanson, C., and Cooper, D. (1990). Development of AIDS in a cohort of HIV-seropositive homosexual men in Australia. *Medical Journal of Australia*, **153**, 260–5.

Videback, A., Christensen, B.E., and Jønsson V. (1982). *The spleen in health and disease.* FADLs Forlag, Copenhagen.

Weiss, L. (1965). The structure of the normal spleen. *Seminars in Hematology*, **2**, 205–28.

Weiss, L. (1974). A scanning electron microscope study of the spleen. *Blood*, **43**, 665–91.

Weiss, L. (1983). The red pulp of the spleen: structural basis of blood flow. *Clinics in Haematology*, **12**, 375–93.

Weiss, L. and Tavossoli, M. (1970). Anatomic hazards to the passage of erythrocytes through the spleen. *Seminars in Hematology*, **7**, 372–9.

Wennberg, E. and Weiss, L. (1969). The structure of the spleen and hemolysis. *Annual Review of Medicine*, **20**, 29–40.

22.5.5 Myeloma and other paraproteinaemias

B. G. M. DURIE and F. J. GILES

Pathological clonal expansion of plasma-cell populations results in a spectrum of disorders. This expansion may be overtly malignant, resulting in myelomatosis, solitary plasmacytoma of bone, extramedullary plasmacytoma, or Waldenström's macroglobulinaemia. A benign pattern of plasma-cell proliferation may result in monoclonal gammopathy of undetermined significance, or primary systemic amyloidosis, or comprise a component of the polyneuropathy, organomegaly, endocrinopathy, monoclonal gammopathy, skin lesions (**POEMS**) syndrome (see Chapter 24.17.1).

Myelomatosis

EPIDEMIOLOGY AND AETIOLOGY

According to data for the years 1984 to 1988 from the United States Surveillance, Epidemiology, and End Results Program, myelomatosis accounts for 2.0 per cent of all malignancies in blacks and 1.0 per cent in whites. The average annual age-adjusted (1970 United States standard) incidence rates per 100 000 are 10.2 for black males and 6.7 for black females, 4.7 for white males and 3.2 for white females. Myelomatosis accounts for 31 per cent of lymphoproliferative malignancies in blacks and 13 per cent in whites. The median age for diagnosis is 69 years for males and 71 years for females, with the average annual age-specific incidence rates increasing sharply with age, independent of gender or race. Similar incidence rates occur in white populations in northern Europe and the United States, with slightly lower rates reported in the United Kingdom, Eastern Europe, South America, India, and Japan. Five per cent of patients are under 40 years of age at time of diagnosis, with a further 10 to 15 per cent being under 50 years. There is a trend toward increasing incidence of myelomatosis within the higher socio-economic groups, with poorer survival correlated with poverty indices. The mortality from myelomatosis has been increasing in recent years, particularly in patients age 55 years or more, with countries that have had the lowest death rates, Greece and Japan for example, showing the largest increase for the years 1970 to 1985. Countries who traditionally had the highest death rates, Norway and Finland for example, have had the lowest rate of increase, with the United Kingdom showing an intermediate rate. The largest percentage increase in mortality has been in the age group 70 to 74 years. As there has been a similar increase in men and women, a common environmental, rather than occupational, exposure is probably responsible. Support for a role of environmental agents in the aetiology of myelomatosis comes from cases occurring among spouses.

The most established risk factors for development of myelomatosis are old age and ionizing radiation, with exposure to both high and long-term low, radiation doses being implicated in atomic bomb survivors, radium dial painters, radiologists, workers in nuclear industry, and atomic-weapons test personnel. No significant association with therapeutic radiation has been demonstrated. Many occupational hazards for myelomatosis have been noted in association with agriculture, including pig, sheep, beef cattle, dairy, and orchard farming, and exposure to grain dust, aflatoxins, and engine exhausts from farm equipment. Exposure to lead vapours, lead liquid, arsenic, cadmium, copper powder, copper fumes, nickel and a variety of other chemicals have been associated with myelomatosis. Associations with employment in the rubber, pulp, paper-making, metal-working, leather-tanning, leather-products, woollen, textile, petroleum, cosmetic, and spray-painting industries have also been demonstrated. Myelomatosis has occurred among siblings in 25 of 37 families with at least two affected members. Other associations include significant links with a family history of autoimmune disorders and degenerative diseases of the nervous system.

While no specific chromosomal abnormality has been linked with myelomatosis, the translocation $t(8;14)(q24 \updownarrow 2)$ has been associated with IgA paraprotein, and abnormalities of chromosome 14 occur in one-third of patients with cytogenetic abnormalities. Associations between the HLA-Cw5 and HLA-Cw2 antigens and the development of myelomatosis have been reported. Increased expression and transcription of the c-*myc* oncogene has been documented in some cases of myelomatosis, and there is a correlation between high *myc* activity in plasma cells and their capacity for self-renewal. The protein products of the c-*myc* and *max* genes dimerize to form a DNA-binding protein, the function of which is currently undefined, as are the roles of the *bcl-1* and *bcl-2* gene products in the development of myelomatosis. Attempts to connect the development of myelomatosis to chronic antigenic stimulation of the immune system, in patients with pre-existing illness for example, have not yielded consistent results.

Although antibody activity, against bacterial antigens or human immunodeficiency virus for example, can be demonstrated by M proteins in less than 1 per cent of patients with myelomatosis, the number of antigenic determinants tested in any given patient is a very small proportion of the potential antigens. The distribution of the immunoglobulin classes in myelomatosis suggests a random origin determined by the relative frequencies of the plasma-cell precursors.

PATHOGENESIS

The origin of malignant plasma cells is unknown. Although myelomatosis is the classical example of a monoclonal neoplasm, in 95 per cent of patients, malignant cells are widely disseminated to the axial skeleton, even at the earliest clinical stages of disease. Plasma cells are rarely numerous in the peripheral blood until myelomatosis enters a terminal phase. An M protein reflects cell clonality, its homogeneity indicating that all the cells which are synthesizing it are descended from a single precursor. The current indications are that plasmablasts in the primary and secondary follicles of lymph nodes, spleen, and Peyer's patches are the progenitors of marrow plasma cells. Plasmablasts represent 0.5 to 1 per cent of peripheral blood mononuclear cells in normal individuals. Histologically, the marrow lesions of myelomatosis appear to be composed almost entirely of plasma cells with many multinucleate forms. Bone-marrow plasma cells have minimal capacity for self-renewal. The occurrence of multiple, spherical, widely disseminated skeletal lesions suggests that cell colonies originate from single, blood-borne precursors. It thus seems that myelomatosis develops when an abnormal clone with limited proliferative capacity arises in a nodal or splenic lymphoid follicle and then seeds multiple marrow sites. However, primary lymph node or splenic disease is very rare in myelomatosis, being seen only in very advances cases of IgD myelomatosis, and although the majority of IgA-producing plasma cells are found in the gut lamina propria, it is never overtly involved in myelomatosis.

Subpopulations of circulating blood lymphocytes in myelomatosis often coexpress plasma-cell and lymphocyte markers, (CD11$_a$, CD19, CD20, CD24, CD10, CD9, CD5, and PCA-1), and include cells bearing surface immunoglobulins identical with the M protein, showing the immunoglobulin gene rearrangement pattern of the myelomatosis plasma-cell clone. These cells may be responsible for the dissemination of myelomatosis from origin to marrow. They have been variously reported as being CD34 positive or negative.

Neoplastic transformation is currently regarded as a multistep process. In order to reconcile this theory with the short time (hours or days) taken for maturation of a plasma cell from a proliferating B cell, it is necessary to postulate that an early initiating mutation takes place in a preplasma-cell phase. The high frequency of expression of myeloid, monocytic, erythroid, or megakaryocytic surface antigens may indicate that early progenitors which are common to both myeloid and lymphoid lineages may suffer the initial genetic insult. In myelomatosis, this mutation must be cryptic, that is, have no overt effect on proliferation. Further complementing (promoting) mutations must then occur at later developmental stages to result in overt disease. It thus seems likely that a pre-plasma-cell compartment of clonogenic myelomatosis cells circulates in the blood and that terminal differentiation occurs only in the micro-environment of the bone marrow.

A key element in the marrow's ability to offer an optimal environment for myelomatosis cells is the compatibility between the cell-adhesion molecules of developing B-lineage cells and the bone marrow matrix and marrow stromal cells. Cells comprising the abnormal circulating B-lymphocyte population in myelomatosis express $CD11_b$, a leucocyte integrin, involved in a haemopoietic-cell/endothelial-cell interactions. $CD11_b$ allows these cells to bind to endothelial layers of vessel walls, a prelude to migration across the endothelial barrier. In addition to $CD11_b$, receptors for extracellular-matrix components are necessary for the loco-motion and extravasation of plasma cells. On the abnormal circulating myelomatosis lymphocytes, these receptors are molecules of the very late antigen (VLA) integrin family in a pattern unique to this population, expressing the $\alpha2$ (laminin/collagen receptor), $\alpha4$, $\alpha5$ (fibronectin receptor), and $\alpha6$ (laminin/collagen receptor) subunits. Abnormal circulating B lymphocytes in myelomatosis have high-density expression of CD44, CD54, and RHAMM homing and motility receptors. Having 'homed' to the marrow, the myelomatosis cells are in a milieu with an optimal local concentration of the cytokine growth factors necessary for differentiation and proliferation.

Bone-marrow plasma cells express CD56 (NCAM), an adhesion molecule that mediates focal clustering of the cells. VLA-4 ($\alpha4\beta1$) (CDw49d), which mediates cell interactions, is strongly expressed on plasma cells and may synergize with CD56 to enhance cell clustering in the vicinity of marrow stromal cells. Stromal cells release interleukin (IL) 1β and monocyte–macrophage colony-stimulating factor (M-CSF), which act as stromal-cell autocrine stimulants, as well as IL-6, granulocyte–macrophage colony-stimulating factor (GM-CSF), IL-7, and IL-11. IL-6 is one of the key myelomatosis-growth cytokines. Some 40 to 60 per cent of myelomatosis cell lines respond to IL-6 stimulation by increased incorporation of ^{3}H-Tdr. GM-CSF, IL-1, granulocyte-stimulating factor (G-CSF), IL-3, and IL-5 are synergistic with IL-6 in stimulating in vitro proliferation of purified myelomatosis cell lines.

Serum IL-6 concentrations are elevated in patients with active myelomatosis in contrast to those of patients with stable myelomatosis or monoclonal gammopathy of undetermined significance, or those of healthy donors. Serum IL-6 is a powerful independent prognostic variable in patients with myelomatosis, being elevated in 35 to 40 per cent of patients at time of diagnosis, and associated with aggressive disease and poor prognosis. IL-6 is a potent inducer of acute-phase proteins. The production of C-reactive protein by human hepatocytes in primary culture is primarily controlled by IL-6. Excess IL-6 production in patients with myelomatosis is mirrored by the serum concentrations of C-reactive protein.

Lytic bone lesions with resultant hypercalcaemia commonly occur in myelomatosis, and osteosclerotic lesions are occasionally seen. Mixed lytic and sclerotic features are more frequently seen in patients with solitary plasmocytoma of bone or POEMS syndrome. Increased osteo-clastic bone resorption is demonstrable in many patients with myelomatosis and in most is related to an increased number of trabecular osteoclasts. Excessive osteoclastic activity may precede overt myeloma by several months or years. In early stages of myelomatosis, abnormal bone remodelling induced by malignant plasma cells generally involves stimulation of both bone formation and destruction. As the myelomatosis progresses, this process is uncoupled and, along with increased osteoclast activity, decreased osteoblastic activity is found in patients with lytic lesions and advanced disease. Progressive suppression of osteoblasts parallels the progression of the myelomatosis.

Many cytokines produced by malignant B lymphocytes, stromal cells, and activated T lymphocytes, including IL-1β, M-CSF, tumour necrosis factor-β (TNF-β), IL-3, and IL-6, have osteoclast-activating properties. IL-6 is constitutively produced by osteoblasts, its production being stimulated by IL-1β and TNF-β. IL-6 stimulates the in vitro generation and bone-resorptive activities of osteoclasts and mediates the bone-resorptive activities of IL-1 and TNF. IL-6 increases natural killer (NK) cell activity and in myelomatosis, unlike the other B-lymphoproliferative disorders, the marrow's NK activity is increased.

While a pivotal role for IL-6 in the pathophysiology of myelomatosis has been established, it is still not clear if it functions mainly as an autocrine or paracrine factor for plasma-cell growth (see Section 6). On balance, current data would support the latter. Malignant plasma cells produce IL-1β, TNF-β, and a functionally active, truncated form of M-CSF. It is currently unclear if fresh myelomatosis cells can produce IL-6.

TUMOUR GROWTH AND PRESENTATION

The pattern of tumour growth in myelomatosis is described mathematically by a Gompertzian model, that is the tumour growth fraction decreases exponentially with time. In this model the absolute number of dividing cells is maximal when the tumour is approximately 37 per cent of its maximum size. Single plasma cells from fresh marrow samples in myelomatosis produce an average of 12 pg of M protein per day. This would imply a total tumour mass in the body at the time of clinical presentation of the order of 3 kg, corresponding to between 0.3×10^{12} and 3.0×10^{12} myelomatosis cells.

Four main aspects of myelomatosis dictate the clinical picture: malignant plasma-cell proliferation, M-protein production, renal failure, and immunodeficiency. Plasma-cell proliferation is largely confined to red bone marrow, with progressive replacement of haemopoietic tissue and tumour extension into the fatty marrow of the long bones. Both diffuse and nodular patterns of plasma-cell infiltration are seen; they result in impairment or failure of bone marrow function leading to anaemia, neutropenia, and thrombocytopenia.

Patients with myelomatosis have a much increased risk of bacterial infection, and some 10 per cent present in this way, often with pneumonia. The traditional dominance of infections due to Gram-positive organisms such as Staphylococcus aureus and Streptococcus pneumoniae has been eroded as Gram-negative sepsis becomes increasingly prevalent. Opportunistic infections by organisms such as Mycobacterium tuberculosis, Pneumocystis pneumoniae, and herpesviruses, although uncommon at presentation, seem to be increasing in incidence in patients with advanced disease. Infection is one of the most common causes of death in myelomatosis and early, intensive intervention is indicated where it is suspected. Fever directly attributable to myelomatosis is said to occur in 1 per cent of patients and may be related to IL-6 production.

Anaemia, usually normochromic and normocytic, is common in myelomatosis and its symptoms may be dominant at time of diagnosis in some 20 per cent of patients. Marrow invasion, the effect of tumour-related inhibitors of erythropoiesis, renal failure, and plasma-volume expansion secondary to M protein are the key factors in its pathogenesis. Current data on serum erythropoietin levels in myelomatosis are inconsistent; some reports suggest that these levels are appropriately raised for the degree of anaemia in those with normal renal function, and inappropriately low only in patients with uraemia, whilst others report inappropriately low levels, in both uraemic and non-uraemic patients.

At presentation, some 60 per cent of patients with myelomatosis have skeletal lytic lesions, with or without osteoporosis, wedging or collapse of vertebral bodies, or pathological fractures; some 20 per cent of patients have osteoporosis alone, and the remainder have no myelomatosis-related radiological abnormality. Localized tumour proliferation and resultant osteoclast/osteoblast abnormalities completely destroy the fine trabeculae in cancellous bone. With further tumour expansion, the nodules encroach on cortical bone, causing punched-out lesions.

The vast majority of patients with lytic lesions have diffuse myelomatosis infiltration of the marrow and often have generalized osteoporosis, involving the long bones and the axial skeleton. Fifteen to 20 per cent of patients have diffuse bone-marrow infiltration with few or no lytic lesions. Because of the concentration of the disease in the axial skeleton, the main effects of osteoporosis and of lytic lesions are in the vertebrae, pelvis, ribs, and sternum. Bone pain, either diffuse or localized, is the predominant presenting symptom in 60 per cent of patients.

Wedging and collapse of vertebral bodies, especially in the mid-dorsal, lower dorsal, and upper lumbar vertebrae, are common. With advanced disease, pathological fractures of the long bones, ribs, and sternum occur. There is no direct relation between severity of pain and the degree of skeletal involvement as assessed radiologically, apart from that associated with the wedging and collapse of vertebral bodies, or gross localized bone destruction. Skull lesions, although often numerous, very rarely cause pain, whereas metastatic cancers of similar radiological appearance are often painful.

Net osteolysis in patients with myelomatosis causes continuing loss of calcium from the skeleton. At presentation, some 25 per cent have an elevated serum calcium, in particular those with extensive lytic bone lesions, often associated with Bence Jones protein-only M proteins. The level of serum alkaline phosphatase remains normal except in the presence of healing fractures. Life-threatening episodes of acute hypercalcaemia leading to severe dehydration and uraemia may occur at any stage. Acute hypercalcaemia is most frequent in patients with generalized osteoporosis and extensive lytic lesions, but may occur before myelomatosis is otherwise clinically apparent.

In a small minority of patients with myelomatosis, plasma-cell infiltration of soft tissues is seen at presentation, and may be found in about 15 per cent of cases at autopsy. The frequency of overt soft-tissue involvement is high in IgD myelomatosis. The most frequent serious consequences of soft-tissue involvement occur with tumour extension beyond the periosteum following complete erosion of the cortex. When this spread is from a vertebral body into the spinal theca, tumour may extend extradurally or may cause compression of the spinal cord by eroding the pia-arachnoid. Rarely, myelomatous deposits occur in other tissues such as the skin, but the majority of instances of skin and subcutaneous involvement seem to be metastatic from extra medullary plasmocytomas. The current literature reports on 21 patients who have presented with skin plasmacytomas as their only site of disease. Extension of tumours intraorbitally occurs frequently if the skull and facial bones are omitted from systemic irradiation fields.

The most serious clinical consequence of M-protein production, particularly that resulting from excessive synthesis of Bence Jones protein, is the development of potentially irreversible renal damage. Twenty-five per cent of patients with myelomatosis are uraemic at presentation, with a further 25 per cent showing overt renal failure as the disease progresses. In a few cases the blood urea will fall to normal levels after rehydration. Without aggressive therapy the prognosis is very poor, and about 70 per cent of those with a blood urea of more than 15 mmol/l or a serum creatinine concentration of more than 200 μmol/l die within 100 days. In over 95 per cent of patients, renal failure is attributable to Bence Jones protein and/or hypercalcaemia.

Bence Jones protein is the only M protein to be produced in approximately 15 per cent of patients with myelomatosis, while the cells of over 80 per cent of the remainder secrete Bence Jones protein and complete Ig proteins. Bence Jones protein consists of monoclonal light chains in a monomeric (molecular weight approx. 22 000) or dimeric (approx. 44 000) form, and enters the renal tubule with the glomerular filtrate. Quantities of up to 50 g may enter the urine daily but in most cases the daily excretion is less than 15 g. Bence Jones protein is precipitated as a viscous mass in the collecting tubules and the distal convoluted tubules, causing obstruction. Proximal to the obstruction the tubule dilates and epithelial cells atrophy. This tubular dysfunction is not by itself sufficient to initiate acute renal failure for it is present in patients with a normal or moderately raised blood urea who have Bence Jones protein. The pathophysiology of Bence Jones protein-related renal failure is not yet well defined. An acute deterioration in function is frequently precipitated by an episode of dehydration. A number of other factors, such as hyperuricaemia, sepsis, disseminated intravascular coagulation, and the use of nephrotoxic antibiotics or cytotoxic drugs, may contribute to its development. Rarely, uraemia is caused by renal-vein thrombosis or direct infiltration by plasma cells or amyloid. There is no convincing correlation with light-chain subtype, although there is some evidence that the more cationic proteins are more damaging.

A particular clinical syndrome, macroglobulinaemia, is associated with the presence of an IgM M protein because it is especially prone to cause hyperviscosity and to act as a cold agglutinin. The intrinsic viscosity of a protein is related to its concentration, size, shape and chemical configuration. The intrinsic viscosity of IgM, which usually exists as a 900 000 Da pentamer, is high relative to that of IgA or IgG, and the hyperviscosity syndrome therefore occurs at relatively lower concentrations, around 40 to 50 g/l. In hyperviscosity associated with IgA, the M protein usually circulates in polymeric form. Polymerization is enhanced by increasing concentration and by the presence of J chains. Hyperviscosity syndrome associated with IgG myelomatosis occurs predominantly at very high M-protein concentrations, although it may do so through the presence of polymers or unusual molecular configurations.

The hyperviscosity syndrome rarely occurs with a relative viscosity of less than 4, commonly at values of 6 or greater. Common components of the syndrome are ocular, haemostatic, and neurological disturbances accompanied by fatigue, malaise or weight loss. Visual disturbances range in severity from mild impairment to abrupt loss of vision. Progression from distension of retinal veins to increasing vessel tortuosity with local constrictions at arteriovenous crossings, areas of beading, and dilation of small venules ('string of sausages' appearance) may lead to a full-blown retinopathy with florid haemorrhages and exudates.

Coagulopathy is common in myelomatosis. With the hyperviscosity syndrome, the bleeding tendency is assumed to be the result of platelet coating by the M protein. This may result in chronic, recurrent bleeding of the gums and upper respiratory and gastrointestinal tracts. The bleeding time is usually prolonged and platelet function tests are abnormal. Neurological symptoms and signs are prominent features of this syndrome; they include headache, fluctuating consciousness, slowed mentation, dizziness, ataxia, vertigo, neuropathies, convulsions, and coma. Plasma volume increases with increasing viscosity, and may compromise cardiac function. A thrombotic tendency in patients with hyperviscosity syndrome may lead to presentation with deep venous thrombosis or pulmonary infarction.

Other effects of M protein contribute in varying degree to the morbidity and mortality of myelomatosis. M-protein production is strongly associated with low serum concentrations of the normal immunoglobulins. In about 70 per cent of patients with IgG myelomatosis at presentation, the serum concentrations of the normal immunoglobulins are less than 20 per cent of normal; this is the case in 40 per cent of patients with IgA myelomatosis, and in 20 per cent of patient with Bence Jones protein myelomatosis. Equally severe immunoparesis occurs in the 1 per cent of patients in whom no M protein is detectable in the serum or urine. Recovery to normal immunoglobulin levels is rarely seen after conventional chemotherapy, even when the concentrations of M protein fall to low levels. Immunoparesis worsens with disease progression. In addition, there is severe suppression of the primary antibody response, the mechanisms of which are not known. Cell-mediated immunity is generally intact but may be impaired, as may granulocyte function and complement activation. These primary immune abnormalities, uraemia, neutropenia, antitumour therapy, multiple blood-component transfusions, indwelling urinary and intravenous catheters and multiple organ failure combine to cause severe immunodeficiency and susceptibility to infection in many patients with myelomatosis.

DIAGNOSIS, STAGING AND PROGNOSIS (PLATES 49, 50)

The criteria for the diagnosis of myelomatosis (Table 1) include the presence of at least 10 per cent abnormal plasma cells in the bone marrow or histological proof of a plasmacytoma, and at least one of the following abnormalities: serum or urinary M protein or osteolytic

Table 1 *Diagnostic criteria for multiple myeloma and monoclonal gammopathy of undetermined significance*

Multiple myeloma
Major criteria
I. Plasmacytoma on tissue biopsy
II. Bone marrow plasmacytosis with >30% plasma cells
III. Monoclonal globulin spike on serum electrophoresis exceeding 35 g/l for IgG peaks or 20 g/l for IgA peaks, $\geq$ 1.0 g/24 h of κ or λ light-chain excretion on urine electrophoresis in the absence of amyloidosis

Minor criteria
(a) Bone-marrow plasmacytosis with 10% to 30% plasma cells
(b) Monoclonal globulin spike present but less than levels in (III) above
(c) Lytic bone lesions
(d) Residual normal IgM < 500 mg/l, IgA < 1 g/l, or IgG < 6 g/l

Diagnosis is established when any of the following are documented in a symptomatic patient with clearly progressive disease. The diagnosis of myeloma requires a minimum of one major plus one minor criterion or three minor criteria that must include (a) + (b), thus:
1. (I) + (b), (I) + (c), (I) + (d) [I + (a) is *not* diagnostic]
2. (II) + (b), (II) + (c), (II) + (d)
3. (III) + (a), (III) + (c), III + (d)
4. (a) + (b) + (c), (a) + (b) + (d)

Indolent myeloma
As per multiple myeloma except:
I. No bone lesions or $\leq$ 3 lytic lesions, no compression fractures
II. M-component levels IgA < 50 g/l < 70 g/l
III. No symptoms or signs of disease, that is:
   (a) Karnofsky performance status > 70%
   (b) Haemoglobin > 100 g/l
   (c) Normal serum calcium
   (d) Serum creatinine < 175 μmol/l (< 20 mg/l)
   (e) No persistent or recurrent infection

Smouldering myeloma
As per indolent myeloma with:
No bone lesions
Bone-marrow plasma cells 10% to 30%

Monoclonal gammopathy of undetermined significance
I. Monoclonal gammopathy
II. M-component levels IgA < 20 g/l, IgG < 35 g/l, < 1.0 g/24 h of κ or λ light-chain excretion on urine electrophoresis
III. Bone-marrow plasma cells < 10%
IV. No bony lesions
V. No symptoms

Table 2 *Myelomatosis: clinical staging system of Durie and Salmon*

Stage I Low myeloma-cell mass ($< 0.6 \times 10^{12}$ cells/m²)
All of the following:
   Hb >10 g/dl
   Serum calcium (corrected) $\leq$ 12 mg/dl*
   Radiographs are normal or show single lesion
M-protein production value of:
   IgG < 5 g/dl
   IgA < 3 g/dl
   Urinary light-chain excretion < 4 g/24 h

Stage II Intermediate myeloma-cell mass ($0.6–1.2 \times 10^{12}$ cells/m²)
Results fit neither stage I nor stage II

Stage III High myeloma-cell mass ($>1.2 \times 10^{12}$ cells/m²)
Any of the following:
   Hb $\leq$ 8.5 g/dl
   Serum calcium (corrected) >12 mg/dl*
   Radiographs show multiple lesions
M-protein production value of:
   IgG >7 g/dl
   IgA >5 g/dl
   Urinary light-chain excretion >12 g/24 h

*Corrected calcium = calcium (mg/dl) − albumin (g/dl) + 4.0.

Subclassification:

A = relatively normal renal function (serum creatinine value 2.0 mg/100 ml);

B = abnormal renal function (serum creatinine value $\geq$ 2.0 g/100 ml).

and quantitation of Bence Jones protein in the urine depend on the demonstration of a monoclonal light chain by immunoelectrophoresis or immunofixation of an adequately concentrated sample from a 24-h urine collection. One of these latter tests should be done on urine from a patient suspected of having myelomatosis even where the sulphosalicylic acid test is negative.

The imunoperoxidase method should be used to detect monoclonal immunoglobulin in plasma cells. A radiological survey of the entire skeleton is mandatory in the diagnosis of myelomatosis. The standard clinical staging system for myelomatosis is that of Durie and Salmon, with a stage I, II, and III differentiation as shown in Table 2.

The finding of destruction of the vertebral pedicles may help to distinguish between the osteolytic bone disease of metastatic carcinoma and myelomatosis, as it is not a feature of the latter. The advent of computerized tomographic (**CT**) scanning and magnetic resonance imaging (**MRI**) has greatly increased the sensitivity of detection of bone disease in myelomatosis. MRI is superior to CT scanning for screening large portions of the vertebral column and spinal canal, and for visualizing soft tissue abnormalities. It clearly defines paraspinal or intraspinal tumour extension. It is of particular value in apparently solitary disease, where it may detect additional sites of involvement, often been missed by other imaging techniques. Traditionally, myelography has been the investigation of choice when patients present with features of cord compression but if there is a complete block to the flow of dye, areas distal to the block will not be visualized. MRI scanning should be done in this situation to screen for additional lesions. MRI can demonstrate imminent cord compression in patients without specific symptoms.

The prognosis for myelomatosis is highly dependent upon the Durie–Salmon stage and various other prognostic factors including serum β_2-microglobulin and albumin levels at time of diagnosis. Other well-established independent prognostic discriminants are degree of renal failure and the plasma-cell labelling index. Data collected in the United States between 1981 and 1987 suggested that whites had a 5-year relative survival rate of 26.3 per cent and blacks a rate of 28.3 per cent. Relative

lesions. Electrophoresis on cellulose acetate membrane is satisfactory for screening the serum to detect M protein, while high-resolution agarose gel electrophoresis has the increased sensitivity necessary to detect smaller quantities of protein. Immunoelectrophoresis or immunofixation or both are confirmatory studies that can also define the immunoglobulin type and its light-chain class. These latter tests should be made whenever myelomatosis, monoclonal gammopathy of undetermined significance, macroglobulinaemia, or amyloidosis are being considered, regardless of a normal-appearing or non-specific electrophoretic pattern. Monospecific antisera to the Fc fragment of IgG, IgA, IgM, IgD and IgE as well as antisera to κ and λ light chains should be employed. Rate nephelometry is the optimal method for quantitation of immunoglobulins. Sulphosalicylic acid should be used to screen urine for protein. The recognition

survival rates for women were higher in both blacks and whites. Recently described, potentially important prognostic factors include: abnormal cytogenetics; serum levels of lactate dehydrogenase, neopterin, osteocalcin, IL-6, or C-reactive protein; H-*ras* expression; the presence or absence of mutations of K- and N-*ras*; and the demonstration of aberrant myeloid, erythroid or megakaryocytic phenotypic markers on malignant plasma cells.

Seventy-five per cent of patients diagnosed with myelomatosis are reported to die 'directly' because of the disorder, this group including patients whose primary cause of death is listed as sepsis, hypercalcaemia, haemorrhage, or renal failure. Causes of death that are arguably not directly due to myelomatosis include 8 per cent of patients who die from 'cardiac' causes, 3 per cent from central nervous events, 2 per cent from other malignancies (including acute leukaemia), 1 per cent from pulmonary emboli, and 0.5 to 1 per cent who commit suicide. In approximately 10 per cent of patients in most series, the cause of death is not specified.

THERAPY

It is important to consider both cytoreduction as well as ancillary treatment necessary to manage complications of the disease. Before proceeding to chemotherapy one must be sure of the diagnosis and need for therapy. This involves the exclusion of early forms of the disease or precursor states, such as monoclonal gammopathy of undetermined significance, which do not require treatment. Increasingly aggressive multidrug regimens are continuously being developed and studied in myelomatosis. This is based on a theoretical sequential process in which M-protein reduction parallels the degree of killing of malignant cells. This fall in M-protein level is used to define the degree of response, which in turn is assumed to define the length of survival. This sequential theory now seems invalid. Reductions in M-protein levels do not seem truly to reflect changes in overall tumour mass. Analysis of current criteria for response and their correlation with duration of survival indicates that the magnitude of regression, as assessed by M-protein reduction, does not correlate in a quantitative way with the anticipated response or survival duration. Thus a 75 per cent regression is not necessarily intrinsically better than a 25 per cent regression, because all of the responses achieved with conventional therapy are partial. Cytotoxic therapy has improved survival by reducing early deaths from complications and by slowing down tumour progression in some patients. The tumour bulk at presentation, intrinsic disease kinetics, and drug sensitivity in individual patients are the major determinants of survival. Multidrug regimens consistently give higher response rates than the traditional melphalan/prednisone combination but this does not translate into prolonged survival.

Induction therapy

In patients with stage I, smouldering or indolent myelomatosis, no specific antineoplastic or immunomodulatory therapy is currently indicated. Patients with stage I, II or III disease that is symptomatic or progressive warrant systemic cytotoxic therapy. Commonly occurring indications for the institution of therapy are bone pain, hypercalcaemia, renal failure, marrow failure, or spinal-cord compression. All patients should be encouraged to drink 2 to 3 litres of fluid daily from time of diagnosis. A combination of melphalan and prednisone (**MP**) is the most widely used induction regimen and no alternative regimen has been convincingly demonstrated to offer superior long-term survival in unselected groups of patients. There are suggestions that patients with a poorer prognosis may benefit from more complex regimens while those with a better prognosis may be optimally treated with MP. There is a need for prospective studies specifically to address this issue. Oral and intravenous melphalan in MP have equivalent impact on survival. Nadir absolute granulocyte counts should be monitored in patients on intermittent oral alkylating-agent therapy. A typical induction regimen is melphalan 6 mg/m^2 and prednisone 100 mg/m^2 daily for 7 days each 28 days for six cycles.

Alternative induction regimens, for example vincristine, Adriamycin, dexamethasone (**VAD**) or vincristine, melphalan, cyclophosphamide, prednisone alternating with vincristine, BCNU, Adriamycin, prednisone (**VMCP/VBAP**), may be of benefit to some patients with particularly aggressive tumours because these regimens may achieve higher overall or faster response rates. VAD is effective and relatively safe in patients with renal failure. Steroid pulses alone as induction therapy may be indicated where marrow function is suppressed. Current induction regimens offer objective-response rates, as defined by the criteria of the Chronic Leukaemic Myeloma Task Force, of 50 to 70 per cent, with more complex regimens tending to give higher rates than MP. Conventional induction therapies are reported to result in median survival times of between 24 and 42 months, a clear improvement over the median survivals of 4 to 10 months achieved before the availability of suitable alkylating agents.

Numerous clinical studies with various α-interferons have demonstrated significant antitumour activity against myelomatosis. A recent review of 12 studies, involving 352 evaluable patients with various dose schedules of different interferon preparations, reported an objective-response rate of 8 to 33 per cent. Overall response rates to single-agent interferon in previously untreated patients are inferior to MP or other cytotoxic regimens. Synergism has been demonstrated *in vitro* between interferon-α and melphalan, cyclophosphamide, anthracyclines, and the MP combination. But though several clinical trials have been made the role of the addition of interferon-α to conventional induction regimens is still not clear.

Maintenance therapy

The majority of patients who achieve an objective response to induction therapy will enter a plateau phase of disease during which clinical assessments indicate a stable tumour burden. Continuing cytotoxic therapy beyond the time of objective response has repeatedly been shown not to prolong survival in myelomatosis. Systemic irradiation using a double hemibody technique as a consolidation procedure has been shown to decrease survival. The introduction of interferon-α as the only agent capable of prolonging the plateau phase has been a major advance in the treatment of myelomatosis.

The ability of interferon-$α_{2b}$ to prolong the duration of plateau phase in patients who have achieved an objective remission with conventional induction therapy has been confirmed in several randomized studies. Maintenance therapy with interferon-$α_{2b}$ should now be offered to all appropriate patients, that is, those who have a 50 per cent reduction of the baseline absolute level of serum or urine paraprotein. Interferon therapy defers relapse by extending the plateau phase by an average of 6 to 9 months.

Consolidation therapy

Allogeneic bone-marrow transplantation has been used as a consolidation procedure in a small number of patients responding to induction therapy. Age restriction (up to 55 years), the need for an HLA-compatible sibling donor, and other demanding criteria mean that the procedure can be offered to few patients with myelomatosis. Complete remissions are achieved in 50 per cent of patients who had responsive disease before marrow transplantation, and 30 per cent of those who were non-responsive. Some 30 per cent of patients die within 100 days of allogeneic transplantation and 40 per cent by 6 months, with current data showing a plateau of actuarial survival of 40 per cent extending from 36 to 76 months. Many of these survivors have evidence of persistent paraprotein production, and whether patients can be 'cured' of myelomatosis by allogeneic bone-marrow transplantation remains unclear. Some of them may have a disorder resembling monoclonal gammopathy of undetermined significance after marrow transplantation. Previously untreated or minimally treated patients who have stage I disease, that is low tumour bulk, have the most durable responses to allogeneic marrow, with a 70 per cent plateau in survival between 6 and 42 months. But these are the patients in whom the early mortality due to the transplant is most difficult to justify. Allogeneic marrow transplantation in patients with progressive disease shows a 30 per cent plateau in survival between 30 and 60 months—very poor results but in an otherwise rapidly fatal disorder. Pre-transplant factors seem to have some predictive value in the response to marrow transplantation but have little clear impact on survival afterwards. Post-transplant factors that predict better long-term survival include achievement of a complete remission and grade I, rather than higher grade, graft-versus-host disease. The role of allogeneic bone-marrow transplantation in treatment of myelomatosis is, therefore, unclear and awaits prospective randomized studies.

Autologous bone-marrow transplantation, using bone marrow and/or peripheral stem cells as rescue therapy, is also being used as a consolidation procedure in patients with myelomatosis. Most conditioning regimens incorporate high-dose melphalan and total body irradiation. Attempts at marrow purging have included the use of antibody/rabbit complement, antibody/momordin, or 4-hydroperoxycyclophosphamide combinations. The apparent lack of an adverse effect on prognosis of even marked plasmacytosis (up to 30 per cent of nucleated cells) within reinfused marrows in autologous transplants indicates a need for more efficient cytoreduction before conditioning, rather than marrow purging. The use of recombinant growth factors has made harvesting of an adequate peripheral blood stem-cell yield a rapid and relatively economic way of performing autologous marrow transplantation. Recombinant growth factors should not be used off protocol in patients with myelomatosis in our present state of knowledge; *in vitro*, both recombinant human GM-CSF and G-CSF can stimulate tumour growth in myelomatosis, and *in vivo* evidence of acceleration of disease by recombinant human G-CSF has been recently reported.

Current data suggest that high initial rates of cell 'kill' can be accomplished with regimens of high-dose alkylating agent alone or with total-body irradiation (autologous or allogeneic marrow transplantation). Complete remission occurs in 25 to 50 per cent of patients. Because of a lack of adequate analyses of prognostic factors and absence of randomized studies, it is impossible to evaluate the true impact of these responses on survival. This is particularly true because late relapses occur despite complete responses after high-dose therapy, and thus the pattern of relapse is not the same as with more conventional chemotherapy. One cannot predict a traditional type of survival plateau after the initial period of stable disease. Much longer follow-up together with careful comparative studies are essential to assess the survival benefit. Current data suggest that there is no further role for high-dose single-drug therapy (e.g. melphalan) unless the agent is given to a level where stem-cell support is necessary. Autologous bone-marrow transplantation has no role in patients with resistant relapse or with a combination of adverse prognostic factors. The present emphasis on the peripheral blood as the source of stem cells, rather than the bone marrow, should be regarded with caution. The peripheral blood contains large numbers of clonogenic myelomatous cells, particularly after growth-factor stimulation, and the best source of stem cells remains to be identified from prospective studies. Similarly, attempts to obtain haemopoietic stem cells, and thereby exclude myelomatous progenitors, on the basis of CD34 positivity, should be subjected to rigorous prospective study; current data suggests that subpopulations of the myelomatous malignant clone may be CD34 positive. Prospective studies comparing traditional induction therapy followed by interferon-α_{2b} therapy with and without consolidation by autologous marrow transplantation are now needed.

In an effort to capitalize on the increased percentage of complete remissions now being achieved either by bone marrow transplantation or chemotherapy/interferon combinations, the number of investigations into postinduction or transplant therapy is increasing. Two studies on the use of interferon-α after autologous marrow transplantation, one randomized, have proved very encouraging. If the British randomized study continues to show positive results, interferon-α_{2b} should become standard therapy after autologous transplantation.

Relapse/refractory therapy

It is of great importance to distinguish between the categories of patient covered by the term relapse/refractory, as the therapeutic approach to, and the prognosis in, each is different. In the first group, which includes up to 50 per cent of patients with myeloma, are those who are truly refractory to first-line chemotherapy. These patients either remain stable, or progress, whilst on chemotherapy. Many patients who remain stable are in a plateau phase at time of diagnosis and do not necessarily have a poor prognosis—indeed, they seem to have a relatively good one. The patients who actively progress while on induction therapy are the truly primarily resistant group, that is they have refractory disease at diagnosis. The second group comprises, those who relapse after an initial response. Relapse may occur while the patient is on or off therapy. If relapse occurs more than 6 months after stopping treatment, the patient is said to have has an unmaintained remission. As myeloma is rarely cured by conventional chemotherapy, all patients who are initially responsive to chemotherapy will eventually relapse if they do not first die of other causes.

It is important to establish in all categories that resistance to chemotherapy is real, not apparent. Some patients respond slowly. The patient may not be receiving adequate amounts of therapy, although this is difficult to demonstrate. It is customary to look for mild myelosuppression 2 weeks after therapy with cytotoxic agents and to increase the dose if it does not occur. Recent data suggest that response rates are similar in patients with an without myelosuppression and the impact of either on survival is unknown.

There are no really satisfactory options for the treatment of truly refractory myelomatosis. No relapse/refractory regimen, either cytotoxic drug or radiation based, consistently achieves a median survival of more than 1 year—most studies record less than 9 months. A relatively effective approach is the use of simple, high-dose glucocorticoid, which is recommended as the second-line treatment for genuinely resistant patients. Response rates of approximately 40 per cent are seen using either one of two alternative regimens: pulsed prednisolone, 100 mg on alternate days, reducing to 50 mg on alternate days when there is a response, or 28-day cycles of dexamethasone, 40 mg orally for 4-day blocks, starting on days 1, 9, and 17. Steroid-related side-effects are a major problem but an important benefit is the lack of myelosuppression.

The VAD regimen is recommended as second-line treatment for patients who relapse on, or within, 6 months of stopping first-line treatment, and response rates are of the order of 75 per cent. Unlike in resistant disease, this regimen is more effective than high-dose steroids alone (40 per cent response rate). It is effective even when other doxorubicin-containing regimens have failed. Regimens such as VBAP can be used as an alternative in relapsing myeloma where VAD is unsuitable or impractical, particularly in relatively asymptomatic patients. Response rates are only 20 per cent with combinations of alkylating agents that do not include doxorubicin.

Currently, systemic radiation therapy in myelomatosis is used either as part of a conditioning regimen before allogeneic or autologous bone-marrow transplantation, or as a double hemibody procedure. Hemibody irradiation has been shown to be an effective, well-tolerated method of therapy in patients with advanced myelomatosis, while current data suggest that double hemibody irradiation gives more durable responses than single hemibody irradiation. The double procedure can be expected to prolong the median survival at least as effectively as the alternative 'salvage' high-dose chemotherapeutic regimens, with equivalent or less morbidity. The entire skeleton must be included within radiation fields for optimum efficacy of double hemibody irradiation.

The great majority of plateau-phase patients will ultimately have evident overt progression of disease. All patients stopping therapy must be closely monitored for the possibility of relapse. A complete battery of tests is necessary at 6-monthly intervals with an annual skeletal survey. Serum M-protein levels may be insensitive for the detection of early relapse. Some 10 to 15 per cent of patients relapse with 'Bence Jones' escape, in which the serum M-protein levels may drop rather than increase at the time of development of relapse. Relapse may develop in an extramedullary site. It is dangerous to rely on single measures for detection of relapse and full, frequent, clinical and laboratory reviews are necessary.

New methods have become available to assess the intrinsic drug sensitivity of myelomatosis to chemotherapeutic agents, including the immunohistochemical detection and quantitation of p-glycoprotein in individual myeloma cells. The presence or absence of increased expression of p-glycoprotein, a 170 000-Da integral membrane-transport glycoprotein, correlates with the presence of multidrug resistance. This form represents resistance to a variety of biological substances, including anthracyclines, vincristine, etoposide, mitoxantrone, mitomycin C and actinomycin D. Increased production of the p-glycoprotein correlates with clinical drug resistance.

Fewer than 5 per cent of patients have detectable p-glycoprotein on the myeloma-cell surface at time of diagnosis. When treated with a single alkylating agent, this remains essentially unchanged. As therapy with anthracycline and/or vincristine is introduced the expression of p-glycoprotein increases. By the time patients are overtly resistant to the VAD regimen, more than 75 per cent now express p-glycoprotein on tumour cells. Thus the increased expression of multidrug resistance in myelomatosis is a phenomenon of cell selection induced by therapy.

Avenues of research to overcome chemotherapeutic drug resistance include increasing dose intensity to increase intracellular drug concentration and using chemosensitizing agents or agents that inhibit p-glycoprotein function. Agents such as verapamil that reverse multidrug resistance bind p-glycoprotein and increase the intracellular accumulation of cytotoxic drugs. Verapamil's cardiovascular side-effects preclude the use of its (S)-optical isomer as a chemosensitizer. Other agents are being studied that might more effectively and safely block the p-glycoprotein system, including R-verapamil, nifedipine, quinine, and the cyclosporins. The development of a transgenic mouse which expresses the multidrug-resistance phenotype in bone marrow cells and is resistant to leucopenia induced by anthracyclines is particularly promising. It should serve as a rapid system to evaluate the bioactivity of potential chemosensitizers.

Treatment of complications
Renal failure
The avoidance of dehydration has been shown to be one of the most important measures in the prevention of renal failure, and patients must maintain a minimal daily fluid intake of 3 litres. Aggressive therapy of hypercalcaemia, early control of disseminated intravascular coagulation, and care when using nephrotoxic drugs all decrease the risk of renal failure. It may be precipitated by the use of intravenous radiographic contrast media; the risk is reduced by ensuring adequate hydration and by using dyes of reduced osmolality.

Allopurinol should be prescribed for at least the first two courses of cytotoxic therapy. Intensification of chemotherapy, with the aim of rapidly controlling light-chain production, is of no benefit in restoring renal function or improving survival. Moderate renal impairment can be completely reversed in many patients by rehydration. It is most likely to be effective when impairment is mild, and is independent of improvement in the underlying myelomatosis. The well-documented relation between renal failure and poor prognosis in myelomatosis is a reflection of the high correlation between renal impairment and a large tumour burden. Prognosis is therefore related to the extent of the myelomatosis rather than to the renal failure. Hypercalcaemia or urinary-tract sepsis need to be aggressively treated. VAD is the induction regimen of choice in the presence of severe renal failure—dose reductions for melphalan are necessary if it is administered intravenously to such patients.

Both peritoneal and haemodialysis have been used successfully in the setting of acute renal failure in newly presenting patients or in those who are rapidly relapsing. Dialysis should be offered to all suitable patients in order to allow time for an adequate trial of antitumour therapy. Plasmapheresis is particularly effective as an emergency measure in patients with acute renal failure secondary to an inability adequately to excrete light chains and is superior to peritoneal dialysis in this circumstance. Plasmapheresis is effective at removing light chains from the blood; this cannot be achieved by haemo- or peritoneal dialysis. The use of plasmapheresis with haemo- or peritoneal dialysis may result in better overall recovery of renal function. Control of the underlying myelomatosis is the key therapeutic goal; reversal of renal failure does not of itself confer survival benefit. However, the use of dialysis or plasmapheresis allows time for chemotherapy to take effect. In patients who are responsive to chemotherapy, renal transplantation should also be considered. The use of long-term dialysis in those patients with unresponsive or progressive disease is more controversial.

Hypercalcaemia
The concentration of serum ionized calcium correlates better with symptoms and signs of hypercalcaemia than does that of the total serum calcium. When assessing the presence of hypercalcaemia it is important to take into account the serum albumin, which is often reduced in myeloma. In addition, occasional patients are seen who are asymptomatic despite very high corrected calcium levels, which may be due to the presence of a paraprotein with high affinity for calcium. In these circumstances it is necessary to measure the ionized calcium fraction, which will be normal.

Vigorous hydration and diuresis are the cornerstones of therapy whenever severe or symptomatic hypercalcaemia is diagnosed in myelomatous patients. Initial therapy of patients with severe hypercalcaemia should consist of rehydration with intravenous saline, with the addition of a loop diuretic such as frusemide after expansion of the intravascular volume. If the patient remains significantly hypercalcaemic after rehydration and diuresis, a specific antiosteoclast agent should be used.

The diphosphonates have superseded other agents such as mithramycin and calcitonin, either because they are more effective or less toxic. Three diphosphonates are currently available, disodium etidronate, disodium pamidronate, and clodronate. The intravenous route is best for giving diphosphonate because its oral absorption is poor and oral therapy is poorly tolerated. Pamidronate is highly effective in the majority of patients. Serum calcium concentrations start to decrease 1 to 2 days after starting the drug, and reach a nadir at 4 to 5 days. Even extremely high concentrations of calcium frequently respond to cytotoxic therapy in newly presenting or relapsing patients. Where basic therapy is inadequate, parenteral mithramycin, diphosphonates, or calcitonin may be indicated. No long-term role has emerged for agents such as the biphosphonates in positively influencing osteolysis in myelomatosis.

Calcitonin is the drug of choice when a very rapid reduction in serum calcium is needed. The serum calcium reaches a nadir at 12 to 24 h but the effect is moderate and brief, and diphosphonate therapy must be started concomitantly. Mithramycin is effective but toxic, causing myelosuppression, hepatitis, and renal damage. Corticosteroids are very effective in hypercalcaemia through their antineoplastic actions, antiosteoclast activity, and their reduction of gastrointestinal absorption of calcium.

Anaemia
Transfusion dependence in myelomatosis is an indication for specific therapy. Anaemia usually improves with response to chemotherapy, but it remains a significant problem in those cases with unresponsive or progressive disease. There is increasing interest in the use of recombinant human erythropoietin as an alternative to blood transfusion in the management of myelomatosis-related anaemia. It offers some patients the potential for considerable improvement in quality of life without the disadvantages of regular red-cell transfusions.

Patients who are minimally or non-responsive to recombinant human erythropoietin tend to have the highest levels of endogenous erythropoietin. Response to the recombinant seems to be independent of reduction in tumour mass by antineoplastic therapy, but may be blunted by sepsis and is minimal in patients with rapidly progressive disease. Occasional patients have significant increases in platelet counts while being treated with recombinant erythropoietin.

Waldenström's macroglobulinaemia

Waldenström's macroglobulinaemia usually presents as a relatively indolent lymphoproliferative disorder with an IgM M protein and without bone lesions. Patients are usually in their 60s when first diagnosed. Fatigue, anaemia, hepatosplenomegaly, lymphadenopathy, and mucosal bleeding are common at diagnosis. Serum viscosity is increased in most patients and the hyperviscosity syndrome, evident in some 70 per cent of patients at some stage of the disease, is severe in some 10 to 30 per cent; bleeding and visual disturbances are the most common manifestations. The M protein in Waldenström's macroglobulinaemia often behaves as a cryoglobulin. Typical signs and symptoms include peripheral vascular disease (Raynaud's phenomenon, acrocyanosis, ulceration and gangrene of the extremities), haemolytic anaemia, vascular purpura, and arthralgia. Waldenström's macroglobulinaemia may involve sites outside the marrow and reticuloendothelial system in some 10 per cent of patients, predominantly with infiltration of pulmonary tissue or the skin. Renal failure is relatively rare, with glomerular lesions being the predominant form of injury.

Anaemia due to plasma expansion, bleeding, and marrow suppression is almost universal at time of presentation of Waldenström's macroglobulinaemia, and may be accompanied by neutropenia and thrombocytopenia. Peripheral lymphocytosis is usually a feature of late disease. The marrow is always involved, usually with a pleomorphic, diffuse infiltrate of lymphocytes, plasmacytoid lymphocytes, and plasma cells. Large, periodic acid–Schiff-positive intranuclear inclusions (Dutcher bodies) may be seen in the lymphoid cells. Platelet function is usually abnormal, with prolonged bleeding times due to defective platelet aggregation and adhesiveness following non-specific coating with M protein. M protein also binds to fibrin, which inhibits aggregation of fibrin monomers leading to bulky, gelatinous, primary clots that are incapable of retraction.

The IgM level required for the diagnosis of Waldenström's macroglobulinaemia has not been standardized and currently ranges from 10 to 30 g/l. The M-protein light chain is found in 75 per cent of patients and 70 per cent have Bence Jones protein. In a Mayo clinic series of 430 patients with an IgM M protein, 56 per cent were associated with monoclonal gammopathy of undetermined significance, 17 per cent with Waldenström's macroglobulinaemia, 7 per cent with non-Hodgkin's lymphoma, 5 per cent with chronic lymphocytic leukaemia, 1 per cent with primary amyloidosis, and 14 per cent with lymphoproliferative disorders including patients with a macroglobulinaemia-like features but having an IgM level of less than 30 g/l.

Median survival in Waldenström's macroglobulinaemia is approximately 6 years. Therapy is not curative. Responses to chemotherapy are always transient. Chlorambucil, melphalan, or cyclophosphamide may control the disorder but rarely produce major remissions. It is not known whether combination cytotoxic therapy is more effective than single agents. In the hyperviscosity syndrome, plasmapheresis is the treatment of choice and may be dramatically effective, as 90 per cent of IgM is intravascular. It is usually necessary to remove 50 per cent of the total plasma volume and some 4 to 6 u of plasma may need to be removed daily until the relative serum viscosity is less than 4. In rare patients with a disease resembling Waldenström's macroglobulinaemia clinically, cytologically, and histologically the M protein is IgG or IgA. The recent introduction of fludarabine and 2-CDA therapy may improve the prognosis.

Solitary plasmacytoma of bone (Fig. 1)

Solitary plasmacytoma of bone may represent a very early stage of myelomatosis. The median age of diagnosis is some 7 years earlier than that for myelomatosis; 70 per cent of patients are males. Although any bone can be involved, solitary plasmacytoma of bone most frequently presents in the axial skeleton, with vertebral presentation in some 35 per cent of patients. The most commonly used diagnostic criteria for solitary plasmacytoma of bone include the presence of a single bone lesion predominantly consisting of plasma cells, negative skeletal survey, normal marrow aspirates and biopsies, and the absence of systemic signs or symptoms that could otherwise be attributed to myelomatosis. With the advent of more sensitive diagnostic techniques such as flow cytometric analysis of marrow and MRI, more cases that would until recently have been diagnosed as solitary plasmacytoma of bone are being categorized as myelomatosis. A serum or urinary M-protein is reported in 24 to 54 per cent of patients. The higher proportion of non-secretory (even on immunofixation) cases is presumed to reflect the relatively lower tumour burden. Immunoparesis is not a feature.

Definitive local radiotherapy using a cobalt-60 device or linear accelerator relieves bone pain and eradicates the lesion in over 90 per cent of patients, with disappearance of M protein in 25 to 50 per cent. A generous margin of apparently uninvolved tissue should be included in radiation fields. At least 10 per cent of irradiated patients have local recurrence and over 70 per cent go on to develop myelomatosis. Variation in diagnostic criteria may account for the apparent variability in rates and times of progression. The median time to the development of myeloma is 2 years, but there is no plateau, and overt myelomatosis can occur decades after initial, apparently successful radiation therapy. The median overall survival of patients with solitary plasmacytoma of bone exceeds 10 years, with up to 20 per cent of patients dying of unrelated causes.

Early progression suggests that the extent of disease may have been underestimated at diagnosis. Immunoperoxidase or immunofluorescent studies should be made at diagnosis in non-secretory patients, in order to have a marker on which to focus screening for progression. The disappearance of M protein after radiotherapy is a good prognostic indicator, with those most at risk of progression being those in whom the M-protein levels remain high after radiotherapy. When progression does occur, the tumour tends to grow slowly and is usually sensitive to chemotherapy. Adjuvant or maintenance chemotherapy after initial radiotherapy has not been shown to slow progression to myelomatosis

Fig. 1 (a) T_1-weighted MRI showing decreased signal intensity in L1 due to solitary plasmacytoma. 1 (b) Short inversion time inversion-recovery (STIR) MRI scan of same lesion.

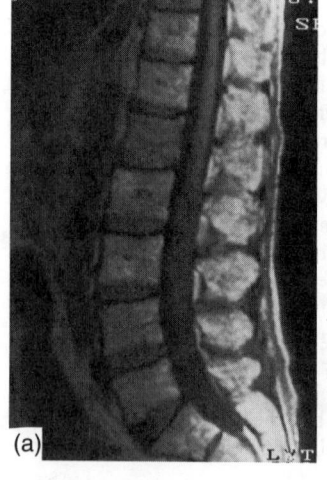
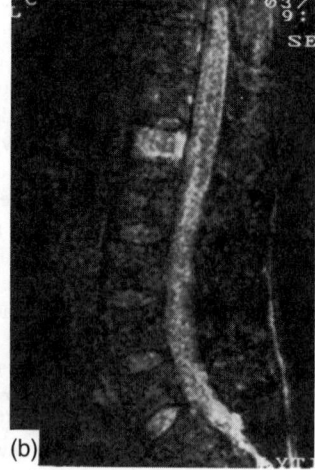

and poses the dual risks of drug resistance and secondary leukaemia. Interferon-α should now be studied as adjuvant therapy in solitary plasmacytoma of bone.

Extramedullary plasmacytoma

Extramedullary plasmacytoma has a natural history distinct from those of myelomatosis and solitary plasmacytoma of bone. The median age at diagnosis is 59 years, with a predominance of males. The most common sites of origin are the subepithelial tissues of the mucous membranes of the oronasopharynx and paranasal sinuses. Others include lung parenchyma, bronchus, thyroid, skin, subcutaneous tissue, and gastrointestinal tract. Local lymph nodes may be involved. In some 10 per cent of patients, extramedullary plasmacytomas are multiple or present in nodes without evidence of a primary site. Treatment consists of local excision and wide-field radiation therapy, which should include regional nodes. Local recurrences occur in up to 30 per cent of cases, but dissemination does not necessarily follow, and most patients with extramedullary plasmacytoma die of unrelated causes as it has a lower rate of conversion to myelomatosis than has solitary plasmacytoma of bone. Disseminated myelomatosis may be diagnosed in the absence of local recurrence. Prognostic factors for conversion are poorly defined but may include the size of the lesion and the presence or absence of an M protein. As with solitary plasmacytoma of bone, adjuvant chemotherapy has not been shown to be of benefit in delaying or avoiding progression to overt myelomatosis.

Monoclonal gammopathy of uncertain (undetermined) significance (MGUS)

An M protein detected without concomitant evidence of an accompanying local or systemic disorder is designated a MGUS. It occurs in about 3 per cent of the normal population over the age of 70 years, and in 1 to 1.5 per cent of the normal population over 50 years. Sixty-five per cent of patients presenting with an M protein do not have an underlying neoplastic disease at diagnosis. In a Mayo Clinic series, 17 per cent of patients developed a lymphoplasmacytic disease at 10 years and 33 per cent at 20 years of follow-up. A serum M protein of more than 3 g/dl is more often associated with progression to neoplasia. The probability of progression is not affected by the heavy-chain isotype. The immunoglobulin levels other than the M protein are more commonly decreased in patients who will develop a lymphoproliferative disease. The presence of a monoclonal light chain is suggestive of a neoplastic process.

The presence of osteolytic lesions favours myelomatosis; however, this population of elderly patients is also at risk of other malignancies that may produce such findings. The plasma-cell labelling index is useful for identifying patients with myelomatosis, but other tests such as serum β_2-microglobulin, plasma-cell J chain or acid phosphatase assays, or levels of CD4 + T cells in the blood are of no value.

In the Mayo Clinic series, the initial haemoglobin level, amount of serum M protein, number of plasma cells in the marrow, and level of normal immunoglobulins did not differ substantially between those whose conditions progressed and those that remained stable. Age, sex, the presence of light chain in the urine, the presence of hepatomegaly or splenomegaly, serum albumin level, and heavy-chain isotype could not be used to predict the course. The combination of C_{219} (a marker for p-glycoprotein) positivity, CD56 positivity and a low plasma-cell labelling index is seen in myelomatosis but very rarely, if ever, in MGUS. It is mainly through the serial measurement of the M-protein level in the serum and urine, and intermittent clinical re-evaluation, that the character of disease can be assessed. The median survival of patients with MGUS is significantly reduced.

REFERENCES

Alexanian, R. et al. (1992). Primary dexamethasone treatment of multiple myeloma. Blood, 80, 887–91.
Attal, M. et al. (1992). Intensive combined therapy for previously untreated aggressive myeloma. Blood, 79, 1130–6.
Baldini, L. et al. (1991). No correlation between response and survival in patients with multiple myeloma treated with vincristine, melphalan, cyclophosphamide and prednisone. Cancer, 68, 62–7.
Bataille, R. et al. (1991). The recruitment of new osteoblasts and osteoclasts is the earliest critical event in the pathogenesis of human multiple myeloma. Journal of Clinical Investigation, 88, 62–7.
Bladé, J. et al. (1993). Alternating combination VMCP/VBAP chemotherapy versus melphalan and prednisone in the treatment of multiple myeloma. Journal of Clinical Oncology, 11, 1165–71.
Boccadoro, M. et al. (1991). Multiple myeloma: VMCP/VBAP alternating combination chemotherapy is not superior to melphalan and prednisone even in high-risk patients. Journal of Clinical Oncology, 9, 444–8.
Buzaid, A.C. and Durie, B.G.M. (1988). Management of refractory myeloma: a review. Journal of Clinical Oncology, 6, 889–95.
Cooper, M.R. et al. (1993). A randomized clinical trial comparing melphalan/prednisone with or without interferon alpha 2b in newly diagnosed patients with multiple myeloma. Journal of Clinical Oncology, 11, 155–60.
Cunningham, D. et al. (1993). A randomized trial of maintenance therapy with Intron-A following high-dose melphalan and ABMT in myeloma. In Proceedings of annual meeting of American Society of Clinical Oncology (Orlando, FL), No.12, P. 364.
Durie, B.G.M. et al. (1990). Prognostic value of pretreatment serum β_2 microglobulin in myeloma: a Southwest Oncology Group study. Blood, 75, 823–30.
Gharton, G. et al. (1991). Allogeneic bone marrow transplantation in multiple myeloma. New England Journal of Medicine, 325, 1267–73.
Gregory, W.M., Richards, M.A., and Malpas, J.S. (1992). Combination chemotherapy versus melphalan and prednisolone in the treatment of multiple myeloma: an overview of published trials. Journal of Clinical Oncology, 10, 334–42.
Jagannath, S. et al. (1992). Low-risk intensive therapy for multiple myeloma with combined autologous bone marrow transplantation and blood stem cell support. Blood, 80, 1666–72.
Johnson, W.J. et al. (1990). Treatment of renal failure associated with multiple myeloma. Archives of Internal Medicine, 150, 863–9.
Kawano, M.M. et al. (1993). Identification of immature and mature myeloma cells in the bone marrow of human myelomas. Blood, 82, 564–70.
Kyle, R.A. (1993). 'Benign' monoclonal gammopathy—after 20 to 35 years of follow-up. Mayo Clinic Proceedings, 68, 26–36.
Ludwig, H. et al. (1991). Interferon alfa-2b with VMCP compared to VMCP alone for induction and interferon alfa-2b compared to controls for remission maintenance in multiple myeloma: interim results. European Journal of Cancer, 27, S4, 40–5.
Mandelli, F. et al. (1990). Maintenance treatment with recombinant interferon alpha 2b in patients with multiple myeloma responding to conventional induction chemotherapy. New England Journal of Medicine, 322, 1430–4.
Miralles, G.D., O'Fallon, J.R., and Talley, N.J. (1992). Plasma-cells dyscrasia with polyneuropathy. The spectrum of POEMS syndrome. New England Journal of Medicine, 327, 1919–23.
Nobuyoshi, M. et al. (1991). Increased expression of the c-myc gene may be related to the aggressive transformation of human myeloma cells. British Journal of Haematology, 77, 523–7.
Oken, M.M. and Kyle, R.A. (1991). Strategies of combining interferon with chemotherapy for the treatment of multiple myeloma. Seminars in Oncology, 18, S7, 30–2.
Österborg, A. et al. (1993). Natural interferon-α in combination with melphalan/prednisone versus melphalan/prednisone in the treatment of multiple myeloma stages II and III. Blood, 81, 1428–34.
Westin, J. et al. (1991). Interferon therapy during the plateau phase of multiple myeloma: an update the Swedish study. European Journal of Cancer, 27, S4, 45–8.

22.5.6 The histiocytoses

V. BROADBENT AND J. PRITCHARD

INTRODUCTION

The histiocytoses are an ill-understood and heterogeneous group of syndromes characterized by an abnormal proliferation of histiocytes. A classification of these conditions was proposed by the Histiocyte Society in 1987 as a basis for diagnosis and management as well as an attempt to standardize nomenclature for research in this field (Table 1). While some of the disorders that are included under this title are undoubtedly malignancies, some of which are described elsewhere, it is quite possible that the histiocytosis in others reflects a reactive state.

In the short account that follows we shall concentrate on the class I histiocytoses and mention briefly the manifestations of the class II and III disorders.

Langerhans-cell histiocytosis

Definition and nomenclature

Langerhans cell histiocytosis is a disorder in which cells with a phenotype similar to that of epidermal Langerhans cells ('**LCH** cells') are found in the dermis similar to that and other organs where they cause tissue damage, possibly through excessive cytokine production. Formerly the disease was known as histiocytosis X but the eponymous term identifies the lesional cell more precisely and distinguishes the condition from other forms of histiocytosis. The terms eosinophilic granuloma, Hand–Schüller–Christian disease and Letterer–Siwe disease are outmoded and should no longer be used.

Pathogenesis

Langerhans cells are derived from haemopoietic stem cells in the bone marrow, and then migrate in the blood to the skin. They are powerful antigen-presenting cells, which secrete interleukin 1 (IL1) and prostaglandin E_2(PGE$_2$) and stimulate T4 lymphocytes to release interleukin 2 (IL2) and γ-interferon (γIFN). An exaggerated cytokine response with its consequent cellular interactions may explain most of the clinical and pathological features of Langerhans cell histiocytosis. The mechanism initiating this process is unknown but current hypotheses implicate either an altered, dysfunctional population of Langerhans cells or an abnormal population of T cells producing trophic cytokines which attract normal Langerhans cells to sites of tissue involvement.

There is still controversy as to whether or not the disease is a malignancy. In situ, Langerhans cell histiocytosis cells proliferate, as judged by 'activation' markers such as CD68, but the fluctuating behaviour of Langerhans cell histiocytosis, with well documented spontaneous regression of widespread disease, suggests a reactive process and flow cytometric studies indicate that lesional Langerhans cell histiocytosis cells are usually diploid. However, recent data strongly suggested that Langerhans cell histiocytosis is a clonal disorder. This finding does not, however, necessarily indicate that Langerhans cell histiocytosis is a 'cancer', because a number of established benign tumours and other conditions (e.g. parathyroid adenoma and atheromatous plaques) are also known to be clonal.

Histology

Diagnostic criteria for Langerhans cell histiocytosis, first proposed by the Histiocyte Society in 1987, are now universally accepted. Early in the disease process, haematoxylin–eosin stained sections show infiltrates of pink-staining histiocytes ('Langerhans cell histiocytosis cells') surrounded by lymphocytes, eosinophils, and occasional giant cells (Fig. 1). Lesional 'Langerhans cell histiocytosis cells' stain positively with

Table 1 *Histiocytosis syndromes—a current working classification*

> *Class I*
> Langerhans cell histiocytosis
>
> *Class II*
> Histiocytoses of mononuclear phagocytes other than
> Langerhans cells:
>   Haemophagocytic lymphohistiocytosis
>   Infection-associated haemophagocytic syndrome
>
> *Class III*
> Malignant histiocytic disorders:
>   Acute monocytic leukaemia (FAB M5)
>   Malignant histiocytosis
>   True histiocytic lymphoma
>
> *Class IV*
> Other histiocytosis syndromes:
>   Sinus histiocytosis with massive lymphadenopathy
>   Xanthogranuloma
>   Reticulohistiocytoma

Adapted from Chu, *et al.* (1987).

S-100, peanut agglutinin, and α-mannosidase. Definitive diagnosis depends on the identification of Birbeck granules—tennis-racquet shaped cytoplasmic inclusion bodies (Fig. 2)—in lesional cells by electron microscopy, or positive CD1a surface antigen staining. These two investigations are best carried out on fresh tissue samples. There is no obvious difference between the histopathological appearance of a single 'eosinophilic granuloma' in bone and progressive, fatal multisystem Langerhans cell histiocytosis. In 'burnt-out' Langerhans cell histiocytosis, fibrosis (e.g. pulmonary fibrosis, cirrhosis) is a prominent histopathological feature.

Incidence

Langerhans cell histiocytosis is more common in children than adults, with a peak age at presentation of 1 to 2 years and a range from birth to old age. The incidence in children under 15 years of age has been estimated to be 3 to 4 per million, but the true incidence of the disease is difficult to assess because: (a) it is probably underdiagnosed and, bone lesions may be symptomless whilst mild skin disease can be misdiagnosed as seborrhoeic eczema and scalp swellings as trauma; (b) its wide clinical spectrum leads it to present to a variety of specialists; and (c), unlike cancer, notification is not obligatory. Males are affected twice as

Fig. 1 Biopsy from skin involved by Langerhans cell histiocytosis. The infiltrate of histiocytes, eosinophils, and lymphocytes traverses the dermo-epidermal junction. In this case, the rash resolved spontaneously (haematoxylin and eosin, ×125).

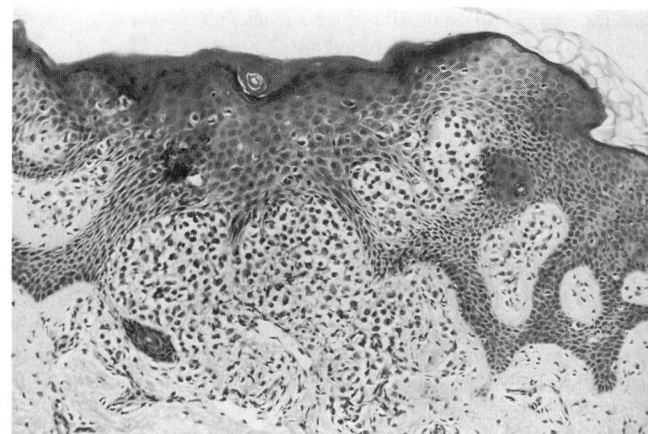

commonly as females. Langerhans cell histiocytosis has been reported in twins and very rarely in other family members but over 99 per cent of cases are sporadic.

Clinical manifestations

GENERAL FEATURES AND PROGNOSIS

The clinical spectrum of the disease is wide and the prognosis varies correspondingly. 'Single (organ) system' disease affects the skeleton, skin, lungs, or lymph nodes, in decreasing order of frequency; in most instances resolution is spontaneous and complete, though there may be residual lung fibrosis. By contrast, when 'multisystem' disease is associated with liver or bone marrow 'dysfunction' (i.e. hypoalbuminaemia or pancytopenia), especially in infants, mortality can be as high as 50 per cent, despite intensive systemic therapy. Between these extremes are patients with multisystem disease but without 'organ dysfunction'; their disease usually responds to systemic therapy but runs a fluctuating course, eventually burning itself out, albeit with residual scarring in one or more organs.

Failure to thrive may be due to such factors as (i) persistent cytokine production due to chronic disease, (ii) occult gut involvement, (iii) growth hormone deficiency, or (iv) treatment with corticosteroids; or to a combination of these factors.

SPECIFIC ORGANS

Organs are listed in order of frequency of involvement

Bone

Painful swelling is the most common presenting feature. Virtually any bone can be affected—skull vault, long bones, flat bones, and vertebrae in decreasing order of frequency. Adjacent soft tissues may be involved, sometimes with ulceration of the overlying skin or mucous membrane. Disease in periorbital bones may cause proptosis and vertebral involvement may cause cord compression. Skeletal radiographs are superior to bone scan in detecting bony lesions. Well-defined osteolytic lesions are typical (Fig. 3) (a sclerotic margin is regarded as evidence of healing) but periosteal reaction may be prominent and mimic the appearance of malignancy.

Skin

In infants, the typical skin rash occurs in the inguinal region and perineum, necklace area, axillary folds, and over the sacrum, and mimics

Fig. 2 Electron microphotograph showing Birbeck 'granules' (arrows) in Langerhans cells from an Langerhans cell histiocytosis skin infiltrate. The 'tennis racket' head and laminar structure of the racket 'handles' is clearly seen.

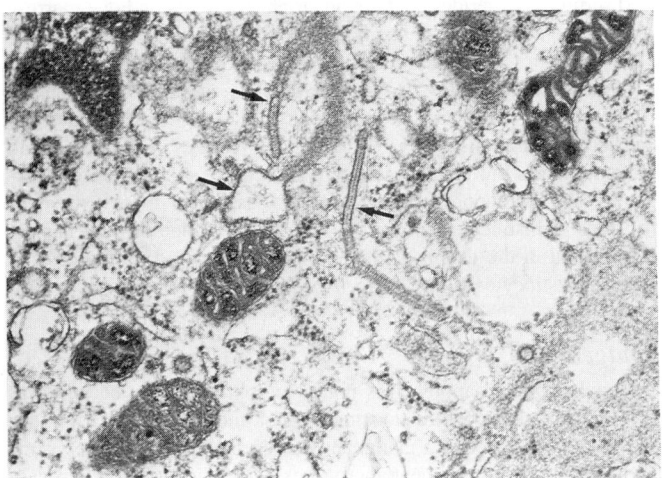

seborrhoeic eczema. Scalp involvement resembles severe cradle cap. Brownish-pink papules with depigmented scars may be found on the trunk (Fig. 4). In neonates the lesions may resemble healing chickenpox with purplish, raised lesions scattered over the trunk, face, soles, and palms. The rash may be purpuric, especially if the platelet count is low.

Reticuloendothelial system

Cervical lymph nodes are most often affected but any group, including mediastinal and abdominal nodes, can be involved. A chronically discharging sinus may form if involved nodes erupt through the overlying skin. The spleen is often enlarged, and may reach an enormous size. Haemophagocytosis may be prominent in these tissues.

Ears

Aural discharge is common and may be caused by otitis externa, owing to extension of skin rash into the auditory canal, or by underlying bony disease. Aural polyps sometimes occur. Careful aural toilet is needed to distinguish these possibilities. Polyps require surgical removal but often grow again unless the underlying bony lesion is treated. Meatal skin disease is treated with topical steroid plus antibiotic ear-drops and, in severe cases, topical mustine hydrochloride (see below). If the middle ear is involved, mastoid disease can mimic mastoiditis. Destruction of the middle ear may cause partial deafness.

Peripheral blood and bone marrow

A mild 'anaemia of chronic disorders' is relatively common. Blood eosinophilia does not occur. The CD4:CD8 ratio in blood is often inverted (2:1). Pancytopenia, usually found in infants presenting with pallor and petechiae or bleeding, and associated with hepatosplenomegaly, is an ominous finding. Bone marrow aspirate shows infiltration with both phagocytic histiocytes and histiocytes typing as Langerhans cells. CDI staining can be successfully done on air-dried bone marrow smears.

Fig. 3 Osteolytic lesion of the humerus in a 5-year-old boy presenting with a painful arm. When the periosteal reaction is as florid as this, the differential diagnosis includes osteomyelitis and malignancy, especially Ewing's sarcoma.

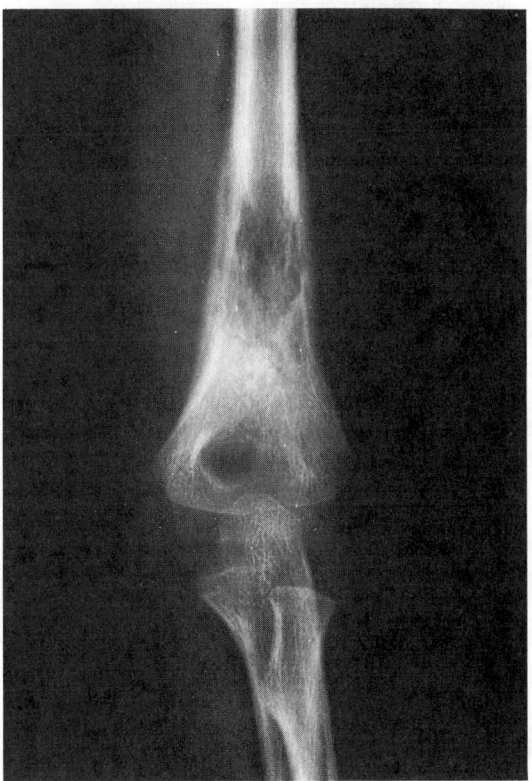

Liver

Liver involvement is often accompanied by reduced hepatic synthesis of albumin and clotting factors (prolonged prothrombin time and/or partial thromboplastin time). Hepatomegaly, and ascites caused by hypoalbuminaemia, are the most common clinical features. Biopsy usually shows periportal infiltration with histiocytes and lymphocytes. Rarely, obstructive jaundice, with a histological picture resembling sclerosing cholangitis, is the presenting feature. 'LCH cells' in the liver rarely contain Birbeck granules. Solitary lesions in the liver parenchyma or porta hepatis may mimic a tumour or abscess. Infiltration of the gallbladder is very rare.

Lungs

Lung disease may be the only manifestation of Langerhans cell histiocytosis in adults and is provoked by smoking. In young children, lung involvement may be symptomless but tachypnoea and rib recession are often seen. The earliest radiological abnormalities are interstitial shadows that cavitate, forming microcysts (best seen on computerized tomographic (**CT**) scan). As the cysts enlarge, bullae form and may rupture, causing pneumothorax. Pleural effusions also occur. Pulmonary function tests show small, stiff lungs with reduced total lung volume and decreased compliance. Diagnosis is confirmed by finding 'LCH cells' in bronchial washings or lung biopsy.

Central nervous system

The pituitary gland, stalk, and hypothalamus are most commonly involved and diabetes insipidus (see below) is the most common presentation. In chronic disease the cerebellar white matter may be involved, causing ataxia, incoordination, and nystagmus. Dural involvement and hydrocephalus can occur as a result of extension of bony disease. A solitary intracerebral deposit may mimic a tumour. Enhanced CT and magnetic resonance imaging (**MRI**) have led to detection of occult disease, especially in the cerebellar white matter. The natural

history of cerebellar disease appears to be variable, some patients deteriorating rapidly and others having stable disease over many years.

Endocrine

Diabetes insipidus may predate the diagnosis of Langerhans cell histiocytosis. Thirst and polyuria developing within 4 years of diagnosis should be assumed to be due to diabetes insipidus and confirmed by appropriate water-deprivation testing with measurement of urinary arginine vasopressin. Gadolinium-enhanced MRI to look for the posterior pituitary 'bright' signal on t_2-weighted images, absent in diabetes insipidus, is an investigation gaining recognition and may also show thickening of the pituitary stalk.

Growth failure in children with Langerhans cell histiocytosis is multifactorial (see above) but up to half of children with diabetes insipidus may have anterior pituitary dysfunction and pituitary function tests are indicated in these patients. Panhypopituitarism may be associated with a mass lesion in the hypothalamus or pituitary stalk.

Gastrointestinal tract

Involvement of oral mucosa, usually adjacent to upper molars, can be seen as broadening of the palatal ridges with a 'granular' appearance of the mucosa. Gum involvement may lead to loss of dental lamina dura and, eventually, 'floating ' teeth. Small-bowel involvement can lead to malabsorption with diarrhoea and failure to thrive, and is probably underdiagnosed. Colonic involvement causes mucous diarrhoea. In both cases, endoscopy is needed for diagnosis.

Other organs

There are isolated reports of involvement of the thyroid, heart, and pancreas.

Diagnosis and evaluation

Definitive diagnosis of Langerhans cell histiocytosis requires the strict histopathological criteria outlined above. Skin and bone biopsy are the usual sources of diagnostic material. Minimal investigations include full blood count, serum bilirubin and albumin, coagulation studies, skeletal survey, chest radiograph, and early-morning urine osmolality. Once evaluated the disease can be catagorized into 'single system' or 'multi-system' Langerhans cell histiocytosis, with or without organ dysfunction. These variables have implications both for prognosis and treatment.

DIFFERENTIAL DIAGNOSIS

Delay in diagnosis is usually due to failure to consider Langerhans cell histiocytosis as a possibility rather than in difficulty in distinguishing it from other diseases. Differentiation from familial or sporadic haemophagocytic lymphohistiocytosis (the second most common form of 'histiocytosis') is relatively easy. Pleocytosis in the cerebrospinal fluid, raised serum triglycerides, and abundant phagocytosis on bone marrow aspirate are characteristic of haemophagocytic lymphohistiocytosis, and do not occur in Langerhans cell histiocytosis. Sinus histiocytosis with massive lymphadenopathy (Rosai–Dorfman disease) should be considered if cervical glands are grossly enlarged. Malignant histiocytosis, which occurs in adults, shares some clinical features with Langerhans cell histiocytosis but is extremely rare and can be distinguished histologically and immunohistochemically. Discussion of these extremely rare forms of histiocytosis, which is beyond the scope of this chapter, can be found in the *Oxford Textbook of Oncology* and, in the case of malignant histiocytosis, in Chapter 22.5.3 of this volume.

Management

A rational treatment approach is not, at present, possible because the cause of Langerhans cell histiocytosis is not understood. Now that the disease is not regarded as a malignancy, aggressive chemotherapy is no longer used. Current treatment approaches reflect the variation in severity and natural history of the disease.

Fig. 4 Skin infiltration of characteristic distribution. Individual lesions are raised brownish-pink maculopapules. The rash is confluent in the groins and there are haemorrhagic areas on the anterior abdominal wall.

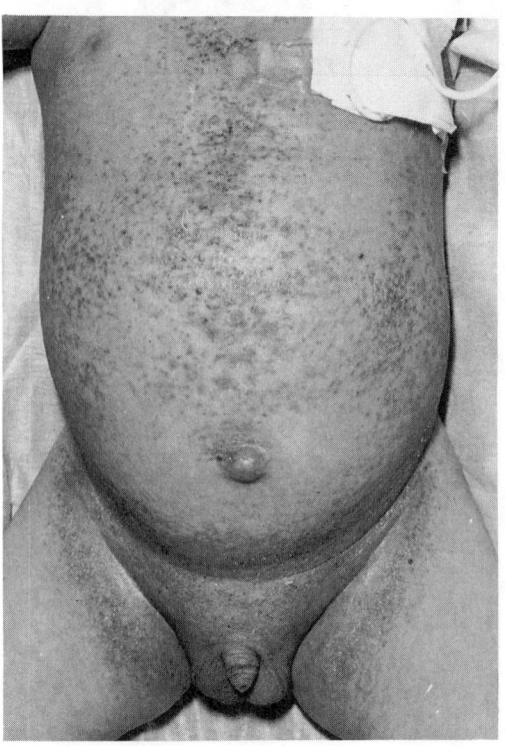

SINGLE-SYSTEM DISEASE

Spontaneous resolution of bony lesions is common and a period of observation is appropriate. Painful or unsightly lumps may require intervention and intralesional corticosteroids (20–80 mg methylprednisolone) (intramuscular depot type) is usually effective. Bony lesions that are inaccessible and might compromise vital organs (optic nerve, spinal cord) may require treatment with low-dose irradiation (7–10 Gy total dose) but this form of treatment should be used only when there is no alternative, to reduce the risk of radiation-induced malignancy. Topical nitrogen mustard (mustine) in a 20 per cent solution, carefully painted on to active skin or aural lesions, is very effective. When disease is confined, clinically, to a single lymph node that is removed for diagnosis, no further treatment is needed. Painful polyostotic disease or massive lymphadenopathy usually responds to a short course of corticosteroids. Indomethacin may be an effective analgesic.

MULTISYSTEM DISEASE

Treatment of multisystem disease is more controversial. Symptomless patients may be managed by careful observation with a real chance of spontaneous resolution. When systemic treatment is required, cytotoxic drugs and corticosteroids, either alone or in combination, have been regarded as 'standard treatment', but no particular regimen has been shown to be superior. Vinblastine and etoposide are most often used, usually alone or with a corticosteroid. A variety of experimental treatments has been used for non-responders. Cyclosporin and allogeneic bone-marrow transplant are promising and interferon-α has also been used.

The management of diabetes insipidus is still controversial. There are reports of response to pituitary irradiation given soon after symptoms (thirst and polyuria) develop. However, laboratory confirmation of the diagnosis is lacking in many instances and it is known that partial diabetes insipidus may remit spontaneously. There are also anecdotal reports of response to etoposide and corticosteroids. In most cases, however, lifelong replacement with DDAVP (1-desamino-8-D-arginine vasopressin) is required.

Late sequelae

The outlook for patients with single-system disease is excellent, with minimal long-term sequelae. The majority of patients will have multisystem disease without organ dysfunction. Mortality in this group is low but about half are likely to have long-term morbidity. Problems include poor dentition, deafness, orthopaedic problems, small stature, diabetes insipidus, cerebellar ataxia, lung fibrosis, and cirrhosis.

Class II disorders

Haemophagocytic lymphohistiocytosis

Haemophagocytic lymphohistiocytosis is a multisystem disorder, more common in children but also seen in adults, in which there is activation or proliferation—or both—of phagocytic histiocytes, chiefly in the spleen, liver, bone marrow, skin, lymph nodes, and central nervous system. The infiltrate also contains many lymphocytes and haemophagocytosis is usually evident. The incidence (around 1:50 000) is similar in males and females but this figure may be an underestimate because the disease is probably underdiagnosed. Haemophagocytic lymphohistiocytosis is considered to be a 'reactive' disorder, not a malignancy. Though the aetiology is unknown, between 30 and 50 per cent of all childhood cases have a genetic basis, with autosomal recessive inheritance. In other patients, including all adults, the disease is 'sporadic'—though often precipitated by infection, especially viral.

In decreasing order of frequency, presenting features are fever, splenohepatomegaly, lymphadenopathy, and neurological abnormalities including altered consciousness, fits, and meningism. Hypertriglyceridaemia, coagulopathy and a decrease in circulating natural killer cells are characteristic blood findings. Etoposide (VP16) is often used for initial treatment and most patients respond. Corticosteroids are also used for their 'anti-inflammatory' action and intrathecal methotrexate often leads to remission of disease in the central nervous system. In a few patients, response to this 'triple therapy' is sustained, but in most cases the disease reappears between 3 and 24 months from diagnosis. Second and third remissions are usually brief and most patients eventually die from 'organ failure' and complicating infection. Because there seems to be an underlying genetic defect manifest in bone-marrow stem cells, a number of centres have recently carried out bone marrow transplantation from histocompatible siblings, mismatched related or matched unrelated donors, after 'conditioning' by combinations of cytotoxic drugs and antibodies such as antileucocyte functional antigen (anti-LFA1). Complete and sustained remissions can be achieved but it is too early to say whether this treatment is actually curative.

Attempts to identify the 'gene' (or genes) for haemophagocytic lymphohistiocytosis have so far been unsuccessful. Even the chromosome location is unknown, at present. Gene localization would provide a crucial tool for identification of predisposed children in families with the inherited form of disease.

Class III disorders

Malignant histiocytosis

In 1939, Bodley Scott and Robb-Smith described several adults with fever, weight loss, generalized adenopathy, hepatosplenomegaly with jaundice, and pancytopenia. They described the pathological process as a 'systematised proliferation of erythrophagocytic histiocytes and their precursors', regarded the disease as distinct from leukaemia and Hodgkin's disease and introduced the descriptive term 'histiocytic medullary reticulosis'. Twenty-five years later, Rappaport suggested the alternative term 'malignant histiocytosis' because he believed that the disorder represented a primary malignancy of histiocytic cells and this rubric gradually replaced 'histiocytic medullary reticulosis'. The Histiocyte Society classification distinguishes between malignant histiocytosis and 'true histiocytic lymphoma' on the rather arbitrary basis that the latter are 'tumoral' processes rather than lesions of poorly cohesive cellularity.

Malignant histiocytosis is probably much less common than previously supposed. In the past, class II disorders—especially those provoked by infection—and large-cell lymphomas were often mistakenly described as 'malignant histiocytosis' but recent histopathological review, using up-to-date immunohistochemical, cytogenetic, and molecular techniques reveals the correct diagnosis. Malignant histiocytosis must be differentiated histopathologically from the more common Ki 1-positive, anaplastic, large-cell lymphoma (usually of T-cell type), reactive 'haemophagocytic disorders', atypical Hodgkin's disease and 'sarcoma' of the interdigitating reticulum cell. To establish the diagnosis, fresh or frozen tissue should show no evidence of rearrangement of Ig- or T-cell receptor genes and the cell should be negative, on immunostaining, for T- and B-cell markers. Positivity for monoclonal macrophage-associated antigens (either on frozen or paraffin-embedded tissue) is needed to clinch the diagnosis. Stains for the enzymes lysozyme and α₁-antitrypsin are unreliable.

Genuine malignant histiocytosis is so rare that it is difficult to be certain of 'typical' presenting features but adenopathy and hepatosplenomegaly seem to be common and neurological involvement occurs. Pancytopenia is probably the most common presenting blood picture but evolution into M4/M5, acute non-lymphoblastic leukaemia has been described. Complete remission and long-term survival can be achieved with combination chemotherapy, including therapy directed at the central nervous system. There is no 'standard' regimen for malignant histiocytosis but, in view of the monocyte/macrophage origin of the disorder, a regimen like that for acute non-lymphoblastic leukaemia (including high dose ara-C, and anthracyclines) seems more logical a strategy than one like that for a non-Hodgkin's lymphoma.

Rosai–Dorfman disease (sinus histiocytosis with massive lymphadenopathy)

This curious chronic reactive disorder was first reported in 1969. A fuller clinicopathological description appeared in 1972. The subcapsular sinuses and the interfollicular areas of affected lymph nodes are grossly distended by massive accumulations of bland-looking, non-Langerhans cell histiocytes, many showing lymphocytophagocytosis. There are also other inflammatory cells and perinodal fibrosis. Apart from lymph nodes, a wide variety of tissues including the central nervous system can also be affected. Aetiology is unknown and immune disturbances in some patients are likely to be a secondary feature. Peak age is around 20 years. Afro-Caribbeans are affected more often than Caucasians and Asians and males more commonly than females. Complete, spontaneous resolution can occur, although the disease lasts longer than a year in most patients. There is no 'standard' treatment but partial responses to corticosteroids, chemotherapy, and radiotherapy are documented. These treatments can be used if there are pressure symptoms or if the patient is distressed by their 'bull neck' appearance, but radiation is best avoided because of the risk of therapy-induced malignancy and, in the case of neck irradiation, hypothyroidism. Survival is probably well over 90 per cent but disease-related fatalities have been recorded.

The most reliable information on this disorder comes from a 'Sinus histiocytosis with massive lymphadenopathy' Registry, collated in New Haven, Connecticut, USA by Professor Rosai and his colleagues. However, as the Registry is not population-based the data may be skewed towards unusual manifestations.

Other class IV histiocytoses

A number of histiocytoses involving the skin, predominantly or exclusively, include juvenile xanthogranuloma, reticulohistiocytoma, and xanthoma disseminatum. There are occasional reports of extracutaneous manifestations; noteworthy is that xanthoma disseminatum may cause diabetes insipidus due to posterior pituitary involvement.

Some histiocytoses defy classification in the current Histiocyte Society system. For instance, cases have been reported with lesional cells that have immunological 'markers' of ordinary histiocytes, but the morphology of dendritic cells. The classification may well need some 'fine tuning' in the future.

REFERENCES

Altman, J. and Winkelmann, R.K. (1962). Xanthoma disseminatum. *Archives of Dermatology*, **86**, 582–96.

Arenzana-Seisdedos, F. *et al.* (1986). Histiocytosis X; purified (T6+) cells from bone granuloma produce interleukin 1 and prostaglandin E₂ in culture. *Journal of Clinical Investigation*, **77**, 326–9.

Basset, F. *et al.* (1978). Pulmonary histiocytosis X. *American Review of Respiratory Disease*, **118**, 811–20.

Broadbent, V., Dunger, D.B., Yeomans, E., and Kendall, B. (1993). Anterior pituitary function and CT/MR imaging in patients with Langerhans cell histiocytosis and diabetes insipidus. *Medical Pediatric Oncology* **21**, 649–654.

Broadbent, V., Gadner, H., Komp, D., and Ladisch, S. (1989). Histiocytosis syndromes in children. II. Approach to the complete clinical and laboratory evaluation of children with Langerhans cell histiocytosis. *Medical Pediatric Oncology*, **17**, 492–5.

Cassady, J.R. (1987). Current role of radiation therapy in the management of histiocytosis X. *Haematogic Oncology Clinics of North America*, **1**, 123–9.

Chu, A. *et al.* (1987). Histiocytosis syndromes in children. *Lancet*, **i**, 208–9.

Dunger, D. *et al.* (1989). The frequency and natural history of diabetes insipidus in children with Langerhans cell histiocytosis. *New England Journal of Medicine*, **321**, 157–62.

Fischer, A., Virelizier, J.L., Arenzana-Seisdedos, F., Perez, N., Nezelof, C., and Griscelli, C. (1985). Treatment of four patients with erythropagocytic lymphohistiocytosis by a combination of epipodophyllotoxin, steroids, intrathecal methotrexate and cranial irradiation. *Pediatrics*, **76**, 263–8.

Foucar, E., Rosai, J., and Dorfman, R.F. (1990). Sinus histiocytosis with massive lymphadenopathy (Rosai–Dorfman disease): review of the entity. *Seminars in Diagnostic Pathology*, **7**, 19–73.

Greenberger, J.S. *et al.* (1981). Results of treatment of 127 patients with systemic histiocytosis. *Medicine*, **60**, 311–38.

Greinix, H.T., Storb, R., Sanders, J.E., and Petersen, F.B. (1992). Marrow transplantation for the treatment of multisystem progressive Langerhans cell histiocytosis. *Bone Marrow Transplantation*, **10**, 39–44.

Henter, J.I., Elinder, G., and Ost, A. for the Histiocyte Society (1991). Diagnostic guidelines for haemophagocytic lymphohistiocytosis. *Seminars in Oncology*, **18**, 29–33.

Jacobson, A.M., Kreuger, A., Hapberg, H., and Sundstrom, C. (1987). Treatment of Langerhans cell histiocytosis with α interferon. *Lancet*, **ii**, 1520–1.

Komp, D.M. (1990). The treatment of sinus histiocytosis with massive lymphadenopathy. *Seminars in Diagnostic Pathology*, **7**, 83–6.

Leblanc, A. *et al.* (1981). Obstructive jaundice in children with histiocytosis X. *Gastroenterology*, **80**, 134–9.

McLelland, J. *et al.* (1990). Langerhans cell histiocytosis; the case for conservative treatment. *Archives of Disease in Children*, **65**, 301–3.

Mahmoud, H., Wang, W., and Murphy, S.B. (1991). Cyclosporine therapy for advanced Langerhans cell histiocytosis. *Blood*, **77**, 721–5.

Pritchard, J. and Malone, M. (1995). In *Oxford Textbook of Oncology* (eds. M. Peckham, H. Pinedo, and U. Veronese). Oxford University Press.

Pritchard, J., *et al.* (eds.) (1994). Proceedings of the Nikolas Symposia on the Histiocytoses. *British Journal of Cancer*, **70**(suppl. XXIII).

Ralfkiaer, E. *et al.* (1990). Malignant lymphomas of true histiocytic origin. A clinical, histological, immunophenotypic and genotypic study. *Journal of Pathology*, **160**, 9–17.

Rappaport, H. (1966). *Tumours of the hematopoietic system. Atlas of Tumour Pathology*, section III, fascicle 8, pp. 48–88. Armed Forces Institute of Pathology, Washington DC.

Rosai, J. and Dorfman, R.F. (1972). Sinus histiocytosis with massive lymphadenopathy. A pseudolymphomatous benign disorder. *Cancer*, **30**, 1174–88.

Sheehan, M., Atherton, D., Broadbent, V., and Pritchard, J. (1991). Topical nitrogen mustard: an effective treatment for cutaneous Langerhans cell histiocytosis. *Journal of Pediatrics*, **119**, 317–21.

Willman, C.L., *et al.* (1994). Langerhans cell histiocytosis (histiocytosis X): a clonal proliferative disease. *New England Journal of Medicine*, **331**, 154–60.

Willman, C.L. (1994). Detection of clonal histiocytes in Langerhans cell histiocytosis: biology and clinical significance. *British Journal of Cancer*, **70**(suppl. XXIII), S29–33.

Yu, R.C., Chu, C., Buluwela, L., and Chu, A.C.(1994). Clonal proliferation of Langerhans cells in Langerhans cell histiocytosis. *Lancet*, **343**, 767–8.

22.5.7 The hypereosinophilic syndrome

C. J. F. SPRY

INTRODUCTION

The discovery that a person has marked eosinophilia is often unexpected. In most people there is a clear explanation, once the clinical features and results of investigations are known. Metazoan parasites are responsible in the majority of patients: hookworms, schistosomes, filaria, and roundworms are the main culprits in endemic areas. In other regions, asthma, hay fever, and drug reactions are frequent causes. When the well-known mechanisms for 'reactive' eosinophilia have been excluded, a search may be necessary for rarer causes such as solid neoplasms, granulomatous and vasculitic diseases, and blood diseases such as chronic myeloid leukaemia and lymphomas. Even when an exhaustive range of investigations has been done, there remains a group of patients with no known cause for their marked eosinophilia. These patients have puzzled clinicians for over 100 years, and have variously been thought to have a malignant disease similar to chronic myeloid leukaemia and have been given cytotoxic drugs, or a non-malignant disease with few problems requiring treatment.

This lack of agreement about a diagnostic category for this group of diseases was resolved in 1968 when it was proposed that they should be classified into a group of their own: the idiopathic hypereosinophilic syndrome. This title made no presuppositions about the nature of the disease process, and it allowed clinicians to reassess the many features of this interesting set of clinical problems. The value of this approach has been shown by several studies in which patients with hypereosinophilic syndrome were found to have a similar range of clinical complications. It encouraged the development of a logical sequence of investigations and long-term approaches to management. It showed that both patients and physicians could relax once dangerous underlying disease processes had been excluded, as the prognosis for most patients with the hypereosinophilic syndrome was often excellent despite the persistence of raised blood eosinophil counts. Since 1975 it has been agreed that the term 'hypereosinophilic syndrome' should be reserved for patients who do not have a malignant disease. This fact alone needs to be better known, as patients have died receiving cytotoxic drugs in an attempt to put them 'into remission'.

DEFINITION OF THE HYPEREOSINOPHILIC SYNDROME

Patients are considered to have the hypereosinophilic syndrome when they have (a) persistent eosinophilia (blood eosinophil counts in excess of 1.5×10^9/l), (b) no demonstrable cause for the eosinophilia after a good quality clinical assessment has been done (e.g. eosinophilia is not reactive as occurs in parasitic, allergic, malignant or other diseases), and (c) one or more of a range of clinical problems (see below). In some patients who have no symptoms, marked eosinophilia is a fortuitous finding. These patients should be investigated in the same way. The diagnosis of the hypereosinophilic syndrome remains a provisional one and ought to be reviewed at intervals. This is because a small number of patients, who are considered initially to have no serious underlying cause for their disease, develop a lymphoma or lymphocytic leukaemia several months or years after presentation. In patients with the hypereosinophilic syndrome, blood eosinophil counts rarely return to normal levels (less than 0.55×10^9/l), even when they are treated with steroids and other drugs that lower the counts in patients with reactive eosinophilia. The diagnosis should be reconsidered if blood eosinophil counts return to normal when steroids are first given. The hypereosinophilic syndrome has been described in many parts of the world and has no clear ethnic predominance.

POSSIBLE CAUSES

By definition, the causes of the hypereosinophilic syndrome are unknown. There are no reports of the syndrome in two members of the same family. The common feature in all patients is inappropriately large numbers of eosinophils in the blood. There are two main ways that this could happen: (i) by an autonomous overproduction of eosinophils and their precursor cells in the bone marrow—in these patients the defects are probably in bone-marrow stem or progenitor cells of the granulocyte lineage; (b) by an appropriate response to excessive peptide growth factors produced in other cells—this includes excessive production of interleukin 5 (**IL-5**) from T lymphocytes in the bone marrow or periphery. Other more subtle possibilities could involve defects in lymphokine production by T cells and other cells, alterations in receptors for the eosinophil-active peptide growth factors, defects in the transduction of signals from growth-factor receptors, and abnormalities of feedback inhibition of growth-factor production. These (and other) possibilities are the subject of current research. High IL-5 levels have been found in serum and high spontaneous levels of IL-5 mRNA have been demonstrated in blood and marrow mononuclear cells from some patients with the hypereosinophilic syndrome. The properties of blood eosinophils from patients with the hypereosinophilic syndrome have been investigated for many years: they are more activated than normal, survive longer in culture, and show an increased capacity to carry out a range of functions

that are otherwise poorly expressed in blood eosinophils from other patients with eosinophilia. There is preliminary evidence that some patients with high levels of IL-5 mRNA in blood mononuclear cells have a more aggressive form of the syndrome.

PRESENTATION AND SYMPTOMS

The hypereosinophilic syndrome is most common in young and middle aged men. The mean age of onset is 37 years. The sex ratio is 9:1 males:females. It is very rare under the age of 12 (fewer than 30 patients reported), and rare after the age of 55 years. In tropical countries, hypereosinophilia in children is usually due to parasitic infections. Children can produce higher blood eosinophil counts than adults, for reasons that are not clear. In areas that are relatively free from parasitic diseases, the discovery of hypereosinophilia in children should lead to a detailed search for an underlying malignant disease, especially a lymphocytic leukaemia.

Many of the symptoms at presentation of the hypereosinophilic syndrome are non-specific: generalized malaise, weight loss, sweating (especially at night), and itching of the lower legs. Other common features are respiratory symptoms (a severe dry cough, mainly at night, wheezing, and a blocked nose), gastrointestinal symptoms (indigestion, abdominal pain, and diarrhoea), musculoskeletal symptoms (painful, swollen large joints, muscle aches, and pains), and neurological features ranging from focal peripheral nerve damage to diffuse cerebral lesions, retinal damage, and even large, focal, central-nervous damage (strokes). The last may be due to embolic events from the heart where thrombi often form over areas of necrosis and fibrosis in the endomyocardium (see Section 15). Some patients have presented with embolic occlusions of the femoral artery. Others have marked alcohol intolerance. Presentation is therefore not confined to haematological specialists; patients may be seen in any of the other major specialities.

Although there may be no abnormal findings on clinical examination, several physical signs may be found in individual patients. The cardiological manifestations are described in Section 15. Splenomegaly is a common finding and in some cases may be marked. Dermatological changes include scratch marks, petechiae, and occasionally ulceration. There may be a firm, generalized lymphadenopathy and some degree of hepatomegaly. Splinter haemorrhages in the nail beds and small retinal haemorrhages have also been described. There have been a few case reports of both peripheral and central nervous involvement, with alterations in sensation and cranial-nerve lesions.

INVESTIGATION

As the hypereosinophilic syndrome is rare, patients are best investigated and managed with the help of centres with experience of this group of disorders. The history, physical examination, and further investigations should include a detailed assessment of possible exposure to parasites and travel to areas of endemic parasitic infection, as many of these (e.g. filariasis, strongyloides, and trichinosis) can persist in asymptomatic forms for years. Clinical evidence for a current or earlier parasitic infection does not exclude a diagnosis of the hypereosinophilic syndrome. Patients may have a prior cause for eosinophilia, and progress later to a disease process in which parasites and allergic diseases appear to be playing no part. Current allergic diseases such as asthma and hay fever are usually obvious. Others require a range of studies to determine whether environmental antigens are causing reactions in the skin, respiratory tract or gut. A total serum IgE assay can be particularly useful as a normal level virtually excludes both parasitic infections and allergic diseases as a cause of persistent eosinophilia. Drug reactions producing eosinophilia may not be obvious when patients have been on treatment for months of years for other conditions. Examples of this are drugs to treat gout, arthritis and inflammatory bowel disease, and diuretics. Unusual reactions to presumed contaminants in food and drink and 'alternative' drugs should also be considered, but it is seldom worth subjecting patients with possible hypereosinophilic syndrome to detailed and expensive allergy tests as the findings are seldom relevant.

During the past 15 years two epidemics of systemic diseases in which eosinophilia was prominent have occurred: the Spanish 'toxic oil syndrome', and hypersensitivity reactions to one preparation of *l*-tryptophan that was first noted in New Mexico. This produced the eosinophilia–myalgia syndrome. Both of these diseases could have been considered examples of the hypereosinophilic syndrome until the epidemic nature of the disease was recognized. Granulomatous and vasculitic diseases, including the Churg–Strauss syndrome and Wegener's granulomatosis, are particularly difficult to diagnose when the lesions do not produce focal symptoms and signs. There is little enthusiasm nowadays for blind biopsies as a rapid way to diagnose vasculitic diseases as they are seldom positive in these circumstances, even when patients are later shown to have this group of diseases. However, focal lesions in the respiratory tract and skin are often used to obtain a tissue diagnosis when the cause of eosinophilia is in doubt. A range of solid tumours, including carcinomas of the lungs, hypernephromas, tumours of the large bowel and cervix, and melanomas, may produce eosinophilia even when they are small. The eosinophil count can then be used as a marker for disease recurrence after treatment.

Eosinophilia is present in patients with a variety of blood diseases including chronic myeloid leukaemia and some with acute lymphoblastic leukaemia. It is a notable feature in the M4EO subgroup of leukaemia where the increase in eosinophils with abnormal morphology may be confined to the bone marrow. There are fewer than 15 reported patients with definite acute eosinophilic leukaemia (although it may be under-reported as I have seen four). Mild to moderate eosinophilia is also often present in patients with lymphomas, but counts in excess of 1.5×10^9/l have been described in fewer than 30 patients. In Hodgkin's disease it is very rare for the blood eosinophil count to rise above 1.5×10^9/l.

When other causes have been excluded and the patient has been investigated as outlined above, the principal investigations in patients suspected of having the hypereosinophilic syndrome should centre on defining alterations in the blood, bone marrow, heart, lungs, and skin, which are the most common sites for tissue injury. As the syndrome is a life-long one, it is sensible to obtain baseline investigations against which to assess changes in the future. In the blood, eosinophils often show a reduced number of granules. This is possibly the most useful single investigation in the hypereosinophilic syndrome, as there are few other diseases in which this occurs. The presence of many structurally abnormal forms points to an aggressive course, which is likely to need steroid treatment. Prominent vacuoles in eosinophils without loss of granules may point to an allergic cause for eosinophilia, such as a drug reaction. It is not generally recognized that blood neutrophil counts are also almost invariably increased in patients with the hypereosinophilic syndrome. It is not known whether the defect also involves neutrophil precursors. Neutrophils may show striking toxic granulation. Markers of clonality have been sought in some centres but they have not proved helpful in defining the syndrome, although they could be useful in showing that eosinophilia was secondary to a T-cell lymphoma. Mononuclear cells in blood smears may be larger and more vacuolated than normal. Platelet counts are low when the marrow is suppressed by eosinophil precursors. Occasionally they are greatly increased, but this should alert the clinician to the possibility that the patient has chronic myeloid leukaemia. When the platelet count is less than 80×10^9/l patients may also be anaemic, although a fall of haemoglobin to below 9 g/dl is unusual in this syndrome.

Marrow biopsies show an increase in all stages of eosinophil differentiation. There are no diagnostic characteristics, but a biopsy may occasionally show features which suggest that the hypereosinophilic syndrome is not the cause of the eosinophilia. In some patients, marrow fibrosis is marked. Chromosome studies have shown abnormal karyotypes in a small number of patients and in them it is likely that the disease will develop into a malignant process. Transformation of the hypereosinophilic syndrome to a leukaemic process does not occur

unless there are features to suggest that the patient has a myeloproliferative disease at presentation. Biopsies of lesions in the skin, liver, and other affected sites show eosinophil infiltration but no diagnostic features. A rare disorder of mucosal ulceration and hypereosinophilia has been described.

TREATMENT

The treatment of the hypereosinophilic syndrome should be directed at improving the patient's symptoms and remedying the complications and tissue damage that can occur. Treatment should not be designed to return blood eosinophil counts to the normal range. This is because eosinophils are among the last cells to disappear from the marrow when it becomes aplastic following aggressive cytotoxic drug treatment or radiation. Similarly, patients with the hypereosinophilic syndrome may become severely anaemic with low platelet counts during cytotoxic drug treatment before blood eosinophil counts enter the normal range. They are then very susceptible to infections. Bone marrow recovery takes place with a return of eosinophils counts to the previously raised level.

Many fit patients in whom eosinophilia is a fortuitous finding require no treatment. There are no trials of treatment of the hypereosinophilic syndrome, but there are many case reports of treatment with a wide range of drugs. Patients with persistent systemic symptoms and/or signs of tissue damage should be treated initially with oral corticosteroid. Many respond well to 15 to 25 mg of prednisolone per day. As the symptoms improve it is usually possible to reduce the dose to a maintenance level of 7 to 15 mg/day. There is no clear merit in giving alternate-day therapy in these patients, and the dose should be taken at one time each day to encourage compliance. If steroids alone are not successful, there are three other possibilities: hydroxyurea, 1 to 2 g daily, vincristine injections, 1.0 to 1.75 mg intravenously once every 2 weeks, or experimental forms of treatment such as interferon-α. Decisions about this should be strongly influenced by the fact that the syndrome is not cured by these drugs, although there may be weeks or months of relative improvement. It follows that treatment should always look to the long term; many of these patients will need treatment for over 15 years. Decisions about which type of drug to use with corticosteroids usually depends on the skills and experience of the medical team caring for these patients. Our preference has been to use vincristine as the second drug. Doses are titrated to ensure that the patients do not develop persistent peripheral-nerve damage, and injections can continue to be given for many years. Bone marrow transplantation should only be considered as an experimental form of treatment in the hypereosinophilic syndrome, in view of the unknown nature of the disease process. There is only one report of it being used. The patient died from complications of the transplant.

Two major complications of the hypereosinophilic syndrome may require specific therapy. These are endomyocardial disease (see Section 15) and thromboembolic disease. Thrombi are treated by either thrombolysis or surgery. Large arterial emboli are best treated surgically. Treatment of endomyocardial clots and microemboli needs careful assessment of potential risks of thrombolytic therapy, but this has been used successfully to clear large intracardiac thrombi. It is not known whether it would be useful in patients with retinal vascular lesions, but (as these are not otherwise reversible) it might benefit them if given early enough.

PROGNOSIS

The prognosis of the hypereosinophilic syndrome is good for many patients. In our series of over 100 patients, half are alive 14 years after onset of their illness. Some have survived for over 25 years, even though they have markedly raised blood eosinophil counts and needed corticosteroid treatment during this time. The main causes of death were thromboembolic disease, central nervous damage, and (rarely) development of a leukaemia. The clinical and haematological course of the hypereosinophilic syndrome is stable for most patients. Once an effective treatment regimen has been found, patients continue for many years with small fluctuations in their symptoms that are usually easily managed by temporary increases in steroid doses.

REFERENCES

Alfaham, M.A., Ferguson, S.D., Sihra, B., and Davies, J. (1987). The idiopathic hypereosinophilic syndrome. *Archives of Disease in Childhood*, **62**, 601–13.

Belongia, E.A., Mayeno, A.N., and Osterholm, M.T. (1992). The eosinophilia–myalgia syndrome and tryptophan. *Annual Reviews of Nutrition*, **12**, 235–56.

Chaine, G., Davies, J., Kohner, E.M., Hawarth, S., and Spry, C.J. (1982). Ophthalmologic abnormalities in the hypereosinophilic syndrome. *Ophthalmology*, **89**, 1348–56.

Chusid, M.J., Dale, D.C., West, B.C., and Wolff, S.M. (1975). The hypereosinophilic syndrome: analysis of fourteen cases with review of the literature. *Medicine (Baltimore)*, **54**, 1–27.

Fauci, A.S., Harley, J.B., Roberts, W.C., Ferrans, V.J., Gralnick, H.R., and Bjornson, B.H. (1982). NIH conference. The idiopathic hypereosinophilic syndrome: clinical, pathophysiologic, and therapeutic considerations. *Annals of Internal Medicine*, **97**, 78–92.

Flaum, M.A., Schooley, R.T., Fauci, A.S., and Gralnick, H.R. (1981). A clinicopathologic correlation of the idiopathic hypereosinophilic syndrome. I. Hematologic manifestations. *Blood*, **58**, 1012–20.

Hansen, P.B., Johnsen, H.E., and Hippe, E. (1993). Hypereosinophilic syndrome treated with alpha-interferon and granulocyte colony-stimulating factor but complicated by nephrotoxicity. *American Journal of Hematology*, **43**, 66–8.

Hardy, W.R. and Anderson, R.E. (1968). The hypereosinophilic syndromes. *Annals of Internal Medicine*, **68**, 1220–9.

Kazmierowski, J.A., Chusid, M.J., Parrillo, J.E., Fauci, A.S., and Wolff, S.M. (1978). Dermatologic manifestations of the hypereosinophilic syndrome. *Archives of Dermatology*, **114**, 531–5.

Keidan, A.J., Catovsky, D., Tavares de Castro, J., and Spry, C.J. (1985). Hypereosinophilic syndrome preceding T cell lymphoblastic lymphoma. *Clinical and Laboratory Haematology*, **7**, 83–8.

Lederman, J., Hasselbalch, H., and Hippe, E. (1988). Alcohol intolerance in the hypereosinophilic syndrome. *Alcoholism* (*NY*), **12**, 147–8.

Leiferman, K.M., O'Duffy, J.D., Perry, H.O., Greipp, P.R., Giuliani, E.R., and Gleich, G.J. (1982). Recurrent incapacitating mucosal ulcerations. A prodrome of the hypereosinophilic syndrome. *Journal of the American Medical Association*, **247**, 1018–20.

Moore, P.M., Harley, J.B., and Fauci, A.S. (1985). Neurologic dysfunction in the idiopathic hypereosinophilic syndrome. *Annals of Internal Medicine*, **102**, 109–14.

Owen, W.F. *et al.* (1989). Interleukin 5 and phenotypically altered eosinophils in the blood of patients with the idiopathic hypereosinophilic syndrome. *Journal of Experimental Medicine*, **170**, 343–8.

Peters, M.S., Gleich, G.J., Dunnette, S.L., and Fukuda, T. (1988). Ultrastructural study of eosinophils from patients with the hypereosinophilic syndrome: a morphological basis of hypodense eosinophils. *Blood*, **71**, 780–5.

Samsoon, G., Wood, M.E., Knight George, A.B., and Britt, R.P. (1992). General anaesthesia and the hypereosinophilic syndrome: severe postoperative complications in two patients. *British Journal of Anaesthia*, **69**, 653–6.

Satoh, T., Sun, L., Li, M.S., and Spry C.J. (1994). Interleukin-5 mRNA in blood and bone marrow mononuclear cells from patients with the idiopathic hypereosinophilic syndrome. *Immunology* (in press).

Schooley, R.T., Flaum, M.A., Gralnick, H.R., and Fauci, A.S. (1981). A clinicopathologic correlation of the idiopathic hypereosinophilic syndrome. II. Clinical manifestations. *Blood*, **58**, 1021–6.

Schooley, R.T., Parrillo, J.E., Wolff, S.M., and Fauci, A.S. (1980). Management of the idiopathic hypereosinophilic syndrome. In *The eosinophil in health and disease*, (ed. A.A. Mahmoud, K.F. Austen, and A. Simon), pp. 323–39. Grune and Stratton, New York.

Silver, R.M. (1992). Eosinophilia–myalgia syndrome, toxic-oil syndrome, and diffuse fasciitis with eosinophilia. *Current Opinions in Rheumatology*, **4**, 851–6.

Slungaard, A., Vercellotti, G.M., Tran, T., Gleich, G.J., and Key, N.S. (1993). Eosinophil cationic granule proteins impair thrombomodulin function. A potential mechanism for thromboembolism in hypereosinophilic heart disease. *Journal of Clinical Investigation*, **91**, 1721–30.

Spry, C.J. (1982). The hypereosinophilic syndrome: clinical features, laboratory findings and treatment. *Allergy*, **37**, 539–51.

Spry, C.J. (1988). *Eosinophils. A comprehensive review, and guide to the scientific and medical literature*. Oxford University Press.

Spry, C.J. (1993). The idiopathic hypereosinophilic syndrome. In *Eosinophils: biological and clinical aspects*, (ed. S. Makino and T. Fukuda), pp. 403–19. CRC Press, Boca Raton, FA.

Spry, C.J., Davies, J., Tai, P.C., Olsen, E.G., Oakley, C.M., and Goodwin, J.F. (1983). Clinical features of fifteen patients with the hypereosinophilic syndrome. *Quarterly Journal of Medicine*, **52**, 1–22.

Wichman, A., Buchthal, F., Pezeshkpour, G.H., and Fauci, A.S. (1985). Peripheral neuropathy in hypereosinophilic syndrome. *Neurology*, **35**, 1140–5.

22.6 Haemostasis and thrombosis

22.6.1 The biology of haemostasis and thrombosis

I. J. MACKIE

The human organism has evolved complex mechanisms to ensure that no massive blood loss follows tissue damage and that circulating blood retains its fluidity, In response to vascular insult, blood around the site of damage is converted from a fluid to a solid state, with the formation of a primary haemostatic plug composed primarily of platelets and fibrin. This response is controlled so that the reaction remains localized and the entire vasculature is not blocked with thrombus. These responses and control mechanisms are known as haemostasis. Thrombosis may occur when there is a disorder or imbalance of the control mechanisms of haemostasis, or when there is an anatomical defect of the vessel wall or circulatory system.

Haemostasis involves the interaction of plasma components (proteins, lipoproteins, hormones), blood cells (platelets, leucocytes, erythrocytes), rheological factors (viscosity, blood flow), and the cells and tissues of the vessel wall. Haemostatic mechanisms cannot be studied in isolation, as there is considerable overlap between the protease cascade systems of the coagulation, fibrinolytic, and complement pathways. There is also an interrelationship between platelet, endothelial cell, and leucocyte function, and haemostatic responses are closely linked with inflammation.

Platelet function

Platelet activation

Damage to the blood-vessel wall disrupts the layer of endothelial cells lining the luminal surface and exposes blood to extravascular tissues. Platelets rapidly adhere to the subendothelial connective tissues and spread across their surface. They secrete their granule contents, which modify vascular tone and recruit more platelets to the site, leading to the formation of an aggregate of cells. ADP released from erythrocytes also contributes to platelet activation and aggregate formation, as does thrombin produced on the surfaces of damaged cells. Activated platelets also provide a procoagulant surface supporting the reactions leading to thrombin generation, and ultimately fibrin is produced, which binds to the platelets and forms a network between them, adding mechanical strength to the platelet plug.

Platelet activation proceeds by the binding of various agents to receptors on the platelet membrane, resulting in phospholipase activation, with consequent production of thromboxane A_2, inositol triphosphate, and diacylglycerol. These substances cause further up-regulation of platelet function, release calcium ions into the cytoplasm, and instigate cytoskeletal processes that cause shape change and degranulation. Integrin and other membrane glycoprotein receptors are made active and bind to various adhesive protein ligands, that link the platelet to adjacent platelets, leucocytes, endothelial cells, and subendothelial matrix components.

Platelet adhesion

One of the earliest events to follow blood vascular damage is the adhesion of platelets to areas denuded of endothelial cells. Adhesion requires specific structural components of the subendothelium, plasma proteins, and receptors on the platelet membrane. Platelets and other cells attach to extravascular matrices by surface receptors, most commonly from the integrin family. The integrins are heterodimeric proteins, each composed of an α- and a β-subunit. There are at least 12 α-subunits and seven β-subunits, but not all αβ combinations appear to be possible, although a few α-subunits can associate with more than one type of β-subunit. Each αβ-integrin complex has a particular ligand specificity and some are more selective than others. Certain matrix proteins such as fibronectin and laminin have multiple integrin receptors on different cell types but these are often specific for different segments of the proteins. Platelets possess several types of integrin receptors as well as some non-integrin receptors that bind adhesive glycoproteins (Table 1).

The major platelet integrin receptor is glycoprotein (**Gp**)IIb/IIIa, which can be activated by a variety of signals including exposure to extracellular matrix proteins such as collagen, and soluble activators such as ADP and thrombin. GpIIb/IIIa is responsible for much of the adhesion of platelets to the extracellular matrix proteins including fibrinogen, fibronectin, and von Willebrand factor. These proteins, as well as vitronectin, have a common tripeptide sequence, Arg-Gly-Asp (**RGD**), which mediates their interaction with GpIIb/IIIa. GpIIb/IIIa is essential for normal platelet aggregation, allowing fibrinogen bridges to form between platelets. The receptor may also be involved in transmembrane signalling, as the αβ complex is associated with underlying cytoskeletal components that modulate platelet shape change.

Platelet integrin receptors (under suitable circumstances) are capable of binding von Willebrand factor, fibrinogen, fibronectin, vitronectin, thrombospondin, collagen, and laminin. The first four of these circulate in plasma, and most of them are stored in the platelet α-granule; all of them, except fibrinogen, are found in the endothelial-cell basement membrane. However, resting, non-activated platelets do not interact with any of the plasma forms of the adhesive glycoproteins, and it is notable that endothelial cells express no adhesive glycoproteins on their luminal surfaces. Platelets exposed to extracellular matrices, fibrin clots, or sol-

uble agents such as ADP or thrombin, rapidly become highly adherent. Thus as soon as damage occurs, platelets attach to the adhesive extracellular-matrix proteins, including those in the endothelial-cell basement membrane, plasma, or those secreted from the platelet α-granule. Plasma adhesive glycoproteins may differ from their counterparts in platelet α-granules or basement membranes; plasma fibronectin has a different structure from other sources of fibronectin, and basement-membrane von Willebrand factor is more highly polymerized and more active with platelets than plasma von Willebrand factor.

A number of adhesive glycoproteins are candidates as mediators of platelet adhesion to the subendothelium, among which are von Willebrand factor, fibronectin, vitronectin, fibrinogen, and thrombospondin; von Willebrand factor is clearly important in platelet adhesion, as congenital deficiency results in a mild to severe bleeding diathesis characterized by a prolonged bleeding time, decreased platelet adhesion, abnormal ristocetin-induced platelet agglutination, and decreased amounts or abnormal molecular forms of von Willebrand factor. The vascular endothelial cell synthesizes and secretes von Willebrand factor directly into the subendothelial matrix as well as into plasma. It is also synthesized by megakaryocytes and stored in platelet α-granules. The protein is a macromolecule, existing as a series of multimers (1500–15 000 kDa), each of which is a polymer of protomers (500 kDa) themselves composed of two identical subunits (250 kDa) held together by disulphide bonds. There are discrete functional domains on the von Willebrand factor molecule, with two separate sites responsible for platelet binding and a further site for binding to collagen fibrils. The platelet membrane has two classes of receptor for the factor, the GpIb/IX complex, and the integrin receptor GpIIb/IIIa, which can also bind other adhesive proteins (Fig. 1; Table 1). Plasma von Willebrand factor does not interact with unstimulated circulating platelets, and for binding to occur either platelets have to be activated or plasma von Willebrand factor must undergo a conformational change. After secretion by endothelial cells, von Willebrand factor binds to the underlying connective tissue matrix, providing an active surface for platelet attachment should the vessel wall be damaged. Such interactions with subendothelial components may cause Ca^{2+}-dependent conformation changes in von Willebrand factor allowing platelet binding, as free ionized calcium mediates platelet adherence in this situation. Alternatively, changes in the environment of the platelet GpIb/IX receptor may occur, perhaps involving activation by proteases and the redistribution of surface charge so that von Willebrand factor can bind; the highly polymerized state of the subendothelial von Willebrand factor may also be critical.

Binding of von Willebrand factor to GpIb/IX may play a part in platelet aggregation as well as adhesion by linking adjacent platelets. The protein also binds to the GpIIb/IIIa complex on the platelet membrane following activation by thrombin or ADP; however, fibrinogen is usually preferentially bound and the role of this interaction is unclear. At the damaged vessel wall, however, the presence of large amounts of von Willebrand factor bound to the subendothelium may cause its local concentration to exceed that of fibrinogen, so that additional binding to GpIIb/IIIa can also occur.

The receptor site for binding of von Willebrand factor to the subendothelium probably involves collagen but other vessel-wall components, such as microfibrillar structures, may support adhesion. Collagen types I, II, and III have been shown to bind von Willebrand factor. The contribution of this protein to platelet adhesion appears to be highly dependent on the shear rate at the vessel wall. At low shear rates similar to those found in large veins and in arteries, adhesion occurs independently of von Willebrand factor and fibronectin appears to play the most significant part, although fibrinogen may also be involved. At high shear rates in the vessel wall, similar to those in capillaries and small arterioles, the residence time of platelets at the subendothelium is short and von Willebrand factor is essential for platelet adhesion. Vitronectin also appears to be important for adhesion at high shear, and can bind to both GpIIb/IIIa and specific vitronectin receptors. Platelet number, viscosity

Table 1 *Platelet membrane receptors involved in adhesive-protein binding*

	Receptor	Subunit	Ligands
Integrins	GpIIb/IIIa	$\alpha_{IIb}.\beta_3$	Fibrinogen, VWF, fibronectin, vitronectin (Vn), (?thrombospondin, collagen)
	Vn receptor	$\alpha_v.\beta_3$	Vitronectin, fibrinogen, fibronectin, VWF, thrombospondin
	GpIa/IIa	$\alpha_2.\beta_1$	Collagen
	GpIc/IIa	$\alpha_5.\beta_1$	Fibronectin
	GpIc'/IIa	$\alpha_6.\beta_1$	Laminin
Non-integrins	GpIb/IX		VWF
	GpIV(IIIb)		Thrombospondin

VWF, von Willebrand factor.

and red-cell count have a linear relation to adherence, which reflects the rheology of high-shear vessels where red cells occupy a central core position and the platelets marginate to the periphery of the blood vessel, thus increasing the contact between platelets and the vessel wall. Recent evidence suggests that platelet adhesion to collagen types I and III in flowing blood is dependent on both von Willebrand factor and fibronectin.

Platelet shape change

After adhering to the subendothelium, platelets spread and cover the exposed connective tissue matrix. In doing so they change from the circulating discoid form to an irregular, elongated cell with cytoplasmic projections. Pseudopod formation appears to result from contractile activity analogous to that in muscle cells and requiring energy. Microfilaments and microtubules are both found in pseudopods and it is thought that the microtubules control recruitment and dissolution of microfilaments. In the early stages of platelet activation, shape change is reversible, but strong stimuli cause the centralization of organelles, degranulation, and release accompanied by irreversible shape change and aggregation. The microtubules form a dense ring around the organelles, which liberate there contents into the channels of the surface connecting system.

Platelet release reaction

Platelets possess two types of storage granule: dense granules that contain nucleotides and serotonin, and α-granules that contain a variety of proteins. Secretion of the platelet granules is thought to occur by fusion of the granule and surface connecting-system membranes in a process requiring membrane labilization, calcium ions, and probably a calcium-dependent phospholipase.

Adenine nucleotides are sequestered in the dense granules mainly as ADP and ATP, in a complex with calcium ions and pyrophosphate, and are not interchangeable with the nucleotides involved in general cell metabolism. A large amount of serotonin is also stored and can be scavenged from plasma. Serotonin acts synergistically with other agents to activate platelets, and is a potent modulator of vascular tone and integrity.

α-Granules contain platelet-specific proteins, such as β-thromboglobulin and platelet factor 4, and others that are normal constituents of plasma, for example fibrinogen, protein S, and factor V (Table 2). β-Thromboglobulin and platelet factor 4 have similar subunit structure, extensive sequence homology, and are complexed to a proteoglycan carrier. Platelet factor 4 interacts with glycosaminoglycans such as heparan sulphate, dermatan sulphate, and chondroitin sulphate, which are components of the endothelial cell surface. It is not surprising therefore

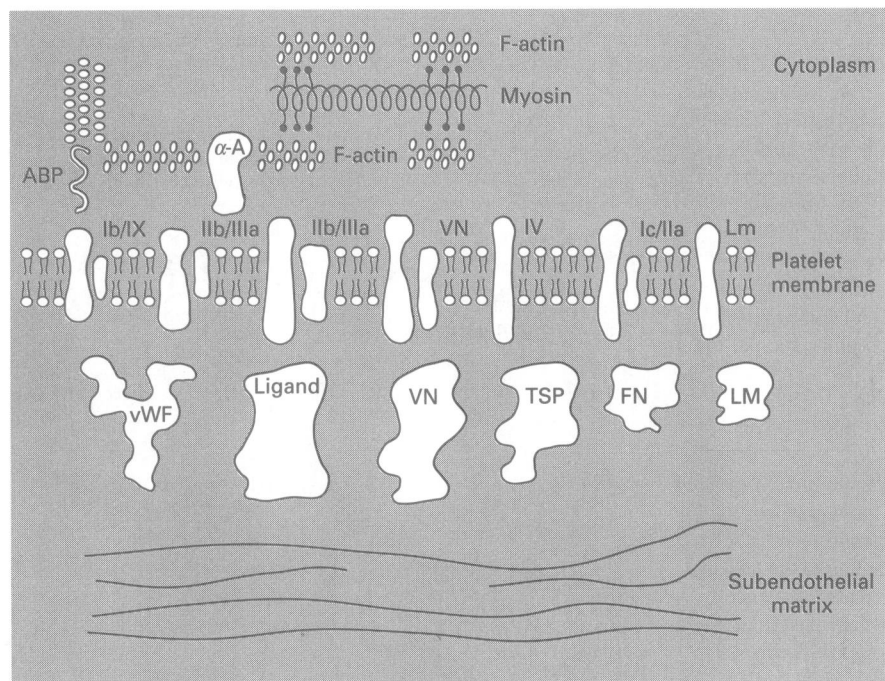

Fig. 1 Platelet adhesion. The platelet membrane phospholipid bilayer contains a variety of glycoprotein receptors to adhesive proteins (indicated by roman numerals, or VN for vitronectin and Lm for laminin receptor). At the cytoplasmic side of the membrane, some of these interact with cytoskeletal components. ABP = actin binding protein; α-A = α-actinin; vWF = von Willebrand factor; VN = vitronectin; TSP = thrombospondin; FN = fibronectin; LM = laminin.

Table 2 *Platelet α-granule proteins*

β-Thromboglobulin
Platelet factor 4
Platelet-derived growth factors
Antiplasmin
α₂-Macroglobulin
α₁-Antitrypsin
Plasminogen activator inhibitor
Fibrinogen
Fibronectin
von Willebrand factor
Thrombospondin
Factor V
Albumin
Protein S

Table 3 *Agents that cause platelet activation*

ADP
Collagen
Thrombin
Thromboxane A₂
Arachidonic acid
Ristocetin
Calcium ionophores
Adrenaline
Serotonin
Vasopressin
Cathepsin G
Prostaglandins G₂ and H₂
Phorbol myristate acetate
Bovine or porcine von Willebrand factor

that platelet factor 4 binds to the endothelium, and the short plasma half-life (less than 3 min) is likely to be due to uptake by the vessel wall. Platelet factor 4 has a strong heparin-neutralizing activity but when bound to the endothelial cell it may be released by heparin. It inhibits the activity of skin and leucocyte collagenases, and the binding of low-density lipoprotein to its cell-surface receptor on fibroblasts, and is chemotactic for monocytes and neutrophils. It may also inactivate the intrinsic system of coagulation, probably by an electrostatic effect, with neutralization of negatively charged surfaces and polysaccharide sulphates. The binding of platelet factor 4 to platelet-membrane receptors enhances aggregation and secretion. Platelet factor 4 may also be involved in controlling the level of natural anticoagulant activity, as it can compete with antithrombin III, heparin cofactor II, and protein C inhibitor for heparinoids. Thrombocytopenic serum contains a factor that causes synthesis of platelet factor 4 in megakaryocytes, so that platelets containing excessive amounts of this protein are produced. α-Granule contents may be liberated by minimal stimuli, and thus provide a further control mechanism, helping to maintain the haemostatic balance in the longer term.

β-Thromboglobulin is a potent stimulator of fibroblast chemotaxis which may be important in wound healing, and it may inhibit prostaglandin I₂ production by endothelial cells.

Platelet-derived growth factor, another platelet α-granule protein, is mitogenic for smooth-muscle cells and when released from platelets at a site where the vessel wall is damaged it stimulates proliferation and migration of smooth-muscle cells in the intima, contributing to the atherosclerotic process. Platelet-derived growth factor may also influence the proliferation of other cell types, and similar substances have been implicated in tumour cell growth and multiplication.

Thrombospondin is the major α-granule glycoprotein, but is also secreted by fibroblasts, endothelial and smooth-muscle cells (which may be induced by platelet-derived growth factor). Thrombospondin is a high molecular-weight adhesive protein with a subunit structure. It is multifunctional and binds to glycosaminoglycans, fibronectin, fibrinogen, plasminogen, histidine-rich glycoprotein, type V collagen, and calcium ions. Thrombospondin associates with cell surfaces and extracellular matrices and facilitates cell–cell and cell–matrix interactions. After platelet activation and release, thrombospondin binds to GpIV on the platelet membrane and behaves as a lectin. It also binds to fibrinogen and promotes or stabilizes platelet–platelet interactions. Thrombin cleavage liberates a heparin-binding domain and increases the affinity for plasminogen and fibrinogen.

Fibronectin is secreted from the α-granule in response to a variety of platelet activators. It is also synthesized by endothelial cells, occurring in large amounts in the basement membrane, and is present in normal plasma. Fibronectin is an adhesive protein that binds to many substances and facilitates cell adhesion and spreading. It is likely that fibronectin is involved in platelet spreading on collagen. Released fibronectin binds immediately to the surface of normal platelets by fibrin-dependent and -independent mechanisms. The GpIIb/IIIa complex may form part of the fibronectin-binding site. During clot formation, fibronectin is covalently cross-linked to fibrin by factor XIIIa, and may have a role in platelet adherence to polymerizing fibrin.

Fibrinogen plays a fundamental part in platelet aggregation following induction by most agonists. ADP-induced aggregation is dependent on the presence of extracellular fibrinogen, which binds to specific membrane receptors on adjacent platelets, thus bringing them into close proximity and causing further platelet activation and aggregate formation. Platelet and plasma fibrinogen appear to be identical; the α-granule source may provide high local concentrations, or present fibrinogen in a more favourable way for aggregation to occur.

Platelet aggregation

Platelet aggregation describes the property of platelets to cohere with one another in a specific process requiring energy, intracellular processes, and initiators. A large number of agents can act alone or together to stimulate platelets and cause their aggregation (Table 3). Aggregation is thought to proceed by at least three different pathways. The first is mediated by ADP released from the dense granules, the second requires the generation of prostaglandin endoperoxides and thromboxane A₂. The third pathway operates independently of ADP release or the generation of thromboxane A₂. One candidate as mediator of the third pathway is platelet aggregating factor. (**PAF**-acether).

Fig. 2 The platelet aggregation. The terminal event in platelet aggregation is thought to be the binding of fibrinogen to glycoprotein IIb/IIIa receptors on adjacent platelets. This fibrinogen bridge may be stabilized by thrombospondin bound to its receptor (GPIV).

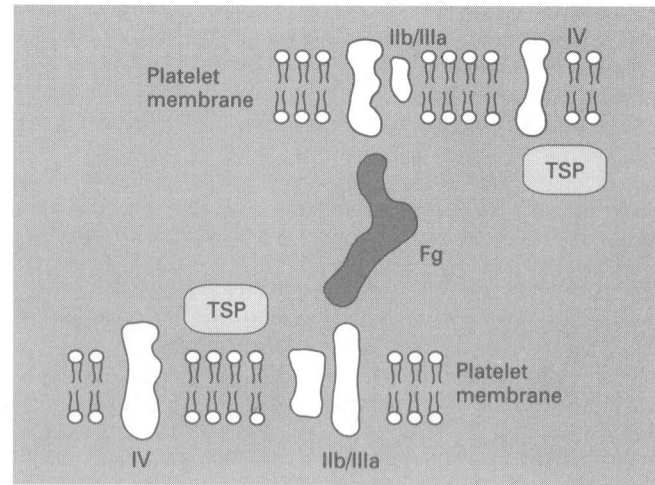

In vivo, perturbed endothelial cells and erythrocytes are probably the main source of ADP, which is supplemented by ADP and serotonin from the platelet dense granules after the release reaction; but several other platelet activators would be present, such as collagen, thrombin, and platelet-derived thromboxane A_2, all of which can act in synergy. In addition, if stress has preceded the haemostatic challenge, adrenaline will have been released, which also up-regulates platelets. ADP probably plays an important part in the secondary aggregation response that follows the activation of adherent platelets at the wound site. There is a specific ADP receptor on the platelet membrane through which ADP down-regulates adenylate cyclase, which thus reduces cAMP levels allowing a generalized activation of cytoplasmic enzymes favouring aggregation and secretion. ADP binding to its receptor also leads to a conformational change in the GpIIb/IIIa receptor on the platelet membrane, so that fibrinogen can bind. Fibrinogen binding along with release of Ca^{2+} into the cytoplasm are essential for aggregation. The platelet fibrinogen receptor is a complex of GpIIb and GpIIIa stabilized by calcium ions; the major GpIIb/IIIa attachment site on the fibrinogen molecule is on the carboxyterminal dodecapeptide of the γ-chain, although a second, weaker site is located on the α-chain of fibrinogen. Fibrinogen is the most likely candidate for the formation of interplatelet bridges during aggregation, and this interaction may well be stabilized by thrombospondin (Fig. 2).

In fact, the GpIIb/IIIa complex may be continuously switching on and off. It appears to cycle between the plasma membrane and the α-granule membrane, probably via the surface connecting system. Megakaryocytes do not synthesize fibrinogen and an uptake mechanism involving the shuttling of fibrinogen bound to GpIIb/IIIa appears to occur in platelets.

Thromboxane A_2 binds to a specific receptor on the platelet membrane and lowers the threshold for release and aggregation. It can also act as a calcium inonophore, and liberates Ca^{2+} from the dense tubular system. It also inhibits prostaglandin E_1 and I_2 stimulation of cAMP production, although there is no effect on basal cAMP levels.

Collagen exists in the vascular subendothelium as four different types with varying subunit composition and properties. These forms are designated types I, III, IV, and V. Types I and III are able to cause platelet adhesion and aggregation, but types IV and V have little effect on platelets. Collagen and thrombin at suitable concentrations cause platelet adhesion, phospholipase activation, and liberation of arachidonic acid from the membrane, as well as granular nucleotide release. The metabolism of arachidonate provides a series of compounds that influence platelet function.

Arachidonic acid metabolism

The rate-limiting step in prostaglandin and thromboxane synthesis is the liberation of arachidonate from the membrane phospholipids. This is brought about by the action of phospholipase C and diglyceride lipase on phosphatidyl inositides; and of calcium-activated phospholipase A_2 on phosphatidyl choline. Once liberated, arachidonate may be converted to a variety of possible products (Fig. 3) by the cyclo-oxygenase and lipoxygenase pathways (ratio approximately 70:30 per cent). In the dense tubular system, arachidonate is converted by 12-lipoxygenase to 12-hydroxy acids (12-L-hydroxy- and 12-L-hydroperoxy-5,8,14-eicosatetraenoic acids; **12-HETE, 12-HPETE**), which may be further modified in neutrophils to give a series of potent bioactive substances known as leucotrienes. The rest of the arachidonate is converted by cyclo-oxygenase to the prostaglandin endoperoxides, prostaglandins G_2 and H_2. A small percentage of these is converted to prostaglandins F_2, E_2, and D_2, but their main fate in platelets is rapid conversion to thromboxane A_2 by thromboxane synthetase. Thromboxane A_2 is an exceptionally potent constrictor of vascular smooth muscle and a strong platelet-aggregating agent.

Although thromboxane A_2 may cause aggregation directly, and release ADP, it is not essential for aggregation. It does lower the activation threshold of other agents and has various effects on calcium-ion flux, liberating calcium from intracellular stores and possibly promoting the influx of extracellular calcium, and along with calcium and calmodulin activates the platelet contractile proteins. It is thought to cause some of these effects by acting as a calcium ionophore, but thromboxane A_2, along with the prostaglandin endoperoxides (which have potent platelet-activating effects in their own right), are also known to phosphorylate myosin light chain and 40 to 47 kDa protein (via protein kinase C).

Thrombin is the strongest of the physiological activators and causes shape change, stimulation of the phosphatidyl inositol cycle, generation of thromboxane A_2, ADP release, and ultimately aggregation. Thrombin has at least two receptors on the platelet surface (GpI and GpV are involved), and binding stimulates either phospholipase-A_2 or phospholipase-C activity.

Phosphatidyl inositol metabolism

Three important messengers are involved in the stimulus–response coupling that follows agonist binding at the platelet membrane—inositol triphosphate, calcium ions, and diglyceride. Diglyceride is produced as a result of the breakdown of phospholipids of the phosphoinositide class (Fig. 4), which are produced by the action of phospholipases when thrombin and other agents activate platelets. Diglyceride is able to acti-

Fig. 3 Arachidonate metabolism.

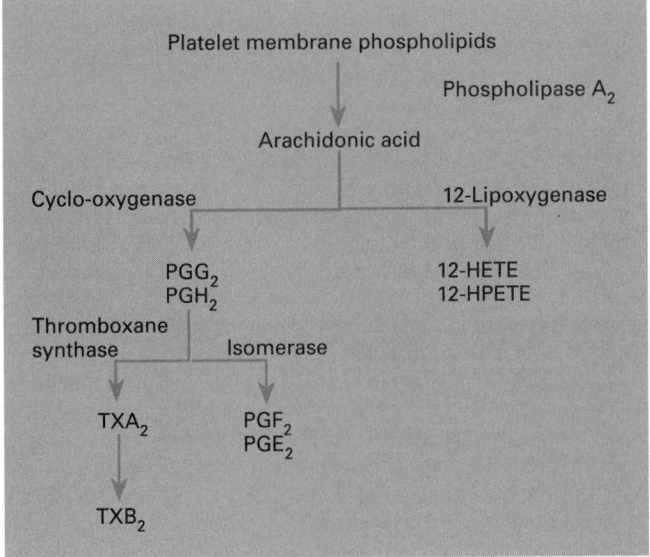

Fig. 4 The phosphatidyl inositol cycle. PLC = phospholipase C; PI = phosphatidyl inositol; PIP = phosphatidyl inositol 4-phosphate; PIP2 = phosphatidyl inositol 4,5-bisphosphate; PA = phosphatidic acid; DAG = 1,2-diacylglycerol; CDPDAG = CDP-diacylglycerol; IP3 = inositol 1,4,5-triphosphate; IP4 = inositol 1,3,4,5-tetrakisphosphate; IP2 = inositol 1,4-bisphosphate; IP = inositol 1-phosphate; 14P = inositol 4-phosphate.

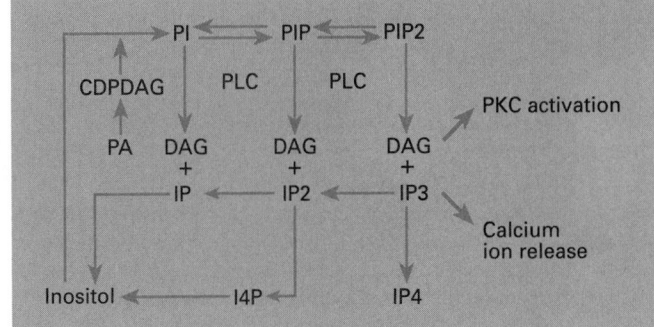

vate protein kinase C, and this enzyme phosphorylates a 40 to 47 kDa protein that appears to be associated with labilization of granules and calcium-ion secretion.

Low concentrations of thrombin capable of inducing platelet shape change activate phospholipase C, which initially cleaves phosphatidylinositol 4′,5′-bisphosphate (**PIP2**) and later phosphatidylinositol, as well as phosphatidylinositol 4′-phosphate, to yield diglyceride and inositol triphosphate. The last has been implicated in the release of calcium from intracellular storage sites in cells and could function similarly with the dense tubular system of the platelet. The cleavage of PIP2 itself may release calcium and increase platelet activation by other mechanisms. An increase in cytoplasmic free calcium-ion concentration leads to the phosphorylation of myosin light chain, with subsequent contraction and granule centralization, as well as several other calcium-mediated events associated with platelet activation.

There are prostaglandin endoperoxide thromboxane A_2-dependent and -independent pathways of Ca^{2+} flux, but the mechanisms are unclear. PIP2 hydrolysis may be involved in calcium mobilization by thromboxane A_2, while inositol triphosphate or lysophosphatidic acid could be responsible for calcium flux through the other pathway. Lysophosphatidic acid also promotes phosphorylation of both the 40–47 kDa protein and myosin light chain. Phosphatidic acid can behave as a calcium ionophore in liposomes and also causes activation of platelets, although some of these effects may be mediated by lysophosphatidic acid.

Platelet calcium control

Platelets contain a high concentration of calcium; about 60 per cent is present in dense granules and can be secreted into plasma, but the cytoplasmic concentration is very low. A small amount of calcium is associated with the plasma membrane and most of the rest is located in the dense tubular system and may be released by thromboxane A_2-dependent and -independent pathways. Calcium is actively taken up by the dense tubular system in a calcium-stimulated, ATPase-driven mechanism. Calcium reuptake is stimulated by cAMP and a cAMP-dependent kinase that phosphorylates a 22-kDa protein. This protein is believed to be analogous to a cardiac muscle protein that activates calcium ATPase, increasing calcium uptake.

Platelet calmodulin regulates Ca^{2+} transport and appears to control the use and availability of Ca^{2+} in the cell. Ca^{2+} forms complexes with this protein, and most of the reactions involving Ca^{2+} are probably controlled by or mediated through calmodulin. The major mechanism for down-regulation of platelet function is the stimulation of adenylate cyclase, which increases the cAMP concentration. Adenylate cyclase is mainly localized in the dense tubular and surface connecting systems and is stimulated by adenosine, prostacyclin, and prostaglandins E_1 and I_2. The action of prostaglandins E_1 and I_2 can be counteracted by thromboxane A_2 and prostaglandin endoperoxides. Adenylate cyclase is inhibited by Ca^{2+}, α-adrenergic agents, and ADP. Cyclic AMP is broken down by phosphodiesterase, which is stimulated by calcium–calmodulin; cAMP inhibits platelet aggregation, fibrinogen binding, secretion, and adhesion to the vessel wall. These effects are probably exerted by inhibiting calcium flux and/or promoting calcium reuptake. Calcium ions activate myosin light-chain kinase, phospholipase C, phospholipase A_2, diglyceride lipase, and promote microtubule polymerization, while cAMP tends to inhibit these, as well as cyclo-oxygenase.

The platelet cytoskeleton

Platelet shape change and release reactions are mediated by the cytoskeleton and related proteins. The cytoskeleton comprises a number of interacting contractile proteins and related enzymes such as actin, myosin, complexes of G-actin (profilin), cross-linkers of actin (actin-binding protein, α-actinin), and filament stabilizers (tropomyosin). Two cyto-

skeletal assemblies can be identified, one important for pseudopod extension, the other for the central contractile process that constricts microtubules and squeezes the granules towards the centre of the platelet. Actin, actin-binding protein and α-actinin are the principal proteins involved in pseudopod extension and the microtubules in the centre of the pseudopod probably add rigidity. Actin–myosin contraction is the basis of the process of centralization but α-actinin is involved. Calmodulin may regulate tubulin assembly and coordinate actomyosin and microtubule systems.

Regulation of the actin–myosin contraction in platelets results from changes in the phosphorylation of the light chain of myosin. Light-chain phosphorylation is caused by myosin light-chain kinase, a calcium–calmodulin-dependent enzyme. Activation of the kinase is triggered by a rise in cytosolic calcium-ion concentration; this leads to the formation of the myosin filaments and their interaction with actin and ATP, producing contractile force. The energy is provided by a magnesium ion-dependent ATPase present in myosin and stimulated by actin. Filaments of actin are attached to the platelet membrane by α-actinin, which binds to the GpIIb/IIIa complex, and actin-binding protein, which when phosphorylated cross-links actin filaments and appears to bind to GpIb. Contraction occurs by actin filaments and myosin rods sliding over one another. Myosin light-chain phosphatase may switch off myosin. In the absence of calcium ions, tropomyosin inhibits the interaction of myosin with actin, and this may be an additional regulatory role of calcium in platelets.

Platelet coagulant activity

Platelets contribute to almost every stage of the coagulation system. They release calcium ions, factors V, XIII, and fibrinogen, as well as fibrinolytic substances and antithrombins. The platelet membrane provides a phospholipid surface on which reactions can occur, and has specific receptors for certain proteins, while others are non-specifically adsorbed to their surface, which results in the acceleration of coagulation reactions.

Platelet membranes have an asymmetrical distribution of phospholipids, with almost all of the acidic (negatively charged) phospholipids such as phosphatidyl serine and phosphatidyl inositol located in the inner leaflet of the plasma membrane. After platelet activation, the acidic phospholipids are translocated to the outer half of the membrane, while phosphatidylcholine moves to the inner half, in a phenomenon known as a 'flip-flop' reaction. This transbilayer movement of phospholipids in the platelet membrane is not well understood, but also occurs in other types of cells such as erythrocytes. One mechanism might be the introduction of intrabilayer inverted micelles. These can be formed by lipids having a conical shape (diacylglycerols and phosphatidic acid), or in the hexagonal phase, that do not develop a bilayer structure. It has been speculated that intermediates of the phosphatidyl inositol cycle cause local disturbance of the bilayer that allows transbilayer movement of phospholipids.

The exposed phosphatidyl serine and other negatively charged phospholipids account for the activity traditionally known as platelet factor 3, by acting as a binding surface for the factor X and prothrombin activation complexes (Fig. 5). The vitamin K-dependent coagulation zymogens bind to the phospholipid surface by virtue of their γ-carboxyglutamic acid residues. This action of platelets can to some extent be mimicked by phospholipid vesicles, but the reaction rate is much lower, suggesting that platelets contribute by additional mechanisms. There is also a translocase enzyme that works in the opposite way and is capable of restoring the acidic phospholipids to the inner leaflet of the membrane bilayer.

Platelets have receptors for a number of clotting factors, including factors XI, IX, VIII, X, and V. Stimulated platelets activate factor XII and factor XI in the absence of calcium. Activated platelets bind factor XI to their membranes in the presence of high molecular-weight kininogen, and it may then be activated by factor XII-dependent and -independent mechanisms. There is evidence that thrombin can activate factor XI at the platelet surface. Factor Xa binds to the platelet surface in a specific and saturable manner that is not dependent on a free active site; the zymogen form does not bind. Binding of factor Xa to washed platelets is dependent on the release reaction, and the receptor is proteolysed by thrombin. The binding of factor Xa appears to be dependent on factor Va, the receptor site for which remains unknown but may involve a cytoskeletal protein.

As well as promoting fibrin formation, platelets possess anticoagulant activities and inhibitors of coagulation and fibrinolytic reactions. Platelets secrete substantial amounts of protein S, which may have local cofactor effects on the platelet membrane. This pool of protein S is released in the free form and may create a local excess over C4BP-bound protein S and thus overcome the competitive inhibition of this inactive form of the protein cofactor. Protein S acts as a cofactor for activated protein C, and promotes the binding of this protein to cell-membrane surfaces, thus localizing the reaction. Activated protein C bound to the platelet surface degrades factors VIIIa and Va, therefore decreasing generation and binding of factor Xa to its receptor, and reducing the rate of thrombin generation. Apart from being a substrate for protein C, factor Va causes a 50-fold enhancement of the rate of protein-C activation by thrombin.

Platelets contain large amounts of plasminogen activator inhibitor 1, although it appears to be in a latent form requiring activation; they also possess α_2-antiplasmin.

During aggregation, platelets produce calpain, which is a calcium-dependent thiol protease that degrades a number of proteins involved in the cytoskeleton and contractile processes. This same protease may

degrade, and reduce the molecular weight of von Willebrand factor, which could limit platelet adhesion, as the higher multimers of that protein possess more adhesive activity. A similar protease cleaves GpIb to liberate glycocalicin, with the result that von Willebrand factor can no longer bind.

Inhibitors of platelet function

Increasing the level of platelet cAMP down-regulates platelet function. Prostaglandins I_2 and E_1 bind to a membrane receptor, which results in stimulation of adenylate cyclase and synthesis of cAMP from ATP. Adenosine and xanthines cause an increase in cAMP levels by inhibiting the enzyme responsible for cAMP degradation, phosphodiesterase. Other substances such as nitric oxide can inhibit platelet function by manipulating cGMP.

Drugs such as aspirin cause the acetylation of cyclo-oxygenase, which results in irreversible inhibition of the enzyme. Certain proteases such as neutrophil elastase and plasmin can proteolytically modify some of the cell-membrane glycoproteins, causing their degradation and/or internalization.

Coagulation cascades

Coagulation factors

Coagulation factors were designated by Roman numerals from I to XIII to avoid the confusion caused by various groups using different names for the same protein. Further numerals have not been assigned to the more recently discovered coagulation proteins, as it is clear that coagulation is a complex mechanism involving a large number of substances. The Roman numerals are used for most of the factors (Table 4), except for factors I, II, and III, which are usually referred to as fibrinogen, prothrombin, and tissue factor, respectively; the name 'calcium ions' is used in preference to factor IV, and factor VI is redundant (it was found to be activated factor V).

The coagulation factors can be divided into enzymes, cofactors, and fibrinogen. The enzymatic coagulation factors generally circulate as an inactive, single-chain, zymogen form and become active after proteolytic cleavage, giving a two chain form with the chains held together by disulphide bonds; this is usually accompanied by the release of a small activation peptide. The light chain, formed from the carboxyterminal region, contains the active site, and the heavy chain from the aminoterminal, contains the structural domains for binding to different cofactors and surfaces. The active forms are usually denoted by a lower case 'a' after the Roman numeral. With the exception of factor XIII, which is a transglutaminase, they are all serine proteases related to trypsin. Some of the coagulation proteins are known as vitamin K-dependent factors (factors II, VII, IX and X, protein C, protein S); there are also other proteins, apparently not involved in haemostasis, that require vitamin K—osteocalcin (an extrahepatic enzyme synthesized in osteoblasts) and enzymes in spermatozoa for example. The vitamin K-dependent proteins are synthesized in the hepatocyte and undergo post-translational modification in a carboxylase reaction. Certain glutamic acid residues in a specific structural domain of the protein undergo carboxylation of their γ carbon atom so that two carboxyl groups are attached, and γ-carboxyglutamic acid is formed. In this reaction vitamin K acts as a coenzyme, the conversion of vitamin K to its epoxide form providing the energy for CO_2 fixation and γ-carboxylation (Fig. 6). The vitamin K epoxide is converted back into active vitamin K by a two-step reductase system. The reduction process is blocked by oral anticoagulants of the coumarin group, which interfere in the normal production of vitamin K-dependent factors. The γ-carboxyglutamic acid (Gla) residues are localized to a discrete region of vitamin K-dependent factors and facilitate the interaction of that region with phospholipids in the presence of calcium ions.

Factors V, VIII, high kininogen, tissue factor, as well as protein S,

Fig. 5 Platelet coagulant activity. Pathways for activation of prothrombin (prothrombinase complex), factor X (tenase complex), and factor XI, on platelet membrane phospholipids.

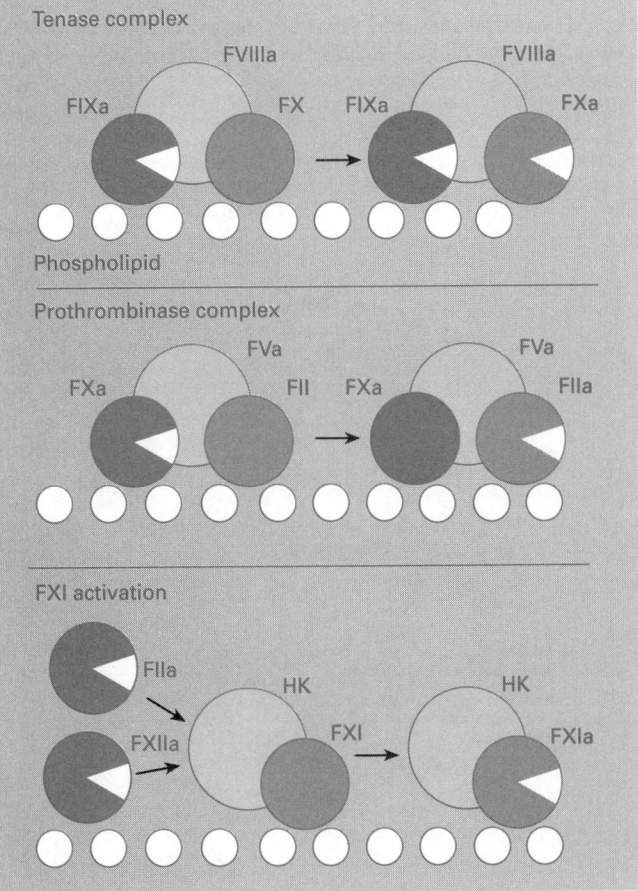

Table 4 *Coagulation factors and Roman numerals*

Factor	Names	M_r	Plasma concentration	Plasma half-life
I	Fibrinogen	340 000	1.5–4 g/l	96–120 h
II	Prothrombin	72 000	1–1.5 μg/ml	72 h
III	Tissue thromboplastin	43 000 (apoprotein)	Tissue bound	
V	Proaccelerin	300 000	10 mg/l	12–15 h
VII	Proconvertin	63 000	500 μg/l	4–6 h
VIII	Antihaemophilic globulin A	200 000	200 μg/l	10–18 h
IX	Antihaemophilic globulin B	55 000	5–10 mg/l	18–30 h
X	Stuart–Prower factor	55 000	10 mg/l	36 h
XI	Plasma thromboplastin antecedent	160 000	5 mg/l	10–20 h
XII	Hageman factor	90 000	40 mg/l	50–70 h
XIII	Fibrin stabilizing factor	320 000	10 mg/l	100–120 h

have no enzyme activity and act as cofactors in the activation of serine proteases.

The tissue factor-mediated pathway of coagulation

Tissue-factor protein is readily identified in the cells surrounding blood vessels, organ capsules, and cells of epithelial surfaces and the nervous system. Tissue factor is present in particularly high concentrations in brain and placental tissues. Monocytes can be stimulated to express tissue factor, and synthesis can be induced by cytokines, growth factors, lipopolysaccharide, antigen–antibody complexes, tumour cells, and anaphylotoxin. Vascular endothelial cells can also be induced to express tissue factor in response to lipopolysaccharide, interleukin 1 (**IL-1**), tumour necrosis factor-α, and vascular permeability factor. Little tissue factor is expressed by cells within the vasculature, but it is present in the subendothelium.

Tissue factor is also exposed after trauma or cell damage, and usually remains localized at the site of injury because it is an apoprotein with a large transmembrane hydrophobic region and only has full activity when associated with membrane lipids. Thus when factor VII binds to tissue factor, the resulting factor X-activating complex remains localized at the cell surface. Factor VII is unusual because the zymogen form appears to have weak proteolytic activity on factor X. Tissue factor acts as a cofactor for the further activation of factor VII to Factor VIIa by factor Xa and the activation of both factor IX and factor X by factor VIIa (Fig. 7). The resultant factor Xa exerts a positive feedback effect by cleaving factor VII to yield factor VIIa, which has enhanced activity on factor X, producing more factor Xa. The factor Xa remains phospholipid bound, and forms a complex with factor V and prothrombin (the prothrombinase complex). Factor Xa cleaves prothrombin to produce thrombin, which is separated from its phospholipid-binding domain and can diffuse away from the phospholipid surface.

The interactions between these coagulation factors are dependent on the presence of calcium ions, which facilitate the binding of prothrombin, factor VII, and factor X to phospholipids. A constant theme in coagulation is the formation of reaction complexes composed of an enzyme, a substrate, a cofactor and an organizing surface (Fig. 8). In these reactions the surface is a phospholipid layer, and the cofactor is tissue factor in the reactions involving factor VII, and factor V in the prothrombinase reaction. The cofactors act by increasing the reaction velocity, while the surface brings the reaction components together, so that a reaction is favoured (the K_m is lowered). The presence of both cofactors and phospholipid surfaces accelerates the reactions several thousand-fold.

Fig. 6 Vitamin K dependent carboxylation. Vitamin K (K) is first converted to a hydroquinone (KH_2) by either a NADPH-dependent or a dithiol (RSH_2)-dependent reductase enzyme. Specific glutamate residues (GLU) are τ-carboxylated (Gla) by a vitamin K dependent carboxylase. During this reaction, the vitamin K hydroquinone is converted to vitamin K epoxide (KO). The latter is converted back to vitamin K.

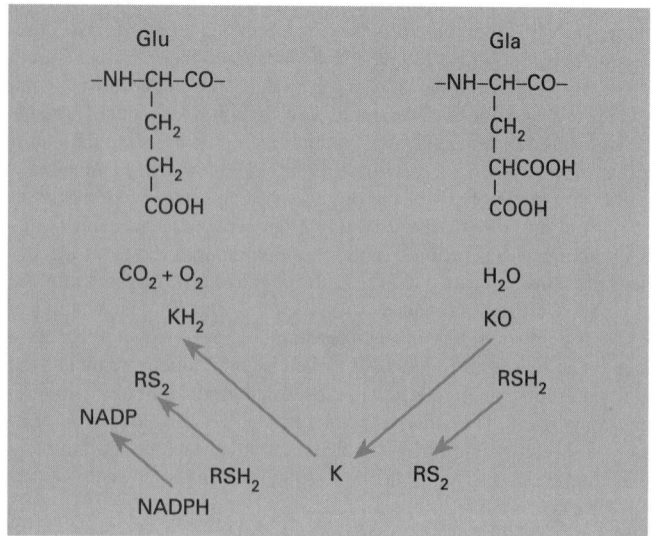

Fig. 7 The coagulation pathways. The coagulation cascade or pathways may be triggered by exposure of blood to foreign or extravascular surfaces, tissue rupture, and exposure of tissue factor, or platelet activation.

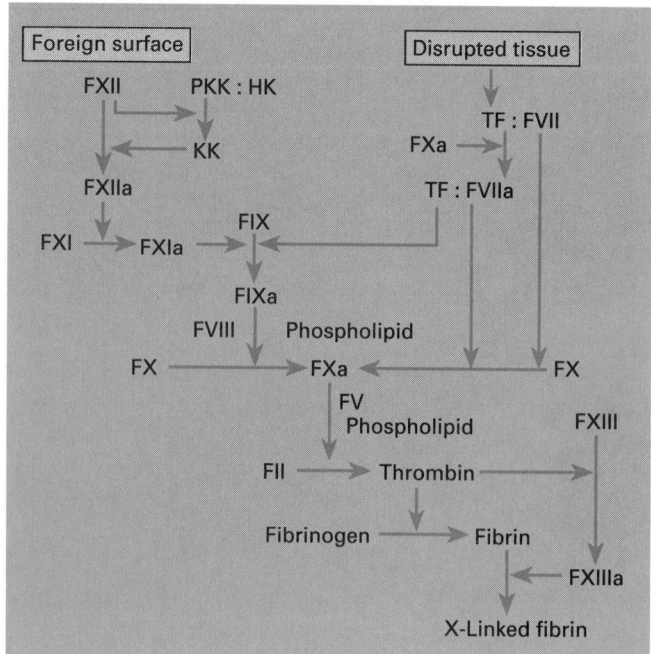

A further action of factor VII is to activate factor IX to factor IXa, which itself can activate factor X. This appears to amplify the response to cell damage and promote a burst of thrombin generation.

The phospholipid-dependent coagulation reactions can take place on the surface of activated platelets, but the membranes of other blood cells as well as endothelial cells are potential surfaces for the reactions to occur. This is a further mechanism to ensure that the reactions leading to fibrin formation remain localized at the site of damage.

When factor Xa accumulates, a complex is formed with a protein known as tissue-factor pathway inhibitor (**TFPI**, EPI, LACI) (Fig. 9). This complex can then form a tetramer with factor VIIa and tissue factor, resulting in the inhibition of factor VIIa and the tissue factor or extrinsic pathway of coagulation. However, activation of factor X by factor IXa (the tenase complex) is not affected. TFPI is released from the endothelium by heparin, and can also be released by platelets. In plasma it exists in a free form, and bound to apolipoprotein a; approximately 50 per cent is lipoprotein bound.

The intrinsic system

There appear to be several mechanisms for the activation of factor XI. It can be cleaved by factor XIIa in the fluid phase, or at negatively charged surfaces; it can also be activated on platelet membranes in factor XIIa-dependent and -independent reactions. The latter may be due to several mechanisms, but the activation of factor XI by thrombin at the platelet surface has recently been described. Thus thrombin formed in an initial rapid burst following the exposure of blood to tissue factor could activate platelets and convert factor XI to factor XIa, and thus trigger the reactions leading to further generation of thrombin. Factor XI is unusual in being a double molecule with two identical chains

linked by disulphide bridges. This appears to be an amplification mechanism, so that two active serine centres are produced from a single interaction with factor XIIa or thrombin. Factor XI circulates as a complex with high molecular-weight kininogen (**HK**), which has surface-binding properties. Proteolytic cleavage of HK removes this binding function, and free factor XI does not readily bind to surfaces. Factor XIa acts on factor IX to produce factor IXa, which forms a complex with factor VIII, factor X, and phospholipid, in the presence of calcium ions, and liberates factor Xa. Thrombin cleaves factors V and VIII and makes them active as cofactors for the tenase and prothrombinase complexes. Prolonged exposure to high thrombin complexes causes further cleavage and inactivation of factors V and VIII. On the platelet surface, thrombin can activate factor XI and cleave several integral platelet-membrane proteins, resulting in platelet activation or up-regulation.

The contact activation pathway

The exposure of factor XII (Hageman factor) to a variety of charged surfaces leads to the expression of its enzymatic activity. It is unclear whether factor XII must be cleaved to become active, or whether a confirmational change resulting from binding at a negatively charged surface can expose the active site. This site of activation can be a foreign surface, collagen fibrils, sulphatides, urate crystals, and exposure to endotoxin. Thus exposure of blood to extravascular tissues or the introduction of foreign materials to the bloodstream can activate the contact system. When factor XII becomes active, it is able to cleave prekallikrein (**PKK**) to yield kallikrein. PKK, like factor XI, circulates as a complex with HK, which acts as a cofactor and facilitates PKK binding at the surface. Kallikrein has a variety of substrates (Fig. 10) including HK, which it cleaves, with the loss of surface-binding capabilities, and liberates the vasoactive peptide bradykinin. Bradykinin can have effects on peripheral resistance, as it releases nitric oxide from the vascular endothelium, which causes relaxation of the smooth muscle and vasodilatation. Kallikrein acts in a positive feedback loop to activate further factor XII to factor XIIa, which can cause more generation of Kallikrein. Further action of kallikrein on α-factor XIIa produces β-factor XIIa, a low molecular-weight fragment that retains the serine centre. These two forms of factor XIIa differ in their properties: the α-form can activate factor XI and PKK, but the β-form does not have the ability to bind to surfaces, and has little activity on factor XI; however, it retains activity on PKK and in some circumstances can activate factor VII (although it is unclear whether this reaction has any physiological relevance). Thus the influence of contact activation becomes diverted from coagulation towards the other pathways that it modulates, i.e. kinin generation, complement activation, and fibrinolysis. Kallikrein is able to activate com-

Fig. 8 Surface mediated coagulation reactions. A constant theme in coagulation is the binding of an enzyme, and its substrate to a surface, which is usually phospholipid. The conversion of substrate into product (an active protease) is catalysed by a cofactor which complexes with the other reaction components.

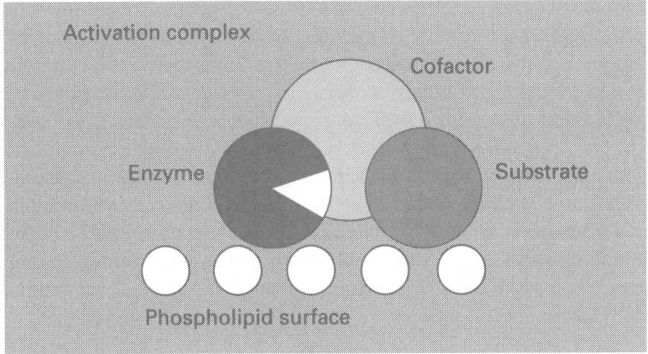

Fig. 9 Tissue factor pathway inhibitor reactions. Tissue factor pathway inhibitor (TFPI) binds to factor Xa and forms a quaternary comlex with factor VIIa and tissue factor, resulting in inhibition of the extrinsic system.

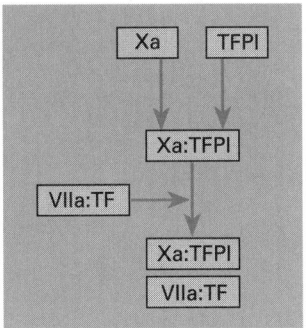

Fig. 10 Contact activation. Factor XII binds to charged foreign or extravascular surfaces and its active site becomes exposed, thus triggering the contact system. HK = high molecular weight kininogen; PKK = prekallikrein; KK = kallikrein.

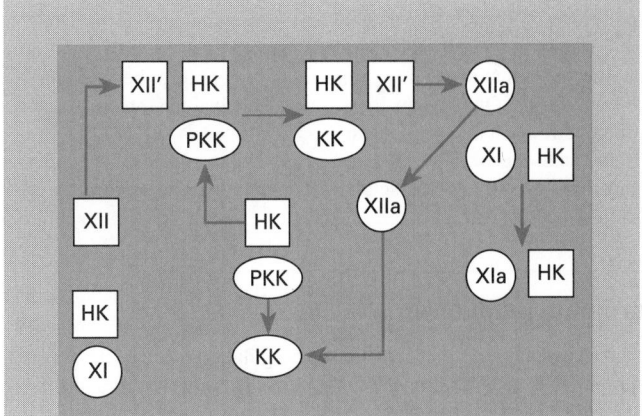

plement by the alternative pathway, and the complement proteins can influence haemostasis in a variety of ways. They may compete for serine protease inhibitors, and C3a and C5a activate neutrophils with the production of NO, and enzymes that promote platelet aggregation and degrade coagulation factors.

Kallikrein can activate plasminogen by three mechanisms: it can directly cleave plasminogen to plasmin, it can activate pro-urokinase type-plasminogen activator to the active two-chain form, and it can activate proactivator.

Kallikrein and factor XIIa are inhibited by C1-esterase inhibitor and to a lesser extent, α_2-macroglobulin. Antithrombin III and protein-C inhibitor are also able to inhibit kallikrein. Factor XIa is inhibited by α_1-antitrypsin and antithrombin III.

Inherited deficiency of factor II, V, VII, X, IX, or VIII usually causes a mild, moderate, or severe bleeding diathesis, while in homozygous factor XI deficiency the patient is only likely to bleed after trauma or surgery. In contrast, factor XII and PKK deficiency are only rarely associated with a haemorrhagic tendency. The contact-activation pathways may only be important for intrinsic coagulation in certain tissues, or at a particular phase of haemostasis, so that deficiency can be compensated for by an alternative mechanism. It is likely that the tissue-factor pathway is important for the early, rapid production of thrombin after tissue damage. The intrinsic system may then take over, initially with activation of factor IX by factor VIIa, and then with factor XI activation by the small amounts of thrombin generated by the extrinsic pathway (or alternatively due to the action of factor XIIa, or other mechanisms). This would give a sustained generation of factor Xa and thrombin.

Thrombin and fibrinogen

Fibrinogen is a large protein with a heterodimer subunit structure. It is composed of two each of three different polypeptide chains, α, β, and γ. They are held together by disulphide bonds near the N-terminal. Thrombin cleaves small peptides (fibrinopeptides A and B) from the α- and β-chains to form fibrin monomer. Fibrin monomer can interact with intact fibrinogen to give soluble complexes, but when sufficient fibrin monomers are formed, they undergo end-to-end polymerization to form long fibrin strands. When a sufficient molecular size is reached, these precipitate to give a solid fibrin clot. However, such a clot lacks tensile strength and would be easily washed away in flowing blood. A system for cross-linking the fibrin polymers to stabilize them therefore exists.

Fibrin-stabilizing factor (factor XIII or fibrinoligase) circulates in a zymogen form with a molecular weight of about 320 kDa and is converted to an active transglutaminase by the action of thrombin. It is composed of two types of subunit, a and b, and possesses two of each type of chain (a2b2). The a subunit contains the active centre cysteine of the transglutaminase, while the b subunit appears to act as a non-catalytic carrier protein. Factor XIII is synthesized in the liver and present in plasma as well as in platelet α-granules. During the activation of factor XIII by thrombin, a small peptide is cleaved from subunit a and a calcium-dependent dissociation of the b subunits occurs, exposing the active centre. Factor XIIIa induces covalent-bond formation between fibrin strands to give dimers between the γ-chains of adjacent fibrin monomers. Then at a much slower rate, polymers form between the α-chains of fibrin. Only when these inter-α-chain links are made does fibrin acquire its stable properties.

Blood cells become trapped in the developing fibrin clot, and the strands bind to and intersperse platelet aggregates as they form to give a primary haemostatic plug.

Thrombin inhibitors

As thrombin plays a pivotal role in the coagulation mechanism, it is not surprising that it has a number of inhibitors. These were originally classified using six Roman numerals, hence the name antithrombin III. This

Table 5 *The serpin superfamily*

Serpin	Target protease
AT-III	Thrombin, factor Xa, kallikrein
Heparin cofactor II	Thrombin, cathepsin G
α_2-Antiplasmin	Plasmin
PAI-1, PAI-2	t-PA, u-PA
PC inhibitor-1 (PAI-3)	APC, kallikrein, t-PA
α_1-Antitrypsin	Neutrophil elastase, factor XIa
Antichymotrypsin	Cathepsin G
C1 inhibitor	C1s, kallikrein, factor XIIa

Abbreviations as in text.

is the only name to have persisted and refers to a protein that is potentiated by heparin and has progressive antithrombin activity. The other numerals referred to the antithrombin activities of fibrin, fibrinogen degradation products, α_2-macroglobulin, and an acquired antibody. A second heparin cofactor (heparin cofactor II, dermatan sulphate cofactor) has been more recently discovered and is discussed below. Antithrombin III is perhaps the main inhibitor of thrombin, but is also an important physiological inhibitor of factor Xa and kallikrein, although it can also complex with most of the other serine protease coagulation factors. It is part of the serpin superfamily of proteins (Table 5), which show extensive sequence homology and have evolved from a primitive ancestral serine protease inhibitor. The serpins form a 1:1 irreversible complex with their target protease, and the complex is subsequently removed from the circulation and catabolized. Other examples of the serpin superfamily are given in Table 5.

The action of antithrombin III is greatly potentiated by heparin, *in vitro* and *in vivo*, when used therapeutically or prophylactically. The physiological counterpart of heparin is probably heparan sulphate, which may be found on the endothelial cell surfaces. Heparin has a specific binding site for antithrombin III and interacts with certain lysine residues in a particular domain of the antithrombin-III molecule. Heparin binding causes a conformational change that opens up the thrombin-binding site in antithrombin III and greatly accelerates the inhibition of thrombin. Heparin also has a specific site that binds to thrombin directly (Fig. 11). Heparin is a highly acidic mucopolysaccharide composed of equal amounts of sulphated D-glucosamine and D-glucuronic acid, interlinked by sulphaminic bridges. Heparin is a mixture of molecules of varying chain length, and some chains are too short to potentiate thrombin inhibition by antithrombin III, as they possess either an antithrombin III-binding site or a thrombin-binding site but not both. Inhibition of factor Xa differs (Fig. 11), as it only binds to the antithrombin III and has no binding site on heparin. Antithrombin III is synthesized mainly

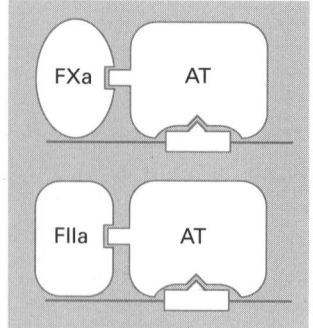

Fig. 11 Antithrombin III and heparin. Heparin contains specific binding sequences for antithrombin III (AT) and thrombin (FIIa), but no binding site for factor Xa (FXa). (Modified from Lane, D., *et al.* (1984). Anticoagulant activities of heparin- oligosaccharides and their neutralization by platelet factor 4. *Biochemical Journal*, **218**, 731, with permission.)

in the liver, but smaller amounts are produced in the endothelial cell, where it is stored as a high molecular-weight complex with a glycosaminoglycan. Low concentrations have also been detected, using immunological techniques, in platelet α-granules. Factor Xa is protected from the action of antithrombin III by phospholipids and factor V.

Heparin cofactor II is also a glycosaminoglycan-dependent thrombin inhibitor with many similarities in structure and function to antithrombin III. However, it shows greater specificity for target proteases and, amongst the coagulation factors, only inhibits thrombin. It is also capable of inhibiting chymotrypsin-like enzymes and can bind to cathepsin G, which may have implications in the haemostatic process. Cathepsin G is released from neutrophils on degranulation and can influence fibrinolysis and cause platelet aggregation.

Antithrombin III and heparin cofactor II are decreased in acute inflammatory disease and shock syndromes. Despite their similar molecular size, antithrombin III is lost through the kidney in nephrotic syndrome, whereas heparin cofactor II is conserved. Heparin cofactor II but not antithrombin III is reduced in malaria and congenital haemolytic defects, suggesting that heparin cofactor II may play some part as a cell-associated thrombin inhibitor, and may have an important role in the prevention of thrombosis. Indeed, it has been shown to have an additive effect to that of antithrombin III for thrombin inhibition at the damaged vessel wall.

Vitronectin, along with platelet factor 4, histidine-rich glycoprotein, and serum amyloid-P component, appears to compete with serpines for heparin binding and neutralizes the acceleration of heparinoids on activity by serpines. Vitronectin appears to protect the enzymes against rapid inactivation. Most plasma vitronectin is in the unfolded form, with no heparin-binding sites exposed, yet it is found in ternary complexes with thrombin and serpines (e.g. antithrombin III, heparin cofactor II). There must be some mechanism responsible for a conformational change in vitronectin during blood coagulation. The ternary complexes are rapidly cleared and metabolized by the liver and vessel wall.

α₂-Macroglobulin can also inhibit thrombin as well as many other proteases of the coagulation, contact, and fibrinolytic systems. It is not a serpine, and although the serine centre of the proteases is masked, it is not covalently bound to the inhibitor as in the serpine family. Fibrin also has an extensive capacity for thrombin inhibition, which has not been well investigated.

The protein C and S system

Protein C and protein S are involved in a pathway that leads to the degradation of the procoagulant cofactors Va and VIIIa. Both proteins are vitamin K dependent, but protein S is unusual as it has no enzymatic activity. It is synthesized in the liver but also released by platelets during activation. It is unclear whether megakaryocytes and endothelial cells have the capacity to synthesise protein S and possess the post-translational enzymes involving vitamin K, or whether they endocytose the protein from plasma.

Thrombin binds to several classes of receptor on the vascular endothelium: one of these is thrombomodulin, a transmembrane protein with an extensive hydrophobic region, which is synthesized and expressed by endothelial cells. Thrombin binds to thrombomodulin with high affinity and thrombomodulin blocks the procoagulant (fibrinogen clotting, factor V activation, and platelet activation) activities of thrombin. The thrombin–thrombomodulin complex binds protein C, which also binds to the membrane phospholipids. The protein C is cleaved by thrombin in a reaction catalysed by thrombomodulin (Fig. 12), to yield activated protein C. This reaction can be catalysed approximately 50-fold by factor Va, but the concentration required to stimulate protein-C activation is greater than that required for platelet-surface prothrombinase activity. The light chain of factor V (the phospholipid- and thrombin-binding region) can inhibit the thrombin–thrombomodulin catalysed activation of protein C. Thus a complex regulatory mechanism exists, whereby factor V is activated by small amounts of thrombin and accelerates the production of further thrombin, but when higher concentrations of factor Va are produced, production of the anticoagulant activated protein C is catalysed. This process is switched off as factor Va is eventually pro-

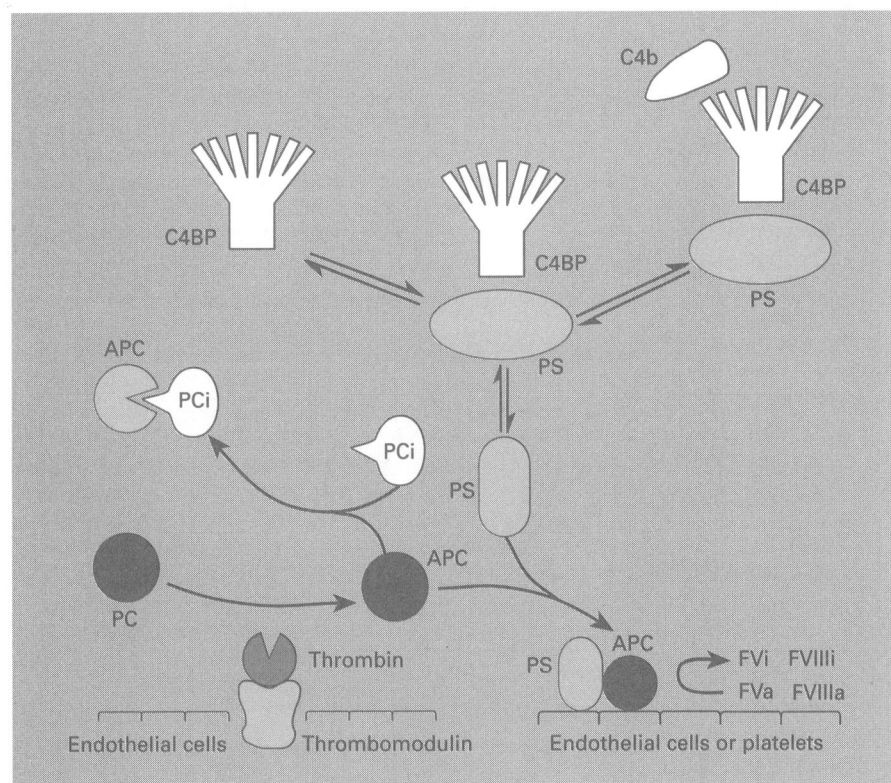

Fig. 12 The protein C anticoagulant system. PC = protein C; APC = activated protein C; PS = protein S; C4BP = C4b binding protein; PCi = protein C inhibitor; FVi = inactivated factor V; FVIIIi = inactivated factor VIII. (Modified from Hessing, M., *et al.* (1991). The interaction between complement component C4b-binding protein and the vitamin K-dependent protein S forms a link between blood coagulation and the complement system. *Biochemical Journal*, **277**, 582, with permission.)

teolysed by activated protein C. Thrombomodulin can also be detected in plasma and has cofactor activity for protein-C activation, but its affinity for thrombin is reduced by approximately 30 per cent. The function of this circulating protein is unknown, and it may be derived from cells after injury or inflammation.

Activated protein C binds to platelet and endothelial-cell membranes by interactions between its Gla residues and membrane phospholipids. The affinity of activated protein C for phospholipid membranes is increased by a cofactor protein S, which catalyses the inactivation of phospholipid-bound factors Va and VIIIa by activated protein C. Factors Va and VIIIa undergo proteolytic cleavage to yield a variety of fragments lacking procoagulant activity.

Activated protein C may be inhibited by several proteins of the serpine family. Protein C inhibitor-1 is probably the main inhibitor, and its action is greatly accelerated by heparin. α_1-Antitrypsin (protein C inhibitor-2) also inhibits protein C in a heparin-independent reaction, and there appear to be other as yet undefined inhibitors of activated protein C in plasma.

Protein S exists in two forms in plasma: 40 per cent of it is free protein and the remainder is complexed with a protein involved in regulating complement activation, C4b-binding protein (**C4BP**). The free and complexed forms of protein S appear to be in equilibrium, but only the free form has activated protein C cofactor activity, although it is unclear whether protein S exists as a procofactor form requiring cleavage for full activity. Cleavage of protein S by thrombin removes the cofactor activity. C4BP is a multimeric protein composed of seven α-chains and one β-chain, linked by disulphide bridges. The protein S-binding site is located on the β-chain, but each α-chain of C4BP has a binding site for C4b, and both proteins can bind to the same molecule of C4BP. Ca^{2+} ions increase the rate of association of protein S and C4BP, and the resulting complex can interact with activated protein C, possibly acting as a competitive inhibitor of free protein S.

Protein S has a high affinity for negatively charged phospholipids, and anchors C4BP to cell membranes. The binding of C4b to C4BP may be a crucial event in the regulation of the C4b:C2a complex (C3 convertase, the classical pathway of complement activation). C4b binding to C4BP accelerates the natural decay of the enzyme C2a from the C4b:C2a complex. C4BP acts as a cofactor to the serine protease factor I in the proteolytic degradation of C4b.

C4BP is also involved in another Ca^{2+}-dependent interaction, with serum amyloid P component (**SAP**). Protein S and SAP bind independently to C4BP, and binding of C4b is not affected. SAP binds to heparin, phospholipid vesicles, and elastin fibrils. In the presence of Ca^{2+} ions, SAP binds with higher affinity to C4BP than to phospholipid. Thus C4BP, SAP, and C4b can bind to phospholipid via protein S, and this may be important in localizing regulatory mechanisms of the protein cascade.

Protein C also modulates fibrinolysis in at least two ways: firstly, by competing with tissue plasminogen activator for inhibitors such as plasminogen activator inhibitor-3, and secondly by reducing release of plasminogen activator inhibitor-1 from the endothelium. Protein C may also modulate the release of tissue plasminogen activator from the endothelium, although there are conflicting data about this.

Fibrinolysis (Table 6)

Fibrin degradation

Fibrin clots are broken down into small fragments and removed by the action of plasmin, which is generated by a variety of mechanisms within the fibrinolytic system. Plasmin is a serine protease produced by limited proteolysis from the zymogen plasminogen by the action of various plasminogen activator enzymes. Plasmin cleaves fibrin at a number of sites, so that progressively smaller fragments or fibrin degradation products are formed (Fig. 13). The first product to be formed is fragment X,

Table 6 *Fibrinolytic proteins*

Protein	M_r	Concentration	Plasma half-life
Plasminogen	92 000	0.2 mg/ml (2 μM)	2 days
t-PA	65 000	5 ng/ml* (80pM)	5 min
u-PA (scu-PA)	54 000	2 ng/ml (40pM)	8 min
PAI-1	48 000	20 ng/ml (400pM)	7 min
PAI-2	60 000	0**	
PAI-3	57 000	2 μg/ml (40nM)	
α_2-Antiplasmin	70 000	70 μg/ml (1μM)	3 days

* Resting, unstimulated levels.

** 250 ng/ml (4nmol) in late pregnancy.

Abbreviations as in text.

and this is proteolysed to give fragments Y and D. Fragment Y is degraded to give a further fragment D and fragment E, which represents the *N*-terminal disulphide knot. These products may then be degraded to progressively smaller forms, which are removed from blood by the reticuloendothelial system. The larger products, X, Y, and D, are able to bind to fibrin monomer and inhibit polymerization, thus interfering with fibrin clot formation. Plasmin also has the potential to cleave fibrinogen, but is usually prevented from doing so by the presence of a large molar excess of its fast-acting inhibitor α_2-antiplasmin, a serpine that forms an irreversible complex with the enzyme, as well as α_2-macroglobulin, and antithrombin III. When cross-linked fibrin clots are lysed, X-oligomers and D-dimers are formed, and these have been used as clinical markers of increased lysis of fibrin, in contrast to non-specific lysis of fibrinogen.

Fibrin, as well as fragments Y, D, and E, increase the rate of plasminogen activation to plasmin, so that once fibrinolysis is initiated it is actually stimulated. Plasmin can decrease thrombin generation by inactivating activated factors V and VIII, and this reaction is potentiated by the presence of phospholipids. Plasmin acts on HK in a similar fashion to kallikrein, and liberates bradykinin.

Some of the fibrin degradation products are known to have chemotactic properties for leucocytes, promote tumour growth, increase vascular permeability, and cause smooth-muscle contraction.

Fig. 13 Fibrin degradation products. Fibrin is degraded by plasmin into a series of degradation products (FDPs), the larger of which are known as fragments X, Y, D, and E. N = amino terminal; C = carboxy terminal; broken line indicates disulphide bonds of the N-terminal disulphide knot. (Modified from Gaffney, P. (1987). In *Haemostasis and Thrombosis*. (ed. A.L. Bloom and D.P. Thomas). p. 233. Churchill Livingstone, Edinburgh, with permission.)

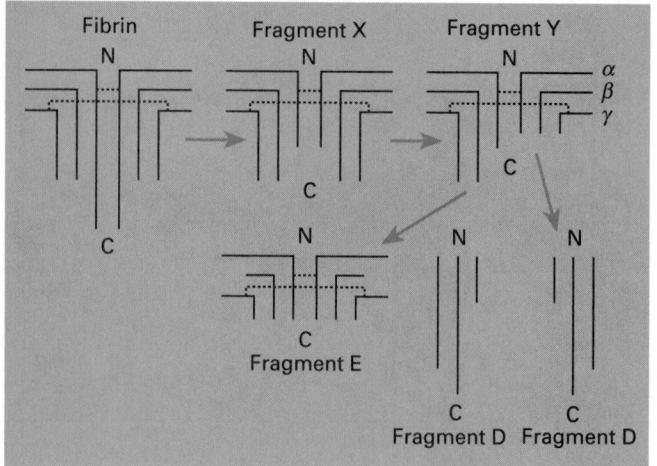

Plasminogen activators and their inhibitors

There are a number of different plasminogen activators, including tissue plasminogen activator (**t-PA**), urokinase-type plasminogen activator (urokinase, **u-PA**), kallikrein, the kallikrein-activated proactivator, and neutrophil elastase (Fig. 14). In addition there are various exogenous activators such as the bacterial enzyme streptokinase, which binds to plasminogen and exposes the active serine centre resulting in plasmin-like activity.

t-PA is synthesized by the vascular endothelial cell and released as a single-chain zymogen form, sct-PA. This zymogen is unusual because it has significant proteolytic activity; proteolytic cleavage to a two-chain form (t-PA, or tct-PA) enhances this activity. t-PA release can be stimulated by exercise and mental stress, venous occlusion, vasodilatation, adrenaline, thrombin and cytokines. In plasma, t-PA is rapidly complexed by various forms of plasminogen activator inhibitor (**PAI**), known as PAI-1, PAI-2, and PAI-3.

The zymogen form of u-PA (scu-PA) is inactive and must be converted to the two-chain form (tcu-PA or u-PA) by kallikrein or plasmin to exert its acivity, which, unlike t-PA, has no requirement for fibrin. u-PA is also found in large amounts in urine (urokinase), from which it was first isolated. u-PA secretion has been demonstrated from fibroblasts, epithelial cells, pneumocytes, and the decidual cells of placenta, but can be secreted by endothelial cells under certain conditions.

PAI-1 is probably the predominant inhibitor in normal plasma; it is released by endothelial cells, but has a wide tissue distribution, and circulates in molar excess over t-PA. Platelets contain significant amounts of PAI-1, accounting for more than 90 per cent of the total blood PAI-1 concentration. However, the endothelium and liver are probably the main sources of plasma PAI-1. The plasma form of PAI-1 is mainly active whereas the platelet form is predominantly latent, although it can be reactivated by denaturation. The rate of inhibition of t-PA and u-PA by PAI-1 is rapid and similar to that of α_2-antiplasmin for plasmin. PAI-1 is bound to the extracellular matrix of the vascular endothelium and may protect it from the digestive action of plasmin.

PAI-2 is primarily a placental protein, and plasma levels are normally negligible, but increase during pregnancy and may be important for haemostasis at the placental interface, during pregnancy and parturition. The inhibitor is also present in peripheral blood monocytes in non-pregnant individuals, and may play a part in controlling cellular and extravascular fibrinolysis. PAI-2 has a lower affinity for t-PA and u-PA than PAI-1.

PAI-3 is found in urine and plasma, but is primarily an inhibitor of activated protein C and perhaps kallikrein and is identical to protein C inhibitor-1. It is unlikely to contribute significantly to the physiological inhibition of t-PA and u-PA. Protease nexin, which is synthesized in fibroblasts, heart muscle, and kidney epithelium, (but is not normally present in plasma), is a weak inhibitor of plasminogen activators.

Plasminogen activation at fibrin surfaces

In normal blood, t-PA is unable to activate plasminogen because of the excess of PAI-1, and the rapid rate of complex formation. Furthermore, any plasmin that was formed would be rapidly inactivated by the excess α_2-antiplasmin. When a fibrin clot forms, t-PA released locally from the endothelial cells binds to the clot with a higher affinity than its interaction with PAI-1. The affinity of t-PA for plasminogen is increased about 400-fold when fibrin is present. Plasminogen has high- and low-affinity lysine-binding sites, which are responsible for binding to fibrin. Thus both t-PA and plasminogen are bound to fibrin and a cleavage occurs resulting in plasmin formation and fibrin degradation. Approximately 40 to 50 per cent of plasma plasminogen is reversibly bound to histidine-rich glycoprotein, which reduces the concentration of plasminogen available for activation. This interaction also depends on the lysine-binding sites of plasminogen. Thrombospondin binds both histidine-rich glycoprotein and plasminogen, and is a non-competitive inhibitor of plasminogen activation by t-PA in the presence of fibrin. In the absence of fibrin, thrombospondin accelerates plasminogen activation by t-PA and may be important in extravascular fibrinolysis. Tetranectin (kringle 4-binding protein) binds plasminogen and accelerates activation by t-PA in the presence of fibrin.

The initial plasmin formed can clip the native plasminogen (Glu-plasminogen) to expose carboxyterminal lysine residues (Lys-plasminogen) for which there are additional binding sites on the fibrin surface. Fibrin is also a cofactor for the conversion of Glu-plasminogen to Lys-plasminogen, and the activation of single-chain u-PA to the active two-chain molecule. Fibrin-bound plasmin is protected from its inhibitor α_2-antiplasmin and can cleave the fibrin clot. As the clot dissolves, the t-PA and plasmin become more accessible to their inhibitors and are complexed. Thus the system ensures that fibrinolysis is localized to the clot that needs to be removed, and native fibrinogen is not proteolysed.

The activation of scu-PA to active u-PA also occurs preferentially on the fibrin surface, not because of fibrin binding but due to the fact that plasmin acts more effectively at that surface and plasmin is a major activator of scu-PA. These mechanisms ensure that fibrinolysis remains localized at the fibrin clot, and plasmin is not freely generated in the circulation.

The cross-linking of fibrin by the action of factor XIIIa masks some of the high-affinity t-PA binding sites. Factor XIIIa also cross-links α_2-antiplasmin to the fibrin clot, decreasing the activation and availability of plasminogen. Thus preformed fibrin clots are more resistant to lysis.

Plasminogen activation at cell surfaces

A variety of cells are able to bind fibrinolytic components such as pro-urokinase, u-PA, t-PA, and plasminogen at specific receptors, as well as accelerating plasminogen activation and protecting the bound plasmin from inactivation by α_2-antiplasmin. The conversion of scu-PA to tcu-PA may occur at the cell surface and plasminogen activation is catalysed more favourably at the cell surface than in solution. In addition, many cells, including monocytes, can up-regulate their expression of plasminogen receptors. Plasminogen is bound by monocytes, lymphocytes, neutrophils, platelets, endothelial cells, hepatocytes and fibroblasts. The binding is dependent on the exposure of the lysine-binding sites of plasminogen. Thrombin stimulation of endothelial cells causes a decline in

Fig. 14 Pathways of plasminogen activation. The various pathways leading to plasminogen activation are shown, as well as the inhibitors involved.

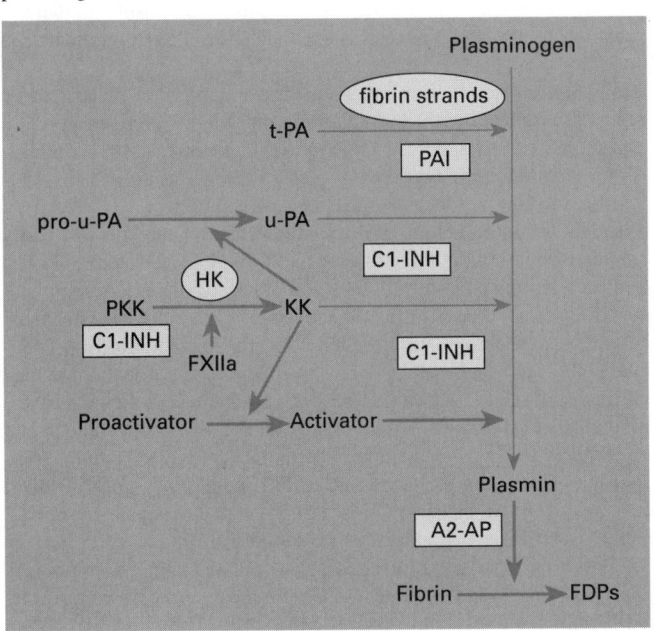

the number of plasminogen receptors, whereas on monocytes, thrombin increases the number of plasminogen-binding sites.

Plasmin has a broad substrate recognition and can cleave a variety of molecules on the cell surface and in the pericellular environment. It will degrade subendothelial matrix constituents, and activate proenzymes and growth factors.

u-PA exists in low concentrations in plasma, and can be inhibited by PAI-1 and PAI-2, and probably functions as an extravascular plasminogen activator. Fibrinolytic enzymes from granulocytes and mononuclear leucocytes are active in inflammatory areas and within tissues in general, probably more so than the enzymes from blood. Mononuclear leucocytes secrete u-PA when in contact with fibrin, but in other circumstances, monocytes can be stimulated by lipopolysaccharide and IL-4 to produce t-PA. There are u-PA receptors on a variety of cell surfaces, including those of monocytes, fibroblasts, epithelial cells, and pneumocytes. Receptor-bound u-PA is catalytically twice as active as fluid-phase u-PA, and needs a 20 times higher molar concentration of monocyte-derived PAI-2 for its inhibition. Whereas t-PA plays an important part in intravascular fibrinolysis, particularly at endothelial surfaces and on fibrin clots, it is likely that u-PA is more important for extravascular fibrinolysis and degradation of subendothelial matrix and other tissues.

Vitronectin may have a regulatory role on the inhibition of t-PA and u-PA by PAI-1. Vitronectin is a major adhesive glycoprotein that circulates in plasma and is present in certain extravascular tissues. It has several types of binding sites, some of which may only be accessible in certain conformations. In its native (folded) form in plasma it does not bind heparin or other glycosaminoglycans, whereas when adsorbed to surfaces it undergoes a conformational transition and the glycosaminoglycan-binding site is exposed. It is possible that transition between these conformations in plasma may be caused by a proteolytic cleavage. Vitronectin has a cell-attachment domain containing the RGD epitope, as do other adhesive glycoproteins. It binds to integrin receptors on platelets, megakaryocytes, and endothelial cells. Vitronectin may bind directly to PAI-1 and other PAIs in the absence of t-PA, and increases the half-life of PAI-1 two-to fourfold.

Vitronectin is able to bind to the subendothelial matrix, and may retain and stabilize PAI-1 released from platelets and endothelial cells. On vessel-wall injury, this PAI-1 becomes accessible and may allow the control of plasminogen activators at these sites to allow an early procoagulant response. The binding of t-PA or u-PA causes dissociation of the PAI-1–vitronectin complex and formation of irreversible plasminogen activator–PAI-1 complexes.Accumulation of t-PA or u-PA in later stages of the response to damage may overcome the local PAI-1 pool. PAI-1 is also a heparin cofactor; both heparin and vitronectin may change the specificity of PAI-1 for its target enzymes t-PA and u-PA, such that thrombin can also be recognized and inhibited.

Neutrophil elastase and fibrinolysis

Plasmin and neutrophil elastase support each other in the degradation of extravascular tissues, each rendering substrates more susceptible to cleavage by the other (sequential digestion). Both neutrophil elastase and cathepsin G are able to degrade fibrin (although they yield different degradation products) and inhibit coagulation by degrading a number of proteins, including factors V, VIII, VII, IX, XII, XIII, HK (cofactor function is removed, but bradykinin-containing region intact), and antithrombin III. Neutrophil elastase is inactivated by complexing with α_2-macroglobulin and α_1-antitrypsin. Neutrophil elastase also potentiates fibrinolysis by modifying plasminogen to a more active form, and inactivating the inhibitors of plasmin and plasminogen activators (C1-inhibitor, α_2-antiplasmin, and PAI-1). Neutrophil elastase and cathepsin G can convert plasminogen to miniplasminogen by removing four of the kringle structures of the plasminogen molecule. Miniplasminogen is converted to plasmin by activators much more rapidly than native plasminogen, and no cofactors are required. The resulting miniplasmin is less sensitive than plasmin to inhibition by α_2-antiplasmin.

Contact activation-mediated fibrinolysis

Kallikrein can activate plasminogen directly, but this reaction is slow, and may not be of physiological importance. However, factor XII and prekallikrein clearly have an important role in fibrinolysis, as contact activation dramatically enhances the rate of dissolution of a fibrin clot, and there is a suggestion that factor XII deficiency may be associated with an increased risk of thromboembolism (preteallikrein deficiency appears to be more rare). The plasma concentration of u-PA is not sufficient to account for the action of kallikrein, and it has long been suggested that kallikrein might act through a proactivator to produce a plasminogen-activating molecule. Such a protein has recently been identified, and awaits full characterization. The contact-mediated pathways of fibrinolysis are controlled by C1-esterase inhibitor and PAI-3. α_2-Macroglobulin can also act as a general inhibitor of fibrinolysis, and can bind kallikrein, factor XIIa, and plasmin.

Haemostatic reactions of the endothelial cell

The endothelial cell interacts with haemostasis at a variety of levels and influences all pathways. The luminal surface possesses anticoagulant and antithrombotic activities, and the endothelial cells synthesize and secrete a variety of substances.

The sulphated proteoglycans, including heparan and dermatan sulphates, are synthesized by endothelial cells and are incorporated into the extracellular matrix. Some of these glycosaminoglycans are also attached to the luminal surface of endothelial cells. Antithrombin III is synthesized in the endothelium as well as the liver and may bind to heparan sulphate on the cell surface, facilitating thrombin neutralization up to fivefold greater than that of commercial heparin plus antithrombin III. This may be due to the more frequent occurrence of the antithrombin III-binding domain in heparan sulphate. The binding of antithrombin III is inhibited by platelet-factor 4, histidine-rich glycoprotein, and vitronectin, which compete with antithrombin III for the heparan sulphate-binding sites. Platelets release an enzyme capable of cleaving the endothelial membrane proteoglycans. In a similar fashion the binding of heparin cofactor II to endothelial dermatan sulphate can be inhibited.

Thrombomodulin provides a specific high-affinity binding site for thrombin on the endothelial surface. It neutralizes the procoagulant activity of thrombin, and the complex may be regulated by internalization. When thrombin is bound to thrombomodulin, its activation of protein C is increased by one thousand-fold. Activated protein C is able to diffuse away from the endothelium and bind to other phospholipid membranes, where it can cleave factors Va and VIIIa in reactions catalysed by protein S.

The vascular endothelium can synthesize and release t-PA and under some circumstances, u-PA, as well as releasing PAI-1. Activated protein C can increase t-PA synthesis and release, and decrease PAI-1 release from the endothelium. The net effect is greater local availability of t-PA to bind to fibrin clots and cause their dissolution.

Platelets do not adhere to the luminal surface of unperturbed endothelial cells, but will bind to damaged and thrombin activated cells. The role of arachidonic acid metabolites and their exchange between platelets and endothelial cells in the maintenance of a thromboresistant surface has been relatively well studied. A major metabolite from endothelial cells is prostaglandin I$_2$ (**PGI$_2$**, prostacyclin), although there may be differential release depending on the site of the endothelial surface. Cells cultured from large vessels have been shown to release abundant PGI$_2$, whereas cells from the microvasculature release very little. Agonists such as thrombin induce an immediate release of PGI$_2$; however, this is short lived because of inactivation of the cyclo-oxygenase enzyme. Release of prostaglandins in response to IL-1 is characterized by a slow onset but is sustained. Cyclic prostaglandin endoperoxides (prostaglandins G$_2$ and H$_2$) released from platelets may be taken up by endothelial cells and rapidly converted to PGI$_2$. The latter is a potent inhibitor of platelet aggregation, adhesion, and secretion, which are mediated by potentiation of adenylate cyclase after binding to a specific platelet-membrane PGI$_2$ receptor. Platelets themselves release a substance that is thought to inhibit PGI$_2$ production, β-thromboglobulin. PGI$_2$ probably acts only as a local hormone, as the plasma half-life is very short.

The initial response of the endothelium to vascular damage may be of a procoagulant nature. Many inflammatory mediators such as thrombin, IL-1, and tumour necrosis factor-α down-regulate anticoagulant mechanisms and fibrinolytic mechanisms, and increase the procoagulant properties. Endothelial cells synthesize tissue factor in response to a variety of agents, in a concentration- and time-dependent, reversible manner. At least 70 per cent of the synthesized tissue factor is expressed in the endothelial cell membrane. An enzyme capable of activating factor XII has also been located in endothelial cell homogenates, and the cells have binding sites for HK, factor IX, and the prothrombinase complex. In addition, factor V is synthesized and bound by the endothelium.

The endothelial cell is the principal site of synthesis of von Willebrand factor. This is produced as a 260-kDa precursor, which undergoes post-translational modification to form a dimer of 220 kDa. These dimers are packaged into high molecular-weight multimers associated with structures known as Weible–Palade bodies, before release into plasma.

Platelet–neutrophil interactions

Neutrophils and platelets interact at different levels, and by several mechanisms, mediated by eicosanoids, nitric oxide, enzymes, and other substances. Thrombin-activated platelets adhere to neutrophils and monocytes in a reaction mediated by GMP-140. This adhesion may modify the activities of both cell types.

Neutrophils utilize certain platelet arachidonate metabolites to increase leukotriene synthesis. Platelet 12-HPETE stimulates neutrophil leukotriene B$_4$ production. Platelets and neutrophils synthesize different types of hydroxy acids (HETE and HPETE), but neutrophils are able to utilize platelet 12-HETE to produce 5-12-diHETE, which cannot be produced by either cell type alone. Neutrophils can produce platelet-activating factor (**PAF**)–acether, which is a potent stimulator of both neutrophils and platelets. A substrate for this synthesis is lysoPAF produced by platelets.

Neutrophils synthesize and release nitric oxide, which inhibits platelet adhesion and aggregation via guanylate cyclase stimulation. Neutrophils possess the inducible form of nitric oxide synthase, which is a calcium-independent enzyme requiring tetrahydrobiopterin as cofactor for the oxidation of L-arginine. It is only detectable after protein synthesis induced by agents such as lipopolysaccharide and interferon-τ.

Neutrophils can also release substances which induce platelet calcium flux, aggregation and secretion, such as the serine protease cathepsin G.

REFERENCES

Bevers, E.M., Comfurius, P., and Zwaal, R.F.A. (1991). Platelet procoagulant activity: physiological significance and mechanisms of exposure. *Blood Reviews*, **5**, 146–54.
Bloom, A.L. and Thomas, D.P. (ed.) (1987). *Haemostasis and thrombosis*. Churchill Livingstone, Edinburgh.
Booth, N. (1992). The laboratory investigation of the fibrinolytic system. In J Thompson (Ed.) *Blood coagulation and haemostasis—a practical guide*, (ed. J. Thompson), pp. 115–50. Churchill Livingstone, Edinburgh.
Coleman, R.W., Hirsh, J., Marder, V.J., and Salzman, E.W. (ed.) (1987). *Hemostasis and thrombosis—basic principles and clinical practice*. Lippincott, Philadelphia.
Faint, R.W. (1992). Platelet–neutrophil interactions: their significance. *Blood Reviews*, **6**, 83–91.
Poller, L. (ed.) (1987 and 1991). *Recent advances in blood coagulation*, Vols. 4 and 5. Churchill Livingstone, Edinburgh. XIVth International Congress on Thrombosis and Haemostasis, New York. (1993) State of the art. *Thrombosis and Haemostasis*, **69**.

22.6.2 Introduction to disorders of haemostasis and coagulation

S. J. MACHIN AND I. J. MACKIE

The normal haemostatic mechanism depends on several overlapping and sequential events including the vessel-wall response to injury, platelet adhesion and aggregation, activation of the coagulation cascade leading to the generation of thrombin and the formation of fibrin, which interdigitates with and reinforces the platelet clump, and finally activation of the fibrinolytic system to complete the repair process. An understanding of the basic physiology and biochemistry of the haemostatic mechanism outlined in the previous section enables the development of a structured approach to the investigation of bleeding and thrombotic defects and treatment of the various resultant disorders. The haemostatic process is carefully balanced so that haemorrhage is promptly arrested and inappropriate thrombosis does not spontaneously occur. The causes of haemostatic abnormalities are numerous and it is essential to have a standardized initial approach to the clinical and laboratory diagnosis of any bleeding or thrombotic tendency.

General approach to the investigation of a bleeding tendency

The initial problem is usually to determine whether bleeding or bruising is due to a local factor, such as a peptic ulcer, or to an underlying haemostatic abnormality. Often a mild abnormality only becomes apparent after trauma or a local precipitating lesion. Any bleeding disorder may be inherited or acquired. This may result from one of six basic mechanisms:

(1) thrombocytopenia;
(2) functional platelet abnormality;
(3) blood vessel defect;
(4) coagulation factor(s) defect;
(5) excess fibrinolysis;
(6) combined defect.

A careful clinical history, drug history, and physical examination should be undertaken; special care must be taken in patients with multisystem disease to recognize any bleeding tendency. In particular, continual oozing from venepuncture and drip sites, extensive petechiae and purpura around pressure areas, and steady blood loss from multiple drainage tubes are often signs of impending haemostatic failure. Generalized purpura, often localized at pressure sites, which if confluent may be accompanied by multiple superficial bruises, usually reflects a failure of platelet function or number (thrombocytopenia) to maintain the integrity of the small blood vessels. Often the cause of the bleeding will be strongly suspected but laboratory tests are always required to make a precise diagnosis and to define the severity of any abnormality.

Most patients with inherited disorders present in childhood, often with a family history of a bleeding tendency and excessive bleeding in response to minor operations, dental extractions, or trauma. However, mild defects may sometimes not present until adult life and occasionally in old age, often as a result of minor trauma or operative procedure. If an inherited disorder is suspected, no effort should be spared to investigate other family members who might also be affected.

Excessive bleeding due to deficiency in the circulating platelet mass or abnormal platelet function can usually be controlled by prolonged local pressure. Generally, platelet bleeding starts immediately after the initiating event but once controlled it does not recur. By contrast, patients with abnormalities of coagulation factors do not bleed excessively after superficial cutaneous lacerations. However, they do produce internal bleeding or deep muscle haematomas, and massive superficial

patient an average of five to six potential carriers are present in the population. Obligate carriers (daughters of haemophiliacs or mothers of a haemophilic child with a maternal history of the disease) can be identified from the family tree. Possible carriers (daughters of carriers, female relatives of haemophiliacs on his maternal side, mothers with one haemophilic son and no family history of the disease) require laboratory investigation in order to determine their carrier status.

Phenotypic assessment of carrier status in haemophilia A can be made by analysis of plasma levels of factor VIII because carriers will, on average, have 50 per cent of the normal female level. As discussed earlier, this method will only identify some 80 per cent of obligate carriers with certainty. The most precise method is to use gene analysis to identify the causative mutation within the patient's factor VIII gene and to then analyse the potential carrier's gene for the same defect. This is now possible in some cases particularly where the chromosome inversion has occurred (see above), and with improving technology is becoming increasingly feasible. Where such techniques are not available, haemophilia gene tracking can be done by DNA polymorphism analysis (see Section 4). Within the factor VIII gene, nine polymorphisms have been described, with varying frequencies throughout the normal population. Six are single nucleotide changes that create (or remove) a restriction-enzyme cutting site (restriction fragment length polymorphisms, or **RFLP**). A seventh is a similar change detectable only with a specific DNA probe and the remaining two are variable-length polymorphisms for the repeated sequence CpA (variable number tandem repeats, or **VNTR**).

Over 90 per cent of females are heterozygous (informative) for at least one of these polymorphisms, and therefore in haemophilia A families the affected gene can be tracked in the majority of cases. Polymorphism analysis has the advantage of being technically simple, especially when PCR based, and is applicable in all families irrespective of the causative gene defect. Disadvantages include occasional non-informativeness, non-availability of key family members, limited use in sporadic haemophilia, and questions of paternity. The establishment of a national database of haemophilia patients and their individual gene defects will eventually lead to direct identification of specific defects in potential carriers, so overcoming the disadvantages with polymorphism analysis outlined above. The technical problems of such procedures, particularly in relation to haemophilia A, mean that this goal is still a few years away.

Haemophilia B

INHERITANCE AND DIAGNOSIS

Haemophilia B is an X-linked deficiency of factor IX and is clinically indistinguishable from haemophilia A. Factor IX functions at the same point in the coagulation system as factor VIII but as a serine protease, which, when activated, activates factor X (in the presence of activated factor VIII, calcium, and phospholipid). The diagnosis is made by measurement of circulating levels of biologically active and/or immunologically detectable protein, the two measurements usually being in agreement, although crm+ haemophilia B is seen overall in about 25 per cent of patients. Carriers of haemophilia B have, on average, 50 per cent of the normal level of factor IX. However, as discussed earlier for haemophilia A, diagnosis of carrier status by factor IX assay is not optimal because only 70 to 80 per cent of obligate carriers have significantly reduced levels.

THE MOLECULAR BASIS OF HAEMOPHILIA B

Factor IX protein

Factor IX is synthesized in the liver as one of the vitamin K-dependent serine proteases and is homologous to coagulation factors II (prothrombin), VII, X, and to protein C. The protein produced within the hepatocyte contains some 454 amino acids. A short signal peptide and a

Table 2 *Haemophilia B database 1992 (Giannelli et al.) 1992*

	Distribution of mutations		
Exon	Domain	Mutants	Unique
1	Signal peptide	4	4
2	Propeptide	41	5
2/3	'Gla' domain	50	32
4	Epidermal growth factor (1)	50	22
5	Epidermal growth factor (2)	24	19
6	Activation peptide	66	29
7	Catalytic domain	29	15
8	Catalytic domain	255	111
		519	237
	Promoter	16	11
	Donor splice sites	20	15
	Acceptor spice sites	13	11
	Cryptic splice	6	4
	Poly(A) site	0	0
		574	278

propeptide, responsible for correct secretion from the cell and for γ-carboxylation (see below), respectively, are cleaved from the aminoterminal end before release from the cell, leaving a 415 amino-acid factor IX protein to circulate in the blood. This mature protein contains several, well-recognized functional domains (listed from amino- to carboxy-terminal): a γ-carboxylated glutamic acid (**Gla**) region containing 12 such residues and involved in phospholipid binding; two epidermal growth factor-like domains; an activation domain cleaved when factor IX is activated by factor XIa; and a serine protease or catalytic domain responsible for converting factor X to Xa (Table 2).

Factor IX gene

This is on the long arm of the X-chromosome at Xq27 and contains eight exons encoding a mRNA of about 1.8 kb. The complete sequence of the gene (33 kb) has been determined and there is a clear relation between the exons and protein functional domains, with, for example exons 2 and 3 encoding the Gla region and exons 7 and 8 encoding the catalytic domain (Table 2)

The genetic basis of haemophilia B

As with most genetic diseases the majority of defects causing haemophilia B have been detected by gene analysis. The factor IX gene is a rather simple gene and has thus lent itself to detailed analysis using the PCR-based procedures discussed above in relation to the factor VIII gene. As a result, several laboratories are reporting that in practically all cases of haemophilia B a genetic mutation can be found within the factor IX gene, or within its promoter regions. Importantly, in almost all these cases the whole of the coding and related regions of the gene have been analysed, thus confirming that the defect found is the causative mutation.

The third edition of the haemophilia B database contains 574 patient entries, not including 29 patients with partial or complete gene deletions or complex rearrangements (as with haemophilia A this last group of patients has a high prevalence of inhibitors to factor IX as a result of replacement therapy). Two hundred and seventy-eight are unique, molecular events, the remainder being repeats. Fifty-five per cent of all entries and 32 per cent of unique mutations involve CpG dinucleotides, confirming, as for haemophilia A, the 'hot-spot' nature of this sequence. Relatively few mutations are recorded as occurring at known functional sites, although mutations at six of the twelve Gla residues are recorded, together with three mutations at the active site, serine 365, and one at the active site, Asp269. As with the factor VIII gene in haemophilia A it is clear that all nonsense mutations cause severe disease, and that most missense mutations resulting in amino acid changes dramatically affect protein stability or release. The distribution of mutations given in the latest database within the eight exons, intron/exon boundaries, and promoter region of the gene are summarized in Table 2. Of the 11 unique mutations in the short 5' promoter region of the gene, 10 give rise to the 'Leyden' phenotype, characterized by the disappearance of the haemophilia after puberty. The effect of these mutations on the expression of the gene thus appears to be negated by the production of adult male hormones. Studies of this region of the factor IX gene have led to several interesting findings on the structure and function of the promoter region.

CARRIER DETECTION AND PRENATAL DIAGNOSIS OF HAEMOPHILIA B

Seven RFLPs have been described within or directly flanking the factor IX gene, and, when all are used, over 90 per cent of females are heterozygous, i.e. informative, for at least one. Because the complete DNA sequence of the gene is known, all are readily detected by PCR-based, DNA amplification procedures. There is, however, considerable ethnic variation in the frequencies of the alleles for most of these polymorphisms and many are not useful in Asian populations. The same is true to a lesser degree for the factor VIII gene polymorphisms discussed above.

The advent of procedures for the detection of factor IX gene mutation that can identify the causative mutation in practically all patients is now having an impact on genetic studies of haemophilia B, particularly in Europe and North America, and RFLP analysis is now less frequently used. In other areas of the world the use of the polymorphism-based gene tracking is still of considerable benefit to affected families.

von Willebrand's disease

INHERITANCE AND DIAGNOSIS

Von Willebrand's disease is an autosomally transmitted bleeding disorder, usually inherited in a dominant fashion. Severe cases are rare though the incidence of mild von Willebrand's disease has been estimated to be as high as 1 per cent in some populations. It is caused by a qualitative and/or quantitative deficiency of von Willebrand factor, a multifunctional, multimeric plasma glycoprotein, of molecular weight from 5×10^5 to 20×10^7, synthesized within vascular endothelial cells and megakaryocytes. Von Willebrand factor has two primary roles in haemostasis. First, it functions in primary haemostasis by binding both to platelets via the glycoprotein (**Gp**) Ib platelet-surface receptor and to exposed subendothelial matrix via an as yet poorly defined collagen type. This has the effect of bringing platelets into contact with exposed subendothelium and initiates the primary haemostatic process. It also mediates in platelet–platelet binding. Any defect in this process, such as defective von Willebrand factor in von Willebrand's disease, will result in poor primary haemostasis and a prolonged skin bleeding time. The second function of von Willebrand factor is to bind to factor VIII and to protect it from destructive proteolysis after its release from the hepatocyte. Only after factor VIII has been activated by thrombin is von Willebrand factor released. As a result of this close association, levels of factor VIII are often reduced in von Willebrand's disease in line with levels of von Willebrand factor when compared to normal plasma levels, although there is a 50 times molar excess of von Willebrand factor.

The diagnosis of von Willebrand's disease is often based initially on a prolonged skin bleeding time, reduced levels of plasma factor VIII, and autosomal inheritance. Qualitative and quantitative assessment of von Willebrand factor is then made both immunologically (as von Willebrand factor antigen) and by a functional test that relies on the ability of the factor to cause normal platelets to agglutinate (aggregate) in the presence of the antibiotic ristocetin. The ristocetin cofactor assay has been shown to be the best assessment of the biological activity of von Willebrand factor in the disease when results are compared with the patient's skin bleeding time and history of bleeding.

In recent years, sophisticated tests have been established to assess the quality of von Willebrand factor in von Willebrand's disease. Of particular importance has been analysis of the multimer structure of von Willebrand factor by gel electrophoretic separation of the multimers and their detection with specific labelled antibodies.

As a result of these studies a phenotypic classification of von Willebrand's disease has developed, as outlined in Table 3. In summary, Type I von Willebrand's disease is characterized by reduced levels of von Willebrand factor (and factor VIII) with no evidence that the von Willebrand factor is abnormal. About 70 per cent of patients with von Willebrand's disease have type I, which is inherited in an autosomal dominant fashion. Type II disease is associated with variant or abnormal von Willebrand factor, characterized by a level of ristocetin cofactor lower than von Willebrand factor antigen and, more importantly, by an abnormal multimer profile. The von Willebrand factor lacks the highest molecular-weight multimers, and the multimeric pattern, which in normal plasma consists of primary bands surrounded by fainter secondary bands, is abnormal. Several studies have demonstrated that the largest multimers of von Willebrand factor are responsible for most of the platelet–subendothelial role of the factor.

Over 10 subtypes of type II von Willebrand's disease have been reported, generally based on differing multimeric patterns of von Willebrand factor. Many of these have been found in single kindred. Of particular interest are types IIA and IIB (see also below). Von Willebrand factor in the former lacks high molecular-weight multimers and shows reduced platelet GpIb binding, while in the latter it also shows a lack of such multimers, but this appears to result from a demonstrable increase in von Willebrand factor–GpIb-binding affinity.

Type III von Willebrand's disease is the rarest form and is autosomally recessive. Affected individuals are either homozygotes or compound heterozygotes and have no detectable von Willebrand factor in either their plasma or platelets. Heterozygotes are usually asymptomatic, although in some cases mild, type I von Willebrand's disease may be present. Several reports have emphasized the fact that in many carriers levels of factor VIII are significantly higher than those of von Willebrand factor.

The fourth type of von Willebrand's disease, von Willebrand Normandy, is characterized phenotypically by von Willebrand factor that shows decreased binding for factor VIII, using enzyme-linked immunosorbent assay-based, factor VIII-binding assays. This variant is clinically asymptomatic in the heterozygous state, which, phenotypically, resembles that for haemophilia A, with levels of factor VIII significantly lower than those of von Willebrand factor when compared to normal plasma levels. Homozygous von Willebrand Normandy disease resembles mild or moderate haemophilia A.

THE MOLECULAR BASIS OF VON WILLEBRAND'S DISEASE

von Willebrand factor protein

Von Willebrand factor circulates in plasma as a series of multimers, each composed of a number of 230-kDa subunits joined initially at the carboxy terminal ends by disulphide bonds to give a dimer, and then at the amino terminal end of the dimers to form multimers of increasing length and size. The primary translation product of the von Willebrand factor gene is a 2813 pre-pro-polypeptide, consisting of a 22 amino-acid signal peptide (necessary for the correct passage of von Willebrand factor through the cell), a 741-residue propeptide and the 2050-residue subunit found in all mature plasma and platelet von Willebrand factor. After cleavage of the signal peptide, pro-von Willebrand factor dimer formation occurs, followed by multimerization via amino terminal-end disulphide bridges. This last process requires the continued attachment to the factor of the propeptide, which is then cleaved after bond formation.

The von Willebrand factor protein has four types of homologous domains (A,B,C, and D), all present in multiple copies, as indicated in Fig. 3. The functional domains of the protein have been identified by

Table 3 *Von Willebrand's disease*

Classification	Characteristics	Genetic mutations
Type I	Reduced vWF, FVIII Normal vWF multimer profile Autosomal dominant	None reported
Type II	Normal or reduced vWF, FVIII Abnormal vWF multimer profile with lack of HMW multimers Autosomal dominant	Point mutations within or close to the GpIb-binding domain of vWF in types IIA and IIB vWd
Type III	Undetectable vWF Low levels of FVIII Autosomal recessive with homozygotes (or compound heterozygotes) only affected Severe bleeding	Partial or complete gene deletions in some cases
Type Normandy	Reduced or normal vWF Reduced FVIII Impaired vWF–FVIII binding Autosomal recessive with heterozygotes generally asymptomatic	Point mutations in FVIII-binding domains

FVIII, factor VIII; Gp, glycoprotein; HMW, high molecular weight; vWd, von Willebrand's disease; vWF, von Willebrand factor.

use of synthetic peptides and specific monoclonal antibodies and are also summarized in Fig. 3. Of the three type-A domains, two (A1 and A3) show a collagen-binding function and both contain an identical-length, intrachain disulphide loop of 185 residues. The A1 domain also contains the only platelet GpIb-binding domain, and also one of the two heparin-binding sites. Von Willebrand factor also binds to platelets via the platelet GpIIb/IIIa complex in common with several other plasma glycoproteins (fibrinogen, fibronectin). This binding is mediated through the tripeptide Arg-Gly-Asp, found towards the aminoterminal end of the von Willebrand factor protein.

The region of von Willebrand factor that binds to factor VIII lies between amino acids 1 to 272. As discussed below, mutations within the gene encoding this region have been identified in patients with von Willebrand Normandy.

von Willebrand factor gene

The gene for von Willebrand factor is found on human chromosome 12 (12p12-pter), although there is also a partial, non-translated pseudogene on chromosome 22, which shows only a 3.1 per cent divergence in sequence to the von Willebrand factor gene. The gene is large and complex, spanning about 180 kb of DNA and containing 52 exons. The pseudogene is 21 to 29 kb in length, covering exons 23 to 34 of the complete gene (amino acids 227 to 1184).

The genetic basis of von Willebrand's disease

Analysis of von Willebrand factor from patients with von Willebrand's disease at a molecular level has not been possible and gene analysis, given its size and complexity, has proved difficult. Southern blotting using complete and partial cDNA probes has identified a few complete

or partial gene deletions in patients with severe type III von Willebrand's disease. However, PCR-based analysis of specific exons encoding known functional domains of the protein, and also RT-PCR (see Chapter 4.1) of von Willebrand factor mRNA from platelets, presumably originating from the parental megakaryocyte, have recently resulted in some interesting findings. To date no defects have been identified in the von Willebrand factor gene of patients with type I disease. Detailed analysis of exon 28, which encodes the A1 and A2 domains of the protein, has revealed missense mutations in almost all patients with type IIA and type IIB studied. The mutations in the type IIB patients are restricted to the loop region of the A1 domain (see above), while those present in type IIA are mainly in the A2 region between residues 742 and 875. In several cases, expression of the putative mutation in mammalian culture using cells transfected with the defective von Willebrand factor gene has shown that the factor produced by these cells shows the expected defective function.

Von Willebrand Normandy is now recognized to be more common than first thought, particularly as its resemblance to the carrier state in haemophilia A has led to the rediagnosis of several families. Five point mutations have, to date, been reported within such families, all within the first 272 residues of the mature von Willebrand factor subunit. It is thought that the missense causing mutations result in changes in the protein conformation leading to reduced binding to factor VIII.

CARRIER DETECTION AND PRENATAL DIAGNOSIS IN VON WILLEBRAND'S DISEASE

Von Willebrand's disease is usually inherited in a dominant fashion and thus carrier detection is not necessary. In some of the milder forms of

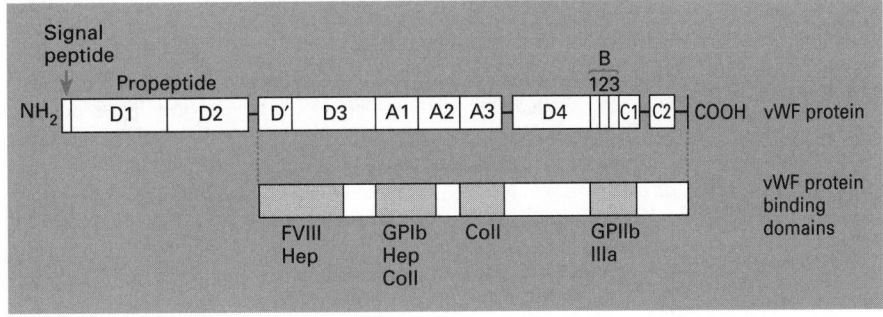

Fig. 3 A diagrammatic representation of pre-pro- von Willebrand factor showing functional domains and regions of homology. FVIII, FVIII binding domain; Hep, heparin binding domain; Coll, collagen binding domain; GPIb, platelet GPIb binding domain; GPIIb IIIa, platelet GPIIb, IIIa binding domain.

the type I disease the phenotypic expression can be variable, and in these cases gene tracking using one or more of the RFLPs within the von Willebrand factor gene (over 30 have been described) can be helpful. Only in type III is recessive inheritance seen and in those rare cases, where the genetic basis of the disease is unknown, heterozygote diagnosis and prenatal diagnosis for a fetus at risk of severe disease can be made. For such genetic studies by far the most informative polymorphic area of the gene is found in intron 40, where at least two VNTR regions composed of four nucleotide repeats can be found, in which, when analysed together result in over 90 per cent of individuals being heterozygous, i.e. informative.

Other coagulation-factor deficiencies

Deficiencies of other factors involved in blood coagulation are rare and are inherited in an autosomal recessive manner. Deficiencies of prothrombin, factor X, factor VII, and factor V usually only result in clinical bleeding in the homozygous or compound heterozygous states. Heterozygotes, rather like carriers of haemophilia A or B, are usually asymptomatic. The genetic basis of the deficiencies has been revealed in a few cases, particularly in relation to factor XI deficiency, which, although rare, is found at a high frequency in Ashkenazi Jews, amongst whom 0.1 to 0.5 per cent are homozygous (9.5–13.5 per cent heterozygous). Heterozygotes are asymptomatic and have a very mild bleeding tendency, while homozygotes (or compound heterozygotes) show a considerable bleeding tendency. Two mutations within the factor XI gene (a change in the intron donor sequence in intron 14, and a nonsense mutation at codon Glu117) account for about half of the genetic changes in the abnormal factor XI genes.

REFERENCES

Asakai, R., Chung, D.W., Ratnoff, O.D., and Davie, E.W. (1989). Factor XI (plasma thromboplastin antecedent) deficiency in Ashkenazi Jews is a bleeding disorder that can result from three types of point mutations. *Proceedings of the National Academy of Sciences* (USA), **86**, 7667–71.

Bloom, A.L. (1994). The management of patients with inherited blood coagulation disorders. In *Haemostasis and thrombosis* (ed. A.L. Bloom, C.D. Forbes, D.P. Thomas, and E.G.D. Tuddenham) pp. 897–917. Churchill Livingstone, Edinburgh.

Giannelli, F. (1989). Factor IX. In *Baillières clinical haematology: the molecular biology of coagulation*, (ed. E.G.D Tuddenham), pp. 821–48. Saunders, London.

Giannelli, F. *et al.*, (1992). Haemophilia B: database of point mutations and short additions and deletions—third addition. *Nucleic Acids Research*, **20**, (suppl. 2027–63).

Mancuso, D.J. *et al.* (1989). Structure of the gene for human von Willebrand factor. *Journal of Biological Chemistry*, **264**, 19514–27.

Peake, I.R. (1992). Registry of DNA polymorphisms within or close to the human factor VIII and factor IX gene. *Thrombosis and Haemostasis*, **62**, 277–80.

Rizza, C.R. (1994). Haemophilia and related inherited coagulation defects. In *Haemostasis and thrombosis*, (ed. A.L. Bloom, C.D. Forbes, D.P. Thomas, and E.G.D. Tuddenham) pp. 819–41. Churchill Livingstone, Edinburgh.

Ruggeri, Z.M. and Ware, J. (1992). The structure and functions of von Willebrand factor. *Thrombosis and Haemostasis*, **67**, 594–9.

Tuddenham, E.G.D. (1989). Factor VIII and haemophilia A. In *Ballières clinical haematology: the molecular biology of coagulation*, (ed. E.G.D. Tuddenham), pp. 849–77. Saunders, London.

Tuddenham, E.G.D. *et al.* (1991). Haemophilia A: database of nucleotide substitutions, deletions, insertions and rearrangements of the factor VIII gene. *Nucleic Acids Research*, **19**, 4821–33.

22.6.5 Clinical features and management of the hereditary disorders of haemostasis

G. F. SAVIDGE

Haemostasis is the complex sequence of biological events that leads to the arrest of haemorrhage following vascular endothelial damage. Two principal and interactive mechanisms are operative in the blood clotting process:

1. Primary haemostasis: in this initial phase, circulating platelets adhere and subsequently aggregate at the site of vessel injury to form a haemostatic platelet plug.
2. Secondary haemostasis: the haemostatic plug is consolidated by the formation of an enveloping fibrin mesh. Commonly known as the coagulation cascade, this mechanism involves a stepped series of reactions whereby specific plasma proteins are converted to serine proteases, leading to the formation of insoluble, cross-linked fibrin.

Genetic defects of one or more components participating in these mechanisms lead to the haemorrhagic symptoms characteristic of the hereditary haemostatic disorders. Diagnosis rests upon a comprehensive history and physical examination, and use of appropriate laboratory screening tests and specific haemostatic assays.

Hereditary disorders of primary haemostasis (Table 1)

The platelet circulates as an inactive, anuclear, non-adherent cell fragment, but on contact with the subendothelial matrix develops pseudopodia and becomes an actively secreting cell, undergoing adhesion, activation, and degranulation, as well as aggregation.

Disorders characterized by platelet adhesion defects

VON WILLEBRAND'S DISEASE (TABLE 2)

This heterogeneous condition is the most common inherited bleeding disorder, with a prevalence of up to 125 per million population. It is characterized by quantitative and/or qualitative abnormalities in platelet, endothelial, and plasma von Willebrand factor that prevent the binding of glycoprotein (**Gp**)Ib to the subendothelial matrix, whereby the bleeding time becomes abnormally prolonged. Low levels of circulating factor VIII may occur due to the absence of von Willebrand factor, which normally acts as a carrier protein and stabilizer for this factor. The complete vWf cDNA has been cloned and the human von Willebrand factor gene spans 178 kb and is interrupted by 51 introns. The von Willebrand factor gene has been localized to the short arm of chromosome 12, and there is a non-functional, partial pseudogene on chromosome 22. Genetic transmission of the disorder is autosomal dominant or recessive depending upon the specific subtype.

The most common clinical symptoms are mucocutaneous haemorrhage, prolonged bleeding after minor trauma or surgical procedures, menorrhagia, and postpartum haemorrhage. Spontaneous bleeding into joints and muscles is unusual, but when it does occur, it is associated with low levels of circulating factor VIII. Severe bleeding is unusual and death from uncontrolled haemorrhage rare. In the common subtypes, symptoms decrease significantly after adolescence with normalization of plasma levels of von Willebrand factor. Von Willebrand's disease is subdivided into severe or mild disease, and treatment is determined by the nature of clinical symptoms and the specific subtype. The diagnosis is based upon the mode of inheritance, screening tests, platelet function

Table 1 *Hereditary disorders of primary haemostasis*

Disorder	Defined defect	Platelet count	Platelet size	Clot retraction	Aggregation studies ADP	Collagen	Ristocetin	Serotonin release
von Willebrand's disease (vWD)	Abnormal von Willebrand factor	N but ↓ in type IIB and pseudo-vWD	Usually N	N	N	N	↓	N
Bernard–Soulier syndrome	GpIb, GpIX, and GpV deficiency	↓	↑	N	N	N	Absent	N
Gray platelet syndrome	Absent α-granules	↓	N or ↑	N	↓	↓	N	↓
Storage-pool deficiency	Reduced number of platelet dense bodies	N	N	N	N but ↓2° aggregation	↓	N	↓
Glanzmann's thrombasthenia	GpIIb–IIIa deficiency	N	N	Absent (type I) ↓ (type II)	Absent	Absent	N	N
Afibrinogaemia	Plasma and platelet fibrinogen deficiency	N or ↓	N	N	Absent	Absent	Absent	N

↑, increased values; ↓, decreased values; N, normal values; Gp, glycoprotein.

Table 2 *Clinical and laboratory features in common von Willebrand's disease (vWD) variants*

Feature	Type I	Type IIA	Type IIB	Type III	Pseudo-vWD
Inheritance	Autosomal dominant	Autosomal dominant	Autosomal dominant	Autosomal recessive	Autosomal dominant
Bleeding time (BT)	Prolonged	Prolonged	Prolonged	Prolonged	Prolonged
vWf: ristocetin cofactor (von Willebrand factor)	Reduced	Reduced	Normal/reduced	Reduced	Reduced
Plasma vWf antigenicity	Reduced	Normal/reduced	Normal/reduced (increased binding to platelets)	Reduced/absent	Normal/reduced
Plasma vWf multimers	Normal	Absent HMW multimers	Absent HMW multimers	Absent/only small multimer band	Absent HMW multimers (bound to platelets)
Platelet vWf antigenicity	Normal/reduced	Absent HMW	Normal	Reduced/absent	Normal
Ristocetin induced platelet aggregation	Normal/reduced	Reduced	Increased at low ristocetin concentrations	Absent	Hyperaggregation
Response to DDAVP	Increase in vWf and factor VIII BT correction	Variable but increase in factor VIII	Variable with intravascular platelet aggregation and thrombocytopenia	None	Intravascular platelet aggregation and thrombocytopenia
Response to vWf replacement therapy	Increase in vWf and factor VIII BT correction	Increase in vWf and factor VIII	Variable thrombocytopenia with increase in vWf and factor VIII	Increase in vWf and factor VIII	Intravascular platelet aggregation and thrombocytopenia

DDAVP, deamino-D-arginine vasopressin; HMW, high molecular weight; RIPA, the factor VIII is of the circulating, functional type.

assays, plasma Factor VIII levels, and measurements of plasma and platelet von Willebrand factor.

Type I vWD

This 'classic' form of vWD, constituting some 75 per cent of all cases, is inherited as an autosomal dominant trait. Reduced levels of plasma von Willebrand factor activity and antigenicity occur, varying from 0.1 to 50 per cent of normal values, with a concordant decrease in circulating factor VIII. No molecular defects have been reported. The bleeding time is variably prolonged and related to clinical severity. Multimers of plasma von Willebrand factor are fully identifiable but in variably reduced concentrations. Multimers of platelet von Willebrand factor may or may not resemble plasma multimers, leading to the subclassification of a platelet concordant form (type IA) and a platelet discordant form (type IB). The therapeutic response to deamino-D-arginine vasopressin (**DDAVP**) in type IA is good, with an increase in plasma von Willebrand factor activity and antigenicity, and in circulating factor VIII levels, with normalization of von Willebrand factor multimers and the bleeding time. In type IB, DDAVP may not correct the bleeding time.

Type II vWD

This entity, comprising some 25 per cent of all of cases vWD, is due to a qualitative defect in von Willebrand factor with discordant reduction in von Willebrand factor and circulating factor VIII by a ratio approximating 1:10. The high molecular-weight multimers of von Willebrand factor are defective due to increased susceptibility to *in vivo* proteolysis, or are structurally abnormal. Type II vWD has at least five subtypes based upon mode of inheritance, von Willebrand factor multimers in plasma and platelets, and platelet reactivity to ristocetin. In type II vWD there is abnormal anodal migration of von Willebrand factor antigen in electrophoretic systems.

Type IIA vWD variant

In type IIA, as in types IID, IIE and IIF, the mode of inheritance is autosomal dominant, while type IIC is autosomal recessive. Mutations have been reported, generally in the 134 amino-acid segment of the von Willebrand factor A2 homologous repeat. Large and intermediate-sized multimers of von Willebrand factor are absent from the plasma and platelets, while biologically inactive, smaller multimers are structurally abnormal. The bleeding time is prolonged and both von Willebrand factor reactivity to ristocetin and ristocetin induced platelet aggregation (RIPA) are undetectable or markedly reduced. Therapeutic response to DDAVP is variable, although plasma levels of von Willebrand factor antigen may increase.

Type IIB vWD variant

Unlike other forms of vWD, type IIB is characterized by increased reactivity between platelet GpIb and the defective von Willebrand factor. Type IIB mutations are clustered within a short segment of the homologous von Willebrand factor A1 domain encoded entirely within exon 28, and the mode of inheritance is autosomal dominant. Platelets aggregate in response to lower concentrations of ristocetin than normal. Plasma multimers of von Willebrand factor are usually of both low and intermediate size, and a normal multimeric pattern in the platelets is diagnostic. The disorder presents with quite severe symptoms and a prolonged bleeding time. DDAVP therapy is mostly contraindicated because the induced release of abnormal but highly reactive von Willebrand factor from the endothelium may cause thrombocytopenia secondary to increased platelet adhesion, intravascular platelet aggregate formation, and accelerated platelet clearance. Type IIB vWD should be considered in the differential diagnosis of thrombocytopenia, as a variant form of type IIb with chronic thrombocytopenia, circulating platelet aggregates, and spontaneous platelet aggregation has been described. Management of symptomatic type IIB patients relies on replacement therapy with von Willebrand factor concentrates, although fresh frozen plasma may be of value in correcting the associated thrombocytopenia.

Type III vWD

Patients with type III vWD are relatively uncommon, but all exhibit very severe bleeding symptoms. Reported genetic defects include several mutations and gene deletions. Transmission is autosomal recessive in homozygotes with no previous family history, or as double heterozygotes if there is type I vWD and consanguinity in the family history. Activity and antigenicity of von Willebrand factor are undetectable in plasma, platelets, and endothelial cells, resulting in bleeding times of many hours. Multimeric analysis of plasma and platelets may show only a single, low molecular-weight band. Circulating levels of factor VIII procoagulant activity (VIII:C) are low, with values approximating those seen in severe/moderate haemophilia A. The clinical picture is one of a combined platelet-adhesion defect and a plasma coagulation-factor deficiency with mucocutaneous haemorrhage and spontaneous muscle and joint bleeding. No increase in von Willebrand factor is detected after DDAVP infusion, and treatment rests with replacement therapy.

Pseudo- or platelet-type vWD

This disorder inherited as an autosomal dominant trait, is characterized by a deficiency of high molecular-weight multimers of von Willebrand factor in the plasma and by enhanced ristocetin induced platelet aggregation. The abnormality is not related to von Willebrand factor but to a defect in the its binding sites on the platelet GpIb–IX complex. Normal von Willebrand factor that is produced in this condition binds to the abnormal platelets and causes aggregation in the absence of ristocetin with the rapid removal of high molecular-weight multimers from the circulation. Bleeding symptoms are relatively mild and are commonly associated with thrombocytopenia. Replacement therapy or DDAVP infusions lead to rapid clearance of high-molecular weight multimers of von Willebrand factor with associated thrombocytopenia, often giving rise to more severe haemorrhagic symptoms than those due to the underlying defect. Platelet infusions in conjunction with replacement therapy may secure satisfactory haemostasis.

vWD with a factor VIII-binding defect

This recently described variant is characterized by the inability of von Willebrand factor to complex fully to circulating factor VIII. The genetic defect in the structure of the factor VIII-binding site on von Willebrand factor is found exclusively in family members with an apparently phenotypic, mild haemophilia but with an autosomal dominant inheritance trait. Haemorrhagic symptoms are mild and induced by trauma, and are related to the circulating factor VIII deficiency. Platelet adhesion is normal because the binding-site defect on the von Willebrand factor molecule does not participate in the platelet subendothelial interaction. Symptomatic management with DDAVP is identical to that in mild haemophilia A.

Therapy in vWD

The aim of treatment in this disorder is to secure haemostasis by correcting the prolonged bleeding time by the provision of adequate levels of functional von Willebrand factor. The cornerstone of treatment of severe vWD is replacement therapy with plasma-derived concentrates containing von Willebrand factor (and factor VIII). In mild cases, DDAVP can be used, while antifibrinolytic and other adjunctive agents may be of value.

Replacement therapy

Cryoprecipitate, used for many years in the treatment of symptomatic vWD, is now no longer recommended in its untreated form, due to the potential risks of viral transmission. Virus-inactivated factor VIII concentrates are generally unsuitable for the treatment of vWD because von Willebrand factor is degraded in the manufacturing process. Two factor VIII concentrates of intermediate purity (Haemate P and BPL 8Y) have, however, been shown to be reasonably effective, and a highly efficacious, purified von Willebrand factor concentrate is currently available. Infusions of 20 to 40 (factor VIII) units/kg factor VIII concentrates or

30 to 45 (von Willebrand ristocetin cofactor) units/kg of purified von Willebrand factor concentrate usually correct the bleeding time for up to 12 h. Plasma factor VIII levels (VIII:C) rise in proportion to the procoagulant factor VIII content of the concentrate administered, but subsequently continue to be maintained for up to 72 h after a single infusion. This secondary transfusion response is a unique feature of vWD, as the infused von Willebrand factor acts as carrier protein for factor VIII, which is produced normally in this disorder. Dosages of factor VIII concentrate for replacement therapy are tailored to circulating factor VIII levels, but for the von Willebrand factor concentrate, measurements of bleeding time and von Willebrand factor reactivity to ristocetin are more relevant. In severe haemorrhagic conditions and for major surgery, twice-daily replacement to maintain normal bleeding times and circulating factor VIII levels (70–100 i.u./dl) is essential for days 1 to 3, with subsequent reduction in the intensity of treatment over 7 to 10 days. Minor surgery and minor bleeding episodes are adequately covered at dosages of von Willebrand ristocetin cofactor of 30 i.u./kg and circulating factor VIII, 10 to 20 i.u./kg body weight. Replacement therapy is indicated in symptomatic patients with type III, and in clinically severe and DDAVP-unresponsive type I and type II variants. In some cases of type III vWD, replacement therapy may induce the formation of alloantibodies to von Willebrand factor, which complicates subsequent management. Concentrates are seldom justified in cases of mild vWD.

Therapy with DDAVP

DDAVP (0.3 µg/kg) as a slow intravenous infusion, or in some cases as a subcutaneous injection, is the treatment of choice in mild type I vWD, and to a variable extent in types IIA, IIC and IID, giving an increase in plasma von Willebrand factor of two to seven times basal values. DDAVP can be given at 8- to 12-hourly intervals for 2 to 6 days, although in some cases tachyphylaxis may occur. As DDAVP also stimulates fibrinolysis, an antifibrinolytic agent (e.g. tranexamic acid) is usually given concurrently. Intranasal DDAVP (300 µg) can be used successfully to treat many type I patients at home with minor haemorrhagic symptoms. Adverse events are uncommon but include facial flushing and hypotension, and also water retention when frequently repeated doses are given. The latter restricts its use in small infants. Benefits of DDAVP treatment in elderly patients with hypertension and cardiac failure should be assessed against possible thrombotic complications. DDAVP is contraindicated in type IIB and in pseudo-vWD because it may cause thrombocytopenia.

Adjunctive therapy

In mild vWD, antifibrinolytic preparations (e.g. tranexamic acid) may be effective as the sole haemostatic agents for minor haemorrhage or minor surgery by inhibition of local fibrinolysis. Local haemostatic agents (e.g. topical thrombin, collagen fleece, and fibrin glue) may be useful in certain circumstances. In women of reproductive age with vWD, an oral contraceptive and tranexamic acid may control menorrhagia. As with other bleeding disorders, aspirin or related platelet-inhibitory agents, dextran infusions for volume replacement, and intramuscular injections should be avoided.

BERNARD–SOULIER SYNDROME

This rare, heterogeneous disorder is transmitted in an autosomal and incompletely recessive fashion, as heterozygotes show mild haematological abnormalities but are clinically normal. The condition is due to a deficiency of the platelet surface glycoproteins GpIb, GpIX, and GpV, abolishing von Willebrand factor-mediated platelet adhesion to the subendothelium. Homozygotes usually have a long history of excessive bleeding with frequent mucocutaneous haemorrhages. Menorrhagia is common. Most patients require blood transfusions at some time, and life-threatening bleeding occurs frequently, with a mortality of 15 per cent.

Key diagnostic features include a mild to moderate thrombocytopenia, with large and occasionally giant platelets due to the absence of the influence of surface GpIb, which normally determines the discoid shape of circulating platelets through its interaction with the platelet cytoskeleton. The bleeding time is grossly prolonged, and substantially more than the thrombocytopenia would warrant. Platelet aggregation to von Willebrand factor and ristocetin, and to bovine von Willebrand factor alone are absent, and abnormal to thrombin due to the associated deficiency of GpV. Levels of plasma von Willebrand factor, platelet nucleotide release, and clot retraction are normal. Demonstration of absent or severely reduced platelet-surface GpIb by fluorescence-activated cell-sorting analysis (**FACS**) using monoclonal antibodies confirms the diagnosis.

A number of reported 'giant platelet' syndromes, some associated with thrombocytopenia, may be confused with the Bernard–Soulier syndrome. These include 'thrombopathic' thrombocytopenia, which is inherited as an autosomal dominant trait, and the 'Montreal' platelet syndrome, where the platelet giantism is attributed to superabundant platelet membranes and abnormal shape change. Other hereditary syndromes such as the May–Hegglin anomaly, stomatocytosis, and autosomal dominant nephritis with deafness (Epstein's syndrome) exhibit similarly abnormal platelet morphology but express functional platelet GpIb. There is no specific treatment for the Bernard–Soulier syndrome but platelet transfusion can be life-saving. The use of this in individual patients should be limited, however, as high-titre alloantibodies can develop in response to the immunogenic surface glycoproteins on infused platelets. In a number of cases of Bernard–Soulier syndrome and May–Hegglin anomaly, DDAVP produces a significant correction of the bleeding time and may be effective in treating minor haemorrhage. Menorrhagia may respond to oral contraceptives and occasionally antifibrinolytic therapy can be helpful.

MISCELLANEOUS PLATELET-ADHESION DISORDERS

Impaired platelet adhesion leading to abnormal bleeding is a common and significant feature of a number of hereditary connective tissue disorders. Mild haemorrhagic manifestations are seen in the Ehlers–Danlos syndrome, osteogenesis imperfecta, pseudoxanthoma elasticum, and in Marfan's syndrome. The diagnosis of these disorders is made almost exclusively on the basis of the characteristic clinical findings rather than on tests of haemostatic function, and no specific therapy is available.

Disorders characterized by abnormal platelet activation

GRAY (GREY) PLATELET SYNDROME

This rare syndrome is characterized by a mild to moderate thrombocytopenia with large platelets, and a moderate to severe bleeding disorder resembling a coagulation factor deficiency. The unusual name was derived from the grey colour of the platelets on Wright-stained blood smears, due to the almost total lack of α-granules in both platelets and magakaryocytes. The severity of symptoms emphasizes the importance of the α-granules and their contents in normal haemostasis. The syndrome is inherited as an autosomal trait and haemorrhage begins in childhood. Platelet aggregation studies show a reduced response to ADP, collagen and to the calcium ionophore A32187, and the impaired release of serotonin on thrombin stimulation may reflect a regulatory role of α-granules in dense-body secretion processes. There is an association between the gray platelet syndrome and myelofibrosis in some kindreds. The severe bleeding may be related to the absence of α-granular platelet factor V, which normally participates in prothrombinase complex formation. For severe haemorrhagic episodes, platelet infusions are necessary, although DDAVP may occasionally shorten the bleeding time.

Storage-pool deficiency

This disorder, inherited as an autosomal dominant trait, is characterized by a moderate bleeding diathesis due to a deficiency in the granule-bound adenine nucleotides, ADP and ATP, associated with a decreased number of dense bodies in the platelets. Cystolic nucleotides involved in platelet metabolism are normal.

The bleeding time is moderately prolonged, and platelet aggregation studies demonstrate a reduced response to ADP and collagen. As ADP rather than ATP is more selectively stored in the dense bodies in storage-pool deficiency, ADP is more markedly reduced, resulting in an ATP:ADP ratio greater than normal. Abnormal platelet levels of adenine nucleotides and reduced release of serotonin confirm the diagnosis. Storage-pool deficiency is associated with a number of unrelated platelet biochemical abnormalities (defects in arachidonic acid metabolism) and with other hereditary disorders. This suggests that dense bodies can be affected by a variety of genetic abnormalities, exemplified in the Hermansky–Pudlak syndrome, the Chediak–Highashi syndrome, the Wiskott–Aldrich syndrome, and the *t*hrombocytopenia with *a*bsent *r*adii (TAR) syndrome. Full platelet support, preferably with HLA-matched platelets, is recommended for severe haemorrhagic symptoms and for major surgical procedures. DDAVP infusions may correct the bleeding time and is useful for minor haemorrhage, while antifibrinolytic agents and oral contraceptives may be useful in menorrhagia.

Disorders characterized by defective platelet aggregation

GLANZMANN'S THROMBASTHENIA

This rare disorder is characterized by moderate to severe mucocutaneous haemorrhages and menorrhagia. Symptoms usually begin in childhood, and pregnancy and delivery represent a severe haemorrhagic risk. Thrombasthenia is inherited as an autosomal recessive trait and a family history often reveals consanguinity, which may account for the remarkably uneven geographical occurrence of the disease in specific regions in the Middle East, southern India, and North Africa. The defect, which may involve either the GpIIa gene or the GpIIIb gene, results in a deficiency or an abnormality of the membrane glycoprotein complex GpIIb–IIIa at both platelet and megakaryocytic levels. As a result, when platelets are activated, fibrinogen cannot bind to the platelet membrane and platelet aggregation does not occur. The bleeding time is prolonged, and platelet aggregation studies demonstrate a deficient response to exogenous or endogenous ADP, collagen, and thrombin, or to any agonist dependent on the induction of the release reaction. Prothrombin consumption and clot retraction are usually reduced.

Two types of thrombasthenia have been classified. In type I, only residual GpIIb and IIIa (less than 10 per cent) are present, the specific platelet antigens PLA 1 (*Zwa*) and its allele (*PLA2*) and (*Lek-a*) are lacking, low levels of intraplatelet fibrinogen are detected, and clot retraction is absent. In type II, although platelet aggregation is absent, 15 to 20 per cent GpIIb–IIIa is expressed and only slightly decreased levels of intraplatelet fibrinogen and PLA-1 antigen can be measured, while clot retraction is normal. Specific diagnosis for the subclassification of Glanzmann's thrombasthenia can be determined by FACS analysis of platelet GpIIb–IIIa and PLA 1, and by measurement of fibrinogen in platelet lysates by enzyme-linked immunosorbent assay.

Treatment of severe haemorrhagic symptoms rests with the administration of HLA-matched platelet concentrates, although the outcome may be variable due to the inhibitory effect of the recipient's defective platelets on infused normal platelets. In life-threatening bleeding, exchange thrombocytopheresis may be of value. Isoantibody formation is seldom observed in clinical practice. DDAVP infusions seldom correct the bleeding time. Antifibrinolytic therapy or topical haemostatic agents may be of value in the treatment of minor bleeding, while oral contraceptives are effective for controlling menorrhagia.

HEREDITARY AFIBRINOGENAEMIA

This rare disorder, which is normally included among the plasma coagulation-factor deficiencies, profoundly affects platelet function and the blood is incoagulable. The condition is inherited as an autosomal recessive or intermediate trait, and family histories of many kindred demonstrate consanguinity. In such cases, fibrinogen is present in only trace amounts in the plasma, although the genes encoding the synthesis of the three fibrinogen chains (Aα, Bβ, and γ) are intact. In terms of primary haemostasis, afibrinogenaemia results in a grossly prolonged bleeding time and absent platelet aggregation to agonists that act through the release reaction. There may also be mild thrombocytopenia. As fibrinogen is the substrate for fibrin, its absence results in profoundly abnormal partial thromboplastin, prothrombin, and thrombin times but a normal thromboplastin generation test and prothrombin consumption. Only trace concentrations (less than 5 mg/dl) of fibrinogen are detected in the plasma, and platelet α-granular fibrinogen is severely deficient. The erythrocyte sedimentation rate in such patients is very low. Hereditary hypofibrinogenaemia probably represents the heterozygous form of afibrinogenaemia or dysfibrinogenaemia.

Afibrinogenaemic patients present with variable severity of mucocutaneous and joint or muscle bleeding, and fetal loss subsequent to implantation. Symptoms may present at birth with bleeding from the umbilical stump, and subsequently may occur after circumcision, during the eruption and loss of deciduous teeth, or after trauma. Wound healing may be defective and spontaneous splenic rupture due to bleeding can occur. Treatment consists of replacement therapy with virus-inactivated fibrinogen concentrates and adjunctive antifibrinolytic therapy. In some cases, DDAVP may correct the prolonged bleeding time and may be useful in treating minor bleeding symptoms. Menorrhagia is well controlled by hormone therapy.

Hereditary disorders of secondary haemostasis

Following platelet-plug formation, thrombin is generated on the surface of the loosely interacting platelets, which catalyses the conversion of fibrinogen to insoluble, cross-linked fibrin. The generation of thrombin by secondary haemostasis involves two major reaction sequences:

1. The activation of factor X to its serine protease counterpart Xa to form the 'tenase complex'. This is achieved through the intrinsic and extrinsic coagulation cascades.
2. Activation of prothrombin (factor II) to its corresponding serine protease thrombin, which converts fibrinogen to fibrin, subsequently cross-linked by factor XIII.

Disorders of the intrinsic coagulation cascade

Hereditary disorders of secondary haemostasis are usually the result of a single plasma-protein deficiency or abnormality, and are all associated with a similar clinical picture. In the following sections the clinical features of haemophilia A, the most common disorder of this kind, will be described in detail. The characteristics of the rarer disorders, and how they differ from haemophilia A, will be outlined for each individual disorder.

HAEMOPHILIA A

This X-linked recessive disorder, recognized as early as the second century AD, is due to a deficiency or abnormality of factor VIII. This factor normally circulates in the plasma expressing both procoagulant activity (VIII:C) and antigenicity, and is bound to von Willebrand factor (see Chapter 22.6.4). In most cases, factor VIII is quantitatively reduced (cross-reacting material (**CRM**) negative) with a proportional decrease in both procoagulant and antigenic factor VIII levels while von Willebrand factor is normal. The incidence of haemophilia A in the population ranges from 1 in 10 000 to 20 000, is rare in the Chinese and uncommon in blacks. Some 5500 patients are currently registered with haemophilia A in the United Kingdom. The fact that the mutation rate for the gene is high (up to 30 per cent) is important because a negative family history does not exclude haemophilia in a child with bleeding symptoms. In any one affected kindred, the expression of the genetic defect is consistent; all affected males demonstrate a similar level of factor VIII deficiency. The most common variant is CRM-positive haemophilia, where non-functional but antigenically normal factor VIII is synthesized. A haemophiliac phenotype may occur in female heterozygous carriers due to skewed X-chromosome inactivation (see Section 4). Affected females may also result from a mating between an affected male and a carrier female, as a consequence of a new mutation, or due to chromosomal abnormalities giving rise to a hemizygous genotype in the female— 45XX/45X mosaicism, 46XY karyotype for example.

Clinical features of haemophilia A

The clinical severity is assessed by the frequency and nature of bleeding, and the level of the procoagulant factor VIII deficiency. Three degrees of clinical severity are recognized:

(1) severe haemophilia, where frequent spontaneous haemorrhage into joints and muscles and severe bleeding after minor trauma occur, and procoagulant factor VIII levels (VIII:C) are less than 1 i.u./dl (under 1 per cent of normal);

(2) moderate haemophilia, where bleeding occurs after minor trauma with few spontaneous symptoms, and the factor VIII levels lie between 1 and 5 i.u./dl;

(3) mild haemophilia, when prolonged bleeding only occurs with trauma or following operative procedures, and where basal levels of procoagulant factor VIII are between 5 and 40 i.u./dl.

Infants with severe haemophilia have low levels of factor VIII at birth because this factor does not cross the placental barrier. It is unusual, however, for haemorrhagic symptoms to occur until the child becomes active. Exceptionally, first-born affected males may develop large cephalohaematomas and occasionally intracranial haemorrhage, particularly if labour is difficult or protracted, or with forceps delivery.

Haemarthroses

Episodic bleeding into joints is common in severe haemophilia. When inadequately treated, these haemarthroses lead to intra-articular pathology, secondary deformity, and eventual crippling. The knee, elbow, and ankle are most commonly affected, although any joint may be involved. Clinical deterioration is directly related to the number of haemorrhages in any one joint. Bleeding occurs from the vascular synovium, and leads to synovial hyperplasia with hyperaemia and a tendency for further bleeding. With repeated haemorrhage, the synovium becomes fibrotic, with cartilage destruction, narrowing of the joint space, subchrondral cyst formation, bone erosion, and osteophyte formation with eventual ankylosis. These features are referred to, collectively, as chronic haemophilic arthropathy.

At the onset of joint haemorrhage, the patient may experience 'tingling' feelings, stiffness, or instability of the joint, evolving into a hot, swollen, and painful joint with restricted movement as blood fills the joint cavity. Inadequate treatment of a severe haemarthrosis leads to muscle wasting in the affected limb and, in some cases, chronic synovial effusion or hypertrophic synovitis. Haemorrhage into one specific joint more than twice a month, or more than three times in a 2-month period, produces a 'target joint'.

Chronic haemophilic arthropathy

The outcome of recurrent bleeding into joints is progressive destruction of articular cartilages and secondary joint degeneration. The degree of arthropathy is classified on clinical and radiological findings, and provides the basis for rational therapy. The history is of importance; the

nature and duration of symptoms, frequency and severity of haemorrhage, pain, swelling or other articular symptoms as related to certain activities or injury, and response to replacement therapy should be determined. Effusions, synovial thickening and bony overgrowth, the range of movement of the joint, and muscle power using the Medical Research Council grading system should be assessed. Radiological evaluation is based on the *Recommendations of the Orthopaedic Advisory Committee of the World Federation of Haemophilia* whereby a joint score can be determined. A 'zero' score indicates no arthropathy while a score of 13 confirms endstage arthropathy. Regular follow-up is essential to assess the efficacy of therapy in relation to disease progression.

Chronic hypertrophic synovitis

Recurrent haemorrhage into specific joints may lead to chronic hypertrophic synovitis. The synovium becomes grossly thickened and the joint swollen due to a painless effusion with adjacent muscle wasting. Although initially the joint has a full range of movement, chronic arthropathic changes are accelerated in the presence of chronic synovitis. This reaction of the synovium is believed to be due to marked hyperplasia of both type A and type B synovial cells in response to recurrent bleeding, and the increased production of synovial fluid containing proteolytic enzymes, which accelerate cartilage destruction.

Haematomata and nerve-compression syndromes

Bleeding into muscles is common, and may lead to pressure necrosis of overlying skin or underlying bone, muscle contractures, and nerve-compression syndromes. The condition presents with pain on movement and later at rest, with swelling. Nerve compression may ensue, with pain, parasthesiae, numbness, motor impairment, and subsequent muscular atrophy. Volkmann's contracture is a consequence of bleeding into the muscular compartment of the forearm. Fibrosis following muscle haematomata is common, particularly in the calf, leading to shortening of the Achilles tendon and progressive walking difficulties. Retroperitoneal haemorrhage and bleeding into the ileopsoas muscle are particularly important because they are common in severe haemophilia, and can be life-threatening. Femoral nerve compression after an ileopsoas bleed can incapacitate a patient with pre-existing haemophilic arthropathy. Correct diagnosis and the rapid instigation of therapy is essential, particularly as ileopsoas haemorrhage often recurs within a few weeks of initial presentation.

Haemophilic cysts and pseudotumours

Inadequate treatment of haematomata may lead to cystic collections of blood that enlarge due to repeated haemorrhage. On reaching a critical size they infiltrate fascial planes, erode adjacent structures, and eventually rupture with life-threatening consequences. Such haematomata can become pseudotumours, which classically arise in the subperiosteum, and lead to periosteal stripping, cortical destruction, and pathological fractures. Pseudotumours in children usually present as involvement of the small bones in the hands and the feet, but in adults may occur at any site, particularly as a progressively enlarging, non-tender mass in the pelvis or lower limbs. Diagnostic difficulties in differentiating pseudotumours from neoplastic musculoskeletal tumours may be resolved by the demonstration of 'daughter cysts' on computerized tomographic magnetic resonance imaging. In children, continuous prophylactic treatment is effective and peripheral pseudotumours resolve satisfactorily. In adults, surgical excision under appropriate factor VIII cover is the treatment of choice. In cases where surgery is not possible, radiotherapy may induce fibrosis and shrinkage of the pseudotumour.

Haemorrhagic symptoms arising in other systems

Bleeding into the central nervous system and the renal and gastrointestinal tracts is common and may be life-threatening.

Next to acquired immune deficiency syndrome (**AIDS**), intracranial haemorrhage is the most common cause of death in haemophiliacs, with a reported incidence of up to 7.8 per cent. In approximately half of these cases there is a history of trauma, and bleeding may be extradural, sub-dural, or intracerebral, although bilateral subdural haematomata are not unusual. Although the mortality rate has dropped to some 30 per cent with modern treatment, over half of the survivors suffer severe neuro-logical sequelae. These figures emphasize the importance of prompt and adequate replacement therapy with neurological observation in all cases of severe haemophilia presenting with seemingly trivial head injuries.

Haemorrhage from the renal tract is common, and either frank or microscopic haematuria occurs in most patients. In many cases, hae-maturia is painless, transient, and clears spontaneously. In others, how-ever, replacement therapy may be required. The indiscriminant use of antifibrinolytic agents in these cases may lead to disastrous conse-quences with ureteric-clot colic, obstruction, hydronephrosis, renal pap-illary necrosis, and renal failure.

Gastrointestinal bleeding is becoming more common, not so much as a symptom of the underlying factor deficiency but as a manifestation of hepatic disease secondary to long-standing hepatitis C infection previ-ously transmitted from blood products. Additionally, it may occur as a result of inappropriate use of non-steroidal anti-inflammatory agents for the management of haemophilic arthropathy. A careful history and the use of screening tests for haemostasis (see Chapter 22.6.2) and hepatic function (see Section 14) facilitate the diagnosis. Bleeding from the mucous membranes of the mouth is common in children with haemo-philia, and poses a specific problem because the mouth and tongue are moist and the haemostatic platelet plug is continually washed away. Treatment with replacement therapy and/or local haemostatic agents is mandatory in such cases because uncontrolled bleeding may lead to respiratory embarrassment.

Laboratory diagnosis

The laboratory diagnosis in haemophilia rests with the appropriate use of coagulation screening tests and the application of specific coagula-tion-factor assays. As with severe deficiencies of any factor in the intrin-sic coagulation cascade, the partial thromboplastin time is prolonged; however, in mild haemophilia, levels of procoagulant factor VIII in excess of 20 to 25 i.u./dl do not lead to such prolongation, and specific assays of procoagulant factor VIII are mandatory for diagnosis.

Diagnosis of severe haemophilia is easy from the characteristic his-tory, physical findings, and very low factor levels. Haemarthroses with progressive disability are rare in hereditary coagulation disorders other than haemophilia A or B. The diagnosis of mild haemophilia is more difficult as a characteristic clinical picture is lacking, and specific factor assays are essential to differentiate between deficiencies of other factors in the intrinsic coagulation cascade, and from von Willebrand's disease. In variant vWD characterized by a defect in the binding of factor VIII the mode of inheritance is critical. In the initial assessment of patients with moderate and mild haemophilia A, the plasma factor VIII response to DDAVP is important because an incremental rise in procoagulant factor VIII after DDAVP provides a safe and highly cost-effective ther-apeutic option for minor haemorrhagic symptoms, and obviates the use of expensive and potentially unsafe coagulation-factor concentrates.

Treatment of haemophilia A
Comprehensive care

The management of haemophilia and other bleeding disorders requires multidisciplinary expertise, as the chronic and diverse nature of these conditions affects many systems, and several complications and unre-lated disorders are consequent to blood-product therapy. The aim of comprehensive care is to offer specialist medical, surgical, and non-medical professional health-care advice to affected individuals and their families. Comprehensive care teams have been developed in several Haemophilia Centres in the United Kingdom and offer 24-h specialist emergency and telephone advisory facilities for patients. A typical core team consists of a general physician/haematologist with a specific inter-est in bleeding disorders, a specially trained haemophilia nurse, an ortho-paedic surgeon/rheumatologist, with access to specialized physiother-apy, a counsellor with skills in AIDS and genetic counselling, and in social work, a paediatrician, and a dentist. Additional members of the team include a psychologist/psychiatrist, and a specialist in infectious diseases. The team is supplemented by full laboratory facilities for phe-notypic and genotypic analyses, and adequate secretarial, administrative, and financial support. Regular follow-up clinics monitor patients' prog-ress with orthopaedic joint scores and clinical measures, and the fre-quency and site of bleeding, dosages of blood products used, and adverse effects of therapy are reviewed. Records are kept of blood-product doses distributed through home-care programmes. Regular clinical and labo-ratory monitoring and extensive counselling are necessary in patients infected with human immunodeficiency virus (**HIV**) and hepatitis C virus. Computerized record-keeping facilitates more cost-effective care, and is invaluable in providing information to Purchasing Authorities.

Factor replacement therapy (Table 3)

Replacement therapy with factor VIII concentrates is the cornerstone of treatment for symptomatic, severe and DDAVP-unresponsive, moderate haemophilia A. Adequate haemostasis is achieved when procoagulant factor VIII values exceed 25 to 30 i.u./dl. Factor VIII concentrates can be given either as on demand therapy for acute bleeding, or as prophy-lactic regimens to prevent haemorrhage. Treatment of haemorrhage is a medical emergency, and prompt replacement therapy is most cost-effec-tive because bleeding is rapidly controlled, the total amount of concen-trate needed to treat the episode is reduced, and progression of secondary musculoskeletal deformities restricted. The need for rapid treatment of haemorrhage has facilitated self-infusion home-care programmes.

Virus-inactivated factor VIII concentrates should be used exclusively for replacement therapy. Untreated cryoprecipitate is not recommended. Concentrates are classified into high-purity and intermediate-purity products based upon the manufacturing technology and their specific activity (procoagulant factor VIII, i.u./mg protein). High-purity products (specific activity greater than 10 i.u./mg) are prepared by immunoaffin-ity or ion-exchange column chromatography of plasma or recombinant-derived source material. Immunoaffinity procedures produce the most purified forms of factor VIII, but human albumin is added to the final products, whether plasma derived or recombinant, to confer stability to the preparations. Intermediate-purity concentrates (specific activity less than 10 i.u./mg) are prepared by conventional plasma fractionation pro-cedures and contain substantial concentrations of contaminating plasma and cellular proteins.

Recent studies have demonstrated that immunoaffinity-purified con-centrates prevent the progressive decline in CD4 lymphocytes seen in HIV-seropositive haemophiliacs treated on intermediate-purity prod-ucts. CD4 lymphocyte abnormalities previously seen in HIV-seronegative patients and attributed to contaminant components present in intermediate-purity products have led to the recommendation that only high-purity products should be used to treat haemophilia patients.

As hepatitis B (**HBV**) is known to be one of the more resistant viruses to current inactivation procedures, all patients who are or could poten-tially receive plasma-derived blood products, and who are seronegative for HBV antibody, should be immunized against HBV.

On-demand treatment and factor VIII dosage

Factor VIII dosage is based upon the observation that 1 unit (i.u.) (defined as that amount of factor VIII in 1 ml of fresh plasma) per kg body weight increases the procoagulant circulating factor VIII (VIII:C) level by 2 i.u./dl (2 per cent). Thus, an infusion of 10 i.u./kg factor VIII in a severe haemophiliac will raise the level to 20 i.u./dl (20 per cent). As the half-life of infused factor VIII is 8 to 12 h, and may be shorter with extensive haemorrhage or with febrile states, repeated doses are often necessary for haemostatic control.

Haemarthroses are adequately treated with 20 to 30 i.u. factor VIII/kg repeated after 12 h, and possibly also at 24 and 36 h. Higher dosages and repeated infusions are necessary when there is pre-existing pathol-ogy in the affected joints and in cases where initial treatment is delayed.

Table 3 *Replacement therapy in haemophilia A and B, and von Willebrand's disease (excluding inhibitors)*

Disorder	Specific therapeutic agent	Major haemorrhage[a]		Minor haemorrhage-[b]		Haemostatic level[c]
		Bolus dose	Maintenance dose	Bolus dose	Maintenance dose	
Haemophilia A (DDAVP-unresponsive)	Factor VIII concentrate	50 i.u./kg	(i) 2 i.u./kg per h continuous infusing for 3–5 days *or* (ii) 25–30 i.u./kg 8–12 hourly, then 10–20 i.u./kg thereafter	20–40 i.u./kg	20–30 i.u./kg every 12 h	100 i.u./dl (major bleeds) 25–30 i.u./dl (minor bleeds)
Haemophilia B	Factor VIII concentrate	60 i.u./kg	10 i.u./kg 12-hourly	30 i.u./kg	10 i.u./kg 24-hourly	60 i.u./dl (major bleeds) 15–35 i.u./dl (minor bleeds)
von Willebrand's disease (DDAVP-unresponsive)	Factor VIII concentrates (intermediate purity)	50 i.u./kg	25–30 i.u./kg 8–12-hourly for 3–5 days, then 10–20 i.u./kg thereafter	20–40 i.u./kg	10–20 i.u./kg 12-hourly	Normalization of bleeding time
	Purified von Willebrand factor concentrate	30–45 i.u./kg (+50 i.u./kg factor VIII concentrate)	30–45 i.u./kg 12-hourly for 1–3 days, then 30–45 i.u./kg thereafter	30–45 i.u./kg	30 i.u./kg daily	Circulating factor VIII and von Willebrand ristocetin cofactor levels 50 i.u./dl

[a]Life-threatening bleeding conditions, major surgery, or major trauma.

Arthrocentesis is seldom indicated. Initial immobilization of the bleeding joint limits the need for analgesia, and isometric exercises followed by active movement, with hydrotherapy or pulsed shortwave, should be started within 48 h. Night splints may be useful to prevent fixed-flexion deformities. In those cases of chronic haemophilic arthropathy where medical management with factor replacement fails to control symptoms of pain, haemorrhage, or progressive restriction of movement, surgery should be undertaken.

Intramuscular haemorrhage usually requires more intensive treatment with doses of 20 to 40 i.u./kg 12-hourly for several days. Complete bedrest is recommended for ileopsoas bleeds. Haematomata are treated actively with ultrasound and pulsed shortwave to induce breakdown and absorbtion of the clot, which may be done safely under adequate haemostatic control, preventing organization and fibrosis with associated contractures. Compression syndromes in the anterolateral and deep posterior compartments of the calf and also the forearm are common. After factor replacement, active physiotherapy reduces swelling and relieves pressure on the nerve. When there is complete loss of neurological function, emergency operative decompression should be undertaken if possible.

The extraction of permanent teeth, and tongue and mouth lacerations, are treated with 20 i.u./kg factor VIII initially and repeated, if necessary, at 12 h. Adjunctive therapy with tranexamic acid for 7 to 10 days prevents clot dissolution, so reducing factor VIII requirements.

Haematuria seldom requires factor replacement, but in persistent cases 20 to 30 i.u./kg factor VIII 12-hourly for 2 to 3 days may clear the urine. Antifibrinolytic agents or protease inhibitors are contraindicated.

For life-threatening bleeds, major surgery, or major trauma a bolus infusion of 50 i.u./kg factor VIII followed by a continuous infusion at 2 i.u./kg per h is the most suitable management. Alternatively, after the bolus, 25 to 30 i.u./kg 8 to 12-hourly may be given with monitoring to maintain the procoagulant factor VIII between 70 and 100 i.u./dl. Continuous infusion therapy for the first 3 to 5 days of treatment is recommended as the most cost-effective form of management.

Home infusion therapy was introduced in the early 1970s and is now the established form of treatment for over half of severely affected, adolescent and adult patients. The patient and his family are trained to infuse concentrates, and are instructed when to treat, how to calculate the correct dosage, and when to request telephone advice or visit the centre. They are also instructed how to dispose of used needles and syringes and how to record blood-product usage. This approach ensures the most prompt treatment for bleeding episodes and is highly cost-effective.

Prophylactic treatment with factor VIII:
(1) Intermittent prophylaxis

Intermittent prophylaxis in severe haemophilia is indicated during rehabilitation after major surgery, in 'target joint' management, and in chronic hypertrophic synovitis. In the treatment of 'target joints' and synovitis, 20 to 30 i.u./kg factor VIII three times weekly for 3 to 6 months may induce improvement by facilitating healing of the synovium, and is highly cost-effective because joint destruction may be prevented. In cases of chronic hypertrophic synovitis that do not respond to conservative management and where either open or arthroscopic synovectomy is considered inappropriate, radionucleide or chemical synovio-orthesis may be done using radiogold, yttrium, or osmic acid by intra-articular injection.

(2) Continuous prophylaxis

Haemophiliac patients after adolescence experience a more benign course of their disease, possibly due to the higher mortality in affected children, the passage through the 'years of discretion' where the patient knows what he can and can't do, and decreased activity as a result of progressive disability. These observations have led to the introduction of continuous prophylactic programmes in children during the years of most frequent haemorrhage, with the objective of providing regular haemostatic cover and thus preventing spontaneous bleeding episodes. Children maintained on continuous prophylaxis with preinfusion levels of procoagulant factor VIII between 1 and 4 per cent achieve as normal a physical, educational, and social development as their unaffected peers.

Follow-up joint scores and bleeding episodes in these cases show significant reductions compared to on-demand treated controls. Factor VIII requirement in a child or adolescent on such therapy varies between 3000 and 7000 i.u./kg per year. Continuous prophylaxis is usually discontinued at the age of 19 to 20 years when the epiphyses have fused, with subsequent adoption of on-demand therapy. Current studies are underway to determine the minimum factor VIII requirement necessary to sustain adequate continuous prophylaxis within reasonable cost containment, and cost–benefit analyses are in progress.

Continuous prophylactic regimens with 20 to 30 i.u./kg factor VIII three times weekly may be more cost-effective than on-demand therapy in many adult patients with progressive arthropathy. The financial benefits of prophylaxis are not just reflected in the reduced unitage of product required, but also in the savings incurred in health-care delivery costs and social benefits by maintaining such patients in full employment.

Complications of replacement therapy

Millions of units of coagulation-factor concentrates derived from hundreds of thousands of litres of plasma from as many individual blood donors may be used to control bleeding in the lifetime of a severe haemophiliac. It is, thus, not surprising that one of the major safety issues in haemophilia care is related to the potential transmission of disease from donor blood/plasma derivatives to the recipient.

The transmission of HIV-1, HCV, and HBV to patients receiving blood products is well recognized, and screening of donated plasma for antibodies to these viruses and virus inactivation of concentrates have been universally adopted. Current virus-inactivation procedures include dry heating, pasteurization, steam and pressure treatment, solvent detergent treatment, and the use of chaotropic agents. For HIV-1 and HCV all these methods seem to be effective, although concerns have been expressed on the transmission of the non-lipid enveloped parvovirus B19, hepatitis A virus (**HAV**) and, more recently, hepatitis E. Pasteurization is generally regarded as the most effective form of virus inactivation based upon the established viral safety of albumin.

Haemophilic patients infected with HIV-1

Between 1980 and 1984, some 1300 patients with haemophilia became infected with HIV-1 in the United-Kingdom, of which more than 300 have died.

Factor VIII requirements in seropositive patients are higher than in seronegative patients of comparable age and severity of the bleeding disorder, due to the increased haemostatic cover necessary for invasive investigations on patients progressing to AIDS, and for the treatment of HIV-associated immune thrombocytopenia. In the latter there is an increased frequency of bruising and 'target joints' when the platelet count falls below 50×10^9/l, and continuous prophylaxis may be needed to control symptoms, while antiviral therapy or splenectomy may be beneficial in the short term. Associated infectious complications of AIDS require increased doses of factor VIII to prevent haemorrhage from sites of infection.

Although seropositive haemophiliacs in older age groups are disproportionately affected and have a worse prognosis with HIV-1 than adolescents, increased survival in all HIV -1 infected patients due to pneumocystis prophylaxis and advances in antiviral, antifungal, and tuberculostatic therapy has resulted in an overall increased usage of high-purity factor VIII concentrates in this category of patients.

Haemophilic patients infected with HCV

On first exposure to untreated factor concentrates the incidence of transmission of non-A, non-B hepatitis in haemophilic patients was almost 100 per cent, and currently some two-thirds of all patients are seropositive for HCV antibody.

Half such patients develop chronic hepatitis, characterized by an asymptomatic but protracted period of elevated transaminases, and at least 25 per cent of these cases proceed to liver failure, mostly due to cirrhosis. There is an established association between chronic hepatitis C infection and hepatocellular carcinoma, although the oncogenic mechanism has yet to be elucidated. Haemophilic patients infected with HCV do not normally have increased factor VIII requirements unless invasive diagnostic procedures are performed, or haemorrhage secondary to liver failure or thrombocytopenia occurs. Other viral infections (e.g. HIV and HAV) when superimposed on chronic HCV-induced liver disease increase morbidity and mortality. Use of interferon-α and possibly ribavirin in the management of HCV hepatitis has been shown to reduce elevated levels of alanine amino transferase and slow HCV RNA production, although there is a high relapse rate when therapy is discontinued. Liver transplantation, which has been successfully done in a few haemophiliac patients with HBV- or HCV-induced hepatic failure, is unlikely to become more popular due to the more widespread use of interferon-α, although it is curative for the underlying haemostatic disorder (macrogene transfer).

Factor VIII inhibitors (antibodies to factor VIII)

One of the most serious complications of blood-product therapy in haemophilia is the development of factor VIII antibodies (usually IgG_1 or IgG_4) as in most cases, conventional replacement with factor VIII concentrate is rendered ineffective through antibody neutralization. Early prevalence figures have been misleading, due to differing ages and levels of severity of haemophilia in the various study groups, previous exposure of patients to blood products of various types, and the varying duration of follow-up and frequency of inhibitor assessment. With the introduction of high-purity factor VIII concentrates, particularly those prepared by monoclonal antibody immunoaffinity of recombinant source material, more structured studies have been made. These have demonstrated that young children with severe haemophilia are at greatest cumulative risk (up to 32 per cent) of inhibitor development after relatively few exposure days (9–15 days). More than 80 per cent of inhibitors have developed before patients have reached the age of 9 years. Monoclonal antibody-purified, plasma-derived or recombinant factor VIII do not demonstrate higher incidence rates of inhibitor formation than earlier-generation blood products, and continuous prophylactic programmes in children have not been shown to alter the incidence of inhibitor formation.

Factor VIII inhibitors are classified on the basis of the basal titre (assessed by the Bethesda assay in Bethesda units (**Bu**) and on their response to challenge with factor VIII concentrate *in vivo* (anamnestic response). Generally two major types of factor VIII inhibitors are encountered: low-titre (less than 10 Bu/ml to human factor VIII) low responders (little if any anamnesis) and high-titre (more than 10 Bu/ml) high responders (inhibitor increase in excess of 10 times basal level on factor VIII challenge). The correct classification of inhibitors is essential because it provides the rationale for effective therapeutic management.

Treatment of inhibitors can be directed at securing haemostasis alone or, additionally, eradicating the antibody. Low-titre, low-responding inhibitors are treated with either human or porcine factor VIII concentrates at a dosage and frequency of infusion high enough to swamp the antibody and achieve haemostatic levels of factor VIII. In those cases where low levels of residual circulating factor VIII are demonstrable, DDAVP may be given to good effect, indicating that endogenous factor VIII is less immunogenic than exogenous material.

In high-titre, high-responding inhibitors, depending on the inhibitor titre and the clinical status of the patient, porcine factor VIII or 'bypassing agents' may arrest haemorrhage. Levels of antibody in excess of 15 Bu/ml directed against porcine material usually render this form of animal factor VIII treatment ineffective. The 'bypassing agents' are human plasma-derived concentrates containing activated coagulation factors, which trigger the coagulation cascades at levels below that at which the inhibitor is operative. These include FEIBA and Autoplex, which contain plasma-derived IXa, VIIa, and modified Xa, and are usually given at a dosage of 100 u/kg 6-hourly. Preliminary data on the recently introduced recombinant factor VIIa concentrate would suggest that it is highly efficacious in securing haemostasis, with a success rate greater than 85 per cent. As inhibitors are usually IgG antibodies of subclass 1 or 4, immunodepletion of the inhibitor with matrix-bound staphylococcal protein A using extracorporeal devices may be attempted before treatment with factor VIII concentrates.

Programmes for induction of immunotolerance for inhibitor eradication in high-titre, high-responding inhibitors, aiming to suppress the antibody-producing clones, have reportedly met with some success. In these programmes, various dosages of human factor VIII, ranging from 100 i.u./kg twice daily to 25 i.u./kg three times weekly have been described. The drawbacks of these regimens are the lack of predictability of patient response and the high cost involved in sustaining factor VIII concentrates for an indefinite time. Success with the regimens is established when no inhibitor levels can be detected and when the factor VIII half-life normalizes so that the patient can be reintroduced to conventional factor-replacement programmes.

DDAVP and adjunctive therapy

As described under von Willebrand's disease, DDAVP (0.3 μg/kg) is the treatment of choice in mild and some cases of moderate haemophilia. Increased procoagulant factor VIII levels of 3.1- to 3.7-fold are usual, peaking some 30 to 50 min after infusion. DDAVP-released factor VIII has a shorter half-life (3 to 6 h) than endogenous factor, possibly due to coexistent release of proteolytic enzymes. DDAVP with an antifibrinolytic agent is the choice for haemostatic cover in mild/moderate haemophiliacs undergoing dental surgery. Additionally, it is effective when given subcutaneously or by intranasal insufflation, promoting its use in home-care programmes.

As adjunctive therapy, antifibrinolytic agents and local haemostatics (e.g. topical thrombin, collagen fleece and fibrin glue sealants) are highly effective in the management of haemorrhage from mucous membranes and in orthodontic/dental procedures for haemophiliac patients. Additionally, such agents reduce the need for repeated factor replacement in many cases, and are highly cost-effective with minor, if any, side-effects.

HAEMOPHILIA B (CHRISTMAS DISEASE)

In 1947, it was recognized that haemophilia represented two different disorders, and in 1952 haemophilia B was distinguished from haemophilia A. Haemophilia B is less common than haemophilia A, with only some 1100 patients currently registered in the United Kingdom. It is inherited as an X-linked recessive trait, with the factor IX gene remote from the factor VIII gene. Spontaneous mutations are uncommon and haemophilia B in women is rare. Three forms of haemophilia B variants have been defined: the common, CRM-positive form with antigenically normal but non-functional factor IX production; a CRM-negative form with a quantitative reduction in factor IX activity and antigenicity; and a variable CRM^R variant where antibody neutralization is proportional to factor IX activity. One unique variant, haemophilia B Leyden is inherited as a CRM-negative form at birth and becomes CRM-positive with advancing age, with factor IX levels increasing from 1 i.u./dl to 15 to 20 i.u./dl during adult life. Factor IX may modulate the extrinsic coagulation cascade as seen in the CRM-positive haemophilia Bm variant, which prolongs the ox-brain prothrombin time and produced an apparent reduction in factor VII levels. Other variants restrict factor IX cleavage on activation (haemophilia B Chapel Hill and factor IX Alabama) or demonstrate abnormal Ca^{2+} binding.

Although severe haemophilia B is proportionally less common than

severe haemophilia A, clinical features of the two disorders are identical. As screening tests for the two haemophilias are similar, diagnosis rests with specific assays for circulating procoagulant factor IX and the thromboplastin generation test. The cornerstone of treatment in symptomatic haemophilia B, irrespective of the clinical severity, rests with virus-inactivated factor IX concentrates. DDAVP is ineffective, and fresh frozen plasma and cryosupernatant are no longer recommended due to low potency and potential virus transmission. Factor IX values of 15 to 35 i.u./dl are adequate to ensure haemostasis in the treatment of muscle and joint haemorrhage, although for major surgery, life-threatening bleeds, and in major trauma, factor IX, 10 i.u./kg 12-hourly, may be necessary after a bolus injection of factor IX, 60 i.u./kg. The dosage of factor IX concentrate differs from factor VIII concentrate in that its half-life is longer (14–20 h) and, that the factor is distributed into the extravascular space due to its low molecular weight. Two types of factor IX concentrates are currently available in the United Kingdom: intermediate-purity prothrombin complex concentrates containing many of the vitamin K-dependent factors, and high-purity concentrates containing only non-activated factor IX. Small but significant concentrations of activated coagulation factors are present in the prothrombin complex concentrates, which may cause thrombosis or disseminated intravascular haemorrhage when given in high doses. The addition of heparin or antithrombin III to these concentrates does not fully eliminate this thrombogenic potential. The current *Recommendations of the U.K. Haemophilia Centre Directors Organisation* propose the exclusive use of high-purity factor IX concentrates for both routine replacement and for surgical haemostatic cover in haemophilia B patients. As factor IX concentrates are obtained from donated plasma, similar constraints with respect to viral safety apply as in the case of factor VIII concentrates. Intermittent and continuous prophylactic programmes are more readily applicable in patients with haemophilia B because the dosages required are lower than in haemophilia A and, due to the longer half-life, factor IX is only required twice weekly to ensure adequate prophylaxis. Inhibitors to factor IX are rare and usually respond to high-dose factor IX therapy.

FACTOR XI DEFICIENCY (TABLE 4)

This disorder, which has a particularly high frequency in people of Jewish extraction, is transmitted as an incompletely recessive autosomal trait either as a major defect in homozygotes (factor XI of less than 20 i.u./dl) or as a minor defect in heterozygotes (factor XI, 15–45 i.u./dl). Clinically, factor XI deficiency presents as a mild bleeding disorder, usually after surgery or trauma, with few if any spontaneous haemorrhages. Mild factor XI deficiency is associated with Noonan's syndrome. In homozygous patients, the partial thromboplastin time is prolonged and specific factor XI assays give values of 3 to 15 i.u./dl. Therapy with factor XI concentrates is available for the treatment of severe haemorrhage, and for surgery or trauma management. Satisfactory haemostasis is secured with factor XI levels of 15 to 20 i.u./dl.

CONTACT FACTOR DEFICIENCIES

Factor XII deficiency is not usually associated with bleeding manifestations, but may predispose to thrombosis due to deficient activation of fibrinolysis, as myocardial infarction and thrombophlebitis have been reported in patients with severe factor XII deficiency. It is inherited as an autosomal recessive trait, and diagnosis is confirmed by demonstration of a grossly prolonged partial thromboplastin time, decreased prothrombin consumption and thromboplastin generation time, and low factor XII values as assessed by specific factor assay.

Prekallikrein deficiency, like factor XII deficiency, is not associated with clinical bleeding but gives rise to abnormal coagulation *in vitro*. In affected patients, variable abnormalities in stress-induced fibrinolysis, chemotaxis, and immediate and delayed inflammatory responses may

Table 4 *Replacement therapy in hereditary disorders other than haemophilia A and B and von Willebrand's disease*

Disorder	Therapeutic product	Bolus dose	Maintenance dose[a]	Haemostatic level[b]
Factor XI deficiency	Factor XI concentrate	10 i.u./kg	5 i.u./kg per day	15–20 i.u./dl
Factor VII deficiency	Factor VII concentrate	10–15 i.u./kg	5–10 i.u./kg 6-hourly	5–10 i.u./dl
Factor X deficiency	Prothrombin complex concentrates	15–20 i.u./kg	10 i.u./kg per day	10–20 i.u./dl
Factor V deficiency	Fresh frozen plasma	20 ml/kg	10 ml/kg every 12 h	15–25 i.u./dl
Prothrombin deficiency (dysprothrombinaemia)	Prothrombin complex concentrates	15–20 i.u./kg	10 i.u./kg per day	40 i.u./dl
Afibrinogenaemia	Fibrinogen concentrate	100 mg/kg	20–40 mg/kg every 48 h	100 mg/dl
Factor XIII deficiency	Factor XIII concentrate	50–70 i.u./kg	50–75 i.u./kg per month	5 i.u./dl
Combined factor V and VIII deficiency	Fresh frozen plasma	20–40 ml/kg	10–20 ml/kg every 12 h	25 i.u./dl for both factors

[a]Dosage required for continued haemostatic control, e.g. in surgery, major trauma, or life-threatening clinical states.
[b]Factor concentration above which haemorrhage is normally arrested.

be observed, reflecting the central role of prekallikrein and factor XII in a variety of other processes apart from contact activation of the intrinsic cascade.

High molecular-weight kininogen deficiency, transmitted as an autosomal recessive trait, is associated with *in vitro* coagulation abnormalities and impaired kinin formation and fibrinolysis. This disorder is not associated with abnormal bleeding.

Disorders of the extrinsic coagulation cascade (Table 4)

FACTOR VII DEFICIENCY

First described as a rare serum prothrombin conversion accelerator (SPCA) deficiency, only 70 per cent of cases have a true factor VII deficiency. It is transmitted as an autosomal recessive trait or as a doubly heterozygous form, and has a high incidence of association with the Dublin–Johnson and Rotor syndromes. Several variants have been described, demonstrating the existence of both qualitative and quantitative abnormalities of factor VII. The diagnosis rests with abnormalities of the ox-brain prothrombin time, and specific assays of activity and antigenicity of factor VII. Clinical symptoms in severe factor VII deficiency closely resemble those of severe haemophilia A, and such patients may be prone additionally to various thromboembolic manifestations. The haemostatic level of circulating factor VII is 5 to 10 i.u./dl. Due to its short half-life (2–4 h), replacement therapy with specific factor VII concentrates 4 to 6 hourly may be indicated for the management of severe haemorrhage or for surgical cover. Mild factor VII deficiency is usually asymptomatic.

FACTOR X DEFICIENCY

This disorder is inherited as an autosomal, incompletely recessive trait and clinically it closely resembles factor VII deficiency. The haemostatic level for factor X is 10 to 20 i.u./dl. Both CRM-positive and CRM-negative variants have been described: in the former the Stypven time can be either normal or abnormal, depending on the kindred type, suggesting extensive genetic polymorphism of this trait. Diagnosis rests with demonstrable prolongation of the partial thromboplastin, and prothrombin, and Stypven times, and reduced factor X activity by specific assay. Although no specific factor X concentrate is available, replacement therapy with prothrombin complex concentrates is usually effective in controlling haemorrhagic symptoms.

Disorders of the common pathway (Table 4)

FACTOR V DEFICIENCY

This uncommon disorder is transmitted as an autosomal recessive trait that presents in its severe form in individuals who inherit the defective gene from both parents. Clinically, the bleeding disorder is usually mild but may vary greatly, and is associated with a high frequency of mucocutaneous haemorrhage and bleeding into the gastrointestinal and genitourinary tracts, and into the central nervous system. Diagnosis rests with the demonstration of prolongation of the partial thromboplastin and prothrombin times, and low factor V levels by specific assay. Remarkably, approximately one-third of patients with severe factor V deficiency have a prolonged bleeding time. As no specific factor V concentrate is available, fresh frozen plasma-replacement therapy usually controls bleeding symptoms when factor V levels are maintained above 15 to 25 i.u./dl.

PROTHROMBIN (FACTOR II) DEFICIENCY

Hereditary hypoprothrombinaemia is very rare and is transmitted as an autosomal recessive trait. Although it usually presents as a mild bleeding disorder, profuse bleeding from the umbilicus is common in affected infants. As with other hereditary disorders of the vitamin K-dependent coagulation factors, there are CRM-positive and CRM-negative variants, the latter being the 'true' hereditary deficiencies. The CRM-positive variants, with diverse non-functional characteristics but antigenically detectable prothrombin, are usually termed the 'constitutional dysprothrombinaemias'. The functional abnormalities include structural defects in prothrombin whereby thrombin is not produced by factor Xa cleavage (e.g. prothrombin Metz) or where Ca^{2+} binding is deficient (e.g. prothrombin San Juan I). The laboratory findings in this disorder include prolonged partial thromboplastin, prothrombin, and Styvpen times. In true inherited hypothrombinaemia, factor II levels are less than 10 i.u./dl, while in the 'constitutional dysprothrombinaemias', they lie between 10 and 50 i.u./dl, as measured by the two-stage prothrombin assay. Treatment relies upon replacement therapy with prothrombin complex concentrates to achieve a haemostatic prothrombin level in excess of 40 i.u./dl.

DISORDERS OF FIBRINOGEN

Hereditary afibrinogenaemia and hypofibrinogenaemia have been previously described under defects in primary haemostasis.

Hereditary qualitative defects in fibrinogen, the dysfibrinogenaemias, are inherited as autosomal dominant or codominant traits, and more than 160 different variants have been reported. In all these disorders, fibrinogen antigenicity is detectable but structural abnormalities may lead to dysfunction of one or more of the three stages involved in the conversion of fibrinogen to cross-linked fibrin by thrombin and factor XIII. These functional abnormalities may result in:

(1) abnormal or retarded enzymatic cleavage of fibrinopeptide A or B from fibrinogen by thrombin;
(2) abnormal or retarded fibrin monomer polymerization;
(3) normal or deficient cross-linkage of fibrin monomers.

As many of the structural defects that arise may disrupt more than one of these stages, several dysfibrinogenaemias demonstrate both abnormal fibrinopeptide release and impaired polymerization of fibrin monomer, while in a number of variants the functional abnormalities have yet to be established.

Clinically, most patients are asymptomatic, particularly as many variants have only been described in the heterozygotic form, that is at least 50 per cent circulating fibrinogen is normal. In less than 30 per cent of cases, the disorder may present with a mild bleeding diathesis, thromboembolic symptoms, impaired wound healing, or a combination of these features. Defective fibrinopeptide release and abnormal fibrin cross-linkage are more commonly associated with haemorrhage.

Prolonged thrombin and reptilase times and low clottable fibrinogen values with normal levels of fibrinogen antigen are characteristic of the hereditary dysfibrinogenaemias, and the partial thromboplastin and prothrombin times are often abnormal. Specialized diagnostic assays include fibrinopeptide A and B to determine release kinetics, sodium dodecyl sulphate electrophoresis to elucidate polymerization and primary cross-linkage abnormalities, and amino-acid sequencing to characterize the primary structure of the abnormal fibrinogen. Haemorrhagic symptoms seldom require treatment, but when necessary virus-inactivated fibrinogen concentrates may be given.

FACTOR XIII DEFICIENCY

Hereditary factor XIII deficiency is a rare condition that is transmitted as an autosomal recessive trait. In homozygotes, the factor XIII A subunit is totally deficient in the plasma and the platelet, while the B subunit is present in the plasma in low concentrations. In heterozygotes, both subunits are detectable but at subnormal levels.

Haemorrhage from the umbilical stump is common in this disorder and may be fatal. Mucosal bleeding is uncommon but cutaneous and muscular haematomata usual. Haemorrhage after surgery or trauma may be severe and protracted, and bleeding into the central nervous system is not uncommon. Affected women demonstrate a greater incidence of spontaneous abortion. Wound healing is often impaired. Diagnosis rests upon clot solubility in 5M-urea and on specific functional assays for factor XIII. Virus-inactivated factor XIII concentrates are available for the treatment of bleeding symptoms, and plasma levels of factor XIII above 5 i.u./dl will secure haemostasis. Because of the long half-life of factor XIII (72–96 h), prophylactic treatment on a 4-weekly basis prevents recurrence of haemorrhagic symptoms.

DISORDERS DUE TO COMBINED FACTOR DEFICIENCIES

Numerous hereditary coagulation disorders involving two or more separate factors have been reported, many involving the presence of abnormal acarboxylated forms of the vitamin K-dependent coagulation proteins.

The most common combined defect, however, involves the inherited deficiency of factors V and VIII, which is transmitted as an autosomal recessive trait involving a double heterozygotic pattern (type I) or a dual abnormality of a combined gene (type II). Although clinically moderate to mild mucocutaneous haemorrhage is common, severe bleeding may occur after surgery or trauma. Prolonged partial thromboplastin and prothrombin times are common, and levels of 5 to 20 i.u./dl factor V and

circulating factor VIII are diagnostic. Treatment with fresh frozen plasma is effective and DDAVP may be useful for minor haemorrhage.

BLEEDING DISORDERS DUE TO HEREDITARY ANTIPROTEASE DEFICIENCIES

Although abnormalities in plasma antiprotease components usually cause thromboembolic symptoms, severe bleeding is not uncommonly associated with hereditary α_2-antiplasmin deficiency. This disorder is inherited as an autosomal recessive trait, and haemorrhage is attributed to premature lysis of fibrin clots. In homozygotes, α_2-antiplasmin levels are less than 10 u/dl. Mild bleeding symptoms occur in heterozygotes. Treatment with antifibrinolytic agents or protease inhibitors is beneficial in some patients.

REFERENCES

Beck, W.S. (ed.) (1991). *Hematology*, (5th edn). Cambridge, MA.
Colman, R.W., Hush, J., Mander, V.J., and Saltzman, E.W. (ed.) (1987). Basic principles and clinical practice. In *Haemostasis and Thrombosis*, (2nd edn). Lippincott, Philadelphia.
Gatti, L. and Mannucci, P.M.M. (1984). Use of porcine factor VIII in the management of seventeen patients with factor VIII antibodies. *Thrombosis and Haemostasis*, **51**, 379–84.
Lusher, J.M. and Kessler, C.M. (ed.) (1991). *Haemophilia and von Willebrand's disease in the 1990's. A new decade of hopes and challenges*, International Congress Series 943. Excerpta Medica, Amsterdam.
Seghatchian, M.J. and Savidge, G.F. (ed.) (1989). *Factor VIII—von Willebrand factor*, Vol. I. CRC Press, Boca Raton, FA.
Seghatchian, M.J. and Savidge, G.F. (ed.) (1989). *Factor VIII—von Willebrand factor*, Vol. II. CRC Press, Boca Raton, FA.
Watson, H.G. and Ludlam, C.A. (1992). Immunological abnormalities in haemophiliacs. *Blood*, **6**, 1–58.

22.6.6 Acquired coagulation disorders

B. J. HUNT

Acquired haemostatic disorders occur, by definition, in patients with no previous bleeding tendency and are secondary to an underlying disease. They are more common than the inherited disorders and are associated with many causes, including multisystem disease, drug therapy, and physiological events such as pregnancy and birth. The disorders may be due to either lack of production and/or excessive loss of haemostatic factors and/or the presence of inhibitory substances. Apart from conditions such as vitamin K deficiency, and in contrast to inherited coagulation disorders, they are usually associated with multiple haemostatic deficiencies involving coagulation factors, physiological anticoagulants, fibrinolysis, platelets and the endothelium (Table 1).

Clinically, the first problem is to recognize a bleeding tendency, after which the abnormalities should be defined by laboratory investigations so that the appropriate therapy is given. The patient should be questioned about a past or family bleeding tendency to exclude a late presentation of a congenital bleeding abnormality such as mild von Willebrand disease, which may not present until the haemostatic system is challenged by surgery or trauma.

A careful clinical history and examination will indicate whether bleeding is due only to local factors such as a peptic ulcer and if an underlying haemostatic defect such as that due to chronic liver disease is a contributory factor. Continued oozing from venepuncture and injection sites, pressure sites, and postoperative drainage tubes is often a sign of haemostatic failure. Paradoxically, areas of cutaneous cyanosis and subsequent gangrene may indicate disseminated intravascular coagulation before excessive bleeding becomes apparent.

Table 1 *Changes in screening haemostatic assays in acquired coagulation disorders*

	PT	PTT	Fibrinogen	Platelet count	FDPs
Liver disease	↑	↑	N/↑↓	↓	sl ↑
Renal disease	↑/N	↑/N	↑	N/↓	sl ↑/N
Disseminated intravascular coagulation	↑	↑	↓	↓	↑
Massive transfusions	↑	↑	N/↓	↓/N	↑/N
Fibrinolytic bleeding	sl ↑	sl ↑	↓	N	↑↑
Oral anticoagulants	↑	↑↑	N	N	N
Heparin	↑	↑↑↑	N	N	N
Idiopathic thrombocytopenic purpura	N	N	N	↓	N

N, normal; ↑, prolonged/elevated; ↓, decreased; sl, slight.
FDPs, fibrinogen degradation products; PT, prothrombin time; PTT, partial thromboplastin time.

Often a bleeding tendency is first suggested by baseline screening tests: prothrombin time (**PT**); the partial thromboplastin time (**PTT**); thrombin time (**TT**); and fibrinogen levels and platelet count (other abbreviations used in this chapter are summarized in Table 2, and in Chapter 22.6.5). If a specific abnormality is suspected, then more exact and sophisticated tests can be done. Haemostatic defects that are not associated with active bleeding do not usually need treatment. Acquired haemostatic abnormalities tend to correct themselves as the underlying disease process resolves, unless the patient has a concurrent congenital bleeding problem, in which case active treatment of the underlying disease is very important in the management.

Haemostasis in the newborn

Because of the fragility of their haemostatic function, bleeding in newborn infants is a complex clinical challenge. Acquired haemostatic disorders are more common than genetic defects, and certain diseases are only encountered at this stage of development; failure to consider them may delay the start of effective therapy. Moreover, the sites of bleeding in an infant are different from those in adults and children in that they are related to perinatal events. They include oozing from the umbilicus, cephalohaematomas, and bleeding after circumcision, from peripheral venepuncture sites, and into the skin. Newborns appear to be at particular risk of intracranial haemorrhage secondary to any bleeding disorder. Due to liver immaturity there is little reserve capacity to respond to haemorrhage, and deficiencies of the vitamin K-dependent factors (II, VII, IX, X, protein C, and S), factors XI, XII, plasminogen and antithrombin III occur regularly. Multiple haemostatic deficiencies such as vitamin K deficiency or disseminated intravascular coagulation can easily develop in association with other disease states.

The constantly changing haemostatic mechanisms in newborns necessitate multiple reference ranges of normal values that are dependent on gestational and postnatal age (Table 2). In children, haemostasis is different from that in adults in that there are higher concentrations of physiological inhibitors such α_2-macroglobulin. Large volumes of blood cannot be obtained for testing and microtechniques must be used.

DISSEMINATED INTRAVASCULAR COAGULATION IN THE NEWBORN

This is a common complication of many diseases of the newborn including the respiratory distress syndrome, asphyxia, trauma, viral and bac-

Table 2 *Haemostasis screening tests and factor assays in premature infants and term infants compared to the normal adult range*

	Premature infants (28–34 weeks)	Term infants (38–41 weeks)	Normal adults
PT (s)	16–20	14–17	12–14
TT (s)	15–24	14–18	12–14
APTT (s)	50–65	40–50	30–40
Factor IX (%)	15–20	20–40	50–200
Factor VII (%)	20–60	35–70	50–200
AT-III (%)	25–35	45–75	80–120

PT, prothrombin time; TT, thrombin time; APTT, activated partial thromboplastin time; AT-III, antithrombin III.

terial infections, hypothermia, and perinatal aspiration of meconium or amniotic fluid. The clinical spectrum is wide; in some it is characterized by haemorrhage or thrombotic complications whereas in others there may be minimal clinical signs.

The diagnosis and management are similar to those of an adult with disseminated intravascular coagulation in that they are dependent on the successful treatment of the underlying condition and the use of replacement therapy if there are bleeding complications (see below).

VITAMIN K DEFICIENCY BLEEDING IN NEONATES

Presentation

Vitamin K deficiency resulting in bleeding in neonates was originally known as haemorrhagic disease of the newborn, but now the term vitamin K deficiency bleeding is used. It can be classified into three patterns of presentation. The classical form of vitamin K deficiency bleeding has an incidence of about 1 in 200 to 400 in the absence of prophylactic therapy. It occurs in breast-fed, full-term infants, usually on the second or third day of life when concentrations of the K-dependent factors normally reach a nadir. Infants present with gastrointestinal bleeding (melaena neonatorum), widespread ecchymosis, bleeding from venepuncture sites, and intracranial haemorrhage. The condition is caused by poor dietary intake of vitamin K as there is little in breast milk (less than 20 μg/l compared with 830 μg/l in formula milk), combined with poor vitamin K synthesis and stores.

The second form of vitamin K deficiency bleeding presents early in the first 24 h of life, usually with serious bleeding such as intracranial haemorrhage. The mothers of these infants have usually taken drugs that interfere with vitamin K metabolism, such as anticonvulsants or warfarin, during the third trimester. The third type occurs later, beyond the first week of life, in infants with malabsorptive diseases, such as cystic fibrosis, α_1-antitrypsin deficiency, hepatitis, and coeliac disease.

Even in the healthy full-term infant population, 20 to 30 per cent of cord blood samples have detectable **PIVKAs** (proteins induced by vitamin K absence or antagonism) indicative of vitamin K deficiency. Most respond to the administration of vitamin K except for the sick, very premature infants whose immature livers have poor synthetic ability.

Management

Prophylactic administration of 1 mg of vitamin K_1 intramuscularly within 24 h of birth was standard practice. However, the route of administration is being reviewed following a report of an association between intramuscular (but not oral) vitamin K_1 in neonates and the later development of childhood cancer. Oral vitamin K_1 is now widely used in the United Kingdom but there have been cases of vitamin K deficiency bleeding in babies who only had a single dose: many were found to have previously unrecognized liver disease. Bottle-fed babies almost never suffer from vitamin K deficiency bleeding presumably because they absorb enough of the 25 to 50 μg of vitamin K taken daily in supplemented milk formulas. Current recommendations are for 3 oral doses of vitamin K_1 in breast fed babies but further research is required to establish the optimal type, frequency, and dose of prophylaxis. There is as yet no licensed oral vitamin K_1 preparation in the United Kingdom.

Certain risk groups, for example those with malabsorptive states such as cystic fibrosis, or children of women receiving anticonvulsants during pregnancy, require additional prophylaxis. Any woman receiving anticonvulsants during the third trimester should receive vitamin K supplements, 5 mg orally per day.

Infants with haemorrhagic complications should receive vitamin K immediately, either subcutaneously or intravenously rather than intramuscularly as this produces a large haematoma.

Vitamin K deficiency disorders

VITAMIN K

Biochemistry

Vitamin K is a fat-soluble vitamin that is a cofactor for the post-translational carboxylation of specific glutamate residues of factors II, VII, IX, and X, as well as protein C and S. This process occurs mainly in the rough endoplasmic reticulum of hepatocytes. γ-Carboxyglutamate residues are necessary for normal coagulation; they bind via calcium ions to phospholipid templates and without them coagulation cannot proceed normally. In the absence of these residues, inactive precursors of factors II, VII, IX, and X (PIVKAs) are released into the circulation.

Sources

Vitamin K exists in two major chemical forms: vitamin K_1 or phylloquinone, produced exclusively by plants, and vitamin K_2 or menaquinones, synthesized by micro-organisms. The major dietary source of vitamin K is K_1. Green, leafy vegetables are the richest source (100–500 μg/100 g). Dietary contributions are made by other vegetables and fruit (1–50 μg/100 g); oils, fats and margarine (1–100 μg/100 g); dairy products (0.5–5 μg/100 g); and bread and cereal products (0.1–10 μg/100 g). The bioavailability of phylloquinone from these foods is unknown but is likely to vary widely, being least efficient from green vegetables and most efficient from processed food. Intestinal bacteria, mainly *Escherichia coli* and bacteroides produce menaquinone but there is little evidence that it is absorbed.

Absorption

The intestinal absorption of dietary phylloquinone is the same as for any fat-soluble vitamin. Intraluminally, vitamin K is solubilized into mixed micelles composed of bile salts and the products of pancreatic lipolysis. The required daily intake of vitamin K is about 0.1 to 0.5 μg/kg. Most of the absorbed vitamin K passes to the hepatocytes, where liver stores are relatively low with a half-life of only a few days. Normal serum concentrations of vitamin K range between 150 and 800 pg/ml.

VITAMIN K DEFICIENCY

Vitamin K deficiency is due to poor dietary intake, malabsorption from the gut, hepatic immaturity or disease, or may be iatrogenic due to oral anticoagulation. Clinically, there may be bruising, ecchymoses, and mucous-membrane bleeding but these symptoms and signs are uncommon unless the PT is greater than 30 s.

In adults, vitamin K deficiency usually occurs in conditions that produce fat malabsorption. Causes include disease of the biliary tree such as fistulae or obstruction (where there is an absence of bile salts in the small intestine); and pancreatic disease, where there is failure to produce pancreatic lipases. Deficiency is especially likely to occur after surgical resection of the small intestine and in coeliac disease. Patients dependent on total parental nutrition require vitamin K supplements. Vitamin K deficiency is potentiated by the use of antibiotic drugs but the mechanisms are unclear. Antibiotics inhibit large-bowel bacterial growth, but

there is no evidence that any vitamin K_2 produced is absorbed from the large bowel.

Laboratory diagnosis

Baseline coagulation tests show prolonged PT and PTT but with a normal TT and fibrinogen levels. Specific assays will show reduced amounts of factors II, VII, IX, and X. Correction of these values, and of the PT and APTT, follows vitamin K administration.

Management

The normal dose to prevent all gastrointestinal causes of vitamin K deficiency is 10 mg intravenously a week. It should be given no faster than 5 mg/min because it can cause anaphylactoid reactions. Four to six hours are required before maximum benefit is obtained. Fresh frozen plasma or prothrombinase complexes will correct the coagulation abnormality immediately.

COUMARIN ANTICOAGULANTS

The clinical indications for oral anticoagulation and the intensity of treatment are discussed in Chapter 22.6.7. Oral anticoagulants, which include coumarin and phenindione derivatives, decrease the availability of vitamin K in the hepatocyte by acting as competitive inhibitors of vitamin K. Consequently, non-functional acarboxyl forms of factors II, VII, IX, X, protein C, and protein S are generated (PIVKAs).

The therapeutic range for oral anticoagulant control is based on the PT, which is itself based on an international normalized ratio (**INR**). This adjusts the PT so that it is expressed as if it had been measured using an international reference thromboplastin and consequently allows for uniform oral anticoagulant therapy. The therapeutic range varies depending on the indication for anticoagulation.

The most common complication of anticoagulant therapy is haemorrhage, which usually results from overdosage. If the INR is greater than 4.5 and there is little or no bleeding, treatment should be withdrawn and then resumed on a smaller maintenance dose once the INR has reached the normal range. If the INR is grossly prolonged and associated with bleeding, a slow intravenous infusion of vitamin K, 0.5 mg, will reverse the prolongation, but the effect does not begin for 6 h, with a maximum at 24 to 36 h. A large dose such as 10 mg is not recommended unless there is life-threatening bleeding because it may prevent effective anticoagulation for up to 2 weeks. With severe haemorrhage, fresh frozen plasma or prothrombinase complexes (factors II, VII, IX, and X) will provide immediate correction of coagulation.

Drug interactions

Many drugs increase the biological effect of oral anticoagulants. It must be remembered that underlying disorders such as diarrhoea, jaundice, or malabsorption may potentiate the effects of anticoagulants by impairing vitamin K absorption.

Some drugs decrease the biological effects of anticoagulants. Several mechanisms are involved, including induction of hepatic microsomal enzymes leading to increased warfarin metabolism. Although these effects do not produce haemorrhage, there is a danger that when these drugs are stopped the current dose of coumarin will exert an excessive effect. An increase in dietary vitamin K intake will also reduce the effect of oral anticoagulants.

Haemostasis and liver disease

AETIOLOGY

Hepatocellular disease can cause serious haemostatic defects, the severity of which is proportional to the extent of liver damage. In chronic hepatic disease there is impaired synthesis of all coagulation factors except for factor VIIIc, which, because it is produced at other sites including lymph nodes and spleen, may be found in normal or increased amounts. Fibrinogen levels are usually normal unless the liver disease is severe. There is inadequate carboxylation of vitamin K-dependent coagulation factors in most patients, despite adequate vitamin K stores. This may be exacerbated by failed absorption of vitamin K due to biliary-tract disease. Platelet dysfunction, attributed mainly to increased levels of fibrin(ogen) degradation products, and thrombocytopenia are common. The cause of the latter is uncertain but it is exacerbated by splenomegaly (hypersplenism) (see Chapter 22.5.4).

Because hepatocytes also synthesize the major inhibitors of coagulation proteins, α_2-macroglobulin and antithrombin III for example, in liver failure their reduction parallels the reduction in coagulation factors. Liver disease can impair clearance of activated coagulation factors, although the mechanisms and cells involved, possibly those of the reticuloendothelial system, are not clearly defined. Due to the diminished clearance of plasminogen activator and plasmin there is an enhanced fibrinolytic state. In some cases of severe hepatic failure the defective synthesis of coagulation factors and excessive fibrinolytic activity are associated with disseminated intravascular coagulation.

Bleeding in liver disease is usually multifactorial in origin. It should be remembered that chronic liver failure induces non-haematological complications that contribute to bleeding. Portal hypertension causes varices that are fragile and easily ruptured, as well as splenomegaly and concomitant thrombocytopenia. Clinically, bleeding is seldom severe except from local lesions such as peptic ulcers, varices, or following liver biopsies and surgery.

In summary, in chronic liver disease there is a complex haemostatic disorder with a precarious *status quo* and limited haemostatic reserve, tending to exacerbate bleeding due to local mechanical effects. Hyperfibrinolysis or overt disseminated intravascular coagulation may complicate the picture.

LABORATORY INVESTIGATION

The simple screening tests (PTT, PT, TT, fibrinogen, and platelet count) will determine whether a patient with liver disease has a major haemostatic problem. Derangement of the baseline tests is common. Usually there is a prolongation of the PT and APTT. In general, the PT is an excellent guide to hepatic function and a reliable prognostic indicator after paracetemol overdose. Deficiency of the vitamin K-dependent coagulation factors (II, VII, IX and X) is reflected in moderately prolonged PT and APTT values.

The TT and fibrinogen levels are normal unless liver disease is severe. The TT is sensitive to a number of abnormalities associated with liver disease including hypofibrinogenaemia, dysfibrinogenaemia (due to an increased sialic acid content of fibrinogen), poor fibrin polymerization due to factor XIII deficiency, and raised levels of fibrin degradation products. Some recommend monitoring the level of factor V in hepatic disease. Because this factor is independent of vitamin K, reduced levels should reflect hepatocellular impairment, but this is probably no more reliable that monitoring with simple screening tests.

An increase in plasma fibrinolytic activity is demonstrated by increased levels of tissue plasminogen activators and fibrin degradation products despite low levels of plasminogen and α_2-antiplasmin.

MANAGEMENT

The patient who is not bleeding, despite abnormal coagulation tests, requires no treatment. It is wise to give vitamin K_1, 10 mg intravenously, if there is evidence of vitamin K deficiency, although, because of ineffective synthesis of coagulation proteins, this may not always improve the PT.

Local management of any local bleeding such as from a gastric or duodenal ulcer, or varices, is crucial. If a patient is bleeding or undergoing an operative procedure the deficient factors can be given in the form of fresh frozen plasma, although complete correction is seldom attained. In the past, prothrombinase complex concentrates (factors II,

VII, IX, and X) were given but this is associated with a thrombotic risk. There is an increased risk of haemorrhage after liver biopsy unless the PT is corrected to within 4 s of the control. If fibrinogen levels are very low, cryoprecipitate or fibrinogen concentrate can be given. Platelet transfusion is useful if there is thrombocytopenia and bleeding, and an infusion of DDAVP (see Chapter 22.6.5) may shorten the bleeding time by temporarily correcting platelet functional abnormalities. If disseminated intravascular coagulation supervenes in liver disease, heparin is of no value; replacement therapy alone is recommended.

During the anhepatic and reperfusion phases of liver transplantation there is increased bleeding due to very high levels of tissue plasminogen activator. Perioperative high-dose aprotinin (an antifibrinolytic agent) has been shown to be beneficial in reducing blood loss. Otherwise fibrinolytic inhibitors are not used in liver disease because they may potentiate intravascular thrombosis.

Renal disease

In renal failure there is an increased likelihood of bleeding. Uraemic patients may develop purpura, epistaxes, gingival bleeding, gastrointestinal haemorrhage, haemopericardium, or intracranial haemorrhage. In general the severity of the bleeding diathesis parallels the degree of uraemia.

AETIOLOGY

The pathophysiology of the bleeding disorder is complex and only partly understood. Abnormalities of platelet function and adhesion are probably the major cause of haemostatic failure. Platelets aggregate poorly, probably due to accumulation of toxic metabolites such as guanidinosuccinic acid and phenolic acid in the plasma. Anaemia contributes to the bleeding tendency by interfering with platelet–endothelial interactions. A selective deficiency of the larger multimers of von Willebrand factor, possibly due to increased proteolytic activity in uraemic blood, results in impaired platelet adhesiveness, contributing to the prolonged bleeding time.

Coagulation factor deficiencies also occur. Deficiency of vitamin K-dependent factors results from malnutrition, antibiotic therapy, or uraemic enteritis. Rarely, factor IX or factor XII deficiencies occur in the nephrotic syndrome, probably due to increased loss in the urine. This is usually diagnosed on the results of laboratory investigations and does not result in bleeding. A low-grade disseminated intravascular coagulation is commonly found in the acute phase of renal disease, at least as evidenced by intraglomerular fibrin deposits.

LABORATORY INVESTIGATIONS

The bleeding time is prolonged due to acquired platelet dysfunction, thrombocytopenia, and anaemia. In most cases the PT, APTT and TT are slightly or moderately prolonged. A disproportionately prolonged APTT may reflect factor IX deficiency, while a long PT and APTT may indicate vitamin K deficiency.

MANAGEMENT

Platelet transfusions have only a temporary effect on the bleeding time because donor platelets acquire the uraemic defect within hours. Infusions of cryoprecipitate or DDAVP also temporarily shorten the bleeding time by increasing the levels of large multimers of von Willebrand factor. Correction of the platelet defects follows haemodialysis. Transfusion of red cells or the administration of erythropoietin shortens the bleeding time in the long term.

In the nephrotic syndrome, thrombosis is more common than bleeding because antithrombin III, protein C, and plasminogen may be lost in the urine. Concomitant prothrombotic changes include increased levels of fibrinogen, von Willebrand factor and factors V, VII, VIII, and X, increased platelet aggregation responses, and decreased fibrinolytic activity due to excess of the plasminogen activator inhibitor-1. The urinary concentration of urokinase also decreases in parallel with the decline in renal function. Furthermore, haemodialysis using heparin has been associated with platelet activation. Administration of antiplatelet drugs can reduce the incidence of thrombosis in chronic renal failure.

Disseminated intravascular coagulation

Disseminated intravascular coagulation is defined as the widespread activation of haemostasis, involving coagulation factors, platelets, physiological inhibitors, fibrinolysis and the endothelium, and the formation of soluble or insoluble fibrin within the circulation. Disseminated intravascular coagulation does not occur *de novo* but is a pathological response to many underlying disorders. Initially the process is compensated but as the haemostatic factors are consumed in diffuse, small-vessel thrombosis, haemostatic failure may develop. In most cases of disseminated intravascular coagulation, bleeding is the major clinical problem; but in an important minority, about 10 per cent, widespread thrombosis is dominant, resulting in tissue ischaemia with multiorgan dysfunction.

The clinical syndrome is extremely variable in severity and often occurs in desperately ill patients. Easy bruising and persistent oozing from venepuncture and intramuscular injection sites and around drainage tubes are often the initial manifestations. This picture can progress to massive mucous-membrane bleeding and, rarely, to the Waterhouse–Friderichsen syndrome (see Section 7). Disseminated intravascular coagulation can be very acute in onset, and overwhelming; total defibrination is associated with profuse bleeding and shock. It is seen most frequently in obstetrics, where postpartum bleeding from the vagina may be catastrophic.

The more common forms of disseminated intravascular coagulation are subacute or chronic. There is a slow depletion of haemostatic components with or without bleeding. If thrombosis is the predominant feature, microthrombotic lesions are often found in the fingers and toes. Other areas of the skin may become involved, with purpura fulminans and/or haemorrhagic bullae (see Section 7). The renal vasculature is usually involved at an early stage, while thrombi in the pulmonary vasculature can cause an acute respiratory distress syndrome and thrombi in the cerebral circulation may cause transient neurological abnormalities. In almost all cases of disseminated intravascular coagulation the diagnosis and management of the underlying disorder lead to restoration of normal haemostasis.

PATHOGENESIS (FIG. 1)

In disseminated intravascular coagulation a powerful and/or persistent trigger activates the haemostatic mechanism. There are four potential, interactive mechanisms:

(1) activation of the extrinsic pathway by the expression of tissue factor on damaged tissues, endothelium and monocytes in trauma, especially surgery, burns and heat stroke, bacterial endotoxin, and by some malignant tumours;

(2) intrinsic-pathway activation by immune complexes, bacterial lipopolysaccharide, or damage to the endothelium exposing negatively charged subendothelium;

(3) platelet activation by bacterial endotoxin, which can induce a membrane defect in platelets—platelet activation also occurs after endothelial damage and thrombin generation;

(4) bypass of the normal mechanisms of activation of haemostasis with direct activation of part of the coagulation cascade—for example, activation of factor X or prothrombin by proteolytic enzymes such as snake venoms.

Other contributory factors may potentiate disseminated intravascular coagulation. The complement system is activated *in vivo* and *in vitro* by the same triggers that activate haemostasis. Some cytokines can cause endothelial procoagulant changes. Blockage of the reticuloendothelial system may occur in liver disease and pregnancy and limits removal of activated clotting factors and fibrin monomers.

Secondary activation of fibrinolysis follows the release of tissue plasminogen activator from the endothelium under the stimulation of thrombin and bradykinin, while plasminogen can also be activated by the contact system. Fibrinolytic activation causes degradation of fibrin into fibrin degradation products, and also fibrinogen into fibrinogen degradation products. Except in fulminant disseminated intravascular coagulation the fibrinolytic system is capable of rapidly lysing large amounts of fibrin as it is formed, and thus maintaining vascular patency. Fibrin degradation products and fibrinogen degradation products inhibit thrombin and fibrin polymerization as well as platelet function, by binding to the platelet membrane. Some patients with severe disseminated intravascular coagulation (DIC) may have no increase in fibrin degradation products due to a poor fibrinolytic response; they tend to have extensive thrombosis and a poor prognosis.

Disseminated intravascular coagulation produces microvascular thrombi with fibrin strands and platelet aggregates, which cause partial blockage of the microcirculation. Red cells are fragmented as they pass

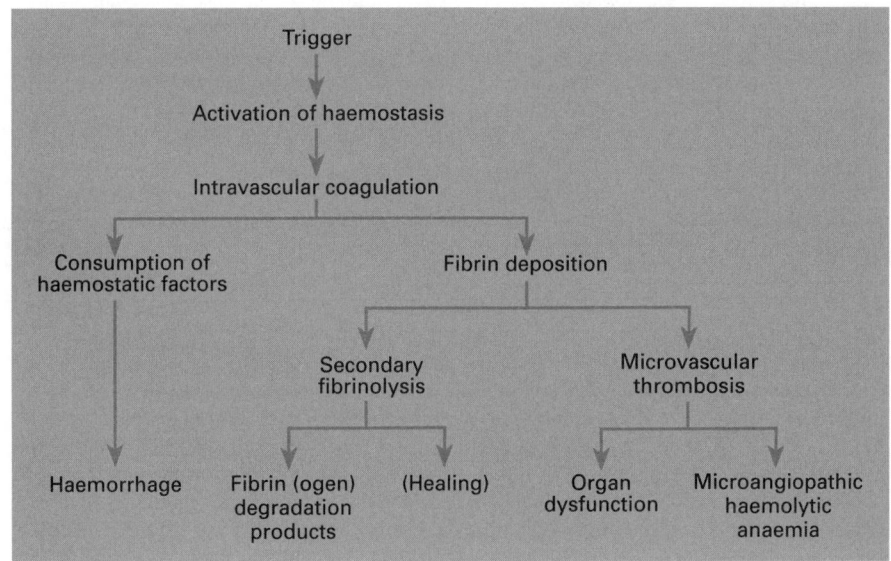

Fig. 1 The pathophysiology of disseminated intravascular coagulation.

Table 3 *Clinical conditions complicated by disseminated intravascular coagulation*

Infections
Septicaemia
Viral
Protozoal (malaria)
Rickettsial

Obstetrics
Abruptio placentae
Amniotic fluid embolism
Placenta praevia
Retained dead fetus
Eclampsia

Malignancy
Carcinoma of stomach, colon, pancreas, breast, lung, especially
    when metastatic
Mucin-secreting adenocarcinomas
Leukaemia, especially acute promyelocytic leukaemia

Shock
Surgical trauma
Burns
Heat stroke

Immunological
Immune-complex disorders
Allograft reaction
Incompatible blood transfusion

Liver disease
Cirrhosis
Acute hepatic necrosis

Miscellaneous
Snake venom
Vascular malformations such as cavernous haemangioma
Fat embolism

over the fibrin deposits, leading to a microvascular haemolytic anaemia in 50 per cent of cases (see Chapter 22.4.13).

AETIOLOGY (TABLE 3)

In hospital practice most cases of disseminated intravascular coagulation are secondary to septicaemia, especially due to Gram-negative bacteria. A severe form of DIC is seen in meningococcal septicaemia, in which widespread haemorrhage, including haemorrhage into the adrenal glands, may be associated with profound shock. This is often fatal and is known as the Waterhouse–Friderichsen syndrome (see Sections 7 and 12).

Obstetric catastrophes are often accompanied by uncontrollable haemorrhage and incoagulable blood. Those most commonly associated with disseminated intravascular coagulation are shown in Table 3. Placental tissue is rich in thromboplastins and it is thought that they are released into the circulation. This occurs against the background of the prothrombotic state of pregnancy, where there are increased coagulation factors, hyperaggregable platelets, decreased fibrinolytic activity (partially due to the production of platelet activator inhibitor-2 by the placenta), and poor reticuloendothelial clearance. In contrast, intrauterine fetal death produces slow, progressive disseminated intravascular coagulation, in which bleeding is a late manifestation, often foreshadowed by deteriorating renal function.

Some neoplasms are associated with a low-grade disseminated intravascular coagulation, especially adenocarcinomas, which may express tissue factor-like activity. In pancreatic carcinoma the release of trypsin may lyse and activate coagulation factors. At presentation, acute pro-

myelocytic leukaemia is associated with a haemorrhagic diathesis, which, in some patients, is attributable to disseminated intravascular coagulation. However, it is now thought that bleeding is more often due to excess fibrinolytic activity (see below).

Worldwide, the most common cause of death due to disseminated intravascular coagulation is from snake-bite envenoming (see Section 8). Most snakes with venom belong to the Viperidae family, which includes vipers, rattlesnakes and adders. In particular *Echis carinatus* (the saw-scaled viper) and *Vipera russelli* (Russell's viper) are found widely throughout the tropical regions of Africa and Asia. *Echis carinatus* produces a venom that directly activates prothrombin, leading to complete defibrination, with death due to haemorrhage in 30 per cent of cases. Russell's viper venom activates factor Xa and also causes non-clotting blood. Many rattlesnake venoms have a thrombin-like effect leading to defibrinogenaemia and thrombocytopenia. The correct treatment is to give the specific antivenom intravenously (see Section 8), if necessary in repeated doses. *Calloselasma (Ankistrodon) rhodostoma* (Malayan pit viper) contains a venom (ancrod) that converts fibrinogen to fibrin by removal of fibrinopeptide A and has been used as an anticoagulant. The presence of shock will exacerbate disseminated intravascular coagulation due to any cause.

LABORATORY FEATURES

Initially, disseminated intravascular coagulation produces few coagulation changes because the liver and bone marrow compensate for the consumption of coagulation factors and platelets. However, if the trigger persists the haemostatic system will eventually fail, the rapidity depending on the strength of the trigger. The main findings are thrombocytopenia (the diagnosis of disseminated intravascular coagulation should not be made unless the platelet count is less than $100 \times 10^9/l$), increased levels of fibrin degradation products, and prolongation of PT, APTT, and TT due to factor deficiencies and the presence of fibrin degradation products. The fibrinogen level is usually reduced, to 0.5–1.5 g/l. Completely incoagulable blood is rare: when encountered it is probably due to the inhibitory effects of fibrin degradation products, which interfere with fibrin polymerization and platelet function. It should be remembered that increased levels of fibrin degradation products are not diagnostic of disseminated intravascular coagulation because they are also increased after surgery and thromboembolic disease.

More sophisticated assays may demonstrate activation of the haemostatic pathway, and the consumption of coagulation factors and physiological inhibitors, especially protein C and antithrombin III. Platelet activation is reflected by increased plasma levels of secretory proteins such as platelet factor 4 and β-thromboglobulin. Markers of haemostatic activity such as thrombin–antithrombin III and plasmin–α_2-antiplasmin complexes may be increased. Levels of von Willebrand factor–ristocetin cofactor activity may be decreased despite normal levels of von Willebrand factor antigen, probably due to the breakdown of the large multimers of von Willebrand factor by proteolytic enzymes.

The blood film may show red-cell fragmentation, evidence of micro-angiopathic haemolytic anaemia.

MANAGEMENT

If the patient is shocked they must be vigorously resuscitated to prevent exacerbation of disseminated intravascular coagulation. It is very important to treat the underlying cause; in obstetrics the rapid evacuation of the uterus can be life saving, and appropriate broad-spectrum antibiotics should be given in septicaemia of unknown cause (see Section 7).

Initial laboratory screening of PT, APTT, fibrinogen level, platelet count and fibrin degradation products is required as a guide to the replacement of blood components. The aim is to maintain the PT and PTT within a ratio of 1.5 of the control values, fibrinogen levels of greater than 1 g/l, and the haematocrit greater than 0.30. Fresh frozen plasma contains near-normal quantities of all of the coagulation factors and inhibitors. Cryoprecipitate or fibrinogen concentrates can be given if fibrinogen levels are disproportionately low. Cryoprecipitate also contains factor VIIIc, von Willebrand factor, factor XIII, and fibronectin. Platelet concentrates should be given if the platelet count is less than $50 \times 10^9/l$.

After haemostatic replacement the screening tests should be repeated, ideally including protein C and antithrombin III levels. Further therapy is given on the basis of the results. Clinical trials suggest that giving antithrombin III and protein C concentrates may be of value in preventing thrombosis because these physiological inhibitors are rapidly consumed.

The use of heparin in disseminated intravascular coagulation has always been controversial. It has been given in an attempt to 'switch off' or inhibit the process that is activating intravascular coagulation, but has only been shown to be beneficial after amniotic fluid embolism or incompatible blood transfusion. As a general guide, if the major clinical problem is bleeding, heparin should only be used after adequate replacement therapy has failed to control the bleeding. However, if thrombosis is predominant, heparin should be used at an earlier stage. A low-dose, continuous infusion of between 500 and 1000 u/h is usual. An infusion of prostacyclin may be helpful in cases in which pathological activation of platelets is a major factor.

Prothrombinase concentrates should not be used as they have prothrombotic effects. Similarly the use of antifibrinolytic agents is not recommended as this may result in failure to remove fibrin thrombi and thus exacerbate thrombotic multiorgan failure.

Hyperfibrinolytic bleeding or primary fibrinolysis

Bleeding may occur if there is excessive generation of plasmin secondary to the release of tissue and urokinase plasminogen activators. Plasmin is a non-specific proteolytic enzyme and will split peptides with arginyl–lysyl amino acid sequences. These include fibrinogen, factors V and VIII, and the first component of complement.

The mechanism of fibrinolysis is not completely worked out, assays are not widely available, and many questions about pathological fibrinolysis remain to be answered.

AETIOLOGY

Some regions, especially prostatic and pelvic tissues, are rich in plasminogen activator, excessive liberation of which may occur during pelvic and prostatic surgery, especially for carcinoma of the prostate. It also occurs during extensive surgery such as cardiopulmonary bypass, and especially liver transplantation, when very high levels of tissue plasminogen activator are thought to be responsible for the bleeding diathesis during the anhepatic and reperfusion phases. Iatrogenic fibrinolytic bleeding can occur through the use of exogenous fibrinolytic activators such as streptokinase or urokinase in the management of thrombosis.

Acute promyelocytic leukaemia is associated with a bleeding diathesis that has not been completely defined, especially as it occurs against a background of bone marrow failure and thus thrombocytopenia. However, the abnormal promyelocytes have granules which release urokinase and other proteases such as elastase. The usual finding of low levels of fibrinogen and increased titres of fibrin degradation products, minimally prolonged PT and PTT, and near-normal levels of antithrombin III, suggesting primary fibrinolytic bleeding rather than disseminated intravascular coagulation as previously thought. Some promyelocytes also have tissue-factor activity. However, the minor fall in coagulation factors suggests that this does not cause disseminated intravascular coagulation in the majority of cases.

LABORATORY INVESTIGATION

Ideally, a global test of fibrinolytic activity such as the euglobulin clot lysis time, fibrin plates (or the use of a thromboelastograph) should be

made. Unfortunately, however, these are not widely available. Levels of fibrin degradation products and fibrinogen degradation products, which can be detected by monoclonal antibodies, are greatly increased. The D-dimer assay is the most commonly used for detection of fibrin degradation products. The differentiation between fibrin degradation products and fibrinogen degradation products may clarify complicated disturbances of haemostasis. More sophisticated tests will reveal decreased concentrations of plasminogen and α_2-antiplasmin, with increased amounts of tissue and/or urokinase plasminogen activators. The PT, PTT, and TT are mildly prolonged due to fibrinogenolysis, with production of large quantities of fibrin degradation products. Factors V and VIII may be normal or moderately reduced, in contrast to disseminated intravascular coagulation. Often it is difficult to exclude disseminated intravascular coagulation, especially as the most useful fibrinolytic assays are complex, time consuming and not widely available.

MANAGEMENT

Treatment with an antifibrinolytic agent should be considered if primary fibrinolytic bleeding is suspected. Tranexamic acid and aminocaproic acid, by acting as competitive inhibitors of plasminogen, are weak antifibrinolytic agents and can be given intravenously or orally. Aprotinin, given as a 500 000 i.u. intravenous bolus, is the most powerful antiplasmin agent available.

The best form of management of acute promyelocytic leukaemia is controversial. Baseline tests should be done and replacement therapy with fresh frozen plasma and platelets instituted as necessary. Trials of heparin, on the assumption that these patients have disseminated intravascular coagulation, have given inconsistent results. The results of preliminary trials of antifibrinolytics are more promising. It is reasonable to give replacement therapy and, if bleeding continues, to give heparin, 500 to 1000 u/h if disseminated intravascular coagulation is suspected, or low-dose antifibrinolytic agents if hyperfibrinolysis is demonstrated. A new form of therapy, transretinoic acid, which is undergoing clinical trials, may correct the defect promptly and limit leukaemic cell growth by causing terminal differentiation of the leukaemic promyeloblasts (see Chapter 22.3.4).

Perioperative bleeding

Continued concerns over the use of donor blood, especially the risk of transfusion-transmitted infection, have rekindled interest in the aetiology and control of perioperative bleeding. Excessive perioperative bleeding can be due to suture deficiency and/or derangement of haemostasis. There is a subset of patients in whom generalized oozing in the surgical field cannot be attributed to bleeding from cut vessels. There is no adequate definition for an 'excessive bleeder' and yet surgeons are convinced that they exist!

The pathogenesis of non-surgical perioperative bleeding is not fully established and in situations where bleeding occurs there are only limited laboratory assays available. Moreover, the investigative approach is often inappropriate. The normal range of laboratory values during surgery should be based what is 'normal' for patients who undergo the same procedure without excessive bleeding, rather than what is 'normal' for the general population.

Perioperative haemostatic changes in simple operations have been poorly researched. Platelet activation, increased fibrinolytic activity, and increased levels of the acute-phase coagulation proteins are thought to reflect the hyperadrenergic state induced by the stress of surgery. In contrast, the complex haemostatic changes of cardiopulmonary bypass have been extensively studied.

CARDIOPULMONARY BYPASS AND BLEEDING

Haemorrhage is one of the most important complications of cardiac surgery. This is especially relevant now that increasing numbers of patients are requiring reoperation or complex procedures such as heart and lung transplantation, and have received anticoagulant, antiplatelet, or thrombolytic therapy before surgery.

Pathogenesis

Cardiopulmonary bypass involves extensive contact between blood and the synthetic surfaces of the membrane oxygenator that result in haemostatic activation. Large doses of heparin are given to the patient prior to bypass (to attain levels of about 3 u/ml), to prevent immediate clotting in the bypass circuit. The mechanism of this haemostatic activation is under review; previously it was thought that direct activation of factor XII by the foreign surface initiated coagulation. New evidence suggests that the main stimulus occurs through the extrinsic pathway, via monocytes which are activated to express tissue factor by the foreign surface. During the bypass operation the activated clotting time (a variant of the whole-blood clotting time) is used to monitor anticoagulant therapy and is maintained above 400 s. At the end of the procedure the effect of heparin is reversed with protamine sulphate; approximately 1 mg of protamine neutralizes 100 u of heparin. Heparin rebound can occur 2 to 6 h later due to the delayed return of sequestered extravascular heparin and release from protamine–heparin complexes. Haemodilution is also a consequence of extracorporeal circulation but the fall in haematocrit and plasma proteins is about 30 per cent and thus not sufficient to cause a bleeding diathesis.

Cardiopulmonary bypass produces platelet fragmentation with consequent thrombocytopenia (unusually less than $100 \times 10^9/l$) and platelet functional abnormalities that include reduced responses to aggregation stimuli, loss of α-granule content, and loss of membrane glycoproteins including glycoprotein (Gp Ib) (the von Willebrand receptor) and Gp IIb/IIIa, mainly a fibrinogen receptor. Scanning electron microscopy shows a rapid transformation from smooth, discoid platelets into activated platelets with pseudopodia. These changes result mainly from hypothermia, mechanical stress, and adhesion to the extracorporeal circuit caused by interaction of Gp IIb/IIIa and the surfaces, which rapidly become coated with fibrinogen. In the patient these platelet changes are corrected by about 3 h postoperatively.

In the past the acquired haemostatic defect has been attributed to the acquired platelet defect; however, it is now clear that fibrinolytic activation is a major cause of excessive bleeding during cardiac surgery. Contact activation, which is maximal on the first passage of blood through the extracorporeal circuit, causes activation of plasminogen. But the main increase in fibrinolytic activity is due to increased release of tissue plasminogen activator, by uncertain mechanisms.

Identification of those at risk of excessive bleeding

Unfortunately there is no test to indicate which patients will suffer perioperative bleeding, unless screening reveals a previously undiagnosed congenital bleeding disorder. A history of previous or familial bleeding, together with a history of previous surgery and current drug therapy, are prerequisites before any surgical procedure. Before cardiac surgery, PT, PTT, and fibrinogen levels should be assayed. A bleeding time will give a guide to platelet function.

Prevention

The search for a pharmacological agent that successfully prevents perioperative bleeding has discarded DDAVP and prostacyclin and yielded aprotinin. A high-dose aprotinin regimen reduces bleeding during repeat cardiac surgery by approximately 80 per cent. Lower doses of aprotinin have produced similar reductions of blood loss. Shorter operating times have also resulted, probably due to a reduction of oozing; the operative fields remain 'bone dry'.

Aprotinin is a basic polypeptide of bovine origin which is a broad-spectrum serine protease inhibitor (serpin) that inhibits trypsin, kallikrein, and plasmin. The currently recommended high-dose regimen maintains aprotinin levels of about 200 kiu/ml in order to inhibit kallikrein and thus limit contact activation by the negatively charged surfaces

of the cardiopulmonary bypass circuit. At this level, aprotinin is also a good antiplasmin agent. Thus by inhibiting plasmin and kallikrein, an activator of plasminogen, it is a powerful antifibrinolytic agent, and this appears to be the main mechanism by which it reduces bleeding for it probably has no effect on the platelet defect. Antifibrinolytic agents such as tranexamic acid, given continuously during cardiopulmonary bypass, also reduce perioperative bleeding, confirming that an antifibrinolytic effect is important.

The thrombotic risks of perioperative aprotinin, especially the maintenance of graft patency after coronary artery grafting, have not been fully defined. Thus, currently, aprotinin is licensed only for cardiac operations with a large risk of perioperative bleeding.

Some of the haemostatic problems associated with extracorporeal circulation have been overcome by the use of heparin-bonded tubing but this is not widely available.

Immediate management of postcardiac surgical bleeding

Initially, the patient should be examined and the rate of filling of the chest drainage tubes checked to ensure that one is not filling more than the others, suggesting a bleeding vessel. A full blood count, PTT, PT, and fibrinogen are helpful, but unfortunately rapid assays of platelet function and fibrinolytic activity (such as a thromboelastograph), which would be particularly useful, are not widely available. A bleeding time will give a guide to platelet function. It has been usual practice to give 6 u of platelets whatever the platelet count, in view of the acquired platelet abnormality. If there is a suggestion of fibrinolytic bleeding 500 000 iu of aprotinin may be given intravenously in the interim whilst waiting for the platelets to arrive.

Massive transfusion

This is defined as transfusion of stored blood of a volume equal or greater than the patient's total blood volume in less than 24 h. Coagulation problems occur in patients with extensive bleeding because of loss of haemostatic factors, consumption in clot formation, dilution with blood products and blood substitutes, and lack of replacement due to inadequate synthesis. However, coagulation factor depletion is not common if stored whole blood is used as replacement therapy. Stored whole blood contains 30 to 40 per cent levels of most coagulation factors, except for factor IX and XII, levels of which fall to 20 per cent, and factor V and VIII, which fall to 10 per cent. However, factor VIII deficiency is partially compensated by increased synthesis and release as part of the reaction to stress.

Modern transfusion practice dictates, however, that an increasing proportion of donor blood is collected for plasma retrieval (see Chapter 22.8.1). Red-cell concentrates are produced that allow for the preservation of red cells with minimal residual plasma. Dilutional reductions in coagulation factors are more likely if these constituents are used, so it is more economical and effective to used stored whole blood, once the need for massive replacement is recognized.

Blood that has been stored for more than a few days is devoid of functioning platelets; dilutional thrombocytopenia should therefore be anticipated during massive blood replacement. However, it is important to appreciate that at least 1.5 blood volumes (i.e. 7–8 l in adults) must be transfused to maintain a platelet count above $50 \times 10^9/l$, or higher if there is evidence of a platelet functional defect. The latter may occur either trauma or massive blood loss. If disseminated intravascular coagulation or blood loss occurs after cardiac surgery, bleeding may occur at a higher platelet count than this, due to an acquired platelet defect. A bleeding time is helpful as supportive evidence of an acquired defect. It should be remembered that each platelet concentrate will provide around 50 ml fresh plasma.

Disseminated intravascular coagulation may supervene, but cannot be predicted. Massively transfused patients do not form a homogeneous group; delayed or inadequate treatment of shock is probably the common predisposing factor, while extensive tissue damage, particularly head injuries, and pre-existing hepatic and renal failure may contribute to a deterioration in haemostasis.

The use of blood substitutes may produce other haemostatic hazards, apart from dilution. Dextrans, and to a lesser extent hydroxylethyl starch, have a fibrinoplastic effect: they accelerate the action of thrombin in converting fibrinogen to fibrin, which makes clots more amenable to fibrinolysis. Both are absorbed on to the platelet surfaces and von Willebrand factor, causing decreased platelet function and an acquired von Willebrand syndrome. Human albumin solution may cause minor depression of protein synthesis in the liver. Gelatins produce few problems, although they decrease plasma fibronectin activity.

MANAGEMENT

It should be remembered that the greatest cause of death in massive transfusion is due to inadequate volume replacement. It is imperative that the prime goal is the treatment of shock; haemostatic changes are a secondary issue and occur late. Transfusion of replacement blood components should be given as necessary according to the monitoring of the screening coagulation tests, aiming to keep the platelet count greater than 50×10^9/l, PT and APTT less than 1.5 times the control value, and fibrinogen concentrations greater than 1.0 g/l.

The place of fresh whole blood place in transfusion is contested. There are no proven advantages of its use over component therapy.

Acquired inhibitors to coagulation factors

In the presence of coagulation factor inhibitors an abnormal APTT (or rarely an abnormal PT) cannot be corrected *in vitro* by a 30-min incubation of the patient's plasma plus an equal volume of normal plasma (called a 50:50 mix test). Because the PT or APTT are prolonged and fail to correct with the addition of normal plasma, this excludes a factor deficiency and implicates a circulating inhibitor. There are two main types: antibodies directed against coagulation proteins and antiphospholipid antibodies.

An antibody may be directed against a specific coagulation protein, either in patients with congenital factor deficiencies or in previously haemostatically normal people. Specific autoantibodies have been reported against factor IX, von Willebrand factor, factors V, XII XIII, and fibrinogen but are extremely rare. They may be associated with lymphoproliferative disorders or following recent blood transfusion. The most common target for inhibitors is factor VIIIc. Approximately 5 to 10 per cent of all patients with haemophilia A develop antibodies against factor VIIIc. Usually they occur after the administration of exogenous factor VIII, which, because of an alteration in the patients own factor VIII molecule, is recognized as a foreign protein (see Chapter 22.6.5).

Factor VIII inhibitors may rarely arise *de novo* in non-haemophiliacs, associated with conditions such as systemic lupus erythematosus and other collagen disorders, penicillin sensitivity, cancer, and inflammatory bowel disease, or in the postpartum period, or in elderly people with no underlying disease. The clinical course is variable but it unusual for fatal haemorrhage to occur, and the antibodies may disappear within months or years.

Most inhibitors are of the IgG class; rarely, IgA and IgM inhibitors are found in patients with paraproteinaemias. The interaction is usually second order, that is one molecule of factor VIII reacts with one molecule of inhibitor. Non-haemophiliac patients with inhibitors cannot be classified into 'strong' and 'weak' responders, as is the case in haemophiliac (see Chapter 22.6.5), because the inhibitors are usually of high titre but an anamnestic response is rarely elicited.

The antiphospholipid antibodies are a heterogeneous group that bind to negatively charged phospholipd. *In vitro*, they may prevent the interaction of coagulation factors with phospholipid that is a necessary part of the template for coagulation reactions. Thus phospholipid-dependent tests such as the PTT are prolonged. Paradoxically, *in vivo* these so-called anticoagulants produce an increased risk of both arterial and

venous thrombosis (see Chapter 22.6.7) and are commonly associated with other autoimmune disorders.

In the rare cases of haemorrhage associated with antiphospholipid antibodies a second haemostatic defect is usually present, such as thrombocytopenia or, occasionally, an acquired prothrombin deficiency due to the production of antiprothrombin antibodies. In addition, uraemia due to associated systemic lupus erythematosus, and treatment with aspirin, may also predispose to haemorrhage.

MANAGEMENT

Treatment is controversial. Considering management of the commonest acquired inhibitor—an acquired F.VIII inhibitor—if there is serious bleeding, high doses of factor VIII can be given to overcome the inhibitor. Alternatively, plasma exchange may be used to remove the inhibitor, or blood products such as porcine factor VIII or factor IX concentrates or activated products can be administered to 'bypass' the need for factor VIII. Steroids and immunosuppressants are unhelpful in the acute situation but are often beneficial in the long-term management of patients with chronic problems.

Isolated factor deficiencies

Factor X deficiency may occur rarely with amyloid disease due to the absorption of factor X to amyloid fibrils. Some patients with amyloidosis also have increased fibrinolysis, probably due to amyloid deposits in the endothelium stimulating the release of tissue plasminogen activator.

Acquired von Willebrand disease is found in hypothyroidism and is relieved by treatment with thyroxine.

REFERENCES

Aoki, N. (1989). Hemostasis associated with abnormalities of fibrinolysis. *Blood Reviews*, **3**, 11–17.
Bloom, A. (19xx). *Thrombosis and haemostasis. A comprehensive textbook of haemostasis.*
Draper, G. and McNinch, A. (ed.). (1994). Vitamin K for neonates: the controversy. *British Medical Journal*, **308**, 867–8.
Hunt, B.J. (1991). Modifying perioperative blood loss. *Blood Reviews*, **5**, 168–76.
Lilleyman, J.S. and Hann, I.M. (ed.) (1992). *Paediatric haematology*. Churchill Livingstone, Edinburgh.
Moia, M. *et al.* (1987). Improvement in haemostatic defect of uraemia after treatment with recombinant human erythropoietin. *Lancet*, **ii**, 1227–9.
Roberts, B. (ed.) (1991). Guidelines for transfusion for massive blood loss. In *Standard haematology practice*, (The British Committee for Standards in Haematology). Blackwell Scientific, Edinburgh.
Shearer, M.J. (1992). Vitamin K metabolism and nutriture. *Blood Reviews*, **6**, 92–104.
Tallman, M. and Kwaan, H.C. (1992). Reassessing the haemostatic disorder associated with acute promyelocytic leukaemia. *Blood*, **79**, 543–53.

22.6.7 Thrombotic disease

M. GREAVES and D. A. TABERNER

INTRODUCTION

A thrombus is defined as a mass composed of blood constituents that forms within a blood vessel. The components—erythrocytes, platelets, leucocytes, and fibrin—vary considerably in proportion, depending upon the stimulus to thrombus formation and the type of vessel involved. Within arteries, thrombi are pale and often friable, having a large platelet component, with fibrin reinforcement but relatively few entrapped erythrocytes. In contrast, venous thrombi are dark and somewhat elastic, with many erythrocytes enmeshed in a fibrin network and only few platelets, forming a red coagulum.

Thrombosis, particularly in arteries, has been underestimated as a clinical problem because the consequences of vascular occlusion, such as myocardial infarction or stroke, or the trigger to thrombosis, malignant disease for example, have tended to receive more attention. Thrombosis has often been regarded as a mechanism rather than a cause of disease, and whilst it is true that thrombus formation is most commonly secondary to some other disease process, it is now apparent that in some conditions a prethrombotic state is a principal underlying abnormality. Certainly this is so in the congenital thrombophilias due to an inherited deficiency of one of the natural anticoagulants, antithrombin, protein C or its cofactor, protein S or due to resistance to activated protein C.

Mechanisms of thrombus formation

Thrombosis arises from the interplay of many influences. Virchow's observation, made over 100 years ago, that the main influences in the pathogenesis of thrombosis are disturbances of the vessel wall, of the blood components, and of the dynamics of flow, have withstood the test of time (Fig. 1).

The role of the vessel wall

The healthy vascular endothelium has a range of antithrombotic properties (Table 1; Fig. 1). They are capable of the modulation and neutralization of the activity of thrombin generated in the vicinity, the lysis of fibrin that is formed by thrombin digestion of fibrinogen, and the inhibition of platelet interaction with the endothelial lining and of aggregation.

Heparan sulphate, a glycosaminoglycan that is intimately associated with the luminal surface of vascular endothelial cells, greatly augments the thrombin-neutralizing activity of plasma antithrombin. In addition, the protein thrombomodulin, which is also a component of the endothelial cell wall, inhibits the procoagulant properties of thrombin and redirects its activity towards an anticoagulant role, in the activation of protein C and thus the neutralization of activated factors VIII and V.

Tissue plasminogen activator, a central component of the fibrinolytic system, is synthesized by, and released from, vascular endothelial cells. It becomes bound on the endothelial surface, along with its substrate plasminogen. This serves to localize fibrinolytic activity for the rapid

Table 1 *Antithrombotic properties of vascular endothelium*

Modulation of thrombin activity
Heparan sulphate
Thrombomodulin

Modulation of platelet reactivity and release of vasodilators
Products of arachidonic acid metabolism:
  Prostaglandin I_2
  12-HODE
Nitric oxide

Activation and localization of fibrinolytic activity
Generation of tPA
Affinity for tPA and plasminogen

12-HODE,; tPA, tissue plasminogen activator.

dissolution of any fibrin generated, whilst protecting against the risks of enhanced systemic fibrinolytic activity.

The metabolism of arachidonic acid, mobilized from membrane phospholipid by phospholipase, is central to one mechanism of platelet aggregation, through synthesis of prostaglandin endoperoxides and thromboxane A_2 within the platelet. In contrast, within the vascular endothelial cell the principal product of arachidonic acid is prostaglandin I_2, a potent inhibitor of platelet activation. It is thought that endoperoxide released from stimulated platelets can also be converted to prostaglandin I_2 by adjacent endothelium, thus limiting platelet adhesive and aggregatory responses. The vasodilator effect of prostaglandin I_2 may also protect against vascular occlusion. The central enzyme involved in arachidonic acid metabolism is cyclo-oxygenase, the activity of which is inhibited by aspirin. Arachidonic acid is also a substrate for a lipoxygenase, one product of this metabolic pathway in the platelet being 13-hydroxyoctadecadienoic acid (13-HODE), which also possesses platelet inhibitory activity.

A potent, local, short-acting vasodilator previously known as endothelium-derived relaxing factor is now known to be nitric oxide. Acting through cGMP it is also capable of the modulation of platelet activation and is physiologically important in the inhibition of vascular occlusion.

The intact vascular endothelium thus possesses a comprehensive range of protective mechanisms that interact to maintain vascular patency. When the vessel wall is breached by trauma, the disruption of endothelial continuity allows platelet accumulation and fibrin generation

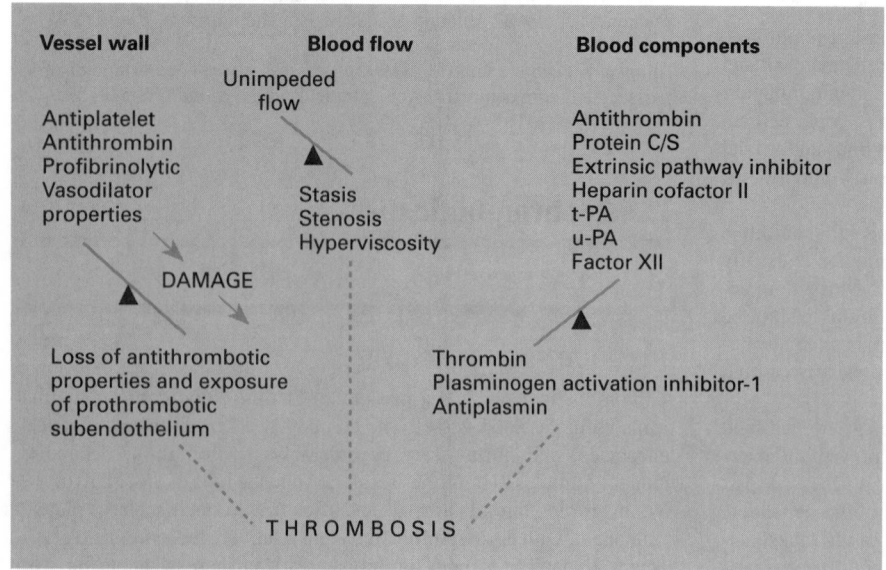

Fig. 1 Virchow's triad and the balance of pro- and antithrombotic factors.

to occur, thus effectively re-establishing vascular integrity. However, where the endothelium becomes damaged through disease, as in ulceration or rupture of an atheromatous plaque, the local loss of the antithrombotic properties of the vessel lining leads rapidly to thrombus formation and occlusion, with consequent tissue hypoxia and, often, infarction.

The role of blood components

The complex interactions between coagulation enzymes, their inhibitors, platelets, and fibrinolytic mechanisms are described in an earlier section. In health, platelet aggregation and fibrin deposition occur only at sites of tissue trauma. Although a background level of coagulation activation may be present, the unopposed generation of thrombin is not permissible. Changes to the components of the system in a direction that favours thrombin generation must contribute to thrombus propagation and ultimate size, although endothelial damage and abnormalities of flow are more important in the initiation of local thrombosis (Fig. 1). In disseminated intravascular coagulation, however, systemic coagulation activation is a major factor in microvascular fibrin deposition.

Clearly, thrombin has a crucial role in haemostasis and thrombosis. It may be generated through the intrinsic coagulation system by exposure of vascular subendothelium or a prosthetic surface, or by contact with platelets activated by ADP or collagen. The rapid generation of thrombin through the extrinsic pathway is initiated by the exposure of tissue factor by vascular damage or through migration of white cells to sites of injury. It is now recognized that the intrinsic and extrinsic pathways are not independent. The factor VII–tissue factor complex activates factor IX as well as factor X, these actions being controlled by an inhibitor–'extrinsic pathway inhibitor'. Feedback loops are also a feature of the system. Also, these pathways may be bypassed, with activation of the common pathway through factor X, for example by protease released from malignant cells or by snake venom. At the endothelial surface the procoagulant effect of thrombin may be neutralized and redirected toward an anticoagulant role, by activation of protein C, as described above. Where the vascular endothelium is deficient, through disease or trauma, the procoagulant pathways will predominate.

Plasmin, the enzyme responsible for clot dissolution by digestion of fibrin, is generated from plasminogen under the control of a system of activators and inhibitors (see above). The fibrinolytic system is capable of the limitation of thrombus to areas that are required for the maintenance of vascular integrity. Thus, at the periphery of a clot, plasminogen (which binds to platelets), when activated to plasmin, results in degradation of platelet surface glycoproteins necessary for adhesion (glycoprotein Ib) and aggregation (IIb/IIIa), thus limiting further recruitment of platelets into the thrombus. Adhesive proteins necessary for platelet interactions—thrombospondin, fibrinogen, and fibronectin—are also attacked. Plasminogen bound to endothelium adjacent to the thrombus is available for activation and thus limitation of clot propagation.

Once fibrin has been deposited, progression of thrombosis is determined in part by the balance between prothrombotic and fibrinolytic activities. Propagation will only occur where there is a powerful thrombogenic stimulus and until a balance is achieved. This balance can be influenced by modulation of the thrombogenic stimulus or fibrinolytic capacity by therapeutic intervention with anticoagulants or thrombolytic drugs as well as by suppression of fibrinolysis in disease. The procoagulant stimulus may be enhanced in several ways in disease states: by exposure of subendothelial or plaque components to provide a potent stimulus to coagulation activation, when platelet activation provides binding sites that enhance thrombin generation; by deficiency of anticoagulant proteins, such as antithrombin; by a reactive increase in the plasma concentration of components of the coagulation cascade, especially fibrinogen; and by inhibition of fibrinolysis.

Most of these prothrombotic changes occur secondarily to another disease or process. Examples are the hyperfibrinogenaemia after trauma, in smokers, during late pregnancy and post partum, and in malignant and inflammatory diseases; and the inhibition of fibrinolysis, most commonly due to increased synthesis of plasminogen activation inhibitor-1 in obese people and in the postoperative state. In the congenital thrombophilias, the procoagulant effect results from a deficiency of, or defective, anticoagulant—antithrombin, protein C, or protein S. Acquired deficiencies also occur, however, in disease. The role of other inhibitors—extrinsic pathway inhibitor and heparin cofactor II—remains to be determined.

The role of disturbed flow

Stasis promotes clot formation by allowing the local accumulation of platelets and activated clotting factors, especially thrombin. Endothelial hypoxia in areas of stasis may also contribute by impairing the antithrombotic functions of vascular endothelium.

In the venous system, stasis occur as a result of immobility and a failure of the muscle pump necessary for forward flow in the deep veins of the lower limbs. In arteries, areas of relative stasis develop distal to the narrowed segments that are most commonly due to the luminal encroachment of atheromatous plaques.

The viscosity of blood is a major determinant of flow. The main contributors are the haematocrit and the concentration of fibrinogen, which determines the viscosity of plasma and also influences the tendency of erythrocytes to aggregate. Thrombotic complications are common in polycythaemia. It is also noteworthy that the plasma fibrinogen concentration is a potent risk factor for coronary and cerebrovascular thrombosis. It may contribute to this risk by its effect on blood viscosity and flow, as well as by its availability for conversion to insoluble fibrin by thrombin and by its cofactor activity in platelet aggregation.

The pathogenesis of arterial thrombosis (Fig. 2)

The arterial system is one of high pressure and rapid flow. Arterial thrombosis almost invariably occurs in association with damage to the vessel wall by atherosclerosis. Whilst arterial disease results in ischaemic symptoms at times of increased oxygen demand, it is super-added thrombosis that produces acute ischaemia and infarction. Even if the antithrombotic control mechanisms are sufficient to prevent vascular occlusion and tissue damage, incorporation of platelets and fibrin into the plaque may none the less result in its growth and thus contribute to the pathogenesis of arteriosclerosis (Fig. 2). Platelets carry growth factors and mitogens in intracellular granules to sites of tissue injury. Their release from platelets incorporated into atheromatous lesions contributes to the accumulation of monocytes and the proliferation of smooth-muscle cells that are the hallmarks of the early vascular lesion.

The principal event leading to thrombus formation is ulceration or rupture of an atheromatous plaque with exposure of subendothelial and plaque material. The generation of high shear stresses beyond a tight stenosis may also initiate thrombosis through endothelial damage and the local generation of platelet agonists, especially ADP and thrombin (Fig. 2).

Platelet adhesion to exposed tissues occurs within seconds, and progress to aggregation leads to the development of a platelet thrombus and release of the vasocontrictors thromboxane A_2 and serotonin. Under high-flow conditions the aggregate may reach a critical size and then disintegrate and embolize, this being more likely in a large-calibre vessel, especially the aortic arch and carotid vessels. Transient cerebral ischaemic attacks are a common result of this process. Similar events in the coronary circulation result in the clinical picture of unstable angina pectoris.

When the platelet aggregate becomes consolidated by fibrin generated through coagulation activation, clot growth results in vascular occlusion and ischaemia. Retrograde propagation continues until limited by anticoagulant and fibrinolytic activities localized in adjacent healthy vascular endothelium. Stasis due to occlusion allows forward clot growth.

This process may possibly be augmented by influences affecting the integrity of the vascular endothelium, such as haemodynamic stress and products of tobacco smoke, as well as those acting on the blood, including increased platelet numbers and reactivity, enhanced coagulation mechanisms, and increased viscosity. Conversely, therapy with aspirin and anticoagulant drugs is partially effective in limiting the progression or prevention of occlusive events.

The pathogenesis of venous thrombosis (Fig. 3)

Stasis is the predominant influence in venous thrombosis. This is supported by the clinical observations that the incidence of postoperative venous thrombosis is proportional to the duration of immobility and that, in hemiplegia, deep venous thrombosis most commonly affects the paralysed leg.

Imaging studies demonstrate that by far the most common site of origin is the deep veins of the calf. Isolated proximal-vein thrombosis is uncommon, unless there has been local vascular injury or compression.

Within the deep calf veins, many thrombi have their origin within the valve pockets, where venous flow is associated with the formation of vortices and local stasis. When the calf pump fails, due to immobility, venous dilatation, raised venous pressure or venous obstruction (Fig. 3), further areas of stasis develop.

Although stasis is central to the pathogenesis of venous thrombosis, under experimental conditions blood within an isolated segment of vein remains fluid for some time. The addition of activated clotting factors rapidly results in clot formation, however. *In vivo*, activated clotting

factors generated at sites of tissue trauma, including operative trauma, or in association with a malignant tumour, enter the circulation and result in fibrin generation in areas of stasis. Again, congenital or acquired deficiencies in the antithrombotic and fibrinolytic mechanisms may accelerate this process. Although platelets may become incorporated into the fibrin mesh, their role in thrombosis under conditions of low shear is a relatively minor one. If conditions are favourable, successive layers of fibrin, with enmeshed red cells and some platelets, are deposited (the lines of Zahn) as propagation occurs.

The mechanism of clot formation in veins accounts for the observed clinical risk factors for venous thromboembolism (Table 2), and the efficacy of physical and pharmacological regimens of prophylaxis against thrombosis as well as the response to therapy with fibrinolytic or anticoagulant drugs.

The consequences of deep venous thrombosis (see also Section 15)

The morbidity associated with acute thrombosis and the risk of pulmonary embolism are the immediate clinical consequences; the postphlebitic syndrome develops later in a proportion of cases. Thrombus confined to calf veins only rarely produces serious early or late morbidity and the risk of death from pulmonary embolism is low. However, at least 20 per cent of untreated calf-vein thromboses progress to the proximal veins of the lower limb and this carries a 50 per cent risk of pulmonary embolism. The postphlebitic syndrome eventually develops in over half of those afflicted by thrombosis in the ileofemoral veins, due to permanent damage to venous valves with or without residual occlusion of major veins, and consequent chronically increased venous pressure (Fig. 4).

Fig. 2 The pathogenesis and consequences of arterial thrombosis.

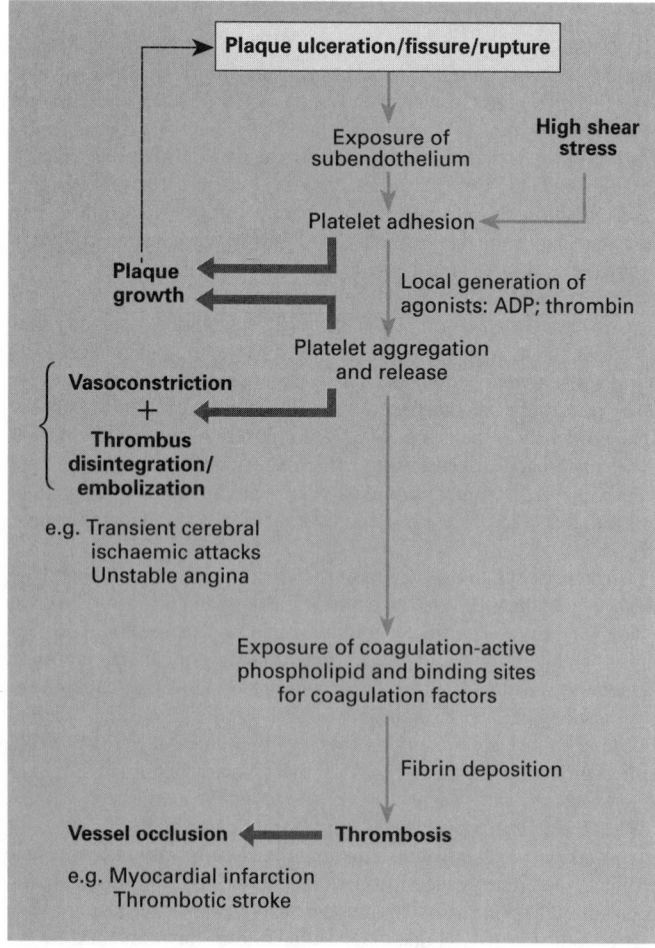

Fig. 3 The pathogenesis of venous thrombosis.

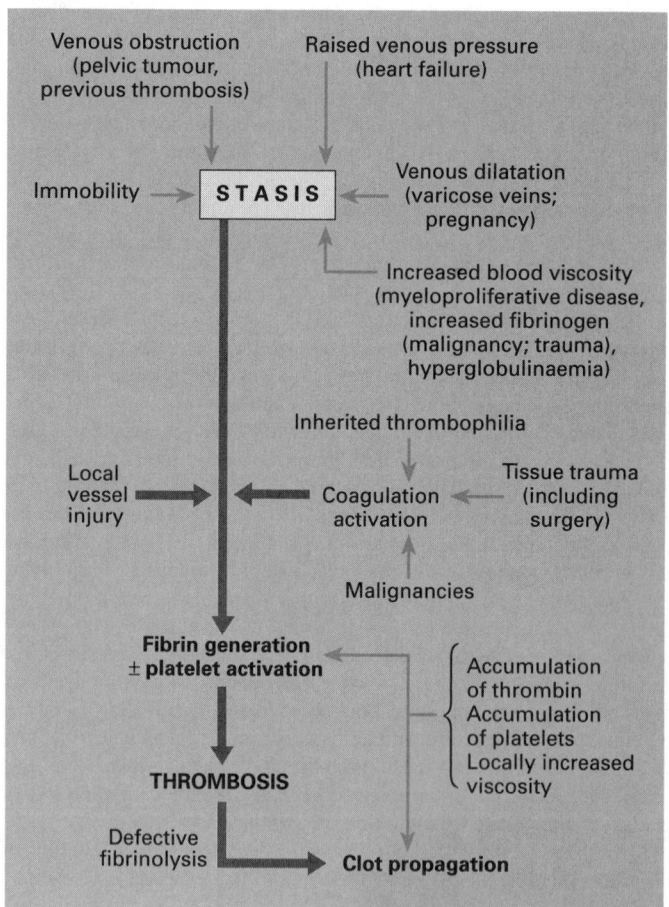

Table 2 *Clinical risk factors for venous thromboembolism*

Immobility

Tissue trauma, including surgery
Myocardial infarction
Pregnancy and puerperium
Oestrogens
Obesity
Varicose veins
Previous deep-venous thrombosis
Congestive cardiac failure
Malignancy
Nephrotic syndrome
Advancing age
Collagen vascular disorders, antiphospholipid syndrome
Hyperviscosity states
Congenital thrombophilia
Therapy with coagulation-factor concentrate containing
   activated factors (II, IX, X concentrate)

Hypercoagulable states

In many instances of thrombotic disease an underlying state of hyper-coagulability appears to be a contributory factor. Occasionally this is due to an inherited defect in the natural anticoagulant mechanisms, the best characterized being deficiencies of antithrombin, protein C or protein S. These disorders account for around 10 per cent of venous thrombosis in people under 45 years of age. More recently resistance to activated protein C due to a mutation in the factor V gene has been described. Instances of a familial thrombotic tendency without deficiency of these anticoagulants are not uncommon, suggesting that there are other disorders of this type which remain to be identified. In homocystinuria, a genetic abnormality of cystathione synthetase is responsible for the development of arterial and venous complications, often at a young age.

More commonly, hypercoagulability is acquired. There is an increased tendency to thrombosis in a wide variety of disorders including malignancy, atherosclerosis, nephrotic syndrome, collagen–vascular disease, primary antiphospholipid syndrome, myeloproliferative disease, paroxysmal nocturnal haemoglobinuria, inflammatory bowel disease, and heparin-induced thrombocytopenia. Microvascular thrombosis is a central feature in disseminated intravascular coagulation, haemolytic

Fig. 4 The pathogenesis of the postphlebitic syndrome.

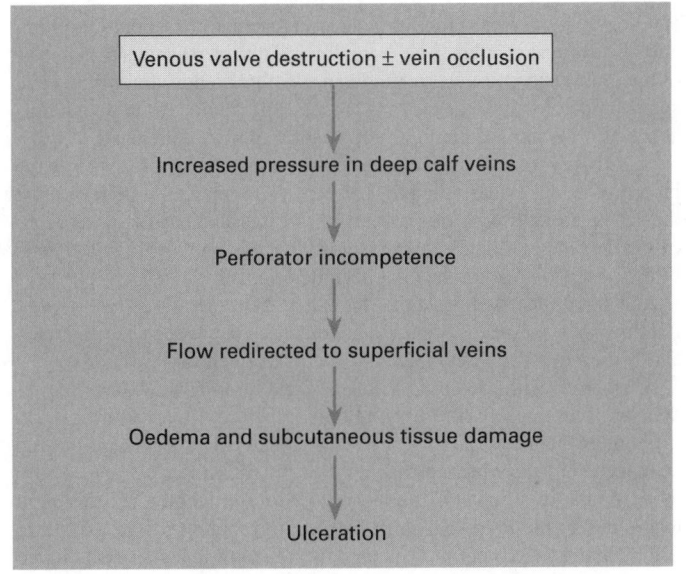

uraemic syndrome, and thrombotic thrombocytopenic purpura. Some additional clinical risk factors for thrombosis were listed in Table 2. These are all acquired hypercoagulable states. In none has a single abnormality of the coagulation or fibrinolytic mechanisms been identified and in some the mechanisms underlying the prethrombotic state are not known.

Inherited thrombotic disorders

The term familial thrombophilia has been applied to a group of disorders in which the increased tendency to venous thromboembolism is due an inherited defect in, or deficiency of, a natural anticoagulant—antithrombin, protein C or protein S or to resistance to activated protein C. Some other familial abnormalities have also been identified, but they are either relatively uncommon or the association with a familial thrombotic tendency is unproven (Table 3).

Antithrombin deficiency

Antithrombin (formerly antithrombin III) is a member of the 'serpin' superfamily, being the major serine protease inhibitor, acting on thrombin, factor Xa, and also factors IXa and XIIa. It is a single-chain glycoprotein of 58 kDa and is synthesized by the liver. The inhibitory effect is through the formation of a 1:1 stoichiometric complex with the enzyme, which involves an active-site serine and a binding domain centred on Arg393 on antithrombin. The rate of enzyme inhibition is enhanced around 1000-fold by heparin, a sulphated polysaccharide, as well as by a heparin-like glycosaminoglycan heparan sulphate, which is present on the vascular endothelium. It is likely that a fraction of plasma antithrombin is bound to heparan sulphate at the luminal surface of the endothelial cell and is thus able to rapidly inactivate any locally generated serine protease.

The association between familial deficiency of antithrombin and thromboembolism was first described by Egeberg in 1965. Inheritance is autosomal dominant. Estimates of the prevalence have been variable, in the range of 1 in 2000 to 1 in 40 000 of the population. The deficiency may be responsible for 2 to 5 per cent of cases of venous thromboembolic disease presenting before the 45th year.

MOLECULAR GENETICS

Protein and cDNA sequencing have revealed that antithrombin shares approximately 30 per cent homology with other serpins such as ovalbumin and α_1-antitrypsin. Although the tertiary structure has not yet been resolved, predictions based on its homology with other serpins, and comparisons with serpins that are also activated by specific sulphated polysaccharides, indicate that the specific heparin-binding site consists of a band of positive charge involving arginine and lysine residues, from which salt bridges may occur with negatively charged sulphate groups of heparin.

The human antithrombin gene has been localized to q23–25 of chromosome 1 and consists of seven exons over 19 kb of genomic DNA. Several polymorphisms have been recognized.

Individuals with antithrombin deficiency are usually heterozygous for the defect. The homozygous condition has been reported and is associated with a severe clinical course. The deficiency can be due to an overall reduction in both immunological and functional levels in plasma (type I) or to a dysfunctional variant (type II). The type II variants are subclassified depending on the presence of altered reactivity with both heparin and thrombin (IIa), thrombin only (IIb), or heparin alone (IIc). This is of clinical significance as the incidence of thrombotic episodes is much lower in subjects heterozygous for a type IIc variant than in other antithrombin-deficient subjects. Type I defects account for 80 to 90 per cent of familial antithrombin deficiencies.

The advent of the polymerase chain reaction and direct sequencing

Table 3 *Familial thrombophilic conditions*

Well-defined disorders	Uncommon disorders	Unproven
Antithrombin deficiency	Dysfibrinogenaemias	Factor XII deficiency
Protein C deficiency		Hypo (dys) plasminogenaemia
Protein S deficiency		tPA deficiency
Resistance to activated protein C		
Homocystinuria		

tPA, tissue plasminogen activator.

techniques has allowed the description of over 30 mutations leading to type I deficiency. Most cause frameshifts and the introduction of early stop codons into the coding sequence of the gene, apparently resulting in a protein that is not secreted or is rapidly removed from the circulation and is therefore undetectable in plasma. In a proportion of type I deficiencies (designated type Ib), low levels of a variant protein are detectable in plasma. An example is antithrombin Utah, which involves a C→T change in codon 407, leading to a substitution in the mature protein at a site that is presumably important for the maintenance of a normal plasma concentration of antithrombin.

Over 20 dysfunctional variants (type II) with defective thrombin inhibitory activity and/or altered heparin affinity have been characterized. They arise from single-base mutations that alter the amino acid sequence of the mature protein. Not all have yet been shown to be associated with an increased thrombotic tendency. In some, a local structural change results, which affects the heparin binding site and impairs heparin binding; in others the mutation results in an altered structure that imposes steric hindrance. Variants with defective thrombin inhibitory activity usually involve mutations of the reactive centre of antithrombin.

CLINICAL FEATURES

Deep venous thrombosis of the lower limb and pulmonary embolism, often recurrent, are the most common presenting features. Thrombosis may also occur in other veins, including the mesenteric, cerebral, portal, and renal vessels, as well as the inferior vena cava. Presentation in pregnancy or during the puerperium is occasionally seen; surgery and immobilization are other precipitating factors. In one-third of cases no precipitating cause can be found for the presenting thrombotic event. Although there are reports of thrombotic stroke and other arterial events in subjects affected by antithrombin deficiency, the association with arterial thrombosis is weak. There is, however, epidemiological evidence that men with plasma antithrombin concentration in the lowest and highest third of the normal distribution are at greater risk of vascular death than those in the middle third.

Presentation before the age of 10 years is rare. However, it is estimated that an asymptomatic heterozygote of 15 years has a 65 per cent risk of developing venous thrombosis by 30 years of age.

A family history is not a reliable guide to antithrombin deficiency because the clinical course in affected family members is variable; also, the condition may arise as a spontaneous mutation.

Protein C deficiency

Protein C is a glycoprotein that circulates as a covalently linked dimer of 62 kDa consisting of a 41-kDa heavy chain and a 21-kDa light chain. It is synthesized by the liver, and, having nine γ-carboxyglutamic acid

residues, is dependent on vitamin K. Activation of the zymogen protein C is by cleavage of a 12-amino acid activation peptide from the amino-terminal end of the heavy chain by thrombin bound to an endothelial cell-surface receptor, thrombomodulin. When activated, protein C, a serine protease, has an anticoagulant function by inhibition of activated factors V and VIII, a process that requires protein S as cofactor, as well as phospholipid. A second effect of activated protein C is profibrinolytic, possibly by binding to plasminogen activation inhibitor-1.

Familial protein C deficiency and its association with venous thromboembolism has been recognized since 1981. It is inherited as an autosomal dominant, although recessive transmission has been suggested in some families in which only homozygotes are clinically affected. The prevalence of the heterozygous state in the general population is a source of controversy. Studies based on subjects presenting with venous thrombosis suggest a prevalence of 1 in 15 000 to 1 in 30 000. However, 1 in 200 to 300 healthy blood donors have been found to have levels consistent with congenital deficiency of protein C. It may be that other, as yet unrecognized, factors play a part in the clinical expression of protein C deficiency. Whether they relate to the protein C gene is not yet known. Clinical studies suggest that the disorder accounts for venous thromboembolic disease in around 4 per cent individuals presenting before the 45th year.

MOLECULAR GENETICS

The human protein C gene has been localized to chromosome 2 and nine exons have been identified. Useful restriction fragment length polymorphisms have been defined.

Analogous to antithrombin deficiency, type I and type II deficiencies of protein C are recognized. Parallel reduction in functional and immunological levels are found in type I deficiency and a relatively greater reduction in functional to immunological activity in type II. In contrast to antithrombin deficiency, in protein C deficiency the clinical manifestations are similar in the two types.

Over 30 different DNA changes within the protein C gene have been identified. Deletions are rare. Point mutations are found in most heterozygotes, mis-sense mutations tending to result in type I deficiency, probably because the abnormal protein is unstable or not secreted, resulting in a reduced plasma concentration. In type II deficiency, mutations that result in disturbance of the function of the γ-carboxylated domain have been noted together with others that affect the function of the serine protease active site.

CLINICAL FEATURES

Heterozygotes for protein C deficiency are prone to venous thromboembolic events, which may be recurrent, mainly deep venous thrombosis of the limbs, and pulmonary embolism. Cerebral venous thrombosis and splanchnic-vein thrombosis may occur. Superficial thrombophlebitis appears to be more common than in antithrombin deficiency. As discussed above, some heterozygotes remain asymptomatic despite plasma protein C levels of less than 50 per cent of normal; it is believed that they have an autosomal recessive form of the disorder, whereas clinically affected individuals have an autosomal dominant form. The genetic basis for this distinction has not been determined.

Anecdotal reports suggest that there may be an increased risk of arterial thrombosis, especially stroke, but this has not yet been substantiated and if present is small compared to the risk of venous thrombosis.

In kindreds with protein C deficiency and thrombosis, 80 per cent of deficient individuals will be symptomatic before 40 years of age. An uncommon manifestation of protein C deficiency is warfarin-induced skin necrosis, where haemorrhagic infarction of the skin occurs, usually over an area of adiposity. It appears to be a thrombotic manifestation that is due to the relatively short half-life of protein C, such that, after administration of a vitamin K antagonist, the plasma level falls at a rate similar to that of factor VII, but in advance of II, IX and X, resulting in a transient hypercoagulable state in the deficient subject.

Homozygous protein C deficiency is very rare. It is phenotypically variable. Most subjects have presented with a syndrome of 'purpura fulminans' within 12 h of birth. Large ecchymoses with purpuric and necrotic skin lesions, disseminated intravascular coagulation, and central nervous thrombosis are typical. Large-vessel thrombosis without skin necrosis may occur. In contrast, some homozygotes with a plasma protein C concentration of less than 10 per cent of normal have remained asymptomatic to adult life.

Protein S deficiency

Protein S is a glycoprotein that circulates as a single-chain species of 70 kDa. Approximately 35 to 50 per cent is bound, in plasma, to C4b-binding protein and only the unbound (free) form is functionally active. Protein S is synthesized by megakaryocytes and vascular endothelial cells, as well as in the liver, and is present in platelet granules. The mature protein has 11 γ-carboxyglutamic acid residues and full synthesis is dependent on vitamin K. Free protein S forms a 1:1 stoichiometric complex with activated protein C on phospholipid surfaces in the presence of calcium and thus has cofactor activity in the inhibition of activated factors V and VIII.

Familial protein S deficiency, with venous thromboembolism, was first described in 1984. It is inherited as an autosomal dominant trait and accounts for around 5 to 8 per cent of cases of venous thrombosis presenting before the age of 45 years.

MOLECULAR GENETICS

The human protein S gene locus is on chromosome 3 and contains two genes, α and β. Only the α-gene is transcribed. It contains 15 exons and has not been fully sequenced. Polymorphisms have been described. The size and complexity of the protein S gene have rendered analysis of the molecular biology of the deficiency more difficult than that of protein C.

Based on assay of free and bound protein S in plasma, three types of deficiency have been defined. In type I deficiency there is a reduction in total protein S, most of which is bound to C4b-binding protein, resulting in reduced free protein S. The majority of these cases appear to result from silent alleles, that is a failure of mRNA production by the defective gene. In type II deficiency, protein S function is impaired, although the total immunoreactive level is normal. Type III deficiency is characterized by an alteration in the binding characteristics between protein S and C4b-binding protein that results in a reduced level of free protein S.

CLINICAL FEATURES

The manifestations are indistinguishable from those in heterozygotes for protein C deficiency, that is venous thromboembolism in various sites. Warfarin-induced skin necrosis has been reported. Again, although stroke, due to cerebral arterial thrombosis, has been recorded, an increased incidence in familial protein S deficiency has not been proven. It seems likely that, in congenital thrombophilia, there may be a minor increase in the incidence of arterial occlusive events in the presence of additional risk factors.

Activated protein C resistance

It has recently been noted that the anticoagulant response to protein C in its activated state is reduced in up to 50 per cent of selected subjects with a personal or family history of thrombosis. Furthermore, resistance to activated protein C is demonstrable in the plasma of up to 5 per cent of healthy individuals. This phenotype is related to a point mutation in the factor V gene (G→A at nucleotide 1691), affected individuals

being heterozygous or homozygous for the mutation. This abnormality may therefore account for the tendency to venous thromboembolism in a very high proportion of subjects.

Dysfibrinogenaemia and thrombosis

Hereditary functionally abnormal fibrinogen has been described in many kindreds but is not a common disorder. It is most usually detected by a prolongation of the thrombin time on screening tests. The majority of defects do not cause symptoms, but around 30 per cent result in a bleeding tendency, some with poor wound healing. Less than 10 per cent appear to be associated with a thrombotic tendency. Although individuals with arterial and venous thrombosis have been reported in over 15 types of dysfibrinogenaemia, in many instances only one family member has been clinically affected. An exception is fibrinogen 'Oslo I', where six of six dysfibrinogenaemic individuals reported a history of venous thrombosis. Overall, the association between dysfibrinogenaemia and thrombotic tendency is weak. Of possible mechanisms, impaired thrombin binding by abnormal fibrin, resistance to lysis by plasmin, and impaired fibrin-mediated plasminogen activation have been proposed.

Other coagulation disorders and thrombosis

Several other abnormalities have been associated with a thrombotic tendency but the relationship appears to be weak or is unproven. Homozygous deficiency of factor XII, a contact factor, produces no haemorrhagic risk, but, possibly due to failure of contact activation of fibrinolysis, may be associated with a thrombotic risk. Whether heterozygotes for factor XII deficiency suffer a thrombotic tendency is disputed.

Dysplasminogenaemia has been described in subjects with thrombosis but clinical problems have usually been restricted to the proband, other affected family members being clinically normal.

Reduced vascular release of tissue plasminogen activator has been reported as a familial disorder, but the vast majority of apparent defects in fibrinolysis in subjects with thrombosis are acquired and often transient. Increased production of plasminogen activation inhibitor-1 is the most frequent cause.

Heparin cofactor II is a plasma inhibitor of thrombin, but, unlike antithrombin it does not inhibit factor Xa. Deficiency has been reported, with thrombotic disease, but the prevalence is similar in healthy subjects and those with a history of thrombosis, and heparin cofactor II deficiency is thus unproven as a risk factor.

Clinical management of inherited thrombophilia

Acute thrombotic events, almost always in the venous system, should be managed in the conventional way, using heparin and an oral anticoagulant drug (see below). In protein C deficiency, and probably protein S deficiency, because of the risk of warfarin-induced skin necrosis, oral anticoagulation should only be commenced after full heparinization and the use of a loading dose should be avoided. Predictably, deficiency of antithrombin results in a degree of heparin resistance and large doses may be required to achieve adequate prolongation of the clotting time. Antithrombin concentrates are available. Although antithrombin replacement therapy is not necessary in most circumstances, it may be justified in life-threatening thrombosis or perhaps in thrombosis complicated by disseminated intravascular coagulation in antithrombin-deficient subjects.

The appropriate duration of oral anticoagulant therapy in familial thrombophilia is controversial. After an apparently spontaneous event, lifelong treatment must be considered. Other factors may influence this decision, including the teratogenic potential of warfarin in women of child-bearing age, and the very variable clinical expression between kindreds in protein C and protein S deficiency states. Where venous thrombosis occurs after trauma or during pregnancy or the postpartum period, long-term anticoagulant therapy may not be justified but particular attention must be paid subsequently to prophylaxis at times of high risk.

Clinically unaffected family members with congenital thrombophilia require counselling, including advice to avoid additional risk factors such as oestrogen-containing oral contraceptives, and on the need for prophylaxis perioperatively and during periods of immobilization. Management of pregnancy is especially difficult. As the risk appears to be greatest in antithrombin deficiency, prophylaxis throughout pregnancy and for 12 weeks postpartum should be considered. Warfarin must not be given during the first trimester and around the time of delivery; many obstetricians now elect to avoid warfarin before the postpartum phase, preferring subcutaneous heparin prophylaxis throughout pregnancy and accepting the as yet unquantified risk of symptomatic osteoporosis. In protein C or S deficiencies, decisions relating to prophylactic anticoagulant therapy in pregnancy will be influenced by the previous obstetric and thrombotic history. Prophylaxis for 12 weeks after delivery is a reasonable option in all cases.

Homocystinuria (see also Section 11)

Homocystinuria is an inborn error of metabolism in which a deficiency of cystathionine synthetase results in an accumulation of methionine and homocystine in the plasma and tissues, and increased excretion of homocystine in the urine. The prevalence is around 1 in 45 000 to 1 in 200 000. It is inherited in autosomal recessive fashion.

The clinical phenotype is variable and includes mental retardation, ectopia lentis, skeletal abnormalities, and a high incidence of venous and premature arterial thrombotic disease. Thrombosis may occur as early as the first year of life. Livedo reticularis may be a feature. A variety of abnormalities of platelets, vascular endothelium, and coagulation have been described, but the pathogenesis of the increased thrombotic tendency remains to be determined. Inhibition of protein C activation by homocystine at the endothelial cell surface has been demonstrated.

The diagnosis and management are considered in Section 11.

Acquired prethrombotic states

The risk of thrombotic complications is variably increased in a range of disease states. In some the pathogenesis has been at least partially determined, for example the possible role of antiphospholipid antibodies in thrombotic manifestations of autoimmune disease. More commonly, the underlying mechanism has not been determined and may be multifactorial.

Thromboembolism is a common complication of trauma, be it accidental or surgical. Pulmonary embolism is an important cause of post-surgical death and is underdiagnosed. Its prevalence is determined by a range of factors, especially the nature and duration of the surgical procedure, and the presence of preoperative risk factors including malignant disease, obesity, increasing age, varicose veins, and a prior venous thromboembolic event. The roles of thrombin generation and stasis in the pathogenesis of venous thrombosis were discussed earlier. Tissue trauma is followed, over a few days, by thrombocytosis and increased platelet reactivity, an increased concentration of plasma factor VIII, and a rise in plasma fibrinogen. Fibrinolysis is suppressed. These changes potentially contribute to the progression of the thrombotic process.

Thrombosis is a common complication of cardiac disease. Pulmonary embolism is frequent in subjects with congestive cardiac failure, and venous thromboembolism and stroke are recognized complications of myocardial infarction and arterial embolism of atrial fibrillation. Again, stasis and immobility are important contributors to the high risk of thrombosis. Furthermore, in the days following myocardial infarction, changes occur in platelets, factor VIII, fibrinogen (and hence blood viscosity), and fibrinolysis analogous to those after tissue trauma.

In patients with malignant disease, there is an increased risk of apparently spontaneous venous thromboembolism, an observation first made by Trousseau in 1868. Postoperative venous thrombosis is also more common, with an increased risk of two- to threefold. Cancer is two to three times more likely to manifest in the 2 years after apparently idiopathic venous thrombosis than in the same period after thrombosis in which another recognized risk factor was apparent at diagnosis. Recurrent thrombosis is even more strongly associated with occult cancer. The risk is, however, not sufficient to warrant intensive invasive investigation of subjects presenting with idiopathic venous thromboembolism if the history and thorough clinical examination, and the results of simple investigations, do not suggest an underlying malignant disease. Whilst immobility, vessel involvement in tumour masses, and reactive increases in fibrinogen and other clotting factors may be contributory, other prothrombotic effects of cancer have been reported. Inappropriate intravascular coagulation may accompany cancer, particularly with mucin-secreting adenocarcinoma. Tumour cells may express tissue factor or induce tissue-factor expression by monocytes. Factor X activators have been described in malignancy. Tumour cells may interact directly with platelets and endothelial cells and may also secrete plasminogen activator inhibitor.

In nephrotic syndrome in adults, arterial and venous thrombosis occurs. It is a rare complication of childhood nephrotic syndrome (see Section 20). Loss of anticoagulants, especially antithrombin, in the urine and platelet hyperactivity may contribute.

Whether there is a specific association between ulcerative colitis and venous thromboembolism is unclear, but thrombotic events may complicate the disease. Thrombotic complications are a major feature of Behçet's syndrome. Superficial thrombophlebitis, deep-vein thrombosis, caval thrombosis, cerebral venous thrombosis, and arterial occlusion, often with aneurysm formation, have been described. The thromboses probably occur in association with vasculitic lesions but reactive increases in fibrinogen and factor VIII may contribute to the prethrombotic state. Antiphospholipid antibodies have been detected in Behçet's syndrome, and may be prothrombotic.

Venous and arterial thrombosis, especially thrombotic stroke, are features of polycythaemia rubra vera and essential thrombocythaemia (Chapters 22.3.8 and 22.3.10). In paroxysmal nocturnal haemoglobinuria, death is frequently due to thrombotic complications (see Chapter 22.3.12). Venous thrombosis may affect the splanchnic circulation as well as limb vessels, hepatic and portal venous thrombosis being prominent features. The mechanisms have not been determined.

Although vascular occlusion in sickle-cell disease is due predominantly to the accumulation of non-deformable sickled erythrocytes in the microcirculation, venous thrombosis has been recorded.

Antibodies to phospholipid and thrombosis

The association between circulating antibody reactive against (mainly negatively charged) phospholipid and thrombotic complications in systemic lupus erythematosus has been recognized for over 40 years. The antibodies may be detected as a 'lupus anticoagulant', as anticardiolipin, or as the 'biological false-positive' test for syphilis, depending upon the apparent phospholipid specificity of the antibodies and the physical presentation of the antigen in the tests. It is concluded that the lupus anticoagulant is present when there is a prolongation of a phospholipid-dependent test of coagulation, such as the activated partial thromboplastin time, without the presence of an inhibitor to an individual clotting factor or a factor deficiency. There is no specific test, but the kaolin clotting time or the dilute Russell's viper venom time, with appropriate controls, are reliable for the detection of lupus anticoagulant. Paradoxically, the presence of the anticoagulant confers an increased thrombotic risk in systemic lupus, and there is no haemorrhagic tendency. Assays for anticardiolipin use purified cardiolipin, a phospholipid present in the inner leaflet of the mitochondrion, in a solid-phase system. Some antibodies react only in one type of assay—coagulation or solid phase—whilst others give positive results in both, with or without positivity in the Venereal Diseases Research Laboratory test.

Table 4 *Situations in which antiphospholipid antibodies may be detected*

Infections
Acute self-limiting infections
Syphilis
Malaria
HIV infection
Hepatitis C

Rheumatic and collagen vascular diseases
Systemic lupus erythematosus
Systemic sclerosis
Rheumatoid arthritis
Temporal arteritis
Psoriatic arthropathy
Sjögren's syndrome

Thrombotic disease
Venous thromboembolic disease
Peripheral arterial occlusion
Microvascular thrombosis
Myocardial infarction and ischaemic heart disease
After coronary artery bypass graft surgery
Valvular heart disease
Renal vascular disease
Pulmonary hypertension

Disorders of the nervous system and eye
Thrombotic stroke
Transient cerebral ischaemia and amaurosis fugax
Sagittal-sinus thrombosis
Ischaemic optic neuropathy
Retinal venous occlusion
Multi-infarct dementia
Chorea
Guillain–Barré syndrome
Transverse myelitis

Obstetric disorders
Recurrent abortion
Fetal growth retardation
Early, severe pre-eclampsia

With medication
Phenothiazines
Procainamide
Hydralazine
Phenytoin
Quinidine

Miscellaneous
Livedo reticularis
Skin ulceration
Autoimmune thrombocytopenia
Autoimmune haemolytic anaemia
Behçet's syndrome
Sickle-cell disease
Intravenous drug abuse

Most individuals with serum that reacts positively for antiphospholipid do not have systemic lupus, but may have a history of thrombosis. However, the antibodies may also appear transiently after tissue trauma, in infections, and as a response to exposure to certain drugs (Table 4). Also, lupus anticoagulant is occasionally responsible for the finding of an unexpected prolongation of the activated partial thromboplastin time in a preoperative coagulation screen. Whether these transient and coincidental lupus anticoagulant/anticardiolipins are of pathogenic significance is open to some doubt, particularly as test positivity is often transient after tissue trauma or infection. The clinical significance of weakly positive tests for anticardiolipin is also open to question.

Antiphospholipids present in women of childbearing age have been associated with a strong tendency to pregnancy failure. Recurrent mid-trimester miscarriage, early pregnancy loss, fetal growth retardation, and the development of severe pre-eclampsia occurring unusually early in gestation have all been observed (see Section 13).

THE PRIMARY ANTIPHOSPHOLIPID SYNDROME (PAPS)

PAPS refers to patients without systemic lupus erythematosus but with positive tests for antiphospholipid with a history of thrombosis and/or recurrent (three or more) miscarriages. Thrombocytopenia may also be present, and is presumably autoimmune. The risk of recurrent thrombosis, both arterial and venous, appears to be high. PAPS thus represents an acquired prethrombotic state with an autoimmune basis.

Thrombosis and antiphospholipid

The prevalence of thrombosis in people who test repeatedly positive for antiphospholipid is difficult to determine, owing to selection bias in published series. In systemic lupus the presence of lupus anticoagulant confers an approximately threefold increased risk of thrombotic complications.

In PAPS, thrombotic stroke is a particularly common manifestation and may be the presenting event. In these individuals, heart-valve abnormalities, sometimes with non-infective vegetations, may be present. The risk of recurrent thrombosis is high. Venous thromboembolism is also common and may occur in relatively unusual sites including the cerebral venous sinuses, portal and hepatic veins, and retinal veins. Small-vessel occlusion may occur. Involvement of dermal vessels may lead to livedo reticularis, first reported in association with thrombotic stroke. Positive tests for antiphospholipid have also been noted in individuals with some conditions without an obvious thrombotic component (Table 4). Whether they are of pathogenic significance, or merely an epiphenomenon, is not yet known.

Intervention is not usually indicated when antiphospholipid is detected incidentally, without thrombotic or obstetric complications. Aspirin, heparin, warfarin, and immunosuppressive agents have been used in the management of recurrent miscarriage and in thromboprophylaxis. Treatment failures are not uncommon and the optimal means of therapy has not been determined. Use of aspirin or warfarin in arterial thrombosis and warfarin in venous thrombosis is logical. In prophylaxis against recurrent miscarriage, aspirin is the usual initial treatment, with introduction of prophylactic doses of heparin where aspirin fails. Corticosteroids have been used but such treatment carries a high risk of maternal morbidity, and efficacy is unproven (see Section 13).

The pathogenesis of thrombosis in PAPS

Cause and effect have not been demonstrated, but a variety of pathogenic mechanisms by which antiphospholipid could result in a prethrombotic state has been postulated. Binding to vascular endothelium, with inhibition of prostaglandin I_2 release, inhibition of fibrinolysis, and interference in the phospholipid-dependent protein C activation, or in the anticoagulant effect of activated protein C have been demonstrated *in vitro*.

Recently, it has been shown that phospholipid may not be the target antigen for many of these antibodies, but a protein on which epitopes become exposed only when the protein itself becomes bound to negatively charged phospholipids. β_2-Glycoprotein I is such a phospholipid-binding protein that also has anticoagulant properties. It is a target antigen for many 'antiphospholipids'. Interaction with phospholipid-bound prothrombin has been demonstrated in some other sera apparently containing 'antiphospholipid'.

Clinical management of acquired prethrombotic states

Arterial and venous thrombotic events are treated with heparin and warfarin (see below). There may be a role for thrombolytic therapy in massive pulmonary embolism and in acute peripheral arterial occlusion (see Section 15). Pharmacological recanalization of the occluded coronary vessel(s) in acute myocardial infarction is now routine, although this is a relatively uncommon site of thrombosis in the acquired prethrombotic states discussed above.

Thromboprophylaxis should be considered in these disorders. The high risk of embolic stroke in atrial fibrillation is a firm indication for long-term oral anticoagulant therapy, but care must be taken in patient selection as the risk:benefit ratio may be narrow in elderly people who may have other complicating disorders predisposing to haemorrhage. Prophylaxis with low-dose subcutaneous heparin (see below) is indicated for the prevention of venous thromboembolism in those immobilized after trauma (including surgery), in acute myocardial infarction, and in those in hospital with congestive cardiac failure. The presence of malignant disease adds to the thrombotic risk. Early mobilization, where medically possible, perhaps with use of graduated compression stockings, is a sensible additional precaution. In general, high awareness of the risk of thromboembolism in these disorders is advisable, with recognition that the presence of additional risk factors such as obesity or varicose veins (Table 2) may compound this risk.

In the presence of antiphospholipid the thrombotic risk appears to be substantial. Anticoagulant therapy may not be indicated when the antibody is an incidental finding, although prophylaxis at times of additional risk is a wise precaution. Venous thromboembolism is treated with heparin and oral anticoagulant and persistence of antiphospholipid may indicate ongoing increased risk with the need for long-term treatment. Thrombotic stroke has a particularly strong association with antiphospholipid and limited data suggest a high recurrence rate. Whether this is influenced by treatment with aspirin or warfarin is unclear, but further events have been recorded in treated subjects. Immunosuppressive therapy should be reserved for situations of anticoagulant failure, or the management of autoimmune manifestations where antiphospholipid complicates a more generalized autoimmune disorder such as systemic lupus erythematosus.

Numerous approaches have been recommended for the prevention of pregnancy failure in women with PAPS (see Section 13). There have been reports of success with aspirin, heparin, corticosteroids, and intravenous high-dose human immunoglobulin, as well as plasma exchange. There are no data from well-conducted clinical trials. Maternal morbidity from hypertension and gestational diabetes mellitus, as well as premature labour, appear to be significant risks of corticosteroid therapy. Subcutaneous heparin carries the risk of maternal osteopenia and the rare complication of severe thrombocytopenia. Until further information becomes available, one approach is to offer low-dose (75 mg daily) aspirin, together with close obstetric observation from confirmation of pregnancy, to women with three or more consecutive episodes of fetal loss and a positive test for antiphospholipid. In the event of failure, heparin prophylaxis (5000 u twice daily, subcutaneously) may be added early in the next pregnancy, with close clinical observation. Corticosteroid and immunoglobulin therapy should perhaps be reserved for those women where pregnancy failure ensues despite aspirin and heparin therapy.

Laboratory screening for thrombophilia

Thorough clinical assessment and simple laboratory investigations will suffice to detect most causes of the prethrombotic state. Screening for inherited thrombophilia is not likely to be cost-effective if applied indiscriminately. However, it is indicated in younger people, particularly in the circumstances listed in Table 5. Identification of a deficiency allows rational decisions to be made about the duration of therapy for thrombotic events. It also leads to identification of affected family members before clinical presentation. Although anticoagulant treatment will not necessarily be indicated, appropriate counselling and recommendations for prophylaxis during periods of high risk, pregnancy and surgery for example, as well as avoidance of other risk factors, are important aspects of management. In screening it must be recognized that the plasma levels

Table 5 *Indications for screening for thrombophilia*

Tests for AT, protein C and protein S	Tests for lupus anticoagulant and anticardiolipin
Venous thromboembolism presenting at < 45 years of age	Venous thromboembolism presenting at < 45 years of age
Recurrent venous thrombosis	Arterial thrombosis presenting at < 45 years of age in the absence of risk factors
Venous thrombosis in an unusual anatomical site	In the investigation of some disorders listed in Table 3, e.g. ischaemic optic neuropathy, chorea, livedo reticularis
Positive family history of thrombophilia	Recurrent (≥3) abortion of unknown cause
	Early, severe pre-eclampsia
	For assessment of thrombotic risk in some cases of SLE

AT, antithrombin; SLE, systemic lupus erythematosus.

of antithrombin and protein C and S can be low in a variety of acquired states (Table 6) and that results on samples taken during an acute event, and whilst on anticoagulant therapy may be misleading. Currently it is recommended that, for antithrombin and protein C, both functional and antigenic assays are made, and, for protein S, both free and bound cofactor are measured.

Screening for antiphospholipid should also be done selectively (Table 5) and a comprehensive laboratory approach employed, which must include a coagulation screening test (activated partial thromboplastin time) as well as a more specific tests (kaolin clotting time or dilute Russell's viper venom time) and an assay for anticardiolipin (these investigations are defined in Chapter 22.6.2).

Anticoagulant and thrombolytic treatment

The various strategies in the treatment and prevention of thromboembolic disease reflect the factors involved in its pathogenesis. Treatment of established disease may involve removing the thrombus. This is the most direct and logical approach, as the thrombus may possibly cause vascular occlusion. The thrombus can be removed pharmacologically by fibrinolysis or physically by catheterization or surgery. Following removal, it is important to inhibit new thrombus formation. To this end, anticoagulants or antiplatelet agents are used, the former primarily for venous disease where thrombi are fibrin rich, the latter for arterial disease where platelet-rich thrombi are found. For venous disease, treatment may rely solely upon anticoagulants. Here, the strategy is to prevent extension of established thrombus while relying on natural fibrinolysis to lyse the existing fibrin-rich thrombus. During anticoagulation, in addition to the prevention of extension of the thrombus, there may be an apparent enhancement of lysis. Thrombus is not biologically static but is continually lysed and renewed, so that anticoagulation by preventing thrombus renewal increases the observed rate of fibrinolysis. However, anticoagulation relies on plasminogen activation by the endothelium to clear and organize the thrombus locally. In such circumstances, resolution will be slow.

Fibrinolytic therapy

The fibrinolytic agents commonly used are plasminogen activators, which activate the proenzyme plasminogen to its active form, plasmin.

Table 6 *Conditions in which acquired deficiency of antithrombin, protein C, or protein S may occur*

Antithrombin	Protein C	Protein S
Liver disease	Liver disease and	Liver disease
Disseminated intravascular	transplantation	Disseminated intravascular
coagulation	Disseminated intravascular	coagulation
Nephrotic syndrome	coagulation	Pregnancy
Protein-losing enteropathy	Cardiopulmonary bypass	Systemic lupus erythematosus
Major surgery	surgery	In association with
Acute thrombosis	Haemodialysis	antiphospholipid antibody
Drugs:	Drugs:	Drugs:
Heparin	Warfarin	Warfarin
Oestrogens	Asparaginase	Cancer chemotherapy
Asparaginase	Cancer chemotherapy	Oestrogens

Although they have the potential for generating plasmin action predominantly on the fibrin contained within a thrombus, they also induce a plasma proteolytic state. The resulting plasminaemia destroys fibrinogen and other circulating clotting factors and may induce serious haemorrhage. This is particularly important if there is an underlying bleeding diathesis or local lesion from which bleeding is likely. For these reasons, in the case of a cerebrovascular accident, intracranial neoplasm, cranial surgery, within 10 days of any form of major trauma to the head, or in uncontrolled hypertension, fibrinolytic therapy can cause intracranial bleeding. After major surgery involving the thorax or abdomen, or with concurrent gastrointestinal lesions, thrombolytic therapy may induce massive haemorrhage. These states are therefore strong contraindications to fibrinolytic therapy. Currently, attempts are being made to develop new plasminogen activators that are more fibrin specific and may prove safer. However, in many of these conditions, haemostasis relies on the integrity of the fibrin plug. Even fibrin-specific agents will still be targeted to such lesions, and an absolutely safe fibrinolytic agent may be impossible to achieve.

Streptokinase and urokinase were the first lytic drugs to be used and they remain in widespread use. Streptokinase is cheaper but is antigenic. Both have low fibrin specificity.

The newer, more expensive agents, tissue plasminogen activator and its recombinant form, acylated plasminogen streptokinase activator complex (**APSAC**), and single-chain urokinase (pro-urokinase, scu-PA) are more fibrin specific. APSAC retains the allergic side-effects of streptokinase (rashes and, rarely, anaphylaxis). Dose-related side-effects, including hypotension, flushing and nausea, are also seen with streptokinase, APSAC, and tissue plasminogen activator.

Fibrinolytic agents may be given locally or systemically. Local delivery via a catheter is particularly useful for peripheral arterial thrombolysis as it allows angiographic assessment of efficacy. For venous thromboembolism, local treatment does not have any advantages, while for myocardial infarction the number of patients requiring treatment and degree of urgency makes intravenous systemic therapy a more practical choice. Suggested dosages are given in Table 7. Laboratory control is not thought to be necessary with such standardized dosage schemes.

When considering fibrinolytic therapy, care should be taken to ensure that the patient warrants such treatment. Objective confirmation of the clinical diagnosis is therefore a prerequisite. For peripheral arterial occlusion the relative merits of surgery and thrombolysis are not clear (see Section 15). During thrombolytic treatment the arteriotomy site for the catheter may bleed and mural thrombi may embolize; in contrast, embolism is rare during lytic treatment for venous disease. Therefore the optimal therapy for peripheral arterial disease is usually decided on an individual basis. In venous thromboembolism, thrombolytic therapy causes more bleeding than does heparin. For deep-vein thrombosis, fibrinolysis, if started early, probably helps preserve valve function. For pulmonary embolism, lytic therapy may give better long-term results, although any benefit is not demonstrable by lung perfusion scanning. Because of the risks of life-threatening haemorrhage many clinicians

prefer heparin therapy in venous thromboembolism except in the situation of massive pulmonary embolism, where thrombolytic therapy may be life-saving. Thrombolytic therapy may also be justified in incipient venous gangrene.

Pulmonary embolectomy is reserved for life-threatening occlusion when the patients are deteriorating on medical management (see Section 15).

In myocardial infarction, prompt lytic treatment provides the most benefit. Intravenous streptokinase, APSAC, and recombinant tissue plasminogen activator all reduce mortality, with a 25 to 30 per cent reduction in the risk of death.

Antiplatelet drugs

Although there has been an interest in the role of antiplatelet agents in thrombotic disease for many years, only recently have clear indications for their use been formulated. Aspirin is of benefit in various groups of thrombotic patients such as survivors of myocardial infarction, and those with unstable angina, transient cerebral ischaemia or ischaemic stroke. Using aspirin, the secondary prevention of myocardial infarction approaches 25 per cent, mortality from vascular accidents can be reduced by one-sixth, and non-fatal stroke by a third (see also Sections 15 and 24). A recent meta-analysis indicates a beneficial effect of aspirin on mortality in all subjects with symptoms of arterial disease.

There is still controversy about the optimal dosage but any dose between 30 and 300 mg appears to be effective; during initial therapy a loading dose of at least 120 mg is required for full effect. There is a slightly increased risk of haemorrhagic stroke and minor bleeding but the buffered or enteric-coated formulations provide good gastrointestinal tolerance. Of other antiplatelet drugs, dipyridamole is widely used but its efficacy is unproven. Ticlopidine appears effective but causes reversible neutropenia and marrow aplasia.

Anticoagulation

Heparin is the drug of choice for rapid anticoagulation because, when given intravenously, its action is immediate. It is usually given by bolus injection followed by continuous infusion, or by intermittent subcutaneous injection. Intermittent intravenous injection is associated with more bleeding than continuous infusion. In contrast, warfarin is given orally and takes 4 days to become fully effective.

When long-term anticoagulation is required, it is usual to start with heparin and then introduce warfarin, continuing heparin until warfarin has achieved a therapeutic level. For distal venous thrombosis, warfarin and heparin are normally started together; while for proximal venous thrombosis and pulmonary embolism, longer periods of heparin may be helpful. Consequently, warfarin may be delayed until 3 to 7 days after starting heparin. A recent study has confirmed the need for hepariniza-

Table 7 *Dose regimens for fibrinolytic agents*

Indication	Streptokinase		Urokinase		Recombinant tissue plasminogen activator		Acylated plasminogen streptokinase activator complex	
	i.v.	Local	i.v.	Local	i.v.	Local	i.v.	Local
Acute myocardial infarction	1 500 000 i.u. over 1 h	10 000–25 000 i.u. as a loading dose then 4 000 i.u./min up to 75 min with angiography	2 500 000 u over 1 h	6000 u/min up to 2 h with angiography	10 mg as a loading dose then 50 mg over 1 h and subsequently 40 mg over 2 h	20 mg over 1 h	30 u over 4–5 min	
Peripheral arterial occlusion	250 000 i.u. as loading dose then 100 000 u/h for 1–3 days		4400 u/kg as a loading dose then 4400 u/kg per hour for 1–3 days	4000 u/min with a total daily dose of up to 1 000 000 u with angiography		0.05–0.1 mg/kg per hour for 1–8 h		
Venous thrombo-embolism	250 000 i.u. as a loading dose then 100 000 u/h for 1–3 days for venous thrombosis and 12–24 h for pulmonary embolism		4400 u/kg as a loading dose then 4400 u/kg per hour for 1–3 days for venous thrombosis and 12–24 h for pulmonary embolism					

tion in addition to oral anticoagulants in the treatment of venous thrombosis; if oral anticoagulants are used alone, recurrence is more likely.

Heparin

Heparin is a glycosaminoglycan composed of chains of alternating residues of D-glycosamine and uronic acid. Its major anticoagulant effect depends on a unique pentasaccharide with a high-affinity binding sequence to the endogenous coagulation inhibitor, antithrombin. After its interaction with heparin, antithrombin undergoes a conformational change that markedly accelerates its ability to inactivate the serine proteases thrombin, factor Xa and factor IXa. Thrombin is most sensitive to this interaction and during inactivation a tertiary complex is formed, heparin binding to both antithrombin and thrombin.

In contrast, the inactivation of factor Xa is achieved by binding to antithrombin without Xa interacting directly with heparin. Low molecular-weight heparin molecules containing fewer than 18 saccharides cannot bind antithrombin and thrombin simultaneously, and hence they lose antithrombin activity although they retain anti-Xa activity.

Heparin cofactor II is also catalysed by heparin but the anticoagulant effect is specific for thrombin and only achieved at high levels of heparin dosage.

Heparins are heterogeneous preparations containing molecules of various anticoagulant pharmacological properties and size; in standard heparin only about one-third have anticoagulant activity. Low molecular-weight preparations show increased anti-Xa as compared to antithrombin activity. This makes potency and hence dosage comparisons between different low molecular-weight formulations difficult. Furthermore, the altered pharmacological properties lead to longer half-lives after subcutaneous or intravenous injection. Low molecular-weight heparins have some advantages over standard heparin: prophylaxis can be achieved with once-daily subcutaneous injections, and they provide better protection against postoperative venous thromboembolism in hip surgery. In other circumstances, standard heparin is satisfactory.

It is usual to inject a loading dose of 5000 of standard heparin intravenously as a bolus when starting full heparinization. Subsequent heparinization is achieved by a continuous intravenous infusion of 24 000 to 32 000 u over 24 h (the lower dose is recommended for patients who have received recent thrombolytic therapy). Patients vary in their response to the anticoagulant effect of heparin so that dose is adjusted depending upon the degree of anticoagulation.

The activated partial thromboplastin time (**APTT**) is the most popular method of monitoring therapy, although more sophisticated assays such as those for anti-IIa or anti-Xa are available. Guidelines for dosage have not yet been standardized. Although APTT reagents differ in their response to heparin, treatment that aims at maintaining the APTT between 1.5 to 2.5 times the average laboratory control value is often used. However, current APTT reagents show increased sensitivity to heparin and higher ratios have recently been recommended. It is wise to seek advice from the local coagulation laboratory on the optimal APTT target range. Monitoring should be started 6 h after induction and continued daily, or more frequently, if response is inadequate or excessive. Overdose responds within a few hours to dose reduction or discontinuation, and in underdosage a further intravenous bolus can be given, as well as increasing the infusion rate. Protamine is rarely required but is prompt and effective in the neutralization of heparin. If bleeding is severe, protamine sulphate should be given in a dose of 1 mg for every 100 i.u. of heparin that have been infused over the previous hour.

Subcutaneous heparin, given 12-hourly in equivalent dosage, can be as effective as intravenous heparin but stabilization to adequate levels takes longer. It is important to test the APTT response at the peak level after injection (usual 2–6 h after injection). For subcutaneous therapy the heparin preparation must be concentrated (e.g. 25 000 i.u./ml): sodium or calcium salts can be used, although with sodium higher levels are obtained. They should also be preservative free to reduce local pain.

Local bruising at the injection sites is common. Twice daily doses of 250 i.u./kg have been recommended, although lower doses (200 i.u./kg) may be required in women over 60 years of age.

Before heparinization a normal baseline prothrombin time and APTT help ensure that there is no important underlying coagulation defect. If the APTT response is excessive, a thrombin time can be measured to confirm that the APTT response is due to excessive heparin and not to any underlying condition such as a lupus anticoagulant (see above). Resistance to the anticoagulant effect of heparin may indicate antithrombin deficiency. Delay in reaching a therapeutic concentration of heparin is associated with a higher incidence of recurrence and extension of venous thrombosis.

Haemorrhage is common with heparin therapy and can occur even when the APTT response is not excessive. Other major side-effects are thrombocytopenia and osteopenia. Thrombocytopenia may be associated with heparin-induced arterial thrombosis. Thrombocytopenia is a dangerous complication and is immune mediated. It occurs more commonly with bovine than porcine heparin and usually 3 to 15 days after starting heparin, unless the patient was previously exposed. It is more common with higher doses and usually resolves within 4 days of stopping the drug. Heparin should be stopped immediately, and if alternative treatment is indicated, warfarin, ancrod, or the heparinoid, lomoparin, should be considered. Re-exposure may be dangerous.

Osteopenia appears to be more likely after long exposure (usually in excess of 6 months and 10 000 u twice daily). This is also a serious side-effect and can cause vertebral collapse. Urticaria and skin necrosis can occur with heparin. In the latter, the histological features suggest a hypersensitivity angiitis.

Oral anticoagulants

Oral drugs are generally used where anticoagulation is to be continued for more than 1 to 2 weeks. The preparation most widely used is warfarin, although the shorter-acting agent nicoumalone, and the longer-acting phenprocoumon, are also in regular use. Phenindione is not recommended because of the high incidence of skin rashes.

Oral anticoagulants compete with the action of vitamin K in the posttranscriptional carboxylation of glutamic acid residues of clotting factors II, VII, IX, and X and the inhibitory proteins C and S. This takes place predominantly in the liver. Warfarin has a plasma half-life of 35 h and it takes about 1 week to achieve a steady anticoagulant effect. Hence, to optimize that effect, heparin and oral anticoagulants should be continued together for 7 days. In practice, heparin is often discontinued earlier when the prothrombin time is at an apparent therapeutic level. During the first few days of oral anticoagulation the defect is predominantly of factor VII, which is rate-limiting in the prothrombin time test. It is uncertain how effective this period of anticoagulation is in preventing thrombus extension. Therefore, for patients with pulmonary embolism or substantial proximal thrombosis, at least 5 days of combined oral anticoagulants and heparin are advisable. This will ensure adequate depression of all the coumarin-sensitive clotting factors before the heparin is discontinued.

The prothrombin time is used to monitor the effect of oral anticoagulants and guide dosage. In order to take into account the variation between laboratories the result is expressed on a common scale as an international normalized ratio (**INR**). The sensitivity of a local method is expressed as the international sensitivity index (**ISI**). This is the slope of prothrombin times obtained with the primary international reference preparation when plotted against local data for prothrombin time on a log scale: INR = (PT ratio) [ISI]. For the majority of therapeutic indications the target range is 2 to 3, but in some instances higher ranges have been recommended. An INR of 3 to 4.5 is currently recommended to prevent systemic emboli in patients with mechanical prosthetic heart valves.

In patients with recurrent venous thromboembolism, in spite of an INR of 2 to 3, higher ranges have also been recommended. A full search

Table 8 *Drugs that interact with the effects of warfarin*

Increase activity	May increase activity	Reduce activity
Alcohol abuse Alcohol Disulfiram	*Antigout agents* Allopurinol	*Antibiotics* Rifampicin
Anabolic steroids Oxymetholone Stanozolol	*Analgesics* Diflunisal Flurbiprofen Mefenamic acid Sulindac Other NSAIDs	*Antiepileptics* Carbamazepine Phenobarbitone Primidone Phenytoin
Analgesics Azapropazone Phenylbutazone	*Anion-exchange resins* Cholestyramine	*Antifungals* Griseofulvin
Antiarrhythmics Amiodarone Propafenone	*Antiarrhythmics* Quinidine	*Barbiturates* *Hormone antagonists* Aminoglutethimide
Antibacterials Aztreonam Cephamandole Chloramphenicol Ciprofloxacin Co-trimoxazole Erythromycin Metronidazole Sulphonamides Trimethaprim	*Antibacterials* Enoxacin Nalidixic acid Neomycin Norfloxacin Tetracyline Other broad-spectrum antibiotics	*Oral contraceptives* *Vitamins* Vitamin K
Antifungals Fluconazole Intraconazole Ketoconazole Micoconazole	*Antidepressants* Fluvoxamine *Anticonvulsants* Phenytoin	
Clofibrates	*Hypnotics* Chloral hydrate	
Hormone antagonists Danazol Tamoxifen	*Lipid-lowering drugs* Simvastatin	
Thyroid hormones	*Ulcer-healing drugs* Sucralfate	
Ulcer-healing agents Cimetidine Omeprazole		
Uricosurics Sulphinpyrazone		

for any underlying cause, particularly neoplasia, could be made. Trousseau's observation, recorded in 1872, of the association between deep-vein thrombosis and cancer must be remembered. Patients who develop deep-vein thrombosis in the absence of identifiable risk factors have an increased likelihood of having cancer.

In arterial disease, aspirin rather than oral anticoagulants is the first choice for therapy. However, if transient cerebral ischaemic attacks continue inspite of aspirin or endarterectomy, oral anticoagulants may be used. In view of the increased risk of cerebral haemorrhage with anticoagulation in cerebrovascular disease, a target INR of 2 to 3 is safer than higher ranges.

Warfarin is advised following myocardial infarction in certain patients who have a high risk of thromboembolism (see Section 15). Continuing anticoagulation, after 3 months, may be required where the left ventricle is diffusely dilated or poorly contracting.

Oral anticoagulants are sometimes used in an attempt to prevent further coronary thrombosis after myocardial infarction. However, the current view is that aspirin is preferred for secondary prophylaxis (see Section 15). If oral anticoagulants are used, INR values in the range 3 to 4.5 are usually advised.

The combination of warfarin and aspirin is potentially dangerous. For patients with very high risk of further arterial thromboembolism, where such a combination may be justified, a high INR must be avoided and the target INR should be low (2–2.5) with very careful anticoagulant control.

During the induction phase of warfarin, daily monitoring is advised, at least for the first few days. This allows the response to be used as a guide to predicting the maintenance dose. Heparin, except in unusually high doses, does not substantially affect the INR. With a normal baseline INR a daily dose of warfarin of 10 mg is recommended for the first 2 days, with lower induction doses if there is an underlying coagulation defect, liver disease, cardiac failure, or in old or unusually small patients. The required maintenance dose varies considerably between patients but is generally 3 to 9 mg/day (mean 5 mg). Weekly testing is advised for the first few weeks, followed by 1 to 2 monthly if compliance and control are good. The hazards must be carefully explained to the patient, who should carry a dosage card that should be shown to all doctors, dentists or pharmacists who deal with them. If there is any change in the patient's condition or medication, the physician should liase with the anticoagulant clinic as more frequent INR testing may be required.

For some patients, control is easy while in others the INR varies without explanation. Drug interaction is a major problem and prescribing requires care and vigilance in warfarinized patients. The chief drug interactions are shown in Table 8: this list is not complete; to ensure that there is no interaction with warfarin requires reference to a drug compendium or an anticoagulant clinic.

Haemorrhage is the main side-effect and omission of dosage with checking of the INR is essential if this occurs. If at an INR of below 5.0, a search for a local cause of bleeding is necessary. For life-threatening haemorrhage, 5 mg of phytomenadione (vitamin K) should be given by slow intravenous injection, together with prothrombin complex concentrate (preparations usually contain factors II, IX, and X). One litre of fresh frozen plasma can be used instead of prothrombin complex concentrate but may not be so effective. For less severe haemorrhage, when overdose is present (INR >5.0) 0.5 to 2 mg of vitamin K by slow intravenous injection or fresh frozen plasma may be required. For overdose without hemorrhage, and if the INR is below 7.0, missing 1 or 2 days' dosage with early review is sufficient. If the INR is above 7.0, even without haemorrhage, reversal with 0.5 mg of vitamin K_1 by slow intravenous injection or fresh frozen plasma should be considered. Caution is required to avoid complete reversal of anticoagulation in subjects with metal prosthetic heart valves.

Other side-effects are very rare. Rashes and alopecia can occur. Skin necrosis is associated with oral anticoagulants, particularly during the induction phase; microscopy shows capillary thrombosis. An association between hereditary protein C or protein S deficiency and coumarin-induced skin necrosis is now recognized (see Fig. 5), although it can occur in the absence of these defects. The mechanism is thought to be an imbalance between the reduction of procoagulant and anticoagulant vitamin-K-dependent factors during the warfarin induction phase, which, combined with the congenital thrombophilia, leads to localized intravascular coagulation in skin capillaries. Adequate heparinization and the use of small induction doses of warfarin minimizes the risk of this complication. It is not thought to be an allergic phenomenon and re-exposure to warfarin is usually safe.

Warfarin should be given for at least 3 months for venous disease, although for postsurgical venous thrombosis 4 to 6 weeks may be adequate (6 months for pulmonary embolism). Recurrent venous thrombosis is considered to be an indication for long-term oral anticoagulants.

Warfarin causes a specific embryopathy and if possible should be avoided in pregnancy (see Section 13). The embryopathy is characterized by chondrodysplasia punctata, nasal hypoplasia, and neurological abnormalities, probably due to fetal haemorrhage. Anticoagulant regimens for pregnant patients reflect a balance between thrombotic and teratogenic effects. The warfarin effect on bone and connective tissue development is maximal 6 to 9 weeks after conception, so subcutaneous heparin is often given for the first trimester. Moderate of doses of heparin are required (e.g. 10 000–12 000 u, twice daily) but even this may be insufficient to protect against thrombosis on mechanical heart valves. Some authorities therefore maintain such patients on warfarin throughout pregnancy. At delivery, the infant may itself be anticoagulated so that heparin is preferred during the last few weeks of pregnancy (e.g. 36–40 weeks). Postpartum, warfarin can be safely used, even with breast feeding, as very little passes into the breast milk. If heparin is used throughout pregnancy there is a risk of oesteopenia.

Prophylaxis for venous thromboembolism (see also Section 15)

Anticoagulants

Pulmonary emboli continue to be a major cause of death in patients in hospital (Table 9). It is not solely a postoperative complication; only 1 in 4 of patients dying from pulmonary emboli in hospital has had recent surgery. In fatal embolism, preceding signs of thromboembolism are

Table 9 *Incidence of venous thromboembolism in hospital patients according to risk group*

	Deep-vein thrombosis (%)	Proximal-vein thrombosis (%)	Fatal pulmonary embolism (%)
Low-risk groups	< 10	< 1	0.01
Moderate-risk groups	10–40	1–10	0.1–1
High-risk groups	40–80	10–30	1–10

Low-risk groups	Minor surgery (< 30 min) with no risk factors except age. Major surgery (>30 min) with age < 40 years and no other recognized risk factor. Minor trauma or medical illness.
Moderate-risk groups	Major general, urological, gynaecological, cardiothoracic, vascular or neurological surgery with age > 40 years or other recognized risk factor. Major medical illness: heart or lung disease, cancer, inflammatory bowel disease. Major trauma or burns. Minor surgery, trauma, or illness in patients with previous deep-vein thrombosis, pulmonary embolism or thrombophilia.
High-risk groups	Fracture or major orthopaedic surgery of pelvis, hip, or lower limb. Major pelvic or abdominal surgery for cancer. Major surgery, trauma, or illness in patients with previous deep-vein thrombosis, pulmonary embolism, or thrombophilia. Lower-limb paralysis (for example, hemiplegic stroke, paraplegia). Major lower-limb amputation.

Fig. 5 Coumarin-induced skin necrosis in a patient heterozygous for protein S deficiency.

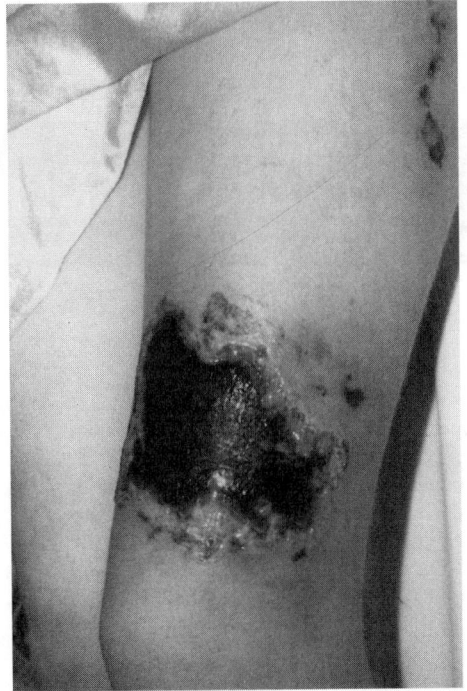

Table 10 *Incidence of deep-vein thrombosis after major general surgery*

	Mean incidence (%) by meta-analysis
No prophylaxis	25.1
Low-dose heparin	8.7
Graduated elastic compression stockings	9.3
Intermittent pneumatic compression	9.9
Dextran	16.6
Aspirin	20.4

often present but not recognized. Serious notice must therefore be taken of any signs or symptoms suggesting venous thromboembolism in patients in hospital. Screening for embolism in asymptomatic individuals, though advocated, is not cost-effective. Routine prophylaxis for moderate-to high-risk patients is recommended, however (see Table 9). The relative merits of the various prophylactic measures available for use after major surgery can be judged from the data in a meta-analysis (shown in Table 10). Low-dose subcutaneous heparin (5000 u 8 to 12 hourly) is widely used and is suitable for moderate- and some high-risk groups. For hip and knee surgery, fixed-dose standard heparin is only moderately effective and adjusted-dose or low molecular-weight heparin give better results. Adjusted-dose heparin requires careful laboratory monitoring and is less convenient than low molecular-weight heparin. Furthermore, low molecular-weight heparin can be given once daily.

General measures

In addition to the use of prophylactic anticoagulants there are a number of general measures that should be carefully instituted in an attempt to further reduce the frequency of venous thrombotic disease, both in hospital and general practice (see also Section 15).

In surgical practice there is now well-documented evidence that the use of elastic stockings in the perioperative period are of genuine value. Other simple measures such as early mobilization, the avoidance of dehydration, and the encouragement of leg exercises postoperatively are also useful. Particular attention should be paid to obesity and, where possible, major efforts at weight reduction should be instituted, particularly before 'cold' surgery. Many of these measures are also relevant to patients with serious diseases who may not be mobile for prolonged periods of time.

It is also important to remember the dangers of venous thromboembolic disease in primary-care practice. There is increasing evidence that long journeys by aeroplane, particularly if associated with dehydration due to excessive alcohol intake, or any other form of prolonged immobilization, increase the likelihood of venous thrombosis. Similarly, patients who stay in bed at home for long periods are at increased risk, particularly those who are exposed to thrombogenic agents, the oral contraceptive pill for example, or who become dehydrated as part of an infective disorder.

REFERENCES

Anonymous (1992). How to anticoagulate. *Drug and Therapeutic Bulletin*, **30**, 7–80.
Bell, W.R. and Marder, V.J.(1987). Fibrinolytic therapy. In *Haemostasis and thrombosis*, (2nd edn), (ed. R.W. Colman, J. Hirsch, V.J. Marder, and E.W. Salzman), pp. 1393–437. Lippincott, Philadelphia.
Bertina, R.M., Koelemann, B.P.C., Koster, T., *et al.* (1994). Mutation in blood coagulation factor V associated with resistance is activated protein C. *Nature*, **369**, 64–7.
Colvin, B.T. and Barrowcliffe, T.W. on behalf of BCSH Haemostasis and Thrombosis Task Force (1993). The British Society for Haematology guidelines on the use and monitoring of heparin 1992: second revision. *Journal of Clinical Pathology*, **46**, 97–103.
Gallus, A.S. (1992). Anticoagulant in the prevention and treatment of thromboembolic problems in pregnancy including cardiac problems. In *Haemostasis and thrombosis in obstetrics and gynaecology*, (ed. I.A. Greer, A.G.G. Turpie, and C.D. Forbes), pp. 319–47. Chapman and Hall Medical, London.
Morris, G.K. (1992). Thrombolytic therapy and myocardial infarction. In *Thrombosis and its management*, (ed. L. Poller and J.M. Thomson), pp. 231–44. Churchill Livingstone, Edinburgh.
Research Committee of the British Thoracic Society (1992). Optimum duration of anticoagulation for deep vein thrombosis and pulmonary embolism. *Lancet*, **340**, 873–6.
Routlege, P.A. and West, R.P. (1992). Low molecular weight heparin. *British Medical Journal*, **305**, 906.
Singer, D.E. (1992). Randomized trials of warfarin for atrial fibrillation. *New England Journal of Medicine*, **327**, 1451–3.
Thromboembolic risk factors (THRIFT) Consensus Group (1992). Risk of prophylaxis for venous thromboembolism in hospital patients. *British Medical Journal*, **305**, 567–74.
Vermylen, J. (1992). Anti-platelet drugs in the prevention of arterial thrombosis. In *Thrombosis and its management*, (ed. L. Poller and J.M. Thomson), pp. 217–30. Churchill Livingstone, Edinburgh.

22.7 The blood in systemic disease

D. J. WEATHERALL

There are few diseases that do not produce some alteration in the blood. Here, some of the haematological changes that accompany and may be the presenting feature of general systemic diseases will be summarized. Many of these topics are discussed elsewhere in this book but they are brought together in order to emphasize how blood changes may give the first indication of the presence of non-haematological disorders. It should be remembered that the haematological consequences of systemic disease vary considerably depending on the age of the patient. Recent reviews which deal specifically with this topic in children and the elderly are cited at the end of this chapter.

Malignant disease

By far the most common haematological finding in malignant disease (Table 1) is the anaemia of chronic disorders, which was described in Chapter 22.4.5. It may occur together with localized or widespread malignancy and is sometimes associated with an elevated erythrocyte sedimentation rate (ESR). It is found in patients with practically every type of carcinoma or reticulosis, is refractory to haematinics, but may respond to successful removal of a primary tumour.

The anaemia of patients with carcinoma, particularly of the gastro-

Table 1 *Principal haematological changes in malignant disorders*

Erythrocytes	
Anaemia of chronic disorders	All forms
Iron-deficiency anaemia	Gastrointestinal; cervix, uterus
Leucoerythroblastic anaemia	Stomach, breast, thyroid, prostate, bronchus, kidney
Microangiopathic haemolytic anaemia	Mucin-secreting tumours; stomach, bronchus, breast
Secondary myelosclerosis	As for leucoerythroblastic; also reticuloses
Selective red-cell aplasia	Thymus, lymphoma, bronchus
Immune haemolytic anaemia	Ovary; lymphoma; other carcinomas
Megaloblastic anaemia	Stomach; rarely others
Sideroblastic anaemia	Myelodysplastic syndrome
Polycythaemia	Kidney, liver, posterior fossa, uterus
Leucocytes	
Leucocytosis	All forms
Leukaemoid reactions	As for leucoerythroblastic anaemia
Eosinophilia	Miscellaneous carcinomas and reticuloses
Monocytosis	All forms
Basophilia	Myeloproliferative disease; mastocytosis
Lymphopenia	Carcinoma, reticuloses
Platelets	
Thrombocytosis	Gastrointestinal with bleeding; bronchus and others without bleeding
Thrombocytopenia	As for the microangiopathies
Acquired thrombocytopathy	Macroglobulinaemia; other paraproteinaemias
Coagulation	
Disseminated intravascular coagulation	Prostate, many others
Primary activation of fibrinolysis	Prostate
Selective impairment of coagulation (see Table 2)	
Thrombophlebitis	All forms
Miscellaneous	
Abnormal proteins-cryofibrinogens	Prostate, others
Fetal proteins	Alpha-fetoprotein—liver and others
	Carcinoembryonic antigen (CEA)—gastrointestinal neoplasms
	Fetal haemoglobin—leukaemia, other tumours
Circulating tumour cells	All forms
Effects of cytotoxic drugs	All forms

intestinal tract, may be complicated by chronic blood loss and superimposed iron deficiency. Chronic bleeding of this type is often associated with a mild thrombocytosis.

DISSEMINATED MALIGNANCY

The most common haematological change with disseminated malignancy is a leucoerythroblastic picture characterized by the presence in the blood of immature myeloid cells together with some nucleated red cells and, sometimes, a mild reticulocytosis. The red cells often show a moderate degree of anisocytosis and poikilocytosis. This finding is very commonly accompanied by the presence of tumour cells in the bone marrow. Clinically, it can cause confusion with the diagnosis of primary myelosclerosis; splenomegaly is unusual in patients with disseminated carcinoma.

Occasionally, widespread carcinoma leads to a leukaemoid reaction with white-cell counts in the range seen in chronic myeloid leukaemia. The differentiation between these two conditions was described earlier (Chapter 22.5.1).

The microangiopathic haemolytic anaemia of disseminated malignancy (Chapter 22.4.13) is most frequently found in association with mucin-secreting adenocarcinoma, particularly of the stomach, breast, and lung.

LESS COMMON FORMS OF ANAEMIA ASSOCIATED WITH CANCER

Autoimmune haemolytic anaemia is sometimes found in patients with an underlying lymphoma. It is much less common in other forms of malignancy except for the association with tumours of the ovary. However, there have been reports of autoimmune haemolysis occurring with a wide variety of tumours, including lung, stomach, breast, kidney, colon, and testis.

Pure red-cell aplasia may occasionally be the presenting feature in a patient with a tumour of the thymus, and there have been occasional reports of this type of anaemia occurring in patients with carcinoma of the bronchus or lymphomas.

Finally, it should be remembered that there is an association between pernicious anaemia and carcinoma of the stomach and a patient may present with a megaloblastic anaemia associated with a malignancy of this type. Sideroblastic anaemias are occasionally found in patients with carcinoma; in one series of 62 patients who presented with a sideroblastic anaemia, 10 were found to have an underlying malignancy.

POLYCYTHAEMIA

The relation between secondary polycythaemia and an underlying neoplasm is discussed in Chapter 22.4.14. It has been found in patients with renal tumours, hepatomas, hamartomas of the liver, uterine fibroids, vascular tumours and cystic adenomas of the cerebellum, and carcinoma of the lung.

CHANGES IN THE PLATELETS AND BLOOD COAGULATION

An otherwise unexplained thrombocytosis may be the first indication of an underlying malignancy. It is important to remember that this is not always associated with chronic blood loss; bronchial carcinoma may present in this way.

Generalized haemostatic failure associated with disseminated carcinoma is considered in detail in Chapter 22.6.6 (Figs 1 and 2).

Some bleeding disorders associated with cancer seem to be due to selective impairment of coagulation. This may result from pathological inhibitors of different parts of the coagulation system or from isolated factor deficiencies. The mechanism is unknown. However, in a patient with a bleeding disorder associated with cancer, which is not characterized by consumption of clotting factors or fibrinolysis, a detailed analysis of the activities of the intrinsic and extrinsic pathways must be made in case a correctable lesion is present (Table 2).

WHITE-CELL ABNORMALITIES

Apart from the leukaemoid reaction mentioned earlier, there are several white-cell changes that should make the clinician think about an underlying malignancy. For example, a persistent monocytosis or eosinophilia may be associated with Hodgkin's disease or with bronchial carcinoma. Persistent lymphopenia may occur in patients with Hodgkin's disease.

Fig. 1 Disseminated intravascular coagulation in association with carcinoma of the prostate. The patient started to bleed extensively from the iliac-crest marrow biopsy site and from venesection sites. Marrow biopsy showed widespread tumour metastases. (Reproduced from Hardisty, R.M. and Weatherall, D.J. (ed.) 1982. *Blood and its disorders*, (2nd edn). Blackwell Scientific, Oxford, with permission.)

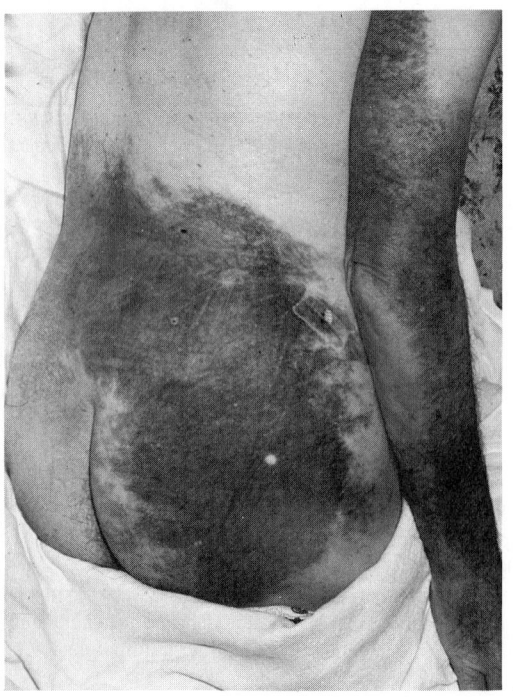

Infection

Most of the important haematological changes in association with infection are considered in Section 7. Just a few points of particular haematological relevance are summarized below.

ACUTE BACTERIAL INFECTION

Most acute bacterial infections are associated with a neutrophil leucocytosis. This may be so marked, and associated with such a 'shift to the left' with production of myelocytes in the blood that the condition may present a leukaemoid type of reaction. Occasionally, however, patients

Fig. 2 Sections prepared from Gardner-needle biopsies from bone marrow infiltrated with neoplastic cells; the primary tumour was in the prostate (H and E stain). (a) ×230, (b) ×920. (Reproduced from Hardisty, R.M. and Weatherall, D.J. (ed.) 1982. *Blood and its disorders.*, (2nd edn). Blackwell Scientific, Oxford, with permission.)

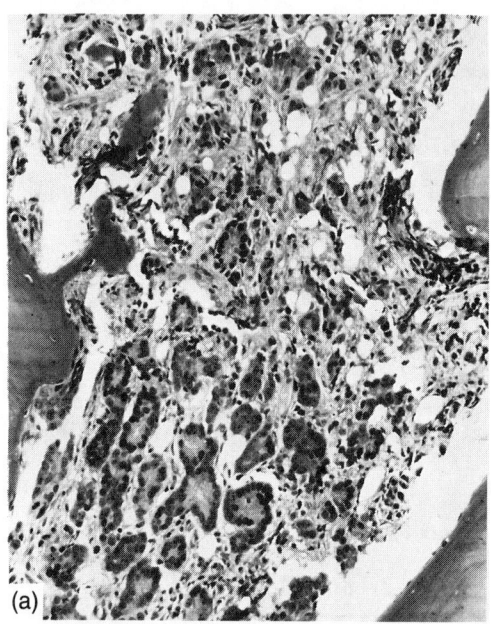

(a)

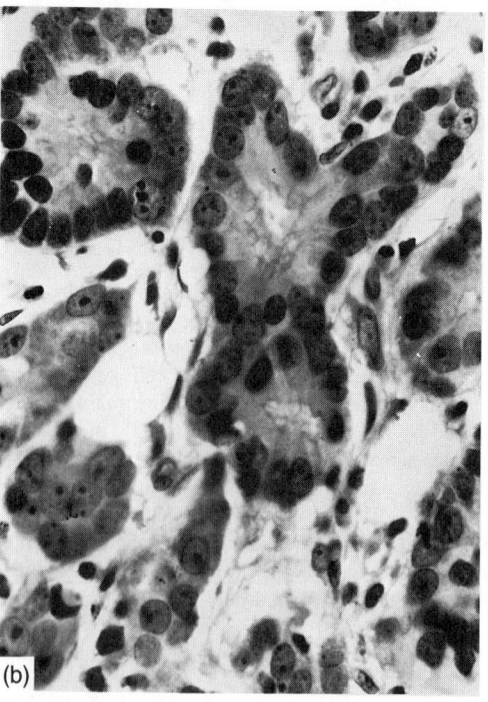

(b)

Table 2 *Selective impairment of coagulation in cancer*

Inhibitors	
Paraproteins	Plasma-cell disorders
Lupus-like	Hodgkin's disease, lymphoma, myelofibrosis, carcinoma
Factor IX inhibitor	Cancer of colon or prostate
Factor VII inhibitor	Bronchogenic carcinoma
Heparin-like	Bronchogenic carcinoma, myeloma
Isolated factor deficiencies	
Factor XIII	Acute leukaemia, chronic myeloid leukaemia
Factor XII	Chronic myeloid leukaemia
Factor XI	Melanoma
Factor X	Myeloma with amyloid
Factor VIII	Macroglobulinaemia, chronic lymphatic leukaemia, Wilms' tumour
Factor V	Chronic myeloid leukaemia, polycythaemia vera

Modified from Goldsmith (1984)

Table 3 *Haematological changes in tuberculosis*

Type of tuberculosis or therapy	Haematological changes
Pulmonary	Anaemia of chronic disorders; iron-deficiency anaemia; Anaemia due to therapy; high ESR
Ileocaecal	Anaemia of chronic disorders; megaloblastic anaemia due to vitamin B_{12} or folate deficiency; high ESR
Cryptic miliary (aregenerative)	Leukaemoid reaction; myelosclerosis;* pancytopenia; Polycythaemia,* anaemia of chronic disorders
Antituberculous drugs:	
PAS or streptomycin allergy	Fever, lymphadenopathy, eosinophilia
INAH, cycloserine	Sideroblastic anaemia
Rifampicin	Thrombocytopenic purpura

* These reports may well represent cases of disseminated tuberculosis in patients with underlying haematological disorders (see text).

are encountered severely ill with acute bacterial infection in whom the neutrophil response seems inadequate, or who may be frankly neutropenic. Although some of them will prove to have an underlying haematological disorder or a debilitating condition such as alcoholism, this is not always the case and a proportion of patients who recover from their infection show no such underlying abnormality subsequently. A marrow examination usually reveals a paucity of mature granulocytes. This clinical picture is particularly common in newborn infants, especially those born prematurely.

Other leucocyte changes are less common in acute infection. Monocytosis has been reported in patients with typhoid fever and sometimes in brucellosis or subacute bacterial endocarditis. In endocarditis a monocytosis may be associated with the presence of undifferentiated reticuloendothelial cells in the blood that show erythrophagocytosis.

Some degree of anaemia is found almost invariably in patients with bacterial infection. It usually presents a picture of the anaemia of chronic disorders. Haemolytic anaemia may occur in severe septicaemias and is usually associated with disseminated intravascular coagulation. Some organisms, *Clostridium welchii* for example, produce an α-toxin that acts as a lecithinase and causes fulminating intravascular haemolysis.

Disseminated intravascular coagulation is a relatively common accompaniment of severe bacterial infection. A number of mechanisms have been suggested, including vascular injury with activation of factor XII or the generation of procoagulants from white cells by the action of endotoxin. Thrombocytopenia is also common in patients with septicaemia. Although this may sometimes reflect disseminated intravascular coagulation, the mechanism is probably more complicated. There may be quite dramatic thrombocytopenia without any other evidence of a consumption coagulopathy. Probably several mechanisms are involved, including suppression of platelet production by the bone marrow, damage to circulating platelets by immune complexes, endothelial damage, and direct interaction of the platelets with bacteria; phagocytosis of bacteria by platelets may be a factor causing the rapid disappearance of platelets from the circulation.

CHRONIC BACTERIAL INFECTION

Chronic bacterial infection is usually associated with the anaemia of chronic disorders. Some particularly interesting haematological changes are sometimes ascribed to tuberculosis (Table 3). While the most common change is a mild, normochromic, normocytic anaemia with a raised ESR, more spectacular blood changes have been reported, particularly in association with disseminated tuberculosis. These clinical pictures

include leukaemoid reactions, pancytopenia, myelofibrosis, and even polycythaemia. The main problem in assessing these associations is whether the reported patients had tuberculous infection or infections due to atypical mycobacteria superimposed on an underlying blood disease, or whether disseminated tuberculosis can occasionally produce a clinical picture similar to leukaemia or a myeloproliferative disease. Unfortunately the answer to this interesting question remains unresolved. In practice any patient who presents with an atypical myeloproliferative disorder, and who is going downhill for no apparent cause, should be investigated for tuberculosis and attempts should be made to grow the organism from bone marrow cultures.

VIRUS INFECTIONS

Some of the haematological changes associated with specific viral infections such as infectious mononucleosis are considered in Section 7. However, it is becoming apparent that haematological changes can occur quite commonly in association with many virus illnesses.

Rubella, acquired in childhood or adult life, is often associated with a leucocytosis and an atypical lymphocytosis. A small proportion of patients develop an acute fulminating thrombocytopenic purpura approximately 4 days after the appearance of the rash. This is usually self-limiting but fatalities have been reported. Thrombocytopenia is also common in infants with congenital rubella, and this condition is also characterized by a non-immune haemolytic episode shortly after birth. Thrombocytopenia has also been reported in association with measles, and in particularly severe forms of rubella and morbilli severe haemorrhagic states due to disseminated intravascular coagulation have been seen. Similar changes occur occasionally in patients with varicella infections.

The haematological changes in infectious mononucleosis are described in Section 7. A very similar picture can occur in patients with cytomegalovirus (**CMV**) infection. In infants with congenital CMV infections there may be striking hepatosplenomegaly with purpura and anaemia. The anaemia is characterized by a haemolytic picture with the appearances of many normoblasts in the peripheral blood. This form of anaemia may last for several weeks and may be associated with severe thrombocytopenia. There are many well-documented cases of an infectious mononucleosis-like disorder occurring after transfusion with fresh blood or after perfusion for open heart surgery. The syndrome usually occurs 1 to 3 months after blood transfusion and is self-limiting, resolving within a few weeks. It is characterized by a moderate rise in temperature, with hepatosplenomegaly, lymphadenopathy, and transient maculopapular rashes. There is a lymphocytosis with a blood picture indistinguishable from that of infectious mononucleosis.

As well as the profound immunological changes that are associated with infections with human immunodeficiency virus type 1 (HIV-1) there is a variety of common haematological problems which are found in patients with AIDS. While lymphopenia is particularly common, neutropenia has been reported to vary between zero and 30 per cent in HIV antibody-positive asymptomatic individuals, and in 20 to 65 per cent of patients with AIDS. Thrombocytopenia occurs in 5 to 20 per cent of asymptomatic HIV-1 infected persons and rises to 25 to 50 per cent in patients with AIDS. Anaemia is also common and bone marrow examination often reveals dyserythropoiesis with a variable degree of erythrophagocytosis. There have been a number of reports of the presence of lupus anticoagulants in the blood of patients with AIDS. In addition to these haematological complications there is the added risk of drug-induced marrow hypoplasia, associated particularly with treatment with zidovudine (AZT).

Haematological complications of infectious hepatitis are rare but when they occur may be extremely severe. Coombs' positive haemolytic anaemia has been reported, and there is now a considerable literature on the occurrence of aplastic anaemia. This disorder seems predominantly to affect young males, and the onset of the aplasia is usually about 9 weeks after the onset of hepatitis. The condition is associated with a mortality in excess of 90 per cent. In those patients who recover, the period to complete haematological normality ranges between 3 and 20 months.

It is becoming apparent that many viruses are capable of provoking severe bleeding due to intravascular coagulation. Why viruses can fire off the coagulation cascade is far from clear. Activation of factor XII due to vascular injury or damage to platelets with the release of coagulants have been suggested as possible mechanisms.

There is increasing evidence that the human parvovirus has a particular affinity for red-cell progenitors. It probably causes transient red-cell aplasia quite commonly but this only gives rise to a symptomatic anaemia in patients who have a markedly shortened red-cell survival. Thus parvovirus infection appears to be responsible for the aplastic crises in patients with sickle-cell anaemia, pyruvate kinase deficiency, or other congenital haemolytic anaemias. Viruses can cause acute damage to the bone marrow in immune-suppressed patients as part of the virus haemophagocytic syndrome (see Chapter 22.5.4).

The haematological changes associated with the virus haemorrhagic fevers are described in detail in Section 7.

PARASITIC DISEASE

The major haematological accompaniments of the parasitic diseases are described in Section 7. Those which produce important haematological changes will be briefly summarized here.

Toxoplasmosis
Congenital toxoplasmosis can produce a condition identical to erythroblastosis fetalis. The clinical picture is of a pale, hydropic infant with a large spleen and liver associated with severe anaemia, thrombocytopenia, and a leucocytosis, often with a marked eosinophilia. In adult life the acquired forms of toxoplasmosis produce a clinical disorder resembling infectious mononucleosis.

Malaria (Plate 53)
Malarial infection produces a variety of haematological abnormalities. The most severe changes occur in association with *Plasmodium falciparum* malaria infection. In acute infections in non-immune individuals there is usually minimal anaemia at the onset of the illness, but during the 2 to 3 weeks after treatment there may be a steady decline in haemoglobin level, the mechanism of which is not yet fully worked out. On the other hand, children or adults with chronic malaria, some degree

of immunity, and low-level parasitaemias, may be severely anaemic at presentation with an inappropriately low reticulocyte count. The bone marrow is often hyperplastic and shows a marked degree of dyshaemopoiesis (Fig. 3) (see also Chapter 22.4.9).

In some patients with severe *P. falciparum* infections there may be marked intravascular haemolysis and haemoglobinuria. Again, the mechanism is not certain, and although some of these patients may be glucose 6-phosphate dehydrogenase deficient, this is by no means the whole story. It has been suggested that some patients with fulminating malaria have disseminated intravascular coagulation, although this is probably uncommon and plays very little part in the pathophysiology of either the anaemia or haemorrhagic phenomenon that occur in this condition. Thrombocytopenia is extremely common in patients with acute malaria but is only rarely associated with evidence of consumption of blood-clotting factors. In most forms of malarial infection there is a neutropenia, and monocytosis has also been described.

There are several interesting haematological manifestations of malaria associated with unusual forms of the disease. In the tropical splenomegaly syndrome there may be anaemia, thrombocytopenia and neutropenia, all secondary to hypersplenism. In the syndrome of congenital malaria, in which the infection is contracted in intrauterine life from the mother, newborn babies have a febrile illness associated with profound anaemia that appears to result from the combination of haemolysis and bone marrow suppression.

Leishmaniasis
Particularly in young children, visceral leishmaniasis, or kala azar, is associated with hepatosplenomegaly, lymphadenopathy, and a pancytopenia. Early in the course of the disease there is often marked neutropenia and the marrow may be grossly infiltrated with parasitized macrophages. The anaemia is due mainly to a short red-cell survival; there is also an inappropriate marrow response and a variable degree of hypersplenism.

Hookworm
The haematological changes of hookworm infestation are described in Chapter 22.4.3. It is one of the most common causes of iron-deficiency anaemia in the world population. During the systemic phase of the illness, when the larvae invade the lungs, there may be a marked eosinophilia. During this phase the bone marrow shows a remarkable increase in the percentage of eosinophilic myelocytes, which may be out of proportion to the eosinophilia observed in the peripheral blood.

Visceral larva migrans
This condition is characterized by striking haematological changes including anaemia, a marked leucocytosis with eosinophilia, and changes in the titre of anti-A and anti-B blood-group antibodies.

Fig. 3 Bone marrow appearances in *P. falciparum* malaria. There is marked dyserythropoiesis with several multinucleate red-cell precursors (Giemsa stain ×800).

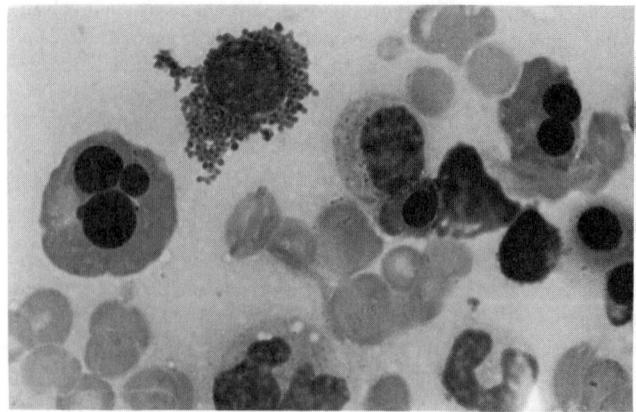

Schistosomiasis

In the chronic phase of *mansoni* and *japonicum* infections there may be severe portal hypertension, splenomegaly, and the typical picture of hypersplenism.

Other trematode infestations, including clonorchiasis and paragonamiasis, are associated with eosinophilia and anaemia. Antibodies to the P$_1$ blood-group antigen may be found in grossly elevated titres in the blood of many patients with acute fascioliasis.

Rheumatoid arthritis and related disorders

In patients with rheumatoid arthritis, anaemia is extremely common. It usually follows the general pattern of anaemia of chronic disorders. It is occasionally complicated by genuine iron deficiency, which may result from a variety of causes including poor diet and chronic blood loss due to the effects of treatment, particularly ingestion of salicylates and non-steroidal anti-inflammatory agents or corticosteroids. Furthermore, it has been found that significant bleeding occurs into actively inflamed joints and it has been estimated that if only two knee joints were affected, the annual blood loss through this mechanism could amount to as much as 2500 ml. It is not certain how much of the iron derived from this blood is available for reutilization for haemoglobin synthesis. The diagnosis of iron deficiency complicating rheumatoid arthritis may not be straightforward; levels of serum iron and iron-binding capacity may be difficult to interpret because of coexisting inflammation, and determination of marrow stores and estimation of serum ferritin may be more helpful. Although the last two are elevated in inflammatory conditions a low level suggests genuine iron deficiency.

There are no particular changes in the neutrophil response in uncomplicated rheumatoid arthritis; a marked leucocytosis may reflect a response to corticosteroid therapy or a superadded infection such as a septic arthritis. The platelet count is elevated in between 20 and 50 per cent of patients with rheumatoid arthritis. The degree of thrombocytosis parallels the degree of activity of the illness and cannot be accounted for on the grounds of associated intestinal blood loss due to drug therapy.

The haematological changes of Felty's syndrome are summarized in Section 18. There is anaemia, thrombocytopenia, and marked neutropenia. Although many of these changes are features of hypersplenism, recent studies on the neutropenia in this disorder indicate that it has a complex basis and that immune destruction of neutrophils may play a major part.

The management of the haematological manifestations of rheumatoid arthritis and Felty's syndrome is unsatisfactory. The anaemia generally reflects the activity of the disease. If there is genuine iron deficiency, iron replacement therapy is indicated. The vexed question of whether intramuscular iron administration has some non-specific effect on the anaemia of rheumatoid arthritis, even in the absence of reduced body iron stores, remains unresolved. Similarly, there is considerable controversy about the best way to manage Felty's syndrome. After splenectomy there is sometimes a dramatic rise in the neutrophil and total leucocyte counts, but this is not always associated with a decreased incidence of infection. Furthermore, some patients show no change in the white-cell count after surgery. At the present time it is difficult to advise about the best approach to the management of this condition; only if there are recurrent, life-threatening infections should splenectomy be done and, because the results are so uncertain, patients require extremely careful surveillance after the operation, and there may be some place for the use of prophylactic antibiotics in those whose neutrophil counts do not respond.

Finally, it should be remembered that there is a variety of haematological changes secondary to drug therapy for rheumatoid arthritis and related disorders. Salicylates may produce chronic blood loss, while drugs containing phenacetin produce methaemoglobinaemia and Heinz-body haemolytic anaemia that may sometimes be preceded by a marked eosinophilia. Phenylbutazone produces pancytopenia, which may be severe and irreversible; this drug has now been discontinued in the United Kingdom. Oxyphenylbutazone and penicillamine may also cause severe marrow depression. The administration of gold occasionally causes marked thrombocytopenia or pancytopenia.

Systemic lupus erythematosus and other collagen disorders

It is quite common for systemic lupus erythematosus (**SLE**) to present with a haematological disorder. This is not the case in the other collagen–vascular disorders.

The most common blood change in SLE is anaemia, which occurs in nearly all patients at some stage of the illness. It is usually a mild anaemia of chronic disorders, which may be complicated by blood loss from analgesics or anti-inflammatory medication, renal impairment, or haemolysis. Acquired autoimmune haemolytic anaemia may be the sole presenting feature in SLE and may antedate the appearance of other typical features by many years. The incidence of this complication varies in reported series but occurs overall in approximately 5 per cent of cases. The Coombs' test is invariably positive with anticomplementary reagents and is positive with anti-IgG during episodes of acute haemolysis. Other forms of anaemia in SLE include those associated with hypersplenism due to splenomegaly, and the occasional occurrence of a hypocellular bone marrow, probably due to involvement of small vessels by the disease process.

The most consistent finding in the white-cell count in SLE is leucopenia, which occurs in up to half the patients at some time during the illness. This is often a combined neutropenia and lymphopenia. Mild eosinophilia occurs occasionally, particularly in association with skin involvement.

A mild thrombocytopenia occurs in 10 to 25 per cent of all cases of SLE. More severe thrombocytopenia, producing a picture almost indistinguishable from idiopathic thrombocytopenic purpura, occurs in a small proportion of patients and may be the sole presenting feature in some. Although early reports indicated that splenectomy might be associated with a flare-up of the systemic symptoms of SLE in patients with thrombocytopenia, this has now been shown to be incorrect.

Another potentially important abnormality of coagulation in patients with SLE is the presence of the so-called lupus anticoagulant. This is a circulating anticardiolipin that is also responsible for the positive Wassermann reaction, the false-positive serological test for syphilis which occurs in this condition. This antibody, which occurs in conditions other than SLE, interferes with the binding of phospholipid to form prothrombin activator and this affects the intrinsic and extrinsic clotting pathways (see Chapter 22.6.7). Although it causes a prolonged partial thromboplastin time, its presence in patients with SLE seems to produce a clotting rather than a bleeding tendency. A significant number of patients who have the lupus anticoagulant have recurrent thrombotic episodes including cerebral thromboses. It is also associated with recurrent spontaneous abortions and, possibly, with 'idiopathic' pulmonary hypertension.

It has been suggested that the lupus anticoagulant inhibits the production of prostacyclin from vessel walls and it may interfere with the release of arachidonic acid from cell membranes. Even more interestingly, it is possible that these antibodies react with complex brain lipids such as sphingomyelin. Early reports of the presence of antibodies of this type in patients with bizarre neurological syndromes such as Jamaican neuropathy and Behçet's disease require further confirmation.

The haematological changes in the other collagen–vascular diseases are much less impressive. They are all associated with the anaemia of chronic disorders. Polyarteritis nodosa may be characterized by an eosinophilia.

The interesting syndrome of polymyalgia rheumatica and temporal arteritis may present to the haematologist (Chapter 22.4.5 and Section 18). There are usually significant haematological changes characterized by a severe anaemia of chronic disorders with a marked elevation of the

ESR. The leucocyte count is usually normal, although there may occasionally be a mild eosinophilia. There is a marked increase in the α_2- and γ-globulins, although this is polyclonal in type. This blood picture can very closely resemble that of multiple myeloma or disseminated malignancy.

Renal disease

Almost all forms of renal disease are associated with haematological changes. However, by far the most important is the severe refractory anaemia that accompanies chronic renal failure.

ANAEMIA

Anaemia is an important and intractable complication of chronic renal failure. The correlation between the blood urea nitrogen and the haemoglobin level is inconsistent. The anaemia has an extremely complex aetiology, which is only partly understood. The red cells of patients with chronic renal disease have a shortened survival, although they survive normally when injected into healthy recipients. Similarly, normal red cells have a shortened survival in uraemic recipients. The nature of the intracorpuscular defect has not been determined. Most red-cell enzymes are present at normal levels and the intracellular level of ATP is elevated. However, changes in membrane function have been demonstrated, in particular decreased activity of the Na^+-K^+ pumps; the toxic substances that cause these changes have not been identified.

In addition to a shortened red-cell survival there is impaired red-cell production in the anaemia of chronic renal failure. The fact that the anaemia of chronic renal failure can be corrected by the administration of recombinant erythropoietin suggests that the ineffective production of this hormone due to renal damage is the major aetiological factor in the anaemia of renal failure. However, using in vitro assays it has been found that the serum from patients on haemodialysis inhibits the proliferation of erythroid progenitors. The suppressive activity is found in serum fractions containing material of molecular weights ranging from 47 000 to above 150 000. Interestingly, patients on continuous ambulatory peritoneal dialysis (CAPD) have higher haemoglobin levels than those on haemodialysis. It is possible this reflects the more effective removal of middle molecular-weight molecules of this type by CAPD. Patients on haemodialysis with low haemoglobin concentrations are more likely to have fibrous replacement of their bone marrow. This has been correlated with secondary hyperparathyroidism, suggesting a role for parathyroid hormone in the bone marrow unresponsiveness and fibrosis (see Chapter 22.3.9).

The anaemia of chronic renal failure may be exacerbated by deficiency of iron resulting from excessive blood sampling, blood loss due to incorrect haemodialysis procedures, or bleeding due to defective platelet function (see below). A small proportion of patients with chronic renal failure develop splenomegaly and hypersplenism. Folate deficiency is found occasionally in patients on haemodialysis. There have been a few reports of nephrosis leading to severe urinary loss of transferrin and hence to a low plasma iron-binding capacity. Some patients with renal disease have chronic inflammatory lesions, which may lead to a superadded anaemia of chronic disorders (see Chapter 22.4.9).

The type of renal lesion is also an important factor in determining the severity of anaemia. For example, the renal failure of polycystic disease of the kidneys is associated with a relatively higher haemoglobin level than other forms of renal failure. Interestingly, the shrunken kidneys of some patients on long-term dialysis programmes develop cysts and this phenomenon is also associated with a rise in haemoglobin level. It seems likely that both these conditions are associated with a relative increase in the output of erythropoietin.

The anaemia of chronic renal failure is normochromic and normocytic unless there is associated iron deficiency. The red cells show characteristic deformities with multiple tiny spicules and contracted poikilocytes.

The capacity of the red cells for oxygen transport does not seem to be impaired. There is often an increased intracellular concentration of 2,3-diphosphoglycerate (2,3-DPG) in response to anaemia and hyperphosphataemia, and the oxygen affinity of haemoglobin is decreased. This right shift in the oxygen dissociation curve may be augmented by uraemic acidosis. However, part of the advantage of the acidosis is cancelled out by the direct effect of low pH on glycolysis and 2,3-DPG production. Intensive dialysis may cause a reduction in the concentration of intracellular phosphate, which has the effect of increasing the oxygen affinity of haemoglobin. This effect may play a part in the so-called dialysis disequilibrium syndrome.

In patients with chronic renal failure who have associated iron deficiency the red-cell indices are typical of this condition; the reduced mean corpuscle haemoglobin and volume (MCV) are corrected by iron therapy.

The bone marrow in chronic renal failure shows normoblastic erythropoiesis but the degree of erythroid hyperplasia is not compatible with the degree of anaemia, indicating suppression of erythropoiesis.

WHITE CELLS

The total and differential white-cell count is usually normal in patients with chronic renal failure. However, the phagocytic activity of granulocytes may be reduced and complement activation by haemodialysis membranes may cause stasis of white cells in the pulmonary circulation with temporary granulocytopenia. Cell-mediated immunity is also depressed.

PLATELETS AND COAGULATION

There is a variety of haemostatic defects in different forms of renal disease. Most forms of renal failure are associated with a bleeding tendency, which is seen in its most florid form in acute renal failure. The main features are purpura, and mucosal and gastrointestinal bleeding associated with abnormal platelet function and a prolonged bleeding time; these changes are reversible by dialysis. Various mechanisms have been proposed, including a direct action of metabolites on platelet function and a disturbance of prostaglandin balance because of a deficiency of a renal factor that modifies or inhibits vascular production of prostacyclin and/or platelet endoperoxide and thromboxane synthesis. The end result of these changes is an abnormality of the control of platelet cAMP causing the platelets to become refractory to aggregation agents. Many conditions that lead to renal failure are also associated with thrombocytopenia. For example, the circulating immune complexes found in patients with acute glomerulonephritis, polyarteritis nodosa or lupus nephritis may be responsible for platelet activation and the release of aggregating agents. Thrombocytopenia may also be aggravated by heparin therapy or the use of immunosuppressant drugs in patients who have received kidney grafts. Mild thrombocytopenia is well recognized in patients with functioning renal allografts. This has also been found to be associated with an inability to clear the immune complexes. Graft rejection is associated with enhanced platelet aggregation and thrombocytopenia.

The nephrotic syndrome is characterized by a marked tendency to thrombosis. This also has a complex pathogenesis. Both platelet aggregation and release reactions have been shown to be enhanced in this condition, and to improve during remission. Protein loss in the urine may also play a part. It has been found that an increased loss of antithrombin III is related to thrombotic episodes. Conversely, coagulation factors IX and XIII are also lost in the urine of patients with a nephrotic syndrome; the deficiency of factor IX may be sufficient to induce bleeding.

The haematological changes associated with the haemolytic uraemic syndrome and thrombotic thrombocytopenic purpura were considered earlier in this section (Chapter 22.4.13).

POLYCYTHAEMIA

The polycythaemias associated with renal lesions and following renal transplantation are discussed in Chapter 22.4.14.

TREATMENT OF THE HAEMATOLOGICAL COMPLICATIONS OF RENAL DISEASE

The management of the anaemia of chronic renal failure, which has been revolutionized by the availability of recombinant erythropoietin, is considered in Section 20. The management of bleeding in patients with acute renal failure is based on correction of uraemia by dialysis and appropriate replacement therapy. Peritoneal dialysis is probably more effective in reversing abnormalities of platelet function, although there is no definite evidence that one form of dialysis is superior to another. If there is severe thrombocytopenia, platelet transfusions should be given.

Gastrointestinal and liver disease

Many of the haematological changes that occur in gastrointestinal and liver disease are described in Section 14. Here we will simply summarize the haematological manifestations of those disorders that present frequently with anaemia or defective haemostasis.

GASTROINTESTINAL BLOOD LOSS

As mentioned earlier in this section, blood loss in excess of 20 ml/day will always result in a negative iron balance and ultimately in iron-deficiency anaemia, the time taken depending on the body stores of iron when the bleeding started.

The haematological picture shows the typical changes of iron-deficiency anaemia, with hypochromic, microcytic red-cell morphology. Occasionally, there are some clues that this blood picture is associated with chronic blood loss. Quite frequently there is a mild to moderate thrombocytosis, and if iron is being taken there may be a dimorphic blood picture (Fig. 4), red-cell polychromasia, and a low-grade reticulocytosis. It is always worth examining the peripheral blood film very carefully as it may give some clue as to the site of the blood loss. For example, the presence of target cells may indicate liver disease, whereas the presence of distorted cells and Howell–Jolly bodies suggests malabsorption due to adult coeliac disease complicated by hyposplenism.

Fig. 4 Peripheral blood picture associated with gastrointestinal bleeding. The red cells show a dimorphic picture with hypochromic and normochromic forms. The platelet count is elevated, a typical finding in bleeding (Giemsa stain ×600).

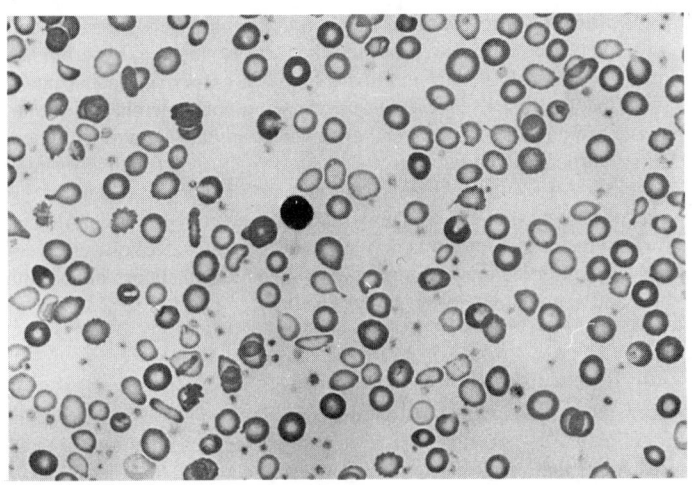

The diagnosis of the site of acute upper intestinal bleeding is considered in Section 14. The investigation of chronic gastrointestinal blood loss may be difficult. First, it is essential to determine whether iron deficiency anaemia is due to a defective intake or due to excessive loss of iron (see Chapter 22.4.4). If gastrointestinal blood loss is suspected the first step is to confirm that this is occurring, by examination of several stool specimens for occult blood. Currently, the most commonly used method is the Haemoccult card which contains a filter paper inpregnated with guaiac, or a similar commercial kit. The peroxidase activity of red blood cells releases a free oxygen radicle from hydrogen peroxide (the developer) which then reacts with the guaiac to produce a blue colour. This test is simple, easy to perform following a rectal examination, and is quick. Nevertheless, it is relatively insensitive, since blood loss must exceed 20 ml daily for 80 to 90 per cent of tests to be positive (the normal loss in a healthy individual is 0.5–1.2 ml daily as measured by ^{51}Cr-labelled red cells). False positive results may result from peroxidase or non-specific oxidants in the diet. Thus in many screening programmes, subjects are requested to omit red meat, fresh fruit, cauliflower, swede, turnip, tomatoes, horseradish, and vitamin C supplements from their diet during the 3 days prior to testing. Non-steroidal anti-inflammatory drugs and aspirin may also give positive results but, since the increased blood loss is in the upper gastrointestinal tract, the haemoglobin is metabolized in the small intestine and is therefore not detected in stools by Haemoccult unless blood loss is considerable. Iron therapy does not affect guaiac-based tests. Many newer tests which are said to be even more sensitive are being developed but their role in clinical practice is not yet established.

Once having established that there is gastrointestinal blood loss the next step is to determine the site. This requires a detailed history and clinical examination as outlined in the introduction to this section. The next step is a careful endoscopy, followed by sigmoidoscopy and colonoscopy. If these investigations do not provide a diagnosis, and there is persistent bleeding, the duodenum and small bowel should be studied radiologically. Occasionally it is necessary to resort to coeliac or superior mesenteric angiography, which may be useful for showing duodenal or ileal varices, bleeding from Meckel's diverticulum or non-specific ulcers of the ileum, small bowel tumours, and vascular lesions. However, small lesions can only be visualized if there is active bleeding at the time of the examination, probably at a rate of at least 0.5 ml min.

INFLAMMATORY DISEASES OF THE BOWEL

A mild anaemia of chronic disorders is a common accompaniment of inflammatory disease of the ileum, caecum, and colon. It is observed frequently in patients with Crohn's disease, ileocaecal tuberculosis, ulcerative colitis, and other forms of proctocolitis. In many of these conditions the anaemia of chronic disorders is often complicated by intermittent blood loss or dietetic iron deficiency. In some cases of extensive Crohn's disease there may be an added factor of malabsorption. Anaemia occurs in about one-third of patients with this condition and occasionally it may be complicated by reduced vitamin B_{12} or folic acid absorption. For example, in one large survey of patients with Crohn's disease, anaemia was present in 79 per cent of the males and 54 per cent of females. Forty-six out of a total of 63 patients had bone marrow biopsies, and of these 39 per cent were megaloblastic. Of this group, 11 were folate deficient, six vitamin B_{12} deficient, and one had both deficiencies. On the other hand, macrocytic anaemia is unusual in patients with ulcerative colitis and the anaemia is usually hypochromic due to blood loss. Interestingly, there have been occasional reports of autoimmune haemolytic anaemia occurring in association with ulcerative colitis; in several cases the autoantibodies showed rhesus specificity.

The anaemia of intestinal inflammatory disease may be made worse by drugs used in its management. Patients who receive salazopyrine for colitis occasionally develop an acute haemolytic anaemia associated with Heinz-body formation. Bone marrow depression may occur in patients receiving immunosuppressive treatment for colitis or Crohn's disease. Ileocaecal tuberculosis may be associated with any of the bizarre haematological manifestations of tuberculosis described above, and it may be complicated by the side-effects of antituberculous drug therapy.

Whipple's disease may produce a clinical picture and blood changes that can mimic several primary haematological disorders. The typical clinical triad of diarrhoea, arthropathy, and enlarged lymph nodes is usually associated with a mild normochromic, normocytic anaemia, a raised ESR, and a polymorphonuclear leucocytosis. Quite often there is associated lymphopenia or eosinophilia. Some cases present less typically, and particularly when the spleen is enlarged the condition may closely mimic a primary reticulosis. Malabsorption of vitamin B_{12} or folic acid may occasionally be encountered in this disorder (see Section 14).

STRUCTURAL DISEASE OF THE STOMACH, AND SMALL AND LARGE BOWEL

The structural changes and resulting abnormalities of absorption associated with gastritis are described in detail in Section 14. Similarly, the various anatomical abnormalities of the small-gut and malabsorption syndromes that lead to vitamin B_{12} and folate deficiency are reviewed earlier in this section. The relation between gastric surgery and iron and vitamin B_{12} metabolism is discussed in Chapters 22.4.4 and 22.4.6.

Most anatomical lesions of the small bowel present to the haematologist as a macrocytic anaemia with a megaloblastic bone marrow due to vitamin B_{12} or folate deficiency or as a refractory iron-deficiency anaemia. Several abnormalities of the small gut are associated with the production of a relatively profuse bacterial flora with subsequent utilization of vitamin B_{12}. These conditions include surgically produced blind loops, strictures, anastomoses between loops of small bowel, fistulae between various sections of the bowel, diverticula of the small bowel, malfunctioning gastroenterostomies, interference of gut motility in conditions such as scleroderma, Whipple's disease, post-vagotomy, and after extensive gut resection, where the disorder may also produce malabsorption. All these conditions are associated with defective vitamin B_{12} absorption, which can be partly corrected by the administration of broad-spectrum antibiotics but not by intrinsic factor.

Megaloblastic anaemia due to intestinal malabsorption is fully reviewed in Chapter 22.4.6. It should be remembered, however, that the malabsorption syndromes may present to the haematologist in other ways. For example, there is a very high incidence of iron-deficiency anaemia in this group and, particularly in childhood, this is the much the more common form of presentation than a megaloblastic anaemia. The peripheral blood changes of hyposplenism are quite frequently associated with an underlying malabsorption syndrome, which itself may also present with a bleeding disorder due to prothrombin deficiency following defective absorption of vitamin K. Patients with malabsorption syndrome frequently have biochemical evidence of vitamin E deficiency; although this may produce a slightly shortened red-cell survival, there is no evidence that vitamin E deficiency alone produces a significant degree of anaemia.

The relation between megaloblastic anaemia, malabsorption and immune diseases of the bowel is considered in Section 14.

LIVER DISEASE

There is usually a moderate degree of anaemia in patients with chronic liver failure (Table 4). The red cells are normochromic or slightly macrocytic with MCV values ranging from 100 to 115 fl. Target cells and a variable degree of polychromasia with a slightly elevated reticulocyte count are often found. The degree of macrocytosis and target-cell for-

Table 4 *Haematological changes in liver disease*

Virus hepatitis
Haemolytic anaemia, hypoplastic anaemia

Chronic active hepatitis
Immune haemolytic anaemia, hyperglobulinaemia

Chronic liver failure
Chronic anaemia is often complicated by:
(a) blood loss and iron deficiency
(b) alcohol, direct effect on marrow
(c) folate deficiency
(d) portal hypertension and hypersplenism
(e) acute haemolytic episodes (e.g. Zieve's syndrome, spur-cell syndrome)
Thrombocytopenia, leucopenia, haemorrhagic diathesis due to:
(a) deficiency of vitamin K-dependent factors
(b) portal hypertension and hypersplenism
(c) increased fibrinolysis
(d) thrombocytopenia

Portal hypertension
Anaemia, leucopenia, thrombocytopenia, bleeding from varices

Obstructive jaundice
Mild anaemia, target-cell formation, masking of hereditary spherocytosis

Tumours
Polycythaemia, leukaemoid reactions, alpha-fetoprotein production

Liver transplantation
Haemorrhagic and hypercoagulable states

mation corresponds reasonably well with the degree of liver failure. The bone marrow tends to be hypercellular with erythroid hyperplasia and macronormoblastic changes.

The actual mechanism of the anaemia of liver failure is uncertain. However, there may be many complicating factors that cause a worsening of the anaemia in this condition. Nutritional folate deficiency is very common in patients with liver disease, particularly the alcoholic form. Secondary iron deficiency is also common and usually results from chronic intestinal blood loss associated with a poor dietetic intake. Interestingly, in patients with severe portal hypertension and cirrhosis, or in those who have undergone portacaval shunt surgery, there may be some increase in iron absorption with marked haemosiderosis of the liver.

A variety of different forms of haemolytic anaemia occur in patients with liver disease. In Zieve's syndrome there is jaundice, hyperlipidaemia, and haemolytic anaemia that follows an excessive alcohol intake (see Chapter 22.4.13). Other forms of haemolytic anaemia may occur. Acute haemolysis has been well documented in patients with viral hepatitis, particularly those who are glucose 6-phosphate dehydrogenase deficient. An acquired haemolytic anaemia with a positive Coombs' test may occur occasionally in patients with chronic active hepatitis. Another form of haemolytic anaemia in liver disease, usually alcoholic cirrhosis, has been observed in which there are marked red-cell abnormalities with burr and spur-shaped forms predominating.

The haematological effects of alcohol

Because excessive consumption of alcohol is so common it is important for clinicians to appreciate the remarkably diverse haematological manifestations that it causes.

Anaemia is particularly common in chronic alcoholics. It has an extremely complex aetiology including a deficient diet, chronic blood loss, hepatic dysfunction, and the direct toxic effects of alcohol on the bone marrow.

Macrocytosis is particularly common in chronic alcoholics. An unexplained macrocytic blood picture should always raise the possibility of alcoholism, although its absence does not rule out the diagnosis. It may be associated with normoblastic or megaloblastic erythropoiesis. In moderately severe alcoholics who are maintaining a reasonable diet it probably reflects the direct toxic action of alcohol on the bone marrow. The normoblasts may show vacuolation or there may be no specific changes on light microscopy. Megaloblastic anaemia is usually seen in severe alcoholics who are poorly nourished, and is due to folate deficiency. While a folate-poor diet is the major factor, there is some evidence that alcohol plays a more direct part in interfering with folate metabolism by an unknown mechanism. It should be remembered that macrocytosis can also occur in alcoholics during a reticulocytosis in response to bleeding or alcohol withdrawal. It may also reflect coexistent liver disease. The occurrence of sideroblastic anaemia in severe alcoholics was mentioned in an earlier chapter (Chapter 22.4.8). It is often associated with a macrocytosis or a dimorphic blood picture and occurs in severe alcoholics. The sideroblastic changes revert to normal after stopping alcohol.

Simple iron deficiency is also found commonly in alcoholics and probably reflects both a poor diet and chronic blood loss due to gastritis or bleeding varices. It may be associated with folate deficiency; the blood film is then dimorphic with macrocytes, microcytes, and hypersegmented neutrophils. Alcoholics with chronic pancreatitis may develop iron loading due to increased absorption.

As well as these changes, which are specific for alcohol, any of the haematological manifestations of liver disease, as described earlier, may be found in alcoholics.

Alcohol also has deleterious effects on the white cells. Severe alcoholics are prone to infection. The neutropenia of alcoholism may reflect both the toxic effect of alcohol on the marrow and folate deficiency. There is also some evidence that alcohol can interfere with neutrophil locomotion and with their ability to ingest foreign material including micro-organisms.

Thrombocytopenia is commonly seen in chronic alcoholics and may occur without accompanying folate deficiency or splenomegaly. Megakaryocytes may be normal or diminished in number. Following withdrawal of alcohol the platelet count usually returns to normal, although it may become markedly elevated for a few days.

Chest disease

(see also carcinoma and tuberculosis, above, and secondary polycythaemia, Chapter 22.4.14).

PNEUMONIA

Most bacterial pneumonias are associated with a neutrophil leucocytosis. Two relatively common forms of pneumonia are associated with more specific haematological changes. In mycoplasma pneumonia, cold agglutinins can usually be detected in increased amounts towards the end of the first week in up to 80 per cent of cases. The cold antibodies are polyclonal IgM and to the red-cell I antigen. Although a positive Coombs' test has been described in these cases, and in most of them there is an increased reticulocyte count, serious haemolysis is rare. Occasionally, the condition is complicated by disseminated intravascular coagulation.

There is increasing evidence that in patients with pneumonia caused by *Legionella pneumophila* (legionnaires' disease) there may be severe thrombocytopenia and, sometimes, lymphopenia. Several cases have been reported to be complicated by disseminated intravascular coagulation.

PULMONARY EOSINOPHILIA (SEE ALSO CHAPTER 22.5.7 AND SECTION 17)

This term refers to a group of disorders that have in common a raised eosinophil count in the peripheral blood in association with pulmonary infiltrates on the chest radiograph. The exact nature of many of the disorders that constitute this syndrome is uncertain. In its simplest form there may be a brief period of respiratory distress in association with eosinophilia. This condition is sometimes called Löffler's syndrome. At the other end of the spectrum there is a severe illness associated with widespread pulmonary infiltrates and eosinophilia, which may culminate with the features of polyarteritis nodosa.

The transient disorder described by Löffler probably represents a heterogeneous group of conditions, which in many cases are associated with parasitic infection. Many parasitic disorders can cause this type of illness, including ascariasis, ankylostomiasis, trichiuriasis, taeniasis, and fascioliasis. A similar condition has been well documented as part of a hypersensitivity reaction to drugs. The most common is *p*-aminosalicylic acid but similar reactions have been observed in patients receiving penicillin, sulphonamides, and nitrofurantoin. A similar clinical picture is associated with the syndrome of allergic alveolitis, including farmer's lung, bird fancier's lung, and a variety of other occupational disorders (see Section 17).

Another condition characterized by a marked eosinophilia with pulmonary infiltrates goes under the general term tropical eosinophilia. There is considerable evidence that this disorder is due to occult filarial infection.

Another well-documented cause of pulmonary eosinophilia is hypersensitivity to fungi, particularly *Aspergillus fumigatus*.

IDIOPATHIC PULMONARY HAEMOSIDEROSIS AND GOODPASTURE'S SYNDROME (SEE SECTION 20)

These disorders occasionally present as a refractory anaemia that has the characteristics of the anaemia of chronic disorders, although it may become markedly hypochromic and microcytic due to chronic blood loss.

Skin diseases

MEGALOBLASTIC ANAEMIA AND THE SKIN

The whole relation between skin disease and megaloblastic anaemia is extremely complex and much of the work in this field is still controversial. The subject is discussed elsewhere (see Chapter 22.4.6).

There is no doubt that a proportion of patients with various dermatoses show evidence of folate depletion, at least biochemically, and in some cases, haematologically. This has been reported in patients with erythroderma, psoriasis, or extensive eczema. There is a well-documented association between malabsorption and dermatitis herpetiformis. Although megaloblastic anaemia is not found frequently in association with disorders of the skin, some patients with these conditions do have mild megaloblastic changes. Although earlier reports suggested that a significant proportion of them had abnormalities of small-intestinal function and structure, leading to the descriptive term 'dermatogenic enteropathy', this concept has been questioned and it is now agreed that a completely flat small-bowel mucosa is rarely seen in these conditions. The relation between dermatitis herpetiformis and malabsorption of the coeliac type seems to be a special case. Several series have shown a high incidence of small-bowel changes of coeliac disease in patients with this condition. Furthermore, there appears to be a high incidence of splenic hypoplasia and many patients show typical haematological changes of defective function of the spleen (see Chapter 22.5.4).

OTHER DERMATOLOGICAL DISORDERS

Several dermatological diseases have a major haematological component. Of particular importance are the systemic mast-cell syndromes (see Chapter 22.3.9), hereditary telangiectasia (see Chapter 22.6.3) and some of the inherited disorders of collagen (see Section 19).

Endocrine disease

PITUITARY DEFICIENCY

A mild, normochromic, normocytic anaemia is very common in patients with anterior pituitary deficiency. The mechanism is not absolutely clear, although the anaemia has many features in common with that of hypothyroidism and is fully responsive to appropriate replacement therapy.

THYROID DISEASE

Hypothyroidism is associated with a variety of haematological changes. Anaemia is common and may be normocytic, microcytic, or macrocytic.

Severe microcytic anaemia in hypothyroidism is most commonly seen in women who have menorrhagia, which is a frequent complication of this condition. Severe macrocytosis in hypothyroidism usually indicates an associated vitamin B_{12} deficiency; there seems to be a genuine association between pernicious anaemia and myxoedema. It has been suggested that mild macrocytosis may occur in hypothyroidism in the absence of vitamin B_{12} or folate deficiency, although published series of studies have shown a remarkable variability in the incidence of this phenomenon. Some patients with severe hypothyroidism have a small proportion of misshapen red cells on their peripheral blood films.

The anaemia of uncomplicated myxoedema is normochromic and normocytic. The mechanism is still uncertain. However, recent studies have shown that T_3, T_4, and reverse T_3 can all potentiate the effect of erythropoietin on the formation of erythroid colonies in vitro. This effect appears to be mediated by receptors with β_2-adrenergic properties. Thus it appears that the thyroid hormones have a direct effect in altering the erythropoietin responsiveness of erythroid progenitors. It has also been suggested that part of the normochromic anaemia of hypothyroidism may be a physiological adaptation to reduced oxygen requirements by the tissues.

Curiously, patients with hyperthyroidism do not have elevated haemoglobin levels. There is some recent evidence that there may be a mild increase in the red-cell mass in hyperthyroidism, but that this is compensated for by an increase in plasma volume. In some patients with severe hyperthyroidism there is a mild anaemia associated with abnormal iron utilization.

ADRENAL DISEASE

A mild, normochromic, normocytic anaemia together with neutropenia, eosinophilia, and lymphocytosis is observed in some patients with Addison's disease. There is a variety of haematological changes following the administration of corticosteroids or endogenous overproduction of these agents. These include granulocytosis, reduced lymphocyte count, involution of lymphatic tissues, and a decrease in the eosinophil and monocyte count.

PARATHYROID DISEASE

Primary hyperparathyroidism is occasionally associated with anaemia, which responds to removal of the parathyroid glands. The relation between parathyroid disease and marrow fibrosis is discussed in Chapter 22.3.9.

DIABETES MELLITUS

The structural changes that occur in the haemoglobin of diabetic patients are discussed in Chapter 22.4.7. There have been recent reports that there may be an increase in the red-cell volume of patients with severe diabetes. The mechanism and significance of this observation remains to be clarified. Severe diabetic acidosis is often associated with a marked leucocytosis, even when there is no underlying infection. Hyperosmolarity impairs neutrophil function, and reduced neutrophil migration has been observed in patients with diabetic ketoacidosis or poorly controlled hyperglycaemia. Because of the high incidence of atheroma in patients with diabetes both platelet function and vessel-wall metabolism have been studied in considerable detail in this condition. Synthesis of prostaglandin I_2 in biopsy specimens of forearm veins is reduced and a variety of changes in platelet reactivity and survival have been observed. The relation of these changes to the vascular disease of diabetes requires further clarification.

Neuropsychiatric disease

ANOREXIA NERVOSA

About a third of patients with severe anorexia nervosa have a mild, normochromic, normocytic anaemia. In patients who are severely malnourished there may be mild neutropenia. There have been reports of the finding of irregularly shaped red blood cells in this condition. The platelet count is usually normal but there may be mild thrombocytopenia and in one study there was a marked increase in the rate of platelet aggregation.

TRAUMA

The brain is rich in thromboplastin activity and acute disseminated intravascular coagulation occurs quite commonly after severe head or brain injury.

MYASTHENIA GRAVIS

The association between myasthenia gravis and pure red-cell aplasia is described in Chapter 22.3.5. An immune neutropenia has also been described as part of the myasthenia–thymoma syndrome.

LESCH–NYHAN SYNDROME

This X-linked recessive disorder is described in detail in Section 11. There have been occasional reports of the development of severe megaloblastic anaemia, presumably resulting from defective nucleic acid synthesis; the condition has been reversed by the administration of large doses of adenine.

ABETALIPOPROTEINAEMIA

This condition is characterized by an ataxic neurological disease, retinitis pigmentosa, fat malabsorption, and the absence of chylomicrons and low-density lipoproteins. It is caused by the failure to synthesize or secrete lipoprotein-containing products of the apolipoprotein B gene. It is characterized by the presence of from 50 to 90 per cent of acanthocytes in the peripheral blood. These are abnormal, spiky red cells, which have a moderately shortened survival. Despite these changes there is only a mild haemolytic anaemia.

ACANTHOCYTOSIS WITH NEUROLOGICAL DISEASE AND NORMAL LIPOPROTEINS (AMYOTROPHIC CHOREA-ACANTHOCYTOSIS)

This syndrome is characterized by marked acanthocytosis associated with a progressive neurological disease, beginning in adolescence or adult life, which includes orofacial dyskinesia, lip and tongue biting, choreaiform movements, sensorimotor polyneuropathy, distal muscle wasting, and hypotonia. Because it has been found to follow both dominant and recessive forms of inheritance it is likely that this is a heterogeneous disorder. The cause is unknown.

Cardiac disease

There are several important haematological manifestions of cardiac disease, all of which are dealt with in more detail in Section 15. The severe haemolytic anaemia that occasionally follows the insertion of prosthetic valves, particularly the aorta, is described in Chapter 22.4.13.

A variety of abnormalities of coagulation are found in patients with cyanotic congenital heart disease. These include thrombocytopenia, low plasma fibrinogen levels, defective clot retraction, a deficiency of factors V and VII, and increased levels of fibrin degradation products. Overall, the severity of these abnormalities correlates with the degree of secondary polycythaemia. The exact mechanism is not known. In addition to the quantitative changes in blood platelets there may also be qualitative abnormalities of platelet function. These include defects in both aggregation and release. They may be associated with a prolonged bleeding time. Again, the mechanism is not understood.

The striking haematological changes that may accompany bacterial endicarditis were mentioned earlier in this chapter. Dressler's syndrome may be associated with the anaemia of chronic disorders, atypical lymphocytes in the peripheral blood, and, certainly in the earlier descriptions of the disease, an eosinophilia of varying degree. Similar changes have been observed in the postpericardiotomy syndrome.

REFERENCES

Boxer, H., Ellman, L., Geller, R., and Wang, C.-A. (1977). Anemia in primary hyperparathyroidism. *Archives of Internal Medicine*, **137**, 588–90.
Castaldi, P.A. (1984). Hemostasis and kidney disease. In *Disorders of hemostasis*, (ed. O.D. Ratnoff and C.D. Forbes), pp. 473–84. Grune & Stratton, Orlando, FA.
Costello, C. (ed.). (1990). Haematology in HIV Disease. *Bailliere's Clinical Haematology*, **3**, 1–218.
Duffy, T.P. (1991). Systemic mastocytosis. In *Hematology basic principles and practice*, (ed. R. Hoffman *et al.*), pp. 1058–62. Churchill Livingstone, New York.
Erslev, A.J. (1995). Traumatic cardiac hemolytic anemia. In *Williams hematology*, (ed. E. Beutler, M.A. Lichtman, B.S. Coller, and T.J. Kipps). McGraw-Hill, New York. In press.
Eschbach, J.W. (1989). The anaemia of chronic renal failure: pathophysiology and the effects of recombinant erythropoietin. *Kidney International*, **35**, 134–48.
Goldsmith, G.H., Jr. (1984). Hemostatic disorders associated with neoplasia. In *Disorders of hemostasis*, (ed. O.D. Ratnoff and C.D. Forbes), pp. 351–66. Grune & Stratton, Orlando, FA.
Hamblin, T.J. (ed.). (1987). Haematological problems in the elderly. *Bailliere's Clinical Haematology*, **1**, 271–596.
Hardcastle, J.D. and Thomas, W.M. (1989) 'Screening an asymptomatic population for colorectal cancer.' In *Ballière's Clinical Gastroenterology*, Vol. 3, No. 3. (ed N. Mortensen) pp. 543–66. Ballière Tindall, London.
Herbert, V. (ed.) (1980). Hematologic complications of anemia in alcoholic patients. *Seminars in Hematology*, **17**, (1 and 2).
Hughes, G.R.V. (1983). The lupus anticoagulant. *British Medical Journal*, **287**, 1088–9.
Ratnoff, O.D. (1984). Hemostatic defects in liver and biliary tract diseases. In *Disorders of hemostasis*, (ed. O.D. Ratnoff and C.D. Forbes), pp. 451–72. Grune & Stratton, Orlando, FA.
St John, D.J.B., Young, G.P., *et al.* (1993). Evaluation of new occult blood tests for detection of colorectal neoplasia. *Gastroenterology*, **104**, 1661–8.
Stockman, J.A.I. and Ezekowitz, A. (1993). Hematologic manifestations of systemic diseases. In *Hematology of infancy and childhood*, (ed. D.G. Nathan and F.A. Oski), pp. 1834–85. Saunders, Philadelphia.
Weatherall, D.J. (1993). Hematologic manifestations of systemic diseases in children of the third world. In *Hematology of Infancy and Childhood*, (ed. D.G. Nathan and F.A. Oski), pp. 1886–904. Saunders, Philadelphia.
Zaroulis, C.G., Kourides, J.A., and Valeri, C.R. (1978). Red cell 2, 3-diphosphoglycerate and oxygen affinity of hemoglobin in patients with thyroid disorders. *Blood*, **52**, 181–5.

22.8 Blood replacement

22.8.1 Blood transfusion

H. H. GUNSON AND V. J. MARTLEW

Blood transfusion has developed from the early discoveries of antigenic differences between the red blood cells of human beings. Several hundred blood-group antigens have now been defined on red cells, leucocytes, and platelets, and they comprise one of the most complex polymorphisms known in man. From this base, increasing knowledge of the physicochemical properties of cellular and plasma components acquired during the past two decades has prepared the way for modern transfusion therapy. The ever-increasing pharmacopoeia of chemotherapeutic agents requires the availability of blood components in order that they may be used to their maximum advantage.

The transfusion of blood and its components must not be undertaken lightly. Although this procedure may have benefits to the patient it also carries hazards, which must be thoroughly understood. It is not possible in the course of this chapter to discuss all aspects of immunohaematology and blood transfusion, and the reader is referred to specialized texts.

Blood-group antigens and antibodies

RED-CELL ANTIGENS

Antigens present on the surface membrane of red cells are developed as a result of gene action or interaction. Sets of antigens may show a relation to each other, and when their inheritance is independent of other sets are regarded as belonging to a blood-group system. Many such systems are known; those encountered most frequently are summarized in Table 1. Some blood-group antigens (e.g. Rhesus (**Rh**)) are confined to red cells, whilst others may be present in the tissues or on the surface of other body cells (e.g. A, B, and Lewis). The physiological function of the red-cell antigens is not known, although some may serve to maintain the integrity of the membrane.

RED-CELL ANTIBODIES

Red-cell antibodies are immunoglobulins, of which there are five classes, IgG, IgM, IgA, IgD, and IgE, each comprising heavy chains, which characterize the immunoglobulin, and light chains (κ and λ), which are common to each type. Blood-group antibodies are principally

Table 1 *Some examples of blood-group systems and their common antigens*

Blood group system	Symbols of common antigens
ABO	$A_1 A_2$ B H
Rhesus	C D E c e
MNS	M N S s
P	$P_1 P_2$
Kell	K k
Lewis	$Le^a Le^b$
Lutheran	$Lu^a Lu^b$
Duffy	$Fy^a Fy^b$
Kidd	$Jk^a Jk^b$
Ii	I i

Table 2 *The immunoglobulin nature of some common blood-group antibodies*

Blood-group antibody	Immunoglobulin
anti-A	
anti-B	IgG + IgM + IgA
anti-Rh	IgG + IgM
anti-K	
anti-k	Usually IgG
anti-Fya	Usually IgG
anti-Jka	IgM and/or IgG
anti-P1	IgM
anti-Lea	
anti-Leb	IgM

Table 3 *The ABO groups, corresponding naturally occurring antibodies, and frequencies in the United Kingdom*

Group of red cells	Antibody in serum	Approximate frequency (UK) (%)
A_1	anti-B	32
A_2	anti-B (+ anti-A_1 in 10%)	10
B	anti-A	8
0	anti-A+ anti-B	47
A_1B	None	2.3
A_2B	None or anti-A_1 (in 25%)	0.7

group systems, ABO(H) and Rh, have the most clinical importance. A brief review of these systems follows, with comments on other systems.

THE ABO GROUPS

The commonly encountered groups in the ABO system and their corresponding antibodies are shown in Table 3. The frequencies of the different groups vary throughout the world; thus group B diminishes in frequency from east to west. The frequencies given in Table 3 are an average for the United Kingdom.

Anti-A and anti-B combine with their corresponding antigens over a wide range of temperatures *in vitro* and can do so readily *in vivo*. It can be appreciated, therefore, that the transfusion of ABO-incompatible blood may lead to the destruction of the transfused cells with, often, serious complications for the patient (see below).

Group O red cells do not bind anti-A or anti-B. It is possible, therefore, to transfuse group O blood to patients of other AB groups. Recourse is taken to this procedure in emergency when time does not permit the determination of the patient's group before transfusion. A cautionary word must be given about this practice. Certain group O individuals have high concentrations of anti-A (and possibly anti-B). These antibodies may attain a level that is sufficient to cause destruction of a proportion of the patient's red cells.

Laboratory investigations (see below) can be made to minimize the undesirable effect of such 'dangerous universal donors'. The frequent use of group O blood, particularly in large quantities, for the transfusion of group A, B, and AB patients should be avoided. Anti-A_1 can be found in group A_2 and more frequently in group A_2B persons. *In vitro*, this antibody is usually reactive only at temperatures considerably lower than 37 °C, and will not cause accelerated red-cell destruction *in vivo*; occasional examples have been found to react at 37 °C, and only in these instances need appropriate blood lacking the antigen be selected for transfusion.

THE RH BLOOD GROUPS

Table 4 illustrates the common Rh groups found in the United Kingdom with their approximate frequencies. The five common antigens known are C, D, E, c, and e. Controversy has existed for decades regarding the mechanism for inheritance of the Rh antigens and four nomenclatures have been proposed. The two shown in Table 4 are in common use.

Patients who have the genotype *rr* do not readily develop anti-C or anti-E and RhD-negative blood is used for transfusion. Fully phenotyped blood is reserved for patients known to have anti-C and/or anti-E. All Rh-positive blood possesses the D antigen. A variant of the D antigen, D^u, is found in a small proportion of whites, and more frequently in blacks. A characteristic of the D^u antigen is its poor reactivity *in vitro*, and this results from the presence of fewer D antigen sites per red cell than normal. It may be a directly inherited characteristic or arise as a result of suppression of D antigen activity by the r' or Ry chromosomes in the *trans* position (see Fig. 1).

The most common antibody encountered in the Rh blood-group sys-

IgG and/or IgM, although those with IgA specificity have been found. Usually IgA antibodies coexist with molecules that are IgG or IgM. The nature of alloantibodies in the common blood-group systems is shown in Table 2. In autoimmune acquired haemolytic anaemia, monoclonal autoantibodies with blood-group specificity may be found, often with the specificity of anti-I, but more commonly IgG polyconal autoantibodies are detected; in a few instances specific IgA autoantibodies have been defined.

The presence of an antibody is usually dependent upon stimulation with the appropriate antigen. Thus a person who is Rh-negative can develop anti-Rh if transfused with Rh-positive red cells. The development of such antibodies results from a complex cellular interaction in the reticuloendothelial system. Antibodies are termed 'naturally occurring' when there is no obvious antigenic stimulus. The mechanism for the development of such antibodies is uncertain, but antigens closely similar to those of blood groups present in bacteria and foodstuffs may be the source. The most common, naturally occurring antibodies belong to the ABO blood-group system.

Antibodies can combine with their corresponding antigen (or possibly closely related antigens when cross-activity occurs). The combination of an antibody with a red cell may result in a change that can be observed *in vitro*. It is in this manner that many of the blood-group systems have been discovered, and is the basis for compatibility testing (see below). Red cells may also be damaged by the binding of antibodies *in vivo*, leading to accelerated destruction. Dependent on the rate and manner of this destruction, incompatible transfusion reactions may occur.

Blood-group systems

Whilst the detection of antibodies to many of the blood-group systems in the serum of a patient may be important in transfusion, two blood-

Table 4 *Common Rh phenotypes and genotypes, and their frequencies in the United Kingdom*

Phenotypes	Most common genotype	Frequency in UK (%)
R$_1$r, CcDee	*CDe/cde*	34
R$_2$r, ccDee	*cDE/cde*	13
R$_1$R$_2$, CcDEe	*CDe/cDE*	13
R$_1$R$_1$, CCDee	*CDe/CDe*	18
R$_2$R$_2$, ccDEE	*cDE/cDE*	3
R$_0$r, ccDee	*cDe/cde*	2
rr, ccee	*cde/cde*	15
r'r, Ccee	*Cde/cde*	1
r"r, ccEe	*cdE/cde*	1

tem is anti-D and is found when RhD-negative persons are subjected to stimulation with RhD-positive red cells; exposure to red cells is a prerequisite because the Rh antigens are confined to human red-cell membranes.

Anti-D can develop in RhD-negative mothers during pregnancy as a result of spontaneous transplacental haemorrhage of fetal RhD-positive red cells. Although transplacental haemorrhage can occur at any time during a pregnancy, and anti-D alloimmunization has resulted from spontaneous or induced abortions in the early weeks of gestation, it is most common at the time of delivery. The administration of anti-D immunoglobulin within 72 h of transplacental haemorrhage (dosage: 250 i.u. (50 µg) up to 20 weeks' gestation and 500 i.u. (100 µg) after 20 weeks or within 72 h of delivery) has greatly reduced the incidence of anti-D alloimmunization. Failures, however, do occur in approximately 2 per cent of patients; approximately one-half of these are because the anti-D immunoglobulin is not given; the remainder are due to inadequate dosage or from too great a delay between the transplacental haemorrhage and the administration of immunoglobulin. The first of the biological causes can be avoided by obtaining an estimate of degree

of haemorrhage by means of a Kleihauer test, which comprises the washing out of haemoglobin in adult cells on a blood film by an acid solution that leaves those containing fetal haemoglobin intact (Fig. 2). Although the standard dose of 500 i.u. (100 µg) will be sufficient to prevent alloimmunization in over 99 per cent of instances, in the remainder dosage should be increased to 125 i.u. (25 µg)/ml of fetal red cells in the maternal circulation. The delay between administration of immunoglobulin and transplacental haemorrhage that leads to a failure to prevent alloimmunisation is usually due to fetomaternal haemorrhage during gestation. Giving two doses of 500 i.u. (100 mg) anti-D immunoglobulin during pregnancy has been recommended to prevent this, but is not universally done.

The inadvertent transfusion of RhD-positive red cells to an RhD-negative person can also result in anti-D alloimmunization. As this can lead to serious Rh-haemolytic disease of the newborn in subsequent pregnancies, efforts should be made to remove these incompatible red cells in women of childbearing age by giving anti-D immunoglobulin intramuscularly in divided doses over 24 h at the dosage of 125 i.u. (25 mg)/ml of transfused red cells. Provided that clearance occurs within 6 to 8 days, alloimmunization is usually prevented. Intravenous preparations of anti-D immunoglobulin have been used to clear incompatible red cells from the circulation. Care must be exercised with this form of treatment, however, because the rapid removal of a large number of red cells can lead to undesirable effects from a significant, rapid haemolysis.

In some women, anti-D may fall to low or even indetectable levels during the course of many years, but antibody production will rapidly respond to further stimulation. Thus, women of unknown group or RhD− should always be given RhD-negative blood; failure to do so may lead to serious, or even fatal, transfusion reactions.

RhD-positive individuals may develop Rh antibodies. Anti-E and anti-c are the most commonly encountered. Such patients should be transfused with blood lacking the corresponding antigen. If anti-E is found in an R$_1$R$_1$ patient it is advisable to transfuse R$_1$R$_1$ blood because such patients also lack c antigen; giving E-negative, c-positive blood (e.g. R$_1$r), although compatible, may stimulate the formation of anti-c.

Fig. 1 Suppression of D antigen activity by the r' (*Cde*) chromosome in the *trans* position.

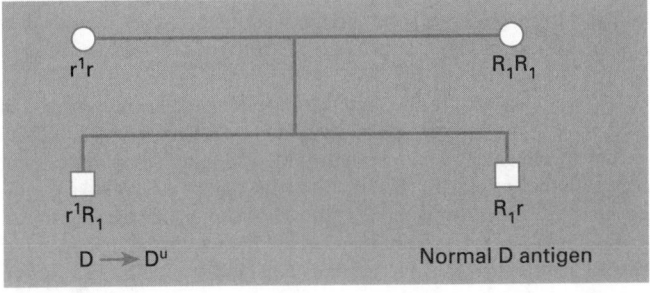

Fig. 2 Appearance of 1 in 100 fetal red cells in the Kleihauer test. The fetal red cells retain their haemoglobin whilst the adult red cells appear as 'ghosts'.

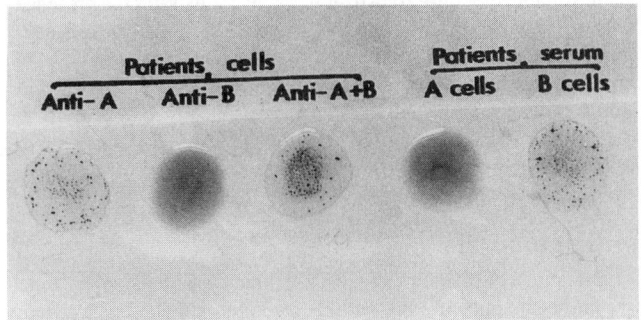

OTHER BLOOD GROUPS

Blood-group antibodies that belong to systems other than ABO and Rh are found in the sera of patients. Some (e.g. Lewis, Ii) are naturally occurring, while others are immune (e.g. Kell, Duffy, Kidd) and in these a history will be elicited of previous transfusion or, occasionally, of previous pregnancies. The selection of appropriate blood for transfusion can be done in the laboratory, and the difficulty in providing blood will depend on the frequency of donors lacking the appropriate antigen.

LEUCOCYTE AND PLATELET ANTIGENS AND ANTIBODIES

Much work has been done on the antigens of leucocytes, and a complex system of human leucocyte antigens (**HLA**) has been defined. These antigens are expressed on lymphocytes and platelets, and possibly also on other leucocytes. Platelets and neutrophils also possess specific antigens. The antigens of the ABO system are also present on leucocytes and platelets.

Leucocyte antigens have been extensively investigated in connection with organ transplantation, but they also have importance in transfusion. Antibodies to leucocytes and platelets may arise as a result of transfusion and pregnancy, and may cause troublesome pyrexial reactions in patients requiring long-term transfusion (see below).

Compatibility tests

In general, all red-cell preparations should be tested for direct compatibility before transfusion. The only exception to this rule occurs in severe haemorrhage when time does not permit testing. In such emergencies, group O, Rh-negative blood is used, and in many hospitals these units of blood are also Kell-negative, and have been screened for lower than average levels of anti-A and anti-B.

The compatibility test comprises the determination of the ABO and Rh group of the patient, and a cross-match of the donor red-cell sample with the serum of the patient. In many laboratories, before non-urgent transfusion, antibody screening tests against a panel of typed red cells are also included.

Whilst the tests themselves are done in the laboratory, compatibility tests begin with the patient. Most transfusion accidents result from clerical errors, with blood being given to a wrongly identified patient. It is important that samples for compatibility tests are taken into tubes labelled correctly with the patient's name, and other identification, address or hospital number for example, and the date of collection. The multiple numbering systems in use in some hospitals are excellent safety procedures; an individual number is placed on the patient's wrist-band, and the same number attached to the specimen bottle, the request form, and any units of blood supplied for the patient. This allows an additional check to be made. Prelabelling specimen tubes for several patients before the collection of the samples is extremely dangerous, and must never be practised. The request form is a valuable document and should be completed fully; adequate clinical information is essential for the staff in the laboratory, and lack of information often leads to unnecessary investigations and frustrating delays.

Grouping, cross-matching, and tests for antibody activity depend upon the characteristics of the reaction, *in vitro*, between a blood-group antibody and its corresponding antigen. A brief review of the principles of these tests is valuable to the understanding of transfusion hazards.

AGGLUTINATION TESTS

Some antibodies have the ability to agglutinate appropriate red cells suspended in saline (0.15 M NaCl) at temperatures up to 37 °C. Many of these antibodies, often referred to as saline agglutinins, are IgM, and common examples are anti-A and anti-B. Fig. 3 is a photograph of the reactivity of group A red cells with anti-A, anti-B, and group O serum (anti-A + B). The serum of this patient agglutinates group B cells and thus contains anti-B; negative reactions can be distinguished by lack of agglutination.

Not all antibodies will agglutinate saline-suspended red cells. However, prior treatment of the red cells with certain proteolytic enzymes (e.g. papain) will effect agglutination. Also, the addition of colloids (e.g. bovine serum albumin) will enable agglutination to occur in some instances. Such antibodies tend to be IgG in nature and common examples are certain Rh antibodies, anti-Kell, and anti-Duffy.

During the past few years it has been found that by reducing the ionic

Fig. 3 Agglutination reactions in the determination of ABO blood group: Group A, see Table 3.

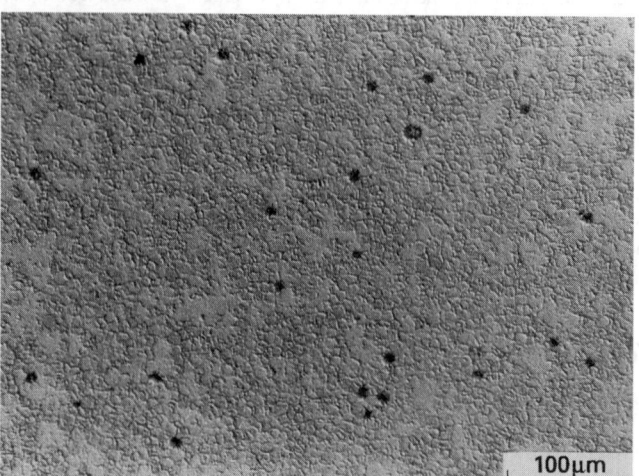

100μm

strength of the reacting mixture of antibody and red cells, antibody will become attached to the red cells more rapidly, that is, the rate of association is increased. This principle has been employed in both blood grouping and cross-matching tests in an attempt to reduce the time involved in these procedures.

THE ANTIGLOBULIN TEST

An antiglobulin serum is raised in animals, usually rabbits, sheep or goats, by injection with human immunoglobulins and complement components. The resultant immune serum is absorbed with normal human red cells to remove species-specific antibodies. Various types of reagents can be prepared. That most commonly used in cross-matching is the broad-spectrum reagent, and contains anti-IgG, anti-IgA, and possibly anti-IgM, together with certain antibodies to complement components, notably antibodies to fragments of C3 and C4. Monoclonal antiglobulin reagents can be prepared from cultured cell lines. This is the preferred method for the preparation of the anticomplement component of the antiglobulin reagent.

When some IgG antibodies bind to red cells suspended in saline, agglutination does not occur. If such sensitized cells are washed to remove contaminating proteins, the antibody immunoglobulin on adjacent red cells may combine with the anti-IgG present in the antiglobulin serum, and agglutination results.

Some blood-group antibodies have the ability to fix complement. Complement comprises a group of nine major components present in plasma of all individuals and activated by certain antigen–antibody complexes to produce an enzyme cascade. If this reaction proceeds to completion via blood-group antibodies, haemolysis of the red cells results. Few examples of blood-group antibodies will produce haemolysis *in vitro*, although certain examples of anti-A and anti-B will do so. More often the complement-fixing antibody causes fixation of C1 to C4. C3 is bound to the red cell as the fragment C3b, which converts rapidly to C3c, C3g, and C3d. It is advantageous to have all these antibodies in the antiglobulin reagent. However, high concentrations of anti-C3d may result in false-positive reactions when the test is used to detect antibodies (i.e. the indirect test), particularly if incubation times in excess of 1 h are used. When the patient's own red cells are sensitized *in vivo* the only complement component on the cells is C3d; thus the same reagent can be used for direct and indirect tests. Some antiglobulin reagents contain anti-C4 but high concentrations are undesirable because they can detect traces of C4 fragments on unsensitized red cells and lead to false-positive results.

IgM antibodies almost always fix complement and the presence of an IgM antibody on a red cell is usually more easily detected by reactivity with anti-complement than with anti-IgM. The latter component is not essential in the antiglobulin serum. Many IgG antibodies fail to fix complement (e.g. anti-Rh) but others have this ability on occasions (e.g. anti-Kell, anti-Duffy). The ability of an antibody to fix complement has a bearing on the rapidity with which incompatible red cells are removed from the circulation (see below).

By using a combination of the serological tests described above in combination with a test cell panel, it is usually possible to determine the specificity of blood-group antibodies present in the patient's serum, and obtain suitable blood for transfusion. Table 5 illustrates the presence of anti-D + anti-Kell in the serum of a group 0 Rh-negative, Kell-negative patient when tested against such a cell panel; antibodies to the other systems that have been defined on these cells have been excluded and cells 4 and 6 would be suitable for transfusion, since they are rr K neg. Cell 8 could also be transfused even though it is E antigen positive (see section on Rh groups).

Hazards of transfusion

The complications of blood transfusion are often classified by their time of onset into acute and chronic, but this results in a degree of overlap.

Table 5 *Example of a serological investigation: detection of anti-D and anti-Kell*

													Compatibility tests			
					Groups of test red cells								Indirect antiglobulin	Agglutination		
														16 °C	37 °C	Albumin
ABO	Rh	MNSs	P_1	Le^a	Le^b	K	Lu^aLu^b	Fy^a	Fy^b	Jk^a	Jk^b					
O	R_1R_1	MMSs	+	+	−	−	− +	+	−	+	−	++++	−	−	+++
O	R_2R_2	MNSs	+	−	+	+	− +	+	+	+	−	++++	−	++	+++
O	R_1R_2	NNss	−	−	+	−	+ −	−	+	+	+	++++	−	−	+++
O	rr	MNSs	+	−	+	+	− +	+	−	−	−	−	−	−	−
O	rr	MMSS	+	−	−	+	− +	−	+	+++	−	++	−	++	++
O	rr	NNSs	−	+	−	−	− +	+	+	+	−	−	−	−	−
O	r′r	MNSs	+	−	−	+	− +	+	−	−	+	+++	−	++	++
O	r″r	MMss	+	−	+	−	− +	+	+	+	+	−	−	−	−

Patient: Group O Rh-negative (rr), Kell-negative

Table 6 *Some potential hazards of transfusion*

Complications of blood transfusion	
Immune	Non-immune

1. Haemolytic
(a) Immediate, e.g., ABO antibodies
(b) Delayed, e.g., Rhesus antibodies
 	
2. Leucocyte antibodies
(a) HLA
(b) antineutrophil, e.g. anti-NAA′
 	
3. Platelet antibodies
(a) HLA
(b) anti-PLA′
 	
4. Plasma allergy
 	
5. Pyrogen response e.g. anti-Iga antibodies
	1. Cardiovascular
	(a) Circulatory overload
	(b) Thrombophlebitis
	(c) Venous thrombosis
	(d) Air embolism
	
	2. Transfusion haemosiderosis
	
	3. Sequelae of massive transfusion
	
	4. Transmission of infection
	(a) Bacterial
	(b) Protozoal, e.g. malaria
	(c) Spirochaetal, e.g. syphilis; yaws
	(d) Viral:
	  (i) Hepatitis A, B, C; non-A, non-B, non-C
	  (ii) Cytomegalovirus
	  (iii) Epstein–Barr virus
	  (iv) HIV-1 and -2

An alternative is to consider possible causes and these fall broadly into two groups, immune and non-immune, as indicated in Table 6.

IMMUNE HAZARDS

Haemolytic

Increased destruction of red cells gives rise to a haemolytic transfusion reaction, which may be immediate or delayed. The usual cause is administration of donor red cells that are incompatible with antibody in the patient's plasma.

Avoidance of this complication is the aim of the major cross-match, which should be done with patient's serum and cells from all units for transfusion. The clinical effect is dependent on several factors, in particular the dose of antigen administered, the quality and quantity of antibody, and the site of lysis.

The dose of antigen is determined by the concentration of antigen per erythrocyte and the amount of blood given. Thus, the consequences of transfusion of group A cells to a group O patient (whose plasma contains anti-A and anti-B) will vary according to the donor's A-antigen status. More extensive destruction of A_1 cells would be expected than of A_2 cells, as the latter have fewer A-antigen sites per cell. Rapid transfusion of a large quantity of incompatible blood may produce little haemolysis initially, because the antibody in the recipient's plasma will be absorbed out by the excess transfused red-cell antigen and the number of antibody molecules per cell insufficient to initiate destruction. Within a few days, however, a sharp rise in antibody production gives rise to enough cell binding for a delayed haemolytic reaction.

There is a tendency for antibodies present in low concentration to cause less red-cell destruction. In certain instances, a recipient may have no detectable antibody before transfusion, although previous exposure to an antigen may have initiated the immune response, leaving the patient 'primed'. Re-exposure to the appropriate antigen, often in the Rhesus or Kidd system, then generates a secondary antibody response and another mechanism for delayed haemolysis in 4 to 7 days. The binding affinity (avidity) of antibody for antigen influences the course of the reaction and is dependent on many factors, such as pH and temperature. In general, those antibodies with low avidity evoke less red-cell destruction.

The liberation of haemoglobin directly into the circulation is a result of intravascular haemolysis, which usually follows complement-mediated, red-cell destruction. Extravascular haemolysis may occur also over a period of days. Red cells are destroyed in the reticuloendothelial system—principally in liver and spleen, but haemoglobinaemia is less common.

CLINICAL FEATURES OF HAEMOLYTIC REACTIONS

Immediate

Rapid intravascular haemolysis of incompatible red cells produces the most severe presentation, with fever, rigors, and haemoglobinaemia. The haemoglobin dissociates into dimers for haptoglobin binding before removal in the liver. Once haptoglobin carrier molecules are saturated, free plasma haemoglobin is oxidized to methaemoglobin. The globin chain dissociates to form methaemalbumin, which may be detected spectroscopically in the Schumm's test. Another means of haemoglobin excretion is via the renal tract but, unfortunately, the attendant red-cell stroma and immune complexes may damage the kidney and contribute to the shock that precipitates renal failure. Skin flushes and chest pain are a consequence of the liberation of vasoactive substance, which may also give rise to disseminated intravascular coagulation.

Delayed

The features of extravascular haemolysis often start after the transfusion has been completed when the patient has been 'primed' by previous exposure to an incompatible antigen. There is a failure of the anticipated rise in haemoglobin, often accompanied by post-transfusion jaundice. Haemoglobinaemia and haemosiderinuria occur less frequently. Sometimes the only indication is a progressive anaemia.

It is not possible to match all the red-cell antigens of the donor with those of the patient. In practice, ABO- and Rhesus-compatible blood is prepared for patients and fortunately few transfusions lead to production of all antibodies. Their incidence increases with exposure to other antigens in pregnancy or repeated blood transfusion. Occasionally, red-cell antibodies may be formed after only one unit of blood, and this risk makes it difficult to justify administration of a single unit to an adult.

Leucocyte antibodies

These may give rise to pyrexial episodes about 30 min from the start of their infusion. They are more commonly found in patients receiving repeated transfusions and they may also occur during pregnancy.

Two sets of antigens may be involved—the general HLA and specific neutrophil systems (e.g. NA[1]; NA[2]).

Reactions resulting from leucocyte antibodies may be avoided by the prior removal of leucocytes by filtration or by the administration of leucocyte-poor blood. Should such patients require granulocyte transfusions, the choice of donors who share major HLA antigens as well as ABO and Rhesus groups may then prevent these unpleasant side-effects. Rarely, anti-NA[1] antibodies produce immune neutropenia about a week after transfusion in the few individuals (2 per cent) who have NA[2] antigens on their neutrophils.

Platelet antibodies

Pyrexial episodes 30 min into a transfusion may also occur as a result of non-specific leucocyte antibodies (anti-HLA) reacting with white-cell contaminants in transfused platelets. The clinical features are identical with reactions to leucocyte antibodies. Rarely, the platelet count may fall about 1 week after transfusion as the donor platelets are destroyed by specific platelet antibodies; anti-PLA[1] occurring in a patient with PLA[2] platelets for example. This is usually a self-limiting condition as transfused platelets disappear within 10 days. Attempts are now being made to prepare platelet concentrates with low levels of leucocyte contamination or leucocytes can be removed by prior filtration.

Plasma reaction

Urticaria may occur as a result of the administration of blood products and is occasionally associated with dyspnoea. These are allergic phenomena, usually relieved by antihistamines in the acute phase. These drugs should be given directly into the patient and not placed in the blood. Certain individuals lack IgA and their introduction to foreign immunoglobulin leads to the development of class-specific anti-IgA. Subsequent transfusions may be complicated by a severe allergic response, with fever, bronchospasm, colic, and hypertension followed by shock. This may be avoided by careful washing of red cells to remove plasma containing IgA or the choice of IgA-deficient donors to provide appropriate blood products.

Pyrogen response

Pyrogens are produced as a result of products of metabolic processes within organisms such as bacteria and viruses. They are often heat-resistant polysaccharides, capable of producing a febrile reaction, and must be excluded from all materials used for transfusion.

NON-IMMUNE HAZARDS

Cardiovascular

Circulatory overload

Rapid infusion of large volumes of fluid increases the workload of the heart. This may precipitate acute left ventricular failure with pulmonary oedema, jugulovenous engorgement, and tachycardia, particularly in the elderly who may already have degenerative vascular disease. This is best avoided by slow transfusion in patients at risk, and prophylactic diuretic therapy where fluid overload is already established.

Thrombophlebitis

Local inflammation is common at the site of intravenous cannulae for transfusion. It may be averted by an aseptic procedure for cannulation, and regular resiting of peripheral lines to avoid infection. It should rarely be necessary to prescribe antibiotics for this problem in an immunocompetent individual.

Venous thrombosis

This is a rare complication of intravenous therapy, more frequently seen where long catheters are in place for some time. Appropriate anticoagulation may be required to prevent subsequent pulmonary embolism from a large thrombosed vein.

Air embolism

A dangerous amount of air (10 ml) may be introduced into the circulation when pressure is applied to a bottle with an airway. This risk has largely been eliminated by the collection of blood in plastic packs that collapse as they empty. Some plasma products (e.g. albumin, intravenous immunoglobulin) are, however, still contained in bottles.

Transfusion haemosiderosis (see also Chapter 27.4.4)

Each 500-ml unit of blood contains approximately 250 mg of iron, while the excretion rate is only 1 mg daily. In the absence of bleeding, iron, from repeated transfusions, accumulates in all tissues, with a predilection for skin, liver, pancreas, heart and gonads, and gives rise to symptoms of haemosiderosis. This will occur in any individual in receipt of transfusion of more than 80 units of red cells, that is, 20 g of iron. In patients with high transfusion requirements (e.g. thalassaemia major), chelation therapy should be undertaken to prevent iron deposition. Desferrioxamine may be given intravenously with blood (usually 1 g per unit transfused). Where an iron overload is established, regular domiciliary subcutaneous therapy is required most nights to prevent further accumulation.

Complications of massive transfusion (see also Chapter 22.6.6)

Massive transfusion is the term used to describe replacement of circulating blood volume by transfusion within 24 h. The amount transfused to achieve this state will therefore depend upon body weight. Such a large volume may give rise to special problems in patients who are usually very ill, as follows.

Hypocalcaemia

This is the consequence of rapid removal of anticoagulant citrate ions from the plasma by circulating cells. A normal adult can withstand 500 ml every 5 min without supplementary calcium, but this facility may be impaired in liver failure or hypothermia. Under these circumstances, 10 ml of 10 per cent calcium gluconate may be injected intravenously with cardiac monitoring under controlled conditions.

Hypothermia

This follows rapid infusion of blood straight from refrigeration at 4 °C and may be avoided by the use of a blood warmer and adequate heating of the patient's room. Prevention of cooling in this way reduces the incidence of hypocalcaemia, acidosis, and potassium accumulation by providing an optimal temperature for metabolic processes to continue in the patient. Great care must be exercised to ensure that the temperature of fluid infused never exceeds 37 °C.

Hyperkalaemia

This rarely complicates transfusion in the adult unless the rate exceeds 150 ml/min or renal function is impaired. There is, however, a steady loss of potassium from red cells with time to 30 mmol/l after 21 days. This is significant in the neonatal period where blood older than 5 days should not be given. For exchange transfusion of neonates, red cells less than 48 h old are preferable to avoid potassium toxicity, although for logistic reasons it is often necessary to extend this period by a further 24 h.

Persistent bleeding

This may arise from one or more of a variety of causes (see Chapter 22.6.6). Stored blood or red cells lack platelets, are depleted of several coagulation factors, and in large volumes have a dilutional effect on the patient's circulation. Furthermore, massive transfusion may itself give rise to disseminated intravascular coagulation with consumption of coagulation factors and platelets. Bleeding postoperatively is a particularly common problem following cardiopulmonary bypass for cardiac surgery, although volumes of blood used may not be truly 'massive'.

In either case, it is advisable to give two units of fresh frozen plasma, and on some occasions platelet concentrate as well, for approximately every five units of stored blood given rapidly. This should be monitored with a coagulation profile before and after transfusion.

2, 3-diphosphoglycerate depletion

There is a downward trend of 2, 3-diphosphoglycerate (**2, 3-DPG**) on storage of blood, which is less marked when citrate phosphate dextrose (CPD) is used as anticoagulant compared with acid citrate dextrose (ACD). 2, 3-DPG is one of the controlling factors in release of oxygen from haemoglobin and this is impaired when 2, 3-DPG falls on storage, leading to one of the few valid reasons for requesting whole blood within a few days of collection. Infusion of excess citrate and lactic acid in red cells contributes to acidosis. This impairs erythrocyte metabolism, but it is rarely necessary to correct the fall in pH with bicarbonate infusion.

TRANSMISSION OF INFECTION

Potentially there are many infectious agents that may be transmitted by blood. However, to minimize transmission, donors are carefully selected. In the United Kingdom, routine screening of all donations is done for *Treponema pallidum*, HBsAg, anti-HCV, and anti-HIV-1 and 2 (see below). Additionally, fractionated plasma products are virally inactivated before issue. Individual infections are described in Section 7.

Treponemal

In the United Kingdom, syphilis is the most common organism in this class transmitted by blood. It does not present a great threat to the recipient's health, as spirochaetes rarely survive for more than 3 days at 4 °C and are sensitive to antibiotic therapy. However, it may present a potential hazard in platelet concentrates stored at 22 °C. All units of blood for transfusion are screened serologically and confirmed positive donors are permanently withdrawn and referred for appropriate specialist follow-up.

Viral hepatitis

Different patterns are recognized clinically and serologically in the transmission of hepatitis.

Hepatitis A is a common childhood disease and is spread by the faeco-oral route. The antigen may be recognized serologically. Its course is normally mild and it is rarely a problem in blood transfusion.

Hepatitis B may be transmitted by transfusion of certain blood and blood products. Its incidence in Western countries is low, and its spread by blood transfusion has been much reduced over the last 20 years by the routine testing of all donations for hepatitis B surface antigen (**HbsAg**), preferably by the sensitive enzyme-linked immunosorbent assay technique. Donors with high levels of hepatitis B surface antibody now contribute specific immunoglobulin for the passive immunization of those at risk of the disease. The implications of hepatitis testing are discussed elsewhere, but all carriers are permanently withdrawn from service as blood donors and should be offered specialist counselling.

Hepatitis C virus (**HCV**) may also cause post-transfusion hepatitis. Its incubation period is shorter than hepatitis B. In most cases, the virus causes jaundice with minimal symptoms. Half will make a complete recovery, but the other half of patients go on to develop chronic active hepatitis and 10 per cent of these progress to cirrhosis.

Hepatitis C antibody screening of all blood donations in the United Kingdom has been routine practice since September 1991, and donors found to have the antibody are withdrawn from service.

Non-A, non-B, non-C hepatitis

There remains a very small number of cases of post-transfusion jaundice of which no evidence of transmitted virus has yet been found.

Epstein–Barr virus

Donations of blood are deferred for 2 years after glandular fever.

Cytomegalovirus

Transfusion of blood, platelets, or leucocytes may transmit cytomegalovirus to susceptible individuals. In normal recipients there is a mild febrile illness with complete recovery. In immunosuppressed patients, however, the organism may give rise to a severe infection with fever and hepatic impairment. This may be avoided by reserving blood free of cytomegalovirus antibodies (20 per cent) for patients at risk, such as neonates, transplant recipients, children with acute leukaemia, and those undergoing open heart surgery. This may be achieved by donor screening or the use of special leucocyte ultrapore filters.

ACQUIRED IMMUNE DEFICIENCY SYNDROME (AIDS) (SEE SECTION 7)

AIDS was described in the early 1980s as the cause of lymphadenopathy, repeated opportunistic infection (e.g. *Pneumocystis carinii*, toxoplasmosis), and unusual malignancy (e.g. Kaposi's sarcoma) occurring in young males amongst the homosexual population in San Francisco.

The venereal association of the disease was realized from the cluster of patients diagnosed, and the condition was later recognized in the recipients of blood products, for example haemophiliacs using factor VIII concentrate from large donor pools prepared before heat treatment, and in intravenous drug users who often share needles.

The human immunodeficiency viruses types 1 and 2 (**HIV-1** and **HIV-2**) have been shown to be the causative agents of AIDS. A high proportion of persons suffering from AIDS have antibodies to HIV in their blood. Screening for this antibody was introduced in the United Kingdom in October 1985 to detect those blood donations from donors who have been exposed to the virus. This significantly increases the safety of transfusion of those cellular and other products that cannot be pasteurized. In addition, donors whose activities may lead to an increased risk of infection are requested not to give blood—homosexuals, intravenous drug users, prostitutes, haemophiliacs, sexual partners of African residents, and sexual partners of any of the above groups for example. Once routine HIV-1 antibody screening had been developed, individuals were discovered in Africa with identical clinical features to those with AIDS but negative HIV-1 serology. Investigation of their blood led to the isolation of the second virus, HIV-2, and all donations in the United Kingdom have been routinely screened to exclude HIV-2 since June 1990.

MANAGEMENT OF TRANSFUSION REACTIONS

Any adverse effects should be thoroughly investigated. The patient must be carefully assessed to determine the specific symptoms and signs of the reaction in relation to the nature and volume of fluid given. Steps must also be taken to institute the necessary laboratory procedures.

Clinical care
All recipients should be carefully observed during their transfusion, with frequent recording of pulse, blood pressure, temperature and urine output. These measurements may give the first indication of the event, and associated symptoms may include rigor, backache, central chest pain, and fever. Early jaundice and haemoglobinuria may also indicate incompatible transfusion. It is most important to monitor urine output carefully throughout. Renal failure is one of the most serious complications; it is caused by the combination of acute haemolysis, shock, and occasionally the consumptive coagulopathy mediated by massive release of complement.

The aim of treatment is to maintain the urine output in excess of 100 ml/h and a normal systemic blood pressure until the reaction subsides. A saline (0.9 per cent) or dextrose infusion (5 per cent) is usually adequate for this purpose, but occasionally when urine output declines, a forced mannitol diuresis may be used to good effect. Fresh frozen plasma may be useful where coagulation factors are being consumed (see above). In the absence of shock, renal failure should be managed as in acute tubular necrosis (see Section 20). If there is any possibility that the blood was infected, appropriate broad-spectrum antibiotics should be given, with proper regard to their side-effects in view of their nephrotoxicity.

Preparation and uses of blood components
The starting material for the preparation of most cellular components is whole blood. In recent years an increasing requirement for certain products has led to their direct procurement by apheresis techniques using cell-separator machines.

RED-CELL PREPARATIONS
The indications for the transfusion of whole blood are now relatively few: procedures requiring cardiopulmonary bypass, vascular surgery, acute haemorrhage exceeding 30 per cent of blood volume, and exchange transfusions. The addition of adenine to the anticoagulant used in collection has increased survival of viable red cells to permit storage up to 35 days at 4 °C.

Red-cell concentrates were introduced as a by-product of the separation of plasma for fractionation, but they have become the treatment of choice for the correction of anaemia and as the first two/three units administered in acute blood loss. Plasma-reduced blood prepared in England and Wales has a haematocrit of 60 to 65 per cent after removal of about 180 ml of plasma and passes readily through the standard blood filter of 170 μm.

In order to achieve national self-sufficiency in plasma, means have been sought to obtain more from each donation using optimal additive solutions. Red cells suspended in a nutrient medium, for example **SAG-M** (saline, 150 mmol/l; adenine, 1.25 mmol/l; glucose 50 mmol/l, with added mannitol) exhibit enhanced viability on storage. The use of 100 ml SAG-M as additive allows an extra 90 ml of plasma to be removed from the red cells. This increases the plasma yield on each unit by 50 per cent and the remaining cells are resuspended in SAG-M for use in the same situations as plasma-reduced blood. Such red-cell preparations are also superior to red-cell concentrates in that flow rates are improved. There appears little disadvantage from the lack of plasma.

LEUCOCYTE-POOR BLOOD (TABLE 7)
This should be given to patients who require regular transfusion over a long period of time in order to prevent febrile reactions to white-cell antibodies. It is necessary to remove 90 per cent of the leucocytes and several methods are available to achieve this target. Freezing is an expensive exercise, but the introduction of micropore filters ($d = 40$ μm) has proved a convenient option. Once red cells have been rendered leucocyte poor by filtration in the laboratory their pack has been entered and they should be transfused as soon as possible, and not later than 12 h after preparation. In recent years, ultrapore filters have been produced for use at the bedside during transfusion. Manufacturers claim that these render products free of white cells and, in some cases, free of cytomegalovirus.

LEUCOCYTES
Harvest from the buffy layer is a tedious manual technique of poor yield. Filtration though scrubbed nylon produces reasonable numbers of leucocytes with impaired function. The best donations are achieved by cell separation from normal individuals pretreated with corticosteroids to boost their counts. Hydroxyethyl starch in the system minimizes neutrophil trapping in the red-cell mass, but donors may only be used for limited number of donations because there is no known excretion route for starch. Some years ago, patients with chronic granulocytic leukaemia were used as a source of neutrophils, but this practice is no longer to be recommended.

Granulocytes are indicated in the treatment of profoundly neutropenic patients (less than 0.5×10^9/l white cells) with bacterial infection unresponsive to antibiotics, and who may be expected to recover in the long term. The minimum course should last 4 days and each daily infusion should contain not fewer than 5×10^9 granulocytes.

PLATELET CONCENTRATES
These may be obtained by removal from whole blood at 20 °C. The separation should be undertaken at the earliest opportunity after collection. The first step is centrifugation of the whole blood to sediment the heavier red cells. Using a closed system the supernatant platelet-rich plasma is transferred to a satellite pack, and centrifuged hard to concentrate the platelets. Two hours are allowed for platelets to disaggregate. They should then be stored at 22 °C and agitated until their issue for transfusion. The shelf-life varies according to the choice of their plastic container. Packs have recently been produced that allow sufficient gaseous exchange to extend the survival of functional platelets from 3 to 5 days.

An alternative technique for the collection of platelets is directly from

Table 7 *Methods of preparation of leucocyte-poor blood and some advantages and disadvantages of each*

Method	% leucocytes removed	Comment
Inverted/differential centrifugation	65–85	Inefficient alone (May be combined with filtration)
Saline washing	80–90	Red-cell loss, slow
Automated batch washing	90–95	Specialized equipment required.
Frozen-thawed	95–99	Expensive apparatus Excellent product
Sedimentation: HES, dextran	90–95	Saline wash extra
Nylon filter	60–70	Unsatisfactory
Cotton-wool filter	95–97	Convenient, if costly

HES, hydroxyethyl starch.

a donor by cell separation; this is known as thrombapheresis. This permits the reinfusion of donor red cells during the procedure, allowing donation more frequently than twice a year. The main advantage of thrombapheresis is the facility for obtaining a recipient 'dose' from one donor instead of from four to six whole-blood donations. This is particularly valuable where the patient exhibits refractoriness to platelet therapy as a result of antibodies, and the pool of suitable donors is small.

The indications for platelet transfusion are to control bleeding in thrombocytopenia and/or thrombocytopathia where disorders of function have been demonstrated *in vivo* (bleeding time) or *in vitro* (aggregation, adhesion etc.). Most clinicians responsible for the care of patients with marrow suppression advocate the use of prophylactic platelet therapy where profound thromobocytopenia is present, (platelets $< 20 \times 10^9$/l) irrespective of haemorrhage. This practice is directed at the prevention of spontaneous bleeding episodes (e.g. cerebral haemorrhage) but may lead to problems of alloimmunization, which then make selected tissue typed the product of choice.

These trends in platelet therapy, in association with more aggressive regimens in chemotherapy and the advances in bone marrow transplantation, have led to marked increases in the use of the concentrate. Objective measurements of therapeutic response are not always helpful, but an increment in the recipient's platelet count is usual in the absence of bleeding, infection, or hypersplenism. Control of bleeding is the most important evidence of effective platelet therapy.

PLASMA FRACTIONS

Plasma is separated from whole blood to provide several different components for clinical use. It is important that a patient is not given cellular components unless these are specifically indicated and this is particularly true in a programme of long-term infusion therapy. Several plasma fractions are in common use.

Fresh frozen plasma

Many coagulation factors are present in this plasma, which is separated from red cells as soon as possible after collection and rapidly frozen below $-30\,°C$. It is valuable in the correction of bleeding due to impaired clotting. Its use is increasing in association with the expansion of facilities for coronary artery bypass grafts, which require cardiopulmonary bypass during surgery, and with advances in other vascular and hepatitic procedures. Guidelines for its use were published in 1992 by the British Committee for Standards in Haematology (*Transfusion Medicine* (1992), **2**, 57–63).

Factor VIII concentrates

Products vary in their factor VIII content and size of donor pool.

Cryoprecipitate

This is prepared by freezing freshly collected plasma, and rapid thawing to precipitate a concentrate of factor VIII and fibrinogen. It is then frozen and stored as cryoprecipitate at $-30\,°C$, containing 70 to 80 i.u. of factor VIII in approximately 5 to 20 ml of plasma. It is no longer to be recommended for the support of inherited coagulation disorders such as haemophilia A or von Willebrand's disease because of its potential for virus transmission. Cryoprecipitates are a valuable source of fibrinogen as well as factor VIII depending on the method of preparation in the treatment of acquired coagulation. They are indicated in certain acquired coagulation factor disorders (e.g. consumptive coagulpathy). The supernatant residues of cryoprecipitate preparation need not be wasted. Stored at $-30\,°C$ it is a valuable source of coagulation factors other than factor VIII, and can replace fresh frozen plasma in the majority of clinical situations.

Lyophilized factor VIII preparations of intermediate or high purity

The raw material for these preparations is cryoprecipitate and further refinements on large donor pools produce concentrates of intermediate or high purity stored at $4\,°C$. The fibrinogen content is inversely proportional to the factor VIII concentration. Produced in batches, they are accurately assayed for coagulation activity and the therapeutic dose may thus be accurately determined. Heat treatment of the dry factor VIII preparations at $80\,°C$ for up to 72 h has been shown to eliminate HIV and HCV. Viruses with a lipid coat (e.g. HIV, HCV) can also be removed by treating the concentrate with a solvent detergent. Intermediate-purity products are rapidly being superseded by high-purity factor VIII concentrate.

Factor IX complex

This is obtained from cryoprecipitate supernatant by fractionation and purification. The product is lyophilized for use in the treatment of Christmas disease. The crude preparation of factor IX contains the clotting factors II, IX, and X. A purified preparation is now available, rendered virally inactive using the same methods as for factor VIII.

Albumin solutions

These are virus free after pasteurization by heating to $60\,°C$ for 10 h.

Zenalb (4.5 per cent) (BPL)

This contains over 90 per cent of the albumin in the plasma, with a final concentration of 45 g/l. It is used to restore blood volume in haemorrhagic shock and burns, and is isotonic.

Zenalb (20 per cent) (BPL)

This is now prepared as a 20 per cent solution in a small volume (100 ml). It is indicated in correction of chronic hypoalbuminaemia in special circumstances of organ failure and fluid overload, for example hepatic insufficiency with ascites. It is relatively low in sodium.

Immunoglobulins

For some years these have been obtained from the plasma known to contain high levels of specific antibodies (e.g. antitetanus, antirubella, antivaricella-zoster, anti-RhD), or from fractionation of normal plasma. There is now considerable activity in the pharmaceutical industry in marketing new intravenous normal immunoglobulins, and many indications for their use have been cited. These preparations are expensive and their applications vary—support of hypogammaglobulinaemia, management of autoimmune disorders such as immune thrombocytopenic purpura, autoimmune haemolytic anaemia for example.

REFERENCES

Harris, J.R. (ed.) (1991). *Blood separation and plasma fractionation*. Wiley, Chichester.

Mollison, P.L., Engelfriet, C.P., and Contreras, M. (1987). *Blood transfusion in clinical medicine*, 8th edn). Blackwell Scientific, Oxford.

Napier, J.A.F. (1987). *Blood transfusion therapy: a problem-orientated approach*. Wiley, Chichester.

Race, R.R. and Sanger, R. (1975). *Blood groups in man* (6th edn). Blackwell Scientific, Oxford.

22.8.2 Marrow transplantation

C. BUNCH

Marrow transplantation is now established as a potentially curative treatment for selected patients with haematological malignancy, aplastic anaemia, and severe congenital haemopoietic and immune deficiencies. Its foundations lie in studies done during the 1950s in which it was found that rats and mice exposed to doses of irradiation sufficient to destroy the haemopoietic system could be saved by infusions of marrow cells obtained from either the animal itself before irradiation (autologous cells), a genetically identical animal (syngeneic cells), or a genetically non-identical animal (allogeneic cells). Rescue with autologous or syngeneic cells proved relatively straightforward but allogeneic transplantation was found to be complicated by the twin problems of graft rejection by immune competent cells remaining in the host, and graft-verus-host disease (**GVHD**)—a progressive and often fatal wasting disease with widespread damage particularly to the skin, liver, gut, and lymphoid system—mediated by immune competent cells within the graft itself (Fig. 1). These problems could be partially overcome by pretransplant immunosuppressive conditioning to prevent rejection, together with post-transplant immunosuppression to modify GVHD. Further progress was made when the importance of the major histocompatibility complex (**MHC**) became apparent, and it was found that allogeneic transplantation can be most reliably done when donor and recipient are siblings who have inherited identical MHC determinants.

Clinical transplantation

Marrow transplantation has been done with increasing frequency during the past 15 to 20 years (Fig. 2). The procedure is straightforward. Marrow is obtained from the donor by multiple aspirations from the iliac bones and sternum under general or spinal anaesthesia. Some 500 to 1000 ml of marrow is collected into heparinized tissue culture medium, and is infused intravenously into the recipient after simple filtration to remove bony particles. The recipient is conditioned before the infusion by high-dose immunosuppressive chemotherapy with or without total-body irradiation to prevent rejection.

In early studies, transplantation was limited to patients with severe aplastic anaemia, which is known to have an otherwise extremely high mortality, and to patients with acute leukaemia in the end stages of their disease who were resistant to chemotherapy and often in poor clinical condition.

In aplastic anaemia, pretransplant conditioning with high doses of cyclophosphamide (200 mg/kg) permitted engraftment in most instances, although subsequent rejection occurred in about one-third of patients. Furthermore, despite sustained engraftment, a number of patients developed fatal infections or GVHD. Nevertheless, about 45 to 50 per cent were successfully transplanted and returned to a normal life, apparently cured.

Patients with acute leukaemia, on the other hand, were treated with high-dose cyclophosphamide (120 mg/kg) and often other cytotoxic agents, together with a single dose of up to 10 Gy total-body irradiation

The data presented in Figs. 2 and 4 of this chapter were obtained from the Statistical Center of the International Bone Marrow Transplant Registry. The analysis has not been reviewed or approved by the Advisory Committee of the IBTMR.

(TBI), a dose that would ordinarily be lethal without a subsequent infusion of haemopoietic cells. Graft rejection was not a problem in this early series, but the overall results were at first sight much less impressive than in aplastic anaemia (Fig. 3), because a large proportion of patients succumbed within the first 3 months from infection and GVHD. Despite this intensive approach to therapy, relapse of leukaemia was common within the first 2 years. After this time, however, the mortality

Fig. 1 Bone marrow transplantation is complicated by a dual immunological barrier, which can be illustrated by transplantation of haemopoietic cells between F₁ hybrid strain and parents. Cells transplanted from an F₁ hybrid offspring to a parent carry antigens inherited from the other parent, which are recognized as foreign and the graft is rejected. On the other hand, a graft from a parent to F₁ offspring is accepted, but immune competent cells with the graft react against the host, which has 'foreign' antigens inherited from the other parent.

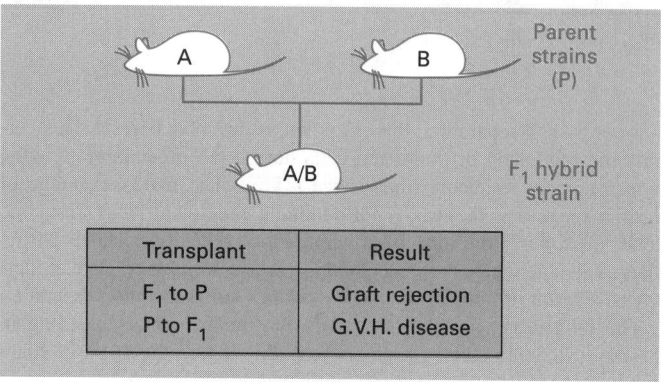

Fig. 2 (a) Annual number of patients receiving allogeneic bone marrow transplants worldwide, 1970–1993. (b) Disease for which allogeneic bone-marrow transplants were performed, 1993.

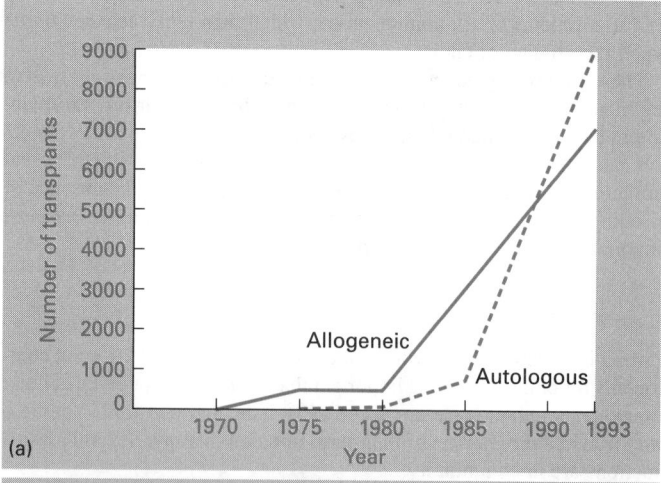

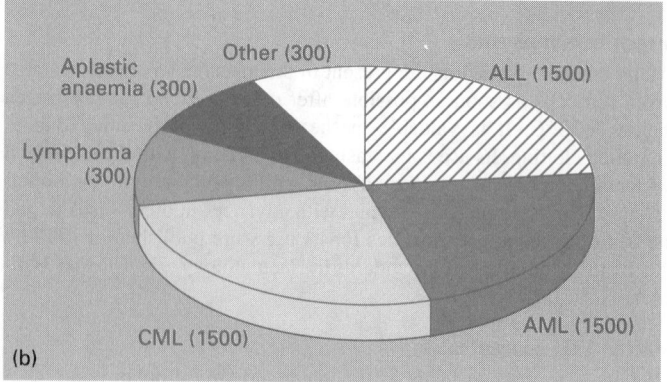

fell dramatically, and some 13 per cent of patients became long-term survivors and most were cured of their disease. These patients would otherwise have died within a few days or weeks had transplantation not been available.

Following this favourable experience, various strategies were adopted in an attempt to improve the overall success rate. It was noted in these early studies that graft rejection occurred more often in patients with aplastic anaemia whose lymphocytes showed *in vitro* evidence of sensitization to donor antigens before transplantation, or in whom the number of cells transplanted was less than average. In most instances this sensitization was thought to result from previous blood transfusion, making a strong case for transplantation to be undertaken as early as possible in the course of the disease—preferably before transfusion becomes necessary. Indeed, the incidence of rejection in patients who have not previous been transfused is very low. The risk of rejection in others can be reduced by more intensive immunosuppression and is virtually eliminated if pretransplant conditioning includes TBI. However, TBI increases the risk of transplantation significantly, and the potential benefit is largely outweighed by a higher mortality from infectious complications and GVHD, although the use of smaller doses of TBI may be equally effective and less toxic.

With the available techniques of marrow harvest, it is difficult to envisage how the number of haemopoietic cells transplanted could be increased. However, animal cross-transfusion and transplantation experiments have demonstrated that haemopoietic stem cells circulate in the blood of these species, and it has been shown that the transfusion of peripheral blood mononuclear cells, collected from the marrow donor for several days after marrow transplantation, can effectively reduce the risk of rejection in sensitized patients. It is not absolutely certain whether these supplementary infusions significantly increase the number of haemopoietic cells transplanted, or whether the addition of large numbers of donor lymphocytes actively interferes with the rejection process. The latter seems more probable as the incidence of chronic (but not acute) GVHD is increased somewhat by this manoeuvre.

Fig. 3 Marrow transplantation for refractory acute leukaemia in relapse. Kaplan–Meier product-limit estimates of percentage survival for the first 110 patients transplanted in Seattle. (Reproduced from Burchenal, J.H. and Oettgen, H.F. ed. (1980). *Cancer: achievements, challenges and prospects for the 1980s.* Grune and Stratton, by kind permission of Dr E. D. Thomas and the publishers.)

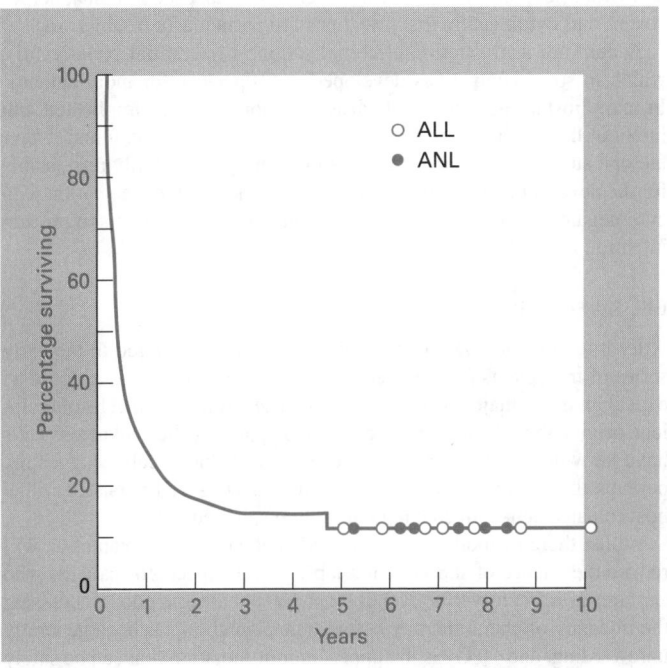

From the initial clinical studies mentioned above it was clear that acute leukaemia could be cured by marrow transplantation. In many instances, failure could be attributed to the patient's poor clinical condition at the time of transplantation or to increased resistance of the leukaemia in the terminal stages of the disease (Fig. 3). Consequently, many centres now elect to transplant during periods of haematological remission in patients who are nevertheless considered unlikely to be cured with conventional treatment. In practice, this means during the first or subsequent remission in acute myeloid leukaemia or 'poor risk' acute lymphoblastic leukaemia, or during the second or subsequent remissions of other patients with acute lymphoblastic leukaemia.

The validity of this approach has been confirmed by several groups. Patients in remission can be in excellent clinical condition and the transplantation procedure is well tolerated. Indeed, the supportive care required during the immediate postgrafting period may be less than that required during intensive induction of remission with conventional chemotherapy. Mortality from infectious complications and acute GVHD appears to be less, particularly in younger patients, and the risk of leukaemic relapse is reduced. The results have been most impressive in acute myeloid leukaemia, possibly because transplants have generally been undertaken earlier in the course of the disease, and currently up to half the patients may expect to become long-term survivors (Fig. 4). However, advances in conventional chemotherapy have also resulted in improved survival, and the advantage of bone marrow transplantation in first remission is less clear-cut. Some groups of patients with acute myeloid leukaemia (such as those with the M3, promyelocytic variant) probably do not benefit from marrow transplantation in first remission.

Complications

Despite this encouraging progress, results are still short of ideal and clearly many problems remain (Table 1). The most pressing of these are GVHD, infection, and relapse of the underlying disease.

GRAFT-VERSUS-HOST DISEASE

Acute GVHD may be seen at any time during the first 2 to 3 months following transplantation. It usually starts as a non-specific maculopapular rash, with or without diarrhoea and biochemical or clinical evidence of liver damage. The rash tends to be generalized, but has a predilection for the face, palms, and soles (Fig. 5). In a proportion of patients, acute GVHD progresses to a fulminant form with a severe exfoliative dermatits, hepatic failure, and a debilitating diarrhoea. Tissue damage is mediated by cytotoxic T lymphocytes of donor origin, which have been activated as a result of disparity of major or minor histocompatibility antigens between donor and recipient.

More recently, with increasing numbers of patients surviving the immediate post-transplantation period, a form of chronic GVHD has been recognized, characterized by a later onset with a progressive sclerodermatous skin reaction (Fig. 5) and, in some patients, liver changes resembling primary biliary cirrhosis. Antibodies may be produced to a variety of tissue antigens, and there are parallels between this form of GVHD and autoimmune disease. It has been suggested that a type of disordered immune reconstitution, with alterations in the proportions of suppressor and helper T cells, may be responsible.

The use of methotrexate after transplantation to prevent GVHD was prompted by earlier animal studies, but has been notably less successful in man, with some degree of GVHD occurring in up to two-thirds of patients. Cyclosporin A, a fungal metabolite with activity against T cells, has been more widely used in recent years. In a randomized study it has been shown to reduce the incidence and severity of GVHD in comparison to methotrexate, but overall survival is similar. Cyclosporin has potentially dangerous side-effects, especially on the kidneys, and must be used with caution. More recent studies indicate that a combination of methotrexate and cyclosporin is more effective than either alone, but with higher degree of toxicity, especially mucositis.

The appreciation that acute GVHD is mediated by mature cytotoxic T cells within the marrow graft has prompted attempts at removal or depletion of T cells from the donor marrow before infusion. Virtually complete T-cell depletion can be achieved by a variety of methods, including physiochemical separation, binding to certain plant lectins, and lysis by monoclonal anti-T-cell antibodies and complement. It has been amply demonstrated that GVHD can largely be prevented by such techniques, but that the advantage is offset by increased risk of graft rejection or subsequent leukaemic relapse.

Treatment of established GVHD is generally unsatisfactory, but the administration of large doses of methyl prednisolone at the first sign of GVHD may successfully abrogate the disease and perhaps prevent the later development of the chronic form. An interesting observation which has become more apparent with improved survival is that patients who had had non-fatal GVHD have a much reduced risk of subsequent leukaemic relapse, suggesting that the graft may exert a useful anti-

Fig. 4 Probability of leukaemia-free survival after HLA-identical sibling bone-marrow transplant for (a) acute lymphoblastic leukaemia, (1987–1992), (b) acute myelogenous leukaemia, (1987–1993), (c) chronic myelogenous leukaemia (1987–1992), according to disease status.

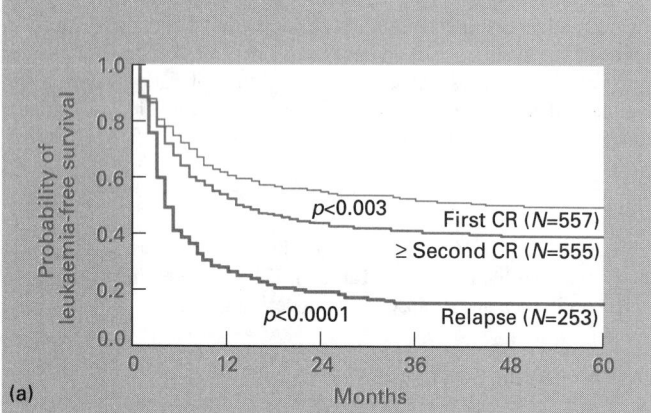
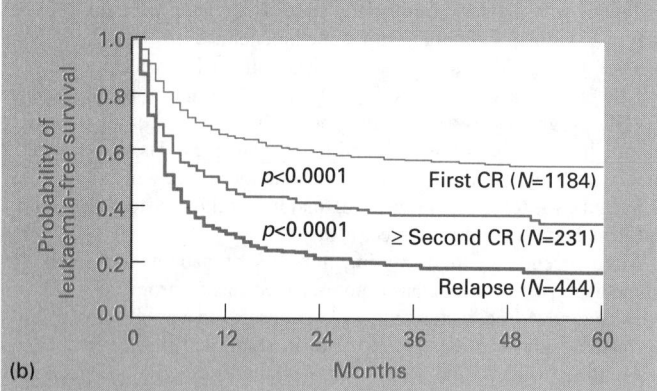
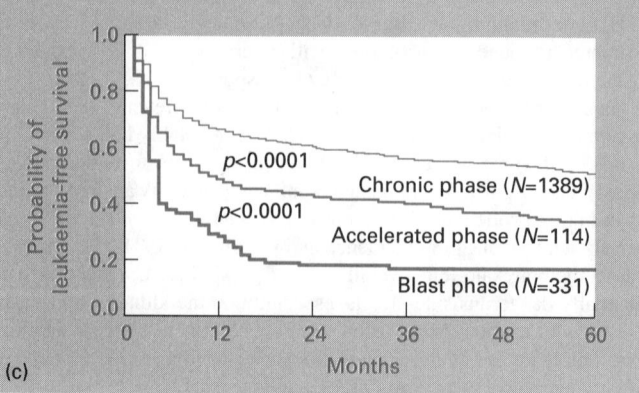

Table 1 *Principal complications of marrow transplantation*

Immediate (days)
Effects of marrow failure:
  Bleeding, infection
Drug toxicity:
  Rashes, cystitis (CY)
  Cardiomyopathy (CY)
  Parotitis (TBI), pancreatitis (TBI)
  Gastrointestinal symptoms (CY, TBI)

Early (weeks)
Failure of engraftment
Graft rejection
Infection: bacterial, fungal, viral
Acute graft versus host disease (GVHD)
Interstitial pneumonitis
Leukaemic relapse

Late (months)
Chronic GVHD
Leukaemic relapse
Infection, particularly herpesviruses and pneumococcal

Long term
Cataracts
Sterility and growth retardation
?new malignant change

CY, cyclophosphamide; TBI, total-body irradiation.

leukaemic effect. A more desirable long-term goal may thus be to temper GVHD rather than to eliminate it altogether.

INFECTION

Infectious complications occur commonly after marrow transplantation and are directly related to the profound immunosuppression that results from pre- and post-transplant conditioning. Reconstitution of the immune system with cells of donor origin takes many months and is considerably delayed by the presence of GVHD; humoral immunity recovers first, but cell-mediated immunity may never completely return to normal, although in the absence of GVHD the risk of infection is not appreciably increased after the first year. Before this time, both bacterial and viral infections may occur, and pneumococcal, pseudomonal, herpes zoster, and cytomegalovirus infections are particularly troublesome.

A common and often fatal complication is interstitial pneumonitis, which in some centres has developed in 50 per cent or more patients. In many instances, cytomegalovirus infection has been implicated, but in about half the patients a causative organism cannot be found. Other factors, such as radiation or drug damage, may be partially responsible for the development of this syndrome. Nevertheless, the association with cytomegalovirus infection is so strong that vigorous attempts to prevent infection or viral reactivation are warranted (see Section 7).

LEUKAEMIC RELAPSE

After infection and GVHD, the chief problem encountered in the early series of transplants for leukaemia was leukaemic relapse. As would be expected, in the majority of instances relapse has involved cells of recipient origin, though in a small number of patients the leukaemic cells have shown the cytogenetic characteristics of donor cells, suggesting perhaps that a transforming agent such as a virus had persisted in the host to cause leukaemic change in the transplanted cells.

Whilst there is good reason to expect that earlier transplantation will reduce the chance of subsequent relapse, the prospects for patients who are already refractory to conventional treatment are less good. Increasing the intensity of chemotherapy before transplantation has been generally unrewarding, and 10 Gy is the upper limit of radiation that can be safely given as a single dose. Attempts to increase the effectiveness of radiotherapy with fractionated TBI at a higher total dose have not shown marked benefit in comparison to single fractions, although fractionated schedules are often preferred for logistic reasons.

LONG-TERM EFFECTS

Apart from chronic GVHD, long-term problems following marrow transplantation have been relatively minor or infrequent. Some patients have developed posterior subcapsular cataracts a few years after TBI. An incidence of 80 per cent has been reported for patients given TBI in a single fraction, with a very much lower incidence when fractionation has been used. With careful follow-up a high incidence of obstructive and restrictive defects in pulmonary function have become apparent. Growth velocity is reduced in children receiving TBI, but not cyclophosphamide alone. This is associated in some with a reduction in the levels of adrenocortical and growth hormones. Most patients can expect to be sterile and premature menopause is common.

Of great concern is the potential risk of subsequent malignant change, as has been occasionally noted following renal transplantation or in patients receiving cytotoxic drugs for other conditions. This has not so far been a significant problem in patients transplanted for haemopoietic disorders, but bizarre lymphoproliferative malignancies have developed in some infants who have been transplanted for immunodeficiency diseases, and occasional cases of glioblastoma multiforme have been reported, generally in patients who had received cranial irradiation before TBI.

Indications for marrow transplantation

The success of marrow transplantation in the treatment of aplastic anaemia and acute leukaemia has led to its use in the management of an increasing number of conditions (Table 2). Because of adverse effects on growth and development, TBI is generally avoided in non-malignant disorders, although less intensive conditioning may fail to eradicate the patient's own, abnormal marrow.

Of particular note are the excellent results of marrow transplantation in chronic granulocytic leukaemia. Originally, transplantation was confined to patients in blast-cell crisis, in whom results were disappointing, but it has more recently been used in the chronic phase of the disease. Interestingly, the high doses of chemotherapy and TBI employed are able to eliminate the neoplastic clone—a feat rarely achieved with conventional treatment. In contrast to acute leukaemia, where conventional chemotherapy can cure a proportion, bone marrow transplantation is the only form of treatment that has been shown to be curative in chronic granulocytic leukaemia and it is currently the treatment of choice for patients with a suitable donor.

The procedure, and in particular TBI, is poorly tolerated by elderly patients, and most leukaemic patients over the age of 45 years are probably best managed by conventional means. The main restriction at the present time is the availability of a suitable donor. The ideal donor would be an identical twin from whom marrow may be transplanted without fear of GVHD and with the prospect of a much more rapid immune reconstitution and correspondingly less risk of infection. More usually, however, transplants are between HLA-identical siblings, although

Fig. 5 Graft-versus-host disease affecting the skin. Early involvement of the trunk, hands, and feet in acute GVHD (a-c). (d) Late changes resembling scleroderma in chronic GVHD.

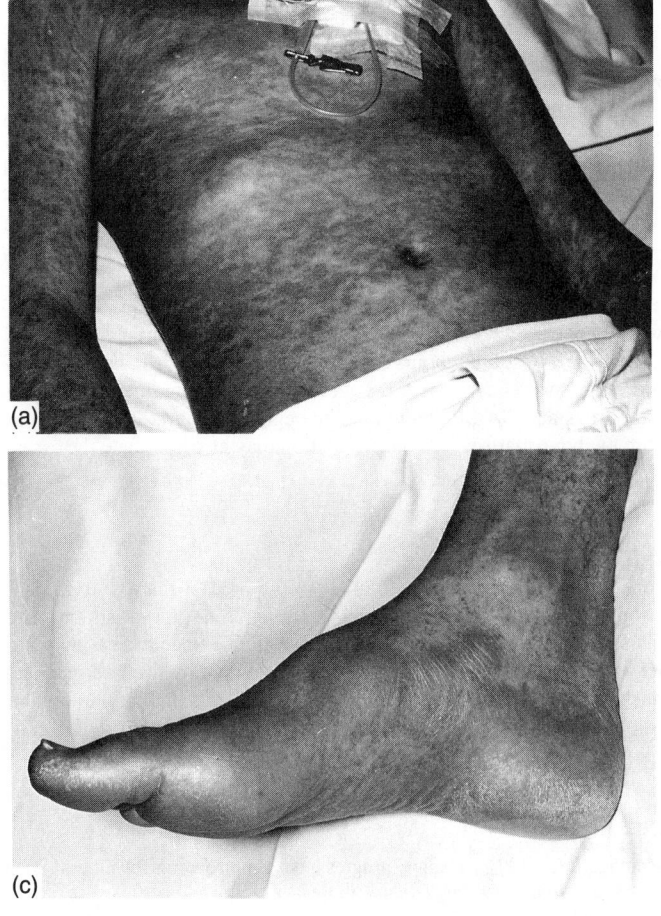

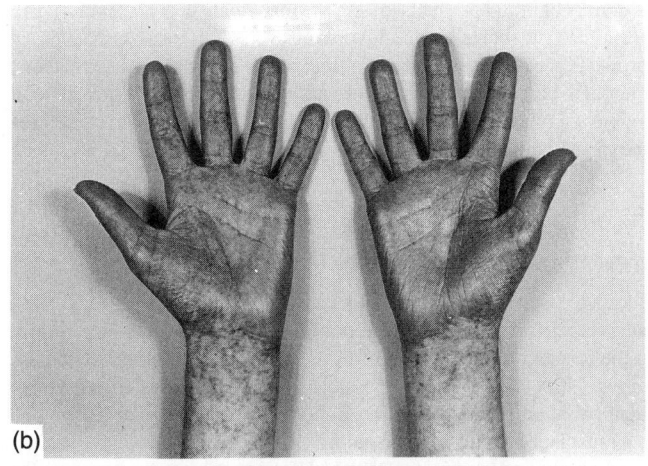

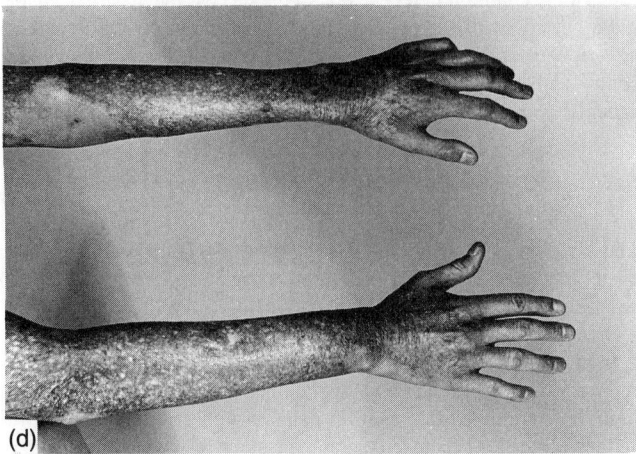

Table 2 *Indications for allogeneic marrow transplanation*

1. Severe aplastic anaemia
Persistent life-threatening agranulocytosis or thrombocytopenia due to failure of production
2. Acute leukaemia
Childhood ALL (good prognosis) in relapse or second remission
Poor prognosis AML and ALL in relapse or first remission
Blast crisis in CGL
3. CGL In chronic phase
4. Congenital immune deficiency disorders, e.g., SCID
5. Congenital haemopoietic disorders
e.g. Chronic granulomatous disease, Wiskott-Aldrich syndrome
Selected patients with thalassaemia for whom long-term transfusion and iron chelation are impracticable

AML, acute myelogeneous leukaemia; ALL, acute lymphoblastic leukaemia; CML, chronic myeloid leukaemia; SCID, severe combined immune-deficiency disease.

occasionally a parent may be a suitable donor, particularly if, because of an unusual degree of homozygosity within the family, he or she is HLA identical with the patient. Minor degrees of incompatibility between a patient and a family-member donor may be acceptable to some transplant centres, but the risk to the patient is greater.

Although marrow transplantation undoubtedly offers the best chance of cure for many patients, it is a hazardous undertaking that may impose severe strain on the patient and family. This is particularly the case when the transplant centre is some distance from the patient's home, as it is –often desirable for the donor as well as other family members to act as donors of blood products during the immediate post-transplant period. The risks and benefits should obviously be fully discussed with the family before a final decision is reached, but care should be taken to approach potential donors before transplantation is suggested to the patient or other members of the family, as this may otherwise create unexpected tensions and pressures within the family.

Extending donor availability
MATCHED, UNRELATED DONORS

Because a suitable family donor can only be found for a minority of patients, attempts to widen the pool of available donors have resulted in the formation of a number of large volunteer panels of individuals of known HLA type. It is now possible to find an unrelated donor who is identical at all HLA loci (A, B, C, D) for up to half of all patients.

Transplants from such matched unrelated donors have become increasingly common in recent years. The success rate has been encouraging, with overall results when donor and recipient are fully matched that are comparable to using an HLA-identical sibling, although morbidity—and thus the overall cost of the procedure—is substantially higher.

AUTOLOGOUS MARROW TRANSPLANTATION

The simplest way of extending the availability of donors is to use the patient's own bone marrow. Autologous transplantation—though not strictly transplantation—has been used extensively over the past 5 to 10 years in patients for whom an alternative donor could not be found.

The basis for autologous marrow transplantation is that the infusion of haemopoietic stem cells itself is in fact a supportive manoeuvre, whilst it is high-dose chemotherapy with or without TBI that is actually curative. It is argued that even in patients with primary bone-marrow malignancy such as acute leukaemia, the number of cells present during complete remission is low, and that any that are inadvertently reinfused following the procedure may be insufficient to cause relapse, or may be eliminated by whatever mechanism the body may have for dealing with small numbers of residual leukaemic cells. Alternatively, techniques may be deployed to purge the harvested marrow of residual leukaemic cells in a manner analogous to T-cell depletion referred to above.

Autologous marrow transplantation is relatively straightforward and is not complicated by GVHD or such serious infections as are encountered after allogeneic transplantation. It is thus easy to see why it has become popular, but difficult to prove or disprove its efficacy. It is virtually impossible to say whether relapse is due to failure to eradicate the disease in the patient, or reinfusion of malignant cells in the harvested marrow, although molecular biological techniques are beginning to shed some light on this. It is equally difficult to prove that a successful outcome could not have been obtained in the individual patient by conventional chemotherapy. Large, randomized, controlled trials are required, though few have been undertaken.

PERIPHERAL BLOOD STEM-CELL TRANSPLANTS

It has been known for some time that very small numbers of haemopoietic stem cells circulate in the peripheral blood, and cross-transfusion and transplantation experiments in animals have demonstrated that these are capable of inducing sustained engraftment in lethally irradiated hosts. It has not, however, been possible to make use of these observations clinically until recently, partly because the proportion of such stem cells is very low, and partly because of concerns that such circulating cells may not be truly pluripotent and thus capable of sustained engraftment in man. It is now known that a pluripotent stem cell resides in a CD 34+ fraction of mononuclear cells, and that CD 34+ cells increase in the peripheral blood during the recovery phase from chemotherapy; the proportions are increased further by administration of granulocyte colony-stimulating factors (**G-CSFs**) such as filgrastim. It is now well established that sufficient cells can be obtained, using a cell separator, over 2 to 3 successive days during the recovery phase from a standard dose of cytotoxic drugs such as cyclophosphamide followed by daily administration of G-CSF. This obviates a need for bone marrow aspiration under general anaesthesia, and has been shown to result in faster engraftment and less requirement for supportive care, especially platelet transfusions. The technique has been enthusiastically embraced as an alternative to autologous bone-marrow transplantation, and preliminary studies indicate that it may also be useful in an allogeneic setting.

Critical studies have not appeared as yet and there are similar concerns about efficacy as for conventional autologous marrow transplantation. It has been argued that it may be the preferable technique in patients with lymphoma who are known to have bone marrow involvement, and possibly also in solid tumours such as breast cancer, where bone marrow metastasis may occur. There is concern, however, that the use of cytotoxic drugs and G-CSF to stimulate the egress of pluripotent stem cells from the bone marrow into the circulation may also stimulate the egress of malignant cells.

Future prospects

Considerable strides have been made in the field of marrow transplantation since clinical studies started in earnest a decade or so ago, and this form of treatment is now becoming available to an increasing number of patients. The problems outlined above are now well defined and much of potential benefit to patients is being learned about the organization of the immune system and its reconstitution with donor cells following a successful engraftment.

REFERENCES

Armitage, J.O. (1994). Medical progress: bone marrow transplantation. *New England Journal of Medicine*, **330**, 827–38.

Bierman, P.J., Vose, J.M., and Armitage, J.O. (1994). Autologous transplantation for Hodgkin's disease: coming of age? *Blood*, **83**, 1161–4.

Blume, K.G. and Petz, L.D. (ed.) (1983). Clinical bone marrow transplantation. Churchill Livingstone, New York.

Bortin, M.M. *et al.* (1993). 1993 progress report from the International Bone Marrow Transplant Registry. *Bone Marrow Transplantation*, **12**, 97–104.

Buckner, C.D. and Clift, R.A. (1984). Marrow transplantation for acute lymphoblastic leukemia. *Seminars in Haematology*, **21**, 43–7.

Forman, S.J. and Zaia, J.A. (1994). Treatment and prevention of cytomegalovirus pneumonia after bone marrow transplantation. Where do we stand? *Blood*, **83**, 2392–8.

Kessinger, A. and Armitage, J.O. (1991). The evolving role of autologous peripheral stem cell transplantation following high dose chemotherapy for malignancies. *Blood*, **77**, 211–13.

Lucarelli, G. *et al.* (1990). Bone marrow transplantation in patients with thalassaemia. *New England Journal of Medicine*, **322**, 417–21.

McDonald, G., Sharma, P., Mathews, D., Shulman, H., and Thomas, E.D. (1985). The clinical course of 53 patients with venocclusive disease of the liver following bone marrow transplantation. *Transplantation*, **39**, 603–8.

Shpall, E.J. and Jones, R.B. (1984). Release of tumor cells from bone marrow. *Blood*, **83**, 623–5.

Storb, R. *et al.* (1984). Marrow transplantation for aplastic anaemia. *Seminars in Haematology*, **21**, 27–35.

Thomas, E.D. (1985). Marrow transplantation for nonmalignant disorders. *New England Journal of Medicine*, **312**, 46–8.

Thomas, E.D. (1992). Bone marrow transplantation: past experiences and future prospects. *Seminars in Haematology*, **19** (suppl. 7), 3–6.

Thomas, E.D. and Storb, R. (1970). Technique for human marrow grafting. *Blood* **36**, 507–515.

Thomas, E.D. *et al.* (1975). Bone-marrow transplantation (first of two parts). *New England Journal of Medicine*, **292**, 832–43.

Thomas, E.D. *et al.* (1975). Bone-marrow transplantation (second of two parts). *New England Journal of Medicine*, **292**, 895–902.

Section 23 *Diseases of the skin*

23 Diseases of the skin

T. J. RYAN

Introduction

The naked survivor as manager

In spite of being the largest, the most visible, and the most social organ of the body, skin is underrated by the medical profession. Many countries have no dermatologists and the skin diseases that are rife in rural areas receive no treatment. People whose skin fails them are unwelcome and die young. What better reason for the *Oxford textbook of medicine* to be the first of its kind to provide adequate space for dermatology. Those who survive skin failure and exposure are not usually in government. Doctors who advise governments have rarely been those who value the skin. There are rare exceptions where dermatologists have been responsible for rational, cost-effective health services.

Dermatology is the study of the skin and so is concerned not only with diseases but with the Greek ideal of beauty, manifested in the confident nude; with the cosmetic as well as disease. This in turn causes the dermatologist to comment on attitudes towards stigma by parents, schoolteachers, spouses, employers, beauticians, nurses, or managers. Whether it be incipient baldness, the wrinkles of ageing, or tattoos, there are cultural factors to be understood, and a decision may have to be made about the cost of not treating. When is ugliness illness; how much is disfigurement worth in a court of law, and on what does the quality of life depend?

Throughout this section, the impairment, disability, and handicap of skin failure will be emphasized, and the reader will be thought of as a member of a team of caretakers of the skin. The dermatologist should be the leader, but often he or she will be absent and others using the chapter may be the givers of advice. When writing a section on dermatology for a general medical textbook, it is usual to concentrate on the skin as it is involved coincidentally with internal disease processes. This section also aims to help the physician who has no dermatological colleague to make the right diagnosis and provide appropriate management of what would normally be regarded as a dermatological condition.

Dermatology is made difficult by its great variety of physical signs. It is an encyclopaedic subject with more than 3000 named entities. Fortunately, fewer than a dozen diseases represent 70 per cent of dermatological practice—acne; bacteriological, viral, and fungal infections; tumours; dermatitis; psoriasis; leg ulcers; and warts.

Every good physician looks at the skin all the time while he is listening to the patient or eliciting physical signs. Whether he recognizes the minutiae that a dermatologist has been trained to see depends not merely on seeing but knowing their significance. Unfortunately, so much of recognition is the naming of physical signs, and dermatologists have accumulated an enormous amount of jargon. Not all of this is necessary for management. In this account uncommon signs have been omitted where their recognition results in no benefit to the patient.

A physician should know enough to recognize a physical sign that is a threat to life, such as a melanoma, the malignant pustule of anthrax, or the eroded blisters in the mouth in pemphigus vulgaris. Otherwise, he should know how to recognize signs that are significant indications of systemic disease such as erythema nodosum, splinter haemorrhages, or arsenical keratoses, and the white macules of tuberous sclerosis.

There is no branch of medicine more dependent on clinical acumen and on previous observations and less dependent on the laboratory. However, in no other branch of medicine is there a requirement for the specialist to be so experienced in histopathology. The value of the information is for sorting out that which is unrecognizable to the naked eye:

it does not often alter the management of the disease. One advantage of the skin biopsy is that it can be sent away to experts, together with a photograph of the clinical lesion.

Where skin disease is the primary cause of severe handicap in countries where the physician is the only doctor, simple measures to give relief should not be neglected simply because the physician claims not to be specially trained in dermatology and has not learned its language.

In spite of the advances in antimicrobials and corticosteroids which have completely altered the nature of skin clinics in technically advanced countries, there is no diminution in the number of patients attending for help with skin problems. There is an increase in skin cancer, in the demand for cosmetic treatment, and in the number of agents in the environment that damage the skin and cause dermatitis. In developing countries the overwhelming demand is for better management of infection of the skin by bacteria and parasites. It does not change for the better because poverty, malnutrition, poor housing, and water shortage are often unsolved.

REFERENCES

Calnan, C.D. and Levene, G.M. (1974). *A colour atlas of dermatology*. Wolfe Medical Books, London.

Goldsmith, L.A. (1991). *Physiology and biochemistry of the skin* (2nd edn). Oxford University Press.

Rook, A., Wilkinson, D.S., and Ebling, F.J.G. (1992). *Textbook of dermatology,* (ed. R.H. Champion, J.L. Burton, and F.J.G. Ebling, (5th edn). Blackwell Scientific Publications, Oxford.

The structure of the skin

The skin consists of the epidermis and its supporting dermis lying on a layer of fat (Fig. 1). It is similar to mucosal surfaces where the surface

Fig. 1 The structure of human skin.

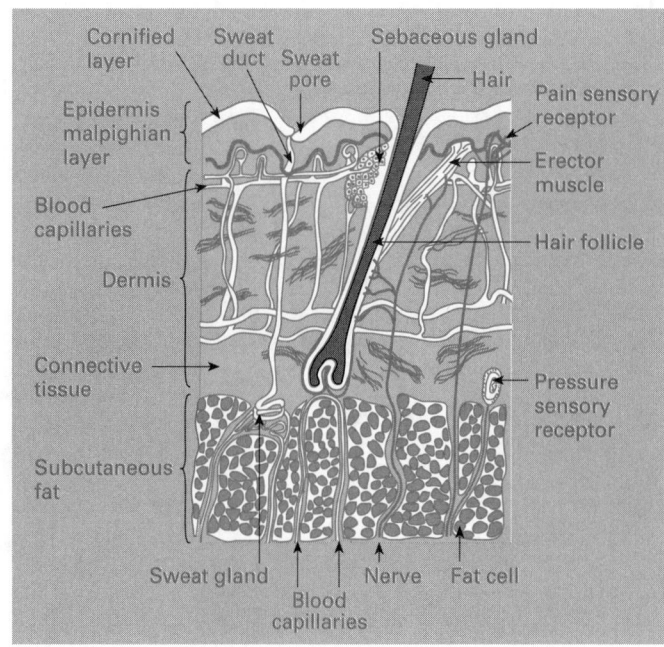

epithelium is separated from its underlying lamina propria by a basement membrane zone which, in turn, is separated from the submucosal fat by the muscularis mucosa.

In man, unlike mucosa or the skin of most animals, the muscle layer lying between the dermis and the underlying tissue is found only in the areola and scrotum. The epithelium gives rise to all the cutaneous appendages. These include the eccrine sweat glands found over the entire cutaneous surface but more numerous in the palms and soles, the apocrine sweat glands found in the axilla, groin, and beneath the breasts, and the hair and oil-producing sweat glands found on the upper chest and back.

The epidermis is a stratified squamous epithelium (Fig. 2) comprising a germinative basal layer which adheres to the basement membrane zone. Through cell division, the basal layer gives rise to successive layers of differentiating cells. Their principal function is to synthesize the insoluble protein, keratin. In the process, these cells ultimately die and are shed from the skin surface. Keratins are the intermediate filaments of the cytoskeleton found in epithelial cells, which serve as a scaffold in these cells and contribute to cell integrity. Subtle changes in the protein molecule can be detected by electrophoresis and, on this basis, over 30 different keratin molecules have been described. Keratins usually exist as a pair of one acidic (type I) and one basic (type II) molecule. The genes coding for type I are localized on human chromosome 17 and for type II on chromosome 12 (Table 1). The keratin changes in its composition as it is carried away from the germinative layer to the spinous layer, to which it provides strength and suppleness.

Keratin antibodies can be detected by immunofluorescent techniques and used to distinguish epithelial cells (keratinocytes) from cells of mesodermal origin (fibroblasts and melanocytes). This can be helpful in clarifying the diagnosis of a spindle cell tumour, for example, as being either squamous cell carcinoma or malignant melanoma.

The epidermis is infiltrated by a number of dendritic cells, including the melanocytes, Langerhans cells, and indeterminate cells. The function of the indeterminate cells is unknown. The epidermal Langerhans cells, derived from bone marrow, are characterized ultrastructurally by a unique cytoplasmic organelle—the Birbeck granule, which internalizes HLA-DR molecules from the cell membrane and is involved in antigen processing. Depletion of these cells, as can be caused by ultraviolet radiation, prevents contact dermatitis mediated by delayed cellular immunity. The same mechanism may play a role in the precipitation of herpes labialis by sun exposure. Pigmentation of the skin is due to melanin fed into the basal keratinocyte rather than that stored within the

Table 1 *Keratin expression*

K14 and K5	Basal cells
K10 and K1	Stratified cells
K18 and K8	Embryo
K17 and K7	Simple epithelia
K16 and K6	Wound healing, proliferation, cancer
K12 and K3	Cornea
K13 and K4	Oesophagus

melanocyte. Skin colour is partly due to the amount and activity of the melanocyte and partly a reflection of how melanin is stored and processed in the keratinocyte. Melanin is produced from tyrosine and dopa and acts as a scavenger of free radicals.

The rich vasculature has a generous reserve to meet the requirements of wounding and repair, so common at the surface. Vasodilatation can increase blood flow by a factor of 100, making it perfectly adapted for thermoregulation. Macromolecules and cells leave the dermis through the lymphatic system, which is initiated in an elastic network at the junction of the upper and middle dermis (Fig. 3). The lymphatic system is responsive to hydrostatic forces and to movement of the solid elements of the dermis by massage or compression. The dermis also supports the extremely complex innervation, so necessary for touch and for sensing danger. The main constituents of the dermis are all secreted by the fibroblast and consists of the collagen and elastic fibrous proteins embedded in the mucopolysaccharide ground substance.

The two functions of basal cells, repair or reduplication and the production of keratin, require that the epidermis should turn over in a controlled way and die in an orderly fashion. The turnover takes about 30 days from the time of reduplication at the basal layer to loss from the surface. The lower layers of the epidermis depend on oxygen for mitosis and migration, but the upper differentiating layers are anaerobic with no mitochondria. The optimal temperature for epidermal metabolism is probably lower than that for most body cells. The energy of the epidermal cells is derived from both lipids and carbohydrates. Current biochemical interest is in the balance between cyclic AMP and GMP and the role of prostaglandins in the control of epidermal cell turnover.

REFERENCES

Goldsmith, L.A. (1991). *Physiology and biochemistry of the skin* (2nd edn). Oxford University Press.

McKee, P.H. (1989). *Pathology of the skin with clinical correlations.* J.B. Lippincott, Philadelphia.

Fig. 2 A section of skin showing epidermis and upper dermis. Note the epidermis and the dermal projections interdigitate. The epidermal cells lose their nuclei as they approach the surface.

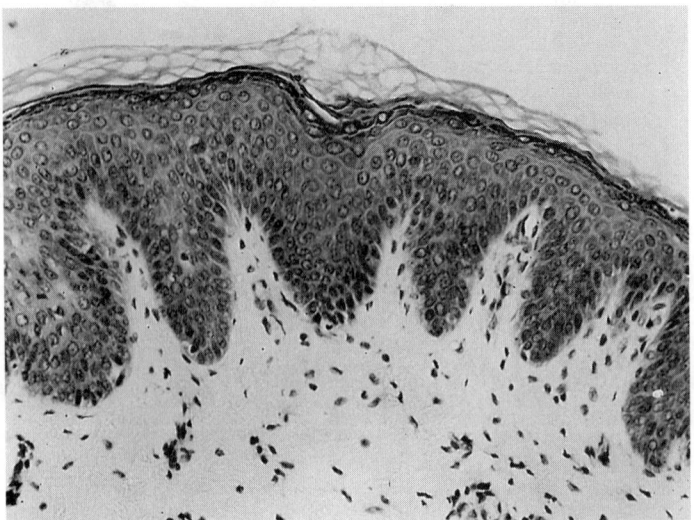

Fig. 3 The lymphatics are the exits from the skin for cells and macromolecules. They control hydrostatic and oncotic pressure and they are one pathway for antigen presentation.

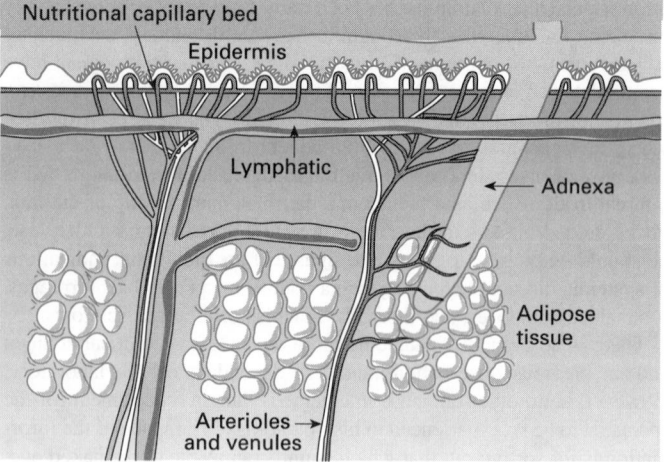

Functions of the skin and 'skin failure'

Like heart failure, respiratory failure, and liver failure, the skin, too, can fail with disastrous consequences. The skin is the largest organ of the body and, being on the surface, it is continuously exposed to injury.

The skin is not only displayed but it is fondled, and together with the hair and nails it is a sexual organ of attraction. It has to be both supple and strong because it is bent, stretched, trodden upon, and compressed, as well as scratched and prodded. It must have a capacity to repair itself rapidly to form a physical barrier impervious to excess water loss or to absorption from the environment. It must resist wear and tear. These functions are impaired in skin diseases which make those affected more vulnerable and less able to reconstitute themselves after damage, as well as causing them social embarrassment.

The skin contains Langerhans cells. These are antigen-presenting cells which detect environmental antigen, travel to the lymph nodes and present the antigen to lymphocytes that are pre-programmed to return to the skin. This network is the primary immunological defence system of the skin and is termed the SALT, analogous to the MALT (mucosal assort lymphoid tissue) found in the bowel. The sensation of pain, so finely mediated by the precise innervation of the epidermis, has a similar warning function, helping us to recognize the environment and to itch in the presence of smaller invaders and to follow this with an accurate scratch response. The skin is capable of presystemic metabolism of drugs and other substances applied topically. It is also capable of forming toxic metabolites. It can synthesize vitamin D from calciferol in the presence of sunlight, and contains the enzyme to metabolize it to a 1,25-dihydroxycholecalciferol. There is an interaction between the cells in the dermis and in the overlying epidermis. This is mediated by cytokines, a number of which have been identified to be important in the skin. These include interleukins 1, 2, 3, 6, 8; interferons α, β, and γ and transforming growth factors (TGFs) α and β. Furthermore, there is a range of peptides, complement factors, eicosanoids, and platelet activating factors present in the epidermis and involved in intracellular communication.

Thus, the epidermis contains very high levels of interleukin-1 (IL-1), 100 000 times greater than the content of most normal tissues. Keratinocytes are the main source, producing it continuously, but more in the presence of ultraviolet light or endotoxin. There is a large intrakeratinocyte preformed pool of IL-1 and a predominantly intracellular inhibitor as a controlling factor competing for receptors, which are normally somewhat few in the epidermis but can be induced by ultraviolet rays, trauma, or γ-interferon.

The dermis supports the epidermis and its adnexa. Like bone, the skin resists distortion. It is subjected to compression and shearing strain and many mechanical stresses are transduced into biochemical signals. It is more supple than bone, and hydrostatic forces or swelling pressure are more finely sensed and distributed.

The dermis is more than a supporting structure. It determines many of the characteristics of the epidermis and controls regional variations. It is an essential inducer and controller of the adnexal organs, such as the hair, sweat, and sebaceous glands, and provides a selective environment whereby hormones such as oestrogen and testosterone can influence some epithelial organs but not others. This is involved in the pathogenesis both of acne and hirsutism as well as androgenic alopecia.

Sexual attraction is an important function on which the fortunes of the cosmetic industry are founded. It is subject to whim and to advertising. The social anthropologist has done much to draw attention to that which denotes sex appeal. Colouring or decolouring, tattooing, distorting, stretching, and, of course, adorning with jewellery and clothing are part of the appeal. All of which add to the demands for the dermatologist as well as for the beautician, tattooist, trichologist, and a host of fringe activities concerned with health. Sex appeal depends on the skin not being too greasy, too matt, or too wrinkled. The white adolescent wants powder to reduce a greasy forehead; the black African wants grease to rid him of any degree of powdery exfoliation. One must have a beauty spot and another must not. The stink of some scents attracts while sweaty feet and rotting shoes repel.

REFERENCES

Goldsmith, L.A. (1991). *Physiology and biochemistry of the skin* (2nd edn). Oxford University Press.

Jarrett, A. (1973–80). *Physiology and pathophysiology of the skin*, Vols 1–7. Academic Press, New York.

Journal of Investigative Dermatology (1980). Analysis of research needs and priorities in dermatology. *Journal of Investigative Dermatology* 73 (Suppl. 5), 514.

McKee, P.H. (1989). *Pathology of the skin with clinical correlations*. J.B. Lippincott, Philadelphia.

Ryan, T.J. (1990). Disability in Dermatology. *British Journal of Hospital Medicine* **46**, 33–6.

The influence of the psyche

It is well known that blushing or cold sweats and pallor are skin reflections of the mind. Any group of students shown an *Acarus* under the microscope will laugh at the sudden awareness of itching it induces in one of their number. But such awareness is typical of the relationship of the mind and the skin. There have been many experiments showing that the acute inflammatory process mediating a weal or any exudation is susceptible to enhancement by anxiety or diminution by relaxation. While a 'neurotic' basis for urticaria, prurigo nodularis, or lichen simplex is no longer overemphasized by terms such as angioneurotic oedema or neurodermatitis, modern Western scientific medicine alone has made such terms unpopular. This is because the influence of the psyche cannot be measured, is mainly subjective, and therefore, by some, is not to be believed. Pavlovian concepts of the neurovegetative are popular among Russian dermatologists. Practitioners of indigenous medicine or fringe medicine, the witch doctor as well as almost every lay person, recognize a link between anxiety and skin disease.

The principal anxieties resulting from skin disease are fear of being infectious, unclean, and, ultimately, unwelcome. If one considers what may happen to a patient with leprosy, such fears are well founded. As with sexually transmitted disease, the upbringing, religious, and social mores of the patient will often determine their reaction to skin disease.

It is surprising how few patients will accept that our largest organ can be defective in its own right or that it and it alone can simply wear out or be worn down like the heels of a leather shoe, which after all is only skin. They will, however, believe that their skin disease is due to a malfunction of the liver, an impurity in the blood, to worry, or to a dietary indiscretion. Such beliefs have to be met with tactful explanation.

One frustration which is experienced far too often by the skin patient is to ask advice or to seek help and to be told that the problem is trivial. So often patients see their problem placed second to an acute emergency and have to accept the correctness of this. However, like all chronic or trivial disease, no one attempts to measure handicap and so the effect it has on the individual is belittled. Not all skin disease is psychosomatic.

The handicap of skin disease

Because patients with skin disease rarely die of it and hardly ever constitute an emergency, the subject of dermatology is a minor speciality. It is not thought essential for medical students to know the subject well and even nursing training may include little of it. As a topic for research it is gaining glamour but attracts funds less easily than cancer, transplants, or CT scanners. Many parts of the world have no dermatological service whatsoever.

Why then should one argue that the need for resources, whether manpower, buildings, or money for research, is greater than previously estimated?

The answer is that the patient with skin disease is at a disadvantage quite as great as those with most other diseases when consideration is given to a person's capacity to achieve the personal and economic independence of his fellows. This may be due to an inherited or acquired constitutional defect but commonly there is also an environmental factor. Writers on handicap refer to the Eastern proverb, 'I wept because I had no shoes, until I met a man who had no feet'.

Dermatologists will know that a man who cannot wear boots because of epidermolysis bullosa or hypersensitivity to agents used in the footwear industry is as disabled as an amputee when the distance he can walk is the measure of his handicap. Personal independence and economic independence constitute the individual's viability as a separate unit.

A human being with skin disease can function like other humans only through his ability to think and communicate. In almost all other respects his functions are threatened.

Common diseases, such as dermatitis and psoriasis, affect the following 'functional specificities' on which personal autonomy depends: (1) to move around in and manipulate the environment; (2) to service oneself; (3) to resist normal stresses and traumas; (4) to groom oneself; and (5) to organize oneself emotionally. Some diseases, such as leprosy, affect other faculties such as sight. To have personal and economic independence it is necessary to perform effectively wherever one finds oneself. Skin diseases which affect the hands and feet prevent the patient from getting out and about or from moving around at home (Figs 4 and 5). Skin disease for a variety of reasons may prevent or threaten the expected care of one's home, self, or family, and it often interferes with education and employment.

The threat to life

Skin disease does sometimes constitute an emergency and may cause death. Fatal melanoma has become much more common especially in young adults. Only accidents are a more common cause of death in males aged between 20 and 30. There is a 10 per cent incidence of metastasis from squamous epithelioma of the lip, a problem which may increase as actinic damage supersedes pipe smoking as a major aetiological factor.

Angio-oedema of the upper respiratory tract is most frightening of dermatological emergencies, accounting for the deaths of most cases of hereditary angio-oedema due to C_1 esterase deficiency. Occasionally other causes of urticaria may be responsible.

Respiratory obstruction is recorded in other diseases such as epider-

molysis bullosa (due to inhalation of 'casts') and in Behçet's disease (due to ulceration of the larynx).

Because the skin is the largest organ of the body and because it is exposed to the environment, many chronic skin diseases cause death by impairing the skin's ability to protect the person from irritants, infective agents and climate, by loss of fluid, or the increased demands on internal organs such as the heart. Blistering disorders, such as pemphigus vulgaris, widespread impetigo, or epidermolysis bullosa, are especially threatening skin diseases.

Erythroderma due to eczema (Fig. 6), psoriasis, or lymphoma commonly results in failure of body temperature control, heart failure, and more rarely, in uncontrollable protein-losing enteropathy. Fluid loss and prerenal failure are important and particularly relevant in hot countries. In the tropics many die from uncontrolled dermatitis and the superinfections which are often associated with it.

Fig. 5 Callus or corn is common in ageing skin and pain can make walking very difficult. The patient is more handicapped than an amputee with a comfortable prosthesis.

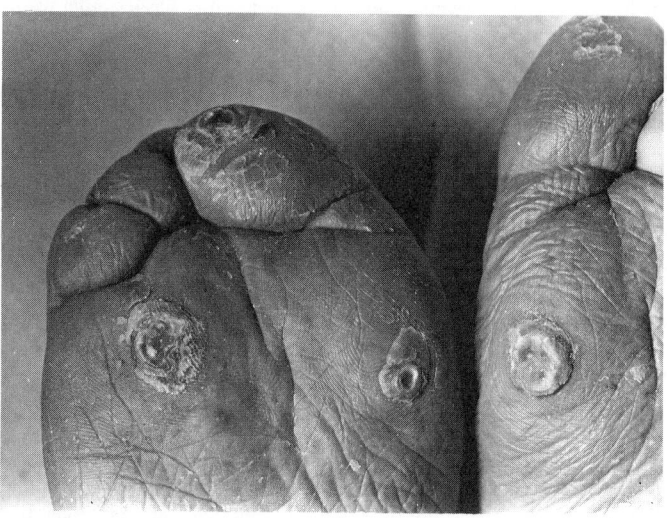

Fig. 4 Psoriasis of the hands interferes with dexterity and makes patients unwelcome in many occupations, such as food handling or public relations.

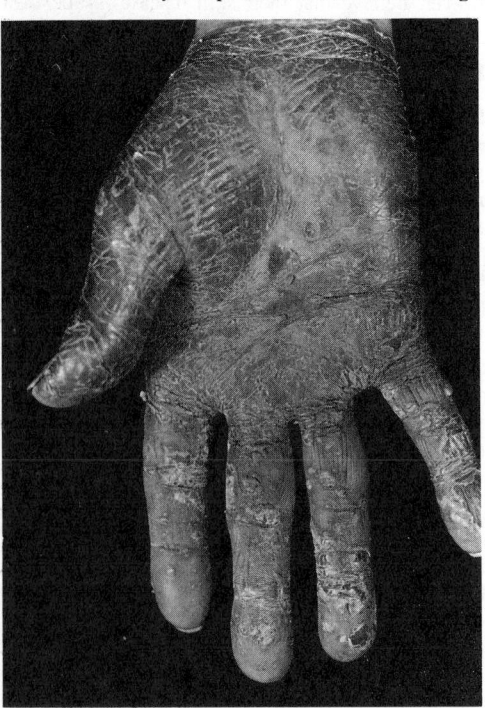

Fig. 6 Some diseases are a threat to life. Exfoliative dermatitis is so because of fluid loss, heart failure, and loss of temperature control. This patient died following perforation of the small intestine while on steroid therapy.

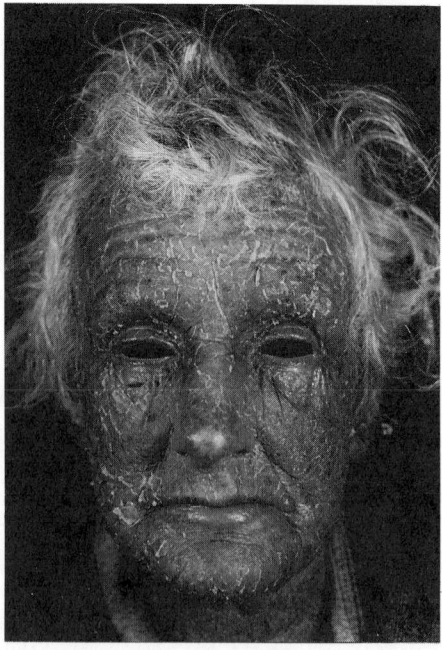

Threatening personal autonomy

Not to be able to resist normal stresses and traumas is a common inconvenience. It accounts for the need for sufferers from atopic eczema, even when in remission, to avoid occupations such as hairdressing, nursing, food handling, and mechanical engineering. For those with a lower intelligence quotient unemployment may be the consequence. Wear and tear of the skin is the most common consequence of work and those who have lowered resistance are unable to work. A severe example of such lowered resistance is epidermolysis bullosa. The Koebner phenomenon, which is the development of skin disease at sites of injury, accounts in part for the common problem of adult psoriasis.

To communicate and to be welcome

Because our skin is on the surface it is there for display. Through it we make contact with others. It is observed and touched. If there are defects in it the observer may not like what he sees and will not touch. Many children with such defects experience insults from other children who refuse to hold hands or play with them. Adults experience more subtle signals which may prevent a normal sex life and interfere with employment (Fig. 7). Isolation causes earlier death.

The greatest handicap of all is to be unwelcome. It matters not whether this is actually so or a belief of the patient without any actual experience of rejection; it is the commonest social effect of skin disease. The whiteness of the skin of vitiligo, the blood on the sheets and scale on clothing and furniture left by the psoriatic are a huge disadvantage. The albino is an outcast in Africa and the severe psoriatic is similarly rejected in the United Kingdom.

The patient with skin disease is unemployable in any job in which he or she is in the public eye or involved in food preparation. For the many whose skin is vulnerable to the minor wear and tear of quite ordinary living, there is a long list of jobs which should be discouraged.

The physician who does nothing to alleviate the handicap of skin disease ignores an appreciable problem which often only a little knowledge and care can do much to remedy.

Prevalence

It is difficult to obtain an estimate of prevalence of skin disease and the extent of the handicap. But an examination of more than 20 000 Americans between the ages of 1 and 74 revealed that 60 per cent had a significant skin condition, actually least frequent among children and most common in the old. In about 10 per cent the condition limited activity and was a physical handicap. Often skin complaints persisted for more than 5 years. Diseases of the hand were the greatest handicap. It has been estimated in the United States that 6.8 million Americans were handicapped in their social relationships because of a skin condition. Diseases of the skin account for almost half of all reported cases of industrial illness in the United States, and the cost of this, estimated by the National Institutes of Health, is more than $2542 billion per annum. In a country which is well endowed with dermatologists, 60 per cent of the skin conditions are in fact dealt with by general physicians. These conditions are the commonest reason for consultation.

REFERENCES

Finlay, A.Y. and Coles, E.C. (1995). The effect of severe psoriasis on the quality of life of 369 patients. *British Journal of Dermatology,* **132,** 236–45.
Jowett, S. and Ryan, T.J. (1985). Dermatology patients and their doctors. *Clinics in Experimental Dermatology* **10,** 246–54.
Jowett, S. and Ryan, T.J. (1985). Skin disease and handicap: an analysis of the impact of skin conditions. *Social Science and Medicine* **20,** 425–9.
Panconesi, E. (1985). Stress and skin diseases. In *Psychosomatic dermatology.* J.D. Lippincott, Philadelphia.
Savin, J.A. and Cotterill, J.A. (1992). Psychocutaneous disorders. In *Text book of dermatology,* (ed. A. Rook, D.S. Wilkinson, and F.J.G. Ebling), pp. 2479–96. Blackwell Scientific Publications, Oxford.

The provision of skin care even when the diagnosis is not known

It is not necessary to know the diagnosis—to give a name to the physical signs—in order to treat the skin, but it is a helpful short cut. The naming of skin disease is like stamp collecting, and it is helpful to match the physical signs to a picture in a book—there are several excellent catalogues of the skin, listed below.

In this account it is assumed that the reader will be able to diagnose very common disorders like dermatitis, psoriasis, acne, leg ulcers, or warts, and the main purpose of the text will be to guide management.

When the physician is faced with physical signs which are familiar to him, such as pigmentation or purpura, and for which the causes are numerous but not on the tip of his tongue, a checklist is provided often with minimal detail. Intermediate are the large number of specific entities known to dermatologists, but described in no more than a paragraph giving principal diagnostic features and the best management.

Most patients like to be given a diagnosis but are happy with general terms such as dermatitis, wart, or birth mark. They hope for management in its broadest sense. They want treatment for itch, stink, scale, or disfigurement, and the general principles of the treatment of these are the same whatever the exact diagnosis. They want to know whether it is an infection, due to something they have eaten, whether it is hereditary or due to something missing from their diet, and whether it is a skin cancer or something to which they are allergic. These problems can be approached in general terms and do not need great diagnostic acumen.

When in doubt, a biopsy should be done. This is not difficult and because one can see exactly what one is biopsying it is possible to identify very small areas which are likely to be diagnostic. Biopsies by dermatologists are small compared to those by surgeons, and the morbidity is very slight and scarring negligible.

A biopsy is not necessarily always a certain answer—very often the combination of histology and a good clinical description provides the final diagnosis. No pathologist should be asked to diagnose without good clinical details.

So much of skin disease in the tropics or in the malnourished, the poor, and badly housed is due to, or complicated by, infection. Bacterial swabs and scrapings for fungus infection should be done even when the suspicion is not high.

As mentioned above, the fear of rejection is great and an important principle of management is a sympathetic hearing. A guide to the ques-

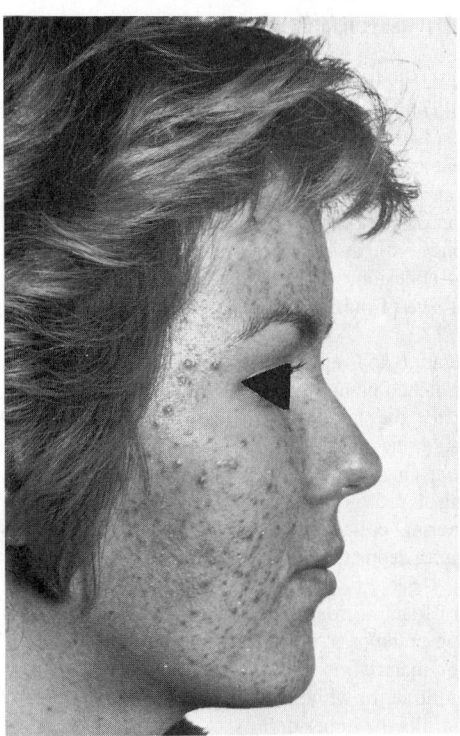

Fig. 7 Acne vulgaris is a cosmetic disability which makes a teenager feel unwelcome and contributes to delinquency.

tioning which makes such a hearing relevant is listed in the next section. Touch is a signal of acceptance. No dermatologist diagnoses from a distance or even from the end of the bed and the texture of the skin and the depth of the lesion is appreciated by touch. Minor procedures like skin scraping for mycelia or an excision biopsy never fail to convince that the problem is being well managed.

The sympathetic listener

The basis of the interview is optimal communication of information. It should not frustrate or cause anxiety and depression. The doctor should be identified and know who is being interviewed and what has been previously diagnosed or prescribed by reading the patient's notes before the interview. Relevant questioning is important because time is so often limited. The following is a suitable basis for such an interview:

1. How long have you had it; exactly when did it start; have you had it before?
2. Which part of your skin was first affected; where were you when it started; what were you doing?
3. How did it progress, to what sites, and what was there before?
4. Does it come and go; how long does each individual lesion last?
5. Does it itch; is it painful, tender, numb?
6. Does it develop blisters or clear fluid?
7. Does anything make it better?
8. Does anything make it worse?
9. What ointments, creams, lotions, or bath oils have you used? Have you had any medicine or injections?
10. Has anyone else you know got it; does it run in your family; do any other diseases like asthma, eczema, or hay fever run in your family?
11. Have you had any previous illnesses?

Do not forget that accurate answers are rare. In rural or tropical climates, particulars about the duration of an ailment are frequently vague.

The examination

Undressing and removal of bandages, and in some countries, even the removal of a hat may be difficult to arrange. One will learn more by looking everywhere and when in doubt, the patient must be undressed. A full examination may include a look at the genitalia and the mouth, but even if the rash is diagnosable at a glance and a history is not obtainable, it is important to speak to the patient. Remember that he has a handicap which responds to a sympathetic hearing as well as to a careful examination.

One should keep looking until something is recognized. Often much of a rash is atypical but somewhere there should be a classical physical sign. Good lighting is essential and, of all lighting, the sun is the best. Many hospitals and clinics in the tropics are purposely placed out of the sun and are too dark for accurate observation. One should not be ashamed to use glasses, or even a magnifying glass. This is essential for nailfold telangiectasia or for recognizing Acarus or crab lice.

Touch assures the patient there is no abhorrence and that contagiousness and uncleanliness are insignificant. Papules are palpable, macules are not. This can be important in, for instance, patch testing in which purely macular responses should be ignored. Compression distinguishes between purpura and telangiectasia. It reveals much about the depth of the lesion and its hardness.

REFERENCE

Ashton, R.E. (1995). Teaching non-dermatologists to examine the skin: a review of the literature and some recommendations. *British Journal of Dermatology*, **132**, 221–5.

Clinical investigation
Skin scrapings for fungal mycelia

Skin scrapings are best taken from moist areas since mycelia in dried scales or in the nails may be too desiccated. Scrapings should be placed on a slide with 10 per cent potassium hydroxide which helps to clear the keratin of extraneous material which obscures the fungus. Gentle heating is helpful. In hot climates the rate of evaporation from potassium hydroxide is such that crystals form and it is best to renew the solution regularly.

Finding parasites

A microscope is essential for the diagnosis of mycelia, lice, and other parasites. Attempting to find parasites in the skin of patients may be difficult, but is often helped by devices. For instance, vaseline placed over the aperture of a 'boil' raised by a bot or tumbu fly may encourage the larvae to expose themselves since they cannot survive without oxygen. If onchocerciasis is suspected, a new itchy papule can be picked up on the end of a needle and quickly snipped and placed in saline and examined under the microscope to see whether microfilariae swim out. Acarus can be picked out of the end of the burrow on the fronts of the wrists and between the fingers.

Wood's light

Wood's light is ultraviolet light (UVA, 360 nm) and is used for recognizing white areas in white skin as in tuberous sclerosis. Fluorescence is also helpful for *Microsporum audouini* and *M. canis,* which fluoresce green. Erythrasma due to *Corynebacterium minutissimum* fluoresces coral red. Porphyrins in teeth or urine fluoresce pink and anaerobes such as *Bacteroides melanogenicus* in wounds and ulcers fluoresce red.

Biopsy

The lesion chosen for biopsy should not be modified by excoriation, therapy, or secondary infection. Small lesions should be totally excised and it is usual to remove skin in the shape of an ellipse along lines of stretch known as Langer's lines. On the face this is equivalent to the wrinkles. It is useful to have diagrams on the wall of the operation room (Fig. 8). In subjects prone to keloids it is best to avoid the sides of the face, neck, sternal region, and shoulders. It is often useful to biopsy the edge of the lesion so that it can be compared with adjacent normal-looking skin. Too much squeezing of the biopsy by forceps makes it impossible to analyse. An appropriate fixative is 10 per cent formalin for at least 12 hours.

Most bleeding is venous since skin is well endowed with venules. It follows that bleeding can be controlled by elevation and by pressure on the skin surrounding the wound.

Inexpensive transport systems have been described so that biopsies can be posted to experts.

The histological report may include the following terms:

Hyperkeratosis: thickening of the horny layer usually resulting from retention and increased adhesion of epidermal cells.

Parakeratosis: cell nuclei in the horny layer usually resulting from a high rate of cell turnover as in psoriasis.

Spongiosis: separation of prickle cells by oedema fluid, i.e. the epidermis looks like a sponge—a feature of eczema.

Acantholysis: loss of cohesion between prickle cells and isolation, and balloon-like appearance of individual epidermal cells, a feature of pemphigus.

Liquefaction: degeneration and rupture of basal cells—characteristic of lupus erythematosus, lichen planus, and erythema multiforme.

Pigmentary incontinence: the shedding of melanin from the epidermis into the dermis following injury to the basal layer.

Elastotic degeneration: changes in dermal collagen which occur in light-exposed and ageing skin. Whorled masses of disorganized elastin-staining fibres replace normal collagen.

Fibrinoid degeneration: deposition of eosinophilic material which resembles fibrin.

Necrobiosis: a type of focal necrosis of collagen which leads to the formation of a palisading granuloma, i.e. macrophages lining up like a fence around the necrotic material.

Lichenoid: a heavy infiltrate of white cells hugs the epidermal interface with the dermis and fills the upper dermis.

Table 2

Disease	Immunofluorescence findings (direct)	Serum (indirect)
Pemphigus	IgG intercellular in the epidermis	Positive in 90%
Pemphigoid	IgG and complement is linear at the dermoepidermal junction	Positive in 70%
Linear IgA dermatosis	IgA is linear at the dermoepidermal junction	Negative
Dermatitis herpetiformis	IgA, granular often complement in dermal papillae	None
Lupus erythematosus	Granular band of IgG or IgM or complement at the dermoepidermal junction	Antinuclear antibodies

Fig. 8 When excising lesions of the skin, it is helpful to follow lines of tension and to be aware of the elasticity of the skin. On the trunk and limbs Langer's lines may be helpful, as in (a), but on the face (b) it is most important to follow the lines of facial expression. The patient should be encouraged to smile and frown in order to ascertain where the wrinkles are and to provide a guide for lines of tension along which biopsies could extend.

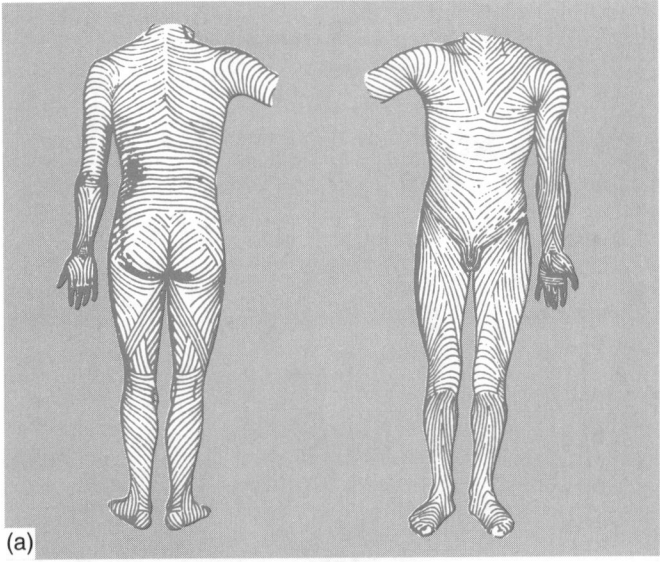
(a)

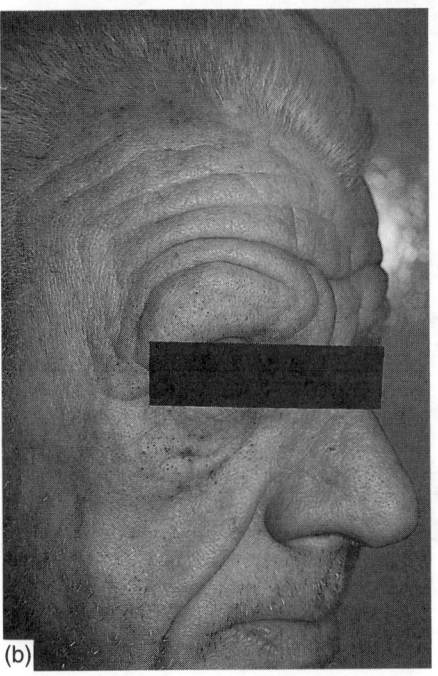
(b)

Immunofluorescence examination: modern immunofluorescence techniques mostly require frozen biopsies, or storage in special transport media, and they cannot be done on fixed or paraffin-embedded material. Immunofluorescence is most useful for bullous disease (Table 2).

REFERENCES

Ackerman, A.B. (1978). *Histologic diagnosis of inflammatory skin diseases,* p. 863. Lea and Febiger, Philadelphia.
Binford, C.M. and Connor, D.M. (1976). *Pathology of tropical and extraordinary diseases,* Vols 1 and 2. Armed Forces Institute of Pathology.
Jones, R.L. and Ponninghaus, J.M. (1982). *Leprosy Review* **53**, 67–8.
Lever, W.E. and Schaunburg-Lever, G. (1992). *Histopathology of the skin,* (7th edn). J.B. Lippincott, Philadelphia.
McKee, P.H. (1989). *Pathology of the skin with clinical correlations.* J.B. Lippincott, Philadelphia
Weedon, D. (1992). *The skin: systemic pathology,* (3rd edn), Vol. 9. Churchill Livingstone, New York.

The basis of rashes

The skin is not a homogeneous organ. It varies in thickness, rate of epidermal turnover, amount and quality of hair, sebaceous glands, or sweat, and in many other qualities. Clearly its components have a structure and some rashes affecting only one of these will have the distribution of that constituent, e.g. hair follicles in folliculitis (Fig. 9), sweat

Fig. 9 Perifollicular hyperkeratosis having the distribution of the hair follicle.

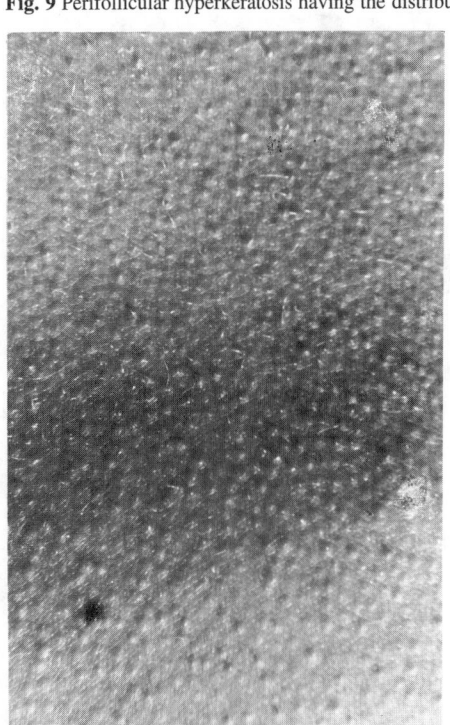

Fig. 10 Distribution of rashes.

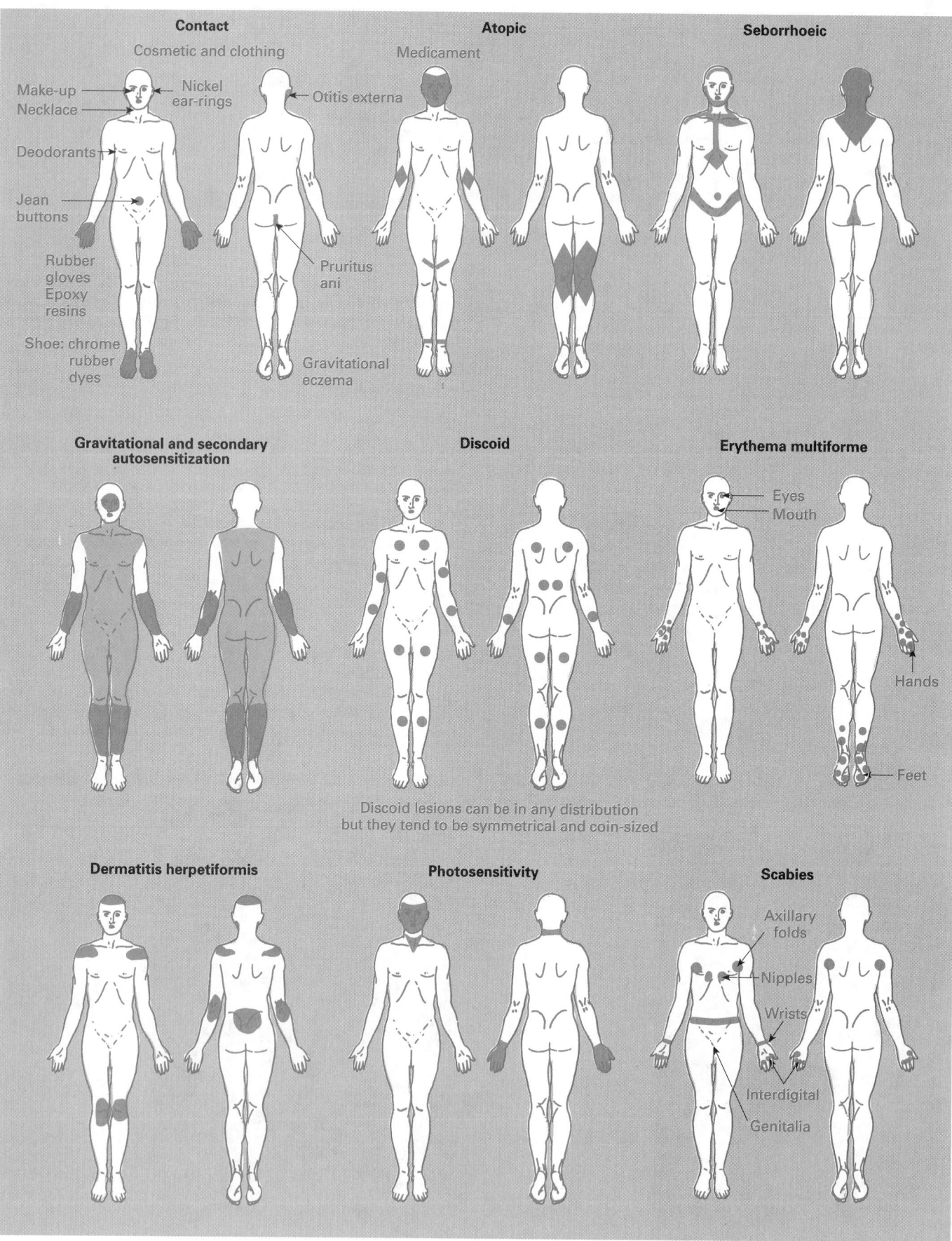

Fig. 10 (continued)

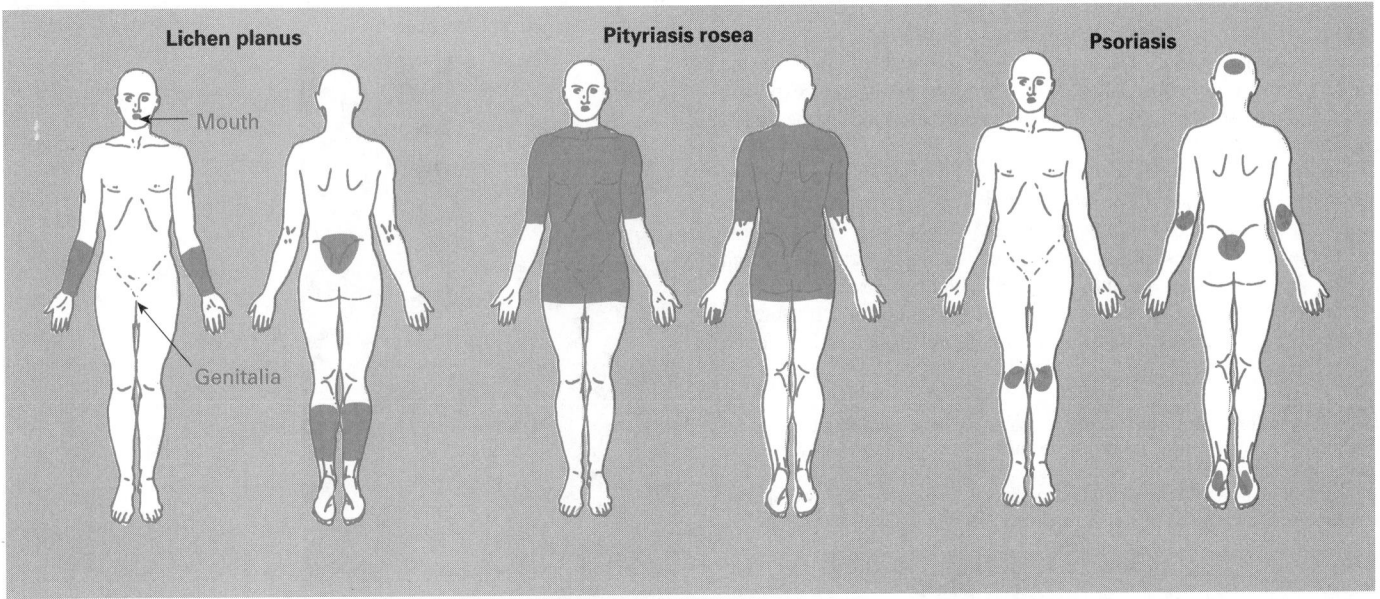

glands in prickly heat, sebaceous glands in acne vulgaris, dermatomes in herpes zoster, or annular and reticulate patterns as in some rashes determined by vascular anatomy.

Inflammation near the surface of the skin usually damages the epidermis so that vesiculation and scaling becomes a feature of the response, whereas deep dermal or subcutaneous inflammation merely produces 'lumps' known as nodules.

The rate of development of the rash is often determined by the type of inflammatory response—oedematous weals or blisters are more acute than white cell infiltration, purpura, or pustules, and ischaemic necrosis and exfoliation are late responses.

The clinician is a detective and in assessing physical signs must know the sequence of events leading up to what he can see. He must look at the distribution of the rash as well as its minutest morphology. Some

Table 3 *Some morphological terms*

A *macule* is flat without change in surface marking or texture—it may be merely redness, purpura, or melanin

A *papule* is a circumscribed, palpable elevation or a thickening of the epidermis or of the upper dermis by infiltration or oedema

A *plaque* is a disc-shaped lesion often as a result of the coalescence of papules

A *nodule* is a circumscribed palpable mass larger than 1 cm in diameter and usually consisting of oedema, malignant or inflammatory cells filling the dermis or subcutaneous tissue. Some are small and painful (Table 4) others are juxta-articular (Table 5)

Vesicles and *bullae* are visible accumulations of fluid (often the lay person uses the term blister to include wealing in which there are no visible accumulations other than swelling). Vesicles are small, while bullae are larger than 1 cm

Annular lesions result from spreading infiltrations or healing centre often with refractoriness due to such factors as raised tissue pressure or scarring preventing vasodilatation or leakiness in the centre of the lesions. Vascular patterns in the skin have a reticular or annular anatomical distribution (Table 6)

Linear lesions are due to external scratches, developmental or anatomical distribution of lymphatics, blood vessels, or nerves (Table 7)

classical distributions are shown in Fig. 10 while Table 3 illustrates some well-known morphological terms and Figs. 11 and 12 show some other shapes.

The concept of endogenous, constitutional, or the host's acting as a receptor for an exogenous and noxious trigger is an important explanation of rashes.

The management of skin disease requires elimination of possible agents causing injury and a recognition and treatment of altered host responses. Thus endogenous rashes tend to be symmetrical, whereas a biting insect does not know about symmetry, and fleas, for example, will produce groups of bites quite indiscriminately. Unlike the rashes of secondary syphilis, the site of the primary chancre is not influenced by host symmetry (Fig. 13). Fungus infections such as cattle ringworm or even the human trichophyton rubrum are frequently more obvious on one side of the body than another, whereas psoriasis is usually exactly symmetrical.

Injury to the skin from contact dermatitis usually has the distribution of contact; in cases due, for example, to mascara, gloves, or shoes, there will be symmetry (Fig. 14), but casually brushing against a noxious plant will produce bizarre asymmetrical patterns. Scratching spares the centre of the back, and a completely clear area between the shoulder blades when the rest of the body is covered with scratch marks (Fig. 15(a)) suggests that the cause of the rash is the injury done by such scratching. *Acarus* seems not to like climbing about in hairy areas so usually spares the head but favours between the fingers, the front of the wrists, or the glans penis.

External irradiation from the sun spares skin beneath the lobes of the ear and under the chin (Fig. 15(b)), whereas an airborne pollen dermatitis will not spare such areas but may have a similar cut off point below the collar. Small islands of normal skin in a generalized erythroderma are characteristic of pityriasis rubra pilaris (Fig. 15).

Recognition of signs of exogenous injury make it easier to eliminate the cause. Unfortunately much skin disease is due to altered host responses and I will call this 'vulnerability'.

Vulnerability

It is a common characteristic in skin disease, and is seen in dermatitis due to the irritants affecting the vulnerable atopic skin. It is seen in the haematogeneous localization of immune complexes or other agents at sites altered by previous injury. It is also seen in the Koebner phenomenon, a term used to describe the development of psoriasis, warts, or lichen planus when the skin is injured to a degree which in most people would not produce more than a temporary wound but in predisposed individuals results in a recognizable skin disease.

Vulnerability is well worth recognizing because it may be possible to treat the predisposition when it may not be possible to eliminate the trigger. Thus, those whose skin breaks down too easily from exposure to unavoidable solvents may be helped to retain their job by the liberal application of emollients.

Recurrent episodes of vasculitis in the legs due to immune complexes may be reduced by more frequent elevation of the legs, supportive bandages, and avoidance of cold environments. Vulnerability in the legs is due to the chronic stress of blood stasis and venous hypertension which can be shown to cause inhomogeneity of capillary vessel patterns and exhaustion of endothelial secretions such as plasminogen activator.

The ecology of the skin with its integrated, well-balanced interaction

Fig. 11 (a) An example of the 'target' lesion of erythema multiforme. (b) Healing of the centre of the lesion is a feature of many skin diseases, including fungus infections and, in this case, psoriasis. See also Fig. 58. (c) Annular erythema in lupus erythematosus with Ro antibody. This pattern of widespread erythema is also observed in association with underlying malignancy.

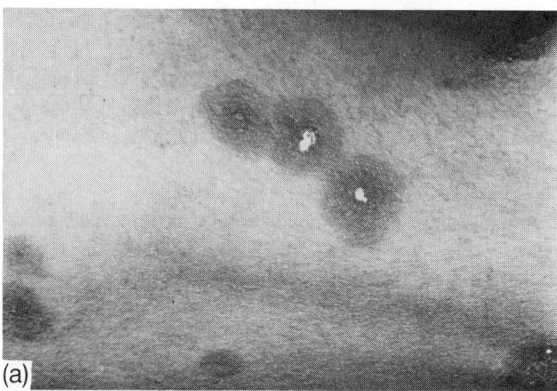

(a)

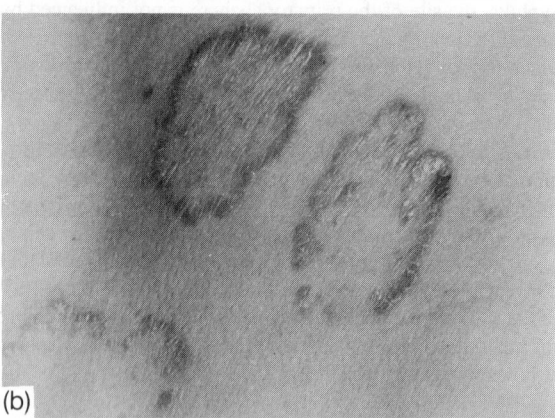

(b)

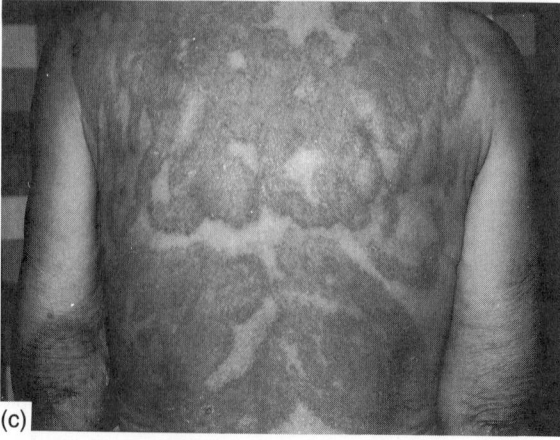

(c)

Fig. 12 Example of a linear distribution, in this case lichen planus. The distribution does not conform to a dermatome and the exact cause of the linear lesions remains largely unexplained.

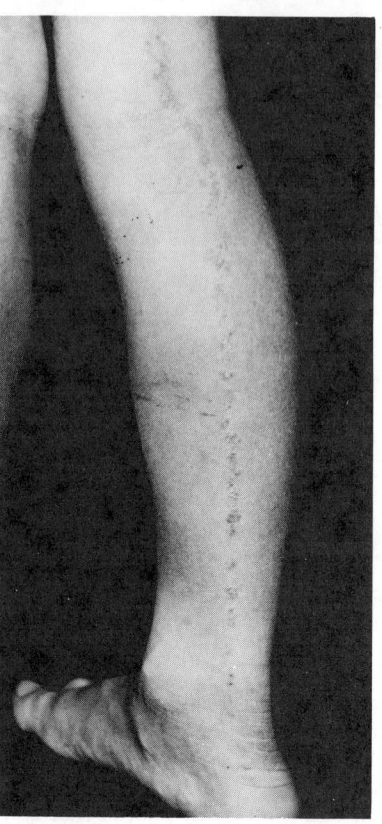

Fig. 13 A primary chancre of the lower left eyelid illustrating how skin diseases due to exogenous causes are often asymmetrical.

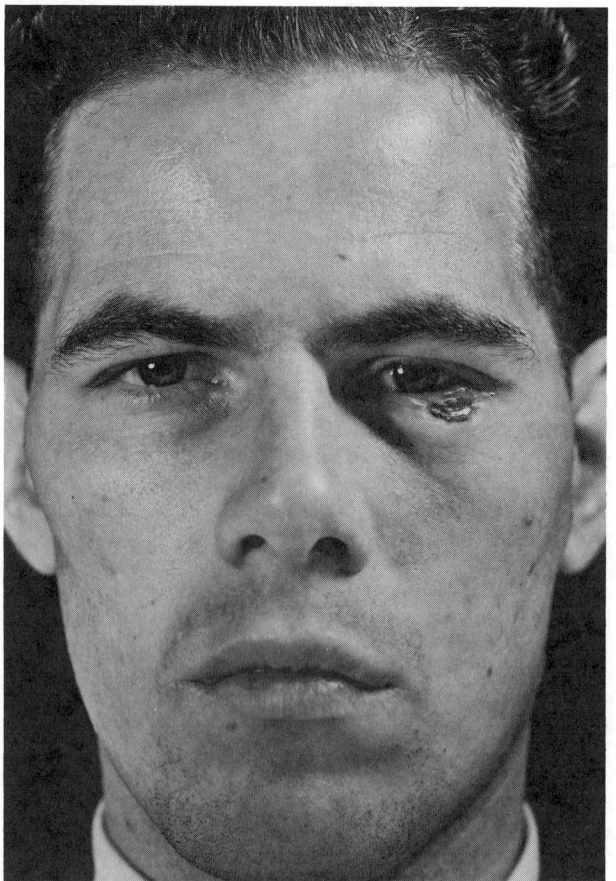

between bacteria and surface secretions also determines the skin's response at the interface with the environment. Erythrasma, pityriasis versicolor, and seborrhoeic eczema are partly constitutional and partly due to exogenous organisms. The seborrhoeic diathesis is poorly understood but such persons seem especially vulnerable to infection by more pathogenic organisms.

Factors determining or modifying skin disease

CHANGES OF SKIN WITH AGE, SEX, AND RACE

Newborn

Birth marks are usually first noticed in the newborn but some, like cavernous haemangiomas, may not be present on the first day. Certain epidermal or pigmented naevi and some neurofibromas do not appear until puberty. Some birthmarks have important diagnostic significance indicating serious systemic disease. Examples are the hypopigmented lesions of tuberous sclerosis (see Fig. 74) and the telangiectatic lesion of the Sturge–Weber syndrome.

Most Caucasian newborn have a pink skin and the vascular immaturity gives rise to flushing, mottling, reticulate markings, and some-

Fig. 14 Occasionally symmetry in the distribution of contact may be due to symmetrical application as in the case of this glove dermatitis.

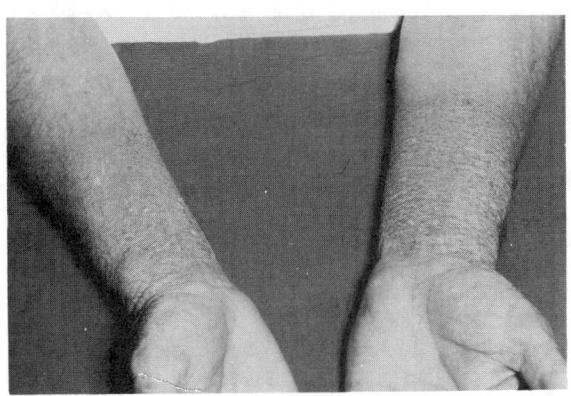

times segmental or one-sided flushing. This immaturity also prevents adequate cooling or heating in extremes of climate. Skin of the newborn is usually oedematous and often inflammation presents as blistering. Papulo-erythematous lesions of the newborn often contain large numbers of eosinophils. Newborn skin is susceptible to infection both from Candida and bacteria such as *Pseudomonas pyocyanea*. (See also dermatoses affecting the genitalia, vesicobullous disease in infancy, and Section 7.)

Puberty

Secondary sexual characteristics develop at puberty and at the same time an increase in susceptibility to apocrine diseases, sweating, and blushing is characteristic. Acne vulgaris is mainly a problem for the teenager. Certain diseases such as ichthyosis and eczema tend to improve while others such as herpes simplex and psoriasis, are more common. Naevi, particularly pigmented ones, tend to become more prominent.

Pregnancy

During pregnancy pigmentation is usually increased, and more hair, spider naevi, and palmar erythema develop. Some naevi, such as neurofibromatosis, become more prominent and certain infections, like perineal warts and candidiasis, are more troublesome. Pruritus, prurigo, blistering disorders such as herpes gestationis, and the rarer impetigo herpetiformis, presenting as pustular psoriasis with hypocalcaemia, are associated with pregnancy.

Old age

Skin diseases in old age are common and reduce the quality of life. Most elderly people have multiple skin problems, including seborrhoeic eczema, intertrigo, and dermatophytosis. Probably the principal characteristic of elderly skin is its inhomogeneity or the increased diversity that develops with age. Some changes are endocrine related, such as hirsutism and baldness. Others are more specifically age-related, like dryness, decreased sweating, or poor healing of superficial wounds. Dry, scaly, rough skin occurs in about 80 per cent of people over the age of 75 and there are disparities in the size and thickness of the epidermis and in its pigmentation. Seborrhoeic warts, actinic injury, Campbell di Morgan spots, and dilatation and derangement of superficial venules are

Fig. 15 (a) The central area of the back is spared from this dermatosis induced by scratching for the simple reason that the patient is not able to reach that site. (b) External irradiation from the sun spares the area beneath the lobes of the ear and under the chin in this case of solar dermatitis. (c) Small islands of unaffected skin scattered throughout a generalized redness and keratoderma are characteristic of pityriasis rubra pilaris.

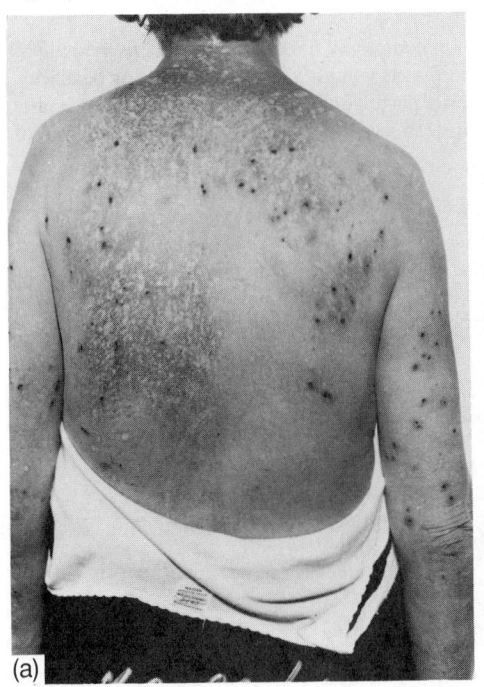
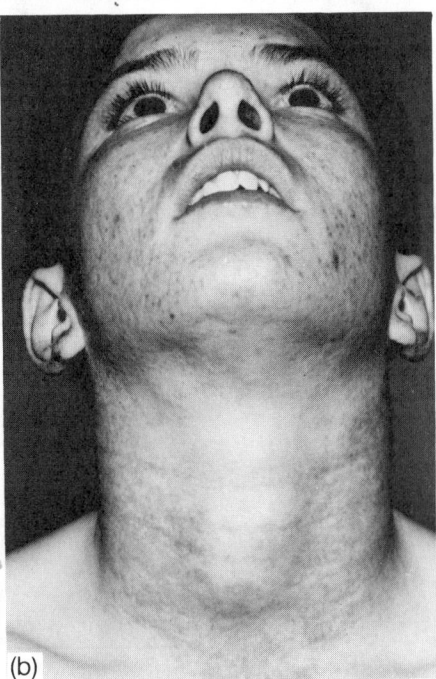
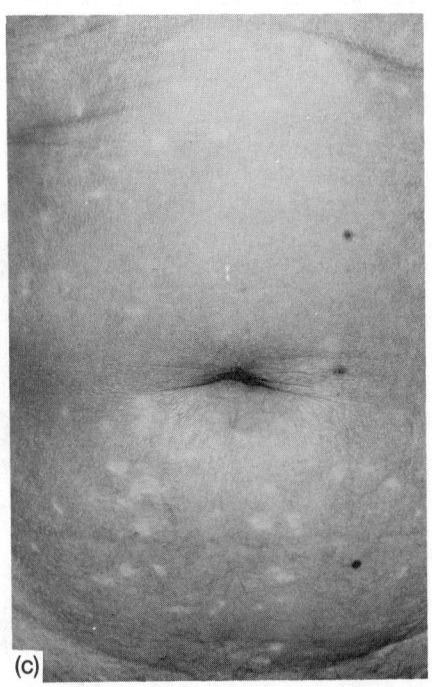

(a) (b) (c)

common features. Some diseases are age-related for reasons which are obscure. These include pruritus, pemphigoid, and lichen sclerosus et atrophicus.

Degenerative disease and the cumulative exposure to solar radiation explains neoplasia of the skin. Degenerative disease of the vascular system explains venous ulcers and arterial ischaemic diseases. In one study after controlling for age, sex, and sun exposure, premature wrinkling increased with years of smoking. Heavy smokers were 4.7 times more likely to be wrinkled than non-smokers.

REFERENCE

Kadunce, D.P., *et al.* (1991). Cigarette smoking: risk factor for premature facial wrinkling. *Annals of Internal Medicine* **114**, 840–4.

Race

Differences in populations are partly explained by genetic factors but so much adaptation to environment occurs that customs and diet may determine some attributes. It is frequently reported that certain diseases are absent in tropical climates but this is probably because they have never been looked for or recognized. In dark skins erythema is violaceous and purpura may be difficult to detect; minor skin problems may not be complained of in the tropics where many neoplastic and inflammatory diseases are so florid and attendance for advice is so often delayed. A move to a more temperate climate is often associated with urbanization which can equally influence the skin. The most easily recognized difference from one person to another is skin colour and the consequences of sun exposure are much reduced in dark skins. Vitiligo is probably more common in the Caucasian races of the Middle East, North Africa, and India. The Japanese seem to develop rather readily a slaty-blue or ashy discoloration of the trunk following inflammatory disease. On the other hand, acne vulgaris is very uncommon in the Japanese and both acne and rosacea seem to be uncommon in the black skin. However, comedone formation due to cosmetics without full-blown acne is common in black skin. Blackness is due to larger and less degradable pigment granules, more evenly dispersed. The stratum corneum of black skin is more compact with higher lipid content and less penetration by irritants. Another easily recognized factor is hair size and shape. Facial hirsutism is rare in Japanese women and relative sparseness of hair is a feature of mongoloid races. On the other hand Mediterranean and some Indian races seem to be particularly hirsute (Fig. 16). The shininess of black skin is partly due to sebum but also thermal stress encourages increased eccrine sweating. Such skins tend to become rather dry when they move to a temperate climate. Scales show up on dark skins. Those with a black skin like to grease it, whereas those with

white skin use powder. Keloids are a considerable problem for the Afro-Caribbean and can sometimes be massive. Susceptibility to infection depends on immunological factors and on previous exposure. As with malaria or syphilis, some populations seem to acquire a genetic resistance to tuberculosis and leprosy.

REFERENCE

La Ruche, G. and Cesarini, J.P. (1992). Histologie et physiologie de la peau noire. *Annales de Dermatologie et de Venerologie* **119**, 567–74.

IS IT CONTAGIOUS (TABLES 4–7)?

One is often asked whether a skin disease is 'infectious'. The questioner means, 'Did I catch it?' 'Can I give it to someone else?' 'Is the treatment of choice a simple antiseptic or antibiotic regimen?' The physician may ask, 'Am I missing something which is a danger to the patients in the rest of the ward or to my nursing staff?'

There are many infections, dealt with elsewhere in this textbook, in which a highly virulent organism has broken the defences of a normally resistant host, but there are also organisms which are usually harmless but occasionally, because of immunosuppression or other changes in the host, produce a rash. Pityriasis versicolor, candidiasis, erythrasma, and trichomycosis axillaris, all discussed in Section 7, are examples. More difficult is the relationship with the staphylococcus or streptococcus which for the most part sit in silence on the skin, but are unwelcome in a ward full of more susceptible patients. Psoriasis is not infectious but the massive exfoliation from such a patient is a great source of cross-infection. The bacterial spread by skin scales is considerable. Few would feel bound to treat every psoriatic for bacterial infection but the same degree of infection in atopic eczema is thought of as a contribution to the disease, perhaps through bacterial allergy.

Pathology from skin infection is more common in hot humid climates, and erosions from scratching, prickly heat, and other infections, such as lice or scabies, predispose to boils and other patterns of pyoderma, especially in the groins and axillae.

The primary pathology of infection is often asymmetrical but an immune response attempting to get rid of it is usually exactly symmetrical and takes 5 to 10 days to develop.

The most difficult diagnostic problem is the viral disease. The hospital doctor is not well placed to recognize its variety. It is the general practitioner called to the patient's home who sees virus disease in its early stages or in its transient phase. It is essential to know what rashes are currently endemic.

Rashes due to infection commonly have an associated fever, lymphadenopathy, coryza, diarrhoea, vomiting, hepatomegaly, or headache. However, the abrupt sterile pustulation of generalized pustular psoriasis (Fig. 17) or the painful deep swelling of delayed pressure urticaria or

Fig. 16 Hair growth on the forehead of an Indian child. This is entirely within normal limits and is of racial origin.

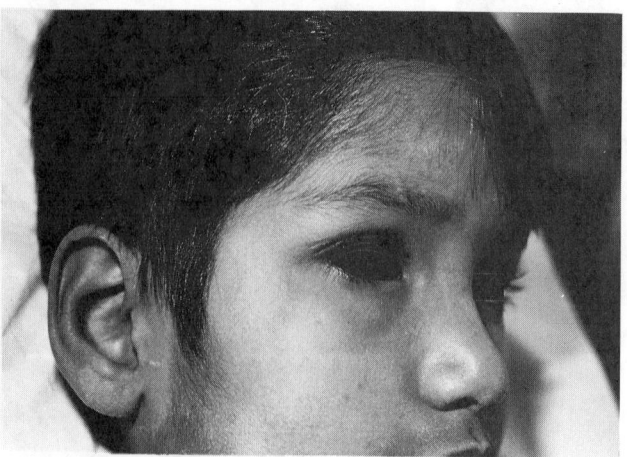

Table 4 *Severe pain on compression of a small dermal papule or nodule is a well-recognized symptom of the following lesions. If there is doubt, excision is the treatment of choice, so that a definitive histological examination can be made*

Glomus	Eccrine spiradenoma
Leiomyoma	Angiolipoma
Neuroma	Chondrodermatitis (of the outer helix)

Table 5 *Juxta-articular nodules*

Rheumatoid nodules	Granuloma annulare
Gouty tophi	Multicentric reticulohistiocytosis
Xanthomata	Synovial cysts, ganglia, or Heberden's nodes

Table 6 *Some annular lesions*

Impetigo	Urticaria
Dermatophytosis	Lichen planus (Fig. 58)
Syphilis	Lupus erythematosus (Ro antibody) (Fig. 11(c))
Leprosy	Purpura
Lupus vulgaris	Seborrhoeic eczema
Pityriasis rosea	Sarcoidosis
Erythemas—toxic, urticarial, and multiforme (Fig. 11(a))	Mycosis fungoides
	Granuloma annulare/multiforme
Psoriasis (Fig. 11(b))	Glucagonoma

Table 7 *Linear lesions with dermatomal distributions include the well-recognized herpes zoster. Many linear lesions follow a pattern which does not exactly conform to innervation or blood supply, especially when it extends the whole way up the leg or arm*

Lichen striatus	Artefacta scratching
Lichen planus[a] (Fig. 12)	Focal dermal hypoplasia
Psoriasis[a]	Incontinentia pigmenti
Epidermal naevi	Papular mucinosis
Darier's disease[a]	Sarcoid[a]
Morphea	Warts[a]
Porokeratosis of Mibelli	Molluscum contagiosum
Contact dermatitis[a]	Syringoma
Phytophotodermatitis	

[a]May be a reaction to a scratch (Koebner phenomenon).

Note: some linear nodules are determined by lymphatic drainage: mycobacteria, sporotrichosis, neoplasm, coccidioidomycosis.

vasculitis will also be accompanied by high fever and a neutrophil leucocytosis, but usually in these non-infectious processes there is no lymphadenopathy. Erythema multiforme, Sweet's disease, and toxic epidermal necrolysis similarly show great systemic effects. Persons with widespread skin disease may not be able to control their body temperature and high fever in such persons is not necessarily a sign of infection.

Good practice when in doubt is to take adequate swabs and specimens for culture and histological examination as well as to treat and touch the patient as his or her comfort requires. Washing of hands suffices for scabies, fungus, and most bacterial diseases as well as warts and syphilis. The principal care is to protect the practitioner against inoculation of the skin when taking scrapings or doing a biopsy. Patients with much exfoliation should not be nursed on a general ward.

Pustules need not be caused by infection, and in psoriasis or an irritant folliculitis from oils, for instance, the primary lesions are always sterile. Vesicles need not be due to viruses since they are a feature of papular urticaria and vasculitis (see Fig. 96). Dark skins exposed to much oil and cosmetics often have a chronic pustular dermatosis of the lower legs which may be sterile.

Humidity is the principal cause of profuse skin infection, and treatment by cooling and drying has always been a standard therapy for an infected eczema. The fact is that drying is promoted by the use of wet dressings and the consequent evaporation. Wet dressings which are occlusive and changed infrequently encourage infection. Ideally they should be changed every 2 to 4 h. Occlusive surfaces such as between the toes, the groins, and the breasts need drying agents such as are commonly present in deodorants (aluminium chloride), or the use of powders. Dry mopping of the ear in otitis externa is similarly helpful.

For the rest, the diagnosis of infection is by a process of exclusion. One aspect of this is a thorough inspection of the skin until the lesions are found that are firmly diagnostic, for instance, psoriasis, lichen planus, or vasculitis, or perhaps conclusive of infection such as the burrows between the fingers in scabies (Fig. 18), or the crab louse in the pubic hair.

In some parts of the world skin clinics are overwhelmed by massive numbers of patients suffering from scabies, staphylococcal and streptococcal infection, and dermatophytosis. The doctor's role in Bombay and Calcutta, for instance, can be compared to that of a good administrator or hygienist attempting to control infections in a large family when it is not possible to treat all members of the family (Fig. 19). Control is impossible because re-infection is inevitable. Desai, in Bombay, believed that soap and water does much to reduce the incidence of common dermatoses but water is too valuable to use for washing when there is a drought.

In Mediterranean countries, ringworm of the scalp would be easy to manage (Fig. 20) were it not that the population explosion provides more children for the infection than it is possible to treat, and subclinical

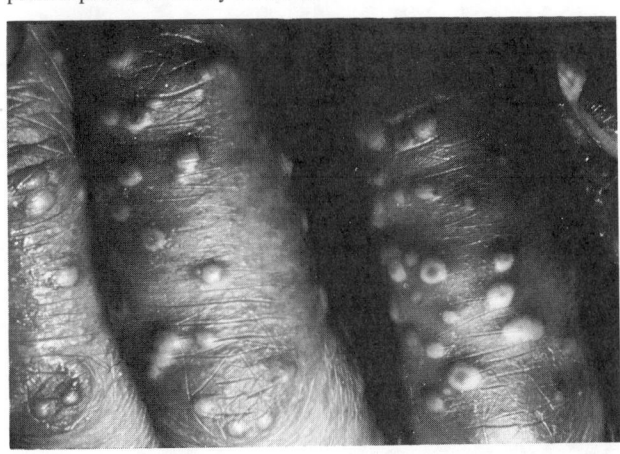

Fig. 17 Pustules are not necessarily due to infection. These pustules are from pustular psoriasis and they are sterile.

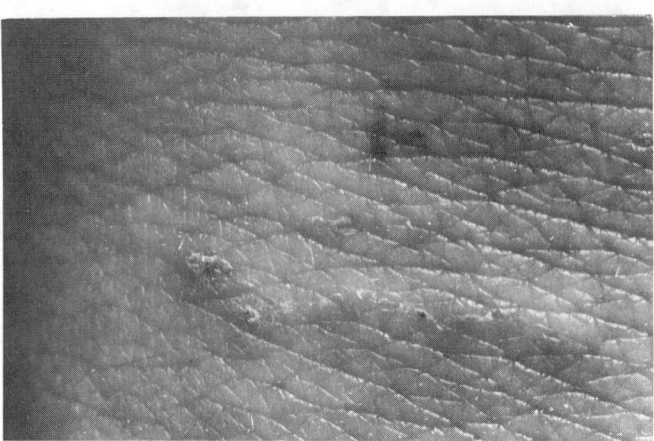

Fig. 18 The diagnostic feature of scabies. The burrow of the mite in the horny layer of the epidermis. The dark spots are the haemoglobin in the belly of the mite.

infections are difficult to recognize. If it is impossible to control head lice in Oxford, the chances of controlling similar infections in Algeria must be very small. Some chronic infections presenting as granulomas are discussed and illustrated later.

IS IT HEREDITARY?

It has long been recognized that many skin disorders, such as eczema and psoriasis, may have a hereditary basis. The concept that some persons have inherent tendencies to develop certain diseases has been supported by studies of the HLA antigens.

Establishing that there has been a strong family history of the disease, especially if environmental factors such as infection can be ruled out, often helps in making a diagnosis. Thus an intensely itchy eczema in an infant is likely to be due to atopy if there are other members of the family affected by asthma or eczema. Most parents or patients will

Table 8 *Common, minor, non-inherited abnormalities*

Accessory nipple
Hypoplastic toenails
Preauricular sinus or skin tag
Overfolded helix
Webbed neck

accept that genetic factors contribute to chronicity and will not expect instant cure.

Each pregnancy carries a 4 per cent risk of congenital malformation and during embryonic life maldevelopment of localized areas of skin can give rise to a variety of developmental defects. Most of the common defects (Table 8) are not inherited but the presence at birth of certain well-recognized lesions, like the hypopigmented macule of tuberous sclerosis (see Fig. 74) or extra, fused (see Fig. 122(b)), or accessory digits, are a feature of some hereditary diseases. Advances in the early recognition of genetic disorders, even *in utero,* and more particularly in the effective use of family planning, have increased the demand for, and application of, genetic counselling. In the Western world fear of transmitting genetic disease is replacing fear of contagion.

With most single-gene conditions, the risk of having another affected child is substantial—more than 1 in 10. This is unfortunately not a field for the non-specialist since subtle variations in the distribution or morphology of a skin rash can determine very different advice. Thus, dominant, sex-linked or recessive forms of ichthyosis or epidermolysis bullosa have distinct differences in pattern.

In some countries, first cousin marriages are very common and even encouraged by local customs, law, and religion. One in four of the offspring of recessive heterozygotes will inherit the defect. It can be calculated statistically that in a family of four children born to such parents, one will be affected in 42.2 per cent of cases, two in 21.1 per cent, three in 4.7 per cent, four in 0.4 per cent, and none in 31.6 per cent. About half the subjects of autosomal dominant disorders listed in Table 9 are new mutants. Autosomal recessive inheritance listed in Table 9 is mostly incompatible with normal physical and mental development and some affected individuals are now more likely to be seen where the standard of nutrition and freedom from infection is high. Xeroderma pigmentosum and albinism are common in countries such as Africa, but affected individuals rarely survive to old age.

The skin and the nervous system are both ectodermal in origin and hence there are many congenital diseases affecting both systems (Table 10).

The concept of clonality has only recently been used to explain some of its most bizarre patterns (Fig. 21(a)) The whorls and linearity of certain naevi are best explained by mosaics and embryological streaming (Happle 1985).

REFERENCES

Happle, R. (1985). *Human genetics* **70**, 200.
Harper, J. (1992). Genetics and genodermatoses. In *Textbook of dermatology,* (ed. A. Rook, D.S. Wilkinson, and F.J.G. Ebling), pp. 305–72. Blackwell Scientific, Oxford

Ichthyosis

Ichthyosis is characterized by a dry and scaling skin. Hereditary forms can always be diagnosed before the age of 5 years and if the disorder is acquired later it usually indicates underlying disease such as carcinoma or Hodgkin's disease. The skin of a severely affected patient is covered by large adherent scales, while fine, white, branny scales characterize mild ichthyosis. Several different types have been described, differentiated by their clinical picture and mode of inheritance.

Fig. 19 Infections such as impetigo are highly contagious and tend to be found in more than one member of the family, as in these triplets.

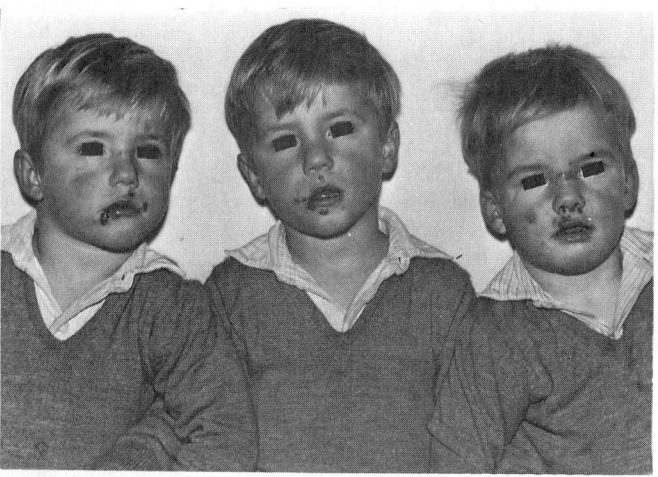

Fig. 20 Multiple exudative lesions due to tinea capitis.

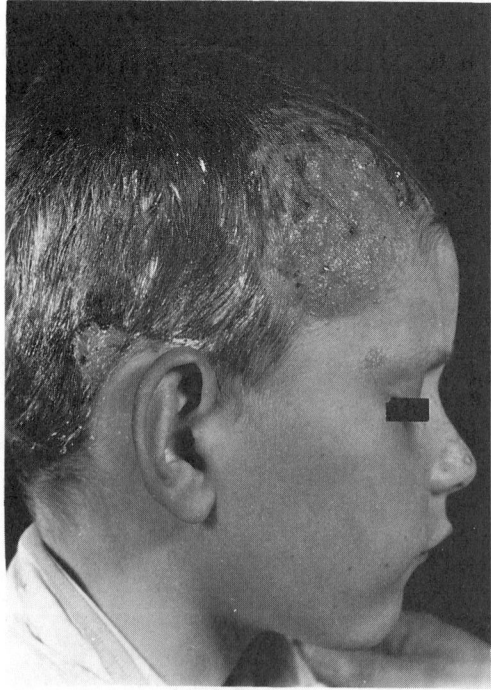

Table 9 *Inherited skin disorders*

Autosomal dominant inheritance	
Neurofibromatosis	Peutz–Jeghers syndrome
Tuberous sclerosis	Monilethrix
Ehlers–Danlos syndrome	Gardner's syndrome
Epidermolysis bullosa	Pachyonychia congenita
Ichthyosis vulgaris	Bullous ichthyosiform hyperkeratosis
Tylosis	Hidrotic ectodermal dysplasia
Benign familial pemphigus	
Darier's disease	
Familial hypercholesterolism	
Autosomal recessive inheritance	
Albinism oculocutaneous	Mal de Maleda
Ichthyosiform erythroderma	Xeroderma pigmentosum
Dystrophic epidermolysis bullosa	Rothmund–Thomson syndrome
Phenylketonuria	Ataxia telangiectasia
Werner's syndrome	Lipoid proteinosis
Acrodermatitis enteropathica	Bloom's syndrome
Chondroectodermal dysplasia	
Sex-linked inheritance	
Ichthyosis	Dyskeratosis congenita
Anhidrotic ectodermal dysplasia	Menkes' syndrome
Chronic granulomatous disease	Angiokeratoma corporis diffusa
Keratosis pilaris atrophica	Aldrich syndrome
Multifactorial, polygenic, and suspected by some	
as being dominant	
Psoriasis	Alopecia areata
Atopic eczema	Acne vulgaris
Hirsutism	Seborrhoeic dermatitis
Skin manifestations of chromosomal disorders	
47 XXY (Klinefelter): leg ulcers, absent beard	
47 XYY: severe nodular cystic acne	
45 XO (Turner): lymphoedema of hands and feet,	
cystic hygroma	
47 XX (XY) + 21 (Down's): vitiligo, alopecia areata,	
ichthyosis vulgaris	

Ichthyosis vulgaris is the most common type and has a dominant form of inheritance. The lower legs are most affected, involvement becoming progressively less towards the head. The skin is dry and scaling, and most patients show a lozenge-shaped pattern resembling crocodile markings. There is usually very evident sparing of the skin of the popliteal spaces, the antecubital fossae, and the creases of the groin. The skin of the palms and the soles shows increased markings—the so-called fortune-teller's nightmare. Perifollicular hyperkeratosis (keratosis pilaris) is also a feature. In some children the ichthyosis is associated with atopic eczema which favours the cubital popliteal fossae, and another common problem in children is the appearance of a dirty neck owing to the retention of skin scales. The dryness of the skin is aggravated by the reduced sebaceous and sweat gland secretion; water evaporates from the epidermal cells because those affected lack the thin film of grease present on the surface of normal skin. There is marked seasonal variation in symptoms and many children are in fact better in the summer, possibly because the skin becomes hydrated as a result of sweating. The characteristic histological appearance is a reduced or absent granular layer, and it has been postulated that the condition results from inadequate shedding rather than overproduction of the horny layer.

Sex-linked ichthyosis is transmitted by clinically unaffected females and is seen only in males. The gene is on the short arm of the X chromosome in the X p22.3 region. A deficiency of steroid sulphatase causes increased cholesterol in all cell membranes. This contributes to reduced cell shedding. Parents and children of males with sex-linked ichthyosis have normal skin but their daughters may transmit the condition to their sons. Affected individuals usually have large, dark scales. Flexures may be involved but the palms of the hands are spared.

Bullous ichthyosiform erythroderma (epidermolytic hyperkeratosis). This rare condition produces a variety of clinical pictures, ranging from local areas of hyperkeratosis of the flexures and periumbilical region to gross involvement of the skin (porcupine man). The palms and soles are usually normal.

Ichthyosiform erythroderma is a rare autosomal recessive trait. It may be present at birth as one of the forms of 'collodion fetus' in which the baby seems to be covered by a film of collodion-like material through which it bursts during the first few days of life. There is a widespread involvement of the skin, including the palms and soles, and no improvement with age (Fig. 21(b)). Ectropion is troublesome.

TREATMENT

There is no known way of stimulating normal sebaceous function in these patients. They should avoid de-greasing their skin with detergents and may be helped by the application of oils and wool fats. Oil or a mixture of emulsifying ointment in hot water (stirred and melted before pouring) may be added to a bath. Creams such as the 10 per cent urea preparation (Calmurid®, Aquadrate®) have a moisturizing effect through their osmotic activity. Sunbathing and exposure to ultraviolet light is usually of value. Etretinate acid 0.5 mg/kg daily has been life-saving in the neonate and clears the scaling within 2 to 4 weeks but soreness of

Table 10 *Disorders of skin and nervous system*

Photosensitivity	
Xeroderma pigmentosum	Retardation, ataxia
Bloom's syndrome	Sometimes retardation
Cockayne syndrome	Retardation, deafness, ataxia
Porphyria	Epilepsy, depression, neuropathy
Hartnup syndrome	Ataxia, retardation
Kloepfer syndrome	Retardation
Pigmentary disorder	
Neurofibromatosis	Acoustic neuroma, retardation, epilepsy
Sneddon's syndrome	Livedo reticularis and arterial stenosis
Tuberous sclerosis	Epilepsy, retardation
Sturge–Weber syndrome	Epilepsy, angioma, retardation
Incontinentia pigmenti	Polymicrogyria, epilepsy, retardation
Chediak–Higashi syndrome	Deafness
Laurence–Siep syndrome	Retardation
Leopard syndrome	Deafness
Hair disorder	
Marinesco–Sjögren syndrome	Retardation, ataxia
Papillon–Lefèvre syndrome	Tremor, retardation
Menkes' syndrome	Retardation, epilepsy
Phenylketonuria	Retardation
Hypoparathyroidism	Epilepsy, retardation
Arginosuccinic aciduria	Epilepsy, retardation
Ichthyosis	
Refsum's disease	Ataxia, deafness, neuritis
Rud's syndrome	Epilepsy, polyneuritis
X-linked	Retardation
Linear sebaceous naevus	
Feuerstein syndrome	Retardation and epilepsy

Fig. 21 Subtle variations in the distribution of a rash may determine the nature of genetic counselling. This scaling is typical of the skin changes in ichthyosis. The involvement of the flexures rules out the common dominant pattern. That palmar changes make ichthyosiform erythroderma (non-bullous) the correct diagnosis. This is a recessive disorder.

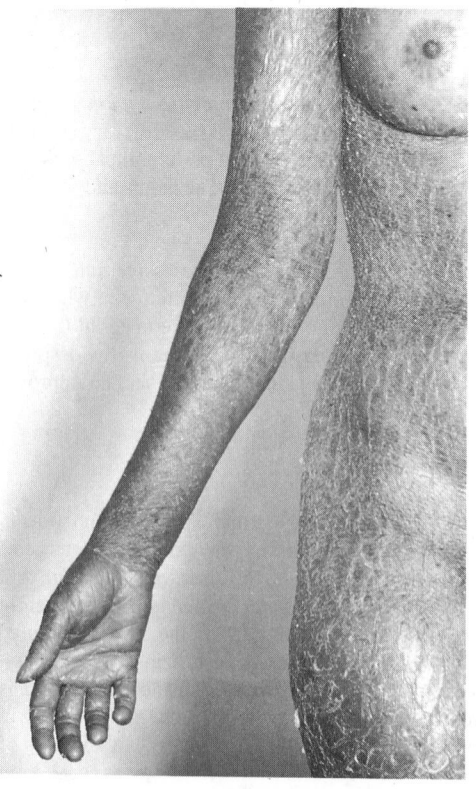

the mouth, eyes, and genitalia as well as erosions of the skin may be unacceptable.

Epidermolysis bullosa

Epidermolysis bullosa was a name given to a group of inherited diseases characterized by the production of blisters in the skin following trauma. The clinical features of the most common of the 16 recorded patterns are given in Table 11. Epidermolysis bullosa may present for the first time in army recruits who are marching with new boots and develop grotesque blistering. There is a tendency for the condition to improve with age.

The dystrophic forms of epidermolysis bullosa are more often recognized at birth. Severe disability may result, repetitive blistering leading to fusion of the fingers and toes, gross scarring, and dystrophy of the nails; there may also be involvement of the mucosa of the mouth and oesphagus, leading to oesophageal stenosis. These epidermal disorders are caused by a collagen type VII defect in the dermis affecting the composition of the basement membrane. There is an increased tendency for neoplasm in the affected scarred areas. The gene locus is linked to the COLYA1 gene on chromosome 3.

In epidermolysis bullosa simplex of the Dowling Meara type, arginine 125 to cystine mutations affect keratin 14.

In epidermolysis bullosa simplex of the Koebner type, a mutation is of the 3542 bp region of chromosome 17, possibly having something to do with the nidogen locus of chromosome 1. The keratin 5 gene is believed to be involved in the Weber–Cockayne type, and there is linkage to the glutamic pyruvic transaminase locus on chromosome 8 in the condition of epidermolysis bullosa simplex described by Ogna.

TREATMENT

There is no specific therapy but much can be done to help these patients by giving them advice on protection and clothing. The very serious

Table 11 *Clinical features of the most common patterns of epidermolysis bullosa*

	Autosomal inheritance	Pathology	Onset	Course	Distribution	Other features
Epidermolysis bullosa simplex	Dominant	Epidermal; clefts through basal cell layer	Soon after birth; may be delayed	May improve with time; worse in warm weather	Feet and hands, also around mouth and trunk	None, no scars
Epidermolysis bullosa simplex of the hands and feet	Dominant	Epidermal; clefts through basal cell layer	Variable	Improves with time; worse in warm weather	Hands and feet, except in babies	None, no scars
Epidermolysis bullosa letalis	Recessive	Junctional; cleft between plasma membrane and basal lamina	At birth	May be mild at onset, usually progressive and fatal; Mild form exists with long-term survivors	Palms, soles, and vermilion border of lips spared	Nail dystrophy; mouth and oesophagus, also respiratory tract, mild atrophy
Epidermolysis bullosa dystrophica (dermolytic bullous dermatosis)	Dominant	Unknown. Increased sulphated glycosaminoglycans	A few days after birth; may be delayed	Relatively mild; improves with time	Extensor surfaces	Scars; nail dystrophy; milia (common); mucous membrane (uncommon)
Epidermolysis bullosa dystrophica (dermolytic bullous dermatosis)	Recessive	Dermal; cleft under basal lamina; Anchoring fibrils absent Increased collagen degradation	At birth	Often severe with deformity and can be fatal; improves with time	Entire skin; even normal-looking skin has an abnormal texture and blisters easily	Scars; nail dystrophy; milia; mouth and oesophagus

blistering that may be seen at birth and which affects the development of the child as a result of the involvement of the oesophageal mucosa can be treated by large doses of prednisolone. Collagenase inhibition by phenytoin or other inhibitors is gaining favour.

Darier's disease and Hailey–Hailey disease

Darier's disease (keratosis follicularis) is an uncommon disorder, first appearing in young adolescence and fluctuating in intensity throughout life. It has an autosomal dominant inheritance carried on chromosome 12 and is characterized by the eruption of small greasy papules, usually on the trunk, extremities, and face which often coalesce to give yellowish-brown scaling sheets. In the groins, perineum, and axillae the lesions may become hypertrophic and liable to secondary infection. Lesions in the mouth are rare but involvement of the fingernails and pitting of the palms and soles is a common accompaniment and the nail change illustrated in Fig. 22 is the commonest.

PATHOLOGY

The characteristic change is loosening of the epidermal cells, usually just above the level of the basal cell. This is probably caused by a defect in the tonofibrildesmosome complex. Isolated epidermal cells may appear round (so-called *corps rond*) with a dark-staining nucleus surrounded by a clear zone, the result of tonofilaments aggregating round the nucleus.

Hailey–Hailey disease (familial benign pemphigus)

This is somewhat similar to Darier's disease and is also inherited as a dominant trait. The flexures are eroded and often there are blisters (Fig.

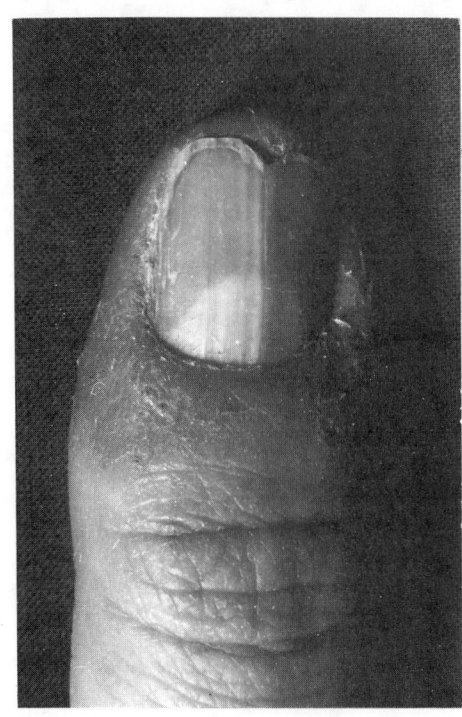

Fig. 22 Minimal signs may be a clue to the diagnosis as in this disease transmitted by a dominant gene. A white line extends from the nailbed to the distal nail plate where there is a 'V'-shaped notch. This is the most common finding of all in Darier's disease, and is present in most affected persons.

23). Sometimes it is extremely difficult to differentiate between the two conditions.

TREATMENT

Darier's disease responds to small doses of etretinate, but for Hailey–Hailey disease there is no effective treatment; controlling secondary infection when present by antibiotic creams and antiseptic lotions may keep the patient comfortable. Hot weather and exposure to the sun seem to aggravate the condition.

IS IT DUE TO MALNUTRITION?

Skin diseases of malnutrition have been termed the dermatoses of the poor. They are common in starving communities but are also seen in those living only on drugs or alcohol, those suffering from malabsorption syndromes, and those debilitated by neoplasia or severe chronic infections. Increasingly, elderly patients suffering from dementia are responsible for more cases in Western urban communities. Poor personal hygiene and lack of, or failure to use, water supplies contribute to some aspects of skin diseases in malnutrition as well as to the infections of both skin and mouth which often accompany them.

The skin is 8 per cent of body weight and uses up about one-eighth of the body's protein; hence it is affected early in malnutrition.

In experimental malnutrition and in studies on humans during the Second World War, dryness of the skin and hyperpigmentation were observed as early signs. At birth, malnutrition is seen as loss of vernix and maceration. The skin is wrinkled and peeling with deficient subcutaneous fat.

Older persons proceed to a mild ichthyosis and the associated hyperkeratosis is often a sign of slow turnover. The dry scale is well knit and retains pigment and histologically may be dense and homogenized. The stratum corneum is unsupple and cracks appear in the horny surface, particularly on the front of the legs (Fig. 24, see also Fig. 126). It is known as eczema craquelée and such eczema that develops is often well marginated, unlike other forms of endogenous eczema.

Most malnutrition is a consequence of mixed deficiencies including protein loss. There is weight loss, weakness, and emaciation. Anaemia, oedema, sore tongue, and dry, thin hair are often featured.

Vitamin A deficiency should be thought of when there is significant dryness of the eye and perifollicular hyperkeratosis. It is the commonest preventable cause of blindness.

Vitamin B deficiency causes a dermatitis that has a seborrhoeic distribution particularly of the nasolabial folds, scrotum, and vulva. The lips are dry, cracked, crusted, or ulcerated; the tongue is sore and smooth.

Nicotinic acid deficiency or pellagra causes the well-known triad of dementia, diarrhoea, and dermatitis. Early signs are prominent sebaceous follicles of the nose. The light sensitivity dermatosis is also exacerbated by heat, friction, or pressure. The erythema is a characteristic dusky brown and the dermatitis is well marginated. In the dark skin the lesions are relatively depigmented but equally well marginated.

Vitamin C deficiency causes perifollicular haemorrhages, painful bruising, or woody oedema of legs. This means in fact that they look oedematous but are hard to the touch. In the dark skin it may appear that the skin is stretched and shiny. Coiled hairs are an early sign but they are common in the normal population especially in the elderly. Swollen and bleeding gums are an important sign but occur only in those with teeth. It should be considered in any non-healing wound.

Protein deficiency is common in all forms of malnutrition, but where it is supplemented by carbohydrate and there is no active starvation, then a characteristic disease is recognizable. In children this is typified by kwashiorkor. Features of protein deficiency include:

(1) erythema as in a second-degree burn;
(2) dry hyperkeratotic hyperpigmented scales;
(3) peeling like enamel paint, cracking like crazy pavement;
(4) it is maximal over pressure areas; and
(5) there is straightening and reddening of the hair.

In some dark skins, raised annular patches of pigmented scales on the trunk are an early sign of malnutrition. It is known as pityriasis rotunda.

Management includes avoiding secondary deficiencies since, by suddenly providing some but not all the necessary foods, conditions like blindness from vitamin A deficiency, may be precipitated. In malnutrition, zinc may be lacking or poorly absorbed. Some improvement in the

Fig. 24 An early and common sign of malnutrition of the skin, especially in the elderly, is cracking of a well-made stratum corneum giving a pattern of eczema craquelée.

Fig. 23 Erosions of the axilla in Hailey–Hailey disease, a benign hereditary pseudopemphigus.

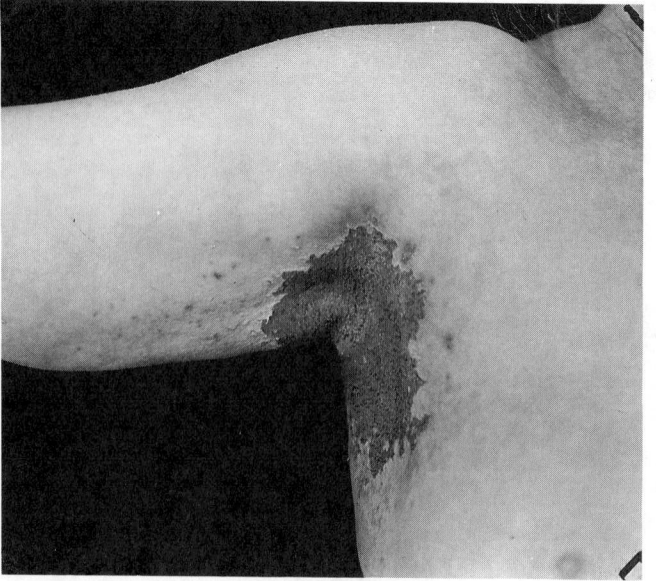

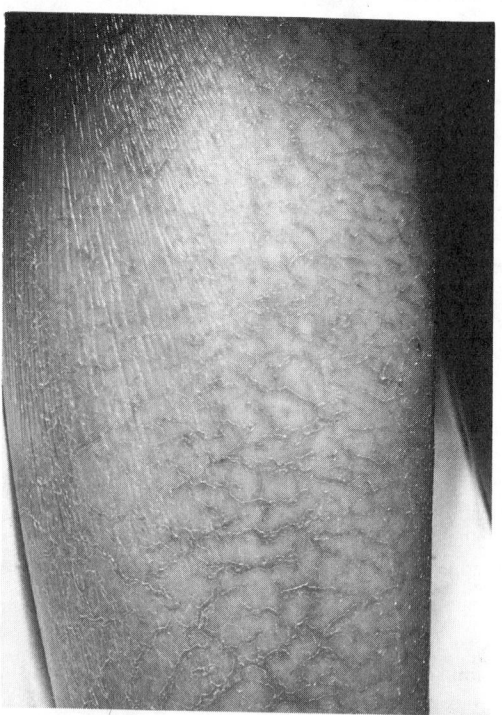

rash of kwashiorkor has been described using local zinc ointments, and prescribing other trace elements such as selenium.

IS THERE AN ASSOCIATION WITH GASTROINTESTINAL DISEASE?

There is a number of associations of skin disease with disease of the gastrointestinal tract. There is no completely satisfactory system for listing these. Many of the skin diseases are discussed more completely in other sections.

Oesophagus

In epidermolysis bullosa bullae are common and occasionally the entire epithelial lining of the oesophagus may be coughed up as a cast. Bullae also occur in pemphigus. Mucocutaneous pemphigoid and epidermolysis bullosa cause eventual scarring. Erosions also develop in lichen planus.

Stiffness and loss of peristalsis occurs in scleroderma often as an early sign. It is best demonstrated by a prone barium swallow. Carcinoma of the oesophagus has been associated with plantar palmar hyperkeratosis (tylosis) in two families. Webbing of the postcricoid region with anaemia is associated with dyskeratosis congenita—an atrophy of the skin and nails.

Stomach

Gastric atrophy and the presence of antibody to the parietal cell are associated with vitiligo and alopecia areata. Carcinoma may present with acanthosis nigricans. Gastric polyposis is associated with perioral and finger lentiginoses in the Peutz–Jeghers syndrome as well as with nail dystrophy and alopecia in the Canada–Cronkite syndrome.

Gastrointestinal bleeding is a consequence of telangiectasia in hereditary haemorrhagic telangiectasia as well as in acrosclerosis with telangiectasia, and rarely also in disorders of elastic tissues such as Ehlers–Danlos syndrome or pseudoxanthoma elasticum. Henoch–Schönlein purpura also causes gastrointestinal bleeding.

Small bowel

Regional ileitis may present with granulomatous swelling of the buccal mucosa or lips as well as with perianal granulomata and fistulae (Fig. 25).

Coeliac disease is associated with dermatitis herpetiformis. Pigmentation and malnutrition of the skin is particularly recorded in Whipple's disease.

Colon

Ulcerative colitis is responsible for many disorders of the skin and mouth in affected patients. Aphthous ulcers are more common. Skin rashes include erythema multiforme, erythema nodosum, and pyoderma gangrenosum. Perianal abscesses and fistulae are also common associations.

Erythema nodosum sometimes progressing to pyoderma gangrenosum occurs more commonly in Crohn's disease of the colon than from ulcerative colitis.

Pancreas

Migratory thrombophlebitis (Trousseau's sign) is more likely to be associated with carcinoma of the pancreas than with any other carcinoma. Acute fat necrosis of the trunk or limbs is a consequence of acute pancreatitis. There is an increased electrolyte concentration in the sweat of patients with mucoviscoidosis.

The glucagonoma syndrome is a recently recognized eruption of necrolytic migratory erythema due to sometimes quite small tumours of the pancreas. The skin lesions are dusky red, annular, and scaly with a vesicopustular element due to epidermal cell necrosis in the most superficial layers of the epidermis. The associations with diabetes mellitus are carotenaemia, moniliasis and dermatophytosis, necrobiosis lipoidica

(see Fig. 139), ulcers and gangrene, insulin lipodystrophy, and xanthoma. Widespread granuloma annulare, pruritus, lichen planus, and psoriasis are probably more common but more data are required to prove this.

Liver

The skin consequences of liver disease includes spider naevi, palmar flush, purpura and bruising, white nails, and clubbing. There is loss of hair in the beard, axillae, and pubic region. Gynaecomastia, acne, Dupuytren's contracture, xanthoma, jaundice, pruritus, and pigmentation are other features.

IS CLIMATE RESPONSIBLE?

Climate is responsible for much skin disease although, in the case of pyoderma or through the effects of famine and drought, its influence is indirect. Food and water supply are dependent on the climate and even if the lack or excess of these is not a direct cause, the management of skin disease requires washing, soaking, and adequate nutrition as well as control of body temperature. Children and the new-born, in particular, are susceptible to the influence of climate.

Humidity explained why, in the rainy season, 70 per cent of lost combat man-days in Vietnam were through skin disease. The distribution of water determines the ecology of many organisms that are parasitic on man, biting insects thriving in the rainy season. Wet clothing can cause severe discomfort, particularly in a boot or around the waist or between the legs while marching. Even in the Arctic, occlusive clothing can accumulate much sweat and make walking impossible. Immersion foot and paddy foot can bring a military campaign to an end. In Kuwait outbreaks of industrial dermatitis were blamed on the absorption of allergens by the skin that become moisturized in certain seasons, while in Scandinavia a low humidity in some factories accounted for drying of epidermis and consequent irritant dermatitis.

Seasonal variations account not only for increased bacterial injury but also for eczema, as for example in the atopic patient sensitive to pollens or the dermatitis due to plants seen so often in market gardeners and florists. Sweaty feet in hot weather increase the dermatitis from foot-

Fig. 25 Perianal granuloma in Crohn's disease.

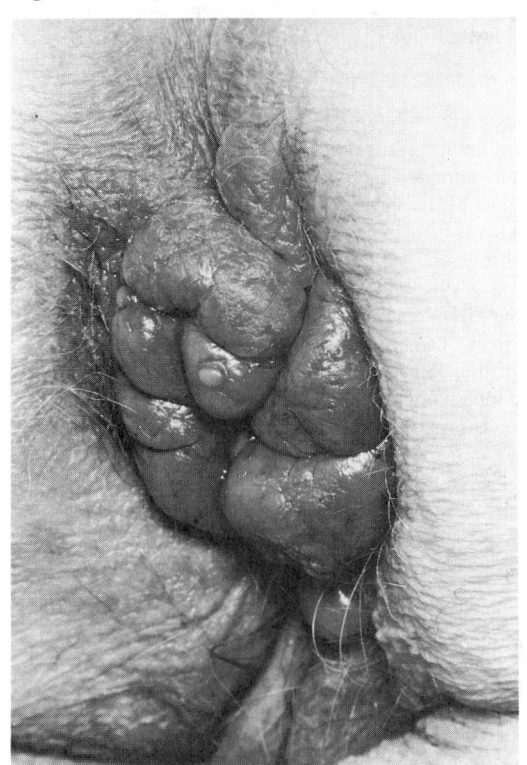

wear, and sweat pore occlusion encourages widespread bacterial infections in extreme heat. The incidence of some disease is influenced by height above sea-level and by the thickness of the atmosphere. One is unlikely to be sun burned at the low level of the Dead Sea but actinic dermatitis is common in Mexico and in the Andes. Many infections are most exuberant at sea-level. At the slightly higher level of 600 to 1500 m, transmission of leishmaniasis and onchocerciasis by flies is more common. Many of the skin diseases caused by infections that have a unique geographical distribution are discussed in the infectious diseases section, e.g. pinta, buruli ulcer, or deep mycoses. In this section they are only mentioned if they are important in differential diagnosis of some physical sign such as depigmentation, wartiness, or blisters.

Cold weather and low humidity predispose to irritant dermatitis and the high incidence of dry skin in hospital is explained by central heating and diminished occlusive clothing. Pediculosis is encouraged when people huddle together to keep warm.

While much is said about changes in the world's climate, less is said about changes in the skin's microclimate. These are brought about by changes in home heating and bed linen, as well as by clothing, including footwear. The skin, like antique wooden furniture, suffers from contemporary Western overheating and the resultant drying out. Dermatitis is one consequence. The second commonest environmental cause of neonatal mortality is hypo- or hyperthermia.

Cold

Frostbite and snow blindness will affect every polar explorer if inadequately protected, but individual susceptibility varies, so that in more temperate climates where the majority do not die of cold, there is a high incidence of skin disease that can be attributed to it. This is due to inadequate protection against minor degrees of cold injury. Vasoconstriction and increased blood viscosity mediate internal disease.

It is often noted that the resident of the United Kingdom has pink cheeks and blue hands to a degree not seen in, for instance, Australia or the United States. This is because of chronic exposure to cooling. In Canada or Scandinavia where the winters are a danger to the unprotected, there would be no such exposure of the schoolchild or teenager as seen during the winter in the United Kingdom where 10 per cent of the population are affected by chilblains, acrocyanosis, Raynaud's phenomenon, and the various manifestations of perniosis, an incidence never approached in most other parts of the world.

Perniosis

Chronic cold causes thickening of the subcutaneous and dermal tissues as in pigs. During the miniskirt era, thighs of girls regularly became fatter in temperature climates. Fat insulates the surface of the skin from the inside, so cooling of the surface is obvious. Chronic cooling causes telangiectasia, which is often perifollicular, and sometimes even angiokeratoma. Pink cheeks are one consequence, but similar changes may be seen over the fat of the calf or upper arm. Cooling causes stasis in the venules so that circulating noxious agents, such as immune complexes and bacteria, are usually localized at such sites.

The anatomy of the skin vasculature is such that cooled skin often shows a pink and blue mottling known as cutis marmorata. If this produces irreversible changes it is then known as livedo reticularis (Fig. 26(a)). Much disease is localized in the venules of such damaged vasculature. Sneddon's syndrome is livedo reticularis and a non-inflammatory stenosis of cerebral arteries.

Chiblains are essentially an ischaemia induced by cold. Pressure from tight clothing often encourages the damage done by cooling (Fig. 26(b)).

Ultraviolet radiation and the sun

The sun emits electromagnetic rays comprising a continuous spectrum of short to long waves. Only a narrow range reacts with photocells in the retina and is visible. Heat is due to infrared and this can be felt. Most short wavelengths which can neither be seen nor felt are filtered out by the Earth's thick atmosphere which includes ozone and water

vapour which screen out these harmful wave bands. As there is less atmosphere on mountain tops the danger of radiation exposure is greater. The content of water vapour in the atmosphere is variable, which accounts for protection from sunburn in winter, cloudy days, the early morning, or late evening sun, and the thick atmosphere of the low-lying Dead Sea in Israel and Jordan. Glass also protects, so that the closed windows of a car will protect even in a tropical desert unless one is sensitive to the longer wave lengths of ultraviolet radiation. Congenital porphyria is, for example, a disease in which it is difficult to protect against sensitivity to long-wave ultraviolet rays.

Ultraviolet rays are classified into three ranges UVB 290 to 320 nm penetrates and is of high energy and hence damages and produces sunburn. UVA (black light 320–400 nm) is of lower energy but it is penetrating and usually it is only damaging in the presence of sensitizers such as drugs, porphyrins, or plant juices. The shortest is UVC, which is non-penetrating, 200 to 290 nm, and accounts for the damage to the

Fig. 26 (a) Chronic vascular disease, especially if inflammatory, summates with the physical effects of cooling to produce livedo reticularis. A non-inflammatory variety associated with cerebrovascular disease is known as Sneddon's syndrome. (b) An equestrian chilblain is due to the combination of the insulating effect of fat and pressure from tight jeans in a young girl riding on a damp and frosty morning.

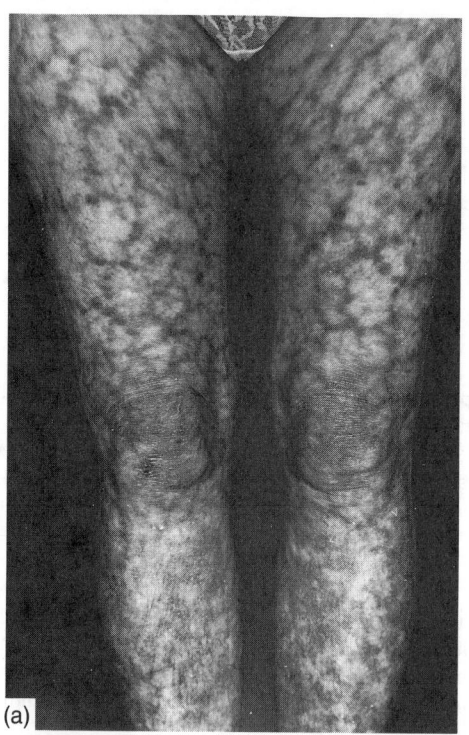
(a)

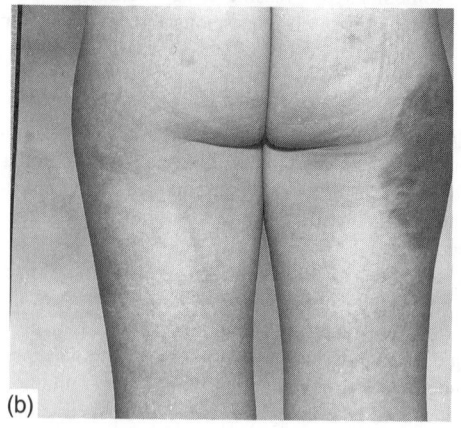
(b)

skin in mountain climbers or from some ultraviolet lamps, especially those used for sterilization.

The diagnosis of ultraviolet damage is determined by recognizing the distribution of the rash as typical of exposure. Thus on the head, nose, and cheeks, which are principally affected, there is often sparing below the eyebrows, under a forelock, beneath and behind the ears, and below the chin (see Fig. 15(b)). The sides and back of the neck are picked out but there is a sharp border to the sun damage where the collar shields the skin from sunlight. Much, of course, depends on the style of clothing as well as on the direction of irradiation, both at work and at play. The backs of the hands and dorsum of the feet are often caught by the sun but there may be some tolerance of such skin previously exposed and tanned so that skin not so tolerant is clearly more damaged. Heat from the sun lowers the itch threshold at sites of vasodilatation. Thus atopic eczema may be aggravated and only partly does such eczema have a light distribution. It is now recognized that ultraviolet rays may produce a subclinical inflammation which summates with subclinical sensitivity of other forms of injury including cold or airborne allergens. The pharmacological mediation of sunburn erythema is partly from prostaglandin generation. Plant dermatitis often produces a rash in the distribution of sun exposure. The condition phytophoto-dermatitis is a rash in the distribution of actual contact with plant juices on which the sun then acts and produces a burn. The pattern of such casual contact is often streaky and bizarre. Some perfumes containing berloque or musk ambrette are also responsible (see Fig. 62).

White skin and the sun

Hats, parasols, long skirts, and shawls as well as shady verandas have over the past 50 years been replaced by bikinis, solariums, and reckless sun worshipping. Even redheads and blondes attempt to brown themselves.

Exposure to sunlight is a major cause of ageing of the skin and of degenerative diseases of the epidermis and dermis that accompany age (Fig. 27). In Australia, South Africa, and the south-western United States solar keratosis, basal cell epitheliomata, chronic solar cheilitis, and squamous carcinoma (Fig. 28) are the commonest cause of referral to the dermatologist (Table 12). Even children are not completely immune and persons who burn easily and still persist in exposing themselves regularly to the sun will inevitably suffer gross changes in their skin, even at an early age. Fortunately, malignancy of the skin based on solar degenerative changes has a low potential for metastases.

Malignant melanoma

The incidence of this tumour is increasing. In Scotland, the incidence rose between 1979 and 1989 by 3.4 to 7.1 per 100 000 in men, and 6.6 to 10.4 per 100 000 in women, and this was mostly observed on the female leg or on the male trunk. Public health campaigns to encourage early recognition results in a fall in mortality due to earlier diagnosis of melanoma as well as decrease in mole counts. This is thought to be an early marker of primary prevention of melanoma, as high melanocytic naevi counts are associated with a greater incidence of melanoma, as is prominent freckling. Naevi increase during childhood, reaching their maximum in early adulthood. The counts have been shown to increase at an earlier age in Caucasians who live closer to the equator where sun exposure is greater. Early recognition is important since it allows the tumour to be detected before it has developed depth. At depth greater than 0.76 mm, the prognosis worsens, from a 95 per cent five-year survival to 80 per cent, and with a tumour thickness greater than 3.5 mm, the prognosis sharply worsens to 40 per cent 5-year survival. Survival from malignant melanoma is determined by early detection and early adequate surgery, and is not influence by chemotherapy. Elective node dissection is declining in popularity and may be replaced by lymphoscintography to detect the draining lymph node basin, followed by a biopsy of the sentinal lymph node or the first port of call of metastatic melanoma. Fortunately, older mutilating surgery has proved no more curative than conservative excision and the current dogma suggests that

the width of the margin should be approximately 1 cm for every mm of depth. It is now virtually certain that the role of sun exposure, and of sunburn in particular during childhood, explains the predilection of this tumour for exposed skin and for depigmented skin. It also explains the geographical distribution. Less than half of emergencies arrive in a previously recognized mole or lentigo (Fig. 29) or in a giant hairy naevus. Giant congenital pigmented naevi become malignant in about 10 per cent of cases. However, opinion is divided as to whether all congenital pigmented naevi should be removed prophylactically. Persons with a family history of multiple pigmented naevi and malignant melanoma, should practice sun avoidance and use sun-screening agents. The most important diagnostic factors are rapid and recent change in growth rate, irregularity of margin, colour, or depth. In addition, the development of a new pigmented lesion after puberty is an important clue. These are illustrated in Plates 1 to 9 and in Fig. 29.

Occasionally, metastatic disease may be the first presentation of melanoma, and to identify the primary lesion it is important to examine the entire cutaneous surface, to look in the eye, inside the mouth, to examine the vulva, and to examine the skin with a Wood's light, as the primary melanoma may have undergone spontaneous regression after giving rise to metastases and only be identified as a hypopigmented patch, using the Wood's light.

Fig. 27 Prominent sebaceous glands and comedo formation in solar elastosis.

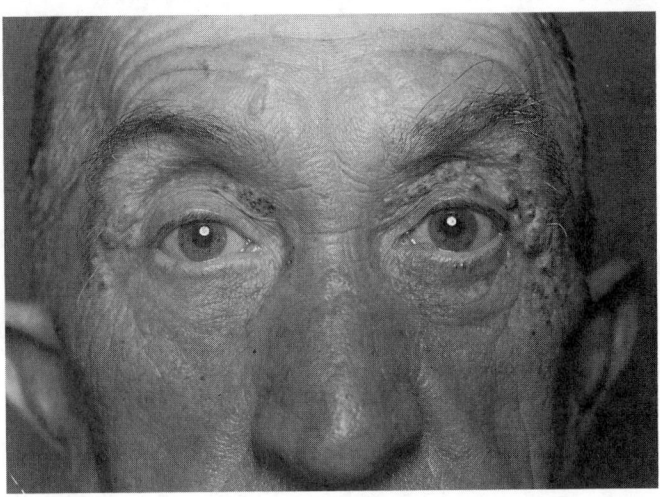

Fig. 28 Squamous epithelioma of lower lip as a consequence of sun exposure.

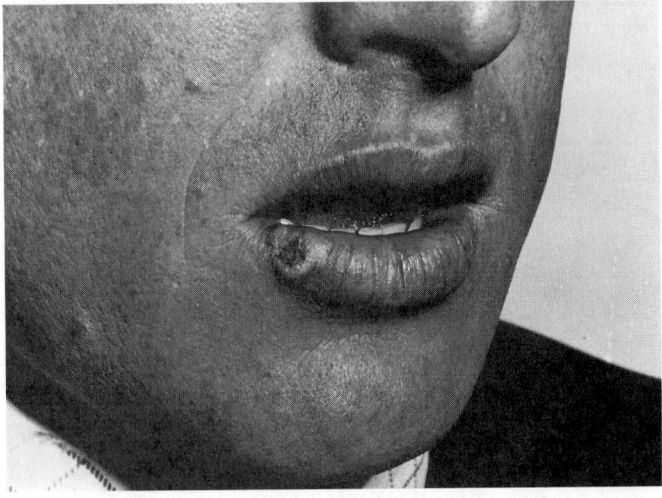

Table 12 *Clinical features of chronic sun exposure*

Elastosis	Less elastic, more fragile, yellowish, furrowed
	Telangiectasia, venous lakes, spider angiomas
	Prominent sebaceous glands (Fig. 27)
	Linear and stellate scars
	Idiopathic guttate melanosis
Keratosis	10 per cent precancerous
	Yellow-brown hyperkeratosis on a red telangiectatic background—the scale is not laminated as in psoriasis but firmly adherent and removal is painful; unlike lupus erythematosus, it bleeds when the scale is removed
	Cutaneous horn common
	Annular lesions frequent
	Bleed easily when scratched
Solar cheilitis	Lower lip
	Yellow-white thickenings
	Scaling and crusting
	Fissuring
Basal cell epithelioma	Central erosion
	Telangiectasia runs over the edge
	Pearl-like border
	Cystic, pigmented, or sclerotic forms
Squamous epithelioma	Indurated beyond the visible margin (Fig. 28)
	Ulcerated, hyperkeratotic, or granulomatous
	Crusted and horny
	Hard, elevated, or undermined edge
Kerato-acanthoma	Rapid growth: 4–6 weeks
	Sharply defined hemispherical
	Central horny core which may leave a crater
	2–12 months disappears spontaneously
	Scarring may be considerable
Bowen's disease	Often single with a well-defined edge
	Usually red scaly or crusted plaques
	Often slightly pigmented
Malignant melanoma	Change in depth of pigmentation (either darkening or loss) irregular notched border
	Growth changes, satellites
	Bleeding, itching, or ulceration
	Family history of atypical multiple pigmented naevi

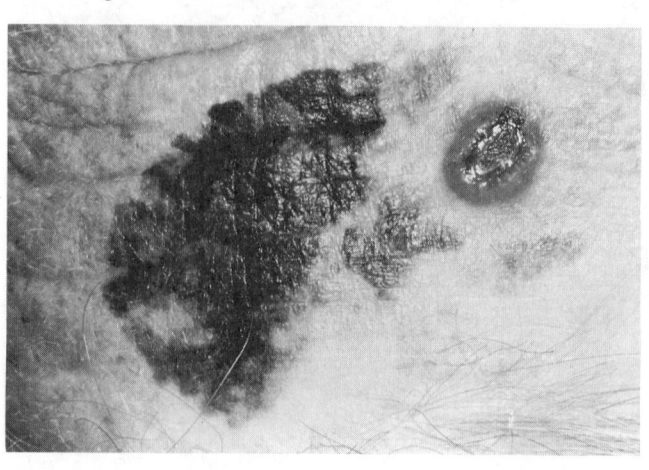

Fig. 29 The features of malignancy in this melanoma are an irregular notched border, variation in colour from red to black, variation in depth, or a history of recent change.

RASHES DUE TO SUN OR ARTIFICIAL LIGHT AND ASSOCIATED ULTRAVIOLET RAYS

Sunburn is initially an erythema at about 6 to 8 h after exposure and may progress to blistering and later peeling; if the exposure is excessive, redness may begin as early as 2 h.

Solar urticaria is an erythema and wealing immediately on exposure to sun, often of sites not habitually exposed to the sun.

Polymorphic light eruption is an altered quality of sunburn. Thus instead of erythema there is itchy papular or eczematous responses about 6 to 8 h after exposure, which may persist for several days (Fig. 30). There are several variants including a lymphoma-like pattern with heavy lymphocytic infiltrates.

Actinic prurigo Sun-induced prurigo shares features with atopic eczema, polymorphic light eruption, and persistent light eruption due to photosensitivity agents in the environment. It is common, and probably genetically determined, in American Indians. It has a chronic course which is only initially seasonal. Urticarial plaques develop a few hours after ultraviolet exposure and are followed by a persistent eczematous rash, not always confined to exposed skin.

Exacerbation or localization of other dermatoses is characteristic of pellagra, Hartnup's disease, lupus erythematosus, Darier's disease, herpes simplex, rosacea, scleroderma, erythema multiforme, actinic lichen planus (psoriasis) sometimes, and lymphocytoma.

Ultraviolet rays may diminish antigen surveillance by reducing the population of Langerhans cells.

Porphyria The rash of exposed areas is a swelling, bruising, or blistering often noticed immediately after exposure (Fig. 31). There is pitted scarring, scleroderma-like thickening (see also Fig. 120), pigmentation, and hirsutes in the more chronic stages. Fragility of the skin is a feature. Bright sun is not a necessity since it is due to the UVA and blue light. Erythropoetic protoporphyria often presents as a burning sensation shortly after exposure to sun.

Fig. 30 Two patterns of altered response to sunburn wavelengths: (a) an eczematous prurigo with excoriations, and (b) a plaque-like form not unlike lupus erythematosus.

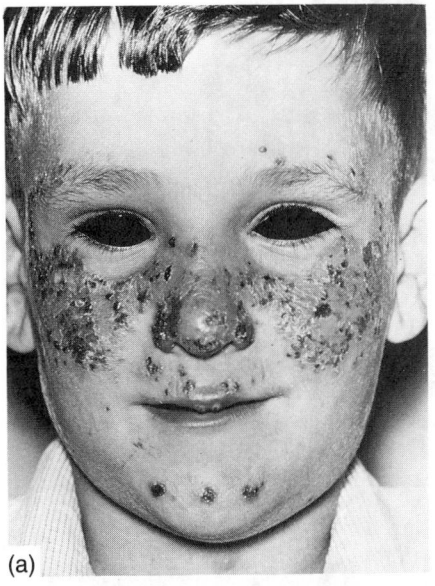

(a)

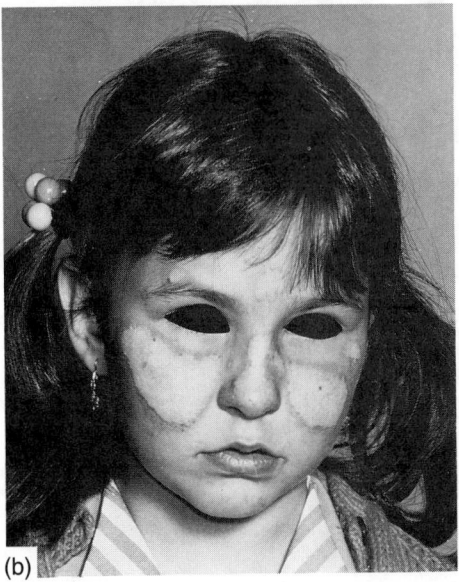

(b)

Drug eruptions These are acute eruptions of erythema swelling or blistering like severe sunburn but not dependent on bright sun since UVA is often responsible. They are often dose dependent as with psoralens in PUVA therapy. Ingestion of a spinach (Atriplex) also causes photosensitivity (see Table 13). Some present only as deep pigmentation.

Xeroderma pigmentosum is the term given to several genetic diseases in which repair of DNA is defective (Fig. 32). Children develop severe redness and swelling up to 72 h after exposure. Chronic injury results in keratosis, telangiectasia, irregularities of pigmentation, and even, in childhood, the early development of cancers and melanomas.

Severe sunburn in infancy must be investigated by fibroblast DNA repair studies because future protection from sun can much reduce the incidence of subsequent malignancy.

There are at least 10 variants with three known different chromosome locations. The mechanisms include a failure of DNA excision repair of ultraviolet-induced thymidine dimers. Variants with postreplication repair defects are described. The incidence of different tumour types is determined by the gene defect.

Persistent light eruption is the term given to sensitivity to light induced by agents previously applied to the skin, often years before. Drugs eliciting light sensitivity are listed in Table 13.

INVESTIGATIONS

The questions asked of the patient should include the family history, drug or food ingestion and exposure to perfumes, and the type of occupation, as well as how and when exposure took place. It is important to know whether glass or cloud is protective.

Although testing to light may be done with a variety of light sources, especially in photobiology units, sunlight is a natural source that can be used by blacking out the skin of the back of the trunk and exposing it by opening 'windows' at 5 min intervals.

Fig. 31 The congenital erythropoietic form of porphyria. The principal feature is fragility and scarring of the skin. Scleroderma and hirsutes with inequalities of pigmentation are other features seen in this child.

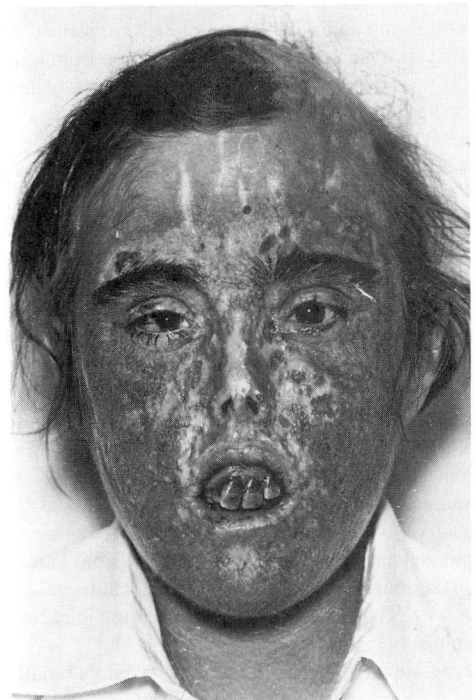

Table 13 *Photosensitivity due to drugs*

Sulphonamides and related chemicals
    Antibacterial group: sulphathiazole, long-acting
       sulphonamides
    Diuretics: chlorothiazide, hydrochlorothiazide, quinethazone
    Antidiabetic: sulphonylureas, carbamides
    Rarely: paraphenylenediamine, procaine group of
       anaesthetics
Antibiotics
    Tetracyclines; tetracycline, dimethylchlortetracycline
       (Ledermycin®)
    Declomycin chlortetracycline (Aureomycin®)
    Griseofulvin
Antiarrhythmic
    Amiodarone
Phenothiazines
    Chloropromazine, promazine, trimeprazine, meprazine,
       promezathine hydrochloride
Other psychotrophic drugs
    Chlordiazepoxide
Antihistamines not of phenothiazine structure
    Diphenhydramine
Antimalarials
    Chloroquine
Occasional, rare, or of historical interest
    Isoniazid, psoralens, stilbamidine 9-aminoacridine, eosin,
       trypaflavine, methylene blue, rose bengal, frusemide,
       nalidixic acid (Negram®)

PROPHYLAXIS

Health education in schools should emphasize that burning in the sun is not related to heat. It is maximal at midday and protection is essential mainly through avoidance by using clothing. Sunscreens are effective if properly used, i.e. they must be applied evenly and thoroughly and well before exposure, but they are not a substitute for avoidance. Frequent uninhibited exposure accumulates almost inevitable and irreversible injury which is only apparent some 20 years later.

MANAGEMENT

The ill-effects of a cool, sunny and windy noon must be explained as well as the relative safety of a hot sunny evening. Protection from light for those with sensitivity to UVB includes advice on the time of day and season likely to be harmful. Most patients can safely take an early morning or late afternoon bathe. Those with severe sensitivities such as xeroderma pigmentosum can be saved from all ill-effects by diligent protection, including clothing. Indeed, clothing and household shade are the best protections for children sensitive to the sun, but a wet T-shirt can transmit ultraviolet rays; tightly woven silks and cottons are more effective than loose weave yarns or wool. Cold wind and other skin allergies should be avoided at the same time as light exposure, and fluorescent lighting should be kept at a distance. Glass windows and certain plastics are protective against shorter wavelengths. Natural pigment and thickening of the epidermis accounts for normal tolerance.

Sun-screening agents include thick pastes or creams such as titanium dioxide; these are popular with skiers but prevent tanning. They are most useful for lip protection. Some have a number indicating the protection factor; the higher the number the better the protection; above 6 is usually advised but severe sensitivity will require double or treble the degree of protection. Sun-screening agents may reflect light and invisible lotions or creams containing para-aminobenzoic acid in 70 per cent alcohol act in in a more complex way. These preparations absorb ultraviolet rays and allow gradual tanning.

β-Carotene and mepacrine are pigments that can be taken by mouth. Mepacrine is probably the most commonly used and can be given 100

mg daily or twice daily. It is chiefly effective against sunburn wavelengths, whereas beta-carotene has been used for longer wavelengths. Aspirin, by inhibiting prostaglandin synthetase, reduces the erythema from sunburn.

Ultraviolet light can be cut out by certain somewhat expensive plastic films (UVethon-C or Y), and hospitals concerned with photosensitivity should have at least one area shielded by such films.

Treatment of the long-term effects of sunlight include the destruction and removal of lesions such as epitheliomata. These can be excised with good cosmetic results since they are often based on loose and inelastic

Fig. 32 The ageing effect of the sun is seen on (a) the neck and (b) the hands of this child with xeroderma pigmentosum, a defect of DNA repair in which sun damage is severe. Although only 9 years old, there is atrophy and inhomogeneity of the epidermal and pigment cells.

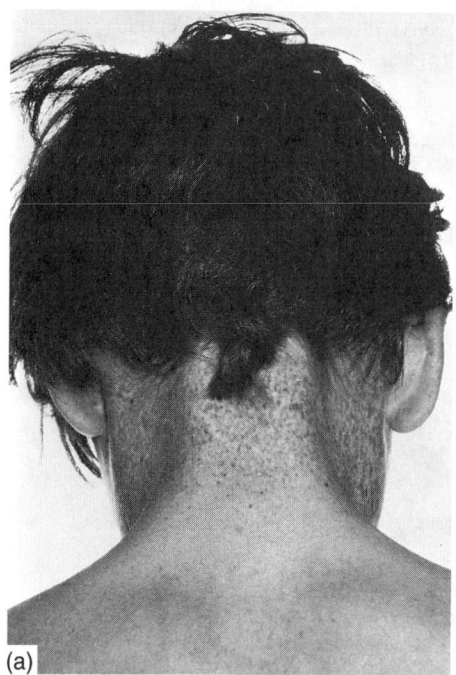

(a)

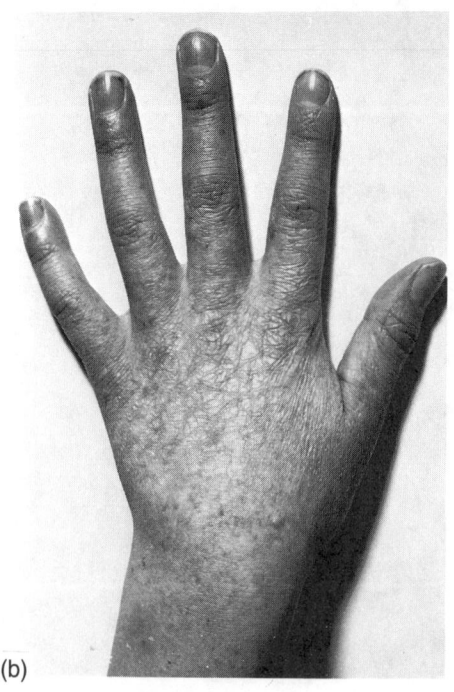

(b)

skin. Curettage with gentle cautery is also effective. Cryosurgery with adequate freezing using liquid nitrogen is often now used. It is the thawing of intracellular ice crystals which destroys the cells. Swelling and blistering is initially troublesome, but provided secondary infection is avoided, scarring should be minimal. 5-Alpha fluorouracil cream is useful for multiple or widespread keratoses that are not suspected of malignant change. The cream is applied once daily and destroys dysplastic cells. Considerable soreness may result after 2 to 3 weeks but new healthy cells repopulate the skin as well as stimulate new ground substance in the upper dermis, diminishing fine wrinkles and, in a sense, rejuvenating the skin.

X-ray is effective in destroying cancer but eventual inequalities in pigment and atrophy or sclerosis often results in a poorer cosmetic appearance than simple excision.

IS IT WHAT I HAVE EATEN? FOOD AND DRUG ERUPTIONS

There is a large folklore and a strong belief that skin disorders are induced by what is eaten. The difficulty of proving this by any skin or *in vitro* test, and the frequency of the idiosyncratic and the rarity of statistical evidence for food hypersensitivity has resulted in swings of the pendulum of medical fashion. Today food allergic disease is taken seriously by many in the medical profession as has always been the case amongst lay people.

It is generally accepted that much of what we eat is antigenic and absorption does occur. Usually allergen is complexed with antibody in the gut wall and tolerance also occurs. It is easy to demonstrate that antibody is made to counteract food allergens and that complexes circulate in the blood as a result of eating. This is not necessarily allergy because resulting inflammation is rare. There is some evidence that the amount of antigen absorbed and complexed is reduced by disodium cromoglycate.

One of the difficulties of interpretation is that hypersensitivity depends on the frequency of ingestion and on the level of tolerance elicited. Infrequent ingestion is more likely to cause allergy than tolerance.

Supporting evidence for food allergic disease comes from the ingestion of medicaments. The public knows well that many drugs taken by mouth can cause a severe generalized eruption, as for instance, sulphonamides at one time commonly elicited.

Both erythema and urticaria can be caused by food. In the atopic, IgE-mediated food allergy is well recognized. It is a contact urticaria when eggs or milk touch the lips, or it is a generalized urticaria and bowel upset when agents such as fish, nuts, or strawberries are eaten. However, in many patients such eruptions may have little to do with allergy but are pharmacologically induced, or at least they are examples of non-allergic intolerance.

Anaphylactoid reactions are either idiosyncrasies in which an individual reacts abnormally to a substance tolerated by most of the population due to some defect in his physiology, or they result from a direct effect or action of a drug on a mast cell, or other cell, often on first exposure to the eliciting substance. Examples of such non-allergic responses include C_1 esterase deficiency and angio-oedema or lactose intolerance and deficiency of lactase, causing diarrhoea.

A high iodine level in a diet induces blistering in dermatitis herpetiformis and exacerbates erythema nodosum leprosum. Sources include iodophors used in dairy cleansing, iodine-containing food supplements and dough improvers in bread, as well as cough mixtures.

Following the development of toxic erythema and purpura in an extensive epidemic amongst eaters of margarine in Holland and Germany, the possibility that food additives could cause a rash has become well recognized. The total number of food additives exceeds 20 000 and an average person eats about 1.5 kg every year. Salicylates and benzoates as well as many colouring agents present in more than 1000 drugs marketed in the United States act in part through the control of prostaglandin metabolism. Ten per cent of persons sensitive to aspirin are also

sensitive to the colouring agent tartrazine. The mechanism, though suspected to be related to prostaglandin metabolism, has yet to be clarified. Table 14 lists common foods containing salicylates, benzoates, and tartrazine. It is confusing that some other types of food allergy, perhaps less dependent on IgE and on the release of histamine from the mast cell, are prevented by prostaglandin inhibitors. 'If one takes indomethacin one can eat anything'!

Careful studies of food additives have led the authors to the conclusion that food with additives is very rarely a danger but food without additives is commonly so. So far as tolerance is concerned, the potentiating effect of psychological tension and unaccustomed or overindulgent eating habits is a probable explanation.

Shellfish and strawberries are well known for not only releasing histamine from mast cells but for causing thrombocytopenic purpura. Usually such agents cause urticaria within hours of ingestion. The response is not consistent since there may be times or forms of presentation of the same food which avoid this effect. Eggs, nuts, chocolate, fish, shellfish, tomatoes, pork, strawberries, milk, cheese, and yeast are common causes of a sudden transient thrombocytopenia, and sensitivity to food in this way is the basis of the thrombo test. A 20 per cent fall in platelet count 1 hour after ingestion occurs in 70 per cent of persons showing allergy to aspirin, barbiturates, and penicillin. In one series 203 out of 215 cases of urticaria had a prolongation of bleeding time from the ear lobe 2 hours after challenge with a drug, chemical, or food. Bitter lemon or tonic water containing quinine is especially well documented.

In atopic eczema and asthma the problem of food allergy is more complex. These patients seem to be more susceptible to histamine release even from non-allergic sources.

The gut of the newborn with atopy is said to be more immature in its handling of foreign protein, or at least it may be that complexing of IgA is less effective and then IgG is brought into play in a manner not usual for the mature gut. This is the basis for the advocation of breast feeding without cows' milk substitution in all babies of atopic parents. Hypoallergic foods are marketed which contain 'predigested' casein and this is a rapidly developing new industry with a strong following. However, minute amounts of antigens from maternal diet are found in breast milk, so one cannot assume that the first experience of dietary antigen is at the time of weaning. Even the fetus is normally supplied by minute samples of the mother's diet. What matters is how much and when.

Another form of food sensitivity is that occurring in nickel-sensitive subjects. Nickel sensitivity is one of the commonest causes of hand dermatitis and there seems little doubt that contamination from metal pots and from some green vegetables can contribute to the eczema in those who are sensitive.

Drug eruptions

The 1975 Boston Collaborative Program of Drug Surveillance observed that adverse reactions accounted for 3 per cent of hospital admissions and 14 per cent of medical resources, and 30 per cent of hospital patients developed adverse reactions. This is an epidemic of modern civilization and is partly due to the abuse of free drugs, particularly where there are health services. In developing countries cheap drugs such as sulphonamides are the commonest cause of adverse reactions. The drugs known to cause disease in the technically advanced countries are slow to be taken off the market and may even be promoted in countries where the drug industry is poorly supervised.

It is wise to assume that any drug can cause any rash, like syphilis, but until there are simple *in vitro* tests for testing human tissue for hypersensitivity which are both reliable and specific, the diagnosis of drug eruptions will depend entirely on clinical judgement. The physician has to decide whether the rash has some other cause by the recognition of physical signs, ranging from the burrows of the acarus in scabies to the herald patch of pityriasis rosea. Then if a drug seems a likely cause, there must be an attempt to decide which of the medications currently prescribed or taken secretly may be responsible.

Drug rashes are essentially blood borne and therefore often have a symmetrical urticarial, erythematous, or purpuric and ischaemic pattern

Table 14 *Colouring- and preservative-free diet (prepared by Karen Ross, John Radcliffe Hospital, Oxford)*

Foods allowed	Foods to be avoided
Meat All types fresh or plain frozen	Manufactured products, e.g. sausages, burgers, tinned meats, etc.
Fish All types, fresh or plain frozen	Manufactured products, e.g. smoked fish, fish fingers, fish in sauces, etc.
Dairy produce Eggs, fresh milk, fresh cream, white cheese[a], natural yoghurt[a]	Dried milks, artificial creams, coloured cheese, cheese spreads, flavoured/fruit yoghurt, ice cream
Fruit Fresh only	Manufactured products, e.g. fruit pie fillings, some tinned fruits
Vegetables Fresh, plain frozen, tinned in salt water only	Manufactured products, e.g. instant potato, tinned vegetable mixes, baked beans, ready mixed salads
Cereals Raw cereals, e.g. rice, sago Flours and homemade flour products, homemade cakes, biscuits, wholemeal bread[a], homemade desserts	Manufactured products including cakes, biscuits, bread mixed, etc. Instant puddings, tinned sponges, custards, blancmanges, dessert mixes Yellow pasta
Beverages Tea, coffee, fresh fruit juices[a], colour-free squashes[a] and fizzy drinks, water, soda water	Fruit squashes and fizzy drinks, malted milk drinks
Preserves Honey[a], homemade jam[a], marmalade[a], lemon curd	Manufactured jams, marmalades, lemon curd
Soups Homemade only	Manufactured tinned and packet soups
Confectionery White mints	Sweets and chocolate
Miscellaneous Salt, pepper, herbs, fresh spices	Pickles, curry powder, bottled sauces, and dressings

[a]May naturally contain benzoic acid or have an added preservative.

Diet sheets of this kind are difficult to compile. The Department of Health and Social Services (United Kingdom) produces a leaflet *Look at the label* which lists all the additives used in foods, and details their corresponding E numbers, enabling identification of their presence in all manufactured foods.

determined by vascular anatomy. Less likely is a 'primary epithelial' reaction in the initial stages and so scaling or even the vesiculation of eczema as a first manifestation of a drug rash would be unusual. The exceptions are well known and include the intraepidermal immunologically induced 'pemphigus' rash of penicillamine, rifampicin, and captopril, especially when the first of these is used to treat rheumatoid arthritis, and the cell-mediated hypersensitivity to epidermal protein and drug haptens in a person previously having a contact dermatitis to a local antihistamine or sulphonamide. The psoriasis-like rash of practolol and various other β-blockers, or the scaly eruption particularly of the scalp from methyldopa, are exceptions.

Nevertheless if a rash looks like eczema, it is probably not caused by a drug. If it is an erythema and urticaria, it may well be. Later stages of the rash are frequently complicated by a secondary epidermal reaction so that diagnosis should be made on the initial manifestation. An increased frequency of adverse reactions to drugs has been reported in HIV-positive patients.

Unlikely or likely drugs

It may be helpful to rule out unlikely offenders such as digoxin, paracetamol, steroids, other hormones, and vitamin and electrolyte supplements. In any drug group there are likely and less likely offenders. Thus of antibiotics, oxytetracycline, nystatin, and erythromycin are not under suspicion but dichlortetracycline is a common cause of a photosensitivity rash, and in infectious mononucleosis ampicillin is almost invariably responsible for a characteristic bright pink maculopapular rash.

To be fair to the drug industry, in rating likelihood one also has to take into account the huge amounts of some drugs that are prescribed without any reactions. In this respect, while one occasionally sees rashes from chlordiazepoxide, diazepam, or nitrazepam, it must be an extremely rare event.

Timing

Timing is useful when trying to establish mechanisms such as anaphylaxis or the Arthus phenomenon. The patient should be asked about previous reactions to drugs. In the absence of such history, and especially if the drugs were new to the patient, it would be unlikely to cause a rash within the first few days of administration. There is an exception to this which may have little to do with recognizing immune mechanisms, and that is the way in which drug eruptions develop in combination with infections. A cough mixture given for a sore throat or co-trimoxazole for some infection or other, especially viral, may produce an extremely severe erythema within 2 or 3 days of the intake. Later administrations on another occasion will cause no trouble. Erythema multiforme or Stevens–Johnson syndrome occasionally occurs surprisingly early after a drug's administration and one suspects that the disease for which the drug was given may have prepared the host in some way.

Where there is a known hypersensitivity to the drug, such as sulphonamides or penicillin, even when the history of the drug rash was decades earlier, the immunological response can be very rapid.

Slow excretion, genetically determined or due to depot injections, are other reasons for slow recovery from an eruption. It is also helpful to realize that for some drugs taken over many years the likelihood of their being the cause of the rash is small, thus the much prescribed phenylbutazone may produce a drug eruption but it does so usually within months of the first prescription. When examining a list of drugs taken by a patient, drugs added within the previous month are the most likely cause of the rash. However, interference with metabolic pathways by drugs may take many months to produce a rash, as for example, isoniazid and the production of pellagra.

Many patients do not admit to taking a drug, perhaps because it was never prescribed but was borrowed from a neighbour or bought over the counter and therefore considered to be harmless. In general drug rashes do not persist after withdrawal of the drug—exceptions include pemphigus from penicillamine.

Transient susceptibility

The best example of susceptibility is urticaria. Many persons with chronic urticaria are susceptible to it for a period of many months, and during that time the rash may be triggered by prostaglandin synthetase inhibitors, such as aspirin or indomethacin. It is possible that certain acute erythemas require both a drug and an infection to provoke the rash, so the underlying disease of the patient should always be taken into account. One suspects that sometimes immune complex diseases from infective organisms are provoked by interference with immunological mechanisms by certain drugs. The particular set of circumstances, which may not recur, would depend on the formation of antibodies, the nature of the infectious organism, and the taking of the drug at that time. Diseases such as psoriasis or dermatitis herpetiformis may go into spontaneous remission and at such time they are less likely to be provoked by drugs. Psoriasis is expected to be made worse by β-blockers, lithium, or chloroquine, but this is unpredictable and not a reason for withholding them. Dermatitis herpetiformis is provoked by iodine so readily that it should be avoided if possible.

Drug allergy is rarely proven but overdosage is a frequent well-established fact due to faulty prescribing, attempted suicide, or altered metabolism as in renal or hepatic failure. Drugs may interfere with metabolism, with hormones, they may be deposited, they may react with sunlight, they may modify the ecology of the skin in respect to infective organisms; they may cause reactivity of certain cells such as the mast cell; they may be cytotoxic and they can act as allergens in the formation of immune complexes, hapten protein complexes, delayed cellular immunity, and a variety of other mechanisms. Some are not understood, such as the effect of halogens on the formation of granulomata (Fig. 33a) and in the causation of an acneiform eruption (Fig. 33(b)). This includes the use of fluoride gel preparations applied to the teeth to prevent dental caries.

Specific drug eruptions

The most common diagnostic problem is a toxic urticated erythema. It begins like measles without the upper respiratory and conjunctival prodromal signs. It usually develops, over a number of hours, as a red indurated papular eruption (Fig. 34) and, unlike urticaria, persists for days, ultimately involving the epidermis and producing scales (Fig. 35). After the first 2 to 3 days the rash tends to be fixed and the principal changes are due to mild bleeding of the skin with overlying slight peeling. This type of rash is usually not seen before at least 8 to 10 days after the ingestion of the drug. Fever and arthropathy may be associated.

Common causes are ampicillin, phenylbutazone, phenothiazine, co-trimoxazole, diazides, and sulphonylureas. Exfoliative dermatitis is the end result of this type of reaction (Fig. 36). Gold, phenylbutazone, indomethacin, allopurinol, hydantoins, sulphonylureas, and para-amino salicyclic acid are causative drugs.

Ampicillin and amoxycillin

Ampicillin rash appears 5 to 14 days after treatment of an infection. Thus the rash is often seen after the course of the drug has been completed. It begins on the extensor aspects of the limbs and has a morbil-

Fig. 33 (a) Iodides and bromides are occasionally responsible for a granulomatous eruption with pseudo-epitheliomatous hypertrophy. Potassium iodide in a cough mixture was responsible for the eruption in this patient. (b) Prolonged administration of iodides or bromides causes a particularly inflammatory form of acne which, although commonly in the distribution of acne vulgaris, may be more widespread. This eruption was due to an iodide-containing 'tonic' for the blood.

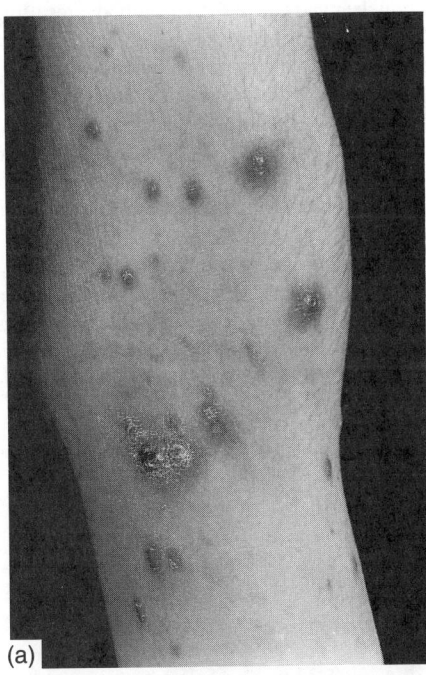

(a)

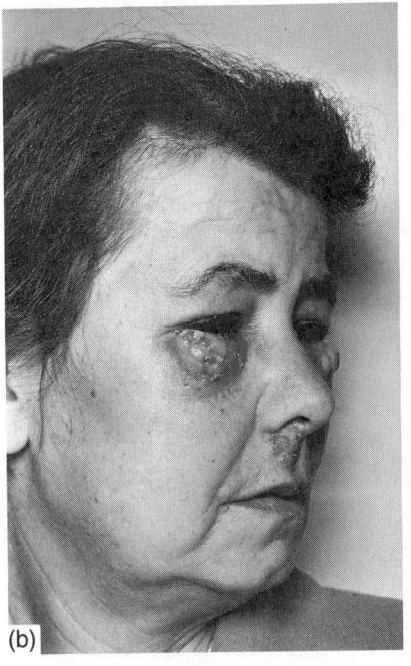

(b)

liform or maculopapular pattern which becomes confluent. It is a bright pink-reddish colour and may become purpuric and desquamate. In the pigmented skin such features are usually recognizable. The rash occurs in 5 to 7 per cent of all recipients and is the usual consequence of prescribing the drug for infectious mononucleosis, cytomegalovirus, or lymphatic leukaemia.

β-blockers

These cause a psoriasiform scaly eruption that may be modified by basal cell necrosis. The high turnover as in psoriasis, with the slowing down that results from such necrosis, gives rise to a hyperkeratotic scale that is more adherent than in psoriasis and often slightly yellowish. The palms and soles, elbows, and knees are particularly favoured (Fig. 37).

Practolol, labetalol, propranolol, and oxprenolol cause a rash which is partly psoriasiform and partly lichenoid and is most marked over bony prominences. There is hyperkeratosis of the palms and soles which is itchy. The rash of practolol develops over several months and, unlike psoriasis, there may be antinuclear and antiepithelial antibody, resulting in damage to the skin and conjunctiva (initially just hyperaemia but later there is sclerosis with shrinkage). Circulating antibody which binds to the intercellular region of guinea-pigs' stratified epithelium can be demonstrated. Eosinophils are sometimes plentiful in the dermis. Most β-blockers merely exacerbate ordinary psoriasis. Remission results from discontinuation.

Lupus erythematosus

Lupus erythematosus, like erythemas or necrotizing vasculitis, are most commonly caused by hydralazine, phenytoin, practolol, penicillamine, and isoniazid. Many other drugs have been incriminated. The drug-induced lupus erythematosus is reversed by withdrawal of the drug, but it recurs when it is readministered. The disease is characterized by anti-

Fig. 35 A later stage of acute drug eruption, in this case due to Myocrisin®, in which the epidermis is reacting to the dermal inflammation by hyperplasia spreading centrifugally to produce an annular scaly lesion with the scale exfoliating in the centre of the lesion and attached to the spreading margin.

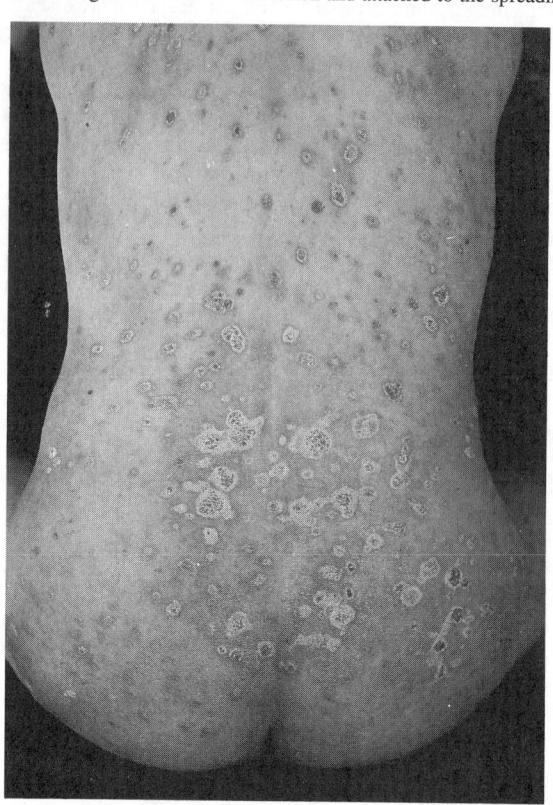

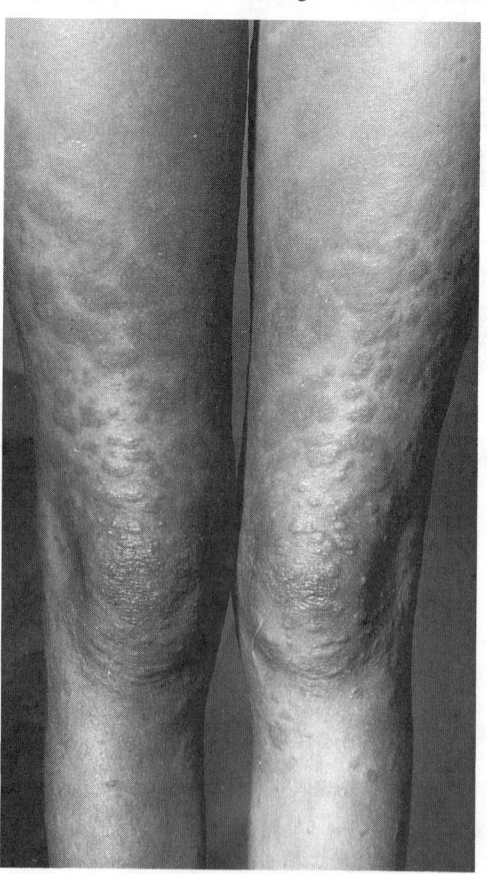

Fig. 34 One of the most common drug eruptions, initially a bright pink papular eruption, symmetrical and becoming confluent. This case is due to ampicillin.

Fig. 36 Severe oedema, crusting, and exfoliation due to dermatitis from arsenicals.

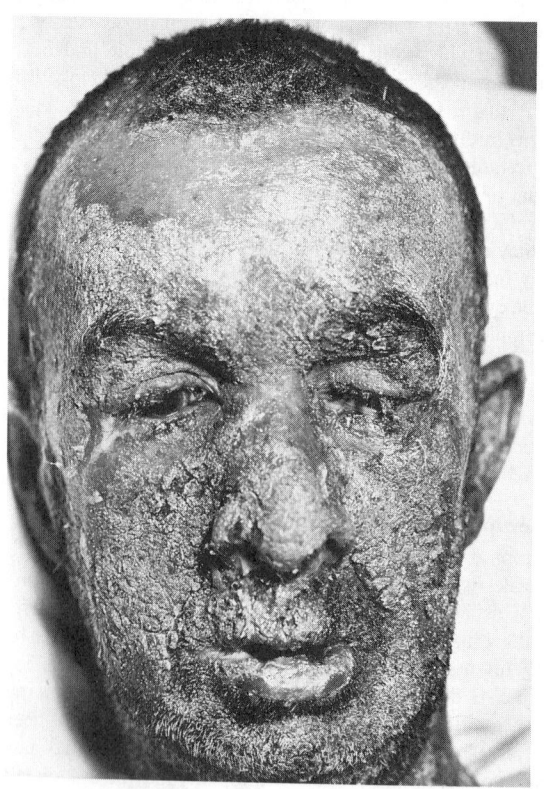

nuclear antibody in high titre with normal DNA binding. Inhibition of C4 underlies the immunological disease induced by hydralazine.

Scleroderma

An epidemic originating from denatured rape-seed oil in Spain caused facial oedema, exanthems, and ultimately a scleroderma-like syndrome.

Photosensitivity

This occurs in light-exposed areas such as the face, neck, forearms, or the dorsum of the feet. It is usually due to long-wave UVA and so glass

Table 15 *Drugs causing fixed drug eruptions*

Phenazone (synonym: antipyrine), dipyrine
Phenolphthalein
Barbiturates: phenytoin
Sulphonamides
Dapsone, iodides
Quinine and derivatives
Tetracyclines
Oxyphenbutazone, pyrazolones
Chlordiazepoxide

and cloud are not necessarily protective. However, photosensitivity does occur more often on a bright spring or summer midday. The resulting phototoxic eruption begins as an erythema and, as with severe sunburn, can become bullous or, as in the case of amiodarone, result in blue-grey pigmentation. The problem drugs are listed in Table 13.

Fixed drug eruption

Although the mechanism is unexplained, the eruption is easy to recognize as it is usually annular and erythematous (Fig. 38), it frequently blisters, and after resolution of the acute phase, may be a dull purple-brown colour caused by macrophage transport of melanin to the dermis. It is fixed in site and whenever the subject takes the causative drug the eruption begins within a few hours and is in exactly the same site as on a previous occasion was affected. The tongue and the glans penis are common sites. The affected area can be transplanted without loss of responsiveness in some cases. In pigmented races very dark pigmentation remains between attacks. Purgatives, blood cleansers and tonics, and many other homely remedies may contain phenolphthalein, which in most countries is the commonest cause. Causative drugs are listed in Table 15.

The investigation of fixed drug eruption is a little easier than for most other drugs since it is safe to test. Many patients are not aware of the significance of many of the drugs they take as analgesics, laxatives, and tonics, and therefore a very searching history is necessary. Others taking indigenous remedies are complicated by their being largely of unknown content and many of the foods we eat have hundreds of unknown constituents. The mechanism of penicillin reactions is discussed elsewhere.

Management of drug eruptions

The best way is to stop the use of all drugs likely to cause the eruptions. Readministration of the drug is possible for most drug eruptions other than those that cause anaphylactic shock, but it is usually at a risk of considerable morbidity and it should be considered only if essential to the patient. Skin tests are not helpful, as a risk of dangerous anaphylaxis, false negatives, and lack of knowledge of the antigen, makes skin testing useless. Penicilloyl polylysine has been found useful for testing for penicillin sensitivity. Where there is a medicament dermatitis due to contact, then patch testing is helpful.

Blood tests are of no help in trying to find which drug is causing the problem. Various tests, such as the reaction of basophil cells or the release of lymphokines from the lymphocyte, have not proved of routine value. Eosinophils may suggest that an eruption is due to a drug, and as mentioned above, a fall of platelets within 1 hour or a prolongation of bleeding time 2 hours after injection is helpful for some urticarial rashes.

Fig. 37 Hyperkeratosis and slight scaling is a feature of the psoriasiform eruption caused by β-blockers.

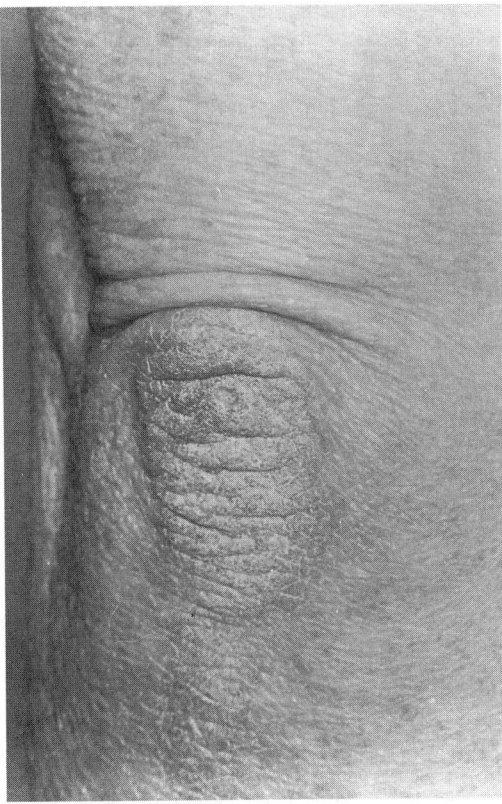

Fig. 38 Fixed drug eruption due to phenolphthalein present in a laxative. Such an eruption characteristically appears within half a day of taking the causative drug and the site affected is the same on every occasion. Violaceous annular lesions are common and may persist for several weeks.

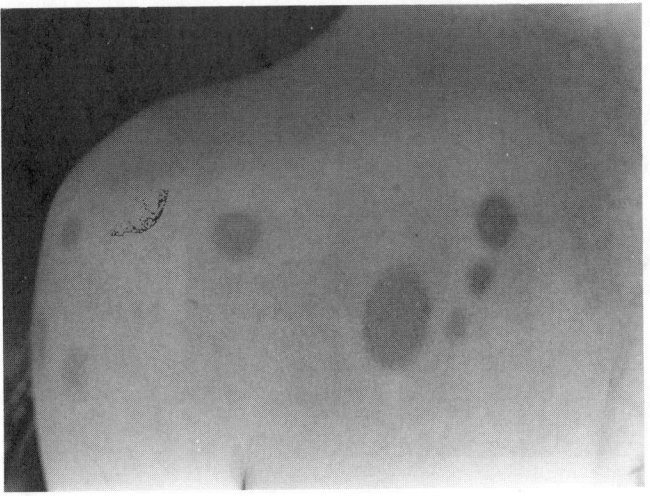

REFERENCES

Ackroyd, J.F. (1985). Fixed drug eruptions. *British Medical Journal* **288**, 1533–4.

Alper, J.C. (1981). Principles of genetics as related to the chromosome disorders and congenital malformations with reference to prenatal diagnosis and genetic counseling. *Journal of the American Academy of Dermatology* **4**, 379–94.

Arndt, K.A. and Jick, H. (1976). Rates of cutaneous reaction of drugs. *Journal of the American Medical Association* **235**, 918–23.

Breathnach, S.M. (1992). Drug reactions. In *Textbook of dermatology,* (5th edn), (ed. A. Rook, D.S. Wilkinson, and F.J.G. Ebling), pp. 2961–3036. Blackwell Scientific Publications, Oxford.

Bergsma, D. (1979). *Birth defects compendium.* Macmillan, London.

Bruinsma, W. (1982). *A guide to drug eruptions. A file of adverse reactions to the skin,* p. 124. Distributed by De Zwaluw, PO Box 21, Oosthuizen, The Netherlands.

Dahl, M.V. (1980). HLA-1A and the skin. In *Year book of dermatology,* (ed. R.L. Dobson and B.H. Thiers), pp. 13–50. Year Book Medical Publishers, Chicago.

Der Kaloustian, V.M. and Kurban, A.K. (1979). *Genetic diseases of the skin,* p. 334. Springer-Verlag, Berlin.

Desai, S.C. (1972). Infections and communicable dermatoses; reflections on the massive morbidity of scabies, pyoderma and mycotic infections. In *Essays on tropical dermatology,* Vol. 2, (ed. J. Marshall), pp. 296–300. Excerpta Medica, Amsterdam.

Du Vivier, A. (1982). Spotting the malignant melanoma. *British Medical Journal* **285**, 671–2.

Ebrahaim, G.J. (1972). The skin in malnutrition. In *Essays on tropical dermatology,* Vol. 2, (ed. J. Marshall), pp. 124–8. Excerpta Medica, Amsterdam.

Emmett, E.A. (1984). The skin and occupational diseases. *Archives of Environmental Health* **39**, 144–9.

Epstein, J.H. (1979). Systemic disease and light dermatology. In *Dermatology update,* (ed. S.L. Moschella), pp. 119–44. Elsevier, New York.

Fitzpatrick, T.B., Eisen, A.Z., Wolff, K., Freedberg, I.M., and Austen, K.F. (1979). *Dermatology in general medicine,* p. 1884. McGraw-Hill, New York.

Gedde-Dahl, T. (1981). Sixteen types of epidermolysis bullosa. *Acta dermatologica* (Suppl. 95), 74–87.

Hanifin, J.M. (1984). Basic and clinical aspects of atopic dermatitis. *Allergy* **52**, 386–94.

Harber, L.C. and Bickers, D.R. (1989) *Photosensitivity: diseases, principles of diagnosis, and treatment.* W.B. Saunders, Philadelphia.

Journal of Investigative Dermatology (1979a). Special issue on aging. *Journal of Investigative Dermatology* **73**, (Suppl. 1), 134.

Journal of Investigative Dermatology (1979b). Infections; *Journal of Investigative Dermatology* **73**, 452–9.

Journal of Investigative Dermatology (1979c). Birth defects and genetic disorders. *Journal of Investigative Dermatology* **73**, 460–72.

Journal of Investigative Dermatology (1979d). Skin reactions to environmental agents. *Journal of Investigative Dermatology* **73**, 501–11.

Lessof, M.H. (1992). Reactions to food additives. *Journal of the Royal Society of Medicine* **85**; 513–15.

Lew, R.A., Sober, A.J., Cook, N., Marvell, R., and Fitzpatrick, T.B. (1983). Sun exposure habits in patients with cutaneous melanoma. A case control study. *Journal of Dermatological Surgery and Oncology* **9**, 981–6.

MacKie, R., *et al.* (1992). Cutaneous malignant melanoma – Scotland 1979–89. *Lancet* **339**; 971–5.

Magnus, I.A. (1976). *Dermatological photobiology. Clinical and experimental aspects.* Blackwell Scientific Publications, Oxford.

Miller, K. (1982). Sensitivity to tartrazine. *British Medical Journal* **285**, 1597.

Orkin, M. (1975). Today's scabies. *Journal of the American Medical Association* **233**, 882–885.

Podell, R. (1985). Unwrapping urticaria. The role of food additives. *Postgraduate Medicine* **78**, 83–97.

Rebello, M., Val, T.F., Garijo, F., Quintana, F., and Berciano, J. (1983). Livedo reticularis and cerebrovascular lesions (Sneddon's syndrome), clinical, radiological and pathological features of eight cases. *Brain* **106**, 965–79.

Rook, A., Wilkinson, D.S., and Ebling, F.J.G. (1992). *Textbook of dermatology,* (5th edn), p. 3160. Blackwell Scientific Publications, Oxford.

Swedlow, A.J. (1979). Incidence of malignant melanoma of the skin in England and Wales and its relationship to sunlight. *British Medical Journal* **282**, 1324–7.

Urbach, F. (1969). *Biologic effects of ultraviolet radiation (with emphasis on skin).* Pergamon Press, Oxford.

Young, A.W. and Miller, L. (1968). Skin problems in the geriatric and general hospital, incidence, scope cause. *Journal of the American Geriatric Society* **16**, 1140–9.

Wall, L.M. and Smith, N.P. (1981). Perniosis: a histopathological review. *Clinical and Experimental Dermatology* **6**, 263–72.

Zachary, C.B., Slater, D.N., Holt, D.W., Storey, G.C.A., and MacDonald, D.M. (1984). The pathogenesis of amiodarone-induced pigmentation and photosensitivity. *British Journal of Dermatology* **10**, 451–6.

Dermatitis

DEFINITION

Dermatitis is the commonest of reaction patterns in the skin. The term is used especially for a reaction of the skin to external injury as in 'industrial' or in 'contact' dermatitis. Eczema has a similar meaning but is used more often for endogenous or constitutional dermatitis.

CLINICAL FEATURES

Dermatitis has both dermal and epidermal components. There are signs confined to the dermis such as swelling, heat, itchiness, tenderness, and redness, but at the same time the epidermis proliferates and therefore thickens and produces scale. The oedema in the dermis extends to the epidermis, swells the cells, and separates them giving the histological appearance of a sponge, known as spongiosis, and frequently this results in vesicles which distinguish dermatitis from other proliferative states of the epidermis such as psoriasis. Acute weeping exudation occurs when the vesicles burst (Fig. 39). In dermatitis itching is usually severe.

The reaction pattern of dermatitis is not homogeneous. It is made up of papular elements of different ages and size sometimes confluent in the centre (Fig. 40) with widely scattered satellite papules or vesicles. The scales are of varied size and broken by excoriation, exudate, and even pinpoint haemorrhages.

A secondary factor prominent in the pigmented skin is loss of melanin or at least failure to retain it in the acute lesion so that the skin is depigmented. In later or more chronic stages the dermis is darkened by 'incontinence' of pigment so that thickened chronic epidermal plaques may contain increased pigment in the underlying dermis. Chronic scratched skin has a brownish violaceous colour due to the combination of pigment, vasodilatation, and epidermal thickening.

Fig. 39 Acute dermatitis is characterized by an oedematous epidermis in which vesiculation, oozing, and crusting are the principal features. The borders are often ill-defined, while the centre of the lesion is confluent.

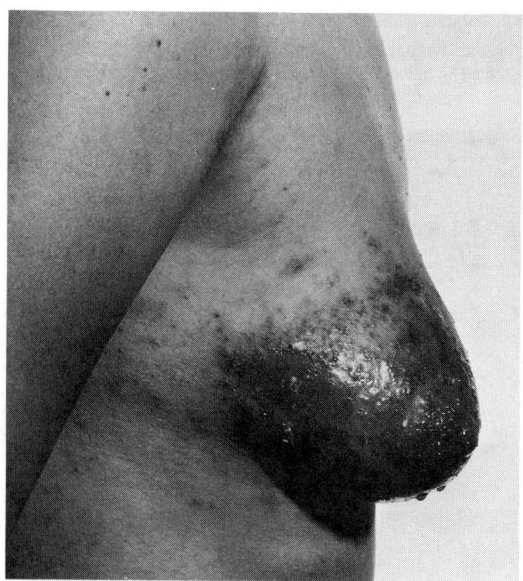

For reasons unknown, dermatitis of the foot frequently provokes a response in the hand. Thus, vesicular eczema of the hands often follows a fungus infection of the feet, and varicose eczema of the lower legs often spreads to the forearms and face.

Contact dermatitis
WEAR AND TEAR OR PRIMARY IRRITANT

Contact dermatitis is one of the greatest public health problems. It particularly affects the hands. Wear and tear, known as irritant dermatitis, is the commonest cause of hand dermatitis. In other words, simple irritation from external agents accounts for by far the greatest proportion of skin disease (and less than one-fifth of such involvement is due to allergy). Indeed in industry, most outbreaks of dermatitis are not due to allergy but due to the introduction of irritants into the work process or changes in the environment such as humidity or excessive drying. Industrial or occupational dermatitis are terms which indicate what may happen to the skin through its everyday exposure.

It is important to distinguish between wear and tear, taking into account different degrees of toughness or vulnerability, and allergic contact dermatitis, since their aetiology and management are different. A skin that is worn is dry and unsupple. Deep cracks occur through the normally resilient and elastic stratum corneum. Underlying epidermal cells and the dermis are no longer protected and the cracks become secondarily infected (Fig. 41).

An irritant can be defined as a chemical that in most people is capable of producing cell damage if applied for a sufficient time and in a sufficient concentration. Fibreglass spicules rubbed into the skin are a typical example (Fig. 42). Many persons at home or in industry are in daily contact with various chemicals over long periods. They work in wet or extremely dry conditions with skin cleaners, alkalis, acids, cutting fluids, solvents and oxidants, reducing agents, enzymes, and medicaments. The skin is also worn and irritated by cold and heat, sun, pressure, scratching, or friction of various kinds from tools or clothing. There are many variables which influence its toughness or vulnerability. It can be immature in the new-born or worn out in the aged. The most important cause of lowered resistance is constitutional disease such as the ichthyotic skin of old age, atopic eczema (Fig. 43), or psoriasis. Heredity of mainly polygenic type influences dermatitis by an effect on the constitution of

Fig. 42 Primary irritant dermatitis due to small spicules of fibreglass at sites of friction following the insulation of a roof.

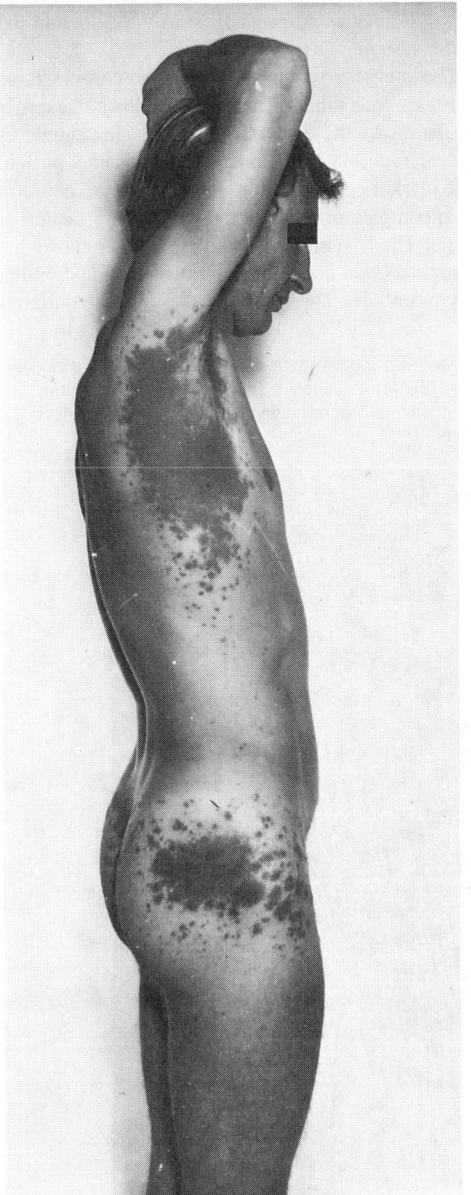

Fig. 40 Dermatitis is comprised of papules which are confluent in the centre and become vesicular or evidently excoriated. Oedema makes the line markings in the skin more prominent. There are satellite lesions beyond an ill-defined border.

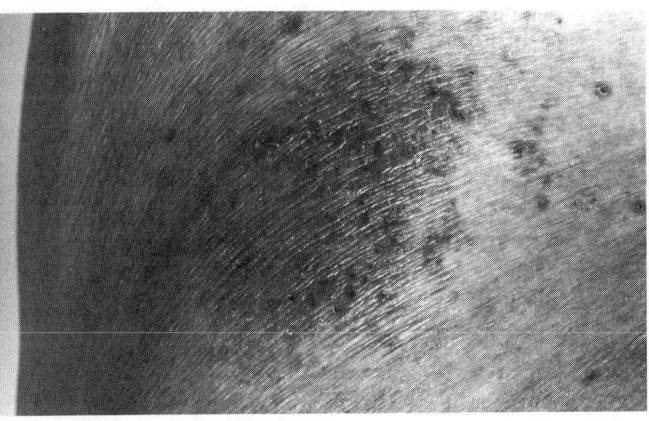

Fig. 41 Chronic dermatitis causes irregular thickening of an inhomogeneous epidermis. The texture of the stratum corneum varies so that it is firmly attached at some points but exfoliates with small scales at others. Loss of moisture causes decreased suppleness, cracking over joints, and exposure of deeper epidermal cells. This causes irritation of the dermis at the bottom of the deep crevasses.

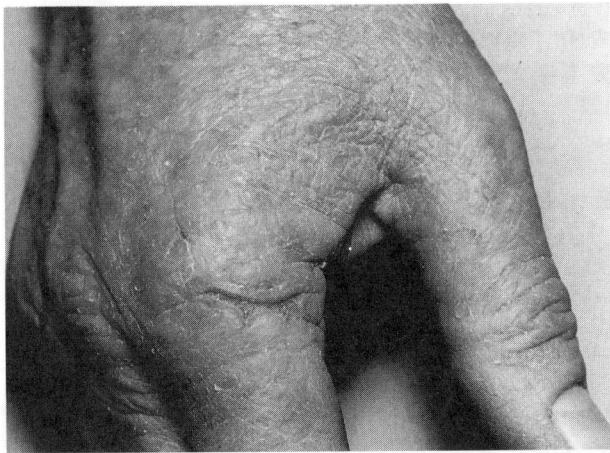

the skin. There is as yet only little evidence in man of a hereditary factor in contact allergic dermatitis, neither HLA studies not twin studies having confirmed such a role in man as compared to animal studies.

CONTACT URTICARIA

This is an acute swelling developing within a few minutes to half an hour of contact with certain agents. In atopic eczema there is an especial susceptibility to this phenomenon but it is also well recognized in non-atopic subjects and is particularly common as a result of the application of cosmetics. Many agents commonly applied to the skin will produce irritation in certain sites, such as the eyelids or scrotum, and this is not always an immunological phenomenon. Agents causing contact urticaria are listed in Table 16. It is increasingly well recognized.

CONTACT ALLERGIC DERMATITIS

Sensitization can occur 7 to 10 days after the first contact with a potent allergen. It is more usually, however, a consequence of many months or years of exposure to small amounts of allergen. Once sensitized, contact with allergen can produce dermatitis within 24 to 48 hours and all areas of the body are equally susceptible. Sensitivity can vary due to the amount of exposure, the degree of penetration of the skin, and the tolerance of the immune system.

It is believed that certain allergens, such as nickel and chrome, have a greater affinity for the skin than others. This is in part due to the easier recognition and assimilation by the epidermal macrophages known as Langerhans cells. The allergen binds to epidermal microsomal protein or to some cell surface marker or to serum proteins which are plentiful in the epidermis. It is a complex of the allergen with such protein that is recognized as foreign. The T lymphocyte ultimately recognizes the complex but the macrophage is a necessary intermediary. Suppression of Langerhans cells by ultraviolet rays diminishes cell-mediated immu-

Fig. 43 Chronically thin and slowly turning-over epidermis results in a closely knit stratum corneum which is firmly adherent but cracks excessively. It is characteristic of elderly, malnourished, or ichthyotic skin. Such skin is less resistant to primary irritants.

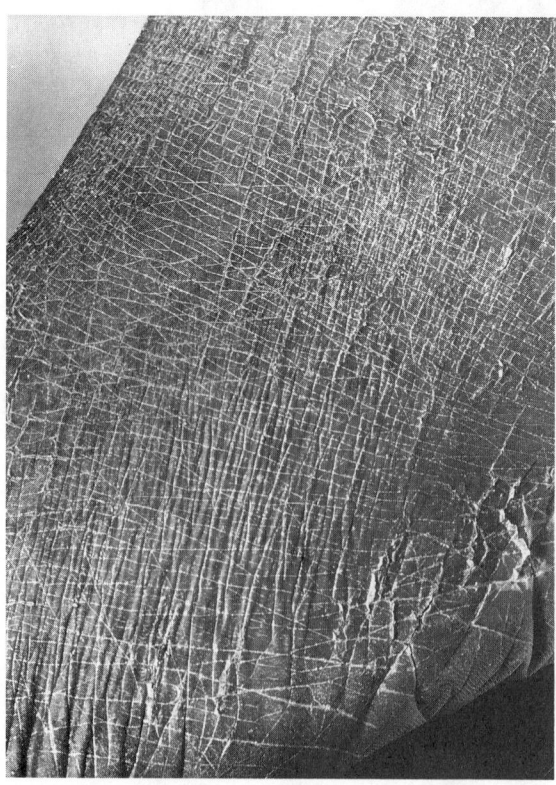

nity. Genetic factors play a part in the recognition process. Once recognized, T-cell proliferation occurs in the paracortical area of the lymph node. On re-exposure sensitized lymphocytes release lymphokines. The mechanisms of lymphocyte stimulation include some role for suppressor and effector cells. The role of antibodies, some of which are clearly specific for the same antigen, is also unknown. The inflammatory reaction resulting from recognition is variable and dependent on other pharmacological agents including secretions from the mast cell and on prostaglandins. Some of the variability of response, such that persons are consequently labelled as more or less allergic, depends on these secondary factors and can be modified by various conditional factors, including anxiety and the hormonal status of the monthly menstrual cycle.

CONTACT DERMATITIS SENSITIZERS

In the following, I will concentrate on some specific groups of sensitizers and irritants:

1. Cosmetics

Cosmetics applied to the skin, although more rarely a cause of dermatitis in technically advanced countries where the industry has worked hard to eliminate allergens, are still a source of much disease in developing countries. Perfumes and preparations containing tars, formaldehyde, and Dowicil are increasingly incriminated, but they are as commonly irritant as allergic.

Vaseline dermatitis in the Bantu is an example. In technically advanced countries, deodorants are a common cause of dermatitis, and in the hair industry, glyceryl monothioglycollate (acid perms) is the most common allergen. Hair bleaches, such as ammonia persulphate, commonly cause immediate, non-immune wealing. When in doubt because the constituents are so complex, cosmetics should be tested by direct application to the skin, but this can give rise to false negative results. Hair dyes are now so common that their relative safety can be expected. However, again in developing countries, the dye paraphenylenediamine may produce an acute dermatitis, often first affecting the eyelids and other aspects of the face before showing much evidence of dermatitis on the scalp.

2. Clothing and textile dermatitis

On the whole this is rare, but clips containing metal are a quite common cause of dermatitis (Fig. 44), e.g. jeans buttons cause dermatitis of the skin below the umbilicus. There is evidence also that the rubber in elastic of many garments is sometimes the cause of dermatitis. Dyes are usually a problem at sites of friction where there is also moisturization by sweat. The majority are azodyes or paraphenylenediamine. In the textile industry chrome and formaldehyde are important agents causing dermatitis.

Fig. 44 Contact dermatitis due to garments containing nickel. The diagnosis is made by observing how the distribution of the rash corresponds to the distribution of the contact with the causative agent.

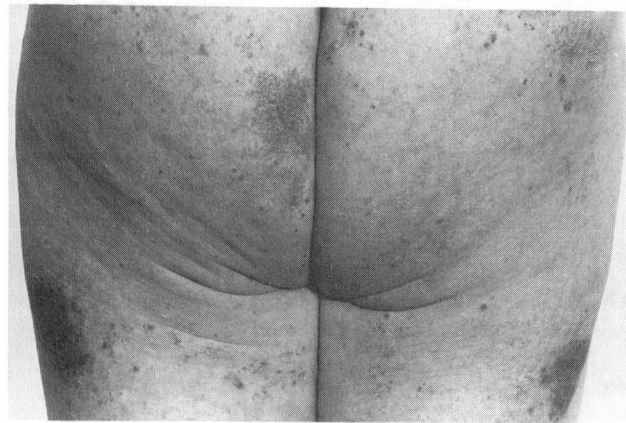

Table 16 *Causes of contact uricaria*

Medicaments	Chemicals	Miscellaneous
Streptomycin	Acrylic monomer and polyacrylic acid	Dander saliva or serum of internal organs of
Penicillin G	Alcohols (ethyl, cetyl, stearyl)	many laboratory animals
Cephalosporins	Aliphatic aldehydes	Egg white or yolk
Neomycin	Alphatic polyamides	Fish and shellfish
Gentamicin	Aliphatic amine hardeners	Various insects giving rise to cotton seed itch,
Bacitracin	Ammonia	copra itch, grocers' itch, millers' itch, etc.
Chlorpromazine	Aminothiazole	Caterpillars, pteropods, schistosomes
Promazine hydrochloride	Ammonium persulphate and potassium salt	Jellyfish
Aspirin	Benzoic acid and sodium benzoate	A glycoprotein in human seminal fluid
Oestrogenic cream	Chlorine	Root vegetables
Cod liver oil	Clothing dyes	Nuts
Horse serum	Citrus fruits	Spices
Tetanus antitoxin	Citraconic anhydride (in guinea-pigs)	Pollens
Diethyl tolbutamide	Cinnamic aldehyde	Exotic woods
Monoamylamine	DMSO	Numerous common weeds
Mechlorethamine hydrochloride	DNCB	α-Amylase
Benzaphone	Detergents with and without enzymes	Flour
Menthol	Formaldehyde	Amniotic fluid and other proteins listed in
Ammoniated mercury	Lindane	Janssens *et al.* (1995)
Arsphenamine	Polysorbate 60	
Emetine	Phenylmercuric proprionate	
Aminophenzaone	Perlon	
Polyethylene glycol	Platinum salts	
Polysorbate 60	Sodium sulphide	
	Sodium dioxide	
	Sorbic acid	
	Terpinyl acetate	
	'Trafuril'	

From Veronica Kirton, private communication.

Shoe dermatitis is commonly due to chrome or to rubber additives such as mercaptobenzothiazole or butyl phenol formaldehyde. Adhesives and dyes may also be responsible. It should be considered in every person with eczema of the feet. It often spares the area between the toes as this is the point at which the shoe is not in contact with the skin. Modern footwear has plasticized toecaps and fails to absorb sweat. Increased sweating encourages shearing strain on the skin, particularly in the athletic child. Frictional dermatitis of the foot is common in such children and is known as juvenile plantar dermatosis.

3. Foods
In the technically advanced countries the handling of animal feeds including antibiotics gives more trouble than the handling of food for human consumption. Elsewhere plants and fruits such as garlic, cinnamon, onion, and lemon or orange cause much trouble, as do shellfish and various species of fish which are sometimes contaminated by algae. This is an important hazard for fisherman and is known as the 'Dogger Bank' itch in the United Kingdom.

4. Plastics
A new and increasingly frequent cause of dermatitis is from acrylic and epoxy polymers or resins. Acrylic accounts for dermatitis from adhesive tape, spectacle frames, bonding agents, dentures, hearing aids, bone cement, artificial fingernails, sealants, printing plates, and inks.

Epoxy resins are used as surface coatings for steel pipes and ships, powder paints, electrical insulation adhesives, construction of concrete and steel buildings, and for the surface of roads and bridges. They are amongst the most potent sensitizers and are active in this respect only during their initial handling. Complete polymerization makes the sensitizing monomer non-available. About 90 per cent of contact dermatitis from epoxy resins is from bisphenol A. Protection in industry depends on common sense avoidance of handling and general cleanliness in the workshop, but volatile epoxy resins affecting the face are difficult to avoid.

5. Rubber
Natural as well as synthetic rubbers require the addition of several agents that are strong sensitizers. They make the rubber more malleable and supple, prevent perishing by oxidization, and some speed up the processes of manufacture.

Accelerators include thiuram, mercaptobenzothiazole, and guanides; antioxidants include monobenzyl ether of hydroquinone. Most cases of rubber sensitivity are from clothing such as rubber gloves, or in industry they are from tyres or rubber linings in the transport industry. Others include the contraceptive sheath, shoes, fingerstalls, masks, particularly in motorbike or scuba-diving pursuits, elastic bands, bicycle or golf-club handles, and rubber sheets or cushions. Anaphylaxis is recorded from Type I sensitivity to rubber latex surgical gloves.

6. Colophony
Rosin is made from pine trees and is used worldwide for paper size adhesives, inks, underseal cables, Elastoplast®, violin rosin, and cosmetics. Some medicaments like Zambuk®, Secaderm® salve, or ilonium, also contain colophony, and it explains contact dermatitis from these agents. It is responsible for about 3.5 per cent of positive patch tests in the London contact dermatitis clinics.

7. Plants and wood
Sensitivity to plants and woods accounts for enormous worldwide morbidity and occasional mortality. Some plants release their allergen only when bruised, others when lightly touched, and others by airborne pollen. Some produce a contact non-allergic urticaria, i.e. immediate stinging, as with the nettle or cowhage; others cause an allergic dermatitis, or even photosensitivity. Many are highly irritant.

In North America the commonest cause is poison ivy. In Europe it is the *Primula obconica*. Both produce a severe streaky blistering eruption from contact allergy mediated by cellular immunity.

The chrysanthemum or ragweed plants, known as the Compositae or daisy family, cause a more diffuse redness and oedema of the face from sesquiterpene lactones. This may look like a photosensitivity and be enhanced by sunlight. Avoidance of the plant may be impossible in those persons whose job depends on contact with it, and is an especial problem where the environment contains it as a common weed. It accounts for mortality in the region of Poona, India where there is the weed *Partheneum hysterophorus*. There the dermatitis builds up into a severe erythroderma with secondary infection and even pseudolymphoma. In those who are suffering from other diseases it may summate and lead to a very severe illness.

Potentially allergenic plants are most numerous in the cashew family, such as poison ivy, poison oak, poison dogweed, elder or sumac, mango, wax, or lacquer trees, and hence in one form or another they are worldwide. Attacks can be aborted by washing within an hour of contact but in some heavily contaminated areas water is in short supply.

When sensitivity is due to the mango or cashew nut, severe oral dermatitis and acute gastrointestinal systems can be troublesome.

Contamination of other agents handled can also cause outbreaks of dermatitis, as has been recorded with articles of clothing, mail, and even from voodoo dolls.

Wood dermatitis is often due to its resins or from lichens, liverworts, and moss, or even its insect parasites are occasionally responsible. It is a severe cause of industrial dermatitis in the furniture industry, but ranges even to mouth dermatitis in children handling wooden toys and it has been noticed also in schools in the music classroom from recorders made of certain woods.

8. Medicaments

The increasing complexity of our environment includes an enormous number of medicaments. Often the constituents in these are unknown. The problem arises particularly where these have been applied repetitively to the skin over a number of years, and therefore it is found in patients with leg ulcers, pruritus ani, or vulvae, and in those suffering from otitis externa. Local anaesthetics, Lanolin and cetylsteacyl alcohols, antibiotics and antiseptics, antifungal compounds, and antihistamines are the most significant groups. Topical corticosteroids are increasingly recognized as relatively common contact sensitizers (hydrocortisone, hydrocortisone-17-butyrate, budesonide).

An example of the importance of recognizing such sensitivity is illustrated by ethylene diamine; this is an increasingly common cause of dermatitis and it is present in certain neomycin nystatin ointment mixtures such as Tri-Adcortyl®. It is also contained in aminophylline suppositories. It is used as a solvent in many industries and is one cause of coolant oil dermatitis. This combination of an industrial use and a medicament may mean that a person may lose his employment as a result of previous use of a medicament. It has serious implications since it is also sometimes used as a preservative of an intravenous medicament, aminophylline, and deaths have been recorded.

9. Metal

Beryllium, used in the manufacture of fluorescent lights, causes skin ulcers, dermatitis, and granulomas. Chrome confers hardness to metals, and dermatitis from it is also common in the tanning industry. It is a contaminator of cement. In industrial countries it is one of the most common sensitizers in men; most obtain their sensitivity from cement but their greatest disability is due to the later inconvenience of not being able to wear leather footwear containing chrome. Ferrous sulphate can be used in cement to convert hexavalent chromium to the less sensitizing trivalent form.

Cobalt sensitivity is commonly found in association with nickel or chrome sensitivity. Jewellery, and possibly metal prostheses for hip replacement, may be responsible.

Nickel is used in various metal alloys, electroplating, enamels, and glass. It is easily absorbed through the skin and its presence in ear-rings and in buttons and clips probably accounts for the high incidence of metal dermatitis in women. There is a general trend towards increased nickel sensitivity and it is a worldwide problem. It contributes substantially to hand dermatitis.

While the handling of money or pots and pans seems not to be responsible, abrasive cleaning of such in washing-up water releases nickel and is a reason for blaming this occupation or for recommending the use of running water.

10. Employment and contact dermatitis

It will be seen from the above that many persons in industry are liable to contact specific types of 'contact dermatitis'. Some industries are particularly susceptible.

Hairdressers During apprenticeship the hands of a hairdresser suffer from the very abnormal wear and tear of frequent shampooing. Atopic subjects almost always break down. Nickel dermatitis is particularly common. When the distribution of the rash affects only the palmar surfaces, contact dermatitis is more likely than irritant dermatitis. The latter commonly affects the more tender dorsa of the hands and between the fingers.

Bakers Dough, sugars, and peels are irritants, and in atopic subjects there is often considerable skin damage from these. Many additives are now used in flour and can cause contact urticaria.

Builders Cement is highly irritant but skin quickly hardens. Severe alkaline burns of the lower legs from calcium hydroxide in wet cement is now well recognized, especially in the amateur using ready-mixed cement.

Chrome dermatitis may be very similar to constitutional patterns including seborrhoeic and stasis eczema, and for this reason anyone in the building industry who has any pattern of eczema should be patch tested.

Agricultural and horticultural workers Fungicides and pesticides carelessly used are frequent causes of dermatitis. This particularly occurs in isolated farms in developing countries.

PATCH TESTING

The principle of patch testing is to apply to the skin the agent to which the patient may be sensitive, but avoiding irritants, and observe its effect on cell-mediated immunity. It involves:

(1) applying the agent on a carrier material such as aluminium foil over filter paper covered by adhesive tape;
(2) using a concentration in white soft paraffin in water or ethyl alcohol which is non-irritant; for most chemicals 0.1 to 1 per cent (in the case of cosmetics or medicaments the concentration used in the whole product is suitable);
(3) applying to the back, which is more consistent in its response than arms or legs, and removing the covering adhesive tape and filter paper 2 h before reading; and
(4) reading at 2 and 4 days.

Most practitioners obtain reagents from Trolab, Karen Trolle-Lassen, Land, Pharm 6B AN, Hansens Alle, 2900 Hellerup, Denmark. These are replaced about every 6 months.

False positives result from sweat gland occlusion, sensitivity to adhesive tape, irritants, and generally increased irritability of the skin, usually due to active eczema, but also from exposure to ultraviolet irradiation.

A positive patch test is a papular and a palpable erythema and may be vesicular (Fig. 45). The internationally agreed standard battery of agents is listed in Table 17.

TREATMENT OF CONTACT DERMATITIS

The level of complaint is often lessened by good industrial relations or a happy home. Those who are well satisfied with life may call their problem merely roughness of the skin; those who are unhappy or dissatisfied may well call their problem dermatitis. Especially in those who have atopic eczema or psoriasis, emotional stress is considered to be a factor worth controlling if possible. Such stresses are often no more than the anxieties and irritations of daily living and employment in a complex society.

Elimination of known irritants or allergens must be attempted but, as in the case of poison ivy in the United States or some of the Compositae in Asia, complete avoidance may be impossible. For less severe allergens, such as chrome or nickel, the skin can settle to a tolerable degree merely by removing obvious sources in clothing or jewellery. Dermatologists interested in good relations in industry or local government can encourage cleanliness and ventilation in working environments and substitute less allergenic materials in industrial processes. It is not always advisable to make a worker change his job; this particularly applies to sensitivity to chrome in the building industry since once sensitized, most other jobs are equally difficult and most sufferers can manage with a little more care at work and with the help of emollients. Anti-inflammatory agents, such as steroid creams, are always of help and can help the affected stay at work, particularly for short periods, such as during the training of the hairdresser or nurse.

Severe chronic allergy can be relieved by immunosuppressive drugs such as azathioprine. For nickel dermatitis where life has become intolerable, chelating agents such as Antabuse® have been used. Nickel-free diets are complicated but much less unpleasant.

The prognosis for contact dermatitis is often good. Thus 30 per cent of nickel dermatitis of the hands is healed in 6 years. Only 25 per cent of apprentice hairdressers with dermatitis of the hands have to change their job. Only rarely, as with certain plant allergies, is the problem a persistent and intolerable problem affecting many persons in the community.

Atopic eczema

This is a constitutional disorder of the skin affecting 1 to 3 per cent of the population. It is one of the most common diseases of childhood and one of the main reasons for loss of work in industry. It accounts for about 50 per cent of hand eczema. It is inherited through several genes

Fig. 45 Contact for about 48 h with the allergen to which the patient is sensitive can be used as a test at any site on the skin. This is the basis of the patch-test reaction. In this case a finger dermatitis due to an allergen in cigarette smoke could be proved by application of the smoked filter paper to the back of the patient.

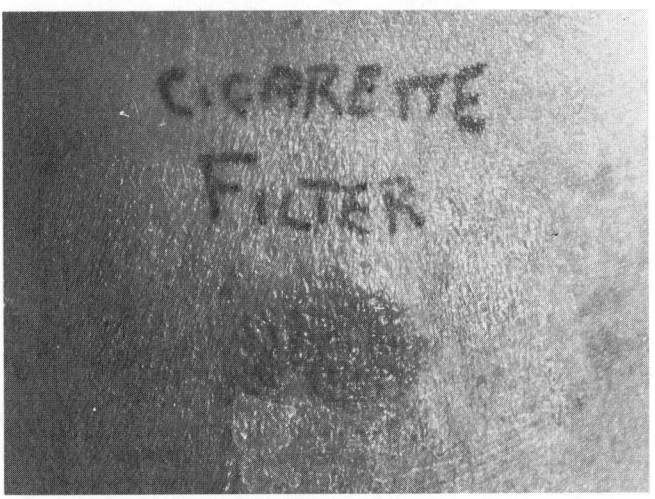

affecting the capacity to produce reagenic antibody reactions to the environment as well as the itch and consequent response to scratching. IgE responsiveness underlying asthma and rhinitis has a dominant inheritance and a location on chromosome 11.

Allergic respiratory disease affects about 50 per cent of eczema sufferers, and 70 per cent of patients are aware of other family members with the disease; for 90 per cent the disorder starts within the first 9 years of life. In the majority, the eczema gradually improves but the skin remains vulnerable to physical and chemical irritants throughout life.

PATHOGENESIS

Atopic disease is essentially a defect in immunology with depressed T-cell function and consequent lack of suppression of some aspects of humoral antibody production.

Atopic dermatitis and the associated elevated IgE is associated with an *in vivo* up-regulation of the interleukin-4 (IL-4), IL-4 receptor pathway, which in turn is under the negative regulatory control of γ-interferon. This may be the explanation of increased atopy in the developed world, as bacterial infections become less overwhelming. Epidemiological studies incriminate urbanization, pollution, central heating, and middle class culture to explain a very much higher incidence in some European cities.

In normal tissues, there is a ratio of 5:1 in β- versus α-adrenergic activity, but in atopics the α-receptors are increased or there is β-adrenergic blockade, reducing the capacity to synthesize cyclic AMP and moderating the responses to β-adrenergic stimulation. This is thought to account both for the eczema and the asthma through an action on lymphocytes. This was first proposed by Szentivanyi in 1968 and he produced experimental models to support the concept. One cannot rule out the possibility that the circulation of lymphocytes through a scratched environment exposes them to a pharmacological cocktail of histamine, eiconosides, and neuropeptides. This same cocktail also bathes the lymph nodes as a consequence of lymphatic massage. Some critics believe that β-adrenergic blockade, if it exists, is due to therapy with sympathomimetic drugs given to the affected patients. For instance, steroid ointments modify such blockade. Infection, too, can have such an effect and many affected subjects have considerable secondary infection. House-mite antigen is increasingly incriminated.

IMMUNOLOGY

Atopic eczema and asthma have long been thought of as 'allergic'. There is no doubt about the altered reactivity to a variety of irritants including allergens. 'Allergic' rhinitis, asthma, and eczema often fluctuate and even alternate, the one improving as the other worsens.

Skin tests by pricking various antigens into the skin result in weal and flare responses that are often multiple and strongly positive. However, there is a poor correlation between the skin test response and the activity of the eczema which may be even in remission in, for example, the hayfever season in spite of strong reactivity to skin testing with grasses.

The role of food allergy is difficult to test accurately in such a fluctuating and multifactorial disease. Neither prick tests nor allergen-specific IgE tests can be used to predict those most likely to benefit from dietary elimination. Exclusive breast feeding is of benefit but not necessarily due to avoidance of factors in the diet. Breast milk contains much IgA. Complete avoidance of cows' milk during the first 6 months of the life of the children of atopic parents is believed to be beneficial but there are nevertheless many who fail to benefit.

Humoral immunity

IgE reagenic antibody is elevated in over 80 per cent of patients with atopic dermatitis, often to over 2000 units/ml, but the significance of this remains uncertain since atopic eczema can occur in agammaglob-

Table 17 *European standard battery of patch tests*

Name	Concentration (%)
1 Potassium dichromate	0.5
2 Paraphenylenediamine dihydrochloride	0.5
3 Thiuram mix	1
Tetramethylthiuram monosulphide	0.25
Tetramethylthiuram disulphide	0.25
Tetramethylthiuram disulphide	0.25
Dipentamethylenthiuram disulphide	0.25
4 Neomycin sulphate	20
5 Cobalt chloride	1
6 Benzocaine	5
7 Nickel sulphate	5
8 Quinoline mix	6
Clioquinol	3
Chlorquinaldol	3
9 Colophony	60
10 Parabens	15
Methyl *p*-hydroxybenzoate	3
Ethyl *p*-hydroxybenzoate	3
Propyl *p*-hydroxybenzoate	3
Butyl *p*-hydroxybenzoate	3
Benzyl *p*-hydroxybenzoate	3
11 Black rubber mix	0.6
N-Isopropyl-*N'*-phenyl-*p*-phenylenediamine	0.1
N-Cyclohexyl-*N'*-phenyl-*p*-phenylenediamine	0.25
N,*N'*-Diphenyl-*p*-phenylenediamine	0.25
12 Wool alcohols	30
12 Mercapto mix	2
N-Cyclohexylbenzothiazylsulphenamide	0.5
Mercaptobenzothiazole	0.5
Dibenzothiazyl disulphide	0.5
Morpholinylmercaptobenzothiazole	0.5
14 Epoxy resin	1
15 Balsams of Peru	25
16 Paratertiary butylphenol formaldehyde resin	1
17 Carba mix	3
1,3-Diphenylguanidine	1
Bis(diethyldithiocarbamato)zinc	1
Bis(dibutyldithiocarbamato)zinc	1
18 Formaldehyde (in water)	1
19 Fragrance mix	8
Cinnamyl alcohol	1
Cinnamaldehyde	1
Eugenol	1
Hydroxycitronellal	1
α-Amylcinnamaldehyde	1
Geraniol	1
Isoeugenol	1
Oak moss absolute	1
20 Ethylenediamine dihydrochloride	1
21*Quaternium 15 (Dowicil 200)	1
22*Primin	0.01

All substances except formaldehyde are incorporated in white petrolatum.

ulinaemia and normal levels are found in many actively eczematous patients. Of course, serum levels need not reflect the level of activity of the IgE surrounding the mast cell in the skin itself. Complexes with antigen and the mast cell are often, after all, the basis of the IgE-mediated weal and flare. There is an increased frequency of the presence of specific reagin (RAST) to numerous allergens in the sera of atopics.

Reactivity of immune system

About 80 per cent of atopics have an excessive reactivity of the immune system. They react to certain foods and to house dust with immediate itching and swelling of the tissues. The agents to which 90 per cent of atopic patients react differ from those usually encountered in allergic disease. They include a number of animal and vegetable proteins from milk, meat, and corn. Eczema itself is most typically a consequence of delayed or cell-mediated immunity but in the case of the atopic skin there seems to be depression of T-cell function leading to a greater susceptibility to viral, bacterial, and fungal infections. Herpes simplex, vaccinia, warts, *Staphylococcus aureus,* and *Trichophyton rubrum* infections are most favoured; 90 per cent of atopic subjects carry *Staphylococcus aureus* in their skin, compared to 10 per cent of normal subjects. Fortunately, the atopic subject is not so susceptible to strains responsible for impetigo, toxic epidermal necrolysis, or furunculosis. There is also decreased reactivity to other common allergens such as poison ivy, *Candida,* or dinitrochlorbenzene (DNCB).

An atopic eczema-like syndrome is also a feature of immune deficiency diseases such as Wiskott–Aldrich syndrome, hyper-IgE syndrome of Buckley, and thymic aplasia, as well as the DiGeorge and Nesselof syndromes which also have high levels of IgE and decreased cell-mediated immunity. It is possible that immaturity of the humoral antibody system results in defective T-lymphocyte regulation, and IgE production is increased as one consequence.

CHARACTERISTICS

The principal characteristics of atopic eczema are described below.

A low itch threshold

Indeed a diagnosis should not be made if there is no history of itching. Besides the usual causes of itching, many minor irritants, such as wool of clothing or changes in climate, cause scratching. Scratching causes excoriations and ulceration as well as thickening of the epidermis and swelling and redness of the underlying dermis. The broken surface is sore and further irritated by soaps, some ointment bases such as sorbic acid, sea-water, or citric fruit juices. It has been found, using intradermal trypsin as a test of itch, that atopics have a prolonged itch reaction, although it may be that other patients with other forms of eczema are similarly affected.

Dry and lined skin

In non-excoriated areas the skin is often dry and lined. This is more obvious in hard water areas with temperate climates. The palms are particularly heavily lined and cause embarrassment even to the fortune teller! About 70 per cent of adult patients have a hand dermatitis and such hand dermatitis usually spares the palms. In adults also, nipple eczema may be a problem during breast feeding. It seems that there is a deficiency in sweating and sebum excretion which leads to chapping, wear, and tear, particularly from solvents or water. In industry, occupational dermatitis from primary irritants is commonly due to an underlying atopic eczema. Other features of atopic dryness are keratosis pilaris which is a perifollicular hyperkeratosis.

Vasodilation of vasculature

In the popliteal and cubital fossae the vasculature too readily vasodilates, heating the skin and hence inappropriately lowering the itch threshold. When scratched, rubbed, or stretched, the skin blanches for a few minutes, beginning 12 to 15 s after injury. This is in part due to upper dermal precapillary shutdown and also to persistent inflammatory oedema. Deeper vessels often dilate so that the skin is warm. This combination of hot but pale skin accounts for the itching as well as the atopic pallor.

CLINICAL FEATURES

Itching is the chief feature and becomes apparent during the first 2 to 6 months of life. The face is usually first affected and scratching begins between the second and third month. Sore lips from licking and chapping as well as conjunctivitis with ectropion are common; 70 per cent of patients have a skin fold or wrinkle just beneath the margin of the lower lid of both eyes (Fig. 46). When the child begins to crawl, the exposed surfaces such as the knees and hands become the most involved. The papules are scratched and become exudative and so secondary infection associated with lymphadenopathy is a common finding. Lymphadenopathy can sometimes be so gross as to lead to suspicion of some dire malignant disease. From 18 months onwards the sites most characteristically involved are the flexures of the elbows, knees, sides of neck, wrists, and ankles (Fig. 47). Local areas of lichenified skin may persist at such sites, and the face, too, may be heavily lichenified. Rubbing of the eyes is not the whole explanation of why keratoconus and anterior subcapsular cataracts are featured in severe cases. Seasonal

influences on the disease are in part climatic, due to sunlight and humidity, but probably even more related are seasonal allergies. Pollen is a feature of spring and early summer, while house dust seems to be a feature of late summer.

ASSOCIATED DISORDERS

Hayfever and asthma occur in 30 to 50 per cent of patients. Drug reactions of the anaphylactic type are more common and abdominal symptoms due to food allergy are frequently described. Contact urticaria is common. Alopecia areata is associated.

Fig. 46 Atopic eczema in an adult, showing the characteristic skin fold of the lower eyelid and the loss of eyebrow hair, as well as the thickening of the skin due to rubbing.

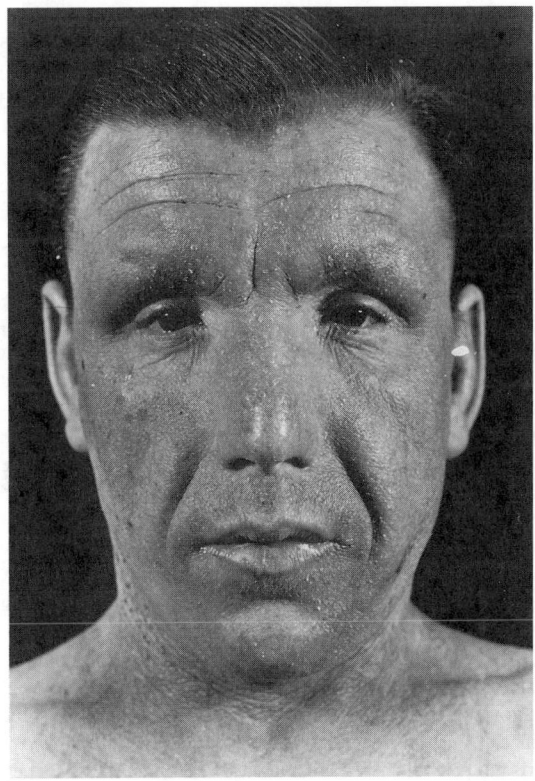

Fig. 47 Typically thickened and excoriated skin of the chronic prurigo of atopic eczema.

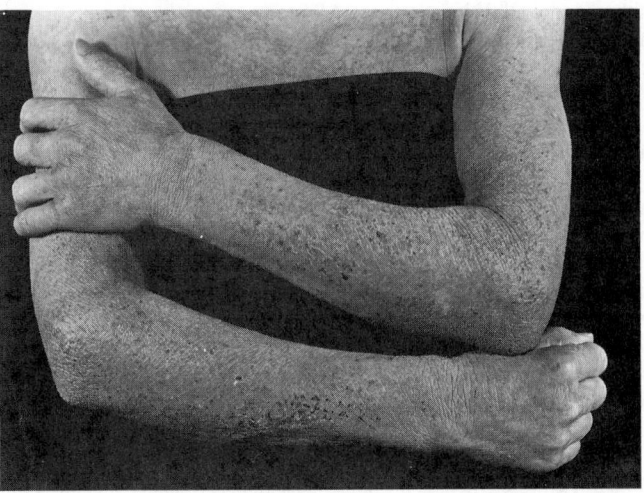

PROGNOSIS

Most children develop their eczema within the first 6 months of life but about one-fifth of patients may have a delayed onset, even into adult life. There is, in general, a tendency for gradual improvement. Complete clearance without breakdown when in contact with skin irritants is unusual but the majority of persons are clear by the time they are teenagers in the absence of major irritants.

MANAGEMENT

This is a multifactorial disease and all factors have to be managed. It is useful for parents to have access both to the doctor and nurse as well as to the literature provided by patient groups. All factors which cause irritation of the skin should be even more avoided in the atopic, and these include various primary irritants such as soap, wool, and extremes of climate. Moisturization of the skin is good but evaporation is bad. Wet wrapping is the application of wet dressings over moisturizing creams. These are then covered by dry dressings. Washing with liberal soap substitutes based on emulsifying ointments is mostly helpful and these are most effective if applied at least four times a day. The common-sense avoidance of jobs in which there is a large amount of primary irritants should be advised. Fortunately smallpox vaccination is no longer compulsory, but it is difficult to avoid the occasional contact with herpes simplex, molluscum contagiosum, and other viruses affecting the skin. If there is an immunological defect, then it remains difficult to know how to remedy this. The role of food allergy is difficult to determine in such a fluctuating and multifactorial disease. While breast feeding is to be recommended for all infants, it may be especially important for babies with a strong family history of eczema. There is evidence that breast feeding may reduce the incidence of atopic eczema by up to two-thirds, though not all authors agree. It is postulated that there is a period of transient immune vulnerability early in life, during which exposure to food antigens, perhaps by complexing with IgG, IgM, and IgE instead of IgA, results in allergic sensitization and the subsequent development of atopic eczema. The effect of breast feeding may be due to its low antigen load compared to cows' milk. Breast milk is also rich in IgA which may modify the absorption of food antigens. Such breast feeding should be for an extra 3 to 4 months, since any supplement exposes the immature gut to foreign protein. Especially to be avoided is any supplement in hospital during the first week of life. Further benefit might be gained by avoiding eggs and cows' milk in the mother's diet, since foreign protein can be transmitted through the mother's milk. Where breast feeding is not possible, milk substitutes are second-best since they are expensive and require care to prevent bacterial contamination. Some paediatricians believe cows' milk should be avoided for 1 year and eggs for 18 months.

Some patients appear to benefit from a regime of antigen avoidance, although not all do so. Neither RAST tests nor skin-patch tests are reliable in selecting patients who are helped by dietary modification, since even those known to benefit from antigen avoidance may not show specifically raised IgE nor positive skin tests.

Elimination diets must be carefully assessed to obtain complete avoidance with, at the same time, adequate nutrition, and since they are not without risk in this respect, they should be reserved for the most severely affected children. Some authors recommend avoidance of egg, chicken, milk, and artificial colouring agents or preservatives. Goat's milk is not now in favour on nutritional grounds. Careful studies of the use of Chinese herbal teas have shown significant improvement in generalized dry eczema in children, but users should be aware of the potential hepatotoxicity of these drinks.

It has to be said that while it seems likely that food allergy plays a role, there is as yet no basis on which to match each patient with a diet that takes into account idiosyncrasy.

Other allergens in the environment that can be shown to be important for some children include the house-dust mite. Avoidance includes eliminating clothing and furniture that are dust collecting and the use of vacuum cleaning rather than brushing. A cold and dry environment discourages the mite.

Topical therapy

Apart from the liberal use of emollients, steroid creams are effective antipruritics (see Tables 32 and 33). There has been some fluctuation in the amount they have been prescribed over the past few years. Certainly there was a period in which overprescription resulted in systemic side-effects as well as local atrophy of the skin. Withholding of steroids, on the other hand, deprives the child of the one effective therapy. Short, sharp bursts of effective therapy with strong steroids may be entirely justified, but prolonged daily usage is bound to lead to complications. Topical steroids are stored in the skin and for this reason once-daily application may be sufficient. It seems an inexplicable fact of life that ringing the changes with ointments is of benefit and a skilled practitioner will always have an alternative cream on which the worried parents can pin their faith. Secondary infection is so common and bacterial allergy is so important that vigorous treatment of infection is justified and systemic antibiotics should be given according to the sensitivities of the bacteria from time to time. Erythromycin is especially valuable; mupirocin, topically, is as effective. The matter of climatic therapy remains unpredictable; undoubtedly a change of climate does effect great improvements in some children. It may be exposure to sunlight or to the sea or to a mountain top.

Severe cases of eczema, as with asthma, may have to be controlled by systemic steroids, either in the form of prednisolone or corticosteroid injections. This may be simply to help the patient over an acute period but a small minority of patients may require long-term therapy for several years. Cyclosporin controls severe eczema but there is little long-term benefit. Traditional herbal remedies are popular and carefully controlled studies have shown some benefits from Chinese medicinal plants.

REFERENCES

Champion, R.H. and Parish, W.E. (1992). Atopic dermatitis. In *Textbook of dermatology,* (ed. A. Rook, D.S. Wilkinson, and F.J.G. Ebling), pp. 589–610. Blackwell Scientific, Oxford.

Emmett, E.A. (1984). The skin and occupational diseases. *Archives of Environmental Health* 39, 144–9.

Epstein, E. (1984). Hand dermatitis: practical management and current concepts. *Journal of the American Academy of Dermatology* 10, 395–424.

4th International Symposium on Atopic Eczema, Bergen (1992). *Acta Dermatol-Venereologica Supplementum* 76, 1–14.

Grandlund, H., Erkko, P., Sinisalo, M., and Reitamo, S. (1995). Cyclosporin in atopic dermatitis: time to relapse and effect of intermittant therapy. *British Journal of Dermatology,* 132, 106–12.

Janssens, V., Morren, M., Dooms-Goossens, A., and Degreef, H. (1995). Protein Contact Dermatitis: myth or reality. *British Journal of Dermatology,* 132, S4–S8.

Kapsenberg, M.L., Wierenga, E.A., Van der Heijden, F.L., and Bos, J.D. (1992). Atopic dermatitis and CD4$^+$ allergen specific Th2 lymphocytes. *European Journal of Dermatology,* 2, 601–7.

Maibach, H. (1987). *Occupational and industrial dermatology,* (2nd edn). Year Book Medical Publishers, Chicago.

Rajka, G. (1989). *Essential aspects of atopic dermatitis.* Springer-Verlag, Berlin.

Renz, H., Jujo, K., Radley, K.O., Dominico, J. Galfand, E.W. and Leung, D.Y. (1992). Enhanced IL-4 production and IL-4 receptor expression in atopic dermatitis and their modulation by interferon gamma. *Journal of Investigative Dermatology* 99, 403–8.

Rycroft, R.J.G. (1992). Occupational dermatoses. In *Textbook of dermatology,* (ed. A. Rook, D.S. Wilkinson, and F.J.G. Ebling). Blackwell Scientific, Oxford.

Sheehan, M.P. and Atherton, D.J. (1994). One year follow up of children treated with Chinese medicinal herbs for atopic eczema. *British Journal of Dermatology,* 130, 488–93.

Sventivanyi, A. (1968). The beta adrenergic theory of the atopic abnormality in bronchial asthma. *Journal of Allergy* **42,** 203–32.

Other patterns of dermatitis

INFECTED DERMATITIS

There is increasing evidence that bacterial allergy plays a part in the development of an eczematous response in the skin. The staphylococcus is particularly responsible. This may play a part in all sorts of eczema but occasionally it is the single cause. This is most frequently seen as a rather well-demarcated patch of eczema with crusting and scaling on an exposed area. There may be small pustules on an advancing edge; it is seen around discharging wounds, around ulcers, and occasionally around a paronychia or in a flexure, subject to sweating and maceration; it is particularly common around the ear or at sites of occlusion such as under a hat band or between the toes. An underlying pediculosis may be one trigger. Black skin seems commonly to develop a similar condition principally affecting the shins. Management includes the use of local antiseptics and wet soaks, or dyes, such as gentian violet, combined with an appropriate systemic antibiotic.

SEBORRHOEIC DERMATITIS

This is an unsatisfactory term but it is a recognizable disease affecting mainly the flexures in the distribution of the head, neck, upper chest, axillae, and groin. The aetiology is unknown but the distribution does appear to be in the areas of sebaceous activity. Breakdown of the skin occurs spontaneously but is activated by bacterial infection and by other primary irritants. There is a strong association with neuroleptic-induced parkinsonism as well as with AIDS. *Pityrosporum orbicularis* may be the responsible pathogen. In AIDS the oval blastosphere is predominant, whereas in pityriasis versicolor, the hyphal form is increased. The most characteristic lesion is a dull or yellowish-red and greasy plaque with a marginated scale. It is most likely to involve hair-bearing areas and particularly the scalp that has considerable dandruff; it spreads on to the face and involves the nasolabial folds and eyebrows. It affects the axillae and groins with well-defined brownish-red scaly areas deep into the folds, on the front of the chest, and in the middle of the back there may be small brown follicular papules covered by greasy scales or multiple discrete patches, or rarely a widespread eruption resembles pityriasis rosea with oval lesions with peripheral scale. Severe cases of seborrhoeic dermatitis develop marked crusting and scaling, particularly of hair-bearing areas and the genitalia. Otitis externa is one manifestation. The disorder tends to recur and may be chronic.

Management includes an attack on local infection and removal of crusts with wet soaks. Preparations, such as vioform hydrocortisone, sulphur, and ichthammol in a variety of water-miscible bases, usually in 1 to 2 per cent concentrations, have been traditionally prescribed. Lithium succinate ointment is recently favoured. Imidazoles control pityrosporum overproduction which is thought to play some part in the diathesis.

NUMMULAR ECZEMA

The main feature of this eczema is that it is discoid or composed of rounded lesions scattered, often symmetrically, over the body. They are intensely vesicular and intensely itchy. They are undoubtedly endogenous, external influence playing little part in their development, although occasionally sensitivity to metals, such as nickel or chrome, may produce a similar picture. Secondary infection is common; sometimes it is as a reaction pattern to a localized primary irritant such as an insect bite.

ASTEATOTIC ECZEMA

This type of eczema is usually associated with drying out of the skin. It is particularly found in the elderly or those suffering from a minor degree of malnutrition (see Figs. 24, 43, and 126). It is seen particularly when there is a change of habitat, as in admission to a centrally heated hospital and enforced nudity. The essential feature is the drying out and cracking of the skin over certain exposed areas, such as the backs of the hands and the fronts of the legs. It gives an appearance of crazy paving with deep fissures. It is aggravated by soaps and other irritants and by scratching. It responds very well to humidifiers and emollients as well as to a weak steroid.

PITYRIASIS ALBA

This is a pattern of eczema quite common in children, often with darker skins, in which a very low-grade dry eczema with shedding of pigment gives rise to a white patch of skin (see Fig. 73). It may be associated with drying out—reduced sebum—around the hair follicles, known as keratosis pilaris.

Pruritus

Pruritus is the term used when itching is the primary complaint unaccompanied by visible evidence of lesions predisposing to itch. Of course, itching is the most prominent symptom in skin disease and tends always to evoke scratching or rubbing (insect bites are the most common cause of pruritic skin lesions). It is subjective and for any one skin disease varies from individual to individual. There are exceptions even to the rule that syphilis never itches. Itch is a sensation largely dependent on superficial nerve endings in an intact upper dermis and epidermis and it is abolished by immersion in water at 40 to 41 °C. It is common in wound healing. It is induced by a number of agents including histamine, bradykinin, bile salts, and proteases, and is potentiated by prostaglandin E. It can be disassociated from pain in hypoalgesia. Central neurological and emotional psychiatric factors control the threshold to itch or pain. Awareness is a complex attribute modifying or intensifying the response to the itch. The itch itself may cause irritability, depression, or the attitude of the masochist who wears a 'hair shirt'. Thinly myelinated nerves in lateral spinothalamic tracts and secondary neurones to the thalamus relay both pain and itch and the cerebral cortex can modify these responses.

Itching is usually worse when the skin is heated to normal body temperature and when there is little else to distract one—a combination common at night. Vasodilatation in the cubital or popliteal fossae partially accounts for the lower itch threshold at such sites in atopic eczema.

The itch of different dermatoses evokes different types of scratching. Urticaria almost never is scratched and usually it is rubbed or pinched perhaps because the exact site of the itch is difficult to pinpoint. Where intense itching is exactly located it is often persistent and deeply excoriated.

Parasites are an important cause of pruritus but those experienced at examining the skin will usually observe primary urticarial or papular lesions in amongst the scratches. Onchocerciasis, trichinellosis, and schistosomiasis cause severe pruritus, usually with marked eosinophilia and well as urticaria, prurigo, and depigmentation. In onchocerciasis, loss of elasticity and the development of a leather-like skin hanging in folds is one consequence.

CAUSES OF PRURITUS (*SINE* SKIN LESIONS)

A common factor is dryness and desiccation of the stratum corneum, common in the elderly and worse in winter.

The threshold of itching is lowered by isolation, including the common accompaniments of ageing such as blindness, deafness, and loneliness. Endogenous depression is often missed in the elderly and should be treated. Paroxysmal itching may originate in the central nervous system and provoke deep scratching which is pleasurable but injurious. It is a feature of cocaine addiction.

Sweat retention also causes intense pruritus such as prickly heat. The intense pruritus of scabies with much excoriation requires a very careful search for burrows especially in well-groomed persons in the early stages of the disease. Head lice may similarly be elusive and the hair rather than the scalp is the principal hiding place; in the early stages the insect lies very close to the scalp. The classical nit is a relatively late stage. Persons recently engaged in insulating their roof with fibreglass suffer from pruritus due to almost invisible spicules of fibreglass (see Fig. 42).

AQUAGENIC PRURITUS

This occurs after contact with water—fresh, salt, or sweat. In some it is from the moment of contact and lasts 15 min. In others, it is less immediate and longer lasting. Some have been helped by acetylcholine or histamine antagonists or by ultraviolet rays. In the elderly, a common similar reaction due to rapid drying out after prolonged hydration is helped by shortening the period of hydration.

GENERALIZED PRURITUS AND SYSTEMIC DISEASE

1. Hepatic disease

Obstructive jaundice causes severe pruritus. It is particularly an early feature of biliary cirrhosis and because bile salts rather than bilirubin are responsible for the itch, the degree of jaundice need not to be great. Indeed, an oestrogen-induced pruritus of pregnancy or from the contraceptive pill often shows little or no jaundice in spite of intrahepatic biliary obstruction, severe pruritus, and a much raised alkaline phosphatase. Chlorpromazine and testosterone can have the same effect. Bile salts in the skin can achieve a relatively higher concentration than may be indicated by serum levels. Bile salts in a concentration of 1 mmol/l cause itching when applied to a blister base. Dihydroxy salts especially chenodeoxycholate are responsible.

2. Blood disease

Iron deficiency also causes itching even when the patient is not anaemic. There is often some thinning of hair. Polycythaemia is frequently associated with itching, particularly after a hot bath and it is believed to be related to blood histamine levels and occasionally to iron deficiency and hence the reported response to iron therapy within 2 to 10 days. Lymphatic leukaemia and Hodgkin's disease are other causes of pruritus often long lasting before it becomes clinically overt.

3. Carcinoma of the internal organs

Carcinoma of the bronchus in particular may present with generalized pruritus.

4. Chronic renal failure

Itching is not a feature of acute renal failure or even of malignant hypertension, however uraemic. In chronic pyelonephritis and chronic glomerulonephritis, the patients usually suffer greatly from pruritus. Haemodialysis does not necessarily relieve it. Parathyroidectomy, for reasons that remain obscure, relieves itching in those in whom removal is necessitated by secondary hyperparathyroidism. The cause of pruritus in renal failure is unknown but dryness of the skin is one factor, and there are also increased numbers of mast cells in the skin.

5. Endocrine disease

Pruritus is sometimes a presenting symptom of diabetes mellitus but mostly this is localized principally to the vulva. About one in ten patients with hyperthyroidism complain of itching. Dry skin in hypothyroidism often itches.

MANAGEMENT OF PRURITUS

Overheating should be avoided as should vasodilators such as alcohol and hot drinks. Calamine lotion is used as a cooling agent. Evaporation is increased by the enhanced surface area provided by the powder. Dryness of the skin should be discouraged by emollients. In hospital a moist microenvironment can be enhanced by the wearing of clothes. Too frequent bathing should be discouraged unless emulsifying ointments are added to the bath as soap substitutes. Bath salts should be avoided. Proprietary bath oils are more cosmetically acceptable but tend to be expensive for regular daily use. The treatment of the cause of the pruritus is obviously indicated where possible. Antihistamines act principally through their sedative effect and they reduce the awareness. Chlorpromazine may reduce the reactivity to the itch. Plasma exchange has been used to control sweats and pruritus. The anion exchange resin cholestyramine, 6 to 8 g daily, or oral activated charcoal helps the pruritus of liver disease and sometimes also its use in chronic renal disease or polycythaemia has been helpful. Suberythema doses of UVB irradiation twice weekly, and even natural sunlight, help pruritus somewhat unpredictably. They have been used to treat the itching of uraemia and of certain acute exanthems such as pityriasis rosea. Hydroxyethyl rutosides (Paroven®) have been advocated in renal failure. The H_2 receptor antagonist cimetidine is sometimes helpful in Hodgkin's disease; 1 per cent menthol and 1 per cent phenol have a mild anaesthetic effect and promote a sensation of cooling. Nails should be kept short and occlusive bandaging may reduce the vicious circle of itch and skin damage.

ARE INSECTS BITING?

Many a cause of prurigo or papular urticaria is due to insects, especially in the rainy season in hot countries. It is a reaction that is not necessarily immediately preceded by the recognition of insect biting and insects without wings are mainly unseen. Flea bites and such like are grouped and since no insect knows how to bite symmetrically, the pattern of scratched lesions can be identified as exogenous. The human flea is found on the skin only transiently and it is the patient's environment that may need to be treated often by agents which are best not applied to the skin.

Cheyletiella mites from dogs, cats, and other pets are picked up by a strip of transparent sticky tape applied to the pet's skin several times, especially where there is any mange from canine scabies. Birds' nests in the eaves may be one source. Stored cereals, fruits, and other vegetables matter sometimes contain mites as does house dust.

In the case of scabies, most of the rash is a hypersensitive response taking about 3 weeks to develop. The characteristic burrows (see Fig. 18) at the front of the wrist and between the fingers or on the areolae of the breasts are not necessarily themselves a cause of pruritus. Widespread scabies has been reported in renal transplant patients receiving azathioprine and prednisolone. Persistent cutaneous granulomas following treatment for scabies or other parasitic infections are not a sign of persistence of the live insects but may be an immune reaction to the dead parts—mouth parts and other insect antigens may cause persistent lesions for more than 3 months in about 20 per cent of patients.

The use of steroid creams has modified the hypersensitivity response so that the appearances of conditions such as scabies may be atypical.

Irritable papules at sites of contact with insects, such as the face, lap, or arms, are a feature of infestation from lap dogs and other pets. These may simulate eczema or dermatitis herpetiformis and, being a hypersensitivity reaction rather than a bite, there are no puncta but necrotic centres may develop.

Delusions of parasitosis are best treated with antipsychotics.

LOCALIZED PRURITUS

Localized intensely itchy areas of skin having no obvious causation are a common problem in the dermatology clinic. The nape of the neck, upper back (Fig. 48), genitalia, lower leg, elbow, and outer thigh are easily accessible sites liable to persistent rubbing and scratching. The injury to the skin results in thickening, purple-brown violaceous coloration due to dilated vessels and postinflammatory pigmentation. The normal line marks of the skin are exaggerated and excoriations are usually numerous. This is termed lichen simplex or neurodermatitis, and the fairly well defined patches cause paroxysms of itching and emotional upsets with anxiety or irritability which are also promoting factors.

Nodular prurigo is an unexplained reaction to scratching, evoking severe very localized pruritus. The nodules are 1 to 2 cm in diameter and scattered over accessible areas. It is sometimes a consequence of a partially resolved more generalized pruritus from atopic eczema or parasite infestation. Freezing with liquid nitrogen is helpful but in pigmented races depigmentation may result.

Local steroids are helpful and anything which protects the skin from scratching may eventually allow healing. Occlusive tape or bandaging is occasionally helpful but secondary infection is a problem, especially in hot countries.

Intralesional injection with triamcinolone causes rapid resolution in some cases but this may be only a temporary response, and where the lesions are large or multiple such inoculation is not without the side-effects of steroid therapy. It is always worth admitting such a patient and treating with traditional dermatological therapies such as tar bandages. A more recent suggestion is that some of these lesions are an immunological response and this has led to therapies as far ranging as azathioprine and thalidomide.

PRURITUS ANI AND PRURITUS VULVAE

Pruritus ani is common in Caucasian adult males. In the negro it is rare except as a manifestation of infestation. An important cause is soiling of the perianal skin. Haemorrhoids, fissures, and fistulae contribute to this. The anal sphincter relaxes in response to anal distension too readily in some sufferers and in others incomplete evacuation of faeces leaves some residual faeces in the folds of the anus. Soft stools are more likely to cause irritation. Diabetes mellitus, trichomoniasis, or candidiasis are amongst the commonest causes of pruritus valvae. In regions where malnutrition is common, pruritus ani and vulvae are rare except as a manifestation of an orogenital syndrome due to vitamin B deficiency. The pruritus is then associated with eczema and angular cheilitis. Reassurance concerning cancer, AIDS or sexually transmitted diseases, as well as avoidance of excessive ritual washing may be coupled with guidance or management of guilt because of extramarital affairs.

Sufferers use a large number of agents to relieve the pruritus some of which cause contact dermatitis. Pruritus vulvae may be caused by sensitivity to the rubber of condoms or spermicidal jelly or even to deodorants. Local anaesthetics and local steroids are much used. The latter encourage secondary infections with fungus or yeasts; these usually spread on to the buttocks and down the thighs.

Fig. 48 Prurigo nodularis is a form of scratched lesion which is very exactly localized. The upper back is a common site for such persistent excoriation.

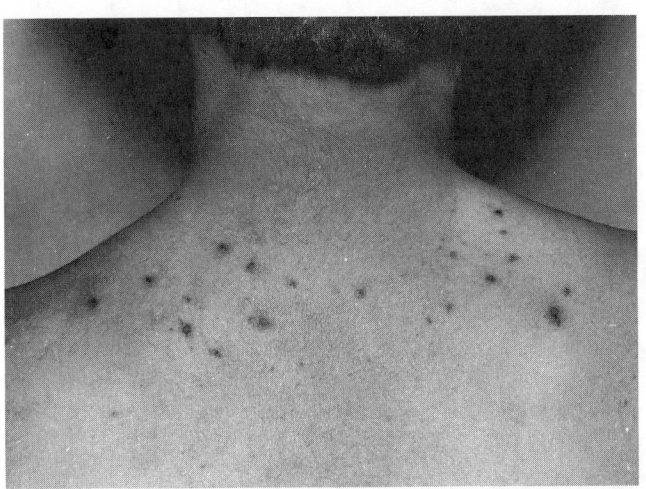

Management includes a thorough examination to exclude the above and there is a need to recognize skin diseases such as psoriasis, seborrhoeic dermatitis, or lichen planus. Lichen sclerosis and atrophicus also usually itches. Threadworm infection is common, especially in children.

Perianal soiling often requires cleaning of the area not only immediately after the bowels have been opened but a hour or two later as well. Weak local steroids often mixed with anticandida or antiseptic agents are the mainstay of treatment. Timodine is a safe example.

REFERENCES

Arnold, H.L. (1984). Paroxysmal pruritus. *Journal of the American Academy of Dermatology* **11**, 322–6.

Greaves, M.W. (1992). Pruritus. In *Textbook of dermatology,* (5th edn), (ed. A., Rook, D.S., Wilkinson, and F.J.G. Ebling), pp. 527–36. Blackwell Scientific, Oxford.

Hampers, C.L., Katz, A.I., Wilson, R.E., and Merrill, J.P. (1968). Disappearance of uraemia itching after sub-total parathyroidectomy. *New England Journal of Medicine* **279**, 695.

Journal of Investigative Dermatology (1979). Pruritis, pain, and sweating disorders. *Journal of Investigative Dermatology* **73**, 495–500.

Salem, H.H., Van der Weyden, M.B., and Young, I.F. (1982). Pruritus and severe iron deficiency in polycythaemia vera. *British Medical Journal* **285**, 91–2.

Savin, J.A. (1992). The skin and the nervous system. In *Textbook of dermatology,* (5th edn), (ed. A., Rook, D.S., Wilkinson, and F.J.G. Ebling), pp. 2469–78. Blackwell Scientific, Oxford.

Shultz, B.C. and Roenigk, H.H. (1980). Uremic pruritus treated with ultraviolet light. *Journal of the American Medical Association* **243**, 1836.

Takkunen, H. (1978). Iron deficiency pruritus. *Journal of the American Medical Association* **239**, 1394.

Psoriasis

In temperate zones psoriasis affects 2 per cent of the caucasian population. It is less common in sunny climates and in pigmented skins. The mode of inheritance is debated, but there is evidence of dominant and polygenic patterns. Two types of inheritance are identified. Type 1 with a strong family history and early onset shows linkage disequilibrium for human leucocyte antigens CW_6, B_{13} and BW_{57}. It affects 30 per cent of patients. It is possibly an IL-Ira gene defect. Type 2 occurs as late onset and is linked with CW_2 and B_{27}.

PATHOGENESIS

The pathogenesis of psoriasis includes a tenfold increase in the speed of epidermal cell proliferation. The cells pass upwards through the epidermis at a faster rate and seem not to have time to produce a horny layer. The cells remain nucleated even when exfoliated. There are numerous problems which beset the measurement of the cell-cycle time in human epidermis. There are the technical difficulties of counting and the exact recognition of different stages of the cell cycle and differentiation. Do all cells in the germinal layer have the potential to divide or is the potential greater in psoriasis? Is the actual cell cycle faster in psoriasis? The answer is probably that the cell cycle is faster and more cells enter the cycle per unit time in psoriasis. The factors inhibiting the cell cycle may be reduced and the factors stimulating are enhanced. The kinetics of the keratinocytes are clearly essential to our understanding of psoriasis. There are many explanations of how the increased turnover is triggered. Probably there is not a single cause, but contributions are made by the neutrophil, which is attracted in large numbers into the epidermis. Streptococcal antigens are cross-reactive with skin antigens and stimulate an autoimmune response. The role of the lymphocyte has long received consideration and has been encouraged by the observations on exacerbations of psoriasis in AIDS, control by cyclosporin and the possible immunosuppressive effects of other effective therapies, such as corticosteroids or PUVA. Psoriasis in AIDS is most pronounced at intermediate levels of immunodeficiency, and is diminished or lost in terminal profound immunodeficiency. At the biochemical level, almost every aspect of cell kinetics is a candidate, including the availability of cyclic AMP, increased cyclic GMP, fatty acid deficiency, eicosanoids, phosphorylating mechanisms, polyamines, putrescine, spermidine, calcium-modulating enzymes, such as calmodulin and vitamin D analogues. How cells stick together and how adhesion is modulated during migration and mitosis introduces many other concepts, ranging through the role of interleukins (IL-1, 2, 6, 8), interferons (γ-IFN), transforming growth factors α and β, and the interaction with proteases, since in psoriasis the proteinase–antiproteinase balance seems to be disturbed. Psoriasis is not merely a disorder of the keratinocyte. Thus arthropody cannot be explained on such a basis. Within the dermis, some would believe that the fibroblast, the mast cell, or even the endothelial cell, are prime targets for whatever it is that fires the psoriatic process. Recent greater understanding of neuropeptides has added them as a potential trigger, since they induce mast cell degranulation and fire interaction between the fibroblast and keratinocyte.

LESION-FREE SKIN

The lesion-free skin in persons with psoriasis is not normal. Psoriasis is more readily induced and various medications such as chloroquine and practolol or lithium can produce a flare-up. There are more cells available for DNA synthesis but, oddly, glycogen levels, so high in the psoriatic lesions, may be less than in normal skin. The dermis is not normal and the earliest signs of any abnormality following injury are infiltration with mast cells and macrophages.

The microvasculature in psoriasis is characterized by tortuous and leaky capillaries, generous protein exudation, and poor clearance through immature lymphatics.

KOEBNER PHENOMENON

The Koebner phenomenon is a term given to psoriasis developing in traumatized skin. After the initial stimulus to repair, the epidermis gradually thickens and there is accentuation of the papillary interdigitations and the rete ridges. There is an early heavy infiltrate by neutrophils forming microabscesses within the epidermis which is preceded by increased mast cells and macrophages in the dermis. High turnover of the epidermal cells results in a less compact and still partially nucleated scale known as parakeratosis.

CLINICAL APPEARANCE

Psoriasis can affect all age groups but has a peak age of onset in the young adult. The commonest lesion is a sharply marginated plaque with silvery scales (Fig. 49). These mask the underlying redness from tortuous convoluted capillaries which lie close to the surface of the skin. The edges of the lesion are usually the most active and there is commonly clearing in the centre (Fig. 50)

Sites most commonly affected are the elbows, knees, and scalp which normally have a higher rate of epidermal turnover. The face is less often affected. Spontaneous fluctuations are common and remissions occur in about one-third of cases per annum. There are several well-recognized patterns and it is important to examine the patient thoroughly until a completely recognizable lesion of psoriasis can be detected. Many lesions and some patterns may be quite atypical especially during the development of psoriasis (Fig. 51), or during its resolution.

Guttate psoriasis

This term is derived from *gutta* meaning a drop. The skin looks as though it has been splashed by the psoriasis. It often follows a streptococcal sore throat or vaccination and is especially common in children. The lesions are scattered over the entire body and tend to be no more than a few millimetres in diameter. They may include the face and are often red slightly scaly spots. They appear less well defined and less obviously covered by silvery scales than in classic types of psoriasis. In the absence of a family history the prognosis tends to be good.

Nummular discoid

This is probably the commonest form of psoriasis and coin-shaped lesions of various sizes (Fig. 52) are scattered over the body in a completely symmetrical distribution. Such lesions are usually well defined and chronic.

Palmar and plantar psoriasis

This may be typical of lesions elsewhere (see Fig. 4) but there is often a modification of the psoriasis due to the nature of the palmar and plantar skin. The scales tend to be more adherent and less silvery and they are more likely to develop deep cracks because of the thickness of the epidermis at these sites (Fig. 53) Neutrophils tend to collect into larger abscesses trapped by the thicker surface layers of the stratum corneum. The sterile pustules so formed are often the most obvious feature. This pattern may be seen as part of a more generalized disease but in many cases it affects only the hands and feet. There is some evidence that it

Fig. 49 A plaque of psoriasis, showing the silvery scales, well-defined border, and predilection for the elbow.

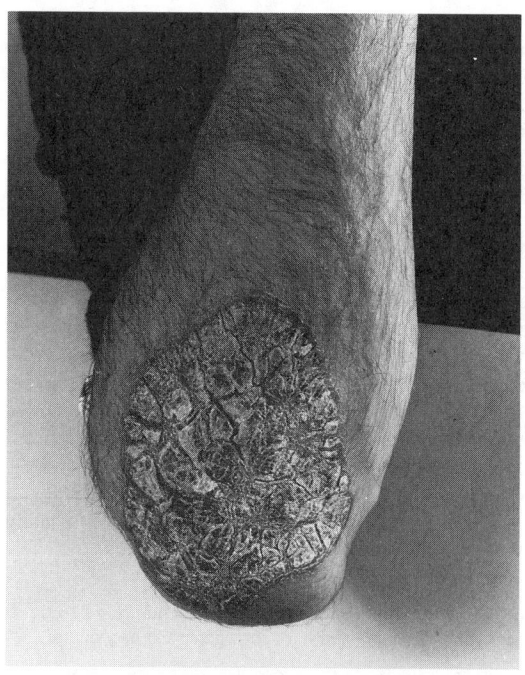

Fig. 50 Psoriasis that is less stable than in Fig. 49. The lesions are erupting and more active at the periphery while healing in the centre.

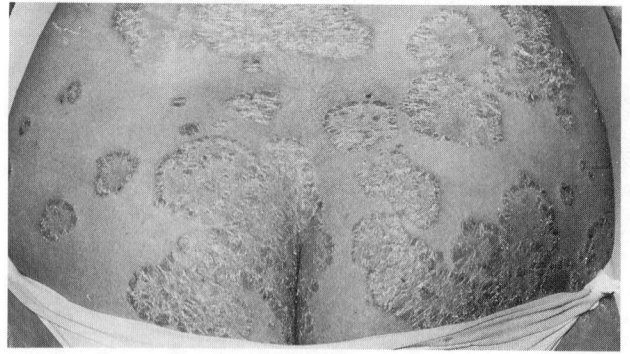

Fig. 51 Still more unstable form of psoriasis, tending to be more exudative and exfoliative and not retaining its rapidly produced scale. While tending to be symmetrical, new ill-defined lesions are erupting. There are some linear lesions on the trunk suggestive of the Koebner phenomenon or reaction to injury of the skin, in this case probably from scratching.

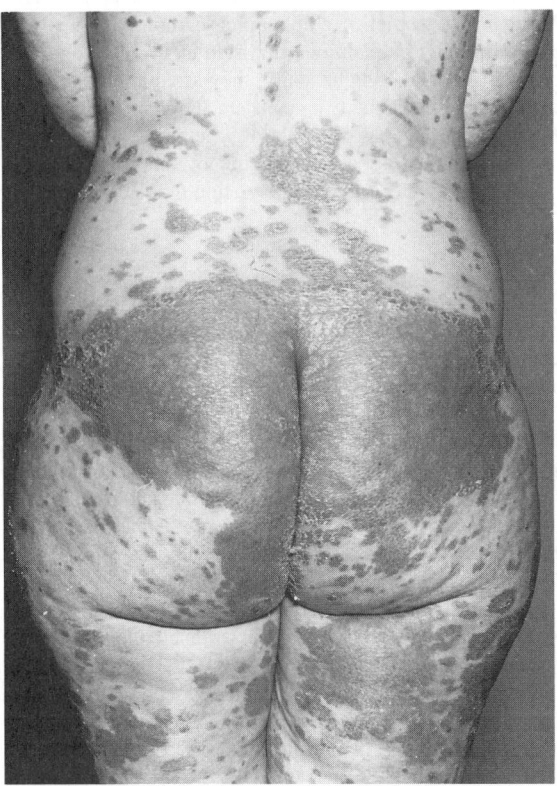

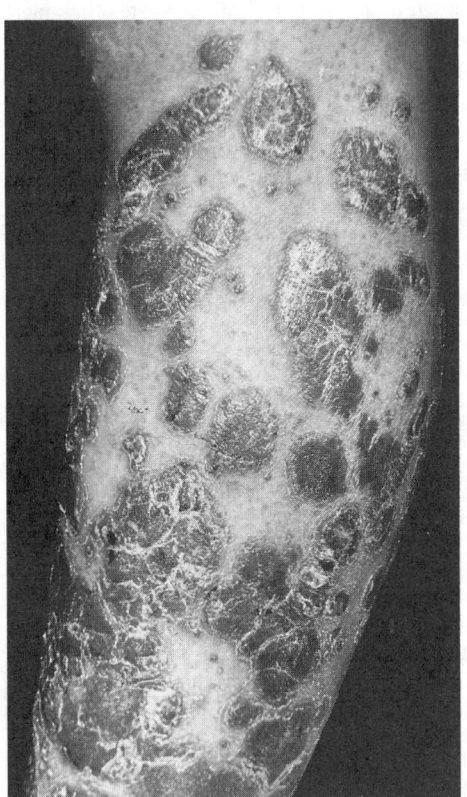

Fig. 52 Discoid lesions still well defined but almost becoming confluent.

is a different disease without the above mentioned HLA associations and without obvious increase in the rate of epidermal turnover. It is an occasional and acute response to infection and is then known as pustular bacterid.

Psoriasis of the nails

Pin-point pitting is usual but can be seen in other disorders affecting nail growth (see Fig. 75). Onycholysis with a salmon-pink discoloration of the base of the uplift of the nail is probably even more characteristic. Sometimes the nail growth is distorted, thickened and friable, and difficult to distinguish from a fungus disorder affecting the nail (see Fig. 78).

Flexural psoriasis

When psoriasis affects the groins, natal cleft, or axillae, it is usually less scaly. The bright red plaques are shiny and liable to cracking and maceration. They may be very well defined.

Erythroderma

This may present as a medical emergency due to fluid loss, septicaemia, or loss of body temperature. The elderly may develop high-output cardiac failure. Oedema is a consequence of capillary leak, low albumin, and heart failure. When psoriasis affects the entire skin there is generalized redness, the well-defined margins are lost and the scales are exfoliated profusely. The erythroderma may be indistinguishable from that found in eczema or lymphoma. When the normal protective function of the skin is lost, bacteraemia is common. The loss of water is difficult to estimate and prerenal failure can develop very rapidly. The vasodilatation and the obstruction to the sweat ducts by the proliferating epidermis results in impaired thermoregulation. Hyperthermia is very common in hot climates; hypothermia can occur in cold climates. Internal organs such as the gut and liver may be impaired and loss of protein both from the skin and the gut is an important complication.

Generalized pustular psoriasis

In this condition, which is relatively rare, waves of bright erythema develop within a few hours with a fever, arthropathy, and leucocytosis.

Fig. 53 Psoriasis of the palms may not have the typical scale. It is sometimes pustular or, as in this case, hyperkeratotic with a tendency to form deep cracks. See Fig. 4.

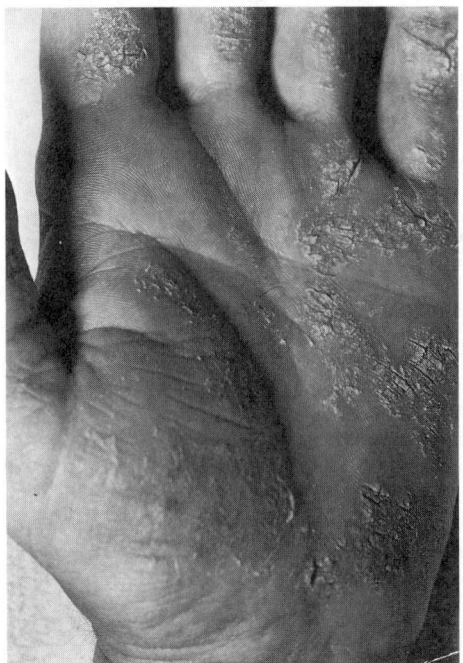

Myriads of pustules (see Fig. 17) quickly develop and equally quickly disappear. This disorder may occur in the absence of a previous history of psoriasis and even occasionally as a viral exanthem. However, most commonly it is only a complication of psoriasis that has been treated by systemic or local steroids. It is an acute rebound phenomenon of steroid withdrawal.

Another rare cause of pustular psoriasis is hypoparathyroidism.

Arthropathic psoriasis

The incidence of polyarthritis in psoriasis is about 7 per cent in hospital series; 4 per cent of all patients with inflammatory polyarthritis have psoriasis. There is a long-standing debate concerning the association of psoriasis with inflammatory polyarthritis; it is not certain whether it is a chance association. Since psoriasis is a common disorder, patients with a positive Rose–Waaler test can have coincidental rheumatoid arthritis. Seronegative arthritis in patients with psoriasis is of three types:

(1) distal arthritis involving the terminal interphalangeal joints of the hands and the interphalangeal joints of the toes with relative sparing of the metacarpophalangeal and metatarsalphalangeal joints;

(2) psoriatic arthritis mutilans which is a severe deforming arthritis involving the multiple small joints of the hands and feet and spine. The hips, cervical, and sacroiliac joints are frequently affected and a complete ankylosing type of spondylitis can occur; and

(3) an indistinguishable or rheumatoid-like type very similar to rheumatoid arthritis.

MANAGEMENT

By far the most disabling aspect of psoriasis is its appearance, and patients' lives can be completely taken over by manoeuvres designed to avoid exposing the affected skin to the public eye. Management includes a sympathetic hearing and often admission to an out-patient or in-patient unit where others are being treated.

The aim is to depress epidermal cell turnover without irreversibly damaging the skin or other organs. The physician is faced with a difficult choice of a cosmetically acceptable therapy in the form of a steroid cream, an antimitotic drug taken by mouth, or use of various forms of irradiation. All such therapies have side-effects and the alternatives, which are preferred on grounds of safety, often tend to be tedious and cosmetically unacceptable. The latter include tar and dithranol preparations.

Local steroids

Steroid creams and ointments are often in practice the first line of treatment because they are so easy to use. A few plaques of psoriasis on the elbows, knees, or scalp may be so treated by daily application, and in about one-third of patients the lesions are controlled within 1 to 2 weeks and remain under control in one-third of those so treated even when the application ceases. The stronger fluorinated steroids or betamethasone valerate are the most effective. One-third of patients need to continue once or twice weekly application and another third show no improvement even with twice daily application. In all those in whom these stronger steroids have to be continued, complications gradually develop. These include skin atrophy, gradual extension of the psoriasis, and greater instability of the skin so that psoriasis erupts whenever the therapy is partially or completely withdrawn. Eventual widespread usage and systemic absorption complicates the increasing addiction of the skin for the stronger steroids. Some such patients show no remission until all such therapy is withdrawn and in a few this can be done without any immediate worsening of the psoriasis but in most there is rapid worsening of their skin condition.

Tar

Tar has been known to be effective and safe for more than 50 years. Follow-up of patients treated with tar between 1917 and 1937, using the Danish Cancer Registry of all cell cancers from 1943 to 1990, found no overall risk of skin cancer. Its smell, colour, and stain make it cosmetically unsatisfactory. Patients should be encouraged to use it because it has no significant side-effects and the clearance of psoriasis is more long lasting. The cruder varieties may be irritant on more vulnerable skin and the more purified varieties of liquor picis carbonis are relatively weak. *National Formulary* preparations are listed in Table 18.

The preparations are applied twice daily; they are diluted by 50 per cent if they are irritant. Occasionally patients are allergic to one or more of the constituents. The general principle of whether to use a lotion, ointment, or paste are discussed later. Acute or inflamed psoriasis responds to ichthammol which has a milder action than coal tar.

Dithranol

Dithranol is more effective than coal tar in the treatment of psoriasis especially if the plaques are large, well-defined, and few in number. It is more irritant, but by diluting it one can usually find a concentration which is acceptable. Once this is so, the concentration can usually be gradually increased. The dithranol is mixed in zinc oxide and salicylic acid paste (Lassar's paste) in a concentration of 0.1, 0.25, 0.5, 1, or 2 per cent. It is irritant to the eyes and genitalia. Weaker preparations are used in the more sensitive occlusive flexures. It is safe in pregnancy.

The non-lesional skin may be protected by vaseline and it is usual to apply dithranol paste accurately to the active parts of the skin lesion. Powdering fixes the paste and a gauze or nylon dressing protects the overlying clothing from its staining property. Patients tolerating this regimen are cleared in about 3½ weeks on average. Staining is inevitable and is a sign of effectiveness. It is short lived. Irritancy like a mild burn is treated by omitting treatment for 1 or 2 days. Various proprietary brands are slightly easier to manage and include vaseline-based preparations and creams or sticks (Table 18). The minute regimen is a system using dithranol 1 to 5 per cent in vaseline and 2 per cent salicylic acid. It is applied only for about 80 min before removal with an oil. It is suitable for those whose employment requires their skin to be free of ointments for most of the day.

Calcipotriol, a vitamin D analogue, is a safe and cosmetically acceptable, effective topical treatment, inhibiting proliferation and enhancing epidermal differentiation. It is applied twice daily at a rate of not more than 100 g/week. It is irritant for about 10 per cent of users. Fish-oil supplements—eicosapentanoic acid capsules for 10 weeks—are helpful for itching.

Phototherapy

Natural sunlight is helpful in about 75 per cent of patients and probably accounts for a decreased incidence of psoriasis in sunny climates. Suberythema doses of UVB are a useful substitute and its effectiveness can be increased by prior bathing in or an application of tar which sensitizes the skin to the UVB.

PUVA therapy was introduced for psoriasis 10 years ago. The combination of long-wave ultraviolet rays (UVA or black light) with eight methoxypsoralen tablets 0.5 mg/kg taken 2 h before exposure produces effective clearance and a bronze skin in most patients. Exposure of 15 to 30 min twice or thrice weekly succeeds in clearing the psoriasis in a month to 6 weeks. Maintenance therapy is weekly or fortnightly. Recurrences are no less frequent than with other forms of therapy. Dryness, atrophy, and other expected changes of irradiation are a consequence. The risk of skin cancer is as yet difficult to estimate but it is not insignificant. In male patients receiving more than 200 treatments, the incidence of squamous cell carcinoma was 30 times greater than that found in the general population in Sweden. Internal cancer was also recorded more frequently. In renal transplant patients, sun-exposure, HLA β mismatching and HLA-DR homozygosity are significantly associated with the risk of squamous cell carcinoma. The risk is especially great in those who have arsenical keratoses or other evidence of previous intake of arsenic.

Climatotherapy is the combination of natural sunlight, or in the case of the Dead Sea, a filtered form of sunlight, with sea salts or other

Table 18 *Topical preparations for the treatment of psoriasis*

Tar preparations
Coal tar solution (liquor picis carbonis)
  20% prepared coal tar ⎫
               ⎬ in 90% alcohol
  10% quillaia ⎭
 Tar bath
 120 ml coal tar solution BP in a 20-gallon bath
Coal tar pomade

Coal tar solution BP	6%
Salicyclic acid	2%
Polysorbate 20	1%
Emulsifying ointment to 100%	

Calamine and coal tar ointment

Calamine, finely sifted	12.5 g
Zinc oxide, finely sifted	12.5 g
Strong coal tar solution	2.5 g
Hydrous wood fat	25.0 g
White soft paraffin	47.5 g

Coal tar and salicyclic acid ointment[a]

Coal tar	2.0 g
Salicylic acid	2.0 g
Emulsifying wax	11.4 g
White soft paraffin	19.0 kg
Coconut oil	54.0 g
Polysorbate 80	4.0 g
Liquid paraffin	7.6 g

Oil of cade pomade
  10% of cade ⎫
                 ⎬ in spirit soap shampoo
  10% triethanolamine ⎭
5% to 15% of cade in olive oil for psoriasis of the scalp
Polytar® shampoo (contains tar, arachis oil, and oleyl alcohol) ⎫ cosmetically
Alphosyl® lubricating cream; special crude coal tar extract 5%, allantoin 2% ⎬ acceptable but
Alphosyl® lotion (contains a vanishing cream base) ⎭ very mild

Lassar's paste
Lassar's paste BNF

Zinc oxide	24%
Starch	24%
Salicylic acid	2%
White soft paraffin	50%

'Stiff' Lassar's paste
 Melting point of soft paraffin 46–49 °C with 15% hard paraffin
'Soft' Lassar's paste
 'Stiff' Lassar's paste and emulsifying ointment in equal parts

Dithranol preparations[b]
Dithranol pomade

Dithranol	0.4%
Liquid paraffin	75.4%
Cetyl alcohol	21.7%
Sodium lauryl sulphate (finely powdered)	2.5%

Dithranol in 'stiff' Lassar's paste (Stanford)

Dithranol	0.1% to 0.4% occasionally stronger
Salicylic acid	0.2% to 0.4%
Hard paraffin	0.5%
Zinc oxide paste	to 100%

Dithranol in 'soft' Lassar's paste (Stanford)

Dithranol	0.5%
Salicylic acid	1.0%
Hard paraffin	5.0%

Plain zinc oxide paste in equal parts of soft paraffin

[a]Cocois® contains sulphur. It is applied to the scalp at night under a swimming cap.
[b]These now include Dithrocream and sticks which are easy to use but not as effective as pastes
Modified from Stankler (1976).

constituents—sulphur, black mud, and bromides—present in different regions. It is effective but no more so than other regimens that provide topical medicaments and mental relaxation. The Dead Sea may be exceptional in the number of its peculiar features such as low humidity, increased atmospheric pressure, filtration of UVB, and minerals in high concentration.

Systemic therapy

ACTH or prednisolone provides short-term control but psoriasis may rebound when it is withdrawn, and the incidence of side-effects, including irreversible vertebral osteoporosis, makes it best avoided if possible. It may be life-saving in generalized erythroderma or pustular psoriasis in the elderly. With good nursing in the absence of heart failure or protein-losing enteropathy, most young people do better to avoid steroids. Methotrexate is the most favoured antimitotic or immunosuppressive agent. Carefully monitored and given intermittently, the serious side-effects of liver fibrosis are slow to develop and may be justified in the older patient. It can be given weekly or fortnightly in intramuscular intravenous form (0.2–0.4 mg/kg). Most oral regimens are also intermittent: 0.2 to 0.4 mg/kg every 1 to 2 weeks taken as tablets with water. Marrow suppression is rarely a problem but fibrosis of the liver is a late complication.

Retinoic acid given orally (0.5 mg/kg daily) is helpful in some more difficult cases and it is the treatment of choice in generalized and pustular psoriasis. It is relatively free of serious side-effects but the effective dose is often a cause of annoying dry mouth, sore lips, and conjunctivitis, as well as skin irritation and erosions, and the high levels of blood lipids induced by the drug are potentially a long-term hazard. It is teratogenic; contraception must be guaranteed for at least 2 years after discontinuing the drug. Hyperostosis is another long-term side-effect.

Cyclosporin is a highly effective treatment of severe psoriasis. The principal side-effects are hypertension and nephrotoxicity. The dose should not exceed 5 mg/kg if these side-effects are to be controlled.

REFERENCES

Camp, R.D.R. (1992). Psoriasis. In *Textbook of Dermatology,* 1391–458. Blackwell Scientific Publications, Oxford. (5th edn), (ed. A. Rook, D.S. Wilkinson, and F.J.G. Ebling), pp.

Heneler, T. and Christophers, E. (1985). Psoriasis of early and late onset: Characterization of two types of psoriasis vulgaris. *Journal of the American Academy of Dermatology* **13,** 450–6.

Kapp, A. (1993). The role of cytokines in the psoriatic inflammation. *Journal of Dermatological Science,* **5,** 133–42.

Kupper, T.S. (1988). The activated keratinocyte: A model for inductive cytokine production by non-bone marrow derived cells in cutaneous inflammatory and immune responses. *Journal of Investigative Dermatology* **94,** 146–50.

Larsen, F.G. (1994). Pharmacokinetics of etretinate and acitretin with special reference to treatment of psoriasis. *Acta Dermato-Venereologica,* Supplement 190, 1–33.

Rosenberg, E.W., Noah, P.W., and Skinner, R.B. (1994). Psoriasis is a visible manifestation of the skin's defense against microorganisms. *Journal of Dermatology* (Japan), **21,** 375–81.

OTHER KERATODERMAS

There are a number of rare scaly disorders of the skin which clinically have a range of patterns lying somewhere between ichthyosis and psoriasis. One of these is pityriasis rubra pilaris; another is ichthyosis hystrix, and others merit the term erythrokeratoderma. The scale is not as silvery or as easily exfoliated as in psoriasis—it is often smaller and more adherent. Most of these disorders are probably inherited, occasionally as a dominant gene but more often as a recessive. Involvement of the face is more characteristic than is the case in psoriasis (Fig. 54). The palms and soles often have a thickened yellow appearance. Nails are less often pitted and quite often show subungual keratosis. A follicular prominence is characterisitc of pityriasis rubra pilaris (Fig. 55); the

extensor surfaces are favoured and so the knees and elbows are often involved, as in psoriasis. Some patterns are present in early childhood, while occasionally it may present for the first time in extreme old age. The latter presentation of pityriasis rubra pilaris is probably acquired through influences other than genetic. The management of these conditions is difficult and, in the case of the erythrokeratodermas, retinoic acid has become the treatment of choice. This is taken by mouth but side-effects of dry mouth and eyes and some soreness of the skin may be sufficiently annoying for the patient to opt for living with his or her disease.

Pityriasis rosea

This not uncommon exanthem is probably due to a virus. The natural history and clustering of cases suggests that it is an infectious disease.

Fig. 54 Pityriasis rubra pilaris, a disorder showing some similarities to psoriasis but differing in its predilection for the face. There is some shrinkage of tissues around the eyes so that ectropion and incomplete closure of the eyelids has developed. This is also a characteristic of the disorder.

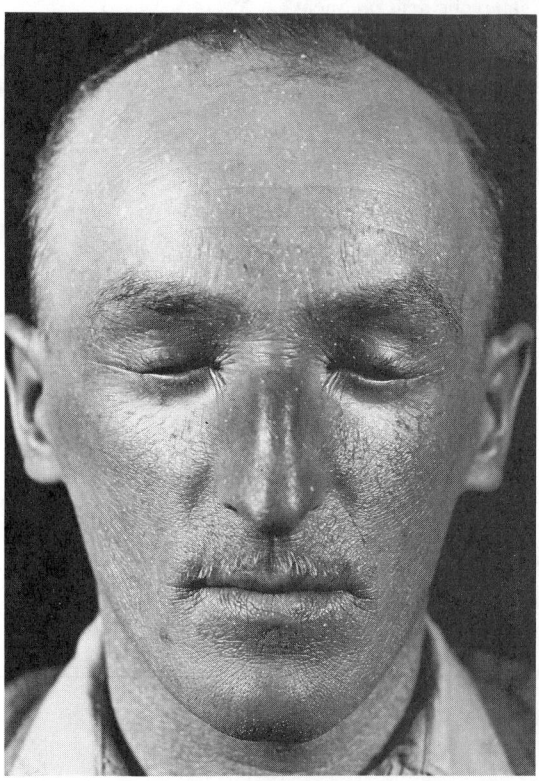

Fig. 55 Pityriasis rubra pilaris is primarily a disorder of the follicular epithelium.

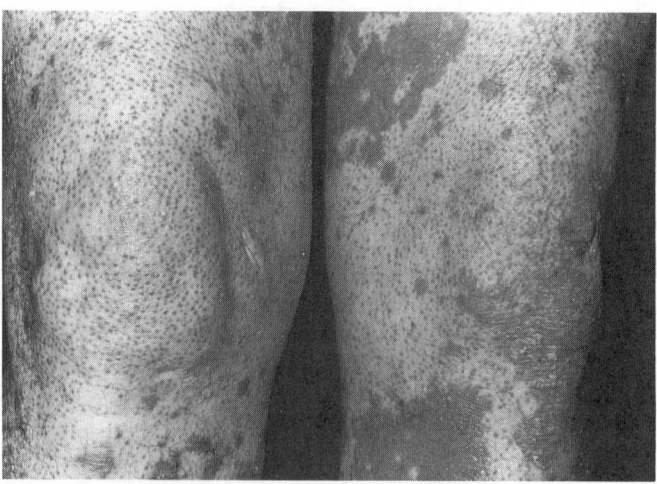

It tends to occur in spring and autumn and in any one individual does not recur. Recurrent or prolonged eruptions of similar nature may be a variant of seborrhoeic eczema. The initial lesion or herald patch is usually on the trunk or proximally on the limbs. It is well-defined, oval, erythematous, and scaly. It precedes the generalized eruption by 3 to 10 days. The rash of pityrisasis rosea is characterized by oval lesions orientated in the line markings of the skin of the trunk. The lesions develop a collarette of scales after 1 week. The rash may spread upwards to the neck and down the arms and legs, usually fading as it reaches below the elbows and knees. It lasts 3 to 6 weeks. Pruritus may be intense. Slight lymphadenopathy and fever rarely accompany the developing rash.

Lichen planus and lichenoid eruptions

Lichen planus and lichenoid eruptions are characterized by violaceous papules which are usually flat-topped and shiny and heal leaving pigmentation. The histology includes damage to the basal layer of the epidermis and an intense infiltration of lymphocytes and a few histiocytes situates immediately below the epidermis (Fig. 56). A T-cell-mediated LD4$^+$ attack on the epidermis may be triggered by viral, drug, or neoplastic processes. Lichen planus thus presents a model for the elimination of damaged and normal keratinocytes. Cytokines, γ-interferon, and tumour necrosis factor β play a critical role. Lymphocytes and keratinocyte molecules subserving adhesion are activated and, in the mouse, lichen planus can be blocked by monoclonal antibodies. The disturbances in the growth of the epidermis that result from this damage range from extreme atrophy with ulceration and almost no epidermal cell turnover to considerable hypertrophy and hyperkersatinization, giving rise to thick nodules meriting the name hypertrophic lichen planus. Most cases are seen between the ages of 30 and 60 and it is extremely rare in children. More erosive forms are seen in the elderly, and pigmented skin tends to develop more hypertrophic varieties.

HLA-A3 and -A5 occur more often in lichen planus than in controls. Graft versus host reactions in the skin that follow bone marrow transplantation often present with an identical pattern of pathology to that of lichen planus. There is some clinical pathological overlap with the appearance seen in lupus erythematosus. Immunofluorescence studies show heavy deposits of fibrin and immunoglobulin but these could be entirely non-specific. There is some evidence of defective carbohydrate metabolism and abnormal glucose tolerance, curves, but the basis of this association still has to be explained. Many drugs produce an identical eruption, i.e. gold and organic arsenicals, antituberculous therapy, chlor-

promazine and related drugs and, more recently, methyldopa and captopril. Lichen planus from contact with colour developers, is well documented, and there is an eczematous form commonly seen on the light-exposed areas, particularly in the Middle East, known as tropical or actinic lichen planus.

CLINICAL FEATURES

The classical lesion is a shiny flat-topped papule (Fig. 57) described as polygonal and violaceous. Small white dots or lines in such papules are due to a mixture of oedema, white cell infiltrate, and disturbance of vasculature. They are termed Wickham striae. The papules may become confluent and heal in the centre, giving rise to annular (Fig. 58) lesions or plaques with varying degrees of epidermal response. This may result in either atrophic skin or extreme hypertrophy. In lesions of mouth or of the glans penis a lacy-white appearance (Fig. 59) is common. Involvement of the hair follicles may give rise to keratosis pilaris and actual destruction of the hair follicle. Thus, lichen planus is one cause of scarring alopecia. Healing of the lesion is often followed by pigmentation due to melanin in the dermis. Warty hyperkeratotic lesions may be very persistent, as may ulceration, particularly of the peripheries or of the mucosa of the mouth. The initial lesions are commonly on the front of the wrists, in the lumbar region, or around the ankles. The palms and soles may be involved, in which case the appearance may even suggest a vesicular eruption. The involvement of the mucosa and tongue, which occurs in anything between 30 and 70 per cent of cases, may extend to the genitalia and perianal area, and it has even been described in the rectum, stomach, and larynx. Severe itching is common. Ridging of the nails is essentially due to cessation of nail growth and produces longitudinal linear depressions.

PROGNOSIS

The mean age of onset is the fifth decade. It may be very explosive or insidious. Most cases clear slowly but two-thirds take up to a year so to

Fig. 57 A black skin affected by the shiny, flat-topped, often polygonal papules of lichen planus.

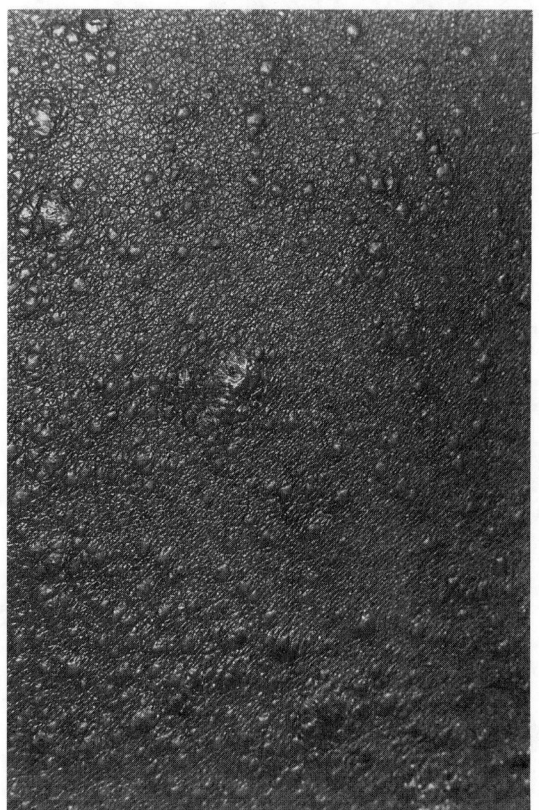

Fig. 56 Lichen planus. There is thickening of the granular layer and necrosis of the basal cell layer. The pale cells at the lower edge of the epidermis are destroyed epidermal cells. The predominant white cell is a lymphocyte. The infiltrate is often confined to the upper dermis.

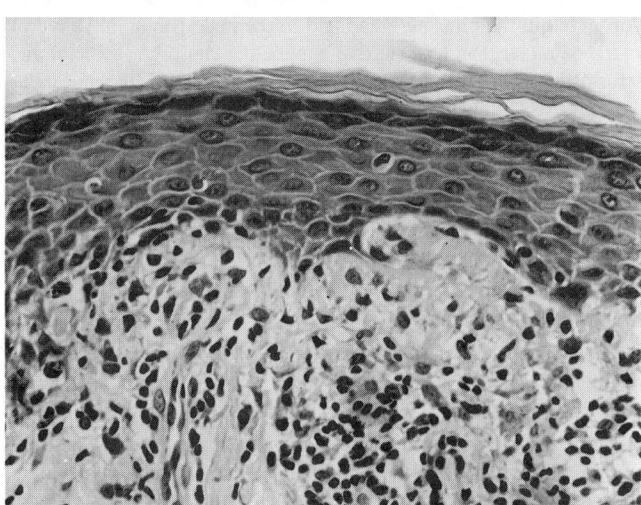

do; 85 per cent of clearance is in 18 months. Mucuous membrane lesions or extremely hypertrophic lesions on the legs often persist for years, and there is risk of squamous epitheliomatous changes, particularly in ulcerated mucosal lesions.

TREATMENT

Treatment is mainly aimed at the relief of the itching, and local steroid creams are perhaps the most effective. Occasionally, for a very severe widespread lichen planus, a course of prednisolone or ACTH is justified. Probably it does not influence the course of the disease but merely its intensity. As with all itching conditions of the skin, cooling evaporating lotions such as calamine lotion may be helpful. Persistent ulcerated lesions can be excised or grafted. In the mouth local steroid creams,

Fig. 58 Lichen planus may heal in the centre, leaving atrophy and pigmentation. The edge is slightly raised; this gives rise to the annular form of the condition.

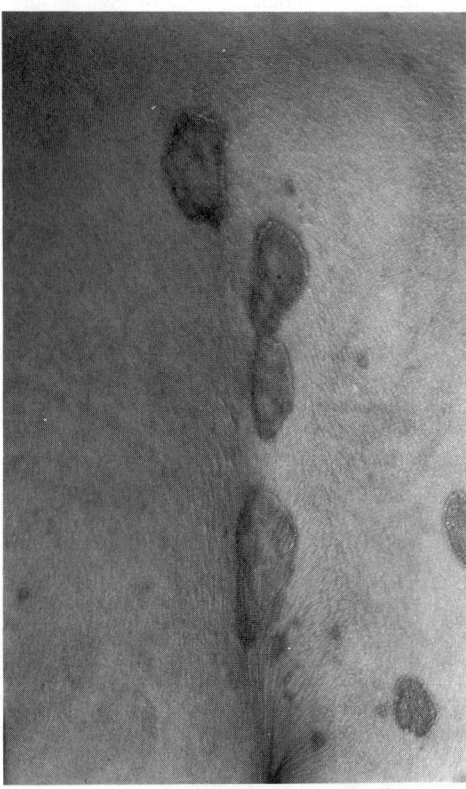

Fig. 59 Lichen planus of the mouth is one cause of mucosal whiteness. Unlike candidiasis the lesions cannot be removed by scraping. They are characteristically 'lacy' in appearance.

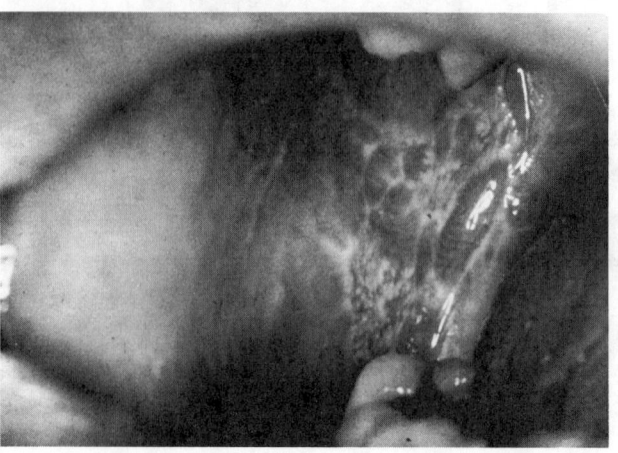

particularly those manufactured for the mouth containing orabase, can be prescribed. A spray such as that used in asthma may be a more convenient way of administering steroid to the mucosa of the mouth, emphasizing that its use is without inhalation.

Acne vulgaris

Acne vulgaris is the most common disease of the skin affecting teenagers and consequently affecting those who are most conscious of their body image.

Acne is a disorder of the pilosebaceous follicles. These are most numerous on the face and upper trunk, hence the distribution of acne.

AETIOLOGY

There are three main processes contributing to acne:

(1) increased sebum excretion;
(2) Pilosebaceous duct obstruction; and
(3) inflammation.

Under the influence of local metabolism of sex hormones, androgens stimulate an increase in the size of the sebaceous glands and hence, more sebum. These large glands themselves produce more androgen metabolites through the activity of 5-α-reductase. One effect of these metabolites is a partnership with resistant bacteria to produce keratinization and hence blockage of the pilosebaceous duct. The organisms responsible are *Propionibacterium acnes*, *Staphylococcus epidermidis*, and *Pityrosporum ovale*. Acne may also be drug-induced, particularly secondary to steroids, iodides, lithium, phenytoin, streptomycin, and isoniazid. Sebum consists of triglycerides, wax esters, squalene, and sterolesters. The fatty acids in sebum are inflammatory and are formed by the lysolytic enzymes of bacteria, even in healthy skin, from unsaturated 14- to 16- or 18-carbon components of the triglycerides. It is possible that acne in the tropics is due to a secondary response in the rate of turnover of the follicular lining, perhaps induced by occlusion under a belt or braces in such a hot environment. The acne of Cushing's disease may also be due to an increased rate of turnover. Chlorinated hydrocarbons also cause acne. Chloracne is an important symptom of poisoning and was present in 168 cases of poisoning in the Seveso disaster. The exact way in which the inflammation is produced is uncertain; the follicle contains fatty acids and bacterial proteases which activate the classical alternative pathway of complement and attract neutrophils.

Sebaceous gland activity is regulated by hormones and, in particular, by androgens from the testes and adrenals, which stimulate, and oestrogens, which seem to suppress activity. In the adult male the glands are normally maximally stimulated and acne is more severe in boys than in girls. The skin itself is a major site for androgenic conversion similar to that observed in the prostate gland and in the male genitalia. Dihydrotestosterone rather than testosterone may be the end-organ effector and it is formed within the target cells where it stimulates lipogenesis as well as mitosis. Eunuchs do not develop acne. Oestrogens reduce the size of sebaceous glands and sebum production is diminished.

There is increasing interest in the role of humoral immunity in the inflammatory process. Circulating immune complexes have been detected in severe acne, as has delayed-type sensitivity and foreign-body-type reactions.

CLINICAL FEATURES

The *closed comedo* is the first stage of acne and appears as tiny white nodules below the surface seen especially when the skin is stretched (see Fig. 7). These may rupture giving rise to irritation of the dermis, i.e. inflamed papules, or form the *open comedo* or blackhead by pushing open the mouth of the follicle (Fig. 60). The black material is melanin; blackheads are blacker in dark skins and white in the albino; the melanin is transferred to the keratinocytes before they are shed into the sebaceous follicle. Acne cysts (Fig. 61) occur as the result of ballooning of the distended follicle, and often the walls of the cyst and hair and sebaceous apparatus are destroyed. Adjacent cysts often form fistulae and sinuses, which rupture, displacing epithelium in the dermis, forming irregular channels or foreign-body reactions.

Atrophic or hypertrophic scars of all types may be seen, and often

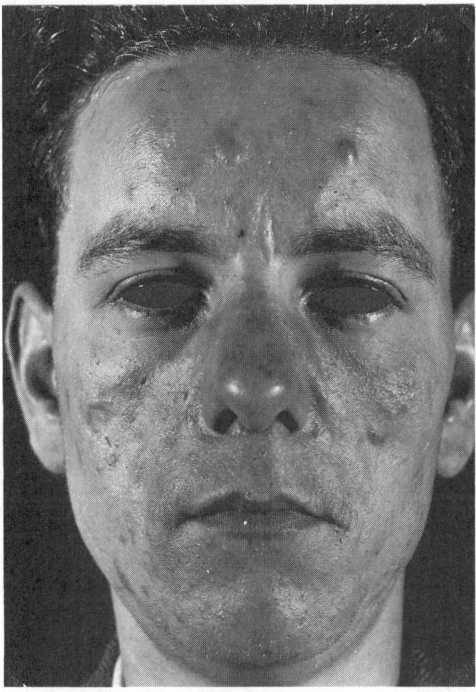

Fig. 60 Greasiness of the skin is a common accompaniment of acne, as is comedo formation, or 'blackheads', as seen on the forehead of this young man. Whether either are wholly responsible for the consequent inflammation and scarring also seen in this photograph is debatable.

Fig. 61 Large cystic lesions are the most disfiguring aspect of acne vulgaris.

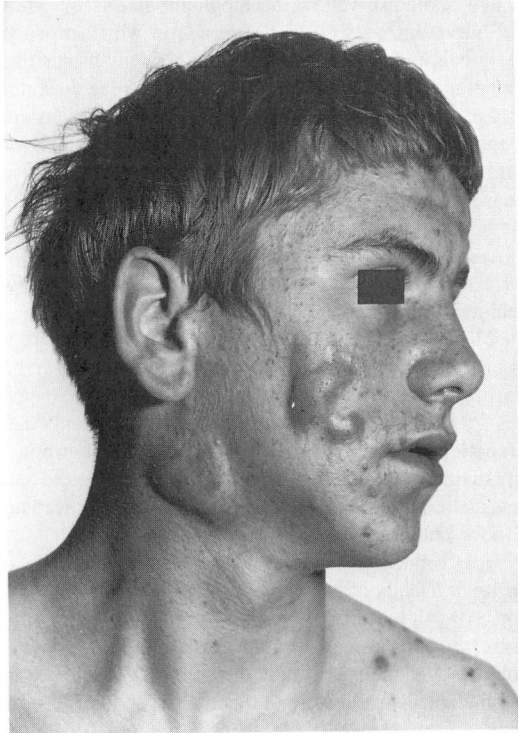

excoriations, picking, and squeezing contribute to the irregularities of pigment and to the epidermal or dermal thickening. Rarely, young males develop suppurative and highly inflamed lesions in the skin over the chest with pain, fever, and accompanying polyarthralgia, probably mediated by immune mechanisms and the activation of complement.

Acne usually presents before the menarche and clears after a few years. A more persistent form—particularly affecting the chin—may be seen in persons up to middle age, especially in women who have premenstrual exacerbations. Most women with adult acne also have the polycystic ovary syndrome.

Neonatal acne is of unknown aetiology; it usually clears within 6 months and is probably due to maternal hormones. Acne is induced by iodides (see Fig. 3(b)) and bromides, steroids, androgens, barbiturates, phenytoin, and phenothiazines.

Cosmetics

In many parts of the world cosmetics contribute to acne and the lesions may be confined to the site of application. Vaseline-type preparations or medicated oil in shampoos in young women with long hair, are a well-known cause.

MANAGEMENT
Local preparations

All local preparations produce some erythema and occasional pustulation before the acne comes under control. Sulphur is a time-honoured agent, producing local irritation and causing peeling. It is helpful for pustules and may not be so good for comedones which precede pustulation, often by several months. Comedones are reduced by retinoic acid and by 10 per cent salicylic acid in ethanol. Sunlight is a popular therapy and it is undoubtedly helpful for some patients. The tanning effect may be a purely cosmetic form of camouflage. However, there is clinical and experimental evidence that in some patients comedones are increased in number after exposure to sunlight.

Long-acting oxidizing antiseptics such as benzoyl peroxide reduce sebum excretion, reduce comedo production, and inhibit *P. acnes in vitro.* They are the topical treatment of choice, are a mild irritant, and produce peeling after several days' application. It is best to start sparingly with 5 per cent and later to increase the amount applied or the concentration to 10 per cent.

Retinoic acid helps the lining cells of the follicle to slough off without plugging the follicle. It is applied in a cream or a lotion or gel, and is indicated for comedones rather than for pustules or cysts. It is irritant and causes redness and peeling. Its effect is not unlike sunburn and should not be used when there is undue sun exposure, either in the summer bather or the winter skier.

Oral therapy

Oral tetracycline is the mainstay of treatment of acne if simple measures have not resulted in clearance. Erythromycin and clindomycin (now usually prescribed as a lotion) are also effective but tetracycline is exceptionally safe. The only side-effect is the discoloration of teeth in the fetus and in children. Anorexia nausea, colic, or vaginal candidiasis are rare. Provided they are taken on an empty stomach, one or two tetracycline tablets taken daily control acne. Rarely Gram-negative folliculitis occurs, particularly around the nose or in persistent cysts. This results in sudden worsening with considerable inflammation and may warrant a course of ampicillin. Severe inflammatory and cystic acne respond to a zinc sulphate citrate complex taken with meals. Acute severe inflammatory disease also responds to prednisolone.

Diet

Studies of the effects of starvation in the obese or the malnourished show little evidence of the effect of diet on acne vulgaris and this is so even in pellagra in which some plugging of the follicles around the nose is an early sign. There may be the individual in whom acne is made worse by chocolate but this has not been shown in trials of larger populations. Nutrition may influence the age of onset of puberty and hence overeating may result in earlier acne.

Acne surgery

Comedo extraction is the expression of a follicle's contents by the application of pressure on the surface often with a special device called a comedo extractor. The benefits of active attack on the lesions counteracting stasis and build up of the contents has to be weighed against the fact that suppression is always incomplete and a tendency to rupture into the dermis may promote inflammation. Cryotherapy destroys the lining of large cysts. Deep sinuses may require externalization. Solitary inflamed lesions benefit from intralesional inoculation of steroids. Persistent acne cysts sometimes resolve with the injection of small amounts of intralesional triamcinolone.

Oestrogen

Oestrogens have to be given in excessive amounts (50 μg or more of ethinyl oestradiol per day in women or 50 mg/day in the male) to have an effect in acne and are now used principally in the most physiological form of therapy, the contraceptive pill.

Acne is made worse by 19-nor-testosterone derivatives in the pill. Cyproterone 17 × acetate up to 100 mg for the first 10 days of the cycle plus ethinyl oestradiol 50 μg for 21 days, is used to block the receptor sites for dihydrotestosterone. This antiandrogen effect works only if the drug is given systemically and no topical preparation has so far found to be of help. Small doses of prednisolone suppress androgen activity.

13-cis-retinoic acid up to 1 mg/kg is the most effective treatment of acne. As a consequence, acne is a problem that is completely controllable. However, vitamin A-type toxicity is usual, including dryness and peeling of the lips and conjunctivae; raised blood lipids, muscle aches, and pains may also occur. The most serious problem is teratogenicity. The drug is incompletely metabolized and can be damaging to the fetus for many months after discontinuing its intake.

Within 3 to 6 months the pilosebaceous gland is much reduced. The side-effects are annoying but it is a safe drug in the short term. Contraception is essential for female patients. The Diane® contraceptive pill, which contains 50 μg ethinyl oestradiol with only 2 mg cyproterone acetate, is partially effective if taken for many months. In resistant cases additional cyproterone acetate taken on days 5 to 14 of the menstrual cycle will improve the effectiveness. Combinations with oxytetracycline show advantages but contraception is less secure. In pregnancy acne can occasionally be severe. The treatment of choice is erythromycin.

REFERENCES

Crow, K.D. (1981). Chloracne and its potential clinical implications. *Clinical and Experimental Dermatology* 6, 243–57.

Cunliffe, W.J. (1989). *Acne*. Dunitz, London.

Darley, M.B. (1984). Recent advances in hormonal aspects of acne vulgaris. *International Journal of Dermatology* 23, 539–41.

Dicken, C.H. (1984). Retinoids: a review. *Journal of the American Academy of Dermatology* 10, 541–51.

Ebling, F.J.G. and Cunliffe, W.J. (1992). Disorders of the sebaceous glands. In *Textbook of Dermatology*, (5th edn), (ed. A. Rook, D.S. Wilkinson, and F.J.G. Ebling), pp. 1699–744. Blackwell Scientific Publications, Oxford.

Journal of Investigative Dermatology (1979). Acne. *Journal of Investigative Dermatology* 73, 434–42.

Rothman, K. and Pochi, P. (1988). Use of oral and topical agents for acne in pregnancy. *Journal of the American Academy of Dermatology* 19, 431–2.

Pigmentation

The most immediately recognizable differences between two persons are often related to skin colour. The social consequences of colour

Table 19 *Localized causes of pigmentation. Light exposed—especially on the face and usually due to increased numbers of normal melanocytes in the epidermis*

Actinic or senile lentigo A common grey/brown macule especially of the face and limbs in middle-aged or older persons, usually due to sun exposure in youth. It is without epidermal changes. Spreading pigmented actinic keratoses show slight verrucous changes and can merge into a squamous cell carcinoma or into a lentigo maligna.

Berloque dermatitis Brown often streaky macules often initially inflammatory with redness, blistering, or scaling at sites exposed to perfumes and sunlight. Several plants may be responsible. The streaky pigmentation may persist for years (Fig. 62).

Freckle-ephelis Small brown macules usually numerous in light-exposed skin of genetically fair, blonde, or red-haired and blue-eyed types.

Lentigo maligna Usually a well-defined irregular brown to black mottled macular lesion especially occurring on the face in old persons. The melanocytes are dysplastic, vacuolated in the epidermis and malignant change is common (see Fig. 29).

Melasma or chloasma Usually brown symmetrical macules of the butterfly area of the face or crossbow pattern on the forehead. It is common in pregnancy or in those on the oral contraceptives containing oestrogen (see Fig. 64).

Xeroderma pigmentosum The patchy macular pigmentation is associated with keratoses, telangiectasia, and malignancies. Basal cell and squamous cell carcinomas and even melanoma are common. Intolerance to the sun results in excessive sunburn often 72 h after exposure. The disorder begins in early childhood, often as a bright erythema and swelling following exposure to the sun. The aetiology is genetic and concerns repair of a defect in DNA, following injury by light (see Fig. 32).

De Sanctis–Cacchioni syndrome Xeroderma pigmentosum, mental deficiency, dwarfism, and neurological disorders.

extend beyond political implications and may be important in health. The principal pigments in the skin include melanin, which is black, phaeomelanin, which is reddish-yellow, haemoglobin and its by-products bilirubin and biliverdin, as well as haemosiderin which produce colours of yellow, green, red, and brown. Longer wavelengths such as red penetrate deeper and are absorbed by melanin. Since blue does not penetrate so deeply it is not absorbed and is reflected back and therefore dermal pigment appears blue—hence blue naevus. All discussions of this subject should begin with racial causes of pigmentation because they are so common, but physical causes are important also, since in the white skin visible tanning may occur in the sun. It is known as immediate darkening when it occurs within minutes of the skin being exposed to sunlight. Over a number of days increased pigment production is associated with epidermal thickening and retention of pigment.

Some pigmented lesions are naevi (Tables 19–21), others result from 'incontinence' of pigment which increases the amount of pigment in the dermal macrophages and is commonly post-inflammatory.

Pigmentation as a feature of systemic illness is most significantly due to endocrine dysfunction affecting the melanocyte stimulating hormone. In countries where malnutrition and infections are common, protein and vitamin deficiency, as well as cachexia from a variety of causes, account for disturbances in the colour of the skin.

'Tinea' or pityriasis versicolor is due to a superficial fungus known as *Malassezia furfur*. It usually affects the upper trunk and may spread on to the neck or on to the arms. The lesions are slightly scaly, off-white, pink, and brown. Pityriasis is the term for a bran-like powdery scale and versicolor implies the variation in the colouring (Fig. 67).

In leprosy, hypomelanosis is a feature of tuberculoid and border-line

Table 20 *Pigmentation more commonly on the trunk*

Acanthosis nigricans   Pigmentation affects the axillae, groins, and there is a velvety thickening of the skin with skin tags. The condition may be benign when associated with obesity and in the young, but in older persons with oral, facial, or hand pigmentation and thickening, it is more often due to an underlying adenocarcinoma. Pruritus may be associated and indicates underlying carcinoma (see Fig. 127).

Becker's naevus   Large, lightly pigmented, and often hairy macular pigmentation affecting a segment of the trunk such as the shoulder or one flank. It is often noticed after puberty for the first time. It is entirely benign (Fig. 63).

Dermatosis papulosa nigra   This is the commonest dark lesion in the Negro and is a papular variety of seborrhoeic warts producing discrete but multiple dark lesions of the face and neck.

Tinea nigra   A localized asymptomatic fungus infection causing a brown or black macular lesion on the palm; sometimes when there is no scaling it may be taken for a lentigo.

Erythrasma   This is due to a corynebacterial infection of the groins, axillae, and in between the toes. On white skin it is light brown, but in dark skin it may produce a lighter or darker hue. Wood's light shows the coral red fluorescence.

Tinea versicolor   This is a flat to slightly elevated scaly papule or reticulate plaque producing either a brownish coloration or depigmentation. It affects the upper trunk and upper limbs and neck (Fig. 67).

Urticaria pigmentosum   These are pigmented lesions due to nests of mast cells in the skin. In children they may be quite large, palpable lesions about the size of a thumb or they may be lentil-sized and numerous. Occasionally, though, there is a diffuse and velvety texture to the skin. The diagnostic feature of the lesion is the wealing that results from scratching.

Café au lait   These lesions resemble large freckles. They are often as large as the thumb or palm. They tend to be oval in shape. There is a variant known as naevus spilus which is speckled with much darker spots. In neurofibromatosis there are usually at least five *café au lait* spots and generalized freckling extends into the axillae (Fig. 65). Very large pigmented macules being unilateral and having serrated edges are characteristic of Albright's syndrome.

Leopard syndrome   Progressive darkening and very numerous lentigos of the trunk and limbs (Fig. 66) is associated with the following denoted by the letters of the word 'Leopard'. Lentigenoses, ECG abnormalities, ocular defects, pulmonary stenosis, abnormalities of genitalia, retardation of growth, deafness.

Peutz–Jeghers syndrome   This consists of polyposis of the small intestine and is associated with numerous small pigmented macules affecting the perioral buccal areas extending quite far beyond the margins of the lips and affecting also the dorsum of the fingers. Note: lentigos of the lips and post-inflammatory pigmentation are in themselves quite common and need not be associated with any internal disorder.

Laugier–Hunziker syndrome   An acquired hyperpigmentation of the lips, oral mucosa, nail bed, fingertips, and genital mucosa, usually sporadic, can be familial.

Table 21 *Disorders of increased pigmentation*

Circumscribed brown[a] hyperpigmentation
  Infection: tinea versicolor: erythrasma
  Café au lait type: Albright's syndrome: neurofibromatosis
  Lentigo type: Leopard syndrome: Peutz–Jeghers syndrome
  Melasma type (chloasma): pregnancy; drugs; idiopathic
  Miscellaneous: acanthosis nigricans; post-inflammatory; stasis; Becker's naevus; fixed drug eruption; urticaria pigmentosa; Minocin-induced (often black)
Generalized brown[a] hyperpigmentation
  Reticulate: naevoid; poikiloderma; dyskeratosis congenita
  Metabolic: haemochromatosis; porphyria; chronic liver disease
  Endocrine and/or autoimmune: Addison's disease: pregnancy; pernicious anaemia; myxoedema; thyrotoxicosis; Felty's syndrome; ACTH and MSH secreting tumour; scleroderma
  Nutritional: malnutrition; malabsorption
  Drugs: antimalarials, tetracyclines, heavy metals, cancer therapeutic agents, phenothiazines, clofazimine (usually reddish-brown), amiodarone, tricyclic antidepressants
  Other types: post-inflammatory; Whipple's disease; catatonic schizophrenia; Schilder's disease
Generalized slate-grey[b] hyperpigmentation
  Haemochromatosis
  Nutritional deficiency
  Drugs: chlorpromazine; Minocin®; gold; silver

[a]Brown: increased melanin in epidermal cells.

[b]Grey, slate or blue: increased melanin in dermis.

Pigmentation by melanin requires the formation of precursor granules known as melanosomes, their melanization, their secretion into keratinocytes, and their transport and often their degradation by the keratinocytes.

DEPIGMENTATION

Leucoderma is a term used for any whiteness of skin, and ranges from a mild hypopigmentation to complete loss of pigment such as characterizes vitiligo. Microbial diseases such as pityriasis versicolor (Fig. 67), leprosy (Fig. 68), and syphilis are important infectious causes of depigmentation. Pinta should be suspected in persons from central or southern America showing a succession of erythematous hyperpigmented lesions progressing to warty or atrophic plaques of depigmented skin. The late stage resembles vitiligo. Naevus anaemicus is a hypovascularity of the skin observed in white skins (Fig. 69). It is not a disorder of melaninization.

Vitiligo

This is a common autoimmune skin disease. The primary defect has not been identified to be necessarily in the melanocyte. Some investigators have observed defective calcium uptake in vitiligo keratinocytes. It is postulated that consequent cell death encourages autoantibodies. The melanocytes are destroyed and the affected skin is totally depigmented. In many parts of the world where skins are deeply pigmented, it is a principal cause of attendances at a dermatology department. It affects up to 1 per cent of the United Kingdom population but 8.8 per cent in India. It presents during the first decade in 25 per cent of those affected. Except in those persons unable to protect themselves from bright sunlight the disability is purely cosmetic, but causes more concern and social handicap than almost any other common disease. However, an association with other autoimmune diseases and a family history of such is found in one-third of cases. The cause is unknown and the melanocyte seems to be damaged by some as yet unidentified antibody or toxin.

tuberculoid types (Fig. 68). Light touch and later pinprick sensation are impaired. There is often lack of sweating and there may be loss of hair. An adjacent enlarged peripheral nerve may be palpable; and this may be mistaken for an enlarged lymph node.

  Pigmentation of the buccal mucosa tongue or fingernails is significant only in white skin since it is a normal finding in dark races.

Fig. 62 Pigmentation due to cosmetic agents. Often initially a dermatitis, it is especially induced by exposure to ultraviolet rays. It tends to have the streaky distribution of application. (a) Neck from eau de cologne; (b) lips from lanolin; (c) also from eau de cologne and sun bathing, the bizarre pattern is characteristic of an exogenous cause.

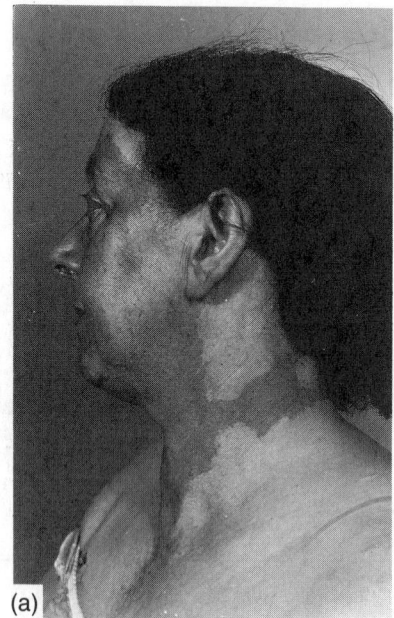

(a)

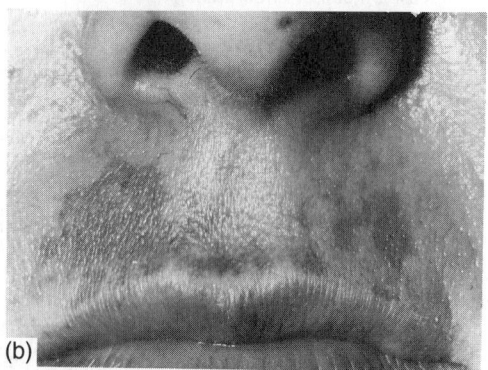

(b)

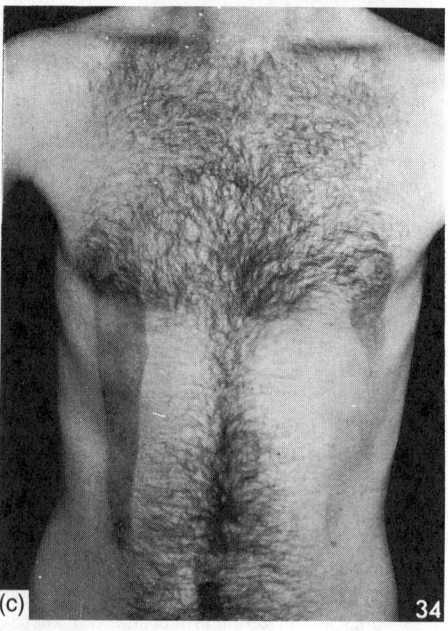

(c)   34

There is a 20 to 30 per cent incidence of vitiligo in those who develop melanoma.

Clinical features

The initial depigmentation is often at sites of trauma, particularly of the knuckles of the hands and sometimes around a naevus (Figs. 70 and 71). The face and neck are usually affected early. In white-skinned persons the first complaint is often in the summer when the unaffected skin is at its darkest from sun exposure. There is usually marked symmetry; the axillary folds and genitalia are commonly affected; the eye is not involved. The depigmentation of the lesion is ultimately total (Fig. 72) and should cause no confusion with the hypopigmentation of diseases such as leprosy. Only in the earlier stages of vitiligo is there hypopig-

Fig. 63 Becker's naevus is due to melanin in the dermis and it is often segmental and usually hairy. It may become overt only after childhood.

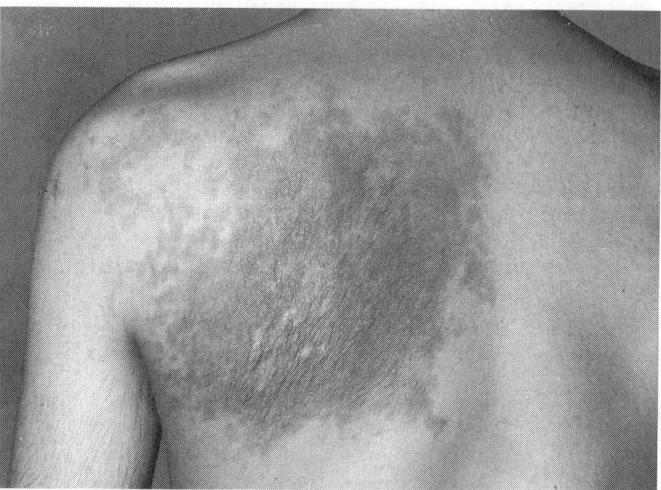

Fig. 64 Crossbow pattern of chloasma in encephalitis, an association that has been described but may be incidental.

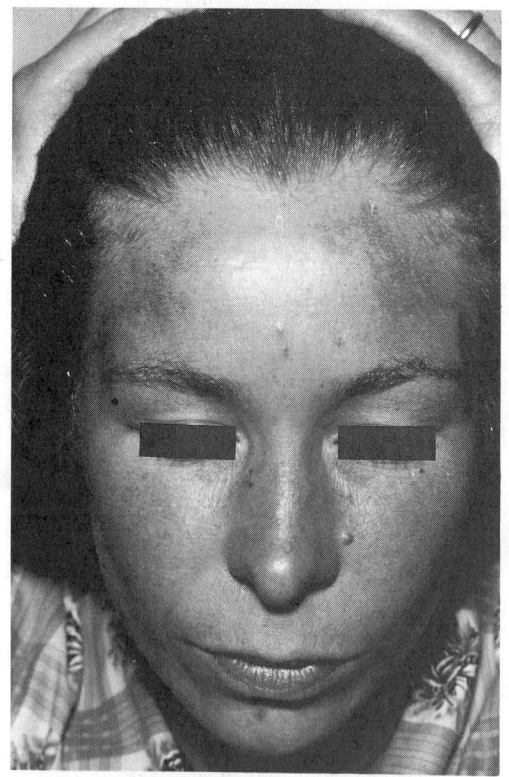

mentation but such areas are never anaesthetic as in leprosy. Pigment may accumulate and be well defined at the borders of the lesion, giving a hyperpigmented edge. Melanocytes of hair follicles are usually unaffected and repigmentation, when it occurs, is often from such sites (Fig. 73).

The clinician should be aware of the likely association of diabetes mellitus, pernicious anaemia, Addison's disease, myxoedema, or thyrotoxicosis. Less than one-third of patients show spontaneous repigmentation. In most the loss of pigment gradually extends. Depigmentation of the vulva, penis, and neck is sometimes persistent and of a localized variety, and need not necessarily progress to generalized vitiligo and should be distinguished from the more atrophic lichen sclerosis of those sites.

Fig. 65 In neurofibromatosis freckles extend into the axilla. This is a diagnostic feature in incomplete penetrance, important in genetic counselling of white-skinned, but less reliable in black-skinned, patients.

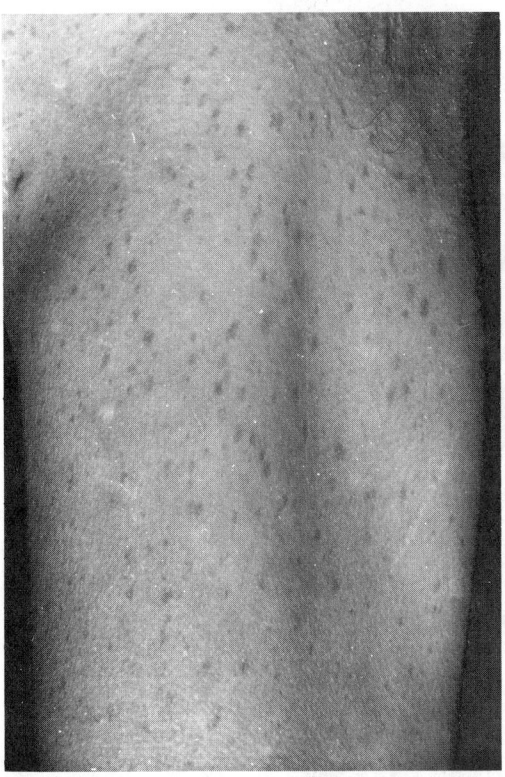

Fig. 66 Syndrome of progessive darkening of numerous lentigos associated with cardiovascular and neurological abnormalities.

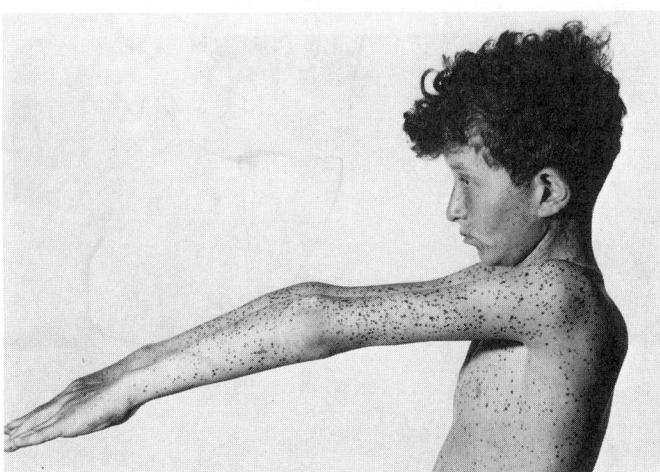

Management

Patients are usually much distressed by the cosmetic disability. It is helpful to explain that there is a 30 per cent chance of spontaneous cure. Offering advice on camouflage with matching of the skin using appropriate mixes gives the patients an opportunity to help themselves, especially on important social occasions. But such camouflage is tedious and difficult to apply effectively for everyday use. There is no special advantage in the purchase of more expensive cosmetics since the basic constituents are cheap. The best effect is achieved from powder and grease mixtures with a powder finish patted gently into the skin after application. Dihydroxyacetone is the basis of many suntan lotions, but again it is difficult to apply satisfactorily without overpigmenting the adjacent unaffected skin.

Patients should be told to avoid occupations which injure the skin, such as playing with animals which scratch. For those whose skin is almost completely depigmented the cosmetic effect of removing the

Fig. 67 Pityriasis versicolor due to the organism *Malassezia furfur* causes redness and slight brownish coloration of very pale, white skin. In dark or sallow skin it causes depigmentation. It favours the upper trunk.

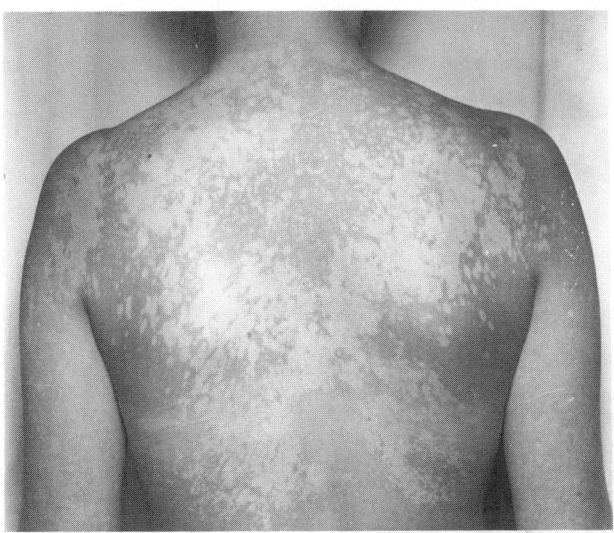

Fig. 68 Hypopigmentation, especially with a hyperpigmented border, should always be tested for loss of sensation. This lesion is typical of tuberculoid leprosy.

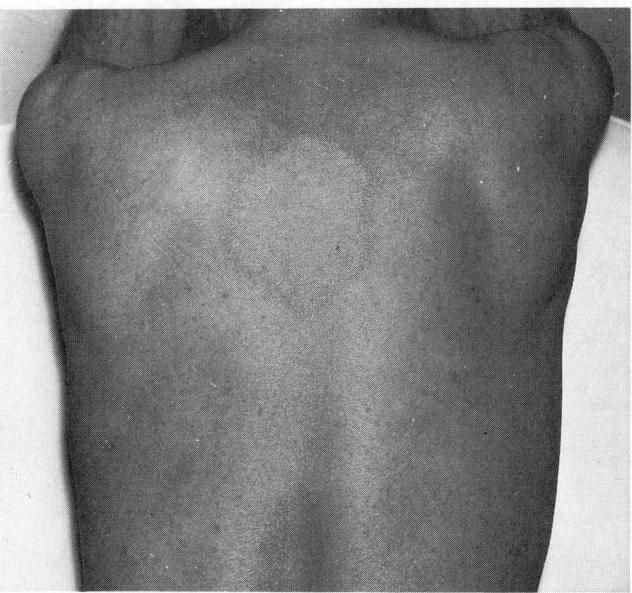

Fig. 69 Not all whiteness is due to loss of pigment. In this case of naevus anaemicus there is decreased vasculature present since birth.

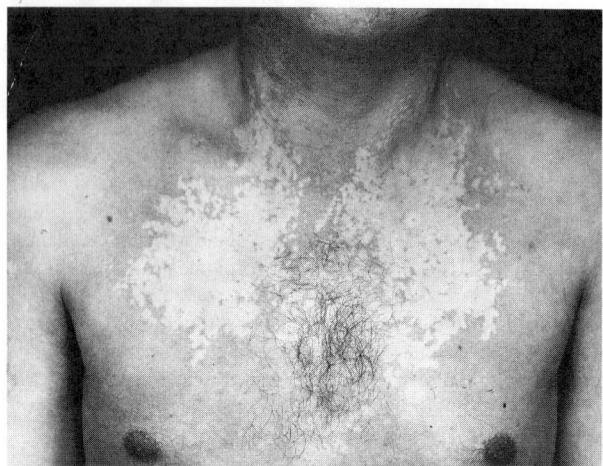

Fig. 70 Vitiligo is complete depigmentation and not merely hypopigmentation; it often begins at sites of minor trauma such as the knuckles. As with all essentially endogenous disorders it is symmetrical.

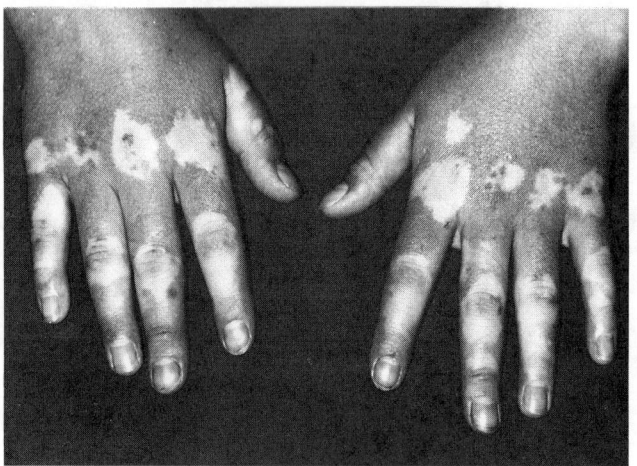

Fig. 71 Vitiligo often begins around a pigmented naevus—a halo naevus.

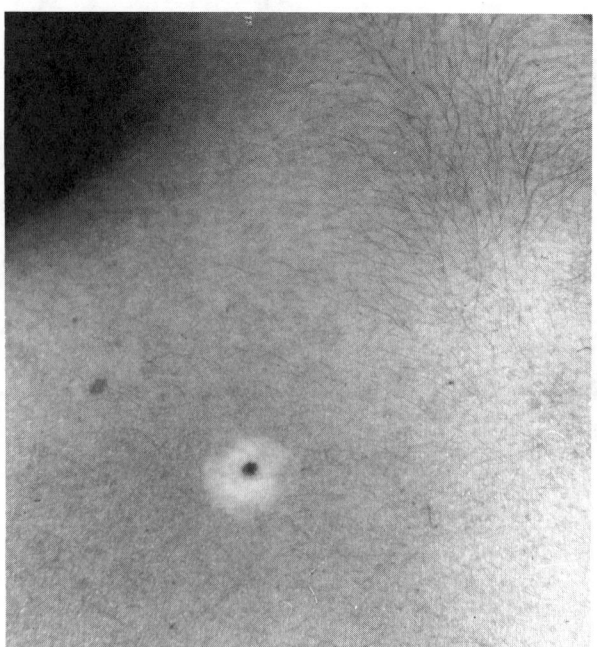

remaining pigment is sometimes preferred. The formulation prepared by Sheffield Royal Infirmary includes the following: hydroquinone 30 g; hydrocortisone BP 6 g; retinoic acid 600 mg; butylated hydroxytoluene 300 mg; and methylated spirit and polyethylene glycol in equal parts to 600 ml.

Psoralens and sunlight are one of the most ancient remedies in medicine and use of UVA (black light) is a recently developed extension of the older remedy. Psoralens, methoxy- or tri-psoralen, are taken by mouth 2 hours before exposure to light or may be applied topically 30 minutes before exposure. The simplest regimen is a combination of meladinin paint and sunlight. It is necessary to test reactivity with short-time exposure and always to expose the skin at the same time of the day in order not to burn the skin by unexpectedly high intensity of UVA. The chances of remission are not much greater than those from natural responses and treatment successes may take 2 to 3 years to accomplish. As might be expected from an autoimmune disorder, local steroid prep-

Fig. 72 (a) The pigment loss in this once dark-skinned woman is almost complete. Satisfactory cosmetic management would be depigmentation of the few residual areas of normal skin. (b) Repigmentation of the skin in vitiligo is usually from the follicles. It is slow, unpredictable, and incomplete.

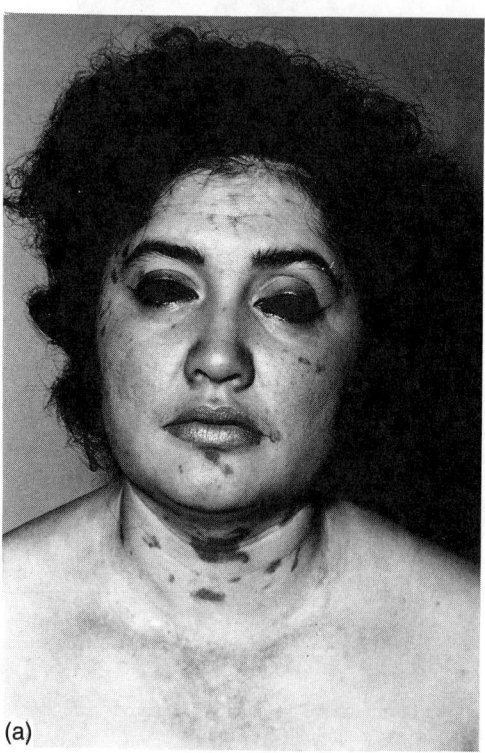

(a)

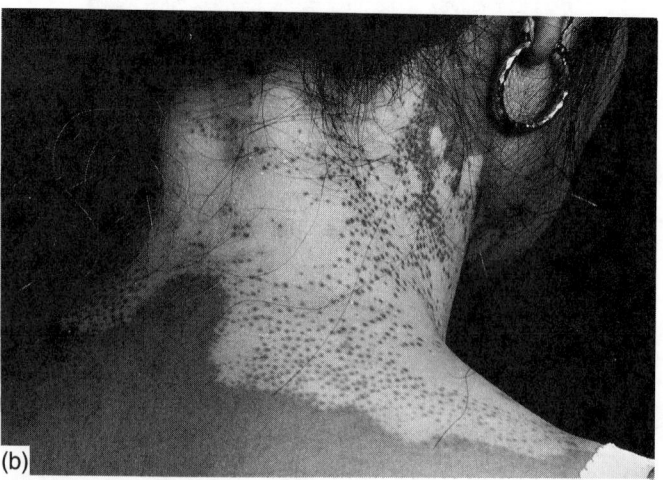

(b)

arations are sometimes helpful. They have been advocated in combination with psoralens but therapeutic triumphs are difficult to assess, and the requirement to use these agents for years rather than days makes side-effects very likely. Local steroids are sometimes used to stabilize a rapidly progressive early stage of the disease. Some Indian practitioners treat cosmetically disabling local patches with light dermabrasion and the application of autologous skin cells from pigmented skin. In that country it is a severe handicap and the writings of Indian practitioners are full of uncontrolled therapies which nevertheless give greater patient satisfaction than that achieved by United Kingdom practitioners who can offer very little for this important disease.

Other forms of depigmentation (postinflammatory)
Chemical depigmentation
A complete loss of melanocytes is a well-recognized effect of certain chemicals—monobenzyl ether of hydroquinone and butyl phenol. The hands are usually first involved and the rubber industry is the commonest source of this problem.

Albinism
This is a group of at least six genetically distinct syndromes determined not by absence of melanocytes but by their inability to synthesize melanin. Since melanin is important not only in the skin but also at such sites as the cochlea and retina, and since also the capacity to transfer organelles other than melanin is sometimes impaired, there are a number of associated defects affecting vision, hearing, and the delivery of lysosomes. In some societies where inbreeding is usual, albinism is common, i.e. San Blas Islands, Tanzania, southern Nigeria. Albinos in many countries are outcast, poor, underfed, and often die from skin cancer.

Complete albinism—autosomal recessive tyrosinase deficiency
Although the melanocytes are in normal numbers, because of a deficiency of tyrosinase no melanin is formed. The hair is white, including the eyebrows and eyelashes, and the iris is pink. There is photophobia, nystagmus, and impaired visual acuity. The principal disadvantage is severe sun damage to the skin so that premature ageing and squamous cell carcinomas are common, especially in summer or if social circumstances require a rural outdoor life. The gene for tyrosinase is mapped at the long arm of chromosome 11q 14–21. A type one variant is cold sensitive and accounts for depigmentation of hair on cold-exposed sites.

Partial albinism—autosomal recessive melanosomal deficiency
Tyrosinase is present in the melanocytes but transfer of melanin to the keratinocytes is defective. The skin is not usually as pale as the complete form and the hair is yellow. Pigment is preserved in some freckles on sun-exposed skin. The eyes are blue but photophobia and nystagmus are usual.

Fig. 73 Pityriasis alba caused by a mild dry eczema. Slightly scaly areas of depigmentation are a common cause of discoloration.

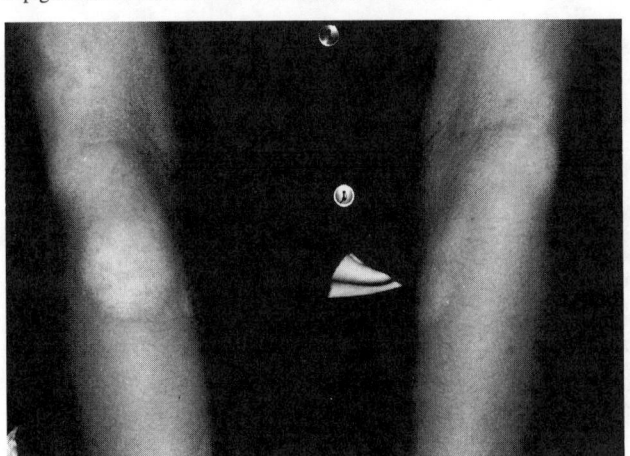

Partial albinism yellow–red mutant variety
This is prevalent in the Amish communities in the United States. Phaeomelanin, the pigment of redhead individuals, requires cystine as well as tyrosine.

Phenylketonuria
This is a cause of whiteness that should not be forgotten, and it results in elevated levels of phenylalanine which competes for tyrosinase.

Cross syndrome
This is an autosomal recessive defect of melanosome formation associated with gingival fibrosis and various maldevelopments of the CNS and eye. Hermansky–Pudlak albinism is associated with an abnormality of platelets which gives rise to bleeding, especially after aspirin.

Chediak–Higashi syndrome
This is an autosomal recessive disorder that gives rise to partial albinism and failure of formation of membrane-bound organelles affecting the melanocytes and the white blood cells, the liver, and the brain cells. It is the human equivalent of Aleutian mink disease. The hair is yellow, and photophobia, nystagmus, and eye translucency are not severe. Affected cells produce giant melanosomes and giant lysosomes. The white cell defect predisposes to severe infection, causing death in children. Hepatomegaly and lymphadenopathy frequently progress to lymphoma.

Piebaldism
This is autosomal dominant absence of melanocytes. It results from a defect in the C-kit proto-oncogene coding for a kinase directing migration. It is present at birth and may be difficult to recognize in fair-skinned individuals. The hands and feet and centre of the back show normal pigmentation. The hair is normal except for a white forelock. The rest of the body shows loss of pigment with no melanocytes. There are islands of residual pigmentation. The condition is inherited as an autosomal dominant and the offspring should be examined at birth with Wood's light.

Waardenburg's syndrome
This is an autosomal dominant disorder in which there is a defect of pigment affecting the cochlea. Deafness is associated with a white forelock as well as bilateral displacement of the medial canthi and fusion of the eyebrows, or at least an unusual facial hair distribution. There is a linkage between pigment, ganglion cells, and cartilage migration.

Tielz's syndrome
This is an autosomal dominant deaf mutism with hypoplasia of the eyebrows and absence of pigmentation.

Vogt–Koyanagi–Harada syndrome
This is a vitiligo including white eyelashes and is associated with bilateral uveitis, alopecia areata, tinnitus, and altered host response to viral meningitis.

Halo naevi
These are characterized by loss of pigment around benign (see Fig. 71) or very rarely malignant melanocytic naevi. It is a common first sign of vitiligo. Antibodies against the cytoplasm of malignant melanoma cells are found in the serum of patients with halo naevi. The naevus need only be removed if there is a progressive enlargement, bleeding, and irregularities of the pigment within the centre of the naevus.

Tuberous sclerosis
The oval macules, which look like a thumb print and are tapered at one end, sometimes known as leaf-like (Fig. 74), are present in about 90 per cent of affected babies. They are easier to see using Wood's light (UVA).

Idiopathic guttate hypomelanosis

This is characterized by small depigmented, sharply defined, often polygonal macules in light-exposed areas. Asymmetrical punctate loss of pigment on the shins and extensor surfaces of the arms is described in young adults from Japan and Brazil.

Post-inflammatory depigmentation

This is probably the commonest cause of leucoderma. Pigmented skin retains less pigment when there is accelerated epidermal turnover as in wound repair, eczema, or psoriasis. The lesions are not as white as in vitiligo and they are sometimes known as *pityriasis alba* (Fig. 73). This is in fact a variant of a dry eczema and causes mild hypopigmentation. It may be sharply circumscribed and have a halo of surrounding inflammation. It is usually slightly scaly and there is follicular prominence due to hyperkeratosis. The cheeks and upper arms are most commonly affected and atopic children are the most frequent sufferers.

In some parts of the world discoid lupus erythematosus is a common cause of depigmentation. It is preceded by the itching, deep violet erythema of light-exposed skin. Hair loss of the scalp is common. This is usually of scarring type.

REFERENCES

Behl, P.N. (1994). *Asian Clinics in Dermatology,* Vol. 1, No. 1. Vitiligo Update. The Skin Institute, Greater Kailash, New Delhi.

Bleehan, S.S., Ebling, F.J.G., and Champion R.H. (1992). Disorders of skin colour. In *Textbook of dermatology,* (5th edn), (ed. A. Rook, D.S. Wilkinson, and F.J.G. Ebling, pp. 1561–622. Blackwell Scientific Publications, Oxford.

Bloch, C.A. (1984). Café au lait spots in colored and Indian children. *South African Medical Journal* **65**, 651–2.

Braverman, I.M. (1970). *Skin signs of systemic disease,* ch. 14. W.B. Saunders, Philadelphia.

Fulk, C.S. (1984). Primary disorders of hyperpigmentation. *Journal of the American Academy of Dermatology* **10**, 1–16.

Nordlund, J.J. (1994). The pigmentary system: an expanded perspective. *Annals of Dermatology (Korea),* **6**, 109–23.

Nordlund, J.J., Halder, R.M., and Grimes, P.E. (1993). Management of vitiligo. *Dermatology Clinics,* **11**, 27–34.

Fig. 74 Typical oval or 'leaf-like' hypopigmented lesions of tuberous sclerosis. They are present at birth.

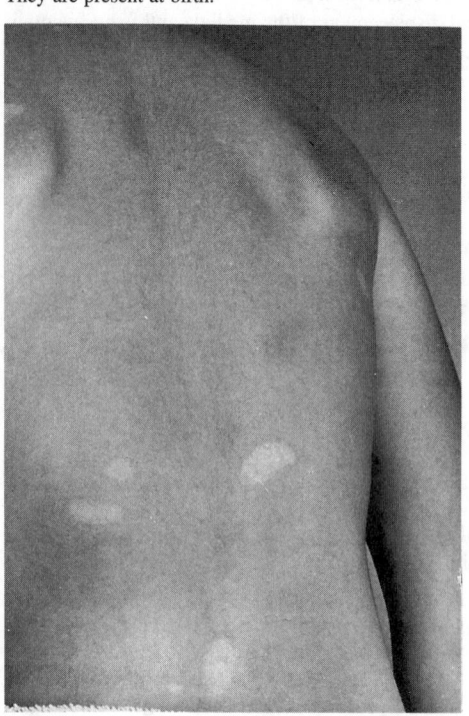

Wasserman, H.P. (1974). *Ethnic pigmentation.* Excerpta Medica, Amsterdam.

Diseases of nails, hair, and sweat glands

Nails and hair adorn. In addition, nails aid the picking up of small objects. The handicap of disease of hair or nails is greatest in those who are most conscious of their contribution to the 'body beautiful'. Beauty is not only in the eyes of the beholder but it is also an image in the mind of the subconscious. Hence most consultations concerning hair are about too much or too little in comparison to the norm for a particular population. Excessive sweating and body odour is also a cause of great distress.

Nails

Nails grow continuously throughout life. Normal fingernails grow at the rate of approximately 1 cm in 3 months and toenails take anything from 9 to 24 months to grow as much. The nails grow more rapidly in psoriasis and more slowly in cold, ischaemia, or severe systemic illness.

Koilonychia is a term for a spoon-shaped depression of the nail plate, sometimes brittle, found in iron deficiency or in overusage of solvents such as nail varnish remover or detergents. It is also a consequence of repetitive trauma such as vibration, or in the case of toenails, from kicking or walking up a hill pushing a trolley, known as rickshaw boy's nail.

Onycholysis is due to premature separation of the nail plate as seen in psoriasis, infection, thyroid disease, and UVA exposure. Trauma from excessive handwashing or keratolytics are other causes.

Clubbing is an increased angle between the nail fold and nail plate and a spongy matrix which is easily depressed. There is also increased curvature of the nail and swelling of the terminal phalanx.

Onychogryphosis is great horny thickening and curving often due to trauma. Sometimes it is a consequence of ischaemia or neglect.

Pits (Fig. 75) are most frequently found in any quantity as a result of psoriasis. Lesser degrees are found in eczema. Fine stippling is seen in alopecia areata and longitudinal pits and thinning are seen in lichen planus.

Ridges or grooves are seen in psoriasis, eczema, and fungus infection. Longitudinal central grooves may be due to habit of picking at the base of the thumb, but occasionally it is idiopathic (Fig. 76). Longitudinal white lines are a feature of the genetic dyskeratoses (Darier's and Hailey Hailey diseases) (see Fig. 22).

Transverse ridges result from injury to the nail fold from infection, as in paronychia or dermatitis (Fig. 77).

Systemic illness interferes with growth and such furrows are known as Beau's lines.

Fig. 75 Pits of the nails are due to very localized accelerations in growth such that the nail keratin is less well knit. In psoriasis such pits are very common.

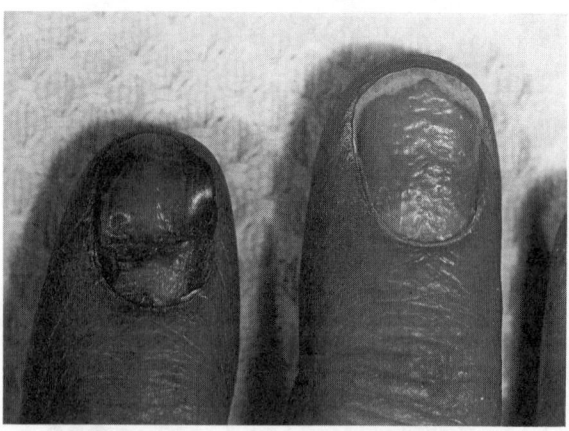

A common cause of nail deformity producing a longitudinal depression is a mucous cyst at the base of the nail. This can be destroyed by cryotherapy or by repeated needling and extrusion of contents over a number of weeks.

Colour changes are listed in Table 22.

PARONYCHIA

This is most commonly due to infection from bacteria and repeated irritation by water and detergents and other agents used by nurses, bar tenders, and bakers. The loss of the natural seal between the nail fold and the nail plate is an important consequence. It is often due to injudicious manicuring. The use of nystatin ointment as a seal applied many times a day before using the hand is an effective therapy, and 3 per cent thymol in chloroform is a broad-spectrum antiseptic used as a paint in this disorder. This is especially useful for discoloration of the nail from *Pseudomonas pyocyanea* which gives rise to a black or green nail. Keeping the hands dry is advisable but difficult to enforce.

TINEA UNGUIUM

This is commonly asymmetrical and the toenails are more involved than the fingernails. Differential diagnosis from psoriasis is often difficult, but psoriasis prefers the fingernails and usually it affects them symmet-

Fig. 76 Longitudinal ridging is usually due to decreased growth, and the nails are often thin and poorly made (idiopathic dystrophy).

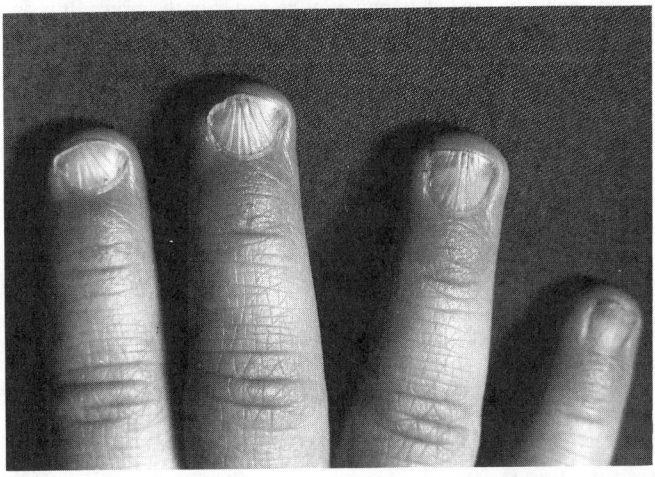

Fig. 77 Transverse white nails, in this case idiopathic, may also indicate arsenical poisoning.

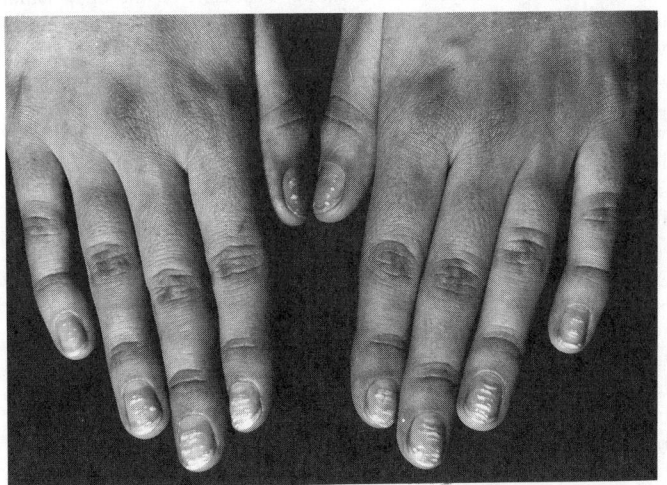

rically and is associated with terminal phalangeal arthritis. Fungus infection usually begins distally, unlike the secondary distortion of a paronychia which affects the nail in the nail bed. Softening and fragility or thickening are further consequences of fungus infection. Microscopic examination of the nail after prolonged soaking of the clippings in 5 to 10 per cent potassium hydroxide should reveal mycelia.

Treatment of toenails is unsatisfactory and should only be embarked upon if the patient complains of the disorder and is prepared to take antifungals daily for very many months. Local fungal preparations are only rarely effective, but amorolfine nail lacquer is a recent improved formulation. Itraconazole, fluconazole, and perhaps most promising terbinafine have greatly improved management but they are given orally and side-effects include hepatoxicity.

REFERENCES

Baran, R. and Dawber, R. P. R. (ed.) (1994). *Diseases of the nails and their management.* Blackwell Scientific Publications, Oxford.

Dawber, R. P. R., and Baran, R. (1992). Disorders of nails. In *Textbook of dermatology,* (5th edn), (ed. A. Rook, D. S. Wilkinson, and F. J. G. Ebling), pp. 2499–532. Blackwell Scientific Publications, Oxford.

Samman, P. D. (1986). *The nails in disease,* (4th edn). Heinemann, London.

Hair

There is no doubt that the majority of hair disorders are associated with changes in other organs, and a complaint of hair loss should be treated with the same seriousness as a cough. The management of a hair problem is in part that of making a diagnosis, but often it is also important to recognize a personality problem.

Up to about 7 months the fetus is covered by long, soft hair. This lanugo hair is shed into the amniotic fluid and may be observed in premature babies, at which stage loss of scalp hair may cause the mother some anxiety. Postnatal hair ranges from short, fine vellus hair covering most of the body to the long, thick terminal hair of scalp and eyebrows. In the adult most hair is of intermediate type and can become coarser when stimulated by local inflammation or by androgens. Suprapubic and axillary hairs are the most easily stimulated, while hair of the beard area and chest requires higher levels of androgen than are normally found in the female. Genetic and racial factors control the response of the hair to androgen. Recent advances in knowledge include evidence that hair growth is mediated not merely by factors in the hair bulb but by cells in the shaft of the hair at the point of attachment of the muscle fibres arrector pili. Drugs or autoimmune processes acting at both sites may influence hair growth.

THE HAIR CYCLE

The life of a hair varies up to about 3 years. Unlike some species which moult periodically, there is little synchrony in the human. Each hair grows at the rate of about 1 cm per month and this is known as the anagen phase. This is followed fairly abruptly by the catagen stage of involution in which the end of the hair forms a club and is shed. This is followed by telogen which is known as the resting stage during which there is no activity. The number of hairs which are shed from the scalp each day ranges from about 50 to 300. The proportion of hairs in anagen in the scalp and beard is greater in spring than in autumn. The lengthening of the eyelashes has been described in AIDS, malnutrition, and in chronic liver disease. There are some 300 000 hairs on the scalp and 1 per cent are in catagen at any one time and the rest are completing their 3-year cycle. When there is a systemic illness or 'shock' or a physiological state such as pregnancy, many of the older hairs may pass into catagen earlier so that a partial moult of longer hairs may occur, often a few weeks later. This is known as telogen effluvium. The hair recovers completely within a few months. Cytotoxic drugs especially cyclophosphamide, inhibit hair growth so that hair loss is a common side-effect.

Table 22 *Colour changes in nails*

Colour change	Cause
Blue black	Subungual haematoma, cytotoxic drugs, Minocin®; pseudomonas infection
	Subungual malignant melanoma
Green	Pseudomonas infection
Brown	Cigarette smoking, potassium permanganate solution, and other dyes
	Chronic renal disease
	Small brown streaks are seen in splinter haemorrhages or thrombi, from trauma, psoriasis, collagen disease, and bacterial endocarditis
	Wider brown streaks are found in subungual melanoma and pigmented benign naevi; these may be exacerbated by Addison's disease
Yellow nails	Slow or distorted growth may result from ischaemia, psoriasis, and fungus infection. If all nails are affected, this may be due to yellow nail syndrome in which there is increased curvature, thickening, and slow growth associated with defective lymphatics. There may be associated pleural effusions
White nails	Hypoalbuminaemia epsecially in cirrhosis, sometimes in renal failure or from cytotoxic drugs. Congenital idiopathic whiteness as an autosomal dominant trait is described. Small white spots are of no significance.
	Transverse white spots are seen with arsenic poisoning, but may be idiopathic while longitudinal streaks occur in Darier's disease (Fig. 22)
Red half moons	Seen in congestive cardiac failure
Blue half moons	Seen in hepatolenticular degeneration or Wilson's disease
Blue nails	Mepacrine

The effect of these drugs can be prevented by cooling the scalp with a tightly fitting ice bag for about 20 min while such drugs are given intravenously.

BALDNESS

Baldness, which for obscure reasons is also called alopecia, has many causes. The most important is physiological sexual maturation. This is due to a shortening of the anagen phase and consequently in an increase of the proportion of hairs in telogen. It is androgen dependent. In its mildest form it is represented by bitemporal recession and occurs in 90 per cent of men and about 80 per cent of women. Frontotemporal loss and thinning of the vertex occurs in 25 per cent of white women by the age of 50 and 60 per cent of men at an earlier age. The commonest pattern is that seen in males and less commonly and severely in females. It begins always as frontal recession exposing the temples and is fol-

lowed variably by gradual thinning of the vertex or the crown. It is age and sex-related; thus both males and females over 80 are commonly bald but males very usually develop baldness early in adult life. A family history of baldness is so common as to make it very likely that there are genetic factors involved. Most important is the influence of testosterone; it is the relative lack of testosterone in young women that accounts for their lessened tendency to develop baldness. Benign baldness of the forehead is associated with normal or slightly raised serum testosterone and a lowering of sex hormone binding globulin. Males castrated before puberty are similarly protected. Hirsuties and baldness go together, so a very hairy chest is a common accompaniment but sexual potency is non-proven. The baldness is initially due to change from terminal to vellus hair but eventually complete follicular atrophy occurs.

EXAMINATION FOR OTHER CAUSES OF HAIR LOSS

The scalp should be examined for evidence of disease such as scaliness, redness, injury, or scarring with its associated loss of follicles (Fig. 79). Severe seborrhoeic eczema, which produces diffuse and excessive dandruff, is often associated with thinning. Psoriasis, on the other hand, tends to leave some scalp unaffected and mostly the hair grows well. In very thick plaques, hair may get broken off or its growth is occasionally inhibited. Lichen planus and discoid lupus erythematosus both destroy the hair follicles and produce respectively a violaceous or red colour as well as scarring. Tinea capitis (see Fig. 20) is a common cause of hair loss in many parts of the world. The acute, painful, boggy, inflammatory swelling of cattle ringworm, known as kerion, is sometimes mistaken for a bacterial abscess, but closer examination would show satellite lesions which are clearly not abscesses. Kerions of the head often heal with scarring and some permanent loss of hair. Equally classic in presentation are groups of children with discoid patches of slightly scaly red areas of broken hairs due to other forms of animal ringworm. Fortunately most adult scalps are resistant to these. It is particularly a problem with children. In many parts of the world *T. violaceum* is responsible in black-skinned children, and *M. canis* in white. White scales and scarring in dark heads is often due to favus. In Africa and the Middle East, favus is due to *T. schoenleinii*. Infection of the scalp with streptococcus

Fig. 78 Severe growth changes of the nail are often a consequence of psoriasis or eczema of the fingertips. The latter may resolve while nail growth disturbance may persist for many months.

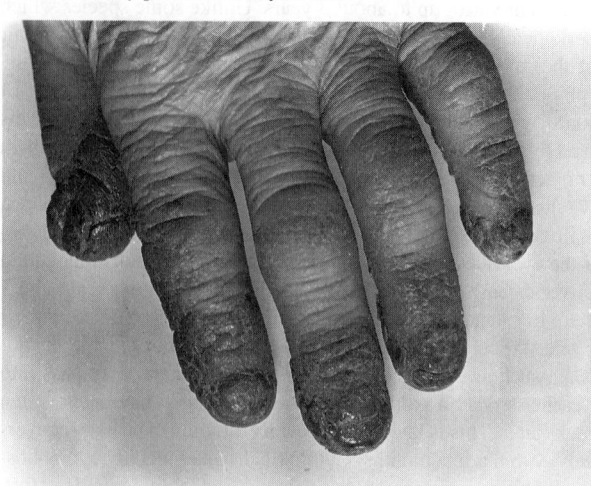

or staphylococcus is common in parts of the world where generalized impetigo is common. The scalp may carry a persistent staphylococcus in persons who scratch or pick at their scalp, sometimes known as 'tycoon scalp'. The rash of secondary syphilis often causes a patchy pattern of hair loss scattered over the scalp like numerous 'glades in a wood'. Loss of eyebrows is a feature of lepromatous leprosy (Fig. 80).

Hair-shaft injury resulting in premature desquamation of inner root sheath is caused by a number of cosmetic procedures, including prolonged traction, permanent waving, or hot combs, which produce burns at the side of the temple area in the Negro attempting to straighten the tightly coiled hair. Scalp massage also damages the hair. Vigorous brushing with old or poor-quality nylon brushes or strong selenium-containing shampoos are other causes of hair loss. The hair becomes more fragile and weathered and breaks at various lengths. Fragility and breaking of the hair is a feature of genetic diseases causing sulphur or cysteine deficiency in the hair. The scalp, too, may be damaged by repetitive hair pulling or twisting or even heating, so one may see redness, scaling, and perifollicular inflammation. Hair pulling or twisting with subsequent breaking is a common habit in infants and in the mentally subnormal, or occasionally in the psychotic (Fig. 81). It is not always consciously done, and if the hair is then eaten there may be little evidence of where the hairs have disappeared to!

Common causes of diffuse hair thinning are iron deficiency, hyperthyroidism, hypopituitarism, severe illness, and drugs such as cyclophosphamide, anticoagulants, and antithyroid drugs, or poisons such as thallium. Temporary thinning is common in those on oral contraceptives.

Rare congenital defects of hair shaft include pili torti, which is a flattened and twisted hair reflecting light unevenly. Menkes' syndrome, which is kinky hair associated with retarded mental and physical development, is associated with copper deficiency.

ALOPECIA AREATA

The cause is unknown and probably it is multifactorial, involving heredity, autoimmunity, stress, infection, and emotional factors in the patho-

Fig. 79 Scarring is an important prognostic feature because hair loss is irreversible. This pattern of hair loss may be due to number of chronic inflammatory processes, including lichen planus.

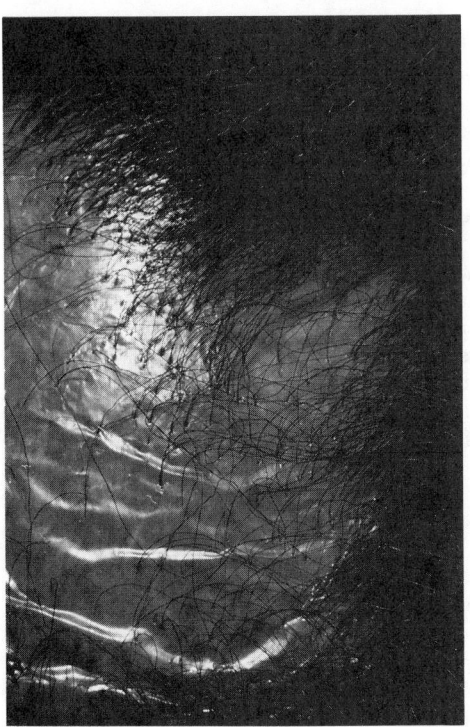

genesis. The hair bulb is infiltrated by CD4 lymphocytes. There are autoimmune associations and response to immuno-modulating therapy. It is not known whether a primary hair-follicle defect invokes this response. It is characterized by localized patches of complete hair loss. At the edges of the lesion there is often a short stubby hair, similar to an exclamation mark, which is due to abortive hair growth (Fig. 82(a)). The scalp may be slightly red but scaling is not a feature. The prognosis of a hair growth within 9 months is good for small patches on the vertex in children, but hair loss at the temples or occiput is less likely to grow well (Fig. 82(b)). New growth is often initially white. A strong family history and an association of atopic eczema or recurrent attacks are not encouraging for a good prognosis. There is an association with vitiligo, thyrotoxicosis myxoedema, pernicious anaemia, and it is common in

Fig. 80 Loss of eyebrows is a feature of lepromatous leprosy. The skin of the face is thickened but the patient may be unaware of the disease, and for this reason the loss of eyebrows could be the first feature about which there is a complaint. Nasal mucosal swelling and erosion is usually obvious.

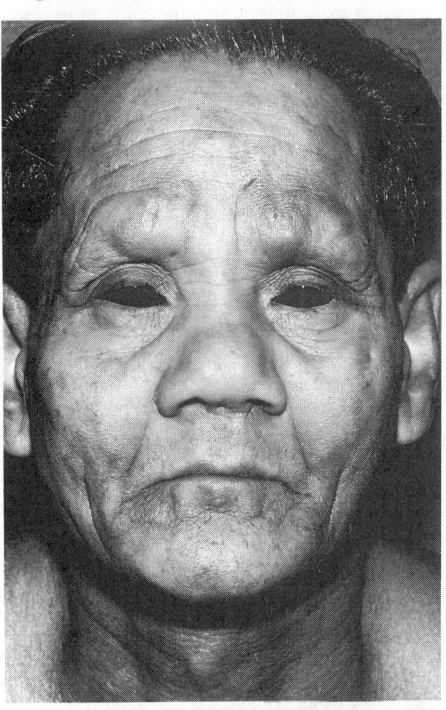

Fig. 81 Trichotillomania, or hair pulling, gives rise to hair loss and the hair length varies because it is broken irregularly. It is a common habit of children, but in the adult it is usually an indication of a personality disorder.

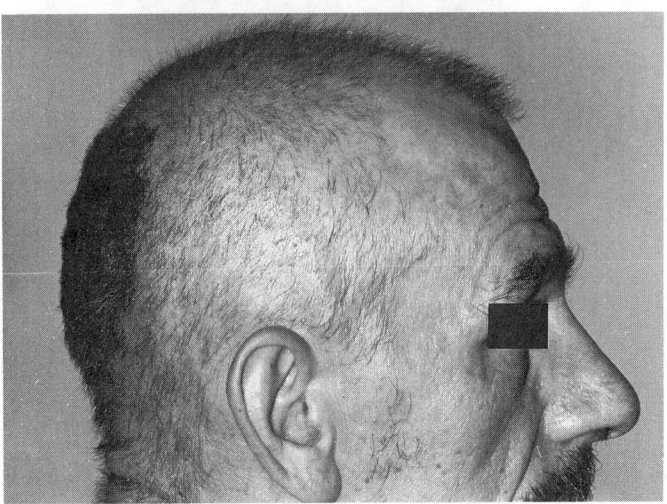

Down's syndrome. An identical picture is a consequence of secondary syphilis. There are large numbers of remedies but none more effective than spontaneous remission. Intralesional steroids encourage local regrowth but atrophy of the scalp is an unpredictable side-effect and the hair often falls out again after a few months.

Coalescence of hair loss gives rise to total scalp alopecia or to universal body alopecia.

DANDRUFF

It is normal to lose small dry scales from the surface of the skin. These tend to be slightly larger in the scalp and show up as white flecks in dark hair or dark clothing. When the skin turns over more rapidly, and in the scalp it normally turns over somewhat faster than in other areas, scales are formed and may even be nucleated. Irritation of the scalp and, in particular, mild infection with a variety of organisms, as in seborrhoeic dermatitis or as with the high rates of turnover in psoriasis, results in excessive dandruff or pityriasis capitis. Most cases respond to regular shampooing twice weekly with preparations containing mild antiseptics or tar. Sulphur or mercury have been incorporated to treat infections.

Fig. 82 (a) Alopecia areata is characterized by abortive hair growth and the formation of a short, stubby, 'exclamation mark' hair at the edge of the area of hair loss. (b) Alopecia of the temple or occiput has a poorer prognosis for regrowth.

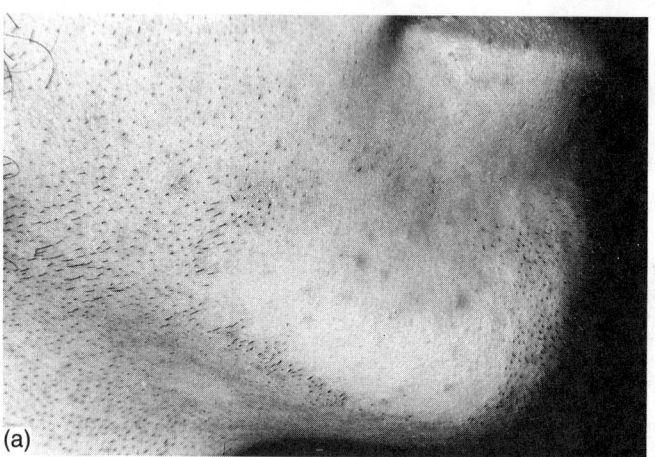
(a)

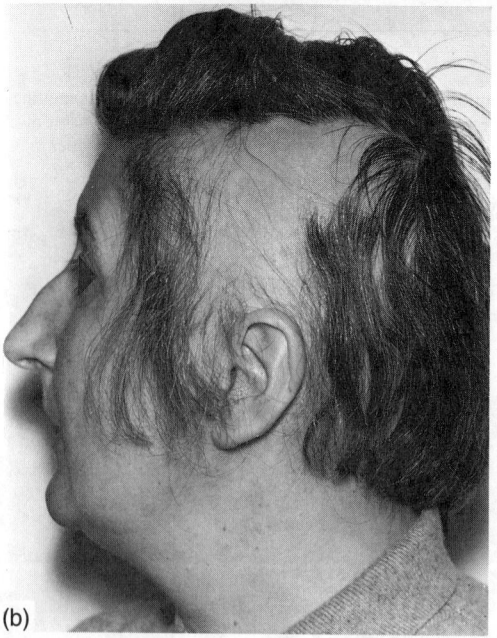
(b)

Table 23 *Hypertrichosis*

Malnutrition
Anorexia nervosa
Early
   Dermatomyositis and scleroderma
   Cutaneous porphyria (see Fig. 31)
   Drugs: diazoxide, minoxidil, phenytoin corticosteroids, cyclosporin
   Various congenital diseases
   Hypertrichosis lanuginosa, either congenital or malignant
Local
   Congenital pigmented naevi
   Spina bifida: faun tail
   Lichen simplex
   Localized chronic inflammation
Endocrine causes of generalized hirsutism
   Polyocystic ovary syndrome
   Idiopathic
   Cushing's syndrome
   Congenital adrenal hyperplasia
   Androgen-secreting tumours
   Hypothyroidism
   Acromegaly

Salicylic acid reduces scaling; a common scalp preparation is *lotio acid salicyl et hydrag perchlor*. The imidazoles are also prescribed.

The scalp is tolerant to strong steroids and there are several spirit lotions containing anti-inflammatory agents, such as Betnovate® or Dermovate®, which are very effective for severe dandruff.

INGROWING HAIRS

The tightly coiled hair of the Negro frequently has difficulty in clearing the follicle and grows into the epidermis at the mouth of the follicle. Eventually ingrowth into the dermis sets up a foreign-body reaction. This is common around the beard area and nape of the neck. Under a hand lens such hairs can be pricked out. Growing a beard often helps to prevent the initial distorted growth pattern.

MANAGEMENT OF HAIR LOSS

This remains unsatisfactory. Hair growth may be stimulated by inducing inflammation in the scalp. High-dose steroids, cyclosporin, and minoxidil have an effect which is often only partial, and loss occurs on withdrawal. It is difficult for both patient and doctor to interpret the many idosyncratic reports of effective therapies. There are several national alopecia societies that provide rational advice.

Wigs are made up of either real or artificial hair. The latter have the advantage of being washable and do not lose their style. However, artificial hair is not as comfortable or as cosmetically satisfactory. For male-pattern baldness, hair pieces may suffice.

Hair transplants are the removal of small, 'punch', full-thickness grafts from the occiput and these are inserted into the bald areas. Fistula formation, scarring, and chronic infection are recorded complications, but for some persons in the public eye the results are regarded as satisfactory.

HIRSUTISM

Hirsutism refers to the male pattern of hair growth and baldness is often associated. It should be distinguished from hypertrichosis which is the growth of terminal hair from vellus hair at sites not normally hairy, such as the forehead in porphyria (Table 23).

A woman with regular menstruation or normal pregnancy and a family history of hairiness is very unlikely to have endocrine disease. Many dark-haired women of India, Wales, and Ireland or of the Mediterranean stock have coarser hair of face, limbs, and trunk than is otherwise observed in Asians or Europeans (see Fig. 16). The Japanese and Chinese are very much less hairy. Many of those who are worried about excess hair are only abnormal because they live amongst persons with an expectation of less hair. Such hirsutism occurs after puberty and can cause great distress in the female and sometimes in the male. After the menopause most women develop coarse hair on the face (Fig. 83). Some normal women may suffer from an enhanced responsiveness of the hair follicles to normal androgen levels in the blood. This is probably due to conversion by the follicle of testosterone into a more active form.

A common cause of hirsutism, also hardly meriting the term 'disease', is due to the secretion of upper limits of normal amounts of testosterone by the ovary. Such women may suffer from seborrhoea, acne, hidradenitis suppurativa, decreased fertility, and male-pattern baldness.

The adrenal gland produces 75 per cent of plasma testosterone. Hyperplasia or tumours are responsible for Cushing's syndrome and the adrenogenital syndrome. In children pseudohermaphroditism due to male-pattern development of the genitalia in a gonadal female will be a feature. In older women marked hirsutism is usually associated with virilism, failure to menstruate, and poor breast development.

Anabolic steroids, anti-oestrogenic drugs, progesterone, and anticonvulsants also cause hirsutism. The polycystic ovary syndrome (Stein–Leventhal) is probably not a single entity and its manifestations vary. Hirsutism is associated with obesity and infertility as well as menstrual disorders. Rarer causes of hirsutism include virilizing tumours of the ovary, gonadal dysgenesis, and Turner's syndrome.

The onset of amenorrhoea, acne, and hirsutism or baldness should merit examination for an enlarged clitoris. This should be followed by plasma testosterone, plasma cortisol, 24-h urinary steroid excretion, and an estimate of pituitary size by skull radiography or scan (Fig. 83).

The development of hypertrichosis or lanugo hair on the face is almost always due to porphyria cutanea tarda or underlying neoplasia.

Treatment

Bleaching with 20 volume hydrogen peroxide makes dark hair on white skin less noticeable. Commercial depilatories are destroyers of hair but not of the hair root. They are highly irritant and many persons find them impossible to use. Various waxes are now available for the legs and arms, some impregnated in gauze which are easy to apply, against the grain, and to pull off with the grain. The abnormally hirsute often require professional electrolysis. The latter is more effective for hairs that have not been repeatedly plucked.

Cyproterone acetate (2 mg daily) is a potent antiandrogen and produces gradual improvement over a period of 6 months to 1 year only if prescribed in the early stages of hair loss of scalp or hair gain on face. Its long-term effects are not known. It is given as a reversed sequential contraceptive with ethinyloestradiol (50 μg daily). Cimetidine and spirolactone may be substituted.

A combination of prednisone and ethinyloestradiol with progesterone is also helpful. The diameter of the hair is a useful measurement for the assessment of response to therapy. Measurement of plucked hair 1 cm above the root should show thickening within the range 40 to 120 μm at the end of 3 months and subsequently at 3 monthly intervals.

REFERENCES

Ginsburg, J. and White, M.C. (1980). Hirsutism and virilism. *British Medical Journal* **i**, 369.

Kvedare, J.C., Gibson, M., and Krusinski, P.A. (1985). Hirsutism: evaluation and treatment. *Journal of the American Academy of Dermatology* **12**, 215–25.

Mitchell, A.J. and Krull, E.A. (1984). Alopecia areata: pathogenesis and treatment. *Journal of the American Academy of Dermatology* **11**, 763–75.

Randall, V.A. and Ebling, J.F.G. (1991). Seasonal changes in human hair growth. *British Journal of Dermatology* **124**, 146–51.

Rook, A. and Dawber, R.P.R. (1991). *Diseases of hair and scalp,* (2nd edn). Blackwell Scientific Publications, Oxford.

Rushton, D.H. (1993). Management of hair loss in women. *Dermatology Clinics* **11**, 47–53.

Savin, R.C. and Atton, A.V. (1993). Minoxidil: update on its clinical role. *Dermatology Clinics* **11**, 55–64.

Shapiro, J. (1993). Alopecia areata. Update on therapy. *Dermatology Clinics,* **11**, 35–46.

Shuster, S. (1984). The aetiology of dandruff and the mode of action of therapeutic agents. *British Journal of Dermatology* **111**, 235–42.

Sweating
APOCRINE

Apocrine glands occur throughout the skin surface in the embryo but subsequently disappear so that they are found in the adults only in the axillae, areolae, and anogenital region. The secretions are formed by the dissolution of apocrine gland cells which are discharged in the hair follicles close to the surface of the skin. They are not active until puberty. Bacterial decomposition accounts for body odour and in the animal kingdom the secretions are important for identity and marking out territorial areas. They are also important sexual organs. All such functions are vestigial in man but body odours are sometimes complained of. Washing with soap and water is the first phase of management. Deodorants reduce the bacterial flora. The eating of garlic and betel nuts should be discouraged since these 'perfumes' are excreted in apocrine sweat. Apocrine sweat is sometimes coloured. If staining is severe and uncontrolled by deodorants, then excision of the glands may be necessary. Retention of apocrine sweat and extreme irritation known as Fox–Fordyce disease is similar to prickly heat. Treatment may include use of topical steroids, destruction with cryotherapy, or excision.

Hydradenitis suppurativa

A chronic activity of the apocrine glands in which disturbance of apocrine flow and sometimes secondary infection gives rise to abscesses,

Fig. 83 Many post-menopausal women develop hirsuties due to altered hormonal balance. Nevertheless one should always be aware of other endocrine causes, as in this patient who has a pituitary tumour

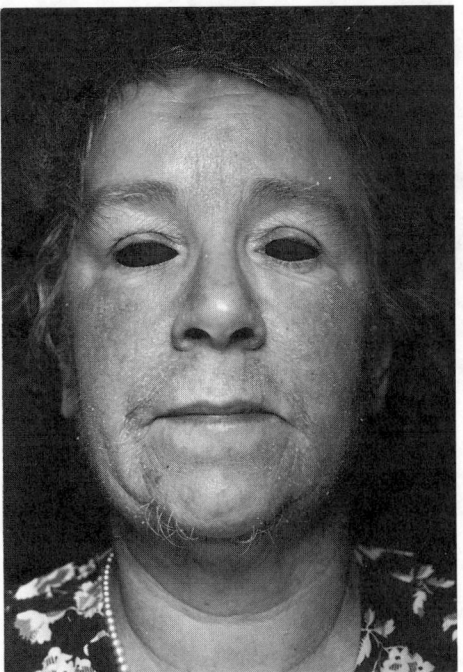

sinuses, and scarring, especially in the axillae and groin. The age of onset, apocrine gland distribution, high levels of serum testosterone, and the presence of comedones also suggest that an endocrine factor, as in acne vulgaris, is important. The early phase of blind boils (Fig. 84) may be responsive to antiandrogens as for hirsuties (see above). Cryosurgery is helpful; courses of antibiotics such as tetracycline three times daily for several weeks are worth trying, but wide surgical excision and grafting is often necessary. When there are acute exacerbations, steroids by mouth may control the eruption. Overuse of deodorants has been blamed for alterations in bacterial flora.

REFERENCES

Mortimer, P.S., Dawber, R.P.R., Gales, M., and Moore, R. (1985). Mediation of hidradenitis suppurativa by androgens. *British Medical Journal* **292**, 245–8.

ECCRINE SWEATING

Humans have about 3 to 4 million sweat glands, equivalent in weight to one kidney. They can secrete at a maximum rate of 2 to 3 litres per hour. The secretory coil produces a plasma-like fluid. Sodium is reabsorbed in the sweat duct.

While eccrine sweat glands occur in all areas, those of the hands, feet, axillae, and face frequently sweat profusely in the absence of general sweating. Man relies on evaporation rather than insulation or panting for protection against a hot environment. Generalized sweating occurs when the body temperature rises and it is a feature of fever as well as thermoregulation in a warm climate, or when the metabolic rate is increased, as in exercise or thyrotoxicosis.

Eccrine sweat glands are largely innervated by unique postganglionic sympathetic fibres that release acetylcholine at the neuroglandular junction. The control centre is in the hypothalamus. It is important to con-

Fig. 84 Axilla showing dusky or violaceous erythema overlying cystic 'blind' boils. The follicular prominence and comedone formation is characteristic of early hydradenitis.

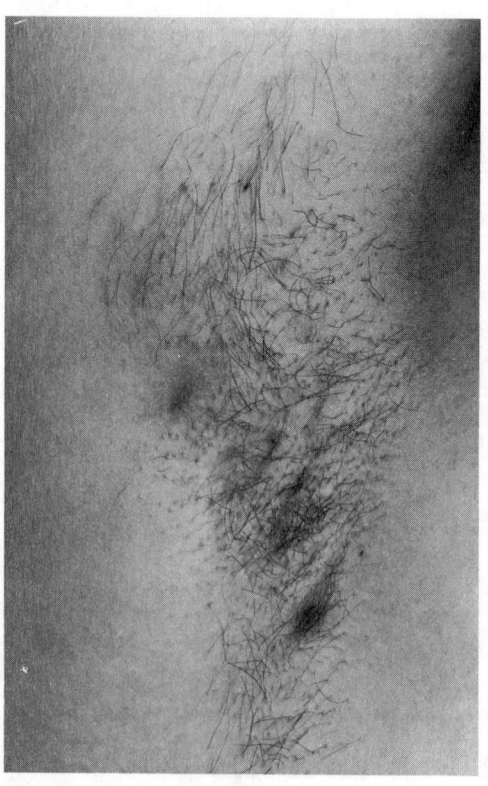

Table 24 *Causes of hyperhidrosis*

Hot weather or room
Exercise
Fever: infection or pyrogen
Fear, anxiety, lie detectors
Thyrotoxicosis, acromegaly, diabetes mellitus
Lymphoma
Cancer
Hypoglycaemia; alcohol intoxication
Nausea
Gustatory
Neurological lesions of the sympathetic nervous system, cortex, basal ganglia, or spinal cord

sider whether the sweating is appropriate for the degree of stimulus (Table 24).

Emotional or anxiety-induced sweating is commonly inappropriate for the degree of anxiety. Many teenagers complain of sweating of the hands and feet and the smell which results from bacterial breakdown of skin and clothing. The fear of being unwelcome increases the anxiety and subsequent sweating. It may summate with thermoregulatory sweating and therefore be worse in hot weather or at a dance. Winter clothing is often more troublesome than the loose garments of summer. Sweating of the hands and feet occurs with acrocyanosis and with some forms of keratoderma.

Segmental, unilateral sweating is often due to irritative lesions of the spine and requires a neurological opinion.

Excessive sweating contributes to tinea pedis and to eczema from footwear.

TREATMENT OF HYPERHIDROSIS

The total daily water loss at rest is about 500 ml but the hyperhidrotic may increase the loss to 12 litres per day or even 3 litres in the first hour. This is faster than it is possible to drink. For this reason it is important to be aware of fluid loss and to restore water and salt in those who are sweating exceptionally.

A sympathetic listener is helpful, as is simple advice on hygiene, washing, keeping cool, and appropriate clothing. The avoidance of obesity, and relaxation if self-conscious are basic points of management. Clothing such as cotton is more appropriate than non-absorbent fibres, and many shoes are now made with linings which prevent absorption and keep the foot and sock wet. Frequent changes of socks prevents bacterial overgrowth, and readjustment of footwear and the wearing of leather shoes or sandals reduces discomfort. Tranquillizers are sometimes helpful and propantheline, 15 mg every few hours, may be helpful or can be reserved for a social occasion; abolition of sweating carries a risk of hyperthermia.

Local therapy

A specific inhibitor of sweating is 20 per cent aluminium chloride hexahydrate in absolute alcohol when it is applied as a saturated solution to the skin. It acts by an effect on the cells at the mouth of the sweat duct. The skin should be as dry as possible and the patient as tranquil as possible since dilution of the saturated solution by sweat causes it to become irritant. It is probably most effective for the axillae when applied at night and maintenance therapy need be only once or twice weekly.

Application of 3 per cent formalin soaks to the soles of the feet for 10 minutes or topical glutaraldehyde 10 per cent solution buffered to pH 7.5 are sometimes helpful. Poldine methylsulphate 3 to 4 per cent in alcohol is another topical agent used on the feet.

Systemic anticholinergic drugs such as propantheline, 15 mg three times daily controls sweating in some patients but dry mouth and blurred vision are side-effects which prove too troublesome for others.

Iontophoresis is a method involving a direct current of low voltage and is a somewhat tedious method of reducing sweating of the hands and feet. Tap-water with or without drugs such as glycopyronium bromide may be used. Injury to the innervation or to the sweat glands themselves is the aim of several techniques for the management of axillary hyperhidrosis. Freezing with liquid nitrogen, if rigorous enough to produce swelling and blistering, destroys the sweat glands, but the necrosis in the axillae is sometimes quite severe. Undercutting with a scalpel causes denervation since only the glands in the apex of the axillae are responsible for most of the sweating. These can also be removed by snipping away the sweat coils on the undersurface of the skin. Excision of an ellipse of skin 4 × 1.5 cm is also effective after mapping the area with 1 per cent iodine in alcohol followed by starch powder. Excision followed by a 'Z' plasty to avoid a linear scar contraction is also recommended. The transverse arm of the Z lies in the apex of the axillae. Cervical lumbar sympathectomy reduces hyperhidrosis of the hands and feet but the risks and irreversibility of the operation have to be weighed against the expected spontaneous resolution of the problem, especially in the teenager.

Hyperhidrosis of the feet is often associated with redness or acrocyanosis and the skin becomes macerated, giving rise to a whitening of the keratin as well as to bacterial contamination which produces pits known as pitted keratolysis.

The multiple asymptomatic pits in the keratin have been blamed variously on corynebacteria, streptomyces, and the organism *Dermatophylus congolensis*. It is common in barefoot persons in the rainy season. The treatment is to dry the feet. Antibacterial remedies are not necessary.

HYPOHIDROSIS

This occurs in the newborn and in premature children in the first month of life and it is seen also in infants from occlusion of the sweat ducts, especially in the flexures of the folds of the skin of the neck. It may result also from exfoliative dermatitis or erythroderma and it is a feature of hypohidrotic ectodermal dysplasia which is a sex-linked recessive disorder. Such patients are usually male and are susceptible to heat stroke and therefore early diagnosis of the affected baby in a hot climate is important. The hair is sparse, dry, fine, and short. The scalp and eyelashes are particularly affected. The skin is smooth and finely wrinkled. The nose is sunken and the teeth conical (Fig. 85). Absence of sweating causes loss of skin moisturization and impaired grip. Examination of the palmar surface of the fingers with a magnifying lens will show the absence of duct orifices.

Miliaria

Miliaria crystallina is a superficial obstruction to sweat glands, producing clear vesicles. This may occur when the sweat produced by the glands exceeds the ability of the duct to absorb it. It is commonly seen with high fever. Deeper obstruction gives rise to red, itchy papules known as prickly heat. It affects one in three persons exposed to hot climates, and while it sometimes begins within a few days of arrival in such a climate it is commonly a problem 2 to 6 months later. Occlusion of the skin by impermeable clothing aggravates it; bacteria may play some part in its generation as well as in one complication, namely staphylococcal abscesses. It is a contributory factor to extreme thermal stress in the unacclimatized. This is also a feature of workers in hot industries with furnaces or in those underground in mines. Relief from sweating even for a few hours is essential. Loose, non-occlusive clothing and exposure of the skin folds as much as possible is beneficial. Vitamin C 1 g daily was advocated by dermatologists in the British Army in Malaysia. It is important to realize that severe hypohidrosis of the trunk and limbs may be missed as a cause of asthenia if the face is sweating. Shake lotions of calamine powder promote cooling by increasing surface area. Localized loss of sweating may be due to tuberculoid leprosy, syringomyelia, and diabetes mellitus.

REFERENCE

Champion, R.H. (1992). Disorders of sweat glands. In *Textbook of dermatology*, (5th edn), (ed. A. Rook, D.S. Wilkinson, and E.J.G. Ebling), pp. 1745–62. Blackwell Scientific Publications, Oxford.

Skin disorders affecting the genitalia

A diagnosis of disorders affecting the genitalia cannot be made without looking. Natural shyness on the part of the patient or lack of zeal on the part of the doctor are common. Racial and religious grounds for incomplete examination must be overcome by appropriate selection of the examiner and chaperoning as well as an interpreter.

It may be inappropriate to delve into the sexual, gynaecological, or medical history and so initial questioning may be limited until an examination has indicated the nature of the disease. A contact dermatitis may require the most detailed and searching questioning.

Many skin conditions of the vulva or penis can be best diagnosed by examining the rest of the skin. For example the knees, scalp, and elbows in psoriasis, the front of the wrists and shins in lichen planus, the mouth in pemphigus, or the neck, breasts, or wrists in lichen sclerosis et atrophicus.

INFECTIONS

Infections are commonly transmitted by sexual intercourse and tend to be associated with vaginal or urinary meatal symptoms. The sexual partner will require treatment. However, in the female some infections may be asymptomatic and this is so with primary chancre, gonorrhoea, chlamydial infections, or trichomoniasis. Where infection is suspected, swabs for culture should be taken from the cervix, urethra, and rectum.

The pubic region is commonly affected by nits and crablice and viral molluscum contagiosum causes smooth pearly umbilicated papules (see Fig. 133).

Fig. 85 Conical teeth, sparse eyelashes, and a sunken nose are clues to hyperthermia. This young boy is affected by the absence of sweat glands known as hypohidrotic ectodermal dysplasia.

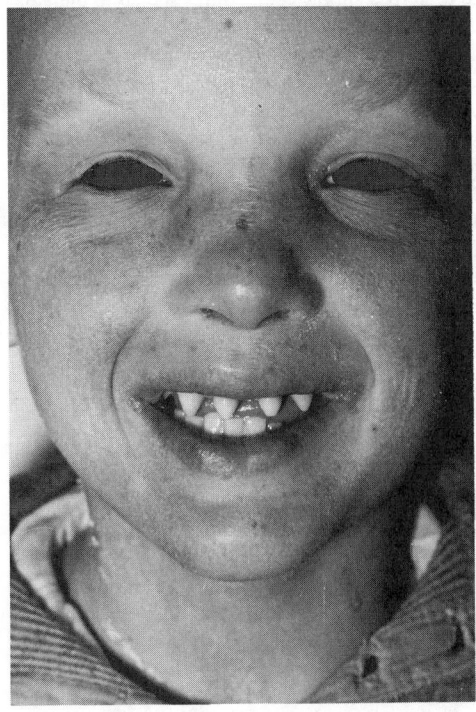

WARTS

Genital warts commonly begin at the introitus and extend forewards or backwards as filiform pink fleshy lesions, often coalescing into velvety or papilliferous masses. They must be distinguished from the moist, flat lesions of syphilis.

Perianal warts are commonly confined to that site. Warts are often transmitted by sexual intercourse and other infectious diseases such as syphilis may be masked. Outlying, more scattered warts on the buttocks, shaft of penis, scrotum, or in the genitocrural folds are less commonly venereal, as are genital warts in infancy or childhood.

Natural immunity to the wart virus is the only certain cure. The easiest therapy is podophyllin 15 to 20 per cent solution in compound tincture of benzoin or spirit. This should be applied to the warts and, depending on the degree of soreness that results in some persons, may be washed off after a few hours. Absorption in the pregnant is recorded as a cause of abortion. An alternative therapy, if available, is cryotherapy. Local or general anaesthetics followed by curettage and cautery or dissection after lifting up of the wart on a bleb of saline is also effective.

Those who have multiple partners should be examined for other sexually transmitted diseases. Women should have cervical smears at regular intervals because of the increased risk of cervical cancer. Wart destruction for cosmetic reasons is the principal role of the dermatologist.

CANDIDIASIS

Pregnancy, diabetes mellitus, and antibiotics predispose to this infection, although a mild degree of non-pathogenic infection is common. White plaques or more diffuse soreness with redness of the vulva or glans penis are common. As part of an intertrigo there is a red flexural rash with a fringe of vesicles, scales, or pustules and more peripheral scattering of satellite lesions. The condition responds to nystatin ointment but clearance of the lower bowel by oral nystatin and treatment of the sexual partner is often necessary. There are now several other effective anticandida agents (see Chapter 7.12.1).

HERPES SIMPLEX

Genital infections due to herpes simplex sometimes spread to the adjacent thigh and buttocks. The infection is commonly a recurrent problem, unlike herpes zoster. The latter may cause confusion but it is clearly unilateral. Specific treatment is unsatisfactory but analgesics and control of secondary infection with antiseptic washes is helpful. Idoxuridine, 5 per cent in dimethyl sulphoxide, is painful to apply but it is especially useful for aborting recurrences where these are frequent and predictable. Where recurrences are associated with a prior rise in temperature aspirin may be tried to abort the fever, as at ovulation or from repeated and recurrent infection. Oral acyclovir prevents recurrences only while taking the drug. Anxieties about viral resistance, long-term side-effects, and rebound infections when the drug is discontinued have not so far proved justified.

NAPPY ERUPTIONS

These are inevitable in the infant but vary in their severity and causation. Urine and faeces can cause maceration and irritation, especially if left in contact with the skin for several hours so that bacteria and Candida have an opportunity to provide ammonia and proteases. The distribution is more nearly that of contact with the nappy so that the genitocrural folds may be spared. The scrotum and labia are often the principally affected sites and a variety of irritants produce sharply defined blisters or ulcers. Abuse may be wrongly suspected. Contact friction with elastic or plastic pants causes well-defined linear marks. In the infant, red, scaly, or sore skin in the genitocrural folds is due to primary skin disease such as seborrhoeic eczema or due to secondary bacterial and Candida infection (Figs 86 and 87). A streptococcal dermatitis gives rise to a well circumscribed painful erythema.

All rashes benefit from bathing and frequent changes of nappy. Soap substitutes such as emulsifying ointments or other greases can be used for cleansing the affected areas. The application of an antiseptic with an anticandida agent like nystatin or miconazole and an antipruritic agent such as hydrocortisone considerably shorten the course of the rash but spontaneous remission is usual. The commonly used ointments are Timodine® or Vioform-Hydrocortisone®. Severe Candida infections may require oral ketoconazole if nystatin is unsuccessful.

Children whose families are known to suffer from atopy may present for the first time with red, scaly, irritated skin in the distribution of the nappy area, which is often very persistent and requires much protective grease and sparingly applied steroid creams.

Diseases that are rare but life-threatening include three that present in the nappy area namely, Letterer–Siwe, acrodermatitis enteropathica, and congenital syphilis. Benign seborrhoeic dermatitis often affects the scalp, axillae, and neck as well as in the nappy area. The child is not usually greatly worried by the rash.

ADULT INTERTRIGO

Obesity and sweating predispose to mixed irritation and infection in the occluded skin under the breast, axillae, and groins. The affected area is moist, red, fissured, and malodorous. Attempts at keeping the site dry and free of excessive infection have been improved by preparations such as miconazole and hydrocortisone, and ZeaSORB® powder acting as a drying agent without too much caking. Washing and gentle drying is the most important therapy. Blind boils and comedones are likely to be due to hidradenitis suppurativa.

Psoriasis in the flexures is usually well defined, bright red, and, unlike at other sites, is non-scaly. It is worth treating initially for 3 days with a strong steroid because this sometimes clears the psoriasis. More often the lesions persist and strong steroids are then harmful since they cause so much atrophy. Hydrocortisone can be used but it is only mildly effective. It is important to protect the skin from excessive infection by regular washing.

Dermatitis of the genitalia is commonly due to contact with the agents listed in Table 25. Some of these are added to the bath and inadequately mixed with the water. There may be a considerable immediate contact swelling from certain deodorant sprays. Infection of mixed type may contribute to the problem. Persistent pruritus and scratching is a very common disorder and produces thickening of the skin and a range of colours from white fissured areas to pigmented and violaceous plaques.

In uncircumcised adult males a persistent reddish brown, somewhat fixed balanitis is heavily infiltrated with plasma cells. This benign condition, known as Zoon's balanitis, is cured by circumcision.

LEUCOPLAKIA VERSUS THE ATROPHY OF LICHEN SCLEROSUS ET ATROPHICUS

This is often confusing and it is possible for the skin of the genitalia to be thinned but nevertheless to be covered by a thickened scale. The lesion of lichen sclerosus is well defined (Fig. 88), white, may have a violaceous border, and small haemorrhagic blisters are common, especially in children, and should not be mistaken for sexual abuse. The perianal areas are always involved, especially in children (Fig. 89). Intractable itching, burning, or soreness of perineum or genitalia is unfortunately common. In young women it usually slowly improves; in older persons it persists. It responds well to high-potency local steroids.

Histologically, lichen sclerosus et atrophicus is characterized by an extremely thin epidermis with a thickened scale and an acellular homogenized upper dermis. By contrast, leucoplakia and lichen simplex are

Fig. 86 Flexural nappy rash with involvement of perineum deep into the body folds suggestive of infection, or seborrhoeic eczema.

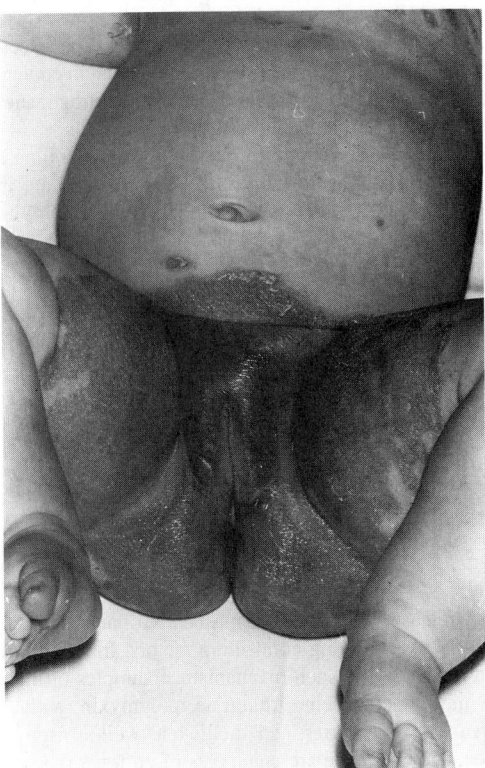

Table 25 *Causes of contact dermatitis affecting the genitalia*

Antiseptics
Fungicides
Ethylene diamine (usually in Tri-Adcortyl®)
Neomycin
Rubber dermatitis (condoms)
Hexachlorophane
Allergens carried on hands (usually also affect eyelids)
Perfumes, antiseptics in soaps and sprays
Wood dusts, oils, fibreglass; irritants according to occupation

Fig. 88 Lichen sclerosis causes tisse-paper-like crinkling or atrophy of the skin. The border is often violaceous but the centre of the lesion is white.

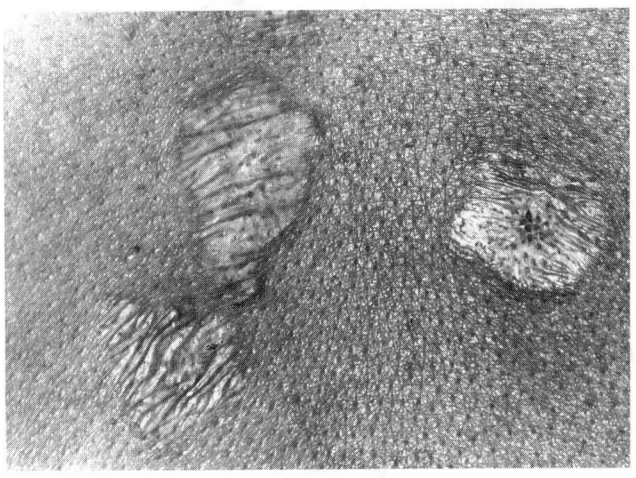

Fig. 89 Lichen sclerosis of the vulva in a child; tends to clear at puberty. In the elderly it is a persistent cause of irritation.

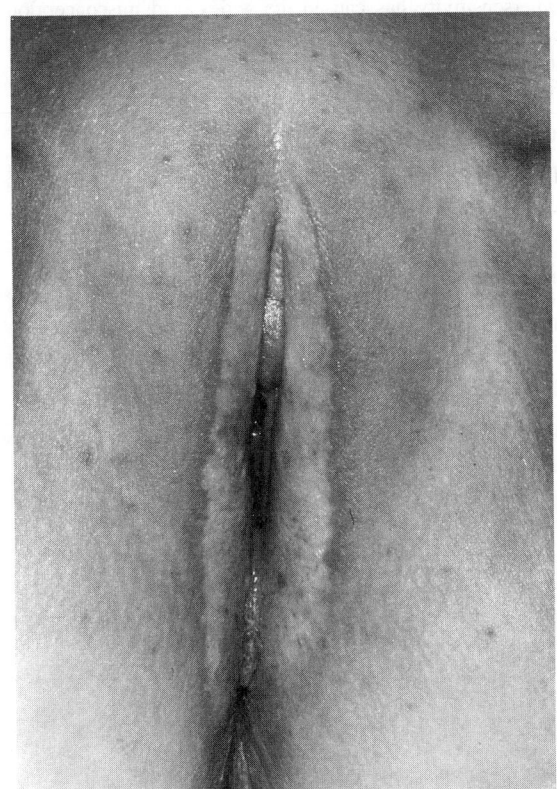

Fig. 87 Sparing of flexures suggests contact with a wet nappy.

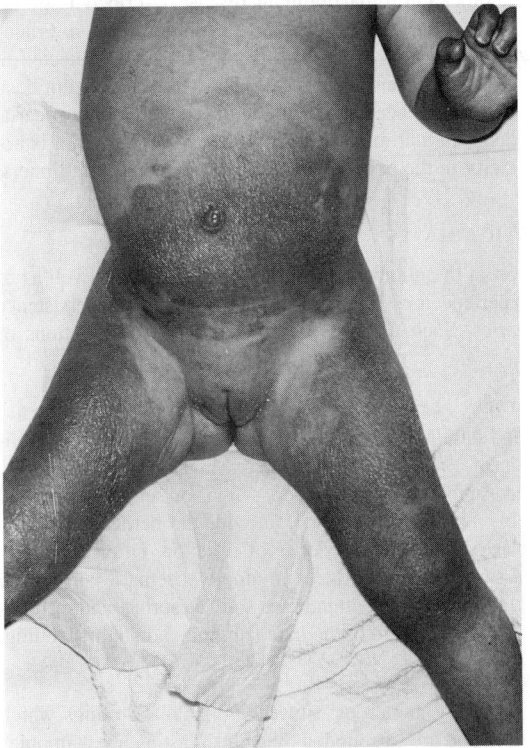

composed of a greatly hypertrophied epidermis and usually thickening of the underlying dermis as well. When in doubt, a biopsy should be performed, but leucoplakia and lichen sclerosus may coexist in as many as 24 per cent of patients. Although lichen sclerosus et atrophicus, especially when damaged by scratching, may develop a squamous cell epithelioma, there is no advantage nor relief of discomfort by prospective vulvectomy.

In the case of leucoplakia, vulvectomy is usually advocated as there is much greater chance of the development of a squamous epithelioma. However, since the skin is predisposed to lichen sclerosus in areas well beyond the genitocrural folds, simple vulvectomy is not a satisfactory treatment for lichen sclerosus itself. Attention to hygiene is important as is exclusion of mixed infections or contact dermatitis. Rarely, perineal discomfort and eczema may be due to vitamin B_2 deficiency.

Well-defined asymmetric plaques of red pigmented skin should be biopsied to exclude intraepidermal carcinoma to which this site is predisposed.

The term kraurosis vulvae is now obsolete since it does not differentiate senile atrophy from the now well-recognized lichen sclerosis.

REFERENCES

Ridley, C.M. (1988). *The vulva*. Churchill Livingstone, London.
Teillac-Hamel, D. and de Prost, Y. (1992). Perianal streptococcal dermatitis in children. *European Journal of Dermatology*, **2**, 71–4.

Urticaria

Urticaria is a transient swelling and/or flushing of the skin. The underlying vasodilatation and accumulation of tissue fluid in the dermis is due to a succession of mediators of inflammation acting mainly on the small blood vessels. The time taken to bring their effects under control varies and thus the inflammatory response varies from the very transient to more persistent inflammation overlapping with vasculitis.

The knowledge that histamine plays a part in immediate-type (anaphylactic) hypersensitivity has caused the widespread misconception that all urticaria must be allergic. A non-immunological pharmacological explanation is more likely in most cases.

IMMUNOLOGY

Allergens of the type commonly incriminated in sufferers from atopic disease are bound to IgE antibodies attached to the surface of the mast cells or basophils whence various mediators are released, including histamine, serotonin, and slow-reacting substance (leucotriene) of anaphylaxis. Allergens causing this include egg white, cows' milk, house dust, dandruff, feathers, and tomatoes. It is commonly of contact type affecting the lips during eating or some other parts of the skin when in contact with animals or house dust. Transfusion reactions and some drug rashes are due to complement fixing antibodies attached to blood cells.

The urticaria of serum sickness, penicillin reactions, the acute illness of systemic lupus erythematosus, and many infectious diseases are in part due to immune complexes of immunoglobulins and allergen with complement activation.

COMPLEMENT ACTIVATION

While complement is activated by immunological reactions, it is also activated enzymatically by proteases such as plasmin when there are insufficient natural inhibitors of this mediator in the serum and tissues. Congenital or acquired deficiencies in inhibitor levels account for some forms of angioedema and for hereditary angioedema in particular. The activation of complement by the alternative pathway may explain some non-familial cases.

HISTAMINE LIBERATORS

Some drugs and foods release histamine from mast cells, or at least make such release more likely by inhibiting controlling factors. Inhibition of prostaglandin activity may be one such mechanism. Examples of mast cell stimulators are morphine, codeine, thiamine, polymyxin, and D-tubocurarine. Bee venom, strawberries, and shellfish as well as aspirin, salicylates, benzoates, and tartrazine are enhancers of an urticarial tendency, bringing it to the fore in susceptible subjects as well as occasionally initiating the eruption.

GENETIC FACTORS

Familial urticaria is a well-recognized phenomenon. Many large families of hereditary angioedema are recorded. The autosomal dominant inheritance is mediated through an absence of C_1 esterase inhibitor. Familial cold urticaria is another autosomal dominant disease described in several families in the United States and others have been described in France and Holland. A low level of chymotrypsin inhibitors was detected in one family. As in atopic eczema, studies of HLA antigen have not been very rewarding. BW35 has been associated with acute ordinary urticaria.

Candidiasis has been incriminated in careful studies, though it is not so important a factor in the experience of the majority of practitioners.

TYPES OF URTICARIA

There is variation in the number, size, and depth of weal as well as of the sensation experienced by the patient. The degree of the persistence of the lesion varies. Such features make up named constellations of physical signs.

Contact urticaria

This is a weal and flare reaction occurring for 20 to 40 min after application to the skin of a number of agents listed in Table 16. Some may be IgE mediated, such as animal dander, saliva, or seminal fluid, but most are probably non-immunological, as with the nettle or jellyfish sting, or the solar or aquagenic varieties of urticaria. Often there is a consequent or associated dermatitis, as in atopic eczema. Many of the ointments used for dermatitis contain bases such as sorbic acid or polyethylene glycol which cause an immediate stinging and slight swelling.

Cholinergic urticaria

This is characterized by numerous, superficial, small swellings which sting, smart, or itch and are surrounded by a blush lasting a few minutes

Fig. 90 Cholinergic urticaria is like blushing brought on by emotion, exercise, or heat. It is transient, lasting no more than about 15 minutes, and may be associated with small, superficial weals with a prominent flush. These tend to sting rather than itch.

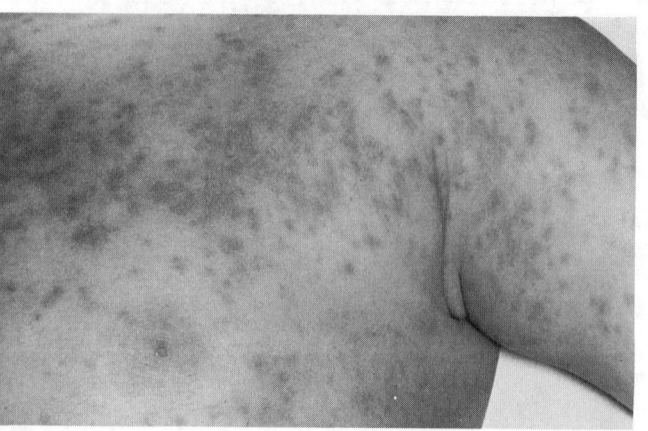

only (Fig. 90). Probably it is mediated by an increase of receptors for acetylcholine from dorsal root nerve endings. The commonest pattern is found in adolescents and young adults and, like blushing, it is brought on by emotion, exercise, or hot baths.

Heat urticaria

This is a rare local response to heat in which histamine is released or complement is activated.

Angio-oedema

This is characterized by a few, deep, large swellings which may be tender and often itch, sometimes preceded by redness, lasting several hours or even days. Proteases such as complement, plasmin, and kinins are incriminated.

Ordinary urticaria or hives

This is characterized by numerous weals of all sizes, and varying degrees of pallor or redness, which itch and last for one or more hours, but not usually more than a day. Successive lesions may account for long illness. Chronic urticaria is arbitrarily defined as continuous or recurrent lesions of more than 3 months' duration. Histamine is the principal mediator. Current evidence supports the view that skin blood vessels have both H_1 and H_2 receptors.

Time of onset

Cholinergic urticaria is like a blush and develops abruptly and instantaneously within minutes of the triggering event. Ordinary urticaria also develops within minutes of the release of the mediator but not all mediators are released instantaneously. Thus foods and certain allergens, or drugs such as aspirin, have to be digested and absorbed. Ordinary urticaria is often difficult to relate to events in the life of the patient for this reason. Delayed onset is a well-recognized phenomenon of some of the physical urticarias. Thus delayed dermographism is the development of redness and slight wealing several hours after scratching the skin. Delayed pressure urticaria is a tender swelling 2 to 12 h after localized pressure injury to the skin. It is possible that the insult localizes noxious agents such as soluble immune complexes, or that mechanisms such as transient ischaemia and release of proteases bring to light homeostatic defects such as deficiency of inhibitors of complement or other proteases.

Physical urticaria

Regardless of the exact mediators released by the injury of the skin, there are several urticarial eruptions determined only by specific physical insults. These include sunlight, cold, heat, pressure, scratch, or stretch.

Solar urticaria is uncommon. A weal develops within 30 s to 3 min exposure to the sun. Tolerance may develop in sites habitually exposed such as the hands and feet. It is important to recognize it by its history and examination, and the differential diagnosis of porphyria, lupus erythematosus, or photosensitivity following drug ingestion has to be considered. In these the urticaria is more persistent, and because the longer, more penetrating ultraviolet rays are responsible, it can occur even on a cloudy day or when the skin is protected from glass, clothing, or sunscreens.

Familial cold urticaria is an autosomal dominant disease in which the rash develops up to several hours after cold exposure from, for example, cold winds, and it usually presents in infancy. Fever and joint pains accompany the rash and there is a leucocytosis. Low levels of a chymotrypsin inhibitor have been demonstrated. It may not be induced by the application of ice to the skin.

Acquired cold urticaria occurs within a few minutes of plunging into cold water or after applying ice to the skin. Mast cells are degranulated and it is one cause of sudden death in young people.

Papular urticaria

This is the only form of urticaria to have a persistent epidermal component. Most often this is due to insect bites, and the epidermis is either damaged directly or by mediators in the upper dermis which evoke an eczematous response so that oedema of the epidermis and a proliferative repair effect results in a typical itchy and persistent papule. Such lesions are usually excoriated, whereas most urticarias are not deeply scratched but merely rubbed. They often blister (see Fig. 100).

Scaling is not a feature of urticaria, and while acute dermatitis and some erythema initially appear to be urticarial the development of scaling immediately excludes such diagnoses.

THE DISTRIBUTION OF THE RASH

Cholinergic urticaria favours the head and upper trunk. Angio-oedema most commonly involves mucocutaneous junctions such as the lips, eyes, and penis. The physical urticarias clearly relate to sites of exposure. Thus solar urticaria affects the face and the dorsum of the hands, or, if tolerance is developed, it occurs at such sites that are exposed for the first time during the summer. Pressure urticaria favours the soles of the feet when walking or digging, or the backs of the thighs or lumbar region when sitting.

Bizarre patterns

Urticaria evolving and resolving inevitably exhibits changing morphology. The redness of the vasodilatation merges with the veiling pallor of the oedema. Healing in the centre and peripheral spread often produces bizarre gyrate or circinate and serpiginous patterns, but they are transient and never scaly, unlike similar patterns in the erythemas or epidermal diseases such as psoriasis.

INVESTIGATIONS

A history is the most effective investigation of urticaria. Intradermal injection of mecholyl (10 μg/0.5 ml saline) reproduces the lesions of cholinergic urticaria. Intradermal histamine, 1 μg in 0.1 ml saline, produces a weal that should disappear within 1 hour. This disappearance is delayed in pressure urticaria and in immune complex disease. The localization of a noxious agent results in a persistent lesion. In practice, avoidance of cause can be advised only if this is recognized after taking a history and examining the patient. The two most helpful investigations are a full blood count and blood sedimentation rate. An eosinophilia should alert one to parasites such as microfilaria or trichiniasis, and a raised blood sedimentation is due to a systemic illness such as sepsis, malignancy, or 'collagen' disease.

Rubbing or scratching of the skin with the fingernail produces a weal and flare in the dermographic subject within 2 min.

A weight of 4 to 6 kg hung for 10 minutes over the shoulder with a bandage or belt, causing a tender swelling 2 to 8 h later reveals delayed pressure urticaria. A biopsy at this stage for immunofluorescence may confirm localization of immune complexes. The white count at the time of the biopsy may show neutrophilia, especially if there is accompanying fever. Absence of C_1 esterase inhibitor in the serum should be looked for in patients with angio-oedema, especially if initiated by minor surgery, associated with abdominal pains, and having other members of the family affected. Complement levels are not a reliable guide to the participation of proteases and hardly influence the management of urticaria.

Chronic urticaria is a known symptom of filariasis and strongyloidosis, but in ascariasis and enterobiasis it occurs if anything more often in controls. Urticaria is such a difficult disease to assess that possible aetiological factors, such as parasitic disease, are worth treating in their own right rather than in the expectation of resolution of the eruption.

About 25 per cent of cases of acute hepatitis B present with urticaria.

Foci of infection as a cause of urticaria are statistically difficult to support but dental and sinus infections continue to be described as aetiological factors based on impressive case histories.

Bleeding time and thrombo test

The urticarial response to food and drugs where the cause is known can be shown to be correlated with a prolonged bleeding time and a fall in the platelet count. This happens within 1 to 2 h of the ingestion of the suspected agent.

BEE STINGS

The stinging bee injects histamine, serotonin, acetylcholine, and kinins. In addition there are proteins to which the subject becomes allergic, including phospholipase A and hyaluronidase. IgE is responsible for the immediate hypersensitivity. Symptoms include pain and swelling, pruritus, urticaria, faintness, asthma, vomiting, and diarrhoea. Cardiac arrhythmia is more likely in the elderly. The generalized reaction is preceded by a pulsating feeling in the ears, tightness in the throat, substernal pain, and fear. Acute anxiety causing hyperventilation or coronary thrombosis should be thought of. Death is actually exceedingly rare. Serum sickness or later joint pains and fever are described, as well as vasculitis and haematuria. Emergency treatment is 0.5 ml of 1/1000 solution of adrenaline injected deeply subcutaneously and repeated in 10 min. Antihistamines and corticosteroids aid recovery. The value of desensitization versus its morbidity is not certain.

WHEN SHOULD URTICARIA BE TAKEN MORE SERIOUSLY?

Urticaria is life-threatening when it is part of anaphylaxis, when angio-oedema involves the upper respiratory tract, or when it is part of the systemic immune complex disease and is associated with more dire pathology such as meningococcal septicaemia or lupus erythematosus. The latter type of urticaria is recognized by its more persistent lesion, lasting at least 1 to 2 days and often tender and ultimately purpuric. It should be remembered that all acute urticaria may be very widespread and be accompanied by joint pains, stomach aches, and fever. However, if the individual lesion lasts for only a few hours it is less likely to be due to a noxious circulating trigger such as immune complex or infective organisms.

MANAGEMENT

Removal of the known physical factor and the known trigger is helpful, but in the majority of cases of chronic urticaria in the adult no cause is found. Some European centres rely on studies of the gastrointestinal tract to reveal *Candida albicans,* Campylobacter, and other infections as possible causes of urticaria. Food, medicines, and infectious or parasitic diseases are the commonest suspected factors, but in Europe and the United States physical urticaria accounts for more than half of the patients in some series. Cold, heat, and solar urticaria often respond to the induction of tolerance by subthreshold desensitization. It is useful to try antihistamines because of much individual variation in response and in the side-effects. Antihistamines are often prescribed in too low a dosage to be effective, and patients should be encouraged to rest at home taking a rather higher dosage. The evidence that skin blood vessels have both H_1 and H_2 receptors has encouraged trials with their antagonists. At present the financial cost and large number of pills that have to be taken every day is a disadvantage. Most H_1 antihistamines are cheap and free of serious side-effects. Drowsiness is often troublesome but the variations in the response are considerable and they are otherwise effective in the majority if taken regularly to prevent the urticaria rather than to treat the existing weals. Long-acting antihistamines are worth trying when short-acting ones fail. The value of combined H_1 and H_2 blockers (4 mg cyproheptadine and 300 mg cimetidine four times daily) remains unproven but like all regimens has some individual successes. Hydrox-

azine (10–25 mg three times a day) is often effective in dermographism or cholinergic urticaria. Nifedipine in conjunction with antihistamines has its advocates. When the urticaria is painful and long-lasting, prednisolone is often effective and need only be given for 2 or 3 days. Avoidance of known triggers of urticaria such as aspirin, tartrazine, benzoate, and other salicylates often requires a rather complex diet (see Table 14).

The acute emergency of upper respiratory obstruction requires the maintenance of the airway, if necessary by intubation or tracheotomy, and administration of oxygen. This should not be delayed while a search is being made for adrenaline and corticosteroids, but if these are quickly available they should be given, as nothing is lost and some benefit may be derived. Adrenaline 1/1000 0.5 ml is given subcutaneously and hydrocortisone 100 mg intravenously.

Management of autosomal dominant hereditary angio-oedema

This should be suspected if there is a family history of angio-oedema or a few long-lasting swellings precipitated by trauma. The signs include a transient erythema followed by the oedema. There is often recurring colicky abdominal pain. The diagnosis should be confirmed by looking for low levels in the serum of alpha-neuro-aminoglycoprotein, C_1 esterase inhibitor (normal 18 ± 5 mg/100 ml).

Prophylaxis includes care to protect against trauma especially in the region of the mouth and neck after dental manoeuvres. Methyltestosterone 10 mg as linguets after breakfast and another when there is a suspicion of developing oedema often aborts attacks. Fresh plasma, containing C_1 esterase, therefore, may be given before surgery or at the initiation of an attack. Unlike other forms of chronic urticaria, adrenaline, antihistamines and corticosteroids are of only a little benefit. Trasylol intravenously is an inhibitor of proteases and is sometimes helpful, as is epsilon aminocaproic acid 12 to 18 g daily in divided dosage. The most effective treatment is danazol. This may be supplemented by fresh plasma during an attack or, if available, C_1 esterase inhibitor concentrate.

REFERENCES

Champion, R.H. (1992). Urticaria. In *Textbook of dermatology,* (5th edn), (ed. A. Rook, D.S. Wilkinson, and F.J.G. Ebling, pp. 1865–80. Blackwell Scientific Publications, Oxford

Czarnetzi, B.M., Meentken, J., Rosenbach, T., and Pokropp, A. (1984). Clinical, pharmacological and immunological aspects of delayed pressure urticaria. *British Journal of Dermatology* **111,** 315–23.

Grattan, C.E.H., Francis, D.M., Slater, N.G.P., Barlow, R.J., and Greaves, M.W. (1992). Plasmapheresis for severe, unremitting, chronic urticaria. *Lancet,* **339,**1078–80.

Gressler, R.B., Sowel, K., and Huston, D.P. (1989). Therapy of chronic idiopathic urticaria and Nifedipine; demonstration of beneficial effect in a double-blind placebo controlled study. *Journal of Allergy and Clinical Immunology* **83,** 756–63.

Henquet, C.J.M., Martons, B.P.M., and Van Vloten, W.A. (1992). Cold urticaria; A clinico-therapeutic study in 30 patients; with special emphasis on cold desensitization. *European Journal of Dermatology,* **2,** 75–7.

Kaplan, A.P. (1984). Exercise induced hives. *Journal of Allergy and Clinical Immunology* **73,** 704–7.

Rubenstein, H.S. (1982). Bee sting diseases, who is at risk? What is the treatment? *Lancet* **i,** 496–9.

Tatnall, F.M., Gaylarde, P.M., and Sarkany, I. (1984). Localized heat urticaria and its management. *Clinical and Experimental Dermatology* **9,** 367–374.

Cutaneous vasculitis

The broadest definition of vasculitis is the response of small blood vessels to injury. No other definition encompasses its great variety, which ranges from a transient increase in permeability or wealing, to coagulation and necrosis of the vessel wall. It is due to agents such as immune complexes, toxins, or to physical stimuli such as cold and heat, as well as impaired perfusion.

The term 'vasculitis' includes many diseases described elsewhere in this book, such as Henoch–Schönlein purpura, polyarteritis nodosa, nodular vasculitis, Wegener's granulomatosis, hypersensitivity angiitis, and allergic granulomatosis. Examples of diseases that are sometimes included within this term are Behçet's syndrome, pyoderma gangrenosum, purpura fulminans, thromboangiitis obliterans, erythema nodosum, chilblains, atrophie blanche, and livedo reticularis. There are many other named variants, the separate recognition of which is no longer helpful, except to communicate with people who have already learned such terms and formed an opinion of what they represent, for example, non-suppurative panniculitis of Weber–Christian.

Vasculitis overlaps with urticaria and with infarction or gangrene. To use some of the older terminology, some authors have described urticaria as the predominant feature of Henoch–Schönlein purpura in children, and there have been a number of more recently described vasculitic syndromes in which urticaria is the only skin manifestation. At the other end of the spectrum necrotizing angiitis and polyarteritis nodosa are labels often given to infarctive or more destructive patterns of vasculitis.

The physical signs of skin disease are more or less recognizable as distinct patterns. The names they have been given are of dubious value when it comes to managing the disease. It is possible to explain these patterns and to decide what aspects of the physical signs are the most useful clues to pathogenesis.

PATHOLOGY AND NOMENCLATURE

When a vessel is injured there follows a response which removes or neutralizes the cause of the injury; this is followed by repair. The response depends on the intensity of the injury, on the efficiency of the inflammation, and on the rate and effectiveness of the repair. Herein lies one of the main reasons why a particular injury does not always produce the same rash. The inflammatory response is a very complex sequence of events (Fig. 91) subject to considerable modification by each individual's particular range of mediators. Important factors explaining variability are local tissue architecture and previous experience. Scarring or even temporary exhaustion of mediators by prior injury alters the sequence of events that follow further injury. Formerly authors used to

describe sites of lowered resistance: we now know that such sites comprise areas of non-homogeneous blood supply with hypoxia, leakiness, and blood stasis as well as exhausted mast cells and endothelial cells undergoing various stages of repair or upgrading of cell wall adhesion factors for white cells. Paralysis of the mononuclear phagocytic system is also important.

This variation in the inflammatory response can be superficial or deep and it is modified by the distribution of the injury—gravitational, light exposed, cold exposed, or at sites of pressure or abrasion; this is one explanation of the physical signs that make up classifiable rashes. It is perhaps not surprising that the French used terms like *maladie trisymptome* or *penta symptome* to describe a rash that had urticarial, purpuric, nodular, pigmented, and necrotic lesions; when morphology was all that could be described it was better not to give an eponymous name to any particular combination of physical signs.

Another reason for the later delineation of different syndromes such as Behçet's triad, cutaneous polyarteritis nodosa, or limited Wegener's granulomatosis was the recognition that vasculitis may be confined to either one or more organs. But this, too, is of dubious value: Behçet described mouth, eye, and genital lesions, but the disease is as often more widespread; Wegener's granulomatosis affects the respiratory tract but skin and kidney are frequently affected.

One other point of debate is the value of the term arteritis. Smooth muscle in the arterial wall is damaged by ischaemia and in most small vessels this is due to vasoconstriction, coagulation, and thrombosis, or to obstructed flow due to more distal vasculitis. Thus malignant hypertension, coagulation, embolism (Fig. 92), thrombotic thrombocytopenia, or vasculitis are often sufficiently appropriate diagnostic terms and are more helpful when considering prognosis, aetiology, or management. The histological diagnosis of arteritis is similarly unsatisfactory. Damaged venules can themselves look like small arteries and even when an artery is clearly involved it is rarely possible in the same section to see the more distal vasculitis responsible for the obstruction to blood flow and consequent ischaemia.

HARMFUL AGENTS RESPONSIBLE FOR VASCULITIS

Immune complexes, infective agents, drugs, food additives, and circulating particulate matter all injure blood vessels. It is probable that these

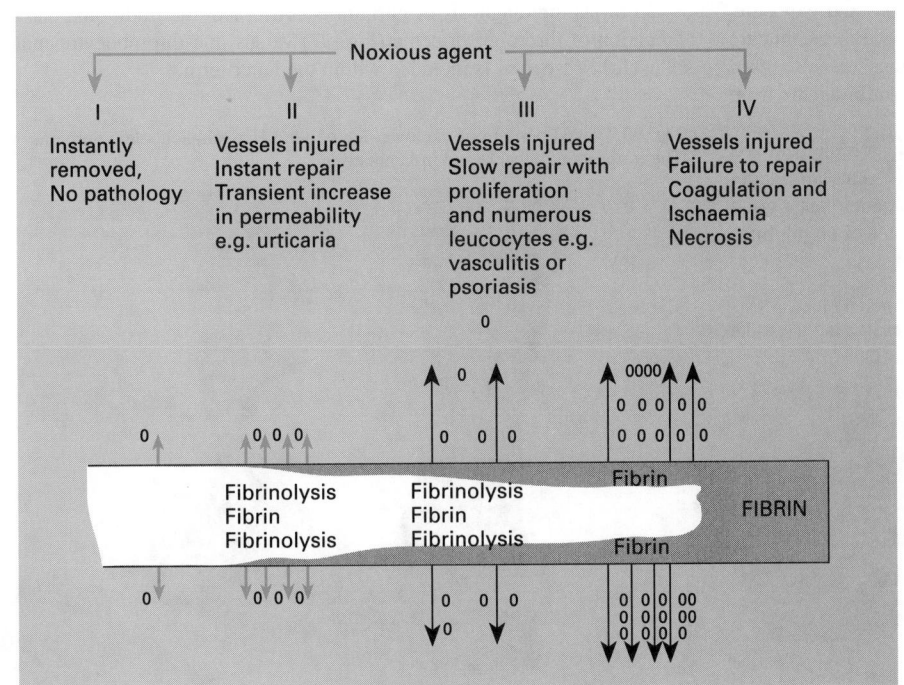

Fig. 91 A spectrum of inflammatory events ranging from a transient wealing or almost physiological permeability through inflammatory neutrophilic infiltration and oedema to complete necrosis of the vessel, due to thrombosis, and coagulation or destruction of its wall.

are present in small amounts in all of us some of the time, but it is likely that the injuries are often so mild as to be imperceptible and quickly repaired.

Immune complexes

The 'defensive' system which clears antigens includes complexing them with antibody and complement to make phagocytosis by macrophages more inevitable. It is a system which is used to remove damaged tissue and it is often difficult to distinguish whether damage preceded or is a consequence of the immune complex. It is the process of complexing that activates complement not the complex itself. Free and poorly complexed antigen may indeed have the greater potential to damage than the well-complexed material. Trapping of antigen in a tissue and its exposure to immunoglobulin and complement is determined by local events having little to do with what circulates in the bloodstream.

Immune complexes follow the ingestion of food, the presence of a fetus in the pregnant, or invasion of the body by parasites such as scabies, or by a neoplasm such as breast cancer, or can be demonstrated in everyone following the most mild of virus infections. For this reason, the mere demonstration of immune complexes is not enough to blame them for coincidental vasculitis. Excess of antigen is released when infections are overwhelming or tissues are broken down by immune attack or neoplasia and sometimes as a consequence of food or drugs.

Immune complexes are mostly harmless but become harmful when they are of certain size and shape or composition. Actual harm is observed only when, and as, they are localized at a site ill-equipped to deal with them and slow to repair the damage done by them.

Often an alteration in host response prevents adequate neutralization of even mildly noxious agents. Recent exposure to similar noxious agents, exhaustion, and insufficient time for recovery of fibrinolytic mechanisms or the phagocytic potential and the secretions of the mononuclear phagocytic system explain why repeated or continuous exposure to harmful agents precipitates vasculitis. Such an explanation most often explains localized recrudescence in the nose, in Wegener's granulomatosis, or in legs affected by gravitational eczema, ulcers, or atrophie blanche. Factors such as severe infection, foods, drugs, diseases promoting coagulation (e.g. hepatitis), and malignancy often alter the inflammatory response and need not act as specific triggers. Immune complexes circulating in a patient known to have disseminated lupus erythematosus may suddenly become damaging when any of these other factors affect the patient. The localization of the defective inflammatory process is often determined by environmental factors: cold exposure, abrasion, or pressure on the skin causing mild stasis and ischaemia are well-known examples met clinically; these conditions are also used experimentally to demonstrate the localization of harmful agents from the bloodstream.

In recent years the discovery of congenital defects in complement and other protease inhibitors has explained why harmful agents are inadequately neutralized in some people; hereditary angio-oedema is a good example of such a disease. There is a congenital absence of an inhibitor of complement but only in certain circumstances is this important. Trauma or infection sets off the sequence of events which in this case includes the activation of complement by plasmin, dependent in its turn upon the secretion of plasminogen activator by damaged endothelium. Normally this is balanced by other inhibitors and by absorption into small amounts of fibrinogen and fibrin.

Local deficiencies in the sequence of events triggered by injury depend upon blood flow and diffusion, not only of activators but also of inhibitors. Injury usually releases activators of fibrinolysis from endothelium and heparin, histamine, and hyaluronidase, amongst other things, from adjacent mast cells. These increase permeability and diffusion but prevent coagulation and the activation of complement. Repeated inoculation of histamine can itself cause vasculitis. It is not always necessary to invoke an immunological mechanism. When the mast cells and endothelium are more or less exhausted and when activating or inhibiting products are released by adjacent epidermal injury the proteases, complement, kinins, and materials like fibrin or C reactive substance occur in sufficient quantities to perpetuate the inflammation and attract white cells in large numbers.

DIAGNOSIS

Almost essential to the diagnosis is purpura (Fig. 93), but an urticarial lesion that is tender, lasts for more than 12 hours, and leaves a slight bruise on resolution falls within the term vasculitis (Fig. 94). The histology of such a lesion often shows more perivascular neutrophils than the common short-lasting urticarial weal. At the other end of the spectrum is obliterative or sclerosing thromboangiitis in which total occlusion of a small vessel often prevents exudation, and because there is no neutrophilic infiltrate, there may not be such acute destruction of the vessel wall. A similar appearance may be observed in DIC (Fig. 95) and in platelet embolic diseases.

Vasculitis affecting deep dermis or fat and subcutaneous tissues most commonly produces a nodule, sometimes with redness or violaceous skin overlying it. Blistering and pustulation, when they occur as manifestations of vasculitis, are usually part of a superficial polymorphic eruption in which at least some of the lesions are palpable purpura, distinguishing the eruption from other more monomorphic blistering diseases. These physical signs are illustrated in Fig. 96. Very heavy infiltration with eosinophils is a feature of eosinophilic cellulitis which is sometimes a reaction to arthropod bites.

So far as the diagnosis of purpura is concerned, the traditional classification of thrombocytopenia (Fig. 97) versus non-thrombocytopenia is useful. Vasculitis is included within the latter term.

Fig. 93 Typical purpura of the lower leg of adult Henoch–Schönlein purpura. The lesions are palpable and inflammatory.

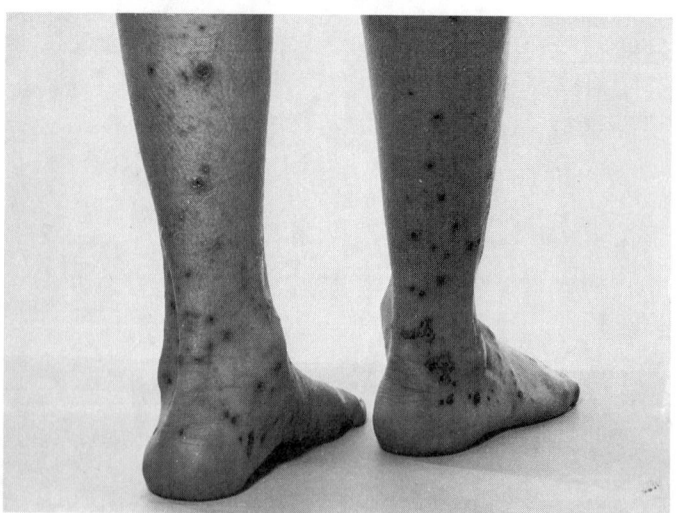

Fig. 92 The white infarct characteristic of embolization or arterial block. Most cutaneous vasculitis that is labelled as arteritis is, in fact, venular, but the white infarct is characteristic of arterial occlusion.

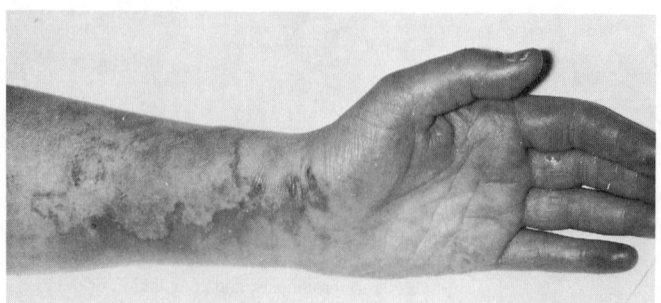

Fig. 94 Typical urticarial initial lesion of vasculitis, often proceeding to purpura and later to necrosis. However, in some types, hypocomplementaemic vasculitis, a persistent urticaria, is the only lesion.

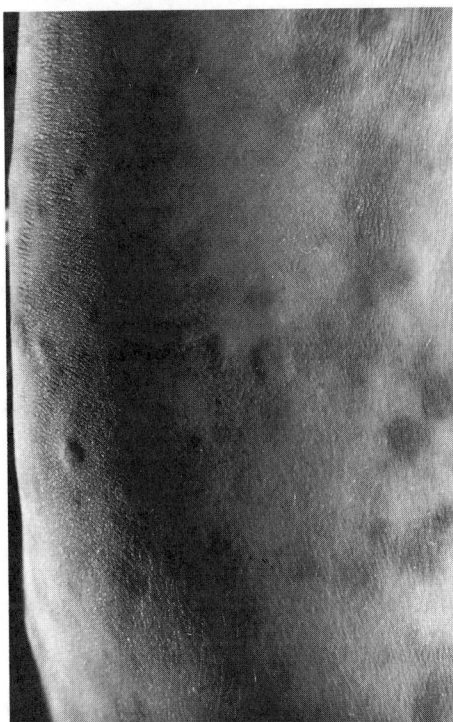

Vasculitis in which immune complexes have played a causative role is more likely to be leucocytoclastic—a term used to describe numerous disrupted neutrophils at the site of the damaged vessel (Fig. 98). It is now well recognized that a mononuclear variety of vasculitis also occurs which is sometimes termed lymphocytic vasculitis and in which complement activation seems less significant but upgrading of cell wall

Fig. 96 The presence of blisters in vasculitis is due to the intensity of the oedema in the upper dermis; sometimes it is due to necrosis.

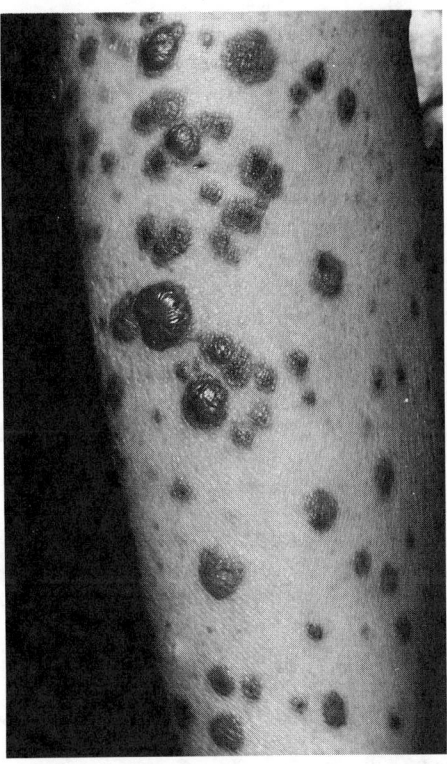

Fig. 95 The blue to black discoloration of the extremities in disseminated intravascular coagulation.

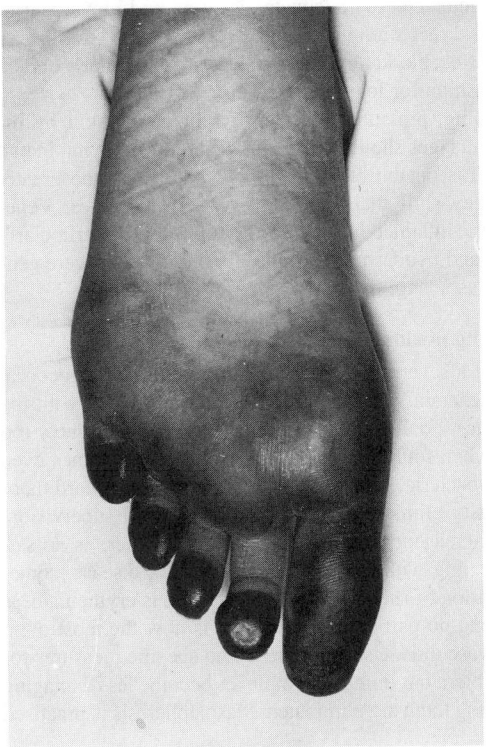

Fig. 97 Bruising or ecchymosis is most commonly due to thrombocytopenic purpura, but it is also a feature of the painful bruising syndrome.

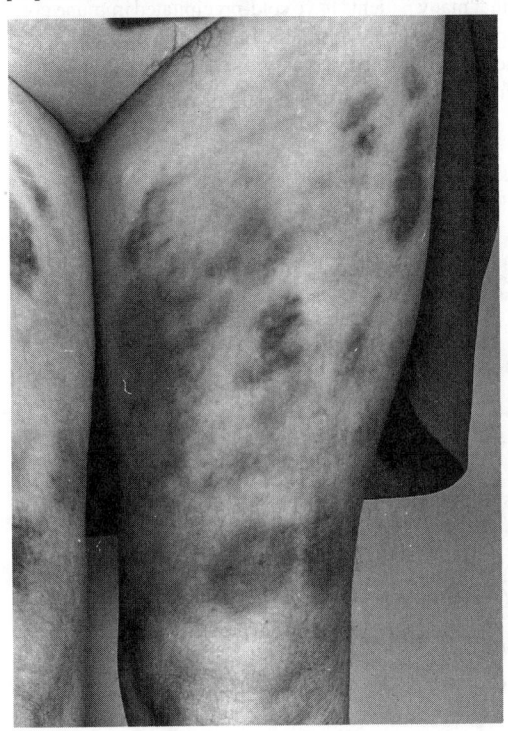

adhesion factors is a response to cytokines and other pharmacological agents, such as histamine. It is a feature of drug eruptions and also of damage to vessels sometimes prior to the deposition of immune complexes, i.e. within 2 h of a cutaneous capillary fragility test. In fact macrophages rather than lymphocytes could be the more injurious infiltrate, depending on the stage of maturation and their secretion. Much of the pathology of vasculitis is that of ischaemia. Whatever the cause of the damage to the vessel, there is usually some impairment of blood flow. Hypoxia and infarction are quite capable of causing equally extensive pathology.

The significance of eosinophils in some forms of vasculitis is not known and they are no guide to prognosis or therapy.

DETECTION OF CAUSE

From the patients' point of view the most worthwhile investigation is that which results in improved management. Specialist units have the additional role of exploration to advance understanding. Certain noxious agents should always be looked for in order to eliminate them. Bacteria are the most important of these: the streptococcal sore throat is still the commonest precursor of vasculitis in children and otitis media, dental caries, cystitis, and sinusitis occasionally play a role; in many countries tuberculosis or leprosy is the commonest cause; bacterial endocarditis and meningococcal septicaemia are often missed. Other treatable infections occasionally causing vasculitis are syphilis, neisseria, rickettsiae, and mycoplasma. Although viruses usually cannot be eliminated, any history of a recent flu-like illness or vaccination may be relevant. Hepatitis B virus is a well-recognized cause.

Lupus erythematosus and rheumatoid arthritis are common causes of immune complex vasculitis. But, as mentioned above, it is the exposure of antigen so that its complexing can activate complement that is important, not the complex itself.

Drugs such as penicillin and sulphonamides have often been incriminated but many other drugs appear less likely to be allergens than modifiers of the host response. Similarly, some foods may act as allergens and others have a more obscure enhancing action. Enquiries should be directed towards headache pills, throat lozenges, purgatives, health foods, any medicine given for a specific illness, and any recent intake of food or drugs to which the patient is known to be sensitive.

It is now clear that many patients have cold-precipitated immune complexes and perhaps even more have soluble immune complexes that are localized by blood stasis due to cold, pressure, vasoconstriction, or prior inflammation. The number of patients in whom an antigen has been

isolated is small and in still fewer has it been possible to eliminate the antigen, except in the case of bacteria sensitive to antibiotics. It is not particularly helpful to find a cryoglobulin; it does not alter management since every patient should be kept warm in any case. One of the difficulties is that it is often the antibody to the infective agent that in its turn becomes recognized as foreign. Infection may initiate this problem but after elimination of the organism the antibody persists as an autoantigen.

FACTORS THAT MODIFY THE INFLAMMATORY RESPONSE

These are very numerous and include any known chronic illness, such as malnutrition, diabetes mellitus, blood disorders, rheumatoid arthritis or other forms of collagen disease, chronic respiratory disease, disorders of the bowels or liver, and hypertension. Malignancy, whether carcinoma or lymphoma, is a not unusual factor and recent surgery, pregnancy, and unusual anxiety are also included.

The mechanisms involved include coagulation and thrombosis, and since these are treatable, a full blood count should always include a platelet count and other simple relevant tests, especially estimation of prothrombin time, fibrinogen titre, and fibrin degradation products.

PROGNOSIS

The difficulty of naming a constellation of physical signs may force the physician to produce labels which traditionally are linked to a poor prognosis. One example is the term polyarteritis nodosa, another Wegener's granulomatosis.

For all patterns it is useful to use the term vasculitis supplemented by the terms 'limited' or 'local' implying a mild process affecting one locale or organ and 'complicated' meaning severe and affecting many organs. Such adjectives, by describing the severity of the disease, give a lead to its management.

MANAGEMENT
Avoid all further injury

This allows healing to take place and prevents further damage to already inflamed tissue. Rest is essential for all acute inflammation but blood stasis should be counteracted by adequate elevation and movement of the limbs. Cold and direct sunlight should also be avoided since both injure the skin and affect blood flow. Female legs are particularly at risk, depending on the fashion for long or short skirts or trousers.

Scratching, pinching, pressure, and constriction of the skin by ill-fitting clothing or bandages should not be allowed. Patients lying in bed will develop vasculitis on the buttocks, elbows, and over the greater trochanter unless they shift their position every few minutes. Venepuncture sites become inflamed in some forms of vasculitis, particularly in Behçet's disease and pyoderma gangrenosum but also in severe generalized leucocytoclastic angiitis.

Eliminate circulating noxious agents especially if antigens

Vasculitis following a severe streptococcal sore throat, meningococcal or gonococcal septicaemia, or tuberculosis should be treated with the appropriate antibiotics. Foci of infection, once so popular, are now too rarely thought of; when found they need elimination, sometimes even by surgery. Certain bacterial diseases, such as bacterial endocarditis or leprosy, are not easily eliminated and require prolonged supervision. Viral diseases are increasingly incriminated but as yet there is no satisfactory way of dealing with them. Immune complex disease, sometimes as a manifestation of rheumatoid arthritis or lupus erythematosus but more often having no particular association, is now the most often suspected cause of vasculitis. Usually there are no specific measures for dealing with the problem but immune complexes become less damaging if the factors localizing them are eliminated. Plasmapheresis is practised

Fig. 98 A damaged vessel surrounded by broken-up neutrophils is typical of the hypocomplementaemic pattern of vasculitis.

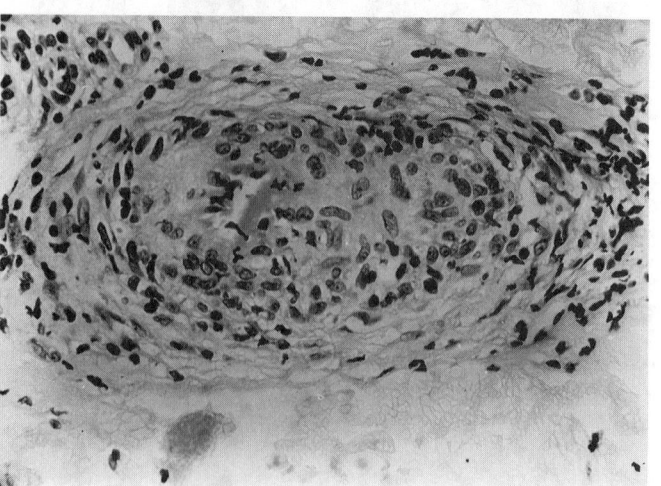

by a few specialized units. Drugs and food thought to be responsible can be omitted.

Provide specific treatment

Acute short-lasting itchy weals often respond to antihistamines. Acute tender swelling due to progressive tissue oedema may need steroids. Painful swollen joints, acute optic neuritis, temporal (giant cell) arteritis, erythema nodosum, tender persistent weals, and tense painful swellings at the edge of pyoderma gangrenosum all usually respond to corticosteroids.

Fulminant vasculitis affecting more than one organ and brought about by a known trigger (allergens, drugs), should be covered by steroids once the cause has been eliminated. Immunosuppressive drugs such as azathioprine, cyclophosphamide, and methotrexate are used as a last resort in persistent chronic vasculitis but they are of doubtful value except in granulomatous forms affecting the lung, in which they are the treatment of choice. Necrosis and gangrene are usually due to ischaemia. While inflammation alone may account for this in small vessels supplying superficial lesions, hypertension, coagulation, and thrombosis, as well as the cause of cardiac or peripheral vascular disease in general, sometimes underlie large areas of necrosis. The causes of vasculitis are also, for the most part, the causes of local or disseminated intravascular coagulation. Heparin is probably the drug of choice when fibrinogen, platelets, and prothrombin have been consumed and fibrin degradation products are raised. It is probably the most useful anticoagulant in malignant disease. Aspirin's anti-inflammatory effect is well known and is particularly effective when platelet aggregation is suspected. Dapsone, enhancers of fibrinolysis, and potassium iodide have had their successes and failures in recurrent nodular forms of vasculitis. Good management includes advice on smoking, oral contraception, high blood pressure, and hyperlipidaemia. The prognosis depends on complications: particularly important are those affecting the eyes, central nervous system, and kidneys. Examination of the eyes for papilloedema and of the urine for red cells, protein, and casts is imperative.

Fig. 99 Tender erythematous swelling on the front of the legs with ill-defined borders is characteristic of erythema nodosum.

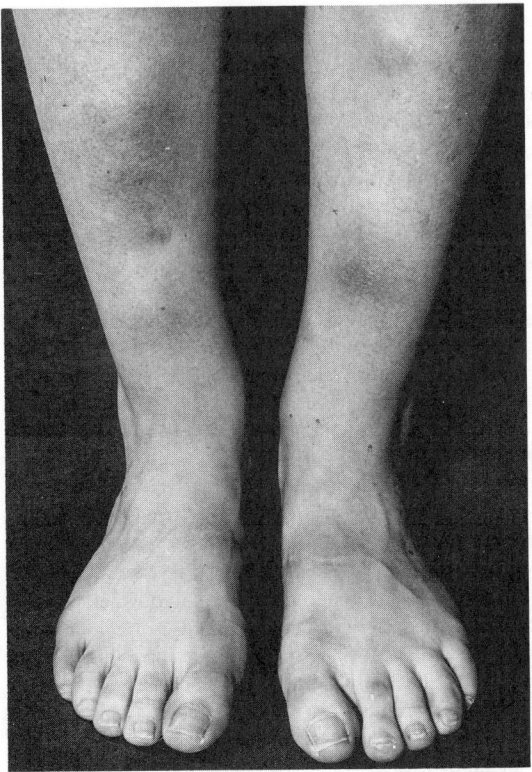

Table 26 *Some causes of erythema nodosum*

Streptococcus	Blastomycosis
Tuberculosis	Coccidioidomycosis
Sarcoidosis	Trichophyton verrucosum
Lymphogranuloma venereum	Ulcerative colitis
Cat scratch disease	Crohn's disease
Ornithosis	Leukaemia
Epstein–Barr virus	Hodgkin's disease
Tularaemia	Sulphonamides
Histoplasmosis	Bromides
Yersinia	Pregnancy and contraceptive pill
Leprosy	

Erythema nodosum

It is convenient to include erythema nodosum under the heading vasculitis though some still prefer to call it panniculitis. There is injury to small blood vessels in the deep dermis and subcutaneous tissue but primary injury to the blood vessels from a noxious agent, such as soluble immune complexes, is difficult to prove: it is characterized by tender red swellings on the front of the shins (Fig. 99) and often also on the thighs and forearms. Bruising is common but necrosis, scarring, and atrophy of the tissues is not a feature.

Erythema nodosum is a reaction pattern to infection (viral, bacterial, and mycotic) and sometimes to drugs. Neoplasia, pregnancy, and sarcoidosis are other causes. The causes are listed in Table 26. By far the commonest is a streptococcal sore throat. Sarcoidosis and tuberculosis are common causes where the incidence of these diseases is high. In teaching hospital practice ulcerative colitis and Crohn's disease are common associations. Worldwide, erythema nodosum is commonly due to lepromatous leprosy. This is a widespread and often very persistent reaction to local antigen and is not typical of erythema nodosum in general. It may become pustular and necrotic. Erythema nodosum is often preceded by or accompanied by fever, malaise, fatigue, loss of weight, and arthralgia. Although it sometimes resolves in 2 to 3 weeks, persistent and recurrent forms over several months may suggest an alternative diagnosis. It is important not to label the disease as polyarteritis nodosa or rheumatic fever, for instance, merely because it is persistent and the patient is ill for several months, or the blood sedimentation rate is unusually high. The number, size, and chronicity of the lesions is variable. They can be few and as large as the hand or multiple and the size of the thumb nail. They can be acute, tender, and last only a few days, or they can be chronic, less tender, and migratory, tending to heal in the centre and spread peripherally as a swollen ring. The more chronic lesions are less red and may be violaceous or any of the colours of a resolving bruise. The front of the leg is a site of poor lymphatic drainage where foreign protein and bacteria are only slowly removed, especially in the deep dermis and adipose tissue. The underlying tibia splints the overlying tissue so that massage of the lymphatics is reduced. Pretibial cellulitis, pretibial myxoedema, and erythema nodosum have similar localizing factors explaining their pathogenesis.

INVESTIGATIONS

A chase for the source of infection should include a history of possible contacts at home and abroad, human or other animal. Chest radiography is essential and the most useful for the diagnosis of sarcoid or tuberculosis. A fall in blood sedimentation rate which is often initially above 100 mm/h is a useful guide to complete recovery.

ANTINEUTROPHIL CYTOPLASMIC ANTIBODIES

During the last decade the detection of antineutrophil cytoplasmic antibodies (ANCA) has become a useful guide to prognosis and management. They occur in those forms of systemic vasculitis such as Wegener's granulomatosis which respond to cyclophosphamide in addition to prednisolone. They may play a part in the pathogenesis of neutrophil induced vascular damage. Subtyping and serum levels provide a guide to disease severity and response to therapy.

TREATMENT

This is one of the diseases in which ultimate recovery is to be expected. While for the first 2 to 3 weeks it is possible to keep the patient at rest and to prescribe acetyl salicylic acid, the difficult period is often several weeks after the initial illness when the patients have to be mobilized. Firm support bandages or stockings give some relief for persistent aching and swelling of the legs. Steroids reduce swelling and fever but do not affect the length of the illness.

Pyoderma gangrenosum

As the name implies this is a necrosis of the tissues often with a heavy neutrophilic infiltrate but it is not primarily an infection, rather it is a reaction pattern in which venous and capillary engorgement, haemorrhage, and coagulation feature prominently. The exact pathogenesis is uncertain. In many cases there is an associated depression of the immune system demonstrable by *in vitro* and clinical tests. Failure of macrophages to respond to tissue injury or to clear noxious agents is another feature. Its associations are an important guide to its possible causation. These include ulcerative colitis, Crohn's disease, particularly of the colon, rheumatoid arthritis, seronegative arthritis with paraproteinaemia, Wegener's granulomatosis, and plasma cell dyscrasias including myeloma. A bullous variety is associated with leukaemia, primary thrombocythaemia, and with myelofibrosis. Nevertheless, up to half of the cases seen in dermatology clinics have no significant association. The clinical features are initially varied but all ultimately become turgid and ulcerate. They include a tender red or blue nodule suggestive of erythema nodosum, vesico pustules, or an acneiform folliculitis. The swollen red or blue edge is often acutely tender; blistering may be considerable, especially in the leukaemic variety. The necrosis follows no particular pattern and, like a carbuncle, may have multiple centres. It is usually undermined, and exuberant granulation tissue sprouts from the base of the ulcer. The calves, thighs, buttocks, abdomen, and face are favoured but no site is immune.

There is considerable toxicity associated with the acute varieties. Dermatologists see the chronic variety which is not obviously associated with underlying disease and in which the general health of the patient is not impaired. The ulcerated lesions are not necessarily tender but they are irregular and persistent often for years. Dermatitis artefacta is often suspected and the personality of the patient disabled for many months may be consequently affected and encourage the suspicion. Synergistic gangrene is one cause of very similar acute pathology. Unlike pyoderma gangrenosum which is often multiple, synergistic gangrene is more clearly associated with a recent wound, such as an operation on the gastrointestinal tract, and the area of gangrene is solitary and an extension of the wound. From any form of pyoderma gangrenosum, aerobic and anaerobic bacterial culture, amoebiasis, tuberculosis, buruli ulcer, and deep fungus infections such as nocardiosis or blastomycosis should be considered.

The treatment of choice is high-dose corticosteroids by mouth. The management of underlying diseases such as ulcerative colitis or leukaemia is essential. Any suspicion of an infective causation such as amoebiasis requires the appropriate investigations and treatment. For cases responding poorly to steroids, dapsone 100 mg daily or clofazimine is worth a try. Colchicine, cyclophosphomide, and cyclosporin have their advocates. There are subacute presentations that respond to locally applied steroids by inoculation or under an occlusive dressing.

Table 27 *Clinical features of Behçet's disease*

Aphthous stomatitis	
Ulceration of genitalia	The triad of Behçet
Iritis and uveitis	
Thrombophlebitis	
Erythema nodosum	
Pustules or folliculitis	Common associations
Arthritis	
Thrombosis of large veins including superior and inferior vena cava and sagittal sinus	
Arterial aneurysms	
Orchitis	
Ulcerative colitis	
Splenomegaly	
Glomerulonephritis (very rare)	
Sjögren's syndrome	

Behçet's disease

The combination of large ulcers in the perineum and mouth with severe iritis and blindness is a distinct syndrome mostly described in Turkey and Israel. In Japan, the ocular manifestations are the most prominent. In many other parts of the world the disease is much less well defined. Even where it is prominent other associated symptoms and signs are common and it is these that seem to present in the United Kingdom. Often in the absence of the full triad of Behçet's description, arthritis and vascular complications such as thrombophlebitis in the legs, are particularly common but there are numerous references to arterial and venous pathology which include large vessels in the thorax or skull (Table 27).

In severe cases ulceration is extensive and deep but mild aphthous ulceration is sufficient to make the diagnosis in the presence of other members of the triad. The classic triad does not always occur together and it is quite common to have to rely on a history of relatively transient mouth, eye, or genital involvement. However, over a number of years it would be unusual for mouth or genital ulceration to be absent if persistent 'vasculitis' or eye signs were due to the disease. The cause of the disease remains unclear but the long-held belief that it is in part genetic is supported by the finding of the HLA-B5 associated with ocular manifestations. A viral aetiology is unproven but this, as well as environmental pollutants, has its advocates.

With vascular complications so common, the search for a basis of thrombosis or coagulation has not distinguished between cause and effect. Certainly fibrinolysis is often grossly impaired, as is platelet aggregation. The finding of circulating soluble immune complexes in Behçet's disease is probably more an indication of tissue damage than of causation.

A peculiar sign shared with pyoderma gangrenosum is the hyperreactivity of the skin to minor injury such as venepuncture. About one-third of patients develop an inflammatory papule or pustule within 24 h of trauma sufficient to damage the small vessels in the dermis.

The treatment of this disease is unsatisfactory. Acute and severe ulceration or iritis should be given the chance to respond to systemic steroids. Some respond rapidly whereas others have a persistent and uncontrolled disease. The same is true of fibrinolytic therapy with phenformin 50 mg twice daily and ethyloestrenol 2 mg four times daily, stanozolol 5 mg twice daily, or streptokinase infusions. Colchicine 1 to 2 mg daily is the latest therapy for which some success is claimed. Minocycline 100 mg daily is worth a trial. It is popular therapy in Japan and South Korea where streptococcal infection is believed to act as an antigen.

REFERENCES

Burrows, N.P. and Lockwood, C.M. (1995). Antineutrophil cytoplasmic antibodies and their relevance to the dermatologist. *British Journal of Dermatology,* **132,** 173–81.

Hickman, J.G. and Lazarus, G.S. (1979). Pyoderma gangrenosum: new concepts, etiology, and treatment. In *Dermatology update,* (ed. S.L. Moschella), pp. 325–42. Elsevier, New York.

Jeannette, C.J. and Falk, R.J. (1994). Vasculitis affecting the skin: a review. *Archives of Dermatology,* **130,** 899–906.

Osler, W. (1914). The visceral lesions of purpura and allied conditions. *British Medical Journal* **i,** 517.

Ryan, T.J. (1976). *Microvascular injury; vasculitis, stasis and ischaemia.* Lloyd Luke, London.

Ryan, T.J. (1992). Cutaneous vasculitis. In *Textbook of dermatology,* (5th edn) (ed. A. Rook, D.S. Wilkinson, and F.J.G. Ebling), pp. 1893–962. Blackwell Scientific Publications, Oxford.

Wiggins, R.C. and Cochrane, C.G. (1981). Current concepts in immunology. Immune complex mediated biologic effects. *New England Journal of Medicine* **304.**

Wolff, K. and Winkelmann, R.K. (1980). *Vasculitis.* Lloyd Luke, London.

Yankey, K.M. and Lawley, T.J. (1984). Circulating immune complexes and their immunochemistry, biology and detection in selected dermatologic and systemic diseases. *Journal of the American Academy of Dermatology* **10,** 711–31.

Vesico-blistering diseases

A vesicle is an elevated circumscribed lesion filled with serum and sometimes blood and pus. It is usually no larger than 0.5 cm in diameter. Above this size a vesicle is called a bulla or blister.

PREDISPOSING FACTORS

These include congenital diseases such as epidermolysis bullosa or metabolic disorders such as porphyria.

CAUSES

Friction or minor knocks can produce blisters in the predisposed or at sites unaccustomed to wear and tear. The hands and feet are most often affected. Friction is increased by damp, sweating skin.

Ischaemia

Prolonged pressure obliterating blood supply for more than 2 h causes damage to the smooth muscle of small arterioles and underlying fat. The epidermis can survive more than 6 hours of ischaemia and in cool skin with a decreased metabolism much longer periods may be survived. The unconscious or those with sensory loss, especially from barbiturate poisoning, are particularly vulnerable but most cases occur from peripheral vascular disease with acute interference of blood supply.

Acute sweat pore occlusion

This occurs especially with fever or in hot climates. Numerous small transparent vesicles are seen especially in the flexures or in parts of the body in which the stratum corneum is unduly thick are usually affected. In the fingers or feet this is called pompholyx.

Burns

Burns can occur from cold (Fig. 100) as in frostbite or from cryotherapy, heat, or ultraviolet irradiation (photosensitivity from plants, porphyria, or pellagra) (Fig. 101). Dermatitis artefacta is often induced by burning the skin; it is clearly self-induced but usually denied and is often a bizarre pattern. Cigarette burns are amongst the commonest induced lesions.

Chemicals

These may be toxic, as from mustard gas or cantharidin. Sometimes an allergic dermatitis from contact also produces vesicles due to separation of the epidermal cells by inflammatory oedema. Plant dermatitis is amongst the most common cause; due to, for example, the primula in Europe and poison ivy in the United States.

Fixed drug eruptions

These can cause erythema and blistering and appear and reappear at the same site whenever the causative drug is ingested; usually there is itching within 6 h of ingestion.

Fig. 100 Urticarial lesions, in this case due to cold; they often blister, especially on the lower legs.

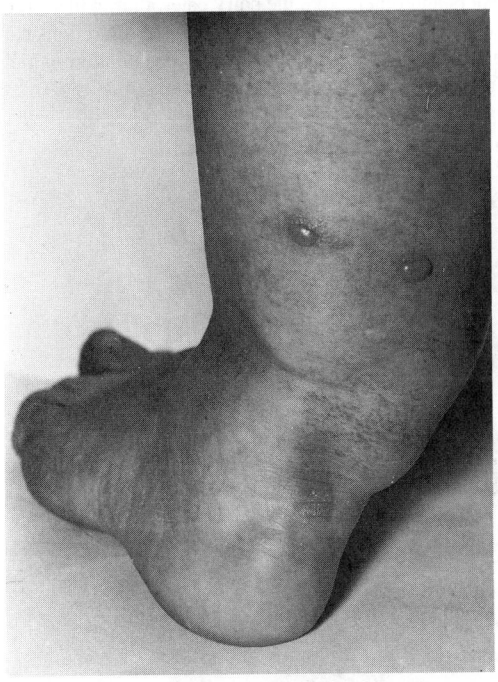

Fig. 101 Blistering on the front of the neck due to an ultraviolet light burn. Self-induced by a home lamp.

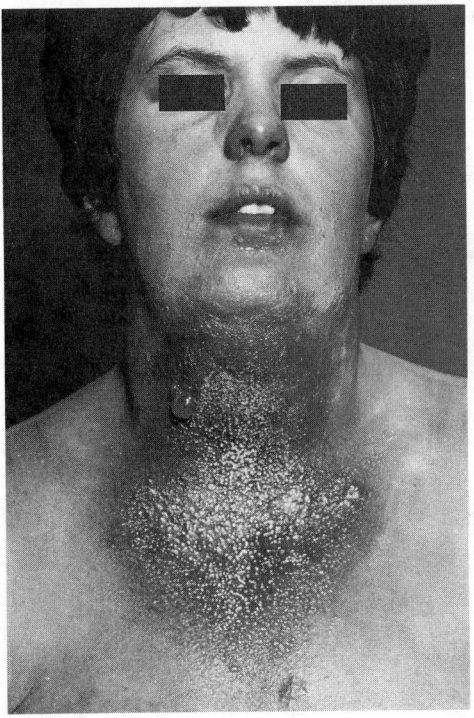

INFECTIONS

(See under appropriate sections.) Viral disorders including herpes simplex (Fig. 102), zoster, chicken pox, and smallpox, or bacterial diseases most commonly cause blisters, particularly the staphyloccus and streptococcus.

Fungus infections commonly present as blistering on the soles of the feet, and insect bites give rise to papular urticaria which often blisters on the lower legs (Fig. 103). Blisters, pruritus, and fever have been described in ornithologists bitten by ticks carried by marine birds on the Middle East coastline. Arthropods, like the brown recluse spider, give rise to necrotic blisters and others, like the hairy caterpillar, will secrete a toxin in its hairs, which can produce blistering. Some infarctions can produce a vasculitis or disseminated intravascular coagulation, which may also present as vesicular or haemorrhagic blisters.

Fig. 102 Blisters on the cheek due to herpes simplex virus.

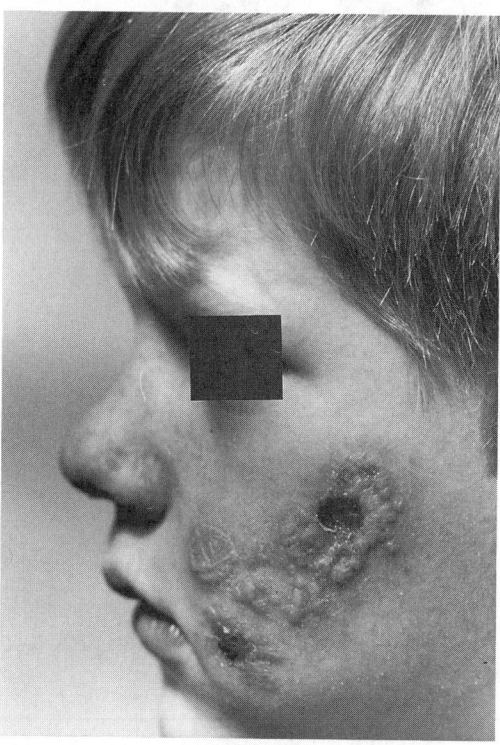

Fig. 103 Typical multiple blisters due to insect bites in the rainy season in India.

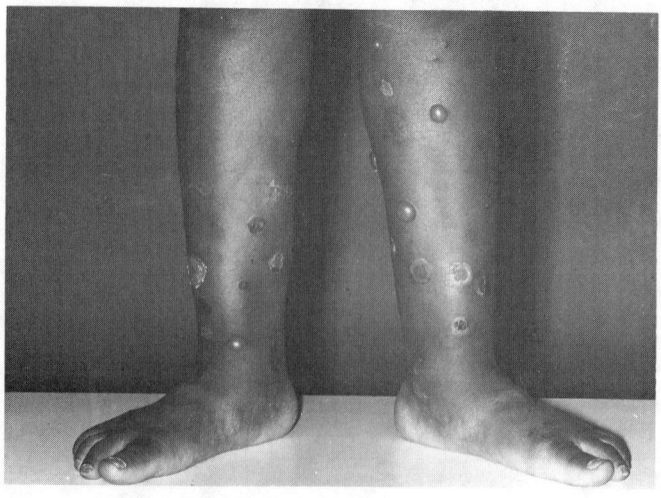

Specific skin disorders

Erythema multiforme

This, as the name implies, can present with a variety of patterns. The classic pattern affects the hands and feet more than the trunk and the lesions have an erythematous and coin-shaped presentation which is more intense and blistering in the centre—a target-shaped lesion (see Fig. 11(b)). Several toxic erythematous eruptions overlap with the classic pattern and sometimes the classic distribution and even the target lesions are missing. Involvement of the mucosa is common so that mouth, eyes, and genitalia may be affected in varying degrees. Where the blistering and mucosal lesions are severe, the disease is termed Stevens–Johnson syndrome (Fig. 104). This is usually associated with high fever and sometimes also anterior uveitis, pneumonia, renal failure, polyarthritis, or diarrhoea.

AETIOLOGY

In 50 per cent of these cases the cause is not known. For the rest the commonest causes are herpes simplex, or other viruses such as orf. Infections such as mycoplasma, streptococcus, typhoid, and diphtheria may be incriminated. Drugs also cause this disorder and sulphonamides are amongst the most common. In fact, any infection and any drug can probably give rise to erythema multiforme, usually after a latent period of 1 to 3 weeks. Other causes include neoplasm and its treatment with drugs or radiotherapy, as well as certain other systemic diseases such as rheumatoid arthritis, lupus erythematosus, or ulcerative colitis. One of the difficulties is the overlap with the other patterns of toxic erythema and their causation. The erythema of pregnancy may sometimes be called erythema multiforme.

PATHOLOGY

There is vacuolar degeneration of the basal cells of the epidermis; vesicles develop between the cells and the underlying basement membrane. There is vasodilation and a lymphocytic infiltrate around the upper dermal vessels.

Fig. 104 Stevens–Johnson syndrome, or severe erythema multiforme, resulting in severe erosions of the mouth and conjunctivitis.

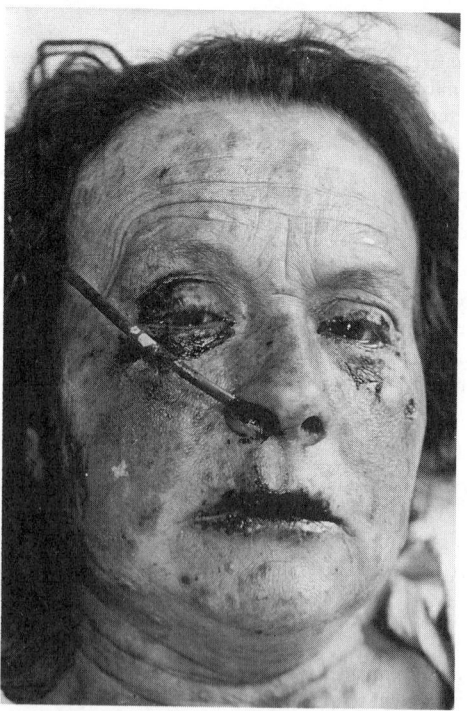

TREATMENT

The cause should be removed if known and systemic steroids should be prescribed if the patient is very uncomfortable and toxic. Recurrent attacks should also be treated by eliminating the cause if known, for instance, treating the earliest stage of the herpes simplex with idoxuridine and avoiding triggers like bright sunlight. Continuous acyclovir therapy is also increasingly recommended. Viral resistance and long-term side-effects of frequent or long-term usage have not so far been demonstrated.

Toxic epidermal necrolysis

This is a rare variety of erythema with acute epithelial necrosis affecting all areas of the skin. This is sometimes called 'scalded skin syndrome' because of its clinical appearance. It is usually acute in onset and may be preceded by various patterns of toxic erythema or blistering. Pressure and shearing stresses on the skin tend to encourage the extension of the blisters. There are two varieties of the disease: the first, originally described by Ritter, is due to a staphylococcus, often phage type 71, and particularly affecting children—the blistering and the resulting erosions are very superficial and they are due to a split at the level of the stratum granulosum; the second is a drug reaction or a toxic consequence of malignant disease or its therapy. The entire epidermis is necrotic. The drugs responsible are sometimes sulphonamides, barbiturates, phenytoin, pyrazolone derivatives, or phenolphthalein, but there are also a number of other drugs more rarely blamed.

Rarer blistering disorders

These include diseases like pemphigus, pemphigoid, and dermatitis herpetiformis. At one time these were all grouped together and their pathogenesis has only recently become clearer. The main distinction is in the level of the blister which determines both clinical and histological features, as pemphigus is an intraepidermal blister whereas the other disorders tend to be subepidermal. The cleavage within the dermis produces dermal inflammation, oedematous papules, infiltration with white cells, as well as bleeding into this blister. The more superficial the blister the more erosive the appearance and the skin lesions may be red and glistening whereas deeper dermal blisters tend to be tense and less easily broken. The type and site of immunoglobulin deposition is a further diagnostic feature (see Table 2).

Pemphigus vulgaris

A blistering condition favouring the mucosa as much as the skin. It is a separation of epidermal cells above the basal layers of the epidermis always in association with an antibody having an affinity with intercellular material in the epidermis. The separated epidermal cell is large, basophilic, and rounded and is termed an acantholytic cell.

AETIOLOGY

The pemphigus antibody will cross the placental barrier and promote neonatal blistering. It is also pathogenic in vitro. The antibody reacts with a specific 85 kDa protein, plakoglobin, and a 130 kDa protein in pemphigus vulgaris, but in pemphigus foliaceous it reacts with a 160 kDa protein, desmoglein. The 130 kDa polypeptide is an epidermal cadherin. Autoantibodies in pemphigus foliaceous bind to an extracellular epitope of desmoglein. The reason why this should cause loss of adhesion in the granular layer remains obscure.

It is assumed to be an autoimmune disease, possibly associated with HLA-A10 and DR4, and is found more commonly in the Jewish race. It is one of the commonest causes of admission to a skin hospital in India. The more superficial variety that affects Brazilians may or may not be a separate, genetically determined reaction pattern. The antibody that binds with complement both in vivo and in vitro is specific for an, as yet unidentified, intercellular material which activates proteases that lyse intercellular adhesive materials. Several investigators have found that the antibody can frequently cause intraepithelial clefting in vitro in human, rabbit, and monkey epithelium. There is an association with thymoma as well as with lymphoma and carcinoma. Not surprisingly, therefore, it occurs with lupus erythematosus and myasthenia gravis.

Penicillamine has been responsible for the development of pemphigus in about 9 per cent of patients treated for rheumatoid arthritis. Captopril and rifampicin as well as meprobamate have also been incriminated.

CLINICAL FEATURES

Erosions of the mucosa of the mouth are the initial problem in more than half the cases. The erosions are often misdiagnosed as mouth ulcers but close examination reveals a friable mucosa with no well-defined aphthous ulcers. Actual blisters may be missed because they are so quickly eroded. On the skin the superficial nature of the blisters also determines that the principal lesion is a more painful erosion and the flaccid blisters quickly burst. The base is red and bleeds easily. The epidermis at the edge of the blister is easily dislodged by sliding pressure (Nikolsky sign). There are many reports of clinical and histological overlap with pemphigus foliaceous or pemphigoid. In all such cases pemiphigus vulgaris proves to be the final diagnosis.

TREATMENT

Corticosteroids are life-saving; without them the disease is one of the most dangerous in dermatology. Very high dosage is required. Prednisolone 120 mg daily is a common starting dose and failure to control the eruption within a week merits doubling of even this high dose. As soon as there are no new blisters the steroids are reduced by large increments about every 3 days. Withdrawal is more gradual below 30 mg daily. Most practitioners now add azathioprine, methotrexate, or cyclophosphamide as a steroid sparing immunosuppressant.

In contrast to the presteroid era cure now seems possible and many patients are off all treatment after 2 years. However, the side-effects of the therapy are considerable. Death from gastrointestinal haemorrhage is not infrequent. Thromboembolic disease is probably a consequence of the disease as much as the therapy. Osteoporosis from the steroids with consequent vertebral collapse is a frequent and irreversible side-effect. Bacterial infection of the eroded skin is inevitable and septicaemia is common. The sore mouth and eroded skin require expert nursing—dressings tend to stick to the skin and removal causes further damage to the skin. Fluids given by mouth should not be strongly osmotic and soft diets should not include particles which lodge under blister roofs or in crevices.

Pemphigus vegetans

This is a reaction to the erosions in which the repairing epidermis becomes hypertrophic and the dermal response is granulomatous. It is common in the axillae and groin and the angles of the mouth and nose (Fig. 105). It may be encouraged by steroid suppression. Small pustules surround the vegetations.

Pemphigus foliaceous

This is a more benign variant of pemphigus in which the blisters are more superficial. The bullae are subcorneal and scaling and crusting may be a principal feature (Fig. 106). The face and upper trunk are most often affected. Localized forms may look more like seborrhoeic warts because of their chronicity and definition. Oral lesions are unusual. Antibodies against intercellular epithelial material are present as in pemphigus vulgaris but basement membrane antibody and antinuclear antibody are also often observed. There is an association with lupus erythematosus and with thymoma and myasthenia gravis.

Fogo selvagem

This is a form of pemphigus foliaceous which is common in rural peanut farms of Brazil. Many members of one family may be involved. Progression to a generalized erythroderma is usual and the mortality is almost 50 per cent. An immunological reaction to an insect vector has been proposed, based on the study of the black fly bites and the hypothesis of cross-reactivity between the epidermal antigens and the antigen of the fly. The mortality in this ethnic group is high due as much to treatment as from the disease. Topical steroids may be preferable to high-dose systemic therapy in those who cannot be closely supervised.

Pemphigoid

The bullae are subepidermal and acantholysis is not a feature. About 80 per cent of patients are over the age of 60. It is about twice as common as pemphigus. There is a specific antibody (usually IgG) for the base-

Fig. 105 Pemphigus vegetans showing the typical granulomatous hypertrophy underlying erosions at the angles of the mouth.

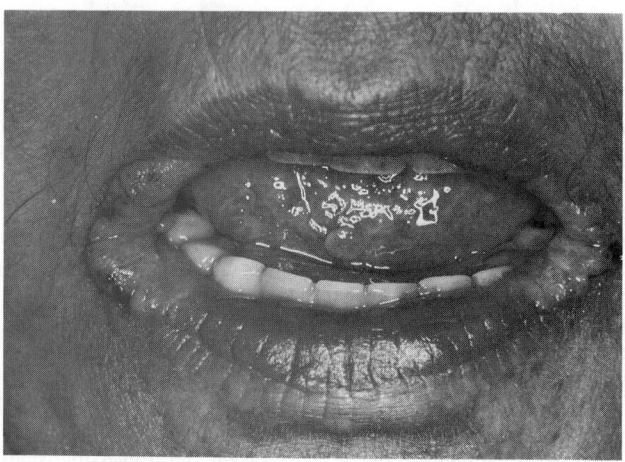

Fig. 106 Pemphigus foliaceous blisters, so superficial that they merely look like crusting of the erosions. In this case it would have to be distinguished from an intertrigo and secondary monilial infection.

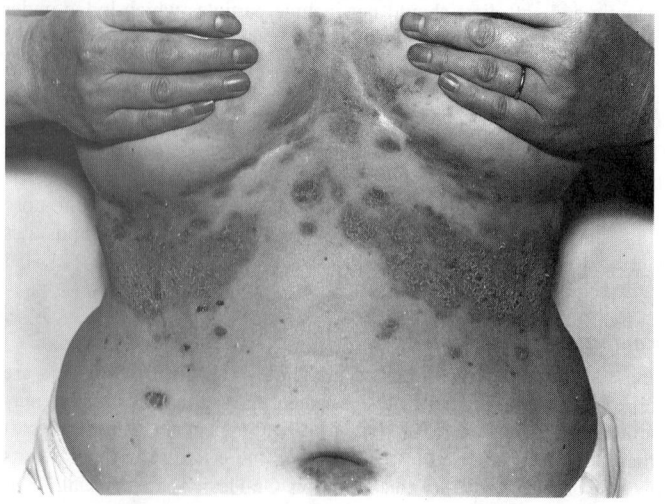

ment membrane zone of the epidermis and this is present in about 70 per cent of patients. Complement is bound *in vivo*. The basement membrane remains in the floor of the bullae in most cases. Two large epidermal polypeptides are the major antigenic target of BP antibodies. The BP230 gene is localized to the short arm of chromosome 6 and BP180 gene to the long arm of chromosome 10. Both proteins are components of the hemidesmosome. BP180 is a transmembrane glycoprotein with an external terminal ectodomain consisting of collagen triple helical domains. It binds keratin to the hemidesmosome.

CLINICAL FEATURES

The initial features of pemphigoid are often non-specific and confusing. It can be eczematous or urticarial. The lesions often begin around a site of damage such as a leg ulcer or burn. After 2 or 3 weeks blisters may erupt abruptly. They favour the flexures and are tense and dome-shaped. They often contain blood. Small blisters in the mouth are rare and tend not to erode as in pemphigus. The patients are distressed by itching, and oedema of the skin may be troublesome, but their general health is usually unaffected.

TREATMENT

The treatment of choice is prednisolone 60 to 80 mg daily until there are no new blisters. Azathioprine, methotrexate, dapsone, or cylophosphamide may be used to allow a lower maintenance dose of the steroid, since morbidity in the elderly is great. Osteoporosis, gastric ulceration, and diabetes mellitus are particularly common complications of steroid therapy. However, complete remission after 1 year is common.

Cicatricial pemphigoid

The cause of this disorder is unknown but the immunology includes autoantibodies to an 180 kDa protein. It is also called benign mucosal pemphigoid. Although mortality is low, it is responsible for great discomfort. It is a disease of older adults and the subepidermal bullae favour the mucosa of the mouth, conjunctiva, and the perineal orifices. The base of the lesions are heavily infiltrated with lymphocytes and plasma cells and there is eventual fibrosis. The adhesions that occur between the bulbar and palpebral conjunctiva result in eventual shrinkage, and entropion is followed by blindness. The skin is less often involved and the lesions are sparse and often heal by scarring. The scalp is more often affected than other sites.

TREATMENT

No treatment is very effective but steroids and azathioprine are usually prescribed.

Dermatitis herpetiformis

This is a vesicobullous disorder associated with the granular deposition of IgA in the dermis and a usually symptomless subtotal villus atrophy of the small intestine. The IgA is believed to be derived from plasma cells in the intestine. As in coeliac disease HLA-A8/DRW 3 is associated and may be responsible for a defective Fc receptor status. It is probable that gluten hypersensitivity results in circulating immune complexes that have an affinity for material in the upper dermis; this is possibly reticulin and the Fc receptor dysfunction impairs the removal by macrophages of the immune material. Histology of the skin shows fibrin, neutrophils, and eosinophils in the dermal papillae.

CLINICAL FEATURES

The eruption is characterized by intensely itchy grouped papular or vesicular lesions that lie on an urticarial or erythematous base. The elbows, knees, sacrum, and shoulders are favoured (see Fig. 10) and the face and scalp are more commonly affected than in the case of pemphigus or pemphigoid. The itchy vesicles are quickly excoriated since this relieves the pruritus. The eruption waxes and wanes sometimes being in remission for many months. However, for most it remains a lifelong disorder.

TREATMENT

Dapsone (100–200 mg daily) or sulphapyridine (0.5 g three times daily) are remarkably effective and can be used as a diagnostic test since itchiness is relieved within 48 h. The maintenance dose should be titrated to suit each patient. It may be as low as 50 mg dapsone weekly. Haemolytic anaemia is common on higher dosage and especially when, in some cases, 400 mg of dapsone is needed daily to control the eruption. A gluten-free diet strictly adhered to controls some but not all patients; 70 per cent can omit dapsone after 2 years of such dieting.

Steroid therapy is strangely ineffective and heparin oddly effective. Inorganic arsenicals (Fowler's solution) is effective and was once very popular, and it is probably justified in elderly patients much troubled by the disease and unable to tolerate dapsone or sulphapyridine.

Juvenile bullous pemphigoid

This is a bullous disorder characterized by a predilection for the face and perineum. Linear IgA is deposited on the basement membrane of the epidermis. It is not associated with enteropathy nor with HLA-A8. The response to dapsone, sulphapyridine, or steroids is unpredictable.

Pemphigoid gestationis

This differs from the common toxic erythema of pregnancy in having large blisters, often periumbilical, beginning as a degeneration of the epidermal cells. It is associated with HLA-B8/DR3 and an IgG_1 autoantibody which avidly binds C3. It is thus a blister above the basement membrane and it is believed to be due to a specific antibody to the basal cell; it is present in the umbilical cord blood and binds with a 180 kDa glycoprotein in the basement membrane of amnion. It occurs during or immediately after pregnancy and usually ceases fairly abruptly within weeks of parturition. It recurs in subsequent pregnancies or as an effect of oral contraceptives.

Other causes of blistering

Lichen planus and lichen sclerosis et atrophicus both rarely blister. Bullous disease and malignancy are a debated association since so much bullous disease occurs in an age group in which malignancy is common. However, individual case histories of uncontrollable bullous disease with atypical immunofluorescence are impressive.

Trophoneurotic blisters are another debated association. The unconscious patient seems predisposed to produce blisters even at sites not affected by pressure or shearing forces. They are subepidermal. This is an important hazard often causing unjustified accusation of mismanagement in the nursing care of such patients.

Diabetes mellitus is a cause of intraepidermal blisters without immunofluorescent material and showing no acantholysis (Fig. 107).

Vesicobullous disorders in infancy
INFECTION

Although infection is the most important cause of bullae in the neonate, such infection is usually contracted during birth. No blisters are seen until at least the second day. However, blisters at birth are described from intrauterine viral infections such as chickenpox or herpes simplex,

and it is also seen in congenital syphilis. Blisters at birth are more usually due to genetic disease such as incontinentia pigmenti, mast cell naevi, or epidermolysis bullosa, the latter more often suggesting widespread absence of skin.

From the second day after birth staphylococcal infections are common and a few days later candidiasis or, in a very sick child, pseudomonas infection may be responsible for blisters. After a few weeks scabies and insect bites should also be considered.

NON-INFECTIOUS
Milia

Forty per cent of full-term infants have scalp, facial, and genital white papules, often grouped and not surrounded by erythema. These are inclusions of epithelial products within the epidermis. They are shed after a few days, but they are also seen in adults after any injury causing blistering (Fig. 108).

Erythema toxicum

This is an almost inevitable papular red rash of the first five days of life and is characterized by infiltrations of the papules by eosinophils. The trunk is mostly affected.

Transient neonatal pustular melanosis

This is commonest in pigmented infants and is initially pustular often at birth, and later develops a scaly collar and thereafter for several weeks there are hyperpigmented macules. No infectious organism has been isolated.

Fig. 107 A haemorrhagic blister on the foot in a patient with diabetes mellitus.

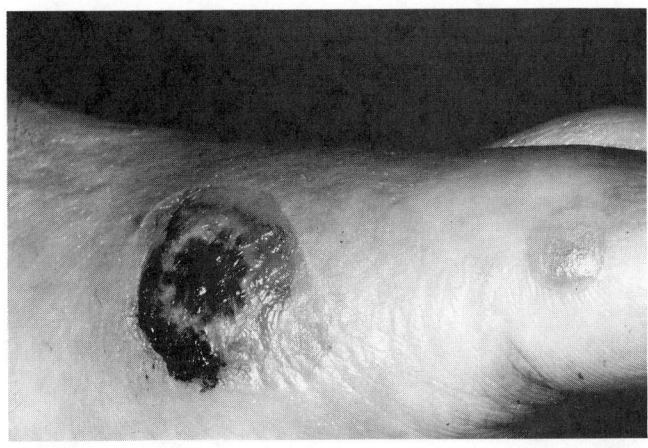

Fig. 108 Milia following a subepidermal blister from a burn.

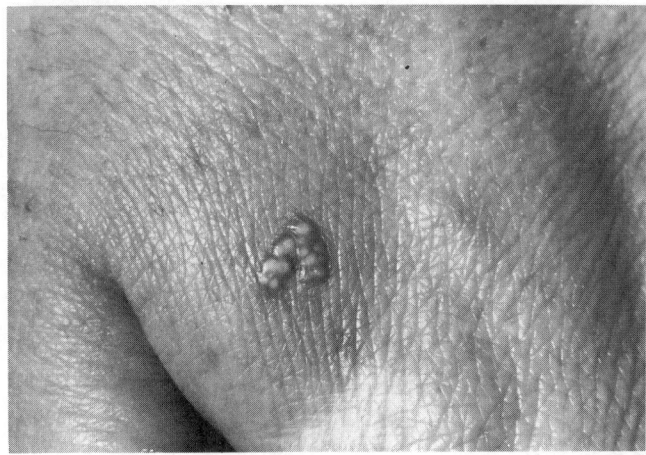

Infantile acropustulosis

Also affects pigmented children and its cause is unknown. It is pruritic and sometimes vesicular and usually affects infants aged 2 to 10 months. It mostly responds to dapsone 2 mg/kg per day.

Miliaris crystallina

There are clear, very superficial and small vesicles occurring without inflammation but as a consequence of sweating. They may be seen when the child is overheated from fever or climate, and affect the flexures, face, and scalp.

Incontinentia pigmenti

Familial cases are lethal to males *in utero* and therefore present in the neonatal girl. The incidence is 2.5 per 100 000. It is due to a translocation between chromosomes X and 10 but sporadic male cases with a different locus are described. There are crops of inflammatory bullae (Fig. 109), often bizarre in pattern, and accompanied or followed by epidermal hyperplasia and disturbance of pigmentation. Nail, hair, eye, skeletal, and CNS changes are common.

Epidermolysis bullosa

There are several genetic varieties (see elsewhere). Features are widespread areas of absent skin or localized to sites of trauma; blisters may be prominent.

Others

Congenital porphyria (Fig. 110), mastocytosis, Letterer–Siwe disease, bullous congenital ichthyosiform erythema, and acrodermatitis enteropathica may all cause blistering.

REFERENCES

Iwatsuki, K., Hashimoto, T., Ebihara, T., Teraki, Y., Nishikawa, T., and Kaneko, F. (1993). Intercellular IgA vesicular-pustular dermatosis and related disorders: diversity of IgA anti-intercellular autoantibodies. *European Journal of Dermatology*, **3**, 7–11.

Jenkins, R.E., Shornick, J.K., and Black, M.M. (1993). Pemphigoid gestationis. *Journal of the European Academy of Dermatology and Venereology*, **2**, 163–73.

Pye, R.J. (1992). Bullous eruptions. In *Rook, Wilkinson, and Ebling's Textbook of Dermatology* (eds. R.H. Champion, J.L. Burton, and F.J.G. Ebling). 5th edn. pp. 1623–74. Blackwell Scientific Publications, Oxford.

Sneddon, I.B. (1980). Bullous eruptions. In *Textbook of dermatology*, 3rd edn, (ed. A. Rook, D.S. Wilkinson, and F.J.G. Ebling), pp. 1441–81. Blackwell Scientific Publications, Oxford.

Tatnall, F.M., Schofield, J.K., and Leigh L.M. (1995). A double blind, placebo-controlled trial of continuous acyclovir therapy in recurrent erythema multiforme. *British Journal of Dermatology*, **132**, 267–70.

Abnormal vascularity of the skin, angioma, and telangiectasia

Patterns of blood vessel development that are inappropriate for the needs of the skin or for thermoregulation include both overgrowth and atrophy. An excess of capillary and venular vessels is a characteristic of wound healing and of many hyperproliferative conditions of the skin such as psoriasis. These usually present as redness and individual vessels cannot be seen by the naked eye. Proliferation is still more extreme in strawberry haemangioma, granuloma telangiectaticum, also known as pyogenic granuloma, and in certain malignancies such as Kaposi's sarcoma or angioendothelioma.

On the other hand, telangiectasia is characterized by the dilatation of individual capillaries or venules so that they are visible to the naked eye. There is little evidence that the endothelial cell is at fault and it is more likely that the basic defect is an atrophy or loss of supporting tissue.

Proliferative vasculature is more unstable than that observed in telangiectasia and the natural history is to resolve, often completely. Vessels and wounds or angiomas are vulnerable and the growing phase may be associated with necrosis as a result of thrombosis secondary to injury to the surface of the skin. Telangiectasia on the other hand has no ten-

Fig. 109 Incontinentia pigmenti blistering and hyperkeratosis of the leg of a female infant.

Fig. 110 Blisters on the lower leg of a child with congenital porphyria. Note also the hypertrichosis. The blister occurred following exposure to sunlight.

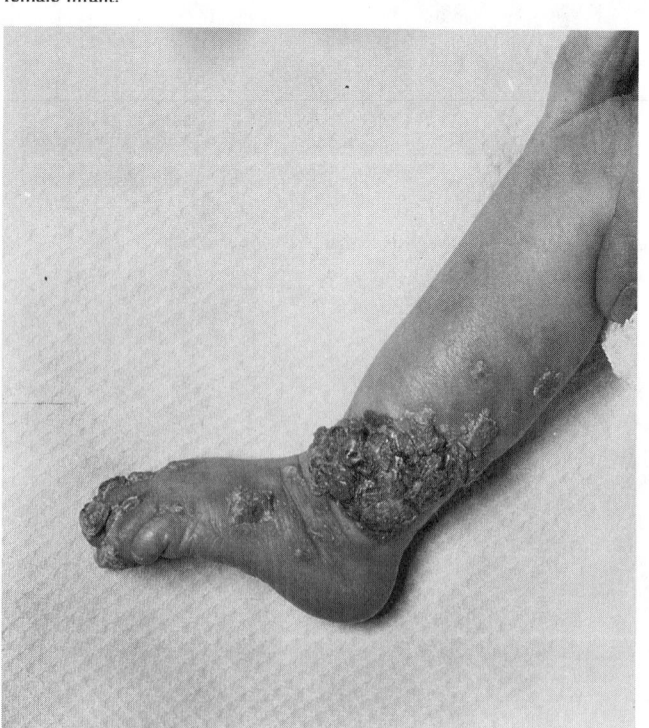

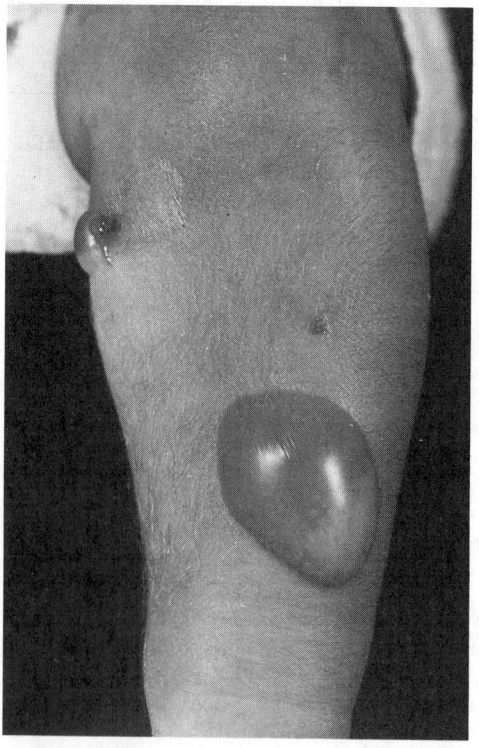

dency to thrombose and the overlying skin rarely ulcerates. The natural history of such dilated vessels is to persist until extreme old age when they may be partially absorbed.

Strawberry naevi

These are almost never present at birth but may be preceded by a small area of blanching observed at birth. From a few days after birth the lesion consists of nests of granulation tissue which proliferate rapidly. After a few weeks the rate of growth becomes less rapid and some vessels become dilated and cavernous. A stable period of no growth often occurs from about 9 months to about 1 year, after which gradual absorption by fibrosis is to be expected. Management consists of reassurance of the parents and emphasis on satisfactory natural resolution (Fig. 111).

Exceptions to this policy include involvement of the eyelid interfering with sight, in which case plastic surgery may be advised. Some large haemangiomata sequester platelets giving rise to a bleeding tendency (the Kassabach–Merrick syndrome). High-dose steroids (3 mg/kg) are life-saving. On withdrawal, rebound overgrowth may be observed, justifying a second or third course. Ulceration of the haemangioma is common, especially in the nappy area and when there is a primary irritant rash. Bleeding is easily controlled by light pressure. The ulceration often accelerates resolution.

Fig. 111 'Strawberry' naevus; (a) a proliferative but benign neoplasia which, after a rapid phase of new growth, stabilizes, and eventually regresses. The lesions often ulcerate if traumatized. In this case, ulceration has hastened resolution but the residual scarring (b) is more than usual.

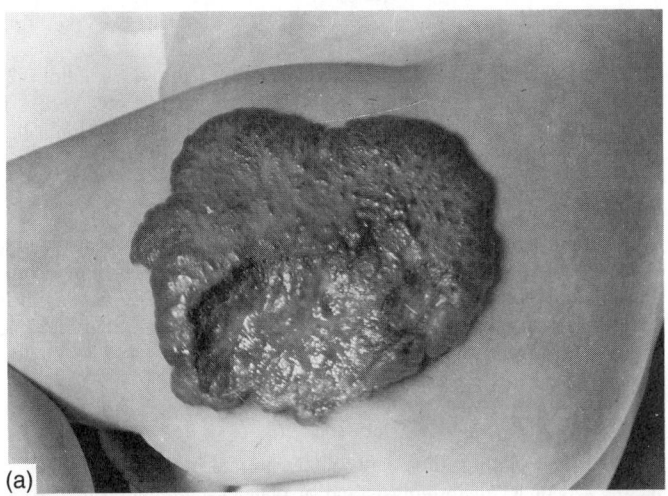

(a)

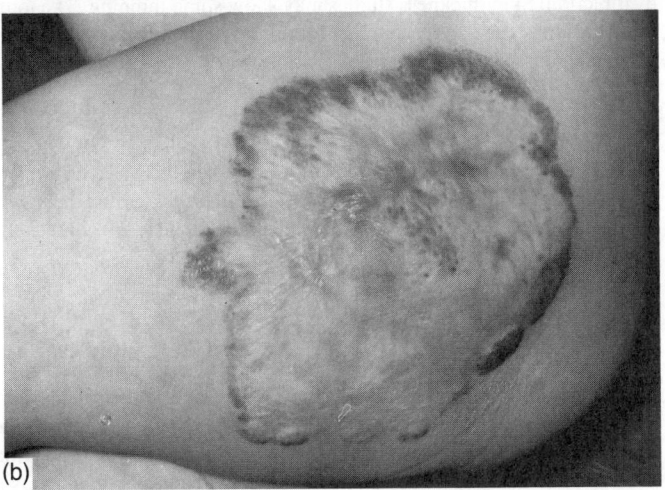

(b)

Sometimes haemangiomata have a deep element in which arteriovenous shunts are a complication. Interference with underlying structures is not common but joint involvement warrants surgical advice and management.

Treatment of haemangiomata has included radiotherapy; more recently, systemic steroids, pressure pads, excision, and, currently, embolization and α-interferon. The latter requires angiographic control and siting of sclerosing adhesives at the appropriate site.

Port wine naevi

This is a pattern of vascular birth mark present at birth and usually segmental. It is unwise to make a prognosis at birth because pale naevi and segmental patterns of erythema may look similar and often fade. The majority of port wine naevi persist for life. Arteriovenous shunts and gravitational stasis often cause some increase in the vasculature in adult life. The nape of the neck is a site in which a pale plaque of macular telangiectasia is present in the majority of normal babies and persists in more than one half of those affected.

Variants of port wine naevi affecting deeper vasculature range from the Klippel–Trenaunay disorder causing enlargement of the limb, to a reticulate and more atrophic pattern associated sometimes with the shortening of the limb. There are developmental patterns of widespread segmental telangiectasia with which asymmetrical gigantism and disturbances of pigment are associated.

Telangiectasia

Telangiectases are enduring dilatations of blood vessels. They are usually less than 1 mm in length and may be point-like or punctate, linear, star-like, spider, or stellate, forming flat, square, oblong, or oval plaques, or mat-like with an eccentric punctum. They blanch completely when they are compressed. Telangiectasia is not new-vessel formation—indeed new vessels in wounds are not unduly dilated.

Telangiectases are probably always secondary to mesenchymal connective tissue dysplasia but can be congenital and naevoid, acquired and genetic, i.e. familial or hereditary, as well as secondary to 'collagen' disease such as lupus erythematosus, scleroderma, or dermatomyositis, or from radiation damage.

All dilatations of small vessels are made worse by blushing, as is seen in rosacea, carcinoid, or due to oestrogen and related hormonal imbalances as in pregnancy or liver disease. They are also made worse by loss of supporting tissue as in steroid atrophy, solar elastosis, ageing (Fig. 112), or Cushing's syndrome.

Telangiectasia is often associated with increased melanin pigmentation and brown spots may be predominant, even in hereditary haemorrhagic telangiectasia, but poikiloderma is a typical example of atrophy, telangiectasia, and pigmentation. Some telangiectasia may be insufficiently dilated to be recognized by the naked eye, and if affecting most of the vessels in an affected area, they may appear as a persistent erythema, for instance, the red cheeks of young children, or some capillary naevi affecting the eyelids, nape of the neck, or forehead known as salmon patches or stork bites. The erythema may be pale pink or deep purple. The darker the lesion the more likely the dilated vessels will be inhomogeneous and some will be visible to the naked eye. Naevoid lesions usually affect well-defined segments of the skin, though not necessarily dermatomal or unilateral (Fig. 113). The best known are naevi affecting the trigeminal nerve (Sturge–Weber) or sometimes an entire limb.

Diffuse polymorphic patterns that develop in childhood or in young adults favor exposed areas such as the face and forearms, probably because sunlight exaggerates connective tissue dysplasia. However, haemodynamic factors such as gravitational stasis of the venous system also play a part, and the distribution of spider naevi may depend on drainage into the superior vena cava. Gravitational stasis particularly determines the patterns of stellate and arborizing telangiectasia on the legs. Five per cent of the population has two to ten telangiectases on the lip, fingers, palms, and soles, and these sites may be involved by grosser patterns of telangiectasia in disease. Dermatomal or unilateral patterns are rare. A high incidence of telangiectasia of up to 40 per cent affecting the trunk is described in aluminium workers. It seems to be associated with the electrolytic processing used in the industry.

Diffuse and acquired patterns of telangiectasia are commonly familial but sporadic cases account for about 20 per cent, even in the well-known hereditary haemorrhagic telangiectasia. A benign variety of this disease is not associated with severe bleeding and is also probably dominant. Telangiectasia confined to the lips may also present a dominant pattern of inheritance. However, no large-scale study has been done to rule out polygenic inheritance in any of these disorders. The haemorrhagic diathesis has been recorded as a dominant gene and many large pedigrees have been described, but even so, 10 per cent of probands with telangiectasia do not bleed. Severe epistaxis and severe bleeding after tooth

Fig. 112 Ageing is accentuated in light-exposed skins. One feature of ageing is poor collagen support of skin vasculature. Telangiectasia is a common consequence.

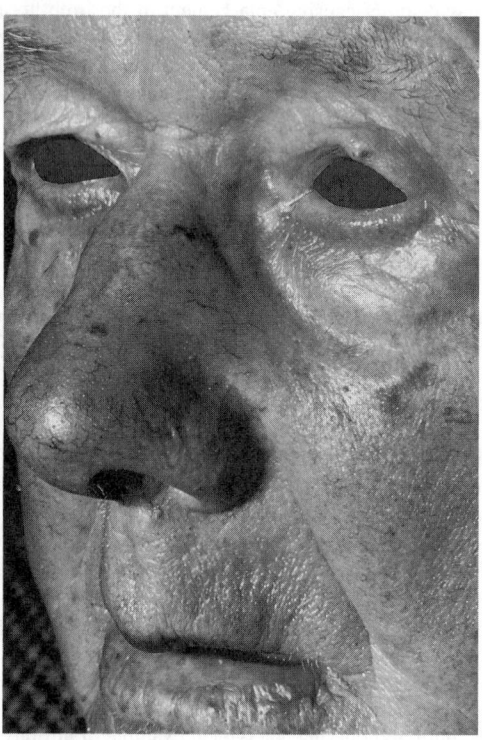

Fig. 113 Segmental telangiectasia of punctate-spider naevoid type.

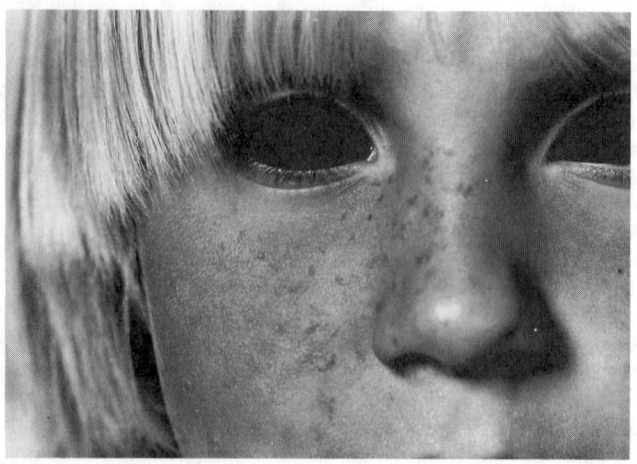

extraction or cuts and even heavy menstrual bleeding are characteristic of hereditary haemorrhagic telangiectasia. Minor but frequent nose bleeds are common with even the benign forms. Arteriovenous shunts are described commonly in association with hereditary haemorrhagic telangiectasia. They result in pulsating nodules of the skin, and in the lung or brain may have severe consequences. They are occasionally seen in the non-haemorrhagic telangiectatic forms of the disease.

HISTOLOGY

The dilated vessels are unremarkable but special studies have helped to show that the vessels are venules, i.e. alkaline phosphatase negative, and they secrete generous amounts of plasminogen activator. Supporting tissue and overlying epidermis is usually atrophic.

TREATMENT

Telangiectases are easy to camouflage with 'covermark' type of preparations but advice may need to be given on its application with respect to the use of cream and powder, blends, and matching of skin colour.

Telangiectases when small and localized can be destroyed by cryotherapy, cautery, electrolysis, or laser therapy. The latter can be endoscopic. The laser specifically burns haemoglobin and it is therefore more successful in the treatment of the larger blood containing dilatations. Sclerotherapy is also possible.

Bleeding should first be treated by the simple first-aid measure of elevation and local pressure. Cautery is most effective only on a dry blanched area controlled by compression. Patients can be taught to inflate a lubricated finger cot tied over the end of a small catheter for the immediate control of severe epistaxis.

Oestrogen therapy

Oestrogen therapy is sometimes advocated, e.g. ethinyloestradiol 0.25 mg daily, and increased to 0.5 mg per day at the end of 4 weeks if epistaxis continues. However, its effectiveness is unproven by controlled trials.

Percutaneous embolization

This is increasingly used to close unwanted vasculature but it requires careful angiographic control and skilled surgeons, and has not overcome the problem of rapid recanalization and opening up of collaterals. It is nevertheless the treatment of choice for severe uncontrolled bleeding from arteriovenous shunts.

INVESTIGATIONS

Bleeding and clotting times are mostly normal but special studies of factor VIII or local fibrinolysis and of platelet aggregation may show dysfunction. Skin thickness studies may show some thinning. The tourniquet test has been advocated as a useful test of the haemorrhagic variant in persons with telangiectasis.

PROPHYLAXIS

Sun, cold, or gravitational stasis all enhance telangiectasia. Bleeding is often first noted after tooth extraction. Alcoholic excesses and the ingestion of aspirin and other prostaglandin inhibitors may precipitate the bleeding problem.

Facial erythema (flushing)

In temperate climates the weather-beaten face of the farmer, or fisherman is largely a reflection of exposure to cold, as are the rosy cheeks and 'shiny morning face' of the school child. The 'butterfly' area of the cheeks and bridge of the nose are sites which pick up thermal irradiation whether hot or cold. Marked telangiectasia of the cheeks in adults is a common consequence of rosy cheeks in childhood. It may be associated with thickening of the subcutaneous tissues.

Rosacea is usually associated with acneiform pustulation and lymphoedema. For unknown reasons a keratitis is sometimes associated. A somewhat similar appearance may be seen in sarcoid, especially the lupus pernio variety in which a diffuse granuloma underlies dilated blood vessels filled with slow-flowing blue blood. Mitral or pulmonary stenosis also causes a persistent malar flush. In discoid lupus erythematosus, telangiectasia (Fig. 114a) is accompanied by atrophy (Fig. 114b), often with well-defined margins and follicular plugging. The borders of the lesions of rosacea and sarcoid tend to be more diffuse. Asymmetry can be a feature of all disorders.

Telangiectasia due to other collagen diseases varies from the redness and oedema of the orbit characteristic of dermatomyositis (Fig. 115) to erythema of the backs of the hands and nailfolds with persistent erythema such that vessels become increasingly inhomogenous, and quite large dilated forms may be observed.

In scleroderma, especially of the adult acrosclerotic variety, telangiectasia in the form of flat macules, often with square or oblong shapes and fairly well-defined margins, are characteristic. Systemic sclerosis of the face usually causes stiffness and tethering of the skin to deeper structures over the nose and loss of suppleness in the perioral skin. There is of course, the associated Raynaud's phenomenon and digital ischaemia.

A plethoric complexion is a feature of superior vena cava obstruction but also of polycythaemia rubra vera and Cushing's syndrome.

Flushing of the face is a common complaint, particularly in the young who may suffer from transient blushing, and in the older age groups it is characterized by persistent rosacea. Carcinoid should be thought of when there is a prolonged blush associated with a bounding pulse,

asthma, abdominal pain, and diarrhoea. Frequent applications of steroids to the face for atopic or seborrhoeic eczema produces gross diffuse telangiectasia and there are often rebound eczematous changes on withdrawal (Fig. 116) and the irritation may be severe. The treatment of this condition is complete withdrawal of all steroids until after 3 to 4 weeks when the condition tends to settle.

Flushing which is neurogenic is accompanied by sweating. Local heating of the oropharynx is one physiological cause. It can be counteracted by sipping iced water. Neurogenic flushing can be dampened by β-blockers. Nocturnal overheating causing restlessness, facial flushing, and rubbing is another contributory factor.

Disorders of collagen and elastic tissue

The metabolism and diseases of collagen are described in Section 19. The fundamental defects are in its chemical structure, its cross-linkage between fibres, and its distribution and quantity.

Signs of collagen disease

These include:

1. Diminished skin thickness and increased transparency so that deeper structures such as veins and nerves are visible and the sclerae are blue.
   There are at least 18 collagen types, hence there are many genetic diseases.
2. Diminished resistance to shear so that the skin splits and tears sometimes even without surface breaks. Purpura is usually associated and healing results in white stellate scars. Cutane-

Fig. 114 In lupus erythematosus—chronic discoid type—(a) telangiectasia and (b) erythema are common. There is follicular plugging and destruction of the skin, resulting in pigment loss and scarring.

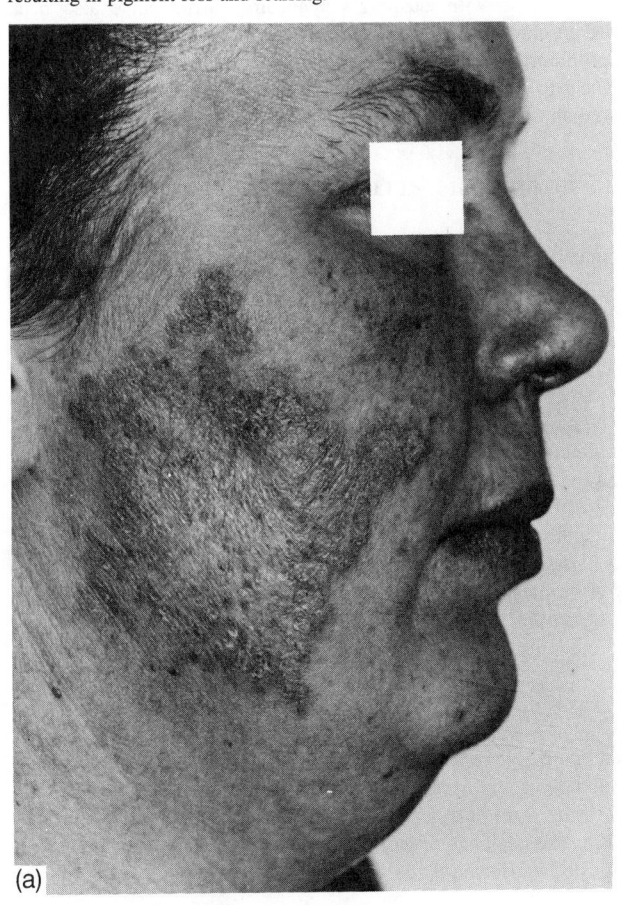

(a)

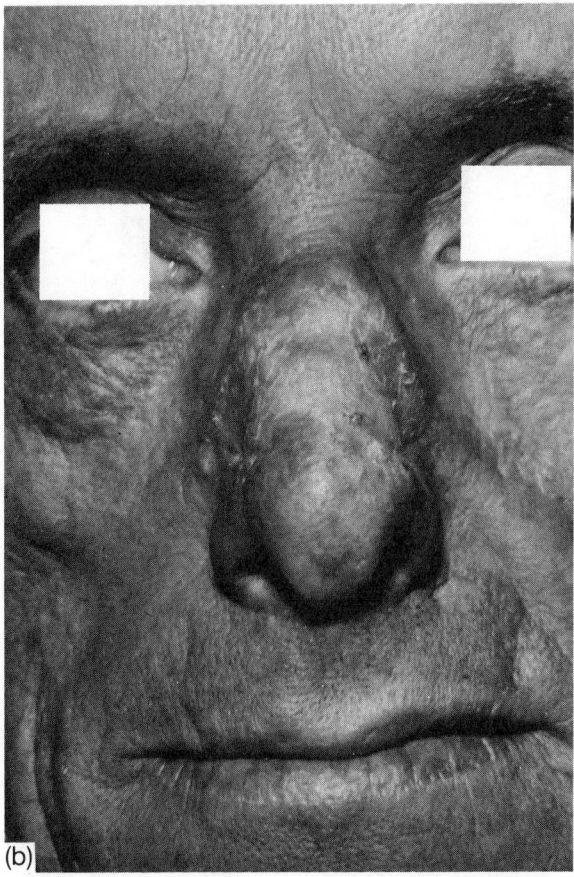

(b)

ous striae are another pattern of stretching of the skin with separation in this case. Diminished resistance of the skin is a feature of age; osteoporosis and rheumatoid arthritis are other recognized associations. Steroids are responsible for both stellate scars and cutaneous striae and this is the case whether they are endogenously produced, as in Cushing's disease, or prescribed for other diseases. Local application of steroid cream is probably now the commonest cause of these changes.

3. Laxity is the failure of the skin to return rapidly to its former state after distortion by stretch. It is in some way caused by degeneration of elastic tissue but changes in water content and

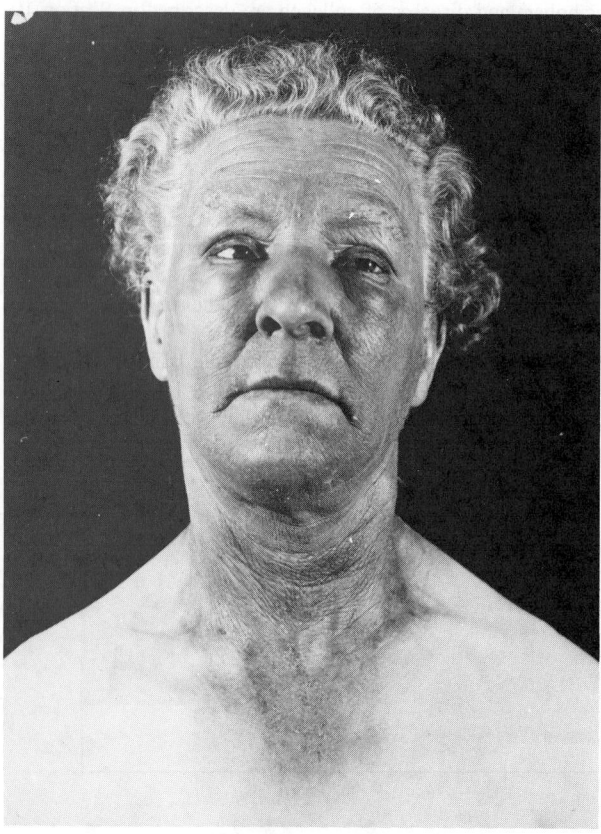

Fig. 115 Bright erythema and oedema of the face, especially periorbitally, is characteristic of dermatomyositis.

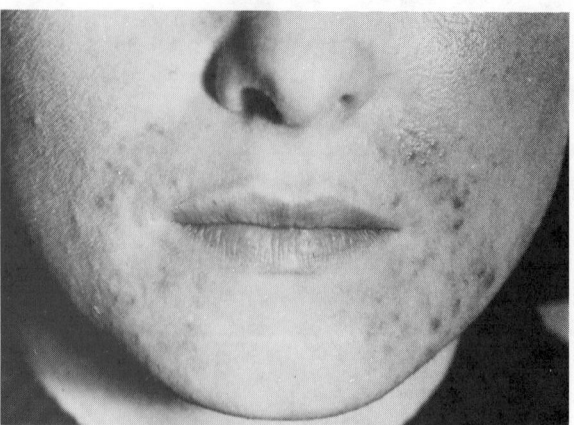

Fig. 116 Perioral dermatitis is a common consequence of the application of fluorinated steroids to the face.

cellularity as well as increased cross-linkage of collagen play some part even when the total collagen is reduced.

Diseases due to defective collagen

SOLAR AND SENILE ELASTOSIS

This affects white-skinned races and especially those employed in agricultural or marine work. Chronic exposure to ultraviolet radiation causes abnormal collagen which has the histological staining characteristics of elastic tissue but not its properties. It is broken and aggregated and contributes to a thickened, yellow, wrinkled skin, especially on the exposed areas in old age. The yellow plaques may be sharply marginated on the face. In the neck deep furrows form a rhomboidal network. The sebaceous glands and ducts are poorly supported, dilated, and patulous, forming giant comedones. On the neck the goose pimple or plucked bird appearance is due to the protection provided by hair follicles shading the dermis against ultraviolet rays. Colloid milium is the abnormal production of a scleroprotein by fibroblasts giving rise to yellowish translucent papules or plaque in light-exposed skin. It may begin in childhood.

STRIAE

These are common but imperfectly understood; stretch is always a factor. The epidermis is thin and elastic fibres are scanty. Striae are seen on the back and thighs of adolescents during growth, especially when there has been a spurt and the child is athletic. It occurs more in girls than in boys. Striae are a feature of pregnancy and affect especially the abdomen and breasts. This is usually due to excessive adrenocortical activity. Incomplete inhibition of fibroblasts causes atrophy of collagen in response to glucocorticoids. When the collagen is ageing or degenerate as follows irradiation or in diseases such as cutis laxa or Ehlers–Danlos syndrome, striae are uncommon and may not appear even in the pregnant or those with Cushing's syndrome. Striae have also been described in chronic infections such as tuberculosis. They are a diagnostic problem only when they are newly formed in which case they may appear to be weal-like and raised. Later they flatten and become bluish-red and still later, white and depressed.

LOCALIZED FIBROSIS, KELOIDS, AND HYPERTROPHIC SCARS

The connective tissue response to cutaneous injury exceeds the limits of the needs for repair appropriate to the degree of injury at that site. This is commonly so a few weeks after injury and gives rise to hypertrophic scars. If the scar continues to hypertrophy and extends beyond the limits of the site of the injured skin, especially after a period of 3 months, since the injury, then it is often termed a keloid. Such scars tend to be more tender than hypertrophic scars. Keloids tend to be familial and are commoner in Negroes. They are rare in infancy and old age and tend to be less severe after the age of 30. Significant factors are the presence of foreign material in the wound and tension. Preferred areas are the ear lobes, chin, neck shoulders, upper trunk, and lower legs. Keloids in their early stages may respond to strong local steroids applied locally or intralesionally. Compression therapy is sometimes helpful, as is cryotherapy in the early stages. Most would now prefer re-excision and radiotherapy to the edges of the wounds.

Ainhum

This is a relatively common disease in Negroes and in Africa especially. Recurrent or chronic fissuring of the digitoplantar fold is followed by fibrosis in the form of a constricting band around the base of the digit (Fig. 117). The peak age of incidence is 30 to 50 years. The most common digit to be affected is the fifth toe.

Fig. 117 Constricting band of sclerosis around the finger—Ainhum.

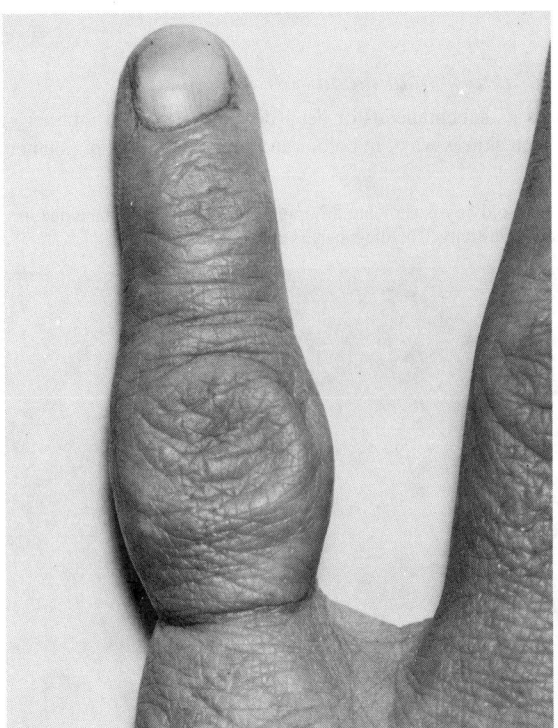

Plastic induration of the penis (Peyronie's disease)

A plaque of firm, fibrous tissue causing painful curvature during erection may be associated with fibrous pads of the hands and feet as well as Dupuytren's contracture.

Pseudoxanthoma elasticum

This is a hereditary disorder of elastic tissue; there are four distinct types:

DOMINANT TYPE I

Small, yellowish papules forming linear or reticulate plaques, which in older persons are soft, lax, and hang in folds, are flexually distributed, especially in the groins, axillae, and neck (Fig. 118). There is a severe degeneration of Bruch's membrane giving rise to the slate-grey, poorly defined 'angioid' streaks forming an incomplete ring or radiating lesions around the optic disc of the retina. There is early blindness. Vascular complications include intermittent claudication and coronary artery disease.

DOMINANT TYPE II

The small, yellowish papules are fewer and flatter. There is increased extensibility of the skin. The vascular and retinal changes are mild. The sclera is blue and there may be a high arched palate and myopia.

RECESSIVE TYPE I

This resembles dominant type I but the vascular and retinal degeneration is mild. Haematemesis is especially common and women are more often affected than men.

Fig. 118 (a) and (b) Yellowish papules and loss of elasticity of the skin of the neck and axillae in pseudoxanthoma elasticum. This may be a clue to gastrointestinal bleeding or even blindness.

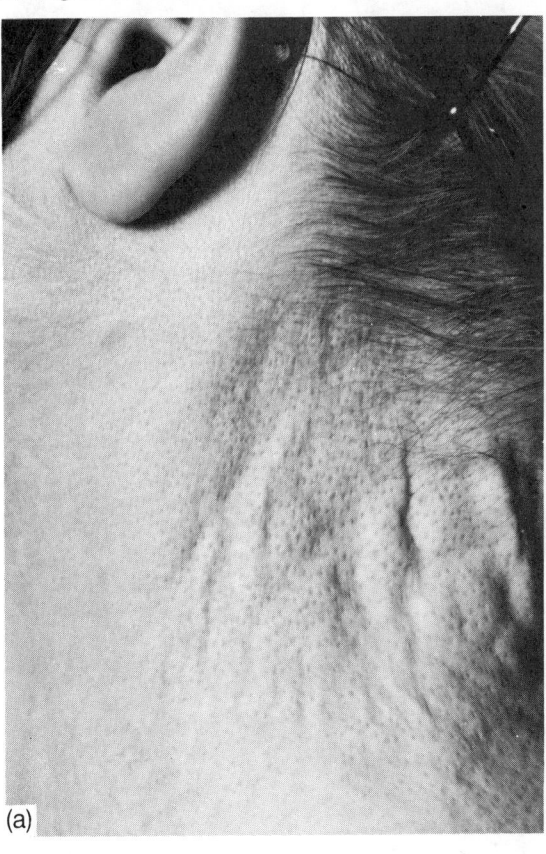
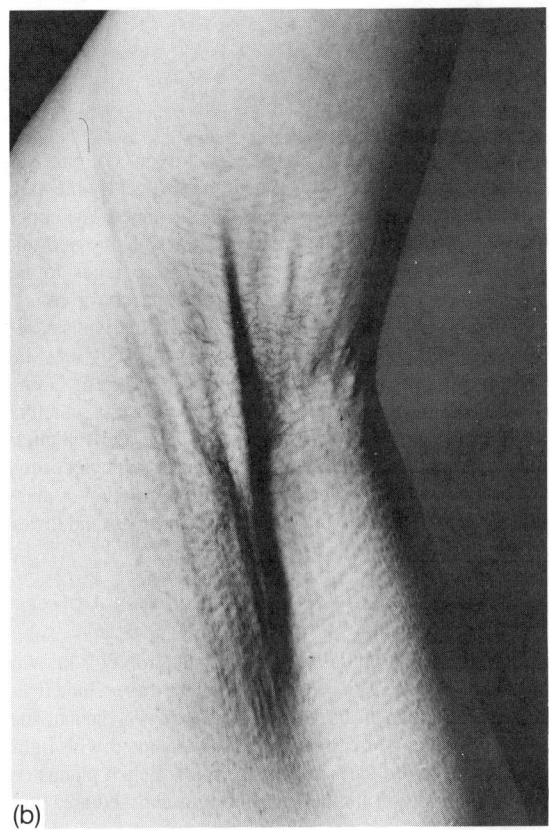

(a)

(b)

RECESSIVE TYPE II

This is a very rare form but the skin changes are extensive and generalized. There tends to be no systemic complications. The pathology of pseudoxanthoma elasticum includes a deposition of calcium on the elastic fibres. The mid-dermal elastic tissue is fragmented and swollen.

Perforating elastoma

This is a condition of degeneration of elastic fibres in the upper dermis with a resulting foreign body reaction and extrusion through the overlying epidermis. This reaction gives rise to papules which develop a central plaque of extruded material. There is a tendency for the formation of annular and serpiginous patterns, particularly over the back and neck region. The disorder is associated with mongolism, Marfan syndrome, Ehlers–Danlos syndrome, pseudoxanthoma elasticum, and osteogenesis imperfecta.

Ehlers–Danlos syndrome: cutis hyperelastica

Ehlers–Danlos syndrome is a rare inherited disorder of connective tissue. More than 10 varieties are recognized, four are clearly dominant and one is X-chromosome linked. It is explained by a gene defect affecting collagen type 1. The condition is usually recognized when the child begins to walk since there is hyperextensibility of the joints. Trivial cuts form gaping wounds and heal poorly. The skin feels soft and can be stretched, particularly over the knees and elbows. Arterial rupture, aortic dissection, and intestinal perforation have been described in severely affected individuals with deletions in the COL 3A1 gene on chromosome 3 affecting the length of collagen type 3.

Cutis laxa

This is a rare disease in which the skin hangs in loose folds owing to loss of elastic tissue. Severely affected individuals have associated pulmonary emphysema. There are both dominant and recessive forms of heredity (Fig. 119).

Atrophy

Atrophy is characterized by thinning, loss of elasticity, loss of hair follicles, and a smooth surface to the skin. When pinched gently the skin produces fine wrinkles and may be compared to tissue paper. The upper dermal atrophy causes poor support to an atrophic vasculature and telangiectasia is often observed. At the same time there tends to be increased pigmentation within the dermis. Atrophy may be a consequence of inflammation following acute bacterial (particularly elastase-producing organisms) infection vasculitis or pancreatitis. It may be widespread as in the chronic scarring of leprosy or onchocerciasis. Some circumscribed atrophies follow an urticarial vasculitic process which is probably due to an infection which destroys elastic tissue. Perifollicular atrophy or postacne atrophy is similarly due to strains of staphylococcus which produce elastase. Syphilis is another cause of destruction of elastic tissue. Non-infectious causes include lupus erythematosus and localized scleroderma with its variants.

POIKILODERMA

The combination of pigmentation, telangiectasia, and atrophy is known as poikiloderma (see Fig. 130). The causes of poikiloderma include irradiation, lymphoma, and collagen diseases such as lupus erythematosus and dermatomyositis. There is a congenital form associated with light sensitivity, skin cancers, and dwarfism. It may follow lichen planus or stasis eczema. It is common on the neck in the light-exposed area and

may be aggravated by cosmetics. It is also described in graft-versus-host diseases.

Deep dermal and subcutaneous atrophy

The skin loses its subcutaneous or deep dermal tissue in a number of conditions. Such skin is waxy in colour and may be yellow, pigmented,

Fig. 119 A 9-year-old boy is showing drooping of the skin of the face due to premature loss of elasticity. The diagnosis is cutis laxa.

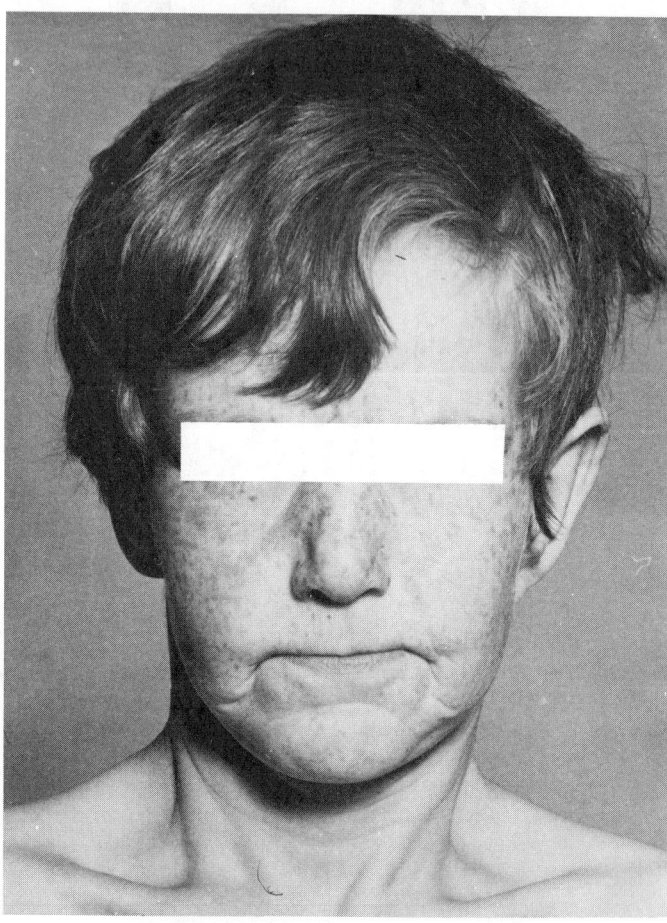

Fig. 120 Scleroderma and loss of finger tissue in porphyria. Hirsutism is also a feature.

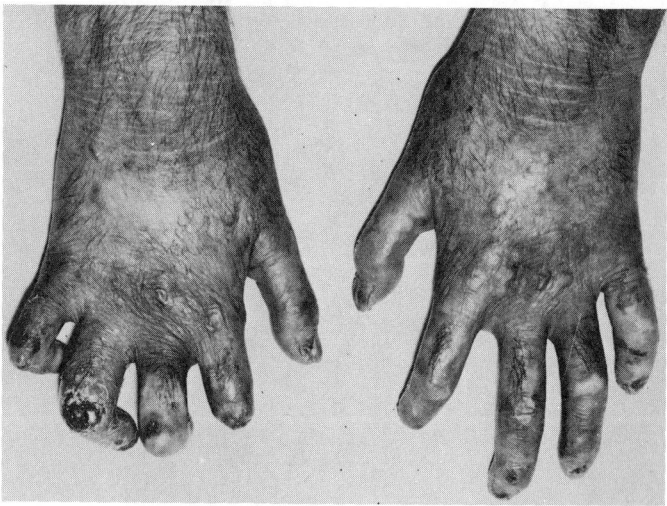

Table 28 *Conditions causing sclerosis*

Scleroderma

Dermatomyositis

Eosinophilic fasciitis (Schulman's syndrome)   This resembles scleroderma but the onset of oedema and induration of the extremities is accompanied by eosinophilia. A variant known as the eosinophil-myalgic syndrome follows the ingestion of L-tryptophan

Scleromyxoedema (lichen myxoedematosus)   A deposition of mucin associated with a paraprotein, an abnormal lambda light chain affecting face, limbs with thickened skin and exaggeration of natural contours or ridges, and flexion of the fingers. The deposition is papular and often linear

Progeria   Associated with alopecia and bird-like facies as well as arteriosclerosis

Porphyria cutanea tarda   The scleroderma is associated with hypertrichosis, skin fragility, blistering and scarring in light-exposed areas (Figs. 21, 110, and 120)

Graft-versus-host reactions   A history of bone marrow or thymus transplant precedes the lichenoid rash and scleroderma

Carcinoid disease and mast cell disorders   The release of serotonin and histamine over a prolonged period is sometimes associated with fibroblast proliferation and sclerosis

Pseudoscleroderma   This is due to infiltration occurring in amyloid, breast carcinoma, leprosy, lipoid proteinosis, mucopolysaccharide storage disorders, myxoedema. Thickening of the tissues is a feature of acromegaly

Scorbutic pseudoscleroderma   In the Bantu this is described as smooth, very dark skin, tightly stretched and hard on the lower aspects of the legs. It has abnormal iron pigment in histological material

---

or bluish with a loss of connective tissue. Deeper vessels may become more obvious so that there is either telangiectasia or obvious cutaneous atrophy and linear stretch marks which are initially red and sometimes protrude above the surface of the skin, but later there is always marked atrophy.

The skin that is atrophic may be tethered to underlying tissue or more obviously scarred. Such skin may feel hard or sclerosed (Table 28).

MORPHEA

Morphea is a localized form of scleroderma with a good prognosis for complete recovery (Fig. 121). It is not associated with any systemic disease. Occasionally a generalized form produces such tightness of the chest wall that breathing may be impaired. The generalized form of morphea also greatly restricts the limbs and a combination of ischaemia and lymphoedema may result in ulceration of the peripheries.

Other causes of deep dermal atrophy include injection of insulin—this is commonly seen on the thighs or arms of diabetics. Anetoderma is a term used for very discrete round idiopathic losses of dermis. Focal dermal hypoplasia is a rare cause of pitted skin usually observed first at birth and associated with eye and bone defects as well as perioral papillomas (Fig. 122).

Hemi- or generalized atrophy of non-inflammatory origin is mainly of unknown aetiology. Partial lipodystrophy is associated with glomerulonephritis and hypocomplementaemia. The Lawrence–Seip syndrome, or total lipoatrophy (with acanthosis nigricans, genital hypertrophy, resistant diabetes, and hepatomegaly), is a condition affecting infants. Atrophie blanche (Fig. 123) is an obliteration of single capillaries in the upper dermis, leading to very localized scarring. The causes are listed in Table 29.

Malignant disease

Infiltrations of the skin presenting as papules, *peau d'orange,* nodules, plaques, or ulcerating tumours of the dermis with destruction of overlying epidermis are a common terminal event of malignancy. Such lesions may arise from localized spread, as from a carcinoma of the breast, and they tend thus to be single or grouped and asymmetrical. More widespread haematogenous spread but with multiple lesions are a still more common terminal event. Certain metastases have diagnostic features and they include the scarring alopecia of breast carcinoma affecting the scalp or the pedunculated tumour of hypernephroma.

In many parts of the world with a high incidence of skin tumours both heredity and environment are determining factors and early diagnosis is rare. Whereas basal cell carcinomas are the predominant skin cancer in the white skin, Africans have a relatively high incidence of squamous carcinoma. Albinism and scarring following burns or other injuries are the main predisposing factors. Malignant melanoma in the African or the black-skinned American is especially a tumour of the feet. There is some evidence that a genetic increase in the number of junctional naevi in the lightly pigmented skin of the foot is a factor. In general, sunlight exposure accounts for the incidence of malignant melanoma in white skins, and exposed areas of skin are most affected.

Factors favouring malignancy

1. The chronic ingestion of inorganic arsenic. This was at one time given as a tonic for anaemia, often as Fowler's solution. It was combined with bromides for epilepsy or chorea and specifically for psoriasis and blistering disorders. It is still prescribed in many parts of the world, although almost obsolete in the United Kingdom and United States. Arsenical contamination of water supplies is recorded in Argentina and Taiwan. It has also been used in arsenical fruit sprays or sheep dips in Europe, and there have been descriptions of contamination of dust in the mines of various parts of the world. Keratoses of the palms and soles are usually persistent and are small, 1 to 3 mm in diameter, round, and hard. Keratoses are one of the few conditions diagnosed by the shaking of the hand. They may progress to squamous carcinoma and should be removed if ulcerated, indurated, or inflamed. Mutant P53 is commonly expressed in solar keratoses and Bowen's disease. The latter and basal epitheliomas (Fig. 124) of the trunk are much more common in chronic arsenically exposed persons. Bowen's disease is a persistent, flat, red, scaly or crusted and pigmented lesion with the features of an intraepidermal carcinoma. Arsenical pigmentation is characterized by a raindrop appearance of areas of paler skin.

2. Skin contact. Prolonged contact on moist skin, such as the scrotum, with coal, soot, and cutting oils may cause malignancy.

3. Radiation. Radiation, especially from ultraviolet B (290–330 nm), is the commonest factor predisposing to skin cancer, and explains its high incidence in Australia, Texas, and South Africa. Glass and thick water vapour are protective. Pigmentation by melanin is the natural protective factor. Albinos are more likely to develop carcinoma of the skin. Ionizing radiation explains the high incidence of carcinoma in the skin of the careless practitioner or research worker using irradiated materials. It is a common cause of baldness following X-ray atrophy in persons treated in the past for tinea capitis or ankylosing spondylitis.

4. Radiant heat. Radiant heat sufficient to produce chronic erythema and pigmentation predisposes to squamous epithelioma, as from the fire brick of the Kangri cancer of Kashmir or the hot water bottle of the chronically discomforted.

5. Scars. Scars from any chronic disease such as lupus vulgaris (Fig. 125), syphilis, burns, epidermolysis bullosa, or leprosy, or even from common stasis ulcer of the skin may all produce malignant change.

6. Lymphoedema. Lymphoedema predisposes to angiosarcomas, a phenomenon described in post-mastectomy limbs but also in congenital lymphoedema.

7. Genetic syndromes. These are rare but distinctive (Table 30). *Gorlin's syndrome* results from an autosomal dominant gene located on chromosome 9q 22:3 q 31, and is characterized by dental cysts, hypertelorism, palmar and plantar pits, bifid ribs, and a great tendency to develop basal cell epitheliomata. The palmar pits are flat, being 1 to 3 mm with a stellate edge. Pseudohypoparathyroidism and medullary blastomata are recorded. P_{53} mutations on chromosome 17 are also associated with epidermal malignancies. *Torre–Muir* syndrome is a condition with multiple sebaceous adenomata and multiple primary malignant tumours of the viscera. *Xeroderma pigmentosum* is a recessively transmitted group of diseases characterized by the progressive development of freckling, telangiectasia, and skin tumours. *Peutz–Jeghers* is discussed elsewhere. There is perioral and finger freckling associated with small intestinal polyps and only occasional malignancy. *Gardner's syndrome* is also a condition of polyposis of the gut, combined with osteomas. *Neurocutaneous syndromes* include the acoustic neuroma (or phaeochromocytoma) in neurofibromatosis. In *tuberous sclerosis* there is an increased incidence of rhabdomyosarcoma.

8. Immunosuppression. There is an increased incidence of skin malignancy in the immunosuppressed. After renal transplantation, warts, keratoses, and skin cancer are common, especially in light-exposed skin.

Signs of underlying malignancy

The three 'P's of pallor, pigmentation, and pruritus are common terminal events in malignant disease but any one can also be a presenting sign. Defective immunosurveillance predisposes to infections such as candidiasis or herpes simplex and herpes zoster. Disseminated intravascular coagulation is a common terminal event of malignancy but may be a presenting sign of lymphoma, leukaemia, or carcinoma of the pancreas. Rarer diseases associated with malignancy include:

1. Acquired ichthyosis in which the skin becomes progressively drier and more scaly. The surface stratum corneum may crack, giving rise to reactive patterns of eczema craquelé (Fig. 126). Increasing scale eventually overlaps with exfoliative dermatitis but, unlike the exfoliative dermatitis due to

Fig. 121 (a) Widespread hardness of the skin and brownish or violaceous plaques that are often atrophic are features of morphea—a localized form of scleroderma. (b) Pseudoscleroderma, identical to morphea, is also a consequence of post-thrombophlebitic fibrosis of the lower limbs.

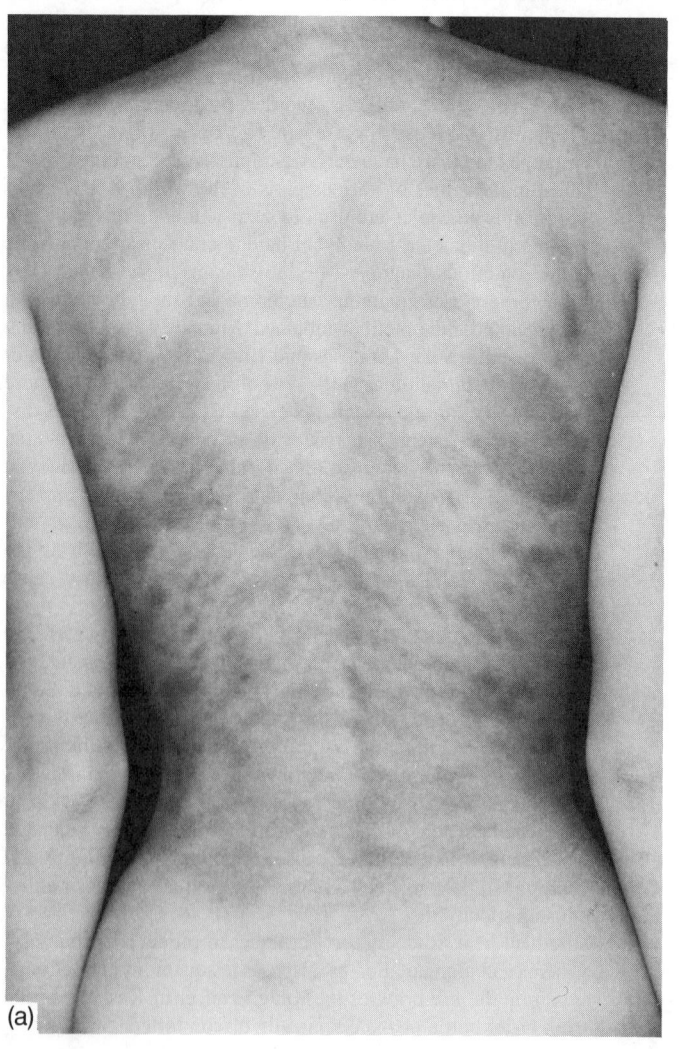

(a)

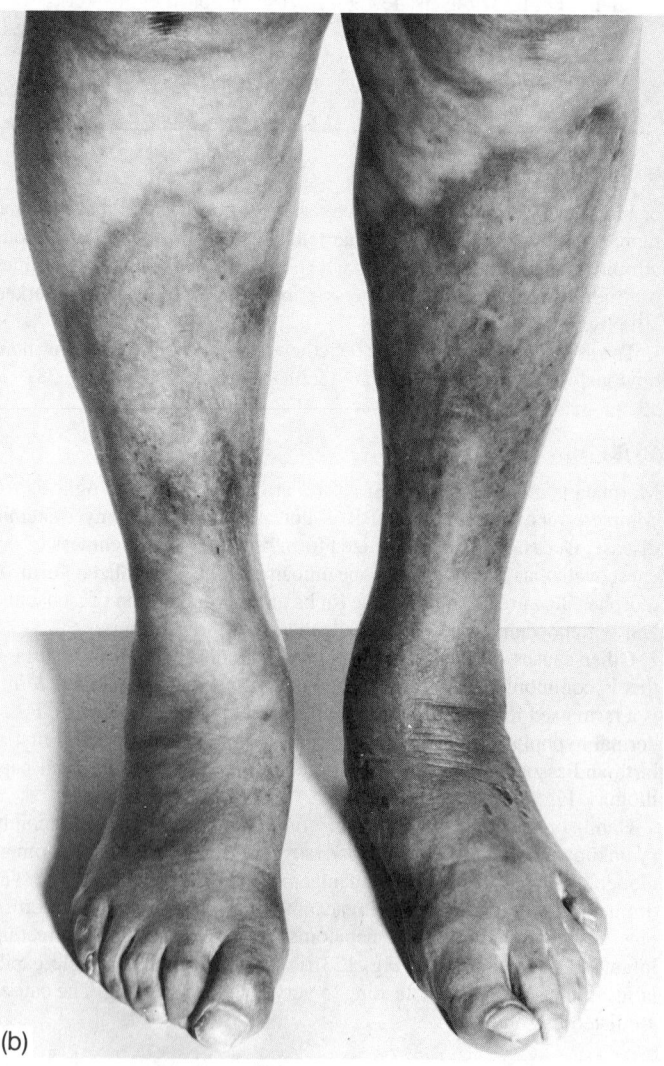

(b)

drugs or psoriasis, the scale is more adherent, i.e. less exfoliative. There is usually accompanying atrophy of the skin.

2. Dermatomyositis is commonly caused by malignancy in the white-skinned adult. In children or in black-skinned Africans it is more often a manifestation of autoimmune (collagen) disease. The muscle weakness is proximal. The skin signs include erythema (see Fig. 115), lichenoid, or psoriaform eruptions, and itching or tenderness may be considerable. Periorbital swelling and redness, as well as a streaky erythema on the backs of the fingers and ragged telangiectatic nailfolds, are other features.

3. Acanthosis nigricans is pigmentation and wartiness of the axilla and groins. There is a velvety brown thickness of the skin of the hands and at mucocutaneous junctions such as the lips (Fig. 127).

4. Acquired hypertrichosis lanuginosa is a generalized increase in terminal hair and should be distinguished from hirsutes which is an increase in hair in sites normally associated with hair growth, such as the chin.

5. Acute onset of multiple irritable seborrhoeic warts is known as the sign of Leser–Trélat.

6. Superficial thrombophlebitis or migrating thrombophlebitis is especially associated with carcinoma of the pancreas.

7. Bullous pyoderma gangrenosum is a feature of leukaemia and myeloma.

8. Bullous disease of erythema multiforme type, or occasionally more suggestive of pemphigoid, is more likely to be associated with malignancy if the oral mucosa is involved or if immunofluorescence studies are negative.

9. Erythema gyratum repens (Fig. 128) is one of many patterns of erythema forming repeated concentric rings. The more bizarre and rapidly evolving the process, the more likely is it to be associated with malignancy. This is particularly so when it is generalized, oedematous, or scaling (see also Fig. 11c).

10. Palmar keratoses are found in association with cancer of the bladder or lung.

REFERENCE

Worret, W.-I.F. (1993). Skin signs and internal malignancies. *International Journal of Dermatology,* **32,** 1–5.

Fig. 122 Goltz's syndrome (focal dermal atrophy), patchy atrophy and (a) pitting of the skin; (b) with syndactyly.

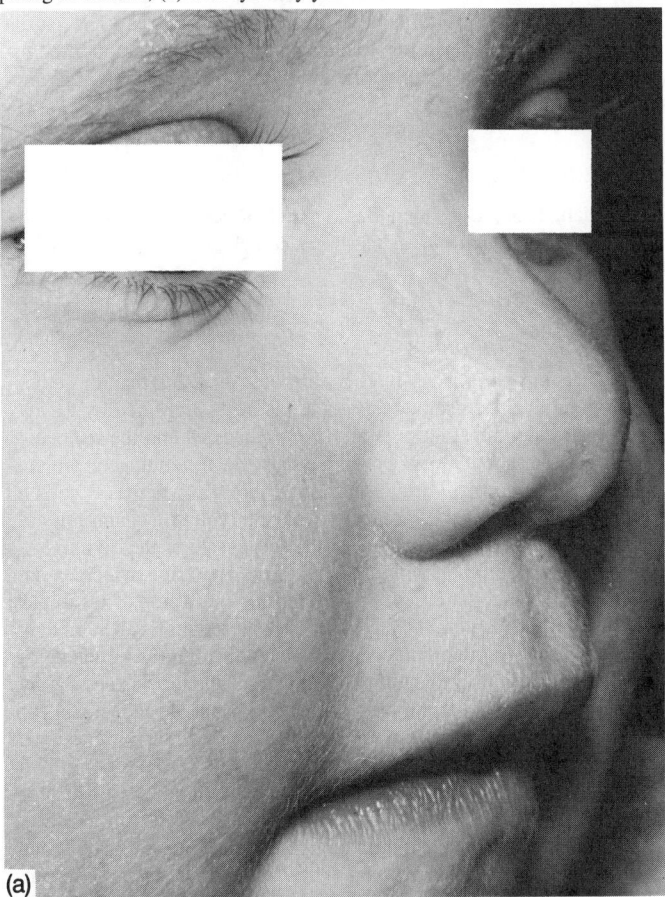

(a)

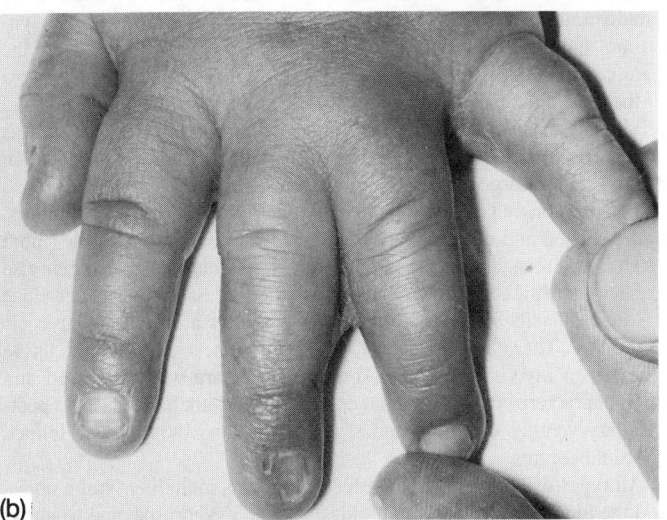

(b)

Fig. 123 Atrophie blanche is an obliteration of the capillaries in the upper dermis, causing sclerosis. Residual vessels are elongated and coiled. They are liable to thrombosis and overlying ulceration is a consequence.

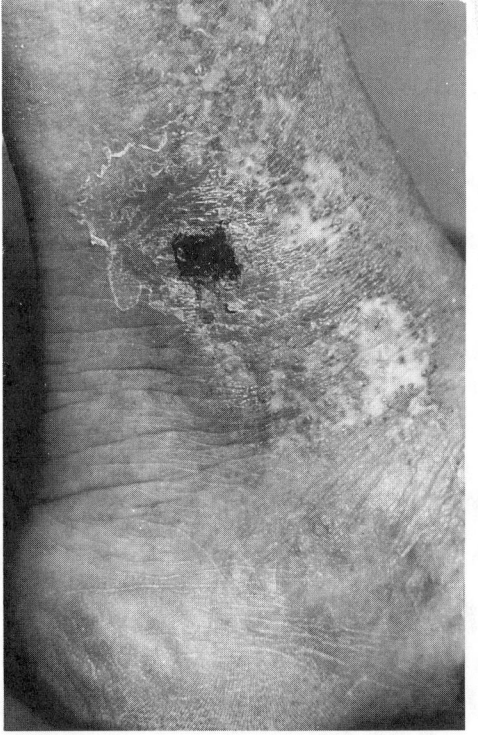

Table 29 *Atrophie blanche: list of associated diseases*

Pigmented purpuric eruptions	Rheumatoid arthritis
Gravitational stasis	Hashimoto's disease
Thrombophlebitis	Sickle-cell anaemia
Thrombo-angiitis obliterans	Anterior poliomyelitis
Polyarteritis nodosa	Sjögren's syndrome
Diabetes mellitus	Capillary naevi
Scleroderma	Drug eruptions
Lupus erythematosus	Trauma, cuts
Dermatomyositis	Carcinoma

Fig. 124 The rolled edge of a basal cell epithelioma of the trunk. In the multifocal superficial form that in this case followed arsenic ingestion many years previously, the edge is less pronounced.

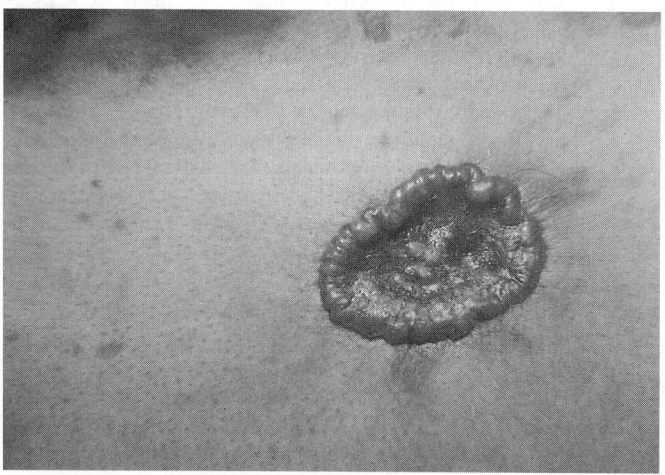

Fig. 125 Lupus vulgaris present for 25 years has resulted in chronic scarring. In this a squamous epithelioma has developed.

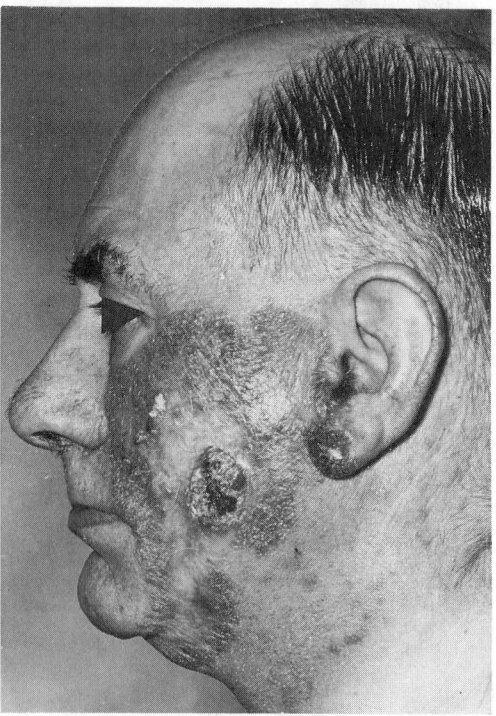

Erythroderma

Causes such as psoriasis, atopic eczema, or drug eruption can usually be diagnosed and appropriate therapy given. It is the acquired erythroderma in the adult that gives most difficulty with diagnosis and has been named the pre-Sézary syndrome. There may be a short or long history of persistent intermittent dermatitis, often with proven evidence of allergy to several agents with which the skin is in contact. Lymphadenopathy and hepatosplenomegaly may be pronounced. The Sézary syndrome of a leucocytosis of circulating T cells may be intermittent or persistent. Sun may be an aggravating factor; IgE levels may be elevated and either atopic eczema or psoriasis may feature in the past history. The skin is thickened and chronically oedematous with a variable degree of palmar plantar keratoderma and alopecia. The histology is of a severe dermatitis, and a frank lymphoma cannot be diagnosed. The partial remissions are only in part due to changes in management, but prednisolone, chlorambucil or azathioprine in low dosage are increasingly prescribed for this syndrome.

REFERENCE

Winkleman, R.K., Buechner, S.A., and Dia-Perez, J.T. (1984). Pre-Sézary syndrome. *Journal of the American Academy of Dermatology* **10**, 992–9.

Cutaneous lymphoma

Few aspects of dermatology have been more confusing than those concerning lymphoma. In some respects it has been simplified by the recognition and identification of B and T lymphocytes and the realization that terms such as reticulosis, pre-reticulosis, and reticulum cell are misapplied. T cells normally traverse through the skin whereas B cells do not. The expression on the keratinocyte of $\alpha3\beta1$ integrin chains possibly explains epidermotropism. The Hassall's corpuscle in the thymus may have features in common with the cells of the epidermis which explain helper T cell, Langerhans cell, and epidermal interaction. The simplest classification into B-cell, T-cell, and non-B and non-T cell lymphoma with a single sub-grouping into small cells, indicating low-grade malignancy, and large cells, indicating high-grade malignancy, is now largely accepted. However, neither morphology nor a panel of monoclonal antibodies have provided a system of identification by which prognosis and treatment can be planned with absolute certainty. CD30 positivity, K_i67 or CD44 negativity are recently described indications of a good prognosis. Large-cell K_i-1 antigen markers have a favourable prognosis.

Enzymic, cytochemical, immunological, monoclonal antibodies, gene rearrangement analysis, functional and ultrastructural methods applied by research workers are not routinely available, but they indicate that conditions in which the epidermis is eczematous, scaly, or crusting are usually infiltrated with T cells, as in mycosis fungoides, Sézary syndrome, and pagetoid reticulosis. Mononuclear phagocytes, including the Langerhans cells and eosinophils, often infiltrate the upper dermis. Most of the purple red tumours showing no involvement of the epidermis and producing sharply demarcated infiltrates in the middle or deep dermis are due to B-cell proliferation. The late tumour stage is reflected in progression to large anaplastic lymphoblastic cells.

The previously labelled reticulosarcomas starting as solitary tumours, dome-shaped and deep red, are now thought to be lymphoblastic, more often B cell than T cell. Such less differentiated blast cells also give rise to heavy infiltrates in the whole dermis and are less inclined to produce the nest of cells within the epidermis which is a feature of mycosis fungoides. There is destruction of blood vessels and fibrous tissue whereas in mycosis fungoides, blood vessels are well preserved and often characterized by prominent epithelioid endothelial cells as in postcapillary venules of lymph nodes. Benign lesions show a well-defined germinal centre.

All types of lymphoma may affect any organ, including lymph nodes and the blood, but mycosis fungoides, Sézary's syndrome, and pagetoid

Table 30 *Classification of cutaneous paraneoplastic syndrome*

Autosomal dominant paraneoplasias	Skin markers	Internal malignancies	Coincidence
Basal cell naevus syndrome (Gorlin)	Multiple BCCs	Brain medulloblastoma	−20%
Birt-Hogg syndrome	Trichodiscoma	Gastrointestinal tract	?
Carney syndrome	Lentigines, blue naevi	Heart myxoma, testes	>75%
Cowden syndrome	Trichilemmoma, fibroma	Breasts, thyroid	70%
Gardner's syndrome	Cysts, osteoma, pigmented ocular fundus	Colon	100%
Howel-Evans syndrome (tylosis)	Palmar plantar keratomas	Oesophagus	100%
Multiple endocrine neoplasia syndrome (MEN 2b)	Neuroma (lips and tongue)	Thyroid, phaeochromocytoma	>85%
Dysplastic naevus syndrome	Multiple dysplastic naevi	Melanoma, testes, eyes	?
Peutz–Jeghers syndrome	Lentigines on lips	Ovaries, testes	rare
Torre-Muir syndrome	Sebaceous tumours	Gastrointestinal tract, lung, urinary	−100%

Modified from Worret (1993).

reticulosis favour the skin and often seem confined to it. The leonine facies is a peculiar feature more often seen in B-cell lymphoma as in chronic lymphatic leukaemia.

During the early stage of mycosis fungoides, the behaviour of the T cell cannot be proven to be malignant and some suggest that it is merely hyper-reactive or over-stimulated. The sources of this stimulus could even be the skin macrophage known as the Langerhans cell. These are increased in number in mycosis fungoides. Exactly when 'over-stimulus' becomes 'lymphoma' has been debated but no conclusions can be reached.

The distinctive cell found in tissues and blood of the Sézary syndrome and in the epidermis of mycosis fungoides a T cell with a usually but not invariably hyperconvoluted cerebri form nucleus. It is also observed in a variety of non-lymphomatous dermatoses and it should be equated more with the 'over-stimulus' concept rather than with malignancy.

CLINICAL FEATURES OF LYMPHOMA

Dermatologists have long grappled with the problem of diseases of the skin which are suspected of culminating, often years later, in a malignancy of the lymphoid tissue. These diseases have features of chronic dermatitis and psoriasis (parapsoriasis) because there is a chronic reaction in the dermis and epidermis which is often indistinguishable from other causes of such a reaction. The feature that causes suspicion is lack of symmetry in an atypical distribution. There is also inhomogeneity within the lesion. Infiltration with white cells suggesting tumour formation is one feature. Another is atrophy or thinning of the dermis, telangiectasia, and pigmentation known as poikiloderma. Persistent superficial dermatitis, previously known as parapsoriasis in plaque (benign type), consists of flat, symmetrical slightly scaly, red patches on the trunk or limbs which persist for years. They are round, oval, or

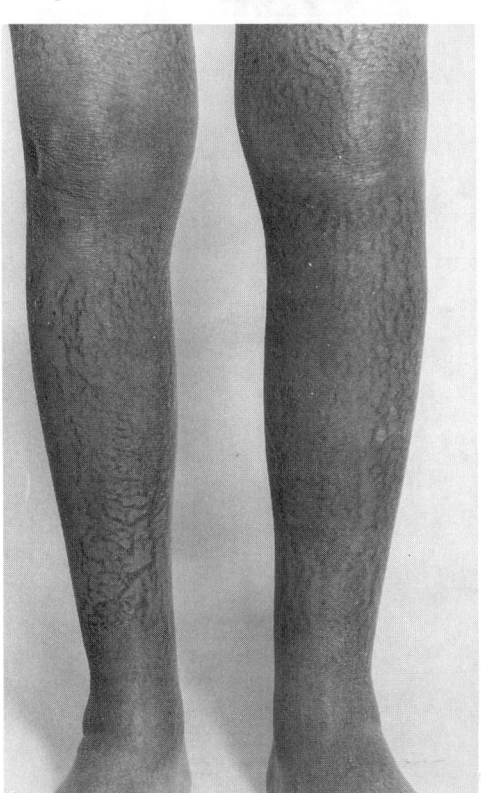

Fig. 126 Eczema craquelée, a consequence of skin malnutrition and an accompaniment and consequence of malignancy.

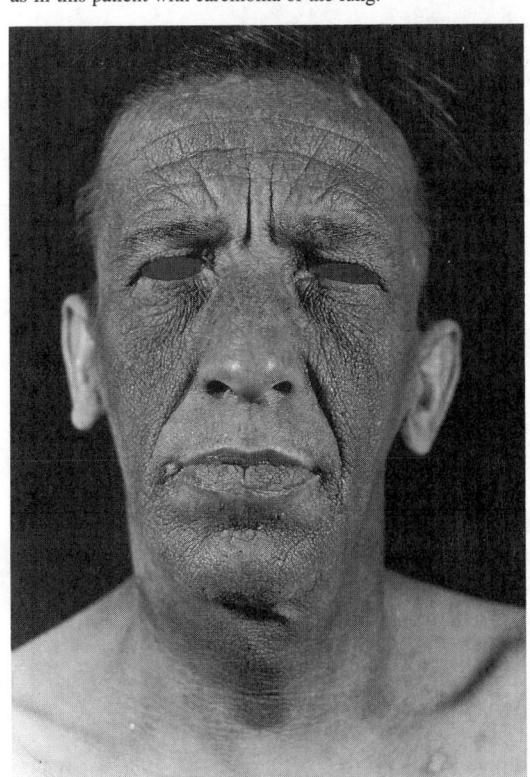

Fig. 127 Acanthosis nigricans; a darkening and thickening of the skin with a tendency to papilloma formation. The angles of the mouth are often involved, as in this patient with carcinoma of the lung.

finger-like and are sometimes yellowish (Fig. 129). This is now thought to be benign.

Poikiloderma atrophicans vasculare, previously known as parapsoriasis (large plaque or lichenoides), resembles radiodermatitis in that there is atrophy, telangiectasis, and reticulate pigmentation (Fig. 130). It favours areas spared exposure to natural sunlight such as the breasts or buttocks. It may be composed of small papules or large plaques of any shape. The expected outcome often many years later is the cutaneous T-cell lymphoma known as mycosis fungoides but Hodgkin's disease is also a possibility.

B-cell lymphoma, when present in the skin, forms firm pink-red or skin-coloured tumours, often in groups coalescing to produce annular or other patterns (Fig. 131).

Lipomelanic reticulosis is a non-specific enlargement of lymph nodes associated with widespread dermatitis or erythroderma.

Mycosis fungoides is initially often no more than a non-specific dermatitis or more commonly poikiloderma atrophicans vasculare. Occasionally it is a tumour from the beginning. The lesions may be symptomless but severe pruritus is common. The affected areas become more infiltrated, scaly, and reddened (Fig. 132). Often they are annular, serpiginous, or have other bizarre shapes. Erythroderma and widespread

Fig. 130 Poikiloderma; atrophy, pigmentation, and telangiectasia, commonly preceding the development of lymphoma in the skin. The clinical appearance is like radiodermatitis.

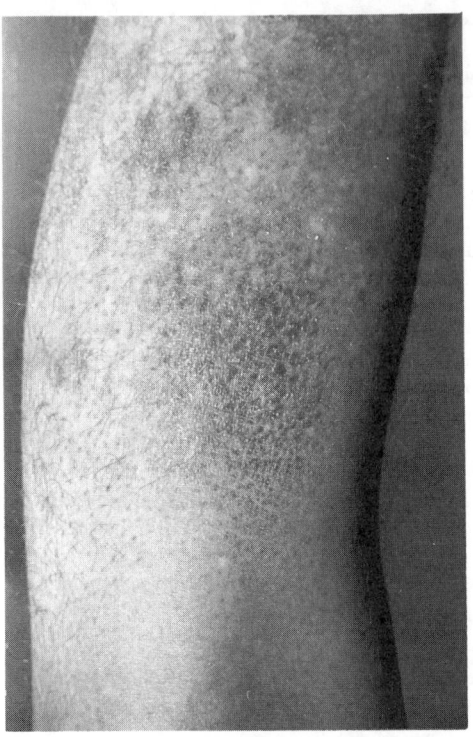

Fig. 128 Erythema gyratum repens in a patient with adenocarcinoma of the colon.

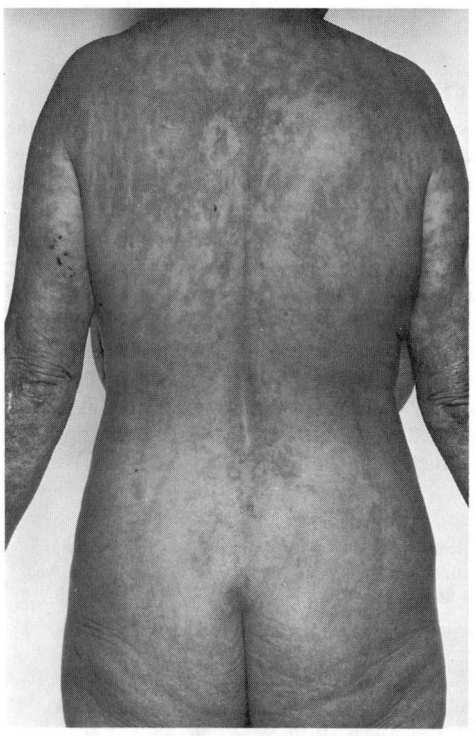

Fig. 131 Fleshy tumours grouped and arising in the dermis without epidermal hyperplasia. This is characteristic of B-cell lymphomas.

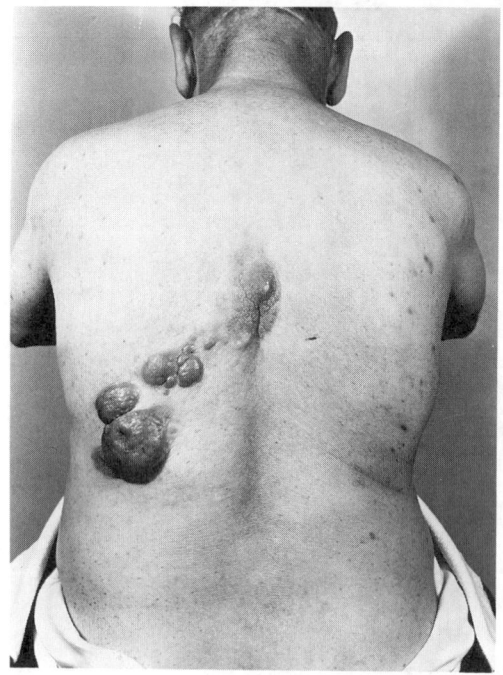

Fig. 129 Lower abdominal, persistent superficial dermatitis (parapsoriasis). These are fixed and persistent digitate (finger-like) patterns, erythematous, and slightly scaly.

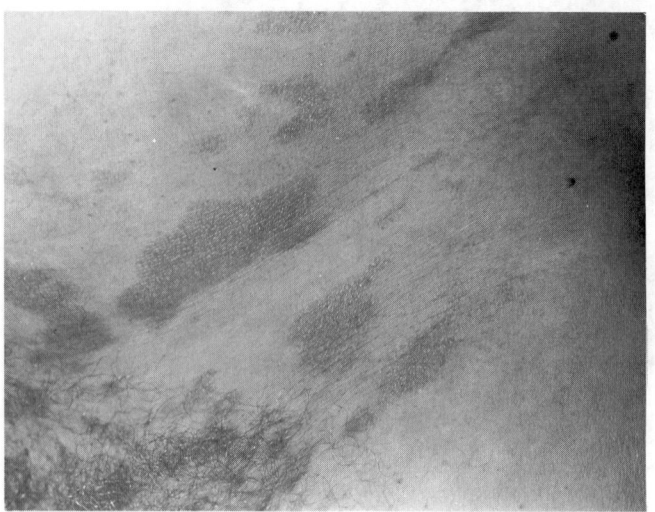

ulceration is the final stage of the disease. The diagnostic histological feature is invasion of the epidermis by atypical lymphocytes, often in clusters—Pautrier abscesses—and a heavy pleomorphic infiltration of the upper dermis hugging the epidermis but causing less necrosis of individual epidermal cells than in lichen planus.

Skin manifestations of Hodgkin's disease include infiltration of the skin with nodules of the disease. Pigmentation and pruritus are common. Prurigo with deep excoriations and secondary infection is one of its most distressing manifestations. Ichthyosiform atrophy as part of the terminal wasting disease is common. The scaling is often as severe as an exfoliative dermatitis but shedding of the scale is less than that of psoriasis. Hair loss, herpes zoster, and rarely erythema nodosum are other complications.

MANAGEMENT OF MYCOSIS FUNGOIDES

The rate of progression is highly variable. There is still no clear picture of the natural history of mycosis fungoides. Samman treated a series of patients conservatively and only 45 of 212 cases died of mycosis fungoides. Most of those who died had tumours, skin ulcers, or palpable lymph-nodes at the time of presentation, and in the absence of these the prognosis tends to be very good. In patients with benign patterns of the disease it is important not to overtreat.

Radiation therapy

Small-field orthovoltage radiation has been standard therapy for many years and it is very useful to control plaques and tumours resistant to other modalities. It is not unusual for patients to require a small dose of radiation to one area only at as little as yearly intervals. Electron beam therapy is recommended for most patients with extensive infiltrated plaques or tumours. A high initial response rate can be expected in a majority of patients but they remain free of disease only for about 3 years.

Topical nitrogen mustard (mechlorethamine, HN$_2$)

This is a useful treatment for patients who have less infiltrated skin lesions. Clinical response may be slow and maintenance therapy may

be required for at least 2 years. The chief side-effect is allergic contact dermatitis, occurring in about 30 to 60 per cent of patients. Desensitization can be attempted but it is difficult to effect. There is some debate as to whether an aqueous or ointment-based preparation is best. It is probable that the ointment-based preparation produces fewer hypersensitivity reactions.

Puva

Several reported series of the good effects of PUVA have resulted in most academic departments using this as a first line of therapy for superficial lesions that are widespread. Penetration of PUVA is limited so that deep tumours are unlikely to be cleared.

Systemic chemotherapy

On the whole this is reserved for palliation in persons with systemic disease and deep tumours. There is usually some initial response. Clearance for more than 1 year is unusual.

REFERENCES

Abel, E.A. (1981). Photochemotherapy for cutaneous T-cell lymphoma. *Journal of the American Academy of Dermatology* **4**, 423–9.
Du Vivier, A. *et al.* (1978). Mycosis fungoides, nitrogen mustard and skin cancer. *British Journal of Dermatology* **99**, 61–3.
Hoppe, R.T. *et al.* (1979). Radiation therapy in the management of cutaneous T-cell lymphomas. *Cancer Treatment Reports* **63**, 625–32.
MacKie, R.M. (1992). Lymphomas and leukaemias. In *Textbook of dermatology*, (5th edn), (ed. A. Rook, D.S. Wilkinson, and F.J.G. Ebling), pp. 2107–34. Blackwell Scientific Publications, Oxford.
Minna, J.D. *et al.* (1979). Report of the committee on therapy for MF and Sézary syndrome. *Cancer Treatment Reports* **63**, 729–36.
Price, N.M. *et al.* (1983). Ointment-based mechlorethamine treatment for MF. *Cancer* **52**, 2214–19.
Samman, P. (1976). Mycosis fungoides and other cutaneous reticulosis. *Clinical and Experimental Dermatology* **1**, 97–214.
Van Vloten, W.A. *et al.* (1985). Total skin electron beam irradiation for cutaneous T-cell lymphoma (mycosis fungoides). *British Journal of Dermatology* **112**, 697–702.
Worret, W.I.F. (1993). Skin signs and internal malignancies. *International Journal of Dermatology*, **32**, 1–5.

Fig. 132 Marked irregular epidermal reactivity is a characteristic response to T-cell lymphoma of the mycosis fungoides type.

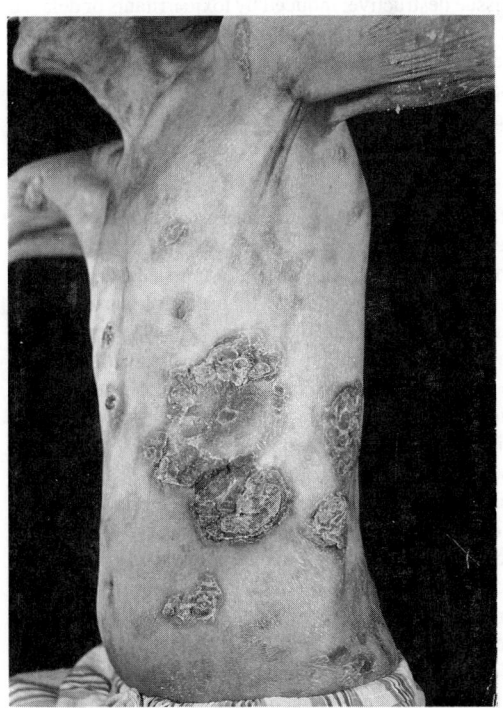

Viral warts

Warts are caused by the papovavirus (see Section 7), which enters the skin through small abrasions, particularly if the skin is moist and warm. Virus is found by electron microscopy in the differentiating cells of the upper epidermis rather than in the proliferating basal cell layer. The incubation period is probably several months. There are a number of strains of wart virus giving rise to different types of warts—common, plantar, mosaic, plane, and anogenital. Molluscum contagiosum is caused by a pox virus (Fig. 133).

The incidence of warts is increased in immunosuppressed patients either from drugs or associated with lymphoma. Cell-mediated immunity is more certainly a factor than humoral immunity. The peak incidence is in children aged 12 to 16 and in recent years in Europe and the United States there seems to be an increase in infection rate compared to Asia, Australia, or Africa.

Trauma may account for the distribution of warts on the hands and feet. Nail biting in children and shaving in men, as well as ill-fitting shoes in adults, are all relevant. Twenty per cent of warts disappear within 6 months and 65 per cent in 2 years. Plane warts and mosaic warts are slow to clear.

Common warts are firm papules with a rough horny surface. They occur singly or coalesce into large masses. The knuckles and nail folds are particularly favoured, as are the knees and, more rarely, the shaft of the penis. They should be differentiated from warty tuberculosis which usually is a solitary plaque with an erythematous border. Granuloma annulare of the knuckles does not have a horny surface. A persistent wart on the toes or fingers may be a reaction to a subungual exostosis. Squamous epitheliomata or keratoacanthoma are usually solitary and found in an older population.

Plane warts are smooth, flat, or slightly elevated affecting the face or back of hands. They may coalesce or form linear lesions in scratch marks. Lichen planus may be difficult to distinguish from plane warts but is unusual on the face and prefers the flexor surface of the wrists as well as the mucosa of the mouth. The histology of plane warts is unexciting, whereas lichen planus shows destruction of the basal cell layer of the epidermis and a heavy infiltrate of mononuclear cells.

Filiform and digitate warts are common in the beard area, on the lips, and in the nasal vestibule.

Plantar warts begin as a small sago grain papule. As it enlarges, paring of the surface with a scalpel distinguishes the wart from the surrounding horny ring of normal epidermis and reveals the small capillaries in the tips of the elongated papillae. Most warts are overpressure points. Clusters of small warts make up a mosaic. A wart which shows numerous thrombosed capillaries and is darker than usual is probably regressing. The fourth interdigital space is a common site for soft corns due to pressure of the little toe on the head of the metatarsal in a tight shoe and in ballet dancers. Soft warts or even condylomata lata have been described at such sites.

TREATMENT

Most human papilloma virus (HPV) infections in the vagina and cervix are not visible to the naked eye but can be identified by painting with acetic acid (3–5 per cent). The demonstration of latent virus is of uncertain biological significance. Infection with HPV is not sufficient to cause cancer and may act as a promoter. There is no successful means of eliminating HPV. Warts should be treated on the basis that they are unaesthetic and uncomfortable.

Spontaneous resolution is to be expected. Overall, 12 weeks is the usual time required to cure warts irrespective of the treatment used and most standard treatments do no better or worse than this. Podophyllin and formalin or salicylic acid are standard therapies.

Podophyllin 10 to 20 per cent in liquid paraffin or in tincture benzoic compound is painted on to anogenital warts and the area is then powdered. The podophyllin is irritant and some persons need to wash it off in 2 h. Others have no such discomfort. It should not be used in the pregnant since absorption sufficient to damage the fetus is a possibility. The treatment is repeated at intervals of 1 to 3 weeks.

Formalin 10 per cent solution can be applied as a soak to multiple warts of the soles of the feet, but dryness and fissuring may be troublesome.

Fig. 133 Molluscum contagiosum: groups of virus-induced papules characterized by a central punctum.

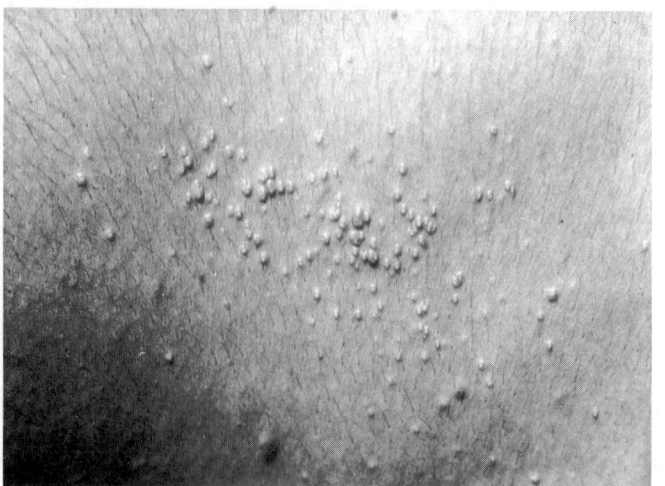

Salicylic acid is the most reliable chemical for treating warts. Paints or plasters containing 20 to 40 per cent salicylic acid are best applied after a 5-min soak with warm soapy water and preferably after removal of excess surface keratin.

Freezing is with liquid nitrogen either in a special spray or by application from a cotton wool bud on the end of an orange stick. The wart should be whitened for at least 20 to 30 sec and blistering is a common consequence.

Local anaesthetic injected into the base of a wart to lift it up from the dermis can be followed by curettage. Compression with the thumb on immediate adjacent tissue prevents bleeding while silver nitrate is applied. The rim of horny tissues around the wart side should be cut away using scissors.

Curettage of molluscum contagiosum may be made painless in the majority of children except at mucocutaneous junctions by the use of a eutetic mixture of local anaesthetics (EMLA) applied under occlusion for 60 min.

REFERENCES

Bunney, M.H. (1980). Viral warts: answering the patients' questions. *Medicine* **31**, 1593–6.
Gissmann, L., Pfister, H., and zur Hausen, H. (1977). Human papilloma viruses (HPV) characterisation of four different isolates. *Virology* **76**, 569–80.
Ling, M.R. (1992). Therapy of genital human papilloma virus infections. *International Journal of Dermatology* **31**, 682–6.
Von Krogh, G. (1979). Warts. Immunologic factors of prognostic significance. *International Journal of Dermatology* **18**, 195–205.

Granulomata and other infiltrations of the skin

A granuloma is a compact accumulation of cells, comprised mainly of monocytes or their variants, macrophages, epithelioid cells, and giant cells. Often there is subsequent fibrosis. Lymphocytes are more numerous in granulomata due to allergens to which the host is sensitive. Degeneration or foreign bodies encourage neutrophil and eosinophil participation.

Granulomata are classified as high or low turnover:

High turnover: tissue destructive; induced by toxic irritants or delayed hypersensitivity; continuous recruitment of macrophages and many mitoses; and epithelioid and giant cells frequent.
Low turnover: space occupying but not destructive; induced by inert (bacterial) and non-degradable irritants; no continued recruitment but long survival of macrophages and few mitoses; and few epithelioid and few giant cells.

The clinical features of granulomata are either space-occupying nodules lying in the dermis or, if close to the surface of the skin, they may be seen as yellow or brownish-red and sometimes translucent areas. The chronic changes in blood supply associated with the lesion cause a bluish colour and sometimes telangiectasia. If they are in the upper dermis, then there may be overlying epithelial hyperplasia or ulceration with extrusion of some of the granulomatous material. On the other hand, thinning of the epidermis may be considerable. In dark skins, pigmentary changes may include hypo- or hyperpigmentation.

A common cause of granulomata is persistent irritation of the skin by external trauma causing ulceration and pseudo-epitheliomatous hyperplasia. Examples include granuloma fissuratum of the ear or nose due to ill-fitting spectacles. The ingrowing toenail, the pilonidal sinus, or the presence of extrafollicular but intradermal hair as is seen in the interdigital clefts of barbers, and cattle or horse dealers are other examples.

Granuloma gluteal infantum is seen in the nappy area due to incomplete resolution of an irritant rash in which steroid creams have been too extravagantly applied. Numerous agents acting as a foreign body incompletely degraded and removed are causes of chronic granulomas in the skin. They include sea urchin spines, silicates, cactus allergen, grit, and various chronic infections such as *Candida albicans, Trichophyton verrucosum* (Fig. 134(a)), coccidioidomycosis, atypical mycobacteria from fish tanks or swimming baths, leprosy (Fig. 134(b)), tuberculosis (Fig. 134(c)), leishmaniasis (Fig. 134(d)), and halogen granulomas (see Fig. 33).

Sarcoidosis

The general features of this disease are discussed in Chapter 17.10.10. Erythema nodosum is the commonest problem. The other skin manifestations are present in about 15 to 25 per cent of cases seen in hospital and are due to accumulations of epithelioid granulomas in the dermis, usually with a free zone sparing the epidermis. It is commoner in black- than in white-skinned patients and in women rather than men. The appearance depends on the level in the dermis and the size and confluence of the lesions. Sarcoid favours scars, even the old ones, and these may suggest keloid formation.

Lupus pernio is a pattern mostly seen in women, in which bluish-red or violaceous swellings present on the nose, cheeks, ears, or hands. The lesions are long-lasting.

The anterior septum and nasal vestibule is commonly involved by granulomatous disease (Table 31 and Fig. 135). It is a site in which epithelial necrosis may occur secondarily to interference with its blood supply.

Micropapular sarcoid consists of yellowish-brown pin-head or pea-sized papules, often grouped and cropping (Fig. 136). Compression with a glass slide removes the reddish vascular dilatation and a translucent yellow lesion, 'the apple jelly', can be observed. This pattern may not be distinguishable from lichen scrofulosorum. In the latter the tuberculin test is strongly positive and the Kveim test is negative. However, in the elderly population of the United Kingdom, cases are increasingly described suspected of tubercular aetiology but in the absence of these confirmatory signs, proved to be questionably sarcoid.

The plaque form is a more diffuse sarcoidosis involving the limbs, shoulders, buttocks, and thighs (Fig. 137). The skin is atrophic and the edges may be serpiginous, suggesting tertiary lues.

The granuloma of sarcoid is a chronic injury to the skin and may evoke a great variety of responses, including scarring alopecia, lupus erythematosus-like epidermal atrophy, ulceration, telangiectasia, hypopigmentation, epidermal hyperplasia, and a psoriasiform plaque or verrucous hypertrophy. Confluence of lesions or healing in the centre gives rise to annular patterns. Histological features of a well-defined epithelioid granuloma are more diagnostic than the clinical picture.

When sarcoid of the skin presents without other subjective or objective evidence of systemic sarcoidosis, the prognosis is good and the patient is unlikely to develop later systemic disease. This may be because the skin lesion is not a manifestation of the tendency to develop sarcoid but is a localized phenomenon in response to an entirely local event. Chest radiography and pulmonary function tests, as well as slit-lamp examination of the eye, should nevertheless be done in every case.

Urticaria pigmentosa or mastocytosis

Mast cells are normally present in the skin but the numbers vary greatly, with up to 80 per mm^3 in the upper dermis. In mastocytosis they are greatly increased in number and may be found as a single isolated mastocytoma or numerous nests scattered over the entire body, i.e. the classic urticaria pigmentosa, or diffusely throughout the entire skin. Occasionally there is systemic infiltration of all tissues including liver, spleen, and bone marrow. A very rare leukaemic variety is also recognized.

The mast cell releases histamine, leucotrienes, and heparin and these

may have systemic effects, but it is increasingly realized that the local contribution is through its secretion of proteases.

In the infant, mastocytosis may present as blisters, but more commonly the lightly pigmented swellings in the skin are noted and observed to swell when scratched or after a hot bath or exercise. Rarely there is a generalized flushing and itching. The condition is most common in the first year of life or at birth and an onset at this age is a good prognosis for eventual complete resolution by adolescence.

In the adult a late onset is associated with diffuse plaques and telangiectasia.

The systemic variety presents in 10 per cent of adult cases causing osteoporosis or osteosclerosis. The spleen may be enlarged and bleeding disorders are the consequence of either thrombocytopenia or from the effects of heparin. Involvement of the gut causes a variety of symptoms including colic and diarrhoea. Right-sided heart failure due to pulmonary hypertension is recorded. Examination of the urine for histamine or prostaglandin D_2 may help to confirm the diagnosis when the skin lesions are absent.

TREATMENT

Treatment is unsatisfactory but the increasing use of H_1 and H_2 antagonists in various combinations is proving beneficial in some cases. The prognosis for eventual resolution is good in children but a solitary or troublesome single lesion in an adult can be excised. The cosmetic appearance of pigmented lesions is helped by sun exposure or by use of UVA and psoralens, but the number of mast cells is not reduced. Disodium cromoglycate helps some patients with systemic mastocytosis. The number of mast cells can be suppressed by high-potency steroids under occlusive dressings.

Cutaneous manifestations of histiocytosis X

The cutaneous lesions of histiocytosis X are small yellow-brown keratotic scaling papules. These coalesce to form a diffuse seborrhoeic dermatitis which is ulcerative, crusting, and purpuric. Granulomatous eroded plaques that are particularly found in the flexures and in the external auditory meatus cause great discomfort. The hair margins are commonly involved. The common association of diabetes insipidus and hepatosplenomegaly are described elsewhere. The diagnosis is confirmed by demonstrating pale-staining histocytes devoid of lipid, which contain the Langerhans cell granule.

Fibrosis, eosinophils, and giant cells are features of a more benign process.

Melkersson–Rosenthal syndrome

This syndrome can be produced experimentally by ligating all the lymphatics at the head and neck. Granulomas of the lips (Fig. 138) and tongue are a consequence of lymphatic stasis and impaired clearance of protein through the normal channels. The triad of facial palsy, enlarged tongue, and chronically swollen lips is difficult to treat. The current hypothesis, supported by some experimental work in rats, suggests that stimulation of macrophages by hydroxyethylrutoside, Paroven®, 200 mg three times daily, may help to clear the protein, but penicillin V is often also prescribed to reduce recurrent episodes of cellulitis.

Granuloma annulare and necrobiosis lipoidica

A partial necrosis of the collagen and the connective tissue cells associated with immunoglobulin and complement deposition results in a lymphocytic and histiocytic response that is known as a palisading granuloma. This is entirely reversible over many months and years in granuloma annulare, but in necrobiosis lipoidica it tends to result in fibrosis and scarring. The association with insulin-dependent diabetes mellitus and AIDS is unpredictable and is to be expected in more widespread

Fig. 134 (a) Chronic granulomas of cattle ringworm: *Trichophyton verrucosum.* (b) The ear involved by lupus vulgaris (tuberculosis); a brownish-red granuloma inducing irritation in the overlying epidermis. (c) The nose is a common site for the granuloma of lepromatous leprosy. (d) Chronic granuloma due to leishmaniasis following a sandfly bite presenting as an ill-defined cresting and wartiness.

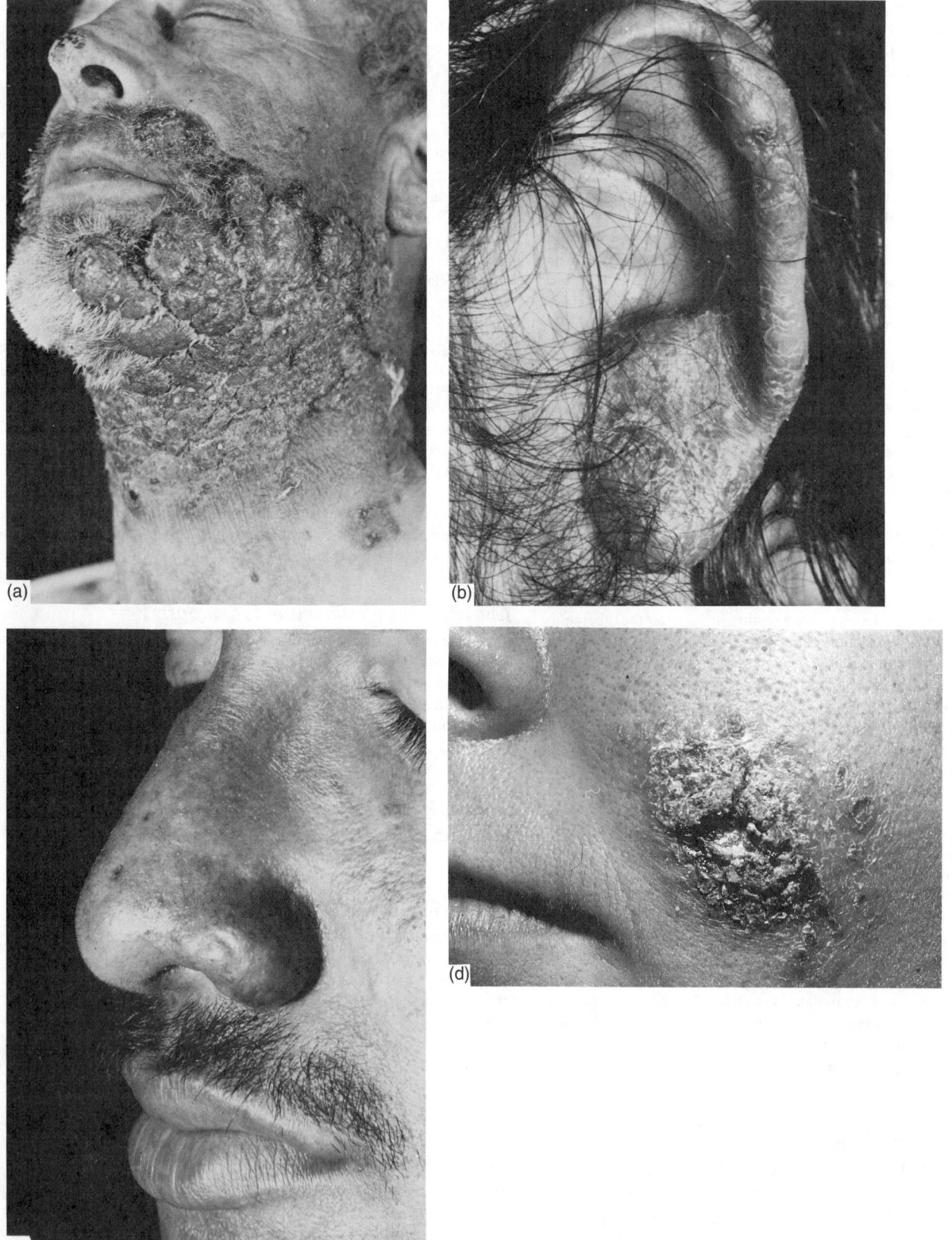

Table 31 *Organisms causing chronic granulomatous disease of the nose; their characteristics, geographical distribution, and the animals they infect*

Disease and causative organism	Geographical distribution	Susceptible animals	Portal of entry and mode of dissemination
Lupus vulgaris: *Mycobacterium tuberculosis* (2.5–3.5 × 0.3 μm) Acid-fast bacillus; alcohol-fast; stains with Sudan black; Gram-positive	Ubiquitous, rare in tropics	Human strain fatal in guinea-pigs; rabbits and mice affected less; *M. bovis* virulent to all; chicken not affected by both strains	Inhalation, ingestion and skin inoculation; lymph and blood-borne spread
Leprosy: *Mycobacterium leprae* (1–8 × 0.2–0.5 μm) AFB less alcohol-fast; not stained by Sudan black; Gram-positive; uncultivatable	Tropics, sub-tropics and endemic in Malta, Cyprus, and countries on the Adriatic, Mediterranean, and Black seas	Ear of hamster, mouse footpad, and armadillo	Undecided; cutaneous? dissemination by blood and nerves
Rhinoscleroma: *Klebsiella rhinoscleromatis* (1.6–2.4 × 0.8 μm) Gram-negative	Central Europe, Russia, China, India, Indonesia, North Africa, Central and South America	Mice	Unknown ?inhalation (upper respiratory tract); localized extension
Venereal syphilis: *Treponema pallidum* (6–15 × 0.9–0.18 μm) Close, rigid (8–20 coils spirochaete); rotar and flexion movements; uncultivatable	Ubiquitous in urban communities	Apes, rabbits, and hamsters	Genital and extragenital, skin and mucosa; transplacental; blood-borne dissemination
Non-venereal endemic syphilis (bejel): same as venereal syphilis; uncultivatable	Arid deserts of Asia and Africa	Apes, rabbits, and hamsters	Mouth (communal drinking, food utensils, and kissing)
Yaws: same as venereal syphilis; uncultivatable	Tropical, humid jungles of Central Africa, Asia, Australia and South and Central America	Monkeys, rabbits, and hamsters	Abrasions or bite in skin by direct contact by vector (hippelates fly); blood-borne dissemination
Mucocutaneous leishmaniasis: *Leishmania brasiliensis* (2–4 × 0.5–2.5 μm)	Endemic in Central and South America (damp forests)	Monkey, dog, guinea-pigs, bat, white rat, squirrel, and hamster	Through a bite by local sandfly (phlebotomus) in skin; dissemination by lymph and blood
Lutz's mycosis: *Paracoccidioides brasiliensis* (10–60 μm diameter); spherical and budding	Brazil, South and Central America, occasionally USA, Italy, Portugal, Morocco, and Bulgaria	Inoculated into guinea-pigs, specific orchitis. In hamsters and mice, dissemination	Undecided? lungs, skin, GI tract, and buccopharyngeal mucosa; blood-borne and lymphatic dissemination
Rhinosporidiosis: *Rhinosporidium seeberi* Dimorphic fungus; sporangium = 2.5-mm diameter; endospores 6–7 μm diamter; uncultivatable	Endemic in India and Ceylon; sporadic elsewhere	Natural infection in nose of cattle and horses; experimental inoculation failed	Unknown.? Direct inoculation in nose; dissemination only 2 cases (blood-borne)
Rhinophycomycosis: *Entomophthora coronata* (5–25 μm diameter) PAS positive; grows better at 25 °C	Tropics and subtropics	Inoculation experiments in young animals failed	Portal of entry unknown? by inhalation
Glanders: *Actinobacillus mallei* Short coccoid, rod-shaped bacillus; Gram-negative	Eastern Europe, Asia Minor, Asia, and North Africa	Natural disease of solipeds; horse, mule, donkey, and occasionally sheep; accidental in man by contact with animals or laboratory material	In animals through the intestinal wall by contaminated fodder with nasal discharge and sputum; dissemination blood-borne

From Kanan and Ryan (1976).

forms or in older age groups of granuloma annulare and in about 75 per cent of necrobiosis lipoidica.

In children, granuloma annulare are commonly on the knuckles (Fig. 139), fingers, and dorsum of the feet. Ears and elbows are quite frequently affected. They may be mistaken for warts but the overlying epidermis, if closely inspected, is rarely papilliferous. The tendency to heal in the centre and spread centrifugally over many weeks gives rise to an annular appearance.

Necrobiosis lipoidica is commonly to be found on both shins (Fig. 140). Widespread forms of granuloma annulare may be often of giant type, forming large violaceous plaques or rings. No treatment is necessary since eventual resolution of granuloma annulare is expected in 75 per cent in 2 years, but intralesional steroids probably speed resolution, particularly sometimes aborting necrobiosis lipoidica.

Fig. 135 Chronic granuloma of the nose due to sarcoid.

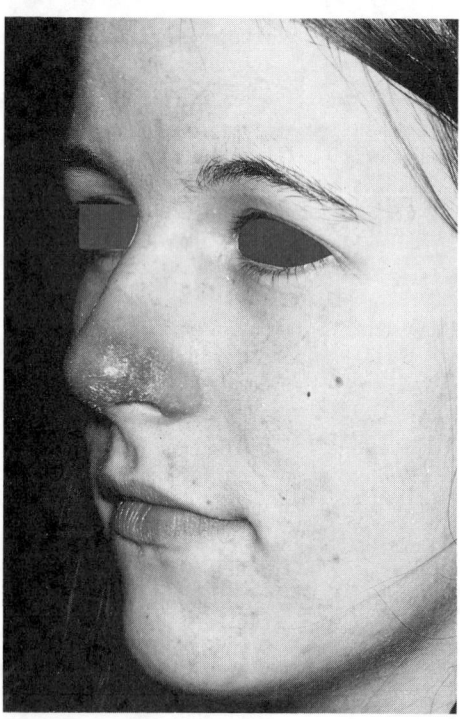

Fig. 136 Grouped brownish-red nodules in the dermis: micropapular sarcoid. This appearance is also compatible with tuberculosis, lichen scrofulosorum variety.

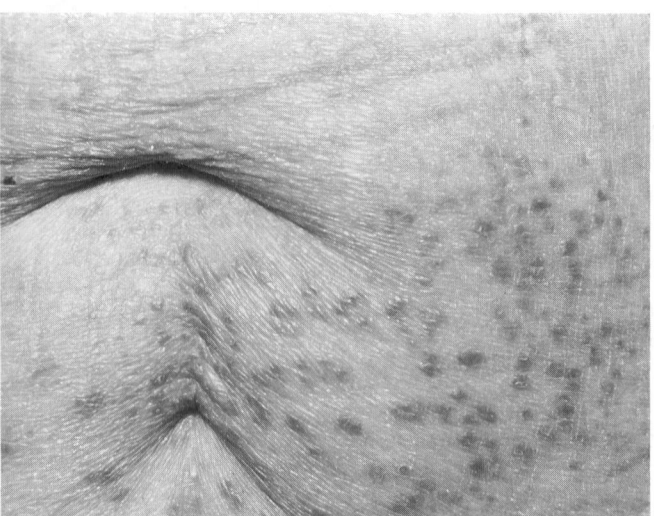

Pretibial myxoedema

Pretibial myxoedema may present acutely as a slightly tender erythema nodosum-like swelling, but more often it is a shiny red and non-tender infiltration of the front of the shins. Chronic forms have the appearance of a local elephantiasis. Classically it is associated with clubbing and exophthalmus and a history and signs of a previous thyroidectomy. Intralesional steroids often encourage resolution of the more acute varieties.

Cutaneous amyloidosis

Systemic amyloidosis is described elsewhere. The features that should suggest the diagnosis in the skin are its waxy appearance and the ease with which purpura develops within the lesions on slight trauma.

Fig. 137 Plaque of sarcoid affecting the skin of the shoulder and causing a brownish-red infiltration with atrophy of the overlying dermis. Unlike lupus vulgaris there is less irritation of the overlying epidermis; it is merely thinned and the scale is due to retention of a well-knit, dried-out stratum corneum.

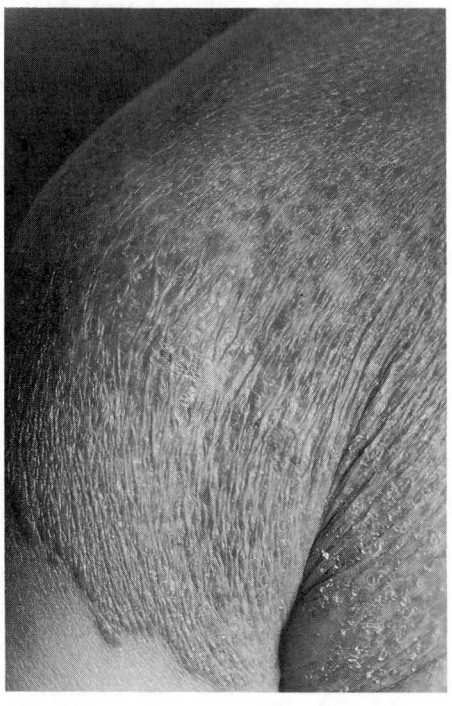

Fig. 138 Granuloma of the lip in which sarcoid and Crohn's disease were part of the differential diagnosis of the Melkersson–Rosenthal syndrome of lymphostasis.

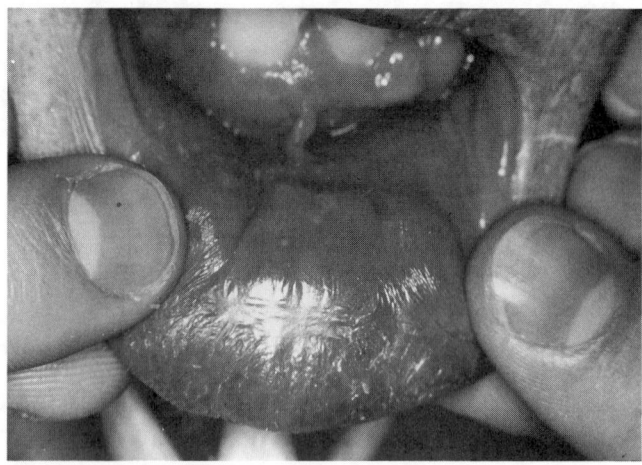

Fig. 139 Papules of granuloma annulare forming a ring around a now healed but previously affected area on the knuckle.

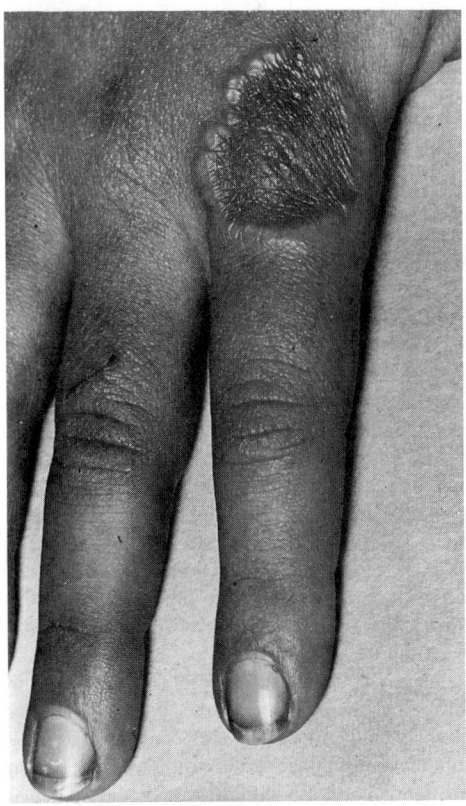

Fig. 140 Necrobiosis lipoidica usually affects the skin of the shins. The yellowish atrophic plaques are associated with diabetes mellitus.

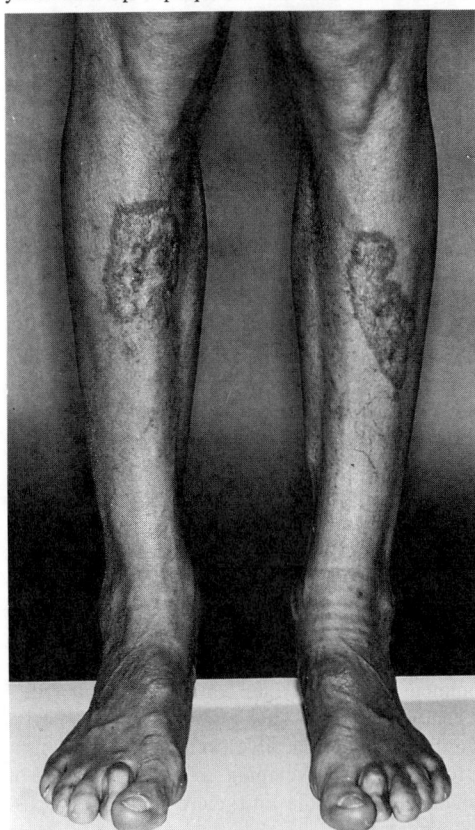

Lichen amyloidosis consists of discrete, firm, hemispheroidal papules. Hyperkeratosis and pigmentation is common, suggesting a waxy infiltrated lichen simplex. The lower legs and outer thighs are involved (Fig. 141). There is no systemic implication.

Macular amyloid is a common pigmented variant affecting the shoulders and back of Asians. It is often in a rippled pattern (Fig. 141(b)). Local high-potency steroids under occlusive dressings have a temporary good effect.

Lipoid proteinosis

Yellowish papules contain hyaline material and are found especially in the eyelids and elbows. The involvement of the vocal cords causing hoarseness from birth is a distinctive feature. Intracranial calcification and epilepsy are associated complications.

Multicentric reticulohistiocytosis

Granulomata are juxta-articular, especially on the fingers, but they also affect the lips, nostrils, and ears. There is an associated polyarthritis and underlying neoplastic disease is frequently associated. The diagnostic features are numerous multinucleated giant cells in the granuloma.

Crohn's disease

This is a well-recognized cause of chronic granulomatous infiltration perianally (see Fig. 25) or in the buccal mucosa.

REFERENCES

Fitzpatrick, R., Rapaport, M.J., and Silva, D.G. (1981). Histiocytosis X. *Archives of Dermatology* **117**, 253–7.

Fig. 141 (a) Lichen amyloidosis commonly affects the shins or outer aspects of the thighs. The brownish, waxy, lichenified skin is pruritic. (b) Rippled pigmentation of macular amyloid.

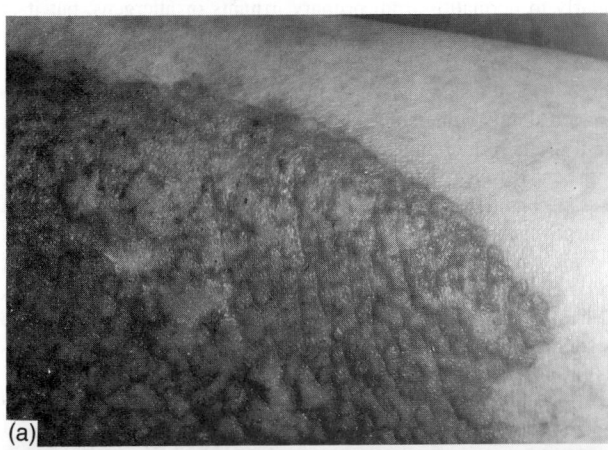

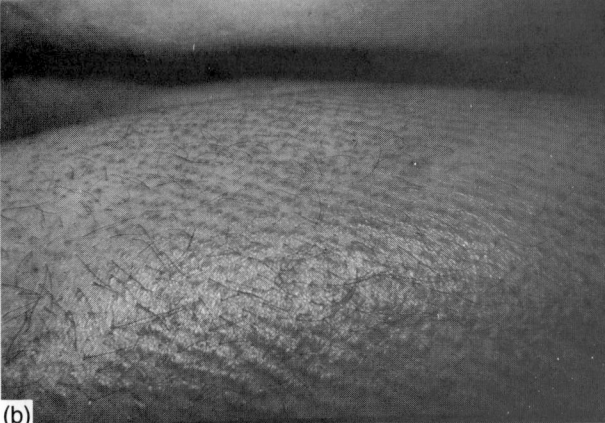

Kanan, M.W. and Ryan, T.J. (1976). The localization of granulomatous diseases. In *Microvascular diseases,* pp. 195–220. Lloyd Luke, London.

Kendall, M.E., Fields, J.P., and King, L.E. Jr (1984). Cutaneous mastocytosis without clinically obvious skin lesions *Journal of the American Academy of Dermatology* **10** (Part 2), 903–5.

Kerdal, F.A. and Moschella, S.M. (1984). Sarcoidosis. *Journal of the American Academy of Dermatology* **11**, 1–19.

Muhlemann, M.F. and Williams, D.R.R. (1984). Localized granuloma annulare is associated with insulin-dependent diabetes mellitus. *British Journal of Dermatology* **111**, 322–9.

Roper, S.S. and Spraker, M.K. (1985). Cutaneous histiocytosis syndromes. *Pediatric Dermatology* **3**, 19–30.

Ryan, T.J. (1978). Lymphatics of the skin. In *Physiology and pathophysiology of the skin* Vol. 5 (ed. A. Jarrett), pp. 1755–808. Academic Press, New York.

Management of skin disease

GENERAL PRINCIPLES

There are several general principles that can be applied to diseases of skin whatsoever their causes.

Acute skin lesions require rest. Limbs should be elevated because this reduces swelling. Dressings should be applied lightly and evenly to the surface and should support the inflamed area without drag or compression. All agents applied to the skin should be no stronger than necessary. It is very easy for instance, to make a potassium permanganate solution too strong or to use poorly mixed and inhomogeneous medicaments. Never apply to the skin any substance the components of which are unknown. This is particularly relevant to indigenous medicine. There is no need for complex mixtures and most agents applied to the skin need to contain a base and only two to three active ingredients. Anyway, a simple agent used well and familiar to the prescriber is always safer than the haphazard prescription of a range of new and poorly tested agents.

Elimination of the cause of the skin lesion is essential. This applies particularly to dermatitis from primary irritants or allergens, but it is also important to know and eliminate infection if possible, but this does not mean attempting to make a chronic ulcer sterile. It is fruitless to attempt to make the skin and its diseases sterile at all times.

Damaged skin is vulnerable skin and every effort should be made to protect it from further injury. Scratching, rubbing, wrongly applied dressings, and unsuitable local medicaments are reasons for worsening of the skin condition and for the impairment of natural defences and repair mechanisms.

Chronic skin conditions are obviously more difficult to cure, and correct diagnosis is even more important than in acute skin conditions which are likely to heal spontaneously if the cause is eliminated. A biopsy for histological analysis is often helpful and where chronic infection is a possibility, bacterial or mycological analysis is clearly indicated.

The handicap of the chronic lesion includes a feeling of being unwelcome, often leading to the accusation of 'unclean' and leading to being 'outcast'. The physician and nurse can sometimes do more to alleviate the skin condition by attention to this aspect of the handicap than by using more specific measures. Sympathetic questioning along the lines indicated earlier will help to relieve the patient's suspicion that one is not interested in the problem. Touching the skin during examination often does more to make the patient feel that the physician cares than any other manoeuvre.

When treating any skin disease, the overall objective is to create the body image which the patient hopes for, and when this fails, to help him to live with his problem and expect less. Every effort should be made to ensure that children remain willing to go to school, adults stay at work, and the old are kept comfortable. Remedies should be convenient and cosmetically acceptable, and if this is not possible, the social support should be that much more intensive. Attention to diet, camouflage measures, and regular careful attention to the skin can be very irksome for the patient, but can be made less so through co-operating with the doctor, nurse, or patient association, for example the obesity clinic supported by a weightwatchers' group.

It is essential that the skin be protected from further injury: short-term gains from the use of powerful remedies must be weighed against possible long-term side-effects. Often the risk is worth taking but it should at least be taken into account. Homely advice such as 'keep warm and out of the sun' and 'rest as much as possible with your feet up' is appropriate for much acute or severe skin disease. Some of the oldest remedies, such as calamine lotion and *British National Formulary* preparations of tar (see Table 18) do least harm, but in chronic skin disease the patient is unlikely to persevere with these unless he is educated and encouraged. This takes time. Remember, patients spend more time listening to other patients in the waiting room than they do with the doctor—and are often in a more receptive frame of mind then. Make sure that the advice given in the waiting room is correct by handing out leaflets and teaching groups of patients, for example with audio-visual aids. Many patients do best with printed sheets of instructions so that they can read at their own pace quietly, without anxiety of the presence of the physician. If appropriate, they should be told that their disease is neither catching nor cancer.

Some skin diseases which are chronic and incurable become easier to tolerate when better understood. Time given to the education of the patient may not reduce morbidity but it increases patient satisfaction and makes them demand less from the service.

The priorities of the patient with skin disease differ from those of the doctor who is treating him. Thus the patient equates severity with social ostracism or the subjective itch rather than with the percentages of body involved or systemic complications. Other people who should be drawn into the management of the patient with skin disease include parents, school teachers, employers, hairdressers, and the sporting fraternity—for example swimming-bath attendants. A school report which refers to weeping sores and scratching which interfere with the work of other children should be a thing of the past.

Patients can be told to live with their disease if given the tools to do so and if people are helpful and understanding. Unfortunately, only too often skin patients find that doctors admit to ignorance and show as little evidence of knowing how to manage their problem as the average doctor at a road accident. Moreover, just as with first aid, the management of common skin ailments is often better understood by the layman—more a reflection on the poor quality of medical education than on public interest in this case.

There are a number of paramedical aids to the management of skin disease which can be of immense value. A high proportion of skin patients are found to be suffering from the stresses of their domestic environment, confused elderly relatives or delinquent teenage children, for example. For these patients the help of a medical social worker is often very successful. The British Red Cross Society in the United Kingdom now provides a 'beauty care' service which has been extended to the provision of camouflage. Patients' associations often provide a great deal of education and support.

In hospital practice in-patient treatment is only occasionally necessary and can be greatly reduced by adequate provision of a good out-patient treatment service. Some departments link this to their in-patient department in order to provide a service outside of the normal convenient department's working hours—it is clearly more convenient for a working man to attend a department which is open in the evening.

Many chronic skin conditions are either hypertrophic or atrophic. Hypertrophic conditions require suppression as is described in the section on psoriasis. Common suppressants are corticosteroids or radiotherapy. On the other hand these are unsuitable for atrophy.

Management of skin disease in technically developed countries usually assumes regular follow-up. In developing countries in Africa or India, or with the nomads of the Middle East, there is almost no pos-

Table 32 *Bases and their properties*

Base	Site for application	Effect	Disadvantage	Examples
Watery and shake lotions (powder in water)	Acutely inflamed, wet and oozing	Drying, soothing, and cooling	Tedious to apply; frequent changes (lessened by polyethylene occlusion); powder in shake lotions may clump	Fuller's earth solution Lotio Terra silica Saline solution BPC Potassium permanganate 1/8000–1/18 000 0.5 acetic acid in water Eusol in chlorinated lime and boric acid solution
Creams	Both moist and dry	Cooling, emollient, and moisturizing	Short bench life; fungal and bacterial growth in base; sensitivities to preservatives and emulsifying agents	Oily cream BP Aqueous cream BP, i.e. variants on water oil, and water mixes
Fatty acid, prophlene, glycol	Both moist and dry	Emollient and moisturizing	May sting when applied; occasional sensitivity to propylene glycol	FAPG base
Ointments	Dry and scaly	Occlusive and emollient	Messy to apply and soils clothing; removed with an oil	Soft white paraffin Vaseline Hydrous wool fat (lanolin) Emulsifying ointment BP
Pastes; powder/ointment mixture	Dry, lichenified, and scaly	Protective and emollient; delays absorption of grease	Messy and tedious to apply (linen or calico needed)	Zinc compound paste BP Lassar's paste BP
Dusting powders	Flexures; may be slightly moist	Lessens friction	If too wet, clumps and irritates	Talc, dusting powder BPC Zinc, starch, and talc dusting powder BPC

sibility of follow-up. Treatments with a high risk of side-effects or exacerbations on withdrawal are not therefore ideal. Because malnutrition and infection is so common, dietary supplements and antibiotics are of value in almost any disease in which the host or constitutional vulnerability is a factor. Health education is always difficult but the mother with children is usually the most receptive pupil.

If it is wet, dry it, and if it is dry, wet it!

LOCAL TOPICAL TREATMENT
The fingertip unit

The fingertip unit is the amount of ointment expressed from a tube with a 5 mm diameter nozzle, applied from the distal crease to the tip of the index finger. One unit weighs 0.49 g and covers 286 cm^2 in males and 0.43 g which covers 257 cm^2 in females. One unit will cover an area equivalent to twice the area of the hand. Four hands is thus equivalent to two finger units, which is equivalent to 1 g.

Drugs are dissolved or suspended in bases which have properties of their own quite independent of the active ingredient. As in Table 32 bases were originally either powder, water, or grease. However, modern processes have prepared bases which are essentially much more complex than this, although still retaining the objectives of the primary agents. Powder may repel water or absorb it and allow further evaporation. Modern powders tend not to cake and abrade the skin as much as the original talc or starch. Watery lotions evaporate and cool as well as wet and dissolve. Various agents, such as alcohol or glycerine, may be added to increase any one of these properties. Creams and emulsions of oil and water (aqueous or milky) or water in oil (butter or oily) are cooling, moisturising, and emollient. Penetration of active agents through the skin is aided by the aqueous (vanishing) oil and water creams. Ointments based on vaseline or paraffin are more occlusive and less quickly absorbed. They are better at softening dry surface scales.

There are various other preparations which are also water soluble, such as macrogels or emulsifying ointment in which a wax or animal fat is mixed with mineral oil. Pastes are powder and oil mixtures, such as talc and vaseline. They are more occlusive and protective. They are useful for slow release at the surface of agents such as dithranol. The addition of an active ingredient to a base often makes it unstable and hence various other agents are added as a preservative or to control pH. Further dilution usually makes the preparation still more unstable and, in other words, shortens its shelf life. Much of the skill in preparing an ointment or cream or paste is in the use of the homogenizer by the pharmacist.

The actions and side-effects of topical steroids are illustrated in Table 33. Tar and dithranol preparations are discussed in the section on psoriasis.

SKIN CLEANING

It is naïve to attempt to sterilize the skin and the consequences of obsessive washing or the use of local antibiotics in the long term are always worse than the original state of the skin. Antibiotic regimens are essential for acute complications such as cellulitis or specific infections such as erysipelas. Washing is important for reducing smell and for removing debris, but this is best done by soaking rather than scrubbing. Soaking is in fact one of the most effective of skin treatments for oozing exudative conditions. Soaps irritate because they are alkaline and degrease. Some patients are sensitive to perfumes and other additives in the soaps. Most skin will tolerate some soaping but in hard-water areas the amounts needed to degrease can cause considerable dryness and cracking of the skin. Soft rainwater or boiled milk should not be despised. Bran is an ancient and harmless water softener. About a pound of bran or oatmeal is tied into a muslin bag and soaked in boiling water. A very thin, starchy emulsion results. The stratum corneum drys, shrinks, and cracks in the cold. Cold water is not good for the skin. The skin that is dry is best treated at body temperature.

Emulsifying ointment is a useful soap substitute; it can be made into 'cakes' of soap or spooned out of a pot and mixed with hot water to soften it. Liberally applied it is a useful softener of crusts.

auditory canal and cerebellopontine angle (Fig. 8). This technique of CT air meatography has been replaced by MRI where this is available.

CT, because of its ease and non-invasive nature, its availability as an outpatient procedure, and its ability to image the brain directly, is the primary neuroimaging investigation in many circumstances. Recognition of the radiation burden imposed by CT, however, and the increase in the availability of MRI, is changing the imaging priorities in most neuroradiological departments.

MAGNETIC RESONANCE IMAGING (MRI)

MRI employs radiofrequency radiation in the presence of a magnetic field to produce images. In certain atomic nuclei an odd number of neutrons, protons, or both results in a spinning electrical charge which, in turn, produces a small magnetic field oriented along the axis of spin. Hydrogen, which contains a single proton, is the most abundant of these nuclei in the human body as a component of water and fat. In MRI, the patient is placed within the bore of a powerful (0.02–2.0 T) magnet,

which causes hydrogen and other magnetic atoms to align along the magnetic lines of force and to precess, that is, wobble like a spinning top, at characteristic (Larmor) frequencies. Application of a radiofrequency pulse perpendicular to the main magnetic field and tuned to the Larmor frequency of hydrogen perturbs the alignment. Once that radiofrequency pulse has ended, these perturbed protons return to their previous position by a process of relaxation. In so doing they generate radiofrequency radiation which forms the basis of the final digital image. The phenomenon of relaxation has two components: T_1, related to surrounding tissue; and T_2, related to adjacent protons. In proton imaging the MR signal is affected by numerous interacting variables which include not only the proton density and the relaxation times but also flow, magnetic susceptibility, diffusion, and perfusion. Image contrast depends on the interaction between all these factors, together with the timing parameters of the radiofrequency pulse and not simply, as in CT, on the attenuation properties of tissue to X-rays. Variations in the timing and composition of the applied radiofrequency pulse allow the operator to exercise control over the influence of each variable on the contrast of the final image (Fig. 9). T_1-weighted images provide high-resolution anatomical detail with excellent delineation of the cerebrospinal fluid pathways. T_2-weighted images are exquisitely sensitive to increases in brain water (Figs 10, 11). The combination of T_1- and T_2-weighted images allows the specific identification of some tissues (Fig. 12), particularly water, fat, and clotted blood (Fig. 13). The various stages of haemoglobin breakdown from oxyhaemoglobin to deoxyhaemoglobin,

Fig. 9 (a) T_1W axial image showing a cystic glioma (arrow). (b) T_2W images at the same level.

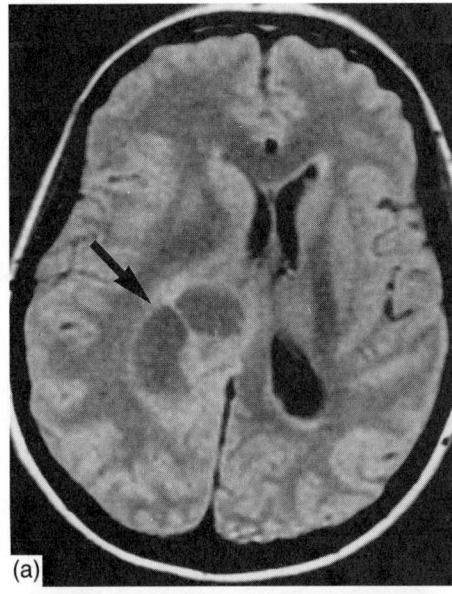

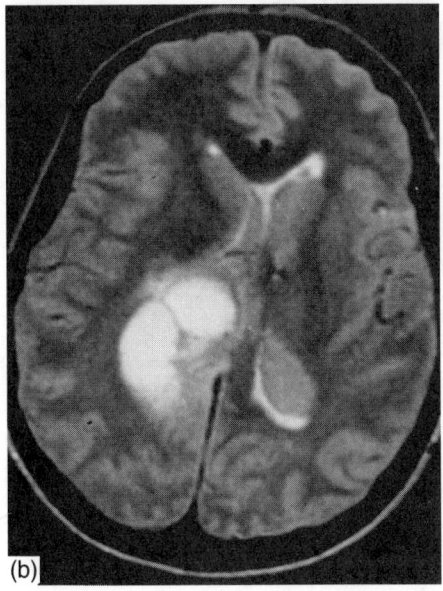

Fig. 10 MRI transaxial (a) T_1W and (b) T_2W images of bilateral occipital infarctions.

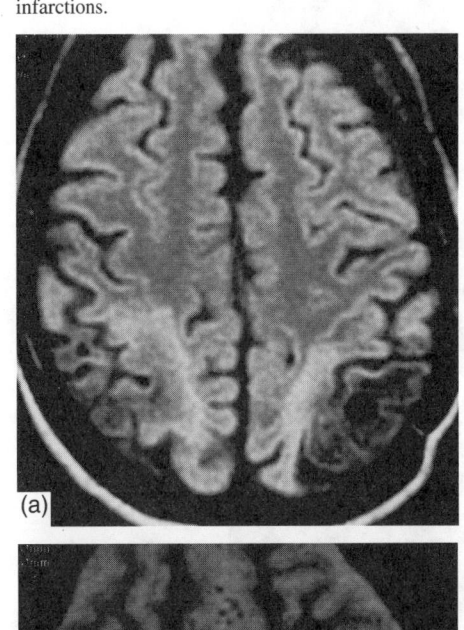

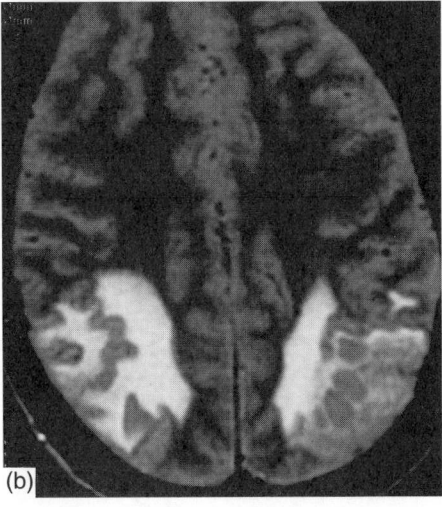

methaemoglobin, and haemosiderin can all be differentiated by their signal characteristics.

Intravenous contrast agents containing gadolinium chelates are paramagnetic and capable of shortening the T_1- and T_2-relaxation times of target tissue, leading to an increase in signal intensity, particularly on T_1-weighted images (Fig. 13). Paramagnetic contrast agents have a similar pharmacokinetic behaviour to iodinated contrast agents, in entering vascular tissues and crossing the damaged blood–brain barrier. They are excreted in a similar way by the kidneys.

The spatial resolution of MRI can be improved by the use of specialized radiofrequency coils placed on the skin surface or in close proximity to the area being imaged. Such coils can transmit and receive radiofrequency pulses, providing a greater signal to noise ratio and improved image quality. Surface coils are used routinely in spinal imaging. Small surface coils can also be used for imaging the orbit and the temporomandibular joints. Spatial resolution can also be improved by modification of the radiofrequency pulse sequences used to acquire the

MR data. Acquisition of data from an entire block of tissue, rather than from a single slice, produces a three-dimensional computer model which can be examined at the MR console. Three-dimensional volume acquisitions allow the operator to 'walk through' the structure, producing high-resolution thin slices in any desired plane, including curved planes (Fig. 14). This technique can provide slices as thin as 1 mm and demonstration of structures which may not be visible on routine MRI. The use of three-dimensional acquisitions also allows the application of sophisticated computerized post-processing techniques, enabling the production of three-dimensional representations which can be of value in the planning of neurosurgical procedures.

Cranial MRI offers considerable advantages over CT and is the more sensitive imaging modality, demonstrating most cerebral disease processes. Cortical bone contains few protons and appears as a signal void on MRI, making it particularly suited to the imaging of lesions adjacent to or within bone. Areas of dystrophic soft-tissue calcification also produce areas of signal void but are often so small or heterogeneous that the signal void cannot be seen on the final image. This uncertainty in the detection of soft-tissue calcification can be a disadvantage, and in

Fig. 11 (a) MRI coronal T_1W image of a patient with early herpes encephalitis (CT was normal). Note the low signal within the left temporal lobe. (b) MRI T_1W transaxial image showing a marked signal change within the affected lobe.

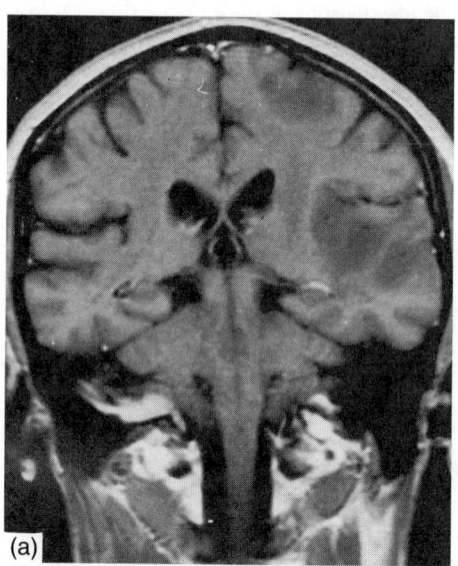

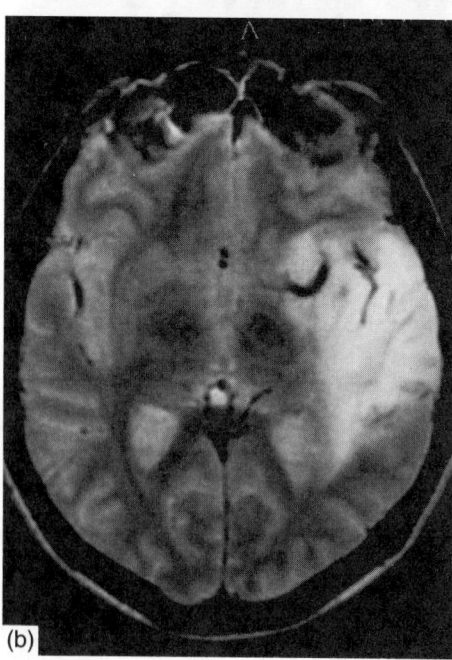

Fig. 12 (a) MRI T_1W image of the same lesion. The low signal intensity confirms a fluid-filled cyst. (b) Postcontrast T_1W image of a pituitary adenoma. The high signal confirms an enhancing solid mass.

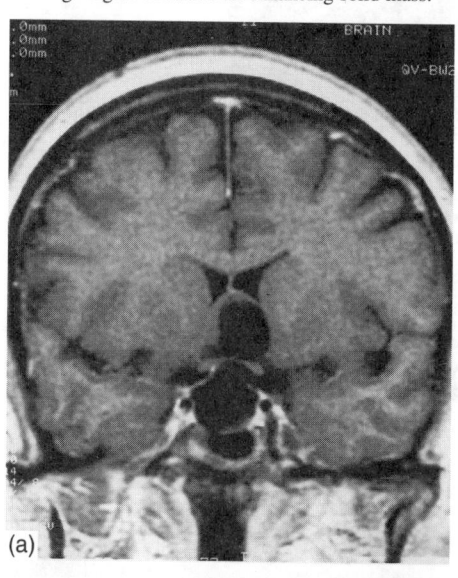

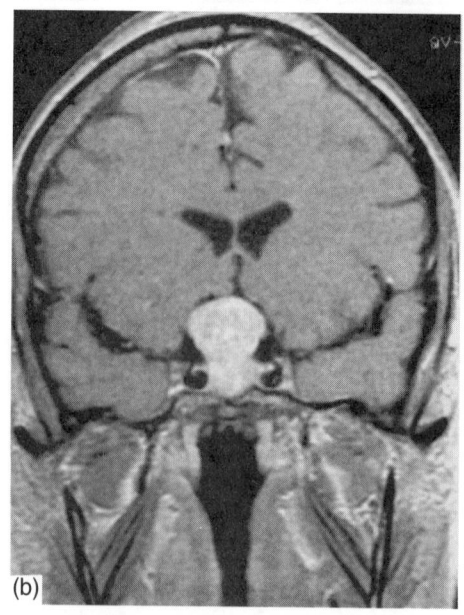

such cases CT may allow more specific tissue diagnosis. MRI incurs no radiation dose, but all patients should be carefully screened for risk factors before they are accepted for MRI. Certain cardiac pacemakers are sensitive to paramagnetic fields and constitute an absolute contra-indication. Small metallic foreign bodies, including some surgical clips, may be displaced by the primary magnetic field. In view of the increasing role of MRI, most neurosurgical vascular clips are now made of non-ferromagnetic materials.

MRI provides the most sensitive method for imaging cerebral tumours and is of particular benefit in the posterior fossa, where images are free of the obtrusive artefacts which may be present on CT images. MRI will detect over 95 per cent of all cerebral masses, but intravenous paramagnetic contrast agents can increase this sensitivity and also provide more accurate delineation. Acoustic neuromas enhance markedly, and postcontrast T_1-weighted images can demonstrate intracanalicular tumours as small as 1 to 2 mm diameter (Fig. 15). The technique is being advanced as a reliable alternative to other procedures in the investigation of sensorineural deafness.

The sensitivity of T_2-weighted images to changes in brain water makes MRI highly sensitive to infective and inflammatory changes in cerebral tissue, enabling identification of encephalitic disorders at a stage when CT is normal (Fig. 11). Most white matter diseases result in abnormalities on T_2-weighted MR images, although areas of chronic gliosis may be best seen on proton density weighted images. MRI will demonstrate demyelinating infarcts in over 95 per cent of patients with multiple sclerosis, but may not provide reliable differentiation between multiple sclerosis and other white matter diseases (Fig. 16). Non-specific microvascular abnormalities in white matter are present in up to 50 per cent of normal subjects over the age of 50 years.

The movement of protons in flowing blood provides the opportunity to image blood vessels. Techniques including phase mapping and magnetic resonance angiography (MRA) for recording and measuring blood flow information are now well established (Fig. 17). MRA provides a non-invasive and radiation-free technique for the investigation of intra- and extracerebral vascular structures without the use of contrast agents. The best technique, for example two- or three-dimensional time of flight or phase contrast, is determined by the area of interest, the flow direction, and the flow velocity. Morphological detail remains inferior to conventional angiography and is, as yet, inadequate for the reliable investigation of any aneurysmal disease or for the planning of endovascular therapy. MRA does provide high-quality images of the main vessels of the neck, and in some centres is becoming the initial investigation of atheromatous, carotid, and vertebral arterial disease. Studies of cerebrospinal fluid flow patterns may help to clarify the aetiology of hydrocephalus and may also be of prognostic value in the preoperative assessment of patients with suspected normal-pressure hydrocephalus.

Techniques of MR imaging are evolving rapidly and several recent innovations hold out the promise of useful clinical applications in the

Fig. 13 MRI T_1W axial image of a cystic ependymoma (a) before and (b) after contrast enhancement. High-signal areas before contrast indicate internal tumour haemorrhage. Low-signal areas correspond to cyst formation. The extent of enhancement indicates tumour tissue. (c) Parasagittal postcontrast T_1W image demonstrates the anatomical relationship of the tumour to the corpus callosum and brain-stem.

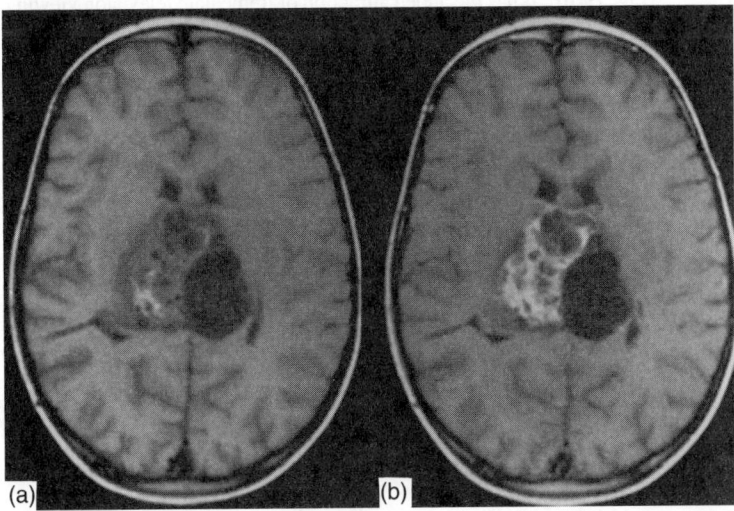
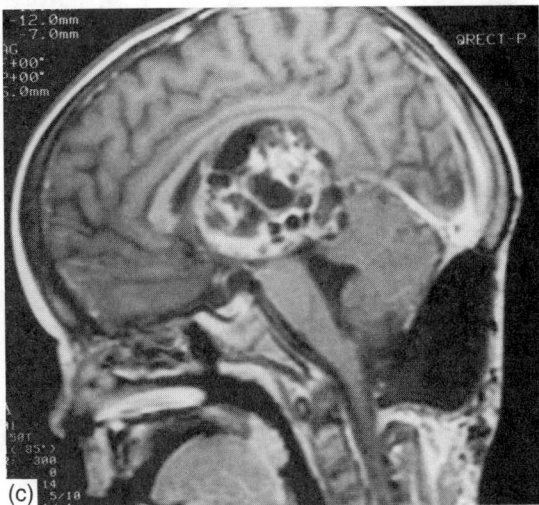

Fig. 14 MRI images from a three-dimensional data acquisition through the brain-stem of a normal patient. Variation in the angle plane of reconstruction allows demonstration of (a) intracranial optic nerves and optic chiasm, (b) third nerve (arrow), and (c) fifth nerve and trigeminal ganglion (arrow).

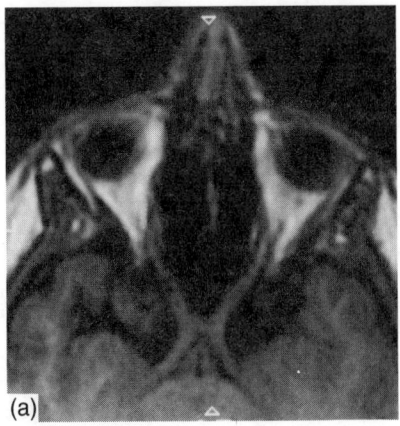
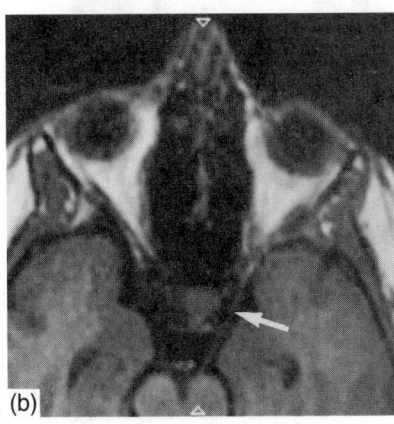
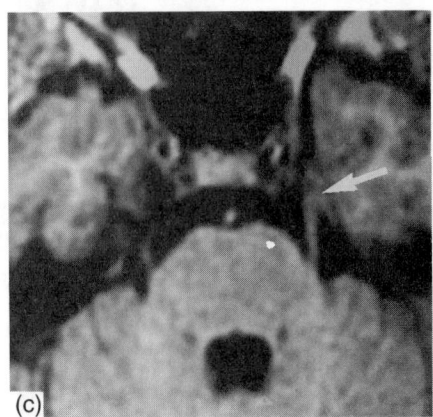

near future. Experimental techniques for the demonstration of proton movement within individual voxels have been used to produce 'diffusion' images of cerebral tissue. Anisotropic diffusion in myelin sheaths has enabled white matter tracts to be imaged selectively. Similar techniques employed to demonstrate perfusion may allow the identification of 'at risk' areas in hypoperfusion states. Photic and motor stimulation together with very rapid image acquisition techniques have been used at 1.5 to 4.0 T to demonstrate regional cerebral metabolic activity without the use of contrast agents. The observed signal changes are considered to be due to a decrease in deoxyhaemoglobin concentration secondary to locally increased cerebral blood flow. Such techniques offer the potential to image functional cerebral abnormalities where morphological change is absent, and thereby extend the role of MRI in the investigation of a wide range of disease states.

CEREBRAL ANGIOGRAPHY

Visualization of the intracranial circulation can be achieved either by percutaneous puncture or selective catheterization of the appropriate carotid or vertebral artery and injection of iodinated contrast. In these circumstances selective catheterization is performed by the Seldinger technique, a percutaneous method of introducing a catheter and flexible guide wire into a peripheral artery. The femoral artery is the most commonly employed and is the safest. Cerebral angiography is a well-estab-

Fig. 15 MRI T_1W (a) unenhanced and (b) enhanced images of bilateral acoustic neuromas. Note two tumours on the right-hand side.

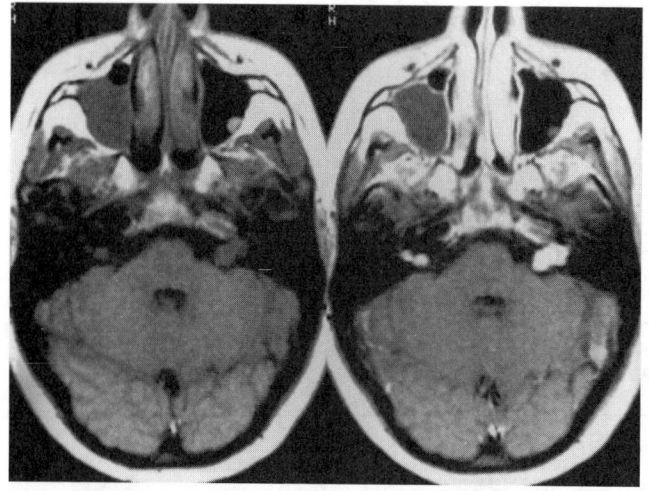

lished technique in departments of neuroradiology for the demonstration of topographical vascular anatomy. Improvement in vascular detail can be achieved by rapid serial film studies with subtraction and radiographic magnification. Subtraction is a photographic or electronic technique whereby the distracting background to a contrast procedure can be removed.

Local and distant displacement of cerebral vessels may permit an anatomical diagnosis, whereas the demonstration of an abnormal circulation can enable a pathological diagnosis to be achieved (Fig. 18). Precise delineation of vascular anomalies and occlusive diseases can only be achieved by angiography. The use of anterior cerebral angiography as a screening method has now been replaced by CT.

DIGITAL FLUOROGRAPHY

Digital fluorography is a technique that provides digitization of the video output of an image intensifier. Although the spatial resolution is not yet as good as with conventional film, electronic subtraction of video frames, together with other image-processing techniques, allows demonstration of intra- and extracerebral vessels by simple intravenous injection of contrast medium. The intravenous technique has particular merit in those circumstances where direct invasion of the arterial system would be hazardous, in the monitoring of intracerebral disease, and in the exclusion of large aneurysms. It is simple to perform and can be carried out on an outpatient basis. A disadvantage is the non-selective nature of the vascular display. Digital fluorography, in association with arterial injection of contrast medium, permits smaller volumes of contrast medium to be used than are necessary in conventional arteriography (Fig. 19(b)). It has the added attraction of immediate television viewing. Both factors are of importance in interventional procedures.

INTERVENTIONAL PROCEDURES

Technical improvements in catheter design and injectable embolic agents have enabled the development of successful endovascular treatments for many intra- and extracranial disorders. A large-bore catheter with its tip in a vertebral internal or external carotid artery allows the introduction of a wide range of specialized microcatheters, which can then be used to introduce embolic materials to dilate vascular stenoses or to dissolve intravascular thrombus. Such microcatheters can be directed by blood flow or steered with a central curved guide wire to gain access deep into the cerebral circulation.

Preoperative embolization of some vascular tumours with embolic particles in the 50 to 200 μm range can greatly simplify subsequent surgical removal (Fig. 20). Such particulate embolization may, however,

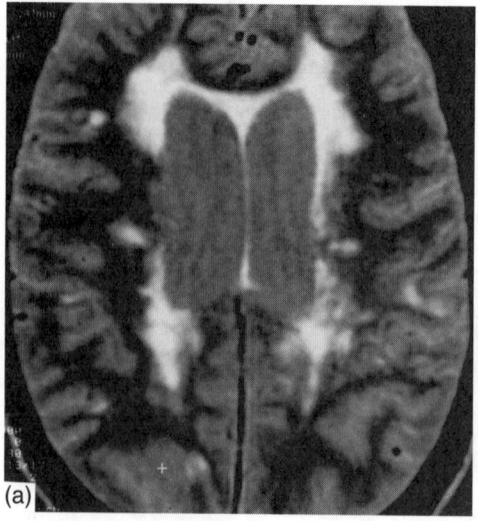

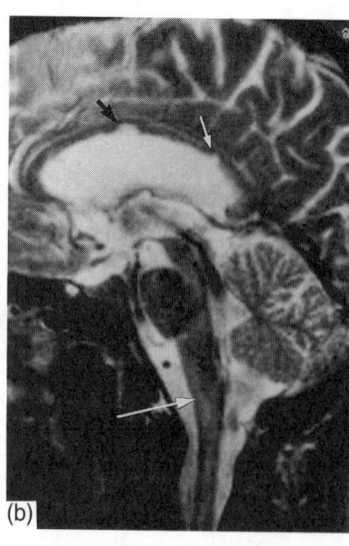

Fig. 16 (a) MRI transaxial T_2W image of extensive periventricular plaques in a patient with multiple sclerosis. (b) Parasagittal T_2W image showing plaques (arrows) within the corpus callosum and lower brainstem.

Fig. 17 (a) MR angiogram showing an atheromatous stricture at the origin of the right external carotid (arrow). (b) MR angiogram of the circle of Willis showing the middle (long arrow) and posterior (short arrow) cerebral arteries.

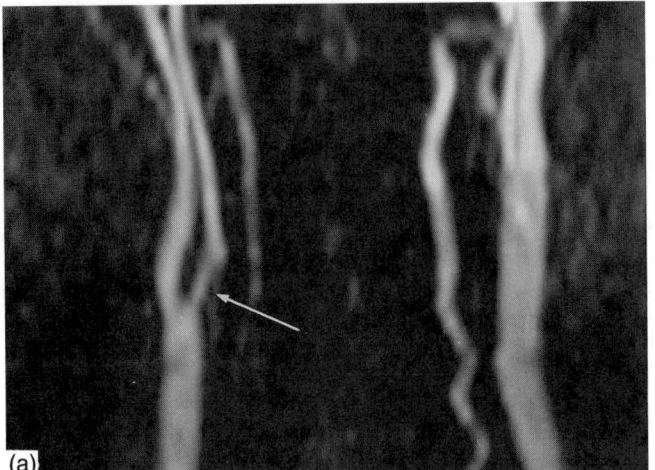

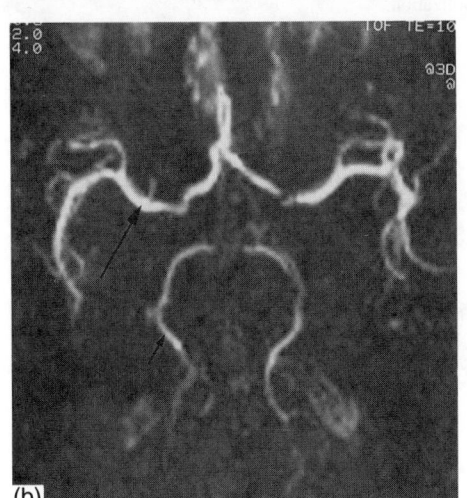

Fig. 18 Subtraction carotid angiogram of a sphenoidal meningioma: (a) arterial phase; (b) capillary phase.

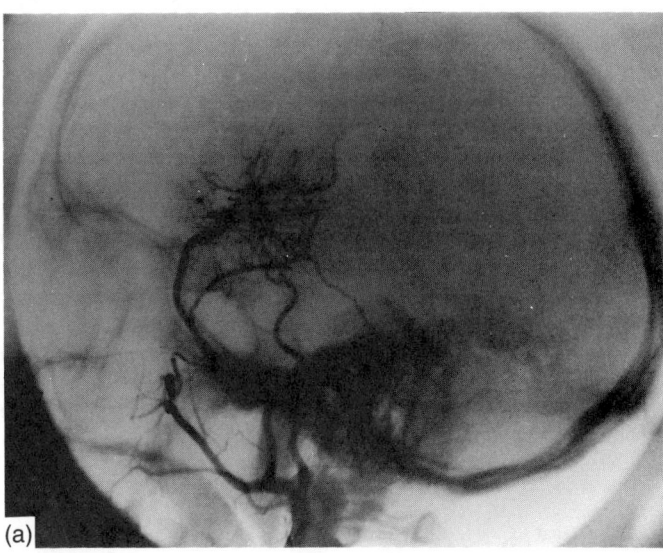

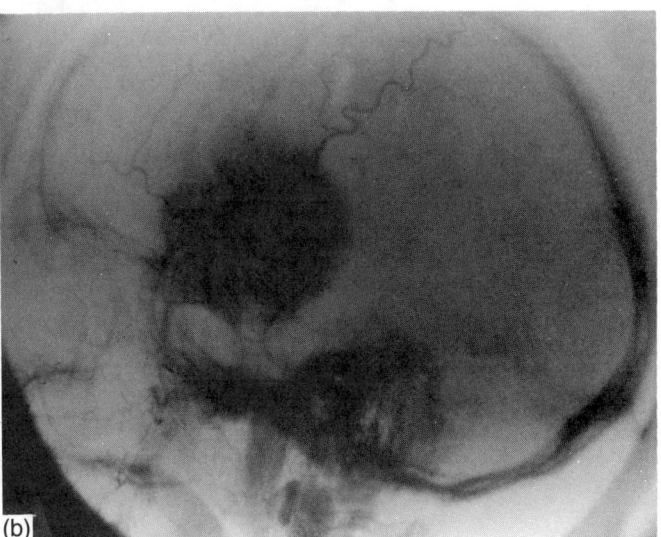

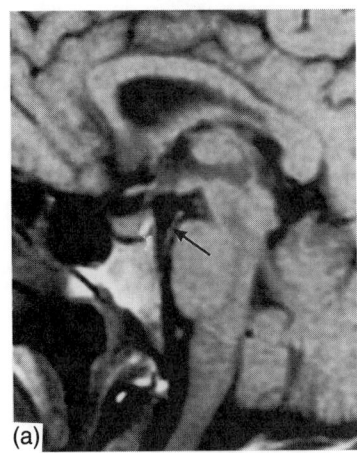

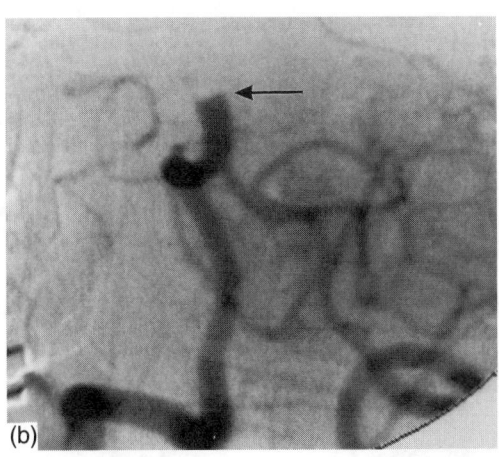

Fig. 19 (a) MRI T_1W image, showing a high signal (arrow) due to thrombus within the terminal basilar artery. (b) Digital subtraction of the posterior circulation, showing complete occlusion of the distal basilar artery immediately above the inferior cerebellar artery origins (arrow).

provide only temporary vascular occlusion and should therefore be performed within 5 days of planned surgery.

Permanent vascular occlusion can be achieved by the injection of polymerizing liquid embolic agents, such as methoxy- and cyanoacrylate, which form the basis of domestic 'superglue'. Superglue embolization is the treatment of choice for many inoperable intracerebral arteriovenous malformations. The aim is to reduce the nidus of the arteriovenous malformation to a size (2 cm) suitable for radiotherapy. Embolization in these circumstances carries a significant risk, is time consuming, expensive, and requires considerable expertise.

Endovascular treatment of cerebral aneurysms involves occlusion of the aneurysm lumen by detachable balloons or by the introduction of small metal coils which promote thrombosis. The techniques are increasingly practised, but results are still unpredictable and the long-term benefits compared with surgical clipping remain uncertain. Endovascular occlusion is of greater value in the treatment of inoperable giant aneurysms and is currently replacing surgical occlusion techniques in the treatment of inoperable cavernous sinus aneurysms.

The use of balloon or laser angioplasty to treat stenotic disease of the carotid and vertebral arteries is increasing. Early concerns that angioplasty would result in propagation of cerebral emboli have not been substantiated. On present evidence, cerebral angioplasty appears to be a relatively safe technique and is the best treatment option in many arteriopathic patients in whom the risks of general anaesthesia are unacceptable.

Angioplasty using microballoon catheters has been used to treat arterial spasm which may follow a subarachnoid haemorrhage. Angioplasty of the middle and anterior cerebral arteries appears to improve the prognosis in patients with severe spasm but carries a small risk of arterial perforation.

Injection of thrombolytic agents is being used increasingly to minimize the damage caused by cerebral arterial emboli. The technique requires superselective catheterization and treatment must be instituted early, preferably within 2 h of the embolic event. Immediate postoperative thrombolysis in patients with cerebral emboli following cardiac bypass procedures can completely reverse the neurological deficit.

Fig. 20 Digital subtraction carotid angiogram of a juvenile angiofibroma: (a) pre-, and (b) postembolization.

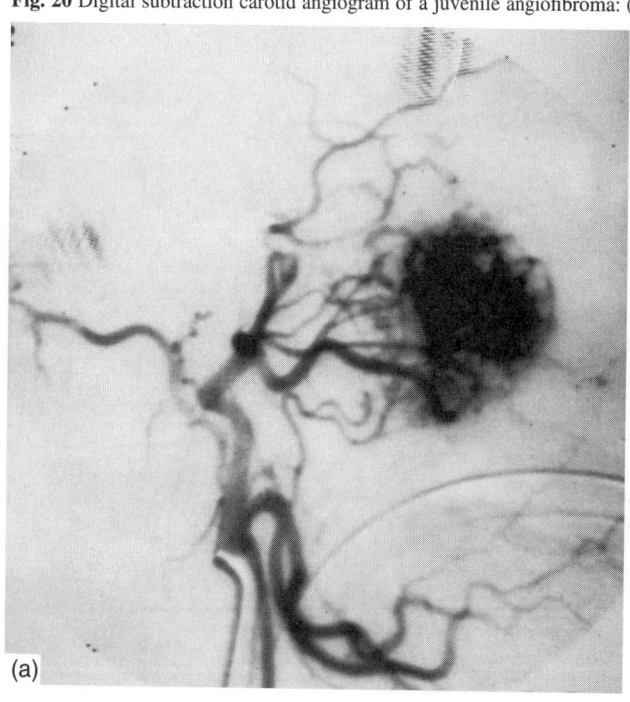

(a)

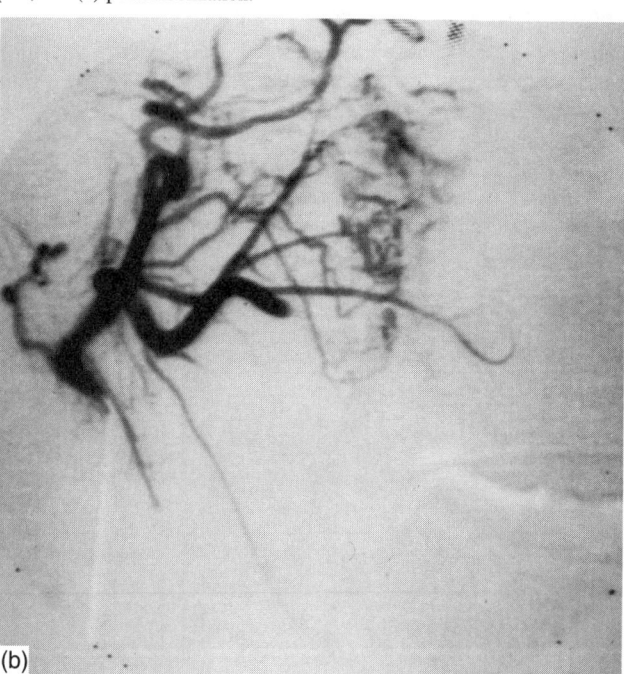

(b)

Fig. 21 Radionuclide scan with ⁹⁹Tc of multiple metastases. Left, anteroposterior projection; right, left lateral projection. (Images by courtesy of Dr H.J. Testa, Manchester Royal Infirmary, United Kingdom.)

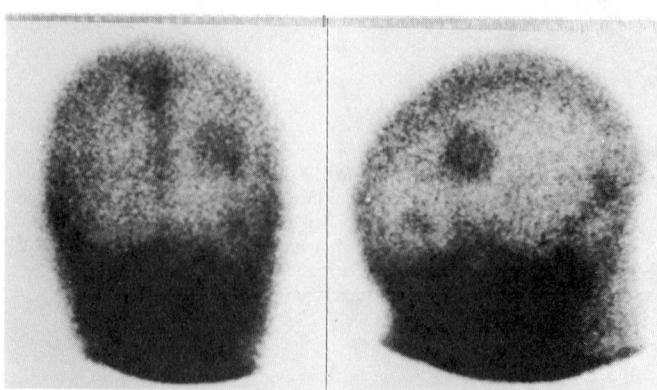

Fig. 22 Transaxial ⁹⁹Tc HM-PAO images: (a) normal; (b) Alzheimer's disease. Note the uniform distribution of tracer in the normal patient and the decreased uptake in the parietal and occipital regions of the patient with Alzheimer's disease. (Images by courtesy of Dr H.J. Testa, Manchester Royal Infirmary, United Kingdom.)

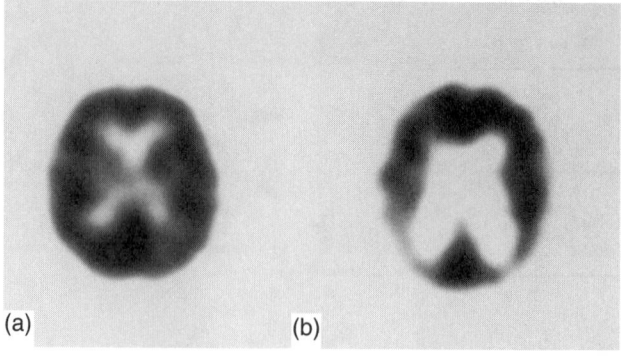

(a)   (b)

Attempts at thrombolysis more than 2 h after the event are associated with a decreasing success rate and an increased risk of cerebral haemorrhage. Thrombolysis is not yet of proven value in spontaneous cerebral thrombosis, because of the time delay between onset and presentation.

ISOTOPE BRAIN SCANNING

Radiopharmaceuticals administered intravenously equilibrate with extracellular fluid and do not normally penetrate the blood–brain barrier. Technetium as $^{99}Tc^m$ in its pertechnetate form is the most commonly used intravenous agent for static brain studies. Detectors in a rectilinear scanner or gamma-camera register activity for normal soft tissue, the major venous sinuses, and some pathological processes within the brain. The normal structures of the brain are not visualized. Only those abnormalities which are vascular or destroy the blood–brain barrier are demonstrated. Radionuclide imaging of the brain is safe, carries little radiation dose, and can be carried out as an outpatient procedure. Its sensitivity depends not only upon the location and size but also on the nature of the abnormality (Fig. 21). A high false negative rate can be anticipated in the posterior fossa and skull base, irrespective of size or histological character, due to overlying activity. Conventional radionuclide imaging suffers significantly from lack of tissue characterization. Zones of cerebral infarction, for example, may, in the first 2 weeks, mimic tumour activity due to uptake of isotope. A number of methods for the measurement of blood flow have been proposed using non-diffusible tracers, such as ^{133}Xe, by inhalation or intracarotid injection, although they are rarely a routine of clinical management. A minicomputer linked to a gamma-camera enables rapid dynamic images (one per second or faster) to be obtained, sorted in digital form, and later processed. Such radionuclide 'angiography' can have value in demonstrating variations in abnormal vascularity.

Modern gamma-cameras can produce images which demonstrate the distribution of radioisotope in a slice of tissue. Single proton emission computed tomography (SPECT) uses computer reformation techniques similar to those employed in CT but also produces images in the standard axial plane. A new class of cerebral agent labelled with single-photon short-lived gamma-emitters (iodo-isopropyl amphetamine (IMP) and hexa-methyl-propoline-amine (**HM-PAO**)), which cross the blood–brain barrier rapidly, provides a means of imaging regional cerebral metabolism. HM-PAO uptake has been used to identify increased neuronal activity responsible for focal epilepsy, to differentiate the variety of atrophic dementing disorders (Fig. 22), and has been employed increasingly as a confirmatory technique in the assessment of brain death.

Positron emission tomography (PET) enables short-lived radioactive isotopes such as ^{11}C, ^{13}N, and ^{15}O to be detected, but usually requires a cyclotron in close proximity. Studies of glucose metabolism and protein synthesis as functions of brain activity are encouraging, particularly in the study of cognitive disorders.

Radionuclide cisternography can be performed with non-lipid soluble materials injected intrathecally. A labelled protein, such as radioactive iodinated serum albumin (RISA), or inorganic chelate, such as ^{169}Yb, is usually used. CT and MR now provide more attractive methods of visualizing both the morphology and dynamics of the cerebrospinal fluid circulation.

Fig. 24 Spinal dysraphism. Note the tethered cord and intramedullary fat. (a) Water-soluble contrast myelography; (b) computer-assisted myelography.

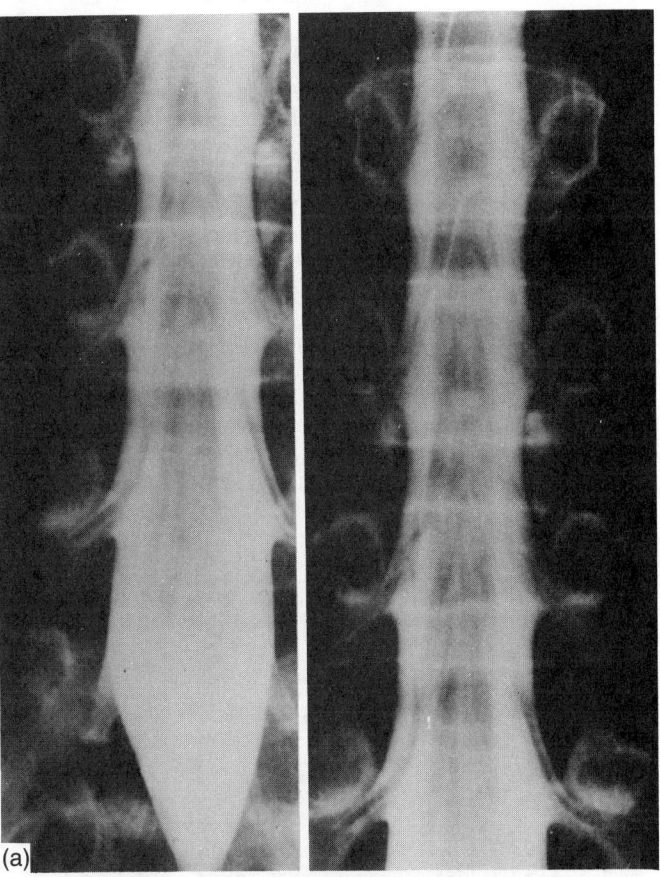

(a)

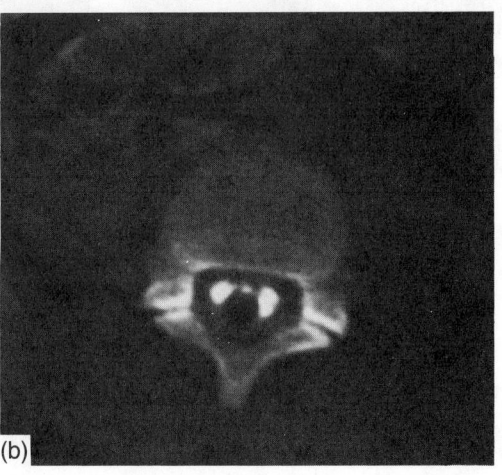

(b)

Fig. 23 Ultrasound transcranial coronal sections of bilateral periventricular haemorrhage with intracranial (small arrow) and intraventricular (large arrow) extension. Note the dilatation of the third and lateral ventricles due to secondary non-obstructive hydrocephalus. (Image by courtesy of Dr S. Russell, St Mary's Hospital, Manchester, United Kingdom.)

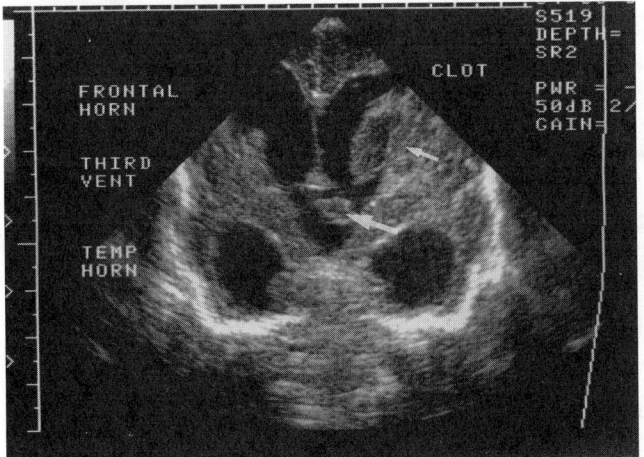

VENTRICULOGRAPHY

Demonstration of the cerebral ventricular system by the introduction of air, iodized oil, or water-soluble iodinated contrast material through a burr hole requires neurosurgical intervention and will only be considered after appropriate consultation. Ventriculography has now been almost completely replaced by CT and MRI but retains a use in the planning of stereotaxic neurosurgical procedures.

PNEUMOENCEPHALOGRAPHY

Demonstration of the ventricular system and subarachnoid spaces by air requires fractional introduction of 25 to 30 ml of air by the lumbar route, with selective positioning of the patient's head to outline the appropriate structures. It should not, except under exceptional circumstances, be performed in the presence of raised intracranial pressure. Pneumo-encephalography has now been replaced by CT and MRI.

ULTRASOUND

Ultrasonic vibrations are produced by passing an electric current through a suitable crystal. The sound-waves thus generated pass directly through homogeneous matter but are reflected back by certain interfaces and detected by the same crystal. This procedure is known as an 'A' scan. A 'B' scan is designed to produce a display of internal structures by controlled movement of the probe and can be obtained in real time. Ultrasound does not employ ionizing radiation and has no hazard but does require considerable operator skill.

An 'A' scan can demonstrate midline intracranial structures and may also reveal the ventricular walls and subdural collections. 'B' and real-time scanning procedures can be used effectively in the cranial cavity through the 'window' of the open fontanelle in infants. In this age group it can have an effective role in the demonstration of ventricular size and the detection of intracerebral haemorrhage in the newborn (Fig. 23). The technique can also be employed operatively in the adult.

Spinal disorders

PLAIN FILMS

Conventional radiography may reveal congenital and acquired bone abnormalities, together with indirect evidence of intervertebral disc disease. In the case of tumour erosion, a significant proportion of a vertebral body must be destroyed before a lesion is detectable. Demonstration of neural or soft-tissue involvement requires more sophisticated techniques.

ISOTOPE BONE SCANNING

The vertebrae are the most frequent sites of skeletal metastases in common cancers. Their detection forms the widest application of skeletal scanning. Several radiopharmaceuticals are available, and their uptake is influenced by the blood supply and mineral turnover of bone. One of the most commonly employed is a technetium-labelled phosphate complex (methylene diphosphonate).

The role of radioisotope bone scanning as a primary screening method in the study of metastatic bone disease in the spine is well established, although many centres now use MRI as a primary investigation. A number of non-malignant conditions, notably degenerative disease and arthritic synovial joints, can give rise to increased isotope activity, and plain films, CT, or MRI may then be necessary as further investigations.

MYELOGRAPHY

Investigation of neural tissue within the spinal canal requires the introduction of a radiographic contrast material into the subarachnoid space. Negative (air) and positive (iodinated) contrast media have been used. Air myelography requires tomography in addition. Iodized oil (Myodil) was once widely used in myelography but is no longer available. The preferred media are now non-ionic, low osmolarity agents which, because of their water solubility and low density, provide a clear outline

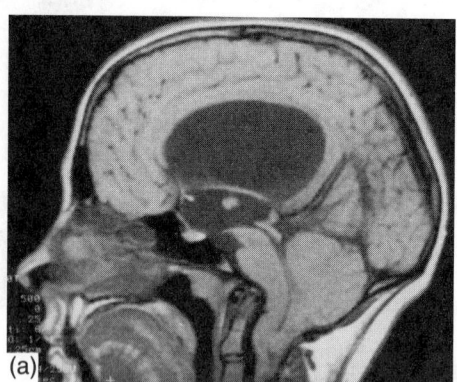

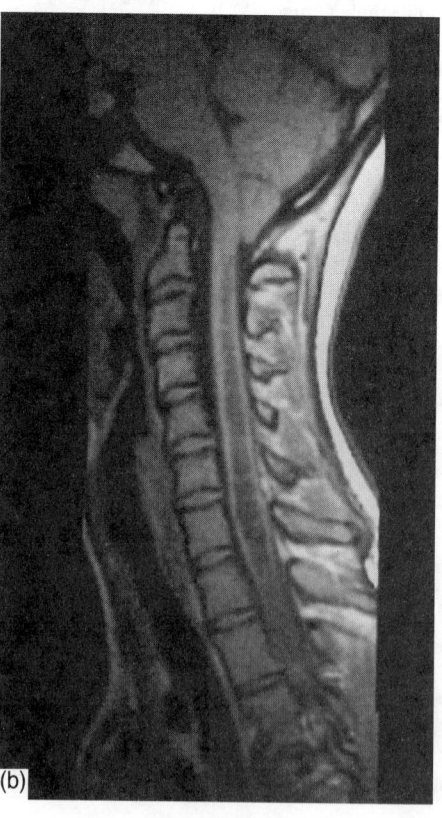

Fig. 25 MRI T_1W parasagittal images of (a) Chiari II malformation—note the prolapse of the medulla and posterior cerebellum through the foramen magnum; (b) syrinx formation throughout the cervical cord.

of the nerve roots and intrathecal contents. Contrast can be introduced by the lumbar or cisternal route. When confined to the lumbar spine, the technique is referred to as radiculography (Fig. 24).

The role of myelography is to obtain accurate anatomical localization of pathological processes in the spinal canal, and to clarify their relationship to the dura (extra- or intradural) and to the spinal cord (extra- or intramedullary).

COMPUTED TOMOGRAPHY (CT) AND COMPUTER-ASSISTED MYELOGRAPHY (CAM)

CT as described above is a non-invasive procedure providing an axial projection of spinal topographical anatomy against a detailed background of paravertebral muscles, vascular structures, and body cavity organs. In particular it provides a more precise identification of the articular configuration of the apophysial joints and their relation to the spinal canal and intervertebral foramina. By its quantitative nature it also has a role in the direct estimation of bone mineral in the axial skeleton.

Computer-assisted myelography (**CAM**) refers to the study of water-soluble contrast medium in the spinal subarachnoid space by CT. The increased sensitivity of CT enables water-soluble contrast medium to be detected in much lower concentrations than would be possible by conventional radiology. When injected by the lumbar route, contrast medium appears in the thoracic spine in 1 h and in the cervical and intracerebral subarachnoid space in 1 to 2 h.

Fig. 27 MRI coronal T_1W image of an intradural thoracic meningioma compressing the spinal cord.

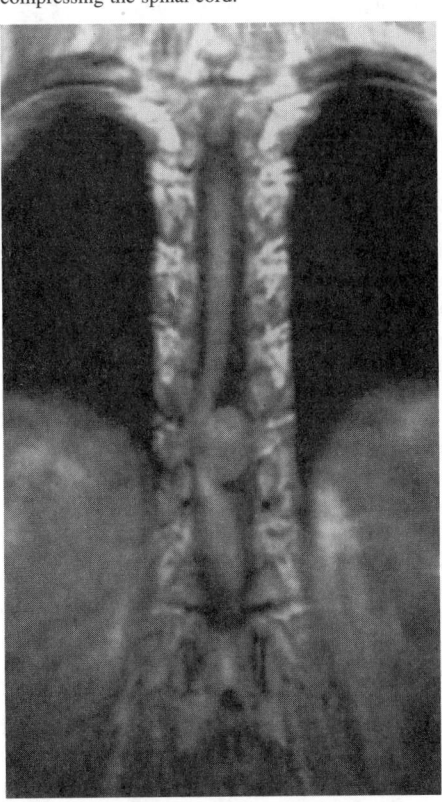

Fig. 26 MRI postcontrast T_1W image of a cystic astrocytoma (arrow) of the upper cervical cord with an extensive tumour syrinx containing debris extending down to the level of C6.

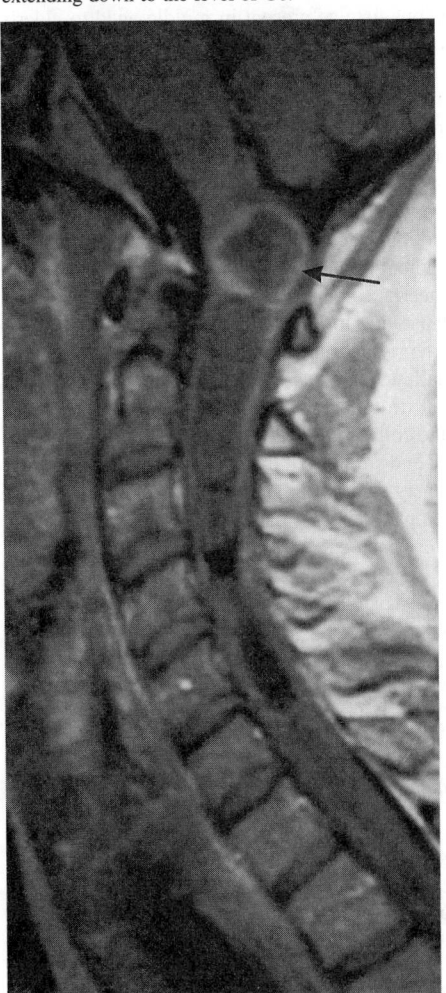

Fig. 28 MR T_2W sagittal section of lumbar spine. Note degenerative intervertebral discs at L4/5, L5/S1, with loss of the normal nuclear signal and disc herniation.

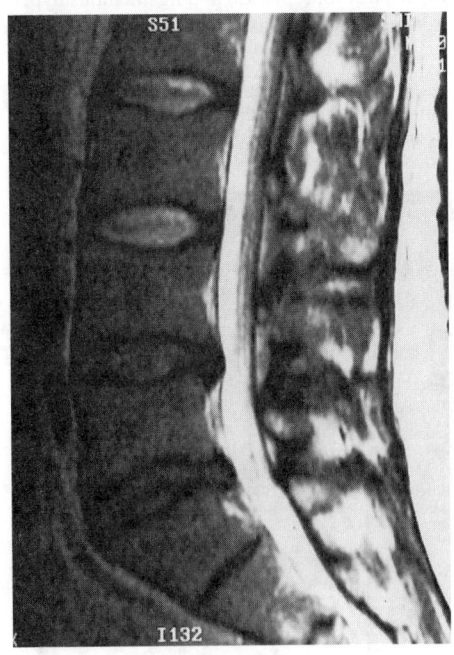

The role of CT and CAM in the evaluation of spinal disorders is increasingly challenged by magnetic resonance imaging.

MAGNETIC RESONANCE IMAGING

MRI offers several major advantages over other techniques in spinal investigation and, where available, has almost replaced myelography, CT, and CAM as the investigation of choice. MRI is non-invasive, incurs no radiation dose, and allows sectional imaging in multiple planes. Surface coils provide high-resolution images with little background noise. Phased array coils enable the whole spine to be imaged. A combination of T_1- and T_2-weighted images provide a degree of tissue characterization not available using other modalities.

Intramedullary lesions are directly visualized by MRI. Their craniocaudal extent can be demonstrated by the use of parasagittal or coronal images. The differentiation between syrinx (Fig. 25) tumour cyst, and solid tumour is relatively straightforward (Fig. 26). Almost all intramedullary spinal tumours enhance following intravenous contrast, and postcontrast T_1-weighted images provide an accurate method of demonstrating the extent of tumour prior to surgery or radiotherapy.

Extramedullary intradural lesions, together with their exact relationship to the spinal cord and the root, are well seen on both T_1- and T_2-weighted images (Fig. 27). Neurofibromas, unlike meningiomas, usually have a high signal. Most extradural spinal lesions cause indentation of the thecal sac, which is well demonstrated on appropriate radiofrequency sequences where cerebrospinal fluid is displayed with a high signal (i.e. white), producing in effect an 'MR myelogram' (Fig. 28). Bone destruction due to neoplastic extradural lesions may be poorly demonstrated on conventional sequences. Out-of-phase gradient echo images can then provide a highly sensitive demonstration of bone marrow invasion and metastatic disease (Fig. 29).

MRI has a special role in the investigation of degenerative spinal disease. Early degenerative disc disease can be identified by loss of the normal high signal from the central nucleus pulposus on T_2-weighted images (Fig. 28). Disc prolapse, disc protrusions, and sequestrated disc fragments are clearly demonstrated. The degree of neural compression can be assessed on both parasagittal and axial images. Spinal canal stenosis and the contribution of facet joint disease and ligamentous hypertrophy can also be assessed accurately. Parasagittal T_1-weighted images

directly demonstrate the neural outlet foramina and the presence of lateral nerve root compression.

SPINAL ANGIOGRAPHY

The main blood supply to the spinal cord is from an anterior and two posterior spinal arteries which run the length of the cord and which are fed by radicular arteries along the entire length of the neural axis. Feeding vessels to spinal vascular anomalies commonly arise at a distance from the lesion, and selective catheterization of multiple vessels is usually necessary. Spinal angiography is valuable in the diagnosis of spinal arteriovenous malformations and of arteriovenous dural fistulae, but has only a limited role in the investigation of spinal tumours.

INTERVENTIONAL PROCEDURES

Endovascular intervention in the spinal canal is limited to embolization of arteriovenous malformations and dural arteriovenous fistulae. Spinal arteriovenous malformations are rare and usually present in early adulthood with slowly progressive neurological deficits. The diagnosis is often suggested by the demonstration of distended spinal veins on myelography or MRI, but angiography is required to confirm the diagnosis and to identify major feeding vessels which might be suitable for embolization. Permanent embolic agents are used following superselective catheterization of the main feeding arteries. Embolic injections can only be made distal to radicular branches that supply the cord, and injection of the vessel which supplies the main radicular spinal artery (Adamkiewicz) is seldom technically possible. Despite these difficulties, spinal arteriovenous malformations are amenable to embolization in the majority of cases.

Spinal dural arteriovenous fistulae present in middle-aged to elderly men. They cause symptoms by vascular compression of the conus medullaris due to gross dilatation of the spinal and extradural veins. Most dural arteriovenous fistulae are fed by a single direct arteriovenous fistula located around one of the lumbar or lower dorsal nerve root sheaths. Embolization is usually technically straightforward, although symptomatic improvement results in only just over 50 per cent of cases.

CT and fluoroscopy can be used to guide biopsy procedures in the spinal column with considerable accuracy. CT biopsy can be invaluable and usually provides sufficient tissue for histological or microbiological analysis and avoids the need for open spinal biopsy.

Painful vertebral collapse due to haemangiomas, venous malformations, or certain neoplasms (lymphoma, leukaemia, and myeloma) can be treated, or at least palliated, by radiologically guided injection of methacrylate bone cement. In this technique, known as vertebroplasty, the trabecular spaces of the collapsed vertebra are filled, thereby improving the structural stability and strength of the affected bone. In carefully selected cases vertebroplasty can halt a benign but destructive process and can provide prolonged pain relief for patients with destructive spinal malignancy.

REFERENCES

Atlas, S.W. (ed.) (1991). *Magnetic resonance imaging of the brain and spine.* Raven Press, New York.

Berenstein, A. and Lasjaunias, P. (1992). *Endovascular treatment of cerebral lesions.* Springer-Verlag, Heidleberg.

Grainger, R.S. and Allison, D.J. (1992). *Diagnostic radiology: an Anglo-American textbook of imaging.* Part 9. *Neuroradiology.* Churchill Livingstone, Edinburgh.

Isherwood, I. (ed.) (1991). Neuroimaging. *Current Opinion in Neurology and Neurosurgery* **4,** (6), 827–66.

Isherwood, I. (ed.) (1992). Neuroimaging. *Current Opinion in Neurology and Neurosurgery* **5,** (6), 841–80.

Sutton, D. (ed.) (1992). *A textbook of radiology and imaging.* Part 7. *The central nervous system.* Churchill Livingstone, Edinburgh.

Woolpert, S.M. and Barnes, P.D. (1992). *MRI in pediatric neuroradiology.* Mosby Year Books, St Louis.

Fig. 29 MRI images of a patient with extensive prostatic metastases. (a) Gradient echo image. (b) Out-of-phase image gradient echo image. Normal vertebral marrow appears as an area of low signal (black), areas of high signal represent metastatic invasion.

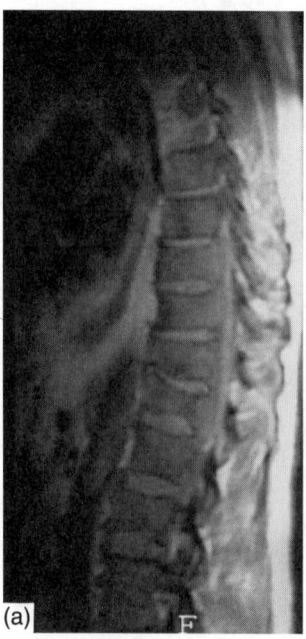
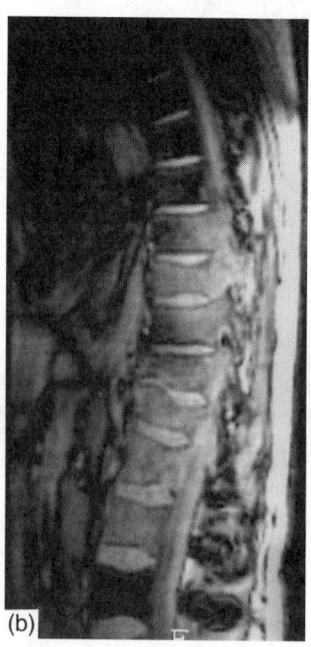

(a)   (b)

changes occasionally lead to confusion, and even disagreement with the histologist. Thus in spinal muscular atrophy motor unit potentials typical of a myopathy may be encountered, while in long-standing collagen muscle disease amplitudes suggestive of chronic partial denervation can occur. A further, sometimes insoluble, problem associated with the latter group of muscle disorders is that of deciding whether increased weakness is due to the condition itself or to an added steroid-induced myopathy.

The cause of weakness may be a clinically evident upper motor neurone disorder but when a lower motor neurone lesion develops in a spastic limb it is often missed until electromyography is performed. Such a combination in a lower limb will confirm a suspected diagnosis of amyotrophic lateral sclerosis.

CHRONIC, FOCAL

Diagnosis depends on the distribution and kind of electromyographical abnormality, and tends to rely more on nerve conduction studies, as when a greatly increased distal motor latency to adductor pollicis shows that small hand muscle wasting is due not to motor neurone disease but to a lesion of the deep palmar branch of the ulnar nerve.

FUNCTIONAL

Psychologically determined weakness shows itself electromyographically in two main forms, the irregularly fluctuating activation of normal motor units which parallels the findings on clinical testing, and the complete paralysis of a muscle group or limb which moves quite normally when the appropriate nerve is stimulated electrically. Foot drop, more often on the non-dominant side, is perhaps the commonest example: an apparently flail and useless foot rises strongly into full dorsiflexion when the common peroneal nerve is stimulated, an event to which the patient's response may be revealing. Conversely, a patient judged to be malingering, hysterical, or merely lazy is sometimes shown by the electromyographer to be suffering from an unrecognized disorder which, if not wholly responsible for the indisposition, may have decided the form it has taken. The forensic importance of such an objective test needs no emphasis.

When all electromyographical findings are normal, the cause of apparent weakness may lie outside the nervous system, as when a tendon is ruptured or of the wrong length, or movement is limited by pain or joint disease.

Wasting

The bulk and strength of muscle may remain normal even when its nerve is undergoing progressive damage, provided that by collateral sprouting the surviving axons can re-innervate and thus preserve the function of denervated muscle fibres. When this compensatory process proves inadequate the muscle will atrophy. Failure to appreciate this point sometimes leads to the erroneous belief that denervation cannot be present because there is no wasting.

Electromyography differentiates wasting due to a lesion of the motor unit, in which motor unit potential abnormality occurs, from disuse atrophy, parietal wasting, and congenital absence of muscle (such as abductor pollicis brevis or pectoralis major) in which it does not. Thus, a bedridden patient with wasted shin muscles may be thought to have disuse atrophy until electromyography reveals compression of the common peroneal nerve which should have been prevented. An unsuspected focal nerve lesion, sometimes responsible for discomfort or distress, may be detected in a limb whose incapacity was thought to be wholly due to a condition such as a stroke.

Wasting near an inflamed joint often has multiple causes: taking the example of the metacarpophalangeal joint in rheumatoid arthritis, thenar wasting may be due to a combination of disuse atrophy associated with pain, inflammatory myopathy, rheumatoid polyneuropathy, and carpal

tunnel compression. Since only the last of these is readily remediable, its recognition by electromyography may be of great benefit.

Frail, elderly people are sometimes unnecessarily referred for electromyography merely because they are thin, but in weight loss due, for example, to thyrotoxicosis, malignant disease, or anorexia nervosa a myopathy may be detected.

Fatiguability

When a patient complains of tiring easily rather than of being continuously weak, repetitive nerve stimulation may result in progressive reduction in the amplitude of the evoked muscle potential, signifying myasthenia gravis. In mild cases this test is insufficiently sensitive and an increase in 'jitter' is sought with the single-fibre needle (see Section 25). Jitter is the variability in time interval between action potentials from single muscle fibres at consecutive discharges of their parent motor unit. An increase occurs in any condition in which neuromuscular transmission is impaired, and over 80 per cent of cases of generalized myasthenia can be diagnosed in this way, considerably fewer of the purely ocular form. Needle electromyography is in any case required in order to exclude conditions which may coexist with myasthenia gravis, such as polymyositis and thyrotoxic myopathy. The Tensilon® (edrophonium chloride) test is useful, but both false negative and false positive results occur.

In the myasthenic syndrome of Lambert and Eaton (see Section 25) repetitive nerve stimulation is the diagnostically decisive test. An initially small evoked muscle potential increases in amplitude by several hundred per cent at rapid stimulation rates.

Entrapment neuropathies

Acute nerve compression has already been referred to. When chronic compression occurs, electromyography must determine not only its level, but how much of the clinical picture is due to block of conduction and how much to axonal degeneration. The higher the proportion of block, the better the prospect of spontaneous recovery. Surgery to relieve compression should ideally be preceded by electromyography in order that a baseline be established by which to judge its results. Failure to relieve symptoms of carpal tunnel compression, for example, may be due to faulty technique or to impaired recovery in the presence of a generalized neuropathy, but if surgery can be shown to have reversed the diagnostic abnormality of nerve conduction, the source of symptoms may lie elsewhere. Anomalous innervation is a rare source of difficulty which electromyography should resolve.

Polyneuropathy

The importance of electromyography in polyneuropathy is threefold: (1) early diagnosis; (2) electrodiagnostic classification (for example, sensory axonal, multifocal demyelinating); and (3) monitoring the natural course or response to treatment.

In the commonest polyneuropathy met with in daily practice, the symmetrical distal involvement of sensory and motor axons, the earliest abnormalities are a reduced sural nerve sensory action potential and a delayed foot muscle F wave. In diabetes these changes often precede subjective awareness of abnormality, while in the neuropathy of alcohol abuse the reverse is true. The diagnosis may be made for the first time when a patient sent for confirmation of carpal tunnel syndrome on one side proves to have not only subclinical compression on the other, but also bilateral subclinical ulnar lesions at the elbows. Such lesions, for which the term 'mononeuritis multiplex' is inappropriate, are simply drawing attention to a symmetrical polyneuropathy which is unsuspected and perhaps even clinically undetectable. Electrodiagnostic classification is achieved by assessment of the distribution of abnormality, the balance of sensory and motor involvement, the degree of slowing of conduction velocity, and the detection of conduction block.

Nerve conduction studies require essentially no co-operation, indeed can be performed if the patient is unconscious. This makes them of special value at the extremes of life, when the history may be poor or unobtainable and physical examination difficult or misleading. Polyneuropathy discovered when there is coma, confusion, or spasticity may raise the possibility of Wernicke's encephalopathy, vitamin B_{12} deficiency, porphyria, or metachromatic leucodystrophy. The important matter of distinguishing axonal from demyelinating polyneuropathies by means of the degree of slowing of conduction has already been mentioned. This is crucial in the identification of the various hereditary neuropathies and their differentiation from such conditions as Friedreich's ataxia and the spinal muscular atrophies.

When systematic nerve conduction studies in upper and lower limbs give normal results in a patient with symptoms suggestive of a polyneuropathy, there are several possible explanations. A neuropathy may indeed be present but is not yet severe enough to give abnormal results with the methods available, or the fibres affected are inaccessible by reason of their small diameter or extremely peripheral situation. Symptoms may, however, be due to an unrecognized pathological process at a proximal level, such as rheumatoid disintegration of the cervical spine, tabes dorsalis, or multiple sclerosis. A patient's fear that he or she has the latter condition may even induce hyperventilation and further complicate the picture. Finally, it may have to be assumed that there is no organic basis for the sensory symptoms.

Electromyography and the surgeon

Apart from its role in the investigation of certain highly specialized organs such as the eye, larynx, bladder, and rectum, there are two main areas of usefulness, the diagnosis and management of nerve compression, already mentioned, and in cases of nerve trauma. When clinical examination suggests that complete nerve degeneration has taken place, such as in the flail arm of the infant with obstetric palsy or the youth injured by a motor cycle accident, electromyography may detect surviving motor units and thus change the prognosis. The electromyographer is often asked whether nerve regeneration is occurring spontaneously, or after nerve repair.

Non-diagnostic uses of electromyography

Electromyographical techniques have found application outside the purely clinical sphere, for example, in the study of toxic and environmental hazards and of the posture of those engaged in heavy static work. The development of aids to rehabilitation is a particularly active field.

REFERENCES

Brown, W.F. and Bolton C.F. (1993). *Clinical electromyography.* (2nd edn) Butterworth-Heinemann, London.

Dawson, D.M., Hallett, M., and Millender, L.H. (1990). *Entrapment neuropathies,* (2nd edn). Little, Brown and Company, Boston/Toronto.

Muscle and Nerve (monthly journal published by John Wiley and Sons).

Payan, J. (1991). Clinical electromyography in infancy and childhood. In *Paediatric neurology,* (2nd edn), (ed. E. Brett). Churchill Livingstone, Edinburgh.

24.2.6 Lumbar puncture

R. A. FISHMAN

INDICATIONS

Lumbar puncture should be performed only after clinical evaluation of the patient and consideration of the potential value and hazards of the procedure. The cerebrospinal fluid findings are important in the differential diagnosis of the gamut of central nervous system (CNS) infections, meningitis, and encephalitis, as well as subarachnoid haemorrhage, confusional states, acute stroke, status epilepticus, meningeal malignancies, demyelinating diseases, and CNS vasculitis. Cerebrospinal fluid examination usually is necessary in patients with suspected intracranial bleeding to establish the diagnosis, although computed tomography (CT), when available, may be more valuable. For example, primary intracerebral haemorrhage or post-traumatic haemorrhage is often readily observed with CT, making lumbar puncture an unnecessary hazard. However, in primary subarachnoid haemorrhage, lumbar puncture may establish the diagnosis when CT is falsely negative. Lumbar puncture is useful to ascertain that the cerebrospinal fluid is free of blood before anticoagulant therapy for stroke is begun. (However, extensive subarachnoid bleeding is a rare complication of heparin anticoagulation, begun several hours after a traumatic bloody tap. Therefore, heparin therapy should not begin for at least 1 h after a bloody tap.) Lumbar puncture has limited therapeutic usefulness, for example, intrathecal therapy in meningeal malignancies and fungal meningitis.

CONTRAINDICATIONS

Lumbar puncture is contraindicated in the presence of infection in the skin overlying the spine. A serious complication of lumbar puncture is the possibility of aggravating a pre-existing, often unrecognized, brain herniation syndrome (for example, uncal, cerebellar, or cingulate herniation), associated with intracranial hypertension. This hazard is the basis for considering papilloedema to be a relative contraindication to lumbar puncture. The availability of CT has simplified the management of patients with papilloedema. If CT reveals no evidence of a mass lesion, then lumbar puncture is usually needed in the presence of papilloedema to establish the diagnosis of pseudotumour cerebri and to exclude meningeal inflammation or malignancy.

Hazards of bleeding disorders

Thrombocytopenia and other bleeding diatheses predispose patients to needle-induced subarachnoid, subdural, and epidural haemorrhage. Lumbar puncture should be undertaken only for urgent clinical indications when the platelet count is depressed to about $50\,000/\mu l$ or below. Platelet transfusion just before the puncture is recommended if the count is below $20\,000/\mu l$ or dropping rapidly. The administration of protamine to patients on heparin, and vitamin K or fresh frozen plasma to those receiving warfarin, is recommended before lumbar puncture to minimize the hazard of the procedure.

COMPLICATIONS

Complications of lumbar puncture include worsening of brain herniation and spinal cord compression, headache, subarachnoid bleeding, diplopia, backache, and radicular symptoms. Headache after lumbar puncture is the most common complication, occurring in about 25 per cent of patients and usually lasting 2 to 8 days. It results from low cerebrospinal fluid pressures due to persistent fluid leakage through the dural hole. Characteristically, pain is present in the upright position and is promptly relieved with a supine position. Aching of the neck and low back are common. The headache is aggravated by cough or strain. Occasionally it is associated with nausea, vomiting, or tinnitus. It is avoided when a small syletted needle is used and if multiple puncture holes are not made. The management of postspinal headache depends upon strict bed rest in the horizontal position, adequate hydration, and simple analgesics. If conservative measures fail, the use of a 'blood patch' is indicated. The technique utilizes the epidural injection of autologous blood close to the site of the dural puncture to form a thrombotic tamponade which seals the dural hole.

CEREBROSPINAL FLUID PRESSURE

The cerebrospinal fluid pressure should be measured routinely. The pressure level within the right atrium is the reference level with the patient in the lateral decubitus position. The normal lumbar cerebrospinal fluid pressure ranges between 50 and 200 mmH$_2$0 (and as high as 250 mm in very obese subjects). With the use of the clinical manometer, the arterially derived pulsatile pressures are obscured but respiratory pressure waves, reflecting changes in central venous pressures, are visible. Low pressures are seen in dehydration, spinal subarachnoid block, following previous lumbar puncture or other cerebrospinal fluid leaks, or may be technical in origin because of faulty needle placement. Increased pressures occur with brain oedema, intracranial mass lesions, infections, acute stroke, cerebral venous occlusions, congestive heart failure, pulmonary insufficiency, and benign intracranial hypertension (pseudotumour cerebri) of diverse aetiology.

CEREBROSPINAL FLUID CELLS

Normal cerebrospinal fluid contains no more than five lymphocytes or mononuclear cells/μl. A higher white cell count is pathognomonic of disease in the central nervous system or meninges. A stained smear of the sediment is needed for an accurate differential cell count. A variety of centrifugal and sedimentation techniques have been used. A pleocytosis occurs with the gamut of inflammatory disorders. The changes characteristic of the various meningitides are listed in Table 1. The heterogeneous forms of neuro-AIDS also are associated with a wide range of cellular responses. Other disorders associated with a pleocytosis include brain infarction, subarachnoid bleeding, cerebral vasculitis, acute demyelination, and brain tumours. Eosinophilia most often accompanies parasitic infections, for example cysticercosis. Cytological studies for malignant cells are rewarding with some CNS neoplasms.

Bloody cerebrospinal fluid due to needle trauma contains increased numbers of white cells contributed by the blood. A useful approximation of a true white cell count can be obtained by the following correction for the presence of the added blood: if the patient has a normal blood count, subtract from the total white cell count (per μl) 1 white cell for each 1000 red blood cells present. Thus, if bloody fluid contains 10 000 red cells and 100 white cells/μl, 10 white cells would be accounted for by the added blood and the corrected leucocyte count would be 90/μl. If the patient's blood count reveals significant anaemia or leucocytosis, the following formula may be used to determine more accurately the number of white cells (W) in the spinal fluid before the blood was added:

$$W = \frac{\text{blood WBC} \times \text{CSF RBC}}{\text{blood RBC} \times 100}$$

(abbreviations: WBC, white blood cells; CSF, cerebrospinal fluid; RBC, red blood cells).

The presence of blood in the subarachnoid space produces a secondary inflammatory response which leads to a disproportionate increase in the number of white cells. Following an acute subarachnoid haemorrhage, this elevation in the white cell count is most marked about 48 h after onset, when meningeal signs are most striking.

To correct cerebrospinal fluid protein values for the presence of added blood due to needle trauma, subtract 0.001 g for every 1000 red blood cells. Thus, if the red cell count is 10 000/μl and the total protein is 1.1 g/l the corrected protein level would be about 1 g/l. The corrections are reliable only if the cell count and total protein are both made on the same tube of fluid.

BLOOD IN THE CEREBROSPINAL FLUID: DIFFERENTIAL DIAGNOSIS AND THE THREE-TUBE TEST

To differentiate between a traumatic spinal puncture and pre-existing subarachnoid haemorrhage, the fluid should be collected in at least three separate tubes (the 'three-tube test'). In traumatic punctures, the fluid generally clears between the first and the third collections. This is detectable by the naked eye and should be confirmed by cell count. In subarachnoid bleeding, the blood is generally evenly admixed in the three tubes. A sample of the bloody fluid should be centrifuged and the supernatant fluid compared with tap water to exclude the presence of pigment.

The supernatant fluid is crystal-clear if the red count is less than about 100 000 cells/μl. With bloody contamination of greater magnitude, plasma proteins may be sufficient to cause minimal xanthochromia; this requires enough serum to raise the cerebrospinal fluid protein concentration to about 1.5 g/l.

Following subarachnoid haemorrhage, the supernatant fluid usually remains clear for 2 to 4 h and even longer after the onset of subarachnoid bleeding. The clear supernatant may mislead the physician to conclude erroneously that the observed blood is due to needle trauma in patients who have had a lumbar puncture within 4 h of aneurysmal rupture. After an especially traumatic puncture, some blood and xanthochromia may be present for as long as 2 to 5 days following the initial puncture. In pathological states associated with a cerebrospinal fluid protein level greater than 1.5 g/l, and in the absence of bleeding, very faint xanthochromia may be detected. When the protein is elevated to much higher levels, as in spinal block, polyneuritis, and meningitis, the xanthochromia may be considerable. A xanthochromic fluid with a normal protein level or a minor elevation to less than 1.5 g/l usually indicates a previous subarachnoid or intracerebral haemorrhage (rarely, the xanthochromia is due to severe jaundice, carotenaemia, or rifampin).

PIGMENTS

Two major pigments derived from red cells may be observed in cerebrospinal fluid, oxyhaemoglobin and bilirubin. Methaemoglobin is only seen spectrophotometrically. Oxyhaemoglobin, released with lysis of red cells, may be detected in the supernatant fluid within 2 h after subarachnoid haemorrhage. It reaches a maximum in about the first 36 h and gradually disappears over the next 7 to 10 days. Bilirubin is produced *in vivo* by leptomeningeal cells following red cell haemolysis. Bilirubin is first detected about 10 h after the onset of subarachnoid bleeding. It reaches a maximum at 48 h and may persist for 2 to 4 weeks after extensive bleeding. The severity of the meningeal signs associated with subarachnoid bleeding correlate with the inflammatory response (the leucocytic pleocytosis).

TOTAL PROTEIN

The total protein level of cerebrospinal fluid ranges between 1.5 g/l and 5 g/l. While an elevated protein level lacks specificity, it is an index of neurological disease reflecting a pathological increase in endothelial cell permeability. Greatly increased protein levels, 5 g/l and above, are seen in meningitis, bloody fluids, or cord tumour with spinal block. Polyneuritis (Guillain–Barré syndrome), diabetic radiculoneuropathy, and myxoedema also may increase the level to 1 to 3 g/l. Low protein levels, below 0.15 g/l occur most often with cerebrospinal fluid leaks due to a previous lumbar puncture or traumatic dural fistula.

IMMUNOGLOBULINS

Although a vast number of proteins may be measured in cerebrospinal fluid, only an increase in immunoglobulins is of diagnostic importance. Such increases are indicative of an inflammatory response in the CNS and occur with immunological disorders, and bacterial, viral, spirochaetal, and fungal diseases. Immunoglobulin assays are most useful in the diagnosis of multiple sclerosis, other demyelinating diseases, and CNS vasculitis. The cerebrospinal fluid level is corrected for the entry of immunoglobulins from the serum by calculating the IgG index (see Table 1). More than one oligoclonal band in cerebrospinal fluid on gel electrophoresis (and absent in serum) is also abnormal, occurring in 90 per cent of multiple sclerosis cases and in the gamut of inflammatory diseases.

GLUCOSE

The cerebrospinal fluid glucose concentration is dependent upon the level of glucose in the blood. The normal range in cerebrospinal fluid is between 2.5 and 4.5 mmol/l in patients with a blood glucose between

Table 1 *Cerebrospinal fluid findings in meningitis*

Meningitis	Pressure (mmH₂O)	Leucocytes/μl	Protein (g/l)	Glucose (mmol/l)
Acute bacterial	Usually elevated	Several hundred to more than 60 000; usually a few thousand; occasionally less than 100 (especially meningococcal or early in disease); polymorphonuclears predominate	Usually 1 to 5, occasionally more than 10	0.2 to 2.2 in most cases (in absence of hyperglycaemia)
Tuberculous	Usually elevated; may be low with dynamic block in advanced stages	Usually 25 to 100; rarely more than 500; lymphocytes predominate except in early stages when polymorphonuclears may account for 80% of cells	Nearly always elevated, usually 1 to 2; may be much higher if dynamic block	Usually reduced; less than 2.5 in 3/4 cases
Cryptococcal	Usually elevated	0 to 800; average 50; lymphocytes predominate	Usually 0.2 to 5; average 1	Reduced in most cases; average 1.7 (in absence of hyperglycaemia)
Viral	Normal to moderately elevated	5 to a few hundred; but may be more than 1000, particularly with lymphocytic choriomeningitis; lymphocytes predominate but may be more than 80% polymorphonuclears in first few days	Frequently normal or slightly elevated; less than 1; may show greater elevation in severe cases	Normal (reduced in 1/4 cases of mumps and herpes simplex)
Syphilitic (acute)	Usually elevated	Average 500; usually lymphocytes; rarely polymorphonuclear	Average, 1	Normal (rarely reduced)
Cysticercosis	Often increased; low with dynamic block	Increased mononuclears and polymorphonuclears with 2 to 7% eosinophilia in about half the cases	Usually 0.5 to 2	Reduced in 1/5 cases
Sarcoid	Normal to considerably elevated	0 to less than 100 mononuclear cells	Slight to moderate elevation	Reduced in 1/2 cases
Tumour	Normal or elevated	0 to several hundred mononuclears plus malignant cells	Elevated often to high levels	Normal or greatly reduced; (low in 3/4 carcinomatous meningitis cases)

Cerebrospinal fluid (CSF) immunoglobulins are commonly increased in all of the above (including carcinomatous meningitis) as well as in multiple sclerosis and CNS vasculitis. CSF immunoglobulins are assessed by the IgG index:

$$\frac{IgG\ (CSF) \times albumin\ (serum)}{IgG\ (serum) \times albumin\ (CSF)}$$

the normal index is less than 0.65.

Oligoclonal bands (by gel electrophoresis) present in CSF but absent in serum are also a measure of abnormally increased CSF immunoglobulins synthesized within the CNS.

4 and 7 mmol/l, that is, 60 to 80 per cent of the normal blood level. Cerebrospinal fluid values between 2.2 and 2.5 mmol/l are usually abnormal, and values below 2.2 mmol/l invariably so. Hyperglycaemia during the 4 h prior to lumbar puncture results in a parallel increase in cerebrospinal fluid glucose. The latter approaches a maximum and the cerebrospinal fluid/blood ratio may be as low as 0.35 in the presence of a greatly elevated blood glucose level and in the absence of any neurological disease. An increase in cerebrospinal fluid glucose is of no diagnostic significance apart from reflecting hyperglycaemia within the 4 h prior to lumbar puncture. The cerebrospinal fluid glucose level is abnormally low (hypoglycorrhachia) in several diseases of the nervous system apart from hypoglycaemia. It is characteristic of acute purulent meningitis, and a usual finding in tuberculous and fungal meningitis. It is usually normal in viral meningitis, although reduced in about 25 per cent of mumps cases, and in some cases of herpes simplex and zoster meningoencephalitis. The cerebrospinal fluid glucose is also reduced in other inflammatory meningitides, including cysticercosis, amoebic meningitis (Naegleria), acute syphilitic meningitis, sarcoidosis, granulomatous arteritis, and other vasculitides. The glucose level is also reduced in the chemical meningitis that follows intrathecal injections, and in subarachnoid haemorrhage, usually 4 to 8 days after the bleed. The major factor responsible for the depressed glucose levels is increased anaerobic glycolysis in adjacent neural tissues and to a lesser degree by polymorphonuclear leucocytes. Thus, the decrease in cerebrospinal fluid glucose level is accompanied by an inverse increase in cerebrospinal fluid lactate level.

MICROBIOLOGICAL AND SEROLOGICAL REACTIONS

The use of appropriate stains and cultures is essential in cases of suspected infection. Tests for specific bacterial and fungal antigens, countercurrent immunoelectrophoresis, are useful in establishing a specific aetiology. DNA amplification techniques using the polymerase chain reaction promise to improve diagnostic sensitivity. Serological tests on cerebrospinal fluid for syphilis include (1) the reagin antibody tests, and (2) specific treponemal antibody tests. The former are particularly ulumbar punctureseful in evaluating cerebrospinal fluid because positive results may occur even in the presence of a negative blood serology. There is no basis for applying the specific treponemal antibody tests to cerebrospinal fluid because these antibodies are derived from the plasma where they are present in greater concentration.

REFERENCE

Fishman, R.A. (1992). *Cerebrospinal fluid in diseases of the nervous system*, (2nd edn). W.B. Saunders, Philadelphia.

24.3 Organization and features of dysfunction

24.3.1 Disturbances of higher cerebral function

J. M. OXBURY and S. M. OXBURY

The pathology underlying disturbances of higher cerebral function may be diffuse, as in Alzheimer's disease, or focal, as in cerebral infarction and small tumours. Diffuse pathology produces dementia with a global impairment of intellect, personality, memory, concentration, and attention. The personality change may lead to social withdrawal, slovenliness, alcohol abuse, sexual aberration, and ultimately to gross personal neglect and wandering. The associated mood change may be apathy, depression, or euphoria. There may be fear and anxiety, particularly when insight is retained. Forgetfulness is particularly common, and indeed a diagnosis of dementia should be questioned if memory function is normal. Disorders of cognition appear as any combination of those described below.

Focal pathology produces more restricted cognitive impairment. The nature of the impairment depends upon the situation of the pathology in the brain. Often there is no change of personality or loss of memory. However, the pathology responsible for a focal disturbance sometimes produces generalized secondary effects as well. For instance, focal tumours can grow to such a size that the intracranial pressure is raised and blood vessels remote from the tumour are distorted. The result is that generalized effects are superimposed on an initially specific disturbance of higher cerebral function, and if consciousness is well preserved, the mental picture may be mistaken for a general dementia.

LOCALIZATION OF COGNITIVE FUNCTION

The concept that higher mental functions (e.g. language, auditory and visual perception, control of voluntary movement) are subserved by specific areas of the brain has a long and contentious history. The notion of localization began with Franz Gall (1758–1828), the founder of phrenology, and grew in stature with contributions from many subsequent workers. The pioneers of the concept tended to overlook both anatomical and clinical facts which did not fit their theories, but their work was of great importance in the development of neuropsychology.

The nineteenth century also witnessed strong criticisms of localization theories. These were voiced particularly by Hughlings Jackson, Henry Head, who branded the localizationists with the contemptuous title of 'diagram makers', and Kurt Goldstein. During the early part of the twentieth century antilocalizationist views also developed from animal experimentation, particularly that of Lashley who proposed the principle of 'mass action', i.e. the generalization that areas of the cortex function as a whole during learning; he added that the most important factor in disrupting learning after a cortical lesion was the extent of the destruction, not its locus.

Recent research on the breakdown of cognitive function in patients with focal cerebral pathology has swung the pendulum back towards a localizationist view, and there is now extensive evidence against the concepts of unification of the mind or notions that different regions of the brain are equipotential for the control of cognitive function. The introduction of radiological structural and functional imaging techniques, initially computerized tomography and more recently positron emission tomography and magnetic resonance, has been a further stimulus to the increased attention to issues of localization in neuropsychology. Coincidentally, an impetus of a different sort has come from the field of cognitive neuropsychology. Here the aim is to create models of behaviour which both explain and have their validity tested by the breakdown of behaviour seen in neurological patients. The weakness of this method is that the model building is often conducted around a single case without regard for details of the nature and location of the underlying pathology. This approach may advance understanding of cognitive systems, but progress in knowledge of brain–behaviour relations will be limited, much as was that of genetics based on mendelian particles prior to an understanding of DNA and the development of molecular biology.

A special emphasis in research has been to explore both the differential function of the left and right hemispheres, demonstrating asymmetries, and functional interconnections within the hemispheres. This is in addition to the time-honoured separation of function in parallel with anatomical division of the brain into lobes (frontal, temporal, parietal, occipital). These anatomical divisions are somewhat arbitrary, but a simplified list of the major cognitive deficits that have traditionally been associated with the different regions of the brain (Table 1) may be helpful as an introduction to the field of behavioural neurology.

CEREBRAL DOMINANCE AND THE ASYMMETRY OF CEREBRAL FUNCTION

First Dax and then Broca, both in the middle of the nineteenth century, noted the relationship between aphasia, right hemiplegia, and left hemisphere pathology. These observations led to the concept of cerebral dominance which in its original form implied that the anatomical bases of language are vested exclusively in one 'major' cerebral hemisphere—usually the left. It has subsequently become clear that the 'minor' hemisphere—usually the right—also has some capacity to subserve language function. Furthermore, it has also become clear that the hemisphere which is 'minor' for language may be 'major' for other non-linguistic abilities such as visuospatial perception. Some cognitive functions seem

Table 1 *Relationship between behavioural impairment and the site of brain pathology*

Lobe	Behavioural deficit	Main hemisphere involved			
		Left	Right	Left=Right	Bilateral
Frontal	Language—aphasia, verbal fluency ↓	+			
	Speech—dysarthria			+	
	Recent memory impaired			+	
	Movement control ↓			+	
	Planning ability ↓			+ <	++
	Disinhibition—social and motor			+ <	++
Temporal	Memory—verbal aspects ↓	+			
	Non-verbal aspects ↓		+		
	Severe amnesia				+
	Music perception ↓		+		
	Language comprehension ↓	+			
	Kluver–Bucy syndrome				+
	Aggression, rage, depression	+			
	Indifference, euphoria		+		
Parietal and occipital	Primary visual–tactile sensation ↓			+	
	Visual discrimination ↓		+		
	Gaze deviation	+	< +		
	Gaze apraxia				+
	Visual disorientation				+
	Visual agnosia				+
	Prosopagnosia				+
	Hemineglect—visuospatial and body		+		
	Topographical disorientation—Major		+		
	Minor				+
	Dressing apraxia		+		
	Constructional apraxia			+	
	Ideomotor apraxia	+			
	Acalculia—Spatial		+		
	Anarithmia	+			
	Finger agnosia	+			
	Right–left disorientation	+			
	Alexia and agraphia	+			

to be particularly affected by damage to the left hemisphere and others by damage on the right, some seem equally affected by damage to either side, and yet others seem to be only markedly affected when there is damage to both sides. Table 1 gives a simplified scheme. There is a complex relationship between cognitive function, laterality of damage, and handedness. Furthermore, a particular skill, for instance the ability to construct three-dimensional structures, may be affected in different ways according to the laterality of the brain damage; similarly, it may be affected by damage situated diffusely, more or less regardless of location, in one hemisphere, whereas it is only affected by damage at a particular locus in the other hemisphere. Therefore the concept of left cerebral dominance has been abandoned, to be replaced by one of complementary specialization with the left mostly subserving language functions and the right mostly visuospatial abilities.

Aphasia

Aphasia is an acquired defect of language function due to brain damage. It is usually manifest in all four language 'modalities'—speech production, speech comprehension, reading, and writing. Aphasia must be distinguished from motor disturbances of voice production such as dysarthria and stuttering (defined below), from poverty of speech due to intellectual impairment, from language abnormalities as in schizophrenia, and from hysterical mutism. A distinction between the terms 'aphasia' and 'dysphasia' is not useful; the former will be used throughout.

Dysarthria is a disorder of speech production arising from dysfunction of the muscles of articulation. The dysfunction can be secondary to damage in the motor system at any point from the cerebral cortex (and then the dysarthria may be associated with aphasia) to the muscles themselves. The precise quality of the dysarthria depends on the site of the pathology and various forms are recognized, for example spastic dysarthria and ataxic dysarthria. Stuttering (stammering) is an abnormality of speech production characterized by hesitancy and repetitions of speech sounds such that the next expected sound is delayed or not produced. The disruption of the proper sequence of activity in the muscles responsible for articulation may be accompanied by grimaces and other tic-like movements of the head, neck, and limbs. The condition may be a manifestation of a motor programming disorder. The possibility of a psychogenic basis has been raised. It is sometimes considered to be associated with incomplete language dominance, and it very occasionally occurs (usually transiently) in association with aphasia.

LATERALITY OF LANGUAGE REPRESENTATION

More than 90 per cent of normal right-handed people have language represented on the left in the sense that left hemisphere damage could make them overtly aphasic but right-sided damage would not do so. Nevertheless, it seems that the right hemisphere of such a person does have some capacity for language. The evidence is derived from a number of sources. First, some degree of language expression and comprehension may return, as may a rudimentary ability to read and write, after complete left hemispherectomy which has occasionally been carried out in adult life as a treatment for tumour. Second, injection of sodium amytal into one internal carotid artery, producing a temporary pharmacological hemispherectomy which allows the non-injected hemisphere to be studied in isolation (the Wada test), may produce aphasic responses from injection on either side in the same patient. Further information regarding the role of the non-dominant cerebral hemisphere in language function has emerged from the studies of patients whose interhemispheric connections have been severed surgically for the relief of epilepsy (Fig. 1). These individuals offer an opportunity to examine left and right cerebral functions independently in the same patient, for the interhemispheric transfer of complex information is abolished after the operation, so that each cerebral hemisphere is restricted to using information gained through its primary pathways. For instance if the patient's eyes are closed, an object which is actively explored by the left hand cannot be recognized by the right and vice versa. Similarly, if these patients are shown printed words for a short time in the left visual half-field (thereby restricting the visual input to the right hemisphere) they can identify, by touching with their left hand, objects corresponding to the words presented, although they cannot as a rule describe them in speech or writing. Studies in split-brain patients have largely confirmed the functional asymmetries of the left and right hemisphere and also the findings which indicate that the right hemisphere does exhibit some degree of linguistic capacity.

HANDEDNESS, CEREBRAL DOMINANCE, AND APHASIA

Early concepts of cerebral dominance held that the dominant hemisphere is contralateral to the preferred hand. This applies to 95 to 98 per cent of right-handers without early childhood cerebral pathology. However, the left hemisphere is also dominant in about 70 per cent of left-handers without such cerebral pathology; about 20 per cent of left-handers have right hemisphere dominance, and in 10 per cent language function is more or less equally distributed between the two hemispheres (bilateral representation). The incidence of left hemisphere dominance may be considerably less than 70 per cent in left-handers who sustained early childhood left hemisphere damage, with the precise figure depending upon the nature and extent of the pathology.

Left-handers as a group are more likely to develop aphasia than right-handers, presumably because a greater proportion of them have bilateral language representation making them liable to the condition regardless of which hemisphere is damaged. However, the left-handers' aphasia tends to be less severe and to recover more rapidly than that of right-handers, and there is some suggestion that language function is more diffusely represented in the left-handers' brain irrespective of which hemisphere is dominant.

LOCALIZATION WITHIN THE LEFT HEMISPHERE

The areas most important for language are shown in Fig. 2. They include the posterior part of the inferior frontal gyrus (Broca's area) located immediately anterior to the primary motor cortical representation for the face, mouth, and tongue, the posterior part of the superior temporal gyrus (Wernicke's area), the inferior parietal lobule including the supramarginal and angular gyri, and the cortex of the frontoparietal operculum.

Fig. 1 Functions separated by surgery: a simplified summary combined from known neuroanatomy, cortical lesion data, and postoperative testing. (Based on Sperry (1974). Lateral specialization in the surgically separated hemispheres. In *Neurosciences 3rd Study Program* (eds. F. O. Schmitt and F. G. Warden). MIT Press, Cambridge, Mass.)

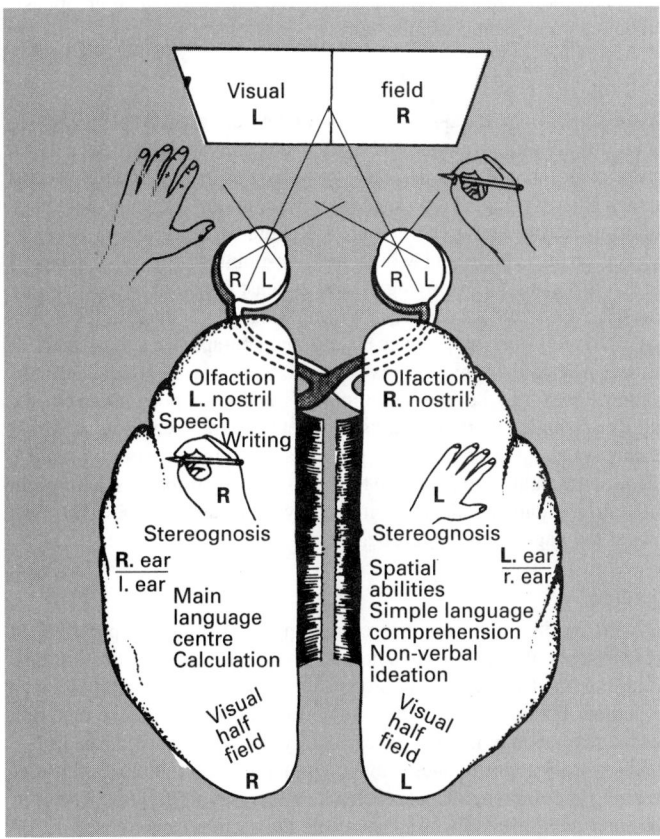

Fig. 2 A lateral view of the left cerebral hemisphere (a) to show the areas important for language functions and the motor area, with a medial view (b) to show the corpus callosum and the primary visual area.

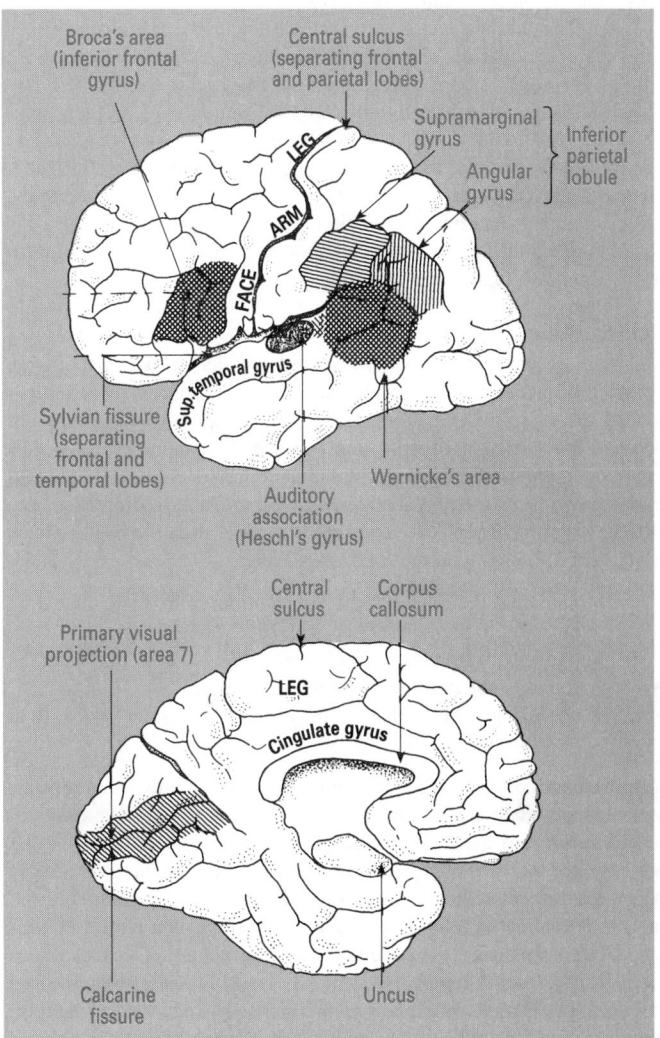

Although these are pre-eminent, sensitive techniques can often detect some linguistic abnormality after damage to other parts of the left hemisphere including subcortical areas.

CHARACTERISTICS OF APHASIA
Spontaneous speech
Difficulty in word finding is a major deficit underlying aphasia and is responsible for many of the characteristic hesitancies and/or circumlocutions. The patient's spontaneous speech may be described as 'fluent' or 'non-fluent'.

Non-fluent aphasia
At its most severe, non-fluent aphasia consists of complete loss of speech and phonation. This is nearly always associated with inability to comprehend anything but the simplest spoken language and with complete inability to read or write. Often there is an associated buccofacial apraxia (a defect of voluntary tongue and palatal movements and of voluntary facial movements, as in whistling or imitating actions such as laughing or blowing, even though all these movements are normal when performed automatically); in the acute phase there may also be an impairment of voluntary swallowing. After some recovery the patient may make phonated but inarticulate utterances or may develop a recurring utterance that is recognizable. The latter is a word, often 'yes' or 'no', or sometimes a phrase. It is produced indiscriminately whenever speech seems necessary, and so it has no meaning for the listener. Sometimes propositional speech may break through for a brief period, particularly in very emotional situations. Occasionally the patient can speak only in an automatic fashion such as swearing.

When the aphasia is less severe, the non-fluent speech is characterized by effortful articulation, a slow rate of word production, and short phrase length. The style is agrammatic, having a telegraphic quality. The language is reduced to a bare minimum by the omission of all those auxiliary and relational words, particularly prepositions, which normally enrich it. Nevertheless, the information content is often high, and adequate meaning can often be conveyed to an attentive listener despite the hesitancies and distorted articulation. Greetings and simple everyday social interactions may be produced quite normally. The quality of writing is similar to that of the spoken language.

Fluent aphasia
This is characterized by spontaneous speech which is abnormal or even completely incomprehensible, not because it is reduced in amount—indeed the rate of word production may be higher than normal—or because it is articulated badly, but because it contains wrong words, non-words, and words arranged in an inappropriate order so that meaning is lost. It is usually accompanied by impaired comprehension. Wrong words have been called paraphasias and various types have been described. These include the following:

- Semantic paraphasia—the substitution of a word related in meaning to the correct one (e.g. cat for dog);
- phonemic paraphasia—the substitution of a word related in sound to the correct one (e.g. tip for top);
- neologism—the substitution of a non-existent word (e.g. brookstruck for broomstick).

In some classifications words containing only one or a few inappropriate syllables are labelled as literal paraphasias if the original word is still recognizable, and the term neologism is then restricted to words that neither exist nor are recognizable. Wrong words can also be simply perseverations of previously used words or random in the sense of having no determinable relationship to other words in the phrase or sentence. Jargon aphasia is the condition where the abnormal characteristics are present to such a degree that speech has very little meaning; the rate of word production, articulation, and prosody (pattern or melody) remain normal. Insight is often lacking, and patients with jargon aphasia may be misdiagnosed as suffering from confusion or an acute psychosis. Careful examination often reveals a right homonomous visual field defect and/or sensory diminution down the right side of the body in addition to the aphasia. Echolalia is a seemingly compulsive repetition of words spoken by others without any apparent understanding of their meaning. Palilalia is repetition reiterated with increasing frequency. Echolalia and palilalia are usually manifestations of diffuse brain disease such as Alzheimer's disease or encephalitis.

Object naming
Most aphasics have some defect of the ability to name objects, although mild aphasia may cause difficulty only with less common objects. This anomia is sometimes the first manifestation of aphasia. It has certain characteristics making it distinguishable from anomia due to other causes such as agnosia. Aphasic anomia is usually independent of the sensory modality through which the object to be named is perceived. Thus a bunch of keys will be equally difficult to name regardless of whether it is shown to the patient, felt tactually, or jangled so that he or she hears them but does not touch or see them. In contrast, the anomia of visual agnosia is restricted to objects presented visually. All but the severest aphasics can describe or indicate the use of objects which they cannot name. Likewise, they usually accept the correct name when it is suggested, rejecting incorrect suggestions, and they can point to the correct object in an array when its name is offered. When an aphasic offers an incorrect name, it is most frequently that of a semantically related object (e.g. table for chair, or hat for coat) or a phonemically related name (e.g. bat for cat, or band for hand). Unusual objects are more difficult to name than common ones.

Speech comprehension
Impaired ability to comprehend speech is a very important functional defect in aphasia. There is little doubt that difficulty in comprehending a statement increases as its linguistic complexity and length increase. As with speech output, confusion may be semantic, phonetic, or syntactic. The bedside analysis of comprehension disturbances is difficult, and a common error is to overestimate the extent to which an aphasic patient can understand what is said.

Writing
Disturbances of writing—agraphia—can be due to a number of causes including aphasia, apraxia, and spatial disorder secondary to parietal lobe damage (Fig. 3). Occasionally agraphia occurs in isolation, but this is rare. The writing of aphasics usually contains the same linguistic abnormalities as their speech. There are grammatical, syntactic, and paraphasic errors, letters and words may be omitted, and misspelling is particularly common. Copying is usually least impaired, writing to dictation more so, and spontaneous writing most of all. Parietal lobe damage, either left or right, produces additional non-aphasic disturbances of writing. The calligraphic form is poor, the lines may be oblique or intersecting, there may be excessive margins and poor positioning on the page, and single letters or groups of letters may be located in isolation. Redundant looping is common, particularly on the letters m, n, and l. These abnormalities may be due to visuospatial disturbances. With right parietal lobe damage all the writing may be located on the right-hand side of the page, with the left being neglected.

Reading
As with writing, abnormalities of reading are usually proportional to other aspects of the aphasia. There are hesitations, word substitutions, omissions, and impaired comprehension. The ability to read aloud is sometimes better preserved than the ability to comprehend the material, but the reverse may happen. Occasionally the disturbance of reading—alexia—is disproportionately severe compared with the abnormality of speaking or comprehending speech and, rarely, severe alexia exists without other manifestations of aphasia (see the section on pure alexia).

Non-linguistic cognitive deficits

These deficits are often associated with aphasia. They may influence considerably the aphasic patient's ability to compensate for the disability and to benefit from therapeutic endeavours, and so they must be recognized.

EXAMINATION OF THE APHASIC PATIENT

A full history must be taken from the patient in so far as the aphasia allows. This provides an excellent opportunity to assess the patient's spontaneous speech, particularly if the aphasia is only mild when it may provide the only abnormalities detectable on clinical as opposed to laboratory examination. It is also essential to take a history from a relative or close friend, particularly if the aphasia is more than mild.

Any previous disturbances such as stuttering or difficulty in learning to read and write should be noted. The language background must be explored. What was the patient's native language? Did he speak foreign languages? Was he a fluent talker or was he always hesitant? Was he a fluent fast reader or was his reading slow and laborious? His education and occupational background must be recorded. Even a mild aphasia will cripple some, such as barristers, whereas in other occupations people may function well despite quite marked aphasia. Hand preferences must be noted, remembering that some people write with the right hand but nevertheless prefer the left, or are ambidextrous, for other activities. A family history of left-handedness should be noted. In those with mixed hand preferences or left-handedness or strong familial sinistrality the usual relationship between aphasia and left hemisphere damage may not obtain.

A scheme for examination is given in Table 2. Much of this consists of looking for abnormalities of the type described in the preceding sec-

Fig. 3 Disturbances of writing. (a) Spontaneous writing of a patient with left hemisphere pathology showing fluent aphasic content and preserved calligraphy. (b) Attempts by a non-aphasic patient with bilateral posterior pathology to write name, alphabet, and digits, showing severe apraxic agraphia.

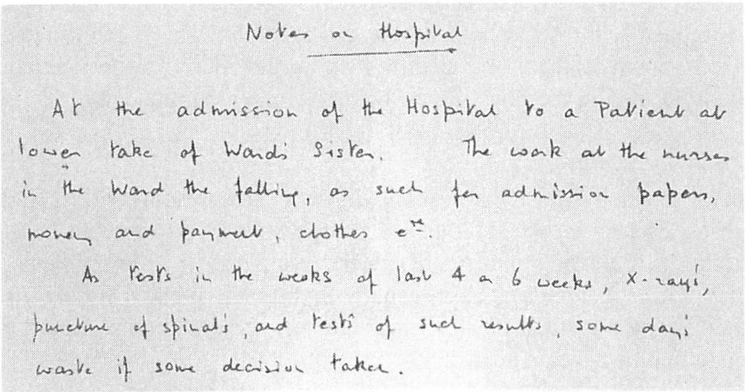

(a)

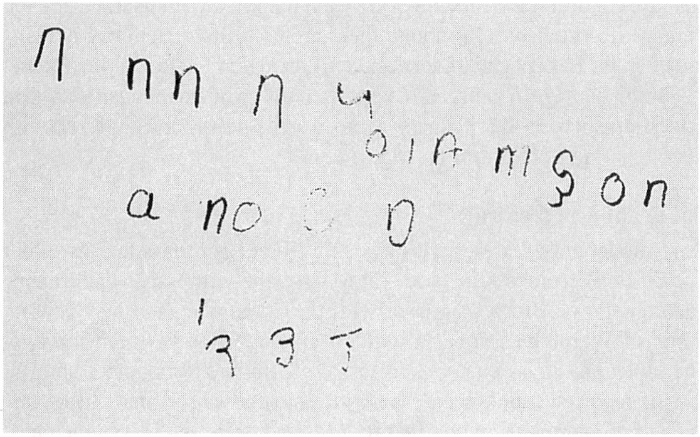

(b)

Table 2 *Examination of the aphasic patient*

History: obtain in full including from a relative/friend (essential if the aphasia is more than minimal)

Spontaneous speech: assess in conversation if possible; note articulation and rhythm, hesitancies and word-finding difficulties, circumlocutions, grammatical errors, paraphasias, and neologisms

Examine patient's ability to:
1 **Name objects** and note frequency/nature of errors (visual presentation as standard, but also auditory/tactile presentation if there is a possibility of agnosia); use clearly identifiable pictures or three-dimensional objects; ask patient to indicate use by words or gesture to establish that the object is recognized
2 **Recite series** (e.g. days of week/months or year) forwards and backwards—errors tend to occur particularly on backward series
3 **Generate words** by saying as many words of a defined character (e.g. beginning with C or names of towns) in a limited time (e.g. 1 min)
4 **Repeat** sentences of varying complexity
5 **Write** name and address and sentences spontaneously and to dictation—note spelling errors, word omissions, calligraphy
6 **Read** a prose passage—note nature and frequency of errors; carry out a written command such as 'close your eyes'

Comprehension: ask patient to point to named objects and to carry out commands (see text)

Other cognitive abilities such as visuospatial, praxis, and memory should be examined at least briefly

Physical examination of other aspects of neurological dysfunction (particularly visual field defect, hemiparesis, and localized sensory change) is very important because aphasia is often associated with other features of left hemisphere pathology.

tion. Comprehension is particularly difficult to determine at the bedside. Some measure can be obtained by assessing the ability to respond correctly to commands of increasing complexity. Thus, with a collection of common objects on a table, the patient may be instructed to carry out commands such as 'close the book' (very simple) and 'close the book, touch the cup, and give me the button' (more complex). With this sort of testing, errors only occur when the aphasia is moderate or severe, and even then they may be due to other factors such as apraxia and memory disorder. A standard test such as the Token Test should be used for milder cases. In this test chips of two different shapes (square and circular), two different sizes (large and small), and five different colours are placed in front of the patient who is given a series of 36 commands which increase progressively in complexity, for example 'touch the yellow square' (simple) and 'together with the yellow circle, take the black circle' (complex). Performance is little affected by mild generalized intellectual deterioration. A quantitative score is obtained (number of correct responses) and the test can be repeated at intervals to assess improvement or deterioration.

CLASSIFICATION AND LOCALIZATION OF APHASIC SYNDROMES

Classification and localization studies have been closely linked to each other in that categories of language disability (the aphasic syndromes) must be defined with some precision if they are to be related to disturbances of specific anatomical structures within the brain. According to current ideas, a rigid doctrine of precisely localized cerebral lesions giving rise to pure forms of aphasia is untenable. Nevertheless, it is generally accepted that aphasic syndromes can be broadly related to the

Table 3 *Geschwind's classification of aphasic syndromes*

Anterior aphasia (non-fluent)
   Broca's aphasia
   Aphemia
   Transcortical motor aphasia

Posterior aphasia (fluent)
   Wernicke's aphasia
   Nominal aphasia
   Transcortical sensory aphasia
   Conduction aphasia
   Pure word deafness

Global aphasia

Disturbances closely allied to aphasia
   Pure alexia
   Pure agraphia
   Alexia with agraphia
   Colour anomia
   Acalculia

occurrence of lesions involving relatively circumscribed regions in the cerebral cortex and their connections.

At present the most widely used classification of aphasia is that proposed by Geschwind (Table 3). He classified disorders of language into two main groups: those resulting from lesions anterior to the Rolandic (central) fissure, and those related to lesions posterior to this fissure. Each of these groups is further subdivided as follows:

- anterior aphasias which are characteristically non-fluent (Broca's aphasia, aphemia, and transcortical motor aphasia);
- posterior aphasias which are characteristically fluent (Wernicke's aphasia, nominal aphasia, transcortical sensory aphasia, conduction aphasia, and pure word deafness).

In addition, the term 'global aphasia' is employed to describe a severe impairment of all aspects of language function. The validity of this classification, which is based on a clinicoanatomical correlation, has gained ground from recent studies which have shown a good correlation between the site of lesions seen on cranial CT scanning and the type of aphasia.

Anterior aphasias
Broca's aphasia (motor/expressive)

This is the most common type of aphasia other than global aphasia. Typically, the patients lose verbal fluency, and there is cortical dysarthria and agrammatism. The speech has a telegraphic quality, and connecting words such as articles, prepositions, and conjunctions are missing. The patient's verbal comprehension is adequate, although not completely normal. The site of the lesion is most frequently at the foot of the third frontal convolution, but usually also involves the cortex of the insula, the lower part of the motor strip, and/or deep structures such as the caudate nucleus and internal capsule. The aphasia may be accompanied by a right facial weakness or hemiplegia but there is usually no visual field defect.

Aphemia

This is considered to be a rare type of aphasia. It presents in the form of mutism or cortical dysarthria. There may be a dysprosody of speech which is an abnormality of rhythm and intonation giving a 'foreign' sound. The patients show no defect in grammar or other aspects of language function, including reading and writing. It is generally difficult to distinguish aphemia from pure Broca's aphasia. A psychogenic cause should always be considered when there is mutism without any specifically aphasic features (i.e. no abnormality of comprehension, reading, or writing).

Transcortical motor aphasia

This is a rare type of aphasia which resembles Broca's aphasia in that there is a marked loss of fluency with no severe deficit of verbal comprehension. It differs from Broca's aphasia in that verbal repetition is significantly less impaired. It has been thought that it arises from the isolation of Broca's area from the remainder of the frontal lobe.

Posterior aphasias
Wernicke's aphasia (sensory/receptive)

This is characterized by a profound loss of the ability to comprehend language. The patients usually have a fluent speech with a marked logorrhoea or press of speech and numerous paraphasias. Not infrequently there are frank neologisms and jargon-type speech. Reading and writing are usually impaired. The lesion is usually found in the posterior aspect of the superior temporal gyrus. The aphasia is often accompanied by a right homonomous visual field defect and right-sided somatosensory changes without hemiparesis.

Nominal aphasia (amnestic/anomic)

The main feature of this disorder is the inability to find the correct name for objects, colours, letters, and numbers. The naming errors are of three main types: circumlocutions (e.g., use in door, instead of key), phonemic errors, and semantic errors. Spontaneous speech is fluent, although there are frequent word-finding difficulties. There are no comprehension deficits. Most frequently the site of the lesion is in the region of the posterior–superior temporal gyrus bordering on the angular gyrus whose involvement may add other deficits, such as reading and spelling difficulties, to the basic pattern. Anomic deficits can also arise from lesions in other parts of the brain, and it is generally agreed that nominal aphasia does not have firm localizing value.

Transcortical sensory aphasia (isolation of the speech area)

In this type of disorder, unlike transcortical motor aphasia, there is a significant comprehension deficit for both spoken and written language. However, the patient can repeat isolated words and sentences without difficulty. Spontaneous speech has the characteristics of fluent aphasia and frequently the patients show marked echolalia. They cannot name objects shown to them and cannot write to dictation. The lesions are usually located in the posterior part of the temporoparietal area.

Conduction aphasia

This is characterized by a striking difficulty in repeating words and phrases. Speech is usually fluent although marked by frequent paraphasias. Verbal comprehension is generally adequate. The lesions associated with conduction aphasia usually involve the perisylvian region, including the arcuate fasciculus which connects the cortex of Wernicke's area to that of Broca's area.

Pure word deafness

This rare condition is characterized by the inability to understand spoken language or to repeat it, although there are no primary auditory defects. However, the patient can understand written material and is able to write. The brain damage usually affects either the primary acoustic area in each hemisphere or the primary acoustic area on the left together with the connecting fibres from the right.

Global aphasia (central)

Many moderately severe aphasics cannot be easily classified as either Broca's or Wernicke's in type. They have the expressive disturbance characteristic of Broca's aphasia with the comprehension loss characteristic of Wernicke's aphasia without disproportion between the two. When the aphasia is severe, speech may be limited to phonated inarticulate or recurrent utterances. There is almost always a marked disturbance of comprehension and inability to read or write. This is the characteristic situation after infarction of the territory supplied by the left middle cerebral artery such that there is involvement of both the cortical area whose damage causes Broca's aphasia and that responsible for Wernicke's aphasia. The aphasia is usually accompanied by a right hemiplegia with sensory loss and there is often a right homonomous hemianopia. The outlook for adequate recovery is poor.

LANGUAGE AND SUBCORTICAL NUCLEI

In recent years, evidence has been amassed indicating that damage to subcortical structures may cause aphasia. This evidence has come primarily from the analysis of patients with subcortical haemorrhages and other naturally occurring lesions, the observation of speech disturbances following stereotactic surgery, and studies of electrical stimulation of various subcortical nuclei.

Thalamus

The aphasia after thalamic haemorrhage or infarction seems very similar to transcortical motor aphasia. There is a significant left laterality effect but aphasia only occurs in a proportion of cases. One explanation is that aphasia is not related to the destruction of a specific nucleus but depends on damage to a particular constellation of nuclei; when this occurs the deficits are likely to be long-lasting. The evidence derived from observations during stereotactic surgery suggests that damage to the left ventrolateral nucleus of the thalamus may be important in the genesis of both receptive and expressive defects. The expressive disorders include alterations of fluency, general hesitation and blocking of language, and naming disturbances.

Basal ganglia

Aphasia has also been reported after ischaemic infarction in the basal ganglia of the dominant hemisphere. The precise pattern of impairment after infarction in the caudate and/or lenticular nucleus is not fully established, but a few patients have features of Broca's aphasia combined with some features of transcortical or nominal aphasia. Stereotactic surgery on the globus pallidus may be followed by reduced accuracy and completeness of oral language formulation and expression; there may also be a reduction of fluency and some impairment of reading and comprehension.

DISTURBANCES CLOSELY ALLIED TO APHASIA

A number of disturbances, some of them rare, are usually regarded as features of damage to the posterior part of the left hemisphere. They are allied to aphasia either because of common underlying neuropsychological mechanisms or because of close overlap between their anatomical substrates.

Alexia with agraphia (cortical, parietal)

The underlying brain damage involves the left angular gyrus. The alexia is severe, so that only an occasional word can be read and the patient makes many errors identifying single letters. The ability to read numbers and music is sometimes preserved. The identification of letters is not aided by tracing them with a finger, which is one way that alexia with agraphia differs from pure alexia. Oral spelling is poor and the patient has great difficulty in identifying words spelt out letter by letter. The agraphia usually matches the alexia so that the patient may even be unable to write some single letters spontaneously or to command. Copying is less impaired but is not normal.

Pure alexia (pure word-blindness)

This syndrome is believed to be due to pathology of the pathway between the primary visual cortex and the left angular gyrus, which is of major importance for reading, such that there is a 'disconnection' between the two areas. The characteristics of the alexia are the same as in alexia with agraphia except that the letters can usually be recognized if traced with a finger (i.e. using somatosensory rather than visual sen-

sory information), and indeed whole words or phrases can be recognized using this strategy. The ability to read numbers and music may or may not be preserved. Oral spelling and the recognition of words spelt aloud are normal. Similarly, writing is normal except for those errors due to the inability of the patients to read back what they have written. Most patients have a right homonomous hemianopia, and some also have colour anomia. Developmental dyslexia is a condition where the ability to read is significantly retarded compared with other aspects of general intellectual development. It is usually detected in childhood or early adolescence. Some children with reading backwardness have unsuspected mental retardation, some have as yet undetected visual or auditory deficit, some have cerebral pathology, some have emotional disturbance, and some simply lack the necessary academic motivation or have been badly taught. A small proportion, more boys than girls, have idiopathic developmental dyslexia for which no cause can be established. They may have a high–normal IQ despite their reading disability, and even if their reading ability becomes adequate with increasing age they may continue to be very poor at spelling.

Colour anomia

This is a bizarre disorder in which patients do not name colours correctly and make errors pointing to named colours, even though they match colours normally and have normal colour vision assessed by the Ishihara pseudoisochromatic plates. Occasional patients have features of visual agnosia, and acalculia is common.

The syndromes of pure alexia and/or colour anomia are usually due to occlusion of the left posterior cerebral artery causing infarction of the left occipital lobe and the splenium of the corpus callosum. However, it occasionally occurs with a glioma of the splenium spreading into the left occipital lobe; then it is often accompanied by severe amnesia.

Pure agraphia (motor)

Agraphia more or less uncontaminated by other features of aphasia has been reported as a manifestation of damage in the parasagittal portion of the left parietal lobe. It may occur as part of a Gerstmann syndrome after damage to the left supramarginal gyrus. It has also been reported after damage to the posterior portion of the left middle (second) frontal gyrus immediately anterior to the motor cortical representation of the right hand.

Gerstmann syndrome

This consists of finger agnosia, right–left disorientation, agraphia, and acalculia. With finger agnosia the patients are unable to name their fingers and can neither indicate nor identify their own or other people's fingers or fingers demonstrated on models. There is not necessarily any impairment of skilled hand movement. In mild cases the thumb and little finger are spared. Severe cases not only have involvement of all the fingers and both thumbs, but also may be unable to name or identify their toes and other parts of the body. The abnormality is almost invariably bilateral and due to left hemisphere damage involving the supramarginal gyrus. The right–left disorientation applies to body parts (of both patient and other people) more than to inanimate objects in extracorporeal space. The pathological significance of Gerstmann syndrome is not clear because the features can be found in various combinations with or without other disturbances such as constructional apraxia, aphasia, and alexia. Indeed, the isolated and complete syndrome is rare.

Acalculia

Impaired ability to calculate can be due to a number of underlying disorders. It is a common early sign of memory failure, as in general dementia, because forgetting the results of the intermediate steps interferes with calculation. Also, aphasia can interfere with the ability to calculate because the patient may fail to comprehend exactly what is required, or may express the results of the calculation in the wrong symbols. Asymbolic acalculia is a disturbance of calculating due to inability to appreciate the meaning of the digit signs or other symbols (e.g. × and +) used in arithmetic. This form of acalculia is closely related to aphasia but may exist without any other manifestation of it. Anarithmia is a primary failure of the ability to calculate even though the meaning of the relevant signs and symbols is understood. Anarithmia and asymbolic acalculia commonly result from damage to the extrastriate cortex of the left occipital lobe. Spatial acalculia can arise from damage to either parietal lobe and produces difficulty with written calculation in particular. This difficulty is secondary to failure to organize the spatial components involved in the calculations. Certain figures or columns of figures may be ignored, or they may be positioned incorrectly and the horizontal and vertical directions may be interchanged with inevitable confusion.

Apraxia

Apraxia is defined as a condition where there is a high level disturbance of voluntary purposeful movements, not attributable to weakness or to incoordination or sensory loss, as usually understood, and not attributable to an aphasic comprehension disorder. Learned skilled movements are performed incorrectly. A rather large number of apraxias have been described. Only ideomotor and ideational apraxia and constructional apraxia will be considered here. Buccofacial apraxia has been mentioned in the section on aphasia, and dressing apraxia will be mentioned in the section on disorders of body perception.

IDEOMOTOR APRAXIA

Ideomotor apraxia is a defect of the ability to mime actions, to imitate how a tool or object would be used, and to make symbolic gestures. Performance improves when using an actual object or tool to demonstrate its use, but even then movement sequences and spatial orientation may be abnormal. Thus the patient may be very defective when, for instance, demonstrating the action of waving good-bye, miming the action of cutting with scissors, or performing the sequential actions of folding a piece of paper, placing it in an envelope, sealing the envelope, and affixing a stamp. The disorder is almost invariably due to posterior left hemisphere pathology, and many apraxic patients are also aphasic. The apraxia can be confined to the left limbs when there is damage to transcallosal fibres crossing to the right hemisphere. Heilman has suggested that the disorder occurs either when the cerebral pathology destroys movement engrams or when it interrupts pathways between the site of those engrams and the motor cortex controlling the limb involved.

He suggests further that movement engrams are located exclusively in the left hemisphere in some people and bilaterally in others (but rarely, if ever, exclusively in the right hemisphere of right-handers). This would explain why apraxia does not occur as often as aphasia with left hemisphere damage even though it rarely occurs in right-handers with damage on the right.

IDEATIONAL APRAXIA

Ideational apraxia is a more severe disorder in that actual use of objects and tools is markedly disturbed, but it is probably not qualitatively distinct from ideomotor apraxia. Many of the patients regarded as having ideational apraxia also have a generalized intellectual deterioration.

CONSTRUCTIONAL APRAXIA

Constructional apraxia is manifest in activities such as building, arranging, and drawing. There is difficulty in assembling parts to make a whole where a spatial component is involved. Patients may complain of symptoms arising from their constructional apraxia. Thus they may no longer be able to perform tasks such as assembling an electric plug, dressmaking, or laying the dinner table. More often the disorder is demonstrated only on clinical examination. Spontaneous drawing and copying is poor (Fig. 4). The patients are unable to copy simple designs with matchsticks. Drawings tend to be smaller than the model and may be crowded into one corner of the page. The lines may be wavy, they may not meet accurately, and they may even be superimposed on the model. There is a tendency to make horizontal and vertical lines oblique. One dimension of the drawing may be unduly prolonged and large parts may be omitted, particularly by patients with right hemisphere damage who ignore the left side (left-sided neglect—see below and Fig 5). There is a general lack of perspective and mirror reversals sometimes occur. Attempts to copy simple designs with matchsticks result in similar abnormalities, and on neuropsychological examination performance on the block design and object assembly subtests of the Wechsler scale is impaired.

Unlike ideomotor apraxia, constructional apraxia can arise from either right or left cerebral hemisphere damage. The right hemisphere damage is usually situated focally in the parieto-temporo-occipital junction area and may also cause left-sided visuospatial neglect, left hemianopia, severe sensory loss down the left side of the body, a tendency to ignore the left side of the body, and sometimes dressing apraxia. The left-sided

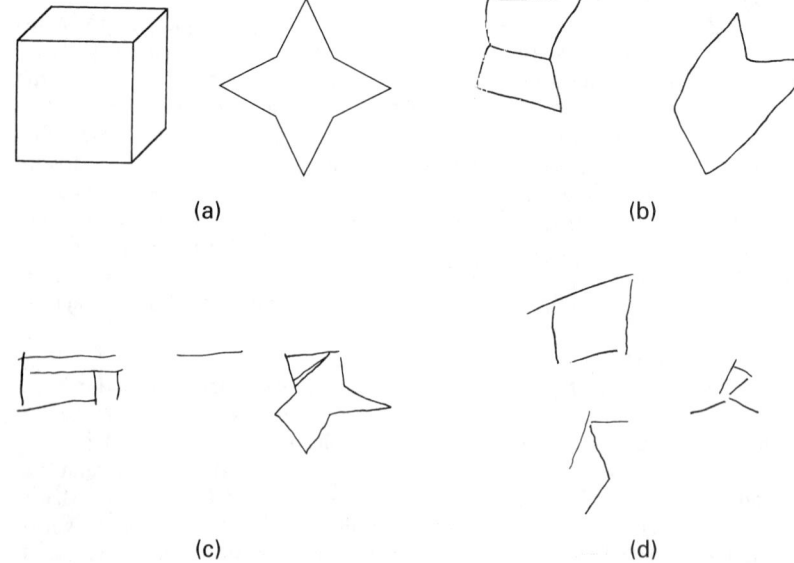

(a)   (b)

(c)   (d)

Fig. 4 Disturbances of drawing. Attempts to copy cube and star (see model (a)) by three patients: (b) with bilateral posterior pathology and severe constructional, ideomotor, and writing apraxia; (c) with early Alzheimer-type dementia and constructional apraxia but other praxis relatively well preserved; (d) with focal right parietal atrophy, severe constructional apraxia, and visuospatial disturbance.

damage tends to be more diffusely distributed in the posterior part of the hemisphere. There have been many attempts to demonstrate that constructional apraxia from right-sided damage is primarily due to a visuospatial disturbance and that with left damage it is primarily an executive disorder, akin to ideomotor apraxia. However, this differentiation has not been established as yet.

Disorders of visual, spatial, and bodily perception

These disorders arise very predominantly in association with damage to cortex in the parieto-temporo-occipital junction area of the right hemisphere, or bilaterally, and only rarely with unilateral left hemisphere pathology (finger agnosia and right–left disorientation as part of the Gerstmann syndrome).

DISORDERS OF VISUOSPATIAL PERCEPTION AND SPACE EXPLORATION

The extent of the right hemisphere 'dominance' in the control of behaviour concerned with visuospatial perception and space exploration at least approaches that of the left hemisphere in relation to language. Vision is a highly developed sense in humans, which is much used in the exploration of environmental space, and it is not surprising that spatial disorders are closely related to high level visual system disorders, particularly of eye movement control and attention.

Unilateral visuospatial neglect

This is a disregard of, and a failure to attend to, one half of external space, almost invariably the left. Patients tend to collide with objects situated on the left and have a marked preference for taking right rather than left turns, so that they may become lost when taking routes from one place to another. They tend to neglect the left side when copying or making free-hand drawings (Fig. 5), although the right side can be drawn very well. Writing may be crowded over on the right-hand side of the page, with the left remaining blank. They may have great difficulty in reading because they neglect the left side of lines or individual words. The disorder is usually associated with a left hemianopia and left-sided sensory loss. Neither of these can be wholly responsible, however, and many patients with one or both do not have clinically detectable neglect. The patients may be aware of their disability but nevertheless be unable to overcome it. Damage to the right inferior parietal lobule seems to be the common anatomical substrate. A left-sided attentional deficit, possibly amounting to neglect, is also described in patients with pathology

Fig. 5 Unilateral neglect. Examples of drawings by patients with right hemisphere pathology and left visuospatial neglect: (a) copies of four pointed star; (b) freehand drawings of daisy and clockface.

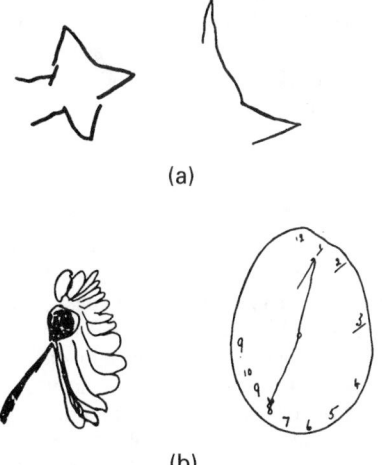

(a)

(b)

confined to the right frontal lobe. When right-sided neglect occurs, associated with left parietal damage, it is only in a minor form and recovers quickly. Neglect can also occur in visual imagery. For instance, when describing a familiar square as seen from one end, buildings to the left may be omitted even though these same buildings are included in a description of the view from the other end when they would be on the right.

Not all patients with neglect show all the symptoms, and it may be that neglect should now be subjected to a nosological classification of the sort that has been applied to aphasia.

Gaze apraxia

This is an inability to direct the eyes towards, and then maintain fixation upon, an object appearing in an intact visual field even though there is no oculomotor palsy and both random eye movements and oculocephalic reflexes seem normal. It is usually associated with biparietal damage and most patients also have visual disorientation.

Visual disorientation

As described by Holmes, visual disorientation is an inability to orient towards and accurately locate objects in space, using vision alone, even though the visual acuity and field seem adequate. It is usually associated with gaze apraxia and damage to both parietal lobes. Judgements of distance, length, and size are faulty, and the patients misreach. Their groping and inability to fixate an object gives the impression that they are blind, but they may recognize objects correctly and may point accurately at sources of sound.

Balint's syndrome

This consists of a combination of gaze apraxia and visual disorientation with simultanagnosia, a condition where visual attention is very restricted such that only one stimulus can be perceived at any one time. Patients with Balint's syndrome have a severe visual disability which can be taken for near blindness. The underlying pathology is usually biparietal infarction secondary to vertebrobasilar or watershed territory ischaemia.

Defective topographical memory or topographical disorientation

This is usually due to bilateral cerebral damage which may not be restricted to the parietal cortex. The patients are unable to remember or describe routes even though they may be very familiar. For instance they may lose themselves in their own homes or in villages where they have spent all their lives. The disorder is usually associated with other features of cognitive impairment, but very occasionally it exists in relative isolation, in which case it may be due to damage restricted to the right posterior parietal and occipital cortex. Such unilateral damage can cause milder disturbances of topographical relationships resulting, for instance, in failure to orient correctly on plans with preserved ability to find and describe routes. In some cases route-finding difficulty arises as part of an agnosic disturbance, such that the patient no longer recognizes the specific features of landmarks and so cannot use them for guidance. This is usually associated with prosopagnosia.

DISORDERS OF VISUAL PERCEPTION

Laboratory studies suggest that patients with posterior right hemisphere damage have more difficulty with complex visual discrimination tasks than do those with similar left-sided damage. However, the majority of patients with clinically recognizable visual perceptual disorders have either focal damage in both hemispheres or diffuse damage.

Visual agnosia

Visual agnosia is a failure to identify objects by sight alone, although sufficient acuity of vision and cerebral function are present and the patient is still able to recognize the objects in question through some other sensory modality such as touch or hearing. The recognition failure results in an anomia which can be mistaken for aphasia. However, the characteristics of the naming failure in visual agnosia are quite different from those of aphasia. The anomia is restricted to objects presented visually, the errors are often bizarre (e.g. 'a coal scuttle' for a telephone) rather than semantic or phonetic confusions, as occur in aphasia, and the correct use of the objects is not described or indicated by mime. Furthermore, the patient often fails to point correctly to named objects. In daily life the recognition failure of visual agnosia leads to abnormal behaviour such as putting jam rather than sugar in tea.

This description of visual agnosia corresponds to 'apperceptive' visual agnosia—a failure to perceive objects, or recognize them, restricted to the visual modality. It differs from optic aphasia which is a typically anomic disorder except that it is restricted to failure to name on visual presentation only, with preserved ability to recognize; thus an object cannot be named on visual presentation, but its use can be described following such a presentation. Optic aphasia is due to pathology located in the posterior part of the left hemisphere and tends to be associated with a right homonomous hemianopia, alexia, and colour anomia.

Disorders of visual perception detectable by laboratory methods are associated with focal posterior right hemisphere pathology. However, the majority of patients with symptoms of visual agnosia have either posterior left hemisphere pathology, with a right homonomous hemianopia and other features of a posterior disconnection syndrome (alexia and colour anomia), or bilateral pathology. An 'associative' visual agnosia has also been described. Here the disorder extends beyond a failure to recognize objects on visual presentation to a state where there is a loss of knowledge, or of the meaning, of objects akin to a semantic memory disorder (see below).

Prosopagnosia

Prosopagnosia is the inability to recognize people from their facial appearance or from photographs. The condition is rare. It may be so severe that even close relatives and old acquaintants are not recognized until they speak or until some characteristic item of their clothing is seen. The disorder can be very disabling. In many patients with prosopagnosia pathology is located more or less symmetrically in the posterior temporal and inferior parietal regions of both hemispheres, particularly ventromedially, and it is usually possible to demonstrate bilateral homonomous visual field defects. However, there is considerable evidence that the right hemisphere plays a major role in processing information about faces, and with magnetic resonance imaging and positron emission tomography it has become clear that prosopagnosia can occasionally be associated with pathology restricted to the right (but not, as yet, the left) occipitotemporal region.

DISORDERS OF BODY PERCEPTION

The higher-order disturbances of body perception, except for the Gerstmann syndrome, affect predominantly the left limbs, just as visuospatial neglect is a predominantly left-sided phenomenon.

Hemiasomatognosia

This is a loss of appreciation of one side of the body, usually the left, resulting from disturbed function of the contralateral parietal lobe. Patients may spontaneously complain that one side of their body, or one limb, feels as if it is not there or does not belong to them. The symptom is usually short lasting and is due to epilepsy, migraine, or a transient ischaemic episode. When there is a basis in permanent pathology, it is usually situated in the right parieto-temporo-occipital region.

Neglect

Neglect of one side is a less transient disturbance. In its most exaggerated form, where there appears to be an almost complete unawareness and occasionally even denial of the existence of one side of the body.

It almost invariably affects the left and is due to extensive right hemisphere damage with superadded confusion. The disturbance is usually combined with a dense hemiplegia. There may be anosognosia, which is a denial that there is any paralysis of the affected limbs. Patients seem convinced that they can and do move these limbs normally and may even seem to think that they had just demonstrated this capacity. The lack of awareness is one factor making rehabilitation of some left hemiplegics very difficult. Severe somatosensory loss, hemianopia, constructional and dressing apraxias, and unilateral visuospatial neglect are often associated with unilateral somatic neglect and anosognosia.

Dressing apraxia

This is a severe and bizarre disturbance of the ability to put on clothes. It almost always arises from right parietal lobe damage. Many patients also have constructional apraxia, left visuospatial neglect, and left hemiasomatagnosia. The patients have great difficulty in orienting individual items of clothing with their bodies. This is not only a left–right and back–front disorientation. There may be great uncertainty about which article goes where; for instance patients may attempt to step into their shirt sleeves or put trousers over their heads.

Frontal lobe damage

Damage to the frontal lobes classically produces a combination of personality change and intellectual deterioration. However, it is not unusual for even extensive damage to be present without detectable symptoms or signs, and this is why slow-growing frontal tumours may remain silent until they have reached a very considerable size. Changes in mood and character include euphoria, impulsiveness, and facetiousness, with apparently decreased anxiety and little concern about the consequences of any actions that are undertaken. Such disinhibition may occur without any evidence of other cognitive impairment. The patient may be fully aware of the disinhibition but nevertheless unable to control it. In contrast, the personality change may produce a depression-like state with decreased initiative and spontaneity.

The cognitive deterioration has been difficult to characterize, particularly in the laboratory. There seems to be a decreased ability for abstract thought and for planning behavior taking into account past experience and future consequences. Perservation of various types is common. The patients may be very distractible and unable to concentrate or keep their attention focused on one topic for more than a short time. This produces an apparent interference with memory. However, frontal damage does not produce amnesia in the strict sense, except perhaps after damage to the cingulate cortex bilaterally. Patients with large frontal meningiomas may be disoriented, hypokinetic, and apathetic; they usually have raised intracranial pressure in addition to damage which probably extends well beyond the frontal lobes. Damage restricted to the prefrontal areas of the left hemisphere can produce what seems to amount to a mild aphasia without articulation defect or paraphasias. It appears as a loss of spontaneity in speaking without a definite difficulty in selecting appropriate words and without impaired comprehension, and may include a marked difficulty in 'fluency' as measured, for instance, by the ability to produce words beginning with a specified letter.

Amnesia

Memory is not a unitary function and various categories are recognized. A useful classification for clinical purposes is given in Table 4.

Explicit memory systems store information that can be consciously accessed and include a major component of a person's knowledge base; the material can be verbalized and discussed. The short-term system retains material for periods measured in seconds or a few minutes at most; for instance this system holds a telephone number from the time that it has been found in a directory until it has been dialled and can be forgotten. The long-term system holds material for periods up to the remainder of the person's life. It is convenient to divide the long-term

Table 4 *Categories of memory*

Explicit (declarative)
    Short-term (working)
    Intermediate
    Long-term
    Episodic
    Semantic

Implicit (procedural)
    Motor and perceptual skills
    Classical conditioning

store into semantic and episodic memory. By semantic is meant knowledge of, for instance, objects, places, words, concepts, etc. Episodic memory is memory for events including autobiographical events. Clearly, episodic and semantic memory must be closely related. Although cognitive psychologists divide memory into short term and long term, for practical purposes there is a need to identify an intermediate memory category for those memories normally held for hours or days, which are of great importance in daily life but are then no longer useful and intuitively do not seem to be retained in a long-term store.

Implicit memory is the information store which enables activities to be carried out more or less automatically without conscious awareness and without the person necessarily being able to explain how they have been achieved. Implicit memory systems include those holding information which determines conditioned reflex responses and allows complex motor acts, such as riding a surf board, to be performed. It may be possible to some extent to verbalize how such complex motor acts are achieved and to subject them to conscious analysis, but it is often impossible to do so fully.

These memory systems depend upon the proper working of multiple cerebral structures, and memory impairment of one sort or another is a common early feature of many brain diseases. The medial temporal lobe structures—including the hippocampus, amygdala, parahippocampal gyrus, and rhinal cortex (Fig. 6)—together with the fornix system, the mamillary bodies, the thalamus, particularly the dorsomedial nucleus, and the cingulate gyri, contribute to a neuronal circuit (Papez circuit) that is of major importance for establishing new semantic and episodic memories, although the actual stores are probably in other parts of the neocortex. Damage to any part of this circuit can cause an anterograde memory disturbance, i.e., defective establishment of new memories commencing at the time of the onset of the pathological process. It may also cause a retrograde memory disturbance manifested by failure to access previously established memories on a temporal gradient, with recent memories being more susceptible to loss than longer established memories. There is reason to assume that damage to the thalamus (including the mamillary bodies), such as in an alcoholic Korsakoff state, causes a longer period of retrograde impairment than does medial temporal lobe damage occurring after herpes simplex virus encephalitis. A progressive and initially selective loss of semantic memory can occur in various degenerative brain diseases, including Alzheimer's disease and Pick's disease. Studies of patients with these conditions have given rise to the suggestion that at least some stores are located in temporal lobe neocortex. It is not clear whether this loss of semantic memory is usually associated with a loss of episodic memory.

Bilateral damage to any part of the Papez neuronal circuit can cause a severe amnesic syndrome. In this condition the anterograde memory disturbance is such that new material can be remembered for only a few seconds, or a few minutes at most, and then only if there is no distraction (i.e. short-term memory is preserved). Beyond this short span new material cannot be learnt, nor events remembered, with the exception that new motor and perceptual skills may be learnt (implicit memory) without the amnesic being able to recall any exposure to the activity. For example the patient may not remember ever having seen a person who

has left the room for 2 or 3 min. There is usually an associated retrograde amnesia, but other aspects of cognition may be entirely preserved. Common causes of severe amnesia are shown in Table 5.

Pathology involving the Papez circuit and/or temporal lobe neocortex on one side of the brain tends to produce a predominantly verbal memory deficit if it is on the left and a non-verbal memory deficit if it is on the right. A verbal memory deficit makes it difficult for patients to remember what has been said to them or what they have read: they forget messages, names, and the contents of conversations, and reading may cease to be a pleasure because they cannot remember further back than a few lines or paragraphs. The deficit is particularly associated with damage to the left hippocampus and amygdala, and the left temporal neocortex, and it may be the presenting feature of a left temporal lobe tumour. The non-verbal memory deficit from right medial temporal lobe damage is much more intangible. Often the symptoms are only minimal, but the defect appears in the laboratory as difficulty in remembering material which cannot be easily verbalized such as spatial location and facial features.

TRAUMATIC AMNESIA

Amnesia is common after head injuries which are severe enough to cause unconsciousness. The duration of post-traumatic amnesia (i.e. the period of severe anterograde memory impairment) is the period between

Fig. 6 The medial aspect of a cerebral hemisphere (a), and a coronal section (b), to show the structures important for memory.

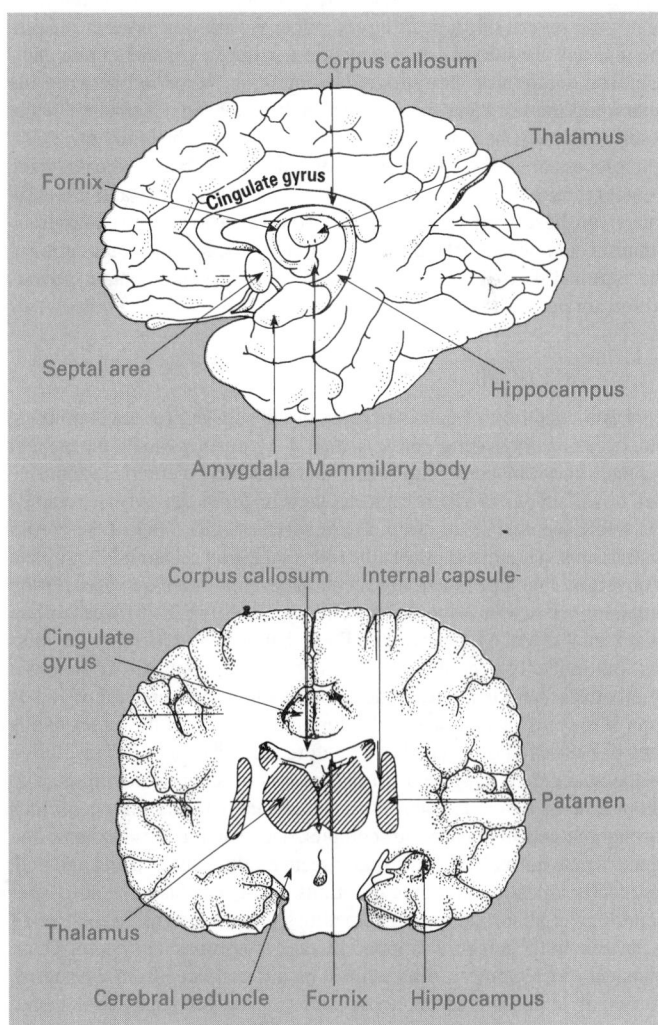

Table 5 *Causes of severe amnesia*

Alcohol (Korsakoff psychosis) and other causes of thiamine deficiency (including inadequate feeding, hyperemesis gravidarum, stomach cancer) leading to cell loss in the thalamic dorsomedial nuclei and the mamillary bodies

Bilateral medial temporal lobe damage including herpes simplex encephalitis and other limbic encephalitides (including non-metastatic carcinomatous), neuronal loss secondary to anoxia/hypoglycaemia/severe convulsions, surgical

Degenerative: Alzheimer's and Pick's diseases may present with very severe memory failure with only minor general deterioration

Vascular: bilateral thalamic infarction, hippocampal infarction secondary to posterior cerebral artery territory ischaemia, bilateral cingulate cortex infarction secondary to anterior communicating artery aneurysm rupture

Pathology around ventricle III: tumours (particularly colloid cysts), chronic meningitis (particularly tubercular), neurosarcoidosis

the injury and the resumption of 'normal' continuous memory. It includes the period of unconsciousness and the subsequent period of confusion; it can also include a further period in which the behaviour seems to be normal, but which cannot be remembered in detail afterwards. The duration of post-traumatic amnesia is one of the better indices of the severity of a head injury. When it lasts for more than 24 h, the injury is classified as severe and there may be permanent brain damage. The duration of the retrograde amnesia is the period between the injury and the last clear memory before it happened. Characteristically it shrinks slowly, becoming shorter as the time since the injury increases. The process of shrinking may take several months, but most cases have a final retrograde amnesia of no more than a few seconds and it is only longer in those with very severe injuries. Occasionally the retrograde amnesia contains an 'island' of memory for events immediately prior to the injury. Likewise, the post-traumatic amnesia may contain periods which are partially remembered.

TRANSIENT GLOBAL AMNESIA

This is a condition of dense amnesia usually lasting for several hours, but occasionally lasting for less than 1 h, during which the patient behaves like somebody with severe amnesia. New memories cannot be laid down and, as in severe amnesia, new material can only be retained for a few seconds or, at the most, minutes, provided that there are no distractions. The attack is usually followed by an apparently complete recovery of memory function, except that events which occurred during it cannot be recalled (laboratory examination within 2 or 3 weeks of an attack may reveal evidence of a mild verbal or non-verbal memory deficit, but this only occasionally persists beyond 6 months). At the onset of an attack there is a retrograde amnesia which may cover a period as long as several years; this shrinks during the course of the attack and is said to be only short immediately before recovery, but after resolution of the attack there may be a permanent loss of a period covering up to about 2 hours before the start of the attack. Patients are fully conscious throughout and may carry out complex acts, such as driving long distances, quite normally. They usually seem mildly confused and agitated, frequently repeating the same questions. Most patients have no further neurological abnormality, but sometimes there are signs suggestive of ischaemia in the territory supplied by the vertebrobasilar system. These transient global amnesic attacks must be differentiated from the automatisms of temporal lobe epilepsy and from psychologically induced

amnesia; an almost identical phenomenon is sometimes seen as part of a migraine attack.

REFERENCES

Hodges, J.R. (1994). *Cognitive assessment for clinicians.* Oxford University Press.
Kapur, N. (1988). *Memory disorders in clinical practice.* Butterworth, London.
McCarthy, R.A. and Warrington, E.K. (1990) *Cognitive neuropsychology: a clinical introduction.* Academic Press, San Diego, CA.
Swash, M. and Oxbury, J. (ed.) (1991). *Clinical neurology,* Vol. 1, pp. 10–59, 71–81. Churchill Livingstone, Edinburgh.

24.3.2 The motor and sensory systems, midbrain, and brain-stem

W. B. MATTHEWS

The motor system

THE LOWER MOTOR NEURONE

The motor unit consists of a number of muscle fibres, ranging from 100 in the facial muscles to 2000 in the quadriceps, supplied by a single fast-conducting alpha motor fibre. These originate from large cells in the anterior horns of the grey matter of the spinal cord and in the somatic motor nuclei of the cranial nerves, and are known as the lower motor neurones. Loss of function of the anterior horn cells, or interruption of their axons, causes weakness or paralysis of the muscles they supply, with loss of stretch reflexes, shown by flaccidity and loss of tendon jerks, and, if paralysis persists, wasting of the muscle due to loss of excitable tissue. The extent and severity of these signs vary with the distribution and speed of onset and duration of the neuronal lesion. Acute destruction of the anterior horn cells causes paralysis of the muscles wholly supplied by the segments involved, but many muscles receive motor fibres from several segments. Gradual reduction in the number of anterior horn cells or their axons does not, at first, cause weakness or wasting, as surviving axons sprout and supply muscle fibres deprived of their nerve supply. The resulting giant motor units are unstable and may fire spontaneously, seen as fasciculation: brief, irregular contractions of parts of the muscle. This is distinct from fibrillation, the spontaneous contraction of single muscle fibres that also occurs in denervated muscles but can only be detected by electromyography. In the peripheral nerves a state of reversible conduction block is a common event, resulting in temporary paralysis without fibrillation or wasting.

THE UPPER MOTOR NEURONE

The main descending motor pathway is derived from neurones in the precentral gyrus. Movements of the foot are controlled by neurones on the medial surface of the hemisphere, and on the lateral surface from above downwards are the areas for the leg, trunk, arm, hand, face, and tongue, although these are not rigidly demarcated centres. Descending axons converge in the posterior limb of the internal capsule and then occupy the middle third of the cerebral peduncle. In the pons the fibres are more dispersed and become concentrated again in the prominent pyramid, from which the name of the pyramidal tract is derived, on the anterior surface of the medulla. Most of the fibres cross at the lower end of the medulla and descend in the lateral columns of the spinal cord. Only a small proportion of the corticospinal fibres synapse directly on lower motor neurones and most terminate on interneurones.

An acute complete lesion of the corticospinal tract causes flaccid paralysis with loss of tendon reflexes. With the passage of time or with a partial or progressive lesion the characteristic effect is spastic weakness or paralysis. Loss of power is accompanied by an increase in stretch reflex activity. In the upper limb the weakness is usually most evident in distal muscles, but movements of the hip joint may be affected when no other loss of power can be found in the lower limb. Loss of fine movements, particularly of the fingers, is often much more prominent than loss of strength. In many complex movements, such as walking, the normal precise sequence of contraction and relaxation of opposing muscles is lost.

The increased resistance to passive movement is more marked in the flexor muscles of the arm and the extensor muscles of the leg. It often has a 'clasp knife' character, in that the resistance suddenly lapses due to reflex lengthening. The tendon reflexes are exaggerated and reflex contractions can often be elicited in muscles other than those usually examined. In the lower limb the knee and ankle jerks may be increased to the point of clonus, where maintained stretch induces an inexhaustible repetitive response. These positive signs are the result of release of spinal reflex activity from some inhibitory effect of the corticospinal pathway.

The normal plantar reflex consists of flexion of all the digits on firm stroking of the lateral side of the sole. In the extensor, or Babinski reflex the big toe dorsiflexes and the other toes fan. This response is reliably found when an upper motor neurone lesion or loss of function is undeniably present, but is far less useful in cases of doubt, when it is often recorded as 'equivocal'. Hoffmann's sign, elicited by flexing and suddenly releasing the terminal phalanx of the middle finger, consists of reflex flexion of all the fingers. It merely indicates increased reflex activity and is not specific for an upper motor neurone lesion.

A curious feature of upper motor neurone lesions is loss of certain cutaneous reflexes. The superficial abdominal reflexes, elicited by stroking the skin in each quadrant are the best known, although a variable, finding, particularly after middle age, but unilateral loss is occasionally a valuable sign.

The leg spastic in extension is an effective prop when walking. In progressive spinal cord disease, however, flexor tone often supervenes. Spasm in the flexor muscles, often painful, leads to permanent flexion at the hip and knee, a posture of great discomfort, in which any residual voluntary power cannot be used.

In the distribution of the cranial nerves an acute upper motor neurone lesion usually causes dysphagia and dysarthria for a few days only. Bilateral lesions cause persistent symptoms with slow tongue movements and often an exaggerated jaw jerk, elicited by a tap on the chin with the mouth half open. This condition is known as pseudobulbar palsy (the 'bulb' being the medulla) to distinguish it from the lower motor neurone bulbar palsy. It is often accompanied by mild limb spasticity, a shuffling gait, and great lability of emotional expression.

An upper motor neurone facial nerve palsy differs in a number of respects from a nuclear or peripheral palsy. The muscles of the upper face are relatively or entirely spared, apparently because of bilateral cortical control. Emotional movements may be affected when forced voluntary movement is virtually intact.

SYMPTOMS

The patients' complaints of weakness and wasting arising from lower motor neurone lesions are seldom difficult to interpret, although the distribution must be precisely determined. Weakness of the pelvic girdle may give rise to a complaint of unsteadiness. The initial complaint in a progressive upper motor neurone lesion may be of loss of use rather than of weakness. If spasticity is prominent, the toes may be scraped on walking, or there may be sudden falls due to loss of extensor tone. In all forms of weakness the complaint may confusingly be of numbness, reflecting the difficulty of subjective distinction between loss of feeling and loss of strength, familiar, in reverse, to anyone who has had a dental block.

OTHER SYSTEMS INVOLVED

The concept of upper and lower motor neurone lesions is a useful clinical approximation that has stood the test of time, but which bears little resemblance to the complexity of the initiation and control of voluntary and reflex movement. The small fusimotor fibres arising in the spinal grey matter are not directly involved in movement but regulate the sensitivity of the muscle spindles. The timing and precision of all forms of movement are controlled largely by the input from these complex sensory organs. Movement is profoundly influenced by both the cerebellum and the extrapyramidal motor system. The effect of disease of these structures can be recognized but the means by which they exert their control are still relatively obscure.

The sensory system

The afferent inflow from skin, muscles, tendons, and joints arises from end organs specifically adapted to respond to appropriate stimuli and also from a non-specific network of cutaneous nerve endings. In the clinical context it is the anatomy of the sensory pathways that is of obvious relevance.

The afferent fibres from the limbs are formed by one branch of the axons of the neurones of the posterior root ganglia, the other branch of which enters the spinal cord. The somatic sensory cranial nerves are similarly organized with equivalent ganglia on the fifth and ninth nerves. The posterior spinal root fibres enter the grey matter where many, apparently concerned with reflex activity, form synapses with interneurones or anterior horn cells. The main afferent stream divides: axons concerned mainly with postural sense and with some aspects of touch, and probably with vibration sense, proceed in the posterior columns of the same side of the spinal cord to the dorsal column nuclei in the medulla, from which arise the secondary sensory axons which decussate and ascend in the medial lemniscus to the thalamus. Fibres concerned with pain and thermal sensation synapse in the posterior horns and the axons of the secondary relay pass upwards for a few segments on the same side before decussating in the centre of the cord and passing up in the lateral columns as the spinothalamic tracts. These lie laterally in the medulla but eventually join the medial lemniscus and enter the thalamus. The sensory relay is continued to the postcentral gyrus and to a wide area of the posterior part of the cerebral hemisphere. Many afferent fibres convey information that does not enter consciousness but is concerned with reflex activity or with the afferent flow to the cerebellum.

The afferent fibres of the trigeminal nerve synapse in the nucleus within the pons and also in the descending nucleus that extends into the cervical spinal cord. Secondary axons cross the midline and ascend with the spinal tracts.

Sensory loss from interruption of a peripheral nerve or posterior root affects all modalities. However, cutting a single posterior root may result in no detectable sensory loss, because of overlap from neighbouring roots. Similarly, the area of sensory loss resulting from a peripheral nerve lesion will be much less extensive than the full distribution of the nerve. Within the central nervous system the separation of the sensory tracts in the spinal cord allows selective loss of different sensory modalities. Pain and thermal sense will be impaired when the spinothalamic tracts are damaged, while lesions of the posterior columns result in loss of postural sense. Sense of touch is distributed between both pathways, the element involved in tickle passing through the spinothalamic tracts. Vibration sense, so valuable to the neurologist, is thought to be conveyed in the posterior columns but is so often impaired in isolation that there is some room for doubt.

Lesions of the parietal cortex may result in loss of all forms of sensation, including that of pain, but sometimes there is severe loss of discriminatory forms of sensation with retention of appreciation of cruder modalities.

SYMPTOMS

Patients' complaints arising from disorders of the sensory system are often difficult to interpret. Loss of cutaneous sensation may be sufficiently obvious, as with the complaint of being unable to feel the feet on the floor or to judge the temperature of the bath water, but other sensory symptoms are less easy to attribute to disturbance of a particular modality and the distinction of positive from negative symptoms is also difficult. The familiar paraesthesiae, 'pins and needles', may apparently result from lesions of the sensory pathways at any level. A complaint that the affected limbs feel too large or that 'they do not belong to me' usually, but not invariably, indicates loss of postural sense, but when the hand is involved the complaint may be merely of 'uselessness'. A sensation as of a tight bandage round the leg is commonly complained of by patients with a lesion of the posterior columns of the spinal cord.

Loss of proprioceptive sensation results in sensory ataxia. Difficulty in maintaining balance is greatly increased when information derived from vision is also lost, leading, on examination, to Romberg's sign, consisting of falling when standing with feet together and eyes closed, and to the complaint of being unable to walk outside after dusk.

Pain may result from disease of the peripheral and, less commonly, of the central nervous system. Compression of a peripheral nerve, or more particularly of a dorsal root, may cause paraesthesiae and pain in the distribution of the sensory fibres. Pain of a peculiarly distressing burning character can arise from lesions of the spinothalamic tract in the spinal cord and brain-stem, and similar and even more persistent pain and dysaesthesia, or unpleasantly altered cutaneous sensation on stimulation, from thalamic lesions. Pain from cortical lesions is usually episodic and a symptom of focal sensory epilepsy.

Subcortical lesions: internal capsule, midbrain, and brain-stem

THE INTERNAL CAPSULE

In the internal capsule the descending motor fibres are condensed into a small space immediately anterior to the similarly narrowly localized ascending fibres. Even relatively small lesions in this area can therefore cause severe hemiplegia of the opposite limbs, the degree of sensory loss depending on the extent of the lesion.

THE MIDBRAIN

Among the crowded tracts and nuclei of the midbrain those that can most readily be identified as contributing to the symptomatology of lesions in this area are the descending corticospinal and corticobulbar tracts, the nuclei of the third and fourth cranial nerves, the reticular formation, and, more speculatively, the red nucleus. The contiguous superior cerebellar peduncles may also be involved. A number of syndromes have been awarded eponymous titles that serve some purpose in the cause of brevity.

Weber's syndrome of a third nerve palsy and crossed hemiplegia is the result of a lesion of the cerebral peduncle involving the third nerve as it leaves the brain. Benedikt's syndrome of a third nerve palsy with involuntary movements of the opposite limbs is thought to result from a lesion of the red nucleus.

A characteristic sign of involvement of the upper midbrain is Parinaud's syndrome which, in its complete form, consists of paralysis of vertical gaze and of convergence. In vestigial form loss of upward gaze is a common feature of increasing intracranial pressure with downward displacement of the midbrain.

Lesions involving the reticular formation have been held responsible for disturbances of conscious level and also for the condition of akinetic mutism in which the patient makes no voluntary movement except of the eyes.

THE PONS AND MEDULLA

The pons and medulla contain nuclei of the fifth to the twelfth cranial nerves, important cerebellar connections, and motor, sensory, and autonomic pathways. Precise localization of lesions is sometimes possible from close study of the physical signs and an intimate knowledge of anatomy, but pathological processes do not always involve the sharply delineated areas depicted in many diagrams. Bilateral, asymmetrical, and discontinuous lesions may produce highly variable signs.

The lateral medullary syndrome of Wallenberg is relatively common. It includes dysphagia and dysarthria (ninth and tenth nerve nuclei), vomiting and hiccup (nucleus ambiguus), and vertigo (vestibular nuclei) combined with cerebellar ataxia of the limbs on the side of the lesion (inferior cerebellar peduncle), ipsilateral Horner's syndrome (descending autonomic fibres), loss of pain and thermal sensation on the face on the side of the lesion (fifth nerve nucleus) and in the opposite limbs (lateral lemniscus). There is no weakness as the pyramidal tracts are spared.

The rare medial medullary syndrome consists of weakness and loss of postural sense in the limbs on the side opposite to the lesion (pyramidal tract and medial lemniscus) and ipsilateral paralysis of the tongue (twelfth nerve nucleus).

Lateralized lesions of the pons similarly give rise to ipsilateral cranial nerve involvement with crossed paralysis or sensory loss as in the Millard–Gubler syndrome of sixth and seventh nerve palsies and crossed hemiplegia. In Foville's syndrome paralysis of conjugate gaze to the side of the lesion is added. An acute centrally placed pontine lesion will cause coma with characteristically extremely contracted pupils.

Certain signs of brain-stem pathology may be encountered in isolation or combined with evidence of widespread disease. An internuclear ophthalmoplegia of the form commonly seen consists of failure of adduction of the eye in conjugate gaze to one or both sides, but with preservation of convergence, indicating that the medial rectus is not paralysed but cannot act in conjunction with the opposite lateral rectus. This results from a lesion of the medial longitudinal bundle connecting the third and sixth nerve nuclei.

The strange condition of palatal myoclonus is associated with degeneration of the ipsilateral dentate nucleus in the cerebellum and the contralateral inferior medullary olive. The palate contracts almost rhythmically once or twice a second, sometimes with an audible click.

The locked-in syndrome results from interruption of the descending and ascending long tracts in the brain-stem. As no speech or movement of the limbs is possible, it is easy to assume that consciousness is lost, but this is not so and such patients readily learn to communicate by using eye-movement signals. This syndrome differs from akinetic mutism where, although the eyes are moved, no communication is possible.

REFERENCES

Bickerstaff, E.R. and Spillane, J.A. (1989). *Neurological examination in clinical practice* (5th edn). Blackwell Scientific Publications, Oxford.

Brodal, A. (1981). *Neurological anatomy in relation to clinical medicine*, (3rd edn). Oxford University Press, London.

Currier, R.D. (1969). Syndromes of the medulla oblongata. In *Handbook of clinical neurology*, (ed. P.J. Vinken and G.W. Bruyn), Vol. 2. North Holland, Amsterdam.

Loeb, C. and Meyer, J.S. (1969). Pontine syndromes. In *Handbook of clinical neurology*, (ed. P.J. Vinken and G.W. Bruyn), Vol. 2. North Holland, Amsterdam.

24.3.3 Subcortical structures—the cerebellum, thalamus, and basal ganglia

N. P. QUINN

The human brain is both proactive and reactive, not only to external stimuli but, via feedback mechanisms, to its own actions. The complexity of these operations calls for subspecialization within the nervous system, so that a deluge of inputs can be integrated semi-automatically and largely subconsciously, freeing consciousness for other things. Such are the tasks of the cerebellum and of the major subcortical nuclei that constitute the thalamus and the basal ganglia. This chapter will consider the anatomy, function, interconnections, and clinical aspects of these structures.

The cerebellum

STRUCTURE AND FUNCTION

The cerebellum occupies the greater part of the posterior fossa, reaching from the tentorium rostrally to the foramen magnum caudally, and lying dorsal to the lower pons and medulla, from which it is separated by the fourth ventricle. Its blood supply is derived from posterior circulation via the superior, anterior inferior, and posterior inferior cerebellar arteries. There are a number of ways in which its components can be classified, and for each there is a 'rule of three'. The cerebellum can be divided into (1) cortex, (2) intrinsic nuclei, and (3) interposed white matter (medullary substance). The cortex comprises three cell layers; from the surface inwards these are (1) the molecular layer, (2) the Purkinje cell layer, and (3) the granular cell layer. The only output cells of the cortex are the Purkinje cells. Inputs to cerebellar cortex comprise either climbing or mossy fibres. The former synapse directly with Purkinje cells. The latter synapse with granule cells in layer 3, whose axons ascend to layer 1 where they form parallel fibres which synapse with Purkinje cell dendrites ascending from layer 2.

The cerebellum can also be divided into (1) archicerebellum (flocculonodular lobe), with largely vestibular inputs; (2) palaeocerebellum (anterior lobe), with largely spinal cord inputs; and (3) neocerebellum (posterior, largest, lobe), with largely pontine inputs from cerebral cortex. A similar way of dividing the midline vermis and the more lateral cerebellar hemispheres and their intrinsic nuclei is into functional 'units' as follows:

(1) the vermal zone, comprising the fastigial nuclei and the midline unpaired portion of cerebellum, projects to vestibular nuclei and controls mainly axial posture, tone and balance, and locomotion;

(2) the paravermal zones, comprising the globose and emboliform nuclei and corresponding cerebellar cortex, project via the contralateral red nucleus and other nuclei of the reticular formation to influence ipsilateral limb tone;

(3) the lateral zones, comprising the dentate nuclei and lateral cerebellar cortex, project via contralateral thalamus on to motor cortex to effect ipsilateral motor co-ordination.

The integrating function of the cerebellum is evident from the fact that afferent fibres (Fig. 1) heavily outnumber efferent ones by about 40 to 1. Connections travel in three cerebellar peduncles, the lower two mainly afferent and the upper one efferent:

(1) the inferior cerebellar peduncle (restiform body) carries spino- vestibulo-, and olivocerebellar fibres and input from other medullary ('precerebellar') nuclei;

(2) the middle cerebellar peduncle (brachium pontis) carries major afferent fibres from the pontine nuclei responsible for relaying and integrating a large input from all areas of the cerebral cortex;

(3) the superior cerebellar peduncle (brachium conjunctivum) contains a few afferent spinocerebellar fibres, but most of its bulk comprises cerebellar efferent fibres which originate in the intrinsic cerebellar nuclei and stream up to the contralateral red nucleus, or through it to the thalamus, heavily to influence thalamocortical, and thence corticospinal, input.

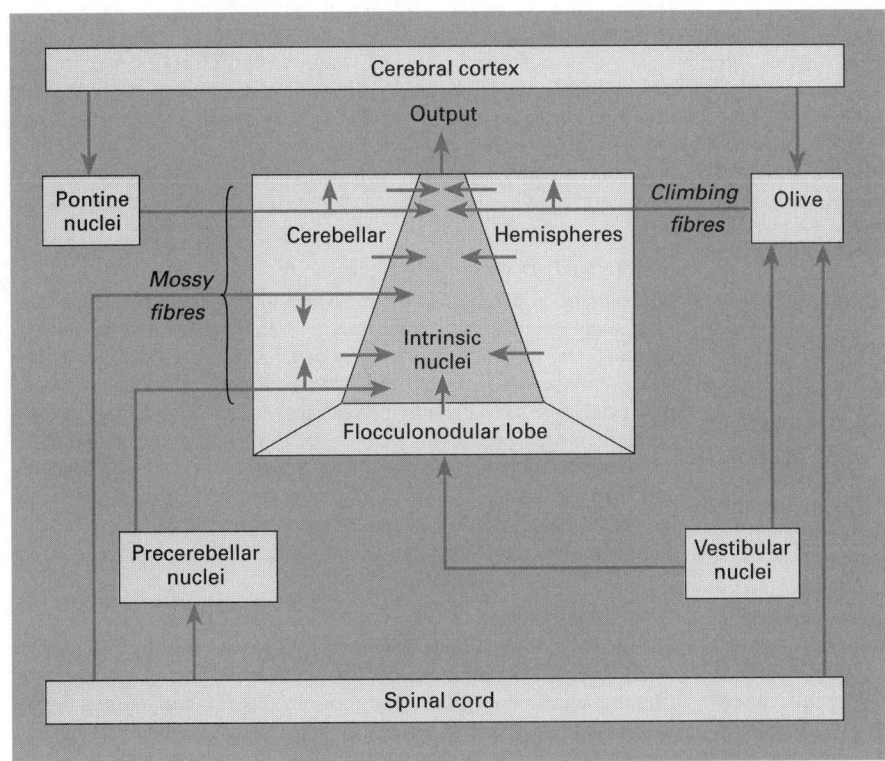

Fig. 1 A simplified diagram showing the principal afferents to cerebellar cortex and to intrinsic cerebellar nuclei. Both mossy (left) and climbing (right) fibre inputs project to both cortex and intrinsic nuclei.

Other cerebellar efferents go to vestibular nuclei and to nuclei in the pontine and medullary reticular formation. These brain-stem efferents provide access to the rubrospinal, vestibulospinal, and reticulospinal tracts.

CLINICAL ASPECTS

There are several theories on the main functions of the cerebellum. Thus:

(1) it may work as a timing device to control the duration and latency of muscle activities;
(2) it may act as a learning device to lay down circuitry for repeating previously performed movements; and
(3) it may act as a coordinator to harmonize and correctly scale the contribution of several brain areas to an intended movement.

The symptoms and signs resulting from lesions of the cerebellum or its pathways in humans have been based on observations in trauma (particularly gunshot wounds), tumour, stroke, and degenerative and demyelinating diseases. A pure cerebellar lesion is progressively less likely in that order.

Midline vermal lesions cause truncal ataxia, often in the absence of limb ataxia. The gait is wide based and particularly precarious on turning or on heel/toe walking. This may occasionally be difficult to distinguish from the gait disorder caused by secondary hydrocephalus, as evidenced by an apparent 'cerebellar ataxia' in a patient with a cerebellar tumour resolving after ventricular shunting without touching the tumour itself. Individuals with large frontal tumours may also present an apparent ataxic gait, accounting for a number of craniotomies performed at the wrong end of the head before good imaging was available. Patients may be unsteady for many reasons, only one of which is ataxia, so the term unsteadiness is preferable where any doubt exists. Unilateral cerebellar hemispheric lesions cause deviation or falling to the ipsilateral side. Unlike a sensory ataxia, cerebellar ataxia is not made particularly worse by shutting the eyes. Patients with pure cerebellar lesions may sometimes inappropriately use the words dizziness or giddiness. If given the alternatives, patients with brain-stem or vestibular problems may admit to be 'dizzy in the head', but those with pure cerebellar problems will often admit to being 'dizzy in the legs' instead. Generally, ataxic patients have more problem going down, and those with weakness going up, stairs.

Disease of cerebellar hemispheres or outflow tracts often causes limb ataxia, which is in fact an amalgam of several components. First, there may be dysmetria (misreaching, or past-pointing) evident in the arms on the finger–nose test or in the legs when the heel is first brought to the opposite kneecap. Secondly, there is the breakdown in force, rate, and rhythm known as dysdiadochokinesia. This can best be sought by asking the patient to tap your hand or a table gently, regularly, and rapidly with his fingers. This breakdown of smooth repetitive movements can even be detected by feel or by sound ('listening to the cerebellum') with the examiner's eyes shut. The third element is intention tremor. Many individuals claimed to have this tremor do not actually have it, the principal error being to use this term to describe a tremor that simply appears or worsens terminally. Thus, many postural tremors are positionally dependent, and some are only seen when the hands are in a given posture, particularly either outstretched or held in front of the nose. Other non-cerebellar tremors may be present, or appear only, during action (action or kinetic tremor). Only if additional signs of cerebellar dysfunction considered above are also present is it reasonable to use the term intention tremor. Such tremor should augment throughout a movement from inception to completion. A particular form of tremor may be produced by lesions strategically placed in a small area between cerebellum, midbrain, and subthalamus. Such 'rubral' (or midbrain or peduncular) tremor combines a tremor at rest with a tremor on posture and an intention tremor on movement. Finally, any judgement concern-

ing possible limb ataxia can only be made after taking into account any weakness, sensory loss, akinesia, or apraxia that is also present.

Cerebellar dysarthria may often simply manifest as slurred speech, as if intoxicated. However, in addition, some patients may have either scanning or explosive speech, due to an inability to modulate its rate, rhythm, and force appropriately. Dysarthria is usually present with lesions of the vermis, whole cerebellum, or its connections, but may be absent if one lateral hemisphere alone is involved. Although cerebellar lesions can certainly reverse hypertonia due to other causes, whether, in man, they actually cause hypotonia as such remains controversial. However, pendular knee jerks (not necessarily due to hypotonia) may occur. Cerebellar lesions may also cause the 'rebound phenomenon' resulting from impaired damping of limbs when suddenly a load is removed or a displacement applied.

Eye movements are frequently abnormal in disease of the cerebellum or its connections. The following may be seen: gaze-evoked, rebound, downbeat, or positional nystagmus; dysmetric voluntary saccades and jerky pursuit; square wave jerks (macrosaccadic oscillations); impaired vestibulo-ocular reflex suppression; and skew deviation. The presence of diplopia usually implies additional pathology outside the cerebellum proper.

The thalamus
STRUCTURE AND FUNCTION

The two thalami sit at the head of the brain-stem, their medial borders largely separated by the third ventricle, but often partially fused as the massa intermedia. Their blood supply derives from the posterior circulation via the posterior cerebral arteries and perforators from the terminal part of the basilar. They constitute the largest nuclear mass in the diencephalon (the others being the hypothalamus and subthalamus), and occupy a strategic position, both anatomically and functionally.

The structure of the thalamus, already complex, is further confused by the existence of different nomenclatures (the one used here is that of Walker). Broadly speaking, there are three nuclear groups (anterior, medial, and lateral). The lateral group is divided into the lateral and ventral masses, each of which contain a number of nuclei. The ventral lateral cell mass is the main region where somatosensory afferents terminate.

The thalamus receives inputs from cerebral cortex, sensory tracts, basal ganglia, and cerebellum. Almost all of its output is to the cerebral cortex, either in the form of reciprocal circuits or of more complex loops (see later) from cortex through other subcortical structures to thalamus and back to cortex again, but there is a small output to the striatum.

Thalamic afferents
Somatic and visceral afferents
Somatic and visceral afferents from the body pass via the medial lemniscus and spinothalamic tract into the ventral posterolateral nucleus caudalis (VPLc), where caudal body parts are represented laterally and rostral parts medially. Input from the face (via trigeminothalamic tracts) pass even more medially into the ventral posteromedial nucleus (VPM). Somatotopic representation is maintained through the connections to the parietal lobe in the form of the sensory homunculus, with legs medially and arms high and face low over the convexity. Taste afferents feed into the ventral posteromedial nucleus parvocellularis, (VPMpc), and hearing and vision into the medial and lateral geniculate bodies, respectively.

Basal ganglia input
The medial globus pallidus (MGP) projects to the centromedian nucleus (CM), to ventral anterior nucleus parvocellularis (VApc), and to ventral lateral nucleus oralis (VLo) and medialis (VLm), and its homologue, the substantia nigra pars reticulata (SNr), to the mediodorsal nucleus (MD) and ventral anterior nucleus magnocellularis (VAmc).

Cerebellar input

Afferents from intrinsic cerebellar nuclei ascend to the ventral lateral nucleus caudalis (VLc), to the ventral posterolateral nucleus oralis (VPLo), and to the adjacent zone x.

Thalamic efferents

All the thalamic nuclei project to cerebral cortex with the exception of important outputs from the intralaminar centromedian-parafascicular nuclear complex to striatum.

CLINICAL ASPECTS

From the above it is clear that, depending on the nuclei involved, thalamic lesions might influence either sensation or motor function, or sometimes both. Most commonly an infarct or haemorrhage (10–15 per cent of all intracerebral haemorrhages) causes contralateral sensory loss or impairment. A small lacunar infarct in the ventral posterolateral nucleus may give rise to a pure sensory stroke, sometimes sparing the face. A larger lesion may cause the thalamic syndrome of Dejerine and Roussy, in which an initial mild and transient hemiplegia is accompanied by persisting superficial and deep sensory impairment, mild hemiataxia, and astereognosis. These are commonly accompanied by choreoathetoid movements and severe, persistent, paroxysmal, often intolerable, pains on the hemiplegic side. When mild, the movements may be pseudoathetotic due to deafferentation; when severe, they suggest that the lesion may extend beyond the thalamus to involve basal ganglia connections. A significant, persisting hemiplegia implies either a large thalamic lesion also involving the internal capsule, or the possibility that the stroke is primarily capsular and not thalamic. A particular form of subcortical aphasia has been described in thalamic lesions.

Finally, surgical lesions are sometimes stereotactically placed in the ventral lateral nucleus caudalis (also known as the ventral intermediate nucleus—Vim in Hassler's nomenclature) to relieve tremor in Parkinson's disease and benign essential tremor, and also rigidity (but not akinesia) in the former. Chronic electrical stimulation of the same area is also effective.

The basal ganglia

STRUCTURE AND FUNCTION

There is no uniform agreement on how many of the subcortical nuclei one should include under the terms basal ganglia and extrapyramidal motor system. However, there is uniform agreement that they at least include the neostriatum (caudate nucleus and putamen, often together called simply the striatum) and the palaeostriatum (the lateral and medial globus pallidus with the latter's homologue, the substantia nigra pars reticulata). The term 'corpus striatum' refers to neostriatum plus palaeostriatum, and lentiform nucleus to putamen plus globus pallidus. The substantia nigra pars compacta and the subthalamic nucleus and the limbic amygdaloid complex of archistriatum should also be considered part of the basal ganglia. The claustrum, substantia innominata, red nucleus, pedunculopontine nucleus, and even the thalamus, are considered in some classifications to be part of the basal ganglia, but will not be dealt with here under that heading.

The putamen lies lateral to the thalamus, separated from it (and from most of the caudate nucleus, except anteriorly) by the internal capsule. The caudate nucleus, whose head lies antero-dorso-medial to the putamen, describes most of a circle as it follows, and progressively tapers with, the lateral ventricles through its body posteriorly, its tail swinging forward until its anteriorly pointing tip terminates in the amygdaloid nucleus. The pallidum lies medial to the putamen but still lateral to the internal capsule, and is divided into lateral (LGP) and medial (MGP) pallidal segments. The substantia nigra lies in the midbrain, transversely above the cerebral peduncles. Its pars reticulata, the termination of the

striatonigral pathway, is homologous with the medial globus pallidus, and its pars compacta (SNc) contains the dopaminergic neurones that form the nigrostriatal pathway. Below the thalamus, medial to the internal capsule and rostral to the midbrain, is the subthalamic nucleus.

Most of the caudate, putamen, and the globus pallidus derive their arterial supply from anterior circulation via the lateral lenticulostriate arteries and branches of the anterior choroidal and anterior cerebral arteries. Like the thalamus, the subthalamic region, and also the substantia nigra, are supplied by posterior circulation.

The basal ganglia and their (inter) connections, rich in neurotransmitters, have been extensively studied. The 'striopallidal complex' receives a wide variety of inputs from cerebral cortex. Its principal output is to the thalamus, which in turn projects back to the cortex to complete a basal ganglia–thalamocortical circuit. However, it is important to note the existence of additional output to the brain-stem in the pallidotegmental tract which terminates in the cholinergic pedunculopontine nucleus. This structure is believed to play an important role in the control of balance and locomotion, and in the maintenance of rigidity. The caudate and putamen are the afferent, and the globus pallidus and substantia nigra pars reticulata the efferent, parts of the striopallidal complex. There is additional dopaminergic input from the substantia nigra pars compacta and the adjacent ventral tegmental area (VTA) in

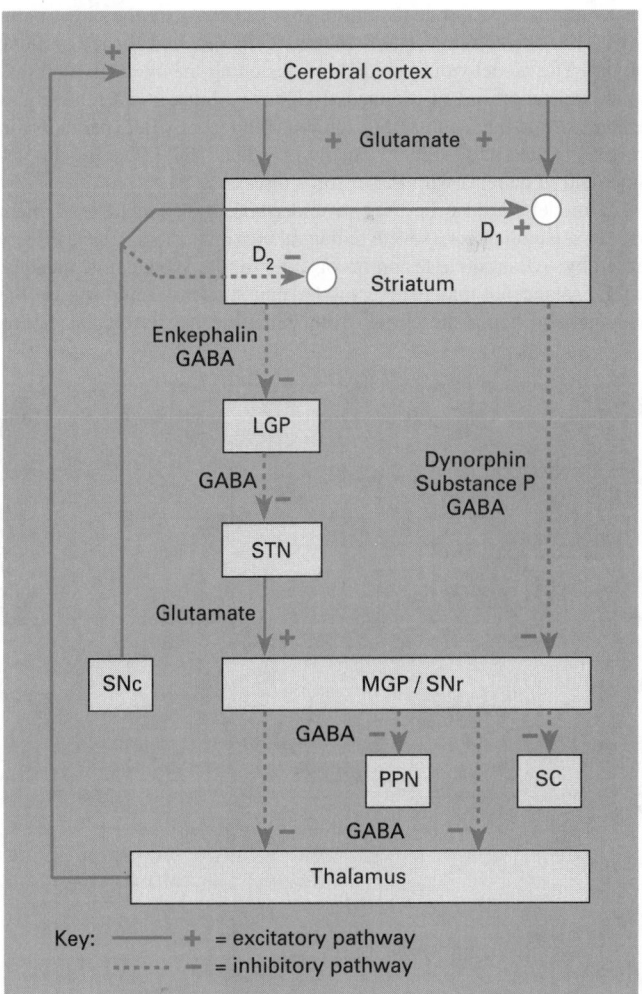

Fig. 2 A simplified schematic diagram showing the principal connections of the basal ganglia. Key: excitatory synapses are indicated by +, inhibitory ones by −. D_1, dopamine D_1 receptors; D_2, dopamine D_2 receptors; LGP and MGP, lateral and medial globus pallidus; STN, subthalamic nucleus; SNr and SNc, substantia nigra pars reticulata and pars compacta; PPN, pedunculopontine nucleus; SC, superior colliculus.

the midbrain which modulates striatal activity. A highly simplified schema concentrating on the motor circuit is presented in Fig. 2.

The massive cortical inputs into the striatum are largely excitatory, using glutamate as a neurotransmitter. Other inputs (not shown) come from the intralaminar thalamic nuclei, amygdala, and dorsal nucleus of the raphe. In the nigrostriatal pathway from the pars compacta, dopamine preferentially stimulates dopamine D_1 receptors to activate neurones of the direct pathway to the medial globus pallidus which contain dynorphin, substance P, and γ-aminobutyric acid (GABA), and are therefore inhibitory. Dopamine D_2 receptor stimulation preferentially inhibits the first neurones of the indirect pathway to the lateral globus pallidus, which contain enkephalin and GABA. These neurones inhibit subthalamic neurones which, in turn, probably using glutamate, excite cells in the medial globus pallidus and the substantia nigra pars reticulata. These in their turn use GABA to inhibit thalamic neurones, which finally complete the loop with an excitatory pathway back to the cortex.

This model can be used to predict the functional consequences of over- or underactivity of individual parts, either in human disease states or in experimental animals. In the latter, 2-deoxyglucose autoradiographic studies can be used to confirm such predictions and validate the model. Thus, the consequences of the loss of substantia nigra pars compacta cells that occurs in Parkinson's disease would be as follows: along the direct pathway there is impaired stimulation of the striatal cells that normally inhibit medial globus pallidus/substantia nigra pars reticulata neurones, so the latter are overactive. Along the indirect pathway, there is impaired inhibition (hence overactivity) of the neurones that inhibit the lateral globus pallidus, which is therefore underactive. However, this leads to less inhibition (hence overactivity) of the subthalamic nucleus (STN), which increases excitatory input to the medial globus pallidus/substantia nigra pars reticulata (already overactive via the direct pathway). This overactivity in turn inhibits thalamic, and thence cortical, activity. The model would predict that lesioning the overactive subthalamic nucleus or part of the medial globus pallidus might relieve parkinsonism, and indeed this has been reported recently in experiments in primates treated with MPTP (1-methyl-4-phenyl-1,2,3,6-tetrahydropyridine) and in patients with Parkinson's disease.

The model can also be used to understand hyperkinetic movement disorders. Hemiballism (severe unilateral proximal chorea) is classically caused by a destructive lesion in, or close to, the subthalamic nucleus. In this instance an underactive subthalamic nucleus would release the thalamus and hence the cortex from inhibition by the medial globus pallidus/substantia nigra pars reticulata, and again this sequence has been confirmed by 2-deoxyglucose experiments in animals.

All that has been mentioned so far concerns motor function, traditionally equated with the function of the basal ganglia. However, as the complexity and diversity of basal ganglia anatomy, circuitry, and function has become apparent, the concept of multiple basal ganglia–thalamocortical circuits has developed. Rather than cortical inputs being simply funnelled through the circuits, some overlapping of cortical input to the striatum does indeed occur, but thereafter the loops are non-overlapping, allowing separate and independent processing throughout the basal ganglia. Five such circuits have been proposed: (1) the motor and (2) the oculomotor, involved in sensorimotor functions of the body and eyes; (3) the dorsolateral prefrontal and (4) the orbitofrontal, involved in cognitive aspects of behaviour; and (5) the anterior cingulate circuit, related to limbic functions. A simplified representation of these loops is given in Fig. 3.

The past decade has also seen considerable advances in our knowledge of striatal anatomy and neurochemistry. Morphological techniques have long demonstrated a variety of striatal neuronal types. These are either projection neurones (spiny medium type I, the vast majority, and large type II), or intrinsic neurones (aspiny types I–III). However, the striatum as a whole seemed rather amorphous until neurochemical markers gave a new perspective. Thus, the medium type I spiny projection neurones are the major targets of nigral dopaminergic transmission, and make synaptic contact with large aspiny cholinergic interneurones. The former cells are selectively lost in Huntington's disease, resulting in a loss of their inhibitory transmitter GABA, together with co-localized metenkephalin or substance P. In contrast, type I aspiny interneurones, containing neuropeptide-Y and somatostatin, and type II aspiny interneurones, containing acetylcholine, are largely spared in Huntington's disease.

It is now recognized that striatal neurones are also organized into a mosaic pattern comprising patches, or striosomes, with high levels of μ opiate receptors and low levels of acetylcholinesterase, suspended in a matrix of cells containing high levels of aceytlcholinesterase, somatostatin, and calbindin. Patch and matrix receive different inputs from midbrain, thalamus, and cortex. In particular, deeper levels of prefrontal or limbic cortex tend to project to striosomes and more superficial layers of sensorimotor cortex to matrix. Patches mainly project to the substantia nigra pars compacta, whereas matrix neurones may take either the direct or indirect route to medial globus pallidus/substantia nigra pars reticulata.

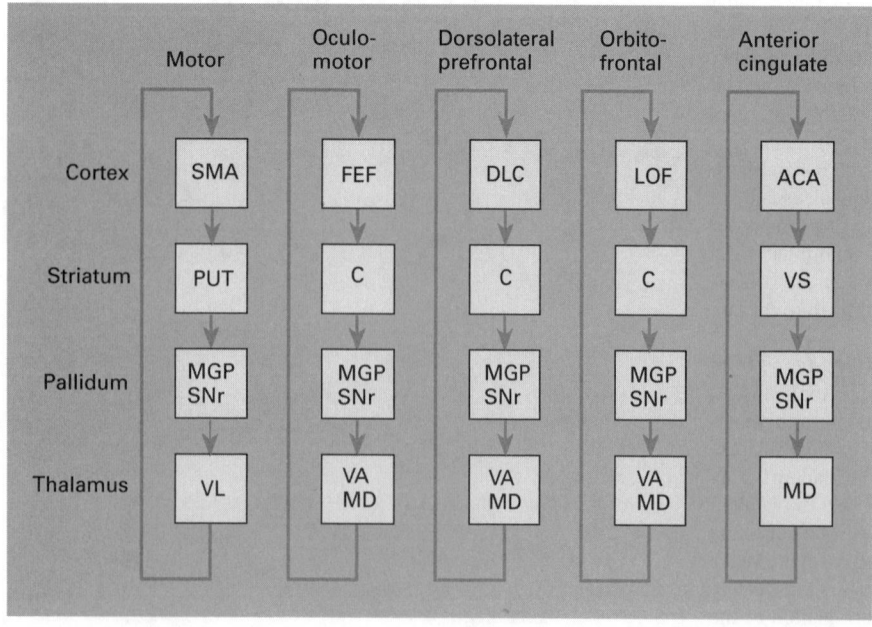

Fig. 3 A highly simplified diagram of proposed basal ganglia–thalamocortical loops (after Alexander *et al.* 1986, with permission). Key: same abbreviations as for Fig. 2, plus: SMA, supplementary motor area; FEF, frontal eye fields; DLC, dorsolateral prefrontal cortex; LOF, lateral orbitofrontal area; ACA, anterior cingulate area; PUT, putamen; C, caudate; VS, ventral striatum; VL, ventrolateral thalamic nucleus; VA, ventral anterior nucleus; MD, mediodorsal nucleus. Segregated parts of the striatum, pallidum, and thalamus convey separate loops.

CLINICAL ASPECTS (SEE ALSO CHAPTER 24.10)

On the basis of the above evidence, we can no longer assume that basal ganglia pathology produces only motor symptoms and signs. Thus, in patients with Parkinson's disease, Huntington's disease, and Steele–Richardson disease, all of which principally (but not exclusively) involve basal ganglia, affective disorder, 'subcortical dementia', or 'frontal lobe deficits' may be seen. Through its projection to superior colliculus, abnormal activity in the substantia nigra pars reticulata may be responsible for some of the eye movement disturbance seen, for example, in Parkinson's disease (delayed latency to onset of voluntary saccades and impaired production of remembered saccades).

Nevertheless, it is a fact that the most striking clinical features of basal ganglia disease remain those in the motor sphere, comprising tremor, rigidity, akinesia, and postural abnormality, as evidenced by Parkinson's disease, and hyperkinetic movement disorders such as chorea and dystonia seen, for example, in Huntington's disease and in levodopa-treated subjects with Parkinson's disease.

The classical tremor of Parkinson's disease is slow (4–6 Hz), pill-rolling, and disappears and diminishes on movement, to reappear once a new posture has been adopted. In traditional animal lesion studies a nigral lesion seems necessary, but not sufficient, to cause this tremor, although it may be seen with virtually a pure nigral lesion in some primates and some humans who have been exposed to MPTP. Of course, the pathology of Parkinson's disease involves more than simply the nigral lesion (although this is far and away the most important). However, no difference in neuropathology between cases of Parkinson's disease with and without tremor (or with and without rigidity) has been noted. A second, faster, postural tremor at around 6 to 8 Hz may also be seen together with, or replacing, the rest tremor of Parkinson's disease. Phenomenologically this can be indistinguishable from essential tremor, for which no pathological substrate has so far been discovered. An action or terminal component may also be seen.

Akinesia is a symptom complex comprising slowness of movement (bradykinesia), poverty of movement, progressive diminution and fatigue of rapid alternating movements, and difficulty in initiating and sequencing movements and in accomplishing simultaneous motor acts. Changes in neuronal discharge relating to movement seem to occur later in the basal ganglia than in the motor cortex. It has therefore been proposed that the basal ganglia are more concerned with using information from a previous movement to set up the premotor areas to select the correct parameters for running subsequent motor programmes. In Parkinson's disease levodopa strikingly reverses much of the akinesia, although sometimes one component, such as bradykinesia, may improve while another, such as poverty of movement, may remain. Thalamotomy or thalamic stimulation do not help akinesia in humans, but stimulation of subthalamic nucleus or medial pallidum, or a selective pallidotomy may do so. (In these situations, high-frequency electrical stimulation effectively temporarily and reversibly disables the function of a small volume of tissue around the tip of the electrode.).

Rigidity almost always accompanies akinesia. Resistance to passive movement is broadly similar in flexion and extension, although somewhat greater in the former to account for the commonly flexed, or simian, posture. It is described as lead pipe or, if there is superimposed tremor (either visible or invisible), as cogwheeling. Abnormalities of the tonic stretch reflex are felt to contribute to its pathophysiology.

As well as akinesia, both tremor and rigidity respond to levodopa. Unlike akinesia, both also respond to thalamotomy, but the lesion needs to be larger for rigidity than for tremor.

Postural instability is another feature of parkinsonism. This is in part due to impairment of anticipatory responses and postural adjustments associated with movement, and problems in controlling body sway. Unlike the above features, this may often be levodopa resistant.

Of the hyperkinetic movement disorders, chorea (in the case of Huntington's disease) and dystonia (when secondary to discernible brain pathology) can be related to basal ganglia disease (see Chapter 24.10).

Although chorea can be produced by lesioning the subthalamic nucleus in intact monkeys, or by chronic dopaminergic treatment of primates with a lesioned nigrostriatal tract, it has not yet proved possible to produce spontaneous chorea in animals solely by making a caudate lesion analogous to that in Huntington's disease. Similarly, although dystonia may be seen in humans after lesions of the putamen (principally), caudate, or thalamus, there is, again, no good animal model, although it can be induced by dopaminergic drugs in MPTP-treated primates.

REFERENCES

Albin, R.L., Young, A.B., and Penney, J.B. (1989). The functional anatomy of basal ganglia disorders. *Trends in Neurosciences* **12**, 366–75. (An excellent synthesis of anatomical and functional aspects of the basal ganglia.)

Alexander, G.E., DeLong, M.R., and Strick, P.L. (1986). Parallel organization of functionally segregated circuits linking basal ganglia and cortex. *Annual Review of Neuroscience* **9**, 357–81.

Carpenter, M.B. (1991). *Core text of neuroanatomy*, (4th edn). Williams and Wilkins, Baltimore. (The best medium-sized all-round textbook of neuroanatomy.)

Crossman, A.R. (1990). A hypothesis on pathophysiological mechanisms that underlie levodopa– or dopamine agonist-induced dyskinesia in Parkinson's disease: Implications for future strategies in treatment. *Movement Disorders* **5**, 100–8.

Gerfen, C.R. (1992). The neostriatal mosaic: multiple levels of compartmental organisation. *Trends in Neurosciences* **15**, 33–9.

Goetz, C.G., DeLong, M.R., Penn, R.D., and Bakay, R.A.E. (1993). Neurosurgical horizons in Parkinson's disease. *Neurology* **43**, 1–7.

Graybiel, A.M. (1989). Dopaminergic and cholinergic systems in the striatum. In *Neural mechanisms in disorders of movement* (ed. A. Crossman and M.A. Sambrook), pp. 3–15. Libbey, London.

Hassler, R. (1959). Anatomy of the thalamus. In *Introduction to stereotaxis with an atlas of the human brain* (ed. G. Schaltenbrand and P. Bailey), pp. 230–90. G. Thieme, Stuttgart.

Marsden, C.D. (1990). Neurophysiology. In *Parkinson's disease* (ed. G.M. Stern), pp. 57–98. Chapman and Hall, London. (A simple, clear, and masterly overview of the physiological mechanisms underlying the clinical features of parkinsonism).

Rothwell, J.C. (1994). *Control of human voluntary movement*. 2nd edn. Croom Helm, London. (A short textbook on the physiology of human motor disorders.)

Walker, A.E. (1938). *The primate thalamus*. University of Chicago Press.

24.3.4 Visual pathways

R. W. Ross Russell

STRUCTURE AND FUNCTION

Each optic nerve has four regions:

(1) the optic disc and nerve head within the globe;
(2) the orbital portion;
(3) the canalicular portion traversing the optic foramen in the sphenoid bone; and
(4) the intracranial portion joining the optic chiasm.

Eighty per cent of the medullated nerve fibres in the optic nerve are axons of small retinal ganglion cells which project to the parvocellular layer of the lateral geniculate nucleus. The remainder are axons of larger ganglion cells which project either to the magnocellular layer of the geniculate nucleus or via small fibres directly to the midbrain. Retinal ganglion cell density is greatest at the central retina and the majority of nerve fibres of all types subserve central vision. Both large and small ganglion cells receive input from cone photoreceptors but only the small ganglion cells subserve colour vision. Each optic nerve is enclosed in a tough dural sheath and the pia arachnoid is continuous with the intra-cranial subarachnoid space.

The blood supply to the orbital portion of the optic nerve is from the ophthalmic and short ciliary arteries with a small contribution from the central retinal artery. The intracranial portion is supplied by numerous small branches from the anterior cerebral and ophthalmic arteries. As the optic nerve approaches the chiasm the axons from the nasal retina (comprising 60 per cent of the total) separate from the remainder and cross to the other side to join the optic tract. Upper and lower fibres in the optic nerve take a slightly different course (see Fig. 1). Axons sub-serving the central parts of the visual field, which occupy the centre of the optic nerve, cross in the posterior portion of the chiasm. The position of the chiasm is variable but it usually lies just above the sella; its most important relations are the pituitary gland below and the cavernous sinuses and carotid arteries on each side. The chiasmal blood-supply comes from small twigs arising from the terminal carotid artery, the anterior cerebral and anterior communicating arteries.

The optic tracts extend from the chiasm to the lateral geniculate nucleus, encircling the cerebral peduncles. In the anterior tract, macular fibres lie medially, but further back they occupy a dorsal position. In the lateral geniculate nucleus, axons from corresponding parts of the two retinas terminate in vertical columns of cells. The majority of axons in the optic tracts synapse at this point, but some bypass the nucleus and proceed to the superior colliculus and midbrain tectum. These are concerned with the pupillary light reflex and with reflex eye movements which orientate the eyes towards the object of interest.

The optic radiation begins in the geniculate nucleus, spreads out to form a wide white-matter tract, and ends in the striate cortex. The upper fibres pass through the parietal lobe on their way to the upper bank of the calcarine fissure; the lower fibres take a longer course through the temporal lobe to end in the lower bank.

The blood supply to the optic radiation is complex; the first part is supplied by the posterior choroidal artery, the upper part of the radiation by the middle cerebral artery, the lower by the posterior cerebral artery.

The primary visual (striate) cortex occupies the medial aspect of the posterior part of each occipital lobe. Much of it is buried in the calcarine fissure. Projections from corresponding half-retinas terminate in a point-to-point fashion in columns of cells precisely arranged in a retinotopic map. Some cortical neurones respond to stimulation from either eye, some from one eye only. Central parts of the visual field have a relatively large cortical representation compared with more peripheral parts. This is situated at or near the posterior pole, while more peripheral parts of the field project more anteriorly.

The columns of neurones in the striate cortex are adapted to detect visual edges and planes; further analysis of visual input in terms of colour, movement, stereopsis, and form analysis is achieved by a series of parallel relays to prestriate cortex in the occipital lobe and also to parietal and temporal lobes. There are two main routes: a superior occip-itoparietal pathway concerned with the detection of movement and localization of visual stimuli and an inferior, or occipitotemporal, route concerned with discrimination of shapes and colours. Further relays to parietal and temporal cortex complete the process of visual recognition and categorization. In these areas extensive transfer of visual informa-tion occurs across the corpus callosum, strict contralateral projection is lost and both hemifields are represented. In addition, some hemisphere specialization is evident at this stage, the non-dominant parietal lobe (normally the right) being concerned with the spatial characteristics of the object, while the dominant parietal and temporal lobes are concerned with recognizing the function and name of the object. Similarly, the right temporal lobe is predominant in the storage and recall of visual memories, while the left has the more important role in verbal memory.

Lesions of the visual pathways (Fig. 2)

OPTIC NERVE

A wide variety of disease processes may affect one or both optic nerves at any point in their course. Anterior lesions within the orbit tend to cause proptosis and ophthalmoplegia in addition to visual loss. Charting of the visual field usually shows a general depression of the field with a relative or absolute central scotoma, but arcuate (fibre-bundle) defects may occur with lesions near the optic disc. Visual acuity is normally depressed and colour vision is affected early. In unilateral lesions the amplitude of the direct pupillary response is reduced on the affected side (relative afferent defect).

In acute cases the optic disc may be swollen, and in long-standing cases it becomes atrophic.

Swelling of the optic disc has a number of causes (Table 1). The term papilloedema is reserved by convention for swelling caused by raised intracranial pressure. This is usually bilateral, causes little interference with vision, and is accompanied by other features of raised pressure, such as headache, vomiting, and diminished conscious level. Visual fields show enlarged blind spots and usually slight peripheral constric-tion. Brief bilateral obscurations of vision are a feature of severe pap-illoedema and may herald permanent visual loss.

Pseudopapilloedema refers to congenital abnormalities which resem-

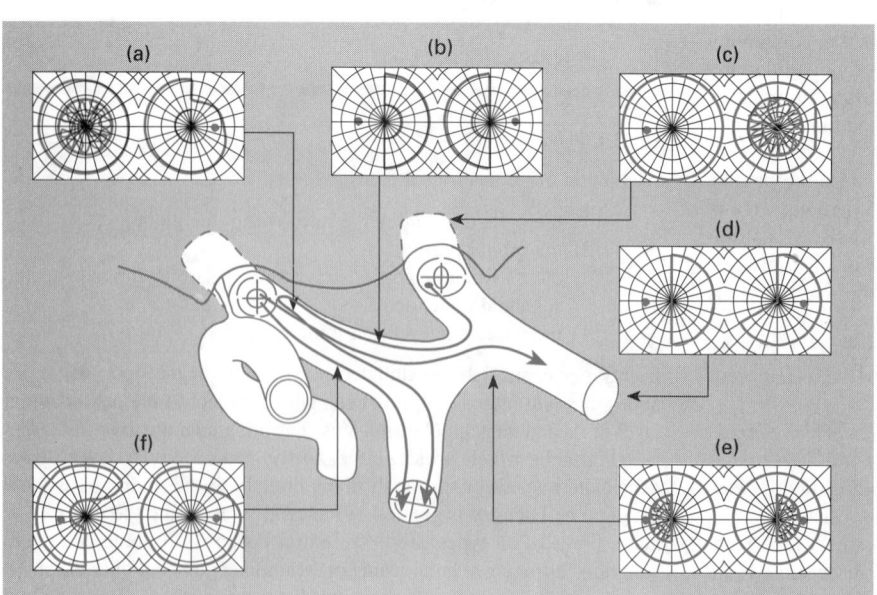

Fig. 1 Optic chiasm and left internal carotid artery viewed from behind to show the arrangement of nerve fibres and the visual field defects produced by lesions at various points. (a) Lesion at junction of optic nerve and chiasm—central scotoma left eye, upper temporal defect right eye (note route taken by lower crossing fibres from right optic nerve); (b) central chiasmal lesion interrupting all crossing fibres—complete bitemporal hemianopia; (c) right optic nerve lesion—general depression of field with central scotoma; (d) lesion of right optic tract—left homonymous hemianopia (incongruous); (e) lesion affecting posterior aspect of chiasm (crossing fibres from central field)—scotomatous bitemporal hemianopia; (f) lesion affecting left side of chiasm—central and nasal field defect left eye, early upper temporal quadrantanopia right eye.

Fig. 2 Lesions of the visual pathways. (a) Orbital meningioma: CT scan of a 45-year-old female patient with progressive proptosis and visual loss in the left eye. (b) Dysthyroid eye disease: orbital axial CT scan of a 34-year-old female patient with bilateral proptosis, papilloedema, and visual loss caused by compression of the optic nerves by swollen and infiltrated ocular muscles. (c) Optic nerve glioma: CT scan of a 14-year-old child with progressive visual loss in the left eye; (i) axial scan through mid-orbit, (ii) sagittal scan through optic nerve. (d) Parasellar meningioma: CT scan of a 50-year-old woman with meningioma arising in the sphenoidal wing and spreading to involve the left optic nerve and cavernous sinus. (e) Pituitary adenoma: MRI scan of a 37-year-old woman with a bitemporal hemianopia caused by upward extension of a prolactin-secreting tumour of the pituitary—the chiasm is stretched over the upper extent of the tumour. (f) Craniopharyngioma: CT san of a 25-year-old man presenting with retardation of growth and sexual development, optic atrophy, and bitemporal hemianopia; the cystic tumour occupies the suprasellar cistern and arises from the hypothalamus; (i) axial scan, (ii) sagittal reconstruction.

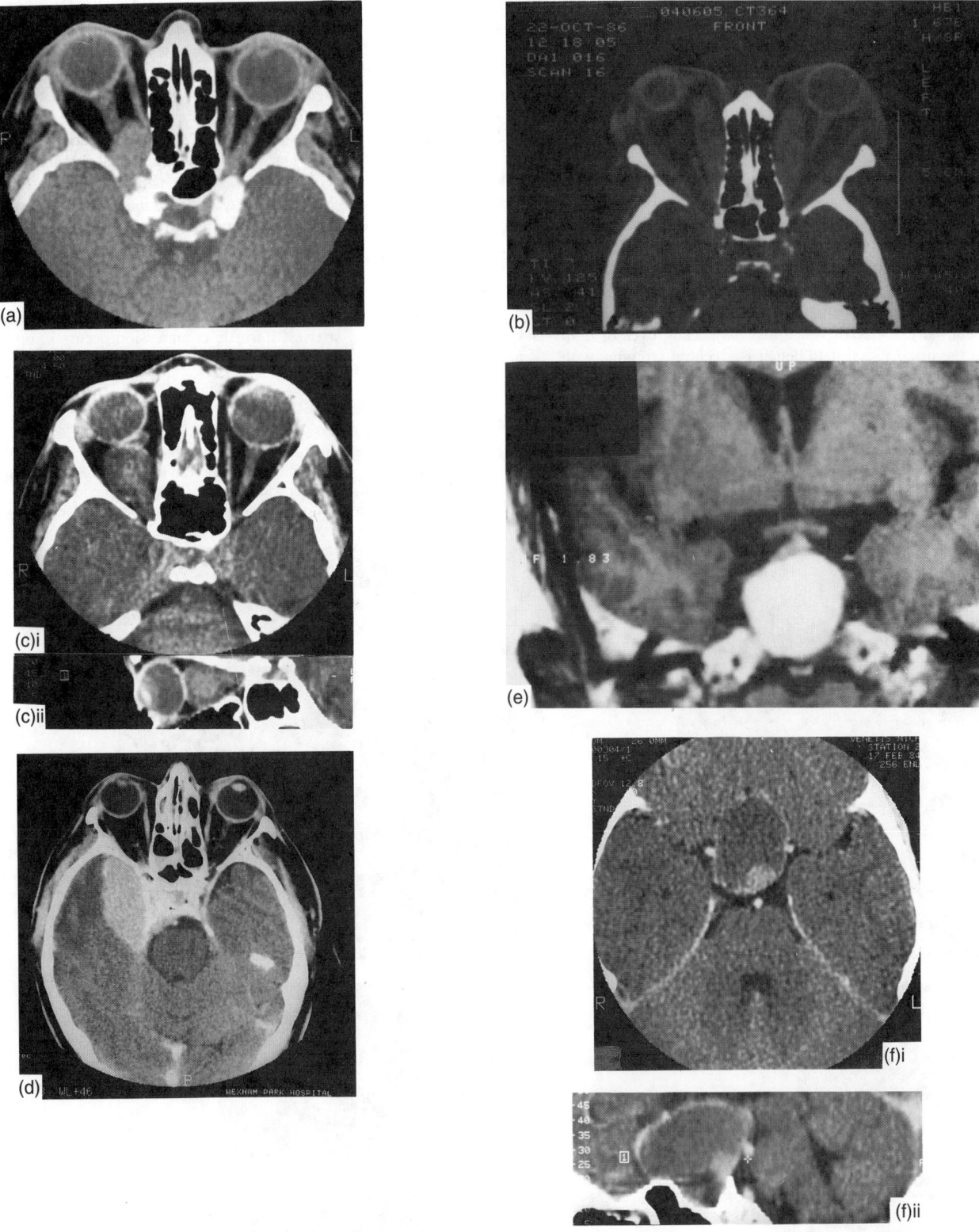

ble papilloedema but occur without raised intracranial pressure. Such a condition is characterized by drusen of the disc; it may be dominantly inherited and may cause progressive field loss and retinal haemorrhage. A pearly excrescence can usually be seen on the disc and a CT scan shows a small calcific deposit which is diagnostic.

Swelling of the disc from demyelination, inflammation, or ischaemia is referred to as papillitis. The characteristics are similar to those of papilloedema but the loss of acuity and visual field is much greater.

Optic atrophy may follow a variety of optic-disc disorders; the disc becomes waxy or white from gliosis, loss of axons, and reduced vascularity. The edges of the disc remain clear-cut and the retinal vessels are normal. If the disc has previously been swollen before optic atrophy supervenes, the edges may be indistinct and the retinal vessels may be sheathed (consecutive optic atrophy).

Demyelinating disease

This is one of the most common optic nerve lesions and usually affects young patients; it is frequently the first sign of multiple sclerosis. Demyelination is patchy, may involve any part of the nerve, and in acute cases the disc may be swollen (papillitis). Atrophy follows at a later stage. Ocular pain is a common accompaniment and is characteristically worse on eye movement. Any degree of visual loss may occur, even of light perception, and the usual visual field deficit is a central scotoma, with particular loss of colour vision. Nerve conduction through demyelinated segments of optic nerve is very sensitive to small changes in temperature and patients often notice a marked deterioration in vision on exercise or external heating (Uthoff's phenomenon). Despite the severity of the initial symptoms, most patients make a good functional recovery over a few weeks. Within 5 years, however, two-thirds will have developed other signs of multiple sclerosis. The cortical evoked potential to a patterned stimulus is markedly delayed (see Chapter 24.2.3) and this abnormality forms the basis of a sensitive test for multiple sclerosis. It may be positive even in patients with no visual symptoms.

Compressive and infiltrating lesions

Compression of the optic nerve by tumour is usually extrinsic and involves the posterior part of the nerve near the optic foramen. Proptosis and ophthalmoplegia may also be present. Meningiomas arising from the nerve sheath or from the margins of the optic canal, lymphomas, plasmocytomas, nasopharyngeal carcinomas, or metastases are the commonest types. Metastatic carcinoma may infiltrate the orbit and cause a progressive painless optic neuropathy without proptosis. In dysthyroid eye disease compression of the nerve may result from grossly enlarged extraocular muscles. Within the skull the optic nerve may be directly compressed or indirectly displaced against the rigid margins of the dura by such lesions as meningioma, pituitary adenoma, carotid aneurysm, or ectatic carotid arteries. Intrinsic compression occurs in optic nerve glioma, a rare tumour of childhood often associated with neurofibromatosis.

Fig. 2 (cont.) (g) Carotid aneurysm: angiogram in a 65-year-old woman with progressive visual loss from a giant suprasellar aneurysm compressing the chiasm. (h) Multiple sclerosis: coronal MRI scan through the frontal lobes of a 28-year-old patient with left optic neuritis; high-signal lesions are seen in the optic nerve and in the hemisphere white matter. (i) Glioma: CT scan of a 45-year-old man with epileptic seizures, left homonymous hemianopia, and dressing dyspraxia; malignant glioma involving the right visual radiation. (j) Infarction: MRI axial scan of a 56-year-old woman with sudden onset of right homonymous hemianopia; there is infarction in the territory of the left posterior cerebral artery caused by embolism from the left atrium.

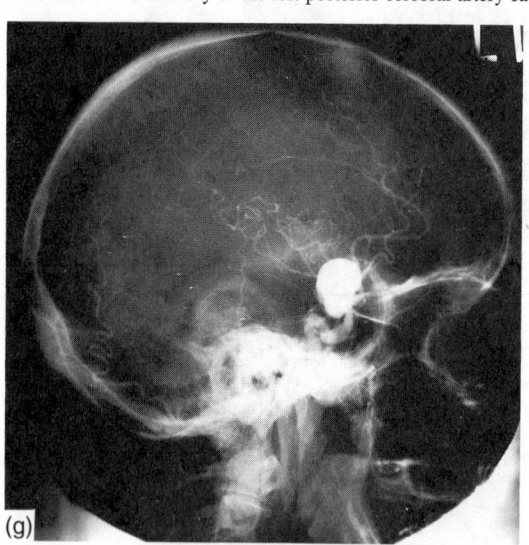
(g)

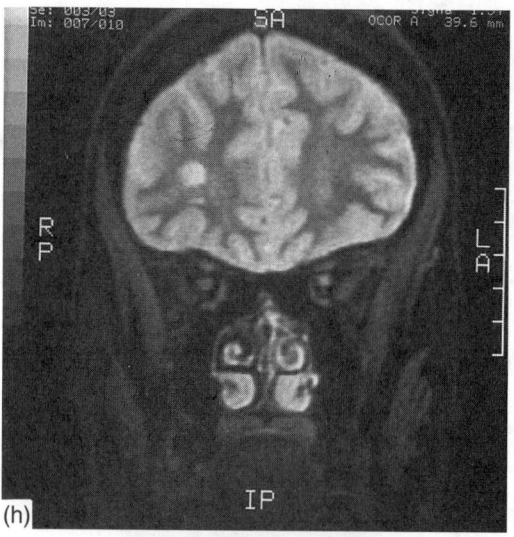
(h)

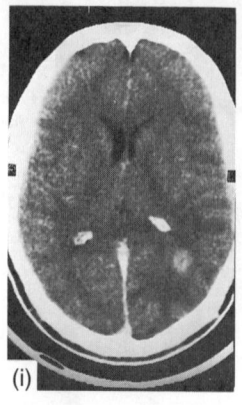
(i)

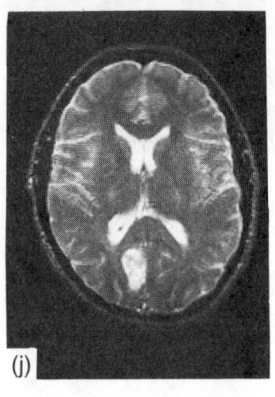
(j)

Table 1 *Swelling of the optic disc; causes and features*

	Congenital	Papilloedema	Papillitis	Ischaemia
Laterality	Either or both	Bilateral	Unilateral	Unilateral
Acuity	Usually normal	Normal until late	Early loss	Usually affected
Colour vision	Usually normal	Normal	Early loss	Early loss
Pupils	Normal	Normal	RAPD[a]	RAPD[a]
Visual fields	Normal/variable loss	Blind spot enlarged	Central scotoma	Altitudinal defect
Disc	Abnormal size, shape vessels	Swollen	Swollen	Swollen, pale
Fundus	May have choroidal pigment	Normal	Normal	Vascular changes
Common causes		Intracerebral, intraorbital tumour, haematoma, venous sinus occlusion, retinal vein thrombosis, CO_2 retention	Optic neuritis	Hypertension, diabetes, arteritis

[a]RAPD, relative afferent pupillary defect.

Inflammatory lesions

Acute or chronic inflammation in the ethmoid or sphenoid sinuses may extend into the orbit and is a rare cause of optic neuritis. Fungal infections such as mucormycosis or aspergillosis, which affect diabetic or immunocompromised patients, tend to occur at this site, as do granulomas of sarcoidosis or Wegener's granuloma. Within the cranial cavity one or both optic nerves may be involved by chronic basal meningitis caused by infections such as tuberculosis, syphilis, or cryptococcosis. The optic nerves may be involved by specific viral infections, such as herpes zoster, or as an immunological reaction following viral infection or vaccination.

Vascular lesions (ischaemic optic neuropathy)

This common condition usually affects elderly patients with degenerative arterial disease or with cranial arteritis. The optic nerve head is a vulnerable area because of its tenuous blood-supply from the posterior ciliary arteries. Loss of vision is rapid and painless, and the optic disc appears swollen and pale. In the non-arteritic variety, visual-field loss is altitudinal and partial, and central acuity may be preserved. In the arteritic type, vision is often lost entirely. Both types show a tendency to involve the other eye after a short interval. High-dose steroid treatment appears to suppress the arteritic process and prevents spread to the second eye, but has little effect in the non-arteritic group.

Toxic and nutritional amblyopias

These disorders are characterized by painless, slowly progressive, bilateral visual loss, showing diminished acuity, central or centro-caecal scotomas, and a variable degree of optic atrophy. They may occur in a setting of generalized malnutrition or with specific deficiency states (e.g. vitamins B_1, B_{12}, or folate deficiency). The syndrome may also follow chronic exposure to a number of toxic substances or drugs, such as alcohol (often in combination with heavy tobacco abuse), ethambutol, isoniazid, halogenated hydroxyquinolines, chlorpropamide, chloramphenicol, streptomycin, D-penicillamine, ergotamine, digitalis, and heavy metals.

Hereditary optic atrophy

There are a number of varieties of inherited optic atrophy, of which the best characterized is Leber's optic neuropathy. This causes severe visual loss in otherwise healthy young patients, beginning in the second decade. About 85 per cent of patients are male and 18 per cent of female carriers are affected. The onset may be acute and unilateral. In the early stages the optic discs may be swollen, with tortuous retinal arterioles and precapillary telangiectasia, but optic atrophy becomes apparent within a few months. The disease is inherited through the female line and the inheritance is consistent with a mutation of mitochondrial DNA.

Three such mutations have been identified in affected families. The disease progresses to severe loss of central vision but seldom causes complete blindness. No treatment has been shown to modify the progress of the condition. Occasional families have shown additional neurological features, such as dystonia, ataxia, or corticospinal tract involvement.

Other types of inherited optic atrophy have been described, following a pattern of dominant inheritance.

OPTIC CHIASM

Axons from the nasal retinas, which decussate in the chiasm, are at particular risk in compressive lesions. Many lesions also affect the uncrossed axons to some degree, and a loss of acuity is the rule, in contrast to lesions of the occipital cortex in which visual acuity is preserved. The classical field defect in chiasmal lesions is a bitemporal hemianopia with a sharp demarcation at the vertical meridian. Most patients have optic atrophy.

Central lesions produce a symmetrical field loss affecting both eyes to an equal extent, but there are two important variations in eccentrically placed lesions: a lesion at the junction of optic nerve and chiasm may cause a central scotoma in the ipsilateral eye and an upper temporal quadrantanopia in the contralateral eye. A lesion affecting the lateral side of the chiasm may cause nasal and central field loss in the ipsilateral eye and upper temporal quadrantanopia in the contralateral eye. Most of the important lesions affecting the chiasm are compressive, and the main features are shown in Table 2.

Pituitary adenomas are the most common type of tumour; they present with painless visual loss, with or without endocrine features. Of the hormone-secreting tumours, prolactinomas are the most frequent, followed by acidophil adenomas causing acromegaly, and by basophil adenomas causing Cushing's syndrome. Non-secreting adenomas or other destructive lesions of the pituitary may present with signs of hypopituitarism.

Meningiomas occur mostly in middle-aged women and present with painless asymmetric visual loss but with no endocrine abnormality. Craniopharyngiomas arise in an embryonic remnant but may present at any age. They are suprasellar rather than within the pituitary fossa, and exhibit hypothalamic signs such as retardation of growth or sexual development, diabetes insipidus, or hypersomnolence. In children they tend to obstruct the third ventricle and to cause hydrocephalus. Aneurysms of the terminal carotid artery produce visual loss by compressing the lateral side of the chiasm. Intermittent pain is usually a feature but rupture and subarachnoid haemorrhage are rare. Other less common lesions which occur in this region include ectopic pinealoma (dysgerminoma), cordoma, intrinsic glioma or hamartoma of the chiasm, microglioma of the hypothalamus, and granulomas such as sarcoidosis.

Table 2 *Lesions of the optic chiasm*

	Occurrence	Visual field	Optic disc	Associated features	Treatment
Pituitary	Adults	Bitemporal hemianopia	Atrophy	Endocrine, prolactin GH[a], ACTH[b]	Surgery, bromocriptine, radiotherapy
Parasellar meningioma	Adults, F > M	Asymmetric bitemporal hemianopia	Atrophy	None	Surgery
Craniopharyngioma	Any age	Bitemporal, homonymous hemianopia	Atrophy, papilloedema (children)	Retarded growth, sexual development	Surgery, radical or palliative, ?radiotherapy
Optic nerve, chiasmal glioma	Children	Variable	Atrophy	Neurofibroma	Very slow-growing, possibly radiosensitive
Carotid aneurysm	Elderly, F > M	Lateral chiasm syndrome	Atrophy (late)	Pain, rarely SAH[c]	Usually conservative ?carotid ligation

[a]GH, growth hormone.

[b]ACTH, adrenocorticotrophic hormone.

[c]SAH, subarachnoid haemorrhage.

Plain radiography of the pituitary fossa no longer has a place in the investigation of pituitary or parasellar lesions, its place having been taken by CT scanning, supplemented in some cases by MRI. Modern CT imaging with enhancement reliably demonstrates and distinguishes adenomas, meningiomas, and craniopharyngiomas. Angiography may be necessary to confirm an aneurysm.

Treatment of chiasmal lesions

A variety of medical and surgical treatments are available for chiasmal compression, depending on the site and size of the tumour, the severity of visual loss, and the type of endocrine disorder. For prolactinomas, bromocriptine has now been shown to decrease tumour size as well as to lower prolactin blood levels, and offers the prospect of long-term medical control. It is possible that somatostatin will provide a similar means of controlling growth-hormone-secreting adenomas (see Section 12).

The classical neurosurgical approach to pituitary and parapituitary tumours is by a subfrontal craniotomy. This is still indicated for meningiomas and for some pituitary tumours with a large upward extension. Craniopharyngiomas may be amenable to radical excision or to a more conservative procedure such as cyst drainage or shunting. For the majority of pituitary adenomas, however, the most satisfactory treatment is trans-sphenoidal excision. This approach carries a lower morbidity than craniotomy and is especially suitable for elderly patients. The risk of recurrence is reduced if surgery is followed by radiation therapy. Although surgery in pituitary tumours is aimed mainly at preventing further visual loss, many patients show a rapid and sustained improve-

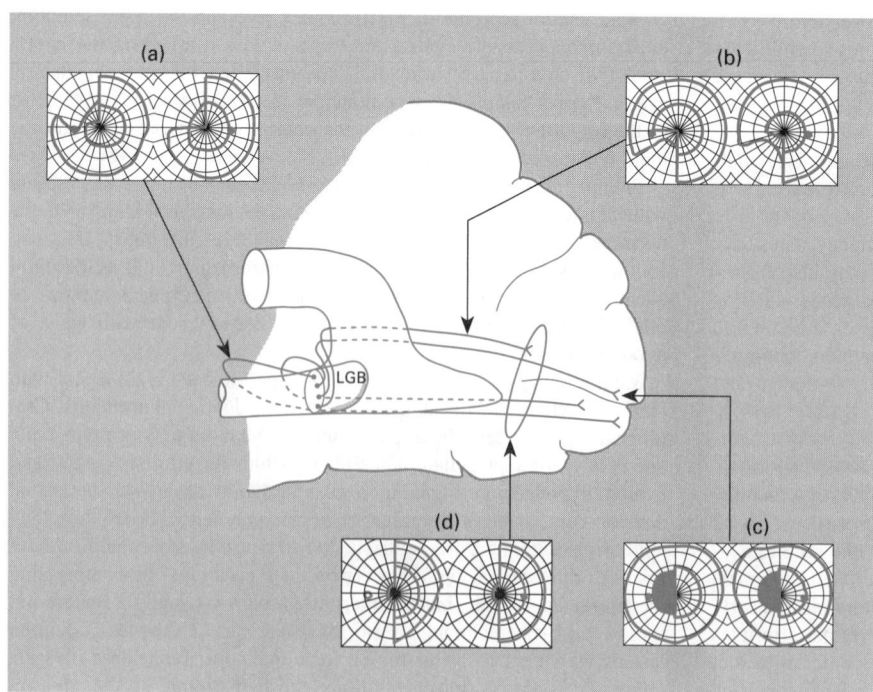

Fig. 3 Right cerebral hemisphere viewed from its medial aspect to show the geniculocalcarine pathway and the visual field defects produced by lesions at various points. (a) Lesion involving the lower fibres of the right optic radiation looping around the temporal horn of the lateral ventricle—left upper quadrantanopia. (b) Lesion involving the upper fibres of visual radiation in the posterior parietal lobe—left lower quadrantanopia. (c) Localized lesion of the calcarine cortex—left homonymous hemianopic scotomas. (d) Subcortical lesion involving the posterior visual radiation—complete left homonymous hemianopia.

ment following surgery, especially if the tumour is soft or haemorrhagic. Lifelong hormone replacement therapy is usually required.

OPTIC TRACT

Lesions of the optic tract are rare, the commonest being craniopharyngioma, an unusually placed pituitary adenoma, or following pituitary surgery. The visual field defect is homonymous but incongruous, i.e. it affects the two eyes to a different extent. Optic atrophy is often present and helps to distinguish this from a hemisphere lesion. There may be an afferent pupil defect in the eye contralateral to the lesion.

OPTIC RADIATION: PARIETAL LOBE

Cerebral tumours are the commonest type of lesion in this area. They are usually malignant gliomas but metastases and meningiomas may also occur. Vascular lesions include spontaneous cerebral haemorrhage and 'watershed' infarction affecting the border zone between the territories of the three main cerebral arteries. All these lesions tend to damage the upper fibres of the radiation, causing a homonymous lower quadrantanopia (Fig. 3(b)). In tumour cases the field defect may gradually enlarge to become complete, and optokinetic nystagmus is frequently lost when following a target to the side of the lesion. In addition to visual loss, there may be features of raised intracranial pressure and of epilepsy. Patients may also show other 'high level' visual perceptual defects, reflecting the different functions of the two hemispheres. Lesions of the dominant hemisphere (usually the left) produce dyslexia, dysgraphia, dyscalculia, right/left disorientation, and finger agnosia. On the non-dominant side, patients show left-sided neglect, geographical disorientation with difficulty in route finding, and dressing apraxia, in addition to a left-sided homonymous hemianopia.

OPTIC RADIATION: TEMPORAL LOBE

Lesions of the posterior temporal lobe may interrupt the lower fibres of the visual radiation, giving rise to an upper homonymous quadrantanopia (Fig. 3(a)). In the dominant hemisphere dysphasia and memory loss may also be present. Intrinsic tumours such as gliomas may show widely variable degrees of malignancy and tend to cause complex partial seizures, a type of focal epilepsy. Patients experience a dreamy state with partial loss of consciousness and with visual hallucinations, formed or unformed, motor automatisms and *déjà vu* (see also Chapter 24.4.1).

Other types of lesion in the temporal lobes are: abscesses originating from the inner ear, arteriovenous malformations, and cavernomas. The visual radiation is also a favoured site for the demyelinating plaques of multiple sclerosis, although these may occur without symptoms. External compression may result from meningioma, aneurysm, and pituitary tumour.

VISUAL CORTEX: OCCIPITAL LOBE

Lesions of the calcarine (visual) cortex give rise to a homonymous hemianopia, often complete, but with preserved central visual acuity (Fig. 3(c)). Usually this is an isolated defect without motor or sensory loss. Pupillary reactions to light are preserved and optokinetic nystagmus is normal to each side. Small lesions may produce congruous scotomatous defects (i.e. exactly the same in each eye). Focal epilepsy may occur in occipital lesions and may consist of unformed visual hallucinations of patterns of angular lines or colours, or of shimmering scotomas similar to the aura of migraine. The great majority of lesions in this area are ischaemic (Fig. 2(j)); the blood supply is from the posterior cerebral artery but the border zone between this territory and that of the middle cerebral artery runs close to the posterior pole. The 'macular sparing', which is a feature of vascular lesions, is probably explained by this alternative source of blood-supply to the posterior pole where the central visual field is represented. Other types of pathology include meningioma, glioma, and abscess. Berry aneurysms in this region are rare but arteriovenous angiomas and other types of vascular malformation, including the Sturge-Weber syndrome, may occur.

Simultaneous or successive occlusion of both posterior cerebral arteries causes a bilateral homonymous hemianopia or cortical blindness. Vision may be lost entirely, but more commonly a small central island of visual field is retained. Pupillary light reactions remain normal. These patients frequently show evidence of damage to other adjacent areas of cerebral cortex in the form of visual hallucinations and amnesia. Some may deny that they are blind (anosagnosia).

Other unusual defects that may occur in patients with bilateral vascular lesions include loss of colour vision (cerebral achromatopsia), loss of facial recognition (prosopagnosia), and visual disorientation, where the patient is unable to judge distance or size and has difficulty following and fixing on objects (Balint's syndrome). These defects usually indicate damage to visual association areas or connecting tracts. True visual agnosia, where the patient retains normal visual perception but is unable to recognize objects or their function, is a very rare defect but may occur, usually as a transient phenomenon in extensive lesions of the dominant hemisphere.

REFERENCE

Glaser, J.S. (1990). *Neuro-ophthalmology*. Harper and Row, Maryland.
Walsh, F.B. and Hoyt, W.F. (1969). *Clinical neuro-ophthalmology*. Williams and Wilkins, Baltimore.

24.3.5 The eighth cranial nerve

P. RUDGE

INTRODUCTION

The eighth cranial nerve has two components, namely, the auditory and vestibular parts. The auditory part of the eighth nerve innervates the cochlear sensory receptors; all the nerve fibres are myelinated and the myelin surrounds the cell bodies as well as the axons. The central auditory pathways are complex with multiple decussations; synapses occur in the cochlear nuclei, superior olivary complex, lateral lemnisci, inferior colliculi, and medial geniculate bodies. There are several cortical areas associated with hearing, including Heschl's gyrus, and a precise tonotopic organization is maintained to this level.

The vestibular nerve innervates two types of receptor, viz. the semicircular canals and the otolith organs (saccule and utricle). Angular acceleration in the three cardinal planes is detected by the semicircular canals, which partially integrate the signal to one of velocity. Linear acceleration (gravity) is detected in the sagittal and coronal planes by the otolith-bearing structures. Exceedingly complex connections between the second-order neurones of the vestibular nuclei pass to the somatic musculature, extraocular muscles, cerebellum, and cerebral cortex. In clinical medicine, connections to the extraocular muscles are the most important as they are concerned with the vestibulo-ocular reflex, which maintains the eye position relative to Earth and derangement of which gives clues to the site of pathology.

In addition to the two major afferent components of the eighth nerve there is an efferent supply to both the cochlear and vestibular end organs. The efferent supply to the cochlea is entirely inhibitory; it arises from the superior olivary complex and supplies the hair cells of both sides. Ninety-five per cent of all the efferent fibres innervate the outer hair cells and may be important in fine tuning of the frequency response. The efferent supply to the vestibular system is both excitatory and inhibitory; its function is unclear.

Symptoms and signs due to dysfunction of the eighth nerve

AUDITORY SYSTEM

Symptoms

Deafness is the cardinal feature of damage to the cochlea or its afferent pathways. Loss of hearing can be unilateral only if the disease process affects the end organ, eighth nerve, or cochlear nucleus. More central lesions cause symmetrical hearing loss, but significant deafness from such lesions is rare. Distortion of hearing is a frequent accompaniment of cochlear loss, as is tinnitus, but neither symptom is confined to such lesions.

Tests of auditory function

The first step in the investigation of a patient who complains of hearing loss is to determine if such a loss exists. This is done by means of pure-tone air conduction audiometry in which pulsed pure tones at octave intervals (approximately 250–8000 Hz) are administered via earphones and the sound pressure level varied. The level at which a tone is just heard is the threshold of hearing for that frequency.

Having determined that the patient does have a hearing loss, it is vital to ascertain by tuning fork tests whether the deafness is conductive or sensorineural. In the normal subject the cochlear hair cells can be stimulated via two routes: air conduction or bone conduction. The first can be tested by placing a tuning fork of 256 or 512 Hz adjacent to the external auditory meatus. The pressure waves set up in the air contained within the external auditory canal causes the tympanic membrane and ossicles to vibrate and transmit the sound waves to the cochlea. Bone conduction can be tested by placing a vibrating tuning fork against the skull which then transmits the signal directly to the hair cells. Since air conduction is much more efficient than bone conduction in normal individuals, a vibrating tuning fork placed adjacent to the external meatus until the sound is no longer detected cannot be heard if it is then placed on the skull. A similar situation exists if a sensorineural hearing loss is present; the abnormality involves the cochlea or its nerve fibres and this does not alter the relative efficiency of transduction of sound waves via the two routes to the cochlea. Conversely, if there is an abnormality of the external canal, such as the presence of wax, or of the ossicles, for example otosclerosis, the efficiency of only the air-conduction route will be impaired. In these circumstances sound will be transmitted more efficiently by bone conduction. To detect this phenomenon clinically, a vibrating tuning fork is placed adjacent to the external meatus until the sound is no longer heard; it is then placed on the mastoid process. The sound will again be detected if a conductive loss is present. This is known as the Rinne test. Similarly, if a vibrating tuning fork is placed on the teeth or forehead in a normal subject, the sound is located at the midline. On the other hand, in a unilateral sensorineural hearing loss the sound is appreciated towards the unimpaired side and with a conductive loss to the impaired side. This is the Weber test.

Having performed these basic clinical tests, it should be clear whether the patient has a conductive or sensorineural hearing loss. Conductive deafness will not be discussed further, as this is the province of the otologist. If sensorineural hearing loss is present, tests of loudness function, adaptation, and speech audiometry will help to differentiate that due to hair cell loss, for example Menière's disease, from that due to retrocochlear lesions such as eighth nerve tumours. The following account is a brief summary of the more commonly used tests.

Tests of recruitment (alternate loudness balance test, loudness discomfort level)

Loudness is a perception; it is partly dependent upon the intensity of the stimulus. In normal subjects a tone of given intensity applied to one ear can be matched for loudness to a tone of similar intensity applied to the other. It might be thought that if a subject has a unilateral hearing loss, a tone would appear to be of similar loudness in the two ears (one normal, the other impaired) if the intensity applied to the impaired ear was greater than that applied to the normal ear by an amount equal to the hearing loss. This is indeed the case in all conductive and some retrocochlear losses, but it does not hold for cochlear impairment, where growth of loudness with intensity is greater than anticipated. This phenomenon is known as recruitment and is the reason why older subjects suffering from presbyacusis ask one to speak up because of their hearing loss only to complain, when their instruction is obeyed, that there is no need to shout!

Recruitment can be assessed by two methods. The first is the alternate loudness balance test. This can only be used in cases of unilateral hearing loss. A tone of given intensity is applied to the normal ear and the patient attempts to match its loudness to a tone of the same frequency applied to the impaired ear. This is repeated at several intensities and frequencies. In cochlear hearing loss, recruitment occurs; indeed in some cases at high intensities the tone appears louder in the impaired ear, so-called over-recruitment. Conversely, in some cases of retrocochlear loss there is no recruitment; there may even be reversal of it, that is the rate of growth of loudness with increasing intensity declines. The second method, applicable to all cases of hearing loss, including those that are bilateral, is to use loudness discomfort levels. In this technique the intensity of a tone is increased until it is unpleasantly loud. This level is remarkably constant in normal subjects and in those with hair cell loss; it occurs at about 100 dB. Loudness discomfort levels are elevated in many patients with retrocochlear lesions.

Tests of tone decay

If a tone is applied to a normal ear at an intensity just above threshold it will continue to be heard indefinitely. In general this also applies to cochlear hearing loss. On the other hand, some patients with a retrocochlear hearing loss are only able to perceive the tone for a short time and its intensity has to be progressively increased for them to regain and maintain perception of the tone. This is known as tone decay, and the amount by which the intensity has to be increased is a measure of it. Tone decay can be marked in some, but not all, retrocochlear lesions.

Speech audiometry

The ability to discriminate phonetically balanced words can be determined by routine speech audiometry in which lists of words are presented at different intensities. From this it is possible to see if there is an intensity at which all the words are correctly identified and to plot an intensity-score graph (a speech audiogram). Although speech discrimination is frequently impaired in cochlear lesions, the impairment is disproportionately greater in retrocochlear disorders. Indeed, with retrocochlear lesions speech discrimination sometimes declines rather than improves at high intensity. This is known as the 'roll-over' phenomenon.

Stapedius reflex

If a high-intensity tone is applied to one ear, the stapedius muscle contracts bilaterally, thereby tensing the tympanic membrane and altering its conductance. The reflex depends upon the cochlea, the eighth nerve for the afferent input, and the seventh nerve for the efferent component, with connections between the two nerves within the brain-stem. In normal subjects a reflex is usually obtained for frequencies of 4 kHz or less at intensities of 85 to 100 dB. If the tone is maintained for 10 s, the reflex contraction shows little attenuation for frequencies of 500 and 1000 Hz, but there is some 'decay' at 2000 and 4000 Hz.

Cochlear hearing loss causes little alteration in the stapedius reflex threshold because of recruitment, and it does not show abnormal attenuation over 10 s. On the other hand, retrocochlear lesions such as acoustic neuromas characteristically raise the threshold of the reflex and cause its pathological 'decay'.

Brain-stem auditory evoked potentials

It is possible to record, via scalp electrodes, neural activity generated in response to a click stimulus by stimulus-locked averaging techniques. A series of components occurring within the first 10 ms arises from the eighth nerve and brain-stem auditory pathways. These are conventionally labelled I (distal auditory nerve), II (proximal auditory nerve and cochlear nuclei), III (trapezoid body or superior olivary complex; some believe that the cochlear nucleus is involved), IV (nuclei of the lateral lemnisci), and V (inferior colliculus) (Fig. 1). Components VI and VII and later waves arise from the diencephalic and cortical structures. Those arising after wave VII are classified by latency into middle and late components.

Brain-stem evoked potentials have proved to be of diagnostic value in two groups of disorders, namely, hearing loss and certain neurological conditions such as multiple sclerosis and coma. We shall confine our discussion to the former. If a click of high intensity is used as the stimulus, the effect of any recruiting hearing loss should be minimized. This is the case in cochlear lesions, for example Menière's disease, where there is little alteration in any of the components of the brain-stem auditory evoked potentials unless the hearing loss is severe (greater than 70 dB). On the other hand, non-recruiting hearing loss due to retrocochlear lesions, such as acoustic neuromas, causes marked changes in the brain-stem auditory evoked potentials: this may take the form of a loss of all components from the affected ear except component I, a marked delay of component V, or a greatly increase I–V interval compared with the normal side. Of considerable interest, however, is the fact that the brain-stem auditory evoked potential recording is frequently abnormal in retrocochlear lesions even if the hearing loss is a recruiting one, suggesting that the initial concept that it is the degree of recruitment that separates peripheral from retrocochlear lesions on brain-stem auditory evoked potential recording is wrong. Be that as it may, the test is extremely valuable (see Chapter 24.2.3).

Electrocochleography

The eighth nerve action potential is small and can be difficult to detect using scalp electrodes. By placing a needle electrode against the medial wall of the middle ear via the tympanic membrane it is possible to record a large eighth nerve action potential as well as the cochlear microphonic and summating potentials. This technique is useful for identifying component I of the brain-stem auditory evoked potentials and also in studying the morphology of component I in a number of conditions, including acoustic neuromata and Menière's disease.

Auditory acoustic emissions (echoes)

In 1978 Kemp found that if a pure tone is applied to a normal ear a mechanical response of similar frequency can be recorded from the external meatus, that is, there is an echo (Fig. 2). It seems that this response is dependent upon an intact cochlear end organ, especially the outer hair cells which, it will be recalled, have a large efferent supply. In clinical practice acoustic emission recording is becoming increasingly important; absence of an echo at a given frequency is good evidence of hair cell dysfunction in the part of the cochlea responding to that frequency. It is important to note that in some patients with eighth nerve tumours the echo is absent, possibly because the mass interferes with the cochlear blood supply, although efferent bundle disruption might be an alternative explanation.

VESTIBULAR SYSTEM

Symptoms

Damage to the vestibular receptors or their neural connections results in a mismatch of input between them (so-called tonus imbalance) and also with the other receptors signalling orientation in space, such as vision, proprioception, and joint position. This results in an unpleasant sensation of imbalance and vertigo which, in extreme cases, causes nausea and vomiting; the patient is reluctant to move and prefers to be in bed. Lesions are usually destructive and their effects are rapidly compensated centrally so that the patient becomes asymptomatic over a period of a few weeks. Exceptionally, compensation, which depends upon brain-stem structures including the olivary nuclei and cerebellum, is incomplete and the symptoms persist.

Nystagmus

Spontaneous nystagmus, which comes in many forms, confuses all clinicians and yet is an extremely useful sign of vestibular dysfunction. We shall begin our discussion with nystagmus in the horizontal plane. Conventionally, the direction of nystagmus is specified by the fast phase.

Fig. 1 Brain-stem auditory evoked potential from a normal subject. A stimulus was given at the arrow. Downward deflection indicates that the vertex electrode is positive relative to the ipsilateral mastoid electrode. The high-pass filter is arranged to accentuate component V. Components I to V arise from the eighth nerve and brain-stem structures (see text). Note: commercial machines vary in their polarity and filter settings.

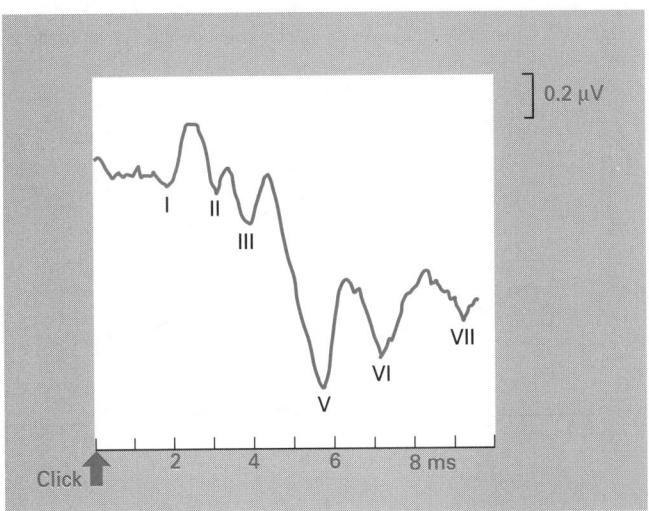

Fig. 2 Oto-acoustic emission from a normal subject. The click stimulus is shown top left. The duplicate (A, B) response is shown below. Note the echo beginning at about 3 ms. The power spectrum of the response is shown top right. The black area is noise obtained by subtracting A from B. The white area is the power spectrum of the cochlear response. A click artefact has been removed in the average trace by applying a rectangular window between 2.5 and 20 ms.

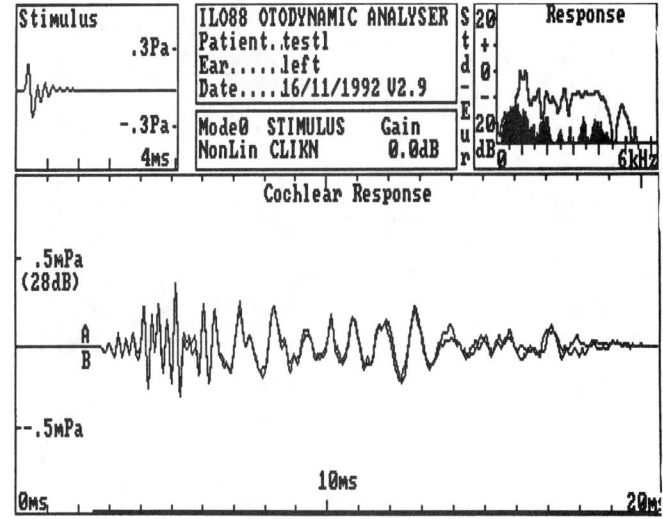

Vestibular nystagmus

The vestibular apparatus and nuclei are paired, one set on each side of the head. The horizontal canals, and the vestibular nuclei with which they connect, drive the eyes as a slow movement towards the opposite side. Thus in the normal subject equal and opposite forces act on the eye muscles, and the eyes remain central. Destruction of one set of vestibular end organs, their nerves or nuclei results in the eyes drifting towards that side as a slow movement (Fig. 3). This phenomenon arises because of the unopposed activity of the intact vestibular apparatus. It is rapidly detected and a counter movement is generated by another system, the saccadic (fast) generator lying in the paramedian pontine reticular formation (PPRF). This saccadic movement to one side is generated by the ipsilateral paramedian pontine reticular formation. Thus in a right-sided vestibular lesion the eyes are pushed slowly to the right by the intact left vestibular system and then are rapidly returned towards the midline under the influence of the left paramedian pontine reticular formation. Repetition of this results in vestibular nystagmus, with its characteristic saw-toothed wave form and fast phase to the side opposite the lesion.

Pulse-step mismatch and gaze-evoked nystagmus

Not all nystagmus is saw-toothed in form. In some cases the slow component is exponential in shape. When the eyes are deviated to one side there are viscous and elastic forces within the orbit opposing the deviation. To obtain a rapid movement (a saccade) it is necessary to innervate the horizontal recti muscles with a pulse of neural activity to overcome the viscous forces within the orbit, and to follow this with an increased tonic innervation (step) to overcome the elastic forces in order to maintain the eye in its eccentric position. This is achieved by burst and tonic cells in the paramedian pontine reticular formation and part of the abducens nucleus; in mathematical terms, the burst response is integrated to achieve tonic deviation. A variety of nystagmoi can be induced by malfunctioning of this system, but all have an exponential slow phase. If there is a mismatch between the pulse and the step (burst/

tonic activity) the pulse being too large, the eyes will drift exponentially towards the midline until a point is reached where the tonic innervation is sufficient to maintain the eccentric position. Each attempt to attain the target will result in the same mismatch and produce a series of usually diminishing saccades followed by an exponential slow phase, that is, nystagmus results. This type of nystagmus typically occurs in the abducting eye of an internuclear ophthalmoplegia.

Gaze-evoked nystagmus occurs when there is a failure of tonic innervation; in mathematical terms, the integrator is leaky. This results in the eyes returning exponentially to the midline after each attempted eccentric fixation. Such gaze-evoked nystagmus is found in a wide variety of conditions, including pontine and cerebellar lesions and after ingestion of drugs, particularly anticonvulsants.

Significance of horizontal nystagmus

Unilateral horizontal nystagmus, especially if its magnitude increases as the eyes are deviated in the direction of the fast phase (Alexander's law), is most commonly due to a peripheral lesion, but can occur with lesions of the eighth nerve or vestibular nucleus. On the other hand, horizontal nystagmus that occurs to both sides at the same time is invariably due to a central lesion.

Removal of optic fixation and recording the eye movements, either with electronystagmography (ENG) or by observing the eyes with an infrared viewer, also helps to differentiate between peripheral and central lesions. Characteristically, nystagmus due to a lesion of the end organ is enhanced by removal of fixation (Fig. 4), whereas that due to a central lesion, including vestibular nuclear lesions, is not. The pathway for this fixation suppression passes from the retina, especially the fovea, via the accessory olivary tract to the cerebellum and thence to the vestibular nuclei. Disruption of this central pathway means that vestibular nystagmus cannot be inhibited fully by fixation; that is, the nystagmus is little affected by removal of fixation. In contrast, if the pathway is intact, fixation inhibition can occur, as in normal subjects, and removal of fixation results in enhancement of the nystagmus, which is some cases is only apparent in darkness.

Disease processes usually damage all three semicircular canals on one side and the effect of this is identical to that of destruction of the horizontal canal alone, since the vertical vectors of the posterior and anterior canals are cancelled, leaving only the horizontal one. Selective damage to part of the semicircular canal system can result in oblique or rotatory nystagmus. In the above discussion it has been assumed that a lesion is a destructive one. If, in fact, it is irritative, the nystagmus is in the opposite sense.

Fig. 3 Diagrammatic explanation of vestibular nystagmus due to destruction of the right vestibular apparatus, nerve, or nucleus. The slow phase is represented on the right, the fast phase on the left, and summation of the two is revealed in the electronystagmogram (ENG) below. VN, vestibular nucleus; PPRF, paramedium pontine reticular formation.

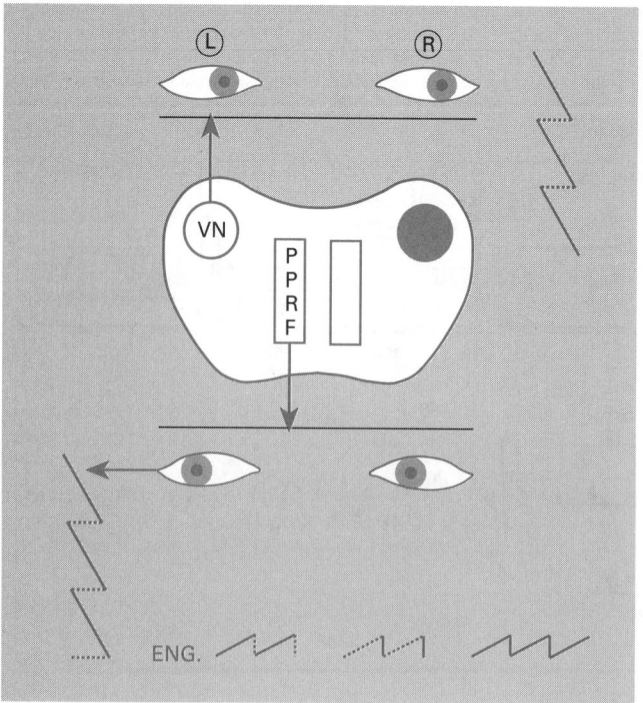

Fig. 4 Nystagmogram following left labyrinthectomy. Note the accentuation of the nystagmus as the gaze is directed towards the fast phase (Alexander's law), and the enhancement of the nystagmus and drift towards the damaged side with removal fixation at D. R, L, eyes deviated to right or left. P, eyes in the primary position.

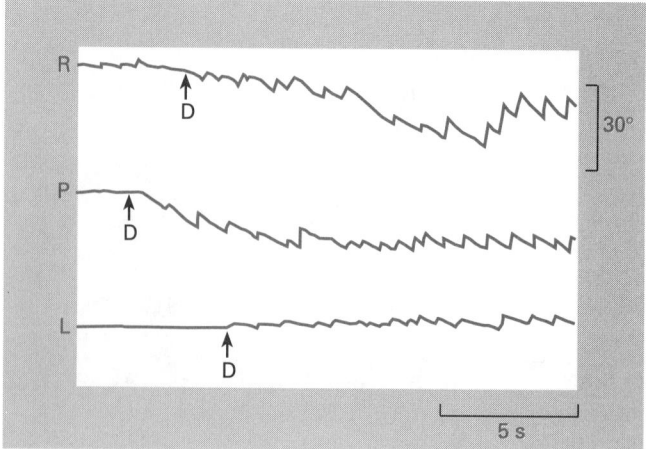

Vertical nystagmus

Although acquired spontaneous nystagmus in the vertical plane is virtually never due to an eighth cranial nerve disturbance, brief mention of it will be made here.

Up-beat nystagmus

The fast phase is upwards. It occurs in patients with lesions in the floor of the fourth ventricle, pontine tegmentum, and perhaps the anterior cerebellum. It rarely occurs in isolation, but is not infrequent in patients with an internuclear ophthalmoplegia.

Down-beat nystagmus

The fast phase is downwards. This is also uncommon. It indicates either a structural abnormality at the level of the foramen magnum, for example cerebellar tonsillar herniation or cerebellar dysfunction, especially an atrophic process. Characteristically, down-beat nystagmus is accentuated when the eyes are moved horizontally 30° to one side or the other. It is also sensitive to the position of the patient; for example, it may only be apparent in the supine position, disappearing when the patient is upright or prone. The importance of this type of nystagmus is that it may indicate the presence of a correctable abnormality.

Torsional clockwise or counterclockwise nystagmus

Rotation about the sagittal meridian is rare, but occurs in central lesions, especially those involving the medial vestibular nucleus, and in patients with cerebellar ectopia associated with syringomyelia.

Positional and positioning nystagmus

Nystagmus induced by altering the position of the head with respect to the gravitational field is known as positioning nystagmus, while that induced the by maintenance of such a position is positional nystagmus.

The best way to examine patients in the clinic is to have them sit on the couch in an upright position with the eyes open and the head rotated to the left or right. The head is grasped by the examiner and the patient instructed to fixate the examiner's forehead while the head is rapidly lowered below the horizontal over the end of the couch. Any nystagmus is noted and the patient then returned to the upright position. This is repeated with the head turned to the opposite shoulder. Basically two types of responses occur, one of which is due to a peripheral defect, the other to a central problem (Table 1).

Benign positional nystagmus

In this form there is a rotatory nystagmus with the fast phase towards the dependent ear—counterclockwise if the right ear is dependent, clockwise if the left ear is dependent. This nystagmus occurs after a latent interval of a few seconds and lasts for 10 to 20 s. It is accompanied by vertigo. On returning to the upright position a lesser nystagmus of opposite sense occurs. Repetition of the test results in an attenuation of the response, this adaptation lasting a number of hours. Classically, there is no nystagmus when the other ear is dependent.

Dix and Hallpike (1952) showed that this type of nystagmus is associated with utricular damage, and Schuknecht (1969) has proposed, on the basis of limited pathological studies, that debris from the damaged utricle collects on the cupula of the posterior semicircular canal, the lowermost part of the vestibular apparatus, such that its mass is greater than normal. The cupula is then sensitive to gravitational pull. When the head is in the inverted position the cupula moves under the influence of gravity and induces nystagmus. The debris rapidly falls from the underside of the cupula which then returns to its normal position and the nystagmus ceases. Repetition of this manoeuvre does not induce further nystagmus since the debris has not had time to reaccumulate on the cupula. Section of the posterior semicircular canal nerve cures the patient, supporting the concept of cupulolithiasis. In most cases, however, conservative therapy with vestibular sedatives or a course of head exercises to disperse the otoconial debris, and advice about head positioning are all that is necessary for this self-limiting condition.

Table 1 *Characteristics of positional nystagmus*

	Benign	Central
Direction	Towards lower ear	Any
Vertigo	++	±
Latent interval	+	0
Adaptation	+	0
Fatigue	+	0

++, severe; +, moderate; ±, slight; 0, absent.

Central positional nystagmus

This form of nystagmus differs from the above in that its direction is not towards the dependent ear; it may be in any direction and is persistent and often unassociated with vertigo. It is frequently produced by positioning on either side. It is thought that this form of nystagmus signifies a central lesion, especially one involving the vestibulocerebellum.

In practice, the vast majority of patients with benign positional nystagmus of classical type have a peripheral and benign lesion (often following head injury, or associated with hypertension or cervical spondylosis), while central positional nystagmus requires investigation to exclude a central nervous system disorder (for example, multiple sclerosis, tumour), although in a substantial proportion of cases no cause will be found.

Gait and stance

Damage to the vestibular apparatus results in an abnormality of stance and gait, since the vestibulospinal tracts carry inadequate information. The patient tends to fall towards the side of the lesion if it is destructive, and veers to that side when walking. These abnormalities are most marked if the eyes are closed and if the lesion is peripheral.

Tests of vestibular function

Nystagmus induced by either visual or vestibular stimuli can help the clinician determine the anatomical site of a lesion. Two vestibular investigations are commonly employed, namely, the caloric test and various rotational tests. Both these techniques examine the integrity of the semicircular canals and their connections. There are no routinely available tests with which to study otolith function.

Direct observation of induced eye movements can be of great value during these tests, especially during the caloric response, but recording of eye movements is invaluable for full assessment of the patient. Electronystagmography (ENG) is the most widely used technique for obtaining a permanent record of the induced eye movement, enabling accurate quantification to be made of nystagmus, saccades, and pursuit. The technique is dependent upon the vector of the corneoretinal potential during the various tests. A more accurate technique is to use a scleral coil, but at present this technique is solely a research one. Infrared recording is also used in some clinics and depends upon the reflection of electromagnetic waves in the infrared spectrum from the corneoscleral junction.

The caloric test

The bithermal binaural caloric test is the only way to assess the function of one horizontal semicircular canal system independently of the other. The head is placed such that the horizontal canal is vertical with the ampulla uppermost (the head is elevated 30° when the patient is lying supine). Irrigation with cold water (30 °C for 40 s) results in a movement of the endolymph away from the ampulla, while hot water (44 °C for 40 s) causes the reverse. Since the afferent nerves of the horizontal canal increase their firing rate with ampullopetal movement, hot water causes nystagmus towards the ipsilateral side and cold water nystagmus to the contralateral side. The duration of the nystagmic response to irrigation is assessed either visually or with electronystagmography; the latter technique enables other variables, such as the slow-phase velocity, to be determined.

Two sorts of abnormality occur. The first is reduced function from one side, known as a canal paresis, and implies unilateral damage to the vestibular apparatus, eighth nerve, or vestibular nucleus. The other type of abnormality is characterized by greater nystagmus in one direction than the other. This is known as a directional preponderance. It occurs with lesions in a wide variety of sites within the CNS, as well as with nerve or end-organ dysfunction. In the case of an acute destructive unilateral vestibular lesion, the directional preponderance is to the side opposite the lesion, that is, in the same direction as any spontaneous nystagmus. The presence of a directional preponderance in these circumstances implies incomplete compensation from such a lesion.

Rotational tests

Rotational tests are conducted by impulsively spinning patients, gradually accelerating them, or sinusoidally rotating them. The advantage of the technique compared with the caloric test is that it is possible to quantify the stimulus and therefore assess the sensitivity of the semicircular canals. The disadvantage is that both horizontal canals are tested simultaneously, one increasing and the other decreasing its firing rate. It is thus not possible to detect unilateral failure convincingly.

The effect of fixation upon nystagmus induced by either the caloric test or rotational stimuli can give important clues to the likely site of a lesion, in the same way as it does in the case of spontaneous nystagmus (see above). An easy way of assessing clinically the effect of fixation on nystagmus induced by rotational stimuli is to ask the patient to fixate a target which is clenched in the mouth and then to rotate the head horizontally in a sinusoidal motion at a fairly low velocity. In normal subjects nystagmus does not occur until the head velocity is 40 or 50 °/s, whereas in patients with a CNS lesion, fixation suppression may be entirely abolished and nystagmus readily elicited even at low velocities.

Optokinetic nystagmus

If a small, striped drum is rotated in front of the patient, nystagmus is induced. The fast phase is in the direction opposite to that of the drum rotation. This task is basically pursuit, and is foveally dependent. In the laboratory the patient can be surrounded by a striped curtain and full-field stimulation administered. This type of nystagmus depends upon the whole retina and is less dependent upon pursuit. Characteristically, optokinetic nystagmus is normal in peripheral compensated lesions, although there may be a directional preponderance if compensation is incomplete. On the other hand, it is frequently abnormal in central lesions, particularly those involving the cerebellum.

Specific disorders of the eighth nerve system

There are many affections of the eighth nerve and we can only cover one or two important ones.

CEREBELLOPONTINE ANGLE TUMOURS

Although all tumours of the cerebellopontine angle are rare, early diagnosis is important since the majority are benign, and morbidity of surgical removal is less if attempted when the tumours are small. About 70 per cent of the tumours are schwannomas, the remainder being meningiomas, epidermoids, neuromas of nerves other than the eighth, and a host of other rare lesions.

Acoustic schwannomas and neurofibromas
Pathology and incidence
Acoustic schwannomas usually arise on the vestibular nerves, especially the superior component. They are sporadic and are not more frequent in

patients with neurofibromatosis type I (NFI, von Recklinghausen's disease). Exceptionally, tumours are bilateral; this only occurs in neurofibromatosis type II (NFII, central neurofibromatosis). No age is exempt, but maximum incidence at presentation is in the fourth and fifth decades, except in the cases of neurofibromatosis type II, when the onset is earlier. The incidence is approximately equal in males and females.

Symptoms
The presenting symptom is typically a progressive hearing loss with unsteadiness. When the tumour protrudes beyond the internal acoustic porus, or arises more centrally, other cranial nerves are involved. The fifth nerve is particularly vulnerable; its involvement causes numbness of the face on the appropriate side. Larger tumours, which compress the brain-stem, cause increasing unsteadiness and, ultimately, in untreated cases, hydrocephalus. Occipital headache is a frequent symptom of acoustic tumours, even before hydrocephalus develops.

Signs
The hearing loss is sensorineural, and in many patients with small tumours it has the features of a cochlear rather than a retrocochlear origin—there is recruitment and reasonably preserved speech reception. Later, as the tumour enlarges, the classical signs of a retrocochlear hearing loss occur. The stapedius reflex is abnormal with elevated thresholds and abnormal decay of the response in a high proportion of cases.

Brain-stem evoked potentials are the best non-invasive auditory functional test for the detection of cerebellopontine angle tumours, especially acoustic schwannomas. Abnormalities, which are found in over 90 per cent of cases, include a total absence of all components beyond wave I or an increased delay of component V on stimulation of the 'tumour' ear, and an abnormally large difference between components V (ITV) or of the I–V intervals (IT I–V) obtained on stimulation of the 'tumour' and 'non-tumour' ears, respectively (Fig. 5). Abnormal brain-stem evoked potentials on stimulation of the normal ear occur with large tumours. Since in Ménière's disease there is little alteration of the brain-stem evoked potential until the hearing loss is severe (> 70 dB), this test has considerable specificity and can be used to separate many cases of peripheral hearing loss from that due to cerebellopontine angle tumours.

Vestibular function is also abnormal in a high proportion of patients. The majority have a canal paresis on caloric testing by the time they present to the clinician. They veer to the side of the lesion and Romberg's test is often positive. Nystagmus develops in all patients at some time during their illness. Initially there is vestibular nystagmus to the

Fig. 5 Brain-stem auditory evoked potential (BAEP) from a patient with a left-sided cerebellopontine angle tumour. Audiogram inset. Note the abnormal morphology of the BAEP obtained from stimulation of the left ear, with marked delay of component V, and a normal response obtained on stimulation of the right ear, i.e. ITV markedly increased.

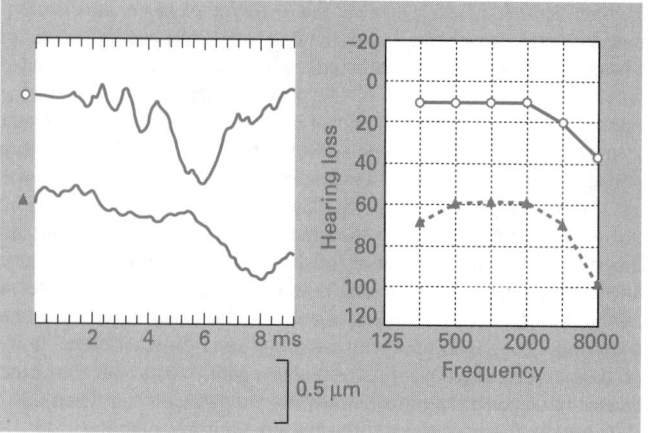

side opposite the tumour; later, when the tumour is large and impinges upon the brain-stem, a gaze-evoked nystagmus towards the side of the lesion is found.

Fifth nerve signs, especially loss of the corneal reflex, are found with large tumours, but, surprisingly, facial weakness is not a prominent sign in many cases. Long-tract signs, especially mild ipsilateral pyramidal features such as hyper-reflexia, are found when the tumours impinge upon the brain-stem.

OTHER TUMOURS

Meningiomas (which are more common in females) and epidermoids are much rarer than acoustic schwannomas, but can mimic the latter. Hearing loss is, in general, less severe and the caloric responses are more frequently normal. The brain-stem evoked potentials from the unimpaired ear are usually normal, even with large tumours.

IMAGING AND TREATMENT

Nuclear magnetic resonance scanning is the best way to demonstrate cerebellopontine angle tumours, especially intracanalicular acoustic tumours. Gadolinium enhancement is essential (Fig. 6). Other techniques, such as computed tomography rarely add information unless imaging of the bone is required.

Surgical removal is the only curative therapy. Morbidity is directly related to the size of the tumour. It is very rare to save hearing, although the seventh nerve can be preserved with modern techniques. Morbidity in terms of hearing loss may be lessened if interoperative brain-stem evoked recording is undertaken. If the tumours are bilateral, it is important to teach the patient to lip-read before operating upon the tumour, if possible.

Fig. 6 Magnetic resonance image of a patient with a right acoustic schwannoma. Above, unenhanced T_1-weighted image; below, gadolinium-enhanced image. The tumour is indicated by an arrow. The image was obtained on a 0.5 scanner, demonstrating that adequate images can be obtained with early generation, low-field machines.

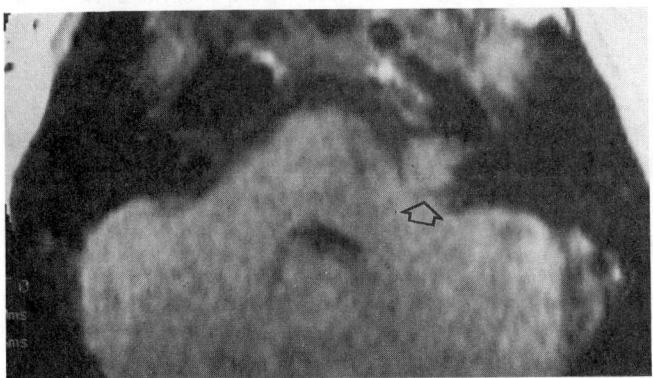

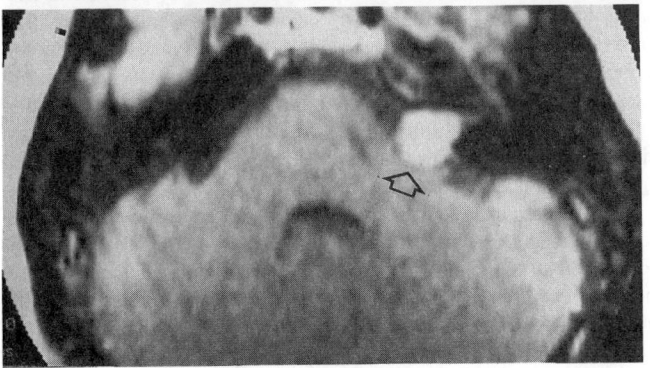

MENIÈRE'S DISEASE

Pathology

Menière's disease is an uncommon condition associated with endolymphatic hydrops involving the pars inferior of the otic capsule. Its cause is unknown. No age is immune, but the peak incidence of the onset of vertigo is in the fourth and fifth decades. Although it appears that females are more frequently affected, there is probably no sexual predominance if only definite cases are considered.

Symptoms

The triad of episodic vertigo, tinnitus, and fluctuating hearing loss are the classical features of Menière's disease. There is often a premonitory symptom of fullness of the appropriate ear. Initially the hearing loss recovers between the attacks, but later it becomes permanent and progressive. Tinnitus is a constant feature which typically increases during the attacks. Vertigo is the most distressing symptom and the patient is usually prostrated with nausea and vomiting. It lasts less than 24 h. The attacks occur in clusters with weeks or months free; the remissions are longer as the disease progresses.

Signs

Characteristically, the hearing loss in Menière's disease is initially of low frequency, but later severe loss (about 60 dB) at all frequencies occurs. Loudness function studies indicate that the hearing loss is peripheral in origin, and in some cases the recruitment can be extremely marked, such that at high intensity the sound seems louder in the impaired than in the good ear, so-called over-recruitment. The hearing loss becomes bilateral in 10 to 25 per cent of patients.

Loss of vestibular function is frequently bilateral. A canal paresis on one or both sides is typical. Nystagmus is seen in all patients during the acute episode and tends to be towards the affected ear at the time of an attack. During the quiescent phase of the disease the nystagmus is often present when fixation is removed, but its direction is variable even in apparently unilateral disease.

Brain-stem auditory evoked potentials are classically normal until the deafness is severe, when there is an increase in latency of the later components. Dehydration tests (for example, giving glycerol), are useful in diagnosis, the pure-tone audiogram typically improving during the test in Menière's disease, but not in other causes of sensorineural hearing loss.

Treatment

A low-salt diet and administration of diuretics is of value in reducing the severity and frequency of attacks of vertigo. Betahistine (8 to 16 mg, three times daily) may also reduce attacks, probably from its action on the stria vascularis. Surgical therapy in the form of saccus decompression has its advocates, although there is no good evidence as to its efficacy.

OTHER VESTIBULAR DISTURBANCES

Episodic vertigo

Many systemic conditions (for example, arteritis, diabetes, hypertension, and genetically determined system degenerations) can cause vestibular or auditory failure. Space does not permit a discussion of these, but the reader is referred to the monographs by Konigsmark and Gorlin (1976), Rudge (1983), and Winter and Baraitser (database) for a detailed discussion of many such disorders.

Mention must be made, however, of that common clinical problem, the patient with episodic vertigo not usually accompanied by deafness. Not all patients with episodic vertigo have Menière's disease. Indeed, the majority do not. An occasional patient has syphilis. Syphilis can mimic Menière's disease completely. An interesting feature of syphilis confined to the eighth nerve system is that the deafness is often progressive in spite of treatment with penicillin. It is mandatory to do fluorescent treponemal antibody tests in anyone presenting with a Ménière's syndrome. Migraine is a disorder that profoundly affects the vestibular system and, to a lesser extent, hearing. Acute attacks of migraine are frequently associated with vestibular abnormalities (vertigo, nausea, and vomiting) and auditory dysfunction (phonophobia), both in the basilar artery form as well as in classical migraine. In addition, patients who have had migraine in the past occasionally develop sporadic vertigo unaccompanied by headache; the cause is unknown.

Vestibular neuronitis is a syndrome of paroxysmal vertigo, first described by Dix and Hallpike (1952). They thought the abnormality was in Scarpa's ganglion and, indeed, the evidence for this has been found at autopsy. The syndrome is, however, common and found particularly in patients with hypertension and following systemic viral infections, where the term 'neuronitis' implies an unwarranted precision of diagnosis. The symptoms result from an episode of vestibular failure of which neuronitis is but one cause.

Finally, we should mention vestibular failure as an uncommon complication of aminoglycoside toxicity, usually in elderly patients with renal impairment. These patients classically complain initially of a visual disturbance with oscillopsia due to loss of the vestibulo-ocular reflex, rather than vertigo or aural symptoms; there is no mechanism that can substitute for the vestibulo-ocular reflex in stabilizing the eyes at high frequencies of head movement (> 1 Hz). Auditory function is usually preserved with the aminoglycosides that are now in clinical use, for example gentamicin. There is no way of detecting incipient vestibular failure due to these agents: careful prescribing and measurement of blood levels of gentamicin is the best precaution, and therapy should be stopped if vertigo occurs, provided alternative antibiotics are available.

Treatment of the vertiginous patient

During an episode of acute vestibular failure, patients are understandably terrified and fear that they are about to die. They require reassurance that they will recover, and should be put to bed and told not to move their heads. Vestibular sedatives such as prochlorperazine (12.5 mg intramuscularly) will be required if the patient is vomiting. Oral therapy can be given as soon as vomiting ceases. A wide variety of such sedatives is available, none of which is ideal; in general, a combination of sympathomimetic and anti-parasympathomimetic drugs is the most efficient way of lessening symptoms, although in clinical practice anticholinergic drugs alone are usually given. Cinnarizine (15 mg, three times a day) or prochlorperazine (5 mg, three times a day) are the most commonly prescribed agents and are moderately effective. Usually, the drugs can be discontinued after 2 to 4 weeks and most patients have recovered completely by this time.

Occasionally symptoms persist. Sometimes this may take the form of benign positional vertigo, for which vestibular sedatives, head exercises, and advice about lying down are all that is required. Other patients are frightened to walk and need vestibular exercises to retrain their vestibular system, using input from other sensory modalities. Some patients are helped by clonazepam, partly because of its sedative properties, but also by its central action on the vestibular system. Such patients may require psychiatric help even though they have a good organic cause for their vertigo.

CONCLUSION

The eighth nerve innervates the two most important sensory organs. Complete loss of the auditory component is a major disaster for any patient, while loss of the vestibular element can be socially and physically crippling. Careful assessment of these two elements is an essential prerequisite for adequate management of the patient who complains of deafness, distortion of hearing, imbalance, or vertigo.

REFERENCES

Brandt, T. and Daroff, R.B. (1980). The multisensory physiological and pathological vertigo syndromes. *Annals of Neurology*, **7**, 195–203.

Dix, M.R. and Hallpike, C.S. (1952). The pathology, symptomatology and diagnosis of certain disorders of the vestibular system. *Proceedings of the Royal Society of Medicine, London* **45**, 341–54.

Eggermont, J.J., Don, M., and Brackmann, D.E. (1980). Electrocochleography and auditory brain stem electric response in patients with pontine angle tumours. *Annals of Otology Rhinology and Laryngology* **89**, (Suppl. 75), 1–19.

Fisher, A., Gresty, M., Chambers, B., and Rudge, P. (1983). Primary position upbeating nystagmus: a variety of central positional nystagmus. *Brain* **106**, 949–64.

Halmagyi, G.M., Rudge, P., Gresty, M.A., and Sanders, M.D. (1983). Downbeating nystagmus: A review of 62 cases. *Archives of Neurology* **40**, 777–84.

Johnson, E.W. (1977). Auditory test results in 500 cases of acoustic neuroma. *Archives of Otolaryngology* **103**, 152–8.

Katz, J. (1972). *Handbook of clinical audiology*. Williams and Wilkins, Baltimore.

Kemp, D.T., Ryan, S., and Bray, P. (1990). A guide to the effective use of oto-acoustic emissions. *Ear and Hearing* **11**, 93–105.

Konigsmark, B.W. and Gorlin, R.J. (1976). *Genetic and metabolic deafness*. W.B. Saunders, Philadelphia.

Korres, S. (1978a). Electro-nystagmographic criteria in neuro-otological diagnosis 1: Peripheral lesions. *Journal of Neurology Neurosurgery and Psychiatry* **41**, 249–53.

Korres, S. (1978b). Electro-nystagmographic criteria in neuro-otological diagnosis 2: Central nervous system lesions. *Journal of Neurology Neurosurgery and Psychiatry* **41**, 214–64.

Leigh, R.J. and Zee, D.S. (1991). *The neurology of eye movements*. F.A. Davies, Philadelphia.

Oosterveld, W.J. (1983). *Ménière's disease*. John Wiley and Sons, Chichester.

Robinson, K. and Rudge, P. (1983). The differential diagnosis of cerebellopontine angle lesions. *Journal of Neurological Science* **60**, 1–21.

Rudge, P. (1983). *Clinical neuro-otology*. Churchill Livingstone, Edinburgh.

Schuknecht, H.F. (1969). Cupulolithiasis. *Archives of Otolaryngology* **90**, 765–78.

Selters, W.A. and Brackmann, D.E. (1977). Acoustic tumour detection with brainstem electric response audiometry. *Archives of Otolaryngology* **103**, 181–7.

Thomas, K. and Harring, M.S. (1971). Long term follow up of 610 cases of Ménière's disease. *Proceedings of the Royal Society of Medicine, London* **64**, 853–66.

Winter, R.M. and Baraitser, M. London dysmorphology database. Oxford University Press.

24.3.6 Other cranial nerves

P. K. THOMAS

The olfactory nerve

Loss of the sense of smell (anosmia) is most commonly encountered as a sequel to head injury and is probably related to severance of the central processes of the neurones of the olfactory mucosa as they pass through the cribriform plate to the olfactory bulb. It is usually permanent. Distortion of olfaction (parosmia) may occur and may be persistent. The sense of smell is occasionally congenitally absent or may be acutely and permanently lost after a coryzal infection. Bilateral anosmia is frequently accompanied by impairment of taste related to reduced detection of the volatile substances that impart flavours to foods. Unilateral anosmia may occur in olfactory groove meningiomas or other subfrontal tumours. This is usually not detected by the patient.

The central connections of the olfactory pathways are complex and include projections to the temporal lobes, hypothalamus, the septal region, and the amygdaloid nuclei. Olfactory hallucinations are well known to occur as a manifestation of temporal lobe epilepsy. Identification of odours may be impaired after bilateral medial temporal lesions and may be defective in multiple sclerosis, possibly as the result of demyelination in the olfactory tracts. Complaints of hypersensitivity of the sense of smell commonly have a psychoneurotic basis and persistent olfactory hallucinations may be reported by psychotic patients. Persistent parosmia is sometimes produced by temporal lobe lesions.

Third, fourth, and sixth cranial nerves

The third, or oculomotor, nerve supplies all the external ocular muscles with the exception of the superior oblique and lateral rectus. It also carries the parasympathetic innervation of the pupilloconstrictor fibres of the iris. A complete third nerve lesion produces a dilated and unreactive pupil, complete ptosis, and loss of upward, downward, and medial movement of the eye. The eye becomes deviated downwards and laterally. Diplopia is only experienced when the lid is held up.

The fourth or trochlear nerve supplies the superior oblique muscle. Following a lesion of this nerve, there is extorsion of the eye when the patient looks outwards. When the patient looks downwards and medially, diplopia is experienced. This is particularly disturbing because of its occurrence on looking downwards and produces difficulty in walking and in descending stairs. The patient may compensate for this by tilting the head to the opposite side.

The sixth or abducens nerve supplies the lateral rectus. A lesion of this nerve causes convergent strabismus, and inability to abduct the affected eye, and diplopia which is maximal on lateral gaze to the affected side.

The third, fourth, and sixth nerves may be affected singly or in combination and the paralysis may be complete or partial. In some instances, the lesion is within the brain-stem, where it may affect either the nuclei or intramedullary portion of the nerve fibres. In older patients, the commonest causes are brain-stem vascular disease and neoplasms.

Extramedullary lesions of the third, fourth, and sixth nerves are more frequent and may occur at any point along their course, either intracranially or within the orbit. A third nerve palsy may develop in the region of the tentorial hiatus as a false localizing sign related to brain-stem displacement produced by supratentorial space-occupying conditions. Unilateral or bilateral sixth nerve palsies may also arise as a consequence of raised intracranial pressure, probably caused by traction, again secondary to brain-stem displacement. These nerves can be involved singly or together in conditions such as chronic basal meningitis or carcinomas of the skull base. Gradenigo's syndrome comprises a sixth nerve palsy and pain of trigeminal distribution. It is produced by a lesion at the apex of the petrous temporal bone. As this syndrome was most commonly infective in origin and related to chronic middle ear disease, it is now encountered considerably less frequently.

The third, fourth, and sixth nerves traverse the cavernous sinus, as do the first and second divisions of the trigeminal nerve. In this situation, they are most commonly damaged by an intracavernous aneurysm of the internal carotid artery. The third nerve is affected more often than the fourth and sixth. The consequent internal and external ophthalmoplegia is frequently accompanied by pain, and sometimes sensory loss and paraesthesiae, in the corresponding frontal region related to compression of the first division of the trigeminal nerve, and occasionally in the cheek from damage to the maxillary division. In the superior orbital fissure syndrome, caused for example by a tumour invading the fissure, a total ophthalmoplegia may result, associated with pain and sensory loss in the distribution of the first division of the trigeminal nerve. The eye is often proptosed because of obstruction of the ophthalmic vein. The Tolosa–Hunt syndrome consists of a painful external ophthalmoplegia related to a granulomatous angiitis. Within the orbit, the third, fourth, and sixth nerves may be affected by conditions such as tumours and granulomas. They may be damaged as a result of trauma at any point along their course and may be affected singly or in combination as part of a cranial neuropathy, of which diabetes, the Miller Fisher syndrome, Lyme borreliosis, and sarcoidosis are the most important examples.

Internal and external ophthalmoplegias are common and this list of causes is by no means exhaustive.

Pupillary abnormalities

Constriction of the pupil (miosis) occurs as a result of paralysis of the sympathetic innervation of the pupillodilator fibres of the iris and may be accompanied by the other features of Horner's syndrome, namely a mild ptosis, and vasodilatation and anhidrosis of the face on the same side. The ocular manifestations may be encountered alone if the damage is restricted to the intracranial portion of the sympathetic plexus around the carotid artery. Raeder's syndrome consists of these components of Horner's syndrome together with involvement of the first division of the trigeminal nerve. It may be caused by tumours of the skull base. Miosis may also be produced by the local action of cholinergic drugs and by morphine and related compounds.

Pupillary dilatation may be caused by lesions of the third nerve, although it is of interest that the isolated third nerve palsies of presumed vascular origin that may occur in diabetes mellitus, in contradistinction to compressive lesions of the nerve, characteristically spare the pupil. Anticholinergic drugs such as atropine and related substances give rise to pupillary dilatation, as does cocaine.

The Argyll Robertson pupil is small, fails to react to light, but constricts on ocular convergence, and, if bilateral, the pupils are frequently unequal in size (anisocoria). The pupil may be irregular in outline and it does not dilate fully in response to mydriatics. Argyll Robertson pupils are almost always related to neurosyphilis but somewhat similar pupils are occasionally encountered in diabetic neuropathy and in some hereditary neuropathies.

The myotonic pupil (Holmes–Adie syndrome) reacts abnormally slowly both to light and on convergence, but particularly so for the response to illumination. A very bright light may be required to demonstrate any pupillary constriction, or if the patient remains in a dark room for some minutes, the pupil slowly dilates. The condition may be unilateral or bilateral and is commoner in women than men. Myotonic pupils may be associated with absence or depression of the tendon reflexes and occasionally with anhidrosis in the limbs.

Trigeminal nerve

The fifth cranial nerve is predominantly sensory in function, but also innervates the muscles of mastication. It emerges from the pons and runs forward to the Gasserian ganglion which is situated in Meckel's cave near the apex of the petrous temporal bone. The three sensory divisions of the nerve run anteriorly from the ganglion. The first or frontal division passes through the cavernous sinus and the superior orbital fissure. Its branches supply sensation to the anterior part of the scalp, the forehead, and the eye, including the conjunctiva and cornea. The second or maxillary division leaves the skull through the foramen rotundum, traverses the infraorbital canal, and supplies the cheek. The mandibular division emerges from the skull through the foramen ovale to reach the infratemporal fossa with the motor root with which it unites to form a single trunk. It is distributed to the lower lip, chin, and the lower part of the cheek, and its auriculotemporal branch supplies part of the ear and temporal area. It also supplies the inner aspect of the cheek and the anterior two-thirds of the tongue, and its lingual branch carries taste fibres from the anterior two-thirds of the tongue which leave it in the chorda tympani to join the facial nerve. It is important that the skin over the angle of the jaw is supplied from the second cervical nerve root, and the absence of this 'trigeminal notch' may be useful in distinguishing hysterical loss of sensation on the face which usually follows the angle of the jaw. The motor root innervates the temporalis muscle, the masseter, the pterygoids, mylohyoid, the anterior belly of the digastric, and also tensor tympani and tensor palati. With unilateral paralysis of the masticatory muscles, the jaw deviates towards the affected side on opening because of the action of the unopposed external pterygoid on the unaffected side.

The trigeminal nerve may be affected by intramedullary lesions, it may be damaged during the intracranial part of its course, or its branches may be compromised extracranially. An acoustic neurinoma may compress the nerve in the posterior fossa or the nucleus of the descending root may be affected by direct compression of the brain-stem by this tumour. Loss of corneal sensation is usually the earliest feature. Reference has already been made to involvement of the nerve in association with damage to the sixth nerve at the apex of the petrous temporal bone (Gradenigo's syndrome), as has involvement of the first and second divisions in the cavernous sinus, or the first division in the superior orbital fissure.

Trigeminal neuralgia

SYMPTOMS

This condition is characterized by paroxysms of intense pain strictly confined to the distribution of the trigeminal nerve. In most cases the cause is unknown. It is generally encountered in individuals over the age of 50. In younger patients it may be due to multiple sclerosis. Rarely, compression of the nerve, for example by tumours in the cerebellopontine angle, is responsible.

The salient feature of the disorder is pain which is usually unilateral and is felt either within the territory of one division of the nerve only, or may involve two adjacent divisions or affect the whole territory of the nerve. Less commonly it is bilateral.

The pain occurs in brief searing paroxysms, each attack lasting only a matter of seconds. The pain is often described as piercing or knife-like. Its intense quality may cause the patient to screw up his face in agony, hence the use of the term *tic douloureux* to describe the condition. The paroxysms may be spontaneous or provoked by movements of the face and jaw, by touching the skin, or by draughts of cold air on the face. Eating and speaking may become extremely difficult. 'Trigger spots' on the skin of the face may be present, the touching of which provokes the paroxysms. The attacks may be followed by less severe pain of a dull, boring character and by tenderness of the skin in the affected area. Fortunately the attacks usually cease at night.

The quality of the pain is characteristic, and when trigeminal neuralgia is present, the diagnosis is not usually missed, especially if a paroxysm is witnessed. The usual mistake is to regard as trigeminal neuralgia pain that is due to some other cause, and since there are many conditions that give rise to facial pain, the opportunities for error are numerous. Pain that is of a continuous character is not trigeminal neuralgia and some other cause must be sought. Absence of provocation by eating, talking, or the touching of trigger spots also makes the diagnosis unlikely. Once the diagnosis is accepted, it is essential to exclude compressive lesions affecting the nerve.

In the early stages, remissions lasting for months or years are usual, but in older patients remissions, if they occur, are likely to be brief. In all cases the remissions tend to become shorter as time goes on, and without treatment the condition persists for the rest of the patient's life.

The distribution of the pain is usually in one or two divisions of the nerve. The first division is rarely affected primarily, but pain may spread into it from the second division. If the pain begins in the second division it may, after a time, affect the third, and vice versa.

TREATMENT

The introduction of carbamazepine revolutionized treatment of this distressing condition. In a high proportion of cases, the paroxysms can be abolished or reduced. A dosage of 200 mg three to five times per day is employed. Ataxia and drowsiness may be troublesome side-effects with higher dosages, and aggravation of ataxia even with modest dosages may impede treatment in cases of multiple sclerosis. Hypersensi-

tivity reactions producing skin rashes or, rarely, bone marrow depression may develop but are, fortunately, uncommon.

If carbamazepine is not successful, or if the patients fail to tolerate it, other drugs such as phenytoin or clonazepam can be tried, but they are rarely effective. In this event, thermocoagulation of the ganglion may have to be considered. This should be undertaken only if the disorder is established so that a prolonged natural remission is unlikely to occur. It should also not be undertaken unless the patient is completely unable to tolerate the disorder, despite analgesics and sedation, and if he is fully aware of the consequences. The persistent analgesia and sometimes dysaesthesiae may subsequently be troublesome, and when the first division is made anaesthetic, damage to the conjunctiva leading to corneal scarring has to be avoided. It may be possible to limit the anaesthesia to the affected area, sparing, for instance, the eye if the first division is not involved in the pain. If thermocoagulation fails, section of the sensory root by a posterior fossa approach employing a microsurgical technique is indicated.

Ophthalmic herpes zoster

In elderly individuals, the fifth nerve is prone to involvement in herpes zoster, the first division being most vulnerable, giving rise to the distressing condition of ophthalmic herpes. The clinical features and treatment of herpes zoster are considered elsewhere (see Chapter 24.2.5). An unfortunate sequel may be visual impairment from residual corneal scarring. Particularly in older subjects, post-herpetic neuralgia may also be a sequel. This gives rise to persistent and unremitting spontaneous pain associated with cutaneous hyperaesthesia in the affected area. Treatment is difficult. Analgesics, sedation, and antidepressive preparations to combat the secondary depression that is frequently present may be of some assistance.

Isolated trigeminal neuropathy

Rarely, a chronic isolated unilateral or bilateral affection of the trigeminal nerve may occur as a manifestation of Sjögren's syndrome or systemic lupus erythematosus, although most cases are idiopathic. Extensive nasal scarring and tissue loss may occur secondary to repeated injury from picking and scratching.

Facial nerve

The seventh cranial nerve is largely motor. The nerve traverses the facial canal in the petrous temporal bone in close relationship to the middle ear and emerges at the stylomastoid foramen. Its branches pass forward through the parotid gland to be distributed to the muscles of the face, including the platysma. Within the petrous bone, a branch is given to the stapedius muscle. The chorda tympani, carrying the taste fibres from the anterior two-thirds of the tongue joins the nerve within the facial canal and a small branch supplies cutaneous sensation to the region of the external auditory meatus. The nerve also carries preganglionic parasympathetic fibres destined for the lachrymal gland.

The distinction between upper and lower motor neurone lesions of the facial muscles is usually easy. In general, with upper motor neurone lesions there is a relative preservation of power in the upper facial muscles, because these have a bilateral innervation from the cerebral hemispheres. There is no loss of tone with upper motor neurone lesions, so that the sagging of the face that is an unsightly feature of lower motor neurone palsy does not occur.

In common with the trigeminal nerve, the facial nerve may be affected by tumours in the cerebellopontine angle. In the past, it was often involved from middle-ear infections. It may be involved in meningeal carcinomatosis, fractures and tumours of the skull base, in a variety of cranial neuropathies, and cephalic herpes zoster, but the most common lesion by far is Bell's palsy. More peripherally, the nerve may be implicated in tumours of the parotid gland.

Bell's palsy

This term describes a usually unilateral facial paralysis of relatively rapid onset related to a lesion of the nerve within the facial canal. Taste may also be affected. It may develop at any age, most commonly between 20 and 50 years, and affects both sexes equally. Its causation is unknown. In the acute stage, the nerve is swollen and compression within the facial canal may contribute to the nerve fibre damage.

The onset is rapid and is frequently heralded or accompanied by aching pain below the ear or in the mastoid region. This clears within a few days and is not present in every case. The paralysis usually reaches its maximum severity after 1 or 2 days but occasionally progresses over the course of several days. Complete paralysis may occur. In the lower face, this may cause a mild dysarthria and some difficulty in eating because of food collecting between the gums and the inner sides of the cheek and the escape of fluid when drinking. The face sags and on smiling is drawn across to the unaffected side. Paralysis of orbicularis oculi renders voluntary eye closure impossible and, particularly in the older subject, ectropion develops. This can result in conjunctival injury from foreign bodies or conjunctivitis. If the paralysis is partial, the lower face is usually affected to a greater extent than the upper.

In the more severe cases, loss of taste over the anterior two-thirds of the tongue is often present, and paralysis of the stapedius muscle may result in a lack of tolerance for high-pitched or loud sounds.

Bell's palsy has to be distinguished from selective lesions of the facial nerve within the brain-stem, in which instance taste will not be affected. A facial paralysis superficially resembling Bell's palsy may occur in multiple sclerosis, in which event evidence of more widespread neurological disease may well be detected on examination, or the history may indicate episodes of neurological disturbance in the past. With respect to peripheral lesions, middle-ear disease requires exclusion. Facial paralysis related to cephalic herpes zoster is discussed below. A lesion of the facial nerve may represent a mononeuropathy from some generalized disorder of which diabetes, Lyme borreliosis, and sarcoidosis are the most important. Bell's palsy is rarely bilateral and the occurrence of bilateral facial paralysis would raise the possibility of the Guillain–Barré syndrome. This may begin with facial weakness, or the weakness may remain restricted to the facial musculature. The occurrence of bilateral facial weakness would also raise the possibility of sarcoidosis.

In approximately 85 per cent of cases of Bell's palsy, the paralysis is the result of a local conduction block within the facial canal without axonal degeneration and this is effectively the situation in all instances of mild weakness. The conduction block is presumably the consequence of segmental demyelination. Providing that such cases do not progress to more severe weakness, all recover fully within a few weeks. In cases where there is total paralysis, a proportion of these will be the result of a conduction block, but in about 15 per cent, axonal degeneration will have occurred. Those with a conduction block will again recover satisfactorily within a few weeks. In patients with a degenerative lesion, recovery has to take place by axonal regeneration. Evidence of re-innervation does not appear in under 3 months and the ultimate recovery is often incomplete or may fail to occur altogether. Synkinesis is frequent after re-innervation so that blinking, for example, results in a simultaneous contraction of the angle of the mouth. Aberrant parasympathetic re-innervation may also occur, leading for instance to gustatory lacrimation ('crocodile tears').

Axons remain excitable distal to the lesion for 3 or 4 days after interruption. It is therefore not possible to be certain from electrodiagnostic tests whether axonal degeneration has taken place until after this time. At that stage, electrical stimulation of the facial nerve at the stylomastoid foramen with brief pulses will still elicit a muscle contraction if the paralysis is due to conduction block, whereas none will be obtained if axonal degeneration has taken place.

In the early stages, the main endeavour of treatment should be to prevent either a partial lesion, or complete paralysis related to a conduction block, progressing to a degenerative lesion. There is some evidence that corticosteroids may be advantageous by reducing oedema in the nerve. Thus it is justifiable to treat all cases with corticosteroids if seen within a few days of onset, providing no contraindication to such treatment exists. A course of a week's duration with an initially high dosage is recommended.

Surgical decompression of the nerve has been advised. To be effective, this would have to be performed at the outset, which is not justifiable as 85 per cent of cases will recover satisfactorily without treatment. So far there are no means of predicting which cases will progress to a degenerative lesion. If this were available, decompression could be undertaken selectively in such cases.

It is helpful to perform electrodiagnostic studies at about 1 week after the onset. If this reveals a degenerative lesion, it is then known that recovery will be delayed. A prosthesis attached to the teeth to elevate the angle of the mouth to reduce facial deformity may be helpful. In patients with severe ectropion, a lateral tarsorrhaphy to protect the eye may be required. Electrical stimulation of the paralysed facial muscles has no effect on the ultimate prognosis.

In those cases in which regeneration fails to occur, operation may be desirable for cosmetic reasons to counteract the facial deformity. The angle of the mouth may be elevated by a fascial sling attached to the temporalis fascia, but the result is never highly satisfactory. Restoration of facial tone may be achieved by anastomosis of the hypoglossal nerve to the facial, but at the expense of denervation of the tongue on that side. Any operation should not be contemplated before an adequate length of time has been allowed for regeneration. This should be of the order of 9 months.

Facial paralysis related to 'geniculate' herpes zoster (Ramsay Hunt syndrome)

Facial paralysis of rapid onset accompanied by severe pain in and around the external auditory meatus and in the throat may accompany 'cephalic zoster'. Vesicles may be detectable in the ear and ulceration in the fauces, or anywhere on the head. Occasionally there is concomitant vertigo, tinnitus, and some deafness with involvement of the eighth nerve ('otic herpes zoster'). Prognosis for recovery of the facial paralysis is less good than in Bell's palsy.

Hemifacial spasm

This consists of a unilateral disturbance affecting the facial muscles, producing irregular clonic or twitching movements of the facial muscles, usually of insidious onset. It most commonly occurs in middle-aged women. There may be a mild degree of facial weakness, but severe paralysis does not occur. Usually no underlying cause is demonstrable. The condition selectively affects the facial nerve, within the brain-stem or in the posterior fossa.

It begins with intermittent twitching of the facial muscles such as around the eye or at the angle of the mouth. These movements gradually become more frequent and extend to involve the rest of the facial muscles, often gradually advancing over the course of some years. If they become severe, the face is contorted by irregular clonic spasms which may keep the eye closed for prolonged periods. The facial distortion is often a considerable embarrassment to the patient, who finds that the spasms tend to be aggravated by emotional stress.

The condition requires to be distinguished from benign fasciculation of the face ('live blood'), which usually occurs around the eyes, related to fatigue or emotional tension, and from the myokymic twitching that is occasionally encountered as a manifestation of multiple sclerosis. The latter consists of a persisting irregular rippling movement of the facial muscles that usually subsides after a week or two. These conditions can be distinguished by electromyography (see Chapter 24.2.5).

No satisfactory treatment is available. If exaggeration by emotional factors is evident, the administration of diazepam or similar preparation may produce a marginal improvement. In severe cases, injections of botulinum toxin may be helpful, although these have to be repeated. Neurosurgical intervention to relieve compression of the nerve by aberrant vessels in its intracranial course has been advocated.

Glossopharyngeal nerve

The ninth cranial nerve leaves the skull through the jugular foramen, closely related to the tenth nerve. It supplies the stylopharyngeus muscle and the constrictor muscles of the pharynx. Parasympathetic fibres are supplied to the parotid gland. Sensory fibres are carried from the posterior third of the tongue, the ear, the fauces, and the nasopharynx, and chemoreceptor and baroreceptor afferents from the carotid sinus.

The glossopharyngeal nerve is rarely affected in isolation. Lesions usually occur in conjunction with involvement of the vagus and give rise to some dysphagia, impaired pharyngeal sensation, and loss of taste over the posterior third of the tongue. It may be affected in the jugular foramen syndrome (Vernet's syndrome), along with the tenth and eleventh nerves, of which glomus tumours or metastatic carcinoma are the commonest causes. The nerve may also be involved in diphtheritic neuropathy and in a polyneuritis cranialis.

Glossopharyngeal neuralgia is a rare form of neuralgia within the distribution of the glossopharyngeal nerve. Its features are otherwise strictly comparable to those of trigeminal neuralgia in the quality and severity of the pain, its occurrence in brief paroxysms, its provocation by actions such as speaking or swallowing, and the remissions in its course. As with trigeminal neuralgia, it is most often encountered in elderly subjects, and the pain may initially be confined to individual branches. Thus it may be felt deep in the ear, related to the tympanic branch, or in the throat, related to the pharyngeal branches.

In treatment, carbamazepine may be effective. In instances of severe pain unrelieved by this preparation, surgical treatment, usually avulsion of the nerve, may be required.

Vagus nerve

The tenth cranial nerve is structurally complex. Within the skull it is joined by the cranial division of the eleventh nerve. It leaves the skull through the jugular foramen. Cutaneous sensory fibres are carried from the external ear and visceral afferent fibres are carried from the pharynx, larynx, trachea, oesophagus, and the thoracic and abdominal viscera. Motor fibres are supplied to the striated musculature of the palate and pharynx and through the external and recurrent laryngeal nerves, to the muscles of the larynx. Parasympathetic fibres are provided to innervate the parotid gland (through the glossopharyngeal nerve), the heart, and the abdominal viscera.

The important symptoms of vagal nerve damage are those relating to pharyngeal and laryngeal innervation. The cells of origin in the nucleus ambiguus of the medulla may be damaged in the lateral medullary syndrome, in motor neurone disease, and in acute bulbar poliomyelitis, leading to dysphagia and dysphonia. Involvement along with the glossopharyngeal nerve in the jugular foramen syndrome has already been mentioned. The recurrent laryngeal nerve may be damaged during operations on the thyroid gland or by tumours within the neck, or within the thorax, usually by carcinoma of the bronchus. The nerve on the left is vulnerable to damage from aneurysm of the aortic arch. Isolated and unexplained lesions of the recurrent laryngeal nerve are not uncommon.

Nuclear or high vagal lesions, as well as involving the larynx, cause palatal and pharyngeal paralysis. If unilateral, there are no symptoms from palatopharyngeal paralysis. The uvula is pulled up to the opposite side on phonation and pharyngeal sensation is impaired on the affected side. With bilateral paralysis, the palate is paretic leading to nasality of the voice and nasal regurgitation of liquids on attempts at swallowing. Bilateral palatopharyngeal paralysis may be encountered in motor neurone disease, bulbar poliomyelitis, diphtheritic neuropathy, and polyneuritis cranialis.

Unilateral intrinsic laryngeal paralysis from lesions of the recurrent nerve may be asymptomatic or give rise to hoarseness of the voice. If the superior laryngeal nerve is also involved leading to paralysis of the cricothyroid muscle, the affected cord lies in a paramedian or cadaveric position. The effects of bilateral lesions of the recurrent laryngeal nerves depend upon the degree of approximation of the vocal cords. Lesions of insidious onset tend to give rise to dysphonia and also to stridor on exertion. In partial lesions, close approximation of the cords may result from selective paralysis of the abductor muscles, giving rise to limitation of the airway and sometimes necessitating tracheostomy. With bilateral lesions involving both the recurrent and superior laryngeal nerves, both cords are paralysed and in the cadaveric position. Phonation is impossible.

Spinal accessory nerve

The spinal accessory portion of the eleventh cranial nerve arises from the upper cervical cord and the lower medulla. The nerve passes through the foramen magnum and joins the cranial portion of the nerve before emerging from the skull through the jugular foramen. The spinal accessory nerve then separates and supplies the sternomastoid and trapezius muscles, the latter also receiving an innervation from the cervical plexus.

The nerve may be affected by lesions in the region of the jugular foramen, but more commonly it is damaged by injuries to the neck or by operations for removal of cervical glands, particularly as it crosses the posterior triangle of the neck. Isolated and unexplained lesions of the nerve are occasionally encountered.

Unilateral paralysis of the sternomastoid usually passes unnoticed by the patient. The muscle does not stand out when the head is turned to the opposite side. Paralysis of the trapezius, on the other hand, causes difficulty in lifting the arm above the horizontal, in shrugging the shoulder and in approximating the scapula to the midline and therefore also in carrying the extended arm backwards. The shoulder droops when the arm is hanging at the side and there is moderate winging of the scapula which is accentuated when the patient attempts to elevate the arm laterally.

The hypoglossal nerve

The twelfth cranial nerve supplies all the muscles of the tongue, both intrinsic and extrinsic. It leaves the skull through the anterior condyloid foramen. A unilateral lesion of the hypoglossal nerve causes weakness and atrophy of the tongue on the affected side. When protruded, the tongue deviates to the affected side. Articulation is unaffected. The nerve may be affected by tumours in the region of the anterior condyloid foramen, or by tumours or penetrating injuries in the neck. If the lesion is the result of a unilateral lower brain-stem lesion, it may be combined with a crossed hemiplegia.

Bilateral lesions give rise to generalized atrophy of the tongue. Protrusion becomes impossible and articulation is disturbed. The commonest cause is motor neurone disease (progressive bulbar palsy). The wasting of the tongue is usually accompanied by fasciculation.

REFERENCES

Adour, W.E.K., et al. (1972). Prednisone treatment for idiopathic facial paralysis (Bell's palsy). New England Journal of Medicine 287, 1268–75.
Asbury, A.K., Aldredge, H., Hershberg, R., and Fisher, C.M. (1970). Oculomotor palsy in diabetic mellitus: a clinicopathological study. Brain 93, 555–66.

Brodal, A. (1965). *The cranial nerves* (2nd edn), Blackwell Scientific, Oxford.

Bruyn, G.W. (1983). Glossopharyngeal neuralgia. *Cephalgia* **3**, 143–9.

Cogan, D.G. (1956). *Neurology of the ocular muscles*, (2nd edn). C.C. Thomas, Springfield.

Cogan, D.G. (1966). *Neurology of the visual system*. C.C. Thomas, Springfield.

Dyck, P.J., Thomas, P.K., Griffin, J.W., Low, P.A., and Poduslo, J.F. (ed.) (1993). *Peripheral neuropathy*, (3rd edn). W.B. Saunders, Philadelphia.

Esslen, E. (1977). *The acute facial palsies. Investigations on the localization and pathogenesis of meato-labyrinthine facial palsies*. Springer Verlag, New York.

Farrell, D.A. and Medsger, A. (1982). Trigeminal neuropathy in progressive systemic sclerosis. *American Journal of Medicine* **73**, 57–61.

Katusic, S., Beard, C.M., Bergstralh, E., and Kurland, L.T. (1990). Incidence and clinical features of trigeminal neuralgia. *Annals of Neurology* **27**, 89–95.

Lecky, B.R.F., Hughes, R.A.C., and Murray, N.M.F. (1987). Trigeminal sensory neuropathy. A study of 22 cases. *Brain* **110**, 1463–86.

Rush, J.A. and Younge, B.R. (1966). Paralysis of cranial nerves III, IV and VI: causes and prognosis of 1000 cases. *Archives of Ophthalmology* **99**, 76–89.

24.3.7 The autonomic nervous system

R. BANNISTER

INTRODUCTION

The autonomic nervous system innervates every visceral organ in the body. It has as complex a neural organization in the brain, spinal cord, and periphery as the somatic nervous system, but remains largely involuntary or automatic. As Claude Bernard put it, 'nature thought it provident to remove these important phenomena from the caprice of an ignorant will'. Langley, who in 1898 first proposed the term 'autonomic nervous system', based his experiments on the blocking action of nicotine at synapses in ganglia. In 1921 Loewi discovered '*Vagusstoff*' which was released by stimulation of the vagus nerve and proved to be acetylcholine. In the same year Cannon discovered that 'sympathin', later shown to be noradrenaline, was produced by stimulation of the sympathetic trunk. The basis was therefore laid for Dale's distinction between cholinergic and adrenergic transmission in the autonomic nervous system.

ANATOMY AND PHYSIOLOGY

The peripheral autonomic nervous system, an efferent system, is made up of neurones which lie outside the CNS and are concerned with visceral innervation. Both sympathetic and parasympathetic systems have preganglionic neurones in the brain and spinal cord arranged as shown in Fig. 1. The afferent limbs of autonomic reflexes may lie in any afferent nerve. The preganglionic sympathetic fibres are myelinated and leave the spinal roots as white rami communicantes and synapse in the ganglia. Unmyelinated postganglionic fibres rejoin the anterior spinal roots by the arrangement shown in Fig. 2, although some sympathetic fibres traverse the ganglia and synapse in more peripheral ganglia, following the arrangement of the parasympathetic fibres.

The transmitter at all preganglionic terminals is acetylcholine which is not paralysed by atropine (the nicotinic effect), whereas the action of acetylcholine at the distal end of the cholinergic postganglionic fibres is paralysed by atropine (the muscarinic effect). Noradrenaline is the principal transmitter for postganglionic sympathetic nerves, the excep-

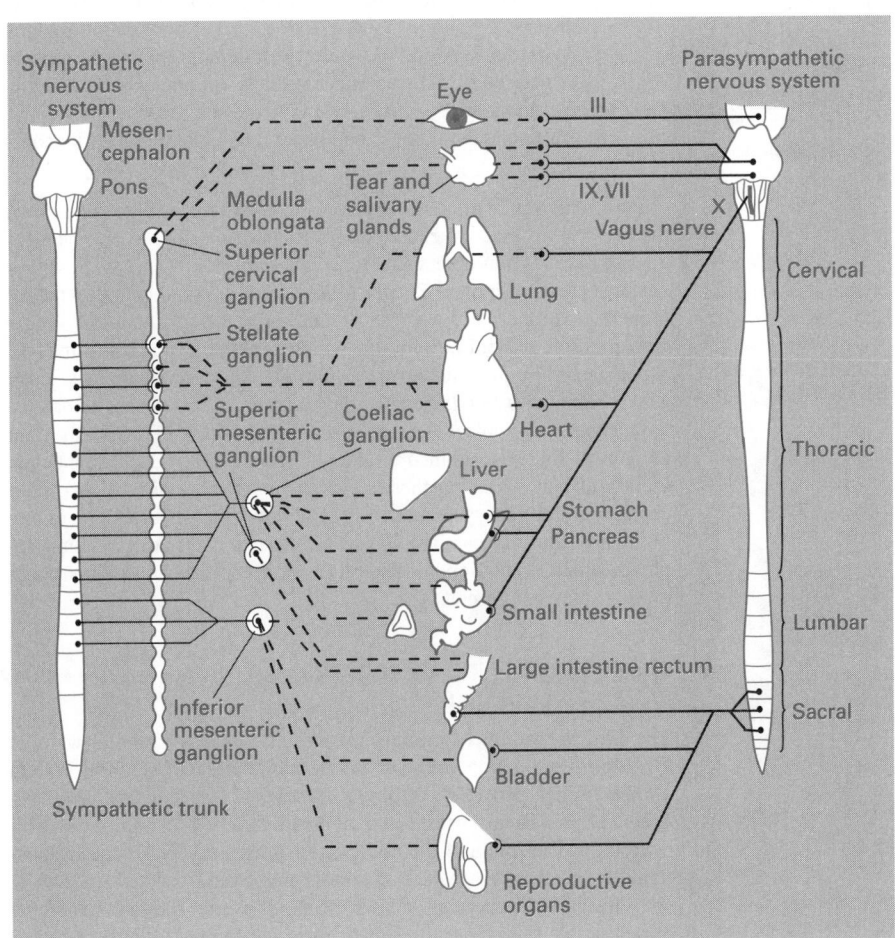

Fig. 1 Peripheral autonomic nervous system. The sympathetic innervation of vessels, sweat glands, and piloerector muscles is not shown. Solid lines, preganglionic axons; dashed lines, postganglionic axons. (Reproduced from Bannister 1992, with permission.)

tions being sudomotor nerves, which are cholinergic in humans; some vasodilator fibres to muscle; and the adrenal medulla, which is innervated by preganglionic (cholinergic) fibres and itself secretes mainly adrenaline. Noradrenaline is stored in the terminals and is released by nerve activity or by sympathomimetic drugs, which may act partly indirectly on the ganglia or more centrally (such as ephedrine and amphetamine) or on the terminals (such as phenylephrine or tyramine). The different actions of noradrenaline and adrenaline are caused by relative effects on different receptors. α-Receptors may be either postsynaptic ($α_1$) or presynaptic ($α_2$, which, when stimulated, decrease the release of the transmitter). β-Receptors mediate vasodilation, especially in muscles, increase the rate and force of the heart with a tendency to arrhythmias, and cause bronchial relaxation. They are further subdivided into $β_1$-receptors, mediating the chronotropic cardiac action of isoprenaline, and $β_2$-receptors, which are responsible for most of the peripheral effects of β-adrenergic stimulation.

The cells of the autonomic nervous system tend to act in conjunction, and this is achieved mainly by specialized intercellular junctions at the ganglion cells which have been demonstrated by electron microscopy and freeze fracture techniques. The autonomic ganglia also contain small intensely fluorescent cells (SIF cells) which contain many peptides, thought to act as modulators and transmitters at synaptic sites. Substance P, vasoactive intestinal peptide (VIP), enkephalins, and somatostatin have all been identified in autonomic ganglia, although their precise role in control of nerve transmission is not yet known.

The previously held notion of a simple antagonism between a sympathetic-adrenergic system, causing rather unselective 'fight or flight' responses, and a parasympathetic-cholinergic system providing tonic activity, has now given way to a new view of a highly selective autonomic nervous system. Although the two systems, in general, have antagonistic functions, there is a subtlety of integrative action at least as complex as that of the somatic nervous system. New transmitters and modulators have been discovered, many still putative, and receptors, both presynaptic and postsynaptic, can be blocked, activated, or modified in their numbers and affinities. New general biological principles have emerged with 'up' and 'down' regulation, by agonists of receptor numbers and affinities, and with the manipulation pharmacologically of presynaptic and postsynaptic receptors by transmitter release, depletion, or blockade.

CLASSIFICATION OF AUTONOMIC DISORDERS (TABLE 1)

A convenient clinical classification of the primary autonomic failure syndromes, cases without known underlying cause, is as follows:

Fig. 2 The autonomic spinal reflex arc. (Reproduced from Bannister 1992, with permission.)

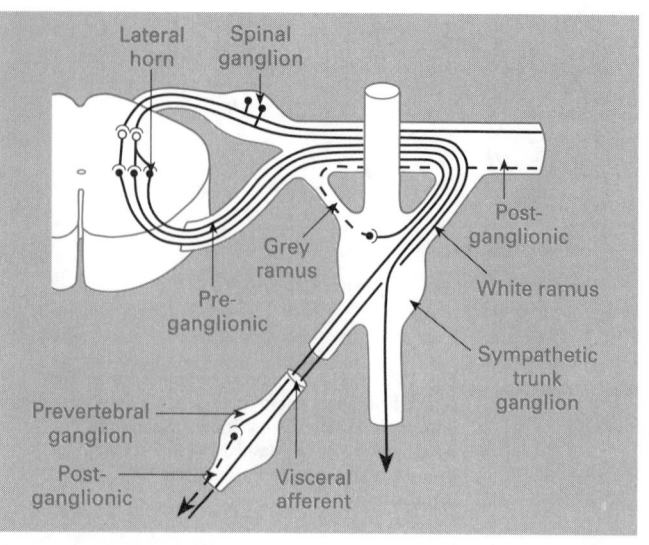

Table 1 *Classification of autonomic disorders (adapted from Bannister and Mathias 1992, with permission)*

Central, primary
  Pure autonomic failure
  Autonomic failure with multiple system atrophy
  Autonomic failure with Parkinson's disease
Central, secondary
  Central brain lesions: craniopharyngioma, vascular lesions
  Infections of the nervous system: tabes dorsalis, Chagas' disease, HIV
  Spinal cord lesions
  Familial dysautonomia
Genetic: dopamine β-hydroxylase deficiency
Distal autonomic neuropathies
  General medical disorders: diabetes, amyloid, porphyria, Tangier disease, Fabry's disease, HIV
  Autoimmune disease: acute and subacute pandysautonomia; Guillain–Barré syndrome; myasthenia; rheumatoid arthritis
Drugs
  Selective neurotoxic drugs: alcoholism, Wernicke's encephalopathy
  Tranquillizers; phenothiazines, barbiturates
  Antidepressants; tricyclics; monoamine oxidase inhibitors
  Vasodilator hypotensive drugs: prazosin, hydralazine
  Centrally acting hypotensive drugs; methyldopa, clonidine
  Adrenergic neurone blocking drugs; guanethidine, bethanidine, debrisoquine
  α-Adrenergic blocking drugs; phenoxybenzamine, labetalol
  Ganglion-blocking drugs; hexamethonium, mecamylamine
  Angiotensin-converting enzyme inhibitors: captopril

1. Pure autonomic failure, without associated neurological disorders.
2. Autonomic failure and multiple system atrophy and a variety of neurological disturbances (usually but not always including parkinsonism).
3. Autonomic failure and apparently classical Parkinson's disease.

Pure autonomic failure occurs alone or as an additional feature in two distinct and well-recognized types of primary neurological degenerative disease, namely multiple system atrophy and Parkinson's disease (see Chapter 24.10). Shy and Drager (1960) described the complex neurological syndrome that bears their name, now called autonomic failure with multiple system atrophy, in which postural hypotension may be accompanied by pyramidal, extrapyramidal, and cerebellar signs. Later a rare variant was recognized in which autonomic failure was associated with apparently typical Parkinson's disease. Cases of clinically pure autonomic failure examined at autopsy show either Lewy intranuclear inclusion bodies, linking these cases to Parkinson's disease, or minor changes of multiple system atrophy. The rare cases of autonomic failure with Parkinson's disease are distinct from cases of multiple system atrophy in which striatonigral degeneration or olivopontocerebellar atrophy, or both, may be present.

CLINICAL FEATURES OF PRIMARY AUTONOMIC FAILURE SYNDROMES

The clinical features of primary autonomic failure are similar whether this is pure autonomic failure or autonomic failure with multiple system atrophy. When the effects of drugs and adrenal insufficiency have been excluded, persistent postural hypotension is almost certainly due to a neurological lesion, and the commonest presenting symptoms of postural hypotension are postural dizziness and fatigue or attacks of loss of consciousness on exercise or after meals. However, the first symptoms of autonomic failure are mild, insidious, and frequently overlooked or misdiagnosed. The patients are all middle-aged or elderly, and males are affected about twice as often as females. In men, impotence and loss of libido are commonly the first symptoms. Patients living in a hot climate may complain of an inability to sweat. Later, the first symptoms of postural dizziness or syncope occur, followed by bladder symptoms including incontinence. The postural attacks may be 'drop' attacks resembling sudden brain-stem vascular dysfunction, but more commonly there is a gradual fading of consciousness over half a minute or so while the patient is standing or walking. A transient ache in the neck radiating to the occipital region of the skull and the shoulders often precedes actual loss of consciousness. Sometimes there are transient visual disturbances, scotomata, or positive hallucinations or tunnel vision, suggesting occipital lobe ischaemia. The patient may then fall to his knees. Experience teaches the patient that after lying flat, recovery and loss of all symptoms including the neck ache will occur within a few minutes. The recovery from such transient neurological symptoms is usually complete and (possibly because the patients have virtually continuous cerebrovasodilation due to years of postural hypotension) occlusive cerebrovascular incidents are rare. The attack differs from the usual 'faint' in that the patient cannot sweat and there is no vagal cardiac slowing. The disease is likely to be progressive for 5 or more years before significant incapacity occurs. Some rare non-neurological presentations occur. A few patients, if treated by bedrest for hypotensive symptoms, develop persistent recumbent hypertension of such severity that they may develop papilloedema with retinal haemorrhages.

In patients with autonomic failure, the ingestion of food results in a number of hormonal, neural, and regional haemodynamic changes which may be linked to a substantial lowering of blood pressure, even in the supine position. This can present a considerable clinical problem. After ingestion of foods, splanchnic vasodilatation occurs, due to vasoactive peptides (possibly somatostatin), which is not counteracted by appropriate haemodynamic adjustments in other parts of the circulation.

The neurological, as opposed to the cardiovascular, features of multiple system atrophy are equally insidious and may precede the cardiovascular features. The most common early signs are of an extrapyramidal disorder in which rigidity is more obvious than akinesis or tremor. The true diagnosis is sometimes dramatically revealed when mild postural hypotension becomes severe on treatment with levodopa or there is unexpected lack of response to levodopa in what appears at first to be a case of Parkinson's disease. In some patients a cerebellar tremor, often with a marked truncal component, is the earliest sign of cerebellar system involvement. The extrapyramidal syndrome may progress and additional symptoms and signs may emerge, including pyramidal signs, muscle wasting, pupillary inequalities, and respiratory abnormalities including sleep apnoea and laryngeal stridor. The order of the development of neurological symptoms is variable. The brain-stem atrophy, with atrophy of the pons, cerebellar peduncles, vermis, and cerebellar cortex, can be demonstrated by computed tomography and by magnetic resonance imaging and positron emission tomography.

TESTING AUTONOMIC FUNCTION

Introduction

Testing autonomic function (Table 2) is complicated by the fact that within each part of the output from the autonomic system partial responses occur and any defects, whether central or peripheral, may be partially corrected by other neuronal, chemical, or hormonal mechanisms. When we add that the lesions caused by disease are often multiple and variable, the task of correlating reflex defects and pathology might seem daunting. However, the cardiovascular system has proved suitable for an analysis of the principles used in testing for autonomic dysfunction, and analysing cardiovascular control is doubly relevant because

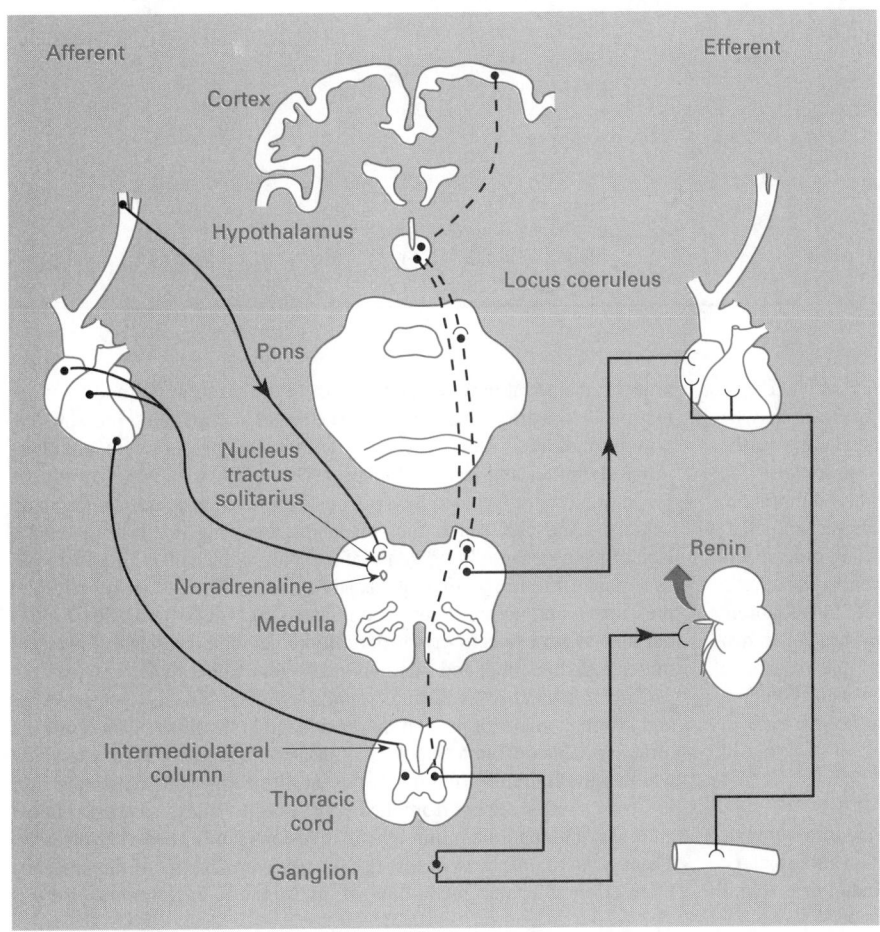

Fig. 3 Diagram of cardiovascular control mechanisms. LC, locus coeruleus; NTS, nucleus tractus solitarius; R, renin. (Reproduced from Bannister and Mathias 1992, with permission.)

Table 2 *Some useful clinical tests of autonomic failure (adapted from Bannister and Mathias 1992, with permission)*

Cardiovascular reflexes

Tests performed and responses:

1. Change of posture: blood pressure and pulse rate monitored while subject is supine and then repeated measurements are made at 60 ° head-up tilt position. Pulse rate and plasma noradrenaline responses to standing. Lower body negative pressure is an alternative to standing

2. Deep breathing: presence or absence of sinus arrhythmia; test of vagal efferent pathway

3. Carotid sinus massage: right and left sides, in turn monitoring cardiac rate and blood pressure; test of vagal efferent pathway. Caution in case of supersensitivity

4. Hyperventilation: for 30 s, causing hypocapnia and fall in blood pressure; response suggests afferent lesion, if baroreflex block

5. Inspiratory gasp: causing reflex vasoconstriction of hands; spinal-cord reflex

6. Stress: causing hypertension and tachycardia; tests of sympathetic efferent pathway.
   (a) handgrip, submaximal sustained for 90 s;
   (b) sudden cortical arousal by unexpected noise;
   (c) mental arithmetic (rapid serial subtraction of 7 from 100);
   (d) cold pressor test—hand immersed in water at 4 °C for 90 s

7. Breath-holding: test of central breathing control; prolonged if vagal afferent dysfunction

8. Valsalva manoeuvre: after a deep inspiration the patient performs a forced expiration for 12 s through a tube connected to a mercury manometer. Most subjects can maintain a pressure of 30 mmHg. In normal subjects there is an increasing tachycardia for the 10 s of sustained forced expiration. Blood pressure falls initially but should cease to fall after the first few seconds if peripheral sympathetic vasoconstriction is normal. On release from blowing there is normally a blood pressure overshoot and a compensatory reflex bradycardia

9. Pharmacological tests:
   (a) plasma noradrenaline at rest and after 30 min standing or tilt;
   (b) pressor response and cardiac slowing to infusion of noradrenaline (or phenylephrine) test of baroreflex sensitivity;
   (c) pressor response and noradrenaline response to infusion of tyramine; test of cytoplasmic stores of noradrenaline;
   (d) cardiac slowing to atropine; test of vagal function

Sweating

1. Response to body heating in order to cause a rise of 1 °C oral or rectal temperature in the course of 90 min. Record sweating and measure hand blood-flow. Test of sympathetic pathway from hypothalamus to periphery

2. Response to brief trunk heating with electric lamp source for 90 s; a reflex response, without involving change of blood temperature, utilizing same efferent pathway as response to body heating

3. Responses to intramuscular pilocarpine; acts directly on sweat glands

4. Pilomotor and sudomotor response to intradermal methacholine; absent with complete postganglionic lesion

Pupillary responses

1. Instillation of 1:1000 adrenaline. Response: dilation after sympathetic postganglionic denervation; no effect on normal pupil

2. Instillation of fresh 2.5 per cent cocaine. Response: dilation of normal pupil; no effect after sympathetic denervation

3. Instillation of fresh 2.5 per cent methacholine. Response: constriction after parasympathetic denervation; no effect on normal pupil

Skin response

Intracutaneous injection of 0.05 ml of 1 per cent 1000 histamine phosphate causes a wheal surrounded by erythema and erythematous flare. The flare of this triple response is an axon reflex mediated by antidromic transmission along sensory fibres

---

postural hypotension is one of the commonest symptoms of defective autonomic function. The homeostatic control of blood pressure may be disturbed by lesions at several levels, from the hypothalamus to the periphery. Figure 3 shows a much simplified diagram of some of the neurological pathways involved in the regulation of blood pressure. There are cortical, limbic, anterior and posterior hypothalamic, and medullary 'centres' at which the input from the carotid sinus and other afferents can be integrated and the output through the vagus and sympathetic system to the heart and blood vessels may be co-ordinated. In autonomic failure the baroreceptors, as feedback transducers in cybernetic terms, do not produce the required responses in the effectors, the resistance and capacity vessels, the heart, and the kidneys. This causes both a change in the 'set point' pressure and an instability in the response to various stresses.

Clinical testing of autonomic function

When a fall of more than some 20 points systolic on standing is found in a patient with symptoms, further investigation is justified and a battery of tests is now available and summarized in Table 2. Radial or brachial artery catheterization will show precisely the postural fall and the fluctuations with various manoeuvres. The finger arterial blood pressure can now be measured non-invasively by an inflatable cuff with a built-in infrared emitter and sensor (Finapres) (Imholz *et al.* 1988). On tilt the blood pressure falls due to lack of constriction in resistance and capacity vessels in muscles and in the splanchnic area (Fig. 4). There is also a lack of the overshoot in phase IV of the Valsalva which normally occurs as a result of reflex peripheral vasoconstriction. The instability of blood pressure in autonomic failure is due partly to lack of baroreflex control but also to supersensitivity of partially denervated vessels to the transmitter noradrenaline, and this may cause recumbent hypertension.

Cardiovascular reflexes, like somatic reflexes, have efferent, central, and afferent connections, and the next stage in the investigation of postural hypotension and a 'blocked' Valsalva manoeuvre is to try to show whether the lesion is afferent or efferent. If the vasoconstrictor response to stress, a reflex arising from the hypothalamus, is lost, as it is in almost all cases of autonomic failure, then the lesion is presumed to be efferent. There is no simple way of testing the afferent pathway in the presence of an efferent lesion. Techniques of investigation have been used combining lower body suction to simulate the effect of posture with neck pressure to 'unload' the carotid baroreceptors and so isolate the contribution of other afferents, including those from low-pressure areas. Further evidence of the lack of sympathetic activity has also been provided by assay of plasma noradrenaline, which is low in patients with autonomic failure and fails to rise on standing (Fig. 5). Patients with pure autonomic failure have a lower resting plasma noradrenaline than autonomic failure with multiple system atrophy, though in neither is there a rise on standing.

A major difficulty is to decide whether the sympathetic efferent lesion is preganglionic or postganglionic or both. This is of practical importance because it affects the degree of denervation supersensitivity and

Fig. 4 (a) Valsalva response in a normal subject, showing blood pressure (upper trace) and cardiac beat-to-beat record (lower trace). (b) Valsalva manoeuvre, showing very abnormal response in autonomic failure. (Records reproduced from Bannister and Mathias 1992, with permission.)

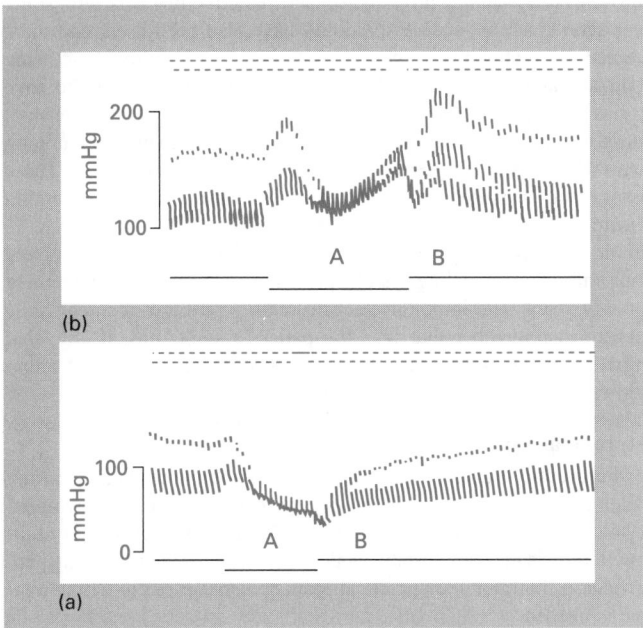

Fig. 5 Effect of tilt on plasma noradrenaline concentration (nmol/l) in patients with autonomic failure (left) and in control subjects (right). R1 and R2 denote recordings following 1 and 2 h of recumbency, respectively. The T recording following a 10 min 60 ° tilt, and the R3 recording a further 1 h of recumbency. (Reproduced from Bannister et al. 1977, with permission.)

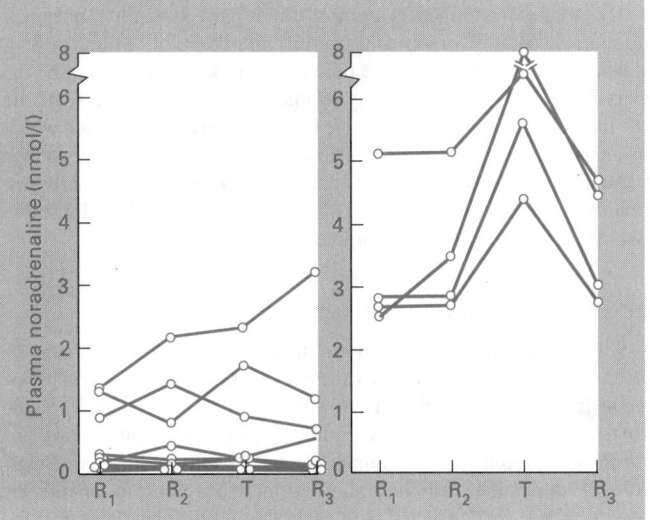

the response to pressor drugs. Following complete postganglionic sympathetic denervation, supersensitivity of vessels to the transmitter noradrenaline occurs, with loss of the response to tyramine. Tyramine acts by releasing noradrenaline from the cytoplasmic pool but not the granular pool, which is accessible to the nerve impulse. All patients with autonomic failure show some supersensitivity to intravenous noradrenaline and there is evidence that this is greater in pure autonomic failure than in autonomic failure with multiple system atrophy.

Such studies in cases of autonomic failure have provided good evidence of an efferent sympathetic lesion which is more postganglionic in pure autonomic failure than in autonomic failure with multiple system atrophy. This sympathetic efferent lesion, affecting resistance and capacity vessels and the heart, is usually more severe than the vagal lesion, shown by lack of sinus arrhythmia. This makes an interesting contrast with the distal diabetic autonomic neuropathy in which the vagal efferent lesion is usually more severe than the sympathetic efferent lesion.

NEUROPATHOLOGY OF PRIMARY AUTONOMIC FAILURE

More than 10 per cent of cases in the Parkinson's Disease Brain Bank in London thought in life to have Parkinson's disease, have been shown at autopsy to have autonomic failure with multiple system atrophy. This illustrates both the difficulty of diagnosis of autonomic failure with multiple system atrophy and the greater frequency of occurrence of autonomic failure with multiple system atrophy than was previously suspected. In almost all patients with autonomic failure and multiple system atrophy carefully studied there has been a reduction by up to 80 per cent in the number of sympathetic preganglionic neurones in the intermediolateral columns of the spinal cord. There have also been brain-stem abnormalities with loss of pigment in the melanin-containing nuclei which are derived from the basal plate of the primitive neural tube, including the substantia nigra, dorsal nucleus of the vagus, the locus coeruleus, and the nucleus tractus solitarius. In patients with autonomic failure with Parkinson's disease, Lewy bodies are found. These are inclusion bodies which contain remnants of melanin from the oxidation of catecholamines. The neurochemical defects in autonomic failure with multiple system atrophy can be distinguished from those of Parkinson's disease. At the limbic–hypothalamic level in autonomic failure with multiple system atrophy there is a marked reduction in noradrenaline involving also the septal nuclei, which is not present in Parkinson's disease. This is supported by the observation of very marked reduction in tyrosine hydroxylase, the rate-limiting enzyme for noradrenaline synthesis, in the hypothalamus, again not present in Parkinson's disease. This observation also correlates with the low cerebrospinal fluid noradrenaline levels in autonomic failure with multiple system atrophy. The associated noradrenaline depletion in multiple system atrophy is likely to be the explanation for the poor response of the extrapyramidal features of multiple system atrophy to dopaminergic agents, which is in marked contrast to Parkinson's disease. There have been few complete pathological studies of pure autonomic failure but some reports show loss of intermediolateral column cells as well as definite ganglionic lesions. This suggests the existence of a more distal process in pure autonomic failure than in multiple system atrophy. In all patients with autonomic failure there is, as might be expected, a reduction of the catecholamine fluorescence of sympathetic nerve endings on muscle blood vessels, and electron microscopy of the endings shows that there is a reduction in the number of small, dense-core noradrenergic vesicles.

THE PATHOGENESIS OF PRIMARY AUTONOMIC FAILURE

The pathogenesis of autonomic failure remains unknown but one possibility is the exposure to a neurotropic virus, against a background of altered immunity. The hypothesis that several different chronic neuronal degenerations have features in common accords well with the current view of autonomic failure and also provides hope that, apart from increasing our understanding about aetiology, early and effective replacement treatment of neurotransmitters might delay secondary anterograde or retrograde cell loss.

DISTAL AUTONOMIC NEUROPATHIES

In contrast to autonomic failure there are also true distal autonomic neuropathies (see Table 1) in which the clinical features resulting from interruption of the efferent autonomic pathways produce certain symptoms and signs which resemble those of autonomic failure. The onset may be more acute, however, and partial or complete recovery may occur. Some of the distal generalized neuropathies secondary to a variety of causes, but with minor autonomic involvement, are described elsewhere in this book, but the methods of investigation and treatment of autonomic features are similar to those described previously for the primary autonomic failure syndromes. There is, however, one distal neuropathy which requires special mention. This is the rare acute or subacute pandysautonomia which may involve either sympathetic or parasympathetic fibres or both. The autonomic defects can be identified as in primary autonomic failure. This disease appears to have an autoimmune basis with a tendency to gradual recovery which may be incomplete. It may be thought of as a variant of the type of autonomic neuropathy which occurs as a feature of the Guillain–Barré syndrome, where autonomic features are often present but rather obscured by the somatic neuropathy (see Chapter 24.17).

TREATMENT OF PRIMARY AUTONOMIC FAILURE SYNDROMES

Orthostatic hypotension

There are several methods, of varying complexity, which can be used to counteract the postural hypotension, but all are in various ways unsatisfactory. Obviously, if the volume into which the pooling of blood takes place on standing is reduced, this will help the patient; or if the volume of blood is increased, then this will also reduce the severity of the postural hypotension. However, because of lack of baroreflexes all patients have a very labile blood pressure, high when lying and low when standing, and relatively low in the morning and after meals and rising towards evening. It is therefore difficult, unless systematic observations are made, to know what blood pressure should be recorded when attempting to compare one form of treatment with another. The most impressive feature of the blood pressure regulation of these patients is their extreme sensitivity to changes in posture.

In autonomic failure it is important not to be overconcerned with a low standing blood pressure if the patient is without symptoms. Patients can sometimes tolerate a standing systolic blood pressure as low as 80 mmHg without dizziness or syncope, probably because their capacity for cerebral autoregulation is better than normal subjects. On lying flat overnight, patients with autonomic failure lose more sodium and fluid than a normal individual. Some are able to release renin normally on head-up tilt and these observations led to the successful introduction of postural treatment by head-up tilt at night. When the patient is made to sleep in a semi-erect position, therefore having a lower blood pressure at night and retaining more fluid and sodium, there is an increase in the body weight, which on a short-term basis can be attributed to an increase in extracellular fluid volume, and the standing blood pressure improves. Almost all patients with postural hypotension due to any form of autonomic failure can be helped by the head-up bed tilt at night. Once patients have experienced the benefits they will usually be ready to tolerate the degree of discomfort this may entail. With certain precautions to avoid hyponatraemia, insufflation of nocturnal intranasal DDAVP can be used to prevent nocturnal fluid loss in these patients, as an alternative to head-up tilt, but as the patients are very sensitive to DDAVP a low dose must be given (from 5–40 µg at bedtime) in hospital in order to ensure that hyponatraemia does not occur, before stabilization on an outpatient basis.

A second line of treatment which is usually helpful is the use of fludrocortisone. In a smaller dose (0.1 mg) than necessary to increase blood volume, fludrocortisone appears to increase the sensitivity of blood vessels to very small amounts of noradrenaline which may still be capable of being released in autonomic failure. There is no reason to believe that effects of this low dose are the result of an increase in blood volume. Larger doses of fludrocortisone do, of course, increase blood volume, but there appears to be an 'escape' effect which occurs after 2 or 3 weeks and so the effect on the blood volume is not as satisfactory as relying on increasing sensitivity to noradrenaline caused by a smaller dose. The use of external support of the leg and trunk with elastic support garments or an 'anti-gravity suit' is unphysiological in that it reduces intrinsic myogenic tone and is rarely of much long-term benefit.

There have been many pressor drugs studied in autonomic failure. These include phenylephrine, which acts directly on sympathetic vascular endings, and ephedrine, which acts indirectly; there have also been trials of combinations of tyramine and monoamine-oxidase inhibitors. The β-blockers, such as propranolol, and selective blockers with some direct agonist action, such as pindolol, have also been used, and there have also been attempts to increase the vasoconstrictor response using the prostaglandin inhibitor, indomethacin. All these drugs tend to have the disadvantage of causing greater relative recumbent hypertension. This is because there are no normal baroreflex mechanisms damping down the rise in blood pressure when the patient is recumbent. These pressor drug mixtures rarely improve the patient's standing blood pressure.

Some patients with pure autonomic failure have continued relatively symptomfree with standing systolic pressures in the region of 80 mmHg for many years. The important fact in treating postural hypotension is therefore to remember that it is the patient's symptoms, if any, that require treatment rather than the mere observation that the standing blood pressure appears to be unusually low.

Postprandial hypotension

The therapeutic approaches to this disabling symptom include taking smaller meals, more frequent meals, less carbohydrate, and avoiding alcohol. An effective drug preventing postcibal hypotension in autonomic failure is the somatostatin analogue, octreotide, a long-acting peptide release inhibitor. For practical management an orally acting analogue is needed.

COURSE OF PURE AUTONOMIC FAILURE

Though the natural history of pure autonomic failure is of a slow progression over some 10 to 15 years, patients with autonomic failure and multiple system atrophy rarely survive longer than 10 years from the diagnosis of the disease. Their downhill course is marked by increasing rigidity, urinary incontinence, and sometimes marked stridor which may require tracheostomy. In some the central disturbance of respiratory control and sleep apnoea may be the final cause of death. Alternatively, the denervation supersensitivity of sympathetic α- and β-receptors of the heart may render patients more liable to cardiac arrhythmias from which they may die. The extrapyramidal features rarely respond to levodopa (in the form of levodopa with a dopamine decarboxylase inhibitor), probably because the central defect of noradrenaline as well as dopamine prevents effective levels of dopamine being achieved.

DOPAMINE β-HYDROXYLASE DEFICIENCY

In 1986 there were the first reports of a new disease—dopamine β-hydroxylase deficiency. Clinically the patients had severe postural hypotension from infancy, with other symptoms and signs of purely sympathetic reflex defects. Investigation showed that there was no recordable noradrenaline or adrenaline in the plasma but there were high levels of dopamine, which is not normally present in significant amounts. These facts pointed to a block between dopamine and noradrenaline in the biosynthetic pathway from tyrosine to adrenaline. This step requires dopamine β-hydroxylase, which is present in the plasma in normal subjects and in patients with other forms of autonomic failure but is not present in any recordable amount in dopamine β-hydroxylase deficiency. Fortunately, there is a synthetic peptide, dihydroxyphenyl-serine (DOPS), which is structurally similar to noradrenaline except that it has a carboxyl group as in dopa (3, 4-dihydroxyphenylalanine). It is therefore acted upon by a non-specific dopa-decarboxylase which is present both intraneurally and in a number of extraneural tissues, including the kidney and liver, and is converted directly to noradrenaline, bypassing the dopamine β-hydroxylase enzymatic stem. This has proved very helpful to the few patients with the disorder so far described.

A locus determining the activity levels of serum dopamine β-hydroxylase has been linked to the ABO blood group gene on chromosome 9. Studies are in progress to clone and sequence the structural gene and the adjacent regulatory regions from individuals expressing high- or low-activity phenotypes in order to establish the nature of the mutation responsible.

REFERENCES

Bannister, R. (1992). *Brain and Bannister's clinical neurology*, (7th edn). Oxford University Press, Oxford.

Bannister, R. and Mathias, C.J. (ed.) (1992). *Autonomic failure: A textbook of clinical disorders of the autonomic nervous system*, (3rd edn). Oxford University Press, Oxford.

Bannister, R., Sever, P., and Gross, M. (1977). Cardiovascular reflexes and biochemical responses in progressive autonomic failure. *Brain* **100**, 327–44.

Craig, I., Porter, C., and Craig, S. (1992). The molecular genetics of dopamine β-hydroxylase. In *Autonomic failure: A textbook of clinical disorders of the autonomic nervous system*, (3rd edn), (ed. R. Bannister and C.J. Mathias), pp. 749–58. Oxford University Press, Oxford.

Fulham, M.J., *et al.* (1991). Computed tomography, magnetic resonance imaging and positron emission tomography with [18F] fluorodeoxyglucose in multiple system atrophy and pure autonomic failure. *Clinical Autonomic Research* **1**, 27–36.

Huang, Y.O. and Plaitakis, A. (1984). Morphological changes of olivopontocerebellar atrophy in computed tomography and comments on its pathogenesis. *Advances in Neurology* **41**, 39–85.

Hughes, A.J., Daniel, S.E., Kilford, L., and Lees, A.J. (1992). The accuracy of clinical diagnosis of idiopathic Parkinsons's disease: a clinicopathological study of 100 cases. *Journal of Neurology Neurosurgery and Psychiatry*, **55**, 181–4.

Imholz, B.P.M., Van Montfrans, G.A., Settels, J.J., Van der Hoeven, G.M.A., Karemaker, J.M., and Wieling, W. (1988). Continuous non-invasive blood pressure monitoring; reliability of Finapres device during the Valsalva manoeuvre. *Cardiovascular Research* **22**, 390–7.

Mathias, C.J., Fosbraey, P., Da Costa, D.F., Thorley, A., and Bannister, R. (1986). Desmopressin reduces nocturnal polyuria, reverses overnight weight loss and improves morning postural hypotension in autonomic failure. *British Medical Journal* **293**, 353–4.

Mathias, C.J., *et al.* (1989). Cardiovascular, biochemical and hormonal changes during food induced hypotension in chronic autonomic failure. *Journal of Neurological Science* **94**, 255–69.

Mathias, C.J., *et al.* (1990). Clinical, autonomic and therapeutic observations in two siblings with postural hypotension and sympathetic failure due to an inability to synthesize noradrenaline from dopamine because of a deficiency of dopamine beta hydroxylase. *Quarterly Journal of Medicine, New Series* **75**, 617–33.

Shy, G.M. and Drager, G.A. (1960). A neurological syndrome associated with orthostatic hypotension. *Archives of Neurology* **3**, 511–27.

24.3.8 Respiratory problems in neurological disease

J. NEWSOM-DAVIS

Breathing may be affected by diseases of the central and peripheral nervous systems, and understanding the principles of its neural control is essential for diagnosis and management. It is of special importance to recognize that the respiratory muscles are under the control of two major systems—the automatic (chemosensitive) and the behavioural (willed)—that are anatomically distinct and whose descending projections compete for control over spinal respiratory motoneurone activity. This section therefore outlines the central control mechanisms and the role of the peripheral respiratory muscles before describing specific disorders and their management. The progressive nature of the disease processes has sometimes led to a pessimistic approach but, as will be seen, in those with chronic peripheral ventilatory failure, therapy can often be effective and rewarding.

Neural mechanisms controlling respiration

The localization of structures generating or mediating the respiratory drive is more important to clinicians than a knowledge of their detailed interaction, which is in any case poorly understood. Figure 1 sets out the broad outline.

THE AUTOMATIC SYSTEM

This system depends primarily on brain-stem structures. It is responsive to chemoreceptive and vagal inputs. Two columns of neurones in the medulla appear essential for rhythm genesis in humans, namely, the nucleus retroambigualis and nucleus tractus solitarius (Fig. 1). The nucleus retroambigualis lies ventrolateral to the nucleus ambiguus, extending from the vagal rootlets rostrally to the upper cervical root caudally. The nucleus tractus solitarius lies ventrolateral to the tractus solitarius. It is largely composed of inspiratory neurones which receive a strong vagal (Hering–Breuer) input. A nucleus in the rostral pons, the nucleus parabrachialis medialis, sometimes known as the pneumotaxic region, is concerned with switching between respiratory phases. The integration of the neural activity of these nuclei, which provides the normally smooth respiratory pattern, is not understood.

The carotid and aortic bodies served by the carotid sinus nerve provide the main hypoxic drive in humans. The hypercapnic drive is mediated mainly by chemoreceptors close to the ventral surface of the medulla which respond to changes in CO_2 via pH changes in the cerebrospinal fluid.

The descending respiratory pathway from the nucleus retroambigualis and nucleus tractus solitarius cross over a relatively wide area in the medulla and descend in the ventrolateral region of the spinal cord (Fig. 1). Bilateral interruption of this pathway above C3 disconnects the automatic system from the respiratory muscles, and spontaneous breathing stops.

THE BEHAVIOURAL SYSTEM

The behavioural system subserves all willed activities involving respiratory muscles, including breath-holding and voluntary deep breathing (for example, vital capacity). Inhibitory and excitatory effects on breathing can be produced by electrical stimulation of different areas of the cerebral cortex, notably the anterior cingulate region and the ventromedial aspects of the temporal lobe. Transcranial magnetic stimulation of the motor cortex in conscious man has recently been shown to excite contralateral inspiratory muscles, predominantly the hemidiaphragm.

The descending pathway for the behavioural system is presumed to lie with the main corticobulbar and corticospinal projections. The latter decussates in the lower medulla and descends in the dorsolateral columns of the spinal cord (Fig. 1), entirely separate from the descending automatic respiratory pathway.

INTERACTION BETWEEN AUTOMATIC AND BEHAVIOURAL SYSTEMS

These two systems interact both at medullary and spinal cord level. In non-REM ('rapid eye movement') sleep, the behavioural system is quiescent, and under these conditions the automatic system operates in functional isolation and breathing is characteristically regular. During wakefulness, the automatic system can be transiently overridden by the behavioural system, most strikingly during breath-holding. The respiratory distress ('breathlessness') occurring at the break point appears to depend on a normally functioning automatic system. Interference with

Fig. 1 Neural organization of breathing (schematic). TS, tractus solitarius; NTS, nucleus tractus solitarius; NA, nucleus ambiguus; NRA, nucleus retroambigualis. Transverse sections are shown for levels A (mid-medulla) and B (upper cervical cord).

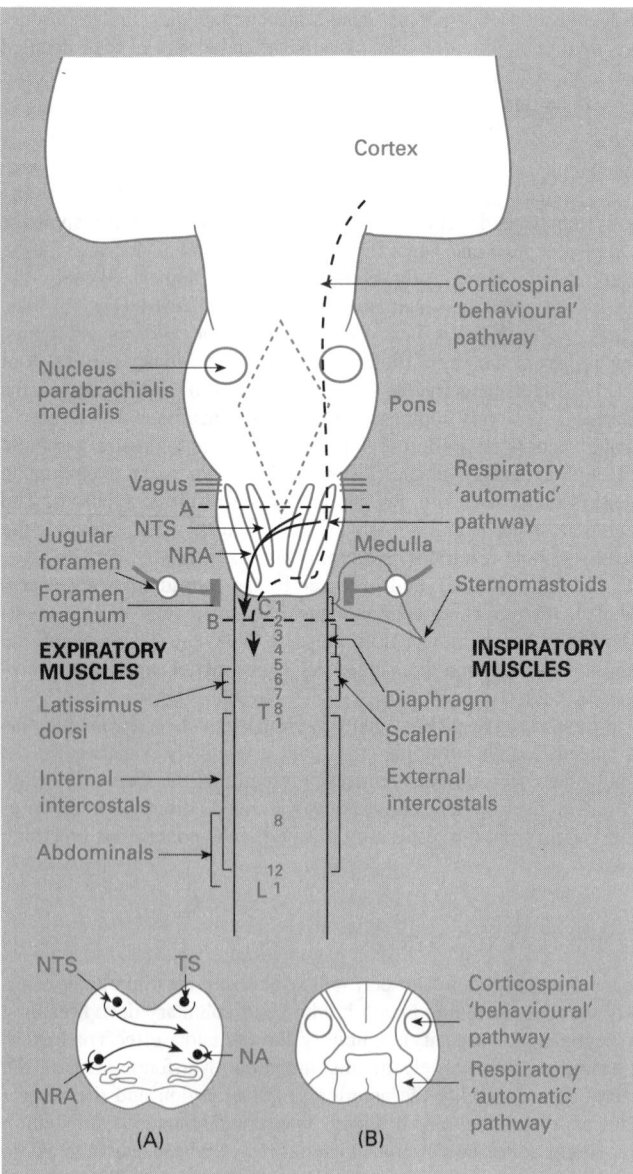

the system by vagal block, or complete interruption of the drive to the respiratory muscle by curarization, abolishes the distress.

In extreme cases, lesions of either the behavioural or automatic systems may leave the other system functioning in anatomical isolation. Destruction of the ventral pons, which results in the 'locked-in' syndrome, disconnects the behavioural system, and breathing becomes 'supernormal' in its regularity. Conversely, disconnection of the automatic system (by destruction of respiratory nuclei, for example) results in very irregular ('behavioural') breathing during wakefulness and cessation of breathing during drowsiness or sleep ('Ondine's curse').

MAJOR PERIPHERAL VENTILATORY APPARATUS

The principal inspiratory muscle is the diaphragm. Downward (inspiratory) movement of the diaphragm is accompanied by outward movement of the abdominal wall, so that the two structures operate in series; this is because the floor and posterior wall of the abdomen are rigid and its contents non-compressible.

Other inspiratory and expiratory muscles are shown in Fig. 1. Accessory inspiratory activity (sternomastoids and scaleni) is particularly evident when other inspiratory muscles are paralysed or when the level of respiratory drive is high.

Central disorders of breathing

CENTRAL RESPIRATORY FAILURE OR INSUFFICIENCY

Lesions affecting the nucleus tractus solitarius, nucleus retroambigualis, or the descending automatic respiratory pathways in the upper cervical cord cause central respiratory failure that can be acute or chronic. The principal pathologies are listed in Table 1.

Clinical features

In acute respiratory failure, patients may report a sense of respiratory unease and may be (justifiably) fearful of sleep. Breathlessness, which as mentioned earlier requires an intact automatic system, is not a feature. Signs of hypoventilation may be present (see below). There is virtually always evidence of brain-stem dysfunction, particularly dysphagia and dysphonia (CN X) and loss of glossopharyngeal sensation (CN IX); hiccup may occur and reflex coughing (for example, during tracheal stimulation) may be depressed. The breathing pattern is abnormal (Fig. 2). During wakefulness, tidal volume and frequency are abnormally variable, and variability increases during drowsiness and sleep, perhaps leading to apnoea. Breath hold may be prolonged, but voluntary control (such as vital capacity) is unaffected.

In chronic respiratory insufficiency, features of persistent hypoventilation ('central alveolar hypoventilation') will be present. These include morning headache, poor sleep, nightmares, daytime somnolence, fatigue, decreased exercise tolerance, cyanosis, polycythaemia, and pulmonary hypertension. These can culminate in right heart failure, seizures, confusion, and coma.

Spinal cord lesions that transect the cord above C3 cause complete loss of automatic breathing. Lower cervical cord lesions allow spontaneous inspiration to continue (via the diaphragm); expiration is largely passive, through the elastic recoil of the ribcage and lungs, but preserved accessory muscle expiratory activity may also be used.

Assessment

In both acute and chronic cases, monitoring the breathing pattern and blood gases (indwelling arterial line or oxymeter) during drowsiness or sleep is crucial. Blood gas measurements during wakefulness are often unhelpful because the contribution of the behavioural system cannot be evaluated. Similarly, the vital capacity (a behavioural manoeuvre) provides no index of the integrity of the automatic system, and even the breathing pattern in wakefulness can be misleading if the subject is trying to breathe 'normally'. Ventilatory response to CO_2 or O_2 will be decreased.

Table 1 *Main neurological causes of respiratory failure*

	Acute	Chronic
Central		
Medulla	Infarct	Congenital
	Haemorrhage	Tumour
	Abscess	Encephalitis
	Encephalitis (e.g. polyomyelitis)	Leigh's disease
	Compression (e.g. cerebellar ectopia)	Motor neurone disease
	Trauma	Multiple sclerosis
	Hypoxia	
	Drugs	
Cervical cord (C1–3)	Compression	Tumour
	Trauma	Compression
		Transverse myelitis
		Multiple sclerosis
Peripheral		
Anterior horn	Poliomyelitis	Motor neurone disease (ALS)
		Spinal muscular atrophy
		Poliomyelitis
Peripheral nerve	Guillain–Barré	Progressive inflammatory polyneuropathy
	Diphtheria	Paraneoplastic neuropathy
	Toxins	
	Porphyria	
Neuromuscular junction	Myasthenia gravis	
	Congenital myasthenia	
	Botulism	
Muscle	Polymyositis	Acid maltase deficiency
	Periodic paralysis	Limb girdle dystrophy
	Metabolic	Dystrophia myotonica
		Polymyositis
		Nemaline myopathy

Fig. 2 Disorders of respiratory rhythm (schematic). Note that irregular breathing associated with a medullary lesion indicates failure of automatic breathing.

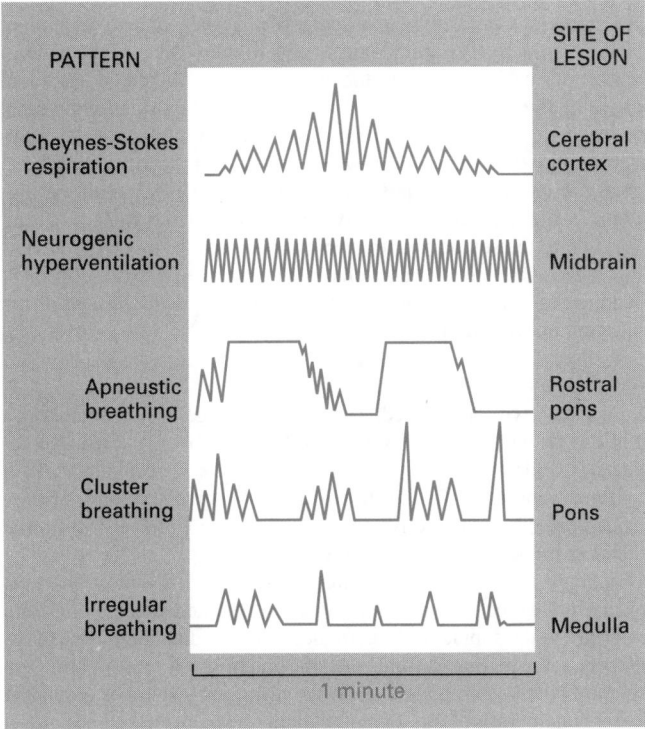

Management

In acute central respiratory failure, immediate intubation and assisted ventilation is usually required while the underlying pathology (Table 1) is identified and appropriate measures taken. Tracheostomy may be needed later, and the possibility of indefinite assisted ventilation has to be accepted. Patient-triggered ventilation is clearly inappropriate. If patients are allowed to breathe spontaneously during wakefulness, a breathing monitor should be used with a suitable alarm system. Phrenic nerve stimulation is potentially usable in these patients, but has not gained general acceptance. Associated dysphagia will require naso-gastric intubation. The impaired cough response makes physiotherapy and tracheal toilet particularly important.

In chronic respiratory insufficiency, nocturnal assisted ventilation will be needed, either by means of a cuirass and pump, or more conveniently by nasal intermittent positive pressure ventilation via a well-fitted nasal mask. Both techniques can be adapted for home use.

DISORDERS OF THE BREATHING PATTERN

This section will deal with disorders of the breathing pattern other than the irregular breathing of central respiratory failure already described. These disorders are not normally associated with hypoventilation. They may help in localizing lesions of the CNS. For the majority, no treatment specifically for the dysrhythmia is indicated (or indeed available).

Cheyne–Stokes respiration

This is characterized by a smoothly incremental and decremental pattern that has a cycle time lasting a minute or more, sometimes with brief intercycle apnoea (Fig. 2). Hyperventilation occurs throughout the cycle. The disorder is a sign of cardiac and/or cerebral cortex dysfunction, not of brain-stem disorder. The two commonest causes are cerebrovascular disease (for example, multiple infarcts) and prolonged circulation time (as in heart failure). The mechanisms contributing to the periodicity are complex but include interference with the 'damping' influence of the cerebral cortex (a behavioural effect) on the automatic system, the effects of pulmonary congestion and hypoxaemia, and the consequences of prolongation in the lung to chemoreceptor transit time.

NEUROGENIC HYPERVENTILATION

This very rare condition is characterized by rapid deep breathing (Fig. 2), a low $PaCO_2$ and normal PaO_2. Neurogenic hyperventilation may follow damage to the midbrain, particularly the periaqueductal grey matter, and has been described in association with brain-stem tumour. It should not be confused with the much commoner hyperpnoea occurring in obtunded patients which arises from pulmonary congestion and vagal reflex stimulation of the automatic system. These patients may also have a low $PaCO_2$ but, by contrast with neurogenic hyperventilation, the PaO_2 is reduced because of pulmonary shunting at poorly ventilated alveoli.

APNEUSTIC BREATHING

Inspiratory or, less commonly, expiratory voluntary breath-holding occurs, which may be prolonged and followed by the breakthrough of rapid rhythmic breathing (Fig. 2). The disorder associates with damage to the dorsolateral rostral pons involving the nucleus parabrachialis medialis.

CLUSTER BREATHING

This irregular breathing pattern lacks the smooth incremental/decremental pattern of Cheyne–Stokes respiration (Fig. 2). Involuntary sighs may be frequent. It occurs with damage to the rostral pontine tegmentum.

EPILEPTIC APNOEA

In view of the strong inhibitory projections from the temporal lobe to respiratory motoneurones, it is not surprising that apnoea occurs in epilepsy and, indeed, can be a cause of death. In rare instances, apnoea may be the sole manifestation of temporal lobe seizures. Diagnosis and management are as for other forms of temporal lobe epilepsy (see Chapter 24.4.1).

HICCUP

A hiccup consists of an intense synchronous diaphragmatic and inspiratory intercostal muscle contraction lasting about 500 ms, followed 30 ms after its onset by glottal closure, which generates the characteristic inspiratory sound and the discomfort. Mean frequency of hiccup is usually less than 30/min. Increasing $PaCO_2$ or breath-holding both reduce hiccup frequency (and may eliminate it); a low $PaCO_2$ increases hiccup amplitude but not frequency. Hiccup occurs in late fetal life and is frequent in the new-born. It seems to be served by a supraspinal mechanism largely distinct from the automatic respiratory system. Its characteristics suggest a gastrointestinal nature; its function (if any) is unknown.

Persistent or frequently recurrent hiccup may occur with neurological disease affecting the medulla in the region of the nucleus tractus solitarius (Table 1), particularly brain-stem tumour, infarction, encephalitis, and occasionally meningitis. It also occurs with metabolic disease such as uraemia and in a variety of thoracic, cardiac, and abdominal conditions, probably mediated via the vagus nerves. 'Pathological' hiccup may continue during sleep, being one of the few involuntary movements to do so. Emotional stimuli (such as shock and sexual intercourse) may end a bout of hiccup.

Management of hiccup can be difficult. Postprandial hiccup either resolves spontaneously or responds to measures that stimulate the pharynx (for example, drinking iced water) or increase in $PaCO_2$ (for example, rebreathing). Nasal mucosal stimulation sufficient to provide sneezing may also abort hiccup, as first reported by Plato (*The Symposium*, 416 BC) whose observations have not always been acknowledged by later authors. Nasopharyngeal stimulation stops hiccup in a high proportion of postoperative cases. When hiccup is secondary to neurological or metabolic disease, none of these methods is likely to provide sustained relief. The wide range of remedies proposed for chronic hiccup implies that none are pre-eminently effective. Chlorpromazine is probably best tried first, as an intravenous bolus. Haloperidol, metoclopramide, clonazepam, baclofen, or anticonvulsants are worth trying in resistant hiccup of neurological origin. Phrenic nerve section, although sometimes undertaken, seems inadvisable because hiccup will continue in other inspiratory muscles and ventilatory capacity may be compromised by the diaphragm paralysis.

PERIPHERAL VENTILATORY FAILURE

Peripheral ventilatory failure is much more common than central failure. It occurs terminally in many patients with progressive neuromuscular disorders, and may be a presenting or prominent early feature in others. The principal causes are listed in Table 1.

Clinical features

Acute ventilatory failure is characterized by anxiety, shortness of breath, tachycardia, and poor sleep, leading to hypoxic confusion, seizure, and coma. Chronic ventilatory failure develops more insidiously and is often overlooked initially. Clinical features of hypoventilation occur (see above). Dyspnoea is often absent at rest and patients may tolerate markedly abnormal blood gases without distress. Seizures may occur during exacerbation of chronic hypoxia.

Clinical assessment

There is accessory muscle activity and often flaring of the alae nasi, particularly in acute failure. Weakness or paralysis of the diaphragm, which can be relatively selective in some disorders (such as acid maltase deficiency), causes breathlessness in the supine posture (orthopnoea); such patients may thus elect to sleep upright. Diaphragm fatigue may contribute to its impaired function.

An important (and often overlooked) physical sign of diaphragm weakness or paralysis is paradoxical (inward) movement of the abdominal wall during inspiration in the supine posture, which comes about because of the in-series coupling between diaphragm and abdominal wall (see above). Gravitational forces increase this effect in the head-down posture (which is usually intolerable for such patients) but decrease it in the upright posture. A further sign of a paralysed diaphragm is the apparently excessive movement of the ribcage during inspiration in the supine posture, which is sometimes misinterpreted as being due to anxiety or as 'functional'. This increased ribcage movement is required to compensate for the passive upward displacement of the diaphragm in inspiration.

Laboratory assessment

Vital capacity will be reduced. The earliest change in blood gases is a fall in $PaCO_2$ with a normal or reduced PaO_2, probably because micro-atelectasis leads to shunting and a reflex increase in respiratory drive. In chronic ventilatory failure, hypoxia and hypercapnia may increase considerably during sleep. Blood gas monitoring (in-dwelling arterial catheter or by percutaneous oxymeter) is necessary.

Diaphragm function is most readily assessed by measuring the vital capacity in the erect and supine postures. A decline when moving from the upright to the supine posture implies selective diaphragm weakness. A 50 per cent reduction is usual when the diaphragm is totally paralysed. Screening (fluoroscopy), particularly in the upright posture, is unreliable in cases where both halves of the diaphragm are paralysed because it cannot readily distinguish between active and passive downward movement of the diaphragm, but it is valuable in the diagnosis of unilateral diaphragm paralysis. Transdiaphragmatic pressure is the best index of diaphragm function, but the measurement is available in only a few special centres. Peak inspiratory pressure provides an index of overall inspiratory force. Measurement of phrenic nerve conduction may occasionally be useful.

Management

Chest infection is common and can be life-threatening. It requires vigorous physiotherapy and early antibiotic treatment (see also Section 17).

In acute ventilatory failure, control of the airway (by, for example, intubation) and assisted ventilation should be immediately undertaken before treatment (when available) is directed to the underlying pathology. If this is unlikely to be corrected within a few days, tracheostomy will be needed.

In chronic ventilatory failure, initial treatment by continuous assisted ventilation corrects daytime blood gases and the systemic consequences of chronic hypoventilation. Improvement can later usually be maintained by assisted ventilation solely at night. This is best achieved by a cuirass jacket attached to a pump, or by nocturnal intermittent positive pressure ventilation, both of which can be used at home. Nocturnal assisted ventilation via a tracheostomy will be needed in some patients. Treatment in this way not only improves or fully corrects daytime blood gases, but also greatly increases the quality of life by reducing fatigue and somnolence. Progressive muscle disease often affects young adults who may have families dependent on them. Nocturnal assisted ventilation usually enables patients to return to work or to take up their previous household activities. It may also greatly relieve the respiratory distress observed in more severely affected patients, particularly those cases of motoneurone disease in whom the respiratory muscles are early and severely involved. The commitment to assisted ventilation is not indefinite because progressive bulbar and respiratory muscle weakness ultimately leads to a terminal chest infection.

NOCTURNAL OBSTRUCTIVE APNOEA

See Chapter 17.4.2 for discussion.

REFERENCES

Adams, L. and Guz, A. (1991). Dyspnea on exertion. In *Exercise: pulmonary physiology and pathophysiology*, (ed. B.J. Whipp and K. Wasserman), pp. 449–94. Marcel Dekker, New York.

Bougousslavsky, J., *et al.* (1990). Respiratory failure and unilateral caudal brainstem infarction. *Annals of Neurology* **28**, 668–73.

Branthwaite, M.A. (1991). Non-invasive and domiciliary ventilation: postive pressure techniques. *Thorax* **46**, 208–12.

Cherniack, N.S. and Longobardo, G.S. (1973). Cheyne–Stokes breathing. *New England Journal of Medicine* **288**, 952–7.

Coulter, D.L. (1984). Partial seizures with apnoea and bradycardia. *Archives of Neurology* **41**, 173–4.

Howard, R.S. (1992). Persistent hiccups. *British Medical Journal* **305**, 1237–8.

Howard, R.S. and Newsom-Davis, J. (1992). Neural control of respiration. In *Neurosurgery: the scientific basis of clinical practice*, (ed. A. Crockard, R. Hayward, and J.T. Hoff), pp. 318–3. Blackwell scientific, Oxford.

Howard, R.S., Wiles, C.M., and Spencer, G.T. (1988). The late sequelae of poliomyelitis. *Quarterly Journal of Medicine* **66**, 219–32.

Howard, R.S., Wiles, C.M., and Loh, L. (1989). Respiratory complications and their management in motor neuron disease. *Brain* **112**, 1155–70.

Howard, R.S., Wiles, C.M., Hirsch, N.P., Loh, L., Spencer, G.T., and Newsom-Davis, J. (1992). Respiratory involvement in multiple sclerosis. *Brain* **115**, 479–94.

Loh, L., Goldman, M., and Newsom-Davis, J. (1977). The assessment of diaphragm function. *Medicine* **56**, 165–9.

Newsom-Davis, J. (1970). An experimental study of hiccup. *Brain* **93**, 851–72.

Plum, F. and Posner, J.B. (1980). *The diagnosis of stupor and coma*, pp. 32–41. F.A. Davis, Philadelphia.

Roussos, C. and Macklem, P.T. (1982). The respiratory muscles. *New England Journal of Medicine* **307**, 786–97.

Shneerson, J.M. (1991). Non-invasive and domiciliary ventilation: negative pressure techniques. *Thorax* **46**, 131–5.

Wedzicha, W. 1992. Nasal ventilation. *British Journal of Hospital Medicine* **47**, 257–61.

24.3.9 Spinal cord

W. B. MATTHEWS

Anatomy

The clinical diagnosis and management of lesions of the spinal cord depend to a large degree on knowledge of its functional anatomy. The diagnosis of these disorders has been greatly facilitated by the use of MRI, CT, and angiography (see Section 24.2).

The spinal cord extends from the foramen magnum to the lower border of the first lumbar vertebra, being enclosed by the arachnoid membrane and the dura mater, both of which extend below the termination of the cord into the sacral canal. The blood supply consists of a posterior system supplying the posterior columns and posterior grey matter, and an anterior system supplying the remainder, including the corticospinal tracts, spinothalamic tracts, and anterior horns of grey matter, separate branches supplying the right and left sides. Both the anterior and posterior spinal arteries receive feeding vessels at many levels, and blood flow may be in a rostral or caudal direction at different levels. The most constant contributions to the anterior spinal artery are from the vertebral arteries and the arteria magna of Adamkiewicz that arises from the tenth left intercostal artery, but even these are subject to much variation and radicular arteries may enter the spinal system at any level.

The main motor and sensory pathways in the spinal cord are described in Chapter 24.3.11 and need only be summarized here. The crossed corticospinal tract lies in the lateral column of the white matter. The posterior columns convey uncrossed fibres serving postural sense and some elements of touch. Fibres serving pain and thermal sensation ascend for a few segments on the side of entry and then cross in the centre of the cord to ascend as the spinothalamic tracts in the lateral and anterior columns of white matter. In close proximity to these are the ascending pathways conveying sensation from bladder and bowel, and descending fibres conveying some degree of voluntary initiation and restraint.

Knowledge of the spinal segments concerned in the reflex arcs of the tendon jerks and cutaneous reflexes commonly elicited in clinical practice is of some assistance in the localization of spinal cord lesions. Some individual variation and spread beyond a single segment must be expected, but in general the pattern is as follows:

C6 biceps and supinator;
C7 triceps;
L4 knee jerk;
S1 ankle jerk;
D7 to D12, superficial abdominal reflexes;
L2 cremasteric;
S1 plantar reflex.

A reflex cannot be obtained if the arc is interrupted by disease of the relevant segment of the spinal cord.

The relationship of the spinal cord segments to the vertebral bodies and palpable spinous processes is of practical importance. In the neck each segment is at the level of the spinous process immediately above; for example, the sixth segment is opposite the fifth spinous process. In the thoracic region the interval progressively widens, the first lumbar segment being at the tenth dorsal vertebral level. The cord terminates at the lower border of the first lumbar vertebra.

From such anatomical approximations it is possible to identify the level and extent of spinal cord lesions. A lesion of the conus medullaris will cause weakness and wasting only of the muscles supplied by the lower sacral segments, mainly the glutei. Sensory loss involves the buttocks and perineum. The anus is patulous and the reflex contraction of the sphincter normally induced by pricking the neighbouring skin is absent. There is no sensation of fullness of the bladder or desire to empty the rectum, and reflex evacuation is also impaired, resulting in a large atonic bladder with overflow incontinence. Sexual function in the male is lost.

A complete transverse lesion of the dorsal cord results in spastic paralysis and loss of all forms of sensation below the level of the segment involved. The segmental organization of cutaneous sensation is shown in Figs. 1 and 2 of Chapter 24.3.11. With partial lesions both motor and sensory deficits are incomplete and, in particular, it is sometimes possible to detect that the major impact is on one side of the cord, producing some elements of the Brown–Séquard syndrome of hemisection of the cord. This consists of spastic weakness on the side of the lesion and loss of pain and thermal sensation on the opposite side, while light touch is little disturbed. A unilateral level, below which some modes of sensation are lost, is often several segments below the level of cord injury. A motor level can sometimes be established in the mid-dorsal region for if the lower abdominal muscles are paralysed, raising the shoulders will pull the umbilicus upwards. The superficial abdominal reflexes may be lost below the level of an obvious lesion, but are too inconstant to be of much diagnostic use.

A lesion of the lower part of the cervical enlargement causes wasting of the hand muscles; while a discrete lesion at the sixth cervical segment results in lower motor paralysis of flexion at the elbow and abolition of the biceps and supinator tendon jerks, with spastic weakness below this level. A complete lesion of the lower cervical cord causes respiratory embarrassment from paralysis of the muscles of the chest wall, while a similar lesion above the fourth cervical segment, the main origin of the phrenic nerves, is incompatible with life without artificial ventilation.

A complete lesion of the cord at any level causes retention of urine with eventual overflow. Incomplete lesions may cause loss of the normal synergy between contraction of the bladder detrusor and relaxation of the sphincter, with resulting urgency and incontinence.

Not all clinical phenomena are readily explicable in simple anatomical terms. For example, reflex activity often appears to be enhanced above the level of a cervical cord lesion, and, conversely, a lesion at the foramen magnum may cause wasting of the hand muscles. This latter confusing effect has been attributed to infarction resulting from obstruction of venous return.

Non-traumatic paraplegia
ACUTE AND SUBACUTE

The patient with sudden or rapidly advancing weakness of the lower limbs presents an urgent problem of diagnosis and management. The presumption is that there is a focal lesion of the spinal cord but other causes such as poliomyelitis and acute polyneuritis, the Guillain–Barré syndrome (Chapter 24.17), must not be forgotten. Confusion is possible as with an acute spinal cord lesion the paralysis may be flaccid, the tendon reflexes absent, and the plantar reflexes unobtainable. A sensory level on the trunk is strong evidence of a spinal cord lesion.

The further distinction must then be made, as quickly as possible, between spinal cord compression and an intrinsic lesion of the cord requiring quite different management. Pain and tenderness over the spinal column, or pain of obvious root distribution, are of little diagnostic value and occur with many non-compressive lesions. Retention of urine is usual and may even distract attention from the weakness of the legs.

Intrinsic lesions
Non-compressive causes of acute myelopathy include multiple sclerosis, acute disseminated encephalomyelitis, viral infection, systemic lupus, Behçet's disease, sarcoidosis, paraneoplastic syndrome, and infarction.

The distinctive features of these diseases, described in the appropriate sections, are usually sufficient to effect diagnosis, although systemic lupus may mimic multiple sclerosis very closely. All except multiple sclerosis and acute postinfective demyelinating or necrotic transverse myelitis are extremely rare causes of acute paraplegia. It is important that the diagnosis of multiple sclerosis is not based on dubious clinical or laboratory evidence of multiple lesions, such as temporal pallor of the optic discs, nystagmus at the extremes of gaze, or paraesthesiae in the fingers. A complete transverse lesion of the cord is more likely to be due to an isolated episode of myelitis than multiple sclerosis, where the lesion is usually incomplete.

Spinal cord compression
In acute paraplegia the following causes of cord compression must be considered: epidural abscess, epidural haemorrhage, cervical spondylotic myelopathy, spontaneous dislocation of the cervical vertebrae in rheumatoid arthritis, arachnoiditis, benign tumour, metastatic tumour, and arteriovenous malformation.

These conditions are described under separate headings. Benign tumours and cervical spondylotic myelopathy much more commonly cause chronic progressive paraplegia but may cause acute paralysis following quite minor trauma.

Management
Urinary retention must be relieved. The level of the lesion must be determined by clinical means. The examination must naturally include a search for possible sources of metastatic lesions or infection.

Lumbar puncture solely for the purpose of examining the cerebrospinal fluid should not be done, as any changes found will not be specific and altering the intrathecal pressure below a spinal cord tumour may precipitate severe paralysis. If the responsible lesion cannot be shown by radiography, CT scanning, or MRI, and compression of the cord is still suspected, then the risk must be taken and a myelogram carried out.

CHRONIC PROGRESSIVE PARAPARESIS

Here again the important distinction is between spinal cord compression and intrinsic lesions. Among the latter, the progressive spinal form of multiple sclerosis is by far the most frequent cause in geographical areas where this disease is common. Other intrinsic diseases that may present in this way include motor neurone disease (Chapter 24.16), hereditary spastic paraplegia (Chapter 24.8), tropical spastic paraplegia, and AIDS myelopathy. The distinctive features of subacute combined degeneration and syringomyelia should prevent diagnostic confusion.

Chronic spinal cord compression is commonly due to benign causes: cervical spondylotic myelopathy, prolapsed dorsal disc, neurofibroma, meningioma, and arteriovenous malformations. A chronic epidural abscess is usually tuberculous and is uncommon where this disease has been largely controlled. Malignant causes include myeloma, chordoma, and glioma. The intramedullary ependymoma is benign and often difficult to diagnose because of the elongated cyst that may form, producing unusual physical signs.

Clinical features of progressive cord compression.
Sensory symptoms usually precede weakness and may be misinterpreted. Root pain is easily recognizable in the cervical region, but when thoracic roots are involved visceral pain may be mimicked. The characteristic pain on movement or coughing may be thought to arise in the chest. Compression of the sensory pathways may cause paraesthesiae or pain in the lower limbs. Cutaneous sensory loss due to involvement of the spinothalamic tracts may show 'sacral sparing' as lamination of

fibres in the tract allows those from lower segments to escape, but this sign is not diagnostic of cord compression.

Motor involvement is usually asymmetrical and, with a cervical cord lesion, classically affects the arm on the side of the lesion, then the ipsilateral leg, the other leg, and eventually the contralateral arm. The degree of sphincter involvement is highly variable.

The principles of establishing the level of the lesion by clinical means are outlined elsewhere, but this must often be only approximate. Lesions may involve several segments asymmetrically and, in life, physical signs do not always accord with the conventional diagrams.

Investigation

To misdiagnose a benign cause of cord compression as multiple sclerosis is a potentially disastrous error. Abnormal visual evoked potentials provide strong, but not wholly conclusive, evidence of relevant lesions beyond the spinal cord which may be more decisively shown by MRI of the head. Plain radiographs should not be neglected, including oblique views of the cervical spine where relevant. The relative values of different forms of imaging are discussed in Section 24.2. MRI of the spinal cord is replacing the need for myelography in many cases. Any cerebrospinal fluid obtained should be sent for analysis, including examination for oligoclonal banding of IgG, characteristically present in multiple sclerosis.

SUBACUTE COMBINED DEGENERATION OF THE SPINAL CORD

This is the commonest and most serious neurological complication of the deficiency of vitamin B_{12} which also results in addisonian pernicious anaemia, (see Section 22). The name refers to the combined degeneration observed at autopsy in the lateral and posterior columns of the spinal cord when the cause and treatment were unknown. Axonal loss is, however, preceded by demyelination, at least potentially reversible, and also involving the peripheral nerves.

Clinical features

The patients are in the age range of pernicious anaemia, that is to say, predominantly middle aged or older. The first symptom is always symmetrical paraesthesiae in the extremities, usually initially in the feet but occasionally confined to the hands. The sensations are often extremely unpleasant. Loss of postural sense causes ataxia in walking and, unless forestalled by treatment, the legs become weak. Examination in the early stages shows distal cutaneous sensory blunting but often severe loss of postural sense in the lower limbs. The ankle jerks may be absent and, at a later stage, the plantar reflexes are extensor. Before treatment was available the disease progressed to severe paraplegia, fatal within a year, but this is no longer seen.

Other neurological effects of vitamin B_{12} deficiency may be present, most commonly moderate loss of mental acuity. Visual impairment, the result of bilateral centrocaecal scotomata, is rare.

Clinical evidence of anaemia may be obvious or entirely lacking. The peripheral blood may be normal and the bone marrow is not always megaloblastic. The serum vitamin B_{12} level is, however, almost always significantly reduced (see Section 22).

The differential diagnosis includes peripheral neuropathy from other causes and, in younger patients, multiple sclerosis. A more common error, however, is simply to dismiss the paraesthesiae and stumbling gait as the inevitable results of advancing age. Tingling in the hands alone may be mistaken for the carpal tunnel syndrome.

Treatment

Hydroxocobalamin, 1 mg, should be injected immediately. In view of the vital importance of minimizing spinal cord damage, unnecessarily large doses are often given; 1 mg repeated daily for a week and thereafter weekly for several weeks before adopting a monthly schedule that must be continued indefinitely to avoid relapse. The response to treatment is,

in general, excellent. Even bedridden patients can be restored to normal walking, and extensor plantar reflexes revert to flexor. Beyond a certain point of disability, however, treatment is unavailing, presumably because of axonal degeneration, but this should now never be allowed to occur. The sensory symptoms can be extremely persistent and a patient rescued from severe disability will continue to complain bitterly of the paraesthesiae. Mental symptoms also respond rapidly but restoration of vision in vitamin B_{12} deficiency amblyopia is less predictable.

SYRINGOMYELIA

The essential lesion implied by this name is the presence of a cavity within the spinal cord. Such a cavity may form part of a cystic tumour, in particular an ependymoma, but the term syringomyelia has been restricted to non-tumourous conditions.

Pathology

The spinal cord contains an irregular asymmetrical cavity, filled with cerebrospinal fluid, extending over many segments, or even its entire length, although usually most extensive in the cervical enlargement. Contiguous structures are destroyed, in particular the anterior horn cells, the sensory fibres decussating within the cord concerned with pain and thermal sensation, and the lateral corticospinal tracts. The syrinx may extend into the medulla.

The abnormality in the spinal cord is frequently accompanied by a congenital abnormality known as the Chiari malformation, in which aberrant cerebellar tissue extends into the cervical spinal canal. Some degree of hydrocephalus is also often present. The significance of these findings is discussed below.

Clinical features

The onset of symptoms is usually in early adult life. The first symptoms usually involve one upper limb, with a combination of wasting of the hand muscles, weakness, and sensory loss, often resulting in painless burns, either from cigarettes or from cooking. Wasting is more extensive than could be accounted for by any single peripheral nerve lesion and is accompanied by loss of tendon reflexes in the arm. Sensory loss, classically of 'dissociated' type with preservation of light touch and proprioception, but loss of pain and thermal sensation, often extends over the whole arm and upper thorax or may be bilateral over the 'cape area'. Scars of painless injuries may provide a diagnostic clue. A Horner's syndrome, or excessive sweating over one side of the face, may indicate involvement of the cervical sympathetic nerve. A mild dorsal scoliosis is almost invariable.

There are many deviations from this classical mode of onset. Pain in the arm may be severe. The corticospinal tracts may be involved at an early stage, causing spastic weakness of the legs, but some abnormal signs will be present in the arms. Although the onset is usually insidious, sudden exacerbations are common, particularly after exertion, coughing, or sneezing.

The symptoms and signs may sometimes remain unchanged for many years but syringomyelia is usually progressive. Wasting of the upper limbs spreads and sensory loss becomes increasingly dense, involving all modalities. The hands may become swollen, and painless ulcers may destroy the digits. Charcot's painless destructive arthropathy often affects the shoulder joints. Spastic paraparesis increases.

Involvement of the medulla, syringobulbia, may occur without evidence of spinal cord disease or, more commonly, as an extension of syringomyelia. The usual pattern of sensory loss includes the peripheral areas of the face, with sparing of the nose and mouth. Damage to the motor nuclei of the lower cranial nerves causes wasting of the tongue, dysphagia, and vocal cord paralysis. Rotatory nystagmus is common.

Diagnosis

In the early stages, syringomyelia must be distinguished from the many other causes of wasting of the hand muscles and, while this may be difficult, the pattern of sensory loss and loss of tendon jerks is usually distinctive. An intrinsic tumour of the spinal cord may produce an identical syndrome.

A diagnosis of syringomyelia is, however, no longer adequate. It is now apparent that in the great majority of cases the cause lies in some obstruction of the outflow of cerebrospinal fluid from the foramina in the roof of the fourth ventricle, most commonly by the Chiari malformation. How this results in an expanding destructive syrinx in the spinal cord is still controversial, but it is probable that the normal vestigial central canal of the cord is distended by cerebrospinal fluid under intermittent pressure and eventually ruptures into the substance of the cord. This may occur suddenly, as the result of a rise in venous pressure, and this accounts for the immediate exacerbations that may follow sneezing. The association with hydrocephalus is also explained by partial obstruction to the flow of cerebrospinal fluid. Other causes of obstruction are less common, the most important being spinal arachnoiditis.

Treatment

Syringomyelia following spinal cord injury is described above. The diagnosis of syringomyelia, its extent and causation, can now be fully displayed by magnetic resonance imaging or, less easily, by myelography and CT scanning. Such investigations are essential for the planning of surgical treatment directed to the relief of obstruction to the flow of cerebrospinal fluid or the draining of the syrinx. The former involves decompression of the posterior fossa and cervical canal. Many ingenious operations have been devised to relieve pressure within the cyst. Surgery is not always indicated and is not always successful, but should certainly be considered when disease is progressive but not yet severely disabling, or when pain is severe. Syringomyelia secondary to arachnoiditis is particularly intractable.

VASCULAR DISEASE

The arteries that supply the spinal cord are not subject to atherosclerosis and ischaemic disease results from more remote causes. Infarction of the spinal cord may result from atheroma or dissecting aneurysm of the aorta, aortic or cardiac surgery, and severe hypotension following cardiac arrest or infarction. Embolism may occur in bacterial endocarditis. A main feeding vessel commonly arises from the tenth left intercostal artery, and surgery in this area can be hazardous. Acute pain at the site of the lesion often occurs at the onset. Paraplegia develops very rapidly and, as the infarct is usually confined to the distribution of the anterior spinal artery, sensory loss is confined to those modalities conveyed in the spinothalamic tracts, pain and thermal sensibility, with sparing of postural sense. A unilateral infarct results in the Brown–Séquard syndrome and occasionally the entire cord is infarcted below a segmental level.

Recovery from incomplete lesions is often unexpectedly good, but severe residual disability may also occur. Transient ischaemic attacks affecting the spinal cord occur rarely in arteriopathic subjects and cause paraplegia for an hour or less.

Haemorrhage within the spinal cord—haematomyelia—is rare. It may occur with rupture of an arteriovenous malformation, as the result of trauma, with disturbances of clotting mechanisms, or for no detectable reason. The onset is usually abrupt but occasionally ingravescent, the symptoms and signs being those of a centrally situated spinal cord lesion.

Thrombophlebitis may cause subacute necrotic myelitis with rapidly developing signs of a usually incomplete cord lesion. This can sometimes be attributed to spread of infection from the pelvis or lower limbs, but often no cause can be found. The prognosis is poor and the condition may spread up the spinal cord in successive episodes.

RADIATION MYELOPATHY

The spinal cord is vulnerable to damage from X-irradiation directed to structures in the neck. The incidence is low and is clearly dose related.

Sensory symptoms in the limbs, often accompanied by Lhermitte's symptom of an electric shock sensation down the spine on flexing the neck, occur soon after exposure and eventually remit. Lhermitte's symptom, if troublesome, can be successfully treated with carbamazepine.

Much more serious is delayed myelopathy, developing from 6 months to 5 years after treatment and resulting in severely disabling progressive paraplegia. The prolonged latent period has not been adequately explained.

MYELITIS

An acute transverse cord lesion may occur as an isolated event following viral infection or inoculation, or for no detectable reason. The outcome varies from complete recovery to permanent paraplegia. A short course of high-dosage intravenous steroids should be given, but this is not always followed by recovery.

Apart from poliomyelitis, direct viral invasion of the spinal cord is uncommon, but myelitis from infection by the Epstein–Barr virus has been reported.

Subacute necrotizing myelitis

This is a rare condition in which the cord lesion is not transverse, involving only one or two segments, but involves the whole cord below an upper level. The paralysis therefore remains flaccid as reflex activity cannot return. There may be successive bouts involving ascending levels. As mentioned above, in some instances the lesion appears to be based on a pre-existing vascular anomaly, but usually no cause can be found. Treatment is ineffective and recovery does not occur.

SPINAL ARACHNOIDITIS

Chronic spinal arachnoiditis may present many years after acute meningitis, and other identifiable causes include subarachnoid haemorrhage, intrathecal steroids, and non-water-soluble contrast media previously used in myelography, but now discarded. The presentation is that of slowly progressive paraplegia or the picture of syringomyelia. Surgical treatment is not effective as the arachnoiditis is usually diffuse.

EPIDURAL HAEMORRHAGE

Haemorrhage into the epidural space is a complication of anticoagulant therapy. The cervical spine is the usual site and haemorrhage should be suspected as the cause of rapidly advancing tetraplegia in a patient on such treatment. Recovery following evacuation of the blood is usually complete.

EPIDURAL ABSCESS

An acute abscess in the spinal epidural space is usually the result of staphylococcal infection, either metastatic or by spread from some contiguous site. Progression of paraplegia is rapid and pain in the back is a constant feature. Fever and a raised white cell count are common. The cerebrospinal fluid may contain an excess of cells but may be normal, and lumbar puncture does not assist diagnosis. Predisposing factors, apart from infection elsewhere, include diabetes, alcoholism, and any cause of immunodeficiency. MRI is the essential diagnostic procedure.

Unfortunately, even with rapid diagnosis and evacuation of the abscess, the prognosis for full recovery must be guarded. Non-surgical management with antibiotics alone has sometimes been successful.

SPINAL CORD TUMOURS

In contrast to the brain, the majority of spinal cord tumours are extrinsic, and many are benign. The neurofibroma arises from the Schwann cells of the spinal roots at any level. It may be part of generalized neurofibromatosis but is usually single. Because of its site of origin, pain of root distribution is a common early symptom. The results of surgical removal, even when spinal cord damage appears to be severe, are remarkably successful and complete recovery is often achieved. The spinal meningioma cannot be distinguished on clinical grounds from a neurofibroma and the results of removal are equally good.

The commonest malignant tumour compressing the cord is metastatic carcinoma, either involving the vertebral body or forming a dense band of meningeal infiltration. The best hope of mitigating the effects of this disaster lie with the immediate intravenous injection of large doses of dexamethasone, precise localization of the tumour, and radiotherapy. Laminectomy is seldom helpful but more radical attempts at removing the tumour may achieve temporary success.

A chordoma, a malignant tumour arising from remnants of the notochord, may arise in the sacral area or, more rarely, in the cervical region.

Intrinsic tumours of the cord are usually malignant but seldom expand rapidly. The most common forms are the astrocytoma and the benign ependymoma. The latter may sometimes form in the filum terminale, causing a cauda equina syndrome but also, most confusingly, papilloedema, attributed unconvincingly to the high cerebrospinal fluid protein level. In this site the tumour may be removed but, for obvious reasons, surgical removal of intrinsic tumours is unavoidably hazardous. Radiotherapy is sometimes unexpectedly successful but, as biopsy of the spinal cord is seldom carried out, histological verification is usually lacking. Multiple sclerosis may cause swelling of the cord visible on myelography.

ARTERIOVENOUS MALFORMATIONS

At the time of diagnosis these lesions consist of a tangled mass of veins containing arterial blood, nearly always on the dorsal surface of the cord, but sometimes involving the dura. The essential lesion, however, is of one or more arteriovenous shunts, presumably of congenital origin.

The clinical presentation is varied. A spinal subarachnoid haemorrhage causes sudden severe pain in the back—the *coup de poignard*—with signs of meningeal irritation and even loss of consciousness. Signs of spinal cord damage are not invariably present. Dural malformations are much less likely to bleed.

More commonly the onset is with paraparesis, often progressive in a stepwise manner, or fluctuating with considerable remissions. Diagnostic confusion may arise, particularly as the symptoms may relapse in pregnancy with subsequent remission, in a pattern shared by meningiomas and often erroneously thought to be typical of multiple sclerosis. A cutaneous angiomatous lesion is sometimes an important clue, and occasionally a pulsatile bruit may be heard over the lesion.

Confirmation of the diagnosis and localization of the vascular shunts prior to treatment by surgery or embolization requires expert and elaborate neuroradiology. How these lesions cause symptoms is not fully known but there are probably elements both of 'stealing' blood from the cord and cord compression, both of which can be relieved by obliterating the shunts and collapsing the arterialized veins. Good results can be obtained if this is done before irreversible damage has been sustained.

CERVICAL SPONDYLOTIC MYELOPATHY

Spondylosis and cord damage due to disc prolapse is discussed in Chapter 24.3.11.

REFERENCES

Byrne, T.N. (1992). Spinal cord compression from epidural metastases. *New England Journal of Medicine* **327**, 614–19.
Dropcho, E.J. (1991). Central nervous system injury by therapeutic radiation. *Neurologic Clinics* **9**, 969–88.
Dyste, G.N., Menezes, A.H., and van Gilder, J.C. (1989). Symptomatic Chiari malformations. An analysis of presentation, management and long-term outcome. *Journal of Neurosurgery* **71**, 159–68.
Esses, S.I. and Morley, T.P. (1983). Spinal arachnoiditis. *Canadian Journal of Neurological Sciences* **10**, 2–10.
Healton, E.B., Savage, D.G., Brust. J.C.M., Garrett, T.J., and Lindenbaum J. (1991). Neurologic aspects of cobalamin deficiency. *Medicine* **70**, 229–45.
Henson, R.A. and Parsons, M. (1967). Ischaemic lesions of the spinal cord: an illustrated review. *Quarterly Journal of Medicine* **36**, 205–22.
Hughes, J.T. (1978). *Pathology of the spinal cord*, (2nd edn). Blackwell, Oxford.
Lipton, H.L. and Teasdale, R.D. (1973). Acute transverse myelopathy in adults. *Archives of Neurology* **28**, 252–7.
Logue, V. (1979). Angiomas of the spinal cord: review of the pathogenesis, clinical features and results of surgery. *Journal of Neurology Neurosurgery and Psychiatry* **42**, 1–11.
Mariani, C., *et al.* (1991). The natural history and results of surgery in 50 cases of syringomyelia. *Journal of Neurology* **238**, 433–8.
Paty, D.W., Blume, W.T., Brown, W.F., Jaatoul, N., Kertesz, A., and McInnis, W. (1979). Chronic progressive myelopathy: investigation with CSF electrophoresis, evoked potentials and CT scan. *Annals of Neurology* **6**, 419–24.
Symon, L., Kuyama, H., and Kendall, B. (1984). Dural arteriovenous malformations of the spine: clinical features and surgical results in 55 cases. *Journal of Neurosurgery* **60**, 238–47.
Teman, A.J. (1992). Spinal epidural abscess. Early detection with gadolinium magnetic resonance imaging. *Archives of Neurology* **49**, 743–6.
Ungar-Sargon, J.Y., Lovelace, R.E., and Brustr, J.C.M. (1980). Spastic paraparesis: a reappraisal. *Journal of Neurological Science* **46**, 1–12.
Vloeberghs, M., Herregodts, P., Stadnik, T., Goosens, A., and D'Haens, J. (1992). Spinal arachnoiditis mimicking a spinal tumour: a case report and review of the literature. *Surgical Neurology* **37**, 211–15.
Zerval, N.T. and Pile-Spellman, J. (1992). Case reports of the Massachusetts General Hospital. *New England Journal of Medicine* **326**, 816–24. (Spinal arteriovenous malformation.)

24.3.10 Spinal cord injury and the management of paraplegia

D. J. GRUNDY

Traumatic spinal cord injury

INTRODUCTION

It is only in the past 50 years that significant progress in the management of spinal cord injury has occurred. Prior to this, a defeatist attitude prevailed and the condition was generally regarded as having a very poor prognosis, death often occurring within a few days from direct effects of the injury or within a few months from pressure sores and urinary tract sepsis. Thus, in 1917, almost 50 per cent of patients died of urinary sepsis within 2 months. The outcome only improved following the work of such pioneers as Guttmann in the United Kingdom and Munro in the United States, who showed that a multidisciplinary approach was required.

The first spinal injuries units in the United Kingdom were established in 1944 to provide comprehensive rehabilitation services for war casualties. Early results were encouraging, with an immediate reduction in morbidity and mortality, but even in the 1960s mortality in tetraplegic patients was 35 per cent. Further advances in treatment have reduced the overall mortality rate in the first year after injury to less than 5 per cent. Early admission to a spinal injuries unit, as well as reducing morbidity and mortality, results in an increased proportion of patients with incomplete spinal cord damage.

A recent study showed that the median survival time for all patients surviving the first year of injury was 32 years. It was greater for those with incomplete lesions and those with low injuries. The causes of death, particularly in incomplete lesions, have moved away from the traditional causes related to spinal cord injury, such as renal failure, and have begun to approximate to the causes of death in the general population. The figures showed that 24 per cent of patients died of urinary tract complications, 23 per cent of cardiovascular causes, and there were 14 per cent respiratory deaths, the latter being more prevalent in tetraplegic patients.

Eighty per cent of spinal cord injuries occur in males. Approximately 50 per cent are due to road traffic accidents and 25 per cent to domestic and industrial injuries, particularly falls down stairs and from ladders or scaffolding. Sporting accidents, such as those occurring from diving into shallow water, rugby, horse riding, and gymnastics account for at least 15 per cent of injuries.

INITIAL MANAGEMENT AT THE SCENE OF INJURY

A casualty with suspected spinal cord injury must be correctly handled, if further neurological damage is not to occur. Diagnosis may be more difficult if the casualty has taken alcohol, drugs, or if a head injury is present. Unfortunately, some patients (5 to 19 per cent in different series) deteriorate neurologically from the time of injury to the time of admission to a spinal injuries unit, because of missed or delayed diagnosis, or inadequate spinal immobilization.

Spinal injury will be suggested by local marking, bruising, or deformity. For example, grazes or lacerations to the face infer that the head was forced backwards, resulting in a cervical hyperextension injury; a gibbus or an increased gap between adjacent spinous processes is associated with a flexion injury to the spine.

The conscious patient with cord damage may complain of neck or back pain, disturbance or loss of sensation, and weakness or flaccid paralysis below a neurological level. In high lesions, diaphragmatic respiration due to intercostal paralysis occurs and in ultra-high lesions with phrenic nerve involvement, assisted ventilation may be necessary from the outset. Sympathetic paralysis in the tetraplegic or high paraplegic patient results in hypotension, bradycardia, and, commonly, priapism.

Having confirmed that the airway is secure, intravenous access is established, in case cardiopulmonary support is required. Clearing the airways of secretions may cause intense bradycardia and occasionally cardiac arrest, due to unopposed vagal action, particularly in hypoxic patients. To minimize this risk, the heart rate must be monitored and atropine and additional oxygen administered prior to pharyngeal suction. Glycopyrronium is preferable to atropine for repeated use.

If the casualty is unconscious, it must be assumed, until radiographs of the whole cervical spine are obtained, that the force rendering the patient unconscious has also injured the cervical spine. The head and neck are stabilized in neutral with a rigid collar, and the trunk must not be flexed or rotated, in case a thoracolumbar injury is present.

The unconscious patient is at risk of aspirating vomit, and therefore the supine position, although protecting the spine and allowing cardiopulmonary resuscitation and rapid assessment of associated injuries, is dangerous unless the casualty is intubated. Orotracheal intubation is relatively safe, if an assistant holds the head and minimizes neck movement. Alternatively, blind oro- or nasotracheal intubation, taking care not to rotate the neck can be performed by an experienced doctor, but it is difficult. The other method of protecting the airway is to 'log-roll' the patient into a modified lateral position, about 70 to 80° from prone, with the head supported in neutral, taking great care not to rotate the spine.

Associated injuries

Almost 50 per cent of patients have other injuries, particularly injuries to the head, chest, and limbs. Thoracic spinal injuries are often associated with multiple rib fractures, haemothorax, pneumothorax, and lung contusion, which further compromise respiration and require urgent treatment.

Spinal shock

The stage of flaccidity with absent reflexes below the level of the lesion—the period of spinal shock—persists for a few hours to several weeks after injury. If the injury has been above the sacral segments of

the cord, the end of spinal shock is denoted by a return of reflex activity below the level of the lesion. The anal and bulbocavernosus reflexes usually return first, followed by the lower limb reflexes. In injuries to the conus medullaris or cauda equina, the reflexes do not return. The plantar response is not always reliable in the diagnosis of acute spinal cord injury.

TRANSFER TO HOSPITAL

A spinal immobilizer, such as a Kendrick extrication device helps to protect the spine during evacuation and transportation to the nearest major accident and emergency department. Hard objects are removed from pockets to relieve pressure. If lying free, the patient should ideally be moved by four people lifting simultaneously, the head, neck, and spine being maintained in the neutral (anatomical) position. The person holding the head and neck directs movement, the second person lifts the shoulders and chest, the third the abdomen and pelvis, and the fourth the legs. Transfer to hospital should be on a firm stretcher, after initial lifting on a 'scoop stretcher' carefully assembled around the casualty.

Tetraplegic and high paraplegic patients are poikilothermic, because sympathetic paralysis results in loss of the usual vasomotor responses to temperature change. Blankets and thermal reflector sheets should therefore be used in cold weather to prevent hypothermia.

Most casualties will be taken to the nearest accident and emergency department but the regional spinal injuries unit should also be contacted so that initial management can be discussed and immediate transfer arranged, unless the patient has multiple injuries or severe respiratory insufficiency.

INITIAL MANAGEMENT AT HOSPITAL (TABLE 1)

A full history, general and neurological examination are essential, particularly because associated injuries are common. Respiratory function is urgently assessed to detect respiratory muscle paralysis and complications of chest injury, such as a pneumothorax or haemothorax, which may require an intercostal drain. Measurements of arterial blood gases and vital capacity are taken, and repeated as necessary. The diagnosis of intra-abdominal injury is difficult in high lesions, because of absent abdominal sensation and loss of the usual signs of peritoneal irritation—tenderness, guarding, or rigidity. Furthermore, paralytic ileus is not necessarily significant as it normally occurs after major trauma and for 2 to 3 days following spinal cord injury. The diagnosis of intra-abdominal injury (or indeed later peritonitis due to acute gastroduodenal stress ulceration with perforation) may therefore be missed or delayed. Occasionally, referred pain to the shoulder from diaphragmatic irritation occurs. If necessary, diagnostic peritoneal lavage should be performed. Intravenous fluids are continued, but oral fluids are withheld for at least 48 h after injury, until normal bowel sounds return. An H_2-receptor antagonist given for 3 weeks minimizes the risk of stress ulceration.

If delay in admission to the ward is likely, the casualty should be placed on a firm pressure-relieving mattress, and 'log-rolled' into the lateral position for 1 min every half hour.

RADIOLOGY

After initial clinical assessment and appropriate resuscitative measures to stabilize the patient, spinal radiographs and a chest radiograph are taken under medical supervision. Further films are taken, depending on the presence or suspicion of associated injuries. In cervical spine injuries, lateral, anteroposterior, and an open mouth view of the odontoid process are necessary. The lateral view is the most important and does not involve moving the patient. The shoulders often obscure the lower cervical spine but careful traction on the arms to depress the shoulders should demonstrate the cervicothoracic junction. If the latter is still not seen, a 'swimmer's' view is recommended, with the arm next to the cassette elevated above the head and the X-ray beam directed through the opposite shoulder. Sometimes lateral tomography may be necessary.

Table 1 *Initial assessment of a patient with a suspected spinal cord injury*

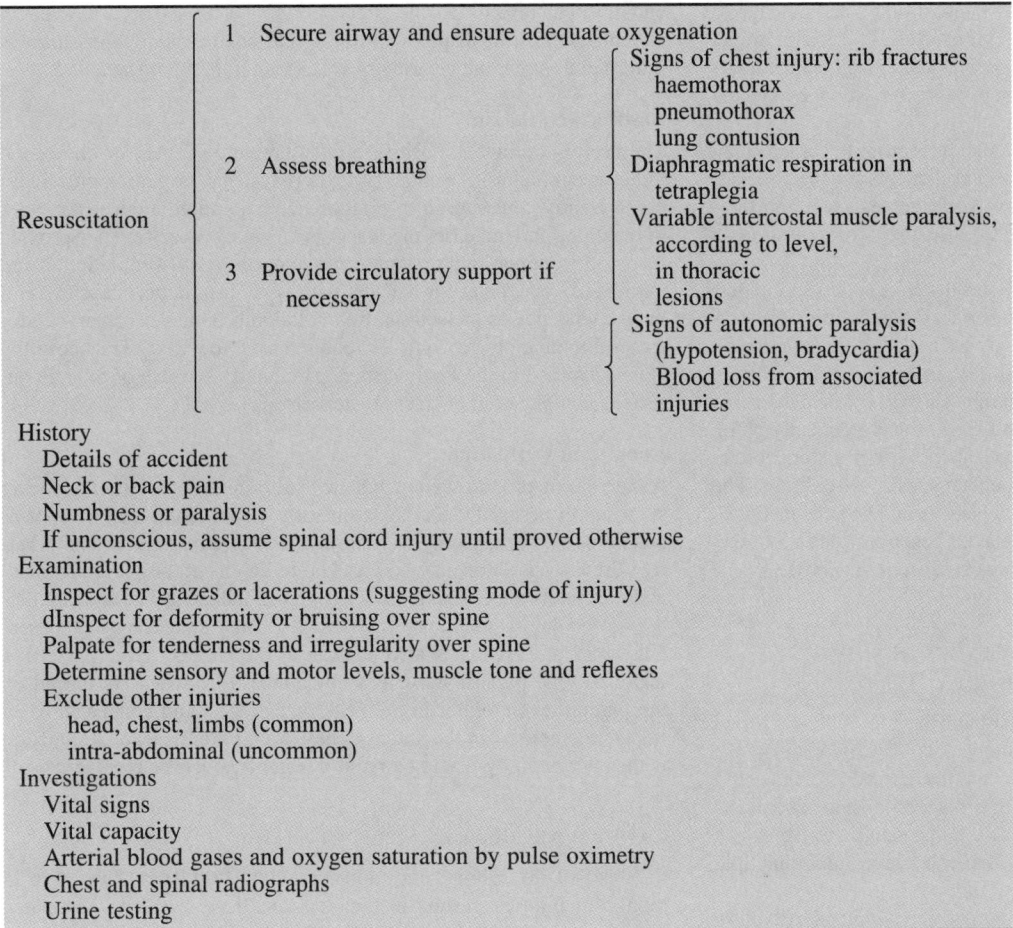

Resuscitation

1 Secure airway and ensure adequate oxygenation

2 Assess breathing
- Signs of chest injury: rib fractures
  haemothorax
  pneumothorax
  lung contusion
- Diaphragmatic respiration in tetraplegia
- Variable intercostal muscle paralysis, according to level, in thoracic lesions

3 Provide circulatory support if necessary
- Signs of autonomic paralysis (hypotension, bradycardia)
- Blood loss from associated injuries

History
  Details of accident
  Neck or back pain
  Numbness or paralysis
  If unconscious, assume spinal cord injury until proved otherwise
Examination
  Inspect for grazes or lacerations (suggesting mode of injury)
  dInspect for deformity or bruising over spine
  Palpate for tenderness and irregularity over spine
  Determine sensory and motor levels, muscle tone and reflexes
  Exclude other injuries
    head, chest, limbs (common)
    intra-abdominal (uncommon)
Investigations
  Vital signs
  Vital capacity
  Arterial blood gases and oxygen saturation by pulse oximetry
  Chest and spinal radiographs
  Urine testing

A cervical spine dislocation normally involves anterior displacement of the upper vertebra on the one below. Anterior displacement of more than half the diameter of the vertebral body denotes bilateral facet dislocation, whereas less than half a vertebral body shift implies unilateral facet dislocation. An increased gap between adjacent spinous processes on the lateral view signifies rupture of the posterior cervical ligamentous complex. Displacement of a spinous process from the midline on an anteroposterior view infers spinal rotation due to a unilateral facet dislocation.

In children, spinal cord injury often occurs without radiological signs of bony damage. Similarly, in older people with cervical spondylosis, a relatively minor hyperextension injury such as a fall on to the face or forehead may produce tetraplegia without evidence of bony injury.

In the thoracic and lumbar spine, anteroposterior and lateral radiographs are taken, but satisfactory views of the upper thoracic spine may be impossible without lateral tomography.

Computed tomography (CT) gives excellent detail of the vertebral column, demonstrates bony fragments in the spinal canal, and sometimes traumatic disc prolapse. With magnetic resonance imaging (MRI), bony detail is limited but the spinal cord itself, and any agent compressing it, is clearly demonstrated.

MANAGEMENT OF THE SPINAL INJURY

The cervical spine

Dislocations can usually be reduced by applying skull calipers and gradually increasing the traction force under radiographic control with the neck in flexion until the facets are disengaged, at which stage the neck is extended and the weights reduced to a maintenance level to splint the spine. Skull traction is continued for 6 to 8 weeks, depending on radiographic evidence of healing. Alternatively, halo traction with subsequent conversion to a halo brace allows early mobilization. Spinal fusion is indicated in some patients with unstable injuries, particularly if the spinal cord lesion is incomplete. In the elderly person with a cervical hyperextension injury, associated with cervical spondylosis but with no fracture or dislocation, traction is unnecessary and the patient should be mobilized early.

Thoracic and lumbar injuries

Injuries of the thoracic and lumbar spine can often be treated conservatively by 'postural reduction', placing a pillow under the lumbar spine to restore and maintain the normal lumbar lordosis, but hyperextension of the spine can cause vomiting, due to the superior mesenteric artery syndrome. Usually after 8 to 12 weeks' bed-rest, the patient is mobilized in a spinal brace. Upper thoracic fractures are splinted by the sternum, but as these injuries are sometimes associated with a sternal fracture, patients can be at risk of developing a flexion deformity of the spine of they are mobilized too quickly. In the lower thoracic and lumbar spine, internal fixation allows early mobilization and is increasingly advocated, particularly if the lesion is incomplete and unstable.

PATTERNS OF INCOMPLETE SPINAL CORD INJURY

Neurological recovery is more likely in an incomplete spinal cord lesion. The commonest incomplete pattern is the anterior cord syndrome, which follows a flexion–rotation or compression force to the spine with dislocation or compression fracture of the vertebral body, and damage to the anterior part of the spinal cord and also often the anterior spinal artery. The resulting injury to the corticospinal and spinothalamic tracts produces loss of power, pain, and temperature sensation below the lesion.

The rare posterior cord syndrome is mainly seen in hyperextension injuries with damage to the posterior vertebral elements and the posterior columns. Although the patient may have good power, pain, and temperature sensation, walking is often difficult, because of profound ataxia due to proprioceptive loss.

The central cord syndrome classically results from a cervical hyperextension injury in older patients with cervical spondylosis. There is often no fracture or dislocation, the spinal cord having been compressed between osteophytes and intervertebral disc anteriorly and thickened ligamentum flavum posteriorly. The centrally situated cervical tracts are most affected, the peripheral lumbar and sacral tracts frequently being partially spared. This often results in a patient with lower motor neurone weakness of the arms and relatively strong but spastic lower limbs. The sacral sparing commonly results in good bladder and bowel function.

Lateral mass fractures of the vertebrae or penetrating injuries may result in a Brown-Séquard syndrome (hemisection of the cord).

RECENT PHARMACOLOGICAL ADVANCES IN THE ACUTE MANAGEMENT OF SPINAL CORD INJURY

Although an American multicentre trial published in 1990 suggested that patients receiving high-dose intravenous methylprednisolone administered within 8 h of injury and continued for 24 h, showed a greater degree of recovery at 6 months than placebo-treated patients, its use has not yet been universally accepted. Its probable mechanism of action is by suppressing the breakdown of membrane by inhibiting lipid peroxidation and hydrolysis at the injury site.

In 1991 a study of GM_1 ganglioside administered within 48 h of injury and continued for an average of 26 days showed an improved neurological outcome, compared to a placebo-treated control group. Gangliosides stimulate growth of nerve cells and regeneration of damaged nervous tissue in animal studies. A larger trial is awaited before it is considered efficacious and safe in treating acute spinal cord injury in humans, but it appears that pharmacological treatment both in the early and later phases of acute spinal cord injury could soon be available.

RESPIRATORY COMPLICATIONS

Respiratory complications are common, particularly in tetraplegic patients who have paralysed abdominal and intercostal muscles, with diaphragmatic respiration. As the phrenic nerve nucleus arises from the C3–5 segments there may be varying degrees of diaphragmatic function, depending on the level of tetraplegia. Furthermore, the neurological level often rises by a spinal segment within the first 48 h of injury, due to cord oedema. This can result in an early deterioration in respiratory function and the need for respiratory support. The reduced respiratory muscle reserve also makes respiratory failure due to muscle fatigue more likely. Abdominal distension due to paralytic ileus must be avoided, otherwise the diaphragm is splinted and respiratory failure may be precipitated, especially in patients with high lesions.

The inability to cough effectively can quickly result in sputum retention and atelectasis, followed by chest infection. Ventilation–perfusion mismatch occurs, with further respiratory impairment.

Hypoxia increases confusion, especially in patients with associated head injuries, and will exacerbate spinal cord injury. Regular chest physiotherapy with assisted coughing is vital, progress being monitored by repeated vital capacity and arterial blood gas measurements, and pulse oximetry. Added oxygen is necessary in the acute stage, and inspired gases must be humidified to prevent secretions becoming viscid

and difficult to clear. Fibreoptic bronchoscopy, performed through an endotracheal tube is a safe procedure if atelectasis occurs, even in patients with cervical spine injuries. Occasionally, minitracheostomy is indicated to assist the clearing of secretions from the trachea.

Assisted ventilation
The use of continuous positive airway pressure (CPAP) or one of the more recent biphasic ventilatory support systems, providing preset levels of positive pressure in inspiration and expiration, reduces the work of breathing and increases the functional residual capacity. They provide respiratory support and may prevent the need for full ventilation, being particularly beneficial for patients with weak inspiratory muscles, who have a tendency to atelectasis. If ventilation becomes necessary, endotracheal intubation may only be required for a few days. Tracheostomy is best avoided in the first instance, particularly because of the rare but serious complication of tracheal stenosis.

Long-term ventilation
An increasing proportion of people with ultra-high cord lesions are being successfully resuscitated at the scene of accident. Some will have complete phrenic nerve paralysis, and require long-term ventilation. A battery-driven ventilator may be attached to an electrically driven wheelchair to enable the patient to have a degree of independence and mobility during the day. Domiciliary ventilation is being increasingly practised. Diaphragmatic pacing is also possible if the phrenic nerve nucleus is intact and the phrenic nerve is stimulatable. Electrodes are placed on the phrenic nerve either in the neck or the chest and connected to an implanted receiver in the anterior chest wall. Phrenic nerve stimulation is then achieved by placing a radio transmitter over the receiver.

CARDIOVASCULAR COMPLICATIONS

Paralysis of the sympathetic thoracolumbar (T1–L2) outflow, seen in high cord injuries, results in hypotension. If there are no associated injuries, a mistaken diagnosis of hypovolaemic shock may be made, resulting in overinfusion and pulmonary oedema. Sympathetic paralysis also results in unopposed vagal action and the risks of bradycardia and cardiac arrest previously mentioned.

The increased intrathoracic pressure occurring during intermittent positive pressure ventilation (IPPV) reduces venous return. It is therefore important to restore fully the circulatory volume of patients with high spinal cord injuries before ventilating them, to avoid a severe fall in cardiac output.

Postural hypotension is often a problem when first mobilizing a tetraplegic patient. Graduated elastic stockings and an abdominal binder help to reduce peripheral pooling. The latter also aids breathing by supporting and, therefore, decreasing abdominal wall compliance, allowing the diaphragm to assume a more normal resting position in the upright posture. If postural hypotension still occurs, 15 to 30 mg ephedrine, administered 20 min before mobilizing, is helpful.

The use of a depolarizing muscle relaxant such as suxamethonium must be avoided from 3 days to 9 months after spinal cord injury, as it will produce sudden hyperkalaemia, with a risk of cardiac arrest. If muscle relaxation is required for endotracheal intubation, the non-depolarizing muscle relaxant pancuronium is safe.

Autonomic dysreflexia
Following spinal shock, patients with cord lesions at T6 and above may develop autonomic dysreflexia, a condition caused by uncontrolled reflex sympathetic activity below the level of the lesion. The precipitating factor is usually bladder distension, due to a blocked catheter or poor bladder emptying. Other causes include bladder calculi, urinary tract infection, a loaded rectum, or anal fissure. The increased reflex sympathetic activity below the level of the lesion results in peripheral vasoconstriction and hypertension, with stimulation of the carotid and aortic baroreceptors. They respond via the vasomotor centre, with

increased vagal tone and bradycardia, but peripheral vasodilation is not possible because stimuli cannot pass distally through the injured cord. The hypertension is, therefore, unrelieved. The patient complains of headache, sweating, and flushing above the level of the spinal cord lesion. Without urgent treatment, intracranial haemorrhage may occur. The patient is sat up, the precipitating cause treated, and 5 to 10 mg nifedipine is given sublingually if necessary. In rare instances parenteral therapy, for example 5 to 10 mg phentolamine intravenously, is required.

Thromboembolic complications

The incidence of deep vein thrombosis following severe spinal cord injury is over 90 per cent, and pulmonary embolism is the commonest cause of death in patients who survive the period immediately following cord injury. Anticoagulants should, therefore, be commenced within 24 to 36 h of the accident, initially using subcutaneous heparin, followed by full anticoagulation with warfarin, unless there are contraindications such as head and chest injuries.

MANAGEMENT OF THE URINARY TRACT (FIG. 1)

The acute stage

During the stage of spinal shock, the bladder is acontractile, and without treatment retention with overflow occurs. Most patients with upper motor neurone cord lesions subsequently develop reflex detrusor activity, but in patients with lower motor neurone cord lesions, or with cauda equina lesions, the bladder will remain acontractile. The bladder is drained by one of three methods.

In patients with multiple injuries, indwelling urethral catheterization is essential for accurate monitoring of the urinary output. Indwelling catheters are associated with an increased incidence of bladder calculi and urinary tract infection, and therefore a daily urinary output of 3 litres is advisable. The risk of calculi is particularly high after injury, due to hypercalciuria associated with paralysis and immobility. A 12FG to 14FG silicone catheter with a 10 ml balloon is recommended.

Suprapubic catheterization has the advantages of indwelling urethral catheterization without the risk of urethral damage, prostatitis, and epididymo-orchitis. In addition, the catheter can be clamped at intervals, to see whether voiding occurs.

Intermittent urethral catheterization is the standard method of early bladder management in spinal injuries units. To permit 6-hourly catheterization, fluids must be restricted initially so that the bladder volume never exceeds 500 ml. After spinal shock ends, reflex detrusor activity may produce voiding in patients with upper motor neurone lesions, and in males a condom and urinary drainage bag are fitted and fluid intake increased. As voiding improves and catheter volumes decrease, the number of catheterizations can be reduced, and discontinued when the residual urine is consistently less than 100 ml. At this stage, the patient has been 'bladder trained' and is managed purely by condom drainage.

Efficient voiding does not necessarily occur however, largely because of detrusor–sphincter dyssynergia, in which the distal urethral sphincter actively contracts during a detrusor contraction, often with incomplete bladder emptying and high intravesical pressures. A large amount of residual urine is likely to be accompanied by recurrent urinary tract infections. Vesicoureteric reflux, hydronephrosis, and pyelonephritis may result, unless the obstruction is relieved.

An intravenous urogram and video-urodynamics are normally performed about 3 months after injury. Video-urodynamics (a study of the pressure–volume relationships of the bladder during slow filling and voiding) will detect early detrusor–sphincter dyssynergia, before renal damage occurs. Further urological follow-up is performed with renal ultrasound and plain abdominal radiography.

Long-term bladder management

Several options are available. Although achieving continence may be desired, the main aim is always to preserve renal function.

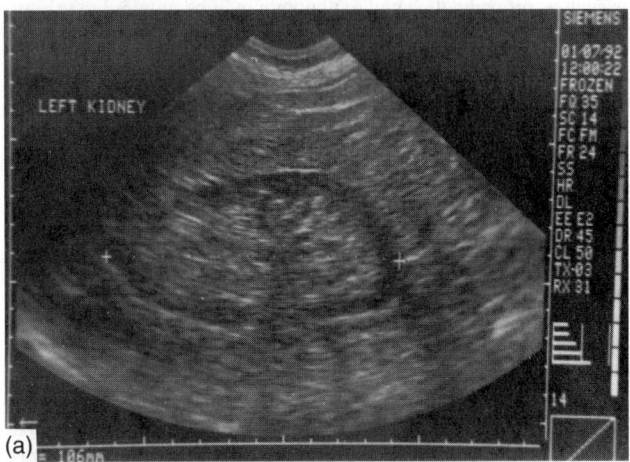

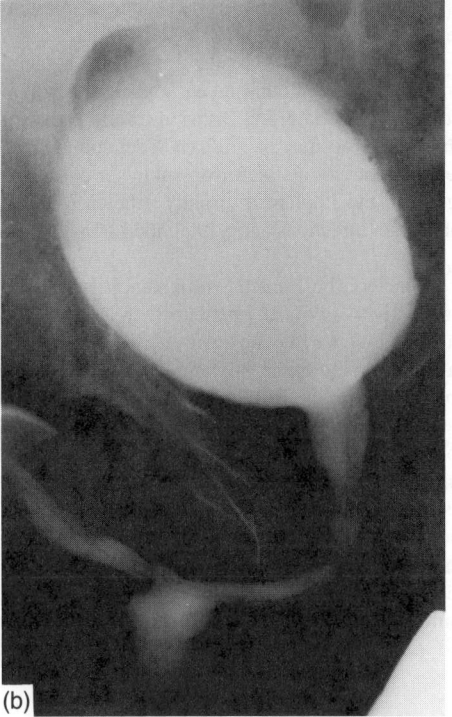

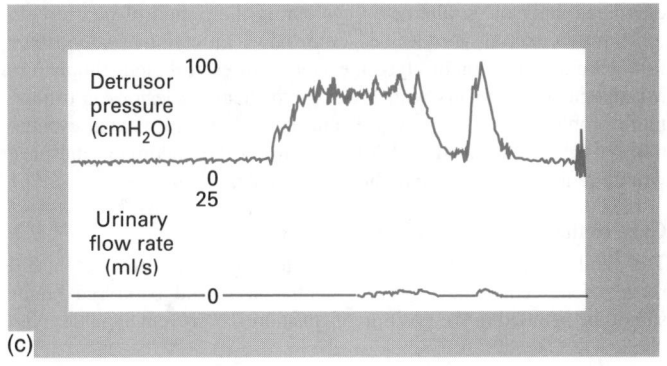

Fig. 1 (a) Renal ultrasound showing generalized thinning of the renal cortex in a 34-year-old tetraplegic patient injured at the age of 15 years. (b) Cystourethogram during micturition shows a tight urethral stricture at the junction of the membranous and bulbar urethra, and a diverticulum in the penile urethra. (c) Cystometrogram shows high-pressure, sustained detrusor contraction, and a poor urinary flow rate, voiding occurring mainly when the bladder (and distal sphincter) is beginning to relax. This is characteristic of detrusor–sphincter dyssynergia.

Most male patients with reflex bladder emptying manage their bladders by condom drainage, but one-third require an endoscopic distal urethral sphincterotomy to achieve satisfactory bladder emptying.

Patients with a non-contractile detrusor are particularly suitable for intermittent self-catheterization, usually performed 6 hourly, once the patient is able to sit up. The ideal is to attain continence between catheterizations. In patients with reflex detrusor activity, anticholinergic drugs such as propantheline and oxybutynin may be required to achieve this by reducing detrusor activity; tricyclic antidepressants such as imipramine also help by increasing bladder outlet resistance, as well as by reducing detrusor activity. Long-term results of intermittent self-catheterization compare favourably with other methods of bladder management.

Indwelling urethral catheterization is convenient in tetraplegic women unable to perform self-catheterization, and in the elderly or frail. In women with contractile neuropathic bladders, expulsion of the catheter may sometimes occur with the balloon inflated, resulting in a dilated urethra. If this happens, the temptation to increase the gauge and balloon size must be resisted, otherwise further urethral damage is likely. A colposuspension may improve continence by tightening the bladder neck and urethra.

Long-term suprapubic catheterization, either alone, or combined with urethral closure (the Feneley procedure) in patients who cannot be rendered continent by colposuspension, has been increasingly performed in recent years. The risk of bladder calculi is similar to that with an indwelling urethral catheter.

Some patients with reflex detrusor activity are suitable for a sacral anterior nerve root stimulator. This is a radiolinked implant attached to the anterior nerve roots of S2, S3, and S4. Division of the posterior sacral nerve roots as part of the procedure increases bladder compliance, and abolishes reflex detrusor activity and detrusor–sphincter dyssynergia. Bladder emptying using the implant is usually efficient, with a diminished risk of urinary tract infections and a likelihood of achieving continence.

The artificial urinary sphincter is best suited to ambulant patients with little or no reflex detrusor activity—typically patients with lower motor neurone lesions. Although continence may be achieved, there is a small risk of urethral erosion and infection of the implant.

There is very little place for urinary diversion with an ileal conduit, due to the high pressure generated in the conduit; the relatively long life expectancy of many spinal cord injured patients would result in a high incidence of renal complications from this procedure in later years.

However, a cystoplasty to create a low-pressure reservoir has its place in selected patients, and is particularly useful when combined with the fashioning of a continent catheterizable stoma, employing the Mitrofanoff principle. This relies on the creation of a small-calibre catheterizing track between the abdominal wall and bladder, often using the appendix as the track. A tunnelled submucosal antireflux anastomosis to the bladder ensures continence.

Bowel care

Immediately after spinal cord injury, the lower bowel is flaccid, but a gentle manual evacuation is usually performed after 48 to 72 h and continued daily or on alternate days during the period of bed rest. In upper motor neurone cord lesions, reflex bowel emptying usually occurs following the insertion of glycerine suppositories or digital stimulation. Management of patients with lower motor neurone lesions is usually more problematical; suppositories are ineffective and manual evacuation, possibly associated with straining using the abdominal muscles, will be required. A high-fibre diet is advisable.

Care of the joints and limbs

The paralysed joints must be passively moved daily, to maintain a full range of movement and prevent contractures, and paralysed hands should be splinted in the position of function. To prevent shoulder pain and stiffness in tetraplegic patients, the arm positions should be changed when the patient is turned.

Heterotopic ossification presents with swelling and induration around a paralysed joint, due to localized osteoblastic activity and new bone formation (Fig. 2). Although of unknown aetiology, local trauma has been implicated. Certainly once the condition occurs, aggressive physiotherapy to the joint should be avoided. Occasionally, gross restriction of movement occurs, but excision of heterotopic bone must be delayed for at least 18 months, until the bone is mature.

Care of the pressure areas

It has been shown repeatedly that the longer the delay in admission of an acutely injured patient to a spinal injuries unit, the greater the incidence of pressure sores. The commonest site for a sore in the acute stage is in the sacral region.

An understanding of safe methods of relieving pressure is essential, if further neurological damage, pressure sores, and joint contractures are to be avoided. Initially, the patient should be turned 2 hourly, usually increasing to 3 hourly after a few days if the skin has not marked on 2-hourly turns. The electrically driven Egerton turning and tilting bed is particularly convenient for patients with multiple injuries. The Stryker frame is also useful but may not be tolerated by tetraplegics when in the prone position because of the adverse effect on breathing. Manual turning methods are satisfactory, as long as the nursing team has the necessary expertise. Paraplegic and tetraplegic patients can be 'log rolled' without danger to the spine. The 'pelvic twist', which consists of a gentle lift and turn of one hip to free the sacrum of pressure, is suitable for many tetraplegic patients, but is contraindicated in paraplegic patients because it rotates the lower spine.

Patients must be warned of the risks of sensory loss and, once mobilized into a wheelchair, they need to inspect their skin regularly, particularly over bony prominences, such as the ischial, trochanteric, and sacral regions, the heels, and malleoli. In patients with established spinal cord paralysis, ischial sores may occur due to excessive interface pressures between the ischial tuberosities and the wheelchair cushion. Patients must be taught to lift in the wheelchair every 15 min, if possible. If patients cannot lift, a specialized cushion should be supplied which allows them to sit in the wheelchair, ideally all day, without producing

Fig. 2 Heterotopic ossification around both hips, 2 years after spinal cord injury.

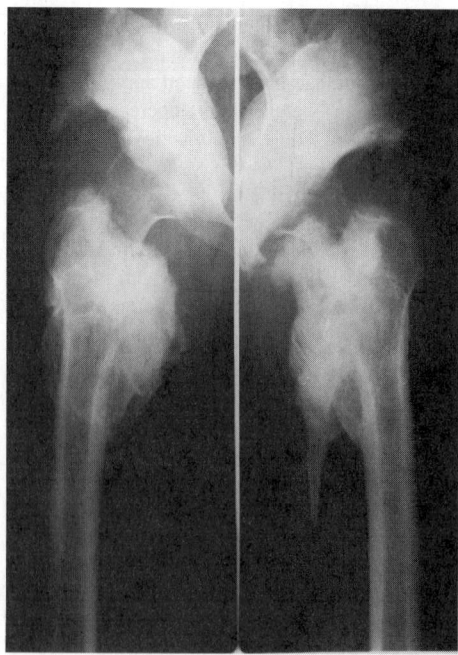

a red mark on the skin. Trochanteric sores are particularly seen in people who sleep on their side and are not adequately turned at night.

If a sore occurs, complete relief of pressure on the region is essential. This usually requires bed rest, with desloughing of the sore by excision of necrotic tissue and the use of desloughing agents. Large sores normally require excision of both the sore and the underlying bony prominence with direct closure or, rarely, the use of a flap.

Spasticity

Spasticity in upper motor neurone cord injuries is often more pronounced in incomplete lesions, and in the presence of irritative foci, such as pressure sores, urinary tract infections, and calculi. Although spasticity maintains muscle bulk, an excessive degree can reduce mobility.

Regular use of a standing frame relieves spasticity and prevents contractures. Spasticity can also be relieved by baclofen and dantrolene sodium, or in resistant cases by motor point injections, local nerve blocks, or neurectomy, for example by obturator neurectomy in severe hip abductor spasticity. Intrathecal 6 per cent aqueous phenol or absolute alcohol blocks are now rarely used, because the conversion of an upper to a low motor neurone lesion affects bladder, bowel, and sexual function. Intrathecal baclofen administered by an implanted reservoir and pump is effective and avoids the drawbacks of the above procedures.

Post-traumatic syringomyelia (Fig. 3)

Occurring in at least 2 per cent of patients following spinal cord injury, the common presenting symptoms are unilateral pain and numbness in the arm with a dissociated sensory loss. Although symptoms may appear a few weeks after injury, they can be delayed for several years. Diagnosis is confirmed by MRI, or CT with myelography. Surgical treatment by insertion of a syringoperitoneal or syringopleural shunt usually relieves the pain, but relief of sensory and motor loss is less predictable.

Psychological and social factors

The psychological trauma of spinal cord injury is huge. In high cord lesions, fear and anxiety is exacerbated by sensory deprivation. Wide mood swings, including anger, depression, and behaviour identifiable with the normal grieving process are common. Long-term decisions must be taken with full participation of the patient, if successful rehabilitation is to be achieved. Most patients wish to return home and many severely disabled people achieve this goal.

Fig. 3 Multilocular syrinx extending from the site of fracture at T4 to the foramen magnum. The patient had loss of pinprick over the left C3 to T1 dermatomes, but no upper limb weakness.

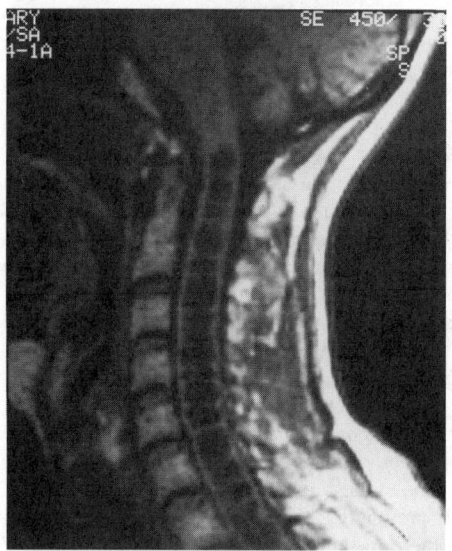

Pain

Pain at or below the level of the neurological lesion is distressingly common, particularly in cauda equina lesions. It often begins a few weeks after injury, and is frequently described as burning or stabbing, and may be continuous or intermittent.

Most patients respond to the distraction of a busy rehabilitation programme, and treatment with tricyclic antidepressants or anticonvulsants. Transcutaneous nerve stimulation, acupuncture, hypnotherapy, and relaxation techniques may also help. Dorsal column stimulation, which probably interrupts the ascending pain pathways and releases endogenous endorphins, may occasionally help, but surgical methods of interrupting pain pathways, such as posterior rhizotomy, spinothalamic tractotomy, and dorsal root entry zone coagulation, are not recommended, as any beneficial effect is likely to be short lasting.

Sexual function

This is generally disturbed unless the cord lesion is very incomplete. Most men with upper motor neurone lesions experience reflex erections, as the parasympathetic connections from S2 to S4 segments of the cord to the corpora cavernosa remain intact. The majority, however, will only ejaculate using artificial methods—by the application of a vibrator to the penis or by rectal electroejaculation.

As the S2 to S4 reflex arc is no longer intact in patients with lower motor neurone lesions, reflex erections are lost, but psychogenic erections and emissions sometimes occur, if the pelvic sympathetic fibres from the T11 to L2 segments (which form the hypogastric nerves) remain connected to higher centres.

In men who cannot otherwise attain erections sufficient for intercourse, intracavernous papaverine, vacuum erection aids, and, rarely, penile implants are useful.

Although the sperm count is usually low, with diminished motility, probably due to continuing non-ejaculation, infection, and raised testicular temperature, seminal fluid quality tends to improve with repeated ejaculation using the vibrator or electroejaculator, or an implanted hypogastric plexus stimulator. Assisted conception techniques, including seminal fluid enhancement, intrauterine insemination, and *in vitro* fertilization have improved the likelihood of fathering children.

In women fertility remains normal, but in lesions above T10 labour may be painless and forceps delivery may be required.

In high lesions there is a risk of autonomic dysreflexia both during ejaculation and labour.

Non-traumatic causes of spinal cord paralysis

Infection of the vertebrae

Vertebral osteomyelitis

The onset of this relatively rare cause of spinal cord paralysis is often insidious with low-grade fever, malaise, weight loss, and spinal pain. Radiographic changes of end-plate erosion, followed by vertebral body destruction may not be detected for 1 to 2 months after the onset of infection. It is therefore not surprising that diagnosis is often delayed.

Vertebral osteomyelitis is more common in males, and in patients with diabetes mellitus and rheumatoid arthritis. In these circumstances, and also with advanced age and a more cephalad level of infection, paralysis is more likely to occur. In recent years, intravenous drug abuse has become increasingly associated with the condition.

The source of infection is mainly the urinary and respiratory tracts, and soft-tissue infections; *Staphylococcus aureus* is the most common pathogen.

Needle aspiration or biopsy is performed to identify the causative organism and 6 to 8 weeks' parenteral antibiotic therapy given, but surgical decompression may also be required.

Tuberculous disease of the spine

This condition, 'Pott's paraplegia', is still a major cause of spinal cord paralysis in many parts of the world, but is now uncommon in Western countries, except in immigrant populations. Prompt administration of antituberculous drugs often results in a major degree of neurological recovery, and urgent surgical intervention is not often required. The condition is discussed in detail in Section 7.

Other causes of non-traumatic spinal cord paralysis

These are discussed in Chapter 24.3.9. The general principles of treatment are as described for the spinal cord injured patient, but the prognosis will depend on the underlying pathology.

Conclusions

Patients require lifelong follow-up, and continuing care and support in the community. Although their injuries have profound physical and emotional effects, it appears that learning to cope with disability gives them special qualities, and an increasing number are achieving independence, working, having children, and integrating back into society.

REFERENCES

Bracken, M.B.,*et al.* (1990). A randomised, controlled trial of methylprednisolone or naloxone in the treatment of acute spinal cord injury: results of the Second National Acute Spinal Cord Injury Study. *New England Journal of Medicine* **322**, 1405–11.

Brindley, G.S. (1986). Sexual and reproductive problems of paraplegic men. In *Oxford Reviews of Reproductive Biology*, (ed. J.R. Clarke), Vol. 8, pp. 214–22. Clarendon Press, Oxford.

Brooks, M.E. and Ohry, A. (1992). Conservative versus surgical treatment of the cervical and thoracolumbar spine in spinal trauma. *Paraplegia* **30**, 46–9.

Brown, D.J. (1992). Spinal cord injuries: the last decade and the next. *Paraplegia* **30**, 77–82.

Carvell, J. and Grundy, D. (1989). Patients with spinal injuries. Early transfer to a specialist centre is vital. *British Medical Journal* **299**, 1353–4.

Donovan, W.H., Carter, R.E., Bedbrook, G.M., Young, J.S., and Griffiths, E.R. (1984). Incidence of medical complications in spinal cord injury: patients in specialised centres compared with non-specialised centres. *Paraplegia* **22**, 282–90.

Ducker, T.B. and Zeidman, S.M. (1994). Spinal cord injury. Role of steroid imaging. *Spine*, **19**, 2281–7.

Eismont, F.J., Bohlman, H.H., Soni, P.L., Goldberg, V.M., and Freehafer, A.A. (1983). Pyogenic and fungal vertebral osteomyelitis with paralysis. *Journal of Bone and Joint Surgery* **65A**, 19–29.

Gardner, B., Theocleous, F., Watt, J., and Krishnan, K. (1985). Ventilation or dignified death for patients with high tetraplegia. *British Medical Journal* **291**, 1620–2.

Geisler, F.H., Dorsey, F.C., and Coleman, W.P. (1991). Recovery of motor function after spinal-cord injury—a randomised, placebo-controlled trial with GM-1 ganglioside. *New England Journal of Medicine* **324**, 1829–38.

Geisler, W.O., Jousse, A.T., Wynne-Jones, M., and Breithaupt, D. (1983). Survival in traumatic spinal cord injury. *Paraplegia* **21**, 364–73.

Grundy, D. and Swain, A. (1993). *ABC of spinal cord injury*, (2nd edn). British Medical Journal, London. (A concise account of the acute treatment and long-term rehabilitation of the spinal cord injured patient.)

Guttmann, L. (1976). *Spinal cord injuries, comprehensive management and research*, (2nd edn). Blackwell Scientific Publications, Oxford. (A classic text, with fascinating detail of the history and evolvement of spinal cord injury management.)

Linsenmeyer, T.A. and Perkash, I. (1991). Infertility in men with spinal cord injury. *Archives of Physical Medicine and Rehabilitation* **72**, 747–54.

Mansel, J.K. and Norman, J.R. (1990). Respiratory complications and management of spinal cord injuries. *Chest* **97**, 1446–52.

Ravichandran, G. and Silver, J.R. (1982). Missed injuries of the spinal cord. *British Medical Journal* **284**, 953–6.

Rossier, A.B., Foo, D., Shillito, J., and Dyro, F.M. (1985). Posttraumatic cervical syringomyelia. *Brain* **108**, 439–61.

Whiteneck, G., Adler, C., Carter, R.E., Lammertse, D.P., Manley, S., Menter, R., Wagner, K.A., and Wilmot C. (ed.) (1989). *The management of high quadriplegia*. Demos, New York. (Describes all aspects of management of high-lesion patients.)

Whiteneck, G.G., *et al.* (1992). Mortality, morbidity and psychosocial outcomes of persons spinal cord injured more than twenty years ago. *Paraplegia* **30**, 617–30.

Woodhouse, C.R.J., Malone, P.R., Cumming, J., and Reilly, T.M. (1983). The Mitrofanoff principle for continent urinary diversion. *British Journal of Urology* **63**, 53–7.

Wyndaele, J.J. (1992). Neurourology in spinal cord injured patients. *Paraplegia* **30**, 50–3.

24.3.11 Disorders of the spinal nerve roots

R. S. MAURICE-WILLIAMS

Anatomy

Each segment of the spinal cord gives off a ventral (motor) and dorsal (sensory) root on each side. These unite in the intervertebral foramina to leave the spinal canal as mixed spinal roots. As the spinal cord ends at the lower border of the L1 vertebra, the lower spinal roots originate from the cord above their corresponding skeletal levels and run an increasingly oblique course before they reach their foramina. The spinal dura, enclosing the spinal subarachnoid space, extends to the middle of the sacral canal, and the leash of roots within it, together with the fibrous band (the filum terminale) which is the continuation of the tip of the cord, form the cauda equina.

There are eight cervical, 12 dorsal, five sacral, and one coccygeal pairs of roots. Each root has motor and sensory fibres which at some levels subserve clinically important tendon reflexes. The roots supplying these are shown in Table 1. The sympathetic outflow leaves the cord via roots D1–L1, while the caudal parasympathetic outflow is via roots S2–S4. The area of skin whose sensation is supplied by a single root is known as a dermatome and the corresponding block of deep tissues is called a sclerotome. Figure 1 shows a dermatome map of the body. The first cervical root contains no cutaneous sensory fibres, so the C2 dermatome adjoins the area of skin supplied by the trigeminal nerve. The overlap of dermatomes and anatomical variation between individuals means that loss of a single root may give rise to a variable sensory loss which may not be detectable clinically. The main motor supply of the different roots is given in Table 2 in terms of movements. Again, there is some variation in anatomy between individuals so that precise localization of a root lesion on the basis of the pattern of motor loss may be difficult. This is especially so for roots C5–8.

The effect of root lesions

In addition to motor, sensory, and reflex loss, irritation or compression of a root may give rise to pain and paraesthesiae in the sensory distribution of that root. Root pain is characteristically made worse by movement of the spine and by actions which cause sudden pulses of pressure in the spinal subarachnoid space, such as coughing or sneezing. Root pain in a limb often has two components: a dull, deep, ill-defined ache thought to correspond to the sensory supply to muscle and bone (the sclerotome) and a sharp, superficial, better-defined pain related to the dermatome of the root.

On a few roots there are important arterial feeders reinforcing the longitudinally running arteries of the spinal cord, mainly the anterior spinal artery; damage to one of these roots may lead to cord ischaemia. A major feeder is usually present on one of the lower cervical roots and on one of the roots of the dorsolumbar junction (the great artery of Adamkiewicz).

Table 1 *Roots involved in tendon reflexes*

Reflex	Roots
Biceps jerk	Cervical 5–6
Supinator jerk	Cervical 5–6
Triceps jerk	Cervical 6–7
Finger jerk	Cervical 7–8
Knee jerk	Lumbar 2–4
Ankle jerk	Sacral 1–2

Table 2 *Main motor supply of roots*

C1–4	Neck muscles (apart from spinal accessory supply to sternomastoid and trapezius)
	Longitudinal spinal muscles
	Diaphragm (C3–5, mainly C4)
C5	Shoulder abductors
C6	Elbow flexors
C7	Elbow extensors
	Wrist flexors/extensors
C8	Finger flexors and extensors
D1	Small hand muscles
D2–D12	Trunk muscles
	Longitudinal spinal muscles
L1	Hip flexors
L2	Hip flexors
	Hip abductors
	Knee extensors
L3	Knee extensors
	Hip flexors
L4	Knee extensors
	Ankle dorsiflexors
	Knee flexors
	Hip extensors
L5	Ankle dorsiflexors
	Dorsiflexor or hallux
	Hip extensors
	Knee flexors
S1	Ankle plantar flexors
	Hip extensors
	Knee flexors

Causes of root lesions

SPINAL DEGENERATIVE DISEASE

This is the commonest cause of a root lesion, usually in the lower lumbar or lower cervical region. It is discussed in detail below.

TUMOURS

Spinal extradural tumours, such as metastatic carcinoma or lymphomas, lying either in the bone of a vertebra or in the fibrofatty epidural space, often produce root compression and root pain. Of the spinal intradural tumours, root pain is most often associated with a neurofibroma which usually originates from a dorsal root. Carcinoma of the lung apex may involve the first dorsal root, producing pain and numbness down the inner surface of the arm, weakness of the small muscles of the hand, and a Horner's syndrome. This clinical picture is known as a Pancoast syndrome. Pelvic or retroperitoneal tumours may involve roots after they have left the spinal canal.

TRAUMA

Rarely, stab and bullet wounds may damage spinal roots. Violent upward or downward movements on the shoulder girdle or the trunk can damage roots contributing to the upper or lower parts of the brachial plexus. The so-called Erb–Duchenne palsy, due to avulsion of the C5 and C6 roots, is caused by forcible depression of the shoulder, as may occur in a difficult delivery, or nowadays more commonly when a person is flung off a motor cycle and lands on the point of his shoulder. Avulsion of the C8 and D1 roots (Klumpke palsy) may follow a fall in which the arm catches on a projection and is jerked upwards violently.

CERVICAL RIB SYNDROME

The C8 and D1 roots run over the surface of the first rib, together with the subclavian artery. All these structures may be compressed if they are elevated at this point by the presence of a cervical rib or a congenital fibrous band running from the tip of a prominent C7 transverse process to the first rib beneath them. Root symptoms from this cause are usually associated with signs of vascular insufficiency in the hand from compression of the subclavian artery. The hand symptoms may be of a Raynaud phenomenon type or multiple lesions due to emboli thrown off from a patch of thrombus within the compressed subclavian artery. A true cervical rib syndrome is rare. In the past it was probably overdiagnosed and confused with root lesions caused by cervical disc protrusions.

NEURALGIC AMYOTROPHY

This is believed to be an inflammatory involvement of C5, C6, and sometimes the C7 roots. It may occur spontaneously or may follow either an infective illness or an immunization injection into the deltoid muscle. Over the course of a few days, pain around the shoulder is followed by weakness and wasting of the muscles supplied by the affected roots. In most cases a good spontaneous recovery occurs over a matter of months. Like the cervical rib syndrome, this may have often

been misdiagnosed in the past in cases of root compression caused by cervical disc protrusions.

ARACHNOIDITIS

Progressive fibrosis of the arachnoid membrane is a rare condition which may involve roots, especially those of the cauda equina. In most cases there has been some clear-cut insult to the arachnoid, perhaps years before, such as spinal infection, radiotherapy, trauma, or surgery. The irritant effects of the oil-based contrast media which were used for myelography until recently are thought to have contributed to many cases, especially if the lumbar puncture for the original myelogram was difficult and caused bleeding into the subarachnoid space.

HERPES ZOSTER (SEE SECTION 7)

The inflammatory process of herpes zoster is based in the dorsal root ganglion and the first symptoms are pain and hyperalgesia in the area supplied by the affected root(s), to be followed a few days later by a skin rash in the corresponding dermatomes. Spread of infection into the anterior horn cells of the cord may produce motor loss in the same segments.

Degenerative disease of the spine

PATHOGENESIS

This condition is the principal cause of lesions of the spinal nerve roots. The term 'disease' is rather misleading for by the age of 60 years the great majority of the population show some radiological evidence of degeneration of the spine. The condition is not necessarily symptomatic and it is perhaps best regarded as a normal ageing process which advances at different rates in different individuals.

The pathological basis of the condition lies in degeneration of the intervertebral discs. These structures act as buffers and fulcra between the vertebral bodies. They permit movement between the vertebrae while cushioning longitudinally acting stress. The discs are thickest at those parts of the spine which are most mobile and which abut fixed sections, namely the lower cervical spine and the lower lumbar spine. In these regions the discs are subjected to the greatest stress and are most prone to symptomatic degenerative change.

In the young adult the nucleus of the intervertebral disc is a tense, well-hydrated structure which holds apart the adjacent intervertebral bodies. Degeneration begins to appear in the third decade and consists of a progressive desiccation and collapse of the nucleus, which may begin to fissure and break up into fragments. By old age the process of fibrosis may lead to what amounts to a fibrous ankylosis between the vertebral bodies. Disc degeneration appears to be a normal wear-and-tear phenomenon and bears only a limited relationship to heavy occupational stress.

Collapse of the disc space leads to a number of secondary phenomena. The annulus of the disc bulges outwards, lifting the periosteum off the vertebral bodies and giving rise to the deposition of marginal osteophytes. The narrowing of the disc space leads to a misalignment of the posterior facet joints, which may accordingly show hypertrophic, osteo-

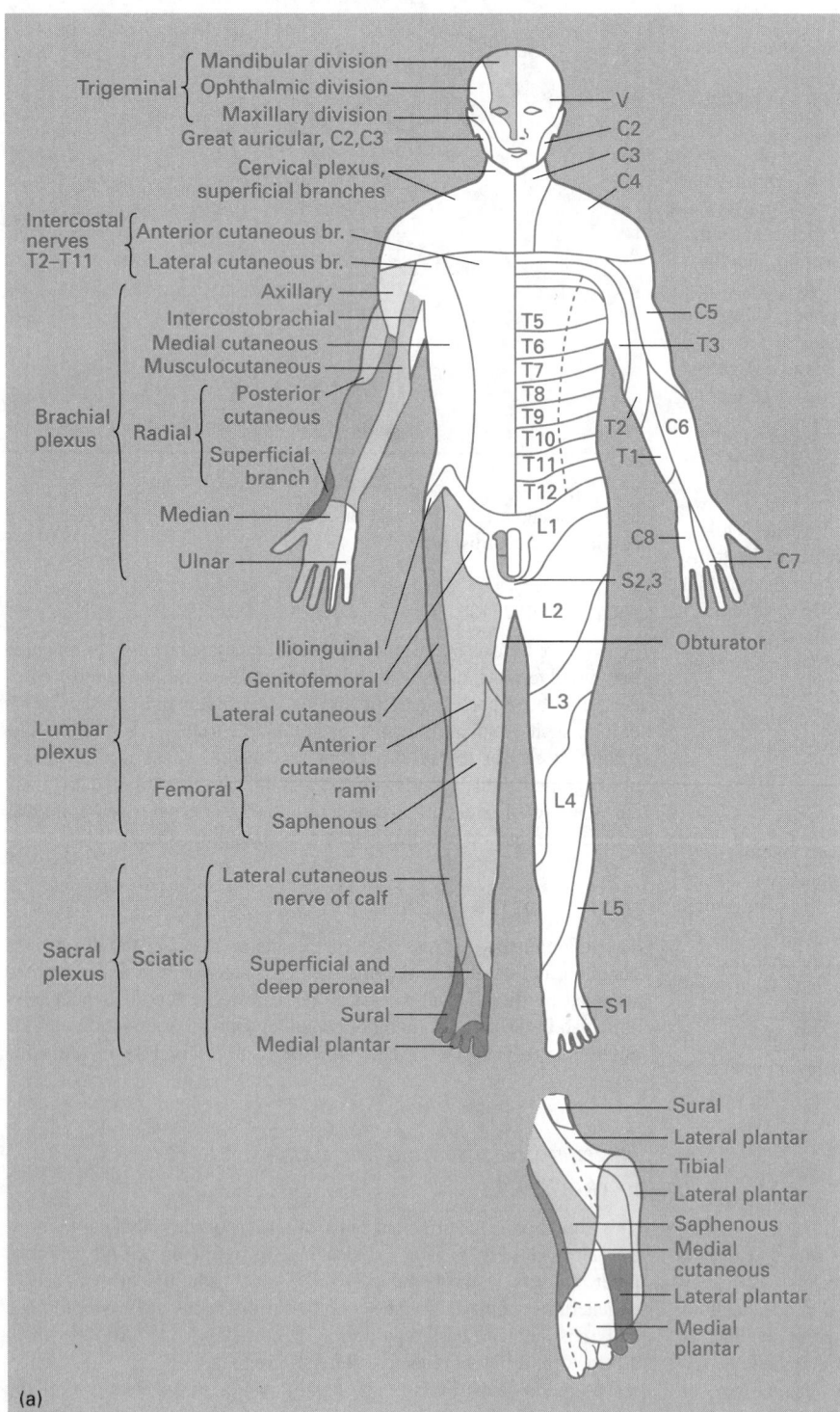

(a)

Fig. 1 Cutaneous areas of distribution of spinal segments and the peripheral nerves. (a) Anterior aspect.

arthritic change. As the vertebral bodies come closer to each other, the posterior longitudinal ligament and the ligamenta flava buckle up. Finally, the disc narrowing and facet joint misalignment may permit some degree of forward or backwards subluxation of one vertebra upon another. This happens most often at the L4/5 level, where the axes of the facet joints in some individuals may permit the development of a forward spondylolisthesis.

All the above changes, osteophytic ridges, swollen facet joints, and concertinaed ligaments, may intrude into the spinal canal and interver-tebral foramina and cause cord or root compression. Collectively these chronic degenerative changes are known as spinal spondylosis. Cervical spondylosis is most marked at the C4/5, C5/6, and C6/7 levels. It may be associated with the development of a myelopathy (see below) or with root compression. The latter occurs in the intervertebral foramina which may be narrowed anteriorly by osteophytes originating from the sides of the intervertebral disc and uncovertebral joints and posteriorly by hypertrophied facet joints. Lumbar spondylosis may lead to narrowing of the lumbar canal and compression of the cauda equina, or to com-

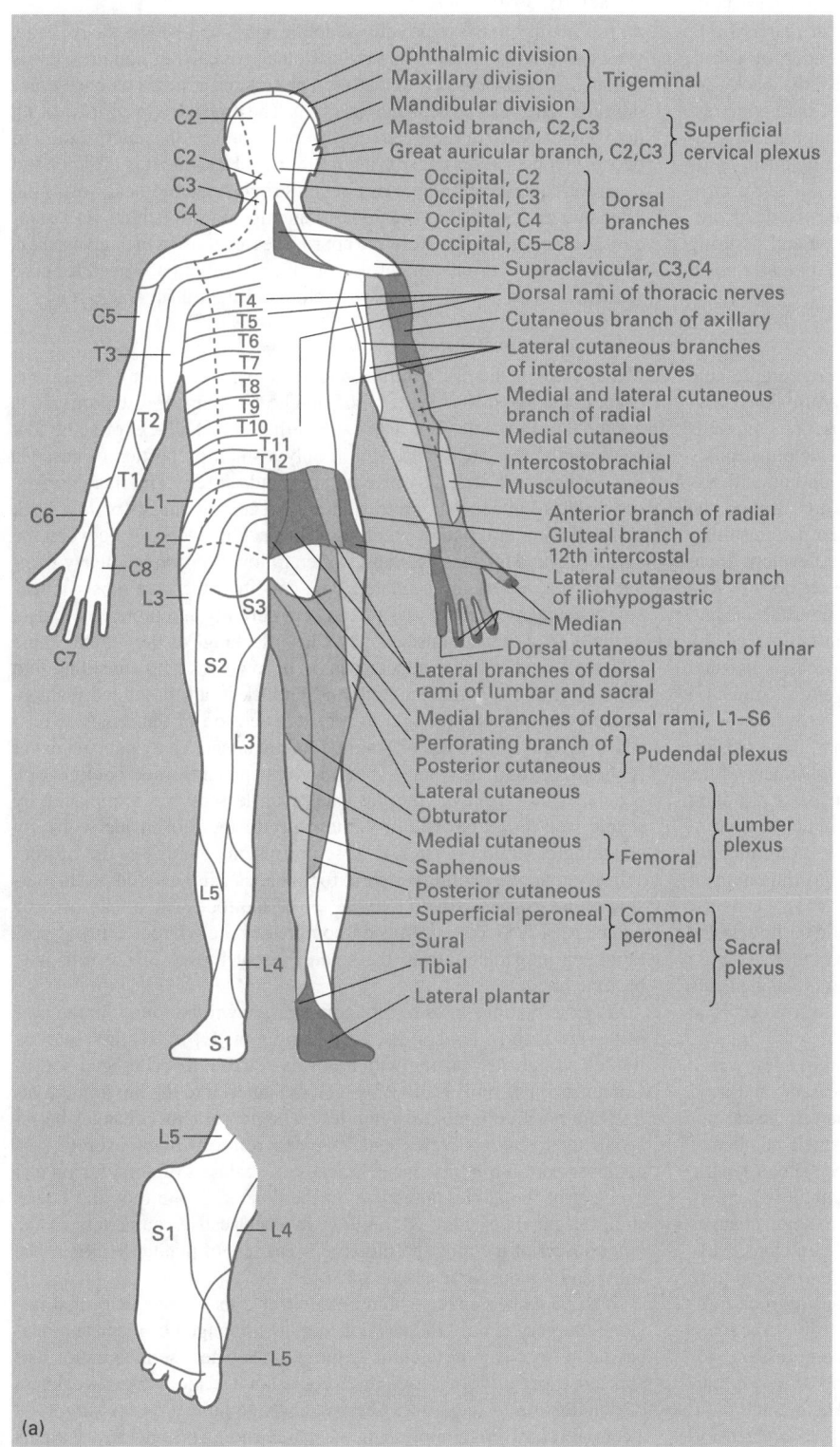

Fig. 1 (cont.) (b) Posterior aspect. (Reproduced from Bannister, R. (1992). *Brain's clinical neurology*, Oxford University Press, with permission.)

pression of individual nerve roots where they lie in the lateral recesses of the spinal canal before they reach their foramina. This so-called lateral recess stenosis results from bulging of the discs in front and the facet joints and yellow ligament behind.

DISC PROTRUSIONS

In addition to the insidious neural compression caused by spondylosis, a more sudden root or cord compression may follow protrusion of an intervertebral disc. A disc protrusion consists of an acute or subacute backwards dislocation of disc substance. It may take the form of a bulge of disc material within an intact annulus or the annulus may tear at one point, permitting extrusion of a free fragment of nuclear material into the spinal canal. The latter event is known as sequestration of a disc. Disc protrusions may occur in any direction, but only the backward protrusions produce symptoms, either by causing root or cord compression or by stretching the highly innervated posterior longitudinal ligament and posterior annulus. The posterior longitudinal ligament tends to reinforce the central part of the posterior annulus and deflects protrusions posterolaterally. Disc protrusions often follow an episode of sudden or unusual exertion, but the underlying degeneration and fissuring of the disc will have been developing silently for some time as a result of normal wear-and-tear strains.

Cervical disc protrusions

These are commonest at the C4/5, C5/6, and C6/7 levels, compressing the C5, C6, and C7 roots, respectively. A symptomatic protrusion occurs most often between the ages of 25 and 50 years. The onset of symptoms is generally over the course of a few days and may occur spontaneously or follow some unusual strain. The first symptom is pain and stiffness in the neck, usually extending into the shoulder or proximal arm on one side in a rather ill-defined fashion. This may be referred pain resulting from stretching of the annulus. As root compression develops there appears a better-defined severe lancinating pain in the territory of that root. With worsening root compression there may be paraesthesiae and numbness in the dermatome of the root and reduction or loss of any tendon reflexes subserved by the root. Marked motor loss is unusual and usually indicates very severe root compression. Painful limitation of some neck movements is almost invariably found.

The main differential diagnoses are median and ulnar nerve palsies, lesions of the rotator cuff of the shoulder joint, and involvement of the lower part of the brachial plexus by an apical carcinoma of the lung (Pancoast's syndrome). The peripheral nerve palsies will not be accompanied by neck and proximal arm pain and they can be confirmed by conduction studies. Shoulder-capsule lesions give rise to limitation of passive movements of the shoulder. An apical lung carcinoma causes a Horner's syndrome from involvement of the sympathetic outflow in the first dorsal root. Many patients diagnosed in the past as suffering from either neuralgic amyotrophy or compression of the lower brachial plexus by cervical ribs or bands may have had root compression from cervical disc protrusions.

In the great majority of cases the symptoms abate within a few weeks with conservative measures—a collar, bed rest if necessary, and mild analgesia. Recurrent attacks are much less common than in the case of lumbar disc protrusions. Surgery is reserved for the small number of patients with an incapacitating degree of pain which persists or recurs, or where severe root compression has led to disabling motor or sensory loss. Recent advances in imaging techniques have led to some changes in the investigations which are preferred by individual clinicians. Nevertheless, CT myelography remains the most satisfactory investigation. It not only serves to exclude unexpected pathology causing root compression, such as a tumour, but also, in the axial views, gives the maximum information about the degree of nerve root compression, for example whether this is caused by a soft disc protrusion or a bony bar. If the pathology is very marked, then MRI scanning and sometimes plain CT scanning may be sufficient before surgery. Surgical decompression

of the root may be carried out from behind (facetectomy or foraminotomy) or from in front. In the latter approach the anterior longitudinal ligament is incised, permitting opening up of the disc space and direct removal of extruded disc material from anterior to the root or spinal cord. On the whole, the results of surgery are extremely good.

A central cervical disc protrusion may give rise to acute or subacute compression of the spinal cord. Young adults are usually affected and an onset after trauma is common. Urgent removal by the anterior route is indicated. A posterior approach via laminectomy is usually more hazardous as it requires mobilization and retraction of the compressed cord.

Dorsal disc protrusions

As the dorsal spine is relatively immobile and is splinted by the rib cage, symptomatic disc protrusions are extremely rare. Root compression is unusual. In most cases a dorsal disc protrusion presents as cord compression. This may be of insidious onset. The protruded material is often hard and calcified and may gradually erode through the anterior dura to become embedded in the spinal cord. Surgical treatment is difficult and hazardous and there is a real risk of catastrophic neurological worsening after surgery, especially if removal is attempted from behind via a standard laminectomy. The preferred approaches are those which give access to the protruded disc from the side or in front without any need for cord retraction, such as a costotransversectomy or the transthoracic route.

Lumbar disc protrusions

Most symptomatic disc protrusions are lumbar and 95 per cent of these occur at the two lowest levels, L4/5 and L5/S1. Lumbar disc protrusions are thought to account for many and perhaps most attacks of acute low back pain and sciatica, although in only a small proportion of cases is the diagnosis confirmed by myelography and surgery. The characteristic course of a lumbar disc protrusion is of recurrent attacks of low back pain radiating into one or other leg. The peak incidence is between the ages of 25 and 50 years. Relapses often follow exertion but heavy manual workers are no more liable to the condition than are those in sedentary occupations. Relapses often occur abruptly and protective spasm of the erector spinae muscles may cause 'locking' of the lumbar spine with severe pain. Initial attacks consist of low back pain spreading into the region of the sacroiliac joint and buttock in an ill-defined fashion. These symptoms are thought to reflect distension of the sensitive posterior annulus and posterior longitudinal ligament. Many patients never progress beyond this stage, but in some patients root compression occurs. If this happens, the low back pain lessens and is replaced by severe well-localized pain in the territory of the root, made worse by coughing or straining. An L4/5 disc protrusion compresses the L5 root some way above its intervertebral foramen, causing pain down the outside of the leg and radiating to the top of the foot, which may become numb. An L5/S1 disc protrusion compresses the S1 root causing posterior leg pain radiating to the sole. The outer edge of the foot may become numb.

On examination, signs of root compression will be found. In the case of the lower three lumbar discs, affecting roots L4 to S1, there will be limited straight-leg raising with a positive stretch test (Lasègue's test). Compression of roots L1 to L3 which run anterior to the hip joint, gives rise to a positive femoral stretch test. The neurological changes correspond to the root affected and vary according to how severely it is compressed. L5 root involvement leads to weakness of dorsiflexion and eversion of the ankle, numbness on the dorsum of the foot and lateral shin, but no reflex loss. S1 root involvement causes numbness of the outer border of the foot and little toe, weakness of plantar flexion at the ankle and a reduced or absent ankle jerk.

Most patients recover within a matter of 2 to 3 weeks with bed rest alone. Surgery is only indicated if there is prolonged or recurrent incapacitating root compression or in those cases where serious motor loss appears, especially if an L4/5 disc protrusion leads to marked weakness of dorsiflexion of the ankle. The one absolute indication for surgery is a central protrusion compressing the cauda equina (see below). Patients with clear signs of root compression do well after operation. Those with back pain as the dominant symptom fare much less well.

Plain radiographs of the lumbar spine and pelvis serve to make sure that an unsuspected tumour or inflammatory lesion is not producing bone destruction, but the plain radiographs are of little value in predicting the level of a symptomatic protrusion. After early adult life most individuals show some degenerative changes on the plain radiograph. Although narrowing of a disc space is often seen, there is very little correlation between this appearance and the occurrence of a clinically significant disc protrusion. At the present time the radiological investigations which give the maximum information about what is going on in the lumbar canal are MRI scanning and CT myelography—that is, myelography succeeded by axial CT scanning before the water-soluble contrast medium has disappeared. CT myelography is especially useful for patients who have already undergone spinal surgery or those where the pathological changes are not especially marked. The disadvantage of CT myelography is that it is not generally practicable to carry it out as an outpatient procedure. The reason for this is that up to 20 per cent of patients may develop post-lumbar headache. Sometimes this can be severe and incapacitating and last for up to several days. It is the general experience that this is most likely to develop in patients with negative myelography, especially if there is a suspicion that there is a neurotic component to the symptoms. Patients and doctors often express anxiety about side-effects from the injection of contrast media. Up until the late 1970s when the oil-based contrast medium, Myodil (known as Pantopaque in North America and on the continent of Europe) was used, this fear had a rational basis, for an inflammatory response of the meninges was by no means uncommon and a small number of patients progressed to severe adhesive arachnoiditis. However, this complication does not occur with the water-based media that are used at the present time.

At operation the root is exposed from behind by laminectomy or by a more limited excision of the yellow ligament and the adjacent bone (fenestration) on one side. A full laminectomy is usually advisable if the main spinal canal is narrow at the point of the disc protrusion, or if there is a large central protrusion, particularly if this is causing cauda equina compression. It is not uncommon to find that the root compression is aggravated by the fact that the lateral angle (lateral recess) of the spinal canal is rather shallow. In such cases it is important to make sure that the nerve root is well uncapped from behind even if this means removing the medial aspect of the facet joint. Once the nerve root has been fully exposed it is retracted to permit removal of any extruded disc material beneath it. The point where the annulus has given way allows an instrument to be inserted into the disc space which is cleared of any loose degenerated material which might protrude in the future. The outcome of surgery depends on case selection, but in approximately 80 per cent of cases the patient is able to resume a normal life with little disability. The outcome of surgery is less satisfactory if there has been previous surgery to the lumbar spine, if back pain rather than sciatica is the predominant symptom, or if the patient is involved in litigation over an accident which has led to the disc protrusion. At one time many surgeons (principally orthopaedic surgeons) advocated a primary fusion of the level at which a disc protrusion had occurred after the protrusion had been removed. This practice, however, has largely disappeared.

Cauda equina lesions

Compression of the cauda equina produces bilateral leg weakness and numbness, loss of sphincter control, and loss of sexual potency. The upper level of the motor and sensory disturbance will be determined by the level of the compressing lesion, but weakness is usually most marked at the ankles and sensory loss is generally most prominent over the sacral dermatomes—the 'saddle' area of the buttocks and perineum. The ankle jerks and anal reflexes are almost lost and, depending on the level of the compression, the knee jerks may also be reduced. Any sphincter disturbance is of a lower motor neurone type with a patulous anus and an 'atonic' bladder which dribbles urine.

The common causes of cauda equina compression are a central lumbar disc protrusion, degenerative spondylolisthesis (most often at the L4/5 level), and a tumour. A mild intermittent compression caused by degenerative stenosis of the lumbar canal leads to a syndrome known as claudication of the cauda equina (see below). Neoplastic compression of the cauda equina is most often due to an extradural malignant tumour such as a metastasis or a lymphoma. Intradural tumours are much rarer but are important clinically because they are often benign. They include neurofibromas, meningiomas, and ependymomas. The last arise from ependymal cells within the filum terminale. The symptoms of a benign tumour of the cauda equina are generally insidious in onset and have often been present for a long time before the diagnosis is made. A characteristic feature is back or root pain which is worse on lying down and is relieved by getting up and walking around. This 'night pain' has a relationship to physical activity which is the reverse of that produced by a disc protrusion.

The cauda equina compression produced by a lumbar disc protrusion is often fairly abrupt in onset. The sudden onset usually reflects complete extrusion of a nuclear fragment through a tear in the annulus into the spinal canal. A past history of attacks of low back pain or sciatica may give a clue to the diagnosis. The cauda equina compression is generally accompanied by excruciating bilateral sciatica in addition to motor and sensory loss below the affected level. Surgery is matter of great urgency if there is to be any chance of neurological recovery.

CLAUDICATION OF THE CAUDA EQUINA AND LUMBAR CANAL STENOSIS

In this condition symptoms of dysfunction of the cauda equina appear on walking or prolonged standing and are relieved by rest. The underlying cause is almost always a congenital stenosis of the lumbar canal which has been made worse in middle age by the development of degenerative change. Bulges of the lumbar discs, infolded yellow ligament, and enlarged facet joints intrude into the constitutionally narrow lumbar spinal canal so that the contained neural structures suffer mild chronic compression. Stenosis may be over several segments of the lumbar spine or at a single level. If the latter, the L4/5 level is most commonly involved. This is normally the narrowest part of the lumbar canal and is also the level most often affected by spondylolisthesis caused by degenerative arthritis of the facet joints.

Symptoms are generally absent at rest and only appear on walking or prolonged standing. On walking there is friction between the nerve roots and the walls of the tight lumbar canal, whereas standing leads to increased extension of the lumbar spine which has the effect of narrowing the lumbar canal further. The irritation of the cauda equina gives rise to pain which spreads from the lumbar spine to the buttocks and down the back of the legs to the feet. Often the pain is accompanied by paraesthesia and numbness which 'marches' over the sacral dermatomes if the patient continues walking or standing. Motor impairment may become manifest as floppiness of the ankles. The differential diagnosis from vascular claudication may be difficult. Both conditions afflict the middle-aged and elderly and may coexist in the same person. Features suggesting claudication of the cauda equina are the 'march' of the pain, its paraesthetic quality, and the fact that on the rest the symptoms may take 5 to 10 min to go away, a much longer period than is required for the symptoms of vascular claudication to evaporate. Sometimes the symptoms disappear more quickly if the patient adopts a position which flexes the lumbar spine such as crouching down on the heels or sitting forward in a chair. The reason for this is that flexion tends to widen the lumbar canal.

There are few physical signs at rest. Root tension signs, such as limited straight leg raising or a positive femoral stretch test, are absent and usually the only neurological deficit to be found is absence of the ankle jerks. However, if the patient exercises until symptoms are produced, root tension signs and a more extensive neurological disturbance may appear. The only treatment is surgery which should be advised if the symptoms are incapacitating. A complete laminectomy with thorough posterior decompression of the compressed neural structures relieves symptoms in the great majority of cases.

Sometimes there may be focal stenosis at a single level, usually the L4/5 level caused by a firm chronic disc protrusion. This by itself may be sufficient to produce symptoms of claudication of the cauda equina. In such cases removal of the protrusion may be enough to relieve symptoms. Recently some neurosurgeons have treated the condition by multiple level bilateral fenestrations preserving the spinous processes and interspinous ligaments. However, it does not seem likely that this less invasive procedure will produce such a satisfactory symptom relief as a full decompressive laminectomy.

Cervical spondylotic myelopathy

In some elderly people the features of a cervical cord disturbance are found to be associated with the changes of cervical spondylosis. These spondylotic changes include chronic disc bulges with posterior osteophyte formation, infolding of the yellow ligament, facet joint hypertrophy, and minor forward or backward slips of one vertebra on the next. All of these changes may impinge on the cervical spinal canal and it is natural enough to suppose that the myelopathy is caused by chronic spinal cord compression, especially as the affected patients tend to have rather narrow cervical canals in addition to superimposed spondylotic changes. However, at operation the degree of spinal cord compression is often found to be relatively slight in relation to the neurological disturbance, and a thorough surgical decompression seldom leads to much neurological recovery. This is in marked contrast to the situation found when the cervical canal is compressed by a long-standing tumour, where cord compression may be very marked before serious neurological disturbance develops and where surgical removal of the compression generally leads to dramatic neurological recovery. To explain this disparity it has been suggested that production of a myelopathy by spondylosis involves more than simple compression. Amongst the other mechanisms that have been postulated are compression of radicular feeding arteries or the anterior spinal artery, and intermittent tractional or frictional stresses from restriction of the normal upward and downward movement of the cervical cord with neck movement.

None of these explanations is entirely satisfactory, and it is possible that in many cases the association between the myelopathy and the spondylosis is based on nothing more than coincidence. It has long been recognized that there is a group of middle-aged and elderly patients with a cervical cord disturbance of obscure origin. Inevitably many of these patients will have cervical spondylosis, which is common enough in that age group.

Two related conditions, in both of which there is an undoubted relationship between degenerative change of the spine and cord damage, must be differentiated from cervical spondylotic myelopathy. One is acute compression of the cervical cord by a soft-disc protrusion. Here compression is indisputably the mechanism involved and surgical removal of the disc protrusion may lead to a gratifying degree of neurological recovery. The other condition is focal spinal cord damage caused by a combination of cervical spondylosis and a hyperextension injury. Extension of the neck, as may happen with a fall forwards on to the face or intubation for anaesthesia, leads to a narrowing of the cervical spinal canal. If the canal is already narrowed by cervical spondylosis, sudden hyperextension may lead to a focal cord contusion. An apparently mild hyperextension injury in an elderly person with cervical spondylosis may lead to severe cord damage in the absence of any cervical fracture or dislocation.

The natural course of cervical spondylotic myelopathy is variable. In a few patients there is progression to severe disability over the course of 2 to 3 years, while in others the disorder advances more insidiously, sometimes with episodes of sudden worsening. The most common course is for an initial period of progression, over a matter of a few months or so, followed by a plateau phase of stabilization which may last indefinitely or even be followed by a phase of spontaneous improvement. The unpredictable natural history makes assessment of the results of treatment difficult to say the least. The advent of cervical CT myelography has revealed that in many patients the compressive lesion is a mixture of a hard osteophytic ridge and a soft-tissue protrusion. The latter component probably accounts for the cases where there is an acute onset or stuttering progression.

The predominant symptoms are tingling and weakness of the hands and stiffness and clumsiness of the legs. Any sphincter disturbance is usually slight, and sphincter control may be preserved even in advanced cases. Physical examination reveals spasticity of the legs with brisk reflexes and extensor plantar responses. There may be slight weakness of hip flexion and ankle dorsiflexion but interference with gait seems to be caused more by spasticity than by weakness. Sensory loss in the legs is generally minimal or absent. Vibration sense may be impaired but loss of joint position sense is unusual. Any loss of light touch or pinprick sensation is usually patchy and ill defined. In the arms, wasting and weakness of the arm muscles is often marked. Again, sensory loss is often mild and may be confined to a patchy paraesthetic numbness of the hands and fingers. The arm tendon reflexes are brisk below the level of the spondylosis and are lost at the level of the apparent cord involvement, either from interruption of the reflex arc within the cord itself or from associated root compression by osteophytes.

The first treatment to be offered the patient is a cervical collar. It is doubtful whether this alters the course of the condition, but at least it can do no harm. Few patients wear the collar consistently or tightly enough to limit movements of the neck to any great extent. A few surgeons will argue that surgery in the earlier stages of the disorder produces the best results, as well it may, as such a course means operating on many patients whose natural history would be mild and self-limiting. Most neurosurgeons reserve surgery for those patients where serious progression occurs despite a collar. Even in such patients caution should be exercised when surgery is offered. Neurological worsening after operation is by no means uncommon and there can be few neurosurgeons who have not experienced catastrophes in treating this condition. Two surgical approaches are available. Where the cord disorder appears to be related to spondylosis at multiple levels, and if there is evidence of some generalized stenosis of the spinal canal, then laminectomy carried over as many segments as is necessary to decompress the cord is carried out. At one time it was a common practice to open the dura and divide the dentate ligaments so as to allow the cord to fall away from anterior osteophytes. However, few surgeons still carry out this procedure. If the spondylotic change impinging on the cord is confined to anterior osteophytes at one or two levels, then an anterior decompression is best. Many surgeons combine the decompression with a fusion at the same levels (Cloward's operation). In this procedure the front of the vertebral column is exposed and a cylinder of the affected disc and adjacent bone is drilled out with a special device. This exposes a circular area of the anterior dura, and disc material and osteophytes can then be removed under direct vision. The space is then fused with a bone graft which is generally taken from the iliac crest. Recently, many neurosurgeons have abandoned the practice of drilling out a cylinder of bone and performing a formal fusion. By clearing the disc space and then cranking it open with a special instrument, it is usually possible to obtain sufficient room to carry out a wide excision of the osteophytes on both sides of the disc space and thus decompress the anterior dura (anterior decompression). This approach is much simpler than a full-blown Cloward's operation and is attended by fewer postoperative problems. The patient can be mobilized immediately without a collar and can often be discharged home within a day or two of operation. There is a wide variation in the reported results of surgery, which may well reflect differences in the selection of patients for operation. On the whole, the results of the anterior operation appear best, especially if the preoperative investigations have shown that the compressive lesion has a large soft-tissue component. This may be because patients selected for an anterior operation are likely to show the best correlation between the level of the spondylotic change and the level of the cord disturbance. In rough terms, 25 per cent of patients improve after surgery, while in about a further 50 per cent the operation is followed by stabilization of the condition. In the remaining patients the disease continues to progress or the patients are actually worse after operation. An unsatisfactory result may reflect inadequate decompression or sometimes the presence of some condition within the substance of the spinal cord which is not fully related to the presence of the spondylotic change.

REFERENCES

Fearnside, M.R. and Adams, C.B.T. (1978). Tumours of the cauda equina. *Journal of Neurology, Neurosurgery and Psychiatry* **41**, 24–31.

Jennett, W.B. (1956). A study of 25 cases of compression of the cauda equina by prolapsed intervertebral discs. *Journal of Neurology, Neurosurgery and Psychiatry* **19**, 109–16.

Kavanagh, G.J., *et al.* (1968). Pseudoclaudication syndrome produced by compression of the cauda equina. *Journal of the American Medical Association* **206**, 2477–81.

Marshall, J. (1955). Spastic paraplegia of middle age. *Lancet* **i**, 643–6.

Maurice-Williams, R.S. (1981). *Spinal degenerative disease*. John Wright and Sons, Bristol.

Monro, P. (1984). What has surgery to offer in cervical spondylosis? In *Dilemmas in the management of the neurological patient*, (ed. C. Warlow and J. Garfield), pp. 168–87. Churchill Livingstone, Edinburgh.

Murphey, F. (1968). Sources and patterns of pain in disc disease. *Clinical Neurosurgery* **15**, 343–51.

Murphey, F., Simmons, J.C.H., and Brunson, B. (1973). Ruptured cervical discs 1939–1972. *Clinical Neurosurgery* **20**, 9–17.

O'Connell, J.E.A. (1951). Protrusions of the lumbar intervertebral discs. *Journal of Bone and Joint Surgery* **33B**, 8–30.

Shaw, M.D.M., Russell, J.A., and Grossart, K.W. (1978). The changing pattern of spinal arachnoiditis, *Journal of Neurology, Neurosurgery and Psychiatry* **41**, 97–107.

24.4 Disorders of consciousness

24.4.1 Epilepsy in later childhood and adult life

A. P. HOPKINS

Definitions

AN EPILEPTIC SEIZURE

Throughout life, neurones interact in an orderly and organized way, as can be revealed by microelectrode recordings within or adjacent to cells, or by cortical or scalp electrodes of relatively large diameter which integrate the changes in voltage generated by large populations of cells. Scalp recordings of this type are known as the electroencephalogram (EEG). The basic event common to all seizures is a paroxysmal discharge of cerebral neurones. Not all paroxysmal discharges result in overt events. For example, the EEG of a man with epilepsy between seizures may well show spikes over one temporal lobe which represent the paroxysmal discharges of neurones. Such events, unaccompanied by any clinical phenomenon, are not generally considered to be seizures. For the definition of a seizure, therefore, it is necessary to add that the paroxysmal discharge of cerebral neurones must be apparent. This may be either to an external observer, as for example in the case of a grand mal seizure, or as an abnormal perceptual experience suffered by the subject, as may occur in a seizure arising, and remaining confined to, one temporal lobe (see below).

Synonyms of seizure in everyday use include the words attack, fit, turn, spell, or, if resulting in jacitation, convulsions. In conversation with patients the word chosen by them can be used, but for general usage it is best to stick to the word 'seizure', qualified by adjectives describing the type of seizure, preferably using the classification recommended by the International League Against Epilepsy. The various types of seizure are discussed later in this chapter.

In older literature, a sudden cerebrovascular event such as an intracerebral haemorrhage was called an apoplectic seizure, but the word 'seizure' now usually implies a paroxysmal discharge of cerebral neurones. One exception is an 'anoxic seizure' (see later in this chapter).

EPILEPSY

For practical purposes, epilepsy may be defined as a continuing tendency to epileptic seizures. For epidemiological purposes, an operational definition of epilepsy is more than one non-febrile seizure of any type. The question of febrile convulsions, and their relation to epilepsy, is discussed below.

Confusions and inconsistencies arise from these definitions. For example, a common reason for referral to neurological clinics is for assessment after an initial seizure. However, a significant minority of patients do not have further seizures. These individuals should not, by definition, be described as having epilepsy until the second seizure occurs. But what of a person who has one seizure at the age of 18, and another at the age of 50? What has the diagnosis been in the intervening 32 years? Or what of a young woman aged 21 who had many seizures during her early teens, but none for the past 5 years? Do we say that she still has epilepsy, or that her epilepsy is in remission, or that her epilepsy has stopped? Certainly, it is known that the chance of her having further seizures is greater than that of someone who has never had a seizure at all, and it cannot, therefore, be said that her epilepsy has definitely stopped.

Some of these inconsistencies are removed if it is realized that an epileptic seizure is just one of the limited ways that the brain can express that it is in trouble. It is a symptom, exactly as breathlessness is a symptom of various types of pulmonary insufficiency. A neuroepidemiologist trying to make sense of the causes and prognosis of epilepsy is in exactly the same position as a respiratory epidemiologist might be if he were trying to assess the prevalence, causes, and prognosis of breathlessness, without accurate diagnostic classifications of the cause of the breathlessness. Unfortunately, most published work does not acknowledge this difficulty, and many papers on the treatment and prognosis of epilepsy group together patients of different ages, with different genetic constitutions, and seizures of different types due to a multitude of different causes.

The second point that might clarify the semantic confusion is to appreciate that any individual can be made to convulse if the stimulus is adequate. A volatile substance, pentylenetetrazol, will induce seizures in virtually 100 per cent of those who inhale it. It would clearly be nonsensical to call such people epileptics. This substance is sufficient to cause everyone to cross the threshold to convulsions. However, the threshold is of different levels for different people, and a stimulus that might be sufficient to cause a seizure in one person will leave another unscathed. Anyone can have a seizure if sufficiently provoked, but the vast majority never do. Those with a low threshold will have a greater tendency to seizures throughout life, a variety of stimuli at different times being sufficient to trigger the seizures.

'EPILEPTICS'

People with epilepsy are understandably reluctant to be called 'epileptics'; many see the term as pejorative, even though analogous terms such as 'diabetics' are often used. None the less, it is right to respect such feelings. However, in communication between doctors, clarity is essential. The use of the terms 'epileptoid' or 'epileptiform' suggest that doctors are trying to conceal from themselves the fact of a seizure. Of course, if there is doubt about a clinical event described or witnessed, then that should be said, accompanied by a full description of what occurred. As to talking to patients, I do not believe that the adjective 'epileptic' as applied to a seizure rather than a person can be avoided. It is to be hoped that the more ready use of the term in everyday discourse, with an increasing realization of just how common seizures are, will rid the word of its pejorative overtones.

The diagnosis can usefully be expanded to a short diagnostic formulation, describing the patient's present age, the age of onset of seizures, the types of seizures suffered, the present frequency of seizures of each type, the presumed causation, the associated features such as mental retardation, and the patient's present social and economic position. For example, it is not much help knowing that 'John Brown is an epileptic'; it is much more useful to know that 'John Brown, a schoolteacher aged 33, had his first of three generalized tonic–clonic seizures at the age of 12, the last being at the age of 31. He has, however, also continued to have frequent complex partial seizures (see below) beginning at the age of 15. These now occur about once a week. His employing education authority does not know of his seizures. The cause of his seizures is not known, but may be related to a presumed meningitic illness at the age of nine'.

Incidence, prevalence, and cumulative incidence of epilepsy

Some bald figures are shown in Table 1; these require considerable elaboration and explanation. Problems arise because of the difficulty in defining epilepsy as described above. Should, for example, a case be considered 'epileptic' until the second seizure has occurred; is a case who has not had a seizure for 3 years still a 'prevalent' case? The prevalence figure of about 500 per 100 000 (0.5 per cent, or 1 in 200 of the population) is that found in a number of European and North American studies when active epilepsy is defined as including those who have had more than one non-febrile seizure within the previous 2 years, and those who are on continuing anticonvulsant medication for more than one non-febrile seizure in the past. As active epilepsy is roughly twice as common in children as in adults, the population figure of 500 per 100 000 is reflected in a prevalence of active epilepsy of about 700 per 100 000 in children under the age of 16 years and about 330 per 100 000 in adults. In developing countries, where there is less good antenatal and obstetric care, bacterial (meningitis) and parasitic (cysticercosis) infections and cranial injury all contribute to cerebral damage with which epilepsy is associated (see below), so that the prevalence is higher.

Figure 1 shows the incidence rates for new cases of epilepsy at different ages. It can be seen that the incidence of new cases is highest in infancy and in old age, but new cases can occur at any age. In this study, the average annual incidence rate for all types of seizures over a period

Table 1 *The epidemiology of epilepsy: figures for a representative population in a developed country*

Annual incidence	72–86 per 100 000[a]
Prevalence	680 per 100 000[b]
Cumulative lifetime incidence	3400 per 100 000[c]
	2030 per 100 000[d]

[a]Hauser and Kurland (1975); includes seizures which, at the time of the surveys, had remained isolated.
[b]Hauser, *et al.* (1991).
[c]Hauser *et al.* (1993).
[d]Goodridge and Shorvon (1983), but see text.

of more than 30 years was found to be 49 per 100 000 per year. It follows that, if an average lifespan is considered to be 70 years, the chances of developing epilepsy is at least 49 × 70/100 000 or about 3.4 per cent. This is what is meant by cumulative incidence—the risk of ever having had a seizure by a specific age. This surprisingly high cumulative incidence (unfortunately confusingly and incorrectly called by some cumulative prevalence) is supported by the findings of a study in Tonbridge, United Kingdom, in which all the medical records of a population of 6000 registered with one general practitioner were inspected. A lifetime incidence of recorded non-febrile seizures of just over 2 per cent was found (Table 1). Bearing in mind that some records are likely to have been incomplete, and the study population was made up of widely different ages, it can be seen that epilepsy is not a rare or unusual disorder, but one that afflicts about 1 in 30 of the population at some time in life. The relationship between incidence, prevalence, and cumulative incidence is shown in Fig. 1.

Another way of expressing the frequency of epilepsy is to consider that on each day in the United Kingdom about 65 people suffer their first seizure. A typical British general practitioner will have under his care about four adults and three or four children who have had a seizure in the past 2 years, and about two adults and two children who remain on anticonvulsants for seizures in the past. In the United Kingdom there are about 136 000 adults and 90 000 children on anticonvulsants at any one time.

Fig. 1 Age-specific incidence rate, cumulative incidence rate, and age-specific prevalence rate of epilepsy. (Reproduced by permission from Hauser *et al.* 1983.)

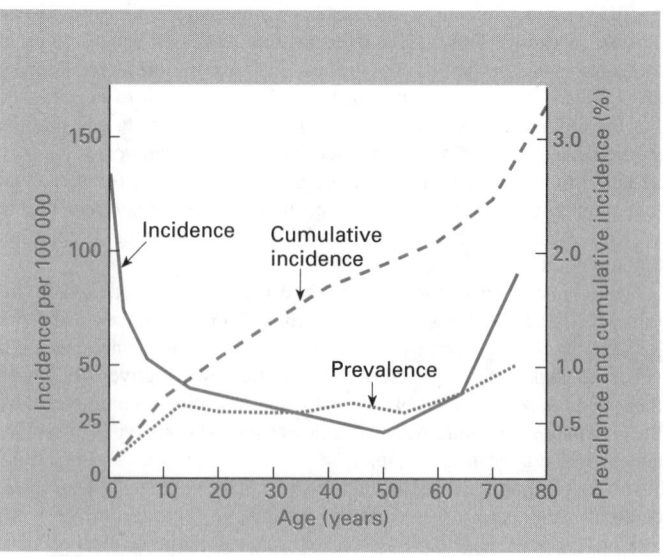

The different types of epileptic seizure

An International Classification of Epileptic Seizures was agreed by a Commission of The International League against Epilepsy in 1981, and revised in 1989 (Table 2). This classification is now used in most scientific communications, but many clinicians regret the passing of the easily understood terms such as temporal lobe seizure and psychomotor seizure. These last have now become complex partial seizures.

Classification of seizure types depends upon an analysis of clinical phenomena observed during the seizure, the changes in the EEG between the seizures, the presumed anatomical substrate and aetiology, and the age of onset. A more detailed description of each type is given below.

Figure 2 illustrates the two main classes of origin of seizure. In the top part of the figure, the hatched area indicates a number of neurones which are in some way abnormal, tending to discharge in paroxysms. They have the facility of driving other neurones to follow their abnormal patterns of discharge. The paths of influence of these abnormal neurones are indicated by the arrows. As long as the discharge remains in one part of the brain, the seizure is said to be a partial seizure. What happens during such a seizure depends upon the site and pattern of discharge of abnormal neurones. In Fig. 2, the abnormal focus is shown in the temporal lobe, by far the commonest site of origin of partial seizures. Clinically observed features of these and other types of partial seizures are described below.

The abnormal discharge may spread, as is shown in Fig. 2(b), through connections linking the two halves of the brain, or, by affecting poorly identified central collections of cells, initiate a generalized seizure discharge. In this case the seizure is said to be a partial seizure which has become secondarily generalized. Some tonic–clonic (grand mal seizures) are of this type.

Figure 2(c) illustrates the second main class of seizure. In this, central collections of cells are themselves in some way abnormal in their behaviour, even though they may seem structurally sound by histological examination. Because of their central position, and the direction and power of their transmissions, a seizure discharge generated within them spreads more or less simultaneously to all parts of the brain. Such a seizure, generalized at onset, is a primary generalized seizure. Typical absences (petit mal absences) and some tonic–clonic seizures (grand mal seizures) are of this type.

TONIC–CLONIC SEIZURES (GRAND MAL SEIZURES, GENERALIZED CONVULSIONS)

Whether the paroxysmal discharge be primary, or secondarily generalized from a cortical focus, the hallmark of a grand mal seizure is disordered muscular contraction. The first phase is known as the tonic phase. The body becomes rigid, and, as it is incapable of maintaining a normal co-ordinated posture, the subject will, if standing, fall to the ground. The chest muscles also contract, forcing the air out through the larynx in an involuntary grunt or cry. The jaw muscles also contract, and the tongue may be bitten. The absence of ventilatory movements and the high oxygen consumption of the vigorously contracting muscles result in the rapid onset of cyanosis. The face becomes suffused by desaturated blood, which is prevented from draining into the thorax by the raised intrathoracic pressure. The normal movements of swallowing are lost, so that saliva may dribble from the mouth. The disordered contraction of abdominal and sphincter muscles may result in incontinence of urine and, occasionally, faeces.

After a brief time in the tonic phase, which may vary from a few seconds to a minute, the seizure passes into a clonic or convulsive phase, with rhythmic contractions of limbs and trunk muscles. The amplitude of these contractions is variable. They continue for a few seconds to a

Table 2 *Classification of epileptic seizures*

I Partial seizures: seizures which start by activation of a group of neurones limited to one part of one hemisphere
  A Simple, without impairment of consciousness. Depending upon anatomical site of origin of seizure discharge, initial symptom may be motor, sensory, aphasic, cognitive, affective, dysmnesic, illusional, olfactory, or psychic. Synonyms include Jacksonian, temporal lobe, or psychomotor seizures according to type
  B Complex partial, with impairment of consciousness
    (a) simple partial onset, followed by impairment of consciousness
    (b) impairment of consciousness at onset: symptoms as in simple, above
  C Partial seizures, either simple or complex, evolving to generalized tonic–clonic seizures; synonym: secondarily generalized seizures. Sometimes seizures become so rapidly secondarily generalized that there is no clinical evidence of partial onset, the only evidence being electroencephalographic

II Generalized seizures: more or less symmetrical, no evidence of focal onset
  A Absence seizures
    (1) Typical absences: abrupt onset and cessation of impairment of consciousness with or without automatisms, myoclonic jerks, tonic, or autonomic components. A 3 Hz spike-and-wave discharge is the usual EEG abnormality for this diagnosis
    (2) Atypical absences: less abrupt onset and/or cessation of consciousness, more prolonged changes in tone, EEG abnormality other than 3 Hz spike-and-wave discharge
  B Myoclonic seizures. Myoclonic jerks, single or multiple
  C Clonic seizures
  D Tonic seizures
  E Tonic–clonic seizures: synonyms: grand mal, major convulsion
  F Atonic or astatic seizures

III Unclassified seizures—as yet undefined

Fig. 2 Origins of different types of epileptic seizure (see text for details).

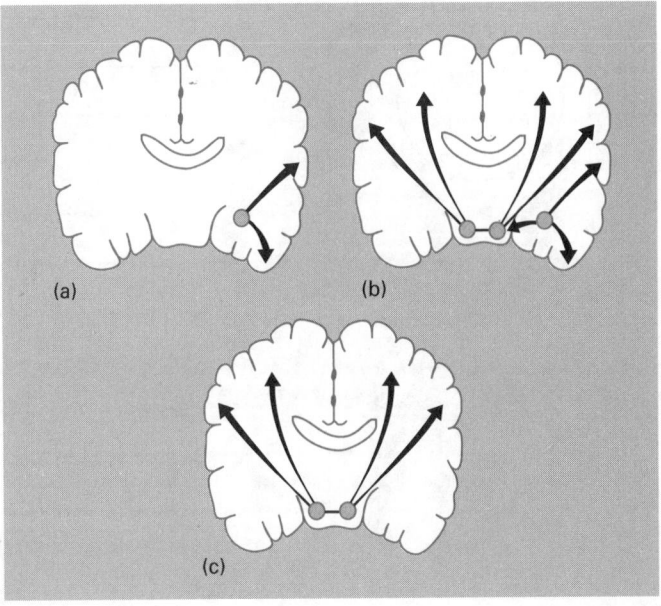

few minutes, after which the subject lies in a deep stupor, which gradually lightens through a stage of confusion into full consciousness. After the seizure the subject may have a headache, and feel generally bruised and battered by the vigorous muscular contractions. Post-ictal confusion must be distinguished from the automatic behaviour of a seizure arising in the temporal lobe (see below).

No bystander behaves very sensibly when he first witnesses a seizure. Relatives of those with epilepsy understandably want to know what they should do during such an attack. If the origin of the tonic–clonic seizure is a partial seizure, there may be sufficient warning for the subject to be helped to a place of safety during the partial phase of the attack, or at least the relative may be able to break the subject's fall. Once on the ground the subject should be turned into the 'coma position'—that is to say into a semiprone position—so that secretions drain from the subject's mouth, rather than into the larynx. Any vomiting that occurs will also find easy egress this way. There is no point in trying to force an object between tightly clenched teeth. The tongue is usually bitten at the onset of the seizure, the airway is not significantly improved by opening the mouth, and damage to the teeth may result from misguided attempts to force a passage. It is, however, useful to give the subject a sharp clap on the back, to drive the tongue forwards. The post-ictal confusion can be minimized by acting calmly, explaining clearly to the subject what has happened, and avoiding calling an ambulance, unless injury has occurred.

TYPICAL ABSENCES (PETIT MAL SEIZURES)

This description should only be given to absence attacks associated with classical 3 Hz spike and wave activity in the EEG (see Fig. 3).

Petit mal is a disorder with onset in childhood, and attacks continuing into adult life are rare. A typical absence attack is very brief, lasting only a few seconds. The onset and termination are abrupt. The child ceases what he is doing, stares, looks a little pale, and may flutter the eyelids. Sometimes more extensive bodily movements occur, such as dropping the head forwards, and there may be a few clonic movements of the arms. Attacks are very commonly provoked by hyperventilation for 3 min or so, and this is well worth testing in the out-patient clinic or during electroencephalography.

The interruption of the normal stream of consciousness is very brief, and the child may be unaware of the attacks, as indeed may be the parents for some time after onset, assuming that the child is just daydreaming.

It is in this type of disorder that the distinction between an EEG abnormality and an overt attack becomes least clear. For example, during the EEG the child may have frequent short bursts of spike-and-wave activity, without any overt clinical concomitant. However, it can be shown that, if tests of abstract reasoning are administered during the course of the recording, the rate of intellectual processing is slower during the time at which the spike-and-wave discharges occur.

Fig. 3 Electroencephalogram of a typical absence seizure. The first 2.5 s of the record are entirely normal. The event begins with a large downward deflection which records eye closure, immediately followed in all channels by a spike-and-wave discharge at a frequency of 3 cycles. The seizure terminates as abruptly as it began. (Record kindly provided by Dr David Fish.)

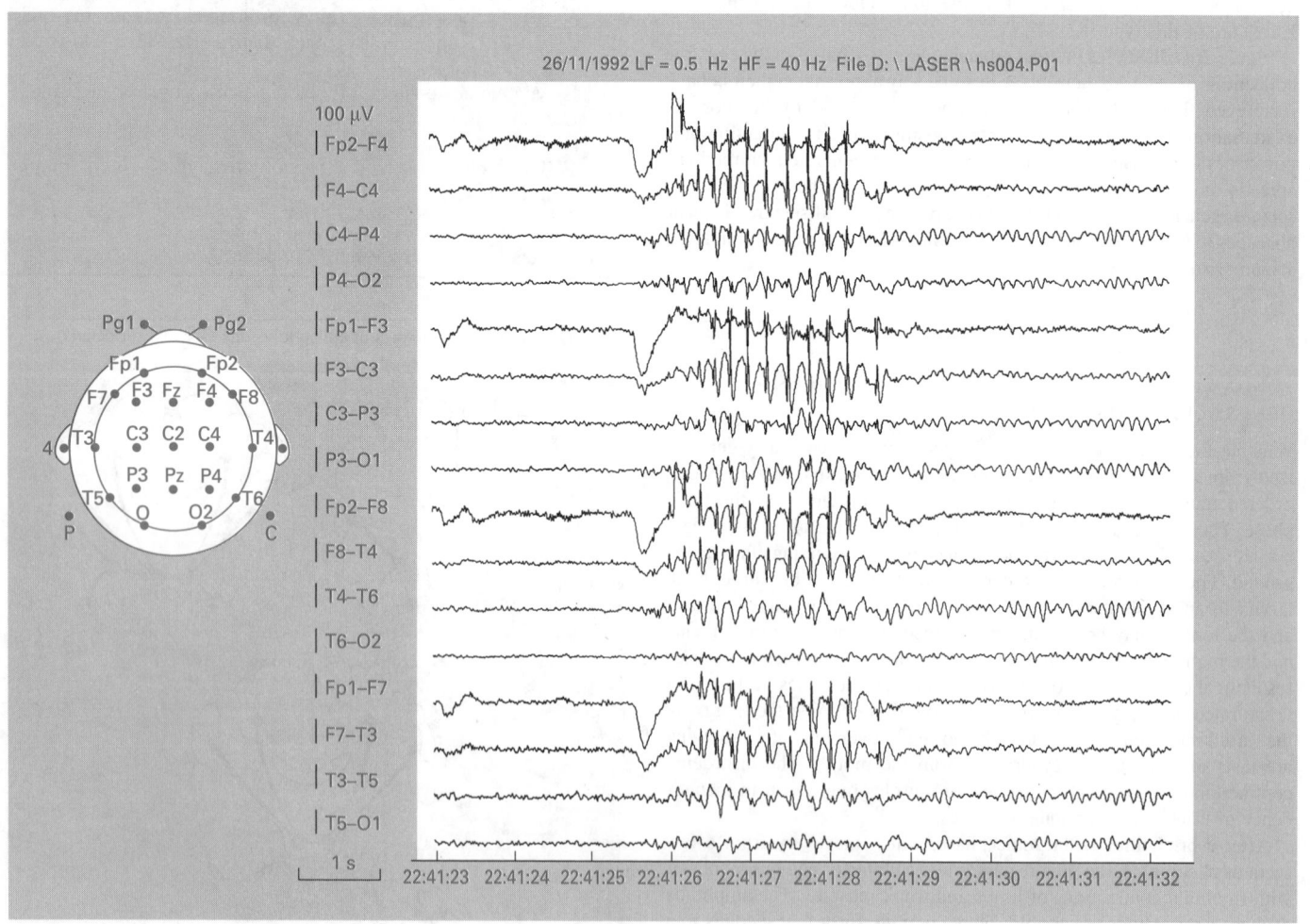

About one-third of all children with petit mal will have one or more tonic–clonic convulsions.

PARTIAL SEIZURES (FOCAL SEIZURES)

Partial seizures reflect a neuronal discharge more or less localized to one part of the brain. The exact internal perception or external manifestation depends upon the site of origin of discharge of the abnormal neurones. If these are in the motor cortex, the initial manifestation will be a contraction of the muscles in the opposite side of the body. Partial motor seizures are most likely to begin at the angle of the mouth, the index finger and thumb, or the big toe. If the seizure discharge then spreads through contiguous layers of cortex, the clinical manifestations march into the homologous parts of the body. A seizure of this type is called a Jacksonian seizure, after one of the neurologists who first described them. These parts of the body are the sites at which seizures most commonly begin, partly because there are many cortical cells assigned to controlling these muscles, which are concerned with the fine tuning of manual skills and facial expression, and partly because their thresholds of excitation are lowest, as judged by direct cortical stimulation.

Another type of partial seizure associated with movement is the versive seizure. Version is usually away from the hemisphere in which the abnormal cells lie, so these seizures are often called adversive. In such an attack the eyes are deviated, followed by the head, and sometimes the whole body may turn on its own axis, often with elevation and abduction of the arm. The site of origin of such seizures is in the posterior frontal region, or, occasionally, the responsible lesion may be in the posterior part of the temporal lobe.

In the partial seizures so far described, there is an overt motor expression of the seizure. However, other groups of abnormal neurones may cause only an abnormal internal event. For example, a somatosensory seizure may result in the subject experiencing only a warmth or tingling in the limbs contralateral to the collection of abnormal neurones in the parietal cortex.

However, by far the most common type of partial seizure is that arising from a discharge of abnormal neurones in the temporal lobe. Such seizures are often called temporal lobe seizures, but more recently have become called complex partial seizures. The classification refers to them as partial seizures with psychic symptoms, or with autonomic symptoms, or with special-sensory symptoms.

The seizure discharge in complex partial seizures is manifested by distortions of consciousness which range from partial loss of awareness, such that the subject is dimly aware of what is going on around him although he may be unable to reply, through to complete inaccessibility, with amnesia for events occurring during the seizure. Even in these, it may be possible to superimpose normal behaviour on the seizure; for example, the subject may be led passively to a chair, so that he can complete the seizure sitting down.

Partial seizures arising in the temporal lobe are often accompanied by stereotyped motor behaviour involving the lower part of the face. Grimacing and sucking movements are quite common, and there may

Fig. 4 Inter-ictal spike and slow-wave complex in a patient with complex partial seizures. The discharges are particularly apparent over the left temporal lobe (T3–T5), but there are also some independent discharges over the right temporal lobe (T4–T6). (Record kindly provided by Dr David Fish.)

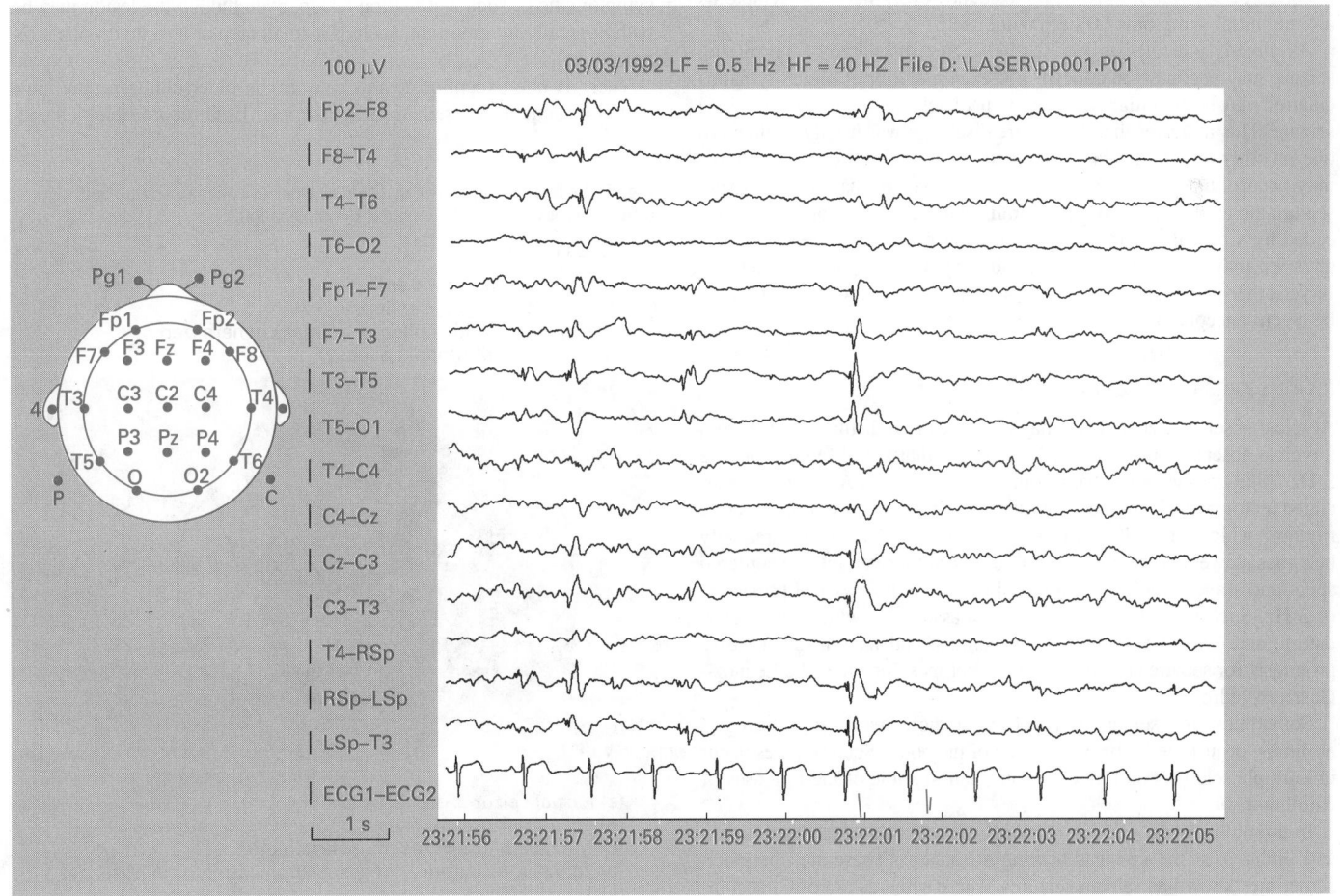

be rotation of the head and eyes as the seizure discharge spreads forwards. Sometimes complex stereotyped behaviour such as undressing may occur, or the patient may be able to continue walking along the road, and indeed crossing streets making appropriate judgements with regard to oncoming traffic, even though he is in the midst of a seizure.

Distorted perceptions during a partial seizure arising in the temporal lobe may give the clue to the correct diagnosis. The subject may report a sense of unreality, even if partially aware of his or her surroundings. The phrase 'déjà vu' is used to describe a sensation that what is happening around him has already occurred at some previous time. The phrase 'jamais vu' is used to describe a perception that what is seen is so unreal that it bears no relation to the subject's previous life events. There may be a pervasive feeling of fear, and dizziness; olfactory and visual hallucinations are not uncommon. The visual hallucinations are sometimes well-formed, so that the subject may recount complex scenes, almost analogous to a film. For example, one 12-year-old boy told me that during some of his partial seizures he was aware of another boy, who was familiar in some way, although he did not know him. He saw this other boy standing the other side of a shower, and the other boy appeared to put his leg under the running water, and then the subject put his leg under the running water alternately. Such hallucinations are quite different from the ill-formed visual flashes and scotomata that may arise from migrainous phenomena, which usually affect the occipital lobe.

A common initial symptom of a partial seizure arising in the temporal lobe is a vague feeling of discomfort in the upper abdomen, which may be accompanied by borborygmi, the discomfort rising to the chest, this then being followed by a sensation of fullness in the head as the seizure continues. Vertigo may be another symptom that occurs during a complex partial seizure arising in the temporal lobe.

The term 'aura' is often used to describe the epigastric sensation, or distorted perception. It must be realized, however, that these symptoms are the initial symptoms of the seizure itself.

As already indicated in Fig. 2, the seizure discharge of any partial seizure may become generalized. For example, a brief olfactory hallucination may be an initial symptom immediately preceding a generalized seizure. This indicates that the seizure discharge was briefly confined to one or other temporal lobe before becoming generalized. All patterns may occur. For example, on some days the patient may have a partial seizure alone, on other days a generalized tonic–clonic convulsion preceded by a partial seizure, and yet on other days the secondary generalization may be so rapid that the initial symptom is not experienced. In yet other patients, the only evidence of focal onset of a seizure may be electroencephalographic (Fig. 4).

RARE TYPES OF SEIZURES

Atypical absences occur. They may be clinically indistinguishable from a typical absence, but show EEG discharges that are different from the 3 Hz spike-and-wave discharge illustrated in Fig. 3. A common associated feature with an atypical absence is known as a 'recruiting epileptic rhythm', which is initially rapid and of low amplitude, but then gradually becomes slower and of higher amplitude. Another variant is disordered spike-and-wave complexes at a rate slower than the classical frequency of 3 Hz. Such variant absences are often associated with mental retardation, and evidence of cerebral dysgenesis, and have a much worse prognosis for seizure control. This is sometimes known as the Lennox–Gastaut syndrome.

Sometimes tonic seizures occur. In these there is a tonic posturing of all limbs, or just the limbs on one side of the body. Such seizures occur in multiple sclerosis on rare occasions, and in some of the lipidoses of childhood.

In infantile spasms, there is a brief sudden flexion of the head, trunk, and limbs, as if the infant is bowing a 'salaam'. These are, therefore, sometimes known as salaam seizures. These seizures are often accompanied by failure of development and progressive retardation (West's

syndrome). The EEG is characteristic, distinguished by irregular high-voltage, diffuse, slow spike-and-wave complexes that are repeated at brief intervals on high-voltage slow background rhythms. Myoclonic epilepsy is considered below.

The different types of epilepsy

In addition to the International Classification of Epileptic Seizures, illustrated in Table 2, there is also an International Classification of Epilepsies and Epileptic Syndromes. The reason for this dual classification is that there are certain clusters of clinical characteristics with common natural histories, even if there may be more than one underlying cause (for example, West's syndrome just mentioned). However, it must be acknowledged that this classification was drawn up largely by paediatric epileptologists, and its usefulness in primary care is doubtful. For example, of 594 cases in the United Kingdom general practice study of epilepsy, two-thirds had to be assigned to various non-specific categories in the classification. Adult neurologists also find the complex classification of little use.

Relationship between seizure type and types of epilepsy

Figure 5 indicates the relationship between seizure types and types of epilepsy. The term 'idiopathic' epilepsy is often used when there is no apparent cause for the seizure. More prolonged EEG recordings, using various activating techniques (see below) and the advent in particular of magnetic resonance imaging (MRI) have shown that many tonic–clonic seizures previously considered to be idiopathic arise from a structural lesion. Partial seizures always arise from some focal area of structural abnormality in the brain, and if such exists, the epilepsy is clearly symptomatic of such a structural lesion, even though the lesion may be pathologically unimportant, such as a small area of atrophy in one temporal lobe.

There is one exception to this rule. Some older children may have partial or generalized seizures, the interictal EEG record being charac-

Fig. 5 The relationship between different types of epileptic seizure and different types of epilepsy. See text for explanation.

Types of epilepsy

(a)+(b) = symptomatic epilepsy
(c)　　 = cryptogenic epilepsy
(d)+(e) = idiopathic epilepsy (primary generalized or
　　　　　constitutional epilepsy)

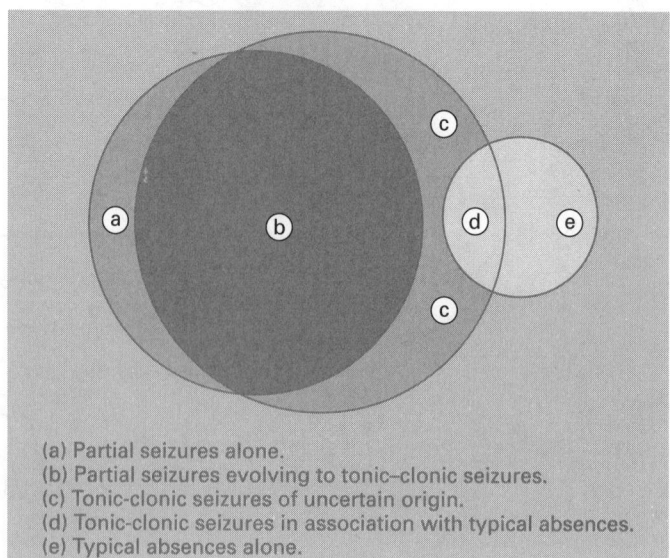

(a) Partial seizures alone.
(b) Partial seizures evolving to tonic–clonic seizures.
(c) Tonic-clonic seizures of uncertain origin.
(d) Tonic-clonic seizures in association with typical absences.
(e) Typical absences alone.

Table 3(a) *Prevalence (per 100 000) of epileptic seizures of different types and different degrees of activity*

Seizure type	Seizure in past 6 months	Seizure in past 2 years	No seizure for 2 years but still on drugs	Seizure at any time in life
Typical absences	7	7	20	240
Partial seizures	130	150	40	2100
Tonic–clonic seizures	90	160	160	1300
Any type of seizure	170	230	100	3400

Sources: right-hand column, Hauser and Kurland (1975); other columns, Hopkins and Scambler (1977).

(b) *Classification of dominant seizure type 6 months after first seizure in the National General Practice Study of Epilepsy (n = 564; all ages)*

	Percentage
Classifiable	91.0
Unclassifiable	9.0
Generalized seizures	39.0
Absences	1.0
Myoclonic	<1.0
Tonic clonic	35.0
Other generalized	2.5
Partial seizures	52.0
Simple	3.0
Complex	11.0
Partial becoming secondarily generalized	27.0
Mixed partial	12.0

Source: Sander, *et al.* (1990).

terized by large spike discharges over the Rolandic area of one hemisphere. Such 'benign childhood epilepsy with centrotemporal spikes' is not associated with any structural lesion, and has an excellent prognosis. It does not fit easily into an understanding of seizures as set out in the foregoing paragraphs.

True idiopathic epilepsy is now known as primary generalized epilepsy. In this type of epilepsy, the seizures are generalized from the onset, either taking the form of tonic–clonic seizures, or typical absences, or just the myoclonus associated with absences. The characteristic 3 Hz spike-and-wave activity, illustrated in Fig. 3, is the hallmark of this type of epilepsy.

Sometimes it is not possible to be certain whether generalized tonic–clonic seizures arise on the basis of primary generalized epilepsy, in which the EEG happens not to have shown any seizure discharge at the time of the recording, or whether, alternatively, the tonic–clonic seizures are very rapidly generalized from a focus which is clinically silent. Such 'cryptogenic' cases should not, however, be called idiopathic.

Table 3 shows the prevalence of seizures of different types and of different degrees of activity. The data are derived from primary care and community based studies. The proportion of seizures that are partial, or of partial onset, is high. In the study by Hopkins and Scambler (1977) 56 per cent of epileptic patients had had partial seizures at some time, and in a further 12 per cent, even though partial seizures by themselves had not occurred, there was clear clinical evidence of partial onset, or EEG evidence of focal onset to the generalized tonic–clonic seizure. Therefore, even without the benefit of imaging studies, there was evidence of a focal and presumably structural origin for the attacks in nearly 70 per cent of the subjects. In the National General Practice Study, 52 per cent of the patients had had partial or partial-onset seizures within 6 months of the onset of their epilepsy. In an adult sample, true idiopathic epilepsy, as defined above, is unusual. The general experience is that, in adult life, the more extensively a minor structural abnormality

is sought by imaging studies in those with epilepsy, the more often one is found. Even if a survey is confined to children of school age, only about 12 per cent are found to have had typical absence (petit mal) seizures, and an even smaller proportion benign partial seizures as described above.

Causes of epilepsy

INHERITANCE

There is good evidence that genetic factors are an important aetiological factor in certain forms of epilepsy. These inherited forms have been estimated to account for at least 20 per cent of all epilepsies. It is useful to distinguish between those conditions in which recurrent seizures are merely one component of a more complex phenotype, and those in which they are an essentially isolated phenomenon. The former are 'single-gene' disorders which display a mendelian pattern of inheritance, whereas the latter nearly all display a 'complex' non-mendelian pattern, indicating the interaction of several genes and environmental factors.

Over 120 mendelian disorders are recognized in which epilepsy occurs in a proportion of patients as a component of the phenotype. They include inborn errors of amino acid metabolism, neurocutaneous disorders such as neurofibromatosis and tuberous sclerosis, and the progressive neurodegenerative conditions such as the ceroid-lipofuscinoses and Unverricht–Lundborg disease or Baltic myoclonus. At least two mitochondrial diseases, myoclonic epilepsy with ragged-red fibres and the mitochondrial encephalomyopathy and lactic acidosis syndrome, are complicated by epilepsy. In some of these conditions the mutated gene and its product are known, and the pathophysiology of seizure generation is at least partially understood. These mendelian disorders collectively amount for a tiny fraction, perhaps 1 per cent of all patients with familial epilepsy.

Most epilepsy syndromes in which recurrent seizures occur in isolation in neurologically and cognitively intact individuals, and which display familial aggregation, have a 'complex' pattern of inheritance. Several difficulties peculiar to epilepsy have confounded attempts to discern mechanisms of inheritance from studies of familial segregation. Even if seizure types can be defined, patients may defy categorization into particular epilepsy phenotypes. Age-dependent penetrance renders diagnosis uncertain in older individuals, and the relationship of EEG abnormalities to epilepsy remains controversial, although it is probable that they do, in certain cases, represent a useful biological marker for the disease.

Nevertheless, studies of several epilepsy phenotypes provide good evidence for a genetic aetiology. These include idiopathic generalized epilepsies such as juvenile myoclonic epilepsy, and the absence epilepsies and idiopathic partial epilepsies, in particular benign childhood epilepsy with centrotemporal spikes. Genetic factors are also clearly important in the causation of febrile convulsions, although some authors would not classify this disorder with the epilepsies. One epilepsy syndrome—benign familial neonatal convulsions—displays mendelian inheritance, segregating in an autosomal dominant manner.

The revolution in molecular genetic methodology has provided new approaches to the investigation of inherited diseases, including epilepsy.

These may allow an understanding of the genetic basis of epilepsy at a molecular level. Two general strategies exist for the application of these techniques to the epilepsies: positional cloning and candidate gene analysis.

Positional cloning is initiated by establishing the map location of the disease gene by linkage analysis. The genomic region containing the disease gene is narrowed down, and molecular cloning techniques are used to identify the gene itself, (see Section 4). Two epilepsy genes have been mapped using linkage analysis: benign familial neonatal convulsions to chromosome 20 and progressive myoclonic epilepsy of Unverricht and Lundborg to chromosome 21. These are both mendelian disorders and the evidence for linkage to specific markers is unequivocal. The more common 'non-mendelian' disorders are more difficult to tackle by this approach. One of these, juvenile myoclonic epilepsy, has been the subject of linkage studies, but present evidence is conflicting. Two studies provided evidence in favour of a gene (designated EJMI) predisposing to juvenile myoclonic epilepsy in the HLA region of chromosome 6p, but a third failed to identify evidence in favour of a gene in this region.

'Candidate' genes for epilepsy include those encoding proteins mediating functions which, if disturbed, could lead to disturbances of neuronal synchrony and clinical seizures, including, for example, those mediating neuronal inhibition, inactivation of excitatory neurotransmitters and ion transport across excitable membranes. The genes encoding voltage-gated potassium channels, mutations of which in the fruitfly cause a phenotype (shaker) with similarities to epilepsy, are an important candidate group. Existing methods allow a rapid search for mutations in these genes in affected individuals. The mitochondrial genome (mtDNA), with its key role in energy generation in the central nervous system, is another 'candidate' gene, and point mutations in mtDNA have been identified as the cause of myoclonic epilepsy with ragged-red fibres and the mitochondrial encephalomyopathy and lactic acidosis syndrome.

Extensive studies of the genetics of epilepsy in man over the past 50 years have established clear evidence for a genetic contribution to its aetiology. The application of new molecular genetic techniques may allow this contribution to be understood at a molecular level: the genes involved, their map location, the proteins they encode, and the mutations which disrupt their function may all be elucidated. New DNA-based diagnostic methods may become available, and entirely new approaches to therapy based on methods to manipulate or prevent the expression of mutant gene products may emerge.

TRAUMA

Penetrating injuries such as those caused by shrapnel or rifle bullets in wartime are a potent cause of epilepsy. However, in civilian life most head injuries are caused by road-traffic accidents and industrial accidents, and result from some deceleration injury to the brain transmitted through the skull without any penetration of the skull itself. Trivial head injuries are one of the commonest causes of attendance at accident and emergency departments, but very few result in the later development of epilepsy.

W.B. Jennett has done a great deal to separate out those factors in a head injury that are most likely to be associated with the subsequent development of epilepsy. In general, head injuries resulting in a long duration of post-traumatic amnesia (that period for which the patient, albeit possibly conscious, is not committing to memory on-going events, even though he may appear to be behaving rationally at that time), although indicating a head injury that is likely to be followed by impairment of cognitive skills and memory, are not particularly likely to be followed by the development of epilepsy unless there is cortical damage, caused either by a depressed fracture, or haemorrhage.

Another factor that Jennett defined as being of considerable importance was the occurrence of a seizure in the first week after a head injury. It may be that such an early seizure is just the marker of an inherited low convulsive threshold. In any event it proved to be a potent predictor of late post-traumatic epilepsy, as is shown in the bar chart in Fig. 6, which lists the incidence (after varying degrees of follow-up) of epilepsy after depressed fractures with various combinations of features. About 70 per cent of those who eventually develop late post-traumatic epilepsy will have had their first late (i.e. later than 7 days) seizure within 2 years. Unfortunately, the evidence is that prophylactic anticonvulsant treatment does not suppress the incidence of late post-traumatic epilepsy.

CEREBRAL DYSGENESIS

There are, of course, other types of brain impairment apart from that caused by road-traffic and industrial accidents. Cerebral palsy and epilepsy are often associated. Traditionally, and still in the minds of many lawyers, 'birth injury' is related to poor obstetric care. However, epidemiological evidence suggests that antenatal factors resulting in varying degrees of cerebral dysgenesis are responsible for most cases of cerebral palsy. With regard to mental retardation, without overt palsy, the prevalence of epilepsy increases progressively with the degree of

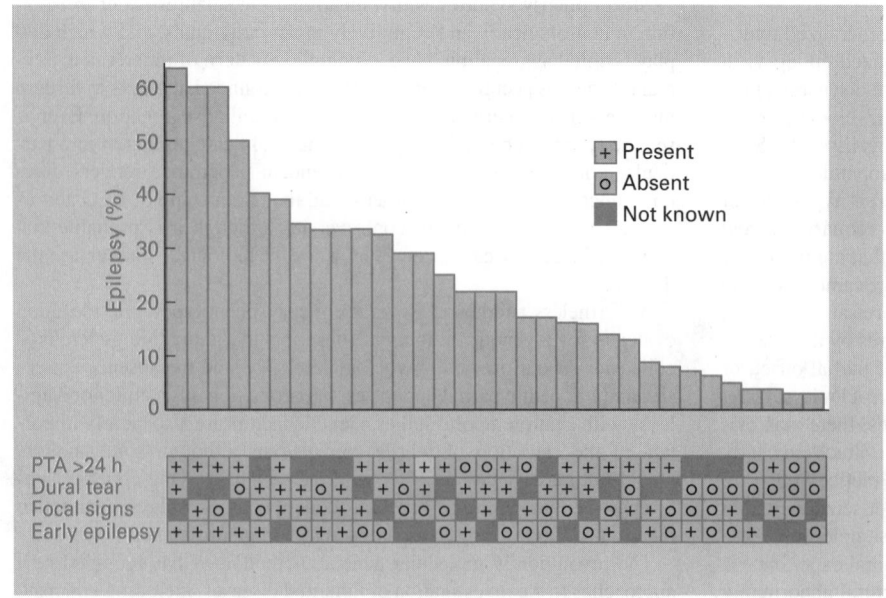

Fig. 6 Incidence of late epilepsy after compound depressed fracture of the skull when three of four factors were known; PTA, post-traumatic amnesia. (Redrawn from Jennett 1975.)

retardation. In those with severe learning difficulties (IQ < 50), the life-time cumulative incidence is at least 30 per cent. Both the seizures and the retardation are common manifestations of an underlying brain dysfunction, due either to metabolic abnormalities, such as lipoidoses or metachromatic dystrophies or to dysplastic conditions in which neuronal embryonic migration is impaired, such as areas of cortical dysplasia or heterotopias or tuberous sclerosis. The Sturge–Weber syndrome and arteriovenous malformations of various types are also prominently associated with epilepsy.

TUMOURS

Older textbooks of medicine stress the need for intensive investigation of patients with 'epilepsy of late onset'. The implication is that epilepsy of late onset is unusual, and frequently due to a tumour, which should not be missed. However, it is now realized, and demonstrated in Fig. 1, that the age-specific incidence curve is more or less flat between the ages of 10 and 59, rising sharply thereafter. The cause of the steep increase in older age is the increasing proportion of patients with seizures due to neuronal degenerations and cerebrovascular disease. Tumours play only a comparatively small part (see Table 4). However, the proportion of cases in whom tumours are the cause does rise with increasing age, reaching 19 per cent between the ages of 50 and 59 in the United Kingdom general practice study. In practice, 'missing' a primary cerebral tumour is not quite so devastating as most non-neurologists would believe. Many cerebral tumours are metastatic, usually from bronchus or breast, and as such are clearly a manifestation of disseminated malignant disease for which treatment is largely ineffective, even if early diagnosis of dissemination is made. Furthermore, the results of surgical removal or irradiation of malignant astrocytomas is disappointing, and in many cases a neurologist will advise against radical operation even if the epilepsy has clearly been demonstrated to be due to tumour. Benign epileptogenic tumours such as meningiomas make up fewer than 5 per cent of all space-occupying intracerebral tumours. The introduction of magnetic resonance imaging and the wide employment of surgery in the management of intractable epilepsy has shown that small areas of focal dysgenesis (hamartomas) may be responsible for seizures. The distinction between an indolent 'tumour' and 'hamartoma' is sometimes extremely difficult.

INFECTIOUS DISEASES

Bacterial meningitis may scar the cortical mantle, resulting in the subsequent development of seizures. Acute bacterial infections in the form of a cerebral abscess may also cause seizures in association with the abscess. Even if the abscess is drained and heals, the thick-walled gliotic scar may well be associated with seizures subsequently. It is for this reason that cerebral abscesses are often excised after they have been drained.

Viral encephalitis may cause seizures during the acute illness, and subsequent seizures after the initial infection has passed. In England the commonest identified cause is the herpes simplex virus. Persistent viral infection such as occurs in subacute sclerosing panencephalitis, in which the measles virus persists after an initial infection, may also be accompanied by generalized seizures and myoclonus.

Echinococcal cysts, cysticercosis, toxocariasis, and toxoplasmosis are, in the United Kingdom, rarer causes of seizures, although some consider that widespread contamination of children's playing fields by *Toxocara canis* is an important cause of epilepsy in childhood. Parasitic infections, particularly cysticercosis, are common causes of epilepsy in Third World countries.

DEGENERATIVE DISORDERS

As already noted, the incidence of seizures increases in old age. They occur in Alzheimer's disease, although usually they are overshadowed by the social and intellectual deterioration.

Table 4 *Identified causes of epilepsy in two studies*

Cause	Study 1 (%)	Study 2 (%)
Perinatal causes/congenital	8.0	n/i
Cranial injury: postoperative	5.5	3
Infections	2.5	2
Vascular	10.9	15
Tumours	4.1	6
Alcohol		7
'Other causes' e.g. Alzheimer's	3.5	6
Total	34.5	39
Idiopathic/cryptogenic	65.5	61

Study 1, Hauser *et al.* (1993); Rochester, Minnesota.

Study 2, Sander *et al.* (1990), 564 cases presenting in general practice between 1984 and 1987.

n/i, no information.

VASCULAR DISEASE

Seizures may result from embolic infarcts. For example, in mitral valve disease, cerebral emboli may be the result of thrombus formation in the left atrium. Furthermore, after replacement of a diseased valve by some types of prosthesis, cerebral embolism may occur after thrombus formation on the new valve. Seizures may also result from emboli following myocardial infarction, from atheromatous emboli in association with carotid artery disease, or from septic emboli in subacute bacterial endocarditis. Occasionally diffuse cerebral anoxia, such as may follow a transient cardiac arrest, may result in subsequent epilepsy.

Imaging studies show a considerable excess of infarcts in the brains of those in whom epilepsy starts later in life, compared to scans of controls matched for age. These infarcts are often deep-seated lacunes, sometimes clinically silent except for the epilepsy. Deep lacunar infarction probably does not in itself cause the seizures, but is merely a marker of more widespread vascular disease.

ALCOHOL

Chronic abuse of alcohol may result in seizures which then continue even if the subject abstains. Seizures also occur sometimes in acute alcohol intoxication and often after abrupt withdrawal of alcohol, as part of the syndrome of delirium tremens (Section 28).

ACUTE SYMPTOMATIC SEIZURES

Apart from the example of acute alcohol intoxication noted above, it is well recognized that some drugs may precipitate seizures. The drugs in everyday use that have been most often incriminated include phenothiazines, tricyclic antidepressants, lignocaine, penicillin, and isoniazid. Other metabolic causes of seizures include hypoglycaemia, most usually induced by exogenous insulin used in the treatment of diabetes; hypocalcaemia, particularly in neonates; and uraemia. Hyperglycaemia has also been reported as a cause of partial seizures. Withdrawal from barbiturates, benzodiazepines, and above all from alcohol, may be associated with seizures.

Other acute symptomatic seizures arise as the result of an acute brain illness, such as meningitis, or herpes simplex encephalitis.

PROPORTION OF EPILEPSY CASES DUE TO DIFFERENT CAUSES

Table 4 illustrates the causes of seizures identified in two studies. Note that an identifiable cause could only be discovered in 34 to 39 per cent of all cases. There has, as yet, been no good population-based study in which every subject has had a magnetic resonance scan, but it is probably that the proportion of cases in which no clear-cut cause was identified would be substantially less in such a study. Both studies illustrated in Table 4 are from developed countries. In less developed countries, the proportion of cases of epilepsy associated with infective causes such as tuberculosis and cysticercosis will be much higher.

Precipitants of seizures

Distinct from the causes of a continuing tendency to seizures are those factors that may precipitate an attack. For example, many patients with epilepsy say that they have more seizures when they are upset or worried; conversely some, particularly those with complex seizures, more if they are relaxed, and if their mind is not concentrating on any particular task. Other precipitants include alcohol and drugs, as already mentioned above, menstruation, lack of sleep, and intercurrent illness. All these precipitants may prove to be very 'personal'. That is to say although staying up late may precipitate seizures the following day in one child, this is not true of every child, and the remote possibility of seizures being caused by everyday events should not be used by parents as an excuse to cocoon their child in a protective web of inaction.

Although lack of sleep may precipitate seizures the following day, drowsiness and sleep may allow seizures to 'escape'. Indeed drowsiness is such a potent activator of abnormal discharges in the EEG that the recordist will often encourage the subject to try to go to sleep during the recording. In some patients with epilepsy, seizures are virtually confined to the hours of sleep. However, one follow-up study of those who said that they had always had nocturnal grand mal showed that approximately one-third of them had an attack during waking hours within the following 5 years.

In some subjects, precipitants of the seizures are so potent and so stereotyped as to warrant the name 'reflex epilepsy'. Many such cases are amongst the curiosities of medicine; for example, the subject who has a seizure only on hearing church bells, or on reading, or on looking at repetitive patterns such as squares of floor tiling. It may be presumed that the perception of such external stimuli results in a particular pattern of neuronal discharge—indeed this is presumably in part how we recognize patterns, tunes, and words. One can only imagine that this particular set of neuronal discharge in susceptible people acts as a specific template which, like a key in a lock, unlooses a seizure.

The commonest type of reflex epilepsy is television epilepsy. This is not due to any malfunction of the set, but seizures may be induced in susceptible children by the normal traverse of the spot down the face of the tube. Such children are most at risk when the screen occupies a considerable proportion of the visual field, as will occur if the size of the screen is large and the child sits close to it. It has been shown that observing the set with one eye covered prevents the occurrence of these seizures.

Differential diagnosis of seizures

A considerable part of the work-load of a neurologist is sorting out 'funny turns' or 'blackouts' of some sort. Before embarking upon antiepileptic treatment, it is therefore essential to ensure that such complaints are due to a paroxysmal discharge of cerebral neurones—an epileptic seizure—and not some other event. What other events have to be considered?

VASOVAGAL SYNCOPE

(See also Chapter 24.4.2 and Section 15)

Vasovagal syncope is distinguished from a seizure principally by the circumstances in which the event occurs. Vasovagal syncope never occurs in bed and rarely in the horizontal position.

Loss of consciousness occurring in crowded trains, waiting at bus stops, or in school assembly, should always be presumed to be syncopal

in nature unless there is clear-cut evidence to the contrary. These are circumstances in which many of us have felt unwell, and may indeed lose consciousness, particularly during adolescence.

The type of symptoms experienced before loss of consciousness may help in reaching the correct diagnosis. For a minute or two before fainting, the subject will usually feel nauseated, cold, and clammy. Vision may 'grey-out' or 'black-out' due to retinal hypoperfusion. It should be noted that a sensation of 'voices being distant' or 'feeling far away' often occurs before syncope, although such phrases may suggest the distorted consciousness sometimes found with complex partial seizures.

If syncope is profound, perhaps because the subject is supported and unable to fall flat, the profound cerebral hypoperfusion may result in a few jerks, and even incontinence. EEGs recorded during such events show no paroxysmal neuronal discharges, but large-amplitude slow waves. The distinction of such 'anoxic seizures' from epilepsy is an important one.

Micturition syncope can be diagnosed by its characteristic history. It occurs when a man gets out of bed at night to pass urine, and, usually just after completing the act of micturition, he suddenly loses consciousness. It has been shown that not only is there the postural fall of blood-pressure resulting from the assumption of the erect posture, but at the onset of micturition there is a reflex vasodilatation in the legs.

CARDIAC SYNCOPE

(See also Chapter 24.4.2 and Section 15)

A falling cardiac output due to a bradycardia or paroxysmal tachycardia may lead to a disturbance of consciousness with symptoms similar to vasovagal syncope, but occurring in circumstances when vasovagal syncope is unlikely, such as while reading quietly in a chair. Exercise in a patient with severe aortic stenosis may also result in syncope. Distinction between such cases and epileptic seizures may be singularly difficult, especially if no bystander observes the pulse during the attack. Holter monitoring may detect transient disturbances of cardiac rhythm, with or without associated neurological disturbances.

The frequency with which such cases are diagnosed depends on the clinic from which the cases are reported, but in at least one series, disturbances of cardiac rhythm were shown to account for about one-fifth of all cases of transiently disturbed consciousness originally believed to be neurological in nature.

TRANSIENT ISCHAEMIC ATTACKS

Transient ischaemic attacks, although causing a focal disturbance of neurological function, are essentially 'negative' phenomena. That is to say they are manifest by an absence of function, usually with little disturbance of consciousness. Jactitation is not seen.

MIGRAINE

(See also Chapter 24.11)

Migraine is another type of transient disturbance of cerebral function in which positive phenomena such as visual hallucinations may occur. However, such hallucinations are virtually always ill-formed, classically scintillating scotomata rather than the formed visual hallucination which may be part of a complex partial seizure. If the area of cortical depressed function is further forward in the hemisphere, then the symptomatology is more like that of a transient ischaemic attack, with weakness, numbness, or disturbance of the functions of language.

NARCOLEPSY AND CATAPLEXY

The relationship, if any, between these fascinating conditions and epileptic seizures is obscure, but the diagnosis is seldom missed once it is thought of. A narcoleptic episode is usually preceded by an intense desire to sleep, however short-lived, against which the subject fights. This is not an initial symptom of any type of epileptic attack.

Furthermore, the association of narcolepsy with cataplexy—the sudden loss of postural tone precipitated by anger or laughter—is so characteristic that little doubt about the diagnosis then remains. It is also worth enquiring about the other rarer associated symptoms of sleep paralysis and hypnagogic hallucinations.

DROP ATTACKS

Drop attacks are not infrequent in middle-aged women. They say that while walking they suddenly fall to their knees, without any disturbance of consciousness. There is no warning of the event, and they are able to get up as soon as they recover their composure. Although many textbooks suggest that vertebrobasilar ischaemia is a cause of these episodes, the distribution of ages and sex affected is so different from that in which arterial disease is found that it is hard to believe that this is really an important factor. Whatever the cause, the attacks usually disappear after a year or two, and it is clear that they have no relation to epilepsy.

NIGHT TERRORS

Night terrors in children may sometimes be mistaken for epileptic attacks. These affect children aged between about 6 and 8 years, who suddenly awaken from a sound sleep, wide-eyed, screaming, and inconsolable. They are amnesic for the events the following morning. They seem to occur just as often in happy children as in children who are not doing well at school or in the family. Fortunately they, too, pass quickly, and once thought of, the diagnosis is quite straightforward.

BREATH-HOLDING ATTACKS

Breath-holding attacks affect much younger children, aged between 1 and 2 years. A typical story is of a child who has some minor injury, or who is crossed in some way so that he becomes suddenly angry, upset, or frightened. He cries vigorously once or twice, and then holds his breath at the end of one expiration. After a few seconds he becomes cyanosed, and then loses consciousness, lying limply. One or two jerks may occur, and then normal respiration and consciousness resume. The association with frustration, rage, or a sudden injury is the most useful pointer to the correct diagnosis. Again, such attacks terminate spontaneously without treatment.

TICS, HABITS, AND RITUALISTIC MOVEMENTS

These usually begin at about the age of 7 or 8 years, and affect principally the upper part of the face, are bilateral, and are not associated with any disturbance of consciousness. Although the child has a compulsion to undertake such movements, they can be controlled, at least for a brief interval, by command. Sometimes infants indulge in repetitive rocking movements of the trunk which are believed to be masturbatory.

VERTIGO

Vertigo, especially if profound, as may be experienced in the course of a paroxysm of Menière's disease, may be mistaken for a seizure. It is true that vertigo may rarely be an initial symptom in a seizure arising from the posterior temporal lobe, but a far more usual cause is peripheral labyrinthine dysfunction.

OVERBREATHING (HYPERVENTILATION)

Anxiety or stress may result, particularly in adolescent girls, in hyperventilation with resulting respiratory alkalosis, decline in the proportion of ionized calcium, and tetanic posturing of the hands and clouding of consciousness. Such symptoms are rapidly relieved by asking the subject to rebreath his or her expired air in and out of a paper or polythene bag.

SIMULATED SEIZURES

Simulated seizures are often a problem in differential diagnosis, especially in those who undoubtedly have some true seizures. Simulated attacks may be used as an attention-seeking device by those with epilepsy, or by siblings or schoolfriends of those with epilepsy. It can be surprisingly difficult to distinguish true from simulated seizures. Perhaps the best guide is that the simulator tends to overplay the seizure, and the temporal coincidence of seizures whenever there is a suitable observer. Features such as injury, tongue-biting, and incontinence can be, and often are, simulated. If serum can be obtained about 20 min after a true seizure, a serum prolactin of four or five times the normal level will be found; the level returns to normal within 24 h. Elevated serum prolactin will be found shortly after true tonic–clonic seizures and complex partial seizures, but not after simulated seizures, nor after true partial seizures arising in parts of the brain other than the temporal lobe.

The investigation of seizures

Once a clinical diagnosis of a seizure has been made, it is reasonable to consider whether any further investigation will be useful. There are three principal reasons for such investigation:

(1) to improve the certainty with which the diagnosis of a seizure is correct (rather than of some other event, as considered above);
(2) to ascertain the type of seizure, which is important when considering appropriate medication; and
(3) to ascertain the cause of seizures, in case treatment of the underlying cause is necessary.

These are three entirely different sets of reasons for investigation. There is no point whatsoever in undertaking a ritual EEG in the case of a man of 35 who has had his first grand mal seizure approximately 7 months after a major head injury. In this clearcut example, the EEG is almost certain to be abnormal in some way, and the recording will not aid either diagnosis of the cause, or future management. Electroencephalography is, however, a useful tool for distinguishing the various types of seizure. Sometimes there may be some confusion between disturbances of consciousness due to typical absences, and disturbances due to complex partial seizures. If abnormalities are seen during the recordings from two patients with such seizure types (and there almost certainly will be a recorded spike-and-wave discharge in someone with frequent typical absences), then a clear-cut distinction between the two types of seizures can be made. This is important not only for the correct choice of therapy (see below) but also for prognosis (see below).

The records illustrated in Figs 3 and 4 show unequivocal abnormalities. A great majority of records from those with epilepsy, however, show changes which are much less open to easy interpretation. There is a danger of over-reporting records, such that minor asymmetries in temporal rhythms are considered to be 'diagnostic'. It must be clearly understood that the EEG does not prove nor disprove the diagnosis of epilepsy. The record can be normal in someone with undoubted epilepsy. There is always the danger that a doctor, hovering on the brink of making a diagnosis of epilepsy, may be tipped into making a 'definite' diagnosis of epilepsy by the presence of marginal abnormalities on the EEG. If the record does show clear-cut paroxysmal activity, then this does lend considerable support to the diagnosis. If the record shows only a minor excess of slower rhythms, and the report reads that the record is 'compatible with epilepsy', then the doctor and his patient are no further forward in establishing any diagnosis.

There is seldom any indication for serial EEG records. Improvement in seizure control is not necessarily accompanied by improvement in any underlying abnormality in the EEG. Furthermore, abnormalities on the EEG in adults have proved to be no predictor of subsequent relapse on stopping anticonvulsant therapy, although in children relapse is somewhat more likely if the EEG is abnormal when the anticonvulsants are discontinued.

Whatever its limitations, the EEG is the generally available method of recording cerebral function. Studies using cyclotron-generated radioactive isotopes (position emission tomography, PET scanning) are of great theoretical interest in so far as they can provide images and direct measurements of local areas of abnormal cerebral metabolism. However, the lack of ready availability of this technique due to the need for a cyclotron is clearly going to confine the method to a few research centres.

In some centres, the technique is proving a useful adjunct to the localization of epileptic foci before surgery; a focus is usually hypermetabolic during a seizure, and hypometabolic in the inter-ictal state. More readily available is single photon emission computer tomography (SPECT scanning), which largely reflects geographical variations in blood flow; again hypometabolic areas can be identified.

At the present time, magnetic resonance imaging (MRI) is the best method of detecting abnormalities of cerebral structure. As scanners become more readily available, it will be difficult to decide which patients should be scanned, and which should not. Clearly, anyone with recent onset of seizures in association with physical signs warrants a scan, as the seizures must be a manifestation of some abnormality of cerebral structure. Also, a subject whose seizures seem difficult to control, or whose seizures change in pattern, should have a scan. As already mentioned, a large proportion of those with epilepsy have seizures arising from a structural abnormality of the brain.

MRI is clearly only available in more developed countries. CT scanning is more widely available, and will show many structural causes of epilepsy—tumours, infarcts, and so on. However, the sensitivity of MRI in detecting small lesions is so overwhelming that there can be no justification for preferring CT scanning if both techniques are available. This is particularly true in the investigation of complex partial seizures arising from a temporal lobe, where CT scanning may be confused by partial volume effects, some pixels containing a mixture of brain and bone of the floor of the middle fossa, or brain and cerebrospinal fluid.

Other radiological investigations are still occasionally employed in the management of epilepsy, but are now really irrelevant. Plain skull radiographs cannot give any information more relevant than that obtained by scanning. Air encephalography is now obsolete. Arteriography may be indicated if scanning has shown evidence of an angioma or a tumour for which operation is being considered.

It is unusual for any test on the blood to be helpful in elucidating the cause of epilepsy in adults. Occasionally, a blood alcohol estimation without warning (but of course with informed consent) may be fruitful, or a serological test for syphilis. However, abnormalities of glucose, calcium, magnesium, or amine metabolism in young children may be revealed by appropriate tests.

Lumbar puncture is only very rarely required in the investigation of epilepsy *per se*, although it may be needed if seizures occur on a background in which meningitis or some other acute illness is suspected.

Direct histological examination of cerebral tissue is not usually undertaken, although it may be justified in exceptional circumstances. However, biopsy of the skin abnormalities associated with tuberous sclerosis or neurofibromatosis may confirm a previously suspected diagnosis. Rectal biopsy may be useful, in so far as abnormal lipids may be deposited in the neurones in the submucosal plexus.

Treatment of epilepsy

PRESCRIPTION OF ANTIEPILEPTIC DRUGS

Seven useful principles of antiepileptic therapy are listed in Table 5. The first point is to reconsider the decision as to whether antiepileptic drugs should be given. It is not unusual to meet subjects with rare seizures occurring at intervals of 3 to 7 years, and in these circumstances many patients quite reasonably prefer to take no medication at all.

Table 5 *The seven principles of antiepileptic drug therapy*

1. Consider the decision: should antiepileptic drugs be given anyway
2. Choose a drug, considering the following factors:
   the seizure type(s)
   age
   the possibility of pregnancy
   interaction with other drugs
   price
3. Give only one drug, except in unusual circumstances
4. Begin the chosen drug in modest dosage
5. Give full information to the patient about:
   the names and alternative names of the drug supplied
   the initial dosage schedule with dates of planned changes in dosage
   the need for compliance with instructions
   adverse effects of the drugs
6. Monitor progress:
   inform subject of date and place of next review
   monitor seizure frequency
   monitor unwanted side-effects of drugs
   monitor blood level of drug
7. Determine policy for termination of treatment

Clearly, the likely social effects of subsequent seizures on employment and on eligibility to hold a driving licence may influence the subjects in this regard.

Most patients will go to their doctor after their first tonic–clonic seizure, and the doctor will then have to decide whether it is worth advising antiepileptic treatment at this stage. Many studies have now shown that most of those who have a first epileptic seizure will have a second one within a year or two (Fig. 7). The greatest risk is within the first few weeks, as indicated by the initial steep part of the curve in Fig. 7. This figure also indicates that drug treatment can reduce the risk, an observation subsequently confirmed by a randomized controlled trial in Italy. However, many patients prefer to take their chances without drugs. Most wish for treatment if a second or subsequent seizures would have serious effects upon their life and work.

CHOICE OF ANTIEPILEPTIC DRUG

The first factor to consider is the type of seizure. It is well worth categorizing the type as accurately as possible, using a combination of clinical history and EEG. Table 6 shows the antiepileptic drugs of choice

Fig. 7 Probability of seizure recurrence after a first epileptic seizure. (Data from the National General Practice Study of Epilepsy, reproduced by kind permission.)

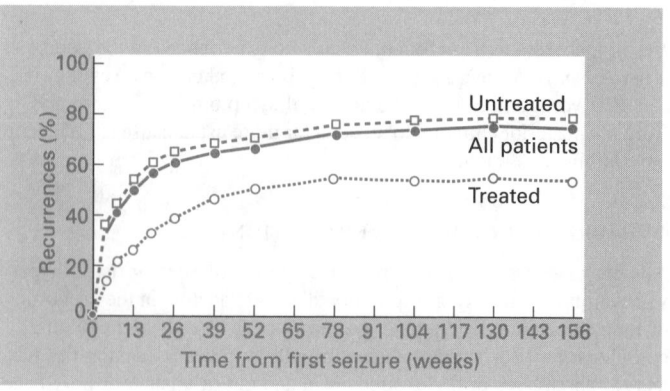

Table 6 *Antiepileptic drugs of choice for seizure types*

Seizure type	Anticonvulsant drugs of choice	Therapeutic levels in serum (μmol/l)[a]	Typical adult dose per day (mg)
Typical absences (petit mal)	Sodium valproate		1500
	(Ethosuximide	285–700	1000
	Clonazepam)		2
Myoclonic and akinetic seizures	Sodium valproate		1500
	(Nitrazepam		10
	Clonazepam)		2
Tonic–clonic seizures (grand mal) in association with typical absences (petit mal)	Sodium valproate		1500
	(Phenytoin	30–80	300
	Phenobarbitone)	65–170	90
Tonic–clonic seizures (grand mal) in association with partial seizures, or partial seizures alone	Carbamazepine	17–42	600
	Sodium valproate		300
	Phenytoin	30–80	
	Vigabatrin		3000
	Lamotrigine		300
	Gabapentin		1200
Infantile spasms	ACTH/prednisone		
	Nitrazepam		
	Vigabatrin		

[a]The level below which therapeutic effects are unlikely to occur and above which toxic effects are likely to occur. Measurement of benzodiazapines and valproate is probably not useful as there is no clear relationship between antiepileptic effect and blood levels. Serum monitoring for lamotrigine, vigabatrin, and gabapentin is not yet routinely available.

for seizures of different types, typical adult dosage per day, and therapeutic levels that represent a reasonable target.

FIRST-LINE DRUGS

Carbamazepine (Tegretol®)

This drug was introduced in the early 1960s and has gained increasingly wide acceptance for the treatment of partial seizures, and for tonic–clonic seizures with partial onset. It is reasonably free of side-effects. A few patients develop a skin rash within a few days of starting the drug. Very rare cases of marrow depression have occurred. Sedation is relatively slight. There is a roughly linear relationship between oral dose and serum level. This means that it is a comparatively simple matter to increase the oral dose based upon a knowledge of past serum levels, without significant danger of intoxication.

Sodium valproate (Epilim®, Depakine®)

This has become the drug of choice for primary generalized epilepsy (typical absences and tonic–clonic seizures associated with typical absences). It is probably as effective as carbamazepine and phenytoin in the management of partial seizures and secondarily generalized tonic–clonic seizures of partial onset.

The drug should be introduced, like all antiepileptic drugs, in a relatively low dosage and increased to a maximum of 2.5 g daily. Many patients are controlled on less than this. There is now good evidence that the clinical effect does not bear any relationship to the serum level, which in any event fluctuates markedly after the ingestion of each tablet. The reason for the disparity between pharmacokinetic and clinical observations has not been established, but suggestions include:

(1) slow penetration of valproic acid at the active site;
(2) an accumulation of an active metabolite with a longer half-life of elimination than valproic acid; and
(3) that the drug may exert its action indirectly via a series of biochemical processes, and accumulation or exhaustion of intermediate compounds will only gradually be affected.

Sodium valproate is usually relatively trouble-free, but a small number of patients develop an acute hepatitic insufficiency. It is impossible to predict who will develop this, but it is clear that the drug should be avoided in those with a history of liver disease, and the manufacturers recommend that tests of liver function should be carried out as the dosage is increased. Unwanted gain in weight may also occur. In high dosage the drug may cause tremor, but this is rapidly relieved by reducing the dose. Even at average doses, however, a significant side-effect is some thinning of the hair. Fortunately the hair regrows even if the drug is continued, but newly produced hair may be unusually curly.

Phenytoin (Epanutin®, Dilantin®)

This is a successful drug for the treatment of tonic–clonic seizures, and to a lesser extent for partial seizures. Because the enzymes responsible for hydroxylating phenytoin may become saturated, a small increment in phenytoin dosage may result in a large increase in serum level. For this reason it is relatively difficult to predict an appropriate increase in oral dosage towards a target serum level, although, now that experience has increased, this can usually be accomplished without major difficulty. Nomograms have been published to aid these calculations.

Phenytoin has significant drawbacks in young people. It causes hirsutism, coarsening of the facies, hypertrophy of the gums, and acne. More unusual side-effects result from the increased hepatic levels of hydroxylating enzymes induced by phenytoin. These enzymes not only hydroxylate phenytoin, but also steroid hormones, including vitamin D. Osteomalacia and rickets may result in rare circumstances, if the subject has a relatively low exposure to sunlight, or a pigmented skin. Oestrogens in contraceptive pills may also be hydroxylated in excess, resulting in inadequate contraceptive protection.

Skin rashes may also occur with phenytoin. Overdosage may result in marked sedation, but sometimes a cerebellar syndrome is seen before significant sedation occurs. Tremor, ataxia, and nystagmus are features of this. Another unusual manifestation of intoxication is chorea. Prolonged phenytoin medication may result in a neuropathy, a cerebellar degeneration, and induction of Dupuytren's contracture.

In spite of this rather alarming list, a great deal is known about this drug, serum levels are relatively easily measured, and many patients have their epilepsy successfully controlled by modest doses. However, most neurologists feel that phenytoin is not a drug of first choice for the management of epilepsy in young women, on account of the hirsutism, acne, and increased risk of pregnancy if oral contraception is used.

OTHER DRUGS

Phenobarbitone

Phenobarbitone is undoubtedly an effective antiepileptic drug, and may be worth a trial if other drugs have failed to control seizures. However, it is certainly not a drug of first choice as older people may become depressed and confused, and children excitable and irritable on this drug. Those in middle-age often state that they feel unpleasantly sedated even on moderate dosage.

Lamotrigine (Lamictal®)

When added on to other regimes where the older drugs are being used to maximum effect, this will result in a useful reduction in seizure frequency (> 50 per cent) in about 25 per cent of patients. However some patients, particularly those with frequent myoclonus, may deteriorate when they begin this drug. A suitable initial dose for an adult is 100 mg/day, increasing to 500 mg/day (less if the patient is on sodium valproate). Adverse events include skin eruptions, sedation, and unexpected exacerbation of seizures, particularly myoclonic seizures.

Vigabatrin (Sabril®)

This is another more recent drug which has a useful effect upon those with intractable epilepsy. About 50 per cent of patients will have their seizure frequency reduced by about 50 per cent. A usual maintenance dose is 1500 mg twice daily. Adverse effects include drowsiness, agitation, and sometimes confusion. Early studies showed that the brains of rats and dogs (but not monkeys) receiving this drug showed extensive intramyelinic oedema.

Gabapentin (Neurontin®)

This drug also has a useful effect on the frequency of partial seizures only partly responsive to the older drugs. Adverse effects include sedation, dizziness, tremor, and unsteadiness.

Primidone (Mysoline®)

Primidone is an effective antiepileptic. This is probably largely because it is metabolized to phenobarbitone, although another metabolite (phenyl-ethyl malonamide) also has antiepileptic activity. If primidone is chosen , it should be commenced at a low dosage, and increased gradually, or else sedation may be severe. Even a quarter of a 250 mg tablet twice a day is not too cautious a beginning for an adult.

Ethosuximide (Zarontin®, Emeside®)

Ethosuximide is a useful drug for absence epilepsy; it may precipitate tonic–clonic seizures in some. It has largely been replaced by sodium valproate.

Clobazam (Frisium®)

Clobazam is a benzodiazepine which has had some reported success in complex partial seizures. Unfortunately, any effect appears often to be relatively short-lived.

Clonazepam (Rivotril®)

Clonazepam is a benzodiazepine which is sometimes used in the management of severe childhood epilepsy, although it is unpleasantly sedative. It may be effective in myoclonic epilepsy when other drugs have failed.

Nitrazepam (Mogadon®)

This benzodiazepine may be effective in controlling myoclonic jerks if these are the only remaining epileptic manifestation of primary generalized epilepsy.

Diazepam (Valium®)

Although effective in the treatment of status epilepticus (see below), this is not an effective antiepileptic for daily use.

Corticosteroids

These are used only in the management of the West syndrome.

USING ANTIEPILEPTIC DRUGS

A greater knowledge of the pharmacokinetics of the various antiepileptic drugs has allowed more rational use. The half-lives of phenobarbitone, phenytoin, and primidone are such that the total daily requirements can be given in one dosage on going to bed at night. The half-life of carbamazepine is significantly shorter, so that the total daily dose should be divided into three, or even four, fractions. The midday dose is often forgotten by schoolchildren and working adults, so this in itself may be sufficient reason to use one of the longer-acting drugs. Sodium valproate has a short half-life as judged by serum levels, but, as already noted above, its biological half-life is much longer.

Table 4 shows some of the other factors, apart from seizure type, that should be considered when choosing an appropriate antiepileptic drug. Fortunately, price is not, in general, a significant problem with any of the older drugs, although of these sodium valproate is by far the most expensive. Even so, a year's treatment with 1500 mg/day will cost £170, compared to about £3 for phenytoin given at a dosage of 300 mg/day. The three recently introduced drugs (lamotrigine, vigabatrin, and gabapentin are substantially more expensive than the older drugs, but in responsive patients may produce a marked improvement in quality of life.

The possibility of pregnancy must certainly be considered when prescribing an antiepileptic drug. Sodium valproate causes teratogenic effects in animals, and valproate should be used only if the likely benefits in severe epilepsy resistant to other drugs outweigh the risks of teratogenicity. However, it has also been shown that epileptic women taking phenytoin are between two or three times more likely to have an abnormal baby than other women. The risk of congenital heart disease is increased by a factor of about four, and of harelip and cleft palate by a factor of about eight. The risks of fetal maldevelopment must be weighed against the risks to the fetus and to the mother of uncontrolled epilepsy. As any fetal damage due to drugs occurs in the first few weeks of pregnancy, perhaps even before the mother realizes that she is pregnant, the decision whether to stop drugs or not has, by default, often already been taken. In this case the mother might as well continue antiepileptic therapy in modest dosage, and protect herself and the baby against the risks of epilepsy.

There is no clear evidence that pregnancy itself increases the frequency of epileptic seizures, although the hormonal changes may have some influence on serum binding of antiepileptic drugs. Epilepsy is therefore virtually never an indicator for termination of pregnancy on medical grounds, although there may be social indications if it is considered that the mother has so many seizures that she is likely to have trouble in caring for the child.

Only one antiepileptic should be given initially, and that drug increased until appropriate levels are found in the serum, or until control of the seizures occurs. Only if this drug fails should another drug be tried, and that preferably in isolation rather than in combination. The interactions between antiepileptic drugs are complex. For example, the levels of carbamazepine are significantly reduced when phenytoin or phenobarbitone is added to a carbamazepine regime, but the ratio of metabolites to parent drug may be increased. There are also important interactions between antiepileptic drugs and other drugs, notably steroid hormones and anticoagulants.

Table 5 stresses the need to give full information to the patient about the names and alternative names of the drugs supplied, and the initial dosage given. Confusion so easily arises that it is well worthwhile taking the trouble to write out the schedule with the dates of changes planned, and to stress that seizure control is much more likely to occur if the patient understands and follows the instructions given. It is always difficult to know how much to say about the unwanted effects of the drugs. A full list of the adverse effects of phenytoin would be so alarming that many patients might refuse to take it if they did not realize how rare many of the adverse effects are. However, the principal effects must certainly be mentioned; in particular, women must be informed of the reduced protection provided by oral contraception while taking phenytoin. The drug induces hepatic hydroxylating enzymes, which also inactivate steroid hormones.

As so many patients with epilepsy are referred to hospital clinics, it is important that the patient, the neurologist, and the general practitioner all realize who is responsible for what aspect of treatment. Failure of compliance is often due to failure of communication, rather than to 'disobedience' of the patient. However, it is worth pointing out to the patient that there is no need to panic if one or two doses of the longer-acting antiepileptic drugs are omitted. The drug is so slowly metabolized that the omission can be easily made up the next day.

Although it is easy to accumulate a mass of redundant data, it is worthwhile asking the patient to record the frequency, type, and severity of his or her seizures, so that any improvement resulting from changes in medication can be observed. As seizures often appear to occur on a random basis, without any obvious precipitant, although sometimes in clusters, there are no adequate statistical methods of handling changes in seizure frequency. Probably the best available method is that of the cumulative sum technique.

One question that patients will undoubtedly want answered is when they will be able to stop treatment. Clearly this depends upon seizure control, but even if immediate control of seizures results, most clinicians will advise continuing antiepileptic medication for approximately 3 years thereafter. Most people whose seizures have stopped view cessation of therapy as the final hallmark of cure, and others are very reasonably concerned about the possible long-term effects of medication, although trouble on this score is unlikely. Unfortunately, even after this long period of freedom, some patients will relapse on continued treatment, but even more will have further seizures if the drugs are withdrawn, even if a period of 2 years is spent in tailing down the dosage. Absence seizures in childhood generally have a good prognosis if drugs are withdrawn in the late teens after a 3-year period of freedom from seizures. Conversely, those who have juvenile myoclonic epilepsy may continue to experience sporadic seizures, sometimes separated by many years, throughout life. In general, the longer the history of seizures and of treatment (with the exception of absence epilepsy), the occurrence of some seizures since starting treatment, and taking more than one antiepileptic drug when withdrawal commences are all unfavourable factors. Conversely, the length of the remission on drugs before withdrawal is attempted is a favourable factor. This evidence comes from a Medical Research Council randomized controlled trial organized by Chadwick. The role of the EEG in predicting relapse is more controversial, but, at least in childhood, an abnormal EEG before withdrawal appears to predict a higher probability of relapse. Most of those relapsing do so within the first year. Unfortunately, the occasional subject relapses shortly after the very last tablet was stopped, suggesting that his or her seizures were controlled by a tiny dose of drug that would not normally be considered adequate for the control of epilepsy.

There may be factors that encourage a patient to continue taking drugs, rather than to try withdrawing them. For example, a trial of managing without therapy may be disastrous if it results in the loss of a driving licence only recently regained. If a decision to withdraw drugs is made, then it seems good sense to reduce the drug gradually over a period of many months.

STATUS EPILEPTICUS

Occasionally seizures may follow each other without remission. If they are generalized tonic–clonic seizures, with major convulsions occurring in sequence without remission, the patient is at risk from death through cardiorespiratory failure. Immediate control of the seizures is necessary. Although diazepam (Valium®) is ineffective in the management of epilepsy on a day-to-day basis, it is a highly effective treatment for the management of status epilepticus. It, or the similar drugs lorazepam or clonazepam, should be given as a bolus intravenous injection as soon as it is clear that the subject is having continuous seizures without remission. A suitable dose of diazepam is 10 mg in 2 ml given over 2 to 5 min. If given more rapidly than this, respiratory depression may occur. Alternatively, a bolus of lorazepam 4 mg intravenously may be given. Prompt treatment in this way may abort what looked likely to be a troublesome episode of status, but if seizures occur again shortly after treatment then one or two further boluses may be given. If these fail, there are several alternative regimes. Phenytoin may be infused intravenously at a dose of 18 mg/kg at a rate of no more than 50 mg/min. This may be done even if the status occurs in a patient already on phenytoin therapy. Alternatively a diazepam, lorazepam, or chlormethiazole infusion may be used. It is certainly best to be familiar with one technique. However, if seizures continue, then the patient should be anaesthetized with propofol or thiopentone, and ventilated until 12 to 24 h after the last clinical or electrically recorded seizure, the dose then being tapered. A cerebral function monitor—a sort of compressed, slow-moving EEG—is extremely useful in the management of these patients.

Absence status or temporal lobe status may also occur, in which the presentation is not with convulsive seizures but with a confusional state, the origin of which may not be readily recognized. The principles of treatment are much the same as recorded above, and again EEG control is useful. Continual focal motor epilepsy is known as epilepsia partialis continua, and is often exceedingly difficult to control, continuing for many days without a significant disturbance of consciousness.

OTHER FORMS OF TREATMENT

There are other methods of treating epilepsy apart from the use of antiepileptic drugs. In cases in which precipitants, such as television, have been clearly been established, patients should be advised to avoid them. However, there are comparatively few occasions in which the precipitant is quite so clear-cut.

Children with epilepsy who are unresponsive to moderate doses of anticonvulsant drugs may benefit from a ketogenic diet. About 70 per cent of the total daily calorie requirement is given as medium-chain triglyceride oil, the remainder as protein and carbohydrate with vitamin supplements.

Surgery may occasionally benefit refractory cases of epilepsy. It is most usually undertaken for refractory temporal lobe epilepsy, and the current view is that more patients would benefit than are being referred for operation. Prolonged and repeated EEG recordings are necessary to show that the epileptogenic lesion is confined to one or other temporal lobe, as bilateral temporal lobectomy is not possible because of the severe amnesic syndrome that results. In the original operation, the anterior 5 cm of the temporal lobe was amputated as a single block containing the uncus, amygdala, and anterior hippocampus. Histological studies of such amputated blocks have furthered our understanding of the genesis of temporal lobe epilepsy. Mesial temporal sclerosis is the commonest lesion found, but occasionally small, previously unidentified tumours or hamartomas or aggregates of abnormal-looking giant neurones are found. The increasing recognition of such dysplastic areas, together with more refined preoperative and intraoperative electrophysiological recordings, has led surgeons to undertake more limited operations confined to the amygdala and hippocampus.

Focal epilepsy can arise from other parts of the brain, and occasionally cortical excision of an epileptogenic focus, such as an angioma or scar following a penetrating head injury, may result in control of previously refractory seizures.

Another surgical approach is to place stereotactic lesions in white matter which is believed to carry epileptic discharges from the diencephalon. Lesions have been placed with moderate success in the lateral thalamus or in the subthalamic field of Forel in an attempt to prevent generalization of paroxysmal discharges from focal lesions.

Studies have been carried out upon the effects of biofeedback in returning the EEG to normal. Although there is no doubt that subjects can learn to increase the amount of alpha rhythm generated, the question of whether they modify seizure frequency is much less certain. Although further research in this field is clearly justified, the present consensus is that EEG biofeedback is an unpredictable treatment which is costly in terms of time and equipment used.

Prognosis and complications of epilepsy

PROGNOSIS

Pessimism about the prognosis of epilepsy derives from hospital and special-clinic surveys. The prognosis of epilepsy as judged from the outcome in community-based samples is much more favourable. The top curve in Fig. 8 indicates the probability of completing a period of five consecutive years without seizures. For example, 6 years after diagnosis 42 per cent of subjects have been seizure-free for 5 years. It is necessary to talk in terms of 5-year remission rates rather than cure, because, analogous to the survival of cases of carcinoma of the breast, subsequent relapse many years after the onset is always possible. The curves in Fig. 8 flatten off with the passage of time. This means that if remission of seizures is not accomplished within the first few years of the onset, subsequent worthwhile remission becomes less likely. For example, although the net probability of achieving a 5-year remission within 10 years after diagnosis was 65 per cent, for patients not in remission 5 years after diagnosis the probability of achieving remission within the next 10 years was only 33 per cent, the same proportion as based on the older surveys of established epilepsy in hospital practice.

Some factors are known to be particularly unfavourable: the combination of complex partial seizures with tonic–clonic seizures, clustering of seizures, injury occurring during tonic–clonic seizures, associated physical signs, and associated learning difficulties are all factors known to be associated with failure to remit.

Fig. 8 Remission of epilepsy. Top curve: probability of completing a period of 5 consecutive years without seizure. For example, 6 years after diagnosis 42 per cent of subjects have been seizure-free for 5 years. Middle curve: the probability of being in remission, at any time, for at least the past 5 years. The difference between the top and middle curve is due to relapse after achievement of a 5-year remission. For example, at 20 years after diagnosis 70 per cent are currently free from seizures and have been for 5 years and a further 6 per cent have had at least one seizure-free period of at least 5 years duration, but have subsequently relapsed. Lowest curve: the probability of being free of seizures for at least 5 years whilst not taking anticonvulsant drugs. In summary, 20 years after diagnosis 50 per cent have been free from seizures without anticonvulsant drugs for at least 5 years. A further 20 per cent continue to take anticonvulsant medication and are also free from seizures. Seizures continue, in spite of medication, in 30 per cent. (Redrawn from Anneger, J.F., Hauser, W.H., and Elveback, L.R. (1979). *Epilepsia*, **29**, 729.)

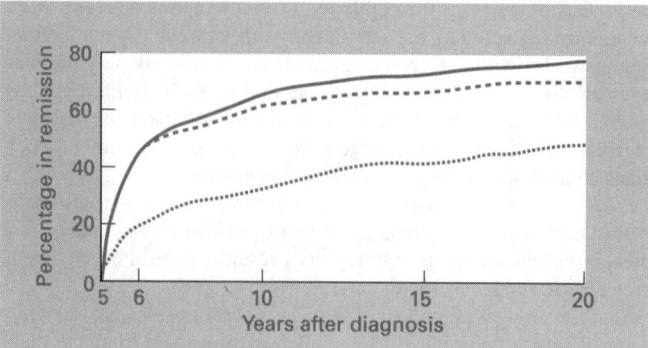

COMPLICATIONS

Clearly there are circumstances in which epilepsy is based upon an underlying and progressive disorder, which gradually assumes more importance than the epilepsy itself. However, there are certain complications which seem to be associated with epilepsy *per se*. First amongst these must be considered the psychiatric disorders associated with epilepsy. People with frequent seizures have a significant reduction in their chances in life. Furthermore, they have to act as their own public relations officers in deciding how much about their epilepsy to reveal, and to whom. Limitations in employment, and usually in driving, reduce earning power, social status, and long-term financial security. Personal relationships with the opposite sex may be spoilt by the fact of epilepsy. Not surprisingly, therefore, many people with epilepsy become unhappy and depressed. Suicide is approximately five times more common in those with epilepsy than in the general population.

If the cause of the epilepsy is antenatal, natal, or early postnatal damage, there may be associated psychological defects in learning, or the epilepsy may be associated with hyperkinesis. A psychotic illness with symptoms similar to those of paranoid schizophrenia may arise in those with temporal lobe epilepsy. Some patients with temporal lobe epilepsy complain of loss of libido and impotence, which may respond to treatment with anticonvulsant drugs.

There is no good evidence that continuing seizures result in a dementing illness. However, prolonged and repeated episodes of status epilepticus may result in cerebral damage occurring through repeated episodes of hypoxia.

Social aspects of epilepsy

Children with epilepsy should, as far as possible, be educated alongside their siblings in normal schools. Clearly, if there are associated difficulties in learning, this would not be appropriate and the child would be better placed at a special school. Occasionally, children with frequent seizures, but with normal intelligence, will do best at a special school for epileptic children, where all members of the staff are trained in, and competent to cope with, the various manifestations of seizures.

Restrictions on activities of children with epilepsy should be few. It is clearly not sensible to allow them to swim alone, nor to climb ropes in the school gym. If bathing alone at home, the depth of the water should be limited. No danger will result from playing the usual sports, such as football or similar games.

Restrictions on adults with epilepsy should also be few. Mothers with epilepsy who have very young children should not bath infants alone, in case they have a seizure during bathtime and the baby drowns.

The question of eligibility to hold a driving licence is particularly important. Obviously there needs to be a balance between protecting other road users from the effects of drivers who may lose control if they have a seizure, and allowing people whose epilepsy is controlled to gain from the advantages that driving confers. Regulations differ in different countries, but in the United Kingdom a period free from all seizures for 1 year is required, or have had an epileptic attack whilst asleep more than 3 years before the date when the licence is granted and shall have had attacks only whilst asleep between the date of that attack and the date when the license is granted. Stricter regulations in the United Kingdom apply to Public Service and Heavy Goods Vehicle Drivers.

Problems concerning employment will certainly arise. Obviously it is not safe to work with heavy moving machinery or at heights. Unfortunately, problems more often arise because of the inability of employers to realize that the vast majority of people with epilepsy have only occasional seizures, and then not often at work. Nevertheless employers may not be willing to accept the 'responsibility' of employing someone with epilepsy, even in a straightforward commercial or office job. For this reason many people with reasonably well-controlled seizures conceal their epilepsy from their employers. In the United Kingdom, someone with epilepsy may consider becoming registered as a disabled person, in order to benefit from the provisions of the Disabled Persons (Employment) Acts of 1944 and 1958, by which employers of more than 20 people in the United Kingdom have a statutory requirement to employ a quota of 3 per cent of their employees from those on the Disabled Persons Register.

ACKNOWLEDGEMENT

The section on the inheritance of epilepsy was kindly provided by Dr Mark Gardiner.

REFERENCES

Anderson, V.E., Hausner, W.A., Leppik, I.E., Noebels, J.L, and Rich, S.S. (1991). *Genetic strategies in epilepsy research.* Elsevier, Amsterdam.

Annegers, J.F., Hauser, W.A., and Elveback, L.R. (1979). Remission of seizures and relapse in patients with epilepsy *Epilepsia* **20**, 729–37.

Goodridge, D.M.G. and Shorvon, S.D. (1983). Epileptic seizures in a population of 6,000. II Treatment and prognosis. *British Medical Journal* **287**, 645–7.

Hart, Y.M., Sander, J.W.A.S., Johnson, A.L., and Shorvon S.D. (1990). National General Practice Study of Epilepsy: recurrence after a first seizure. *Lancet* **336**, 1271–4.

Hauser, W.A. and Kurland, L.T. (1975). The epidemiology of epilepsy in Rochester, Minnesota, 1935 through 1967. *Epilepsia* **16**, 1–66.

Hauser, W.A., Annegers, J.F., and Anderson, V.E. (1983). Epidemiology and the genetics of epilepsy. In *Epilepsy* (ed. A.A. Ward *et al.*). Raven Press, New York.

Hauser, W.A., Annegers, J.F., and Kirkland, L.T. (1991). Prevalence of epilepsy in Rochester, Minnesota: 1940–1980. *Epilepsia* **32**, 429–45.

Hauser, W.A., Annegers, J.F., and Kirkland, L.T. (1993). Incidence of epilepsy and unprovoked seizures in Rochester, Minnesota: 1935–1986. *Epilepsia* **34**, 453–68.

Hopkins, A., Shorvon, S.D. and Cascino, G. (1995). *Epilepsy.* Chapman and Hall, London.

Hopkins, A. and Scambler, G. (1977). How doctors deal with epilepsy. *Lancet* **i**, 183–6.

Jennett, W.B. (1975). *Epilepsy after non-missile head injuries.* Heinemann, London.

Sander, J.W.A.S., Hart, Y.M., Johnson, A.L., and Shorvon, S.D. (1990). National General Practice Study of Epilepsy: newly diagnosed epileptic seizures in a general population. *Lancet* **336**, 1267–71.

The First Seizure Trial Group. (1993). Randomised clinical trial on the efficacy of antiepileptic drugs in reducing the risk of relapse after a first unprovoked tonic-clonic seizure. *Neurology,* **43**, 478–83.

24.4.2 Syncope

L. D. BLUMHARDT

DEFINITION

Syncope is a brief loss of consciousness which results from an acute reduction in cerebral blood flow (from the Greek, *synkoptein*, to cut or break). It is the commonest cause of recurrent episodes of disturbed consciousness.

PATHOPHYSIOLOGY

Although there is a seemingly endless list of causes and predisposing factors (Table 1), the sequence of reflex events which, once triggered, result in syncope, is relatively constant. Loss of consciousness (probably due ultimately to hindbrain ischaemia) results from a sudden reduction in cerebral perfusion as the compensatory mechanisms fail, due either to a reflex reduction of venous return to the heart, or to the inadequate

Table 1 *Causes of syncope and predisposing/trigger factors*

Common faints (Vasovagal syncope)	Prolonged standing
	Sudden postural change
	Warm, stuffy environment
	Emotion
	Pain
	Extreme fatigue
	Alcohol
	Hunger
Postural hypotension	Elderly
	Convalescence
	Drugs
	Orthostatic hypotension
Valsalva mechanism	Wind instruments
	Defaecation
	Weight-lifting
Micturition syncope	Nocturnal micturition
	Alcohol
Cough syncope	Chronic obstructive airways disease
	Smoking
Carotid sinus disease	Atherosclerosis
Cardiac syncope arrhythmias	Sinus node disease (sick sinus syndrome)
	Tachyarrhythmias
	Bradyarrhythmias
structural	Hypertrophic cardiomyopathy
	Valvular stenosis
	Pericarditis (constrictive)
	Atrial myxoma
Anoxic ('vagal') seizures (non-epileptic)	Pain
	Emotion
Hypovolaemia	Haemorrhage
	Protein loss
	Acute sodium/water loss
	Addison's disease
	Burns
Areflexic (paralytic) postural hypotension	Diabetes
	Polyneuropathy
	Tabes dorsalis
	Shy–Drager syndrome
	Drugs
	Quadriplegia
Metabolic	Hypoxia
	Hypoglycaemia
Hyperventilation	Anxiety
Vertigo	Vestibular disease

response of the heart when increased demands require an increased cardiac output.

In the common faint (vasovagal syncope), the reduced venous return is caused mainly by a sudden reflex reduction in the resistance of peripheral blood vessels with pooling, particularly in the abdomen and lower limbs. There is generally some associated, but less important slowing of heart rate (hence the term vasovagal which was originally coined by Sir Thomas Lewis), but in some individuals, an exaggerated reflex bradycardia or even sinus arrest due to vagal hyperactivity may be the dominant factor in reducing cardiac output (cardio-inhibitory syncope). This is a particular feature of loss of consciousness arising from painful pressure on the eyeball (oculocardiac reflex). In cough syncope, the high intrathoracic pressures generated by violent coughing (which may exceed 250 mmHg) are transmitted to the extrathoracic baroreceptors, triggering a reflex fall in cardiac output. Similar events underlie syncope associated with the Valsalva manoeuvre and possibly also contribute to the rare defaecation syncope. The proposed mechanisms responsible for carotid sinus syncope include hypersensitivity of the baroreceptors in a diseased carotid sinus and possibly contributions from an exaggerated vagal response or oversensitivity of the sinus node. In syncopes associated with swallowing, a vagally induced bradycardia may be triggered by stretching of the oesophagus (swallow syncope), or by very cold stimuli ('ice-cream syncope'). In other subjects, critical cardiac slowing can be provoked by rectal stretching (e.g. proctoscopy, prostatic massage). In micturition syncope the mechanism in susceptible subjects is thought to be a combination of the sudden loss of the vasopressor effect of a full bladder, postural hypotension, and high nocturnal vagal tone (NB, not increased intrathoracic pressure caused by straining).

CLINICAL FEATURES

Many subjects experience a characteristic sequence of premonitory symptoms (presyncope). A typical history may include 'dizziness', sweating, nausea, sensations of warmth or cold, and bilateral blurring of vision. There may also be tinnitus, receding sounds, weakness, increased salivation, urgency of micturition, vomiting, or diarrhoea. These symptoms may be proffered in almost any combination and any, or all, may be missing. It is important to distinguish symptoms of dizziness, giddiness, 'muzziness', or lightheadedness from vertigo (rotational element) which does not occur in syncope. An eye witness may report on the sweating, restlessness, excessive yawning, slow sighing respiration, and facial pallor. In some individuals, the loss of consciousness is abrupt and without warning, whereas in others presyncope may vary from a very brief period of a few seconds to a slow development over several minutes. With sufficient warning, some subjects may be able to prevent the syncope by lying down and elevating their legs, but many are either unaware of this possibility, or are unable to invoke it in time.

If no preventative action is taken, syncope may then follow, with a sudden loss of consciousness and a collapse with loss of muscular tone. Depending on the circumstances of the syncope, injuries may occur. If the bladder is full, there may be incontinence. During the attack the tone is limp or floppy (no stiffness, rigidity, or tongue biting) and the patient is usually motionless. In some subjects there may be some flickering of the eyelids and perhaps an occasional irregular anoxic twitch or jerk of the limbs may be seen. The pulse is often difficult to feel, but may be noted to be thready, rapid, or slow. If the anoxia is profound, the patient may vomit or be doubly incontinent. If a recumbent posture does not result from the fall, a secondary anoxic seizure may occur (convulsive syncope) and is commonly mistaken for epilepsy. Unless there is a secondary head injury (complicated syncope), or a secondary tonic-clonic seizure, there is usually rapid recovery of awareness within a minute or two, with no subsequent confusion or disorientation. Sweating and profound waxy pallor due to intense vasoconstriction in the skin may persist well after recovery. If the patient gets up too quickly, a further episode of syncope may occur.

MAIN VARIANTS OF SYNCOPE

Vasovagal syncope

The common faint usually occurs for the first time in childhood or adolescence and recurs in well-recognized situations (for example, with venepuncture, dental procedures, at the sight of blood, sudden emotions, acute pain, prolonged standing in assembly or church or stuffy crowded areas). There is almost invariably a postural element, faints occurring when standing or sitting and rarely when lying (pregnancy). Convalescence, sleep deprivation, hypoglycaemia, anaemia, postural hypotension, drugs, blood loss, cardiac or vascular disease, may all predispose the susceptible subject to fainting. Although there is often a recrudescence later in life, caution should be exercised in diagnosing simple faints when they occur de novo in the elderly, as syncope may be the presentation of a cardiac arrhythmia (check for a prior history of fainting in typical situations).

Susceptibility to fainting is widely variable, and some individuals will experience syncope only in association with particular triggers. The diagnosis is usually easy when intense pain such as abdominal colic, glossopharyngeal neuralgia, migraine, or diagnostic manipulations such as oesophagoscopy, bronchoscopy, venepuncture, or rectal examination provoke attacks. It may be more difficult when a severe episode of vertigo due to vestibular disease triggers a syncopal event.

Micturition syncope

The occurrence at night, during or shortly after micturition, is highly characteristic of this condition which, contrary to a surprisingly widespread misconception, is not a complication of prostatism, occurring mainly in healthy men (peak incidence in third and fourth decades). Some of these individuals also suffer from vasovagal syncope. Elderly men with postural hypotension and vascular disease and, rarely, young women may be afflicted by this condition. The treatment is to advise sitting down to micturate at night and to delay standing up after micturating, although these precautions are not always effective.

Cough syncope

This condition is usually associated with chronic obstructive airways disease and smoking. A severe bout, or even a very forceful single cough, is followed by a collapse with brief loss of consciousness. There may be jerks or twitches during cough syncope and the differentiation from epilepsy is important. The eye-witness account is often critical. Treatment is directed towards the chest disease and education of the patient and relatives into the mechanism and its possible avoidance. Posterior fossa lesions with medullary compression can present in a similar way.

Carotid sinus syncope

This is a rare but important cause of syncope because it is potentially curable. The diagnosis should be considered in patients whose blackouts are associated with head-turning, a tight collar, or even the pressure and posture associated with shaving, particularly in elderly patients with atherosclerotic vascular disease, hypertension, or diabetes. It may also occur in patients with infiltrating cervical tumours or after cervical irradiation. If suspected, gentle sequential unilateral carotid sinus massage carried out with electrocardiogram (ECG) control for 6 s per side may result in a conduction block or cardiac arrest. Most would accept an asystole of more than 3 s in this situation, but the diagnostic criteria are somewhat controversial. Denervation of the carotid sinus or cardiac pacing is usually effective.

Cardiac syncopes

These can be divided into syncopes caused by outflow obstruction from the left ventricle, and syncopes due to disorders of cardiac rhythm. An inability to increase the cardiac output as required, for example, during excercise or sexual activity, may cause syncope in hypertrophic cardiomyopathy, aortic stenosis, restrictive pericarditis, left ventricular insufficiency, or atrial myxoma. However, it is more common, even when structural heart disease exists, for the loss of consciousness to be caused by an arrhythmia. Syncope may be sudden with no warning (for example, with heart block or sinus arrest) or there may dizziness, palpitations, dyspnoea, or chest pain (for example, with tachyarrhythmias). The symptoms may closely mimic those of complex partial seizures which can themselves generate secondary cardiac arrhythmias. After transient cardiac arrest there may be marked facial flushing as the cardiac output is restored. The clinical presentation of a patient, often elderly, with a slow pulse and syncopal attacks has long been recognized (Stokes–Adams syndrome) and may be due to atrioventricular block, ventricular tachycardia, fibrillation, or standstill. Similar attacks occur with sinus node disease (sick sinus or tachycardia–bradycardia syndrome) and with the long QT syndrome (see Section 15).

Reflex ('vagal') anoxic seizures

This particular form of reflex cardiac arrhythmia can be regarded as one end of the spectrum of fainting disorders. The condition is frequently misdiagnosed as epilepsy. In its most common form, a child (the condition can persist into early adult life) has faints which are triggered by minor trauma such as a painful knock in the playground, but there is complicating rigidity, pallor, twitching, and sometimes incontinence. There is usually a rapid recovery with little if any confusion. Simultaneous ECG and electroencephalogram (EEG) recording shows that the mechanism is a cardiac asystole followed by generalized high-amplitude slow activity in the EEG (secondary anoxic features) without epileptic phenomena. Similar attacks can be provoked by ocular pressure. Treatment, if necessary, is with long-acting atropine preparations.

Postural hypotension

Elderly or convalescent patients may be subject to falls of blood pressure on postural change, particularly after prolonged sitting or lying. Many different drugs, including diuretics, antihypertensives, L-dopa, major tranquillizers, antidepressants, and calcium antagonists, may play an important or primary role. Areflexic or 'paralytic' postural hypotension and syncope may complicate, or even be the presenting symptoms, of serious diseases affecting the autonomic nervous system, such as idiopathic orthostatic hypotension, extrapyramidal diseases, tabes dorsalis, polyneuropathies, and high spinal cord lesions. Some otherwise healthy individuals are peculiarly sensitive to mild postural hypotension. A lordotic posture may contribute to syncope, for example, in subjects standing at attention on a parade ground, and the inflicted is often a young male. Loss of consciousness can be abrupt or with only a very brief warning of loss of vision or lightheadedness.

Diagnostic approach

The key to the diagnosis of syncope often lies in the history of the immediate circumstances of the collapse and the events leading up to it. A past or family history of similar events, perhaps in more obvious circumstances, will often provide the diagnosis. Is there a factor favouring syncope, such as the previous initiation of drugs or a prolonged erect posture or postural change? Was there a Valsalva factor present (for example, the playing of a musical instrument) or an emotional or painful episode? Were there existing background factors favouring syncope, such as convalescence, tiredness, or the presence of cardiac disease, anaemia, or blood loss? The history of the attack needs to be built up in considerable detail and an eye-witness account obtained of the events immediately before, during, and after the loss of consciousness. Was the patient's muscle tone appropriately limp? There should be no tongue-biting, rigidity, or rhythmic tonic-clonic movements suggesting seizure activity. If a seizure has occurred despite appropriate circumstances for a syncope, a careful history will often establish that the posture of the patient after the fall did not allow restoration of adequate cerebral perfusion (for example, the subject was propped up in a confined space) so that a secondary anoxic seizure (convulsive syncope) is the correct diagnosis, rather than epilepsy. The presence of injuries (apart from tongue-biting) do not particularly favour a diagnosis of epilepsy, but confusion is unlikely after syncope unless there was a complicating head injury.

Young men who collapse in the bathroom or on their way back to the bedroom at night are at risk of misdiagnosis, particularly if a secondary convulsive syncope has occurred. These circumstances should alert the clinician to the possibility of micturition syncope. With cough syncope the patient is often peculiarly 'amnesic' for the attacks which he does not associate with his otherwise frequent cough, but an eye-witness account will clarify the sequence of events and the correct diagnosis. Associated medical disorders such as chronic bronchitis (cough syncope), cardiac disease (Stokes–Adams attacks), or atherosclerosis (carotid sinus disease) may provide the main diagnostic clue to the aetiology.

MANAGEMENT

Simple faints require counselling and education for patients and relatives into the avoidance of predisposing situations and triggers, and into the measures to be taken during a presyncopal episode. Apart from a blood count if anaemia is suspected, or a blood sugar estimation if hypoglycaemia is a possibility, patients seldom require investigation unless there are other abnormalities suggested by the history and examination. Investigating every patient with syncope is expensive and produces a low yield of positive results. Syncopal episodes ocurring *de novo* in adults without obvious trigger factors or associated with exercise may require cardiological investigation with ECG, Holter monitoring, treadmill tests, and, perhaps, sophisticated measures such as intracardiac conduction studies. Structural heart disease or heart failure should be excluded. Where epilepsy is a possibility, an EEG and perhaps simultaneous ECG and EEG monitoring may be indicated.

REFERENCES

deBono, D.P., Warlow, C.P., and Hyman, N.M. (1982). Cardiac rhythm abnormalities in patients presenting with transient non-focal neurological syndromes. *British Medical Journal* **284**, 1437–9.

Eberhart, C. and Morgan, J.W. (1960). Micturition syncope. *Journal of the American Medical Association* **174**, 2076–7.

Jaeger, F.J., Maloney, J.D., and Fouad-Tarazi, F.M. (1990). Newer aspects in the diagnosis and management of syncope. In *Cardiology update*, (ed. E. Rappaport). Elsevier, New York.

Kapoor, W.N., Karpf, M., Maher, Y., Miller, R.A., and Levey, G.S. (1982). Syncope of unknown origin. The need for a more effective approach to its diagnostic evaluation. *Journal of the American Medical Association* **247**, 2687–91.

Kapoor, W.N., Peterson, J., and Karpf, M. (1986). Defecation syncope. *Archives of Internal Medicine* **146**, 2377–9.

Leatham, A. (1982). Carotid sinus syncope. *British Heart Journal* **47**, 409–10.

Levin, B. and Posner, J.B. (1982). Swallow syncope: report of a case and review of the literature. *Neurology* **22**, 1086–93.

Lewis, T. (1932). Vaso-vagal syncope and the carotid sinus mechanism. *British Medical Journal* **1**, 873–6.

Lipsitz, L.A. (1983). Syncope in the elderly. *Annals of Internal Medicine* **99**, 92–105.

Proudfit, W.L. and Forteza, M.E. (1959). Micturition syndrome. *New England Journal of Medicine* **260**, 228–31.

Sharpey-Schafer, E.P. (1953). The mechanism of syncope after coughing. *British Medical Journal* **ii**, 860–3.

Sharpey-Schafer, E.P. (1956). Syncope. *British Medical Journal* **1**, 506–9.

Stephenson, J.P.B. (1978). Reflex anoxic seizures (''white breath holding''): non-epileptic vagal attacks. *Archives of Disease in Childhood* **43**, 193–200.

Sugrue, D.D., Wood, D.L., and McGoon, M.D. (1984). Carotid sinus hypersensitivity and syncope. *Mayo Clinic Proceedings* **59**, 637–40.

24.4.3 Narcolepsy and related sleep disorders

C. D. MARSDEN

DEFINITION

Described by Gelineau in 1880, narcolepsy is defined as 'a syndrome of unknown origin that is characterized by abnormal sleep tendencies, including excessive daytime sleepiness and often disturbed nocturnal sleep, and pathological manifestations of REM (rapid eye movements) sleep. The REM sleep abnormalities include sleep-onset REM periods and the dissociated REM sleep inhibitory processes, cataplexy, and sleep paralysis. Excessive daytime sleepiness, cataplexy, and less often sleep paralysis and hypnagogic hallucinations are the major symptoms of the disease'. (Definition drafted by the First International Symposium on Narcolepsy 1975.)

AETIOLOGY

The cause of narcolepsy is unknown. Symptomatic narcolepsy is very rare; occasional cases have been attributed to encephalitis lethargica or multiple sclerosis. Idiopathic narcolepsy occurs in between 20 and 50 per 100 000 of the population. Between 10 and 40 per cent of patients with narcolepsy give a history of a similar disorder amongst other family members, and about a quarter describe a parent as affected. The most likely mode of inheritance is autosomal dominant with variable penetrance. Virtually all patients with narcolepsy express the major histocompatibility antigens HLA-DR2 and DQw1, compared with about a quarter of normal controls. This confirms the genetic origin of this disease and links it with the short arm of chromosome 6.

No convincing pathological or biochemical abnormality has been found as yet in patients suffering from narcolepsy, but neurophysiological studies have revealed a disturbance of sleep mechanisms. Normal sleep begins with a change in the electroencephalogram (EEG) from the fast activity characteristic of wakefulness to increasingly slower frequencies. After about 90 min or so of early sleep, short (10–15 min) periods occur in which REM take place, accompanied by cessation of bodily movement, loss of all muscle tone, and a tendency to dream. Between three and six periods of REM sleep occur during the average night, each period becoming progressively longer, so that the total duration of REM sleep corresponds to about 20 to 25 per cent of total sleep time. Light sleep in patients with narcolepsy very commonly commences with a period of REM sleep and this abnormality is believed to be responsible for sleep paralysis, due to inhibition of movement and loss of muscle tone, and hypnagogic hallucinations. Daytime sleep attacks also commonly commence with a period of REM activity, and the sudden falling attacks characteristic of cataplexy may also be associated with bursts of REM activity. These neurophysiological abnormalities point towards an abnormal dissociation between the brain-stem mechanisms responsible for maintaining wakefulness due to activation of the cerebral cortex, and other parallel brain-stem mechanisms responsible for generating REM activity and maintaining muscle tone. Why there should be disordered control of REM sleep in narcolepsy is not known, but animal experiments suggest that sleep mechanisms are under the control of brain-stem reticular formation pathways utilizing monoaminergic neurotransmitters. This may explain why drugs influencing cerebral monoamines, such as amphetamines and tricyclic antidepressants, are used to treat the disorder.

CLINICAL SYMPTOMS

The narcoleptic tetrad consists of excessive daytime sleepiness with sleep attacks (narcolepsy), episodes of sudden falling associated with emotion (cataplexy), sleep paralysis, and hypnagogic hallucinations. Virtually every patient develops excessive daytime sleepiness and sleep attacks, about two-thirds experience cataplexy, about a third suffer hypnagogic hallucinations, and about a sixth have sleep paralysis. Approximately one-third of patients experience all four symptoms.

Excessive daytime sleepiness and sleep attacks

These are the hallmark of narcolepsy. On average, patients will report between two and six attacks of falling asleep each day, but some may experience up to 20 or 30 episodes. Each attack lasts, on average, around 10 or 30 min, but sometimes they may be as brief as a minute or as long as 2 h. Attacks are common after heavy meals, alcohol, and monotony, and in warm rooms or while travelling or driving. Of course, the normal person may fall asleep in these circumstances, but the hallmark of narcolepsy is the bizarreness of the situations in which the patient may drop off to sleep. Thus, narcoleptics may fall asleep over their meals, dropping into the soup, may nod off while standing, during intercourse, and

even while driving the car or flying an aeroplane. Patients describe such episodes as irresistible and are quite overwhelmed by their sleepiness. Many have to give up going out in the evening to friends, and find it pointless to watch a film or television. In females, the severity of narcolepsy may be linked to the menstrual cycle. Night-time sleep frequently is disturbed in narcolepsy. Apart from the problems of sleep paralysis and hypnagogic hallucinations, excessive sleep during the day frequently leads to shorter deep sleep at night, although the total time spent in REM sleep is usually normal. Overall, most narcoleptics do not sleep excessively throughout the whole 24-h period.

Cataplexy

This describes an abrupt but reversible paralysis into which a narcoleptic patient may be precipitated by emotional events. The severity of cataplectic attacks can vary from total paralysis with collapse to the ground, to lesser degrees in which the jaw sags and the head drops. Consciousness is preserved throughout the attack, but the patient may see double. Attacks usually last for a few seconds, but may be prolonged for as long as 10 min. They occur more frequently at times of stress, fatigue, or after heavy meals. Laughter and anger are the commonest triggers, but elation or any other intense emotion may be sufficient to precipitate an episode. A stimulus may come from something heard or seen, or may arise while listening to music, reading a book, or even just remembering a happy or emotional event. The excitement of a successful athletic activity, such as a fine stroke at cricket or tennis, or even the thrill of sexual intercourse, may prompt an episode. The frequency of cataplectic attacks is very variable, but some patients may have many attacks each day. Cataplexy tends to improve in adult life.

Sleep paralysis

In sleep paralysis the patient becomes totally unable to perform a voluntary movement despite remaining alert and aware. It may occur either on falling asleep (hypnagogic) or on awakening (hypnapomic). During an episode the patient is powerless to move, speak or even open his eyes, although he is fully aware of his condition and can recall it completely afterwards. Naturally, such episodes may cause extreme terror particularly if they are accompanied by vivid and frightening hallucinations. The patient may feel as though he is dying, and since he cannot move, is terrified of being buried alive. An episode rarely lasts more than 10 min, and usually much less. Episodes tend to be infrequent and to improve with age.

Hypnagogic hallucinations

These almost always involve visions, which may consist merely of simple coloured forms, still or in motion, or may take the shape of animals or persons. Frightening or erotic scenes are quite common. Noises, voices, or melodies occur less frequently. Psychic hallucinations, taking the form of an impression that somebody is present, can be particularly distressing. The narcoleptic frequently experiences these hallucinations as vivid and real, making them all the more terrifying.

While sleep attacks, cataplexy, sleep paralysis, and hypnagogic hallucinations form the core of the narcoleptic tetrad, these patients also experience other symptoms. Particularly distressing are periods of automatic behaviour, lapses of memory, and 'blackouts'. In such episodes, for which the patient has little or no memory, he may continue activity which does not require extensive skill, but may make frequent mistakes. Many patients have experienced such episodes while driving, and most have developed automatic behaviour in social situations. Simple questions are answered appropriately, but if the conversation requires more thought, the patient may respond with inappropriate or meaningless sentences. Such episodes may occur daily and cause great difficulties. In almost every respect they represent the automatic behaviour with amnesia characteristic of nocturnal sleepwalking. In view of the many and bizarre symptoms encountered in narcolepsy, a proportion of patients may become considerably disturbed by their illness. A secondary reactive depression or anxiety state is not uncommon, and may add to the symptomatology. In evaluating psychiatric symptoms, the effects of drug treatment must also be taken into account.

COURSE

Narcolepsy beings in adolescence or in early adulthood, and is lifelong; remissions are very uncommon. Around 60 per cent of cases commence between 15 and 30 years of age, but a few start before the age of 10 years or up to the age of about 50 years. Sleep attacks are the first symptom in 90 per cent of cases, but a few patients begin with cataplexy or hypnagogic hallucinations. Once established, excessive daytime sleepiness and sleep attacks never cease completely during the patient's lifetime, but cataplexy tends to become less of a problem as the patient becomes older.

DIFFERENTIAL DIAGNOSIS

The excessive daytime sleepiness and sleep attacks characteristic of narcolepsy are difficult, on occasion, to distinguish from the range of normal. The best index of pathological sleepiness is an unambiguous history of inappropriate daytime sleep episodes. The bizarre situations in which narcoleptics fall asleep are diagnostic, and most patients will give a history of blackouts and automatic behaviour if questioned carefully. If there is any doubt, a history of cataplexy settles the issue.

Problems in diagnosis arise in separating narcolepsy and its associated features from epilepsy, in distinguishing cataplexy from other causes of drop attacks, and in separating excessive daytime sleepiness and sleep attacks from other causes of pathological sleep.

Sleep attacks may be mistaken for minor fits, hypnagogic hallucinations and night terrors for nocturnal seizures or temporal lobe partial complex seizures, and cataplectic drop attacks for akinetic seizures. Periods of automatism in narcolepsy also may be indistinguishable from post-epileptic automatic behaviour; in both situations the patient is in a state of being able to move around in a relatively normal manner, but is at the same time lacking in understanding or purpose, and subsequently cannot clearly recall what occurred during that period. A similar state is characteristic of transient global amnesia, sometimes due to ischaemia in posterior cerebral arterial territories.

Many structural lesions of the central nervous system may cause pathological drowsiness, but this seldom resembles narcolepsy and the other features of this illness do not occur. Drugs are not known to cause true narcolepsy. Structural lesions in the hypothalamus may cause periodic somnolence and hormonal disturbances, but they do not cause classical narcolepsy.

Narcolepsy may be distinguished from the other conditions causing excessive daytime sleepiness (hypersomnia) by its characteristically short duration (1–30 min), irresistible sleep attacks, and by the presence of cataplexy, sleep paralysis, and hypnagogic hallucinations, which do not occur in the other hypersomniac states. The last cause longer (hours to days or even weeks) periods of sleep without the other features of the narcoleptic tetrad.

Symptomatic hypersomnia

This occurs in a range of organic brain diseases, including encephalitis, toxic or metabolic encephalopathies, tumour, vascular or traumatic brain damage. Sleep, as distinct from coma from which the patient cannot be awakened, frequently is more-or-less continuous in these conditions.

Functional hypersomnias

These are periodic. The sleep attacks may last one to several hours, with attacks occurring most days (short cycle), or may last a day to several weeks, with attacks occurring at intervals of a month to several years (long cycle). Patients with either short-cycle or long-cycle hypersomnias are normal between attacks. Other functional hypersomnias are associated with respiratory disorders during sleep, so-called sleep apnoea. Four short-cycle periodic functional hypersomnias are recognized.

Idiopathic hypersomnia is characterized by excessive prolonged night-time sleep, extreme difficulty in awakening, signs of 'sleep drunkenness' on awakening, and prolonged periods of sleep during the day. Such patients may sleep 15 or even 20 h a day if not disturbed. The condition is hereditary in as many as one-third to one-half of patients.

Neurotic hypersomnia may occur in some hysterics or 'faint hearted' neuraesthenic individuals, and a complaint of excessive tiredness is common in depression

Nocturnal myoclonus syndrome is characterized by short bouts of muscle jerking at night, which disturb sleep. This is accompanied by extreme restlessness of the legs, and is often associated with daytime sleepiness. A nocturnal dose of clonazepam may help.

Sleep apnoea is characterized by cessation of breathing during sleep, which causes extreme restlessness with frequent respiratory pauses and snoring during night sleep, and by daytime drowsiness and irritability (see Section 17). Such a syndrome may occur:

(1) in those with severe obesity, chronic alveolar hypoventilation, right heart failure, and polycythaemia (pickwickian syndrome) (see Chapter 22.4.14);

(2) in those with upper respiratory tract obstruction due, for example, to prognathism, acromegaly, goitre, tonsillar and adenoidal hypertrophy, or laryngeal stenosis;

(3) in those with muscle or neuropathic disease affecting respiratory muscles (myopathies, myotonic dystrophy, motor neurone disease);

(4) in those with brain-stem disease (tumour, stroke, encephalitis) which cause failure of respiratory drive (central sleep apnoea). Developmental failure of brain-stem respiratory mechanisms can occur ('Ondine's curse').

The diagnosis is established by polygraphic recording of sleep which shows periods (at least 30 of 10 or more seconds duration in 7 h of sleep) of apnoea, associated with a fall in arterial oxygen saturation. Such patients are chronically tired during the day, complain of headache and irritability, and have excessive daytime sleep and automatic behaviour. Untreated it can lead to pulmonary and systemic hypertension, cardiac arrhythmias, and sudden death. Weight loss, surgical correction, and nocturnal continuous transnasal positive airways pressure may help. This condition is considered further in Section 15. Tracheostomy may be required to restore normal sleep.

Long-cycle periodic functional hypersomnia is rare, and may or may not be accompanied by excessive eating (Kleine–Levin syndrome). Such patients, most commonly young adult males, begin to overeat prodigiously (bulimia), become irritable, restless, and hypersexual, and then fall into a deep sleep for a day to a few weeks, during which time they awake to attend to toilet needs and can be aroused to eat. On awakening they are amnesic for that period, but rapidly return to normal behaviour and sleep patterns, and remain free of attacks for months or years. Another cause of recurrent hypersomnia at intervals longer than a day is periodic disruption of the normal sleep–wake cycle, as may occur in air crews and shift workers.

TREATMENT

Narcoleptic sleep attacks and excessive daytime sleepiness are, in many cases, greatly improved by the regular use of amphetamines (5–40 mg daily), or mazindol (2–8 mg daily). Despite the possible misuse and unwanted effects of such stimulants on chronic use, at present they are the only effective drugs available. In fact, although some patients develop tolerance, and require progressively higher dosage, addiction in narcoleptics is very uncommon. These drugs do not affect cataplexy, but tricyclic antidepressants such as chlormipramine (10–150 mg nightly) may abolish both cataplexy and sleep paralysis. Chlormipramine can be used safely with amphetamines or other stimulants, but blood pressure should be monitored.

REFERENCES

Guilleminault, C. (1987). Obstructive sleep apnea syndrome in children. In *Sleep and its disorders in children*, (ed. C. Guilleminault), pp. 213–24. Raven Press, New York.

Guilleminault, C. and Dement, W.C. (ed.) (1978). *Sleep apnea syndromes*. Alan Liss, New York.

Guilleminault, C., Dement, W.C., and Passouant, P. (ed.) (1976). *Narcolepsy*. Spectrum Publications, New York.

Kales, A. and Kales, J.D. (1984). *Evaluation and treatment of insomnia*. Oxford University Press.

Moore-Ede, M.C., Czeisler, C.A., and Richardson, G.S. (1983). Circadian time-keeping in health and disease. *New England Journal of Medicine* **309**, 469–76.

Parkes, J.D. (1981). Daytime drowsiness. *Lancet* **ii**, 1213.

Parkes, J.D. (1985). *Sleep and its disorders*. W.B. Saunders, Philadelphia.

Parkes, J.D. (1986). The parasomnias. *Lancet* **2**, 1021–4.

24.4.4 Coma

M. J. G. HARRISON

The emergency measures to be investigated when a patient presents in coma are considered in detail in Section 16. This section describes the subsequent neurological assessment and how a diagnosis is arrived at.

Consciousness is maintained by activity of the reticular formation of the brain-stem (Fig. 1). It follows that coma may be due to the global suppression of neuronal function or to the presence of a focal lesion in the brain-stem. The latter may be an intrinsic lesion such as an infarct, or may be secondary to the compressive effects of an enlarging mass (Fig. 2). After the essential first steps in the care of the unconscious patient—maintenance of an airway, correction of fluid balance problems, assessment of life-threatening injuries or cardiopulmonary problems (see Section 16)—the history-taking and examination must be geared to the task of distinguishing global and 'metabolic' causes of coma from those of brain-stem origin. It is particularly important to detect those whose declining conscious level is due to secondary compression of the brain-stem, since they may need neurosurgical relief of the expanding mass in the supratentorial compartment.

HISTORY

The history may provide important clues. A fit may have been witnessed and the coma prove to be only that seen transiently after a grand mal attack, or the patient may have fallen to the ground holding his head as though struck down by severe headache, suggesting subarachnoid haemorrhage. An empty pill bottle or a history of depression may suggest a drug overdose, and a history of diabetes prompts consideration of ketotic or hypoglycaemic coma. Vague mental symptoms and headaches over the previous weeks should raise suspicions of a tumour that is now causing coma by brain-stem compression. A telephone call to relatives and medical attendants can be highly revealing and cost effective.

CLINICAL ASSESSMENT

General examination

This may provide useful clues to the aetiology of coma. Fever suggests meningitis or metabolic coma complicating infection, hypothermia, hypothyroidism, or primary hypothermic coma. Hypertension may be due to cerebral causes or hypertensive encephalopathy may explain clouded consciousness. Hypotension can be a clue to septicaemia or to hypovolaemia or loss of left ventricular function. Cyanosis, pallor, or the cherry-red colour of carboxyhaemoglobin will suggest metabolic problems, and trauma may be obvious from bruises and lacerations, a black eye, or blood behind the ear-drum.

Level of coma

Documentation of the level of coma is important since progressive deterioration suggests brain-stem compression. By contrast, most patients with metabolic causes of coma or an intrinsic brain-stem lesion have a stable or improving level of awareness. To detect subtle changes in the level of consciousness requires careful description of the patient's response to specific stimuli. Words such as 'semicoma' are to be avoided as they are inexact and mean different things to different observers. The coma scale of Jennett and Teasdale is in general use and overcomes these difficulties (Table 1). It records the best level of response of eyelids, speech, and limb movement to verbal request, shouts, and painful stimuli. Deterioration can be detected readily, even when different observers are responsible for the sequential examination. For example, a patient whose eyes opened when he was spoken to and replied in a confused way has obviously deteriorated when his eyes only open to a painful stimulus, and the verbal response consists only of a groan.

Focal signs

The presence of a hemiparesis suggests the possibility of a cerebral hemisphere mass lesion as the cause of the coma. Its presence must be inferred in the unconscious patient from observation of asymmetries; of the face during expiration, of spontaneous limb movements or tone, and of responses to painful stimuli. If a decorticate or decerebrate posture develops symmetrically in response to painful stimuli, no localizing significance is implied. If, however, the responses are asymmetrical, for example flexion of one arm and extension of the other, then the latter

Fig. 1 Schematic representation of the role of reticular formation in the brain-stem in maintenance of an aroused state of the cerebral hemispheres.

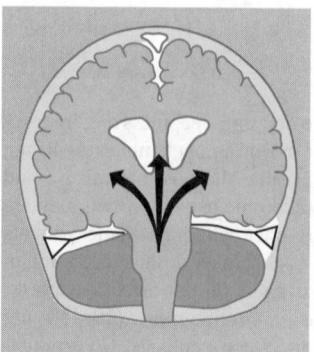

Fig. 2 Illustration of herniation of the temporal lobe (small arrow) and displacement of the upper brain-stem (large arrow) resulting from an intracranial mass whether extra or intracerebral.

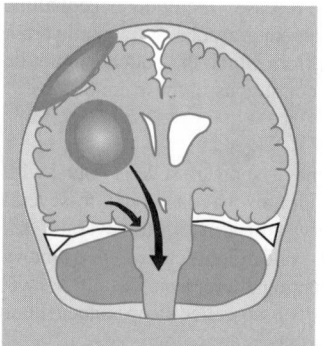

Table 1 *Glasgow coma scale*

Eyes open	Spontaneously	4
	To speech	3
	To pain	2
	Never	1
Best verbal response	Orientated	5
	Confused	4
	Inappropriate words	3
	Incomprehensible sounds	2
	None	1
Best motor response	Obeys commands	6
	Localizes pain	5
	Withdrawal	4
	Flexion to pain	3
	Extension to pain	2
	None	1

Table 2 *Diagnosis of coma*

Diagnostic category	Diagnostic features
A. 'Metabolic'	Normal pupil responses
	Normal or absent eye movements depending on depth of coma
	Suppressed Cheyne–Stokes, or ketotic respiration
	Symmetrical limb signs usually hypotonic
B. Brain-stem: intrinsic	From outset: Abnormal pupil responses
	Abnormal eye movements
	Abnormal respiratory pattern
	Cranial nerve signs
	Bilateral long tract signs
C. Brain-stem: compression	Papilloedema
	Hemiparesis
	Progressive: Loss of pupillary responses
	Loss of eye movements
	Abnormal respiratory pattern
and/or	Long-tract signs
	Appearance of 3rd nerve palsy

side showing the more primitive reaction is 'hemiparetic'. Rarely, asymmetries result from hypoglycaemia, hyponatraemia, or hepatic failure. Most will prove to reflect structural lesions in the cerebral hemisphere, or brain-stem.

Eye signs (see Section 16)

A key part of the examination concerns the assessment of the pupillary responses and eye movements. If these brain-stem functions are normal, the cause of coma is likely to be metabolic or due to a diffuse disease. Structural damage to the brain-stem, on the other hand, whether local or secondarily provoked, manifests itself by loss of pupil reflexes and abnormalities of eye movement. Herniation of the temporal lobe over the free edge of the tentorial opening causes compression of the third cranial nerve so a unilaterally dilated fixed pupil is indicative of the presence of a compressing mass lesion. Central herniation of the brainstem through the tentorial hiatus reflects a pressure gradient between a supratentorial mass-containing compartment and the posterior fossa. Such a pressure gradient is dramatically and dangerously increased by ill-advised lumbar puncture. Central herniation causes progressive brain-stem compression with sequential loss of pupil responses, and abnormalities of eye movements passing from a stage of readily elicitable symmetrical horizontal eye movements to a stage of dysconjugate eye movements or unilateral paralysis of gaze, and finally to total immobility of the eyes. Eye movements in the unconscious patient are tested by counter rolling of the head or by cold-water syringing of the external auditory meati to cause a unilateral suppression of tonic vestibular input to brain-stem gaze centres. Patients in deep metabolic coma may show total loss of eye movement but will retain the pupil reflexes. With central herniation pupil reflexes are lost as the eye movements become abnormal or are lost. Anoxia may cause large, fixed pupils with coma due to diffuse neuronal damage.

Respiration

Little has been said about respiratory patterns since these are of limited diagnostic value. Deep breathing suggests acidosis, as in diabetic coma, regular but shallow breathing suggests depression by drug overdose, and Cheyne–Stokes breathing has no diagnostic significance. All other departures from a normal pattern, if not due to respiratory disease, suggest some brain-stem compromise.

DIAGNOSIS OF TYPE OF COMA AND CAUSE

The distinction between the three broad categories of coma can thus be made by bedside observations (Table 2). Associated clinical features, and special investigations such as electroencephalography (EEG) and computed tomography (CT) scans are then needed to make specific diagnoses (Table 3). If the coma appears to be metabolic in type but no

systemic disorder or drug overdose has been diagnosed, the cerebrospinal fluid should be examined. Both meningitis and subarachnoid haemorrhage may cause coma, and neck stiffness is often missing when conscious level is depressed. (If there are focal signs, or if papilloedema is detected, a lumbar puncture is contraindicated until after CT, magnetic resonance imaging (MRI), or EEG, and angiography have excluded a mass lesion). Other investigations that may be needed when the diagnosis is in doubt include arterial blood gases, urea, electrolytes, liver function tests, osmolarity, cortisol, and thyroid studies. The blood sugar should always be measured as delayed correction of hypoglycaemia can cause severe permanent neurological disability. The EEG can be helpful in detecting encephalitis, especially that due to *Herpes hominis*, some kinds of metabolic coma such as that due to hepatic encephalopathy, and status epilepticus.

If a focal lesion is suspected, a CT scan or MRI is needed to see if there is a surgically accessible problem such as a subdural haematoma or meningioma. In the posterior fossa, cerebellar haemorrhage may cause a rapidly evolving coma due to local pontine compression. This may cause unilateral ataxia at an early stage but may have to be recognized by the presence of a unilateral paralysis of horizontal eye movement in the absence of a matching hemiparesis, in a patient whose conscious level is declining. Surgery is indicated for all but the smallest haematomas. Pontine haemorrhage causes coma with loss of horizontal eye movements and pin-point pupils that may still just react to a bright light. There are bilateral long-tract signs and the patients often develop hyperpyrexia. Surgery is rarely possible. Massive cerebral haemorrhage causing coma is also usually inoperable.

RELATED CONDITIONS

Confusional state

Patients suffering from an acute confusional state have a short attention span and are distractable. They often appear perplexed or bewildered and have difficulty in following questions and commands. Their mem-

Table 3 *Causes of coma*

Metabolic	Drug overdose	Hepatic failure
	Ischaemia/hypoxia	Hyponatraemia
	Diabetic	Hypercalcaemia
	Hypoglycaemia	Sepsis
	Cardiac failure	Alcohol
	Respiratory failure	Wernicke's encephalopathy
	Renal failure	Carbon monoxide poisoning
Diffuse intracranial disease	Head injury	
	Meningitis	
	Subarachnoid haemorrhage	
	Encephalitis	
	Epilepsy	
	Hypertensive encephalopathy	
	Cerebral malaria	
Cerebral hemisphere lesions (with brain-stem compression)	Cerebral infarct	
	Cerebral haemorrhage	
	Subdural haematoma	
	Extradural haematoma	
	Abscess	
	Tumour	
Brain-stem lesion	Brain-stem infarct	
	Brain-stem haemorrhage	
	Tumour/abscess	
	Cerebellar infarct/haemorrhage	

ory is poor and they have some problems with orientation. They tend to misinterpret what they see. The acute onset of such a state with some variable drowsiness and inattentiveness is usually due to toxic metabolic conditions, and the diagnosis depends on defining the underlying physical condition. Purely psychiatric causes of confusion, and dementia in its early stages, do not affect the level of awareness, so identification of drowsiness is all-important in the distinction.

Delirium

This, too, is usually due to toxic/metabolic problems such as alcohol or barbiturate withdrawal and hepatic failure, or encephalitis. It may be seen during recovery from head injury. There is disorientation, confusion, and reduced attention as in confusion but the picture is more florid with agitation, irritability, and fear, and the disorientation is more profound. Complex delusions are often seen with prominent visual hallucinations (auditory hallucinations are more often seen in psychoses).

Locked-in syndrome

If patients have a paralysis of vocalization and speech, and of movement of the face and limbs, they may appear unconscious when in fact they are not. They may be able to feel pain. Often the patients have had damage to the ventral pons or medulla, for example due to multiple sclerosis or a stroke. Communications can usually be established. They can blink or perhaps make some vertical eye movement which can be coded as 'yes' and 'no' in order that they may signal their wishes and converse in a limited way. A similar incapacity may occur with myasthenia gravis or the Guillain–Barré syndrome but its evolution does not give rise to the same problems of knowing that the patient is alert and of undiminished intellect. An EEG can help to show an alert state, reactive to external stimuli.

Akinetic mutism

This superficially resembles the locked-in state with a patient who is mute and immobile, although apparently alert. No communication can be established, however, and the patient is doubly incontinent. The usual cause is bilateral frontal lobe damage or diffuse anoxic damage, or a small lesion in the reticular formation.

Psychogenic unresponsiveness

Mutism and a lack of response to the environment may also be seen in primary psychiatric conditions such as catatonia, depression, and hysteria. In these situations the pupil responses are normal, and caloric stimulation of the ears provokes nystagmus in the normal subject. The EEG shows a responsive wakeful pattern. (By contrast, patients with akinetic mutism of organic origin have an EEG dominated by slow wave activity.)

Chronic vegetative state (see Chapter 24.4.5)

Prolonged survival after severe head injury or anoxic insult may lead to the development of this state. There is no evidence of recovery of higher function but cycles of wakefulness appear. Some patients are akinetic but some are not. Their eyes may open to verbal stimuli. Spontaneous respiration and maintenance of blood pressure ensures continuation of life, until death from complications such as bronchopneumonia. At autopsy the brain-stem is relatively spared, the forebrain showing extensive damage. The cortex usually shows laminar necrosis.

PREDICTING OUTCOME IN NON-TRAUMATIC COMA

The prognosos is poor if the coma persists for more than 6 h. Recovery after non-traumatic coma is unlikely if pupil responses and cranial reflexes are still lost at 24 h, if the best motor response at 3 days is worse than withdrawal to pain, and if spontaneous roving eye movements do not return by 7 days. The severity of coma as judged by the Glasgow coma scale is predictive as is aetiology. Drug-induced coma has the best outlook, anoxia, ischaemia, and stroke the worst, with other metabolic causes occupying an intermediate position. Unfortunately, in individual cases prediction is less than precise and caution has to be exercised.

REFERENCES

Bates, D. (1991). Defining prognosis in medical coma. *Journal of Neurology Neurosurgery and Psychiatry* **54**, 569–71.
Bates, D. (1993). The management of medical coma. *Journal of Neurology, Neurosurgery and Psychiatry*, **56**, 589–98.

Plum, F. and Posner, J.B. (1980). *Diagnosis of stupor and coma*, (3rd edn). F.A. Davis, Philadelphia.

Sacco, R. L., Van Goot, R., Mohr, J. P., and Hauser, W. A. (1990). Non-traumatic coma. **47**, 1181–4.

Shewman, D.A. and De Giorgio, C.M. (1989). Early prognosis in anoxic coma. *Neurologic Clinics* **7**, 823–43.

24.4.5 Brain death and the vegetative state

B. JENNETT

Cardiopulmonary resuscitation and intensive care are now commonplace in acute hospitals in developed countries and when used to avert a temporary threat to life they can result in complete recovery and long survival. But the price paid for these successes can be to prolong the process of dying from a few minutes to many days in a large number of other patients; and to leave a few to survive for months or years in the vegetative state, which some have described as a living death. This price can be too high unless there is wider recognition of when it is appropriate to initiate, to continue, or to withdraw technological interventions that will not save worthwhile life. The problem is not a small one. The American hospital that pioneered 'Do not resuscitate' orders found 10 years later that no less than a third of patients who died there had had one or more attempts at cardiopulmonary resuscitation. In the United Kingdom, where intensive care beds are much fewer than in the United States, there are estimated to be at least 2000 cases of brain death each year; there must be many more that have prolonged attempts at resuscitation without being formally recognized as brain dead. There are likely to be more patients in these states in the future unless clear rules are established for withholding resuscitation from certain patients and in others for abandoning it once it is recognized that brain failure is irreversible. Fortunately there is no longer any dearth of data from which to derive reliable criteria for recognizing brain death and the vegetative state. Society is now sending clear signals to its doctors in both the United Kingdom and the United States that it expects them to try to avoid undignified persistence with technology when no benefit can come from it. We may not be able to anticipate the occurrence of these artefacts of nature that are the byproducts of technological innovation; but we can at least take steps to see that they do not persist any longer than necessary once they have been reliably recognized.

Much of the controversy about brain death, now largely resolved, arose from misconceptions about the nature of death. Only when concepts of death are clarified can criteria consonant with them be accepted with confidence. The first concept is that death is a process and not an event, that organs cease to function in several sequences, and that what is regarded as the time of death is arbitrary rather than actual. Death is when the body as a whole ceases irreversibly to function, but this does not imply that all organs (let alone all cells) have already 'died'. Consider the common sequences by which the process of death can occur. Most often the heart fails first and within minutes hypoxia causes brain-stem failure; the respiratory drive then stops and breathing ceases. Much less often respiratory failure is primary; the brain-stem then fails but the heart can go on beating for 15 to 30 min. Although resuscitation from cardiac or respiratory arrest may be completely successful, it is sometimes too late to save the cerebral cortex, which is more vulnerable to hypoxia than the brain-stem; the patient then survives in a vegetative state. This may also result from severe head injury without cardiorespiratory arrest having occurred. Sometimes resuscitation is too late for even the brain-stem to survive, yet the heart continues to beat, because the myocardium is more resistant to hypoxia than the brain-stem. Much more often this combination of a dead brain, mechanically maintained ventilation, and a spontaneously beating heart (the syndrome of brain

death) results from a primary intracranial catastrophe. Breathing stops from brain-stem dysfunction but mechanical ventilation is established in the hope that the intracranial crises will be reversible. On occasions it is and prompt respiratory resuscitation is then rightly recognized as having been lifesaving. It is when the brain failure cannot be reversed that the outcome of these worthy efforts is brain death.

BRAIN DEATH

The crucial lesion is irreversible loss of function of the brain-stem with subsequent lack of downward drive to maintain respiration, and of upward activation of the cerebral cortex by the ascending reticular pathways. Except when systemic hypoxia has been the initial insult the cerebral cortex may be structurally intact and islands of electrical activity may be detected on EEG. However, this makes no difference to the inevitability of spontaneous cardiac asystole within a few days of death of the brain-stem. Early definitions of brain death (for example, in the Harvard criteria of 1968) implied that the whole nervous system was dead with a flat EEG and absence of all motor activity. But the spinal cord is more resistant to hypoxia and is unaffected by intracranial catastrophes that wreck that brain-stem—so spinal reflexes often persist after brain death. Indeed, reflex limb movements frequently become more active if ventilation is maintained for more than 24 h after the brain-stem has ceased to function. It has been suggested that uncertainties might be dispelled if the nomenclature were changed to brain-stem death; but the term brain death is difficult to displace after a quarter of a century.

What matters for practical purposes is that if the brain-stem is dead, the brain is dead. And if the brain is dead, the person is dead. As long ago as 1970 the State of Kansas enacted the first brain death law, and Finland led the Europeans a year later. By 1983 all but 16 American States had such a law and six of the exceptions had legal precedents for accepting death of the brain as indicating legal death. Britain is less liable to look to lawyers for leadership in such matters and it was the Medical Royal Colleges' Memorandum in 1979 that stated that death should be declared when brain death is diagnosed, not at the later time when the heart stops. This removes any ambiguity about the action of the doctor who discontinues ventilation after diagnosing brain death. He is simply stopping doing something useless to someone who is already dead; that is different from withdrawing support from someone who is hopelessly ill so as to allow death to occur.

Causes and frequency of brain death

Data about the epidemiology of brain death have come from studies of organ donation, although this applies to only a subset of such patients.

About half the cases of brain death in the United Kingdom follow head injury, respiratory failure occurring after hours or days of intensive treatment. This may be due to brain-stem distortion from a compressing intracranial haematoma that can be surgically evacuated, but more often it results from a combination of brain swelling and reduced cerebral perfusion. About a third of cases of brain death are associated with spontaneous intracranial haemorrhage, either ruptured aneurysm in a younger person or hypertensive haemorrhage in older patients. Brain death is particularly likely when a recurrent subarachnoid haemorrhage occurs in a patient who is waiting in hospital for investigation or for surgery, for it is then that a ventilator is at hand. The remaining cases of brain death follow failure to control a variety of intracranial conditions (e.g. tumour or infection), or from cardiopulmonary resuscitation necessitated by extracranial events. Systematic study of brain death in the United Kingdom has revealed that three-quarters of the cases occur in non-teaching hospitals that do not have a neurosurgical unit. The criteria for diagnosing brain death therefore need to be widely applicable; they should not depend on neurosurgeons or neurologists, nor on investigations that are available only in specialist regional centres.

Criteria for diagnosis

Undue emphasis on the final confirmation that no residual brain function persists has sometimes distracted attention from the stepwise process of diagnosing brain death, in which these tests are only the last stage. Indeed the most important step is the first one, satisfying the preconditions. These require that the patient be apnoeic and in deep coma due to irreversible structural damage to the brain, and this implies that reversible causes of brain-stem depression have been adequately excluded. It is usually obvious that structural brain damage has occurred—there has been a recent head injury or a classical history of spontaneous intracranial haemorrhage or of some less acute intracranial condition. Establishing the irreversibility of such brain damage depends on failure to improve with the passage of time and after the correction of factors such as systemic hypotension and hypoxia, and raised intracranial pressure. Other factors that can cause temporary absence of brain-stem function are depressant drugs (including alcohol), neuromuscular relaxant drugs, and physiological factors such as hypothermia and gross metabolic imbalance. The first two of these may complicate cases of structural brain damage but it is only in a minority of cases that serious doubts arise about confusing factors. For example, when a patient is found unconscious and no satisfactory history can be discovered it may be necessary to undertake formal screening for drugs; also to delay the diagnosis of brain death until sufficient time has passed for the exclusion of all temporary causes of brain-stem depression.

The tests applied to indicate lack of brain-stem function are simple to carry out and to interpret. There should be no response of the pupils to light, of the eyelids to corneal touching, of the facial muscles to pain, of the throat muscles to movement of the endotracheal tube, or of the eyes to syringing of each external auditory meatus with ice-cold water (the caloric or vestibulo-ocular reflex). Only when there has been a negative response to all of these is the final crucial test applied—to verify that there is still apnoea. There must be no respiratory movement after disconnection from the ventilator for long enough to allow the $PaCO_2$ to rise to 60 mmHg, oxygenation being maintained by delivering 6 l/min of oxygen down the endotracheal tube. It is usual to require that all these tests are repeated to exclude any possibility of observer error; the interval before repeating the two tests need be no more than half an hour, provided that the preconditions were fully satisfied before undertaking tests for the first time.

The validity of these criteria has now been tested in thousands of cases. It was several years before clinicians were confident enough to disconnect the ventilator once brain death had been diagnosed and experience from many places is that the heart always stops within 14 days, usually within 2 to 4 days. However, the concept of brain death is still not readily grasped even by all doctors and nurses, only a tiny minority of whom ever encounter it. Moreover, the notion that the beat of the heart is the signal of life, which took root when the stethoscope was invented 150 years ago, dies hard. Taken together with a certain public disquiet about organ transplantation, particularly of the heart, this led during the 1970s to the suspicion that doctors might sometimes be tempted to diagnose brain death prematurely, in their eagerness to secure donor organs. The fact is that few brain-death cases lead to organ donation, as transplant surgeons frequently complain. If transplantation were superseded as a means of treating organ failure there would still be decisions to make about discontinuing ventilators in brain-dead patients in every acute hospital in the land. However, during the 1970s sporadic reports appeared in the lay press of patients who had recovered after supposedly having been brain dead, and this reached a climax on BBC television in 1980. In the event this led to a reaffirmation of the brain-death criteria that the Royal Colleges had originally published in 1976 and to clarification of the situation in a second edition of the Code of Practice of the Health Departments in the United Kingdom. Since then there has been much wider acceptance of the concept of brain death and of the propriety of making an early diagnosis and of then withdrawing ventilation.

None the less, it remains important to be sensitive to the misunderstandings that can arise in what is still a delicate area of decision-making in medicine. Perhaps the commonest situation is when a family is told soon after an acute episode of brain damage that the outcome is 'almost hopeless'. Resuscitation of such patients is sometimes successful, otherwise it would not be undertaken; but by that time relatives may themselves have raised the matter of organ donation. Rather than replying that such an offer is welcome but premature, doctors or nurses may be drawn into discussing the procedures that would be involved if brain death did occur. It is easy to see how it may then appear as though 'they nearly took his kidneys'. The same can happen when depressant drugs are not at first suspected but with the passage of time brain-stem depression proves to have been temporary. Occasionally doctors unfamiliar with brain death consider it as a possible explanation for other unresponsive states, such as the vegetative state. But the activity of the brainstem should rule out any serious question of confusion. Sometimes a brain-dead patient is suspected by naive bystanders of being still alive, because of the persistence of spinal reflexes—a misunderstanding to anticipate by ensuring that all witnesses of this phenomenon have it explained to them.

The best safeguard against such embarrassment is a well-written set of guidelines in the hands of experienced doctors—two of whom should always be involved in the diagnosis. Experience is more important in assessing the preconditions than in applying the brain-stem tests. Time is the other safeguard—time to satisfy the preconditions, to establish the diagnosis, and to ensure that the state is not reversible. This time varies widely according to the circumstances; at least 6 h is needed to satisfy the preconditions and 12 to 24 h is more usual. Least time is required when a patient with a known lesion develops a crisis (for example, recurrent subarachnoid haemorrhage after angiography has already disclosed the lesion); most time is needed for the patient found in coma with no history but a suspicion of drug ingestion.

In the past some clinicians have sought diagnostic support from laboratory investigations designed to show either arrest of the cerebral circulation or the absence of cerebral electrical activity. Circulatory tests are complex and not without risk, whereas EEG is more often available and involves no hazard. But critics maintain that EEG is irrelevant and potentially misleading because it reflects activity in the cerebral cortex and not in the brain-stem, and because securing an isoelectric recording can be technically difficult in the electronically active environment of an intensive care unit. Criteria used in the United Kingdom for the diagnosis of brain death specifically state that EEG is not required, whereas more recent American recommendations emphasize that its use there is optional. However, in 1984 two-thirds of American neurosurgeons and neurologists questioned were still using EEG as a criterion. In contrast to the United Kingdom, where national guidelines have been enforced since 1976, a third of these American doctors in 1984 did not support the case for national standards, although guidelines had been published in 1981. The current state of practice and the law in regard to brain death worldwide has been reviewed by Pallis (1990). Guidelines for determining brain death in children after the first week of life were published by a task force in the United States in 1987. It recommended that under the age of 1 year confirmatory laboratory tests should be used. These cautioned against diagnosing brain death in the first 7 days of life and the Royal Colleges in the United Kingdom declared in 1988 that organs should not be taken in the first 7 days of life.

Action after diagnosis of brain death

There is now wide acceptance of the concept that when the brain is dead the person is dead. It can help to clarify the situation for nurses and relatives if a death certificate can be issued before discontinuing the ventilator. Some doctors are still reluctant to make this diagnosis explicitly and then to act logically and legally by disconnecting the ventilator. The useless ventilation of brain-dead patients wastes resources for intensive care, deprives the patient of death with dignity, needlessly prolongs the distress of relatives, and is bad for the morale of nursing staff. Moreover, the opportunity to offer organs for transplantation is lost because gradual circulatory failure makes such organs useless for donation. It would be of benefit to bereaved families, nurses, and other patients if doctors shared a greater readiness to recognize brain death and then to act appropriately.

THE PERSISTENT VEGETATIVE STATE

This term was introduced in 1972 by Jennett and Plum to describe the clinical condition resulting from loss of function in the cerebral cortex with a functioning brain-stem. Because of the latter, vegetative patients breathe spontaneously and are not ventilator-dependent; another difference from brain death is that they can survive for many years, if adequately fed and nursed. The commonest cause of vegetative survival after acute brain damage is severe head injury, the mechanism being severe diffuse axonal injury severing the subcortical connections over a wide area. In some traumatic cases, however, secondary hypoxic brain damage is a contributing factor. Most non-traumatic cases result from severe hypoxia/ischaemia of the brain following cardiac arrest, near drowning, or strangulation, while a few result from severe hypoglycaemia in diabetics. At autopsy after these metabolic insults neocortical necrosis is found with widespread loss of cortical neurones. Intracranial infection is as common a cause as asphyxia in children. Whereas this term was initially applied to survivors after acute brain damage, it is now recognized that this clinical syndrome can also occur in the end-stage of Alzheimer's disease or multi-infarct dementia and in some infants born with devastating congenital cerebral defects. After acute traumatic and non-traumatic damage leading to vegetative survival there is progressive degeneration over many months of nerve fibres remote from the site of initial damage, demonstrable by special stains at autopsy, and reflected during life in progressive enlargement of the ventricles and subarachnoid spaces as visualized by CT or MRI. EEG findings are variable but there is usually loss of evoked cortical responses to somatic stimuli. Positron emission tomography shows severe depression of glucose metabolism in cortical grey matter, to levels found only in experimental deep barbiturate narcosis.

In practice, however, the diagnosis depends on characteristic clinical features recorded by skilled observers over a period of time. The patient has long periods of spontaneous eye opening (hence the inappropriateness of calling this condition irreversible or prolonged coma). The eyes may briefly follow a moving object and the head turn reflexly to a sudden noise that produces a startle reaction. All four limbs are paralysed and spastic, with only reflex posturing and withdrawal. The face may grimace and groans be heard, but never words. There is no psychologically meaningful response to external stimuli or any learned behaviour—no evidence of a working mind. It is concluded that although awake these patients are not aware, and do not suffer distress or pain. They need to be distinguished from patients with a locked-in syndrome who are aware and can communicate by their only remaining motor power, namely by blinking or eye movements.

Patients in a vegetative state for some time can still make some recovery. A substantial number of traumatic cases gain independence after 1 month in a vegetative state, and a few after 3 months, with children more likely to recover. Some other regain some degree of consciousness to become severely disabled and dependent. Although there are occasional reports of a limited degree of later recovery it is generally agreed that after 1 year the vegetative state can be considered permanent. Once this stage is reached ethical and economic questions arise about whether it is wise to maintain life-sustaining treatment. There is good evidence that many people regard survival in this state as worse than death, in that it is an undignified existence of no benefit to the patient and is distressing to the family. Yet survival for 10 to 20 years or more is possible with adequate feeding and nursing.

Several groups have declared that it is appropriate to let such patients die by withdrawing tube feeding. In the United States many cases have been brought before the courts, including one to the Supreme Court, seeking permission to withdraw tube feeding. These courts have all agreed to this and have indicated that judicial review should no longer be necessary before such action, unless there is some dispute between the involved parties. At the end of 1992 the first case legally tested in Britain came before the High Court, the Court of Appeal, and the House of Lords, and withdrawal of life support was unanimously declared to be lawful. This is in line with developments in medical ethics and practice in recent years that emphasize the importance of withholding or withdrawing treatment that does not benefit a patient, as well as that to which the patient does not consent. Incompetent patients, such as those in a vegetative state, can best ensure that their preferences about treatment are respected by making an advance directive (living will and/or appointing a proxy decision-maker). Recent pressure to encourage patients with various conditions to make such directives have been increased in both the United States and the United Kingdom by the highly publicized spectacle of vegetative survivors having to go to the highest courts in the land before death is allowed to come.

REFERENCES

Brain death

Black, P.M. and Zervas, N.T. (1984). Declaration of brain death in neurosurgical and neurological practice. *Neurosurgery* 15, 170–4.

Conference of Medical Royal Colleges and their Faculties in the United Kingdom (1976). Diagnosis of brain death. *British Medical Journal* 2, 1187–88.

Conference of the Medical Royal Colleges and their Faculties in the United Kingdom (1979). Diagnosis of death. *British Medical Journal* 1, 322.

Conference of the Medical Royal Colleges and their Faculties in the United Kingdom (1988). *Report of Working Party on organ transplantation in neonates.* DHSS, London.

Gentleman, D., Easton, J., and Jennett, B. (1990). Brain death and organ donation in a neurosurgical unit: audit of recent practice. *British Medical Journal* 301, 1203–6.

Gore, S.M., Cable, D.J., and Holland, A.J. (1992). Organ donation from intensive care units in England and Wales: two year confidential audit of deaths in intensive care. *British Medical Journal* 304, 349–55.

Health Departments of Great Britain and Northern Ireland (1983). *Cadaveric organs for transplantation: a code of practice, including the diagnosis of brain death.* HMSO, London.

Jennett, B. (1981). Brain death. *British Journal of Anaesthesia* 53, 1111–19.

Jennett, B. and Hessett, C. (1981). Brain death in Britain as reflected in renal donors. *British Medical Journal* 283, 359.

Pallis, C. (1983). *ABC of brain death.* British Medical Journal, London.

Pallis, C. (1990). Brain stem death. In *Handbook of clinical neurology: head injury,* (ed. R. Braakman), Vol. 57, pp. 441–96. Elsevier, Amsterdam.

President's Commission for the Studies of Ethical Problems in Medicine (1981). Guidelines for the determination of death. *Journal of the American Medical Association* 246, 2184–6.

Report of Special Task Force (1987). Guidelines for the determination of brain death in children. *Pediatrics* 80, 298–9.

Vegetative state

Ashwal, S., *et al.* (1992). The persistent vegetative state in children: a report of the Child Neurology Society Ethics Committee. *Annals of Neurology* 32, 570–6.

British Medical Association. (1993). *Guidelines on treatment decisions for patients in the persistent vegetative state.* Annual Report, Appendix 7, British Medical Association, London.

Council on Ethical and Judicial Affairs of the American Medical Association (1990). Persistent vegetative state and the decision to withdraw or withhold life support. *Journal of the American Medical Association* 263, 426–30.

Institute of Medical Ethics (1991). Working Party Report on withdrawing life supporting treatment from patients in a vegetative state after acute brain damage. *Lancet* 337, 96–8.

Jennett, B. (1991). Vegetative state: causes, management, ethical dilemmas. *Current Anaesthesia* 2, 57–61.

Jennett, B. (1992). Letting vegetative patients die. *British Medical Journal* **305,** 1305–6.

Jennett, B. and Dyer, C. (1991). Persistent vegetative state and the right to die: the US and Britain. *British Medical Journal* **302,** 1256–8.

Jennett, B. and Plum, F. (1972). Persistent vegetative state after brain damage. *Lancet* **i,** 734–7.

President's Commission for the Study of Ethical Problems in Medicine (1983). *Deciding to forego life-sustaining treatment: ethical, medical and* *legal issues in treatment decisions.* US Government Printing Office, Washington.

Statement of a Multi-Society Task Force (1994). Medical aspects of persistent vegetative state, *New England Journal of Medicine*, in press.

Walshe, T.M. and Leonard, C. (1986). Persistent vegetative state. Extension of the syndrome to include chronic disorders. *Archives of Neurology* **42,** 1045–7.

24.5 Pain: pathophysiology and treatment

J. W. SCADDING

This chapter considers the mechanisms of chronic pain and suggests guidelines to the various forms of treatment. Pain is the most common symptom in medicine, usually a signal to the development of some potentially damaging lesion. Pain always merits treatment but the underlying cause of persistent pain must always be sought. For the majority of pains, adequate symptomatic treatment is relatively easily achieved, but in certain circumstances pain becomes an intractable problem, either because of incurable underlying disease, or because it is due to damage to the peripheral or central sensory nervous system, or, occasionally, because it is a manifestation of unrecognized psychiatric disturbance.

DEFINITION

Pain may be defined as an unpleasant sensation that is perceived as arising from a specific region of the body and is commonly produced by processes that damage, or are capable of damaging, bodily tissue. The second part of this definition refers to pains that are within everyone's experience and is termed nociceptive pain, that is pain due to a peripheral tissue cause signalled by an intact nervous system. This contrasts with the less common, but important, disorders that comprise neuropathic pain, that is pain due to damage to the nervous system itself (Table 1). Neuropathic pain is invariably more difficult to treat than nociceptive pain, for two reasons. First, because many of the causes produce irreversible damage to either the peripheral or central nervous system (CNS), and, secondly, because the mechanisms responsible for neuropathic pain are quite different to those of nociceptive pain and are less well understood. Thus, although the incidence of neuropathic pain is much less than that of nociceptive pain, neuropathic pain is commonly intractable.

Perception of pain

The amount of pain experienced in response to a particular stimulus may be modified by several factors. These include the circumstances in which the injury is sustained, anticipation of pain, past experiences of pain, and psychological factors such as mood and state of distraction. The experience of pain may change over short periods of time while the initiating lesion remains unchanged. These observations suggest that nervous impulses responsible for the experience of pain may be substantially altered at various levels in the nervous system. A number of sites of modulation have now been identified, both in nociceptive and neuropathic pain, although the means by which these endogenous control mechanisms are activated are only partly understood.

Peripheral mechanisms of nociception

TYPE OF FIBRE AND SENSATION

Fast-conducting myelinated sensory fibres (conduction velocity 30–100 m/s) have receptors with low thresholds, while slow-conducting myelinated A delta fibres (conduction velocity 4–30 m/s) and unmyelinated afferents (conduction velocity less than 2.5 m/s) have receptors that are activated by noxious stimuli. Selective stimulation of single afferents by microneurography in man shows that large-fibre activation causes pressure or tickling sensations; A delta and larger C-fibre activation cause brief sensations often described as pricking, and activation of slower C fibres causes diffuse severe pain, often with a burning quality.

HYPERALGESIA AND CHEMICAL SENSITIZATION OF RECEPTORS

Hyperalgesia, that is, an exaggerated response to stimuli above the normal pain threshold, often results from tissue damage. Both peripheral receptor sensitization and secondary central sensitization contribute to hyperalgesia.

Receptor sensitization

Substances mediating inflammation, including bradykinin, 5-hydroxytryptamine (5HT), histamine, and prostaglandins released in response to injury, are extremely algesic. They act synergistically to lower the threshold of C fibres and increase their activity. Prostaglandins, which play a particularly important potentiating role in pain and inflammation, are fatty acids formed from arachidonic acid derived from phospholipids in cell membranes. Corticosteroids inhibit the formation of arachidonic acid from phospholipids, a basis for their anti-inflammatory and analgesic action. Arachidonic acid is converted to prostaglandins and prostacyclins through a series of intermediate compounds, the initial step being the formation of endoperoxides through the action of cyclo-oxygenase. Aspirin, indomethacin, and other non-steroidal anti-inflammatory drugs (NSAIDs) inhibit this enzyme.

Central sensitization

When there is prolonged nociceptor activation in the periphery, dorsal horn cells in the spinal cord may change in the way they are activated. Those that are normally only activated by nociceptors begin to respond to low-threshold afferents, so that innocuous peripheral stimuli may evoke painful sensations. Such activity is probably in part the basis of allodynia (all types of stimuli produce painful sensation) and hyperpathia (summation of pain sensation with repetitive stimulation and pain persisting after cessation of stimulation).

Table 1 *Causes of neuropathic pain*

Peripheral nerve
  Trauma
    Entrapment neuropathies
    Partial or complete transection: causalgia, amputation, and
    stump pain
    Painful scars
    Post-thoracotomy
  Other mononeuropathies and multiple mononeuropathies
    Diabetic
    Malignant nerve/plexus invasion
    Ischaemia
    Radiation plexopathy
    Connective tissue disease (rheumatoid arthritis, systemic
     lupus erythematosus, polyarteritis nodosa)
  Polyneuropathies

Diabetic	Alcoholic
Nutritional	Amyloid
Fabry's disease	Isoniazid
Subacute myelo-optic neuropathy	
Idiopathic	

Root and dorsal root ganglion

Prolapsed disc	Post-herpetic neuralgia
Arachnoiditis	Trigeminal neuralgia
Root avulsion	Tumour compression
Surgical rhizotomy	

Spinal cord

Complete transection	Dysraphism
Hemisection	Vitamin B$_{12}$ deficiency
Compression/contusion	Syphilitic myelitis
Syrinx	Surgery
Multiple sclerosis	cordotomy
Tumours	commissural
	myelotomy
Arteriovenous malformation	Lissauer's tract section

Brain-stem

Wallenberg's syndrome	Multiple sclerosis
Syrinx	Tuberculoma
Tumour	

Thalamus

Infarction	Surgical lesions in ventroposterior medialis/ ventroposterior lateralis
Haemorrhage	Tumours

Cortical and subcortical

Infarction	Tumour
Arteriovenous malformation	Trauma

Central nervous system

DORSAL HORN

The dorsal horn is now recognized as having a crucial role in pain processing. The complex cellular organization allows the responses of individual cells to afferent stimulation to be markedly altered both by impulses in other afferents and also by descending impulses from the brain.

Anatomy and physiology

The dorsal horn is a laminated structure. The most superficial layer, lamina 1 (substantia gelatinosa), contains small neurones in an area devoid of myelin. These cells receive the terminals of many nociceptive

afferents and project into lamina 2, where more cells also receive low-threshold afferent input. Receptive field sizes and responses of these cells vary greatly, some showing prolonged responses to brief afferent stimulation, others rapidly habituating (novelty detectors), and others showing large changes in receptive field shape and size over minutes or hours. Lamina 3 contains similar small cells to lamina 2, with an extensive network of dendrites extending into this lamina from the deeper ventral laminae. The cells in laminae 3 and 4 respond mainly to low-threshold afferents. Lamina 5 contains neurones of a wide dynamic range, responding to a variety of low- and high-threshold stimuli. Their receptive fields often comprise a central area in which all types of stimuli cause excitation and a larger outer region in which the cells only respond to noxious stimulation. Some lamina 5 cells respond to convergent, somatic, and visceral high-threshold afferents, a possible substrate for referred pain (see below). The cells in lamina 6 respond to high- and low-threshold cutaneous afferents and low-threshold muscle afferents, the modality of the response being under descending control. Cells with complex responses are found in lamina 7 and project into the spinothalamic tract.

The increasing complexity of afferent responses in the deeper laminae of the dorsal horn indicates that these laminae receive input not only directly from the periphery but also from the laminae dorsal to them. This arrangement lends itself to modulation by a number of influences, including segmental, descending, and ascending.

Segmental control

Modulation of a noxious input by non-noxious counterstimulation afferent at the same spinal segmental level is a long-established means of relieving both acute and chronic pains. Experimental evidence indicates that the therapeutic action of counterstimulation is mediated at the level of the dorsal horn. For example, high-frequency, low-amplitude electrical stimulation of the type used in transcutaneous electrical nerve stimulation (TENS) reduces the firing of dorsal horn cells responding to a noxious input gradually over several minutes. This inhibition is mediated by interneurones, which are of great interest particularly because of their peptide and opiate content and thus the potential for targeted pharmacological manipulation. These interneurones are probably mainly situated in lamina 2 and are connected to similar neurones in neighbouring segments via the Lissauer tract, which may thus have the function of influencing the excitability of interneurones over several adjacent segments of the cord (juxtasegmental control).

Descending control

Stimulation of certain sites in the brain-stem can produce profound analgesia, the most effective being the periaqueductal grey and the medullary nucleus raphe magnus. The periaqueductal grey projects to the nucleus raphe magnus which, in turn, projects to the spinal cord via the dorsolateral funiculus, terminating in the dorsal horn. A second important descending pathway originates in the locus coeruleus and projects to the dorsal horn.

SPINAL CORD PHARMACOLOGY

Neurotransmitters in primary sensory neurones

Several peptides have been identified in afferent C fibres and their terminals in the dorsal horn, and there is strong evidence that some at least have a neurotransmitter function. They include substance P, vasoactive intestinal polypeptide, somatostatin, cholecystokinin-like peptide, and angiotensin. In addition, glutamate and aspartate are widespread in the dorsal horn and have excitatory actions. Substance P is present in about 20 per cent of dorsal root ganglion cells and their terminals in laminae 1 and 2. Only noxious peripheral stimuli cause its release. Application of substance P to dorsal horn neurones produces a delayed but prolonged depolarization, unlike the pattern of the dorsal-horn cell response to natural peripheral stimulation. It thus seems unlikely that substance P acts as a classical rapid neurotransmitter, and more likely that it modulates dorsal horn responses over longer time periods when co-released with another transmitter. Other peptides may have a similar function.

Capsaicin, the pungent extract of red pepper, desensitizes C fibres, depletes substance P, and abolishes cutaneous inflammation induced by chemical irritants (mediated by axon reflexes in afferent C fibres). Topical application of capsaicin is useful in the treatment of some hyperalgesic states, particularly post-herpetic neuralgia.

Endogenous opiates and modulation of spinal cord activity

The presence of specific opiate receptors and their ligands, the endorphins, was demonstrated only 20 years ago, but several receptor subtypes with different opiate affinities have now been identified. Opiate receptors and endorphins are widely distributed in the nervous system, including the terminals of some primary sensory neurones, laminae 1 and 2 of the dorsal horn, the medullary raphe nuclei, periaqueductal grey, locus coeruleus, basal ganglia, hypothalamus, and pituitary. Several endorphins have been identified, of which β-endorphin is a relatively stable compound, possibly having a 'gain control function' such as that suggested for substance P, contrasting with the enkephalins which are unstable and thus more likely to be classical neurotransmitters.

Enkephalin is present in high concentration in laminae 1 and 2 of the dorsal horn, where there are also many other opiate receptors. Application of morphine or enkephalin on to dorsal horn neurones reduces responses to noxious afferent stimulation but has no effect on the response to low-threshold afferent stimulation, indicating a presynaptic and selective inhibition of noxious input, possibly mediated via opiate receptors on the terminals of afferent C fibres. A reduced release of substance P from primary afferent terminals following opiate application supports this idea. These and other experimental observations provide a scientific rationale for the use of spinal opiates for pain relief.

Pharmacology of descending control

Experimentally, electrical stimulation in either the periaqueductal grey/nucleus raphe magnus or the locus coeruleus reduces dorsal horn cell responses to noxious primary afferent stimuli, and microinjection of opiates into the periaqueductal grey or nucleus raphe magnus will produce similar effects, which are reversed by naloxone. Both the periaqueductal grey and the nucleus raphe magnus contain high concentrations of opiate receptors and enkephalins, so, taken together, these observations indicate that this is an opiate-dependent endogenous pain control mechanism. However, it has been shown that 5HT and noradrenaline are the neurotransmitters involved in the pathway from the nucleus raphe magnus to the dorsal horn, and the projection from the locus coeruleus to the dorsal horn is noradrenergic. Both intrathecal 5HT and noradrenaline have been demonstrated to produce analgesia in experimental situations, and epidural clonidine (an α_2-agonist) has an analgesic effect in man.

Visceral and referred pain

Pain from deep tissues, including visceral pain, is different from superficial pain, particularly in terms of localization and quality, and it serves different functions. The importance of rapid and accurate localization for cutaneous noxious stimuli has an obvious protective function in terms of removal from the potentially injurious situation. The function of deep and visceral pain is usually immobilization because escape from the stimulus is not a possibility. Thus, exact localization and immediacy of pain sensation are not issues of such importance. Visceral pain is often poorly localized, leading to diagnostic difficulties.

In contrast to cutaneous nociceptive afferents, it is difficult to identify specific visceral nociceptors and show clear stimulus intensity–response relationships in many organs and tissues. Severe distension of the biliary duct or urinary bladder can be shown experimentally to activate certain classes of unmyelinated afferents which probably have a nociceptive function. In relation to joint-capsule receptors, the situation is much

more akin to cutaneous afferents, in that in inflammation, A delta and C fibres clearly show sensitization and may become continuously active in chronically inflamed joints. In skeletal and cardiac muscle, some unmyelinated C afferents are particularly, but not exclusively, stimulated by ischaemia.

Most visceral afferents terminate on cells in laminae 1 and 5 in the dorsal horn where there is always convergence with somatic afferents. Certain severe types of visceral stimulation will activate these dorsal horn neurones, and can be shown to produce ascending impulses in spinothalamic tract neurones.

REFERRED PAIN

A common accompaniment to pain of visceral origin is referred pain. Indeed, referred pain may be the predominant or only complaint of pain, and may even be associated with cutaneous hyperalgesia and underlying muscle tenderness, causing potential diagnostic difficulties. For example, although most patients experiencing acute myocardial infarction complain of central chest pain with or without radiation, some will only report anterior neck pain and pain in the left arm. Usually the areas of referred pain from a particular organ and the associated cutaneous hyperalgesia, if present, are reasonably constant from patient to patient, conforming approximately to a spinal segmental distribution, although this pattern of distribution of referred pain is more predictable with muscle pain than with pain arising from the viscera.

Mechanisms of referred pain

The most likely explanation for referred pain is the deep and visceral afferent convergence with somatic input to dorsal horn cells, so that input from either source is capable of stimulating activity in spinothalamic neurones. Because the brain frequently receives nociceptive information from somatic structures and only rarely from the viscera, it localizes the pain to the relevant somatic structure. When a nociceptive input arises from the viscera, the brain may then have difficulty in localizing the source of the pain, which may be projected to the somatic structures normally activating that part of the spinothalamic tract. Differences in patterns of nociceptive input between somatic and visceral structures may help in identifying the source of pain as being visceral.

The explanation of the cutaneous hyperalgesia and muscular tenderness sometimes associated with referred pain is more difficult. Visceral pain may lead to reflex somatic muscle contraction which then produces tenderness and its own secondary nociceptive input. A further possibility is that a reflex increase in efferent sympathetic activity induced by the pain may lower the threshold of cutaneous and muscle nociceptors. Other manifestations of increased sympathetic outflow secondary to visceral pain and leading to autonomic disturbances are commonly observed. The most striking evidence of such a sympathetic efferent sensitization of nociceptors occurring in normal skin and muscle occurs in reflex sympathetic dystrophy, in which sympathetic block may temporarily relieve the hyperalgesia and muscle tenderness (see below).

Spinothalmic tract origins and thalamic terminations

The spinothalamic tract is an almost completely crossed tract. There are four types of spinothalamic tract neurones, including some responding only to non-noxious stimuli, which arise from laminae 4 and 5 in the dorsal horn; some which are purely proprioceptive, arising from deep laminae; neurones of wide dynamic range in lamina 5, responding to noxious and non-noxious stimuli; and neurones responding only to noxious stimuli, arising from laminae 1 and 2.

Near to the thalamus, the spinothalamic tract divides into a larger part, which terminates in the lateral ventroposterior nucleus, and a smaller medial part, which terminates in the parafascicular and intralaminar nuclei.

Travelling with the spinothalamic tract are the spinoreticular and spinomesencephalic tracts. The spinoreticular tract contains neurones which project to nuclei in the medullary reticular formation, including the nucleus raphe magnus, and thence to the medial group of thalamic nuclei. The spinomesencephalic tract contains similar neurones and projects to the midbrain reticular formation, the superior and inferior colliculi and the periaqueductal grey, and from there to the medial thalamic nuclei.

THALAMIC PROJECTIONS: FUNCTIONAL ASPECTS

There are thus two main subdivisions of the spinothalamic tract, one being a direct pathway to the main thalamic sensory nucleus (the ventroposterior nucleus) where there is overlap with the terminations of the medial lemniscus. This has a somatotopic organization and the main rostral projection is to the primary somatosensory cortex. This arrangement is well designed to subserve the sensory discriminative functions of pain, that is localization, duration, and type of noxious stimulus.

The other part of the spinothalamic tract, to the intralaminar and medial groups of nuclei is supplemented by the polysynaptic projections from the medulla and midbrain via the spinoreticular and spinomesencephalic tracts. The neurones in this part of the thalamus have no somatotopic organization and characteristically have very wide receptive fields. The rostral projection is very diffuse and includes the frontal lobe and limbic neocortex. It is likely that this part of the pain pathway subserves the affective and autonomic components of pain.

Further endogenous pain modulating mechanisms

In addition to segmental and descending influences on the onward transmission of nociceptive information acting at the level of the dorsal horn, two other mechanisms are probably also of clinical importance.

ASCENDING CONTROL

The medial thalamus, receiving part of the spinothalamic tract together with the spinoreticulothalamic and spinomesencephalothalamic tracts, has many enkephalin-containing terminals and high concentrations of opiate receptors. In addition, there are many 5HT-containing terminals in the medial thalamus which exert an inhibitory action on cells responding to noxious stimuli.

DIFFUSE NOXIOUS INHIBITORY CONTROL

It is a frequent clinical observation that pain in one part of the body may suppress pain arising in another part. It has been shown experimentally that the response of dorsal horn cells to a noxious input can be reduced by a separate distant noxious input at another spinal segmental level, while the response to low-threshold afferent stimulation is unaltered, indicating a presynaptic inhibition. This mechanism has been termed diffuse noxious inhibitory control. It is absent in spinal animals, with destruction of the nucleus raphe magnus, or with 5HT depletion, and it is reversible with naloxone. These findings strongly suggest that diffuse noxious inhibitory control is mediated via opiate-dependent brain-stem pathways and the descending 5HT-mediated projection from the nucleus raphe magnus to the dorsal horn.

CONTROL OF PAIN-MODULATING MECHANISMS

Little is known about the circumstances that normally activate segmental, descending, and ascending inhibitions and diffuse noxious inhibitory control. Primary, afferent, large-fibre input is clearly important in segmental control and the juxtasegmental inhibitory influence mediated by Lissauer's tract. It has been shown that descending control also depends to some extent on primary afferent fibre activity. For example, the discharge of periaqueductal grey of neurones can be provoked by peripheral nerve stimulation. Naloxone leads to an increase in dorsal horn cell response to peripheral noxious stimulation, indicating the presence of a tonically active, opiate-mediated analgesic mechanism. Much remains to be learnt about the activation of these various endogenous analgesic systems, although therapeutic enhancement of some is already possible. In addition to methods such as electrical stimulation at various sites, both peripheral and central, the location of endogenous opiates, 5HT, and noradrenergic pathways, with demonstrated physiological significance in relation to analgesia, begins to provide a rational basis for treatments such as opiate therapy and offers hope for increasingly selective interventions in future.

Neuropathic pain

DEFINITION

The term neuropathic pain is used here to embrace all pain due to lesions of the sensory pathway, both peripheral and central. Some prefer to make a division into peripheral, neuropathic, and central pain syndromes, but as it is increasingly clear that major central changes may result from peripheral nerve lesions and that the pain in these situations is, at least in part, generated by altered central mechanisms, it is arguably better simply to use the term neuropathic pain and qualify it by description of the initiating cause.

The many causes of neuropathic pain are shown in Table 1. Taken together, those conditions affecting the primary sensory neurone (including the dorsal root ganglion and dorsal root) are much more common than the central causes. Malignant disease is a relatively unusual cause of neuropathic pain. However, the majority of the non-malignant conditions listed are not amenable to complete and permanent cure. Neuropathic pain is thus a severe chronic affliction for many patients.

DEAFFERENTATION

The amount of sensory loss with neuropathic pain is variable, even within a single diagnostic category. The degree of deafferentation shows no direct relationship to the severity of the pain. However, it is helpful to assess the degree of deafferentation for three reasons. First, the greater the deafferentation the more likely it is that central nervous system mechanisms are important in generating the pain. Secondly, methods of counterstimulation, such as transcutaneous electrical nerve stimulation, are less likely to be effective if there is significant deafferentation; and thirdly, any treatment that is likely to increase already severe deafferentation may make the pain worse.

CLINICAL FEATURES OF NEUROPATHIC PAIN

The major clinical features of neuropathic pain are given in Table 2. Unlike nociceptive pain, a focus of damage in peripheral tissues often can not be demonstrated. The quality of the pain is different and outside the patient's previous experience of pain, making it difficult to describe. There are often paroxysmal shooting or shock-like pains in addition to continuous background pains. Changes in emotional state and fatigue may cause the pain intensity to vary over short periods. The onset of neuropathic pain may be immediate following the initiating cause, but is often delayed. For example, it is characteristic for thalamic pain to develop at an interval of 2 or 3 months following thalamic infarction, and myelopathic pain may take many months to develop following spinal cord trauma. Neuropathic pain and associated hyperalgesia, allodynia, and hyperpathia are not necessarily confined to the territory of an affected nerve or root but may radiate widely, indicating secondary central involvement, and this can cause diagnostic difficulty. However, there is often a clear anatomical correlation of pain and sensory abnormality, and the presence of sensory loss is particularly helpful in distinguishing neuropathic from nociceptive pain.

Abnormalities of local or regional sympathetic activity are common in association with neuropathic pain, particularly with peripheral nerve lesions, but may also occur with root, cord, or thalamic lesions. The

Table 2 *Clinical features of neuropathic pain*

Quality of pain: often burning, raw, aching, gnawing
Additional paroxysmal, shock-like pains
Pain associated with some sensory impairment
Associated allodynia, hyperalgesia, and hyperpathia are
  common
Sympathetic dysfunction is common, particularly with
  peripheral nerve lesions
Sometimes associated with changes of reflex sympathetic
  dystrophy
The onset of pain may be immediate or delayed
Pain intensity is often markedly altered by fatigue and emotion

possible role of abnormal sympathetic outflow in producing or maintaining neuropathic pains, and the therapeutic implications, are discussed below.

MECHANISMS OF PAIN IN PERIPHERAL NEUROPATHY

Morphometric studies in nerve biopsies from patients with a wide variety of neuropathies have shown that earlier ideas that pain might result from an imbalance in the distribution of fibre sizes in peripheral nerves are no longer tenable. Although there are painful neuropathies in which small fibres are selectively preserved, there are others in which loss of large fibres rarely leads to pain (for example, uraemic neuropathy). Review of the clinical evidence indicates that pain seems to be related to the acuteness of degenerative change and preferential involvement of small fibres by the underlying disease process (for example, small-fibre diabetic neuropathy and amyloid neuropathy), particularly when there is also marked regenerative activity in the nerves.

In some mononeuropathies there is tenderness at the site of the nerve lesion which is due to local inflammation and structural abnormality in the nerve. This is pain signalled by the nervi nervorum and is thus nociceptive rather than neuropathic in type. To what extent this mechanism of pain is relevant in polyneuropathies is uncertain.

Ischaemia can be shown to provoke readily pain and paraesthesiae in certain situations, for example carpal tunnel syndrome, and it is likely that ischaemia is a contributory factor in some neuropathies, for example diabetic mononeuropathy and the mononeuropathies associated with connective tissue disease which have a microangiopathic basis.

Abnormal sympathetic activity is certainly important in maintaining causalgia. Sympathetic block may relieve pain and associated allodynia and hyperpathia in patients with causalgia and other types of post-traumatic neuralgia, whether or not there are signs of abnormal sympathetic function in the affected limb.

These clinical observations have been supplemented by the results of experimental studies on a variety of nerve lesions, ranging from nerve section with neuroma formation to mild lesions producing reversible demyelination. The following abnormal properties of relevance to pain have been documented:

1. Injured peripheral nerve axons generate impulses at the site of damage. This is most marked in axotomized, sprouting, regenerating sensory fibres, and affects all myelinated and unmyelinated fibre classes.
2. Marked mechanical sensitivity develops in damaged fibres. The clinical counterpart of this is the Tinel sign, producing paraesthesiae and pain radiating in the distribution of the injured nerve.
3. Regenerating fibres develop an α-adrenergic sensitivity which increases their ectopic discharges. A non-synaptic interaction between noradrenergic sympathetic efferent fibres and sensory fibres can be demonstrated in regions of nerve damage. This property provides an explanation of the therapeutic effect of

sympathetic block in causalgia and other post-traumatic neuralgias.

4. Ischaemia, anoxia, increased extracellular potassium, and certain peptides present in unmyelinated fibres in peripheral nerves have also been shown to excite the abnormal impulse activity in damaged nerve fibres.
5. Warming tends to increase ectopic impulse activity in myelinated fibres, while cooling has a similar effect on C fibres, possibly of relevance to the cold hyperalgesia which is a frequent feature of painful peripheral nerve lesions.
6. Local anaesthetic silences all ectopic impulse activity arising from areas of nerve damage. In experimental situations, local corticosteroids, glycerol, phenytoin, and carbamazepine all reduce abnormal activity. However, their action in clinical settings is generally disappointing, (other than intracisternal glycerol in trigeminal neuralgia).
7. In addition to the sympathetic sensory interaction, other interactions also occur between fibres in nerve injury. Ephaptic transmission, that is a tight electrical coupling between fibres, has been demonstrated experimentally, but never convincingly shown in man. Another type of interaction has been termed 'crossed after discharge', in which afferent activity in a group of fibres may induce activity in neighbouring sensory fibres. Again, there is, as yet, no direct evidence that this property exists in man.
8. In addition to the impulse generation at the site of injury, ectopic impulses also arise proximally in the region of the dorsal root ganglion cell. Ongoing activity from nerve damage, mechanical sensitivity, and activity arising from the dorsal root ganglion have all been recorded in single fibres in human nerves by microneurography.
9. Finally, in different experimental situations there is great variability in the magnitude of these various properties, together with clear species and even strain differences. This may help to explain the enormous clinical variability in the experience of painful symptoms following peripheral nerve damage in different patients, and points to the possibility of similar clinicopathophysiological variability following central nervous system lesions in relation to pain.

CENTRAL NERVOUS SYSTEM REACTION TO PERIPHERAL NERVE DAMAGE

Some symptoms and signs associated with peripheral nerve injury cannot be explained on the basis of these abnormal peripheral properties and implicate secondary changes in the central nervous system. These include the almost immediate onset of pain and associated sensory abnormalities in some patients (for example, causalgia in some patients following gunshot wounds) which develop before the peripheral abnormalities outlined above have had time to develop. Allodynia, hyperpathia, and reflex sympathetic changes may all extend beyond the territory of the affected nerve and indicate central factors.

Central sensitization

When there is prolonged nociceptor activation in the periphery, dorsal horn cells may change their activation characteristics. Cells normally activated by nociceptors begin to respond to low-threshold afferents, so that innocuous peripheral stimuli may evoke painful sensations, and this may gradually increase over time. Such activity could contribute to allodynia and hyperpathia.

Reduced inhibitions

The normal presynaptic dorsal horn inhibitions of small-fibre activity, discussed above, become less effective after certain types of nerve damage, and some postsynaptic inhibitions are also less powerful. Furthermore, dorsal horn neurones that lose their afferent input completely show disinhibited high-frequency bursting discharges, relevant to clinical situations such as brachial plexus avulsion and post-herpetic neuralgia.

Cell death

After nerve damage causing a severe painful afferent input, there may be trans-synaptic death of dorsal horn cells. It may be that this only occurs in situations where there are also reduced inhibitions, and the mechanism by which such cell death occurs is uncertain.

Taken together, all this evidence shows that peripheral nerve damage is capable of producing marked central changes, some of which may become irreversible. Any therapeutic interventions, particularly peripheral, are then bound to have, at best, a limited effect.

Reflex sympathetic dystrophy and causalgia

CLINICAL FEATURES

Reflex sympathetic dystrophy describes a group of conditions, the common features of which include pain, allodynia, hyperpathia, sudomotor and vasomotor changes, and dystrophic changes which may affect both soft tissues and bone, leading to major loss of function in the affected limb. When dystrophic changes are marked, it is sometimes called Sudeck's atrophy. Thus defined, reflex sympathetic dystrophy embraces a number of disorders such as algodystrophy, post-traumatic osteoporosis, acute atrophy of bone, and neurovascular dystrophy. There are many causes, but little is known about the reasons for the development of reflex sympathetic dystrophy in only a tiny minority of patients with the various conditions listed in Table 3, nor the pathogenesis of the changes. Diagnostic criteria are not even fully agreed, and although there are abnormalities on investigations such as isotope bone scanning, the diagnosis remains a clinical one. The condition may be self-limiting and mild, but in some cases it is relentlessly progressive, leading to a painful, very sensitive, useless limb.

Causalgia means burning pain. Some use the term to refer only to such pain when associated with partial lesions of major limb nerves. In this situation there is nearly always accompanying allodynia, hyperpathia, and vasomotor and sudomotor abnormalities, and it thus fulfils the criteria for reflex sympathetic dystrophy. The same type of burning pain and other features are often present with other causes of reflex sympathetic dystrophy. It is thus probably best to use the term 'causalgia' simply to describe burning pain and not to link it with any particular cause, especially since there is no pathophysiological justification for doing so at the moment.

PATHOGENESIS

The pathogenesis of reflex sympathetic dystrophy is uncertain. The often widely radiating allodynia and hyperpathia are mediated by large afferent myelinated fibres and, in many patients, can be temporarily relieved by sympathetic blockade. This implies that the normal terminals of undamaged low-threshold afferent fibres may become sensitized to noradrenaline. According to the most popular model of reflex sympathetic dystrophy, a vicious circle develops. The initiating painful cause leads to noxious input to the spinal cord, which, by an unknown mechanism, leads to reflex sympathetic activation via sympathetic, preganglionic neurones in the intermediolateral column of the spinal cord. This increases sympathetic efferent postganglionic activity which, again by some undetermined mechanism, is capable of sensitizing the terminals of undamaged primary afferent fibres in the periphery, lowering their threshold to stimulation, leading to an increased afferent barrage, in this way completing the vicious circle. In addition, there would need to be central sensitization, in order for the increased afferent input to be perceived as painful. Sympathetic block would break the vicious circle by removing the peripheral sensitization of primary afferent terminals.

Table 3 *Causes of reflex sympathetic dystrophy*

Peripheral tissues
    Soft-tissue injury, including infection
    Fasciitis, tendinitis, bursitis, ligamentous strain
    Fractures and dislocations
    Arthritis
    Deep venous thrombosis
    Arterial thrombosis
    Immobilization

Peripheral nerve and dorsal root
    Peripheral nerve trauma
    Brachial plexus lesions
    Post-herpetic neuralgia
    Root lesions, particularly trauma

Central nervous system
    Spinal cord lesions, particularly trauma
    Head injury
    Cerebral infarction
    Cerebral tumour

Idiopathic

Problems with this theory include the absence of any explanation for the rarity of reflex sympathetic dystrophy and the lack of effect of sympathetic block in some patients. Indeed, sympathetic block may temporarily exacerbate the pain in some patients. It seems likely that there is considerable pathophysiological variation within what we currently recognize clinically as reflex sympathetic dystrophy.

TREATMENT

Simple analgesia is rarely effective. Strong analgesics, including opiates, often have only marginal effect. Sympathetic block may sometimes dramatically relieve the symptoms. If so, a series of blocks combined with physiotherapy may be sufficient to gradually reverse the condition. In refractory cases, prolonged analgesia by epidural local anaesthetic infusions together with physiotherapy may be successful. There have been no adequately controlled trials of any treatment of reflex sympathetic dystrophy, but there are reports of improvement with systemic corticosteroids, NSAIDs, calcitonin, antiepileptic drugs, calcium-channel blockers, and tricyclic antidepressants. However, in severe cases of reflex sympathetic dystrophy none of these drugs may be effective, and other modalities, such as electrical stimulation and psychological measures, are also without effect. Despite all efforts, there remains a small number of patients with truly refractory reflex sympathetic dystrophy.

Requests for amputation by patients should be resisted because of the high risk of the development of phantom limb pain, although there is some evidence that the incidence of stump and phantom pain may be reduced if good analgesia can be produced prior to amputation for 2 or 3 days by spinal block and maintained peroperatively and for a period postoperatively.

All patients suspected of having or developing reflex sympathetic dystrophy should be urgently referred to a pain clinic since there is evidence that early treatment may prevent the development of severe reflex sympathetic dystrophy.

Pain due to central nervous system (CNS)

The CNS lesions that lead to neuropathic pain usually involve the spinothalamic tract or its rostral thalamoparietal projection (Table 1). Within the thalamus, lesions causing thalamic pain (usually infarcts) involve the main sensory nuclei, which receive both the medial lemniscal pathway and part of the spinothalamic tract. Pure dorsal column lemniscal system lesions do not cause chronic neuropathic pain, although cervical dorsal column lesions, most commonly demyelinating plaques may provoke a Lhermitte symptom which can have an unpleasant quality.

There is usually sensory impairment accompanying central neuropathic pain although loss may be subtle and is often of dissociated spinothalamic type. As with peripheral neuropathic pain, there is no clear correlation between the severity of the pain and the degree of sensory loss.

SPINAL CORD LESIONS

Pain from spinal cord lesions may be localized, unilateral, or bilateral, but is often diffuse and widespread below the level of the lesion. It is sometimes particularly severe in the perineum. The pain is usually continuous and may have an aching, stinging, burning, cramping, or vice-like quality. Superimposed focal or diffuse paroxysmal pains are common. Both the ongoing and paroxysmal pains are usually unprovoked but either may be exacerbated by movement, fatigue, or emotion.

BRAIN-STEM LESIONS

Vascular lesions affecting the pons and medulla are the commonest brain-stem lesions leading to pain. Multiple sclerosis, tumours, syrinx, and tuberculoma are occasional causes. Lesions confined to the midbrain do not cause pain. The older therapeutic operations of medullary spinothalamic tractotomy and trigeminal tractotomy can both result in severe pain and are thus no longer performed.

THALAMIC LESIONS

Pain was originally described as part of the thalamic syndrome by Dejerrine and Roussy in 1906. The whole syndrome comprised superficial and deep hemianaesthesia, sensory ataxia, intractable pain, mild hemiplegia, and sometimes choreo-athetosis. It is almost always caused by infarction, with haemorrhage and arteriovenous malformation being occasional causes and, very rarely, tumours involving the thalamus. Therapeutic surgical lesions in the main thalamic sensory nuclei may lead to thalamic pain and the naturally occurring lesions causing thalamic pain always produce damage predominantly in these nuclei, with sparing of the medial and posterior nuclei.

CORTICAL AND SUBCORTICAL LESIONS

Lesions rostral to the thalamus leading to pain are extremely rare but vascular lesions, trauma, and tumours are recorded causes. Pain has also been observed after therapeutic parietal cortectomy for intractable pain (not an operation now performed) and after hemispherectomy for severe epilepsy with infantile hemiplegia, or for the treatment of tumour.

MECHANISMS OF NEUROPATHIC PAIN DUE TO CNS LESIONS

Hyperactivity of cells

The hyperactivity of deafferented dorsal horn cells has already been discussed. In addition, it is now known that dorsal rhizotomy may produce a similar disinhibition of cells in the ventrobasal complex of the thalamus, demonstrating that lesions may cause changes at distant rostral levels. Direct recordings made in thalamic explorations in patients with thalamic or myelopathic pain have shown neurones with high-frequency bursting discharges.

Altered sensitivities of cells

Psychophysical observations have been made in small numbers of patients undergoing thalamic explorations prior to lesioning or stimulating procedures for intractable pain and in patients with movement disorders without pain, providing control observations. In patients with movement disorders and with intractable nociceptive pain, stimulation of the spinothalamic tract or ventrobasal complex only rarely produced pain and burning sensations, in contrast with patients suffering from neuropathic pain in whom pain and burning sensations could be evoked by stimulation at multiple sites, referred to the contralateral side and felt within the area of the patient's ongoing neuropathic pain. Similar sensations could be provoked by stimulation of the spinothalamic tract in the mesencephalon or in the rostral thalamic projections and in the somatosensory cortex, always referred to the region of the patient's ongoing pain.

This is further evidence that a lesion at a relatively caudal level in the nervous system may induce rostral changes in parts of the nervous system not directly involved by the initiating lesion. The activity of some cells becomes altered in such a way that the sensation evoked by activity in these cells is perceived abnormally as pain. The mechanisms by which these changes occur, particularly at rostral levels, is largely obscure, but the implications in terms of treatment, particularly neuroablative, are clear.

Endogenous opiates and neuropathic pain

There is little evidence that endogenous opiate mechanisms for pain suppression are activated by neuropathic pain. Therapeutic trials of periaqueductal grey electrical stimulation seem to be much more effective for nociceptive pain than for neuropathic pain. Furthermore, systemically administered opiates produce good relief of neuropathic pain in only a small proportion of patients, in contrast with nociceptive pain which usually responds well.

SYMPATHETIC ACTIVITY AND NEUROPATHIC PAIN DUE TO CNS LESIONS

Temporary peripheral sympathetic blocks may sometimes relieve neuropathic pain due to CNS lesions, suggesting that sympathetic block may act by reducing or altering part of the afferent input, leading to therapeutic secondary central effects. However, the majority of patients with pain due to CNS lesions show no response to sympathetic blockade and there are no reports of patients with a good result from temporary sympathetic blockade, achieving lasting analgesia with permanent sympathectomy.

THERAPEUTIC IMPLICATIONS

It is thus clear that many possible sites of pathophysiological change can develop after damage to somatosensory pathways. How these all interact is uncertain, although the multiplicity of possible sites of abnormality may be an important factor in explaining the great variation in the development of pain with either a peripheral nerve or CNS lesion. It is also now clear why many of the neuroablative treatments advocated in the past for the treatment of chronic neuropathic pain have, at best, only a temporary effect, and may themselves lead to neuropathic pain, which can develop years later. This has led to a shift of emphasis towards therapeutic stimulation procedures. A small minority of patients are considered for neuroablative procedures, almost exclusively patients with cancer pain in whom overall prognosis is very limited.

Psychological aspects of pain

Psychological factors are often of great importance in chronic pain. Failure to recognize and attempt to deal with these, which may be contributing considerably to the production and maintenance of the patient's chronic pain, will invariably lead to an unsatisfactory outcome. Individual responses to pain vary enormously, particularly the degree to which pain leads to loss of normal functioning. Leaving aside the question of intensity of pain, which is clearly of major importance, at least five other factors need to be considered. The first is the perceived significance of the pain to an individual. For example, a sprained ankle, although very painful, has a clear cause and a reasonable guarantee of recovery, whereas persistent headache may raise fears of cerebral tumour and may be associated with much more severe loss of function. Secondly, differences in underlying psychological make-up and personality have an important influence. This is particularly true for anxious subjects, who demand more analgesia and whose behavioural decompensation is often greater than normal. Thirdly, environmental factors in the patient's social, domestic, or work life may have a powerful effect on the experience of pain and its effect on functioning. Fourthly, cultural factors may be of importance. Permissible and even expected pain behaviours in one society may be alien and unacceptable in another. Linked with this, pain behaviour is learnt over a long period in childhood and adolescence, and there may be a variety of individual and unusual circumstances within families which lead to abnormalities of behavioural reaction to pain. Finally, secondary gain from medical attention, the effects of drugs or other treatment, the necessity to maintain a particular behavioural pattern with impending medicolegal proceedings, and the maintenance of unemployment and disability benefits may all become factors which greatly influence the complaint of pain and its effect on functioning.

Some assessment of these factors is thus essential in the overall evaluation of patients with chronic pain. Often patients are either unwilling to discuss psychological factors or are unaware of them, in contrast with their readiness to discuss the somatic aspects of their pain.

There has been much controversy about the personality traits which may predispose certain subjects to develop chronic pain. The main problem with studies on patients attending pain clinics is that they have often had their pain for a considerable time and this has had an effect in altering their psychological state. Obtaining adequate control observations for many types of painful state is extremely difficult. None the less, certain psychological factors do seem to predispose patients to develop chronic pain. Common psychological abnormalities present in patients with chronic pain include depression, loss of libido, sleep disturbance, fatigue, reduced activity, and somatic preoccupation.

PSYCHIATRIC FACTORS WHICH PREDISPOSE TO THE DEVELOPMENT OF CHRONIC PAIN

Patients with major depression are more common amongst chronic pain patients than in the normal population. Pre-existing depression impairs the ability of patients to cope with chronic pain. The pain intensifies the depression, which in turn, leads to increased complaints of pain. Overemphasis on the treatment of the somatic element of the depressed patient's pain and failure to recognize and treat the depression will lead to an unsatisfactory outcome of treatment.

SOMATIZATION DISORDER

This refers to a chronic condition, starting before the age of 30 and often earlier, in which patients present with numerous somatic symptoms at different times, associated with an unshakeable certainty that they have serious underlying disease. Pain is a very frequent complaint in this group of patients. It usually takes several years for the disorder to become obvious and it is under-recognized. Treatment is always difficult, but the diagnosis should at least lead to a more careful and selective approach to the investigation of further new symptoms.

CONVERSION DISORDER

In this condition there are again complaints for which no underlying somatic basis is evident. These patients tend to have only one symptom and this may be chronic pain, unlike patients with somatization disorder who often have multiple symptoms. Other distinguishing features include a relative indifference to the complaints and their effects, and

provocation by a particular event of great emotional significance to the patient. Treatment of the symptoms will be of very limited benefit and only with recognition of the underlying emotional problem and appropriate psychiatric treatment can cure be achieved.

HYPOCHONDRIASIS

This refers to an undue concern about the presence of underlying serious disease, often a particular disease over many years, for example, cancer. The patient complains excessively about trivial symptoms and becomes extremely anxious but not physically incapacitated, in contrast with some patients with somatization disorder, and many patients with conversion disorder. Again, successful treatment of pain in this group of patients often requires expert psychiatric help.

PSYCHOGENIC PAIN

This category, as distinct from the above conditions, may be questioned. However, in some patients pain develops as a way of dealing with feelings of guilt, often rooted in feelings of an aggressive nature, or guilt about inadmissible or unacceptable sexual feelings. Early childhood experiences are thought to be important. Improving the painful symptoms in such patients requires expert and often prolonged psychiatric treatment, and is extremely difficult since the abnormal psychological pattern is often deep-rooted, having its origin in early childhood experiences.

Guidelines to treatment of chronic pain

It is beyond the scope of this chapter to describe treatment of the many individual pain syndromes for which referral to a pain clinic is made. Table 4 lists some of the more common problems. It can be seen that some of these demand joint management with an appropriate specialist. There are often continuing diagnostic problems in such patients and periodic review of the cause of the pain is essential. Multidisciplinary pain clinics consist of a core staff that includes an anaesthetist, physiotherapist, occupational therapist, and psychologist, but the availability of other specialists, particularly a neurologist and a psychiatrist, is important.

LOCAL MEASURES

Counterstimulation
Most pains are localized and local measures should always be attempted in the first instance, although a combination of local and systemic treatment may be necessary. Regardless of the type of pain, whether nociceptive or neuropathic, counterstimulation techniques may be helpful. These simple and effective methods are all too often neglected in favour of systemic drug treatment, which tends to cause side-effects.

Heat and cold
Many intractable musculoskeletal pains respond to heat, which can be delivered by a heat pad or radiant heat. Neuropathic pains tend to be exacerbated by cold but an exception is post-herpetic neuralgia in which regular application of cold packs for 20 min may reduce troublesome allodynia for up to several hours.

Vibration and ultrasound
Both nociceptive and neuropathic pains may respond to these simple measures, of which vibration is the more practical on a long-term basis since it can be used regularly by the patient at home. None the less, ultrasound regularly for several weeks may have a lasting effect, for example in post-herpetic neuralgia.

Transcutaneous electrical stimulation (TENS) and acupuncture
TENS, acting by segmental inhibition, has been shown to be effective in a wide range of different chronic pains, but is probably more effective

Table 4 *Conditions commonly seen in pain clinics*

Musculoskeletal pains
   Chronic non-inflammatory degenerative arthritis, particularly
     spinal
   Poorly defined pains: fibromyalgia

Mixed musculoskeletal and root pains
   Low back and leg pains
     radiating lumbar pains
     root pain
     failed back surgery
     arachnoiditis
   Neck pain with brachalgia
     musculoskeletal pain
     root pain
     failed neck surgery

Post-herpetic neuralgia

Painful mononeuropathies
   Trauma
   Persistent pain with entrapment

Painful polyneuropathies, particularly small-fibre neuropathies

Other neuropathic pains
   Thalamic pain
   Myelopathic pain, particularly after trauma
   Brachial plexus avulsion

Difficult headaches and facial pain

Chronic perineal pain, without obvious local cause

Psychiatric conditions
   Somatization disorder
   Psychogenic pain

for neuropathic than nociceptive pains. TENS may produce analgesia over a wider area than can be accounted for on the basis of segmental inhibition, and this is probably due to the diffuse noxious inhibitory control mechanism already discussed. A trial period of 2 to 3 weeks, with the patient experimenting with different electrode placements, is essential before concluding that TENS is unhelpful.

Acupuncture probably works by segmental inhibition and by diffuse noxious inhibitory control. The latter is more marked with the noxious counterstimulation of acupuncture than with TENS.

Cerebrospinal fluid endorphin levels are raised by acupuncture but not by TENS, and TENS-induced analgesia is not reversed by naloxone. Thus, although diffuse noxious inhibitory control may be partly opiate-mediated, TENS appears to induce a type of diffuse noxious inhibitory control that does not depend on opiate mechanisms.

Topical local anaesthetic

Simple lignocaine ointment, although poorly absorbed, is sometimes helpful in areas of severe allodynia and hyperpathia, particularly in some patients with painful scar syndromes, tender amputation stumps, and post-herpetic neuralgia.

Topical capsaicin

Capsaicin (0.075 per cent) may also be effective in these situations, probably through its action of desensitizing afferent C fibres for long periods. However, it may produce intolerable burning pain in some patients.

Local anaesthetic injections and spinal opiates

Local anaesthetic blocks to peripheral tissues, peripheral nerves, or roots may be useful in three ways. First, the origin of a particular pain may be more accurately defined. Secondly, injection into a peripheral trigger point, for example in muscle, may reduce widely radiating pain and offer effective treatment with one or a series of injections; and thirdly, in the case of neuropathic pain due to peripheral nerve or root lesions, failure to relieve all the pain with an adequate peripheral nerve or root block indicates an element of secondary central pain, which will be less amenable to peripheral measures. There is some evidence that lesions including trigger points in muscle, painful scars, and peripheral nerve lesions such as neuromas may respond better to a combination of local anaesthetic and corticosteroid. However, in some patients the tissue disruption caused by local injections may exacerbate pain.

Epidural injection of a local anaesthetic, with or without an opiate, can produce analgesia over a wide area. Its use in obstetric analgesia and other operative treatment is well established. In relief of chronic pain, single or repeated epidural injections may have a partial, lasting effect in some patients. The use of highly lipid-soluble opiates such as fentanyl ensures rapid local absorption into neural tissue in the region of needle or catheter tip, producing good analgesia, with less risk of drug spread. Thus, the epidural route may be safely used throughout the spine, though with caution in the cervical region due to the greater risk of producing respiratory depression. Low back pain with root pain not amenable to surgery, arachnoiditis, and brachalgia with neck pain may respond to such treatment.

A further development in the treatment of pain of non-malignant origin is the epidural infusion of a local anaesthetic and an opiate over periods of 2 to 3 weeks. In some patients a period of analgesia thus obtained may produce a degree of long-lasting or even permanent pain relief following the block, although often the pain returns to its former level within days or weeks.

A variable degree of motor block is produced by epidural analgesia, together with loss of bladder and bowel control, although it is usually possible to titrate the amount of drug used to produce localized unilateral sensory blockade which causes minimal motor deficit and spares sphincter function. Epidural or intrathecal infusion of opiate over long periods has proved useful in the management of pelvic pain due to cancer.

Injection of very low concentrations of morphine into the third ventricle may produce profound analgesia, associated with a low risk of respiratory depression. This procedure has been advocated for the relief of bilateral pain due to cancer affecting the neck and skull base, and may prove to have wider application.

Sympathetic blocks

Intravenous injection of the short-acting sympathetic blocker, phentolamine, has some value in indicating which patients have sympathetically maintained pain and in predicting the response to other types of sympathetic block, either local anaesthetic block of cervical and lumbar sympathetic ganglia or intravenous regional guanethidine block (IVRG). IVRG, given by the Bier's block technique, either in the arm or leg, produces partial sympathetic blockade for several days. For sympathetically maintained pain associated with peripheral nerve lesions, there is sometimes a cumulative analgesic effect from a series of such blocks. The results of permanent sympathectomy, produced either surgically or chemically with phenol, are often disappointing for reasons that are not entirely clear. An additional danger of phenol sympathectomy is damage to the nearby brachial and lumbosacral plexuses, which is often associated with severe pain. For these reasons, repeated temporary sympathetic blocks are preferable.

SYSTEMIC DRUGS

Simple analgesics, NSAIDs and weak opiates

Simple analgesics (such as paracetamol and aspirin) the NSAIDs, weak opiates (including codeine, dihydrocodeine, and dextropropoxyphene), partial opiate agonists (such as buprenorphine) mixed agonist antagonist drugs (for example pentazocine), and strong opiates may have a beneficial effect in nociceptive pains. Long-term therapy may be limited by side-effects and, in the case of opiates, there are additional problems of habituation and addiction. Careful clinical judgement must be applied to the use of any analgesic drug over long periods. All these analgesics are much less effective for neuropathic pains. None the less, many patients with neuropathic pains, both of peripheral and central origin, will report some lasting analgesia, and many will wish to take simple analgesics or weak opiates on a long-term basis. The prescription of morphine and other strong opiates should always be resisted in patients with pain of non-malignant origin.

Psychotropic drugs: antidepressants, minor tranquillizers, and neuroleptic drugs

Depression is a common accompaniment to chronic pain and lowers tolerance to pain. Antidepressant treatment will help depressed patients whatever the type of pain. The tricyclic antidepressants have an enhancing effect on the descending bulbospinal 5HT-mediated analgesic pathway to the dorsal horn, and thus theoretically have an analgesic action independent of any antidepressant effect. An analgesic effect of amitriptyline has been shown convincingly in some neuropathic pains, notably post-herpetic neuralgia. However, zimolidine, a tricyclic with a greater serotoninergic effect than amitriptyline, is less effective, and the newer, selective, serotonin re-uptake inhibitor drugs have not been shown to be superior to amitriptyline in their analgesic effect.

Benzodiazepines such as diazepam, oxazepam, and chlordiazepoxide may be helpful for short-term relief of anxiety and of muscle spasm associated with some pains. However, sedation, dysphoria, dependence, and severe withdrawal effects in some patients limit their use in chronic pains. This is particularly true for lorazepam.

Neuroleptic drugs have often been advocated for the treatment of neuropathic pains but, in the absence of clear evidence of useful effect in controlled studies, these drugs are best avoided in view of their extrapyramidal effects. An exception is chlorprothixene, which is occasionally helpful in a variety of neuropathic pains and which does not produce extrapyramidal effects at the doses used (up to 45 mg/day).

Antiepileptic drugs

Antiepileptic drugs have no effect in nociceptive pains. With the exception of the remarkably specific effect of carbamazepine in trigeminal neuralgia, antiepileptic drugs are also disappointingly ineffective in neuropathic pains. Although claims have been made for carbamazepine, phenytoin, valproate, and clonazepam in a variety of neuropathic pains, positive results have, on the whole, only emerged from poorly controlled short-term trials.

Sympathetic blocking drugs

Other than phentolamine, neither α- nor β-blockers have been shown convincingly to have any long-term analgesic effects in chronic pain.

Membrane-stabilizing drugs

Intravenous infusions of lignocaine at doses as small as 1 mg/kg have been shown to reduce neuropathic pain and associated allodynia and hyperpathia, but this is not a practical long-term treatment. Mexiletine, which can be taken orally, has local anaesthetic-like membrane-stabilizing properties and has been shown to have a short-term analgesic effect in painful diabetic peripheral neuropathy. However, long-term treatment in this and other neuropathies and a variety of central neuropathic pains has no demonstrable analgesic effect.

ROLE OF SURGERY IN THE TREATMENT OF CHRONIC PAIN

The indications for surgical treatment for chronic pain are now very limited. These indications, and comments about particular problems with lesions at different levels, are discussed here.

Peripheral neurolysis

The risks of producing neuropathic pain with neurolytic procedures are high. Partial percutaneous intercostal neurectomy by radiofrequency lesioning may relieve pain due to malignant invasion of the chest wall. The same technique will reduce the allodynia of post-herpetic neuralgia, but will tend to increase deafferentation and may lead to increased pain. Neurolysis for other benign sensory mononeuropathies, such as meralgia paraesthetica, may provide short-term analgesia but usually results in later development of a different and worse pain. In addition, the sensory loss itself may be poorly tolerated. The combination of sensory loss and pain is known as anaesthesia dolorosa and is particularly a problem on the face, caused by neurolytic procedures used in the treatment of trigeminal neuralgia.

Rhizotomy

Surgery to dorsal roots has the theoretical advantage of selectively lesioning sensory fibres, but operations on several adjacent roots may be necessary, as the noxious input from most peripheral causes is rarely confined to a single dorsal root. The resulting sensory loss is usually unacceptable. Although rhizotomy has been advocated for the relief of conditions such as occipital neuralgia and coccydynia, short-term results are unpredictable and the risk of producing a new type of chronic neuropathic pain are high.

Dorsal root entry zone lesions

The dorsal root entry zone lesion devised by Nashold was based on the observation that deafferented dorsal horn neurones show disinhibited activity. This is of relevance to conditions such as post-herpetic neuralgia and brachial plexus avulsion. Thermocoagulation or laser lesions are made in the superficial layers of the dorsal horn in the deafferented spinal segments. As with other neuroablative procedures, the extent of the lesion is hard to control, and a degree of ipsilateral pyramidal weakness is common, indicating a lesion extending much deeper than the dorsal horn. Brachial plexus avulsion pain is now the only agreed indication for this operation, although there may be a role in myelopathic pain associated with paraplegia. In post-herpetic neuralgia there is an unacceptably high incidence of severe motor deficits, and this, together with variable success in achieving analgesia, has led to most centres abandoning the operation for this condition.

Anterolateral cordotomy

Section of the spinothalamic tract in the anterolateral quadrant of the cord, usually now performed by a percutaneous radiofrequency heat lesion at C2 level, is useful in relieving contralateral cancer pain. Analgesia may be short-lived, so the procedure is only indicated for patients with a prognosis of months at most. The complication rate in experienced hands is remarkably low.

Thalamotomy

There have been many attempts to produce lasting analgesia by selective lesioning within the posterior and medial thalamic nuclei, to which a large part of the spinothalamic tract projects. Lesions within the intralaminar group produce the best analgesia and have been recommended for chronic intractable pain, both nociceptive and neuropathic. However, the analgesia often lasts only a few months and new dysaesthesiae related to the operation may develop.

Leucotomy

Analgesia may result following leucotomy, which destroys frontothalamic connections. Patients report that their pain is still present but it does not distress them in the same way. Unfortunately, analgesia can only be achieved at the expense of a change in personality.

CNS STIMULATION

Dorsal column stimulation

Direct stimulation of the dorsal columns has the advantage over TENS of giving stimulation over a much wider area. Dorsal column stimulation is only effective when the region of the patient's pain is covered by the stimulation and this is often technically difficult to achieve. Moreover, in many patients good initial results are not sustained over long periods, for reasons that are not always clear. Dorsal column stimulation may be particularly useful in unilateral lower limb pain, for example persistent lumbosacral root pain after failed back surgery or when arachnoiditis is present. Segmental inhibition at dorsal horn level is a possible mechanism of the action of dorsal column stimulation, as is more rostral inhibition at the thalamic level. Dorsal column stimulation does not raise endorphin levels in the cerebrospinal fluid and the analgesia induced is not naloxone reversible.

Periaqueductal grey stimulation

Stimulation of the periaqueductal grey and its rostral extension to the level of the third ventricle in the hypothalamus, the periventricular grey, activates descending opiate-mediated analgesic pathways, and has been used in the treatment of intractable pain in man. However, it is technically difficult, and spread of stimulation often leads to side-effects, including nystagmus and other oculomotor disorders, nausea, vertigo, dyspnoea, anxiety, and panic. Overstimulation causes habituation and loss of effect. Periaqueductal grey stimulation is relatively ineffective in neuropathic pain. It is currently little used.

Thalamic stimulation

Stimulation in the main thalamic sensory nuclei may produce analgesia, probably due to a gating mechanism, similar to TENS and dorsal column stimulation. It has been used for both intractable nociceptive and neuropathic pains, including thalamic pain. CT-guided stereotactic techniques permit accurate placement of electrodes and, in contrast to thalamotomy, the risk of damage to the nearby internal capsule and other structures is acceptably low. However, as with all types of neural stimulation, the results are unpredictable and analgesia is often short-lived.

PSYCHOLOGICAL MEASURES

Leaving aside the psychiatric disorders associated with pain discussed above and which call primarily for psychiatric treatment, psychological

intervention has a role in the management of other chronic pain problems. At a basic level, careful explanation of the nature of the problem and, particularly with neuropathic pain of non-malignant origin, reassurance that the pain does not indicate ongoing progressive tissue damage, is very important. Getting patients to accept some responsibility for their pain and its treatment is often the first step towards the patient gaining control over the pain and its effects. Involving the patient in measures such as TENS further promotes the feeling of control over their pain.

In addition to these simple approaches, other helpful psychological interventions include relaxation therapy, biofeedback, and cognitive and behavioural methods, which form the basis of many pain-management programmes. Hypnosis has a limited role in the treatment of chronic pain but may be successful in susceptible individuals.

REHABILITATION

The importance of rehabilitation for patients with chronic pain cannot be overemphasized. For many, their pain has been the major focus of their lives for long periods and the effects far reaching in terms of limitation of work and other activities and impact on personal relationships. At all levels, energetic multidisciplinary efforts are needed to rehabilitate patients with chronic pain, many of whom also face other physical and sometimes psychological disabilities. Detailed discussion of rehabilitation is beyond the scope of this chapter, but one point is worth emphasizing. When any pain-relieving procedure, however temporary, is successful, it is essential that the use of the affected painful part begins immediately. Thus, with sensory or sympathetic blocks, the physiotherapist should be present to start passive and active movements straight away. Analgesia alone is insufficient to regain function and unless strenuous immediate efforts are made, rehabilitation is likely to fail.

REFERENCE

P.D. Wall and R. Melzack (eds). (1994). *Textbook of pain*. 3rd edn. Churchill Livingstone, Edinburgh.

24.6 Cerebrovascular disease

C. P. WARLOW

Cerebrovascular disease includes disorders of the vascular system which cause ischaemia, infarction or haemorrhage in the brain. In most developed countries this is the third most common cause of death, after coronary heart disease and cancer, and is responsible for much physical and mental disability in the elderly. In the British National Health Service about 5 per cent of the budget is devoted to stroke care.

DEFINITIONS

Many terms used to describe cerebrovascular disease are confusing but two are generally accepted: a transient ischaemic attack is an acute loss of focal cerebral or monocular function with symptoms lasting less than 24 h and which, after adequate investigation, is presumed to be due to embolic or thrombotic vascular disease. A stroke (or cerebrovascular accident) is a rapidly developing episode of focal, and at times global (applied to patients in deep coma and to those with subarachnoid hae-

morrhage), loss of cerebral function, with symptoms lasting more than 24 h or leading to death, with no apparent cause other than that of vascular origin; the main pathological types of stroke are cerebral infarction, primary intracerebral haemorrhage, and subarachnoid haemorrhage. These two rather rigid definitions have an indistinct boundary in clinical practice because the 24-h time limit separating stroke from transient ischaemic attack is entirely arbitrary. There are many patients whose symptoms resolve in a matter of days and who therefore have had, by definition, a stroke, even though there is no persisting neurological disability; along with transient ischaemic attacks, such episodes, if ischaemic rather than haemorrhagic, are sometimes referred to as reversible ischaemic attacks and their pathogenesis, investigation, and treatment are the same as for transient ischaemic attacks. However, the differential diagnosis of brief neurological attacks lasting minutes or hours is different from more prolonged episodes lasting days, and transient ischaemic attacks, unlike some mild strokes, are never caused by primary intracerebral haemorrhage.

Epidemiology

The annual incidence of stroke in developed countries is about two per 1000 population, but the exact figure depends on the age structure of the population because the incidence rises steeply with increasing age (Fig. 1). Other reasons for differences in incidence between and within countries are differences in diagnostic criteria, whether only first-ever strokes or all strokes are being analysed, and perhaps the year of the study because the incidence of both cerebral infarction and primary intracerebral haemorrhage is falling in some countries. The prevalence of stroke is about 5 per 1000 population. The annual incidence of transient ischaemic attacks is about 0.5 per 1000 population, and so about 25 000 new cases per annum present to doctors in the United Kingdom.

Until the introduction of computed tomography (CT) scanning, the understanding of cerebrovascular disease was hampered by the impossible task of differentiating intracranial haemorrhage, with the exception of subarachnoid haemorrhage, from cerebral infarction on the basis of just the clinical symptoms and signs. Nowadays, as a rough estimate, it is known that about 80 per cent of strokes are due to cerebral infarction, 10 per cent to primary intracerebral haemorrhage, and 10 per cent to subarachnoid haemorrhage. In Japan and China, the proportion due to primary intracerebral haemorrhage is rather higher.

Epidemiological studies have identified various risk factors for stroke, which are similar to those for coronary heart disease. Hypertension is the most important, both for cerebral infarction and primary intracerebral haemorrhage. The risk of stroke increases with increasing blood pressure in both sexes and at all ages; this risk about doubles with each 7.5 mmHg rise in diastolic blood pressure. Interestingly, there is much less difference in the incidence of cerebral infarction between males and females (Fig. 1) than there is for myocardial infarction. Other risk factors for cerebral infarction include heart disease of any kind, atrial fibrillation, transient ischaemic attacks, peripheral vascular disease, diabetes mellitus, smoking, high blood cholesterol, high blood fibrinogen, factor VII coagulant activity, heavy alcohol consumption, cervical arterial bruit, poor maternal and infant health, and social deprivation. The contraceptive pill increases the risk of stroke by about three times. It is claimed that by identifying the important risk factors for stroke in an asymptomatic population it is possible to identify the 10 per cent from which 50 per cent of the subsequent cases of stroke will emerge. Indeed, stroke is distinctly unusual in an individual without one or more risk factors for vascular disease.

Fig. 1 Age- and sex-specific incidence of first-ever in a lifetime stroke in Oxfordshire, 1981–86. About 25 per cent occur under the age of 65, 50 per cent below the age of 75, and 50 per cent above the age of 75.

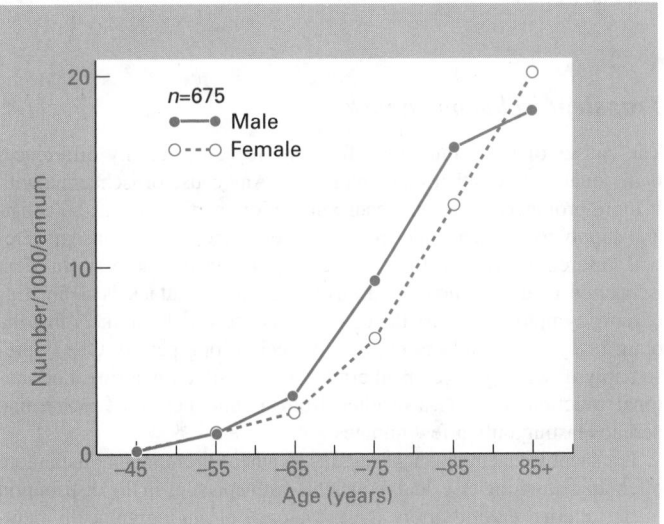

Although the effect of racial and genetic factors is not fully known, there are some well-known but rare familial causes of stroke (Table 1)

The blood supply to the brain

Because most strokes are the result of cerebral infarction, which is caused by an impaired blood supply to the brain, it is important to be familiar with the anatomy of both the extracranial and intracranial arterial supply and the way in which it is affected by atheroma, the commonest disorder of arteries in the developed world. The brain has a particularly rich blood supply which is derived from four main arteries: the left and right internal carotid and vertebral arteries (Fig. 2). The internal carotid artery supplies the eye through the ophthalmic artery and then divides into the anterior and middle cerebral arteries which supply the anterior two-thirds of the cerebral hemisphere, the basal ganglia, and the internal capsule regions (Fig. 3). The vertebral arteries unite to form the basilar artery, whose branches supply the brain-stem and cerebellum, which then divides into the two posterior cerebral arteries supplying the posterior one-third of the cerebral hemispheres (Fig. 3). The carotid arterial systems are interconnected by the anterior communicating artery and are linked with the vertebrobasilar system by the posterior communicating arteries so forming the circle of Willis at the base of the brain (Fig. 4). In many individuals parts of this arterial ring are hypoplastic and fewer than half are of the standard pattern. None the less, it can form, unless affected by disease, an excellent collateral channel for blood to the brain if one or more of the four main extracranial arteries is occluded. Other potential collateral channels may also become functionally important: branches of the internal carotid artery and external carotid artery anastomose with each other around and within the orbit; anastomoses between arterial branches in the cortex; meningeal anastomoses, since the dura is supplied by the internal and external carotid arteries and vertebral arteries; and there are various anastomoses between the major arteries in the neck.

Cerebral blood flow is autoregulated to ensure a constant supply of blood to the brain between mean systemic blood pressures of approximately 60 and 160 mmHg. Within this range a rise in blood pressure is met by intracranial vasoconstriction, and a fall by vasodilatation. However, outside these limits cerebral blood flow follows perfusion pressure: ischaemia occurs if the systemic blood pressure falls, and vasogenic oedema and ultimately hypertensive encephalopathy if it rises. These limits within which autoregulation is effective are set higher in patients with chronic hypertension who will, therefore, experience ischaemia at a higher level of systemic blood pressure than normotensive individuals. However, a patient with sustained hypertension, and whose autoregulation is set higher, is less likely to sustain cerebral damage and hypertensive encephalopathy than a normotensive patient when there is an acute increase in blood pressure (e.g. during eclampsia).

When the brain is damaged by stroke or other diseases, focal areas may no longer autoregulate normally and blood flow will follow fluctuations in systemic blood pressure, while the reactivity to arterial $P\text{aco}_2$ is often impaired as well (under normal circumstances an acute rise of 1 mmHg in $P\text{aco}_2$ increases cerebral blood flow by 5 per cent). These abnormalities are unpredictable and presumably depend on the age of the brain lesion and exactly where flow is being considered in relation to that lesion.

Cerebral blood flow falls with increasing levels of haematocrit, even through the commonly accepted normal range. However, this is not so much because the high haematocrit increases whole-blood viscosity, but because the higher oxygen carrying capacity of high haematocrit blood allows a lower cerebral blood flow for the same oxygen delivery.

THE PATTERN OF ATHEROMA

Atheroma is a generalized disorder of large and medium-sized arteries affecting, clinically or subclinically, the blood supply to many organs

Table 1 *Some causes of 'familial' stroke*

Vascular anomalies	Vascular malformation
	Saccular aneurysm
	Hereditary haemorrhagic telangiectasia
Connective tissue anomalies	Ehlers–Danlos syndrome
	Pseudoxanthoma elasticum
	Marfan's syndrome
	Polycystic kidney disease
	Mitral leaflet prolapse
Haematological diseases	Haemophilia and other coagulation factor deficiencies
	Sickle-cell disease
	Antithrombin III deficiency
	Protein C deficiency
	Protein S deficiency
Others	Familial hypercholesterolaemia
	Cerebral amyloid angiopathy (Icelandic form)
	Neurofibromatosis
	Tuberous sclerosis
	Homocystinaemia
	Fabry's disease
	Migraine
	Cardiac myxoma
	Von Hippel–Lindau syndrome
	Mitochondrial cytopathy

Fig. 2 The arterial blood supply to the brain and eye. Places most often affected by atherothrombosis are shown as white indentations into the arterial lumen.

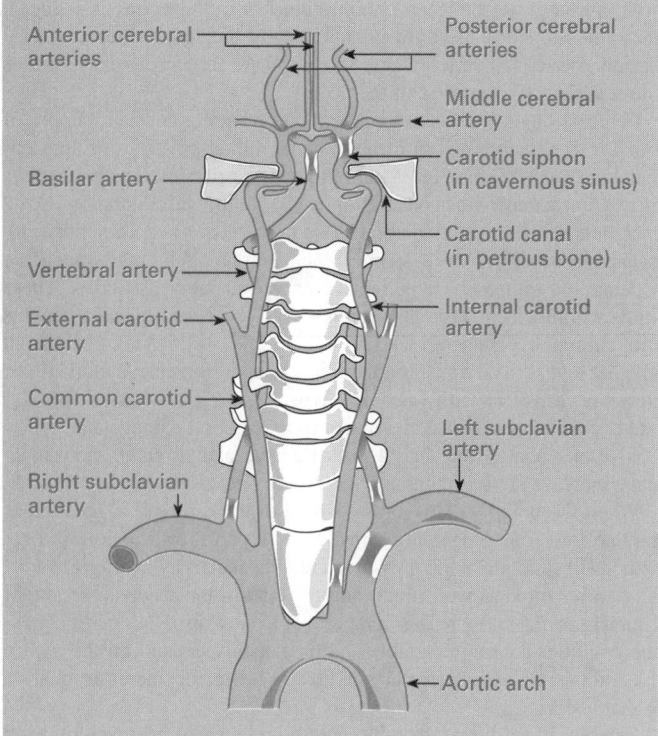

and parts of the body. It tends to occur at points of arterial branching and tortuosity, which are sites of haemodynamic stress on the arterial wall, turbulent blood flow, and blood stasis. It is more extensive in hypertensive than normotensive individuals. The common sites of atheroma in the arteries supplying the brain are shown in Fig. 2 and the most important are the bifurcation of the common carotid artery into the internal and external carotid arteries, the carotid siphon within the cavernous sinus, the origin and termination of the vertebral arteries, the basilar artery, the circle of Willis, the proximal portions of the three cerebral arteries, the origin of the major arteries from the aorta, and the arch of the aorta itself. It is remarkable how free of atheroma certain areas can be, particularly the internal carotid artery between its origin and the siphon.

Thrombosis occurs on atheromatous plaques which have ulcerated as a result of plaque fracture, necrosis, or intraplaque haemorrhage, and also in areas of turbulent or sluggish blood flow in relation to atheromatous stenotic areas which are severe enough to have an important haemodynamic effect. Thrombi may occlude arteries, embolize to distal sites, be lysed, become incorporated into the plaques themselves, or propagate proximally and/or distally. The whole process of atherothromboembolism may be at different stages in different arteries, or even along one artery of the same individual. It is this underlying pathology which is the single most common cause of cerebral ischaemia and infarction. It is important to stress the close relationship between atheroma in arteries supplying the brain, coronary artery atheroma, and arterial disease in the periphery; a patient with clinically manifest disease in one area will almost certainly have subclinical, or clinically manifest, disease in other areas.

Transient ischaemic attacks

The causes of ischaemia and infarction are identical, any differences being quantitative rather than qualitative. Any cause of ischaemia will, if more prolonged or severe, cause infarction, particularly if the collateral supply to the ischaemic area is inadequate, while any cause of cerebral infarction will, if less severe or prolonged, cause a transient ischaemic attack. Although a transient ischaemic attack is defined as causing symptoms for less than 24 h, it is exceedingly unlikely that the brain or eye is actually ischaemic for such a long period. One is presumably observing the clinical effects of reversible impairment of neuronal function which has resulted from a short period of ischaemia, perhaps lasting only a few minutes.

Transient ischaemic attacks are due to atherothromboembolism more often than anything else, and in patients with episodes in the distribution of the internal carotid artery the prevalence of angiographically demonstrated disease of the artery is about 50 per cent. However, the heart

(Table 2) is also a particularly potent source of emboli to the brain, eye, and elsewhere; about 30 per cent of patients with a transient ischaemic attack have a potential, if not a definite, cardiac source of embolism, the most common being non-rheumatic atrial fibrillation, and in perhaps 20 per cent of patients with a transient ischaemic attack embolism from the heart is the actual cause of the attack. Like lacunar ischaemic stroke (see below), some transient ischaemic attacks are due to small vessel disease within the brain. Others may be due to embolism from atherothrombosis affecting the aortic arch. A transient fall in blood pressure (e.g. due to postural hypotension, vasodilators or other hypotensive drugs, cardiac

Table 2 *Cardiac sources of embolism (in anatomical sequence)*

Paradoxical embolism from the venous system
  Atrial septal defect
  Ventricular septal defect
  Patent foramen ovale
  Pulmonary arteriovenous fistula

Left atrium
  Atrial fibrillation
  Sinoatrial disease
  Myxoma
  Interatrial septal aneurysm

Mitral valve
  Rheumatic stenosis or regurgitation
  Infective endocarditis
  Non-bacterial thrombotic (marantic) endocarditis
  Prosthetic valve
  Mitral annulus calcification
  Mitral leaflet prolapse
  Libman–Sacks endocarditis

Left ventricular mural thrombus
  Acute myocardial infarction
  Left ventricular aneurysm
  Cardiomyopathy
  Myxoma
  Blunt chest injury

Aortic valve
  Rheumatic stenosis or regurgitation
  Infective endocarditis
  Non-bacterial thrombotic (marantic) endocarditis
  Prosthetic valve
  Calcification and/or sclerosis
  Syphilis

Congenital cardiac disorders
  (particularly with right to left shunt)

Cardiac surgery

Fig. 3 The areas supplied by the anterior cerebral artery (a), middle cerebral artery (b), and the posterior cerebral artery (c) in horizontal slices through the brain. The dark shadowing represent the minimal territories and the light shadowing the maximal territories. (Adapted with permission from Dr Albert van der Zwan.)

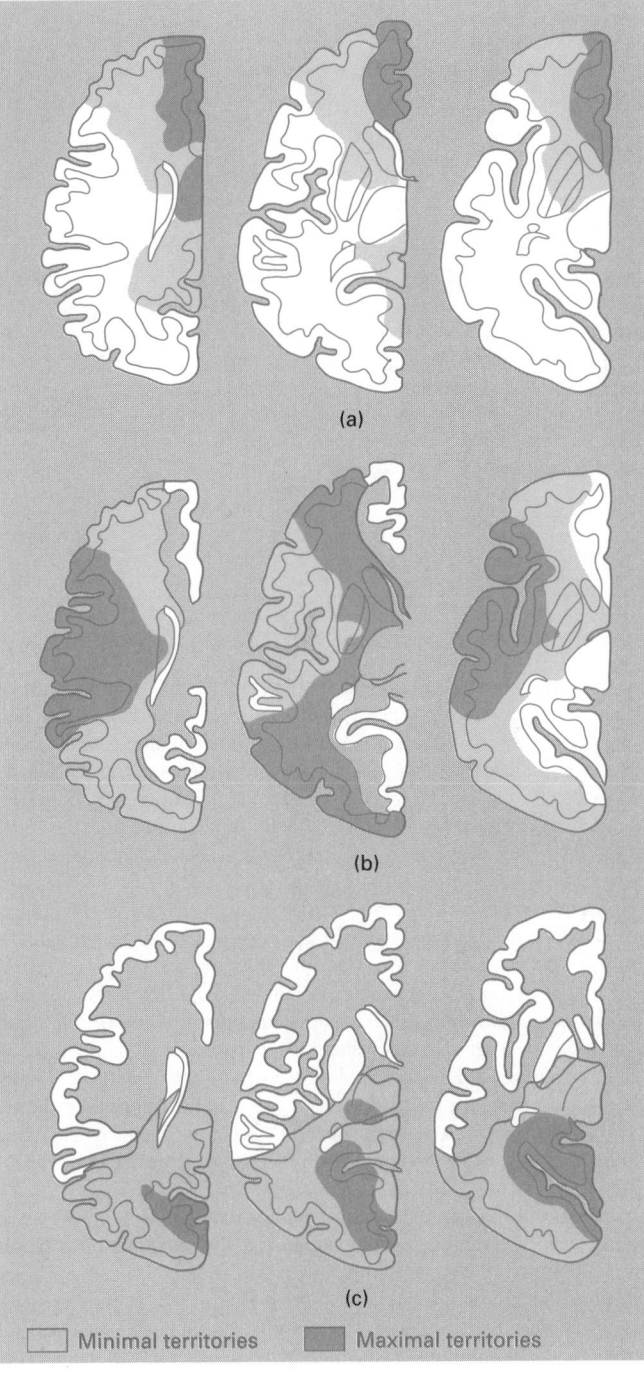

(a)

(b)

(c)

☐ Minimal territories   ■ Maximal territories

Fig. 4 The circle of Willis as seen at the base of the brain in relation to the optic chiasm.

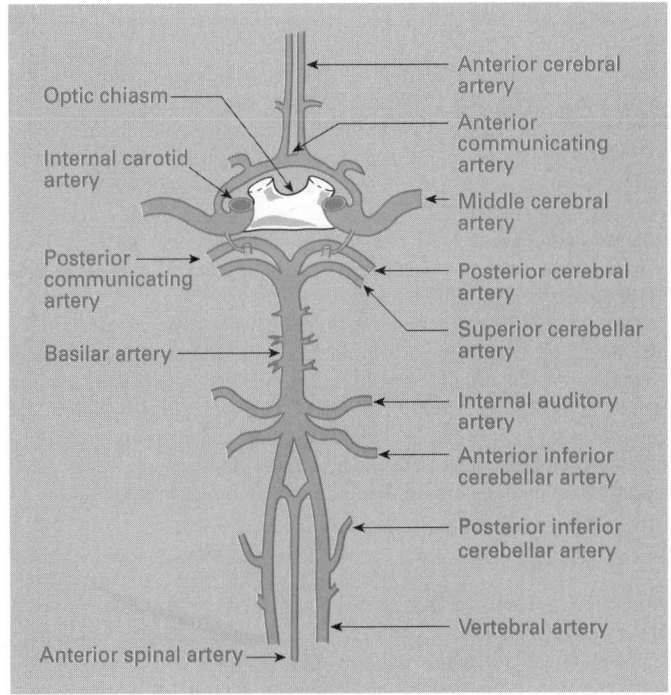

Table 3 *Causes of arterial disease*

Atheroma	Dissection
	Trauma
Intracerebral small-vessel disease (lipohyalinosis,	Cystic medial necrosis
microatheroma)	Fibromuscular dysplasia
	Inflammatory arterial disease
Inflammatory vascular disease	Marfan's syndrome
Giant-cell arteritis	Pseudoxanthoma elasticum
Systemic lupus erythematosus	Ehlers–Danlos syndrome
Systemic vasculitis	Infective arterial disease (e.g. syphilis)
Sarcoid angiitis	
Behçet's disease	Congenital
Progressive systemic sclerosis	Fibromuscular dysplasia
Rheumatoid disease	Loops, coils, etc.
Sjögren's syndrome	Aneurysms
Relapsing polychondritis	
Takayasu's disease	Infections
Isolated granulomatous angiitis of the nervous system	Tonsillitis, pharyngitis
Malignant atrophic papulosis (Kohlmeier–Degos disease)	Cervical lymphadenitis
Buerger's disease	Endarteritis obliterans due to tuberculosis, syphilis, bacterial or fungal
	meningitis etc.
Trauma	Herpes zoster
Penetrating injuries of the neck	Mucormycosis
Blow to the neck	
Cervical manipulation	Miscellaneous
Yoga	Homocystinaemia
Cervical rib	Angioendotheliosis
'Whiplash' injury	Neoplastic invasion of the arterial wall
Tonsillectomy	Irradiation
Strangulation	Embolism from extra- or intracranial aneurysm sacs
Atlantoaxial dislocation/instability	Fabry's disease
Fractured clavicle	Inflammatory bowel disease
Fractured base of skull	Migraine
Angiography	Drug abuse
	Mitochondrial cytopathy
	Binswanger's disease
	Nephrotic syndrome
	Fat embolism
	Fibrocartilagenous embolism

arrhythmia, hot bath, heavy meal, etc.) can cause transient ischaemic attacks but only if one or more arteries to the brain (or eye) is extremely stenotic or occluded, or there is a focal area of defective autoregulation as a result of previous ischaemic damage. In general, a fall in blood pressure causes non-focal neurological symptoms such as faintness, bilateral dimming of vision, and generalized weakness. The pathogenesis of transient ischaemic attack in the vertebrobasilar distribution has been less well studied but is probably similar to that in the carotid distribution although haemodynamic rather than embolic causes may be more common, and, very occasionally, distortion of the vertebral arteries by cervical spondylosis is relevant.

About 5 per cent of patients with a transient ischaemic attack have rare forms of arterial disease (Table 3) or a haematological disorder (Table 4). It is important to emphasize that the pathogenesis of transient ischaemic attacks is heterogeneous and, even though the majority of episodes may well be due to embolism, the emboli themselves can consist of any combination of platelet aggregates, fibrin, calcific debri from heart valves, and cholesterol debris from atheromatous plaques.

CLINICAL FEATURES

A transient ischaemic attack starts abruptly and is not normally related to any particular activity. The attack may be single, recurrent but infrequent, or repetitive, and involve one or more parts of the brain or eye. On occasions transient ischaemic attacks can be remarkably stereotyped.

The symptoms usually all appear within a matter of seconds, with no spread from one part of the body to another, and depend on which part of the brain or eye is ischaemic. It can be difficult to elucidate the exact location of ischaemia in an individual patient, depending as it almost always does on a history taken after recovery. However, it is important to divide transient ischaemic attacks into carotid and vertebrobasilar distribution events if carotid surgery is a consideration (see below).

Ischaemia in the carotid territory may cause weakness in the contralateral face, arm, hand, or leg in isolation or in various combinations; numbness or paraesthesiae in a similar distribution; language disturbance if the dominant hemisphere is affected; dysarthria, but usually only in association with facial weakness; and transient monocular blindness (amaurosis fugax) in the ipsilateral eye. Ischaemic amaurosis fugax may involve the whole visual field of one eye or only the top or bottom half of the field and is often described like a blind, curtain, or shutter obscuring vision over a matter of seconds. It is important to realize that amaurosis fugax is a symptom, not a disease, and has several causes (Table 5).

Ischaemia in the vertebrobasilar territory may cause hemiparesis or hemisensory disturbance, bilateral blindness or a homonymous hemianopia, diplopia, vertigo, vomiting, dysarthria, dysphagia, ataxia, a bilateral motor deficit, or a bilateral sensory deficit. Thus, in patients with only unilateral motor or sensory symptoms it is impossible to be sure which arterial distribution has been affected unless there is some other

Table 4 *Haematological causes of cerebral ischaemia or infarction*

Sickle-cell disease
Polycythaemia rubra vera
Essential thrombocythaemia
Acute or chronic leukaemia
Thrombotic thrombocytopaenic purpura
Paroxysmal nocturnal haemoglobinuria
'Hyperviscosity' syndromes
  Multiple myeloma
  Waldenström's macroglobulinaemia
Severe anaemia (probably causes only transient cerebral
  symptoms)

Table 5 *Causes of transient monocular blindness (i.e. amaurosis fugax)*

Retinal ischaemia (i.e. transient ischaemic attack)
Papilloedema
Glaucoma
Uhthoff's phenomenon in retrobulbar neuritis
Retinal haemorrhage
Retinal detachment
Retinal venous thrombosis
Intraorbital tumour
Macular degeneration
Caroticocavernous fistula
Intracranial arteriovenous malformation
Reversible diabetic cataract
Retinal migraine?

symptom which definitely suggests carotid or vertebrobasilar ischaemia (such as dysphasia or diplopia, respectively).

Symptoms during a transient ischaemic attack may, by definition, last up to 24 h but are normally over in a matter of minutes, or perhaps an hour, and ischaemic amaurosis fugax rarely lasts more than 5 min. The rate of recovery is usually slower than the onset of the symptoms.

Some patients have a mild headache during or after a transient ischaemic attack and there may be chest pain or palpitations at the onset of an attack in the rare case with severe cerebral arterial disease precipitated by a cardiac arrhythmia. It is extremely unusual to lose consciousness and then, to make the diagnosis of transient ischaemic attack, there must be some additional focal neurological feature. Vertigo, dizziness, diplopia, faintness, dysarthria, unsteadiness, or confusion as isolated symptoms can be to due to thromboembolism in the vertebrobasilar territory, but are often caused by something else, such as a drop in systemic blood pressure, sudden head movement, or labyrinthine disorders. Therefore, transient ischaemic attack should never be diagnosed if there are only such symptoms in isolation.

Drop attacks

The patient, typically a middle-aged or elderly woman, suddenly falls to the ground, usually while walking, sometimes while standing. Consciousness may be lost for a fraction of a second so that the patient does not remember the actual fall. Considerable injury can result. In most patients no cause is found, there is no particular evidence of vascular disease, the attacks resolve and there are no long-term consequences.

Transient global amnesia

For a matter of a few hours there is profound loss of ability to remember any new information and there is usually retrograde amnesia as well, sometimes stretching back many years. The patient is fully conscious, knows his or her name, and is able to continue normal activities such as eating, walking, or even driving. He or she cannot recall what they have just done or what has just been said and so often repetitively ask the same question about such matters. Recovery is normally complete, but memory for the duration of the attack itself is not regained. This syndrome of transient global amnesia is very rarely caused by vertebrobasilar ischaemia affecting the temporal lobes or thalamus bilaterally through their posterior cerebral arterial supply. Occasional cases are epileptic, particularly if the attacks are frequently repeated and last less than an hour. In the vast majority of patients, however, no cause at all is found and the prognosis is very good, certainly much better than after a transient ischaemic attack, although sometimes the attacks do recur.

Subclavian steal

Subclavian steal is a rare syndrome in which, as a result of stenosis or occlusion of the subclavian artery proximal to the origin of the vertebral artery, any increased metabolic demand of the arm musculature during ipsilateral arm exercise is met by retrograde blood flow down the vertebral artery to cause symptoms of brain-stem ischaemia, particularly 'dizziness'. There is always a difference between the two radial pulses and unequal systolic blood pressures between the two arms, usually greater than 30 mmHg. Often there is a bruit in the supraclavicular fossa over the affected subclavian artery.

DIFFERENTIAL DIAGNOSIS

Transient ischaemic attacks may be caused by any kind of arterial (Table 3), cardiac embolic (Table 2), haematological (Table 4), or other disease leading to transient ischaemia of the brain or eye. They must be differentiated from migraine and focal epileptic seizures on the basis of an adequate history, if necessary from a witness as well as the patient. The aura of migraine is a spreading and slowly intensifying phenomenon and the symptoms are usually positive (e.g. scintillating scotomata). The aura characteristically reaches a maximum within about 5 min, lasts 20 to 30 min, and is usually, but not always, followed by severe headache, often with nausea and vomiting. Focal seizures also normally causes positive symptoms, particularly twitching, jerking, or dysaesthesiae, which spread or march up one limb and from one limb to another on the same side over a minute or so. Rare causes of transient focal neurological disturbances include structural brain disorders such as a tumour, subdural haematoma, arteriovenous malformation, and giant aneurysm, but these are very unusual effects of such lesions; malignant hypertension; hypoglycaemia; severe anaemia; the paroxysmal symptoms which sometimes occur in multiple sclerosis; peripheral nerve lesions; labyrinthine disorders such as Menière's disease; and somatization which curiously is more likely to involve the left than right side of the body.

PHYSICAL SIGNS

If the patient happens to be examined during an attack, then the signs appropriate to the ischaemic part of the nervous system will be found. But usually the patient is examined after the attack, when there should be no abnormal neurological signs; if there are, then some, perhaps only trivial, neurological damage has occurred. Whether or not abnormal physical signs are found also depends on the time since the attack and on the competence of the examiner. It is important to examine carefully the arterioles in the retina for any evidence of embolization (Fig. 5): platelet emboli appear as white bodies passing through the circulation, calcific fragments of heart valve as dense white deposits which often obstruct the retinal circulation near the disc margin, and cholesterol emboli as refractile and glittering yellow particles more peripherally, particularly at arteriolar branching points. Of considerable importance is examination of the vascular system, with a search for bruits over the carotid and subclavian arteries, absent or diminished foot pulses, femoral bruits, the pulses and blood pressure in both arms, and any signs of ischaemic or valvular heart disease. The site of various bruits in the neck is shown in Fig. 6, and their causes in Table 6.

INVESTIGATIONS

Investigations are directed towards the diagnosis of transient ischaemic attacks and excluding other causes of transient focal neurological attacks; finding the cause of the attack; defining risk factors for vascular disease in general; and the management of any associated vascular disease (Table 7).

Computed tomography (CT) (or magnetic resonance imaging (MRI)) excludes most structural intracranial disorders, but these are found unexpectedly in very few cases (well under 5 per cent). On CT about 25 per cent of patients have an area of infarction relevant to the transient ischaemic attack, even though clinically the symptoms lasted less than 24 h, but this does not alter management. If there is any reason to believe that there is a relevant cardiac source of embolism, then chest radiography and echocardiography, followed by further appropriate cardiological investigation, are required, i.e. clinical signs of a potential cardiac source of embolism, ischaemia in more than one arterial territory, a young patient with no risk factors for, or evidence of, arterial disease. On the whole, 24-h monitoring of the electrocardiogram (ECG) is unnecessary unless the patient also complains of transient non-focal neurological symptoms, such as a faintness or giddiness, or the transient

Fig. 5 A cholesterol embolus (black arrow) at the bifurcation of a retinal arteriole. Cholesterol emboli are yellow, refractile bodies which usually impact at arteriolar branching points without necessarily obstructing blood flow.

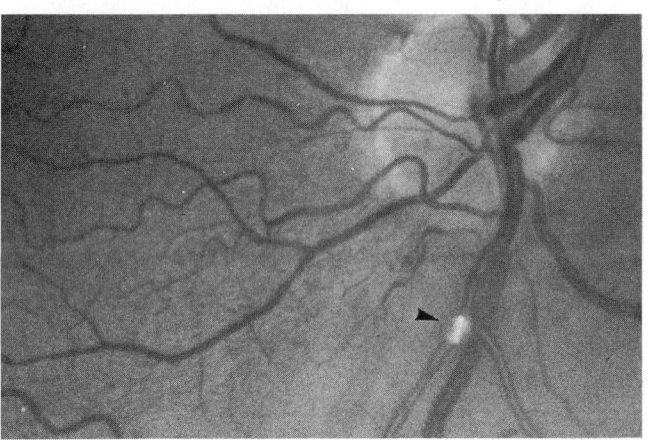

Fig. 6 The sites of maximum intensity of arterial bruits in the neck. Bruits behind the angle of the jaw may be due to either internal or external carotid origin stenosis, while bruits in the supraclavicular region may be due to stenosis of the subclavian or vertebral arteries.

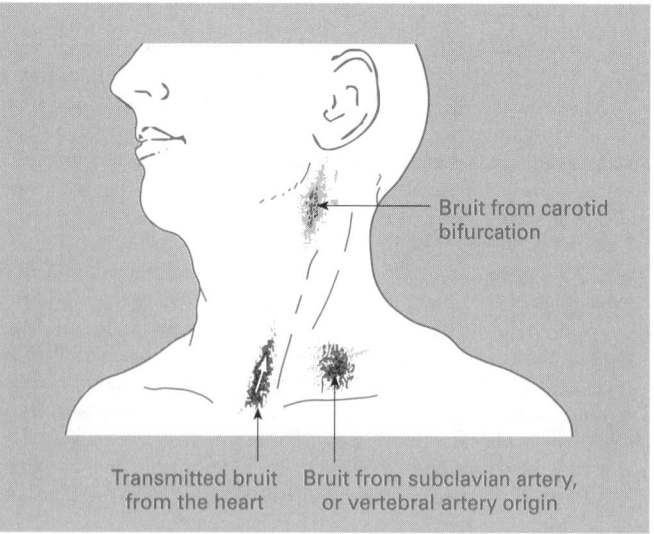

Transmitted bruit from the heart   Bruit from subclavian artery, or vertebral artery origin

Bruit from carotid bifurcation

Table 6 *Causes of cervical bruits*

Arterial disease
  Internal carotid artery origin stenosis
  External carotid artery origin stenosis
  Subclavian stenosis
  Vertebral artery origin stenosis

Transmitted bruit from arch of aorta, or heart

Increased blood flow
  Anaemia
  Thyrotoxicosis
  Fever
  Intracranial arteriovenous malformation
  Occlusion of contralateral internal carotid artery
  Goitre

Venous hums in the supraclavicular region

Benign arterial bruits in young adults

focal neurological symptoms are associated with chest pain or palpitations. Electroencephalography is not particularly helpful.

Imaging the cerebral circulation

The diagnosis of transient ischaemic attack is clinical and does not depend on the result of arterial imaging, which is to delineate the anatomy of arterial lesions which are appropriate to the symptoms and potentially amenable to carotid surgery, and then only in patients who are fit enough and willing to consider such surgery. The first step is real-time ultrasound imaging of the carotid bifurcation, combined with Doppler analysis of blood flow (so called Duplex, Fig. 7) to eliminate patients with little or no stenosis from the dangers of carotid angiography (about 1 per cent permanent stroke risk). For patients with carotid stenosis or possible occlusion, selective intra-arterial carotid angiography (by conventional or digital techniques) is then performed to demonstrate the symptomatic internal carotid artery in the neck and the intracranial circulation. Tightly stenosing lesions at the origin of the internal carotid artery (Fig. 8) are operable (see below), whereas intracranial lesions and internal carotid artery occlusion (Fig. 9) are not. The presence of a carotid bruit makes the likelihood of internal carotid artery stenosis high but, even without a bruit, there can be extreme stenosis with very low blood flow. Conversely, there can be a bruit, even in the presence of a relatively normal or occluded internal carotid artery, due to external carotid artery stenosis, or transmitted from the aortic valve or aortic arch. The absence of a carotid bruit should not, therefore, discourage one from Duplex if subsequent surgical intervention for carotid disease might be indicated. Palpating the carotid artery in the neck is not very useful because it is usually the common or external carotid pulsation that is being felt; if there is no pulsation at all then the common carotid artery is occluded. Conceivably, magnetic resonance angiography will replace conventional X-ray angiography—and its inherent risks—within the next few years.

MEDICAL TREATMENT

Transient ischaemic attacks are, by definition, short lasting and are seldom frequent or worrying enough to require treatment in their own right. However, the risk of stroke is about 12 per cent in the first year and then 7 per cent per annum, that of myocardial infarction or cardiac death is also about 7 per cent per annum, and of 'stroke, myocardial infarction, or vascular death' is about 10 per cent per annum. The excess risk of stroke in these patients is seven times that of the background population. Individual patients at highest risk are those with frequent transient ischaemic attacks, the elderly, claudicants, those with severe carotid stenosis, or with left ventricular hypertrophy.

Table 7 *Investigations recommended in cases of transient ischaemic attack (TIA)*

Investigation	Treatable disorder detected
Baseline tests for most TIA patients	
Full blood count	Anaemia, polycythaemia, leukaemia, thrombocythaemia
Erythrocyte sedimentation rate	Vasculitis, infective endocarditis, hyperviscosity
Plasma glucose	Diabetes, hypoglycaemia
Plasma cholesterol	Hypercholesterolaemia
Syphilis serology	Syphilis, anticardiolipin antibody
Urine analysis	Diabetes, renal disease
Electrocardiogram	Left ventricular hypertrophy, arrhythmia, conduction block, myocardial ischaemia or infarction
Non-routine investigations	
Electrolytes (if on diuretics)	Hyponatraemia or hypokalaemia
Urea (if hypertensive)	Renal impairment
Thyroid function (if in atrial fibrillation)	Thyrotoxicosis
Chest radiography	Enlarged heart, calcified valve, pulmonary arteriovenous malformation
Cranial CT/MRI	Structural brain lesion
Carotid ultrasound	Carotid stenosis
Echocardiography	Cardiac source of embolism
24-h ECG	Cardiac arrhythmia
Activated thromboplastin time, dilute Russell viper venom time, anticardiolipin antibody	Antiphospholipid antibody syndrome
Antinuclear antibodies	Systemic lupus erythematosus
Serum protein electrophoresis	Myeloma
Haemoglobin electrophoresis	Sickle-cell trait/disease
Electroencephalogram	Epileptic seizures
Protein C, protein S, antithrombin III	Deficiency
Plasma/urine amino acids	Homocystinaemia
Cerebrospinal fluid	Neurosyphilis, multiple sclerosis, infective endocarditis
Temporal artery biopsy	Giant-cell arteritis
Blood cultures	Infective endocarditis
Cardiac enzymes	Acute myocardial infarction

Fig. 7 Real-time ultrasound (lateral image) of a normal carotid bifurcation. The common carotid artery (small arrow with tail) bifurcates into the internal (arrows without tails) and external (large arrow) carotid arteries. (Reproduced by courtesy of Dr Pierre-Jean Touboul.)

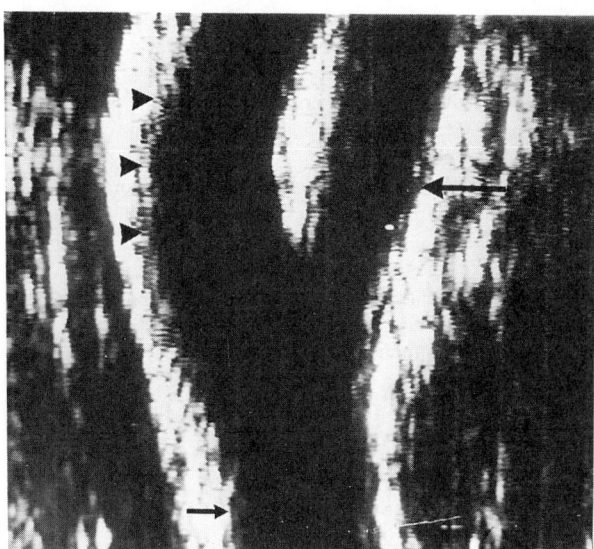

The most important issue in the management of transient ischaemic attacks is, therefore, reduction in the risk of stroke and coronary events, which can occur within hours, days, weeks, or years of the transient ischaemic attack. It is, therefore, logical to start any treatment as soon as the diagnosis is made, even if there has only been one attack. It is important to control treatable and causal vascular risk factors, particularly hypertension and cigarette smoking. The phase V diastolic blood pressure should be gradually lowered to about 100 mmHg, first by non-pharmacological means and then, if necessary, with drugs. In elderly patients, or those with severe arterial stenosis, it is important to use drugs cautiously because of the possibility of side-effects, particularly cerebral hypoperfusion and postural hypotension. It is probably helpful to control very abnormal glucose tolerance even if there are no symptoms of diabetes; reduce excessive weight if possible, to encourage exercise, and to lower the blood cholesterol by dietary changes unless it is very high (> 7.5 mmolar), when cholesterol-lowering drugs may be needed.

Long-term aspirin reduces the odds of serious vascular events by about one-fifth, similar to the reduction in other high risk vascular disease patients (Fig. 10). The dose is 150 mg daily, provided there are no contraindications such as peptic ulceration, but if there is indigestion then enteric-coated preparations are available, or a lower dose can be given but no lower than 75 mg daily, or there is the second-choice antiplatelet drug, ticlopidine (250 mg twice a day). It is conceivable that antiplatelet drugs increase the risk of intracranial haemorrhage which counteracts some of their beneficial effect in reducing the risk of cerebral infarction. If, as is sometimes the case, aspirin does not control very frequent transient ischaemic attacks then it is reasonable to try formal oral anticoagulation, which can be tailed off and replaced by aspirin a few weeks after the attacks stop. If the transient ischaemic attacks do not stop, either the diagnosis is wrong or the treatment is ineffective, in which case it should be reconsidered and perhaps stopped.

Patients with a definite major cardiac valvular source of embolism (such as mitral stenosis, a prosthetic valve, or dilating cardiomyopathy) should be anticoagulated indefinitely to prevent further intracardiac fibrin formation, particularly if atrial fibrillation is also present; the INR

Fig. 8 Lateral view of a selective carotid angiogram to show stenosis at the origin of the internal carotid artery (white arrow) just past the bifurcation of the common carotid artery (black arrow).

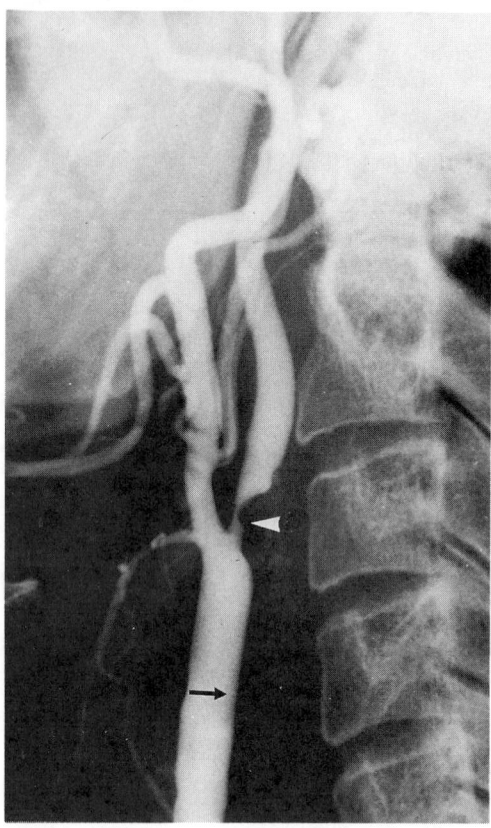

Fig. 9 Lateral view of a selective carotid angiogram to show occlusion of the internal carotid artery at its origin (arrow with tail). The external carotid artery is stenosed (arrow). It is always possible to distinguish the internal from external carotid artery because the latter has several branches in the neck, whereas the former does not.

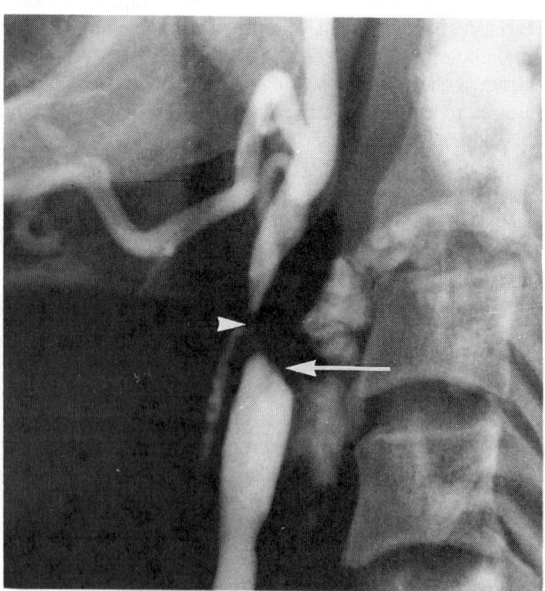

should be kept at about 3.5. If transient ischaemic attacks occur within days or weeks of an acute myocardial infarction, anticoagulation is only required for a matter of 3 to 6 months. Patients with non-rheumatic atrial fibrillation should be anticoagulated, but if this is not practical or too risky they should be given aspirin.

SURGERY

For patients who have recovered from a carotid ischaemic event, the removal of any tightly stenosing atherothrombotic lesion at the origin of the symptomatic internal carotid artery by carotid endarterectomy is logical because such a lesion is likely to cause stroke by embolism to the brain, or a reduction in cerebral blood flow if the stenosis is extreme. This logic now has the unambiguous backing of randomized trials which have shown that the more severe the stenosis is (above about 70 per cent diameter reduction of the arterial lumen) the greater the probability of ipsilateral ischaemic stroke without surgery and, therefore, the more worthwhile is the inevitable risk of surgery, which must be less than 5 to 10 per cent stroke and/or death. However, carotid endarterectomy should only be done in centres with adequate experience and where the risk is kept under continuous review. Carotid occlusion is inoperable.

Subclavian stenosis or occlusion causing subclavian steal can be dealt with by a variety of vascular surgical procedures which usually abolish the symptoms. Frequent vertebrobasilar transient ischaemic attacks due to vertebral stenosis or occlusion can occasionally be reduced in frequency by vascular surgical procedures in the neck.

Cerebral infarction

Cerebral infarction usually causes the clinical picture of stroke but occasionally there may only be a transient neurological deficit for less than 24 h (i.e. a transient ischaemic attack), or even no symptoms at all. The underlying pathogenesis is, like transient ischaemic attack, mostly atherothromboembolism, or embolism from the heart, and any difference between ischaemia and infarction is one of degree; a process which causes ischaemia must, if prolonged, eventually cause infarction, particularly if the potential collateral blood supply is compromised by preexisting disease. A fall in systemic blood pressure does not normally cause focal cerebral infarction unless a focal area of brain is already ischaemic, is supplied by an extremely stenotic artery, or is critically dependent on a collateral blood supply from a stenotic artery. Prolonged hypotension or anoxia normally causes widespread cerebral infarction and, if the patient survives the circulatory catastrophe, this infarction is often found to have occurred in the boundary zones between arterial territories (see below).

Cerebral infarcts are pale at first but may become haemorrhagic, particularly if the infarct is large. Infarction is associated with surrounding cerebral oedema and in large supratentorial infarcts the amount of 'swelling', and thus occupation of space, is extensive enough to cause transtentorial herniation (Fig. 11). This then causes secondary midbrain haemorrhage due to distortion and rupture of small penetrating vessels, and sometimes occipital infarction due to compression of the posterior cerebral artery against the edge of the tentorium. Cerebral oedema associated with an infarct takes a few days to develop to its maximum and then gradually resolves in 3 to 4 weeks.

CLINICAL FEATURES OF ISCHAEMIC STROKE

The symptoms, signs, duration, and severity of stroke due to cerebral infarction are very varied and depend on the location and extent of the lesion (Table 8). It can be difficult, and is not really always necessary, to relate the clinical picture exactly to embolic occlusion (or occasionally thrombosis) of a particular artery, because the state of the collateral blood supply as well as individual variation in vascular anatomy are of

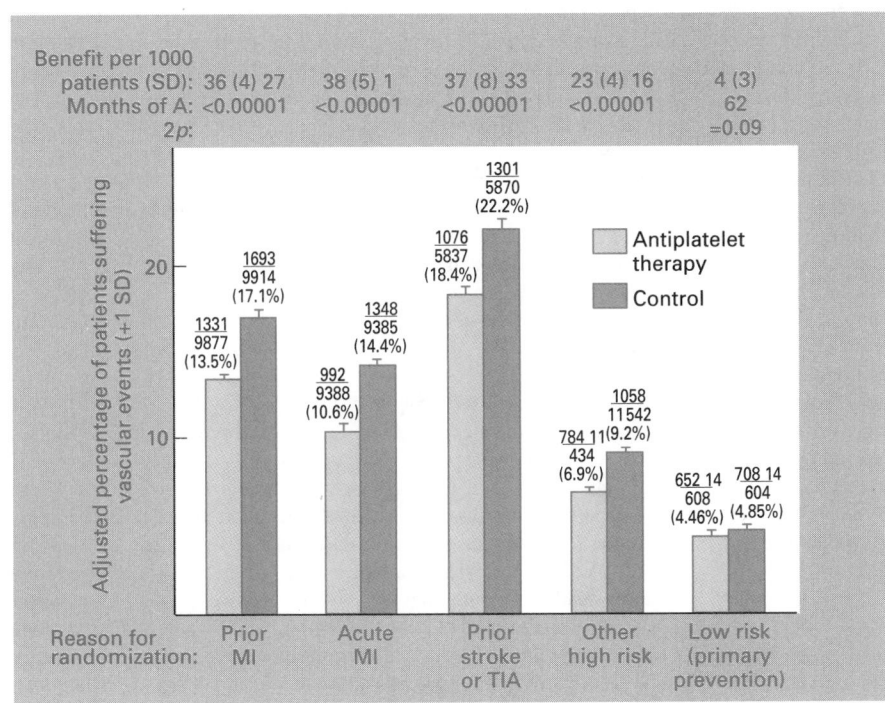

| Benefit per 1000 patients (SD): | 36 (4) 27 | 38 (5) 1 | 37 (8) 33 | 23 (4) 16 | 4 (3) |
| Months of A: 2*p*: | <0.00001 | <0.00001 | <0.00001 | <0.00001 | 62 =0.09 |

Fig. 10 Absolute effects of antiplatelet therapy on serious vascular events (myocardial infarction, stroke, or vascular death) in all main high risk categories of trial and in low risk (primary prevention). Months of A = means of scheduled antiplatelet duration. No trial lasted under 1 month. (Figure reproduced by permission of the British Medical Journal and the Antiplatelet Trialist's Collaboration.)

Fig. 11 Coronal section of a fixed brain to show a large infarct in the distribution of the right middle cerebral artery. The whole of the right cerebral hemisphere is swollen with oedema and there is downward herniation of the thalamus and mamillary bodies (closed arrow) and herniation of the cingulate gyrus across the midline (open arrow) below the falx. The right lateral ventricle is compressed and distorted (arrow without tail). Note the loss of demarcation between the cortical grey and underlying white matter in the swollen hemisphere. (Reproduced by courtesy of Dr Richard Greenhall.)

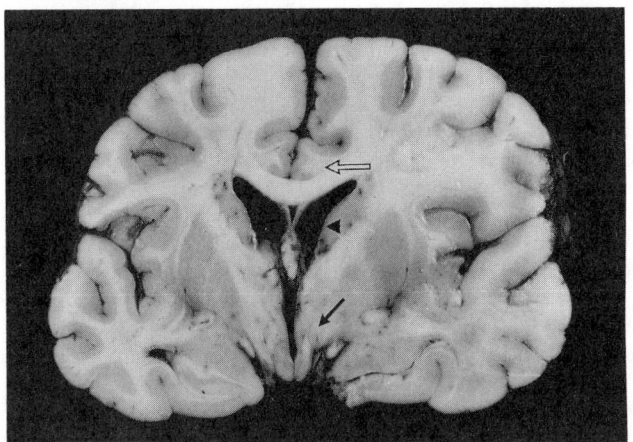

Table 8 *The distribution of the subtypes of cerebral infarction in the Oxfordshire Community Stroke Project*

Total anterior circulation infarction		15%
Partial anterior circulation infarction		35%
Lacunar infarction		25%
Pure motor stroke	50%	
Pure sensory stroke	5%	
Sensory motor stroke	35%	
Ataxic hemiparesis	10%	
Posterior circulation infarction		25%

bosis, but further embolization, haemorrhage into infarcted brain, or cerebral oedema, and these possibilities are difficult, if not impossible, to distinguish with any degree of certainty.

Cerebral hemisphere infarcts

Infarction in one cerebral hemisphere may cause contralateral hemiparesis or hemiplegia, hemisensory loss, or homonymous hemianopia. The motor and/or sensory disturbance may involve the entire side of the body, the upper limb, the face and the upper limb, both limbs, occasionally the leg alone, and rarely just the face. A small cortical infarct may cause clumsiness of the hand, or only of some of the fingers of one hand. To begin with, any hemiplegia tends to be flaccid with diminished deep tendon reflexes, albeit with an extensor plantar response, but within days or weeks spasticity and increased reflexes gradually appear. Lesions in the dominant hemisphere are likely to impair language function (speaking, reading, or writing) while in the non-dominant hemisphere may cause visuospatial problems, such as constructional or dressing apraxia. If the parietal lobe is affected, there is a tendency for the patient to ignore the contralateral side of the body; asterognosis; sensory inattention; sensory loss to all modalities; or just isolated loss of joint position sense. To begin with the head and eyes may be turned towards the side of the lesion but this usually resolves in a few days. Dysarthria tends to be in proportion to the extent of any facial weakness. Initially there is often some contralateral palatal weakness and dyspha-

very great importance in determining whether arterial occlusion causes infarction rather than ischaemia and, if so, how extensive it is. At one extreme it is possible to occlude the internal carotid artery without any symptoms but, at the other extreme, if the circle of Willis is compromised by arterial disease, the whole ipsilateral cerebral hemisphere can undergo infarction.

The onset of symptoms is normally quite sudden, or occurs during sleep, but there may be worsening in a subacute or stepwise fashion over a few hours; occasionally the clinical picture develops over a matter of several days but very rarely over a few weeks. An increase in the neurological deficit over a few hours or days is sometimes referred to as stroke-in-evolution but the cause may not only be propogating throm-

gia. Headache is quite common, but not usually very severe. Epileptic seizures are unusual but can be an early, or more often late, complication of cerebral infarction (less than 5 per cent of patients). If the infarct is extensive, and particularly if transtentorial herniation occurs, consciousness is impaired and Cheyne–Stokes or some other abnormality of the respiratory pattern develops.

It is helpful to identify patients who have infarcted the whole of their middle cerebral artery territory, usually because of middle cerebral artery occlusion as a result of embolism from the heart or proximal site of atherothrombosis. Total anterior circulation infarction is recognized by a combination of weakness, with or without a sensory deficit, of two out of three body areas (arm, leg, face) plus a homonymous hemianopia plus new higher cerebral dysfunction (e.g. dysphasia, apraxia). If the patient is drowsy, then one has to assume the hemianopia and cognitive deficit. On the other hand, patients with partial anterior circulation infarction, likely due to embolic occlusion of a branch of the middle cerebral artery or the anterior cerebral artery, are recognized by having only two of the three features of total anterior circulation infarction or new higher cerebral dysfunction alone, or a motor/sensory deficit restricted to one body area or part of one body area, or a predominantly proprioceptive deficit.

Lacunar infarction

Small deep infarcts (usually less than 1.5 cm in diameter) in the basal ganglia, thalamus, internal capsule, cerebral peduncle and pons are called lacunes. Higher cortical function is normal and the patient is conscious. Such patients can usually be recognized by a number of characteristic clinical syndromes:

Pure motor stroke

Complete or incomplete weakness of one side of the body, involving the whole of two out of the three body areas (face, upper limb, leg). Sensory symptoms, but not signs, may be present and there may be dysarthria and sometimes dysphagia.

Pure sensory stroke

Sensory symptoms and/or sensory signs (but not impaired joint position sense alone) in the same distribution as pure motor stroke.

Sensory motor stroke

A combination of pure motor and pure sensory stroke.

Ataxic hemiparesis

A combination of hemiparesis and ipsilateral cerebellar ataxia, often with marked dysarthria, clumsiness of the hand, and unsteadiness.

Most lacunar infarcts are thought to be caused by disease of the small perforating vessels within the brain substance. There is tortuosity, lipohyalinosis, and disorganization of the vessel wall. It is these damaged vessels that may form microaneurysms (Charcot–Bouchard aneurysms) which rupture to produce either small localized haematomas or massive intracerebral haematomas (see below). Therefore, lacunar syndromes are usually caused by small-vessel disease leading to a small deep infarct, but they can occasionally be caused by embolism to the same vessels, and certainly to small intracerebral haematomas in the same part of the brain.

Brain-stem infarction

Infarction in the brain-stem tends to cause a rather complicated neurological deficit, which is hardly surprising given the fact that all the ascending and descending pathways are close together at this point. Hemiparesis, hemiplegia, tetraparesis, tetraplegia, and unilateral or bilateral sensory loss can all occur. In addition, there may be a disturbance of gaze or extra-ocular muscles palsies, dysphagia, dysarthria, hiccups, ataxia, Horner's syndrome due to a lesion involving the descending sympathetic pathways, deafness, vertigo, vomiting, periodic breathing, and respiratory arrest particularly during sleep. An extensive brain-stem infarct can result in the locked-in syndrome in which, despite being conscious, the patient is unable to move anything except perhaps the eyelids, or the eyes in the vertical plane, and can neither speak nor swallow.

It is important to remember that thromboembolism within the vertebrobasilar arterial system may cause not only brain-stem infarction but also occipital infarction, with a hononymous hemianopia or even cortical blindness due to ischaemia in the posterior cerebral arterial supply. The term posterior circulation infarction therefore applies to patients with an occipital, brain-stem, thalamic, or cerebellar infarct (in any combination).

Boundary zone (or watershed) infarction

A profound but transient fall in systemic blood pressure usually causes syncope (i.e. faintness or unconsciousness) or generalized weakness; if it continues for some minutes, an epileptic seizure can occur. More prolonged hypotension of the sort that occurs after cardiac arrest, massive blood loss, or the overenthusiastic use of hypotensive drugs can cause massive cerebral infarction, leading to the persistent vegetative state or death, or, sometimes, to infarction between arterial territories, particularly in the parieto-occipital region, which is the boundary zone between the middle, anterior, and posterior cerebral arteries. Boundary zone infarction in this area is commonly bilateral and the symptoms include cortical blindness or visual disorientation, associated with a visual field defect and often memory impairment. Internal carotid artery occlusion, or very severe stenosis, may predispose to unilateral boundary zone infarction, even when there is a relatively small drop in systemic blood pressure, in the subcortical boundary zone (between the territories of the lenticulostriate perforating arteries and the superficial cortical branches of the middle cerebral artery) or in the anterior boundary zone (between the territories of the anterior and middle cerebral arteries).

Boundary-zone infarction can be recognized partly by the distribution on CT and partly by the circumstances of the stroke (i.e. when a fall in blood pressure is likely and/or there is severe carotid arterial disease).

Cerebral infarction and migraine

Occasionally cerebral infarction with a persistent neurological deficit occurs during a migrainous episode. This is possibly due to arterial narrowing caused by oedema of the vessel wall rather than vasospasm. It probably only occurs in patients with migraine with aura, and the neurological deficit has a similar clinical pattern to the transient neurological symptoms during the previously experienced auras.

Stroke and pregnancy

Stroke occurs most often in the last trimester of pregnancy or in the puerperium. However, this is rare; about 30 cases/100 000 deliveries in the United Kingdom. The middle cerebral artery is the most frequently occluded vessel, but the cause is unknown since there appears to be no underlying arterial disease. Some cases could be due to paradoxical embolism from thrombosis in the venous system of the legs or pelvis. Intracranial venous thrombosis is another cause.

Cortical venous and/or dural sinus thrombosis (i.e. intracranial venous thrombosis)

Thrombosis of the cortical veins and/or dural sinuses is a much less common cause of cerebral infarction than arterial disease, and occurs as a result of local conditions affecting the cortical veins or dural sinus, or systemic disorders (Table 9). Venous infarcts are commonly haemorrhagic. The clinical picture can be like cerebral hemisphere infarction caused by arterial occlusion but epileptic seizures and impaired consciousness are more common and raised intracranial pressure develops rapidly if the dural sinuses become obstructed. Cortical venous and sinus thrombosis may propagate widely to produce a catastrophic encephalo-

Table 9 *Causes of intracranial venous thrombosis*

Local conditions affecting the cerebral veins and sinuses directly
Head injury (with or without fracture)
Intracranial surgery
Local sepsis (sinuses, ears, scalp, mastoids, nasopharynx)
Subdural empyema
Bacterial meningitis
Tumour invasion of dural sinuses
Dural or cerebral arteriovenous malformation
Catheterization of jugular veins for parenteral nutrition, etc.
Systemic disorders
Dehydration, hypernatraemia
Septicaemia
Pregnancy and the puerperium
Oral contraceptives
Haematological disorders (Table 4)
Inflammatory vascular disease (Table 3)
Diabetes mellitus
Congestive cardiac failure
Inflammatory bowel disease
Androgen therapy
Antifibrinolytic drugs
Non-metastatic effect of extracranial malignancy
Nephrotic syndrome

Table 10 *General complications of stroke*

Respiratory	Pneumonia
	Inhalation
	Pulmonary embolism
Cardiovascular	Myocardial infarction
	Cardiac failure
	Cardiac arrhythmia
	Neurogenic pulmonary oedema
Infections	Pneumonia
	Urinary
	Skin
	Septicaemia
Metabolic	Vomiting
	Dehydration
	Electrolyte imbalance
	Hyperglycaemia
	Renal failure
Mechanical	Spasticity
	Contractures
	Malalignment/subluxation/frozen shoulder
	Falls and fractures
	Osteoporosis
	Ankle swelling
	Peripheral nerve pressure palsies
Others	Pressure sores
	Depression, anxiety, apathy
	Epileptic seizures
	Deep venous thrombosis
	Acute gastric ulceration
	Incontinence of urine/faeces

pathic illness with similar features to severe viral encephalitis. Isolated sagittal or transverse dural sinus thrombosis is one cause of the benign intracranial hypertension syndrome. The diagnosis is increasingly being made by MRI rather than conventional angiography. Treatment with anticoagulation seems to be both effective and surprisingly safe, even if there are haemorrhagic venous infarcts. Thrombosis of the cavernous sinus is rare but is usually due to pyogenic or fungal infection spreading from the face, sinuses, or nasal space; the symptoms include unilateral orbital pain and swelling, proptosis, visual loss, papilloedema, and often palsies of the third, fourth, fifth, and sixth cranial nerves.

DIFFERENTIAL DIAGNOSIS OF CEREBRAL INFARCTION

The clinical picture of stroke, either due to cerebral infarction or indeed to primary intracerebral haemorrhage, is characteristic and the diagnosis depends not so much on where the lesion is thought to be, but on the sudden onset in a patient with no recent history of head injury. Usually the patient is over the age of 50 and has one or more vascular risk factors or diseases (such as hypertension or angina). It is important to consider the possibility of a chronic subdural haematoma, or drug overdose, in an unconscious patient with few or no focal signs, and without a good history of a sudden onset. Encephalitis, cerebral abscess, sudden deterioration in a patient with a cerebral tumour, multiple sclerosis, peripheral nerve lesion, hypoglycaemia, and somatization can all usually be excluded after an adequate history, clinical examination, and straightforward investigations. In acute stroke, like in other severe acute illnesses, there is often transient hypertension, fever, hyperglycaemia, glycosuria, and a neutrophil leucocytosis. Sometimes there are arrhythmias and ischaemic changes on the electrocardiogram (but not the classical development of Q waves as in myocardial infarction), making it difficult to know if cerebral infarction has occurred as a result of embolism from left ventricular mural thrombus overlying an acute myocardial infarct. In any stroke patient it is important to remember that there are rare but often treatable underlying causes (Tables 2, 3, and 4).

COMPLICATIONS

The most important local complication of cerebral infarction is the development of cerebral oedema, which impairs, possibly only tempo-

rarily, local blood flow and neuronal function over a wider area than just the infarct and, if extensive, causes transtentorial herniation. There are a number of general complications of acute paralysis which include bronchopneumonia, particularly if consciousness or swallowing are impaired; venous thromboembolism; pressure sores and septicaemia; urinary infection, particularly if catheterization is necessary, and eventually uraemia; contractures in spastic limbs; frozen shoulder; cardiac rhythm disturbances; and mood disorder (Table 10). Death in the first week is almost always due to the infarct itself and the effects of cerebral oedema, but later it is more often due to one of the general complications, particularly pneumonia.

INVESTIGATIONS

These are the same as in patients with transient ischaemic attacks, but tempered by the age of the patient, the likelihood of recovery, and the chance that they will influence the immediate and long-term management. The most reliable way in which primary intracerebral haemorrhage can be differentiated from cerebral infarction is by an unenhanced CT scan within hours of stroke onset; neither the clinical picture nor the absence of blood in the cerebrospinal fluid rules out primary intracerebral haemorrhage. The high density of an intracerebral haematoma appears at once, although after it has resolved (in a matter of weeks and possibly only days if the haematoma is small) the scan may become normal or show only a low-density area very similar to that after cerebral infarction (Fig. 12). The characteristic low-density appearance of infarction usually takes a day or two to appear clearly (Figs. 13 and 14) although subtle loss of brain density can be apparent within hours of onset. Small infarcts less than about 0.5 cm in diameter, particularly in the posterior fossa, are not visible on CT but are much more readily imaged by MRI (Fig. 15). MRI is not, however, so good as CT at detecting primary intracerebral haemorrhage soon after stroke onset and, in any event, it is not very practical in restless and confused patients, even when it is available. Ideally, stroke patients should never be anticoagulated nor even exposed to antiplatelet drugs unless a CT scan has been done first to exclude primary intracerebral haemorrhage. Indications for CT scanning are summarized in Table 11.

Cerebral angiography is not usually indicated during the acute phase of cerebral infarction since the result is unlikely to influence the immediate management, and the procedure itself can make the patient worse. In a young patient there is an argument for urgent angiography, particularly if there is a possibility of traumatic arterial dissection with medicolegal implications, but usually it is best left until any recovery is well under way when it will be easier to decide whether carotid surgery is likely to be indicated. There are no reliable angiographic criteria for distinguishing between arterial embolism and thrombosis.

The cerebrospinal fluid may need to be examined if there is a possibility of encephalitis, neurosyphilis, or multiple sclerosis. It is not helpful in ruling out primary intracerebral haemorrhage which can, if small, be confined within the brain without any blood leaking into the cere-brospinal fluid. After stroke there are no more than 100 white blood cells per mm³ unless there have been septic emboli to the brain.

PROGNOSIS

Recovery, to some extent, is the rule after cerebral infarction unless the stroke is severe enough to cause death. Sudden death (i.e. within an hour of the onset of symptoms) is very rarely due to cerebral infarction or any other form of cerebrovascular disease except spontaneous subarachnoid haemorrhage. Most of any recovery occurs in the first 3 months but may not be absolutely complete for something like 1 or 2 years. The immediate prognosis is particularly poor if there is any impairment of consciousness. Case fatality is about 20 per cent at 1 month for stroke in general, but much higher after primary intracerebral haemorrhage than cerebral infarction (Fig. 16). Of the survivors from stroke, about a half recover completely, or more or less completely, while the rest are dis-

Fig. 12 CT scan of intracerebral haemorrhage: (a) at 4 days poststroke the haematoma is clearly shown as a high-density area in the right basal ganglia region (arrow); (b) by 12 days the high-density area is less obvious; and (c) at 18 days poststroke the high-density area has been replaced by a low-density area (arrow) which, without knowledge of the previous scan, might easily be mistaken—and is too often misleadingly reported—as infarction.

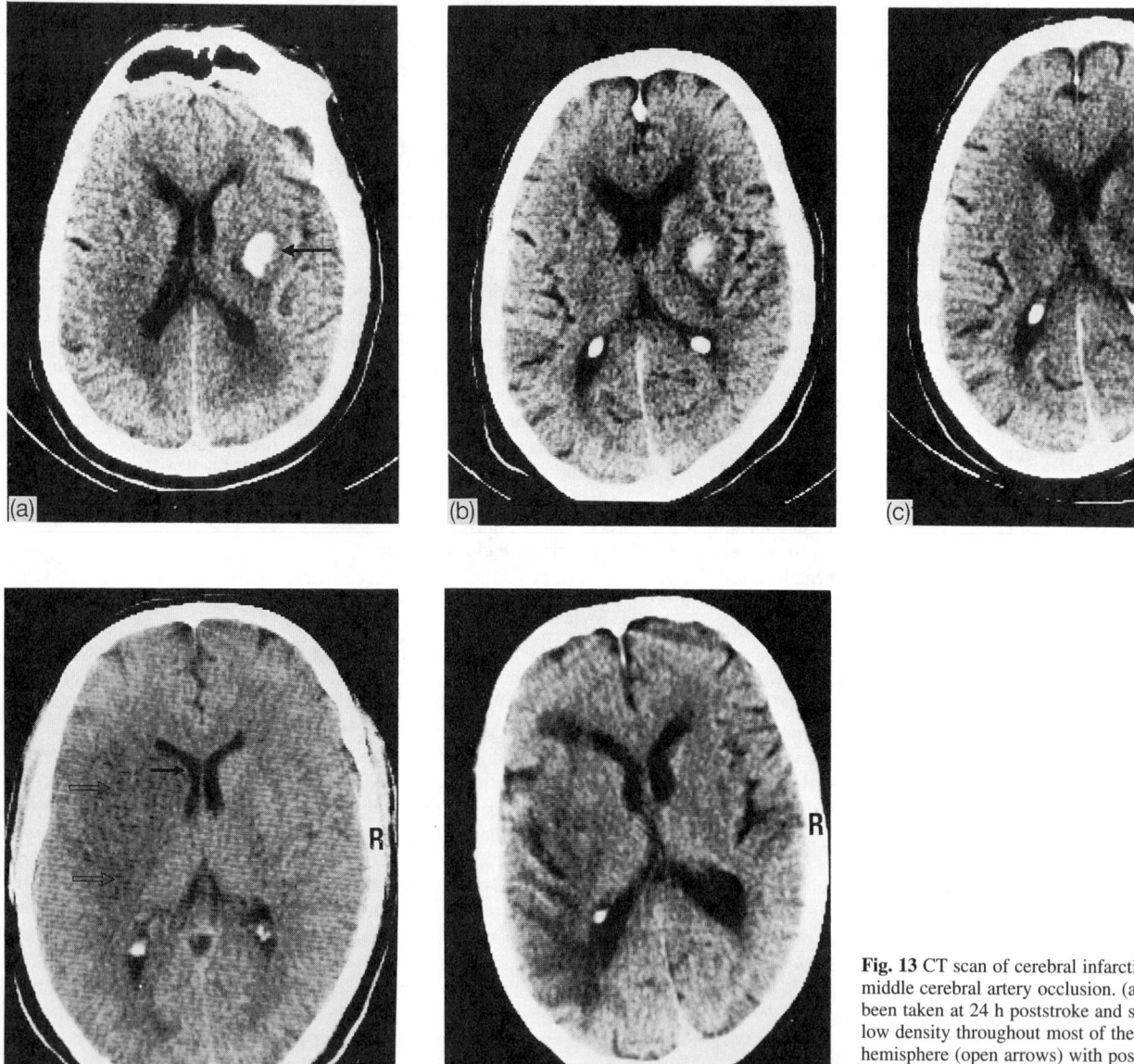

Fig. 13 CT scan of cerebral infarction due to left middle cerebral artery occlusion. (a) The scan has been taken at 24 h poststroke and shows a vague low density throughout most of the left cerebral hemisphere (open arrows) with possible compression of the anterior horn of the left lateral ventricle (closed arrow). (b) Three weeks poststroke, the low-density area of infarction is sharply defined.

abled to some degree. However, there are considerable differences between the different types and subtypes of stroke (Fig. 16). Good prognostic factors for recovery of function include young age, urinary continence, rapid improvement, mild stroke, and no perceptual or cognitive disorder.

TREATMENT

There is little that medical treatment and nothing that vascular surgery can do to alter the immediate outcome after cerebral infarction. In theory the reduction of cerebral oedema by mannitol, glycerol, or dexamethasone should be useful, but there have been no adequate clinical trials. Thrombolysis causes intracerebral haemorrhage and this risk may not be outweighed by the potential benefit, if any. Aspirin is currently being

Fig. 14 CT scan of a lacunar infarct in the region of the posterior limb of the left internal capsule (arrow). This scan was performed 3 days after the onset of stroke. If it had been done 4 weeks after the stroke, the appearances would have been consistent with either an old haemorrhage or an old infarct.

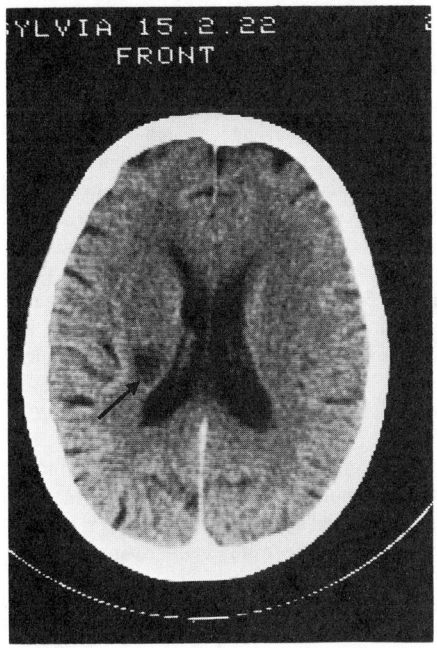

Fig. 15 An axial T$_2$ weighted MR image of the posterior fossa to show a small infarct (large black arrow) due to occlusion of the right vertebral artery (open arrow). The left vertebral artery is open and normal (smaller black arrow). The infarct was invisible on CT.

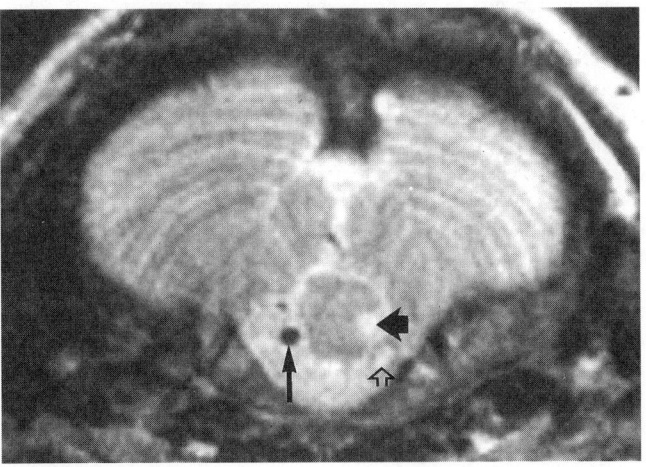

Table 11 *Indications for CT scan in acute stroke*

Uncertain diagnosis with the possibility of non-stroke intracranial pathology, particularly cerebral tumour or subdural haematoma. This situation usually only arises if there is uncertainty over the details of the symptom onset and the time course of the neurological deficit

The patient is taking, or may need to take, antihaemostatic drugs (anticoagulants, antiplatelet drugs, thrombolytics). To distinguish reliably between primary intracerebral haemorrhage and cerebral infarction, the scan should be performed as soon as possible, preferably within hours of stroke onset. A normal scan or hypodense lesion more than 2 or 3 weeks poststroke does not exclude a haemorrhagic origin

Cerebellar stroke

Subarachnoid haemorrhage

Uncharacteristic deterioration after the first 24 h, making non-stroke intracranial pathology rather more likely

Mild carotid distribution stroke possibly suitable for carotid endarterectomy

Young patient

Fig. 16 Outcome at 1 year in the 675 first-ever stroke patients in the Oxfordshire Community Stroke Project by (a) pathological type and (b) clinical subtype of ischaemic stroke. TACI, total anterior circulation infarct; PCAI, partial anterior circulation infarct; LACI, lacunar infarct; POCI, posterior circulation infarct; CI, cerebral infarction; PICH, primary intracerebral haemorrhage; SAH, subarachnoid haemorrhage.

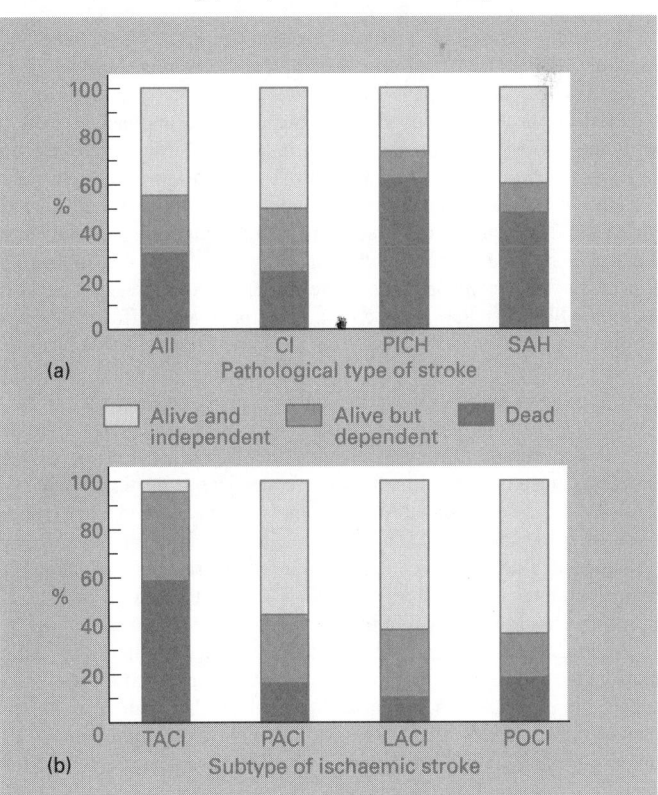

evaluated. Heparin has been recommended for stroke-in-evolution, although there have been no convincing trials and, since some cases may be due to haemorrhage into infarcted brain or even to primary intracerebral haemorrhage from the beginning, this treatment is not normally to be recommended. It is important to remember that there are many other reasons for stroke patients to deteriorate, and some are potentially reversible (Table 12).

If there is a definite major cardiac source of embolism the patient should probably be anticoagulated in an attempt to inhibit further embolization, provided of course there is no CT scan evidence of intracerebral haemorrhage (see discussion of anticoagulation in patients with transient ischaemic attacks above). Anticoagulants are contraindicated in infective endocarditis because of the risk of haemorrhage from mycotic aneurysms which form when the arterial wall is weakened by bacterial infection spreading from an infected embolus. Anticoagulation in acute embolic stroke always carries some risk because of the possibility of haemorrhage into infarcted brain, so there is a dilemma between anticoagulating too early and causing haemorrhagic transformation of the infarct and too late after further embolization has occurred. It is perhaps advisable to use an oral anticoagulant and achieve full anticoagulation over a matter of a few days.

Cerebral infarction often causes transient hypertension which settles without treatment. If the patient is taking hypotensive drugs, they should normally be continued. If the systolic blood pressure is greater than about 240 mmHg, it is probably best to reduce it, but slowly over a matter of days, and with extreme caution, because not only is there loss of normal cerebral autoregulation in and around infarcts, but in chronic hypertension autoregulation is set higher so that rapid and extreme reduction of blood pressure can lead to a catastrophic fall in cerebral blood flow and more extensive cerebral infarction. Surprisingly, no adequate trials of the speed and extent to which the blood pressure should be manipulated have yet been done.

Naturally, if a reversible underlying cause for cerebral infarction is found, then the appropriate treatment should be used; for example, corticosteroids for giant-cell arteritis, antibiotics for bacterial endocarditis, etc. Analgesics, tranquillizers, antiemetics, laxatives, and antispastic drugs all have their place in the relief of the appropriate symptoms.

The complications of cerebral infarction are often preventable and treatable (Table 10). Chest physiotherapy and care of the airway, particularly in unconscious patients and those with difficulty in swallowing, will reduce the risk of pneumonia which, if it occurs, can be treated with antibiotics. Occasionally intubation and tracheostomy are needed in patients who cannot protect their airway due to impaired brain-stem reflexes, but who are otherwise expected to have a reasonably good prognosis. Nasogastric tube feeding is used for adequate hydration and electrolyte balance in patients who cannot swallow, and later for feeding if necessary. Good nursing should prevent pressure sores. Early physiotherapy will reduce the risk of contractures, pain, and stiffness in hemiplegic limbs and leads naturally on to active physical rehabilitation. Urinary catheterization is often avoidable in males for whom an appliance is a better alternative, but in females it may be necessary so that the skin can be kept dry to reduce the chance of pressure sores. Cardiac arrhythmias should be treated on their merits but are not normally a problem. Since cerebral infarcts can become haemorrhagic, it is uncertain whether deep venous thrombosis in the legs and pulmonary embolism should be prevented, or even treated, with antithrombotic drugs, but the benefit of high-dose heparin followed by oral anticoagulation for major pulmonary embolism probably outweighs the risks. Epilepsy, if it occurs, should be treated in the normal way.

Vigorous rehabilitation is essential from as early in the illness as is reasonable, and may include physiotherapy, occupational therapy, and speech therapy if there is dysphasia. Stroke clubs, day-centre care, health visitors, key workers, district nurses, and help from enthusiastic volunteers all have their place. For some patients there may be a need for specific retraining for work and also advice concerning sexual activity, which can normally be resumed without any particular danger. For sec-

Table 12 *Causes of neurological deterioration after stroke*

Local	Extension of thrombus
	Recurrent embolism
	Recurrent haemorrhage
	Haemorrhagic transformation of the infarct
	Cerebral oedema
	Brain shift and herniation
	Hydrocephalus
	Epileptic seizures
General	Hypoxia (pneumonia, pulmonary embolism, cardiac failure)
	Hypotension (cardiac failure, cardiac arrhythmia, septicaemia, pulmonary embolism, dehydration, pneumonia, drugs, bleeding, or perforated peptic ulcer)
	Infection (chest, urine, septicaemia)
	Dehydration, hyponatraemia
	Hyper- or hypoglycaemia
	Sedatives/hypnotics
	Depression

ondary prevention, risk factors for vascular disease should be minimized in a similar way as in patients with transient ischaemic attacks, and aspirin given. There is little doubt that the adequate treatment of hypertension after stroke will reduce the risk of recurrence, and fears that any such treatment will, by causing low pressure, lead to cerebral infarction are unfounded provided drugs are used carefully and overt postural hypotension avoided.

In the United Kingdom up to 50 per cent of stroke patients are treated at home by their general practitioners and it is uncertain whether hospital treatment in a non-specialist unit confers any particular benefit unless the domestic circumstances make home nursing impossible. However, units specifically for the acute care and subsequent rehabilitation of stroke patients may well reduce both case fatality and morbidity, and undoubtedly increase the understanding of stroke and make the running of adequate clinical trials to assess potential treatments easier. It is astonishing how many treatments have been suggested for cerebral infarction and yet how few adequate trials have been undertaken. Any hospital-based stroke service should ideally extend into the community and include an early diagnostic component with appropriate neuroradiological back-up, and a nursing and rehabilitation component.

Multi-infarct dementia

Multi-infarct dementia is defined as a deterioration in previously normal mental function due to cerebral ischaemia and infarction. It is a less common cause of dementia than Alzheimer's disease. The main distinction between the two conditions is that in multi-infarct dementia the progression tends to be in a series of more or less sudden 'steps', because it is due to repeated episodes of ischaemia or infarction, some of which may cause overt strokes. It is a more likely cause of dementia than Alzheimer's disease if there is hypertension, focal neurological symptoms or signs, focal or lateralizing features on the electroencephalogram, vascular bruits, and reduced regional cerebral blood flow. It is, however, impossible to delineate these two main causes of dementia very precisely during life, and it could be argued that, since there is no specific treatment for either, there is no particular advantage in distinguishing one from the other in routine clinical practice.

Some believe that Binswanger's disease (chronic progressive subcortical encephalopathy or leucoaraiosis) is a distinct nosological entity causing slowly progressive dementia and unsteadiness of gait in late middle age, punctuated by transient ischaemic attacks and stroke-like episodes. The patients are often hypertensive and there is patchy or diffuse loss of the periventricular cerebral white mater, which is shown on CT scan or MRI, with or without ventricular dilatation and lacunar infarcts. Normal pressure hydrocephalus is an important differential diagnosis because it is treatable.

Cerebrovascular disease seldom causes a well-defined parkinsonian syndrome but, when widespread, is a common cause of pseudobulbar palsy.

Spontaneous intracranial haemorrhage

About 20 per cent of strokes are due to intracranial haemorrhage, which usually occurs as a result of rupture of a saccular aneurysm or an arteriovenous malformation, or hypertensive vascular disease. Rarer causes are listed in Table 13. The site of bleeding may be destroyed as a result of the haemorrhage which is usually into the subarachnoid space from a saccular aneurysm and directly into the brain (primary intracerebral haemorrhage) from hypertensive vascular disease or a vascular malformation. There can be blood in both sites after intracranial haemorrhage from any cause.

PRIMARY INTRACEREBRAL HAEMORRHAGE

Not every patient with primary intracerebral haemorrhage has hypertension and microvascular disease affecting the small arteries perforating the brain substance; sometimes the rupture of vascular malformations or other rare disorders may be responsible. However, Charcot–Bouchard aneurysms on the small perforating arteries do tend to occur where haemorrhage is common (the basal ganglia, thalamus, cerebellar hemisphere, pons, and subcortical areas) and their rupture is thought to explain the majority of cases. Haemorrhage in the cerebral hemispheres outside the basal ganglia region (so-called lobar haemorrhage) is less likely to be due to hypertensive vascular disease than to one of the other causes mentioned above. Sometimes primary intracerebral haemorrhage is multiple (Table 14). A haematoma may cause transtentorial herniation in the same way as cerebral infarction.

Clinical features

Clinically, it is difficult, if not impossible, to distinguish reliably between primary intracerebral haemorrhage and cerebral infarction unless a substantial amount of blood has entered the cerebrospinal fluid, via the ventricles and/or the surface of the brain, in which case meningism develops. Headache and coma occur in both cerebral haemorrhage and infarction, and are not very reliable differentiating features. However, severe headache and coma within a few hours of onset is unusual in cerebral infarction. The symptoms, signs, investigations, differential diagnosis, and general management of infarction and haemorrhage are similar, but with some important exceptions which need to be discussed separately below.

Cerebellar haematoma

This condition, although rare, is important because surgical treatment can be life-saving and survivors may have remarkably little neurological disability. The patient presents with sudden occipital headache, dizziness, truncal ataxia, rapid reduction in consciousness, a gaze palsy to the side of the lesion, ipsilateral facial weakness, and often raised intracranial pressure due to acute obstruction of cerebrospinal fluid flow. Cerebellar signs cannot normally be elicited unless the patient is conscious. Any hemiparesis is mild although bilateral extensor plantars are common. Sensory signs are unusual. The diagnosis is confirmed by CT scan (Fig. 17).

Angiography

Cerebral angiography is unnecessary if a haematoma has been demonstrated by CT scanning and the patient is extremely ill or seriously

Table 13 *Causes of spontaneous intracranial haemorrhage*

Hypertension (chronic, acute)	Vascular tumours
	melanoma
Aneurysms	malignant astrocytoma
saccular	oligodendroglioma
atheromatous	medulloblastoma
mycotic	choroid plexus papilloma
myxomatous	hypernephroma
dissecting	endometrial carcinoma
	bronchogenic carcinoma
Vascular malformations	choriocarcinoma
arteriovenous	
venous	Drug abuse
cavernous	
telangiectasis	Infections
	herpes simplex
Cerebral amyloid angiopathy	leptospirosis
	anthrax
Haemostatic failure	
haemophilia and other	Scorpion bite
coagulation disorders	
thrombocytopenia	
thrombotic thrombocytopenic purpura	
anticoagulation	
therapeutic thrombolysis	
antiplatelet drugs	
polycythaemia rubra vera	
essential thrombocythaemia	
sickle-cell disease	
paraproteinaemias	
disseminated intravascular coagulation	
renal failure	
liver failure	
snake bite	
Inflammatory vascular disease (Table 3)	
Haemorrhagic transformation of cerebral infarction	
Intracranial venous thrombosis (Table 9)	
Moyamoya syndrome	
Carotid endarterectomy	
Posterior fossa surgery	
Alcoholic binge	

Table 14 *Causes of nearly simultaneous and multiple intracerebral haemorrhages*

Cerebral amyloid angiopathy
Metastases (Table 13)
Haemostatic defect
Intracranial venous thrombosis
Inflammatory vascular disease
Vascular malformations
Malignant hypertension
Multiple haemorrhagic infarcts
Head injury
Drug abuse

disabled. However, if the patient has recovered useful function, is normotensive, and not particularly elderly or compromised by some other disease, angiography may reveal a cause for the haemorrhage which is potentially treatable by surgery, for example an arteriovenous malformation or an aneurysm which has bled directly into the brain substance rather than into the subarachnoid space. Both these lesions, if large, may be suspected on CT scanning if contrast material is used to reveal the abnormal vascularity (Fig. 18). An arteriovenous malformation may cause a cranial bruit, which is usually best heard by auscultation over the orbits, and there may be a history of epilepsy.

Medical treatment

Naturally, anticoagulants are contraindicated. It is not certain whether aspirin worsens the outcome after cerebral haemorrhage but, since it undoubtedly leads to a haemostatic defect, it is probably best avoided. If a patient's course is complicated by pulmonary embolism, it is unclear whether the benefits of anticoagulation are outweighed by the risks of making the cerebral haemorrhage worse. Medical treatment and rehabilitation are otherwise the same as for patients with cerebral infarction (see above). If a patient survives, the recovery and long-term prognosis are often remarkably good.

Surgical treatment

The evacuation of a haematoma, particularly if it is superficial, is a tempting surgical possibility, but whether this increases the chance of recovery is uncertain. Some surgeons operate on haematomas acutely but there have been no clinical trials to support such a policy. A more widely accepted indication is in the patient whose conscious level is deteriorating, usually because of brain shift and transtentorial herniation. Surgery will not improve the situation in a deeply unconscious patient nor in one who is improving and has only a mild neurological deficit. Surgical evacuation and/or ventricular drainage is the treatment for cerebellar haemorrhage unless spontaneous recovery is already occurring.

Spontaneous subarachnoid haemorrhage

Most patients have ruptured an intracranial saccular aneurysm; about 5 per cent have bled from an arteriovenous malformation, and a few have rare causes of intracranial haemorrhage (Table 13). In about 15 per cent of patients no cause can be identified, particularly in those with a restricted haemorrhage around the midbrain, and in this group the prognosis is particularly good.

The clinical picture is distinctive and not easily confused with stroke due to cerebral infarction or primary intracerebral haemorrhage. The onset is with sudden headache, usually but not always severe, which is

Fig. 17 Cerebellar haematoma. On the left the CT scan through the posterior fossa shows the haemorrhage as a large white area (arrow). On the right, the CT scan is through the lateral ventricles to show their enlargement due to obstruction of cerebrospinal fluid flow from the ventricular system by the haematoma in the cerebellum, and blood has spread from the haematoma through the ventricular system into the lateral ventricles (arrow).

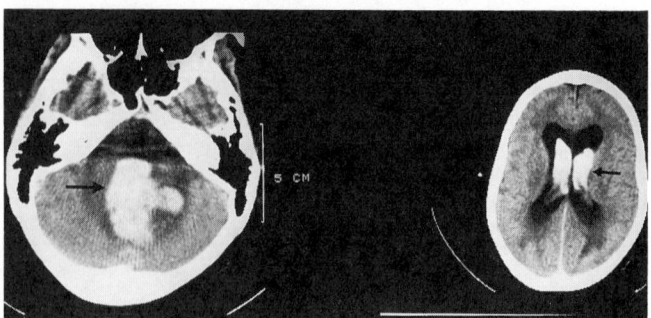

often occipital and radiates over the head and down the neck, sometimes down as far as the back or legs as blood tracks down the spinal canal. Consciousness is often impaired or lost transiently at the onset and if the haemorrhage is extensive the patient remains comatose. Vomiting is quite common and occasionally epileptic seizures are an early feature. Meningism develops, but sometimes not for several hours, and there are no signs of focal neurological damage unless bleeding has also occurred into the brain substance, or unless there is an oculomotor palsy due to pressure from a posterior communicating artery/distal internal carotid artery aneurysm. The patient is very often irritable, confused, photophobic, and drowsy for several days, and the headache may persist for weeks. Arteriovenous malformations may occasionally be diagnosed clinically if there is a cranial bruit. A rapid rise in the intracranial pressure at the onset of a subarachnoid haemorrhage is probably the cause of the subhyaloid haemorrhages which are often observed in the fundus.

The diagnosis can be most easily confirmed by early CT scan, which almost always shows blood in the cerebrospinal fluid pathways (Fig. 19) and perhaps a collection of blood in relation to the ruptured aneurysm or arteriovenous malformations. If a CT scan is not easily available or

Fig. 18 CT scan after intravenous contrast injection to show the typical appearance of a large intracerebral arteriovenous malformation. The abnormal vasculature in the right occipital lobe (large arrow) and a large draining vein (small arrow) are enhanced.

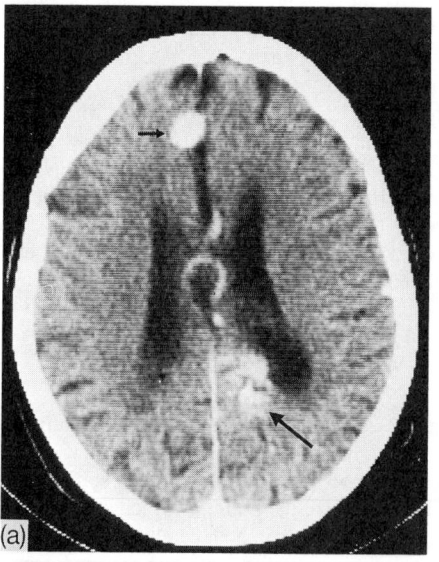
(a)

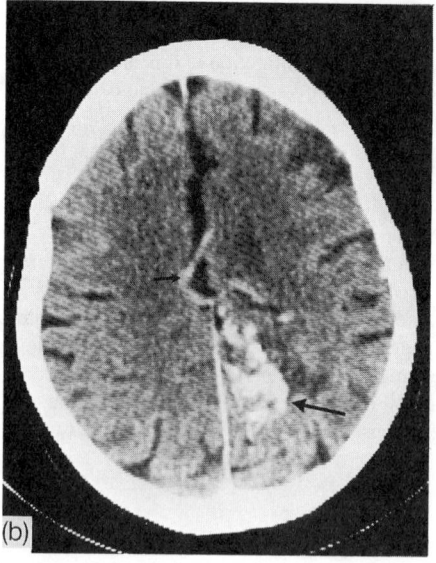
(b)

is normal, then lumbar puncture is mandatory and the cerebrospinal fluid will be bloodstained. If the haemorrhage is more than about 12 h old, the cerebrospinal fluid becomes xanthochromic due to altered blood pigment. Clearly, if there is any clinical difficulty distinguishing between subarachnoid haemorrhage and acute meningitis, then the cerebrospinal fluid should be examine at once. The CT scan and cerebrospinal fluid become normal within 2 or 3 weeks of the onset.

The complications of subarachnoid haemorrhage are similar to those of cerebral infarction and primary intracerebral haemorrhage. In addition, organized blood clot in the subarachnoid space may cause obstruction to cerebrospinal fluid flow and thus acute hydrocephalus. This is common and often asymptomatic, but it may lead to a deterioration in the patient's conscious level a few days or weeks after the onset of the haemorrhage, when progress has otherwise been satisfactory. This complication can be easily diagnosed by CT and then treated with ventricular drainage procedure. Occasionally the disturbance of cerebrospinal fluid flow may not present until some years after the subarachnoid haemorrhage and the clinical picture is then of normal pressure hydrocephalus. Vasospasm is discussed below.

INTRACRANIAL SACCULAR ANEURYSMS

These develop on the medium-sized arteries at the base of the brain and the common sites are at the distal internal carotid/posterior communicating artery origin (30 per cent), the anterior communicating artery complex (40 per cent), and at the bifurcation of the middle cerebral artery (25 per cent). The basilar artery is a less common site (5 per cent). About 25 per cent of cases have multiple aneurysms. The aneurysms vary from a few millimetres to several centimetres in diameter. Some aneurysms may be congenital but others develop in adult life, probably as a result of atherosclerosis and hypertension. Various associated conditions may be present (Table 15). Aneurysmal rupture can be caused by sudden increases in blood pressure during strenuous exercise, lifting, defaecation, and coitus. Many aneurysms remain asymptomatic and are found in 2 per cent of routine necropsies. A few grow to a large size and present as a space-occupying lesion.

VASCULAR MALFORMATIONS

Arteriovenous malformations

These are congenital vascular anomalies which vary greatly in size from a few millimetres to several centimetres in diameter. They consist of

Fig. 19 Unenhanced CT scan showing blood (white areas) in the subarachnoid space and between the frontal horns of the lateral ventricles (arrow) where an anterior communicating artery aneurysm has ruptured.

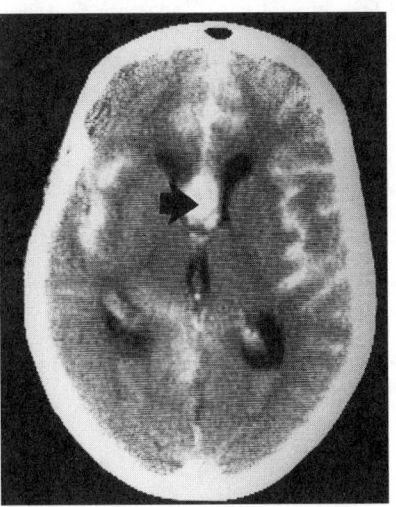

Table 15 *Associations of intracranial saccular aneurysms*

Polycystic kidney disease*
Fibromuscular dysplasia
Cervical artery dissection*
Coarctation of the aorta
Intracranial vascular malformations*
Marfan's syndrome*
Ehlers–Danlos syndrome*
Pseudoxanthoma elasticum*
Hereditary haemorrhagic telangiectasia*
Moyamoya syndrome
Klinefelter's syndrome
Progeria

*Can be familial

convoluted masses of blood vessels which are fed by large arteries and drained by increasingly large veins as time goes by. They may present with epilepsy, subarachnoid haemorrhage, primary intracerebral haemorrhage, and rarely as a space-occupying lesion or with headache. In infants they may occasionally cause high-output cardiac failure. Early death (about 10 per cent) and risk of rebleeding is much less than after rupture of a saccular aneurysm, but the neurological damage is usually more extensive. However, even after several recurrent haemorrhages, patients may survive for many years with remarkably little disability.

There are other less common vascular malformations involving the brain. Telangiectases are made up of groups of dilated capillaries. They may be associated with the Osler–Rendu–Weber syndrome (see Section 22) and occasionally rupture, although this is very unusual. Cavernous malformations (angiomas) form circumscribed collections of blood-filled spaces. They may be associated with similar lesions elsewhere in the body and can be familial. They may present with epilepsy, but rarely rupture. Haemangioblastomas are tumours of angioblastic origin which consist of vascular channels and spaces, and tend to form cysts. They can be multiple and are usually found subtentorially, often in the cerebellum, medulla, or even the spinal cord, and present as a space-occupying lesion. Bleeding is unusual, although polycythaemia may occur. They are often associated with anomalies elsewhere in the body: haemangioblastoma of the retina; cysts of the pancreas and kidneys; hypernephromas and tumours of the suprarenal glands. The association of these lesions is known as the von Hippel–Lindau syndrome which is autosomal dominant in many cases. Finally, in the Sturge–Weber syndrome there may be extensive capillary–venous malformations affecting one hemisphere, particularly the parieto-occipital region, associated with a characteristic wavy pattern of subcortical calcification. There is usually an associated port-wine stain on the ipsilateral face and there may be associated glaucoma. Epilepsy is the main clinical manifestation.

MANAGEMENT OF SUBARACHNOID HAEMORRHAGE

About 25 per cent of patients die within 24 h of aneurysmal subarachnoid haemorrhage. Another 25 per cent die in the first month (usually due to recurrent haemorrhage, or infarction as a consequence of vasospasm) and 50 per cent survive for longer, but still with a risk of rebleeding (about 2 per cent per annum). The first week is the time of maximum risk of rebleeding so, if possible, neurosurgical intervention to clip the aneurysm should be as soon as possible. However, the risk of surgery is unacceptably high if the patient is unconscious or has a severe neurological deficit. If the patient is conscious with little or no deficit, then four-vessel angiography should be undertaken to delineate the site of the bleeding (Figs 20, 21) and surgery carried out soon afterwards.

Vasospasm and secondary cerebral infarction may occur in relation to, and even at a distance from, the aneurysm-bearing artery and is one explanation for the high risks of surgery in ill patients. The cause of vasospasm is unknown but is probably to do with some constituent of the blood in the subarachnoid space.

If an arteriovenous malformation has bled and is surgically accessible, it should probably be removed. Ligation of the feeding vessels has little or nothing to offer since the arteriovenous malformation will be revascularized by vessels too small to be seen on the preoperative angiogram.

Fig. 20 Anteroposterior view of a right carotid angiogram to show a middle cerebral artery aneurysm (arrow).

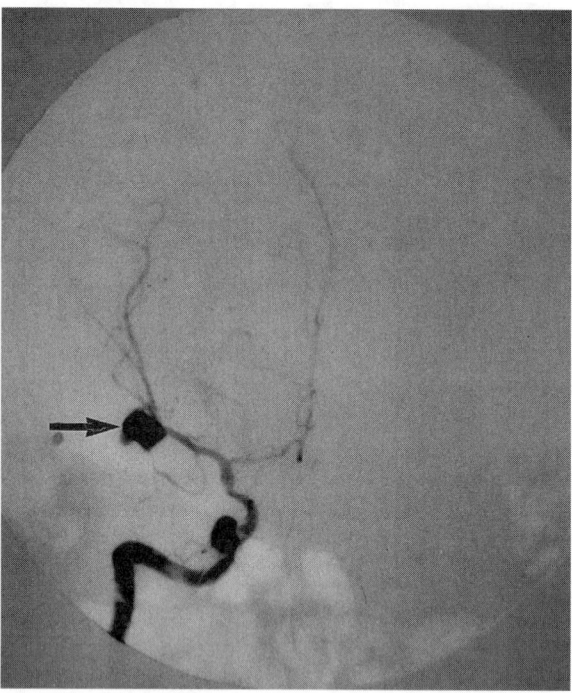

Fig. 21 Carotid angiogram to show an arteriovenous malformation (black arrow) which is fed from the middle cerebral artery (open arrow).

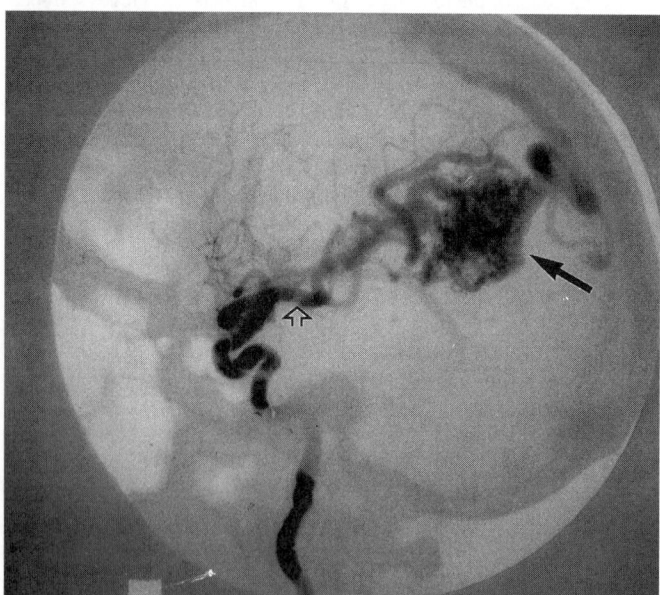

Embolization and radiotherapy have been suggested but, like surgical removal, there have been no adequate clinical trials.

From the medical point of view, cautious control of severe hypertension is wise, and occasionally cardiac rhythm disturbances or even acute neurogenic pulmonary oedema require appropriate treatment. Naturally, analgesia for the headache and sedation if the patient is very irritable are useful. Antifibrinolytic drugs reduce the risk of rebleeding by inhibiting the lysis of the fibrin clot plugging the ruptured aneurysm, but do not improve the overall prognosis, probably because the risk of vasospasm is increased. Prophylactic nimodipine reduces the risk of vasospasm after aneurysmal subarachnoid haemorrhage. Bedrest for a few weeks is usually recommended, but there is an increasing tendency gently to mobilize patients when the headache has resolved.

The prevention of stroke

Since the medical and surgical treatment of stroke is usually so unrewarding, it is sensible to concentrate considerable efforts on stroke prevention. There are two ways in which this may be achieved: primary prevention in asymptomatic individuals and secondary prevention in patients who have already experienced a transient ischaemic attack or stroke. Primary prevention must, at the moment depend, on the detection and adequate treatment of hypertension, reducing the average blood pressure in the population by dietary means (more exercise, reduce weight, less salt, and reduce heavy alcohol consumption) and the reduction of cigarette-smoking. Manipulation of diet to reduce cholesterol levels on a large-scale population basis is likely to be difficult to achieve, but is still worth attempting. The use of antithrombotic drugs such as aspirin in asymptomatic individuals has been suggested, but randomized clinical trials, notably among many thousand British and American doctors, do not support this. Anticoagulation or aspirin reduce the risk of stroke in patients with atrial fibrillation. The secondary prevention of ischaemic stroke has already been dealt with under the management of transient ischaemic attacks.

Asymptomatic carotid stenosis is fairly common in the elderly, and, although carotid endarterectomy may reduce the risk of stroke, this risk is not really high enough to justify the risk of the surgery itself. Asymptomatic stenosis, and indeed asymptomatic cervical bruits, are a marker for ischaemic heart disease as well as for cerebrovascular disease and, as such, point to the need to control vascular risk factors.

REFERENCES

Barnett, H.J.M., Mohr, J.P., Stein, B.M., and Yatsu, F.M. (1992). *Stroke: pathophysiology, diagnosis, and management*, (2nd edn). Churchill Livingstone, New York.

Caplan, L.R. and Stein, R.W. (1993). *Stroke: a clinical approach*, (2nd edn). Butterworths, Boston.

Ebrahim, S. (1990). *Clinical epidemiology of stroke*. Oxford University Press.

Hankey, G. and Warlow, C.P. (1994). *Transient ischaemic attacks*. W.B. Saunders, London.

The Management of Patients with Stroke. (1993). A report of a working group of the National Medical Advisory Committee, Scottish Office Home and Health Department HMSO, Edinburgh.

Vermuelen, M., Lindsey, K.W., and van Gijn, J. (1992). *Major problems in neurology: subarachnoid haemorrhage*. W.B. Saunders, London.

Warlow, C.P. (1993). Disorders of the cerebral circulation. In *Brain's diseases of the nervous system* (10th edn) (ed. J.W. Walton), pp. 197–268. Oxford University Press.

Warlow, C., Sandercock, P., Wardlaw, J., *et al.* (1996). *The practical management of stroke*. Blackwell, Oxford.

24.7 Dementia

24.7.1 Introduction

J. R. HODGES

Definition

Dementia is now defined as 'a syndrome consisting of progressive impairment in two or more areas of cognition (i.e. memory, language, visuospatial and perceptual ability, thinking and problem-solving, personality) sufficient to interfere with work, social function, or relationships, in the absence of delirium or major "non-organic" psychiatric disorders (e.g. depression, schizophrenia)'.

This definition differs from those previously used in that the term 'global impairment in intellectual function' has been removed, and replaced by a more refined description of the cognitive deficits. This change has allowed dementing disorders to be diagnosed with more accuracy and at an earlier stage. Although a global or diffuse loss of higher cerebral function is the eventual fate of patients with dementing illnesses, the vast majority of cases begin with more circumscribed deficits. The requirement for impairment in two or more cognitive domains excludes patients with isolated cognitive deficits such as aphasia, or amnesia (e.g. Korsakoff's syndrome), but allows a diagnosis of dementia to be made before the patient reaches a state of gross generalized mental decay. The contrasting features of dementia and delirium, and the patterns of deficit associated with various types of dementia and will be discussed below.

Epidemiology and causes of dementia

Dementia is, predominantly, a disorder of later life. The true prevalence and incidence has not been fully established since there have been few comprehensive community-based studies, but as an approximate figure, 5 to 8 per cent of all people above the age of 65 suffer from some degree of dementia. However, this figure hides the dramatic increase with advancing age; the prevalence doubles every 5 years above the age of 65, reaching over 20 per cent in 80-year-olds. It has been estimated that there are approximately 1 million sufferers in Britain and over 4 million in the United States, a third of whom are severely incapacitated by their disease. Women are affected more than men even when adjustment is made for the increased longevity of women.

A very large number of neurological diseases can cause dementia, as shown in Table 1, but most of these are very rare. Many of the conditions listed, such as multiple sclerosis, systemic lupus erythematosus, and the inherited metabolic disorders, cause dementia, but almost invariably in the setting of other neurological symptoms or signs. Alzheimer's disease is by far the commonest cause of dementia; most epidemiological surveys find that between 50 and 70 per cent of cases are due to Alzheimer's disease. Recent studies, however, indicate that two other primary degenerative conditions which previously would have been subsumed within the rubric of Alzheimer's disease, namely diffuse cortical Lewy body disease and focal lobar atrophy (or Pick's disease), appear to be relatively common, perhaps accounting for up to 25 per cent of cases previously diagnosed as Alzheimer's disease. Vascular dementia remains the second commonest cause, accounting for 20 to 30 per cent of cases, although its prevalence appears to be falling. The term vascular dementia encompasses a number of separate disorders, the commonest being multi-infarct disease secondary to atherosclerosis of the extra- and intra-

cranial arteries. Of the inherited disorders which may present as dementia, Huntington's disease is the most common. Unfortunately, curable diseases still account for only a small minority of cases—around 10 to 20 per cent in hospital-based series, but a much smaller proportion of unselected community-based cases.

Patterns of cognitive impairment: cortical versus subcortical dementia

A recently proposed division, which has proved theoretically and practically useful, is between those diseases which affect primarily the cerebral cortex and those which have their major pathological impact on subcortical structures (i.e. the basal ganglia, thalamus, and deep white matter). This classification highlights two facts. First, diseases that affect diverse cerebral structures can result in cognitive dysfunction; and, secondly, that the pattern of cognitive deficits seen in patients with different types of dementia may be strikingly different. The reason for the intellectual impairment in cortical diseases is obvious since the cerebral cortex is clearly associated with higher cerebral function. The critical role of subcortical structures has been realized more recently. The cortex, particularly the prefrontal area, is interconnected with subcortical nuclei and, therefore, diseases affecting the subcortical nuclei may have their impact by functionally deactivating an otherwise normal cortex. Table 2 contrasts the major features of cortical and subcortical dementias.

CORTICAL DEMENTIAS

Alzheimer's disease is the prototypical example of a cortical dementia in which disturbances of memory, language, praxis, visuospatial, and perceptual abilities predominate. Marked impairment in memory is always the earliest feature; this amnesic deficit results from a failure to lay-down (encode) new memories and, to a lesser extent, to recall older memories. Within the domain of language, aphasia occurs fairly early in the course of the disease; the semantic (word meaning) component of language is selectively affected, causing word-finding difficulty in spontaneous conversation, impaired object naming on formal tests, difficulty understanding the meaning of less common words, and a marked reduction in the exemplars produced on category fluency testing (also called controlled word association in which the patient is asked to generate as many examples from a given category, such as animals or vegetables, in 1 min). Visuospatial deficits, apparent on constructional tests, and perceptual deficits, causing visual agnosia, are also common. The attentional deficit and general slowing of cognitive processes which characterizes the subcortical dementias are not seen, at least early in the course of the disease. Likewise, personality and social conduct are well preserved in the initial stages.

Creutzfeldt–Jakob disease is another form of cortical disease which causes a rapidly progressive dementia, often resulting in death within months of presentation. The cognitive features of this condition have not been well characterized, but severe memory impairment and aphasia are usually present and some patients develop cortical blindness. Myoclonus is present in 80 per cent of cases.

SUBCORTICAL DEMENTIAS

In subcortical dementias, such as Huntington's disease and progressive supranuclear palsy (Steele–Richardson–Olszewski syndrome), impairment in attention and frontal 'executive' function (i.e. planning, prob-

Table 1 *Causes of dementia*

Primary degenerative diseases
  Alzheimer's disease
  Pick's disease (focal lobar atrophy)
  Huntington's disease
  Parkinson's disease
  Diffuse cortical Lewy body disease
  Progressive supranuclear palsy (Steele–Richardson–
    Olszewski syndrome)
  Striatonigral degeneration
  Corticobasal degeneration
  Olivopontocerebellar degeneration
  Progressive myoclonic epilepsies
 	
Vascular diseases
  Multi-infarct disease secondary to atherosclerotic disease of
    extracranial vessels or cardiac emboli
  Hypertensive encephalopathy
  Binswanger's disease (subcortical arteriosclerotic
    encephalopathy)
  Vasculitides: systemic lupus erythematosus, polyarteritis
    nodosa, Behçet's disease, giant-cell arteritis, isolated CNS
    angiitis
  Primary cerebral amyloid (congophilic) angiopathy
 	
Infections
  AIDS dementia complex
  Progressive multifocal leucoencephalopathy ⎤ associated
  Cerebral toxoplasmosis   ⎬ with immune
  Cyptococcal meningitis   ⎦ compromise
  Creutzfeldt–Jakob and other prion-related diseases
  Syphilis
  Subacute sclerosing panencephalitis and progressive rubella
    panencephalitis
  Whipple's disease
 	
Neoplastic causes
  Primary intracerebral tumours: frontal gliomas crossing the
    corpus callosum (butterfly glioma), posterior corpus
    callosal or midline (thalamic, pineal, third ventricle)
    tumours, cerebral lymphoma, etc.
  Extracerebral tumours: frontal meningiomas, posterior fossa
    tumours (acoustic neuroma) causing hydrocephalus
  Multiple cerebral metastases
  Malignant meningitis
  Non-metastatic (limbic) encephalitis
	Other non-neoplastic space-occupying disorders
	  Chronic subdural haematoma
	  Normal pressure hydrocephalus
	
	Chronic intoxications
	  Alcoholic dementia
	  Heavy metals: lead, mercury, manganese
	  Carbon monoxide poisoning
	  Drugs: lithium, anticholinergics, barbiturates, digitalis,
	    neuroleptics, cimetidine, propranolol
	
	Acquired metabolic disorders and deficiency states
	  Cerebral anoxia
	  Chronic renal failure
	  Portosystemic encephalopathy
	  Hypothyroidism
	  Cushing's disease
	  Addison's disease
	  Panhypopituitism
	  Hypoglycaemia (chronic or recurrent)
	  Hypoparathyroidism
	  Vitamins B_{12}, B_1, folic acid deficiency
	
	Inherited metabolic diseases which may present with dementia
	  in early adult life
	  Wilson's disease
	  Porphyria
	  Leucodystrophies: adrenoleucodystrophy, metachromatic
	    leucodystrophy, globoid cell leucodystrophy
	  Gangliosidoses
	  Niemann–Pick disease
	  Cerebrotendinous xanthomatosis
	  Adult onset neuronal ceroid-lipofuscinosis (Kufs' disease)
	  Mitochondrial cytopathies
	  Subacute necrotizing encephalopathy (Leigh's disease)
	
	Miscellaneous
	  Multiple sclerosis
	  Sarcoidosis
	  Sickle-cell disease
	  Macroglobulinaemia
	  Recurrent head injury, dementia pugilistica

lem-solving, self-initiated activity) predominate. Patients appear mentally slowed down (or bradyphrenic). Change in mood, personality, and social conduct are very common, resulting often in an indifferent, withdrawn state. Spontaneous speech is reduced and answers to questions are slow and laconic. Memory is moderately impaired due to reduced attention with poor registration of new material, but the severe amnesia which typifies Alzheimer's disease is not seen in the early stages. Features of focal cortical dysfunction, such as aphasia, apraxia, and agnosia, are characteristically absent, but visuospatial deficits are consistently present.

The term subcortical dementia has now been applied to a range of basal ganglia and white matter diseases (see Table 3). Of these, most research has focused on the degenerative basal ganglia disorders, but recent studies indicate that the dementia associated with primary human immunodeficiency virus (HIV) infection of the nervous system also conforms to a pattern of subcortical dementia. Neuropsychological complications of multiple sclerosis are much more common than previously supposed and also resemble the prototype of subcortical disease.

The focal lobar atrophies (Pick's disease) present a potential problem for this classification, particularly when the frontal lobes are selectively

involved. In this variant, often called dementia of frontal-lobe type, there is progressive and often striking atrophy of the frontal cortex, yet clinical and neuropsychological features traditionally associated with cortical dementia are absent; patients present instead with an insidious change in personality, behaviour, and social conduct; cognitive testing shows deficits in frontal 'executive' functions. Within the cortical–subcortical dichotomy, these features epitomize subcortical dementia. This apparent contradiction can be resolved if it is remembered that the subcortical dementias have their impact by deactivating the frontal cortex. Hence it is entirely consistent that subcortical and frontal pathologies should present with similar clinical syndromes; indeed, some authors have used the term frontostriatal dementia to encompass both.

MIXED CORTICAL–SUBCORTICAL DEMENTIAS

It should be emphasized that not all dementing disorders fit neatly into the cortical–subcortical dichotomy. In multi-infarct dementia, for instance, the lacunar lesions which are largely responsible for the cognitive impairment, preferentially involve the basal ganglia, thalamus, and adjacent white matter, resulting in a subcortical syndrome. How-

Table 2 *Contrasting features of cortical and subcortical dementia*

Characteristic	Cortical dementia	Subcortical dementia
Speed of cognitive processing	Normal	Slowed down (bradyphenic)
Frontal 'executive' abilities[a]	Preserved in early stages	Disproportionately impaired from onset
Memory	Severe amnesia	Forgetfulness
	Recall and recognition affected	Recognition better
Language	Aphasic features	Normal except dysarthria and reduced output
Visuospatial and perceptual abilities	Impaired	Impaired
Personality	Intact until late	Typically apathetic and inert
Mood	Usually normal	Depression common

[a]Planning, problem-solving, initiation, etc.

Table 3 *Major causes of subcortical dementia*

Degenerative
  Progressive supranuclear palsy
  Huntington's disease
  Parkinson's disease
  Striatonigral degeneration
  Olivopontocerebellar degeneration

Vascular disorders
  Multi-infarct dementia (lacunar state)[a]
  Binswanger's disease

Metabolic
  Wilson's disease

Demyelinating disease
  Multiple sclerosis
  Leucodystrophies
  AIDS dementia complex

Miscellaneous
  Normal pressure hydrocephalus

[a]Cortical features often coexist.

ever, larger-vessel strokes frequently coexist which cause cortical features (aphasia, apraxia, etc.).

The recently recognized condition of diffuse cortical Lewy body disease also illustrates this point. Lewy bodies are the pathological hallmark of Parkinson's disease, but in Parkinson's disease they are confined, very largely, to the substantia nigra. In diffuse cortical Lewy body disease, however, these same intraneuronal inclusions are widely distributed in cortical and subcortical structures. The behavioural features are also in keeping with mixed cortical and subcortical pathology; attentional and frontal 'executive' deficits are prominent, but there are also marked visuoperceptual and memory impairments. Visual hallucinations and fluctuations in cognitive performance also characterize this disorder.

Differential diagnosis

PSEUDODEMENTIA

This term has been used to describe two distinct disorders—depressive pseudodementia and hysterical pseudodementia. Of these, the former is more common and represents the most important treatable cause of memory failure. Depressive pseudodementia is almost invariably a condition of the elderly. The patient presents with complaints of poor memory and concentration but usually denies overt symptoms of depression.

Clues to the diagnosis are biological features of depression (particularly a disturbed sleep pattern and loss of appetite), low energy, pessimistic and ruminative thoughts, and a lack of interest in work or hobbies. The onset is usually relatively acute or subacute over weeks or months. A past or family history of affective disorder can be an important marker. On bedside cognitive assessment, attention is impaired and performance on tests of memory and of frontal executive function is patchy and often inconsistent. Language output may be sparse but paraphasic errors are not seen. Responses to questions are often 'don't knows'. Even after detailed neuropsychological testing it may be impossible to distinguish true dementia from depressive pseudodementia; as a general rule, if any of the above symptoms or signs are present a psychiatric opinion should be sought.

Patients with hysterical pseudodementia present with a fairly abrupt onset of memory and/or intellectual impairment. They typically appear unconcerned. Unlike organic amnesic disorders, the memory loss is worse for salient personal and early life events. Loss of personal identity is very common. There is usually an identifiable precipitant (such as bereavement, marital or financial problems, or recent offending) as well as a past psychiatric history. Patients may show features of the so-called 'Ganser syndrome', the core symptom of which is the giving of bizarre approximate answers. For instance, when asked 'How many legs does a cow have', they reply three or five. As in other hysterical conversion states, there may be an underlying organic disorder which has been grossly exaggerated at a conscious or subconscious level.

DELIRIUM (ACUTE CONFUSIONAL STATE)

This clinical syndrome is characterized by the abrupt onset of marked attentional abnormalities, clouding of consciousness, disorders of perception, thinking, memory, psychomotor activity, and sleep–wakefulness cycle, and a marked tendency to fluctuations in cognitive performance and behaviour. The features of dementia and delirium are contrasted in Table 4. It should be noted that a disturbance in attention is the most consistent abnormality: patients are unable to sustain attention to external stimuli, are distractable and easily lose the thread of conversations. Severe disorientation in time is invariable. Thinking ability is drastically affected and delusions are common. Illusions and hallucinations are also a frequent feature, particularly in the visual domain. Patients may be restless, excitable, and hypervigilant. Alternatively, they may be excessively sleepy, but most commonly patients oscillate between these extremes, with a tendency to be more aroused and restless at night. Delirium occurs most frequently in the elderly. Those with the beginnings of dementia are particularly vulnerable. The potential causes are legion and include any form of metabolic disturbance, intoxication by drugs and poisons, drug and alcohol withdrawal states, infections both intra- and extracranial, head trauma, epilepsy (postictal states and non-convulsive status), raised intracranial pressure, subarachnoid hae-

Table 4 *Differential diagnosis of delirium and dementia*

Characteristic	Delirium	Dementia
Onset	Acute or subacute	Insidious and chronic
Course	Fluctuating with lucid intervals, often worse at night	Stable over the course of the day
Duration	Hours to weeks	Months to years
Consciousness (response to environment)	Clouded	Clear
Attention	Impaired with marked distractability	Relatively normal
Orientation	Almost always impaired for time; tendency to mistakes on place and person	Impaired in later stages
Memory	Impaired	Impaired
Thinking	Disorganized, delusional	Impoverished
Perception	Illusions and hallucinations common, usually visual	Absent in early stages, common later
Speech	Incoherent, hesitant, slow or rapid	Aphasic features common
Sleep–wake cycle	Always disrupted	Usually normal

morrhage, and focal brain lesions, particularly if the right hemisphere is involved. The prognosis clearly depends on the aetiology, but if the underlying cause is cured then return to baseline performance can be expected.

ISOLATED HIGHER CEREBRAL FUNCTION DISORDERS

Occasionally patients with focal cognitive deficits are mistakenly diagnosed as demented. This is perhaps most common in those with fluent Wernicke's type aphasia who often have no other signs and are erroneously thought to be confused. Clearly, any significant degree of language disorders precludes verbal memory testing, and formal neuropsychological assessment is required to evaluate non-verbal intelligence and memory. Occasionally patients with visual agnosia, resulting from posterior cerebral lesions, may be misdiagnosed, as may patients with the amnesic syndrome in which memory is severely impaired but other aspects of cognitive function are relatively unaffected (causes include alcoholic Korsakoff's syndrome, diencephalic damage from bilateral paramedian thalamic infarction or tumours of the third ventricle, and medial temporal lobe damage following herpes simplex virus encephalitis, surgical resection, head injury, cerebral anoxia, or posterior cerebral artery territory strokes).

Assessment of suspected dementia

There are two questions to be asked when assessing patients with suspected dementia. First, does the patient fulfil the criteria for a diagnosis of dementia and can other potential causes of cognitive impairment (discussed above) be confidently excluded? Secondly, if so, what is the likely cause of the dementia? The first question can, in most cases, be answered using basic clinical skills, namely history taking and bedside cognitive testing. The second requires a careful neurological examination and additional investigations, which might range from the fairly elementary to the elaborate. Since Alzheimer's disease is responsible for the majority of cases of dementia, one of the fundamental goals is to decide whether there are any symptoms or signs which are not typical of Alzheimer's disease. It is, therefore, essential to have a firm grasp of the usual pattern of deficits found in patients with Alzheimer's. Some of the commoner clinical features which should alert one to alternative diagnoses are listed in Table 5.

HISTORY

History taking is the cornerstone of patient evaluation. As well as obtaining a history from the patient it is essential to question a close relative or other informant. This should be done without the patient being present; many patients with dementia are unaware of their failings, or at least of their extent, and, more importantly, the informant may be understandably reluctant to reveal potentially embarrassing details in front of the patient. The earliest observed problems (e.g. memory loss, personality change, etc.) should be established, as well as the subsequent course of the illness. The pattern and rate of decline (insidious, stepwise, fluctuating, rapidly progressive, etc.) is important. In all cases, the narrative account should be supplemented by questions designed to probe specific domains of cognitive function. A checklist is given below. It is obviously important to probe both the patient and the informant for any symptoms suggestive of focal neurological deficits or raised intracranial pressure. In this regard, it is noteworthy that patients are frequently unaware of even quite marked involuntary movements. A particular note should be made of any symptoms suggestive of past cerebrovascular events (transient ischaemic attacks or stroke) and of risk factors for thromboembolic disease. Alcohol intake, in terms of units per week, tobacco usage, and all medications should be carefully documented. In younger patients, or those with other unusual features, the possibility of immunocompromise from the acquired immunodeficiency syndrome (AIDS) must be considered and appropriate enquiries made concerning potential past exposure to infection. In all patients, the state of health, or cause and age of death of first-degree relatives should be recorded and specific enquiries made regarding any family history of neurological or psychiatric disease.

COGNITIVE FUNCTIONS: SUGGESTED AREAS OF ENQUIRY

Memory
- anterograde: recall of new information in day-to-day life (e.g. messages, appointments, family news, etc.), repetitiveness
- retrograde: past personal and public events

Language
- output: word finding, grammar, word errors (paraphasias)
- comprehension
- reading and writing ability

Table 5 *Clinical features which suggest diagnoses other than Alzheimer's disease*

Young age (< 65 years)	Huntington's disease, infections (e.g. AIDS, SSPE), inherited metabolic disorders (e.g. Wilson's disease), vasculitides, neoplasia
Rapid progression (weeks or months)	Neoplasia, infections, Creutzfeldt–Jakob disease
Personality change early in course	Pick's disease, subcortical dementias, frontal tumours
Early onset incontinence	Tumours, normal pressure hydrocephalus
Cardiac disease, past TIA or stroke	Cerebral vascular disease (multi-infarct dementia)
Symptoms of raised intracranial pressure	Tumours, subdural haematoma
Fluctuating performance	Subdural haematoma, vascular dementia
Immunocompromise	Infections (e.g. PML, toxoplasmosis), primary intracerebral lymphoma
Systemic illness	Metabolic disorders, neoplasia, infections, vasculitides
Family history of dementia or involuntary movements	Huntington's disease, inherited metabolic diseases
Anosmia	Frontal meningioma
Eye movement abnormalities	Progressive supranuclear palsy, multiple sclerosis, mitochondrial cytopathies
Ocular signs	Syphilis, Wilson's disease, raised pressure
Myoclonus	Creutzfeldt–Jakob disease, SSPE, postanoxia, myoclonic epilepsies
Gait disturbance	Normal pressure hydrocephalus, tumours, progressive supranuclear palsy, Huntington's disease

Abbreviations: AIDS, acquired immunodeficiency syndrome; SSPE, subacute sclerosing panencephalitis; PML, progressive multifocal leucoencephalopathy; TIA, transient ischaemic attack.

Numerical skills
- handling money, shopping, dealing with bills

Visuospatial and perceptual abilities
- dressing
- spatial orientation and route finding
- recognition of objects, colours, and people

Thinking and problem-solving

Personality and social conduct

Symptoms of depression

Delusions and hallucinations

EXAMINATION

All patients presenting with dementia require a full neurological examination. Clues to possible diagnoses are listed in Table 5. Cognitive evaluation is also mandatory, and should include assessment of orientation, concentration/attention, reasoning, memory, language, numerical skills, praxis, and visuospatial ability. This qualitative assessment of cognition should be supplemented with a quantitative score. Of the many available brief assessment instruments, the Mini-Mental State Examination (see Table 6) is the most widely standardized and validated. A score of 24 out of 30 was originally suggested as the lower limit of normal, but it has been repeatedly shown that performance on even this simple test is influenced very considerably by age and by educational attainment. Hence, a young adult with university level education should perform flawlessly, whereas a normal elderly subject who left school at age 14 may score as low as 22 or 23. With this proviso, the Mini-Mental State Examination provides a reasonable screening instrument and is particularly useful for grading and monitoring the severity of dementia. However, patients with early Alzheimer's disease can score normally on this test. Furthermore, this and similar tests are notoriously insensitive to frontal lobe dysfunction and to the deficits seen in patients with subcortical dementing syndromes (see above). In these cases, and in others in whom there is any doubt about the diagnosis, it is essential to obtain a formal neuropsychological assessment.

INVESTIGATIONS

The minimum investigations for a newly presenting patient with dementia are shown in Table 7. The main indication for performing a computed tomography (CT) scan is to exclude hydrocephalus and benign tumours. Where resources are limited, scanning should be reserved for cases with atypical features. The extent of further investigations will depend on the patient's age, the presence of specific features in the history and examination, and the results of preliminary screening investigations. Cerebrospinal fluid examination is recommended in young patients, and in those in whom there is any doubt about the diagnosis. Electroencephalography is particularly valuable in cases of suspected Creutzfeldt–Jakob disease. Functional brain scanning by means of positron emission tomography or single photon emission tomography can be helpful in difficult cases; in Alzheimer's disease, characteristic bilateral temporoparietal changes are present which contrast to the focal frontal or temporal lobe hypoperfusion found in the focal lobar atrophies (Pick's disease)—the perfusion deficits in degenerative disorders are secondary to the reduced metabolism in affected brain regions; vascular dementia is associated with perfusion deficits which correspond to vascular territories. Very occasionally brain biopsy is required in young patients who defy diagnosis by other means.

Treatable causes of dementia
NORMAL PRESSURE HYDROCEPHALUS

The classical presentation of normal pressure hydrocephalus is a triad of cognitive impairment, gait disturbance, and incontinence. The cog-

Table 6 *The Mini-Mental State Examination*

	Score
Orientation	
Year, month, day, date, season	_____/5
Country, county, town, hospital, ward (clinic)	_____/5
Registration	
Examiner names three objects (e.g. orange, key, ball)	
Patient asked to repeat the three names.	
Score one for each correct answer	_____/3
Then ask the patient to repeat all three names three times	
Attention	
Subtract 7 from 100, then repeat from result, stop after 5: 93, 86, 79, 72, 65	
Alternative if patient makes errors on serial subtraction: spell 'world' backwards: D L R O W	
Score best performance on either task	_____/5
Recall	
Ask for the names of the objects learned earlier.	_____/3
Language	
Name a pencil and a watch	_____/2
Repeat 'No ifs, ands, or buts'	_____/1
Give a three-stage command. Score one for each stage (e.g. 'Take this piece of paper in your right hand, fold it in half, and place it on the chair next to you.')	_____/3
Ask patient to read and obey a written command on a piece of paper stating: 'Close your eyes'	_____/1
Ask patient to write a sentence. Score correct if it is sensible and has a subject and a verb.	_____/1
Copying	
Ask patient to copy intersecting pentagons	
Score as correct if they overlap and if each has five sides	_____/1

Total score	_____/30

Table 7 *Recommended investigations in dementia*

Routine
Full blood count and ESR
Biochemical profile: urea or creatinine, electrolytes, calcium, liver function
Serum vitamin B_{12} and folate
Thyroid function
Serological tests for syphilis
Chest radiograph
CT scan

Other tests which may be indicated in certain cases
  EEG (e.g. Creutzfeldt–Jakob disease and SSPE)
  Functional brain imaging: SPECT
  CSF examination (e.g. infections, malignant meningitis, etc.)
  Screening for cardiac sources of emboli
  Immunological tests for vasculitides (e.g. SLE)
  Slit-lamp examination for Kayser–Fleischer rings and caeruloplasmin estimation (Wilson's disease)
  Specific blood and/or urine tests for inherited metabolic disorders
  Cerebral biopsy

Abbreviations: CSF, cerebrospinal fluid; CT, computed tomography; EEG, electroencephalography; ESR, erythrocyte sedimentation rate; SLE, systemic lupus erythematosus; SPECT, single photon emission tomography; SSPE, subacute sclerosing panencephalitis.

proportion to the degree of cortical atrophy, sometimes accompanied by periventricular low-density changes.

Patients with ventricular enlargement should be referred to a neurosurgeon for consideration of insertion of a ventricular shunt. Prior to permanent shunting, intracranial pressure monitoring is usually performed. In patients who subsequently respond to shunting, pressure monitoring reveals spontaneous periodic waves with a frequency of 0.5 to 2 min—so-called B waves—for a minimum of 5 per cent of the day. A variety of CSF circulation tests, including radio-isotope cisternography, metrizimide cisternography, and CSF infusion studies, have been used but are not usually necessary. A trial of lumbar puncture with removal of 25 to 50 ml of CSF has been advocated, but a negative response does not exclude a diagnosis of normal pressure hydrocephalus. Ventricular shunting remains the definitive treatment. In patients with the full clinical triad, a useful improvement with shunting occurs in up to 70 per cent of cases, with full recovery in a third. Those with a short history, the typical gait disturbance, an identified aetiology, and in whom imaging shows small sulci, respond best to shunting. The results are very poor in patients with dementia alone. The complications of surgery are not inconsiderable and include subdural haematomas, shunt infection, pneumonia, epilepsy, intracerebral haemorrhage, and pulmonary emboli. Most series report a mortality rate of 2 to 12 per cent and a morbidity rate of up to 50 per cent.

CHRONIC SUBDURAL HAEMATOMA

This treatable complication of head injury can present with subacute dementia, often associated with symptoms of raised intracranial pressure. Focal signs may be present. Fluctuations in conscious level or in cognitive performance are characteristic. It commonly occurs in individuals prone to recurrent head trauma (alcoholics, the elderly, epileptics). Those with coagulation defects are also at high risk. On CT scan a chronic subdural haematoma is seen as a peripheral mass lesion of varying signal intensity. Treatment is by surgical evacuation except in cases with very small collections without significant mass effect. Recurrence is fairly common, occurring in 10 to 40 per cent of cases, and patients may require further drainage procedures, but the long-term outcome is usually excellent.

nitive profile is that of subcortical dementia with prominent psychomotor slowing. The gait disorder is best described as an apraxia and patients may show the pathognomonic 'glued-to-the-floor' sign when they stand and first attempt to walk. Others merely show a wide-based unsteady gait with a tendency to fall. Despite these abnormalities of gait, there are usually few, if any, pyramidal or extrapyramidal signs when examined on the bed. Urinary incontinence is a late and variable feature of the condition.

Isolated measurement of cerebrospinal fluid (CSF) pressure at lumbar puncture led to the erroneous belief that the intracranial pressure in these patients was normal. In fact, they show periods of intermittently raised pressure due to raised CSF outflow resistance, usually at the level of the arachnoid villi. The known causes include prior head injury, subarachnoid haemorrhage, and meningitis. Despite full investigation, however, in many cases there is no identifiable cause. The screening investigation of choice is the CT scan, which shows ventricular enlargement out of

BENIGN TUMOURS

Patients with subfrontal meningiomas typically present with an insidious change in personality and other features of a frontal lobe syndrome. Examination may reveal anosmia or unilateral visual failure with optic atrophy. Occasionally relatively benign midline tumours, such as colloid cysts of the third ventricle, and non-secretory pituitary tumours may present with cognitive impairment secondary to hydrocephalus.

METABOLIC AND ENDOCRINE DISORDERS

Virtually any acquired metabolic derangement (e.g. hyponatraemia, uraemia, hepatic failure, etc.) can cause cognitive impairment, but the features are almost invariably those of delirium (acute confusional state) rather than dementia. Chronic hypocalcaemia and recurrent hypoglycaemia may result in a dementia, sometimes accompanied by ataxia and involuntary movements. Endocrine disorders, however, more frequently cause dementia, although overt psychiatric symptoms often coexist. Hypothyroidism sometimes presents with prominent complaints of mental slowing, apathy, and poor memory. The psychological symptoms of Addison's disease and hypopituitism are very similar, and in all of these disorders, the overall picture is more like that seen in subcortical than in cortical dementias (see above). Cushing's syndrome is frequently associated with psychiatric symptoms (depression, paranoid delusions) and may rarely present with a dementia.

DEFICIENCY STATES

In untreated pernicious anaemia, secondary to vitamin B_{12} deficiency, the classical features of subacute degeneration of the spinal cord and peripheral nerves are accompanied by a progressive low-grade dementia. It is, however, extremely unusual for the cognitive features to predominate. Cases of dementia without the other neurological manifestations are even rarer. Folic acid deficiency may cause mild cognitive dysfunction but this hardly ever amounts to a true dementia. Severe thiamine (vitamin B_1) deficiency results in the Wernicke–Korsakoff syndrome. In the acute stages, there is delirium. If it is not promptly treated, a chronic amnesic syndrome may ensue.

INFECTIONS

Primary CNS infection with HIV is now the commonest cause of early onset dementia in some parts of the world. The encephalopathy, known as the AIDS-dementia complex, which develops early in the course of the disease, may be the sole manifestation. It is characterized by poor concentration, psychomotor slowing, personality change, and other features of a subcortical dementia. Investigations reveal increased CSF protein, pleocytosis, and oligoclonal bands. White matter changes may be seen on CT scan and are more obvious on magnetic resonance imaging. Treatment with azidothymidine can improve the cognitive deficits. Patients with AIDS are also at risk from a number of opportunistic infections, including cerebral toxoplasmosis, cryptococcal meningitis, and progressive leucoencephalopathy, which can all present with rapidly progressive dementia. Neurosyphilis is now a rare cause of dementia but should be considered in patients with other neurological features (seizures, dysathria, ptosis, pupillary abnormalities, tremor, pyramidal signs, ataxia, etc.). Specific serological tests are positive and the CSF shows an increase in protein and pleocytosis. Treatment with penicillin may result in some improvement.

REFERENCES

Adams, R.D., Fisher, C.M., Hakim, S., Ojemann, R.G., and Sweet, W.H. (1965). Symptomatic occult hydrocephalus with 'normal' cerebrospinal fluid pressure. A treatable syndrome. *New England Journal of Medicine* **273**, 117–26.

Brown, R.G. and Marsden, C.D. (1988). Subcortical dementia: the neuropsychological evidence. *Neuroscience* **36**, 1179–85.

Bulbena, A. and Berrios, G.E. (1986). Pseudodementia: facts and figures. *British Journal of Psychiatry* **148**, 87–94.

Byrne, E.J. (1992). Diffuse Lewy body disease. In *Recent advances in psychogeriatrics*, (ed. T. Arie), pp. 33–43. Churchill Livingstone, Edinburgh.

Cooper, B. (1991). The epidemiology of dementia. In *Psychiatry in the elderly* (ed. R. Jacoby and C. Oppenheimer), pp. 574–85. Oxford University Press.

Cummings, J.L. (ed.) (1991). *Subcortical dementia*. Oxford University Press.

Cummings, J.L., Miller, B., Hill, M.A., and Neskes, R. (1987). Neuropsychiatric aspects of multi-infarct dementia and dementia of the Alzheimer type. *Archives of Neurology* **44**, 389–93.

Folstein, M.F., Folstein, S.E., and McHugh, P.R. (1975). Mini-mental state: a practical method for grading the cognitive state of patients for clinicians. *Journal of Psychiatric Research* **12**, 189–98.

Gibb, W.R.G., Luthert, P.J., Janota, I., and Lantos, P.L. (1989). Cortical Lewy body dementia: clinical features and classification. *Journal of Neurology, Neurosurgery and Psychiatry* **52**, 185–92.

Hodges, J.R. (1994) *Cognitive assessment for clinicians: a practical guide*. Oxford University Press.

Hodges, J.R. (1994). Pick's disease. In *Dementia* (ed. A. Burns and R. Levy). pp. 739–53. Chapman and Hall, London.

Huber, S.J., *et al.* (1986). Cortical versus subcortical dementia: neuropsychological differences. *Archives of Neurology* **43**, 392–4.

Jorm, A.F., Korten, E., and Henderson, A.S. (1987). The prevalence of dementia; a quantitative integration of the literature. *Acta Psychiatrica Scandinavica* **76**, 465–79.

Lishman, W.A. (1987). *Organic psychiatry: the psychological consequences of cerebral disorder* (2nd edn). Blackwell Scientific, Oxford.

Neary, D. (1990). Non Alzheimer's disease forms of cerebral pathology. *Journal of Neurology, Neurosurgery and Psychiatry* **53**, 927–31.

Oxbury, J.M. (1991). Dementia: introduction. In *Clinical neurology*, (ed. M. Swash and J. Oxbury), pp. 112–19. Churchill Livingstone, Edinburgh.

Pickard, J.P. (1991). Normal pressure hydrocephalus. In *Clinical neurology*, (ed. M. Swash and J. Oxbury), pp. 151–64. Churchill Livingstone, Edinburgh.

Rossor, M. (1991). The dementias. In *Neurology in clinical practice*, (ed. W.G. Bradley, R.B. Daroff, G.M. Fenichel, and C.D. Marsden), pp. 1407–41. Butterworth-Heineman, Boston.

Sagar, H.J. and Sullivan, E.V. (1988). Patterns of cognitive impairment in dementia. In *Recent advances in clinical neurology No. 5*, (ed. C.J. Kennard), pp. 47–86. Churchill Livingstone, Edinburgh.

Sahakian, B.J. (1991). Depressive pseudodementia in the elderly. *International Journal of Geriatric Psychiatry* **6**, 453–8.

24.7.2 Alzheimer's disease

M. N. ROSSOR

Alzheimer's disease accounts for between 50 and 70 per cent of cases of dementia, either alone or in combination with vascular disease. The eponym followed the description in 1907 of a woman in her early fifties with a progressive dementia and behavioural disturbance. At autopsy neurofibrillary tangles and senile plaques were demonstrated throughout the cerebral cortex. Initially the term 'Alzheimer's disease' was reserved for presenile cases but current usage encompasses all cases of dementia with neurofibrillary tangles and senile plaques, irrespective of the age at onset. There is, however, increasing evidence of heterogeneity and under this rubric there may be a number of different diseases.

EPIDEMIOLOGY

One in five people over 80 years of age will develop dementia, of which Alzheimer's disease is the most common cause. However, it is not confined to the elderly and cases may present in patients as young as 30.

Age is the biggest risk factor, followed by a family history. The high prevalence in the elderly results in many cases having a family history, but clear autosomal dominant pedigrees account for perhaps only 5 to 10 per cent of cases, a small proportion of which are associated with mutations in the amyloid precursor protein (APP) gene (see below). Individuals with trisomy 21 (Down's syndrome) also develop Alzheimer histopathological changes in their third and fourth decade, attributable to an extra copy of the APP gene. Significant head injury is a risk factor in some studies, and there is evidence that increased aluminium exposure might predispose to Alzheimer's disease. The role of aluminium in dialysis encephalopathy is well established but its contribution to Alzheimer's disease is controversial.

PATHOLOGY

Macroscopically there is cortical atrophy, particularly affecting the temporal lobes and hippocampus. The histopathological hallmarks of Alzheimer's disease are neurofibrillary tangles and senile plaques (Fig. 1). Neurofibrillary tangles are intraneuronal argentophilic inclusions found within the cell body, which on electron microscopy consist of paired helical filaments. The latter have a central core of the microtubule-associated protein, tau, which is involved with microtubule assembly. The tau of paired helical filaments is in an abnormally phos-

Fig. 1 (a) Neurofibrillary tangles (arrowheads) and senile plaques (arrows) in Alzheimer's disease. Modified Bielschowsky stain, ×300. (By courtesy of Professor P. Lantos, Institute of Psychiatry.) (b) βA4 peptide deposition in a senile plaque (arrow) and in the wall of a blood vessel (arrowhead) in Alzheimer's disease. Immunocytochemistry: ABC method, ×800. (βA4 antibody kindly provided by Professor B.H. Anderton, Institute of Psychiatry.)

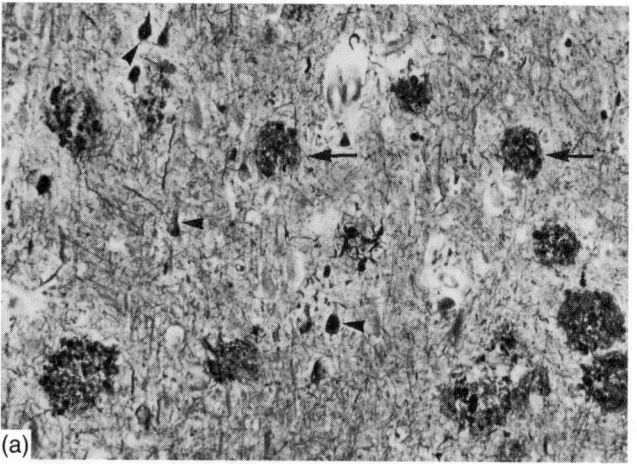

(a)

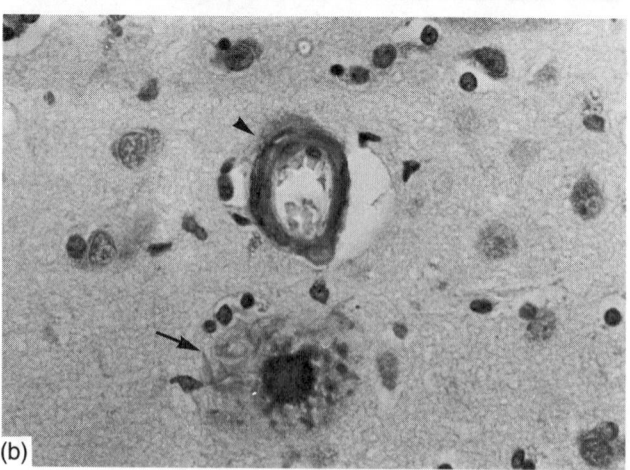

(b)

phorylated state which causes abnormalities of microtubule aggregation and subsequent collapse of the cytoskeleton. Ubiquitin is also found in association with neurofibrillary tangles and, as with other inclusions such as Lewy bodies, antiubiquitin immunostaining is a useful histological adjunct. The presence of ubiquitin probably represents an attempt by the cell to degrade the abnormal protein. Neurofibrillary tangles are found particularly within the pyramidal cells of layer 3 in the neocortical association areas, hippocampus, amygdala, and certain subcortical nuclei which have diffuse connections to the cortex, such as the nucleus basalis of Meynert and the nucleus raphe. It is suggested that neurofibrillary tangles form in cell bodies whose axons and dendrites are involved in senile plaque formation. Hirano bodies and granulovacuolar degeneration are also intraneuronal features and are found particularly in the hippocampus. Lewy bodies are seen in a proportion of cases of Alzheimer's disease, not only in the substantia nigra but also more widely throughout the cerebral cortex. Neuropil threads are filamentous structures on silver staining scattered throughout the neuropil with a similar, but not coterminous, distribution to neurofibrillary tangles. Ultrastructurally they also consist of paired helical filaments and straight filaments.

Classical senile plaques consist of a central core of amyloid protein with a rim of dystrophic argentophilic neurites. In the centre of the amyloid core aluminosilicate deposition occurs, although the extent to which aluminium is abnormally deposited in the Alzheimer brain is controversial. The amyloid protein within senile plaques is the same as that deposited within cerebral blood vessels, which results in the congophilic or amyloid angiopathy. This protein, of 39 to 43 amino acids, tends to form insoluble fibrils due to prominent β-pleated secondary structure which confers the amyloid properties; it is referred to as β-amyloid, βA4 peptide, or Aβ protein. It is derived from a much larger, 770 amino acid transmembrane molecule, the amyloid precursor protein. β-Amyloid may be deposited as preamyloid plaques without fibril formation which can be demonstrated by specific immunostaining. This has led to the hypothesis that plaques commence with deposition of preamyloid, progressing to a fibrillary amyloid core, with the subsequent formation of a dystrophic neuritic rim which is identified as the classical senile plaque. This model is supported by autopsy studies in trisomy 21 Down's syndrome, in which deposition of preamyloid deposits commences in adolescence. However, not all preamyloid deposits follow this pattern; in the cerebellum, for example, there are no associated neuritic plaques. Senile plaques are distributed widely throughout the brain and can be seen in all layers, but are particularly prominent in the hippocampus and association areas of the neocortex. The amyloid angiopathy in Alzheimer's disease is variable but can be prominent, and in some instances is associated with microscopic haemorrhage. In hereditary cerebral haemorrhage with amyloidosis of Dutch type, neurofibrillary tangles and neuritic plaques are absent but angiopathy is prominent and leads to recurrent cerebral haemorrhage. Clinically significant cortical haemorrhage is rare in Alzheimer's disease.

Neuronal loss is also regionally selective, and the large pyramidal cells of the cerebral cortex and the neurones of subcortical nuclei, such as the nucleus basalis of Meynert, are particularly vulnerable; it is believed that cells containing neurofibrillary tangles are those that die. Additional white matter changes may relate to the neuronal loss or to the additional vascular effects of the amyloid angiopathy. In general, the histopathological changes are more severe in cases of younger onset. Postmortem studies of neurotransmitter markers have revealed evidence of selective deficits which reflect the selective vulnerability of particular neuronal systems. The most consistent is a cholinergic deficit reflecting damage to the subcortical–cortical projection from the nucleus basalis of Meynert. The activity of the cholinergic biosynthetic enzyme choline acetyltransferase is reduced, with relative preservation of the muscarinic class of postsynaptic cholinergic receptors. However, this is not the only ascending projection system to be involved, with 5-hydroxytryptamine (serotonin) and, to a lesser extent, noradrenergic markers also reduced. The pyramidal neurones of the cortical association network utilize glutamate as a transmitter, which is more difficult to measure as it constitutes part of the metabolic pool. However, measures of glutamate uptake indicate that this system is particularly vulnerable, more so than the inhibitory cortical transmitter, γ-aminobutyric acid (GABA). A variety of coexistent cortical neuropeptides, such as somatostatin, are also reduced. These changes in neurotransmitter markers are seen to be a consequence of either cell loss or early dysfunction, rather than as a primary abnormality in the disease. Nevertheless, they are important in developing strategies for symptomatic treatment based on neurotransmitter replacement.

PATHOPHYSIOLOGY

Recent work on familial Alzheimer's disease has provided important insights into the possible pathophysiological mechanisms. Three different single-point mutations and one double mutation have been reported in the APP gene in individuals with histologically proven familial Alzheimer's disease (Fig. 2). These cases are very rare, but since the histological and clinical features appear to be identical, an understanding of the molecular pathology might be generalized to the common sporadic disease. Mutations in the APP gene focus attention on β-amyloid deposition as the key event. The amyloid precursor protein is normally metabolized either by an endosomal–lysosomal pathway which can liberate Aβ moieties or by a secretase pathway which results in cleavage within the Aβ domain adjacent to the cell surface. Soluble Aβ protein can also be generated as an apparent normal product of amyloid precursor protein metabolism, although its physiological role is not known. There is evidence that the molecule is toxic if it is in the aggregated fibrillary form of β-amyloid rather than the soluble form. The toxicity may relate to disruption of calcium homeostasis and enhancement of the toxicity of glutamate, which might also explain the formation of neurofibrillary tangles since the hyperphosphorylation of tau is calcium dependent. This amyloid hypothesis would explain the rare familial Alzheimer's disease APP mutation and also trisomy 21 Down's syndrome in which there is an extra copy of the APP gene. Head injury, a risk factor for Alzheimer's disease, causes marked up-regulation of APP expression and, theoretically, could initiate a cascade of amyloid-dependent Alzheimer histopathological change. However, to what extent the amyloid hypothesis will explain other familial Alzheimer's disease pedigrees, many of which are linked to chromosome 14, or the more common sporadic disease is far from clear. The association of late onset disease with the apolipoprotein E$_4$ genotype has been related to interaction both with amyloid and tau.

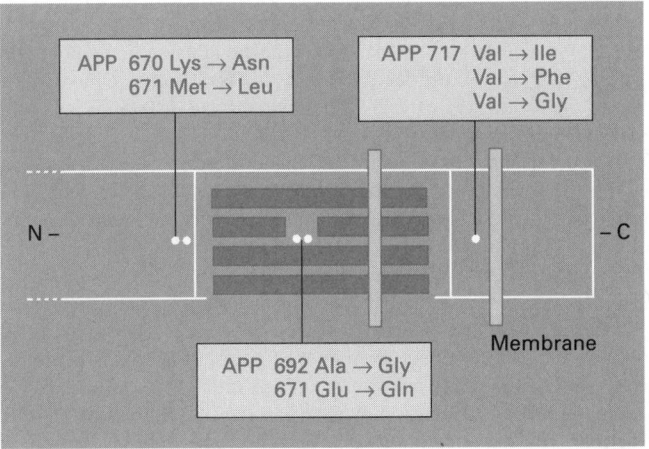

Fig. 2 Ideogram of the amyloid precursor protein molecule, showing sites of mutations associated with familial Alzheimer's disease. The shaded area indicates the Aβ domain.

SYMPTOMS AND SIGNS

Disturbance of higher cortical function dominates the clinical picture, and the pattern of deficits reflects the distribution of the histopathology, namely hippocampus, temporal lobe, and neocortical association areas. Memory impairment is a prominent and early feature, particularly of episodic memory, with relative preservation early in the disease of short-term memory as assessed by the digit span. There is some suggestion that remote memory may be relatively preserved. Language is often impaired with some word-finding difficulty and comprehension deficit, but repetition is usually preserved early in the disease, reminiscent of transcortical sensory aphasia. Although most patients are relatively fluent, some may show an early fall in verbal output. Visuospatial difficulties, and impairment of topographic memory, are a frequent early feature and patients will often get lost when out on their own. In some patients, dressing apraxia is a prominent deficit and, in others, more obvious dyspraxic and agnosic difficulties may develop. Frontal lobe features tend to emerge within the context of a more generalized cognitive impairment. Relative preservation of vocabulary may allow some patients to maintain a social façade for some considerable time, but closer questioning reveals their profound cognitive impairment. Insight is often lost, and occasionally a marked anosognosia can lead to problems with management.

Psychiatric problems are common and many patients develop depression early in the disease. This can be particularly difficult since depressive pseudodementia is an important differential diagnosis of early Alzheimer's disease. Delusions occur in approximately 15 per cent and can be a source of considerable distress for the caregivers. Hallucinations have a similar frequency and are usually visual; often the caregiver may misinterpret perceptual errors by the patient as hallucinations. As the disease progresses speech output is reduced and the patient becomes totally dependent. Seizures occur late in the disease and myoclonus is prominent in some patients. Incontinence is rare until late, in contrast to frontal lobe dementia. Death is usually due to bronchopneumonia, and the median expectancy from diagnosis is approximately 7 to 10 years, but variation in the natural history is considerable.

Examination is normal early in the disease apart from the disturbance of higher cortical function. Increased tone is seen as the disease progresses and is usually of gegenhalten type, but some patients have prominent extrapyramidal features with cogwheeling. Primitive reflexes with rooting, sucking, and grasp reflexes tend to occur late, in contrast to frontal lobe dementia. Pyramidal signs and gait disturbance are rarely seen.

A number of subtypes of Alzheimer's disease have been recognized on clinical grounds. The original distinction between presenile Alzheimer's disease and senile dementia of the Alzheimer type is now seen to be artificial, but nevertheless there are some differences associated with age. Thus the neurochemical deficits are greater with a younger onset, but this may in part reflect a threshold effect, in that more severe deficits are required in the younger brain before dementia is apparent. Familial Alzheimer's disease as a group tends to be younger, but most researchers have selected early-onset families due to the censoring of pedigrees in late-onset disease. Myoclonus tends to be prominent in familial Alzheimer's disease and within this group there is further evidence of clinical and neuropathological heterogeneity, which may reflect the allelic and genetic heterogeneity. Thus within the APP mutation group, there are four mutations associated with Alzheimer's disease and two with congophilic angiopathy. There is genetic heterogeneity, with a substantial group of early familial Alzheimer's disease linked to markers on chromosome 14. Later-onset familial Alzheimer's disease shows neither APP nor chromosome 14 linkage but an association with apoliprotein E$_4$ genotype.

Some Alzheimer patients have early and prominent extrapyramidal features with cogwheel rigidity, bradykinesia, and some gait disturbance. These probably overlap with diffuse Lewy body dementia, and a combination of plaques, tangles, and cortical Lewy bodies may be found at autopsy. Onset with focal deficits can, in some cases, be striking; this is most commonly dysphasia but patients have presented with a hemiparesis and profound unilateral cortical sensory loss. Instances of early-onset dementia with prominent cerebellar and pyramidal features have also been reported with Alzheimer histopathology.

INVESTIGATION

There are no specific diagnostic tests for Alzheimer's disease. Standardized clinical criteria, such as the National Institute of Neurological and Communicative Diseases and Alzheimer's Disease and Related Disorders Association criteria, provide approximately 70 per cent accuracy, higher in research studies. Neuropsychological assessment is important to establish the extent and pattern of deficit and to help exclude a depressive pseudodementia. Routine blood tests and cerebrospinal fluid examination are normal. The EEG shows early diffuse slowing, in contrast to frontal lobe dementia and Pick's disease in which it tends to be normal. Neuroimaging is essential to exclude other causes, such as a space-occupying lesion or hydrocephalus. CT is adequate for this and will frequently show cortical atrophy, but MRI may show more specific regional atrophy involving the hippocampus and temporal lobe; in the elderly patient white matter ischaemic changes are frequently found. Quantitative functional imaging to demonstrate regional metabolism using positron emission tomography with either oxygen-15 or fluorodeoxyglucose shows a characteristic pattern of posterior biparietal bitemporal hypometabolism. Although non-quantitative, a similar pattern of relative posterior hypometabolism can be demonstrated by single photon emission computed tomography (SPECT). Cerebral biopsy will provide a definitive diagnosis in most cases, but is not indicated unless alternative treatable diagnoses, such as cerebral vasculitis, are considered.

TREATMENT AND MANAGEMENT

There is no specific treatment to arrest the disease process. Neurotransmitter replacement strategies are being developed which have concentrated on the cholinergic deficit. Anticholinesterases have shown some benefit in research trials, and tetrahydroaminoacridine (tacrine) has been licensed in the United States and some European countries. Treatment of individual symptoms is important and includes management of any depressive illness, agitation, and troublesome hallucinations. Small doses of neuroleptics may be beneficial, but can cause severe exacerbation of extrapyramidal features in patients with coexistent Lewy body disease. Maintenance of good general health is important since systemic illness such as intercurrent infections, or cardiac failure, can cause deterioration in cognitive state, as can concomitant drugs and alcohol. Simple orientation strategies with labelling of rooms can be valuable. Explanation and prognosis is important for the family, even if an early definite diagnosis is difficult, and contact with caregiver associations should be offered. Patients will need to inform the appropriate driving licence authorities, although decisions about driving vary between individual patients. Appropriate legal arrangements also need to be made for management of the individual's financial affairs.

REFERENCES

Burns, A. and Levy, R. (1992). *Clinical diversity in late-onset Alzheimer's disease*, Maudsley Monographs 34. Oxford University Press.
Citron, M., *et al.* (1992). Mutation of the β-amyloid precursor protein in familial Alzheimer's disease increases β-protein production. *Nature* **360**, 672–4.
Corder, E.H., *et al.* (1993). Apolipoprotein E$_4$ gene dose affects the risk of Alzheimer's disease in late onset families. *Science* **261**, 921–3.
Goate, A., *et al.* (1991). Segregation of a missense mutation in the amyloid precursor protein gene with familial Alzheimer's disease. *Nature* **349**, 704–6.
Goedert, M., Wischik, C.M., Crowther, R.A., Walker, J.E., and Klug, A. (1988). Cloning and sequencing of the cDNA encoding a core protein of the paired helical filament of Alzheimer's disease: identification of the microtubule-associated protein tau. *Proceedings of the National Academy of Sciences USA* **85**, 4051–5.
Hansen, L., *et al.* (1990). The Lewy body variant of Alzheimer's disease: a clinical and pathologic entity. *Neurology* **40**, 1–8.
Hardy, J. and Higgins, G.A. (1992). Alzheimer's disease: The amyloid cascade hypothesis. *Science* **256**, 184–5.
Kang, J., *et al.* (1987). The precursor of Alzheimer's disease amyloid A4 protein resembles a cell-surface receptor. *Nature* **325**, 733–6.
Khachaturian, Z.S. (1985). Diagnosis of Alzheimer's disease. *Archives of Neurology* **42**, 1097–105.
Knapp, M.J., *et al.* (1994). A 30-week randomised controlled trial of high-dose tacrine in patients with Alzheimer's disease. *Journal of the American Medical Association*, **271**, 985–91.
McKhann, G., Drachman, D., Folstein, M., Katzman, R., Price, D., and Stadlan, E. (1984). Clinical diagnosis of Alzheimer's disease: Report of the NINCDS/ADRDA workgroup under the auspices of the Dept. of Health and Human Services Task Force on Alzheimer's disease. *Neurology* **34**, 939–44.
Mayer, R.J., Landon, M., Laszlo, L., Lennox, G., and Lowe, J. (1992). Protein processing in lysosomes: the new therapeutic target in neurodegenerative disease. *Lancet* **340**, 156.
Murphy, M. (1992). The molecular pathogenesis of Alzheimer's disease: clinical prospects. *Lancet* **340**, 1512–15.
Rossor, M.N. (1992). Familial Alzheimer's disease. In *Unusual dementias*, (ed. M.N. Rossor), pp. 517–34. Ballière Tindall, London.
Schellenberg, G.D., *et al.* (1992). Genetic linkage evidence for a familial Alzheimer's disease locus on chromosome 14. *Science* **258**, 668–71.
Whitehouse, P.J. (ed.) (1993). *Dementia*. F.A. Davis, Philadelphia.

24.7.3 Pick's disease (focal lobar atrophy)

J. R. HODGES

HISTORY AND DEFINITION

In 1892 Arnold Pick reported a 71-year-old man with progressive mental deterioration and unusually severe aphasia who at autopsy had marked atrophy of the cortical gyri of the left temporal lobe. Pick drew attention to the fact that progressive brain atrophy may lead to symptoms of local disturbance (i.e. aphasia). In subsequent papers, he described further patients with temporal and/or frontal lobe atrophy, stressing the respective progressive language and behavioural disturbances associated with focal atrophy of these areas.

A few years later, in 1910, Alzheimer recognized histological changes in patients with focal lobar atrophy distinct from those found in the form of cerebral degeneration later associated with his name. Alzheimer described both argyrophilic intracytoplasmic inclusions (Pick bodies), and diffusely staining ballooned neurones (Pick cells) in such cases. However, these characteristic changes are not seen in all patients with focal atrophy and this has led to considerable confusion in the literature regarding the use of the label 'Pick's disease': some authors have reserved the diagnosis for cases with Pick cells and/or Pick bodies; others have included patients with lobar atrophy even if these specific neuropathological changes were absent. Since there is no evidence that patients with or without specific histological changes differ clinically, neurologically, or radiologically, I have defined Pick's disease as a clinical syndrome characterized by the combination of (1) clinical features suggestive of progressive dysfunction of temporal and/or frontal lobes, and (2) radiological or pathological confirmation of focal atrophy.

There are, therefore, two main variants of Pick's disease (or focal lobar atrophy) which reflect the region of the brain which is predominately involved; the first, referred to as 'dementia of frontal lobe type', is better known. The other clinical syndrome of progressive aphasia associated with left temporal lobe atrophy is less widely recognized.

EPIDEMIOLOGY

The true prevalence of Pick's disease in the community has not been established. It is clearly much less common than Alzheimer's disease, but recent studies have shown that it is not as rare as was supposed. Estimates of the ratio between Pick's and Alzheimer's disease, derived from clinicopathological hospital-based surveys, range from 1:5 to 1:20. It affects younger patients than does Alzheimer's disease. The peak age of onset is 45 to 65. Occasional patients with onset as young as the 20s are reported. In most series, men and women are represented equally. Although there are well-documented families in which Pick's disease is inherited with an autosomal dominant pattern of inheritance, overall the genetic aspect has been exaggerated; at least three-quarters of cases are sporadic.

PATHOLOGY

Macroscopically, the defining characteristic of Pick's disease is the striking topographical limitation of the cortical atrophy. In severely affected cases, the frontotemporal regions appear profoundly atrophied, producing thin, 'knife-edged' gyri and deep, widened sulci. In approximately one-half of cases there is frontotemporal atrophy; in a quarter, frontal lobe atrophy predominates; and in a quarter the temporal lobe (particularly the anterior part), bears the brunt. The atrophy is also often asymmetric and more frequently involves the left hemisphere.

Microscopically, there is intense neuronal loss in the atrophic areas, with cortical and subcortical gliosis. Pick bodies, argyrophilic intracytoplasmic inclusions consisting of non-membrane-bound accumulations of filaments in an irregular granulovacuolar matrix, are seen in a minority (around 20 per cent). Pick cells, expanded globular neurones, are found in about one-half of cases.

A number of attempts have been made to subdivide cases according to histological features, for instance, into those with and without inclusions. In general, there is a close relationship between clinical features and the region of involvement, but the exact histological findings bear little relationship to the clinical phenomena.

The consistent decline in cholinergic markers (acetylcholinesterase and choline acetylesterase) found in the neocortex in Alzheimer's disease is not present, but alterations in pre- and postsynaptic serotonergic markers have been reported.

CLINICAL FEATURES

Two main presentations, which mirror the topography of neuropathological change, can be identified, but often features of the two coexist.

Dementia of frontal lobe type

Patients with frontal lobe atrophy present with changes in personality and behaviour, consisting of impaired judgement, a lack of initiation, and difficulty with planning. There is often indifference to domestic and occupational responsibilities, and carelessness in appearance. Social conduct may deteriorate. Facetiousness, inappropriate jocularity, and hypomanic behaviour may also be observed. Many patients are restless. Obsessive-compulsive behaviour is fairly common, rarely more overt psychiatric phenomena such as delusions and hallucinations are seen. Many patients with frontal dysfunction may acquire a label of functional psychiatric disease, because despite gross behavioural changes other aspects of cognition are typically preserved in the early stages. They also characteristically obtain normal scores on simple mental test batteries such as the Mini-Mental State Examination (see Chapter 24.7.1).

Language dysfunction is an early, but subtle, finding in many patients with frontal type dementia and consists of factually empty speech which is reduced in quantity. The articulatory and grammatic aspects of language are typically preserved. Impairment of naming (anomia) is often present but repetition is normal. Many patients develop spontaneous echolalia (a tendency to repeat the examiner's last phrase). Finally, muteness supervenes.

Memory is relatively spared in the early stages, but as the disease advances, it is affected. Motor, sensory, and reflex function remain normal throughout. Occasional patients develop extrapyramidal syndromes with akinesia and rigidity. Myoclonus and epilepsy are rare.

Progressive aphasia

The outstanding clinical manifestation of temporal lobe involvement in Pick's disease is an aphasia syndrome which presents with reduced vocabulary and a severe deficit in naming with meaning-based (semantic) errors, such as clock for watch or dog for lion. The progressive anomia in these patients is not simply a linguistic or word production deficit, but reflects a fundamental loss of semantic memory (or knowledge). Eventually the impairment in semantic memory may be so profound that patients often fail to recognize even very common objects and animals, a condition known as associative agnosia. This clinical syndrome of progressive semantic memory loss has, therefore, been called 'semantic dementia'. Semantic memory is the term applied to the component of long-term memory which stores our knowledge about things in the world and their interrelationship and general facts, as well as words and their meaning. In contrast, other aspects of language competency are usually strikingly preserved; speech production remains fluent, grammatically correct, and well articulated. Unlike patients with Alzheimer's disease, these patients have relatively good day-to-day (episodic) memory, arithmetic ability, and visuospatial skills, at least in the early stages.

A different form of primary progressive aphasia was recently delineated by Mesulam, who described patients with a gradual loss of expressive abilities in which the sound-based (phonological) and grammatical aspects of language production are selectively affected, leading to non-fluent, distorted, agrammatic, and poorly articulated speech with multiple phonemic paraphasic errors (sitter for sister, fencil for pencil). In contrast to the cases described above, word comprehension and object recognition are preserved. These patients with non-fluent aphasia progress slowly to a state of complete mutism. They show selective atrophy of the perisylvian language area of the dominant hemisphere and rather variable histological changes at autopsy.

Patients with severe temporal lobe involvement may develop the Klüver–Bucy syndrome, which consists of emotional placidity, a prominent tendency to place things in the mouth (hyperorality), constant environmental exploration, hypersexuality or altered sexual orientation, and changes in dietary habits with bulimia or even pica. The syndrome, which is caused by amygdalar damage, was first described in monkeys after bilateral anterior temporal lobectomy. A similar complex is seen in humans with extensive bilateral temporal lobe damage from a variety of causes, including herpes simplex encephalitis, trauma, and Pick's disease.

PROGNOSIS AND MANAGEMENT

The time course of progression is highly variable. Some patients deteriorate very rapidly, reaching a state of advanced dementia within a year of diagnosis, others progress very slowly. The average duration of the disease is around 5 to 10 years. At the present time there is no specific treatment.

ASSESSMENT

The diagnosis of Pick's disease (focal lobar atrophy) is based on a combination of clinical, neuropsychological, and neuroimaging assessment. Table 1 compares the features of Pick's and Alzheimer's disease.

The pattern of neuropsychological deficits will depend on whether the disease is mainly frontal or temporal. In early cases involving the frontal lobes, general intellect will typically be normal. Likewise, tests of memory and visuospatial function may show no significant abnormality. By contrast, tasks aimed at specific evaluation of the frontal lobes (i.e. problem-solving, set-shifting, etc.) will show marked impairment. With dis-

Table 1 *Contrasting features of Pick's disease and Alzheimer's disease*

	Pick's disease	Alzheimer's disease
Age of onset (years)	45–65	Usually > 65
Presenting features	Frontal type: Personality change Lack of planning, organization, etc. Antisocial behaviour Obsessive–compulsive behaviour Reduced verbal output Temporal type: Progressive fluent aphasia (semantic dementia) Klüver–Bucy syndrome	Frontal features are a late development Rarely severe Very rare
Memory	Preserved until late	Severely affected from onset
Visuospatial and perceptual skills	Preserved until late	Impaired early in course
Mental test batteries (e.g. MMSE)	Often normal	Impaired score
Imaging: CT scan or MRI	Frontal and/or temporal lobe atrophy	General atrophy
SPECT or PET hypoperfusion	Frontal or temporal	Bilateral temporoparietal

Abbreviations: CT, computed tomography; MMSE, mini-mental state examination; MRI, magnetic resonance imaging; PET, positron emission tomography; SPECT, single photon emission computed tomography.

ease progression, intellectual ability deteriorates along with memory, but visuospatial functions are characteristically normal, even late in the disease.

In temporal lobe cases, a selective decline in the semantic (word meaning and usage) aspects of language occurs. This is most evident on tests of naming, word comprehension (such as pointing to pictures of objects in response to their spoken name), and category fluency (in which subjects are asked to produce as many examples as possible from defined categories, such as animals, within 1 min). As with frontal cases, performance on tasks dependent on the parietal and occipital lobes, such as visuospatial and perceptual skills, remain normal until very late in the disease.

The most significant advance in premorbid diagnosis has come from functional brain imaging. As opposed to the characteristic bilateral temporoparietal deficit in cerebral blood flow and metabolism seen in early Alzheimer's disease, in Pick's disease there is focal reduction in frontal and/or temporal perfusion on single photon emission computed tomography or positron emission tomography scanning.

Computed tomography (CT) scanning may show frontal lobe atrophy, but the temporal lobes are poorly seen on conventional CT scans because of the orientation of scanning and artefacts from the temporal bones. Magnetic resonance imaging (MRI), especially with coronal or horizontally orientated cuts, can demonstrate striking focal temporal lobe atrophy, as illustrated in Fig. 1.

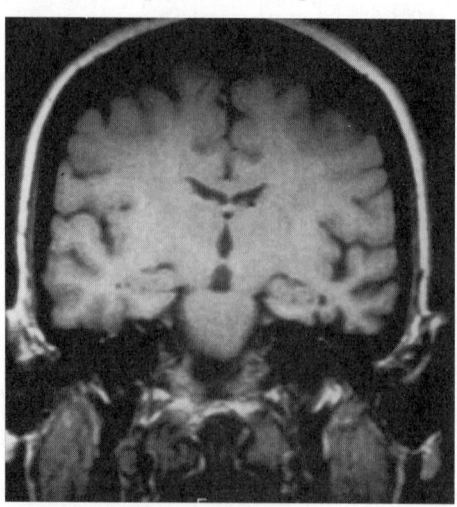

Fig. 1 T$_1$-weighted MRI scan in the coronal plane of a patient with progressive semantic memory impairment presenting with a fluent aphasic syndrome. Note the selective atrophy of the left temporal lobe.

REFERENCES

Corsellis, J.A.N. (1976). Ageing and the dementias. In *Greenfield's neuropathology* (eds. W. Blackwood and J.A.N. Corsellis), pp. 796–848. Year Book Medical Publishers, Chicago.

Cummings, J.L. (1991). Pick's disease. In *Clinical neurology* (ed. M. Swash and J. Oxbury). Churchill Livingstone, Edinburgh.

Gustafson, L. (1987). Frontal lobe degeneration of non-Alzheimer type. II. Clinical picture and differential diagnosis. *Archives of Gerontology and Geriatrics* **6**, 209–23.

Hodges, J.R. (1993). Pick's disease. In *Dementia*, (ed. A. Burns and R. Levy). pp 739–52. Chapman and Hall, London.

Hodges, J.R., Patterson, K., Oxbury, S., and Funnell, E. (1992). Semantic dementia: progressive fluent aphasia with temporal lobe atrophy. *Brain* **115**, 1783–806.

Knopman, D.S., *et al.* (1989). The spectrum of imaging and neuropsychological findings in Pick's disease. *Neurology* **39**, 362–8.

Mesulam, M.M. (1982). Slowly progressive aphasia without dementia. *Annals of Neurology* **11**, 592–8.

Miller, B.I., *et al.* (1991). Frontal lobe degeneration: clinical, neuropsychological, and SPECT characteristics. *Neurology* **41**, 1374–82.

Neary, D., Snowden, J.S., Northern, B., and Goulding, P. (1988). Dementia of frontal lobe type. *Journal of Neurology, Neurosurgery and Psychiatry* **51**, 353–61.

Orrell, M.W. and Sahakian, B. (1991). Dementia of frontal lobe type. *Psychological Medicine* **21**, 553–6.

Pick, A. (1892). Uber die Beziehungen der senilen Hirnatrophie zur Aphasie. *Prager Medicinische Wochenschrift* **17**, 165–7. Introduced and translated by D. Girling and G.E. Berrios, *History of Psychiatry*, in press.

Poeck, K. and Luzzatti, C. (1988). Slowly progressive aphasia in three patients: the problem of accompanying neuropsychological deficit. *Brain* **111**, 151–68.

Sparks, D.L. and Markesbery, W.R. (1991). Altered serotonergic and cholinergic synaptic markers in Pick's disease. *Archives of Neurology* **48**, 796–9.

Tissot, R., Constantinidis, J., and Richard, J. (1985). Pick's disease. In *Handbook of clinical neurology*, Vol. 2, (ed. J.A.M. Frederiks), pp. 233–46. Elsevier Science Publishers, Amsterdam.

Weintraub, S., Rubin, N.P., and Mesulam, M.-M. (1990). Primary progressive aphasia. Longitudinal course, neuropsychological profile and language features. *Archives of Neurology* **47**, 1329–35.

24.7.4 Prion diseases

J. COLLINGE

The prion diseases are neurodegenerative conditions which affect both humans and animals and which have been known as the spongiform encephalopathies, slow virus diseases, or transmissible dementias. Creutzfeldt–Jakob disease, Gerstmann–Sträussler–Scheinker syndrome, and kuru represent the traditionally recognized human conditions. These diseases are transmissible to experimental animals by inoculation and are, in the case of the familial forms of the human prion diseases, also transmitted in an autosomal dominant fashion. The prion diseases are biologically unique in this regard. For many years these diseases have been an intense and controversial area of research interest because of the unique properties of the transmissible agent, or prion. The need for a clearer understanding of these rare human diseases has been highlighted by the epidemic of a prion disease amongst cattle herds in the United Kingdom (bovine spongiform encephalopathy) and the potential threat to human health that this could pose.

AETIOLOGY

Historical background

The first disease of this group to be recognized was scrapie, a naturally occurring disease of sheep and goats, which has been known in the United Kingdom for over 200 years. It was demonstrated to be transmissible between sheep by experimental inoculation, following long incubation periods, in 1936. It was assumed that some type of virus must be the causative agent and Sigurdsson coined the term 'slow virus infection' in 1954. There was considerable interest in the 1950s in an epidemic of a neurodegenerative disease, kuru, characterized principally by a progressive ataxia, amongst the Fore linguistic group of the Eastern Highlands of Papua New Guinea. Subsequent fieldwork suggested that kuru was transmitted by ritualistic endocannibalism. In 1959, Hadlow drew attention to the similarities between kuru and scrapie at the neuropathological, clinical, and epidemiological levels. A landmark in the field was the subsequent demonstration of the transmission, by intracerebral inoculation with brain homogenates, of kuru to the chimpanzee by Gajdusek and colleagues in 1966. This work led to the concept of the 'transmissible dementias'. Creutzfeldt–Jakob disease was successfully transmitted in 1968. Creutzfeldt–Jakob disease was a term introduced by Spielmeyer in 1922, drawing from the earlier case reports of Creutzfeldt and Jakob, and was used in subsequent years to describe a range of neurodegenerative conditions, many of which would not meet modern diagnostic criteria for this disease. The new criterion of transmissibility allowed diagnostic criteria for Creutzfeldt–Jakob disease to be assessed and refined.

Both the animal and human conditions share common histopathological features. The classical triad of spongiform vacuolation (affecting any part of the cerebral grey matter), neuronal loss, and astrocytic proliferation may be accompanied by amyloid plaques. As a result of this spongiform vacuolation, these diseases also became known as the spongiform encephalopathies. Gerstmann–Sträussler–Scheinker syndrome was transmitted to experimental animals in 1981.

Creutzfeldt–Jakob disease occurs principally as a sporadic disorder, although around 15 per cent of cases occur in a familial context. Gerstmann–Sträussler–Scheinker syndrome is usually familial. Extensive epidemiological studies in the 1970s and 1980s confirmed the apparently random distribution of cases of Creutzfeldt–Jakob disease (with the exception of three ethnogeographical clusters which will be discussed later), with an incidence of 0.4 to 1 case/million/year. There was no evidence that the incidence of Creutzfeldt–Jakob disease was related to local scrapie prevalence, Creutzfeldt–Jakob disease being as common in countries which have been free of scrapie for many years, and also there was no excess of Creutzfeldt–Jakob disease in those particularly exposed to scrapie as a result of their work. There was therefore no epidemiological evidence that Creutzfeldt–Jakob disease was caused by environmental exposure to infective material, with the exception of the rare iatrogenic cases (discussed later).

The nature of prions

The nature of the transmissible agent in these diseases has been a subject of heated debate for many years. The initial assumption that the agent must be some form of virus was challenged both by the failure to demonstrate such a virus directly (or indeed any immunological response to it) and by evidence indicating that the transmissible agent showed remarkable resistance to treatment expected to inactivate nucleic acids (such as ultraviolet radiation or treatment with nucleases). Such findings had led to suggestions as early as 1966 by Alper and others that the transmissible agent may be devoid of nucleic acid. Pattison and also Griffith had suggested in 1967 that the transmissible agent may be a protein. Progressive enrichment of brain homogenates for infectivity resulted in the isolation of a protease-resistant sialoglycoprotein, designated the prion protein (PrP), by Prusiner and coworkers in 1982. This protein was the major constituent of infective fractions and was found to accumulate in affected brains and sometimes to form amyloid deposits. The term prion (from *pro*teinaceous *in*fectious particle) was proposed by Prusiner in 1982 to distinguish the infectious pathogen from viruses or viroids. Prions were defined as 'small proteinaceous infectious particles that resist inactivation by procedures which modify nucleic acids'.

The protease-resistant PrP extracted from affected brains was of molecular mass 27 to 30 kDa and became known as PrP 27–30. At the time, PrP was assumed to be encoded by a gene within the putative slow virus thought to be responsible for these diseases. However, in 1985 it was demonstrated that PrP was in fact encoded by a single-copy chromosomal gene and was therefore host encoded. PrP 27–30 is derived from a larger molecule of molecular mass 33 to 35 kDa, designated PrP^{Sc} (denoting the scrapie isoform of the protein). The normal product of the PrP gene, however, is protease sensitive and designated PrP^C (denoting the cellular isoform of the protein). No differences in amino acid sequence between PrP^{Sc} and PrP^C have been identified. PrP^{Sc} is known to be derived from PrP^C by some post-translational process. The precise nature of this modification has yet to be determined.

While arguments for the provocative notion that the transmissible agent may be an abnormal isoform of a host-encoded protein rested largely on the inability of workers to demonstrate significant co-purifying nucleic acids, such arguments would obviously remain controversial. Positive evidence that the prion may consist principally (or entirely) of PrP^{Sc} has now been provided by a remarkable series of experiments which followed from the identification of pathogenic mutations in the PrP gene in 1989 in both familial Creutzfeldt–Jakob disease and Gerstmann–Sträussler–Scheinker syndrome. Given that familial Creutzfeldt–Jakob disease and Gerstmann–Sträussler–Scheinker syndrome showed a clear autosomal dominant pattern of disease segregation, PrP, mapped to the short arm of chromosome 20, was an obvious candidate gene. The initial demonstration of linkage of Gerstmann–Sträussler–Scheinker syndrome to a missense variant in PrP has now been followed by the identification of a whole family of PrP mutations in the inherited forms of these conditions. These mutations are only seen in at risk or affected individuals from these families, not in the normal population. Strong statistical evidence therefore supported the idea that these were pathogenic mutations. Prusiner and colleagues were able to demonstrate in 1990 that an analogous mutation to that identified in Gerstmann–Sträussler–Scheinker syndrome produced spontaneous neurodegeneration in transgenic mice, establishing directly the pathogenicity of this DNA variant. Furthermore, brain tissue from such spontaneously ill animals appears to be able to transmit the disease to normal animals by inoculation. The familial forms of these diseases are therefore autosomal dominant mendelian disorders in addition to being horizontally transmissible to experimental animals by inoculation. These diseases are biologically unique to date in this respect. Such appreciation that PrP mutations produce spontaneous neurodegeneration in humans which is then transmissible by inoculation (and the modelling of this phenomenon in transgenic mice) argues persuasively that PrP, or rather an abnormal isoform of PrP, is the central component of the infectious agent.

How then can PrP^{Sc} replicate, and how is it that a disease can be both transmitted vertically in the germline and also be infectious? Recent work in transgenic mice and human molecular genetics strongly supports a model based on the importance of a direct interaction between PrP molecules. The idea is that PrP^{Sc} may, by dimerization or more complex interaction with PrP^{C}, act as a template, thereby catalysing the conversion of PrP^{C} to PrP^{Sc}. The failure to identify differences between PrP^{C} and PrP^{Sc} with respect to known post-translational modifications suggests that the difference between the two isoforms of PrP may be conformational (Fig. 1(a)). PrP^{Sc} therefore, when inoculated into a recipient, sets off a chain reaction of conformational change with progressively more of the cellular PrP^{C} being sequestered in the abnormal and protease-resistant isoform, which accumulates and interferes with cellular function. It is then suggested that the effect of PrP mutations is to render the mutant PrP^{C} inherently unstable such that the conversion to PrP^{Sc} occurs spontaneously at some time during the lifetime of the individual, then setting off the chain reaction of conversion as before (Fig. 1(b)). Once initiated, brain tissue from such inherited cases could then pass on this process to a normal individual by inoculation. Such a disease model, although unprecedented, does not challenge fundamental biological principles. PrP is produced by the host PrP gene normally. The prion does not need an independent genome, rather prion replication occurs by catalytic modification of cellular PrP. Although such a model of pathogenicity is novel, a closely analogous situation has now been described with respect to the tumour suppresser protein p53. Mutations in p53 can result in p53 adopting an abnormal, and biologically inactive, conformation. It has been demonstrated that co-translation of mutant and wild-type p53 leads to the wild-type protein adopting the abnormal conformation. This is thought to explain how mutation of one copy of the p53 gene can lead to inactivation of the p53 produced by the normal allele and thereby allow tumours to develop.

A key piece of supporting evidence for the above model is the finding that the large majority of cases of classical sporadic Creutzfeldt–Jakob disease are homozygous with respect to a common protein polymorphism in PrP. Residue 129 of PrP can be either methionine or valine and while in the normal caucasian population the gene frequencies are estimated as 38 per cent methionine homozygotes, 11 per cent valine homozygotes, and 51 per cent heterozygotes, nearly all classical sporadic cases of Creutzfeldt–Jakob disease are either methionine or valine homozygotes. This importance of PrP sequence homology is further emphasized by the observation in some families with inherited prion diseases that the age at onset is later in individuals heterozygous at codon 129 as compared to homozygotes. Since all the inherited cases to date are autosomal dominant conditions associated with coding mutations in PrP, they are all heterozygotes with respect to the mutation. This may also have the effect of interfering with the protein–protein interaction discussed above and contributing to the much more prolonged clinical course seen in the inherited cases than in sporadic Creutzfeldt–Jakob disease (where the interacting PrP molecules are identical).

An unresolved issue in prion biology is the explanation of the existence of different strains of prions in experimental scrapie. The existence of such strains, with distinct and stable incubation times and which result in characteristic pathology in mice, is difficult to explain in terms of a protein only model. To accommodate the existence of strains, it has been suggested that PrP^{Sc}, while sufficient for infectivity, may associate with a small cellular nucleic acid or 'co-prion' which confers strain phenotype. Recent experiments, showing that strain type, as well as infectivity, is resistant to treatments which inactivate nucleic acids, make such a model unlikely. Many different glycosylation patterns of PrP have been identified and this may represent a mechanism for strain variability. It is known that different neuronal populations can glycosylate proteins differently. Therefore it could be that a specifically glycosylated form of PrP would replicate most favourably (as the degree of structural homology would be most similar) in a specific population of neurones, resulting in a characteristic progression of disease both anatomically and temporally.

What then is a prion disease and how is it best defined? The biology of these conditions is advancing remarkably quickly and it is important at this stage not to be dogmatic in such definitions. In the case of the inherited prion diseases, the identification of a pathogenic PrP mutation represents the clearest aetiological marker; however, these constitute

Fig. 1 (a) Diagrammatic representation of a possible mechanism of prion replication. The disease-related isoform PrP^{Sc} (fully shaded symbols) forms a dimer with the normal cellular isoform, PrP^{C} (lightly shaded symbols). It is proposed that PrP^{Sc} catalyses a conformational change in PrP^{C}, leading to the progressive accumulation of the protease-resistant PrP^{Sc}. (b) In the inherited prion diseases it is proposed that the mutant PrP^{C} may be inherently unstable, and change spontaneously to PrP^{Sc} at some stage in the lifetime of an individual. Once PrP^{Sc} is generated the chain reaction of conformational change can then proceed as in (a), where PrP^{Sc} was introduced by inoculation.

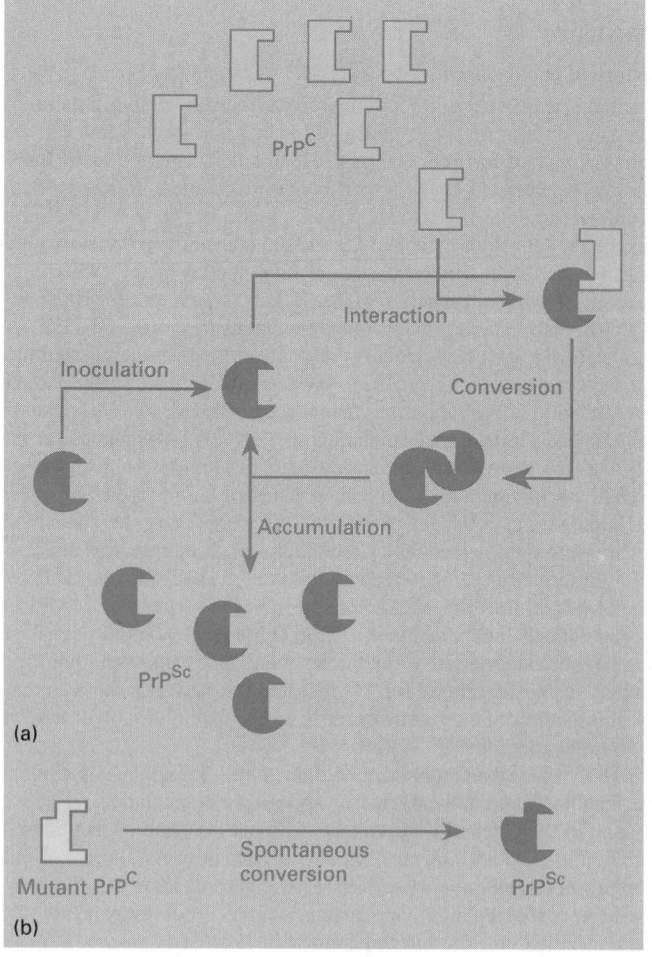

only a minority of cases. In all the prion diseases, protease-resistant PrP can be demonstrated either by immunohistochemical identification of PrP amyloid or by immunoblotting of brain homogenates. We cannot assume that all prion diseases will be experimentally transmissible. This is particularly important in the case of the inherited forms, where the mutation may render the prion produced in such cases more difficult to transmit to wild-type animals as the protein–protein interaction involved would be between heterologous molecules. Transmission from such cases may require the use of transgenic mice expressing an homologous PrP. The process suggested to account for prion propagation may not be unique to PrP. Many other proteins may show such an effect. However, to be as transmissible, such proteins, like PrP^{Sc} would need to be sufficiently stable in the environment (and in the gastrointestinal tract) to reach their cellular target in another host. The detection of other hypothetical prion diseases may therefore only be possible in specific experimental conditions. Once the precise molecular mechanism of the production of PrP^{Sc} is determined, it may be possible to produce a more precise definition of prion disease based on principles that may be of significance for other neurological and non-neurological disorders.

CLINICAL FEATURES

The human prion diseases have been classically divided into Creutzfeldt–Jakob disease, Gerstmann–Sträussler–Scheinker syndrome, and kuru. With the advances in our understanding of the aetiology of these conditions it now seems more appropriate to divide the human prion disease into inherited, sporadic, and acquired forms (see Table 1) with Creutzfeldt–Jakob disease, Gerstmann–Sträussler–Scheinker syndrome, and kuru now seen as clinicopathological syndromes within a wider spectrum of disease.

Kindreds with inherited prion disease have been described with phenotypes of classical Creutzfeldt–Jakob disease, Gerstmann–Sträussler–Scheinker syndrome, and also with other neurodegenerative syndromes, including fatal familial insomnia. Some kindreds show remarkable phenotypic variability which can encompass cases like both Creutzfeldt–Jakob disease and Gerstmann–Sträussler–Scheinker syndrome, as well as other cases which do not conform to either of these phenotypes. Cases diagnosed by PrP gene analysis have been reported which are not only clinically atypical but which lack the classical histological features entirely. Significant clinical overlap exists with familial Alzheimer's disease, Pick's disease, frontal lobe degeneration of non-Alzheimer type, and amyotrophic lateral sclerosis with dementia. Although classical Gerstmann–Sträussler–Scheinker syndrome is described below, it now seems more sensible to designate the familial illnesses as inherited prion diseases and to then subclassify these according to mutation (see Table 2).

Acquired prion diseases include iatrogenic Creutzfeldt–Jakob disease and kuru. Kuru is described in detail in Chapter 24.7.5.

Sporadic prion diseases at present consist of Creutzfeldt–Jakob disease and atypical variants of this disease (which may be classified as Creutzfeldt–Jakob disease on the basis of transmissibility to primates). Cases lacking the characteristic histological features of Creutzfeldt–Jakob disease have been transmitted. As there is at present no equivalent aetiological diagnostic marker for sporadic prion diseases as in the inherited diseases it cannot yet be excluded that more diverse phenotypic variants of sporadic prion disease exist, which may not be as easily transmissible to primates as the cases with classical spongiform encephalopathy.

Creutzfeldt–Jakob disease

The core clinical syndrome of Creutzfeldt–Jakob disease is of a rapidly progressive multifocal dementia, usually with myoclonus. The onset is usually in the 45 to 75 year age-group, with peak onset between 60 and 65 years. The clinical progression is typically over weeks, progressing to akinetic mutism and death often in 2 to 3 months. Around 70 per cent of cases die in under 6 months. Prodromal features, present in around

Table 1 *Human prion diseases*

Type	Examples	Aetiology
Acquired	Kuru	Cannibalism
	Iatrogenic CJD	Accidental inoculation
Sporadic	CJD	May represent somatic
	Atypical CJD	PrP gene mutation or rare spontaneous conversion PrP^C to PrP^{Sc}
Inherited	Familial CJD	Germline mutation
	GSS	
	Fatal familial insomnia	
	Various atypical dementias	

CJD, Creutzfeldt–Jakob disease; GSS, Gerstmann–Sträussler–Scheinker syndrome; PrP, prion protein.

Table 2 *Human inherited prion diseases*[a]

Inherited prion disease (PrP Leu$_{102}$)
Inherited prion disease (PrP Val$_{117}$)
Inherited prion disease (PrP Asp$_{178}$)
Inherited prion disease (PrP Ser$_{198}$)
Inherited prion disease (PrP Lys$_{200}$)
Inherited prion disease (PrP Arg$_{217}$)
Inherited prion disease (PrP 96 bp insertion)
Inherited prion disease (PrP 120 bp insertion)
Inherited prion disease (PrP 144 bp insertion)
Inherited prion disease (PrP 168 bp insertion)
Inherited prion disease (PrP 192 bp insertion)
Inherited prion disease (PrP 216 bp insertion)

[a]Suggested notation: inherited prion disease (PrP mutation); bp, base pair; PrP, prion protein.

one-third of cases, include fatigue, insomnia, depression, weight loss, headaches, general malaise, and ill-defined pain sensations. In addition to mental deterioration and myoclonus, frequent additional neurological features include extrapyramidal signs, cerebellar ataxia, pyramidal signs, and cortical blindness. Routine haematological and biochemical investigations are normal, although occasional cases have been noted to have raised serum transaminases or alkaline phosphatase. There are no immunological markers and acute-phase proteins are not elevated. Examination of the cerebrospinal fluid is normal, although raised neuronal-specific enolase, indicating a loss of neurones, has been proposed as a useful marker. Neuroimaging with computed tomography (CT) or magnetic resonance imaging (MRI) is useful to exclude other causes of subacute neurological illness, but there are no diagnostic features, cerebral and cerebellar atrophy may be present. The most useful investigation is the electroencephalogram (EEG) which may show characteristic pseudoperiodic sharp wave activity. Prospective epidemiological studies have demonstrated that cases with a progressive dementia, and two or more of the following—myoclonus; cortical blindness; pyramidal, cerebellar, or extrapyramidal signs; or akinetic mutism in the setting of a typical EEG—nearly always turn out to be confirmed as histologically definite Creutzfeldt–Jakob disease if neuropathological examination is performed. Neuropathological confirmation of the disease is by demonstration of spongiform change, neuronal loss, and astrocytosis. PrP amyloid plaques are usually not present in Creutzfeldt–Jakob disease, although protease-resistant PrP, seen in all the currently recognized prion diseases, can be demonstrated by immunoblotting of brain homogenates. Genetic susceptibility to Creutzfeldt–Jakob disease has been demonstrated in that most classical cases of this disease are homozygous with respect to a common protein polymorphism of PrP (see above). Atypical forms of Creutzfeldt–Jakob disease are well recognized. Around 10 per cent of cases of Creutzfeldt–Jakob disease have a much more prolonged clinical course, with a disease duration of over 2 years. These cases may represent the occasional occurrence of Creutzfeldt–Jakob disease in individuals heterozygous for PrP polymorphisms.

Iatrogenic Creutzfeldt–Jakob disease

While prion diseases can be transmitted to experimental animals by inoculation, it is important to appreciate that they are not contagious in humans. Documented case-to-case spread has only occurred by cannibalism (kuru) or following accidental inoculation with prions. Such iatrogenic routes include the use of inadequately sterilized intracerebral electrodes, dura mate, and corneal grafting, and from the use of human cadaveric pituitary-derived growth hormone or gonadotrophin. These cases are rare, but a careful history of such exposure should be sought in suspected cases. Interestingly, cases arising from intracerebral or optic inoculation manifest clinically as classical Creutzfeldt–Jakob disease, with a rapidly progressive dementia, while those resulting from peripheral inoculation present frequently with a progressive ataxia initially, reminiscent of kuru. Unsurprisingly, the incubation period in intracerebral cases is short (19–46 months for dura mater grafts) as compared to peripheral cases (typically 15 years or more). There is evidence for genetic susceptibility to iatrogenic Creutzfeldt–Jakob disease. There is an excess of codon 129 homozygotes, in particular valine 129 homozygotes, in iatrogenic cases arising from pituitary hormone therapy. It has been argued that valine 129 PrP may be more susceptible to conversion to the disease-related isoform than methionine 129 PrP, and therefore that valine 129 homozygotes may be particularly susceptible to acquired prion diseases.

Epidemiological studies have not shown an increased risk to those of particular occupations who may be exposed to human or animal prions, although individual cases of Creutzfeldt–Jakob disease in two histopathology technicians, a neuropathologist, and a neurosurgeon have been documented.

Gerstmann–Sträussler–Scheinker syndrome

This presents classically as a chronic cerebellar ataxia with pyramidal features, with dementia occurring later in a much more prolonged clinical course than that seen in Creutzfeldt–Jakob disease. The mean duration is around 5 years, with onset usually in either the third or fourth decades. Histologically, the hallmark is the presence of multicentric amyloid plaques. Spongiform change, neuronal loss, astrocytosis, and white matter loss are also usually present. Numerous kindreds with this syndrome, from several countries (including the original Austrian family described by Gerstmann, Sträussler and Scheinker in 1936), have now been demonstrated to have mutations in the PrP gene (see below). Gerstmann–Sträussler–Scheinker syndrome is an autosomal dominant disorder which can now be classified within the spectrum of inherited prion disease.

Inherited prion diseases

The identification of one of the pathogenic PrP gene mutations in a case with neurodegenerative disease allows not only molecular diagnosis of an inherited prion disease but also its subclassification according to mutation (see Table 2). Pathogenic mutations reported to date in the human PrP gene consist of two groups: (1) point mutations within the coding sequence, resulting in amino acid substitutions in PrP; (2) insertions encoding four to nine additional copies of an octapeptide repeat present in a tandem array of five copies in the normal protein.

Inherited prion disease (PrP leucine 102)

This mutation has been demonstrated in kindreds in the United States, United Kingdom, Germany, Italy, and Japan, including the original kindred reported by Gerstmann, Sträussler, and Scheinker in 1936. Pro-

gressive ataxia is the dominant clinical feature, with dementia and pyramidal features. However, marked variability both at the clinical and neuropathological level has now been reported. A family in which marked clinical features characteristic of amyotrophic lateral sclerosis are additionally present has been reported. Neuropathologically, PrP immunoreactive plaques are generally present.

Inherited prion disease (PrP valine 117)

Present in three families from France, the United States, and the United Kingdom, with presenile dementia associated with pyramidal signs, parkinsonism, pseudobulbar features, and cerebellar signs. Neuropathologically, PrP immunoreactive plaques are usually present.

Inherited prion disease (PrP asparagine 178)

First described in Finnish kindreds with a characteristic phenotype of Creutzfeldt–Jakob disease, this mutation has also been demonstrated in Italian and French families with fatal familial insomnia. Fatal familial insomnia is characterized by progressive untreatable insomnia and dysautonomia. Later, these patients develop dementia. Histologically, fatal familial insomnia is characterized by selective thalamic degeneration. Spongiform change is seen in a few cases and protease-resistant PrP has been demonstrated by immunoblotting. It is not, as yet, clear if these represent two distinct phenotypic manifestations of PrP asparagine 178 in different families, or whether, as seems more likely by comparison with the other inherited prion diseases, both phenotypes will be seen in individuals from the same kindred and therefore represent parts of a spectrum of codon 178 disease.

Inherited prion disease (PrP serine 198)

This variant has been described in a family with presenile dementia, ataxia, and parkinsonism. Histologically, numerous neurofibrillary tangles are present, as in Alzheimer's disease, in addition to PrP amyloid plaques. Transmissibility to experimental animals by inoculation has not yet been demonstrated in this condition.

Inherited prion disease (PrP lysine 200)

This was first described in families with Creutzfeldt–Jakob disease. Affected individuals develop a rapidly progressive dementia with myoclonus and pyramidal, cerebellar, or extrapyramidal signs. The duration of illness is usually less than 12 months. EEG shows the characteristic appearances of Creutzfeldt–Jakob disease. Interestingly, this mutation accounts for the three main ethnogeographical clusters of Creutzfeldt–Jakob disease (amongst Libyan Jews, in Slovakia, and also in Chile). However, with genetic screening, atypical forms of this condition are now being detected. This mutation shows incomplete penetrance. Elderly unaffected carriers of the mutation have been reported. Individuals homozygous for the mutation are phenotypically indistinguishable from heterozygotes, demonstrating that this condition is a fully dominant disorder.

Inherited prion disease (PrP arginine 217)

Reported in a single Swedish family, the presentation is with dementia followed by gait ataxia, dysphagia, and confusion. Histologically, neurofibrillary tangles are very prominent, as seen with inherited prion disease (PrP serine 198). Transmissibility to experimental animals has not yet been demonstrated in this condition.

Inherited prion disease (PrP 144 bp insertion)

This subtype of inherited prion disease shows remarkable phenotypic variability both at the clinical and histological level. Affected individuals develop (usually with onset in the third to fourth decade) a progressive dementia associated with a varying combination of cerebellar ataxia and dysarthria, pyramidal signs, myoclonus, and occasionally extrapyramidal signs, chorea, and seizures. The dementia is often preceded by depression and aggressive behaviour. Some cases have a longstanding personality disorder, characterized by aggression, irritability, antisocial and criminal activity, and hypersexuality which, in some individuals, is present from early childhood, long before overt neurodegenerative disease develops. The histological features vary from those of classical spongiform encephalopathy (with or without PrP amyloid plaques) to cases lacking any specific features of these conditions. Age at onset in this condition can be predicted according to genotype at the polymorphic codon 129. Since this pathogenic insertional mutation occurs on a methionine 129 PrP allele, there are two possible genotypes for affected individuals, methionine 129 homozygotes or methionine 129/valine 129 heterozygotes. Heterozygotes have an age at onset about a decade later than that of homozygotes. Transmission to experimental animals has not yet been demonstrated.

Other insertion mutations

Families with mutations consisting of four, five, seven, eight, and nine extra PrP octarepeats have been described, in addition to the six extra repeat insertion described above. A number of these families have atypical neurodegenerative syndromes with marked intrafamilial variability.

Presymptomatic testing and genetic counselling

The availability of direct gene tests for the inherited forms of these diseases allows presymptomatic testing of unaffected but at-risk family members, and also allows the possibility of antenatal testing. In some families it may also be possible to determine whether a gene carrier will have an early or late onset of disease by codon 129 genotyping. Most of the inherited prion diseases show, to date, no evidence of incomplete penetrance, although experience with some of these is still very limited. A notable exception is inherited prion disease (PrP lysine 200) in which elderly unaffected gene carriers have been identified. In many respects the counselling situation resembles that of Huntington's disease and it seems reasonable to adopt the same counselling protocols established for the latter. It is important to appreciate that performing PrP gene analysis for diagnostic purposes may have important consequences for other family members and, ideally, such issues should be discussed with the family prior to testing. Following identification of a mutation, the family should be referred for genetic counselling, and testing of asymptomatic individuals should not be performed until this has been done and full informed consent obtained.

BOVINE SPONGIFORM ENCEPHALOPATHY

This novel bovine disease was first recognized in British cattle in 1986 and rapidly reached epidemic proportions. Epidemiological studies indicated that this was due to the practice of using dietary supplements prepared from the rendered carcasses of sheep, a proportion of which would have been scrapie contaminated. Such dietary exposure to prions probably also caused earlier epidemics of captive animals, including transmissible mink encephalopathy and chronic wasting disease of mule deer and elk, as well as the newly recognized feline spongiform encephalopathy (of domestic cats) and prion diseases of various zoo species. Most of the infectivity in bovine spongiform encephalopathy, as in the other prion diseases, is found in CNS or lymphoreticular tissue. Attempted transmissions using muscle have been negative. Therefore, it seems unlikely that beef represents, or represented, any hazard. Since November 1989 a ban on the use of bovine offal (such as brain) has been in force. However, a window of risk clearly occurred from before recognition of the bovine spongiform encephalopathy epidemic until such comprehensive bans were initiated and, clearly, some infective material entered the human food chain. Whether or not such exposure results in transmission of bovine serum encephalopathy to humans remains to be determined. This will depend on the dose individuals were exposed to and on the effectiveness of the 'species barrier' (transmission of prion disease across mammalian species occurs but only with difficulty and often only following long incubation periods). The effectiveness of the bovine–human barrier can be addressed to some extent using transgenic mice expressing human prion proteins. At the moment it seems most unlikely that bovine spongiform encephalopathy would produce epidemic disease in humans. That some cases will result cannot, however, be excluded at this stage.

PROGNOSIS

All the prion diseases currently recognized are relentlessly progressive and invariably fatal. No current treatment affects outcome. The duration of illness is usually measured in months in the case of sporadic Creutzfeldt–Jakob disease, but in some of the inherited prion diseases may be 20 years or more. General supportive care for the patient and family is all that can currently be offered, with admission to hospital in the latter stages. The rapid advances in the molecular biology of these diseases does, however, lead to realistic possibilities of therapeutic approaches. Such approaches may include agents with selective binding properties for PrP^{Sc} or the application of gene targeting methods to interfere with PrP gene expression.

REFERENCES

Brown, P., Cathala, F., Raubertas, R.F., Gajdusek, D.C., and Castaigne, P. (1987). The epidemiology of Creutzfeldt–Jakob disease: conclusion of a 15-year investigation in France and review of the world literature. *Neurology* **37**, 895–904.

Buchanan, C.R., Preece, M.A., and Milner, R.D. (1991). Mortality, neoplasia, and Creutzfeldt–Jakob disease in patients treated with human pituitary growth hormone in the United Kingdom. *British Medical Journal* **302**, 824–8.

Cathala, F. and Baron, H. (1987). Clinical aspects of Creutzfeldt–Jakob disease. In *Prions: novel infectious pathogens causing scrapie and Creutzfeldt–Jakob disease*, (ed. S.B. Prusiner and M.P. McKinley Academic Press, San Diego. pp. 467–509.

Collinge, J. and Palmer, M.S. (1992). Prion diseases. *Current Opinion in Genetics and Development* **2**, 448–54. (Brief review of recent advances with recommended references.)

Collinge, J., *et al.* (1991). Presymptomatic detection or exclusion of prion protein gene defects in families with inherited prion diseases. *American Journal of Human Genetics* **49**, 1351–4. (Paper describing the use of PrP gene analysis in genetic counselling.)

Collinge, J., *et al.* (1992). Inherited prion disease with 144 base pair gene insertion. II: Clinical and pathological features. *Brain* **115**, 687–710. (Detailed description of a large kindred with inherited prion disease illustrating the marked phenotypic heterogeneity.)

Hsiao, K., *et al.* (1991). Mutation of the prion protein in Libyan Jews with Creutzfeldt–Jakob disease. *New England Journal of Medicine* **324**, 1091–7. (Report of cases with the codon 200 disease which accounts for the three main ethnogeographical clusters of Creutzfeldt–Jakob disease.)

Medori, R., *et al.* (1992). Fatal familial insomnia, a prion disease with a mutation at codon 178 of the prion protein gene. *New England Journal of Medicine* **326**, 444–9.

Palmer, M.S. and Collinge, J. (1992). Human prion diseases. *Current Opinion in Neurology and Neurosurgery* **5**, 895–901. (Short review focusing on clinical aspects.)

Prusiner, S.B. (1991). Molecular biology of prion diseases. *Science* **252**, 1515–22. (Detailed review of biology of prion diseases.)

Prusiner, S.B., Collinge, J., Powell, J., and Anderton, B. (ed.) (1992). *Prion diseases of humans and animals*. Ellis Horwood, London. (A comprehensive review of current research with detailed historical reviews.)

24.7.5 Kuru

M. P. ALPERS

Kuru has historical importance as the first of the human spongiform encephalopathies to be shown to be transmissible, thereby opening up this whole field for investigation.

Epidemiology

Kuru is a disease similar to Creutzfeldt–Jakob disease, but with cerebellar ataxia as the progressive dominant feature rather than dementia. Creutzfeldt–Jakob disease is normally a sporadic encephalopathy with an annual incidence throughout the world of about 1 per million, although it is not uncommonly found as familial or spatiotemporal clusters, a small number of which have been proven to be iatrogenic. Kuru is a similar transmissible encephalopathy, which reached epidemic proportions in the Okapa district of the Eastern Highlands of Papua New Guinea, in which the mechanism of transmission was the local practice of endocannibalism. The original sporadic case which occasioned the outbreak is presumed, from the testimony of local informants, to have occurred in the region in the early part of this century. The highlands were totally unknown to the outside world until 1930 and specific administrative contact with the people of the Okapa area was not made until the 1950s.

When kuru was first investigated by medical science in 1957 the total annual mortality from the disease was about 200, with a disease-specific mortality rate of 3 per cent per annum in the groups with the highest incidence. The disease affected adult women in the main and children of both sexes: only 2 per cent of cases at the time of first investigation were in adult males. Female age-specific mortality rates from kuru were, in some age groups, as high as 20 per cent per annum, and most deaths in women occurred from the disease. Subsequent epidemiological investigation has shown a striking decline in kuru incidence with progressive elimination of the disease from the younger age groups; the cohort born since 1960 has grown up completely free of the disease. The epidemiological patterns are all explained by transmission of an infectious agent, not normally contagious, through the practice of endocannibalism, which ceased in the region around 1956 and was certainly finished by 1960; women, with their attendant young children, but not men, partook of infectious bodily organs at the mortuary feasts which were held to honour the dead. The current incidence of the disease of the order of 5 patients per annum, all of whom are aged 40 or more, is consistent with transmission by cannibalism before 1956 and an incubation period of 40 years or more. It is anticipated that this epidemic focus of the disease will eventually die out. It is hard to estimate how long this will take since the rate of decline of kuru incidence has been slowing and the longevity of people living in the region has been increasing; if the incubation period may, in some instances, be of the same order as the human lifespan, the occasional new case may continue to occur in progressively older people for many more years.

Aetiology

Kuru was first transmitted to chimpanzees in 1965. The remarkable properties of the causative agent are still being worked out. In physicochemical properties the kuru agent is similar to the agents of Creutzfeldt–Jakob disease, Gerstmann–Sträussler–Scheinker syndrome, and

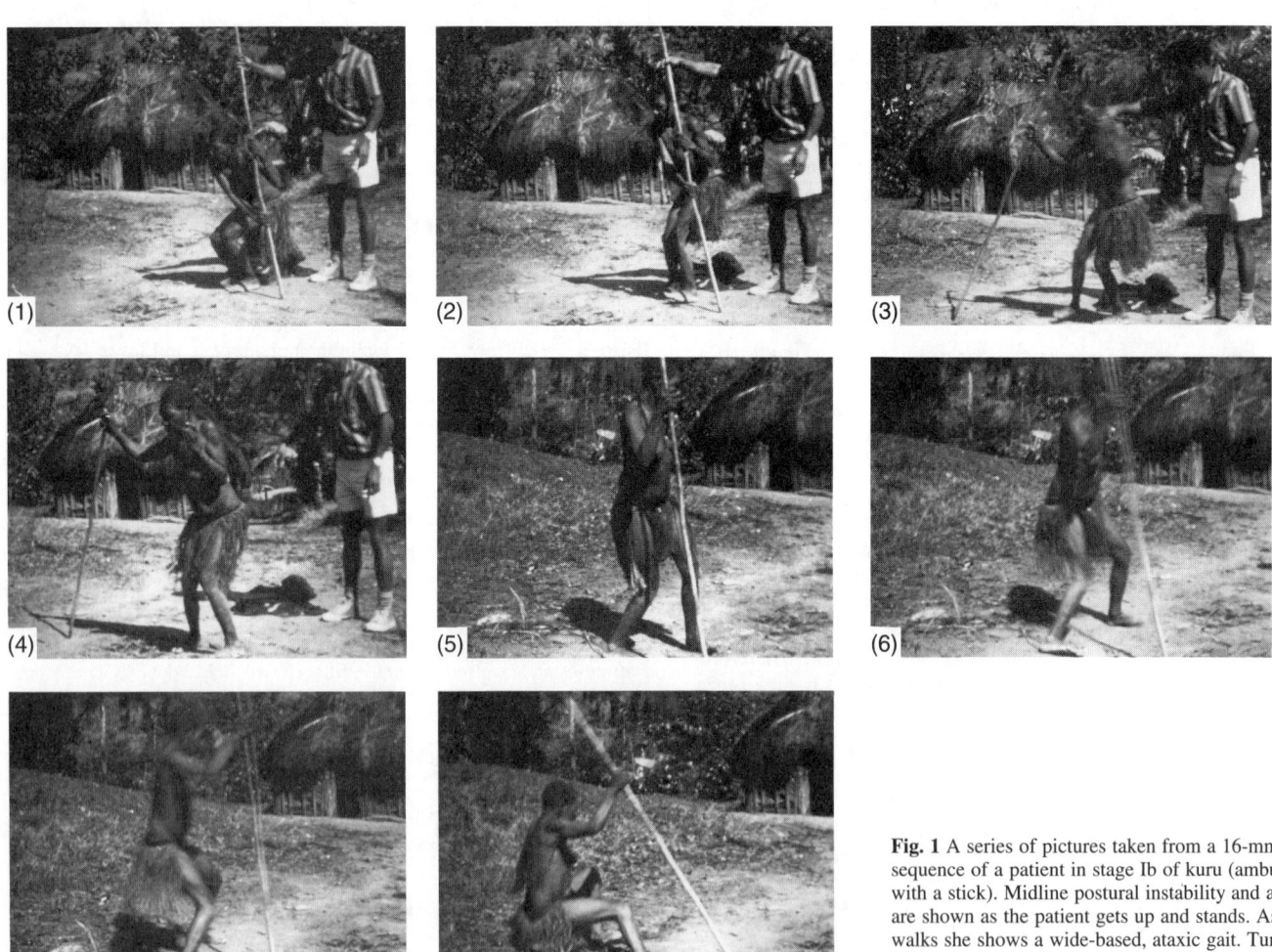

Fig. 1 A series of pictures taken from a 16-mm movie sequence of a patient in stage Ib of kuru (ambulatory with a stick). Midline postural instability and astasia are shown as the patient gets up and stands. As she walks she shows a wide-based, ataxic gait. Turning, even with the aid of a stick, leads to severe unsteadiness and loss of balance.

scrapie with all its congeners (see Chapter 24.7.4). The incubation period shortens after the first experimental passage to a new host, and may be profoundly affected by host genes; within a single system it is dependent on inoculation dose.

The clinical course of kuru has been found to be essentially the same in all patients, and all ages were affected. The wide age range depended both on variable age at transmission and variation in the length of the incubation period. Transmission to females, but not males, over a wide range of ages explains the strong predominance of females among adult patients seen in the past. From the cases in young children it is known that the incubation period can be short (in this context, a small number of years). From the residual patients seen in recent years it is known that the incubation period can be long (at least of the order of 40 years, although the final determination has yet to be made). Kuru is not transmitted vertically. It is postulated that the first case in the region was a sporadic case of Creutzfeldt–Jakob disease. Subsequent cases were acquired through ingestion or inadvertent inoculation of infectious material.

Either peripheral transmission of the agent or its own inherent conformation determined the clinical form of the disease in kuru; it is relevant that a kuru-like ataxic disease results from iatrogenic peripheral transmission (as with growth hormone), in contrast to iatrogenic cerebral transmission (as from infected electrodes), which produces the usual dementing clinical syndrome of Creutzfeldt–Jakob disease. The conformation of the protein agent presumably takes a 'kuru form' and induces a similar change in the cellular prion (PrP) protein to establish the infectious kuru isoform of PrP, which breeds true within the same host system. As with the other prion agents, replication of the normal cellular isoform of PrP is coded for by the host *PrP* gene. The change to the infectious prion form involves the conformational transition from α-helices to β-sheets, which allows their polymerization and the deposition of insoluble β-pleated amyloid proteins. These may appear as rods or highly organized plaques. For some reason this endstage does not occur in every case of kuru but, when it does, the striking amyloid plaques first described by Klatzo are found.

As would be predicted from the fact that kuru is an acquired form of prion disease, or transmissible amyloid encephalopathy, none of the mutant codons in the *PrP* gene which predispose to the inherited forms of prion disease have been found in kuru patients. However, it is still not known whether polymorphisms in the *PrP* gene or other host genes which modify susceptibility to acquired disease occur in the Fore people, making them particularly susceptible to the transmission of kuru.

Pathology

The pathology of kuru, as with Creutzfeldt–Jakob disease, is characterized by neuronal degeneration and loss, with ballooning of neurones both in the cell body and in processes, where the vacuoles appear as spongiform change; by marked astrocytic hypertrophy and proliferation, with gliosis; by lack of inflammatory response; and, in about 70 per cent of cases, by the deposition of amyloid plaques. The latter are of a particular kind, with radiating filaments from a central core, and are called kuru plaques; they have the same form in both kuru and Creutzfeldt–Jakob disease. Although plaques are widespread and numerous in some patients with kuru, in others plaques are not found at all. The most advanced pathological changes in kuru are found in the cerebellum, although the whole of the brain is affected. The only macroscopic change found in the brain is atrophy of the vermis. Specific pathological changes have not been detected in other organs. The diseases of which kuru is a member have also been called the subacute spongiform encephalopathies, but although spongiform change is characteristic of the disease which follows experimental transmission, it may not be found in all kinds of primary disease; in kuru, which is an acquired disease, spongiform change is invariably found.

Clinical features

Clinically, the disease is confined to the central nervous system, with major effects on the motor systems, predominantly the cerebellum. The cardinal feature of the disease is progressive cerebellar ataxia, the gradual worsening of which marks the clinical evolution of the disease. This has been divided into three stages: ambulatory, sedentary, and tertiary. There are usually prodromal symptoms of headache, aching limbs, joint pains, and, less frequently, double vision. The onset of the disease proper is marked by midline trunkal instability and astasia, titubation, and ataxia of gait (Fig. 1). Astasia is the principal early and diagnostic sign, confirmed by the progression of the cerebellar disease through an inexorable subacute course to death. The disease is invariably fatal with an average duration of about 12 months (and a range of 3 months to 3 years). Its clinical characteristics have not changed since it was first investigated.

The disease follows the same course in all age groups but the duration tends to be shorter in younger patients. Dysmetria and static and kinetic cerebellar tremors are found. Incoordination affects all motor activity, including extraocular movements and emotional expression; strabismus may occur, but nystagmus is not found. Progressive dysarthria and dysphagia occur. Hypotonia and weakness may be found, but paralysis is not seen, not even terminally. There is no sensory loss.

Apart from the cerebellar signs there is evidence of involvement of other motor systems and cortical dysfunction. Spasticity and hyperflexia with marked clonus are characteristic of the late second and early third stage of the disease, but plantar responses remain flexor and abdominal reflexes are intact. Extrapyramidal features of athetosis and chorea and, occasionally, parkinsonian tremors may be found; usually these signs occur during a restricted period in the development of the disease, but in a few cases are florid and persistent. During the third stage there may be diencephalic, pseudobulbar, and bulbar signs, and signs of cortical dysfunction, such as grasp reflexes, primitive snout reflexes, and, in some cases, dementia. In the majority of patients dying of kuru, dementia is conspicuous by its absence, a major difference from Creutzfeldt–Jakob disease. However, in a small proportion of patients dementia, together with ataxia, is part of the set of progressive features, and such cases resemble closely the ataxic form of Creutzfeldt–Jakob disease. Kuru is probably best regarded as a rare form of the syndrome of Creutzfeldt–Jakob disease. Gerstmann–Sträussler–Scheinker disease resembles kuru closely but with a more prolonged course. Death in kuru finally occurs from intercurrent infection or from medullary involvement by the progressive neuropathological process.

REFERENCES

Alpers, M.P. (1968). Kuru: implications of its transmissibility for the interpretation of its changing epidemiologic pattern. In *The central nervous system, some experimental models of neurological diseases*, (ed. O.T. Bailey and D.E. Smith), pp. 234–51. Williams & Wilkins, Baltimore.

Alpers, M.P. (1992). Kuru. In *Human biology in Papua New Guinea: the small cosmos* (ed. R.D. Attenborough and M.P. Alpers), pp. 313–34. Clarendon Press, Oxford.

Alpers, M. and Gajdusek, D.C. (1965). Changing patterns of kuru: epidemiological changes in the period of increasing contact of the Fore people with Western civilization. *American Journal of Tropical Medicine and Hygiene* **14**, 852–79.

Gajdusek, D.C. (1977). Unconventional viruses and the origin and disappearance of kuru. *Science* **197**, 943–60.

Gajdusek, D.C., Gibbs, C.J., Jr, and Alpers, M. (1966). Experimental transmission of a kuru-like syndrome to chimpanzees. *Nature* **209**, 794–6.

Klatzo, I., Gajdusek, D.C., and Zigas, V. (1959). Pathology of kuru. *Laboratory Investigation* **8**, 799–847.

Prusiner, S.B. and McKinley, M.P. (ed.) (1987). *Prions: novel infectious pathogens causing scrapie and Creutzfeldt–Jakob disease*. Academic Press, San Diego.

Prusiner, S., Collinge, J., Powell, J., and Anderton, B. (ed.) (1992). *Prion diseases of humans and animals*. Ellis Horwood, London.

24.8 Inherited disorders

P. K. Thomas

There are many genetically determined neurological disorders, and others in which a genetic predisposition can be detected. Inherited disorders of the extrapyramidal system, peripheral nerves, and muscle, and those aminoacidurias that are associated with neurological involvement, are considered elsewhere, as is the question of genetic predisposition in the aetiology of conditions such as developmental abnormalities of the nervous system, epilepsy, migraine, Alzheimer's disease, and multiple sclerosis.

HEREDITARY ATAXIAS

The classification of the hereditary ataxias remains a matter of controversy. A spinocerebellar degeneration may develop in disorders with a known metabolic basis. This category includes abetalipoproteinaemia (see Section 11), ataxia telangiectasia and xeroderma pigmentosum (see Section 23). The majority of the inherited cerebellar and spinocerebellar degenerations are at present of unknown causation. In general these can be divided into examples of early onset (under the age of 20 years), which are usually of autosomal recessive inheritance and of which Friedreich's ataxia is the commonest example, and the later onset cases of cerebellar degeneration that are most often dominantly inherited.

Early onset hereditary ataxias

Friedreich's ataxia

This disorder is an example of a spinocerebellar degeneration and is dominated by progressive ataxia with an onset in childhood or adolescence. The condition is inherited as an autosomal recessive trait and affects males and females approximately equally. The responsible gene has been mapped to the long arm of chromosome 9 in the region of q13–q21. Degeneration of the larger dorsal root ganglion cells occurs with consequent loss of the larger myelinated fibres in the peripheral nerves and degeneration of the dorsal columns. Degeneration is also evident in Clarke's column, in the spinocerebellar tracts, and in the corticospinal pathways. There is variable loss of Purkinje cells in the cerebellum.

The average age of onset is 11 to 12 years. The initial symptom is almost invariably ataxia of gait, although foot or spinal deformity may antedate this. At first it is noted that the child walks awkwardly with a tendency to stumble and fall readily; in cases of early onset, walking may never have been normal. As the disease progresses, the gait slowly becomes more irregular and clumsy. The patient walks on a broad base and tends to lurch from side to side. Involvement of the upper limbs develops later, at first giving rise to clumsiness of fine movements, subsequently for all movements. A coarse intention tremor becomes obvious. The trunk is also affected, leading to oscillation of the body when standing or sitting unsupported. A regular tremor of the head (titubation) occasionally appears. Nystagmus is present in about one quarter of the cases. Dysarthria of cerebellar type develops and may become severe enough to make speech almost unintelligible.

Initially weakness is not obtrusive, but this develops as the disease advances, beginning in the legs and later involving the upper limbs. It results from degeneration in the corticospinal pathways and tends to vary in severity between cases. The plantar responses become extensor, but tone is not usually increased because of the accompanying disturbance of the afferent fibres from muscle spindles. There may be mild wasting of the anterior tibial and small hand muscles related to loss of

anterior horn cells. Bladder and bowel function is usually unaffected.

Loss of the larger dorsal root ganglion cells leads to impairment of joint position sense, vibration sense, and to some extent of touch–pressure sensibility, initially distally in the legs. The impairment of proprioception superimposes a sensory element in the cerebellar ataxia. The tendon reflexes are depressed or absent.

Apart from occasional nystagmus, the ocular movements are usually intact. The pupils are unaffected. Optic atrophy is present in about one-third of cases and 10 per cent develop sensorineural deafness.

Associated skeletal deformities are common, in particular foot deformities (pes cavus and pes equinovarus) and kyphoscoliosis. Contractures of the knees may develop in the later stages. Electrocardiography demonstrates widespread T-wave inversion and ventricular hypertrophy in nearly 70 per cent of patients. Echocardiography may suggest the presence of hypertrophic obstructive cardiomyopathy, but these findings are not specific and the ECG is a more sensitive investigation for the detection of cardiomyopathy. The ECG changes are present early in the disease and tend not to be associated with symptoms. Cardiac failure occurs late and is usually precipitated by supraventricular arrhythmias.

Although progressive dementia is not a feature of the disease, reduced intelligence is present in some cases. There is an increased incidence of diabetes mellitus in Friedreich's ataxia (10 per cent).

The disease is slowly progressive, the average age of death being in the latter part of the fourth decade. The foot and spinal deformities may require orthopaedic correction. Ultimately patients become bedridden. Death is usually from an intercurrent infection with associated cardiac failure.

Other early onset hereditary ataxias

A genetically distinct disorder that resembles Friedreich's ataxia is recognizable but has a more benign prognosis. The condition has a similar age of onset, is also of autosomal recessive inheritance, but exhibits preserved tendon reflexes and is not associated with cardiac abnormalities or diabetes. Further rare disorders in this category include progressive myoclonic ataxia (Ramsay Hunt syndrome) in which a spinocerebellar degeneration is associated with myoclonic epilepsy, and a cerebellar degeneration that is accompanied by hypogonadism.

Later onset hereditary ataxias

The category of Marie's delayed cerebellar atrophy was introduced to describe cases of hereditary ataxia with a later onset than Friedreich's ataxia in which the symptoms develop during the third or fourth decades of life or later. It is clear that Marie collected together a heterogeneous group of disorders, but his description served to emphasize the broad subdivision of the hereditary ataxias into the early and later onset groups.

Autosomal dominant cerebellar ataxia

This comprises the main group of disorders within the adult onset hereditary ataxias. The age of onset ranges from the third to the fifth decades and represents the area in which there is most diagnostic confusion. Much of this stems from the fact that the clinical manifestations vary considerably between individuals within families, and between families, so that the existence of a wide range of separate disorders has been claimed. In type I spinocerebellar ataxia (SCA1) linkage analysis has located the gene to 6p22–p23. A trinucleotide repeat expansion has been identified in this region in affected individuals, the longest abnormal allele being observed in cases of juvenile onset. In other families the disorder maps to chromosome 12q23–q24.1 (SCA2) and 14q24.3–q31 (SCA3), and in further families linkage to all three of these loci has been excluded. The occurrence of a slowly progressive cerebellar ataxia with dysarthria, intention tremor in the upper limbs, and an ataxic gait is the salient clinical feature. However, many of these patients show additional clinical manifestations that include dementia, optic atrophy, ophthalmoplegia, and extrapyramidal rigidity, which occur in varying combinations. Machado–Joseph disease, the dominantly inherited cerebellar degeneration associated with ophthalmoplegia and other features in Portuguese families originating in the Azores, maps to the same locus as SCA3. Pathologically these dominantly inherited cerebellar ataxias have been equated with olivopontocerebellar atrophy, although it is clear that the neuropathological changes are more widespread than this, and that the pattern of the neuropathological change also varies between individuals within the same family.

Other late onset cerebellar degenerations

A late cortical cerebellar degeneration that develops at around the fifth decade of life was defined by Marie, Foix, and Alajouanine. It is typified by a predominantly gait and truncal ataxia related to degeneration of the cerebellar vermis. Rare late onset dominantly inherited cerebellar degenerations, such as one associated with deafness and myoclonus, have been described. Many instances of late onset cerebellar ataxia, particularly those without ophthalmoplegia or optic atrophy, are probably nongenetic.

HEREDITARY SPASTIC PARAPLEGIA

Hereditary spastic paraplegia can be subdivided into a 'pure' form (Strümpell's disease) and others in which a variety of other features coexist. Strümpell's disease may display either an autosomal dominant or autosomal recessive inheritance. It may present during childhood or even with delayed motor development in infancy; in other cases the onset is retarded until adult life. It gives rise to difficulty in walking because of weakness and spasticity in the legs. The tendon reflexes are exaggerated and the plantar responses are extensor. In cases of early onset, foot deformity may be present. Some patients show a mild degree of cerebellar ataxia and sensory impairment in the legs of posterior column type. The disease progresses slowly and may later affect the upper limbs. Precipitancy of micturition or urinary incontinence may occur. Pathologically there is degeneration of the corticospinal pathways in the lateral columns of the spinal cord and some fibre loss in the gracile fasciculi.

With regard to treatment, if there is severe spasticity, this may be alleviated to some extent by baclofen or dantrolene orally. Continuous intrathecal administration of baclofen by an infusion pump is helpful in selected cases. The precipitancy of micturition may be improved by propantheline. Surgical correction of foot deformities is sometimes required.

Genetically distinct disorders in which a spastic paraplegia is associated with other clinical features include the Sjögren–Larsson syndrome, a recessively inherited condition which combines congenital ichthyosis and oligophrenia with a childhood onset spastic paraplegia, and the dominantly inherited disorder in which the paraplegia is associated with distal amyotrophy in the limbs resembling peroneal muscular atrophy.

DISORDERS OF LIPID METABOLISM

(See also Section 11.)

Neurolipidoses

The lipidoses constitute a group of disorders characterized by the intracellular accumulation of a variety of different lipids. Some predomi-

nantly involve the nervous system; others primarily affect the reticuloendothelial system, but may also involve nervous tissue. They may be classified in terms of the particular lipid that is stored.

Niemann–Pick disease

This consists of a group of four recessively inherited disorders in which there is an accumulation of lipid in 'foam cells' in the reticuloendothelial system. In types A and B, sphingomyelin accumulates, related to a deficiency of sphingomyelinase, the gene for which maps to chromosome 11. In type B, progressive mental deterioration and hypotonic paralysis in association with hepatosplenomegaly appear in the first 6 months of life, leading to death before the age of 3 years. Cherry-red spots are present at the maculae in 50 per cent. Type B does not affect the nervous system. Types C and D resemble type A but the storage material consists of cholesterol and neutral lipids. Sphingomyelinase activity is normal.

Glucosyl ceramide lipidosis (Gaucher's disease)

Three variants exist, all recessively inherited, characterized by hepatosplenomegaly related to the accumulation of glucosyl ceramide in histiocytes as a consequence of a deficiency of the enzyme glucocerebrosidase. The type 1 adult onset form does not affect the nervous system but types 2 and 3, with an infantile and juvenile onset respectively, and a more rapid progression, display widespread cerebral involvement.

Gangliosidoses

These comprise a group of recessively inherited disorders in which there is a combination of progressive dementia, epilepsy, and visual failure. They are related to defective ganglioside degradation. Several GM_1 gangliosidoses exist and are the result of an inherited deficiency of acid β-galactosidase. In the infantile form, which maps to chromosome 3p14.3, there is a generalized storage of GM_1 ganglioside affecting the brain, the viscera, and the skeleton. The onset is at birth or in early infancy, and initially is manifested by a failure to thrive and by hepatosplenomegaly. Later, mental and motor deterioration becomes evident, and a cherry-red spot may be present at the macula, related to retinal degeneration. Skeletal abnormalities, including abnormal facial features, have led to the condition being referred to as the 'pseudo-Hurler syndrome'. Death takes place before the age of 3 years. A juvenile onset variant also exists.

The GM_2 gangliosidoses involve the storage of GM_2 gangliosides, which are largely confined to the nervous system. In the type 1 variety (Tay–Sachs disease), the disorder usually begins within the first 6 months of life. It is encountered most frequently in Ashkenazi Jews. Initially there is retardation of development which is followed by progressive dementia, hypotonic weakness, and blindness. There is a cherry-red spot at the macula. Later, seizures occur and terminally generalized spasticity develops. Death generally takes place in the fourth year of life. The disorder is related to an inherited deficiency of hexosaminidase A and the gene has been localized to chromosome 15q23–q24. Carrier detection is possible by a serum assay, and mass screening programmes have been undertaken in some countries. Antenatal diagnosis by amniocentesis is also possible. There is no specific therapy. The type 2 form (Sandhoff's disease) is similar clinically but involves a combined deficiency of hexosaminidase A and B. A form with juvenile onset also exists, as do phenotypes presenting as spinal muscular atrophy, spinocerebellar degeneration, or as a dystonic syndrome. The gene is localized on chromosome 5q13.

Neuronal ceroid lipofuscinosis

Under this heading are grouped a number of rare disorders in which retinal degeneration, progressive dementia, epilepsy, spasticity, and ataxia occur in various combinations. The age of onset may be infantile (Santavuori), late infantile (Jansky–Bielschowsky), juvenile (Spielmeyer–Vogt), or adult (Kufs). Eponyms abound: the late infantile and juvenile cases are often collectively termed Batten's disease. There is neuronal storage of lipopigment, but the molecular basis for these disorders has not been established. The gene for the juvenile form has been localized to chromosome 16p12.1.

Leucodystrophies

These disorders are characterized by a diffuse disintegration of white matter in the central nervous system and sometimes also by segmental demyelination in the peripheral nerves. The cell bodies of the neurones are generally spared, although both myelin sheaths and axons show destruction in the white matter lesions.

Metachromatic leucodystrophy (sulphatide lipidosis)

The most common variant is the late infantile type which usually begins in the third year of life with weakness and ataxia in the limbs. Subsequently a progressive dementia supervenes, seizures may occur, and in some instances optic atrophy develops. The tendon reflexes may be depressed or absent in those patients in whom peripheral nerve involvement is prominent. Nerve conduction velocity is reduced. Death sometimes occurs after a course of a few months, sometimes of as much as 5 or 6 years. Terminally the affected children are demented, with a spastic tetraplegia, and are often blind.

The term metachromatic leucodystrophy is derived from the presence of galactosyl sulphatide in the affected tissues. This stains metachromatically with dyes such as cresyl violet and toluidine blue. It may be demonstrated within cells in fresh specimens of urine and also within Schwann cells and macrophages in biopsies of the peripheral nerves or rectal wall. The disorder, which maps to chromosome 22q13–13qter, is inherited in an autosomal recessive manner, and is due to a deficiency of aryl sulphatase A. This can be demonstrated by assay on leucocytes.

Juvenile and adult onset forms of metachromatic leucodystrophy are also encountered, but are rare. Prenatal diagnosis by amniocentesis and assay of aryl sulphatase activity on cultured amniotic fibroblasts is possible in both the late infantile and juvenile forms. Variants related to multiple sulphatase deficiency and to deficiency of activator protein also occur.

Globoid cell leucodystrophy (Krabbe's disease)

This derives its title from the presence of large multinucleate cells containing galactosylceramide in areas of white matter damage. The condition begins at the age of 3 or 4 months as a failure to thrive. Developmental regression then becomes evident and the tendon reflexes are lost. As the disease advances, generalized hypertonus appears, together with various types of seizure, and optic atrophy. Death often occurs in the first year of life or may be delayed into the second year. There are also rare late onset cases.

The peripheral nerves are affected, biopsies showing segmental demyelination and inclusions within Schwann cells. Nerve conduction velocity is reduced.

The disorder is inherited in an autosomal recessive manner and is due to a deficiency of galactosylceramide β-galactosidase. It maps to chromosome 14q21–q31. This may be demonstrated by assays in leucocytes or serum.

Adrenoleucodystrophy and adrenomyeloneuropathy (see Chapter 24.10)

Amongst a group of conditions that give rise to widespread demyelination in the brain with an onset during childhood, cases of adrenoleucodystrophy can be separated by virtue of X-linked inheritance and associated adrenal insufficiency with features resembling Addison's disease. The disorder maps to chromosome Xq28. The affected boys exhibit a progressive illness characterized by the development of dementia, cortical blindness, ataxia, and spastic weakness in the limbs. A myeloneuropathy is sometimes the presenting deficit, as well as other phenotypes. Manifesting female carriers may show a mild spastic paraparesis or adrenal insufficiency.

Other rare demyelinating conditions

Pelizaeus–Merzbacher disease is an X-linked recessive disease that appears in early infancy. It maps to chromosome Xq22. Affected males

develop ataxia and spasticity. It is due to the defective production of proteolipid protein in central myelin. Canavan's disease also develops in early infancy, is of autosomal recessive inheritance, and gives rise to progressive mental deterioration and megalencephaly associated with spongy degeneration of the white matter. It is related to a deficiency of aspartoacylase. Affected children show excessive urinary excretion of N-acetylaspartic acid. Prenatal diagnosis is possible.

Fabry's disease (α-galactosidase A deficiency)

(See also Section 11.)

This condition, otherwise known as angiokeratoma corporis diffusum, is an inborn error of glycosphingolipid metabolism. Neutral glycosphingolipids are deposited in various tissues as a consequence of a deficiency of the enzyme α-galactosidase A. The disorder is inherited in an X-linked recessive manner and maps to chromosome Xq21.33–q22. Affected hemizygous males develop a mild peripheral neuropathy which is manifested by the occurrence of severe pains in the extremities, often beginning in childhood. Cerebrovascular lesions also occur, either cerebral infarction or haemorrhage. Non-neurological features include corneal opacification, punctate angiectatic lesions over the lower trunk, buttocks, and upper legs, and cardiac and renal lesions. Heterozygous females may display mild manifestations, most usually corneal opacification.

Hereditary lipoprotein deficiency

(See also Section 11.)

The occurrence of peripheral neuropathy in hereditary high density lipoprotein deficiency (Tangier disease) is discussed in Section 11. Hereditary abetalipoproteinaemia (Bassen–Kornzweig disease) is a recessively inherited disorder in which a spinocerebellar degeneration may develop with features that bear some resemblance to Friedreich's ataxia. Other manifestations of this uncommon disorder include intestinal malabsorption, pigmentary retinal degeneration, and the presence of acanthocytes in the peripheral blood (see Section 22). In addition to the absence of serum low-density lipoproteins, the serum cholesterol level is substantially reduced. There is evidence that the development of the neurological lesions may be prevented by the administration of vitamin E, the absorption of which from the gut is impaired. A spinocerebellar degeneration has also been described in individuals homozygous for hereditary hypobetalipoproteinaemia, a genetically separate condition.

Isolated vitamin E deficiency

A spinocerebellar syndrome resembling Friedreich's ataxia has been described in recent years due to vitamin E deficiency in the absence of generalized fat malabsorption. Its precise mechanism has not yet been established. The disorder is of autosomal recessive inheritance and maps to chromosome 8q. Treatment is by vitamin E replacement.

NEUROCUTANEOUS SYNDROMES

This category encompasses a number of disorders in which a variety of neurological disturbances is associated with cutaneous abnormalities.

Neurofibromatosis

Two major forms of this disorder exist. Both are of autosomal dominant inheritance. The gene for type 1 neurofibromatosis (NF1, von Recklinghausen's disease) is on the proximal long arm of chromosome 17 at q11.2. The gene product neurofibromin is a member of the GTPase-activating family of proteins. The disorder has a wide range of manifestations, the most constant of which are focal areas of hyperpigmentation (café-au-lait spots), multiple neurofibromas, and Lisch nodules on the iris. Six or more café-au-lait spots are necessary for them to be considered abnormal. Axillary and inguinal freckling is frequent. The cutaneous fibromas are of varying dimensions and can be extremely numerous. At times, giant plexiform neuromas develop in which there is extensive subcutaneous overgrowth of neurofibromatous tissue. Massive mediastinal, pelvic, or retroabdominal plexiform neurofibromas can occur, as well as cervical paraspinal tumours and astrocytomas of the optic nerve, cerebellum, or brain-stem. Malignant change occurs in a small proportion of peripheral neurofibromas. Mental retardation due to diffuse cortical dysgenesis is encountered in at least 10 per cent of patients. Other manifestations include congenital glaucoma, phaeo-chromocytoma, spinal deformity, pathological fractures of limb bones with malunion and pseudoarthrosis, and local gigantism of a limb. The neurofibromas are composed of proliferated Schwann cells and fibro-blasts in a collagenous matrix through which course nerve fibres in an irregular manner.

Most cases of NF1 require no treatment. Neurofibromas causing pressure symptoms may necessitate excision and others may merit removal for cosmetic reasons. Rapid expansion of a tumour, the development of pain and loss of neural function, will suggest malignant change. This most often occurs during adolescence or in young adults. The development of hypertension will require investigation for phaeochromocytoma, and spinal deformity may need orthopaedic attention. The gene product merlin has homology with proteins at the plasma membrane/ cytoskeleton interface. The gene for type 2 neurofibromatosis (NF2, central neurofibromatosis) has been mapped to chromosome 22q12.2. This disorder is characterized in particular by bilateral acoustic neurinomas (Fig. 1) but tumours may occur on other cranial nerves or spinal roots and also paraspinally. Meningiomas and gliomas may develop. A further feature is the occurrence of juvenile posterior subcapsular lenticular opacities.

Segmental neurofibromatosis affecting a restricted area of the body may be due to somatic mutation.

Tuberous sclerosis (Bourneville's disease, epiloia)

The features of this condition are mental retardation, epilepsy, and the occurrence of characteristic skin lesions. The disorder is dominantly inherited, but may be transmitted by individuals who are asymptomatic and who show only minimal clinical evidence of the disease. Isolated cases are frequent, comprising as many as 80 or 90 per cent of index cases. Many of them probably represent new mutations: others are transmitted by gene carriers with trivial manifestations. Genetic heterogeneity has now been established, with separate loci on chromosomes 9 (**TSC**1) and 16p13.3 (**TSC**2). The gene TSC2 has been identified and its product, called tuberin, has the structure of a GTPase activating protein.

The earliest cutaneous lesions are irregular foliate areas of depigmentation over the trunk. These patches are readily identified when viewed under ultraviolet illumination using a Woods lamp. Adenoma sebaceum

is a second type of skin lesion which develops over the cheeks in a 'butterfly' distribution and on the forehead (Fig. 2). Multiple small warty elevations appear which histologically are fibromatous and not adenomatous. Finally, a 'shagreen patch' may be present over the lower back. This consists of an area of elevated roughened skin with a yellowish tinge which has been likened to shark skin.

The cerebral changes give rise to mental retardation evident in early life which may be static or involve a slowly progressive cognitive decline, often complicated by behaviour disorder. Epilepsy with recurrent generalized or focal seizures may occur in association with mental retardation or in individuals of normal intelligence. The cerebral lesions, which are demonstrable by CT scanning or MRI, are typified by nodular or tuberous masses composed of proliferated glial cells and enlarged distorted neurones. They may become calcified. They are found scattered throughout the cerebral cortex and also extend into the ventricles to produce an appearance that was considered to resemble 'candle guttering' when seen in pneumoencephalograms. Gliomas sometimes arise in these lesions.

Retinal tumours, termed phakomas, may be present, and cardiac rhabdomyomas occasionally arise as well as hamartomas of the lungs and kidneys. Polycystic disease of the kidneys may also be associated.

Treatment consists of control of the epilepsy and the management of the mental retardation and behaviour disorder. Many of the more severe cases require institutionalization.

Cerebelloretinal haemangioblastosis (von Hippel–Lindau disease)

This condition comprises the occurrence of vascular tumours in the retina and within the central nervous system, most commonly in the cerebellum and spinal cord. The inheritance is autosomal dominant in pattern. The disorder maps to chromosome 3p26–25.

The retinal lesions consist of angiomatous vascular malformations. The cerebellar lesion is a haemangioblastoma, often cystic, which may slowly expand and present with features of a cerebellar tumour. It may require surgical treatment. Such tumours may be associated with polycythaemia, related to the production of erythropoietin or similar substance by the tumour. Haemangioblastomas may occur in the spinal cord and rarely in the cerebral hemispheres.

The skin is not involved but other tissues outside the nervous system

Fig. 2 Adenoma sebaceum in a patient with tuberous sclerosis.

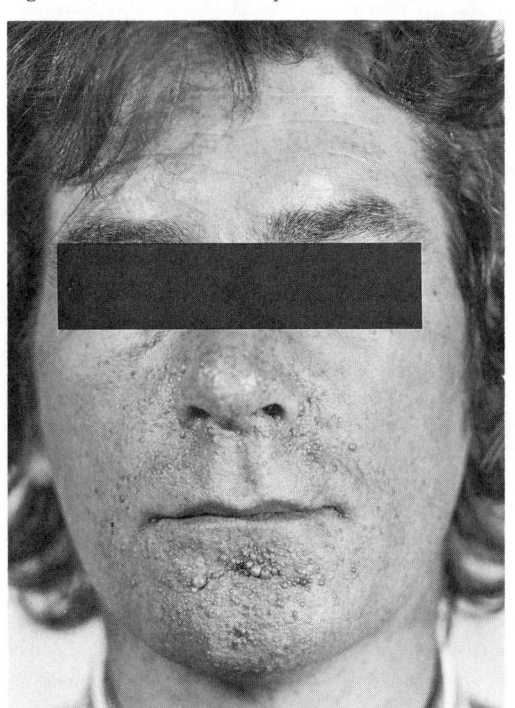

Fig. 1 CT scan showing bilateral acoustic neurinomas in a patient with type 2 neurofibromatosis. She also had an astrocytoma of the thoracic spinal cord.

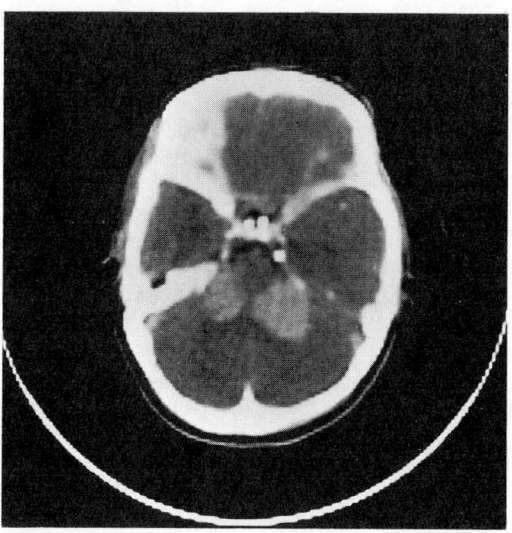

may be implicated, including the development of haemangioblastomas of the pancreas, kidney, and adrenal glands, which may be associated with the presence of multiple cysts. Hypernephromas can occur.

It should be emphasized that the majority of cerebellar haemangioblastomas are non-genetic.

Ataxia telangiectasia (Louis-Bar syndrome)

The inclusion of this disorder with the neurocutaneous syndromes depends upon the coincidence of a progressive cerebellar degeneration with cutaneous vascular lesions. The inheritance is of autosomal recessive type and the gene is localized on chromosome 11q22.3–q23.1. Ataxia begins in early childhood and choreoathetosis and oculomotor apraxia appear later. Telangiectasia of the conjunctivae is present as a relatively early feature and later becomes evident in the pinnae, over the face, and in the limb flexures. Some patients show an immunoglobulin deficiency and recurrent infections, or the development of malignancies may complicate the clinical picture. Defective DNA repair after X-irradiation is demonstrable in cultured skin fibroblasts. Affected children usually become unable to walk by the age of 12 years and death occurs during the second or sometimes third decade of life.

HEREDITARY MYOCLONIC EPILEPSIES

(See also Chapter 24.10.)

A number of conditions exist in which generalized epileptic seizures and myoclonus are associated with a progressive degenerative neurological disorder occurring on a genetic basis.

Lafora body disease

This is the most clearly defined form of progressive myoclonic epilepsy. It consists of a combination of major seizures, myoclonus and progressive dementia with an onset in late childhood or early adolescence, and death usually before adult life is reached. Cerebellar signs may appear later in the illness. The condition is characterized by the presence of intracellular inclusion bodies found most consistently in neurones of the cerebral cortex and in the cerebellar dentate nuclei. They are also detectable in the liver and in skeletal muscles, both of which are convenient sites for biopsy in order to establish the diagnosis. These Lafora bodies are composed of a polyglucosan. The disorder is caused by an autosomal recessive gene. Treatment is directed towards control of the epilepsy.

Less well-characterized disorders with a more prolonged time course in which epilepsy and myoclonus are associated with ataxia are progressive myoclonic ataxia (Ramsay Hunt syndrome) and progressive familial epilepsy of Unverricht–Lundborg type (Baltic and Mediterranean myoclonus). Lafora bodies are not present. The gene for Unverricht–Lundborg disease has been mapped to chromosome 21q22.3. Myoclonus and ataxia, along with other features, may be encountered in mitochondrial disease (see Section 25).

Sialidosis

The cherry-red-spot-myoclonus syndrome is an autosomal recessive disorder with an onset in late childhood, adolescence, or early adult life that combines action myoclonus with ataxia, cherry-red spots at the maculae, and cataracts. Childhood dysmorphic sialidosis is a similar disorder with an onset in early childhood in which mental retardation, myoclonus, and ataxia are associated with coarse facial features and other dysmorphic changes. Both are related to a deficiency of sialidase.

The myoclonus in these inherited disorders may respond to treatment with clonazepam or to piracetam in high dosage. 5-Hydroxytryptophan is less effective than in postanoxic action myoclonus.

HEREDITARY SPINAL MUSCULAR ATROPHIES

The hereditary spinal muscular atrophies constitute a group of disorders that involve a selective degeneration of anterior horn cells and sometimes also of the lower cranial nerve motor nuclei. They can be classified in terms of the pattern of involvement and the age of onset. Only the more common varieties will be described.

Hereditary proximal spinal muscular atrophy

Acute infantile spinal muscular atrophy (Werdnig–Hoffmann disease) almost always begins within the first year of life. It may have a prenatal onset and is one cause of the 'rag-doll' child syndrome of hypotonic muscle weakness in infancy. Progressive proximal muscular weakness and wasting, later becoming generalized and involving the bulbar musculature, usually lead to death before the age of 4 years. Cases with prolonged survival also occur (chronic childhood form). In hereditary juvenile proximal spinal muscular atrophy (Kugelberg–Welander disease) the onset is during childhood after the age of 2 years or as late as adolescence. The involvement of the proximal limb and trunk musculature mimics limb girdle muscular dystrophy, but fasciculation may be observed. The course is relatively benign, but progressive disability in adult life occurs in some cases; others remain relatively mildly affected. All three forms are of autosomal recessive inheritance and have been mapped to chromosome 5q12.2–q13.3. They appear to be due to allelic genes.

X-linked bulbospinal neuronopathy

This disorder, otherwise known as Kennedy's syndrome, consists of the development, commonly in the third or fourth decades, of progressive limb weakness, and, later, a bulbar palsy. Contraction fasciculation of the facial muscles is usually present. Muscle cramps and upper limb postural tremor are often evident from early adult life. About 50 per cent of cases show gynaecomastia and some have diabetes mellitus. The disorder is due to a trinucleotide repeat expansion within the androgen receptor gene on the proximal long arm of the X chromosome at q21.3–q22.

OTHER MISCELLANEOUS DISORDERS

A wide variety of other rare inherited conditions exist, of which the following deserve brief mention.

Hereditary optic neuropathy

Dominantly inherited juvenile optic neuropathy

This disorder gives rise to the insidious bilateral onset of optic atrophy during childhood with either mild or severe loss of vision. A central or centrocaecal scotoma may be detected. Electroretinography and visual evoked potentials demonstrate no loss of retinal receptors and suggest that the lesion affects retinal neuronal elements. There are no associated neurological abnormalities.

Leber's hereditary optic neuropathy

This disorder typically gives rise to acute or subacute bilateral visual loss in males between the ages of 18 and 30 years, although earlier and later ages of onset may be encountered. It may remain monocular for months or years. Initially there is enlargement of the blind spot and later this increases to involve central vision, producing a large centrocaecal scotoma. In the acute phase there is swelling in the nerve fibre layer around the optic disc with tortuous retinal arterioles and peripapillary telangiectases. Later the disc becomes atrophic. In affected females the age of onset tends to be later and a multiple sclerosis-like syndrome may develop. The disease is only transmitted by females and has recently been shown to be due to mitochondrial DNA mutations.

Mucopolysaccharidoses

(See also Section 11.)

The mucopolysaccharidoses constitute a group of disorders related to deficiencies of specific lysosomal enzymes, involving an accumulation in various tissues of acid mucopolysaccharides and gangliosides, and the presence of mucopolysaccharides in the urine. In both the recessively inherited Hurler's syndrome and the X-linked recessive Hunter's syndrome, the skeletal and other manifestations may be accompanied by mental retardation and pigmentary retinal degeneration. A spastic weakness in the limbs may develop in Hurler's syndrome. Mental retardation is also seen in the recessively inherited Sanfilippo's syndrome. Entrapment neuropathies are a feature in some forms, related to the skeletal changes.

Subacute necrotizing encephalopathy (Leigh's syndrome)

Typically this label is applicable to a fatal encephalopathy that develops during the first 2 years of life with variable combinations of mental retardation, seizures, optic atrophy, cerebellar ataxia, and central respiratory failure associated with lactic acidosis. Pathologically there are necrotic lesions in the brain-stem and a prominence of small blood vessels. Haemorrhage does not occur. The distribution of the lesions bears some resemblance to Wernicke's encephalopathy. Later onset cases with similar pathological changes occur. The disorder is genetically heterogeneous. Some are of probable autosomal recessive inheritance and related to deficiencies of the pyruvate dehydrogenase complex. Others are examples of mitochondrial encephalomyopathy.

Progressive neuronal degeneration of childhood with liver disease (Alpers–Huttenlocher syndrome)

This disorder, which is probably of autosomal recessive inheritance, begins at 3 to 15 months of age with developmental delay and failure to thrive. Recurrent vomiting and hypotonia are common, followed by intractable seizures. Death occurs at 10 to 90 months. Pathologically there is extensive neuronal loss and astrocytosis, particularly in the cerebral cortex, and fatty degeneration, cell loss, and fibrosis in the liver. An unidentified biochemical defect is assumed.

Infantile neuroaxonal dystrophy (Seitelberger's disease)

This is a rare, probably recessive condition that develops between the ages of 1 and 3 years and gives rise to progressive motor weakness from both upper and lower motor neurone deficits. It maps to chromosome 22q13–qter. Optic atrophy also occurs and death usually ensues before the end of the first decade. Degenerative changes are present in the brain and the spinal cord, the most striking feature of which is the occurrence of large axonal swellings in the grey matter of the brain and spinal cord.

Menkes' syndrome ('kinky' or 'steely' hair)

Menkes' syndrome is an X-linked recessive disorder in which developmental regression begins within a few months of birth. The gene locus is at Xq12–q13. Muscle hypotonus or hypertonus and seizures appear and are associated with abnormal hair. The scalp hair is sparse, stubbly, and greyish in colour. When examined under magnification, the hairs are seen to be twisted and display partial breaks. The serum copper and caeruloplasmin levels are low and the condition probably results from defective copper absorption from the gut. Prenatal diagnosis is possible.

Lesch–Nyhan syndrome

This is an X-linked recessive disorder (see also Chapter 24.10 and Section 11) related to the absence of an enzyme of purine metabolism, hypoxanthine-guanine phosphoribosyl transferase. It maps to chromosome Xq25–q27.2. The salient features are overproduction of uric acid and consequent hyperuricaemia which are associated with various behavioural and neurological manifestations, including mental retardation, self-mutilation, choreoathetosis, pyramidal signs, and spasticity in the limbs. The neurological abnormalities develop in childhood and death usually occurs in the second or third decade from renal failure. Allopurinol may reduce some of the non-neurological consequences of the hyperuricaemia, but no treatment influences the neurological abnormalities, the mechanism of which is not understood. Prenatal diagnosis and carrier detection are available.

Cockayne's syndrome

This is of autosomal recessive inheritance and consists of the development in childhood of dwarfism, microcephaly, progeria, mental retardation, cataract, pigmentary retinopathy, and ataxia. There is cutaneous sensitivity to ultraviolet light. The cerebral changes are those of a leucodystrophy. A demyelinating neuropathy coexists.

REFERENCES

Baraitser, M. (1990). *The genetics of neurological disorders*, (2nd edn). Oxford University Press.
Bundey, S. (1992). *Genetics and neurology*, (2nd edn). Churchill Livingstone, Edinburgh.
Emery, A.E.H. and Rimoin, D.L. (1990). *Principles and practice of medical genetics*, (2nd edn). Churchill Livingstone, Edinburgh.
Harding, A.E. (1984). *The hereditary ataxias and related disorders*, Churchill Livingstone, Edinburgh.
Harding, A.E. and Deufel, T. (1992). *Inherited ataxias*, Raven Press, New York.
Martin, J.B. (1993). Genetics in neurology. *Annals of Neurology*, **34;** 757–773.
Rosenberg, R.N., Prusiner, S.B., DiMauro, S., Barchi, R.L., and Kunkel, L.M. (eds) (1993). *The molecular and genetic basis of neurological disease.* Butterworth-Heinemann, Oxford.

24.9 Demyelinating disorders of the central nervous system

D. A. S. COMPSTON

Clinicians usually suspect demyelination when symptoms and signs, arising from damage to white matter tracts within the central nervous system, develop subacutely in young adults; and the diagnosis of multiple sclerosis—by far the commonest demyelinating disease in man—becomes probable when these episodes recur and affect different parts of the brain and spinal cord. Demyelinating disease is also the basis for many of the neurological syndromes triggered by infectious illness and vaccination. The clinical manifestations of demyelination are not specific and identical symptoms are seen in other disorders affecting the same parts of the nervous system.

Cellular neurobiology

Neuropathology

Perivascular inflammation occurs as the initial abnormality in the lesions of multiple sclerosis, isolated focal demyelination, and acute disseminated encephalomyelitis. In most situations, these evolve into plaques characterized by demyelinated axons and an increased number of astrocytes. Demyelination, without perivascular inflammation, also occurs in central pontine myelinolysis and in the heterogenous group of conditions known as dysmyelinating disorders.

Inflammatory demyelination of the central nervous system depends upon penetration of the blood–brain barrier by activated lymphocytes. This brings the full repertoire of cellular and soluble immune mediators to the abluminal surface of cerebral blood vessels, but microscopic changes in the acutely inflamed brain are limited to intense perivenular mononuclear cell infiltration and haemorrhage, without demyelination. Plasma cells accumulate in more mature lesions, and macrophages are seen to contact oligodendrocytes or their myelin lamellae, which split, vacuolate, and fragment. Occasionally, nerve fibres are remyelinated in acute lesions, known as shadow plaques, in which oligodendrocyte-like cells resynthesize thin layers of myelin with short internodes around the naked axons. Chronic lesions are characterized by oligodendrocyte depletion, astrocytic overgrowth, demyelination, few inflammatory cells, and some axonal loss. Plaques are commonly found adjacent to venous networks around the ventricles, and in the corpus callosum, the optic nerve, brain-stem, and cervical cord. Inflammatory changes also occur in the retina, which is devoid of myelin, and in peripheral nerves.

In the Marburg variant of hyperacute multiple sclerosis, large confluent zones of demyelination are associated with extensive axonal loss and surrounding oedema but little inflammation; similar pathological appearances are seen in diffuse cerebral sclerosis (Schilder's disease), sometimes with central cavitation, in the cerebrum, brain-stem, and cerebellum. In Devic's disease, the brunt of the disease is borne by the optic nerves and spinal cord, but demyelination is usually not confined to these parts. In central pontine myelinolysis, a single, sharply outlined focus of myelin destruction occurs in the rostral part of the pons, indiscriminately involving all myelinated pathways but sparing nerve fibres; demyelination is sometimes observed outside the pons but there is no inflammation.

Glial development and myelination

Glia consist of astrocytes, oligodendrocytes, and microglia. Oligodendrocytes synthesize and maintain myelin sheaths in the central nervous system, ensheathing short segments of neighbouring axons. Fully differentiated oligodendrocytes neither proliferate nor migrate and do not

Fig. 1 (a) An oligodendrocyte, cultured *in vitro*, contacting and myelinating short segments of four neighbouring nerve fibres or axons. (b) An oligodendrocyte process undergoing phagocytosis by an activated microglial cell, *in vitro*.

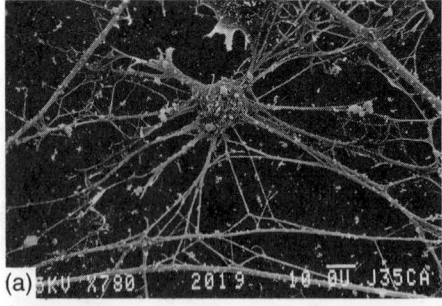

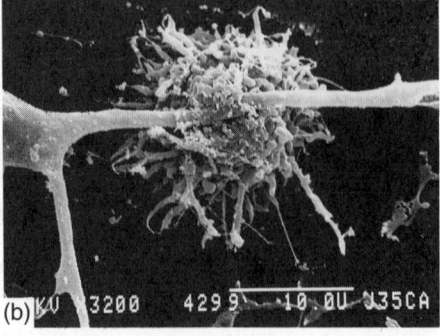

successfully remyelinate exons after injury; *in vitro* studies suggest that oligodendrocytes are uniquely vulnerable amongst glia to injury by inflammatory mediators. Astrocytes provide a physical structure for the nervous system, define its external limits, contribute to formation of the blood–brain barrier and contact the nodes of Ranvier. It is uncertain whether each function is performed by the same cell type, and separate astrocyte lineages probably exist within the human brain: *in vitro* studies of rodent glia indicate that oligodendrocytes are derived from bipotential precursors which, under growth factor control, differentiate either into oligodendrocytes or those astrocytes (type 2) which contact axons at the node of Ranvier.

These glial progenitors have the potential to divide, migrate, and differentiate; taken with the characterization of growth factors which orchestrate glial development, the identification of adult bipotential progenitors in the mature rodent brain and the detection of oligodendrocyte precursors in the adult human nervous system are exciting recent discoveries, sustaining the hope that endogenous glial repair and remyelination might be possible if the growth factor environment of the developing brain could be restored after injury of the mature nervous system (Fig. 1).

Inflammation and the brain

Traditionally, the brain has been regarded as protected from circulating inflammatory mediators by the blood–brain barrier and considered to lack its own immune repertoire; yet the central nervous system frequently suffers immunologically mediated tissue injury. The blood–brain barrier is made up by cerebral endothelial cells surrounded by a basement membrane around which the foot processes of type 1 astrocytes and microglia establish tight junctions. Inflammatory injury of the blood–brain barrier occurs when activated immune cells alter the expression of cell surface adhesion molecules and become entangled within the microvillar processes of cerebral endothelia; cytokines alter the expression of vascular addressins on endothelia, which interact with ligands on the surface of circulating activated inflammatory cells and assist their migration into the brain.

Infiltration by activated inflammatory cells occurs irrespective of antigen specificity; cells which recognize brain antigen persist and establish inflammatory foci within the nervous system, whereas others are removed by apoptosis. Cellular traffic across the blood–brain barrier non-specifically allows a variety of potentially pathogenic molecules to assemble on the abluminal surface of cerebral vessels, creating conditions which cause tissue injury by cellular and soluble immune mediators. In fact, the central nervous system does possess its own immunocompetent cells. These microglia are derived from bone marrow macrophages; they express receptors for a variety of ligands which enable contact to occur with opsonized target cells; in demyelinating disease, inflammatory events culminate in microglial digestion of oligodendrocytes and myelin.

Isolated demyelinating syndromes

Multiple sclerosis is characterized by demyelinating events which recur and are disseminated throughout the nervous system. In other situations, demyelination is focal and monophasic, but even in these cases imaging studies show that a high proportion of patients have more than one lesion. The distinction between multiple sclerosis and the various isolated demyelinating disorders can therefore reliably be made only when more than one episode has occurred, affecting two or more sites, and not merely on the basis of anatomical dissemination of lesions.

ACUTE DISSEMINATED ENCEPHALOMYELITIS

Typically, acute disseminated encephalomyelitis follows 14 days after an infectious illness. The disorder is usually cerebral, resulting in focal neurological deficits, fits, and drowsiness. In some cases, the manifestations are confined to the brain-stem, optic nerves, or spinal cord. These cases are not rare. A proportion of patients recovering from the initial attack subsequently relapse and their illness cannot then be distinguished from the encephalitic presentation of multiple sclerosis. In some patients, although the illness remains monophasic, separate sites are involved sequentially over several weeks but the disorder does not recur and differs from multiple sclerosis in this important respect.

The hyperacute form of acute disseminated encephalomyelitis (Hurst's disease) starts with headache and progresses over hours to disorientation, confusion, drowsiness, and coma; events move quickly and the illness often proves fatal before the diagnosis has been established. The combination of pyrexia and a marked cerebrospinal fluid pleocytosis with a predominantly neutrophil response mimics pyogenic infection of the central nervous system, but the course is uninfluenced by antimicrobial treatment. Occasionally, the clinical and pathological features of acute haemorrhagic leucoencephalitis are focal and mimic rapidly expanding tumour or herpes simplex encephalitis.

Formerly, acute disseminated encephalomyelitis affected 1:1000 children with exanthematous illnesses, the risk being slightly higher following pertussis and scarlet fever than measles and rubella; with vaccination, these illnesses are less common, as is acute disseminated encephalomyelitis, and a high proportion of cases now occur without identification of the provocative agent. About 50 per cent of postvaricella cases present with a pure cerebellar syndrome. A greater variety of causative organisms has been implicated in adult-onset acute disseminated encephalomyelitis, but in both groups a presumptive diagnosis often has to be made in the absence of preceding infection; recently identified causes include echovirus, coxsackie and herpes viridae, mycoplasma, borreliosis, and cases associated with acquired immunodeficiency syndrome.

Headache, drowsiness, meningeal irritation, signs of systemic infection, focal or generalized fits, and combinations of lesions indicating damage to the cerebrum, optic nerves, brain-stem, or spinal cord evolve over the course of a few days; the cerebrospinal fluid contains a mixture of polymorphonuclear cells and lymphocytes with raised protein and a slight reduction in glucose; oligoclonal bands may be present. Although there is an appreciable mortality, the majority of patients survive, albeit with persistent neurological deficits; the outcome probably is influenced by the early use of high-dose steroids. Magnetic resonance imaging shows changes similar to those occurring in multiple sclerosis, but the lesions are more extensive and symmetrical; they persist long after recovery of the clinical illness. Some patients develop new lesions after evolution of the presenting episode, indicating continuing disease activity, and the diagnosis of multiple sclerosis then becomes more likely.

Postvaccinial encephalomyelitis has become a rare disorder and the definitive series were collected several decades ago following the need to vaccinate large numbers of individuals against smallpox. The illness develops within 21 days of vaccination, with a skin rash and systemic symptoms, followed by cerebral or myelitic signs which usually recover spontaneously, in due course.

OPTIC NEURITIS

Optic neuritis presents with pain on eye movement, followed by blurred vision which evolves over hours or days, sometimes to complete blindness; there may be selective loss of colour vision and flashes of light (phosphenes) on eye movement. The pain disappears within a few days; vision improves in 90 per cent of patients over months but defects of colour perception frequently persist. Optic neuritis may present with progressive visual failure but in this situation care must be taken to exclude compression of the anterior visual pathway. Transient visual loss, mimicking optic neuritis, also occurs in ischaemic optic neuropathy, sarcoidosis, or Eales' disease, and a family history should be taken since the presentation of visual failure in Leber's hereditary optic neuropathy is similar to bilateral sequential optic neuritis in men. The lesion

responsible for optic neuritis can be imaged *in vivo*, and inflammation within the intracanalicular portion of the nerve is associated with delayed or incomplete recovery of vision. Correlations between imaging, symptoms, and neurophysiological changes indicate that the visual deficits in optic neuritis arise at the time of altered blood brain–barrier permeability; they are associated with conduction block and precede demyelination or axonal degeneration.

The frequency with which the optic nerve is involved in multiple sclerosis leads to anxiety in the informed patient that an episode of optic neuritis is likely to be the first manifestation of multiple sclerosis. The risk is highest in the first 5 years but the proportion of cases having recurrent demyelination increases thereafter and life-table analysis suggests that up to 80 per cent of cases eventually develop multiple sclerosis. In children, optic neuritis is commonly bilateral, and recurrent demyelination affecting other parts of the nervous system rarely occurs; bilateral simultaneous optic neuritis in adults, although less common than in children, also carries a low risk of conversion to multiple sclerosis. Recurrent optic neuritis is associated with an increased rate of conversion and the risk is marginally higher in females than males. Periventricular white matter abnormalities demonstrated by magnetic resonance imaging are found in more than 60 per cent of patients with optic neuritis, and the risk of developing multiple sclerosis is substantially increased for those having two or more such lesions at presentation; the presence of oligoclonal bands on cerebrospinal fluid electrophoresis during the acute phase is also a significant risk factor.

TRANSVERSE MYELITIS

The spinal cord is vulnerable to inflammatory damage but, as with acute disseminated encephalomyelitis in adults, the precipitating cause is often not identified. Acute necrotizing myelitis causes rapidly progressive flaccid areflexic paraplegia with anaesthesia and loss of sphincter control. The intensity of inflammation results in severe pain with meningism, pyrexia, and systemic symptoms. The condition mimics cord compression; the cerebrospinal fluid changes resemble pyogenic or tuberculous infection of the central nervous system. For these reasons, treatment with high-dose corticosteroids, which may usefully influence mortality and limit long-term disability, may be withheld. Acute necrotizing myelitis has recently been described in association with herpes virus infection, and as a complication of acute lymphocytic leukaemias, lymphoma, carcinoma, and acquired immune deficiency syndrome.

Transverse myelitis presents with pain at the site of the lesion, followed by weakness in the legs, sensory symptoms, and sphincter involvement. The weakness increases and the clinical picture is that of spinal shock, features which are rarely seen in acute cord lesions due to multiple sclerosis; sphincter control is lost but, unlike patients with multiple sclerosis, there is usually difficulty in emptying rather than filling the bladder. The need to exclude a structural abnormality in patients with transverse myelitis means that many patients undergo radiological investigation which may demonstrate cord swelling. The spinal fluid shows an increased mononuclear cell count, numerically intermediate between the marked pleocytosis of acute necrotizing myelitis and the marginal abnormalities seen in multiple sclerosis; total protein is raised and oligoclonal bands may be present on electrophoresis, but the glucose is usually normal. Transverse myelitis is more common in adults than in children; there is a high frequency of persistent disability but a much lower conversion to multiple sclerosis than following optic neuritis. There is frequently no preceding history of infection but recognized causes include infection with herpes zoster and simplex type 2, hepatitis A, cytomegalovirus, toxoplasmosis, and schistosomiasis.

DEVIC'S DISEASE

Devic's disease is characterized by massive confluent demyelination in the anterior visual pathway, together with equally severe spinal cord damage, occurring simultaneously or sequentially and in either order, the episodes usually separated by weeks or months. Demyelinating disease often follows the Devic pattern in Japanese, where multiple sclerosis is otherwise rare, and some series of patients with Devic's disease in northern Europe have emphasized the low conversion rate to multiple sclerosis; however, the majority of European patients with bilateral simultaneous optic neuritis and transverse myelitis show manifestations of widespread demyelination and multiple events occur in due course. In those cases that follow a biphasic course without further manifestations of demyelination, the cause is rarely identified but cases are described complicating pulmonary tuberculosis.

Multiple sclerosis

Aetiology

The aetiology of multiple sclerosis involves an interplay between genetic and environmental factors. It is a disease of northern Europeans and occurs less frequently in other racial groups. Within the United Kingdom, the disease is more prevalent in north-east Scotland than in other parts; the regional prevalences in North America match patterns of migration from northern Europe, and correlate inversely with the distribution of Americans of African origin. In South Africa, multiple sclerosis occurs more commonly in English-speaking Whites than in Afrikaaners or Coloureds but is not seen in native Africans; in Australia and New Zealand the disease is rarely diagnosed in Aborigines or

Maoris but occurs commonly in those of European origin. The lifetime risk of multiple sclerosis in northern Europeans—about 1:800—increases to 1:50, 1:20, and 1:3 for the offspring, siblings, and monozygotic twin partners of affected individuals, respectively (Fig. 2).

Susceptibility to multiple sclerosis is polygenic. Candidate genes include class 2 alleles of the histocompatibility complex (DRB1.1501, DRB5.0101, DQA1.0102, DQB2.0602); preliminary evidence suggests that germline variations in the variable regions of the T-cell receptor β-chain and the immunoglobulin heavy chain also increase the risk of multiple sclerosis. Heritability may, in time, be shown to result entirely from the contribution of genes which restrict the immune response, and the claim that, in some populations, inherited differences in the structure of myelin also contribute to susceptibility has not been confirmed.

The distribution of multiple sclerosis cannot be explained only on the basis of population genetics. In White South Africans and in Australia, prevalence rates are half those documented for many parts of northern Europe and there is a gradient in frequency, both in Australia and in New Zealand, which does not follow genetic clines. Multiple sclerosis occurs at a low frequency in Caribbeans but the risk increases substantially in their first-generation descendants raised in the United Kingdom. Conversely, the risk is higher for English-speaking Whites migrating into South Africa as adults than in childhood.

Prospective studies have demonstrated that new episodes of demyelination are more likely to occur following viral exposure, but no one triggering agent has been identified. The risk of developing multiple sclerosis is increased for individuals who are exposed to measles,

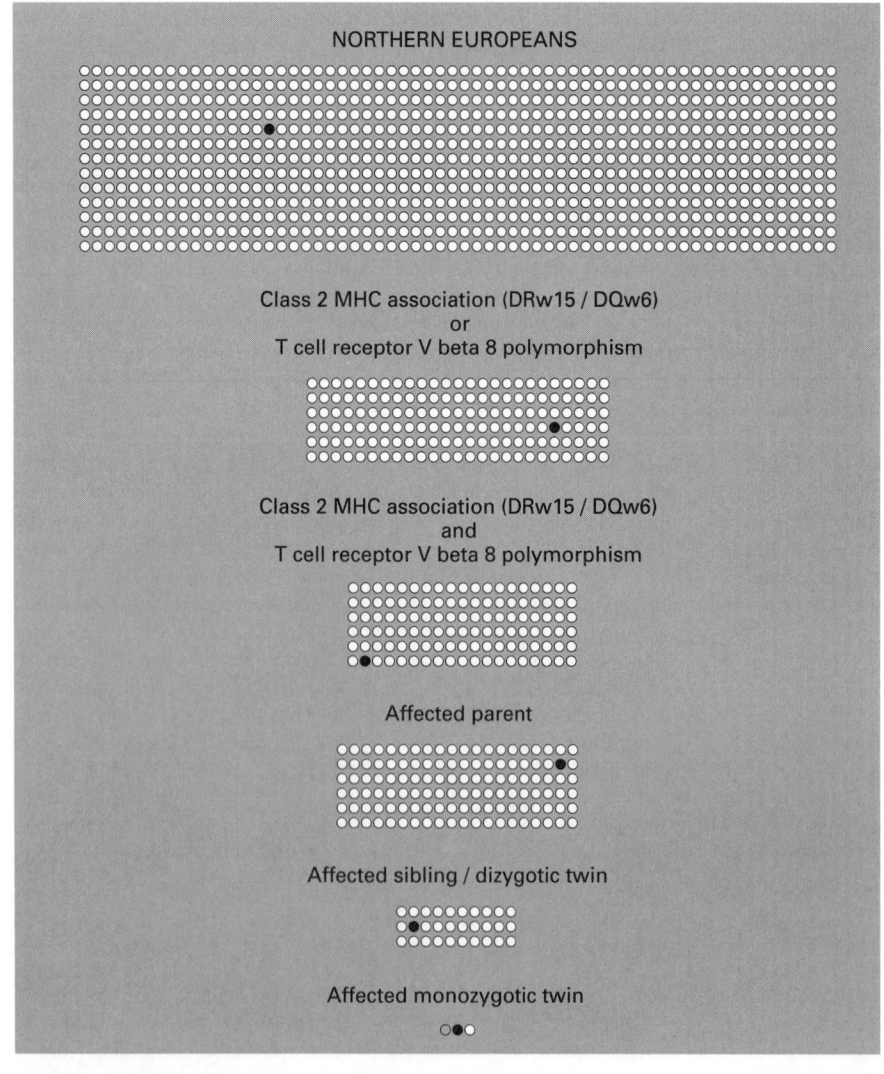

NORTHERN EUROPEANS

Class 2 MHC association (DRw15 / DQw6)
or
T cell receptor V beta 8 polymorphism

Class 2 MHC association (DRw15 / DQw6)
and
T cell receptor V beta 8 polymorphism

Affected parent

Affected sibling / dizygotic twin

Affected monozygotic twin

Fig. 2 The lifetime risk of developing multiple sclerosis for northern Europeans, individuals with one or more candidate susceptibility gene products, and those already known to have an affected relative.

mumps, rubella, and Epstein–Barr virus infection relatively late in childhood or adolescence. These studies do not implicate any one of these agents as the exclusive cause of multiple sclerosis but suggest that a narrow and age-linked period of susceptibility to viral exposure exists in those who are constitutionally at risk of developing the disease.

Pathophysiology

Myelin injury blocks saltatory conduction through myelinated axons. Partially demyelinated pathways cannot transmit fast trains of impulse; depolarization may cross the lesion but at reduced velocity, accounting for the characteristic delay in arrival of evoked potentials. Partially demyelinated axons discharge spontaneously, causing unpleasant distortions of sensation and facial myokymia; and increased mechanical sensitivity results in movement-induced phosphenes and the electric sensation provoked by neck flexion (Lhermitte's symptom). Increased temperature sensitivity explains the temporary increase in symptoms after exercise or immersion in hot water; and transmission between neighbouring partially demyelinated axons results in paroxysmal symptoms of demyelination such as trigeminal neuralgia or tonic brain-stem seizures. Physiological principles do not fully account for the dynamics of symptom onset and recovery; some arise from pathways that are not yet demyelinated and little is known about the contribution that remyelination makes to recovery of function.

Clinical symptomatology

SPECIAL SENSES

Involvement of the visual pathways is almost invariable and most commonly affects the optic nerve (see above); the postchiasmal visual pathway is occasionally involved, resulting in hemianopic field defects. Deafness occurs in multiple sclerosis, occasionally at presentation. Feelings of unsteadiness are common; and acute brain-stem demyelination causes severe positional vertigo, vomiting, ataxia, and headache. Taste may be subjectively abnormal but aguesia is rarely described.

MOTOR SYMPTOMS AND SIGNS

Impaired mobility affects the majority of patients with multiple sclerosis, usually as a result of spinal disease; movements are slow, weakness differentially affecting extensors in the arms and flexors in the legs, and there are the expected signs of upper motor neurone lesions. Spasticity may be more problematic than weakness and all aspects of immobility are frequently complicated by fatigue. Cerebellar involvement causes incoordination of speech, bulbar control, eye movements, the individual limbs or balance, usually in combination with corticospinal damage. Damage to the superior cerebellar peduncle or red nucleus produces a disabling proximal wild flinging tremor, and many other movement disorders have been described. Lower motor neurone signs occur when there is extensive demyelination adjacent to the dorsal root entry zone.

SENSORY SYMPTOMS AND SIGNS

Altered sensation occurs at some stage in nearly every patient with multiple sclerosis. Damage to the posterior columns in the cervical cord produces tight, burning, twisting, tearing, or pulling sensations, which are usually painful; associated loss of proprioception severely compromises function. Spinothalamic tract involvement leads to loss of thermal and pain sensation. Non-specific tingling without accompanying signs is often described and the commonest physical sign found in the absence of symptoms is impaired vibration sense in the legs.

Demyelination of the dorsal or lumbar segments of the spinal cord produces paraesthesiae and numbness in the legs, ascending to the trunk, and sometimes associated with sacral sparing, although a characteristic sensory syndrome seen in patients with multiple sclerosis is numbness of the perineum and genitalia with disturbed sphincter function.

AUTONOMIC INVOLVEMENT

Autonomic symptoms occur in many patients with multiple sclerosis. Bladder symptoms are most common in women whereas impotence occurs frequently in males. Loss of inhibition of reflex bladder emptying, normally mediated by cholinergic neurones that contract the detrusor and relax the internal sphincter, results in urgency and frequency, with incontinence when combined with immobility. With conus lesions, the problem is impaired bladder emptying. Failure to fill and empty may coexist, resulting in detrusor contractions against a closed sphincter.

Impaired control of the rectal sphincter is much less of a problem than failure of emptying. Some impotent males with multiple sclerosis retain reflex erections, in which case psychogenic factors are often invoked; others have erectile failure due entirely to spinal cord disease. Mechanical difficulties, spasticity, altered sensation, skin excoriation, and in-dwelling catheters affect sexual performance in both sexes.

EYE MOVEMENTS

Abnormalities of eye movement are extremely common in multiple sclerosis and often occur in the absence of symptoms. Weakness of the lateral rectus, or an internuclear ophthalmoplegia, produces double vision; the latter may coexist with gaze paresis to produce the 'one and one-half' syndrome. Visual instability (oscillopsia) occurs most commonly in the context of bilateral internuclear ophthalmoplegia or downbeating nystagmus, and with ocular flutter and opsoclonus. Asymptomatic disorders of eye movement include gaze paretic nystagmus and the replacement of smooth pursuit conjugate movements by jerky saccades.

OTHER BRAIN-STEM MANIFESTATIONS

Facial weakness, indistinguishable from Bell's palsy, occurs in patients with multiple sclerosis, alone or association with other signs of brain-stem disease, including hemifacial spasm and diffuse rippling of muscle fibres (myokymia). Extensive brain-stem demyelination disturbs consciousness and respiratory drive.

Paroxysmal symptoms, resulting from ephaptic transmission, include trigeminal neuralgia, paroxysmal dysarthria and ataxia with a clumsy arm, complex disturbances of sensation (including bursts of pain, sensory distortion, itching), hiccup, and tonic brain-stem seizures producing painful tetanic posturing of the limbs for seconds or minutes.

COGNITIVE AND AFFECTIVE SYMPTOMS

Defects of visual and auditory attention occur in multiple sclerosis, sometimes at an early stage, and these are also detectable in patients with isolated demyelinating lesions; an overall impairment in intelligence quotient relates more to duration of disease, and onset of the progressive phase, affecting memory by comparison with language skills. Specific cognitive deficits due to hypothalamic involvement, including the Korsakoff state and Kleine–Levin syndrome, are sometimes seen. Psychotic behaviour is rare but depression occurs more frequently than in patients with comparable neurological disability; hypomania is occasionally seen but should not be confused with pathological laughter and crying, arising from loss of central inhibition of facial and bulbar reflexes in association with extensive brain-stem disease.

RARE MANIFESTATIONS OF MULTIPLE SCLEROSIS

The list of rare clinical manifestations includes massive cerebral lesions, aphasia, headache, fever, movement disorders, epilepsy, hypothalamic and pituitary symptoms, respiratory failure, sympathetic involvement, behavioural and psychiatric disease, and peripheral neuropathy. Narcolepsy, Sjögren's syndrome, ankylosing spondylitis, and autoimmune disease have periodically been associated with multiple sclerosis.

Clinical course

Eighty per cent of patients present with relapsing/remitting disease, episodes occurring at random frequency and for an unpredictable period, but averaging about 0.5/year and decreasing with time. Later, a high proportion of patients enter a slowly progressive phase of the disease, but in 20 per cent the illness is progressive from onset. Life expectancy is at least 25 years, and a high proportion of patients die from unrelated causes. Recovery from each attack is invariably slower than onset, and may be incomplete. In about 5 per cent of patients, a latent period of more than 20 years occurs between the presenting and the next episode.

The spinal cord bears the brunt of progressive multiple sclerosis, but optic nerve, cerebral, and brain-stem disease may also deteriorate slowly. Primary progressive spinal disease is the usual mode of presentation when multiple sclerosis develops beyond the fifth decade. Secondary progressive multiple sclerosis tends to affect whichever system has been involved during the relapsing phase. Progression may follow directly upon a severe relapse and be interrupted by further episodes.

About 25 per cent of patients have multiple sclerosis in a form which is not disabling. Benign disease usually occurs in young females with predominantly sensory symptoms and complete recovery from individual episodes. Conversely, in 5 per cent relapses occur frequently and do not recover, leading rapidly to disability and early death; and up to 15 per cent become severely disabled within a short time. Occasionally patients die acutely from respiratory failure when the medulla is affected and from massive cerebral demyelination.

Two per cent of patients with multiple sclerosis present before the age of 10 years, and 5 per cent before 16 years of age; even so, there is reluctance to make the diagnosis in children. The presentation is often similar to that seen in adults, although an encephalitic onset mimicking acute disseminated encephalomyelitis is well recognized.

Prognosis

The prognosis is relatively good when sensory or visual symptoms dominate the illness; conversely, motor involvement, especially when co-ordination or balance are disturbed, has a less good prognosis. The outlook is also poor in older-onset patients and these are often males. Frequent, prolonged relapses with incomplete recovery and a short interval between the initial episode and first relapse carry a worse prognosis, but the main determinant of disability is onset of the progressive phase.

Nine per cent of infections occurring in patients with multiple sclerosis are followed by relapse, and 27 per cent of new episodes are related to infection. The risk of relapse is increased in the puerperium. The available evidence suggests that trauma does not precipitate new symptoms or influence the course of multiple sclerosis. Physical manifestations of the disease are inevitably coped with less well in the context of emotional stress, but this does not otherwise influence the disease.

Investigation

Investigations are required in patients suspected of having multiple sclerosis when the clinical findings are insufficient for establishing the diagnosis; they are used to demonstrate anatomical dissemination of lesions and provide evidence for intrathecal inflammation. Conditions that mimic demyelinating disease may also need to be excluded.

ELECTROPHYSIOLOGY

Demyelination can be detected in clinically unaffected pathways using visual, auditory, somatosensory, central motor, and event-related potentials; their latencies are characteristically delayed, whereas, except in acute lesions, the amplitude is unaffected. Evoked potentials add little in situations where the pathway under investigation is clinically affected and their role as an adjunct to diagnosis has largely been replaced by imaging techniques.

IMAGING

Low-density lesions, corresponding to areas of demyelination, may be seen using contrast-enhanced computed tomography, and these occasionally have the appearances of cerebral tumour or abscess, but this technique is insensitive compared with magnetic resonance imaging (Fig. 3). More than 95 per cent of patients with clinically definite multiple sclerosis have periventricular lesions, and more than 90 per cent also show discrete white-matter abnormalities, each corresponding to areas of histological damage. Gadolinium enhancement of these lesions signifies altered permeability of the blood-brain barrier and indicates that they are of recent origin. The lesions are not specific and similar changes occur with inflammatory or vascular lesions and with advancing age. Focal demyelination can be imaged in the optic nerve, brain-stem, and spinal cord.

The evolving lesion starts with increased blood–brain barrier permeability which lasts for up to 4 weeks and precedes the onset of T_2-weighted magnetic resonance changes. These lesions may disappear altogether, but reactivation is sometimes seen, the cycles lasting about 8 weeks. The periventricular lesions, which best characterize multiple sclerosis, correlate with areas of persistent demyelination, the signal arising from increased water content associated with astrocytosis. A mixture of new, evolving, and recovering lesions may be seen in an individual patient at any one time. Magnetic resonance lesions occur about 15 times more frequently than new clinical events. There is no change in the frequency of new lesions as patients switch from the relapsing to the progressive phases of the disease, and the number or volume of lesions does not correlate with disease severity or the course, but there is less cerebral involvement in patients who present with primary progressive disease compared with those having comparable disability from secondary progression.

Imaging is not necessary for diagnostic purposes in patients with a history of relapsing disease and signs indicating involvement of multiple sites within the central nervous system. The major practical use is in the investigation of individuals with isolated demyelinating lesions, recurrent episodes at a single site, or progressive disease affecting the spinal cord. In all these situations the requirement is to exclude a structural lesion, especially since these can present with relapsing symptoms. Magnetic resonance imaging has now almost replaced invasive radiology of the cord by myelography. Imaging any region of the nervous system, clinically affected in isolation, will reliably exclude a structural lesion that might mimic multiple sclerosis and may show changes consistent with focal demyelination, but will not distinguish the syndromes of isolated demyelination from multiple sclerosis. Once the clinically affected part has been negatively screened for a structural lesion, the

Fig. 3 Magnetic resonance imaging in a patient with multiple sclerosis, showing periventricular abnormal T_2-weighted signals.

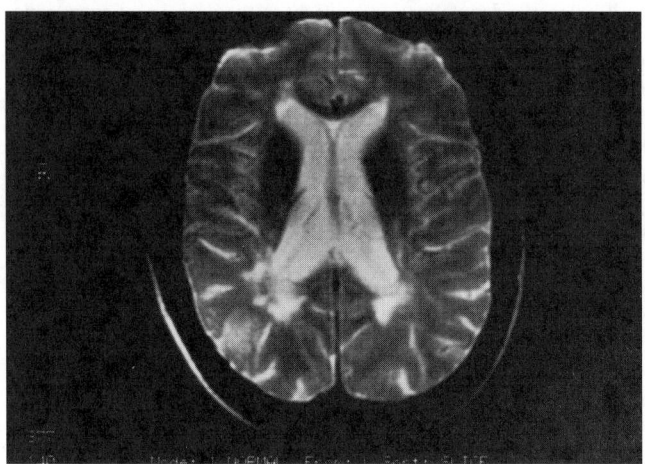

diagnosis of multiple sclerosis also requires the demonstration of cerebral periventricular lesions, ideally with evidence for lesions of different ages provided by gadolinium enhancement.

CEREBROSPINAL FLUID

Cerebrospinal fluid analysis provides information, which is complementary to imaging abnormalities, in patients suspected of having multiple sclerosis. The cell count rarely exceeds 50 lymphocytes/mm³, even during periods of clinical activity, and is normal in more than 50 per cent of patients. There is a rise in total protein with a specific increase in the immunoglobulin concentration and the presence of oligoclonal bands on protein electrophoresis in more than 90 per cent of cases, after correction for leakage of serum proteins through the blood–brain barrier, providing evidence for synthesis of immunoglobulin within the central nervous system. As with the imaging abnormalities, these are sensitive but not specific. The specificity of antibodies appearing in spinal fluid remains largely elusive; some are directed against components of the oligodendrocyte cell body or its myelin membranes, and others against extrinsic antigens, including viruses, but collectively these antibodies only account for a minority of the bands.

In each clinical situation a number of additional investigations will be required to exclude conditions that mimic multiple sclerosis.

Differential diagnosis

The commonest error in clinical practice is to make the diagnosis of multiple sclerosis in patients with progressive spinal disease in whom a structural lesion has not been adequately excluded. Lesions at the foramen magnum are particularly well placed to cause confusion through appearing to produce evidence for independent spinal and brain-stem lesions. Errors also arise with progressive or relapsing manifestations of brain-stem or spinal arteriovenous malformations.

Care must be taken in the diagnosis of multiple sclerosis when several members are affected within one family. Hereditary spastic paraplegia mimics familial multiple sclerosis, and this should also be considered in isolated cases of progressive spastic paraplegia when pyrimidal manifestations occur in isolation and with disproportionate spasticity. Other familial disorders that are confused with multiple sclerosis include the hereditary ataxias and adult-onset leucodystrophies; pedigrees with affected males and maternal inheritance may be examples of X-linked adrenoleukodystrophy, and individuals with the phenotype of multiple sclerosis occur in families with the clinical and genetic features of Leber's hereditary optic atrophy.

Clinical, immunological, and imaging abnormalities indistinguishable from multiple sclerosis occur with granulomatous and vasculitic diseases of the brain, especially the cerebral variant of systemic lupus erythematosus, which usually occurs in the absence of systemic manifestations or informative serology. Sarcoidosis may present with clinical involvement of the central nervous system, typical magnetic resonance and cerebrospinal fluid abnormalities, and without pulmonary or cutaneous manifestations; uveitis also occurs in multiple sclerosis and so is not necessarily a useful discriminator. Orogenital ulceration in a patient with the clinical manifestations of multiple sclerosis suggests the diagnosis of Behçet's disease.

Alternative diagnoses need to be considered when multiple sclerosis is diagnosed in Africans or Orientals in whom progressive spinal disease, sometimes with visual involvement, is more probably due to human T-cell leukaemia virus-1 (HTLV-1)-associated tropical spastic paraplegia.

Direct infections of the nervous system can mimic the isolated demyelinating syndromes and multiple sclerosis. These include tuberculous and other chronic meningitides, the neurological manifestations of acquired immunodeficiency syndrome, and Lyme disease; borreliosis can also cause a chronic or relapsing disorder of the central nervous system, but this is usually preceded by the characteristic painful poly-radiculitis and facial palsy that epitomizes Lyme disease. Similarities between multiple sclerosis and neurosyphilis should not be forgotten in the context of opportunistic infection complicating HIV infection. The age distribution and clinical manifestations usually make it easy to distinguish subacute combined degeneration of the spinal cord from multiple sclerosis, but focal spinal lesions, accompanied by Lhermitte's symptom, occur in B_{12} deficiency.

The high public profile which multiple sclerosis currently enjoys leads many individuals with vague sensory symptoms or dizziness to consider the diagnosis, but they are easily reassured and these transient symptoms not accompanied by physical signs can usually be dismissed; they differ from the syndromes fabricated by individuals seeking the dignity of a neurological diagnosis in the setting of neurotic or psychiatric disease, which are much more difficult to manage.

Treatment of demyelinating disease

Caution is usually observed in recommending treatment in patients with multiple sclerosis since no agent has yet proved effective at altering the long-term course of the disease, and a significant proportion of affected individuals remain free from disability over several decades. However, treatments that modify existing symptoms and accelerate the rate of recovery from relapse are often used in the management of individual patients.

THE TREATMENT OF ACUTE RELAPSE

Since the natural history of relapse is for spontaneous recovery, treatment is not required for every exacerbation. Corticosteroids, preferably given as high-dose intravenous methylprednisolone, shorten the duration of relapse and have fewer complications than steroids given orally or by the intramuscular route, even when multiple courses have been administered. Improvement starts during or soon after a 3 to 5 g course of methylprednisolone given by daily intravenous infusion over several days. Intravenous methylprednisolone reduces tissue oedema in areas of acute inflammation and temporarily alters the permeability of the blood–brain barrier; immunological effects include a reduction in macrophage activity.

THE TREATMENT OF SYMPTOMS

Many manifestations of multiple sclerosis can be improved symptomatically. Patients with urinary symptoms due to spinal cord involvement often achieve reasonable bladder emptying by abdominal pressure or perineal stimulation, and tolerate mild incontinence; urgency or frequency respond well to drugs that include anticholinergic activity (oxybutynin or propantheline), but when detrusor and sphincter function become uncoupled, causing impaired bladder emptying with failure to fill, the preferred treatment is intermittent self-catheterization, which is easily adopted by motivated patients with adequate vision and arm function, and ensures complete bladder emptying, often with unimagined advantages to social activities and sleep. Permanent use of a catheter is preferable to dribbling incontinence, with its attendant risks of skin excoriation. Constipation should be managed by dietary alteration and the use of bulk laxatives, avoiding agents that act directly on the bowel wall.

Sexual function is frequently impaired in males with spinal demyelination. Potency can be restored by self-administered cavernous injections of papaverine, and more complicated techniques for stimulating ejaculation can be used to ensure fertility in impotent males who wish to have children.

Altered mobility in multiple sclerosis results from weakness, impaired co-ordination, spasticity, fatigue, or loss of proprioception. Tremor can be managed by partial physical restraint or the use of β-blockers and occasionally with isoniazid, primidone, and dopamine receptor blockade; stereotactic neurosurgical procedures have been used to stabilize one arm in patients who can no longer manage basic aspects of daily living. Unsteadiness due to altered vestibular input may improve with the use of a vestibular sedative. Fatigue handicaps not otherwise disabled patients, and some success has been claimed for amantadine hydrochloride, but the fatigue often proves refractory to treatment. Weakness and spasticity contribute differentially to immobility in patients with multiple sclerosis, depending on which spinal pathways are most affected. The relief of spasticity can aggravate weakness and paradoxically reduce mobility, since patients may depend on increased muscle tone in order to stand. High-dose intravenous methylprednisolone, baclofen, dantrolene sodium, or tizanidine each have some effect on spasticity and they are indicated in individuals with preserved muscle strength, or those with painful spasms who no longer attempt to stand or walk; these agents can be used in combination since many act at different sites involved in the maintenance of muscle tone. Spasticity can be relieved by intrathecal baclofen, using a delivery pump, or, ultimately, by surgical interruption of the reflex pathways or tenotomy, but these techniques must be regarded as irreversible.

The paroxysmal manifestations of multiple sclerosis are usually very responsive to treatment; tonic brain-stem seizures stop abruptly with the use of carbamazepine or other anticonvulsants which increase membrane stability, and these also help in patients with trigeminal neuralgia and more refractory forms of pain due to spinal demyelination. These unpleasant sensations are influenced by alterations in mood and respond to antidepressants.

INFLUENCING THE COURSE OF MULTIPLE SCLEROSIS

Attempts to influence the course of multiple sclerosis are based on the logic that tissue injury is immunologically mediated. Immune stimulation with γ-interferon is known to increase disease activity. Immune suppression stabilizes the clinical course in rapidly progressive multiple sclerosis, but adverse effects are common, the benefits are rarely maintained and are of a magnitude which is not necessarily useful for the individual patient.

A meta-analysis of trials using azathioprine confirms the statistically significant but individually limited role of this well-tolerated immunosuppressive agent. The majority of patients requesting treatment which might alter the course of the disease still receive azathioprine, with some theoretical justification and modest success, but there is no evidence that the efficacy of azathioprine can be enhanced by combination therapy or the additional use of methylprednisolone.

Cyclosporin influences progression of the disease, relapse rate, and severity, but only in doses which are poorly tolerated. By comparison with azathioprine, which is well tolerated but of limited benefit, cyclosporin is probably effective but associated with unacceptable adverse effects, at least in multiple sclerosis, and neither agent can be recommended for the majority of patients. Plasma exchange has been used, in the hope of matching the benefits achieved in other inflammatory disorders, but usually as an adjunct to immunological treatment and with no evidence for any useful additive effect.

Similar problems have characterized the evaluation of cyclophosphamide in patients with multiple sclerosis. Following initial reports of improvement in patients with chronic progressive disease, dose-ranging studies have confirmed the potential toxicity of cyclophosphamide, but repeated low-dose monthly pulsed therapy may steer a course between efficacy and toxicity. A comparison between intravenous cyclophosphamide given with oral corticosteroids, and oral cyclophosphamide, or alternate-day prednisolone and weekly plasma exchange, showed no difference in outcome between groups. Nevertheless, many neurologists would still use pulsed cyclophosphamide in the rapidly deteriorating individual for whom therapeutic inactivity is mutually unacceptable to patient and doctor. Promising results have been obtained in the treatment of multiple sclerosis using β-interferon. After 3 years, treated patients with relapsing disease showed a one-third reduction in new clinical epi-

sodes but without any effect on disability or the course of the disease; however, a 60 to 70 per cent reduction in the rate of accumulation of new lesions, identified by magnetic resonance imaging, was also detected.

In view of the partial benefits of immune suppression in patients with multiple sclerosis, alternative means of interfering with the sequence of events that leads to tissue injury, using agents that have much more radical, but precise, immunological effects than the non-specific immunosuppressants that are routinely available, should not be neglected. Monoclonal antibodies that lyse T lymphocytes or block their function, engineered so as to minimize anti-idiotypic responses (by hybridizing murine variable with human constant immunoglobulin regions), have been used in preliminary and uncontrolled studies, but with anecdotal success; this appears to be the most promising novel therapeutic approach for the immediate future.

Central pontine myelinolysis

Central pontine myelinolysis is not rare. A high proportion of cases first described had metabolic disturbances resulting from alcohol abuse, but the condition occurs in association with Wernicke's encephalopathy, non-alcoholic cirrhosis, Wilson's disease, after hepatic transplantation, as a complication of uraemia and haemodialysis, after prolonged vomiting, and following diuretic therapy. In each of these situations, affected individuals are usually hyponatraemic before the onset of neurological symptoms. This observation has led to the hypothesis that central pontine myelinolysis results from over zealous correction of a low serum sodium. Pontine damage correlates both with the degree of hyponatraemia and rate at which this is corrected; starting levels of less than 110 mmol/l or rates of correction of greater than 2 mmol/l/h substantially increase the risk of central pontine myelinolysis. Rapid changes in sodium are better tolerated in acute than chronic hyponatraemia; pontine myelinolysis is occasionally seen as a result of rapidly corrected hypernatraemia.

The illness affects pathways placed centrally within the pons and spreads centrifugally. The fully evolved clinical picture is of flaccid paralysis with facial and bulbar weakness, disordered eye movements, loss of balance, and altered consciousness. Features of hyponatraemia, such as epilepsy, are not usually present since pontine demyelination follows correction of the serum sodium. Prognosis depends on the underlying metabolic disorder; with stabilization of the serum sodium and management of bulbar failure, neurological recovery is often complete and the condition does not recur spontaneously.

The clinical features are distinctive and present no diagnostic difficulties unless the reduction in serum sodium has been overlooked; the acute changes of central pontine myelinolysis can be imaged, and persistent abnormal signals are seen after clinical recovery.

Diffuse sclerosis

Diffuse cerebral sclerosis describes a group of metabolic diseases affecting cerebral white matter. Of those originally included, sudanophilic diffuse sclerosis, Pelizaeus–Merzbacher disease, Krabbe's diffuse sclerosis (globoid cell leucodystrophy), Canavan's diffuse sclerosis (spongy degeneration of the white matter), Alexander's disease, and metachromatic leucodystrophy are all dysmyelinating disorders with characteristic microscopic findings, clinical features, and genetically determined enzyme defects.

SCHILDER'S DISEASE

Schilder's disease is characterized by sharply demarcated areas of demyelination distributed posteriorly in the cerebral hemispheres, with glial proliferation and axonal sparing. It occurs in childhood but is rare; many previously designated male cases had adrenoleukodystrophy. Some experts retain the view that Schilder's disease is an exceptionally severe variety of multiple sclerosis occurring in childhood or early adult life.

The illness usually begins insidiously in a previously healthy child, with intellectual impairment and gait disturbance. Visual impairment, mental deterioration, epilepsy, aphasia, weakness, and incoordination of the limbs all occur at an early stage, but the usual clinical course is the development of cortical blindness with progressive spastic weakness of the limbs. Discriminative sensation is impaired, with loss of postural sensibility, but cutaneous sensation is also involved. The mental changes are those of progressive dementia with generalized or focal seizures occurring at any stage. The disease is progressive and usually fatal within 1 or 2 months, although temporary remissions lasting years may occur. There is no treatment other than symptomatic control of convulsions.

The early onset of blindness with progressive dementia and spastic paralysis presents a distinctive clinical picture, but intracranial tumour needs to be distinguished when the symptoms and signs are unilateral and if there is papilloedema. The electroencephalogram is of value in making the distinction from subacute sclerosing panencephalitis. Imaging shows extensive areas of white matter low attenuation in both cerebral hemispheres but these are not specific. Slowed motor nerve conduction due to peripheral nerve involvement occurs in Krabbe's disease and metachromatic leucodystrophy; metachromatic granules can be detected in the urine and leucocyte arylsulphatase is reduced in the latter, but not in diffuse sclerosis.

Adrenoleukodystrophy (see also Section 11)

An important group of disorders is characterized by saturated fatty acid deposition in all lipid-containing tissues as a result of defective very-long-chain fatty acyl-CoA synthetase activity in peroxisomes, which allows membrane-like cytoplasmic inclusions to accumulate in brain tissue. The diagnosis is made by ultrastructural examination of nerves biopsied from skin or conjunctiva.

Four related syndromes share this biochemical abnormality; childhood adrenoleukodystrophy and adult-onset adrenomyeloneuropathy are sex linked, whereas neonatal adrenoleukodystrophy and Zellweger's syndrome are autosomal recessive disorders.

Sex-linked childhood adrenoleukodystrophy presents with behavioural disturbance, dementia, and epilepsy, followed by involvement of special senses and motor systems. Although a significant proportion of children later develop adrenal insufficiency, Addison's disease may precede the neurological manifestations by several years.

Adrenomyeloneuropathy presents in adult men with spastic paraparesis and sensory loss in the legs; attention is drawn to an unusual cause for this otherwise common neurological problem by the associated peripheral neuropathy, but the diagnosis is frequently overlooked if adrenal insufficiency is not apparent at presentation. Identification of the peroxisomal defect in easily sampled body tissues has led to the description of cases with obscure clinical manifestations; these include focal cerebral lesions, Klüver–Bucy syndrome, dementia, spinocerebellar degeneration, and olivopontocerebellar atrophy. Mild spastic paraparesis with sphincter involvement and peripheral neuropathy may occur in obligate heterozygote female carriers with elevated very-long-chain fatty acids. The gene for X-linked adrenoleukodystrophy has been mapped to Xq28, close to that for glucose 6-phosphate dehydrogenase deficiency and colour blindness.

Autosomal recessive adrenoleukodystrophy presents in infancy with seizures, hypotonia, retardation, retinal degeneration, and hepatic involvement; females are more commonly affected than males. Although the clinical manifestations and mode of inheritance are similar in neonatal adrenoleukodystrophy and Zellweger's syndrome, these are thought to be separate disorders.

The treatment of adrenoleukodystrophies has not been very rewarding; erucic acid reduces plasma very-long-chain fatty acid concentration albeit without influencing the clinical course.

REFERENCES

Berman, M., Feldmann, S., Alter, M., Zilber, N., and Kahana, E. (1981). Acute transverse myelitis: incidence and aetiologic considerations. *Neurology* **31**, 966–71.

Birk, K., Ford, C., Smeltzer, S., Ryan, D., Miller, R., and Rudick, R.A. (1990). The clinical course of multiple sclerosis during pregnancy and the puerperium. *Archives of Neurology* **47**, 738–42.

Callanan, M.M., Logsdail, S.J., Ron, M.A., and Warrington, E.K. (1989). Cognitive impairment in patients with clinically isolated lesions of the type seen in multiple sclerosis. *Brain* **112**, 361–74.

Canadian Cooperative multiple sclerosis study group (1991). The Canadian cooperative trial of cyclophosphamide and plasma exchange in progressive multiple sclerosis. *Lancet* **337**, 441–6.

Compston, D.A.S. (1991). Genetic susceptibility to multiple sclerosis. In *McAlpine's multiple sclerosis*, (ed. W.B. Matthews), pp. 301–19. Churchill Livingstone, Edinburgh.

Duquette, P., *et al.* (1987). Multiple sclerosis in childhood: clinical profile in 125 patients. *Journal of Pediatrics* **111**, 359–63.

Ebers, G.C., *et al.* (1986). A population based study of multiple sclerosis in twins. *New England Journal of Medicine* **315**, 1638–42.

Fenichel, G.M. (1982). Neurological complications of immunisation. *Annals of Neurology* **12**, 119–28.

Hammond, S.R., *et al.* (1988). The epidemiology of multiple sclerosis in three Australian cities: Perth, Newcastle and Hobart. *Brain* **111**, 1–25.

Hickey, W.F. (1991). Migration of hematogenous cells through the blood brain barrier and the initiation of CNS inflammation. *Brain Pathology* **1**, 97–105.

IFNB Multiple Sclerosis Study Group. (1993). Interferon beta-1b is effective in relapsing-remitting multiple sclerosis. 1. Clinical results of a multicenter, randomized, double-blind, placebo-controlled trial. *Neurology*, **43**, 655–61.

Kermode, A.G., *et al.* (1990). Breakdown of the blood brain barrier precedes symptoms and other MRI signs of new lesions in multiple sclerosis. *Brain* **113**, 1477–89.

McDonald, W.I. (1986). The pathophysiology of multiple sclerosis. In *Multiple sclerosis*, (ed. W.I. McDonald and D.H. Silberberg), pp. 112–33. Butterworth, London.

Miller, D.H., Ormerod, I.E.C., Rudge, P.R., Kendall, B.E., Moseley, I.F., and McDonald, W.I. (1989). The early risk of multiple sclerosis following isolated acute syndromes of the brainstem and spinal cord. *Annals of Neurology* **26**, 635–9.

Miller, H.G., Stanton, J.B., and Gibbons, J.L. (1956). Parainfectious encephalomyelitis and related syndromes. *Quarterly Journal of Medicine* **25**, 427–505.

Miller, R.H., ffrench Constant, C., and Raff, M.C. (1989). The macroglial cells of the rat optic nerve. *Annual Review of Neuroscience* **12**, 517–34.

Moser, H.W., Moser, A.E., Singh, I., and O'Neill, B.P. (1984). Adrenoleucodystrophy: survey of 303 cases: biochemistry, diagnosis and therapy. *Annals of Neurology* **16**, 628–41.

Mumford, C., Wood, N., Kellar-Wood, H., Miller, D.H., Thorpe, J., and Compston, D.A.S. (1994). The British Isles Survey of Multiple Sclerosis in twins. *Neurology* **44**, 11–15.

Olerup, O. and Hillert, J. (1991). HLA class II-associated genetic susceptibility in multiple sclerosis: a critical evaluation. *Tissue Antigens* **38**, 1–15.

Paty, D.W., Li, D.K.B., and The IFNB Multiple Sclerosis Study Group. (1993). Interferon beta-1b is effective in relapsing-remitting multiple sclerosis. MRI results of a multicenter, randomized, double-blind, placebo-controlled trial. *Neurology*, **43**, 662–7.

Prineas, J.W. (1985). The neuropathology of multiple sclerosis. In *Handbook of clinical neurology*, (ed. P.J. Vinken, G.W. Bruyn, and H.L. Klowans), Vol. 3(47), pp. 213–57. Elsevier Science Publishers, Amsterdam.

Sadovnick, A.D., Baird, P.A., and Ward, R.H. (1988). Multiple sclerosis; updated risks for relatives. *American Journal of Medical Genetics* **29**, 533–41.

Sandberg-Wollheim, S., Bynke, H., Cronqvist, S., Holtas, S., Platz, P., and Ryder, L.P. (1990). A long term prospective study of optic neuritis: evaluation of risk factors. *Annals of Neurology* **27**, 386–93.

Sibley, W.A., Bamford, C.R., and Clark, K. (1985). Clinical viral infections and multiple sclerosis. *Lancet* **i**, 1313–15.

Sibley, W.A., Bamford, C.R., Clark, K., Smith, M.S., and Laguna, J.F. (1991). A prospective study of physical trauma and multiple sclerosis. *Journal of Neurology Neurosurgery and Psychiatry* **54**, 584–9.

Sterns, R.H., Riggs, J.E., and Schochet, S.S. (1986). Osmotic demyelination syndrome following correction of hyponatraemia. *New England Journal of Medicine* **314**, 1535–42.

Tyler, K.L., Gross, R.A., and Cascino, G.D. (1986). Unusual viral causes of transverse myelitis: hepatitis A virus and cytomegalovirus. *Neurology* **36**, 855–8.

Yudkin, P.L., *et al.* (1991). Overview of azathioprine treatment in multiple sclerosis. *Lancet* **338**, 1051–5.

Weinshenker, B.G., *et al.* (1989). The natural history of multiple sclerosis: a geographically based study. 2. Predictive value of the early clinical course. *Brain* **112**, 1419–28.

24.10 Movement disorders

C. D. MARSDEN

Diseases of the extrapyramidal motor systems cause either a loss of movement (akinesia) accompanied by an increase in muscle tone (rigidity), or abnormal involuntary movements (dyskinesias) often accompanied by a reduction in muscle tone. The akinetic–rigid syndrome, called parkinsonism, and the dyskinesias represent opposite ends of the spectrum of movement disorders.

Akinetic–rigid syndromes

Parkinson's disease

DEFINITION

A disease with insidious onset, usually in the second half of life, characterized by slowly progressive akinesia, rigidity, postural abnormality, and tremor (Fig. 1). Described by James Parkinson, a Hoxton practitioner, in 1817, as the 'shaking palsy', the symptoms of Parkinson's disease have now been established as due to striatal dopamine deficiency consequent on death of the substantia nigra. The pathology in the substantia nigra consists of loss of pigmented neurones in the zona compacta, with eosinophilic inclusions, called Lewy bodies, in remaining neurones.

AETIOLOGY

The cause of Parkinson's disease is unknown. A similar akinetic–rigid syndrome with characteristic tremor was a common aftermath of the worldwide epidemic of encephalitis lethargica that occurred 60 years ago (1918–30) (postencephalitic parkinsonism). Neuroleptic drugs (such as reserpine, phenothiazines, and butyrophenones) also may produce the same clinical picture (drug-induced parkinsonism) by blockade of striatal dopamine receptors.

Parkinsonism may also be the main feature of a number of other degenerative diseases of the central nervous system, but other abnormalities point to the diagnosis of these various syndromes of 'parkinsonism-plus' (Table 1). They include progressive supranuclear palsy, multiple system atrophy, and corticobasal degeneration, which are discussed later.

Parkinsonism also may be apparent in any diffuse brain disease causing generalized cerebral damage. In addition to dementia, paralysis, and other signs of widespread brain damage, an akinetic–rigid syndrome occurs in many such cases. In some patients, Lewy body degeneration extends from the brain-stem pigmented nuclei to the cerebral cortex, to cause diffuse Lewy body disease, which causes dementia and parkinsonism. Parkinsonism also may be evident in Alzheimer's disease and cerebrovascular disease, but also occurs in many other such conditions (Table 2). 'Arteriosclerotic parkinsonism' is a term that has created confusion. That parkinsonism occurs as part of the symptomatology of cerebrovascular disease is not in doubt, but vascular brain damage is not a cause of pure Parkinson's disease, for the substantia nigra is strikingly resistant to stroke. Isolated focal lesions of the substantia nigra, due to trauma, tuberculoma, and tumours, do cause contralateral hemi-parkinsonism, but such cases are exceedingly rare.

Parkinson's disease is a common disorder with a prevalence of about 1 in 1000, rising to 1 in 200 in the elderly. It occurs worldwide in all ethnic groups (although perhaps less frequently in China and Africa), in all social classes, and is slightly more common in men than in women. Hereditary factors are not evident in the majority of cases, but about 5 to 10 per cent of patients give a history of the same illness in other family members. Evidence of dominant inheritance occurs in some rare families, and the genetic data have been taken to suggest the influence of a dominant gene with poor penetrance. However, recent studies of identical twins have failed to find high concordance when one twin is

Fig. 1 Reproduction of a photograph showing Paul Richer's '*statuette pathologique*' of a patient with Parkinson's disease.

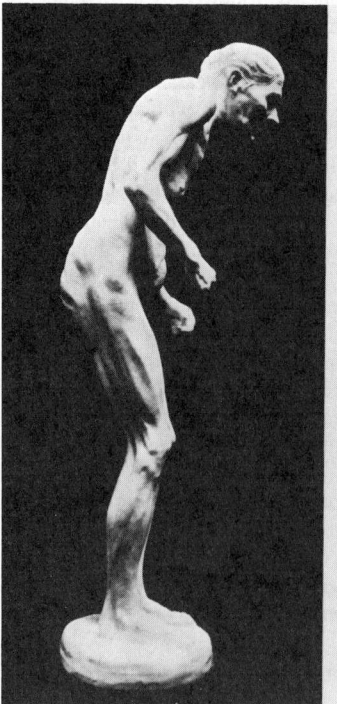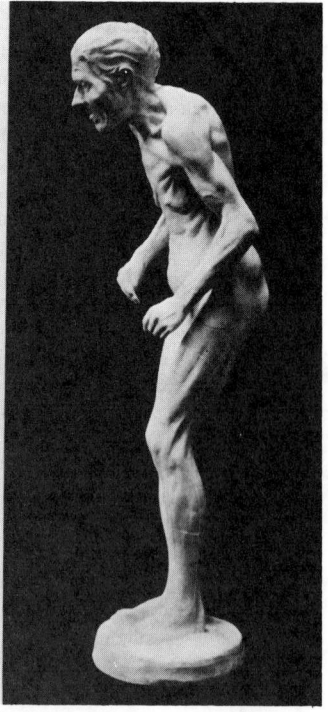

Table 1 *Causes of akinetic–rigid syndrome in adults*

Pure parkinsonism	Parkinsonism-plus
Parkinson's disease	Progressive supranuclear
Drug-induced parkinsonism	palsy
Postencephalitic parkinsonism	Multiple system atrophy
MPTP toxicity	olivopontocerebellar
Other toxins (e.g. manganese	degeneration striatonigral
carbon monoxide)	degeneration autonomic
	failure
	Corticobasal degeneration
	Parkinsonism-dementia-
	ALS syndrome (Guam)
	Basal ganglia calcification

Abbreviations: ALS, amyotrophic lateral sclerosis; MPTP, 1-methyl-4-phenyl-1,2,3,6-tetrahydropyridine.

Table 2 *Diffuse brain diseases causing multifocal dementia in adults, in which elements of parkinsonism also may occur*

Common	Rare
Alzheimer's disease	Pick's disease
(including senile dementia)	Creutzfeldt–Jakob disease
Diffuse Lewy body disease	Manganese poisoning
Multi-infarct dementia	Neurosyphilis
Binswanger's disease	Cysticercosis
Congophilic angiopathy	Communicating hydrocephalus
Head injury (e.g. boxers)	
Cerebral anoxia	

affected with Parkinson's disease. This suggests that heredity alone is not responsible for the condition.

Extensive studies have failed to identify any viral agent responsible for Parkinson's disease, and attempts to suggest that all cases are due to residual effects of encephalitis lethargica have been discredited. Parkinson's disease neither occurs in, nor can be transmitted to, animals, which perhaps do not usually live long enough to be at risk of such an illness.

Toxins can cause human parkinsonism. Certain drug addicts in California, in the course of synthesizing a heroin substitute, meperidine, inadvertently produced a contaminant, 1-methyl-4-phenyl-1,2,3,6-tetrahydropyridine (MPTP). Within a few days of intravenous injection of this compound, they developed acute severe parkinsonism, similar in nearly all respects to the idiopathic disease. This has led to an intensive search for similar environmental toxins, but none has been identified as yet. MPTP is not itself the active toxin; it is converted in brain by monoamine oxidase B into 1-methyl-4-phenyl-pyridinium (MPP^+), which is trapped in dopamine (more than noradrenaline) neurones by the normal dopamine reuptake system. Within dopamine neurones, MPP^+ binds to neuromelanin and is concentrated within mitochondria. MPP^+ poisons complex I of mitochondrial respiratory activity to cause cell death, a process that may involve oxidative stress and the production of free radicals.

PATHOLOGY

Anatomical

The essential pathological abnormality is loss of pigmented neurones in the pars compacta of the substantia nigra (Fig. 2). These neurones, which contain neuromelanin, project to the caudate nucleus and putamen (neostriatum), and employ dopamine as their neurotransmitter. The adjacent pigmented ventral tegmental area, which projects dopaminergic axons

to mesolimbic and cortical regions also degenerates. Other pigmented brain-stem nuclei are also affected, including the noradrenergic locus coeruleus.

In all cases of Parkinson's disease the degenerating pigmented brain-stem neurones contain eosinophilic inclusion bodies, Lewy bodies, which are characteristic of the disease. Lewy bodies are found also in about 4 per cent of brains from patients without parkinsonism dying of other causes; these may be patients with subclinical Parkinson's disease, for 80 per cent of the zona compacta must degenerate before clinical symptoms appear. Lewy bodies are found not only in pigmented neurones, but also in other areas, including the cerebral cortex, the substantia innominata, the lateral grey horns of the thoracic cord, and even in sympathetic ganglia. Their origin is unexplained.

Biochemical (Table 3)

In 1960 Ehringer and Hornykiewicz discovered profound loss of dopamine in the striatum (putamen more than caudate) and substantia nigra of patients dying with Parkinson's disease. Loss of dopamine in the caudate nucleus and putamen correlates with the extensive cell loss, atrophy, and glial scarring in the substantia nigra, the damage being more severe and diffuse in postencephalitic patients than in those with idiopathic Parkinson's disease. There is a close correlation between the extent of nigral cell loss, the degree of depletion of striatal dopamine, and the severity of akinesia.

It is necessary to lose something of the order of 50 to 60 per cent of

Fig. 2 The pathology of Parkinson's disease. Top, medium power and bottom, higher power photomicrographs of midbrain from a normal subject (left) and from the brain of a patient with Parkinson's disease (right). The normal substantia nigra contains many densely staining dark pigmented nerve cells, running as a vertical band deep to the cerebral peduncle. Few pigmented cells are left in the Parkinsonian substantia nigra (haemotoxylin and eosin).

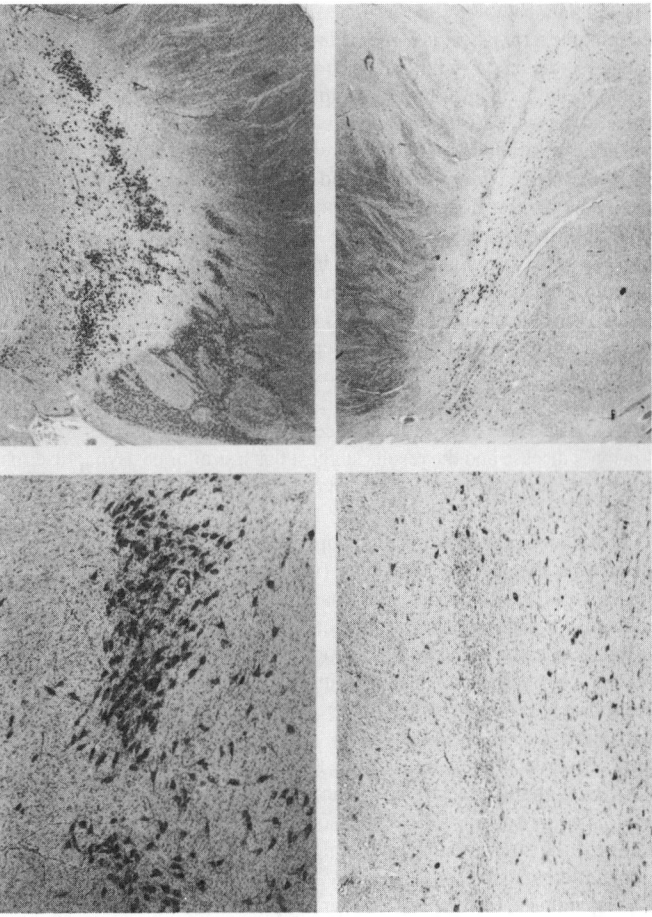

Table 3 *Neurotransmitters and their enzymes in the striatum in Parkinson's disease*

	Control	Parkinson's disease	
Dopamine (μg/g)	5.37	0.50	9%
Homovanillic acid (μg/g)	11.40	2.06	18%
DA/HVA ratio	2.1	4.1	
Dopa decarboxylase (nmol/ 100 mg/h)	432	32	7%
Tyrosine hydroxylase (nmol/ 100 mg/h)	36	8	22%
Monoamine oxidase (nmol/ 100 mg/h)	1520	1650	normal
Catechol-*O*-methyl transferase (nmol/100 mg/h)	24	20	normal
5-Hydroxytryptamine (μg/g)	0.32	0.14	44%
Noradrenaline (μg/g)	1.29	0.52	40%
Choline acetyltransferase (μmol/g/h)	49	37	75%
Glutamic acid decarboxylase (μmol/100 mg protein/h)	4.7	3.9	normal

DA/HVA, dopamine/homovanillic acid.

Mean values are shown for putamen, except for noradrenaline which was measured in nucleus accumbens.

All differences were statistically significant at $p < 0.05$ or less, except where indicated by 'normal'.

Data from Hornykiewicz *et al.*, McGeer and McGeer (quoted in Marsden and Fehn, 1982, 1987, 1994).

nigral neurones, and to deplete the striatum of about 80 to 85 per cent of its dopamine content, for frank symptoms of Parkinson's disease to appear. The pathology of the illness, focusing on nigral cell loss in the zona compacta, is progressive. It is assumed that there must be a prolonged period of asymptomatic striatal dopamine depletion until the critical level for appearance of symptoms is reached. During this asymptomatic period, several mechanisms attempt to compensate for the loss of the nigrostriatal dopamine pathway. The concentration of the dopamine metabolite, homovanillic acid, falls below that of the transmitter itself; the ratio of homovanillic acid to dopamine increases, suggesting that the turnover rate of dopamine has increased. A second compensatory mechanism involves changes in the sensitivity of the postsynaptic receptors on which dopamine acts in the striatum. Lesions of the nigrostriatal system in animals leads to denervation supersensitivity of the postsynaptic striatal dopamine receptors. This is evidenced by both an enhanced pharmacological response to dopamine agonists, and an increase in the number of receptors measured by ligand-binding techniques. The latter have been applied to the brains of patients with Parkinson's disease and the results suggest that a similar postsynaptic dopamine receptor supersensitivity may exist at least initially in such patients.

Most brain areas containing dopamine are affected in Parkinson's disease. In the nucleus accumbens (which in man forms an inferior part of the head of the caudate nucleus identified by a high noradrenaline content), dopamine concentrations are reduced to some 42 per cent of normal, in comparison to a reduction of caudate nucleus dopamine to 36 per cent and putamen dopamine to 9 per cent of control values, respectively. Some areas of the cerebral cortex also contain dopamine, and there is a severe depletion in the parolfactory gyrus (Broadmann area 25). It is tempting to associate this change in the cortical dopamine systems with the affective disturbances and psychic changes that can be seen in some patients with Parkinson's disease.

Since the striatal dopamine depletion is due to degeneration of the dopaminergic nigrostriatal pathway, the intraneuronal enzymes required for dopamine synthesis also are markedly diminished. Thus, the activity of L-aromatic amino acid decarboxylase (dopa decarboxylase), an intraneuronal enzyme responsible for the conversion of dopa to dopamine, is strikingly low in the nigrostriatal regions of the parkinsonian brain. Likewise, the rate-limiting enzyme, tyrosine hydroxylase, responsible for conversion of tyrosine to dopa, is also depleted in dopamine-containing brain regions.

In addition to the crucial changes in brain dopamine in Parkinson's disease, less marked depletion of noradrenaline and 5-hydroxytryptamine has been noted. Studies on acetylcholine activity of postmortem brain samples suggest that cholinergic neurones in the striatum are relatively well preserved in Parkinson's disease. However, a reduction in cerebral cortical choline acetyltransferase, a marker of cholinergic neurones, has been described particularly in those with dementia. This reflects loss of cholinergic neurones in substantia innominata which project to cerebral cortex. Changes in the enzyme glutamic acid decarboxylase (GAD) responsible for synthesis of γ-aminobutyric acid (GABA) have been demonstrated in Parkinson's disease; GAD concentration is reduced in the substantia nigra and cerebral cortex. The major striatal output pathways utilize GABA as their neurotransmitter, and the changes in nigral GAD may represent some functional reduction in activity of these pathways, for levodopa therapy restores glutamic acid decarboxylase levels back towards normal. Specific binding of [³H]-GABA is also altered in Parkinson's disease; there is a striking reduction in the number of GABA binding sites in the substantia nigra, with normal levels in the caudate nucleus, putamen, and cerebral cortex. Since the GABA striatonigral pathway synapses, at least in part, on dopaminergic nigral neurones, this loss of nigral GABA binding is interpreted as due to loss of nigral dopamine nerve cells containing the GABA receptors. There is also loss of certain peptide neuronal systems in the basal ganglia, particularly those containing enkephalins and substance P.

SYMPTOMS

The onset is insidious and in 70 per cent of patients the presenting feature is tremor, which usually commences unilaterally. Parkinsonian tremor is present at rest, is decreased by action, is increased by emotion or stress, and disappears during sleep. The arms are most often affected initially, but tremor may spread to involve the face, jaw, and legs. It is due to rhythmical alternating contraction in opposing muscles at a frequency of 4 to 6 Hz (Fig. 3). In the arm it characteristically causes

Fig. 3 Recordings of tremor with accelerometers placed on the right arm (above) and the left arm (below) in (a) a patient with enhanced physiological tremor of the outstretched arms (frequency 9–10 Hz); (b) a patient with benign essential tremor with the arms outstretched (frequency 7 Hz);(c) a patient with left-sided Parkinson's disease at rest (frequency 5 Hz); and (d) a patient with severe cerebellar disease and marked intention tremor attempting to touch his nose with the right hand (frequency 2–3 Hz). All recordings are of 4 s duration. (By courtesy of Dr M. Gresty.)

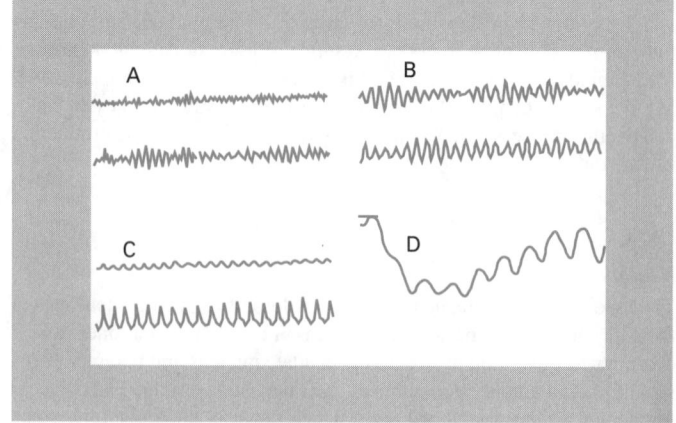

rhythmic pronation/supination and 'pill-rolling' of the opposed thumb and fingers. Occasionally tremor may be more evident on posture and movement, particular in the initial stages of the illness, when it is at a faster frequency of 6 to 7 Hz. Rigidity is appreciated by the patient as stiff muscles, and by the examiner as a plastic resistance to passive movement, equal in opposing muscle groups and constant throughout the range of manipulation. Rigidity affects all muscles, but is most marked in the neck and trunk, and in proximal muscles at the shoulder or hip. When tremor coexists, the smooth plastic nature of rigidity may be broken up by rhythmic catches (cogwheel phenomenon). Akinesia refers to the poverty (hypokinesia) and slowness (bradykinesia) of movement so characteristic of Parkinson's disease. It is not merely the effect of rigidity, for stereotaxic thalamotomy (see below) can abolish limb rigidity without improving akinesia. There is a delay in initiation of movement, a slowness in execution of voluntary movement, and a loss of normal automatic movements, such as those of emotional expression and blinking. Postural changes include generalized flexion of the limbs, neck, and trunk, and postural instability causing falls.

These four cardinal signs of Parkinson's disease—tremor, rigidity, akinesia, and postural changes—contribute to the many typical features and disabilities of the illness (Fig. 1). The face is strikingly bland and mask-like. The voice loses volume and normal modulation of tone to become soft and monotonous. The bent, flexed patient walks with slow, small steps, without swinging the arms; it may be difficult to start walking ('freezing'), but once in motion the pace may quicken and the patient may be unable to stop ('festination'). They may 'freeze' into immobility when passing through a door or around furniture. While standing, a push may lead to falling or tottering in the direction of displacement until the patient falls, or comes into contact with a solid object. They sit immobile and flexed like a statue. Getting out of a chair and turning over in bed may be impossible. The handwriting becomes small (micrographia), tremulous, and untidy (Fig. 4). Rapid movements of the hands and feet are impaired. Eating, washing, and toilet demands become increasingly difficult.

While objective sensibility is unimpaired, patients often complain of fatigue, pain, and discomfort, and of hot or cold sensations. Vision, hearing, taste, and smell are normal. Eye movements are unaffected, except for paralysis of convergence, some limitation of up-gaze, and loss of speed of voluntary saccades. The pupils are normal. The eyelids may be tremulous (blepharoclonus) and spasms of eye closure (blepharospasm) may occur. Drooling of saliva is common, due to failure to swallow, and dysphagia may occur. Constipation is universal; urinary frequency and urgency are frequent complaints. Excessive sweating and a greasy skin (seborrhoea) contribute to the facial appearance. Some patients develop postural hypotension. The tendon reflexes and plantar responses are normal.

Most patients have normal intellectual function initially, although some defects of cognitive abilities attributable to frontal lobe functions may be detectable; slowness of thought processes (bradyphrenia), and slight difficulties with memory and word retrieval ('tip of the tongue' phenomenon) may be evident. Subsequent drug therapy may provoke mental disturbances and, with the passage of time and progression of the disease, a proportion of patients develop organic mental changes. Depression is very common, affecting 30 per cent or more, and often antedating the appearance of obvious physical symptoms. The commonest mental consequence of drug therapy is a toxic confusional state, but other behavioural disturbances, such as a schizophreniform psychosis or isolated hallucinosis with insight, can occur. Many patients complain of more severe slowness of thought and defects of memory in the later stages of the illness, and a proportion (perhaps 20 per cent) finally develop a frank global dementia. The latter may be due to the coexistence of Alzheimer's disease in this elderly population, or to diffuse Lewy body disease. The appearance of dementia in a patient with Parkinson's disease warrants full investigation to exclude other treatable causes.

NATURAL HISTORY

The mean age of onset of Parkinson's disease is about 55 years. Onset under 40 years is rare, but thereafter the incidence rises exponentially with increasing age. Most patients localize the onset of symptoms to one or other side, but progression to bilateral signs and disability is the rule. Symptoms and signs confined to one side (hemiparkinsonism) is uncommon. In most patients the disease progresses inexorably, with increasing difficulty in speaking, eating, washing, dressing, standing, and walking. Eventually, in those most severely affected, the patient becomes chair- or bed-bound and anarthric. Many patients, however, remain reasonably active, but with increasing restrictions, until they die from other causes. The rate of progression is very variable. Prior to the advent of levodopa therapy, death occurred on average about 9 years after the onset of symptoms (Fig. 5); the range varied from benign par-

Fig. 4 Samples of handwriting and spiral drawings from (a) a 50-year-old woman with benign essential tremor, (b) a 38-year-old man with Parkinson's disease, and (c) a 20-year-old boy with torsion dystonia (who attempts to write COLLEGE).

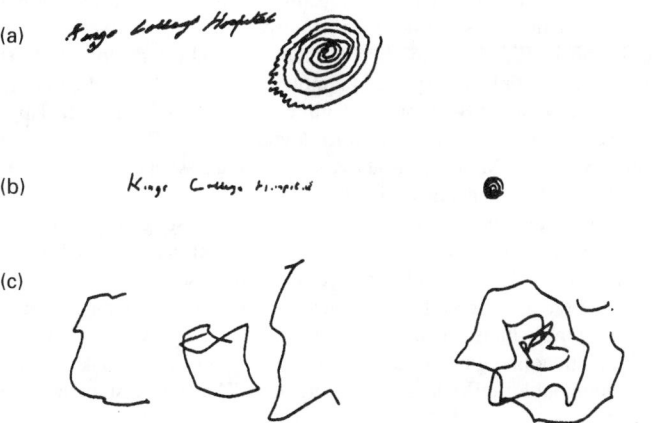

Fig. 5 The impact of levodopa therapy on Parkinson's disease. A hypothetical concept of the effects of chronic levodopa treatment. The underlying pathology (of unknown cause) is believed to progress over many years irrespective of therapy. After an initial period it becomes severe enough to cause symptoms. Before levodopa, pathological changes and disability progressed to cause death on average about 9 years after onset. Levodopa therapy results in considerable initial symptomatic improvement, but no change in pathology. Despite some loss of benefit after a few years of treatment, life expectancy is prolonged, but this means that new aspects and consequences of the progression of the disease are likely to emerge. (Reproduced from Marsden and Parkes, *Lancet*, 1977, **i**, 349, with permission.)

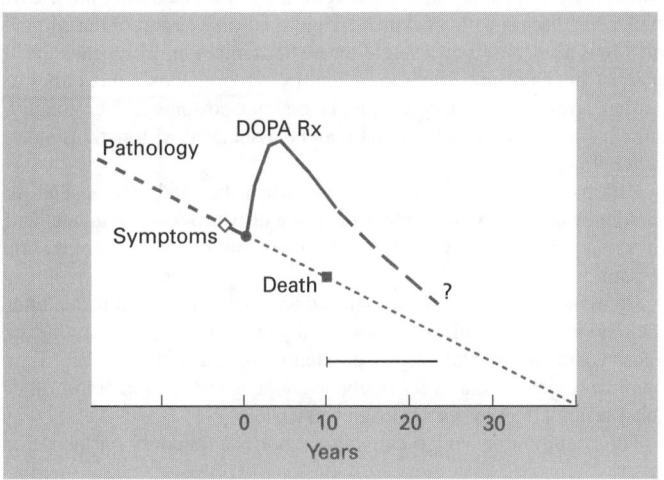

kinsonism with little or no progression over 30 years or more, to malignant parkinsonism with death in 1 or 2 years from onset. Mortality was some three times that expected in a general population of the same age and sex. Death was usually from vascular diseases, bronchopneumonia, or intercurrent neoplasia. Older treatments did not influence the prognosis of idiopathic Parkinson's disease, but it is likely that levodopa therapy has prolonged life expectancy. Indeed, a number of studies have now shown that with present-day treatment the patient with Parkinson's disease is likely, on average, to live as long as unaffected people of the same age.

DIAGNOSIS (SEE TABLES 1 AND 2)

The combination of tremor, rigidity, akinesia, and postural abnormality constitutes the syndrome of parkinsonism. A history of encephalitis lethargica in the 1920s or 1930s (the epidemic then ceased), plus additional features characteristic of the sequelae of encephalitis lethargica, indicate the diagnosis of postencephalitic parkinsonism. These include spasms of eye deviation, often with compulsive thought (oculogyric crises), pupillary abnormalities, and dyskinesias such as torsion dystonia. About 80 per cent of patients with postencephalitic parkinsonism developed their symptoms within 10 years of infection. Postencephalitic parkinsonism was a more benign disease, and only about 25 per cent of patients were severely disabled after 20 years of illness.

A history of intake of neuroleptic drugs indicates drug-induced parkinsonism, which remits in 95 per cent of cases slowly over weeks or months when the offending drug is withdrawn. Drugs that may cause parkinsonism include not only the antipsychotic neuroleptic agents used to treat schizophrenia, but also antiemetics such as phenothiazines and metoclopramide, and some calcium-blocking agents. All these drugs are dopamine receptor antagonists.

A number of other degenerative diseases affecting the basal ganglia may produce a parkinsonian syndrome, but other distinctive features give the clue to the true diagnosis (Table 2). In general, these conditions show little or no response to treatment with levodopa or dopamine agonists. A gaze palsy for voluntary and following eye movements, particularly when down-gaze is affected, with preserved vestibulo-ocular reflex eye movements, indicates progressive supranuclear palsy (see below). A cerebellar ataxia or cerebellar atrophy on CT scan, and orthostatic hypotension with other features of an autonomic neuropathy, point to multiple system atrophy (see below). Severe rigidity of a limb, with apraxia and myoclonus, suggests corticobasal degeneration (see below).

The presence of frank dementia and pyramidal signs indicate a widespread disease such as diffuse Lewy body disease, Alzheimer's disease, or cerebrovascular disease such as multi-infarct dementia. The latter most commonly occurs in long-standing sufferers of poorly controlled hypertension and often is characterized by the additional presence of a pseudobulbar palsy with emotional incontinence and a distinctive gait which is upright, short-stepped, and military (*marche à petit pas*). Diffuse brain disease with an akinetic–rigid syndrome as part of the clinical picture is also caused by a single severe head injury, or by repeated head injury ('punch drunk' syndrome), and by cerebral anoxia due either to cardiac arrest or secondary to carbon monoxide poisoning. Occasionally, calcification of the basal ganglia may be associated with parkinsonism (see below).

Parkinson's disease is the diagnosis when the syndrome appears in middle or late life without other evidence of neurological damage, and in the absence of any history of provoking drugs or encephalitis lethargica.

Hemiparkinsonism may be confused with hemiplegia, but in the latter the tendon reflexes will be pathologically brisk, the abdominal reflexes absent, and the plantar response extensor on the affected side. True hemiparkinsonism may very rarely be due to a cerebral tumour or other focal lesion affecting the opposite hemisphere.

The condition of benign essential tremor is commonly mistaken for Parkinson's disease. However, in benign essential tremor, which is often inherited, the tremor is postural and other signs of parkinsonism are absent, for there is no true rigidity or akinesia. However, postural tremor of the outstretched hands may be the initial or only feature of Parkinson's disease, and in some patients it is exceedingly difficult to decide initially on the true diagnosis. In general, such patients will have developed obvious other signs of Parkinson's disease within about a year of the onset of their tremor.

Depression may pose diagnostic problems. Patients with profound psychomotor retardation due to severe depression often exhibit a superficial resemblance to those with Parkinson's disease, particularly with their sad, expressionless face, bowed posture, and immobility. Many patients with the earliest symptoms of Parkinson's disease are misdiagnosed as depressed, which indeed they may well be.

Finally, a proportion of patients with Parkinson's disease present with generalized ill-health, fatigue, restlessness, sleep difficulties, bizarre sensory symptoms, or non-specific neurasthenia. The diagnosis may be exceedingly difficult in such patients unless the impassive face, the stooped posture, and the short-stepped gait with failure to swing the arms are spotted early on in the interview.

TREATMENT

The treatment of Parkinson's disease involves the use of drugs, physical therapy, and occasionally surgery.

Drug treatment

Until 1967, when oral levodopa was introduced, treatment was with anticholinergic drugs and stereotaxic surgery. Levodopa is now the best therapy available, and stereotaxic surgery is only rarely indicated. Levodopa is converted into dopamine in the brain by the enzyme dopa decarboxylase, thereby restoring striatal dopamine action. Less than 5 per cent of an oral dose of levodopa reaches the brain; the rest is metabolized by dopa decarboxylase in gut wall, liver, kidney, and cerebral capillaries. This peripheral decarboxylation can be prevented by the addition of a selective extracerebral decarboxylase inhibitor, such as carbidopa or benserazide, which themselves do not penetrate into the brain. Levodopa combined with carbidopa (Sinemet®) or benserazide (Madopar®) is now the treatment of choice when levodopa is indicated. Such combined therapy requires a lower dose of levodopa for optimal benefit, and results in a quicker therapeutic response and a lower incidence of those side-effects that are due to the formation of levodopa metabolites outside the brain. These include nausea and vomiting, cardiac dysrhythmias, and, at least in part, postural hypotension. The main side-effects of combined therapy are dyskinesias and psychiatric disturbances. Both are dose-dependent are remit when the drug dosage is reduced.

Initiation

Sinemet® or Madopar®, which appear similar in potency and side-effects, do not affect the underlying pathology or cause of Parkinson's disease; they are equivalent to a substitution therapy for striatal dopamine deficiency. It is not necessary to use such drugs in every patient on diagnosis. Either Sinemet® or Madopar® is indicated if disability is severe, or if it fails to respond to simple therapy. In the mild case, the monoamine oxidase B inhibitor selegiline (Eldepryl®), 5 mg twice daily, has been shown to delay the need for levodopa. Selegiline prevents the neurotoxicity of MPTP (see above) and decreases the catabolism of dopamine, which generates oxidative stress; both actions are due to inhibition of monoamine oxidase B. Therefore it was suggested that selegiline might actually slow the rate of progression of Parkinson's disease, but there is no definite evidence that this is the case.

An anticholinergic such as benzhexol, 2 or 5 mg tablets or orphenadrine, 50 mg tablets, three to eight times daily, may be beneficial initially. Anticholinergics cause peripheral parasympathetic blockade with a dry mouth, blurred vision, and constipation. They may also precipitate glaucoma and urinary retention, and a toxic confusional state, so generally should be avoided in the elderly. Small doses should be used initially and gradually increased. Alternatively, in a mild case, amantadine hydrochloride, 100 mg twice or three times daily, may be effective. Amantadine, originally introduced as an antiviral agent, is slightly more powerful than anticholinergics, but less effective than levodopa. However, it causes few side-effects, mainly ankle oedema and the skin rash, livedo reticularis. In high dosage it can provoke a toxic confusional state or fits.

If disability warrants levodopa therapy, Sinemet® or Madopar® should be started in small dosage and gradually increased over a period of weeks to the maximum tolerated, or until adequate therapeutic benefit has been obtained. Nausea and vomiting are less common with these combined preparations than with plain levodopa, and if vomiting occurs it can usually be prevented by taking the drug after meals, prefaced by an antiemetic such as domperidone. The commonest dose-limiting side-effects are dyskinesias and mental disturbances and the aim should be to keep the patient free of these complications. The usual starting dose of Sinemet® (each tablet of Sinemet-275 contains 250 mg levodopa and 25 mg carbidopa) is half a tablet twice or three times daily. The average optimum dose is 3 to 4 tablets daily. The elderly are particularly sensitive to levodopa, and Sinemet-110 (containing 100 mg levodopa and 10 mg carbidopa) may be used. Sinemet-plus (containing 100 mg levodopa and 25 mg carbidopa) has also been introduced to provide adequate carbidopa intake for those on low doses of levodopa. For Madopar® the starting dose is one Madopar-125 capsule (which contains 100 mg levodopa and 25 mg benserazide) twice or three times daily. The average optimum dose is 2 to 4 capsules daily of Madopar-250 (which contains 200 mg levodopa and 50 mg benserazide). Maximum dosage of Sinemet-275 is about 6 to 8 tablets daily, and of Madopar-250 about 5 to 8 capsules daily, but some patients require even more than this. Other formulations of Sinemet® and Madopar® include Sinemet LS® (containing 50 mg of levodopa and 12.5 mg of carbidopa) and Madopar-62.5 (containing 50 mg of levodopa and 12.5 mg of benserazide), which may be useful in those who are very sensitive to these drugs. Recently, longer-acting delayed-release formulations of both drugs have been introduced (Sinemet® CR and Madopar® CR), which may prove valuable.

Maintenance

The response to levodopa therapy usually is obvious. In those who fail to obtain adequate benefit, the addition of an anticholinergic drug or/ and amantadine may give added improvement.

In those who do respond, approximately two-thirds will experience some loss of benefit after two to five years of treatment (Fig. 5). Those patients who do deteriorate while on long-term levodopa therapy do so in one of two ways. Some experience a progressive recurrence of their parkinsonian disability, particularly akinesia and postural instability with freezing and falls. Such patients usually are elderly and frequently show signs of dementia as well. Such a progressive loss of benefit and deterioration is very difficult to reverse. Increasing the daily dose of levodopa often causes toxic confusional states without the added benefit. A few such patients may gain renewed relief by switching to a directly acting dopamine agonist such as bromocriptine (see below), but mental side-effects are common with these drugs.

A number of patients with Parkinson's disease deteriorate rapidly in the face of an intercurrent infection, particularly urinary tract infections which are common, or incidental surgery, which should be avoided unless absolutely necessary. Following such a dramatic relapse, it may be a matter of weeks or months before such a patient regains their previous response to levodopa and their usual mobility.

Other patients on long-term levodopa therapy, particularly the younger individuals, develop fluctuations in mobility throughout the day associated with the appearance of levodopa-induced dyskinesias. Such fluctuations initially take the form of end-of-dose deterioration or the 'wearing-off' effect. When levodopa is first started, each dose usually lasts for a matter of 4 h or so. With the passage of years, the duration of action of each dose of the drug shortens to as little as 1 or 2 h. On the usual three or four times daily regime, this means that patients begin to experience a recurrence of disability, particularly immobility, prior to the next dose. At this stage, the correct management is to take an adequate levodopa dose at more frequent intervals. Such patients may require to take levodopa every 2 h or so, or may benefit from the longer-acting forms of Sinemet® CR and Madopar® CR.

Unfortunately, many of those with end-of-dose deterioration cannot be controlled adequately by such dose adjustments, or go on to develop other types of fluctuation in response. Typically, levodopa-induced dyskinesias become more severe, either at the peak time of levodopa action or biphasically prior to and at the end of action of each dose. In addition, the swings from mobility (with dyskinesias) to immobility (with distress and sometimes tremor and rigidity) become more frequent and abrupt, hence the description of this problem as the 'on–off' effect, for it can be like switching a light on and off. Such swings also become increasingly unpredictable and variable, quite unrelated to the timing of levodopa dosage, so that the patient may 'yo-yo' from mobility to immobility many times a day.

The management of severe 'on–off' problems, which usually occur in the younger patient with preserved intellect, is exceedingly difficult. Once stabilized on optimum timing of levodopa dosage, consideration should be given to adding a directly acting dopamine agonist such as bromocriptine (Parlodel®). The latter is employed widely as a dopamine agonist in endocrinological practice, but much larger doses are required in Parkinson's disease. Bromocriptine is about as effective therapeutically as levodopa, and has a similar range of unwanted effects, although psychiatric complications may be more common, and it is much more expensive. However, bromocriptine can be of value in those experiencing 'on–off' problems. It is introduced at a dose of 2.5 mg nightly and gradually built up by 2.5 mg increments to a three or four times daily regime normally totalling about 20 to 40 mg daily. Levodopa dosage must be reduced concomitantly for the effects of the two drugs are additive. Other newer dopamine agonists are lisuride and pergolide (Celance®), which act, like bromocriptine, directly on dopamine receptors, and which have similar side-effects. Some prefer to use these directly acting dopamine agonists rather than levodopa when disability requires dopamine replacement therapy. However, many patients do not gain adequate benefit when directly acting dopamine agonists are given alone. Another strategy which promises to reduce the risks of long-term complications of levodopa therapy is to combine levodopa in low dosage with a directly acting dopamine agonist from the start.

Unfortunately, some patients who develop severe 'on–off' phenomena during chronic levodopa therapy eventually become resistant to all conventional forms of treatment. Such patients may benefit from the use of apomorphine injections to rescue them from severe off periods, or continuous apomorphine infusions subcutaneously to maintain mobility. Another recent development has been the stereotaxic implantation of fetal substantia nigra into the striatum, but this is still in the experimental stage.

Surgery

In the 1950s and early 1960s, stereotaxic surgery was employed widely to treat Parkinson's disease. The initial target was the globus pallidus, but subsequent experience showed that the most favourable site was in the ventrolateral nucleus of the thalamus. A small lesion at that site was created mechanically, electrolytically, or thermally. Such a stereotaxic thalamotomy could abolish rigidity and tremor in the opposite limbs, but unfortunately did not relieve the disabling akinesia and postural instability. Both were found subsequently to respond to levodopa, at least initially, so by the early 1970s most centres were doing few or no stereotaxic operations for Parkinson's disease. Today, the operation is reserved for the uncommon patient with early Parkinson's disease, whose tremor is severe, resistant to drug therapy, and so disabling as to prevent work. However, new surgical techniques, such as continuous thalamic stimulation, are being reconsidered.

Physical therapy and aids

Parkinson's disease produces a wide range of functional locomotor disabilities, many of which can be helped by sensible aids. An initial assessment by the physiotherapist and occupational therapist will identify each individual patient's particular problems. Special training can then be given to help eating, washing, dressing, and walking. Intensive training may aid equilibrium and restore effective gait patterns, and the physiotherapist can teach a simple sequence of useful exercises for use at home. Advice on shoes ('slip-on' with sliding soles, not rubber), the use of 'Velcro®' rather than zips, feeding utensils with built-up handles, and other aids is invaluable. A visit to the patient's home will allow assessment of the need for structural alterations such as hand rails in the bathroom and lavatory, raising the toilet seat, removal of door sills, provision of high chairs (patients with Parkinson's disease find great difficulty in getting out of the usual low soft chair or sofa), removal of scatter rugs which slip, and provision of rubber mats. Sticks and other walking aids often are not very useful to patients with Parkinson's disease, but can be tried. Regular physiotherapy is not warranted, but reassessment if circumstances change or disability increases is essential. The advice of a speech therapist may be of value to those with communication difficulties.

Management of specific problems

Many particular problems arise in the treatment of Parkinson's disease and pose difficult management decisions.

Psychiatric illness

Toxic confusional states are common in Parkinson's disease, and may be due to drug overdosage or intercurrent acute illness, such as infection with fever. In practice, if no obvious other condition is apparent, it is wise to assume that drugs are the cause, for any of those employed to treat Parkinson's disease may provoke delirium. In those taking multiple drug therapy, amantadine may be stopped first, then the dose of anticholinergics can be halved, and subsequently these drugs can be withdrawn. Finally, if confusion persists, it is reasonable to decrease levodopa intake gradually until either the mental state clears, or immobility gets worse. For reasons that are not clear, it may take some days or even weeks for such a patient to regain mental clarity. Some never do, and it is apparent that this acute toxic confusional state was superimposed upon an underlying dementia, which should be investigated in its own right.

Psychotic behaviour, disrupting home life or ward routine, is common in such patients. Conventional neuroleptic drugs are best avoided in Parkinson's disease, because they antagonize dopamine action, but they may have to be used. In fact, the noisy disruptive parkinsonian may be calmed without deterioration in his mobility by a judiciously chosen dose of thioridazine (Melleril®) or other neuroleptic. Such drugs also may be of value for night sedation of those with reversed sleep rhythm.

Depression has been noted as very common in Parkinson's disease, often demanding treatment. Conventional monoamine oxidase inhibitors are quite contraindicated for they interact with levodopa to cause severe hypertension. However, tricyclics such as amitriptyline (Tryptizol®) can be used in the usual way, and their anticholinergic properties may add a little antiparkinsonian action. A large nocturnal dose of a sedative antidepressant such as amitriptyline (50–150 mg) often gives a gratifying night's sleep, and may prove of more value than benzodiazepine hypnotics in patients with Parkinson's disease. Newer, less sedative antidepressants with little peripheral anticholinergic action, may also be used. If severe depression does not respond to adequate antidepressant drug therapy, electroconvulsive treatment may be used without fear of complications. Indeed, electroconvulsive treatment by itself may pro-

voke considerable, but transient, improvement in the physical symptoms of Parkinson's disease.

Levodopa treatment has been associated with provocation of a wide range of psychiatric symptoms. Enhanced sexual desire and prowess was overestimated and exaggerated by the press, but levodopa can occasionally unmask latent sexual deviant behaviour; such tendencies disappear when the dose of the drug is reduced. Likewise, reversible mania may appear. A very distinctive acute, but reversible, visual hallucinosis, often with delusions, in the setting of clear consciousness, preserved insight, and intact thought is also not uncommon. In general, all such side-effects remit if levodopa dosage is reduced.

Intercurrent physical illness

Patients with Parkinson's disease are of an age when other illness may strike, to pose a number of difficulties.

The mobility of a patient with Parkinson's disease may deteriorate dramatically if influenza, a chest infection, or urinary tract infection occurs. Indeed, any sudden unexplained deterioration in such a patient should prompt a careful search for some such infective illness. Levodopa replacement therapy should be continued, via a nasogastric tube if necessary, throughout any intercurrent illness. Stopping levodopa will soon provoke a severe loss of mobility, with respiratory restriction and risk of deep vein thrombosis.

Many of the warning symptoms of other illness are already present in patients with Parkinson's disease. Constipation, for example, is universal; it is due to a combination of immobility, dietary restriction, neglecting roughage and liquid, and anticholinergic drug therapy. However, a definite change in bowel habit should be investigated as usual. Likewise, urinary hesitancy with frequency and urgency may occur in Parkinson's disease, but may also be due to infection, prostatic hypertrophy, or prolapse. In general, it is best to undertake appropriate investigation for such symptoms rather than blame them on Parkinson's disease, although this may turn out to be the case. This is particularly true of weight loss, which may be frightening in some individuals with rapidly progressive Parkinson's disease.

A recent myocardial infarct poses a problem in a patient with Parkinson's disease, for levodopa can provoke cardiac arrhythmias mainly due to metabolism to vasoactive amines. Combination of levodopa with a selective extracerebral decarboxylase inhibitor, as in Sinemet® and Madopar®, goes some way to avoiding this problem, by preventing levodopa metabolism. However, it is unwise to commence levodopa therapy in the month after a new myocardial infarct, particularly as the increased mobility may provoke extra strain. Levodopa, in combined form, can be continued in those already on treatment who have a myocardial infarct, but the dose can be reduced during any period of bed-rest.

A few other symptoms occur sufficiently often in Parkinson's disease to warrant mention. Ankle oedema due to immobility (and amantadine) is unsightly but not usually serious. Postural hypotension, sometimes exacerbated by drug therapy, rarely causes symptoms, and requires no treatment unless it does. Seborrhoea may be severe, causing dandruff and dermatitis, and conjunctivitis, leading to sore, red eyes and crusted lids, may require local therapy. Salivation is particularly unpleasant, leading to dribbling. Anticholinergic drugs may help, and improved swallowing produced by levodopa therapy may avoid the problem.

Drug interaction

Patients with Parkinson's disease often require other drugs to control other illnesses. No interactions between antiparkinsonian drugs and the following have been noted: anticoagulants, benzodiazepines, tricyclic antidepressants, digoxin, diuretics, trinitrin, propranolol, antiarrhythmic drugs, antibiotics, thyroxine, and hypoglycaemic agents.

Diabetic control is not altered usually. Hypotensive therapy with α-methyldopa (Aldomet®) leads to an increase in levodopa-induced side-effects, for α-methyldopa inhibits dopa decarboxylase. Propranolol (Inderal®) or other β-adrenergic antagonists probably are the drugs of choice to treat hypertension for they also slightly benefit parkinsonian tremor.

Levodopa should never be given with a conventional monoamine oxidase inhibitor, and the directly acting sympathomimetic amines contained in bronchodilators and some cold remedies are best avoided due to the risks of paroxysmal hypertension.

The fact that neuroleptics, all of which are dopamine antagonists, may cause deterioration in Parkinson's disease and may reverse the beneficial actions of levodopa, has already been noted. Phenothiazines, butyrophenones, and thioxanthenes are best avoided if possible, as is papaverine, included in many so-called cerebral vasodilators, for it too is a dopamine antagonist.

Pyridoxine (vitamin B_6) is a cofactor for decarboxylase, so enhances metabolism of plain levodopa. Many combined vitamin preparations contain pyridoxine and may reverse the beneficial actions of plain levodopa. However, pyridoxine can be given with Sinemet® or Madopar®.

Surgery

Patients with Parkinson's disease may require surgery for other illnesses, but the need should always be balanced against the risks. Some patients deteriorate severely after anaesthesia and enforced bed-rest, and may never make up the lost ground. If surgery is essential, then levodopa therapy should be continued up to the night of the operation. The morning dose is omitted, but treatment is restarted as soon as the patient can swallow. In those with prolonged postoperative difficulties, levodopa can be given via a nasogastric tube, or apomorphine by injection.

Other akinetic–rigid syndromes in adults

PROGRESSIVE SUPRANUCLEAR PALSY

Definition

In 1964 Steele, Richardson, and Olszewski described a syndrome with similarities to parkinsonism, but with an additional characteristic and diagnostic abnormality of voluntary eye movement. The illness is progressive and is characterized by akinesia, axial rigidity, postural imbalance, dysarthria, a supranuclear paralysis of voluntary vertical eye movements, and mental changes, with onset in middle or late life.

Aetiology

The cause of progressive supranuclear palsy is not known. It is a rare sporadic disease. Males are affected more than females, and no familial cases have been described. Onset usually is in the fifth to seventh decades.

Pathology

There is widespread neuronal loss and gliosis in the brain-stem, affecting particularly the globus pallidus, substantia nigra, subthalamus, red nucleus, tectum and periaqueductal grey matter, and dentate nucleus. Such affected nerve cells contain neurofibrillary tangles. The cerebral cortex, however, is unaffected and senile plaques do not occur.

Symptoms

The illness most commonly presents either with imbalance or visual symptoms. The latter consist of difficulty with reading or coming down stairs, because both demand voluntary downward gaze, and vertical gaze characteristically is impaired. The patient cannot voluntarily look up and down, nor follow an object moved in the vertical plane (Fig. 6). But a full range of vertical eye movements can be elicited reflexly by rapid posturing of the head (the doll's eye manoeuvre). Horizontal eye movement also is similarly affected, but usually later than vertical eye movement. The earliest signs of impairment of eye movement is a breakdown of swift, smooth, rapid voluntary movement into short, jerky, repetitive saccades. The characteristic profound and early involvement of vertical gaze is accompanied by a typical dystonic extension of the neck, and a fixed wide-eyed stare. The patient looks around by moving the head, rather than the eyes.

Imbalance and unexplained falls are a common early complaint. At this stage the patient also will exhibit characteristic axial rigidity of neck, trunk, and proximal limb muscles, and poverty of movement, particularly of whole-body movement. Speech is dysarthric, as in a pseudobulbar palsy, and swallowing may be impaired. Dystonic postures and other abnormal movements, including tremor, may occur. Akinesia and rigidity are evident, but power is preserved, as is sensation; the tendon reflexes are brisk and the plantar responses may be extensor.

Mental function is impaired. The patient may give an impression of dementia, with difficulty in memory and loss of intellectual power. Careful examination, however, reveals that memory and intellect are better than is apparent at first sight, provided the patient is given adequate time to formulate answers. This impairment of mental processes, characterized by mental slowness and inefficiency on tests sensitive to frontal lobe dysfunction, has been termed 'subcortical dementia'.

Natural history

The disease is relentlessly progressive, the patient becoming bedridden and anarthric, leading to death in 5 to 7 years.

Fig. 6 Defective ocular movements in progressive supranuclear palsy. The patient, a 67-year-old man, can voluntarily look to left and right (upper panels), but cannot voluntarily look down or up, or follow a moving object (a pen) down or up (middle panels). However, when the head is passively extended or flexed, a full range of reflex vertical eye movement is achieved (lower panels).

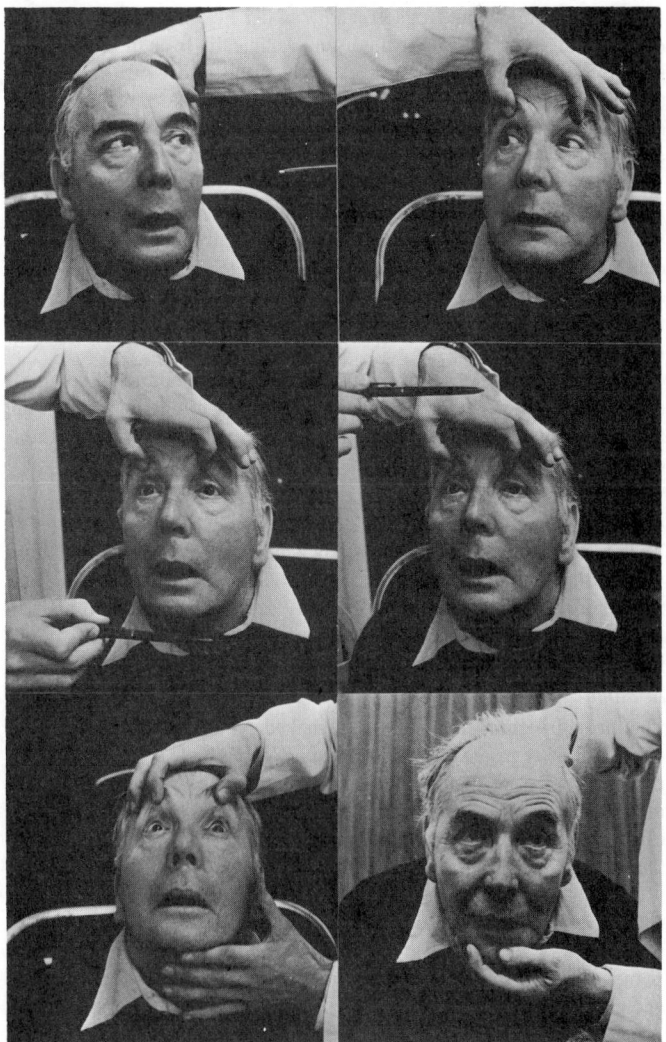

Diagnosis

The crucial diagnostic feature is the supranuclear gaze palsy. However, eye movements may also be abnormal in patients with other types of parkinsonism. Progressive supranuclear palsy is diagnosed with confidence only when down-gaze is affected, but this may occur late in the illness, and such a disorder of eye movements is not specific for Steele–Richardson–Olszewski disease.

Treatment

There is no effective treatment for this condition, which usually does not respond to levodopa or other dopamine agonists, although such drugs are worth trying. Amantadine and anticholinergic drugs also occasionally may help.

MULTIPLE SYSTEM ATROPHY (SEE ALSO CHAPTER 24.3.7)

Definition

Three separate conditions are included in this category, olivopontocerebellar atrophy, striatonigral degeneration, and autonomic failure.

The term 'olivopontocerebellar degeneration' was given by Thomas and Dejerine to an isolated case of ataxia in middle life, with widespread degeneration affecting particularly the cerebellar cortex, inferior olives, and pontine nuclei. In contrast to the familial cerebellar ataxia associated with olivopontocerebellar degeneration originally described by Menzel in 1891, such sporadic cases also may exhibit an akinetic–rigid parkinsonian syndrome, with additional degeneration in the striatum and substantia nigra, and autonomic failure.

In 1961 Adams, van Bogaert, and Van der Eeken described a group of middle-aged patients indistinguishable clinically from those with Parkinson's disease, but with severe cell loss and gliosis in the striatum (especially the putamen) and substantia nigra. Many such patients, however, also exhibit the pathological changes of olivopontocerebellar atrophy and develop autonomic failure.

In 1960 Shy and Drager drew attention to a syndrome characterized by autonomic failure with severe postural hypotension, and often akinesia and rigidity. Pathologically such cases exhibited extensive loss of cells in the intermediolateral nuclei of the lateral horns in the spinal cord; these cells are the preganglionic sympathetic neurones. In addition, there often was severe cell loss and gliosis in the olivopontocerebellar and striatonigral regions.

Thus three clinical syndromes, cerebellar ataxia due to olivopontocerebellar degeneration, Parkinsonism due to striatonigral degeneration, and autonomic failure overlap, and share a common widespread pathology, which Oppenheimer has named multiple system atrophy.

Aetiology

The cause of this disease, which may account for 10 per cent of those with parkinsonism, is unknown. Nearly all cases are sporadic. Both sexes are affected and symptoms usually begin in middle age.

Pathology (see Table 4)

Anatomical

The most striking abnormality to the naked eye in olivopontocerebellar degeneration is gross shrinkage of the pons and middle cerebellar peduncles due to loss of pontine nuclei and of their transverse fibres. In the medulla there is loss of neurones in the inferior olives and of their olivocerebellar fibres. The cerebellar cortex has lost Purkinje cells, but the deep cerebellar nuclei are preserved.

In striatonigral degeneration there is gliosis and extensive loss of neurones in the caudate, and especially in the putamen, and in the substantia nigra.

In autonomic failure there is widespread neuronal loss in caudate nucleus, substantia nigra, locus coeruleus, inferior olives, Purkinje cells, dorsal vagal nucleus, Onuf's nucleus, and intermediolateral column of

Table 4 *Sites of pathology in different basal ganglia degenerations*

	Parkinson's disease	Progressive supranuclear palsy	Multiple system atrophy
Cerebral cortex	(+)	−	(+)
Striatum	(+)	(+)	+
Globus pallidus	(+)	++	−
Subthalamus	(+)	++	−
Pigmented nuclei	++	++	+
Pontine nuclei	−	(+)	+
Inferior olives	−	(+)	+
Purkinje cells	−	(+)	+
Dentate nucleus	−	++	−
Intermediolateral columns	(+)	(+)	+
Sympathetic ganglia	+	?	−
Pyramidal tracts	−	+	+
Cellular change	Lewy body	Neurofibrillary tangle	Glial cytoplasmic inclusions

++, Always or nearly always affected; +, commonly affected; (+), occasionally affected; −, seldom if ever affected.
After Oppernheimer quoted in Quinn (1994).

the thoracic cord, the latter being held responsible for the sympathetic failure.

Recently, specific inclusions have been described in affected neurones and glia.

Biochemical

The main neurochemical findings described in multiple system atrophy are: a considerable loss of dopamine in the caudate and putamen, nucleus accumbens, and substantia nigra (to between 5 and 50 per cent of normal); a profound reduction of noradrenaline, particularly in the nucleus accumbens, septal nuclei, hypothalamus, and locus coeruleus (to between 10 and 27 per cent of normal); a general reduction in glutamic acid decarboxylase in cerebral cortex, brain-stem, and cerebellum (to between 1 and 48 per cent of normal); and a similar generalized reduction in choline acetyltransferase in most brain areas examined (to between 10 and 47 per cent of normal). The changes in dopamine and noradrenaline reflect degeneration in the substantia nigra and locus coeruleus, but the changes in glutamic acid decarboxylase probably were due to the prolonged anoxic mode of death. In contrast, choline acetyltransferase is largely unaffected by antemortem factors and probably reflects extensive loss of cholinergic neurones.

Clinical features

Olivopontocerebellar degeneration presents as a progressive cerebellar ataxia of gait and arms, accompanied by dysarthria and, often, nystagmus. In addition, there may be pyramidal signs, akinesia, and rigidity.

Striatonigral degeneration presents as a parkinsonian syndrome indistinguishable from that of Parkinson's disease, although cerebellar atrophy may be evident on CT or MRI brain scans.

Autonomic failure presents as postural (orthostatic) hypotension, urinary incontinence, loss of sweating, sexual impotence, akinesia and rigidity, and sometimes tremor and severe dysarthria. Serious respiratory stridor and sleep apnoea may develop.

With time and progression of the disease, patients become increasingly disabled by an akinetic–rigid syndrome with profound postural imbalance, and by severe postural hypotension and urinary incontinence. The intellect is usually spared. Death occurs within some 10 years.

The clinical features of autonomic failure are described in detail in Chapter 24.3.7.

Diagnosis

Multiple system atrophy may be confused with any of the other causes of a progressive cerebellar syndrome, including cerebellar tumour, other spinocerebellar degenerations, multiple sclerosis, and the cerebellar ataxia that may be associated with myxoedema, a remote neoplasm, or alcoholism.

Striatonigral degeneration is usually misdiagnosed as Parkinson's disease, but does not respond to treatment.

Orthostatic hypotension may be due to drugs, diabetes, or other causes of an autonomic neuropathy, including amyloid. Most difficult is to separate orthostatic hypotension with an akinetic–rigid syndrome due to multiple system atrophy from Parkinson's disease due to Lewy body degeneration with postural hypotension. Other features of an autonomic neuropathy, however, do not occur in Parkinson's disease. Denervation of the anal and urethral sphincter, which can be detected by electromyography, due to degeneration of neurones in Onuf's nucleus, occurs in multiple system atrophy and may be diagnostic.

Treatment

Unfortunately, there is no effective therapy for multiple system atrophy. The akinetic–rigid parkinsonian features do not usually respond to levodopa replacement therapy as well as they do in Parkinson's disease. Indeed, many patients with multiple system atrophy are resistant to dopamine agonists or anticholinergic drugs. Amantadine may be of benefit.

Postural hypotension may be helped by elastic stockings, a G-suit, and fludrocortisone combined with head-up tilt at night.

The treatment of autonomic failure is considered in detail in Chapter 24.3.7.

CORTICOBASAL DEGENERATION

Aetiology and pathology

This condition, which occurs sporadically in middle or late life, has only been recognized recently. It is characterized pathologically by atrophy of the frontal and parietal cortex, and of the striatum, globus pallidus, subthalamus, substantia nigra, and other brain-stem nuclei. Cell loss in these areas is accompanied by gliosis, and remaining neurones may be swollen and achromatic, similar to those seen in Pick's disease; but there are no Pick bodies or Lewy bodies. The cause is unknown.

Symptoms

The onset is insidious and the course progressive. Common early features are clumsiness of one limb, usually the arm, due to a mixture of rigidity, akinesia, and apraxia. The affected limb may exhibit uncontrollable wandering (the alien limb), spontaneous and reflex myoclonic jerks, dystonia or a jerky tremor, and sensory loss. This motor deficit spreads to involve other limbs, balance and gait become impaired, speech becomes dysarthric, and a supranuclear palsy of gaze appears. Frontal release and pyramidal signs are common. The intellect and language usually remain intact until the later stages of the illness, which leads to death within some 7 to 10 years. There is no effective treatment.

CEREBRAL ANOXIA

Aetiology and pathology

Severe cerebral anoxia, whether its cause be cardiac arrest, carbon monoxide poisoning, or pure anoxic anoxia, may cause disproportionate damage to the basal ganglia, leading to bilateral necrosis of the striatum or globus pallidus. While the effects of damage to the cerebral cortex are apparent immediately, those resulting from basal ganglia destruction may appear days or up to about a month after the insult, and thereafter, for reasons that are not clear, the syndrome may progress.

Table 5 *Causes of akinetic–rigid syndrome in childhood*

Hereditary	Other
Wilson's disease	Drugs
Dopa-responsive dystonia-parkinsonism	Athetoid cerebral palsy
Hallervorden–Spatz disease	
Progressive pallidal atrophy	
Juvenile Huntington's disease	
Pelizaeus–Merzbacher disease	
Ataxia telangiectasia	
Lesch–Nyhan disease	

All the hereditary diseases of childhood affecting the basal ganglia also may cause abnormal involuntary movements such as torsion spasms and, sometimes, chorea.

Symptoms

After the episode of cerebral anoxia, the patient may recover from the initial coma, only to relapse over the next few weeks into an increasingly severe akinetic–rigid state with profound dysarthria and dysphagia. The arms characteristically are flexed while the legs are extended, all limbs showing dystonic posturing and athetoid movements of the fingers and toes.

Progression to death may occur, but the condition can arrest or even improve, and levodopa sometimes helps.

BASAL GANGLIA CALCIFICATION

Many elderly brains at necropsy show a mild degree of calcification in the striopallidal structures, most evident in the globus pallidus, without symptoms in life. Such asymptomatic brain calcification is found in about 0.5 per cent of CT scans of elderly subjects.

About 20 to 30 per cent of those with widespread calcification of the basal ganglia and other structures, including the dentate nucleus, exhibit neurological symptoms and signs, which include an akinetic–rigid parkinsonian syndrome, dyskinesias such as chorea, and sometimes epilepsy, ataxia, and dementia.

Some patients with symptomatic basal ganglia calcification have previously had radical thyroid surgery, and others have idiopathic hypoparathyroidism or pseudohypoparathyroidism. Other causes include cerebral irradiation and mitochondrial disease. Many such patients, however, including some familial cases, have no demonstrable endocrine or metabolic disorder.

AKINETIC–RIGID SYNDROMES IN CHILDHOOD

The causes of an akinetic–rigid syndrome in childhood or adolescence are quite different from those responsible for a similar syndrome in middle or late life (Table 5).

Many children with Huntington's disease present with the Westphal variant of the disease, namely an akinetic–rigid syndrome. Other hereditary conditions, such as Wilson's disease, Hallervorden–Spatz disease, progressive pallidal degeneration, and Pelizaeus–Merzbacher's disease, also may present as parkinsonism in childhood or early adult life, usually with other dyskinesias, such as dystonia and chorea, and cognitive impairment.

Wilson's disease will be described in detail, for it is a treatable and preventable cause of extrapyramidal (and liver) disease in childhood, adolescence, and young adult life. Brief notes follow on the other rare disorders. Certain other rare diseases of childhood also may present with such extrapyramidal disorders, and brief notes on these conditions, such as ataxia telangiectasia and the Lesch–Nyhan syndrome, are also included at this point for they enter into any differential diagnosis of a movement disorder in a child.

WILSON'S DISEASE (SEE ALSO SECTIONS 11 AND 14)

Definition

A rare, often familial, progressive disease of the central nervous system and liver due to a disorder of copper metabolism, causing copper retention and toxicity. It is important because it is treatable.

Aetiology

Wilson's disease, or hepatolenticular degeneration, occurs in male or female siblings, but not parents or children, indicating autosomal recessive inheritance. The gene responsible for Wilson's disease lies on chromosome 13. Homozygotes develop the disease, while heterozygotes are symptomless. One primary defect appears to be a congenital deficiency of the copper-carrying plasma protein, caeruloplasmin, but this is not the critical abnormality. A small minority (5 per cent or so) of patients with Wilson's disease have normal plasma caeruloplasmin concentrations, while some asymptomatic heterozygotes (10–20 per cent) have low levels. Caeruloplasmin normally binds 98 per cent of the copper present in serum. Defective biliary excretion of copper, in the face of normal copper absorption, is probably the crucial defect.

The deficiency of caeruloplasmin is associated with low serum copper concentration, but excessive deposition of copper in the brain, cornea, liver, and kidneys, and excessive output of copper in the urine. The copper deposition leads to damage to neurones in the brain and to liver and kidney.

Pathology

In the brain, the globus pallidus and especially the putamen (together known as the lenticular nucleus, hence the name hepatolenticular degeneration) are strikingly affected, but the cerebral cortex and other basal ganglia structures are also damaged. The liver shows portal cirrhosis.

Symptoms

Wilson's disease presents to neurologists as a behaviour disturbance, an akinetic–rigid syndrome and with a variety of dyskinesias; or it presents to hepatologists with the complication of acute hepatitis or chronic cirrhosis. Onset is usually in childhood or adolescence, but may be delayed as late as the fifth decade of life. The first symptoms of the disease frequently lead to psychiatric referral with conduct disorders, personality change, or frank psychotic disturbance. Common initial neurological symptoms include tremor of any type, dysarthria and drooling (Fig. 7), chorea, dystonic spasms and posturing, or akinesia and rigidity. Without treatment, progression is inevitable, with dementia, increasingly severe dysarthria and dysphagia, and increasing akinesia, rigidity, and dystonia, leading to contractures and immobility. Vision, hearing, and sensation are not affected, and the tendon reflexes and plantar responses are usually normal. Fits may occur in a minority of cases.

A Kayser–Fleischer ring may be seen in the cornea with the naked eye and is always present in those with neurological symptoms when looked for with a slit-lamp. It consists of a ring of greenish-brown copper pigment deposited around the margin of the cornea in Descemet's membrane. A 'sunflower' cataract, due to copper deposition in the lens, may also be seen. Copper deposition in the nailbeds produces blue lunulae, while copper deposits in the kidney may produce selective proteinuria and aminoaciduria.

Clinical evidence of liver disease may occur without neurological symptoms and signs. In those with neurological deficit, there can be no clinical evidence of liver damage, but a history of hepatitis or jaundice may be obtained and the liver often will be found to be damaged on investigation. Hepatic coma and gastrointestinal haemorrhage due to varices may occur. Without treatment the disease is usually fatal in 5 to 14 years from the onset.

Investigation

Any child or young adult presenting with any form of dyskinesia or akinetic–rigid syndrome, or with unexplained liver disease, should be investigated to exclude Wilson's disease. In an established case, relatives must also be screened to allow treatment before neurological or liver damage occurs.

Abnormality of liver function and aminoaciduria should be sought for, and the cornea examined by slit-lamp. Serum copper usually is low (<12 μmol/l or 90 μg/100 ml) and serum caeruloplasmin is low (<0.2 μmol/l or 20 μg/100 ml) or absent. Urinary copper excretion is high (usually more than 0.2 g/24 h), but other liver diseases can increase urinary copper excretion and any condition causing proteinuria may be associated with hypercupruria. These investigations may be normal in some patients, but liver biopsy content of copper is almost always in excess of 250 μg/g dry weight (normal <55 μg/g). Specialized studies of the metabolism of radioactive copper may aid diagnosis in difficult cases. However, in neurological cases the absence of a Kayser–Fleischer ring on slit-lamp examination of the eye, and a normal content of copper in a liver biopsy exclude the diagnosis. Brain CT or MRI often shows cerebral atrophy and degenerative changes in the basal ganglia.

Treatment

Penicillamine (dimethylcysteine) has superseded BAL (dimercaprol) and calcium EDTA (ethylenediaminetetraacetic acid; versene) as the treatment of choice to chelate and remove the excess copper in the body. D-Penicillamine in a dose of 1.0 to 1.5 mg daily is given for life. Discontinuation leads to a relapse. A small dose is given initially and gradually increased until biochemical studies indicate an adequate and sus-

Fig. 7 The facies of a 20-year-old man with severe Wilson's disease, causing a severe pseudobulbar palsy with marked dysarthria and dysphagia, as well as a generalized akinetic–rigid syndrome. A Kayser–Fleischer ring is just evident around the periphery of the cornea, especially on the right.

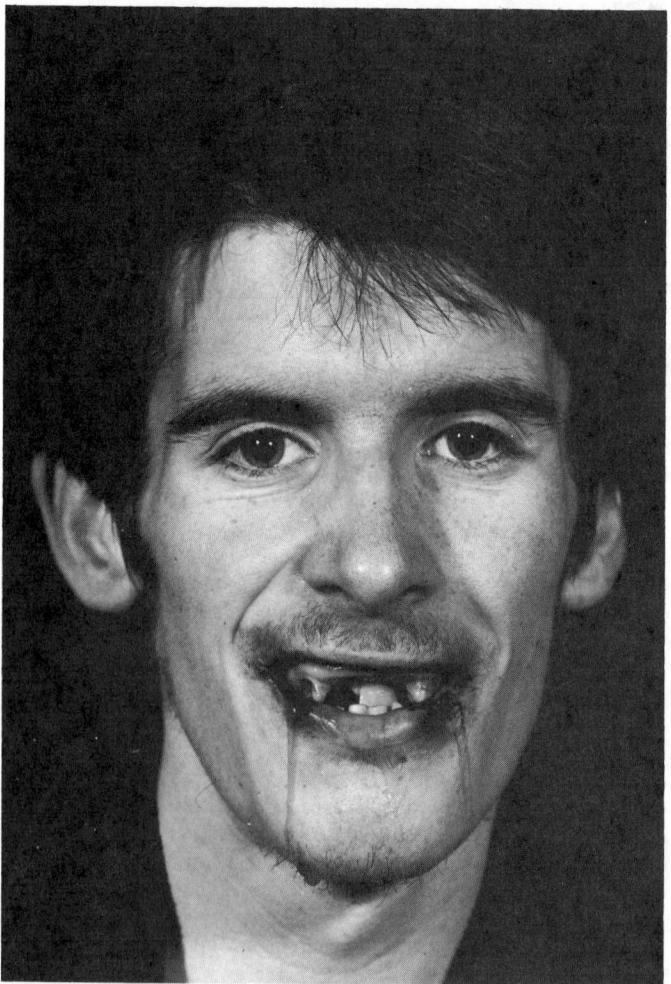

tained negative copper balance. Penicillamine may cause skin rashes, proteinuria, and marrow depression, in which case alternative therapy such as triethylene tetramine (trientene) is indicated. Potassium sulphide and zinc supplements inhibit copper absorption and may be useful adjuncts, and a diet low in copper should be advised. Those with neurological symptoms may deteriorate to begin with after starting treatment, and it may take many months for improvement to occur. However, if treated early enough, the disease can be completely controlled and the affected individual rendered normal, both mentally and physically.

HALLERVORDEN–SPATZ DISEASE

In 1922, Hallervorden and Spatz described a very rare, often familial, condition of childhood in which iron-containing pigment is deposited, particularly in the globus pallidus and zona reticulata of the substantia nigra. Large oval spheroids, probably containing mucoprotein, are found in these pigmented areas, and are thought to be degenerating axons.

A family history is obtained in less than a quarter of cases, usually affected siblings, indicating autosomal recessive inheritance. Similar neuroaxonal dystrophic changes also can be caused by exogenous agents in animals, such as vitamin E deficiency.

Clinically, the condition presents as progressive rigidity, initially in the legs with a characteristic equinovarus foot deformity (club foot), later of the arms. Dystonic movements of the affected limbs are common, as is dysarthria and dementia. The illness does not respond to treatment and most children die by early adult life.

PROGRESSIVE PALLIDAL ATROPHY

In 1917, Ramsay Hunt described a very rare syndrome of progressive parkinsonism with onset in childhood or adolescence ('juvenile parkinsonism'). One such patient came to necropsy and showed severe degeneration of the globus pallidus, with other changes in the striatum. Subsequently, similar cases have been reported with variable degeneration of the globus pallidus, subthalamic nuclei (pallidoluysian degeneration), and pyramidal pathways (pallidopyramidal degeneration).

Many patients have a family history suggesting inheritance usually as an autosomal dominant trait, but sometimes the illness only appears in siblings.

Clinically, the condition presents in childhood or adolescence with a progressive parkinsonian syndrome, including akinesia, rigidity with rest tremor, with preserved intellect and sensation, but often with pyramidal signs and sometimes with dystonia and torsion spasms. The parkinsonian features may respond to levodopa therapy.

PELIZAEUS–MERZBACHER DISEASE

A rare demyelinating leucodystrophy of unknown cause, histologically distinct from Krabbe's disease, metachromatic leucodystrophy, and adrenoleucodystrophy, inherited as an autosomal recessive or sex-linked recessive trait. The illness characteristically presents in the first decade of life with progressive dementia, gross nystagmus, and ataxia, and sometimes optic atrophy and spasticity, often with fits. Extrapyramidal features may also be prominent, particularly dystonic postures and torsion spasms, and finally an akinetic rigid state. Most patients with childhood onset die before the age of 20 years, but a few cases with onset in adult life and slower progression have been recorded.

ATAXIA TELANGIECTASIA

Madame Louis-Bar in 1941 described an illness, apparently inherited as an autosomal recessive trait, characterized by the gradual appearance in early childhood of ataxia, parkinsonian features, and abnormal movements such as chorea or torsion spasms. In addition, dysarthria, nystagmus, a supranuclear gaze palsy and oculomotor apraxia evolve, associated with hypotonia and areflexia. Intelligence is preserved until later

Table 6 *Causes of tremor*

Rest tremor
  Parkinson's disease
  Postencephalitic parkinsonism
  Drug-induced parkinsonism
  Other extrapyramidal diseases
Postural tremor
  Physiological tremor
  Exaggerated physiological tremor, as in:
    thyrotoxicosis
    anxiety states
    alcohol
    drugs (e.g. sympathomimetics, antidepressants, valproic acid, lithium)
    heavy metal poisoning (i.e. mercury—the 'hatter's shakes')
  Structural neurological disease, as in:
    severe cerebellar lesions ('red nucleus tremor')
    Wilson's disease
    neurosyphilis
    peripheral neuropathies
  Benign essential (familial) tremor
  Orthostatic tremor
Intention tremor
  Brain-stem or cerebellar disease, as in:
    multiple sclerosis
    spinocerebellar degenerations
    vascular disease
    tumour

in the illness, which is slowly progressive. Telangiectasia develops in the conjunctiva, pinna of the ear, face, and limb flexures, but may not appear until after the age of 5 years. Such children are very prone to infection, particularly respiratory infection, for they also exhibit immunological deficiencies, characteristically hypogammaglobulinaemia with gross loss or absence of IgA.

LESCH–NYHAN SYNDROME (SEE ALSO SECTION 11)

A rare condition, apparently inherited as a sex-linked recessive trait, with onset in infancy or early childhood with progressive abnormal movements such as chorea and torsion spasms, mental retardation, spasticity, and characteristically a tendency to self-mutilation as the child grows older. Diagnosis is established by the finding of a raised serum uric acid, due to deficiency of hypoxanthine-guanine phosphoribosyltransferase. Uric acid renal calculi may develop, so treatment with allopurinol is justified, although the reduction is serum uric acid levels does not prevent neurological deterioration.

The dyskinesias

Most abnormal involuntary movements may be classified into one of five main categories: tremor, chorea, myoclonus, tics, and dystonia. Each type of dyskinesia may be caused by a variety of diseases. In some patients the dyskinesia is accompanied by other neurological deficits or some other clue as to the cause; in others, the involuntary movements occur in isolation and constitute the illness. Nearly all dyskinesias disappear in sleep, are made worse by anxiety and stress, and are improved by relaxation.

Tremor is a rhythmic sinusoidal movement of a body part, due to regular rhythmic muscle contractions. The common causes of tremor are shown in Table 6.

Chorea consists of a continuous flow of irregular, jerky, and explosive movements, that flit from one portion of the body to another in random sequence. Each muscle contraction is brief, often appearing as a fragment of what might have been a normal movement, and quite unpredictable in timing or site (Fig. 8). The common causes of chorea are shown in Table 7.

Myoclonus consists of rapid shock-like muscle jerks, often repetitive and sometimes rhythmic. The common causes of myoclonus are shown in Table 8.

Tics are similar to myoclonic jerks in appearance, but are repetitive, stereotyped movements that can be mimicked voluntarily and can be held in check by an effort of will at the expense of mounting inner tension. Simple tics are confined to a few muscles; complex tics may involve more co-ordinated quasi-purposeful movements. The common causes of tics are shown in Table 9.

Dystonia consists of sustained spasms of muscle contraction which distort the limbs and trunk into characteristic dystonic postures—the twisted neck (torticollis), flexed (antecollis) or extended neck (retrocollis), the arched back (lordosis) or twisted back (scoliosis), the hyperpronated arm, and plantar-flexed inverted foot. Such dystonic spasms typically occur on willed action (action dystonia). Dystonic spasms may be intermittent, producing dystonic movements, which may be repetitive to give a rhythmic character, or sustained to hold a fixed dystonic posture. The common causes of torsion dystonia are shown in Table 10.

There is confusion between the use of the terms dystonia and athetosis, which are employed interchangeably. Dystonia literally means any abnormality of muscle tone, but most neurologists employ it to describe movements and postures instantly recognized as dystonic. The term dystonia frequently is qualified as torsion dystonia, to emphasize the twisted nature of the abnormal postures. Many patients with torsion dystonia, whatever its cause, not only have abnormal postures, but also abnormal involuntary movements. They may be called dystonic (torsion spasms), if they affect proximal joints (axial torsion dystonia), or athetoid, if they affect the fingers and toes. The term athetosis was introduced originally to describe the sinuous, writhing digital movements that may follow a stroke. Subsequently, athetosis became synonymous with one type of cerebral palsy, resulting from brain damage due to anoxia or kernicterus at birth. Such babies typically are floppy, exhibit delayed motor milestones, and sometime before the age of 5 years develop athetoid abnor-

Table 7 *Causes of chorea*

Sydenham's chorea
    Variants include: chorea gravidarum, chorea caused by
       contraceptive pill
Huntington's disease
    Variants include: senile chorea, juvenile chorea, Westphal
       variant
Benign hereditary chorea
Neuroacanthocytosis
Symptomatic chorea
    Thyrotoxicosis
    Systemic lupus erythematosus
    Polycythaemia rubra vera
    Encephalitis lethargica
    Hypernatraemia
    Hypoparathyroidism
    Subdural haematoma
Drug-induced chorea
    Neuroleptic drugs
    Anticonvulsants
    Contraceptive pill
    Alcohol
Hemiballism (hemichorea)
    Stroke
    Tumour
    Trauma
    Post-thalamotomy

mal movements. The whole syndrome is known as athetoid cerebral palsy, or simply athetosis.

Many of the diseases known to cause the various dyskinesias shown in Tables 6 to 10 are discussed elsewhere. However, a number of conditions in which the dyskinesia is the major feature of the illness will be described here.

Tremor

BENIGN ESSENTIAL (FAMILIAL) TREMOR

Definition

An illness characterized by postural tremor of the arms and head, often inherited as an autosomal dominant trait, which presents at any age and is usually only slowly progressive causing mild disability.

Aetiology

The cause of benign essential tremor, which may appear in childhood, adolescence (juvenile tremor), early adult life, or old age (senile tremor), is unknown. A positive family history is obtained in over half of such patients and the pattern of inheritance in such families indicates an autosomal dominant trait.

Pathophysiology

No pathological or biochemical abnormality has been identified in benign essential tremor, but few cases have come to necropsy. The condition may well represent some instability in the many feedback neuronal loops that control the posture of the hands, head, and other parts of the body. A defect of cerebellar control has been identified recently.

Everyone has a physiological tremor of the outstretched hands, at about 8 to 12 Hz, due to summation of the many factors which combine to generate an oscillation at this frequency (Fig. 3). Such factors include:

(1) the tendency for motor units to start firing at about 8 Hz, which is below the natural tetanic fusion frequency of human muscle (about 12 Hz);

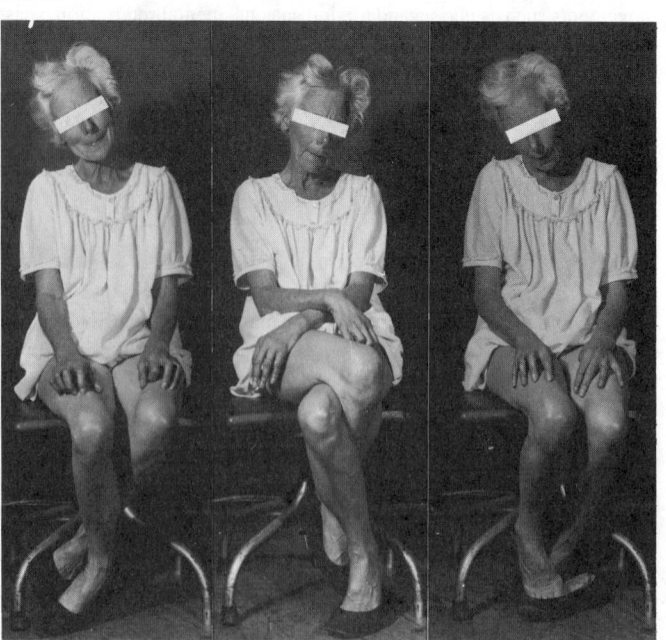

Fig. 8 Chorea due to polycythaemia rubra vera in a 57-year-old woman. The characteristic fleeting choreic movements are captured in these three sequential frames.

pain from the upper cervical spine and posterior fossa is referred principally to the occiput and neck via the upper three cervical nerves. Supratentorial and infratentorial tumours can cause frontal headache by causing obstructive hydrocephalus which distends the lateral ventricles, displacing blood vessels in their walls. Terminally, coning causes pain referred to the neck as the cerebellar tonsil impacts.

Few headaches fail to evoke some anxiety, which can distort and magnify the primary clinical features.

REFERRED PAIN AND MUSCLE CONTRACTION HEADACHE

The orbits, paranasal sinuses, and teeth cause pain referred via branches of the trigeminal nerve to the forehead and temple. Sinusitis and toothache are commonplace examples, but glaucoma, orbital cellulitis, and cavernous sinus thrombosis may produce referred frontotemporal pain. Secondary involuntary contraction of scalp and facial muscles further complicate the picture, causing a secondary generalized 'tension headache' which may obscure the primary source.

Primary tension headache is psychogenic; its mechanisms are not wholly understood. Stretching of pain-sensitive nerve endings within muscle fascicles and compression and traction of scalp blood vessels are considered important. Infiltration of lignocaine temporarily relieves the pain which is transmitted in the trigeminal and upper cervical nerves.

CRANIAL NEURALGIAS

'Idiopathic' trigeminal and glossopharyngeal neuralgias are thought to be due to an irritative lesion of these nerves, often microvascular compression by tortuous posterior fossa vessels which cause strictly anatomical localization of the pain (see Chapter 24.3.6). When these neuralgias result from multiple sclerosis, or extrinsic compression, the quality of pain is similar.

Post-herpetic neuralgia is a classic example of pain secondary to an inflammatory irritative lesion, although its prolonged course is thought to be due to a 'central component' related to facilitation of pain circuits in the reticular formation and its input to the thalamus.

Apart from these localized cranial neuralgias, the position of headache is no indication of its origin. Vascular, throbbing pain is aggravated by vasodilators, alcohol, exertion, and by coughing or straining. Typical of migraine, these factors are not specific since a vascular or hydrodynamic headache may herald a tumour or hydrocephalus.

The trigeminovascular reflex (Fig. 1)

This mechanism is probably common to many different causes of headache. On the afferent side there is a 'centre' in the upper cervical cord. Pain fibres descend in the spinal root of the trigeminal nerve to C2 where they converge with afferents from C1 to C3 on second-order neurones. This provides a pain pathway from head to neck and vice-versa. The raphe nuclei and locus coeruleus project rostrally to the cortex, and caudally as part of the endogenous pain control circuit. Stimulation of these brain-stem nuclei and of the trigeminal complex increases extracranial blood flow by reflex connection with the parasympathetic part of the facial nerve—via the greater superficial petrosal nerve, sphenopalatine and otic ganglia. This constitutes a link between neural and vascular mechanisms, the fashionable 'trigeminovascular reflex'.

Antidromic stimulation of trigeminal fibres on blood vessels causes extravasation of plasma in the dura. Plasma extravasation is thus stimulated by perivascular sensory fibres which release neurokinin A, calcitonin G-related peptide, and substance P. Stimulation of the trigeminal nerve also produces measurable increases in these peptides in the venous

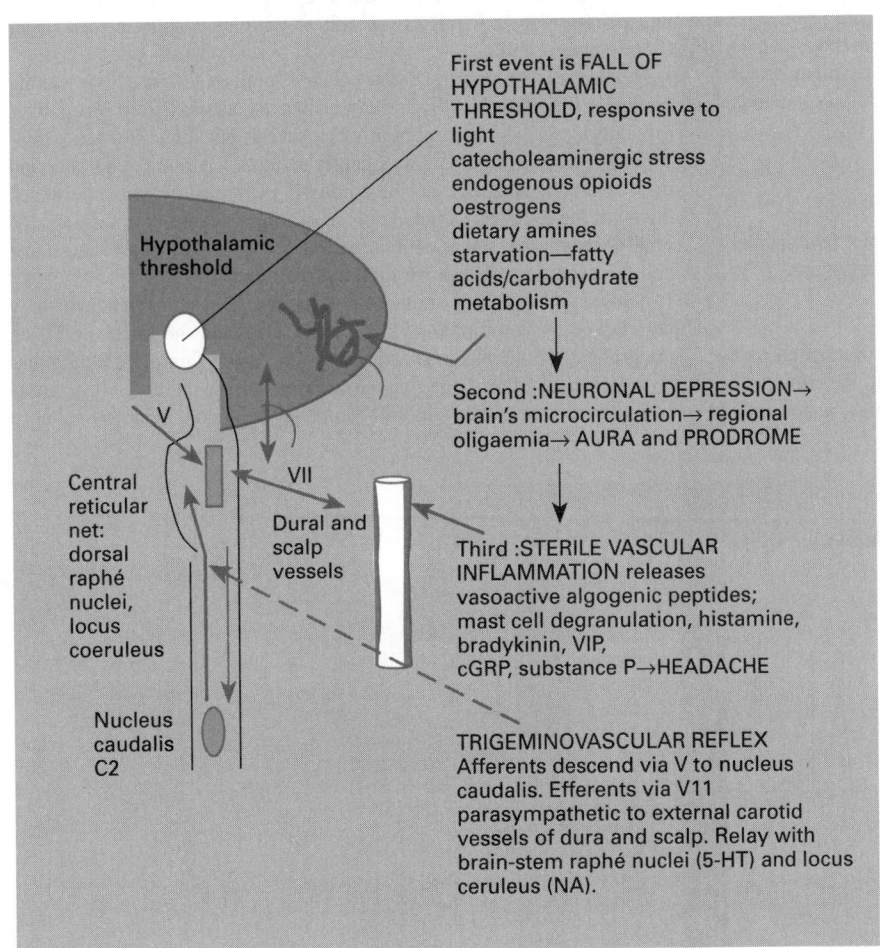

First event is FALL OF HYPOTHALAMIC THRESHOLD, responsive to light
catecholeaminergic stress
endogenous opioids
oestrogens
dietary amines
starvation—fatty acids/carbohydrate metabolism

Second :NEURONAL DEPRESSION→ brain's microcirculation→ regional oligaemia→ AURA and PRODROME

Third :STERILE VASCULAR INFLAMMATION releases vasoactive algogenic peptides; mast cell degranulation, histamine, bradykinin, VIP, cGRP, substance P→HEADACHE

TRIGEMINOVASCULAR REFLEX Afferents descend via V to nucleus caudalis. Efferents via V11 parasympathetic to external carotid vessels of dura and scalp. Relay with brain-stem raphé nuclei (5-HT) and locus ceruleus (NA).

Hypothalamic threshold

Central reticular net: dorsal raphé nuclei, locus coeruleus

Nucleus caudalis C2

Dural and scalp vessels

V

VII

Fig. 1 Hypothetical mechanism of classical migraine.

sinuses. 5-Hydroxytryptamine ($5HT_1$) agonists (ergotamine, sumatriptan) bind to receptors and constrict dural and pial vessels and impede plasma extravasation. The prejunctional action of 5HT receptors on trigeminovascular axons mediates the antimigraine effects of ergot and sumatriptan.

However, the initiating stimulus, or cause of the attack, is not always evident, and the importance of the trigeminovascular reflex remains unclear.

Migraine

DEFINITION

Classic migraine: synonym migraine with aura (20 per cent of patients)

This is a paroxysmal disorder with headaches, often unilateral at the onset, associated with nausea, anorexia, and often vomiting; it is preceded or accompanied by visual, sensory, motor, or mood disturbances, and is often familial.

Common migraine: synonym migraine without aura (75 per cent of patients)

This refers to similar paroxysmal headaches without the aura. Both types of attack may occur at various times in the same patient.

It is common for migraine sufferers to have tension headaches between their migraines: these should be identified to prevent misdirected treatment.

Migraine variants

Occur in 5 per cent of patients.

PREVALENCE

Migraine is common, affecting approximately 20 per cent of women and 15 per cent of men at some time in their lives. However, many attacks are not incapacitating, and half the sufferers may never seek medical attention.

CLINICAL FEATURES

The frequency of attacks varies from 1 to 2/week to a few sparsely scattered over a lifetime. Daily headaches are never migrainous.

Childhood

The earliest attacks are before the age of 10 years in a third of patients. These may be missed if the child is unable (clearly) to describe headaches and strange visual and sensory experiences; or may be concealed by labels of 'bilious attacks', 'periodic syndrome', or 'acidosis'. Affected children may simply appear pale, ill, limp, and inert, complaining of ill-localized abdominal pain. Headache is usually present, vomiting is common, and there may be a fever of up to 38.5 °C. Mesenteric adenitis and appendicitis are important considerations, although a past history of self-limiting episodes is a helpful pointer to abdominal migraine.

Adults

Over 80 per cent of migraineurs have their first attacks before the age of 30 years, and the diagnosis should be viewed with suspicion in anyone over 40. Some subjects have only a few attacks in a lifetime; most have several attacks each year. Promises of remission at the menopause are often ill-founded, although attacks tend to lessen after the age of 50 years, when headache may disappear, leaving attacks of aura alone (Fig. 2). Remission occurs in 70 per cent of pregnancies. Exacerbation, or complicated migraine with infarction, may result from oral contraceptives.

The prodrome is of cerebral, probably hypothalamic origin. It refers to vague yawning, euphoria, unbridled energy, or depression and lethargy, sometimes with craving or distaste for various foods, in the 24 h before the headache.

The aura is usually visual. Flashing lights, zig-zag castellations, balls, or filaments of light may start peripherally and spread centripetally, or centrally spreading centrifugally. Fragmentation, jig-saw appearances, with or without central scotomata (like frosted glass), micropsia, and metamorphopsia (Alice in Wonderland syndrome) are common. Vague blurring is not migrainous. Aurae typically last 30 min and are succeeded by headache. Attacks may start with numbness and tingling of one or both hands, or of the face, lips, and tongue. The spread of paraesthesiae is slow over many minutes and should not be confused with the more rapid march of jacksonian epilepsy. Weakness, clumsiness, and occasionally a hemiparesis with or without dysphasia may occur (hemiplegic migraine).

Headache is commonly, but not always, unilateral. It starts on waking or during the day, but less often can waken victims from sleep. It is typically described as throbbing or pulsating, but there is often a nonspecific dull ache, and not infrequently patients complain of a tight band or pressure. This should not be confused with tension headache which does not have the paroxysmal course of migraine and is not associated with photophobia, phonophobia, neurological aura of classic migraine, and the accompanying prostration and vomiting.

Nausea and vomiting often occur at the height of pain. Headache may be relieved by vomiting, and sleep often terminates headache and is an integral part of the attack. Diarrhoea, chills, pallor, faintness, fluid retention, and, rarely, facial bruising may complicate the picture. All vigorous activities are shunned; light and sound aggravate the symptoms, hence

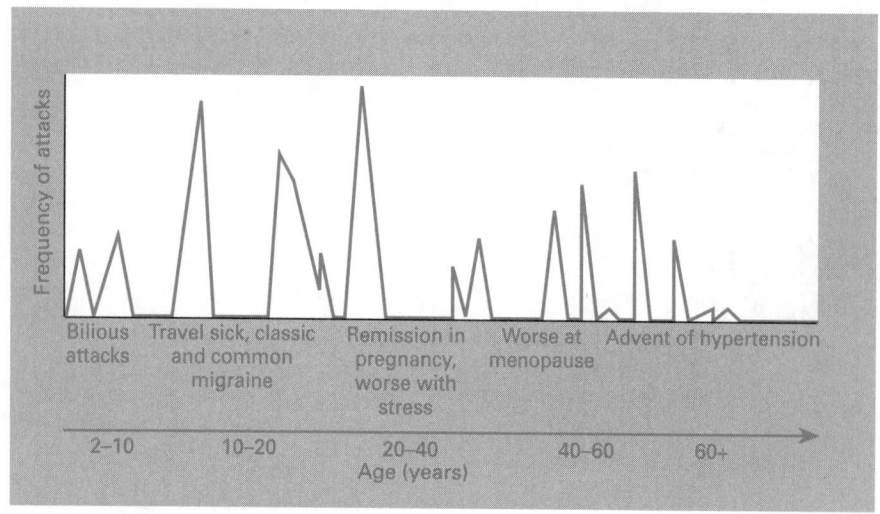

Fig. 2 Scheme of life pattern of attacks of migraine.

the retreat to bed in a dark room. Many attacks end gradually after 24 to 48 h, but attacks in children often last only 2 to 6 h.

Attacks may worsen in menopausal women, but generally the frequency and intensity of headaches diminish after middle age. The headache may disappear completely, attacks presenting with teichopsiae and no headache ('migraine sine cephalgia'). The mechanism is uncertain. Indeed, the apparent onset of migraine in the elderly implies atherosclerotic, thromboembolic disease.

AETIOLOGY

The phasic pattern and diversity of precipitating agents (Table 2) support the notion of a cerebral rather than a primary vascular disorder. Genetic factors operate in 70 per cent of patients, but there is no simple mendelian pattern. Distended scalp and intracranial dural arteries with increased pulsation and the release of vasoactive pain-producing peptides are related to the pain. Cerebral symptoms of the aura may be initiated by depression of neuronal activity (theory of Leão) with secondary spreading regional oligaemia (Fig. 2).

Food idiosyncrasies, food allergies, red wines, specific dietary amines (for example, tyramine) and omission of food are occasional precipitants but not causes. Remissions in 70 per cent of pregnancies and aggravation by menstruation and oral contraceptives tell of the ill-understood but important role of hormonal factors. Worsening by emotional stress and fatigue is the most important aggravating factor but is not causal. Serotonin derived from platelets is depleted in the aura; other biochemical anomalies of opioids, prostaglandins, and diverse peptides are reported, but provide no general explanation.

Migraine is determined by a primarily cerebral (neural) mechanism with a fluctuating threshold which determines the timing and pattern of attacks. A neural trigger activates the trigeminovascular reflex (see above) and releases vasogenic amines from blood vessel walls which cause painful, pulsatile distension.

The cerebral mechanism is responsive to mood, emotions, tiredness, relaxation, and hormonal changes, as well as to peripheral stimuli, such as bright lights, noise, and possibly atmospheric changes. Its threshold is susceptible to hypothalamic function which, in turn, is modulated by seasonal patterns, diurnal and biological clocks, and by hormonal factors—seen in the worsening when the subject is on oral contraceptives and the remission in pregnancy in many patients.

Personality and variations of mood and behaviour also reflect and influence the pattern of attacks and remissions.

TREATMENT

Assessment of the patient's habits, work, personality, and stresses is important. Known precipitants should be sought, if necessary with the aid of a diary, and should be eliminated when possible (Table 2). The patient's recognition of stressful patterns and the acceptance of an essentially benign disorder will achieve some benefit. Good rapport enhances reassurance and facilitates the marked placebo effect of all therapy which often confounds the analysis of drug trials.

Symptomatic treatment

This is offered for individual attacks (Table 3). Rest, dark, and quiet, where practicable, are supplemented by simple analgesics (paracetamol 1 g, or aspirin 0.6 g) or non-steroidal anti-inflammatory drugs, such as naproxen, 500 mg. The addition of caffeine and spasmolytics add to expense but not to benefit. Codeine, 15 to 30 mg, may enhance pain relief. Analgesics should be taken immediately the attack begins, then repeated 4 to 6 hourly as needed. Absorption is improved by taking aspirin or paracetamol with, or 10 min after, metoclopramide (10 mg) or domperidone (10 to 20 mg). These drugs are useful both in relieving gastric stasis and as antiemetics. If vomiting is severe, suppositories of domperidone, prochlorperazine, or chlorpromazine are valuable. Ergotamine is effective in 50 per cent of cases, but is badly absorbed orally and should be given by suppository or by inhalation (Medihaler-Ergo-

Table 2 *Common migraine precipitants*

Anxiety
Relaxation after stress
Exercise (especially football)
Change in sleep pattern
Bright lights
Fasting (missing a meal)
Alcohol
Specific food intolerance
Oral contraceptives
Menstruation

tamine®, 0.36 mg/puff). If a single dose does not work, it should not be repeated. Ergotamine has no place as a prophylactic and when overused leads to habituation with ergotamine-induced headache. This can be confused with migraine status; when suspected, ergotamine should be withdrawn.

Sumatriptan is a selective 5HT₁ agonist (similar to ergotamine) causing vasoconstriction and reduced plasma extravasation in dural vessels. A dose of 6 mg subcutaneously or 100 mg orally provides prompt and effective relief of all symptoms in 60 to 70 per cent of patients, but headache rebounds in one-third of patients. This expensive treatment can be repeated.

Such symptomatic measures improve rather than cure most attacks; demands for injections of opioid analgesics should be resisted.

Prophylaxis

Prophylaxis should be attempted if attacks occur more often than twice each month. Acupuncture, hypnosis, and biofeedback techniques are successful in certain subjects, but claims for their general application should be viewed with scepticism. Prophylactics aim to reduce the frequency, but none is a panacea. In patients with exacerbations related to stress or anxiety, amitriptyline, 50 to 100 mg at night introduced gradually, is often effective. Which of its actions—sedative, antidepressant, antiserotoninergic, or calcium-channel blockade—is implicated is not known. Propranolol, atenolol, and metoprolol give adequate reduction in about 60 per cent of cases, and are most effective in the tense or hypertensive subject with tachycardia and overt physical signs of autonomic 'overdrive'. Their action depends on upregulation of other receptors coupled to intracellular messengers, reflex vasoconstriction, reduced sympathetic outflow, membrane stabilizing action, and reduced platelet activation releasing serotonin.

Serotonin (5HT) inhibitors are valuable in 60 to 70 per cent of patients. Cyproheptadine, 4 mg three times a day, inhibits calcium channels and serotonin and histamine activity. Pizotifen, 0.5 mg three times a day or 1.5 mg at night, is moderately effective and free of hazards other than sedation and weight gain. Methysergide, 1 to 2 mg three times a day, is the most potent of this group but should be used only under hospital supervision in courses not exceeding 3 to 4 months. Pleural, pericardial, and retroperitoneal fibrosis are rare but serious side-effects which may result from more prolonged use; they usually regress when the drug is stopped. Myocardial and peripheral vascular ischaemia are uncommon complications. Calcium antagonists (Flunnarizine*, verapamil) and sodium valproate have been established as useful prophylactics in recent trials.

Menstrual migraine

Migraine occurring exclusively with menstruation is uncommon, but may be relieved by oestrogen patches or implants. Migraine, between menstrual periods but worse with menstruation, is common (35 per cent) but usually resistant to diuretics and hormonal manipulation.

---

* Flunnarizine is not marketed in the United Kingdom, but is widely available in the United States and Europe.

Table 3 *Treatment of migraine*

Avoid	Prophylactic*	Symptomatic

Physical factors
  Bright light
  Fasting
  Fatigue
  Irregular sleep
Dietary
  Individual precipitants
  ?Tyramine (e.g. cheese)
  ?Phenylethylamine (e.g. chocolate)
  Alcohol
    Sodium nitrate
  Monosodium glutamate
	Cyproheptadine, pizotifen, propranolol,
	    methysergide, amitryptiline
		Oral
		  Aspirin or paracetamol with metoclopramide,
		    sumatriptan
		Rectal
		  Suppository ergotamine, suppository
		    chlorpromazine
		Inhalation
		  'Medihaler' ergotamine
		Intramuscular[d]
		  Codeine, chlorpromazine, or prochlorperazine

* If migraine frequency is greater than twice a month.

[d] Very rarely needed.

Cluster headache

(Synonyms: migrainous neuralgia, Harris's syndrome, Horton's syndrome.)

CLINICAL FEATURES

This is a distinctive clinical syndrome separable from migraine, which predominantly affects men (10:1). It begins at any age, most often between 20 and 50 years, and is characterized by daily bouts of unilateral headache of great severity lasting 30 to 120 min. The brevity, severity, lack of aura and vomiting, occurring daily in clusters lasting usually for 4 to 16 weeks clearly separate it from migraine. The pain is boring, aching, or stabbing and is centred on one orbit with radiation to the forehead, temple or cheek, and jaw ('lower-half headache'). It characteristically strikes at night, an hour or so after sleep, and may recur during the day, often at the same time ('alarm-clock headache').

In many cases the ipsilateral eye becomes red and bloodshot, watering profusely. The nostril may be blocked or may run. A transient Horner's syndrome is seen in 25 per cent of cases and occasionally this persists. Restlessness, crying, and head-banging betray the frightening severity of the pain, and, in contrast to migraine, most patients get out of bed and pace the floor, even taking nocturnal walks. Alcohol and other vasodilators are important precipitating factors: nitroglycerine has been used as a provocative test—a typical attack following within an hour of a sublingual 0.5 mg tablet. Clusters last for 1 to 4 months, although occasionally the condition continues for a year or more—chronic migrainous neuralgia. Remissions are complete but the clusters usually recur every year or two.

AETIOLOGY

The cause is unknown, and elevated blood histamine levels during attacks are of uncertain significance. Autonomic involvement is shown by the Horner's syndrome, and segmental mural oedema of the carotid syphon has been shown at angiography. Investigation is rarely necessary, since cluster headache in typical form is seldom symptomatic of other cranial lesions. The quality, timing, duration, and distribution of pain separate it from trigeminal neuralgia, migraine, and other cephalgias. There is no family history, and it is uncommon for a patient to have both migraine and cluster headache. There is an unexplained high incidence of peptic ulcer.

TREATMENT

The essence of treatment is prevention. During clusters ergotamine is given 1 hour in anticipation of daytime attacks, and just before getting into bed for nocturnal attacks. Suppositories are the most useful preparation. Control is excellent in 75 per cent of patients and the drug is stopped each Sunday to see if the cluster recurs; if so, ergotamine is continued for a further week, until the cluster ends. If ergot is unsuccessful, sumatriptan 100 mg orally, methysergide 1 to 2 mg three times a day, or verapamil 40 to 80 mg three times a day are useful alternatives. Oxygen 5 to 10 l/min for 10 min at the onset is effective, but β-blockers and pizotifen are not. Lithium can be used in the chronic variant if other methods fail. In intractable cases, a 'crash course' of corticosteroids may provide dramatic relief of symptoms.

Tension headache

(Synonym: muscle contraction headache.)

Tension headache is the most common of human complaints. It constitutes 70 per cent of referrals to a 'Headache Clinic' and in random samples of healthy subjects over 90 per cent volunteer one or more previous attacks of recognizable tension headache. In most instances it is a short-lived complaint with obvious preceding cause: overwork, lack of sleep, or an emotional crisis. This is entirely benign and is recognized by patients as 'normal headaches'.

Rarely, it can present in acute form as an emergency; the headache has usually built up over a few hours, but has become very severe. The patient looks ill, anxious, and pallid with tachycardia; the picture may simulate subarachnoid bleeding, especially if there is photophobia and a stiff neck. There are no other signs, the victim is afebrile, but lumbar puncture is occasionally necessary to exclude meningeal irritation by blood or infection. More often the emotional basis is obvious and recovery ensues quickly after reassurance, analgesia, and a brief period of sedation.

CHRONIC TENSION HEADACHE

The chronic is very much more common than the acute syndrome. It is encountered by physicians in all branches of clinical practice. The pain is diffusely felt all over the head. It is, however, often located on the vertex, or may start in the forehead or in the neck. Some patients describe several points of pain which they describe with a single finger, usually in both temples or over the crown. It may radiate over the glabella on to the bridge of the nose, or from the temples into the jaws. It is commonly bilateral, but there are cases where the pain is unilateral.

The quality of the pain is characteristic. Patients complain of a sense of pressure, a feeling of tightness or as if a heavy weight were pressing down on the crown. 'A tight band like a skullcap' or 'as if a clamp or vice was squeezing my head' are common descriptions. Some are at pains to relate 'it is not really a pain, but a pressure'. The symptoms may also seem to originate from inside the cranium: 'as if my head is bursting' or 'about to explode'. A 'creeping' sensation (formication) may be felt under the scalp, or a sense of sharp knives or needles driven in, burning hot, may be related by other patients.

Tension headache is a daily occurrence, in contrast to the periodic and paroxysmal attacks of migraine. It is worse as the day goes by, whereas migraine commonly presents on waking. Visual disturbance and vomiting do not occur, although nausea may accompany the pain.

Most patients continue their normal work during tension headache. Patients are not photophobic and confined to bed in a darkened room—as in migraine. Symptoms continue for months or years without evident deterioration of general health. They are worse when the victim is tired or under pressure at work, and in the face of personal or domestic stresses. Most sufferers have insight into these relationships so that a carefully taken history usually clarifies both the diagnosis and the relevant aggravating circumstances.

Clinical examination may appear to be superfluous in the face of such distinctive symptoms, but it is of great importance. Most patients are frightened, emotional, and anxious. They harbour fears of brain tumours, hypertension, and of 'clots in the brain'. A thorough examination is of the utmost therapeutic value and provides a rational basis for effective reassurance. It is my practice to enquire specifically about fears of serious brain disease, whether the fears are voiced by the patient or not. 'Television illnesses' are not infrequently 'contagious', as are those suffered by relatives and acquaintances; these too need careful appraisal.

TREATMENT

Treatment is most effective when the history is short. To cure such headaches after 10 or more years is a daunting and often unsuccessful task. The main step is to try to identify the events which determined the onset. These are often forgotten, or perhaps suppressed, yet repeated enquiry at subsequent consultations will often unravel the apparent mystery, the consequent knowledge being sufficient to explain the cause to the patient. No amount of superficial reassurance will eradicate tension headache if its origins are obscure and the complex psychological mechanisms deriving from the source are untreated. Similarly, sedatives, tranquillizers, and tension-relieving drugs will be of limited value unless the psychological aberration is adequately handled. When the history is short and if a cause is exposed, drugs are unnecessary if reassurance is adequate. In the common situation where daily pain has persisted for years, the prognosis is less predictable, but short courses of benzodiazepines for 4 weeks or amitriptyline may be helpful and will secure the occasional 'cure'.

Latent depression presenting as tension headache is easy to overlook. Early morning insomnia, negativism, guilt, and diurnal mood swings are suggestive. The headache is worse in the morning (resembling that of raised pressure), and a cause for the misery is often inapparent. Full doses of tricyclic antidepressants or fluoxetine, if necessary administered on an inpatient basis, are needed. The prognosis is good.

Headaches as a symptom of intracranial disease

Confronted by a patient with headaches, the major clinical responsibility is to exclude a structural or dynamic cause. Any expanding mass can cause headache.

CHARACTERISTICS OF RAISED-PRESSURE HEADACHE

Its location is non-specific, though when a progressive headache starts to involve the neck, tonsilar coning is imminent. The headache is:

(a) worse in the morning;
(b) aggravated by sitting up or standing, and relieved by lying down;
(c) aggravated by coughing, straining, and vomiting;
(d) relieved by aspirin or paracetamol in the early stages (in contrast to psychogenic headache);
(e) associated with vomiting and eventually by papilloedema and progressing focal signs. By the stage of stupor and hemiplegia with a dilated (Hutchinson's) pupil, diagnosis has been delayed too long.

Acute headache

Headaches of abrupt onset may signify trauma, spontaneous intracranial haemorrhage, hydrocephalus, or acute meningeal irritation at any age; the elderly are not immune. The most common cause is acute meningeal irritation due to subarachnoid haemorrhage or to meningitis—bacterial or viral (rarely fungal or malignant). An abrupt onset, fever, neck stiffness, and Kernig's sign accompany the obvious severe pain, vomiting, and photophobia. Cerebrospinal fluid examination is mandatory if infection is considered, provided that an abscess mass or haematoma have been first excluded.

Computed tomography (CT) (or magnetic resonance imaging (MRI)) scan is usually the first investigation to exclude a mass lesion, haematoma, or hydrocephalus, each of which precludes lumbar puncture. Subarachnoid haemorrhage may be shown, but can be missed by CT in up to 20 per cent of patients on admission. When a mass lesion is excluded, lumbar puncture may be necessary to examine the cerebrospinal fluid for subarachnoid bleeding and meningitis. Acute migraine and tension headache can rarely produce a meningitic picture, diagnosable by exclusion.

Acute headache should be distinguished from the common and totally benign 'exploding head syndrome' in which patients are alarmed by a sudden, momentary, very loud noise in the twilight stage of sleep. Acute headache, sometimes severe, and lasting between 30 min and 24 h, may occur with sexual orgasm—'coital cephalgia'. It has a male to female ratio of 5.4:1 and there is a history of migraine in 47 per cent of cases. It recurs with intercourse for several months. Propranolol (40–80 mg) before intercourse is effective, and can be withdrawn after a month's freedom from the symptom.

Atypical facial pain

This label conceals a number of cases with chronic face-ache whose cause we do not understand. If the history is taken cursorily, they are often mistaken for the distinctive trigeminal neuralgia. Patients present a characteristic and clinically recognizable pattern. They are mostly women aged between 30 and 50 years, with a dull constant aching pain in one, or both cheeks. It has no trigger factors, but is worse with fatigue and under mental duress. It is continuous, although often sparing sleep, and may radiate into the ear, forehead, and jaw. There are no physical signs, and often there is no overt evidence of depression. Occasionally the onset can be related to some grave personal hurt or Freudian 'slap in the face'. With reassurance and a prolonged course of tricyclic drugs or monoamine-oxidase inhibitors many patients obtain lasting relief.

TEMPOROMANDIBULAR PAIN

Although patients with rheumatoid and osteoarthritic changes on radiographs of their temporomandibular joints commonly have no pain, myofascial pain dysfunction is a common cause of complaint in young adults. Modern opinion tends to discount overclosure of the joint or malocclusion, but favours a neuromuscular dysfunction causing spasm and fatigue of masticatory muscles. The importance of misplaced portions of the articular cartilage shown on CT and MRI is uncertain. The syndrome is of aching in front of the ear, worse with jaw opening and accompanied by clicks and clunks—signs not uncommon in asymptomatic people. The quality and relation of pain to chewing and jaw opening distinguish it from trigeminal neuralgia (Chapter 24.3.6); radiographs exclude sinus disease and neoplasm. Anxiety and latent depression are important factors, but despite extensive investigation, treatment is based on reassurance and symptomatic analgesia. Many remit spontaneously and after a decade of study, one expert's view is 'the best therapy . . . in most cases appears to be the least'. None the less, correction of a gross disorder of dental bite may be worthwhile; a trial injection of steroids and lignocaine, 2 per cent, into the joint, will afford striking relief in some patients. A course of tricyclics such as amitriptyline can provide substantial benefit in some sufferers.

Post-traumatic headache

Headache following injury is a common complaint. In most circumstances a knock on the head will cause local bruising and abrasions no different from those resulting from a kick on the shin; local pain subsides in a few days without sequelae. The emotional vulnerability of the head and the common recourse to medicolegal compensation complicate both symptoms and mechanisms. Many victims of severe head injury, with post-traumatic amnesia of 24 h or more wake up with no headache. Similarly, the headache of patients after major craniotomy seldom lasts more than 3 to 7 days. The commonest complaints are heard from those with minor injury, often without loss of consciousness.

Minor head injuries are those with: a loss of consciousness lasting less than 20 min; Glasgow coma scale 13 to 18 (see Chapter 24.4.4; and a stay in hospital of less than 48 h.

The crucial importance of strict definition is emphasized by the vague and often subjective complaints of plaintiffs. Their genuine nature has been supported by claims of cognitive deficits present in even the mildly injured with brief unconsciousness and post-traumatic amnesia. In contrast, there is clear evidence that the majority of such cases leave hospital within a few days, have no organic signs, recover quickly, and return to work without further complaints. This is particularly true of those suffering injury during contact sports, many victims continuing the game, or returning to normal activities the next day without ill effect.

Assessment of symptoms and disability: the post-traumatic syndrome

The main concern of physicians is the assessment of the significance of symptoms and disability (Table 4). Headaches persist without accompanying neurological signs, but often with a collection of intrinsically subjective symptoms often referred to as the post-traumatic syndrome.

The complaints are forgetfulness, irritability, slowness, poor concentration, fatigue, dizziness (usually not vertigo), somnolence, intolerance of alcohol, light and noise, loss of initiative, depression, anxiety, loss of interests, and impaired libido. The number of complaints is often inversely related to the severity of the injury.

The failure of doctors to provide complete reassurance shortly after injury is important in determining patients' fears of brain damage or subdural haematoma; it may also delay return to work and induce morbid anxiety. Headaches are either localized to the site of trauma, often with local scalp tenderness, or, like tension headaches, are diffuse, aching or tight and heavy. They are resistant to analgesics, and investigations in these patients are unwarranted and unrevealing. Anxieties, phobias, loss of self-esteem, resentment, and depression are genuine accompanying features in some cases, and serve to induce or to aggravate headache. Deliberate exaggeration or malingering in other cases is motivated by the quest of financial gain. In litigants there is great pressure from Union officials and legal advisers, which together with the common delay in legal settlement contrive to prolong and exaggerate the symptoms. Headaches generally improve when the patient returns to normal work, and often, although not invariably, disappear when satisfactory settlement is attained.

Headache in the elderly

In addition to the causes of headache already discussed, certain syndromes feature more prominently in the middle-aged and elderly, although age is not a diagnostic barrier.

CERVICOGENIC HEADACHE

Cervicogenic headache refers to head pain referred from cervical spondylosis (see Chapter 24.3.11). It is undoubtedly common, with pain on one or both sides of the neck radiating to the occiput, but also to the temples and frontal region. It may be a dull 'toothache' pain, worse in the morning when the neck has been badly positioned at an angle on misplaced high pillows during sleep. It may last throughout the day and

Table 4 *Assessment of symptoms and disability following head injury*

1. Initial pain, suffering, loss of work
2. Estimate of severity: hospital attendance and treatment
3. Persisting organic symptoms
4. Persisting psychological symptoms
5. Disability related to:
   (a) Work prospects and capability
   (b) Domestic activities
   (c) Quality of life
   (d) Loss of earnings

be aggravated by neck movement. It is a rather nondescript pain, with no accompanying vomiting and no physical signs other than marked restriction of lateral flexion and rotation of the neck. Such signs are common, however, in those without headache, and thus are of limited value. Vague and intermittent symptoms of tinnitus, dizziness, and visual disturbance are sometimes attributed to compression of the vertebral arteries traversing the foramina transversaria, but this is unproven speculation. It is probable that the pain arises from the posterior zygapophyseal joints and related ligaments as the result of osteophytes; irritation of the C2 nerve root or of the greater occipital nerves are important contributory factors which may respond well to local injection of lignocaine and hydrocortisone. Immobilization in a collar is often used but seldom very effective. Manipulation endangers the vertebral arteries and is contraindicated.

GIANT-CELL ARTERITIS (SEE ALSO SECTION 18)

(Synonyms: cranial or temporal arteritis)

This condition, rarely seen under the age of 60 years, is important as an eminently treatable cause of headache, but also as a preventable cause of blindness and strokes. Headache is generalized or may be sited over an engorged, reddened tender superficial temporal or occipital artery. It is aching, throbbing, or felt as sharp stabs of pain, often worse at night. The history is usually short (of a few weeks' duration); the patient is unwell with muscle aches and pains in the shoulder and pelvic girdle muscles (polymyalgia rheumatica) and there may be fever, sweats, and masseter claudication (see Section 18). Visual involvement (50 per cent of patients) is due to an ischaemic optic neuropathy which presents with unilateral blindness or with a branch retinal occlusion. It is irreversible. Posterior cerebral artery lesions cause a hemianopia.

Ophthalmoplegia is due to ischaemic lesions in the third, fourth, or sixth cranial nerves, and diplopia may be the presenting sign, before the onset of headache and malaise: hence the importance of early diagnosis. The disease also affects the vertebral arteries, and less often the carotids, and may present as a stroke or transient ischaemic attack. Some have a normochronic anaemia and one-third of patients have antineutrophil cytoplasmic antibodies (ANCA). Cytotoxic eosinophil granule proteins may contribute to the necrotic lesions and the development of thrombi. Every elderly subject with recent headaches should be suspected of harbouring this condition. Serial erythrocyte sedimentation rates (usually 80–120 mm/h) supplemented by an adequate biopsy of the clinically affected scalp vessel, which should be serially sectioned, will prove the diagnosis. Biopsy is indicated in the uncertain case with a borderline erythrocyte sedimentation rate or plasma viscosity of 30 to 50 mm/h. Steroid therapy will avert blindness in almost every case, and should be started immediately the patient is seen and the erythrocyte sedimentation rate or plasma viscosity taken. It does not affect biopsy changes for at least 48 h. The initial dose of 60 mg prednisolone is quickly reduced as symptoms abate and the erythrocyte sedimentation rate or plasma viscosity falls; the maintenance dose of 5 to 10 mg/day is usually reached within a month or two and is governed by clinical progress and erythrocyte sedimentation rate measurements. Late relapses are common and treatment is continued for many years, with very gradual reductions by 1 mg per month only when the patient and the ESR have been normal for over 2 years. In many, small doses are necessary for life, as proved by relapse when the dose of prednisolone is reduced.

Atypical presentations which should prompt assiduous investigation include: (1) patients with minimal headache; (2) an initially normal erythrocyte sedimentation rate; (3) fever of unknown origin; (4) psychiatric symptoms of hallucinations, depression, and 'confusional states'; and (5) isolated third or sixth nerve palsy.

HYPNIC HEADACHE

This is a curious headache, seen mainly in the over 60s. Patients are woken by pulsating headache, sometimes accompanied by nausea, at the same time, one to three times each night. This occurs most nights, lasts about 30 min and may coincide with REM sleep. But it differs from chronic cluster headache in the respect of age, generalized location, and absence of autonomic features. There are no physical signs and the disorder is benign. The response to lithium, 300 mg at night, is often spectacular.

REFERENCES

Cawson, R.A. (1984). Pain in the temporomandibular joint. *British Medical Journal* **2**, 1857–8.

Dalessio, D.J. (ed.) (1993). *Wolff's headache and other head pains* (6th edn). Oxford University Press.

Feinmann, C., Harris, M., and Cawley, R. (1984). Psychogenic facial pain: presentation and treatment. *British Medical Journal* **288**, 436–8.

Hall, S., *et al.* (1983). The therapeutic impact of temporal artery biopsy. *Lancet* **2**, 1217–20.

Hopkins, A. (1988). *Headache. Problems in diagnosis and management.* Saunders, London.

Lance, J.W. (1993). *Mechanism and management of headache* (5th edn). Butterworth-Heinemann, Oxford.

Lance, J.W. (1991). Migraine. In *Clinical neurology*, (ed. M. Swash and J. Oxbury), Vol. **1**, pp. 336–50. Churchill Livingstone, Edinburgh.

Leading article, (1982). Classification of headache. *Lancet* **2**, 1318.

Merskey, H. (1982). Pain and emotion: their correlation in headache. *Advances in Neurology* **33**, 135–43.

Pearce, J.M.S. (1984). Migraine: a cerebral disorder. *Lancet* **2**, 86–9.

Pearce, J.M.S. (1987). Neural aspects of migraine. In *Migraine*, (ed. J.N. Blau), pp. 247–65. Chapman Hall, London.

Pearce, J.M.S. (1991). Tension Headache. In *Clinical neurology*, (ed. M. Swash and J. Oxbury), Vol. **1**, pp. 331–6. Churchill Livingstone, Edinburgh.

Pearce, J.M.S. (1992). Headaches. *Medicine International* **98**, 4086–91.

Pearce, J.M.S. (1994). Headache. *Journal of Neurology, Neurosurgery and Psychiatry*, **57**, 134–44.

Sacks, O. (1991). *Migraine, evolution of a common disorder*, (2nd edn). Faber and Faber, London.

24.12 Intracranial tumours

P. J. TEDDY

Introduction

As in all other parts of the body, intracranial tumours may be benign or malignant, primary or secondary. However, perhaps more than at any other site, management of tumours within the cranial cavity is influenced as much by their exact location and by the potential adverse effects of treatment on surrounding normal tissue as by the degree of malignancy of the neoplasm itself. Most primary tumours of the brain in adults occur above the tentorium cerebelli and must be considered generally to be malignant. The intracranial tumours of childhood differ considerably from the adult forms in terms of distribution within the brain, histological characteristics, and prognosis.

Incidence and distribution

Autopsy findings suggest that intracranial tumours comprise approximately 8 per cent of all primary neoplasms. The annual incidence in the United Kingdom is about 5 per 100 000 of population. Metastatic lesions account for about 25 per cent of all intracranial tumours found at autopsy. In children the central nervous system is the second most common site for primary tumours and about 70 per cent of childhood intracranial neoplasms are infratentorial. Intracranial tumours represent the sixth most common form of neoplasm in adults, of which 70 per cent occur above the tentorium. Cerebral gliomas rarely occur in the first two decades of life but the incidence then steadily increases. They are twice as common in males as in females. Meningiomas and schwannomas occur mainly in women and are rare in childhood. Medulloblastoma, cerebellar astrocytoma, and true pineal tumours occur mainly in childhood. There appears to be an increased incidence of craniopharyngioma and pineal germinoma in Japan, ependymoma in India, and medulloblastoma in Europe and North America. Otherwise, geographical distribution of intracranial tumours is probably even throughout the world.

Aetiology and associated lesions

It has been estimated that the risk of developing an intracranial tumour of any type is marginally greater in close relatives of patients with known cerebral gliomas. There have also been occasional reports of families having a high incidence of various intracranial tumours but no clear-cut pattern of inheritance of the development of isolated intracranial neoplasm has been demonstrated. Von Recklinghausen's disease (neurofibromatosis) is associated with optic and hypothalamic glioma, schwannomas of various cranial nerves, most commonly the eighth, and intracranial meningiomas. Tuberose sclerosis is associated with periventricular glioma, and von Hippel–Lindau disease with cerebellar haemangioblastoma which have a tendency to recur. Earlier beliefs that head injury or glial scarring increased the risk of glioma have not been substantiated, but meningiomas have occasionally been reported as occurring directly below the site of focal injury to the skull. Transplant and other patients receiving immunosuppressive therapy have been shown to have an increased risk of intracranial lymphoreticular neoplasms. Some patients have been shown to develop local meningiosarcoma or glioma following local irradiation of the scalp for ringworm or high-dose irradiation for pituitary neoplasms.

Pathology

Primary intracranial tumours may be derived from the skull itself, from any of the structures lying within it, or from their tissue precursors. They may be divided into tumours of neurectodermal origin (derived from the neural tube, neural crest, and ectoderm) and those of other cell types (see Table 1). It is better to avoid assessing malignancy of primary intracranial tumours on histological grounds alone or on their propensity to metastasize outside the CNS. Primary tumours may involve almost all parts of the brain, are not limited by sulci, and may cross the midline

Table 1 *Classification of intracranial tumours*

Tumour type	Cells/site of origin	Cellular precursor	Site of predilection
Astrocytoma	Astrocytes	Neural tube	Cerebral hemisphere, cerebellum, brain-stem, optic pathways
Glioblastoma	Astrocytes		Cerebral hemisphere
Oligodendroglioma	Oligodendrocytes		Cerebral hemisphere
Ependymoma	Ependymal cells	Neural tube	Lateral and IV ventricle
Colloid cyst			III ventricle
Choroid plexus papilloma			Lateral and IV ventricle
Medulloblastoma	Neurones	Neural tube	IV ventricle, cerebellar vermis
Ganglioneuroma			
Ganglioglioma			
Pinealoma	Pinealcytes	Neural tube	Pineal gland
Pineoblastoma			
Neurofibroma		Neural crest	Cranial nerves
Schwannoma	Schwanna cells		VIII and V nerves
Meningioma	Arachnoid cap cells		Dural surface, ventricles
Craniopharyngioma	Epithelial cells	Ectoderm	Hypothalamus, III ventricle
Cholesteatoma			
Chordoma		Notochord	Clivus
Germinoma	Germ cells		Pineal gland
Teratoma		Germinal layers	Pineal gland
Microglia	Uncertain		Cerebral hemisphere
Sarcoma	Connective tissue		Meninges
Glomus tumour	Glomus jugulare		Glomus jugulare
Pituitary adenoma	Adenohypophyseal cells		Pituitary gland
Haemangioblastoma	Uncertain	?Vascular	Cerebellum
Secondary tumours	Bronchus, breast, kidney, thyroid, melanoma, large bowel, leukaemia, lymphoma		Cerebral hemisphere, cerebellum, meninges
Tumours of the skull	Cholesteatoma, osteoma, chordoma, osteoblastoma, bone cysts, myeloma, oesteosarcoma Secondary tumours		
	Nasopharynx, breast, prostate, bronchus, thyroid		

in corpus callosum, hypothalamic, or thalamic regions. Equally, however, histologically benign lesions may involve vital structures, rendering tumour management much more difficult than some of their more malignant counterparts. Histologically low-grade gliomas may undergo rapid and frank malignant change after many years of slow progression. Metastases outside the CNS from primary tumours are rare but do occur, particularly with medulloblastoma. Widespread dissemination through the brain and spinal cord is seen in cases of medulloblastoma, ependymoma, and pineal germinoma. The spread occurs along the pial or ependymal surfaces or through the cerebrospinal fluid. Leukaemic or carcinomatous deposits on the meninges may also disseminate widely through the cerebrospinal fluid pathways (see Section 22).

An estimate of degree of malignancy of neurectodermal tumours is often made by histological grading such as in the Kernohan or WHO scales (see below). This differentiation is at best an approximation as the tumours may be extremely heterogeneous and tissue sampling made by very limited biopsy. An estimate of malignant propensity and growth rate of the tumour may often be made more accurately by observing the clinical progress of the patient. A comprehensive list of intracranial tumours, together with their cells of origin, is given in Table 1 and the classification and frequency of occurrence of the more common intracranial tumours in Table 2. Note that although the term 'glioma' may be used loosely to describe all tumours derived from neural tube, and

particularly those of glial cell, origin (astrocytes, oligodendrocytes, and ependyma), its everyday use is usually confined to tumours of astrocytic origin, i.e. astrocytoma and glioblastoma.

ASTROCYTOMAS

These are the most common primary intracranial tumours. They are derived from the supportive astrocytic framework of the brain. They were commonly graded between I and IV in terms of malignancy but this scheme has now been replaced by the WHO histological typing of tumours of the central nervous system (1993). They are now classified as being either astrocytoma, anaplastic astrocytoma, or glioblastoma, on a scale of increasing malignant tendency. This new classification has a far better correlation with survival than the old grading system and distinction among the three groups is histologically firm, depending on the presence of mitoses, endothelial cell hyperplasia, and necrosis. Supratentorial astrocytomas in children have been thought to be more benign than their adult counterparts, but recent evidence suggests that this is not the case. The benign astrocytomas of childhood arise in either the optic nerve or chaisam, the hypothalamus, or the cerebellum. Within the cerebellum they are generally cystic and the cyst wall contains a well-circumscribed solid component of variable size. The solid part of the tumour secretes a yellowish glairy cyst fluid. Such lesions are usually

Table 2 *Incidence of commoner intracranial tumours*

Tumour	Overall percentage incidence	Most common ages of presentation
Astrocytoma and glioblastoma (adults)	38	40–60 years
Astrocytoma (childhood)	Approximately 50 per cent of childhood primary intracranial tumours	6–12 years
Oligodendroglioma	3	30–60 years
Ependymoma	3	6–12 years, occasional in adults
Medulloblastoma	3	5–15 years, occasional in adults
Schwannoma	8	40–70 years
Meningioma	18.5	40–60 years
Craniopharyngioma	2	5–60 years, above half in children
Haemangioblastoma	9	10–20 years
Pituitary adenoma	10	Adult life
Metastatic	4, but 25 per cent of all intracranial tumours at autopsy	
Miscellaneous	1.5	

very slow-growing and curable by complete removal, although some are frankly malignant and show a tendency to recur. The so-called piloid astrocytomas which involve the optic pathways and hypothalamus are slowly growing but, because of their position, are difficult to remove.

Low-grade astrocytomas in the cerebral hemispheres in both adults and children may remain well circumscribed for many years or show only slowly progressive infiltration accompanied by few clinical symptoms. Some undergo patchy calcification but others undergo change to a more malignant form after long periods of apparent quiescence.

Malignant astrocytomas are seen in the brain-stem, usually of children and adolescents, and produce enlargement of the brain-stem itself ('megapons'). Disturbances of gait, conjugate gaze, and lower cranial nerves are common but, interestingly, obstructive hydrocephalus is usually a late complication.

In adults, malignant astrocytomas are found most frequently in the cerebral hemispheres. They are rapidly growing, diffusely infiltrating, and commonly undergo central necrosis. The most malignant forms are often designated glioblastoma multiforme. Malignant gliomas commonly induce considerable oedema in the surrounding 'reactive' brain (see Fig. 1).

OLIGODENDROGLIOMA

These are usually slow-growing tumours with a very long history (10–15 years) and occur almost invariably in adults. They may show patchy calcification. Eventually they tend to undergo differentiation to become indistinguishable from malignant astrocytoma. When the tumour abuts the ventricle it has a tendency to seed throughout the ventricular system, and when adjacent to the surface of the brain may spread over the pia.

EPENDYMOMAS

These are predominantly tumours of children or young adults and arise in the walls of the fourth or, less commonly, the lateral ventricle. They are occasionally malignant, when they may disseminate widely through cerebrospinal fluid pathways.

MEDULLOBLASTOMAS

These are highly malignant tumours, usually arising in the roof of the fourth ventricle and infiltrating locally into the cerebellar vermis. They occur most commonly in the first decade of life and rarely beyond the mid-teens. They have a tendency to metastasize, not only through the

cerebrospinal fluid pathways but also outside the CNS to involve bone, bone marrow, and lymph nodes. Theories have been advanced that widespread dissemination of ependymoma and medulloblastoma may occur after posterior fossa surgery and ventricular shunting, but the evidence for this is dubious.

PINEAL TUMOURS

Pineal and parapineal tumours are a mixed group and the natural history of the individual components is uncertain since surgical access to them is often limited or hazardous, and many have therefore been treated by a shunt procedure and irradiation without biopsy. The group includes teratomas, so-called pineal gliomas, true pinealomas, and germinomas, the latter being the most common form. Some teratomas are ectopic in that they develop in the floor of the third ventricle and spread to the

Fig. 1 Contrast CT scan, showing typical 'butterfly' malignant glioma (arrow A) spreading across midline in posterior corpus callosum. Note compression and displacement of the lateral ventricle (B).

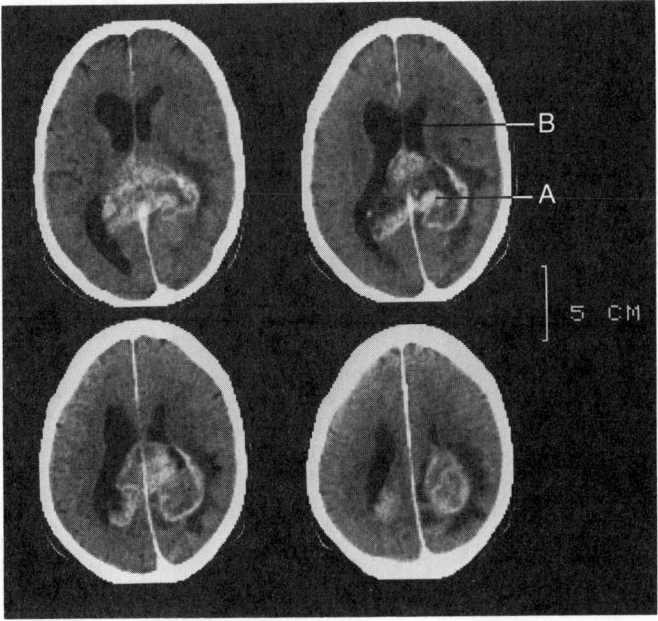

parapineal region. Pineal tumours quite often spread within cerebrospinal fluid pathways including the spinal canal. Histologically, germinomas resemble ovarian dysgerminoma and seminoma and have a marked preponderance in males.

SCHWANNOMAS

These lesions are derived from Schwann cells of the neural sheaths and are known as neurilemmomas and neurinomas as well as by the common misnomer of neuroma. They are benign and usually arise on the vestibular branch of the eighth nerve or less commonly on the trigeminal nerve, and rarely on the vagal group. They are usually very slow-growing but can reach an enormous size with consequent pressure effects on surrounding structures. Bilateral eighth nerve schwannomas have been found in association with von Recklinghausen's neurofibromatosis.

MENINGIOMAS

These tumours arise from the arachnoid covering the brain, particularly from the arachnoid villi, and are thus commonly found close to the major dural venous sinuses. They arise most often from the dura of the falx (parasagittal), the sphenoid wing, the convexity of the cerebral hemispheres, and from the olfactory nerve in the anterior fossa. However, they derive from any dural compartment and may be found on the tentorium, in the suprasellar region and even within the lateral ventricle. They are mainly adult tumours, occurring between the ages of 40 and 50 years, and are occasionally multiple. Most are benign but, incompletely removed, have a tendency to recur. Some are frankly malignant and recur rapidly even after apparently complete removal. Meningiosarcomas may form pulmonary metastases. Rare cases of meningioma occurring entirely outside the skull have been reported. One of the 'malignant' forms of vascular meningioma is a haemangiopericytoma (a type of tumour that also occurs elsewhere in the body with a tendency for recurrence, and ultimately metastasis).

Meningiomas tend to involve the skull close to the site of dural origin invoking a focal endostosis or occasionally an exostosis. Sometimes there will be osteal hypertrophy and sclerosis overlying the tumour and this is generally seen in the meningioma *en plaque* of the sphenoid wing. The form and consistency of meningiomas varies considerably. Microscopically they may be endothelioma-like masses comprising epithelial-like cells arranged in sheets or islands separated by vascular connective

Fig. 2 Contrast CT scan. Large bifrontal meningioma (A) with surrounding oedema (B).

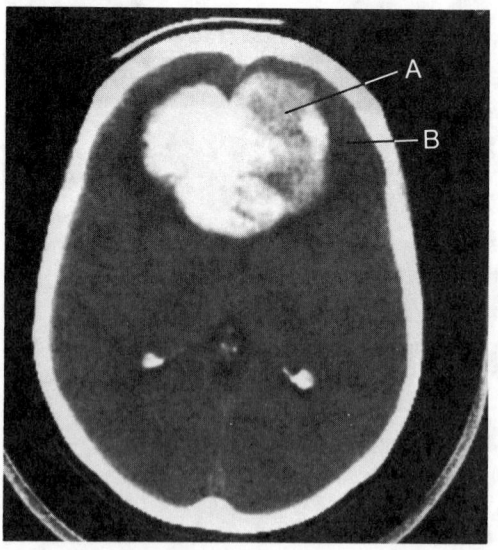

tissue trabeculae and forming whorls which are often hyalinized and calcified to form so-called psammoma bodies. Some present a more fibroblastic appearance. The more vascular tumours may produce erosion of the skull at the point of tumour attachment to the dura. Meningiomas are usually benign and slow-growing but may reach an enormous size before presentation, particularly when adjacent to relatively silent parts of the brain (Fig. 2). They tend to form a nest in the brain and have a relatively clear arachnoid plane between tumour capsule and surrounding cortex. The more indolent lesions may calcify or even ossify. Even when entirely benign, the position of some meningiomas makes them either inoperable or amenable only to partial excision. This is particularly true of those which involve the cavernous and sagittal sinuses or surround the proximal part of the internal carotid artery.

CRANIOPHARYNGIOMAS

These tumours, which are found both in adults and children, are formed of epithelial cell remnants in the region of the pituitary stalk. It was thought that they represented a persistent form of Rathke's pouch but this theory has been questioned. Although considered to be a congenital anomaly, they may grow extensively, causing compression of the optic nerves and chiasm, obstruction of the third ventricle with subsequent hydrocephalus, and may expand into the pituitary fossa with resultant hypopituitarism. They may even grow in a far more widespread manner towards the cavernous sinus, under the frontal and temporal lobes, and occasionally into the posterior fossa. About 50 per cent of craniopharyngiomas are calcified and may be identified on skull radiographs as speckled areas of calcification above the posterior clinoid process. A few tumours may be confined within the pituitary fossa itself. They may be wholly or partially cystic; the cyst contains fluid with many cholesterol crystals which have a typical shimmering appearance.

PITUITARY ADENOMAS (SEE ALSO SECTION 12)

These are the most common neoplasm of the pituitary gland and, although usually benign, they range in size from small growths entirely limited to the adenohypophysis to giant forms. They may have large suprasellar components, or extend laterally to involve the cavernous sinus or beyond into the basal cisterns and under the frontal and temporal lobes (invasive adenoma). Adenocarcinomas of the pituitary are extremely rare and resemble metastatic lesions.

Pituitary adenomas are divided into secreting and non-secreting tumours and, although the differentiation into chromophil and chromophobe adenomas still pertains, immunofluorescent techniques and electron microscopic studies are progressively changing classification in simple histological terms. The non-secretory adenomas comprise cells of variable size and morphology, ranged as simple masses or in a trabecular pattern. The secretory adenomas contain many types of cell dependent upon the cellular precursor from which they are derived. They may produce prolactin, growth hormone, and adrenocorticotrophic hormone. The abnormalities produced by the secretory tumours include Cushing's syndrome, acromegaly or gigantism, and hyperprolactinaemia. The non-secretory tumours may compress normal pituitary tissue and produce hypopituitarism.

Both non-secretory and secretory tumours may also produce effects through space occupation, the commonest sequel being compression of the optic chiasm from below. Occasionally the tumours can become big enough to occlude the third ventricle and produce an obstructive hydrocephalus.

COLLOID CYSTS

Colloid cysts occur in the third ventricle, always at its anterior end. They are rare tumours and occur predominantly in young adults. They are benign, probably arising from ependyma in the region of the tela choroidea. They comprise a capsule with an epithelial lining and usually contain glairy mucoid material with debris of desquamation. The cells lining the cyst sometimes have cilia. Although these masses may present slowly with evidence of progressive dementia or mental changes, they more often present with acute episodes of loss of consciousness. This is thought to be related to their acting intermittently as a ball valve with obstruction of the foramen of Munro. Occasionally they may be large enough to completely fill the third ventricle and even obstruct the entrance to the aqueduct.

CHOROID PLEXUS PAPILLOMAS

These frond-like tumours are usually benign and arise, predominantly in the first decade of life, in the lateral and fourth ventricles. Very occasionally they arise in the third ventricle. They may reach an enormous size (see Fig. 3) and produce symptoms by mass effect through obstructive hydrocephalus or by excessive secretion of cerebrospinal fluid. Occasionally they are malignant and may seed through the cerebrospinal fluid pathways. Even when benign, their rich vascularity may make surgical treatment extremely hazardous. Histologically they are papillary outgrowths identical with normal choroid plexus.

GANGLIONEUROMAS AND GANGLIOGLIOMAS

These are rare, well-circumscribed tumours occurring mainly in children and found predominantly in the floor of the third ventricle. They may contain a mixture of two cell types derived from both neuronal and astrocytic components surrounded by fibrous connective tissue, and they are often partially cystic. They are fairly indolent and tend not to recur if removal is complete.

CHOLESTEATOMAS

These are developmental inclusion lesions in which epithelial remnants are incorporated into deeper layers. They include epidermoid and dermoid cysts. The epidermoid cysts have a thin connective tissue capsule and contain material rich in cholesterol from the breakdown of keratin which is shed by the desquamating epithelial cells. Dermoid cysts may also contain follicles, sebaceous glands, and sweat glands. These rare tumours are found predominantly in the cerebellopontine angle and in the parasellar region. They have a tendency to recur, for whereas the contents of the cyst (pearly-white degenerative material) is easy enough to remove, the capsule is thin and adherent to many of the surrounding structures. Failure to remove the whole capsule results in further desquamation of cells and a gradual accumulation of the contents of the cyst.

CHORDOMAS

Chordomas arise from remnants of the primitive notochord. Intracranial chordomas arise therefore from the clivus and sella turcica. They contain clear cells surrounded by connective tissue trabeculae and are usually lobulated tumours. They may be locally invasive with bony erosion despite usually being benign. One of the chief problems in their treatment is their inaccessibility.

HAEMANGIOBLASTOMAS

These tumours are seen in older children and young adults and are most commonly found in the cerebellum. They constitute about 2 per cent of all intracranial tumours. Rarely, they are found within the medulla or above the tentorium. Most are single but they may be associated with retinal and renal or pancreatic cysts and occur in families—von Hippel–Lindau disease. Haemangioblastomas are occasionally solid but much more commonly cystic, containing a small mural nodule attached to the inner wall of the cyst (see Fig. 4). The cyst fluid is a golden-yellow colour and the solid nodule cherry red. The nodule contains multiple small capillaries, reticulin fibres, and clear cells. Their true origin is uncertain but they are commonly regarded as being vascular tumours. They are usually benign and the solitary lesions generally do not recur if complete removal is effected. The familial forms tend to recur more frequently. Occasionally, they are associated with ectopic erythropoietin production and polycythaemia (see Section 22).

GLOMUS JUGULARE TUMOURS

These are very rare neoplasms arising from the jugular body in the adventitia of the jugular bulb. The mass grows into the middle ear and may present as a pulsating vascular lesion at the external auditory meatus. In about half the cases growth is into the posterior fossa and presents as a cerebellopontine angle mass. The tumours are similar to those of the cartoid body with large clear cells in a connective tissue framework and a very rich vascular supply. They may secrete serotonin.

CEREBRAL LYMPHOMAS

Tumours originally identified as reticulum cell sarcoma and microglioma are now recognized as being lymphomas of the CNS; they may

Fig. 4 Contrast CT scan of posterior fossa. Solid nodule (A) within typical cyst cavity (B) of haemangioblastoma.

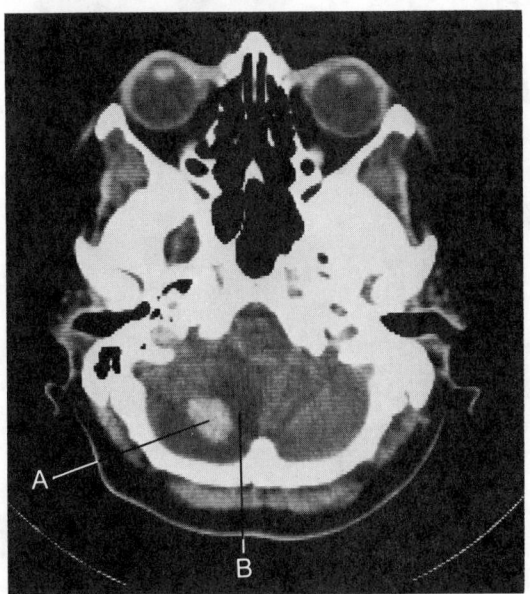

Fig. 3 Contrast CT scan, showing large choroid plexus papilloma in right lateral ventricle (A). Associated hydrocephalus (B).

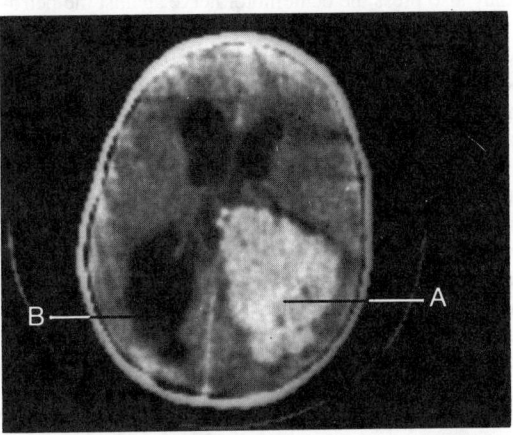

be primary or secondary. They are being identified more frequently and may occur in immunosuppressed patients. They may be indistinguishable from other forms of intracranial tumour on CT scan or MRI. This provides one very good reason for obtaining a histological diagnosis of tumours recognized on scans, even in cases where the prognosis seems gloomy.

True microglial cells in the brain are CNS representatives of the monocyte/phagocyte system and there is no known tumour representative of this system in the CNS.

Intracranial metastases

Although the incidence of secondary intracranial neoplasm is only about 4.5 per cent of all intracranial tumours in neurosurgical practice, these secondary tumours represent about 25 per cent of the total in autopsy studies. They may occur in the skull or involve any structure within the cranium. Although they most commonly occur in the cerebral hemispheres or cerebellum, the brain-stem, meninges, or cranial nerves may be involved. They are usually multiple (see Fig. 5), variable in size, and well circumscribed, but the differentiation between tumour and surrounding brain is not always clear. They are variable in consistency and the greater use CT scanning has demonstrated that haemorrhage into these tumours occurs more frequently than was once thought. The cellular appearance is usually that of the primary source, but the origin of the more anaplastic tumours and those exhibiting severe necrosis can be difficult to determine. The most common primary tumours are those of bronchus and breast, followed by malignant melanoma, renal carcinoma, and various carcinomas of the alimentary tract. Thyroid carcinoma, although rare, also metastasizes to brain. Retinoblastomas of childhood may infiltrate the subarachnoid space, as may leukaemic and lymphomatous deposits. Malignant lymphoma and melanoma may be seen as primary neoplasms within the intracranial cavity. Infiltration of the meninges by carcinoma, leukaemia, and lymphoma may produce a malignant meningitis often associated with lower cranial nerve palsies owing to infiltration around the brain-stem.

Fig. 5 Contrast CT scan. Multiple metastatic deposits (arrows A), each surrounded by an area of cerebral oedema (B).

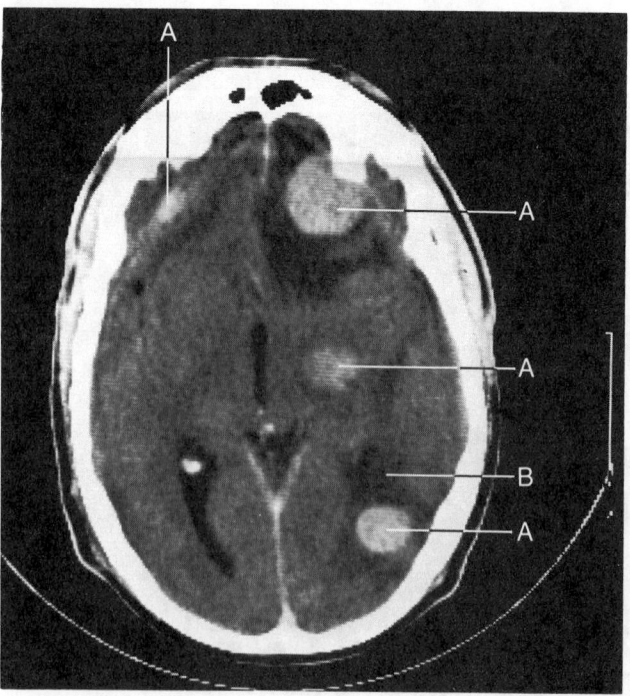

Pathophysiology

The pathological effects of any enlarging intracranial neoplasm and the speed with which they progress will depend upon the morphological characteristics of the mass, its rate of growth, its anatomical location, the neural tissues which it compresses, distorts or invades, its capacity to induce oedema of the surrounding brain, and the displacement or obstruction of fluid components (blood and CSF) within the cranium. The effects may be local or generalized, or both.

By infiltrating or compressing normal structures close to the site of the mass, tumours produce focal neurological deficits. Irritation of the cerebral hemisphere may result in epilepsy, and infiltration of the dura may lead to local pain and to meningeal irritation. Increase in the size of the mass within the effectively fixed volume of the skull will lead to a rise in intracranial pressure. Of all these effects the latter is usually the most important in terms of precipitating rapid irreversible deterioration.

For practical purposes the skull may be considered as a closed rigid box containing three principal elements, the brain, cerebrospinal fluid, and blood. Any increase of the volume of these elements will lead to a rise in intracranial pressure but this may be offset initially by compensating mechanisms. For instance, a slowly enlarging tumour may increase the volume of the cerebral contents but be compensated for by a reduction in the volume of cerebrospinal fluid which becomes squeezed out of the compressed lateral ventricles and the basal cisterns. Clearly, the compensatory mechanisms will be more effective if the factors increasing pressure are only slowly progressive. The pressure–volume curve relating to intracranial pressure is not linear but exponential, so that the effects of increased volume due to a slowly growing tumour may be compensated for over a long time without undue rise in pressure. A point is then reached at which reduction in cerebrospinal fluid volume, brain displacement, and perhaps reduction in cerebral perfusion can no longer be compensated for as efficiently. At this point even small rises in volume will produce substantial rises in intracranial pressure.

As intracranial masses increase in size, other phenomena occur which are of great significance in terms of brain function and which may prelude rapid clinical deterioration (see Figs 6 and 7). Axial displacement of the brain at the foramen magnum, when the cerebellar tonsils are driven through this aperture, is commonly seen with masses in the posterior fossa. This cerebellar tonsillar herniation is known as coning. The term has been extended to include axial and lateral displacement of the brain at the level of the hiatus. A unilateral hemisphere mass may displace towards the unaffected side, causing the medial part of the temporal lobe (the uncus) to be pushed into the tentorial hiatus. Lateral displacement of the brain combines with the uncal herniation to force the contralateral cerebral peduncle against the free edge of the tentorium. Conduction in the fibres traversing the compressed peduncle becomes impaired, leading to a false localizing sign with ipsilateral hemiparesis (Kernohan's notch phenomenon). Lateral displacement producing tentorial herniation may also press the oculomotor nerve against the petroclinoid ligament and stretch it by virtue of downward displacement of the posterior cerebral artery around which it hooks. This will result in pupillary dilatation and fixation which may be reversible in the early stages but which may become irreversible if the blood supply to the nerve is impaired.

Supratentorial masses may also depress the tentorium and displace the contents of the posterior fossa downwards so that the cerebellar tonsils herniate through the foramen magnum. Deformation of the brainstem distorts arteries which penetrate it and with severe brain-stem distortion infarcts and haemorrhages may occur which may be fatal. With incipient tentorial and tonsillar herniation a further change in pressure differential between the supratentorial and infratentorial or infratentorial and spinal compartments may be catastrophic. Lumbar puncture must therefore be strictly avoided until a suspected intracranial mass lesion has been excluded.

Papilloedema is most probably caused by the effects of increased intracranial pressure transmitted to the cerebrospinal fluid in the optic nerve sheath. However, even very large, slowly growing intracranial masses can present without demonstrable papilloedema. This may relate anatomically to differing degrees of patency of the optic nerve sheaths. Papilloedema will be absent in cases in which optic atrophy has already supervened.

Prolonged raised intracranial pressure may result in erosion of the base of the skull, so that patients present with cerebrospinal fluid rhinorrhoea or meningitis. Extensive erosion of the pituitary fossa can occur, especially in cases of severe hydrocephalus, and the posterior clinoid process will be eroded. Chronic raised pressure may also cause focal erosions of the inner table of the skull and lead to a 'thumb-printing' pattern on skull radiography.

Clinical features

Despite their adverse nature, all intracranial tumours will present in one of (or in a combination of) three ways: raised intracranial pressure, focal neurological deficits, or epilepsy.

Focal epileptic seizures may, in their own right, be of localizing value. The neurological deficit will depend to a large extent upon the site of the tumour, and raised intracranial pressure may be a function of the tumour mass itself, of reactive oedema in the surrounding brain, and of obstructive hydrocephalus. More generalized systemic disturbances may

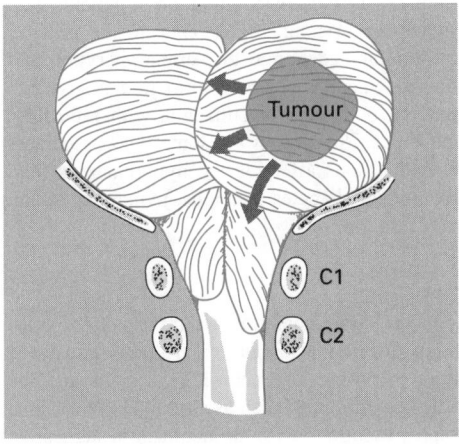

Fig. 6 Herniation of cerebellar tonsils. (Reproduced from Jefferson, *Oxford Textbook of Medicine*, 1st edn.)

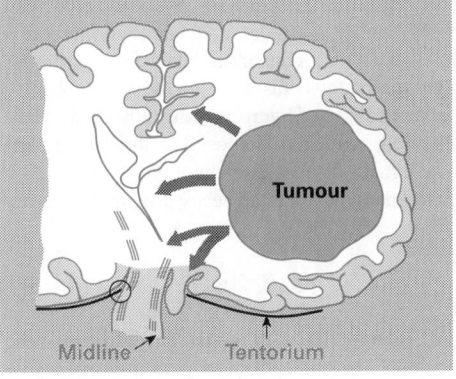

Fig. 7 Diagram of inferior aspect of the brain with a left temporal tumour. The arrow shows the uncus compressing the oculomotor nerve. Note also how descent of the posterior cerebral artery stretches the nerve. (Reproduced from Jefferson, *Oxford Textbook of Medicine*, 1st edn.)

be evident, particularly in cases of hormone-secreting tumours of the pituitary and in metastatic disease. Neck stiffness and pain in patients with intracranial tumour can be caused either by local infiltration of the meninges or by tonsillar herniation.

RAISED INTRACRANIAL PRESSURE

Evidence of raised intracranial pressure is, perhaps, the most ominous feature of intracranial mass lesions and should prompt urgent investigation. The cardinal symptoms are those of headache, vomiting, and drowsiness. The headaches may come on at any time of day but characteristically occur early in the morning or wake the patient from sleep. This is due, in part, to relative CO_2 retention during sleep with cerebrovascular dilatation and further increase in intracranial pressure. The headaches may be increased by stooping or coughing and are generally recognized as being different in character from headaches suffered previously, even in patients who have a past history of migraine. The headache may be accompanied by vomiting which may partially relieve the headache. Headaches are seldom of localizing value, although tumours of the posterior fossa may produce occipital and upper cervical pain. Evidence of neck stiffness in conjunction with nuchal pain in the patient with a suspected intracranial mass lesion requires immediate investigation.

Vomiting sometimes occurs as an isolated symptom or precedes headache by many months, particularly in cases of fourth ventricular tumour.

Two sinister symptoms of raised intracranial pressure are failing vision and deterioration of the level of consciousness. Papilloedema is present in only about half of all patients with intracranial tumours. However, chronic papilloedema may result in enlargement of the blind spot and defects of central vision, and ultimately leads to episodes of transient blindness (visual obscurations). These attacks are often exacerbated by coughing, straining, or stooping. Prolonged raised intracranial pressure may produce complete visual failure when optic atrophy supervenes.

In the early stages, alteration of the level of consciousness may be noticed by relatives and friends simply by increased lethargy, tiredness, and somnolence. More severe degrees of raised pressure associated with brain-stem distortion and tentorial or tonsillar herniation may lead to dramatic deterioration in conscious level and require prompt attention.

In infants raised intracranial pressure can present with failure to thrive, lethargy, head clutching, and vomiting, and be associated with an increasing head circumference and a tense bulging fontanelle. In older children there may be separation of the sutures of the skull vault and on percussion the skull may give a 'cracked pot' note.

FOCAL NEUROLOGICAL DEFICITS

These are legion owing to the variability of type and site of intracranial tumours and only a few specific syndromes associated with the more common tumours can be described here.

In general, lesions involving the cerebral hemisphere produce mental and behavioural changes when the frontal lobes are involved, contralateral hemiparesis when the (posterior frontal) motor cortex is involved, contralateral cortical sensory impairment and homonymous hemianopia with parietal lesions, disturbance of memory, mood, and sometimes hemianopia or quadrantanopia with temporal lesions, and dysphasia with lesions of the temporofrontal or temporoparietal areas of the dominant hemisphere. Tumours of the brain-stem commonly present with disorders of ocular movement, balance, and motor impairment. Cerebellar hemisphere lesions produce limb ataxia and central cerebellar lesions produce gait ataxia. Tumours compressing or invading the visual pathways may produce visual failure or field defects. Masses within the cerebellopontine angle produce evidence of brain-stem and cerebellar compression and affect specifically the cranial nerves V, VII, VIII, and sometimes the vagal group. Tumours of the non-dominant frontal and anterior temporal lobe and those within the anterior one-third of the corpus callosum or within a ventricle may be manifest purely by symptoms and signs of raised intracranial pressure without focal deficit. Bifrontal lesions may result in intellectual deterioration with memory loss and urinary incontinence, and those involving the third ventricle and hypothalamus can cause hormonal and metabolic changes together with raised intracranial pressure through obstructive hydrocephalus.

Two facets of neurological examination are frequently overlooked or improperly performed by inexperienced clinicians; testing the sense of smell and assessing visual fields. There are probably many patients who have been diagnosed as having simple dementia whose large olfactory groove meningiomas have been missed for want of simple tests of sense of smell. Smell may also be lost in cases of extrinsic tumours invading through the floor of the anterior cranial fossa.

Apart from the effects of papilloedema, vision will be impaired when masses stretch or compress the optic nerves and chiasm, or when tumours interrupt some, or all, of the optic radiations in one hemisphere. Chiasmal lesions are classically regarded as producing a bitemporal hemianopia, and while this is very commonly the case, the deficit is often asymmetric, producing obvious symptoms in one eye whereas the other eye shows changes demonstrable only by refined field testing. When the optic radiations are involved, either the right or left halves of both visual fields are affected (homonymous hemianopia). Temporal lesions affect chiefly the contralateral upper quadrants, and parietal lesions the contralateral lower quadrants. A surprising degree of visual loss may occur without the patient being aware of the deficit; for example, unilateral visual loss may remain unnoticed until the healthy eye is obscured for some reason, or road-traffic accidents may occur through loss of peripheral vision. Visual field and acuity deterioration is particularly hard to demonstrate in children.

Tumours of the midbrain may produce complex disorders of eye movement (internuclear ocular palsies). Isolated third nerve palsy may be nuclear in origin but is more likely to be peripheral and associated with uncal herniation. Unilateral or bilateral sixth nerve palsy may occur, and is rarely of localizing value. It is usually a secondary effect of raised intracranial pressure when displacement of the brain presses the nerve against the anterior inferior cerebellar artery. Tumours in the pineal region compress the dorsal midbrain, resulting in failure of upward gaze and abnormal pupillary reactions (Parinaud's syndrome).

Disorders of fifth nerve function are usually manifest as either numbness or pain in the face in one or more divisions of the sensory root. The commonest site for tumours to affect fifth nerve function is in the region of the pons, most particularly meningiomas or schwannomas in the cerebellopontine angle. Occasionally both sensory and motor impairment of the trigeminal nerve is seen with intrinsic pontine lesions.

Peripheral facial nerve lesions are sometimes associated with tumours in the base of the skull, but facial weakness is more commonly seen with tumours of the cerebral hemispheres which extend deeply into the brain and involve the internal capsule. Acoustic schwannomas may greatly stretch the facial nerve but facial weakness is usually a very late sign.

The vast majority of schwannomas of the eighth nerve arise on the vestibular division and present with unilateral sensorineural hearing loss (see also Chapter 24.3.5). This is accompanied by diminished or absent caloric responses (cold water applied to the external ear will normally stimulate the lateral semicircular canal and produce nystagmus with the fast component away from the irrigated ear). Downward enlargement of the tumour may impair ninth and tenth cranial nerve function, posterior enlargement affects the cerebellum and produces truncal and limb ataxia, and medial enlargement may encroach upon fifth nerve and brainstem, producing sensory impairment in the face and long tract signs. Acoustic nerve tumours are often seen in late middle age and elderly patients, in whom the significance of dementia, deafness, and ataxia is not always appreciated.

Eleventh and twelfth cranial nerves are affected by tumours of the base of the skull, such as chordomas, or by other large tumours of the posterior fossa which project towards the foramen magnum.

EPILEPSY (SEE ALSO CHAPTER 24.4.1)

Only some 10 per cent of adults presenting with late-onset epilepsy (after age 25 years) will prove to have an intracranial supratentorial neoplasm. However, the diagnosis should at least be suspected, particularly in cases of focal epilepsy in which the character of the attacks changes. Epilepsy occurs in about 30 per cent of cases of supratentorial tumour and the type of fit may give some idea as to the site and nature of the tumour. Gustatory or olfactory attacks imply an intrinsic tumour within the medial temporal lobe, whereas focal attacks, particularly of sensory type starting in the foot or lower limb, are strongly indicative of a falcine or parasagittal meningioma. Sometimes apparently idiopathic attacks may precede other symptoms suggestive of intracranial tumours by many years, and give a clue as to the true natural history of the tumour. This is particularly the case in oligodendrogliomas, but with the faster growing malignant astrocytomas there may be only a few weeks between the onset of fits and the appearance of other neurological abnormalities.

OTHER SYMPTOMS AND SIGNS

It is important when dealing with cases of suspected behavioural change or memory impairment to obtain a full history from relatives or close friends of the patients and not to rely on the patients for an accurate description of their symptoms. The changes may be subtle and go unrecognized or ignored by the patient. Relatives can comment more accurately on increased aggression, lethargy or neglect, failure to cope at work, and memory disorder. Expressive dysphasia may sometimes be mistakenly described as confusion and receptive dysphasia as deafness and it is important to distinguish these by simple clinical testing.

More generalized systemic disturbances may be seen in patients with intracranial metastases when the systemic signs relate to the primary neoplasm. Non-secretory pituitary adenomas and craniopharyngiomas may produce hypopituitarism, whereas secretory tumours may give rise to acromegaly and gigantism, or hyperprolactinaemia with infertility, galactorrhoea, and amenorrhoea. Pinealomas are sometimes associated with precocious puberty and lesions affecting the hypothalamus (e.g. craniopharyngioma) may produce diabetes insipidus, hyperphagia, and disorders of temperature regulation.

Differential diagnosis

The symptoms associated with intracranial tumours are usually of gradual onset so that the major differential diagnoses are other causes of raised intracranial pressure or progressive neurological signs and fits rather than causes of abrupt deterioration such as stroke. However, one catch is that of meningioma presenting in a stuttering fashion suggestive of transient ischaemic attacks or incomplete stroke. The differential diagnosis of intracranial neoplasm includes chronic subdural haematoma, which is not always associated with known head injury and is often attended by a fluctuating level of consciousness; cerebral infarction; cortical venous thrombosis; benign intracranial hypertension, which normally presents in young women and, although headache, papilloedema and sixth nerve palsy may be seen, is not associated with drowsiness; cerebral abscess which is usually associated with infection of the sinuses and middle ear or with congenital heart disease; herpes simplex encephalitis; granulomatous disease, including syphylitic gumma and tuberculoma; and causes of hydrocephalus other than those associated with neoplasm (e.g. aqueduct stenosis). Patients who are already known to have malignant disease elsewhere who present with neurological symptoms should not be assumed necessarily to have intracranial metastases.

Investigations

The speed of progression of symptoms with particular reference to the presence of raised intracranial pressure will determine the urgency of investigation and whether hospital admission is required. Non-radiological investigation may include formal plotting of visual fields in cases of suspected optic nerve or chiasmal compression, caloric testing, audiometry, and measurement of brain-stem evoked potentials in cases of possible acoustic tumour, full endocrine assessment for cases of suspected pituitary adenoma, and serological and haematological investigation to help exclude syphilis and other bacterial infection.

Electroencephalography has a limited role to play in the diagnosis of cerebral tumour. It may be useful in certain cases of focal epilepsy and, together with sphenoidal recordings, may be of particular value in temporal lobe seizures in children. In these cases it may demonstrate a single focus for the fits in the mesial temporal lobe and indicate whether temporal lobectomy or hippocampectomy would be beneficial.

Chest radiography is mandatory in all cases of suspected intracranial tumour to exclude primary neoplasm or tuberculosis.

SKULL RADIOGRAPHS

Plain radiographs of the skull may show evidence of raised intracranial pressure in both adults and children (erosion of the dorsum sellae, 'copper beating' of the skull vault, and separation of the sutures). Calcification is commonly seen in oligodendrogliomas, in virtually all cases of craniopharyngioma of childhood, and in about half the adult cases with this particular neoplasm. Calcification of the pineal in children is highly suggestive of pineal tumour. Unilateral tumours of the cerebral hemispheres may displace a calcified pineal gland.

Hyperostosis or bony erosion of the skull can occur immediately adjacent to meningiomas, and acoustic schwannomas commonly erode the internal auditory meatus. In such cases tomography of the petrous bones or an MRI scan is indicated.

RADIO-ISOTOPE BRAIN SCAN

This investigation is now rarely used. Although it may reveal between 50 and 75 per cent of supratentorial neoplasms, it is of little value in detecting posterior fossa masses.

MAGNETIC RESONANCE IMAGING (MRI) AND COMPUTED TOMOGRAPHY (CT) SCANNING

Although MRI is unlikely to replace CT scanning completely in the investigation of intracranial mass lesions, it is of great value in demonstrating small multiple metastases, basal intracranial tumours, differentiating tumour from demyelination, and defining tumour masses within an area of cerebral oedema. It is now the investigation of choice in planning operations for intracranial tumours, although in some instances it is particularly useful to have both MRI and CT. MRI is usually carried out with both T_1- and T_2-weighted images and proton-density scans. Contrast enhancement with gadolinium is particularly useful in diagnosing malignant meningitis (see Fig. 8).

Even if MRI is available, some patients are unable to undergo this investigation because of claustrophobia, previous intracranial surgery involving the insertion of ferrous materials (usually older-type aneurysm clips), or because they have cardiac pacemakers. MRI is also less useful in calcified lesions, but it is particularly good for distinguishing bleeds into tumours as opposed to primary intracerebral haematomas.

With contrast-enhancement CT, over 95 per cent of intracranial tumours may be demonstrated with a resolution of around 2 mm, depending on the density of the tumour compared with the surrounding brain. CT scanning will also show whether the tumour is solid or partially cystic, and will show the amount of lateral shift produced by the tumour mass and surrounding oedema. Tumour size may not always be accurately assessed as there may be difficulty in differentiating between solid components of low-grade infiltrative gliomas and the surrounding reactive oedema of the brain itself. Tumours often have peripheral reactive hyperaemia, and when the neoplasms are partially necrotic they show

up as ring-enhancing lesions with low-density centres. Under these circumstances it may be impossible to differentiate a tumour from a cerebral abscess by CT, although MRI can usually make this differentiation. Finally, both CT scan and MRI will demonstrate the presence of obstructive hydrocephalus associated with intracranial masses.

CEREBRAL ANGIOGRAPHY

Prior to CT scanning this was the investigation of choice for confirming the diagnosis of cerebral tumour. It is now mainly used as an adjunct to scanning to exclude arteriovenous malformation, in the preoperative embolization of very vascular tumours, and as a preoperative investigation to demonstrate the blood supply of tumours and their relationship to important vascular structures nearby. If MRI is not available, then the venous phase of angiography may be useful in planning operations on parasagittal meningiomas in which the sagittal sinus may be involved.

Management

Except for cases in which age or general medical condition preclude operation, most intracranial tumours will require some form of surgery, either to obtain a histological diagnosis, to palliate and help to control fits or neurological symptoms, or to achieve total removal. With malignant tumours radiotherapy is often used in conjunction with a surgical procedure (see Table 3). Medical treatment is largely supportive and symptomatic in the absence of any specific antitumour agent.

IMMEDIATE TREATMENT

The principal features associated with intracranial neoplasms which require urgent investigation and treatment are raised intracranial pressure, particularly when associated with deteriorating level of consciousness and/or failing vision and epileptic fits. Fits should be aborted promptly with 10 mg intravenous diazepam, or if this fails, 10 ml of intramuscular paraldehyde (adult doses). It is important to establish the cause of raised intracranial pressure and the only certain way of doing this is by carrying out a CT or MRI scan. Raised pressure associated with tumour mass and surrounding reactive oedema may be reduced by giving intravenous frusemide or 20 per cent w/v solution of mannitol (200 ml over about 15 min). Intravenous dexamethasone (12–16 mg) may also be used in extreme cases.

Corticosteroids may also be used in rather less urgent cases when, for

Fig. 8 Coronal MRI of brain with gadolinium enhancement, showing extensive hemisphere intrinsic tumour with surrounding cerebral oedema and meningeal infiltration.

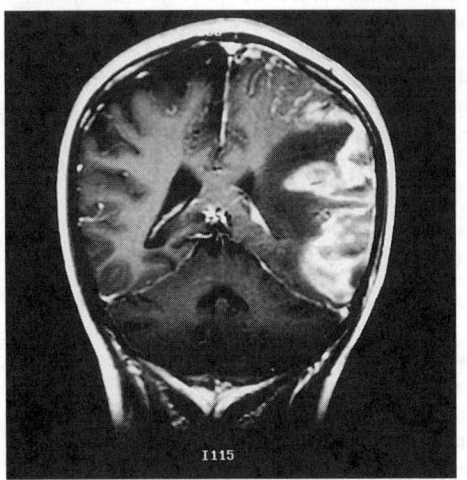

Table 3 *Treatment and prognosis of the more common intracranial tumours*

Tumour	Commonest surgical procedure	Effect of radiotherapy	Prognosis
Glioblastoma	Biopsy or partial removal	Minimal	Less than 20 per cent 1-year survival rate
Astrocytoma	Biopsy or subtotal removal, decompression	Variable, average of 10 per cent increase in survival	Up to 50 per cent 5-year survival rate reported
Oligodendroglioma	Biopsy or subtotal removal	Given for 'recurrent' tumour; marginal effect	55 per cent 10-year survival rate; tend to undergo malignant change
Cerebellar cystic astrocytoma	Complete removal	Not generally used	Over 70 per cent recurrence-free
Ependymoma	Radical removal, possibly with shunt	Variable, probably sensitive	30–40 per cent 5-year survival rate
Medulloblastoma	Radical removal, possibly with shunt	Whole neuraxis irradiation improves survival	Average survival about 1 year, recent reports much more favourable
Haemangioblastoma	Complete removal, possibly with shunt	Not generally used	15 per cent recurrence; excellent prognosis if totally removed
Meningioma	Complete removal	Minimal effect	10 per cent recurrence after 'total' removal; occasionally frankly malignant
Acoustic schwannoma (neuroma)	Complete removal	Not used	Excellent prognosis if totally removed; high rate of recurrence with subcapsular removal
Craniopharyngioma	Complete removal or subtotal removal	Given after subtotal removal; claims of less than 10 per cent 5-year recurrence	10 per cent 5-year recurrence after total removal, but high risk of endocrine dysfunction
Pituitary adenoma	Transnasal microadenectomy; transfrontal craniotomy for mainly suprasellar tumours; total removal by trans-sphenoidal or transethmoidal routes	Given for invasive or recurrent tumour Variable response, probably beneficial	About 12 per cent recurrence after surgery and radiotherapy

Tables 2 and 3 are derived from tables published in *Medicine International* and reproduced with kind permission of Medical Education (International) Ltd.

example, an intracranial mass has been shown on CT scan to be associated with cerebral oedema and there has been slow progression of neurological signs. Dexamethasone (4 mg six-hourly) may produce symptomatic relief by reducing brain swelling and may make subsequent surgery safer. If there is doubt as to whether a mass lesion may be an abscess or neoplasm, steroids should be avoided until a diagnosis has been firmly established.

Raised intracranial pressure from obstructive hydrocephalus requires some form of ventricular drainage procedure or ventricular shunting. Once this has been done, fuller investigation may be undertaken rather less urgently and elective surgery planned as required.

Severe headaches should be treated with codeine or dihydrocodeine but other opiate analgesics are generally contraindicated because of their tendency to depress respiration, conscious level, and pupillary responses. Vomiting may be controlled with metaclopramide or cyclizine.

SURGICAL TREATMENT

Surgery is aimed, whenever possible, at obtaining as complete a removal as is feasible without producing neurological deficit. Benign tumours which are surgically accessible and not involving important structures such as brain-stem, basal ganglia, or major vessels are curable by complete surgical excision. At operation, however, a balance might have to be struck between potential cure from a risky complete excision, and accepting the possibility of recurrence over many years by leaving small

fragments of tumour and preserving vital structures. Tumours in which complete excision is most commonly attempted include meningiomas, colloid cysts, neurofibromas, schwannomas, and pituitary adenomas. Most supratentorial tumours are removed at craniotomy, the exact approach being dictated by the site of the tumour. Pituitary adenomas are removed trans-sphenoidally, transethmoidally, or transcranially. Adenomas with a large suprasellar component, particularly when associated with compression of the chiasm or optic nerves, have traditionally been removed at craniotomy. However, even very large pituitary adenomas may now be removed effectively by the trans-sphenoidal route, with better preservation of functioning pituitary tissue and minimal risk of postoperative epilepsy.

Gliomas of the frontal, temporal, and occipital poles might seem curable by lobectomy with a line of excision well behind the apparent limits of the tumour as judged on the CT scan or, more accurately, MRI. However, even in these circumstances histological examination often shows tumour cells to be present right up to the line of excision, implying that removal has not been complete. The benefit of this procedure is a good internal decompression and, with the more slowly growing neoplasms, a considerable remission of symptoms. Lobectomy is most appropriate to polar tumours in patients with evidence of raised intracranial pressure but few focal neurological signs.

Complete removal of single metastatic lesions is often well worth while. Even in those cases in which prolongation of life cannot be achieved, the quality of the survival time is often improved, sometimes remarkably so. For instance, patients who are completely incapacitated by vomiting and ataxia related to a metastasis in the cerebellum can achieve almost complete alleviation of these symptoms by excision of the mass.

The decision to attempt complete surgical removal is particularly difficult in some cases of craniopharyngioma. These tumours have a great tendency to recur if incompletely removed and the best chance of cure is to obtain as complete a removal as possible followed by radiotherapy. However, radical removal is often attended by severe hypothalamic and pituitary dysfunction and the endocrine deficits may be so debilitating as to make life intolerable for the patient.

Similarly, the best chance of long-term survival in cases of medulloblastoma and ependymoma is as complete a macroscopic removal as possible followed by radiotherapy. Attempts at complete excision in these cases are usually limited by risk of damage to structures in the floor of the fourth ventricle. Nevertheless, complete excision should be the aim whenever possible.

Malignant gliomas infiltrate diffusely and it is rarely possible to excise them completely. The aim of surgery is to remove the maximum amount of tumour possible without producing or adding to neurological deficit. At operation a good internal decompression can often be obtained and at the same time provide the theoretical advantage of reducing tumour bulk to make for more effective radiotherapy. The decision to embark upon subtotal resection depends upon the age and general medical condition of the patient, the consistency of the tumour as judged by CT scan or MRI (tumours with small, solid components and large cysts may be readily decompressed), and the site of the lesion itself. Superficial tumours in the non-dominant hemisphere may be amenable to more radical surgery than those deeply placed within the dominant hemisphere.

With the advent of CT scanning and MRI it was thought that sufficient definition could be achieved to recognize with total confidence intracranial neoplasms and to distinguish them from other pathology. Despite advances in scan technology, there may still be difficulty in differentiating abscess, benign tumour, or malignant neoplasm. For these reasons it is preferable in almost all cases to obtain a tissue diagnosis by biopsy. This may be carried out through a burr-hole with needle biopsy, by stereotactic procedures, or by craniotomy. However, the mass may be lying in the basal ganglia, thalamus, or brain-stem, in which case even needle biopsy could be detrimental. CT scan or MRI-guided stereotactic biopsy is now a far simpler procedure than the older operations using contrast ventriculography, and it provides a far safer and more accurate method of obtaining samples of tumour for histology. It should now be the method of choice for sampling intracranial tumours in all but the most superficial and largest lesions.

Even so, there are definite risks of stereotactic biopsy in some deep-seated tumours, notably in the brain-stem. It might then be reasonable to give radiotherapy without a tissue diagnosis, or simply to follow up the patient by serial scanning and to operate only if raised intracranial pressure supervenes or if the risk of producing surgical neurological deficit becomes more balanced in the face of progressive neurological signs.

Other surgical procedures include ventriculoatrial and ventriculoperitoneal shunting, or the insertion of a temporary ventricular drain in cases of obstructive hydrocephalus associated with posterior fossa or third ventricular tumours. This may be carried out as a prelude to definitive surgery or used as a palliative procedure in cases which are deemed inoperable. Large tumour cysts are sometimes drained by burr-hole aspiration or by the insertion of a drain and reservoir system which allows frequent tapping of the cyst fluid and administration of local chemotherapy.

RADIOTHERAPY

The usual method of irradiating intracranial tumours is to give external irradiation to the site of the tumour in fractionated doses over a period of about 6 weeks. Improved techniques over the past few years reduced many of the unwanted side-effects of cranial irradiation, although lethargy, hair loss, and minor radiation damage to the scalp are seen almost invariably.

Benign tumours are generally insensitive to irradiation, and histologically benign mengiomas which have been treated only by partial excision are not influenced by postoperative radiotherapy. Irradiation is frequently given in cases of malignant meningioma which have a tendency to recur rapidly even after complete excision, but such treatment has yet to be shown to be of any great value.

The tumours showing the greatest sensitivity to radiotherapy are medulloblastoma and pineal germinoma. Ependymomas and cystic astrocytomas of the cerebellum show variable sensitivity but postoperative radiotherapy is generally advised, particularly if surgical excision is judged not to have been complete. Medulloblastoma, ependymoma, and pineal germinoma are treated by whole neuraxis irradiation (brain and spinal cord) because of their tendency to disseminate through CSF pathways. Even with complete removal and high-dose irradiation the prognosis with medulloblastoma has always been considered poor (about 30 per cent 2-year survival) but more recent reports suggest that up to 80 per cent 5-year survival rates can be achieved in this manner.

Craniopharyngioma, optic glioma, and hypothalamic gliomas are usually irradiated, most frequently following some form of surgery. Potential radiation damage due to the visual pathways, pituitary, and hypothalamus, however, has to be balanced against a low risk of recurrence in cases in which there has been complete surgical excision. Cases of pituitary invasive adenoma which have been treated by partial surgical excision are generally given postoperative radiotherapy. Similarly, certain forms of metastatic tumour may be given postoperative irradiation when the primary tumour is known to be radiosensitive.

The role of radiotherapy in the treatment of malignant gliomas is uncertain. Many trials have been carried out comparing the role of radiotherapy, chemotherapy, and surgery in their treatment, but despite claims to the contrary there is no definite evidence that radiotherapy significantly extends or improves the quality of life in patients with high-grade glioma. In patients whose general condition is good and who are shown to have a tumour which is amenable to some form of surgery and to be histologically grade I or II, the treatment of choice is (subtotal) resection with postoperative external radiotherapy. There have been reports of a mean increase in survival time of up to 10 per cent using postoperative irradiation. The prognosis with higher-grade tumours is much less favourable (see Table 3).

Despite the available evidence, there is a natural tendency to submit patients with known malignant gliomas to radiotherapy on the basis that they are young, are in otherwise good health, and have a family to support. Nevertheless, one must consider that if life expectancy is very short, it is often preferable for the patient to spend this time in family surroundings rather than attending hospital appointments. It is under these circumstances that frank, honest discussion with the patients and their relatives is essential and a policy of management decided as a result of a combined and agreed decision by both physicians and family.

Neuroradiotherapeutic techniques which hold some promise for the future include stereotactic radiosurgery (which has been found to be of some benefit in the early treatment of small, deep-seated gliomas and arteriovenous malformations) and boron/neutron capture irradiation. This latter method involves subtotal tumour resection and systemic administration of boron which is preferentially taken up by tumour tissue. The primed tumour remnant is then bombarded with neutrons.

CHEMOTHERAPY

Various forms of chemotherapy may have a place in the treatment of secondary deposits within the brain (e.g. cis-platinum in the treatment of seminoma; the nitrosoureas, vincristine, and procarbazine in secondary lymphoma) but there is no real evidence as yet to suggest that chemotherapy has any major role to play in the treatment of primary intracranial tumours. The management of cerebral leukaemia and lymphoma is considered further in Section 22.

PROGNOSIS AND LONG-TERM MANAGEMENT

The prognosis relating to most of the common intracranial tumours is given in Table 3. Patients with glioblastomas have a mean survival time of only 6 to 12 weeks from presentation. Patients with low-grade tumours have a mean survival of about 9 months following surgery and radiotherapy, although there have been reports of up to 50 per cent 5-year survival in grade I cases.

Meningiomas, apparently completely resected, are still associated with a 5 to 10 per cent recurrence rate within 10 years, and this rises to over 20 per cent symptomatic recurrence if fragments of tumour are known to have been left behind. Cerebellar astrocytomas and haemangioblastomas are associated with a good prognosis after complete removal, although occasionally cerebellar astrocytoma may act in a more malignant fashion. Fourth ventricular ependymoma has a poor prognosis if incompletely removed; the prognosis of medulloblastoma has already been described. The generally accepted recurrence rate of craniopharyngioma following radical surgery and irradiation is about 25 per cent within 5 years, but some reports suggest a less than 10 per cent recurrence rate. Radical treatment, however, may lead to severe morbidity despite increased survival time. Acoustic schwannomas will recur if incompletely removed, but their growth rate is usually slow and in a few elderly patients with large tumours it may be preferable to accept this risk of slow recurrence and opt for a subcapsular resection. In all other instances radical removal should be attempted.

Patients with intracranial tumours, particularly those associated with large amounts of cerebral oedema, are generally kept on steroid medication throughout their course of surgery and on a lower dose during their course of radiotherapy. They will need to be warned about the potential side-effects of steroids. Some patients with malignant gliomas or with inoperable recurrent tumour who have some evidence of raised intracranial pressure but without rapidly progressive focal deficit may also be treated with dexamethasone. However, the long-term use of steroids in these instances should be avoided as they certainly become less effective after a few weeks.

Patients should also be warned of the possible social consequences of their tumour and its treatment, with particular reference to driving. Patients with benign supratentorial lesions who have undergone major surgery will normally be banned from driving in the United Kingdom for 1 year following operation even if they have suffered no fits. Drivers of heavy goods vehicles may well have their licences withdrawn permanently. Patients who have suffered fits will normally have their licences revoked for a period of 2 years following the last seizure. Those patients who have malignant intracranial tumours may have to have these general rules applied more cautiously. Following major supratentorial craniotomy most surgeons will advise continuing treatment with anticonvulsant agents for 1 to 2 years.

REFERENCES

Blackwood, W. and Corsellis, J.A.-N. (eds) (1976). *Greenfield's neuropathology*. Edward Arnold, London.

Courville, C.B. (1967). Intracranial tumours. Notes upon a series of three thousand verified cases with some current observations obtaining to their mortality. *Bulletin of the Los Angeles Neurological Society*. **32**, Suppl. 2.

Northfield, D.W.C. (1973). *The surgery of the central nervous system*. Blackwell Scientific Publications, Oxford.

Teddy, P.J. (1983). Intracranial tumours. *Medicine International*. **31**, 1456–60.

Weller, R.O., Swash, M., McLelland, D.L., and Scholtz, C.L. (1982). *Clinical neuropathology*. Springer Verlag, Berlin.

Youmans, J.R. (ed.) (1982). *Neurological surgery*, (2nd edn), (6 vols). W.B. Saunders, Philadelphia.

24.13 Benign intracranial hypertension

N. F. LAWTON

Synonyms

Pseudotumour cerebri. Idiopathic intracranial hypertension.

Definition

Benign intracranial hypertension is a syndrome of raised intracranial pressure occurring in the absence of an intracranial mass lesion or enlargement of the cerebral ventricles due to hydrocephalus. The synonyms pseudotumour cerebri and idiopathic intracranial hypertension have both been preferred because the outcome is not invariably benign. Although rarely life-threatening, the rise in intracranial pressure may result in permanent visual loss due to optic nerve damage.

Incidence

Benign intracranial hypertension is a rare disease. The incidence is approximately 1/100 000 in the general population but rises to 19/100 000 in obese women of childbearing years. The disease is certainly more common in females, the preponderance over males ranging from 3 : 1 to 8 : 1. Although benign intracranial hypertension may occur in infants and the elderly, it is primarily a disease of young women between the ages of 17 and 44 years. Very rarely, benign intracranial hypertension is familial and may occur in more than one generation.

Clinical features

It is the hallmark of benign intracranial hypertension that presenting symptoms and signs are those of raised intracranial pressure alone. The diagnosis should not be entertained in the presence of neurological features which suggest a focal lesion. Furthermore, there is a remarkable preservation of consciousness and intellectual function rarely encountered in patients with mass lesions or hydrocephalus. A history of epilepsy, either generalized or focal, virtually excludes the diagnosis of benign intracranial hypertension, although seizures may occur in the small group of patients with venous sinus thrombosis (see below). Preservation of cerebral function also distinguishes benign intracranial hypertension from viral or bacterial meningoencephalitis. Patients with benign intracranial hypertension routinely present to outpatient departments and not as medical emergencies.

HEADACHE

This is the most common symptom and is present to some degree in virtually every case. Characteristically the headache is typical of raised intracranial pressure. It is then generalized, throbbing, worse on waking, and aggravated by factors which temporarily increase CSF pressure such as straining, coughing, or changing posture. Not infrequently, however, headache is mild and non-specific so that the distinction from common tension headache may be difficult. At presentation headache has usually been present for weeks, although sometimes for months. Although up to 50 per cent of patients complain of nausea, typical early morning projectile vomiting is rare.

OBESITY

Amongst the medical conditions associated with benign intracranial hypertension, obesity is sufficiently common to be a characteristic feature. Up to 90 per cent of patients in reported series are overweight, although a history of rapid weight gain immediately prior to the onset is unusual.

PAPILLOEDEMA

This is a virtually universal finding and the importance of fundus examination in every patient with headache cannot be overemphasized. Papilloedema is usually moderate and may be unilateral. Occasionally the appearance of the optic discs may be equivocal, and fluorescein angiography is indicated to demonstrate the characteristic leakage of dye in true papilloedema.

The classical symptom of papilloedema, which is not specific to benign intracranial hypertension, is a transient obscuration of vision, often described as a fleeting greyness, a halo, or a more vivid episode of 'Catherine wheels' lasting for a few seconds. Obscurations may be provoked by straining or a change in posture, but may also occur spontaneously. Persistent blurring of vision may also occur and patients may describe scotomata in the field of vision associated with optic nerve damage. Occasionally sudden and permanent loss of vision results from infarction of the optic nerve.

Visual obscurations, persistent blurring, or scotomata are reported by 30 to 70 per cent of patients.

VISUAL FIELD DEFECTS

Visual field analysis is the essential investigation in the examination and follow-up of patients with benign intracranial hypertension. The most common defects are enlargement of the blind spots, generalized constriction of the fields, and scotomata caused by optic nerve damage. There may be a predilection for visual field loss in the inferior nasal quadrants.

DIPLOPIA

About 30 per cent of patients complain of horizontal diplopia due to VIth nerve palsy which may be bilateral. The cause is a false localizing sign of raised intracranial pressure.

Figure 1 shows a typical patient with benign intracranial hypertension who presented with a 6 week history of headache, visual obscurations and diplopia, but without any disturbance of consciousness.

Aetiology

In the majority of patients with benign intracranial hypertension no cause can be identified. A wide variety of clinical associations have been reported, but in many instances may have occurred by chance. Preceding minor head injury and intercurrent infections come into this category. Furthermore, the known associations are rare with the exceptions of obesity and the predilection for females. Heredity, vitamin deficiency, and drugs are each a factor in less than 2 per cent of cases.

DURAL SINUS THROMBOSIS

Prior to the advent of antibiotics, benign intracranial hypertension was frequently associated with chronic middle-ear disease complicated by dural sinus thrombosis. The term 'otitic hydrocephalus' was coined to describe this syndrome on the erroneous assumption that ventricular enlargement was present.

Although true 'otitic hydrocephalus' is now rare, the syndrome of benign intracranial hypertension may still occur following venous thrombosis in dural sinuses or in the extracranial jugular system. Sinus thrombosis may complicate pregnancy, the use of oral contraceptives, venous occlusive disease due to hypercoagulability states, or mediastinal obstruction. Sinus thrombosis should be suspected clinically when the onset of headache is sudden and accompanied by focal signs or impaired consciousness. In the majority of patients, however, venous obstruction

Fig. 1 Bilateral papilloedema and left nerve palsy in benign intracranial hypertension (patient looking to the left). (Reproduced with permission.)

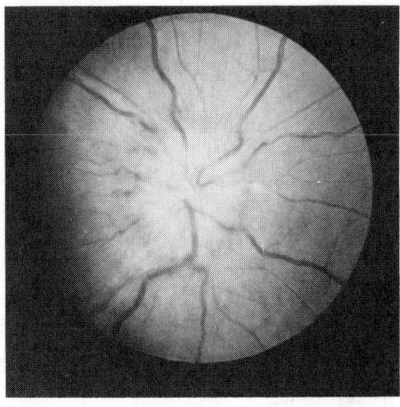

Right fundus

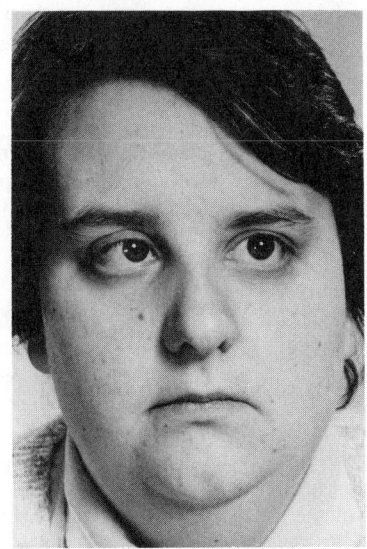

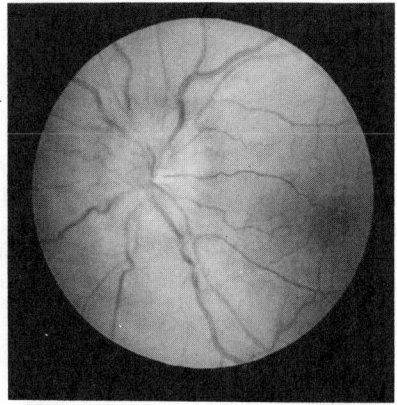

Left fundus

is not the predisposing cause and the cerebral venous system is normally patent.

MENSTRUAL DISORDERS

Apart from the complication of venous thrombosis, benign intracranial hypertension is associated with pregnancy *per se*. It is not clear whether an association with menstrual irregularity is more than would occur by chance in obese young women. An association with menarche has been reported.

In spite of the clinical associations which suggest an underlying disorder of female endocrinology, hormonal studies have not shown a consistent abnormality. The pituitary–adrenal axis is intact and occasional abnormal responses may be due to obesity rather than benign intracranial hypertension. Thyroid function and prolactin secretion both appear to be normal. CSF vasopressin levels are raised, but this is not specific and may occur in a variety of neurological diseases. Reports of a specific increase in CSF oestrone, which might link benign intracranial hypertension with obesity because adipocytes are the major source of oestrone, have not been confirmed.

DEFICIENCY STATES

A rare cause of benign intracranial hypertension in children is hypovitaminosis A due to generalized nutritional deficiency or malabsorption. In such cases the condition responds specifically to vitamin A supplements. Interestingly, poisoning with vitamin A due to excessive consumption of fish or animal liver may cause benign intracranial hypertension.

DRUG-INDUCED BENIGN INTRACRANIAL HYPERTENSION

Both tetracycline and the retinoids isotretinoin and etretinate, which are vitamin A derivatives, may cause benign intracranial hypertension during long-term treatment for acne. These drugs should not be used in combination. Other drugs occasionally responsible for the syndrome include nalidixic acid, nitrofurantoin, and lithium. Corticosteroids may lead to benign intracranial hypertension during their withdrawal after chronic treatment.

EMPTY SELLA

It has been suggested that this association in about 4 per cent of cases is caused by raised intracranial pressure in combination with incompetence of the diaphragma sellae. The theory is supported by the finding of raised pressure at lumbar puncture in some patients with empty sella, suggesting chronic benign intracranial hypertension as the underlying cause. Clinical hypopituitarism does not occur, but occasionally the empty sella may harbour a prolactinoma.

Pathogenesis

The mechanism by which intracranial pressure rises is poorly understood and the contribution of various factors controversial. Since the intracranial contents are housed in a rigid container, an increase in CSF pressure may result from an increase in blood volume, swelling of the brain parenchyma, or an increase in the CSF volume due to overproduction or malabsorption.

INCREASE IN BLOOD VOLUME

Measurements of cerebral blood volume based on the clearance rate of injected isotope indicate an increase in this volume which reverts to normal as benign intracranial hypertension remits. However, the increase in cerebral blood volume would only account for a volume increase in intracranial content of approximately 1 per cent, and would not be sufficient to produce a sustained rise in CSF pressure. It is generally held, therefore, that increased blood volume plays a minor role, and may indeed be secondary to the rise in intracranial pressure.

SWELLING OF THE BRAIN PARENCHYMA

Direct evidence of a swelling due to cerebral oedema is slight. A single report of oedematous changes in biopsied brain has not been confirmed since neither biopsy nor surgical decompression are indicated in current management. However, the tendency for the ventricles to be small may indicate an increase in cerebral volume.

If cerebral oedema is a significant factor, it is almost certainly due to leakage from the cerebral vascular bed rather than transudation of CSF from the ventricular system. The computed tomography (CT) scan in benign intracranial hypertension does not show the periventricular leakage of CSF that occurs in hydrocephalus. Although there is currently no direct evidence for vasogenic cerebral oedema, this factor cannot be ignored, because it is the only mechanism for raised pressure which does not anticipate some degree of hydrocephalus.

INCREASED PRODUCTION OF CSF

Indirect measurements do not suggest that this is a significant factor. Tripling the volume of CSF by saline infusion into the subarachnoid space of normal subjects produces only a small rise in the CSF pressure.

DECREASED ABSORPTION OF CSF

A defect of CSF absorption is widely regarded as the important factor in the pathogenesis of benign intracranial hypertension. Apart from those cases in which there is dural sinus thrombosis, it is assumed that the defect lies in the arachnoid villi of the superior sagittal sinus where the bulk of CSF absorption takes place. The delayed clearance of radioiodinated human serum albumin from the ventricular system after injection into the lumbar subarachnoid space is indirect evidence of reduced CSF absorption. Simultaneous cannulation of the superior sagittal sinus and the subarachnoid space has shown increased resistance to CSF absorption in the majority of cases. Finally, vitamin A deficiency in rats and cows produces a rise in intracranial pressure associated with diminished absorption of CSF and histological changes in the arachnoid villi which are reversible with vitamin A supplements.

The absence of hydrocephalus in benign intracranial hypertension has been sited as an objection to the theory of reduced CSF absorption. It is probably more significant, however, that sinus thrombosis may cause the syndrome of benign intracranial hypertension by preventing CSF absorption, and is similarly associated with normal or small cerebral ventricles.

Investigations

The diagnosis of benign intracranial hypertension can only be confirmed by measurement of CSF pressure, but in suspected cases it is essential to exclude a mass lesion or hydrocephalus before proceeding to lumbar puncture.

RADIOLOGY

The plain skull radiograph shows changes of raised pressure in only 5 per cent of cases. The pituitary fossa may be enlarged, reflecting an association with the empty sella syndrome.

Characteristically, CT scanning shows small and slit-like cerebral ventricles which may increase in volume as benign intracranial hypertension resolves. A similar appearance is seen on magnetic resonance (MR) imaging. Sagittal sinus thrombosis may be visualized on CT scanning as the characteristic 'empty delta' sign due to clot within the sinus. Angiography is usually required, however, if sinus thrombosis is suspected clinically. Currently the preferred technique is by digital subtraction angiography following intravenous contrast injection, but MR angiography promises to avoid the need for contrast injection.

CSF PRESSURE

At lumbar puncture the opening pressure is greater than 200 mm CSF but it is important to note that in simple obesity CSF pressure may be as high as 250 mm CSF. The diagnostic significance of CSF pressure must therefore be correlated with the clinical picture. In the few patients whose CSF pressure is equivocal, continuous monitoring may demonstrate intermittent peaks of raised pressure.

CSF ANALYSIS

The composition of the CSF in benign intracranial hypertension is entirely normal, and the presence of white cells or a raised protein concentration cast serious doubt on the diagnosis. An exception to this rule is the rare syndrome resembling benign intracranial hypertension which occurs in association with postinfective polyneuropathy and with spinal tumours. Both conditions may lead to raised intracranial pressure with papilloedema and normal sized ventricles but a marked rise in CSF protein.

Management

There is good evidence that anticoagulation with heparin is effective in the treatment of acute sinus thrombosis, emphasizing the importance of angiographic diagnosis in this small group of patients. With the further exception of rare cases due to drug treatment, the management of benign intracranial hypertension is aimed at the symptomatic reduction of intracranial pressure to protect vision and relieve headache. The methods available are difficult to evaluate because of the high spontaneous remission rate and the lack of controlled trials. Choice of treatment is further complicated by the absence of reliable risk factors for visual loss. In particular, the height of the CSF pressure at diagnosis is of no prognostic significance.

In the past, repeated therapeutic lumbar puncture every 2 to 5 days has been shown to reduce CSF pressure temporarily and may occasionally lead to spontaneous remission. When acute medical treatment is indicated, however, it is now usual practice to prescribe prednisolone (40–60 mg daily). This regime is effective in relieving headache and visual obscuration due to papilloedema. However, steroids are unsatisfactory as long-term treatment because of their complications, especially in obese young females. For this reason diuretics are widely used in patients with mild symptoms. Acetazolamide or a thiazide diuretic may relieve headache, but the efficacy of diuretics in preventing slowly progressive visual loss is unproven.

Because of the limitations of medical treatment, an increasing number of patients are treated surgically, progressive visual field loss and unrelieved headache being the indications for operation. Because of the difficulty of tapping small cerebral ventricles, a lumboperitoneal shunt is usually favoured. Unfortunately, the technical failure rate of lumbo-peritoneal shunts is high and surgical revision may be required in up to 20 per cent of patients. For this reason the alternative operation, in which the optic nerve sheath is decompressed, has recently been revived, particularly in North America. This procedure produces rapid improvement in papilloedema, occasionally in both eyes after unilateral surgery. It is not clear whether long-term improvement is due to the creation of a CSF fistula into the orbit or fibrosis of the meninges preventing transmission of the high CSF pressure to the optic nerve head. However, headache is often unrelieved by this procedure, and lumboperitoneal shunting may not be avoided. There is also a risk of further visual loss postoperatively.

Currently it would seem reasonable to begin treatment with diuretics, reserving steroids as a temporary medical treatment in patients with severe symptoms. If surgery becomes necessary, lumboperitoneal shunting is the logical procedure, with resort to optic nerve sheath decompression in the event of repeated shunt failure.

Although the efficacy of weight loss *per se* has not yet been established, a weight-reducing diet is recommended in obese patients.

PREGNANCY

The major threat is to the fetus and the rate of spontaneous abortion is increased. Spontaneous remission of benign intracranial hypertension during pregnancy has been the rule, although the number of reported cases is small. It would seem reasonable to begin treatment with diuretics, although steroids and shunt operations may occasionally be required.

Prognosis

Benign intracranial hypertension is a chronic condition in most patients but spontaneous relapse and remission of symptoms is common. There is evidence that raised intracranial pressure may be found at follow-up lumbar puncture in patients whose symptoms have been in remission for several years. Mortality from benign intracranial hypertension is nil in most series, although an underlying sagittal sinus thrombosis may occasionally lead to a fatal outcome. Permanent visual loss occurs in up to 50 per cent of patients and is a significant disability in 10 per cent. Because the choice of treatment is determined primarily by progression of optic nerve damage, serial visual field analysis is the important yardstick of clinical progression.

REFERENCES

Ahlskog, J.E. (1982). Pseudotumour cerebri. *Annals of Internal Medicine* **97**, 249–56.

Corbett, J.J. and Thompson, H.S. (1989). The rational management of idiopathic intracranial hypertension. *Archives of Neurology* **46**, 1049–51.

Janny, P., Chazal, J., Colnet, G., Irthum, B., and Georget, A. (1981). Benign intracranial hypertension and disorders of CSF absorption. *Surgical Neurology* **15**, 168–74.

McComb, J.G. (1983). Recent research into the nature of cerebrospinal fluid formation and absorption. *Journal of Neurosurgery* **59**, 369–83.

Rush, J.A. (1980). Pseudotumour cerebri: clinical profile and visual outcome in 63 patients. *Mayo Clinic Proceedings* **55**, 541–6.

Sergott, R.C., Savino P.J., and Bosley, T.M. (1988). Modified optic nerve sheath decompression provides long term visual improvement for pseudotumour cerebri. *Archives of Ophthalmology* **106**, 1384–90.

24.14 Head injuries

G. M. TEASDALE

Each year in the United Kingdom one million head-injured patients attend hospital. Fortunately most injuries prove to be mild: 80 per cent of patients have not even been 'knocked out', only one in five is admitted to hospital and most of these stay for less than 48 hours. Nevertheless, some 5000 patients die each year and many others survive with mental disability. In a proportion of these cases outcome could have been improved by either more prompt or more effective recognition and treatment of secondary complications of the injury.

Many head-injury victims are young adult males and head injury is a leading cause of death and long-lasting mental disablement in the productive years of life. More than half of the more severe injuries are caused by road traffic accidents; other frequent causes are falls and assaults, often also related to alcohol intake.

The pathology of head injury

SCALP AND SKULL INJURY

A scalp laceration is present in about 40 per cent of patients who attend hospital but a skull fracture is found in only 1.5 per cent. Although each feature can indicate the location and severity of impact on the head, this is less important diagnostically than the contribution they make to establishing that a head injury has occurred—if a history is not available—and the clue they provide to the risk of subsequent complications. The excellent healing of the scalp after surgical toilet and closure reflects its generous blood supply, but this can sometimes result in a laceration bleeding so profusely that shock ensues. This risk is highest in children or elderly people with extensive scalp injuries.

A skull fracture is described by several features. (1) Location: the vault of the cranial cavity; the posterior fossa; or the base of the skull. (2) Shape: linear (fissure) or comminuted into fragments. (3) If the fragments are depressed inwards. (4) If it is open, or compound, i.e. associated with a local wound which creates a passage between the exterior and the interior of the cranial cavity.

TRAUMATIC BRAIN DAMAGE (TABLE 1)

A certain amount of brain damage is sustained at the time of injury and in a closed, non-missile injury is the result of shear strains occurring within the head at the moment of impact. More important than such primary damage, at least from the point of view of early management, are the complications which lead to secondary brain damage. In a severe injury it is common for more than one disorder to be present; indeed the interactions between the various pathophysiological processes illustrated in Fig. 1 can pose the greatest threat to the brain, with ischaemia being the most important final mechanism in most cases.

Primary traumatic brain damage

Diffuse axonal injury results when the shear strains between different parts of the brain cause distortion, stretching, and even tearing of the axons in the white matter of the cerebral hemispheres and brain-stem. The tiny neuronal lesions that result are distributed widely and diffusely and it is now believed that the number of these lesions and whether or not they are reversible or permanent, are the main determinants of the initial severity of a head injury. Clinically their characteristic feature is an immediate impairment of consciousness. In its most mild form, this may be restricted to a transient loss of awareness and memory for a few

Table 1 *Traumatic brain damage*

Primary (impact) damage
Diffuse: axonal injury
Focal: cortical contusion and lacerations

Secondary complications
Extracranial: hypoxia, hypotension
Intracranial: haematoma, infection

Consequences of complications
Brain swelling, raised intracranial pressure
Brain shift
Hypoxic/ischaemic brain damage

minutes classically referred to as 'concussion'. At the other extreme the patient may be in profound and prolonged coma. Diffuse white matter lesions are also thought to underlie many of the symptoms and much of the disability that follows when consciousness is ultimately recovered.

Contusions and lacerations are found focally, predominantly in the cerebral cortex. Whatever the site of a blow on the head, the subsequent contusions are located maximally on the undersurfaces of the frontal and temporal lobes, and are due to displacement of the brain and contact with the sharp bony ridges at the base of the skull. The concept of a 'contrecoup' distribution of injury, i.e. maximal opposite to the point of impact on the skull, is now thought to be invalid. A blow struck violently with a sharp instrument may produce a compound depressed fracture with a contusion directly underlying the wound.

When contusions occur in an eloquent area of the cortex there may be focal neurological signs in the acute stage. Contusions in the frontal and temporal lobes also may contribute to the changes in personality and mental state and the epilepsy that can follow a head injury.

Secondary brain damage

Secondary brain damage develops after a delay and should be treatable or preventable. The damage to the brain is ultimately the result of ischaemia, secondary to inadequate delivery of oxygen, and is usually either

Fig. 1 Interactions between impact brain damage and the complications leading to secondary ischaemic brain damage.

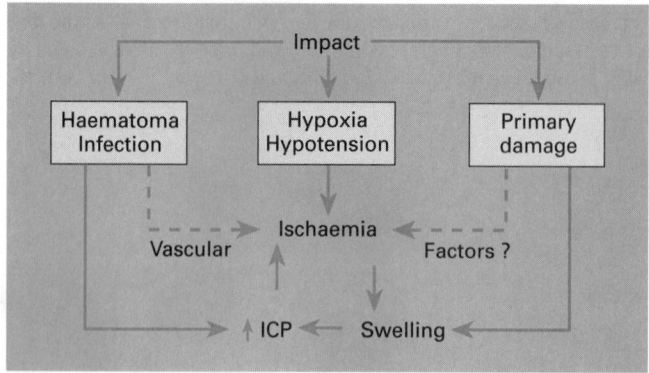

Table 2 *Causes of hypoxia or hypotension after a head injury*

Hypoxia
Airway obstruction
Chest injuries (fractures, flail chest, haemo/pneumo/thorax)
Chest infection and pulmonary collapse
Lung shunting
Fat emboli
Adult respiratory distress syndrome
Neurogenic pulmonary oedema (rare)

Hypotension
Multiple injuries with blood loss
Associated spinal cord injury
Excessive bleeding from scalp, from a base of skull fracture,
    or, in an infant, with an extradural clot
Myocardial injury or infarct

Table 3 *Risks of an intracranial haematoma in adult head injured. Patients assessed at the time of first hospital attendance*

	Percentage of head injuries	Risk of a haematoma
No skull fracture		
Fully oriented	91	1 in 6000
Not oriented	7	1 in 120
Skull fractured		
Fully oriented	1	1 in 30
Not oriented	1	1 in 4

a consequence of impaired oxygenation of the blood or an inadequate cerebral blood flow. The difference between the systemic arterial pressure and the intracranial pressure (ICP) is termed the cerebral perfusion pressure. Either a low blood pressure or a high ICP may threaten cerebral blood flow, and a combination is particularly dangerous.

Normally the brain copes with reductions in blood oxygenation or in cerebral perfusion pressure by adjusting the cerebral circulation to maintain adequate blood flow and oxygenation. Primary brain damage interferes with this autoregulatory mechanism so that flow may become dependent on the perfusion pressure, therefore, the brain is even more vulnerable after a head injury.

EXTRACRANIAL COMPLICATIONS

The most important complication of the immediate loss of consciousness characteristic of a head injury is airway obstruction and/or inadequate ventilation. So long as consciousness is impaired, and especially if a patient has other serious injuries, several factors may lead to hypoxia or hypotension (Table 2). Hypoxia and hypotension are particularly likely to occur during the transport of a patient between different departments in a hospital or between two hospitals. Brief episodes are also common even while the patient is receiving intensive care, but may not be detected unless continuous monitoring is employed.

INTRACRANIAL COMPLICATIONS

Traumatic intracranial haematoma

Although only 1 in 500 patients attending hospital develops intracranial bleeding, the supposed unpredictability of this complication is responsible for the treacherous reputation of head injuries.

An extradural haematoma is usually associated with a skull fracture and is the result of bleeding between the site of the fracture and the underlying dura.

Intradural haematomas are more common (three out of four cases). The bleed may be into the subdural space or within the brain itself (intracerebral haematoma); in a third of cases there is a combination of subdural bleeding, cortical laceration, and intracerebral haemorrhage, the so-called 'burst' frontal or temporal lobes. Many patients have a skull fracture but intradural clots often are not closely related to the fracture as are the extradural clots.

Blood vessels giving rise to a traumatic intracranial haematoma probably are damaged at the time of injury, but some time is needed before the size of the haematoma is sufficient to exhaust the brain's capacity to compensate for a space-occupying lesion. There then ensues a combination of shift and mechanical distortion of the brain and also an impairment of cerebral blood flow secondary to the rise in intracranial pressure. The most important clinical characteristic of the resulting cerebral ischaemia is a deteriorating level of consciousness.

The interval between injury and deterioration is usually measured in hours, or days, but may be as short as a few minutes, or occasionally as long as a few weeks. During this period the patient is rarely completely well, most have persisting confusion or altered consciousness as a result of a degree of primary damage.

Risk of a haematoma

During this 'silent' interval information about the presence or absence of a skull fracture and whether or not the patient is fully conscious can be used to estimate the risk of the patient later developing a haematoma. (The data for an adult are shown in Table 3; the risks in children are slightly lower but show the same pattern.) More profound degrees of impairment of consciousness carry much greater risks. Even without a fracture, persisting coma carries a risk of a haemotoma of 1 in 4.

Infection

Meningitis and brain abscess are complications of either a compound depressed fracture of the vault of the skull, or an open fracture of the base of the skull. In the latter case, where the fracture runs into the paranasal air spaces, the clue to the risk of infection is the presence of a leak of cerebrospinal fluid from the nose (rhinorrhoea) or from the ears (otorrhoea). Other signs of a basal fracture are corneal or conjunctival haemorrhage without a posterior limit, a black eye on both sides, and bruising developing behind the ear (Battle's sign). Sixty per cent of cases are due to the pneumococcus but a wide variety of organisms can be responsible. Infection may develop several days, weeks, or sometimes years after the injury.

Brain swelling

The damaged brain around a contusion or underneath a blood clot may become progressively swollen; this can also occur diffusely in one or both cerebral hemispheres. The cause may be a vascular engorgement or true oedema, i.e. an accumulation of water. Oedema and engorgement may be less common than previously believed. They seem to occur often as a response to an injury, rather than being a primary mechanism in producing damage.

Other neurological complications

Other structures that may be injured in a head injury include the cranial nerves (especially the olfactory, optic, occulomotor, facial, and auditory nerves), and, in severe injuries, the pituitary gland and hypothalamus. Deafness and dizziness may also be caused by damage to the structures of the middle and inner ear, either as a result of the initial forces of the injury or a fracture of the base of the skull.

Management in the acute stage

RESUSCITATION (SEE ALSO SECTION 16)

The ABC of resuscitation is the priority in those patients who arrive at hospital in coma, or who have multiple injuries. The *airway* must be cleared and maintained free from the earliest possible moment. As a temporary measure this may be achieved by placing the patient in the

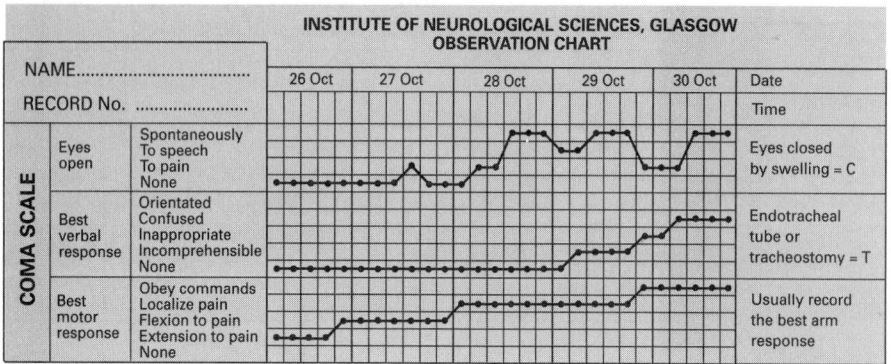

Fig. 2 Chart showing Glasgow Coma Scale recorded on a patient progressively recovering from a diffuse primary head injury. (Reproduced by kind permission of the *Journal of The Royal College of Physicians*.)

semiprone position; later the use of oropharyngeal or endotracheal tubes may be necessary. If *breathing* proves inadequate, particularly as judged by abnormal blood gas values, mechanical ventilation may be necessary. Restoration of an adequate *circulation* is essential; hypotension is rarely the result of a head injury alone and should be a signal to search for serious extracranial injuries.

DIAGNOSIS

In a patient with impaired consciousness an accurate initial diagnosis can be difficult but it is important to discover the answers to two questions. Has the patient had a head injury? Has the patient had only a head injury? Common errors include the misdiagnosis of a head-injured patient as being 'drunk' or suffering from a stroke, or the overlooking of major injuries elsewhere in the body in a patient with an obvious head injury.

Assessing brain damage and its evolution

Changes in the level of consciousness are more important than focal neurological signs and provide an overall index of brain dysfunction and damage. Repeated assessments of the degree of altered consciousness provide a guide to the initial severity of brain damage and to the pattern of recovery. When a patient has suffered only primary damage, a steady improvement can be anticipated; if the patient's consciousness does not improve, and particularly if there is deterioration, the occurrence of secondary damage should be suspected.

It is therefore important to learn as much as possible about the immediate effects of the injury on conscious level and to reassess consciousness frequently. Communication of such information between nurses and doctors, and with doctors in other hospitals is an essential part of management and this task has been made simpler by the use of the Glasgow Coma Scale (see Chapter 24.4.4). This assesses three aspects of consciousness: eye opening, verbal, and motor responses, and can be readily and clearly charted (Fig. 2). Its use in coma is described in more detail in Chapter 24.4.4 and Section 16. Comparisons of the movements and power of the limbs can be useful clues to focal damage, but tendon and plantar reflexes are rarely helpful. Changes in the response of the pupil to light are an important sign of dysfunction of the third cranial nerve and of developing intracranial shift and brain-stem compression.

Radiological investigations (Fig. 3)

A skull radiograph can provide helpful information because the finding of a fracture greatly increases the risk of intracranial complications. Fractures of the vault are readily shown in radiographs but fractures in the base of the skull can be difficult to detect because some bones are paper thin and others extremely thick and dense. Suspicion should be raised by the finding of intracranial air or fluid levels in the paranasal air sinuses.

A skull radiograph is not needed for all head injuries, and clinical criteria that help to select patients for radiography are shown in Table 4. Whenever there is a question of multiple injuries, additional plain radiographs of the cervical spine, chest, and pelvis should be taken.

Computed tomography (CT) scanning

CT scanning (Fig. 4) can detect only the more severe forms of primary brain damage but its ability to show very clearly the presence of a haematoma has transformed the management of head injuries. Selection of patients for CT scanning is discussed below.

Intracranial pressure (ICP) monitoring

ICP monitoring is used in some units in the management of more severe injuries. Many of the complications of head injury cause a rise in ICP and monitoring can provide early warning of their development and so direct appropriate management.

Fig. 3 Examples of radiographs of head-injured patients showing (a) Linear fissure fracture crossing the course of the posterior branches of the middle meningeal vessels. (b) A depressed comminuted fracture of the skull vault.

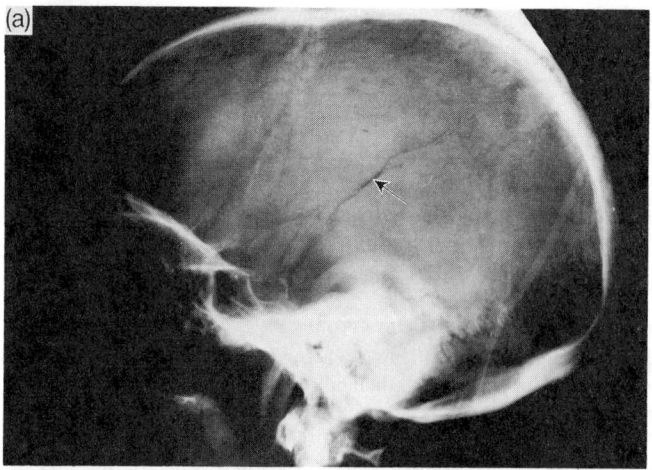

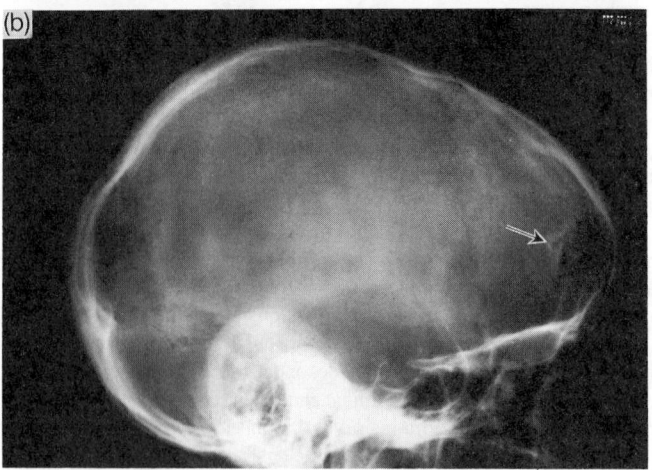

Table 4 *Guidelines for the performance of a skull radiograph in a recently head-injured patient*

Clinical judgement is necessary but the following criteria are helpful:

1. Loss of consciousness or amnesia at any time
2. Neurological symptoms or signs
3. Cerebrospinal fluid or blood from the nose or ear
4. Suspected penetrating injury
5. Scalp bruising or swelling
6. Difficulty in assessing the patient (i.e. alcohol intoxication, epilepsy, children)

MANAGEMENT OF INTRACRANIAL COMPLICATIONS

Intracranial haematoma

Until recently the diagnosis of an intracranial haemorrhage rested mainly upon finding evidence of deteriorating responsiveness. This led to the admission of many patients for observation in hospital for 1 to 2 days, most of whom proved not to have a haematoma. In practice there is not a characteristic sequence of changes in consciousness, and delayed recognition of deterioration allows secondary degree brain damage to develop. The capacity of CT scanning to enable diagnosis before deterioration becomes advanced and before cerebral compression becomes irreversible has provided the opportunity for more effective intervention. CT scanning often involves transfer to a neurosurgical unit and it is therefore necessary to select patients most likely to benefit.

The data about a skull fracture, the patient's initial conscious level, and the risk of a haematoma (Table 3) provide a basis for guidelines about which patients may merit admission for observation, which can be sent home, and those for whom CT scanning should be arranged without delay. Tables 5 and 6 show the guidelines used in the West of Scotland; essentially similar criteria have been put forward by a national group of neurosurgeons and accepted by a Government working party and it is expected that their use will improve the results of management of head injuries.

The outcome of operation for an extradural haematoma is usually good, with a mortality of 10 to 15 per cent. Although an intradural clot is more often associated with primary brain damage and mortality is 30 to 40 per cent, prompt evacuation is also usually followed by recovery.

Depressed skull fracture

Open fractures of the vault of the skull require surgical debridement and closure both of the skin and of the dura. The latter forms a very good barrier to subsequent infection. If the operation is carried out within the

Fig. 4 Computed tomographic images of head injury. (a) Small areas of bleeding (white lesions) in the basal ganglia and brain-stem (arrowed) of a patient with severe diffuse axonal injury. (b) Contusions in the cortex of frontal and temporal lobes. (c) An extradural haematoma. (d) Subdural and intracerebral (arrowed) bleeding.

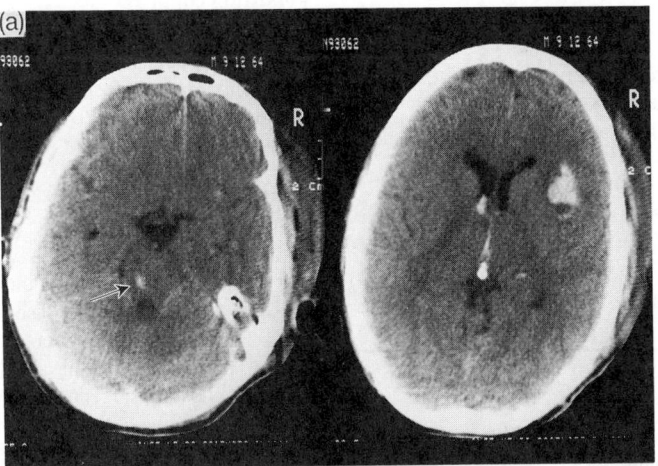

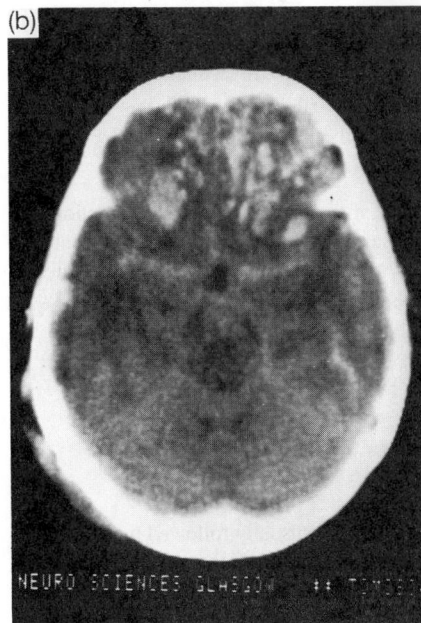
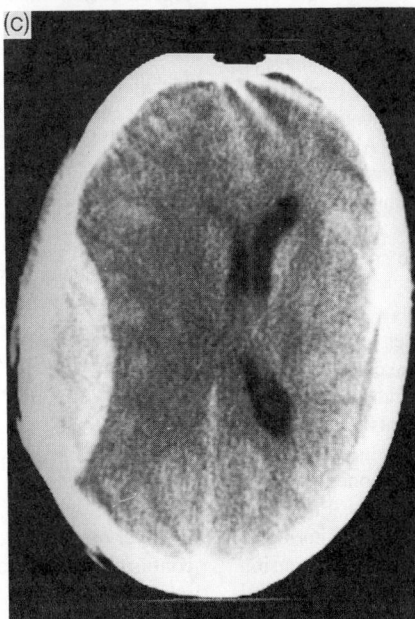
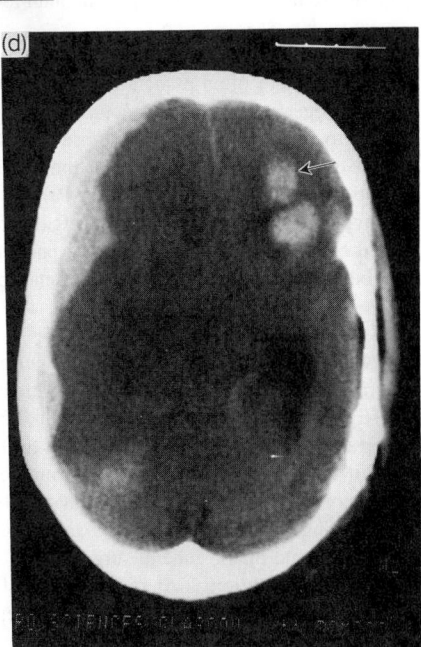

Table 5 *Guidelines for admission of adult head-injured patients to hospital*

1. Confusion or any other depression of the level of consciousness at the time of examination
2. Skull fracture
3. Neurological symptoms or signs
4. Difficulty in assessing the patient, e.g. alcohol, epilepsy
5. Other medical conditions, e.g. haemophilia
6. The patient's social conditions or lack of a responsible adult/relative

   Post-traumatic amnesia or unconsciousness with full recovery is not necessarily an indication for admission

   Patients sent home should receive advice to return immediately if there is any deterioration

Table 6 *Guidelines for consultation with a neurosurgeon about a head-injured patient*

1. Fractured skull
   with confusion or worse impairment of consciousness or
   with focal neurological signs or
   with fits, or
   with any other neurological symptoms or signs
2. Coma continuing after resuscitation—even if no skull fracture
3. Deterioration in level of consciousness or other neurological signs
4. Confusion or other neurological disturbances persisting for more than 6–8 h, even if there is no skull fracture
5. Compound depressed fracture of the vault of the skull
6. Suspected fracture of base of skull (CSF rhinorrhoea or otorrhoea, bilateral orbital haematoma, mastoid haematoma) or other penetrating injury (gunshot etc.)
   Patients in categories 1–3 should be referred urgently

   NOTE: In all cases the diagnosis and initial treatment of serious extracranial injuries take priority over transfer to the neurosurgical unit

first 24 h the risk of infection is minimal, but heavily contaminated wounds are treated with prophylactic antibiotics.

Cerebrospinal fluid leakage and basal fracture

Such injuries are often associated with substantial primary damage to the brain but many of these fractures heal spontaneously. Therefore it is usual to delay operation and to close the fistula only in patients whose cerebrospinal fluid leak persists for more than a week. Although there is controversy about their value, most British neurosurgeons recommend prophylactic antibiotic treatment during this period. Penicillin is administered because of its efficacy against pneumococcus, and sulphadimidine because of its ability to penetrate into the cerebrospinal fluid.

Multiple injuries

It is vital to diagnose and treat these injuries in order to stabilize the general condition of the head-injured patient. This takes priority over investigation and operation on intracranial injuries and is particularly important in victims of high-speed road traffic accidents. On the other hand, it is best to avoid extensive definitive surgery, e.g. for internal fixation of major limb fractures, which can often be postponed for some days, during which time simple external fixation suffices. Prolonged anaesthesia and major general surgery interfere with the monitoring of the patient's condition. If there is extensive bleeding with hypotension or if the anaesthetic agent raises the intracranial pressure, additional

Table 7 *Guidelines for patients in coma or with possible multiple injuries*

1. Assess for respiratory insufficiency, for shock, and for internal injuries, especially after a high-velocity injury, e.g. a road traffic accident
2. Perform: (*a*) chest radiograph; (*b*) blood gas estimation; (*c*) cervical spine radiograph; (*d*) other investigations as relevant
3. Appropriate treatment may include:
   Intubate (e.g. if airway obstructed or threatened)
   Ventilate (e.g. cyanosis, $Pao_2 < 60$ mmHg, $Paco_2 > 45$ mmHg
   Commence IV infusion (1500 ml/24 h)
   Mannitol, only after consultation with neurosurgeon
   Application of cervical collar or cervical traction
   Immobilization of fractures, treatment of internal injuries
4. If accepted for transfer the patient should be accompanied by personnel able to insert or to reposition an endotracheal tube, and to initiate or to maintain ventilation

brain damage may be incurred. Table 7 shows the recommendations given to hospitals in the West of Scotland for the assessment and management of patients in coma or with multiple injuries prior to transfer to the neurosurgical unit.

Persisting coma

This carries risks of respiratory dysfunction and infection, fluid and electrolyte imbalance, nutritional deficiency, joint contractures, bedsores, and urinary infection. The avoidance of these usually entails management in a well-staffed and equipped intensive care unit (see Section 16).

Ventilation

This is necessary in patients whose respiratory dysfunction threatens adequate oxygenation. This may be the result of inadequate ventilation, due to airway obstruction or thoracic injury, for example, or of inadequate gas exchange—atelectasis from aspiration of blood or gastric contents. Hyperventilation lowers cerebral blood volume and hence intracranial pressure, but can also reduce cerebral blood flow so that ischaemia develops; it is now used selectively and as briefly as possible.

Osmotic agents

Agents such as mannitol or frusemide are given intravenously to remove water from the brain and effectively lower intracranial pressure. They can be useful in producing a temporary improvement, e.g. to buy sufficient time to allow definitive intracranial investigation, but repeated doses lose efficacy and may result in hypovolemia with reduced cerebral perfusion pressure, as well as leading to electrolyte imbalance.

Drugs

Drugs that have been used with the aim of preventing or ameliorating brain damage include corticosteroids (in the expectation of reducing cerebral oedema) and barbiturates (to depress cerebral metabolism). Although experimentally effective when given before an injury, recent clinical studies have shown conclusively that these treatments are not of value and they carry risks of increased infection and hypotension. More specific 'neuroprotective' drugs are now under trial.

Late sequelae and disability after head injury
AMNESIA

Recovery from altered consciousness is usually followed by a period of confusion and loss of memory. The time from the injury to the restoration of on-going memory is referred to as post-traumatic amnesia

(PTA) and its duration provides a good index, albeit in retrospect, of the severity of brain damage. Some loss of memory for events immediately prior to the injury is common but such retrograde amnesia is usually relatively brief and shrinks as time passes.

POSTCONCUSSIONAL SYMPTOMS

Even an apparently mild injury can be followed by a variety of symptoms, including headache, dizziness, failure of concentration, and impairment of memory. Because physical signs may be lacking, and any abnormalities are often subtle, the basis of these symptoms has been in debate. There is now evidence that periods of loss of consciousness of even as little as 5 min can result in diffuse axonal brain damage. This has provided a valid basis for many complaints, especially when they develop within the first few days after an injury. In many patients the symptoms resolve spontaneously, if sometimes slowly, but they can be perpetuated by premature return to 'stressful' work or by other causes of anxiety or depression. When there is a gap of some weeks between the injury and the onset of 'postconcussional' symptoms, it is likely that psychological factors are prominent in their generation.

DISABILITY AFTER SEVERE INJURY

Prolonged loss of consciousness in the early stage increases the risk of persisting disabilities, and these are almost invariable when post-traumatic amnesia has been longer than a month. Obvious physical deficits, such as hemiparesis and ataxia, are less common and much less important than changes in mental function, and particularly in memory and personality. Assessment of outcome after head injury should therefore be directed to overall social reintegration as shown in Table 8.

POST-TRAUMATIC EPILEPSY (SEE ALSO CHAPTER 24.4.1)

Epilepsy occurring within 1 week of a head injury is distinguished from that developing later, which is more likely to recur. The main pointers to the risk of late epilepsy are the presence, in the acute stage, of an intracranial haematoma, a compound depressed skull fracture, particularly with dural laceration, and amnesia for more than 24 h. If any of these are present, the patient should be advised to seek the approval of the Department of Transport before recommencing driving. The treatment of post-traumatic epilepsy should be with conventional anticonvulsant drugs. Prophylactic treatment may be considered appropriate if the risk is judged to be very high, but compliance is often poor unless or until a seizure occurs.

CHRONIC SUBDURAL HAEMATOMA

A fluid collection of blood between the dura and the brain can follow even a relatively mild head injury, particularly in the elderly, alcoholics, or those with impaired coagulation function. In about half of cases no injury is recalled. Symptoms may occur hours or even months after the injury. If the condition follows a severe head injury with unconsciousness, the patient may recover consciousness only to lapse into coma again. In more chronic cases the course is typically fluctuating. Particularly in the elderly, however, the trivial injury is frequently forgotten. The commonest symptom is headache and, as the condition worsens, vomiting. The condition may cause considerable diagnostic difficulty in the elderly, particularly if it presents with mood changes, irritability, urinary incontinence, or drowsiness, all of which may be mistakenly attributed to senescence. The commonest neurological signs are pupillary inequality, and long track signs with motor limb asymmetry and, occasionally, an extensor plantar response. Dysphasia occurs in about a fifth of patients. Fits are less common although they occurred in approximately 5 to 10 per cent of cases in one large series.

This condition should be suspected in any patient who deteriorates after an initial period of improvement after a head injury or who presents

Table 8 *Glasgow scale of outcome after severe head injury*

Death	Most occur in the first week but may
Vegetative state	be delayed several months. Spontaneous breathing and eye opening and 'sleep-wake' cycles present but no sign of psychologically mediated responses; do not speak; do not obey commands
Severe disability	Conscious, speaking, some have no physical disabilities but mental changes predominate in making a person dependent for survival in society, e.g. cannot shop, cannot go on public transport
Moderate disability	Independent, but are unable to resume fully preinjury activities; may work but in a reduced capacity
Good recovery	Able to resume preinjury life-style, even if mild residual neurological deficits are present

with an unusual neurological picture at any age. In the majority of cases, the condition can be diagnosed by CT scanning although, because the subdural collection may be isodense at some stage during its evolution, the interpretation can be difficult. Isotope scanning is also accurate in about 90 per cent of cases. The treatment of choice is to evacuate the haematoma through burr holes. It is possible that very small collections can be allowed to resolve under careful surveillance. It has also been suggested that corticosteroids may have a place to play in mild cases, although this remains uncertain; subdural haematoma should never be treated without expert neurosurgical advice. A review of recent results showed that the overall mortality was 6 per cent, which seems to have changed little following the advent of CT scanning. Another 5 per cent showed severe disability while the outcome was good in 89 per cent of cases. Importantly, the prognosis was not related to age and therefore this condition should be sought for and treated actively in all age groups.

HYDROCEPHALUS

Hydrocephalus very occasionally results from an obstruction of the cerebrospinal fluid pathways and should not be confused with the passive *ex vacuo* ventricular enlargement which occurs with cerebral atrophy after a severe head injury. This can be brought about by fibrosis, a sequel to bleeding in the early stages, and such patients may be greatly benefited by insertion of a ventriculoperitoneal shunt in order to divert the cerebrospinal fluid flow.

BRAIN DAMAGE AFTER BOXING, POST-TRAUMATIC ENCEPHALOPATHY

It has been recognized for many years that certain boxers developed a syndrome characterized by forgetfulness, irritability, dysarthria, pyramidal damage, and ataxia. This occurred particularly after a long but unsuccessful career—prompting the term 'punch drunk'. Although in some cases the deterioration appeared to be simply an acceleration of normal ageing processes, in others it progressed more rapidly. In such cases a specific accentuation of damage in the hippocampus and mamillary bodies has been suggested by postmortem studies.

There is clinical evidence that repeated minor head injuries in many other sports (e.g. riding) may also cause cumulative brain damage, and there is now great concern that sports' participants should be warned of this risk. Although it is customary to advise a person who has been 'knocked out' to refrain from sport for some time, it is not known for how long this should be, or indeed if it will ever be 'safe' again.

REFERENCES

Adams, J.H., Graham, D.I., Scott, G., Parker, L.S., and Doyle, D., (1980). Brain damage after fatal non-missile head injury. *Journal of Clinical Pathology* **33**, 1132–45.

Anon (1984). Guidelines for initial management after head injuries in adults. *British Medical Journal* **288**, 983–5.

Brooks, N., *et al.* (1984). *Closed head injury. Psychological, social and family consequences.* Oxford University Press.

Fenton Lewis, A. (1983) *The management of acute head injury.* Harrogate Seminar Report 8, Department of Health and Social Security, London.

Jennett, B. and Teasdale, G. (1981). *Management of head injuries.* F.A. Davies, Philadelphia.

Teasdale, G. and Jennett, B. (1974). Assessment of impaired consciousness and coma. *Lancet* **ii**, 81–4.

Teasdale, G.M., *et al.* (1990). Risks of acute traumatic intracranial haematoma in children and adults: implications for managing head injuries. *British Medical Journal* **300** 363–7.

24.15 Clinical presentation of infections of the nervous system

24.15.1 Bacterial meningitis

D.W.M. CROOK, PRIDA PHUAPRADIT, AND D.A. WARRELL

Bacterial meningitis, also known as pyogenic, purulent, or cerebrospinal meningitis, is an inflammation of the leptomeninges with infection of the cerebrospinal fluid (CSF) within the subarachnoid space of the brain and spinal cord, and the ventricular system.

Anatomy of the subarachnoid space

In the absence of pathological blockages, bacteria entering the subarachnoid space at any point can spread over the surface of the brain and into the perivascular spaces of Virchow Robin. After reaching the basal cisterns they can pass through the foramina of Luschka and Magendie into the fourth ventricle, and thence through the cerebral aqueduct of Sylvius to reach the third ventricle, and through the interventricular foramina of Monro to the lateral ventricles. Subdural empyema (pachymeningitis interna) or effusion complicating leptomeningitis can also spread freely because the arachnoid membrane and dura matera are almost entirely separated. By contrast, because of the tight application of the dura mater to the periosteum of the skull, epidural collections of pus are localized. In the spinal column, however, the epidural space is loose and contains fat, permitting the extension of a posterior spinal epidural abscess over several vertebral segments. Within the subarachnoid space and intraventricular system, infection may produce blockages of CSF circulation, especially at the various foramina or in the aqueduct, causing obstructive hydrocephalus or spinal block. If reabsorption of CSF across the subarachnoid granulations is prevented by a subarachnoid haematoma or empyema or thrombosis of the intracranial veins and venous sinuses, communicating hydrocephalus will result. In patients with meningitis, intracranial hypertension may be the result of cerebral oedema, the ventricular dilatation of hydrocephalus, or subdural or epidural collection of pus. Obstructive hydrocephalus and intracranial collections of pus carry a special risk of producing brain herniation after lumbar puncture.

Because they cross the inflamed basal meninges, the cranial nerves and cerebral arteries may be damaged. Cranial nerves may be compressed by intracranial hypertension (VI) or brain herniation (III) or suffer ischaemic damage from vasculitis.

Acute bacterial meningitis

CLASSIFICATION

Pyogenic bacterial meningitis occurs in a number of clinical situations, each of which is associated with a particular pattern of infecting organisms, clinical presentation, management, and outcome. Spontaneous meningitis is the most important category and can be divided into neonatal meningitis or meningitis of childhood and adulthood. Posttraumatic meningitis follows neurosurgery or fracture of the skull. Device-associated meningitis occurs particularly in association with cerebrospinal fluid shunts and drains. Infection may also be considered as community acquired or nosocomial (hospital acquired) (Table 1).

AETIOLOGICAL AGENTS AND EPIDEMIOLOGY

The bacterial species that cause meningitis vary by geographical region and according to the categories mentioned above. Age and local social conditions also have a major influence on the attack rate and mortality of spontaneous meningitis.

Neonatal meningitis is usually caused by three species; group B streptococci *(Streptococcus agalactiae),* K1 capsulate *Escherichia coli* and *Listeria monocytogenes.* A wide range of other organisms has been reported to cause the disease. Infection mostly occurs in the postpartum period, but can occur as late as 6 weeks after birth. Prolonged rupture of membranes and low birth weight are two major risk factors.

Spontaneous community-acquired meningitis in children (under 14 years of age) is usually caused by *Neisseria meningitidis, Streptococcus pneumoniae,* and *Haemophilus influenzae.* However, national implementation of conjugated *H. influenzae* type b (Hib) capsular vaccine immunisation programmes by many countries during the 1990s will produce a dramatic reduction and near disappearance of Hib meningitis. The highest attack rate of all three bacterial species is in children under 1 year of age and falls off rapidly with increasing age. The decrease in susceptibility to infection by these organisms with increasing age results from the acquisition of protective immunity, mainly as a result of nasopharyngeal carriage.

In adults, spontaneous community acquired meningitis is usually caused by *N. meningitidis* and *Strep. pneumoniae* which account for approximately 70 to 80 per cent of the cases. *Listeria monocytogenes,* aerobic Gram-negative bacilli (such as *E. coli), H. influenzae* and *Staphylococcus aureus* cause most of the remaining cases (see Table 2). The attack rate of *N. meningitidis* meningitis is usually low (1–5 cases/10^5 persons/year) and considered endemic, but occasionally the incidence

Table 1 *Predisposing factors in 404 single episodes of spontaneous adult bacterial meningitis, Massachusetts General Hospital, Boston, USA, 1961–88*

Factor	Community acquired (N = 253) (%)	Nosocomial (N = 151) (%)
Actute otitis media	19	1
Chronic otitis media	7	0
Sinusitis	12	4
Pneumonia	15	8
Endocarditis	7	1
Head injury[a]		
Recent	5	13
Remote	4	0
Recent neurosurgery[a]	0	68
Neurosurgical device[b]	1	32
Altered immune state	19	31
Diabetes mellitus	10	6
Alcoholism	18	5
Cerebrospinal fluid leak	8	13
None of the 13 factors	25	8

[a]Recent denotes head injury or neurosurgery within 1 month of the onset of meningitis; remote, more than 1 month before the onset of meningitis.

[b]Neurosurgical devices included ventriculostomy, ventriculoperitoneal or ventriculoatrial shunt, lumbar epidural catheter, lumboperitoneal catheter, and dorsal-column stimulator.

(Reproduced from Durand *et al.* (1993), with permission.)

Table 2 *Causative organisms in spontaneous single episodes of adult meningitis, Massachusetts General Hospital, Boston, USA, 1962–88*

Organism	Community acquired (N = 253) number (%)	Nosocomial (N = 151) number (%)
Strep. pneumoniae	97 (38)	8 (5)
Gram-negative bacilli	9 (4)	57 (38)
N. meningitidis	35 (14)	1 (1)
Streptococci	17 (7)	13 (9)
Enterococcus	0	4 (3)
Staph. aureus	13 (5)	13 (9)
L. monocytogenes	29 (11)	5 (3)
H. influenzae	9 (4)	6 (4)
Mixed bacterial species	6 (2)	10 (7)
Coagulase-negative staphylococci	0	13 (9)
Other	4 (2)	5 (3)
Culture negative	34 (13)	16 (11)

Percentages do not always total 100 because of rounding.

(Reproduced from Durand *et al.* (1993), with permission.)

of the infection may increase and even reach epidemic proportions (for example, >300 cases/10⁵ persons/year). Crowding is thought to play a role in the epidemics occurring in military recruits, South African miners, and other groups of people crowded together in closed environments. The attack rate of *N. meningitidis* disease may increase secondarily to epidemics of influenza A. However, the precise origin of the major epidemics affecting countries such as Brazil in the 1970s and regions such as sub-Saharan Africa remains unexplained. The bacterial capsule plays a role in determining the pattern of invasive disease caused by *N. meningitidis*. Capsulate serogroups A, B, and C occur sporadically and cause outbreaks of invasive disease, while serogroups Y, W, Z, W-135, and 29-E cause only occasional cases.

The attack rate of *Strep. pneumoniae* meningitis (1–2 cases/10⁵ persons/year) is remarkably constant around the world. It increases in patients of advanced age (>70 years). A high proportion of pneumococcal cases exhibit an associated infected focus. Otitis media or sinusitis is found in approximately 30 per cent of cases and pneumonia in up to 25 per cent. Hypogammaglobulinaemia (primary or secondary, for example nephrotic syndrome and chronic lymphocytic leukaemia), sickle-cell disease, and previous trauma to the skull (see below) are risk factors for developing pneumococcal meningitis.

Strep. suis (Group R haemolytic streptococcus) serotypes 2, 4, and 14 is an important cause of meningitis (and rarely infective endocarditis) in the Far East (Hong Kong, Thailand) and in other countries, related to occupational contact with pigs or pork. In Holland, the incidence of *Strep. suis* meningitis among abattoir workers and pig breeders was 3.0/100000 per year and it is now the commonest cause of bacterial meningitis in Hong Kong. Possible routes of entry include skin abrasions found in 40 per cent of patients and upper respiratory and gastrointestinal tracts.

Listeria monocytogenes accounts for few cases of meningitis, with an attack rate of approximately 0.2 to 0.4 cases/10⁵ persons/year or 1 to 5

per cent of the cases of meningitis. Increased attack rates have been associated with contaminated foods such as unpasteurized soft cheeses, pâté, and poorly refrigerated pre-cooked chicken. People at the extremes of age, pregnant women, and those with altered host defence from prolonged immunosuppression with corticosteroids or alkylating agents such as azothiaprine are at increased risk of listeriosis. *Staphylococcus aureus* causes 1 to 5 per cent of the cases with spontaneous meningitis and usually occurs in association with infective endocarditis. Spontaneous cases of *H. influenzae* meningitis, both capsule type b and noncapsulate strains, account for up to 5 per cent of adult cases of meningitis. Aerobic Gram-negative (for example *E. coli*) meningitis occurs especially in the aged, debilitated, and diabetic. The source in these infections is usually thought to be the renal tract.

Post-traumatic meningitis occurs in patients who have sustained trauma to the skull or spine (for example skull fracture) or who have undergone head and neck or spinal surgery. It usually arises in association with a CSF leak and soon after injury, but may occur many years after the trauma. The risk of developing meningitis is as high as 25 per cent with clinically apparent CSF leak. The aetiology depends on whether the infection is acquired nosocomially or in the community. The majority of hospital-acquired infections are caused by aerobic Gram-negative bacilli, such as *E. coli*, *Klebsiella pneumoniae*, other Enterobacteriaceae, *Acinetobacter* spp. and *Pseudomonas* spp. (see Table 2). Less commonly, *Strep. pneumoniae*, *H. influenzae*, *Staph. aureus*, and other normal upper respiratory tract flora cause meningitis in patients in hospital. Post-traumatic meningitis acquired in the community is caused mainly by *Strep. pneumoniae* (>90 per cent) and *H. influenzae*. Various other bacterial species have been reported as rare causes of post-traumatic meningitis.

Device-associated meningitis is a well-recognized entity and occurs in patients with CSF drains and CSF shunts. Most infections are nosocomial and are caused by coagulase-negative staphylococci (50–60 per cent) and *Staph. aureus* (15–30 per cent). Aerobic Gram-negative bacilli, *Streptococcus* spp., *Corynebacteria* spp., and *Propriobacterium acnes* are encountered. These infections usually present within a few months of inserting the device. Occasionally, *Strep. pneumoniae*, *N. meningitidis*, and *H. influenzae* are responsible.

Recurrent meningitis is an unusual (<10 per cent of meningitis), but well-recognized clinical category. Such cases frequently have either an underlying anatomical defect (for example, CSF leak or spina bifida) or an immunological defect. The immune deficiencies that most often predispose to recurrent meningitis are hypogammaglobulinaemia and complement deficiencies.

PATHOGENESIS

The acquisition and mode of invasion of the CSF vary with the type of meningitis. However, once infection is established, the inflammatory injury and pathophysiology are remarkably similar in all types of meningitis.

The organisms that cause neonatal meningitis are acquired by the baby from the vagina and perineum during delivery, or from the environment soon after birth. The three main infecting species, *Strep. agalactiae* (group B streptococci), *E. coli*, and *L. monocytogenes*, invade the host, cause septicaemia, and, as a result, produce meningitis. An unusual feature of the *E. coli* and a large proportion of the *Strep. agalactiae* strains (capsular types K1 and III, respectively) is that their capsules consist of polysialic acid. The remarkable association of this unusual type of capsule with two strains causing this disease suggests a role in the pathogenesis of neonatal meningitis.

The organisms that cause spontaneous meningitis, *Strep. pneumoniae*, *H. influenzae*, and *N. meningitidis*, are acquired by person-to-person spread. Colonization is the essential first step before invasion. Asymptomatic carriage implies a stable and well-adapted relationship between microbe and host. Fortunately, this is the usual outcome. Invasion and infection of the host resulting in disease represents a rare and potentially catastrophic breakdown in the relationship between the bacterium and host. Invasion of the host is particularly likely to occur early after acquisition of the organism, before the host has developed protective immunity. Carriage is sufficient to produce immunity and resistance to disease. The greatest risk of disease, therefore, is in the first few years of life, at a time when the non-immune host first encounters these pathogens. The precise anatomical site of invasion is not known for all three pathogens. Animal studies suggest that for *H. influenzae* meningitis the nasopharynx is the probable site of systemic invasion. Invasion is associated with escape into the bloodstream of a single organism that multiplies and produces septicaemia. Bacteria then gain access to the CSF in a proportion of these bacteraemic cases. Invasion of the CSF is probably dependent on the concentration of organisms in the blood and on the species causing bacteraemia (for example, bacteria such as enterococci can cause high-intensity bacteraemia under some conditions but the organisms seldom enter the CSF, whereas *N. meningitidis*, *H. influenzae*, and *Strep. pneumoniae* frequently invade the CSF). The choroid plexus, a highly vascular tissue, is probably the site of CSF invasion. Once organisms have entered the CSF and multiplied, purulent meningitis is inevitable.

Organisms causing post-traumatic meningitis gain access to the CSF by direct invasion through an anatomical defect. Bacteraemia, which is common, is secondary to the meningitis. Shunt-associated meningitis is caused mainly by organisms that colonize the skin and contaminate the surgical wound and prosthetic material at the time of surgery. The infected shunt becomes coated with a film of adherent bacteria, commonly referred to as a biofilm. Organisms forming a biofilm are not susceptible to clinically achievable levels of antibiotic. Such infections are usually incurable unless the foreign material is removed.

Once bacteria have gained access to the subarachnoid space they multiply in the CSF relatively uninhibited by host defences. Neutrophils, which rapidly accumulate in the infected CSF, have little inhibitory effect on the growth of the infecting bacteria in experimental animals. Complement is found in such low concentrations in CSF that it is unlikely to have an antibacterial effect. Investigation of the mediators of this inflammatory response is incomplete, but studies of pneumococcal and *H. influenzae* meningitis have identified important features of this inflammatory reaction. The pneumococcal cell wall has been shown to be a potent inducer of inflammation. This reaction can be attenuated with cyclo-oxygenase inhibitors, and so prostaglandins are believed to

be important. The role of cytokines in the CSF has not been fully elucidated in this type of meningitis. However, the pneumococcal cell wall is a potent inducer of systemic interleukin-1 (IL-1), but not of tumour necrosis factor (TNF). The exact role of these mediators in pneumococcal meningitis remains unresolved. The main bacterial component responsible for inducing inflammation in *H. influenzae* type b is lipopolysaccharide (LPS or endotoxin), a potent inducer of cerebrospinal fluid TNF and IL-1 which have been shown to mediate the inflammatory response in the subarachnoid space. There is a suggestion of a dose–response effect between lipopolysaccharide and the inflammatory mediators, and so interventions which release lipopolysaccharide may exacerbate the inflammatory reaction. It has also been suggested that certain antibiotics which produce enhanced lipopolysaccharide release may temporarily exaggerate the inflammatory reaction in a type of Jarisch–Herxheimer reaction.

The inflammatory reaction in meningitis is associated with a number of major alterations in the normal physiology of the CNS. First, permeability of the blood–brain barrier increases. This is best measured by the increased penetration of the CSF by albumin. Also, antibiotic penetration of the CSF is greatly enhanced. Secondly, increased intracranial pressure results from cerebral oedema secondary to an accumulation of interstitial fluid, and communicating hydrocephalus is caused by decreased CSF re-absorption and cellular swelling secondary to cell injury. Thirdly, a vasculitis may affect mainly the large vessels traversing the subarachnoid space. This vascular injury may not only disrupt the normal autoregulation of cerebral blood flow; but, in severe cases, the vessel may become obstructed with thrombus, causing a cerebral infarct. The major impact of increased intracranial pressure and vasculitis is decreased cerebral perfusion, causing general hypoxic brain injury.

PATHOLOGY

There is diffuse acute inflammation of the pia-arachnoid, with migration of neutrophil leucocytes and exudation of fibrin into the CSF. Pus accumulates over the surface of the brain, especially around its base and the emerging cranial nerves, and around the spinal cord. The meningeal vessels are dilated and congested and may be surrounded by pus. Pus and fibrin are found in the ventricles and there is ventriculitis, with loss of ependymal lining and subependymal gliosis. Dilatation of the ventricular system may result from obstructive or communicating hydrocephalus. Other abnormalities include subdural effusion or empyema, septic thrombosis of the cerebral venous sinuses, subarachnoid haematomas, compression of intracranial structures as a result of intracranial hypertension, and herniation of the temporal lobes or cerebellum. Gross changes, such as pressure coning, which would provide an obvious cause of death, are rarely found. In some cases death may be attributable to related septicaemia (Fig. 1), although the familiar finding of bilateral adrenal haemorrhage (Waterhouse–Friederichsen syndrome) may well be a terminal phenomenon rather than a cause of fatal adrenal insufficiency as was once imagined. Patients with meningococcal septicaemia may develop acute pulmonary oedema. Myocarditis was a common finding in some series of patients. Histological appearances were of an acute interstitial myocarditis, occasionally with myocardial necrosis and thrombosis of small arterioles. Pericarditis and pericardial effusion were features, particularly of group C meningococcal infections. Myocarditis and Waterhouse–Friederichsen syndrome also occur, less frequently than in meningococcal septicaemia, in septicaemia caused by *H. influenzae*, pneumococcal, streptococcal, and staphylococcal infections.

CLINICAL FEATURES

Acute bacterial meningitis carries a mortality in untreated patients of between 70 and 100 per cent. Delay in treatment greatly increases the risk of permanent neurological sequelae. The early diagnosis of this condition is, therefore, a formidable challenge to clinical acumen, but it is clear from our own experience and from the medical literature that early clinical suspicion of meningitis may be impossible in many cases, especially in neonates and small children. When meningitis is secondary to infection elsewhere, such as pneumococcal pneumonia or *H. influenzae* otitis media, the presenting symptoms may be those of the original infection. The incubation period is only a few days. Progression is occasionally so rapid (*N. meningitidis*) that the patient becomes comatose within a few hours after the first symptoms. Early manifestations include non-specific malaise, apprehension, or irritability, followed by fever, usually without rigors, headache, myalgias, and vomiting. Convulsions occur in infants and children and meningitis must always enter into the differential diagnosis of childhood febrile convulsions. Photophobia, drowsiness, or more severe impairment of consciousness usually develop later. Headache quickly becomes more severe and is the dominant symptom. In older children and adults the symptoms most suggestive of meningitis are irritability, severe headache, and vomiting, but in the case of meningococcal infection, diarrhoea is a common non-specific symptom and the vasculitic rash is a crucial sign. An early symptom of meningococcal septicaemia is pain in the calves.

There is rarely any doubt that the child or adult with meningitis is severely ill and distressed. Meningism is best elicited by gentle passive flexion or rotation of the neck with the patient lying supine. If patients can shake their heads vigorously they are unlikely to have meningitis. To elicit Kernig's sign the lower limb is flexed at the hip. The patient with meningism will resist extension of the knee by contracting the hamstring muscles. Brudzinski's neck sign is best elicited while the patient sits up in bed with the legs stretched out. Gentle flexion of the neck will induce a compensatory flexion of the hips, knees, and sometimes the upper limbs. Later, the patient with marked meningism lies in a characteristic position with the neck and back fully extended (Fig. 2) as in tetanic opisthotonos. Local causes of neck stiffness, such as local sepsis (for example in the nuchal muscles), cervical spondylitis (particularly common in the elderly), temporomandibular arthritis, dental problems, and pharyngeal lesions, should be considered. Meningism is not uncommon in patients without meningitis who have other febrile conditions such as pyelonephritis. Meningism may be reduced or absent in patients who are immunosuppressed. The optic fundi should be examined as a prelude to lumbar puncture. Papilloedema is suggestive of cerebral oedema or an intracranial space-occupying lesion such as a cerebral abscess or a subdural or epidural collection of pus. The absence of papilloedema does not, however, exclude cerebral oedema and, if in doubt, and computer-assisted tomography is available, that investigation must precede a lumbar puncture. Retinal vein pulsation excludes intracranial hypertension. Hypertensive retinopathy will suggest hypertensive encephalopathy, and subhyaloid haemorrhages a subarachnoid haemorrhage. Patients with meningococcal meningitis associated with meningococcal antigenaemia have a petechial rash (Fig. 3) which may appear first on the shins or volar surface of the forearms. Petechiae may be visible on the bulbar and tarsal conjunctivae (Fig. 4) and palate. An identical rash is occasionally seen in patients with echovirus type 9, leptospirosis, *Staphylococcus aureus, Strep. pneumoniae, Strep. suis* (see Plate 2) *H. influenzae, Salmonella typhi,* and other infections, especially in those associated with infective endocarditis. The brownish or reddish geometrical, vasculitic rash of fulminant meningococcaemia is unmistakable (Figs 5 and 6) and, characteristically, the toes and fingers become necrotic (Fig. 7). There is associated profound hypotension, shock with peripheral cyanosis, and spontaneous systemic bleeding. Herpes labialis is commonly seen in all forms of bacterial meningitis, because a fever is the rule and recurrences are provoked by fever (see Figs 2 and 8). Physical examination must exclude otitis media, sinusitis, mastoiditis, and nasopharyngeal and other possible sites of sepsis. In patients with recurrent bacterial meningitis, a search should be made for a congenital dermal sinus, which is usually in the midline between head and coccyx and is often marked by a tuft of long hairs. Watery discharge from the nose or ears should be collected and tested for glucose; the possibility of a basal skull fracture with cerebrospinal fluid leak should be excluded.

Cranial nerve lesions may become evident as the disease progresses. The commonest are VI (Fig. 8), III, VII, VIII, and II. Patients who become unconscious (meningoencephalomyelitis) may lose all signs of

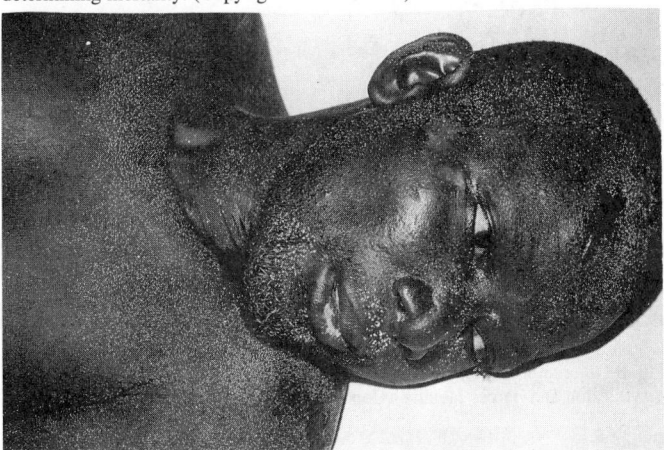

Fig. 1 Nigerian patient with pneumococcal meningitis and septicaemia who developed 'urea frost' and later died of renal failure. This illustrates the importance of septicaemic complications outside the central nervous system in determining mortality. (Copyright D.A. Warrell.)

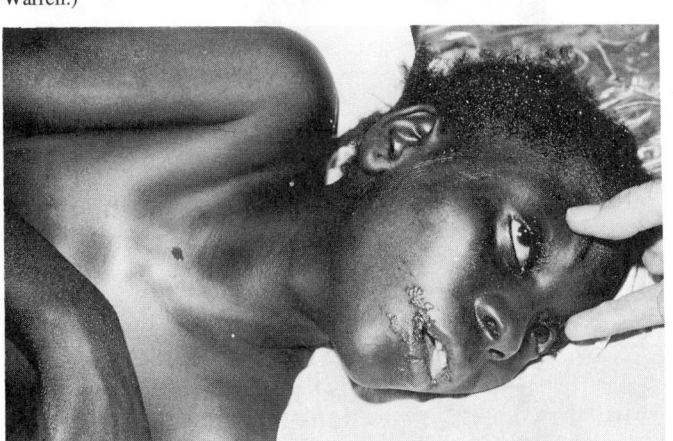

Fig. 2 Nigerian girl in coma with severe meningococcal meningoencephalitis. Note head retraction, dysconjugate gaze, and herpes labialis. (Copyright D.A. Warrell.)

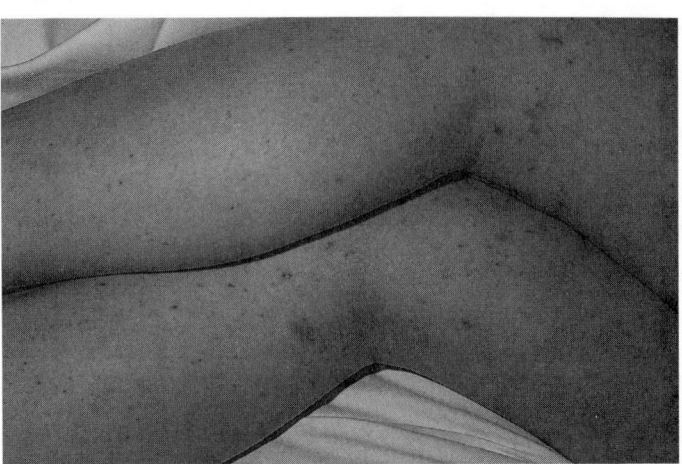

Fig. 3 Cutaneous petechiae in a patient with acute meningococcal meningitis. (Copyright D.A. Warrell.)

Fig. 4 Conjunctival petechiae in a Nigerian boy with meningococcal meningitis. (Copyright D.A. Warrell.)

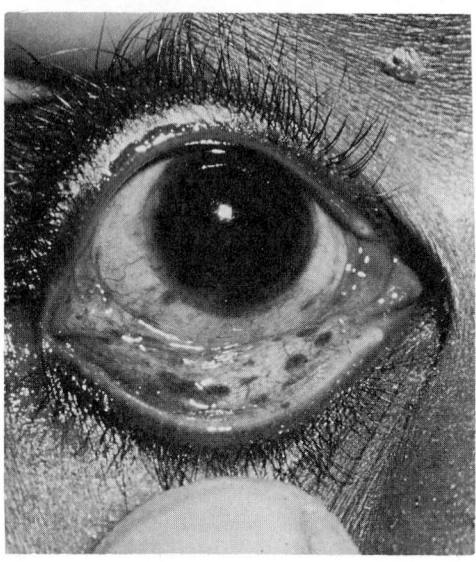

Fig. 5 The rash of meningococcal septicaemia in an English child.

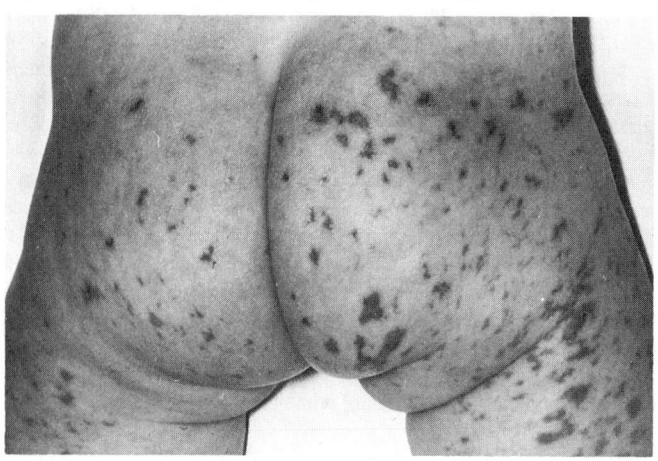

Fig. 6 Healing vasculitic rash in a Vietnamese boy with meningococcal meningitis and meningococcaemia. (Copyright D.A. Warrell.)

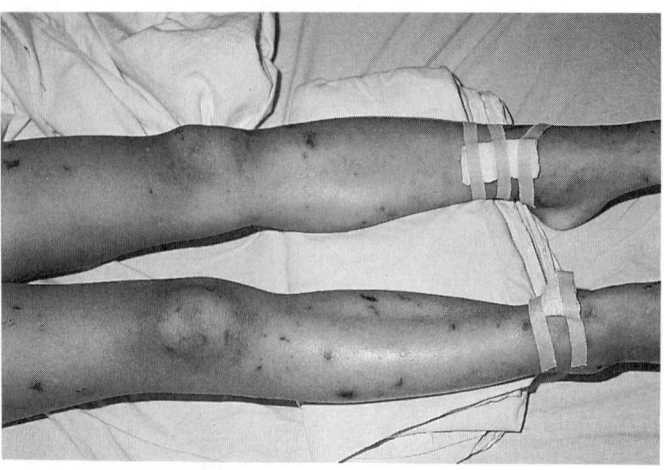

meningism and develop focal neurological signs, focal epileptiform convulsions, dysconjugate gaze, upper motor neurone signs, and involuntary movements. Vascular lesions may produce hemiparesis or quadriparesis, speech disorders, and visual field defects. Bilateral sensorineural deafness develops early, 2 to 9 days after the start of symptoms, in the majority of patients with *Strep. suis* type 2 meningitis. Initially associated with tinnitus and vertigo, this may progress to complete deafness within 24 h. Bacteria probably invade the cochlea via the cochlear aqueduct from the subarachnoid space to produce suppurative labyrinthitis and acute deafness. Associated clinical features of *Strep. suis* meningitis include third nerve palsy, septic arthritis (Plate 1) and purpuric skin lesions (Plate 2).

Papilloedema, with or without other symptoms and signs of intracranial hypertension (vomiting, coma, high blood pressure, bradycardia, etc.) and localizing neurological signs, suggests a subdural effusion or empyema. This is particularly common in children under 2 years old with *H. influenzae* meningitis.

Neonates and infants

Meningitis is particularly difficult to diagnose in this age group. Infants may become irritable or lethargic, stop feeding, and are found to have

Fig. 7 Gangrene of the fingers in a man with fulminant meningococcaemia. Eventually, three of his limbs had to be amputated. (Copyright D.A. Warrell.)

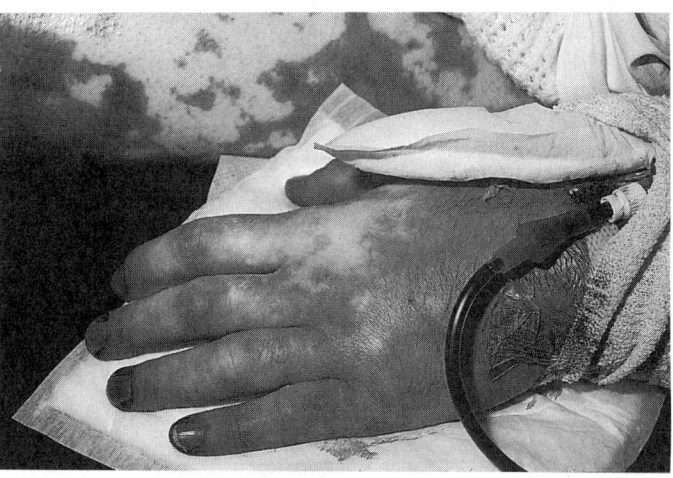

Fig. 8 Nigerian man recovering from meningococcal meningitis. Note right VI nerve lesion and herpes labialis. (Copyright D.A. Warrell.)

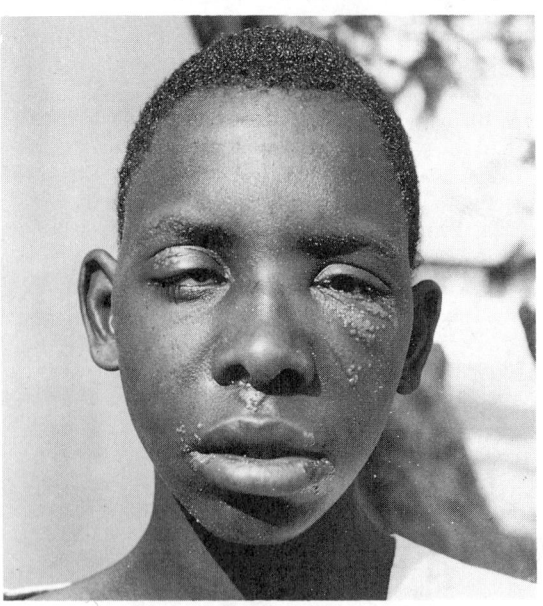

a bulging fontanelle, separation of the cranial sutures, meningism, and opisthotonos, and they may develop convulsions. These findings are uncommon in neonates, who sometimes present with respiratory distress, diarrhoea, or jaundice.

Post-traumatic meningitis

This is often indistinguishable clinically from spontaneous meningitis. However, in obtunded or unconscious patients who have suffered a recent head injury, few clinical signs may be present. A fever and a deterioration in the level of consciousness or loss of vital functions may be the only signs of a meningitis. Finding a CSF leak adds support to the possibility of meningitis in such patients, but a leak may be undetectable in many cases.

Infections of CSF shunts

Patients may present with clinical features typical of spontaneous meningitis, especially if virulent organisms are involved. The more usual presentation is insidious with features of shunt blockage such as headache, vomiting, fever, and a decreasing level of consciousness. Fever is a helpful sign, but is not a constant feature and may be present in as few as 20 per cent of cases. Shunts can be infected without causing meningitis, in which event the features of the infection will be determined by the distal site of the shunt. Shunts terminating in the venous system produce a disease similar to chronic right-sided infective endocarditis together with glomerulonephritis (shunt nephritis). Distal infection of shunts draining into the peritoneal cavity produces peritonitis.

DIAGNOSIS

Examination of cerebrospinal fluid

Analysis of a sample of CSF is crucial for the diagnosis of meningitis. The main risk of lumbar puncture is fatal pressure coning. This risk is greatest in patients with space-occupying lesions or post-traumatic cerebral oedema. In cases with spontaneous meningitis it is fortunately a rare complication, but caution should be exercised when contemplating spinal puncture. Patients with clinical features suggesting raised intracranial pressure (for example papilloedema, loss of retinal vein pulsation, focal neurology, bradycardia, and coma) should be examined by CT or MRI of the head, if available, to exclude a space-occupying lesion or severe cerebral oedema. In meningitis, the CSF opening pressure is usually raised (>200 mm of CSF), and occasionally it is markedly raised (>500 mm of CSF), suggesting the potential danger of pressure coning. Other contraindications to lumbar puncture include local skin sepsis at the site of puncture and any clinical suspicion of spinal cord compression.

Microscopic examination of CSF for white cells, red cells, and organisms; the measurement of glucose and protein; and culture are important investigations in a case of possible meningitis (see Table 3). A raised CSF white cell count is present in the majority of cases with bacterial meningitis but, rarely, the count may be normal (<6 wbc/μl, all lymphocytes). A majority of cases (>90 per cent) present with a count of >100 wbc/μl. The white cell differential count is helpful. Most cases (>80 per cent) have >80 per cent neutrophils. A predominance of lymphocytes is occasionally found and is reported especially in early bacterial meningitis and in association with L. monocytogenes infection. Red blood cells and xanthochromia are sometimes present. A wide range of non-bacterial infections and non-infectious conditions lead to pleocytosis of the CSF. In this respect, early viral meningitis, parameningeal septic foci, meningeal or cerebral tumours, cerebral infarction, chemical meningitis, aseptic meningitis complicating immunoglobulin replacement, cerebral vasculitis, and demyelination may be indistinguishable from bacterial meningitis.

Detection of bacteria in CSF confirms the diagnosis of bacterial meningitis. Gram staining of the CSF will reveal organisms in 50 to 80 per cent of cases. Gram stain appearance of bacteria may be characteristic of a particular species, but caution must be exercised for up to 10 per cent of smears are misinterpreted. It is prudent, therefore, to administer

Table 3 *Initial cerebrospinal fluid values in 493 episodes of adult bacterial meningitis in the Massachusetts General Hospital, Boston, USA, 1962–88*

Variable	Community acquired (N = 296) (%)	Noscomial (N = 197) (%)
Opening pressure (mm of water)		
1–139	9	23
140–299	52	52
300–399	20	11
≥400	19	15
White-cell count per mm		
0–99	10 (13)	17 (19)
100–4999	61 (59)	65 (62)
5000–9999	15 (15)	11 (12)
≥10000	13 (13)	7 (8)
Percentage of neutrophils		
0–19	2	2
20–79	19	31
≥80	79	66
Total protein (mg/dl)		
0–45	4	6
46–199	40	42
≥200	56	52
Glucose <40 mg/dl	50	45
Gram-positive	60	46
Culture positive	73	83

(Reproduced from Durand *et al.* (1993), with permission.)

appropriate empirical therapy initially and to change to specific therapy only when the infecting organism has been isolated and identified. Culture of organisms has a sensitivity of approximately 80 per cent in untreated cases. Organisms are much less often recovered from partially treated cases. Isolation of an organism is not only helpful in establishing the diagnosis, but allows the identification and susceptibility testing of the aetiological agent. The culture result can also be used to decide on the need for antibiotic prophylaxis, contact tracing, and other public health control measures.

Measurement of CSF glucose is helpful in making the diagnosis of bacterial meningitis. A glucose concentration of <40 mg per cent is considered low and is found in 50 to 70 per cent of cases. In many cases, glucose may even be undetectable. As the CSF glucose concentration is a function of the serum glucose, a more reliable measure of hypoglycorrhachia (low CSF glucose) is the ratio of serum to CSF glucose concentration. A ratio below 0.31 for glucose concentrations of simultaneously obtained serum and CSF indicates hypoglycorrhachia. A few other conditions may lead to a reduced CSF glucose. They are: tuberculous, syphilitic, parasitic, fungal, or mumps meningitis, herpes simplex encephalitis, carcinomatous meningitis, meningeal sarcoidosis, post-subarachnoid haemorrhage, severe systemic hypoglycaemia, and rare forms of central nervous system vasculitis.

An elevated CSF protein concentration is a common, but non-specific, finding. Similarly, measurement of CSF lactate is sensitive, but non-specific for meningitis. A range of rapid bacterial antigen tests may be helpful in detecting the presence of bacterial capsular polysaccharide antigens of pneumococci, meningococci, H. influenzae and group B streptococci. These tests reach a sensitivity and specificity of 90 per cent or greater for detecting specific causes of bacterial meningitis. The detection of bacterial lipopolysaccharide by the Limulus lysate assay has been suggested by some authorities.

The interpretation of the CSF test results depends on the clinical presentation and course of the disease. Acute viral meningitis is the most common differential diagnosis of bacterial meningitis. The CSF in viral

Table 4 *Recommended immediate antimicrobial treatment by general practitioners in cases of suspected meningococcus meningitis/septicaemia*

Antimicrobial	Route	Adults and children 10 years and over	Children 1–9 years	Infants less than 12 months
Benzylpenicillin	IV/IM	1.2 g	600 mg	300 mg
Cefotaxime	IV/IM	1.0 g	500 mg	250 mg
Chloramphenicol	IV	1.0 g	500 mg	250 mg

meningitis typically contains a preponderance of lymphocytes, <1000 wbc/µl, and a normal glucose. Fortunately, most patients with acute bacterial meningitis will exhibit a combination of clinical and CSF findings sufficiently characteristic to allow reliable diagnosis. However, in many cases, it may be impossible to distinguish between aseptic meningitis, chronic meningitis, partially treated bacterial meningitis, and early acute bacterial meningitis. In these circumstances it may be necessary to initiate empirical antibiotic treatment. Depending on the clinical course of the patient, it may also be necessary to repeat the spinal tap which may reveal the diagnosis (for example chronic meningitis). However, it is important to appreciate that CSF abnormalities secondary to bacterial meningitis, such as neutrophil pleocytosis, low glucose, and raised protein, may persist for a week or longer, but there should be a progressive improvement in these variables with appropriate treatment. Since the pleocytosis and hypoglycorrhachia typical of acute bacterial meningitis persist for a number of days after starting treatment, it is often possible to diagnose partially treated meningitis despite negative Gram stain and culture.

Other tests

Blood cultures should be obtained on all patients with suspected meningitis, as the aetiological agent may be grown. Radiological imaging of the central nervous system may be helpful. CT scanning can indicate whether or not a shunt is obstructed. Skull fractures or parameningeal septic foci (for example, sinusitis, spinal epidural abscess, or brain abscess) may also be detected on scanning.

DIFFERENTIAL DIAGNOSIS

Meningeal irritation is seen in many acute febrile conditions, especially in children. Local infections of the nasopharynx, cervical lymph nodes, muscles, and spine may produce convincing neck stiffness. Tetanus may be easily confused with meningitis if the persisting rigidity and recurrent spasms are not noticed. In all these conditions the CSF will be normal. Subarachnoid haemorrhage can present with sudden headache, neck stiffness, and deteriorating consciousness, and a less dramatic progression of symptoms is seen in patients with some intracranial tumours. Tuberculous and cryptococcal and other fungal meningitides usually develop more slowly than acute bacterial meningitis. They may be distinguished by examining CSF. Cryptococci and free-living amoebae may be mistaken for lymphocytes in the CSF unless an India ink preparation is examined to reveal the capsule of cryptococcus and the characteristic movements of amoebae. Aseptic meningitis comprises a large number of conditions, many of them caused by viruses in which there are clinical signs of meningism and the CSF is found to be abnormal. This group includes partially treated bacterial meningitis and the chemical meningitides, resulting from the introduction of irritants into the subarachnoid space (contrast media, antimicrobial agents, and contaminants of lumbar puncture and spinal anaesthesia). The CSF glucose concentration may be very low. Discharge of a tuberculoma may produce a sterile tuberculin reaction and the discharge of the contents of a craniopharyngioma or epidermoid cyst into the CSF can also cause chemical meningitis. Lead encephalopathy may present with meningism, lymphocyte pleocytosis, and an increase in CSF protein.

Recurrent purulent meningitis

This usually suggests a congenital or traumatic defect providing access to the subarachnoid space, such as congenital occult spina bifida or fracture of the base of the skull. A CSF leak may be apparent in about 50 per cent of the cases with post-traumatic recurrent meningitis. The head trauma may have occurred many years earlier and a connection with the subarachnoid space may be clinically inapparent. *Streptococcus pneumoniae* and *H. influenzae* are the predominant aetiological agents for community-acquired cases. Gram-negative aerobic bacilli or *Staph. aureus* are the main causes in nosocomial cases.

Rarely, recurrent meningitis may arise from episodes of recurrent sepsis of a parameningeal focus (for example, sinusitis or mastoiditis) or from a complement deficiency. Deficiency in a number of the components of the complement pathway has been detected in patients with recurrent meningitis. *Neisseria meningitidis* meningitis caused consecutively by different serogroups is the usual presentation in these cases.

Mollaret's meningitis (benign recurrent aseptic meningitis or benign recurrent lymphocytic meningitis) is mentioned here because it is an important differential diagnosis of recurrent bacterial meningitis. It is a sporadic condition presenting between the ages of 5 and 60 years. The symptoms are typical of acute meningitis—malaise, fever, vomiting, neck stiffness, convulsions, and coma. There is complete spontaneous recovery, usually within a few days, and symptom-free intervals lasting from a few days to years. About half the patients develop other neurological disturbances including hallucinations, diplopia, cranial nerve lesions, and signs of an upper motor neurone lesion. Pleocytosis is usually less than 3000/µl, with a predominance of lymphocytes, monocytes, and large endothelial ('Mollaret's') cells, but occasionally neutrophils are in the majority. The CSF protein is mildly increased, with increased gammaglobulin. CSF glucose concentration may be decreased. Recently, evidence of Herpes simplex type 1 and 2 has been obtained, using PCR. Other causes of recurrent meningitis include Behçet's syndrome, Vogt–Koyanagi–Harada syndrome, sarcoidosis and systemic lupus erythematosus, and undiagnosed viral meningitis (for example, that due to encephalomyocarditis virus).

MANAGEMENT

Bacterial meningitis progresses rapidly and has a high mortality. Antimicrobial treatment must therefore be started as soon as possible after the diagnosis is suspected clinically. This is vitally important in meningococcal meningitis/septicaemia. If this condition is suspected by the practitioner (and in Britain the first doctor the patient meets is usually the general practitioner), the patient should without delay be given benzylpenicillin (intravenous or intramuscular (IV/IM)), cefotaxime (IV/IM), or chloramphenicol (IV), preferably after a blood culture has been taken (Table 4). These drugs should be carried by general practitioners in their emergency bags. Antigen may still be found in the CSF later in hospital. Patients with no papilloedema or lateralizing neurological signs that suggest a space-occupying lesion, and with no other contraindications (see above), should be lumbar punctured immediately. Antimicrobial treatment should then be started, based on clinical assessment, before the results of the CSF examination are known.

Table 5 *Empirical treatment of meningitis*[a]

Type	Drug	Dose		Duration
Neonatal	Ampicillin plus aminoglycoside (e.g. gentamicin) or cefotaxime	Dose depends on age		Until organism is isolated OR 2 weeks
Spontaneous meningitis				
Childhood	Cefotaxime	200 mg/kg/day divided IVI	6 hourly	Until organism is isolated OR 2 weeks
	Chloramphenicol plus	100 mg/kg/day divided IVI	4 hourly	
	Penicillin or	200 mg/kg/day divided IVI	4 hourly	
	Ampicillin	200 mg/kg/day divided IVI	4 hourly	
	Ceftriaxone	100 mg/kg/day given IVI	1 daily	
Adult	*Prevalence of intermediate penicillin-resistant organisms low and Staph. aureus unlikely*			
	Penicillin	2.4 g IVI	4 hourly	
	Prevalence of chloramphenicol-resistant organisms low and Staph. aureus unlikely			
	Chloramphenicol	1 g IVI	6 hourly	Until organism is isolated OR 2 weeks
	Prevalence of intermediate penicillin-resistant organisms > 5% and Staph. aureus likely			
	Cefotaxime or	2 g IVI	4 hourly	
	Ceftriaxone	2 g IVI	12 hourly	
	High prevalence of penicillin-resistant pneumococci (MIC > 1 mg/ml)			
	Vancomycin	1 g IVI	12 hourly (measure levels)	
	Underlying immunosuppression, pregnancy or age > 65 years			
	Ampicillin plus	2 g IVI	4–4 hourly	Until organism is isolated OR 3 weeks
	cefotaxime or	2 g IVI	4 hourly	
	ceftriaxone	2 g IVI	12 hourly†	
Post-traumatic meningitis				
Community acquired	Treat as for spontaneous meningitis in adults			Until organism is isolated OR 2 weeks
Nosocomial	*Probability of Pseudomonas spp. high*			
	Ceftazidime	2 f IVI	8 hourly	Until organism is isolated OR 3 weeks
	Probability of Pseudomonas spp. low			
	Cefotaxime or	2 g IVI	4 hourly	
	ceftriaxone	2 g IVI	12 hourly†	
Shunt-associated meningitis				
Insidious onset	Vancomycin	1 g IVI and 5–10 g intrathecally	12 hourly 48–72 hourly	Until organism is isolated OR 2 weeks
Acute onset	Treat as for nosocomial post-traumatic meningitis			

[a]Empirical treatment should be started immediately the diagnosis is made, and in this table does not take into account Gram stain or antigen test results. Cultures of blood can usually be obtained before antibiotics are given. If CSF has not already been sampled, it should be obtained as soon as possible after starting treatment.

IVI, intravenous injection; MID,

†Once the patient is improving and stable, 2 g IVI may be given once a day.

Table 6 *Specific treatment of meningitis*

Type	Drug	Dose		Duration
Pneumococcal (choice of drug depends on susceptibility tests)	Penicillin or	2.4 g IVI	4 hourly	
	chloramphenicol or	1 g IVI	6 hourly	
	ceftriaxone or	2 g IVI	12 hourly	2 weeks
	cefotaxime or	2 g IVI	4 hourly	
	vancomycin	1 g IVI	12 hourly	
Meningococcal	Penicillin or	1.4 g IVI	4 hourly	
	chloramphenicol or	1 g IVI	6 hourly	
	ceftriaxone or	2 g IVI	12 hourly	7 days
	cefotaxime	2 g IVI	4 hourly	
Haemophilus influenzae	Chloramphenicol or	1 g IVI	6 hourly	
	ceftriaxone or	2 g IVI	12 hourly	14 days
	cefotaxime	2 g IVI	4 hourly	
Gram-negative bacillary (e.g. *E. coli*)	Ceftriaxone or	2 g IVI	12 hourly	3–4 weeks
	cefotaxime	2 g IVI	4 hourly	
Pseudomonas aeruginosa	Ceftazidime	2 f IVI	8 hourly	3–4 weeks
Listeria monocytogenes	Ampicillin plus	2 g IVI	4 hourly	3 weeks
	gentamicin or	1 mg/kg IVI	3 hourly	2 weeks
	trimethoprim/ sulphamethoxazole*	5 mg/kg trimethoprim IVI	12 hourly	3 weeks
Staphylococcus aureus	Flucloxacillin or	2 mg IVI	4 hourly	4 weeks
	naficillin	2 mg IVI	4 hourly	

*Trimethoprim/sulphamethoxazole is formulated in a fixed ratio of one part trimethoprim and five parts sulphamethoxazole.

Antimicrobial treatment

Successful antimicrobial treatment of meningitis (Tables 5 and 6) depends on the agent's crossing the blood–brain barrier and achieving a concentration of more than tenfold the minimum bactericidal concentration in the CSF (a level which predictably sterilizes the subarachnoid space). Before the aetiological agent has been isolated, empirical treatment that will be effective against the likely bacterial causes should be started immediately the diagnosis is made. Once the pathogen has been isolated, specific treatment can be substituted for the empirical regimen based on the susceptibility of the isolate.

Empirical regimens (Table 5) depend on the clinical circumstances of the case and the local pattern of aetiological agents and their antibiotic susceptibility patterns. Neonatal meningitis is largely caused by group B streptococci, *E. coli* and *L. monocytogenes.* Initial treatment, therefore, should consist of an aminoglycoside and penicillin or ampicillin; alternatively, a third-generation cephalosporin, preferably cefotaxime, and penicillin or ampicillin should be used.

In the community, children are at risk of meningitis caused by *N. meningitidis, Strep. pneumoniae* and, rarely in Hib-vaccinated children, *H. influenzae.* The following three regimens are accepted as effective: ceftriaxone, cefotaxime, or chloramphenicol plus ampicillin. Spontaneous meningitis in adults is usually caused by *Strep. pneumoniae* or *N. meningitidis;* however, in older patients (>50 years) and chronically immunosuppressed patients, there is an increased risk of *L. monocytogenes* and infection caused by Enterobacteriaceae (for example *E. coli*). Therefore, in younger adults, penicillin (2.4 g intravenously 4 hourly) alone should be adequate; alternatively, cefotaxime or ceftriaxone can be used; but in older and immunosuppressed patients penicillin or ampicillin alone or in combination with cefotaxime or ceftriaxone should be used. In all age groups, patients presenting with features of meningococcaemia should immediately receive penicillin (for example 2.4 g or 4 million units) parenterally. *Strep. suis* meningitis should be treated with penicillin, or in the rare penicillin-resistant cases, with ampicillin.

Community-acquired post-traumatic meningitis is caused mainly by *Strep. pneumoniae, H. influenzae,* and a wide range of other bacterial species. Cefotaxime (2 g intravenously 6 hourly), ceftriaxone (2 g intravenously daily), or chloramphenicol (1 g 6 hourly) plus ampicillin (2–3 g intravenously 6 hourly) should be given. Nosocomial post-traumatic meningitis is mainly caused by multiresistant hospital-acquired organisms such as *Klebsiella pneumoniae, E. coli, Pseudomonas aeruginosa,* and *Staph. aureus.* Depending on the pattern of susceptibility in a given hospital unit, ceftazidime (2 g intravenously 8 hourly), cefotaxime, or ceftriaxone should be chosen. If *P. aeruginosa* infection seems likely, ceftazidime is the preferred antibiotic.

Device- and shunt-associated meningitis is caused by a wide range of organisms, including methicillin-resistant staphylococci (mostly coagulase-negative staphylococci) and multiresistant aerobic bacilli. Cases with shunts and an insidious onset are probably caused by organisms of low pathogenicity, and empirical therapy is a less urgent requirement. However, when antibiotic treatment is given, vancomycin, both intravenously (1 g intravenously 12 hourly) and via the shunt (10 mg) should be administered and levels measured. In cases with an acute presentation, a third-generation cephalosporin such as cefotaxime, ceftazidime (which has anti-pseudomonal activity), or ceftriaxone plus vancomycin intravenously and via the shunt or drain should be given. The infected shunt or drain should be removed immediately in most cases.

Once the aetiological agent has been isolated and its susceptibilities determined, the empirical treatment should be changed, if necessary, to an agent or agents specific for the isolate (Table 6). The optimal duration of treatment has not been determined by rigorous scientific investigation; however, treatment regimens that are probably substantially in excess of the minimum necessary to achieve cure have been arrived at through wide clinical experience.

General management and treatment of complications

General treatment

In the conscious patient, the severe headache may need treatment with opiates and the associated pyrexia may require treatment with antipyretics or cooling with tepid sponging or fanning. Many patients are unconscious and should be managed accordingly. Their airway should be maintained and they may need intubation to protect the airway and maintain ventilation. A urethral catheter should be inserted.

The associated septicaemia in patients with meningitis may result in septicaemic shock. These patients require careful monitoring and treatment of shock. A combination of fluid administration to expand the intravascular volume, pressors, and inotropic support is needed. Multiple end-organ failure may develop requiring intensive medical support, including ventilation and renal dialysis.

Treatment of complications

Raised intracranial pressure is a serious complication of meningitis. Clinically, altered consciousness, poorly reactive unequal or dilated pupils, cranial nerve palsies, bradycardia, and hypertension suggest its onset. Various measures can be used to lower a raised intracranial pressure, including the elevation of the head of the bed to 30°, administration of mannitol, and endotracheal intubation and mechanical hyperventilation. These measures may be used to maintain an adequate perfusion pressure monitored by continuous intra-arterial and intracranial pressure monitoring. The effect of these measures on the outcome of patients with raised intracranial pressure have not been evaluated systematically. The role of corticosteroids in reducing intracranial pressure remains unresolved and no consistent approach to their use is accepted.

The use of corticosteroids aimed at reducing the sequelae of meningitis has received support from a number of studies. The most pronounced effect has been the reduction of deafness in children infected with H. influenzae and treated with cefuroxime (a less effective cephalosporin for meningitis than cefotaxime or ceftriaxone). In three recent studies of bacterial meningitis (mainly H. influenzae) in children treated with ceftriaxone, dexamethasone (0.4 mg/kg 12 hourly for 2 days intravenously starting 10 min before the first dose of antibiotic) reduced the incidence of neurological and audiological sequelae. Studies in Cairo suggested that dexamethasone reduced significantly the mortality and incidence of permanent sequelae in adult patients with pneumococcal meningitis.

Seizures occur in as many as 40 per cent of patients with meningitis and subclinical fitting should be considered in patients with persisting coma. Prophylactic anticonvulsant might be justified in pneumococcal meningitis. Rapid control of seizures can be achieved by administrating intravenous diazepam or lorazepam. Phenytoin should be used for the longer-term control of seizure activity. Severe cases that fail treatment

with these antiepileptic agents should undergo endotracheal intubation and receive high-dose phenobarbitone.

Many patients with meningitis develop hyponatraemia as a result of the syndrome of inappropriate antidiuretic hormone secretion (SIADH), such cases may require fluid restriction. Complications such as cerebral venous sinus thrombosis and cavernous sinus thrombosis may occur, but may be difficult to detect. Anticoagulants or fibrinolytics may be used in such patients with the hope of improving the outcome (Chapter 24.6).

PROGNOSIS AND SEQUELAE

In Europe and North America the overall mortality of meningitis caused by N. meningitidis is about 7 to 14 per cent; for H. influenzae, 3 to 10 per cent; Strep. pneumoniae, 15 to 60 per cent; and for group B streptococci and L. monocytogenes meningitis, above 20 per cent. The mortality is much higher in the very young and old, and in patients with debilitating illnesses. A study in Zaria, Nigeria, demonstrated that the mortality of pneumococcal meningitis was 32 per cent in patients who were fully conscious on admission, 40 per cent in those who were confused, 54 per cent in semiconscious patients, and 94 per cent in those who were comatose.

Permanent neurological sequelae include mental retardation, deafness and other cranial nerve deficits, and hydrocephalus. The reported incidence of sensorineural deafness after meningitis ranges from 5 to 40 per cent. A large proportion recover within a few months. Neisseria meningitidis and H. influenzae are the main causes of this complication. Permanent deafness occurs in more than 50 per cent of patients with Strep. suis meningitis. It may be bilateral, complete, and associated with vestibular involvement. Haemophilus influenzae appears to be the major cause of acquired mental retardation in the United States. This complication is found in 30 to 50 per cent of children who have suffered from H. influenzae meningitis.

PREVENTION

Vaccination

Vaccines to the three major pathogens causing community-acquired meningitis are available. Haemophilus influenzae type b capsular conjugate vaccines are in wide use and are dramatically reducing the incidence of H. influenzae type b meningitis. In Finland conjugate vaccines appear nearly to have eliminated Hib invasive disease. The capsular polysaccharide vaccines directed at N. meningitidis (serogroups A, C, Y, and W135) and Strep. pneumoniae (23 valent) are less effective than Hib vaccine, especially in children under 2 years of age. No effective vaccine exists for N. meningitidis serogroup B. Vaccination of groups of adults at high risk, such as close contacts, military recruits, and migrant miners in Africa, has been highly effective in preventing meningococcal meningitis caused by serogroups A and C. Mass vaccination of large populations (for example, with Hib vaccine) with meningococcal and pneumococcal vaccine is not deemed cost effective. However, with the development of improved conjugated meningococcal and pneumococcal vaccines, active vaccination of the age group at highest risk, young children between 6 months and 4 years of age, may be cost effective.

Chemoprophylaxis

The attack rate of meningitis is higher in the immediate contacts of an index case of meningococcal (up to 1000–fold) or H. influenzae type b meningitis (500-fold only in children under 4 years of age) than in the population at large. The administration of rifampicin or ciprofloxacin eliminates the carrier state and is assumed to eliminate the risk of secondary cases of meningitis. A major preventive effect of sulphadiazine chemoprophylaxis has been shown in large outbreaks of meningococcal meningitis among military recruits; however, meningococci are now frequently resistant to sulphonamides. Rifampicin and ciprofloxacin are assumed to produce a similar effect. Close adult contacts of meningo-coccal disease are given either rifampicin 300 mg twice a day for 2 days or a single dose of ciprofloxacin 750 mg orally (ciprofloxacin is still avoided in children, but is now accepted for prophylaxis). Contacts of *H. influenzae* type b disease (including adults) are given rifampicin for 4 days, and Hib vaccine is given to unvaccinated children less than 4 years old. However, in those countries where Hib vaccination has been implemented, the need for chemoprophylaxis is under review. Doctors, nurses, and other health care workers need not be given chemoprophy-laxis unless they have given mouth to mouth resuscitation.

Although antibiotics are administered prophylactically to many cases of skull fracture with CSF leak, there is no evidence of benefit. Surgical closure of the leak is the only effective means of preventing meningitis in such cases. However, since many acute leaks heal spontaneously, this is necessary only in cases with large defects or in cases of recurrent meningitis.

The prevention of device-associated meningitis relies on rigorous infection control. Ventricular and lumbar drains should be removed as soon as possible. Shunt insertion should be performed adhering to strict aseptic technique, and surgical antibiotic prophylaxis may also help reduce shunt infection.

Tuberculous meningitis

EPIDEMIOLOGY

Tuberculous meningitis has been a major problem and cause of death in developing countries. Human *Mycobacterium tuberculosis* is respon-sible for most cases. In Western countries, the incidence of tuberculous meningitis has fallen in parallel with tuberculosis as a whole. For exam-ple, in the late 1940s there were 2000 cases/year in England and Wales, accounting for 10 to 20 per cent of cases of bacterial meningitis; but by the early 1970s this had fallen to less than 4 per cent.

In Britain, immigrants from Pakistan, India, Africa, and the West Indies are now the most likely to contract the disease. Most cases of tuberculous meningitis are in young children but primary infection can be acquired at a later age and, in recent years, a larger proportion of patients with tuberculous meningitis have been adults. The disease is uncommon, but severe, in pregnant women.

Recently there has been an increase in the incidence of tuberculosis in many parts of the world and this is related to the epidemic of human immunodeficiency virus (HIV) infection. HIV-infected patients with tuberculosis are at increased risk of meningeal involvement. In some areas of endemic tuberculosis, tuberculous meningitis is an important complication in patients with HIV infection.

PATHOGENESIS

Small caseous microtubercles develop in the brain, meninges or, less commonly, in the bones of the skull and vertebrae close to the meninges. This infection has seeded through the bloodstream from the primary lesion or a site of chronic infection. Many patients develop miliary tuberculosis at the stage of haematogenous spread. Infection of the meninges results from rupture of a microtubercle with discharge of tuberculoprotein and mycobacteria into the subarachnoid space. In the sensitized (tuberculin-positive) patient, this event will be marked by an episode of fever and meningeal irritation caused by the intrathecal tuber-culin reaction. Subacute inflammation, especially of the basal meninges, then develops, producing cranial nerve lesions, cerebral arteritis causing infarction, impairment of CSF absorption, or obstruction to the CSF circulation causing hydrocephalus, and, in the spinal cord, spinal arach-noiditis, producing multiple radiculopathy or myelopathy.

PATHOLOGY

Meningeal miliary tubercles may be found on the brain surfaces of most victims of miliary tuberculosis. They are usually few in number and

occur in the region of the sylvian fissure, while there may be larger caseous plaques deeper in the sulci. The brains of patients dying of tuberculous meningitis are usually oedematous. A mass of thick, greyish exudate encases the base of the brain, filling the basal cisterns. Within the ventricular system there is ependymitis with a similar exudate chok-ing the choroid plexus. The exudate consists of lymphocytes, plasma cells, giant cells, and foci of caseation, but mycobacteria are usually scanty. At the base of the brain the cranial nerves and the internal carotid artery and its branches are trapped and damaged by the exudate. Arteries are obliterated by an endarteritis, with resulting ischaemia and infarction of superficial areas of the brain, internal capsule, basal ganglia, and brain-stem. There is congestion and phlebitis of the meningeal veins. Both the inflammatory exudate and the arteritis are probably a delayed hypersensitivity reaction to the tuberculoprotein. Some degree of hydro-cephalus develops in most cases. Usually the hydrocephalus is com-municating in type and is caused by obliteration of the basal cisterns. Less commonly, blockage of the foramina of Luschka and Magendie in the fourth ventricle, or the aqueduct, causes obstructive hydrocephalus. The exudate may extend into the spinal cord, enveloping the nerve roots and spinal cord and producing spinal arachnoiditis and spinal block.

CLINICAL FEATURES

Symptoms of meningitis are preceded by 2 to 8 weeks of non-specific prodromal symptoms less likely to raise the suspicion of tuberculous meningitis. This phase of vague malaise, irritability, insomnia, lethargy, anorexia, headache, abdominal pain, vomiting, and behavioural changes may develop after a head injury, surgical operation, or common child-hood infection such as measles, influenza, or otitis media. The impli-cation is that meningeal infection is precipitated by these conditions. By the time patients have developed obvious symptoms and signs of men-ingitis, the disease is well advanced. Patients usually have low-grade fever, but severe pyrexia can occur. Half of the patients will have symp-toms and signs of tuberculosis in the lungs or elsewhere. Rarely, tuber-culous meningitis presents dramatically with an acute encephalopathy with severe headache, neck stiffness, vomiting, and seizures, mimicking acute bacterial meningitis, viral encephalitis, and subarachnoid haemorrhage.

During the second stage there is evidence of meningeal irritation (headache, vomiting, neck stiffness), cranial nerve damage, developing hydrocephalus, and cerebral endarteritis. Infants are irritable with opis-thotonos and a tense fontanelle. Cranial nerve lesions, seen in 25 per cent of cases, involve one or more of the following: II, III, IV, VI, VII, and VIII. The pupils may be dilated, unequal, and unresponsive, and many patients develop a squint from abducens nerve palsy (Fig. 9). Fundal examination reveals papilloedema in 40 per cent and sometimes evidence of optic atrophy. Choroid tubercles are occasionally seen (Fig. 10). Bilateral visual failure with optic atrophy is a feature of arachnoid-itis in the cistern of the optic chiasm. Raised intracranial pressure, a common and serious complication of tuberculous meningitis, results from obstruction of the CSF circulation in the basal cisterns by the exudates or, less commonly, obstruction of the outlets of the fourth ventricle. Increasing headache, vomiting, and impairment of conscious level are mainly the result of intracranial hypertension rather than the meningeal irritation. Hydrocephalus, which often accompanies the increased intracranial pressure, is common and should be suspected in all patients with tuberculous meningitis. They often have severe head-ache, ocular palsy, pyramidal signs in the lower limbs, and incontinence of urine. If left untreated, the patients become stuporose or comatose and develop signs of brain-stem damage, such as decerebrate rigidity, irregular breathing, and impairment of brain-stem reflexes. About 20 per cent of the patients develop focal neurological signs such as hemiparesis, hemianaesthesia, aphasia, and hemianopia. These are the results of cere-bral infarct, caused by the arteritis. Convulsive disorders are common in children but rare in adults. About 10 per cent of the patients develop symptoms and signs of spinal arachnoiditis (Fig. 11) which vary from radicular pain, radicular weakness of the lower limbs and urinary retention, to paraplegia with sensory loss on the trunk. The syndrome of inappropriate secretion of antidiuretic hormone (SIADH) is common in patients with severe tuberculous meningitis. It produces impairment of consciousness, but decerebrate rigidity or other signs of brain-stem damage are not found. Other uncommon neurological abnormalities include internuclear ophthalmoplegia, hemichorea, and hypothalamic disorders leading to loss of control of blood pressure and body temperature and diabetes insipidus.

HIV-infected patients with tuberculosis are at higher risk of developing the meningitis than non-HIV-infected patients. In HIV-infected patients peripheral, intrathoracic, and intra-abdominal lymphadenopathy is more common, but the clinical manifestations of tuberculous meningitis do not seem to be modified by the HIV infection.

DIAGNOSIS

Full blood count is usually normal, but marked leucocytosis of more than 20 000/μl may be found occasionally in tuberculous meningitis and miliary tuberculosis. Examination of CSF is crucial. Lumbar puncture does not seem to be subject to the same dangers as in acute bacterial meningitis and, apparently, lumbar puncture has been repeated safely as a treatment of raised intracranial pressure in patients with tuberculous meningitis even when there is papilloedema. CSF opening pressure is raised in the majority of patients, but it may be low or fall in those developing block from spinal arachnoiditis. The CSF is clear or slightly turbid, and may form a spider's web clot on standing. The mechanism of the cobweb formation is unclear, but it does not appear to be caused by the high protein concentration. In patients with spinal block the fluid

may be xanthochromic with a very high protein concentration and may quickly form a jelly (Froin's syndrome). Total cell counts range between 10 and 1000/μl. Both lymphocytes and neutrophils are present and the latter can be as high as 70 per cent of the total. In 90 per cent of the patients the white cell count is less than 500/μl. Rarely, the cell count exceeds 1000/μl. The CSF glucose concentration of the initial CSF sam-

Fig. 10 (a, b) Tuberculous choroiditis in a 23-year-old Thai girl. (Copyright Prida Phuapradit.)

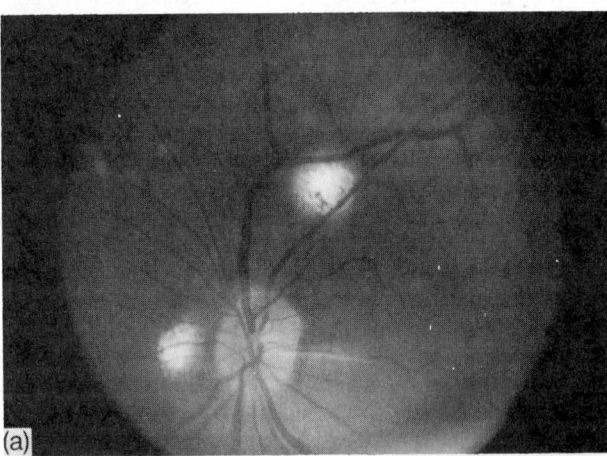

(a)

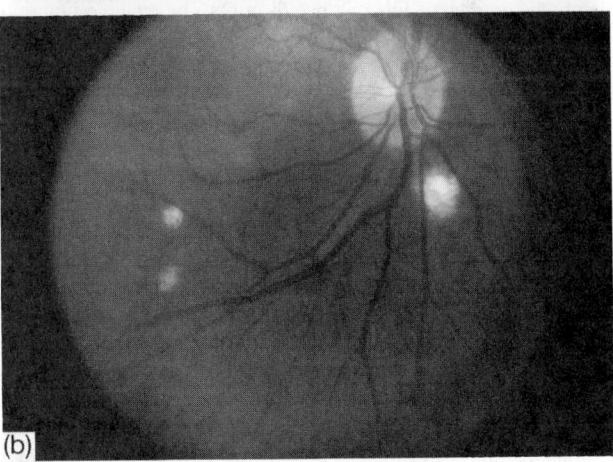

(b)

Fig. 9 Bilateral VI nerve palsies in a Thai girl with tuberculous meningitis. The cervical node biopsy was positive for acid-fast bacilli. (Copyright Prida Phuapradit.)

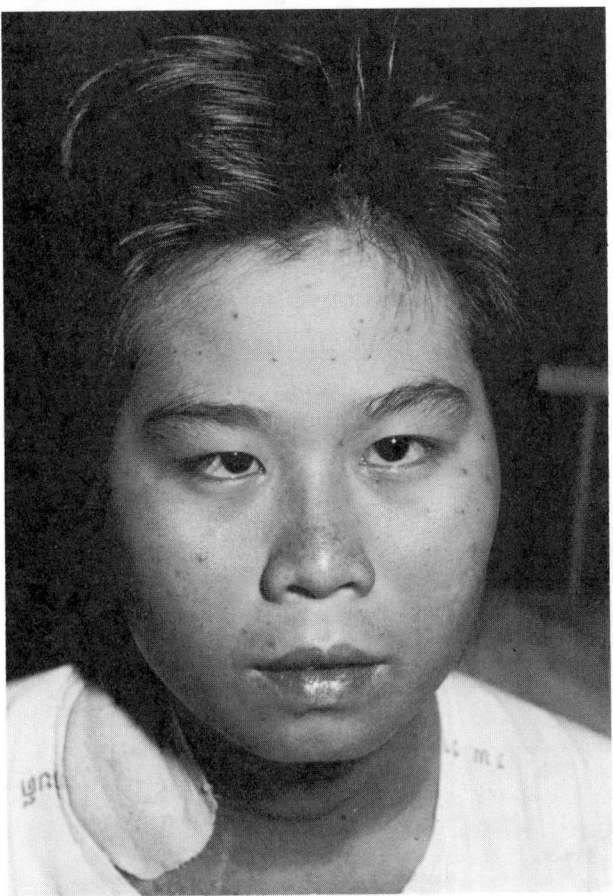

Fig. 11 Spinal arachnoiditis revealed by myelography in a Thai patient with tuberculous meningitis. (Copyright Prida Phuapradit.)

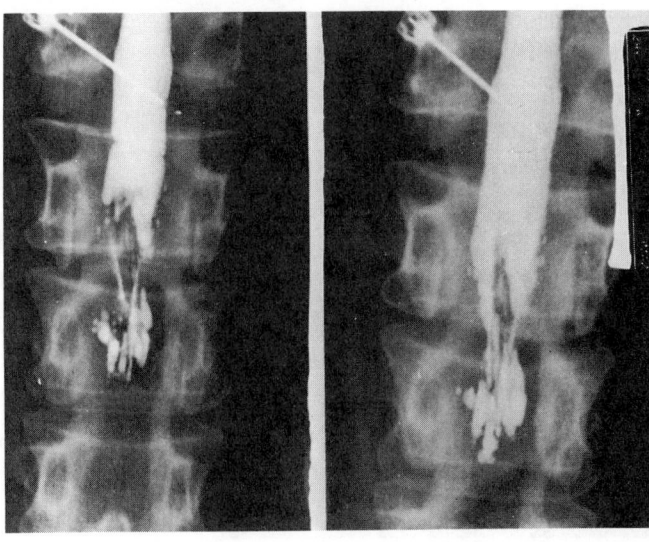

ple is low in about 90 per cent of the patients. Although non-specific, this finding is of great practical use, because it is a simple test which differentiates tuberculous meningitis presumptively from most cases of viral meningitis. Indeed, tuberculous meningitis must be strongly suspected in any patient who presents with lymphocytic meningitis and a low CSF glucose concentration. Protein concentration of the CSF is usually raised and ranges from normal to 5 g/l. Levels of more than 5 g/l suggests a spinal block. Success in detecting tubercle bacilli in CSF by acid-fast, auramine, or fluorescent staining can, in some hands, be increased from the usual average of 10 to 20 per cent by centrifuging a large volume of CSF (10–20 ml) and carefully examining the sediment under a microscope. Repeated lumbar punctures increase the chance of finding tubercle bacilli and of observing the characteristic changes in CSF composition. Marked neutrophil pleocytosis of the CSF may be seen transiently in association with abrupt deterioration of the headache, increased neck stiffness, and fever, suggesting bacterial meningitis. The phenomenon is self-limited and is thought to be the result of a rupture of a microtubercle into the subarachnoid space. Culture of mycobacteria is successful in 10 to 90 per cent of cases. Specimens other than CSF (for example sputum, gastric washings in children, urine, etc.) should also be cultured. As it would take up to 2 months or longer for the mycobacteria to grow in the cultures, a number of methods for rapid diagnosis of tuberculous meningitis have been developed. The bromide partition test is not of practical use, because it lacks specificity and is abnormal in other types of meningitis and even in cerebral malaria. It is no more useful than the CSF glucose concentration. Tests for detecting membrane antigen of tubercle bacilli in CSF by enzyme immunoassay and latex particle agglutination are disappointing because they are not reproducible and do not have sufficient sensitivity and specificity to be of clinical use. Detection of tuberculostearic acid (a lipid component of the mycobacterial cell wall) in the CSF by gas chromatography and mass spectroscopy is highly specific and sensitive, but the apparatus is very expensive and technically too complicated for clinical use. At present, detection of the genome of *Mycobacterium tuberculosis* in the CSF by polymerase chain reaction (PCR) is specific, sensitive, and practical in the rapid diagnosis of tuberculous meningitis. CSF specimens are suitable for PCR, even if they are kept at room temperature for a few weeks, and in developing tropical countries, CSF specimens can be sent from rural areas to a centre with a PCR facility. A search for evidence of tuberculosis elsewhere in the body is useful. Chest radiographs are normal in about half of the patients, and military mottling is seen in only a minority. CT scans are useful in detecting the complications of tuberculous meningitis. Communicating hydrocephalus and its characteristically enhanced basal exudates can be demonstrated by CT scans

in about 80 per cent of the patients (Fig. 12). They may also reveal a cerebral infarct secondary to the arteritis or associated tuberculomas (Fig. 13).

Cell-mediated immunity should be assessed. The tuberculin test is positive in 50 to 95 per cent of patients with tuberculous meningitis. Reactivity is suppressed in debilitated or immunosuppressed patients. Serological tests for HIV infection and a CD4 cell count should, if possible, be performed in every case.

DIFFERENTIAL DIAGNOSIS

Although a few patients with tuberculous meningitis present acutely, the majority show a subacute or chronic progression. Clinically, the differential diagnosis should include cryptococcal meningitis, and various subacute or chronic meningitides, including partially treated bacterial meningitis, parameningeal infections, neoplastic and granulomatous infiltrations of the meninges (for example carcinomas, leukaemias, lymphomas, sarcoidosis), and cerebral tumours. Fungal meningitides (Cryptococcus, Coccidioides, Histoplasma, Candida) may present like tuberculous meningitis. Other conditions which have caused confusion in particular clinical or geographical settings are meningovascular syphilis, toxoplasma meningitis in immunosuppressed patients, notably in AIDS, cysticercosis, amoebic meningoencephalitis, African trypanosomiasis and schistosomal myelopathy. In most of these cases, CSF examination, including cytology, India ink preparation, immunodiagnostic tests (for example cryptococcal latex agglutination), serological tests and microbial cultures, will allow differentiation.

TREATMENT

The untreated mortality of tuberculous meningitis is close to 100 per cent. Full treatment must be started when the diagnosis is suspected on clinical grounds, immediately after adequate samples have been taken for microscopy, culture, and immunodiagnosis. Choice of antituberculosis drugs has been based mainly on pharmacokinetic and antibacterial properties of the drugs. Isoniazid, pyrazinamide, ethionamide, and cycloserine are freely distributed into the CSF. Penetration is limited, but still adequate during the first few months of the meningitis, in the case of rifampicin, ethambutol, and streptomycin. *p*-Aminosalicylic acid should not be used because it does not enter the CSF. At least two drugs to which the organism is sensitive should be used. However, during the first 2 months intensive chemotherapy with three or four antituberculosis drugs should be given, because the impairment of the blood–brain barrier during the active stage of meningitis allows most antituberculosis drugs to enter the CSF in amounts sufficient to kill the organism, and

Fig. 12 CT scan with enhancement showing thick basal exudate and hydrocephalus. (Copyright Prida Phuapradit.)

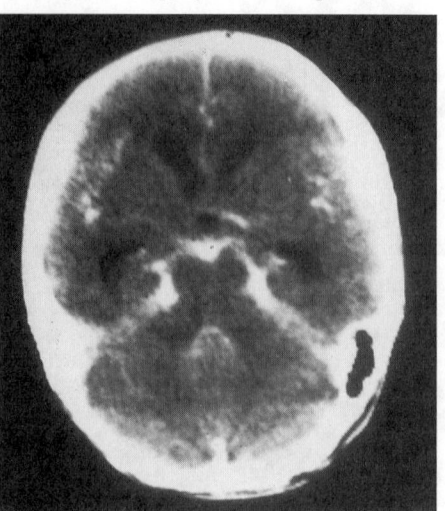

Fig. 13 CT scan with enhancement of a patient with tuberculous meningitis showing multiple tuberculomas developing near the basal cisterns. (Copyright Prida Phuapradit.)

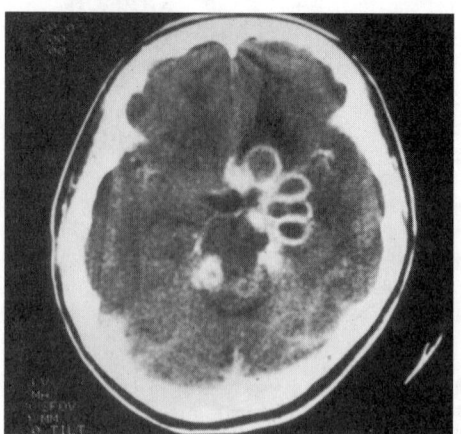

offers a good chance of eliminating mycobacteria from the CSF after a short period of treatment. The combination of isoniazid and rifampicin for 12 months, with pyrazinamide and streptomycin during the first 2 months, is an effective regimen which has been widely used. In adults daily single doses of 300 mg of isoniazid, 600 mg of rifampicin, and 1500 mg of pyrazinamide provide adequate levels in the sera and CSF of patients with active tuberculous meningitis. Higher doses of these drugs are not necessary and may result in a higher incidence of hepatotoxicity. The incidence of adverse reactions of antituberculosis drugs in tuberculous meningitis is acceptable and is similar to that encountered in the treatment of pulmonary tuberculosis.

In countries where rifampicin cannot be afforded, triple therapy with isoniazid, pyrazinamide, and streptomycin should be tried. Tuberculous meningitis in HIV-infected patients should be similarly treated as the meningitis in those not infected. Responses to treatment and the outcome of tuberculous meningitis are similar in the two groups. Drug-resistant isolates of *Mycobacterium tuberculosis,* which have been found increasingly, poses problems in the treatment now and in the future. Ethionamide, kanamycin or amikacin, and cycloserine should be considered in this situation. Development of new effective antituberculosis drugs is urgently needed.

Response to antituberculosis chemotherapy is slow, particularly in patients who are not given corticosteroids. There may be an increase in temperature and CSF protein concentration and transient neutrophil pleocytosis during the first 2 months after starting optimal chemotherapy. However, some signs of clinical improvement are usually seen within the first few weeks. Early clinical evidence of response is an improvement of the headache, sense of general well-being and a decrease in the elevated intracranial pressure. A rapid return to normal in CSF composition within a few days virtually excludes the diagnosis of tuberculous meningitis, in which case antituberculosis treatment should be stopped. Usually it would take at least a few weeks to a few months for the cells, CSF glucose, and protein to return to normal. In some patients the high protein concentration persists.

'Trial' of chemotherapy is justified when there is clinical suspicion of tuberculous meningitis, particularly when diagnostic facilities are limited. Treatment should be continued for 12 months unless there is rapid improvement in the patient's condition and CSF composition, suggesting another cause for aseptic meningitis. In some severely ill patients who present acutely with features of acute bacterial meningitis (for example neutrophil pleocytosis) but in whom initial laboratory results are not helpful, it may be necessary to initiate 'blind' treatment for acute bacterial and tuberculous meningitis simultaneously. In these, fortunately rare cases, isoniazid, rifampicin, and streptomycin or ethambutol, together with penicillin or a third-generation cephalosporin, can be given.

TREATMENT OF COMPLICATIONS

The complications of tuberculous meningitis are common and some are often serious enough to cause severe morbidity and death in spite of active treatment with antituberculosis drugs. Increased intracranial pressure, found in about 90 per cent of the patients and often associated with communicating hydrocephalus, is usually caused by the basal arachnoiditis. Less commonly, it is caused by diffuse cerebral oedema with small lateral ventricles. In these patients conservative treatment with repeated lumbar punctures in combination with acetazolamide, with or without frusemide, and corticosteroids should be tried. Within the first 4 to 6 weeks of treatment, the CSF pressures of the majority of the patients return to normal and the transependymal oedema (periventricular lucency on the CT scan) disappears. However, the sizes of the ventricles usually remain unchanged during the first 4 to 6 weeks of treatment. This is a state of arrested hydrocephalus. In general it would take up to 6 months for the ventricular size to return to normal. Intrathecal hyaluronidase, which has a potential to resolve the basal exudates, has been shown to be beneficial in the treatment of commu-

nicating hydrocephalus and spinal arachnoiditis in a few centres. If these conservative measures fail, surgical treatment will be needed for the hydrocephalus. Patients with communicating hydrocephalus who are very ill with impairment of consciousness should receive early temporary external ventricular shunting. Shunt surgery, as a first-line treatment, should be reserved for patients with non-communicating hydrocephalus.

Corticosteroids might be expected to reduce the inflammatory reaction and the fibrotic organization of exudate in the brain and spinal cord. A recent, large, controlled trial has demonstrated that dexamethasone increases survival and decreases sequelae in children with severe tuberculous meningitis. Corticosteroids should be given to patients with hydrocephalus, threatened or established spinal block, visual failure from optochiasmic arachnoiditis, those who develop focal neurological signs caused by arteritis, and the severely ill. The usual regimen is intramuscular dexamethasone (16 mg/day in adults and 0.5 mg/kg/day in children) in divided doses, or oral prednisolone 60 mg/day for adults, 2 mg/kg/day for children, given in a tapering course over 3 to 6 weeks. There is no evidence that corticosteroids interfere with the penetration of antituberculosis drugs into the CSF. Intrathecal injection of corticosteroids is unnecessary.

Fluid, electrolyte, and acid–base disturbances are common, the result of vomiting, inadequate fluid intake, and SIADH. Progressive loss of vision caused by fibrosing exudate around the optic chiasma may respond to surgical decompression. Cerebral tuberculomas may occasionally develop during the course of the treatment of tuberculous meningitis. Characteristically the lesions are thick-walled nodules of small or moderate size in clusters, and develop in the surface of the brain near the basal cisterns, such as the interpeduncular cistern and cistern of the optic chiasm (Fig. 13). They should be treated conservatively and the response to antituberculosis treatment assessed by CT scan. Biopsy or surgical intervention is not necessary and may be harmful. Tuberculomas usually respond very slowly to antituberculosis drugs and it usually takes at least 24 months or longer for the lesions to disappear. Nursing care is very important during the acute illness when there are the usual problems presented by unconscious patients and during the prolonged phase of convalescence and rehabilitation. Anticonvulsants are often needed, especially in children.

PROGNOSIS AND SEQUELAE

In Western industrialized countries, the mortality of tuberculous meningitis is still high, at about 15 to 30 per cent, and in developing countries it remains between 30 and 50 per cent. The prognosis is worst and the risk of sequelae highest in those admitted in coma with signs of brain-stem damage, in the very young and very old, pregnant women, and those with malnutrition or other diseases. The outcome of tuberculous meningitis in HIV-infected patients is similar to the tuberculous meningitis in patients without HIV infection. There are permanent sequelae in 10 to 30 per cent of survivors. Intellectual impairment is especially common in infants and young children. As many as 60 per cent of patients who have seizures during the illness will suffer recurrences. Up to 25 per cent of survivors will have cranial nerve deficits, including blindness, deafness, and squints. Ten to 25 per cent of survivors have some residual weakness after hemiparesis or paraparesis. About 10 per cent of patients develop CSF spinal block at some stage of the illness, but this will recover completely in at least half of them. Occasionally neurological deficit may progress or appear months after the illness as the subarachnoid exudate becomes fibrotic and calcified.

PREVENTION (SEE ALSO CHAPTER 7.11.22)

BCG vaccination at birth reduces the risk of infection by at least 80 per cent, but this seems to vary in different countries. It is recommended for all infants born into communities where tuberculosis is prevalent, including Asians living in Britain and expatriates living in tropical countries. To prevent the development of tuberculous meningitis in household contacts of newly diagnosed cases of pulmonary tuberculosis, prophylaxis with isoniazid 10 mg/kg daily for 6 to 12 months is recommended for all Mantoux-positive children under the age of 5 years.

REFERENCES
Acute bacterial meningitis

Bisno, A.L. (1989). Infections of central nervous system shunts. In *Infections associated with indwelling medical devices,* (ed. A.L. Bisno and F.A. Waldvogel), pp. 93–109. Washington.

Christie, A.B. (1980). *Infectious diseases: epidemiology and clinical practice* (3rd edn), pp. 605–46. Churchill Livingstone, Edinburgh.

Durand, M.L., *et al.* (1993). Acute bacterial meningitis in adults. *New England Journal of Medicine* **328**, (1), 21–8.

Girgis, N.I., Farid, Z., Kilpatrick, M.E., and Bishai, E. (1990). Dexamethasone for the treatment of children and adults with bacterial meningitis. *Reviews of the Infectious Diseases* **12**, 963–4.

Gray, L.D. and Fedorko, D.P. (1992). Laboratory diagnosis of bacterial meningitis. *Clinical Microbiological Reviews* **5**, (2), 130–45.

Hardman, J.M. and Earle, K.M. (1969). Myocarditis in 200 fatal meningococcal infections. *Archives of Pathology* **87**, 318–25.

Kay, R., Cheng, A.F., and Tse, C.Y. (1995). *Streptococcus suis* infection in Hong Kong. *Quarterly Journal of Medicine,* **88**, 39–47.

Mollaret, P. (1977). La meningite endothelio-leucocytaire multirecurrente benigne. *Revue Neurologique* **133**, 225–44.

Moxon, E.R., *et al.* (1974). *Hemophilus influenzae* meningitis in infant rats after intranasal inoculation. *Journal of Infectious Diseases* **129**, 154–62.

Rathore, M.H. (1991). Do prophylactic antibiotics prevent meningitis after basilar skull fracture? *Pediatric Infectious Disease Journal* **10**, 87–8.

Schaad, U.B., *et al.* (1993). Dexamethasone therapy for bacterial meningitis in children. *Lancet* **342**, 457–61.

Scheld, W.M., Whitley, R.J., and Durack, D.T. (1991). *Infections of the central nervous system*. Raven Press, New York.

Tedder, D.G., Ashley, R., Tyler, K.L., and Levin, M.J. (1994). Herpes simplex virus infection as a cause of benign recurrent lymphocytic meningitis. *Annals of Internal Medicine,* **121**, 334–8.

Tugwell, P., Greenwood, B.M., and Warrell, D.A. (1976). Pneumococcal meningitis: a clinical and laboratory study. *Quarterly Journal of Medicine* **45**, 583–601.

Tuberculous meningitis

Alarcon, F., Escalante, L., Perez, Y., Banda, H., Chacon, G., and Duenas, G. (1990). Tuberculous meningitis: short course chemotherapy. *Archives of Neurology* **47**, 1313–17.

Bateman, D.E., Newman, P.K., and Forster, J.B. (1983). A retrospective survey of proven cases of tuberculous meningitis in the Northern Region, 1970–1980. *Journal of the Royal College of Physicians of London* **17**, 106–10.

Berenguer, J., *et al.* (1992). Tuberculous meningitis in patients infected with the human immunodeficiency virus. *New England Journal of Medicine* **327**, 668–72.

Donald, P.R. and Seifart, H.I. (1989). Cerebrospinal fluid concentrations of ethionamide in children with tuberculous meningitis. *Journal of Pediatrics* **115**, 483–6.

Girgis, N.I., Farid, Z., Kilpatrick, M.E., Sultan, Y., and Mikhail, A. (1991). Dexamethasone adjunctive treatment for tuberculous meningitis. *Pediatric Infectious Disease Journal* **10**, 179–83.

Kaojarern, S., Supmonchai, K., Phuapradit, P., Mokkhavesa, C., and Krittiyanunt, S. (1991). Effect of steroids on cerebrospinal fluid penetration of antituberculosis drugs in tuberculous meningitis. *Clinical Pharmacology and Therapeutics* **49**, 6–12.

Parsons, M. (1988). *Tuberculous meningitis. A handbook for clinicians.* (2nd edn). Oxford University Press.

Phuapradit, P. and Vejjavjiva, A. (1987). Treatment of tuberculous meningitis: role of short-course chemotherapy. *Quarterly Journal of Medicine* **62**, 249–58.

Schoeman, J.F., le Roux, D., Bezuidenholt, P.B., and Donald, P.R. (1985). Intracranial pressure monitoring in tuberculous meningitis: clinical and computerized tomographic correlation. *Developmental Medicine and Child Neurology* **27**, 644–54.

Schoeman, J.F., Donald, P., van Zyl, L., Keet, M., and Wait, J. (1991). Tuberculous hydrocephalus: comparison of different treatments with regard to intracranial pressure, ventricular size and clinical outcome. *Developmental Medicine and Child Neurology* **33**, 396–405.

Shankar, P., Manijunath, N., Mohan, K.K., Prasad, K., Shriniwas, M.B., and Ahaja, G.K. (1991). Rapid diagnosis of tuberculous meningitis by polymerase chain reaction. *Lancet* **337**, 5–7.

Visudhiphan, P. and Chiemchanya, S. (1989). Tuberculous meningitis in children: treatment with isoniazid and rifampicin for twelve months. *Journal of Pediatrics* **114**, 875–9.

24.15.2 Viral infections of the central nervous system

D. A. WARRELL and P. G. E. KENNEDY

Viruses invade and damage the central nervous system in two ways: directly, by infecting the leptomeninges, brain, and spinal cord and, indirectly, by inducing an immunological reaction resulting in para- and postinfectious syndromes. In both cases, the terms meningitis, encephalitis, and myelitis are used alone or in combination. Meningitis implies inflammation of the meninges without alteration of consciousness, convulsions, or production of focal neurological abnormalities; in encephalitis there is impairment of cerebral function, usually with an altered state of consciousness and often with convulsions and focal neurological signs; while myelitis indicates involvement of the spinal cord. Chronic and 'slow' viral infections of the central nervous system are dealt with elsewhere (see Chapters 7.10.31 and 24.3.8).

VIROLOGY

There is considerable geographical and seasonal variation in the kinds of viruses causing meningitis, myelitis, and encephalitis; but, compared with bacterial infections of the central nervous system, there is less variation with age and immunocompetence.

Enteroviruses are responsible for 80 to 90 per cent of diagnosed cases of viral meningitis. Almost all the serotypes have been implicated in sporadic cases, and outbreaks have been associated with coxsackieviruses A7 and 9, all the coxsackie B types, and many of the echoviruses, especially 4, 6, 9, 11, 14, 16, and 30. Mumps is responsible for about 10 to 20 per cent of cases of viral meningitis. Other less common causes include herpes zoster, herpes simplex (predominantly type 2, HSV-2), measles, adenoviruses, Epstein–Barr virus and, in the United States, togaviruses, such as St Louis, eastern and western equine encephalitides, and bunyaviruses, such as California (La Crosse) encephalitis viruses.

Polioviruses are almost the only cause of viral 'paralytic' myelitis throughout the world, but coxsackie A7 (AB IV) has caused occasional small outbreaks and other coxsackie A and B viruses, echoviruses, and enterovirus 70 have caused sporadic cases. Herpes zoster, paralytic rabies, Epstein–Barr, and *Herpes simiae* B viruses can cause myelitis or ascending paralysis, and HSV-2 can cause lumbosacral myeloradiculitis.

Viruses causing encephalitis vary from country to country. Japanese (B) encephalitis virus is the most widespread human togavirus infection in the world and is the major cause of encephalitis throughout Asia. In Thailand there are, on average, 1500 cases each year, with 370 deaths. In North America, herpes simplex virus is the most common cause of sporadic fatal viral encephalitis, followed by the California encephalitis group, St Louis encephalitis virus, herpes zoster, enteroviruses, mumps, and measles. In the United States herpes simple encephalitis has an estimated incidence of 2.3/million population each year; HSV-1 accounts for 95 per cent of cases; HSV-2 causes encephalitis mainly in neonates and those who are immunosuppressed, such as transplant patients and those with human immunodeficiency virus (HIV) infection. In the United Kingdom, mumps is the most frequently diagnosed viral cause of encephalitis, followed by echoviruses, coxsackieviruses, measles, herpes simplex virus, herpes zoster virus, Epstein–Barr virus, and adenoviruses (especially adenovirus 7). Louping ill is the only indigenous arthropod-borne virus infection in Britain and has caused a few cases of encephalitis (see Section 7). In many developing countries rabies is an important cause of viral encephalitis. Other regional causes are Rift Valley fever virus in Africa and the Middle East, arenaviruses (Junin, Guanarito, Sabiá, Lassa, and Machupo) in Latin America and Africa, Marburg and Ebola viruses in Africa, and Colorado tick fever virus in North America.

Postinfectious encephalomyelitis most commonly follows measles, vaccinia, varicella, rubella, mumps, and influenza. Guillain–Barré syndrome, a sensorimotor polyneuropathy (Chapter 24.17) has been associated with infections by Epstein–Barr virus, cytomegalovirus, coxsackie B, and herpes zoster virus. Nervous-tissue vaccine against rabies may give rise to postvaccinal encephalitis (see below) while vaccination against rabies, influenza, and smallpox has been complicated by Guillain–Barré syndrome.

Immunodeficient patients are particularly vulnerable to some viral infections. Those with depressed cell-mediated immunity (Hodgkin's disease) may develop herpes zoster encephalitis and cytomegalovirus may cause a subacute encephalitis in patients with acquired immunodeficiency syndrome (AIDS). In children or adults with hypogammaglobulinaemia, enteroviruses, including live attenuated polio vaccine, may produce a progressive and fatal meningoencephalitis. Progressive multifocal leucoencephalopathy, a chronic and fatal papovavirus infection in patients with impaired cell-mediated immunity is described below. HIV infection of the brain and meninges may be responsible for acute meningoencephalitis at the time of seroconversion and subacute chronic encephalopathies and dementia in patients with AIDS (see Chapter 24.15.3).

EPIDEMIOLOGY

Many viral infections of the central nervous system occur in seasonal peaks or as epidemics, while others, such as herpes simplex encephalitis, are sporadic. Epidemics of Japanese encephalitis occur in the summer or rainy season because of the abundance of the vector mosquitoes (principally *Culex tritaeniorhynchus*) which have been infected by first feeding on the bird (cattle egrets, herons) or mammal reservoir species. Indigenous children and non-immune (immigrant) adults are most susceptible. Tick-borne encephalitides occur in spring and early summer when the ticks are most active. Mumps encephalitis is commonest in the late winter or early spring, while enterovirus infections occur most often in the summer and early autumn. Rodent-related encephalitides, such as the arenaviruses, are most common when the rodent population is at its peak, either in the fields (Machupo and Junin viruses) or in the home (lymphocytic choriomeningitis virus). The zoonotic viral infections survive periods of cold weather, during which the invertebrate–vertebrate cycle is suspended by 'overwintering' in their arthropod vectors or hibernating vertebrate reservoirs.

Invasion of the central nervous system seems to be a rare event in most viral infections. In the case of some togavirus infections, such as Japanese encephalitis, there may be only one case of encephalitis for every 500 to 1000 asymptomatic infections. The eastern equine encephalitis virus produces a much higher proportion of encephalitic cases than other togaviruses.

Infections by many neurotropic viruses are most frequent and severe in children or in the elderly. Herpes simplex encephalitis affects all age groups but shows peaks of incidence in those aged between 5 and 30 years and above 50 years. When HSV-2 invades the central nervous system it is likely to cause a benign lymphocytic meningitis in adults, but in neonates it usually produces a severe encephalitis. Among mosquito-borne epidemic encephalitides, California encephalitis is most common in children, St Louis encephalitis in the elderly, while eastern and western equine encephalitis and Japanese encephalitis viruses affect both the very young and the elderly. Postinfectious encephalitis is most frequent in children, for it complicates the common childhood exanthematous infections. It is the most common demyelinating disease in the world.

PATHOGENESIS

This subject has been reviewed thoroughly by Johnson (1982), Mims and White (1984), and Tyler and Fields (1988). Most viral infections reach the central nervous system from the primary site of infection and multiplication via the bloodstream. Viruses inoculated through the skin include those transmitted by arthropods, rabies virus, herpes simplex virus, *Herpes simiae* B, and lymphocytic choriomeningitis virus. Arthropod-borne viruses are presumed to replicate in local lymph nodes, vascular endothelium, and circulating fixed macrophages, in order to sustain viraemia. Rabies virus multiplies locally in the cytoplasm of muscle cells before entering peripheral nerves. Viruses which enter through the respiratory tract (for example measles, mumps, varicella) or gut (enteroviruses) multiply in local lymphoid tissue before they enter the bloodstream. Viraemia is a feature of most viral infections, yet invasion of the central nervous system is rare in most of them. The explanation for this is not known, but the CNS contains a number of intrinsic physical barriers to infectious agents such as viruses. These include the blood–brain barrier with its 'tight junctions', the presence of virus-resistant cells, and the absence of lymphatic drainage. Non-specific mechanisms at or near the site of virus entry, such as gastric acidity and cilia in the respiratory tract, also play a protective role. In the case of rabies, herpes simplex and herpes zoster viruses, the virus enters the central nervous system through the peripheral nerves. Although the subarachnoid space surrounding the olfactory nerves projects through the cribriform plate and is directly beneath the nasal mucosa, this route of infection seems to be extremely rare in humans and has been proven only in a few cases of inhaled rabies virus infection and herpes simplex encephalitis. Virus has been inoculated directly into the central nervous system by infected corneal transplant grafts (rabies) and infected brain surface electrodes (Creutzfeldt–Jakob disease). Herpes simplex encephalitis may complicate primary herpes simplex virus infection in children and young adults, but in most cases of herpes simplex encephalitis the cause is thought to be reactivation of latent virus (HSV-1) in the trigeminal nerve, autonomic nerve roots, or brain.

Some viruses, such as the enteroviruses and mumps, usually infect the meninges rather than the parenchyma of the central nervous system, whereas others, such as the togaviruses, usually cause encephalitis. Johnson (1982) has emphasized the selective vulnerability of different neural cells to different neurotropic viruses. Examples are the predilection of polioviruses for motor neurones of the anterior horns of the spinal cord and rabies for neurones of the limbic system and cerebellar Purkinje cells. The pathological effects of viral infections on the central nervous system include:

(1) the destruction and phagocytosis of neurones (neuronophagia) as a result of either viral invasion *per se* or immune lysis;
(2) demyelination;
(3) inflammatory oedema with the compressive effects of raised intracranial pressure; and, in some cases,
(4) vascular lesions.

In rabies, a universally fatal encephalitis, the relatively mild degree of neuronolysis has always puzzled neuropathologists. However, recent work suggests that rabies virus may produce its devastating effects by interfering with neurotransmission at central as well as peripheral cholinergic junctions. This virus also produces severe systemic effects, perhaps as a result of its centrifugal spread (for example in the case of myocarditis and cardiac arrhythmias) or its focal effects on vasomotor and respiratory centres in the brain-stem (Chapter 7.10.15).

Postinfectious encephalitis and Guillain–Barré syndrome are thought to result from sensitization to central and peripheral myelin, respectively. The animal model for the former is experimental allergic encephalomyelitis which can be produced in a variety of animals following immunization with myelin basic protein. A similar animal model for Guillain–Barré syndrome is known as experimental allergic neuritis. It is uncertain how the preceding viral infection induces this autoimmune response. In the case of postvaccinal encephalomyelitis resulting from nervous tissue antirabies vaccines, the explanation is more obvious, as these vaccines contain myelin from the animal in which the virus was grown.

Various host immune responses to viruses play a crucial role in combatting infection. Such responses may be directed either against the virus particle or the virus-infected cell, and may be humoral or cell-mediated. An important local immune response at infected surfaces is provided by IgA antibody, which is present in secretions in the gut, saliva, and respiratory tract. This is important, for example, in the early stages of poliovirus infection where the antibody neutralizes the virus by combining with viral surface proteins. The systemic viral infection may also be limited by means of circulating IgG and IgM antibodies, which can neutralize the virus in a variety of different ways. Immune responses may also occur locally within the CNS, where local synthesis of immunoglobulins, sometimes in an oligoclonal pattern, in response to virus infection may be evident. Such antibody elevations may be of considerable diagnostic value (see below). Under certain conditions immune responses to viruses may themselves set in train immunopathological processes leading to disease. This may occur in a number of different ways, such as through the deposition in blood vessels of immune complexes formed between antiviral antibody and viral antigen. In other cases, such as lymphocytic choriomeningitis virus infection, the induction of virus-specific cytotoxic T lymphocytes is itself responsible for the production of encephalitis.

PATHOLOGY

Meningitis

The basal leptomeninges, ependyma, and choroid plexus are infiltrated with mononuclear cells but the parenchyma is normal. In mumps meningitis there may be exfoliation of ependymal cells.

Poliomyelitis

Virus is distributed widely throughout the brain and spinal cord, possibly even in non-paralytic cases, but usually the only cells to suffer chromatolysis and phagocytosis are motor neurones in the anterior horns of the spinal cord, medulla, and grey matter of the precentral gyrus.

Encephalitis

Most viral encaphalitides are characterized by lymphocytic infiltration of the meninges and perivascular cuffing (Virchow–Robin spaces) in the cortex and underlying white matter, by lymphocytes, plasma cells, histiocytes, and some neutrophils, and proliferation of microglia with formation of glial nodules. Neuronolysis and demyelination are variable in their degree and location. Infected neurones may show characteristic inclusion bodies in their nuclei (measles, herpes simplex virus, and adenoviruses) or cytoplasm (Negri bodies in rabies). Microhaemorrhages and foci of necrosis may be found.

Herpes simplex encephalitis

The special features of this condition are gross cerebral oedema and severe haemorrhagic and necrotizing encephalitis, which is often asymmetrically localized to the inferior and medial parts of the temporal lobe, the insula and the orbital part of the frontal lobe. Histological sections show eosinophilic Cowdry type A intranuclear inclusions with margination of chromatin in neurones, oligodendrocytes, and astrocytes, inflammatory and haemorrhagic perivascular reactions, but no demyelination. Cowdry type A inclusions are also found in herpes zoster virus and cytomegalovirus encephalitides. The unique cerebral localization of herpes simplex encephalitis has not been satisfactorily explained, but is probably the result of viral spread along specific neural pathways rather

than differential susceptibility of particular cell populations. Although a popular theory is that herpes simplex virus spreads along olfactory pathways to the base of the brain and temporal lobes, it is also possible that virus may spread from the trigeminal ganglia through sensory fibres innervating the dura near these regions. The last mechanism is consistent with confirmed observations that HSV-1 is present in latent form in the trigeminal, superior cervical, and vagal ganglia in a high proportion of normal individuals, irrespective of whether they have a history of mucocutaneous herpes infections ('cold sores'). Although in the latter case latent HSV-1 may be reactivated by a multitude of different stimuli, such as sunlight, fever, trauma, and stress, the actual mechanisms underlying herpes simplex virus latency and reactivation in the nervous system are not yet fully understood. Even if herpes simplex encephalitis is indeed caused by the reactivation of virus which has remained latent in the trigeminal ganglia, the fact that it is relatively so rare despite the almost ubiquitous asymptomatic infection in humans has still to be explained.

Japanese (B) encephalitis

Microscopical appearances are typical of other viral encephalitides: there is oedema, congestion, and focal haemorrhages of the brain and meninges, and perivascular cuffing, neuronophagia, and glial nodules of the brain parenchyma. Neuronolysis and neuronophagia are unusually widespread in the cerebral cortex, thalamus, basal ganglia, brain-stem, cerebellum (where there is marked destruction of Purkinje cells) and the spinal cord. Viral antigen is localized to neurones, especially in the brain-stem and thalamus

Postinfectious encephalomyelitis

This is a perivenous microglial encephalitis with demyelination. Fibrinoid necrosis of arterioles is an associated lesion in a more severe form designated acute haemorrhagic leucoencephalitis

CLINICAL FEATURES

Meningitis

A prodromal influenza-like illness, followed by a brief remission of symptoms is typical of lymphocytic choriomeningitis viral infection and some outbreaks of enteroviral meningitis (for example echo 9) but in most cases of viral meningitis, symptoms start suddenly. As with bacterial meningitis, there is fever, headache, a stiff neck, and vomiting, especially in children. Compared with bacterial meningitis, headache is less severe and tends to be frontal or retrobulbar (eye movements may be painful) and neck stiffness is less marked. Nausea, anorexia, abdominal pain, myalgias, and sore throat are particularly common in enteroviral meningitis. Myalgia is particularly severe with coxsackie B infections. As in acute bacterial meningitis, infants usually present with vague irritability and a tense fontanelle and young children with fever and irritability or lethargy. Conjunctival injection, pharyngitis, and cervical lymphadenopathy may be found. Macular or petechial exanthems or enanthems are seen with coxsackie A and B and echovirus infections (especially echo 9). Vesicles on the hands, feet, and mouth have been reported with coxsackie A16 and enterovirus 71 infections. By definition, the level of consciousness is normal in simple meningitis. Neurological features include vertigo, nystagmus, cerebellar ataxia, facial spasms, and involuntary movements.

The specific cause of viral meningitis may be suggested by characteristic signs outside the nervous system, such as genital or rectal vesicles in the sexually active age group (HSV-2), herpes zoster skin lesions, swelling in the parotid region (mumps and occasionally coxsackie, lymphocytic choriomeningitis, and Epstein–Barr viruses), orchitis (mumps and lymphocytic choriomeningitis virus) and arthritis (lymphocytic choriomeningitis virus). However, potentially helpful features, such as gastrointestinal symptoms associated with enteroviral infections and parotitis associated with mumps, may be completely absent in patients with meningitis.

Fig. 1 Paralytic poliomyelitis in a 3-year-old Thai child. Note systemic illness and paralysis of right arm. (Copyright D.A. Warrell.)

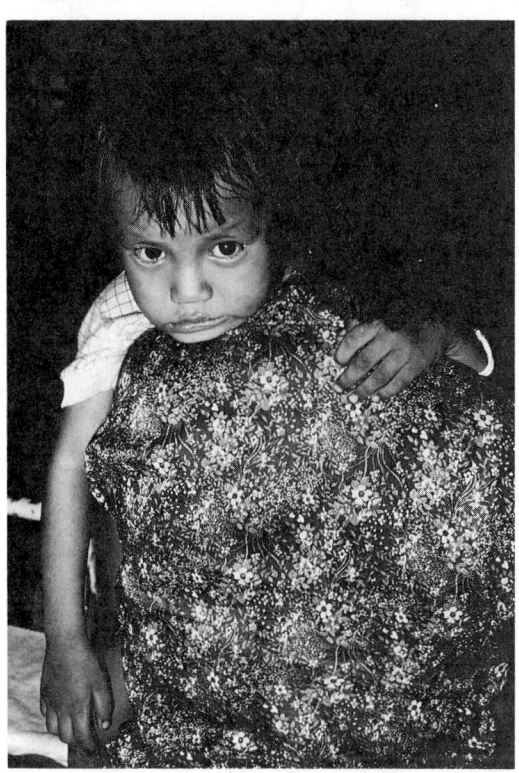

Paralytic poliomyelitis

The infection (see Chapter 7.10.13) is acquired by droplet spread from the respiratory tract or by the faecal–oral route. The 'minor illness', coinciding with viraemia, is a non-specific episode of influenza-like symptoms—fever, headache, sore throat, malaise, and mild gastrointestinal symptoms—which resolves in a few days. Most of those infected have no further symptoms but, in a minority, the 'major illness' follows, sometimes after a few days' remission of symptoms. The features are those of viral meningitis: muscle pain, spasms, and sensory disturbances may precede or accompany the development of lower motor neurone (flaccid) paralysis. Any combination of motor unit deficits may be seen (Fig. 1). It is most unusual for paralysis to extend after the first 3 days or after the temperature has fallen (Fig. 2). Respiratory and bulbar paralysis is life-threatening. Encephalitis is rare. The commonest causes of death are aspiration and airway obstruction, resulting from bulbar paralysis, and paralysis of respiratory muscles. Disturbances of respiratory and cardiac rhythm, thought to be the result of damage to medullary vasomotor and respiratory centres, are extremely uncommon. Other complications include impaired control of body temperature and blood pressure, gastrointestinal haemorrhage, aspiration pneumonia, and paralysis of the bladder and bowel.

Encephalitis

Most patients with viral encephalitis present with the symptoms of meningitis (fever, headache, neck stiffness, vomiting) together with altered consciousness, convulsions, and sometimes focal neurological signs, signs of raised intracranial pressure, or psychiatric symptoms.

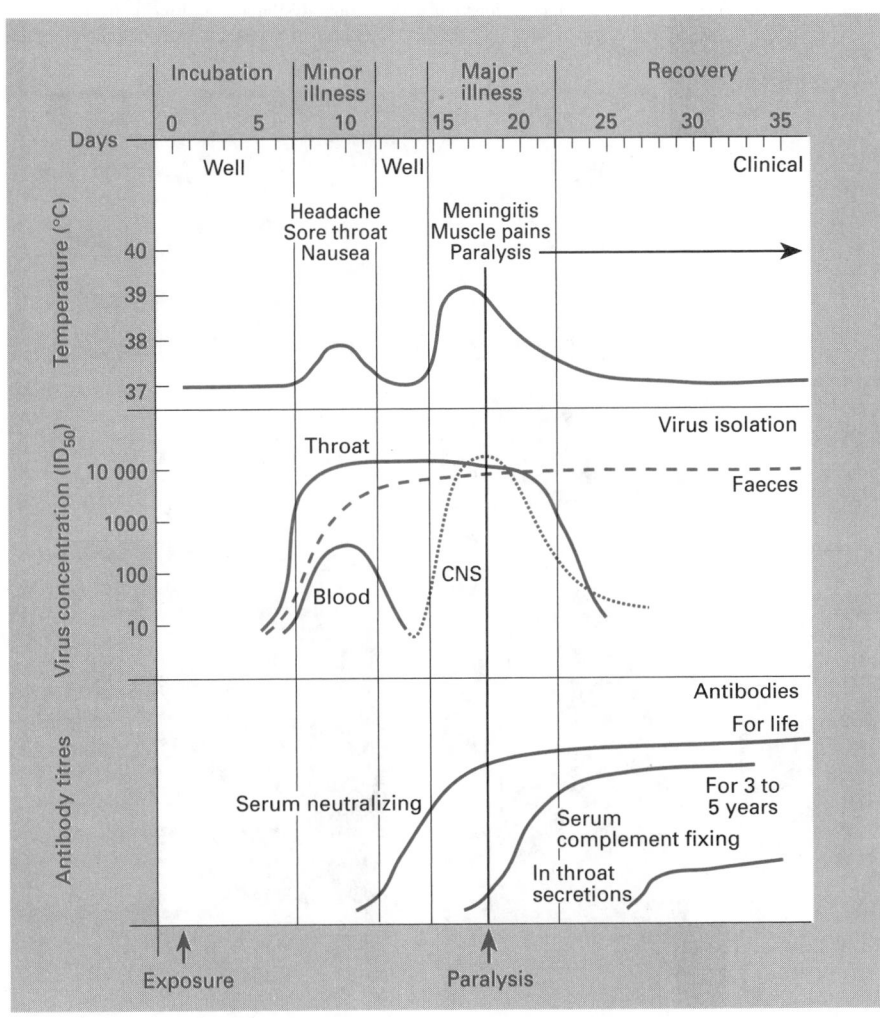

Fig. 2 The course of a paralytic poliomyelitis infection. (Reproduced from Christie, 1981, *Medicine International*, **1,** 139. Adapted from Bodian, D. (1957). *Mechanisms of infection with polio viruses.* In *Cellular biology, nucleic acids, and viruses.* New York Academy of Sciences, by permission.)

Herpes simplex encephalitis

This is a relatively common sporadic encephalitis that may occur in any age group. The origin of the virus is almost always unknown. The majority of cases are presumed to be due to reactivation of latent virus, possibly HSV-1 from the trigeminal ganglion. In neonates herpes simplex encephalitis is caused by HSV-2.

As well as the usual clinical features of a severe viral encephalitis, patients with herpes simplex encephalitis have symptoms related to the focal nature of the encephalitis (frontal and temporal cortex and limbic system). These include behavioural abnormalities, olfactory and gustatory hallucinations, anosmia, amnesia, expressive aphasia, and temporal lobe seizures. Herpetic skin or mucosal lesions are rarely found, except in the case of acute genital HSV-2, or proctitis, and a past history of 'cold sores' does not affect the chances of the infection being due to herpes simplex virus. Effects of cerebral oedema are unusually severe. Patients usually lapse into coma towards the end of the first week and most deaths occur within the first 2 weeks. This condition is also considered in detail in Chapter 7.10.2.

Japanese (B) encephalitis

After an incubation period of 7 to 14 days, patients develop non-specific prodromal symptoms (fever, headache, malaise, and nausea) lasting 2 to 3 days. Neurological symptoms begin suddenly with increasing headache, deteriorating level of consciousness, and generalized convulsions, which may result in status epilepticus. There is meningism and mask-like facies, with upper motor neurone signs or a myelitic pattern, cranial nerve lesions (for example lower motor neurone VII), ataxia, involuntary movements (Fig. 3), and, in severe cases, prolonged coma, hemi- or quadriparesis, decerebrate rigidity, and respiratory failure. Fever persists for 6 to 7 days and, in survivors, neurological symptoms last for 1 to 2 weeks. Case fatality rate is 50 per cent in those over 50 years old, but less than 20 per cent in children. Most deaths occur in the first 7 to 10 days from respiratory failure, aspiration pneumonias, intracranial hypertension, and uncontrolled seizures. Up to 50 per cent of survivors suffer from intellectual impairment, psychiatric problems, persistent epilepsy, or a vegetative state with spastic quadriparesis and evidence of basal ganglia involvement, such as dystonia of the limbs and trunk, rigidity, and tremor (Fig. 3)

Postinfectious encephalomyelitis

Sudden convulsions, coma, fever, or pareses appear 10 to 14 days after the start of vaccination (vaccinia or nervous tissue rabies vaccine) or after infection with measles, varicella, rubella, mumps, or influenza. In the case of measles, varicella, and rubella, encephalitic symptoms develop 2 to 12 days after the rash has appeared, and in mumps before or after parotid swelling. Involuntary movements, cranial nerve lesions (VII, III), pupillary abnormalities, nystagmus, ataxia, and upper motor neurone signs are common

DIAGNOSIS

Clinical and epidemiological details

The time of year, known current epidemics, the patient's age, occupation, and countries or states visited recently may help to narrow down

Fig. 3 Japanese (B) encephalitis in Anuradhapura, Sri Lanka. (a) Comatose female patient showing symmetrical chorioathetotic movements of the upper limbs; (b) comatose child showing dystonic movements of the upper and lower limbs; (c) convalescent child, conscious but with residual dystonia of all four limbs; (d) convalescent child with floppy head and involuntary movements of all four limbs; (e) convalescent boy with residual weakness of the neck flexors. (By courtesy of Dr D.T.D.J. Abeysekera.)

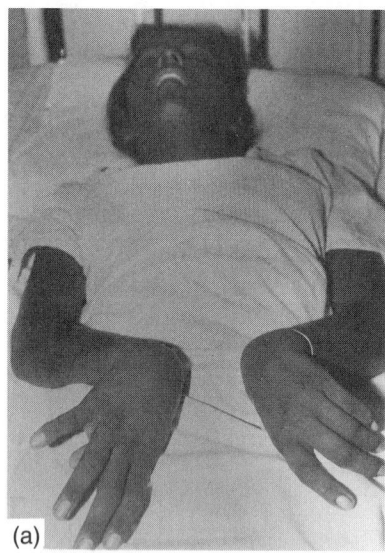
(a)

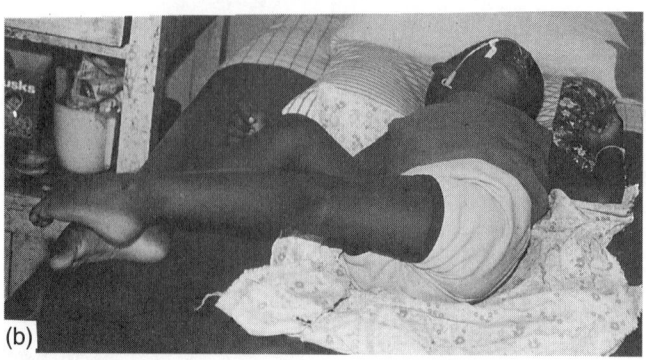
(b)

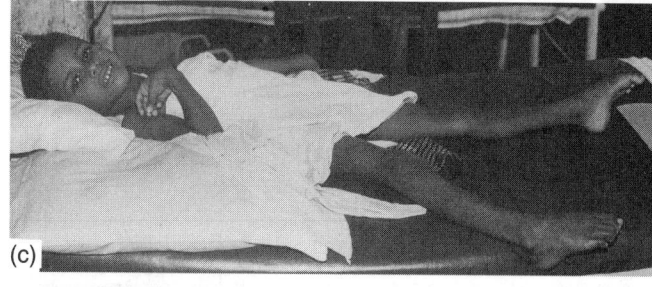
(c)

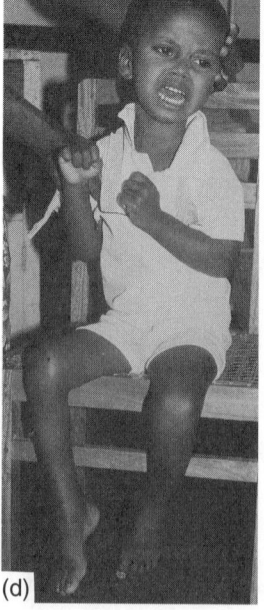
(d)

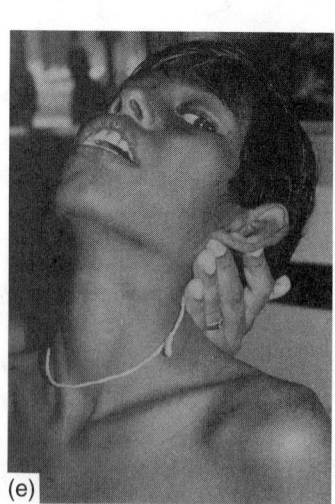
(e)

the possibilities. A specific diagnosis may be suggested by distinctive clinical features of the encephalitis itself (for example hydrophobia in rabies, temporal lobe features in herpes simplex encephalitis) or of the associated infection (for example mumps parotitis; measles rash; skin and mucosal lesions of herpes viruses; and gastrointestinal symptoms associated with enteroviral infections).

Laboratory investigations

These should aim to demonstrate a specific viral agent (particularly important for the potentially treatable herpes virus infections) or exclude potentially treatable non-viral causes of meningitis or encephalomyelitis (Table 1). The most important investigation is examination of the cerebrospinal fluid (CSF). Contraindications to lumbar puncture are the same as in acute bacterial meningitis (Chapters 24.2.6 and 24.15.1). If there are lateralizing neurological signs or evidence of raised intracranial pressure, a CT scan should be performed to exclude an intracranial mass lesion before contemplating a lumbar puncture. CSF pressure is increased especially in herpes simplex encephalitis, where there is intense cerebral oedema. Pleocytosis ranges from tens to thousands of cells/μl. Lymphocytes and other mononuclear cells predominate, except in the early stages of some infections (for example enteroviruses, herpes simplex encephalitis). CSF contains erythrocytes or is xanthochromic in haemorrhagic encephalitides such as herpes simplex encephalitis and acute necrotic leucoencephalitis. Protein concentration is usually increased in the range of 50 to 150 mg/dl with an increasing proportion of IgG as the disease progresses. Leakage of serum IgG into the CSF and intrathecal IgG synthesis, indicated by a monoclonal band, are responsible. CSF glucose concentration is usually normal or increased towards the level in a blood sample taken simultaneously, but low levels are occasionally reported, especially in mumps and lymphocytic choriomeningitis virus infections. Measurement of lactate, C-reactive protein, lactic dehydrogenase, creatine kinase (CK-BB), muramidase, and various cytokines in the CSF have not proved helpful in distinguishing viral from other infections. CSF examination may be misleading if it is normal, as it is at the first examination in 10 to 15 per cent of patients with herpes simplex encephalitis, if there is a predominantly neutrophil pleocytosis, or if the glucose concentration is low. Myelin basic protein may be found in the CSF of patients with positive infective encephalomyelitides.

Virology

A specific virus can be implicated in 70 to 75 per cent of cases of lymphocytic meningitis and 30 to 40 per cent of patients with meningoencephalitis (Table 2). At appropriate stages of the illness, a rapid diagnosis by direct immunofluorescence may be made of herpes simplex virus (skin and brain), herpes zoster virus (skin lesion scrapings), rabies (skin sections and brain), measles (nasopharyngeal aspirate), and some non-viral causes such as Rocky Mountain spotted fever (skin). Electron microscopy of skin lesions will identify a herpes virus. Some viruses can be isolated from the CSF (for example mumps, enteroviruses, lymphocytic choriomeningitis virus, Central European encephalitides, Louping ill, and HIV). Virus cultured from a distant site may help with the diagnosis (for example polio and other enteroviruses from stool, or arthropod-borne viruses from blood culture) but they may not be related to the neurological symptoms (for example, cytomegalovirus from the pharynx or urine, herpes simplex virus from skin or mucosa or adenovirus seen in stool by electron microscopy). Specific viral IgM can be detected in serum for mumps, Epstein–Barr virus, cytomegalovirus, or measles, or, using a μ-capture technique, in the CSF for Japanese encephalitis virus. The method is being used increasingly for IgM to other viruses. A viral diagnosis is often delayed until a rising convalescent antibody titre is found by an appropriate technique. This is usually the case for mumps, coxsackie, and most arthropod-borne viruses.

A significant recent diagnostic advance has been the introduction of the polymerase chain reaction (PCR) technique. Using PCR, which greatly amplifies the amount of viral nucleic acid in the test sample, it has been possible, for example, to identify herpes simplex virus in the CSF of suspected cases of herpes simplex encephalitis within a short time of the onset of symptoms. PCR is likely to be used for the early diagnosis of a wide variety of CNS viral infections in the future (Table 2).

Brain biopsy

For the rapid diagnosis of some viral encephalitides there is at present no substitute for brain biopsy. Electroencephalography, computerized tomographic (CT) or magnetic resonance imaging (MRI) scans, angiography, or technetium scans can help to direct the surgeon towards the affected area of brain. Failing this, a biopsy of the medial or inferior surface of the temporal lobe is most likely to yield the diagnosis. Opinion is divided about the safety and importance of this procedure.

Imaging of the brain and spinal cord

CT and MRI scans of the brain and spinal cord are proving extremely useful for the diagnosis of the site, nature, and extent of mass lesions and associated oedema, sub- and epidural empyemas, meningitis, cerebritis, and ventriculitis, the presence of intracranial hypertension, hydrocephalus, cerebral and brain-stem herniation, demyelination, and other anatomical abnormalities (see Chapter 24.2.1).

CT scans are superior for bony details and calcifications, are quicker to perform and are less dependent on the patient being able to lie motionless. Repeated CT scans may carry a risk of causing cataracts. The resolution of MRI is greater for parenchymal lesions but this cannot be done in patients with pacemakers and may be dangerous in those with metal clips in cerebral blood vessels.

DIFFERENTIAL DIAGNOSIS

Viral infections of the CNS must be distinguished from the many other conditions which produce similar clinical features and CSF abnormalities (Table 1). The differential diagnosis of viral meningitis includes the other causes of aseptic meningitis, such as partially treated bacterial meningitis, tuberculous meningitis, spirochaetal infections (leptospirosis, borreliosis, Lyme disease, and syphilis), fungal, amoebic, neoplastic, granulomatous, and idiopathic meningitides. Viral myelitides must be distinguished from other causes of transverse myelitis and the Brown–Séquard syndrome. These include spinal compression by tumours, abscesses, helminths or their ova, or vertebral disease.

The differential diagnosis of paralytic poliomyelitis includes postinfectious and other immunopathic polyneuroradiculopathies, such as Guillain–Barré syndrome and Landry's ascending paralysis; metabolic neuropathies such as acute porphyria; paralytic rabies; neoplastic polyradiculopathies; and rarities, such as tick paralysis and *Herpes simiae* B virus infection. The lack of objective sensory loss in poliomyelitis usually distinguishes it from these other entities.

The differential diagnosis of viral encephalitis includes other infective encephalopathies—bacterial, fungal, protozoal, and parasitic; intracranial abscesses and neoplasms; toxic and metabolic encephalopathies; and heat stroke. The diagnosis of 'viral encephalitis' should not be made too hastily, as it may condemn the patient with concealed cerebral malaria or some other curable encephalopathy to delayed treatment or even death.

TREATMENT

Antiviral chemotherapy

Acyclovir (Zovirax®) and, to a lesser extent, vidarabine (cytosine arabinoside) have proved effective in treating herpes simplex encephalitis. This subject is discussed in Chapter 7.10.2. The nucleoside analogue acycloguanosine (acyclovir, Zovirax®) is only taken up by cells infected by herpes simplex virus and is therefore non-toxic to normal, uninfected cells. In view of this remarkable lack of serious toxicity, treatment can be started as soon as herpes simplex encephalitis is suspected clinically. Although there is still some controversy in the United States regarding the role of brain biopsy in herpes simplex encephalitis, virtually all

Table 1 *Causes of aseptic meningitis[a], with or without encephalitis or myelitis, other than viruses and postinfectious/postvaccinal syndromes*

Cause	Diagnostic clinical feature or investigation
Bacteria	
Acute bacterial meningitis (partially treated)	Cerebrospinal fluid (CSF) antigen detection (CIE, LA), repeated CSF examination
Intracranial/spinal abscess or empyema	Physical examination (exclude otitis media, trauma, dermoid sinus, etc.), radiographs, CT/MRI scans, myelogram
(parameningeal infections)	
Brucella	CSF, blood culture, serology
Cat scratch disease bacillus	Warthin–Starry stain skin and lymph-node, skin test
Mycobacteria	CSF microscopy, LA, culture; Mantoux test, chest radiograph
Mycoplasma	CSF + serum IgM (IFA)
Spirochaetes	
Leptospira	Serology
Relapsing fevers	Blood smear, mouse inoculation
Lyme disease	Serology (EIA, IFA), culture, skin biopsy, CSF IgG (EIA IFT)
Syphilis	Serology (FTA-ABS) serum and CSF
Spirillum minus	Microscopy of wound or lymph-node aspirates, mouse inoculation
Rickettsiae	
(Rocky Mountain spotted fever, murine, epidemic, scrub typhus)	Serology (Weil–Felix), skin biopsy IFT (RMSF)
Fungi	
Blastomyces	CSF culture, EIA, demonstration at other sites, lung, skin, biopsy
Candida	CSF culture (repeated)
Coccidioides	CSF-CFT, culture, microscopy
Cryptococcus	CSF India ink, LA—beware false positive with surface condensate on agar
Histoplasma	CSF culture (repeated), demonstration at other sites, blood smear (buffy coat) serum, urine, CSF antigen detection (RIA)
Protozoa	
Amoeba (Acanthamoeba, Naegleria)	CSF microscopy (fresh wet preparation + India ink), culture
Malaria (cerebral)	Blood smears
Toxoplasma	(Immunocompromised patients—AIDS) CSF animal inoculation, serology, brain biopsy
Trypanosomiasis (African and South American)	Blood smear (buffy coat), lymph node aspirate, CSF microscopy, and IgM, serology, xenodiagnosis
Helminths	
Angiostrongylus cantonensis	CSF larvae, eosinophilia
Cysticercosis	CT/MRI scan, radiographs, examination for subcutaneous cysts, CSF-CFT, histology
Gnathostoma spinigerum	Cutaneous migratory swelling, CSF eosinophilia
Hydatid disease	Casoni test, serology, CT/MRI scan, radiographs
Paragonimus	CSF ova, eosinophils, serology, CT/MRI scan or skull radiograph, histology
Schistosomiasis	Low transverse myelitis, ova in urine or stool, CT/MRI scan, CSF eosinophilia, myelogram, histology
Sparganosis	Histology, CT/MRI scan
Strongyloides stercoralis	(Immunocompromised patients) larvae, ova in stool, duodenal fluid, etc.
Behçet's syndrome	Clinical syndrome
Carcinomas, cysts, leukaemias, lymphomas	CSF cytology, evidence of condition elsewhere
Chemical	Recent lumbar puncture, spinal anaesthesia, myelography, isotope cisternography
Drugs	Non-steroidal anti-inflammatory agents, immunomodulators, antimicrobials (e.g. trimethoprim)
Kawasaki's disease	Clinical features, echocardiography, coronary angiography, etc.
Lead encephalopathy	Blood lead, blood smear, urinary coproporphyrins
Mollaret's meningitis	Recurrence, CSF 'Mollaret's' cells (PCR for HSV)
Sarcoidosis	Histology, Kveim test, Mantoux test, serum Ca^{2+}, angiotensin-converting enzyme
Systemic lupus erythematosus and other collagen/vascular diseases	Antinuclear antibodies, DNA antibodies, lupus erythematosus cells
Vogt–Koyanagi–Harada syndrome	Clinical syndrome
Whipple's disease	Clinical features, jejunal histology

[a]Aseptic meningitis: CSF pleocytosis but no bacteria stainable by Gram's method and no growth on standard bacterial culture media.

CFT, complement fixation test; CIE, countercurrent immunoelectrophoresis; EIA, enzyme immunoassay; FTA-ABS, fixed Treponema antigen-antibody slide test; IFA, immunofluorescent antibody; LA, latex agglutination; RIA, radioimmunoassay; RMSF, Rocky mountain spotted fever.

Table 2 *Specimens for the virological diagnosis of acute meningitis or meningo-encephalomyelitis (after Johnson 1982; Jackson and Johnson 1989)*

	Specimens for virus isolation/identification						Serology	
	Throat swab	Stool	CSF	Blood	Other specimens	PCR CSF	Acute	Convalescent
Adenovirus	+ +ᵃ	+	−		?ᵇ	?ᵇ	+	
Arenavirus								
Lymphocytic choriomeningitis	−	−	+ + +	+		?ᵇ	+	+ 2–3 months
Enteroviruses								
Polioviruses	+	+ + +	−	−		+ +ᶜ,ᵈ	+	+
Coxsackie and echovirusesᶠ	+	+ + +	+ + +	−		+	+	+
Herpesviruses								
Cytomegalovirus	−	−	−	−	Urineᵃ	+	+ᵃ	+
Epstein–Barr	+ᵃ	−	−	−		+	+ᵃ	+
Herpes simplex								
type 1	+ᵃ	−	+	−	Brain	+ + +	+ᵃ	
type 2	−	−	+	−	Vesicular fluid	+	+ᵃ	+
Herpes simiae (B)	−	−	−	−	Vesicular fluid	−	+ᵃ	+
Herpes varicella/zoster	−	−	+	−	Vesicular fluid	+ᵇ	+ᵃ	+
Mumps	+ + +	−	+ +	−	Saliva, urine	?ᵇ	+	+
Rhabdoviruses								
Rabies	−		+	−	Skin biopsy, saliva, brain	?ᵇ	+	+
Retroviruses								
HIV-1	−	−	+	+ + +		+ + +ᵉ	+ + +	−
HIV-2	−	−	+	+ + +		?	+ + +	−
HTLV-1	−	−	+	−		+	+ + +	−
Togaviruses	−	−	+	+ +		+ᵉ	+	+

ᵃIsolations or antibody responses may represent non-specific activation.

ᵇToo few data to indicate general usefulness in diagnosis.

ᶜAlso serum/blood.

ᵈAlso stool.

ᵉAlso brain tissue.

ᶠSome Coxsackie A serotypes (especially A1-6) cannot be grown on cells.

clinicians in the United Kingdom now start therapy with acyclovir routinely without attempting to confirm the diagnosis by brain biopsy. Acyclovir has also been used for herpes zoster virus encephalitis, but there is no convincing evidence for its efficacy in cytomegalovirus infections of the CNS. The rare but very dangerous encephalomyelitis caused by *Herpes simiae* B virus should be treated with acyclovir (see Chapter 7.10.5). Ribavirin is effective against some RNA viruses, such as those causing Lassa fever, haemorrhagic fever with renal syndrome, and possibly Argentinian haemorrhagic fever, Rift Valley fever, and Congo Crimean haemorrhagic fever.

Interferons have been used by intravenous, intrathecal, or intraventricular routes in the treatment of rabies, herpes zoster virus, and other herpes virus encephalitides, but have not proved effective.

Hyperimmune plasma given within 8 days of the start of symptoms has reduced the mortality of Argentinian haemorrhagic fever (Junin virus) from 20 to 30 to 1 to 3 per cent. Hyperimmune human globulin has also proved effective in the treatment of Congo Crimean haemorrhagic fever.

Supportive treatment

Corticosteroids have been used in most of the viral encephalomyelitides, both in an attempt to combat cerebral oedema (especially in herpes simplex encephalitis) and for their other anti-inflammatory effects. Convincing evidence of benefit, from controlled trials, is lacking, but the immunosuppressive effects of corticosteroids have not led to obvious clinical deterioration, except perhaps in some cases of diffuse myelitis. Corticosteroids or adrenocorticotrophic hormone (ACTH) have also been used for postinfectious and postvaccinal encephalomyelitides, but the evidence for their efficacy is not convincing. Severe intracranial hypertension should be treated with intravenous mannitol or mechanical hyperventilation. Nursing and general care are the same as for acute bacterial meningitis (Chapter 24.15.1) and tuberculous meningitis. Seizures must be controlled with prophylactic phenytoin, fever lowered by cooling, respiratory failure treated by mechanical ventilation, and attention given to fluid, electrolyte, and acid–base balance. Hyponatraemia is attributable to inappropriate secretion of antidiuretic hormone in some cases.

Paralytic poliomyelitis

Most authorities recommend rest and even mild sedation during the preparalytic stage of the 'major illness', because of the suspicion that exercise increases paralysis. The severe muscle pains and spasms reported from some parts of the world are treated with mild analgesic, such as salicylate, and with hot-water bottles. During the phase of developing paralysis, patients must be observed closely and, if possible, assessed objectively for the development of life-threatening bulbar and respiratory paralysis. Those with weakness of swallowing should be nursed on their sides to prevent aspiration. The need for a cuffed tracheostomy tube may be avoided by careful positioning, frequent observations, and suction. Indications for mechanical ventilation are a progressive decline in ventilatory capacity to less than 30 to 50 per cent of normal, hypoxaemia, or gross disturbances of respiratory rhythm (Cheyne–Stokes respiration, long apnoeic intervals, etc.) suggesting damage to the respiratory centres. Respiratory weakness without bulbar paralysis may be treated in a tank respirator or rocking bed, which do not require tracheostomy. However, patients with severe or rapidly progressing respiratory paralysis need urgent tracheostomy and intermittent positive pressure ventilation. Overventilation must be avoided. Assisted ventilation may be required for long periods, but attempts should be made to wean patients off the ventilator as soon as their condition becomes stable. Severe fluctuations in body temperature and blood pressure, reminiscent of those in severe tetanus and rabies, may require intensive care. The paralysed patient may have to lie in bed for many months and will develop complications of this prolonged immobilization. These include bed sores, osteomalacia, hypercalciuria leading to renal calculi, recurrent urinary tract infections resulting from chronic urethral catheterization, respiratory infections and contractures of muscles and tendons leading to severe musculoskeletal deformities which will require orthopaedic correction. Some of these can be prevented by passive movement of joints and splinting. Physiotherapy and psychological support are needed during the prolonged phase of rehabilitation.

PROGNOSIS AND SEQUELAE

Viral meningitis has an excellent prognosis, but some patients with HSV-2 infection have recurrent attacks with spinal cord or nerve root involvement. Case fatality rates of some viral encephalomyelitides are as follows: rabies, 100 per cent; herpes simplex encephalitis (untreated), 40 to more than 75 per cent (highest in neonates and those over 30 years old); eastern equine encephalitis, 50 per cent; Japanese encephalitis, 10 to 40 per cent; measles, 10 to 20 per cent; varicella, 10 to 30 per cent; western equine encephalitis, 8 per cent; St Louis encephalitis, 3 per cent; California encephalitis, Venezuelan encephalitis, and mumps, less than 1 per cent. The mortality of paralytic poliomyelitis increases from 5 per cent in young children to more than 20 per cent in adults. Postinfectious and postvaccinal encephalomyelitides carry case fatalities of 15 to 40 per cent.

Neurological sequelae are found in 5 to 75 per cent of survivors of Japanese encephalitis and herpes simplex encephalitis, and are especially common in infants. They include mental retardation, loss of memory, speech abnormalities (including subtle expressive aphasias), hemiparesis, ataxia, dystonic brain-stem and cranial nerve lesions, recurrent convulsions, and various behavioural and personality disturbances. Sequelae are common with postinfectious encephalomyelitis. An unusual sequel to paralytic poliomyelitis developing after an interval of many years is a condition characterized by progressive muscle weakness and wasting, which has some similarities to motor neurone disease.

PREVENTION

Prophylactic vaccination against poliomyelitis and measles has virtually eradicated encephalitides caused by these viruses in many communities. Postexposure rabies vaccination has also proved effective in preventing rabies encephalitis, and human diploid cell strain vaccine is used increasingly for pre-exposure prophylaxis. A formalin-inactivated adult mouse brain vaccine is manufactured in Osaka for Japanese encephalitis. It appears to be effective and carries a very low risk of objective neurological complications (one in a million courses). Vaccines for use in humans have been prepared against a number of other arthropod-borne viruses (for example European tick-borne encephalitis).

Hyperimmune immunoglobulin has been used for prophylaxis (and in some cases attempted treatment) of measles, herpes zoster virus, HSV-2, vaccinia, rabies, and some other infections in high-risk groups.

Immunocompromised patients, such as those with leukaemia, who are household contacts of a case of herpes zoster virus infection, should be given prophylactic hyperimmune globulin and, if they develop skin lesions, they should be treated with acyclovir to prevent development of severe disease.

Interferons have been used with some success to prevent herpes virus infections, such as cytomegalovirus in high-risk groups such as renal transplant recipients. However, the evidence does not yet justify their recommendation.

Caesarean section before rupture of the membranes in a full-term pregnant woman with genital herpes may prevent HSV-2 encephalitis in the neonate. If the herpetic lesions are discovered during or after vaginal delivery, topical acyclovir should be applied to the eyes of the neonate, as they are the most likely portal of entry.

Control of animal vectors and reservoirs: arthropod-borne viral encephalitides can be prevented by avoiding or controlling the arthropod vectors (for example by the use of mosquito nets, insect repellents, insecticides, etc.), by attempting to control the numbers of wild vertebrate reservoir species, or by immunizing domestic animals, such as horses (eastern and western equine encephalitides) and pigs (Japanese encephalitis). To control rabies, the principal wild mammalian vectors can be reduced in numbers or they can be immunized (for example, wild foxes have been immunized by distributing oral vaccine in bait). Domestic dogs and cats can be vaccinated. To prevent the viral encephalitides transmissible from laboratory animals (for example, lymphocytic choriomeningitis from mice and rats, *Herpes simiae* B from monkeys) their quarantine, handling, and housing should be strictly controlled.

Reye's syndrome

Reye's syndrome is an acute encephalopathy affecting children between the ages of 2 and 16 years. It is rapidly fatal in 10 to 40 per cent of cases. The defining characteristics are sudden impairment of consciousness, increase in serum aminotransferase concentrations (or, if a biopsy is done, a fatty liver), and the exclusion of other diseases. Symptoms develop a few days after varicella or an upper respiratory tract or gastrointestinal illness. Clusters of cases (median age 11 years) have been associated with influenza B epidemics, while sporadic cases (median age 6 years) have followed varicella, coxsackie, dengue, and other viral infections. Recent studies in the United States have suggested an association between Reye's syndrome and the use of salicylates, but not of paracetamol, during the preceding viral illness. This has led the Committee on Safety of Medicines to recommend that aspirin should not be given to children under 12 years of age, unless specifically indicated for childhood rheumatic conditions. Aflatoxin has been implicated in Thailand. In the United States, the annual incidence of Reye's syndrome in those under 18 years old is 0.42 per 100 000 urban dwellers and 1.8 per 100 000 rural and suburban dwellers.

The child is nauseated and retches or vomits for 1 or 2 days before becoming confused or comatose and requiring admission to hospital. Most are afebrile and have hepatosplenomegaly but no jaundice at presentation. Fever develops later. The CSF is usually normal or contains a few mononuclear cells. Irritability, extreme agitation, aggression, and delirium are succeeded by coma and death in 2 to 3 days. Decorticate and decerebrate posturing and convulsions may be partly attributable to hypoglycaemia, which occurs in the majority of cases. There is rapid neurological deterioration with loss of pupillary and oculovestibular reflexes, evidence of increased intracranial pressure, deepening coma, and death. Neurological sequelae are common in survivors. Blood ammonia is increased above the normal limit of 48 µg/dl in almost all cases. The characteristic histological abnormality is fatty droplets in the liver cells. Mitochondrial abnormalities, but no inflammatory changes, have also been seen in neurones and hepatocytes.

The differential diagnosis includes acute hepatic encephalopathy, especially associated with poisoning, infective encephalopathies such as cerebral malaria (usually distinguishable by positive blood smear) or bacterial, viral, and fungal meningoencephalitides (distinguished by characteristic CSF abnormalities).

There is no specific treatment, but mortality can be reduced by treating hypoglycaemia, cerebral oedema, respiratory failure, fluid and electrolyte disturbances, and other complications. These measures are also considered in Chapter 24.15.1.

Other viral infections or disorders in which viruses may play a role in the pathogenesis of neurological disease

Subacute sclerosing panencephalitis

This disorder (see also Section 7) is a form of subacute encephalitis affecting children and young adults due to persistent infection with the measles virus. The cumbersome title, usually abbreviated to SSPE, is derived from the conditions formerly known as subacute sclerosing leucoencephalitis and inclusion-body encephalitis, now known to be the same disease.

AETIOLOGY

An infective cause was long suspected and there is now conclusive evidence to incriminate the measles virus. Measles virus antibody titres are extremely high in blood and CSF, measles antigen has been demonstrated in the brain, and the virus has sometimes been isolated, but only with difficulty. Most affected children have had measles at an unusually early age and there is a mean interval of some 6 years between infection and the onset of encephalitis. The disease can occur in children vaccinated with live measles virus, but the risk is much lower than that following the natural disease.

The measles virus in subacute sclerosing panencephalitis appears to be incomplete as the matrix (M) protein required to attach the nucleocapsid to the cytoplasmic membrane prior to budding is deficient or absent. It is not known whether the absence of M protein from the brain is the result of an abnormality of the virus or of the host, and, if the latter, whether inborn or acquired. It is thought that during the long symptom-free interval between infection and appearance of disease, viral material accumulates, eventually leading to cell damage. The paradox of high antimeasles antibodies, except against M protein, and persistent virus has not been fully explained. The comparatively early age of clinical measles in affected children, often below the age of 2 years, may indicate that the immature immune system permits entry and persistence of the virus in the brain.

PATHOLOGY

As its name implies both grey and white matter show the changes of encephalitis, with perivascular cuffing and more diffuse cellular infiltration, neuronal loss and myelin destruction, with variable glial scarring or sclerosis. Acidophilic nuclear inclusion bodies are never profuse and may not be detected. No visceral lesions are found.

CLINICAL FEATURES

In the great majority, the onset is in the first two decades but young adults may also be affected. The disease is twice as common in boys as in girls. Incidence has fallen sharply in countries where measles vaccination is at a high level; the annual incidence in England and Wales has fallen from 20 to around 5. Subacute sclerosing panencephalitis remains relatively common in parts of eastern Europe, Egypt, and the Lebanon. No convincing predisposing factors have been identified and, in particular, immunosuppressed children are not at special risk but may occasionally develop acute measles inclusion-body encephalitis.

The speed of onset is extremely variable, but there is usually a prolonged period of altered behaviour, mild intellectual deterioration, and loss of energy and interest, often misinterpreted as sloth or neurosis. After some weeks or months increasing clumsiness or the appearance of focal neurological symptoms draws attention to the organic nature of the disease. Periodic involuntary movements then appear, the commonest form being myoclonus, consisting of a stereotyped jerk or lapse of posture involving the limbs, often asymmetrically, occurring every 3 to 6 s. The myoclonus may result in sudden falls which are occasionally the presenting symptom. Visual signs may be prominent, with papilloedema, retinitis, optic atrophy, or cortical blindness. Choroidoretinal scarring is present in 30 per cent of cases. In other cases the onset is relatively abrupt with no recognizable prodromal stage. There is no fever or other evidence of systemic infection.

Further progression is marked by intellectual deterioration, rigidity and spasticity, and increasing helplessness. Some 40 per cent die within a year but a similar proportion survive for more than 2 years. A period of apparent arrest is common and in some patients, particularly at the upper end of the age range, substantial remission and prolonged survival occur. Even in such cases there may be radiological evidence of continued cerebral damage and it is probable that the disease is always eventually fatal.

INVESTIGATION

There is no significant pleocytosis in the cerebrospinal fluid and total protein is not increased, but there is evidence of intrathecal synthesis of immunoglobulin and oligoclonal bands of IgG. The measles antibody titres in blood and CSF are usually raised to high figures, but occasionally overlap control values. In established disease, the electroencephalogram (EEG) shows highly characteristic periodic discharges, synchronous with the myoclonus, but persisting in the absence of the movements. Computerized tomographic (CT) scan shows low-density white matter lesions and cerebral atrophy.

TREATMENT

There is no effective treatment for subacute sclerosing panencephalitis. The antiviral agent inosiplex, 100 mg/kg daily by mouth in divided doses, possibly prolongs survival, particularly in older patients with disease of slow onset, but adequately controlled trials are naturally difficult to mount. Interferon given by intraventricular catheter has been reported to induce partial remission.

Progressive multifocal leucoencephalopathy

This disease is caused by opportunistic infection by papovaviruses, most commonly JC virus and SV40. A high proportion of normal adults have antibodies to the former and the agent appears to be ubiquitous. The reservoir of SV40 is in monkeys and the agent was apparently transmitted in early types of poliomyelitis vaccine, without evident ill-effects. These viruses are potentially oncogenic but non-pathogenic for humans unless the immune system has been compromised.

Progressive multifocal leucoencephalopathy thus occurs in patients already affected by such conditions as lympho- or myeloproliferative diseases, sarcoidosis, and other chronic granulomatous diseases or, more recently, AIDS, and also in those therapeutically immunosuppressed. Most patients are over 50 years old but, with the spread of AIDS, younger people are being affected, with a male preponderance, and the disease is no longer rare.

PATHOLOGY

The virus particularly invades the nuclei of the oligodendroglia and, as a result, there is demyelination of the white matter of the cerebral hemisphere, spreading from numerous foci. The cerebellum and brain-stem are less often involved and the spinal cord is spared. Abnormal giant forms of oligodendrocytes are seen microscopically with eosinophilic inclusions, and arrays of intranuclear virus particles can often be identified by electron microscopy. JC virus antigen can be identified by immunofluorescence or immunohistochemistry. DNA probing has revealed unintegrated virus in oligodendrocytes, astrocytes, endothelial cells, and in extraneural organs such as kidney, liver, lung, spleen, and lymph nodes.

CLINICAL FEATURES

The onset is usually with progressive signs of a focal lesion of one cerebral hemisphere; limb weakness, aphasia, or visual field defect such as homonymous hemianopia. More widespread signs gradually develop, leading to personality changes, intellectual deterioration, dysarthria or fluent aphasia, and bilateral weakness. Fits are rare. There is no systemic evidence of infection. Spontaneous temporary arrest or partial remission are common but eventual progression causes death in 6 to 12 months, although much more chronic cases are on record, with survival, exceptionally, to 5 years.

INVESTIGATION

The CSF is normal apart from occasionally mild elevation of protein and slight pleocytosis, and is not under increased pressure. The EEG shows a bilateral excess of slow activity. The CT scan may at first show little abnormality, but eventually large, non-enhancing, low-density lesions appear in the cerebral white matter. MRI is more sensitive. Serum antibodies are of no diagnostic help but the response in the CSF has not been fully evaluated. The diagnosis can be confirmed only by cerebral biopsy, but it is essential that white matter is included in the specimen. This may be important to distinguish lymphoma and, rarely, herpes simplex encephalitis involving white matter.

TREATMENT

No treatment is of proven value, but cytosine arabinoside has sometimes appeared to induce partial remission.

Progressive rubella panencephalitis

This extremely rare disorder (see also Section 7) may follow congenital rubella or rubella in early childhood. It evolves insidiously some 10 years after the original illness and is characterized by progressive mental retardation with behaviour changes, fits, ataxia, spasticity, optic atrophy, and macular degeneration. Pathological changes are those of encephalitis with perivascular infiltration. The CSF may show a slight rise in white cell and protein content, elevation of gammaglobulin and of anti-rubella antibodies to an extent greater than the rise in the serum level, suggesting local production of antibody within the CNS. The EEG may show changes similar to those seen in subacute sclerosing panencephalitis due to measles virus. The mechanism responsible for the appearance of this disorder is unknown and there is no effective treatment.

Vogt–Koyanagi–Harada syndrome

The cause of this rare syndrome is thought to be inflammatory autoimmune reaction to an unidentified viral infection. The disorder affects tissues having a common embryological origin, the uvea and leptomeninges and the melanoblasts, ocular pigments and auditory labyrinth pigments originating from the neural crest. The dermatological features consist of patchy whitening of eyelashes, eyebrows, and scalp hair, alopecia, and vitiligo. Neurological manifestations include meningo-

encephalitis, raised intracranial pressure, neurosensory deafness, tinnitus, nystagmus, ataxia, ocular palsies, and focal cerebral deficits. Ocular features are those of uveitis with pain and photophobia, more generalized inflammation of the eye, retinopathy, and impaired visual acuity. The condition tends to be self-limiting but may result in serious permanent ocular and neurological deficits. Steroids and immunosuppressive drugs have been used and are said to arrest the progression of at least some features of the disorder.

Epidemic neuromyasthenia

The existence of this disorder, sometimes known as epidemic or benign myalgic encephalitis ('ME'), is denied by some, but it appears to be an increasing medical problem sometimes following viral infection (see Chapter 7.19.4). Its main features are said to be headache, fever, muscle pains, and psychiatric disturbances such as lassitude, depression, and possibly hysterical reactions. Symptoms of upper respiratory infection and lymphadenopathy may occur. Transient oculomotor palsies, peripheral weakness, altered reflexes, and altered sensation have been recorded in some patients said to be suffering from this disorder. The cerebrospinal fluid is normal. Abnormal lymphocytes have been seen in the peripheral blood films in some patients but no specific infective agent has been isolated, although enteroviruses, notably coxsackie B virus, have been implicated in some people with this condition (see Chapters 7.10.13 and 7.19.4).

Viral causes of psychiatric illness

Mental changes are common in patients with encephalitis. Influenza, infectious mononucleosis, and infectious hepatitis are sometimes followed by psychiatric sequelae, in particular a depressive reaction. Psychosis following encephalitis lethargica was reported on occasions.

Other possible virus infections in which the nervous system is involved

Acute disseminated encephalomyelitis is considered in Chapter 24.9. Reye's syndrome is discussed above and Behçet's syndrome in Chapter 18.11.8. Mollaret's meningitis is discussed in Chapter 24.15.1.

REFERENCES

Aurelius, E., Johannson, B., Skoldberg, B., Staland, A., and Forsgren, M. (1991). Rapid diagnosis of herpes simplex encephalitis by nested polymerase chain reaction assay of cerebrospinal fluid. *Lancet* **337**, 189–92.
Behan, P.O. and Behan, W.M.H. (1988). Postviral fatigue syndrome. *Critical Reviews in Neurobiology* **4**, 157–78.
Boos, J. and Esiri, M.M. (1986). *Viral encephalitis: pathology, diagnosis and management*. Blackwell Scientific Publications, Oxford.
Brown, F. and Wilson, G. (ed.) (1984). *Topley and Wilson's principles of bacteriology, virology and immunity*, (7th edn), Vol. 4. Edward Arnold, London.
Christie, A.B. (1980). *Infectious diseases: epidemiology and clinical practice*, (3rd edn). Churchill Livingstone, Edinburgh.
Corey, L. and Spear, P.G. (1986). Infections with herpes simplex and viruses. *New England Journal of Medicine* **314**, 686–91, 749–57.
Griffiths, J.F. (1985). SSPE and lymphocytes. *New England Journal of Medicine* **313**, 952–3.
Ho, D.D., *et al.* (1985). Isolation of HTLV-III from cerebrospinal fluid and neural tissues of patients with neurological syndromes related to the acquired immunodeficiency syndrome. *New England Journal of Medicine* **313**, 1493–7.
Jackson, A.C. and Johnson, R.T. (1989). Aseptic meningitis and acute viral encephalitis. In *Handbook of clinical neurology*, Vol. 12 (56), *Viral dis-*

eases, (eds. P.J. Vinken, G.W. Bruyn, H.L. Klawans, and R.R. Mc-Kendall), pp. 125–48. Elsevier, Amsterdam.

Johnson, R.T. (1982). *Viral infections of the nervous system.* Raven Press, New York.

Johnson, R.T., *et al.* (1985). Japanese encephalitis: immunocytochemical studies of viral antigen and inflammatory cells in fatal cases. *Annals of Neurology* **18**, 567–73.

Kennedy, P.G.E. (1990). The role of molecular techniques in studying viral pathogenesis in the nervous system. *Trends in Neuroscience* **13**, 424–31.

Kennedy, P.G.E. (1990). The widening spectrum of infectious neurological disease. *Journal of Neurology Neurosurgery and Psychiatry* **53**, 629–32.

Kennedy, P.G.E. and Johnson, R.T. (1987). *Infections of the nervous system.* Butterworths, London.

Krupp, L.B., Lipton, R.B., Swerdlow, M.L., Leeds, N.E., and Llena, J. (1985). Progressively multifocal leukoencephalopathy: clinical and radiological features. *Annals of Neurology* **17**, 344–9.

Mims, C.A. and White, D.O. (1984). *Viral pathogenesis and immunology.* Blackwell Scientific Publications, Oxford.

Pattison, E.M. (1965). Uveomeningoencephalitic syndrome (Vogt–Koyanagi–Harada). *Archives of Neurology* **12**, 197–205.

Price, R.W. and Plum, F. (1978). Poliomyelitis. In *Handbook of clinical neurology*, (eds. P.J. Vinken, G.W. Bruyn, and H.L. Klawans), Vol. 34, pp. 93–132. North Holland, Amsterdam.

Resnick, L., di Marzo-Veronese, F., and Schupbach, J. (1985). Intrablood–brain barrier synthesis of HTLV-III-specific IgG in patients with neurologic symptoms associated with AIDS or AIDS-related complex. *New England Journal of Medicine* **313**, 1498–504.

Scheld, W.M., Whitley, R.J., and Durack, D.T. (ed.) (1991). *Infections of the central nervous system.* Raven Press, New York.

Townsend, J.J., *et al.* (1975). Progressive rubella panencephalitis – late onset after congenital rubella. *New England Journal of Medicine* **292**, 990–3.

Tyler, K.L. and Fields, B.N. (1988). Pathogenesis of viral infections. In *Virology*, (ed. B. Fields *et al.*) (2nd edn), pp.191–239. Raven Press, New York.

Whitley, R.J., *et al.* (1986). Vidarabine versus Acyclovir therapy in herpes simplex encephalitis. *New England Journal of Medicine* **314**, 149.

24.15.3 Neurological manifestations of infection with human immunodeficiency virus type 1

R. K. H. PETTY AND P. G. E. KENNEDY

Neurological features are common during infection with HIV-1 (human immunodeficiency virus type I) (Table 1). This virus is a member of the lentivirus group of retroviruses and is trophic for two cell lineages; the macrophage–monocyte cell line (and their CNS equivalent, the microglial cell) and T-helper lymphocytes; neurological manifestations result from the combined infection of these two cell lineages (see Section 7).

The course of disease can be divided into three periods: primary infection; an asymptomatic period during which certain immunologically mediated disorders may occur; and, finally, a stage at which disorders related to the macrophage infection and the acquired immunosuppression occur. The general clinical features occurring during infection are described in Section 7. The neurological manifestations will be discussed along temporal and pathogenetic lines.

Primary infection illness

An illness probably occurs in the majority of individuals at the time of primary infection. In most cases this is like 'glandular fever' but in a minority, of the order of 10 per cent, neurological symptoms develop.

MENINGITIS

The most frequent manifestation is an aseptic meningitis. The cerebrospinal fluid shows a lymphocyte pleocytosis, and infectious virus can be isolated from the fluid. There are no neurological features of this illness which distinguish it from other viral meningitides, although general features of any accompanying illness resembling 'glandular-fever' may do so (Section 7). A few patients develop an associated cranial mono- or polyneuropathy, most often involving the seventh cranial nerve, and this should clearly raise the suspicion of an HIV-1 seroconversion illness.

ENCEPHALITIS

A smaller number of patients develop encephalitis, again clinically indistinguishable from other viral encephalitides, with a mild cerebrospinal fluid lymphocytosis (20–30 lymphocytes/mm³) and an electroencephalogram (EEG) consistent with an encephalitis. Virus can again be isolated from cerebrospinal fluid in some patients and may allow diagnosis prior to seroconversion, which may be delayed for 6 months or even longer after infection. A full recovery can be expected from both meningitis and encephalitis over about 2 to 3 weeks.

These illnesses are clear indications of early CNS invasion by HIV-1. It is not yet clear, however, whether early invasion occurs in all patients, being symptomatic in only a minority, or whether those with early symptomatic disease differ in some way from the remainder. These early CNS features may predispose to later CNS disease and more rapid disease progression. The role of azidothymidine (AZT), an antiretroviral agent, at this stage is also uncertain; there is no evidence that the use of this agent affects subsequent virus isolation or antibody titres.

RARE MANIFESTATIONS

Rarer manifestations associated with seroconversion have included case reports of isolated cerebral angiitis and acute rhabdomyolysis which were fatal, transverse myelitis and neuralgic amyotrophy in which partial recovery occurred, and a Guillain–Barré-like inflammatory neuropathy associated with full recovery.

Neurological manifestations of asymptomatic infection

Patients then enter what has been termed the asymptomatic phase. It is now clear that at this stage of infection there are ongoing immunological abnormalities, with falling peripheral blood CD4 lymphocyte and high CD8 lymphocyte counts with polyclonal elevations in serum immunoglobulins and defects in T-cell responsiveness (see Section 7). These immunological changes are presumed to be associated with the immunologically mediated disorders which are seen at this stage of disease. These include thrombocytopenic purpura, the presence of a lupus-anticoagulant-like activity, and seronegative arthropathies as well as neurological disorders.

ASEPTIC MENINGITIS

A chronic aseptic meningitis can be demonstrated in up to 40 per cent of patients. There is a mild cerebrospinal fluid pleocytosis, rarely in excess of 100 lymphocytes/mm³, with a slightly raised protein and hypergammaglobulinaemia. The cerebrospinal fluid sugar is normal. Oligoclonal banding can be detected in cerebrospinal fluid and these proteins have anti-HIV-1 specificity. Postmortem studies on patients who have died during this period, largely drug addicts, have shown a lymphocytic meningitis, not associated with detectable HIV-1. The existence of these cerebrospinal fluid changes in a high proportion of otherwise asymptomatic patients must be borne in mind when interpreting the results of cerebrospinal fluid examinations undertaken for whatever reason at all stages of infection.

Table 1 *Neurological manifestations of HIV-1 infection*

At time of seroconversion
  Meningitis
  Encephalitis
  Cranial mono- and polyneuropathy
  Rare:
    Angiitis
    Rhabdomyolysis
    Transverse myelitis
    Neuralgic amyotrophy
    Acute inflammatory polyneuropathy
Asymptomatic period
  Aseptic meningitis
  Polymyositis
  Chronic inflammatory demyelinating polyneuropathy
  Subclinical axonal sensory neuropathy
  Unproven:
    Acute inflammatory polyneuropathy
    Intellectual impairment
Symptomatic HIV-1 infection (AIDS)
  Direct effects of HIV-1
    HIV-1 associated cognitive–motor complex
    Peripheral neuropathy
    Myopathy
    Myelopathy
  Infection
    Toxoplasmosis
    Cryptococcal meningitis
    Mycobacterial disease
    Neurosyphilis
    Progressive multifocal leucoencephalopathy
    Herpesvirus group, especially cytomegalovirus
  Tumours
    Primary cerebral lymphoma
    Secondary Kaposi's sarcoma
    Secondary systemic lymphomas
  Cerebrovascular diseases
    Bacterial endocarditis
    Non-bacterial endocarditis

POLYMYOSITIS

An inflammatory necrotizing myopathy may occur and is clinically indistinguishable from polymyositis. Patients present with a painful proximal myopathy evolving over months, with elevated serum creatine kinase levels, and an electromyogram (EMG) showing myopathic changes. Muscle biopsy, essential for diagnosis, shows muscle fibre necrosis with CD8+ lymphocytic infiltrates, and macrophages which may stain for HIV-1 antigen. Nemaline rods are often prominent, and an inflammatory infiltrate is not universal. These features have raised the question as to whether this disorder should be regarded as polymyositis, or a distinct necrotizing myopathy unique to HIV-1. The pathogenesis is obscure; HIV-1 has not been detected in muscle cells. Treatment with prednisolone in the doses used for polymyositis, may produce a good clinical response and there is no evidence that it causes an increased risk of subsequent opportunistic infections or accelerates the decline in immunological function.

INFLAMMATORY NEUROPATHIES

There is an increased incidence of chronic inflammatory demyelinating polyneuropathies in patients positive for HIV-1, but it is unclear whether this is the case for acute inflammatory demyelinating polyneuropathy (Guillain–Barré syndrome). The clinical presentation of both disorders is identical to that in HIV-1 seronegative subjects. Nerve conduction studies confirm a demyelinating neuropathy, but cerebrospinal fluid examination shows, in addition to a mild elevation of the protein content, a mild pleocytosis, distinct from cases of Guillain–Barré syndrome. This may reflect a differing pathogenesis or a feature of the subclinical chronic lymphocytic meningitis referred to earlier. Nerve biopsy shows demyelination with an inflammatory infiltrate of CD8+ lymphocytes and macrophages. Patients may recover spontaneously but treatment with plasmapheresis or gammaglobulin has been reported to be beneficial.

SUBCLINICAL INTELLECTUAL DECLINE

The occurrence of subclinical intellectual decline remains unproven, and abnormalities that have been described in the asymptomatic phase are subtle. Frank dementia does not appear to occur in the absence of severe systemic immunosuppression. It might be anticipated in view of the clear evidence for early CNS invasion by HIV-1 that some changes may be identifiable. There is emerging neuropathological data (largely from drug-abusing populations) for a chronic lymphocytic meningitis with associated perivascular mononuclear cell infiltrate, sometimes of sufficient intensity to be termed vasculitis, and, in addition, diffuse white matter pallor with astrocytosis and microglial proliferation occurring in neurologically normal patients. HIV-1 could be demonstrated in a minority of these lesions, and it has been suggested that these changes are the basis for the leucodystrophy and vascular mineralization seen later in established HIV-1 encephalitis (see below). In addition, virus can be isolated from cerebrospinal fluid in asymptomatic patients, and this presumably reflects continuing replication in the brain. Cranial CT and MRI data also suggest that early atrophy occurs in a proportion of otherwise neurologically normal patients.

However, there is no correlation between these pathological and radiological findings and the neuropsychological deficits recorded by some workers in the asymptomatic period, and it has proved difficult to demonstrate progression of these changes. Defects have included abnormalities in verbal memory, information processing, and event-related potentials (most often P300). Other workers have found no evidence of early intellectual decline, nor abnormalities in neurological function, when seropositive patients were compared with well-matched controls. These subtle subclinical abnormalities, detected in a proportion of patients, may date from as early as the seroconversion illness. Some longitudinal studies have suggested progression of these changes with time in asymptomatic patients but this is not universally accepted.

SENSORY NEUROPATHY

There is more definite evidence using sensory threshold testing for a subclinical sensory axonal neuropathy developing during the asymptomatic phase, and this has been linked to patients with relatively higher CD4+ and lower CD8+ lymphocyte counts. It is unclear whether this is a forerunner of the axonal sensorimotor neuropathy that occurs in patients with the acquired immunodeficiency syndrome (AIDS) (see below).

It has been suggested that all patients presenting with the disorders mentioned above should now be offered screening for HIV-1 infection. This must remain up to individual practitioners and be based on the patient's age, the local epidemiology of HIV, and the estimated risk, but in reaching these decisions it must be borne in mind that early diagnosis of infection allows prophylactic therapy and azidothymidine to be offered to patients in the anticipation of an improved quality of life, as well as possibly reducing the risk of further spread of infection.

Neurological manifestations of AIDS

Neurological features are very common when peripheral blood CD4+ lymphocyte counts fall to levels around 500/mm^3. It is important to recognize that many of the neurological disorders occur at predictable levels of immunosuppression (as judged by the peripheral blood CD4 cell count); cerebral toxoplasmosis is unusual with CD4 counts in excess of 150 to 200/mm³, for example.

Some 80 to 90 per cent of patients with AIDS will develop neurological symptoms of some form, 50 per cent have neurological disability, and up to 20 per cent present with a neurological AIDS-defining illness. All levels of the neuraxis can be affected; disease mechanisms are diverse but can be divided broadly into opportunistic infections, neoplasms, and diseases thought to be directly related to HIV-1 infection of the CNS. When seeing these patients it is important to recall that in this disease Occam's razor does not apply; multiple diagnoses and pathologies are the rule. Furthermore, immunosuppression may alter the presentation of disease. It is also important to recognize that a division between focal and diffuse cerebral dysfunction, while helpful, does not always hold true in AIDS; toxoplasmosis, for example, may give rise to a diffuse necrotizing encephalopathic syndrome without focal features, and HIV-1 encephalitis may be associated with a picture suggestive of focal neurological disease. Finally, in treating patients it is important to identify local disease patterns; the incidence of both toxoplasmosis and cryptococcal disease vary widely across the United States and Europe, and reported series may not necessarily apply to one's own practice.

DISEASES DUE DIRECTLY TO HIV-1 INFECTION

HIV-1-associated cognitive–motor complex

Intellectual impairment of some degree is frequent in advanced HIV-1 disease. This is related, in many patients, to such factors as intercurrent systemic disease, infections, drug effects, depression, and malnutrition, but there remain some in whom progressive deterioration occurs with associated neurological findings and no identifiable cause can be found. The pattern is often 'subcortical' (see below) and terms such as 'AIDS-related organic brain disease', 'HIV-1-associated dementia', and the 'AIDS dementia complex' have been used to describe this syndrome. It is important to recognize that this is a clinical syndrome, possibly with a variety of pathophysiological mechanisms, associated with a range of pathological features. The term HIV-1-associated cognitive–motor complex (HCMC) will be used here as it makes no assumptions about pathogenesis, and is the currently recommended term for this clinical syndrome. The incidence of HCMC is not certain. Early cross-sectional studies, which suffered from selection bias, suggested figures up to 70 per cent, but more recent data suggest an incidence of 10 per cent or possibly less in patients with AIDS.

Neuropathology and pathogenesis

Nonspecific abnormalities, including atrophy and diffuse gliosis are found in the vast majority who progress to AIDS. A leucoencephalopathy characterized by diffuse pallor with myelin loss and phagocytosis, and a reactive astrocytosis, often most marked in the centrum semiovale, is seen in up to 40 per cent of cases. In some cases these changes are multifocal, suggesting a vasculitic component. Multinucleate giant cells may be seen in association with this process.

HIV-'encephalitis', seen in up to 40 per cent of cases is unique to HIV-1 infection, and is characterized by multinucleate giant cells with multifocal perivascular macrophage infiltration, and microglial nodules made up of large numbers of microglia and macrophages containing HIV-1. These are most commonly seen in white matter, brain-stem, and basal ganglia. In addition, patients have recently been shown to have reduced neuronal cell populations in the frontal cortex, not necessarily in association with either of the changes described above. The overall pattern of neuronal loss within the brain is still being evaluated, but this loss has not been found in asymptomatic seropositive patients.

Finally, it is important, when ascribing causation in HCMC, to recognize that these changes are superimposed on other findings in all autopsies of patients, including cytomegalovirus encephalitis (25–69 per cent), toxoplasmosis (20–60 per cent), tumours including primary cerebral lymphoma and non-Hodgkin's lymphoma (5 per cent or more), and infarcts (up to 20 per cent), one or more of which will complicate the diagnosis in the majority of patients.

It is also recognized that while there is an overall relationship between advanced HCMC and both the HIV-1-specific giant-cell encephalitis and the white matter changes, all three may occur independently, and none of these processes is precisely correlated with the clinical state of the patient; some clearly demented patients have had minimal evidence of CNS involvement at autopsy and some with striking neuropathological abnormalities had not been thought to be demented in life. These disparities have led to speculation about the underlying pathogenetic mechanisms in these disorders. The most widely held hypothesis is that HIV-1 infection of monocytes leads, by their trafficking through the brain, to infection of CNS macrophages and thence microglial cells.

In the early stages of disease, replication rates are slow and there is little or no pathological change in the CNS. As immunosuppression progresses, two processes occur; first, an increased productive infection of CNS microglial cells, and secondly, infective processes within the CNS occurring as a result of immunosuppression and which result in the entry of further infected monocytes and macrophages into the CNS, thereby increasing the virus load. It is suggested that the latter as well as the presence of activated macrophages and microglia lead to the observed clinical features and neuropathology by a variety of mechanisms. These include the action of viral proteins themselves, especially gp120, which has been shown in vitro to be toxic to neuronal cultures, resulting in cell lysis. Viral proteins may also act as false neurotransmitters (gp120 has similarities to vasoactive intestinal polypeptide (VIP)). Lymphokines, such as α-tumour necrosis factor, may cause demyelination, and other products of macrophage activation, such as quinolinic acid, are toxic to CNS myelin, and, again, act as excitotoxins. Viral proteins have been identified, although not consistently, in cerebral vascular endothelial cells, and this infection may disrupt the blood–brain barrier, with resultant neuronal dysfunction. There is evidence that co-infection of the CNS with other agents, such as cytomegalovirus, may enhance HIV-1 replication rates and thus enhance the damage that occurs by the mechanisms mentioned above. Hitherto, there is no convincing in vivo evidence of direct HIV-1 infection of either glial cells or neurones.

Clinical factors

The initial symptoms are non-specific and include slowness of thought, often with a degree of social withdrawal and general loss of interest. This is slowly progressive over months and neuropsychological studies indicate a primarily 'subcortical' pattern of impairment; bradyphrenia, poor concentration, attentional defects, impairment of visuomotor tasks, and memory impairment. Symptoms of focal cortical dysfunction such as agnosias, aphasia, and apraxias are unusual. Later, neurological signs emerge, including abnormal eye movements, spasticity, ataxia, and movement disorders. Terminally ill patients are mute, vegetative, paraparetic, and incontinent. The illness usually progresses to severe dementia in a few months. There are no studies clearly linking the dementia to any of the minor abnormalities of intellectual functioning which may occur during the asymptomatic phase of infection discussed earlier. There are no diagnostic tests, since imaging, cerebrospinal fluid examination, and EEGs show only non-specific changes, and the diagnosis is one of exclusion of drug toxicities, deficiency states, poisoning, infections, tumours, and depressive illness. The HCMC occurs in the context of severe immunosuppression and the diagnosis should be made with great caution earlier in the course of disease, when alternative explanations should be sought.

There are no proven therapies for the HCMC in adults, with only temporary and modest improvement in neuropsychological parameters following treatment with azidothymidine or other antiretroviral agents. This may reflect a general improvement in well-being rather than a direct effect on the primary disease process. A single retrospective study from

The Netherlands has suggested a decreased incidence in the HCMC following the introduction of azidothymidine, and some longitudinal studies support its use in HCMC. In addition, azidothymidine penetration into brain and cerebrospinal fluid is poor and the optimal dosages required are not yet clear, and may be higher than those currently used in the treatment of AIDS. In paediatric cases there is more evidence for a clinically useful response: the reason for this difference is not clear.

HIV-1-related myelopathies

There are three distinct myelopathies described in HIV-1 disease. First, a vacuolar myelopathy in which the neuropathological features are similar to those of subacute combined degeneration of the cord with posterior and lateral column white matter vacuolation. The clinical features include a subacute, progressive, spastic, ataxic paraparesis, often with an apparent truncal sensory level, and the diagnosis depends on the exclusion of compressive lesions or a chronic meningitic process. An abnormal cerebrospinal fluid methylation ratio, as seen in vitamin B_{12} deficiency, has been described, but there is no evidence of vitamin B_{12} deficiency and the cause remains obscure. The changes are not associated with the HIV-1 encephalitis or leucoencephalopathy and this appears to be a distinct disorder. It is of interest that similar change has been described rarely in patients not infected with HIV-1 who have been become immunosuppressed through other mechanisms.

Secondly, degeneration restricted to the gracile tracts with a consequent deafferenting gait ataxia may follow dorsal root ganglion necrosis, which has been linked in some patients with cytomegalovirus infection.

Finally, the HIV-1-specific multinucleate giant-cell changes characteristically seen in the brain may extend into the spinal cord; this occurs much more often in children than in adults. The clinical features are again non-specific and the diagnosis is one of exclusion.

HIV-1-related peripheral nerve disease

The third major disease process linked directly to HIV-1 is a diffuse axonal sensorimotor neuropathy. This may develop in the asymptomatic phase, but with the advent of severe immunosuppression a clinical neuropathy becomes much more common, affecting 50 per cent or more patients on clinical grounds and up to 90 per cent on neurophysiological grounds. The cause of this neuropathy is unclear; pathological studies show a distal axonopathy with proximal macrophage infiltration of the peripheral nerve. At this stage of disease patients have often lost considerable weight, are on multiple drug therapy, and may be infected with a number of organisms, all of which may be pathogenetic factors. The symptoms are of slowly progressive distal dysaesthesias with sensory loss followed by weakness and areflexia. The sensory symptoms may lead to disability, although it is unusual for patients to become unable to walk because of weakness alone. Autonomic symptoms may occur, presumably reflecting small-fibre involvement, evidence for which can be detected in up to 50 per cent of patients. Treatment is difficult, and involves the management of the potentially reversible causes mentioned earlier. There are anecdotal reports of symptomatic improvement with the introduction of antiretroviral agents such as azidothymidine, but often treatment is directed toward providing symptomatic relief with drugs such as carbamazepine or phenytoin, or with other techniques such as transcutaneous nerve stimulation.

HIV-1 myopathy

Diffuse muscle wasting is an almost universal finding in advanced AIDS. In many patients this reflects cachexia associated with neoplasia and multiple infections, but there is evidence for a discrete HIV-1-related myopathy. This may be distinct from AZT myopathy referred to below, and the inflammatory myopathy that occurs during the asymptomatic period. Patients present with proximal myalgia, weakness and elevated serum creatine kinase levels. The EMG may show myopathic changes, and biopsy reveals myofibre degeneration, cytoplasmic bodies, nemaline rods, and myofibrillar loss. The aetiology of this myopathy and its precise relationship to the other myopathies described in HIV-1

infection remains uncertain. At a practical level, a myopathy should be suspected in any patient with muscle weakness, or in whom a diagnosis of 'slim disease' or 'HIV wasting syndrome' is made. If the patient is receiving AZT, the drug should be withdrawn, and, if there is evidence of inflammatory change on biopsy, a trial of steroids should be considered.

Infectious diseases in AIDS

TOXOPLASMOSIS

Toxoplasmosis due to reactivation of latent infection is the most common opportunistic CNS infection in patients with AIDS in the United Kingdom occurring in some 10 to 15 per cent, and occurring in higher numbers in France and the southern United States. It usually develops when the CD4+ cell count falls to 150/mm^3 or less. The presentation is usually a slowly evolving mass lesion with appropriate neurological signs, most frequently hemipareses and ataxia with accompanying fever, headache, and seizures. Fulminant cases may present with a diffuse encephalopathy without focal signs. The diagnosis depends on a combination of the clinical picture with neuroimaging to demonstrate single or multiple ring enhancing lesions by CT scanning, ideally using a double dose of contrast agent, or by MRI scanning where available. The latter technique demonstrates multiple lesions in a higher proportion of patients. Management is difficult. In patients with a compatible story and multiple lesions it is usual to treat for toxoplasmosis and await a clinical response, which should be apparent within the first week, in the hope of avoiding a brain biopsy. If there is severe brain swelling, dexamethasone, 12 to 16 mg/day in divided doses, may be given but may lead to improvement in patients with abscesses due to other organisms. In those with an atypical story or a single lesion on CT, some clinicians still treat expectantly for toxoplasmosis and only perform biopsies in those patients who do not respond, while others advocate primary biopsy. In this situation, postmortem and brain biopsy studies indicate high error rates; progressive multifocal leucoencephalopathy and lymphoma are the most frequently misdiagnosed conditions. There are no proven alternative methods of confirming a diagnosis of toxoplasmosis; serology in blood and cerebrospinal fluid is not helpful, with a high incidence of both false positives and negatives, while the use of the polymerase chain reaction (PCR) (see Section 5) to identify toxoplasmosis DNA in blood or cerebrospinal fluid is of unproven value. Furthermore, because of brain swelling a lumbar puncture is contraindicated in many patients.

First-line therapy is with a combination of pyrimethamine (50–100 mg/day) and sulphadiazine (4 g/day), with folinic acid (20 mg/day). With this regime a response rate of over 80 per cent can be expected. Subsequent lifelong prophylaxis with pyrimethamine (25 mg/day) and sulphadiazine (2 g/day) is mandatory because microscopic evidence of continuing encephalitis can be seen in all treated patients, and without secondary prophylaxis, relapse is common. Adverse reactions are frequent, however. Alternative therapies include clindamycin (2–4 g/day) with pyrimethamine, and other novel macrolides such as clarithromycin, azithromycin, or atovaquone. In some areas, toxoplasmosis is now so common that primary prophylaxis is being evaluated (along the same lines as for *Pneumocystis carinii* pneumonia) for patients who are seropositive for toxoplasmosis at an early stage of disease. Clindamycin alone appears to be too toxic, and pyrimethamine with or without dapsone is under evaluation. There is some preliminary evidence that toxoplasmosis prophylaxis may be a useful 'side-effect' of the use of co-trimoxazole as *Pneumocystis carinii* pneumonia prophylaxis.

CRYPTOCOCCAL MENINGITIS

Cryptococcus neoformans may produce either a chronic meningitic illness or, less commonly, hydrocephalus or a cryptococcoma. Prevalence varies worldwide and in the United Kingdom some 5 to 10 per cent of patients will develop cryptococcal meningitis. Clinical features may be typical of a chronic meningitis, with fever, headache, and a stiff neck, but patients may present with malaise alone, cranial neuropathies, or seizures. Hydrocephalus may lead to drowsiness. Diagnosis is by cerebrospinal fluid examination, after CT scanning to exclude hydrocephalus. This may be acellular and the protein and sugar content may also be entirely normal. The diagnosis relies on demonstration of organisms in the cerebrospinal fluid or detection of cryptococcal antigen in blood and/or cerebrospinal fluid. The polymerase chain reaction is being evaluated as a method of early and rapid diagnosis. Treatment is difficult, with no agents of proven value and 75 per cent three-month survival rates from diagnosis. Standard therapy in patients without AIDS is a combination of amphotericin B (0.25–1.5 mg/kg/day) with flucytosine (100–200 mg/kg/day). However, both are toxic and fluconazole (200 mg/day) has been advocated as an alternative. Overall, only 40 to 50 per cent of patients show a clinical response, and alternative regimes such as itraconazole have not been shown to be superior. High relapse rates in those who do respond mean that long-term treatment is necessary; and here fluconazole (200 mg/day orally) has been shown to be superior to weekly intravenous amphotericin B (1 mg/kg/week).

OTHER BACTERIAL INFECTIONS

Other bacterial infections of the CNS are less common. Mycobacterial disease due to either tubercle bacilus or atypical mycobacteria (especially *Mycobacterium avium intracellulare*) is a major problem in central Africa, where 60 per cent of the population has been exposed to tubercle bacillus. The disease is similar to that in the non-immunosuppressed populations but with a higher incidence of extrapulmonary tuberculosis and a more rapid course. The diagnosis of tuberculous meningitis may be difficult because few organisms are present, (the cerebrospinal fluid is normal in 10 per cent of patients) and treatment is along conventional lines. Relapse, off treatment, is common. Overall, mortality is of the order of 20 per cent, being higher in those with a blood level of CD4 lymphocytes less than 200 mm³. These infections may be a greater problem in the future; there has been a 16 per cent increase in cases of tuberculosis in the United States since 1985, with associated rises in drug resistance. Atypical mycobacterial infections affect over 50 per cent of patients dying of HIV-1. Meningitis or intracranial involvement may occur but is usually overshadowed by the systemic features. Diagnosis is by biopsy or culture, and treatment options are very limited (see Section 7).

SYPHILIS

The incidence of neurosyphilis is increasing in the United States, where it is found in about 1.5 per cent of patients. Progression to tertiary symptoms may be unusually rapid, and occasionally treponemal serology may revert to negative with advancing immunosuppression. Clinical features alone, such as dementia, or a meningitic illness, do not allow a clear distinction from other disorders, and so it is essential to maintain a high index of suspicion of this treatable illness. The diagnosis relies on the demonstration of positive specific treponemal serology in the cerebrospinal fluid. It is important to recall that the polyclonal stimulation of B cells in HIV-1 infection leads to a high rate of false positive reagin tests for syphilis (such as the VDRL test). Penicillin remains the first-line therapy, and a more aggressive regime than in the HIV-1-negative population is advocated: penicillin G, 2.0 to 4.0 megaunits, 4 hourly for 10 to 14 days.

PROGRESSIVE MULTIFOCAL LEUCOENCEPHALOPATHY

Progressive multifocal leucoencephalopathy is a rapidly progressive demyelinating disorder related to infection of oligodendrocytes by a papovavirus (JC virus) and occurs in 2 to 5 per cent of patients with AIDS, being the AIDS-defining illness in some 50 per cent of these patients. This agent is ubiquitous, with the majority of the population showing evidence of infection by adult life. The site of latency is unknown, but immunosuppression is associated with a productive infection, possibly in B cells. Oligodendrocyte infection then occurs, although it is unclear how the agent gains access to the CNS. Virus particles can be recognized in oligodendrocyte nuclei, and infection leads to cellular lysis, demyelination, and reactive astrocytosis. The clinical features reflect this process with hemi- and parapareses, ataxia, hemianopias, and, thereafter, dementia. Diagnosis is only possible with brain biopsy, although cranial MRI scanning may back a clinical suspicion, showing widespread areas of abnormal T_2 signal in white matter. The polymerase chain reaction has demonstrated the virus in brain, but less frequently in the cerebrospinal fluid. Progressive multifocal leucoencephalopathy usually develops along with severe immunosuppression but there cases have been reported when patients had in excess of 500 CD4 cells/mm³. In these latter patients it is now recognized that, in contrast to the disease in patients not infected with HIV-1, arrest or regression of the process may occur, with survival for over 1 year. This more benign course is associated with a prominent perivascular inflammatory reaction. There is no proven treatment, with anecdotal reports only of a symptomatic response to azidothymidine and cytarabine, given either intravenously or intrathecally. The overall prognosis is poor, with a 15 per cent one-year survival. There are reports of a remitting and relapsing disease with symptoms similar to those of multiple sclerosis in which MRI and cerebrospinal fluid examination also show indistinguishable features. It is not yet clear whether this represents progressive multifocal leucoencephalopathy, the simple coincidence of two common diseases, a new disease, or is another manifestation of the altered immune state in HIV-1 infection resulting in a higher incidence of true multiple sclerosis.

OTHER VIRAL INFECTIONS

Other intercurrent viral infections include those of the herpesvirus group. Varicella-zoster virus may produce shingles, which is often disseminated or multidermatomal. Treatment with acyclovir is advised in order to avoid further dissemination of infection. Herpes viruses 1 and 2 may give rise to meningitis or encephalitis but these are uncommon in patients infected with HIV-1.

Cytomegalovirus is an important pathogen in AIDS. Disseminated reactivation with virus detectable in blood, urine, and cerebrospinal fluid is usual with advanced disease, and this can lead to multiorgan pathology. Most frequently infected are the lung and retina. Mono- or binocular visual loss occurs subacutely. Any part of the retina may be involved but at the time of presentation the posterior pole is usually involved. Examination reveals a granular, white, swollen, haemorrhagic retinitis, leaving an avascular necrotic retina, with later optic atrophy. In contrast to Toxoplasma and Candida retinitis, there is little vitritis or uveitis. Untreated, this leads rapidly to permanent loss of vision. Treatment with ganciclovir (5 mg/kg twice a day, for 21 days) results in an arrest of the retinopathy in over 80 per cent of cases. Ganciclovir is toxic (especially in combination with azidothymidine), and foscarnet (≤ 200 mg/kg/day, depending on renal function, for 21 days) may offer an alternative, although the evidence for efficacy is not as compelling as with ganciclovir and there is a slower response time and more frequent relapses. Maintenance therapy is essential in order to avoid relapse of the ocular disease.

Cytomegalovirus is also implicated in the pathogenesis of a rapidly progressive necrotizing lumbosacral radiculopathy which usually occurs in the context of advanced HIV-1 immunosuppression. Patients frequently have evidence of active cytomegalovirus infection in other organ systems and present with the evolution over days of a cauda equina syndrome; back pain, ascending hypo- and dysaesthesias, weakness, and urinary retention. The upper limbs are usually spared but there are reports of involvement of the arms in untreated cases. The cerebrospinal fluid shows a polymorphonuclear pleocytosis, often up to 1000/mm^3. The protein is raised and the cerebrospinal fluid sugar may be lowered. Cytomegalovirus can be cultured from the cerebrospinal fluid. EMG studies show acute denervation, and at post-mortem examination cytomegalovirus has been demonstrated in ventral and dorsal roots. Spinal cord involvement may occur and may result in a spinal sensory level. Aggressive and early treatment with ganciclovir is essential for recovery of function.

The role of cytomegalovirus in other neuropathies associated with HIV-1 infection is less certain; cases of mononeuritis multiplex, a rare manifestation of HIV-1 infection, have been recognized, with endoneurial necrosis and demonstration of cytomegalovirus inclusions in peripheral nerves, and with symptomatic responses to ganciclovir. It is important to recognize that some of these cases present as a confluent mononeuritis multiplex, mimicking a peripheral neuropathy. Other workers have reported a diffuse burning/dysaesthetic peripheral neuropathy evolving over months in association with active cytomegalovirus infection elsewhere, and have suggested that this was related to cytomegalovirus infection of the dorsal root ganglion.

Epstein–Barr virus has been implicated in the aetiology of AIDS-related primary cerebral lymphoma; tumour cells have been shown to express viral RNAs associated with Epstein–Barr virus-induced lymphocyte transformation, as well as a latent Epstein–Barr virus membrane protein also implicated in lymphomagenesis. There is also evidence for an increased rate of development of Burkitt's lymphoma among children infected with HIV-1 in central Africa.

CNS TUMOURS IN AIDS

Primary CNS lymphoma, which must be distinguished from systemic immunoblastic lymphoma and Burkitt's lymphoma, occurs with severe immunodeficiency and, with improving general care, is now seen in 2 per cent of cases in the United States, where it is predicted to become more common than gliomas in the general population. In addition, systemic lymphoma or, less often, Kaposi's sarcoma may metastasize to the CNS. Diagnostic accuracy is improving; many earlier cases were diagnosed only at postmortem examination. Patients present with non-specific features, including headache, intellectual blunting, or seizures, and less commonly with focal neurological signs. CT and MRI scans show abnormalities in the majority of these patients but may be normal, with a diffuse infiltrating tumour, and are non-specific even when abnormal. Biopsy is usually undertaken to exclude treatable intercurrent infection. The prognosis is very poor, with most patients dying within 2 months from diagnosis, either from other illnesses or from the direct effects of the tumour. There are reports of response to a combination of radiotherapy and aggressive chemotherapy, but the overall state of the patient must be taken into account in making therapeutic decisions at this stage of the disease.

CEREBROVASCULAR DISEASES

The incidence of cerebrovascular complications during HIV-1 infection is unclear. Pathological studies report that up to 20 per cent of patients have infarctions or haematomas; clinical studies suggest a lower frequency. These differences may reflect selection bias and variations in pathological technique. The most common condition is embolization from infective endocarditis in intravenous drug users and marantic endocarditis in others, bleeding into tumours, and haemorrhage in haemophiliac patients. There remains, however, a group of patients with otherwise unexplained ischaemic infarction, and it has been suggested that these events may reflect coagulation abnormalities that may occur with HIV-1 infection (see Section 22), including thrombotic thrombocytopenic purpura or the presence of the lupus anticoagulant. Rarer causes include the cerebral angiitis which may follow trigeminal zoster, and the endarteritic complications of syphilis and the chronic meningitides.

DRUG-RELATED NEUROLOGICAL TOXICITY IN AIDS

Drugs used specifically in HIV disease may also lead to neurological problems. Azidothymidine may cause a myopathy characterized by muscle pain, proximal weakness and wasting, with elevations of the serum creatine kinase level. Biopsies have shown a range of abnormalities, including myofilament loss, microvacuolation, and mitochondrial accumulations in the peripheries of fibres. The last changes may be related to the inhibition of the mitochondrial γ-DNA polymerase, which will thus lead to impairment of mitochondrial protein synthesis, defective mitochondrial function, and mitochondrial proliferation in an attempt to restore cellular energy metabolism. This myopathy appears to be related to the total dose of azidothymidine used, and is often associated with haematological toxicity. These complications respond to withdrawal of the drug, although this may take up to 1 or 2 months. Some patients show a response to steroids, and some authors doubt the existence of a distinct azidothymidine myopathy, but the morphological changes described above and the response to drug withdrawal would appear to define a syndrome.

Novel antiretroviral drugs, including dideoxyinosine (ddI) and dideoxycytosine (ddC), are being used (increasingly) and both may produce a reversible, painful distal axonal sensory neuropathy, which is dose related; it is common with doses of ddC over 0.18 mg/kg/day, and ddI over 12.5 mg/kg/day.

Other drugs used in HIV-1-related diseases may be toxic; for example, the motor neuropathy associated with dapsone, and seizures associated with ciprofloxacin and foscarnet.

PAEDIATRIC MANIFESTATIONS OF INFECTION WITH HIV-1

Globally, an estimated 500 000 children are thought to be infected with HIV-1. Most are exposed to the virus *in utero* and about 40 per cent of at-risk fetuses become infected. Serological diagnosis is not possible in early infancy because of the presence of maternal antibody which may persist for up to 10 months, and in rare cases as long as 18 months. Alternative diagnostic techniques are under evaluation, including the polymerase chain reaction. The neurological patterns of disease differ from those of the adult in that opportunistic infections such as toxoplasmosis, cryptococcal meningitis, and progressive multifocal leucoencephalopathy are rare, but there is a higher risk of bacterial infection, and neurodevelopmental abnormalities occur in up to 90 per cent of children infected *in utero*. These take the form of developmental delay, loss of milestones, microcephaly, and pyramidal signs and seizures. Imaging studies show atrophy often associated with a calcifying leucoencephalopathy and basal ganglia calcification. This encephalopathy appears to respond to azidothymidine, with recovery of motor milestones, but, as in adults, the disease is eventually relentlessly progressive. There are pathological differences, with vascular and perivascular mineralization, intimal proliferation, and with microglial nodules and multinucleate giant cells occurring in 75 per cent or more of brains. A vacuolar myelopathy is rare but extension of the encephalitis into the spinal cord is more common than in adults. A final distinction is that peripheral neuropathies are very much less common, at least on clinical grounds, in the paediatric population than in adults.

The pattern of disease seen in haemophiliacs, many of whom are currently in the paediatric population, appears to depend on the age of infection; those infected after the age of 5 to 10 years have an adult pattern of disease.

REFERENCES

Berenguer, J., *et al.* (1992). Tuberculous meningitis in patients infected with the human immunodeficiency virus. *New England Journal of Medicine* **326**, 668–72.

Connolly, S., *et al.* (1994). Long latency event-related potentials in asymptomatic Human Immunodeficiency Virus type 1 infection, *Annals of Neurology*, **35**, 189–96.

Cornblath, D.R., Griffin, J.W., McArthur, J.C., Kennedy, P.G.E., Witte, A.S., and Griffin J.W. (1987). Inflammatory demyelinating neuropathies associated with human T-cell lymphotrophic virus type III infection. *Annals of Neurology* **21**, 32–40.

de la Monte, S., *et al.* (1988). Peripheral neuropathy in the acquired immunodeficiency syndrome. *Annals of Neurology* **23**, 485–92.

Epstein, L.G. and Gendelman, H.E. (1993). Human immunodeficiency virus type 1 infection of the nervous system: pathogenetic mechanisms, *Annals of Neurology*, **33**, 429–36.

Everall, I., *et al.* (1993). A review of neuronal damage in human immunodeficiency virus infection: its assessment, possible mechanism and relationship to dementia. *Journal of Neuropathology and Experimental Neurology*, **52**, 561–6.

Fuller, G.N., *et al.* (1993). Nature and incidence of peripheral nerve syndromes in HIV infection. *Journal of Neurology, Neurosurgery and Psychiatry*, **56**, 372–81.

Gillespie, S.M., *et al.* (1991). Progressive multifocal leucoencephalopathy in persons infected with human immunodeficiency virus, San Francisco, 1981–1989. *Annals of Neurology* **30**, 597–604.

Glass, J.D., *et al.* (1993). Clinical-neuropathologic correlation in HIV-associated dementia. *Neurology,* **43**, 2230-7.

Gray, F., *et al.* (1992). Early brain changes in HIV infection: Neuropathological study of 11 HIV seropositive, non-AIDS cases. *Journal of Neuropathology and Experimental Neurology* **51**, 177–85.

Gray, F., *et al.* (1993). Early central nervous system changes in human immunodeficiency virus (HIV)-infection, *Neuropathology and Applied Neurobiology*, **19**, 3–9.

Lange, D.J. (1994). Neuromuscular diseases associated with HIV-1 infection. *Muscle and Nerve*, **17**, 16–30.

McAllister, R.H., *et al.* (1992). Neurological and neuropsychological performance in HIV seropositive men without symptoms. *Journal of Neurology Neurosurgery and Psychiatry* **55**, 143–8.

McArthur, J.C., *et al.* (1993). Dementia in AIDS patients: incidence and risk factors, *Neurology,* **43**, 2245–52.

Navia, B.A., *et al.* (1986). Cerebral toxoplasmosis complicating the acquired immunodeficiency syndrome: clinical and neuropathological findings in 27 patients. *Annals of Neurology* **19**, 224–38.

Petito, C.K., *et al.* (1985). Vacuolar myelopathy pathologically resembling subacute combined degeneration in patients with the acquired immunodeficiency syndrome. *New England Journal of Medicine* #312, 874–9.

Rudge, P. (ed.) (1992). *Neurological aspects of human retroviruses.* Baillière, London.

Saag, M.S., *et al.* (1992). Comparison of amphotericin B with fluconazole in the treatment of acute AIDS-associated cryptococcal meningitis. *New England Journal of Medicine* **326**, 83–9.

Sidtis, J.J., *et al.* (1993). Zidovudine treatment of the AIDS dementia complex: results of a placebo-controlled trial. *Annals of Neurology*, **33**, 343–9.

Vago, L., *et al.* (1993). Reduced frequency of HIV induced brain lesions in AIDS patients treated with Zidovudine. *Journal of AIDS*, **6**, 42–5.

24.15.4 Intracranial abscess

P. J. TEDDY

Intracranial abscesses may occur within the extradural or subdural space or may be intracerebral. Occasionally abscesses exist in more than one tissue plane. Intracerebral abscesses and subdural abscesses may rupture into the subarachnoid space and be accompanied by meningitis, and intracerebral pus may rupture into the ventricular system and produce ventriculitis.

Incidence

A neurosurgical unit in the United Kingdom serving a population of about 3 million would expect to treat about 12 cases of cerebral abscess a year and about five cases of subdural empyema unrelated to trauma or previous surgery. Extradural abscesses are rather less common.

Aetiology

Extradural abscesses are usually related to focal osteomyelitis of the skull, mastoiditis and nasal sinusitis, penetrating injuries of the skull, and are a rare complication of craniotomy. They are occasionally found in combination with subdural empyema and as a complication of infected dermal sinuses of the scalp.

Subdural empyema is related most commonly to infection of the paranasal sinuses and middle ear. Other causes include septicaemia related to cyanotic congenital heart disease, lung abscess, trauma and intracranial surgery.

The most common intracranial abscess is found within the intracerebral compartment, with about 60 per cent related to middle-ear infection and 20 per cent to frontal sinusitis. Other established causes are septicaemia related to congenital heart disease with a right-to-left shunt, lung abscess, bronchiectasis, penetrating injuries of the head, and bacteraemia following tooth extraction. In about 10 per cent of cases no primary source of infection can be identified. Owing to their strong connection with sinus and middle-ear disease, most intracerebral abscesses are found within the frontal or temporal lobes, or within the cerebellum. Infection disseminated through the bloodstream from more distant sites may result in multiple abscesses in any part of the brain. Cerebellar abscess is almost exclusively related to middle-ear infection but about 60 per cent of abscesses associated with middle-ear disease are found within the temporal lobe. Frontal sinusitis is most commonly related to frontal-lobe abscess or subdural empyema. In infants, subdural empyema most often occurs as a secondary infection following bacterial meningitis.

Indirect spread of infection from distant sites is probably venous, either by embolic spread through venous pathways or by extension of venous thrombosis with pyogenic infections.

Microbiology

Some 15 years ago up to 30 per cent of cultures of pus from intracranial abscesses might have been expected to show no growth. This percentage has dropped considerably owing to better methods of culture and identification of obligate anaerobic micro-organisms. The demonstration of such anaerobes in intracranial abscesses and the institution of appropriate therapy has probably been a major factor in the decline in mortality from cerebral abscess during this period.

The most common organisms associated with subdural empyema are aerobic, anaerobic, and microaerophilic streptococci, *Staphylococcus aureus*, and *Bacteroides* species. In infants with subdural empyema secondary to bacterial meningitis the principal organisms are *Haemophilus influenzae, Neisseria meningitidis*, and *Streptococcus pneumoniae*. Even in these cases anaerobic organisms may yet be shown to be present in apparently sterile cultures.

Cerebral abscesses associated with otitis media, mastoiditis, and nasal sinusitis usually show a mixed growth of anaerobes and aerobic organisms including anaerobic and microaerophilic streptococci and bacteroides. *Streptococcus viridans* and *Staph. aureus* are frequently seen. Infections from distant sources also show mixed growths and usually include anaerobic and microaerophilic streptococci, Staphylococci, Klebsiella, and sometimes actinomycosis and pseudomonads. *Listeria* species tend to produce areas of focal cerebritis rather than true abscess.

Pathology

Infection within an accessory air sinus or the petrous bone may cause an area of localized osteitis just above the dura, which can then spread intracranially. Initially it may be entirely confined to the extradural space, but will eventually penetrate the dura and spread subdurally or, if the adjacent arachnoid is stuck to the inflamed patch of dura, then it will spread into the subarachnoid space to give meningitis. If the subarachnoid space has been obliterated, it may penetrate the brain to produce initially a focal cerebritis. Usually after about 10 days the area of cerebritis becomes enclosed within an area of gliotic brain, and after about 3 weeks a firm capsule forms around the pus. Large intracerebral abscesses may rupture into the ventricular system, thus producing a ventriculitis. Thick-walled abscesses are most commonly associated with penetrating injuries of the skull and with middle-ear or mastoid disease, whereas infection from the frontal sinuses, and those associated with congenital heart disease and haematogenous spread from distant foci, are more often thin-walled.

Cerebral abscesses are usually surrounded by areas of oedematous brain, which may exert a considerable mass effect. An extradural empyema is seldom large, but subdural abscesses may be extremely extensive, with the pus flowing over the convexity of the brain to reach the space between the falx cerebri and the medial surface of the hemisphere. This feature is important in terms of treatment. Cerebral abscesses may be either single or multiple, and the single abscess is often multilocular.

Clinical features

The clinical features of intracranial abscess will depend upon the site, size, and number of lesions, and involvement of neighbouring structures such as the cerebral ventricles and the venous sinuses. The signs are therefore legion, but the diagnosis should be considered in any case where there is an obvious primary source of infection associated with evidence of either raised intracranial pressure, focal neurological signs, epileptic seizures, or meningeal irritation, or any combination of these.

Extradural abscess may be difficult to detect clinically, but is sometimes manifest by severe unremitting localized headache in association with sinusitis or mastoiditis. Patients with subdural empyema frequently appear toxic with a swinging pyrexia, severe headache, a depressed level of consciousness, contralateral hemiparesis, papilloedema, meningeal irritation, and seizures. There is usually an accompanying frontal sinusitis with tenderness of the forehead and redness and swelling of the eyelids, or mastoiditis or scalp infection. Of patients with intracerebral abscess about 70 per cent will present with headache, 60 per cent with impaired consciousness, 40 per cent with a hemiparesis, and 30 per cent with seizures. The focal neurological signs will depend upon the site of the abscess, with temporal-lobe lesions producing an early superior homonymous quadrantanopia together with dysphasia if the dominant temporal lobe is involved. There may also be a brachiofacial weakness. Cerebellar abscesses are accompanied by ipsilateral limb ataxia and hypotonia, and by nystagmus. Blood-borne abscesses often seed to the parietal region and produce little in the way of early focal neurological signs.

As with any mass lesion the most pressing symptoms and signs associated with intracranial abscesses are those of raised intracranial pressure, namely, headache, vomiting, and impaired conscious level, often, but not invariably, accompanied by papilloedema.

Diagnosis

Despite advances in antimicrobial therapy and radiological investigations, intracranial abscess remains a disease with a high mortality and morbidity. Outcome is closely related to the conscious level prior to operative treatment, and one major factor contributing to morbidity is late diagnosis. The development of massive cerebral oedema with brain-stem compression, secondary ventriculitis or meningitis, and missed multiple lesions also contribute to a high morbidity.

If a brain abscess is suspected, predisposing sources of infection, including possible distant sites, should be carefully sought, as intracranial abscesses derived by haematogenous spread are often more fulminating in their course than those associated with local cranial disease. If CT is available, scans of the skull base, including views of the mastoids and other skull sinuses, should be performed. Otherwise, skull radiography with sinus views are necessary. Chest radiographs should be performed.

The investigations of choice for all forms of suspected intracranial abscess are either computed tomography (CT) scanning, with and without contrast, or magnetic resonance imaging (MRI).

CT will normally demonstrate both extradural and subdural empyema, may demonstrate diffuse cerebritis in early cases, and will normally show intracerebral abscesses as ring-enhancing lesions with low attenuation centres (see Figs 1 and 2). Nevertheless, there are pitfalls, particularly in the early stages both of subdural empyema and of cerebral abscess. Subdural empyema may initially be fairly thinly spread over the cerebral cortex, producing relatively little midline shift, and may be virtually isodense with brain on CT. Under such circumstances, contrast

Fig. 1 Contrast scan showing massive right-sided multilocular subdural empyema secondary to a pansinusitis (arrow A). Note cerebral oedema (B) and displacement of ventricular system (C). The child made a complete recovery after evacuation of the pus and antimicrobial therapy.

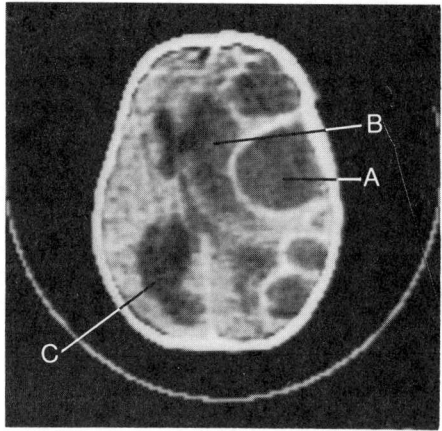

Fig. 2 Contrast CT scan showing large right frontal cerebral abscess (A) with surrounding oedema (B) and ventricular compression (C).

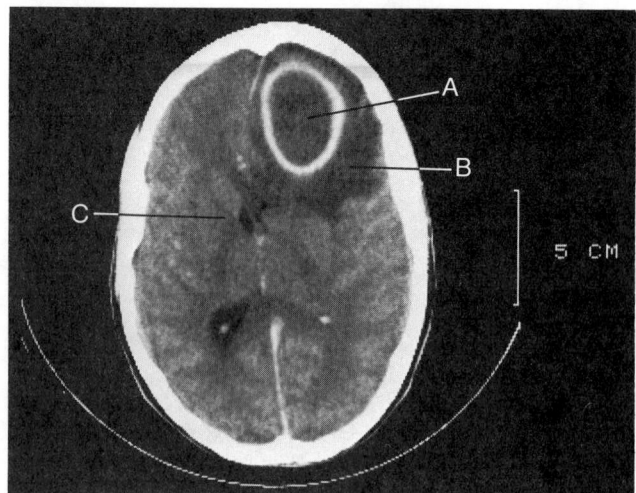

enhanced MRI (particularly with coronal views) is of great value. If MRI is not available, then sinus radiographs may be of particular importance. If the patient is not too ill, the CT scan could be repeated after a few days, but if the scan appearances are doubtful and MRI not available, cerebral angiography may demonstrate displacement of peripheral vessels.

In acute cases, if there is a high index of suspicion of subdural empyema and the patient is too ill to be transferred to distant centres for MRI, then exploratory burr-holes should be performed even in the presence of an apparently normal CT scan.

Patients suspected on CT scan as having an area of cerebritis adjacent to sinus or middle-ear disease, should have a scan repeated after a few days. Both plain skull radiography and CT scan may demonstrate free gas when gas-forming organisms are present.

The principal differential diagnoses in an intracranial abscess are meningitis, subdural haematoma, and intracranial tumour. It is not always possible to differentiate between intracerebral abscess and tumour on CT scan, particularly when there is an appearance of ring enhancement, and it is largely for this reason that the biopsy of suspected cerebral tumour is advocated in nearly all such cases. MRI scan, however, tends to show a low signal capsule on T_2-weighted images and may be helpful in making this differentiation.

One obvious concern is to differentiate between bacterial meningitis and intracerebral abscess. Both may present with pyrexia, neck stiffness, and with some focal signs, but if there is any evidence whatever of raised intracranial pressure, or any other supportive evidence of cerebral abscess, a lumbar puncture should be strictly avoided until a neurosurgical opinion has been sought. Lumbar puncture in the presence of cerebral abscess can lead to tonsillar or tentorial herniation, and in any event, the cerebrospinal fluid can be entirely normal.

Management

Management of intracranial abscess is essentially treatment of the abscess itself and treatment of the underlying cause. Except in a few cases of multiple or inaccessible abscess, and the occasional patient whose general medical condition is such that surgery is precluded, treatment of the intracranial infection requires evacuation of pus and high-dose intravenous antibiotic therapy.

Although there is evidence that serial CT scanning and more effective antimicrobial therapy has reduced the mortality and morbidity of intracranial abscesses over the past decade, the single main factor in securing a good outcome is early diagnosis. Early management includes taking specimens for blood culture and culture of any extracranial infective lesion, setting up an intravenous infusion, administration of anticonvulsant agents and, in cases of grossly depressed level of consciousness and massive cerebral oedema seen on CT scan, giving intravenous dexamethasone.

Pus from the suspected primary site of infection should be collected immediately and both aerobic and anaerobic cultures obtained. The intracranial pus must be similarly cultured. Antimicrobial treatment, using massive intravenous doses, should be commenced immediately without waiting for the culture report, and subsequently changed in the light of the sensitivity findings. The antimicrobial regime should include penicillin (4 megaunits four-hourly), metronidazole, ampicillin, and either gentamicin or chloramphenicol depending on the likely source of infection and the infective agent. Intravenous antimicrobials should be continued for at least 1 week before reverting to oral medication.

Most supratentorial abscesses can be sterilized by aspiration through a burr-hole, and the direct instillation of antibiotics is sometimes employed. Aspiration must usually be repeated several times, but in about 30 per cent of cases a single aspiration will suffice. Once the abscess is sterile, the capsule will shrink and finally form an irregular gliotic scar within the brain. Shrinkage of the abscess must be checked by serial CT scan. Subdural empyema should be evacuated through a

craniotomy rather than burr-holes, as very often the pus can spread widely, and particularly alongside the falx cerebri. Extradural empyema is evacuated through a burr-hole or through a craniotomy for larger collections.

Cerebellar abscess, when diagnosed early, may be aspirated through a burr-hole, but immediate total excision is often recommended because the small volume of the posterior cranial fossa leaves little latitude in terms of tonsillar herniation and death. Some superficial supratentorial abscesses with thickened capsules may be excised rather than aspirated, and in a few cases in which there is extensive brain swelling and continuing tentorial herniation, excision through a craniotomy might similarly be advised. In cases of otitis media and frontal sinusitis, mastoidectomy or drainage of the frontal sinus should be performed in conjunction with a neurosurgical procedure. Where there is osteitis the infected skull bone should also be removed.

Prognosis

Until fairly recently the mortality figure for intracranial abscess stood between 30 and 50 per cent. The use of serial CT scanning to localize the lesion and to show that surgical treatment has been successful, improved microbiological investigation, and antimicrobial therapy have all combined to reduce the mortality rate to around 10 per cent, but the main problems remain those of late diagnosis and resistant bacteria. Even with an otherwise good outcome, epilepsy may continue in about 30 per cent of cases, particularly in patients with temporal-lobe abscess and subdural empyema.

REFERENCES

Alderson, D., Strong, A.J., Ingham, H.R., and Selkon, J.B. (1981). Fifteen year review of the mortality of brain abscess. *Neurosurgery* **8**, 1–6.

Bannister, G., Williams, B., and Smith S. (1981). Treatment of subdural empyema. *Journal of Neurosurgery* **55**, 82–8.

De Louvois, J., Gortvai, P., and Hurley, R. (1977). Bacteriology of abscesses of the central nervous system: a multicentre prospective study. *British Medical Journal* **ii**, 981.

Garfield, J. (1978). Brain abscesses and focal suppurative infections. In *Infections of the nervous system.* Part 1. *Handbook of clinical neurology*, Vol. 33, (ed. P.J. Vinken and G.W. Bruyn), pp. 107–47. North Holland, Amsterdam.

Jefferson, A.A. and Keogh, A.J. (1977). Intracranial abscesses: A review of treated patients over 20 years. *Quarterly Journal of Medicine* **46**, 389.

Stapleton, S.R., Bell, B.A., and Uttley, D. (1993). Stereotactic aspiration of brain abscesses: is this the treatment of choice? *Acta Neurochirurgica– Wien*, **121** (1–2), 15–19.

Youmans, J.R. (ed.) (1982). *Neurological surgery*, (2nd edn), (6 vols). W.B. Saunders, Philadelphia.

24.15.5. Neurosyphilis

R. J. GREENWOOD

INTRODUCTION

In the United Kingdom, only 89 new cases of neurosyphilis were reported during 1982. Neurosyphilis is thus now a rare disease in the United Kingdom, seen at most only once or twice a year by practising neurologists. These figures are not reflected by experience in the United States where, in 1985, it was calculated that the incidence of neurosyphilis in California was twice that of amyotrophic lateral sclerosis, and about half that for multiple sclerosis. This difference is also seen in the number of new cases of early and late syphilis: in England and Wales 3564 cases were reported in 1982, a figure that had changed little in the previous 25 years, falling to between 1538 and 1305 from 1987 to 1990; whereas in the United States the number of new cases has increased six- or sevenfold since its nadir in the late 1950s, about 50 000 cases being reported in 1990.

Despite the current rarity of neurosyphilis, early recognition remains of paramount importance, since treatment with penicillin before the onset of irreversible neurological damage so effectively produces a cure. An expectation that patients will present with textbook features of neurosyphilis is thus both seldom rewarded and clinically irrelevant; diagnosis should be established before the classic features of tabes dorsalis, general paresis, or meningovascular syphilis are apparent. That this occurs was demonstrated by a prospective study which showed that, of 251 new cases of neurosyphilis presenting between 1965 and 1970, 43 per cent were discovered incidentally, 24 per cent presented with fits, 11 per cent with strokes, 8 per cent with 'dizziness', and 2 per cent with personality change. All these symptoms were well recognized before the antibiotic era, and the concept that 'modified' or 'atypical' neurosyphilis is produced by incidental exposure to antibiotics seems to this author to be misleading. Concurrent human immunodeficiency virus (HIV) infection produces an increased frequency of accelerated or resistant disease, particularly in immunocompromised subjects, with more frequent ocular changes.

Clinical features and natural history (see also Section 7)

CNS invasion by *Treponema pallidum* occurs within the first few weeks or months of primary infection. During this period the majority of patients are neurologically normal. In many patients with untreated primary or secondary syphilis, 41 per cent in one recent study, there are minor cerebrospinal fluid abnormalities comprising a slight elevation of cells or protein or positive serology, usually specific rather than nontreponemal. This is asymptomatic neurosyphilis.

If untreated, by the end of the secondary stage of syphilis these cerebrospinal abnormalities have resolved in the majority of patients. One to two per cent of patients develop an acute meningitis, while only 5 to 10 per cent go on to develop tertiary (meningovascular) or late (general paresis or tabes dorsalis) neurosyphilis: in one study only 6.5 per cent of patients with untreated syphilis developed symptomatic neurosyphilis (Fig. 1).

The disease, whether acquired congenitally or later in life, can be regarded as a meningovasculitis, which may occasionally be acute but is usually more or less chronic. Thus, in some patients there is early emphasis on the leptomeningitis and arteritis of meningovascular neurosyphilis. In others the meningitic element is less obvious and parenchymal degeneration predominates. The factors contributing to this great variation in clinical expression are not understood.

MENINGEAL AND VASCULAR NEUROSYPHILIS

Within the first 10 to 12 years of infection a sequence of histopathological change can be seen. Various combinations of a subacute or chronic diffuse leptomengitis, subpial parenchymal degeneration in the brainstem and cord, and inflammation of the media and adventitia of large and medium-sized vessel walls with intimal fibroblastic proliferation (Heubner's endarteritis obliterans) develop and may lead to vascular occlusion with infarction. Thus serological tests are essential in young patients presenting with meningitis, stroke, isolated cranial nerve palsies, papilloedema of uncertain cause, acute vertigo or recent sensorineural deafness. The onset of symptoms may be gradual rather than abrupt, sometimes preceded by several weeks of headache or personality change.

Acute syphilitic meningitis usually occurs within 2 years of infection. Patients are usually afebrile, and meningeal irritation may be obvious clinically or evident only upon lumbar puncture. There may be a considerable cerebrospinal fluid lymphocytosis, although in the acute stage polymorphs may predominate and occasionally a low cerebrospinal fluid sugar is found. Other features of secondary syphilis should be sought, especially the rash and hepatomegaly or evidence of disordered liver function. Characteristically, cranial nerve palsies occur, especially of nerves III, VI, VII, and VIII, sometimes bilaterally; optic disc swelling or fits may be seen. Less commonly, arteritic infarction in the brain or spinal cord occurs, or the basal or vertex elements of the meningitis cause hydrocephalus. Treatment is usually successful, provided it is begun early.

Chronic meningovascular neurosyphilitic syndromes result from pathological emphasis upon leptomeningeal fibrosis. Thus chronic basal meningitis may result in hydrocephalus and involvement of a variety of cranial nerves, including the optic nerves and chiasm. Hypothalamic disturbances may occur. Leptomeningitis may cause headache, drowsiness, and focal cortical symptoms, including fits. At spinal cord level the chronic leptomeningitis is usually accompanied by a subpial demyelination (the syphilitic halo). Syphilitic meningomyelitis is accompanied by symptoms of patchy root irritation and appropriate radicular wasting and weakness, for example, sciatica and foot drop. If presentation is mainly that of a very slowly progressive paraparesis with little sensory loss, then the spastic paraparesis of Erb results. Localization of the leptomeningitis to the cervical region produces an amyotrophic meningomyelitis in which there is obvious wasting, usually asymmetrical, of arm muscles and neck extensors, often with few sensory symptoms and little pain. Initial presentation with wrist drop may occur. Combined leptomeningeal and dural thickening (hypertrophic pachymeningitis) occurs particularly in the cervical region. Dorsal roots are involved and sensory symptoms and pain in the arms are prominent. These cord syndromes may be confused with motor neurone disease but generally do not produce the widespread fasciculation and wasting usually seen in that condition.

Large and medium-sized arteritic occlusions may occur independently or may accompany leptomeningeal disease. Any vessel may be involved, especially the middle and posterior cerebral arteries, producing results similar to those seen after arteriosclerotic occlusion, although often in younger patients. Angiography reveals multifocal narrowing of

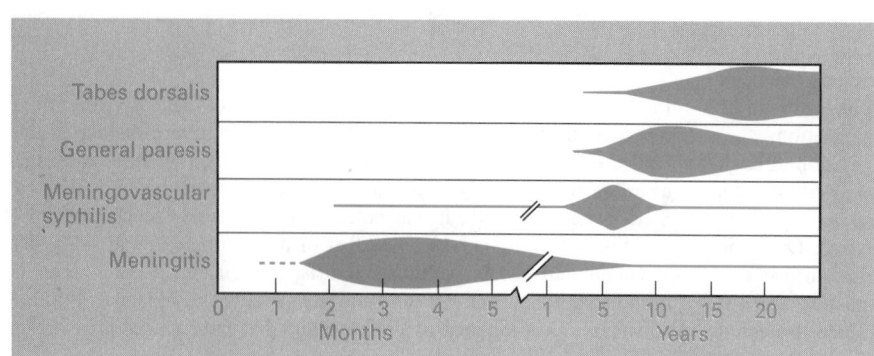

Fig. 1 Approximate interval between primary infection and symptomatic neurosyphilis by type (after Hook and Marra 1992).

the intradural vessels resembling that seen in other forms of cerebral vasculitis.

Isolated gummas are very uncommon, although they still occur. They consist of focal granulomatous meningeal thickening, including the dura, and produce symptoms by space occupation. Surgical excision in addition to penicillin may be required.

GENERAL PARALYSIS OF THE INSANE

General paralysis of the insane is a subacute, progressive meningo-encephalitis which occurs 5 to 20 years after infection. Macroscopically there is a granular ventricular ependymitis and atrophy, especially of the frontal and temporal lobes, over which the meninges are thickened and in which numerous spirochaetes are usually seen. Their persistence for many years after infection and their anatomical localization remain unexplained. Microscopic changes are similar to those seen in other forms of subacute encephalitis, such as sleeping sickness. Presenting symptoms are often vague, as in any dementing illness, consisting of ill-defined personality changes with irritability and forgetfulness, headaches, weight loss, and poor concentration and work record. Behaviour gradually deteriorates as memory, insight, and judgement are progressively impaired. Dress, personal appearance, and social behaviour become inappropriate. Alcohol excess, vagrancy, sexual aberration, and various psychotic delusions may occur, although a simple dementia is most often seen. Classic grandiose delusions are uncommon. Fits, sometimes with transient focal neurological deficits, may accompany deterioration, or occasionally herald it. Motor signs gradually appear until the 'insane' patient becomes 'generally paralysed', mute, and incontinent. Death usually occurs from intercurrent infection.

Physical signs usually appear after at least some degree of mental deterioration. Commonly seen signs are relaxed and expressionless faces; tremor of the face, tongue, and lips, and often of the whole body; a slurred and tremulous dysarthria; pupillary abnormalities, often of Argyll Robertson type; and, with time, an increasingly severe quadriparesis. Tabes dorsalis may coexist (taboparesis).

TABES DORSALIS

Presentation of tabes dorsalis 10 to 25 years after infection is usual, although the interval may be much longer. Histology reveals atrophy of the central processes of the dorsal root ganglion cells mainly in lumbar and lower thoracic, rather than cervical, roots. Dorsal column degeneration is probably a secondary phenomenon. There may be mild, diffuse leptomeningeal thickening and also cranial nerve degeneration. The pathogenesis of tabes still remains uncertain.

Presentation with the triad of lightning pains, ataxia in the lower limbs, and sphincter dysfunction due to bladder hypotonia is common. These symptoms are often accompanied by pupillary abnormalities, of Argyll Robertson type, loss of knee and ankle jerks and of vibration, position, and deep pain sensation in the legs; the last is often tested by squeezing the Achilles tendon (Abadie's sign). Similar symptoms and signs in the arms are much less common. The gait is broad-based, slapping, and worsened by eye closure (rombergism). Lightning pains strike at right angles to the limb like a needle stab. Other dysaesthesiae, sometimes radicular in distribution, occur in the limbs and trunk, and although superficial sensation is relatively preserved, areas of reduced sensibility to pinprick over the shins, sternum, inner sides of the forearms, and butterfly area of the face (Hitzig zones) are well recognized. Crises of pain and dysfunction in various viscera may occur; gastric crises, the commonest, may cause epigastric or shoulder-tip pain with or without vomiting, or vomiting without pain. Fluid levels may be seen on plain abdominal radiography. Charcot joints, usually in the legs or lumbar spine, perforating foot ulcers, muscular hypotonia, ptosis, optic atrophy, colonic distension as well as a large bladder and impairment of genital sensation, or coexisting general paralysis of the insane (taboparesis) may also be present.

NEURO-OPHTHALMOLOGICAL FEATURES

Argyll Robertson described the pupillary changes occurring in neurosyphilis in 1869. They may be seen in any form of the disease but most commonly occur in tabes and often provide confirmation of the diagnosis. When fully developed, the pupils are completely unreactive to light but constrict briskly to accommodation–convergence (light–near dissociation). They are small and irregular and there is often a poor response to sympathetic stimulation or mydriatics. Purely unilateral changes are very rare, in contrast to tonic pupils. The poor pupillary dilatation, iris atrophy, and pupillary irregularity are probably the result of local ocular disease, the miosis and light–near dissociation the result of subependymal gliosis in the periaqueductal midbrain tegmentum. This lesion may also be the cause of the bilateral ptosis that contributes to the 'tabetic facies'. Other pathology in this area may result in light–near dissociation and occasionally miosis as well as ptosis, but not in the local ocular elements. It is frequently forgotten that partial unresponsiveness to light, or mid-position or even large pupils rather than miosis, may be seen, as may tonic pupils.

Optic nerve involvement may result from inflammation and arteritis of the optic nerve itself in meningovascular disease, either secondary or tertiary, and may subacutely produce a central scotoma with significant visual loss (optic neuritis). A papillary vasculitis with disc swelling but without much visual loss (optic perineuritis) may also occur in secondary syphilis. Early treatment of these two disorders, especially the latter, is usually effective. By contrast, tabetic optic atrophy, which may occur alone or herald accompanying tabes, usually evolves slowly, starting unilaterally before involving both eyes. Histologically there is degeneration of the intracranial optic nerves and chiasm and infiltration of the surrounding pia-arachnoid. A variety of field defects may be found, but a constriction of peripheral fields with a central or paracentral scotoma is usual. Treatment is often relatively ineffective.

Laboratory diagnosis

Serological tests for syphilis divide into those that detect antibodies against lipoidal antigens secondary to treponemal–host interaction (reagins) and those detecting antigens derived from *Treponema pallidum*.

BLOOD SEROLOGY

The Venereal Disease Research Laboratory test (VDRL) is the most often used reaginic test and relies on flocculation of a suspension of cardiolipin, lecithin, and cholesterol antigen by the patient's serum. It is quantifiable, titres greater than 1 in 8 being good evidence of active infection. Lower titres, which may occur in active disease, are also seen as biological false-positive reactions in collagen disease, febrile illnesses, following immunization, or in leprosy, old age, pregnancy, or drug addiction. In up to 40 per cent of active cases of neurosyphilis, usually in late disease, the serum VDRL is negative, as it may be in patients with the acquired immunodeficiency syndrome (AIDS).

The specific antitreponemal tests, of which the TPHA (*Treponema pallidum* haemagglutination test) and FTA-ABS (fluorescent treponemal antibody in serum from which treponemal group antibodies have been previously adsorbed using non-pathogenic treponemes) are the most commonly used, are positive in nearly all cases with active disease, whether early or late. These are non-quantified tests but are both more sensitive and specific than reaginic tests; positive reactions are also found in yaws and usually persist after adequate treatment of syphilis, when the VDRL titre falls and becomes negative; biological false-positive reactions are uncommon but have been recorded in association with abnormal serum globulins. Negative specific blood serology virtually excludes active disease except possibly in patients with HIV; only very rarely in active disease is cerebrospinal fluid serology positive with specific blood serology negative.

If specific blood serology is positive, cerebrospinal fluid examination may be used to identify symptomatic non-luetic neurological disease, and irrelevant 'burnt out' or treated neurosyphilis. Estimation of specific IgM antibodies in serum and cerebrospinal fluid to confirm active disease, either acquired or congenital, may be useful but is not widely available.

CEREBROSPINAL FLUID

Cerebrospinal fluid specific serology is virtually always positive in active disease, and frequently remains so after adequate treatment or in burnt-out tabes, whereas the VDRL often becomes negative. A positive specific serological test is thus not a good indication of active disease, whereas a positive cerebrospinal fluid VDRL is more likely to indicate active neurosyphilis, especially in titres over 1 in 8. False-positive cerebrospinal fluid FTA-ABS tests occasionally occur, but the cerebrospinal fluid TPHA and VDRL are specific for neurosyphilis.

Further information is obtained from the cerebrospinal fluid cell count and protein concentration. Active neurosyphilis of any kind usually produces an increase in cells of up to about 200/mm mononuclear cells, mainly lymphocytes with some reactive and plasma cells, and a rise in cerebrospinal fluid protein concentration to about 2 g/l. Both these parameters are usually normal if the disease is inactive and are the most sensitive indicators of the effects of treatment. Neurosyphilis also causes a rise in cerebrospinal fluid IgG, and electrophoresis of cerebrospinal fluid often shows an elevation of cathodal IgG, which may be diffuse or banded. These changes may persist despite treatment and do not necessarily indicate active disease.

Treatment

Treatment in the early stages of any form of neurosyphilis often fully reverses the disease. If treatment is delayed, progressive changes may be only partially reversible. Patients with signs of neurosyphilis but with an unreactive cerebrospinal fluid, as is seen in late tabes, will not improve with treatment and may deteriorate. In recent years there have been very occasional reports of neurosyphilis developing after penicillin treatment, usually given as benzathine penicillin for early syphilis, and particularly in patients also infected with HIV.

Argument remains about exact regimes that should be adopted to treat all cases of neurosyphilis. Active neurosyphilis demands treatment that is effective beyond doubt and repeat cerebrospinal fluid examination to ascertain cure. Spirochaetocidal cerebrospinal fluid penicillin levels are produced by aqueous penicillin G (12–24 mIU intravenously daily for 10–15 days). Procaine penicillin (2.4 mIU intramuscularly daily) with oral probenecid (2 g daily), or 3 g twice daily of oral amoxycillin with probenecid, for 14 days may also be used.

Benzathine penicillin should be avoided unless compliance is problematic. Patients allergic to penicillin should be given oral tetracycline in a dose of 500 mg 6 hourly for three 15-day courses at monthly intervals. Corticosteroid cover (for example, prednisolone, 40 mg daily) for the first 3 days of treatment, penicillin starting after 24 h of steroids, should be given to prevent a Herxheimer reaction. This consists of malaise, fever, headache, and arthralgia, and sometimes worsening of local disease, which is usually temporary; it is most likely to occur in general paralysis of the insane. A longer course of steroids in optic atrophy may be helpful.

The cerebrospinal fluid cell count should return to normal within 3 months, the protein within 6 months. This response should be checked, particularly after treatment that does not include penicillin, by repeat lumbar puncture at 6 weeks and 3 months after completion of therapy, and thereafter at 6-monthly intervals until cells and protein have been normal on two consecutive occasions. The VDRL titre usually decreases and may become normal and IgG and electrophoresis may revert, but specific serology frequently remains positive.

Symptomatic treatment may be required for confusion, ataxia, Charcot joints, or urinary retention. Lightning pains may be treated with carbamazepine or phenytoin, gastric crises with subcutaneous adrenaline solution BP (0.5 ml of 1:1000). Sexual partners should be checked, especially those with whom the patient associated at the probable period of early infection.

REFERENCES

BMJ, editorial (1978). Modified neurosyphilis. *British Medical Journal* **2,** 647–8.

Clark, E.G. and Danbolt, N. (1955). The Oslo study of the natural history of untreated syphilis. *Journal of Chronic Disease* **2,** 311–44.

Currie, J.N., Coppeto, J.R., and Lessel, S. (1988). Chronic syphilitic meningitis resulting in superior orbital fissure syndrome and posterior fossa gumma. *Journal of Clinical Neuro-ophthalmology* **8,** 145–55.

Dewhurst, K. (1969). The neurosyphilitic psychoses today. A survey of 91 cases. *British Journal of Psychiatry* **115,** 31–8.

Department of Health (1979–1991). *On the state of the public health.* The annual report of the Chief Medical Officer of the Department of Health. Her Majesty's Stationery Office, London.

Feraru, E.R., Aronow, H.A., and Lipton, R.B. (1990). Neurosyphilis in AIDS' patients: initial CSF VDRL may be negative. *Neurology* **40,** 531–3.

Fletcher, W.A. and Sharpe, J.A. (1986). Tonic pupils in neurosyphilis. *Neurology* **36,** 188–92.

Harner, R.E., Lawton-Smith, J., and Israel, C.W. (1968), The FTA-ABS test in late syphilis. *Journal of the American Medical Association* **203,** 545–8.

Heathfield, K.W.G. and Aldren Turner, J.W. (1951). Syphilitic wrist-drop. *Lancet* **2,** 566–9.

Holmes, M.D., Brant-Zawadski, M.M., and Simon, R.P. (1984). Clinical features of meningovascular syphilis. *Neurology* **34,** 553–6.

Hook, E.W. III and Marra, C.M. (1992). Acquired syphilis in adults. *New England Journal of Medicine* **326,** 1060–9.

Hooshmand, H., Escobar, M.R., and Kopf, S.W. (1972). Neurosyphilis. A study of 241 patients. *Journal of the American Medical Association* **219,** 726–9.

Joffe, R., Black, M.M., and Floyd, M. (1968). Changing picture of neurosyphilis: report of seven unusual cases. *British Medical Journal* **1,** 211–12.

Johns, D.R., Tierney, M., and Feisensten, D. (1987). Alteration in the natural history of neurosyphilis by concurrent infection with the human immunodeficiency virus. *New England Journal of Medicine* **316,** 1569–72.

Jordan, K.G. (1988). Modern neurosyphilis – a critical analysis. *Western Journal of Medicine* **149,** 47–57.

Katz, D.A., Berger, J.R., Duncan, R.C. (1993). Neurosyphilis: a comparative study of the effects of infection with human immunodeficiency virus. *Archives of Neurology*, **50,** 243–9.

King, A., Nicol, C., and Rodin, P. (1980). *Venereal diseases*, (4th edn). Baillière Tindall, London.

Loewenfeld, I.E. (1969). The Argyll Robertson pupil, 1869–1969. A critical survey of the literature. *Survey of Ophthalmology* **14,** 199–299.

Lukehart, S.A., Hook, E.W., Baker-Zander, S.A., Collier, A.L., Critchlow, C.W., and Handsfield, H.H. (1988). Invasion of the central nervous system by *Treponema pallidum*: implications for diagnosis and treatment. *Annals of Internal Medicine* **109,** 855–62.

Luxon, L., Lees, A., and Greenwood, R.J. (1979). Neurosyphilis today. *Lancet* **1,** 90–3.

Martin, J.P. (1925). Amyotrophic meningomyelitis (spinal progressive muscular atrophy of syphilitic origin). *Brain* **48,** 153–82.

Merritt, H.H., Adams, R.D., and Solomon, H.C. (1946). *Neurosyphilis.* Oxford University Press, New York.

Moore, J.E. and Hopkins, H.H. (1930). Asymptomatic neurosyphilis. VI. The prognosis of early and late asymptomatic neurosyphilis. *Journal of the American Medical Association* **95,** 1637–41.

Musher, D.M., Hamill, R.J., and Baughn, R.E. (1990). Effects of human immunodeficiency virus (HIV) infection on the course of syphilis and the response to treatment. *Annals of Internal Medicine* **113,** 872–81.

Poole, C.J.M. (1984). Argyll Robertson pupils due to neurosarcoidosis: evidence for site of lesion. *British Medical Journal* **289,** 356.

Schoth, P.E.M. and Waters, E. Ch. (1987). Penicillin concentrations in serum and CSF during high-dose intravenous treatment for neurosyphilis. *Neurology* **37,** 1214–16.

Simon, R.P. (1985). Neurosyphilis. *Archives of Neurology* **42**, 606–13.

Spillane, J.D. (1975). *An atlas of clinical neurology* (2nd edn). Oxford University Press.

Tramont, E.C. (1987). Syphilis in the AIDS era. *New England Journal of Medicine* **316**, 1600–1.

Vatz, K.A., *et al.* (1974). Neurosyphilis and diffuse cerebral angiopathy: a case report. *Neurology* **24**, 472–6.

Wang, A.M., Barriger, T.K., and Wesolowski, D.P. (1991). Intracranial gamma mimicking a tuber cinereum tumour. *Computerised Medical Imaging and Graphics* **15**, 57–60.

Wilner, E. and Brody, J.A. (1968). Prognosis of general paresis after treatment. *Lancet* **2**, 1370–1.

24.16 The motor neurone diseases

M. DONAGHY

INTRODUCTION

The motor neurone diseases result from selective loss of function of the lower and/or upper motor neurones controlling the voluntary muscles of the limbs or bulbar region. The term 'motor neurone disease' is best used to describe a family of diseases within which there is an extensive differential diagnosis; in the past the term has been used synonymously with amyotrophic lateral sclerosis, the most serious of these diseases. Precise diagnosis is essential for advising patients about prognosis, for identifying those diseases with genetic implications, and to offer immunosuppressant therapy to some patients with some acquired lower motor neurone syndromes.

In practice, differential diagnosis requires clinical and electrophysiological classification as to whether the disease involves the upper or the lower motor neurones, or both. This anatomical differentiation is augmented by the age of onset, the rate of deterioration, and familial occurrence (Table 1). Sensation and cognition are normal on simple clinical assessment in the motor neurone diseases.

The clinical signs of lower motor neurone involvement consist of muscle wasting, fasciculations, and flaccid weakness. The tendon reflexes are often retained until profound denervation or fibrous replacement have affected the muscle. Fasciculations are visible flickerings within the muscle belly, which are insufficient to produce joint movement; electromyography shows that they correspond to simultaneous discharge of all the muscle fibres within a diseased motor unit. Nerve conduction studies will exclude peripheral neuropathy (Chapter 24.17). Electromyography helps to distinguish denervation from myopathy (Chapter 24.2.5). Muscle biopsy is often required to exclude myopathy, particularly in syndromes causing slowly progressive proximal weakness.

Upper motor neurone involvement produces spasticity, clonus, extensor plantar responses, and weakness. The abdominal reflexes are often preserved in motor neurone diseases involving the upper motor neurone. This contrasts with their loss in spinal cord disease due to tumours, compression, or demyelinating disease. Sphincter control and sexual function are usually preserved in motor neurone disease, although trunk and abdominal wall weakness may make excretion slow and awkward.

Motor neurone diseases are incurable for the most part, and therefore treatment must aim to overcome, or minimize, the various sources of disability. Malnutrition due to dysphagia can be circumvented by nasogastric tube feeding or gastrostomy. Various forms of assisted respiration offset respiratory muscle weakness, including continuous positive airways pressure via a facial mask. Limb spasticity can be reduced by baclofen, dantroline, or diazepam. Wheelchairs and arm appliances may overcome inadequate limb function. Electronic communication devices should be supplied to those whose speech is incomprehensible. Amitriptyline may help contain the embarrassing emotional lability of pseudobulbar palsy. Housing and workplace modifications can allow patients to maintain independence despite their disability.

Table 1 *Classification of the motor neurone diseases*

Combined upper and lower motor neurone syndromes
  Amyotrophic lateral sclerosis
    sporadic (A,E)
    familial adult onset (*D) (A)
    familial juvenile onset (*R) (C)
Lower motor neurone syndromes
  Proximal hereditary motor neuronopathy:
    acute infantile form (Werdnig–Hoffmann) (*R) (I)
    chronic childhood form (Kugelberg–Welander) (*R) (I, C)
    adult onset (*R) (A)
    adult onset (*D) (C,A)
  Hereditary bulbar palsy
    with deafness (Brown–Violetto–van Laere) (*) (C,A)
    without deafness (Fazio–Londe) (*R) (C)
  X-linked bulbospinal neuronopathy (*) (A,E)
  Hexosaminidase deficiency (*R) (C,A)
  Multifocal motor neuropathies (A,E)
  Postpolio syndrome (E)
  Postirradiation syndrome (A,E)
  Monomelic, focal, or segmental spinal muscular atrophy (A)
Upper motor neurone syndromes
  Primary lateral sclerosis (A,E)
  Hereditary spastic paraplegia (*D) (A,E)
  Lathyrism (A)

*, inherited disorder: D, dominant; R, recessive.

Age of onset: I, infantile; C, childhood; A, adult (15–50 years); E, elderly (more than 50 years).

COMBINED UPPER AND LOWER MOTOR NEURONE SYNDROMES

Amyotrophic lateral sclerosis

Amyotrophic lateral sclerosis occurs worldwide, usually with an incidence of 1 to 1.5 per 100 000 population and a prevalence of 4 to 6 per 100 000. It is commoner in men and the incidence increases with advancing age; it is unusual before the fifth decade of life. The cause of the common sporadic form of amyotrophic lateral sclerosis is quite unknown. Its incidence is particularly high in areas of the western pacific, particularly in Guam and the Japanese Kii Peninsula, where it tends to occur in younger adults and can be associated with dementia or parkinsonism. Autosomal dominant inheritance is evident in approximately 5 per cent of patients with adult-onset amyotrophic lateral sclerosis and is associated with superoxide dismutase gene mutations in some. It tends to begin earlier in adulthood and may involve minor sensory symptoms. A rare juvenile-onset autosomal recessive form of amyotrophic lateral sclerosis with prominent bulbar involvement has been described from North Africa.

Pathology

Lower motor neurones are lost from clinically affected areas of the spinal cord and brain-stem. Surviving neurones may show intracytoplasmic inclusions (Bumina bodies) and proximal axonal accumulations of neurofilaments (spheroids). The motor cortex is depleted of Betz cells and the pyramidal tracts degenerate. It is increasingly recognized that other populations of neurones can also degenerate in motor neurone disease, even though this is not usually evident clinically. These include peripheral sensory neurones and Clarke's column neurones, and up to 10 per cent of patients may eventually develop a mild dementia, often of frontal lobe type. These recent findings show that amyotrophic lateral sclerosis is either a generalized neurodegenerative disorder, in which the motor neurones take the vast brunt of the disease, or that it overlaps sometimes with other neurodegenerations. However, for the practical purpose of clinical diagnosis early in the disease, amyotrophic lateral sclerosis should be regarded as having purely motor manifestations.

Clinical features

At presentation, patients either have bulbar or spinal symptoms, although both usually become evident as the disease progresses.

The bulbar form causes dysphagia, dysphonia, and inhalation of foodstuffs due to weakness of the tongue, pharynx, and larynx. The tongue is wasted, weak, and fasciculating, palatal movements are reduced, and the ability to cough explosively is lost due to vocal cord paralysis. This bulbar palsy is usually accompanied, or even preceded, by varying degrees of pseudobulbar involvement. The tongue is spastic and immobile with 'hot potato' speech and difficulty in containing emotional responses such as laughing or crying. Ventilatory respiratory failure may develop due to weakness of diaphragm and intercostal muscles. Occasionally, amyotrophic lateral sclerosis can present with dyspnoea. Diaphragm weakness can be detected clinically by noting that the upper abdomen is drawn inwards, rather than outwards, during the second half of inspiration. Furthermore, the forced vital capacity is substantially lower when the patient is lying down compared to standing, because the liver's weight no longer aids diaphragmatic descent.

The spinal form of amyotrophic lateral sclerosis usually presents with wasting and weakness of one limb, usually as intrinsic hand muscle wasting or foot drop. Asymptomatic involvement of other limbs is often evident on examination. It is diagnostically important to demonstrate combined upper and lower motor neurone signs in at least two limbs. Wasted fasciculating muscles also exhibiting clonus or hyperreflexia are a helpful finding. With time, the limbs become useless due to progressive denervation. Patients become wheelchair- or bed-bound, or are unable to use their arms for grooming or feeding. Despite enforced recumbency, decubitus ulcers are relatively unusual because autonomic regulation of skin blood flow and secretion is unaffected. Sphincter control is not affected, although practical difficulties in excretion may result from immobility, and because abdominal wall weakness prevents intra-abdominal pressure being raised to aid excretion.

Prognosis

Amytrophic lateral sclerosis progresses relentlessly, both in the severity and the extent of muscular involvement. Death commonly results from ventilatory respiratory failure, from choking, or from inhalational pneumonia; malnutrition often contributes. The median survival from first symptoms in those with bulbar onset is approximately 20 months, with only 5 per cent surviving 5 years. The alternative diagnosis of X-linked bulbospinal neuronopathy should be considered in these long survivors. The median survival for those with spinal onset is approximately 29 months, with nearly 15 per cent surviving 5 years. Although a subacute and reversible syndrome resembling spinal amyotrophic lateral sclerosis has been described, this is so extraordinarily rare that it should not influence the physician's prognostications.

Differential diagnosis and investigation

A diagnosis of amyotrophic lateral sclerosis is usually depressingly obvious on simple clinical grounds. Often only electrophysiological investigation is necessary to confirm denervation and to exclude a potentially treatable myopathy or demyelinating neuropathy. Sometimes upper motor neurone involvement is not clinically demonstrable, particularly in patients with absent Babinski responses due to severely denervated toe extensor muscles. Such cases may be clarified by measuring central motor conduction following electromagnetic stimulation of the brain. If patients present with the combination of arm denervation and upper motor neurone signs in the legs, the cervical spinal canal should be imaged with magnetic resonance scanning or myelography in order to exclude a compressive lesion, most often spondylitic radiculomyelopathy.

The usual diagnostic problem lies in differentiating amyotrophic lateral sclerosis from other motor neurone diseases. A lack of upper motor neurone involvement should raise the possibility of alternative diagnoses. The postpolio syndrome causes slow deterioration in limb or bulbar function some decades after acute poliomyelitis. X-linked bulbospinal neuronopathy is much more slowly progressive than bulbar amyotrophic lateral sclerosis; grimacing usually evokes characteristic lower facial contractions; gynaecomastia, diabetes mellitus, or abnormal sensory nerve conduction are often evident; and other male family members may be affected. Multifocal motor neuropathy or neuronopathy usually develops insidiously, predominantly affecting the arms, may be associated with paraproteinaemia or antiganglioside antibodies, and may involve motor nerve slowing or conduction block. Adult-onset proximal hereditary motor neuronopathy is very slowly progressive, with early and symmetric involvement of proximal muscle, and rarely involves bulbar muscles.

Telling the diagnosis

Doctors or relatives are sometimes tempted on compassionate grounds not to tell patients about their diagnosis of amyotrophic lateral sclerosis. When patients eventually detect this conspiracy of secrecy it can lead to serious loss of trust at a time when death looms and trustworthy relationships are of inestimable value. When given the opportunity, patients usually indicate that they wish to know the name of the disease and the likely outcome, and they may even wish a detailed discussion of likely modes of death. Of course, questions should be answered honestly, although sometimes it may be preferable to discuss them in stages with the spouse present so as to soften the blow early on in the course of the disease. Once a patient has been told the diagnosis, the doctor must address the particular issues presented by that patient's own brand of amyotrophic lateral sclerosis before the patient becomes upset by the summary information which he may glean from lay reference books.

Treatment

No treatment is known to cure amyotrophic lateral sclerosis. Yet much can be done to overcome disability and alleviate distress by the care team of speech therapist, physiotherapist, occupational therapist, social worker, and physician. The Motor Neurone Disease Association is often able to provide equipment promptly. Severe dysphagia is most effectively treated by percutaneous endoscopic gastrostomy. Preferably the patient or their carer should have good hand function and vision so that they can change nutrient bags at home. If video-swallow shows that cricopharyngeal spasm is responsible for dysphagia, cricopharyngeal myotomy may help. Speech failure can be circumvented by computer-assisted communication devices operated through an appropriate modality, such as pressure, blowing, head-nodding, or blinking, depending upon which muscles remain strong. Decisions regarding the advisability of instituting assisted respiration pose complex practical and ethical dilemmas. Patients with diaphragm weakness and nocturnal dyspnoea may be helped by continuous positive airways pressure delivered by a facial mask. Endotracheal intubation and ventilation are rarely recommendable in a disease causing such ubiquitous irreversible weakness.

LOWER MOTOR NEURONE SYNDROMES

These forms of motor neurone disease generally follow a much more benign course than amyotrophic lateral sclerosis. They include syndromes previously described as spinal muscular atrophy and progressive muscular atrophy. Differential diagnosis within the lower motor neurone syndromes depends principally upon attention to the age of onset, the pattern of the weakness, and a possible family history.

Proximal hereditary motor neuronopathy

Acute infantile form (Werdnig–Hoffmann disease)

This is one of the most common fatal autosomal recessive disorders of children. The disease frequency of approximately 1:25 000 in England results from a gene frequency of 1:160. Before the age of 6 months, babies become inactive, weak, hypotonic, feed poorly, and slow to attain motor milestones. They may be born with limb deformities, and, in retrospect, fetal movements have often been absent or sparse. The tongue is weak and may fasciculate. Head control is poor and the infant's areflexic and proximally wasted limbs tend to assume a frog-like position. Respiratory movements are decreased, with prominent involvement of intercostal muscles. Half the infants die by 6 months, and almost all have succumbed by 18 months, usually to respiratory complications.

Chronic childhood form (Kugelberg–Welander disease)

This form develops at any time from infancy to the early teens. It is also autosomal recessive, may be genetically heterogeneous, and may commence discordantly within families. It may resemble Werdnig–Hoffmann disease if the onset is early, but follows a comparatively benign course. More than 90 per cent of patients are able to walk or to sit unsupported at some time, although these abilities are often lost eventually. Tongue involvement occurs in only half the patients, and significant dysphagia is unusual. Some patients develop respiratory insufficiency as a result of intercostal muscle involvement. The proximal limb weakness and wasting is only slowly progressive and may stabilize spontaneously. Those with severe early weakness often develop secondary spinal and joint deformities. The prognosis varies, although survival into middle age is usual. It is important, although initially difficult, to differentiate those with infantile onset and no family history from Werdnig–Hoffmann disease.

Adult-onset forms

The autosomal recessive adult form starts from 15 to 60 years of age, usually in the fourth decade. Slowly progressive proximal limb weakness ensues, but significant disability for walking usually does not occur until the sixth or seventh decade. Life expectancy is only slightly reduced. Distal muscles can be involved too; the tendon reflexes are usually lost, but bulbar involvement is uncommon. The lack of upper motor neurone signs or of bulbar involvement, and the rather indolent progression distinguish this from amyotrophic lateral sclerosis.

Autosomal dominant forms are rare, and fall into two groups, with onset in childhood and in early middle age, respectively. The limb weakness is predominantly proximal. Bulbar involvement does occur, although it is unusual. The childhood form may stabilize at adolescence and some patients retain walking ability into middle or old age. The adult-onset form causes more severe disability. The lack of upper motor neurone signs distinguishes these conditions from hereditary amyotrophic lateral sclerosis.

X-linked recessive bulbospinal neuronopathy (Kennedy syndrome)

This disorder occurs only in men, with onset in the third to fifth decades of life. It is due to a mutation causing increased length CAG repeat sequences within the androgen receptor gene. Molecular genetic analysis now forms the basis of a diagnostic test. Weakness usually first affects hand or pelvic girdle muscles and the bulbar symptoms may not be evident until 20 years later, if at all. Fasciculations are usually visible in the limb, tongue, and facial muscles. Characteristically, muscle contractions around the chin are induced by pursing the lips or grimacing. The disorder is only slowly progressive. Most patients survive into their seventh or eight decades, except when bulbar involvement is unusually severe. The disorder is often misdiagnosed as amyotrophic lateral sclerosis until the unusually slow deterioration is questioned. Unlike amyotrophic lateral sclerosis, there are no upper motor neurone signs and patients commonly show gynaecomastia, diabetes mellitus, and absent sensory nerve action potentials.

Hexosaminidase deficiency

Autosomal recessive GM_1 gangliosidosis presents a variable neurological picture, occasionally as a pure motor neurone syndrome due to lower and, rarely, upper motor neurone involvement. More usually these are combined with other neurological abnormalities, such as cerebellar ataxia or dementia. Hexosaminidase assays should be reserved for those patients with early onset of unusual motor neurone disorders, particularly Ashkenazi Jews.

Hereditary bulbar palsy

The Brown–Vialetto–van Laere syndrome presents in the teens with bilateral sensorineural deafness, followed some years later by bulbar, facial, limb, and sometimes respiratory muscle, weakness. Fazio–Londe disease is a bulbar palsy of childhood, without deafness, and respiratory muscle involvement may lead to death within a few years. It is usually inherited as an autosomal recessive trait.

Monomelic, focal, or segmental motor neuronopathies

This condition is also known as chronic asymmetric or focal spinal muscular atrophy, or monomelic motor neurone disease. Although most commonly described from Japan and Asia, it is seen regularly elsewhere in the world. It usually occurs sporadically and most patients are young adult males. It presents with distal wasting and weakness of one hand or forearm. This progresses steadily for the first 2 years before either stabilizing, or settling to a slow rate of subsequent progression. Initially there may be concern that this is the first presentation of amyotrophic lateral sclerosis, but the expected upper motor neurone and bulbar involvement fail to materialize, and spread to other limbs is unusual. Nerve conduction studies are necessary to exclude focal entrapment neuropathies, or multifocal motor neuropathy with conduction block. Magnetic resonance imaging of the cervical spine will detect syringomyelia or other spinal cord disease.

Postirradiation motor neurone syndrome

This may follow months or years after the lower thoracic and upper lumbar spine are included in irradiation fields treating testicular tumours or lymphoma. It usually affects both legs, or occasionally one, but spares the sphincters and sensation. It is painless, and electrophysiology does not reveal the myokymic discharges, or abnormal sensory nerve action potentials of irradiation plexopathy. The normal imaging of the lumbosacral plexus and cauda equina, and the absence of pain, exclude tumour recurrence.

Postpolio syndrome

After two or more decades, very slowly progressive weakness may affect muscles previously involved by acute paralytic poliomyelitis. Although this predominantly affects the limbs, approximately half the patients also have mild choking or dysphagia. The sluggish deterioration, lack of upper motor neurone involvement, and previous history serve to distinguish postpolio syndrome from amyotrophic lateral sclerosis. Electromyography reveals the giant motor units typical of extensive re-innervation during recovery from previous acute poliomyelitis.

Multifocal motor neuropathy and neuronopathy

Patients with these conditions may present at any stage of adult life with multifocal and slowly progressive muscle weakness for as long as 20 years. The clinical picture is immensely variable. Distal limb muscles are mainly involved, often notably asymmetrically. The first symptoms and most severe weakness usually affect the arms. Reflex loss is generally restricted to affected muscles. The condition is neurophysiologically heterogeneous, ranging from muscle denervation to multifocal conduction block in motor nerves, and occasionally a diffusely demyelinating pure motor peripheral neuropathy. Serum antibodies to GM$_1$ gangliosides are detectable in at least half the patients, but are not of proven pathogenetic significance. This antibody assay presently lacks specificity since positives are sometimes found in other neurological diseases. Paraproteinaemia is common, particularly IgG. These motor neuropathies usually progress insidiously, sometimes in a stepwise manner, and occasionally spontaneous remissions occur. It is important to detect the subgroup of patients with multifocal motor conduction block, or with diffuse demyelinating neuropathy, because improvement may follow immunosuppressant therapy. Although cyclophosphamide is reportedly effective, its use should be reserved for those patients with severely disabling and progressive weakness. High-dose intravenous human immunoglobulin therapy can produce dramatic temporary improvement. Unfortunately, steroid therapy does not improve multifocal motor neuropathy, and may precipitate further deterioration.

UPPER MOTOR NEURONE SYNDROMES

The pure upper motor neurone syndromes are the rarest forms of motor neurone disease. They should be considered only after magnetic resonance imaging has excluded structural or demyelinating disease of the spinal cord, foramen magnum, or brain. Spasticity is often severe in the purely upper motor neurone diseases, but unfortunately antispasticity medications are often relatively ineffective. Rarely, similar upper motor neurone syndromes may be seen with syphilis, Lyme disease, and human T-cell leukaemia virus (HTLV-1) infection.

Primary lateral sclerosis

This rare sporadic form of motor neurone disease has an average age of onset of 50 years, and slow progression thereafter for an average of 15 years. The clinical features are all attributable to symmetric degeneration of the upper motor neurones destined for the spinal cord and bulbar motor neurones. Spasticity and weakness usually commence insidiously in the legs and ascend ultimately to involve the bulbar muscles. Less commonly, patients present with an isolated spastic dysarthria, a symptom of pseudobulbar palsy. Pseudobulbar emotional lability may be distressing for these patients, given their normal cognition, and it often responds well to amitriptyline. Bladder function is generally preserved, at least until the later stages. Electromyography does not reveal the muscle denervation to be expected in predominantly upper motor neurone forms of amyotrophic lateral sclerosis. Magnetic resonance imaging may reveal atrophy of the precentral gyrus motor cortex, reflecting loss of the Betz cells from which the pyramidal tract originates. Central motor conduction is notably delayed following electromagnetic stimulation of the motor cortex.

Autosomal dominant 'pure' familial spastic paraplegia

Various forms of slowly progressive symmetric spastic paraparesis may be inherited, most usually on an autosomal dominant basis with onset in the fourth to sixth decades. The degree of leg spasticity often outweighs the severity of the weakness. Bulbar involvement is very rare, and arm function may be well preserved despite severe leg involvement. The condition is slowly progressive. It may remain asymptomatic in some family members, coming to light only when a familial basis for

the disease is sought. Sphincter control is not impaired, but sexual impotence can develop.

Lathyrism

Neurolathyrism is a spastic paraparesis caused by regular consumption of the chickling pea vetch (*Lathyrus sativus*) for some months. It is endemic in parts of India and may be epidemic in times of famine. Patients present either subacutely or chronically with a spastic paraparesis and a characteristic scissoring gait in which the balls of the feet take most of the weight. Once it has developed, neurolathyrism is usually not progressive, but little or no recovery occurs even after chickling pea consumption ceases.

REFERENCES

Cochrane, G. and Donaghy, M. (1993). Motor neuron disease. In *Neurological rehabilitation*, (ed. R.J. Greenwood, M.P. Barnes, T.M. MacMillan, and C.D. Ward), pp. 571–85. Churchill Livingstone, Edinburgh.
Gregory, R.P., Mills, K.R., and Donaghy, M. (1993). Progressive sensory nerve dysfunction in amyotrophic lateral sclerosis: a prospective clinical and neurophysiological study. *Journal of Neurology*, **240**, 309–14.
Donaghy, M. *et al.* (1994). Pure motor demyelinating neuropathy: deterioration following steroid therapy and improvement with intravenous immunoglobulin. *Journal of Neurology, Neurosurgery and Psychiatry*, **57**, (in press).
Harding, A.E. (1993). Inherited neuronal atrophy and degeneration predominantly of lower motor neurons. In *Peripheral neuropathy*, (3rd edn), (ed. P.J. Dyck, P.K. Thomas, J.W. Griffin, P.A. Low, and J.F. Poduslo), Ch. 55. W.B. Saunders, Philadelphia.
Howard, R.S., Wiles, C.M., and Loh, L. (1989). Respiratory complications and their management in motor neuron disease. *Brain* **112**, 1155–70.
La Spada, A.R., Wilson, E.M., Lubahn, D.B., Harding, A.E., and Fischbeck, K.H. (1991). Androgen receptor gene mutations in X-linked spinal and bulbar muscular atrophy. *Nature* **352**, 77–9.
Ludolph, A.C., Hugon, J., Dwivedi, M.P., Schaumburg, H.H., and Spencer, P.S. (1987). Studies on the aetiology and pathogenesis of motor neuron diseases. I Lathyrism: clinical findings in established cases. *Brain* **110**, 149–66.
McShane, M.A., Boyd, S., Harding, B., Brett, E.M., and Wilson, J. (1992). Progressive bulbar paralysis of childhood. A reappraisal of Fazio–Londe disease. *Brain* **115**, 1889–900.
Olney, R.K., Aminoff, M.J., and So, Y.T. (1991). Clinical and electrodiagnostic features of X-linked recessive bulbospinal neuronopathy. *Neurology* **41**, 823–8.
Pestronk, A., *et al.* (1990). Lower motor neuron syndromes defined by patterns of weakness, nerve conduction abnormalities, and high titres of antiglycolipid antibodies. *Annals of Neurology* **27**, 316–26.
Pringle, C.E., Hudson, A.J., Munoz, D.G., Kiernan, J.A., Brown, W.F., and Ebers, G.C. (1992). Primary lateral sclerosis. Clinical features, neuropathology and diagnostic criteria. *Brain* **115**, 495–520.
Rosen, D.R., *et al.* (1993). Mutations in Cu/Zn superoxide dismutase gene are associated with familial amyotrophic lateral sclerosis. *Nature* **362**, 59–62.
Sobue, I., Saito, N., Ilda, M., and Ando, K. (1978). Juvenile type of distal and segmental muscular atrophy of upper extremities. *Annals of Neurology* **3**, 429–37.
Sonies, B.C. and Dalakas, M.C. (1991). Dysphagia in patients with the post-polio syndrome. *New England Journal of Medicine* **324**, 1162–7.
Tandan, R. and Bradley, W.G. (1985a). Amyotrophic lateral sclerosis: Part 1. Clinical features, pathology, and ethical issues in management. *Annals of Neurology* **18**, 271–80.
Tandan, R. and Bradley, W.G. (1985b). Amyotrophic lateral sclerosis: Part 2. Etiopathogenesis. *Annals of Neurology* **18**, 419–31.

24.17 Peripheral neuropathy

P. K. THOMAS

PATHOPHYSIOLOGICAL CONSIDERATIONS

The peripheral nerves consist of bundles (fascicles) of unmyelinated and myelinated axons that have their cell bodies in the anterior horns, dorsal root ganglia, or autonomic ganglia. The fascicles are surrounded by a lamellated sheath, the perineurium, which provides a diffusion barrier that separates the intrafascicular or endoneurial compartment from the extracellular tissues. Peripheral nerve trunks usually consist of several fascicles bound together by the mainly collagenous epineurial connective tissue. The nutrient vessels connect with a longitudinal anastomotic network of arterioles and venules in the epineurium. This in turn communicates through perforating vessels with a longitudinal intrafascicular capillary anastomotic network. This anastomotic system is extremely efficient: experimentally it is very difficult to produce ischaemia of nerve trunks by ligation of nutrient vessels. The occurrence of an ischaemic neuropathy, therefore, implies widespread vascular insufficiency. A blood–nerve barrier, comparable to the blood–brain barrier, exists in peripheral nerves (except in the sensory and autonomic ganglia). This, in conjunction with the diffusion barrier provided by the perineurium, probably regulates the composition of the endoneurial connective tissue fluid and thus the ionic environment of the nerve fibres.

All nerve fibres, whether myelinated or unmyelinated, are closely related to satellite cells, the cells of Schwann. There is evidence that they may provide metabolic support for the axons, which often extend for very considerable distances from their perikarya. In myelinated fibres the myelin segments are derived by the spiralling of Schwann cell surface membrane around the axons. The axon is exposed at the nodes of Ranvier, which represent the gaps between adjacent myelin segments. Conduction in unmyelinated axons takes place by the spread of a continuous wave of depolarization, the action potential, that migrates along the axolemma. In myelinated fibres, because of the high electrical resistance of the lipid in the myelin lamellae, the generation of the action potential is restricted to the region of the nodes of Ranvier. Conduction is therefore saltatory, jumping from one node to the next by local currents that traverse the axon and the extracellular tissue fluid. By this means, conduction velocity is increased from about 1 m/s in unmyelinated axons to 60 to 70 m/s in the largest myelinated fibres in human nerves.

The majority of the synthetic mechanisms in neurones are sited in the cell bodies. Synthesized materials are then transported down the axons to the termination of the fibres by an active transport system. This involves a fast system with a rate of about 400 mm/day, and a slow system, in which the structural proteins travel, at 1 to 2 mm/day. The system is bidirectional: apart from the two anterograde fluxes, there is a retrograde system transporting materials, including neurotrophic factors, back from the periphery to the cell body. The retrograde system may be involved in the regulation of protein synthesis in the cell body and probably carries the signal for chromatolysis which ensues on transection.

Disorders of peripheral nerve function can be categorized in terms of the site of the primary disturbance. Conditions that lead to the death of the neurone as a whole, with the loss of the cell body and the axon, are categorized as neuronopathies. Conditions that have a selective effect on axons are termed axonopathies. A selective effect on axonal conduction is seen in poisoning with tetrodotoxin, which blocks the sodium channels at the nodes. Axonopathies may be focal or generalized. Focal axonopathies occur as a result of insults such as trauma or ischaemia. Axonal interruption leads to wallerian degeneration below the site of the injury. Recovery has to take place by axonal regeneration which is a slow process: the rate of axonal regeneration is about 1 to 2 mm/day.

Generalized axonopathies often lead to a selective degeneration of the distal portion of the fibres which then extends proximally. The axons are said to 'die back' towards the cell bodies. This pattern is seen in many toxic neuropathies and neuropathies due to nutritional deficiency. It has been suggested that in these conditions the axonal breakdown may result either from interference with enzymes involved in glycolysis, and which provide the metabolic energy for axonal transport mechanisms, or from cofactor deficiency or inactivation. As the enzymes are synthesized in the cell body and then transported down the axons, the further the distance from the cell body the greater will be the likelihood of the occurrence of metabolic insufficiency. This probably accounts for the distal distribution of many such neuropathies, as longer axons will be more vulnerable. Recovery again has to take place by axonal regeneration. In many distal axonopathies that involve the peripheral nervous system, not only does the degeneration affect the distal parts of the motor and sensory axons in the periphery, but the terminal parts of the centrally directed axons derived from the dorsal root ganglion cells also degenerate. Thus degeneration may be found in the rostral portions of the posterior columns. This process has been referred to as central-peripheral distal axonopathy. Neuropathy from iminodipropionitrile blocks the slow axonal transport system and leads to large swellings in the proximal parts of the axons that contain aggregations of neurofilaments (proximal axonopathy).

Other neuropathies primarily affect the myelin, either directly, or through an interference with Schwann cell function. The consequence is a selective demyelination with relative preservation of axonal integrity. This may be restricted to the region of the nodes of Ranvier (paranodal demyelination) or involve whole internodal segments (segmental demyelination) with consequent conduction block. The selective myelin damage may occur, for example, as the result of a cell-mediated attack on myelin by sensitized mononuclear cells, which is the likely explanation of the Guillain–Barré syndrome. Another instance is in diphtheritic neuropathy where the demyelination is considered to be secondary to an interference with Schwann cell protein metabolism. Local compression by a tourniquet also gives rise to selective damage to myelin through mechanical effects, although more severe pressure also causes axonal interruption. In diffuse demyelinating neuropathies, the distribution of the clinical effects, as for distal axonopathies, is often maximal peripherally. Presumably, this is a statistical effect: the longer the nerve fibre, the more likely will it be that it develops a region of demyelinating conduction block.

Recovery after paranodal or segmental demyelination occurs by remyelination. Initially, the newly formed myelin is thin, which results in abnormally slow conduction velocity. Such reductions in conduction velocity may be focal, for example in relation to localized myelin damage in entrapment neuropathies, or widespread as in the Guillain–Barré syndrome or the inherited demyelinating neuropathies. In the latter, motor nerve conduction velocity is sometimes reduced to 10 m/s or less.

Finally, in other neuropathies the nerve fibres may be secondarily damaged by processes that primarily affect the connective tissues of nerve or the vasa nervorum. Usually a combination of demyelination and axonal loss occurs.

CLINICAL CATEGORIES OF NEUROPATHY

Mononeuropathy, multifocal neuropathy, and polyneuropathy

Peripheral neuropathies may be divided into two broad categories depending upon the distribution of the involvement. The first category comprises lesions of isolated peripheral nerves or nerve roots termed mononeuropathy or multiple isolated lesions termed multifocal neuropathy (multiple mononeuropathy or 'mononeuritis multiplex'). The lesions in a widespread multifocal neuropathy may summate to produce a symmetrical disturbance, but the history or a careful examination may indicate the involvement of individual nerves. Isolated or multiple isolated peripheral nerve lesions arise from conditions that produce localized damage, such as mechanical injury, nerve entrapment, thermal, electrical, or radiation injury, vascular causes, granulomatous, neoplastic, or other other infiltrations, and nerve tumours.

Secondly, there may be a diffuse and bilaterally symmetrical disturbance of function which can be designated polyneuropathy. When such a process affects the spinal roots, or affects the roots and the peripheral nerve trunks, the terms polyradiculopathy and polyradiculoneuropathy are sometimes employed. In general terms, polyneuropathies result from causes that act diffusely on the peripheral nervous system, such as metabolic disturbances, toxic agents, deficiency states, and certain instances of immune reaction. Isolated nerve lesions may sometimes be superimposed upon a symmetrical polyneuropathy, as a consequence, for example, of pressure lesions in a patient confined to bed. In certain polyneuropathies, there is an abnormal susceptibility to pressure lesions.

SYMPTOMATOLOGY

Weakness or paralysis may be due either to conduction block in the motor nerve fibres or to axonal degeneration. Conduction block is related to demyelination with preservation of axonal continuity (neurapraxia). Recovery may occur by remyelination and may be rapid and complete. This can be the situation in localized nerve lesions, for example 'Saturday night' paralysis of the radial nerve, or in more widespread polyneuropathies, such as in acute idiopathic polyneuropathy (Guillain–Barré syndrome). If axonal interruption takes place, axonal degeneration occurs below the site of interruption. The muscle weakness is accompanied by denervation atrophy and electromyographic signs of denervation. In a reversible process, recovery has to take place by axonal regeneration which is often slow and incomplete. An important recovery mechanism in conditions in which muscles become partially denervated is re-innervation of denervated muscle fibres by collateral sprouting from the remaining intact axons.

In generalized symmetrical polyneuropathies, the muscle weakness and wasting are commonly peripheral in distribution with an onset in the lower limbs. This results in bilateral footdroop and a 'steppage' gait in which the affected individual lifts his feet to an abnormal extent to avoid catching his toes against the ground. Involvement of the upper limbs begins with weakness and wasting of the small hand muscles and usually weakness of the finger and wrist extensors before the forearm flexor muscles are affected. At times, a symmetrical involvement of the proximal musculature in the limbs occurs in polyneuropathies, for example in the Guillain–Barré syndrome or porphyric neuropathy. Fasciculation due to spontaneous contraction of isolated motor units is most often a feature of anterior horn cell disease but may be encountered in peripheral neuropathies, as may muscle cramps. Postural tremor, mainly affecting the upper limbs and resembling essential tremor, may be seen in patients with chronic demyelinating polyneuropathies with slow conduction velocity. This 'neuropathic tremor' is most often encountered in type I hereditary motor and sensory neuropathy, chronic inflammatory demyelinating polyneuropathy, and paraproteinaemic neuropathy. A rare manifestation of peripheral neuropathy is the occurrence of continuous repetitive discharges in motor nerve fibres leading to generalized muscular rigidity or 'neuromyotonia' (Isaacs' syndrome, continuous motor unit activity syndrome).

Loss of the tendon reflexes is a frequent accompaniment of a peripheral neuropathy, and usually first affects the ankle jerks. In assessing the clinical findings, it is important to remember that the ankle jerks may be lost in later life, probably as a result of senile changes in the peripheral nerves.

Sensory symptoms and sensory loss in symmetrical polyneuropathies are usually distal in distribution, giving rise to the 'glove and stocking' pattern of involvement. Only rarely is a proximal pattern encountered. The sensory loss may affect all modalities or be restricted to certain forms of sensation. If the loss is restricted, two broad patterns are discernible. In the first, the impairment predominantly affects joint position sense, and vibration and touch-pressure sensibility, corresponding to a predominant loss of function in the larger myelinated nerve fibres. Loss of postural sensibility may lead to sensory ataxia in the limbs and to 'pseudoathetosis', that is, involuntary movements, most often of the fingers and hands, that occur, for example, when the patient holds his arms outstretched with his eyes closed. In the second pattern of selective sensory loss, pain and temperature sensibility are predominantly affected, often associated with loss of autonomic function, corresponding to a predominant loss of small myelinated and unmyelinated axons. 'Trophic changes' may complicate peripheral neuropathies. The most important factor in their genesis is the loss of the protective effect of pain sensation with the consequent development of persistent ulceration or more extensive tissue loss, most commonly in the feet, and neuropathic joint degeneration.

Paraesthesiae are a frequent feature in peripheral neuropathy. These are usually of a tingling nature ('pins and needles'), but may involve thermal sensations, most often with a burning quality. The paraesthesiae may be aggravated by touching or rubbing the skin. Stimuli that are normally not painful may acquire an unpleasant quality (allodynia) and painful stimuli may give rise to an excessive or hyperpathic response, in which the stimulus, for example a pinprick, is abnormally intense. With repeated stimulation at the same site, the pain that is felt may spread widely and reach an intolerable intensity. An unusual symptom encountered most often in uraemic neuropathy is that of 'restless legs' (Ekbom's syndrome). The affected individuals experience sensations in the feet and legs that they find difficult to describe but which are temporarily relieved by movement of the feet and legs. Ekbom's syndrome may also occur in the absence of any detectable disease process.

Spontaneous pains of an aching or lancinating character may complicate a number of generalized polyneuropathies. Severe paroxysms of lancinating pain occur in trigeminal neuralgia, but here the responsible lesion may well lie within the central nervous system. Causalgia constitutes a particularly troublesome painful syndrome, most often following gunshot wounds injuring the median nerve, the lower trunk of the brachial plexus, or the tibial nerve. It is a severe persistent pain, often with a burning quality that is characteristically aggravated by emotional factors. Sympathectomy relieves a high proportion of such cases.

Disturbances of autonomic function are occasionally the salient abnormality in a peripheral neuropathy, as in the Riley–Day syndrome, or they may accompany other manifestations, and can be observed both with localized peripheral nerve lesions and in generalized neuropathies.

DIAGNOSIS AND INVESTIGATION

The history and physical examination frequently indicate that the disturbance has affected the peripheral nerves. If confirmation is required, this may usually be obtained by nerve conduction studies. Conduction may be examined in motor and sensory nerve fibres, and can give evidence of both localized and generalized neuropathies. Severely reduced conduction velocity may occur as a result of segmental demyelination or because of conduction in regenerating axons of small calibre after axonal degeneration.

Examination of the cerebrospinal fluid is not commonly of value in the diagnosis of peripheral neuropathies, although the substantially elevated protein content that often occurs in the Guillain–Barré syndrome may be helpful, as may inflammatory changes in some neuropathies.

Nerve biopsy is rarely required in establishing the existence of a peripheral neuropathy, but may be of diagnostic value in establishing the cause of the neuropathy, particularly in conditions that affect the vasa nervorum or neural connective tissues, or in 'storage' disorders.

Individual nerves

PHRENIC NERVE (C$_{2-4}$)

This nerve innervates the diaphragm. When the diaphragm is totally paralysed, the normal protrusion of the upper abdomen during inspiration is lost, or is replaced by retraction. Radiographically, paralysis may be detected by unilateral or bilateral elevation of the diaphragm in a chest radiograph and its failure to descend on inspiration. The phrenic nerve may be involved in its course through the neck or thorax by wounds, or tumours such as bronchial carcinoma, and it is sometimes affected in idiopathic brachial plexus neuropathy (neuralgic amyotrophy).

NERVE TO SERRATUS ANTERIOR (C$_{5-7}$)

The serratus anterior acts as a fixator of the scapula, holding the scapula against the chest wall when forward pressure is exerted by the arm. It is involved in forward movement of the shoulder as in a rapier thrust and in elevation of the arm, when it rotates the scapula. When serratus anterior is paralysed in isolation, the position of the scapula is normal at rest but if the extended arm is pushed forwards against resistance, 'winging' of the scapula becomes evident. The vertebral border, particularly in its lower portion, stands away from the chest wall. The nerve to serratus anterior may be involved in penetrating wounds, but usually in association with damage to the brachial plexus. It may be injured by forcible depression of the shoulder. Serratus anterior weakness is a common component of idiopathic brachial plexus neuropathy (neuralgic amyotrophy) and it is not infrequently encountered as an isolated and unexplained lesion.

BRACHIAL PLEXUS

The brachial plexus may be affected by penetrating wounds of the neck, in fractures and dislocations of the shoulder and clavicle, as a result of traction on the arm, by pressure from an aneurysm or a cervical rib, and by neoplastic involvement.

Traction lesions

Traction on the arm may result in damage to the plexus itself or may lead to avulsion of the spinal roots from the cord. If the roots are avulsed, sensory nerve action potentials will be preserved if recorded from affected fingers despite total anaesthesia, and the histamine flare response will be preserved in anaesthetic skin. This follows from the fact that the nerve fibres are interrupted proximal to the dorsal root ganglia and therefore the peripheral sensory axons do not degenerate.

In severe traction lesions, commonly encountered in current medical practice as a result of motorcycle accidents, the whole of the plexus may be damaged. With forcible downward displacement of the shoulder, as when someone is thrown forwards and the shoulder strikes against an obstacle, only the upper part of the plexus, involving the contribution from the fifth and sixth cervical nerve roots, may be damaged. This may also be encountered as a birth injury from traction on the head, or on the trunk in a breech presentation (Erb's palsy), and rarely in anaesthetized patients during operation or in individuals carrying heavy rucksacks. Selective injury to the lower part of the plexus involving the contributions from the eighth cervical and first thoracic nerve roots occurs as a result of traction with the arm extended, as when an individual falls from a height and tries to save himself by hanging on to a ledge. It may also occur as a birth injury following traction with the arm extended (Klumpke's paralysis), but is less common than upper plexus damage.

Selective damage to the upper portion of the plexus (C$_5$ and C$_6$ roots or upper trunk) results in paralysis of deltoid, biceps, brachialis, brachioradialis, and sometimes supraspinatus, infraspinatus, and subscapularis. If the roots are avulsed from the cord, the rhomboids, serratus anterior, levator scapulae, and the scalene muscles will be affected. The arm hangs at the side, internally rotated at the shoulder, with the elbow extended and the forearm pronated in the 'waiter's tip' position. Abduction at the shoulder and flexion at the elbow are not possible. The biceps and brachioradialis jerks are lost. Sensory loss affects the lateral aspect of the shoulder and upper arm and the radial border of the forearm. Selective paralysis of the lower brachial plexus (C$_8$ T$_1$) results in paralysis of all the intrinsic hand muscles and a consequent claw-hand deformity, weakness of the medial finger and wrist flexors, and sensory loss along the medial border of the forearm and hand and over the medial two fingers. Cervical sympathetic paralysis, giving rise to Horner's syndrome, is frequently associated.

When the spinal roots are avulsed from the cord, regeneration is impossible and intractable spontaneous pain may be a highly troublesome sequel. Where the injury is distal to the dorsal root ganglia, lesions of the upper portion of the brachial plexus recover more satisfactorily than lower plexus lesions. The value of surgical repair is still a controversial issue. In the Erb's form of birth injury, weakness of abduction at the shoulder and flexion at the elbow often persist, although there may be little residual sensory loss. Full recovery takes place in about a third of the cases. It is less likely to occur with lower plexus injuries or if the whole plexus is involved. Early recognition and the application of measures to reduce the risk of joint contractures are important. Surgical treatment is of no value.

Thoracic outlet syndromes

The contribution of the eighth cervical and first thoracic roots to the brachial plexus may be damaged by angulation over an abnormal rib or, more usually, a fibrous band arising from the seventh cervical vertebra and attached to the first rib. Although local structures such as the tendon of scalenus anterior may be involved in the production of symptoms, the isolation of a separate 'scalenus anterior syndrome' or of 'costoclavicular compression' is not justified. The subclavian artery may be affected by cervical ribs giving rise to aneurysmal dilatation and vascular symptoms such as Raynaud's syndrome and embolic phenomena, but the simultaneous occurrence of both neural and vascular phenomena is rare.

Damage to the lower part of the brachial plexus leads to weakness and wasting of the small hand muscles, and of the medial forearm wrist and finger flexors. Occasionally, there is selective wasting of the thenar pad in the hand, mimicking to some extent the appearances of the carpal tunnel syndrome. Numbness, pain, and paraesthesiae occur along the inner border of the forearm and hand, extending into the medial two fingers. The pain tends to be provoked by carrying heavy articles in the hand on the affected side. Horner's syndrome may be a feature. Nerve conduction studies are helpful when there are difficulties in distinguishing a cervical rib syndrome from a lesion of the ulnar or median nerves on clinical grounds. Surgical removal of the rib or fibrous band often leads to abolition of the pain and paraesthesiae, but recovery of power in the small hand muscles is frequently disappointing.

Neoplastic involvement

Tumours may arise locally in the brachial plexus, such as neurofibromata in von Recklinghausen's disease (type I neurofibromatosis) or a solitary neurinoma, or the plexus may be invaded by tumours arising in other structures. In the latter eventuality the commonest situation is involvement of the lower part of the plexus by an apical carcinoma of the lung (Pancoast's syndrome), which gives rise to wasting and weakness of the small hand muscles and of the medial forearm wrist and finger flexors, pain and sensory loss affecting the medial border of the forearm and hand, and cervical sympathetic paralysis. Other tumours that may invade the brachial plexus include carcinoma of the breast and malignant lymphomas affecting the lymph glands in the root of the neck.

Neuralgic amyotrophy

This condition was not clearly differentiated from the other painful paralytic disorders of the shoulder and upper arm, such as root compression from disc prolapse, until the Second World War. It has been described in a variety of terms, including 'idiopathic brachial plexus neuropathy' and 'paralytic brachial neuritis'. It may follow immunizing procedures, in particular the administration of antitetanus serum, or operations, or occur without recognizable antecedent event. Occasionally brachial plexus neuropathy is encountered in several members of a family, suggesting autosomal dominant inheritance with variable penetrance.

The disorder develops acutely with intense pain in the shoulder region which may take some weeks before it subsides completely although generally it ceases after a few days. Paralysis of the muscles of the shoulder girdle becomes evident within a day or two of the onset of the pain, sometimes also of the arms or of the diaphragm. It may be unilateral or bilateral and may be associated with sensory loss. More distal upper limb muscles may at times be affected, as may the phrenic nerve and, occasionally, the recurrent laryngeal nerve. The cerebrospinal fluid is consistently normal. The affected muscles show electromyographic evidence of denervation, but recovery is usually ultimately satisfactory. Not all cases recover fully and recurrences may occur.

The pattern of muscle involvement and sensory disturbances suggests that the condition affects the brachial plexus in a patchy manner. An immune reaction is assumed but not established. The condition takes the same course whether or not it follows an immunizing procedure. Corticosteroids do not influence either the initial pain or the ultimate outcome.

Post-irradiation brachial plexus neuropathy

Brachial plexus damage may occur as a sequel to radiotherapy for breast carcinoma or other tumours in the neck. The onset of symptoms is usually several years after treatment, but may be within months. It can be difficult to distinguish from tumour recurrence but is less likely to be painful. Magnetic resonance imaging may be helpful.

RADIAL NERVE (C$_{5-8}$)

The long course of the radial nerve and its position in relation to the humerus make this nerve unusually susceptible to external compression. It is a continuation of the posterior cord of the brachial plexus. In the upper arm it supplies triceps and anconeus and the skin on the back of the arm through the posterior brachial cutaneous nerve. The lateral aspect of the lower part of the upper arm is supplied by the lower lateral brachial cutaneous branch and the dorsal aspect of the forearm by the posterior antebrachial cutaneous nerve. Muscular branches of the radial nerve innervate brachioradialis and extensor carpi radialis longus and brevis. The superficial branch of the nerve is its continuation. It descends along the radial border of the forearm and supplies the skin over the dorsum of the hand and the thumb, index, and middle fingers. The deep branch winds around the lateral aspect of the radius, passes through the supinator, which it supplies, and innervates the extensor digitorum, extensor digiti minimi, extensor carpi ulnaris, and often extensor carpi radialis brevis. Its continuation is the posterior interosseus nerve which supplies the abductor pollicis longus, extensor pollicis longus and brevis, and extensor indicis.

The nerve may be injured in wounds of the axilla so that the paralysis includes triceps, resulting in loss of extension at the elbow. The most frequent type of injury is compression of the nerve in the middle third of the arm against the humerus. This is encountered as 'Saturday night paralysis' in which an individual falls asleep when intoxicated with his upper arm over the arm of a chair. Triceps is spared, but brachioradialis,

supinator, and all the forearm extensor muscles are paralysed. Sensory impairment is limited to the dorsum of the hand. Commonly the lesion consists of a localized conduction block (neurapraxia) so that muscle wasting does not occur and a muscle response can be obtained on stimulation of the nerve below the level of the lesion. Recovery is complete within a matter of weeks. A cock-up wrist splint may be helpful while recovery is awaited. At times, there is some associated axonal degeneration so that electromyographic evidence of denervation is detectable and recovery is correspondingly delayed.

Many muscles not supplied by the radial nerve work at a disadvantage when the wrist and finger extensors are paralysed. These defects must not be mistaken for signs of injury to other nerves. Owing to the flexed position of the wrist, gripping is impaired, but if the power of the wrist and finger flexors is tested with the wrist extended, it can be shown to be normal. The action of the interossei in abducting and adducting the fingers is also feeble when the wrist is flexed, but full power is demonstrable if these muscles are tested with the hand resting flat on a table.

The deep branch of the nerve may be injured distal to the supinator muscle. This muscle is, of course, spared, together with brachioradialis and the radial wrist extensors, and there is no sensory loss. A lesion of the posterior interosseus nerve gives rise to weakness confined to abduction and extension of the thumb and extension of the index finger.

AXILLARY NERVE (C$_{5,6}$)

This is a branch of the posterior cord of the brachial plexus. It supplies deltoid and teres minor and the skin over deltoid through the upper lateral brachial cutaneous nerve. It may be damaged in injuries to the shoulder and the chief symptom is an almost complete inability to raise the arm at the shoulder. In the past, it was sometimes injured by pressure from a crutch ('crutch palsy').

MUSCULOCUTANEOUS NERVE (C$_{5,6}$)

This nerve is rarely damaged alone, but may be involved in injuries to the brachial plexus. It supplies coracobrachialis, biceps, and brachialis and the skin over the lateral aspect of the forearm through the lateral antebrachial cutaneous nerve. Flexion at the elbow is still possible by brachioradialis, but is weak, and sensation may be impaired along the radial border of the forearm.

MEDIAN NERVE (C$_{6-8}$ T$_1$)

The median nerve arises from the medial and lateral cords of the brachial plexus and descends with the brachial artery through the upper arm, entering the forearm deep to the bicipital aponeurosis. It has no muscular branches above the elbow. It supplies all the muscles in the anterior aspect of the forearm except flexor carpi ulnaris and the medial half of flexor digitorum profundus. The main trunk of the nerve supplies pronator teres, flexor carpi radialis, palmaris longus, and flexor digitorum superficialis. Through the anterior interosseus branch, it also supplies flexor pollicis longus, the lateral aspect of flexor digitorum profundus, and pronator quadratus. The main trunk passes deep to the flexor retinaculum of the wrist and its recurrent muscular branch supplies abductor pollicis brevis, opponens pollicis, and contributes to the innervation of flexor pollicis brevis. It also supplies the lateral two lumbrical muscles and the skin of the lateral aspect of the palm and the lateral three and a half digits over their palmar aspects and terminal parts of their dorsal aspects.

Lesions of the forearm

The median nerve may be injured in the region of the elbow or compressed at the level of the pronator teres muscle. Entrapment neuropathies in the upper forearm, however, are uncommon. Occasionally the anterior interosseus branch is involved in isolation.

Complete lesions of the median nerve at the elbow give rise to paralysis of pronator teres, the radial flexor of the wrist, the long finger flexors except the ulnar half of the deep flexor, most of the muscles of the thenar eminence, and the two radial lumbricals. In brief, there is an inability to flex the index finger and the distal phalanx of the thumb, flexion of the middle finger is weak, and opposition of the thumb is defective. The appearance of the hand has been described as simian; it shows ulnar deviation, the index and middle fingers are more extended than normal, and the thumb lies in the same plane as the fingers.

In more detail, pronation is incomplete and defective. The patient attempts to overcome this by rotating the whole limb at the shoulder. Paralysis of the wrist flexors is evident when attempts are made to flex against resistance. The tendon of flexor carpi ulnaris stands out alone and the hand goes into ulnar deviation. Flexion of the fingers is good in the ulnar two fingers, although weaker than normal. The index finger cannot be flexed, and the middle finger only incompletely. Flexion at the metacarpophalangeal joints is possible in all fingers, including the index, and flexion at these joints with extension at the interphalangeal joints is accomplished by the interossei and lumbricals. If the proximal phalanx of the thumb is immobilized, it will be found that flexion of the terminal phalanx is abolished because of paralysis of flexor pollicis longus. Paralysis of the thenar muscles gives rise to defective abduction and opposition of the thumb. By means of the abductor, the thumb can be drawn into the palm, but as the radial fingers cannot be flexed or the thumb opposed, it is impossible to place the tip of the thumb on the fingers.

Sensory loss is evident over the lateral three and a half digits and the lateral aspect of the palm, although individual variations occur. There is almost complete anaesthesia over the two terminal phalanges of the index and middle fingers. This degree of sensory loss, combined with the motor deficit, renders the thumb and index fingers almost useless and makes paralysis of the median the most serious single nerve lesion in the upper limb.

Vasomotor and trophic changes often ensue. The skin in the distribution of the median nerve tends to become reddened, dry, and atrophic. The pulp of the affected fingers becomes atrophic and ulceration occasionally develops in the tip of the index finger. The nails may become white and atrophic.

After a total transection of the nerve in the region of the elbow, even with a satisfactory surgical repair, recovery is slow and rarely complete, particularly with respect to the innervation of the hand.

With partial lesions of the median nerve in the arm or forearm, causalgia may be a troublesome consequence. This most often follows gunshot wounds. The pain develops at any time from a few hours to 45 days after the injury. The pain is severe and unremitting, frequently of a burning or smarting quality. Upon this may be superimposed severe paroxysms of pain provoked by touching or jarring the limb or by emotional factors. Vasomotor and sudomotor changes may be associated. The skin usually becomes dry and scaly, but excessive sweating may be a feature. The patient adopts a protective attitude towards the limb, so that fixation of the joints of the fingers and wrist may develop, together with atrophic changes in the skin and subcutaneous tissue. About 80 per cent of cases of true causalgia are relieved by sympathectomy. Untreated, the pain gradually subsides over months or years.

Lesions at the wrist

The superficial situation of the median nerve at the wrist renders it liable to injury in lacerations sustained by falling against a window with the hand outstretched or in suicidal attempts. It may also be damaged as an occupational hazard by individuals who exert repeated pressure on the butt of the hand.

Much the most common lesion at this site is the carpal tunnel syndrome, in which the median nerve is compressed as it passes deep to the flexor retinaculum. The usual presentation is with acroparaesthesiae. These consist of numbness, tingling, and burning sensations felt in the hand and fingers, the pain sometimes radiating up the forearm as far as the elbow or even as high as the shoulder or root of the neck. The

paraesthesiae are sometimes restricted to the radial fingers, but may affect all the digits as some fibres from the median nerve are distributed to the fifth finger through a communication with the ulnar nerve in the palm. The attacks of pain and paraesthesiae are most common at night and often wake the patient from sleep. They are then relieved by shaking the hand. The hand tends to feel numb and useless on waking in the morning but recovers after it has been used for some minutes. The symptoms may recur during the day following use, or at times if the patient sits with the hands immobile. Such symptoms of acroparaesthesiae may persist for many years without the appearance of symptoms of median nerve damage. In other patients, weakness of the thenar muscles develops, particularly of abduction of the thumb, and is associated with atrophy of the lateral aspect of the thenar eminence (Fig. 1). Sensory loss may appear over the tips of the median innervated fingers. Occasionally patients present with symptoms of median nerve deficit in the hand without attacks of acroparaesthesiae having occurred, or motor and sensory signs may be discovered incidentally in the absence of symptoms, particularly in older individuals.

The symptoms are usually characteristic. If confirmation is required in atypical cases, this can generally be obtained by nerve conduction studies. In patients who are experiencing frequent attacks of acroparaesthesiae, the symptoms may be reproduced by inflating a sphygmomanometer cuff around the arm above arterial pressure for two minutes. At times percussion over the carpal tunnel may elicit a Tinel's sign, or symptoms may be provoked by hyperextension of the wrist or sustained flexion (Phalen's sign).

The majority of cases occur in middle-aged and often obese housewives. In younger women it is commonly associated with excessive use of the hands, and it may develop in males after unaccustomed use of the hands, such as in house-painting. In these instances, tenosynovitis of the flexor tendons is responsible. It may also be caused by tuberculous tenosynovitis at the wrist or involvement of the wrist joint in rheumatoid arthritis. It may develop as a consequence of osteoarthritis of the carpus, perhaps related to an old fracture. Other predisposing causes are pregnancy, myxoedema, acromegaly, and infiltration of the flexor retinaculum in primary and hereditary amyloidosis.

In cases in which muscle weakness and wasting, or sensory loss, are present when the patient is first seen, treatment should be decompression

Fig. 1 Thenar wasting in a patient with the carpal tunnel syndrome.

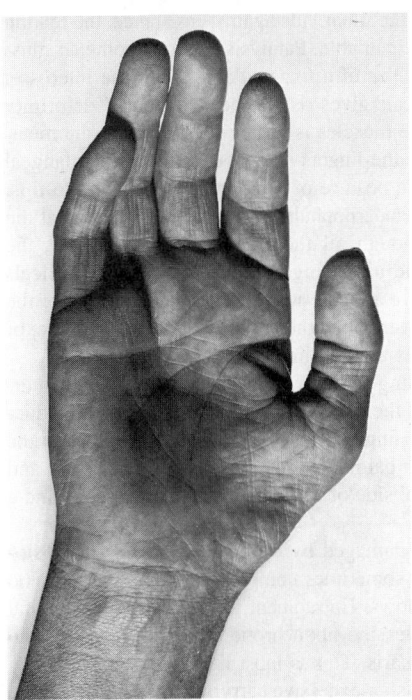

of the nerve by section of the flexor retinaculum. In patients with acro-paraesthesiae alone and in which the cause is probably tenosynovitis at the wrist, reduction in the amount of activity engaged in with the hands may be sufficient to allow the symptoms to subside. Injection of the carpal tunnel with a long-acting corticosteroid preparation may give temporary relief. Splinting of the wrist to reduce movement during the day may also be useful. If the symptoms persist despite conservative measures, decompression is then advisable.

The majority of patients with acroparaesthesiae are relieved by decompression. In patients with sensory impairment and cutaneous hyperaesthesia, such symptoms may persist for prolonged periods and if denervation of the thenar muscles has been present for any length of time, recovery may not occur.

ULNAR NERVE ($C_{7,8}T_1$)

This nerve arises from the medial cord of the plexus, usually with a contribution from the lateral cord. It descends in the medial side of the upper arm, passes around the elbow in the ulnar groove and enters the forearm under an aponeurotic band between the humeral and ulnar heads of flexor carpi ulnaris. It then runs superficial to flexor digitorum profundus to the wrist and enters the hand between the pisiform bone and the hook of the hamate, superficial to the flexor retinaculum. After penetrating the hypothenar muscles, its deep branch crosses the palm and ends in the flexor pollicis brevis.

In the upper arm, branches arise that supply flexor carpi ulnaris and the medial part of flexor digitorum profundus. In the forearm, the dorsal branch arises that winds around the ulna and supplies the skin over the dorsal aspect of the hand and the medial one and a half fingers. In the hand, a superficial branch supplies palmaris brevis and the skin over the medial aspect of the palm and the medial one and half fingers. The deep branch, after supplying the hypothenar muscles, innervates the interossei, the third and fourth lumbricals, the adductor pollicis, and part of flexor pollicis brevis.

Lesions at the elbow

Total paralysis from lesions at this level, including the branches to flexor carpi ulnaris and flexor digitorum profundus, gives rise to wasting along the medial side of the forearm flexor mass. There is weakness of flexion of the fourth and fifth fingers. If the proximal portions of these fingers are held immobilized, flexion of the terminal phalanges is not possible. When the hand is flexed to the ulnar side against resistance, the tendon of flexor carpi ulnaris is not palpable. Paralysis of the hypothenar muscles abolishes abduction of the fifth finger. Paralysis of the interossei and the medial two lumbricals gives rise to the 'claw-hand' deformity (Fig. 2). The action of these muscles is to flex the fingers at the metacarpophalangeal joints with the fingers extended at the interphalangeal joints. In the claw hand, the posture of the fingers is opposite to this, namely, extension of the metacarpophalangeal joints with flexion at the interphalangeal joints. Although all the interossei are paralysed, the defect is seen mainly in the ulnar fingers since the radial lumbricals supplied by the median nerve are still active. The long extensors of the fingers, being unopposed, overextend the proximal joints, and the flexor digitorum superficialis flexes the proximal interphalangeal joints.

In the hand, there is wasting of the hypothenar muscles, of the interossei, and the medial part of the thenar eminence. Movements of abduction and adduction of the fingers are weak, as is adduction to the extended thumb against the palm. Sensory loss affects the dorsal and palmar aspects of the medial side of the hand and the medial one and a half fingers.

The ulnar nerve may be damaged by dislocations or fracture dislocations at the elbow and is sometimes compressed in individuals who habitually lean on their elbows. Entrapment may occur in the cubital tunnel as the nerve underlies the aponeurotic band between the two heads of the flexor carpi ulnaris. This is most likely to occur in heavy manual workers or if there is an excessive carrying angle at the elbow,

as may occur following a previous malunited supracondylar fracture of the humerus ('tardy ulnar palsy'). The medial wall of the cubital tunnel is formed by the elbow joint; osteoarthritis of the elbow can lead to osteophytic encroachment on the tunnel and compression of the ulnar nerve. In the cubital tunnel syndrome, the ulnar nerve is often palpably enlarged in the ulnar groove and for a short distance proximally. Ulnar nerve lesions are not infrequent in leprosy. Here the enlargement of the nerve tends to be maximal at a little distance above the elbow.

When it is suspected that the nerve has been subjected to repeated compression at the elbow, surgical transposition to the front of the medial epicondyle should be considered. If the nerve is compressed in the cubital tunnel, decompression by slitting the aponeurosis may suffice.

Lesions at the wrist or in the hand

Damage to the nerve at the wrist will spare the dorsal branch, so that cutaneous sensation over the dorsum of the hand and fingers is spared. A lesion just proximal to the wrist will give rise to sensory impairment on the palmar aspect of the hand and fingers alone, and weakness of all the ulnar-innervated intrinsic hand muscles. A slightly more distal lesion spares the superficial branch of the nerve and therefore produces no sensory deficit. Finally, damage to the deep palmar branch spares the hypothenar muscles, but causes weakness of the other ulnar-innervated small hand muscles. Lesions at the wrist or in the hand are usually the result of compression by ganglia or by repeated occupational trauma. Damage to the deep palmar branch, for example, may be caused by firm pressure from a screwdriver or drill. If occupational pressure is the cause, recovery follows cessation of the precipitating cause. Should improvement fail to occur after an appropriate interval, surgical exploration to establish whether a ganglion is present is merited.

It is not always easy on clinical grounds to decide whether the lesion is at the elbow or the wrist. Compression of the nerve in the cubital tunnel, for example, may spare the branches of the flexor carpi ulnaris and flexor digitorum profundus. In these circumstances, nerve conduction studies may be helpful, as they may in distinguishing between

Fig. 2 Claw-hand deformity in a patient with an ulnar nerve lesion.

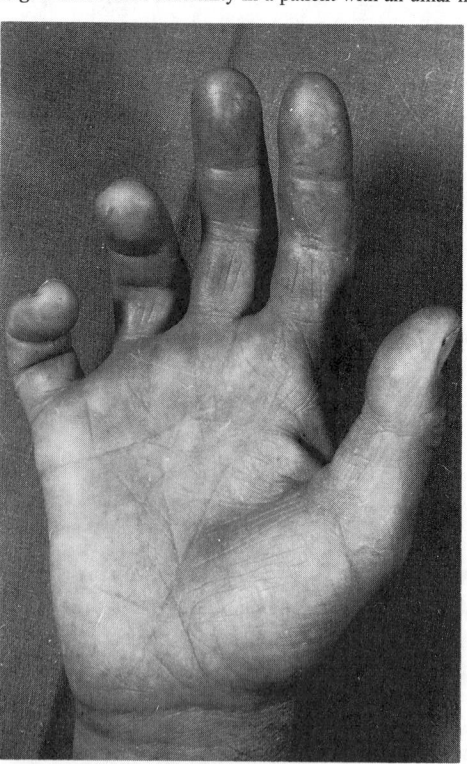

lesions of the ulnar nerve and damage to the eighth cervical and first thoracic spinal roots.

LUMBOSACRAL PLEXUS

Lesions of the lumbosacral plexus are not common. The plexus may be involved in pelvic malignancy, such as from carcinoma of the cervix, bladder, prostate, or rectum, or be the site of a local neural tumour. It may be compressed by a haematoma in patients receiving anticoagulant therapy or suffering from haemophilia, or be involved in fractures of the pelvis. The lumbosacral cord may be compressed against the rim of the pelvis by the fetal head during parturition, with consequent weakness of the anterior tibial and peroneal muscles, and sensory impairment in the distribution of the fourth and fifth lumbar dermatomes. The superior gluteal nerve may also be affected. Recovery is initially good but may not be complete. Rare instances of idiopathic lumbosacral plexus neuropathy are encountered, comparable to the corresponding disorder that affects the brachial plexus.

FEMORAL NERVE (L_{2-4})

This nerve arises from the lumbar plexus, crosses the iliac fossa between the psoas and iliacus muscles, and enters the thigh deep to the middle of the inguinal ligament. In the iliac fossa it supplies the iliacus, and in the thigh, pectineus, sartorius, and quadriceps femoris, and anterior cutaneous branches to the front of the thigh. The continuation of the femoral nerve is the saphenous which supplies the skin over the medial aspect of the lower leg as far as the medial malleolus.

Damage to the femoral nerve causes weakness of knee extension, wasting of the quadriceps, loss of the knee jerk, and sensory impairment over the front of the thigh and in the distribution of the saphenous nerve. With a proximal lesion, there may also be weakness of hip flexion from paralysis of iliacus.

The femoral nerve may be injured in fractures of the pelvis or femur, in dislocations of the hip, and at times during operations on the hip. It may be involved by psoas abscesses, tumours, or implicated in wounds of the thigh. It is commonly involved in large psoas muscle haematomas in haemophiliacs (see Section 22). Owing to the rapid dispersion of the branches in the thigh, partial lesions are common from wounds at this site. The nerve to quadriceps is most often injured. The resulting paralysis causes considerable difficulty in walking as the knee cannot be locked in extension and gives way, especially when descending stairs. The saphenous nerve is sometimes damaged in operations for the treatment of varicose veins.

OBTURATOR NERVE (L_{2-4})

The nerve emerges from the lateral border of psoas, crosses the lateral wall of the pelvis, and enters the thigh through the obturator foramen where it supplies gracilis, adductor longus and brevis, adductor magnus, obturator externus, and sometimes also pectineus, and the skin over the lower medial aspect of the thigh.

Damage to the obturator nerve results in weakness of adduction and internal rotation at the hip, pain in the groin, and sensory impairment on the medial part of the thigh. The nerve may be involved in neoplastic infiltration in the pelvis and can be damaged by the fetal head or by forceps during parturition.

LATERAL CUTANEOUS NERVE OF THE THIGH ($L_{2,3}$)

This nerve arises from the lumbar plexus, passes obliquely across the iliacus and enters the thigh under the lateral part of the inguinal ligament. It supplies the skin over the anterolateral aspect of the thigh.

Meralgia paraesthetica is an entrapment neuropathy resulting from compression of this nerve as it passes under the inguinal ligament. It is more common in men, who are often obese, and may be unilateral or bilateral. The symptoms consist of numbness in the territory of the nerve combined with tingling or burning paraesthesiae provoked by prolonged standing, or following excessive walking. Weight reduction may be helpful and in many instances the condition subsides spontaneously. Decompression of the nerve is rarely necessary.

SCIATIC NERVE ($L_{4,5}$ S_{1-3})

The sciatic nerve enters the thigh through the sciatic notch. It is composed of the tibial and peroneal divisions which are usually bound together within a common sheath. It descends the posterior aspect of the thigh, initially deep to gluteus maximus and supplies semitendinosus, semimembranosus and the long head of biceps through its peroneal division. It separates into the tibial and common peroneal nerves in the lower thigh, which supply all the muscles below the knee, and both nerves contribute to the formation of the sural nerve.

Total interruption of the sciatic nerve gives rise to foot drop. Walking is possible, but the patient cannot stand on the toes or the heel of the affected foot and the ankle is unstable. All movement below the knee is paralysed. If the injury is in the upper thigh, flexion of the knee is also weak. The skin is completely anaesthetic over the entire foot except for the medial border which is supplied by the saphenous nerve. Pressure sores may develop. The anaesthesia extends upwards on the posterolateral aspect of the calf in its lower two-thirds. Joint position sense is abolished in the foot and toes. Beyond this area of complete anaesthesia, there is a wide zone in which sensibility may be diminished. Sweating is absent on the sole and dorsum of the foot, but is preserved on the medial side. The ankle jerk is lost but the knee jerk is retained.

The sciatic nerve may be involved in pelvic tumours or injured by fractures of the pelvis or femur. After the radial and ulnar, it is implicated in gunshot wounds more frequently than any other nerve. Partial injury of the tibial division may be followed by causalgia. Incomplete lesions of the nerve may be caused by pressure of the nerve against the hard edge of a chair in individuals who fall asleep while intoxicated. Similar lesions may occur in diabetic subjects, in whom the peripheral nerves are more susceptible to pressure neuropathy.

The syndrome of root pain and sciatica is considered in Chapter 24.3.11.

TIBIAL NERVE ($L_{4,5}$ S_{1-3})

After separating from the peroneal division of the sciatic nerve in the lower thigh, this nerve passes through the popliteal fossa and enters the calf deep to gastrocnemius through the fibrous arch of soleus. It descends through the calf to the medial side of the ankle, passes beneath the flexor retinaculum, and divides into the medial and lateral plantar nerves. It supplies the popliteus, all the muscles of the calf, and through the plantar nerves, the small muscles of the sole of the foot and sensation to the sole.

When the nerve is interrupted, the patient is unable to plantarflex or invert the foot, or flex the toes. He cannot stand on the ball of the foot. Paralysis of the interossei leads to a claw-like deformity of the toes. Sensation is lost over the sole. Causalgia may arise after partial lesions. Injury to the distal portion of the nerve by a penetrating injury or deep wound of the calf gives rise to paralysis of the intrinsic muscles of the foot but spares the muscles acting at the ankle. Sensation is lost on the sole of the foot and this may be accompanied by pain. If the injury is distal to the origin of the branches to flexor hallucis longus and flexor digitorum longus, the lesion may escape detection since paralysis of the small foot muscles and sensory loss over the sole may be overlooked.

The tibial nerve is occasionally compressed under the flexor retinaculum (tarsal tunnel syndrome), usually precipitated by osteoarthritis or post-traumatic deformities at the ankle or by tenosynovitis. Burning pain and tingling paraesthesiae occur in the sole, usually following prolonged standing or walking. The condition is generally unilateral. Careful examination may demonstrate wasting of the intrinsic muscles in the medial aspect of the foot, and sensory impairment over the sole. Nerve conduction studies may be diagnostically helpful. Treatment is by surgical section of the flexor retinaculum.

Painful neuromas sometimes develop on the digital branches of the plantar nerves. These give rise to the syndrome of Morton's metatarsalgia in which pain occurs in the anterior part of the foot on standing. A localized area of tenderness is detectable on palpation. The condition is relieved by excision of the neuroma.

COMMON PERONEAL NERVE (L$_{4,5}$ S$_{1,2}$)

After separating from the tibial division of the sciatic nerve in the lower part of the thigh, this nerve descends through the popliteal fossa, winds around the neck of the fibula, and divides into its superficial and deep branches. The superficial peroneal nerve passes down in front of the fibula, supplies peroneus longus and brevis, and emerges in the lower leg, supplying the skin on the lateral aspect of the lower leg. It crosses the extensor retinaculum and supplies the skin on the dorsum of the foot and the second to the fifth toes. The deep peroneal branch continues to wind around the fibula, pierces the anterior intermuscular septum, and descends on the anterior interosseous membrane. It innervates tibialis anterior, extensor hallucis longus, extensor digitorum longus, and peroneus tertius. It passes deep to the extensor retinaculum where it supplies the extensor digitorum brevis and the skin of the adjacent sides of the first and second toes.

Damage to the common peroneal nerve is more frequent than injury to its two branches because of its vulnerable superficial position at the neck of the fibula. It gives rise to foot drop with paralysis of dorsiflexion and eversion at the ankle and of toe extension. Cutaneous sensation is impaired over the lateral aspect of the lower leg and ankle and on the dorsum of the foot.

The common peroneal nerve may be compressed at the neck of the fibula by habitual sitting with the legs crossed, prolonged squatting, pressure during sleep or while anaesthetized, and various other events. It can be damaged by traction caused by fractures of the tibia and fibula and is sometimes damaged by ischaemia in the anterior tibial compartment syndrome. Paralysis caused by external pressure frequently gives rise to a local conduction block (neurapraxia) with satisfactory recovery within a few weeks. If electromyography indicates that nerve degeneration has taken place a foot drop support should be provided while axonal regeneration is awaited.

SURAL NERVE (L$_5$ S$_{1-2}$)

This arises from the sciatic nerve and descends to the back of the calf, winds around to the lateral side of the ankle, and reaches the lateral border of the foot. It supplies the skin in this distribution. Sensory impairment occasionally results from pressure on the nerve as it lies in a superficial situation in the back of the calf.

Generalized neuropathies

NEUROPATHIES RELATED TO METABOLIC AND ENDOCRINE DISORDERS

Diabetes mellitus

A significant degree of peripheral neuropathy develops in about 15 per cent of patients with diabetes, although a substantially greater number either have minor symptoms without signs, or evidence of a subclinical neuropathy either on clinical examination or on the basis of abnormalities of nerve conduction. In general, the neuropathies that appear can be divided into symmetrical sensory polyneuropathies and autonomic neuropathies on the one hand, and isolated peripheral nerve lesions or multifocal neuropathies on the other. Mixed syndromes are common.

The commonest form is a mild symmetrical sensory polyneuropathy, giving rise to numbness and tingling paraesthesiae in the toes and feet and less often in the fingers. Aching or lancinating pains in the feet and

legs, particularly at night, may be a troublesome feature. Examination reveals loss of vibration sense in the feet, depression of the ankle jerks, and mild distal cutaneous sensory impairment. More rarely a more severe sensory neuropathy develops, sometimes referred to as 'diabetic pseudotabes'. Loss of pain sense results in perforating ulcers on the feet and neuropathic joint degeneration, particularly in the toes and in the tarsal joints; impaired postural sense gives rise to an ataxic gait. An acute painful diabetic neuropathy also occurs that predominantly affects the lower limbs. The onset is often associated with poor diabetic control and precipitate weight loss ('diabetic neuropathic cachexia').

Autonomic neuropathy frequently accompanies the sensory neuropathy and may be the salient manifestation. It rarely occurs in isolation. Pupillary disturbances usually take the form of a reduced response to light. Gustatory sweating on the face is probably due to aberrant regeneration. Anhidrosis may occur distally in the limbs; if it is extensive and also affects the trunk, heat intolerance may result. Symptoms referable to the alimentary tract include dysphagia from oesophageal involvement, episodes of vomiting related to gastric atony, and episodic nocturnal diarrhoea, often alternating with periods of constipation. Those related to the genitourinary system include impotence, retrograde ejaculation, and bladder atony with difficulty in voiding and urinary retention with overflow. Vascular denervation sometimes results in postural hypotension, and cardiac denervation may be demonstrable by an elevated resting heart rate and the absence of beat-to-beat variation with respiration.

Isolated nerve lesions tend to occur more commonly in elderly diabetic subjects. At times they develop insidiously, at others they have an abrupt onset with pain. Of the cranial nerves, the nerves to the external ocular muscles, particularly the third, and also the facial nerve, are the most often affected. In contradistinction to the effects of compression of the third nerve by a carotid aneurysm, the pupillary innervation is often spared. In the limbs, the lesions tend to occur at the common sites of compression or entrapment. It seems likely that diabetic nerve exhibits an excessive vulnerability to damage from pressure.

Diabetic amyotrophy represents a particular example of a multifocal neuropathy that develops usually in elderly obese diabetics. It consists of an asymmetrical proximal motor syndrome that affects the anterior thigh muscles and hip flexors, and sometimes also the anterolateral muscles of the lower leg. Less commonly it is symmetrical. Its onset may be acute or insidious and is often accompanied by pain, particularly at night. There is generally little or no associated sensory loss. The knee jerks are usually depressed or absent.

The causation of diabetic neuropathy is uncertain. It tends to occur more often in poorly controlled diabetics, but the correlation is not close. It may occur for the first time on initiation of treatment with insulin, or be the presenting symptom in maturity onset diabetes. There is evidence to suggest that diabetic microangiopathy is important in the genesis of isolated nerve lesions. Probably metabolic factors are more important in the origin of the symmetrical polyneuropathies, but their nature is uncertain. An increased concentration of sorbitol secondary to hyperglycaemia may be involved in causing nerve fibre dysfunction.

Focal peripheral nerve lesions and diabetic amyotrophy, if of acute onset, often recover adequately, as does acute painful diabetic neuropathy when satisfactory control is achieved. The symmetrical sensory and autonomic neuropathy, once established, recovers less satisfactorily, even with good diabetic control. Correcting the hyperglycaemia by continuous subcutaneous insulin infusion or pancreatic transplantation will stabilize the neuropathy. Trials of aldose reductase inhibitors to reduce sorbitol accumulation have, so far, not given clear evidence of improvement in neuropathy.

Care of the feet is vitally important in diabetic sensory neuropathy, to prevent the development of chronic ulceration. Pain may sometimes be helped by carbamazepine, tricyclic antidepressants, phenothiazines, or mexiletine. Postural hypotension can be improved by raising the head of the bed at night or by support bandages to the legs; more severe cases may require treatment with fludrocortisone. Gastroparesis may respond to metoclopramide, domperidone, or erythromycin; persistent vomiting may necessitate a Roux-en-Y gastroenterostomy. Diabetic diarrhoea can be helped by low-dosage tetracycline or diphenoxylate, loperamide, or codeine phosphate. Diabetic cystopathy can be managed in the earlier stages by regular voiding and cholinergic treatment with bethanechol. Urinary tract infections should be treated promptly. Bladder neck resection can be useful in carefully selected cases. Penile papaverine injections can be employed for erectile impotence. Silicone implants should be avoided because of the risk of infection.

Amyloidosis

The various forms of amyloid disease are described in Section 11. The peripheral nerves may be involved in primary amyloidosis and in amyloidosis related to myeloma. There are also several dominantly inherited forms of amyloid neuropathy, the most important being the Portuguese type (see later). Isolated lesions may occur from the infiltration of amyloid into nerves or from compression of the median nerve in the carpal tunnel because of deposits in the flexor retinaculum. More strikingly, a generalized neuropathy may develop. It begins with selective loss of pain and temperature sensation in the feet and later in the hands. Motor involvement, loss of tendon reflexes, and impairment of other sensory modalities occur later. Autonomic involvement is an early feature, causing impotence, postural hypotension, bladder atony, and disturbances of alimentary function. Amyloid deposits are present in the peripheral nerve trunks, which may be enlarged, and in the dorsal root and sympathetic ganglia.

No treatment influences the progress of the neuropathy except possibly in the inherited form. The spontaneous pains are sometimes improved by carbamazepine. Care must be taken to prevent damage to the anaesthetic feet, lower legs, and hands. Autonomic symptoms may require treatment as described for diabetic neuropathy.

Uraemia

Uraemic neuropathy did not become a clinical problem until the advent of treatment of endstage renal failure by haemodialysis. It occurs in patients with severe chronic renal failure. It was most often seen in patients under treatment with periodic haemodialysis but is now much less frequently a problem. The symptoms are usually predominantly sensory, with numbness and tingling paraesthesiae in the feet. 'Restless legs' (Ekbom's syndrome) are often a conspicuous feature (see Section 25). A distal motor neuropathy may be associated and occasional cases are purely motor. The condition is improved by increased haemodialysis and more dramatically by renal transplantation. A retained metabolite is assumed to be the cause, but this has not so far been identified.

Myxoedema

Compression of the median nerve in the carpal tunnel in myxoedema has already been discussed. Rarely a generalized mixed motor and sensory neuropathy develops. This improves on treatment of the hypothyroidism.

The slow contraction and relaxation observed in the tendon reflexes is not due to a disturbance of peripheral nerve function, but to an alteration in the contractile mechanism of the muscle fibres.

Acromegaly (see Section 12)

The occurrence of the carpal tunnel syndrome in acromegaly has also been mentioned. A rare manifestation of this condition is a sensorimotor polyneuropathy in which the peripheral nerves are thickened because of an overgrowth of the neural connective tissues. A similar neuropathy is occasionally observed in pituitary gigantism.

Critical illness polyneuropathy

A generalized polyneuropathy involving widespread axonal degeneration may be encountered in patients in intensive care units with sepsis and multiple organ failure. The neuropathy is discovered when attempts are made to wean them from the ventilator. The precise cause of this condition which has been termed critical illness polyneuropathy is unknown. Slow recovery occurs.

Other metabolic disorders

It has been claimed that a generalized peripheral neuropathy may be caused by either acute or chronic hepatic failure, but this is probably uncommon. A mild painful sensory neuropathy is occasionally encountered in primary biliary cirrhosis, sometimes related to xanthomatous deposits in the cutaneous nerve trunks. A motor neuropathy is a rare sequel to severe recurrent hypoglycaemia.

TOXIC NEUROPATHIES

Industrial and environmental substances

Acrylamide

This substance is now widely employed industrially. The monomer is neurotoxic and causes peripheral neuropathy with mixed motor and sensory features. Ataxia is prominent and is possibly the result of concomitant cerebellar damage. Axonal degeneration affecting the periphery of the fibres occurs and slow recovery takes place on cessation of exposure.

Arsenic

Arsenical poisoning is occasionally seen as a result of accidental or homicidal ingestion of insecticides containing arsenic, or from indigenous medicines in India. Gastrointestinal symptoms develop after acute ingestion, followed by a mixed sensory and motor neuropathy after 1 to 3 weeks. Desquamation of the skin of the feet and hands takes place after about 6 weeks and white lines (Mees' lines) appear in the nails. With ingestion of smaller quantities on a chronic basis, gastrointestinal symptoms are less obtrusive and a slowly progressive neuropathy makes its appearance. The skin may become generally pigmented or show focal 'raindrop' pigmentation, and hyperkeratosis of the palms of the hands and soles of the feet may appear.

Slow recovery in the neuropathy occurs with removal from exposure. Chelating agents are of value in treating the non-neurological complications, but it is uncertain whether they are effective for the neuropathy.

Lead

Lead neuropathy is now a rare occurrence in Britain, although it was encountered as a consequence of the contamination of drinking water by lead pipes in old buildings. Subclinical neuropathy may be detectable in lead workers. It remains a hazard in certain parts of the world from the use of lead glazes in pottery. Lead neuropathy is predominantly motor, typically giving rise to wrist and foot drop. The 'lead colic' that may occur is probably a manifestation of autonomic involvement. Other features of lead poisoning that may be associated include a sideroblastic anaemia and a 'lead line' on carious teeth. The neuropathy improves on cessation of lead intake; the utility of treatment with BAL, edetate, or penicillamine is uncertain.

Mercury

Exposure to inorganic mercury salts and to organic mercurial compounds may lead to neurological damage, as in 'Minamata disease' which was related to consumption of fish contaminated by organic mercury. Dementia, cortical blindness, and ataxia occur, together with sensory changes in the limbs attributed to a sensory neuropathy, although how far these have a peripheral origin is uncertain. Historically, a peripheral neuropathy was an important component of 'pink disease' which was caused by the administration of mercury-containing purgatives.

Thallium

This is present in certain pesticides and rodent poisons and was formerly used as a depilatory agent. Accidental or homicidal poisoning is occasionally encountered. Abdominal pain and diarrhoea are followed after 2 or 5 days by the development of a mixed motor and sensory neuropathy which is often painful. Evidence of central nervous system damage may be present with behaviour disorder, optic neuropathy, and choreiform movements. Alopecia develops later, after about 2 or 3 weeks, and renal damage may be produced. Diethyldithiocarbamate, which binds thallium, has been employed in treatment.

Triorthocresyl phosphate (TOCP)

This substance is used industrially as a high-temperature lubricant. Outbreaks of a sensorimotor neuropathy, often accompanied by evidence of CNS damage, occur periodically, usually as a consequence of the contamination of cooking ingredients or utensils. The original description was in relation to illegal liquor distillation (ginger jake paralysis) in the United States during the prohibition era. In more recent years, a large outbreak occurred in Morocco from the use of contaminated cooking oil. Recovery is slow and often incomplete.

Other industrial substances

Carbon disulphide, used in the manufacture of rayon, occasionally gives rise to a mild sensory neuropathy. Neuropathy may occur as a result of industrial exposure to the organic solvents n-hexane and methyl n-butyl ketone. The former is also encountered as a consequence of 'glue-sniffing'; n-hexane, which has an intoxicant action, has been used as a solvent in certain glues. Other industrial agents causing neuropathy are ethylene oxide and methyl bromide. Trichlorethylene (or an impurity) has caused trigeminal neuropathy.

Iatrogenic

Cisplatin

This platinum derivative (cis-diamminedichloroplatinum) is used in the treatment of malignancy, including carcinoma of the ovary. A predominantly sensory neuropathy that recovers poorly may develop after the administration of several courses. Ototoxicity is more frequent, causing high-tone deafness and tinnitus.

Isoniazid

A mixed motor and sensory neuropathy may be produced by isoniazid and is more likely to occur in individuals who acetylate the drug slowly. The neuropathy is related to an interference with pyridoxine metabolism. Axonal degeneration occurs in the peripheral nerves. The neuropathy recovers slowly on cessation of administration of the drug and may be prevented by giving pyridoxine, which does not interfere with the antituberculous action of the isoniazid.

Nitrofurantoin

Excessively high blood levels of this preparation, as may occur in patients with reduced renal function, can cause a mixed motor and sensory neuropathy.

Vincristine

A neuropathy will occur in all subjects if sufficient amounts of this cytotoxic agent are administered. Mild sensory symptoms and loss of tendon reflexes may have to be accepted if a satisfactory therapeutic effect of the drug is to be achieved. If the neuropathy advances, bilateral weakness of the extensors of the wrist and fingers develops, followed by more widespread weakness. The neuropathy improves satisfactorily if the drug is withdrawn or if the dosage is reduced.

Other substances

Less important drugs that may give rise to neuropathy are almitrine, amiodarone, dapsone, disulfiram, gold, metronidazole, misonidazole, nitrous oxide (with a myelopathy) perhexilene, suramin and zimeldine. A mild sensory neuropathy may develop after prolonged administration of phenytoin, and neuropathy was one of the complications produced by thalidomide. Pyridoxine, if taken in large doses, as 'megavitamin therapy', causes a sensory neuropathy.

DEFICIENCY NEUROPATHIES

Beri beri neuropathy (see also Section 10)

This disorder is predominantly encountered in populations subsisting on diets composed largely of polished rice, but a similar neuropathy may be observed in other malnourished communities. Thiamine deficiency is probably involved, but a deficiency of other vitamins of the B group may also be implicated. A distal motor and sensory neuropathy develops which is frequently accompanied by spontaneous aching pain in the extremities, cutaneous hyperaesthesia, and tenderness of the soles of the feet and calves. Involvement of the recurrent laryngeal nerves may lead to hoarseness of the voice. The neuropathy may be associated with a cardiomyopathy ('wet beri beri'). Thiamine deficiency is established by the finding of reduced erythrocyte transketolase activity. This enzyme requires thiamine as a cofactor.

Axonal degeneration occurs in the peripheral nerves and slow recovery ensues with vitamin replacement.

Strachan's syndrome

Strachan's syndrome, originally described in Jamaica but also observed in other parts of the world under conditions of nutritional deficiency, is characterized by the combination of a painful sensory neuropathy with amblyopia and at times deafness, in association with an orogenital dermatitis. It is assumed to be due to B vitamin deficiency, but the precise deficit has not been identified.

Alcoholic neuropathy

This always occurs on a background of nutritional deficiency. The dietary intake of the alcoholic is high in carbohydrates and low in vitamins. Moreover, alcoholics are known to have a reduced capacity to absorb thiamine. A direct toxic effect of alcohol on peripheral nerves may also be involved. The clinical features of alcoholic neuropathy are similar to those of beri beri. Other deficiency states may coexist, such as the Wernicke–Korsakoff syndrome. Improvement may take place with vitamin replacement, but it is beset with the usual difficulties met in treating alcoholic patients.

Pyridoxine deficiency

Attention has already been drawn to the fact that isoniazid neuropathy is related to an interference with pyridoxine metabolism. Pyridoxine deficiency may contribute to the neuropathy that occurs in nutritional deficiency states, and possibly accounts for the mild neuropathy of pellagra.

Pantothenic acid deficiency

Experimental deficiency of pantothenic acid in human volunteers is known to give rise to a sensory neuropathy, and the administration of pantothenic acid has been reported to alleviate the 'burning feet' syndrome which sometimes develops in deficiency states.

Vitamin B$_{12}$ deficiency

Vitamin B$_{12}$ deficiency from whatever cause, may be responsible for the development of a distal sensory neuropathy, with 'glove and stocking' sensory loss and paraesthesiae, and areflexia, either in isolation or in association with a myelopathy or other central nervous system manifestations. Haematological changes are not always present. The peripheral neuropathy improves more satisfactorily with treatment than the central disturbances. This condition is considered in detail in Chapter 24.3.9.

A peripheral neuropathy is one component of Nigerian ataxic neuropathy, in which the other features are posterior column degeneration, sensorineural deafness, and optic atrophy. It has been suggested that an interference with vitamin B$_{12}$ metabolism by cyanide derived from cassava in the diet, combined with nutritional deficiency, may be responsible.

Chronic severe vitamin E deficiency has recently been established as a cause for peripheral neuropathy in combination with a spinocerebellar degeneration. This may occur in abetalipoproteinaemia, and isolated vitamin E deficiency, both of autosomal recessive inheritance, and in congenital biliary atresia, cystic fibrosis, and occasional adults with chronic intestinal malabsorption.

INFLAMMATORY AND POSTINFECTIVE NEUROPATHIES

Leprous neuropathy
Peripheral nerve involvement in leprosy is considered in Section 7.

Guillain–Barré syndrome (acute idiopathic inflammatory polyneuropathy)
The Guillain–Barré syndrome is characterized by a polyneuropathy that develops over the course of a few days up to maximum of 4 weeks. Cases that progress for up to 8 weeks (subacute Guillain–Barré syndrome) are probably distinct. An identifiable infection may precede the onset of the neuropathy by 1 to 3 weeks. This is commonly an upper respiratory tract infection or an infection with an enterovirus, Epstein–Barr virus, or mycoplasma. More recently, *Campylobacter jejuni* has been recognized as an important cause, as has human immunodeficiency virus (**HIV**) infection. Other cases may follow surgical operations. In approximately 40 per cent of cases no antecedent event is identifiable.

The neuropathy may be ushered in by severe lumbar or interscapular pain. Motor involvement usually predominates over sensory loss and may be of a proximal, distal, or generalized distribution, and in severe cases affects the respiratory musculature. Distal paraesthesiae in the limbs are common and, if sensory loss occurs, it tends to affect tactile, vibratory, and postural sensibility. The cranial nerves may be affected, in particular the facial nerves, but bulbar involvement also occurs sometimes. A complete 'locked-in' state may develop. Autonomic disturbances may be associated, including bladder atony, ileus, hypertension (possibly the result of denervation of the carotid sinus), and orthostatic hypotension. Associated central nervous system involvement is occasionally encountered, particularly after infectious mononucleosis, and such cases are sometimes excluded from the Guillain–Barré syndrome as such. Papilloedema sometimes develops, possibly related to impaired cerebrospinal fluid resorption because of the elevated protein content. Further variants are a combination of an external ophthalmoplegia, ataxia, and tendon areflexia (Miller Fisher syndrome), or diffuse cranial nerve involvement (polyneuritis cranialis), as possibly are instances of acute sensory neuropathy or pandysautonomia.

Nerve conduction studies reveal evidence of demyelination in most cases, but at times the findings indicate an axonopathy ('axonal' Guillain–Barré syndrome), as is seen in the acute motor neuropathy that occurs as an annual epidemic in children in northern China. The cerebrospinal fluid protein is usually raised, often to a substantial degree, but it may be normal, particularly in the early stages. The cell content is usually normal, but there may be a mild lymphocytic pleocytosis; this is more likely to occur in cases related to HIV infection or infectious mononucleosis. Histologically, the abnormalities are maximal in the spinal roots but also occur diffusely throughout the peripheral nerves. In the demyelinating form, focal perivascular accumulations of inflammatory cells are associated with segmental demyelination of the nerve fibres and relative preservation of axonal continuity. Recovery occurs by remyelination. The disease probably represents a cell-mediated hypersensitivity reaction in which myelin is stripped off the axons by mononuclear cells. Whether antibody-mediated demyelination is also involved is not yet established. Severe axonal loss may be a 'bystander effect' or represent direct axonal damage in cases of axonal Guillain–Barré syndrome.

Most cases of the Guillain–Barré syndrome recover satisfactorily within weeks or months. Severely affected patients, particularly those that require assisted respiration and in whom extensive axonal degeneration occurs, recover slowly and often show residual muscle weakness. Occasional patients have recurrences, which are sometimes multiple.

Although widely employed in the past, controlled trials of treatment with corticosteroids have shown no beneficial effects. Plasma exchange and high-dose intravenous human immunoglobulin have both been shown to improve the rate of recovery if given before the nadir of the disease. Because of significant morbidity, particularly with plasma exchange, and cost, these forms of treatment are best reserved for more severe cases. Such patients may require extensive support in an intensive care unit because of respiratory failure and autonomic dysfunction.

Chronic inflammatory demyelinating polyneuropathy
Instances of peripheral neuropathy occur that resemble the Guillain–Barré syndrome in that the neurological involvement is predominantly motor and the cerebrospinal fluid protein level is elevated, but which pursue either a chronic relapsing or chronic progressive course. They are also associated with widespread demyelination in the spinal roots and peripheral nerves and with inflammatory infiltrates. Nerve conduction velocity is usually markedly reduced and multifocal conduction block may be evident. Cases with localized involvement, most often of the brachial plexus, are occasionally encountered. Both the generalized and focal cases may respond to treatment with corticosteroids, plasma exchange, high-dose intravenous human immunoglobulin, or cytotoxic drugs. The response is less satisfactory in the chronic progressive cases.

Patients have recently been identified with a chronic multifocal motor neuropathy with persistent conduction block associated with GM1 ganglioside antibodies. They probably represent a variant of chronic inflammatory demyelinating polyneuropathy. They may respond to immunosuppressive therapy or plasma exchange.

Lyme borreliosis
Lyme borreliosis is a multisystem disease caused by a tick-borne spirochaete, *Borrelia burgdorferi* (see Chapter 7.11.30). The peripheral nervous system is frequently affected both during the phase of early disseminated infection and during the late stage. Cranial neuropathies or an acute or subacute radiculoneuritis characterize involvement in the early stages, and a mild, predominantly distal neuropathy characterizes the late stage. Nerve biopsies show perivasculitis and nerve fibre degeneration, but spirochaetes are not identifiable. Laboratory diagnosis is based on the detection of specific antibodies to *B. burgdorferi* but seronegative cases occur, as may false positive reactions. Treatment, which is with doxycycline and amoxycillin, may therefore have to be given on clinical suspicion of the disease.

Human immunodeficiency virus infection (see Chapter 24.15.3)
A variety of neuropathies may be related to HIV-1 infection, particular types tending to occur in different phases of the disease. Characteristically, the Guillain–Barré syndrome or chronic inflammatory demyelinating polyneuropathy occur at the time of seroconversion, when the patient is otherwise well, and a multifocal vasculitic neuropathy occurs in the early symptomatic stage. A distal, often predominantly sensory and painful neuropathy occurs mainly in the later AIDS phase, and an aggressive lumbosacral polyradiculoneuropathy from cytomegalovirus infection is encountered in advanced cases. Neuropathy may also occur in patients with human T-cell leukaemia virus (**HTLV-1**) infection. The treatment of HIV infection is discussed in Section 7.

Sarcoid neuropathy
Sarcoidosis (see Section 17) may give rise to a multifocal neuropathy with a particular tendency to involve the facial nerves, or to a generalized neuropathy. The neuropathy may be restricted to the cranial nerves (polyneuritis cranialis). Evidence of involvement of other systems is not always present and sarcoid tissue may or may not be detectable on nerve biopsy.

Diphtheritic neuropathy
The neuropathy of diphtheria (Section 7) is caused by the exotoxin which produces segmental demyelination by interfering with Schwann

cell function, probably by affecting protein synthesis. The nerves are not invaded by the bacteria.

Palatal weakness tends to develop after 2 to 3 weeks following pharyngeal diphtheria, and local muscle paralysis after a similar interval following cutaneous diphtheria. Paralysis of accommodation and sometimes of the external ocular muscles appears after an interval of 4 to 5 weeks. A generalized predominantly motor neuropathy of distal distribution may develop after 5 to 7 weeks. In severe cases the respiratory muscles are affected, but if death occurs it is usually as a result of an associated myocarditis.

NEUROPATHY IN AUTOIMMUNE CONNECTIVE TISSUE DISORDERS

Peripheral nerve involvement may be encountered in a wide range of the 'collagen-vascular' disorders. Polyarteritis nodosa characteristically gives rise to a multifocal neuropathy, often with considerable pain. Wegener's granulomatosis may similarly be associated with a florid neuropathy and, in both instances, the peripheral nerve damage is related to necrotizing angiitis of the vasa nervorum. Such changes may also occur in rheumatoid arthritis in association with a florid multifocal neuropathy; at other times, a less aggressive neuropathy is observed, either in the form of a distal sensory neuropathy or one restricted to the digital nerves. Entrapment neuropathies also occur in rheumatoid arthritis, for example median nerve compression in the carpal tunnel, related to articular or tendon sheath changes.

An ataxic sensory neuropathy related to a sensory ganglionitis can complicate Sjögren's syndrome. A clinical constellation that combines a distal sensory neuropathy with a trigeminal sensory neuropathy, and myotonic pupils with the sicca syndrome is particularly characteristic. A multifocal neuropathy can also be seen in patients with Sjögren's syndrome.

The neuropathy of polyarteritis nodosa or rheumatoid arthritis may respond to corticosteroids or cyclophosphamide. The neuropathy of Sjögren's syndrome is largely refractory to treatment.

NEOPLASTIC AND PARANEOPLASTIC NEUROPATHY

Peripheral neuropathy may develop as a non-metastatic complication of carcinoma, most often bronchial or gastric, or lymphoreticular proliferative disorders. The precise mechanism of production of the neuropathy is uncertain. The neuropathy may antedate the discovery of the carcinoma by as much as 2 or 3 years. In relation to carcinoma of the bronchus, the neuropathy may be purely sensory, either subacute or chronic, often with troublesome distal dysaesthesiae, or mixed sensory and motor. The sensory neuropathy is associated with circulating anti-Hu antibodies. The Guillain–Barré syndrome may be encountered in Hodgkin's disease and in chronic lymphocytic leukaemia, and a subacute, mainly motor neuropathy in relation to lymphoma. Non-metastatic carcinomatous neuropathies may regress following removal of the underlying tumour, or may remain unaffected.

Direct invasion of cranial nerves or spinal roots may occur in cases of malignant infiltration of the meninges and of the cervical and lumbosacral plexuses from local malignancies. Infiltration of peripheral nerve trunks is seen most commonly from malignant lymphomas.

PARAPROTEINAEMIC NEUROPATHY

A sensory or sensorimotor polyneuropathy related to benign monoclonal paraproteins (monoclonal gammopathies of undetermined significance) has emerged in recent years as an important cause of late onset neuropathy. The neuropathy is usually demyelinating, with features similar or identical to chronic inflammatory demyelinating polyneuropathy. A postural upper limb tremor is often a prominent feature. The paraprotein is most commonly an IgM, less frequently IgG or IgA. The IgM paraproteins can be demonstrated on surviving myelin sheaths in nerve biopsies,

where they are probably acting as demyelinating antibodies. Neuropathies associated with IgG or IgA paraproteins may respond to corticosteroids, immunosuppressive drugs, or plasma exchange; the response in IgM paraproteinaemic neuropathy is disappointing. Although a distal sensorimotor and often painful axonal neuropathy may be associated with myeloma, a demyelinating neuropathy accompanied by a dermato-endocrine syndrome may be encountered, referred to as the Crow–Fukase or POEMS syndrome (polyneuropathy, organomegaly, oedema, M protein, skin changes). Neuropathies are most often related to osteosclerotic myeloma.

Multifocal, predominantly lower limb neuropathy may be caused by single or mixed cryoglobulins in myeloma, lymphoma, systemic lupus erythematosus, rheumatoid arthritis, or Waldenström's macroglobulinaemia. They may be the result of vasculitis produced by the deposition of immune complexes in the walls of the vasa nervorum, or to intravascular precipitation of the cryoglobulin. These neuropathies occasionally respond to treatment either with immunosuppressive or cytotoxic drugs, or to repeated plasma exchange.

GENETIC NEUROPATHIES

Porphyria (see also Section 11)

A predominantly motor neuropathy may complicate acute attacks in the autosomal dominant disorders, acute intermittent and variegate porphyria and hereditary coproporphyria, and in the recessively inherited δ-aminolaevulinic acid dehydratase deficiency. It tends to affect the proximal muscles to a greater extent. There may be associated sensory loss which, although sometimes distal in distribution, can affect the trunk and the proximal portions of the limbs. The tendon reflexes are lost, with occasional paradoxical sparing of the ankle jerks. Accompanying autonomic features include abdominal pain and vomiting, tachycardia and hypertension; mental confusion, psychotic behaviour, and epilepsy may be associated.

The explanation of the neurological damage has not been established. Axonal degeneration occurs in the peripheral nerves so that recovery is slow and often incomplete.

Attacks may be provoked by a variety of drugs, including barbiturates, sulphonamides, and the contraceptive pill, and by alcohol, probably by enzyme induction in the liver (see Section 14).

Treatment with oral or intravenous glucose, or by infusions of laevulose or haematin, has been shown to reduce the urinary excretion of porphyrin precursors, but a beneficial effect on the neurological disturbances has not been established.

Familial amyloid polyneuropathy

A number of inherited amyloid neuropathies have been recognized, related to point mutations in the gene for transthyretin, formerly known as prealbumin, which is on chromosome 18. The commonest is the Portuguese type where there is a valine → methionine substitution in the transthyretin molecule. The neuropathy begins with the involvement of small nerve fibres, leading to a distal loss of pain and temperature sensation and autonomic failure. Spontaneous pain is often a feature and a mutilating acropathy frequently develops. The onset is commonly in the fourth or fifth decades and the disorder is slowly progressive, leading to death within about 10 years. Transthyretin is produced mainly in the liver and early reports suggest that liver transplantation may halt the progression of the disease. In other types of hereditary amyloid neuropathy with differing clinical features, the amyloid is derived from a variant apolipoprotein A1 (Iowa form) or plasma gelsolin (Finnish form).

Hereditary motor and sensory neuropathy, types I and II and X-linked (Charcot–Marie–Tooth disease, peroneal muscular atrophy)

Hereditary motor and sensory neuropathy (**HMSN**) types I and II usually present during childhood or adolescence with difficulty in walking or because of foot deformity. The deformity is most commonly pes cavus associated with clawing of the toes and sometimes with an equinovarus position of the foot. Muscle weakness tends to affect the lower leg muscles and may give rise to a bilateral foot drop with a 'steppage' gait. The muscle wasting is often restricted to below the knees, producing a 'stork leg' appearance (Fig. 3). Weakness and wasting of the small hand muscles may appear later. The tendon reflexes become depressed or lost, and there is a variable degree of distal sensory loss. Progress of the disease is slow and cases with little disability or who are asymptomatic are common.

In the commoner type I families, there is a diffuse demyelinating neuropathy. The onset is most frequently in the first decade. Foot deformity and scoliosis occur more often than in type II HMSN. Sensory loss and ataxia tend to be greater and generalized tendon areflexia is usual. Weakness in the hands appears earlier. The peripheral nerves may be thickened. Cases with ataxia and upper limb tremor are sometimes referred to as the Roussy–Lévy syndrome. They are not genetically distinct. The onset in the type II form, which is an axonal neuropathy, is most often in the second decade but it may be delayed until middle or even late adult life. Inheritance in both types I and II HMSN is usually autosomal dominant. The disorder in some families with HMSN I maps to chromosome 1 (HMSN Ib) and is now known to be due to mutations in the gene for myelin protein P_O. In most families the disorder (HMSN Ia) is caused by a segmental duplication of chromosome 17 which includes the gene for peripheral myelin protein 22 (PMP 22). X-linked dominant HMSN is uncommon. The clinical features resemble HMSN I but female carriers are asymptomatic or only mildly affected. The disorder is now known to be due to mutations in the gene for connexin 32, a gap junction protein.

Nerve conduction velocity is severely reduced in type I cases, moderately reduced in the X-linked form, and either normal or only slightly reduced in HMSN II.

Affected individuals may be helped by the use of orthotic appliances and sometimes by surgical correction of foot deformity or tendon transfer.

Hereditary motor and sensory neuropathy, type III (Dejerine–Sottas disease)

Although the term Dejerine–Sottas disease has been used more widely in the past, it should now be restricted to a disorder that produces a slowly progressive mixed motor and sensory polyneuropathy with an onset in childhood, often accompanied by ataxia. Inheritance is usually autosomal recessive. There is hypomyelination and extensive demyelination in the peripheral nerves, and there may be accompanying hypertrophic changes (concentric Schwann cell proliferation), a type of pathological change that was formerly termed hypertrophic interstitial neuropathy. Striking enlargement of the peripheral nerve trunks is detectable on palpation, or may even be visibly evident.

Refsum's disease

This is a rare disorder inherited as an autosomal recessive trait that gives rise to a mixed motor and sensory polyneuropathy accompanied by a variety of other clinical features, including ataxia, anosmia, pigmentary retinal degeneration, pupillary abnormalities, deafness, cardiomyopathy, and ichthyosis. The presentation is usually during adolescence or early adult life and the course may be steadily progressive or relapsing. The the peripheral nerves become thickened and display hypertrophic changes. Nerve conduction velocity is usually severely reduced.

The disorder is due to an inability to metabolize phytanic acid, a long-chain fatty acid, which accumulates in the blood and tissues. It is largely of dietary origin and clinical improvement may be achieved with diets low in phytanic acid. For acute episodes of deterioration, plasma exchange is effective.

Hereditary sensory neuropathies

Predominantly sensory neuropathies may occur with either an autosomal dominant or recessive inheritance. The symptoms in the latter instance are usually present from birth; in the former they generally develop

Fig. 3 Patient with type I hereditary motor and sensory neuropathy (Charcot–Marie–Tooth disease) showing symmetrical distal lower limb muscle wasting.

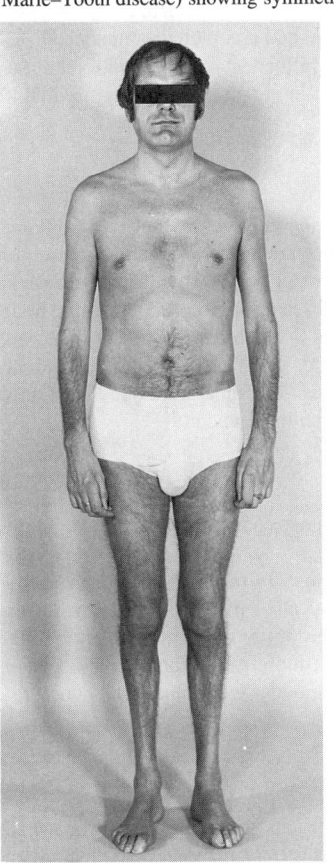

Fig. 4 Chronic foot ulceration and deformity in a case of hereditary sensory neuropathy.

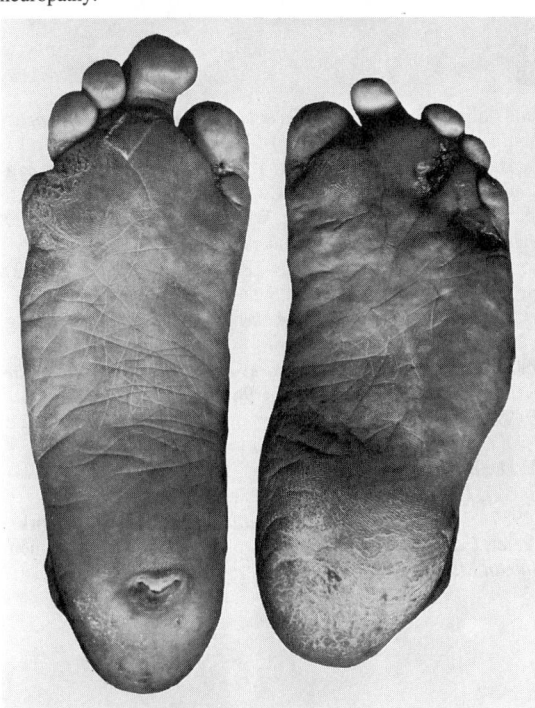

during the second or third decades. In both, the sensory loss often leads to a mutilating acropathy, with neuropathic joint degeneration and chronic cutaneous ulceration, particularly of the feet (Fig. 4). A further rare recessive neuropathy combines congenital insensitivity to pain and anhidrosis. Most cases of 'congenital insensitivity to pain' are probably examples of small-fibre neuropathies.

Familial dysautonomia

Otherwise known as the Riley–Day syndrome, this recessively inherited disorder is encountered most often in Jewish populations. There is an aplasia of peripheral autonomic neurones that leads to a variety of symptoms, including absence of tears, unexplained pyrexia, cutaneous blotching, and episodic sweating attacks. These symptoms are present at birth and are accompanied by congenital insensitivity to pain related to an associated sensory neuropathy. In early infancy there is usually difficulty in feeding because of poor sucking, and repeated episodes of pneumonia. Later, stunted growth and often kyphoscoliosis become evident. The disorder has been mapped to chromosome 9.

Other hereditary neuropathies (see also Section 11)

Peripheral nerve involvement occurs in metachromatic and globoid cell leucodystrophy and adrenomyeloneuropathy, in Fabry's disease, and in hereditary lipoprotein deficiency (Tangier disease and hereditary abetalipoproteinaemia). Certain families show an inherited liability to pressure palsies with autosomal dominant inheritance. Nerve fibres show focal regions of myelin thickening (tomacula) and are related to deletions on chromosome 17 affecting the gene for PMP 22. Giant axonal neuropathy is a rare autosomal recessive disorder with an onset in childhood, characterized by segmental axonal enlargements containing accumulations of neurofilaments. Affected children usually have abnormally curly hair.

CRYPTOGENIC NEUROPATHY

Despite extensive investigation, the cause of a substantial number of peripheral neuropathies remains unknown. This applies in particular to examples of chronic progressive axonopathies, some of which may be instances of late-onset type II hereditary motor and sensory neuropathy. A careful family history in such cases may reveal evidence of undetected neuropathy in relatives. Follow-up in other cases may disclose underlying malignancy.

REFERENCES

Asbury, A.K. and Gilliatt, R.W. (1984). *Peripheral nerve disorders. A practical approach*. Butterworths, London.

Dawson, D.M., Hallett, M., and Millender, L.H. (1990). *Entrapment neuropathies*, (2nd edn). Little, Brown and Co., Boston.

Dyck, P.J., Thomas, P.K., Asbury, A.K., Winegrad, A.I., and Porte, D. (1987). *Diabetic neuropathy*. W.B. Saunders, Philadelphia.

Dyck, P.J., Thomas, P.K., Griffin, J.G., Low, P.A., and Podulso, J. (1993). *Peripheral neuropathy*, (3rd edn). W.B. Saunders, Philadelphia.

Hughes, R.A.C. (1990). *Guillain–Barré syndrome*. Springer Verlag, London.

Kimura, J. (1980). *Electrodiagnosis of diseases of nerve and muscle. Principles and practice*, (2nd edn). F.A. Davis, Philadelphia.

Lundborg, G. (1988). *Nerve injury and repair*. Churchill Livingstone, Edinburgh.

Schaumburg, H.H., Berger, A.R., and Thomas, P.K. (1991). *Disorders of peripheral nerves*, (2nd edn). F.A. Davis, Philadelphia.

Stewart, J.D. (1987). *Focal peripheral neuropathies*. Elsevier, New York.

Suter, U. and Patel, E.I. (1994). Genetic basis of inherited peripheral neuropathies. *Human Mutation*, **3**, 95–102.

24.17.1 The POEMS syndrome

J. G. G. LEDINGHAM

INTRODUCTION

The acronym POEMS was first suggested by Bardwick and his colleagues in 1980 as an appropriate label to describe a syndrome variably combining peripheral neuropathy, organomegaly, endocrinopathy, monoclonal gammopathy, and skin changes. The term is now widely used but synonyms include the Crow–Fukase syndrome, Takatsukis syndrome, and PEP (polyneuropathy endrocrinopathy and plasma cell dyscrasia).

The cause(s) of this rare syndrome is quite obscure and the major features are not all present in individual cases. It is probably more common in the Japanese race, but this perception may be a reflection of the frequency of reporting the disease from Japan. The commonest and earliest manifestation is undoubtedly the characteristic neuropathy, and most would agree that the diagnosis should not be made in its absence. A number of disorders not included in the acronym have now been reported to coincide with the syndrome more often than can be attributed to chance (see below).

Peripheral neuropathy

A progressive sensorimotor polyneuropathy is found in nearly all cases of the syndrome and is the most common presenting feature. Beginning distally, it characteristically spreads proximally; involvement of respiratory muscles has been described but pain is unusual and cranial nerve or autonomic dysfunction are not features. There is usually an increase in the protein content of the cerebrospinal fluid, sometimes exceeding 200 mg/100 ml without abnormality in cell counts. Motor and sensory nerve conduction velocities are much reduced, and biopsy of nerve tissue shows segmental demyelination and axonal degeneration. Antibodies to myelin-associated glycoproteins have been detected in some cases in the presence of an IgM paraprotein, and complement-mediated damage to nerves has been postulated. Papilloedema, usually with increases in cerebrospinal fluid pressure, is common and has been reported in 40 to 60 per cent of cases.

Organomegaly

The organ most commonly found to be enlarged is the liver (in some 80 per cent) and splenomegaly has been detected in around a quarter of cases. Lymphadenopathy is common (60 per cent) and in many cases the pathology is that of Castleman's disease (angiofollicular lymph node hyperplasia (see Chapter 22.5.3); this can be either of the hyaline vascular or plasma cell type, in the latter case associated with systemic symptoms and often a poor prognosis. The enlarged nodes are found most commonly in the mediastinum and abdomen.

Endocrinopathy

Gonadal dysfunction is the commonest endocrine association in the POEMS syndrome, with amenorrhoea a feature in nearly every case reported in women of child-bearing age. In males gynaecomastia, impotence, or both affect some 70 per cent of patients. Hypothyroidism, with or without increased plasma levels of thyroid stimulating hormone, has also been a common association; more rarely there have been reports of adrenocortical insufficiency, glucose intolerance, and hyperproactinaemia.

Monoclonal gammopathy

Monoclonal increases in immunoglobulins, more commonly IgG than IgA, have been reported in 60 per cent to 75 per cent of patients with

Table 1 *Recognized associations with the POEMS syndrome*

Oedema, pleural effusions, and ascites
Polycythemia leucocytosis and thrombocythaemia
Fever and malaise
Raynaud's phenomenon
Clubbing of the fingers
Dilated cardiomyopathy
Proteinuria and microangiopathic changes in renal glomeruli
Flushing resembling the carcinoid syndrome
Otherwise unexplained premature peripheral vascular
  calcification

other manifestations of the POEMS syndrome. In contrast to the pattern which is characteristic of myeloma, when kappa light chains predominates over lambda in a ratio of 2 : 1, excess of lambda is more common in the POEMS syndrome and has been reported in some 80 per cent of cases. These immunoglobulin abnormalities have been associated with a variety of myelomatous lesions in bone. These may consist of solitary, usually painless, sclerotic lesions, which have been reported in some 60 per cent of cases. So-called ring lesions, with areas of peripheral sclerosis surrounding a central lucency, have also been reported, but the classical lucent areas of multiple myeloma are less common. Biopsy of affected areas of bone often show an excess of monoclonal plasma cells, but routine bone marrow examination shows such increases in plasma cells in only about 40 per cent of cases.

There have also been a few examples of polyclonal increases in immunoglobulins associated with other manifestations of the POEMS syndrome in patients who have apparently been exposed to organic solvents or other chemicals.

Other features

A number of much less frequent associations have now been described and are listed in Table 1. Some combinations of these features may coincide with the finding of high titres of antinuclear antibodies and/or rheumatoid factor. Given the multisystem involvement in most cases of the POEMS syndrome, the differential diagnosis with systemic lupus erythematosus can sometimes be particularly difficult.

TREATMENT

Case reports of remission following removal or irradiation of local bone lesions suggest that at least in some cases a product(s) of abnormal plasma cells may play a central role in causing the syndrome. Interleukin-6 has been a suggested, but not proven, mediator in some cases.

More commonly there is a need for drug therapy and a large variety of agents have been reported to have been used successfully. There are many reports of moderate to excellent responses to high-dose steroid therapy. Other agents used include azathioprine, cyclophosphamide, chlorambucil, cytosinarabinoside, thioguanine, and even tamoxifen and recombinant interferon. Given a large number of anecdotal case reports of the value or otherwise of these individual agents, it is probably sensible to start treatment with a combination of prednisolone (40–60 mg/day) and azathioprine (2–2.5 mg/kg/day) or a similar dose of cyclophosphamide. The response to treatment has been very variable. Many cases do very well for a number of years. Others do not, and this is perhaps a reflection of the heterogeneity of the disease which we can only recognize at the moment by description, with almost no understanding of pathogenesis.

REFERENCES

Bardwick, P.A., Zvaifler, N.J., Gill, G.N., Newman, D., Greenway, G.D., and Resnick, D.L. (1980). Plasma cell dyscrasia with polyneuropathy, organomegaly, endocrinopathy, M protein and skin change, the POEMS syndrome. *Medicine (Baltimore)*, **59**, 311–22.
Case records of the Massachusetts Hospital (1992). *New England Journal of Medicine* **327**, 101–421.
Jackson, A. and Burton, I.E. (1990). A case of POEMS syndrome associated with essential thrombocythaemaemia and dermal mastocytosis. *Postgraduate Medical Journal* **66**, 761–7.
Mandler, R.N., Kerrigan, D.P., Smart, J., Kuis, W., Viliger, P., and Lotz, M. (1992). Castleman's disease in POEMS syndrome with elevated Interleukin-6. *Cancer* **69**, 2697–703.
Miralles, G.D., O'Fallon, J.R., and Talley, N.J. (1992). Plasma cell dyscrasia with polyneuropathy. The spectrum of POEMS syndrome. *New England Journal of Medicine* **327**, 1919–23.
Mizuiri, S., *et al.* (1991). Renal involvement in POEMS syndrome. *Nephron* **59**, 153–6.
Murphy, N. and Schumaker, H.R. (1992). POEMS syndrome in systemic lupus erythematosus. **19**, 796–9. *Journal of Rheumatology*
Shimpo, S. (1968). Solitary plasmacytoma with polyneuritis and endocrine disturbances. *Japanese Journal of Clinical Medicine* **26**, 244–56.

24.18 Developmental abnormalities of the nervous system

D. GARDNER-MEDWIN

INTRODUCTION

In about 1 per cent of all births the baby has a malformation of the nervous system. About 2 per cent of schoolchildren are mentally retarded, and at least 3 per cent of school-leavers have some form of neurological handicap.

Developmental disorders are defined by the coexistence and mutual effects of a pathological lesion or function and continued growth and development. Primary agenesis or early destruction of a structure is followed by abnormal development or dysgenesis of related ones. The extent to which this happens is greatest during embryogenesis, but it occurs in an anatomical sense at least to the age of 2 years, and all

neurological lesions in early life have effects on the functional and social development of children for as long as their personalities and the patterns of their lives continue to grow.

Down syndrome, spina bifida and the fragile-X syndrome are the commonest entities, but several hundred different anomalies and syndromes contribute to the remainder, and a variety of genetic defects, noxious agents and accidents, most of them poorly understood, may interfere with the complex development of the nervous system before or after birth. Ideally it should be equally possible to classify the developmental disorders according to the clinical features, or the pathology, or the developmental processes involved, or the causation. In practice, none of these is wholly feasible. A variety of causes may give the same

Table 1 *Brain development and malformations*

Postovulatory stage	Developmental process	Some related malformations
	Gametogenesis	
Preconception to 3 days	Gametogenesis, early cell division	Chromosome anomalies
		Mutant genetic disorders
	Embryogenesis	
15–17 days	Neural plate	None, or lethal
18–30 days	Notochord present	Induction disorders—vertebral clefts;? chordomas;? teratomas;? holoprosencephaly
22–24 to 40 + days	Forebrain and optic vesicles appear; cerebral hemispheres form	Holoprosencephaly
24–26 days	Anterior neuropore closes	Anencephaly
26–32 + days	Neural crest cells proliferate	? Neurocutaneous syndromes; ? Sturge–Weber syndrome
26–28 days	Posterior neuropore closes	Spina bifida
28–32 days	Spinal nerve roots form	Thalidomide intoxication
30 days to 25 weeks (especially 10–18 weeks)	Neuronal and vascular proliferation	Primary microcephaly;? megalencephalies;? embryonal cell tumours
7–20 + weeks	Neuronal migration	Lissencephaly, 3rd–6th month; Zellweger syndrome;? fetal alcohol syndrome; agenesis of corpus callosum, 10–15 weeks; ? craniopharyngiomas.
		Destruction causes hydranencephaly and polymicrogyria
4–8 weeks	Cerebellar vermis forms	Dandy–Walker syndrome; Joubert syndrome
	Later fetal development	
20 weeks to 4 years	Glial proliferation	Fetal malnutrition; secondary microcephaly
18 weeks to 2nd decade (mainly 32 weeks to 2 years)	Myelin formation	Amino acid disorders and leucodystrophies
18 + weeks to 4 + years	Synapse formation	? Phenylketonuria; secondary 'deprivation' syndromes

Table 2 *Some causes of prenatal malformations*

Cause	Effects or examples
Parental balanced translocation	Chromosome disorders
Microdeletions	Angelman, de Lange syndromes
Single gene defects	For example, Crouzon, Meckel, Aicardi, Zellweger syndromes
Low maternal age	? Septo-optic dysplasia; cerebral palsy
High maternal age	Down syndrome
High paternal age	Genetic mutations
Radiation	Microcephaly, retardation, cerebellar defects
Trauma	For example, amniocentesis, failed abortion, maternal hypotension
Maternal fever	Retardation + dysmorphism
Exogenous toxins	For example, thalidomide, alcohol, organic mercury
Endogenous toxins	
Maternal	Maternal phenylketonuria or diabetes
Fetal	For example, Zellweger syndrome
General nutritional deficiency or placental insufficiency	Microcephaly, retardation; predisposes to perinatal asphyxia
Specific nutritional deficiency	Iodine deficiency (endemic); ? vitamins and neural tube defects
Intrauterine infection	Cytomegalovirus, rubella, etc.
Death of a twin	Microcephaly, encephalomalacia in the survivor

clinical or pathological effect, and the timing of an insult is usually more important than its nature in determining its outcome. In the past decade an increasing number of malformation syndromes have been found to be caused by genetic microdeletions. Nevertheless in most developmental malformations the cause is unknown and, while the origin of some may be dated to a particular stage of embryogenesis, the defects in others clearly span long periods of development. Tables 1 and 2 illustrate some known associations but classification in this chapter is arranged on a clinical and anatomical basis.

Neurological assessment of a patient with a developmental disorder of the nervous system should be designed to identify:

(1) the site of the lesion(s);
(2) the nature of the pathology;

Table 3 *Causes of severe mental retardation*[a]

	Moser and Wolf (1971) IQ < 70[b]	Turner (1975) IQ < 50[c]
Metabolic and genetic disorders	4.2	11.6
Down syndrome	17.0	[18]
Other chromosome anomalies	1.7	1.1
Multiple anomaly syndromes	5.9	2.7
Congenital CNS malformations	4.7	3.9
Prenatal infections	2.8	1.9
Postnatal infections	3.9	5.3
Perinatal encephalopathies	17.4	11.9
Postnatal trauma, etc.	1.9	1.9
Unknown, with neurological signs	20.2 ⎱ 39.3	⎱
with fits but no signs	3.0 ⎰ (63% male)	41.7 ⎰
without fits or neurological signs	16.1 ⎰	
Others	1.3	—

[a]Figures (per cent) adapted from original data.

[b]1378 residents of a state institution (IQ < 50 in 78%); all ages.

[c]1000 children assessed for IQ < 51; Down's syndrome separately estimated.

(3) the nature and degree of the handicapping effect on the patient and his family;

(4) the genetic recurrence risk for other members of the family; and

(5) any opportunity for specific treatment.

Therapy to alleviate or circumvent handicap is possible in all cases, whether it is aimed at developing the skills of the patient or, in the most profoundly handicapping disorders, at providing relief for the parents and family who are the principal sufferers in such a situation.

Mental retardation

Mental retardation or intellectual impairment is defined as permanent impairment of intelligence necessitating special care or training; in severe impairment the person is incapable of independent life or of protecting himself from exploitation. For educational purposes children are classified as having 'learning disability' whether moderate or severe. The IQ lies in the range 50–69 or below 50, respectively. Profound learning disability implies an IQ below 30. Among school children the prevalence rates for moderate learning disability lie between 15 and 25 per 1000, for severe between 3 and 4 per 1000. In addition, many children suffer from lesser degrees, and often specific patterns, of learning difficulties requiring special help at mainstream schools.

Severe mental retardation occurs almost equally frequently in all socio-economic groups. It is usually associated with identifiable cerebral pathology (Table 3). Moderate handicap is more rarely so; some cases represent the lowest part of the range of normal human intelligence, others have minimal pathology. To polygenic hereditary factors in families of low intelligence are added the effects of deprivation of intellectual stimulation or training, the inculcation of maladaptive patterns of behaviour, and in some families, the effects of poor nutrition, emotional deprivation, or frank non-accidental injury.

The responsibilities of the doctor to this major section of our society lie in three main areas:

(1) the early diagnosis of mental retardation and its differential diagnosis from other causes of delayed or deviant development;

(2) the recognition of specific causes of mental retardation and the provision of genetic counselling and, if possible, treatment;

(3) the recognition and management of any associated handicaps involving impaired vision, hearing, behaviour, motor skills or epilepsy.

Retardation may be predicted at birth if a major associated malformation syndrome or microcephaly are recognized. However, certain abnormal-looking babies, for example with the Treacher–Collins syndrome, Moebius syndrome, or certain craniofacial dysostoses may be expected to have normal intelligence. Other children 'at risk' of handicap because of adverse factors in their gestation or birth, or severe cerebral symptoms in the newborn period, must be assessed at intervals and given special stimulation and support until their developmental status declares itself. These children, and those others who come to attention because of delay in the attainment of normal motor, language, and behaviour skills, must not be judged to be intellectually retarded until alternatives, especially deafness, specific motor or language handicaps, infantile autism, emotional deprivation, and chronic illness have been excluded. Developmental assessment techniques may be used to screen the population for children who are delayed; the analysis of the nature and degree of their handicaps requires repeated assessment by a skilled team over a prolonged period of infancy, coupled always with stimulation, provision of opportunities for learning, and repeated assessment of the response to this intervention.

Once mental handicap is identified or suspected, its cause should be sought. In most large-scale reviews 20 to 40 per cent of cases are of unknown cause, and of the remainder about two-thirds originate before birth and one-third are acquired in the perinatal period or later. A detailed history of the gestation and birth (preferably from the obstetric notes) may reveal 'risk factors'; a search for dysmorphic features may provide clues, not only to specific syndromes but sometimes to the timing of a lesion in relation to embryogenesis. Abnormalities of stature and of head growth are further clues in many cases. At this stage a search of one of several books or databases on dysmorphic syndromes may prevent the need for extensive investigation. Otherwise the depth of investigation of a child with mental handicap will depend on the clinical findings, but is usually designed to identify congenital infections, chromosome anomalies, and those of the deletion syndromes or inborn errors of metabolism that are compatible with the clinical picture. Some of the amino acid disorders and mucopolysaccharidoses may present with featureless retardation. Clinical features necessitating wider investigation for metabolic errors include:

(1) regression in development;

(2) progressive microcephaly or megalencephaly;

(3) deteriorating epilepsy;

(4) progressively abnormal neurological signs;

(5) intermittent neurological deterioration, especially during infections or fasting;

(6) suggestive ocular, skeletal, abdominal, skin, or hair abnormalities;

(7) a suggestive family history.

In males with featureless and unexplained mental retardation, the fragile-X syndrome and preclinical Duchenne muscular dystrophy should be excluded.

Treatable (or partially treatable) causes of mental retardation are few and are usually indicated by progressive or fluctuating symptoms. Examples are congenital hypothyroidism, phenylketonuria, galactosaemia, and some of the vitamin-responsive neurometabolic disorders (see Section 11), compressive disorders, especially hydrocephalus, bilateral subdural haematomas or craniosynostosis, and some epileptic syndromes in which chronic minor status may occur.

Specific learning disorders

Mild or subtle handicaps are more common, are recognized later and are often less well managed than severe ones. A child with intelligence 'within the normal range' but well below the rest of the family, and the child with normal overall intelligence but a specific learning disorder, mild motor handicap, or behavioural disorder may suffer the impatience and misunderstanding of parents and teachers. If they come to medical attention at all such symptoms as dyslexia, clumsiness, or hyperkinesis may be falsely elevated to the status of diagnoses. In such circumstances the search for physical signs of neurological dysfunction must be extended beyond the routine of the neurologist by a clinical psychologist willing to analyse defects of perception or concentration, disconnection of sensorimotor function, etc. This provides a starting point for a search for the underlying pathology, and for planning remedial education. The aetiology of specific learning disorders is rarely identifiable with certainty. Genetic factors and prenatal or perinatal risk factors should be critically examined before being accepted as relevant. Epilepsy or a past history of cerebral trauma, encephalitis, or meningitis are found in a minority. Cognitive problems are occasionally the presenting symptom of subacute sclerosing panencephalitis or of adrenoleucodystrophy, Huntington's chorea, or other progressive genetic encephalopathies; in unusual cases follow-up to rule out progressive disorders is wise. There is an increased incidence of congenital apraxia in sex chromosome reduplication disorders.

Infantile autism

This is a particular form of deviant and delayed development characterized in 1943 by Kanner. Autistic children look normal, even graceful, but their severe language disorder and lack of emotional rapport or even eye contact, are major barriers to communication. Solitary and orderly, often distressed by change in routine, they treat people as objects, sometimes favourite objects, and words as meaningless sounds. Speech and gesture are absent at first, or at best echoes and stereotyped. About half develop useful speech by the age of 5 years, but no conversation. Play is repetitive, joyless, unimaginative, and ritualistic but sometimes mechanically skilful. Spinning objects and toe-walking are common habits. Adaptive behaviour is often seriously retarded though sometimes nearly normal; 40 per cent have IQs below 50 and 30 per cent above 70. About 25 per cent develop epilepsy, usually in adolescence. Ten per cent become partially independent as adults.

Most autistic children are abnormal from birth; in a few language and behavioural regression occur in the second year after an initial normal period of development. In such children, neurodegenerative disease, Rett syndrome, the epileptic aphasia syndrome, minor status epilepticus, and psychosis enter the differential diagnosis.

Autistic behaviour is sometimes seen in deaf children or those with severe language disorders; here it seems to result from barriers to communication. It is also frequent, but not constant, in certain clinicopathological entities, especially tuberose sclerosis and the fragile-X syndrome. Indeed it may always be secondary and non-specific and pure autism, *sui generis*, may not exist; but the typical behaviour occurs without evident cause so often that it remains a useful nosological concept until its aetiology is better understood. No consistent neuropathological or biochemical changes are found, although cerebellar hypoplasia and arginylsuccinase deficiency or minor abnormalities of purine metabolism are described in a few cases. The incidence is 0.2 to 0.4 per 1000, and is higher in boys than girls. Sibs, other than monozygotic twins, are rarely affected.

Asperger syndrome is an analogous behavioural syndrome, possibly a variant of autism, with mildly impaired or normal intelligence, usually affecting boys. Those affected tend to be late to walk and talk and remain rather clumsy. They are typically more socially inept than aloof, friendless, more unaware than uncaring of the feelings of others, literal and pedantic in manner, with intense but narrow interests often involving feats of memory rather than of comprehension. The pathogenesis is unknown.

In both syndromes, recognizing the nature of the problem brings support for the parents and directs individually tailored special education towards mitigating the generally poor social prognosis.

Chromosome anomalies*

Down syndrome (trisomy 21)

This is the most frequent single cause of mental retardation. It contributes 20 to 30 per cent of the total population prevalence and in most large mental retardation hospitals about 15 to 20 per cent of the patients have Down syndrome. The familiar facies can be recognized in Renaissance paintings, yet the first case description was in 1846 by Seguin, 20 years before the account by Langdon Down. In 1959, 3 years after the normal number of human chromosomes had been established as 46, an extra G chromosome was discovered in Down syndrome by Lejeune and by Jacobs and their colleagues.

Trisomy 21 due to non-disjunction (see Chapter 4.3) accounts for all but 8 per cent of cases. The rest are the result of translocations, usually to group F or G chromosomes, or rarely of parental mosaicism. The resulting neuropathology is not very obvious, but the brain weight is low with relative hypoplasia of the superior temporal gyri and the cerebellum. There is a simple gyral pattern, and the density of cortical neurones and the number of synapses are reduced.

The natural incidence is about 1.5 per 1000 live births in most races. It rises exponentially with increasing maternal age (0.38 per cent at age 35 years, 3.75 per cent at age 46 years). There is some evidence that maternal hypothyroidism is an occasional predisposing factor. Studies of spontaneous abortuses suggest that two-thirds of trisomy 21 fetuses fail to survive to term. The increasing use of amniocentesis to screen for chromosome anomalies in mothers over the age of 35 has resulted in a decline in the incidence.

CLINICAL FEATURES

The major clinical features are a round, flat face with slightly upslanting palpebral fissures, Brushfield spots on the iris, epicanthus, brachycephaly, short stature especially affecting the limbs, small hands and fingers, small fifth middle phalanges, clinodactyly, transverse palmar creases, a prominent fissured tongue, hypoplastic ears, and infantile hypotonia. Certain dermatoglyphic anomalies (more than eight digital ulnar loops, and distal axial triradii) are characteristic. Redundant skin folds over the

---

* The nomenclature of chromosome abnormalities is described in Chapter 4.3.

nape, and hypotonia may be prominent at birth. The development of walking is delayed and throughout life the gait remains broad-based; the speech is usually dysarthric and hoarse. Strabismus, nystagmus, and myopia are common.

The usual range of IQ in Down syndrome is 20 to 80, in most cases being between 35 and 55. The rare mosaic cases are often brighter.

Practical self-help skills, personal affection, a sense of humour, mimicry, and musical appreciation are relatively well-preserved, while abstract thought and number sense are very poor. A decline in IQ is sometimes observed in late childhood or subsequently. Institutionalization or hypothyroidism are sometimes responsible, but dementia associated with the pathology of Alzheimer's disease is also a frequent and specific complication even in childhood but more often after the age of 30 years. This seems to be related to the location on chromosome 21 of the amyloid precursor protein gene (one of several genes, mutations of which predispose to Alzheimer's disease).

Few adults survive beyond 50 years.

COMPLICATIONS

Neurological complications in childhood include centrencephalic epilepsy in up to 10 per cent of cases, infantile spasms being particularly associated with subsequent profound handicap. Occasionally spinal cord compression, due to atlantoaxial dislocation, causes a sudden or progressive tetraparesis.

Severe complications may occur in infancy as a result of some common associated malformations, especially congenital heart disease (in nearly 40 per cent of cases), duodenal atresia (2.5 per cent), or imperforate anus (0.7 per cent). The cardiac defects in decreasing order of frequency are atrial and ventricular septal defects, tetralogy of Fallot, and patent ductus. Respiratory obstruction by adenoids in a hypoplastic pharynx, and aspiration pneumonitis are common. Acute myeloblastic leukaemia in the new-born and lymphoblastic leukaemia in older children are both relatively frequent, but transient leukaemoid responses are a common source of error; together they affect 1 per cent of all cases of Down syndrome. Acquired autoimmune hypothyroidism is a frequent association. Most girls are subfertile, but pregnancy can occur; males are sterile. A distressing complication in adult life is corneal clouding consequent upon keratoconus.

Difficult decisions about treating life-threatening complications must often be made in early life. However, a half-hearted approach to the management of heart disease or epilepsy, for example, often results in more disabling and difficult symptoms later. Problems which are not likely to be fatal are best treated promptly and effectively both to avoid distress to the child and to support the parents in their attempts at an unequivocal approach to making his life as worthwhile as possible. Most children with Down syndrome are brought up by their families, in later life their relatively good social skills often make hostel accommodation and sheltered employment successful.

Prevention depends upon the screening of 'elderly' mothers by amniocentesis or chorionic villus biopsy, and genetic counselling after checking both parents, and, if necessary, other relatives for balanced translocations. A low level of maternal serum alphafetoprotein is a potentially useful marker for Down syndrome and a normal level may reduce the need for amniocentesis in lower-risk pregnancies.

Other trisomies

Trisomy 13 and trisomy 18 are not infrequent malformation syndromes at birth, but are almost always lethal. The following rarer trisomies are compatible with survival into adult life.

In Trisomy 22 intelligence may be normal, though most cases are mentally handicapped. The usual features are cleft palate, iris colobomas, preauricular appendages and sinuses, anal atresia, and congenital heart disease, but there is much variation. Many survive to adult life. Affected relatives are common, so karyotyping and counselling the family are important.

Trisomy 8 and normal/trisomy 8 mosaic Here intelligence varies from normal to severe subnormality. Extra vertebrae, dolichocephaly, hypertelorism, a thick drooping lower lip, dysplastic ears, bulbous nose, high-arched palate, absent patellae, deep palmar and plantar creases, thick skin, and congenital heart disease occur. Agenesis of the corpus callosum is found in most, if not all, cases. Increased muscle tone and joint stiffness may develop later.

Trisomy 9p is characterized by retardation, short stature, microcephaly, hypertelorism, prominent nasal bridge and globular tip, simple ears, small fingers (especially the fifth), and hypoplastic nails.

Neurological aspects of the sex chromosome aneuploidies

Mental retardation occurs in a few cases of Klinefelter syndrome (XXY syndrome), in which the average IQ is less than 10 points below controls, and with increasing frequency and severity in the XXXY and XXXXY syndromes. Apathy, lack of emotion, and fatigue are common, and hypotonia, specific learning difficulties, tremor, and congenital apraxia have been associated with these disorders, though not consistently. Men with XYY or XYYY are usually only mildly retarded if at all, but these anomalies have been associated with antisocial behaviour. Girls with Turner syndrome (45X) are generally of average intelligence without neurological symptoms, but a rather consistent impairment of performance skills compared with normal verbal skills is found, together with defective number sense, and right–left disorientation (see also Chapter 4.3).

Deletion syndromes and other structural chromosomal defects

Major deletions of parts of chromosomes are generally fatal before birth or in infancy. Small deletions, while presumably more often compatible with survival, are more difficult to demonstrate. Grouchy in 1963 described a patient with 18p−. Shortly afterwards Lejeune and his colleagues described the first patients with the cri du chat syndrome, in which quite large deletions of the short arm of chromosome 5 (5p−) are compatible with survival at least into the sixth decade. The syndromes associated with the deletions 4p−, 13p−, 18q−, and 21p− were identified in the 1960s. With improved banding techniques, quite small deletions, duplications, and chromosomal structural defects were found to be associated with previously well-known syndromes, such as the Prader–Willi syndrome and, most importantly, with certain cases of X-linked mental retardation which were not identified as comprising a recognizable entity until the discovery of the fragile site on the X chromosome which now gives the syndrome its name. The developments in molecular genetics in the past 10 years have realized earlier predictions that many familiar malformation syndromes would be found to be caused by chromosomal deletions, and no doubt others remain to be discovered. Most deletions, are sporadic *de novo* mutations, but in certain circumstances simple Mendelian inheritance may make them resemble single gene defects. The examples that follow are some of the deletion syndromes with implications beyond the period of early childhood.

CRI DU CHAT SYNDROME (5P−)

This occurs in about one in 50 000 births. Some cases are familial with a balanced translocation of the deleted fragment in one parent. Mental retardation is usually profound, but may be so mild as to comprise a selective learning disorder, the degree of retardation correlating broadly with the size of the deletion. The other cardinal features are remarkably constant: short stature, a mewing cry in the early years of life and distorted laryngeal anatomy, microcephaly, a wide nasal bridge, epicanthus, sometimes hypertelorism and micrognathia. Neonatal feeding and respiratory difficulties are frequent. About 30 per cent of cases have congenital heart defects. Many cases reach adulthood.

α-THALASSAEMIA AND MENTAL RETARDATION (SEE ALSO SECTION 22)

Two distinct syndromes combine these features. Attention was first drawn to them by the discovery in red blood cells of inclusions of haemoglobin H, but in the second syndrome these are not always detectable.

In one syndrome significant anaemia and moderate, rather featureless mental retardation are associated with a deletion in the α-globin gene complex at 16p13.3. Only one parent of each case carries the α-thalassaemia trait.

The other syndrome causes only a mild anaemia, but severe mental retardation, and no deletion is present in the α-globin gene. The inheritance is X-linked and the gene, now identified as *XH2*, codes for a transcription factor that is expressed from early fetal life. Hypotonia and small abnormal genitalia at birth, delayed walking, and failure to develop speech or continence are associated with a characteristic facies (small palpebral fissures, telecanthus, hypoplasia of the mid-face and nasal bridge, anteverted nostrils, widely spaced incisors, protruding tongue), microcephaly, and short stature.

ANGELMAN SYNDROME

Formerly called the 'happy puppet' syndrome because of the characteristic happy smile, gales of inappropriate laughter, jerky movements, and wide-based apraxic gait, this always causes severe retardation without speech but with some ability to sign; other features are microcephaly, tongue protrusion, prognathism, epilepsy (often resistant and occurring in clusters) in over 80 per cent, and a characteristic electroencephalogram (EEG) (spikes and rhythmic slow waves on eye closure). It is nonprogressive and usually sporadic, with an incidence of about 1 in 20 000.

A *de novo* 15q11–13 deletion of the maternally derived chromosome is found in at least two-thirds of cases; a few others display uniparental disomy, deriving both copies of chromosome 15 from the father, and the remainder are assumed to have a point mutation in the maternal gene. In this last group sibs may be affected. The same 15q11–13 deletion, when it affects the paternally derived chromosome, causes the quite different Prader–Willi syndrome (see below). The differential pathogenesis of these two phenotypes remains an enigma.

DE LANGE SYNDROME

This disorder is distinguished by severe retardation, short stature, low-pitched cry, microcephaly, hirsutism, synophrys, long eyelashes, small anteverted nose, small hands and feet, and various minor skeletal anomalies. It is usually sporadic. Chromosomal deletions, duplications or translocations have been found at or near 3q26.3 in several cases.

PRADER–WILLI SYNDROME

The presenting problem is severe neonatal hypotonia with swallowing difficulties, usually requiring tube-feeding for several days or weeks. The typical facies may be recognizable in infancy with experience (Fig. 1(a)), and the ulnar border of the hand is abnormally straight. The genitalia are hypoplastic, often with cryptorchidism. Despite the hypotonia, muscle paralysis is not a feature and muscle biopsy reveals only immature muscle development. In later life short stature, small hands, and feet, severe obesity (evident from about 9 to 15 months) and retardation (in the IQ range 20 to 90, usually 50 to 80) are the major features (Fig. 1(b)). The severe hyperphagia requires stringent calorie restriction for

its control. Non-insulin-dependent diabetes is a frequent complication. Other minor endocrine anomalies are probably secondary to the obesity rather than causal. A defect in lipolysis has been suggested. Most cases arise *de novo*, and the risk of recurrence in sibs is under 2 per cent. A population incidence of one in 20 000 is possibly an underestimate. *De novo* 15q11–13 deletions of the paternally derived chromosome 15 are found in most cases and about half of the remainder have monoparental disomy for the maternally derived chromosome, the converse of the situation found in Angelman syndrome (see above).

RUBINSTEIN–TAYBI SYNDROME

Here there is retardation (usually severe), short stature, retarded bone growth, microcephaly, high arched palate, beaked nose, low-set ears, broad thumbs and toes, and various other less constant anomalies, including agenesis of the corpus callosum. It is a sporadic disorder probably caused by a microdeletion at 16p13.3.

THE FRAGILE-X SYNDROME

This major cause of mental retardation, possibly accounting for 10 to 15 per cent of all cases, was identified as recently as 1969 (see also Chapter 4.3). The fragile site at Xq27.3 (near the tip of the long arm of the X chromosome) can be demonstrated cytogenetically only with difficulty, using special conditions of low concentrations of calf serum, thymidine, and folate in the culture medium. Routine karyotyping, even with banding techniques, is of no value in excluding it. The fragile site cannot always be found even in affected siblings of proven cases, and occasionally it is found in normal males. However, molecular genetic techniques have identified the mutation as an increase in the number of CGG repeats in one exon of the gene. The normal exon contains 15 to 50 repeats of this sequence, a 'small insert' bringing the number to 70 to 200 constitutes a premutation, while greater numbers of CGG repeats become methylated and then give rise to both cytogenetic and clinical manifestations in males, and often also in heterozygous females. Mothers (but not fathers) with premutations tend to have offspring with larger inserts. These findings explain some of the previously enigmatic features

Fig. 1 Prader–Willis syndrome. The same patient aged (a) 3 weeks, (b) 5 years; severe infantile hypotonia, later moderate retardation and obesity.

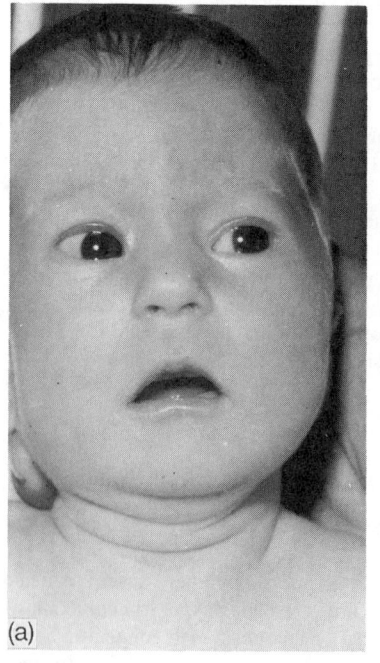
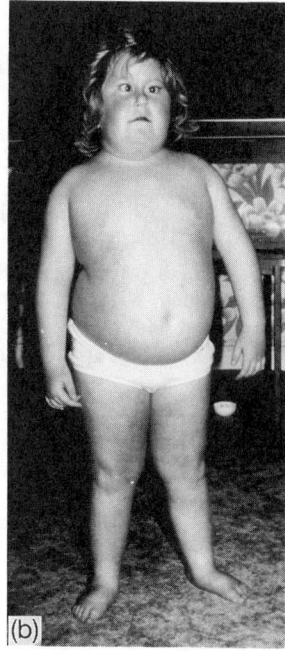

of the inheritance (including the variable manifestation in females and the occasional transmission by unaffected males) and, moreover, provide a means of accurate carrier detection and prenatal diagnosis (see also Chapter 4.3).

The clinical diagnosis is not easy. The IQ is in the range 20 to 80, usually 35 to 60. Affected adult males are of normal stature but typically have high foreheads, large mandibles, prominent ears (Fig. 2) and, most characteristically, large testes, but these findings are not consistent. Neurological examination is usually normal but tremor, apraxia, and a broad-based gait are occasionally recorded. Stuttering repetitive speech is common. Epilepsy occurs in about 20 per cent of cases. Affected young boys are even less easy to recognize. Macro-orchidism is often absent; the average birthweight and head circumference are slightly increased. Female carriers of the gene may themselves be retarded though most are normal. Turner found that 7 per cent of non-specific retardation among females in the IQ range 55 to 75 was associated with heterozygosity for the 'fragile X'. Evidence about the true incidence is still insecure, probably somewhat less than 1 in 1000 males and 1 in 2500 females.

The neuropathology is subtle—synapse structure is slightly abnormal with paucity of dendritic spines.

Complex malformation syndromes

Numerous rather specific syndromes are recognized, mostly representing single gene defects and together contributing about 5 per cent of cases of mental retardation. The following are a few of the most frequent, or theoretically important, ones.

AICARDI SYNDROME

Here the main features are mental retardation, infantile spasms and later epilepsy, multiple lacunar retinal defects, agenesis of the corpus callosum, and independent electrical activity of the two hemispheres in the EEG. The disorder is confined to girls (and is probably X-linked dominant lethal in males).

Fig. 2 Fragile-X syndrome: a boy with severe mental subnormality and macro-orchidism. (By courtesy of Dr M. Bhate.)

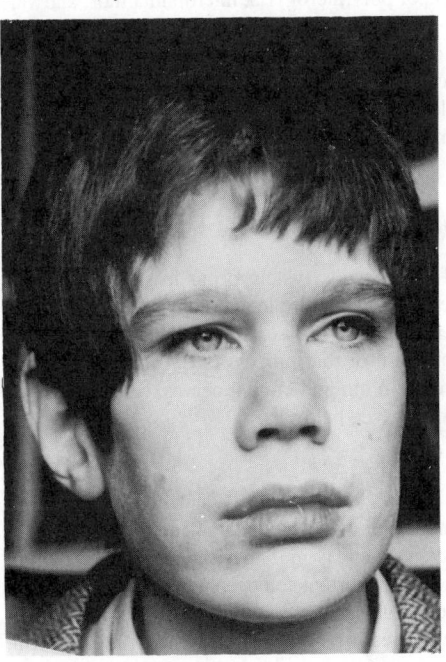

COCKAYNE SYNDROME

The features are mental retardation, short stature, deep-set orbits, microcephaly, retinal pigmentation, sensorineural deafness, photosensitive rash, later peripheral neuropathy, and ataxia. Cerebral calcification and leucodystrophy may be seen on CT scan. Cultured cells, including amniocytes, show failure of RNA and DNA synthesis after UV light exposure. A defect in DNA ligase may be responsible. Chromosomal deletions at 10q21 have been found in some cases, but inheritance is usually autosomal recessive.

COFFIN–LOWRY SYNDROME

In this disorder there is severe retardation, moderate growth retardation, downslanting eyes, hypertelorism, small maxilla, wide nose, short sternum, scoliosis and vertebral anomalies (on radiography), large soft hands, tapering fingers, tufted distal phalanges (also on radiography), and lax ligaments. It is of X-linked recessive inheritance; mothers may have scoliosis and the finger anomalies. The gene is located at Xp22.

SMITH–LEMLI–OPITZ SYNDROME

This comprises mental retardation, low birthweight, failure to thrive, irritability, microcephaly, severe hypotonia (central), anteverted nose, ptosis, broad maxillary alveolar ridges, cryptorchidism and hypospadias in males. It is of autosomal recessive inheritance. There are multiple anomalies of cerebrum, cerebellum, and spinal cord. Exceptionally for a malformation syndrome, there is a specific biochemical marker, the accumulation in blood of 7-dehydrocholesterol.

SOTOS SYNDROME (CEREBRAL GIGANTISM)

This is shown by mild to moderate retardation, high birthweight, macrosomia in childhood but advanced bone age and early epiphyseal fusion, megalencephaly, large hands and feet, high forehead, slight downslant of eyes, characteristic facies, impaired co-ordination, increased incidence of febrile convulsions, and often scoliosis. It is sporadic, and probably of autosomal dominant inheritance confined to new mutants.

WILLIAMS SYNDROME (SEVERE INFANTILE IDIOPATHIC HYPERCALCAEMIA)

Here there is moderate or mild retardation, 'elfin facies', and supravalvular aortic stenosis. Hypercalcaemia may be severe in infancy but does not persist. There is early failure to thrive and vomiting. The retardation affects speech less than perceptual and motor skills. The disorder is sporadic and the aetiology and significance of the hypercalcaemia are unknown. Absorption of calcium is increased and sensitivity to vitamin D may be a factor. Restriction of calcium and vitamin D intake is useful in the hypercalcaemic phase of the disease, but not curative.

ZELLWEGER (CEREBROHEPATORENAL) SYNDROME

Features of this disorder are profound retardation, severe central hypotonia, areflexia, feeding difficulties, high forehead, flat facies, hepatomegaly, cirrhosis and sometimes liver failure, multiple small renal cysts, and often early seizures. Survival is usually under 6 months. The neuropathological features are micropolygyria, pachygyria, and defects of neuronal migration. The underlying defect is total absence of the peroxisomes in all body cells and consequently of all peroxisomal enzyme activity. Thus patients fail to metabolize phytanic acid, pipecolic acid, or very-long-chain fatty acids (with carbon chain lengths of 24–26 atoms) and fail to synthesize plasmalogens. This uncommon disorder deserves mention as a rare example of a cerebral malformation caused

24.19 Metabolic and deficiency disorders of the nervous system

C. D. MARSDEN

The brain depends on glycolysis and respiration to synthesize its energy needs. An adequate supply of glucose and oxygen depends upon cerebral blood flow which, under normal resting conditions, is about 50 ml per 100 g/min, an amount equal to 15 to 20 per cent of the resting cardiac output. Each 100 g of brain of the normal human utilizes about 0.31 mol (5.5 mg) of glucose per minute. In the basal fasting state the brain's consumption of glucose almost equals the total amount the liver produces. Under normal conditions, glucose consumption varies from region to region of the brain, depending upon local functional changes. The brain contains only small stores of glucose and glycogen such that if blood supply is abruptly cut off, normal function can only continue for 2 to 3 min. If the brain is deprived of both glucose and oxygen, as occurs in cardiac arrest, normal energy metabolism can only continue for about 10 to 15 s.

General metabolic disorders

HYPOGLYCAEMIA

Hypoglycaemic coma is difficult to diagnose, and dangerous. In any case of coma, stupor, or confusion of unknown cause, blood should be drawn for glucose analysis and insulin levels, and then 25 g of glucose (with thiamine) should be administered intravenously. Such an injection can do no harm and may save life.

The commonest cause of hypoglycaemia is insulin overdose, or excessive hypoglycaemic drug intake. Hyperinsulinism due to an adenoma of islets of Langerhans in the pancreas is uncommon, as is hypoglycaemia due to pre-diabetes or a retroperitoneal sarcoma. Hypoglycaemia may also occur in alcoholism and liver disease, after gastric surgery, and in a variety of rare metabolic conditions.

Hypoglycaemia usually presents in one of four manners: (1) as an organic toxic confusional state, sleepy confusion, bizarre behaviour, or mania; (2) as unexplained coma with brain-stem dysfunction, including decerebrate spasms and neurogenic hyperventilation, but with preserved oculocephalic reflexes and pupillary responses; (3) as a stroke-like illness with focal deficit; and (4) as epilepsy. Hyperinsulinism, very rarely, also causes predominantly motor peripheral neuropathy.

Hypoglycaemia is established by measurement of blood glucose concentration, and by clinical response to intravenous glucose replacement. Hyperinsulinism is difficult to diagnose on occasion, but can be established by satisfying the criteria for Whipple's triad, namely symptoms of hypoglycaemia, associated with a low blood sugar and a disproportionately high serum insulin, and clinical response to glucose replacement. A 72-h fast, measuring morning blood sugar and insulin levels, will detect nearly all pancreatic islet cell adenomas (see Section 11).

ANOXIA

Cerebral anoxia may be due to insufficient cerebral blood flow, reduced oxygen availability, reduced oxygen carriage by the blood, metabolic interference with the utilization of oxygen, or combinations of these events.

A brief period of global ischaemic anoxia causes syncope. If the episode is prolonged, myoclonic jerks or tonic–clonic seizures may occur. If longer still, there may be a period of confusion and residual amnesia.

Acute severe prolonged anoxia is commonly due to cardiac arrest, resulting from heart disease, cardiac surgery, or anaesthetic catastrophe. Carbon monoxide poisoning, usually suicidal, also damages the brain by anoxia.

Acute anoxia rapidly leads to loss of consciousness, generalized fits, dilated pupils, and bilateral extensor plantar responses. If oxygen deprivation lasts longer than a few minutes, permanent or prolonged but reversible brain damage occurs. Even more severe anoxia may lead to irreversible coma with flaccidity and loss of all reflex function except heart beat and tendon jerks. Pupils remain fixed and dilated and the electroencephalogram (EEG) is flat on repeated examination. (Drugs and hypothermia may cause a flat EEG, but recovery is possible.) Such patients may be said to have suffered irreversible brain death if all signs of brain-stem function are absent on repeated examination over 12 to 24 h (see Chapter 24.4.5). Other, less severely affected, patients show partial recovery of reflex function, such as pupillary responses, reflex eye movements, and muscle tone, and may breathe spontaneously. However, no sign of consciousness or intelligent response to the external world occurs, and they may remain in such a 'persistent vegatative state' for months or years. Lesser degrees of anoxia may cause transient coma with recovery of consciousness but with residual dementia, amnesic syndrome, pseudobulbar palsy and other pyramidal signs, gait ataxia, and incontinence. Some of these patients may be severely disabled by action myoclonus, that is dramatic muscle jerking on attempted movement. These residual deficits following prolonged cerebral anoxia with survival may be permanent, but in other patients they gradually recover. In general, the potential for recovery following cerebral anoxia is considerable over months or years. An optimistic prognosis is justifiable in the early stages, and the final outcome can never be predicted with certainty, except in those with unequivocal evidence of cerebral death.

In a small number of patients apparent recovery from an acute anoxic insult is followed some weeks or months later by delayed postanoxic encephalopathy. The patient recovers, but days or weeks later relapses with increasing irritability, apathy, and confusion. An akinetic-rigid syndrome with or without dystonia then emerges and the condition may progress over a matter of some weeks or months. Often, these neurological changes are first mistaken for psychological disorder, until frank neurological signs clarify the diagnosis. The cause of delayed postanoxic deterioration is not clear, but pathologically there is a diffuse, severe, bilateral white matter degeneration in the hemispheres and in the basal ganglia.

Subacute or gradual anoxia may occur in severe anaemia, heart failure, pulmonary disease, or exposure to high altitude ('mountain sickness'). It produces inattentiveness, fatigue, headache, and intellectual deterioration, followed by memory difficulties and ataxia.

Cerebral anoxia is also the main cause of neurological symptoms in a number of other systemic conditions. Disseminated intravascular coagulation (see Section 22) resulting from platelet aggregation and fibrin formation, can be produced by a number of illnesses, including sepsis, and malignancy. Patients complain of headache and difficulty in concentration, vertigo, blurred vision, and speech difficulties. Such confusion and disorientation may progress to stupor and coma with focal or generalized signs of brain disturbance. Spontaneous bleeding is common, in the form of petechiae in the skin or optic fundus, purpura, and even intracranial haemorrhage. Cerebral malaria (see Section 7) is a complication of infection with *Plasmodium falciparum*, and should always be borne in mind as a cause of unexplained coma in patients recently returning from an infective area. Most patients describe chills and fever for a few days prior to the onset of lethargy, stupor, and finally coma. The diagnosis is established by finding the parasite in fixed smears of the blood. Fat embolism follows severe trauma, particularly to the limbs, but may also be a complication of burns and other severe system disturbance. Multiple pulmonary microemboli of fat may lead to progressive hypoxia and respiratory failure. Multiple cerebral microemboli produce confusion, lethargy, stupor, and finally coma. Symptoms often begin hours to days after the original injury, and are accompanied by fever and hyperventilation. A characteristic petechial rash usually develops over the upper half of the body on the second to third day after injury. There may also be fundal haemorrhages. The respiratory features range from the appearance of linear streaks radiating from the hilar region or patchy opacities on the chest to the fully developed adult distress syndrome (see Section 16). Clotting abnormalities range from mild thrombocytopenia to acute disseminated intravascular coagulation (see Section 22). Management consists of correcting hypoxia, in severe cases with positive end-expiratory pressure (PEEP), and correction of the coagulation disorder (see Section 16). Cardiac surgery, at least in the earlier days of bypass pump oxygenation, produced frequent transient neurological damage in many patients. Improvements in technique, such as the introduction of filters in blood perfusion lines to remove debris, have greatly reduced neurological complications of the procedure. However, some patients still come round from the anaesthetic with signs of diffuse or focal brain damage. If they survive the acute episode, the prognosis usually is good.

Metabolic complications of organ failure

HEPATIC FAILURE

Patients with liver disease of whatever cause (see Section 14) may develop acute hepatic coma or a more chronic form of hepatic encephalopathy with behavioural disturbance and other neurological symptoms.

Acute hepatic coma

This occurs with massive liver necrosis due to severe hepatitis or poisons such as paracetamol. In other patients, who may have relatively well-preserved liver function but extensive portal–systemic shunts, coma may be precipitated by a sudden intake of nitrogenous substances as occurs with gastrointestinal bleeding, infections, or high-protein diets. Confusion, apathy, and lack of concentration, or occasionally excitement requiring sedation, are rapidly followed by stupor and coma in a matter of a few hours or days. Characteristic findings are asterixis ('liver flap'), in which the outstretched hands show postural lapses, and hepatic foetor. Chorea and pyramidal signs may appear as the patient lapses into coma. Decerebrate posturing is common at this stage, and focal deficits such as hemiplegia may occur. Nystagmus, conjugate deviation of the eyes, skew deviation, and even disconjugate eye movements may be evident, but reflex eye movements and pupillary responses are preserved, until the patient becomes totally unresponsive and dies. Paroxysmal and later persistent high-voltage triphasic slow waves are present in the EEG until death is imminent. Many metabolic abnormalities may contribute to the cause of hepatic coma, including hyperammonaemia (more than 145 μmol/l or 200 mg/dl), which results from the products of intestinal digestion bypassing the urea-synthesizing mechanisms of the liver. However, hypoglycaemia and hyperventilation producing a respiratory alkalosis are also almost always present. Altered amino acids and neurotransmitters (especially γ-aminobutyric acid), formation of toxic amines such as octopamine, and short-chain fatty acids, have also been incriminated. Intravascular coagulation occurs, as do other coagulation defects, leading to secondary vascular damage to the brain. Hepatic

coma carries a high mortality, but if the patient can be kept alive, liver regeneration and recovery may occur. Treatment includes sterilizing the bowel, correction of metabolic and bleeding abnormalities, the administration of lactulose, and haemoperfusion or other techniques to remove toxins.

Chronic hepatic encephalopathy

This refers to the development of changes in intellect, cognitive function, and consciousness, often accompanied by other neurological signs (such as tremor or chorea, an akinetic-rigid syndrome, ataxia, or even spastic paraparesis) occurring in those with chronic liver failure, and particularly in those with extensive portal-system anastomoses. The exact nature of the substances responsible for chronic hepatic encephalopathy has not been established. Characteristically, the disorder fluctuates, with episodes of marked confusion, excitement, or frank hepatic coma. In addition, intellectual changes, parkinsonism, ataxia, or spasticity may gradually progress. Treatment consists of a low-protein diet and antibiotics to sterilize the gut, and the administration of lactulose.

RENAL FAILURE

Renal failure (see Section 20) is associated with a variety of neurological complications. Uraemic encephalopathy was common before the use of dialysis. Patients become progressively drowsy, stuporose, and finally lapse into coma. Hyperventilation, multifocal myoclonus, tremor, asterixis, tetany, and generalized fits are common. Eye movements and pupillary reactions are not affected. Uraemia, metabolic acidosis, hyperkalaemia, disorders of calcium, sodium, and water balance, and hypertensive encephalopathy all contribute to the clinical picture. Dialysis rapidly reverses the metabolic abnormalities of uraemia, but the encephalopathy may take days to clear. Some patients develop the dialysis disequilibrium syndrome during correction of their uraemic abnormalities. Rapid correction of the metabolic changes leads to the emergence of asterixis, myoclonus, delirium, generalized convulsions, stupor, and even coma. Dialysis dementia occurred in a proportion of those dialysed for years with fluid having a high aluminium content. Such patients, after 3 to 7 years of dialysis, begin to develop speech disturbance, intellectual and cognitive abnormalities, convulsions, myoclonus, and sometimes focal neurological abnormalities. Other complications of chronic renal failure include myopathy due to chronic hypocalcaemia, a peripheral neuropathy which may be resistant to dialysis, and Wernicke's encephalopathy due to chronic dialysis without vitamin supplements. Patients with renal disease are particularly prone to develop toxic complications of drugs normally excreted in the urine, as for example a peripheral neuropathy due to nitrofurantoin, labyrinthine damage due to streptomycin, or optic atrophy due to ethambutol.

RESPIRATORY FAILURE

Hypoventilation due to lung disease (see Section 17) or neurological disorder can lead to encephalopathy or coma. Hypoxaemia, hypercapnia, congestive heart failure, systemic infection, fatigue due to laboured respiration, and nocturnal sleep apnoea all contribute to the syndrome. Serum acidosis by itself probably is not the important factor, since alkali infusions without ventilatory support do not improve cerebral function in these patients. They develop dull, diffuse headache, accompanied by progressive drowsiness, stupor, and coma. Eye movements and pupillary reactions are normal. However, a small proportion of such patients develop ophthalmic venous distension and papilloedema. Most exhibit asterixis and multifocal myoclonus but epileptic fits are unusual. Respiratory encephalopathy may begin gradually, or may be precipitated by infection or sedative drugs. All such patients hypoventilate, and those with obstructive emphysema gasp and puff. Oxygen therapy in these circumstances may be dangerous, for by removing the hypoxaemic drive to respiration, it may lead to lethal hypercapnia. If low concentrations of oxygen cause respiratory depression, assisted ventilation may be necessary.

Metabolic disorders due to endocrine disease (see Section 12)

DIABETES MELLITUS

Diabetes causes a wide variety of neurological disturbances. Stupor or coma may be produced by hyperosmolality, ketoacidosis, lactic acidosis, hypoglycaemia occurring spontaneously (pre-diabetes) or due to treatment, uraemia, or hypertensive encephalopathy. Transient ischaemic attacks and stroke due to cerebral arteriosclerosis and hypertension are common in diabetics. Peripheral nerve damage may occur in established diabetics, or may be the presenting feature of the illness (see Section 9). Single painful nerve lesions (mononeuritis) such as isolated ocular nerve palsies, Bell's palsy, a lateral popliteal nerve palsy, or an intercostal neuropathy, are common, and may result from haemorrhage or infarction of the nerve. A carpal tunnel syndrome or an ulnar nerve palsy may result from the undue susceptibility of peripheral nerves in diabetes to pressure palsies. Mononeuritis multiplex may occur. Diabetic amyotrophy refers to a proximal motor neuropathy causing the subacute weakness and wasting, often with pain, affecting quadriceps muscles, usually asymmetrically. It is probably due to ischaemia or haemorrhage in the femoral nerve or lumbosacral plexus. A distal symmetrical peripheral neuropathy in diabetes may take the form of a mild asymptomatic sensory neuropathy with loss of vibration sense in the feet and absent ankle jerks. Less commonly, there is severe and progressive sensorimotor neuropathy affecting the legs before the arms. Autonomic neuropathy is common, producing impotence, diarrhoea, loss of sweating, and abnormal pupils. The latter may be irregular, and unreactive to light, mimicking Argyll Robertson pupils. Autonomic neuropathy causes orthostatic hypotension, syncope, and sometimes abrupt cardiac arrest in diabetics.

CUSHING'S SYNDROME

Spontaneous hyperadrenalism is most often due to adrenal tumour, but occasionally occurs with a basophil pituitary adenoma, as after adrenalectomy for breast cancer. Iatrogenic hyperadrenalism due to prolonged excessive steroid administration causes similar neurological symptoms. Cushing's syndrome frequently leads to an encephalopathy often manifest by behavioural changes such as elation or depression. Frank psychotic disturbance may occasionally be accompanied by headache and papilloedema, and may progress to stupor or coma. Cushing's syndrome also may be associated with proximal myopathy, which can be severe and painful.

ADDISON'S DISEASE

Hypoadrenalism due to adrenal failure causes hypotension, hyponatraemia, hyperkalaemia, and often hypoglycaemia as well. Patients with untreated Addison's disease complain of weakness and lassitude, and stupor or coma may be precipitated by surgical procedures or other acute illness. Attacks of periodic paralysis may occur, associated with hypokalaemia. A peripheral neuropathy is rare. Addisonian crisis may be accompanied by generalized convulsions, which are attributed to hyponatraemia and water intoxication. Benign intracranial hypertension with papilloedema and a proximal myopathy may also occur.

MYXOEDEMA

Hypothyroidism may present as a toxic confusional state, psychosis, or dementing illness. Infection, trauma, exposure to cold, or sedation may provoke hypothermic coma. Episodic encephalopathy has been reported in patients with thyroiditis. Myxoedema is associated with the peculiar failure of relaxation of muscle (pseudomyotonia) which produces prolonged tendon jerks, and sometimes muscle cramps, pain, and stiffness. Muscle hypertrophy (Hoffmann's syndrome) is rare. The carpal tunnel syndrome may occur due to deposits of myxoedematous tissue around the median nerve of the wrist, and rarely this may cause a peripheral neuropathy. Occasionally myxoedema may present as an ataxic syndrome, suggesting cerebellar disease.

THYROTOXICOSIS

The symptoms of hyperthyroidism include anxiety, tremor, tachycardia, and insomnia. Chorea or mania may occur. A severe proximal myopathy is common, and occasionally myasthenia gravis or hypokalaemic periodic paralysis occurs. Dysthyroid eye disease may occur in hyperthyroid or euthyroid patients. Diplopia due to superior rectus weakness is the most common initial symptom, but the condition may progress to external ophthalmoplegia with proptosis and chemosis.

Metabolic disorders due to ionic or acid–base abnormalities

HYPONATRAEMIA OR 'WATER INTOXICATION'

Sodium is the most abundant serum cation, so that hyponatraemia (see Section 20) is almost always the cause of hypo-osmolality. Serum osmolality is approximately equal to double the serum sodium concentration plus 10, provided glucose and urea levels are normal. Normal serum osmolality is 290 ± 5 mosmol/kg; serum osmolality below about 260 or above about 330 mosmol/kg is likely to produce cerebral changes. Hyponatraemia means that body water is increased relative to solute, resulting in water excess in the brain. Rapid changes in serum sodium osmolality produce much greater neurological effects than does slowly developing chronic hyponatraemia. Hyponatraemia occurs in renal disease, as a result of excessive intravenous water infusions, due to excessive diarrhoea, vomiting, or sweating, or may result from the inappropriate secretion of antidiuretic hormone that occurs in bronchial carcinoma, diffuse brain disease resulting from head injury, meningitis or encephalitis, subarachnoid haemorrhage, or focal hypothalamic damage due to neoplasm or infection. Patients with hyponatraemia become confused and restless, and develop asterixis, multifocal myoclonus, generalized convulsions, stupor, and coma. Symptoms may appear when the plasma sodium drops below about 120 mmol/l, and fits and coma usually are associated with plasma sodium values below 110 mmol/l. A few patients with chronic hyponatraemia may develop the syndrome of central pontine myelinolysis. Treatment is by water restriction; infusions of hypertonic saline are rarely required.

HYPERNATRAEMIA

The common cause of hyperosmolality is diabetes, producing severe hyperglycaemia. Hyperosmolality due to hypernatraemia is rare, except in those who dehydrate in hot climates. Chronic uncompensated water loss in untreated diabetes insipidus may result in mild hypernatraemia, but such patients only develop severe hypernatraemia if they fail to drink. Patients with simple diabetes insipidus usually maintain thirst, but if intercurrent illness leads to excessive water loss and restricted water intake, they may become dehydrated, drowsy, stuporose, and unconscious. Simple diabetes insipidus may be due to pituitary surgery, trauma, or pituitary tumours. If pathology extends into the hypothalamic region, not only may secretion of antidiuretic hormone be deficient, but thirst regulation may also be abolished. Hypothalamic damage causing severe hypernatraemia may occur in large pituitary tumours, craniopharyngiomas, hypothalamic tumours, sarcoidosis, or Hand–Schüller–Christian disease. Loss of thirst in such patients often precipitates hypernatraemic coma with serum sodium rising above 160 to 170 mmol/l.

Hypernatraemia may also occur as a result of severe water depletion, particularly in children with intense diarrhoea.

HYPERCALCAEMIA (SEE SECTIONS 12, 19, AND 22)

A high serum calcium concentration may be due to primary hyperparathyroidism, immobilization, sarcoidosis, vitamin D intoxication, or multiple bony metastases. Symptoms include anorexia, nausea, vomiting, intense thirst, polyuria, and polydipsia. Muscle weakness, lassitude, and a mild encephalopathy are common. The latter may produce delusions and changes in mood so that many such patients are initially treated for a psychiatric condition. A toxic confusional state with lethargy and stupor, sometimes with generalized or focal seizures and papilloedema also may occur.

HYPOCALCAEMIA (SEE SECTION 12)

Reduced serum calcium concentration may be caused by parathyroid or thyroid surgery, chronic renal failure, or chronic anticonvulsant drug treatment. It also occurs in primary idiopathic hypoparathyroidism (when the serum parathormone level is low), and in pseudohypoparathyroidism (in which the serum parathormone level is normal or high, and there is no response to parathyroid hormone; skeletal deformities and dysmorphism also are present). Pseudopseudohypoparathyroidism is a syndrome with similar skeletal and dysmorphic abnormalities but normal serum calcium and parathormone levels. Hypocalcaemia causes neuromuscular irritability, tetany with a positive Chvostek's sign, and a mild encephalopathy. Severe degrees of hypocalcaemia produce generalized convulsions, psychotic behavioural disturbances, stupor, and coma. Raised intracranial pressure with papilloedema may occur. Hypocalcaemia commonly is misdiagnosed as mental retardation, dementia, or epilepsy. Skin changes and cataracts are characteristic. Calcification in basal ganglia on skull radiograph or CT scan may be evident. Rarely, basal ganglia calcification may be associated with extrapyramidal disorders.

MAGNESIUM

Renal disease may impair the ability to excrete magnesium, which is cardiotoxic. Hypomagnesaemia, due to inadequate intake or excessive renal or gastrointestinal loss, causes secondary hypocalcaemia.

ACID–BASE DISTURBANCES

Systemic acidosis and alkalosis (see Section 20) occur in many diseases causing metabolic coma, but of the four disorders of acid–base balance (respiratory acidosis and alkalosis, and metabolic acidosis and alkalosis) only respiratory acidosis acts as a direct cause of stupor and coma. Hypoxia associated with respiratory acidosis may be important in producing neurological abnormalities. Metabolic acidosis may be important in producing neurological abnormalities. Metabolic acidosis, by itself, usually only causes delirium or, at most, drowsiness. The reason why even severe disorders of systemic acid–base balance usually do not interfere with the function of the brain is that it possesses powerful mechanisms for protecting its own acid–base balance, including respiratory compensation, changes in cerebral blood flow, and cellular buffering in nervous tissue. Coma in metabolic acidosis due to diabetic ketosis or hyperosmolality, lactic acidosis, uraemia, alcohol poisoning, or intake of ethylene glycol, methyl alcohol, or paraldehyde is usually due to associated metabolic abnormalities or direct effects of other toxins in these conditions. Severe respiratory acidosis produces a reduction in alertness parallel to the degree of acidosis. Respiratory alkalosis, although constricting cerebral arterioles and decreasing cerebral blood flow, rarely interferes with cerebral function. A patient in coma with respiratory alkalosis due to hyperventilation, has some other condition such as sepsis, hepatic disease, pulmonary infarction, or salicylate over-

dose. Even severe metabolic alkalosis only produces a confusional state rather than stupor or coma.

ALCOHOL

Alcohol hits the nervous system in many ways. Some are the result of acute or chronic poisoning, while others are a consequence of associated vitamin deficiency. We are not concerned here with the acute effects of alcohol, such as drunkenness and delirium tremens, but with the neurological consequences of chronic, excessive alcohol intake.

THE WERNICKE–KORSAKOFF SYNDROME

Aetiology

Inadequate intake of thiamine, of whatever cause, may lead to foci of marked hyperaemia with multiple small haemorrhages effecting particularly the upper brain-stem, hypothalamus, and thalamus adjacent to the third ventricle, and the mamillary bodies. Histologically there is a proliferation of dilated capillaries with perivascular haemorrhage in these areas. The extent of such pathology can vary considerably from case to case, and may be associated with evidence of alcohol-induced damage to the cerebral cortex, cerebellum, and peripheral nerves.

Such pathology can be produced in animals by a diet deficient in thiamine. Thiamine deficiency can be demonstrated in patients with the Wernicke–Korsakoff syndrome, and administration of thiamine can reverse many of the symptoms and signs of this syndrome. Thiamine and its pyrophosphate are cofactors to at least four enzymes, pyruvate decarboxylase, α-ketoglutarate dehydrogenase, the branched-chain ketoacid decarboxylase system, and transketolase. Thiamine deficiency results in reduced conversion of pyruvate to acetyl CoA, causing elevated plasma and tissue pyruvate levels, with decreased flux through the Krebs cycle, reducing ATP production, and impairing energy supply. In addition, there is a shortage of acetyl groups for biosynthesis.

Alcoholism with an inadequate diet is the commonest cause of the Wernicke–Korsakoff syndrome today. Malnutrition in prisoners of war, or at times of famine, may also be responsible. Chronic vomiting, for example, during pregnancy or due to gastrointestinal disease, system malignancy, prolonged intravenous feeding and anorexia nervosa, are rarer causes.

Clinical features

The onset may be insidious or subacute with increasing lethargy and inattentiveness, which develops into a typical confusional state with disorientation in time and place, loss of memory, and altered consciousness. Ophthalmoplegia develops with diplopia. The most common eye signs are nystagmus on lateral or vertical gaze, sixth-nerve palsies, or defects of conjugate gaze. Retinal haemorrhages may occur. Most alcoholic patients will also have signs of a peripheral neuropathy, and many exhibit ataxia. Untreated, the patient lapses into stupor and then coma, and dies. Hypothermia may appear.

In less acute cases, or in those recovering from the acute confusional phase, the characteristic features of the Korsakoff psychosis or amnesic syndrome will appear. The patient has a gross defect of memory for recent events, such that new information cannot be retained for more than a matter of minutes or hours. The patient is disorientated in time and place, but alert. Despite the severe defect of recent memory, he or she can recall events in the remote past. Gaps in memory are filled by giving imaginary and often graphic accounts of events (confabulation). Many patients who recover from a severe episode of Wernicke–Korsakoff syndrome are left with such an impaired recent memory that they can only function by writing all essential information into a book to replace their defective memory.

Diagnosis

Diagnosis is essentially clinical. The cerebrospinal fluid is usually normal, although the protein may be slightly raised. A computer tomography (CT) brain scan is normal, but it is worth remembering that alcoholics who fall often have subdural haematomas. Demonstration of reduced red cell transketolase activity, or of raised plasma pyruvate levels, are often invalidated by intake of food as soon as the patient comes under supervision.

Treatment

The Wernicke–Korsakoff syndrome must be considered in any individual with unexplained confusion, stupor, or coma, particularly in the presence of eye signs, a peripheral neuropathy, or a history of alcoholism or excessive vomiting. Thiamine should be given to all such patients. Usually this is in the form of combined vitamin B and C by an injection containing 250 mg of thiamine. Such high-potency vitamin injections should be given daily until oral vitamin B complex preparations can be taken.

A particular problem arises commonly in the emergency department when cases of stupor or coma of unknown cause are admitted. All such patients should be given high-dose thiamine and glucose parenterally. The risk is if glucose is given without thiamine to a patient with the Wernicke–Korsakoff syndrome, for this leads to rapid deterioration and death. Those who are thiamine deficient cannot handle the glucose load. The emergency-room doctor always needs two syringes in this situation, one with glucose, the other with thiamine.

Effective treatment will restore consciousness and reverse eye signs, but unfortunately the Korsakoff amnesia syndrome frequently does not resolve. The earlier the treatment, the better the chances of recovery, so suspicion or possibility of this diagnosis is a medical emergency.

ALCOHOLIC PERIPHERAL NEUROPATHY (SEE ALSO CHAPTER 24.17.)

Aetiology

As with the Wernicke–Korsakoff syndrome, thiamine deficiency is thought to play an important role in the production of the peripheral neuropathy associated with chronic alcoholism. Pathologically the picture of peripheral nerve damage is very similar to that seen in beri beri. There is predominantly axonal neuropathy of the 'dying back' type, affecting the somatic and sometimes the autonomic nerves. However, pure thiamine deficiency may not be the sole cause of such a neuropathy. Other vitamin deficiencies may contribute, and a direct toxic effect of alcohol on peripheral nerves may occur.

Clinical features

Alcoholic peripheral neuropathy predominantly involves sensory nerves, producing distal paraesthesiae in the feet, followed by the hands, and characteristic pain. The latter may be intense and agonizing. Squeezing the calves or scratching the soles of the feet may cause severe discomfort. At a later stage, weakness and wasting of the distal muscles of the legs and arms follows. Tendon reflexes are lost. Evidence of autonomic neuropathy may be seen in abnormal pupillary reactions and tachycardia, although postural hypotension is rare and the sphincters are usually spared.

Treatment

Alcohol must be proscribed and high-potency vitamin B given parenterally for some 10 days and then orally. The prognosis depends on how early treatment is commenced. Symptoms may take weeks to subside, but in more severe cases recovery may take many months or may be incomplete.

Alcoholic cerebellar degeneration

Some alcoholics may develop a relatively pure syndrome of ataxia, with a progressive unsteadiness of gait and of leg movements, with little or no involvement of the arms. Speech is not affected, and nystagmus is not present. Many such patients also have evidence of alcoholic peripheral neuropathy. Pathologically there is degeneration of the cerebellar cortex, particularly of the Purkinje cells, and also of the olivary nuclei. Changes in the cerebellum characteristically affect the anterior and superior parts of the vermis and hemispheres. This complication of alcoholism does not seem to be due to thiamine deficiency. However, withdrawal of alcohol and vitamin replacement can lead to recovery.

Alcoholic dementia (see Section 27)

In the past, there has been much debate over whether alcoholism produces dementia. However, it is now clear that a large proportion of those who habitually take excessive alcohol develop cognitive deficits. These can vary from mild changes to severe diffuse global dementia. They are associated with evidence of atrophy of the cerebral cortex and enlargement of the cerebral ventricles on CT brain scan.

The dementia has the usual features of change of personality, loss of memory, impairment of intellectual capacity, and emotional instability. Such patients commonly fail at work or in marriage. The gradual drift into destitution is only too well described in the literature and recognized on the streets. Head injuries in alcoholic bouts and epilepsy may occur and contribute to the overall final picture. The fully developed case of the 'down and out' is an antisocial demented individual, with dysarthric speech, tremor, an ataxic gait, and a peripheral neuropathy, who still clutches to the bottle and a bag of residual belongings.

The dementia of alcoholism is not directly related to thiamine deficiency alone. Treatment by withdrawal of alcohol, if possible, and vitamin replacement can lead to improvement. Indeed, some degree of reversal of evidence of cerebral atrophy on CT brain scan can be seen after 'drying out'. However, the prognosis is generally poor, not least because of the difficulties of persuading such people to stop drinking.

Marchiafava–Bignami disease

This rare disease was first described in Italian drinkers of crude red wine, but occurs in other alcoholics. It presents as a subacute dementing illness, which progresses rapidly to fits, rigidity, and paralysis, culminating in coma and death within a few months. Pathologically there is widespread demyelination and axonal damage in the corpus callosum and the central white matter of the cerebral hemispheres, as well as in the optic chiasma and middle cerebellar peduncles.

Central pontine myelinolysis

This is another rare disease, occurring in alcoholics and a number of other illnesses, including severe liver and renal disease, and other metabolic disturbances. A common association is with hyponatraemia, and rapid attempts to correct serum sodium by parenteral fluids. The disease is characterized by a rapidly progressive flaccid or spastic quadriplegia, with involvement of bulbar muscles to produce dysarthria and dysphagia. Consciousness and eye movement may remain intact. At worst the patient may be unable to speak or swallow, or to move any muscle except those of the eyes. Death is common, but remarkable recovery may occur.

Alcoholic myopathy

Acute alcohol poisoning can produce a dramatic toxic myopathy. There is severe pain, muscle tenderness, oedema, and weakness, which may be associated with myoglobinuria, renal damage, and hyperkalaemia. A subacute painless myopathy resolving after withdrawal of alcohol has also been described.

Tobacco–alcohol amblyopia

Another uncommon complication of alcohol occurs in combination with strong tobacco. The patient develops sudden or subacute bilateral visual failure, associated with bilateral centrocaecal scotomas. The condition has been attributed to cyanide in tobacco causing a disorder of vitamin B_{12} metabolism. Visual failure and optic atrophy may occur in patients with pernicious anaemia, particularly those who smoke. A related condition is tropical amblyopia, occurring in Africa. This has been related to excessive consumption of cassava root containing cyanide. Treatment of these conditions is with hydroxycobalamine injections.

OTHER DEFICIENCY STATES

Vitamin B$_{12}$ and folic acid deficiencies are considered in Chapter 24.3.9 and in Section 22. Other B-group vitamins are discussed in Section 10. Vitamin A and E deficiency is also discussed in Section 10.

REFERENCES

Metabolic diseases
Arieff, A.I. (1985). Aluminum and the pathogenesis of dialysis encephalopathy. *American Journal of Kidney Diseases* **6**, 317–21.
Auer, R.N. (1986). Progress review: hypoglycemic brain damage. *Stroke* **17**, 699–708.
Biasioli, S., *et al.* (1986). Uremic encephalopathy: an updating. *Clinical Nephrology* **25**, 57–63.
Bulens, C. (1981). Neurologic complication of hyperthyroidism. *Archives of Neurology* **38**, 669–70.
Butterworth, R.F. and Layrargues, G.P. (ed.) (1989). *Hepatic encephalopathy, pathophysiology and treatment.* Humana Press, Clifton, New Jersey.
Cogan, M.G., Covey, C.M., Arieff, A.I., Wisniewski, A., and Clark, O.H. (1978). Central nervous system manifestations of hyperparathyroidism. *American Journal of Medicine* **65**, 563–630.
Haussain, M. (1970). Neurological and psychiatric manifestations of idiopathic hypoparathyroidism: Response to treatment. *Journal of Neurology Neurosurgery and Psychiatry* **33**, 153–6.
Hetzel, D.J. (1981). Fulminant hepatic failure. *Anaesthesia and Intensive Care* **13**, 277–82.
Krieger, D.T. (1972). The central nervous system in Cushing's syndrome. *Mount Sinai Journal of Medicine* **39**, 416–28.
Lester, M.C. and Nelson, P.B. (1981). Neurological aspects of vasopressin release and the syndrome of inappropriate secretion of antidiuretic hormone. *Neurosurgery* **8**, 735–40.
Marks, V. and Rose, F.C. (1981). *Hypoglycemia.* Blackwell Scientific, Oxford.
Plum, F. and Posner, J.B. (1984). *Diagnosis of stupor and coma,* (3rd edn). F.A. Davis, Philadelphia.

Raskin, N.H. and Fishman, R.A. (1976). Neurologic disorders in renal failure. *New England Journal of Medicine* **294**, 143–8, 204–10.
Sanders, V. (1962). Neurologic manifestations of myxoedema. *New England Journal of Medicine* **266**, 547–52, 559.
Summerskill, W.H.J., Davidson, E.A., Sherlock, S., and Steiner, R.E. (1956). The neuropsychiatric syndrome associated with hepatic cirrhosis and an extensive portal collateral circulation. *Quarterly Journal of Medicine* **25**, 245–66.
Wilkinson, D.S. and Prockop, L.D. (1976). Hypoglycaemia: effects on the nervous system. In *Handbook of clinical neurology*, Vol. 27, (ed. P.J. Vinken and G.W. Bruyn), pp. 53–78. Elsevier North Holland, New York.

Alcohol
Charness, M.E., Simon, R.P., and Greenberg, D.A. (1989). Ethanol and the nervous system. *New England Journal of Medicine* **321**, 442–54.
Harper, C. (1983). The incidence of Wernicke's encephalopathy in Australia – a neuropathological study of 131 cases. *Journal of Neurology Neurosurgery and Psychiatry* **46**, 593–8.
Harper, C., Giles, M., and Finlay-Jones, R. (1986). Clinical signs in the Wernicke–Korsakoff complex: a retrospective analysis of 131 cases diagnosed at necropsy. *Journal of Neurology Neurosurgery and Psychiatry* **49**, 341–5.
Lishman, W.A. (1981). Cerebral disorder in alcoholism: syndromes of impairment. *Brain* **104**, 1–20.
Reuler, J.B., Girard, D.E., and Cooney, T.G. (1985). Wernicke's encephalopathy. *New England Journal of Surgery* **312**, 1035–8.
Ron, M.A. (1977). Brain damage in chronic alcoholism: neuropathological, neuroradiological and psychological review. *Psychological Medicine* **7**, 103–12.
Ron, M.A., Acker, W., Shaw, G.K., and Lishman, W.A. (1982). Computerized tomography of the brain in chronic alcoholism. *Brain* **105**, 497–514.
Victor, M., Adams, R.D., and Collins, G.H. (1971). *Wernicke–Korsakoff syndrome.* F.A. Davis, Philadelphia.

24.20 Neurological disorders due to physical agents

C. D. MARSDEN

More detailed accounts of the conditions described here can be found in Section 8. The discussion below summarizes the main neurological features.

HEAT STROKE

Heat stroke occurs in both young people undertaking excessive exercise in unaccustomed heat, and in older people or those taking anticholinergic drugs (for instance, those with Parkinson's disease) exposed to high temperatures. Anything that interferes with sweating may provoke heat stroke. Usually, such patients become agitated and confused, before passing into stupor or coma, often with generalized convulsions. The patient's skin is usually hot and dry, and there is tachycardia and hypotension. Death due to circulatory collapse occurs unless the patient is rapidly cooled. Some patients who survive heat stroke are left with permanent neurological complications, including amnesia, dysarthria, ataxia, dementia, and hemiparesis. Occasionally, polyneuropathy may complicate hyperthermia.

Malignant hyperthermia

This is a rare disorder of muscle metabolism characterized by a sudden fulminating unexpected increase in body metabolism and temperature in patients exposed to anaesthetics. High fever, respiratory and meta-

bolic acidosis, and diffuse muscular rigidity occur in susceptible individuals given anaesthetic agents such as halothane or succinylcholine. Malignant hyperthermia occurs as a result of an abnormality of muscle metabolism which is inherited as an autosomal dominant trait. It affects approximately 1 in 20 000 patients exposed to anaesthesia (see Section 8).

HYPOTHERMIA

Accidental hypothermia follows prolonged exposure to cold on mountains or in water. Hypothermia may also occur in the elderly without food and heating, and in myxoedema or hypopituitarism. A low body temperature also occurs in metabolic coma due to hypoglycaemia and drug overdose, particularly with barbiturates, phenothiazines, or alcohol. The hypothermic patient gradually lapses into confusion, stupor, then coma. Respirations are slow and shallow, shivering is usually absent, the pulse is very slow, and blood pressure may be unmeasurable. Such patients are sometimes thought to be dead when first seen. Body temperature is usually less than 32.2 °C.

DECOMPRESSION SICKNESS

This condition ('the bends') affects deep-sea divers, tunnel workers operating in a pressurized atmosphere, and amateur scuba divers unaccustomed to depth. It is due to release of bubbles of nitrogen into the blood during a too-rapid decompression, causing gas emboli and microinfarction in the nervous system. That a sudden reduction in pressure may cause liberation of gas bubbles is familiar to all who remove the top of a carbonated drink. Since nitrogen is especially soluble in body fat, it is liberated in large amounts in the nervous system, and fat men are more liable to decompression sickness than those of thinner habitus. Neurological symptoms include hemiplegia, paraplegia, visual disturbance, and vertigo. Any neurological symptoms indicate the need for urgent recompression in a compressed air chamber, with subsequent controlled slow decompression. Neurological recovery is usually slow, but may be complete. A persistent myelopathy may occur.

ELECTRICAL INJURY

Electrocution may be immediately fatal due to cardiac arrest. Less severe electrical shocks cause local burns and tissue necrosis. Changes in the nervous system are most likely to occur when the current has been applied to the skull. A severe electric shock causes immediate coma. Lesser shocks may lead to severe pain associated with hemiplegia, a flaccid paraplegia or tetraplegia, or peripheral nerve damage. Such acute neurological complications of electrical injury may disappear after about 12 h, but some are permanent. Delayed effects of electric shock have been recorded, including a delayed myelopathy and neuropathy, not unlike motor neurone disease.

RADIATION INJURY

Damage to the nervous system may be produced by radiotherapy directed at cerebral or spinal tumours, or may occur incidentally as a result of radiation employed to treat tumours elsewhere, such as those of the neck, ear, or breast. Radiation myelopathy may develop acutely during radiotherapy concentrated in the region of the cord, or may appear much later. Acute radiation myelopathy is usually transient and recovers within a matter of weeks. However, a slowly progressive paraparesis or tetraparesis may occur within 1 to 4 years after a course of radiation in the region of the cord. Weakness, spasticity, and sensory loss gradually develop, usually with sphincter impairment, and progress inexorably. The dose of radiation nearly always exceeds 40 Gy and is usually of the order of 60 to 80 Gy. Radiation encephalopathy follows similar large doses applied to the head as, for example, have been employed in the treatment of pituitary tumours. Radiation necrosis may cause swelling, producing the appearances of a tumour, or multifocal white matter degeneration. The effects of such changes may not appear for months or years after the irradiation. Irradiation in the region of the optic nerves or brachial plexus very occasionally may cause delayed optic atrophy or brachial neuropathy. Delayed radiation necrosis appears to be mainly the result of vascular damage with ischaemic change. There is no known treatment. This topic is discussed in Section 19.

REFERENCES

Burns, R.A., Jones, A.N., and Robertson, J.S. (1972). Pathology of radiation myelopathy. *Journal of Neurology Neurosurgery and Psychiatry* **35**, 888–98.

Davis, J.C., Tager, R., Polkovitz, H.T., and Workman, R.D. (1971). Neurological decompression sickness. *Aerospace Medicine* **42**, 85–94.

Jellinger, K. and Sturm, K.W. (1971). Delayed radiation myelopathy in man. *Journal of Neurological Science* **14**, 389–93.

Mehta, A.C. and Baker, R.N. (1970). Persistent neurological deficits in heat stroke. *Neurology, Minneapolis* **20**, 336–40.

Petty, P.G. and Parkin G. (1986). Electrical injury to the central nervous system. *Neurosurgery* **19**, 282–4.

Stefanini, M. (1975). Heat stroke. In *Handbook of clinical neurology: injuries of the brain and skull*, Part 1, (ed. P.J. Vinken and G.W. Bruyn), Vol. **23**, pp. 669–82. Elsevier, New York.

24.21 Neurological complications of systemic diseases

M. J. G. HARRISON

Many multisystem diseases and neoplastic conditions produce striking neurological complications. In some the cause is attributable to a vasculitis (collagenosis), in others to granulomatous infiltration (sarcoidosis), or to metastatic invasion (neoplasm). Often the mechanism of neurological damage is poorly understood, for example, in the case of the so-called non-metastatic complications of malignancies.

In most situations diagnosis depends on the identification of a well-established systemic disorder, but the neurological involvement can sometimes be the presenting feature, or even be the only clinical manifestation. Some understanding of the likely and unlikely syndromes that may be encountered is important.

Autoimmune rheumatic diseases (collagenoses)

These may affect the central or the peripheral nervous system, the underlying damage often being from microinfarction due to a vasculitis affecting small vessels. A combination of neurological signs implicating both the central nervous system and the peripheral nervous system in the same patient at the same time should raise suspicions of one of these disorders. In the CNS the combination of signs of a diffuse disorder or encephalopathy plus some focal signs is suggestive, and in the peripheral nervous system a patchy neuropathy or mononeuritis multiplex is equally suspicious of a vasculitis.

SYSTEMIC LUPUS ERYTHEMATOSUS (SEE ALSO SECTION 18)

This is probably the commonest of the so-called autoimmune rheumatic diseases and most often affects women of childbearing age. It is especially common in North American and West Indian Negro women. From one-third to one-half of the patients have neurological problems, mostly due to involvement of the CNS by a vasculitis affecting small vessels (>100 μm in diameter). Such vessels show fibrinoid necrosis and proliferative wall thickening. However, microinfarcts are sometimes found at post-mortem without an associated vasculitis. The role of deposition of antigen–antibody complexes, for example in the choroid plexus, is uncertain.

Osler described recurrent attacks of hemiplegia in a young physician who later developed nephritis, and such stroke-like episodes in the cerebral hemispheres or brain-stem are not uncommon. More usual, however, and perhaps affecting 50 per cent of victims, are mental changes. These may take the form of depression, mania, or a schizophrenic-like psychosis with hallucinations, paranoia, and even catatonia. The mental state may be difficult to distinguish from a steroid psychosis if the patient is on steroids for systemic features of the disease. Formal psychometry reveals cognitive impairment in as many as 66 per cent of patients.

Focal electroencephalogram (EEG) changes, 'ischaemic' white matter lesions on magnetic resonance imaging (MRI), and an abnormal cerebrospinal fluid are helpful pointers to CNS lupus.

Seizures ultimately occur in up to 1 in 3 cases, probably due to microinfarcts. They may respond to steroids. Confusion is possible when an epileptic patient develops a drug-induced systemic lupus erythematosus syndrome due to anticonvulsants.

Chorea is also well described and is indistinguishable from that due to rheumatic fever or associated with the use of an oral contraceptive agent. It is associated with antiphospholipid antibodies (see below).

Microinfarction in the cord may rarely produce a rapidly evolving paraplegia with sensory level and sphincter involvement. The cerebrospinal fluid sugar content may be low. There is usually little recovery. The tendency for microinfarction to occur in the brain-stem, spinal cord, and optic nerve sometimes produces a multiple sclerosis-like picture, and the cerebrospinal fluid may contain oligoclonal IgG. The systemic features of the disease with arthritis, skin lesions, alopecia, pleurisy, Raynaud's phenomenon, and nephritis make the distinction.

Rarer involvement of the peripheral nervous system may produce a neuropathy that may take one of several forms (Fig. 1). Microinfarction of peripheral nerves can produce a mononeuritis multiplex or cause a diffuse neuropathy. Rarely, a rapid onset is reminiscent of a Guillain–Barré neuropathy. Polymyositis may need to be distinguished from a steroid myopathy by electromyography (EMG), creatine kinase assay, and biopsy. A more-than-chance association with myasthenia gravis has been described.

Diagnosis

EEGs are commonly, although non-specifically, abnormal, and the cerebrospinal fluid often has an excess of cells and an elevated protein content even when there is no clinical evidence of meningism. Cerebrospinal fluid levels of complement may be depressed, but the hope that they would be an accurate marker of disease activity has not been substantiated. Computed tomography (CT) scans may show infarcts or haemorrhage or, more commonly, simple atrophy. Regional oxygen metabolism measured by positron tomography has been reported to show patchy disturbances in cerebral lupus but this has yet to be confirmed.

Magnetic resonance imaging may reveal small lesions of high signal intensity on T_2-weighted images. These are predominantly in the white matter and similar to the lesions of multiple sclerosis. They are often subcortical rather than periventricular in site, however, and do not show the radial orientation more often seen in multiple sclerosis.

The diagnosis remains essentially a clinical one, with multisystem involvement and anti-double-stranded DNA and cardiolipid antibodies. It should be suspected if a patient shows signs of both peripheral and central nervous system disturbances. The prognosis for CNS involvement, which is usually seen in the first year of disease, is initially good. Conservative measures are advised for all but the severest complications. In severe cases corticosteroids are usually combined with cytotoxic agents, and plasmapheresis may be tried.

Complications of systemic lupus erythematosus

These may affect the CNS. Thus renal failure may cause headache, confusion, drowsiness, tremor, myoclonic jerking, and fits. Hypertension may be responsible for focal signs, or headaches, fits, and coma due to hypertensive encephalopathy. A tendency to infection includes the possibility of meningitis, and emboli may occur from the heart affected by Libman–Sacks endocarditis. Two haematological complications have important neurological sequelae.

Antiphospholipid antibodies (see also Sections 13, 18 and 22)

These antibodies are not uncommon in patients with lupus. They may also be seen in patients with livedo reticularis, frequent miscarriages, and thrombotic episodes who do not have other features of lupus. The antiphospholipid syndrome causes thrombotic phenomena due to the presence of the so-called lupus anticoagulant. This misnamed protein affects the prothrombin complex and prostacyclin synthesis, giving rise to deep vein thromboses, pulmonary embolism, and cerebral infarction. It should be sought in young stroke victims, especially those with a history of other thrombotic events or miscarriages. Lifelong antithrombotic treatment is required. Warfarin is usually prescribed, except during pregnancy when heparin or aspirin and prednisone are preferred.

Thrombotic thrombocytopenia purpura (see also Sections 20 and 22)

This rare condition, which may complicate systemic lupus erythematosus, is probably due to immune complex formation. It causes a thrombocytopenic purpura, haemolytic anaemia, neurological abnormalities, fever, and evidence of renal disease. Ninety per cent of cases have neurological symptoms and signs, although these are often fleeting in nature. Frequent seizures, fever, and coma occur terminally, when the autopsy reveals widespread small-vessel occlusions in the brain. The course of the disease is usually aggressive although some patients have been kept alive for a few years by the use of immunosuppression, antiplatelet agents, and plasmapheresis.

POLYARTERITIS NODOSA (SEE ALSO SECTION 18)

This rare but serious disease is characterized by fibrinoid necrosis of the media, extending to involve the adventitia and intima. The intense inflammatory response that is also seen in all three layers of the walls of small and medium-sized arteries may be secondary. Weakened areas of the necrotic wall may lead to aneurysm formation (hence 'nodosa'). The vasculitis causes thromboses, infarctions, and haemorrhage. Most patients are male and have fever, malaise, arthritis, abdominal pain, renal disease, hypertension, and pulmonary involvement in some combination or other.

Neurological complications are common. Some 50 per cent of patients have a peripheral neuropathy, and at autopsy as many as 75 per cent may show signs of involvement of the vasa nervorum. A mononeuritis multiplex, often presenting with a peroneal nerve palsy causing foot drop, may be the first sign of the disease. Individual nerve lesions may come on over a few hours and follow a relapsing and remitting course. The neuropathy is commonly more motor than sensory in its manifestations and affects the legs more than the arms. Less commonly, a diffuse and symmetrical mixed polyneuropathy may develop which is often

Fig. 1 Claw hand deformity due to combined median and ulnar nerve lesion in a case of vasculitis ? SLE.

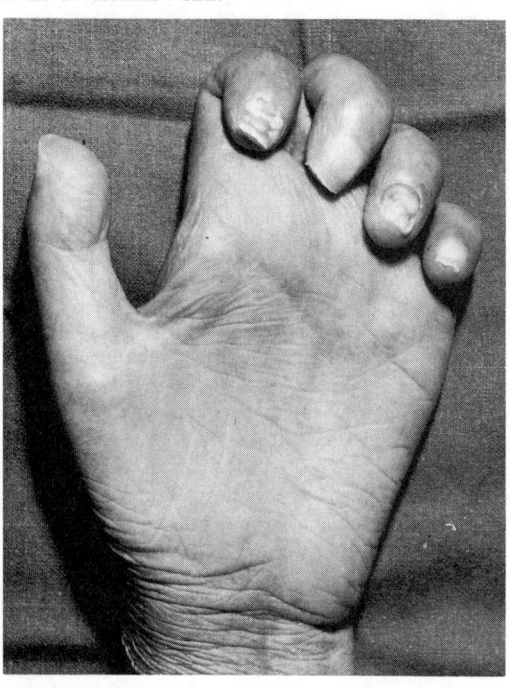

accompanied by weight loss and anorexia. A subclinical neuropathy may be detected by nerve conduction studies or biopsy. Rarely, patchy sensory loss is seen due to damage to small cutaneous nerves.

Muscle pain is reported by many patients, due either to a polymyalgia rheumatica-like syndrome or to polymyositis, with elevated creatine kinase levels and a biopsy finding of arteritis and microinfarcts. Some biopsies prove normal, however, due to the patchy nature of the changes.

Central nervous system manifestations are protean and tend to wax and wane. Organic psychoses, dementia, seizures, and focal lesions may result from vessel occlusions, and subarachnoid or cerebral haemorrhage may be seen. A meningeal illness with or without cranial nerve palsies can occur with a cellular cerebrospinal fluid. The cord is rarely affected due to thrombosis of spinal arteries.

The diagnosis of polyarteritis nodosa may be suggested by fever, weight loss, purpura, arthritis, proteinuria, red cell urinary casts, abdominal pain from bowel ischaemia, and renal failure. The erythrocyte sedimentation rate may be raised and there is usually a leucocytosis. Biopsy confirmation may be obtained from muscle, nerve, or kidney. Polymyositis and the mononeuritis multiplex may respond to steroids but the response is unpredictable. Involvement of the CNS implies a poor outlook, but is uncommon.

SCLERODERMA (SEE ALSO SECTION 18)

This collagenosis mainly affects females. It is rare, with something like 2.7 per million per year new cases appearing in the United Kingdom. It is often more severe in Negroes. There is a widespread and progressive sclerosis affecting the skin, lungs, kidneys, upper gastrointestinal tract, and myocardium. Raynaud's disease and painful stiffness of the hands are frequent early features, together with fatigue and headache. Over 5 per cent of patients develop oesophageal motility disturbances and many have reticular shadowing on chest radiograph. Progressive pulmonary hypertension and right heart failure may develop late in the disease. Renal involvement is common and carries a poor prognosis. However, progression is not the rule, and in some patients scleroderma may even regress.

It has been estimated that between 10 and 15 per cent of patients with scleroderma have a form of myositis. This is manifested by the development of proximal muscle weakness. Wasting and weakness of neck muscles is often striking. Creatine kinase levels may be elevated, and EMG studies show abnormalities of motor units, together with insertional activity and fibrillation potentials. Steroids are indicated. In other patients, creatine kinase levels are unremarkable and EMG findings suggest a myopathy rather than a myositis, in which case steroids are less likely to be helpful.

Cranial nerve lesions may also develop, with trigeminal sensory loss and pain being the commonest findings. This develops insidiously and may be accompanied by a facial nerve lesion mimicking a Bell's palsy. Trigeminal neuropathy may even be the presenting feature before skin changes are obvious. These cranial nerve lesions may be due to perineural sclerosis or a microangiopathy. A peripheral neuropathy like that seen in rheumatoid arthritis, and a stroke due to progressive narrowing of the cervical carotid artery are rare complications. Dementia, and a pseudotabetic picture due to posterior column degeneration have also been described.

RHEUMATOID ARTHRITIS (SEE ALSO SECTION 18)

Assessment of neurological complications is made difficult by pain and deformity due to joint disease. Muscle wasting and weakness may be due to disuse as well as to neuropathy, and EMG studies may be needed to make such distinctions.

As many as one in three patients develop true muscle weakness. In some cases this is due to steroid myopathy with type II fibre atrophy, although the same histological appearance may be found in patients who have never been given steroids ('rheumatic myopathy'). Less com-

monly, biopsies show an inflammatory myositis. Commonest of all is a minimal histological change, the pathogenesis of which is not fully understood.

Occasional patients, especially those with the cutaneous stigmata of vasculitis, develop a peripheral neuropathy. This is usually predominantly sensory in nature and most obvious in the legs, but it occasionally produces distal weakness and wasting as well as impairment of all modalities of sensation. Victims have usually had long-standing arthritis and have skin nodules, vasculitic skin lesions, weight loss, and fever, and high titres of rheumatoid factor. Many more patients manifest nerve compression syndromes, for example, of the median nerve in a carpal tunnel compromised by rheumatoid changes in the carpus and flexor tendons, or the ulnar nerve at a disorganized elbow. Muscle wasting in the hand may thus be due to disuse associated with destructive joint changes, median or ulnar neuropathy, or peripheral neuropathy, the distinction being aided by EMG and nerve conduction studies. Pallis and Scott brought to general attention an unusual digital neuropathy in victims of rheumatoid arthritis. Sensory testing may reveal loss of pinprick sensation restricted to one side of a finger.

The prognosis for peripheral nerve involvement tends to be good for those with solitary nerve lesions, although surgical decompression may be required. Some recovery of the predominantly sensory neuropathy can occur, but the severe mixed neuropathy, or a mononeuritis multiplex, appears to be a reflection of an aggressive vasculitic form of the disease. Such patients commonly succumb to septicaemia or the effects of coronary or mesenteric arteritis.

Serial radiographs of the cervical spine show that patients seropositive for IgM rheumatoid factor, especially females on steroids, tend to develop atlanto-axial or subaxial subluxation (Fig. 2). These changes, and vertical movement of the odontic peg, result from disruption of ligaments and decalcification of the bones (for example, of the occiput). Such involvement of the cervical spine may only cause the appearance of brisk reflexes in the upper limbs, but in the late stages of the disease

Fig. 2 Lateral radiographic view of the cervical spine of a patient with long-standing rheumatoid arthritis showing atlantoaxial dislocation with wide separation of the arch of the atlas and the odontoid peg (by courtesy of Dr M. Chapman).

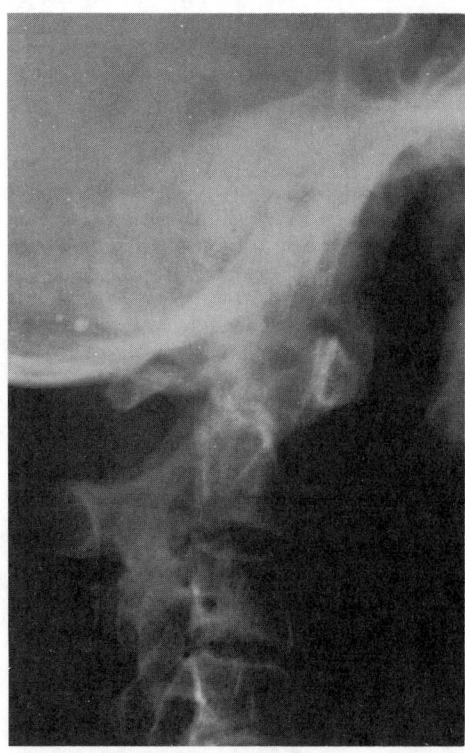

a dangerous myelopathy may develop. The patients may then present with a paraplegia or with atrophy of hand muscles and painless sensory loss in the hands. Root pain over the occipital region (C2) is also common. If the odontoid is displaced upwards, nystagmus and dysarthria may be added to the picture of high cord compression. Immobilization externally or internally is essential, but is difficult and often hazardous.

Very rarely, the CNS is affected by vasculitis causing epilepsy, cognitive change, or focal signs. Alternatively, the same picture can be due to rheumatic nodules.

SJÖGREN'S SYNDROME

Lymphocytic infiltration may develop in the lacrimal and salivary glands of patients with a connective tissue disorder, usually rheumatoid arthritis or systemic lupus erythematosus. Others have no such underlying disease. Keratoconjunctivitis sicca (dry eyes) may be accompanied by xerostoma (dry mouth) and salivary gland enlargement. Ninety per cent of these patients are female. An associated arteritis may cause an isolated trigeminal neuropathy, as seen in progressive system sclerosis, and some 10 per cent of patients develop a mild distal sensory neuropathy. Psychiatric disturbances are the commonest manifestation of CNS involvement.

From some centres more florid CNS disease mimicking multiple sclerosis has been reported, but this has not been the experience in the United Kingdom.

Sarcoidosis (see also Section 17)

This systemic disease is defined pathologically by granulomatous formation in many organs. A granulomatous meningoencephalitis underlies most of the neurological features, although confluent granulomas may rarely produce a mass lesion in the CNS.

Early in the course of the disease there may be cranial nerve lesions or a neuropathy. The second and seventh nerves are most often affected, and sarcoidosis should always be suspected in cases of bilateral Bell's palsy and optic neuritis. Dysphagia, deafness, and vocal cord paralysis may be seen. These individual nerve lesions tend to be transient. The diagnosis is suggested by the presence of concurrent intrathoracic or ocular disease, such as uveitis or lacrimal gland swelling. Because of the granulomatous changes in the meninges, root lesions may also be seen. The cerebrospinal fluid is commonly abnormal, with a lymphocytic pleocytosis, elevated protein, and, in about a third, a reduced glucose level. Oligoclonal IgG may be found, raising suspicions of multiple sclerosis.

Late in the disease the CNS may be involved, especially in the hypothalamic–pituitary areas, with diabetes insipidus, amenorrhoea, and somnolence. Before biopsy, hemisphere masses may be indistinguishable from a glioma. Such CNS involvement is usually chronic. When it occurs without systemic disease the diagnosis depends on the CT or MRI (Fig. 3) scan appearances, cerebrospinal fluid changes, and a Kveim test, which is positive in 75 per cent of cases. Biopsy of the liver, lymph nodes, or muscle, even though the last is usually asymptomatic, can also be diagnostic. Occasional patients develop myopathy when muscle biopsies reveal granulomata.

Steroids are always worth trying, but their effects are unpredictable. As suggested, the prognosis for peripheral nerve lesions is better than that for involvement of the cord or brain.

System sarcoidosis may also cause neurological symptoms by causing hypercalcaemia. Confusion, irritability, or proximal muscle weakness may occur, which must be distinguished from the effects of neurosarcoidosis *per se*.

Behçet's syndrome (see also Section 18)

Behçet, a Turkish dermatologist, described the triad of relapsing oral and genital ulcers with uveitis. Arthritis and skin changes such as ery-

thema nodosum are also frequent and the nervous system is involved in 10 to 25 per cent of patients. The neurological complications also tend to relapse and remit so that the differential diagnosis is often between Behçet's syndrome and multiple sclerosis. Behçet's syndrome is more likely than multiple sclerosis to produce a hemiplegia or pseudobulbar palsy, and to be associated with an elevated erythrocyte sedimentation rate and occasionally with a slight lymphocyte pleocytosis in the cerebrospinal fluid. There are also likely to be systemic symptoms, with a fresh crop of mouth and genital ulcers, joint pains, uveitis, and vascular thrombosis at the time of each neurological relapse. Recurrent brainstem episodes may also be confused with recurrent strokes. The pathological changes responsible for focal neurological changes include necrosis and demyelination with scarring. Some vessels also show an inflammatory cell infiltration. Other presentations with, for example, headache and papilloedema, reflect the occurrence of a meningoencephalitis or cerebral venous thrombosis. The cerebrospinal fluid often shows a pleocytosis. There are no specific tests, the cornerstone of diagnosis being a long history of mouth and genital ulcers and uveitis, as neurological complications are usually a late feature of the syndrome. Patients may have to be asked directly about ulcers as many have become accustomed to them as part of their normal lives. CT, MRI, and single photon emission tomography (Fig. 4) may show non-specific lesions or masses. Once the diagnosis of the neurological type of Behçet's syndrome is made, treatment with steroids should be tried. Few patients die of their neurological involvement.

Wegener's granulomatosis (see also Section 18)

This is a rare form of necrotizing vasculitis of the upper and lower respiratory tract with granuloma formation, usually accompanied by glomerulonephritis. Ulceration of the nasal mucosa often occurs and patients present with haemorrhagic sinusitis or pulmonary infiltration. The chest radiograph shows diffuse infiltrates or nodular opacities often mimicking metastases. The diagnosis can be made by biopsying the nasal mucosa, lung, and kidney. The nervous system is affected in some 25 per cent of cases. The vasculitis causes damage in the CNS or to the cranial nerves or peripheral nerves when it produces the picture of a mononeuritis multiplex. Less commonly, direct spread from the nasopharynx may affect the orbit or cause cranial nerve lesions. Modern treatment combines steroids with cytotoxic agents, usually cyclophosphamide.

Fig. 3 MRI scan, showing multiple small foci of enhancement on T_1-weighted images after the injection of gadolinium-DTPA in a patient with symptomatic cerebral sarcoidosis.

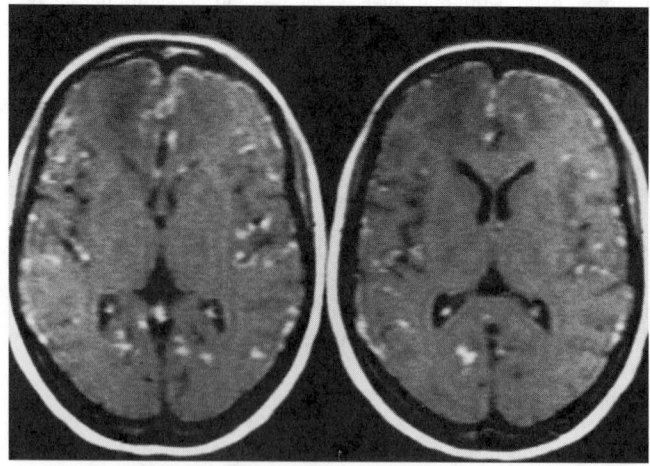

Malignancy (see Section 6)

As many as 1 in 5 patients with generalized cancer develop evidence of involvement of the nervous system. Metastases often develop in the brain or in the epidural space, and at death some 10 to 20 per cent of cancer victims have a cerebral metastasis (Fig. 5). Other patients develop neurological problems as a result of their antineoplastic treatment, whether this is by radiation of chemotherapy. In a third group neuro-

Fig. 4 Single photon emission tomography after injection of ⁹⁹Tcᵐ-hexamethylpropylene oxime in a patient with Behçet's disease, showing marked asymmetry of regional cerebral blood flow in the posterior fossa due to a recent left-sided brain-stem lesion.

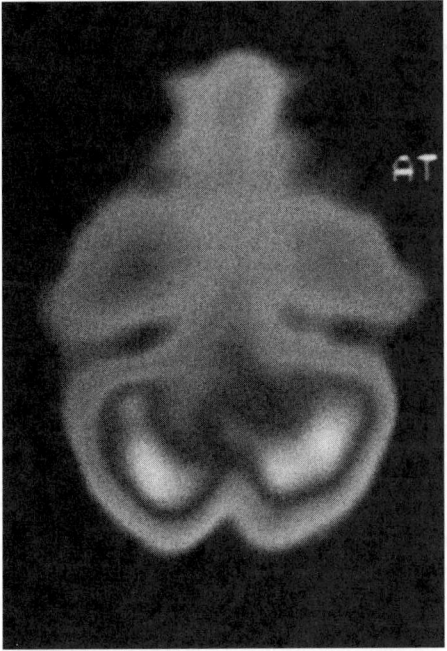

Fig. 5 Radionuclide brain scan after an injection of ⁹⁹Tcᵐ glucoheptonate showing multiple metastases from carcinoma of the breast (by courtesy of Dr P. Ell).

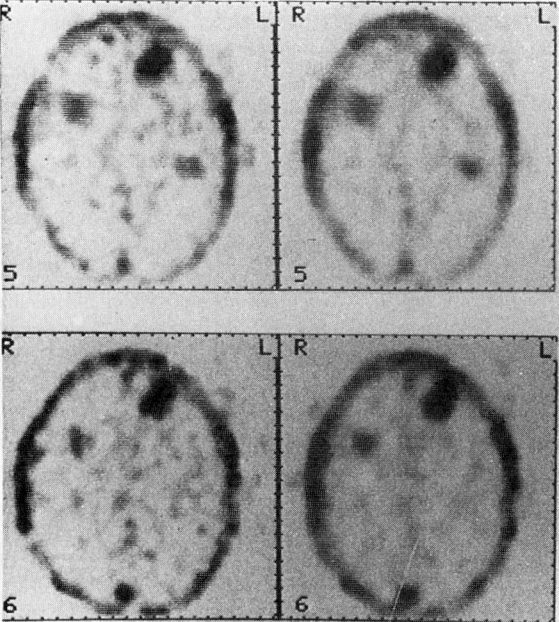

logical features are unrelated to the spread of malignant tissue. In these the mechanism is poorly understood, although some are due to opportunistic infections in the immunodeficient patient. Others are known as 'non-metastatic' complications or the 'remote effects' of cancer on the nervous system. Both lymphomas and cancers produce these manifestations but there are important differences.

LYMPHOMA (SEE ALSO SECTION 22)

Generalized lymphomas rarely cause intracerebral deposits but spinal cord compression from epidural masses arises in up to 5 per cent of cases. Local back pain is usual, often accompanied by root pain. Most patients have a deposit between mid-cervical and mid-thoracic levels. At first the only signs may be of lost abdominal reflexes and extensor plantars and the diagnosis needs to be made by myelography or MRI at this early stage to obtain the best results from treatment by steroids and radiotherapy. Later, sensory loss, weakness, and sphincter damage develop, sometimes acutely with flaccidity and areflexia from spinal shock. Once paralysis is marked there is little chance of recovery.

Although cerebral masses are rare, nasopharyngeal or orbital deposits are not uncommon, especially in non-Hodgkin's lymphoma (Fig. 6). Patients present with a proptosis or with nerve palsies. A local mass must be demonstrated clinically or radiologically to distinguish an extra-cranial lesion from a lymphomatous meningitis which may also cause cranial nerve palsies. In the latter case headache and vomiting are usually prominent and cytology of the cerebrospinal fluid is diagnostic. If no diagnostic cells are seen, myelography or MRI sometimes shows nodules. Such patients need radiotherapy and intrathecal chemotherapy. A CT scan should precede the lumbar puncture if at all possible.

Opportunistic infections are common in the lymphomata, causing meningitis with or without hydrocephalus or brain abscess. Listeria, herpes zoster, Cryptococcus, Toxoplasma, coccidiomycosis, and Aspergillus all need consideration, with appropriate bacteriological or virological study of the cerebrospinal fluid and search for antibodies. A peculiar invasion of the white matter with papova-like virus may cause a progressive unilateral then bilateral hemisphere disorder with visual disturbance, hemiparesis, and mental change. CT scans show non-enhancing low-density changes in the white matter, and MRI shows areas of high signal on T_2-weighted images which have no mass effect.

This condition (progressive multifocal leucoencephalopathy) is rapidly fatal in most instances (Fig. 7) (see also Chapter 24.15.2). Alter-

Fig. 6 CT scan showing a soft tissue mass in the left side of the nasopharynx obliterating the air passages. The patient had presented with a sixth nerve palsy. Biopsy confirmed that the nasopharyngeal tumour was a non-Hodgkin's lymphoma.

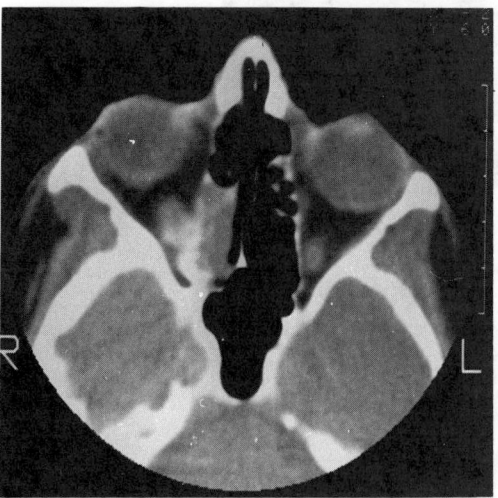

natively, an encephalitic illness with mental changes, sometimes amounting to dementia or a severe amnesic state, may occur. Although there are inflammatory changes, sometimes concentrated on the limbic area, no infective agent has yet been identified in these patients. Fits suggest the rare alternative possibility of an intracerebral lymphomatous mass.

Several other non-metastatic complications may be seen in patients with a lymphoma. A subacute cerebellar ataxia may cause severe disability within a few months. Various types of peripheral neuropathy are encountered, ranging from an acute Guillain–Barré-like illness to a mixed neuropathy indistinguishable from that due to diabetes mellitus. Asymmetrical wasting with weakness and fasciculation is particularly associated with lymphoma; anterior horn cell loss is responsible and there is some associated dorsal column change, although sensory loss is slight. A subacute sensory neuropathy with disabling loss of position sense can also occur, and is due to mononuclear cell infiltration and cell loss in the dorsal root ganglia. Polymyositis and a necrotizing myelopathy are other paraneoplastic syndromes that may be seen.

Primary CNS lymphoma was an uncommon brain tumour until the advent of the acquired immunodeficiency syndrome (AIDS). Since the first description of this syndrome in 1981 an increasing number of B-cell tumours have been reported, affecting only the CNS. Headache, seizures, mental changes, and focal deficits prove on CT or MRI to be due to mass lesions. Biopsy is needed for diagnosis. The lesions are sensitive to radiation therapy but most patients are severely immuno-suppressed and their prognosis is poor.

CARCINOMAS

Metastases

In the case of carcinoma, intracerebral metastases (Fig. 5) predominate, affecting as many as 20 to 40 per cent of patients with carcinoma of the bronchus, for example. Almost any primary tumour may metastasize to the brain and, as survival lengthens with modern treatment, more unusual tumours are appearing as causes of cerebral secondaries. The most common sources of cerebral metastases are tumours of the lung, breast, testes, and skin (melanoma). The presentation is indistinguishable from that of a primary intracerebral tumour until scans show a second or third lesion. Multiple deposits are more common than single ones,

Fig. 7 MRI T_2-weighted scan, showing large area of high-intensity signal in the white matter of the left cerebral hemisphere due to biopsy-proven progressive multifocal leucoencephalopathy in a case of AIDS.

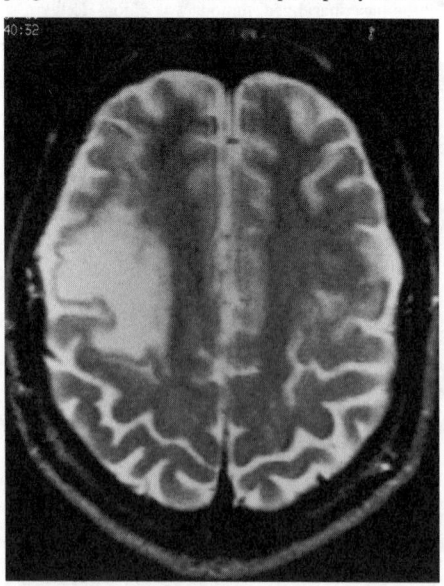

and the brain is rarely the only site of metastatic spread. Isotope scanning, CT, and MRI are all reliable investigations. Surgery may be indicated for a solitary posterior fossa deposit to relieve vertigo and vomiting, and radiotherapy and steroids may add several months of good-quality life in other selected cases.

Occasionally the deposits are in the skull base, with cranial nerve palsies, or in vertebrae, with secondary spinal cord compression. In the latter case plain spine films will often show an eroded pedicle. However, MRI or myelography is usually needed to plan treatment.

Radiotherapy and steroids are indicated for such a patient if the tumour is radiosensitive, although a laminectomy may be needed, especially if signs progress under treatment or if there is no tissue diagnosis. A carcinomatous meningitis causing multiple cranial nerve palsies may also occur as described for lymphomas. Opportunistic infections also occur although progressive multifocal leucoencephalopathy is rare.

Non-metastatic complications

Non-metastatic complications are more common. For example, a subacute progressive ataxia, which often causes severe disability, may develop, particularly in cases of carcinoma of the bronchus, breast, and ovary. A peripheral neuropathy not infrequently develops terminally, especially in patients with carcinoma of the bronchus. Limb weakness can be due to cachexia or a neuropathy, or a mixed picture may develop in which some of the features look myopathic (proximal weakness) and some neuropathic (absent ankle jerks). The fact that a particular syndrome is due to an underlying neoplasm may be suggested by combinations of neurological features such as lost ankle jerks from a neuropathy, and extensor plantar responses, all in a patient with a cerebellar syndrome. A subacute myelopathy may cause paraparesis and needs to be distinguished from cord compression (by MRI or myelography).

Polymyositis, with or without dermatological changes, sometimes proves to be associated with a neoplasm, particularly in males over the age of 50 years. Proximal muscle weakness is accompanied by pain and muscle tenderness, although the latter diagnostic features may be missing. EMG changes, an elevated creatine kinase, and a high erythrocyte sedimentation rate may be confirmatory but the diagnosis is finally dependent upon a muscle biopsy, which reveals muscle cell damage and inflammatory cell infiltration. Corticosteroids may be indicated, the prognosis being good in the short term for suppression of the myositis but dominated in the longer term by the underlying malignancy. Muscle atrophy may, alternatively, be due to cachexia.

Rarely, a syndrome of fatiguable weakness is seen. This is the Eaton–Lambert syndrome (see Section 25), in which an autoimmune process affects the release of acetylcholine quanta at the neuromuscular junction. Patients have a myasthenic-like weakness, usually affecting limb rather than eye muscles, in contrast to most cases of myasthenia gravis. The diagnosis may be suggested clinically by the finding that depressed or absent reflexes are enhanced by prior voluntary contraction of the muscle. This effect is best demonstrated, however, by repetitive nerve stimulation with recordings of the evoked muscle action potential, which may increase two- to sixfold. Power may be improved by oral doses of guanidine (see Section 25).

Some cancer patients develop an encephalomyelitis which affects the limbic areas (with amnesia, hallucinations, and epilepsy), the spinal cord, or dorsal root ganglia with a sensory ataxia, as described with lymphomas. These syndromes may be accompanied by a cellular response in the cerebrospinal fluid. There is no specific treatment. Antibodies to dorsal root ganglia and Purkinje cells have been identified in individual cases and these encephalitic complications may well prove to be due to immunological processes. Opsoclonus (chaotic eye movements) and myoclonus may complicate neuroblastoma in children.

Vascular disease (stroke) can be due to marantic endocarditis, especially with carcinoma of the lung. Echocardiography may reveal vegatations, and cerebral angiography may reveal branch occlusions. Heparin is indicated if the patient's progress is sufficiently favourable.

MULTIPLE MYELOMATOSIS (SEE ALSO SECTION 22)

This disorder very commonly involves vertebrae, with back pain and cord compression, usually with a sensory level. The diagnosis is made by an elevated erythrocyte sedimentation rate and alkaline phosphatase, and by protein electrophoresis and bone marrow biopsy. Hypercalcaemia from myeloma, or from multiple carcinomatous bony metastases, may itself cause symptoms either of muscle weakness or of lethargy, drowsiness, confusion, or delirium. Symptoms are likely with a corrected calcium level of 3.5 nmol and almost universal at 4.0 nmol. Myeloma patients also develop a peripheral neuropathy, even when the myeloma is restricted to a solitary bone. Amyloidosis may complicate myeloma and cause a painful small fibre neuropathy with autonomic changes, and distal pain and temperature loss. If the myeloma protein causes a hyperviscosity syndrome, mental confusion and clouding of consciousness may be accompanied by visual disturbance due to retinal haemorrhages and exudates.

BRACHIAL PLEXUS LESIONS

Carcinoma of the breast also affects the brachial plexus by local infiltration. A painful progressive paralysis of the arm develops. It has to be distinguished from radiation damage to the plexus after radiotherapy to axillary nodes. The latter may be painless and more often affects upper roots (C5/6) than lower (C8/T1). EMG findings and imaging may help in the distinction, but sometimes this requires surgical exploration.

LEUKAEMIA (SEE ALSO SECTION 22)

As treatment of leukaemia increases survival, more patients develop involvement of the nervous system. Leukaemic cells may be found in the walls of veins, the arachnoid, and in the brain parenchyma. Some patients have multiple episodes of neurological involvement, and relapses may occur when the patient is in complete systemic remission. The brain is a sanctuary for leukaemic cells as chemotherapy may fail to cross the blood–brain barrier. This problem has led to prophylactic treatment of the asymptomatic CNS, for example, in children with acute lymphatic leukaemia, when a combination of radiotherapy and intrathecal cytotoxic drugs is often employed.

Involvement of the CNS by leukaemia represents a serious advance in the disease and carries a poor prognosis. A meningeal picture is commonest with headache, drowsiness, vomiting, papilloedema, and neck stiffness. The cerebrospinal fluid pressure is elevated, as is the cell count, and the glucose level may be low. It is important that the nature of the

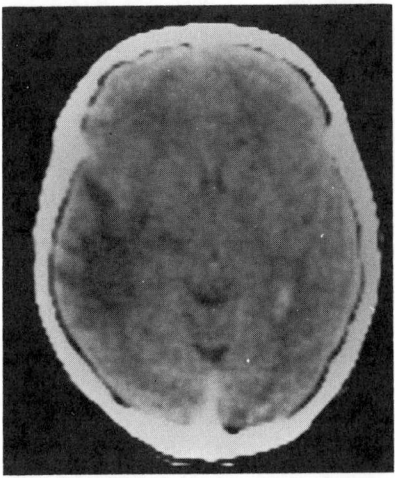

Fig. 8 CT scan showing low-density area in the left hemisphere due to radionecrosis after radiotherapy to the parotid bed. The patient presented with temporal lobe epilepsy.

cerebrospinal fluid cells be identified. A leukaemic patient may have leukaemic cells in the cerebrospinal fluid with infiltration of arachnoid and dura, but equally might be suffering from a superadded viral meningitis, due to herpes zoster, for example, in which case the cells are mature lymphocytes. A CT scan may show hydrocephalus due to meningeal block.

Cerebral haemorrhage is a common terminal event and is associated with high blood white cell counts and, sometimes, with the presence of intracerebral leukaemic nodules. Multiple haemorrhages tend to occur in the cerebral white matter, often associated with a general bleeding tendency due to thrombocytopenia.

Infiltration can cause cranial nerve or peripheral nerve lesions and a 'non-metastatic' neuropathy can occur. There is a common problem of an encephalopathy with lethargy, confusion, and drowsiness which may have a variety of causes. Intracranial hypertension from meningeal infiltration and hydrocephalus, hyperviscosity from very high white cell counts, subdural haematoma from a bleeding tendency, diffuse intravascular coagulation with multiple infarcts, and progressive multifocal leucoencephalopathy are all possible and are best distinguished by CT scanning or MRI.

Finally, patients with leukaemia are vulnerable to opportunistic infections, especially fungal meningitis and brain abscess.

COMPLICATIONS OF TREATMENT

Damage to the brachial plexus during radiotherapy to the axilla in patients with cancer of the breast has already been mentioned. Similar damage to the pelvic plexus may develop after treatment of the cervix or lower bowel.

Radiotherapy can also damage the spinal cord either transiently in the few weeks after a course of treatment, when Lhermitte's sign develops, or much more rarely a progressive cord syndrome may develop 6 months after irradiation. Such radiation necrosis of the cord can be fatal and is resistant to treatment, although steroids may be tried. Aggressive treatment of carcinoma of the larynx or bronchus is often responsible. Metastatic compression must be excluded by MRI or myelography.

Radiation necrosis can also occur in the brain (Fig. 8). Sometimes this causes a swollen mass that behaves clinically like a tumour and may be indistinguishable from a new tumour or tumour recurrence before biopsy. If it produces a mass effect, surgical excision is needed. Other patients develop a demyelinating or atrophic lesion, which may cause epilepsy, memory loss, somnolence, or brain-stem signs, depending on the treatment field. These changes are best defined by MRI. The risk of radionecrosis depends on the total dose and fraction size, it being unwise to exceed 200 cGy to the brain per treatment.

Of the drugs used in cancer patients, several cause a peripheral neuropathy, for example cisplatinum and vincristine. The latter regularly causes areflexia after as little as 5 mg, and after about three injections the patients complain of paraesthesiae in the fingers. Weakness is often prominent in finger extensors, and autonomic fibre damage may produce postural hypotension. The changes are reversible if the drug is stopped early in the development of the symptomatic phase. Methotrexate is neurotoxic, causing cerebellar ataxia, epilepsy, and impaired intellectual development when given intrathecally in combination with radiotherapy in the prophylaxis against CNS involvement in childhood leukaemia.

REFERENCES

Systemic lupus erythematosus

Feinglass, E.J., Arrett, F.G., Dorsch, C.A., Zizic, T.M. and Stevens, M.B. (1976). Neuropsychiatric manifestations of systemic lupus erythematosus diagnosis, clinical spectrum and relationship to other features of the disease. *Medicine* **55**, 323–39.

Kaell, T., Shetty, M., Lee, B.C.P., and Lockshin, M.D. (1986). The diversity of neurologic events in systemic lupus erythematosus. *Archives of Neurology* **43**, 273–6.

Sigal, L.H. (1987). The neurologic presentation of vasculitic and rheumatologic syndrome: a review. *Medicine* **66**, 157–80.

Polyarteritis nodosa

Cohen, R.D., Conn, D.L., and Ilstrup, D.M. (1980). Clinical features, prognosis and response to treatment in polyarteritis. *Mayo Clinic Proceedings* **55**, 146–55.

Scleroderma

Clements, P.J., *et al.* (1978). Muscle disease in progressive systemic sclerosis. *Arthritis and Rheumatism* **21**, 62–71.

Farrell, D.A. and Medsger, T.A. (1986). Trigeminal neuropathy in progressive systemic sclerosis. *American Journal of Medicine* **73**, 57–62.

Teasdell, R.D., Frayhan, R.A., and Schulman, L.E. (1980). Cranial nerve involvement in systemic sclerosis (scleroderma). A report of 10 cases. *Medicine* **59**, 149–59.

Rheumatoid arthritis

Nabaro, K.K., Schoena, W.C., Baker, R.A., and Dawson, D.M. (1978). The cervical myelopathy associated with rheumatoid arthritis: analysis of 32 patients – with 2 post-mortem cases. *Annals of Neurology* **3**, 144–51.

Nakano, K.K. (1975). The entrapment neuropathies of rheumatoid arthritis. *Orthopedic Clinics of North America* **6**, 837.

Pallis, C.A. and Scott, J.T. (1965). Peripheral neuropathy in rheumatoid arthritis. *British Medical Journal* **1**, 1141–7.

Neoplasms

Henson, R.A. and Ulrichm, H. (1982). *Cancer and the nervous system*. Blackwell Scientific Publications, Oxford.

Posner, J.B. (1989). In *Neurology and general medicine*, (ed. M. Aminoff), pp. 341–64. Churchill Livingstone, New York.

Rogers, L.A., Cho, E.-S., Kempin, S., and Posner, J. (1987). Cerebral infarction from non-bacterial thrombotic endocarditis. *American Journal of Medicine* **83**, 746–56.

Sarcoidosis

Delaney, P. (1977). Neurologic manifestations in sarcoidosis. *Annals of Internal Medicine* **87**, 336–45.

Luke, T.A., Stern, B.J., Krumholz, A. and Johns, C. (1987). Neurosarcoidosis: the long term clinical course. *Neurology* **37**, 461–3.

Matthews, W.B. (1965). Sarcoidosis of the nervous system. *Journal of Neurology Neurosurgery and Psychiatry* **28**, 23–9.

Behçet's syndrome

Lehner, T. and Barnes, C.G. (ed.) (1979). *Behçet's disease*. Academic Press, London.

O'Duffy, J.D. and Goldstein, N.P. (1976). Neurologic involvement in seven patients with Behçet's disease. *American Journal of Medicine* **61**, 170–8.

Wegener's granulomatosis

Drachman, D.A. (1963). Neurological complications of Wegener's granulomatosis. *Archives of Neurology* **8**, 145–55.

Wolf, S.M., Fauci, A.S., Horn, R.G., and Dale, D.C. (1974). Wegener's granulomatosis. *American Journal of Medicine* **81**, 513–25.

Section 25 *Disorders of voluntary muscles*

25.1 Introduction

J. WALTON

The anatomy and physiology of muscle

Voluntary muscle is made up of muscle fibres, each of which is a multinucleate cell containing myofibrils, sarcoplasm, and discrete intracellular organelles including mitochondria, ribosomes, and the sarcotubular system. Each fibre is enclosed within a sarcolemmal sheath beneath which muscle nuclei are situated and each has a motor endplate in which the nerve fibre terminates. The sarcolemma consists of three layers, of which the innermost is the plasma membrane, the middle layer the basement membrane, and the outer layer is collagen.

The plasma membrane, 10 nm thick, is a lipoprotein bilayer. It is differentially permeable to various ions; this helps maintain the contrast in ionic composition of the intracellular and extracellular fluids which is responsible for the resting membrane potential of the muscle fibre (see below). The permeability of the membrane is altered in several diseases. The amorphous basement membrane, about 50 nm thick, acts as a microskeleton, becoming more specialized in the motor endplate region where it contains the enzyme acetylcholinesterase, which degrades acetylcholine (ACh).

Under normal conditions muscle fibres never contract singly; the functional unit of activity is the motor unit, which comprises the group of fibres supplied by a single anterior horn cell and its axon. Discharge of an anterior horn cell causes simultaneous contraction of all of its muscle fibres. The individual muscle fibres that make up a motor unit are often widely separated within the muscle. The electrical activity that accompanies contraction of a motor unit, and which can be recorded electromyographically, depends upon many physical factors, including the characteristics of the recording electrode and of the muscle examined. In the biceps brachii of a healthy young adult, a motor unit action potential gives a di- or triphasic wave with a duration of 5 to 8 ms and an amplitude of not less than 250 μV, but there is considerable normal variation in form, amplitude, and duration. It is probable that many so-called motor unit potentials are produced not by contraction of the muscle fibres of the entire unit but by the summated electrical activity of a proportion of the component fibres, which constitute a subunit.

In 1934 Dale first demonstrated that transmission of the nerve impulse at the myoneural junction is dependent on ACh. Synaptic vesicles in the motor nerve terminal contain packets of ACh, which is released continuously to give small depolarizations (miniature endplate potentials) in the nerve terminal; these can be recorded with a microelectrode. When an action potential reaches the nerve terminal, calcium ions (Ca^{2+}) enter it from the extracellular space and many packets of ACh are released synchronously. Once released, the ACh diffuses through the synaptic clefts to combine with receptors on the fibre membrane. These receptors (AChR) are highly concentrated in terminal expansions of the postsynaptic junctional folds of the plasma membrane, with a packing density of 10^4 μm^2. The AChR molecule is about 11 nm long and 8.5 nm in diameter, spans the lipid bilayer of the membrane and protrudes 5.5 nm above its surface. It has a molecular weight of about 250 000 and is composed of five glycosylated polypeptide subunits. In normal, mature muscle the ACh receptors are localized to the endplate but, after denervation of a muscle fibre, extrajunctional receptors are formed. The arrival of the nerve action potential causes a localized depolarization of the muscle fibre membrane, giving rise to an endplate potential. When the endplate potential reaches a critical size, an action potential is induced, which travels from the endplate along the fibre surface membrane. At rest, the inside of the membrane is some 80 mV negative with respect to the outside, but as the action potential passes, the polarization of the membrane reverses, so that the inside of the fibre becomes positive. This reversal of polarity is caused by increased sodium permeability. The wave of excitation spreads into the fibre substance via a transverse system of tubules (the T-system); the resulting release of calcium ions in the sarcoplasmic reticulum initiates contraction of the fibrils.

The unit of structure of the myofibril is the sarcomere, extending from one Z-line (situated in the midst of the I-band) to the next (Fig. 1). Attached to each Z-line are thin filaments of actin, which interdigitate with thicker myosin filaments, the latter corresponding to the dark (birefringent) A-bands (Fig. 2). In cross-section, each myosin filament is surrounded by a hexagonal array of actin filaments; the actin and myosin filaments are joined by molecular cross-bridges. During contraction,

Fig. 1 The dimensions and arrangement of the contractile components in a muscle. The whole muscle (a) is made up of fibres (b) which contain cross-striated myofibrils (c, d). These are constructed of two types of protein filaments (e), put together as shown in Figure 2. (Reproduced from Huxley and Hanson (1960), with permission.)

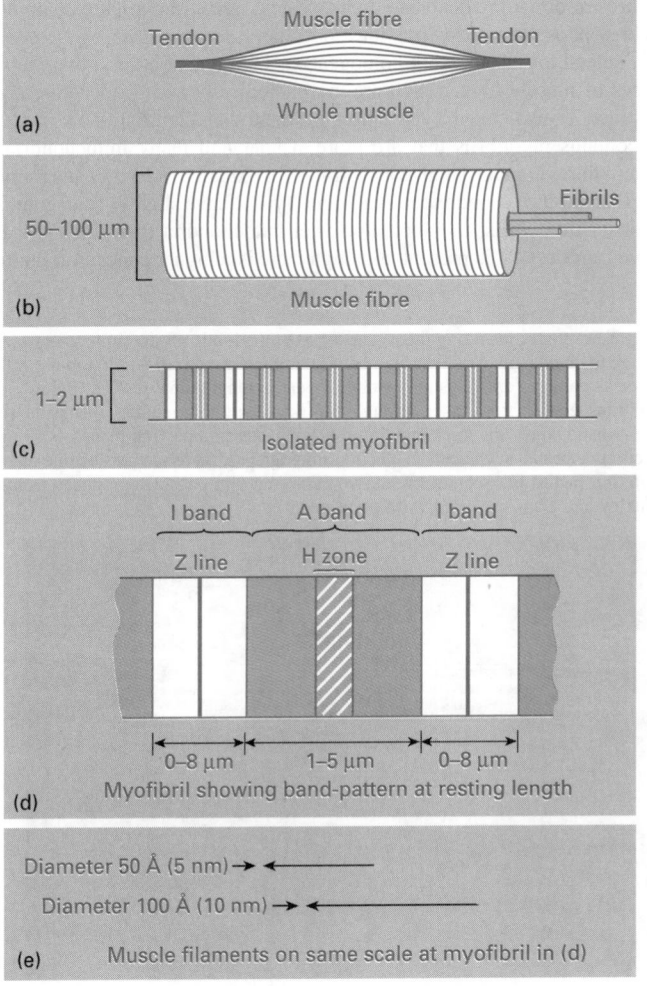

Table 1 *Histochemical and physiological characteristics of the three major muscle fibre types*

	Fibre type		
	1	2A	2B
Enzyme reactions			
NADH-tetrazolium reductase and SDH	+++	++	+
Myofibrillar ATPase			
pH9.4	+	+++	+++
pH4.6	+++	–	+++
pH4.3	+++	–	–
Phosphorylase	+	+++	+++
Physiological properties			
Twitch speed	Slow	Fast	Fast
Fatigue resistance	+++	++	+
Nomenclature			
Peter *et al.* (1972)	Slow-twitch Oxidative	Fast-twitch Oxidative-glycolytic	Fast-twitch Glycolytic
Burke *et al.* (1971)	S (slow contracting)	FR (fast contracting, fatigue resistant)	FF (fast contracting, fast fatigue)

From Walton, J.N. and Mastaglia, F.L. (1980).

these cross-bridges repeatedly disengage and re-engage at successive sites and the actin and myosin filaments slide upon one another so that the myofibril shortens. The biochemical changes accompanying this process are complex, but creatine phosphate is broken down in the presence of calcium to creatine and phosphate, and adenosine triphosphate (ATP) is broken down to adenosine diphosphate (ADP). The release of high-energy phosphate bonds provides much necessary energy.

Skeletal muscles are not homogeneous but contain at least two main types of muscle fibre, which are morphologically and histochemically distinct. The so-called Type 1 fibre is slightly smaller than the Type 2; it contains myofibrils that are more slender and many mitochondria. These fibres contain a high concentration of oxidative enzymes and more fat than do the second type. The larger Type 2 have slightly coarser and broader myofibrils, they contain fewer mitochondria than the Type 1 fibres and less fat is present, although there is a higher concentration of

glycogen and of enzymes, such as phosphorylase, which are concerned with anaerobic metabolism. In man, all skeletal muscles contain an admixture of Type 1 and Type 2 fibres, so that in sections stained histochemically a checkerboard pattern is seen. Physiologically, the Type 1 fibres are concerned largely with the maintenance of posture, and contract and relax relatively slowly. Type 2 fibres, by contrast, contract more rapidly (fast-twitch fibres). Subdivision of Type 2 fibres into Types 2a and 2b is also possible on the basis of their intensity of staining with the myofibrillar ATPase reaction at different pHs (Table 1). Type 2a fibres show inhibition of ATPase activity at pH 4.6 and a relatively higher content of oxidative enzymes than the Type 2b fibres, which inhibit ATPase activity only at pH 4.3 (Fig. 3). Both subtypes are physiologically fast-twitch fibres but, with their greater oxidative metabolic activity, the Type 2a fibres are more fatigue-resistant than the Type 2b fibres.

The two major fibre types are also distinguishable through the prop-

Fig. 2 Diagram illustrating the arrangement of the kinds of protein filaments (thick filaments–myosin, thin filaments–actin) in a myofibril. At the top are three sarcomeres drawn as they would appear in longitudinal section. Below are transverse sections taken through the H-zone and through the other parts of the A-band where the thick and thin filaments interdigitate. The plane of section determines whether, in electron micrographs, there seem to be one or two thin (actin) filaments between two thick (myosin) ones. (Reproduced from Huxley and Hanson (1960), with permission.)

Fig. 3 A transverse section of normal human skeletal muscle stained for the myofibrillar ATPase reaction after preincubation at pH 4.6. The Type 1 and 2a and 2b fibres are labelled. In the more usual myofibrillar ATPase reaction at pH 9.4, the Type 1 fibres stain light and the Type 2 fibres dark. In this so-called reverse ATPase reaction, however, at pH 4.6, the 2a and 2b fibres are easier to distinguish. Magnification ×150. (Kindly supplied by Dr Margaret Johnson.)

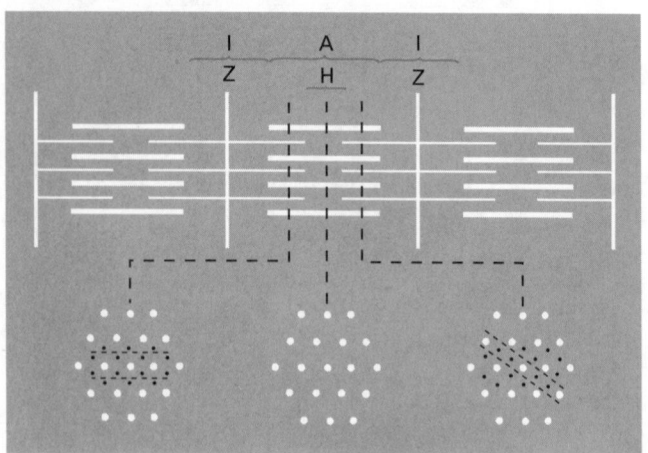

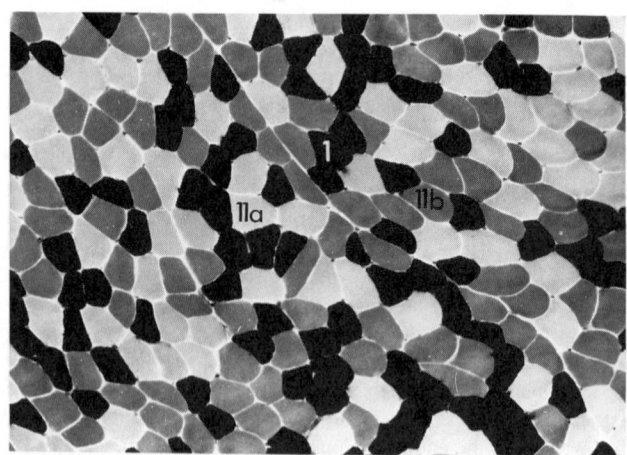

erties of their myosin light chains and through their tropomyosin and troponin content, the respective proteins in Type 1 and Type 2 fibres being immunochemically distinct. The motor nerve controls not only the physiological behaviour but also the histochemical structure of the fibres; transposition of the motor nerve from a group of 'fast' fibres to a group of 'slow' ones in animals may reverse their physiological and histochemical characteristics. It follows that all muscle fibres being supplied by a single motor neurone are of the same histochemical type and that, in a sense, therefore, we can talk of Type 1 and Type 2 neurones. Hence, when a muscle has been partially denervated, as in spinal muscular atrophy (see Section 24), surviving neurones may sprout, grow out into the muscle, and then adopt denervated muscle fibres which, on being reinnervated, form groups of muscle fibres, which are all of the same histochemical fibre type (fibre type grouping; Fig. 4).

Finally, certain drugs that act at the neuromuscular junction should be mentioned. ACh is broken down by cholinesterase, which is present in the subneural apparatus of the endplate and can be demonstrated histochemically. Curare acts on the postjunctional membrane and reduces or prevents the depolarizing effect of the ACh. Drugs like neostigmine destroy cholinesterase and allow ACh to accumulate. Guanidine hydrochloride and 4-amidopyrine act by increasing the ACh output. Initially ACh produces muscular contraction through depolarization of the fibre membrane, but if it accumulates in excess, depolarization persists and may then block the action potential (depolarization block). Whereas drugs like curare and gallamine compete with ACh for the endplate receptors and are thus known as competitive inhibitors, decamethonium and suxamethonium produce muscle paralysis first as a result of depolarization block, but later also cause competitive block, and so are said to have a 'dual' action.

General comments on muscle disorders

As diseases of the spinal cord, anterior horn cells, and peripheral nerves that affect muscle have been dealt with earlier, this section will deal only with those disorders that primarily affect voluntary muscle. The term 'myopathy' can be used to define any disease or syndrome in which the patient's symptoms and/or physical signs can be attributed to pathological, biochemical, or electrophysiological changes involving the muscle fibres or the muscular interstitial tissues, and in which there is no evidence that the symptoms are secondary to disordered function of the central or peripheral nervous system. This group includes many genetically determined diseases, others of metabolic origin, and yet others in which the disease process is inflammatory.

Clinical nosology

Pain, muscular weakness, and fatiguability are the most important symptoms of muscle disease. Muscle cramps occurring in the elderly, particularly at night, are common and may be relieved by a nocturnal dose of quinine or phenytoin; in younger individuals cramp can follow unaccustomed exertion but is sometimes a manifestation of metabolic disease. Spontaneous muscle pain at rest can occur in inflammatory disorders, but pain experienced on exertion generally implies either muscle ischaemia or a metabolic disorder such as hypothyroidism, or deficiency of phosphorylase or of one of the many other enzymes concerned with the degradation of glycogen or lipid in muscle. There is also an uncommon syndrome of benign exertional muscle pain for which no cause has yet been identified, while pain in the calf muscles following effort may be an early manifestation of increased muscle tone (spasticity), occurring, for example, in early multiple sclerosis. Every physician with an interest in muscle disease sees patients who complain bitterly of diffuse muscular pain induced by effort, which greatly restricts their activity but for which no physical or biochemical cause can at present be demonstrated. Some such individuals are obsessional and introspective and their symptoms may be of emotional origin, although treatment with tranquillizing drugs is only rarely helpful. But in other, similar, cases one can only conclude that the patient may be suffering from an as yet unidentified metabolic disorder; unfortunately symptomatic treatment with analgesic and relaxant drugs is often of little if any benefit and the symptoms may prove to be both persistent and disabling. One rare cause is myosin ATPase deficiency, in which pain can be partially relieved by verapamil.

Muscle weakness is the predominant symptom of most forms of myopathy. It is important to judge its distribution and tempo of development. Proximal muscle weakness in the upper limbs results in difficulty in lifting the arms above the head, and in the lower limbs difficulty in climbing stairs and in rising from the floor or a low chair. In most genetically determined disorders of muscle, weakness develops gradually over months or years; a more rapid onset suggests that the patient more probably has an inflammatory or metabolic myopathy. Periodic attacks of weakness with complete recovery in between strongly suggest one of the periodic paralyses. Fatiguability is characteristic of myasthenia gravis and myasthenic syndromes. The term implies that muscle weakness increases with exercise; many patients say that the more they exert themselves the weaker they become, or that weakness increases towards the end of the day. The family history is also important; if blood relatives are affected, a genetically determined disorder of muscle is probable.

On physical examination, general examination is important as there may be changes in the eyes, skin, lymph nodes, or viscera indicating that the patient's muscular weakness is but one manifestation of a systemic multisystem disease. On examining the muscular system, the presence of atrophy, hypertrophy, or fasciculation may be of diagnostic value, as may the presence of muscular contractures and skeletal deformity. Fibrillation (the spontaneous contraction of single muscle fibres) is an electrical phenomenon that can be recorded electromyographically from denervated muscle, but cannot be seen through the skin. Fasciculation (the spontaneous contraction of individual muscle fasciculi) is seen most often in patients with anterior horn cell disease; it is uncommon in primary muscle disease but occurs rarely in polymyositis or thyrotoxic myopathy. Coarse fasciculation, particularly in the calf muscles, is a benign phenomenon and may occur in normal individuals. When such benign fasciculation is widespread and accompanied by hyperhidrosis, this is often called myokymia. However, this term has also been applied to an intermittent twitch of the lower eyelid often observed in normal individuals when fatigued ('benign myokymia of the lower eyelid') to a curious continuous rippling movement of the

Fig. 4 A transverse section of human skeletal muscle obtained by biopsy from a patient with spinal muscular atrophy stained for the myofibrillar ATPase reaction after preincubation at pH 4.6. There is extensive evidence of fibre type grouping, particularly of the Type 1 fibres, resulting from reinnervation. Magnification ×150. (Kindly supplied by Dr Margaret Johnson.)

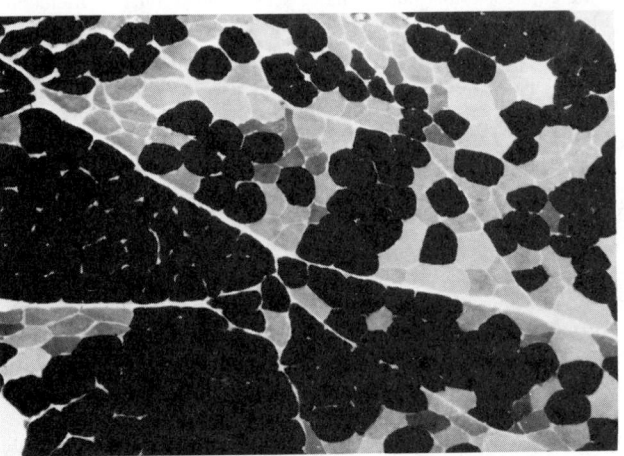

muscles of one side of the face ('facial myokymia', usually of unknown aetiology but occasionally due to multiple sclerosis), and also to a rare syndrome (also called 'neuromyotonia' or 'continuous muscle fibre activity and spasm') in which coarse fasciculation is associated with muscular spasms, with delayed relaxation resembling myotonia (see below), and with continuous activity, which can be recorded electromyographically, in affected muscles.

Delayed muscular relaxation after contraction or following percussion of a muscle is the most prominent feature of myotonia, a diagnosis that can be confirmed electromyographically (see Section 24), but in hypothyroidism both muscular contraction and relaxation are slowed and the time-course of the tendon reflexes is slower than normal. Myoidema is the formation of a localized ridge, lasting a few seconds after local percussion of a muscle; this type of ridge is electrically silent and the phenomenon is seen particularly in patients with malnutrition or cachexia due to malignant disease, although it can also occur in hypothyroidism. Physiological contracture differs from pathological contracture with permanent shortening of muscles and tendons due to fibrosis in chronic muscle disease, and is a reversible shortening of muscle lasting for some minutes after exercise; it is seen in muscle phosphorylase deficiency (McArdle's disease) and in related disorders of glycogen breakdown. Direct myotactic irritability is the reflex contraction that occurs in the belly of a muscle when it is percussed or stimulated mechanically. As with the tendon reflexes, this reflex response can be accentuated by anxiety but is particularly striking in patients with tetany and hypocalcaemia.

The response of muscle to stretch, i.e. muscle tone, is also of diagnostic value. Increased tone (spasticity or rigidity) implies disease in the central nervous system, but many primary disorders of muscle cause reduced tone (limpness or hypotonia); differential diagnosis of these disorders may be difficult in infancy. Palpation of muscles is also helpful. Tenderness can imply inflammation and an abnormally firm consistency can imply infiltration with fat, connective tissue, calcium, or even the presence of a neoplasm, but muscle tumours are rare and localized swellings usually imply either haematoma formation, rupture of a tendon, herniation of muscle tissue through its covering fascia, or, more rarely, a muscle infarct (as in polyarteritis nodosa) or severe local inflammation (as in tropical or pyogenic myositis or localized nodular myositis).

The examination of muscle power is sufficiently important almost to warrant a chapter to itself. Careful testing of the power of individual muscles, with quantitative assessment, is an important facet of the clinical examination. Different diseases show different patterns of muscular involvement; selective atrophy and weakness of certain muscles with sparing of others may give an important clue to the nature of the illness. The tendon reflexes in muscle disease are usually diminished or lost when the muscles subserving them are involved in the disease process. In general, however, in muscular dystrophy the tendon reflexes disappear early, in myasthenia gravis and polymyositis they often remain unexpectedly brisk even in the presence of substantial weakness, and in the myopathy of metabolic bone disease they are often exaggerated, even in very weak muscles.

Diagnostic methods

When muscular involvement is but one part of a systemic inflammatory or metabolic affliction, many investigations, including blood counts, erythrocyte sedimentation rate, serum electrophoresis, and estimation of serum electrolytes and of calcium and phosphorus, may be relevant and, where considered important, will be mentioned below in relation to specific disease entities. In any patient suffering from muscular weakness it is first necessary to determine whether the weakness is secondary to disease primarily involving other tissues or organs. If this can be excluded, the next step is to determine whether the pathological process lies in the lower motor neurone, at the myoneural junction, or in the muscle itself. The techniques of most value in providing this informa-

tion, in distinguishing between neuropathic and myopathic disorders on the one hand and between specific myopathic conditions on the other, are electromyography (see Section 24); biochemical techniques, of which serum enzyme studies are among the most important; muscle biopsy; and DNA recombinant studies.

BIOCHEMICAL DIAGNOSIS

In the various endocrine myopathies to be described below, many tests related to the diagnosis of individual endocrine disorders may be required. In the periodic paralysis syndromes, in addition to serial estimations of serum potassium and measures designed to precipitate attacks for diagnostic purposes, there are cases in which sodium and potassium output in the urine, and even sodium and potassium balance, may need to be measured. In patients with generalized muscle pain and weakness, myoglobin must be sought in the urine, while in individuals suffering muscle pain after effort, it may be necessary to exclude some forms of glycogen storage disease by measuring lactate in venous blood distal to a tourniquet before and after a period of ischaemic work. Estimations of phosphorylase, of other glycolytic enzymes and of AMP deaminase in muscle biopsy samples may then be needed. The identification of other glycogen storage disorders involving muscles that do not cause exertional pain may necessitate estimations of total glycogen content of muscle and of other enzymes like acid maltase. Similarly, in a lipid storage myopathy it may be necessary to measure total muscle lipids, individual fatty acids, carnitine or specific enzymes such as carnitine palmityl transferase. The mitochondrial myopathies are so complex that many sophisticated biochemical techniques may be needed when a muscle disorder is found to be associated with a mitochondrial abnormality (see below).

In many forms of muscle disease there may be excessive creatinuria or diminished creatinuria, but these findings are non-specific, as is the occasional amino aciduria. The serum aldolase and transaminases (aminotransferases) may be substantially raised in various forms of myopathy, but the most useful serum enzyme in the diagnosis of muscle disease is unquestionably creatine kinase (CK) (normal < 75 i.u/l). In early or preclinical cases of muscular dystrophy of the Duchenne type, a 300-fold increase in the serum activity of CK is often found; changes of similar magnitude sometimes occur in acute and subacute polymyositis. Less striking rises are observed in patients with other more indolent forms of myopathy and the more benign varieties of muscular dystrophy. In some endocrine and metabolic myopathies and in the benign congenital myopathies, serum CK activity is often normal, as it may be in patients with muscular weakness secondary to disease of the anterior horn cell or motor nerve. However, in the chronic spinal muscular atrophies (such as the Kugelberg–Welander syndrome), and in some cases of motor neurone disease, the continual and recurrent process of denervation and reinnervation of muscle fibres, combined with the trauma to which weak muscles are subjected through use, can produce secondary myopathic change so that in such cases serum CK activity is often considerably increased. These changes may also produce myopathic potentials in the EMG in some areas of partially denervated muscle and appearances suggesting myopathy in some parts of muscle biopsy sections; these findings may lead the unwary erroneously to diagnose a primary myopathy.

MUSCLE BIOPSY

While it is usually possible by studying sections of muscle obtained by biopsy to distinguish between muscular atrophy secondary to denervation on the one hand and that resulting from a primary myopathy on the other, differential diagnosis between the various forms of myopathy is much less exact. Modern techniques, including intravital endplate staining, histochemistry, immunochemistry, and electron microscopy, have also added precision to histological diagnosis. Thus 'fibre type grouping' (large groups of fibres of uniform histochemical type) is usually diagnostic of chronic denervation atrophy (see Fig. 4). The histological features of muscular dystrophy are similar in all varieties of the disease, though varying in severity. The most common are marked variations in fibre size, fibre-splitting, central migration of sarcolemmal nuclei, patchy atrophy of muscle fibres, nuclear chains, segmental areas of necrosis within fibres with phagocytosis of necrotic sarcoplasm, and sarcoplasmic basophilia with enlargement of sarcolemmal nuclei showing prominent nucleoli (indicating regeneration); there is also infiltration by fat cells and connective tissue. In subacute or chronic polymyositis, the changes may be similar, but signs of muscle fibre destruction and repair (necrosis, phagocytosis, and regeneration) are usually more striking and widespread; in addition, there are often interstitial or perivascular infiltrations of inflammatory cells such as lymphocytes or plasma cells. In dermatomyositis there is often less necrosis of fibres but perifascicular fibre atrophy and evidence of vasculitis are more common. Perivascular collections of lymphocytes (lymphorrhages) are occasionally seen in myasthenia gravis and thyrotoxic myopathy, but generally in the endocrine myopathies histological changes are non-specific. Striated annulets (*ringbinden*), in which striated myofibrils encircle transversely cut muscle fibres, are common in biopsies from patients with myotonic dystrophy, in whom chains of nuclei within muscle fibres can be prominent; there may also be peripheral masses of palely staining homogeneous sarcoplasm (sarcoplasmic masses). These, too, are non-specific and have been noted in patients with muscular symptoms due to myxoedema.

Immunocytochemical techniques using monoclonal antibody stains to locate specific proteins such as dystrophin (totally absent in Duchenne dystrophy, partially in the Becker variety and in manifesting carriers of the Duchenne gene) have added much to diagnostic precision (Fig. 5), as has staining for specific enzymes such as cytochrome oxidase (deficient in some cases of mitochondrial myopathy). Subsets of infiltrating cells such as T lymphocytes can also be identified with appropriate stains.

Vacuolar change in muscle fibres, if widespread, usually indicates storage of abnormal metabolites and is particularly striking in glycogen storage disease. Specific stains for glycogen (e.g. PAS), before and after diastase digestion, are then helpful in identifying the stored material. Similarly, stains for neutral lipid such as Oil Red O or Sudan Black B will usually identify the abnormal storage of fat seen, for example, in the myopathy of carnitine deficiency (Fig. 6). In frozen sections stained for oxidative enzymes such as NADH diaphorase, dark rings or clumps at the periphery of Type 1 muscle fibres indicate abnormal mitochondria and the internal architecture of the fibres is often deranged ('ragged-red fibres') (Fig. 7); the abnormal mitochondria are seen more clearly in sections examined in the electron microscope (see Fig. 8). The electron microscope has also identified 'rimmed vacuoles', which have a dis-

Fig. 5 Antidystrophin immunolabelling in tissue sections using a monoclonal antibody (Dy4/6D3) to the rod domain of dystrophin. Visualization of label is by the indirect immunoperoxidase technique with a haematoxylin counterstain. (a) Normal adult human skeletal muscle showing clear immunolabelling at the periphery of all muscle fibres. (b) Duchenne muscular dystrophy (DMD) patient aged 5 years showing complete absence of labelling for dystrophin. (c) Becker muscular dystrophy (BMD) patient aged 17 years showing overall decrease in dystrophin immunolabelling and some intrafibre variation in labelling intensity. (d) Manifesting DMD carrier showing dystrophin 'positive' and 'negative' fibres and some with intermediate labelling intensity. All magnifications ×250. (Kindly supplied by Dr Louise Nicholson and reproduced from Walton (1993) with permission.)

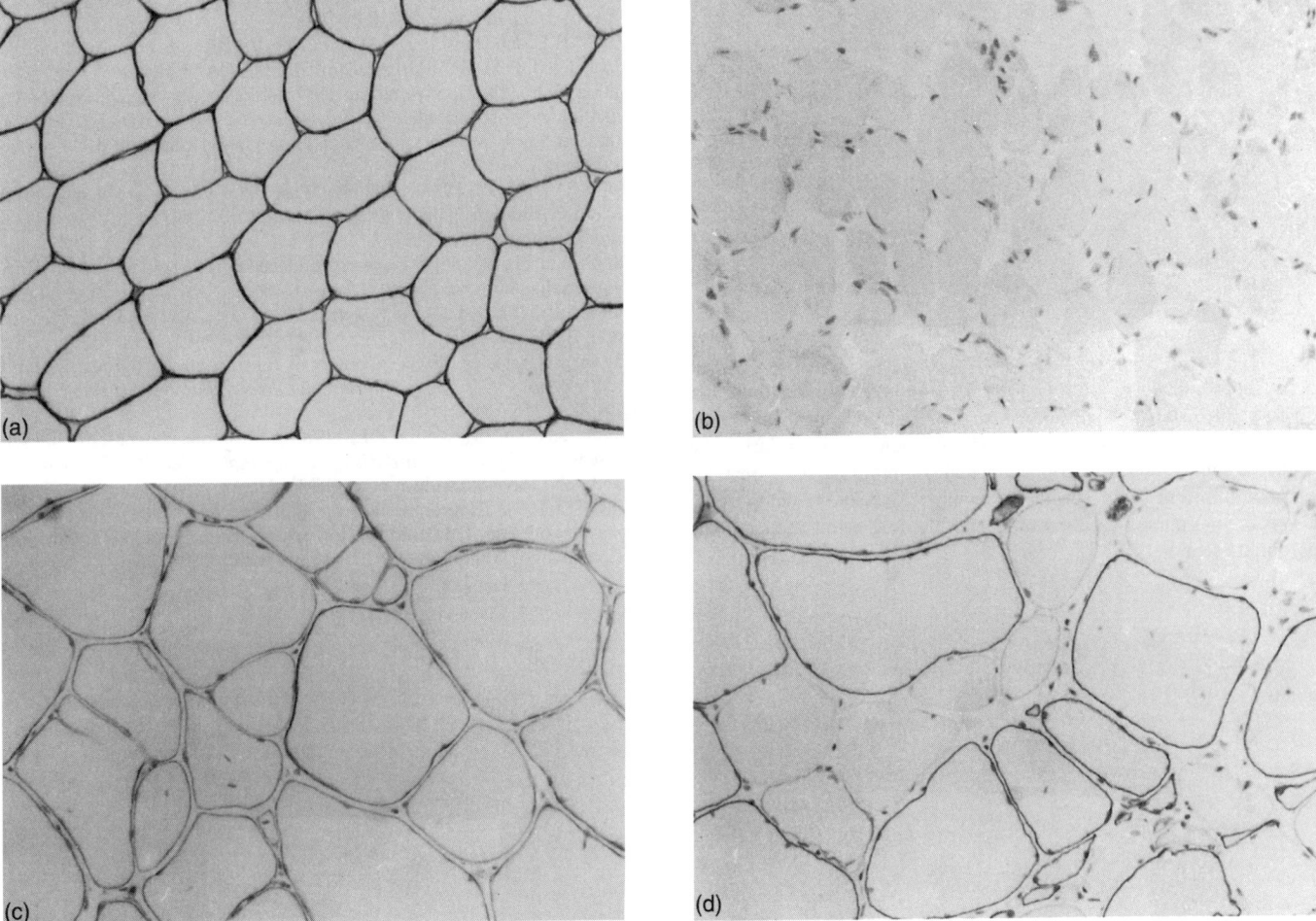

Fig. 6 A transverse section of human skeletal muscle obtained from a patient with carnitine deficiency and stained with Sudan black B. The massive accumulation of neutral fat, especially within the Type 1 fibres, is evident. Magnification ×196.

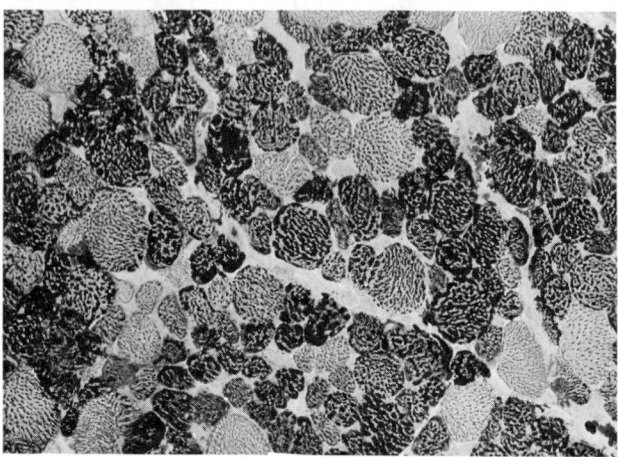

Fig. 8 A transverse section of a biopsy specimen obtained from one quadriceps muscle in a patient with mitochondrial myopathy showing arrays of paracrystalline inclusions in the damaged mitochondria. Bar = 1 μm. (Kindly supplied by Dr Michael Cullen.)

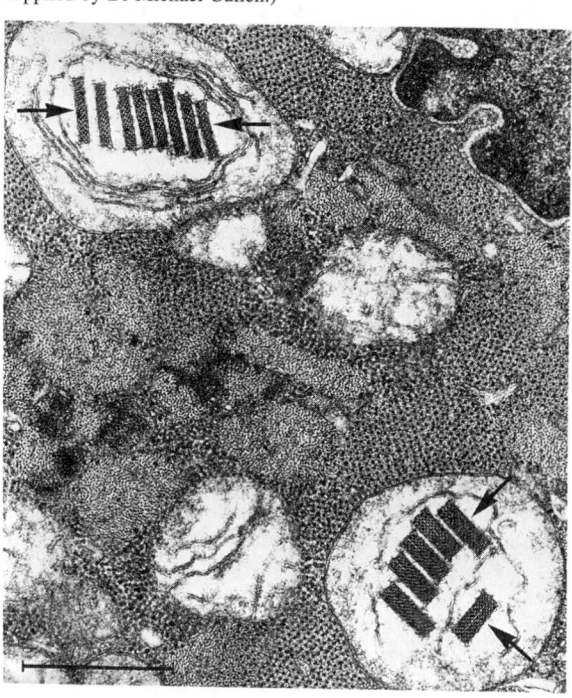

Fig. 7 A transverse section of skeletal muscle obtained from a patient with a mitochondrial myopathy, stained for the NADH-TR reaction. The Type 1 fibres are darkly stained and show the typical reticulated appearance of so-called 'ragged-red fibres' with massive clumping of mitochondria, particularly in many fibres just deep to the sarcolemma. Magnification ×384. (Kindly supplied by Dr Margaret Johnson.)

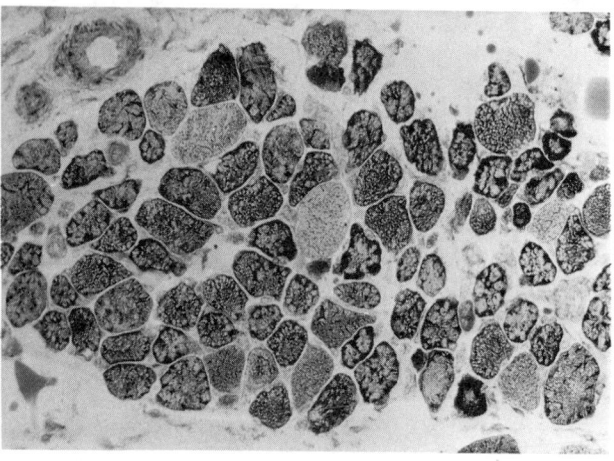

REFERENCES

Dale, H. (1934). Chemical transmission of the effects of nerve impulses. *British Medical Journal*, **ii**, 835–837.

Huxley, H.E. and Hanson, J. (1960). In *The structure and function of muscle*, Vol. 1 (ed. G.H. Bourne). Academic Press, New York.

Landon, D.N. (1992). Skeletal muscle—normal morphology, development and innervation. In *Skeletal muscle pathology*, 2nd edn. (ed. F.L. Mastaglia and Lord Walton of Detchant), pp. 1–94. Churchill Livingstone, Edinburgh.

Taylor, D.J., *et al.* (1988). CA²+-ATPase deficiency in a patient with an exertional muscle pain syndrome. *Journal of Neurology, Neurosurgery and Psychiatry*, **51**, 1425–33.

Walton, J.N. (1981). Diffuse exercise-induced muscle pain of undetermined cause relieved by verapamil. *Lancet*, **i**, 993.

Walton, J.N. (Sir John) (1987). *Introduction to clinical neuroscience*, 2nd edn. Baillière Tindall, London.

Walton, J.N., *et al.* (1993). Disorders of function in the light of anatomy and physiology. In *Brain's diseases of the nervous system*, 10th edn. pp. 28–32. Oxford University Press.

Walton, J.N. and Mastaglia, F.L. (1980). The molecular basis of muscle disease. In *The molecular basis of neuropathology* (ed. R.H.S. Thompson and A.N. Davison). Edward Arnold, London.

Wray, D. (1994). Neuromuscular transmission. In *Disorders of voluntary muscle*, 6th edn. (ed. Lord Walton of Detchant), pp. 139–78. Churchill Livingstone, Edinburgh.

tinctive appearance and are found in inclusion body myositis and in a rare form of distal myopathy. Less striking vacuolar change is often seen in biopsies taken from patients with periodic paralysis during the attacks. In some rare benign congenital and non-progressive myopathies described in recent years, special stains may be needed to demonstrate the specific morphological abnormalities which will be mentioned in the appropriate sections.

25.2 The muscular dystrophies

J. WALTON

While muscular dystrophy can be defined as genetically determined primary degenerative myopathy, several other rare myopathies to be referred to later are also genetically determined but are not regarded as muscular dystrophies in the accepted sense of the term.

Classification

Classification is the only safe guide to prognosis and genetic counselling; the most satisfactory clinicogenetic classification of the 'pure' muscular dystrophies based upon current knowledge is:

(1) X-linked muscular dystrophy:
(a) severe (Duchenne);
(b) benign (Becker);
(c) benign with early contractures (Emery–Dreifuss);
(d) benign with acanthocytes (McLeod syndrome);
(e) scapuloperoneal (rare).

(2) Autosomal recessive muscular dystrophy:
(a) limb-girdle (usually scapulohumeral, rarely pelvifemoral);
(b) childhood type, resembling Duchenne;
(c) distal type;
(d) congenital muscular dystrophy.

(3) Autosomal dominant muscular dystrophy:
(a) facioscapulohumeral;
(b) scapuloperoneal;
(c) late-onset proximal (limb-girdle);
(d) benign early onset with contractures (?Bethlem, ?Emery–Dreifuss type);
(e) distal;
(f) ocular;
(g) oculopharyngeal.

Although this classification is comprehensive, some cases that are difficult to fit into any of the groups described still emerge.

Aetiology

Powerful evidence now suggests that in Duchenne dystrophy there is a defect in the plasma membrane of the muscle fibre, and that this allows the uncontrolled entry of calcium. This in turn causes areas of hypercontraction of myofibrils and activation of calcium-activated neutral proteases, leading to muscle fibre necrosis. In 1987 the gene responsible for Duchenne dystrophy was isolated in the Xp 21 region of the X chromosome. It is one of the largest genes known in human genetics, with a length of almost two megabases. The genes for Duchenne and Becker dystrophy are allelic. Their clinical expression depends, at least in part, upon the number and extent of deletions within the gene. However, some patients with Duchenne dystrophy do not have deletions and in them the disease is presumed to result from a point mutation. Identification of the gene led to isolation of the missing gene product, a protein named dystrophin, which is totally absent in almost all cases of Duchenne dystrophy and much reduced in those of the Becker variety. Dystrophin forms a vital structural component of the skeletal muscle fibre membrane; its absence or deficiency renders the plasma membrane incompetent, leading to the fibre breakdown process outlined above. Now that the gene responsible for X-linked Emery–Dreifuss muscular dystrophy has been located on the distal part of the long arm of the X chromosome (Xq 28), that for facioscapulohumeral dystrophy has been found to be on chromosome 4, that for limb-girdle dystrophy on chromosome 15, and that for myotonic dystrophy on chromosome 19; more information about missing and abnormal gene products in these and in the other dystrophies is emerging, yielding additional information about pathogenesis.

The muscular dystrophies are comparatively rare, but occur worldwide, affecting all races; the Duchenne type is the most common, with an incidence of between 13 and 39 per 100 000 live births. Its prevalence has been estimated to be 2.48 per 100 000, while that of the benign Becker type is about 2.38 per 100 000 (these patients live much longer–the cumulative birth incidence of the latter condition is about one-third that of the Duchenne type). Some varieties are more common in certain parts of the world than others (see below).

Pathology

The pathological changes observed in dystrophic muscle have been outlined above in the section on muscle biopsy. The specific histological hallmark of early Duchenne dystrophy is that in transverse sections of muscle stained with haemalum and eosin, scattered opaque hyalinized fibres (due to myofibrillar hypercontraction as described above) are prominent. The other dystrophic features, including segmental necrosis, regeneration, and subsequent random variation in fibre size, etc. are less prominent at first but appear later as in other forms of dystrophy. For reasons that remain unclear, perivascular cellular infiltrates are not uncommon in the facioscapulohumeral variety. In Duchenne dystrophy and, to a much greater extent, in the Fukuyama variety of congenital dystrophy, various forms of cerebral dysgenesis are often found, while some degree of cortical atrophy with cerebral ventricular dilatation is common in myotonic dystrophy.

Electromyography (also see Section 24)

Electromyography reveals volitional activity characteristic of any form of myopathy, and spontaneous activity is usually absent on recording from relaxed, resting muscle, although spontaneous fibrillation and positive sharp waves are occasionally recorded, especially in more rapidly progressive cases.

Symptoms and signs

The symptoms and signs of the disease depend upon the muscles first involved by the disease and upon its rate of progression. Weakness of pelvic girdle muscles gives slowness in walking, inability to run, frequent falling, difficulty in climbing stairs or in rising from the floor, and eventually accentuation of the lumbar lordosis with a characteristic waddling gait. Climbing up the legs on rising from the floor (Gowers' sign) is characteristic but not specific, as it occurs in any disorder in which pelvic girdle muscles are weak. Involvement of the shoulder girdles gives a sloping appearance with a tendency for the scapulae to rise prominently when the patient abducts the arms. Many use trick movements by placing one hand beneath the other elbow so as to lift the hand to the face or head. Facial weakness, as in facioscapulohumeral dystrophy, causes inability to whistle, difficulty in pouting the lips or in closing the eyes, while distal weakness in the extremities (as seen in the distal variety) causes weakness of grip and of fine finger movement, and foot-drop. Contractures are common in all forms of dystrophy in the later stages, but are seen especially in the Duchenne type. They are due to weakness developing in muscles whose antagonists remain powerful (this causes the equinovarus deformity of the feet seen in advancing cases of the Duchenne type, causing patients to walk on their toes; the anterior tibial muscles are weak while those of the calf remain powerful). Contractures are also accentuated by postural factors in patients confined to a wheelchair, when biceps and hamstrings usually shorten. The most important clinical feature of all forms of dystrophy is that muscles are picked out selectively. Although there are differences in the patterns of weakness and wasting seen in the various subvarieties, it is common in the upper limbs to find that the serrati and pectorals are weak and atrophic, as are biceps and brachioradialis, while deltoid and triceps remain relatively unaffected. In the lower limbs, quadriceps and anterior tibials are usually involved first, and the calf muscles are spared, but in limb-girdle cases the hamstrings and quadriceps are often affected equally.

The severe X-linked Duchenne type

Although this condition is due to an X-linked recessive gene, about half of the affected boys are isolated cases, and in about one-third the disease is presumed to have resulted from a new mutation occurring in the ovarian cells of the mother or maternal grandmother.

The condition usually first becomes apparent towards the end of the third year with slowness in walking, frequent falling, and difficulty in climbing stairs. However, muscle biopsies obtained in the first few weeks of life in preclinical cases (younger brothers of affected boys, identified at birth by serum creatine kinase estimation) show that the pathological process is active even at birth and many affected boys walk late (at 18 months of age or later). Nevertheless, early symptoms and signs (even though readily recognizable to parents who may have seen them in an older child) are very difficult for the doctor to detect. It is important to consider this possibility in young boys who walk late or develop walking difficulty in early life, when estimation of the serum creatine kinase will always be advisable. Enlargement of the calf muscles and sometimes of quadriceps and deltoids occurs in about 90 per cent of cases at some stage, but later disappears. This phenomenon, often called pseudohypertrophy, is more often due to true hypertrophy of unaffected muscle fibres. Most patients deteriorate steadily and become unable to walk by about the age of 10 years, but apparent improvement may occur between the ages of 5 and 8, when the rate of deterioration is outstripped by the processes of normal development. When the boy is confined to a wheelchair, progressive deformity with skeletal distortion and atrophy occur. Death usually results from inanition, respiratory infection, or cardiac failure. With improved management, including the prevention of scoliosis and early treatment of complications (including assisted ventilation to control chronic alveolar hypoventilation, in appropriate cases) many sufferers now survive into their late twenties. Some affected boys waste progressively, but others become obese; macroglossia and absence of some incisor teeth are occasionally seen. The intelligence quotient is 10 per cent or more lower than in a group of control children of comparable age and sex. Skeletal atrophy may so affect the shafts of long bones that they fracture on minimal trauma. Involvement of cardiac muscle is invariable, though not clinically detectable at first; the ECG typically shows tall R waves in the right precordial leads and deep Q waves in the limb and left precordial leads.

The benign X-linked (Becker) type

In this disorder the onset of the disease is usually between 5 and 25 years, it may be transmitted by affected males through carrier daughters to their grandsons, there is often an initial phase of generalized muscular hypertrophy before weakness and wasting of pelvic and later of shoulder girdle muscles develops; most patients become unable to walk 25 years or more after the onset. Cardiac involvement is usually absent, contractures and skeletal deformity occur late, and many patients, though severely disabled, survive to a normal age.

The Emery–Dreifuss type

This uncommon X-linked dystrophy is due to a gene lying on the Xq 28 region of the long arm of the X chromosome, linked to the gene for Factor VIII. Muscular weakness and wasting is most prominent in humeroperoneal distribution, the onset is between 5 and 15 years of age, there is slow progression with the early development of contractures (especially in the neck, knees, and ankles) and of cardiac involvement causing conduction abnormalities (many patients eventually require a pacemaker).

The X-linked scapuloperoneal type

While scapuloperoneal muscular atrophy is usually neurogenic rather than myopathic, and more often dominant than X-linked, families in which the condition was clearly myopathic and X-linked have been described. The condition resembles the Emery–Dreifuss variety but is almost certainly a different disease.

McLeod myopathy

This rare X-linked disorder of the Kell erythrocyte antigen system, causing acanthocytosis, is due to a gene lying on the short arm of the X chromosome. Affected individuals show increased serum creatine kinase activity and a subclinical non-specific myopathy with histological changes in muscle biopsy specimens superficially resembling those of muscular dystrophy.

Neonatal screening

Using the luciferase technique for serum creatine kinase estimation on a single drop of blood on a filter paper, it is possible to identify at birth (with subsequent confirmation from a venous blood sample) those newborn male infants who will subsequently develop Duchenne muscular dystrophy. Many now favour the performance of such a test on all newborn males in order to identify preclinical cases of the disease, partly to prevent the birth of a second affected male before the disease has been diagnosed in the first-born and partly to achieve early diagnosis in the hope that gene therapy (see below) will soon become available. Surveys suggest that most women would wish to know soon after birth whether their child was to develop a handicapping disorder.

Developments in molecular genetics, carrier detection, prenatal diagnosis, and embryo research

In a family in which the gene for Duchenne or Becker dystrophy is known to have been transmitted, any sister of a dystrophic boy will have a 50:50 chance of being a carrier; if she is, half her sons will be affected and half her daughters will also be carriers. In families in which an isolated case is presumed to have resulted from a new mutation, the probability of carrier status in the sister of a dystrophic boy is much less and will depend, of course, upon whether the mutation arose in his mother's or his grandmother's ovary (in the latter case his mother would be a carrier). Some carrier females do show minor (and some more severe) clinical, biochemical, and histological evidence of muscular dystrophy (manifesting carriers) due to uneven lyonization of the X chromosome.

For many years, serum creatine kinase estimation, using Bayesian methods to determine the probability that a young woman is or is not a carrier, was the most reliable means of carrier detection and was best carried out on adolescent girls. Many carrier females so detected decided not to have children; others preferred selective abortion of male fetuses identified by amniocentesis at about 14 weeks. However, the situation has been transformed since discovery of the Duchenne gene. The use of DNA restriction fragment length polymorphisms (RFLPs) linked to the gene has made accurate carrier detection possible in many families; the method is about 98 per cent accurate in informative families. However, the use of complementary DNA probes and the polymerase chain reaction still detects only about 65 per cent of mutations; linkage analysis is only helpful in families with known carriers and not in those with isolated affected males. Possibly the comparison of dystrophin abnormalities by immunofluorescence and immunoblot analysis, and dystrophin staining (which demonstrates mosaic staining in manifesting carriers) of muscle biopsy samples may prove to be one of the best techniques for carrier detection.

Following the introduction of chorionic villus biopsy as an alternative method of sexing the fetus (a procedure possible at 8 to 9 weeks and with fewer complications than amniocentesis), prenatal diagnosis in male fetuses using RFLPs has made it possible to embark upon a programme of selective abortion of affected male fetuses only. Of even greater importance is that following the passage into law of the Human Fertilization and Embryology Act in the United Kingdom in 1990, allowing experiments under licence upon the conceptus or pre-embryo in the first 14 days after fertilization, in vitro fertilization of ova harvested from a female carrier with her husband's sperm can be followed by embryo biopsy and by pre-implantation diagnosis. This will allow female carriers of the gene responsible for Duchenne and Becker dystrophy to have unaffected male and non-carrier female children.

Limb-girdle muscular dystrophy

This form of the disease occurs equally in the two sexes and usually begins in the second or third decade of life, although it can occasionally first appear in middle life. It is the least well defined of the more common forms of dystrophy; indeed it has been suggested that many cases so diagnosed have been cases of Becker dystrophy, manifesting carriers of the Duchenne gene, or were suffering from spinal muscular atrophy, polymyositis, or metabolic myopathy. Some who prefer to talk of the 'limb-girdle syndrome' have questioned whether a specific limb-girdle variety of muscular dystrophy exists, while others have suggested that it should be divided into scapulohumeral and pelvifemoral subvarieties. Certainly, in most cases and families the condition is due to an autosomal recessive gene, now localized to chromosome 15. However, in some families showing onset in adult life inheritance is clearly autosomal dominant, and dominant inheritance has also been reported in a family showing early onset with the rapid development of contractures (so-called Bethlem myopathy) and often with cardiomyopathy reminiscent of that seen in Emery–Dreifuss dystrophy. The exact status of the 'rigid spine syndrome', in which contractures develop in the posterior cervical and paraspinal muscles and often at the elbows and knees, almost invariably in males, in the second decade, and in which there is evidence of a generalized mild myopathy, is still uncertain. Hence the situation remains confused and will only be clarified when it proves possible to determine whether the limb-girdle variety embraces just one or two or several different disease entities.

In about half the cases muscle weakness begins in the shoulder girdle muscles and may not involve the pelvic girdle for many years, but in the remainder, pelvic girdle muscles are first involved and weakness affects the shoulders within about 10 years. Enlargement of calf muscles is not uncommon. Sometimes muscular weakness and wasting are asymmetrical initially and occasionally the disease process arrests temporarily, but most patients are severely disabled within 20 years of the onset.

The course of the disease is generally more benign in those in whom upper limb muscles are first involved. Contractures and skeletal deformity occur late but progress more rapidly when the patient is confined to a wheelchair. Most sufferers are severely disabled in middle life and many die before the normal age.

Childhood muscular dystrophy with autosomal recessive inheritance

The existence of this comparatively rare variety has been confirmed by the occasional occurrence of muscular dystrophy superficially resembling the Duchenne type in young girls and occurring in families in which parental consanguinity made autosomal recessive inheritance likely. This form is clinically similar to the Duchenne type, but more benign. It is also, as a rule, more benign than the true Duchenne dystrophy which can occur in girls with Xp 21 chromosomal translocation. This variety of the disease, although rare in the United Kingdom and North America, is much more common in the Middle East and North Africa. The onset may be in the second year or as late as the fourteenth, but is most often in the second half of the first decade. Progression is comparatively slow and patients usually become unable to walk in their early twenties, but sometimes as early as 15 years or as late as 40 years. The pattern of weakness is similar to that found in typical Duchenne dystrophy and most patients die in middle life.

Congenital muscular dystrophy

This rare disorder presents with severe, generalized muscular hypotonia, which is noted from birth and is accompanied by relatively non-progressive muscular wasting and weakness. Many affected children have widespread contractures suggesting arthrogryposis multiplex congenita. Occasionally the weakness increases rapidly after birth and the disease terminates fatally within the first year of life, but in most cases it seems relatively non-progressive. Few affected patients are ever able, however, to sit or stand unsupported and the prognosis is uniformly unfavourable. Diagnosis from spinal muscular atrophy of infancy can only be made with confidence by EMG, serum enzyme studies, and muscle biopsy. The occasional involvement of sibs confirms that this rare disorder may be due to an autosomal recessive gene. It can be distinguished from the benign congenital myopathies to be discussed below, first by its severity and secondly by the fact that the histological changes in muscle biopsy specimens are similar to those observed in other forms of muscular dystrophy.

Two relatively specific subvarieties have been identified. In the hypotonic-sclerotic variety (Ullrich's syndrome) there is a non-progressive congenital myopathy with slender muscles, proximal contractures, severe distal hypotonia and hyperextensibility, relative sparing of facial muscles, prominence of the calcaneus, a high arched palate, hyperhidrosis, and normal intelligence. The Fukuyama variety is due to an autosomal recessive gene; it is about half as common in Japan as the Duchenne type but uncommon in other countries. The principal features are progressive muscular dystrophy of early onset, severe mental retardation and epilepsy. The muscle shows changes similar to those of Duchenne dystrophy; the brain shows multifocal cerebral and cerebellar dysplasia, micropolygyria, aberrant fascicles of myelinated fibres, and general pallor of myelin with gliosis of white matter.

Facioscapulohumeral muscular dystrophy

This variety, inherited by an autosomal dominant mechanism and due to a gene now located on chromosome 4, occurs equally in the two sexes and can begin at any age from childhood until adult life but is usually first recognized in adolescence. Facial involvement, with a typical pouting appearance of the lips and difficulty in closing the eyes, is apparent early and is accompanied by weakness of shoulder girdle muscles with bilateral scapular winging and wasting of the pectorals. Muscular enlargement is uncommon; in the lower limbs the anterior tibial muscles are often first involved, causing bilateral foot-drop. In many patients the disease runs a prolonged course with periods of apparent arrest, so that contractures and skeletal deformity develop late. However, in some the condition progresses more rapidly and severe accentuation of the lumbar lordosis is seen early; but in others the disease is abortive and, once certain muscles have been affected, the spread of weakness seems to cease. Most affected individuals survive and remain active to a normal age. Heart muscle is not involved and the range of intelligence is normal. As in limb-girdle muscular dystrophy, it is clear that in some few cases with an atypical clinical syndrome the disease process is neuropathic (spinal muscular atrophy) rather than myopathic. In some myopathic cases, inflammatory cell infiltrates in muscle biopsy sections are unexpectedly common, but there is no clinical improvement on treatment with steroids.

Diagnosis depends upon serum enzyme and EMG studies but especially upon muscle biopsy; the recent localization of the gene makes it likely that the use of RFLPs will soon enable diagnosis to be even more precise.

Recently an association between this form of dystrophy and sensorineural deafness and mental retardation, retinal telangiectasia, exudation, and detachment (Coats' syndrome) in some affected individuals and families has been reported. Facial diplegia and sensorineural hearing loss in early infancy may even be presenting features. The significance of these inconstant associations is still uncertain but early diagnosis of hearing loss and retinal disease is important so that appropriate treatment can be given.

Distal muscular dystrophy

Distal muscular dystrophy (also known as the Welander type) is rare in Britain and in the United States, but is not uncommon in Sweden. It is generally inherited as an autosomal dominant trait, usually beginning between the ages of 40 and 60 years and involving both sexes. Weakness begins in small hand muscles and in the anterior tibials and calves, but eventually spreads to proximal muscles, unlike the pattern seen in peroneal muscular atrophy, with which it is most often confused. In Sweden the condition is comparatively benign, but sporadic cases observed in other countries tend to be more severe and rapidly progressive.

Recently a distal form developing in young adults, of autosomal recessive inheritance, has been recognized; the disease process, resembling Duchenne dystrophy histologically but not clinically, first affects the gastrocnemii, solei and anterior tibials, spreading to the thighs and glutei later; in the arms there is moderate weakness of forearm muscles but the small hand muscles are spared. This variety must be distinguished from another variety, also of autosomal recessive inheritance, in which there is progressive muscle fibre atrophy and loss with characteristic rimmed vacuoles containing concentric lamellar bodies but without fibre necrosis and regeneration. This type is more severe, involves flexor muscles in the upper limbs more often than extensor, and may be associated with cardiomyopathy.

The ocular and oculopharyngeal varieties

Involvement of the external ocular muscles is uncommon in most varieties of muscular dystrophy but can occur in dystrophia myotonica (see Chapter 25.4). In the past, patients who developed ptosis and progressive limitation of ocular movements without significant diplopia were usually identified as cases of progressive nuclear ophthalmoplegia, but Kiloh and Nevin interpreted the histological changes as myopathic. They concluded that progressive external ophthalmoplegia was a form of muscular dystrophy, which they called ocular myopathy. Sporadic cases and others occurring in families showing either autosomal recessive or dominant inheritance were reported. Later it was found that patients with this syndrome who also had signs of nervous system involvement and retinal pigmentation (the Kearns–Sayre syndrome) had widespread mitochondrial pathology in muscle and brain.

It is now evident that a mitochondrial myopathy is responsible for many, but not all, cases of progressive external ophthalmoplegia. A few such patients have spinal muscular atrophy with loss of neurones from the oculomotor nuclei and others peripheral neuropathy. While the term ocular myopathy, or muscular dystrophy, is losing popularity, it remains the most satisfactory description for a few otherwise unexplained cases of progressive external ophthalmoplegia.

The same conclusion can be drawn in relation to oculopharyngeal myopathy, a term introduced by Victor et al. in 1962 to identify patients with progressive external ophthalmoplegia of late onset associated with dysphagia. Some cases are sporadic but autosomal dominant inheritance has been reported in several extensive kindreds, many of French–Canadian ancestry. Certainly, at autopsy the condition is myopathic but, as in ocular myopathy, some cases have mitochondrial pathology whereas many others simply show moth-eaten and whorled or atypical ragged-red fibres with rimmed vacuoles. The external ophthalmoplegia commonly develops at between 40 and 50 years of age but is rarely symptomatic, whereas the dysphagia becomes progressively more troublesome and mild weakness of facial, neck, and proximal limb muscles is usually present.

Treatment

While long-term treatment with steroid drugs such as prednisone has been shown to result in a marginal reduction in the rate of deterioration in patients with Duchenne dystrophy, most authorities now feel that the side-effects and disadvantages of such treatment outweigh the advantages, and at present no form of drug treatment is generally recommended in any form of muscular dystrophy. However, much invaluable work has been done, in Duchenne dystrophy in particular, in defining the pattern of clinical progression and the effects of supportive therapy, and similar efforts have been made in other chronic neuromuscular disorders. Complications such as respiratory infection may require antibiotics, physiotherapy, and even suction. Hope for the future rests in gene therapy, with the objective of replacing a missing gene product, such as dystrophin, within diseased muscle either in early infancy in affected individuals identified as neonates (or even in utero) or at least as early as possible in the course of the disease. Myoblast transfer, which can reinstate dystrophin in deficient muscle in the mdx mouse and in the extensor digitorum brevis of boys with Duchenne dystrophy is unlikely to become an effective treatment because of the problem of delivering a sufficient number of myoblasts to a sufficient number of muscles to have a clinical effect, even if the problem of rejection can be completely overcome. The calcium antagonists flunarizine and nifedipine have been shown to be ineffective, although diltiazem seemed to have a slight beneficial effect. And while chronic, low-frequency electrical stimulation of the quadriceps in boys with Duchenne dystrophy may produce a slight increase in strength, this method seems unlikely to find an established place in treatment.

Moderate physical exercise can help delay the march of weakness and the development of contractures. A regular exercise programme should be started soon after diagnosis under the supervision of a physiotherapist and subsequently continued at home. Passive stretching of tendons (such as the Achilles), which tend to shorten, is also useful but night splints are even better. Light spinal supports are helpful in delaying scoliosis but it is now clear that in many cases spinal fusion (the Luque operation) is much more effective in the long term and should be undertaken prophylactically when there is a high risk of a rapidly evolving curve and of a restrictive lung syndrome. Calipers and standing frames can help many patients walk for longer than they would otherwise be able to do. Surgical division of the Achilles tendons in selected cases, a procedure long regarded as being contraindicated, and certain other surgical procedures, may also be beneficial provided these are followed by immediate mobilization of the patient in walking plasters or calipers. When cramps in the calf are troublesome in Becker dystrophy, gastrocnemius fasciotomy may be helpful. Immobilization of patients with muscular dystrophy is in general to be avoided as far as ever possible as this frequently causes deterioration. Radical surgery may help patients with Duchenne dystrophy to walk for two or three years longer than they would otherwise do, but many at this stage take to a wheelchair with relief and the time may come when adjustment to a wheelchair life may be preferred. Many types of appliance are of great value in improving the quality of life at all ages, and the advice of a skilled occupational therapist may be invaluable.

It has long been believed that, in a progressive disease like muscular dystrophy, assisted respiration in the terminal stages was unjustified for fear of 'striving officiously to keep alive'. But now it is clear, especially in the presence of scoliosis, that respiratory insufficiency may cause hypoventilation and hypercapnia with attendant symptoms of alveolar hypoventilation (headache, lethargy, and drowsiness) comparatively early. In some obese patients with Duchenne dystrophy, obstructive sleep apnoea may occur and in patients with other neuromuscular disorders, including various congenital myopathies, cases of myotonic dystrophy and motor neurone disease, severe respiratory insufficiency due to diaphragmatic weakness may develop while the patient is still ambulant. When the vital capacity falls below 700 ml, the patient's life is in danger. Often hypoventilation is at its worst during sleep. Methods of giving ventilatory support in such cases include the rocking bed, the cuirass ventilator or positive pressure respiration via a face mask, while inspiratory resistive training may be of temporary benefit. However, in most cases of Duchenne dystrophy, and in those with similar respiratory difficulties due to neuromuscular disease, overnight intermittent positive pressure ventilation via the mouth using a face mask may produce a dramatic improvement in alertness and in the quality of life and longevity.

Not least in importance is the psychological management of patients, who may demand considerable reserves of patience and understanding on the part of parents, doctors, nurses, and social workers. Optimism and encouragement, however unjustifiable in the face of continuing deterioration, are greatly needed and long-term psychological support and counselling by trained and experienced workers may be required.

Course and prognosis

This has been mentioned in relation to the individual subvarieties of the disease.

REFERENCES

Arahata, K., *et al.* (1989). Dystrophin diagnosis: comparison of dystrophin abnormalities by immunofluorescence and immunoblot analysis. *Proceedings of the National Academy of Science of the USA*, **86**, 7154–58.

Arahata, K., *et al.* (1989). Mosaic expression of dystrophin in symptomatic carriers of Duchenne's muscular dystrophy. *New England Journal of Medicine*, **320**, 138–42.

Becker, P.E. and Kiener, F. (1955). Eine neue x-chromosomale Muskeldystrophie. *Archiv für Psychiatrie und Nervenkrankheiten*, **193**, 427–428.

Ben Hamida, M., Fardeau, M., and Attia, N. (1983). Severe childhood muscular dystrophy affecting both sexes and frequent in Tunisia. *Muscle and Nerve*, **6**, 469–80.

Brooke, M.H., *et al.* (1989). Duchenne muscular dystrophy: patterns of clinical progression and effects of supportive therapy. *Neurology*, **39**, 475–81.

Bushby, K.M.D., Thambyayah, M., and Gardner-Medwin, D. (1991). Prevalence and incidence of Becker muscular dystrophy. *Lancet*, **337**, 1022–24.

Cullen, M.J. and Fulthorpe, J.J. (1975). Stages in fibre breakdown in Duchenne muscular dystrophy. An electron microscopic study. *Journal of the Neurological Sciences*, **24**, 179–200.

Cullen, M.J., Johnson, M.A., and Mastaglia, F.L. (1992). Pathological reactions of skeletal muscle. In *Skeletal muscle pathology*, 2nd edn. (eds. F.L. Mastaglia and Lord Walton of Detchant), pp. 123–84. Churchill Livingstone, Edinburgh.

Edstrom, L., Thornell, L.-E., and Eriksson, A. (1980). A new type of hereditary distal myopathy with characteristic sarcoplasmic bodies and intermediate (skeletin) filaments. *Journal of the Neurological Sciences*, **47**, 171–90.

Edwards, R.H.T. and Griggs, R.C. (1994). The medical and psychological management of neuromuscular disease. In *Disorders of voluntary muscle*, 6th edn. (ed. Lord Walton of Detchant), pp. 837–50. Churchill Livingstone, Edinburgh.

Emery, A.E.H. (1992). *Duchenne muscular dystrophy*, 2nd edn. Oxford University Press, Oxford.

Fukuyama, Y., Kawazura, M., and Haruna, H. (1960). A peculiar form of congenital progressive muscular dystrophy: report of fifteen cases. *Paediatria Universitatis, Tokyo*, **4**, 5–8.

Galasko, C.S.B. (1994). The orthopaedic management of neuromuscular disease. In *Disorders of voluntary muscle*, 6th edn. (ed. Lord Walton of Detchant), pp. 851–77. Churchill Livingstone, Edinburgh.

Gardner-Medwin, D. and Walton, J.N. (1994). The muscular dystrophies. In *Disorders of voluntary muscle*, 5th edn. (ed. Lord Walton of Detchant), pp. 543–94. Churchill Livingstone, Edinburgh.

Greenberg, C.R., *et al.* (1988). Gene studies in newborn males with Duchenne muscular dystrophy detected by neonatal screening. *Lancet*, **ii**, 425–27.

Kiloh, L.G. and Nevin, S. (1951). Progressive dystrophy of external ocular muscles (ocular myopathy). *Brain*, **74**, 115–43.

Mastaglia, F.L. and Walton, J.N. (Lord Walton of Detchant) (eds.) (1992). *Skeletal muscle pathology*, 2nd edn. Churchill Livingstone, Edinburgh.

Miller, R.G., Chalmers, A.C., Dao, H., Filler-Katz, A., Holman D., and Bost, F. (1991). The effect of spine fusion on respiratory function in Duchenne muscular dystrophy. *Neurology*, **41**, 38–40.

Mohire, M.D., Tandan, R., Fries, T.J., Little, B.W., Pendlebury, W.W., and Bradley, W.G. (1988). Early-onset benign autosomal dominant limb-girdle myopathy with contractures (Bethlem myopathy). *Neurology*, **38**, 573–80.

Mokri, B. and Engel, A.G. (1975). Duchenne dystrophy: electron microscopic findings pointing to a basic or early abnormality in the plasma membrane of the muscle fibre. *Neurology*, **25**, 1111–20.

Nicholson, G.A., Gardner-Medwin, D., Pennington, R.J.T., and Walton, J.N. (1979). Carrier detection in Duchenne muscular dystrophy: assessment of the effect of age on detection rate with serum-creatine-kinase activity. *Lancet*, **i**, 692–694.

Nicholson, L.V.B., Johnson, M.A., Gardner-Medwin, D., Bhattacharya, S., and Harris, J.B. (1990). Heterogeneity of dystrophin expression in patients with Duchenne and Becker muscular dystrophies. *Acts Neuropathologica*, **80**, 239–50.

Nonaka, I., Sunohara, N., Ishiura, S., and Satoyoshi, E. (1981). Familial distal myopathy with rimmed vacuole and lamellar (myeloid) body formation. *Journal of the Neurological Sciences*, **51**, 141–55.

Nonaka, I., Une, Y., Ishihara, T., Miyoshino, S., Nakashima, T., and Sugita, H. (1981). A clinical and histological study of Ullrich's disease (congenital atonic-scleurotic muscular dystrophy). *Neuropediatrics*, **12**, 197–208.

Panegyres, P.K., Mastaglia, F.L., and Kakulas, B.A. (1990). Limb girdle syndromes: clinical, morphological and electrophysiological studies. *Journal of the Neurological Sciences*, **95**, 201–18.

Skinner, R., Emery, A.E.H., Scheuerbrandt, G., and Syme, J. (1982). Feasibility of neonatal screening for Duchenne muscular dystrophy. *Journal of Medical Genetics*, **19**, 1–3.

Swash, M. and Schwartz, M.S. (1988). *Neuromuscular diseases: a practical approach to diagnosis and management*, 2nd edn. Springer, London.

Swash, M., Schwartz, M.S., Carter, N.D., Heath, R., Leak, M., and Rogers,

K.L. (1983). Benign X-linked myopathy with acanthocytes (McLeod syndrome). Its relationship to X-linked muscular dystrophy. *Brain*, **106**, 717–33.

Victor, M., Hayes, R., and Adams, R.D. (1962). Oculopharyngeal muscular dystrophy. A familial disease of late life characterised by dysphagia and progressive ptosis of the eyelids. *New England Journal of Medicine*, **267**, 1267–72.

Walton, J.N. (Lord Walton of Detchant) (ed.) (1994). *Disorders of voluntary muscle*, 6th edn. Churchill Livingstone, Edinburgh.

Walton, J.N. and Nattrass, F.J. (1954). On the classification, natural history and treatment of the myopathies. *Brain*, **77**, 169–231.

Weatherall, D.J. (1989). Gene therapy. *British Medical Journal*, **298**, 691–93.

Yates, J.R.W., *et al.* (1986). Emery–Dreifuss muscular dystrophy: localisation to Xq27.3 qter confirmed by linkage to the factor VIII gene. *Journal of Medical Genetics*, **23**, 587–90.

25.3 The floppy infant syndrome

J. WALTON

Generalized muscular hypotonia in infancy can be due to many causes, including cerebral palsy, mental retardation, various metabolic disorders, cerebral degenerative disease, and a number of neuromuscular conditions. Spinal muscular atrophy (Werdnig–Hoffmann disease) is an important cause and in such cases the hypotonia is usually profound and widespread, there is generalized areflexia, respiratory muscle weakness, and often fasciculation of the tongue. The diagnosis can be confirmed by EMG and muscle biopsy. This condition, of grave prognosis, may be mimicked by congenital muscular dystrophy, as described above.

Benign congenital or infantile hypotonia

This term is often used to identify those floppy infants in whom hypotonia is not shown to be the result of any specific metabolic disorder, nor secondary to mental handicap or disease in the central or peripheral nervous system; in such cases full investigation, including EMG and muscle biopsy, may fail to demonstrate any specific abnormality of the muscle fibres other than, in some cases, an overall decrease in their diameter. Sometimes all the muscle fibres seem to be of one uniform histochemical type, suggesting a disorder of muscle differentiation, but these cases are rare. In yet others there is a marked disproportion in number and size between the fibres of different histochemical types (congenital fibre type disproportion). The aetiology of the latter condition is unknown but it usually improves progressively with increasing age.

Differential diagnosis is made more difficult by the fact that the clinical course of spinal muscular atrophy in infancy and childhood is very variable. Three clinical variants have been described (see Section 24) and all appear to be due to a gene lying on chromosome 5q12–q14. Arthrogryposis multiplex congenita, a syndrome of widespread muscular weakness, wasting, and hypotonia with contractures of the extremities, which is present from birth, can be due to congenital muscular dystrophy, fetal spinal muscular atrophy, congenital peripheral neuropathy, or excessive intrauterine pressure.

Undoubtedly, the syndrome of benign congenital or infantile hypotonia is one of multiple aetiology. Some patients demonstrating similar diffuse hypotonia in early infancy, show improvement later, although the muscles remain weak, slender, and hypotonic throughout life, and these cases may be regarded as examples of 'benign congenital myopathy', even though the EMG and muscle biopsy findings in such individuals are often non-specific. Some such patients are found to be suffering from apparently specific, though benign, disorders of muscle, which will now be mentioned.

Central core disease

In 1956 Shy and Magee described a family in which affected children did not walk until the age of 4 years. There was widespread muscular hypotonia and muscle biopsy revealed large muscle fibres, most of which showed one or sometimes two central cores, which had different staining properties from the other fibrils. The central core was shown to be devoid of oxidative enzymes and of phosphorylase activity, and seemed to be non-functioning. The condition is probably due to an autosomal recessive gene and runs a benign course, but its pathogenesis is obscure and X-linked recessive inheritance has also been described.

In a clinically similar syndrome, multiple cores (multicore disease) can be found in the affected muscle fibres, while in yet others minicores are present. Multicore and minicore disease are usually of autosomal dominant inheritance. The gene for central core disease lies on chromosome 19q and is linked to that for malignant hyperpyrexia.

Nemaline myopathy

This is another congenital and relatively non-progressive myopathy in which collections of rod-shaped bodies are found within the muscle fibres, usually lying beneath the sarcolemma. These patients often show evidence of diffuse myopathy, but also facial weakness, a high arched palate, prognathism of the lower jaw, and skeletal changes resembling those of arachnodactyly, although none of the other stigmata of Marfan's syndrome are present. Examination of muscle from such cases with the electron microscope has shown that the subsarcolemmal rods appear to be due to a selective swelling and degeneration of Z-bands with consequent destruction of myofilaments in the adjacent part of the muscle fibre.

Even though the condition runs a benign course in most patients, there are rare severe cases causing death in infancy, and progressive respiratory insufficiency is not uncommon. No specific treatment is available but nocturnal nasal ventilation and vigorous treatment of respiratory infection, along with control of skeletal deformity, may all improve the prognosis.

Fingerprint body myopathy, tubular aggregates, and other rare congenital myopathies

Other forms of myopathy associated with non-progressive muscular weakness in infancy and early childhood have also been described in recent years, one showing hypertrophy of Type 2 fibres with fingerprint-like inclusions demonstrated with the electron microscope in the Type 2 fibres, another demonstrating widespread tubular aggregates in all fibres. Other rare causes of infantile hypotonia include 'reducing body myopathy', 'sarcotubular myopathy', 'cytoplasmic body myopathy', and 'benign autophagic myopathy'. The mitochondrial and lipid storage (see Chapter 25.9) myopathies can also present with hypotonia and developmental delay. The nature and specificity of these ultrastructural changes remain in doubt.

Myotubular or centronuclear myopathy

In 1966 Spiro, Shy and Gonatas reported the case of a 9-year-old child suffering from a form of Möbius syndrome characterized by facial diplegia, external ocular palsies, a decrease in muscle mass, moderate symmetrical muscle weakness, and poor development of all limb muscles. Most muscle fibres contained central nuclei, often lying in chains; the appearances in the muscle were similar to those of the myotubes seen in normal fetal muscle in the early months of intrauterine life. These fibres are, however, in several respects different from fetal myotubes; nevertheless the condition seems to represent an example of cellular developmental arrest. It usually runs a benign course, with progressive improvement, but occasional severe cases with death in early infancy have been reported. By contrast, complete recovery has also been reported. In many families the condition appears to be due to an autosomal recessive gene but dominant inheritance has been described and late clinical onset of the myopathy is also seen rarely.

While it is still uncertain whether all of the syndromes mentioned are specific disease entities, within the difficult field of 'benign congenital myopathy' advances are occurring rapidly and many new and apparently specific structural abnormalities of the muscle fibre are being demonstrated by modern techniques in children with congenital hypotonia and developmental delay.

REFERENCES

Barth, P.G., van Wijngaarden, G.K., and Bethlem, J. (1975). X-linked myotubular myopathy with fatal neonatal asphyxia. *Neurology*, **25**, 531–36.

Campbell, M.J., Rebeiz, J.J., and Walton, J.N. (1969). Myotubular, centronuclear or pericentronuclear myopathy? *Journal of the Neurological Sciences*, **8**, 425–43.

Dastur, D.K., Razzak, Z.A., and Bharucha, E.P. (1972). Arthrogryposis multiplex congenita. Part 2: Muscle pathology and pathogenesis. *Journal of Neurology, Neuro-surgery and Psychiatry*, **35**, 435–50.

Engel, A.G. (1988). Metabolic and endocrine myopathies. In *Disorders of voluntary muscle*, 5th edn. (ed. Sir John Walton), pp. 811–68. Churchill Livingstone, Edinburgh.

Engel, A.G., Gomez, M.R., and Groover, R.V. (1971). Multicore disease: a recently recognized congenital myopathy associated with multifocal degeneration of muscle fibres. *Mayo Clinic Proceedings*, **46**, 666–81.

Engel, A.G., Angelini, C., and Gomez, M.R. (1972). Fingerprint body myopathy: a newly recognized congenital muscle disease. *Mayo Clinic Proceedings*, **47**, 377–88.

Fardeau, M. (1991). Congenital myopathies. In *Skeletal muscle pathology*, 2nd edn. (eds. F.L. Mastaglia and Lord Walton of Detchant), pp. 237–81. Churchill Livingstone, Edinburgh.

Gardner-Medwin, D. (1994). Neuromuscular disorders in infancy and childhood. In *Disorders of voluntary muscle*, 6th edn. (ed. Lord Walton of Detchant), pp. 781–836. Churchill Livingstone, Edinburgh.

Hudgson, P., Gardner-Medwin, D., Fulthorpe, J.J., and Walton, J.N. (1967). Nemaline myopathy. *Neurology*, **17**, 1125–42.

Jerusalem, F., Engel, A.G., and Gomez, M.R. (1973). Sarco-tubular myopathy: a newly recognized, benign, congenital, familial muscle disease. *Neurology*, **23**, 897–906.

Kalimo, H., *et al.* (1988). X-linked myopathy with excessive autophagy: a new hereditary muscle disease. *Annals of Neurology*, **23**, 258–65.

Mastaglia, F.L. and Walton, J.N. (Lord Walton of Detchant) (eds.) (1992). *Skeletal muscle pathology*, 2nd edn. Churchill Livingstone, Edinburgh.

Patel, H., Berry, K., MacLeod, P., and Dunn, H.G. (1983). Cytoplasmic body myopathy: report on a family and review of the literature. *Journal of the Neurological Sciences*, **60**, 281–92.

Shy, G.M. and Magee, K.R. (1956). A new congenital non-progressive myopathy. *Brain*, **79**, 610–21.

Spiro, A.J., Shy, G.M., and Gonatas, N.K. (1966). Myotubular myopathy. *Archives of Neurology*, **14**, 1–14.

Walton, J.N. (1957). The limp child. *Journal of Neurology, Neurosurgery and Psychiatry*, **20**, 144–54.

Yuill, G.M. and Lynch, P.G. (1974). Congenital non-progressive peripheral neuropathy with arthrogryposis multiplex. *Journal of Neurology, Neurosurgery and Psychiatry*, **37**, 316–23.

25.4 Myotonic disorders

J. WALTON

Myotonia is the continued active contraction of a muscle after the cessation of voluntary effort or stimulation; an electrical after-discharge accompanies the phenomenon in the EMG. Clinically it is best demonstrated as slowness in relaxation of the grip or by persistent dimpling after a sharp blow on a muscle belly, e.g. in the thenar eminence or tongue. It is due to an abnormality of the muscle fibre, as it persists after section or blocking of the motor nerve, and after curarization. It is associated with low chloride conductance in the muscle fibre membrane.

Myotonia appears in three hereditary syndromes, mainly of autosomal dominant inheritance, namely myotonia congenita, dystrophia myotonica, and paramyotonia. The three conditions breed true and are plainly different diseases. While dystrophic changes occur in certain muscles in dystrophia myotonica, these disorders are more closely related to each other than to the muscular dystrophies. There is a close relationship between paramyotonia on the one hand and the periodic paralyses on the other.

In a rare syndrome variously called one form of myokymia, pseudomyotonia, neuromyotonia, the myotonia–myokymia–hyperhidrosis syndrome and a syndrome of continuous muscle fibre activity and spasm, a phenomenon similar clinically but electrically different from myotonia is associated with myokymia (benign coarse fasciculation), cramps, hyperhidrosis, and sometimes muscle wasting. Its nature is little understood, though recent evidence strongly suggests an autoimmune aetiology, but the impaired relaxation in these cases, like that of myotonia, seems to be relieved by phenytoin and related remedies (see below).

Myotonia can also be produced experimentally by drugs such as diazocholesterol, dichlorophenoxyacetic acid, triparanol or clofibrate, rarely by propranolol and other β-adrenergic agents. Clinically it may rarely be a symptomatic phenomenon in polyneuropathy, polymyositis, and motor neurone diseases, but it must then be distinguished from electrical 'pseudomyotonia', which is quite different from the EMG of true myotonia and which occurs in a variety of metabolic myopathies and denervating diseases.

negative myasthenia gravis – evidence for plasma factor(s) interfering with acetylcholine receptor function. *Annals of the New York Academy of Science*, **681**, 529–38.

Willcox, N., Schluep, M., Ritter, M.A., Schuurman, H.J., Newsom-Davis, J. and Christensson, B. (1987). Myasthenic and nonmyasthenic thymoma.

An expansion of a minor cortical epithelial cell subset? *American Journal of Pathology*, **127**, 447–60.

Willcox, N. and Vincent, A. (1988). Myasthenia gravis as an example of organ-specific autoimmune disease. In *B lymphocytes in human disease* (ed. G. Bird and J.E. Calvert), pp. 469–506. Oxford University Press.

25.8 Metabolic and endocrine myopathies

D. HILTON-JONES

This section deals with those disorders of voluntary muscle that are thought to arise either as the result of a primary or secondary disturbance of muscle intracellular metabolism, or to involve disordered ion flux, although in many cases precise mechanisms have yet to be defined.

The term metabolic myopathy is applied most frequently to those disorders in which there is a primary defect, usually an enzyme deficiency, in the biochemical pathways associated with energy generation (ATP synthesis). This group includes the extremely important mitochondrial disorders, which have risen over the last 20 years from relative obscurity to being recognized as providing some of the most common examples of primary metabolic myopathy seen in clinical practice, and which are discussed in detail elsewhere (Chapter 25.9).

Endocrine myopathies and nutritional and toxic myopathies, including drug-induced myopathies, can be considered as secondary metabolic myopathies.

Altered membrane sodium conductance in the primary periodic paralyses, and altered chloride conductance in myotonia congenita relate to disturbed ion channel function. The mechanism of disordered calcium homoeostasis in malignant hyperthermia remains uncertain but may relate to dysfunction of the ryanodine receptor, which is involved in calcium release in the sarcoplasmic reticulum.

Primary metabolic myopathies

The major energy currency of living cells is adenosine triphosphate (ATP). Whereas in most organs the rate of ATP utilization is fairly constant, in voluntary muscle the change from rest to strenuous activity may increase the demand on ATP generation several thousand-fold. If that demand is not met, contractile failure (i.e. fatigue or weakness) will develop and may be accompanied by destruction of muscle fibres. In many of the primary metabolic myopathies it is often assumed that exercise-induced symptoms relate to failure of ATP generation, and although this is probably not always correct it is a useful generalization. Whilst exercise-induced symptoms are often a striking feature of this type of metabolic myopathy, they are not always present. Some patients develop a chronic progressive myopathy.

The major fuels providing energy for ATP generation in skeletal muscle are glycogen, fatty acids, and glucose (Fig. 1). Their relative contributions depend upon the state of nutrition and, more importantly, the level and duration of exercise. A gross over-simplification of these pathways aids understanding of the clinical features of the different forms of metabolic myopathy.

At rest the major fuel source is circulating free fatty acids, with a lesser contribution from circulating glucose. Small amounts of ATP may be generated directly from glycolysis but far more important is the production of the energy-rich electron carriers reduced nictotinamide adenine dinucleotide (NADH) and reduced flavine adenine dinucleotide (FADH$_2$) from glycolysis, fatty acid β-oxidation, and the Krebs' cycle. Transfer of their electrons to molecular oxygen through the electron transport chain of the mitochondria releases energy for the generation of ATP (oxidative phosphorylation)

The increased demand on ATP generation during early strenuous exercise cannot be met by these oxidative pathways. The resting blood flow provides inadequate delivery of oxygen and substrate, and compression of blood vessels by the contracting muscle exacerbates the problem. ATP is therefore generated by the breakdown of muscle fibre stores of glycogen. The relative lack of oxygen leads to increasing levels of NADH and pyruvate. NADH build-up would inhibit glycolysis, and thus ATP generation, and is avoided by the reduction of pyruvate to lactate, explaining the lactic acidosis seen in disorders of oxidative metabolism.

Adaptive processes occur as exercise continues; muscle blood flow increases, the respiratory rate rises, and free fatty acids are mobilized from adipose stores. Glycogen stores in muscle are depleted and circulating free fatty acids, with a much lesser contribution from circulating glucose, become the main energy source.

Certain deductions can be made from the above that are largely borne out in clinical practice. Disorders of glycogen and glucose metabolism may be asymptomatic at rest but produce symptoms in early exercise. If low levels of exercise can be sustained symptoms might improve as fatty acid oxidation increases ('second wind' phenomenon in McArdle's disease). Disorders of fatty acid metabolism, insufficient to cause symptoms at rest, are likely to be exposed by sustained exercise and fasting. The central role of oxidative phosphorylation explains why disorders of the respiratory chain may be symptomatic at rest. The clinical presentation will also depend upon whether the enzyme defect is restricted to skeletal muscle or is more generalized. Systemic features may dominate in disorders of β-oxidation and in mitochondrial disorders, but are absent in McArdle's disease as the defective enzyme is muscle-specific.

DISORDERS OF GLYCOGEN AND GLUCOSE METABOLISM (SEE ALSO SECTION 11)

Several of the glycogenoses show significant skeletal muscle involvement. The major pathways of metabolism, and the enzymes associated with these disorders, are shown in Fig. 2. They are autosomal recessive disorders, except for phosphoglycerate kinase deficiency which is X-linked recessive. In most of these disorders the serum creatine kinase is elevated, massively so after exercise-induced muscle damage.

Acid maltase deficiency (Type II glycogenosis)

Acid maltase is a lysosomal enzyme not directly involved in energetic pathways, and exercise-induced symptoms are absent. In the infantile form (Pompe's disease) there is widespread organomegaly as well as skeletal muscle involvement, and death occurs by the age of 2 years due to cardiac or respiratory failure. The adult form is of considerable importance and has probably been underdiagnosed. The most obvious feature is a slowly progressive, painless, proximal myopathy. Diaphragmatic involvement is very common and a significant number of patients first present with symptoms of respiratory failure. Nocturnal assisted ventilation alleviates symptoms and may prolong survival for many years. Muscle biopsy is usually suggestive, showing glycogen-containing vacuoles, but the definitive diagnosis is established by enzyme assay in muscle, fibroblasts or leucocytes, or by demonstrating glycogen granules by PAS staining in lymphocytes on a peripheral blood film.

There is an intermediate juvenile form, with limited survival.

Myophosphorylase deficiency (type V glycogenosis – McArdle's disease)

Onset of symptoms is usually in childhood and the cardinal features are pain, weakness, and stiffness of muscles early in exercise, relieved by rest. Strenuous exercise may induce painful electrically-silent muscle contractures. Muscle fibre breakdown is reflected in myalgia and myoglobinuria (dark red urine), which, if severe, may cause renal failure. If low levels of activity are maintained symptoms may ease ('second wind' phenomenon), as circulating free fatty acids and glucose become available as alternative fuels.

Progressive proximal weakness frequently develops and is sometimes the mode of presentation in late-onset cases.

Failure of lactate generation during ischaemic forearm exercise is consistent with the diagnosis, but not specific, and may give a misleading result if the enzyme deficiency is partial. The definitive diagnosis is established by demonstrating absence of phosphorylase staining, or by enzyme assay, on muscle biopsy.

Debrancher enzyme deficiency (Type III glycogenosis, Cori–Forbes disease)

In infancy and childhood the main features of this disorder are hepatomegaly, hypoglycaemia, and failure to thrive. During adolescence muscle symptoms become more prominent. A small group of patients first present in adult life with muscle symptoms, but may give a history of a protruberant abdomen in childhood. Both exercise intolerance and a slowly progressive proximal myopathy are present.

It has recently been recognized that most patients develop a potentially fatal cardiomyopathy.

The ischaemic forearm test shows impaired lactate generation, muscle biopsy shows glycogen accumulation, and administration of glucagon fails to produce a hyperglycaemic response. Enzyme assay can be performed on muscle, liver, erythrocytes, and leucocytes.

Phosphofructokinase deficiency (Type VII glycogenosis, Tarui's disease)

The clinical picture is very similar to that of myophosphorylase deficiency, but deficiency of phosphofructokinase in erythrocytes leads to

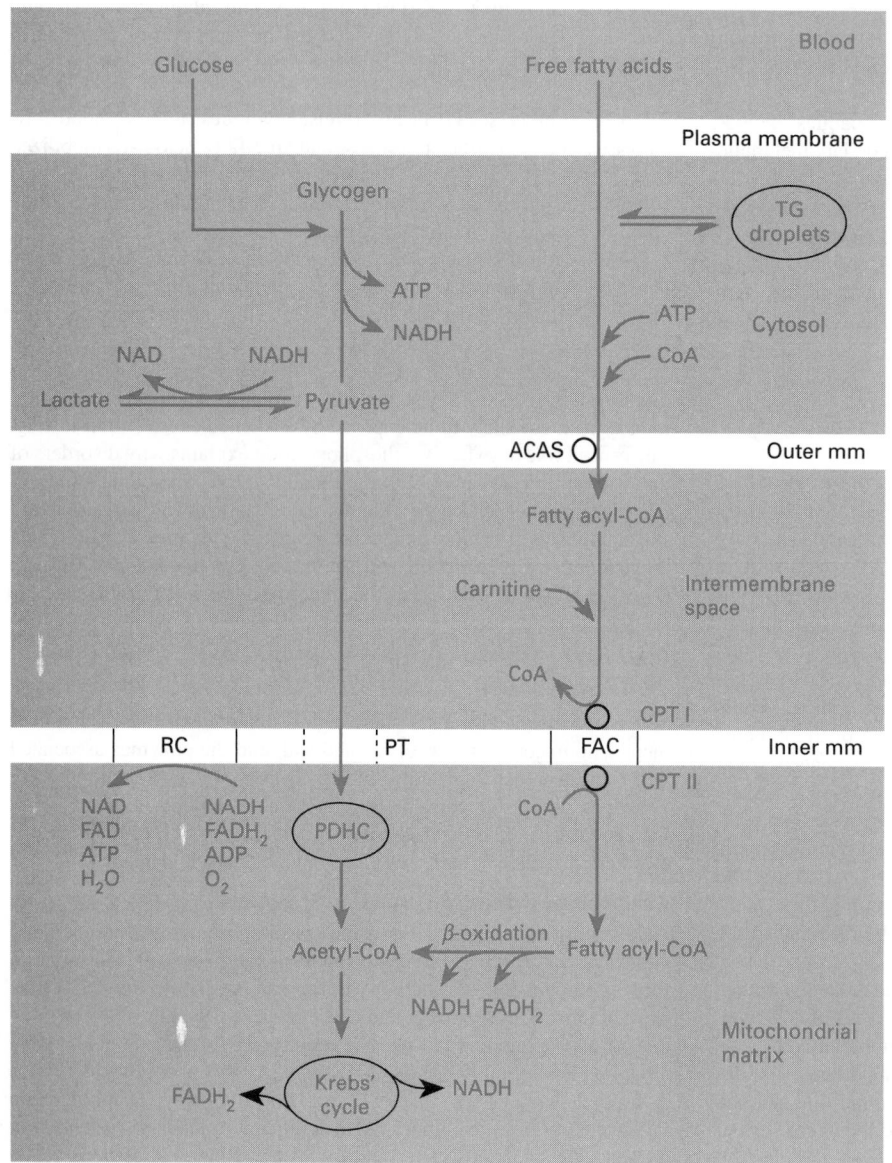

Fig. 1 Major pathways associated with energy production in skeletal muscle. ACAS, acyl-CoA synthetase; ADP, adenosine diphosphate; ATP, adenosine triphosphate; CoA, coenzyme A; CPT, carnitine palmityl transferase; FAC, fatty acyl-carnitine; FAD, flavin adenine dinucleotide; FADH$_2$, reduced FAD; mm, mitochondrial membrane; NAD, nicotinamide adenine dinucleotide; NADH, reduced NAD; PDH, pyruvate dehydrogenase complex; PT, pyruvate translocase; RC, respiratory chain; TG, triglyceride.

the additional features of haemolytic anaemia and gout. Diagnosis is established by enzyme assay in muscle.

Defects of distal glycolysis

Deficiencies of phosphoglycerate kinase, phosphoglycerate mutase, and lactate dehydrogenase have been described recently. All three are associated with exercise intolerance and myoglobinuria. It is highly likely that other defects of glycolysis causing similar symptoms remain to be discovered.

Treatment

There is as yet no specific treatment for any of the disorders described above. Attempts at dietary manipulation have generally proved unsuc-

Fig. 2 Pathways of glycogenolysis and glycolysis. Enzymes known to be associated with particular clinical syndromes are shown.

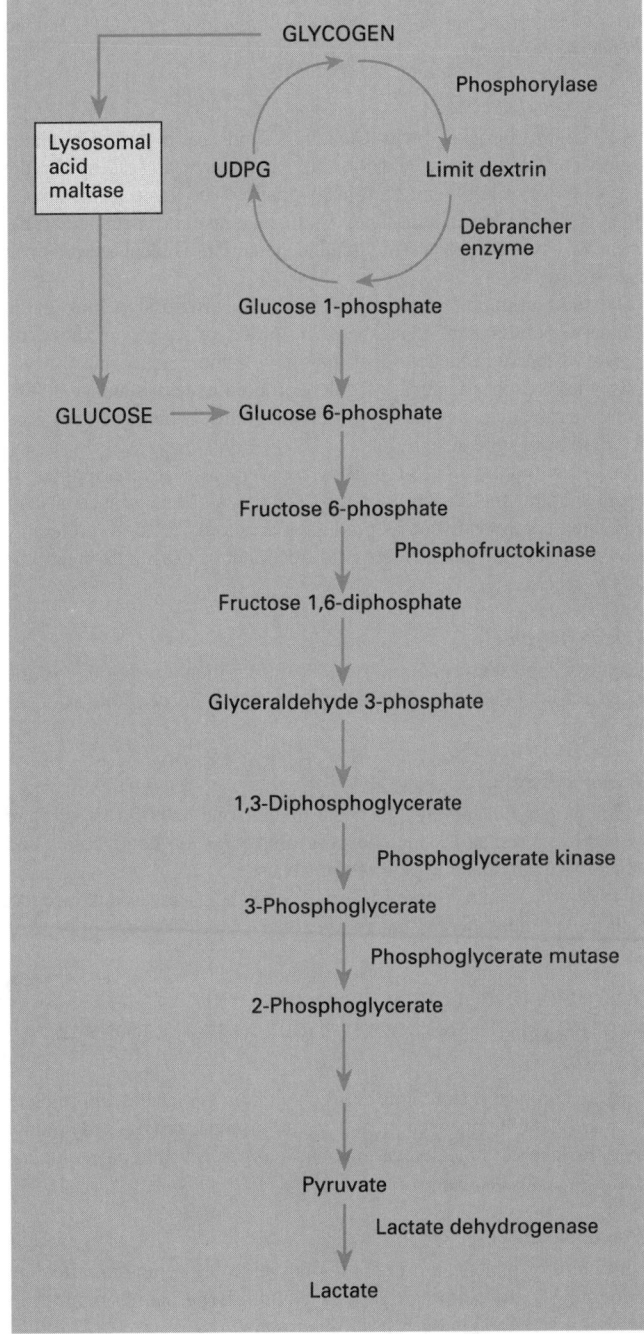

cessful. Patients must be aware of the risk to renal function from myoglobinuria, and try to avoid intense exercise.

DISORDERS OF LIPID METABOLISM

Unlike glycolysis, lipid metabolism is entirely dependent upon oxidative processes, and there is a close relationship between the disorders described below and defects of the mitochondrial respiratory chain (see Chapter 25.9) For example, lipid accumulation in muscle is a common histological feature in respiratory chain disorders.

Free fatty acids, mainly from the blood but also from triglyceride droplets stored within muscle fibres, are a major fuel at rest and during sustained exercise (see Fig. 1). They are converted to fatty acyl-coenzymeA (CoA) at the outer mitochondrial membrane which, within the mitochondrial matrix, can undergo β-oxidation. A transport system involving carnitine and the enzyme system carnitine palmityl transferase (CPT) is required to enable fatty acyl-CoA to cross the inner mitochondrial membrane. Defects involving carnitine, CPT, and β-oxidation have been described.

Carnitine deficiency

Muscle carnitine deficiency, causing fluctuating weakness and lipid storage, and systemic carnitine deficiency causing weakness and recurrent, often fatal, Reye-like episodes, have been described. It has become apparent that in most cases of so-called systemic carnitine deficiency, and perhaps even in some purely myopathic cases, the carnitine deficiency is secondary to another metabolic disorder, most commonly defects of β-oxidation or of the mitochondrial respiratory chain.

Defects of β-oxidation

Many enzyme deficiencies have been described, but clinical features are limited. They may present in the neonatal period with hypotonia, hypoglycaemia, cardiomyopathy, failure to thrive, and early death. Later-onset cases develop Reye-like crises, muscle weakness, and cardiomyopathy. Such defects may be a cause of some cases of sudden infant death syndrome. Secondary carnitine deficiency is common. A high carbohydrate and low fat diet may help.

Carnitine palmityl transferase deficiency

This rare disorder shows male predominance. Symptoms are precipitated by sustained exercise (e.g. a route march) or prolonged fasting, and consist of muscle pain followed by myoglobinuria, which may cause renal failure. The diagnosis may be suggested by showing impaired ketone body production during fasting, but is proven by enzyme assay in skeletal muscle. A high carbohydrate, low fat diet may reduce the number of attacks.

Myoadenylate deaminase deficiency

Deficiency of myoadenylate deaminase has been suggested as a cause of exercise induced myalgia, weakness, and cramps, but its exact status remains controversial. The enzyme catalyses the reaction AMP→IMP + ammonia. Theoretically, this reaction may aid ATP production by removing AMP and increasing flux through the adenylate kinase reaction 2ADP→ATP + AMP. The diagnosis is established by showing a lack of rise in plasma ammonia during the ischaemic forearm exercise test and by histochemical demonstration of absent enzyme activity.

ENDOCRINE MYOPATHIES

Weakness is a common symptom in many endocrine disorders. The mechanisms are generally poorly understood, the myopathy responds to treatment of the underlying hormonal disorder, and extensive investigation of the myopathic component is rarely required. The commonest pattern is limb-girdle weakness.

Thyroid disorders (see also Section 12)
Thyrotoxicosis
Typically, weakness develops shortly after the onset of other thyrotoxic symptoms, and 80 per cent of patients have demonstrable weakness at presentation. The shoulder girdle muscles tend to be involved before the pelvic musculature. Muscle atrophy is usually slight. Asymmetric and distal weakness, myalgia, cramps, and fasciculations are rare findings.

The serum creatine kinase level is usually normal. Electromyography shows features consistent with muscle disease. The myopathy responds to treatment of the thyrotoxicosis.

Thyrotoxic periodic paralysis
Most cases have been reported in individuals from the Orient, with a strong male predominance. The clinical features closely mimic those of familial hypokalaemic periodic paralysis, and the attacks cease when the patient is rendered euthyroid. The onset of paralytic attacks usually follows the development of hyperthyroid symptoms.

Graves' ophthalmoplegia
The classic features of this condition include eyelid lag, retraction, and swelling, and progressive swelling of the extraocular muscles and orbital soft tissues leading to proptosis and diplopia and, in severe cases, corneal ulceration, papilloedema, and optic atrophy. An extremely important and often missed variant is the patient who presents with minimal diplopia only.

In mild cases X-ray computer tomography is useful for detecting extraocular muscle swelling. Simple tests of thyroid function may be normal. Estimation of antithyroglobulin and antimicrosomal antibodies, and performance of a thyrotrophin releasing hormone (TRH) stimulation test may be required. Thyroid stimulating immunoglobulins are present in most patients.

If thyrotoxic, the patient should be rendered euthyroid. Lid retraction may respond to topical 10 per cent guanethidine. Persisting major eye problems may require high dose prednisolone, plasma exchange, or orbital decompression. Tarsorrhaphy protects the cornea.

Thyroid disease and myasthenia
Patients with myasthenia gravis have an increased incidence of thyroid disease, including hyperthyroidism, hypothyroidism, Hashimoto's thyroiditis, and increased antibodies to thyroglobulin or microsomal fractions. Thyroid disease may predate or follow the onset of myasthenia and must be considered as a cause of deterioration in an otherwise stable patient with myasthenia. Some 5 per cent of patients with myasthenia will develop thyroid disease, but only about 0.1 per cent of thyrotoxic patients develop myasthenia.

Hypothyroidism
Hypothyroid myopathy may be asymptomatic but mild weakness is probably present in most patients. Even in the absence of weakness the serum creatine kinase level is often markedly elevated. Slow relaxation of the tendon jerks may be present in isolation. Muscle pain and cramps are common. In children, the combination of hypothyroidism (cretinism), weakness, and muscle hypertrophy is referred to as the Kocher–Debre–Semelaigne syndrome. In adults, Hoffman's syndrome describes the combination of hypothyroidism, weakness, muscle hypertrophy, cramps, and myoedema (the formation of a localized ridge of muscle following direct percussion). They probably represent variants of the same disorder.

All hypothyroid myopathic symptoms respond to thyroxine replacement.

Pituitary–adrenal axis disorders
Clinically, the most important of these is iatrogenic steroid myopathy.

Acromegaly
Proximal weakness, pelvic more than shoulder girdle, is present in about one-half of patients and common complaints include tiredness, weakness, and myalgia; muscle wasting is slight. Serum creatine kinase levels are normal or slightly elevated. Normalizing growth hormone levels improves the myopathy, but recovery may be incomplete.

Hypopituitarism
Growth hormone deficiency in childhood impairs muscle and skeletal development proportionately; weakness is not usually a feature. In adults, panhypopituitarism causes generalized weakness and fatigue, which usually responds to thyroxine and cortisone replacement therapy.

ACTH excess
ACTH excess, from a functioning pituitary adenoma or from ectopic production, is usually associated with high glucocorticoid levels, producing pituitary or ectopic Cushing's syndrome. Weakness is common and thought to relate to glucocorticoid excess. Weakness may occur in Nelson's syndrome, in which there is a high level of ACTH but no glucocorticoid excess.

Glucocorticoid excess
The myopathy associated with Cushing's syndrome is probably related to glucocorticoid excess, and the clinical features are essentially the same as those of iatrogenic steroid myopathy. The 9α- fluorinated steroids, including dexamethasone, triamcinalone, and betamethasone, appear to have the greatest myopathic potential. Topical steroids can cause myopathy.

The most common picture is of a slowly progressive limb-girdle weakness, pelvic more than shoulder girdle, often accompanied by myalgia. The drug-induced form may have a more acute onset. Myopathy without other features of glucocorticoid excess is unusual. The serum creatine kinase is usually normal and muscle biopsy shows nonspecific type II fibre atrophy.

Steroid withdrawal is followed by recovery over several months. If steroid therapy for the primary disorder has to be continued a nonfluorinated compound such as prednisolone should be used, preferably on an alternate-day basis. Successful treatment of Cushing's syndrome leads to recovery.

Conn's syndrome
Weakness is present in about 75 per cent of patients and is due to the associated hypokalaemia. Secondary hypokalaemic periodic paralysis may occur.

Addison's disease
Weakness, fatigue, and myalgia occur in up to one-half of patients. Rare myopathic presentations include progressive flexion contractures and secondary hyperkalaemic periodic paralysis.

The serum creatine kinase is normal or slightly increased. Glucocorticoid replacement therapy is curative.

DISORDERS OF CALCIUM, VITAMIN D, AND PARATHORMONE METABOLISM (SEE ALSO SECTIONS 12 AND 19)

There are complex interactions between vitamin D metabolism, calcium and phosphate homoeostasis, and parathormone activity. Myopathy occurs in several clinical situations, but the precise pathophysiological mechanisms are unclear.

Osteomalacia
In one-third of patients weakness is the presenting symptom, affecting predominantly the pelvic girdle musculature. Bone pain is prominent. The serum creatine kinase is usually normal.

The pain responds fairly rapidly to vitamin D treatment, but the weakness recovers more slowly.

Primary hyperparathyroidism

Myalgia, stiffness, and complaints of fatigue are common, but overt weakness is rare. Symptoms resolve when the underlying parathyroid adenoma is removed and serum calcium levels fall.

Renal osteodystrophy

Endstage renal failure is frequently accompanied by a predominantly pelvic girdle myopathy, sometimes with buttock and thigh pain. Symptoms respond to dialysis, transplantation, or vitamin D treatment.

Dialysis osteodystrophy

Some patients undergoing dialysis develop a severe myopathy with bone pain, fractures, and vitamin D resistance. It probably relates to aluminium toxicity.

Ischaemic myopathy

Rarely, a painful ischaemic myopathy with arterial narrowing due to calcium deposition complicates renal failure. Skin ulceration and bowel infarction may also occur.

NUTRITIONAL AND TOXIC MYOPATHIES

Whilst malnutrition causes muscle wasting, specific myopathic effects of nutritional deficiencies are uncommon, a notable exception being vitamin D deficiency, discussed above. Myopathies due to ingested toxins are common and include alcoholic and drug-induced myopathies.

Alcoholic myopathies

Chronic alcoholics may develop subacute or slowly progressive proximal muscle weakness with mild wasting, mainly affecting the lower limbs. It is still debated whether this is myopathic, neuropathic or both, and whether the cause is a direct toxic effect of alcohol or a secondary phenomenon, perhaps relating to malnutrition. Abstinence may lead to recovery.

Much more dramatic is acute alcoholic myopathy, which usually occurs during a binge. There may be widespread cramps, pain, and weakness but the most striking feature is the development of extremely painful muscle swelling, which may be localized or generalized. Myoglobinuria presents a threat to renal function and hyperkalaemia may be present in severe cases. The serum creatine kinase is elevated and muscle biopsy shows acute necrosis. Recovery, which may be incomplete, occurs over several weeks.

Vitamin E deficiency

Vitamin E deficiency probably causes a myopathy, but interpretation is confused by the presence of additional neurological problems including neuropathy and ataxia.

Drug-induced myopathies

Drug-induced neuromuscular disorders are common, under-recognized and under-reported. Numerous drugs have been implicated, several mechanisms are responsible (Table 1), and some drugs can affect both muscle and peripheral nerve (e.g. vincristine, D-penicillamine, perhexiline).

ION FLUX DISORDERS

Several myopathic disorders are known to be associated with altered ion flux and, in some, specific ion channel defects have been identified.

Periodic paralysis

Marked hypokalaemia and hyperkalaemia from whatever cause may produce weakness or paralysis (secondary periodic paralysis). The pri-

Table 1 *Drug-induced myopathies*

Focal damage/fibrosis	Intramuscular opiates antibiotics paraldehyde
Necrosis	Heroin Clofibrate Epsilon aminocaproic acid
Myoglobinuria/rhabdomyolysis	Heroin Methadone Amphetamines Barbiturates Diazepam Isoniazid Carbenoxolone Phenformin Amphotericin B
Inflammatory myopathy	Procainamide D-Penicillamine L-Dopa
Hypokalaemic weakness	Diuretics Carbenoxolone Liquorice Purgatives
Subacute or chronic painless proximal myopathy	Corticosteroids Chloroquine β-blockers
Myasthenic syndrome	D-Penicillamine Aminoglycoside antibiotics
Malignant hyperthermia	Suxamethonium Cyclopropane Halothane Enflurane Ketamine

mary periodic paralyses are familial, usually dominantly-inherited, disorders characterized by recurrent attacks of paralysis, and which have previously been subdivided into hyperkalaemic, hypokalaemic, and normokalaemic forms on the basis of changes in the serum potassium level during attacks. Recent evidence has shown that the primary defect is an abnormality of muscle membrane sodium conductance, which in the hyperkalaemic form is due to a mutation of the adult skeletal muscle sodium channel. The molecular basis of hypokalaemic periodic paralysis has not yet been determined, but does not involve the same gene locus.

Hypokalaemic periodic paralysis

Attacks usually start in the second decade and then vary in frequency from daily to years between episodes. Weakness may be present on waking or develop during the day, typically in response to a heavy carbohydrate meal or during rest after strenuous exercise. The weakness involves legs more than arms, proximal muscles more than distal, and may be asymmetrical. Bulbar and respiratory muscle weakness is rare. Attacks last from hours to several days. The tendon reflexes may be depressed or lost during an attack. Permanent and progressive proximal weakness often develops by middle age.

The serum potassium level typically falls during an attack, but not necessarily outwith the normal range. If diagnostic doubt remains an attack may be precipitated by administration of glucose and insulin.

Acetazolamide (up to 1.5 g daily) is the treatment of choice to prevent attacks. Acute attacks respond to oral potassium.

Apparently-identical attacks may occur in association with thyrotoxicosis and resolve when the patient is rendered euthyroid.

Hyperkalaemic periodic paralysis

Attacks tend to start at an earlier age than in the hypokalaemic form, and do not last as long. Precipitants include cold, fasting, rest after exercise, pregnancy, alcohol intake, and potassium loading. Readily utilized carbohydrate sources, such as a sweet drink, may abort an attack. A progressive proximal myopathy may also develop. Myotonia is present in some patients (see below).

The serum potassium level may rise during an attack, but the change is often slight.

Mild attacks respond to carbohydrate ingestion. Kaliuretic diuretics usually prevent attacks.

Paramyotonia congenita

Paramyotonia congenita describes a dominantly-inherited condition characterized by cold-induced weakness and muscle stiffness (paramyotonia), and which is sometimes accompanied by periodic paralysis. The relationship between this disorder and primary hyperkalaemic periodic paralysis has been much debated, but recent evidence has shown that hyperkalaemic periodic paralysis, hyperkalaemic periodic paralysis with myotonia, paramyotonia congenita, and paramyotonia congenita with periodic paralysis are allelic disorders involving the tetrodotoxin-sensitive adult skeletal muscle sodium channel.

MYOTONIA CONGENITA

Autosomal dominant and recessive forms of this condition are recognized. Onset tends to be earlier in the dominant form but both usually become apparent in childhood. There is muscle stiffness, worse after rest and exacerbated by cold; minimal or no weakness, readily demonstrable percussion myotonia; and muscle hypertrophy, which tends to be more marked in the recessive form.

Electrophysiological evidence pointed to a disorder of muscle membrane chloride conductance and recent evidence suggests that different mutations of the skeletal muscle chloride channel may cause dominant or recessive myotonia.

MALIGNANT HYPERTHERMIA

The main features are a rapidly rising body temperature and generalized muscular rigidity during anaesthesia. Additional features include skin mottling, cyanosis, tachypnoea, tachycardia, cardiac dysrhythmias, and autonomic instability. Attacks in susceptible individuals may be triggered by suxamethonium and anaesthetic agents (halothane, cyclopropane, enflurane, ketamine). A similar, but probably different, disorder may be associated with heat stroke.

Attacks are life threatening. Treatment consists of withdrawal of the offending agent, general supportive measures and intravenous dantrolene (2 mg/kg body weight).

Disturbed calcium homeostasis underlies the attacks, with excessive calcium iron influx into the sarcoplasmic reticulum. The molecular basis remains uncertain. A candidate gene is that for the calcium channel (ryanodine receptor), on chromosome 19, but cosegregation studies suggest genetic heterogeneity.

The disorder is inherited as an autosomal dominant trait. Screening for susceptibility involves muscle biopsy and *in vitro* testing for a reduced contractile threshold to halothane and caffeine. False positive results are common but false negative results appear to be very rare. It is hoped that specific molecular biological tests will soon become available.

MYOGLOBINURIA

Myoglobin is a protein that acts as an oxygen store within skeletal muscle fibres. Myoglobinuria causes dark brown/red discoloration of the

Table 2 *Causes of myoglobinuria*

Metabolic	Glycogenoses
	Carnitine palmityl transferase deficiency
	Severe electrolyte disturbance
Excessive activity/temperature	Marathon running
	Military training
	Status epilepticus
	Malignant hyperthermia
	Neuroleptic malignant syndrome
Drug and toxins	Several drugs (See Table 1)
	Venoms and animal toxins
Infection	Viral
	Toxic shock
	Clostridial infection/ gangrene
Ischaemia and trauma	Crush
	Coma
	Any cause of severe ischaemia
	Compartment syndromes
	Electric shock
Inflammatory myopathies	Dermatomyositis/ polymyositis

urine and the main concern is that the protein can cause renal tubular necrosis, and thus renal failure. Numerous disorders are known to be associated with myoglobinuria (Table 2). In the metabolic disorders the presumed mechanism is failure of substrate utilization or supply when energy demands increase during exercise or starvation. In other disorders there is disruption of the plasma membrane. Apparently idiopathic cases are probably due to an unidentified metabolic defect or infection.

Rhabdomyolysis is considered further in Section 20.

REFERENCES
General

Engel, A.G. and Banker, B.Q. (ed) (1986). *Myology.* McGraw-Hill, New York.

Brooke, M.H. (1986). *A clinician's view of neuromuscular diseases*, 2nd edn. Williams and Wilkins, Baltimore.

Walton, J.N., Karpati, G., and Hilton-Jones, D. (eds.) (1994). *Disorders of voluntary muscle*, 6th edn. Churchill Livingstone, Edinburgh.

Metabolic myopathies

Angelini, C. (1990). Defects of fatty-acid oxidation in muscle. *Balliere's Clinical Endocrinology and Metabolism*, **4(3)**, 561–82.

Barsy, T. and Hers, H-G. (1990). Normal metabolism and disorders of carbohydrate metabolism. *Balliere's Clinical Endocrinology and Metabolism*, **4(3)**, 499–522.

Layzer, R.B. (1990). Muscle metabolism during fatigue and work. *Balliere's Clinical Endocrinology and Metabolism*, **4(3)**, 441–59.

Endocrine myopathies

Fells, P. (1991). Thyroid-associated eye disease: clinical management. *Lancet*, **338**, 29–32.

Ruff, R.L. and Weissmann, J. (1988). Endocrine myopathies. *Neurologic Clinics*, **6(3)**, 575–92.

Weetman, A.P. (1991). Thyroid-associated eye disease: Pathophysiology. *Lancet*, **338**, 25–8.

Nutritional and toxic myopathies

Argov, Z. and Mastaglia, F.L. (1994). Drug-induced neuromuscular disorders in man. In *Disorders of voluntary muscle*, 6th edn (ed. J.N. Walton, G. Karpati, and D. Hilton-Jones), pp. 989–1029. Churchill Livingstone, Edinburgh.

Ion flux disorders

Ebers, G.C. *et al.* (1991). Paramyotonia congenita and hyperkalemic periodic paralysis are linked to the adult muscle sodium channel gene. *Annals of Neurology*, **30**, 810–16.

Fontaine, B. *et al.* (1990). Hyperkalemic periodic paralysis and the adult muscle sodium channel α-subunit gene. *Science*, **250**, 1000–2.

Fontaine, B., *et al.* (1991). Different gene loci for hyperkalemic and hypokalemic periodic paralysis. *Neuromuscular Disorders*, **1(4)**, 235–8.

Gronert, G.A. (1980) Malignant hyperthermia. *Anesthesiology*, **53**, 395–423.

Koch, M.C., *et al.* (1992) The skeletal muscle chloride channel in dominant and recessive human myotonia. *Science*, **257**, 797–800.

MacLennan, D.H., *et al.* (1990). Ryanodine receptor gene is a candidate for predisposition to malignant hyperthermia. *Nature*, **343**, 559–61.

Myoglobinuria

Penn, A.S. (1986). Myoglobinuria. In *Myology* (ed. A.G. Engel and B.Q. Banker), pp. 1785–805. McGraw-Hill, New York.

25.9 Mitochondrial myopathies and encephalomyopathies

A. E. HARDING

DEFINITION

The term mitochondrial myopathy or encephalomyopathy is applied to a clinically and biochemically heterogeneous group of diseases that often exhibits major mitochondrial structural abnormalities in skeletal muscle. Ragged red fibres, containing peripheral and intermyofibrillar accumulations of abnormal mitochondria and seen with the modified Gomori trichrome stain, are the morphological hallmark of these disorders. These were initially observed in patients presenting with syndromes of chronic progressive external ophthalmoplegia (PEO) and/or proximal myopathy, often with weakness induced or enhanced by exertion. They were then described in children and adults with complex multisystem disorders predominantly or exclusively affecting the central nervous system (CNS). The diseases present with psychomotor retardation, dementia, pigmentary retinopathy, ataxia, seizures, movement disorders, stroke-like episodes, deafness, and peripheral neuropathy in various combinations. Involvement of other systems, such as the heart, endocrine glans, and haemopoietic tissues, also occurs.

AETIOLOGY

Biochemistry

Many patients with mitochondrial encephalomyopathy have a pathological increase in serum lactate concentration during and after exercise, suggesting a defect of aerobic metabolism in muscle mitochondria, and defects of the mitochondrial respiratory chain have been demonstrated in the majority of cases investigated. The main products of oxidation of pyruvate and fatty acids in the mitochondrial matrix are carbon dioxide and NADH. NADH is the principal substrate for the four respiratory chain enzyme complexes (I–IV), which are embedded in the inner mitochondrial membrane. Electrons from NADH (and $FADH_2$) pass along the electron transfer chain, gradually releasing energy, which pumps protons across the inner membrane. This process utilizes oxygen and creates an electrochemical proton gradient across the inner membrane. The latter drives the production of ATP from ADP and phosphate by the enzyme complex ATP synthase (complex V) bound to the inner mitochondrial membrane. This energy is also used to transport pyruvate and other mitochondrial enzyme substrates, and nuclear encoded mitochondrial proteins, into the mitochondrial matrix.

Studies of respiratory chain function and oxidative phosphorylation in muscle have identified a variety of defects in patients with mitochondrial encephalomyopathy, involving single or multiple respiratory chain complexes, all of which are associated with a wide range of clinical syndromes.

Genetics

The mitochondrial respiratory chain has the special characteristic of being encoded by two genetic systems, mitochondrial DNA (mtDNA) as well as nuclear genes. Mammalian mitochondria each contain five to ten circular DNA molecules, which are double stranded and about 16.5 kilobases (kb) in length. Mitochondrial DNA encodes for 13 of the 67 or so subunits of the mitochondrial respiratory chain and oxidative phosphorylation system: seven subunits of complex I; cytochrome *b* (complex III); subunits I, II and III of cytochrome oxidase (complex IV); and subunits six and eight of ATP synthase. The nuclear genome encodes the remaining polypeptides in the respiratory chain and controls their transport into the mitochondrion. Replication, transcription, and translation of mitochondrial genomes are also dependent on nuclear products, although mitochondrial DNA encodes its own translation system in the form of two ribosomal RNAs and 22 transfer RNAs (tRNAs). The coding function of mitochondrial DNA and its mode of transmission led to the hypothesis that the defects of this genome could cause mitochondrial encephalomyopathy. As a constituent of the ovum's cytoplasm, mitochondrial DNA is exclusively maternally transmitted. The majority of patients with mitochondrial encephalomyopathies do not have a history of affected relatives, but when individuals are affected in more than one generation, maternal transmission to offspring is far more frequent than paternal transmission.

Several different types of mitochondrial DNA defects have been reported in patients with mitochondrial encephalomyopathy (Table 1). The most common is a single large deletion, varying between about 1.5 and 9 kb in length. Deleted mitochondrial DNAs coexist with normal molecules in the muscle and, sometimes, other tissues of patients; they are rarely detectable in blood. Patients with such deletions do not have affected relatives and it seems most likely that deletions originate during oogenesis in the patients' mothers. Duplications of mitochondrial DNA have also been described, and these probably represent deleted dimers. In contrast to patients with deletions, those with point mutations of mitochondrial DNA commonly have affected relatives with either a similar or less severe phenotype. Again, mutant mitochondrial DNA coexists with normal mitochondrial DNA in variable proportions in different tissues, a situation known as heteroplasmy.

No defects of the nuclear genome causing specific respiratory chain subunit deficiencies have been reported, although it is likely that these

Table 1 *Mitochondrial DNA defects in mitochondrial encephalomyopathies*

Defect	Disease
Primary mitochondrial DNA defects	
Large single deletions/duplications (sporadic)	PEO, Kearns–Sayre syndrome
Point mutations (may be maternal FH)	
in tRNA genes (bp):	
8344, 8356	MERRF*
3243, 3250, 3271	MELAS/other encephalomyopathies*
3260	myopathy/cardiomyopathy*
in reading frame:	
8993	Neurogenic weakness, ataxia, RP*
Mitochondrial DNA defects secondary to presumed nuclear mutations	
Multiple deletions (AD)	PEO, myopathy, deafness, neuropathy
Depletion (varies between tissues) (AR)	Myopathy/encephalopathy/renal/hepatic failure

*Detectable in blood samples and hence a useful screening test; there are other less common mutations.
AD, autosomal dominant; AR, autosomal recessive; bp, base pair; FH, family history; MELAS, mitochondrial encephalopathy, lactic acid, and stroke-like episodes; MERRF, myoclonic epilepsy with ragged red fibres; PEO, progressive external ophthalmoplegia; RP, retinitis pigmentosa;

exist. Two defects of mitochondrial DNA thought to be secondary to nuclear genetic abnormalities have been described. In one, multiple mitochondrial DNA deletions are inherited as an autosomal dominant trait. This is thought to be due to a defect of a nuclear gene involved in mitochondrial DNA replication. In the second, there is a variable degree of mitochondrial DNA depletion in different tissues and this appears to be an autosomal recessive trait. Overall, primary defects of mitochondrial DNA account for 65 per cent of patients with mitochondrial encephalomyopathy. There is more correlation between clinical features and mtDNA defects than is the case in relation to biochemical lesions, as will be discussed below.

CLINICAL FEATURES

The clinical presentations of mitochondrial encephalomyopathy are diverse, but can be divided into four broad categories.

Infantile lactic acidosis

This is the most severe phenotype and characteristically comprises a floppy baby with failure to thrive and developmental delay. Lactic acidosis is the clue to diagnosis, although respiratory chain deficiencies are not the only cause of this syndrome; others include pyruvate dehydrogenase deficiency and β-oxidation defects. There may be non-neurological features, including defective haematopoiesis, renal tubular acidosis, and cardiac failure. Biochemical studies tend to show complex I, IV, or multiple, defects. The genetic basis of this clinical presentation is so far poorly defined. In a group of patients with pancytopenia, exocrine pancreatic and hepatic failure (Pearson's syndrome), there is a deletion of mitochondrial DNA that is easily detected in blood. Others with multisystem disease have been shown to have depletion of mitochondrial DNA in some tissues, the degree and distribution of this determining phenotype, which may include myopathy, encephalopathy, renal dysfunction, and hepatic failure. Muscle biopsies from infants with mitochondrial encephalomyopathy tend to show cytochrome oxidase deficiency, as demonstrated by histochemical staining, rather than ragged red fibres. In some cases this is reversible, indicating a good prognosis. It is thought that this reflects the existence of specific isoforms of cytochrome oxidase subunits in relation to different phases of development.

Progressive external ophthalmoplegia and the Kearns–Sayre syndrome

Progressive external ophthalmoplegia has insidious onset and usually develops during childhood or adolescence, giving rise to ptosis and lim-

itation of eye movements in all directions of gaze. Fatigue, a 'salt and pepper' type of retinopathy, and proximal limb weakness are common associated features, and the presence of retinopathy points to a diagnosis of mitochondrial encephalomyopathy. Progressive external ophthalmoplegia has quite a wide differential diagnosis including myasthenia gravis, thyroid eye disease, congenital myopathy, and oculopharyngeal dystrophy. The last is generally of adult onset and of autosomal dominant inheritance; dysphagia is common whereas this is relatively unusual in mitochondrial encephalomyopathy.

The Kearns–Sayre syndrome (KSS) is defined by progressive external ophthalmoplegia and pigmentary retinopathy with onset before the age of 20 years, with one or more of the following features: ataxia, an increased cerebrospinal fluid protein concentration (> 1 g/l) and cardiac conduction defects. Other features may occur, such as diabetes, hypoparathyroidism, short stature, and deafness. Many patients with mitochondrial encephalomyopathy have progressive external ophthalmoplegia and some but not all of the elements of Kearns–Sayre syndrome indicating that progressive external ophthalmoplegia, progressive external ophthalmoplegia 'plus', and Kearns–Sayre syndrome are part of a spectrum of disorders, and this concept is supported by genetic data. Deletions of mitochondrial DNA in muscle are observed in 80 to 90 per cent of patients with Kearns–Sayre syndrome, a similar proportion of those with progressive external ophthalmoplegia and retinopathy, and about half of those with progressive external ophthalmoplegia alone. Patients with a similar phenotype occasionally have tandem duplications of mitochondrial DNA. All patients with Kearns–Sayre syndrome and the majority of those with progressive external ophthalmoplegia are sporadic cases, which reflects the association with a mitochondrial DNA deletion in many cases. However, some patients with progressive external ophthalmoplegia have the 3243 base pair point mutation (see Table 1), and if this is the case there may be maternal inheritance. In some families where progressive external ophthalmoplegia is dominantly inherited, patients have multiple, different, mitochondrial DNA deletions. The genetic defect underlying progressive external ophthalmoplegia and progressive external ophthalmoplegia 'plus' syndromes has not been established in all patients with mitochondrial encephalomyopathy.

Myopathies

A relatively small proportion (about 15 per cent) of patients with mitochondrial encephalomyopathy have limb and facial weakness alone, sometimes with accompanying ptosis but no restriction of extraocular movements. Such patients sometimes have retinopathy. The muscle weakness is usually enhanced by exertion and associated with elevation of serum lactate concentrations which increases after exercise. Complex I deficiency is common in this group. There may be a family history suggesting either maternal or autosomal recessive inheritance. The genetic basis of this syndrome is largely unknown, although it has been observed with the 3243 base pair point mutation or a further mutation at position 3260, which is associated with additional cardiomyopathy.

Encephalomyopathies

Within mitochondrial encephalomyopathy syndromes are two that are clinically very distinctive, namely myoclonic epilepsy with ragged red fibres (MERRF) and mitochondrial encephalopathy, lactic acidosis and stroke-like episodes (MELAS). However, these account for less than one-half of patients with encephalomyopathies and there is substantial overlap between them in some cases. The cardinal features of MERRF are myoclonus, epilepsy, and ataxia. Onset is most commonly in the second and third decades of life. Associated features include deafness, muscle weakness, dementia, optic atrophy, neuropathy, and multiple lipomas. Seizures are often photosensitive and include absences or drop attacks, as well as generalized tonic–clonic seizures. The myoclonic jerks are also induced by noise or bright lights and electrophysiologically have the features of cortical reflex myoclonus. Biochemical studies of muscle tend to show a generalized reduction of respiratory chain enzyme activity. This syndrome is particularly commonly maternally inherited and this reflects the presence of a point mutation of mitochondrial DNA at position 8344 in approximately 80 per cent of cases. Genetic studies have shown that index cases have the cardinal triad of myoclonus, epilepsy, and ataxia, but maternal relatives with the mutation may be asymptomatic or have partial expression of the phenotype such as deafness and/or epilepsy alone. Within families there is some correlation between the proportion of mutant mitochondrial DNA and clinical severity. The differential diagnosis of progressive myoclonic ataxia and epilepsy is wide and includes other genetic neurodegenerative disorders such as Lafora body disease and Unverricht–Lundborg disease.

Patients with the MELAS syndrome classically present in childhood or early adult life with recurrent stroke-like episodes. These often have migrainous elements with headache, vomiting, and visual disturbance and the neurological deficit is frequently heralded by a focal seizure. Hemiparesis or hemianopia persist for days to months and usually leave minor residual disability; after numerous episodes the cumulative effects are disabling, leading to dementia, quadriparesis, cortical blindness, and ataxia. Other features such as short stature, peripheral neuropathy, deafness, and progressive external ophthalmoplegia are common. Complex I deficiency is the most common biochemical defect. About half of patients have affected maternal relatives, and 80 per cent of patients with this syndrome have a point mutation of mitochondrial DNA, again in a tRNA gene at position 3243. As is the case with the 8344 (MERRF) mutation, maternal relatives with the mutation may have a less severe phenotype (e.g. deafness, muscle weakness), or may be clinically unaffected. Muscle weakness does not occur in some patients, and not all have ragged red fibres. Unlike the MERRF mutation, the 3243 mutation is associated with a much wider phenotype, and the proportion of mutant mitochondrial DNA is not closely correlated with clinical severity. Stroke-like episodes occur in only about 50 per cent of patients with this mutation and some have progressive external ophthalmoplegia and/or myopathy alone, or deafness, ataxia, and dementia of adult onset. Diabetes appears to be particularly common in association with this mitochondrial DNA defect, and in some large kindreds it appears to give rise to diabetes and/or deafness without neurological disease.

A maternally transmitted syndrome of neurogenic muscle weakness, ataxia, and retinitis pigmentosa is associated with a point mutation of mitochondrial DNA, which is unusual in that it is in a protein coding gene (ATPase subunit 6) rather than a tRNA gene. Leigh's syndrome, defined as progressive or relapsing brain-stem dysfunction with char-acteristic pathology is the most severe phenotype of this genetic defect, and this also applies to the 8344 base pair mutation.

DIAGNOSIS

The differential diagnosis of mitochondrial encephalomyopathy syndromes is wide, particularly in those with CNS involvement. This diagnosis should be considered in children and adults with multisystem CNS disease of unclear origin. Apart from the more obvious phenotypes such as progressive external ophthalmoplegia, MERRF, MELAS, and Leigh's syndrome, combinations of ataxia, dementia, or epilepsy, together with features such as short stature and deafness, are particularly suggestive of mitochondrial disease. In possible encephalomyopathy syndromes it is logical to perform mitochondrial DNA analysis of blood samples as a screening investigation, as this is relatively non-invasive. In the vast majority of symptomatic patients with the 3243 and 8344 base pair mutations these are detectable in blood, although the proportion in muscle is usually higher. If these analyses are negative, histochemical analysis of a muscle biopsy is the most useful investigation. Apart from ragged red fibres, there is usually also evidence of focal cytochrome oxidase deficiency, again detected histochemically. However, ragged red fibres are not present in the muscle of all patients with predominant CNS involvement. Ragged red fibres are occasionally observed in small proportions (less than 3 per cent) in normal elderly subjects or in other muscle diseases including muscular dystrophies and polymyositis.

An increase in blood and cerebrospinal fluid lactate concentrations, particularly after exercise, is common in mitochondrial encephalomyopathy, but this is not always the case and the controlled exercise required is difficult for disabled patients. Plasma creatine kinase is often normal or only mildly elevated, and electromyography may be normal in patients with encephalopathies. In such cases, computerized tomography and magnetic resonance imaging show a wide range of abnormalities, including multifocal low density lesions, cerebral and cerebellar atrophy, and calcification of the basal ganglia. Such abnormalities are particularly frequent in the MELAS syndrome. More widespread tissue involvement may be demonstrated by the ECG, echocardiography, and renal, endocrine and liver function tests.

PROGNOSIS

Prognosis is determined largely by age of onset and degree of CNS involvement. It is worst in patients with infantile lactic acidosis, who may not survive infancy, and encephalopathies such as MELAS developing in childhood. In those with progressive external ophthalmoplegia alone, disability may be minimal and life expectancy normal. If there is progressive external ophthalmoplegia and retinopathy, annual electrocardiograms should be performed to detect the development of cardiac conduction defects, which may require a pacemaker. Patients with weakness enhanced by exertion are particularly susceptible to lactic acidosis precipitated by exercise, alcohol, and intercurrent infection, although this applies to some extent to all patients with a respiratory chain defect. This needs treatment with slow infusion of sodium bicarbonate. On the whole, treatment of these disorders is disappointing. Steroids and respiratory chain cofactors such as ubiquinone, menandione and ascorbic acid, although the subject of several anecdotal encouraging reports, have not been demonstrated to show convincing long term improvement. Respiratory chain dysfunction may be associated with secondary carnitine deficiency, and carnitine supplements may improve symptoms of muscle weakness in such patients.

REFERENCES

Attardi, G. and Schatz, G. (1988). Biogenesis of mitochondria. *Annual Review of Cell Biology*, **4**, 289–333.

Ciafaloni, E., *et al.* (1992). MELAS: Clinical features, biochemistry, and molecular genetics. *Annals of Neurology*, **31**, 391–8.

DiMauro, S., Bonilla, E., Zeviani, M., Nakagawa, M., and DeVivo, D.C. (1985). Mitochondrial myopathies. *Annals of Neurology*, **17**, 521–38.

Hammans, S.R., Sweeney, M.G., Brockington, M., Morgan-Hughes, J.A., and Harding, A.E. (1991). Mitochondrial encephalopathies: molecular genetic diagnosis from blood samples. *Lancet*, **337**, 1311–13.

Hammans, S.R., *et al.* (1993). The mitochondrial DNA transfer RNA^{Lys}A→G$^{(8344)}$ mutation and the syndrome of myoclonic epilepsy with ragged red fibres (MERFF): relationship of clinical phenotype to proportion of mutant mitochondrial DNA. *Brain*, **116**, 617–32.

Hatefi Y. (1985). The mitochondrial electron transport and oxidative phosphorylation system. *Annual Review of Biochemistry*, **54**, 1015–69.

Holt, I.J., Harding, A.E., Cooper, J.M., Schapira, A.H.V., Toscano, A., Clark, J.B. and Morgan-Hughes, J.A. (1989). Mitochondrial myopathies: Clinical and biochemical features of 30 patients with major deletions of muscle mitochondrial DNA. *Annals of Neurology*, **29**, 600–8.

Marsden, C.D., Harding, A.E., Obeso, J.A., and Lu, C-S. (1990). Progressive myoclonic ataxia (the Ramsay Hunt syndrome). *Archives of Neurology*, **47**, 1121–7.

Moraes, C.T., *et al.* (1989). Mitochondrial DNA deletions in progressive external opthalmoplegia and Kearns–Sayre syndrome. *New England Journal of Medicine*, **320**, 1293–9.

Munnich, A., *et al.* (1992). Clinical aspects of mitochondrial disorders. *Journal of Inherited Metabolic Disease*, **15**, 448–55.

Petty, R.K.H., Harding, A.E. and Morgan-Hughes, J.A. (1986). The clinical features of mitochondrial myopathy. *Brain*, **109**, 915–38.

Rotig, A., *et al.* (1990). Pearson's marrow-pancreas syndrome. A multisystem mitochondrial disorder in infancy. *Journal of Clinical Investigation*, **86**, 1601–8.

Tatuch, Y., *et al.* (1992). Heteroplasmic mtDNA mutation (T→G) at 8993 can cause Leigh disease when the percentage of abnormal mtDNA is high. *American Journal of Human Genetics*, **50**, 852–8.

Tritschler, H.-J., *et al.* (1992). Mitochondrial myopathy of childhood associated with depletion of mitochondrial DNA. *Neurology*, **42**, 209–17.

Wallace, D.C. (1992). Diseases of the mitochondrial DNA. *Annual Review of Biochemistry*, **61**, 1175–212.

Zeviani, M., *et al.* (1991). Maternally inherited myopathy and cardiomyopathy: association with a new mutation in the mitochondrial DNA t-RNA$^{Leu(UUR)}$. *Lancet*, **338**, 143–7.

Zeviani, M. (1992) Nucleus-driven mutations of human mitochondrial DNA. *Journal of Inherited Metabolic Disease*, **15**, 456–71.

25.10 Tropical pyomyositis (tropical myositis)

D. A. WARRELL

DEFINITION

The term tropical pyomyositis should be restricted to primary muscle abscesses arising within skeletal muscles. This condition must be distinguished from abscesses extending into muscle either from subcutaneous sites following infection through the skin, or from osteomyelitis or suppuration originating in tissues other than muscle.

GEOGRAPHICAL OCCURRENCE

Tropical myositis has been reported from most parts of tropical Africa, Malaysia, Thailand, Indonesia, Oceania, Central and South America, and the Caribbean. It is common in many tropical countries, accounting for 4 per cent of admissions to a hospital in Uganda and for 2.2 per cent of all surgical admissions to a hospital in eastern Ecuador. In temperate climates, pyomyositis is extremely rare, but a few cases have been described, including some with immunosuppression resulting from HIV infection, asplenia, and Felty's syndrome.

AETIOLOGY

Staphylococcus aureus is the organism most commonly cultured from the abscesses. *Streptococcus pyogenes* (usually group A) is responsible for a few cases, but tropical pyomyositis must be distinguished from streptococcal necrotizing myositis (also known as peracute streptococcal pyomyositis or spontaneous streptococcal gangrenous myositis) which is more fulminant and diffuse and has a very high mortality (see Section 7). Other isolates have included *S. pneumoniae*, *Haemophilus influenzae*, *E. coli*, and *Pseudomonas* species. The strikingly different incidence of pyomyositis in tropical and temperate countries has not been explained. In Africa and South America, the condition appears to be relatively more common in indigenous peoples. A history of preceding trauma to the affected muscle is obtained from more than 20 per cent of patients in most series. It has been suggested that, by analogy with

osteomyelitis, a muscle haematoma provides a nidus for blood-borne infection. A number of predisposing causes has been suggested: preceding viral infection (for example an arbovirus), general debilitation, and nematode infections—particularly toxocariasis, *Lagochilascaris minor*, and filariasis. None has been supported by convincing evidence, but sickle-cell disease may be a genuine predisposing cause in a minority of cases. Most of the abscesses associated with helminth infections should not be termed pyomyositis as they are inter- rather than intramuscular. For example, *Dracunculus medinensis* can give rise to deep intermuscular abscesses secondarily infected with *Staphylococcus aureus*.

PATHOLOGY

The abscesses may be large, are usually loculated, and are situated within skeletal muscles beneath the deep fascia. Histologically, there is focal muscle necrosis with an infiltration of mononuclear cells and inflammatory oedema.

CLINICAL FEATURES

Tropical pyomyositis can occur at any age but its highest incidence is in the second decade. It is more common in males. The earliest symptom is pain and tenderness of the affected muscle. Any of the skeletal muscles may be involved, but those of the trunk and lower limbs are the most commonly affected. Usually there is a single localized abscess, but multiple abscesses in distantly separated muscles can occur. At an early stage, an ill-defined tender and thickened area may be palpable in the muscle. Later, a localized, very tender, and hot swelling is palpable. There may be redness and oedema of the overlying skin, but the skin is not primarily involved. The swelling is usually non-fluctuant and there is no local lymphadenopathy. Symptoms and signs usually develop over a few days. Peripheral leucocytosis is not invariable. Eosinophilia is frequently described but is usually common in the populations most affected by tropical pyomyositis. In spite of considerable muscle destruction at the site of the abscess, serum concentrations of muscle enzymes may not be elevated, but in some cases there is myoglobinaemia, myoglobinuria, and acute renal failure. Complications are uncommon and consist of spread of infection from the affected muscle to other structures such as joints, resulting in septic arthritis; to the pleural cavity, resulting in empyema; or by haematogenous spread to the heart valves. Mortality of hospitalized cases is said to be less than 1.5 per cent.

DIAGNOSIS

The differential diagnosis is from pus tracking from abscesses in other organs and tissues, muscle haematomas, torn muscles, certain highly vascular or necrotic tumours of connective tissue or muscle (such as rhabdomyosarcoma), and the inflammatory and allergic swellings resulting from the migration of helminths such as Loa loa, Gnathostoma, Paragonimus, and sparganum. Staphylococcus aureus is usually cultured from the pus, but blood cultures are positive in less than 5 per cent of cases. Ultrasound and CT scans are useful for localizing abscesses and guiding needles for diagnostic and therapeutic aspiration.

TREATMENT

Full surgical exploration, debridement, and drainage is essential. Because the abscesses are usually loculated, needle aspiration is inadequate. Parenteral treatment with a β-lactamase resistant penicillin (flucloxacillin) should be started immediately, but if group A Streptococcus is cultured, benzyl penicillin is the drug of choice.

REFERENCES

Anand, S.V. and Evans, K.T. (1964). Pyomyositis. *British Journal of Surgery* **51**, 917–20.

Chiedozi, L.C. (1979). Pyomyositis: review of 205 cases in 112 patients. *American Journal of Surgery* **137**, 255–9.

Echeverria, P. and Vaughan, M.C. (1975). 'Tropical myositis'. A diagnostic problem in temperate climates. *American Journal of Diseases of Childhood* **129**, 856–7.

Fanney, D., Thomas, L.C., and Schwartz, E. (1982). An outbreak of pyomyositis in a large refugee camp in Thailand. *American Journal of Tropical Medicine and Hygiene* **31**, 131–5.

Gibson, R.K., Rosenthal, S.J., and Lukert, B.P. (1984). Pyomyositis: increasing recognition in temperate climates. *American Journal of Medicine* **77**, 768–72.

Horn, C.V. and Master, S. (1968). Pyomyositis tropicans in Uganda. *East African Medical Journal* **45**, 463–71.

Kerrigan, K.R. and Nelson, S.J. (1992). Tropical pyomyositis in eastern Ecuador. *Transactions of the Royal Society of Tropical Medicine and Hygiene* **86**, 90–1.

Levin, M.J., Gardner, P., and Waldvogel, F.A. (1971). 'Tropical' pyomyositis. An unusual infection due to *Staphylococcus aureus*. *New England Journal of Medicine* **284**, 196–8.

Marcus, R.T. and Foster, W.D. (1968). Observations on the clinical features, aetiology and geographical distribution of pyomyositis in East Africa. *East African Medical Journal* **45**, 167–76.

Smith, P.G., Pike, M.C., Taylor, E., and Taylor, J.F. (1978). The epidemiology of tropical myositis in the Mengo districts of Uganda. *Transactions of the Royal Society of Tropical Medicine and Hygiene* **72**, 46–53.

Traquair, R.N. (1947). Pyomyositis. *Journal of Tropical Medicine and Hygiene* **50**, 81–9.

Section 26 *The eye in general medicine*

26 The eye in general medicine

P. FRITH

The significance of disorders of the eye in general medicine

Because the eye may be involved in so many diseases, it is essential that clinicians familiarize themselves with the major ocular manifestations of systemic disorders, learn how to examine the eye and, in particular, become proficient using an ophthalmoscope. The pattern of disease in the eye may often point to the diagnosis of a particular systemic disorder, while in some cases an ocular complication may need urgent and specific treatment.

Common clinical manifestations of ocular disease (Plates 1–20)

RED EYE AND THE SLIT LAMP

Although the red eye is often an isolated problem there may be a systemic association. The pattern of redness suggests a possible diagnosis and there may be other features to help confirm this, as shown in Table 1. A more detailed description of the findings in iritis and scleritis is given later in this section. The slit lamp gives a stable, magnified, well-illuminated view of the eye surface and shows the specific features of some types of conjunctivitis, the detail and staining pattern of corneal lesions, and cells diagnostic of uveitis within the eye chambers. Glaucoma may be diagnosed by finding raised eye pressure.

DRY EYE

Mild dryness of the eyes is common in the elderly population but if lack of tears is severe or occurs in younger patients there may be a systemic cause, particularly if there is also dryness of the mouth (sicca syndrome). Sicca with an identifiable systemic association is called Sjögren's syndrome, as with rheumatoid arthritis, systemic sclerosis, or mixed connective tissue disease and sarcoidosis. Patients with dry eyes complain of gritty discomfort and the eyes may be red or sticky with discharge. The Schirmer test and characteristic findings with the slit lamp are described under Rheumatoid arthritis below. Symptoms may be improved by using artificial tear drops but the patient with severely dry eyes has a miserable problem which can be very difficult to manage and carries the risk of eventual sight loss.

LOSS OF VISION

If there is no obvious external cause for poor vision the ophthalmoscope is invaluable, but before reaching for this it is important to have a clear history of the visual problem and to assess some simple signs. Visual acuity should be measured in each eye, even if only with a newspaper but preferably with a Snellen chart at 6 m, using glasses or a pinhole to correct for any error of focus. If there is a focal retinal problem such as oedema or haemorrhage giving distortion or loss of central vision, the patient may be able to draw their defect in relation to fixation and this is a good guide to the size and position of a lesion near the fovea. The symmetry of alternate direct pupil responses to a bright light (the relative afferent pupil test) should also be carefully examined as major impairment of vision in one eye compared with the other gives an asymmetrical response which has a limited number of important causes within the retina or optic nerve (Table 2).

The ophthalmoscope

The direct ophthalmoscope gives least trouble if a good modern instrument is used, viewing as close as possible to the patient. The optic nerve head is usually visible through an undilated pupil, but it is impossible to assess the retina reliably without using dilating drops. It is better practice to use drops than to avoid them and to use a short-acting drop (tropicamide 1 per cent in single-dose formulation is recommended, acting within about 15 min and lasting about 2 h) which carries almost no risk of precipitating an acute rise in eye pressure. The pupil should not be dilated if the patient has an acute neurological or neurosurgical problem such as subarachnoid haemorrhage, coma, or recent head injury, in which pupillary reaction is an important observation. The posterior retina is visible with the direct ophthalmoscope, as in diabetic and hypertensive retinopathies, but parts further forwards in the peripheral retina are best seen with the indirect ophthalmoscope or with the slit lamp and special lenses. The central fovea is seen if the patient looks directly into the light, and in diabetic retinopathy the area temporal to the fovea should also be examined. If the view is clouded there may be opacity in the lens or vitreous which is best seen by standing back and adjusting the light to focus on the pupil margin to give a red reflection against which opacities stand out as clumped black shadows, especially if the pupil is dilated.

Retinal changes

Retinal haemorrhages have a variety of shapes, depending on their depth within the retina. Superficial flame-shaped haemorrhages, though not unique to hypertension, dictate that blood pressure should be measured. Deeper dot and blot haemorrhages suggest diabetes (particularly if temporal to the macula), vein occlusion (particularly if unilateral or localized), or a haematological disease (particularly if bilateral). Haemorrhage in front of the retina, lying just behind the vitreous (subhyaloid), forms a dense focus which may sediment into a characteristic flat-topped shape which is typical of bleeding from new vessels (as in diabetes or after retinal vascular occlusion), secondary to a haematological abnormality, or to trauma (including non-accidental injury). The amount of damage caused by haemorrhage depends on its site and severity. Most are asymptomatic and resolve if the cause is treated, but vision falls if the fovea is involved or if blood leaks into the vitreous itself, causing 'floaters' or mistiness of vision.

Pale retinal lesions are subtly diverse. Hard exudates (Plate 2) are shiny and take a variety of forms; if in circles (circinate) this strongly suggests diabetes with foci of retinal vascular leakage. A star of exudate forms around the fovea with resolving retinal oedema, as in treated hypertension or papilloedema. The most common lesions confused with exudates are retinal drusen (Plate 3), which are more uniform and discrete and usually scattered around the retina or congregated close to the fovea. Cotton-wool spots (Plate 1) are fluffy pale patches indicating microvascular closure. They are swollen nerve fibre axons and are always significant, though there are many causes (Table 3). Retinal infiltrates look like cotton-wool spots but they are cellular, and cells spilling into the overlying vitreous are visible with the slit lamp. Infiltrates are uncommon but important as they may indicate foci of infection (as in active toxoplasmosis or cytomegalovirus retinitis), sarcoidosis, Behçet's

Table 1 *Findings in the red eye*

Cause	Features	Associations
Conjunctivitis	Redness of conjunctiva, both eye and inside lids Sticky discharge almost always Discomfort rather than pain or photophobia Follicles may be visible	Bacterial or viral Sicca
Episcleritis	Redness of eye only, may be overall or sectorial Not sticky Discomfort rather than pain Common Not serious and no threat to sight Systemic cause sometimes identified	Systemic inflammatory
Scleritis	Redness as for episcleritis but may be intense and bluish Pain which may be intense Uncommon Serious disorder with threat to sight Systemic disorder often present	Rheumatoid arthritis Wegener's granulomatosis
Iritis (anterior uveitis)	Redness mostly around the cornea, may be bluish Pain and photophobia usual Corneal precipitates may be visible Pupil small and may festoon on dilating	Sarcoidosis Ankylosing spondylitis Behçet's disease Some infections
Corneal lesion (keratitis)	Redness often sectorial and adjacent to corneal lesion Pain photophobia and watering usual Fluorescein staining will highlight	Herpes virus infection Vasculitis
Acute glaucoma	Redness of the entire eye, often bluish Pain may be intense and vomiting common Uncommon Cornea steamy Eye feels cricket-ball hard Pupil dilated, oval and fixed	Dilating drops (rare with tropicamide)

Table 2 *Some causes of a relative afferent pupil defect*

Central retinal artery occlusion
Ischaemic optic neuropathy, as in giant cell arteritis
Optic neuritis
Extensive retinal detachment
Advanced unilateral glaucoma
Optic nerve compression

Table 3 *Some causes of cotton-wool spots*

Accelerated hypertension
Diabetes
Retinal vein occlusion (sometimes)
Microemboli or hyperviscosity
Acute pancreatitis
Vasculitis
HIV retinopathy

syndrome, or, rarely, ocular lymphoma. Discrete punched-out scars suggest healed foci of inflammation of the retina and underlying choroid, of which the most common cause is Toxoplasma.

Pigmentation is frequent around the optic nerve head and often forms around scars. Benign naevi which are pigmented and flat are quite common, but occasionally a raised area represents a malignant melanoma of the choroid. Scattered and clumped peripheral pigment may be characteristic of retinitis pigmentosa (accompanied by night blindness) or retinal pigment epithelial hyperplasia (associated with polyposis coli).

Fluorescein angiography

This technique is useful to define the type and severity of retinal vascular disease, including diabetic retinopathy. It is usually uneventful but occasional patients have an allergic or even anaphylactic reaction, and there are reports of fatalities. Fluorescein dye is injected into the antecubital vein and circulates via the lungs and heart to the retina, filling the vessels in a sequence which is photographed as a series. The dye demonstrates patterns of perfusion and non-perfusion, both in the retina and in the underlying choroidal circulation, outlines abnormalities of the vessels such as microaneurysms, and identifies sites of leakage indicating damage to retinal vessels or the formation of new vessels. The angiogram gives valuable diagnostic information and indicates if and where laser treatment is needed.

Visual fields

If ophthalmoscopic findings are normal, the visual fields should always be examined as it is surprisingly easy for large defects to go unnoticed by patients. A central or altitudinal (top or bottom of field) defect suggests pathology in the retina or optic nerve, whereas a bitemporal defect draws attention to the optic chiasm, and a homonymous defect to the visual path posterior to the chiasm. With bilateral occipital infarction there may be difficulty in defining the visual loss and pupil reactions are normal. If it proves difficult to account for poor vision in one eye, reconsider whether there is a defect of focus or an amblyopic (lazy) eye because of squint or refractive error in childhood: the first should improve with a pinhole device but the second will not.

The eye in diagnosis of inherited conditions (see also Section 4)

The eye is quite frequently involved in genetic disease. Sometimes the changes are obvious without using magnification or special equipment, but in other cases the slit lamp or the indirect ophthalmoscope may be needed for careful examination of the cornea or lens, or to visualize the periphery of the interior eye. Even babies may be examined at the lamp or with the ophthalmoscope, although a general anaesthetic may be

Table 4 *Eye findings in some inherited disorders*

Eyelid	
Epicanthus	Turner's (XO), trisomy 18 (Edward's), Down's deletions 13q, 18, 4p, 5p
Ptosis	Kearns–Sayre, myotonic dystrophy, Turner's (XO) 13q deletion
Conjunctiva	
Conjunctival telangiectasia	Osler–Weber–Rendu, Louis-Bar, Sturge–Weber, Fabry's fucosidosis
Pingueculae	Gaucher's
Cornea	
Kayser–Fleischer ring (copper)	Wilson's
Corneal dystrophy (verticillata)	Fabry's
Corneal crystals	Cystinosis
Corneal clouding	Mucolipidoses, mucopolysaccharidoses, Lowe's, X-linked ichthyosis, tyrosinaemia, Tangier, trisomy 18
Thickend corneal nerves	Multiple endocrine neoplasia type 2b
Keratoconus	Down's
Iris	
Iris tremor (iridodonesis)	Marfan's
Lisch nodule	Neurofibromatosis type I
Iris transillumination	Albinism
Aniridia (absent iris)	Wilms' tumour/11p deletion
Coloboma (cat eye)	Trisomy 22
Brushfield spots	Down's
Lens	
Lens dislocation	Marfan's, homocystinuria, ectopia lentis
Lenticonus	Alport's
Cataract, infantile	Galactosaemia, galactokinase deficiency, Down's, Lowe's
Cataract, childhood	Skeletal, chromosomal, and dermatological syndromes
Cataract, adult	Myotonic dystrophy, Wilson's, neurofibromatosis type II, Fabry's mannosidosis
Retina	
Retinal angioma	Von Hippel–Lindau, Sturge–Weber
Retinal phakoma	Tuberous sclerosis, neurofibromatosis type I
Angioid streaks	Pseudoxanthoma elasticum
Retinal dysplasia	Norrie's, incontinentia pigmenti
Macular abnormality	Batten's, Farber's, Gaucher's
Macular cherry-red spot	Sialidosis, Niemann–Pick, Tay–Sachs
Pigmentary retinopathy	Usher's, mitochondrial myopathy (some), Refsum's, Kearns–Sayre, abetalipoproteinaemia, Hurler's, Laurence–Moon–Biedl
Retinal pigmented patches	Gardner's
Retinal gyrate atrophy	Hyperornithinaemia
Retinoblastoma	13q deletion
Retinal vascular anomaly	Fucosidosis
Retinal crystals	Cystinosis, oxalosis, Alport's
Sclera	
Blue sclera	Osteogenesis imperfecta
Thinned sclera	Ehlers–Danlos
Pigmented sclera	Alkaptonuria
Glaucoma	Neurofibromatosis type I, Sturge–Weber

needed and may be combined with taking biopsy material. Some ocular features of inherited conditions are given in Table 4.

Some genetic disorders are important enough to warrant screening of families to detect the phenotype as early as possible for genetic counselling, Marfan's syndrome, neurofibromatosis type I, Von Hippel–Lindau, and myotonic dystrophy, for example. There are a few inherited conditions in which eye features are found in patients at risk of developing malignant tumours.

MARFAN'S SYNDROME

Most patients with Marfan eye features are affected from early childhood and almost all of them have reduced vision or squint at the time of screening. A minority develop progressive changes which manifest later in life. The most common finding is of a myopic and astigmatic error of focus which may be deduced in older patients from their spectacle lenses. The slit lamp often shows that the ocular lens is dislocated, usually upwards and temporally, and that the iris trembles slightly with small eye movements (iridodonesis) because it is poorly supported by an abnormally mobile lens. Rarely, the lens may dislocate completely and lie free in the back chamber, occasionally the front. The dislocated lenses are best retained even though they produce a marked error of focus. Careful correction of focus can improve vision dramatically in early childhood and may prevent permanent amblyopia. Even if the lenses are central and stable, an abnormally enlarged eyeball may produce myopia in Marfan patients, often of high degree. The main differential diagnoses in a patient with dislocated lenses are isolated ectopia lentis (lacking other Marfan features) and homocystinuria (with Marfanoid habitus). There is also a significantly increased incidence of retinal detachment and of glaucoma.

NEUROFIBROMATOSIS TYPE I (SEE ALSO SECTION 24)

The vast majority of patients (estimated at over 90 per cent by the age of 6 years in one large series) who carry this relatively common dominant gene will have Lisch nodules of the iris, visible using the slit lamp.

These are raised, often yellowish or brown, and almost always multiple. They must be distinguished from the extremely common simple, flat iris freckle. Other ocular signs may be found, particularly corneal, retinal, or orbital neurofibromas or schwannomas. There is an increased incidence of glaucoma. The screening for and management of intracranial tumours associated with neurofibromatosis type I, including optic nerve or chiasmal gliomas, is controversial. Neurofibromatosis type II is associated with cataract of the posterior subcapsular type.

VON HIPPEL–LINDAU'S DISEASE

Retinal angiomas occur in about two-thirds of patients with this dominant gene, developing by the teens or twenties, when they may be the presenting and sole feature, as other features may emerge in later years. The angiomas are usually multiple and bilateral. They are most often found in the mid-peripheral retina and so may be visible with dilatation of the pupils using the direct ophthalmoscope, although screening with the indirect ophthalmoscope is advised. The angioma starts as a very small lesion no bigger than a microaneurysm which progressively enlarges, developing dilated and tortuous feeder and draining retinal vessels. Early peripheral angiomas may be destroyed by laser treatment, preferably before they bleed or detach the retina. These patients need prolonged eye follow-up. Occasional angiomas occur on or beside the optic nerve head (juxtapapillary) where they may affect vision early in their development and are particularly difficult to treat.

MYOTONIC DYSTROPHY (SEE ALSO SECTION 25)

The typical eye finding is a particular type of lens change with multiple small, scintillating, and brilliantly coloured crystalline opacities in the lens cortex, visible only by slit-lamp examination. The number and prominence of opacities vary between different members of the same family so it is worth examining them all by slit lamp.

THE EYE IN DIAGNOSIS OF INHERITED PREMALIGNANT CONDITIONS (SEE ALSO SECTIONS 4, 6, AND 12)

A few uncommon inherited conditions associated with the development of malignant tumours have significant eye features. The least uncommon is Gardner's syndrome, in which pigmentation at the level of the deep retinal pigment epithelium is associated with polyposis coli. The retinal lesions are dark patches (best seen with the indirect ophthalmoscope) which are multiple and usually bilateral. The condition is dominant so it is worth screening the fundi of those at risk. Absence of the iris (aniridia) is associated in between a quarter and a third of patients below the age of 3 years with Wilms' tumour of the kidney, especially if there is a chromosome 11p deletion. Deletion of chromosome 13q may be associated with retinoblastoma which is then inheritable as a dominant trait with high penetrance, and such patients may also develop other tumours such as osteosarcomas. Multiple endocrine neoplasia syndrome type 2B, inherited as a dominant trait and associated especially with thyroid gland malignancy and with marfanoid habitus, is associated with enlarged corneal nerves (visible using the slit lamp) and sometimes with neuromas of the conjunctivae, thickened eyelids, and dry eyes (see Section 12). Patients with von Hippel–Lindau disease may also develop renal malignant tumours.

The eye in systemic inflammatory diseases

Systemic inflammatory disorders may be associated with changes in the external or internal eye. The eye disease may be an early warning of a flare in systemic activity, and in some the pattern of eye inflammation may suggest the underlying diagnosis. In a minority, the eye disorder in its own right may need systemic treatment to prevent loss of sight.

SARCOIDOSIS (SEE ALSO SECTION 17)

Sarcoidosis may involve the eye at many sites and the pattern is sometimes characteristic enough to suggest or support the diagnosis. There are usually symptoms but occasionally asymptomatic conjunctival granulomas may provide easily accessible tissue for biopsy, so it is always worth carrying out a slit-lamp examination.

External eye findings

Sarcoid granulomas may occur in the eyelids or conjunctiva. They are solid, raised, of variable size, often clustered and characteristically yellowish in colour. It is simple to biopsy them at the slit lamp using only topical anaesthetic drops but 'blind' biopsy of a normal looking conjunctiva is not fruitful. The most common differential diagnosis, to be distinguished on clinical grounds, is a granuloma from a meibomian cyst. Dry eye is common in sarcoid, causing symptoms of grittiness, positive Schirmer's test, fluorescein staining of the cornea, and, sometimes, enlarged lacrimal glands. Lacrimal with salivary enlargement is typical of Mikulicz's syndrome, of which sarcoid is one common cause, with lymphoma or infection as the important differential diagnoses.

Uveitis

Iritis (anterior uveitis) is the most common feature. It is usually bilateral and recurrent and it may be severe and damaging. In the acute stages the eye is red and painful, often with photophobia. The typical slit-lamp finding is large, greasy (like mutton-fat) precipitates on the internal surface of the cornea. Granulomata may be visible in the iris or at the pupil margin. Repeated attacks of iritis may be associated with cataract, glaucoma, or calcified corneal band keratopathy, particularly if there is also hypercalcaemia.

Inflammation further back in the eye (posterior uveitis) causes cells to appear in the vitreous, which the patient often notices as floaters. These may obscure the view of the fundus and may aggregate into characteristic strands or round 'snowballs'. Granulomata may form in the retina or choroid, visible as pale foci behind a haze of cells. Vision may be further impaired by oedema, which commonly leaks from inflamed retinal vessels and collects around the fovea, threatening sight permanently. In sarcoidosis, inflammation of the retinal vessels characteristically affects the retinal branch veins, which look dilated, irregular, and, later, sheathed. Inflammatory cells may cluster around the veins and fluorescein angiography shows leakage into and through the vessel wall in a segmental pattern. The branch veins may occlude, causing focal retinal haemorrhages. This appearance, of an occlusive retinal phlebitis, strongly suggests sarcoidosis; the most important differential diagnoses are Behçet's syndrome or an 'idiopathic' retinal vasculitis in which systemic features are absent both on presentation and follow-up.

Neuro-ophthalmic involvement

Sarcoid-related inflammation or granuloma can also affect the optic nerve, causing the clinical picture of optic neuritis, sometimes with an enlarged nerve on scanning, as with the other cranial nerve palsies of neuro-sarcoid. Occasionally, sarcoid granulomas behind the eye may produce signs of an orbital lesion.

Management (see Section 17)

Corticosteroids are the mainstay of treatment, given topically for anterior and systemically for posterior eye lesions. Most eyes respond but recurrent or chronic inflammation can still damage the eye, with significant threat to vision in the long term, though registrable blindness is uncommon.

BEHÇET'S SYNDROME (SEE CHAPTER 18.11.8)

Inflammation of the internal eye (uveitis) is one cardinal and important clinical feature helping to define Behçet's syndrome. The inflammation may be anterior (iritis) or posterior (particularly involving the retinal vessels as a retinal vasculitis), although in most patients both sites are involved at some stage and attacks are characteristically recurrent. These episodes damage the eye progressively and there is a serious risk of blindness. In parts of the world where the disease is most often found, particularly in Japan and Turkey, it is the most common cause of uveitis. The incidence in northern Japan is about 1 per 10 000 population, of whom roughly 75 per cent have ocular inflammation at some stage. Some surveys suggest a blindness rate in the individual eye of 50 per cent within 5 years of the onset of the first attack.

In some populations those most at risk of eye disease are males with the HLA-B5 haplotype, particularly the BW51 subtype, but neither seems to apply to populations of the United Kingdom or the United States. The disease is most common in the northern parts of the Japanese islands and the incidence in American immigrants of Japanese parentage is lower than expected from these rates.

Clinical features

Ocular disease is usually bilateral, although there may be a gap of many years between sequential involvement of the two eyes. Anterior uveitis (iritis) is common and may present. Attacks are typically acute, with pain, redness of the eye, and photophobia. In some brisk attacks, white cells may sediment in the anterior chamber to form a visible level, or hypopyon, which is characteristic of, although not unique to, Behçet's (Plate 16). Occasionally hypopyon may form in an eye that does not look inflamed. Attacks settle spontaneously, sometimes quite rapidly, but the eye may be damaged in the process and it is best to treat topically, in short intensive courses, with corticosteroid drops and dilatation of the pupil. Even with prompt treatment of each attack the eye may develop a cataract or high pressure (glaucoma), with threat to vision.

Inflammation at the back of the eye typically involves the retinal vessels, causing a retinal vasculitis which particularly involves capillaries and branch veins; inflammatory cells spilling into the vitreous give rise to floaters. The inflamed vessels commonly leak and may cause foveal oedema with a fall in visual acuity, sometimes with distortion of central vision, and risk of permanent foveal damage. Occlusion of inflamed branch veins causes haemorrhages (Plate 15) and cotton-wool spots, and the affected retina becomes atrophic. Vision is permanently affected if occlusion involves the fovea. Fluorescein angiography documents the type and extent of vascular changes and is a guide to the severity of leakage and closure. With recurrent attacks, the retina gradually dies, vessels become sheathed, and the optic nerve head atrophies. Neovascularization may occur, as in the ischaemic diabetic eye, and give rise to vitreous haemorrhage with the risk of retinal detachment. Acute retinal infiltrates (probably polymorph leucocytes) which form white, fluffy patches may occur, often unrelated to branch vessels, with cells in the overlying vitreous visible using the slit lamp. These settle spontaneously but are an indicator of active inflammation and are strongly suggestive of Behçet's eye disease.

Long-term management

Management of recurrent eye disease is difficult. There are few controlled studies of large numbers of patients, and no form of immunosuppression, either singly or in combination at a level tolerated long term, will prevent attacks. In limiting damage, systemic corticosteroids are the mainstay in the acute attack. Longer term, agents such as azathioprine, chlorambucil, colchicine, or cyclosporin A seem to be helpful, but the impact on blindness rates is so far unassessed and, in most patients, ocular attacks break through treatment eventually.

GIANT-CELL ARTERITIS (SEE CHAPTER 18.11.7)

Involvement of the optic nerve head circulation is the characteristic complication of this disorder. Because the phenomenon is ischaemic, visual loss, when it occurs, is irretrievable. It is difficult to assess the risk to vision of the patient presenting with features of the disorder elsewhere, although once patients are receiving adequate systemic corticosteroid

treatment the risk seems to fall appreciably and blindness is rare. In patients presenting with visual loss, the risk of further progressive loss in that eye or involvement of the second eye is high and it is fully justified to give these patients high initial doses of corticosteroids until the symptoms, erythrocyte sedimentation rate, and/or C-reactive protein level are controlled. This usually takes days rather than weeks. Thereafter, the problems of reducing steroid dose are the same as for the systemic disorder. In the rare patient in whom there is evidence that the second eye is already involved at presentation, it is justified to commence methylprednisolone intravenously. Temporal artery biopsy is valuable in helping to confirm the diagnosis and the need for continued treatment in patients with visual loss, bearing in mind that some elderly patients have structural and not arteritic ischaemic optic neuropathy, which may be associated with headache but with normal erythrocyte sedimentation rate and C-reactive protein level.

Clinical features of eye involvement

Loss of vision may come on overnight or may evolve rapidly during the daytime. Occasionally, there are episodes of transient visual loss in the preceding weeks or days. Established loss may be partial at the beginning, and may involve either the top or bottom half of the visual field, but often becomes total. The optic nerve head is characteristically pale and swollen (Plate 19), but sometimes the vascular occlusion is behind the immediate nerve head which then appears to be normal. Because the onset is usually unilateral and the loss of nerve function considerable, there is almost always a significant relative loss of afferent pupil response compared with the normal eye. Occlusion of the central retinal artery, producing a pale retina and cherry-red foveal spot, is uncommon but well documented. Patients with visual loss often have pain and tenderness in the temple, and jaw claudication is characteristic.

TAKAYASU'S ARTERITIS (SEE CHAPTER 15.13)

This inflammatory disorder involving large arteries can cause an aortic arch syndrome with raised erythocyte sedimentation rate, although, unlike giant-cell arteritis, typically in young patients. There may be amaurosis fugax or the established retinal vascular changes of chronic ocular ischaemia (see below) (Plate 17), sometimes with characteristic anastomoses at the optic nerve head. Scleritis or iritis may also occur.

WEGENER'S GRANULOMATOSIS (SEE SECTION 18)

Episcleritis is very common in the active stages and many patients notice that their eyes become red when the disease flares up. Occasionally there is a painful scleritis (Plate 18) which may involve the cornea (sclerokeratitis) with the risk of corneal thinning or even perforation. In the acute stages not only is the eyeball fiery red but the slit lamp shows infiltrates of inflammatory cells in the peripheral cornea. The eye responds poorly to topical treatment and may require systemic immunosuppression in its own right, particularly for sight-threatening sclerokeratitis.

In patients in whom the disease is limited to the upper airway, the orbit may be involved, usually secondary to disease in the adjacent sinuses, but sometimes as an isolated site. Granuloma behind the eye produces proptosis which is usually painful and may involve cranial nerves, including the optic nerve with an acute threat to vision (Plate 12). Most of these patients have a positive ANCA test though the titres may be low. Many respond to immunosuppression but may require high doses for local control.

POLYARTERITIS NODOSA (SEE SECTION 18)

Inflammation of the eye coat may cause episcleritis, scleritis, or keratitis, with cells characteristically infiltrating the peripheral cornea. Complications may be severe, and may require systemic immunosuppression. The retinal vessels may be involved, with or without hypertensive changes, and branch arteriolar closure is characteristic. Uveitis is not a feature.

RELAPSING POLYCHONDRITIS (SEE SECTION 18)

This disorder is associated with inflammation of the eye coat, similar to rheumatoid arthritis, or the interior. Roughly half the patients will have eye features at some stage. Episcleritis and scleritis are most common and there may be severe corneal features similar to Wegener's granulomatosis and polyarteritis. Uveitis and retinitis also occur and the eye may be dry (Sjögren's syndrome). Ischaemic optic neuropathy is also documented.

SYSTEMIC LUPUS ERYTHEMATOSUS (SEE CHAPTER 18.11.3)

Uveitis is not associated with systemic lupus erythematosus, though episcleritis causes a red eye in some patients and may occur with flare-ups of systemic activity. Scleritis is uncommon. Retinal vascular occlusions (particularly venous but sometimes branch arterial) may be linked with the development of antiphospholipid antibody. A distinct form of retinopathy with cotton-wool spots should be distinguished from hypertensive changes. The spots represent nerve fibre microinfarcts due to capillary closure and are associated with active vasculitis. Occasional patients develop an ischaemic optic neuropathy with acute irretrievable loss of vision. Some, particularly those with mixed connective tissue disease, have dry eyes (Sjögren's syndrome). In patients with cutaneous lupus the eyelids may be involved: lid oedema is quite common and the lower lid margins may occasionally develop scarring inflammatory plaques.

DERMATOMYOSITIS (SEE CHAPTER 18.11.6)

External eye features, with purple coloration of the eyelids and oedema of the lids and conjunctiva, are typical of dermatomyositis. Less common is retinal ischaemia with microinfarcts, arising from closure of small retinal vessels.

KAWASAKI'S DISEASE (SEE CHAPTER 18.11.9)

Bilateral non-suppurative conjunctivitis is a cardinal feature of Kawasaki's syndrome, characteristically found in young children. Other features include fever, rash, changes in the other mucosae and nails, and lymphadenopathy. Cells may be found in the front chamber (mild iritis) and in the cornea (keratitis) using the slit lamp. The eyes do not need specific treatment. The aetiology is unknown but is presumed to be infective.

Inflammatory eye disease associated with neurological disorders (see also Section 24)

MULTIPLE SCLEROSIS

Uveitis can occur in association with multiple sclerosis, one study finding a high prevalence of low-grade, subtle changes, such as sheathing of the peripheral retinal veins, sometimes associated with inflammatory cells within the vitreous, in patients with optic neuritis. Fluorescein angiography showed that the retinal veins might be inflamed and leak, similar to the cerebral perivenous pathology. This is of particular interest as the retina itself does not usually contain myelin. The association of similar ocular and neurological features occurs in sarcoidosis and in Behçet's syndrome, but in these patients the degree of eye inflammation is usually more marked.

VOGT–KOYANAGI–HARADA SYNDROME

This curious and uncommon clinical syndrome comprises a central nervous disorder, usually deafness or meningoencephalitis with a lymphocytosis in the cerebrospinal fluid in the acute stages, with uveitis, usually bilateral and panuveal. It is found almost exclusively in oriental patients and there are HLA associations. Inflammatory cells collect within the retinal pigment epithelium and may cause fluid detachment of the retina or deeper layers, associated with reduced vision. The disease responds to systemic corticosteroids but often relapses if the dose is reduced. In the chronic phase there may be cutaneous features, particularly depigmentation of skin, hair, or eyelashes (poliosis).

COGAN'S SYNDROME

Cogan's syndrome is a rare disease of young adults, especially males, in which eye inflammation is associated with deafness or vestibular dysfunction. There may be associated proximal aortitis or inflammation of medium-sized arteries. There is usually a keratitis with patchy cell infiltration in the corneal stroma. Later the cornea vascularizes, as in syphilitic keratitis. Some patients have anterior uveitis, inflammation of the eye coat, or retinitis. The aetiology is unknown. The disorder is responsive to systemic (or, in the case of the eye, topical) corticosteroids, which may prevent total deafness if given early enough.

Ocular features of bowel disease (see also Section 14)

INFLAMMATORY BOWEL DISEASE

Crohn's disease may be accompanied by ocular inflammation, which may cause episcleritis, scleritis, or uveitis. Corneal or retinal inflammation is uncommon. Episodes of episcleritis may be associated with an exacerbation of the bowel disorder. Eye involvement is less common in ulcerative colitis.

PANCREATITIS

Acute pancreatitis may be associated with an ischaemic retinopathy and acute visual loss. The typical findings include retinal oedema with microinfarcts (cotton-wool spots), and fluorescein angiography shows closure of branch retinal arterioles and capillaries with patches of retinal non-perfusion. Recovery is related to severity. The cause is unknown but the retinal closure may be related to intravascular aggregation of leucocytes in the acute attack.

WHIPPLE'S DISEASE

This rare disorder is characterized by the association of a malabsorbing enteropathy with arthritis, ocular inflammation, and neurological changes. The eye features include retinal haemorrhages, diffuse retinal and choroidal vasculitis with cells in the vitreous, or corneal inflammation (keratitis). Neurological features include cranial nerve palsies, papilloedema, and brain-stem involvement. It is important to recognize the disorder because there is a specific curative treatment, without which the clinical course is inevitably downhill. The diagnosis is confirmed by small bowel biopsy which shows characteristic rod-shaped inclusions in foam cells in the lamina propria, believed to represent micro-organisms within macrophages. The main ocular differential diagnoses are sarcoidosis and Behçet's disease.

The eye in disorders of the joints (see also Section 18)

The concurrence of eye and joint disease may suggest a particular diagnosis, and the pattern of eye involvement will help to narrow the field. Some disorders are associated with inflammation of the external coat, as episcleritis or scleritis which may occasionally lead to loss of vision, or of the eye itself. Others are associated with inflammation of the eye internally, with iritis or posterior uveitis. Either type of eye disease, if severe enough, may need systemic immunosuppression in its own right.

RHEUMATOID ARTHRITIS

This is the prototype of a joint disease associated with involvement of the external eye. For some patients the eyes are their major problem and there is a significant risk of loss of vision, although bilateral blindness is, fortunately, rare. Severe eye disease may be very difficult to treat effectively.

The most common, dry eye, or keratoconjunctivitis sicca, appears to result from autoimmune damage to lacrimal tissue with lymphocytic infiltration and destructive fibrosis. The eyes are uncomfortable and gritty, and easily become sticky due to low-grade lid infection and poor flushing of the eye surface. The signs include reduced wetting on a Schirmer's test, which is worth doing as a rough guide to the severity of dryness. Small filter-paper strips are folded and hooked over the outer lower eyelids without topical anaesthetic and left for 5 min, after which the level of wetting is measured in millimetres. Less than 5 mm confirms dryness, and more than 10 mm makes significant dryness unlikely. Staining of the conjunctiva, particularly of the surface exposed between the eyelids, may be useful; it is positive with fluorescein if epithelial cells are shed, and with Rose Bengal if epithelial cells are degenerate. Rose Bengal should be used with caution in very dry eyes as it irritates the eye and can be painful. The symptoms of dryness may respond to topical tear substitutes containing methyl cellulose (the most common is hypromellose) which should be used as often as the patient finds helpful, even up to hourly. In some patients filaments of adherent mucus may disperse with topical acetyl cysteine treatment. Severe dry eye is best managed by a specialist who may find other helpful strategies and keep a watch for complications, particularly corneal ulceration. Other systemic conditions associated with sicca (Sjögren's syndrome) include systemic sclerosis, mixed connective tissue disease, lupus erythematosus, and sarcoidosis.

Episcleritis

This is common in rheumatoid patients. It is recognized by redness of the eyeball, either focal (perhaps with a local nodule) or diffuse, without pain or stickiness (Plate 17). It is usually self-limiting, though it may accompany a flare-up in systemic activity. In some patients attacks eventually merge into scleritis. Conjunctival nodules have the same histological pattern as rheumatoid skin nodules although biopsy should be avoided. If treatment is required, symptoms may improve with non-steroidal anti-inflammatory agents.

Scleritis

On the other hand, scleritis is much more serious and is usually found in patients with active vasculitis. The cardinal symptom is pain, and the eye is usually red and boggy (Plate 18), although if inflammation involves the back part of the eyeball (posterior scleritis) there may be few signs to help in diagnosis. Occasionally the inflammatory process spreads from the posterior eye into the internal eye or to the orbit. Any rheumatoid patient with a painful eye should be referred for specialist assessment, even if the eye is white. Scleritis is an ischaemic vasculitic process involving the vessels which supply the sclera. It responds best to systemic immunosuppression with corticosteroids or cytotoxic agents and poorly to topical or non-steroidal anti-inflammatory agents. Treatment may need to be pulsed intravenously to control the acute attack. Untreated, scleritis may result in scleral thinning and even perforation of the eyeball.

Corneal changes

In rheumatoid arthritis, corneal changes are an important cause of visual loss. The cornea may become thinned or vascularized and may ulcerate

or even perforate. The disease often reflects a combination of active inflammation with poor function of the dry eye surface. Patients are rarely suitable for corneal grafting.

ANKYLOSING SPONDYLITIS

This is the prototype joint disease associated with uveitis. Most cases of acute anterior uveitis (iritis) seen in an eye casualty department will never have an identifiable cause and it is best to reserve investigation for those patients who have symptoms or signs of a systemic disorder. Ankylosing spondylitis is the most common association and all young patients with iritis, particularly men, should be asked about pain and stiffness of the spine or sacroiliac joints. They may have typical findings on radiography of lumbar spine or sacroiliac joints, and the HLA-B27 haplotype. About a third of patients with ankylosing spondylitis will develop eye features at some stage.

The disease presents as a painful, aching, photophobic eye which becomes red. The signs are best seen with the magnification of the slit lamp, which shows the cells diagnostic of iritis floating in the front chamber and sedimented on the back surface of the cornea, particularly on the lower half (keratic precipitates) (Plate 14). These attacks of inflammation rarely damage the eye, but the back of the iris may become stuck to the front of the lens (posterior synechiae), often in the constricted position. Dilating the pupil may break most or all of these adhesions and it is important to continue dilating drops until inflammation has settled, so that the pupil remains large and the iris is eventually mobile. The cells clear quite rapidly with topical corticosteroid treatment which should be tailored to the severity of the attack and monitored until inflammation has subsided. Treatment can usually be tailed off over about 2 weeks. Severe or neglected attacks may take longer to settle. Patients with ankylosing spondylitis should be warned that iritis may be recurrent and should be treated early and effectively in each attack. It is reasonable for the non-ophthalmologist or the patient to start topical treatment with both steroid and dilator for a typical recurrent attack, but to report as soon as possible for slit-lamp assessment. With this regime secondary complications are rare and vision usually remains good.

REITER'S SYNDROME

Conjunctivitis is common in the early stages of Reiter's syndrome and is usually a self-limiting sterile inflammation, although occasional patients have chlamydial conjunctival infection. The patient will give a history of red sticky eye near the onset of the other symptoms. Later iritis may develop; the features and management are similar to those of ankylosing spondylitis. Occasional patients with Reiter's develop posterior uveitis, scleritis, or corneal involvement. The other differential diagnoses of arthritis with conjunctivitis or iritis include gonococcal infection, Behçet's syndrome, or psoriatic disease; with intestinal involvement, inflammatory bowel disease, or even Whipple's disease.

JUVENILE CHRONIC ARTHRITIS

Some children with inflammatory arthritis develop eye inflammation which can come to dominate the clinical picture and threaten vision. Most at risk are those with chronic arthritis of the seronegative pauci-articular type (perhaps involving only one digit or an ankle), especially younger patients, girls, and those with a positive antinuclear antibody test. There is usually a low-grade recurrent iritis, over several months or years. The problem is compounded by lack of symptoms or of redness of the eye in the early stages; these patients should be screened by slit-lamp examination, as cells appear in the front chamber when inflammation is active. Untreated, the inflammation can damage the cornea, lens, and aqueous drainage structures, causing band keratopathy, cataract, and glaucoma. With topical treatment, complications may be avoided, although some patients still lose useful vision. Other causes of iritis in children include sarcoidosis and early ankylosing spondylitis.

Vascular occlusion

Occlusion of small central or branch vessels in the retina is a common cause of permanent visual loss, especially in elderly patients. The event can also be a valuable warning of vascular disease elsewhere, particularly in the cerebral circulation. Most episodes are associated with degenerative vascular disease, and many risk factors are common to both arterial and venous occlusions. An underlying systemic disorder is more likely in younger patients, particularly those with previous occlusion in the eye or elsewhere (Tables 5 and 6).

RETINAL ARTERY OCCLUSION

Retinal arterial occlusions, whether of central or branch vessels, are almost always embolic, with a source downstream in the carotid system (either in the neck or intracranially) or in the heart. As with a stroke, the onset is usually abrupt and loss of function marked and permanent once the retina has infarcted. The extent of visual loss depends on the area involved; if the central artery occludes, loss of vision is profound, whereas branch occlusion causes a corresponding defect in the field of vision which often has a horizontal (altitudinal) edge which the patient may be able to define. Prognosis for recovery of vision is poor, but the outlook for the other eye is good unless there is an underlying systemic cause.

Amaurosis fugax (see also Chapter 24.6)

Some patients have prior attacks of transient retinal ischaemia which usually cause brief episodes of blindness limited to one eye, amaurosis fugax. Most attacks last for a few seconds, some up to a few minutes but rarely longer, and although total loss of vision is common, sometimes there is partial loss of the upper or lower half of the field, like a blind moving up or down. Most attacks are painless and there are rarely associated symptoms. There may be a history of cerebral transient ischaemic attacks elsewhere in the carotid territory. Occasionally, emboli have been seen to pass through the retinal circulation during an attack, moving from central to branch arterioles, where they often disperse. Recovery from attacks is usually complete.

Clinical findings

The ophthalmoscopic findings depend on the time between onset and examination. Within minutes the infarcted retina swells and becomes opaque, except at the fovea where a 'cherry-red' spot appears as the intact underlying choroidal circulation shows through. Whitening may affect all the retina or just the territory of an occluded branch artery. This appearance persists for days or weeks and then subsides, leaving a thinned retina and narrowed, often sheathed, vessels (Plate 4). The optic nerve head may atrophy over the following months as the nerve fibres die. If much of the retina is infarcted, there is a defect in the afferent pupil response compared with the normal eye, a sign which persists when others have subsided. Emboli may be visible at any stage, either in the central vessel or within branch vessels, often at a bifurcation (Plate 5). The appearance of the embolus may suggest its origin; most are small, glistening white or yellow pieces of cholesterol from atheromatous plaque. Larger, round, solid white emboli, which usually lodge proximally within or near the disc in the larger vessels, may have come from a calcified heart valve, whereas fibrin and platelet emboli from thrombosed plaque or cardiac thrombus may look dark or grey.

Associated findings include a carotid bruit (relevant if on the same side), and heart murmurs or dysrythmias, particularly atrial fibrillation. There may be absent pulses or bruits at other sites. The patient may be hypertensive. Rarely there may be signs of a systemic vasculitis.

Table 5 *Associations with retinal vein occlusion*

Hypertension	
Diabetes	
Smoking	
Hyperlipidaemia	
Haematological	Raised cell or platelet count, hyperviscosity such as myeloma
Glaucoma	
Clotting tendency	Antiphospholipid syndrome, deficiency of protein S, C, or antithrombin III
Vasculitis	Sarcoid, Behçet's

Table 6 *Systemic associations with retinal artery occlusion*

Vascular embolic	Atheroma—commonly carotid bifurcation, carotid siphon, or aortic arch
	Paradoxical embolus (rare)
Cardiac	Thrombus from left atrium or ventricle, AF, MI, cardiomyopathy, myxoma
	Mitral valve prolapse (mechanism not known)
	Aortic valve degeneration or prosthesis
	Endocarditis
Vasculitis	Behçet's, polyarteritis, SLE, syphilis
	Giant cell arteritis (in a minority with this disorder)
	Takayasu-type aortitis
Sickle-cell disease	

AF, atrial fibrillation; MI, myocardial infarct; SLE, systemic lupus erythematosus.

Investigation and management

In the acute stages no treatment is worthwhile apart from firm ocular massage which might dislodge an unstable central embolus. Retinal fluorescein angiography will demonstrate arterial closure but is not necessary if the clinical picture is typical. General vascular risk factors are sought by assessing blood sugar, lipids, and renal function. A full blood count is important, as although haematological disorders are rarely solely responsible for arterial occlusions, they may contribute to risk. Hypertension should be controlled. An electrocardiogram may reveal a recent 'silent' infarct as a source of thrombus. If carotid surgery might be feasible, carotid Doppler ultrasound study is a useful screening test for significant atheromatous disease at the bifurcation, even in the absence of a bruit. Investigations for vasculitis or a sickling disorder may be relevant in some patients. Giant-cell arteritis is an occasional cause if the retinal rather than ciliary branches of the ophthalmic artery are occluded; the erythrocyte sedimentation rate or C-reactive protein level should be checked in elderly patients.

Management is directed at reducing risk factors such as smoking, hypertension, and obesity. The indications for carotid surgery will vary in different circumstances and are discussed in Section 15. Patients unsuitable for surgery may tolerate long-term aspirin.

RETINAL VEIN OCCLUSION

Retinal venous occlusion, in contrast to arterial, usually occurs *in situ*. Although most are related to age, hypertension or diabetes, other important risk factors include glaucoma, haematological disorders, and, occasionally, systemic inflammation. The onset of symptoms is not as abrupt as an arterial event and commonly occurs overnight, so that the patient wakes with blurred vision. The hallmark is the appearance of retinal haemorrhages in the affected sector; with a central vein occlusion they are scattered throughout the fundus with a very characteristic 'bloodstorm' pattern, often with some cotton-wool spots (Plate 6). With a less complete block the appearance may be more subtle, with sparse scattered haemorrhages, but vision may still fall due to oedema collecting at the fovea. With occlusion of a branch vein, usual at an arteriovenous crossing, there is a wedge-shaped sector of haemorrhage in the area of drainage, with the apex pointing to the optic disc. Vision in the affected eye may improve, depending on the state of the fovea, and the outlook for the opposite eye is good if risk factors are minimized. If the retina is ischaemic, there is a risk of forming new vessels, as in diabetes, which may be prevented by laser treatment. The acute signs of occlusion may persist for many weeks or months, as curly shunt vessels develop at the disc or in the peripheral retina.

Investigation and management

All patients should have their blood pressure, blood sugar, blood count, and erythrocyte sedimentation rate measured, and should be referred for ocular pressure measurement as glaucoma is a treatable risk factor. Screening by protein electrophoresis, blood viscosity, or clotting studies, including antiphospholipid antibodies or lupus anticoagulant, may be relevant in younger patients, particularly if the changes are recurrent, bilateral, or associated with thrombosis elsewhere. Other possibilities include sarcoidosis or Behçet's disease, particularly if the slit lamp shows inflammatory cells within the eye. General risk factors such as blood pressure, smoking, and obesity also need to be tackled. There are no studies of the benefit of long-term aspirin in the patient with venous occlusion.

CHRONIC OCULAR ISCHAEMIA

Eye ischaemia associated with vessel stenosis anywhere from the aortic arch to the ophthalmic artery causes a typical constellation of symptoms and signs. The eye is often painful and red with reduced vision. With the slit lamp, eye pressure is found to be low and there are dilated vessels on the iris with a protein flare in the front chamber. There may be cataract but if the retina is visible the retinal vessels are dilated and tortuous, often with haemorrhages. Retinal or disc new vessels may form, with the risk of vitreous haemorrhage. The syndrome is important, particularly in younger patients when it may suggest the diagnosis of a rare congenital or acquired proximal arterial occlusion, particularly Takayasu's arteritis. In the older patient with a remediable stenosis, surgery may save and even improve vision.

OCCLUSION OF VESSELS SUPPLYING THE OPTIC NERVE

Giant-cell arteritis may be associated with acute ischaemia of the optic nerve, as is discussed above. The disease occludes the ciliary rather than the central retinal branches of the parent ophthalmic artery. Some patients have non-inflammatory occlusion associated with atheroma. Rarely, acute optic nerve ischaemia, which may be bilateral, is associated with shock following catastrophic haemorrhage, usually postpartum or gastrointestinal. The prognosis for recovery of vision is poor.

Hypertension (see also Section 15)

In the hypertensive patient it is important to look carefully at the retina as the changes will help to decide if treatment is necessary, if it is adequate, or if it is needed urgently. Grading is a useful guide to the severity, but rather than rely only on a grading system it is best if the features are also described and roughly sketched, as this is a more accurate way of assessing both immediate and longer-term change. As detection and treatment of hypertension have improved, the incidence of severe retinopathy has declined, but it is important to remember that blood pressure high enough to damage renal and cerebral vessels is best recognized by looking carefully at the retinal vessels. There may be no symptoms, as the vision is normal in most patients, even those with more severe retinopathy. It is unwise to be dogmatic about levels of blood pressure likely to be associated with severe retinal changes, but as a guide, the diastolic pressure is usually 110 mmHg or higher at some stage and there is almost invariably proteinuria. In populations with the benefit of good screening and treatment for raised blood pressure, severe retinopathy is particularly associated with secondary hypertension, and hence needs careful investigation. In some patients the retinal changes are asymmetrical, although they are rarely unilateral, and sometimes there is marked narrowing or occlusion of the internal carotid on the side with less-pronounced retinopathy. On the other hand, unilateral haemorrhages are more often a sign of retinal vein occlusion than of hypertension.

USING THE OPHTHALMOSCOPE

In the less urgent case, to decide if treatment for hypertension is necessary or adequate, it may be possible to assess the larger retinal vessels and several arteriovenous crossings without using dilating drops. It is not easy to assess vessel calibre and quality without being familiar with the normal appearance, so experience of normal fundi is also important. On the other hand, if the problem is more urgent and the blood pressure has risen quickly or to high levels, particularly with proteinuria, it is best to dilate the pupils with a short-acting agent such as tropicamide (1 per cent), which acts within about 15 min and is conveniently dispensed in single-dose units. Unless the pupils are dilated it is easy to miss or to underestimate the retinal changes. It is helpful to have a bright halogen bulb in the ophthalmoscope, and the vessels and any haemorrhages may be seen best with the green or 'red-free' filter in the instrument, which darkens them.

Particular attention should be directed at the major vessel trunks above and below the macula, which lies temporal to the optic nerve head, as these are the areas most likely to be affected by the haemorrhages or cotton-wool spots which indicate acute changes. The optic nerve head should be inspected to decide if the margins are blurred or heaped, indicating disc oedema. If the patient's vision has deteriorated, ask if straight lines are distorted or if there are patchy areas of blurring close to fixation, as these symptoms suggest oedema or haemorrhage at the central fovea. In patients with recent onset of such symptoms and significant hypertension, it is mandatory to give dilating drops and to examine the fovea by asking the patient to look straight into the ophthalmoscope light. Foveal involvement warrants particularly urgent reduction in blood pressure if the retina is to recover.

CLASSIFICATION OF HYPERTENSIVE RETINOPATHY

In the 1940s, when ophthalmoscopes were reliable but treatment of high blood pressure was not, a classification of hypertensive retinal change was developed. Key features in the fundi were found to be an important indicator of prognosis and it was well recognized that patients with the changes of 'malignant' retinopathy had a high mortality if the blood pressure could not be lowered; 90 per cent of 197 patients with uncontrolled malignant hypertension were dead within a year of presentation in a study carried out in London in 1958. Perhaps the best known is the Keith–Wagner classification:

Grade 1 Mild narrowing or sclerosis of retinal arteries
Grade 2 Moderate to marked narrowing or sclerosis with light reflex and arteriovenous crossing changes
Grade 3 In addition, haemorrhages or cotton-wool spots
Grade 4 In addition, swelling of optic nerve head (papilloedema) or retina

Grades 3 and 4 are indicative of severe, accelerated, or 'malignant' retinopathy. It is now realized that it is not necessary to have papilloedema to qualify for this severity, and agreed that disc swelling is an unreliable feature in assessing urgency for treatment; the prognosis is similar for both grades 3 and 4.

INDIVIDUAL FEATURES OF HYPERTENSIVE RETINOPATHY AND THEIR EVOLUTION

The non-acute changes in hypertension are similar to those found with ageing but they may be more pronounced or appear at an earlier age if the blood pressure is also raised. The arterioles are narrowed, either generally or focally, and may be irregular or tortuous. The wall may be thickened, showing an increase in reflected light which is described as 'copper' or 'silver wiring' (the lighter silver appearance is thought to suggest more advanced thickening). There may be nipping at the arterio-venous crossings so that the arteriole appears to cause local constriction of the underlying vein. These long-standing changes often persist with treatment of hypertension, but it is reassuring to see them stabilize. In contrast, younger patients with an acute rise in blood pressure often show marked narrowing of retinal arterioles, sometimes with focally narrowed segments, and these changes reverse rapidly with treatment.

The more acute and severe retinal changes indicate either leakage or closure of smaller vessels. Flame haemorrhages are common in acute hypertension, particularly around the vessel trunks above and below the macula, temporal to the optic disc. These indicate leakage of blood from fine superficial capillary branches supplying the nerve fibre layer. The more numerous the haemorrhages, the more severe the retinopathy. Bleeding deeper in the retina forms larger, more blot-like haemorrhages. If these occur throughout the fundus or just in a wedge-shaped sector based on an arteriovenous crossing, they probably represent a retinal vein occlusion, either of the central or a branch vein. If blot haemorrhages are profuse in both fundi, remember to check the blood sugar as well as the blood pressure, and consider a haematological disorder if the blood pressure is not dramatically high and the patient is not diabetic. Haemorrhages resolve over the weeks following treatment of the blood pressure. Only foveal haemorrhage is likely to cause a permanent reduction in vision.

A few flame haemorrhages are an early warning in hypertensive patients, but a more alarming sign is the appearance of cotton-wool spots which indicate closure of vessels within the same areas. These are a significant indicator of more severe retinopathy (Plate 11). They are no longer called 'soft exudates' as the changes they represent are intracellular. If capillaries supplying the nerve fibres close, small infarcts occur, the patch of ischaemia causes stasis of axoplasmic flow and the intracellular contents pile up to distend and opacify the fibres, producing the pale, fluffy appearance of the cotton-wool spot. Microinfarcts are not unique to hypertension but they are always significant and the severity of closure is roughly related to the number of spots. It is a reassuring sign if the spots gradually resolve in the weeks following treatment. Spots in the absence of an elevated blood pressure suggest an inflammatory vasculitis such as systemic lupus or polyarteritis.

The retinal vessels are normally impermeable but hypertensive damage causes disruption of tight junctions so that fluid, protein, and lipid leak from the vessels into the retina. These are removed by macrophages and processed into shiny hard exudates which may persist for many months. Hard exudate implies leakage has been present for more than a matter of days. They are common in resolving hypertensive retinopathy and may form a characteristic star around the fovea or near the optic disc. In hypertension, exudate rarely forms in the ring-shaped (circinate) pattern typical of diabetes in which the leakage is deeper, more focal, and more long-standing.

Swelling of the optic nerve head (papilloedema) implies hypertensive damage to the supplying vessels or may rarely suggest raised intracranial pressure in patients with headache attributable to hypertension. Changes in the retina probably reflect what is happening in similar-sized vessels in the brain and there may be cerebral oedema in severe cases. In such patients sudden reduction of blood pressure may cause acute loss of vision which may be irreversible, and there is also risk of precipitating a stroke.

HISTOPATHOLOGY

An experimental model of hypertensive retinopathy in primates with renovascular clamps has shown the histopathological changes responsible for the clinical appearances. The pattern produced depends not only on the height of blood pressure but also on its rate of rise. Disruption of endothelial cells or tight junctions has been demonstrated in the early phases of severe retinopathy, followed by damage to the vessel wall, causing closure, sometimes with fibrinoid necrosis or frank thrombosis of small vessels. These changes are more pronounced if the blood pressure rises acutely and to high levels.

FLUORESCEIN ANGIOGRAPHY

The vascular pattern in the human retina can be seen in life using fluorescein angiography, which confirms the phases of leakage and closure in severe retinopathy, although it is rarely necessary to use this technique in hypertensive patients. It is less invasive to document and follow the improvement with treatment using the ophthalmoscope, perhaps with retinal photography. In the occasional patient with visual loss, the angiographic appearance may be helpful to show the cause and to give a prognosis. In patients with vasculitis the angiogram may show characteristic focal narrowings or patchy leakage from the vessel wall.

NON-RETINAL EYE CHANGES IN HYPERTENSION

Some patients with severe hypertension develop more pronounced loss of vision secondary to occlusive changes in the vessels supplying the optic nerve head or in the choroid underlying the retina itself. These changes are most common in patients with eclampsia or renal failure. The tissues become swollen and pale and the retina may even become detached by fluid accumulating under it. Choroidal infarcts mature into permanent scars with spots or streaks of pigment in the more peripheral parts of the fundus. Rarely, patients with secondary hypertension may have eye manifestations of a genetic disorder such as neurofibromatosis type I, von Hippel–Lindau, or Sipple's syndrome (see above).

Diabetes (see also Chapter 11.11)

Retinopathy is the most common and the most serious eye complication in diabetes. In some cases the threat of blindness is paramount and in industrial countries diabetic retinopathy is the commonest reason for blind registration in the younger adult population. Retinal screening is essential, as early treatment, preferably before symptoms appear, can avoid blindness, even though laser treatment is at best damage-limiting. It is still not clear why some patients are more prone than others to develop severe retinopathy, although this becomes more common as patients survive longer. All doctors can play a part in educating diabetics about eye care.

Particularly in older patients, retinal disease may be compounded by cataract, glaucoma, retinal vein occlusion, and cranial neuropathies, including, occasionally, an ischaemic optic neuropathy. The physician needs to understand the threats to vision, to be able to explain them to the patient, to implement screening, and to decide when to refer for specialist advice.

PATHOLOGICAL CHANGES IN THE DIABETIC RETINA

It is unclear why the retina is so commonly affected by diabetes whereas cerebral capillaries appear to be spared. Histologically, both in man and in experimental diabetic animal models, the earliest change in the retinal capillaries is basement membrane thickening, which is associated with an increase in the amounts of laminin and type IV collagen. Pericytes surrounding the capillaries are reduced in number and are eventually lost, a change which is pronounced in retinal but not in brain capillaries. Endothelial cells degenerate and may either be lost or may proliferate, forming microaneurysms which herniate through the defective capillary wall. Such lesions allow leakage of blood and plasma into the retina as the normally impermeable endothelium is disrupted. Later, small vessels may occlude, with formation of small collateral channels at the edges of enlarging avascular areas. Abnormal capillaries here or on the optic nerve head may bud to form tufts of new vessels (neovascularization). These new vessels often grow forwards into the vitreous itself and, as they are fragile, may bleed spontaneously in front of the retina or into the vitreous.

The biochemical basis for these events is not clear. Basement membrane thickening may be related to glycosylation of proteins and increase in monokine activity. Some changes (in some but not all animal studies) are prevented by giving aldose reductase inhibitors early on. There is some evidence that endothelial cells are regulated by pericytes and, in turn, may have a function in controlling local fibroblast growth factors. There appear to be haemodynamic changes, with retinal hyperperfusion in the earlier stages, as in the kidney. The stimulus for the formation of new vessels is uncertain and studies of soluble angiogenic factors are inconclusive. Insulin-like growth factors might be involved and might explain why proliferation is rare before puberty.

INCIDENCE, PROGRESSION, RISK FACTORS, AND PROGNOSIS FOR DIABETIC RETINOPATHY

Patients understandably often ask about the risk of losing vision and it is difficult to give a reliable answer. There are few large studies and their results depend on the population included. The definition of blindness is not uniform and, even if it were, the impact of different degrees of visual loss will depend on the individual patient. Macular damage will impair detailed vision but navigational function is kept, whereas vitreous haemorrhage or retinal detachment associated with proliferative disease can cause extensive loss. Usually both eyes are at similar risk. The likelihood of progression and the risk to vision depend on many factors, including age, the type and duration of diabetes, and the patient's current retinal findings.

An epidemiological study undertaken in Wisconsin in the 1980s involved a sample of nearly 2500 from a diabetic population of 10 000. Patients were divided into three groups: A, younger than 30 years of age at diagnosis and using insulin; B, older than 30 years at diagnosis using insulin; and, C, 'older' patients not using insulin. Retinopathy was detected and graded photographically and the groups were treated according to current practice and followed for 4 years. The overall prevalence of any retinopathy was 50.1 per cent, although only 2.2 per cent had high-risk features for severe visual loss. These were optic disc new vessels, either larger tufts which had not necessarily bled or smaller tufts which had, or larger tufts of new vessels elsewhere in the retina which had bled. In the 'younger' group, the prevalence of moderate visual impairment was 1.4 per cent, and of legal blindness, 3.2 per cent.

Overall, the incidence within 4 years in the entire population of any retinopathy was 40.3 per cent and of proliferative retinopathy with features of high risk to sight was 2.4 per cent. Results of their 4 year follow-up for blindness varied a great deal between the groups, tending to be worse, as perhaps expected, with increasing age, longer duration of diabetes, and more severe initial retinal changes. The overall 4 year incidence for the population, giving current laser treatment as appropriate and taking into account both eyes, was 9.4 per cent for significant visual impairment and 2.3 per cent for legal blindness. The risk was zero in patients before puberty, rising to 24 per cent in both elderly patients with severe macular exudates and in younger patients with high-risk proliferative features. The major reason for failure of follow-up was death.

Some risk factors for the development or progression of retinopathy emerge from a number of studies. Crucially, the relationship to quality of diabetic control as judged by glycosylated haemoglobin levels is still unclear, although it is recognized that tightening diabetic control can lead to formation of microinfarcts temporarily. A large multicentre randomized controlled trial (Diabetes Control and Complications Trial or DCCT) of 1400 type 1 diabetic patients has begun, with planned 10 year follow-up in the late 1990s. Results published in 1993 showed a reduced risk for the development of retinopathy in the intensively-treated groups. Duration of diabetes is the most important risk factor identified: in the younger-onset patients in the Wisconsin study, proliferative changes developed in only 3 per cent by 10 years from diagnosis but in 56 per cent by 30 years. Some racial groups such as Pima Indians and Mexican Americans have a higher incidence, although genetic factors such as relationship to HLA type are controversial. Relation to blood pressure and smoking are non-proven but proteinuria does correlate in some studies. Pregnancy may accelerate existing changes, although the emergence of new proliferation is rare (7 per cent in one study). It should be remembered that the severity of retinopathy is correlated with mortality so that in the Wisconsin study in younger onset patients 6 year survival was 96 per cent with no retinopathy, but fell to 66 per cent if they had proliferative retinal changes.

CLINICAL FINDINGS

Retinopathy, particularly macular oedema, may be the presentation first leading to a diagnosis of diabetes, particularly in elderly patients in whom exudates are more common. Many diabetics complain also of an acute change in focusing during the early days of treatment, which settles as the blood sugar stabilizes.

Most diabetic patients have good vision despite significant retinopathy. Only if the foveal part of the macula is affected will vision fall, with blurring, difficulty in reading, or distortion of straight lines. Such maculopathy tends to be a progressive problem, and with time the fovea is permanently damaged. With ischaemic changes and proliferative disease, symptoms of vitreous haemorrhage may occur, a small bleed causing multiple small floaters like a cloud of insects, and a larger one producing a veil effect or more profound acute deterioration in sight. Most vitreous haemorrhages clear but repeated bleeding gradually destroys vitreous clarity and may distort and eventually detach the retina, often irretrievably.

The early 'background' signs in the retina are microaneurysms, seen as small, round red dots. Sparse scattered haemorrhages in dot or blot pattern and a few hard exudates may form (Plate 7), particularly temporal to the macula. Fluorescein angiography will distinguish 'small red lesions' as due to microaneurysms or dot haemorrhages, but is rarely justified at this stage. The ophthalmoscopic findings at later stages depend on the predominant pathology, with either leakage or ischaemia, or a combination of both.

With leakage from foci of abnormally permeable capillaries, hard exudates form as macrophages process the leaked fluid into lipid and protein residues. These may have a characteristic ring or 'circinate' form around a leaking focus at the centre—a pattern which is rarely found in hypertensive or other non-diabetic retinopathies. If oedema or frank exudate forms near the fovea, retinopathy is moving into the 'exudative' or 'maculopathy' phase and vision is threatened (Plate 8). At this stage, focal laser burns applied to leaking lesions may prevent progression, preferably before vision becomes poor. Screening should aim to find patients at risk of macular damage who should be referred for assessment (and perhaps fluorescein angiography) to decide if laser treatment is needed. Exudates may be seen close to the fovea but oedema is more difficult to detect with the direct ophthalmoscope. Any patient with a fall in vision of two Snellen lines acuity should be referred if vision cannot be improved with a pinhole or correcting lenses.

Ischaemic changes are more sinister and may be recognized from characteristic features which may appear singly or together, even before

Table 7 *Practical screening programme for diabetic retinopathy*

Retinopathy type	Prognosis*	Action	Treatment appropriate	Rescreen interval
None	0.3	Rescreen	Optimize risk factors	2–3 years
Background	3	Rescreen	Also warn to report symptoms	1 year
Exudative	20	Refer	Focal laser	3–6 months
Ischaemic	30	Refer	Observe closely	3 months
Proliferative	50	Refer	Panretinal laser	Monthly until regress

*Approximate percentage of untreated eyes likely to be blind in 5 years.

the formation of frank new vessels. These include massed blot haemorrhages, dilatation/beading/looping or tortuosity of the larger retinal veins, or the appearance of multiple cotton-wool spots which represent microinfarcts in the retinal nerve fibre layer. This appearance can resemble retinal vein occlusion and a fluorescein angiogram may be needed to distinguish between the two. Later, areas of budding from small dilated vessels at the edge of ischaemic areas appear as intraretinal microvascular abnormalities, best seen with an experienced eye and a red-free (green) filter in a good ophthalmoscope with a bright halogen bulb.

Some of these buds adjacent to ischaemic areas progress to frank tufts of new vessels in the peripheral retina ('new vessels elsewhere' or NVE). New vessels most commonly form on the optic nerve head itself ('disc new vessels' or DNV) and the skill in screening lies in detecting such early tufts (Plate 9). They often have a looped appearance and clustered fronds. Any patient with suspected new vessels should be referred early and assessed for laser treatment. A survey by the National Eye Institute in the United States in the 1970s showed that the risk of visual loss depends on the site and size of new vessels, so that patients with small tufts of peripheral new vessels which had not bled had a risk of severe visual loss of 6.7 per cent within 2 years, whereas in those with larger new vessels on the optic disc which had already bled the risk rose to 37 per cent in 2 years. New vessels visible with the slit lamp may also form on the iris (rubeosis), bringing the risk of glaucoma. Patients with cataract or persistent vitreous haemorrhage in whom it is difficult to see the retina should also be referred, as surgery may be needed to improve both vision and quality of screening.

PRACTICAL SCREENING PROGRAMMES

The skill of screening lies in detecting significant oedema or exudate threatening the fovea and in identifying patients at high risk of developing new vessels so that these may be detected at the earliest possible stage.

Ideally, all diabetics should have a retinal examination at presentation and then annually, unless they are both younger than 30 years of age and free of retinopathy, in which case an interval of 3 to 5 years until rescreening is acceptable. Pregnant diabetics and those with early exudation or ischaemia should be screened every few months. Table 7 outlines a practical programme. Screening should include the measurement of visual acuity at 6 m with correcting glasses or pinhole to detect macular oedema in particular, plus dilating the pupils (ideally with tropicamide 1 per cent) before inspection of both fundi. It is important to include the area of retina temporal to the macula. Some centres screen photographically, preferable to no screening but inferior to careful fundoscopy. Who should screen may be a dilemma and the team might include a general practitioner, optometrist, diabetic physician, and hospital ophthalmologist. Records and recall need to be organized to integrate screening the eye with other sites.

TREATMENT OF DIABETIC RETINOPATHY

Medical management is directed at improving risk factors and should include control of blood sugar and lipids, weight, and smoking. Control

of hypertension is important. Possible benefits of aspirin are not substantiated.

Leakage affecting the fovea may be reduced by laser treatment, either focally to identified sites of leakage or using a grid pattern of burns carefully applied around the fovea. The number of burns needed is relatively small, usually fewer than a hundred. Patients whose vision deteriorates often mistakenly attribute this to the treatment, though in practice the risk of secondary macular scarring is small.

Proliferative retinopathy is treated by destroying the peripheral retina which is presumed to be ischaemic by applying thousands of laser burns outside the disc and macular areas (Plate 10). This is exacting and may need to be done over several sessions. If the vessels do not regress, retreatment is necessary until they do so. Direct coagulation of the vessels themselves is rarely successful. The treatment can cause constriction of peripheral visual field and a degree of night blindness.

How far does effective treatment reduce the risk to vision? There is no precise answer, as the measured outcome will depend on the population, criteria for treating, and the efficiency of screening. In patients with macular oedema, in the relatively short term an estimated two-thirds will have arrest of progression by focal or grid treatment. With proliferative retinopathy it is estimated that the incidence of visual loss can be reduced by about 60 per cent if treatment is given early enough.

Surgical treatment for opaque vitreous and retinal distortion or detachment is, in most cases, a salvage measure appropriate only for selected patients. Patients with irretrievably poor vision need advice about low-vision aids and the services of a specialist social worker to marshal help for home or work-place.

OTHER VISUAL COMPLICATIONS

Diabetes accelerates the development of cataract which therefore occurs at a younger age by an average of 5 years. Lens surgery is no different from the usual procedure and most diabetic patients are suitable for lens implantation, but the postoperative complication rate is higher than in non-diabetics.

Diabetes is a risk factor for retinal vein occlusion and this possibility should be remembered if retinal haemorrhages appear acutely or within a sector in one eye. Ischaemia related to some vein occlusions increases the risk of glaucoma and reduces the likelihood of return of good acuity.

Chronic glaucoma is more common in diabetics, and patients with severe ischaemia may develop intractable rubeotic glaucoma secondary to neovascularization of aqueous drainage channels in the front chamber. Measurement of eye pressure should be included in the screening programme for diabetic patients and can be undertaken by most 'high street' optometrists.

Palsies of cranial nerves III, IV, or VI, which are often painful, may cause double vision. This may improve within weeks of onset and can be managed by patching one eye, but persistent cases may be reviewed by an orthoptist. Some patients develop an acute ischaemic optic neuropathy with a pale swollen optic nerve head and poor vision. Patients who suffer a stroke may have homonymous hemianopia.

Rarely, lipaemia retinalis may be seen in association with the hyper-triglyceridaemia of acute ketoacidosis, sometimes with the patient in coma and the diabetes previously undiagnosed: the major retinal vessels appear pink or white with opalescent fat. The appearance is reversible with metabolic control and vision remains normal. Another incidental but sometimes striking finding in diabetics is 'asteroid hyalosis' of the vitreous with multiple small white suspended opacities, often, surprisingly, without symptoms.

Infectious diseases (see Section 7 for individual diseases)

Eye complications occur in some patients with a systemic infection and it is a pity to miss the clues which may be found, particularly if an unusual infection has characteristic features. Occasionally eye involvement may threaten vision, and management of the eye itself is then important. Occupation, travel, immunosuppression, and other risk factors, such as sexually transmitted infections and intravenous drug abuse, all have relevance to a likely diagnosis in the eye, as elsewhere.

Two particular constellations deserve special mention. In the United Kingdom, marked conjunctival inflammation with conjunctival haemorrhages is usually due to adenovirus infection, but if the patient is systemically ill with a fever, rash, and red eyes this is suggestive of measles or, occasionally, of meningococcal or disseminated gonococcal infection. In other parts of the world, borrelial (relapsing fever) or rickettsial infections should be added to the differential diagnoses. Conjunctivitis with marked local lymphadenopathy (oculo-glandular syndrome) may be due to infective causes such as adenovirus or chlamydia, and less commonly to mumps.

Organisms from the eye surface can be identified from swabs but those inside the eye are identified from their pattern of involvement and it is rarely necessary to aspirate material from inside the eye. Similarly, treatment for superficial eye infections is a topical antimicrobial, given as drops or ointment, whereas a systemic regime is needed for internal infection, when the choice is partly dictated by penetration into the eye cavities. Rarely, drugs should be given by injection directly into the vitreous to supplement systemic treatment with high intraocular levels.

BACTERIAL INFECTIONS

The most common bacterial eye infection is simple conjunctivitis, usually caused by Staphylococcus, Haemophilus, or Pneumococcus. All respond to topical chloramphenicol as drops (hourly for the first 24 h and then three times daily for several days), with ointment at night. Cellulitis around the eye is not uncommon and is usually caused by the same organisms, Haemophilus being particularly common in children. The first-line regime is systemic amoxycillin or flucloxacillin. Spread of infections to the orbit behind the eye is an ophthalmic emergency and the patient should be hospitalized for investigation and intravenous antibiotic treatment.

Metastatic endophthalmitis is an important infection in which blood-borne bacteria seed to the internal eye. The most common sources are meningeal, urinary, and endocardiac, with the most likely organisms Neisseria, streptococci, or staphylococci. Bacillus cereus is common in association with intravenous drug abuse and unusual organisms can occur in the immunosuppressed. Infection inside the eye causes progressive reduction in vision, usually with pain, and the cells and debris, found within either or both eye chambers, blur the ophthalmoscopic view, though a pale chorioretinal focus of infection may be visible. Cultures, particularly of blood, urine, and perhaps cerebrospinal fluid are necessary, and tapping of the internal eye for vitreous microscopy and culture is justified in some cases. In subacute bacterial endocarditis, retinal haemorrhages and microembolic infarcts are common, classically in the form of a white-centred Roth spot.

In parts of the world where mycobacterial infections are endemic the eye may be involved. Ocular tuberculosis is uncommon and is associated usually with indolent granulomatous uveitis, either of the iris or choroid. In contrast, the eye is frequently involved in leprosy and ocular leprosy has a high incidence of complications which may cause blindness,

including a specific iritis in the multibacillary (lepromatous) form, with which cataract is also common, and corneal scarring from exposure associated with facial palsy and/or reduced corneal sensation. Eye protection and hygiene are very important.

Syphilis is associated with many different eye changes, depending on the stage. Uveitis or neuroretinitis occur in the secondary stage, and the optic neuropathy and Argyll Robertson pupils of the tertiary stage are well known and still occur. Congenital syphilis is associated with interstitial keratitis and a salt-and-pepper retinopathy. In leptospiral infections the eye signs may be a diagnostic clue. Leptospirosis icterohaemorrhagica commonly causes a conjunctivitis at the onset (when the association with fever and jaundice is suggestive of the diagnosis) and there may be a late uveitis. Lyme disease in its later stages is possibly a cause of inflammation at several ocular sites.

Occasionally specific eye signs are found in rare bacterial infections. The gonococcus causes a marked purulent conjunctivitis in the newborn or in those sexually exposed. Tularaemia is occasionally associated with a severe granulomatous conjunctivitis with local lymph node enlargement (in the United Kingdom consider this in meat-handlers and lab workers especially). Botulism is associated with paralysis of the ocular muscles, sometimes with autonomic signs, for which a differential diagnosis in certain parts of the world would be diphtheria. Brucellosis can cause optic neuritis or uveitis (consider this especially in slaughterhouse or farm workers). Whipple's disease, caused by an unidentified organism, possibly an actinomycete, is associated with retinal vasculitis and cranial nerve palsies (see above). Actinomycetes can infect the tear canaliculi. Rarely, Nocardia can infect the internal eye, usually causing focal chorioretinal infection.

Chlamydial eye infection
Trachoma

This is the most common chronic conjunctivitis worldwide and is important as a preventable cause of blindness. It is estimated that at least 600 million people are infected, of whom about 6 million are blinded. Chlamydia trachomatis serotypes A–C cause a chronic conjunctivitis with follicles that look like pale grains of soft rice in the conjunctiva. This produces scarring of the lids associated with inturning of eyelashes which may accelerate corneal scarring. The clinical findings are characteristic but diagnosis may be helped by seeing inclusions in conjunctival scrapes or by culturing the organism from swabs. WHO recommendations for control of potentially blinding trachoma infection are topical tetracycline ointment twice daily for 7 days repeated at intervals six times a year, or six once-a-month doses of oral doxycycline, 5 mg/kg, annually.

In industrialized countries, the genital serotypes of Chlamydia cause inclusion conjunctivitis, usually seen in the new-born or young sexually active. Genitourinary symptoms are often absent but the diagnosis is important as specific systemic treatment is needed and sexual contacts should be traced. The eye is red and usually very sticky, with lymphoid follicles often found in the conjunctiva lining the eyelids. Diagnosis may be confirmed by microscopy of a conjunctival scrape or by swab culture. The infection is usually persistent and only responds partially to topical chloramphenicol. Systemic tetracycline or erythromycin with topical tetracycline is effective treatment.

VIRAL INFECTIONS AND THE EYE

The most common viral infection is adenovirus conjunctivitis, usually caused by types 3, 4, 7, 8, or 19 in a highly contagious form which may be epidemic. The eye is acutely red and uncomfortable but with scanty discharge. Lymphoid follicles may be visible in the conjunctiva lining the eyelids and the preauricular node may be enlarged. Symptoms may continue for some weeks but recovery is usually uneventful and treatment rarely necessary. The most important differential diagnosis is chlamydial infection, in which eye discharge is more pronounced.

Herpes simplex

This can also cause conjunctivitis in the primary episode, as well as lid infection, which may be severe in eczematous patients, eczema herpeticum. More commonly it is involved in recurrent attacks, causing corneal ulceration in the characteristic dendritic pattern. Recurrences, especially if a topical corticosteroid is given, can result in corneal scarring and poor vision. Varicella-zoster virus is also an important eye pathogen and can cause many unpleasant complications, including corneal ulceration, iritis, and glaucoma, as well as delayed cranial nerve palsies, including the optic nerve. It is important to refer cases of shingles involving the ophthalmic division of the fifth cranial nerve to the eye department of a hospital if there is any sign of eye involvement, as evidenced by redness or impairment of vision. All members of the herpes virus group can cause retinal infection, particularly in the immunosuppressed. Simplex and zoster infections occasionally cause acute retinal necrosis, a severe and blinding disorder which progresses rapidly and responds poorly to systemic antiviral therapy. This is rarely seen with primary varicella infection.

Cytomegalovirus

This also causes progressive retinitis with characteristic haemorrhages and patchy retinal necrosis (see below). In transplant patients, cytomegalovirus infection may respond to reduction of immunosuppression.

Epstein–Barr virus

This virus may occasionally be associated with inflammation of the conjunctiva, episclera, iris, or lacrimal gland, but not with retinitis.

Other viral infections associated with conjunctivitis include varicella, influenza, mumps, rubella, and measles. Measles may also cause a scarring corneal inflammation which is an important cause of blindness in undernourished children. Internal eye inflammation is less common in viral infections other than the herpes group, but iritis is characteristic of mumps. Neuro-ophthalmic problems are found particularly in subacute sclerosing panencephalitis and may occur occasionally with other viral agents. Congenital rubella and varicella are associated with cataract and retinopathy in infancy. Among the pox group, molluscum contagiosum, cowpox, and orf can cause lid infection.

FUNGAL INFECTIONS

Indolent fungal infection of the cornea occurs occasionally in wearers of contact lenses, and in diabetics. Internal fungal infection is metastatic, usually due to *Candida albicans* and associated with immunosuppression, irradiation, intravenous drug abuse, and poorly controlled diabetes. Cells are found in either chamber; small, dense, white 'snowballs' are seen in the vitreous. There may be white foci of infection visible in the choroid and overlying retina but retinal haemorrhage is uncommon. The diagnosis is usually made clinically, but may be confirmed by vitreous biopsy, at which time an antifungal agent can be instilled into the eye, once microscopy confirms the diagnosis. The differential diagnosis of a white focus with a hazy vitreous full of cells includes toxoplasmosis, intraocular lymphoma, sarcoid and tuberculosis, or another low-grade infection.

Fungal infection in the tissues around the eye and in the orbit is rare but characteristic of invasive mucormycosis. This occurs in the same predisposed groups as for Candida, particularly debilitated patients during treatment for haematological malignancies or those with severe diabetic ketoacidosis. The infection spreads rapidly and often involves the vascular supply, producing characteristic tissue necrosis, in particular blackening of the hard palate. Medical treatment alone is usually unsuccessful and should be combined with surgical removal of necrotic tissue.

In endemic parts of the world, in particular the Mississippi basin, it is believed that *Histoplasma capsulatum* produces a characteristic multifocal scarring chorioretinal infection, with an appearance known as 'histo spots'.

RICKETTSIAL INFECTION

Petechial haemorrhage of the conjunctiva and retinal haemorrhages are characteristic of rickettsial infection.

PROTOZOAL INFECTIONS

Toxoplasma gondii has a predilection for the retina and underlying choroid. It is usually a congenital infection, the mother acquiring the primary infection in pregnancy. In certain parts of the world, particularly France and Brazil, there is a very high rate of Toxoplasma infection and the organism is a common cause of intraocular inflammation. The primary scarring focus in the eye may involve the macula or optic nerve head and result in congenitally poor vision. More commonly, an asymptomatic scar reactivates later in life, producing cells in the vitreous which may spill forwards into the anterior chamber. An inactive scar may be visible in the second eye. The patient usually presents with blurring of vision often describing 'floaters'. The diagnosis is based on the clinical findings together with serology. The optimum management is still not resolved by adequate trial, but it is usually recommended to treat acute flares as early as possible with combined systemic clindamycin and corticosteroid for a period of several weeks, under specialist ophthalmic supervision. In some infants there may be the associated features of cerebral toxoplasmosis.

Retinal haemorrhages are commonly found in patients with cerebral malaria, and are a poor prognostic sign. Neuro-ophthalmic complications are occasionally reported. There are a few reports of retinal toxicity (of the 'bull's-eye' type) in patients taking regular, long-term chloroquine for malaria prophylaxis, and associated with chloroquine abuse.

Cutaneous leishmaniasis of the eyelids (with ulcers or nodules) occurs in endemic areas. Retinal haemorrhages are common in visceral kala-azar, particularly with associated anaemia.

Trypanosomiasis in Africa is occasionally associated with corneal inflammation. In South America, oedema of the eyelids, lacrimal gland, and local lymph nodes may occur in the weeks following a periocular bite transmitting *Trypanosoma cruzi*, which causes Chagas' disease. This is known as Romaña's sign.

Acanthamoeba can cause an indolent and potentially blinding corneal infection, found almost exclusively in contact lens wearers or after contaminated corneal trauma.

Pneumocystis choroidal infection is discussed below.

INFESTATIONS

In some parts of the world parasitic infestation is common. Characteristic eye features may help in diagnosis and in some cases vision may be threatened.

Onchocerciasis is endemic in parts of equatorial Africa and central America and can cause high rates of blindness in the adult population (see Section 7). Adult worms produce microfilariae which lodge particularly in the choroid, causing a gradually progressive destructive and scarring chorioretinitis. Optic atrophy and sheathed retinal vessels are common features in the late stages, and in some areas corneal inflammation and scarring are common, and uveitis may also occur. The diagnosis is made from skin snip microscopy for filariae, though they are sometimes visible in the cornea or front chamber using the slit lamp. The management of onchocerciasis is discussed in Section 7.

In communities with a large domestic dog population, *Toxocara canis* infection can affect the internal eye, forming a visible mass, usually beneath the retina, with uveitis and, sometimes, whitening of the pupil. An important differential diagnosis is a tumour such as retinoblastoma.

Some adult worms invade the eye surface. Loa loa may be felt by the patient and maybe visible beneath the conjunctiva over the eyeball, from where it can be removed. In Japan, the fly-transmitted 'oriental eye worm', Thelazia, occurs in the conjunctival sac. In Thailand especially,

Gnathostoma infection affects the eyelids or internal eye, where the larvae may be visible with the slit lamp.

In pork-eating cultures, trichinosis due to *Trichinella spiralis* infestation may involve the extraocular muscles, causing pain and periorbital oedema with orbital signs of proptosis and defective eye movements. There may be internal eye involvement.

In southern China and other parts of South-East Asia, sparganosis may be associated with contact with frogs or water infected with tapeworm larvae. In some cultures there may be direct inoculation into the eye from the use of frog skin as an eye poultice. The organism causes conjunctivitis with marked swelling and itching, and orbital infection can cause proptosis and blindness.

In cysticercosis, the larval form may be visible inside the eye in either chamber, looking like a motile pearl. Posterior uveitis and retinitis may occur, and the larvae may form a mass similar to Toxocara. Orbital involvement is rare. In Echinococcus infection, orbital cysts, sometimes calcified, may occur in patients with hydatid disease.

Trematodes such as *Schistosoma haematobium* may affect the eye surface as an urticarial conjunctivitis associated with egg deposition, but the interior of the eye is rarely involved.

In sheep-farming areas, particularly in the Mediterranean, Central America, and Africa, the external eye may be infected with the maggots of sheep flies, a condition called ophthalmomyiasis externa. Less commonly, the maggots may invade the eye or orbit.

HUMAN IMMUNODEFICIENCY VIRUS INFECTION AND AIDS (SEE PLATE 20)

Signs within the eye are common in patients infected with human immunodeficiency virus (HIV), particularly in the later stages of the acquired immunodeficiency syndrome (AIDS). The most important complications are associated with infection, the pattern of which may point to the diagnosis. The retina is the most common site, although the optic nerve head may also be involved. The only definitive means of making a diagnosis in life is by retinal biopsy, which is rarely justified, so the clinical findings are crucial. The pattern of infection is often different from that seen in non-immunosuppressed patients. In particular, the cell response within the eye is much scantier. The organisms are commonly facultative intracellular parasites. The agents vary between different AIDS subpopulations; cytomegalovirus retinitis is the most commonly found condition in homosexual patients in the United Kingdom and United States but is rarely found in their haemophiliac counterparts or in African patients, whereas non-specific retinopathy and herpes zoster are more common in Africans. If an effective treatment exists, as for cytomegalovirus infection, this may preserve sight in what is often a bilateral and therefore potentially blinding condition.

Non-specific AIDS retinopathy

Many patients with HIV infection develop features of retinal microvascular disease, but it is not possible to identify a particular infective pattern or to isolate an organism from the retina, even in cases which come to autopsy. Cotton-wool spots are common from a relatively early stage of HIV infection and there may also be haemorrhages or white-centred Roth spots and microaneurysms. There may be closure and sheathing of the peripheral retinal venous branches and, occasionally, microvascular closure around the fovea, which produces loss of vision. It is unclear what causes these changes—possibly high fibrinogen levels or deposition of immune complexes. This retinal pattern is common in African patients, particularly children. The changes are unresponsive to ganciclovir therapy but may improve with systemic corticosteroid or zidovudine treatment.

Cytomegalovirus retinitis

This is the most common ocular complication in sexually acquired HIV infection in the United Kingdom and United States, affecting about one

in five patients; it usually emerges in the later stages of AIDS when the CD4 T-cell count is low. The typical appearance is patchy areas of pale, crumbled-looking retina with associated scattered haemorrhages (Plate 20), sometimes said to look like the cheese and tomato of pizza. The patches, which are usually bilateral, may appear anywhere in the retina, although they are most common around branch vessels. They represent areas of replicating cytomegalovirus with oedematous and necrotic retina and some cells, mostly neutrophils and macrophages, although the cell response within the eye cavity is usually scanty. The patches spread contiguously from their borders and, untreated, can be seen to enlarge over the course of several days. As the retina progressively dies there will be eventual blindness, often within weeks of the onset. The average life expectancy of AIDS patients with cytomegalovirus retinitis is about 6 months.

The differential diagnosis of pale areas of retina associated with haemorrhage includes branch retinal vein occlusion (usually a single patch) or, much less commonly, other infections such as toxoplasmosis (more cell response in the cavity), early acute retinal necrosis (more confluent and very rapidly progressive), Candida (no haemorrhage), or Cryptococcus. Definitive diagnosis is difficult and culture and serology are helpful only to discourage a diagnosis if repeatedly negative.

Retinal infection with cytomegalovirus can be suppressed by an adequate dose of ganciclovir or foscarnet, and the lesions then become atrophic with resolution of the pale and haemorrhagic features and halting of the advancing edges. The usual regime for ganciclovir is an induction course for 2 to 3 weeks of twice daily intravenous doses at 5 mg/kg. The dose should be reduced progressively if there is renal impairment. This is followed by a maintenance regime of 5 mg/kg daily (or of 6 mg/kg on 5 out of every 7 days) given intravenously, usually via an indwelling intravenous line. The most important complication is bone marrow suppression. To avoid toxicity, ganciclovir may be given by direct injection into the eye (vitreous) but this is rarely justified as the injections must be repeated weekly and the cytomegalovirus infection is usually in both eyes and also present elsewhere in the body. Breakthrough of retinitis is common and is treated by repeating the induction course of ganciclovir or by switching to foscarnet. The regime for foscarnet is tailored to renal function and to retinal response.

Spread of retinitis will occur if treatment is interrupted and will often smoulder on during the treatment course; in many patients there is frank breakthrough from the agent after several weeks and it may be necessary to increase the dose or to change from one agent to the other. Patients with cytomegalovirus retinitis should be under ophthalmic supervision as it is important to assess the lesions by indirect ophthalmoscopy, preferably with serial retinal photographs, to document progression at the edges of lesions. Patients should also be monitored for side-effects of treatment. With adequate treatment, the majority of patients should have useful remaining vision, at least in one eye, at the time they die.

Herpes zoster and simplex

In younger African patients, HIV infection is the commonest cause of herpes zoster ophthalmicus. The skin lesions are often widespread, and secondary eye complications are frequent and often severe. Retinal infection causes rapidly spreading retinal death (also called acute retinal necrosis) with pale oedematous areas which lack the crumbled texture and the haemorrhages characteristic of cytomegalovirus retinitis. There is often involvement of the optic nerve with optic neuritis and there may be encephalitis. Loss of vision can be rapid and bilateral, within days if untreated. Treatment with acyclovir, initially intravenous, may halt spread within the retina, but the infection usually escapes control.

Syphilis

Syphilis in HIV infection may cause iritis or optic neuritis, which are often bilateral. There may be retinitis with a vitreous cell reaction and abnormal cerebrospinal fluid findings or other signs of neurological involvement. The non-specific treponemal serology may be negative, so specific tests must be done. Treatment of eye complications should be with benzathine penicillin, initially intravenous, with a regime suitable for CNS infection, otherwise there may be progression or relapse of ocular problems (see Section 24).

Toxoplasmosis

Chorioretinal involvement with Toxoplasma occasionally occurs in HIV-infected patients and the appearance may be atypical, although focal choroidal lesions with cells in both chambers should suggest the diagnosis. Another unusual feature is a granulomatous iritis in which Toxoplasma cysts are found in the iris, with a higher-than-usual organism load. The eye features may be a clue to accompanying optic neuritis or encephalitis. Treatment is recommended with clindamycin without systemic or topical corticosteroids.

Pneumocystis pneumoniae

This organism may occasionally cause a multifocal chorioretinitis with multiple pale, rounded patches visible beneath the retina. The infection is most common in patients maintained on inhaled pentamidine for pulmonary infection.

Mycobacteria

Rarely, atypical mycobacteria may cause a choroiditis without specific features.

Fungi

Cryptococcus is the most likely fungal agent to infect the eye, usually in the choroid, particularly if there is associated optic nerve or meningeal involvement. Candida infection is rare in the HIV group unless associated with indwelling intravenous cannulae or drug abuse.

Blood disorders (see Section 22)

Retinal changes are probably more common than is supposed in haematological disorders, and even if vision is normal it is wise to look at the retina carefully, as the changes are a guide to the severity of the underlying disease and there may also be specific diagnostic clues. The signs are easily missed unless the pupils are dilated. The changes are usually bilateral and are likely to be a compound of several factors, including the level of anaemia, degree of hyperviscosity, any bleeding or clotting tendency, and, possibly, complications of infection or therapy.

Hypoxia of the retina causes the veins to enlarge and in some cases to become tortuous with arteriovenous nipping and scattered retinal haemorrhages. Hyperviscosity causes similar changes but haemorrhages are often more widespread. The picture of bilateral retinal haemorrhages always suggests a blood disorder and it is wise to check the blood count, erythrocyte sedimentation rate, and plasma protein electrophoresis. Marked hypoxia, particularly if it is acute, may cause cotton-wool spots (microinfarcts) to appear, in addition to haemorrhage. The compound picture of hypoxia and hyperviscosity with haemorrhage and infarcts is sometimes called 'slow flow' or 'stasis' retinopathy.

Retinal haemorrhages can occur in pure anaemia, particularly if acute, although they tend to be more profuse and larger if there is also hyperviscosity or a bleeding tendency. The size and shape of the haemorrhage depends on its depth within the retina. Superficial haemorrhages are flame-shaped whereas those in the deeper layers tend to be blotchy, as they spread more. White-centred haemorrhages, sometimes called Roth spots, may occur in a variety of conditions, including leukaemia and hyperviscosity. Haemorrhages will not cause symptoms unless they involve the fovea, when the patient may describe a patch of blurred central vision. With severe bleeding, the blood may leak in front of the retina to form a dense rounded, often boat-shaped, subhyaloid blotch, and leakage into the vitreous causes symptoms of floaters or clouding of vision with an obscured ophthalmoscopic view.

BLEEDING DISORDERS

Bleeding may occur in the eyelids, on the eye surface, or inside the eye in patients with a bleeding tendency. Suggestive patterns include pronounced or repeated subconjunctival haemorrhage, hyphaema with blood settling within the front chamber, and vitreous haemorrhage. Such bleeding may be either spontaneous or after minor trauma or eye surgery. In haemophilia, bleeding around or inside the orbit may compress the optic or other cranial nerves.

HYPERCOAGULABLE STATES

Disorders encouraging thrombosis, including deficiency of protein S, protein C, or antithrombin III, are associated with retinal vascular occlusion, in the veins more often than the arteries. Closure of vessels within the choroid may also affect vision if fluid exudes to detach the retina, and this pattern is particularly suggestive of thrombotic thrombocytopenic purpura or diffuse intravascular coagulation. Occlusion of retinal veins or arteries also occurs in patients with systemic lupus erythematosus and lupus anticoagulant or antiphospholipid antibodies. Vascular closure may occasionally involve the optic nerve head, causing amaurosis fugax or a frank ischaemic optic neuropathy with a pale, swollen disc and poor vision. It is worth doing a full screen of clotting tests on a patient with retinal vein thrombosis if there is also another site involved, if the episodes are multiple, or if there is a family history of juvenile thrombosis at any site.

MYELOMA AND RELATED MONOCLONAL GAMMOPATHIES

Retinopathy due to hyperviscosity may progress to an established retinal vein occlusion, and the diagnosis of myeloma should be excluded in any patient with bilateral retinal haemorrhages if hypertension and diabetes are excluded. The retinal changes may reverse slowly over several months with treatment of the myeloma and this is an important aspect of management. A minority of patients have more specific eye findings with deposition of abnormal protein as crystals in the cornea or within cysts in the peripheral retina. Occasionally the retina detaches as protein-rich fluid collects beneath it. Plasmacytomas may rarely present with a neuro-ophthalmic problem.

LEUKAEMIAS

Retinopathy is probably common in both acute and chronic leukaemias, but only a minority will have visual symptoms. Occasionally, it may be the presenting symptom. The retinal haemorrhages are non-specific (Plate 13), although white-centred ones are characteristic and represent a focal collection of white cells. Rarely, if the white cell count is very high there may be frank infiltration of the retina or optic nerve head, causing pale, fluffy areas, and cells may spill into the vitreous. The retina may detach. Cotton-wool spots are common and these microinfarcts are likely to be present also in the brain. Chronic leukaemias may cause a slow flow picture from chronic retinal hypoxia. Often the retinopathy will improve as the condition is treated. Occasionally, particularly in acute lymphoblastic leukaemia, collections of cells may form a mass, either in the orbit causing proptosis, within the eyelid, or on the iris, masquerading as iritis. Rarely, the iris may be involved in a relapse of treated leukaemia. Ocular infiltrations may respond to radiotherapy. Eye complications may also occur from associated infections which may be exotic (such as orbital mucormycosis), or from therapy both with drugs and radiotherapy. Bone marrow transplantation is associated with cataract and dry eye, and in some patients with conjunctival scarring due to graft versus host disease.

LYMPHOMA

Lymphoma may occur around or even inside the eye, either in isolation, as part of a disseminated disease, or in relapse. The tumours may involve one or both eyes. They are usually of the non-Hodgkin type and are often low grade. B-cell lymphomas typically form firm swellings in the eyelid or conjunctiva (where their appearance is said to resemble smoked salmon) and may also be found in the orbit or causing neuro-ophthalmic signs. T-cell tumours may involve the internal eye, particularly the iris or choroid. A rare form of lymphoma, ocular reticulum cell sarcoma or 'histiocytic' lymphoma, presents in the eye with cells which can masquerade as uveitis, usually with a pale mass just visible in the choroid or retina through a cloudy vitreous. These monoclonal cells may spread from or to the brain, often the frontal or temporal lobes, so cranial scanning is necessary. The diagnosis may be made by vitreous biopsy with immunocytochemistry of the cells obtained. The various ocular forms of lymphoma usually respond to local radiotherapy, although late complications may occur locally, such as dry eye, cataract, and radiation retinopathy.

SICKLING DISORDERS

Minor eye features are common in the sickling haemoglobinopathies and they may help in diagnosis. Major eye features occur in less than half the patients and are more common in patients with haemoglobin SC disease and sickle-cell thalassaemia (SThal) than in patients homozygous for haemoglobin S (SS). Blindness in one eye occurs in a minority, even in SC patients, and bilateral blindness is rare. As trials have suggested early treatment improves prognosis, it is important to screen the retina of selected high-risk patients. The risk of both types of glaucoma is increased, both acute and painful or chronic and painless. Other eye features are rare, including orbital infarction or pneumococcal ophthalmitis. In addition, patients may suffer a stroke affecting the visual field.

Conjunctival changes

Conjunctival signs are found in all types but they are more marked in SS than in SC patients. The small conjunctival vessels develop linear, saccular, or comma-shaped dilatations, which are more prominent in children and after topical phenylephrine drops. Their severity correlates with the number of irreversibly sickled cells in the peripheral blood.

Retinal changes

Bleeding into the retina causes a round 'salmon patch' to appear. As the blood resolves over several weeks, haemosiderin is left as iridescent spots in the superficial retina. Deeper haemorrhages damage the underlying retinal pigment layer and a 'black sunburst' scar forms permanently. These bleeds are usually asymptomatic and not a threat to sight.

Sickling in the terminal branches of the retinal arterioles produces signs of variable severity in about 50 per cent of patients. Their prevalence is related to age as most new vessels form between the ages of 10 and 25 years, with a low incidence after the age of 40. Blindness peaks in haemoglobin SC patients between the ages of 20 and 30 years. Severe retinal ischaemia causing formation of new vessels is about twice as common in SC and SThal than in SS patients. The risk of blindness is related to the number and size of new vessels with the risk of vitreous haemorrhage, which distorts, tears, and may detach the retina.

The important areas of vessel closure in the peripheral retina can rarely be seen with the direct ophthalmoscope so the patient must be screened after dilating the pupils using the indirect ophthalmoscope or an accessory lens at the slit lamp. Changes are most common in the superior temporal sector of the eye. The earliest sign of peripheral ischaemia is closure of arterioles (stage I) with a paler background and narrow white vessels. If these areas extend and become confluent, anastomotic loops form (stage II), preceding frank new vessel tufts (stage III). As the tufts grow forwards into the vitreous they often look like coral 'seafans'. Fluorescein angiography shows new vessels leaking fluorescein profusely in the same way as diabetic new vessels, and their size can be assessed before or after treatment. Many new vessel tufts will autoinfarct, even if not treated, presumably due to blockage of the feeder arteriole with sickled cells. They will not then bleed but others may form, so the patient has avoided immediate treatment but still needs to be observed. New vessels on the optic nerve head, as found in diabetes, are rare.

There are no symptoms until the vitreous haemorrhage (stage IV). If the haemorrhage is small, there will be a sudden shower of many small floaters, like 'midges'. If large, there is sudden marked cloudiness with a poor red reflex on fundoscopy. If the retina is distorted or detached (stage V) there may be flashes of light and a visual field defect. Occasionally there may be loss of central vision, either gradual with macular ischaemia or sudden with a haemorrhage into the fovea or a central retinal artery occlusion. Curiously, retinal vein occlusion is not associated with sickling.

Screening and treatment

Retinal screening should be carried out annually for patients between the ages of 20 and 30, especially those with haemoglobin SC and SThal disease. If new vessels are detected, they should be reassessed every few months, and if they do not autoinfarct and their size increases, or if vitreous haemorrhage occurs, local scatter laser treatment around the vessels should cause them to regress. Trials of laser treatment have shown a significant impact on early blindness rates. The ophthalmologist may also tackle the feeders of persistent vessels directly using laser, or operate on detached retina, but surgery carries a risk of profound ischaemia and glaucoma or acute retinal vascular occlusion. These complications may also follow eye trauma or systemic use of a carbonic anhydrase inhibitor.

Disorders of the thyroid (see also Chapter 12.4)

Eye signs in disorders of the thyroid are common. Some are directly related to thyroid hormone imbalance and may be an important clue to the diagnosis. Others are associated with an immunological disorder affecting both the thyroid (Graves' disease) and orbital tissues. In the United Kingdom, thyroid-related disease of the orbit is the most common cause of protrusion of the eye, proptosis or exophthalmos, terms which are synonymous. Many endocrinologists refer to 'Graves' ophthalmopathy' or 'ophthalmic Graves' disease' because of the association of eye changes with autoimmune thyroid dysfunction.

The eye changes vary in severity in each patient and at different times during the course of the disorder, which may persist for several years. Cosmetic problems and eye discomfort are common, but occasionally there is also a threat to vision which may present acutely as an emergency. The evolution of eye signs is often independent of the thyroid disease, as the patient may be euthyroid, hyperthyroid, or hypothyroid when the eye disease is first noticed and correction of the hormone imbalance may have little impact on eye features. A particularly common pattern is for orbital disease to appear in a patient who has become hypothyroid after treatment for hyperthyroidism.

PATHOGENESIS AND TISSUE PATHOLOGY

It is likely that the orbital disorder is autoimmune, with infiltration of the eye muscles by T cells. What attracts the cells is uncertain; antibodies to orbital tissue may be involved and there seems to be cross-reactivity of T cells with both thyroid and eye muscle membranes, but the exact sequence of events is still unclear. It is possible that fibroblasts are stimulated by T cells to produce mucinous material and oedema within muscle or fat, with eventual fibrosis and atrophy.

CLINICAL FEATURES

Werner proposed a classification which highlights the range of severity of eye features, although few patients progress logically through it: Class 0, signs and symptoms both absent; Class 1, signs without symptoms; Class 2, both symptoms and signs of soft tissue involvement; Class 3, proptosis indicating orbital involvement; Class 4, eye muscle involvement with double vision; Class 5, corneal involvement; Class 6, optic nerve involvement with loss of vision.

Eyelid and surface signs

The eyelids may be swollen in both hyper- and hypothyroidism. In hyperthyroid patients this is typically most pronounced on waking; the upper lids may be retracted so that white sclera appears above the upper cornea and the upper lid may lag behind the eyeball on rapid downgaze, so that this white area briefly becomes more pronounced (lid lag). The lid retraction makes the patient appear to stare, and blinking may also be reduced. With inflammation or congestion within the orbit, the eye may become congested, with redness and swelling of the conjunctiva, particularly over the tendon insertions of the lateral rectus muscles which are visible when the patient looks inwards. Conjunctival swelling varies from mild to severe. In patients with discomfort, a characteristic pattern of inflammation of the superior conjunctiva and cornea may be seen which stains with Rose Bengal.

Exophthalmos

Protrusion of the eye causes white sclera to appear below the lower corneal margin. In thyroid disease protrusion is often asymmetrical, but there are usually bilateral signs. Protrusion can be estimated with an exophthalmometer, using a mirror to look tangential to the corneal surface and superimposing a millimetre scale which measures from the bony rim of the orbit. These measurements are notoriously difficult to standardize but give a useful impression of the degree of symmetry and progression of proptosis.

If protrusion is severe, and particularly if there is also upper lid retraction, the lids may not cover the cornea on blinking and there is risk of corneal damage from poor wetting and exposure of the eye surface. Corneal abrasion, ulceration, and even perforation can develop rapidly; the patient with a protruding eye and impaired blinking, especially with pain or fluorescein staining of the cornea, should be treated as an ophthalmic emergency.

Even more alarming is loss of vision in the exophthalmic patient, as the optic nerve may be compressed by expanded orbital tissues. Paradoxically, orbital pressure may be highest in those without proptosis, as protrusion tends to have a decompressing effect. The vision is generally blurred, almost always in one eye at first, often most pronounced in the centre, perhaps with a frank central scotoma, and loss of colour definition is common. There may be a relative afferent pupillary defect. The optic nerve head may look swollen and there may also be wrinkling of the coat of the eye visible with the ophthalmoscope. Scanning will show enlarged muscles.

Double vision

Some limitation of eye movement causing diplopia is common with significant orbital pathology. The inferior recti are most commonly involved. The typical pattern of double vision is vertical, worse on waking, and on looking upwards due to restriction of lengthening of the swollen inferior rectus in the 'up and out' position.

Eye pressure

Ocular pressure is commonly raised if there is involvement of the eye muscles, and the pressure may rise when the patient looks up. The high pressure is usually well tolerated but some patients need topical treatment.

DIAGNOSIS

Laboratory investigations for thyroid disorder (both functional and immunological) should be carried out, though they are normal in some patients who otherwise have typical eye disease. Scans, especially coronal views, will usually show enlargement of ocular muscles bilaterally. Only a few conditions mimic thyroid eye disease in having bilateral if asymmetrical signs, and the clinical finding of upper lid signs is particularly helpful in suggesting thyroid disease. One rare differential diagnosis is orbital pseudotumour or myositis (which is characteristically more painful). Another is a caroticocavernous arteriovenous fistula, in which case a bruit may be present. There are neuroradiological methods which help to distinguish between these conditions.

MANAGEMENT OF THYROID-RELATED EYE DISEASE

Cosmetic problems are not easily solved. In some patients upper lid retraction responds to guanethidine drops but patients rarely tolerate these for long. Orbital surgery is rarely justified, but surgery to the upper lid is sometimes worthwhile. Discomfort is notoriously difficult to treat, although simple artificial tear drops may be tried. The response of orbital disease to immunosuppression has never been subjected to trial but this is generally thought to be justified only in emergency. Double vision is best managed initially with a plastic Fresnel prism stuck onto a spectacle lens, as the prism can be easily altered to adjust to what is often a changing pattern. Stable double vision may need a permanent spectacle prism or surgery, or sometimes improves with botulinum toxin injection into eye muscles. Corneal exposure may need a lateral tarsorrhaphy, when the eyelids are stitched together at the outer corner to narrow the gap between them. More urgent corneal covering may be achieved by taping the lids or putting in a single lid suture under local anaesthetic. Optic nerve compression needs urgent orbital decompression, which may be achieved medically with high-dose systemic corticosteroid treatment. The response is rapid, as with reduction in intracranial pressure with brain tumours, but is often partial and so surgery may be needed to remove bone from the orbital walls. Orbital radiotherapy may have a place for severe cases.

PARATHYROID DISORDERS

Hyperparathyroidism producing hypercalcaemia may cause deposition of calcium in the external eye tissues, particularly in the cornea, as a band keratopathy. This opacity stretches horizontally in the gap exposed between the eyelids, beginning at the margins and spreading inwards, often with a lacy appearance. Symptoms of red and gritty eyes are common.

Hypoparathyroidism (and also pseudohypoparathyroidism) is associated with lens opacities due to hypocalcaemia. Small white or coloured crystals lying beneath the lens capsule may be severe enough to interfere with vision. Rarely, papilloedema may occur with increased intracranial pressure which reverses with correction of the low calcium.

MULTIPLE ENDOCRINE NEOPLASIA SYNDROME

The type 2b subgroup of this rare autosomal dominant condition is associated with prominent corneal nerves, easily detected using the slit lamp. Occasionally frank neuromas of the conjunctiva or thickened eyelids are seen.

Ocular drug toxicity and screening

Blindness is a rare side-effect of therapy and only a few drugs require ophthalmic screening. Visual loss can occur in some cases of poisoning.

ANTIMALARIALS

Chloroquine

This drug carries a small but definite risk of toxicity to the retina, particularly to the macula, causing a disturbance of pigmentation in a 'bull's eye' pattern, a diffuse concentric ring around the fovea. The risk is usually dose-related and is very rarely seen below a total dose of 100 g of chloroquine base (equivalent to a regular daily dose of 500 mg chloroquine phosphate for 6 months). Rarely, a patient may show an idiosyncratic reaction early in treatment, so the drug must be stopped if vision falls within the first few weeks. Most reports of toxicity are in patients with a small body mass taking large doses for long periods to control inflammatory joint or skin diseases. Significant visual loss is rare in patients taking long-term choroquine in lower doses for malaria prophylaxis, although there is a risk in patients who abuse chloroquine.

Patients should be warned of the low risk of toxicity and told that the early symptoms are usually found on reading, especially small print. Typically, small scotomas close to fixation give the impression that letters are missing in part of each word. They should report these symptoms, stop taking the drug, and attend for testing. Screening should entail a base-line assessment before or soon after starting the drug, which should include measurement of visual acuities (particularly for reading type), macular sensitivities (of the Dicon type), or testing the central 10° of field with a 3 mm red target at 1 m on a tangent screen, and inspection of the macula of each eye after dilating the pupil, ideally with photographs at base-line for future comparison. Follow-up is recommended at intervals of 6 to 12 months. Maculopathy is usually reversible in the early stages.

Hydroxychloroquine

This seems to carry a much lower risk of retinal damage and monitoring is recommended at present only for those patients regularly taking more than the standard dose of up to 400 mg daily. Patients should be reassured of what seems to be an extremely low risk to sight.

ETHAMBUTOL

Toxicity is rare at doses of 15 mg/kg or less and is usually related to total dose, and therefore least likely in the first 6 months of treatment. Occasional reports exist of idiosyncratic toxicity in the weeks after starting treatment and patients with typical symptoms should stop taking the drug immediately. The clinical picture is that of an optic neuropathy, similar to optic neuritis of the demyelinating type. Patients should be warned of the low risk but asked to monitor and report any change in visual clarity or particularly in colour vision. Monitoring of visual acuity, colour vision (100 Hue test), and optic disc appearance (for swelling or atrophy) is suggested, and should be repeated at least once every 2 months while on treatment. Patients with previous optic nerve damage or with renal failure are at greater risk. The early changes usually recover if the drug is stopped.

CORTICOSTEROIDS

Systemic corticosteroids can cause lens opacities, typically beneath the back capsule (posterior subcapsular) where they tend to produce light scatter and glare even if not very dense. Opacities may be seen with the slit lamp or using the ophthalmoscope set to catch the red reflex in focus, particularly if the pupil is dilated. They are almost invariably suitable for routine surgery when the patient becomes significantly handicapped. As they are irreversible and not amenable to other therapy, it is not worth screening patients routinely.

OTHER OCULAR DRUG TOXICITIES

Many drugs are potentially toxic to the eye or visual path and there are several monographs on the subject. A few important toxicities are given in Table 8.

EYE SIGNS IN POISONINGS

Quinine poisoning carries a significant risk of blindness due to acute damage to the retina and optic nerve head, and ethyl alcohol (found in some antifreeze preparations) also damages the optic nerve. Ingestion

Table 8 *Some drugs with ocular side-effects*

Tetracyclines	Benign intracranial hypertension
Tigason®	Dry eye, sometimes conjunctival scarring
Tamoxifen	Retinopathy
Vincristine	Optic neuropathy

of raw cassava may also cause blindness. All of these will produce impaired pupil response to light.

Anticholinesterases (organophosphorus compounds), used mostly in pesticides, cause pupillary constriction due to parasympathetic stimulation in the acute stages of intoxication, but vision is not affected. Opiate use or abuse is also associated with pupillary constriction. Poisoning with atropine-like compounds or ingestion of nightshade berries causes dilatation of the pupils.

The external eye is vulnerable to applied agents. The most important include ammonia, alkalis (including lime, cement, and plaster), acids, and some riot-control agents. The important primary treatment is prolonged irrigation (using tapwater or milk if necessary) and then referral for specialized management.

Blindness worldwide

Accurate figures for the number of blind people do not exist and the only certainty is that they exceed official estimates, given as 45 million worldwide. One of the problems is to define blindness: the World Health Organization suggests a binocular vision of Snellen 6/60 incapacitates for working, but perhaps two-thirds of those estimated blind have worse vision which prevents even self-sufficiency. Some causes are preventable and some treatable but the feasibility of these measures may be limited, particularly in poor populations.

TRAUMA

Physical or chemical injury to the eye is a common cause of visual loss in populations with poor prevention and treatment. Easily available emergency eye surgery and antibiotics are mainstays for saving vision.

CATARACT

There is no known method of preventing cataract and it remains the most common cause of blindness in populations with limited surgical services. As the lens ages its protein structure changes and the lens becomes more opaque. Poor diet, dehydration, diabetes, and perhaps sunlight are all thought to accelerate lens ageing. Even if medication were available to retard cataract formation, there would be formidable problems in administering this long term on a large scale. In some populations the cataract problem is compounded by the complications of primitive surgical 'couching' or dislodging of the lens within the eye. Implanting artificial lenses is impractical in many countries and even if surgery is successful the correction by spectacles needed after surgery is often unsatisfactory. At present, attention in poorer countries is focused on organizing the training and deployment of mobile surgical teams to achieve large numbers of operations in the most effective way possible.

GLAUCOMA

This is an imprecise and unpredictable condition which often needs long-term medical treatment. In some patients progression is controlled permanently by surgery to improve drainage of aqueous fluid within the eye. Nerve fibres within the rim of the optic nerve head are damaged by relatively high intraocular pressure and impaired blood supply. The central cup of the nerve head enlarges progressively and visual field is irretrievably lost long before central acuity is affected, so the early stages are usually asymptomatic and painless. Even in wealthy populations screening for early glaucoma is difficult and some patients will progress to blindness despite all efforts. Those most at risk have a first-degree relative with glaucoma or have diabetes.

AGE-RELATED MACULAR DEGENERATION

The central retina around the fovea has an extraordinarily high metabolic turnover and in some patients the efficiency of recycling metabolic products fails, with deposition of abnormal material in the retina and breakdown of tissue integrity. Drusen may form around the fovea, and although they do not impair vision themselves they may herald the onset of aberrant vessels which grow into the fovea from the choroid beneath. These vessels may leak and often bleed, forming a scar which may have a 'disciform' shape which permanently damages the fovea. The patient loses detailed central vision, although peripheral vision allows them to navigate independently. Only a few patients at an early stage are ever likely to benefit from laser coagulation.

DIABETIC RETINOPATHY

This remains an important cause of blindness in younger patients in populations with relatively well-organized health care. Impaired vision arises either from macular damage due to vascular leakage or from the more widespread complications of ischaemia and proliferation of new vessels, or from both together. Major problems are the organization of effective screening programmes for diabetic patients and the deployment of laser treatment. It is estimated that over 50 per cent of blindness in diabetics is potentially preventable by laser if given early enough.

TRACHOMA

This chronic scarring conjunctivitis, due to infection with *Chlamydia trachomatis*, is described above. Blindness occurs in populations who have poor eye hygiene and repeated infection borne by flies. Immunity does not develop, so vaccination is not feasible and the only effective means of control is by intermittent topical or systemic treatment with tetracycline. Surgery for established scarring is less effective on a mass scale.

VITAMIN A DEFICIENCY (XEROPHTHALMIA)

This is a particularly tragic cause of blindness. It most commonly affects young children, may destroy the whole eye, and is preventable by eating foods which are often available but not included in the diet because of ignorance. Lack of vitamin A causes dryness and keratinization (xerosis) of the conjunctiva and cornea, with characteristic dry foamy Bitot's spots. The cornea softens (keratomalacia), ulcerates, may perforate, and becomes infected, often resulting in endophthalmitis. Vitamin A is found in many green, leafy vegetables or those coloured yellow or orange. Prevention is by education about diet or by supplementing with oral vitamin A. Measles keratitis compounds the risk of corneal scarring in malnourished children.

ONCHOCERCIASIS

Onchocerciasis is estimated to cause blindness in 1 million people, with a devastating effect in endemic areas where large numbers of adults in the population are navigationally blind and dependent on their children. The microfilarial disease is transmitted by the bite of blackfly which breed in fast-flowing rivers (river blindness). Visitors to endemic areas should be screened for infection on return (see above).

LEPROSY

Blindness is very common in chronic leprosy due to a combination of corneal anaesthesia and exposure from facial palsy so eye hygiene and protection are vital for these patients. The multibacillary form is often associated with a destructive iritis and secondary cataract.

REFERENCES

Inherited conditions

Morse, R.P., *et al.* (1990). Diagnosis and management of infantile Marfan syndrome. *Pediatrics* **86**, 888–95.

Renie, W.A. (ed.) (1986). *Goldberg's genetic and metabolic eye disease*, (2nd edn). Little, Brown and Company, Boston/Toronto.

Systemic inflammatory diseases

Aiello, P.D., *et al.* (1993). Visual prognosis in giant cell arteritis. *Ophthalmology* **100**, 550–5.

Charles, S.J., *et al.* (1991). Diagnosis and management of systemic Wegener's granulomatosis presenting with anterior ocular inflammatory disease. *British Journal of Ophthalmology* **75**, 201–7.

Ozyazgan, Y., *et al.* (1992). Low dose cyclosporin A versus pulsed cyclophosphamide in Behcet's syndrome. *British Journal of Ophthalmology* **76**, 241–3.

Rothova, A., *et al.* (1989). Risk factors for ocular sarcoidosis. *Documenta Ophthalmologica* **72**, 287–96.

Stafford-Brady, F.T., *et al.* (1988). Lupus retinopathy. *Arthritis and Rheumatism* **31**, 1105–10.

Syners, B., *et al.* (1990). Retinal and choroidal vaso-occlusive disease in SLE associated with antiphospholipid antibodies. *Retina* **10**, 255–60.

Wechsler, B. (1992). Behcet's disease (editorial). *British Medical Journal* **304**, 1199–200.

Vascular occlusion

Elman, M.J., *et al.* (1990). The risk for systemic vascular diseases and mortality in patients with central retinal vein occlusion. *Ophthalmology* **97**, 1543–8.

Hypertension

McGregor, E., *et al.* (1986). Retinal changes in malignant hypertension. *British Medical Journal* **292**, 233–4.

Diabetes

Diabetic Retinopathy Study Group (1981). Photocoagulation treatment of proliferative diabetic retinopathy: clinical application of DRS findings. *Ophthalmology* **88**, 583–600.

Early Treatment of Diabetic Retinopathy Study Research Group (1985). Photocoagulation for diabetic macular oedema. *Archives of Ophthalmology* **103**, 1796–806.

Forrester, J.V., *et al.* (1993). The role of growth factors in proliferative diabetic retinopathy. *Eye* **7**, 276–87.

Klein, R., Klein, B.E.K., and Moss, S. (1989). The Wisconsin Epidemiologic Study of Diabetic Retinopathy: a review. *Diabetes and Metabolism Reviews* **5**, 559–70.

Rohan, T.E., *et al.* (1989). Prevention of blindness by screening for diabetic retinopathy: a quantitative assessment. *British Medical Journal* **299**, 1198–201.

The DCCT Research Group. (1986). The Diabetes Control and Complications Trial: Design and methodologic considerations for the feasibility phase. *Diabetes* **35**, 530–45.

The Diabetes Control and Complications Trial Research Group. (1993). The effect of intensive treatment of diabetes on the development and progression of long-term complications in insulin-dependent diabetes mellitus. *New England Journal of Medicine,* **329**, 977–86.

Thompson, J.R., Du, L., and Rosenthal, A.R. (1989). Recent trends in the registration of blindness and partial sight in Leicestershire. *British Journal of Ophthalmology* **73**, 95–9.

Infectious diseases

Chignell, A.H. (1992). Endogenous *Candida* endophthalmitis. *Journal of the Royal Society of Medicine* 85, 721–4.

Holland, G.N. (1992). AIDS and ophthalmology: the first decade (editorial). (1992). *American Journal of Ophthalmology.* **114**, 86–95.

Koppe, J.G. and Rothova, A. (1989). Congenital toxoplasmosis. A long term follow-up of 20 years. *International Ophthalmology* **13**, 387–90.

Spalton, D.J. (1990). Lyme disease (editorial). *British Journal of Ophthalmology* **74,** 321–2.

Studies of Ocular Complications of AIDS Research Group (1992). Mortality in patients with AIDS treated with either Foscarnet or Ganciclovir for CMV retinitis. *New England Journal of Medicine* **326,** 213–20.

Blood disorders

Cohen, S.B. *et al.* (1986). Review of ocular features of sickle cell haemoglobinopathies. *Ophthalmic Surgery* **17,** 57.

Fox, P.D., *et al.* (1991). Influence of genotype on the natural history of untreated proliferative sickle retinopathy. *British Journal of Ophthalmology* **75,** 229–31.

Thyroid

Monro, D. (1993). Thyroid eye disease. (editorial) *British Medical Journal* **306,** 805–6.

Ocular drug toxicity

Fraunfelder, F.T. (1989). *Drug-induced ocular side effects and drug interactions,* (3rd edn). Lea and Febiger, Philadelphia/London.

World blindness

Foster, A., *et al.* (1992). Epidemiology of childhood blindness. *Eye* **6,** 173–6.

Section 27 *Psychiatry in medicine*

27.1 Introduction

M. G. GELDER

This section gives an account of psychiatric disorders that commonly present to physicians. The account is selective because psychiatry deals with many issues that seldom arise in medical wards, for example the care of patients with chronic schizophrenia. The account focuses on practical issues of diagnosis and management, but deals only briefly with aetiology and epidemiology. Child psychiatry and mental handicap are excluded because this textbook does not deal systematically with diseases of children. The topic of dependence on drugs and alcohol is not presented here but in Section 28. For a more comprehensive account of psychiatry readers are referred to the *Oxford Textbook of Psychiatry* or a similar postgraduate text for psychiatrists.

The detection of psychiatric disorder in physically ill patients

It has been shown repeatedly that psychiatric disorder is common among physically ill patients, but frequently goes undetected by physicians. Thus, when reliable standardized interviews and strict diagnostic criteria are used, about 20 per cent of medical inpatients are found to have psychiatric disorders, of which only half are detected by the physicians caring for the patients. Most of these disorders are emotional disorders or complications of alcohol abuse. Rates of psychiatric disorder vary between medical specialities; they are high, for example, in gastro-enterology clinics.

For several reasons it is important to detect psychiatric disorders in the physically ill. First, severe psychiatric disorders may worsen if not treated promptly, and some may carry a risk of suicide. Second, moderately severe disorders may be less hazardous, but may seriously reduce compliance with medical treatment and thereby delay recovery from physical illness. Third, mild disorders may increase the distress of physical illness. For all these reasons it is important to detect psychiatric disorder in medical patients and to give appropriate treatment.

Why is the detection rate low? Psychiatric symptoms may go unnoticed because they are more difficult to detect in physically ill than in physically healthy patients, and because some physicians do not enquire about them in a systematic and routine way. There are several reasons why psychiatric symptoms are more difficult to detect in patients who have a physical illness. First, the symptoms may be mistaken for a normal emotional reaction to physical illness – patients may be thought to be understandably despondent when in fact they are suffering from a depressive disorder. Second, some of the symptoms characteristic of psychiatric disorder are also symptoms of physical disorder, for example insomnia, lack of energy, and weight loss. Third, psychiatric patients who are depressed or apathetic may remain unnoticed because they are quiet and compliant.

Some physicians do not ask routinely about psychiatric symptoms because they believe that questioning will upset the patient. These reservations are usually greatest when asking patients with malignant disease about hopelessness and tearfulness, and also when asking patients about suicidal ideas. Such enquiries are not distressing if made sensitively, and if the physician leaves enough time to listen sympathetically to the answers. Questions about feelings may induce an immediate reaction of weeping and other signs of distress, but if the physician responds in a sympathetic and unhurried way, patients generally feel relieved to be able to express their feelings and share their concerns. Questions about suicide do not increase the risk of suicide; on the contrary they make patients feel that their distress has been understood, which in turn makes them less hopeless and less likely to attempt suicide.

Mental state examination in medical work

The full mental state examination used in psychiatry is detailed and elaborate. In other branches of medicine it is generally more appropriate to use a shorter interview focusing on disorders of mood and cognition. This brief routine interview can be expanded to include disorders of thinking and perception when appropriate (for example when there is a severe disturbance of behaviour suggesting delirium or acute schizophrenia). If the brief examination indicates the possibility of a severe mental disorder it is important to interview another informant, such as a relative or close friend of the patient. This importance of this further interview is that some patients do not recognize the nature or extent of their abnormal behaviour, and the full picture can be revealed only by an additional informant.

A useful routine is to ask all patients about mood disorder, with particular reference to low spirits, worry, and tension; loss of interest and low energy; and difficulty in sleeping. Useful questions include: 'How are your spirits?' 'Have you been worrying more than usual?' 'Have you been feeling tense and unable to relax?' The second and third questions are examples of closed questions; that is, the answers can be simply 'Yes' or 'No'. If the answer to such a question is 'Yes', the interviewer should ask for recent examples. Questions about orientation and memory may be resented by patients with a normal mental state; it is usually evident when such questions must be asked, because the possibility of impairment of orientation or memory has been suggested by the patient's responses during the medical history. If necessary, questions about memory can be introduced by explaining that such enquiries are routine.

As an alternative to asking screening questions for psychiatric disorder when taking the medical history, it can be valuable to use a standardized written questionnaire that is completed by the patient. Questionnaires of this kind can be used not only to detect psychiatric symptoms but also to assess the severity of an emotional disorder. Several valid and reliable questionnaires are available, of which the General Health Questionnaire is particularly useful for medical patients. Such questionnaires have been used widely with medical patients and have proved acceptable and informative.

Reactions and disorders

There is a useful diagnostic convention that normal emotional responses to adverse circumstances (including those associated with physical illness) are called emotional reactions, and that abnormal responses are called psychiatric disorders. The distinction between normal and abnormal responses is made on two criteria. The first is a commonsense judgement about the amount of distress that most patients experience in similar circumstances. A degree of depression or anxiety is a normal response to physical illness, to pain or to other kinds of physical discomfort, to the unfamiliar surroundings of hospital life, and to uncertainty about the future. Physicians who see many patients within their specialty are usually better placed than a psychiatrist to judge whether a psychological reaction to a particular physical illness is normal or abnormal, especially if the illness is uncommon. The second criterion is that an abnormal reaction can be identified as a clinical syndrome with a specific pattern of symptoms. Psychiatric syndromes are usually not difficult to recognize. Physicians should be able to detect the majority of syndromes, but psychiatric advice should be sought in doubtful cases.

When to obtain psychiatric advice

When a psychiatric disorder has been diagnosed, its severity should be assessed. Severity is judged by the intensity of the patient's distress, and by the intensity and nature of the symptoms (for example, in depressive disorders extreme severity is indicated by delusions and hallucinations). These points are considered further when the various psychiatric syndromes are reviewed in subsequent sections. If the diagnosis is certain and the disorder is not severe, the physician may initiate treatment or ask the family doctor to do so. In other cases he may refer the patient to a psychiatrist.

Estimates vary, but it is likely that 5 to 10 per cent of patients admitted to medical wards would benefit from referral to a psychiatrist. The main indications for referral are: uncertainty about the psychiatric diagnosis; the psychiatric disorder not responding to treatment prescribed by the physician; a disorder of great severity, particularly when there may be a risk of suicide or of harm to other people; and behaviour that is disruptive and not controlled by simple measures. These points are taken up in subsequent sections.

REFERENCES

Gelder, M.G., Gath, D.H., and Mayou, R. *Oxford textbook of psychiatry*. Oxford University Press.
Goldberg, D., Benjamin, S., and Creed, F. (1987). *Psychiatry in Medical Practice*. Tavistock Publications, London.
Kaplan, H.I. and Sadock, B.J. (1989). *Comprehensive textbook of psychiatry*, (5th edn). Williams and Wilkins, Baltimore.
Leff, J.P. and Isaacs, A.D. (1990). *Psychiatric examination in clinical practice*, (3rd edn). Blackwell Scientific Publications, Oxford.

27.2 Psychiatric disorders as they concern the physician

27.2.1 Reactions to stressful events

M. G. GELDER

Physicians see many patients who have emotional and physical symptoms as reactions to stressful events. Some of these reactions are abnormal and are classifiable as psychiatric disorders. Most are normal reactions to adversity; they are not pathological but they are distressing and require help.

Reactions to stressful events have three elements: an emotional response, a physical response, and psychological responses that reduce the impact of the stressor. The emotional response may be anxiety or depression or both, and the physical response varies accordingly. The physical response associated with anxiety is autonomic arousal and increased muscle tension; the physical response associated with depression is fatigue and lethargy.

The psychological responses that serve to reduce the impact of stressful events are mechanisms of defence and coping strategies. *Mechanisms of defence* are of several kinds, of which the most important are denial and regression. *Denial* is the exclusion from awareness of distressing information; this response is shown, for example, by patients who have been told that they have cancer but who continue to behave as if unaware of the diagnosis. When it occurs immediately after exposure to stressful events, denial is adaptive because it reduces the impact; when it continues beyond this early stage, denial is maladaptive because it prevents the person from taking necessary steps to resolve the problems or adapt to them. *Regression* is the adoption of behaviour appropriate to an earlier stage of life, usually dependence on others. Regression is common in physical illness. In the acute stage of illness this response can be adaptive by enabling the patient to accept nursing care, but if persistent it prevents the patient from playing an active part in recovery.

Coping strategies may also be adaptive or maladaptive. Adaptive coping strategies include working out solutions to problems and coming to terms with circumstances that cannot be changed. Maladaptive strategies include the excessive use of alcohol or drugs to relieve distress. Some strategies are adaptive in the early stage of responding to stress, but

maladaptive if continued for long; an example is the avoidance of stressful situations.

There are three kinds of reaction to stressful events: acute reactions, adjustment reactions, and post-traumatic stress disorders. These reactions are described next. The special features of reactions to physical illness, to terminal illness, and to bereavement are described in Section 27.3.

Acute reactions to stress

An acute reaction to stress is the emotional response to brief stressful events. The symptoms are anxiety, depression, irritability, poor sleep, difficulty in concentration, restlessness, and symptoms of autonomic arousal such as palpitations and tremor. Physicians see these reactions in people admitted to hospital in stressful circumstances, or in the relatives of the seriously ill. Usually an acute stress reaction resolves within a few days as the stress subsides or the person comes to terms with it.

Treatment

Usually the emotional response can be reduced by encouraging the person to talk about the stressful experience and by giving appropriate reassurance. If the reaction is severe, an anxiolytic or hypnotic drug may be needed but should be prescribed for only 2 or 3 days. If the stressful event was very distressing it may be necessary to help the patient to talk about it several times, and to release emotions.

Adjustment disorder

An adjustment disorder is the emotional response to prolonged stressful circumstances such as a serious illness. The symptoms of an adjustment reaction resemble those of an acute reaction to stress, namely anxiety, depression, irritability, poor sleep, and symptoms of autonomic arousal. The response lasts longer than an acute reaction because the stress is more prolonged. Patients may avoid stressful situations, or may deny knowledge of the seriousness of their situation even though it has been explained clearly. Such responses may protect the patient from developing high levels of anxiety or depression and may be adaptive in the early stages, but if persistent they may prevent the patient from coming to terms with the problem.

Treatment

This is directed to helping the normal processes of adjustment. Problem-solving counselling is used to reduce denial and avoidance, and to encourage resolution and acceptance of the new situation. Drug treatment is seldom needed, but occasionally a benzodiazepine drug is helpful for a few days to improve sleep and to reduce anxiety enough to allow the person to concentrate better on the problems, and to find ways of adjusting to them. Bereavement and reactions to terminal illness are special kinds of adjustment disorder. These are described in Chapter 27.3.2.

Post-traumatic stress disorder

Post-traumatic stress disorder is an intense, prolonged, and sometimes delayed reaction to an exceptionally stressful event such as a major road accident, rape, or other severe physical experiences. This kind of reaction may affect anyone, but the risk is greater if the stressful experience is extremely severe, if the person under stress is in childhood or old age, or if the person has had a psychiatric disorder in the past. The clinical picture of post-traumatic stress disorder has three sets of features:

1. Anxiety, depression, irritability, poor concentration, and insomnia, often with panic attacks and sometimes episodes of aggression.
2. Intrusive daytime images ('flashbacks') and nightmares of the stressful events, together with difficulty in recalling the events at will.
3. Detachment, diminished interest, and inability to feel normal emotions.

These symptoms usually resolve within a few months but occasionally persist for years.

Treatment

This is similar to that for adjustment disorder. The patient is helped to talk about the events frequently, and to release pent-up emotions on each occasion. Treatment is generally less successful for post-traumatic stress disorder than for acute reactions to stress or adjustment disorders. Even with skilled and persistent counselling the response of established cases is often limited. It has been suggested that counselling given immediately after the event reduces the frequency and severity of these persistent disorders, but there is no convincing evidence to support this claim.

REFERENCES

Davidson, J. (1992). Drug therapy for post-traumatic stress disorder. *British Journal of Psychiatry*, **160**, 309–14.
Gelder, M.G., Gath, H., and Mayou, R. (1994) *Concise Oxford textbook of psychiatry*. Oxford University Press, Oxford.

27.2.2 Anxiety and obsessional disorders

M. G. GELDER

Anxiety disorders

Physicians see many anxious patients. Usually the anxiety is a normal reaction to the stressful circumstances of physical illness, that is an acute reaction to stress or an adjustment disorder (see Chapter 27.2.1). In a few cases, however, the severity and duration of the anxiety are out of proportion to the stressful circumstances. These abnormal states are called anxiety disorders. They present to physicians because the symp-

Table 1 *Physical symptoms of anxiety*

Cardiovascular	Palpitations Awareness of missed beats Discomfort in the chest
Respiratory	Overbreathing Sense of dyspnoea
Gastrointestinal	Dry mouth Difficulty in swallowing Epigastric discomfort Excessive wind Frequent or loose motions
Genitourinary	Frequent or urgent micturition Failure of erection Amenorrhoea Menstrual discomfort
Neuromuscular	Tremor Aching muscles Pricking sensations Headache Dizziness, tinnitus

toms resemble those of physical illness. It is important, therefore, that physicians should be able to recognize and arrange appropriate treatment for anxiety disorders.

Anxiety disorders are of three kinds: generalized anxiety disorders, in which anxiety is continuous; phobic anxiety disorders, in which anxiety is episodic and occurs in relation to specific stimuli; and panic disorder, in which anxiety is episodic without any consistent relationship to external stimuli. Although anxiety disorders differ in these ways, the symptoms of anxiety are the same in all three. These symptoms will be described in relation to generalized anxiety disorder.

GENERALIZED ANXIETY DISORDER

Clinical picture

The patient's appearance is characteristic: the expression is strained, the posture is tense, and there may be tremor and motor restlessness.

The patient often complains of one or more physical symptoms that result from autonomic arousal and increased tension in skeletal muscles. Such symptoms are numerous but can be grouped conveniently into cardiovascular, respiratory, gastrointestinal, genitourinary, and neuro-muscular symptoms (see Table 1).

Some anxious patients overbreathe and thus cause faintness, tinnitus, palpitations, precordial discomfort and (in severe cases) tingling in the extremities as well as carpopedal spasm.

The patient always has psychological symptoms but may not volunteer them because of a belief that they are normal reactions to physical symptom such as palpitations. These psychological symptoms include fearful anticipation, inner restlessness, irritability, and poor concentration. The latter may lead to complaints of poor memory, although memory is normal in this disorder. Many patients have persistent worrying thoughts that they are seriously ill, or that their relatives are unwell or liable to an accident. Other features are difficulty in falling asleep, and wakening during the night. These sleep disturbances contrast with the early morning wakening which is characteristic of depressive disorder.

Aetiology

The causes of generalized anxiety disorder are not fully understood. The concordance of anxiety disorder has been reported to be greater in monozygotic than in dizygotic twins. Such a finding suggests genetic causes, but the studies did not distinguish clearly between the three types of anxiety disorder, and it is therefore not clear how far the results apply to generalized anxiety disorder.

There is a widely held view that insecure relationships in childhood can predispose to anxiety disorder in later life. To test this idea long-term follow-up studies are needed, but are lacking because of the difficulty of carrying them out. Generalized anxiety disorders are precipitated by stressful life events, especially those that threaten the person's future security. In generalized anxiety disorder the autonomic nervous system is overactive, whilst responses to stressful stimuli habituate more slowly than in the normal population.

Differential diagnosis

Generalized anxiety disorder has to be distinguished from physical illness and from other psychiatric disorders. Anxiety disorder can present with symptoms resembling physical illness, whilst some physical illnesses are accompanied by marked anxiety symptoms. When a patient complains of physical symptoms of anxiety such as palpitations or epigastric discomfort, the correct diagnosis can usually be reached by enquiring about other symptoms of the syndrome of generalized anxiety disorder, and by carrying out appropriate physical investigations. Thyrotoxicosis, phaeochromocytoma, and hypoglycaemia may present with symptoms resembling anxiety. Any other physical illness may be accompanied by marked anxiety if the patient has a special reason to fear its outcome, for example if a relative died after developing similar symptoms.

Several psychiatric disorders can present with anxiety symptoms. Depressive disorder is the most frequent, but senile dementia and schizophrenia may also come to notice in this way. The correct diagnosis can usually be made by careful enquiry for symptoms of the other disorder, for example low mood and early morning wakening as symptoms of depressive disorder, or memory impairment as the cardinal symptom of dementia. Another important cause of symptoms resembling anxiety disorder is alcohol withdrawal, occurring after a bout of heavy drinking or in a dependent person (see Chapter 28.3.4).

Prognosis

Generalized anxiety disorders often recover slowly; without treatment about three-quarters persist up to 3 years. The outcome is worse when the history is long, stressful circumstances are persistent, and the personality is abnormal.

Treatment

Treatment is mainly psychological. It should begin with an explanation that physical symptoms of anxiety are an exaggeration of the normal response to stressful events and not evidence of bodily disease. The patient should be encouraged to deal with any stressful problems, and helped to come to terms with any that cannot be resolved. If symptoms persist, anxiety management (see Chapter 27.4.2) is usually helpful; this treatment can be provided by a psychiatrist or a clinical psychologist. If patients hyperventilate when anxious, they should be shown how to terminate the acute episode by rebreathing expired air from a paper bag to restore normal alveolar concentrations of carbon dioxide. To prevent further episodes patients can practise slow, controlled breathing which is timed by tape-recorded instructions.

If these psychological treatments are not available, if the patient does not respond to them, or if the symptoms are very severe, drug treatment may be needed. Benzodiazepines produce rapid relief of anxiety but should not be prescribed for more than 3 or 4 weeks because they may cause dependence when taken for longer. β-Adrenergic agonists are useful to control severe palpitations and tremor, but do not have a direct anxiolytic effect. Care should be taken to observe the contraindications to the use of β-adrenergic antagonists (notably heart block, a history of bronchospasm, metabolic alkalosis, and prolonged fasting), and to follow the manufacturer's guides to usage.

Antidepressants have both anxiolytic and antidepressant actions. They do not cause dependency and the anticholinergic side-effects of tricyclics are seldom troublesome in the doses required to control generalized anxiety (about 75 mg per day of amitriptyline). These drugs are useful for chronic generalized anxiety disorders that have not responded to anxiety management.

PHOBIC ANXIETY DISORDER

The symptoms of phobic anxiety disorder resemble those of generalized anxiety disorder. The difference between the two conditions is that the symptoms of phobic anxiety disorder occur intermittently and in relation to specific situations, whilst the symptoms of generalized anxiety disorders are more frequent and prolonged. Phobic patients tend to avoid situations that provoke symptoms, and this avoidance may limit their ability to work or deal with social situations.

There are three types of phobic disorder: simple phobia, social phobia, and agoraphobia. Physicians are most likely to encounter these conditions when the patient complains of episodes of severe physical symptoms of anxiety, such as paroxysms of tachycardia, episodes of dizziness or shortness of breath.

Simple phobia

In this disorder the symptoms are greatly exaggerated common fears, such as fears of enclosed spaces, injections, or heights. Physicians are most likely to encounter patients with phobic anxiety provoked by some aspect of medical investigation or treatment, for example injections or enclosed spaces (as in scanning procedures). Treatment with behaviour therapy (see Chapter 27.4.2) is usually successful.

Social phobia

In this disorder patients experience severe anxiety when they feel themselves to be under critical scrutiny, for example in business meetings or social gatherings. Sometimes the anxiety is related to specific actions, such as eating a meal or writing in the presence of another person. The symptoms resemble those of other anxiety neuroses, but blushing, trembling, nausea, and frequency of micturition are particularly frequent. Socially phobic patients are preoccupied with the belief that others are observing them in a critical way, although they realize that this belief is irrational. Some patients seek advice about physical symptoms that they experience when anxious, for example urinary frequency or urgency of defecation.

Social phobia usually begins with an initial anxiety attack in a social situation; subsequent episodes seem to arise through processes of conditioning. Treatment is with behaviour therapy (Chapter 27.4.2).

Agoraphobia

Agoraphobic patients become severely anxious when they leave home, enter crowded places, or are in situations that they cannot leave easily. They may experience any of the physical symptoms of anxiety, but palpitations are particularly common, and often accompanied by the fear that a heart attack will follow. Fears of fainting are also common. These fears may lead agoraphobic patients to consult physicians in the early stage of the disorder and to seek reassurance about their physical health. Agoraphobic patients restrict their activities to avoid situations that provoke anxiety. This avoidance maintains the disorder. Some patients become virtually housebound.

Agoraphobia usually begins with a panic attack in a situation, which is subsequently associated with anxiety. The first attack may be associated with stressful life events, or may occur spontaneously as in panic disorder (see below). Phobic disorder is them maintained by avoidance and by anxious concerns about the effects of anxiety on physical health (for example, fears that repeated tachycardia will cause heart disease). Treatment is with cognitive behaviour therapy in which emphasis is placed on returning to situations that have been avoided. If this treatment is not available, symptoms can often be reduced with imipramine prescribed as for panic disorder (see below).

PANIC DISORDER

In this disorder there are sudden episodes of severe anxiety which are not provoked by external stimuli (a point of difference from phobic disorders). The symptoms may be any of those described under generalized anxiety disorder. Palpitations are particularly common; they often cause patients to seek advice from physicians and cardiologists because of fears of serious heart disease. Understandably in the past cardiologists referred to this condition as disorderly action of the heart, or effort syndrome. In panic disorder anxiety is not associated regularly with the same situations, but occurs unpredictably. For this reason patients do not develop the marked avoidance that characterizes phobic disorders.

Aetiology

Patients with panic disorder react excessively to agents that increase central adrenergic activity (e.g. yohimbine). They also have irrational fears that anxiety symptoms will be followed by a medical emergency such as a heart attack. These two factors interact to set up a vicious circle: thus, anxiety leads to physical symptoms, which activate fear of physical illness, which leads to more anxiety, which eventually leads to a panic attack.

Prognosis

When the condition is of recent onset, patients often recover if the benign nature of the anxiety symptoms is explained and the fears of physical illness are dispelled. When the condition has lasted more than 6 months, it is likely to persist for years.

Treatment

Panic attacks can be controlled with high doses of benzodiazepines, but prolonged treatment may lead to dependency. Imipramine, a tricyclic antidepressant drug with anxiolytic properties, is effective and does not cause dependency. The drug has to be given in high dosage, and causes more side-effects than do benzodiazepines. The effective dose is greater than the dose usually given for depression; thus 150 to 200 mg per day, or even higher doses, are given provided that cardiac and other medical systems are normal. When first prescribed for panic disorder, imipramine may cause apprehension and sleeplessness. For this reason a small starting dose should be used; for example 10 mg per day for 3 days, increased by 10 mg every 3 days to a dose of 50 mg per day, and then by increments of 25 mg per week to the final dose. Imipramine should be continued for 6 months and then withdrawn gradually. About one-third of patients relapse and need further treatment with imipramine or with cognitive therapy.

Cognitive therapy is an alternative treatment, which can be given by a clinical psychologist, or a psychiatrist. It is designed to change the fears of physical symptoms that contribute to the panic attacks (see above). The patient is helped to recognize the irrational basis of the fears and to control them. The results of cognitive therapy are similar to those of imipramine, and the relapse rate may be lower.

Obsessive compulsive disorder

The main features of obsessive compulsive disorder are thoughts that intrude repeatedly and insistently into the patient's awareness and are recognized by the patient as irrational. The thoughts are usually associated with repetitive behaviours (rituals). Patients feel ashamed of the symptoms and may not reveal them to a physician treating a coincident physical disorder. Admission to hospital or an investigation may reveal the condition by provoking the patient's obsessional symptoms (for example fears of contamination), and consequent anxiety.

CLINICAL FEATURES

The syndrome of obsessional neurosis comprises obsessional thoughts, rituals, anxiety, depression, and depersonalization. Obsessional thoughts are usually about unpleasant themes, which patients try to exclude from their minds, but without success. A common theme is that of spreading disease by touching objects and thereby contaminating them. Other obsessional thoughts are fearful preoccupations about illness ('disease phobias'), often cancer or venereal disease. Other kinds of obsessional thought are ruminations (repeated internal debates, often about unanswerable metaphysical questions), and thoughts of performing dangerous or embarrassing acts (e.g. to jump from a height or shout blasphemies in church). Obsessional rituals (also known as compulsive rituals) include behaviours such as repeated handwashing or arranging objects in a particular way, and mental activities such as the repeated counting of objects.

AETIOLOGY

Obsessional disorders often begin at a time of increased stress, although they may persist long after the stress has ceased. There may be a genetic predisposition but the data from twin studies is not conclusive. Amongst patients with obsessional disorders some have an obsessive personality (see Chapter 27.2.5) but this association is not invariable. Various psychological theories have been proposed to explain the condition, but none is convincing.

DIFFERENTIAL DIAGNOSIS

Obsessional neurosis may be mistaken for an anxiety neurosis or depressive disorder when there is a mood change and when the patient does not disclose the obsessional symptoms. Some obsessional thoughts are so unusual that schizophrenia is suspected; careful and repeated examination for characteristic features of schizophrenia usually leads to the correct diagnosis. All these diagnostic distinctions may be difficult and may require a psychiatric opinion.

PROGNOSIS

Amongst obsessional disorders of recent onset, about two-thirds improve within a year. The rest usually run a fluctuating course for many years, often with long periods of partial or complete remission.

TREATMENT

When obsessional disorders are mild and of recent onset, usually the only requirements are supportive treatment and encouragement not to give way to rituals. Any associated depressive disorder should be treated with an antidepressant drug, because improvement in a depressive disorder is often accompanied by improvement in obsessional symptoms. More persistent obsessional disorders should be assessed by a psychiatrist. Some patients respond to 5-HT uptake blocking drugs (see Chapter 27.4.1), although many relapse when the drugs are withdrawn. Most patients improve with a form of behaviour therapy known as response prevention, but mild residual symptoms are common. Dynamic psychotherapy is rarely beneficial. In the past, a few intractable cases have been treated by psychosurgery but the long-term results are not known to better those of intensive and prolonged treatment with behaviour therapy and drugs.

REFERENCES

Coryell, W. and Winokur, G. (1991). *The clinical management of anxiety disorders*. Oxford University Press, New York.
da Rosa Davis, J. and Gelder, M.G. (1991). Long term management of anxiety states. *International Review of Psychiatry*, **3**, 5–17.
Kennerley, H. (1990). *Managing anxiety: a training manual*. Oxford University Press, Oxford.
Nutt, D. and Lawson, C. (1992). Panic attacks: A neurochemical overview of models and mechanisms. *British Journal of Psychiatry*, **160**, 165–178.

27.2.3 Psychiatric conditions with physical complaints

M. G. GELDER

The term somatization denotes the expression of psychological distress as bodily complaints and the seeking of medical help for these complaints. Somatization disorders are disorders in which somatization occurs. Somatization can be either an acute response to stressful events, or persistent. *Acute somatization* is common. Amongst patients who attend general practitioners with stress reactions, anxiety disorders, or depressive disorders, many complain of physical rather than psychological symptoms. This aspect of somatization is discussed in the sections dealing with these three syndromes. Acute somatisation also presents with conversion symptoms (Chapter 27.2.4).

Persistent somatization is of four main kinds: somatization disorder, hypochondriasis, dysmorphophobia, and psychogenic pain. These disorders are referred to collectively as somatoform disorders. In the United States conversion disorder is classified as a somatoform disorder but in the International Classification of Diseases it is classified separately.

Somatization disorder

Patients with somatization disorder complain of multiple, recurrent, and often changing physical symptoms for which no physical cause can be found. The patient is not satisfied with appropriate investigation and reassurance and their complaints continue or change to another symptom, which can be of any kind. Common complaints are regurgitation, belching, nausea, and abnormal skin sensations. Patients with somatization disorder are extremely persistent in seeking further help and investigation.

The cause of somatization disorder is not known. Some patients have grown up with parents who were excessively concerned about illness, but this family background is not invariable. Some patients have long-standing difficulties in personal relationships. Occasionally there is a primary cause, for example a depressive disorder, but in most patients there is no clear cause.

There is no specific psychological treatment for somatization disorder. It is important that the access of patients to medical advice and to investigations should be kept within reasonable limits, which are agreed and adhered to by the physician and general practitioner. Psychiatrists can sometimes help in formulating this plan of management, and in excluding a primary depressive disorder as a cause of the symptoms, but they can seldom provide more specific and effective treatment.

REFERENCES

Bass, C.M. (1990). Assessment and management of patients with functional somatic symptoms. In *Somatization: Physical symptoms and psychological illness* (ed. C. Bass), pp. 40–72, Blackwells, Oxford.
Escobar, J.I., Burham, M., Karno, M. *et al.* (1987). Somatization in the community. *Archives of General Psychiatry.* **44,** 713–18.
Goldberg, D., Gask, L., and O'Dowd, T. (1989). The treatment of somatization: Teaching techniques of reattribution. *Journal of Psychosomatic Research*, **33,** 689–95.
Smith, R.G., Monson, R.A., and Ray, D.C. (1986). Psychiatric consultation in somatization disorder. *New England Journal of Medicine*, **314,** 1407–13.

Hypochondriasis

Hypochondriasis is an illness preoccupation that persists despite reassurance based on appropriate medical investigation. In medical practice hypochondriacal concerns are met frequently in patients who have no psychiatric disorder; severe and persistent hypochondriasis is usually associated with psychiatric disorder or personality disorder.

CLINICAL FEATURES

Hypochondriacal concerns take many forms, but they usually relate to physical disease or the appearance of the face or body. Concerns about disease are often associated with awareness of a normal bodily sensation such as forceful heart action, flatulence, or minor aches and pains, which are interpreted as symptoms of undetected disease. Other concerns relate to normal variations in appearance such as pigmented areas in the skin or benign lumps. Preoccupations with cancer or AIDS are common. These preoccupations persist despite repeated reassurance based on appropriate and thorough investigation. They often cause great distress. Some patients are concerned with a single symptom and a single disease, others have a series of changing concerns.

AETIOLOGY

Hypochondriasis may be provoked by stressful events. In mild cases there may be no associated psychiatric disorder, but in some severe and persistent cases there is a depressive, anxiety, or obsessional disorder. Occasionally, hypochondriacal complaints are the first evidence of schizophrenia or dementia. Most other cases of severe and persistent hypochondriasis are associated with a personality disorder. There is no single personality type, but obsessional and paranoid traits occur frequently.

TREATMENT

When hypochondriasis is mild and related to stress, it usually subsides when the stressful circumstances pass and the patient is given reassurance. When hypochondriasis is secondary to a psychiatric disorder, it usually improves when the primary disorder has been treated successfully. If the personality is abnormal, treatment is difficult.

Patients with persistent hypochondriasis often demand repeated investigations, but these demands should be resisted when appropriate investigations have been completed. Repeated discussions of the complaints are seldom helpful and should be replaced, if possible, by discussion of any stressful life problems. Whilst showing sympathy, the doctor should indicate clearly that the patient's distress is recognized but that firm rules are needed about the frequency and length of interviews. Many patients request repeated reassurance from their families as well as from doctors; family reassurance usually prolongs the condition, so relatives should be helped to resist such requests. Some patients check the functions or appearance of their bodies; this behaviour should be discouraged because it maintains hypochondriacal concerns.

Special care is needed when a patient believes that a supposed physical illness exonerates them from personal failure. If this psychological defence is removed, the patient may fall into a state of despair, which is more serious than the hypochondriasis.

Review by a psychiatrist can be helpful in identifying the minority of hypochondriacal patients with a depressive or other psychiatric disorder. The psychiatrist may be able to suggest ways of managing some patients, but there is no established treatment for primary hypochondriasis. As hypochondriasis confers no protection against physical illness, some hypochondriacal patients eventually develop a serious medical condition. For this reason, new symptoms should be investigated as carefully in these patients as in any others.

REFERENCES

Barsky, A.J. and Klerman, G.L. (1983). Over-view: Hypochondriasis, bodily complaints and somatic styles. *American Journal of Psychiatry*, **140,** 273–83.

Barsky, A.J., Wyshak, G., and Klerman, J.L. (1990). Transient hypochondriasis. *Archives of General Psychiatry*, **46**, 746–52.

Kellner, R. (1985). Functional somatic symptoms and hypochondriasis: A survey of empirical studies. *Archives of General Psychiatry*, **42**, 821–33.

Pilowsky, I. (1970). Primary and secondary hypochondriasis. *Acta Psychiatrica Scandinavica*, **46**, 273–85.

Dysmorphophobia

Dysmorphophobia is a persistent and inappropriate concern about the appearance of the body, for example the shape of the nose or ears. The intensity of the conviction varies, but in some people it is delusional. In these cases it is important to search for signs of schizophrenia, which is an occasional cause of this symptom. In most cases, however, no associated psychiatric disorder is present. The condition is seen mainly by plastic surgeons and dermatologists; the cause is unknown. Psychological treatment seldom lessens the concerns of patients who receive plastic surgery; whilst some patients are satisfied, many continue to be dissatisfied with their appearance. It is not easy to predict the outcome of surgery, but a joint assessment by a psychiatrist and a surgeon is often helpful.

REFERENCE

Hay, G. (1970). Dysmorphophobia. *British Journal of Psychiatry*, **116**, 399–406.

Psychogenic pain

Psychogenic pain may be experienced in any part of the body, but the head, neck, and lower back are the common sites. Psychogenic pain is most often associated with depressive disorders and anxiety disorders (in the latter pain may be associated with increased muscle tension). Pain may also be a symptom of dissociative disorder. Whenever psychogenic pain has been diagnosed, there should be careful follow-up to exclude an organic disorder.

Diagnosis depends on taking a careful history of the quality, site, and timing of the pain; these features can then be compared with the features of pain with organic causes. At the same time an enquiry should be made to elicit any symptoms of the relevant psychiatric disorders. Although descriptions of psychogenic pain are often vague and dramatic, such descriptions should not influence the diagnosis because they depend more on the patient's personality than on the cause of the pain.

Attempts have been made to identify the characteristics of pain-prone patients but the results are not convincing. It is not known why complaints of pain are made by some emotionally disturbed people but not by others. It has been suggested that pain may be provoked by pent-up anger or guilt. This explanation is not convincing in general, but may apply to some patients.

PROGNOSIS

The prognosis of psychogenic pain is that of the associated psychiatric disorder.

TREATMENT

If there is a psychiatric disorder, it should be treated in the usual way. Otherwise, the patient should be helped to reduce any stressors or internal conflicts, and should be encouraged to live as normal a life as possible despite the pain.

REFERENCE

Feinmann, C. Harris, M., and Cawley, R. (1974). Psychogenic pain: Presentation and treatment. *British Medical Journal*, **228**, 436–8.

Table 1 *Principal dissociative symptoms**

Motor symptoms	Seizures
	Paralysis
	Aphonia and mutism
	Tremor
	Tics
	Disorders of gait
Sensory symptoms	Anaesthesia
	Paraesthesia
	Pain
	Deafness
	Blindness
Mental symptoms	Amnesia
	Pseudodementia
	Fugue
	Stupor

*Motor and sensory symptoms are called conversion symptoms in the American Classification (DSMIV).

27.2.4 Dissociative disorder

M. G. GELDER

Dissociative disorder is the term used in the International Classification of Diseases to refer to the syndrome previously called hysteria. In dissociative disorder, signs and symptoms resembling those of organic disease occur in the absence of corresponding physical pathology. These signs and symptoms are caused not by malingering but by psychological processes of which the patient is not completely aware. The symptoms may resemble those of physical disease or those of organic psychiatric disorder. In the International Classification of Diseases both types of symptom are called dissociative disorder. In the United States, however, it is the convention to restrict the term dissociative disorder to symptoms resembling psychiatric disorder, while the term conversion disorder is applied to symptoms resembling physical disorder. The term dissociative denotes failure to integrate different aspects of mental activity, for example to integrate the intention to move a limb with the processes that initiate movement. The term conversion derives from the notion of mental distress being converted into physical symptoms. In addition to unexplained physical symptoms, three features characterize dissociative disorder: the disorder begins in stressful circumstances; there is 'secondary gain', that is, the symptoms enable the patient to avoid stressful circumstances; and there is 'belle indifference', that is, an apparent lack of distress about the physical symptoms.

It is often extremely difficult to be certain that organic disease has been excluded as a cause of dissociative symptoms. For this reason, the diagnosis of dissociative (or conversion) disorder should be made with great caution, and should be regarded as provisional until appropriate follow-up has confirmed the absence of physical pathology.

CLINICAL FEATURES

Dissociative symptoms are of many kinds (Table 1). The most frequent symptoms are those that resemble disease of the nervous system; despite the resemblance, they differ from the features of organic disease of the nervous system in several important ways. Sometimes the differences are gross; for example a patient may report inability to move a limb, but examination may reveal active but opposed contraction of extensor and flexor muscles. Sometimes the difference is less obvious; for example there may be a discrepancy between the distribution of the patient's sensory impairment and the distribution of sensory impairment associated with any possible neurological lesion.

Some dissociative symptoms require special comment. *Dissociative seizures* differ from epileptic seizures in that the patient may appear inaccessible, but does not lose consciousness; convulsive movements lack the regular, stereotyped form seen in epilepsy; and there is no incontinence, cyanosis, injury, or biting of the tongue. It is sometimes difficult to distinguish between complex partial seizures and dissociative seizures; in these cases ambulatory monitoring of the EEG during a seizure helps to decide the diagnosis.

Difficulty in swallowing without an identified organic cause is occasionally due to a dissociative disorder ('globus hystericus'), but it is more often due to an undetected organic lesion. For this reason, physical investigation should be particularly thorough before the diagnosis of dissociative disorder is made, and follow-up should be especially careful.

Amnesia is the most frequent dissociative mental symptom. It differs from amnesia caused by organic disease in affecting the recall of distant memories as much as the recall of recent ones. In dissociative memory disorder, there may be denial of awareness of personal identity (in memory disorder due to organic causes, amnesia occurs only as part of a severe general intellectual deterioration). Diagnosis can be difficult because dissociative memory disorder may occasionally be provoked (for unknown reasons) by organic brain disease at a stage when there are no localizing neurological signs. Dissociative memory disorder may also follow a head injury, and may occur in epilepsy and multiple sclerosis.

The term *dissociative pseudodementia* is applied to a syndrome in which patients respond to tests of general intellectual functions with answers that are wrong but systematically related to the question (e.g. $7 + 3 = 11$; $8 + 5 = 14$). The syndrome is rare, but has been described in patients with parietal lobe lesions; hence the diagnosis of dissociative pseudodementia should be made cautiously. Systematic wrong answering can also be due to malingering.

The term *compensation neurosis* refers to psychologically determined physical or mental symptoms occurring when there is an unsettled claim for compensation. Although the condition has been grouped with hysteria in the past, few cases are due to dissociative disorder. Most are prolongations of physical disability that are induced by a variety of psychological and social factors. These factors include but are not restricted to the unsettled claim.

The term *epidemic hysteria* refers to the spread of dissociative symptoms among a group of people, usually members of a closed social group such as a school or hostel, often at a time of stress for the group. Usually the epidemic begins when a member of the group has a definite or suspected physical illness which alarms the others. A few people then develop dissociative symptoms resembling those of the primary case. Other members of the group become anxious, and progressively more people become affected.

DIFFERENTIAL DIAGNOSIS

Many of the important points have been mentioned above. The difficulties in distinguishing dissociative disorder from undiagnosed organic disease are so great that the diagnosis of hysteria should generally be regarded as provisional until adequate follow-up has been carried out. When in doubt it is helpful to consider four points. First, dissociative disorder occurs in response to stress; if no stressors can be identified the diagnosis of dissociative disorder is less likely. The finding of stressful circumstances, however, does not add to the evidence for dissociative disorder because such circumstances are often associated with organic disease by chance. Second, secondary gain is invariable in hysteria and its absence is against the diagnosis. The presence of secondary gain, however, does not add to the evidence for dissociative disorder because the limitations imposed by physical illness sometimes result in patients avoiding stressful situations. Third, 'belle indifference' (apparent lack

of distress) is a non-specific symptom not restricted to dissociative disorder. Fourth, dissociative disorder seldom occurs for the first time in patients over the age of 40 years. By paying attention to these four points many errors of diagnosis can be avoided.

Dissociative disorder has to be distinguished from two kinds of behaviour. The first is malingering, in which symptoms are produced by deliberate deception and for obvious gain; the second is factitious disorder in which symptoms are produced deliberately for reasons that are related to complex psychological problems. Malingering is uncommon except in prisons or the armed services, or occasionally in legal claims for compensation. Malingering cannot be sustained consistently for long periods; but the symptoms and signs of dissociative disorder persist when the patient believes they are unobserved. In practice, the distinction is less clear-cut because some patients with dissociative disorder exaggerate their symptoms deliberately, especially when they think that the doctor is unsympathetic. Factitious disorder is considered in a separate section below.

PROGNOSIS

Most dissociative disorders of recent onset recover quickly, but when symptoms have lasted for a year they usually persist for several more. As explained already, physical disease is often missed in patients who are thought to have dissociative symptoms. In one series from a specialist neurological hospital, one-third of patients diagnosed as having 'hysteria' developed an organic disease during 7 to 11 years of follow-up.

TREATMENT

Treatment is along simple practical lines. First, information should be given to the patient about the steps that have been taken to exclude physical pathology. Second, an unhurried explanation should be given of the nature and origins of the condition. It is not enough to leave the patient with a list of conditions that have been ruled out; the patient should understand that the symptoms have arisen in response to stress, by a dissociation of psychological functions. This process can be explained as a difficulty in exerting voluntary control over movement, or in integrating sensory input. This explanation requires time and can seldom be given effectively in the course of a busy ward round.

After this explanation, the focus of concern should be directed away from the symptoms to the stressful problems that provoked them. In helping the patient to resolve these problems, the form of counselling known as problem-solving should be used. The patient should be assured that the physical symptoms will improve. It is often useful to arrange physiotherapy to encourage mobility or restore sensory awareness. Further psychological treatment should focus on ways of dealing with stressful problems more effectively in the future. As explained above, it is important to confirm the diagnosis by follow-up; for this purpose observations should be as unobtrusive as possible to ensure that the patient is not made more anxious by them.

More complex psychological treatment is seldom more effective than these simple measures. In dynamic psychotherapy patients with dissociative disorder readily produce memories of traumatic experiences in earlier life, but few show lasting benefit from such treatment.

REFERENCES

Mersky, H. (1979). *An analysis of hysteria.* Bailliere Tindall, London.
Slater, E. and Glithero, E. (1965). A follow-up of patients diagnosed as suffering from hysteria. *Journal of Psychosomatic Research*, **9**, 9–13.
Toone, B.K. (1990). Disorders of hysterical conversion. In *Somatization: Physical symptoms and psychological illness*, (ed. C. Bass). pp. 207–34. Blackwells, Oxford.

27.2.5 Malingering and factitious disorders

M. G. GELDER

Malingering is the deliberate and fraudulent production of physical of psychological symptoms with the motive of financial gain or other reward. Malingering is seen most often in prisoners or members of the armed forces who wish to avoid some duty that is required of them, or in people who are attempting to obtain financial compensation for supposed injury or illness. Malingering should be diagnosed only after full investigation.

The term *factitious disorder* refers to the deliberate production of physical or psychological symptoms when there is no obvious material gain of the kind seen in malingering. Instead the gain is psychological, and often related to complex abnormalities of personality. Both malingering and factitious disorder need to be distinguished from dissociative disorder (see Chapter 27.2.4), in which physical or psychological symptoms bring some advantage to the patient but are produced unconsciously, not deliberately. The distinctions between the three disorders depend on judgements by the physician as to whether there is clear benefit to the patient, and whether or not the patient has deliberately produced the symptoms. Often these judgements can be made without difficulty, but sometimes they are very difficult. Some factitious disorders consist of a single symptom, for example recurring skin lesions (dermatitis artefacta), bruising, or self-induced fever. Some patients deliberately aggravate a true physical illness, for example by preventing the healing of varicose ulcers.

The term *dermatitis artefacta* refers to skin lesions that the patient produces deliberately but without admitting it. Another well recognized form of factitious disorder is the production of artefactual fever by falsifying thermometer readings. Both conditions are usually episodes in a long history of emotional difficulties arising from a disorder of personality.

The most extreme form of factitious disorder is *Munchausen's syndrome*, a rare disorder in which patients present repeatedly with dramatic symptoms that suggest the need for urgent medical or surgical treatment. Munchausen's syndrome was described first by Asher in 1951, and was named after Baron Munchausen whose extravagant fabrications and restless wanderings had been described by Rudolph Raspe in 1787. The name has been criticized because Baron Munchausen did not present the clinical picture now named after him, but no alternative name has been generally accepted.

Munchausen's syndrome is more common in men than women, and usually begins before middle age. The patient feigns an acute and urgent illness and gives a plausible and often dramatic history, which is subsequently found to be false. There may be spurious physical signs, for example self-induced bleeding from the urinary or gastrointestinal tract, or haematemesis caused by ingested blood. When a full history has been compiled, it is usually found that the patient has been admitted many times to different hospitals, often far apart, and that the patient has usually discharged himself before investigations could be completed.

The presenting symptoms fall into several groups, including: (1) acute abdominal symptoms, which are sometimes accompanied by the deliberate ingestion of foreign bodies, complaints of severe abdominal pain, and requests for powerful analgesics; (2) episodes of bleeding from the urinary tract or gastrointestinal tract; (3) neurological symptoms; (4) repeated lesions of the skin; (5) simulated symptoms of cardiac or respiratory disease. Some patients have the scars of multiple operations, including laparotomies and sometimes craniotomies. The personality is often characterized by failure to make close relationships, aggressive behaviour, restlessness, and extreme forms of lying.

Patients usually arrive in the emergency department of a hospital during the night or at weekends, when they are less likely to be seen immediately by senior staff. They go to great lengths to deceive staff, giving false names and addresses and withholding information about previous hospital admissions. The assessment of these patients can be very difficult, not least because they may at times develop physical disease after some years of feigning ill health. These patients often have detailed medical knowledge and give histories which, although false, are extremely convincing.

The aetiology of Munchausen's syndrome is not known. The patients go to extreme lengths to imitate illness with no obvious motive for doing so. These features strongly suggest a profound disorder of personality. The nature and origins of this disorder can seldom be determined because patients avoid giving accurate information about their past. Although some patients attempt to get powerful analgesics, most are not addicted to drugs. Those who obtain opiates by simulated illness could have done so in other ways. When an accurate history can be obtained, it often reveals a severely disrupted childhood with parental abuse or neglect and sometimes prolonged hospital treatment.

The management of these patients is difficult. Psychiatric treatment is rarely effective, and the patients seldom remain in hospital long enough to receive it. After physical disease has been excluded, the immediate treatment is to tell the patient of the findings, though not in a confrontational way which would only increase hostility and lack of cooperation. Help should be offered for any social problems that can be identified, but most patients refuse it. If the patient agrees, a psychiatric opinion can be obtained; this may throw more light on the complex motivation for the behaviour, but is unlikely to result in effective treatment that the patient will accept.

REFERENCES

Adnan, R.P., Fanci, A.S., Dale, D.C. Herzeberg, J.H., and Wolff, S.M. (1979). Factitious fever and self induced infection: A report of 32 cases and a review of the literature. *Annals of International Medicine*, **90**, 230–42.

Asher, R. (1951). Munchausen's syndrome. *Lancet*, **i**, 339–40.

Fabisch, W. (1980). Psychiatric aspects of dermatitis artefacta. *British Journal of Dermatology*, **102**, 29–34.

Reich, P. and Gottfried, L. (1983). Factitious disorders in a teaching hospital. *Annals of International Medicine*, **99**, 240–7.

Sussman, N. and Hyler, S.E. (1985). Factitious disorders. In *Comprehensive textbook of psychiatry*, (5th edn). (ed. H.I. Kaplan and B.J. Saddock). Williams and Wilkins, Baltimore.

27.2.6 Personality and its disorders

M. G. GELDER

The term personality refers to the enduring characteristics of an individual that are shown as ways of behaving in a wide variety of circumstances. Personality is important to physicians because it determines ways in which patients react to illness and treatment. When the personality is so abnormal as to cause suffering to the person or to other people, the person is said to have a personality disorder.

CLINICAL FEATURES

There are many different kinds of personality and personality disorder and only those of special interest to the physician will be described here (a comprehensive account is given in the *Oxford textbook of psychiatry*).

Obsessional personality

People with obsessional personality have rigid views, adapt poorly to change, and expect high standards of performance from themselves and others. They readily feel guilt, are often moralistic, and do not enjoy themselves easily. Some obsessional people are indecisive, seek more and more advice, and worry about a decision once made. Although outwardly courteous and eager to please, obsessional people often harbour unexpressed feelings of irritation or anger. They do not respond well to the changes imposed by illness, and they may find it difficult to make choices about treatment. They are irritated by small deviations from a care-plan, and may harbour unexpressed indignation at failures to reach their own unrealistic standards.

Histrionic (hysterical) personality

This personality is characterized by self-dramatization and a shallow, self-centred approach to relationships. When ill, histrionic people may appear demanding, selfish, and inconsiderate. They may describe symptoms in a demonstrative way and may show extremes of emotion. This combination of features is sometimes called 'hysterical overlay'.

Paranoid personality

People with this kind of personality are markedly sensitive, touchy and suspicious. They distrust other people, and are secretive, argumentative, and ungrateful. Such people take offence easily and yet behave in ways that invite rebuffs. People of this kind make difficult patients. They seem constantly ungrateful for efforts to help them, and they may complain about their treatment unreasonably and for a long time.

Schizoid personality

People with schizoid personalities are emotionally cold, introspective, and unduly self-sufficient. They appear aloof and ill at ease in company, and do not make friends easily. When ill, schizoid people underplay their suffering and confide little in their doctors. Their lack of warmth and their social awkwardness make it difficult for doctors to discover their real concerns.

Antisocial personality disorder

This disorder is also called psychopathic personality. There are four important features of this kind of personality: impulsive actions, lack of guilt, failure to make loving relationships, and failure to learn from experience. Antisocial people are heartless and aggressive, and may be cruel and violent. They are often inadequate parents, and may neglect or abuse their children. These antisocial qualities may be obvious, or masked by superficial and deceptive charm. Antisocial people lack consistent goals, and seek immediate gratification rather than long-term achievement. They often break the law. Their behaviour is often made worse by overindulgence in alcohol or drugs. When ill, antisocial people are difficult and demanding patients. They often expect immediate help, but generally avoid taking responsibility for themselves, and fail to comply with long-term plans for treatment. When frustrated they may become angry and at times dangerous. Doctors can offer only as much care as the patient will allow at the time, whilst keeping in touch with the patient and watching for problems in the family over a long period. In this way, even if the patient cannot be helped, at least harmful behaviour to others be reduced.

Other types of personality and personality disorder

Several other kinds of personality and personality disorder are recognized but are of less concern to physicians and will therefore be mentioned briefly. Affective personality disorder is characterized by persistently low mood or, less often, persistently elevated mood. People with cyclothymic personalities have alternations of mood: when their mood is high they may take on new tasks and responsibilities with enthusiasm; when their mood becomes low they see these tasks as stressful burdens. Explosive personality disorder has two features of the antisocial personality – readiness to anger and aggressive acts – but not the other abnormal features. People with asthenic personality disorder are weak-willed, easily led, and lack vigour; they have many dissatisfactions, often about their health or medical care, but do little to help themselves.

AETIOLOGY

The causes of personality disorder are uncertain. The available evidence is reviewed in *The Oxford Textbook of psychiatry*, and will not be considered here.

DIFFERENTIAL DIAGNOSIS

Personality disorder is diagnosed when there is a continuous history of abnormal behaviour from the teenage years. In contrast, mental disorders start after a period of normal psychological functioning. Two circumstances may give rise to difficulty in diagnosis. First, in adolescence abnormal behaviour may occasionally be due to a mental disorder. Second, in response to stressful circumstances people with abnormal personalities may exhibit behaviour suggestive of mental disorder. This problem arises mainly when people with paranoid or antisocial personalities respond with behaviour resembling that of schizophrenia. In doubtful cases a psychiatric opinion should be sought.

PROGNOSIS

Patients with personality disorders show little response to treatment. Over the years, however, they may recognize their limitations and may adapt their lives accordingly. They may then present fewer problems to their families and doctors.

TREATMENT

Even with intensive psychological treatment only small changes occur in most personality disorders. It is usually realistic to help the patient to find a way of living that leads to few problems. This adaptation may take several years. The requirement is for a commonsense approach provided by whichever doctor the patient trusts most, who may be a physician caring for a chronic medical illness. A psychiatric assessment may help to determine whether the patient is one of the few patients who could benefit from psychotherapy. Psychiatric management may be helpful when a patient with personality disorder shows an abnormal reaction to stressors. Otherwise psychiatrists can do little more than other doctors for personality disorders.

REFERENCES

Gelder, M.G., Gath, D.H., and Mayou, R. Personality disorder. *Oxford Textbook of Psychiatry*. Oxford University Press.
Vaillant, G.E. and Perry, J.C. Personality disorders. In *Comprehensive textbook of psychiatry* (ed. H.I. Kaplan, A.M. Freedman, and B.J. Sadock). Williams and Wilkins, Baltimore.

27.2.7 Eating disorders

C. G. FAIRBURN

Introduction

The term 'eating disorders' is generally used to refer to two closely related psychiatric syndromes, anorexia nervosa and bulimia nervosa. These disorders share many features and together they are a major source of psychiatric morbidity amongst young women. Anorexia nervosa has long been recognized, with particularly good descriptions being published in the last century (Fig. 1). In contrast, the first series of patients with bulimia nervosa was described as recently as 1979.

Anorexia nervosa

DEFINITION

Three features are required to make a diagnosis of anorexia nervosa. The first is the active maintenance of an unduly low weight: the definition of what constitutes low varies – 15 per cent below the expected weight for the person's age, height, and sex is a widely used figure. The low weight is achieved by a variety of means, including strict dieting or fasting, excessive exercising and, in some, self-induced vomiting. Patients with diabetes mellitus may underuse or omit insulin. Whilst the low weight may be the most striking feature, it is the second feature that is most distinctive. This is the presence of certain characteristic attitudes to shape and weight. These are sometimes described as the 'core psychopathology' and they are pathognomonic of anorexia nervosa and bulimia nervosa. Various expressions have been used to describe them, including the 'relentless pursuit of thinness' and a 'morbid fear of fatness'. These concerns are far more intense than the dissatisfaction with shape and weight experienced by many young women today. The third diagnostic feature is amenorrhoea (in postmenarchal females who are not taking an oral contraceptive).

DISTRIBUTION

Anorexia nervosa is largely confined to women aged between 10 and 30 years and to Western countries in which thinness for women is considered attractive. Estimates of the incidence of the disorder range from 0.24 to 14.6 per 100 000 female population per annum and it seems that the incidence has increased in recent decades. Estimates of the prevalence of the disorder amongst adolescent girls, the group most at risk, range from 0.2 to 1.1 per cent. The disorder is rarely encountered among men (less than 10 per cent of cases are male) and it is also uncommon among non-whites. The social class distribution seems to be uneven, with an over-representation of cases from the upper socioeconomic groups.

DEVELOPMENT OF THE DISORDER

The onset of anorexia nervosa is usually in adolescence, although prepubertal cases are encountered and occasionally the disorder does not begin until adulthood. Often it starts as normal adolescent dieting, which then gets out of control. As the dieting intensifies, weight falls and physiological and psychological features characteristic of semistarvation develop. Additional methods of controlling shape and weight may be adopted at any stage. The characteristic attitudes to shape and weight do not tend to develop until slightly later on.

Fig. 1 A patient of Sir William Gull's before and after treatment (21 April 1887 and 14 June 1887). (Reprinted with permission from Ryle, 1936.)

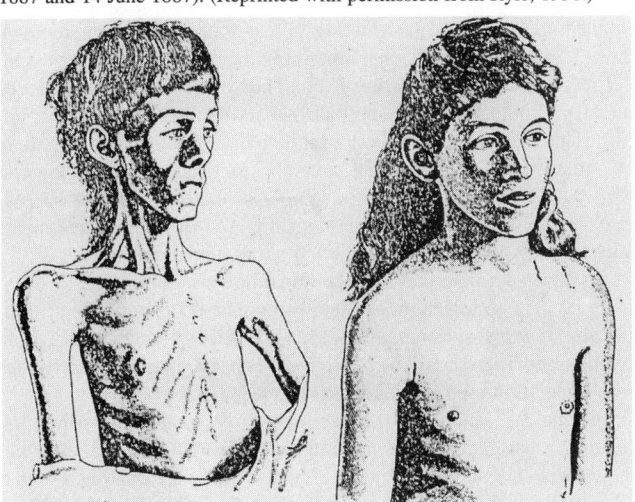

GENERAL CLINICAL FEATURES

The weight loss is mainly achieved through a severe reduction in food intake. The amount consumed may be very small and some patients fast at times. Typically the range of foods eaten is restricted with foods viewed as fattening being avoided. Except in long-standing cases, appetite persists and for this reason the term 'anorexia' is not appropriate. Frequent intense exercising is common and adds to the weight loss. Laxative and diuretic misuse and self-induced vomiting may also be practised, particularly by those patients whose control over eating occasionally breaks down. This happens in about one-third of the patients, but the amount eaten is often not truly large.

Accompanying the abnormal eating habits is the so-called body image disturbance. This takes various forms. It may include a perceptual component such that all, or parts, of the body are seen as larger than their true size, and an attitudinal component characterized by an intense dislike of the body or parts of it. Neither feature improves as weight is lost: indeed, both tend to get worse.

Depressed mood, lability of mood, irritability, anxiety, and obsessional symptoms related to eating are all common features. In more chronic cases there may be hopelessness and thoughts of suicide. There is preoccupation with thoughts about food, eating, shape, and weight, and concentration may be impaired. Outside interests tend to decline as weight is lost and social withdrawal may be marked.

PHYSICAL FEATURES

The physical abnormalities seen in anorexia nervosa have been the subject of much interest. Earlier this century the disorder was mistakenly attributed to pituitary insufficiency, and more recently, and again probably mistakenly, it has been suggested that there might be an underlying primary hypothalamic disorder. The main argument for such a disorder rests upon two observations: first, in a small proportion of patients, menstruation ceases prior to weight loss; and second, restoration of a healthy weight is not always accompanied by the resumption of regular menstruation. However, it is likely that in both these instances the endocrine disturbance responsible for the menstrual dysfunction is secondary to dieting or overexercising, as both are known to affect menstruation and both often precede the onset of weight loss and persist following weight gain.

SYMPTOMS AND SIGNS

Many patients with anorexia nervosa have no physical complaints. However, systematic enquiry often reveals heightened sensitivity to cold and a variety of gastrointestinal symptoms such as constipation, fullness after eating, bloatedness, and vague abdominal pains. Other symptoms encountered include restlessness, lack of energy, low sexual appetite, and early morning wakening. In females who are not taking an oral contraceptive, amenorrhoea is by definition present. Occasionally patients complain of infertility.

On examination, the degree of emaciation may be striking. Growth may be stunted in those with a prepubertal onset and there may be failure of breast development. Unlike patients with hypopituitarism, axillary and pubic hair is preserved and there is no breast atrophy. A fine downy lanugo hair may be present on the back, arms and side of face. Typically the skin is dry and the hands and feet are cold. Blood pressure and pulse are low. There may be dependent oedema.

ABNORMALITIES ON INVESTIGATION

Endocrine abnormalities

Many of the abnormalities have been reproduced in studies of the physiological effects of dieting and are reversed by the restoration of healthy eating habits and a normal weight. Luteinizing hormone releasing hormone (LHRH) secretion is impaired, and as a result levels of luteinizing hormone (LH), follicle stimulating hormone (FSH) and oestradiol are low. There is an immature pattern of luteinizing hormone release. The luteinizing hormone response to LHRH is reduced, but the follicle stimulating hormone response is normal or exaggerated.

Hypothalamic disturbance is also evident in the delayed thyrotrophin (thyroid stimulating hormone; TSH) response to thyrotrophin releasing hormone (TRH). In addition, there is reduced peripheral conversion of thyroxine (T_4) to tri-iodothyronine (T_3), and an increased conversion of thyroxine to inactive reverse tri-iodothyronine. These changes are seen in other chronic illnesses. Thyroxine levels are in the low normal range, whereas tri-iodothyronine levels are depressed. Clinical evidence of hypothyroidism includes sensitivity to cold, constipation, dry skin, and bradycardia.

Plasma cortisol levels are raised and the normal diurnal variation is lost. These changes are due in part to the increased half-life of cortisol seen in starvation and in part to a relative increase in cortisol production. Growth hormone levels are also increased, another secondary effect of starvation. Prolactin secretion is normal.

Haematological changes

A normocytic normochromic anaemia is found in a minority of patients and is sometimes attributable to a low intake of iron or folate. Mild neutropenia is common. The erythrocyte sedimentation rate (ESR) is often low (see Section 22).

Other metabolic abnormalities

Hypercholesterolaemia is frequently present. The mechanism is not understood. Increased serum β-carotene may also be found and reflects increased dietary intake. Life-threatening hypoglycaemia occurs very occasionally, and may not present typically due to an impaired sympathetic response. Electrolyte disturbance is found in those who vomit frequently or misuse large quantities of laxatives or diuretics.

Other abnormalities

Cranial computerized tomography has revealed enlargement of the cortical sulci and cisternes and dilatation of the ventricles. This appears to be reversible and has been termed 'pseudoatrophy'.

In long-standing cases, osteopaenia and osteoporotic fractures are not uncommon and are thought to be secondary to the oestrogen deficiency and low weight. The extent to which the bone loss is reversible has yet to be established.

Delayed gastric emptying and a prolonged gastrointestinal transit time are common and may account for the complaints of fullness after eating, bloatedness, and constipation. Acute gastric dilatation is a rare complication that can be provoked by episodes of overeating or over-vigorous attempts at refeeding.

AETIOLOGY

Predisposing factors

Dieting appears to be a general vulnerability factor for both anorexia nervosa and bulimia nervosa. It is a common precursor, and the two disorders are largely confined to countries in which dieting amongst young women is common. However, whilst many young women diet, few develop an eating disorder. Therefore other aetiological factors must operate. These include a family history of an eating disorder, obesity, and depression. The fact that eating disorders run in families is particularly well established: anorexia nervosa is about eight times more common in the female first degree relatives of anorectic probands than in the general population. The results of twin studies suggest that this vulnerability may be in part genetic in nature. The personal histories of these patients often include reports of long-standing low self-esteem and extreme perfectionism. The finding that communication between family members is often disturbed is difficult to interpret because it has not been established whether the disturbance predates or follows the onset of the eating disorder.

Maintaining factors

As food intake decreases and weight is lost, there are secondary physical and psychological changes, some of which perpetuate the disorder. For example, delayed gastric emptying will tend to result in fullness even after eating small amounts, and social withdrawal may contribute by isolating the person from his or her peers. Those who have been overweight are understandably pleased with the weight loss and may be complimented on it, and many patients report that exerting strict self-control over their behaviour is rewarding in its own right. Sometimes refusing to eat also has gratifying effects within the family.

Assessment

Few patients with anorexia nervosa refer themselves for treatment. Usually they are persuaded to seek help by concerned relatives or friends, and as a consequence they attend somewhat reluctantly.

Careful history-taking from both the patient and, if at all possible, from an informant will make the diagnosis clear. It will be evident that the low weight has been achieved through the patient's own efforts and is associated with the characteristic core psychopathology. No physical tests are required to make the diagnosis. Similarly, unless there are positive reasons to suspect another physical condition, no tests are required to exclude other medical disorders. Excluding the presence of coexisting depressive disorder can be difficult, however, as many depressive symptoms are a known consequence of semistarvation. To make this diagnosis it may be necessary to wait until body weight has been restored to a healthy level. It is more straightforward to exclude the possibility that a depressive disorder is the sole diagnosis because the core psychopathology of anorexia nervosa is not present in depression and the weight loss is rarely self-induced.

Some patients present complaining of features associated with anorexia nervosa rather than the disorder itself. For example, they may present with gastrointestinal symptoms, amenorrhoea or infertility, or with depressive or obsessional symptoms. However, once the weight loss has been identified and it has been found to be self-induced, the diagnosis should be clear.

Whilst physical tests are not required for diagnostic purposes, all patients with anorexia nervosa should have a thorough physical examination and whatever investigations are indicated on the basis of the findings. The electrolytes should be checked of all those who frequently vomit or misuse significant quantities of laxatives or diuretics (see bulimia nervosa).

Management

Patients with anorexia nervosa vary. Some present with short histories and are willing and able to change; others have an entrenched disorder and resist all attempts to help them.

In principle, there are two aspects to treatment. One is establishing healthy eating habits and a normal weight, and the second is the removal of those factors that have been maintaining the disorder. Both are essential. The normalization of eating habits and weight is mainly achieved through a combination of commonsense advice and nutritional counselling. This may be achieved on an inpatient, daypatient, or outpatient basis. Addressing the factors that have been maintaining the eating disorder generally involves the use of more specialized treatments such as family therapy and cognitive behaviour therapy. Both these treatments require training and are best conducted on an outpatient basis.

Drugs have a limited role. Short-acting minor tranquillizers may occasionally be used to lessen the anxiety some patients experience prior to eating and, if depressive symptoms persist following weight restoration, antidepressant drugs should be prescribed. Tube feeding and intravenous hyperalimentation are rarely indicated.

Occasionally it is appropriate to use drugs to stimulate the resumption of regular menstruation. Most patients whose weight has reached a reasonable level and who are eating healthily restart menstruating within 6 to 12 months. If this does not happen, either clomiphene or LHRH are usually effective in inducing menstruation. It is not appropriate to use these drugs with patients who are underweight or who are eating abnormally. Instead, their eating disorder should be addressed.

The initial phase of treatment

There are four aspects to this phase of treatment.

Forming a collaborative therapeutic relationship

This is especially important in patients who are reluctant attenders.

Educating the patient

Patients need to learn about the clinical features of anorexia nervosa, the factors relevant to its development and maintenance, and the importance of weight gain. Certain popular books may be recommended.

Agreeing that there is a need for weight gain

A major goal is to establish the need for weight gain. In doing so, it is also important to emphasize that weight restoration is only one part of treatment, albeit a necessary one.

Deciding upon the treatment setting

Most patients with anorexia nervosa may be managed on an outpatient basis. Some need an initial period of daypatient or inpatient treatment followed by outpatient care. Outpatient treatment is not appropriate if the patient's physical health is a cause for concern, or if the patient is depressed and at risk of suicide. Physical indications for admission include a weight below 70 per cent of the expected weight for the person's age, height, and sex, rapid weight loss, and the presence of medical complications such as massive oedema, severe electrolyte disturbance, and significant intercurrent infection. Under these circumstances admission should be to a general medical ward or a psychiatric unit with good access to general medical help. Partial or full hospitalization is also indicated if no progress is being made with outpatient care or there are no outpatient facilities nearby.

Not infrequently, inpatient treatment is indicated, but the patient does not want to be admitted. Under these circumstances, unless immediate hospitalization is essential, two options are available: either management on a daypatient basis or a brief trial of outpatient treatment. If the latter option is chosen, patients should be asked to demonstrate that they can gain weight at a reasonable rate (about 1 kg per week). It should be agreed that if they do not succeed, they will come into hospital. A small number of patients refuse admission even though their life is in danger. In such cases compulsory hospitalization must be seriously considered.

Inpatient treatment

Admission may be to a general or psychiatric hospital. In either case it is a great advantage if the ward staff are experienced in the management of these patients. Weight restoration may be achieved in either setting, but with a psychiatric admission it is easier to make arrangements for the other forms of treatment needed to maximize the chance that progress will be maintained following discharge.

Within a few days of admission, patients should be introduced to the consumption of regular meals and snacks consisting of between 1000 and 1500 kcal a day; and, if possible, by the end of 2 weeks these should be of a normal quantity and composition, consisting of about 2000 kcal a day. However, it is important to note that over-rapid refeeding is dangerous because it may result in severe fluid retention, cardiac failure, or acute gastric dilatation. A target weight gain of about 1 kg per week should be set with the patient and staff monitoring the weight gain each morning. As between 3000 and 5000 kcal a day are likely to be required to achieve this rate of weight gain, average-sized meals and snacks will not be sufficient. It is the author's view that the best solution is to supplement the patient's diet with energy-rich drinks rather than additional food. Supplements of this type seem preferable to encouraging them to overeat, which does little to help establish healthy eating habits and may increase the risk that they develop bulimia nervosa.

The target weight range should be one at which the patient is eating healthily and not dieting, and one at which normal physiological functioning is restored. Once patients enter the target range, the energy-rich drinks should be phased out, leaving them consuming a diet sufficient to maintain their weight. At this stage patients should be given full control over their eating and they should be encouraged to shop, cook, and eat out with friends and family. Unless considerable effort is put into this phase of treatment, the risk of relapse after discharge is considerable.

Running concurrently with weight restoration should be other forms of therapy. At first, straightforward support is often best, but once the patient's mental state begins to improve, more specific treatments may be introduced including family therapy and cognitive behavioural procedures.

With an inpatient regime of this type, body weight is usually restored to a healthy range within 2 to 3 months and the patient discharged 2 to 4 weeks later. The transition from inpatient to outpatient care should be carefully planned.

Daypatient treatment

There is increasing interest in the use of daypatient treatment in place of full hospitalisation for all but the most ill patients. A comprehensive treatment programme can be provided, including supervised eating and weight gain, whilst patients remain based in their usual social environment. The hope is that daypatient treatment will be found to be associated with a reduced risk of relapse following discharge. This has not yet been established.

Outpatient treatment

This may be the sole form of treatment or it may follow a period of inpatient or daypatient care. Various approaches are used from simple support and encouragement through to sophisticated forms of individual and family therapy. There has been so little research on the overall management of anorexia nervosa that firm recommendations cannot be made. There is evidence to suggest that family therapy should be used with young patients, and there is interest in using cognitive behavioural techniques with those who are older. (The cognitive behavioural approach is described in outline in the section on bulimia nervosa.)

Course and outcome

For some, anorexia nervosa is a relatively benign self-limiting disorder; for others, up to one-quarter of sufferers, it may lead to death or chronic disability. Few consistent predictors of outcome have been identified, the exceptions being a long history and late onset, both of which are associated with a poor prognosis. The presence of a low body weight, bulimic episodes, self-induced vomiting or laxative abuse, and a history of premorbid psychosocial problems, also tends to be associated with a poor outcome.

Whilst at least half the patients recover in terms of their weight and menstrual function, the disturbed attitudes to shape and weight often persist and eating habits may remain disturbed. Up to one-quarter of the patients develop bulimia nervosa. Standardized mortality ratios have been reported between 1.36 and 6.01, the deaths being either a direct result of medical complications or due to suicide. The most recent follow-up studies have been obtaining lower mortality figures suggesting that the rate is falling. The outcome in males appears to be essentially the same as that in females.

Bulimia nervosa

DEFINITION

Three features are required to make a diagnosis of bulimia nervosa. The first is the presence of frequent bulimic episodes. By definition, these 'binges' involve the consumption of unusually large amounts of food, given the circumstances, and a sense of loss of control at the time. The second is the use of extreme behaviour to control body shape and weight. This behaviour resembles that used by patients with anorexia nervosa, although self-induced vomiting and laxative or diuretic misuse are much more common. The third feature is the presence of attitudes to shape and weight similar to those found in anorexia nervosa.

There are some patients with anorexia nervosa who have bulimic episodes similar to those of patients with bulimia nervosa and are therefore potentially eligible for both diagnoses. In practice both diagnoses are not given: instead, the diagnosis of anorexia nervosa is given precedence over that of bulimia nervosa.

DISTRIBUTION

People with bulimia nervosa are somewhat older than those with anorexia nervosa, most presenting in their twenties, and they have a broader social class distribution. The disorder is rarely seen in men.

There has been considerable interest in the prevalence of the disorder. Amongst young women in Britain and North America the rate is between 1 and 2 per cent, with the great majority of cases not having come to medical attention. Whilst there are no satisfactory data on the incidence of bulimia nervosa, it seems that the disorder has become more common over the past 25 years. In all countries in which anorexia nervosa is found, there has been a dramatic upsurge in the number of cases of bulimia nervosa: from being viewed as an unusual variant of anorexia nervosa, it is now the most common eating disorder encountered in psychiatric practice (Fig. 2).

GENERAL CLINICAL FEATURES

There are marked similarities between the clinical features of bulimia nervosa and those of anorexia nervosa. The patients share the same extreme concerns about shape and weight and engage in the same methods of weight control. However, two features distinguish bulimia nervosa from anorexia nervosa: first, the body weight of most patients is in the healthy range; second, there are frequent bulimic episodes. These binges are a source of great shame, they are kept secret and, in the

Fig. 2 Annual rates of referral to an eating disorder centre in Canada (Clarke Institute of Psychiatry and The Toronto General Hospital). Reprinted with permission from Garner and Fairburn, 1988.

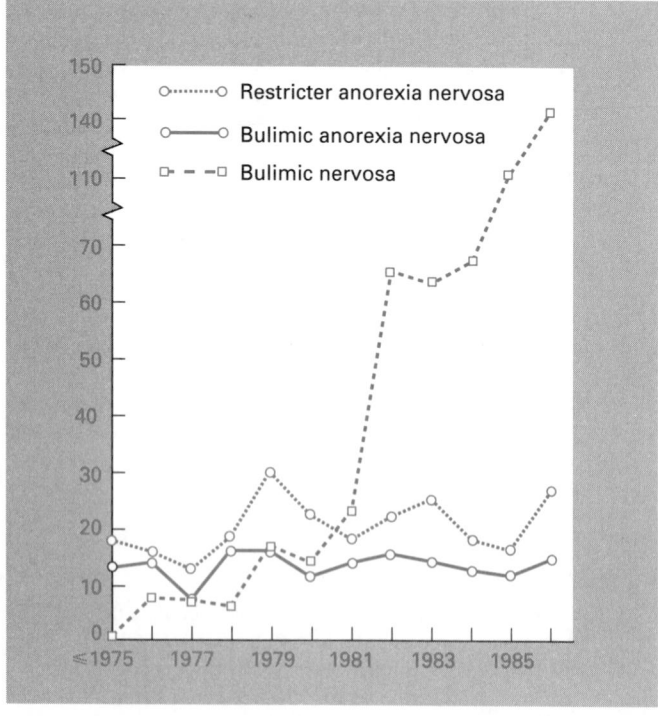

majority of cases, they are followed by self-induced vomiting or the taking of laxatives. Contrary to the impression given by the popular term 'carbohydrate craving', the proportion of carbohydrate eaten is not remarkable: the distinctive feature is the overall amount of food consumed, on average about 3000 kcal per episode. Some bulimic episodes are extremely large and carry the risk, albeit remote, of acute gastric dilatation or rupture. Between episodes, the patients restrict their food intake in much the same way as patients with anorexia nervosa.

Depressive and anxiety symptoms are also a prominent feature, more so than in anorexia nervosa. A significant minority have problems with alcohol or drugs.

PHYSICAL FEATURES

The majority of patients have few physical complaints. Those most commonly encountered are irregular or absent menstruation, weakness and lethargy, vague abdominal pains, and toothache. On examination, appearance is usually unremarkable. Salivary gland enlargement may be present: typically, this involves the parotids and gives the patient's face a slightly rounded appearance. Sometimes it is associated with a raised serum amylase level, the increase being in the salivary isoenzyme. The underlying pathophysiology is not understood. In those who vomit there may be calluses on the dorsum of the dominant hand (Russell's sign) due to the fingers being used to stimulate the gag reflex. Also, there may be significant erosion of the dental enamel particularly on the lingual surface of the upper front teeth. A minority of patients, particularly those who take large quantities of laxatives or diuretics, have intermittent peripheral or facial oedema.

ABNORMALITIES ON INVESTIGATION

Of most importance is the electrolyte disturbance which is encountered in about half those who vomit or take laxatives or diuretics. Metabolic alkalosis, hypochloraemia, and hypokalaemia are the most common abnormalities and they may account for the weakness and tiredness (and on rare occasions hypokalaemic paralysis) experienced by some patients. The overall picture may resemble Bartter's syndrome and has been termed 'pseudoBartter's syndrome', as it is self-inflicted and usually reversible. Severe electrolyte disturbance is encountered occasionally, particularly low potassium levels, but even when it is long-standing there may be surprisingly few accompanying symptoms. Despite concern about possible cardiac arrhythmias, nephrogenic diabetes insipidus, and the suggestion that chronic hypokalaemia may induce changes in the renal proximal tubular cells, aggressive treatment of this type of chronic electrolyte disturbance is rarely appropriate: instead, it should be monitored but the focus kept on the treatment of the eating disorder itself.

Endocrine abnormalities may be present. These resemble those in anorexia nervosa, but they are not as severe. They are thought to be secondary to the strict dieting and they are probably reversible given that the menstrual disturbance responds to the successful treatment of the eating disorder. There have been recent reports that ovarian morphology is abnormal in a high proportion of cases. This is also likely to be reversible.

AETIOLOGY

Many patients with bulimia nervosa give a history of disturbed eating stretching back into adolescence, and about one-third have previously fulfilled diagnostic criteria for anorexia nervosa. Most of the remainder started with an anorexia nervosa-like picture although the weight loss was not of sufficient magnitude to allow the diagnosis to be made. Given this sequence of events and the fact that the two conditions are so similar, it may be assumed that most factors of relevance to the aetiology of anorexia nervosa are also relevant to the aetiology of bulimia nervosa. Nevertheless, it seems that some factors may specifically increase the risk of developing bulimia nervosa rather than anorexia nervosa. These include vulnerability to obesity, affective disorder, and substance abuse, the rates of all three disorders being increased amongst the relatives of these patients.

ASSESSMENT

Most people with bulimia nervosa are ashamed of their eating habits and keep them secret for many years. Like those with anorexia nervosa, when they present for help they may complain of features associated with the disorder rather than the disorder itself. For example, they may present with gastrointestinal or gynaecological symptoms, depression, or substance abuse. Under these circumstances making the correct diagnosis may be difficult because there are rarely any clear pointers to the eating disorder.

Those patients who present complaining of the eating disorder are generally referred to psychiatrists, and, unlike those with anorexia nervosa, they are usually eager to receive treatment. Assessment is straightforward and the diagnosis can be made with little difficulty. As with anorexia nervosa, no physical tests are needed to make the diagnosis. However, the electrolytes should be checked of all those who frequently vomit or misuse large quantities of laxatives or diuretics.

TREATMENT

The treatment of bulimia nervosa has been the subject of much research. It is clear that the great majority of patients may be managed on an outpatient basis. Full or partial hospitalization is indicated under four unusual circumstances: first, if the patient is either too depressed to be managed as an outpatient or there is a risk of suicide; second, if the patient's physical health is a cause for concern; third, if the patient is in the first trimester of pregnancy, because there is some evidence that the spontaneous abortion rate may be high; and fourth, if the eating disorder proves refractory to outpatient care. If hospitalization is indicated, it should be brief and serve as a preliminary to outpatient care.

PSYCHOLOGICAL TREATMENT

The most effective treatment for bulimia nervosa is a specific form of cognitive behaviour therapy. This is a specialized psychological treatment that aims to modify not only the disturbed eating habits but also the disturbed attitudes to shape and weight. It usually involves about 20 sessions over 5 months and results in substantial improvement in all aspects of the psychopathology. The techniques used include the following: the daily self-monitoring of relevant thoughts and behaviour; education about eating, shape and weight; the use of self-control procedures to help establish a pattern of regular eating; the gradual introduction of avoided foods into the patient's diet; and so-called cognitive restructuring procedures designed to identify and challenge problematic thoughts and attitudes.

PHARMACOLOGICAL TREATMENT

Antidepressant drugs are the only pharmacological treatment to have shown promise. They result in a decline in the frequency of overeating and an improvement in mood, but the effect is not as great as that seen with cognitive behaviour therapy and, more importantly, it is often not maintained. These drugs cannot be recommended as a first line treatment. Appetite suppressants have no beneficial effect.

OTHER APPROACHES

Some patients respond to brief educational treatments and self-help manuals probably have a role. For this reason a 'stepped care' approach to treatment delivery has been proposed in which treatments are provided sequentially according to need. This approach involves a simple treatment being used initially and moving on to more complex ones only if the patient fails to respond.

COURSE AND OUTCOME

As yet little is known about the course of bulimia nervosa. Some of the cases identified in community surveys appear to be relatively benign in that they are short lived. In contrast, patients who are referred for treatment often present with long histories and previous unsuccessful attempts at treatment. Most respond well to cognitive behaviour therapy with the changes being maintained for at least the following 12 months. There have been no studies of long-term outcome. The evidence to date suggests that the disorder tends to 'breed true'; that is, it rarely evolves into anorexia nervosa or any other psychiatric disorder.

PREGNANCY AND CHILDREARING

There is growing concern about the effects of eating disorders on pregnancy and childrearing. This topic has come to the fore with the emergence of bulimia nervosa because pregnancy does not often occur in the course of anorexia nervosa. In general it seems that eating disorders tend to improve during pregnancy, but the amount of weight gained may be abnormal. The impact on the fetus has yet to be established, although there have been reports of intrauterine growth retardation and low birth weight. Childrearing is influenced in some cases with adverse effects on both infant feeding and growth.

Atypical eating disorders

In addition to anorexia nervosa and bulimia nervosa, various 'atypical eating disorders' are encountered: indeed, they make up over one-third of all referrals. They have not been well characterized. Most common are disorders resembling anorexia nervosa or bulimia nervosa but not quite meeting their diagnostic criteria, either because one or more features is absent or because the features are not of sufficient severity, or both. In addition, there are people with eating problems distinct from anorexia nervosa and bulimia nervosa. For example, there are those who vomit when anxious, and people who have difficulty eating or swallowing in public. Both these groups should be classed as having an anxiety disorder and treated accordingly. There is another group who stop eating as a way of bringing attention to themselves. Such people generally have major personality difficulties. In common with those with anxiety disorders, they do not show the attitudes to shape and weight that are characteristic of patients with anorexia nervosa and bulimia nervosa. Their management needs to focus on resolving the problems that brought about their refusal to eat, rather than on the disturbed eating itself.

REFERENCES

Brownell, K.D. and Fairburn, C.G. (1995). *Comprehensive handbook of eating disorders and obesity.* Guildford, New York.

Cooper, P.J. (1993). *Bulimia nervosa: A guide to recovery.* Robinson, London.

Fairburn, C.G., Marcus, M.D., and Wilson, G.T. (1993). Cognitive behaviour therapy for binge eating and bulimia nervosa: A comprehensive treatment manual. In *Binge eating: Nature, assessment and treatment* (ed. C.G. Fairburn and G.T. Wilson). Guilford, New York.

Garner, D.M. and Fairburn, C.G. (1988). Relationship between anorexia nervosa and bulimia nervosa: Diagnostic implications. In *Diagnostic issues in anorexia nervosa and bulimia nervosa*, (ed. D.M. Garner and P.E. Garfinkel). Bruner/Mazel, New York.

Garner, D.M. and Garfinkel, P.E. (ed). (1985). *Handbook of psychotherapy for anorexia nervosa and bulimia nervosa.* Guilford, New York.

Kaplan, A.S. and Garfinkel, P.E. (1993). *Medical issues and the eating disorders.* Brunner/Mazel, New York.

Mitchell, J.E., Specker, S.M., and de Zwaan, M. (1991). Comorbidity and medical complications of bulimia nervosa. *Journal of Clinical Psychiatry*, **52,** (10, suppl.), 13–20.

Newman, M.M. and Halmi, K.A. (1988). The endocrinology of anorexia nervosa and bulimia nervosa. *Neurologic Clinics*, **6,** 195–212.

Palmer, J.L. (1988). *Anorexia nervosa*, (2nd edn). Penguin, London.

Russell, G.F.M. (1979). Bulimia nervosa: An ominous variant of anorexia nervosa. *Psychological Medicine*, **9,** 429–48.

Ryle, J.A. (1936). Anorexia nervosa. *Lancet*, **October 17th**, 893–9.

Sharp, C.W. and Freeman, C.P.L. (1993). The medical complications of anorexia nervosa. *British Journal of Psychiatry*, **162,** 452–62.

Strober, M. (1991). Family-genetic studies of eating disorders. *Journal of Clinical Psychiatry*, **52,** 9–12.

Stunkard, A.J. (1993). A history of binge eating. In *Binge eating: Nature, assessment and treatment* (ed. C.G. Fairburn and G.T. Wilson). Guilford, New York.

27.2.8 Affective disorders

D. H. GATH

Affective disorders are those in which a change of mood is the central feature of the syndrome. The mood change may be depression, elation, or rarely a combination of the two.

Depressive disorders

Physically ill patients are often depressed. Often this depression is a normal reaction to the circumstances of illness but sometimes it is a symptom of a depressive disorder. It is important to identify these depressive disorders, which can complicate the management of physical illness, cause suffering and, in severe cases, threaten life. Physicians also encounter patients with depressive disorders when they seek their help for symptoms such as tiredness or weight loss. For these reasons, it is important that physicians should be able to detect and treat depressive disorders.

Depressive disorders are common in the general population: the one year incidence is about 1 to 2 per thousand for men and three times this figure for women. Among physically ill patients the rates are higher, although many cases are unrecognized by physicians because depressed mood is dismissed as a normal reaction to the physical illness, and other symptoms of the depressive disorder have not been elicited.

CLINICAL FEATURES

The central features of a depressive disorder are low mood and impaired capacity for enjoyment shown in social withdrawal and loss of interest in work and hobbies (Table 1). These features are accompanied by two other groups of symptoms. The first group, known as biological symptoms, are reduced energy, sleep disturbance with early morning waking, a worsening of symptoms in the first part of the day ('diurnal variation'), loss of appetite and weight, constipation, low libido, and amenorrhoea. Some patients seek medical help for one or more of these symptoms rather than the mood disorder. The second group, known as cognitive symptoms, are hopelessness and pessimistic thoughts about the future, ruminations about death as a release from suffering and suicidal ideas, and guilty preoccupations.

Other symptoms, which are common but less specific to depression (and therefore of less value in diagnosis), include irritability, anxiety, and poor concentration with consequent poor recall. (True memory disorder does not occur in depressive disorder.)

The patient's facial appearance is of sadness with downturned corners of the mouth and vertical furrows of the brow, and the posture is stooped. Movements and speech are slow and the tone of the voice is monotonous. Occasionally these outward signs of depression are lacking and in

Table 1 *Principal features of depressive disorders*

Low mood
Reduced energy and activities
Loss of enjoyment
Early morning wakening
Diurnal mood variation
Loss of appetite and weight
Complaints of constipation
Loss of libido
Amenorrhoea
Pessimistic thoughts
Guilty recollections
Suicidal ideas

Table 2 *Variations in the clinical picture of depressive disorder*

Anxiety symptoms
Somatic symptoms
Worsening of physical complaints
Failure to comply with medical treatment
Brief depressive episodes
Excessive use of alcohol

these cases it is easy to miss the depressive disorder unless systematic enquiries are made about all the symptoms that make up the syndrome. Other atypical features include restlessness instead of retardation, overeating instead of weight loss, and excessive somnolence instead of insomnia.

Delusions and hallucinations may be present in a severe depressive disorder and, when this happens, the condition is called a psychotic depression. Depressive delusions are concerned with guilt, worthlessness, serious illness, and poverty. Sometimes the delusions are persecutory and in this case patients generally regard the supposed persecution as something they have brought upon themselves; an attitude that contrasts with that of schizophrenic patients who are resentful or angry. Hallucinations are usually of words or phrases that confirm the ideas of guilt and worthlessness (for example a voice saying that the patient is wicked). When delusions and hallucinations are present, suicide risk should be assessed most carefully because it is usually increased, and psychiatric advice should be obtained promptly.

VARIATIONS OF THE CLINICAL PICTURE

Anxiety symptoms

In depressive disorders of mild intensity anxiety symptoms are often present in the form of generalized anxiety by day, early onset insomnia, and phobias. When these anxiety symptoms are more obvious than those of depression, a mistaken diagnosis of anxiety disorder may be made if the mental state is not examined systematically (Table 2).

Somatic symptoms

Some patients complain of tiredness, malaise, poor appetite, constipation, or aches and pains, rather than depressed mood. These patients have the style of thinking that is part of a depressive disorder and interpret these symptoms in a pessimistic way as evidence of serious illness. This depressive thinking makes it hard to reassure these patients who often seek further opinions, or become convinced that they are terminally ill and beyond hope. If the mental state is examined, the correct diagnosis can usually be made.

Worsening of physical complaints

Depressed patients are less able to tolerate discomfort that they endured previously and may seek fresh help for long-standing problems of back pain, osteoarthritis, or bronchitis. If the physical condition is unchanged, the possibility of a physical illness should be considered.

Failure to comply with medical treatment

Depressed patients who lack energy and feel hopeless may neglect the treatment of concurrent physical illness such as diabetes or hypertension. Failure to comply with treatment in a patient who has previously complied well, suggests the possibility of a depressive disorder.

Brief depressive episode

Usually a depressive disorder persists for several months but a few patients have repeated episodes of severe depression lasting for a few days with normal mood between. These brief depressive episodes are difficult to control. Specialist advice should be obtained.

Excessive use of alcohol

Some depressed patients try to improve their mood by taking alcohol. Although there may be a brief lessening of distress, the longer-term effect of alcohol is to increase the mood disorder. Depressive disorder should be considered in cases of excessive drinking.

AETIOLOGY

Family and twin studies have shown that genetic factors are important causes of depressive disorder but linkage studies have not yet identified a relevant gene. Separation from the mother in childhood may predispose to depressive disorder by making the person more vulnerable to adverse circumstances in adult life. This increased vulnerability is reflected in personality; there is no single predisposing personality type but traits of low self-esteem and persistent pessimism are important. Epidemiological studies indicate that depressive disorders are provoked by stressful life events, especially the loss of a close relationship by separation or death. Other physical illnesses can act as a non-specific stressor but influenza, glandular fever, and Parkinson's disease are particularly associated with depressive disorder. There is evidence that the adverse effect of stressful events is less when people have a confidante with whom they can talk about their problems.

Neuroendocrine challenge tests have shown diminished 5-HT function in depressive disorder, and this finding is consistent with the observation that drugs that increase 5-HT function have antidepressant effects. The recent discovery of several subtypes of 5-HT receptor has led to further studies to identify which subtype is involved in depressive disorder. 5-HT$_2$ receptor function appears to be important but the mechanisms have not been worked out fully.

A causal role for endocrine abnormalities is suggested by associations between depressive disorder and Cushing's syndrome and hyperparathyroidism, and with the mood changes associated with the menstrual cycle and childbirth. Such associations could be caused by the action of hormones on neurotransmitter function. Cortisol secretion is increased in depressive disorder and the increase may not be a simple reaction to stress since it involves a change in the diurnal pattern of secretion of cortisol. However this change is not specific to depressive disorder occurring also in some cases of mania, schizophrenia, and dementia.

DIFFERENTIAL DIAGNOSIS

For the physician there are four main diagnostic issues: (1) to distinguish depressive disorder from normal feelings of sadness in physically ill patients; (2) to detect depressive disorder in patients with unexplained physical symptoms; (3) to distinguish depressive disorder from other psychiatric disorders as a cause of physical symptoms and of dementia; and (4) to identify depressive disorder as a cause of excessive use of alcohol.

From normal sadness

This distinction is made by enquiring about other symptoms of a depressive disorder (see Table 2). Biological symptoms are particularly significant, and, although uncommon, psychotic symptoms are even more important. When there is uncertainty, another person who knows the patient may describe features that the patient has not revealed such as loss of energy and diurnal variation

As a cause of unexplained physical symptoms

The first step is to identify the symptoms of the syndrome of depressive disorder. The second step is to establish whether the physical symptoms preceded or followed the depressive symptoms. If the physical symptoms came first it is likely that depressive disorder is secondary to a physical illness rather than the primary problem.

From other psychiatric disorder

When anxiety symptoms are prominent the other symptoms of a depressive disorder may be overlooked. It is important, therefore, to enquire about depressive symptoms when patients complain of anxiety. Some depressed patients complain of poor memory and, when this happens, the possibility must be considered that the primary disorder is dementia, and the depression is secondary. Sometimes the correct diagnosis can be made by determining whether memory disorder preceded or followed the mood change, and by testing memory (depressed patients concentrate badly but remember normally when concentration is ensured). Despite careful observations it is often difficult to be certain of the diagnosis and specialist advice may be needed.

As a cause of alcohol abuse

Some patients with depressive disorder take excessive alcohol to obtain temporary relief of their symptoms. Diagnosis can be difficult because excessive use of alcohol leads to depressed mood, and disturbs sleep. The correct diagnosis may be reached by finding out whether depressed mood preceded or followed the excessive use of alcohol, and systematic examination for other symptoms of a depressive disorder (see Table 2). Often, diagnosis is not certain until the patient has been persuaded to abstain from alcohol for several days.

PROGNOSIS

Most untreated depressive disorders last for 3 to 9 months, although a few persist for several years. Younger patients usually recover completely but in old age residual symptoms are more frequent. Recurrence is common, the risk increasing with the number of previous episodes. A careful history of previous episodes of depression, not all of which may have been treated, is an essential guide to prognosis. Patients with depressive disorder have an increased risk of suicide: 10 to 15 per cent of patients with severe and recurrent depressive disorder eventually die by suicide.

TREATMENT

Most depressive disorders can be managed successfully by physicians but it is important to identify those who require treatment by a psychiatrist. The principal indications for referral to a specialist are: (1) severe depressive disorder especially with hallucinations or delusions, and severe biological symptoms including failure to eat and drink adequately; (2) high suicide risk, or difficulty in assessing suicide risk; (3) failure to respond to treatment by the physician; and (4) relapsing or recurring disorder.

All patients require simple psychological management starting with an explanation that the condition is an illness not a sign of personal failure (Table 3). Easily understood information should be given about the nature of the illness and the good prospect of recovery. Patients should be helped to deal with current problems but exploration of past problems is not appropriate during the acute state of the illness. The

Table 3 *Treatment of a depressive disorder*

Psychological management (see text)
Antidepressant drug
If no response
check compliance
check social factors
increase dose
If continued non-response consider*
adding lithium
changing to monoamine oxidase inhibitor
ECT (electroconvulsive therapy)

*These decisions are usually taken by a specialist.

more severe the depressive disorder, the more the patient should be relieved temporarily of responsibilities and encouraged to live from day to day rather than worry about future difficulties.

If the depressive disorder is mild, these simple measures may be all that is required until spontaneous recovery takes place. However, in most cases of depressive disorder an antidepressant drug should be prescribed. There are many such drugs, which differ in their side-effects but not their therapeutic effects. A commonly used drug is the tricyclic antidepressant amitriptyline, which is well tried and inexpensive. Its sedative side-effect is useful in promoting sleep (the drug is usually given as a single dose at night), but anticholinergic side-effects may be troublesome. To reduce side-effects the starting dose is less than the therapeutic dose and is increased slowly as a degree of tolerance develops (the manufacturer's doses should be followed). Dry mouth, difficulty in visual accommodation, and constipation are among the most frequent side-effects. Anticholinergic effects are likely to cause difficulties for patients with prostatic enlargement or glaucoma. Alternatives to amitriptyline are described in Chapter 27.4.1.

Whatever drug is used there is a delay of usually about 2 weeks before a therapeutic effect occurs. Patients should be warned of this delay and supported during the waiting period. Patients should be warned also of the sedative effect of most of these drugs, especially in relation to driving motor vehicles, the use of machinery at work, and their additive effect with alcohol.

If there is no response within 3 weeks, a check should be made that the medication is being taken (depressed patients may comply poorly because of apathy or hopelessness, or because of unpleasant side-effects). Social factors, such as marital problems, may account for slow recovery and should be enquired into again if they were denied at the first assessment. There is generally no benefit from changing to another antidepressant unless side-effects made it impossible to give a full dose of the first drug and the new drug has a different profile of side-effects. The exception is that monoamine oxidase inhibitors are sometimes effective for patients who have failed to respond to a tricyclic or related antidepressant.

If these measures are ineffective, response to the antidepressant may be augmented by adding lithium carbonate (see Chapter 27.4.1) but this combined treatment is usually initiated by a psychiatrist. Electroconvulsive therapy may be effective in patients who do not respond to combined medication and is valuable in urgent cases because it acts more rapidly than antidepressant drugs (Chapter 27.4.1).

When recovery has taken place drug treatment is continued to prevent relapse, usually for 6 months. Recurrence may be prevented either by prolonging the antidepressant drug beyond 6 months, or by the use of lithium carbonate or another 'mood regulator' (see Chapter 27.4.1).

Mania and manic depressive disorder

Mania is characterized by elevated mood, increased activity, and self-important ideas. When these features are severe, the condition is called

Table 4 *Principal features of mania*

Elevated mood
Increased energy and activity
Expansive ideas
Impaired insight
Reduced sleep
Increased appetite
Increased libido

mania, when mild to moderate it is called hypomania. People who experience mania at one time in their lives usually have a depressive disorder at an other time. This sequence is called manic depressive disorder or bipolar affective disorder (bipolar referring to the opposite 'poles' of mania and depression). Surprisingly, a few patients show features of both mania and depression at the same time (e.g. increased activity with depressive ideas); such patients are said to have a mixed affective disorder.

States of mania are much less common than depressive disorders. Estimates of the annual incidence of manic depressive (bipolar) disorders in the population vary from about 10 to 15 per 100 000 among men and 10 to 30 per 100 000 among women.

CLINICAL FEATURES

The principal features of the syndrome of mania are summarized in Table 4. As noted above they are elevated mood, increased activity, and self-important ideas. Most patients are inappropriately cheerful, but a few are irritable instead. Sleep is reduced, with early wakening, but despite this manic patients wake energetic and refreshed. Behaviour is uninhibited; patients make extravagant purchases or enter into unsound business schemes. In a medical ward, interfering, noisy, or restless behaviour draws attention to the problem, although at first this behaviour may be related to personality rather than illness. Appetite for food and sexual desires are increased. Speech is rapid with rapidly changing topics of conversation ('flight of ideas'), which reflects both a rapid flow of ideas, easy distraction, or the ready use of puns and rhymes. Grandiose ideas are common; less often there are delusions of grandeur, for example, the belief that the patient is a religious prophet or a person destined to play an important role in public life. Because manic patients seldom have insight into the morbid nature of these experiences, it is difficult to obtain their collaboration with treatment.

AETIOLOGY

Family and twin studies show the importance of genetic factors but no linkage has been established to a particular gene. Some episodes are provoked by stressful events, others occur spontaneously. Cyclothymic personality is associated with bipolar disorder but childhood experiences seem to be less important than in depressive disorders (see above). The mechanism of the shift between mania and depression in bipolar cases is not understood.

DIFFERENTIAL DIAGNOSIS

When the behaviour of a physically ill patient becomes disturbed, an important differential diagnosis is between mania and delirium (Chapter 27.2.10); the correct diagnosis can usually be made by determining whether there is presence of clouding of consciousness which is characteristic of the latter. It is sometimes difficult to distinguish mania and acute schizophrenia but this uncertainty seldom causes problems for the physician since the immediate treatment of the two conditions is much the same (see Chapter 27.2.9), and subsequent management is usually by a psychiatrist.

PROGNOSIS

Without treatment, moderate and severe mania lasts usually for a few months, although mild cases may recover more quickly. Although patients recover eventually recurrence is frequent, in the form either of a manic or a depressive disorder.

TREATMENT

Treatment of mania is with drugs and psychological management. It is important to avoid responding to uninhibited behaviour or irritable mood as if it were directed deliberately at the doctor, rather than a symptom of illness because such a response is likely to increase the abnormal behaviour. An antipsychotic drug such has haloperidol will usually control symptoms within a few days. The advice of a psychiatrist should be obtained at an early stage because further treatment of the mania may be difficult and the phase of mania may be followed by severe depression. Further information on initial treatment is given in the sections on the treatment of emergencies (Chapter 27.4.3) and drug treatment (Chapter 27.3.4). After more than one episode of mania lithium carbonate is often prescribed to prevent further recurrence (Chapter 27.4.1).

REFERENCES

Gelder, M.G., Gath, D.H., and Mayou, R. *Oxford textbook of psychiatry*. Oxford University Press.

Hawton, K.E. (1981). The long-term outcome of psychiatric morbidity detected in general medical patients. *Journal of Psychosomatic Research*, **25**, 237–43.

Paykel, E.S. (ed.) (1992). *Handbook of affective disorders*, (2nd edn). Churchill Livingstone, Edinburgh.

Paykel, E.S. and Priest, R.G. (1992). Recognition and management of depression in general practice: Consensus statement. *British Medical Journal*, **305**, 1198–1202.

27.2.9 Schizophrenia

M. G. GELDER

Schizophrenia is the most severe form of functional mental disorder. It affects mainly thinking and perception. Some patients have only a single episode of illness, but most have either recurrent episodes or chronic illness. The care of schizophrenic patients is a major part of the work of psychiatrists. Schizophrenia presents to physicians less often. It may do so in several ways, for example: (1) the disorder may be provoked by a physical illness; (2) a patient with chronic schizophrenia may present with a physical disorder; or (3) occasionally a schizophrenic patient has the delusion that they are physically ill. Because the involvement of physicians with schizophrenia is small, the present account is brief. (For more comprehensive accounts see the *Oxford textbook of psychiatry*, and the references listed at the end of this section).

The annual incidence of schizophrenia is between 0.1 and 0.2 per 1000; because many cases become chronic, the 1-year prevalence is much higher, at about 3 per 1000 of the population.

Clinical features

The clinical picture of schizophrenia is very varied, but two well-recognized syndromes can be described: (1) an acute syndrome with delusions, hallucinations, and disordered thinking ('positive' symptoms); and (2) a chronic syndrome with apathy, slowness, and social withdrawal ('negative' symptoms).

Table 1 *Common symptoms of schizophrenia*

Acute syndrome
   persecutory and grandiose delusions
   auditory hallucinations
   thought disorder
   abnormal affective responses
   disordered behaviour

Chronic syndrome
   apathy
   slowness
   social withdrawal
   any acute syndrome

Table 2 *Diagnostic ('first rank') symptoms of schizophrenia*

Hearing thoughts spoken aloud
'Third person' hallucinations
Hallucinations in the form of a commentary
Somatic hallucinations
Thought withdrawal or insertion
Thought broadcasting
Delusional perception
Feelings or actions experienced as made or influenced by
   others

ACUTE SYNDROME

Delusions in schizophrenia are commonly persecutory ('paranoid') or grandiose (Table 1). These kinds of delusion, although frequent in schizophrenia, are found in other psychiatric disorders and are not valuable in diagnosis. Certain other delusions are less common, but are seldom seen in other psychiatric disorders and therefore more valuable in diagnosis. As shown in Table 2, these diagnostic delusions (often called 'first rank' symptoms) are as follows: the delusion that the patient's thoughts are being transmitted to other people ('thought broadcasting'), the delusion that thoughts are being taken out of the patient's head ('thought withdrawal'), the delusion that some of the patient's thoughts have been implanted by an outside agency ('thought insertion'), and the delusion that the patient's actions are being controlled by an outside agency. Another first rank symptom, delusional perception, is the attribution of a very odd significance to a normal percept; for example, a schizophrenic patient may believe that the positioning of a chair indicates that they are about to be harmed by persecutors.

Hallucinations are of several kinds. Auditory hallucinations are among the most frequent symptoms of schizophrenia. They may be experienced as noises, or voices uttering words, phrases or conversation. The voices may seem to speak to the patient. Two or more voices may seem to discuss the patient; this kind of hallucination is known as a 'third person' hallucination because the voices refer to the patient as 'he' or 'she'. Third person hallucinations differ from other auditory hallucinations in that they seldom occur in disorders other than schizophrenia. They therefore have the most diagnostic value. Other kinds of hallucination particularly characteristic of schizophrenia (although found infrequently) are hearing one's own thoughts spoken aloud as if by another person, and hallucinations of bodily sensations. Visual hallucinations and those of taste, smell and bodily sensations also occur in schizophrenia, but they are less common than auditory hallucinations.

Disorders of thinking in schizophrenia are varied and complicated. They cannot be detected reliably and are therefore not a good guide to diagnosis. For this reason they will not be described in detail. The main feature is lack of logical connection between ideas. The disorder of thought is reflected in the patient's speech, which is vague and difficult to follow, and which becomes more obscure as the interviewer seeks to clarify the reasoning. *Abnormal emotional responses* may be of several kinds: lack of emotional response ('flattened affect'), depressed or elevated mood, or inappropriate emotional responses (e.g. laughing in response to sad news). *Behavioural disorders* in acute schizophrenia include withdrawal from social situations, oddity of manner, or noisy or disruptive acts. Memory and consciousness are not impaired, and therefore disorder of these functions (other than apparent memory problems due entirely to poor concentration) should prompt a search for an organic cause of the patient's symptoms.

Occasionally the first evidence of schizophrenia is a concern about physical health. A few schizophrenic patients experience somatic hallucinations of uncomfortable feelings in the chest, abdomen, or genital regions, and they may seek the advice of physicians about these sensations. Often the true nature of the problem is revealed by eliciting the patient's ideas about the cause of the symptoms. This question may reveal that hallucinatory sensations are being interpreted in a delusional way. For example, sensations in the vagina may be ascribed to the actions of unknown people who are having intercourse with the patient during sleep; or hallucinatory sensations in the abdomen may be ascribed to malefactors. If available, a relative or other informant should be interviewed and asked about the patient's abnormal behaviour or ideas. For cases of this kind the opinion of a psychiatrist is usually required.

CHRONIC SCHIZOPHRENIA

The main features are apathy, slowness, and social withdrawal. Delusions, hallucinations, and disordered thinking may also occur; they are similar to those of acute schizophrenia, but generally less prominent. Depressive symptoms are frequent in chronic schizophrenia (and may be exacerbated by treatment with antipsychotic drugs).

As in acute schizophrenia, memory and consciousness are not impaired in the chronic syndrome (except sometimes for difficulty in remembering age and past dates); if impairment is found, an organic cause should be considered, which may be either primary or superimposed on pre-existing schizophrenia.

Aetiology

Studies of families point strongly to a genetic cause of schizophrenia; for example, the rates of schizophrenia are consistently higher among monozygotic than among dizygotic twins, whilst the adopted away children of schizophrenic parents have rates of schizophrenia similar to those of children brought up by their own schizophrenic parents. Imaging studies of living patients show abnormalities in the temporal lobes of the brain, whilst neuropathological investigations after death confirm abnormalities in the parahippocampal areas, and also suggest that these changes may have originated before birth. These findings have led to the suggestion that an abnormality of brain development predisposes to schizophrenia.

Whatever the nature of the predisposing causes, the precipitating factors for schizophrenia are stressful life events and occasionally physical illness. Life events are also important causes of relapse after a first episode of schizophrenia.

Drugs that reduce the positive symptoms of schizophrenia have in common the property of reducing dopaminergic transmission in the brain. It does not follow, however, that schizophrenia is caused by excessive dopamine function (similarly anticholinergic drugs control the symptoms of parkinsonism but the primary disorder is not of cholinergic transmission).

At present these and other findings cannot be integrated into a convincing simple aetiological hypothesis, and it is not known whether all cases have the same aetiology. It would not be surprising if there were more than one cause of the complicated and variable behavioural syndrome of schizophrenia.

Differential diagnosis

Diagnosis is not difficult in most established cases of schizophrenia, but in first episodes, diagnosis may be very difficult, and usually requires the advice of a psychiatrist. When the patient is overactive and excited, schizophrenia has to be distinguished from mania; when the patient is withdrawn, the differential diagnosis is depressive disorder. In either case the correct diagnosis can be made if there are the characteristic delusions, hallucinations, and other mental phenomena of the schizophrenic syndrome, as described above. Some patients show the phenomena obviously, but others hide their symptoms to the extent that the clinician needs considerable skill to discover them. For the physician the issue of diagnosing schizophrenia is likely to arise when a physically ill patient develops abnormal behaviour; it is then particularly important to distinguish schizophrenia from an acute organic psychiatric disorder especially a drug induced state, complex partial seizures, or encephalitis, and (rarely) cerebral syphilis (see Chapter 24.15.5). Of the drug-induced states, the condition caused by excessive use of amphetamine most closely resembles schizophrenia, but the effects of taking LSD or very large amounts of cannabis can present diagnostic problems. Alcoholic hallucinosis (see Section 28) may also resemble schizophrenia. When long-standing and frequent complex partial seizures arise in the temporal lobe, some patients develop a mental disorder with persecutory delusions, which is very difficult to distinguish from schizophrenia (see Chapter 27.2.10). Finally, it may be difficult to distinguish between personality disorder and schizophrenia starting insidiously in a young person. The physician will usually need the advice of a psychiatrist in making any of these diagnostic distinctions.

Prognosis

It is difficult to predict the outcome during a first episode of schizophrenia. As a broad generalization, about a quarter of patients with a first schizophrenic illness make a lasting recovery, about a quarter develop a chronic disorder, and the rest have repeated illnesses with varying degrees of recovery between episodes. Prognosis tends to be better when there is a sudden onset, a definite precipitant, and prominent affective symptoms. A prompt response to immediate treatment also suggests a favourable long-term outcome. About 10 per cent of schizophrenics die by suicide: the risk is particularly great in younger patients with sufficient insight to appreciate the likely effects of the illness on their hopes and plans. While it is usually possible to identify patients with an increased long-term risk of suicide, it is very difficult to anticipate when a suicide attempt will be made.

Treatment

The long-term care of schizophrenic patients is complicated and involves complex arrangements for rehabilitation for working with families. This care is described in textbooks of psychiatry. The physician is more likely to be concerned with two specific aspects of treatment: the control of symptoms in an emergency and the continuation of drug treatment for chronic schizophrenic patients admitted to hospital for treatment of a medical illness. The treatment of acute symptoms is described in the section on psychiatric emergencies (Chapter 27.4.3), and only maintenance drug treatment will be considered here.

Clinical trials have shown that symptoms can be kept under control and relapse can be prevented if patients with chronic schizophrenia receive long-term treatment with an antipsychotic drug. Many schizophrenic patients fail to take oral medication regularly; therefore the drugs are often given by intramuscular injection of a long-acting preparation, every 2 to 4 weeks, in a schedule and dosage established for each patient. A physician may need to continue this treatment while the patient is in hospital. If there is reason to do otherwise the advice of a psychiatrist should be obtained.

Frequently, schizophrenic symptoms cannot be controlled without provoking extrapyramidal side effects. Antiparkinsonian drugs will usually reduce these side-effects but anticholinergic drugs should not be given to every patient because they may increase the risk of tardive dyskinesia (a late and sometimes irreversible effect of prolonged treatment with antipsychotic drugs).

If physical illness is associated with an increase of schizophrenic symptoms it is usually better to give additional oral rather than intramuscular medication. Suitable drugs include chlorpromazine if a sedating effect is required, and trifluoperazine if not (see Chapter 27.4.1 for further information about antipsychotic drugs).

Paranoid states

Paranoid delusions are concerned with a changes in the patient's relationships with other people. Usually the delusions are concerned with persecution. The term paranoid is often used as a synonym for persecutory; as a technical term, however, it includes beliefs about love, jealousy, and the supernatural, as well as persecution. Paranoid delusions are usually a symptom of schizophrenia, severe depressive disorder, delirium, dementia, or a disorder induced by drugs or alcohol. Occasionally, paranoid delusions occur when there is no evidence for these other conditions; the patient is then said to have a paranoid state. Sometimes the latter proves to be the early stage of one of the other conditions, when other symptoms become evident with time. Other paranoid states are transient reactions to stressful events or physical illness ('acute paranoid reactions'). In a small but important group of paranoid states, the paranoid symptoms persist without the emergence of symptoms of an underlying disorder; in this group the delusions are often concerned with persecution, jealousy, or erotic themes. These conditions will not be reviewed here; it should be stressed, however, that these delusions – especially those of jealousy – may lead to dangerous behaviour towards other people. For this reason, the patient should usually be assessed by a psychiatrist.

The main symptoms of an acute paranoid reaction are paranoid delusions (usually persecutory) and hallucinations. Often the patient does not reveal any delusion at first and may not be recognized as mentally ill until a sudden irrational act draws attention to the disorder. Some patients, for example, suddenly appear terrified and attempt to run away from the medical ward; and some patients attack a person they believe to be their persecutor; others demand to leave the hospital before the appointed time.

Acute paranoid reactions are more frequent in people with touchy, suspicious personalities. These reactions are also more likely when patients have a reduced awareness of their surroundings: for example because they are deaf, or unable to see when their eyes are bandaged as part of ophthalmic treatment, or when they are isolated from other people because in need of intensive care. A small minority develop a paranoid reaction during ordinary medical treatment.

Acute paranoid reactions are usually brief, lasting usually a few days or sometimes a few weeks. Acute symptoms can generally be controlled quickly with an antipsychotic drug, prescribed as for acute schizophrenia. An important step in treatment is counselling to help the patient to regain contact with reality and to reconsider their paranoid ideas. With this treatment most patients can remain on the medical or surgical ward, but a brief admission to a psychiatric ward may be necessary.

REFERENCES

Bebbington, P. and McGuffin, P. (ed.) (1988). *Schizophrenia: The major issues*. Heinemann, London.
Gelder, M.G., Gath, D., and Mayou, R. *Oxford textbook of psychiatry*. Oxford University Press.
Roberts, G.W. (1991). Schizophrenia a neuropathological perspective. *British Journal of Psychiatry*, **158**, 8–17.

27.2.10 Organic (cognitive) mental disorders

R. A. MAYOU

This section reviews the general characteristics of organic (cognitive) psychiatric disorders caused by cerebral pathology or dysfunction and their management. Associations with particular physical conditions are described in the following section and in other chapters (for example, epilepsy).

Table 1 lists the main types of organic mental disorder. Delirium and dementia are syndromes associated with widespread disturbance of cerebral function. The former is characterized by impairment or clouding of consciousness, is often of acute onset, and is frequently reversible. Dementia is usually a more chronic condition and only a minority of cases are reversible. In addition to these general syndromes there are number of more specific neuropsychiatric disorders.

It is important to be aware that it is not uncommon, especially in the elderly, for delirium to complicate a pre-existing dementia and result in a dramatic (although potentially treatable) deterioration in thinking and behaviour.

Delirium

Delirium is a varied syndrome in which the cardinal characteristic of disturbance of consciousness is accompanied by widespread cognitive symptoms and behavioural changes including disturbances of attention, perception, thinking, memory, behaviour, as well as effects on emotions and sleep (Table 2). Delirium is often transient and is characteristically fluctuating. The symptoms are likely to be particularly severe at night, when sensory input is reduced and orientation more difficult to maintain. The main symptoms are listed in Table 2. Agitated and disturbed delirious patients are more conspicuous but less common than those who are quietly confused and whose management usually causes little difficulty.

Table 1 *Types of organic mental state*

Delirium
Dementia
Amnesic disorder
Organic mood disorder
Organic anxiety disorder
Organic delusional disorder

Table 2 *Delirium: clinical features*

Impairment of consciousness (clouding) and attention
Fluctuating course
Changes in cognition
disorientation
memory impairment
perceptual disturbance (misinterpretations, illusions, hallucinations)
language disturbance (incoherent, irrelevant, perseveration)
Emotional symptoms
depression
irritability
apathy
Disturbed behaviour
agitation
overactivity
underactivity
Abnormality of sleep–wake cycle

Table 3 *Some causes of delirium*

Cerebral disease and injury
Epilepsy
Alcohol intoxication and withdrawal
Drug intoxication and withdrawal
Metabolic conditions
Infections
Vitamin deficiency

EPIDEMIOLOGY

Delirium may occur at any age but is especially common in the elderly. Because it occurs in association with severe illness, it is extremely common amongst general hospital inpatients, especially those aged over 60 and those recovering from acute illness or major surgery. Delirium often goes unremarked on medical wards, with only the most disturbed and agitated patients attracting specific attention.

AETIOLOGY

Many conditions can cause delirium (Table 3). Predisposing factors apart from the nature of the physical condition include age, pre-existing dementia, unfamiliar surroundings, and lack of information. Characteristically, patients are more likely to be disturbed when away from their own homes and separated from their family. Impersonal wards, ever-changing staff and ill-understood investigations and treatment all make delirium more likely. Alcohol withdrawal is a frequent cause both of emergency attendance and of delirium developing during a hospital admission.

DIFFERENTIAL DIAGNOSIS

Delirium needs to be distinguished from dementia and from acute psychotic illnesses. It may be difficult to distinguish complaints of subjective confusion occurring in psychotic illnesses from the clouding of consciousness of delirium and a specialist opinion may be necessary.

MANAGEMENT

Diagnosis is based upon the clinical features and on the history. Patients are often unable to give any coherent account and it is essential to obtain information from relatives and, if in hospital, the ward staff, whose observations of behaviour are often particularly helpful. The diagnosis does not depend upon identifying a specific physical cause, but treatment does and appropriate physical investigations should proceed in parallel. Occasionally no physical cause is ever found but this should not cause doubt about the diagnosis if there are clear clinical features. Assessment of predisposing factors in the patient's situation is essential.

If delirium is not associated with significant distress or with management problems, there is little need to consider specific treatment. However, it is always necessary to make special efforts to explain to the patient what is going on, to repeat information as frequently as is necessary and also to explain the nature of the disorder to relatives.

In more severe delirium, a more elaborate treatment plan is necessary. The emphasis should be on general measures rather than psychotropic drug treatment, although this is indicated if the patient is acutely distressed or is behaving in a manner that is causing difficulties for carers. The minimum effective amount of medication should be used and doses should be reviewed regularly over a period of days, so as to avoid erratic drug regimes in which the patient varies from being oversedated to being distressed and disturbed should be avoided.

Management of an acutely distressed patient is described in Chapter 27.4.3. Further treatment is usually with a regular regime of oral (tablet or syrup) haloperidol, an effective antipsychotic drug that does not have

Table 4 *Dementia: clinical features*

Memory impairment
Cognitive impairment affecting
disorientation
new learning
comprehension
language
Emotional impairment
anxiety
irritability
depression
lability
Behavioural impairment
disorganized, inappropriate, distractible
neglect of social conventions
self-neglect
Neurological impairment
aphasia
agnosia
agraphia
Perceptual impairment
illusions
hallucinations
Thinking–delusions
Insight–impaired

Table 5 *Some causes of dementia*

Degenerative
Alzheimer's disease
multiple sclerosis
Parkinson's disease
normal pressure hydrocephalus
Huntington's chorea
Space occupying lesions
tumour
chronic subdural haematoma
Traumatic–severe head injury
Infections
postencephalitis
syphilis
Vascular–multi-infarct dementia
Toxic–alcohol
Anoxia
cardiac arrest
carbon monoxide poisoning
Vitamin lack–B_{12}
Endocrine–hypothyroidism

sedative cardiovascular side-effects of phenothiazines. However, the latter is a useful alternative for agitated patients and when haloperidol is ineffective. Treatment regimes for patients with alcohol withdrawal and other substance abuse syndromes are described in Section 28.

Dementia (see also Section 24)

Dementia is a syndrome resulting from brain disease, usually chronic or progressive, in which there is generalized impairment of higher cortical functions, including memory, thinking, orientation, comprehension, learning, language, and judgement; consciousness is not impaired. The cognitive deficits are frequently accompanied by emotional symptoms and by changes in behaviour (Table 4). There are many causes of dementia but it is most common in the elderly with Alzheimer's disease and cerebrovascular disease (Table 5).

Table 6 *Management of dementia*

Aim to maintain patient in as normal as possible surroundings
Consistent repeated explanation and simple behavioural measures
Practical help
Support for the family
Minimum medication
Offer holiday and respite care

MANAGEMENT (TABLE 6)

Management of a patient with dementia is directed towards identifying the small minority with treatable causes and to more general measures to enable the patient to have a full a life as possible and to provide the family with support necessary to manage what may be a demanding and distressing burden.

Investigation should be no more than necessary to identify a treatable cause, and may include thyroid function, serum vitamin B_{12}, skull radiographs and computer tomography scan (see Section 24). More intensive investigations may be necessary in younger patients in whom the chances of an uncommon treatable cause are greater. Psychological testing is of limited use in diagnosis but maybe of value in monitoring changes over time.

The aim of medical and social care is to enable the patient to live in as independent and normal a setting as possible (Table 6). This is preferably the patient's home or that of another member of the family. Some form of residential care may be necessary in the later stages of dementia. Hospital admission is generally required only for the management of complications, for holiday relief, and for nursing care of very advanced dementia. Whatever the setting, practical measures to reduce difficulties in everyday living are essential. These include keeping changes to a minimum and arranging as simple and familiar daily routine as possible. Relatives need to know the nature of the patient's condition, the prognosis, and the ways in which they can help. They may need practical as well as emotional support. Domiciliary welfare services such as home help, and meals on wheels are important.

As the condition worsens, day centre or day hospital attendance, or holiday admissions to relieve relatives are required. Careful planning, which gives relatives the assurance that further help will always be available when needed, can greatly prolong a relative's ability and willingness to care for the patient.

There is a rather limited role for psychotropic medication. Antidepressants are occasionally useful in the management of depressed mood in the early stages of dementia. Small doses of hypnotics and antipsychotic drugs can be valuable in calming agitation and associated behavioural disturbances. Memory aids and specific psychological treatments of inappropriate behaviours are sometimes useful. Measures directed towards reducing disorientation, such as a clear ward layout, a simple routine, and continuity of care by one or two staff members, are important.

Specific organic syndromes

Table 1 lists a number of specific syndromes that do not cause global psychological severe impairment, and that may or may not be associated with evidence of neurological deficit.

AMNESIC DISORDER

This uncommon disorder (also known as Amnestic or Korsakov's syndrome) is characterized by impairment of short term memory without altered consciousness, general intellectual deterioration, or perceptual abnormality. It is commonly accompanied by confabulation. The clinical picture is characteristic in that the patient appears articulate and aware but gradually reveals an inability to remember information for more than a few seconds. The most frequent cause of organic memory disorder is thiamine deficiency, most often due to chronic alcoholism but occasionally to prolonged vomiting, and starvation.

The neuropathological basis is usually a lesion in the posterior hypothalamus or nearby midline structures, the common factor to all pathologies being damage to the limbic system.

ORGANIC PERSONALITY DISORDER

Localized cerebral damage may lead to changes in personality without evidence of cognitive damage. Occasionally personality change is the first sign of a cerebral lesion and uncharacteristic behaviour should suggest the possibility of an organic mental state.

ORGANIC MOOD DISORDER

Depression may be a direct result of a number of physical disorders, such as some primary brain diseases (for example, multiple sclerosis and Parkinson's disease) and endocrine disorder. However, it is often very difficult to distinguish organic mood disorder from depression arising as either a psychological reaction to physical illness or coincidentally. Treatment of the underlying physical cause can be expected to relieve the depression. Antidepressants are often effective, whatever the aetiology.

ORGANIC ANXIETY DISORDER

Several conditions can cause organic anxiety disorder, including hyperthyroidism, hypoglycaemia, and phaeochromocytoma. The treatment is that of the underlying cause.

DELUSIONAL DISORDER

A schizophrenia-like delusional disorder is a rare complication of temporal lobe epilepsy and other brain diseases. Management is often difficult but follows the general principles for psychotic disorder.

Aspects of differential diagnosis
ORGANIC OR FUNCTIONAL?

It may be difficult to distinguish between functional and organic psychiatric disorder, especially when an organic disorder presents in the emergency department with disturbances of behaviour and thinking in the absence of obvious neurological symptoms or signs. It is sensible to consider a possible organic cause in every case of psychological or behavioural disturbance, and especially when there are atypical features. Psychiatric causes are not identified solely by exclusion of organic causes but on positive evidence of psychological aetiology since organic causes may be undetectable in the early stages of illness.

The points in favour of an organic cause of disturbed behaviour are: cognitive disorder preceding mood or other disorder, specific cognitive defects, neurological signs, and symptoms not typical of functional disorder.

In affective disorder and schizophrenia there may be an impression of impairment of cognitive functions. A common diagnostic problem is presented by so-called depressive pseudodementia. In this syndrome, a depressed patient complains of poor memory and performs poorly on cognitive tests, thus giving the appearance of dementia. The patient's difficulty in remembering occurs because poor concentration leads to inadequate registration. A history from another informant may show that the depressed mood preceded the cognitive problems. Careful memory testing may show that the poor performance on tests is due to lack of interest and motivation rather than impaired intellectual functions. These patients are retarded and usually unwilling to co-operate in the inter-

Table 7 *Delirium versus dementia*

Delirium	Dementia
Acute onset	Insidious onset
Fluctuating course	Stable or progressive
Impaired consciousness	Normal consciousness
Thinking disorganized	Thinking impoverished
Perceptual disturbance common	Perceptual disturbance
Alertness usually impaired	uncommon
	Normally alert

view; in contrast, patients with dementia are usually willing to reply to questions but make mistakes.

DELIRIUM OR DEMENTIA?

Delirium is an acute reversible condition, dementia is a chronic disorder (Table 7). The two syndromes may occur together, especially in the elderly. When this happens the underlying dementia may be overlooked or, alternatively, the reversible acute stage may not be detected or treated. Sometimes the longstanding dementia becomes apparent only after successful treatment of the more recent delirium. As shown in Table 7 delirium can usually be diagnosed correctly by an acute onset, fluctuating course, impaired consciousness, and disorganised thinking. Perceptual disturbance is more frequent and alertness more often impaired in delirium.

27.2.11 Mental disorders of old age

R. J. JACOBY

Mental disorders in the elderly are of the greatest importance for a number of reasons:

1. Demographic trends in developed countries have resulted in a marked increase in the number of elderly persons, especially the very old.
2. This age group is particularly prone to debilitating mental illness.
3. Presentations of mental illness in the elderly may differ from those at younger ages and therefore go unrecognized.
4. The pattern of morbidity differs from younger patients; the elderly suffering much more from organic disorder – delirium and dementia.
5. Mental and physical illness often go hand in hand, the one sometimes masking the other.

In this last regard, surveys of elderly patients admitted to non-psychiatric beds in general hospitals show high rates of mental disorder of various sorts. Surveys in the community also demonstrate high morbidity increasing with age. For instance, the prevalence of dementia is about 7 per cent in those aged over 65 but approaches 20 per cent in those over 80. Community rates for depression in the elderly are less easy to determine because of difficulties in defining a case. For serious depressive illness the prevalence is about 2 to 3 per cent, but for pervasive depressive symptoms it is around 12 per cent. There are no valid data for the community prevalence of late paraphrenia (schizophrenia-like psychosis) but this group constitutes approximately 10 per cent of admissions to psychogeriatric beds. The closure of large mental institutions in most developed countries has resulted in a greatly increased number of elderly patients in the community suffering from chronic schizophrenia that began much earlier in their lives.

Assessment

There are no shortcuts in the assessment of mental disorder in the elderly. Factors to be considered first are the setting in which the patient is examined and his/her ability to provide information. Assessment in the patient's own home can give invaluable clues about premorbid adjustment, activities of daily living, and even causes of an abnormal mental state – a waste bin full of empty whisky bottles being just one example. If patients are to be assessed in general hospital wards it should be done in the privacy of a side-room if possible. Many elderly patients are unable to give a history. It is essential always to find reliable informants, even if this means disturbing a neighbour or making an out-of-town telephone call. Doctors examining patients outside hospital should carry appropriate equipment. For example, a low reading thermometer, a sphygmomanometer, and sugar detection urine sticks can each prove invaluable at home in detecting the cause of mental disturbance.

Examination of the mental state of an elderly person is essentially the same as for any adult, but with different points of emphasis. More attention is paid to the level of consciousness, particularly subtle clouding or fluctuations throughout 24 h. For patients with suspected dementia a full cognitive examination must be made. It is frequently necessary for this to be carried out in several brief sessions because patients become easily fatigued and unable to co-operate. Tired or inattentive patients may fail a test that they might otherwise have been able to perform satisfactorily. Systematic evaluation of all higher cerebral function deficits, such as memory, praxis, language, and others, is essential. On general hospital wards or home visits the routine administration of standardized questionnaires is of value as an alerting mechanism to morbidity and for audit but is not a substitute for full evaluation. Examples of such tests are the Mental Test Score (MTS), Abbreviated Mental Test Score (AMTS) and the Mini-Mental State Examination (MMSE). The Mini-Mental State Examination is often preferred because it assesses, directly or indirectly, a wider range of higher cerebral functions.

Because the capacity to live independently is frequently compromised in the elderly and becomes the crucial determinant of social outcome, it is essential to assess the patient's ability to perform activities of daily living (ADL) – dressing, feeding, toilet care and so on. Impairment in activities of daily living may reveal dyspraxia or agnosia that has not been disclosed by more formal clinical tests of cognitive function. The informant's account is particularly important here, as the patients' assessment of their own abilities may be quite misleading.

Delirium

The clinical features of delirium are described in Chapter 27.2.10. Although a major cause of mental disturbance in the elderly, especially in general hospital wards, delirium is frequently missed because it is not thought of. The elderly are particularly susceptible for two reasons. First, they more commonly suffer from the physical disorders that cause delirium: hypoxia, infections, toxicity (especially from drugs), and metabolic and CNS disorders. Second, many elderly patients have a decreased cerebral reserve because of incipient or overt dementia. It follows that an underlying physical cause for delirium must be sought assiduously as it is generally more important to treat this than the mental symptoms. Physical illnesses causing delirium can be relatively minor. For example, a urinary tract infection can account for marked and reversible disturbance, especially in patients with mild or moderate dementia. A further point is that because the elderly generally suffer high physical morbidity they tend to receive more prescribed medication. Single or multiple drugs, as well as drug withdrawal effects, are potent causes of delirium. Management is essentially that of the underlying cause and psychotropic drugs should be avoided if possible. However, short-term treatment of mental symptoms and behavioural disturbance with a neuroleptic, such as haloperidol, is sometimes unavoidable to allow medical treatment to proceed unhindered, e.g. preventing an intravenous infusion or urinary catheter from being pulled out.

Dementia

The importance of dementia lies not only in the great suffering it causes to patients but also in the demands it makes upon family carers and the medical and social services. The great majority of cases are due to Alzheimer's or cerebrovascular disease, although other causes such as cortical Lewy body and Parkinson's disease, frontal and Pick's dementia may be more common than has hitherto been appreciated. The clinical features of the dementia syndrome are described in Section 24 and in Chapter 24.2.10. It should be stressed that global impairment is required for diagnosis and that memory loss alone, of which the elderly frequently complain, is not a sufficient criterion. Accurate diagnosis is of great importance because treatable or arrestable causes may be discovered, management can be planned and implemented, carers (family and professional) are greatly helped by having a clearer understanding of the process affecting the patient and the likely course of future events, and knowledge of the underlying conditions is accrued and advanced. Whilst diagnosis is defined by cognitive deficits – such as dysphasia and agnosia – rational management requires an appreciation of their practical implications; for example, ensuring nutrition in a patient with dyspraxic inability to feed herself. Patients should be maintained at home for as long as possible, not only for humane reasons but because they will usually have lost the capacity to become familiar with and adapt to a new environment. This is best achieved through a continuing partnership between clinicians, family carers, and local statutory and voluntary social services. Such interagency co-operation and discussion facilitates access to community services, which include those brought to the patient – meals, nursing, bathing, house cleaning – and day care away from home. Intercurrent illness should be treated along with other medical problems, such as urinary and faecal incontinence, which are due more commonly to urinary tract infections and impaction, respectively, than to the underlying disease processes of dementia. Particular attention must be given to principal carers, most frequently spouses or adult daughters but sometimes unrelated neighbours, who show high levels of psychiatric morbidity themselves due to their burden of care. The clinician who repeatedly evaluates and balances the patient's increasing impairment against the stress upon carers will be able to judge if and when to advise that the patient moves temporarily, for respite, or permanently into some form of institutionalized care. The principles of terminal care are discussed in Section 32.

Affective illness

DEPRESSION

Depressive illness in the elderly does not differ fundamentally from that in earlier life, varying from mild dysthymia to major psychosis with high risk of suicide. There are, however, some differences of emphasis. Psychosocial factors are as important but genetic loading is usually lower in patients with late onset depression. Cerebral organic change is more common in late onset cases.

Psychomotor retardation is frequent, as in younger patients, but anxiety and agitation are also characteristic. Delusions of guilt and unworthiness are typical but hypochondriacal or nihilistic beliefs also often occur. Histrionic or other bizarre behaviour, which is out of premorbid character, is also seen. These features can sometimes make differentiation between depression and late paraphrenia difficult. Furthermore, patients with severe depression often perform badly on cognitive tests, which may lead to a wrong diagnosis of organic dementia, so called 'depressive pseudodementia'. Hypochondriacal delusions together with anorexic weight loss can be mistaken for physical illness, such as cancer. Some patients may even deny low mood (masked depression), but the presence of other typical affective symptoms and a favourable response to antidepressant treatment reveal the correct diagnosis. It is important for the clinician not to miss a treatable depression in patients, such as those with severe physical illnesses, who appear to have a good reason to be unhappy.

The elderly are vulnerable to the unwanted effects of psychotropic drugs but respond well to standard antidepressants. Less toxic tetracyclics or selective serotonin reuptake inhibitors (SSRIs) are often preferred. However, tricyclics, such as amitriptyline and imipramine, are highly effective if care is taken to observe the general principle of prescribing psychotropic drugs to the elderly, namely small initial doses increasing slowly to lower therapeutic doses than are given to younger patients. The elderly also respond well to electroconvulsive therapy (ECT), which is regarded by many as the treatment of choice for deluded and/or suicidal patients. Advanced age, dementia, and physical infirmity are not contraindications to electroconvulsive therapy. After recovery from an episode of major depression antidepressant treatment should be continued for at least 2 years, if not indefinitely.

MANIA/HYPOMANIA

Manic illness, which accounts for about 5 per cent of psychogeriatric admissions, is usually less florid than in younger patients. Mixed manic and depressive pictures have been described as typical but are probably not more common in old age than before. Cerebral organic disease is found in a high proportion of cases. Diagnosis is sometimes difficult to make because patients may present with a rather non-specific psychosis, or one mimicking an organic delirium. It is therefore particularly important to enquire about a previous history of affective illness. Secondary mania is also seen. This is defined as a first onset in close temporal relationship with a physical illness or drug treatment in patients with no previous history of affective disorder. Elderly manic patients respond well to treatment with neuroleptics and lithium carbonate in the acute phase. Lithium is also widely used to prevent relapse. Here, frequent monitoring of renal and thyroid function is essential, and the serum lithium level should be maintained at the lower end of the therapeutic range, i.e. around 0.6 mmol/l.

PARANOID DISORDERS

Paranoid ideas, usually but not invariably of persecution, are common in the two major groups of mental illness in old age – dementia and affective disorder. In dementia they tend to be transient, variable, and unsystematized. In affective disorder they are usually mood-congruent, for example persecution deserved because of guilt. Persecutory ideas are also seen in paranoid personalities and acute paranoid reactions, but late paraphrenia is the main paranoid syndrome of old age, equivalent to paranoid schizophrenia of earlier adult life. The following aetiological factors have been reported consistently in late paraphrenia:

(1) a high female to male ratio (up to 7:1);
(2) a family history of schizophrenia intermediate between the general population and younger schizophrenic patients;
(3) social isolation and poor premorbid interpersonal relationships;
(4) low marriage and fecundity rates compared with age-matched peers;
(5) long standing deafness.

The clinical picture is sometimes indistinguishable from early onset paranoid schizophrenia but the patient usually presents with a few simple delusions and associated auditory hallucinations. For example, the patient may complain of hearing the neighbours plotting to do them harm, or impugning their sexual virtue. Response to neuroleptic medication is good and most are able to return to their premorbid level of adjustment. However, delusional beliefs are not necessarily extinguished but become encapsulated, which means set aside or compartmentalized and not permitted to intrude into so many aspects of mental and daily life, as happens during the acute phase of illness. Adherence to treatment, preferably with the help of a community psychiatric nurse, is essential because relapse is usual on stopping medication.

NEUROTIC, PERSONALITY, AND OTHER DISORDERS

These are subjects that are too complex to discuss briefly and the reader is advised to refer to specialist texts. Some general principles can be stated. It is essential to differentiate lifelong neurosis from neurotic symptoms of first onset in old age because the latter, predominantly anxiety and phobia, are most likely to indicate an underlying depressive illness. Elderly patients with lifelong neurosis have frequently adapted to their disability in spite of continued suffering. Mild and moderate lifelong personality deviations are common but severe disorders are occasionally encountered, such as the senile squalor (Diogenes) syndrome, which can require compulsory removal from home under mental or public health legislation. Illicit drug taking is rare among the present generation of elderly but abuse of prescribed drugs, notably benzo-diazepines, is common. Alcohol abuse is increasingly appreciated by psychiatrists as an important cause of mental and social disability in the elderly.

REFERENCES

Folstein, M.F., Folstein, S.E., and McHugh, P.R. (1975). 'Mini Mental State'. A practical method for grading the cognitive state of patients for the clinician. *Journal of Psychiatric Research*, **12**, 189–98.

Jacoby, R. and Oppenheimer, C. (1991). *Psychiatry in the Elderly*. Oxford University Press.

27.2.12 The patient who has attempted suicide

H. G. MORGAN

This section is concerned with deliberate acts of self-harm not leading to death, whether involving physical means, drug overdosage, or poisoning with non-ingestants, and is carried out in the knowledge of their potential harm. Such episodes of self-harm constitute the most common cause of acute hospital medical admission in females and are second only to ischaemic heart disease in males. Self-harm is most commonly in the form of drug overdosage.

The term 'deliberate self-harm', which refers to self-poisoning or injury, will be used here rather than 'attempted suicide' because a conscious wish to die is present in only a minority of these patients. Soon after the event of self-harm only one-third of women and a half of men admitted to hospital claim that they had wanted to die, and even fewer regret that they had failed to kill themselves. The assessment and management of patients who have 'attempted suicide' encompasses a much wider remit than that of suicide risk, although it is of great importance to be able to recognize the minority who represent failed suicides and who may present significant on-going risk of suicide in the immediate future.

Description

EPIDEMIOLOGY

Deliberate self-harm is most frequent in young adults, and it occurs more often in females than males at all ages except in the elderly (Fig. 1). For some ten years beginning in the early 1960s its incidence increased rapidly in countries throughout the Western hemisphere. During the 1970s the incidence continued to rise but much more slowly, to reach a peak in 1979. The incidence in each sex then declined, especially in females, to stabilize at slightly lower levels. The selectively high incidence in teenage females has become less striking. It is more prevalent in social classes 4 and 5, tending to be concentrated in those parts of urban areas where social problems abound, particularly in local authority

housing estates. In certain city centres the annual incidence of deliberate self-harm in young adult females may reach 1.6 per cent, exceeding by a factor of 9 that found in middle class suburbia.

METHOD

The most frequent method is some kind of drug overdosage (90 per cent). Psychotropic drugs (minor tranquillizers/sedatives 15 per cent, antidepressants 10 per cent) feature prominently and these are usually obtained through medical prescription. In contrast, analgesics such as salicylates and paracetamol (30 per cent) are commonly obtained without prescription at retail chemists. Poisons and gassing are each used in less than 1 per cent of cases. Self-injury usually in the form of skin laceration with or without drug overdosage occurs in about 5 per cent of all episodes of attempted suicide presenting to hospitals. Concomitant alcohol intake within the previous 6 h has been reported in 50 to 66 per cent of men and in 25 to 45 per cent of women.

Causes

Personality disorder with its attendant chronic social disruption is seen in 25 to 50 per cent of persons admitted to hospital after deliberate self-harm, and many of these also have long-standing problems caused by alcohol abuse. Florid psychotic mental illness, which is found in only a small minority (12 per cent), most commonly occurs as some form of depressive disorder, although no diagnostic category is exempt. Each episode is usually accompanied by marked anxiety and depressive symptoms, which often subside rapidly after the event, but these usually persist unchanged in patients who have harmed themselves in the context of an established mental disorder, or when the psychosocial reaction to the event is adverse.

Many episodes of deliberate self-harm appear to be impulsive acts by vulnerable persons who have become emotionally upset in response to some kind of disturbing event; the intention being either to seek temporary oblivion or to achieve some change in the situation, perhaps by appealing to others through an act that highlights the degree of personal distress. Conscious suicidal intent, even when present, is often transient and barely enters into the conscious reasoning of the person concerned. However, an important minority of patients who survive are in fact failed suicides. In these particular patients, who are more likely than the others to be suffering from some form of mental illness, the suicide risk may

Fig. 1 Admission rates for suicide in Edinburgh, 1988–9.

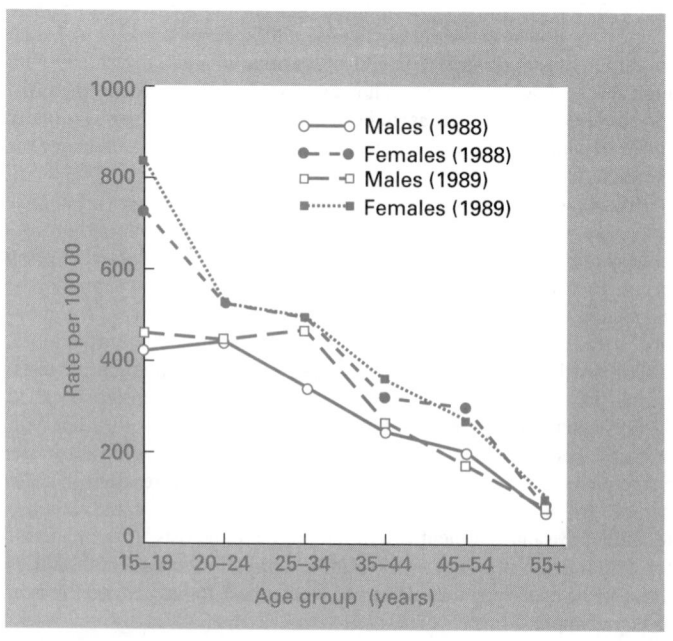

well continue after the event: their reliable identification is an important part of clinical assessment.

Some kind of upsetting life event appears to be important in about two-thirds of cases. Most commonly this takes the form of disharmony with a person who is important to the patient. Other factors that are seen less frequently include problems concerned with work, financial matters, or physical health. Evidence suggests that unemployment, particularly if it is prolonged, may increase the risk of deliberate self-harm. Lack of close support and a sense of loneliness is reported by about half of all such patients admitted to hospital. In the United Kingdom the rate in ethnic minority groups was until recently lower than in the host community, but in some areas the incidence has now become greatest in Asian women.

The possible reasons for the dramatic increase in incidence of deliberate self-harm since the early 1960s are complex. Its appeal effect may have increased, particularly in the case of overdoses of non-prescribed analgesics in adolescents. Changes in the prescribing of psychotropic drugs may also be important, as there has been a marked increase in the quantity of prescriptions for these drugs during the period in which the incidence of deliberate self-harm has increased. Also, the types of drug used in deliberate self-poisoning reflect quite clearly the general pattern of medical prescribing. The risk during treatment with psychotropic drugs is probably increased when medication is used merely to relieve symptoms without any attempt being made to resolve concomitant upsetting events. An increase in the prevalence of relationship difficulties, as indicated by a rise in the rate of divorce, and more widespread use of alcohol, may be other factors related to the increased incidence of deliberate self-harm since the 1960s.

Assessment

Adequate assessment of deliberate self-harm depends upon full and reliable information and, whenever possible, other relevant informants should be interviewed as well as the patient. A detailed evaluation of social and interpersonal factors is necessary, as well as a clinical assessment. Some patients are unwilling to discuss personal matters and suicidal ideas openly, a few are suspicious because of psychotic ideas, and aggressive behaviour may have arisen from a toxic confusional state due to the overdose of drugs. Good interview technique is needed to surmount all these problems.

The main immediate risks are: physical complications, a further episode of non-fatal self-harm, or suicide, and hazards concerning dependent children or other family members. These should all be evaluated and dealt with urgently where necessary.

PHYSICAL COMPLICATIONS

Physical treatment is discussed in Sections 8 and 16. In this account only a few obvious points need to be considered. First aid treatment is of the utmost importance particularly for the unconscious patient before transfer to hospital, maintenance of an adequate airway at this time being a paramount consideration. Only a few (4 per cent) need to be admitted to an intensive care unit, and less than one-quarter are unconscious for more than 24 h. Few specific antidotes are available and effective care for most overdose patients depends almost entirely upon good basic nursing techniques and appropriate physiotherapy.

SUICIDE RISK

Most deliberate self-harm patients are interviewed in the hospital ward as soon as they are able to discuss matters fully and clearly, usually a day or so after the event. The detection of the minority who are failed suicides is an important immediate objective. This is a difficult and uncertain task, but it is helped by the fact that the social and clinical correlates of completed suicide tend to be different from those of

Table 1 *Clinical and social factors associated with increased risk of suicide*

Massive drug overdosage posing major physical risk
Extensive deep lacerations
Use of potentially lethal agent (e.g. firearm)
Precautions to avoid discovery and to succeed in killing self
Detailed planning
Increased age
Male sex
Recent bereavement, separation, or divorce
Unemployment
Social isolation, alienation
Incapacitating physical disability and illness
Depressive illness
Other mental illness (organic brain disorder, schizophrenia, drug addiction)
Personality difficulties (especially poor impulse control and social difficulties)
Epilepsy complicated by mood disorder

patients whose deliberate self-harm does not have a fatal outcome. Factors associated with increased risk of suicide are listed in Table 1.

Assessment of risk involves the compilation of an overall picture of individual and environmental/relationship factors, both current and from the past. The factors listed in Table 16 are not necessary for suicide to occur, but merely represent an important checklist of those that have been shown to have a positive association with increased suicide risk. They are particularly useful as indicators of caution whenever overall assessment suggests that such risk is not significant. The essential element of suicide risk assessment must be the precise clinical picture and weighting of individual risk factors, which will vary from one patient to another.

INTERVIEWING THE SUICIDAL

There is no evidence that open discussion will in any way increase the risk of suicide, and indeed a common error is failure to enquire about such risk adequately. However, the enquiry must be made appropriately: a brusque, challenging, and unsympathetic approach is hazardous, particularly in tense angry patients who are liable to react with dangerous impulsive behaviour.

Continued suicidal motivation may not be easy to assess by interview, and it is necessary to be aware of the potential pitfalls as well as ways of circumventing them. Assessment should ideally be performed without interruption in a quiet situation where it is possible to talk in private and without hurry. The patient usually shows varying amounts of depression, despair, anger, or frustration and may express an unwillingness to talk about personal feelings. There may also be reluctance to discuss the act of self-harm because this provokes, guilt, shame, and the fear of adverse consequences. Assessment of the mental state should be directed particularly to the detection of the characteristic clinical features of depressive illness. These include overt depression of mood, tearfulness, disorders of thinking such as poor concentration, ideas of futility, and morbid self-blame. Biological changes such as insomnia, reduced libido, poor appetite, and weight loss are important features of a severe depressive illness, although suicide risk can be significant even in their absence.

If the patient appears despairing and hopeless, it is appropriate to signify recognition of this in a sympathetic and reassuring way at an early stage in the interview. Such a comment can be an important first step in overcoming the feelings of isolation and alienation which are so characteristic of suicidal persons. Discussion of suicidal ideas should be entered upon carefully. A useful sequence of questions, which leads gradually up to discussion of suicidal ideas, their severity, and associ-

Table 2 *Interview sequence of topics in assessing suicidal motivation*

Hope that things will turn out well
Get pleasure out of life
Feel hopeful from day to day
Able to face each day
See point in it all
Ever despair about things
Feel that it is impossible to face next day
Feel life a burden
Wish it would all end
Wish self dead
Why feel this way (e.g. be with a dead person, life bleak, morbid guilt)
Thoughts of ending life. If so, how persistently
Thought specifically about method of suicide (means readily available)
Ever acted on them
Feel able to resist them, anything make them disappear
How likely to kill self
Ability to give reassurance about safety, e.g. until next appointment
Circumstances likely to make things worse
Willingness to turn for help if crisis occurs
Risk to others

ated risks is listed in Table 2. Continuing suicidal ideas must of course always be taken seriously.

A suicidal person may exhibit marked hour to hour fluctuation in the degree of overt distress, and some who are risk may at times appear to be free from symptoms. This is particularly likely in those who are admitted to hospital and thereby removed from the life problems which led to despair. Those with continued suicidal intent often show anger and resentment towards either their situation or other people, and they may appear unco-operative or unreasonable as well as depressed and despairing. When the clinical picture is of this mixed kind it is important not to underestimate the suicide risk.

More than half of those who actually commit suicide turn to others for help in the weeks preceding their death, and they communicate their suicidal ideas openly before killing themselves. It is therefore wrong to believe that people who talk about suicidal ideas never end their lives. It is also rash to dismiss such comments as mere threats or manipulation, unless the patient is well known to the doctor and such an interpretation is wholly consistent with previous behaviour. Even then such a judgement can be mistaken. A high proportion of individuals who have severe suicidal intent are ambivalent about ending their lives and may temporarily recover hope. This may lead an unsuspecting interviewer into a false sense of optimism. Occasionally a person at serious risk of suicide conceals the fact because of the belief that no help is likely to be effective. When a person who denies suicidal ideas has behaved in an inconsistent manner, such as having left a suicide note, or having engaged in serious life-endangering behaviour, particular care should be taken not to accept this denial too readily.

NON-FATAL REPETITION

Another risk which requires immediate assessment is that of a further non-fatal act of self-harm. The patient may talk openly about wishing to repeat the act and such statements should never be dismissed lightly, particularly when upsetting life events that led up to the episode remain unresolved or are even made worse by it, for example by increasing the hostility of other people. Other correlates of non-fatal repetition include a long history of psychiatric disturbance suggestive of personality disorder, abuse of alcohol or drugs, and a previous history of deliberate self-poisoning or injury.

OTHERS AT RISK

The welfare of dependents such as children should always be assessed carefully. There is some evidence of an increased incidence of child abuse in persons who carry out acts of deliberate self-harm.

Management

During the initial period in an accident and emergency department or medical ward the emphasis of treatment must of course be upon physical risk and complications. Nevertheless, from the beginning the hazard of suicide and non-fatal repetition should not be forgotten. The degree of risk should be decided in every case and if any doubt exists psychiatric advice should be obtained immediately. It has long been recognized that the degree of physical risk correlates poorly, if at all, with the severity of suicidal ideation. In view of this, inpatient overnight admission to allow thorough assessment next day has been the commended practice in the management of all deliberate self-harm patients. Discharge home from the accident and emergency department should always be a matter of great caution, although it seems that considerable numbers have in recent years been managed in this way. It should be remembered that adolescents in particular may be difficult to assess thoroughly in an accident and emergency department. Once the degree of risk is decided it should be clearly understood by all those concerned with the patient's care. Particular attention should be given to prevent any access to hazards such as open stairs and windows. It is the hospital's responsibility to ensure that such patients are nursed only in situations where their safety can be reasonably assured. The number of nursing staff available is important and the need should be reviewed frequently. Patients who have taken drug overdoses may be noisy and unco-operative as a result of confusion induced by drugs or disinhibition due to concomitant alcohol intake, often compounded by personality difficulties. Such patients are not always those most welcome in medical wards. Each hospital ward should have a clear code of practice concerning the levels of supportive observation required according to the degree of perceived suicide risk. These may vary from a nurse remaining with the patient at all times in the case of severe risk, through graded levels of care to unrestricted movement within the ward when risk is judged to be minimal. It is wise initially to nurse in bed all patients who are admitted to medical wards following deliberate self-poisoning or injury, no matter how trivial the physical risk may be, at least until thorough psychiatric assessment has provided a full evaluation of the immediate risk of suicide or non-fatal repetition. Physical hazards in the ward itself should always be kept in mind in order to ensure that the environment is sufficiently safe when suicide risk is high.

About one-fifth of deliberate self-harm episodes necessitate admission to a psychiatric ward, usually because of florid mental illness, continuing risk of self-harm, or a worsening social situation. A very small number (1 per cent) may have to be admitted under a compulsory legislative provision when the immediate risk of suicide is very serious, and the patient is mentally ill and unwilling to accept help. In the United Kingdom this situation most commonly involves a Section 2 Assessment Order of the 1983 Mental Health Act. This requires an application by (or on behalf of) the nearest relative together with two medical recommendations, one of which must be made by a recognized specialist in psychiatry.

About a quarter of patients admitted to medical wards because of deliberate self-harm are returned to and remain in the care of their general practitioners. Approximately a half are given appointments in psychiatric outpatient clinics but only a half of these attend. Such low compliance with treatment is a major problem, and it has many possible causes, which may include a reluctance to look at underlying causes once symptoms have settled and the crisis has blown over, or simply an unwillingness to become a psychiatric patient. The treatment that is offered needs to be perceived by the patient as valid, relevant, and feasible if it is to be accepted readily. A problem-solving approach is a good example: this clarifies the principal difficulties faced by the patient, and identifies mutually agreed steps in resolving them. The use of contract techniques in achieving the goals can be particularly helpful. Poor communication with key other persons may require conjoint work, and it may be necessary to involve other agencies, such as social services, particularly when the welfare of dependents such as children or elderly persons is relevant.

ONGOING SUICIDE RISK

When a serious depressive disorder is the underlying cause of the suicidal behaviour, antidepressant medication may be needed or even physical treatment, such as electroconvulsive therapy. However, psychotropic drugs alone are never an adequate safeguard against the risk of suicide. There is evidence that persons who later proceed to commit suicide are often prescribed such drugs for long periods in dosages too low to be effective. Sometimes it is necessary to support a suicidal person as an outpatient over a long period, especially when intensive treatment in hospital has not produced a complete resolution of the problems, for example when there are intractable social or interpersonal difficulties. Correct interview techniques should include appropriate concern, sympathy, and non-judgemental attitudes of the therapist and a refusal to share the patient's feeling of despair. Provision of 'hotline' contact for vulnerable individuals can be useful either with the medical services or one of the voluntary agencies such as the Samaritans, which undoubtedly makes contact with persons who are in serious crisis and who by the usual criteria are at risk of suicide. The principle of befriending, which is followed by the Samaritans, is sound. Close collaboration between statutory and voluntary initiatives of this kind should be strongly encouraged.

PREVENTION OF NON-FATAL REPETITION

During the subsequent year about a quarter of patients repeat one or more non-fatal acts of self-harm, particularly within the first 3 months. There may merely be a further single episode, or a chronic pattern of repeated episodes is resumed, and this may cluster around acute episodes of stress. The likelihood of repetition is greater when the person has made one or more previous attempts. This is one reason why patients seen after the first overdose should be particularly encouraged to accept further help in the hope that this will prevent the development of a repetitive pattern subsequently. Although the provision of intensive psychiatric and social work has not been shown to have a significant effect on the rate of non-fatal repetition, nevertheless thorough clinical assessment can draw attention to problems for which the family doctor would have provided help had the patient sought it in the usual way. In planning treatment, it is advisable to take into account the style of help the patients prefer: some wish to attend their general practitioner, others think psychiatric help more relevant to their problems. There is now some evidence to suggest that open access to help as opposed to fixed appointments may reduce the incidence of non-fatal repetition.

REFERENCES

Department of Health (1992). *The health of the nation: A summary of the strategy for health in England.* White Paper Cm. 1986. HMSO, London.
Hawton, K. and Catalan, J. (1987). *Attempted suicide. A practical guide to its nature and management*, (2nd edn). Oxford University Press.
Morgan, H.G. (1979). *Death wishes. The understanding and management of deliberate self-harm.* Wiley, London.
Paykel, E.S. and Priest, R.G. (1992). Recognition and management of depression in general practice: Consensus statement. *British Medical Journal*, **305**, 1198–1202.

27.3 The relationship between psychiatric disorders and physical illness

27.3.1 Psychological factors and the presentation and course of illness

C. BASS

INTRODUCTION

Psychological and social factors are major determinants of the presentation of illness to doctors. They may also have a primary role in the onset and course of physical illness. Illnesses caused by unhealthy patterns of behaviour, such as smoking, overeating, and excessive alcohol consumption are well documented. What is not so clearly established is whether more specific psychological factors are involved, such as response to life stress and personality traits. This chapter begins with the psychosocial aspects of presentation, and goes on to consider the aetiological significance of psychological and social factors in the onset and course of illness. The effects of psychosocial intervention in certain physical illnesses will also be described.

Determinants of consultation

A number of psychological and social factors may promote consultation with doctors. For example, the frequency, severity, and location of symptoms, stressors in the social environment, family attitudes, and the coexistence of an emotional disorder can all influence what is called 'consulting behaviour'.

Although most people suffer some abnormal sensations much of the time, only a few will take these sensations to doctors for advice. Health diary surveys reveal that the symptoms recorded most frequently are not those that are most commonly reported. For example, in primary care headache is more common than chest pain, yet consultation rates for chest pain are relatively higher. This probably reflects the extent to which chest pain causes concern to patients (and doctors) in our culture.

Women report more acute illness and are greater users of health care services than men of similar age. Women report higher symptom rates even after pregnancy, gynaecological disorders, and breast disease are taken into account. This suggests that women have a greater concern with health, a tendency towards 'introspection' and increased risk of emotional disorders. In addition to this differential sex ratio, broader cultural patterns of illness consulting have been described. For example, one study in New York contrasted the dramatic accounts of symptoms given by Italian Americans with the more stoical response of Anglo-

Saxons. These differences may be a consequence of different family atmospheres and cultural factors at play during the patient's formative years.

Psychological precursors of physical illness

PERSONALITY TRAITS

Clinicians and research workers continue to try to identify personality traits that predispose to illness. The chief difficulty with this approach is that the links almost always have to be made retrospectively. Most interest has focused on what has been called 'type A' personality, a group of traits characterized by impatience, hostility, and 'time-urgency'. In earlier prospective studies, individuals with these characteristics were found to have significantly higher rates of coronary heart disease than their type B counterparts. These personality traits are thought to encourage the appraisal of situations as more stressful, or to prompt behaviours that produce elevated sympathetic and neuroendocrine responses. The resulting physiological reactivity is thought to place a strain on the cardiovascular system and thereby increase the risk of heart disease.

LIFE EVENTS

There have been many accounts of sudden death following unexpected psychological stress. The cause of death is assumed to be an acute myocardial infarction or cardiac arrhythmia, and there is sufficient evidence to attribute many of these cases of sudden cardiac death to psychophysiological factors.

More recently research has concentrated on the nature of the situation or event preceding the onset of illness, along with those long-term personality factors that might render an individual especially sensitive to that situation. For example, there is a significant excess of severely threatening life events before the onset of stroke. It is possible that these stressful events accelerate the arteriosclerotic process, possibly by increased blood pressure or by increasing blood viscosity or coagulability. Certain types of life events have also been implicated in the onset of peptic ulcer, i.e. those in which an important life goal is frustrated by the occurrence of the stressor. An example of such an event is a person's repeated unsuccessful attempts to sue a builder for faulty work.

Current theories propose a series of chains of circumstances, each linking the external situation to the particular physical disorder via the specific characteristics and responses of the individual along the lines shown in Figure 1.

If the emotional response to life events is of sufficient intensity, the disorder may be 'functional' and involve less organic pathology. For example, in Figure 2 the patient may complain to a doctor because their perceptions of physical abnormalities and pain have been heightened by the intensity of the emotional response. This is an important illustration

Fig. 1 Proposed model linking external stressors (life events) to a physical disorder via specific predispositions.

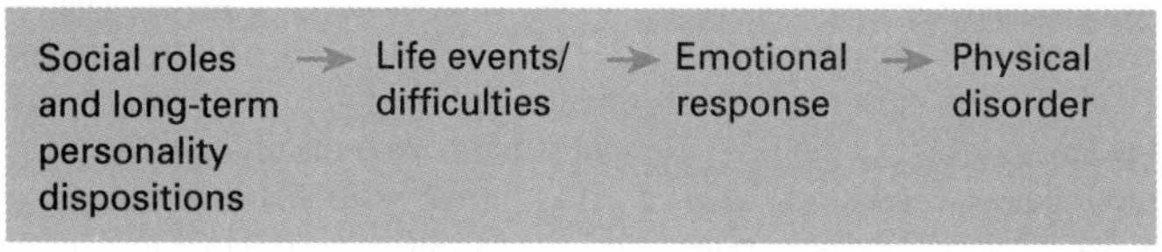

Social roles and long-term personality dispositions	→	Life events/ difficulties	→	Emotional response	→	Physical disorder

Fig. 2 Proposed link between life events, psychological distress, and the perception of bodily sensations.

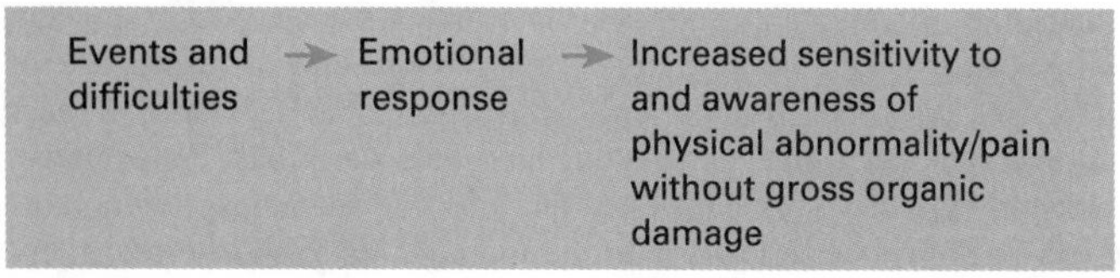

Events and difficulties	→	Emotional response	→	Increased sensitivity to and awareness of physical abnormality/pain without gross organic damage

of the way in which psychological distress influences perceptions of bodily complaints and, in turn, consultation with doctors (see above).

The most persuasive evidence for such a link is the association between life event stress and the onset of a variety of 'functional' illness complaints including unexplained abdominal pain and functional dysphonia, and the recognition that the stressors involved are very similar to those implicated in the onset of emotional disorders.

In another model (Fig. 3), it is less the emotional response and its intensity than the physiological concomitants of this response leading to organic changes that play the critical intervening role in bringing the subject into treatment. A ventricular arrhythmia is an example of such a physiological event.

These models are crude, but they illustrate the crucial interaction between social factors, personality dispositions, and life events that influence the experience and presentation of illness. Complex combinations of the two models are also certainly possible, and there is no reason why both, albeit with different relative importance, may not contribute to the presentation of illness.

Psychosocial factors and the course of illness

There is also strong evidence for the effects of psychological and social variables on the course and recovery from physical illness. For example, habitually anxious patients with peptic ulcers report greater pain, have more postoperative infections and experience more chest complications than less anxious patients. Similarly, the amount of time off work for symptoms of chronic obstructive airways disease is not predicted by standard measures of illness severity (e.g. FEV_1 and PCO_2), but is highly correlated with a combination of psychological variables.

There has been an enormous amount of interest in identifying the mechanisms by which psychological and social factors might be related to the vulnerability and progression of cancer. Patients with certain personality attributes are more likely to avail themselves of early screening for cancer. This is clearly important because early detection and treatment are major determinants of survival. It is less clear, however, whether there is an association between the experience of adverse life events and difficulties and recurrence of certain cancers.

Psychological treatment and physical illness

HEART DISEASE

A number of interventions designed to alter type A behaviour have been shown to reduce the recurrence of myocardial infarction. Another recently completed study appears to have shown that a number of comprehensive 'lifestyle' changes led to regression of even severe coronary atherosclerosis after only 1 year, without the use of lipid-lowering drugs. Although it was not possible to state which component of the intervention (dietary change, exercise, stress reduction, or social support) led to the objective changes in coronary atherosclerosis, further studies examining the impact of psychosocial interventions in the progression of heart disease are warranted.

CANCER

There has been growing interest in the possibility that psychosocial treatment may extend survival time among cancer patients. Women with metastatic breast cancer randomized to weekly group therapy for a year

Fig. 3 Proposed link between life events, psychological distress, and tissue damage, e.g. mental stress can promote ventricular ectopy.

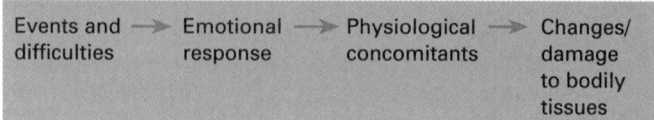

Events and difficulties	→	Emotional response	→	Physiological concomitants	→	Changes/ damage to bodily tissues

have been shown to live significantly longer than those who receive routine treatment, by an average of nearly 18 months. In this important study the emphasis of treatment was on improving communication with family members and doctors, facing and mastering fears about death and dying, and controlling pain and other symptoms. Further studies are required to establish whether the observed differences in survival were a consequence of improved social support or other factors, such as improved compliance, diet, or immune and neuroendocrine function. Nevertheless, both this and the cardiovascular studies demonstrate that psychosocial interventions have a powerful impact on the course of medical illness.

Conclusions

There is little doubt that emotional factors can exert a powerful influence on the onset and course of physical illness. In some instances these may outweigh the extent and influence of any coexisting physical disorder. The application of these ideas to primary prevention is, at present, limited. In established illness, however, there is evidence that psychological management improves the medical outcome, especially in coronary heart disease and certain cancers.

The clinical applications of these research findings are, as yet, undeveloped, but enquiry into recent stresses should be an essential part of the interview when any patient presents new symptoms or a new episode of illness. Clinicians should also encourage patients to avoid unnecessary stressful activities and social isolation and, whenever possible, to participate in exercise. Furthermore, there is a need for doctors to understand the psychological and social determinants of consultation and compliance, so that they can encourage attendance of those who need care and ensure that they obtain the maximum benefit from medical treatment. There is much research evidence to show that compliance is greater when there is a good relationship between patient and doctor, and the patient's role in treatment is explained clearly. Patient handouts, which contain basic information about the illness, medication, and advice for the family, are likely to enhance compliance.

REFERENCES

Harris, T.O. and Brown, G.W. (1989). The LEDS findings in the context of other research: An overview. In *Life events and illness*, (ed. G.W. Brown and T.O. Harris), pp. 385–438. Unwin Hyman, London.

Lloyd, G.G. (1991). *Textbook of general hospital psychiatry*. Churchill Livingstone, Edinburgh.

Ornish, D., *et al.* (1990). Can lifestyle changes reverse coronary artery disease? The lifestyle heart trial. *Lancet*, **336**, 129–33.

Spiegel, D., Bloom, J.R., Kraemer, H.C., and Gottheil, E. (1989). Effect of psychosocial treatment on survival of patients with metastatic breast cancer. *Lancet*, **ii**, 888–91.

27.3.2 Emotional reactions in the dying and the bereaved

R. A. MAYOU

Hospital staff can do much to prevent and relieve distress associated with dying and bereavement. To achieve this, they need some knowledge of the common emotional symptoms and their causes, and of the principles of care. The psychological processes defence mechanisms and copying strategies and the symptoms in response to threat (mainly anxiety) and to loss (mainly depression) are similar for all major stresses, including those described in the previous section on emotional reactions to physical illness.

Distress in the dying

This section (which should be read in conjunction with Section 32) is mainly concerned with patients whose dying is prolonged, rather than those who die rapidly as a result of acute illness. The most common emotional symptoms shown by such patients are depression and anxiety, which frequently include fear of suffering and the unknown, guilt at being a burden to others and abandoning family, and anger directed towards relatives, hospital staff, and to God. This distress and uncertainty may cause difficulty in discussing feelings and practical issues with the family.

DEFENCE MECHANISMS

Those who are dying may use a variety of psychological defence mechanisms to ward off distressing thoughts and feelings, and thereby to assimilate the prospect of dying gradually without overwhelming distress. Variations in the level of denial account for inconsistent behaviour in which dying patients sometimes appear to accept the illness but later behave as if they knew nothing about it. Dependency on other people is inevitable and appropriate. However, a few patients show exaggerated dependency, relinquishing all responsibility; at the other extreme, patients stubbornly resist help although obviously needing it. Displacement is a method of dealing with powerful emotions by displacing them onto others; for example, displacing anger about the fatal illness onto medical staff or relatives. Whilst reducing the patients distress such mechanisms may cause greater distress for others and interfere and prevent appropriate behaviour and treatment.

Causes of emotional distress in the dying patient

The causes of emotional symptoms can be grouped under three headings: physical, psychological, and problems in communication.

PHYSICAL

Emotional distress is often related to physical symptoms, such as pain, nausea, vomiting, and breathlessness or to the fear of such symptoms. It may also be a symptom of delirium. Medication (for example, steroids) and threatening and unpleasant physical treatments, such as radiotherapy and chemotherapy, are also frequent causes of emotional symptoms.

PSYCHOLOGICAL

The threat of physical suffering and the unknown, as well as of the possibility of being abandoned by other people, such as relatives, friends or medical staff are obvious causes of distress. The fear of isolation, loneliness, or abandonment is often strong and may be aggravated by the fear of being a burden to other people. Depression can be understood as a mourning over many losses, the loss of family and friends, a role in society, and life itself. Feelings of anger are sometimes justifiably evoked by neglect or mismanagement by relatives or medical staff; but more often anger is irrational, as an expression of the patient's feeling of helplessness and frustration. The extent to which these emotional reactions emerge in the individual patient will be determined in part by previous personality, especially the capacity to withstand stressful events. Understandably, older patients are generally more reconciled to dying, whilst young adults are especially disturbed by the prospect of leaving young dependent children.

PROBLEMS IN COMMUNICATION

Difficulties in communication are a considerable cause of emotional distress. These difficulties occur because other people are uncertain how to talk to dying patients, and so withdraw from them, leaving them

Table 1 *Elements of psychological management*

Relief of distressing physical symptoms – pain, nausea, breathlessness, etc.
Good relationship with doctor and other hospital staff
Counselling relatives
Enabling death in most appropriate surroundings
Symptomatic relief of emotional distress

Table 2 *Features of normal grief*

Phase 1	Numbness lack of feeling crying disbelief, denial somatic: sighing, choking, abdominal emptiness
Phase 2	Full reaction sadness anger insomnia fatigue guilt social withdrawal preoccupation with the dead person
Phase 3	Resolution ability to think of past with pleasure regained interest in activities new relationships normal sleep sadness at anniversaries and other reminders of dead person

feeling isolated. It is particularly distressing when patients and their families feel unable to communicate openly with one another. This often occurs because each is uncertain what the other knows about the diagnosis and prognosis. They draw back from one another, and the resulting loss of intimate contact is frightening and painful. It also prevents them from discussing future plans realistically. In the absence of good communication, an impending death may cause marital strain, particularly if a marriage has been disturbed in the past.

Giving the diagnosis

Patients have a right to know what is wrong, but how much they are told should depend on how much they want to know and are able to understand. Some patients are too ill for discussion; others want to know themselves, but do not want their relatives to know. (Frequently patients indicate they do not want explicit information.) In the early stage of a serious illness, especially when a cure may be possible, there is little reason to insist on giving full details of the diagnosis and possible prognosis to a patient who has been given ample opportunity to ask further questions but has not done so. Unrealistic reassurance should be avoided. In the later stage of illness, most patients are generally aware of the outlook of their condition and both want and need information.

It is important to be straightforward, avoiding conspiracy with relatives to conceal the truth. There are advantages in seeing the patients and a close relative together but this may not be possible. The doctor should begin by checking what is already known. Information should be given stage by stage, allowing the recipients to absorb what has been said and to ask questions. It is essential to explain positive features, such as the opportunity for effective palliative treatment and a promise to treat unpleasant symptoms. Unrealistic reassurance should be avoided. Some patients and relatives give clear indications they do not want the diagnosis and implications spelt out. Their wish should usually be respected but denial leading to inappropriate behaviour should be explored gently.

Principles of care

It is very important that people are able to die in appropriate surroundings close to their family. Home is often the right place for the patients and relatives, on other occasions a hospice with specialist nursing care may be indicated. It is the doctor's responsibility to help the family make the best arrangements. All hospital units should develop clear policies for the care of the dying and of their relatives.

The prevention and treatment of emotional distress in the dying patient should be directed towards its three main causes: physical, psychological, and distorted communication (Table 1). As much emotional distress is determined by physical causes, it is essential that physical symptoms such as pain, nausea, vomiting, and breathlessness are treated adequately. Dying patients need to know that, if they suffer physical distress, effective medical treatment is available.

The basic requirement for treatment of psychological factors is a good relationship with patients in which they feel free to talk about their illness and feelings. Understandably, doctors find that talking to dying patients is difficult. A fundamental principle is to leave most of the talking to patients. If doctors are willing to listen compassionately, patients will usually be encouraged to talk about their feelings and prob-

lems. Letting patients talk in this way has several advantages. First, it makes them feel valued and accepted rather than abandoned. Second, by allowing them to set the pace on any potentially disturbing subject, it reduces distress. Third, by listening to the cues offered by patients, the clinician can gauge when to intervene. Relatives need to be fully involved and helped by separate counselling. Psychiatric disorder, depression, anxiety, and delirium are all common and can frequently be helped by psychiatric treatment.

Bereavement

Grief is the normal response to the loss of a loved person and similar psychological reactions occur following other forms of loss, such as the break up of a relationship. The psychological processes are also similar to those seen in depressive illness, in which the feeling of loss is a central feature.

It is important that clinicians understand the features of grief, so that they can offer help and because they need to identify a small minority who suffer more severe atypical grief or psychiatric illness. In general practice, the rates of consultation for both emotional and physical symptoms are greatly increased in the months after bereavement. Hospital doctors are most frequently concerned with immediate responses of relatives and friends.

TYPICAL GRIEF

Although the underlying features of grief are similar in different cultures there are considerable differences in the way they are expressed. Many cultures are both more demonstrative in their grief and more supportive to the bereaved than is usual in many developed nations. After bereavement there is usually a stage of numbness followed by the characteristic full reaction and then by then gradual adaptation and recovery to normal function (Table 2).

Phase 1: Shock

This stage, in which the defence mechanism of denial is prominent, usually lasts a few hours or days, and sometimes up to 2 weeks. The patient is largely free of distress and acts as if nothing has happened, apparently, not fully realizing the death has occurred. This feeling of emotional numbness can be helpful at a time when there are usually many special arrangements to be made. There may be bouts of crying and also somatic symptoms. Occasionally there is inability to express any emotion.

Phase 2: Full reaction

This stage of distress and preoccupation with the deceased begins in hours or days of the death and may last for several months. The symptoms, which are described more fully below, are most intense within the first 4 to 6 weeks. Thereafter, there is gradual improvement, spasms of grief can occur at any time precipitated by events, people, or places that bring back memories of the dead person. However, grief is likely to be more prolonged following the death of a spouse and especially following the death of a child.

Grief is especially more likely to be severe if the relationship was ambivalent, there is a feeling of responsibility for the death, there is a history of previous difficulty of coping with losses, and there is a lack of emotional or practical support or if there are major social and financial difficulties.

Phase 3: Resolution

As the more intense feelings of grief diminish, there is resumption of activities and interests, and most people recover from a major bereavement within 1 to 2 years. Despite continuing sadness, especially when reminded by anniversaries or other events, energy and interests increase and it becomes possible to look back on the past with pleasure.

The specific features of typical grief can be described under three headings: (1) psychological changes; (2) social changes; and (3) physical symptoms.

PSYCHOLOGICAL CHANGES

These include depressed mood, preoccupation with memories more systemic of pain, perceptual disturbances, and behavioural anomalies. The bereaved person experiences many of the features of depression, including sorrow, tearfulness, pessimism or despair, loss of interest in work and other activities, a sense of futility, self-neglect, anorexia, and poor sleep. There is often considerable lability of mood. Guilt is highly characteristic in grief, bereaved people accusing themselves of neglecting the deceased or reproaching themselves for minor omissions. Suicidal inclinations may occur and are usually associated with self reproachful ideas of being responsible for the death, or with the belief that life has now little to offer. Insomnia is also common occurring with some frequent severity in up to 80 per cent of bereaved people.

There may be intense preoccupation with memories of the dead person. These include visual mental pictures, perceptual disturbances (including illusions of seeing the dead person and hallucinations of seeing or hearing the dead person). Up to 50 per cent of bereaved people experience the feeling the dead person is present, though not perceived. This is usually described as comforting. There is often a tendency to talk about the lost person at great length, or to idealize them and disregard their faults.

Restlessness and disorganized overactivity are frequent. Some bereaved people wander repeatedly from home, as if attempting to escape from the distress. Others do the opposite, returning to places associated with the deceased, such as their old haunts, the hospital where the person died, or the cemetery, other practices include clinging to the dead persons belongings.

SOCIAL CHANGES

These commonly involve withdrawing from social contact, and sometimes rejection and consolation. There may be a disconcerting loss of warmth and compassion to other people, with resentment and irritability, or even open hostility to relatives, friends, doctors, clergymen, or God. Grief usually impairs working capacity for a period of weeks.

Table 3 *Atypical grief*

Lack of distress
Delayed onset
Prolonged cause
Excessive intensity
Distorted (prominent guilt, overwhelming preoccupation with memories, anger, etc.)
Psychiatric disorder

Table 4 *Management of grief*

Immediate
    break news gently and slowly
    allow opportunity for questions
    offer information and advice
    consider hypnotic for a few days

Later
    offer opportunity for discussion
    give information about counselling and self-help group
    practical help
    be alert to atypical grief

PHYSICAL SYMPTOMS

The most common physical disturbances are those of autonomic disturbance occurring in bouts lasting 20 minutes to an hour. They include tightness in the throat, choking sensations with shortness of breath, sighing, and an empty feeling in the abdomen. Symptoms resembling those of the dead person's final illness are frequent. Mortality is increased following bereavement. The suicide rate is elevated during the year after the loss and death from other causes is also more frequent.

Atypical grief

Atypical grief in which the course or characteristics are exaggerations of normal grief (Table 3) is common and is an indication for extra help (see below). Psychiatric disorder, especially depression, is considerably more frequent than expectation in the months after bereavement. Such illnesses are diagnosed by standard criteria but depressive illness can be especially difficult to distinguish from severe grief. It is more severe, may occur as an obvious deterioration of the normal progress of grief and is more prolonged. Suicidal ideas may occur and there is a lack of even transient pleasure or interest in everyday life.

Helping the bereaved

Most people cope with grief with the help of their family, friends, the clergy, and with support from their primary care doctor and clinical team. Occasionally additional measures are needed. The main indications being abnormally severe or prolonged grief, especially with excessive grief or self-blame. Help may take the form of counselling, which has broad aims of supporting the bereaved person through the period of mourning, and of helping to accept unaccustomed feelings, to readjust to an environment in which the deceased is missing, and to establish new patterns of contact and new relationships. Doctors frequently have to tell relatives that a loved person has died (Table 4).

The first step thereafter in counselling is to befriend the bereaved person and to encourage them to express their feelings of grief. Reassurance about the psychological and physiological accompaniments of normal grief, encouragement to review the lost relationship and to take stock of the present way of life lead to discussion of new directions. Such counselling may be provided by doctors and social workers, but also by voluntary workers from organizations for the bereaved. The

There are far fewer specialists in sexual medicine in the United Kingdom than in the United States, where multidisciplinary clinics for people with sexual problems exist. Some psychiatrists and psychologists specialize in this area of work, particularly for people with sexual problems that are primarily psychological in aetiology. The Relate organization in the United Kingdom has a large number of counsellors training in treating sexual problems. Some urologists take a broad interest in male sexual dysfunctions, not just in the use of intracavernosal injections. Sexual problems resulting from endocrine disorders are best managed by endocrinologists or other medical practitioners specializing in sexual medicine.

PREVENTION

The physician should be particularly concerned with preventing sexual problems consequent on physical illness. Here, awareness of disorders likely to cause sexual difficulties, and willingness to offer appropriate advice are essential. Myocardial infarction provides a good example. The patient can be reassured that sexual intercourse is no more stressful than other moderate physical activity and that it is probably best to resume this aspect of the relationship gradually after 4 to 6 weeks, Sexual activity is best avoided soon after a heavy meal, drinking alcohol, or when tired or anxious. The male superior position should not be used initially because of the extra energy expenditure involved in supporting body weight. If angina occurs during sexual intercourse, this may be prevented by taking a short-acting coronary vasodilatory 10 min beforehand. Both partners should be present when such advice is being provided. Using relatively simple counselling and advice such as this physicians can undoubtedly do much to prevent sexual problems after physical illness.

REFERENCES

Bancroft, J. (1989). *Human sexuality and its problems*, (2nd edn). Churchill Livingstone, Edinburgh.
Friedman, J.H. (1978). Sexual adjustment of the postcoronary male. In *Handbook of sexology* (ed. J. LoPiccolo and L. LoPiccolo), pp. 373–86. Plenum Press, New York.
Hawton, K. (1985). *Sex therapy: A practical guide*. Oxford University Press.
Higgins, G.E. (1978). Aspects of sexual response in adults with spinal cord injury: A review of the literature. In *Handbook of sexology* (ed. J. LoPiccolo and L. LoPiccolo), pp. 373–86. Plenum Press, New York.
Rosen, R.C. and Leiblum, S.R. (1992). *Erectile disorders: Assessment and treatment*. Guilford Press, New York.
Schover, L.R. and Jensen, S.B. (1988). *Sexuality and chronic illness: A comprehensive approach*. Guilford Press, New York.

27.4 Aspects of treatment

27.4.1 Psychopharmacology in medical practice

P. J. COWEN

Because psychotropic drugs are widely used in medical practice, most clinicians are likely to have under their care a number of patients receiving treatment with psychoactive medication (Table 1). Practitioners, therefore, need to have an understanding of the uses and side-effects of psychotropic drugs, particularly of the way in which such medication can interact with drugs used to treat other medical disorders.

The majority of psychotropic drugs are prescribed for the treatment of depressive and anxiety disorders. This reflects the frequency of these conditions in both primary care and general hospital settings; accordingly, drug treatment for anxiety and depression will often be instituted by general practitioners and hospital clinicians. Similarly, while the principal use of antipsychotic drugs is in the treatment of schizophrenia, such agents are also used frequently in general hospitals in the management of organic psychoses. Finally, while treatment with mood stabilizing drugs, such as lithium, will generally be initiated by psychiatrists, patients receiving long-term therapy may well require treatment for coexisting medical disorders where a knowledge of the effects of lithium on different body systems and its liability to produce adverse drug interactions will be required.

Drug overdose

The effects of deliberate or accidental overdosage of psychotropic drugs will also involve physicians (see Chapter 8.2.10). Related to this is the general point that when prescribing psychotropic drugs, particularly for depressed patients, the risk of overdose should always be considered. If such a risk is present the practitioner should: (1) ensure that medication is dispensed in small amounts; (2) consider asking a close relative to supervise the medication; (3) use a relatively non-toxic drug, if possible.

Pharmacokinetic factors

Most psychotropic drugs are highly lipophilic and are well absorbed from the gastrointestinal tract. They are metabolized by the liver to water-soluble derivatives, which are eliminated by the kidney. The half-life of psychotropic drugs will be prolonged in patients with hepatic or renal impairment. Where psychotropic medication is added to other drug treatment the possibility of drug interaction must be considered. Alcohol potentiates the sedative effects of many psychotropic agents and should be avoided during treatment. Sudden discontinuation of psychotropic drugs, particularly tranquillizers, antidepressants, and perhaps lithium, can cause withdrawal symptoms such as insomnia, anxiety, and affective disturbance. Where possible, therefore, the dose of medication should be tapered under supervision.

Compliance with treatment

In psychotropic drug prescribing, compliance is an even greater problem than in general therapeutics. Psychoactive drugs frequently have unpleasant side-effects and, while side-effects are experienced early in treatment, several days may elapse before a therapeutic response is evident. In addition, patients may not see the need for treatment, or believe that it can help them. Careful explanation, supplemented by written instructions, can help ensure that necessary medication is taken.

Antidepressant drugs

TRICYCLIC ANTIDEPRESSANTS

Pharmacology

Tricyclic antidepressants inhibit the neuronal uptake of 5-hydroxytryptamine (5-HT) and noradrenaline. These acute pharmacological actions are followed by a cascade of secondary changes in monoamine and other neurotransmitter receptors. It is believed that the antidepressant effects of drug treatment are caused by these secondary adaptive changes.

Table 1 *Classification of clinical psychotropic drugs*

Name	Examples of classes	Indications
Antipsychotic	Phenothiazines Butyrophenones Substituted benzamides	Acute treatment of schizophrenia and mania, prophylaxis of schizophrenia
Antidepressant	Tricyclic antidepressants Monoamine oxidase inhibitors Selective 5-HT uptake blockers	Major depression (acute treatment and prophylaxis), anxiety disorders, obsessive compulsive disorder (5-HT uptake blockers)
Mood stabilizer	Lithium Carbamazepine	Acute treatment of mania. Prophylaxis of recurrent affective disorder
Anxiolytic	Benzodiazepines Azapirones (buspirone)	Generalized anxiety disorder
Hypnotic	Benzodiazepines Cyclopyrrolones (zopiclone)	Insomnia

Principal drugs

These are amitriptyline, clomipramine, desmethylimipramine, dothiepin, doxepin, imipramine, nortriptyline, and protriptyline.

Indications and use

Tricyclic antidepressants are still the most widely prescribed drug treatment for the management of depressive illness, but their use, particularly in less severe depressive states, is giving way to newer compounds that are better tolerated (see below). However, none of the newer antidepressants is more efficacious than the tricyclics and their therapeutic activity in more severely ill patients is not as well established. For this reason, unless there are specific contraindications, tricyclic antidepressants should be preferred in depressed inpatients or in those with marked melancholic features.

Depressed patients with prominent sleep disturbance and anxiety should be treated with a sedating antidepressant such as amitriptyline; for other patients, less sedating compounds such as imipramine or desipramine can be used. In order to obtain tolerance to side-effects it is usual to begin treatment at a low dose, for example 50 mg of amitriptyline at night, and to increase the amount over about 1 to 2 weeks to the usual therapeutic dose, which ranges between 75 and 200 mg daily for amitriptyline and imipramine. Tricyclic antidepressants have long half-lives and a single daily dose taken at night is usually appropriate. Patients should be warned about side-effects because this helps ensure compliance in the early stages of treatment. They should also be advised that a clear therapeutic response may not appear for up to 2 to 4 weeks. If treatment is successful it is usual to continue the antidepressant for 4 to 6 months at the original dose if tolerance allows. This reduces the risk of early relapse. Some patients with recurrent depressive illness require long-term prophylactic treatment with antidepressant drugs.

Side-effects

As well as inhibiting the uptake of noradrenaline and 5-HT, tricyclic antidepressants possess antagonist properties at a variety of neurotransmitter receptors, including muscarinic cholinergic receptors, α_1-adrenoceptors and H_1-histamine receptors. These receptor antagonist effects account for much of the adverse effect profile of tricyclics, particularly, of course, their anticholinergic properties (Table 2). Tricyclics also possess membrane stabilizing effects that underlie their most serious side-effect of cardiotoxicity. This can be particularly problematic in tricyclic overdose, where ingestion of less than 1 g may sometimes prove fatal.

Drug interactions

Tricyclic antidepressants antagonize the hypotensive effects of adrenergic neurone blockers and clonidine but can be safely combined with

Table 2 *Some adverse effects of tricyclic antidepressants*

Pharmacological action	Adverse effect
Muscarinic receptor blockade (anticholinergic)	Dry mouth, tachycardia, blurred vision, glaucoma, constipation, urinary retention, sexual dysfunction, cognitive impairment
α-Adrenoceptor blockade	Drowsiness, postural hypotension, sexual dysfunction, cognitive impairment
Histamine H_1-receptor blockade	Drowsiness, weight gain
Membrane stabilizing properties	Cardiac conduction defects, cardiac arrhythmias, epileptic seizures
Other	Rash, oedema, leucopenia, elevated liver enzymes

thiazides, β-blockers, and angiotensin converting enzyme (ACE) inhibitors. The ability of tricyclics to block noradrenaline uptake can lead to hypertension with systemically administered noradrenaline and adrenaline.

NEWER ANTIDEPRESSANTS

Principal drugs

These can be classified as follows: (1) selective 5-HT uptake inhibitors (SSRIs), fluoxetine, fluvoxamine, paroxetine, sertraline; (2) modified tricyclic, lofepramine; (3) monoamine receptor antagonists, mianserin, trazodone.

Pharmacology

The actions of selective 5-HT uptake inhibitors are essentially confined to inhibition of 5-HT uptake. Their use is associated with a sustained increase in brain 5-HT neurotransmission. In contrast, the tricyclic compound, lofepramine, mainly inhibits noradrenaline uptake. It also possesses anticholinergic properties, but to a lesser extent than amitriptyline. Mianserin and trazodone lack 5-HT and noradrenaline-uptake-inhibiting properties. They both act as antagonists at certain 5-HT receptor subtypes and at α_1-adrenoceptors. All these compounds, including lofepramine, lack the cardiotoxicity of conventional tricyclic antidepressants. They are, therefore much safer in overdose.

Table 3 *Pharmacological actions and adverse effects of some newer antidepressants*

	Dose (daily) (mg)	Adverse effects
5-HT uptake inhibitors		
fluoxetine	20–60	Nausea, vomiting, anxiety, insomnia, headache, reduced appetite, sweating, skin rash, extrapyramidal movement disorders (rare), generalized allergic reaction (rare), seizures (rare)
fluvoxamine	100–300	
sertraline	50–200	
paroxetine	20–50	
Modified tricyclic		
lofepramine	140–210	Anxiety, insomnia, dry mouth, constipation, seizures (rare)
Sedating antidepressants		
trazodone	150–300	Cognitive impairment, postural hypotension, priapism (rare), cardiac arrhythmias (rare).
mianserin	30–120	Cognitive impairment, weight gain, postural hypotension, bone marrow depression (rare), seizures (rare)

Indications and use

The newer antidepressants should be used in patients where the use of tricyclic antidepressants is contraindicated because of their anticholinergic and cardiotoxic effects. In addition, some patients unable to tolerate a clinically effective dose of a tricyclic may find one of the newer drugs causes fewer side-effects. The lack of sedation associated with the selective 5-HT uptake inhibitors and lofepramine can be beneficial in outpatients striving to carry out their usual activities. Unlike tricyclics, selective 5-HT uptake inhibitors do not stimulate appetite and may therefore be appropriate in patients in whom weight gain would be undesirable. Finally, in patients where the risk of overdose cannot be minimized, the newer drugs may be preferred because of their lower acute toxicity.

Side-effects

The clinical profiles of the newer antidepressants are shown in Table 3. The major distinction between compounds is whether or not they are sedating. The sedating antidepressants have the advantage of improving sleep at an early stage but may impair cognitive function, while the reverse is true for selective 5-HT uptake inhibitors and lofepramine. Like tricyclic antidepressants, the newer compounds appear to lower seizure threshold to some extent, though this effect may be least with trazodone. The SSRIs have rarely been implicated in the development of extrapyramidal disorders such as akathisia and parkinsonism.

Drug interactions

The selective 5-HT uptake inhibitors slow the metabolism of numerous other drugs including warfarin, antipsychotic agents, and tricyclic antidepressants. Dangerous interactions, characterized by 5-HT neurotoxicity, have been reported between SSRIs and monoamine oxidase inhibitors (MAOI). This may be particularly problematic with fluoxetine, whose active metabolite norfluoxetine has a half-life of at 7 to 10 days. At least 5 weeks should therefore elapse between stopping fluoxetine and prescribing monoamine oxidase inhibitor. Selective 5-HT uptake inhibitors may also produce neurotoxicity in combination with lithium. Trazodone and mianserin may increase the sedative effects of other centrally acting drugs. The interactions of lofepramine are similar to those of other tricyclic antidepressants.

MONOAMINE OXIDASE INHIBITORS (MAOIS)

Pharmacology

Monoamine oxidase inhibitors block the enzyme, monoamine oxidase, which deaminates the neurotransmitters, 5-HT, noradrenaline, and dopamine. Monoamine oxidase exists in two forms, known as type A (which deaminates noradrenaline and 5-HT) and type B (which preferentially deaminates dopamine and tyramine). Conventional monoamine oxidase inhibitors irreversibly deactivate both type A and type B monoamine oxidase. This has two main consequences of importance for monoamine oxidase inhibitor use; (1) there is a potential for serious food and drug interactions; and (2) the consequent drug and food restrictions need to be continued for 2 weeks after cessation of monoamine oxidase inhibitor treatment so that new monoamine oxidase can be synthesized.

Recently a new monoamine oxidase inhibitor, moclobemide, has been introduced. Moclobemide differs from conventional monoamine oxidase inhibitors in that its inhibition of monoamine oxidase is reversible and it selectively inhibits type A monoamine oxidase only. This leads to an increase in brain noradrenaline and 5-HT but other amines such as tyramine are much less affected. These factors make moclobemide much less likely than the older monoamine oxidase inhibitors to produce adverse food and drug interactions, which gives it a significant safety advantage. However, current clinical experience with moclobemide is still somewhat limited and accordingly the discussion below will focus on the conventional monoamine oxidase inhibitors.

Principal drugs

These are isocarboxazid, phenelzine, tranylcypromine, and moclobemide.

Indications and use

Conventional monoamine oxidase inhibitors are rarely used as a first choice of antidepressant except where a patient is known to have responded to them in the past. They are accordingly usually reserved for subjects who have failed to respond to tricyclic antidepressants or electroconvulsive therapy, where a very useful antidepressant effect can often be achieved. Monoamine oxidase inhibitors may also be more effective than tricyclics in atypical depressive states characterized by mood reactivity, hypersomnia, hyperphagia, and excessive sensitivity to real or imagined rejection. In addition, some forms of bipolar depression, with features of anergia and hypersomnia respond better to monoamine oxidase inhibitors than to tricyclics.

Phenelzine and tranylcypromine are the two most commonly prescribed monoamine oxidase inhibitors. The usual therapeutic dose for phenelzine is between 30 and 90 mg daily. As with tricyclic antidepressants, patients should be informed about side-effects and advised that a therapeutic response from monoamine oxidase inhibitors may not be apparent for 3 to 4 weeks. Once a response is obtained, it is usually necessary to continue treatment for several months.

Side-effects

Monoamine oxidase inhibitors may cause the following side-effects. Central nervous system: dizziness, muscular twitching, insomnia, confusion, mania. Cardiovascular: tachycardia, postural hypotension, hypertension. Other: dry mouth, blurred vision, impotence, peripheral oedema, hepatocellular damage, leucopenia.

Food and drug interactions

The major hazard of conventional monoamine oxidase inhibitor treatment is through interaction with indirect sympathomimetics, that is, agents that release noradrenaline from nerve endings. The usual source of the interaction is tyramine in certain foodstuffs, especially cheese and meat extracts. Tyramine is usually metabolized by monoamine oxidase in the gut wall and liver but in patients taking monoamine oxidase inhibitors large amounts may enter the systemic circulation, resulting in hypertension and even cerebrovascular accidents. Similar adverse effects have been reported when sympathomimetic drugs, such as amphetamine or ephedrine, are administered to patients taking monoamine oxidase inhibitors. As the latter drug, or its derivatives, are frequently present in cold cures, patients must be warned against self-medication. Hypertensive episodes resulting from interaction of sympathomimetic drugs and monoamine oxidase inhibitors are best treated with an α_1-adrenoceptor antagonist, such as phentolamine. If this is unavailable, intramuscular chlorpromazine is an alternative. Monoamine oxidase inhibitors also produce important interactions with other commonly used drugs including opiates, insulin, and oral hypoglycaemics. Except in special circumstances, combination with tricyclic antidepressants is best avoided. Combination with clomipramine and selective 5-HT uptake inhibitors can cause a 5-HT neurotoxicity syndrome and is contraindicated.

From the foregoing it will apparent that conventional monoamine oxidase inhibitors should only be prescribed to patients capable of adhering to the necessary dietary restrictions. Written instructions listing prohibited foods should be provided. No additional medication should be given until the possibility of adverse drug interaction has been excluded.

Moclobemide

Controlled studies have shown that the reversible type A monoamine oxidase inhibitor, moclobemide, is effective in the treatment of major depression. Moclobemide is well tolerated, although insomnia and nausea may occur. Unlike conventional monoamine oxidase inhibitors, moclobemide does not cause significant interaction with tyramine; adverse drug interactions also seem to be less likely. However, caution is recommended when prescribing with opiates and, until further data is available, combined use with selective 5-HT uptake inhibitors and sympathomimetic agents should be avoided. Because of the reversible nature of moclobemide's interaction with monoamine oxidase and its short half-life (about 3 h), normal monoamine oxidase activity is restored within a day of stopping treatment.

While moclobemide appears to be effective in the treatment of uncomplicated major depression, it is not yet clear whether its antidepressant effect will match that of phenelzine and tranylcypromine in patients resistant to tricyclic antidepressants. Similarly it is not yet known whether moclobemide will be effective in the treatment of patients with atypical depression.

Mood stabilizing drugs

LITHIUM

Pharmacology

Lithium salts have effects on receptor transduction systems, particularly the turnover of phosphoinositols, that may prevent excessive intracellular signalling. Lithium also produces marked increases in some aspects of brain 5-HT function.

Indications and use

The main use of lithium is in the prophylaxis of recurrent affective disorders, especially manic depressive illness. Lithium is also used in

Table 4 *Some adverse effects and interactions of lithium*

Central nervous system	Drowsiness, lethargy, headache, memory impairment, fine tremor
Cardiovascular system	Conduction defects (rare)
Gastrointestinal system	Nausea, vomiting, diarrhoea
Genitourinary system	Polydipsia, polyuria, nephrogenic diabetes insipidus
Endocrine system	Hypothyroidism (T4 ↓ TSH ↑), hyperglycaemia, hyperparathyroidism
Other	Leucocytosis, skin rash, weight gain
Drug interaction (lithium level ↑)	Diuretics, non-steroidal anti-inflammatory drugs, metronidazole, erythromycin
Signs of toxicity (plasma level > 1.5 mmol/l)	Nausea, vomiting, coarse tremor, drowsiness, dysarthria, seizures, coma, renal failure, cardiovascular collapse

T$_4$, thyroxine; TSH, thyroid stimulating hormone.

the acute treatment of mania but is less immediately effective than antipsychotic medication, particularly in the presence of psychotic symptoms. Depressed patients unresponsive to antidepressant drugs often show benefit when lithium is added to their antidepressant drug treatment.

The excretion of lithium is from the body is critically dependent on the kidney and since there is little margin between therapeutic plasma levels of lithium (0.5 to 1.0 mmol/l) and those causing toxicity (> 1.5 mmol/l) the introduction of lithium therapy should be preceded by a clinical and laboratory assessment of renal function. Renal function tests should include urine analysis and estimations of plasma creatinine and electrolytes. A creatinine clearance test should be performed if there is any suggestion of impaired renal function.

Patients should initially be treated with 400 to 800 mg daily of lithium carbonate. It is usually preferable to administer the whole daily dose at night. Slow release preparations of lithium are available but their pharmacokinetics *in vivo* are very similar to those of the standard preparation. Dosage should be adjusted every 5 to 7 days on the basis of plasma lithium determinations obtained approximately 12 h after the last dose. For prophylaxis of recurrent mood disorders plasma levels of 0.5 to 0.8 mmol/l are usually satisfactory; however, some patients, particularly those with an acute manic episode may require higher levels (0.8 to 1.0 mmol/l). Most patients achieve adequate plasma levels on dosages of lithium carbonate between 800 and 1600 mg daily, and following this the lithium requirement is usually remarkably stable. In the absence of clinical indications it is usually sufficient to check lithium levels every 2 to 3 months and repeat renal function tests every 6 months. Lithium can also cause hypothyroidism, so thyroid function tests should be performed prior to treatment and at 6-monthly intervals thereafter. If necessary lithium can be combined with thyroxine replacement therapy.

Side-effects

Many patients suffer from a fine tremor and nausea; diarrhoea may occur, especially at the start of treatment (Table 4). Some degree of thirst and polyuria is often present, and a few patients develop nephrogenic diabetes insipidus. These latter effects are probably caused by lithium blocking the effect of antidiuretic hormone (ADH) on the renal tubule. Most patients taking lithium have a demonstrable impairment of tubular concentrating ability, although this is rarely of clinical significance. Glomerular function is not usually affected by lithium, although, following lithium toxicity, glomerular damage and interstitial fibrosis have been reported. From current evidence it seems unlikely that long-term use of lithium within therapeutic plasma concentrations results in irreversible renal damage.

Up to 80 per cent of the lithium filtered by the renal glomerulus is reabsorbed by the proximal tubule. Conditions such as diarrhoea and excessive sweating, which decrease body sodium, result in increased lithium reabsorption by the renal tubule leading to elevated plasma lithium levels.

Drug interactions

Thiazide diuretics, through their effect on sodium excretion, increase lithium reabsorption and can produce lithium toxicity unless the dose of lithium is reduced and plasma concentrations carefully monitored. It is said that loop and potassium sparing diuretics are unlikely to alter lithium clearance but it is prudent, nevertheless, to monitor lithium levels when using these drugs. Plasma lithium levels may also be increased by concomitant administration of non-steroidal anti-inflammatory drugs, and a similar effect may be produced by metronidazole and erythromycin. While the effects of lithium on cardiac conduction are usually considered benign, the effects of cardiac glycosides on conduction may be potentiated. Finally lithium may increase the liability of antipsychotic drugs to cause extrapyramidal movement disorders.

Lithium toxicity

Acute lithium toxicity usually appears at plasma levels above 1.5 mmol/l. Early signs are coarse tremor, drowsiness, and dysarthria. Higher plasma concentrations (> 2.5 mmol/l) can lead to seizures, coma, and death. Lithium toxicity is therefore a potentially fatal disorder and any suspicion of intoxication should lead to immediate withdrawal of lithium treatment and close monitoring of serum lithium and plasma electrolyte and creatinine concentrations. Severely ill patients with high serum lithium levels may require dialysis.

CARBAMAZEPINE

Pharmacology

Like certain other anticonvulsant drugs, carbamazepine blocks neuronal sodium channels. The relation of this effect to its therapeutic actions in affective disorder is uncertain. Similarly to lithium, carbamazepine facilitates some aspects of brain 5-HT neurotransmission.

Indications and use

Carbamazepine is effective in the acute treatment of mania and in the prophylaxis of bipola
r affective disorder. It is used in patients who have difficulty tolerating or who do not respond to lithium therapy. It is possible in the latter patients for carbamazepine to be combined with lithium.

The dose range of carbamazepine employed to treat affective illness is similar to that used in the treatment of seizure disorders, although it is advisable to titrate the dose according to clinical response. Plasma level monitoring may be used to help avoid toxicity. Initial treatment should be with 100 mg of carbamazepine twice daily and the dose increased according to tolerance over the next 2 to 4 weeks. The effective dose range in the treatment of bipolar disorder is generally between 600 and 1200 mg daily, although some patients may require higher doses.

Side-effects

Dizziness, drowsiness, and nausea are common early in treatment, particularly with rapid dose titration, but tolerance to these effects usually occurs. Persistent ataxia and diplopia may indicate toxic plasma levels. A moderate degree of leucopenia is often seen during carbamazepine treatment and agranulocytosis may develop occasionally. For this reason it is prudent to monitor white cell counts well as carbamazepine levels

during treatment. Skin rashes are also quite common. Other rarer adverse effects include low plasma sodium concentrations and liver cell damage. Circulating thyroid levels may be lowered by carbamazepine treatment but thyroid stimulating hormone (TSH) levels generally remain in the normal range and clinical hypothyroidism is unusual. Carbamazepine can impair cardiac conduction and should be used with caution in patients with cardiovascular disease.

Drug interactions

Carbamazepine increases the metabolism of a number of other drugs including tricyclic antidepressants, haloperidol, oral contraceptive agents, warfarin, and other anticonvulsants. A similar mechanism may underlie the decline in plasma carbamazepine levels sometimes seen during continued treatment. Carbamazepine levels may be increased by erythromycin, and some calcium-channel blockers such as diltiazem and verapamil. Reversible neurotoxicity has been reported when carbamazepine has been combined with lithium.

Antipsychotic drugs

PHARMACOLOGY

Antipsychotic drugs, also known as major tranquillizers or neuroleptics, are a group of agents of varied structure that have in common the ability to block dopamine receptors in the central nervous system. It is likely that the antipsychotic effect of major tranquillizers is caused by blockade of dopamine receptors in mesolimbic and mesocortical brain regions. However, while the dopamine receptor blockade occurs within hours of drug administration, a useful clinical response may not occur for days and sometimes weeks after the start of treatment.

PRINCIPAL DRUGS

These are chlorpromazine, clozapine, haloperidol, flupenthixol, fluphenazine, loxapine, pimozide, risperidone, sulpiride, thioridazine, and trifluoperazine.

INDICATIONS AND USE

Antipsychotic drugs are used mainly in the management of schizophrenia. They are also used to treat mania and sometimes given to depressed patients who have psychotic symptoms or who are particularly agitated. Antipsychotic drugs are also used in the management of disturbed behaviour arising from other causes, for example, confusional states, but their use as non-specific tranquillizing agents should be limited to short-term use if possible because of potentially serious side-effects.

In the treatment of acute confusional states, haloperidol, in doses of 1.0 to 5.0 mg is often helpful. This can be administered either orally or parenterally and the dose repeated after an hour if the patient remains disturbed. Cardiovascular and respiratory side-effects are unlikely with haloperidol but acute dystonias can occur and should be treated appropriately (Table 5). Thioridazine is popular for the treatment of confused elderly patients but its anticholinergic properties may worsen orientation and memory. Finally it is worth noting that certain groups of demented patients (particularly those with Lewy body type dementia) may suffer severe extrapyramidal effects from comparatively low doses of antipsychotic drugs.

The treatment of patients with schizophrenia or mania with antipsychotic drugs requires careful monitoring and persistence because the full therapeutic response may be delayed for some weeks and the dose of antipsychotic drug required may vary considerably from patient to patient and also within the same patient at different stages of the illness. Generally for a young person with an acute psychosis, up to 1000 mg a day of chlorpromazine may be necessary, this dose being achieved gradually over several days, while sedative and hypotensive side-effects

Table 5 *Extrapyramidal disorders and antipsychotic drugs*

Disorder	Description	Treatments employed
Dystonic reaction	Involuntary muscle contraction, especially face and jaw, occulogyric crisis	1. Benztropine (1–2 mg IM or IV) 2. Diazepam (10 mg iv)
Akathisia	Sense of subjective motor restlessness, continual pacing	1. Reduce dose of antipsychotic drug 2. Benztropine (1–6 mg daily) 3. Propranolol (40–120 mg daily) 4. Diazepam (10–30 mg daily)
Parkinsonism	Rigidity, bradykinesia, tremor	1. Reduce dose of neuroleptic 2. Benztropine (1–6 mg daily)
Tardive dyskinesia (late onset)	Choreoathetoid movements, especially tongue, lips and jaw	1. Withdraw antipsychotic drug 2. Sulpiride 3. Calcium channel blocker
Neuroleptic malignant syndrome (rare)	Fever, muscular rigidity, coma, death	1. Discontinue neuroleptic 2. Intensive care support 3. Bromocriptine 4. Dantrolene

decrease. In patients with cardiovascular disease, treatment with haloperidol in doses up to 30 mg daily is safer. All antipsychotic drugs are subject to first-pass metabolism so parenterally administered medication produces a proportionally greater effect. If a patient has responded to an antipsychotic drug it is usual to continue the medication for a number of months into remission. Frequently it is necessary to administer medication on a long-term basis to prevent relapse, in which case the use of long-acting intramuscular preparations will improve compliance. The decanoates of fluphenazine, flupenthixol, and haloperidol are most commonly used.

SIDE-EFFECTS

Movement disorders

Through their blockade of brain dopamine receptors, antipsychotic drugs produce a variety of movement disorders that can mimic signs of basal ganglia disease (Table 5). Many patients, for example, may exhibit symptoms of parkinsonism very similar to those of the idiopathic disorder (although tremor is less prominent). A side-effect that appears early in treatment is acute dystonia, which can present with abnormal postures or dramatic muscular spasms involving the face and limbs. Laryngeal spasm with respiratory distress can also occur. A history of recent antipsychotic drug use can help avoid misdiagnoses (it is not unusual, for example, for such reactions to be viewed as 'hysterical'). Another movement disorder that patients find very distressing is akathisia, which is a state of motor restlessness often with agitation and dysphoria. Distinguishing this reaction from symptoms arising from the underlying psychiatric disorder may not be easy.

All these movement disorders may be treated by a reduction in dosage of the antipsychotic drug or by the introduction of anticholinergic medication such as benzotropine. However, anticholinergic drugs should not be prescribed routinely with antipsychotic medication because of the risk of abuse for their euphoriant effects. Later in treatment tardive dyskinesia may develop. This consists of involuntary repetitive movements usually involving the tongue and lips though other parts of the body may be involved. Tardive dyskinesia may be associated with supersensitivity of postsynaptic dopamine receptors in the basal ganglia; at present this disorder cannot be treated easily and anticholinergic medication may make it worse. If possible the antipsychotic drug should be stopped but this decision is often difficult because of the risk of relapse of the psychiatric disorder. Of the available antipsychotic drugs, sulpiride, risperidone, and clozapine (see below) are least likely to cause movement disorders.

Neuroleptic malignant syndrome

A rare but potentially very serious reaction to antipsychotic drugs is the neuroleptic malignant syndrome (Table 25). This is characterized by fever, rigidity and altered consciousness, together with tachycardia and labile blood pressure. Laboratory investigations usually reveal a leucocytosis together with markedly raised levels of creatinine phosphokinase. Antipsychotic drug treatment should be withdrawn immediately if the neuroleptic malignant syndrome is suspected. Management in an intensive care facility may be needed to deal with cardiovascular, respiratory, and renal complications. Treatment with dopamine receptor agonist, bromocriptine, and the antispasticity agent, dantrolene, appears to be beneficial.

Other side-effects

Antipsychotic drugs, especially chlorpromazine and thioridazine, can produce a variety of side-effects due to blockade of muscarinic receptors and α-adrenoceptors. These include drowsiness, psychomotor impairment, confusion, tachycardia, postural hypotension, blurring of vision, precipitation of glaucoma, dry mouth, constipation, urinary hesitancy, and impaired sexual function. Other side-effects include, endocrine: elevated prolactin levels, amenorrhoea, and galactorrhoea; skin: rashes, pigmentation, and photosensitivity (especially phenothiazines); other: precipitation of seizures, hypothermia (especially chlorpromazine), cardiac arrhythmias (pimozide), weight gain, cholestatic hepatitis, leucopenia, and retinitis pigmentosa (thioridazine in doses > 800 mg daily).

Drug interactions

Antipsychotic drugs potentiate the effects of other central sedatives. They may delay the hepatic metabolism of tricyclic antidepressants and antiepileptic drugs leading to increased plasma levels of these latter agents. The hypotensive properties of chlorpromazine and thioridazine may enhance the effects of antihypertensive drugs.

CLOZAPINE

Clozapine is pharmacologically distinct from other antipsychotic drugs in that it is a weak dopamine D_2 receptor antagonist but binds strongly to the 5-HT$_2$ receptor subtype. A significant proportion (perhaps about 50 per cent) of patients refractory to conventional antipsychotic drugs may derive clinical benefit from clozapine treatment. Interestingly, negative symptoms of schizophrenia, such as apathy and amotivation, which are frequently refractory to conventional antipsychotic drugs, may also respond. However, the use of clozapine is associated with a significant risk of leucopenia (about 2 to 3 per cent), which can progress to agranulocytosis. Weekly white cell counts during treatment are mandatory and with this intensive monitoring the early detection of leucopenia can be followed by immediate clozapine withdrawal and reversal of the low white cell count. While this procedure makes progression to agranulocytosis very unlikely, fatalities due to clozapine-induced agranulocytosis have been reported despite the use of this monitoring system. In severe and intractable schizophrenia, however, the use of clozapine may be justified.

Clozapine is less likely than other neuroleptics to cause extrapyramidal movement disorders and does not increase plasma prolactin. However, its use is associated with hypersalivation, drowsiness, postural hypotension, weight gain, and hyperthermia. Seizures may occur at higher doses. It is usually recommended that clozapine be used as the sole antipsychotic agent in a treatment regime and clearly it is wise to avoid concomitant use of drugs, such as carbamazepine, which may also lower white cell count.

RISPERIDONE

Risperidone is a benzisoxazole derivative that is a potent antagonist of dopamine D_2 and 5-HT$_2$ receptors. Placebo-controlled trials have shown that risperidone is at least as effective as haloperidol but causes fewer extrapyramidal movement disorders. It may also produce a greater amelioration of depressive symptoms. There are indications from the controlled studies that risperidone may be of benefit in the treatment of negative symptoms of schizophrenia, but further investigations will be needed to determine the significance of this effect for clinical practice.

Risperidone has some antagonist activity at α_1-adrenoceptors but is generally not sedating. It has, however, been reported to cause postural hypotension. Other side-effects that are observed include insomnia, anxiety, and headache.

Antianxiety agents
BENZODIAZEPINES

Pharmacology
Benzodiazepines enhance the action of the neurotransmitter, γ-aminobutyric acid (GABA), in the central nervous system, by binding to a specific benzodiazepine receptor located in a complex with a GABA receptor and a chloride ion channel. The pharmacological effects of benzodiazepines are attributed to facilitation of GABA neurotransmission.

Principal drugs
These are alprazolam, chlorazepate, diazepam, flurazepam, lorazepam, lormetazepam, nitrazepam, and temazepam.

Indications and use
The prescription of benzodiazepines is now decreasing following concern about their liability to produce dependence. For most anxiety-related disorders, alternative therapies are available and it is recommended that the drug treatment of anxiety and insomnia should be limited to a few weeks duration. The major indication for the use of benzodiazepines is to help patients in a crisis when anxiety and insomnia are causing functional impairment and reducing ability to cope. Patients should be advised that drug treatment will be of short duration to help them manage their immediate difficulties. All benzodiazepines have hypnotic and anxiolytic properties. The major distinction of clinical importance is their length of action. Derivatives with a 3-hydroxy group such as temazepam are metabolized by the liver to inactive glucuronides and have shorter half-lives; such drugs are suitable hypnotics because of their lack of hangover effect. Other benzodiazepines, for example diazepam, have long half-lives and are metabolized to active compounds. These drugs may used for the treatment of anxiety either in the

form of regular dosing, or on the now preferred 'as required' basis with an agreed maximum daily dose.

Side-effects and interactions
Benzodiazepines have a low acute toxicity. Their adverse effects are extensions of their clinical effects and include the following: drowsiness, psychomotor impairment, dizziness, ataxia, and paradoxical aggression (rare). Benzodiazepines potentiate other central sedatives, particularly alcohol. The effects of benzodiazepines are potentiated by cimetidine.

Patients who have taken clinical doses of a benzodiazepine for more than a few months may show a withdrawal syndrome when the medication is stopped. In many respects this syndrome resembles an anxiety state but perceptual disturbances and dysphoria may also occur. It is thus apparent that benzodiazepines can cause physical dependence and although the withdrawal syndrome is less severe than that seen following cessation of barbiturates, patients frequently find it extremely difficult to stop their medication. A gradual reduction is usually best. Generally, withdrawal from a long-acting benzodiazepine is easier than from a short-acting preparation. If patients taking short-acting benzodiazepines have difficulties withdrawing, a switch to a long-acting preparation may be helpful.

OTHER DRUGS THAT INCREASE BRAIN GABA FUNCTION
Zopiclone
Zopiclone is a cyclopyrrolone derivative that binds to a site close to the benzodiazepine receptor and thereby facilitates brain GABA function. Zopiclone is indicated for the short-term treatment of insomnia and is claimed to be less likely than benzodiazepine hypnotics to produce tolerance and withdrawal effects. These proposals, however, have yet to be fully evaluated.

Chlormethiazole
Chlormethiazole also binds at the GABA receptor complex but its clinical effects resembles barbiturates rather more than benzodiazepines in that it can cause serious respiratory depression in overdose, particularly in combination with alcohol. In fact, chlormethiazole is a popular treatment to ameliorate the symptoms of alcohol withdrawal but should be used in short courses to prevent the development of dependence. Because of its short half-life (4 to 5 hours), chlormethiazole is also used as a hypnotic in the elderly; dependence in this age group has not been reported.

DRUGS ALTERING MONOAMINE FUNCTION
Buspirone
Buspirone is a 5-HT receptor agonist, structurally unrelated to benzodiazepines. It is effective in the treatment of generalized anxiety disorder (less so in patients previously exposed to benzodiazepines) but has a slow onset of action (1 to 3 weeks). Unlike benzodiazepines buspirone does not cause significant sedation or cognitive impairment and at present appears unlikely to cause dependence. It does not have hypnotic properties. Side-effects include nervousness, dizziness, and headache.

Other drugs
Tricyclic antidepressants, selective 5-HT uptake inhibitors and monoamine oxidase inhibitors are effective in the management of patients with anxiety syndromes characterized by frequent panic attacks. Alprazolam is also used for this purpose but carries the general disadvantages of benzodiazepine treatment. Obsessive compulsive disorder is also classified as an anxiety disorder, although benzodiazepines are not an effective treatment. In fact, the drug treatment response of patients with obsessive compulsive disorder is rather specific in that clear superiority over placebo has been demonstrated only for drugs such as the selective

5-HT uptake inhibitors and clomipramine that potently inhibit the uptake of 5-HT.

REFERENCES

Chou, J.C.-Y. (1991). Recent advances in the treatment of acute mania. *Journal of Clinical Psychopharmacology*, **11**, 3–21.

Cowen, P.J. (1992). New antidepressants: have they superceded tricyclics. In *Practical problems in psychiatry: some clinical guidelines* (ed. K.E. Hawton and P.J. Cowen). Oxford University Press.

Davis, J.M. (1991). Treatment of schizophrenia. *Current Opinion in Psychiatry*, **4**, 28–33.

Eison, A.S. and Temple, D.L. (1986). Buspirone: A review of its pharmacology and current perspectives on its mechanism of action. *American Journal of Medicine*, **80**, (3b), 1–9.

Goodman, W.K., McDougle, C.J., and Price, L.H. (1992). The pharmacotherapy of obsessive compulsive disorder. *Journal of Clinical Psychiatry*, **53** 4 (suppl.), 29–37.

Goodwin, F.K. and Jamison, K.R. (1990). Maintenance medical treatment. In *Manic depressive illness*, pp. 665–724. Oxford University Press.

Kane, J., Honigfeld, G., Singer, J., and Meltzer, H. (1988). 'Clozaril Collaborative Study Group'. Clozapine for the treatment resistant schizophrenic: A double blind comparison with chlorpromazine. *Archives of General Psychiatry*, **45**, 789–96.

Lader, M. and Herrington, R. (1990). *Biological treatments in psychiatry*. Oxford University Press.

Marder, S.R. and Van Putten, T. (1988). Who should receive clozapine? *Archives of General Psychiatry*, **45**, 865–7.

Nutt, D.J. and Glue, P.W. (1989). Monoamine oxidase inhibitors: Rehabilitation from recent research. *British Journal of Psychiatry*, **154**, 287–91.

Paykel, E.S. (1989). Treatment of depression: the relevance of research to clinical practice. *British Journal of Psychiatry*, **155**, 754–763.

Potter, W.Z., Rudorfer, M.V., and Manji, H. (1991). The pharmacologic treatment of depression. *New England Journal of Medicine*, **325**, 633–42.

Reynolds, G.P. (1992). Developments in the drug treatment of schizophrenia. *Trends in Pharmacological Sciences*, **13**, 116–21.

Rudorfer, M.V. and Potter, W.Z. (1989). Antidepressants: a comparative review of the clinical pharmacology and therapeutic use of the newer versus the older drugs. *Drugs*, **37**, 713–38.

Tyrer, S.P. and Murphy, S. (1987). The place of benzodiazepines in psychiatric practice. *British Journal of Psychiatry*, **151**, 719–23.

Wood, A.J. and Goodwin, G.M. (1987). A review of the biochemical and neuropharmacological actions of lithium. *Psychological Medicine*, **17**, 579–600.

27.4.2 Psychological treatment in medical practice

M. G. GELDER

Psychological treatment varies in complexity between the simple support and explanation, which form a part of good medical care, and elaborate forms of psychotherapy carried out by specialist psychotherapists. The present account is restricted to an outline of the kinds of psychological treatment most likely to be of value for patients encountered by physicians. These treatments are supportive therapy, problem solving counselling and crisis intervention, and certain cognitive and behaviour therapies. Brief mention will be made also of dynamic psychotherapies. The simplest of these psychological measures can be carried out by the physician, some of the others can be given by another member of the medical team – often a social worker or nurse specialist – while the rest require referral to a psychiatrist, a clinical psychologist, or a psychiatric nurse-specialist. A fuller account will be found in the *Oxford textbook of psychiatry*.

THE VALUE OF LISTENING AND GIVING INFORMATION

Before considering specific methods of psychological treatment, note should be taken of the value of allowing patients to express their worries and to find out about the illness and its effects. Many mildly anxious or depressed patients need no more help than a simple interview of this kind. Surveys of patients have shown that most wish to receive a fuller explanation of the nature of the illness, the results of tests, the purpose of medication, the length of time they may be off work, and whether any lasting disability is to be expected. Although physicians try to provide this information, they do not always allow enough time to find out what patients want to know and whether they have understood what they have been told.

Information should be in simple language, avoiding technical terms, but complete; doctors often underestimate patients' capacity for understanding medical matters. Extra care is needed when giving information to a person from another culture who may hold different views about illness or treatment. Because anxious people remember little of what they have been told, important points should be repeated or put in writing to be read later.

Reassurance should be offered only after finding out the patient's concerns in some detail and it should be realistic and truthful. It is important, of course, to find out what others may have told the patient so that the advice does not appear contradictory or, if it is different, that the reasons for the alternative view are explained. Relatives as well as patients, may need advice and reassurance and it is not uncommon to find that a patient's excessive anxiety does not subside until the relatives have been reassured.

SUPPORTIVE COUNSELLING

As explained above, advice and reassurance from the physician can relieve many of the psychological problems encountered in physically ill patients. However, some patients require more than one interview to talk over their concerns about the illness and its effects. This supportive counselling can be carried out by the physician or may be delegated to a nurse counsellor who has experience of the problems associated with physical illness: this arrangement is sometimes adopted for example for patients after myocardial infarction, or for patients requiring a colostomy.

Supportive counselling does not involve technical procedures; the main requirements are an understanding of the effects of illness on every life, an ability to listen, and sufficient time. Patients are encouraged to collaborate fully with the plan of medical treatment and discover the ways of making use of their remaining capacities.

In supportive counselling, as in every other kind of psychological treatment, care is needed to ensure that patients do not become too dependent on the counsellor. Excessive dependency may cause unnecessary distress for the patient, unreasonable demands on the doctor to prolong interviews, and unreasonable calls for help. Dependency is avoided when the relationship between the patient and the counsellor is clearly professional, and the patient understands that the counsellor is equally concerned about other patients. It is helpful to explain the team work involved in care so that feelings of dependency are directed to the group of staff and not to an individual. A careful watch should be kept carefully for early signs of dependency such as inappropriate ways of claiming attention. If such signs are observed, they should be discussed with to the patient and the limits of a professional relationship pointed out.

Problem solving counselling and crisis intervention

Problem solving counselling is a more structured treatment designed to help patients to find solutions to problems that are causing distress. The aim is to help patients deal with problems themselves, not to do this for them; in this way they are more likely to deal effectively with future problems without help. Problem solving counselling can be learnt quickly and used by physicians, or carried out by nurses or social workers. There are four stages. First, patients are encouraged to list and define their current problems. This alone often helps people who feel overwhelmed by their illness and other problems. Second, patients select a problem to work on, are helped to consider possible ways of dealing with this problem, and are encouraged to choose a solution likely to succeed. Third, patients are encouraged to carry out the first part of the chosen plan and to report the result. These activities are presented as experiments in which an attempt that proves unsuccessful not a failure but as a source of information leading to a more effective plan. This approach is important for patients who are demoralized as a result of persistent ill health and social difficulties. Fourth, when the first problem has been solved, another is chosen and the process is repeated. This simple but systematic counselling has been shown in randomized clinical trials to be as effective as drug treatment for the patients with anxiety and depression treated in primary care and it is equally suitable for use in hospital practice.

When problem solving counselling is used for patients whose life problems have suddenly become overwhelming it is called crisis intervention. Suitable patients include those who have taken a drug overdose as a form of deliberate self-harm. These patients are usually in a state of high emotional arousal when first interviewed, and before problem solving counselling can be started it is usually necessary to reduce arousal by allowing the patient to talk about their feelings. As in the treatment of patients who are not in crisis, it is important to emphasize that the patient is not just resolving the present crisis but also learning a general approach that can be used should there be future problems.

COGNITIVE BEHAVIOUR THERAPY

This type of psychological treatment corrects ways of thinking and behaving that delay recovery from certain psychiatric disorders. There are many different cognitive–behavioural treatments, each designed for a specific disorder or group of disorders. These specific treatment procedures are based on research showing which ways of thinking and behaviour prolong each of the several kinds of disorder that are treated in this way. The techniques most relevant to patients treated by physicians are for anxiety disorders and for bulimia nervosa. Cognitive behavioural treatments are provided by psychiatrists, clinical psychologists, and some nurse specialists. Readers requiring a more comprehensive account should consult the book by Hawton et al. (1989).

Relaxation training

Relaxation training is a part of most programmes of 'stress management'. There are several techniques, some of which concentrate solely on the relaxation of skeletal muscles, while others include concentrating on the calming mental images. Research has shown that these procedures bring about significant reductions in the physical accompaniments of anxiety, for example they lower muscle tension, heart rate, and blood pressure. No significant differences have been found between the outcomes of different types of relaxation procedure. To be effective, the exercises should be repeated daily, but it is often difficult to persuade patients to comply with this requirement. Some patients persist more with methods such as yoga that have a philosophical aspect which interests them, as well as the training in relaxation. If regular practice can be ensured, relaxation training is an effective treatment for some patients with stress related anxiety and tension symptoms.

Anxiety management

Anxiety management combines relaxation training with procedures for the control of the kinds of worrying thoughts that have been shown to prolong anxiety symptoms, for example fears that palpitations are a forerunner of serious heart disease. These thoughts are not usually dispelled by a simple explanation that, for example, palpitations are a normal part of an anxiety response and are not caused by heart disease. However, specific cognitive procedures, involving behavioural experiments to challenge patients' beliefs, result in changes in these beliefs which lead to an effect on anxiety comparable with that of anxiolytic drugs.

Exposure treatment

Exposure treatment is used for phobic anxiety disorders in which patients habitually avoid situations that provoke anxiety. Research has shown that avoidance prolongs the disorder because it prevents the deconditioning and cognitive relearning that normally brings fear reactions to an end. The principles of treatment are simple: patients are encouraged to enter relevant situations repeatedly, and to remain there until the anxiety response has died away. This second point is of great importance, because to leave before this point can exacerbate rather than relieve symptoms. Exposure is usually combined with the anxiety management techniques described above. Exposure has shown in randomized controlled trials to be an effective treatment for phobic disorders.

Cognitive therapy for panic disorder

This technique is used to reduce the fear of physical symptoms of anxiety that research has shown to be the cause of persistence of panic disorder (see Chapter 27.2.2). Patients are helped to recognize these fears (of which they are usually incompletely aware), and their role in producing panic is explained. Their fears are then modified using cognitive therapy techniques and patients are encouraged to practise new ways of thinking about the early symptoms of anxiety. Controlled trials have shown that this treatment is as effective as drug therapy for panic disorder and may lead to a lower rate of relapse.

Response prevention

Response prevention is used to treat obsessional disorder. The basis of treatment is the observation that although obsessional rituals give immediate relief from the distress caused by obsessional thoughts they also prolong the disorder. The suppression of rituals is known as response prevention. To be effective the control should continue for about an hour (shorter periods are usually ineffective) and should be repeated many times. Patients are helped to control rituals and to observe the benefits starting with the least severe rituals and in the circumstances in which the urge to perform the ritual is weak. Treatment continues in situations in which the urge is to perform the ritual is stronger (e.g. for hand-washing rituals, after dirtying the hands). Randomized controlled trials have shown that response prevention is an effective treatment for obsessional patients with rituals. The minority of patients who have obsessional thoughts without rituals cannot be treated effectively with these methods, but many respond to drug treatment.

Cognitive behaviour therapy for bulimia nervosa

Cognitive behaviour therapy for bulimia nervosa is intended to restore regular meal times (instead of an alternation between severe dieting and over-eating), and to change the patient's beliefs and attitudes. The latter are usually low self-esteem and an unjustified conviction of being fat and ugly. These beliefs are modified by cognitive techniques, which in principle are concerned with questioning their basis, and suggesting alternative ways of dealing with feelings of worthlessness. (In practice the treatment is more complex and needs special training.) Cognitive behaviour therapy has been tested in randomized controlled clinical trials and found to be effective, for bulimia nervosa.

BRIEF DYNAMIC PSYCHOTHERAPY

This term describes a group of treatments for emotional disorders and difficulties in relationships which seek to discover the connections between the current problems and events in earlier life and to help the patient gain more control of feelings. Although it usually lasts for about 6 months the treatment is described as 'brief' to distinguish it from longer methods of psychotherapy such as psychoanalysis. There are several ways of carrying out dynamic psychotherapy (originating in the work of Freud, Jung, Klein, and others) but these variations of technique have not been shown to affect the outcome.

Brief dynamic psychotherapy is most useful for patients with recurrent anxiety or depression or relationship difficulties, associated with feelings of worthlessness or other problems resulting from disturbed family relationships in childhood. Dynamic psychotherapy has been used for some medical disorders when these are exacerbated by the emotional problems mentioned above. Two randomized controlled trials have shown that dynamic psychotherapy has positive results with two conditions in which psychological factors appear to exacerbate the disorder in some cases, namely asthma and irritable bowel syndrome, but further studies are needed to confirm these findings.

It is reasonable to consider brief dynamic psychotherapy for patients whose medical condition appears to be exacerbated repeatedly by anxiety, depression, or suppressed anger and when these emotions arise mainly from the patient's psychological make-up rather than from the circumstances of life. The advice of a psychiatrist should be obtained on the suitability for this treatment which may be carried out by a psychiatrist, or a specialist psychotherapist.

REFERENCES

Bloch, S. *An introduction to psychotherapies.* Oxford University Press.
Catalan, J., Gath, D.H., Anastasiades, P., Bond, S.A.K., Day, A., and Hall, L. (1991). Evaluation of a brief psychological treatment for emotional disorders in primary care. *Psychological Medicine*, **21**, 1013–18.
Guthrie, E., Creed, F., Dawson, D., and Tomenson, B. (1991). A controlled trial of psychological treatment for the irritable bowel syndrome. *Gastroenterology*, **100**, 450–7.
Hawton, K., Salkovskis, P.M., Kirk, J., and Clark, D.M. (1989). *Cognitive Behaviour Therapy for Psychiatric Problems; a Practical Guide.* Oxford University Press.
Rosser, A.M. and Guz, A. (1981). Psychological approach to breathlessness and its treatment. *Journal of Psychosomatic Research*, **25**, 439–47.

27.4.3 Psychiatric emergencies

R. A. MAYOU

This section covers urgent psychiatric problems that may require immediate action by the physician. They include acute psychiatric and behavioural disturbance, in which there is insufficient time to obtain specialist help, and also less dramatic problems, encountered in emergency departments or elsewhere in the general hospital, that require immediate decisions about management, for example severe anxiety, alcohol withdrawal, and refusal of medical treatment.

Whatever the problem, the patient should be interviewed calmly so that a good relationship is established and information obtained about symptoms, past history, personality, and observations made of behaviour and mental state. In an emergency a systematic approach may be difficult but time can be saved and mistakes avoided if this can be achieved. Many emergencies become less urgent and bewildering if dealt with in a calm and deliberate way. Although it is not always possible to make an accurate diagnosis, it is not always necessary since the treatment of disturbed behaviour is similar whatever the cause.

General considerations

THE DISTURBED PATIENT

Before seeing a disturbed patient as much information as possible should be obtained from medical notes and from informants such as relatives, nursing staff, and police. Table 1 lists some of the psychological and

Table 1 *Some causes of disturbed behaviour*

Anxiety, fear
Alcohol or drug abuse and withdrawal
Personality disorder
Delirium (acute organic stage, confusional state)
    side-effects of treatment
    hypoglycaemia
    epilepsy
    head injury
    encephalitis and meningitis
Dementia
Schizophrenia and paranoid psychoses
Affective disorder: depression and mania

Table 2 *Management of violence*

Ensure adequate help and medication is immediately available
Make sure you can retreat rapidly. Do not take risks
Do not let the patient feel trapped
Listen to the patient, talk calmly, and do not argue
Do not try to restrain patient in any way unless you have adequate support
If there are medical indications for restraint, act quickly and effectively but with minimum force.

physical causes of disturbed behaviour. The list includes several important physical causes that are easily missed, especially if there is a history of psychiatric, alcohol, or drug problems that might deflect attention from organic causes.

Whenever possible disturbed patients should be interviewed in a room that is private and has a telephone and emergency bell with other staff available close by. Having obtained as much information as possible from the case notes and from others, the doctor should try to take a history, observe behaviour, and perform a physical examination. Many disturbed patients are frightened or angry: when these feelings are understood and taken seriously the disturbed behaviour often becomes less. The approach to the patient should be friendly and time should be spent at the beginning of the interview listening, explaining, and reassuring. Occasionally medication is necessary to calm the patient (see below). When the disturbed behaviour has settled a full physical examination and appropriate investigation should be carried out.

THE VIOLENT PATIENT

The causes of aggressive behaviour and the assessment are the same as those for other disturbed behaviour. Whenever there is the threat of violence, the doctor should be sure that adequate but unobtrusive support is available before approaching the patient (Table 2). The doctor should always be ready to listen, sympathize, and, if necessary, make sensible compromises. Extreme caution is, of course, required with any patient thought to possess any kind of offensive weapon and in such cases it is often best to ask the police to intervene. Staff should always avoid single-handed restraint or actions, such as a physical examinations suggesting that physical contact is intended, unless the purpose has been clearly understood and agreed by the patient.

If restraint cannot be avoided, it should be accomplished quickly by an adequate number of people using the minimum of force. Medication, such as parenteral haloperidol or chlorpromazine, should always be available. The use of such medication may provide the only way to calm the patient so as to carry out a physical examination or obtain further information.

EMERGENCY DRUG TREATMENT OF DISTURBED OR VIOLENT PATIENTS

This section is concerned with immediate management, (fuller information about drug treatment is given in Chapter 27.2.2). For a patient who is moderately frightened, diazepam (5 to 10 mg) may be useful. For a more disturbed patient, rapid calming is best achieved with 2 to 5 mg of haloperidol intramuscularly, repeated if necessary every 30 min or every hour up to 20 mg in 24 h. Occasionally larger doses are required, but it is desirable to obtain a specialist opinion from a psychiatrist.

When the patient has become calmer, regular oral doses of haloperidol, probably three to four times a day, should be started, preferably as syrup or tablets. The exact dosage requires regular review and depends on the patient's weight and general physical state, and on the initial response to the drug. Regular nursing observations of behaviour, conscious level, and blood pressure are necessary during tranquillization. Extrapyramidal side-effects may require treatment with an antiparkinsonian drug (see Chapter 27.4.1). Chlorpromazine (75 to 150 mg intramuscularly) is a useful alternative to haloperidol but more likely to cause hypotension.

STUPOR

In psychiatry the term stupor denotes a condition in which the patient is immobile, mute, and unresponsive but appears to be fully conscious, usually because the eyes are open and following external objects. (The term is also sometimes used by physicians to refer to impaired consciousness.) It may be due either to neurological or psychiatric conditions. The most common psychiatric causes of stupor are severe depressive disorder, hysteria, and schizophrenia (catatonia). As a patient in stupor stops eating and drinking, energetic management is necessary and the opinion of the psychiatrist should be obtained.

Thorough neurological examination and assessment is always necessary, even if the patient has a history of psychiatric disorder. A psychiatric diagnosis should be made only when tests of cerebral hemisphere and brain-stem function have been found to be normal. Information from other informants is essential to establish the onset, nature and cause of the condition.

THE PATIENT WHO REFUSES TREATMENT FOR PSYCHIATRIC DISORDER

If a patient has a severe mental illness that threatens life or safety and also impairs the ability to give informed consent, it may be appropriate for the doctor to seek legal powers of compulsory assessment and treatment. The doctor must be familiar with the local legislation and its application to clinical practice. In England and Wales, provision for such action is made in the Mental Health Act (1983), and other countries have comparable legislation. Powers for compulsory treatment of a mental disorder do not give the right to treatment of any concurrent physical disorder. However, successful treatment of any concurrent psychiatric disorder often results in the patient being able to give informed consent for the treatment of the physical illness at a later stage.

THE PATIENT WHO REFUSES MEDICAL TREATMENT

Patients may be unwilling to accept medical treatment for many reasons. Frequently they do not understand what is happening, or are angry and frightened; sometimes, however, their decision is well considered and rational. It is only very occasionally that the cause is a mental illness that interferes with the patient's ability to make an informed decision, and it is only this small minority which need to be referred to a psychiatrist. If the patient has a psychiatric disorder, compulsory treatment of this condition may be possible but, as explained above, this does not give any right to treat the accompanying physical illness, though as the psychiatric disorder improves, the patient's consent may be obtained.

When a patient refuses medical treatment the doctor should explain the proposed treatment and why it is needed, try to relieve any anger or anxiety that is hindering understanding, and discuss any worries and possible misconceptions. In this way, it is usually possible to agree a reasonable plan of medical care, although a degree of compromise may be needed. However, it has to be accepted that some patients will refuse treatment even after full discussion, and it is, a fundamental right of a conscious, mentally competent adult to do so. When this happens the doctors should keep a careful record of what they have tried to do, and whenever possible should ask the patient to sign a declaration of refusal to accept medical advice.

In many countries it is accepted that the doctor in charge of the patient has the right to give immediate treatment in life-threatening emergencies without the patient's consent. If doctors have to do this, they should if possible obtain supporting opinions from other medical and nursing colleagues and from the patient's relatives. They should kept detailed records of the reasons for their decision.

SOMATIC SYMPTOMS WITHOUT PHYSICAL CAUSE

Somatic symptoms for example abdominal pain, chronic fatigue, chest pain, without significant physical cause are very common in medical practice (see Table 4) and may present as emergencies. Some of these patients also have an undoubted physical illness and are often said to have 'functional overlay'. Such complaints should always be taken seriously as 'real' medical problems. Mild cases usually respond to authoritative reassurance after thorough history taking and examination. It is important not only to reassure that there is no serious physical cause but also to explain the cause of the symptoms and allow the patient to ask questions. It is sensible to encourage follow up assessment for further advice, discussion and reassurance.

A small proportion of patients present repeatedly with recurrent functional physical complaints. Although proper history taking and examination is necessary on each occasion, it is a mistake to order further investigations or specialist advice unless there are clear medical indications.

VICTIMS OF TRAUMA

Survivors of major accidents and other trauma and people who have suffered bereavement or other emotional shocks may be dazed, numbed, or distressed, and present as emergencies. They may also describe unpleasant intrusive memories of the trauma, which may be severe enough to be diagnosed as post-traumatic stress disorder (see Chapter 27.2.1) They require sympathy and reassurance, and assistance with immediate practical problems. It is useful to talk through distressing thoughts and fears and also give the patient and relatives advice leaflets to read when they return home. An anxiolytic hypnotic can be helpful. Patients should be advised to seek further help from their doctor if they continue to suffer intrusive memories or anxiety.

Victims of violence may find it difficult to discuss the distressing event and particular sensitivity is needed to help them do this and to express their feelings. The risk of further violence (for example in the home) should be reviewed; immediate referral to a social worker may be necessary. After the emergency, further help may be needed from the general practitioner or from a self help group.

A particular problem is the management of victims of rape or other sexual assault. Apart from treating injuries, doctors should record any evidence that may be needed for subsequent legal proceedings. They should give the victim advice about possible venereal disease or pregnancy and, with the victim's permission, they should talk to her relatives or close friends. The victim should be given the opportunity to talk about the experience and their feelings with an experienced and sensitive member of staff and also encourage to talk to relatives or friends. Follow-up advice should be offered. Some hospitals have special services

Table 3 *Causes of acute anxiety*

Lack of understanding and misunderstanding of what is
  happening
Fear of physical illness and its treatment
General anxiety, panic, and phobic anxiety neurosis
Post-traumatic
Alcohol withdrawal
Drug intoxication and withdrawal
Specific medical illness, e.g. thyrotoxicosis, hypoglycaemia
Hyperventilation
Agitated depression

Table 4 *Somatic symptoms without physical cause*

Simulated symptoms
  malingering
  factitious disorder
    specific simulated symptoms
    Munchausen syndrome
'Functional' symptoms
  transient fear of illness responding to reassurance
  misinterpretation of physiological processes or minor
    pathology
  somatic symptoms of a primary psychiatric disorder
  hypochondriacal personality

for rape victims and many hospitals are able to refer to a local rape crisis organization with special expertise in providing help.

The emergency department should be prepared to offer psychological and social help to victims and to staff as a part of disaster planning. This means identifying experienced staff who can be called upon to provide immediate help and to organize follow-up care.

Psychiatric syndromes as causes of emergencies

ORGANIC MENTAL DISORDERS

Acute and chronic organic mental disorders may cause agitation, aggressive, or erratic behaviour. The characteristic behavioural and cognitive symptoms are usually easily recognized (see Chapter 27.2.10), but in the absence of a clear history or obvious physical signs, a functional psychiatric illness may be diagnosed in error. Doctors should always be suspicious that odd, out-of-character behaviour is a sign of an organic mental disorder, and they should be prepared to undertake full physical examination and assessment.

It is wise to assume that any patient who is exhibiting disturbed behaviour and is elderly or has physical illness, may have an organic mental disorder until proved otherwise. Careful psychiatric assessment may reveal fluctuating disorientation or cognitive functions that seem impaired is judged by what is known of the patient's normal functioning.

As explained in the section on organic mental disorders, treatment is primarily medical. Confused patients require consistent nursing care, with repeated reassurance and explanation from a few familiar nurses. It may be useful to nurse the patient in a single room with some light at night. Regular visits from close family and friends are helpful. Modest dosages of a benzodiazepine hypnotic or a tranquillizer (such as haloperidol or a phenothiazine) are valuable in the management of agitation, restlessness and disturbed behaviour. Regular but flexible dosage regimes are preferable to the intermittent treatment of crises.

STATES OF ACUTE ANXIETY AND PANIC

Many medical patients are tense and worried and some suffer more severe anxiety, which is distressing and interferes with medical care. Table 3 lists some of the common causes. Most are easily recognized; all that is required is sympathetic discussion, encouragement, and reassurance. When anxiety is a response to acute stress, benzodiazepines can be helpful either as night sedatives or an anxiolytics. However, the prescription of these drugs should not be prolonged after the emergency has passed. Panic attacks are a common cause of presentation in the emergency department. Once diagnosed (see Chapter 27.2.2) they should be treated as described above. Hyperventilation responds to slow breathing or rebreathing into a paper bag.

CONVERSION AND DISSOCIATIVE DISORDER

Patients with acute onset of symptoms such as paralyses, sensory impairments, and amnesias are occasionally seen as emergencies. Possible

such symptoms of conversion and dissociative disorder (hysteria) require full medical examination and appropriate special investigations. The doctor should always bear in mind that some cases originally diagnosed as conversion or dissociative disorder are later found to have physical illness, and that physical illness can occur in patients with a history of recurrent hysterical symptoms. Once conversion or dissociative disorder is suspected, the exclusion of organic disorder must be accompanied by a search for a psychological explanation of the patient's symptoms. Admission to hospital may be necessary for further assessment and for treatment.

Symptoms of acute onset often recover quickly. Resolution is helped by thorough assessment and sympathetic and authoritative reassurance, and by avoiding anything that might reinforce the symptoms. The patient should not be confronted but rather given face-saving opportunities for improvement. As with other forms of emotional disorder, psychological treatment directed to underlying emotional difficulties is important and patients should be offered outpatient follow-up.

SIMULATED ILLNESS (TABLE 4)

Malingering is the faking of illness for obvious rewards (e.g. to obtain narcotics, taking time off work, or to gain compensation). Suspicions should be raised by inconsistencies in the patient's account of the symptoms and of previous medical treatment and vagueness about addresses and the names of doctors and other informants. The diagnosis can be confirmed only the patient's confession, and careful history taking and gentle confrontation are often effective in securing this.

Factitious disorder covers the dramatic but rare Munchausen syndrome seen in emergency departments, and the much more frequent simulation of particular symptoms such as bleeding skin lesions and pyrexia. It differs from malingering in bringing no obvious external reward for the fabrication of symptoms. Although the grosser syndromes of recurrent faking and pathological lying are notably resistant to all forms of psychological treatment, patients exhibiting them should be confronted tactfully and offered referral to a psychiatrist. Patients with less extreme and more specific forms of simulated illness are somewhat more likely to respond to psychological treatment. It is essential to avoid angry confrontations but the patient should gently be made aware of the doctors suspicions and offered the opportunity to discuss them. Even though patients are often unwilling to admit to their behaviour it may be possible to agree on an appropriate management plan.

ALCOHOL PROBLEMS (SEE SECTION 28)

The numerous physical disorders that arise directly from abuse of alcohol are described in Chapter 28.2.3(a). Problems arising from acute intoxication or withdrawal may present as emergencies. In such cases thorough physical assessment is always required. Emergency departments should have a clear positive management policies for managing noisy and potentially violent drunks. Facilities for withdrawing alcohol ('detoxification') should also be available and rapid access to specialist services. Every patient with a drinking problem should be given advice on stopping drinking and information on how to obtain further help.

Acute intoxication

Medical examination is necessary to exclude other important causes of actively disturbed behaviour, for example epilepsy and hypoglycaemia. It is occasionally necessary to offer the patient the opportunity of several hours of recovery within the emergency department.

Withdrawal symptoms

Acute withdrawal symptoms of tremor, nausea, and sweating occur 6 to 8 h after stopping drinking or reducing alcohol intake and may be a cause of presentation to the emergency department or of the onset of symptoms shortly after admission for treatment of physical illness. The much less common and more dramatic syndrome of delirium tremens (see Section 28) occurs 48 to 72 h after stopping or reducing alcohol. Definite signs of delirium tremens are always an indication for hospital care; it is important to be aware of the dangers of fits, hyperthermia, and circulatory failure.

In less severe cases withdrawal can be managed outside hospital but the abrupt discontinuance of alcohol usually requires tranquillizers, dispensed daily so as to avoid overdoses or other misuse. It is important to be flexible about dosage, adjusting it to the clinical state. Diazepam is valuable in a basic regime of 10 mg four times/day for 3 days; 10 mg three times/day for 2 days; 5 mg twice/day for 2 days. Many doctors prefer chlomethiazole, although there is a considerable risk of dependence, which means it is contraindicated outside hospital. A basic regime is 1.5 g three times/day for 2 days; 1 gm three times/day for 2 days; 0.5 mg three times/day for 1 day. In view of the possibility of liver damage phenothiazines should be avoided.

DRUG DEPENDENCE (SEE SECTION 28)

Drug-related problems may present as violence, withdrawal problems, demands for drugs, and feigned illness (e.g. renal colic) as an attempt to obtain drugs or psychiatric problems. Doctors should have a policy of refusing to prescribe addictive drugs to unknown patients who present themselves as needing emergency supplies. The management of withdrawal is described in Chapter 28.3.4.

Any suspicion of drug misuse should lead to a careful history and physical examination with efforts to check the genuineness of the history and testing of urine and blood for the presence of drugs. Management depends on the nature of the drug and the circumstances of consultation. Overnight hospital admission is required for drug-dependent patients who are brought to hospital after an overdose or who are disturbed enough by flashbacks or a 'bad trip' to require care. For the latter, reassurance and the prescription of non-controlled drugs is often an effective temporary measure in relieving the patient's anxiety. Chronic use of illicit drugs may lead to psychiatric illnesses which require specialist assessment and care.

Section 28 *Alcohol and drug-related problems*

Introduction

Drug and alcohol problems are every doctor's business. They are considered in this section in four parts. An opening group of chapters considers assessment and diagnosis, and the importance of vigilance during everyday clinicl practice. In the second part the opportunities (often missed) for secondary prevention are considered, with attention not only to simple screening measures, but also to brief interventions that can easily be implemented. The third part covers the special complications that may result from alcohol and drug use, and the responses that may be initiated. Finally, in the fourth part, a series of chapters looks at the drug- and alcohol-related problems and crises that may confront the clinician in his or her work, accompanied by an exploration of the types of clinical management.

28.1 Assessment and diagnosis

28.1.1 Drug problems as every doctor's business

G. EDWARDS

The editors of this section, and their contributors, share a background of specialism in problems of substance abuse. Their approach is aimed at helping doctors more effectively to deal with these problems as encountered in wide arenas of practice.

The job of this introductory contribution is to signpost the detailed contributions which follow, and draw out certain general principles which cut across the individual statements.

Mind-acting drugs and their misuse: essential knowledge

DRUGS OF CONCERN

The drugs in this group are all in some way rewarding to the drug taker. Many of them are to a degree reinforcing, in that their use builds up a habit of further use. Many, but not all, of these drugs can give rise to a habit of such strength as to deserve the designation of dependence (see below). Throughout this chapter the word drug will be used generically for substances from within all the groups characterized below. In the following simple classification, drugs within any given family are likely to produce rather similar effects, involve the same biological systems as substrate for their actions, show cross-tolerance, and if this particular class gives rise to withdrawal symptoms, the syndrome will show common class features.

Opiates

These include the opium-derived drugs, morphine and codeine, the semisynthetic heroin, and synthetic opiates such as methadone, pentazocine, and palfium®. Opiates have a high dependence potential and give rise to extremely unpleasant but not fatal withdrawal symptoms.

General depressants

These include the barbiturates, the benzodiazepines, chloral, and paraldehyde, and very important, alcohol. Withdrawal symptoms from depressants can be distressing, benzodiazepine withdrawal can give rise to protracted disturbance, and withdrawal from alcohol can result in life-threatening illness.

Stimulants

Stimulants include plant products such as cocaine and coffee, and synthetics such as the amphetamines and appetite suppressants. Withdrawal from stimulants generally does not result in severe physical disturbance, but there can be a sense of lethargy and depression.

Hallucinogens

Hallucinogens include LSD and mescaline. These drugs can give rise to acute mental disturbance and sometimes to intermittent and quite prolonged 'flashback' experience. They do not give rise to dependence nor to withdrawal symptoms.

Volatile organic substances

These include anaesthetic gases, petrol, toluene, butane, fluorinated hydrocarbons found in aerosol propellants, and amyl nitrite. They have in common the ability to produce acute intoxication and sometimes transient sensory distortion or hallucination. Intoxication or associated consequences can cause immediate death. Dependence potential varies with substance type, is usually low, and withdrawal symptoms are not marked.

Substances with mixed or atypical properties

Several substances do not fit conveniently into any of the groups listed above, often because of an action that crosses group boundaries. Thus cannabis has both depressant and, in higher doses or idiosyncratically, hallucinogenic effects. Nicotine has both stimulant and depressant effects. MDMA (Ecstasy) is an amphetamine derivative with stimulant and hallucinogenic properties.

DRUG TOLERANCE

Increased clearance (metabolic tolerance) is usually less important than CNS tolerance: the general meaning of tolerance is that a greater quantity of the drug than previously is needed to obtain the same effect. Cross-tolerance implies that one drug will relieve withdrawal associated with cessation of another. The potential clinical significance of tolerance can be seen, for example, in opiate dependence, where a patient may be capable of taking more than, say, 600 mg pure heroin a day while still working as a garage attendant. That kind of tolerance carries implications for substitute medication, and the likely intensity of distress if withdrawal is untreated. However, tolerance is quickly lost with abstinence, and a patient who is unaware of this fact may die of accidental overdose on resumption of drug taking at a high previous dose.

WITHDRAWAL STATES

Treatment of withdrawal requires exercise of clinical skills, and these issues are discussed in Chapter 28.3.4.

DRUG DEPENDENCE

This is discussed in Chapter 28.1.3. Dependence is a learnt habit which becomes self-perpetuating and which can be difficult to eradicate. The learning can come about through the direct reinforcing effect of the drug, or through learning processes connected with relief or avoidance of withdrawal. To distinguish between 'psychological' and 'physical' dependence makes little sense: dependence is a psychophysiological state.

DRUG-RELATED PROBLEMS

The concept of a drug-related problem is again fully discussed in Chapter 28.1.3, but emphasis may usefully be given to the following facts.

1. Problems affect the user but, commonly, may also affect others (passive smoking, the deformed child of the cocaine-using or alcohol-drinking mother, the victim of the drunk driver).
2. They can be in the physical, psychological, or social spheres.
3. Problems can be chronic disease processes, or an acute problem. Alcohol is involved in about 50 per cent of deaths due to road accidents, 30 per cent of drownings, 40 to 50 per cent of deaths through fire, and about 30 per cent of deaths incurred through falls.

ROUTES OF ADMINISTRATION

The drugs with which we are concerned can be taken into the body by different routes, and the doctor needs to be aware of the implications. First, the following statement summarizes the general relationships between route of use and risk of dependence: injection (very high dependence risk); smoked or inhaled (very high); sniffed or snorted (quite high); eaten (lower); chewed (low). Thus, tobacco used to be chewed (low dependence risk) or sniffed as snuff (fairly high risk), but is now almost universally smoked, with a high dependence risk (pipes, cigars, cigarettes). The introduction of a new technology for delivery can radically alter the dependence risk for a given drug: coca leaves as chewed in the Andes carried minimal risks of dependence, but when the alkaloid was extracted from the leaves and used by sniffing, injection, and most recently by smoking ('crack' or 'freebase' cocaine), the risk arose of destructive epidemics. Secondly, routes of administration are important because of their toxic associations: a chewed drug can give rise to oral cancer (tobacco), as can a swallowed drug (alcohol); a smoked drug can cause lung disease through contaminants (smoking and bronchial carcinoma); injected drugs carry the risk of overdose or transmission of infection through shared equipment (see Chapter 28.3.1).

WHY PEOPLE USE MIND-ACTING DRUGS

The reasons for starting to use a drug, continuing to use it, or using it in a given pattern or dose, are always multiple. The nature of the drug is certainly important, as is availability. Price must be taken into the reckoning: taxation of alcohol and tobacco are potentially potent public health measures, but price also affects consumption of illicit drugs. Sociocultural factors, general social attitudes and informal controls, and the quality of the social environment, bear on the likelihood of drug taking, as do family structure, family drug-taking, and failure in family support. Peer approval and sub-cultural influences which encourage and support drug use, and teach methods of acquisition and techniques of use, are a significant causal factor. Genetic predisposition plays a role in vulnerability to drinking, but is not a significant factor with other drugs. Personal motivation for drug use can be enormously varied and can include sedation or relief of anxiety, depression or pain; enjoyment of experimentation, thrill seeking, or the lack of alternative pleasures and rewards, and the symbolic value attaching to drug use or to being a drug user may be important (being 'cool', being a hippie). Personality can contribute to vulnerability, but there is no evidence for a unique 'addictive personality'. When in a society the use of a given drug is statistically deviant (heroin for instance in the United Kingdom, as opposed to cannabis), personality disorder is likely to show an association with use of that drug. Underlying mental illness of any kind may be of clinical significance—excessive drinking may, for instance, be a self-medication for an anxiety state, or a sequel to brain damage or dementia.

Drug problems: necessary attitudes

A doctor's attitude to any type of problem or patient, including drugs and drug taking, may affect the quality of the care that is likely to be given. The leading role that the medical profession has taken over post-war years in patient education and public action on cigarette smoking, provides persuasive evidence of what professional action can achieve, once it is accepted that the problem is a medical one. It may be significant that some of the earliest and most seminal epidemiological studies of smoking mortality were conducted among doctors, a strategy which accidentally but potently brought the problem home to the profession. If further progress is to be made with alcohol and illicit drugs, the following attitudes will have to be corrected by medical school teachers and the profession as a whole.

THE BELIEF THAT SUBSTANCE PROBLEMS ARE RARE AND THEREFORE MEDICALLY UNIMPORTANT

Drug problems, broadly defined to encompass licit as well as illicit substances, are a heavy burden in general practice, and almost every hospital department (see particularly Chapter 28.3.2). Alcohol problems can, for instance, present in neonates as a fetal alcohol syndrome, to the geratologist as a fracture; to the neurologist as brain damage; to the cardiologist as hypertension or cardiomyopathy; to the gastroenterologist as hepatitis, cirrhosis, or pancreatitis; in the casualty department as any kind of trauma, or as hypoglycaemia in the child who has sipped the cherry brandy; to the skin clinic with an exacerbation of psoriasis; to the X-ray department with unexplained old multiple rib fractures. Alcohol can be associated with presentations as mundane as the beer-drinker's obesity and as exotic as pseudo-Cushing's disease. Twenty to 25 per cent of patients in general hospital wards have an alcohol problem. The United States Epidemiologic Catchment Area study found a lifetime prevalence of DSM-III alcohol abuse or alcohol dependence, of just under 1 in 4 for men and 1 in 22 for women.

Table 1 reminds us that although advances have been made in curbing the cigarette habit, smoking remains prevalent: smoking continues as the largest single preventable cause of premature death. Although illicit drugs are less demanding on medical services because they are less prevalent than licit drugs, simple prevalence figures alone do not reflect adequately the burden on services, nor the significance of regional and demographic variations. In some socially deprived areas of the United Kingdom up to 1 in 10 young men will have used opiates. The entry in the table for psychotropic misuse also needs careful interpretation: benzodiazepine use has a much higher prevalence than that indicated in the table if women and the middle-aged are considered, and benzodiazepines have now become a common street drug.

NEGATIVE STEREOTYPES

Diagnoses will be overlooked, compassion withdrawn, or patients rejected, if medical attitudes to the drug taker are tainted by stereotype. Sadly, there is ample research evidence to show that such stereotypes exist, and can adversely affect the quality of patient care. For instance, the doctor who believes that all 'alcoholics' are middle-aged male vagrants will overlook the fact that the 23-year-old woman presenting at the outpatient clinic has an alcoholic myositis. The belief that all illicit drug takers conform to the picture of 'the junkie' was never true, and certainly does not represent today's reality. Most of these stereotypes are, of course, negative in complexion, a way of distancing our patients from ourselves.

Table 1 *Prevalence estimates for misuse of licit substances in adults aged over 18 years*

	Male (%)	Female (%)
Alcohol		
Over safe limits, no complications	13	7
Over safe limits, with problems	7	2
Over safe limits, with dependence	5	2
Smoking	33	30
Benzodiazepines		
Continued daily use	2.5	5

ATTITUDES AND OPTIMISM

One reason why doctors have in the past sometimes found it difficult to muster the necessary commitment to meet the challenge set by drugs, comes from the professional belief that the outlook for drug problems is hopeless. The cirrhotic will, within that perspective, inevitably go out from the ward and drink himself to death, every heroin-dependent patient is bent on his or her own destruction, too many patients start smoking again after their coronary occlusion. Drug problems are therefore seen as unrewarding to treat, as self-inflicted wounds beyond the doctor's cure, and if they are anyone's medical business the responsibility lies not with the generality of doctors but with specialists.

This gloomy caricature of medical pessimism sufficiently reflects prevalent attitudes to deserve serious attention. It is a caricature composed of misapprehensions. There are at least two points to be made in refutation.

First, not all members of the target population are all extreme cases, but include people suffering varying degrees of damage from substance abuse. Secondly, there is ample evidence from controlled research to demonstrate that brief interventions given in the community can significantly influence cigarette smoking, drinking over safe limits, and even established alcohol dependence (see Section 28.2). Simple advice in those circumstances is proven good medicine. There are few other ways in which a doctor can, in passing, week after week, produce tangible health benefit on so large a scale. Controlled research on efficacy of advice given to illicit drug users is not available, but there can be little doubt that doing something tangible, giving informed advice or appropriate routeing to a community drug team or other specialized help, is, likely to be better medicine than pessimistically doing nothing.

Pessimistic attitudes are unwarranted and are bad medicine. The doctor who believes that he or she is helpless in the face of such issues will encourage and multiply the patient's own sense of helplessness.

Alcohol, illicit drugs, and tobacco: the needed skills for good clinical practice

The skills that a doctor working in any type of general or specialist medical setting must be able to deploy to deal with alcohol, tobacco, and other drugs include the abilities to win confidence, ask questions, use laboratory tests, build motivation, give advice, monitor progress, and make appropriate referrals as necessary. Treating drug problems involves motivating and empowering patients to believe in the possibility of making their own healthy choices and changes. The basics of this kind of work are fully discussed in Chapter 28.2.1, with a particular focus on alcohol, but the same kind of approach may be varied and is then widely applicable to other types of substance.

In essence, the challenge here is that of learning very worthwhile skills which are to some extent special, but which are rooted in traditional aspects of the doctor–patient relationship and good practice. The result of this kind of work is to invite the doctor to think about, define,

refine, and sharpen his or her basic ability to use himself or herself effectively as motivator and communicator. The doctor is personally the therapeutic agent, and accuracy, warmth, and empathy are the necessary qualities. Learn how to use these skills for 5 to 10 min with the next patient on the ward who needs to reduce their drinking, and in doing so you will have developed valuable skills applicable to many other types of health-related behavioural problems.

Drug problems in the medical profession

Up to now this chapter has talked about doctors and patients as if they were distinct categories of person. However, alcohol and other drug problems are common in the medical profession, run across the age spectrum, and can affect general practitioners and doctors in every type of hospital practice. Better awareness of the nature of the dangers might enhance self-protection, and in particular medical students should be taught that it is unwise for a doctor in any circumstances to prescribe potentially dangerous psychoactive drugs for self or family members. Similarly, there should be discussion of the vulnerability to excessive drinking which may arise through professional stress and career pressures if alcohol is seen as an acceptable coping mechanism. While hoping that fuller and more open discussion of these issues will, over time, make drug problems less common in the medical profession, there is also meanwhile a need to develop a better capacity to recognize a substance problem that a colleague is experiencing, and offer early, informed, firm, and sympathetic help. Perhaps the recognition that substance problems are no respecters of persons or professions may in some way serve further to persuade doctors that alcohol, other drugs, and tobacco, raise pervasive issues that must be taken seriously by the whole profession. Thus even enlightened self-interest suggests that the medical profession would do well to enhance its ability to recognize and deal with the everyday issues that are discussed in this section.

28.1.2 Assessing substance use and misuse

M. FARRELL, I. B. CROME, and J. STRANG

Introduction

The assessment of alcohol, drug, and smoking behaviour requires a degree of attention and time that few doctors feel able to spend on it. Usually, insufficient effort is given to eliciting in detail the patterns of alcohol and drug consumption. Doctors generally doubt whether patients will be accurate about this aspect of their behaviour. This may be the case, but in most instances a thorough and detailed history will provide sufficient detail for a comprehensive assessment of the impact of substance use on overall physical, psychological, and social well-being. Hospital doctors are increasingly aware of the need to suspect that presenting complaints may be alcohol- or drug-induced. Conditions such as pancreatitis and liver cirrhosis will prompt all doctors to take a more detailed drinking history, and evidence of human immunodeficiency virus (HIV) or hepatitis B will raise the possibility of injecting drug use.

Both patients and doctors frequently feel that the assessment interview should be directly relevant to the presenting complaint, and doctors are reticent about asking detailed questions about people's private lives such as drug use and sexual behaviour. However, it is only by the routine inclusion of such enquiries that a clinician can feel reasonably confident. Such a line of questioning should not be a random event prompted by the physical appearance of a particular individual.

Spotting the opportunity for a brief intervention

Many studies have demonstrated the power of the brief intervention in modifying smoking and drinking behaviour. When they present with a health problem, patients may be especially receptive to the consideration of modification of other aspects of the health-related behaviour. Part of the skill in enquiring about alcohol, drug, and tobacco consumption is to maintain a cool, clinical and non-judgemental attitude which aims to help patients to assess their substance use and to determine whether they suspect there is any adverse health risk related to their behaviour.

It is vital that the ambivalence associated with substance use be fully appreciated. For instance, when heavy smokers declare that smoking has not harmed their health the clinician should avoid falling into the trap of attempting to convince them that it has. It is likely that most people who drink and smoke heavily or use other drugs have contemplated or even attempted giving it up. Some remain abstinent, but others will be successful for a period of time, and then relapse. Subtle encouragement can nudge such a person in the direction of change. Studies of smokers divide them in to three groups:

(1) 'pre-contemplators'—people who are smoking and do not think they are at risk and are not planning to stop;
(2) 'contemplators'—smokers who are concerned about the health risks and are considering quitting; and
(3) 'active quitters'—those who are actively attempting to stop smoking.

People may move between these categories and can move from being an 'active quitter' to a 'contemplator'. A similar model has been applied to alcohol and drug use and it can be helpful to categorize patients in this way. Thus, if someone is a 'pre-contemplator' the key task would be to shift them to being a 'contemplator', and if a person was contemplating change the task would be to facilitate the shift into action.

Assessing need

Assessment varies considerably according to the substance involved. An individual who smokes nicotine is usually dependent on it. The pattern of alcohol consumption varies a lot more, with less than 10 per cent of drinkers being dependent. Thus, there is a need to clarify this in more detail for alcohol, and similarly with benzodiazepines, opiates, and cocaine. The detection of alcohol, opiate, or benzodiazepine dependence is important for planning appropriate ward management of such individuals. All may require detoxification and general medical management. If dependence is undetected, acute withdrawal syndromes and attendant medical and ward problems may arise.

SCREENING

The case for screening is made in Chapter 28.2.1. If regular screening is conducted, it can be a helpful educational tool that doctors can use to assess how good they are at detection.

Asking the right questions

A checklist of questions on alcohol to be included in drug-history taking is provided below. Ideally, junior doctors should use this protocol in any individual with an alcohol- or drug-related problem. The aim of the interview should be to determine the nature of substance use and misuse, the degree of alcohol or drug dependence, and the level of alcohol- or drug-related problems. The most reliable answers will be about the drugs used most recently. If the patient can co-operate, a detailed history of what was consumed in the previous 24 h will give a good indication of the nature of the problem. This should be checked against the patient's description of a typical drinking day. A detailed picture of such a day provides a vignette of the patient's life-style and gives a good indication of how much alcohol or drug consumption dominates his or her life. Patients may describe early morning waking with withdrawal symptoms and the pursuit of alcohol or other drugs to restore equilibrium. It is then essential to obtain a longitudinal or panoramic history of the pattern of alcohol or drug consumption, from initiation, to the development of

regular habits, the transition to daily and to heavy substance use, and the pattern of 'binge use', along with the evolution of related problems. Hidden within these histories will be episodes when patients have grappled with the problem and temporarily changed their behaviour. Such episodes may be useful evidence of future capacity for change.

The assessment should reveal whether a patient is dependent and estimate the severity of dependence. While the doctor may focus on alcohol or drug use as the problem, it is important to remember that the patient may not view the substance use as a problem but more as a recreational activity. Sensitive enquiry about personal, family, financial, and occupational problems may reveal a complex web of interrelated problems. The patient can be helped to put the problems in order of importance and to begin to address them sensibly.

Alcohol history

1. Personal history and developmental history: childhood disruption, educational achievements, employment history, marital and sexual history. Are any major factors in these life events influenced by the patient's alcohol consumption?
2. Family history: enquire whether parents or close relatives had alcohol problems. Alcohol problems are four times more common in those with a positive family history.
3. Drinking history:
   (a) alcohol consumption (units) in the past 24 h;
   (b) average alcohol consumption (units) in the past month;
   (c) average alcohol consumption (units) in the past 6 months. (1 unit = 1 glass of table wine = 1/2 pint of beer = 1 measure of spirits = 1 measure of sherry. Standard bottle of spirits = 32 units; standard bottle of wine = 8 units; can of extra-strong lager = 4 units.)
4. Drinking career:
   (a) Age of:
       first ever drink
       regular weekend drinking
       regular evening drinking
       regular lunch-time drinking
       early morning drinking;
   (b) withdrawal symptoms: anxiety, tremor, night sweats or morning nausea, convulsions;
   (c) other features of dependence: tolerance, compulsion to drink, salience of drink-seeking behaviour, rapid reinstatement after abstinence;
   (d) delirium tremens;
   (e) periods of abstinence.
5. Alcohol related problems:
   (a) physical, e.g. gastritis, hepatitis, cirrhosis, neuropathy, pancreatitis;
   (b) psychological, e.g. anxiety, depression, phobias, delusions, suicidal ideation or suicide attempts, hallucinations, jealousy, paranoid ideation, eating disorders;
   (c) social, e.g. marital, sexual, occupational, or financial.
6. Other drug use: type of drug, frequency of use, and route of use.
7. Previous treatment history: general practitioner or specialist alcohol treatment service, medication.
8. Forensic history: drinking and driving, or drunk and disorderly offenses.
9. Present lifestyle: marital, occupational, and leisure activities, social support network, non-drinking social network.

DRUG HISTORY

1. Personal, developmental, and family history: will provide information on developmental disruption such as time spent

in care, early loss of parents, and history of alcohol or drug problems in family.

2. Drug-taking history:
   (a) drug use in the past 24 h;
   (b) drug use in the past month.

3. Drug-using career:
   (a) age at first drug use for each individual drug;
   (b) age for regular drug use for each drug;
   (c) age of dependent drug use; note milestones of loss of control;
   (d) routes of drug use; oral, inhaled, intravenous;
   (e) periods of abstinence.

4. Injecting history, should cover first injecting episode in detail with particular reference to the sharing of injecting equipment:
   (a) first time injected;
   (b) duration of injecting;
   (c) daily frequency of injecting;
   (d) knowledge about HIV transmission;
   (e) injecting sites: arms, legs, groin, neck, local injecting site problems;
   (f) source and use of sterile injecting equipment.

5. HIV risk:
   frequency of sharing injecting equipment;
   person shared with, partner, friend, or dealer;
   knowledge on method of cleaning contaminated equipment;
   sexual risk-taking behaviour.

6. Treatment history and other periods of abstinence.

7. Forensic history: previous court cases and prison sentences, and specifically enquire about pending court cases.

8. Present lifestyle: marital, occupational, general aspects of lifestyle, in particular non-drug-using support networks, non-drug-using leisure activities.

Smoking history

Patients tend to provide highly accurate descriptions of their volume of cigarette smoking. The evolution of a pattern of smoking tends to be straightforward. So far, nicotine consumption has not been a source of occupational or marital stress; however, with the advent of strong workplace smoke-free policies and a general taboo on nicotine consumption it is likely that there will be more frequent reports of people's nicotine consumption disrupting their pattern of working or leisure activity. The key questions to explore are:

(1) the motivation to stop smoking;
(2) description of previous efforts at quitting;
(3) average daily cigarette consumption; and
(4) time from waking to smoking first cigarette as indicator of nicotine dependence.

Integrating information

A full assessment provides a more quantified and structured diagnostic approach to the problem of alcohol and other drugs. Careful integration between these data and other psychiatric history formulation is desirable in view of the recognizable psychiatric morbidity among people with alcohol and drug problems.

There is, however, little predictive validity or prognostic indicators to assess individual cases, apart from the general impression that high occupational status and a good social support network are more conducive to positive treatment outcomes.

Assessments may be most useful in attempting to ensure that an individual patient is appropriately matched to treatment. People who have not had previous treatment should initially have outpatient-based, low-intensity community treatment. However, other psychiatric or medical problems may alter overall treatment requirements. There is considerable evidence that patients listen to the advice of the doctor. Time spent listening to patients and putting into order what may be a chaotic picture of substance misuse may be the most valuable tool in promoting change.

REFERENCES

Bernadt, M., Mumford, J., Taylor, C., Smith, B., and Murray, R.M. (1982). Comparisons of questionnaire and laboratory tests in the detection of excessive drinking and alcoholism. *Lancet*, **1**, 325–8.

Edwards, G. (1987). *The treatment of drinking problems*. Blackwell, Oxford.

Glass, I.B., Farrell, M. and Hajek, P. (1991). Tell me about the patient: history taking and formulating the case. In *International handbook of addictions*, (ed. I.B. Glass). Routledge, London.

Prochaska, J. and Di Clemente, C. (1983). Stages and processes of self change of smoking: towards a more integrative model of change. *Journal of Consulting and Clinical Psychology* **451**, 390–5.

Strang, J., Bradley, B., and Stockwell, T. (1989). Assessment of drug and alcohol use. In C. Thompson (ed) *Instruments of psychiatric research*, (ed. C. Thompson). John Wiley and Sons, Chichester.

28.1.3 Diagnoses and classifications: Substance problems and dependence—what is the difference?

I. B. CROME

The focus of this section is on what a physician needs to know about definition, classification, and diagnosis of substance problems. Who are addicts? What is a substance problem? Why do you need to know? These questions are not only of conceptual and theoretical importance, there are practical implications. Diagnostic clarity can facilitate communication between professionals and the public, consolidate prognostic predictive power and treatment outcome, and form a basis for elucidating aetiology and natural history.

Contributions to the history of definition in the addictions have come from the medical profession, scientists, social scientists, and patients themselves. Habitual drunkenness, dipsomania, chronic alcoholism, morphinismus, and inebriety were some of the forerunners of the term addiction. Addiction originates from the Latin word which describes debtors, who, by virtue of their relationship to their creditors, were slaves to them. 'Pendere', however, means to hand down and thus dependence implies a condition of being beholden to, subordinate to, or reliant upon.

Since the early 1950s the debate on definition and classification has centred around the World Health Organization, which, in 1976, proposed the concept of alcohol-dependence syndrome, which combined physical and psychological dependence. This definition also distinguished alcohol-related problems (or problem drug-taker). It is thus a biaxial rather than a unitary concept. The consensus is that this term is less pejorative than 'drunkard', 'druggie', 'dope fiend', or even substance abuse.

In order to place the issues in the discussion in perspective, it is useful to consider a few brief case histories.

Mr A, a 31-year-old, separated, unemployed accountant, presented to a specialist problem drinking clinic. He was referred by a neurologist as he had complained of tremor and difficulty in walking. His γ-glutamyl transaminase was 483 IU/l (normal < 35). He was wheeled into the consulting room by his younger sister, the only family member with whom he remained in contact. He had begun to drink socially at the age of 15, and by the age of 24 people began to comment on the amount he was drinking and the money he was spending on alcohol. At about this time he began to experience withdrawal symptoms. He had been unemployed for 3 years, and had married in 1988 but separated in 1989. A year previously he had been admitted to hospital with jaundice, alcoholic hepatitis, alcohol-induced withdrawal fits, cerebellar degeneration, and impotence. He continued to drink at least a bottle of whisky each day, and spent most of the time alone. His financial state was parlous and he was faced with eviction from his flat. He was once more admitted to hospital where he was detoxified and attended group and individual therapy. Investigations revealed cerebral atrophy. He was ambivalent about attending Alcoholics Anonymous and abstinence as a goal. He drank while on the ward, and discharged himself.

Dr B is a 37-year-old, twice-divorced general practitioner who referred herself to a drug-dependence unit. She had become concerned about her own use of amphetamines for slimming while she was director of a private obesity treatment clinic. She felt she was on the verge of becoming out of control in her use and might succumb to cocaine. Although she did drink, this was only occasional. She was a heavy smoker. Her investigations demonstrated a positive urine screen for amphetamines. She managed to stop using amphetamines and cigarettes of her own accord and without any obvious symptoms. For many months thereafter she experienced volatile moods, punctuated by episodes of wrist-slashing with underlying poor self-esteem and apathy. It became apparent that this reflected the complex and difficult relationships with her parents. In particular she felt neglected by her mother. She alluded to sexual abuse as an additional issue. She lived in chaos during this time, finding it impossible to organize herself. She became heavily involved in recovery groups and primal therapy. She engaged in supportive psychotherapy, although she was initially very resistant to this form of help. However, over several years she gained confidence, has a more structured lifestyle, is more able to tolerate relationships with her family, and is thinking of a gradual return to work.

Mr C is a 35-year-old man who presented to the drug dependence Unit requesting injectable opiates. He was referred from a genitourinary clinic where he had been diagnosed as being HIV positive, with weight loss, lymphadenopathy, Candida infection, and evidence of a falling CD4 count. He appeared persistently depressed, apathetic, and socially withdrawn. He refused to attend a general psychiatric clinic (specializing in patients with HIV) for his psychological symptoms, and would only attend a specialist HIV clinic when he was acutely ill. He was resistant and negative about all other offers and suggestions, e.g. respite care, reduction of injectable medication, Narcotics Anonymous groups, and other organizations. He wanted prescribed oral methadone changed to tablets as he claimed the linctus gave him stomach pains. He said he required more prescribed injectables as he was having to use even more illicit injectable medication because of withdrawal symptoms. He refused the opportunity to test the dose he required. There was some speculation from the dispensing pharmacy as to whether he was selling his drugs. He was living alone supported by his girlfriend and social services. His major activity appeared to be collecting his medication at the clinic. He claimed he was too exhausted to do anything else.

Mr D was a 35-year-old gay teacher who had been diagnosed as being HIV positive and was referred by the genitourinary medicine unit. Since the time he was diagnosed he had noticed that he was drinking up to six units a day whereas two units were usual for him. He was aware that this habit could escalate, and he presented to the clinic saying he wanted help to stop. He thought he was psychologically dependent. He was still finding that drinking made him relaxed and helped him to sleep, but he drank in the evenings with meals. He never drank in the morning and denied withdrawal symptoms. He was using no other drugs and his lifestyle was otherwise stable. He was involved with a number of activities and groups relating to his HIV infection and found this support invaluable. Physically he appeared fit. He attended the first appointment, then failed to attend follow-up. Six months later he once more presented with a story that he had managed to abstain and cut down but was drinking six units a day again. This time he admitted that he felt depressed.

Table 1 *Features of the alcohol dependence syndrome (1976)*

Narrowing of the drinking repertoire
Increasing severity of dependence is marked by increasingly stereotyped drinking with little day-to-day variability of beverage choice; drinking is scheduled so as to maintain a high blood alcohol level

Salience of drink-seeking behaviour
Increasing severity of dependence is marked by the individual granting highest priority to maintaining alcohol intake, with a failure of negative social consequences to deter drinking behaviour

Increased tolerance
Increasing severity of dependence is marked by the individual functioning at blood alcohol levels that would incapacitate the non-tolerant drinker. In later stages, the individual begins to lose previously acquired tolerance because of liver damage, ageing and/or brain damage

Repeated withdrawal symptoms
With increasing severity of dependence, the individual manifests more frequent and severe withdrawal symptoms; four key symptoms are tremor, nausea, sweating, and mood disturbance

Relief avoidance of withdrawal symptoms
With increasing severity of dependence, the individual drinks earlier in the day and may even awaken in the middle of the night to drink

Subjective awareness of a compulsion to drink
With increasing severity of dependence, the individual experiences a sense of 'loss of control' or impaired control over alcohol intake and a subjective sense of craving or desire to drink. Cues for craving may include the feeling of intoxification, withdrawal, affective discomfort, or situational stimuli

Reinstatement after abstinence
With increasing severity of dependence, the individual feels 'hooked' within a few days of starting to drink, and drinking will revert to the old stereotyped pattern. The six elements of the syndrome rapidly reappear

Thus, although 'addiction' has been and is commonly used, more precise definitions were seen to be mandatory. The term substance abuse describes the consumption of mind-altering chemicals, be they licit or illicit, for example alcohol, nicotine, opiates, amphetamines, cocaine, cannabis, LSD, ecstasy. Substance misuse indicates actual or potential harm resulting from use of a substance, whereas substance-related problems or alcohol-related disabilities are the gamut of adverse physical, psychological, and social problems directly or indirectly consequential upon excessive drinking or drug taking or substance dependence. These are described in detail in other sections.

As can be seen from Tables 1 and 2, the dependence syndrome is an interrelated cluster of cognitive, behavioural and physiological symptoms. The dependence syndrome was outlined in the original provisional description as follows:

Increased tolerance

This refers to the fact that a person will need more of the drug to maintain the effect. A severely dependent person can tolerate doses of drug which may be fatal to a drug-naïve individual. Tolerance to alcohol, for example, can also decrease at a very advanced stage of the process.

Repeated withdrawal symptoms

This refers to the development of symptoms when the drug is withheld. Type, timing, and severity of symptoms vary for different drugs. Central nervous system depressants lead to anxiety, tremor, nausea and vomit-

Table 2 *Substance use disorders criteria for DSM-III-R, DSM-IV, and ICD-10; adapted from Rounsaville et al. (1993) with permission*

DSM-III-R dependence (3 items required)
  (1) substance often taken in larger amounts or over a longer period than the person intended
  (2) persistent desire or one or more unsuccessful efforts to cut down or control substance use
  (3) a great deal of time spent in activities necessary to get the substance, taking the substance, or recovering from its effects
  (4) frequent intoxication or withdrawal symptoms when expected to fulfil major role obligations at work, school, or home
  (5) important social, occupational, or recreational activities given up or reduced because of substance use
  (6) continued substance use despite knowledge of having a persistent or recurrent social, psychological, or physical problem that is caused or exacerbated by the use of substance
  (7) marked tolerance
  (8) characteristic withdrawal symptoms
  (9) substance often taken to relieve or avoid withdrawal symptoms
DSM-III-R abuse (1 item required)
  (1) continued use despite knowledge of having a persistent or recurrent social, occupational, psychological, or physical problem that is caused or exacerbated by use of the psychoactive substance
  (2) recurrent use in situations in which use is physically hazardous
DSM-IV dependence (3 items required)
  (1) tolerance, as defined by either of the following:
    (a) a need for markedly increased amounts of the substance to achieve intoxication or desired effect
    (b) markedly diminished effect with continued use of the same amount of the substance
  (2) withdrawal, as manifested by either of the following:
    (a) the characteristic withdrawal syndrome for the substance
    (b) the same (or a closely related) substance is taken to relieve or avoid withdrawal symptoms
  (3) The substance is often taken in larger amounts or over a longer period than was intended
  (4) there is a persistent desire or unsuccessful efforts to cut down or control substance use
  (5) a great deal of time is spent in activities necessary to obtain the substance (e.g., visiting multiple doctors or driving long distances), use the substance (e.g., chain-smoking), or recover from its effects
  (6) important social, occupational, or recreational activities are given up or reduced because of substance use
  (7) the substance use is continued despite knowledge of having a persistent or recurrent physical or psychological problem that is likely to have been caused or exacerbated by the substance (e.g., current cocaine use despite recognition of cocaine-induced depression, or continued drinking despite recognition that an ulcer was made worse by alcohol consumption)
  Specify if: with physiological dependence: evidence of tolerance or withdrawal (i.e., either Item 1 or 2 is present) without physiological dependence: no evidence of tolerance or withdrawal (i.e., neither Item 1 nor 2 is present)
DSM-IV abuse (1 item required)
  (1) recurrent substance use resulting in inability to fulfil major role obligations at work, school, or home
  (2) recurrent substance-related legal problems
  (3) continued substance use despite having persistent or recurrent social or interpersonal problems caused or exacerbated by the effects of the substance
  (4) recurrent substance use in situations in which it is physically hazardous
ICD-10 dependence (3 items required)
  (1) a strong desire or sense of compulsion to use a substance or substances
  (2) evidence of impaired capacity to control the use of a substance or substances. This may relate to difficulties in avoiding initial use, difficulties in terminating use, or problems about controlling levels of use
  (3) a withdrawal state or use of the substance to relieve or avoid withdrawal symptoms, and subjective awareness of the effectiveness of such behaviour
  (4) evidence of tolerance to the effects of the substance
  (5) progressive neglect of alternative pleasures, behaviours, or interests in favour of substance use
  (6) persisting with substance use despite clear evidence of harmful consequences
ICD-10 harmful use (1 item required)
  (1) clear evidence that the use of a substance or substances was responsible for causing actual psychological or physical harm to the user

ing, sweating, fits, and delirium. Stimulant drugs lead to depression, fatigue, and sleepiness.

Subjective awareness of compulsion to drink or take drugs

Also known as 'craving', this describes the overwhelming subjective sense of the need to obtain drugs. The person is constantly preoccupied with thoughts and feelings centred on the desire to take action in order to satisfy the urge to take drugs.

Salience of drug-seeking behaviour over all other activities

Drug taking becomes the all-important major priority in the person's life. Social and occupational obligations and responsibilities become secondary, no matter what the consequences.

Narrowing of the drug-taking repertoire

The pattern varies and becomes less flexible. A person who, at one time, could vary the amount, type, and timing of drink or drug consumed, becomes increasingly rigid, if what is required is available. This stereo-typed pattern might become more chaotic if dependence is very severe and the person takes whatever is available.

Reinstatement after abstinence

This refers to the phenomenon where a person who has, at one time, developed dependence manages to abstain for a given period, but who then begins drug taking once more. This time round, dependence will develop very much more quickly than before.

The 'alcohol dependence syndrome' has provided the theoretical basis for the *Diagnostic and Statistical Manual* (DSM) of the American Psychiatric Association's diagnosis of substance-related disorders. As can be seen from Table 2, DSM-IV identifies seven criteria (three or more of which must be met to make a diagnosis). The DSM systems and ICD-10 differ in that:

  (1) ICD-10 has a harmful abuse category which is more narrowly defined than the abuse category in DSM-III-R and DSM IV;

(2) ICD-10 item 1 (craving or compulsion) is not a component of DSM;

(3) ICD-10 only includes physical and psychological harm, not social and legal consequences for harmful use; and

(4) ICD-10 has fewer, more broadly defined dependence criteria.

ICD-10 contains detailed clinical guidelines and research diagnostic criteria, whereas DSM was originally designed for clinical and educational purposes. DSM is the main system used to diagnose and classify psychiatric disorders in the United States and thus now has research utility. Thus ICD-10 and DSM are not identical, although there is high agreement between the two systems for a dependence diagnosis. There is very low agreement for abuse and harmful use diagnoses. DSM-IV abuse category is enlarged to include a wider range of social problems than DSM-III.

A further elaboration of the dependence syndrome concept has been to grade it according to mild, moderate, or severe degrees of severity. This dimensional (rather than categorical) approach stresses variation or heterogeneity amongst individuals. A number of questionnaires have been developed to quantify degree or severity of drug or alcohol dependence and level of related problems.

The framework described above has had important implications for public health strategies. It has highlighted the need for identification and assessment, and the value of brief intervention for the majority of patients with substance problems who present as medical out-patients. Only a minority will need to be referred on to appropriate specialists.

It can be argued that the dependence syndrome concept has contributed significantly to description and measurement of substance problems, and perhaps less to prognosis and treatment outcome and to an understanding aetiology and natural history.

However, the development of a set of diagnostic criteria enhances the generalist's ability to differentiate between substance use, substance misuse, substance-related problems, and dependence. Thus, it is of major importance to appreciate that patients need not be severely dependent and still be seriously affected by substance problems.

As will be discussed elsewhere, such competence enlarges the repertoire of treatment options available to the physician. Brief interventions have been shown reliably to be feasible and effective for harmful substance use, even in situations where contact between physician and patient is short.

To return to the case histories. Mr A's case history gives a clear picture of withdrawal symptoms. In addition, he manifests numerous related disabilities of a social (financial, marital, accommodation, employment) and physical (brain and liver damage) nature. He has a severe degree of dependence.

Dr B, in contrast, reported no withdrawal experiences. She managed to terminate use, and denied the desire to use substances. She claimed she had not developed tolerance, and substance use did not drive her to neglect her interests. Her psychological problems were long-standing both prior to and following her self-detoxification. She did not, therefore, meet a harmful use or a dependence diagnosis. She did suffer difficulties in adjusting to many life situations, for example her inadequate functioning in marital, social, and occupational situations. Poor self-esteem precipitated volatile moods, apathy, frustration, and impulsive behaviour, including drug seeking. As a result she was unemployed, lived alone, and had unsatisfactory sexual relationships.

In the case of Mr C, although it was highly likely that he was dependent on opiates, certain proof, especially of the degree to which he might be dependent, eluded those involved in his care as he refused to submit himself for thorough assessment. He had a range of the social, psychological, and physical disabilities related to a combination of intravenous injecting and subsequent HIV infection. He has demonstrated certain evidence of harmful use, but circumstantial evidence of dependence.

Mr D admitted to episodic difficulty in controlling his level of use and resisting the desire to drink. He found he had to drink more for the same effect. At first he did not recognize that he was depressed, but once he accepted that he was, he appreciated that it was a factor causing his drinking, rather than consequential. Mr D demonstrates at least three features of the dependence syndrome, which is likely to be moderately severe.

REFERENCES

American Psychiatric Association. (1994). *Diagnostic and Statistical Manual of Mental Disorders*. 4th edn. Washington, DC.

American Psychiatric Association (1987). *Diagnostic and statistical manual of mental disorders*, (3rd edn, revised). American Psychiatric Association, Washington, D.C.

Bien, T.H., Miller, W.R., and Tonigan, J.S. (1993). Brief interventions for alcohol problems: a review. *Addiction*, **88**, 315–36.

Edwards, G. (1992). Taking substance misuse seriously. *Health and Hygiene*, **13**, 146–57.

Edwards, G. and Gross, M.M. (1976). Alcohol dependence: a provisional description of a clinical syndrome. *British Medical Journal*, **1**, 1058–61.

Erickson, C.K. (1992). A pharmacologists' opinion – alcoholism: the disease debate needs to stop. *Alcohol and Alcoholism*, **27**, 325–8.

Institute of Medicine (1990). *Broadening the base of treatment for alcohol problems*. National Academy Press, Washington DC.

Rounsaville, B.J., Bryant, K., Babor, T., Kranzler, H., and Kadden, R. (1993). Cross-system agreement for substance use disorders: DSM III-R, DSM-IV and ICD 10. *Addiction*, **88**, 337–48.

Royal College of Physicians (1987). *A great and growing evil*. Tavistock, London.

World Health Organisation (1978). *Mental disorders: glossary and guide to their classification in accordance with the Ninth revision of the international classification of diseases*. Geneva: World Health Organisation.

World Health Organisation (1987). *Tenth revision of the International Classification of diseases*, Chapter V(F), *Mental, behavioural and developmental disorders*. World Health Organization, Geneva.

28.2 Brief interventions for prevention

28.2.1 Screening and brief intervention

P. D. ANDERSON

The focus of this section is on screening and brief intervention for hazardous and harmful alcohol consumption. However, the same principles and techniques apply for other substances, including drugs and tobacco.

The continuum of alcohol consumption and alcohol problems

It is now recognized that both alcohol consumption and alcohol problems exist within continua. Alcohol consumption ranges from no or light consumption through to heavy consumption and alcohol problems range from no problems through to substantial or serious problems. This understanding of a continuum has led to new definitions of alcohol consumption and problems. Hazardous alcohol consumption can be defined as a level of alcohol consumption or pattern of drinking that is likely to result in harm should present drinking habits persist. Harmful alcohol consumption is the consumption of alcohol which is causing harm to the psychological or physical well-being of the individual.

The continuum of response to alcohol problems

Just as there is a continuum of both alcohol consumption and alcohol problems, so there is a continuum of responses to alcohol problems, ranging from primary prevention through brief interventions to specialized treatment.

The clinician in the general hospital and the physician in general practice are in ideal settings to offer screening and brief interventions for hazardous and harmful alcohol consumption. Screening instruments have been developed and considerable evidence has accumulated that demonstrates the effectiveness of brief interventions for hazardous and harmful alcohol use in both general practice and hospital. The World Health Organization's multicentre trial of brief intervention procedures designed to reduce the risks associated with hazardous alcohol use demonstrated that men who received 5 min of advice to reduce their alcohol consumption reported 38 per cent less alcohol consumption at 6 months follow-up, while the control group reduced its typical daily consumption by 10 per cent.

SCREENING

Recognizing hazardous alcohol consumption.

QUALITY FREQUENCY QUESTIONNAIRES

Standard questions provide a proven, simple, and reliable method of finding out how much a patient drinks. Simply asking patients 'How much do you drink?' tends to elicit responses such as 'not a lot', or 'just occasionally'.

To help work out the amount of alcohol that your patient drinks each week (in units, where one unit contains about 10 g of alcohol and equals half a pint of beer, lager, or cider, a single measure of spirits, or a glass of wine, sherry, or vermouth) ask the following questions: 'On average, how many days a week do you have an alcoholic drink?'. 'On average, on a day when you have had an alcoholic drink, how much do you usually have as half pints of beer, lager, cider, glasses of wine, sherry, or vermouth, and singles of spirits.' By adding up the number of units of alcohol on a typical drinking day and multiplying this number by the number of drinking days a week gives an estimate of the patient's total weekly alcohol consumption. The amount of alcohol should be recorded in the medical notes.

Quantity frequency questionnaires can be used to obtain quantitative information about alcohol intake. They contain questions on the usual frequency of drinking in a certain period of time (a week or a month), the type of alcoholic drink taken, and the usual quantity of each drink consumed per day. From this information the average weekly alcohol intake can be calculated (Fig. 1). Quantity frequency questionnaires have high test–retest reliability and substantial validity when compared with drinking diaries. As a screening instrument for hazardous alcohol consumption in general practice settings, quantity frequency questionnaires have a sensitivity of 70 per cent, a specificity of 76 per cent, and a positive predictive value of 78 per cent. It is important to offer options of high alcohol intake.

DRINKING DIARIES

Retrospective 7-day drinking diaries are the best way to ascertain the amount of alcohol consumption. However, as screening instruments they are more complicated and time consuming than the completion of quantity frequency questionnaires, although they give more accurate information about alcohol consumption than the latter. The reliability of the diary method has been estimated to be at least 90 per cent. Under-reporting on questionnaire completions of alcohol consumption has been studied. Respondents tend to underestimate frequency of drinking and to overestimate the quantity consumed on a typical drinking occasion. Deliberate under-reporting of alcohol consumption may occur because

Fig. 1 Quantity frequency questionnaire to measure alcohol consumption.

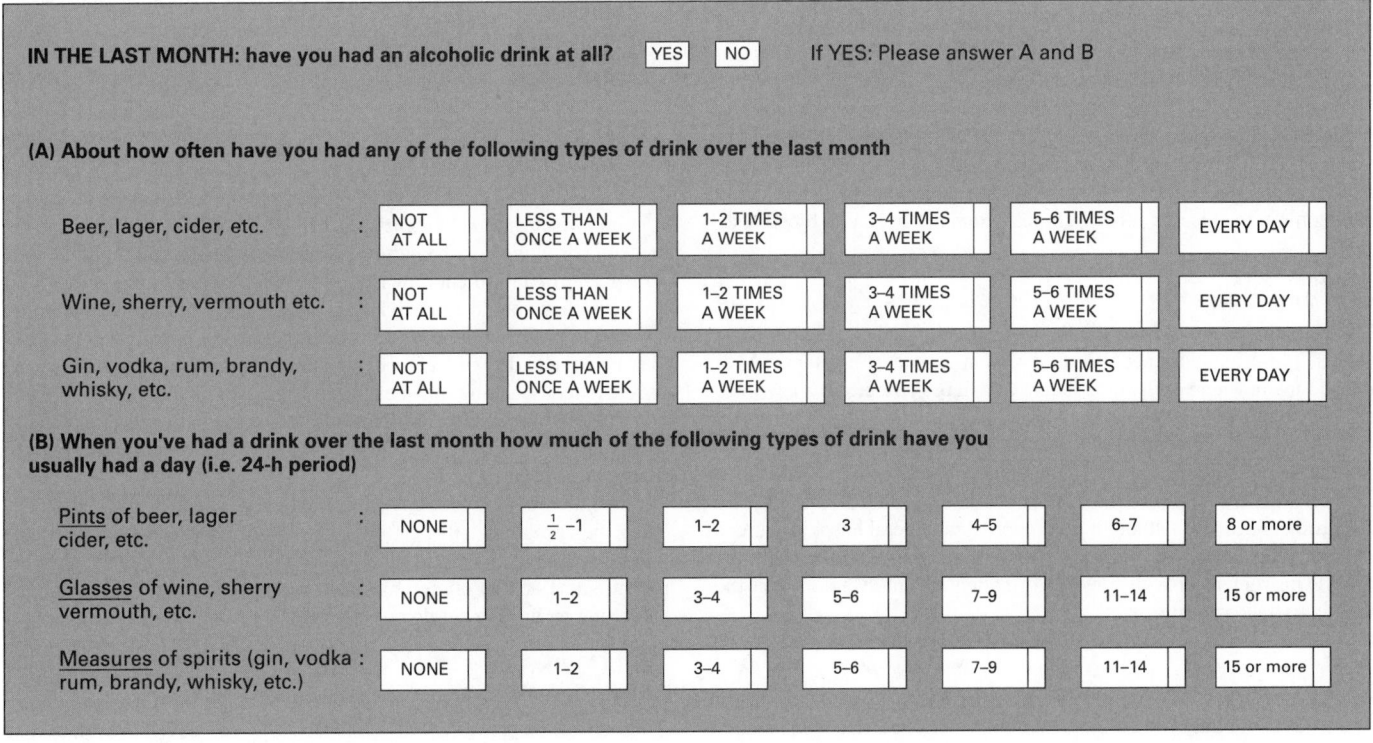

of stigma associated with excessive alcohol use and its behavioural effects. There is some evidence that increased levels of reporting may be found when interviewer contact is reduced or eliminated. Computerized interviewing techniques have been shown to result in increased self-reported consumption levels when compared to personal interviews.

ALCOHOL METERS

Alcohol meters measure the breath ethanol concentration. They are the same as those used by the police in roadside checks. A considerable number of heavy drinkers are missed by the alcoholometer because they have not actually been drinking shortly before the breath test. Alcoholmeters therefore probably have limited usefulness as screening instruments, although they can be used to give an estimate of blood alcohol levels in accidents or casualty departments.

Recognizing harmful alcohol consumption

ALCOHOL USE DISORDERS IDENTIFICATION TEST (AUDIT)

The World Health Organization (WHO) has developed a simple instrument to screen for persons with early signs of alcohol-related problems. The WHO core screening instrument consists of 10 simple questions (Fig. 2). Seven have been chosen as the most representative of the following areas:

(1) alcohol dependence and black-outs (four questions);
(2) negative alcohol reactions (one question);
(3) alcohol problems (two questions).

Three additional questions on alcohol consumption have also been included. As indicated by the AUDIT questions shown in Fig. 2, each item is scored by checking the response category that comes closest to the patient's answer. A score of eight or more produces the highest sensitivity and is used as the cutoff point. In general, high scores on the first three items in the absence of elevated scores on the remaining items suggests hazardous alcohol use. Elevated scores on items 4 through 6 imply the presence or emergence of alcohol dependence. High scores on the remaining items suggest harmful alcohol use.

The validity of the instrument has been calculated using hazardous alcohol consumption as the criterion for a positive case. This was defined as a mean daily alcohol intake of 40 g or more for men or 20 g or more for women. The sensitivity had a mean value of 80 per cent. The sensitivity was higher in men than in women. The specificity had a mean value of 89 per cent. It was higher in women than in men. The positive predictive value had a mean value of 60 per cent, and the predictive value of a negative result a mean value of 95 per cent. The instrument had an additional screening programme procedure that included a two-question trauma history, a brief clinical examination, and a blood test.

Other measures of psychosocial consequences of drinking

These include the 25-item Michigan Alcoholism Screening Test (MAST) and its shortened 10-item version and the four-item CAGE questionnaire where each of the letters CAGE is a letter from a key word from each of the four items. The CAGE is a more sensitive instrument than the MAST questionnaires for identifying the individual with drinking problems in general hospital and general practice populations. Two or more positive replies to the CAGE questionnaire are said to identify the problem drinker. Although it is reported in general hospital settings to have a high sensitivity (85 per cent) and specificity (89 per cent), the CAGE instrument provides less information for intervention than the longer AUDIT instrument.

Biological markers

The most commonly used biological markers of excessive alcohol consumption are mean cell volume and γ-glutamyl transpeptidase. Of these,

γ-glutamyl transpeptidase is a better predictor than mean cell volume. Although the mean cell volume is related to alcohol consumption, a raised mean cell volume is very unreliable as a screening instrument. The proportion of heavy drinkers who have mean cell volume over 98 fl ranges somewhere between 20 per cent and 30 per cent, and the false-positive rate is between 4 and 6 per cent.

There is a positive relationship between alcohol consumption and γ-glutamyl transpeptidase levels. Increased γ-glutamyl transpeptidase activity in the serum can be observed after a few weeks of alcohol intake. Following reduction in drinking, serum γ-glutamyl transpeptidase levels rapidly fall, returning to normal levels within 2 to 4 weeks. The rise of the enzyme in the serum is primarily due to hepatic enzyme inductions. Nevertheless, γ-glutamyl transpeptidase is not very good as a screening instrument. The proportion of heavy drinkers with a raised level, more than 50 IU/l, is about 50 per cent. The false-positive rate is between 10 to 20 per cent. Other causes of a raised γ-glutamyl transpeptidase level include other diseases of the liver, biliary tract, and pancreas. The most important use of γ-glutamyl transpeptidase is for monitoring changes in alcohol consumption.

Brief intervention for hazardous alcohol consumption

Hazardous alcohol consumption is best defined as a consumption of 350 g (35 units) or more per week for men and 210 g (21 units) or more per week for women. Studies have shown that a 5 min advisory session is effective in reducing hazardous alcohol consumption. Firm but friendly advice should be given to cut down. The patient should be reassured that they are not thought to be an 'alcoholic', but that if they go on drinking at the current rate, health damage, and work and personal problems are likely to develop.

The harm that can arise from too much drinking can be explained. These include raised blood pressure, headaches, stomach upsets, anxiety and depression, sexual difficulties, overweight, sleep problems, poor concentration, poor work performance, accidental injuries, liver disease, hangovers, cancers, irritability, and financial worries.

The positive reasons for drinking less can be pointed out. These include: less risk of accidents, high blood pressure or liver disease; possible reduced weight; improved concentration and a clear head; fewer hangovers, headaches, and stomach upsets; sounder sleep and less tiredness generally; more energy and time for new activities; fewer arguments and rows with friends and family; more pleasure out of sex; a new sense of being in control of life and feeling fitter; if trying for a baby, improved chance of success for both men and women; and extra cash.

A patient's ultimate target should be to keep well below the weekly limits of 210 g (21 units) of alcohol for men and 140 g (14 units) of alcohol for women. Some people will want or need to abstain altogether. It is important that the patient agrees that the target is realistic, and for someone drinking very heavily, a higher interim target might be set with a longer-term aim to cut down further.

The patient should be encouraged to keep a regular drinking diary as a way of measuring progress and sticking to new limits. If there is time, the last 7 days' drinking can be gone through, working backwards from the current day, noting down each day's drinking in units of alcohol and working out the weekly total. This will help make sure the patient understands how to use the diary and give him or her a baseline from which to assess progress.

The patient's motivation will be strengthened if it is made clear that his or her progress will be followed. Self-help booklets are available which can supplement the doctor's advice. These booklets give the patient some advice on getting ready for cutting down on alcohol and some tips on how to cut down on alcohol.

Brief intervention for harmful alcohol consumption

An alternative approach, which has recently been developed, should be applied for patients with harmful alcohol consumption. This approach,

Fig. 2 World Health Organization Core Screening Instrument.

Tick the number that comes closest to the patient's answer.

1. How often do you have a drink containing alcohol?

| (0) NEVER | (1) MONTHLY OR LESS | (2) TWO TO FOUR TIMES A MONTH | (3) FOUR OR MORE TIMES A WEEK | (4) FOUR OR MORE TIMES A WEEK |

2.* How many drinks containing alcohol do you have on a typical day when you are drinking?
[CODE NUMBER OF STANDARD DRINKS]

| (0) 1 OR 2 | (1) 3 OR 4 | (2) 5 OR 6 | (3) 7 OR 8 | (4) 10 OR MORE |

3. How often do you have six or more drinks on one occasion?

| (0) NEVER | (1) LESS THAN MONTHLY | (2) MONTHLY | (3) WEEKLY | (4) DAILY OR ALMOST DAILY |

4. How often during the last year have you found that you were not able to stop drinking once you had started?

| (0) NEVER | (1) LESS THAN MONTHLY | (2) MONTHLY | (3) WEEKLY | (4) DAILY OR ALMOST DAILY |

5. How often during the last year have you failed to do what was normally expected from you because of drinking?

| (0) NEVER | (1) LESS THAN MONTHLY | (2) TWO TO FOUR TIMES A MONTH | (3) FOUR OR MORE TIMES A WEEK | (4) FOUR OR MORE TIMES A WEEK |

6. How often during the last year have you needed a first drink in the morning to get yourself going after a heavy drinking session?

| (0) NEVER | (1) LESS THAN MONTHLY | (2) MONTHLY | (3) WEEKLY | (4) DAILY OR ALMOST DAILY |

7. How often during the last year have you had a feeling of guilt or remorse after drinking?

| (0) NEVER | (1) LESS THAN MONTHLY | (2) MONTHLY | (3) WEEKLY | (4) DAILY OR ALMOST DAILY |

8. How often during the last year have you been unable to remember what happened the night before because you had been drinking?

| (0) NEVER | (1) LESS THAN MONTHLY | (2) MONTHLY | (3) WEEKLY | (4) DAILY OR ALMOST DAILY |

9. Have you or someone else been injured as a result of your drinking?

| (0) NO | (2) YES, BUT NOT IN THE LAST YEAR | (4) YES, DURING THE LAST YEAR |

10. Has a relative or friend or a doctor or other health worker, been concerned about your drinking or suggested you cut down?

| (0) NO | (2) YES, BUT NOT IN THE LAST YEAR | (4) YES, DURING THE LAST YEAR |

* In determining the response categories it has been assumed that one 'drink' contains 10 g alcohol. In countries where the alcohol content of a standard drink differs by more than 25 per cent and 10 g, the response category should be modified accordingly.

Record sum of individual item scores here _____.

Table 1 *The menu of strategies*

1. Opening strategy: lifestyle, stresses, and substance use
2. Opening strategy: health and substance use
3. A typical day/session
4. The good things and the less good things
5. Providing information
6. The future and the present
7. Exploring concerns
8. Helping with decision-making

which is widely liked by doctors in general hospital and general practice settings, is called brief motivational interviewing and is based on the fact that ambivalence about patients changing their alcohol consumption is a common problem in health-care consultations. Doctors are used to speaking to patients about the need to drink less. However, since the most common form of consultation involves the delivery of medical advice controlled by the doctor, negotiations about reducing harmful drinking frequently take the form of persuasion. Although giving advice about reducing harmful drinking clearly works with some patients, as demonstrated by research, success rates could be higher.

One problem with giving advice about drinking alcohol is that many patients are not ready to change and thus direct persuasion may push the patient into a position of defensiveness.

Ambivalence is a common and normal experience. For people with a drinking problem, there is a conflict between indulgence and restraint, each having pros and cons associated with it. The intensity with which people experience this conflict varies a great deal and appears to increase as the person approaches decision-making. The most effective way to help the patient is to explore this conflict and to encourage patients to express their reasons for concern and the arguments for change.

Patients with harmful alcohol consumption are at different ends of a continuum with respect to their readiness to change. At one end of the continuum are patients who are not at all ready to consider change. Towards the other end are those in the process of decision-making and actual change, while those in the middle are in a state of ambivalence about their drinking. Amongst excessive drinkers in hospital, 29 per cent were found not to be ready for change, 26 per cent were ready to change, and 45 per cent were ambivalent. People can move backwards and forwards along this continuum. Helping them move forward, even if they do not reach a decision to change, let alone make a change, is an acceptable outcome of a consultation. If a doctor talks to patients as if they were further along the line than they really are, resistance will be the likely outcome. The first task of the doctor is therefore to establish the patient's degree of readiness for change and to then select a strategy appropriate to this level of motivation.

There is a menu of eight strategies, each of which takes 5 to 15 min to work through, (Table 1).

As the doctor moves down the menu, so the strategies require greater readiness to change from the patient. While strategies towards the top of the menu can be used with almost all patients, those towards the bottom can only be used with the smaller number of patients who are making a decision to change. Strategies 1 and 2 are opening strategies. Strategies 3 and 4 provide a solid platform of rapport and help the doctor understand the patient's life circumstances. Further progress down the menu depends upon the readiness to change. If the patient openly expresses concern, strategies 7 and 8 can be used. However, if the patient appears unconcerned about their drinking, strategies 5 and 6 should be used.

OPENING STRATEGY: LIFESTYLE, STRESSES, AND ALCOHOL USE

This strategy involves talking generally about the person's current lifestyle and stresses and then raising the subject of alcohol with an open question like 'Where does your use of alcohol fit in?'.

OPENING STRATEGY: HEALTH AND ALCOHOL USE

This strategy is particularly useful in hospital and general practice settings when the doctor thinks that alcohol use is causing health problems. A general enquiry about health is followed by a simple open question like 'Where does your use of alcohol fit in?' or 'How does your use of alcohol affect your health?'

A TYPICAL DAY/WEEK/SESSION

The functions of this strategy are to build rapport, to help the patients talk about current behaviour in detail within a non-pathological framework and to assess in more detail their degree of readiness to change. Because the doctor makes no reference to problems or concerns it is particularly useful to patients who seem not ready to consider change. It is also a useful starting point for other more ready patients, since it helps the doctor understand the context of the behaviour in question and can produce a wealth of information relevant to assessment.

A typical day/week or session is identified and the doctor begins as follows: 'Can we spend the next 5 to 10 min going through this day from beginning to end. What happened, how did you feel, and where did your use of alcohol fit in. Let's start at the beginning.' The goal is simply to follow the patient through a sequence of events, focusing on both behaviour and feelings, with simple open questions being the main input from the doctor.

THE GOOD THINGS AND THE LESS GOOD THINGS

This strategy helps build rapport, provides information about context, and enables an assessment of readiness to change to be made. It approaches the exploration of concerns, although it avoids using terms like 'problem' or 'concern'. The patient can be asked 'What are some of the good things about your use of alcohol?' or 'What do you like about your use of alcohol?' Then the patient is asked 'What are some of the less good things about your use of alcohol?' or 'What do you dislike about your use of alcohol?' Once both questions have been answered, the doctor should summarize the good things and the less good things in 'you' language. For example, 'So, using alcohol helps you relax, you enjoy doing this with friends and it helps when you are really feeling fed up. On the other hand you say that you sometimes feel controlled by alcohol and on Monday mornings you find it difficult to do anything at work.'

PROVIDING INFORMATION

Giving patients information is a routine task of doctors. Crucially, however, the way in which information is given can affect how the patient responds and reacts. There are three phases of giving information: the readiness of the patient to receive information, its provision in a neutral and non-personal way, and asking the patients' reaction with an open question like 'What do you make of this?' At the outset it is useful to seek permission from the patient to give information, using a question like: 'I wonder, would you be interested in knowing more about the effect of alcohol on health?' Information is best provided in a neutral and non-personal way, in general by referring to what happens to people, rather than to the particular patient.

THE FUTURE AND THE PRESENT

This strategy can only be used with patients who are at least concerned to some degree about their drinking. A focus on the contrast between the patient's present circumstances and the way the patient would like to be in the future may uncover a discrepancy which can be a powerful motivating force. A useful question is 'How would you like things to be different in the future?' The doctor can then focus on the present by asking 'What is stopping you doing these things you would like to do?'

and 'How does your use of alcohol affect you at the moment?' This often leads directly to an exploration of concerns about alcohol use and the issue of changing drinking.

EXPLORING CONCERNS

This is the most important strategy of all since it provides the framework of eliciting from the patient their concerns about their drinking. It can only be used with patients who do not have concerns and therefore cannot be used with someone who is not considering change. After following the patients answers to the opening question 'What concerns do you have about your use of alcohol?', the strategy simply involves summarizing the first concern and then asking 'What else, what other concerns do you have?' and so on until all concerns have been covered. The strategy ends with a summary which highlights not only these concerns but also the positive benefits of alcohol use expressed by the patient; this is done to bring out the contrasting elements of the patient's ambivalence.

Part of the patient's conflict involves wondering what it would be like if a change in drinking were to take place. Therefore, a similar strategy can be constructed around concerns about changing. The opening question would be something like: 'What concerns do you have about reducing your use of alcohol?'

HELPING WITH DECISION-MAKING

This strategy can only be used with patients who indicate some desire to make a decision to change. The outline of the strategy is as follows. Patients should not be rushed into decision-making. Options for the future should be presented rather than a single course of action. What other patients have done in a similar situation can be described. It should be emphasized to the patient that 'you are the best judge of what will be best for you'. Information should be provided in a neutral non-personal manner. Failure to reach a decision to change is not a failed consultation. Resolutions to change often break down. The patient should understand this and be told that future contact should take place even if things go wrong. Commitment to change is likely to fluctuate. The doctor should expect this to happen and empathize with the patient's predicament.

This patient-centred approach to negotiating behaviour change is a new skill for many doctors. Although it is more time consuming, a patient-centred approach is more effective than simply giving advice and, thus, in the long run will be of more benefit to the patient.

Finally, it should be said that the brief interventions described in this section are designed for those patients with hazardous and harmful alcohol consumption. Patients who show signs of dependence or serious physical illness as a result of their alcohol consumption will require a different approach, which may need abstinence as the goal of intervention and referral to a more specialized service.

REFERENCES

Anderson, P. (1991). *Management of drinking problems*. WHO Regional Publications, European Series, No 32. World Health Organization Regional Office for Europe, Copenhagen.

Bien, T.H., Miller W.R., and Scott Tonigar, J. (1993). Brief interventions for alcohol problems: a review. *British Journal of Addiction*, **88**, 315–36.

Institute of Medicine (1990). *Broadening the base of treatment for alcohol problems*. National Academy Press, Washington.

Miller, W.R. and Rollnick, S. (1991). *Motivational interviewing. Preparing people to change addictive behaviour*. The Guilford Press, New York.

Rollnick, S., Heather, N., and Bell, A. (1992). Negotiating behavioural change in medical settings: the development of brief motivational interviewing. *Journal of Mental Health*, **1**, 25–37.

Watson, R.R. (ed.) (1989). *Diagnosis of alcohol abuse*. CRC Press, Florida.

World Health Organization (1992). *AUDIT, The Alcohol Use Disorders Identification Test. Guidelines for use in primary health care*. (WHO/PSA/92.4). World Health Organization, Geneva.

World Health Organization (1992). *Project on identification and management of alcohol-related problems. Report on Phase II: A randomized clinical trial of brief interventions in primary health care*. (WHO/PSA/91.5). World Health Organization, Geneva.

28.2.2 Harm reduction

J. STRANG and M. FARRELL

Focus on improving health

Harm reduction has been brought to the fore by human immunodeficiency virus (HIV) infection, but its relevance is much wider. Underlying much of the current debate about possible harm-reduction strategies there exists a new clarity of vision about the goals of individual and public interventions (and hence the measures we may incorporate to gauge the extent of success of these interventions)—the goal of these interventions is the reduction of individual and public harms. The harms in question may vary between substances, populations, and countries, and the weightings we assign to different harms will vary with the ebb and flow of public and scientific debate: hence the advent of HIV/AIDS has led to a 'promotion' of injecting drug use within our hierarchy of concerns. Thus the United Kingdom Advisory Council on the Misuse of Drugs concluded that 'the spread HIV is a greater danger to individual and public health than drug misuse: accordingly, services which aim to minimise HIV risk behaviour by all available means should take precedence in development plans'.

The consideration has been broadened so as to include the non-dependent injector or the ex-injector, and the planning of treatment programmes has included consideration of approaches that target the injecting behaviour quite specifically. The Advisory Council on the Misuse of Drugs recommended that 'we must therefore be prepared to work with those who continue to misuse drugs to help them reduce the risks involved in doing so, above all the risk of acquiring or spreading HIV'. By accepting that some drug use will continue, it becomes possible for us to consider a wider range of possible inventions—such as advice on effective cleaning of infected needles and syringes, or the provision of clean needles and syringes from pharmacists or special syringe exchange schemes, or the establishment of health screening and hepatitis B immunization programmes amongst these high-risk populations. Our tolerance of imperfection thereby increases the extent of therapeutic opportunity. The aim is quite simply the identification and promotion of strategies that will lead to reductions in specified harms.

Although the recent debate about harm-reduction strategies has been provoked by concerns about HIV/AIDS, it is important that this consideration should go much further.

Broadening of constituency

A harm-reduction approach requires consideration of the broader population of drug takers. The general practitioner or hospital doctor who only identifies alcohol or drug abuse when it is the presenting feature, will miss many opportunities for effecting individual and public health benefit at an early stage. Neither HIV nor hepatitis B or C are transmitted by the drug of abuse nor by dependence on the drug, and there are instances in which they have been transmitted on a single occasion of injecting or of unprotected sex. Certain drugs of abuse seem to be particularly associated with HIV transmission (particularly crack cocaine), and both sexual and injecting HIV risks are greater amongst heroin addicts with higher scores of severity of dependence. However, only a minority of problem drinkers or drug takers are identified as such and are in contact with specialist treatment services. Hence the public health benefit from harm-reduction measures is likely to be most reliant on the clinical acumen of doctors working in a non-drug-specialist setting, through whom the greatest gains will be made by identification and intervention with the patient who is not otherwise identified as having an alcohol or drug problem.

Examples of harm-reduction measures that can be easily implemented

With alcohol, sensible drinking limits are proposed—especially for the pregnant woman. The clinician will find himself/herself involved in providing advice about levels of alcohol intake, as part of the management of peptic ulcer or hepatitis as well as with the patient with an identified alcohol problem. The publication of sensible drinking limits is essentially a pragmatic approach to the harm that results from the alcohol intake. Likewise, with alcohol and driving, no alcohol intake is undoubtedly the best option, but it is hoped that the chosen levels may be more acceptable and more widely followed, even though they may be second best. Indeed, the recent debate about a protective effect of alcohol consumption on cardiovascular disease is to do with balancing the benefits and harms—hence avoiding an absolute approach to being either 'for' or 'against'.

In the case of tobacco, the introduction of filter cigarettes and low-tar cigarettes represent attempts at harm-reduction measures, and the recent development of nicotine replacement systems is an attempt to separate a major psychoactive drug from some of the accompanying products that are responsible for much of the long-term morbidity and mortality. Ceasing tobacco intake entirely is the best solution, when achievable; but there may well be widespread public health benefit from the wider adoption of a compromise measure of nicotine substitution.

The heroin addict may be offered detoxification or may be recruited into an oral methadone maintenance programme—an acceptance of the continued dependent drug use while effecting a move away from injecting, with the rationale being similar to that used for nicotine replacement therapy. Oral methadone maintenance programmes have become widespread in some countries such as the United States and Australia, while they are non-existent in other countries (for example, India and France) and they have not been developed as a formal system in the United Kingdom (where most such prescribing is not in the context of a formal maintenance programme). The merits of this approach (particularly in terms of reduced injecting and reduced HIV infection and transmission) have recently been reviewed in the United States and Australia, and are currently under review in the United Kingdom.

For the injecting drug user, advice has been provided in the United Kingdom by the Departments of Health, with information to be given to drug users on cleaning of injecting equipment (contained within the *Guidelines of good clinical practice in the management of drug misuse*). In the United States, such programmes are often referred to as 'bleach and teach' campaigns, with the information being passed on from one injector to the next. In the United Kingdom, there has been much investment in needle and syringe exchange schemes, accompanied by a marked increase in the willingness of community pharmacists to be involved in over-the-counter sales of needles and syringes. Recent guidelines on infectious diseases identify injecting drug users and their sexual partners as a target population for hepatitis B testing and immunization: so far, this is not widely provided, but the brief contact that the hospital doctor or general practitioner may have during an acute admission may be an excellent opportunity to test for past infection and to commence an immunization programme against hepatitis B if the patient is seronegative.

For the patient who is HIV positive or has chronic hepatitis B infection, each point of occasional contact is an opportunity to review the patient's physical status and establish another point in the immunological surveillance. For such patients, the early identification of changes in these parameters will draw the attention of both patient and clinician to, for example, needed prophylactic treatment or the early treatment of opportunistic infections.

28.2.3 Physical complications

28.2.3(a) Physical complications of alcohol misuse

T. J. PETERS

No organ, pathological process, or system is immune from the deleterious effects of acute or chronic alcohol misuse. For each system discussed, these are subdivided into acute effects requiring immediate action to minimize the local toxicity and into chronic conditions in which alcohol abstention with nutritional support is the primary objective. Clearly, the natural history of an alcohol misuser will be punctuated by a series of acute episodes against a background of chronic toxicity.

Central nervous system

The range of alcohol-related neurological disorders well illustrates the acute–chronic inter-relationships referred to above. Table 1 lists the principal syndromes.

ACUTE INTOXICATION

Ethanol is a CNS depressant and was used for centuries as an anaesthetic, albeit a relatively unsatisfactory one. It directly and indirectly (via fluidizing effects on the cell membrane) interferes with γ-aminobutyric acid receptor function, predominantly disinhibiting frontal cortical control. The progression of the acute intoxification effects listed in Table 1 correlates broadly with blood/breath/urine alcohol levels, although the correlation is closest with the former. It should be noted that chronic alcoholics are likely to have much higher blood alcohol levels than normal social drinkers for the same clinical picture. Females and minors will generally exhibit these features at significantly lower ethanol levels: euphoria, 25 to 50 mg%; incoordination, 50 to 100 mg%; ataxia, 100 to 200 mg%; stupor, 200 to 400 mg%; coma, 400 to 900 mg%.

The clinical features are self-evident, but it must be stressed that accompanying causes of apparent intoxication are common and must be actively excluded or treated. Thus, a comatose alcoholic may have hypoglycaemia, head injury (subdural haematoma), or systemic infection, contributing to, or overwhelming, the alcohol toxicity. Serial measurements of blood/breath alcohol are useful in monitoring these patients, as well as having medicolegal implications. The strong possibility of accidental or intentional overdose of licit or illicit drugs, including methanol, should always be considered. Urgent toxicological analyses are essential in suspected cases. Mild to moderate intoxication usually requires little specific treatment. Close observation for signs of deterioration, unconsciousness, sedation, and re-hydration are appropriate. Use of naloxone and other detoxification remedies is not recommended at present.

Alcoholic coma

This is a serious disorder, with a mortality rate approaching 5 per cent. Admission to hospital is essential for maintenance of vital functions, particularly respiratory integrity. Inhalation of vomitus is frequently fatal due to anoxaemia from acute respiratory distress (Mendelson's syndrome). Careful clinical examination, together with a full medical history from a partner where possible, must be performed to exclude other conditions, both acute and chronic, to which alcohol misusers are particularly prone, namely trauma, cerebral haemorrhage, meningitis and septicaemia, cardiovascular failure, hepatic failure, and gastrointestinal haemorrhage. Full investigation of suspected complications, including imaging procedures, metabolic profiles, viz. electrolytes, glucose, ammonia, lactate, blood gases, and toxicology screens, should be performed. Close clinical monitoring and the use of intravenous glucose solutions, respiratory and cardiovascular support, and, in serious cases,

Table 1 *Alcohol-related neurological disorders*

Acute intoxication (euphoria, incoordination and ataxia, confusion, stupor, and coma)
Withdrawal syndromes (blackouts, nightmares/terrors, tremulousness, epileptiform seizures, hallucinosis, delirium, tremors)
Nutritional deficiency syndromes (Wernicke–Korsakoff syndromes, cerebellar degeneration, peripheral neuropathy, pellagra, amblyopia)
Miscellaneous disorders (cerebral atrophy—dementia, central pontine myelinolysis, Marchiafava–Bignami syndrome, neuromyopathy, fetal alcohol syndromes)

haemo- or peritoneal dialysis will avoid many of the tragedies that occur. It is essential that following recovery the patient is not just promptly discharged, possibly with the telephone number of an alcohol treatment agency, but that he or she is fully assessed, both medically and psychiatrically, and an alcohol misuse treatment and re-education programme initiated. This is likely to involve a variety of agencies, both voluntary and statutory, and should involve medical/psychiatric follow-up, as appropriate. Failure to undertake these measures will almost invariably lead to continuation and progression of the alcohol/drug misuse.

WITHDRAWAL SYNDROMES

These are serious disorders occurring in chronic alcohol misusers with clear evidence of alcohol dependence who will have been abusing alcohol heavily on a regular basis for 5 to 10 years. It is still somewhat controversial as to whether the period of abstinence precipitates the syndromes (majority view), or whether cessation of drinking is the first event in the syndrome itself. It is important to recognize the prodromal symptoms of withdrawal, as prompt treatment should prevent the full-blown syndrome.

The patient will show anxiousness, tremulousness, and irritability, often complaining of the 'shakes' or 'jitters', nausea, vomiting, and, more specifically, nightmares, night-terrors, or blackouts. The symptoms occur most frequently 12 to 36 h after abstinence. In the more serious forms overt epileptiform seizures occur. In some patients the fits may be Jacksonian and in others show features of temporal lobe epilepsy. It should also be noted that alcohol intoxication may precipitate fits in patients with idiopathic or secondary (for example, following head injury) epilepsy. Alcohol withdrawal ('rum') fits differ from alcohol-associated epilepsy in that they occur during abstinence, do not show typical electroencephalogram evidence of epilepsy, and may be precipitated by photic stimulation (for example, flickering television screens). Treatment is with chlordiazepoxide in preference to chlormethiazole and carbamezepine for overt seizures. Conventional anticonvulsants (such as phenytoin) are less effective.

Although minor withdrawal syndromes and planned detoxification programmes can often be managed, either at home by the general practitioner with suitably trained nursing care or at a hospital outpatient clinic, a short period of admission, often to a medical rather than a psychiatric ward, is often the best approach. Monitoring of vital clinical signs, avoidance of metabolic consequences (for example, lactic or keto-acidosis, hypoglycaemia, hyponatraemia, and other electrolyte disturbances), and preliminary psychosocial assessment should be undertaken. Seriously disturbed patients with alcoholic hallucinosis will require psychiatric care, preferably in a general hospital setting.

It is important to note that these most dramatic of alcohol-related syndromes may be associated with underlying medical problems. Surveys of alcoholics referred to psychiatric in- and outpatient departments reveal that approximately three-quarters have a significant medical problem requiring investigation, assessment, and treatment. In addition, because of the serious consequences of the failure to prevent Wernicke–Korsakoff syndrome, it is routine practice to administer a parenteral

vitamin preparation, rich in thiamine (such as Parentrovite ®) to all such patients.

NUTRITIONAL DEFICIENCY SYNDROMES

Although the application of multiple biochemical and haematological tests to alcohol misusers will show evidence of deficiency of one or more nutrients in a significant number of patients (25–50 per cent), it is only in a small proportion that this is clinically and pathologically significant. None is more important, however, than the Wernicke–Korsakoff syndrome. The syndrome may be subdivided into the neurological disorder, Wernicke's disease, and the psychiatric, Korsakoff syndrome. Although one or other clinical pictures may predominate, there is frequently considerable overlap and progression between these two disorders. Both have a common pathology, with severe neuronal loss in the mamillary bodies, with associated lesions in and around the aqueduct and fourth ventricle. Lesions of the vermis and anterior cerebellar lobules occur frequently.

The biochemical basis of the pathology has been shown to be due to thiamine deficiency. Wernicke's disease patients display the triad of ophthalmoplegia, most commonly nystagmus and impaired ocular abduction; ataxia most predominantly of cerebellar type; and a confusional state. The latter predominates in the Korsakoff syndrome, and is characterized by both behavioural and mental function disorder. The patient shows apathy for mental and physical activity, and impaired awareness and concentration with deranged perceptual functions. Some patients show a clinical picture complicated by features of withdrawal syndrome. The classical Korsakov amnesic syndrome, which may persist after vitamin replacement and prolonged abstinence, comprises severe antegrade and retrograde amnesia with confabulation and lack of insight, and is a serious condition, with a poor long-term prognosis.

The clinical findings may be complex or dominated by a single clinical feature. Clinical evidence of vitamin deficiency (for example, oral or labial inflammation), cardiovascular disorder (such as hypotension), high output cardiac failure (for example, beri beri), and peripheral neuropathy may assist in alerting one to the diagnosis. Diagnosis is confirmed by assays of the thiamine-dependent erythrocyte enzyme, transketolase, where enzyme activity is often reduced to half normal values. More discriminatory is the observation that enzyme activity can be restored by prior incubation of the red cell homogenate with thiamine pyrophosphate. The earlier test in which an abnormal rise in venous pyruvate following a glucose load is now considered obsolete. It is important not to delay treatment with thiamine, both oral and parenteral, while waiting for the results of the biochemical investigations.

Alcoholic cerebellar degeneration

This is an important, but rare, complication of chronic alcohol abuse, caused mainly by prolonged spirit drinking accompanied by a poor nutritional intake. There is gross ataxia, particularly of the lower limbs, due to atrophy of the anterosuperior lobules and vermis of the cerebellum. Histopathologically, there is Purkinje cell loss. Modern imaging techniques, particularly magnetic resonance imaging (MRI), may demonstrate cerebellar atrophy. The syndrome is probably part of the clinical spectrum of the Wernicke–Korsakoff syndrome and may, at least at the early stages, before the degeneration is apparent macroscopically, respond well to thiamine treatment.

Peripheral neuropathy

This is a common finding in alcohol abusers, and ranges from purely subjective symptoms of paraesthesia to a severe distal combined sensorimotor neuropathy. The neuropathy is due to a variable combination of vitamin deficiency and chronic alcohol toxicity. The lower limbs are usually involved more severely and more frequently than the upper limbs: cranial nerves are rarely involved. Loss of tendon reflexes occurs in approximately half the patients. Foot and wrist drop, distal muscle weakness and wasting, and positive signs on detailed sensory testing may occur. It is useful to distinguish the neuropathy with secondary muscle wasting from the common proximal muscle metabolic myopathy described in Section 25. This latter does not have a nutritional or neuropathic component to its pathogenesis. The neuropathy may be confirmed and assessed quantitatively by neurophysiological studies.

Assessment of vitamin deficiency by erythrocyte enzyme assays, viz. transketolase (thiamine), aspartate aminotransferase (pyridoxine), and glutathione reductase (riboflavin), will usually show a multiple deficiency, particularly if the more sensitive *in vitro* activation studies are performed.

Treatment by immediate parenteral vitamin supplements and a successful abstinence programme with physical rehabilitation will usually lead to considerable, if not complete, recovery, but this may take many months. Note also that alcohol misusers are candidates for other forms of neuropathy (for example, carcinomatous, viral, traumatic, and vascular nerve damage).

Pellagra

Pellagra is an unusual complication of alcohol misuse with a quite inadequate vitamin intake, particularly of niacin and of trytophan-containing proteins. The disorder is not uncommon in the Third World, where combined vitamin and protein deficiency in raw-spirit drinkers occurs. Mental symptoms with cognitive and mood impairment (depression), chronic diarrhoea (dysentery), pigmented inflammatory skin lesions on sun-exposed areas (dermatitis), and other nutritionally related symptomatology are the typical findings. Diagnosis is supported by assays of urinary nicotinic acid and its metabolites and demonstration of amino acid deficiencies, most notably tryptophan. Treatment is by multiple vitamin replacement, principally oral nicotinic acid or, if necessary, parenteral nicotinamide, in addition to a high-protein diet, particularly of animal-derived proteins.

Alcohol–tobacco amblyopia

This is a rare, but important, complication of alcohol misuse, combined with nutritional deficiencies, including vitamin B_{12}. It is most likely a complication of optic neuritis with impaired visual acuity and visual field defects, and usually improves with multiple vitamin therapy.

MISCELLANEOUS DISORDERS

Cerebral dementia

This is a frequent finding in chronic alcohol abusers: this may be only discernible on detailed psychological testing, or may progress to severe dementia with dilated ventricles and marked cortical atrophy, most strikingly demonstrated by computed tomography (CT) and MRI scanning. It is claimed that alcohol abuse is one of the most common causes of pre-senile dementia. The pathogenic mechanism appears to be an alcohol-mediated neuronal loss. Interestingly, abstinence can be accompanied by both cognitive and neuroradiographic improvement.

Central pontine myelinolysis

This is a rare, but often fatal, disorder associated with alcohol misuse, in which there is extensive demyelination of the pons. The patient has quadriplegia with psuedobulbar palsy and often other features of CNS damage. The lesions may be demonstrated strikingly by MRI scanning. The pathogenic mechanism is unclear, but several cases have been reported in patients with hyponatraemia, particularly with rapid changes in electrolyte levels.

Marchiafava–Bignami syndrome

This is due to alcohol-associated demyelination of the corpus callosum, and occurs in adult male alcoholics with a varied clinical picture indicating multiple cortical dysfunction. Neuroradiographic imaging can demonstrate the lesions, which are often associated with other features of alcohol-related CNS damage.

Fetal alcohol syndrome

This is considered to be the commonest single cause of mental handicap. Maternal alcohol misuse within the first 4 weeks of conception is associated with craniofacial abnormalities, including micro-ophthalmia, elongated mid-face, long upper lip with a poorly developed philtrum, and CNS involvement with intellectual impairment and development delay. Alcohol misuse at other stages of pregnancy may be accompanied by intellectual deficit, auditory and visual deficits, specific learning difficulties, and hyperkinetic syndromes in infancy. Maternal alcohol misuse can also be associated with a variety of cardiovascular, hepatic and musculoskeletal defects in the infant. The pathogenic mechanism is unclear and several hypotheses have been proposed, apart from ethanol itself. These include acetaldehyde formed in the placenta, protein–calorie malnutrition, associated vitamin and zinc deficiency, and a synergism, with heavy tobacco usuage. Clearly, prevention is a major public-health challenge.

REFERENCES

Charness, M.E., Simon, R.P., and Greenberg, D.A. (1989). Ethanol and the nervous system. *New England Journal of Medicine* **321**, 442–54.

Higgins, E.M., and du Vivier, A.W.P. (1992). Alcohol and the skin. *Alcohol and Alcoholism* **27**, 595–602.

Ishak, K.G., Zimmerman, M.J., and Ray, M.B. (1991). *Alcoholism—Clinical and Experimental Research* **15**, 45–66. Alcoholic liver disease: pathologic, pathogenetic and clinical aspects. **15**, 45–66.

Laitinen, K., and Valimaki, M. (1991). Alcohol and bone. *Calcified Tissue Research* **49**, (Suppl.), 570–3.

Martin, F., Ward, K., Slavin, G., Levi, J., and Peters, T.J. (1985). Alcoholic skeletal myopathy, a clinical and pathological study. *Quarterly Journal of Medicine* **218**, 233–51.

Peters, T.J., and Edwards, G. (ed.) (1994). Alcohol misuse. *British Medical Bulletin* **50**, No. 1.

28.2.3(b) Physical complications of drug abuse

D. A. HAWKINS

Drug users have always suffered considerable morbidity with, in particular, increased susceptibility to various infections such as subcutaneous abscesses, cellulitis, pneumonia, septicaemia, and endocarditis. More recently, the advent of the human immunodeficiency virus (HIV) epidemic has focused attention on the viral infections that are most efficiently transmitted by contaminated injecting equipment. These include the retroviruses HIV-1, HIV-2, HTLV-1, HTLV-2, and also the hepatitis viruses B, C, and D. In addition, the importance of sexual transmission of these viruses in drug users and their partners must not be forgotten; although the efficiency of this mode of transmission varies markedly among the different viruses.

Immunosuppression due to HIV infection will, of course, aggravate the severity of many of the infective complications of drug use. Thus, various studies have shown increased morbidity and mortality in HIV-seropositive users with, for example, endocarditis, compared to an HIV-seronegative comparison group.

While considering the complications below, remember that one of the aims of drug treatment services is to promote a more health-conscious drug-using population. Clearly, it may be preferable for an individual to become drug free, but this may not be immediately achievable, or sustainable, and more modest goals such as non-injecting drug use or the use only of sterile injecting equipment can be just as important. Access to medical care should be promoted as this may be the stimulus to a favourable change in behaviour.

Technique-specific hazards

Technique-specific hazards are complications due to the mode of drug administration. Those associated with injecting are the most serious and are often related to poor sterile and injecting technique. However, complications may also occur, despite careful aseptic precautions, from normal skin flora or contamination of the supplied drug. Guidelines have been issued for cleaning injecting equipment, should sterile 'works' not be available. However, no technique (other than perhaps autoclaving) is guaranteed to be effective against all possible pathogens, and so this should just be considered a 'harm-reduction' not a 'harm-elimination' procedure.

Infections

SOFT TISSUES

Commensal skin flora such as *Staphylococcus aureus* and *Streptococcus pyogenes* may infect an injection site, leading, quite commonly, to cellulitis and thrombophlebitis. Management may require antibiotic therapy, with incision and drainage if localized abscess formation develops. Larger abscesses may lead to extensive skin ulceration requiring debridement and, possibly at a later stage, skin grafting. Occasionally, abscess involvement of muscle can lead to the development of the serious complications of necrotizing fasciitis and myositis.

SEPTICAEMIA

It is likely that bacteraemia commonly accompanies injecting episodes but this is usually contained by the immune system. However septicaemia may develop and at times lead to endocarditis. Thus any users with a pyrexia of unknown origin should be suspected of a septicaemic illness. Appropriate cultures should be performed prior to therapy with parenteral broad-spectrum antibiotics. Systemic fungal (particularly candidal) infection may occur, either due to contaminated heroin or to the lemon juice used to dissolve the drug. Candidal ophthalmitis is a serious complication and early systemic antifungal therapy, such as amphotericin, should be instituted if this is suspected.

It has been postulated, with some laboratory support, that many of the drugs used by addicts may suppress the immune system, although hard clinical evidence for this is lacking. Other factors including nutrition, mode of administration, and adulteration of drugs are likely to be important. Thus, in the specific case of HIV-positive drug users the continued injecting of street drugs appears to lead to more rapid decline in the immune system and thus, progression to AIDS. This acceleration is not evident in drug users on methadone substitution and may, in part, be related to a more chaotic lifestyle and poor diet.

ENDOCARDITIS

It has been estimated that about 2 per cent of injecting drug users per year develop infected heart valves. Drug users with endocarditis are more likely to be younger, have acute disease, previously normal cardiac valves, and tricuspid valve involvement than other groups. HIV-positive users, may have an even wider variety of, often multiple, infecting organisms. The commonest organism is *Staphylococcus aureus* which is found in about two-thirds of cases. *Streptococcus viridans*, accounts for another 20 per cent and there is an important contribution from Gram-negative bacilli, such as *Pseudomonas* species, and various fungi. Patients usually present with a brief illness, fever, a varying heart murmur, and a history of infection elsewhere. Tricuspid involvement with shedding of emboli into the pulmonary circulation may, in addition, lead to dyspnoea, cough, haemoptysis, and pleuritic chest pain.

Mortality is generally low (less than 5 per cent) with early identification of the causative organism(s) and appropriate therapy. However, surgical replacement of valves is sometime necessary, particularly when there is candidal or Pseudomonas infection. Prognosis is also poorer with left-sided involvement and after recurrent attacks due to continued injecting.

HEPATITIS

There are many causes of hepatitis in injecting drug users, but the most important are the hepatotropic viruses B, D, and C. There may be no history as some infections with these agents are mild or asymptomatic. Hepatitis may also be a feature of other systemic viral infections, such as Epstein–Barr virus and cytomegalovirus, and mild hepatitis has recently been shown to occur in some patients with acute HIV-1 seroconversion illnesses.

Worldwide seroprevalence studies for markers of hepatitis B infection show that some 50 to 80 per cent of injecting drug users have been exposed. Chronic carriers make up about 5 to 10 per cent, and further transmission, both sexually and parenterally, is a common event as the virus is often present in very high copy number in blood and other body fluids. Immunosuppression due to HIV increases the proportion of chronic carriers. In view of the long-term sequelae with chronic liver disease, cirrhosis, and liver cell carcinoma, immunization should be offered to all susceptible drug users. An active immunization programme would also reduce the transmission of the hepatitis delta virus (HDV) as this is a defective RNA virus which requires the presence of hepatitis B to replicate. It may, thus, coinfect or superinfect carriers of hepatitis B virus, and often will cause an exacerbation of the hepatitis.

The diagnosis of hepatitis C virus (HCV) infection has recently been facilitated by the development of a number of assays including antibodies to recombinantly expressed HCV antigens and detection of HCV RNA in serum by the polymerase chain reaction. Application of these tests to drug-using populations worldwide has shown a consistent, remarkably high, seroprevalence level. This high seroprevalence may occur in areas where HIV prevalence is low, possibly reflecting either an earlier presence, but perhaps, also, more ready transmission of HCV, by a significant level of persistent viraemia. Thus, in Glasgow, 85 per cent of injecting drug users have markers of HCV infection, whereas under 2 per cent are HIV-1 seropositive. Sexual transmission to a non-injecting partner is said to be low, but this may be higher if coexistent infection with HIV is present (however published studies are discordant). HCV is important as a substantial proportion, possibly over 50 per cent of carriers will go on to develop chronic liver disease, including hepatocellular carcinoma, although this may take several decades. Treatments with interferon and ribovarin are under investigation.

PULMONARY

Inhalation of drugs maybe associated with acute bronchospasm, but the most common lung problem in drug users is bacterial pneumonia. This is attributable to heavy cigarette-smoking and, in the more chaotic users, general debilitation associated with the lifestyle. Pulmonary tuberculosis is also more common (although in the United States this risk is boosted by the ethnic origin of many of the drug users). Recurrent bacterial pneumonia and pulmonary tuberculosis contribute significantly to HIV morbidity and mortality in HIV-positive users and in January 1993 were classified as AIDS diagnoses by the Communicable Disease Center (CDC) in Atlanta.

A pneumothorax may result from inadvertent penetration of the lung when injecting into neck veins. Other uncommon complications may be related to inert particulate matter, such as talc, reaching the vascular bed and leading to pulmonary hypertension or granulomatosis.

ORTHOPAEDIC

Septic arthritis most commonly results from septicaemia spread, but may also occur from direct infection or extension from an adjacent abscess.

Osteomyelitis may arise in a similar way, but is usually caused by emboli from a distant infected focus, common sites of involvement being the thoracic and lumbar vertebrae.

RENAL

Glomerulonephritis developing in long-term injectors is probably related to infective causes, such as staphylococcal and other bacterial infections or chronic hepatitis B infection. Recently, hepatitis C has been found to be associated with cryoglobulinaemia and membranoproliferative glomerulonephritis.

Other complications of injection

VASCULAR

Long-standing injecting drug users frequently have problems with venous access, and may become quite ingenious in their search for veins. Repeated episodes of lymphangitis often associated with 'skin popping' may cause lymphatic obstruction. The resultant chronic lymphoedema is characteristically seen on the back of the hand, and this may persist long after the cessation of drug use.

Injecting into the femoral vein runs the risk of deep venous thrombosis with possible serious sequelae of pulmonary emboli or venous gangrene. Anticoagulation should be instituted. In addition, local decompression of an expanding abscess may be required if contributing to the venous occlusion.

Arterial occlusion may occur with inadvertent arterial injection. The latter may damage the vessel wall at the needle entry point, or there may be vasospasm locally, due to irritant materials, or peripheral embolism of injected particular matter. Additional arterial problems may be infected false aneurysms, which are infected haematomas at the site of needle puncture. Sometimes infected aneurysms develop at a distance from the injection site, when they are termed mycotic aneurysms. Emergency surgical extirpation of a blockage may be required. However, surgical management may be initially expectant in cases of vasospasm or peripheral embolism using heparin, low molecular weight dextran infusions, or sympathetic nerve blockade. The intense pain of ischaemic lesions is difficult to control in dependent drug users. Appropriate pain relief is best discussed jointly by medical and surgical teams and the substance misuse service.

Substance-specific complications

It can be seen from the above section that mode of administration of a drug, particularly injecting, is often the major factor in causing morbidity. Clearly, the nature of the injected material contributes to a variable extent. This may relate to the presence of adulterants used to cut the drug, or the use of crushed tablets, or to processing of gel capsules (such as temazepam) which are not supposed to be injected.

The following paragraphs deal with the complications that are mainly related to the specific substances; these may be due to dose-related toxicity or other adverse reactions.

OPIATE OVERDOSE

Opiate overdose may be deliberate or may occur when using a drug of unexpected purity. In addition, accidental overdose is often associated with a period of abstinence, and thus reduced tolerance. Such a potentially dangerous situation often arises when ex-drug-using prisoners are released from custody. Prisoners should be specifically advised about this as part of their prison education and rehabilitation programmes.

Opiates may be the cause of coma, when there are signs of respiratory depression and pin-point pupils. If suspected, the specific opiate antagonist naloxone (0.4–2.0 mg) should be administered intravenously, and

subsequent reversal may be quite dramatic. However, caution must be exercised as sometimes patients relapse due to the longer duration of action of the self-administered agonist drugs, such as methadone. Observation should thus be continued for a period of at least 24 h.

Poor response suggests the use of other additional CNS depressant drugs, and patients should be supported in intensive care as long as necessary.

STIMULANTS (AMPHETAMINES, ECSTASY, AND COCAINE)

Ecstasy is the popular name for 3,4, -methylene-dideoxymethamphetamine, a synthetic amphetamine derivative. It has a number of similar side-effects, including anorexia, tachycardia, paranoia, irritability, depression, and bruxism (grinding of teeth). However, severe reactions are unpredictable and appear to be precipitated by concurrent physical exertion. Thus its use as a 'dance' or 'rave' drug has led to a number of deaths as well as convulsions, collapse, hyperpyrexia, disseminated intravascular coagulation, rhabdomyolysis, and acute renal failure. The risk of hyperthermia is well recognized by drug agencies, and appropriate advice to those who use the drug is to wear loose clothing, to drink liquids to facilitate thermoregulation, and to stop dancing when feeling exhausted. Indeed, some clubs provide 'chill-out' rooms with seating and non-alcoholic liquids to help cooling.

Management is urgent for the acutely ill and includes control of convulsions, measurement of core temperature, rapid rehydration, and acute cooling measures.

The catalogue of complications associated with cocaine use is extensive and these have been well documented in American studies of patients attending emergency rooms. They include myocardial infarction, cardiac arrythmias, hypertension, cerebrovascular accidents, seizures, and hyperthermia. Other medical complications of cocaine depend in part of the mode of administration. Thus, inhalation of freebase 'crack cocaine' may cause pulmonary damage, and there is the well-known association of mucosal damage and even perforation with intranasal administration.

SEDATIVES

Most habitual users of benzodiazepines and barbiturates present problems with management of intoxication or withdrawal. These should be dealt with according to standard protocols. Most patients survive overdosage with supportive measures only.

VOLATILE SUBSTANCES

These include butane gas (lighter fluid, aerosols), solvents, toluene, dry-cleaning fluid, typewriter correction fluid, glues, and fire extinguisher contents. Users are often children, and the greatest risk is of a sudden death associated with cardiac arrhythmias during an episode of sniffing. Other dangers are due to asphyxia when using a plastic bag over the face, inhalation of vomit, or fatal accidents when intoxicated. Many agents are highly flammable and severe burning injuries occur.

ALCOHOL

See Chapter 28.2.3(a) for discussion.

Other behavioural aspects that may lead to physical harm

The lifestyle associated with the acquisition of illicit drugs understandably increases the risk of trauma and contact with the criminal justice system. Sexual activity may be disinhibited with almost any drug, and less attention paid to safer sex and the risk of HIV, hepatitis, and other more traditional sexually transmitted infections. Sex may be exchanged directly or indirectly for drugs. Data from the United States suggest that female crack cocaine users run a particularly high risk of being HIV seropositive. In order to minimize the risks of these additional sources of infection-related morbidity, it is important for those looking after drug users to maintain close links with family planning services and sexually transmitted disease clinics. Furthermore, obstetric and neonatal morbidity is raised in drug users, and early attendance at antenatal clinics should be encouraged to allow the stabilization of drug use.

Conclusions

The recent change in the CDC classification in America which will soon be followed in Europe, will allow the extent of morbidity and mortality associated with HIV infection in drug users to be recorded more clearly. The likelihood of considerable heterosexual spread of HIV in many Western countries is uncertain, but, clearly, heterosexual drug users are an important contributory factor to the equation and action on the points made above may reduce the risk.

The HIV epidemic has increased attention given to the physical complications of drug use. These risks must continue to be well publicised in the hope of reducing initiation to the more harmful practices. However, drug misuse will continue, and so education about reduction of risks is likely to be the most effective policy.

REFERENCES

Banks, A. and Waller, T.A. (1988). *Drug misuse: a practical handbook for GPs*. Blackwell Scientific Publication, Oxford.
Barr, L.C. (1988). The surgical complications of drug abuse. *Surgery* **60**, 1420–4.
Boag, F., *et al.* (1992). Abnormalities of liver function during HIV seroconversion illness. *International Journal of STD and AIDS*, **3**, 46–8.
Brettle, R., Farrell, M., and Strang, J. (1990). The clinical manifestations of HIV in drug users. In *AIDS and drug misuse*, (ed. J. Strang and G. Stimson). Routledge, London.
Buehler, J.W. and Ward, J.W. (1993). A new definition for AIDS Surveillance. *Annals of Internal Medicine*, **118**, 390–2.
Cregler, L. and Mark, H. (1986). Medical complications of cocaine abuse. *New England Journal of Medicine* **315**, 1495–500.
Farrell, M. (1991). Physical Complications of Drug Misuse. In *International Handbook of Addiction Behaviour*. (ed. I. Glass), Routledge, London.
Frieden, T.R., *et al.* (1993). The emergence of drug-resistant tuberculosis in New York City. *New England Journal of Medicine* **328**, 521–6.
Henry, J.A. (1992). Ecstasy and the dance of death. *British Medical Journal* **305**, 5–6.
Johnson, J.R., *et al.* (1993). Membranoproliferative glomerulonephritis associated with hepatitis C virus infection. *New England Journal of Medicine*. **328**, 465–70.
UK Health Departments. (1991). *Drug Misuse and Dependence Guidelines on Clinical Management*. HMSO, London.

28.3 Problems and crises for the clinician

28.3.1 Complications of drug use, particularly injecting drug use

R.P. BRETTLE

INTRODUCTION

The use of recreational drugs incurs a number of complications which include the excessive or withdrawal effects of the drugs themselves as well as a number of associated medical conditions. The medical conditions associated with injection drug use (IDU) vary from, for instance, asymptomatic abnormalities of pulmonary function tests, to life-threatening infections or immunological problems such as polyarteritis nodosa. IDU-related human immunodeficiency virus (HIV) injection has not only widened the spectrum of disease in drug users but has also increased the frequency of some existing conditions.

Drug use, and IDU in particular, is not well quantified because in most countries it is an illegal activity. In Edinburgh during 1983–84 the prevalence of opiate-related IDU was estimated at 0.6 per cent for those between the ages of 15 and 35. Before HIV, perhaps up to 50 per cent of narcotic-related deaths were the result of drug excess, while nearly 60 per cent of admissions to hospitals were related to infection, one-third as a consequence of acute viral hepatitis. Health service workload related to IDU is considerable; around 1 per cent of admissions to hospital, twice the usual general practice consultation rate (7/year versus 3.25/year) and 0.1 to 0.6 per cent of consultations at accident and emergency facilities (60 per cent related to the effects of drugs, 8 per cent to trauma, 10 per cent to other medical conditions, and 21 per cent to infections, although less than 1 per cent were as a consequence of serious infection).

Non-infection-related complications of IDU

The medical complications of IDU which are not related to infection are summarized in Table 1.

FREQUENCY

As with IDU itself, quantification of the complications of IDU is difficult and may well be underestimated, because the drug use is often not declared. A pre-HIV survey of admissions in the 1970s to a specialized medical inpatient unit of a New York Hospital devoted to drug addiction revealed that although nearly 60 per cent of admissions were due to infection, 21 per cent were for general medical conditions: diabetes, 7.5 per cent; pulmonary disease, 6 per cent; cardiovascular disease, 4 per cent; and gastrointestinal disease, 3.5 per cent. The pulmonary problems noted were pulmonary fibrosis (obstructive or restrictive), carcinoma of the lung, chronic bronchitis, pleural effusion, pulmonary emboli, and bronchial asthma. Heavy cigarette smoking was regarded as a probable cause of many of the problems, although the injection of inert material was also thought to be a contributing cause of the pulmonary fibrosis. The cardiovascular problems included congestive heart failure, cardiomyopathy, and viral pericarditis. The gastrointestinal disorders included ulcers, gastritis, small bowel dysfunction, and cirrhosis.

The survey of narcotic-related deaths in New York in the 1950s that found nearly 50 per cent of the deaths were related to drug excess, also noted that 20 per cent were due to infections and 18 per cent to medical conditions (including 7 per cent because of respiratory problems other than pulmonary oedema and drug overdose). A few of the lungs studied contained microscopic granulomas of the foreign-body type, which were thought to have occurred because of a reaction to injected foreign particulate matter which adulterates 'street heroin'. Particles of cotton fibres

only a small quantity should be given and the patient referred either to their general practitioner or to the relevant specialist out-patient clinic for fuller assessment.

MISCELLANEOUS DRUG ABUSE

A proportion of patients abuse other psychoactive drugs, not usually associated with addiction. These include anticonvulsants and, in particular, the antiparkinsonian drugs used to counter the side-effects of neuroleptic drugs. The patient may be known to have a history of psychosis, but the abuse of these drugs for their stimulant properties often exacerbates the underlying mental illness. Hence even if a diagnosis of mental illness is known, it is undesirable to replace 'lost' antiparkinsonian drugs unless there are clear signs of untreated side-effects.

Engagement in treatment

Many drug abusers have no contact with health or other caring agencies unless an emergency problem arises. Ambivalence, ignorance of available facilities, and the often secret nature of drug-abuse problems contribute to this. There is often great fear associated with approaching statutory services, and drug-abusing parents may believe their children will be removed or placed on the Social Services Child Protection Register.

Staff in the accident and emergency department may therefore become a vital link between drug abusers and services, encouraging addicts to seek treatment for their dependence over and above the problem that has precipitated hospital attendance. To facilitate the referral process, staff need to have ready access to, and knowledge of, local advice and treatment agencies. Some regional drug problem teams publish comprehensive directories of services within their region, and national directories are also available. If the accident and emergency department is in a hospital with a drug unit on site, it is mutually beneficial to establish liaison and referral procedures.

Data collection and statutory requirements

The strategic response to drug-abuse problems depends on information and knowledge of their scale and nature, both locally and nationally. The situation is never static and inevitably data are inaccurate and patchy. Health services as a whole have a role in data gathering but only addiction to certain drugs was centrally recorded via the Home Office Addicts Index, and then only if the drug user was seen by a doctor. It is essential that accident and emergency department doctors comply with the statutory notification regulations, but in addition, regional health authorities have now established substance abuse databases. For these, information is collected on anonymous forms, covering any drug-abuse problem, and is not restricted to addiction to the notifiable drugs. The extent to which regional database forms are in operation in accident and emergency departments may vary between Health Regions, but for convenience combined substance use regional database and Home Office Notification Forms are now in use.

With the enlarging scope of recreational and experimental drug use, and the development of 'designer drugs', the accident and emergency department is in the front line of coping with the adverse effects, and there may be few sources of detailed knowledge of the pharmacological and physiological actions of these new drugs. Good record-keeping will assist in increasing knowledge, and at all times a urine sample should be collected for toxicological analysis for any attender who is suspected of having a drug-abuse problem. Although the result of analysis is not likely to be immediately available for the accident and emergency department doctor, it can prove extremely useful to others who may be involved in the follow-up or continuing care of the patient.

REFERENCES

Bedi, A.R. (1987). Alcoholism, drug abuse and other psychiatric disorders. In *Alcohol and drug abuse,* (ed. R.E. Harrington, G.R. Jacobson, and D.S. Benzer), pp. 346–84. Warren H. Green Inc., St. Louis, Missouri.

Brettle, R., Farrell, M., and Strang, J. (1990). Clinical features of HIV infection and AIDS in drug takers. In *AIDS and drug misuse: the challenge for policy and practice in the 1990s,* (ed. J. Strang and G.V. Stimson). Routledge, London.

Drug misuse and dependence. Guidelines on clinical management (1991). HMSO, London.

Ghodse, A.H. (1976). Drug problems dealt with by 62 London casualty departments. *British Journal of Preventative and Social Medicine* **30,** 251–6.

Ghodse, A.H. (1977). Casualty departments and the monitoring of drug dependence. *British Medical Journal* **1**, 1381–2.

Ghodse, A.H. (1978). The attitudes of casualty staff and ambulance personnel towards patients who take drug overdoses. *Social Science and Medicine* **12,** (5a), 241–6.

Ghodse, A.H. (1989). *Drugs and addictive behaviour: guide to treatment.* Blackwell Scientific Publications, Oxford.

Ghodse, A.H., Sheehan, M., Stevens, B., Taylor, C., and Edwards, G. (1978). Mortality among drug addicts in Greater London. *British Medical Journal* **2**, 1742–4.

Ghodse, A.H., Stapleton, J., Edwards, G., and Edeh, J. (1987). Monitoring changing patterns of drug dependence in Accident and Emergency Departments. *Drug and Alcohol Dependence* **19**, 265–9.

Glass, I.B. and Marshall, J. (1991). Alcohol and mental illness: Cause or effect. In *Addiction behaviour handbook* (ed. I.B. Glass), pp. 152–62. Routledge, London.

Kessel, N. and Grossman, G. (1961). Suicide in alcoholics. *British Medical Journal,* **2**, 1671–2.

Maxwell, D. (1990). Medical complications of substance abuse. In *Substance abuse and dependence,* (ed. A.H. Ghodse and D. Maxwell), pp. 176–203. Macmillan Press, London.

28.3.6 The pregnant drug abuser

C. GERADA

Extent of the problem

The past two decades have seen a rise in the number of women who abuse illicit drugs such as heroin and cocaine. At present one-third of all notified addicts are women, 80 per cent of whom are within their childbearing years. While general ill-health, low weight, and decreased libido act as inhibitors of fertility, the drugs themselves do not. The number of drug users who become pregnant is unknown as many go completely undetected through the antenatal services. Nevertheless, an increasing number of women who abuse drugs are presenting for care, sadly often late in their pregnancy or in labour.

The nature of the danger

The effects on drugs on both mother and fetus can be considered to be directly or indirectly related to the drug ingested.

DRUG DEPENDENT

The properties (pharmacokinetics) of the drug

All drugs are able to cross the placenta to some extent. Factors such as lipid solubility, low molecular weight, and ability to bind to certain plasma proteins enhance this transfer.

Teratogenicity

The evidence that drugs such as opiates, LSD (lysergic acid diethylamine 25), amphetamine, and benzodiazepines produce an increase in congenital malformations is conflicting and confusing, not least because users of illicit drugs seldom can be certain of the drug actually ingested. An increase in genitourinary and neural defects have been reported to be more frequent in babies of cocaine-using mothers.

DRUG INDEPENDENT

Route and pattern of drug use

Drugs taken by an intravenous or intramuscular route cross the placenta more easily than drugs taken orally. Drugs taken by the oral route may undergo significant first-pass metabolism in the liver, reducing their ability to cross the placenta. Intravenous drug use also places the mother and child at increased risk through complications related to the injecting and the sharing of injecting equipment.

Variable absorption through the nasal mucosa following inhalation ('chasing the dragon') may reduce levels reaching the fetal circulation and hence cause less damage to its development, unless the quantity taken is correspondingly increased.

Gestation of pregnancy

The fetus is most susceptible to structural damage early in development. Drugs taken in the later stages of pregnancy (days 55–term) are more likely to affect growth or cause neonatal addiction and subsequent withdrawal. Drugs taken during labour can also affect the infant. Diazepam taken by the mother during labour can still be detected in the blood of the newborn 10 to 18 days after delivery. Cocaine may be excreted by the newborn for 5 days and methadone may persist for a week of more.

Maternal well-being

Complications of drug abuse are confounded by social adversity such as homelessness and poverty. General neglect and late presentation for health care, poor nutrition, intercurrent infections, cigarette smoking, complications due to dirty and shared needles, together with erratic and chaotic life-styles, predispose drug users to a wide variety of health problems and increases the likelihood of complications of pregnancy. Encouraging women into treatment can reduce some of these complications.

Complications of drug use

(See Table 1.)

OBSTETRIC AND MEDICAL COMPLICATIONS

Drug-abusing women are at higher risk of obstetric, medical, and fetal complications, thereby increasing perinatal morbidity and mortality. Cocaine use in pregnancy is particularly hazardous. Cocaine acts as a vasoconstrictor, which decreases the blood flow to the placenta and increases uterine contractibility. The increased rate of spontaneous abortion, abruptio placentas, and premature labour found in cocaine-using pregnant women is consistent with the pharmacological actions of cocaine. Onset of labour can occur after a single intravenous injection of cocaine.

FETAL AND INFANT COMPLICATIONS

General

The most common fetal complications are those of prematurity and intrauterine growth retardation. Studies in the United Kingdom have reported prematurity rates of between 20 and 33 per cent. Sudden intrauterine withdrawal from heroin can result in premature delivery or intra-

Table 1 *Complications of long-term drug use*

Obstetric complications
    Abruptio placentas
    Amnionitis
    Eclampsia
    Placental insufficiency
    Postpartum haemorrhage
    Premature labour
Medical complications
    Anaemia
    Chronic bronchitis (especially if the drug is inhaled)
    Malnutrition
    Sexually transmitted diseases
    Urinary tract infections
Fetal complications
    HIV/AIDS
    Intrauterine addition
    Intrauterine growth retardation
    Neonatal addiction and withdrawal
    Neonatal death
    Prematurity
    Still birth

uterine death. Opiates also have a direct effect on intrauterine growth, giving rise to small-for-dates babies even when factors such as infrequent antenatal care and smoking are controlled for. Cerebral infarction, possibly related to excessive vasoconstriction, occurs with increased frequency in babies born to cocaine-abusing mothers.

Neonatal dependence and withdrawal

Neonates regularly exposed to drugs *in utero* may become physically dependent. The infant may suffer physical withdrawal symptoms if the drug is suddenly withdrawn. The severity of the abstinence (withdrawal) syndrome will be determined by the specific drug/s involved, dosage used, timing of the dose before delivery, and the maturity of the infant. Before birth withdrawal is characterized by an increase in fetal movements, which women report as occurring approximately 30 min to 1 h before they feel any withdrawal symptoms themselves. After delivery the infant may undergo a withdrawal reaction (usually within 24–48 h). The infant may be jittery and irritable. Other symptoms include sneezing, feeding disorders, vomiting, and diarrhoea. Severe withdrawal can lead to death through generalized seizures or electrolyte imbalance. The symptoms, in varying degrees, can persist (especially in babies born to crack/cocaine-using mothers) for up to 10 weeks.

Withdrawal reactions are more idiosyncratic in infants born to heroin users.

Neonatal transmission of HIV

The majority of women infected with human immunodeficiency virus (HIV) in the United States are intravenous drug users, with women making up about 10 per cent of currently known cases of acquired immunodeficiency syndrome (AIDS). Paediatric HIV infection is acquired largely from the mother, either *in utero* or at birth; the relative risk of vertical transmission has been estimated to be between 15 and 40 per cent.

Long-term effects

The long-term effects on infant development of drug abuse during pregnancy are beyond the scope of this chapter. Nevertheless, differences in growth, neurobehavioural development, and in mental and motor development have been found in the infants born to heroin- and cocaine-using mothers.

Management of the pregnant drug user

GENERAL AIMS

The general principles of treatment are to:

(1) identify possible drug-using women;
(2) provide antenatal and health care;
(3) advise reducing all illicit drugs, replacing with a prescribed substitute if available (see below);
(4) coordinate management with a multidisciplinary team.

It should now be routine practice to ask women presenting for antenatal care about illicit and prescribed drug use.

The overall goals of treatment are regular attendance for antenatal care, safe delivery of the infant, and the withdrawal of mother and child off drugs. Given the high relapse rate of addiction, the first goal is not always possible. Keeping the women in contact via low-dose prescribing may be a more realistic option as it decreases additional illicit drug use, increases stability, and enables closer monitoring of the pregnancy. Equally, women enrolled in treatment programmes usually have better antenatal care, less anaemia, and better general health, even if still using illicit drugs.

HIV

There is no evidence that infection with HIV *per se* affects the outcome of the pregnancy, although complications such as premature labour are more likely if the woman has developed AIDS. Continued intravenous drug use increases these complications significantly, hence further evidence that attracting women into treatment and helping to reduce illicit drug use can play a major part in outcome.

MANAGEMENT OF DEPENDENCE (SEE TABLE 2.)

Opiates

Methadone mixture BNF 1 mg/ml is the substitute drug of choice for opiate users. It is relatively long acting, and herefore minimizes the likelihood of peaks and troughs in the circulation. Methadone also reduces craving and withdrawal, and hence should reduce illicit drug use. It is also unlikely to be injected.

An initial dose, ranging between 20 and 40 mg, should be given depending on the patient's drug history, in particular length of habit and claimed daily use of heroin. Doses can be adjusted daily, depending on reported maternal withdrawal symptoms and signs. After stabilization, a reducing programme should be devised, usually involving 2.5 to 5 mg methadone reductions per week. Reduction can occur at any time, but ideally should be in the second trimester (14–28 weeks). If reduction is carried out in the first trimester a spontaneous abortion may erroneously be attributed to the reduction. If the woman presents after 30 weeks of pregnancy it may be impossible to implement a stabilization and withdrawal programme in the time available. These women should receive a stable dose of methadone until delivery.

Stimulants

Stimulants such as Ecstasy and cocaine do not produce major physical dependence. In these situations, it is best to advise gradual daily reduction of the drug rather than substitute with other stimulant drugs.

Benzodiazepines

Long-acting diazepam should be substituted for other benzodiazepines and steady withdrawal can then be achieved by small weekly reductions. Temazepam capsules must never be prescribed to drug users because of their potential misuse through injection.

IN LABOUR

Women who have received antenatal care should undergo routine assessment and management of their labour and delivery. There is no indi-

Table 2 *Rationalization of drug use: hierarchy of aims*

1. Stabilize illicit drug use
2. Replace illicit drugs with prescribed oral equivalent
3. Stabilize oral licit use
4. Gradual detoxification to either:
   (a) low-dose maintenance, or
   (b) complete reduction

cation for withholding analgesia, in addition to their daily methadone dose, in these patients. Epidural anaesthesia is not contraindicated.

The drug abuser presenting in labour is an obstetric emergency because of the substantial increase in low birth weight babies, premature delivery, and babies undergoing severe withdrawal. Although methadone is the drug of choice for opiate-dependent women, in emergencies a shorter-acting agent, such as diamorphine or morphine, may be required.

Narcan® must not be given to the newborn baby as its use may induce severe withdrawal symptoms. Paediatric units differ as to management of the infant, but many observe the infants for signs of withdrawal in the first 72 h.

POSTNATALLY

Breast-feeding

Methadone and heroin are excreted into breast milk, albeit not in sufficient quantities to be harmful to the infant. Methadone entering breast milk may actually prevent withdrawal symptoms in addicted infants.

The contribution of breast-feeding to neonatal infection is difficult to establish. HIV has been isolated from breast milk, and several cases of infection attributed to breast-feeding have been reported.

Breast-feeding should be recommended to HIV-positive women in areas where infectious diseases and malnutrition are the main causes of infant deaths. In other areas formula milk should be advised.

Contraception

Detoxification and withdrawal from illicit drugs results in increasing well-being, better weight gain, increased libido and return of normal menstrual functions, all of which improve fertility. Pre-existing liver damage may contraindicate the combined oral contraceptive pill. However, injectable long-acting progestogen (Depo-Provera®), which bypasses the liver, is safe. Barrier methods of contraception should be encouraged with regards to safer sex in addition to other methods. Intrauterine devices can be used, except if the women is HIV positive or has pelvic inflammatory disease.

Hepatitis

The postnatal period provides an opportunity to immunize against hepatitis A and B and rubella and perform cervical cytology screening.

FOLLOW-UP

Pregnancy and delivery of drug-using women are a small but visible and professionally time-consuming part of a much larger problem. Follow-up studies have shown that as many 25 per cent of children born to drug-using women will be adopted or fostered away, with many more of the children being involved in criminal behaviour. It is important to provide continuing care to mother and child.

REFERENCES

Centres for Disease Control (1989). *AIDS weekly surveillance report–United States*. 20 February.
Chasnoff, I.J. (ed.) (1986). *Drug use in pregnancy: mother and child*. MTP Press, Lancaster, UK.

Chasnoff, I.J., Chisum, G.M., and Kaplan, W.E. (1988). Maternal cocaine use and genitourinary tract malformations. *Teratology* **37**, 201–4.

Department of Health, Scottish Office; Home and Health Department, Welsh Office (1991). *Drug misuse and dependence. Guidelines on clinical management.* Report of a medical working group. HMSO, London.

European Collaborative Study (1991). Children born to women with HIV-1 infection: natural history and risk of transmission. *Lancet* **337**, 253–60.

Hawkins, D.F. (ed.) (1983). *Drugs and pregnancy. Human teratogenesis and related problems.* Churchill Livingstone, Edinburgh.

Johnson, M.A., and Johnstone, F.D. (eds) (1993). *HIV injection in women.* Churchill Livingstone, UK.

Kolar, A.F., Brown, B.S., Haertzen, C.A., and Michaelson, B.S. (1994). Children of substance abusers: the life experiences of children of opiate addicts in methadone maintenance. *American Journal of Drug and Alcohol,* **20**, 159–71.

Koonin, L.M., *et al.* (1989). Pregnancy associated deaths due to AIDS in the United States. *Journal of the American Medical Association* **261**, 1289–94.

van Baar, A. (1991). *The development of infants of drug dependent mothers.* Swets and Zeitlinger BV, Amsterdam. Alan Liss, New York.

World Health Organization (1987). *Special programme of research, development and research training in human reproduction and special programme on AIDS.* Report of a meeting on contraceptive methods and HIV infection. World Health Organization, Geneva.

28.3.7 Management of pain in the drug abuser

A. C. DE C. WILLIAMS AND M. GOSSOP

Physicians are often uncertain about the correct procedures for the management of pain in known or suspected drug abusers. This uncertainty leads to inadequate treatment of real pain as often as to the overprescription of drugs. However, there are simple principles of good practice which can be applied when dealing with these issues.

Drug abusers may suffer from many conditions that cause pain. Not the least of these are the illnesses associated with human immunodeficiency virus (HIV) infection and acquired immunodeficiency syndrome (AIDS). Drug abusers, like other patients, are entitled to competent treatment of their medical problems. United Kingdom Department of Health guidelines state that 'All doctors have a responsibility to provide care for both the general health needs of drug misusers and their drug related problems'; and that 'Drug misusers have the same entitlement as other patients to the services provided by the NHS'.

Whereas drug abusers who present with pain are undoubtedly challenging, they can be managed using established principles of pain treatment. There is no reason to depart from good clinical practice with such patients, and when treatment does not succeed in relieving pain, pain specialists can be helpful in exploring treatment options, including those not involving the prescription of opiates.*

PAIN AND PAIN RELIEF

Pain cannot be observed or measured directly; the best measure is the patient's report. Clinical impressions of the likely nociception from physical problems may not be reliable; indeed, they may be incorrect. The severity of pain is often not proportional to the extent of physical findings. Because the patient's report is central to assessment, this creates problems when the patient has an agenda other than pain relief.

Patients who are suspected of requesting pain relief in the absence of serious pain in order to obtain opiates are a source of annoyance to many doctors. However, the incorrect identification of such cases may occur

*The term opiate is used throughout to refer to both natural and synthetic opioids.

as a result of 'pseudoaddiction', in which a patient's response to consistently inadequate analgesia resembles the exaggerated display of pain behaviour and hostile demands for opiates associated with the covert opiate abuser. In general, the risk of iatrogenic addiction among medical patients treated with opiates has been found to be very small.

Pain is a complex psychophysiological experience. Psychological state, beliefs about pain, and the likelihood of relief, all influence the patient's experience and report of pain and its severity. Patients generally find pain more bearable when its significance is clear, and when they are assured that it can be relieved. Providing accurate information in a reassuring manner about the likely course and severity of pain and discomfort can significantly reduce the distress and discomfort of the patient.

The measurement of pain requires separate assessment of sensory and affective components. This may be done using numerical or visual analogue scales. Such scales usually require the patient to rate pain intensity and pain distress between the marks of 'no pain' to 'pain as bad as it can be', and 'no distress' to 'distress as bad as it can be' (or similar). Relief can also be measured on a suitably labelled scale ('no relief' to 'total relief'). The McGill Pain Questionnaire, a series of adjectives endorsed by the patient, gives scores for different components of pain. Recording of change in pain over time should include other relevant factors such as activity and the use of analgesics and other pain-directed strategies.

The goals of pain treatment with any patient should be clearly specified. These may extend beyond relief of pain and of concomitant distress to the recovery of patients' function in terms of work, leisure, and social activities. Assessment of disability attributable to pain is complicated, and except where reduction of disability is the main focus of treatment, numerical or visual analogue scales of the extent of interference with, or disruption of, their normal life-style by the pain are adequate.

PAIN RELIEF WITHOUT OPIATES

Non-opioid analgesics, such as paracetamol/acetaminophen, aspirin, or non-steroidal anti-inflammatory drugs (NSAIDs), can be used with the opiate-abusing patient. Other agents include local anaesthetics, used for neural blockade, short or long term; and for neuropathic pains in particular, anticonvulsant and heterocyclic (tricyclic) antidepressant drugs, the latter in lower doses than used in the treatment of depression. Steroids may also be used in the treatment of rheumatological problems. Benzodiazepines have no essential place in pain relief, and because of their considerable potential for abuse, should be avoided.

Ready and Edwards (1992) offer guidelines for good practice in the treatment of acute pain, using pharmacological and non-pharmacological treatments for pain in a variety of conditions. Common chronically painful conditions in patients with HIV/AIDS include rheumatological problems; peripheral neuropathies; chest, abdominal, and oropharyngeal pain related to carcinoma or infection; and skin pain due to sarcoma, pressure sores, or infection. Many patients with these conditions can be treated with non-opiate analgesics. Cardiac pathology in cocaine users, who may also abuse other drugs, may lead to chronic chest and back pain.

PAIN MANAGEMENT

Pain management is a rehabilitative approach whose components may be learned through a variety of methods, from self-help texts to in-patient programmes. Pain management techniques can be used alongside interventions for pain relief, and in general wards or in the community, by liaison with specialist staff. Forms of relaxation may be taught which can reduce muscle tension, and biofeedback may enable the patient to recognize the association between stresses, such as worrying thoughts or conflict with others, and muscle tension, and to learn how to control it. Strategies of distraction, visualization, and self-reassurance can considerably enhance the effects of relaxation. All of these require practice in calmer times to be useful in crises.

When physical activity is associated with increased pain, regular pacing of activity, with frequent changes of position and activity, can improve the patient's control of pain intensity. Overactivity and strain in an unfit patient, followed by prolonged rest, contribute to further loss of condition. Pacing enables the patient to plan and to carry out plans reliably within his or her limitations, returning to moderate physical exercise, social activity, and even work. In addition, by making activity level time-contingent rather than pain-contingent, it reduces the patient's monitoring of pain level. It also constitutes a graded exposure programme to feared activities, consistent with standard psychological treatment, and improves confidence in managing pain.

Non-pharmacological options for pain reduction may also include physiotherapy (and home exercise programmes); transcutaneous nerve stimulation (TENS); and acupuncture. However, the more chronic the condition, the more important it is to address patients' function if pain relief alone does not improve this.

Cognitive and behavioural therapy for anxiety and for depression can usefully be incorporated where appropriate, even with patients with very limited life expectancy. Reducing the distress and overall suffering of the patient will improve the management of pain, whatever techniques are used to address the pain directly.

OPIATES FOR PAIN RELIEF

Where the prescription of opiates is required, liaison with drug-abuse specialists is recommended. For cases in which the patient is physically dependent upon opiates, and because of the relevance of tolerance and cross-tolerance, an assessment should be carried out to determine the presence and extent of dependence. Precise, objective methods for determining the degree of physical tolerance are not available. However, dependent patients are unlikely to hide their addiction, especially if its relevance to treatment is explained by the doctor.

Assessment of physical dependence usually begins with self-reported drug use, paying attention to typical daily doses and variations in daily dose. The probability of self-reported doses should be checked against known patterns of drug use (tolerant users may be taking doses considerably greater than therapeutic doses); this may be done, for instance, by phone with a local drug-treatment agency. Variations in the purity of street heroin make accurate estimates of morphine equivalents problematic.

For patients who are tolerant to the effects of opiates, prescribing should be at a sufficient dose to cover both the dependence and the pain. For drug abusers who are not physically dependent and have not developed tolerance, normal therapeutic doses should be used. There may be considerable variation between individuals in the blood levels of a given dose of the same drug. Observation should be made of the patient's response to medication during the initial stages of treatment. Where signs of sedation occur, doses should be reduced accordingly. In the event of more serious overdosage or respiratory depression, naloxone may be used to reverse these effects. Where pain, distress, or withdrawal symptoms are reported, increased doses should be considered. The deliberate underprescribing of opiates or giving a placebo, except in a properly conducted trial, should be avoided. Either may undermine the therapeutic alliance.

The patient may be given methadone for pain relief, with doses increased to cover pain if the patient is already maintained on methadone, observing and titrating the dose according to the patient's response (see above). Agonist–antagonist combinations such as pentazocine, or partial agonists such as buprenorphine, may precipitate withdrawal and should be avoided. Any opiate agonist can be used with methadone, and, as in the non-addicted patient, increased until satisfactory analgesia is attained, or until limited by side-effects. Many opiate addicts will also have liver disease and the unpredictable effects of hepatic dysfunction on the pharmacokinetics of opiates should be noted.

For some cases, a slow-release morphine compound may be used. This is standard practice in palliative care and is provided time-contingently not as required, and with a provision for 'rescue' doses. Opiates may be delivered subcutaneously, intravenously, or spinally, offering more control to the clinician and bypassing the possibility of abuse. The use of continuous intravenous or subcutaneous infusion by a microprocessor-controlled syringe pump (patient-controlled analgesia), although expensive in equipment, allows patients, within overall dosage limits programmed into the pump by the clinician, to titrate their own analgesia, and often results in lower overall doses than when provided in traditional ways.

To minimize the exploitation of opiate prescriptions by the drug-abusing patient, one person should be responsible for pain relief, and for negotiating and recording plans and changes with the patient. In such a role, a clinician can educate the patient about the problem, aiming for better adherence, and less anxiety (and related drug abuse). Shared decisions for dealing with behaviours suggestive of abuse, such as 'loss' of drugs or of prescriptions, apparent alteration of prescriptions, obtaining treatment from other sources without agreement, or presentation to emergency services requesting more opiates, allow consistent limits to be observed by staff, if not necessarily by patients.

Properly prescribed, opiates can offer great benefits in relief from pain, to some extent from anxiety and distress, and, as tolerance develops to sedative effects, the possibility of more normal functioning. Prescribing opiates in ineffective quantities, as required rather than time-contingently, or delivery at longer than optimal intervals (often the decision of nursing staff), achieves little, increases the patient's anxiety, and makes for a struggle for control between patient and staff.

Opiophobia is a term that has been used to describe the unusual behaviour of clinicians who often depart from good principles of practice and ignore textbooks in favour of underprescription, affected by mistaken beliefs about addiction, and pressure from statutory restrictions. Poor management of acutely painful crises (as in sickle-cell disease) increases patients' fear of such episodes, and encourages patients to hoard analgesics, seek multiple consultations, and to show other behaviours associated with drug abuse. One study of patients with sickle-cell disease showed that many believed that staff treating their pain underestimated its severity.

In painful but not life-threatening conditions, the cost-benefit balance of long-term opiate prescription may be more controversial, and there is doubt about its efficacy, particularly for neuropathic pains. Chronic pain may in some cases be well controlled on a steady dose of opiates, but many chronic pain patients take opiates without significant improvement in pain or function. A patient presenting with chronic pain who demands potent opiates should be re-evaluated. The patient who seems preoccupied with the pain and requests ever-increasing doses of opiates needs help in addressing the causes of distress; these may include catastrophic beliefs about the meaning of the pain, or about inability to cope with it. The agreement of goals between doctor and patient, and the time course for trial of any drug, is recommended. Return of function, with or without pain relief, may best be achieved by pain management techniques.

Existing principles and procedures for the treatment of pain provide useful techniques and strategies with which to tackle the difficult problems presented by the drug-abusing pain patient. Physicians should be alert to additional but avoidable problems which may be caused by misconceptions and fears about opiate users held by many clinical staff.

REFERENCES

Brody, S.L., Slovis, C.M., and Wrenn, K.D. (1990). Cocaine-related medical problems: consecutive series of 233 patients. *The American Journal of Medicine* **88**, 325–31.

Department of Health (1984). *Guidelines of good clinical practice in the treatment of drug misuse.* DHSS, London.

Department of Health (1991). *Drug misuse and dependence: guidelines on clinical management.* HMSO, London.

Gossop, M. and Green, L. (1988). Effects of information on the opiate withdrawal syndrome. *British Journal of Psychiatry* **83**, 305–9.

Kluger, M. and Owen, A. (1990). Patients' expectations of patient controlled analgsia. *Analgesia* **45**, 1072–4.

Lebovits, A.H., *et al.* (1989). The prevalence and management of pain in patients with AIDS: a review of 134 cases. *Clinical Journal of Pain* **5**, 245–8.

McQuay, H.J. (1989). Opioids in chronic pain. *British Journal of Anaesthesia* **63**, 213–26.

Melzack, R. (1975). The McGill Pain Questionnaire: major properties and scoring methods. *Pain*, **1**, 275.

Moorey, S. and Greer, S. (1989). *Psychological therapy for patients with cancer*. Heinemann, Oxford.

Morgan, J.P. (1989). American opiophobia: customary underutilization of opioid analgesics. In *Advances in pain research and therapy,* Vol. 11 (ed. C.S. Hill and W.S. Fields), pp. 181–9. Raven Press, New York.

Murray, N. and May, A. (1988). Painful crisis in sickle cell disease: patients' perspectives. *British Medical Journal* **297**, 452–4.

Portenoy, R.K. and Payne, R. (1992). Acute and chronic pain. In *Comprehensive textbook of substance abuse,* (ed. J.H. Lowinson, P. Ruiz, and R.B. Millman), pp.691–721. Williams and Wilkins, Baltimore.

Ready, L.B. and Edwards, W.T. (ed.) (1992). *Management of acute pain: a practical guide*. IASP Publications, Seattle.

Rowe, I.F., *et al.* (1989). Rheumatological lesions in individuals with human immunodeficiency virus infection. *Quarterly Journal of Medicine* **73**, 1167–84.

Schofferman, J. (1988). Pain: diagnosis and management in the palliative care of AIDS. *Journal of Palliative Care* **4**, 46–9.

Stimmel, B. (1989). Adequate analgesia in narcotic dependency. In *Advances in pain research and therapy,* Vol. 11 (ed. C.S. Hill and W.S. Fields), pp.131–8. Raven Press, New York.

Wall, P.D. and Melzack, R. (ed.) (1994). *Textbook of pain,* (3rd edn). Churchill Livingstone, Edinburgh.

28.3.8 Caring for the HIV-positive drug user

J. Strang and M. Farrell

SEIZING THE OPPORTUNITY

The immunocompromised HIV-positive drug taker is not only more likely to be infected with a variety of agents, but is also more likely to suffer more serious sequelae from these infections. For such a patient, opportunistic infections (such as herpes simplex) may not only herald the onset of acquired immunodeficiency syndrome (AIDS), but may actually hasten the progression of the disease process. Many such patients will not be in regular contact with any specialist HIV or drug service, and may not have a regular GP. Much of the observed morbidity (and mortality) amongst the populations of HIV-positive drug takers is eminently responsive to treatment, and is of a form which could reasonably be provided by doctors without special AIDS expertise, or at least on a 'shared care' basis.

RECONCILING PUBLIC HEALTH AND PERSONAL HEALTH PERSPECTIVES

Concern about the spread of HIV infection amongst injecting drug users, and, through their sexual behaviour, into the wider population has lead to increasing attention being paid to public health strategies for the management of drug misuse, and, in particular, for any approaches which may reduce the extent of contaminated sharing of injecting equipment.

The *AIDS and drug misuse* report from the Advisory Council on the Misuse of Drugs (1988) stated that: the spread of HIV is a greater danger to individual and public health than drug misuse: accordingly, services which minimise HIV risk behaviour by all available means should take precedence in development plans. However, this should not be taken as a reason to discard one's concern about the injecting drug use: rather, concerns should become more focused and should lead to particular attention being paid to personal health and public health approaches which may lead to reductions in the extent of sharing of needles and syringes.

Substantial reductions in the extent of sharing of injecting equipment have already occurred amongst injecting drug users and the doctor should look for new opportunities to promote a complete move away from injecting or further substantial reductions in sharing. It is particularly important to promote these changes amongst the HIV-positive patient, not only on public health grounds, but also to reduce the likelihood of further infections or immunosuppression which may hasten the HIV disease process.

IS THE HIV-POSITIVE DRUG USER A SPECIAL CASE?

Intravenous drug abuse is associated with its own morbidity and mortality. Injecting drug users are more likely to suffer from a variety of pathologies than a non-drug-abusing age-matched population. Some of this increased morbidity and mortality will be associated with the direct effects of the drugs themselves (for example, damage to brain or liver from alcohol, barbiturates, etc.; or the immunosuppression of opiates) which may be compounded by the poor attention to nutrition and hygiene in these generally disadvantaged populations. However, recent attention has particularly focused on the mortality and morbidity associated with blood-borne viruses such as HIV and hepatitis B. The proportional contributions of these different influences is the subject of much current debate, and will vary by city, by population, by prevailing seroprevalence, and hence by year. An interesting observation is that levels of reported morbidity amongst HIV-negative drug users have increased: for example, tuberculosis is now reported four times as frequently amongst New York heroin addicts who do not have AIDS (compared with data predating AIDS awareness).

MAINTAINING CONTACT AND MAXIMIZING BENEFIT

Much importance has been attached to strategies for identifying the injecting drug user at risk of HIV infection (or already HIV positive) and for maintaining contact with such individuals. However, this must be accompanied by attention to the extent to which the individual and society benefit from this contact. What should the doctor be seeking to achieve by establishing and maintaining contact with the drug taker? In managing the HIV-positive drug user, there is a fortunate confluence of public and individual health goals, with a need to reduce as far as possible the extent of continued sharing of injecting equipment and of unprotected sex. In considering the individual drug taker, the doctor must also seek to promote reductions in any injecting, and will need to pay attention to the general health of the patient.

Tuberculosis is seen more commonly amongst the drug-taking population, and active clinical tuberculosis develops more frequently among HIV seropositive drug misusers. As yet this has not become a marked feature of care of the HIV-positive drug user in the United Kingdom, due to the different prior levels of protection against tuberculosis. Drug abusers may develop clinical tuberculosis or other bacterial pneumonia at a stage when they may not satisfy Center for Disease Control criteria for AIDS.

For reasons that are not yet clear, Kaposi's sarcoma is extremely rare amongst the heterosexual drug-using HIV-positive population.

The relationship between co-infection with hepatitis B virus, C virus, and delta fragment, and a previous or simultaneous infection with HIV has not yet been clarified. However, immunization against hepatitis B is an appropriate precaution for the hepatitis B virus-negative, HIV-positive drug abuser. It has now been clearly established that antiviral treatment (for example, zidovudine) can be given successfully to both ex-drug users and current drug users, with the most reliable attendance being seen amongst those simultaneously receiving a substitute opiate prescription.

Table 1 *Drugs-related and HIV-related problems*

Symptom	Drug-related[a]	HIV-related
Shortness of breath	Heroin-precipitated asthma, bacterial pneumonia, endocarditis, chronic bronchitis	Pneumocystis pneumonia, TB
Cough	Bacterial pneumonia, endocarditis, chronic bronchitis	Pneumocystis pneumonia, TB
Cyanosis	Bacterial pneumonia, endocarditis, chronic bronchitis	Pneumocystis pneumonia
Fever	Injection abscess, septicaemia, pneumonia, endocarditis	Pheumocystis pneumonia, TB
Rash		
Small blood spots	Septicaemia, endocarditis	Thrombocytopenia
Bruises at injection site	Leakage from injection, arterial injection	Thrombocytopenia
Itchy spots	Formication associated with amphetamines or cocaine	Allergy, seborrhoeic dermatitis
Abscesses	Missing injection, leakage from injection (especially barbiturates and crushed tablets), infected injection material	Susceptibility to bacterial infection
Sores around mouth	Poor diet, nasal ulceration from snorting cocaine	Chronic cold sores (herpes)
Sore mouth	Poor diet	Cold sores, thrush, oral leucoplakia
Weight loss	Poor diet, anorexic effect of amphetamines or cocaine	CDC IVa, TB, other infections
Vomiting	Opiate withdrawal, septicaemia	Infection, gastric irritation, side-effect of treatment
Diarrhoea	Opiate withdrawal	Cryptosporiadiosis
Flu-like sympotms	Opiate withdrawal, septicaemia, endocarditis	CDC III/IVa
Sweating	Opiate withdrawal, septicaemia	CDC III/IVa, TB
Night sweats	Insufficient opiate cover	CDC III/IVa
Loss of vision	Endocarditis, local injection, candida infection of eye	Cytomegalovirus infection
Confusion	Drug use, pneumonia, endocarditis, meningitis	Meningitis, toxoplasmosis, etc.
Fits/episodic loss of consciousness	Drug overdose, bacterial meningitis, withdrawal (alcohol, barbiturates, benzodiazepines), cocaine-induced fit	Meningitis, toxoplasmosis, etc.
Paralysis	Nerve damage from infection	CDC III/IVa

[a]The term 'drug-related' is used broadly to include those problems associated with route of administration.

CDC, Centers for Disease Control; TB, tuberculosis.

OVERLAP OF DRUG AND HIV SYMPTOMATOLOGY

Lists of signs and symptoms indicative of advancing HIV disease are often difficult to interpret in the drug taker. Night sweats, diarrhoea, vomiting, and occasional flu-like symptoms are frequently reported by the opiate addict, and weight loss, abscess or fever may have no direct relevance to the assessment of HIV status. Consequently the clinician must be alert to the possible drug-related as well as HIV-related origin of the observed signs and symptoms (see Table 1).

WHAT IS THE PRESENT HIV STATUS?

The drug taker of unknown HIV serostatus

For the injecting drug taker who does not know his or her HIV serostatus and has chosen not to be tested, it is extremely important to emphasize the need for change in injecting and sexual behaviour as if the individual were HIV positive. There is a danger that the drug taker, who may previously have blotted out unpleasant realities with drug use, may blot out the reality of the HIV risk to themselves and others by continued drug use accompanied by a hope that all is (and will continue to be) well. The decision not to be tested must not be seen as an endorsement of the previous behaviour.

The previously undiagnosed HIV-positive drug taker

Receiving a positive HIV test result will be a profoundly traumatic event, as for any other patient. By previous consideration and preparation of the circumstances and available supports, it is possible to increase the likelihood of a constructive outcome to the imparting of this information. At this point of crisis, the injecting drug taker may be more-than-usually receptive to an opportunity for either detoxification or ces-

sation of any further injecting (for example, coinciding with entry into an oral methadone maintenance programme). Great attention should be paid to planning beyond the immediate period, so as to ensure continuity of care and benefit. This can be particularly important when the doctor is attending the patient within a short-term context (for example during a brief hospital admission), and the doctor may need to help with referral to new services (arranging for future care from a general practitioner, and arranging referral to a drug clinic).

The asymptomatic HIV-positive drug taker

The goal here is to extend the asymptomatic period as far as possible by avoiding any further infection or behaviour which may promote the HIV disease process. Fortunately these changes will also succeed in reducing the likelihood of any onward transmission of the virus to sexual or injecting partners. In initiating a new treatment approach (for example, the prescribing of substitute drugs), attention must be paid to the longer-term impact on risk behaviours, so as to avoid therapeutic stagnation with inadvertent preservation of continued lower levels of risk behaviour. While it is an important first step to have enabled a reduction in risk to the individual patient and his or her contacts, it is essential to look beyond this initial therapeutic gain to identify the next intermediate treatment goal.

During this asymptomatic phase, there should be immunological monitoring of the patient so that the level of vigilance can be increased as the markers indicate the imminent onset of active disease. When the CD4 count drops to near 200, when there is the appearance of p24 antigen, or when there is loss of the p24 antibody, then the frequency of appointments should be increased so that opportunistic infections can be treated as early as possible. Prophylactic aerosolized pentamidine may be commenced to prevent (or at least delay) the onset of pneumocystis pneumonia.

The symptomatic HIV-positive drug taker

At this stage, the patient is vulnerable to those opportunistic infections which are especially associated with AIDS as well as to the more commonly encountered infections. Special attention to AIDS-linked pathologies must not take away from the need for identification and thorough treatment of more orthodox infections.

28.3.9 The needs of the alcohol/drug user in custody

A. MADEN

Substance abuse is the most common health problem encountered in prison and offender populations. Prevalence rates vary according to the diagnostic criteria used, but, if cannabis use is excluded, over 10 per cent of men and 23 per cent of women serving a prison sentence in England and Wales report drug dependence at the time of their offence. Opiates account for most cases, followed by amphetamines and cocaine. The type of offence is a poor guide to the likely presence of drug dependence, as most drug users are sentenced for acquisitive offending, with a minority convicted of possession or supplying. Epidemiological links between drugs and crime are well established but causal relationships are complex. Most drug users report offending in order to finance their habit, but offending often precedes the onset of drug dependence, and both crime and drug use are most prevalent in areas that have high levels of poverty and social deprivation. The links between crime and drug use are irrelevant to the doctor treating the drug user in custody, as intervention is justified by the principle of harm minimization. In contrast to the United States, drug dependence in the United Kingdom does not have a statistical association with violent offending.

Problem drinking also affects a substantial minority of prisoners, from 10 to 50 per cent, depending on the criteria used. Alcohol misuse in prisoners covers a spectrum similar to that seen in other populations, from the vagrant, homeless, petty offender through to the professional criminal. Again, causal relationships are difficult to unravel.

The principles of assessing and treating the drug or alcohol user in custody are the same as in other situations but they must be modified to take account of the custodial environment and legal concerns. The importance of these factors changes as an inmate progresses through the criminal justice system, so the needs of the substance abuser can best be described in the early, middle, and late phases of time spent in custody.

On reception into custody

For all prisoners, this is the time of highest risk for psychiatric morbidity and mortality, usually from suicide. The transition from freedom to imprisonment brings isolation from social supports. Anxiety is increased by impending legal proceedings and the fear of victimization within prison. The substance abuser has the added fear of withdrawal symptoms.

The clinical and medicolegal components of the doctor's task can never be entirely separated. The immediate clinical priorities are the assessment and treatment of withdrawal symptoms, and other complications of substance abuse. The medicolegal priorities are the assessment of fitness to be detained and fitness to be interviewed by police. These assessments depend on the degree of intoxication or the severity of withdrawal symptoms and the extent to which they can be treated without impairing cognitive function. There are no generally accepted criteria for fitness to be detained or interviewed.

This work is complicated by the circumstances in which it is carried out, often within a police station. All actions may be scrutinized by a court, sometimes after a delay of years, so scrupulous record-keeping is essential. The time for interview and examination may be limited, the premises unsuitable because of noise or lack of privacy and the patient may be uncooperative and threatening. It is the doctor's responsibility to ensure that conditions allow him to carry out his work adequately and safely. Any difficulties should be noted, along with the steps taken in an attempt to resolve them.

The doctor should begin all interviews by introducing himself, explaining his role and the purpose of the interview. If the doctor is likely to prepare reports for the court, the defendant should be informed of this, and warned that the interview is not confidential and that he is not obliged to answer any questions.

HISTORY

Background information, particularly about the nature of the charges, should be obtained in advance whenever possible, so that the initial interview can focus on medical issues.

After a full introduction, the interview may begin with an enquiry as to whether the prisoner has any complaints about the way the police or prison authorities have dealt with him. This serves the dual function of recording at an early stage allegations which may become the subject of proceedings at a later date, and establishing the doctor's role in the protection of his patient's interests.

In addition to a thorough alcohol and drug history, needle-sharing, tattooing, sexual promiscuity, and prostitution (both male and female) may have relevance for HIV risk. Alcohol abuse is common in violent and sexual offenders, and both may predispose to self-harm, as may the threat of a long sentence. Most people who harm themselves in custody have a prior history of self-harm in other circumstances.

Past experience of treatment may influence future recommendations. It may also indicate past complications of substance abuse or reveal other, coexisting psychiatric disorder. Reported difficulty in coping with previous imprisonment suggests that further problems are likely. A family and social history may reveal isolation and a lack of potential visitors, increasing the risk of self-harm. Women entering custody often have additional worries about the care of dependent children.

PHYSICAL AND MENTAL STATE EXAMINATION

General physical inspection may reveal systemic or localized complications of substance abuse. Offenders, especially heavy drinkers, are often the victims of violence and may also have sustained injuries at arrest, including head injury.

Mental state examination aims to confirm the diagnosis of substance dependence or abuse, detect withdrawal symptoms, and exclude other psychiatric disorder. Severe alcohol withdrawal or drug intoxication must be distinguished from other causes of acute organic syndromes. Depression may be a consequence of stimulant withdrawal or a result of adverse circumstances, so questions about suicidal thoughts and intent are essential; negative and positive findings must be adequately recorded. Personality disorder is commonly associated with substance abuse but its presence should not be assumed, nor should it be disregarded when present. Chronic low self-esteem, self-mutilation, poor anger control, and unsatisfactory or violent relationships will influence the possibilities for treatment. Psychosis may accompany drug intoxication or withdrawal and may be indistinguishable from functional psychosis. Substance abuse complicates some cases of chronic schizophrenia and increases the chances that the patient will come into conflict with the law.

SPECIAL INVESTIGATIONS

Blood or urine samples confirm drug use. Quantitative measures of alcohol can be of great medicolegal importance.

MANAGEMENT

The management of withdrawal syndromes is determined by the particular characteristics of the drug, but the custodial setting can create additional problems. Doctors may face demands to prescribe excessive quantities of drugs, or there may be an institutional ethos which resists all demands for medication. Neither attitude is justified. Institutions should develop a policy on prescribing and drug withdrawal regimes, which can be implemented with minimal variation and reduce confrontation. Occasionally, the complications of drug withdrawal can be life-threatening, in which case the aim is to secure urgent transfer to hospital.

Many substance abusers will be released on bail after a short period in custody. Further treatment should be offered, through liaison with other agencies. The impact of being arrested will lead some users to re-evaluate their substance abuse and it is important that they are made aware of treatment options.

THE COURT REPORT

The report should give a diagnosis where appropriate and discuss possible treatment options. Questions of retribution and punishment should be left to the court. The United Kingdom Criminal Justice Act 1991 allows for the treatment of drug or alcohol problems as a condition of a probation order. Treatment need not be within a hospital setting, so a knowledge of local treatment agencies is essential, as is liaison with the probation service.

Serving a sentence

SUBSTANCE ABUSE WITHIN PRISON

The extent of drug use and sexual behaviour within prisons is a matter of debate on which there is little hard evidence. The doctor working in prison must be aware of the possibility of drug intoxication and the need for HIV counselling.

It has been suggested that the risk of HIV transmission within prison may be reduced by the provision of condoms, syringes, or cleaning materials, or maintenance prescribing. None of these approaches has been widely adopted in English prisons. As they have implications for prison discipline, they are subject to institutional policies, rather than being left to the discretion of individual doctors.

TREATMENT FOR SUBSTANCE ABUSERS WITHIN PRISON

A basic package of counselling and advice should be available to all substance abusers. The artificial environment of prison limits what can be achieved and there is doubt about the extent to which change will generalize to behaviour in the outside world. Therefore, in British prisons, the emphasis is on throughcare and preparation for release. Most prisons have groups run by Alcoholics and Narcotics Anonymous, and other groups may be organized by prison or probation officers, often oriented towards health education. The prison doctor may have an organizational or supervisory role, although the main responsibility falls on the probation service.

A more specialized form of treatment, based on the principles of a therapeutic community, is available for a minority of substance abusers. It is most suitable for prisoners with acknowledged personality difficulties and existing facilities (at HMP Grendon and the Wormwood Scrubs Annexe) are oversubscribed and cater for serious offenders serving long sentences, with violent and sexual offenders predominating.

Preparation for release

Release from prison presents a high risk of relapse. The stress of rebuilding a life in the outside world is combined with a return to the setting of previous drug use, renewed contacts with other drug users, and the loss of supports established within prison. Deaths due to overdose are common and all former users should be warned of the dangers of a reduced tolerance. Pre-release training schemes address this and other issues relating to drugs and alcohol. Invitations to drug treatment agencies to visit prisons encourage links that may be maintained after release.

Medical reports are influential in parole decisions and, in the past, substance abuse was likely to reduce an inmate's chances of parole. In fact, it can provide an opportunity for a period of statutory supervision in the community, prior to full release. Voluntary contact with the probation service may continue after this time.

REFERENCES

Collins, J.J. (1982). *Drinking and crime: perspectives on the relationship between alcohol consumption and criminal behaviour.* Tavistock, London.

Farrell, M. and Strang, J. (1991). Drugs, HIV and prisons. Time to rethink current policy. *British Medical Journal* **302;** 1477–8.

Maden, A., Swinton, M. and Gunn, J. (1992). A survey of pre-arrest drug use in sentenced prisoners. *British Journal of Addiction* **87,** 27–33.

Smith, R. (1984). *Prison health care.* British Medical Association, London.

Section 29 Forensic medicine

29 Forensic medicine

B. Knight

Forensic medicine, also known as 'legal medicine' or 'medical jurisprudence', is an amalgam of many separate disciplines. Indeed, it may be said that it encompasses the whole of medical practice because every speciality in medicine has medicolegal aspects.

Unlike the rest of clinical medicine, forensic medicine varies considerably according to the geographical jurisdiction in which it is practised, because the legal systems vary greatly from country to country, and even within the same country, as in the United Kingdom, where the laws and practice in England and Wales vary considerably from Scotland and, to a lesser extent, from Northern Ireland. Many areas of the world, especially those in the Commonwealth, have legal systems closely akin to the United Kingdom, although as time goes on the divergence becomes greater. It is therefore almost impossible to write on forensic medicine in a universal way, although there is a substantial core that is common to virtually all jurisdictions.

Forensic medicine consists of two major portions, that in which medical science is applied to the administration of justice (both criminal and civil) and that in which the law impacts upon the practice of medicine. In the context of this book, it is the latter topic that is more important to clinicians and will be concentrated upon in this chapter.

Forensic pathology

This is the part of forensic medicine that gains most publicity, both in the media and in the memories of doctors from their undergraduate teaching. Although tuition in the legal aspects of medicine is far more important to the practising clinician, the recollection of lectures giving lurid details of homicides with appropriately gruesome photographs tend to remain with the undergraduate for life!

Forensic pathology is the application of autopsy pathology to the examination of the dead. Although death certification, etc. will be discussed later, in general deaths due to criminal action, or that are sudden, suspicious, or obscure, come to a medicolegal autopsy. The function of the forensic pathologist is to enumerate the injuries where present, to ascertain the cause of death, to assess the contribution of natural disease to death and to interpret the wounds or other unnatural processes that may have caused or contributed to death. Other functions include estimating the time since death, identifying the body and a number of other matters related to judicial requirements.

Forensic pathologists may be aided in their work by a variety of other disciplines, some purely clinical. The assistance of a radiologist in child abuse deaths, missile injuries and in the identification of skeletal remains is important. The forensic odontologist frequently assists in the identification of decomposed or skeletalized remains, by matching the dentition with known dental charts: the recognition and matching of bite marks, especially in child abuse and sexual assaults, is another aspect of forensic dentistry. Toxicologists, microbiologists, virologists, and histologists also play a supporting role in many autopsy situations. An anatomist or forensic anthropologist can be of considerable assistance in ageing, sexing, and otherwise identifying skeletal remains.

Medicolegal autopsies fall into two main categories: the greater number comprise sudden unexpected deaths, usually due to cardiovascular disease, together with accidents, suicides, and industrial diseases. In the United Kingdom these are usually dealt with by hospital histopathologists acting for the coroner or, in Scotland, the Procurator Fiscal. The much smaller group of criminal, suspicious, or obscure deaths are dealt with in England and Wales by the Home Office pathologists, who are drawn either from the small cadre of university forensic pathologists or from hospital histopathologists, who by training and experience have considerable forensic expertise.

However, as stated earlier, this aspect of forensic medicine, fascinating though it is, has little day-to-day relevance to practising clinicians, either in hospital or general practice. The most important fact that these doctors must appreciate in the forensic context, is when to report a death for medicolegal investigation because of some unusual or undetermined circumstance. Unfortunately, most doctors have an understandably low threshold of suspicion and many deaths that should be so investigated fail to be notified early enough or even at all.

The doctor's duties after a death

Although the procedure to be described is that of England and Wales, most jurisdictions have a broadly similar requirement. First, the doctor must ensure that the fact of death is confirmed. This is a clinical exercise rather than a legal one and consists of the confirmation that cardio-respiratory functions have ceased irreversibly. The particular problem of brain-stem death in patients on a ventilator will be discussed later.

In most deaths, the marker of the moment of death is cardiac arrest and this must be confirmed by the doctor by auscultation of the heart, as depending upon the radial or even carotid pulse in a moribund patient is often unreliable. Even listening over the apex for heart sounds may be difficult near the point of death and prolonged use of the stethoscope may be required before a decision is made that the heart has finally stopped. Listening for the cessation of respiratory function is less reliable, but attempting to hear air entry over the trachea with a stethoscope may be used. The older traditional tests, such as feathers or mirrors before the mouth or strings tied around the finger, should be relegated to medical history! Rarely, electrocardiograph tracings might be needed. Probably the nearest simulation of death was given by barbituate intoxication, but fortunately these are rarely seen these days, due to the voluntary limitation of prescription of these dangerous drugs.

When the fact of death has been confirmed, the time and date should be recorded in the clinical notes. The doctor then has to decide whether or not he or she is in a position to issue a death certificate or report the case for medicolegal investigation. In England and Wales, between one-quarter and one-third of deaths are reported to coroners, usually with a withholding of a death certificate, although in strict law, the doctor who has attended the patient in their last illness is statutorily obliged to give a death certificate. However, if the cause of death is thought to be unnatural or is unknown, then it is futile for the doctor to provide such a certificate, this function being taken over by the coroner.

If the doctor was in attendance upon the patient during the 14 days preceding death, is confident of the cause of death and that the cause was natural, then he or she must provide a death certificate on the forms issued by the Registrar General. Although commonly called 'The Death Certificate' it is actually the 'Medical Certificate of the Cause of Death'. This must be transmitted to the Registrar of Births and Deaths within 5 days of issue, usually taken personally by the near relatives of the deceased. The book of certificates has a counterfoil for the doctor's own records and a further tear-off strip called 'Notice to Informant', which must be handed to the next-of-kin.

The form of the certificate is self-explanatory but the most important part is the box that contains the cause of death. This is printed in the international format of the World Health Organization, being divided into Part I, the disease or condition leading directly to death and Part II, other significant conditions contributing to the death but not related to the disease or condition causing it.

Part I is further subdivided into (a), (b), and (c). These are causally linked in a consecutive order, so that (a) is due to (b) which is due to (c). In other words, the basic pathological disease process is always the lowest line of Part I. It is not necessary that all lines be completed and a perfectly acceptable cause of death would be '1(a) Coronary atherosclerosis'.

The death certificate must avoid undesirable terms that have no aetiological usefulness, such as 'heart failure, syncope, coma'. Useful instructions are given inside the covers of the books of certificates issued by the Registrar General.

Unfortunately, the standard of accuracy of death certification is very poor, the medical causes of death being frequently incorrect. Additionally, the way in which the available information is displayed on the face of the certificate is frequently illogical and unhelpful. This defeats the object of national mortality statistics, which have a considerable public health and preventive medicine role.

Following deaths that are not to be reported to the coroner, some clinicians will request a postmortem examination. This is to be held only for clinical purposes to determine the *extent* and not the *nature* of disease. By definition, if a doctor does not know the cause of death, they cannot request a clinical autopsy to find out, because the very fact of doubt about the cause makes it a case reportable to the coroner.

Where a clinical autopsy is to be carried out, it is preferable to await the result of the pathologist's findings before completing the death certificate, as an appreciable proportion of cases reveal a different cause of death to that which was forecast by the clinicians. Many surveys have shown a discrepancy rate of 20 to 50 per cent between the presumed cause and the cause discovered at autopsy.

REPORTING TO THE CORONER

There is no particular duty upon a doctor to report death to the coroner, other than that placed upon every citizen. The only persons statutorily obliged to report deaths to the coroner are the local Registrars of Births and Deaths and certain officials, such as the governors of prisons. However, it is conventional that doctors voluntarily report deaths to the coroner wherever the circumstances so indicate. It is better for the doctor, where there is doubt as to whether a death should be reported, to seek the advice of the coroner, the coroner's officer, or a senior pathologist.

The following deaths should be reported to the coroner, usually via the coroner's officer, a policeman, or a civilian who handles the administrative work of the coroner:

1. Where the deceased was not attended in their last illness by a doctor. Here, if another doctor is called to certify the fact of death or in the mistaken impression that medical treatment or resuscitation can be given, this doctor is in no position to issue a certificate and must report the death to the coroner. This often applies to emergencies, to accident and casualty officers, and to deputizing services.
2. Where the deceased was not seen by a doctor either after death or within the 14 days prior to death. The alternative of not seeing the body after death should never occur, as only a tiny minority of deceased persons are now not viewed after death by a doctor. In every other country it is mandatory that the body be seen after death, and this may soon be enforced by legislation in the United Kingdom. The 14-day rule causes a considerable number of deaths to be reported to the coroner, even though another doctor has seen the deceased within the past fortnight. A frequent occurrence in general practice is that one partner attends a patient regularly but when on holiday or

ill, another partner or assistant takes over. Deaths occurring during this period are usually reported to the coroner, who in these circumstances may decline to take on the case and direct the doctor to issue a certificate.
3. Where the cause of death is unknown.
4. Where death appears to be due to industrial disease or poisoning. On the face of the death certificate there is a box that must be ticked if the doctor thinks that occupation or industrial disease has contributed to the death. This automatically makes it a case reported to the coroner.
5. Where death may have been unnatural or caused by violence, neglect, or abortion, or attended by suspicious circumstances. This rather wide category includes death that may have been due to medical treatment and potentially medical negligence.
6. Where death has occurred during operation or before recovery from an anaesthetic.

It is a convention with many coroners, although not a legal requirement, that deaths occurring within 24 h of emergency admission to hospital be reported. Similarly, many coroners will require deaths that occur within 24 h of surgical operation or other significant medical intervention, and certainly an anaesthetic, to be reported.

Any death that is thought potentially to be related to a medical procedure, either diagnostic or therapeutic, should be reported to the coroner. Whether to do this is the doctor's decision, but it is always preferable to err on the safe side when in doubt. For example, a patient who dies suddenly with a presumed pulmonary embolus, 1 week after a surgical operation, should be reported to the coroner, as this is likely to be related to the surgical event. Similarly, deaths following an accident, however remote in time, should be reported. Many such deaths, especially following fractured femur in old people are not reported, even though the possibility of pulmonary embolism, chest infection, or other post-traumatic or postoperative complication may be likely.

Once a death is reported to the coroner, no further action should be taken by the doctor. Although a death certificate may be provided if the relatives insist, Box A on the back of the certificate should be signed to indicate that the case has been reported to the coroner and thus the Registrar of Births and Deaths cannot register the death until they hears from the coroner about the final outcome. Similarly, an autopsy cannot be requested and cremation forms cannot be issued in a coroner's case, as this is the function of the coroner on Form E. As discussed below, the donation of organs for transplantation cannot be implemented if the death is reported to the coroner, without the consent of the latter.

Transplantation and human tissue act

In the United Kingdom, the donation of cadaver tissue and organs for transplantation together with clinical autopsies is regulated by the Human Tissue Act (1961). With the exception of corneae, organs are now taken with the minimum warm ischaemic time, i.e. with a beating heart up to the moment of harvesting. Thus virtually all cadaver donation must come from patients on artificial ventilation who have been declared brain-stem dead. There is a Code of Practice issued by the Department of Health, based upon the recommendations of the Royal Colleges, which should be followed as a model procedure for organ donation.

An organ donor must be irreversibly unconscious, unable to maintain spontaneous respiration, and must be shown to have irreversible brain-stem death. Persons with systemic infections, tumours other than primary brain neoplasms, renal disease, and severe atherosclerosis are unsuitable for organ or tissue donation apart from corneae. The medical team providing care for the patient must be seen to be distinct from the transplant team and, until brain-stem death is certified, nothing should be done to the patient for the purposes of donation that would not have been done in the normal course of treatment. However, there is no objection, and indeed it may be essential, that when blood samples are taken for diagnostic purposes, a portion is retained for tissue-typing in anticipation of transplantation. When death is found to be an inevitable outcome, the transplant team should be alerted but by this time the relatives should have been informed of the impending death and their attitude to donation explored. When a donor card has been left by the patient, this constitutes sufficient legal authority for transplantation, but it is obviously good practice and courtesy to discuss the procedure fully with the relatives.

The consent of the coroner or Procurator Fiscal in Scotland must be obtained before organs are taken from a case that is reportable to the coroner: sometimes permission will be withheld if the death is due to criminal action, although the opinion of the forensic pathologist may be sought by the coroner in individual cases.

The Human Tissue Act (1961) provides that the person lawfully in possession of the body after death (usually the Health Authority or one of their servants, including consultants) may authorize the removal of tissues if the person during their lifetime expressed the wish for this to occur. The display of a signed donor card fulfils this purpose. If no such permission is available, then removal may be authorized if the person lawfully in charge of the body, having made such reasonable enquiry as may be practicable, has no reason to believe that the deceased had ever expressed any objection to donation and that the surviving spouse or any surviving relative has made no such objection. Unlike the consent form for clinical autopsy, there is usually no specific document for this purpose, but the clinicians must be satisfied that no such objections exist and should record this in the hospital notes or the check list recommended by the Code of Practice. The actual removal of donor organs must be made by a fully registered practitioner who is specifically charged with determining that life is extinct.

As virtually all organs are obtained from brain-stem-dead patients on ventilation, a strict regime for determining brain-stem death must be observed. The Code of Practice, based upon the pronouncements of the Conference of Royal Colleges and Faculties of the United Kingdom lays down that:

1. The inevitable deep coma must be shown to be due to natural disease and not to the effect of hypothermia, depressant drugs, or metabolic or endocrine disturbances.
2. Spontaneous respiration must be inadequate or absent and neuromuscular blocking agents and other drugs must be excluded as a cause of such apnoea.
3. The diagnosis of the fatal condition must be known and be due to irreversible brain damage.

The diagnostic tests for brain-stem death are set out in the Code of Practice and consist of absent brain-stem reflexes, including fixed unresponsible pupils, absent corneal reflexes, absent vestibulo-ocular reflexes, absent motor responses in cranial nerves, absent gag reflex after stimulation of the trachea, and no respiratory movements when the patient is disconnected from the ventilator after the aterial $P\text{CO}_2$ level has been shown to exceed 50 mmHg.

The tests should be made by two doctors to ensure permanent absence of response. It is usual for the test to be repeated at least once, unless the diagnosis of gross brain damage is patently obvious, such as a severe head injury. The persistence of spinal reflexes is not relevant in the diagnosis of brain-stem death and the use of electroencephalography or cerebral angiography, etc. is also not considered vital in British practice. Testing should be carried out with a body temperature of not less than 35 °C, as hypothermia may mimic brain-stem death.

Although the majority of transplanted organs in Britain are obtained from cadaver donation, the use of living donor material is strictly controlled both by the Human Tissue Act and by the Human Organ Transplant Act (1989). The latter Act is to prevent commercial exploitation of live donors and, in summary:

1. Prohibits any payment for donating organs, including any negotiation or advertising for this purpose.

2. The removal or transplantation of any organ or tissue from a living person, unless they are genetically related, within certain fixed limits is prohibited, unless specific consent is obtained. The Act lays down certain serological tests to establish the degree of relationship.
3. A regulatory authority must give permission to doctors who wish to transplant from live donors who are not within the prescribed limits of genetic relationship and a new registration system has been established.

Medical negligence

Unfortunately, complaints by patients about their medical care have escalated very considerably, both in the United States and in other developed countries. Many such complaints are dealt with by the machinery of the National Health Service in the United Kingdom, both in hospital and general practice, and only a proportion proceed to civil litigation for damages. Of these, only a very small proportion, (probably about 5 per cent) actually reach courts of law, as the vast majority are settled out of court, because the plaintiff (patient) gives up the action voluntarily, because the patient's claim is found to have no substance in law, or because the (defendant) doctor's actions are obviously indefensible. It is only the more evenly balanced cases, where no agreement between the parties can be made, that are required to go before a judge for decision.

Although doctors can leave the legal aspects of such unfortunate events to their protection and defence societies, a brief overview of the legal situation helps the doctor to understand the process. Before a patient can succeed in a civil action against a doctor, three criteria must be satisfied:

1. That the doctor had a duty of care to the patient.
2. That there was a breach of this duty either by an act of commission or omission.
3. That the patient suffered physical, financial, or damage mental.

A duty of care is set up very readily and depends merely upon the intention of the doctor to act in a healing capacity, i.e. to diagnose and/or treat another person. That person need not be aware of the doctor's existence (as during an emergency upon an unconscious patient) nor need there be any contractual or financial agreement between them. Once a doctor assumes a caring role in relation to a patient, the duty of care is established. The only exceptions are where the doctor is acting in an administrative capacity or is performing a contractual duty for another party, such as a medical examination for an insurance policy or during a legal examination as a police doctor, etc.

The breach of the duty is self-explanatory and covers the whole range of medical practice. The most difficult part of establishing or denying negligent action is in differentiating a true accident or a genuine error of clinical judgement from a failure to discharge a proper duty of care, which is negligent. The only way in which the matter can be resolved is by peer review, in which other knowledgeable doctors of the same seniority and in the same speciality, give their opinion as to whether the actions or omissions of the accused doctor were in line with current medical practice. It should be noted that such peer opinions need not be unanimous, as there is such a broad range of differing practice in the medical profession. As long as a substantial body of practice approves the actions of the doctor, that is sufficient to validate the behaviour under dispute.

Finally, the patient must suffer damage, as the whole object of legal actions for negligence is to restore the patient as far as possible to the situation he or she was in before the effects of negligence. Thus, if there are no deleterious effects, no compensation can be claimed. Unfortunately, the compensation is termed 'damages', which may be confused with 'damage', which is the mental or physical disadvantage resulting from the negligence. Where no such damage develops, then there is no need for any legal remedy. For instance, if a general practitioner was negligently late in attending a call to a patient, who subsequently died, no damage would accrue if it could be shown that the earlier intervention of the doctor would have made no difference to an inevitably fatal outcome.

RISK MANAGEMENT IN MEDICINE

As already outlined, the majority of untoward events in medical practice are not negligent but are either pure accidents or errors of clinical judgement that could have been made by any doctor of that rank in that particular situation. The differentiation, which is often extremely difficult or even impossible, may not be known even to the doctor and, therefore, no admission of negligence should be made to the patient or their relatives at or soon after the event, this being a matter for the medical defence and protection societies and their lawyers. However, this is certainly not to say that the doctor should not express regret and sympathy for the event, which is quite different from acknowledging blame. One of the major factors in avoiding legal actions for negligence is the maintenance of the doctor–patient relationship. A significant number of negligence actions commence after a breakdown of this relationship and very many patients or their relatives will be forgiving and not initiate complaints where a sympathetic doctor expresses regret (although not admitting culpability) and shows a sympathetic and helpful attitude.

A number of general precautions, which mitigate against the likelihood of allegations of negligence, should be borne in mind by doctors throughout their clinical practice. Of course, different specialties have markedly different risk rates: the most vulnerable specialist is the obstetrician, mainly in relation to claims that brain-damaged babies who develop cerebral palsy were the result of negligence during childbirth, although recent scientific evidence has cast doubt on the proportion of such tragedies that are truly due to intrapartum factors.

The surgical professions are also in the front line of vulnerability. Accident and emergency departments are at the cutting edge of medical intervention and consequently suffer a high incidence of complaints, even though the emergency situation may be a frequent and legitimate explanation for untoward events.

Neurosurgery and cosmetic surgery are also high risk specialties, the latter particularly because the expectations of patients, especially in the private sector, may be unduly high. Anaesthesia is also a high-risk speciality, whereas dermatology, pathology, and psychiatry are less exposed, although no section of medicine is immune from complaint.

As protective measures, the most urgent requirement is for every doctor to have the constant support of an expert organization, which will provide specialized medical and legal advice and indemnity against legal costs and damages. In the United Kingdom and much of the world, including the Commonwealth and parts of Europe, the three British protection and defence societies, which are non-profit making mutual organizations, offer a unique service without which a doctor is risking professional ruination. Even though, since 1990, doctors in the National Health Service hospitals have financial indemnity provided by the state, this does not extend to general practice or private practice and does not cover any doctor outside their contractual employment with the Health Service. It does not cover issues of professional misconduct, coroners' inquests, disputes with employers, and a whole range of other matters other than the strictly limited indemnity within the hospital. In other countries, where these societies are not available, commercial insurance has to be obtained, often at great cost and without the expert medical component that is provided by the British orrganizations.

The second defensive mechanism apart from the maintenance of excellent doctor–patient relationship mentioned earlier, is the keeping of good clinical records. Many accusations of negligence are sustained not because they were true, but because the doctor's notes failed to contain any indication that some alleged omission was in fact performed. This is particularly true of emergency admissions and general practice visits, where the urgency of a situation overtakes the making of contemporaneous notes, although these should have been completed afterwards at the earliest opportunity. Notes should never be altered, especially when it is obvious on later inspection that the alteration or addition was made with the object of filling a gap in the record. Illegibility, the use of unintelligible abbreviation, and the inclusion of pejorative or even defamatory remarks all contribute to the difficulties of defending a doctor against allegations of malpractice.

CATEGORIES OF NEGLIGENCE

A famous judge once said that 'the categories of negligence are never closed', indicating that every new technique that is developed is a further potential source of error. In a chapter such as this, it is impossible even to begin cataloguing the danger areas, but the following occur with such depressing frequency that they should be particularly guarded against:

1. Failure or delay in attending a patient, usually in general domiciliary practice. Although the decision to attend is that of the doctor, failure to do so where serious or fatal complications occur, especially to children, is a common cause of complaint leading to negligence actions or even to disciplinary actions for professional misconduct.
2. Surgical errors include operating on the wrong patient because of confusion of names and notes, or operating upon the wrong limb, digit or even organ of the correct patient due to errors over left-, or right-sidedness of the lesion.
3. The sources of error in orthopaedic surgery and accident and emergency units are legion, but often concern fractures, either the missing of an actual fracture, especially the scaphoid bone or missing a severe head injury due to a lucid interval followed by serious or fatal consequences. Although it is not mandatory to obtain radiographs for every lesion seen in a casualty department, strict criteria for radiography must be established and maintained.
4. In operative surgery, usually in the abdomen, the retention of instruments and swabs is a 'hardy annual' in the annals of medical negligence.
5. Numerous actions occur in obstetrics and gynaecology over brain damaged infants following childbirth, and also for complications of termination of pregnancy, hysterectomy, and failed sterilization. Similarly, failed vasectomy in males is commonly dealt with by the protection societies.
6. On a more routine basis, many problems arise from the giving of injections and the introduction of needles and other invasive procedures for diagnostic or therapeutic purposes. Injections of the wrong substances, such as potassium chloride instead of water as a diluent, the wrong dosage of a whole range of drugs and the hazards of intrathecal injections make it mandatory for every doctor to consider carefully what is in a syringe before committing this to parenteral administration.
7. The operating theatre is naturally a focus for potential errors, apart from the retention of objects in operation sites mentioned above. Anaesthetic mishaps, usually hypoxic in nature or due to failure to monitor the patient adequately are regularly the source of expensive litigation. Errors in transfusion, paresis from splints, and burns from diathermy add to the list of operating room hazards.
8. As well as the more technical errors listed above, many complaints arise from failure of communication between doctors, so that the patient suffers because diagnostic or therapeutic information fails to be transmitted from one section of the caring team to another, usually between hospital and general practitioner or between different partners in a general practice. Once again the keeping of adequate records is a common thread running through many mishaps.

Examination of sexual offences

Although in the United Kingdom the examination of the victims of sexual offences is largely the province of the police surgeon or 'forensic physician', on some occasions a gynaecologist or Accident and Emergency doctor may be requested to carry out this duty. In other countries the procedure varies and, in many areas, virtually any doctor might be involved in such examinations.

Where serious injury has occurred, almost inevitably a hospital clinician, usually a gynaecologist will be involved. As now recommended for the examination of suspected child sexual abuse, a police surgeon together with the appropriate clinician (gynaecologist or paediatrician) might well conduct a joint examination. This is an extremely onerous duty and not one to be undertaken lightly. In areas where there is a police surgeon or a formal Rape Centre, then it is unlikely that any other doctor will be asked on an occasional basis to examine the victims of alleged sexual abuse. However, there are areas of the country where no experienced police surgeon is available or where other factors make it mandatory for the victim to come to a hospital, where the hospital staff will inevitably become involved in the procedure. Some guidelines can be offered for the conduct of an examination, although it is emphasized again that this is a specialized task and, wherever possible, should be left to those with considerable experience.

Because of the highly unsatisfactory circumstances of former years, arrangements have been set up, in the United Kingdom and other advanced countries for special 'rape suites', either in hospitals or police stations, where such examinations can be carried out with the minimum of embarrassment, indignity, and discomfort to the women concerned. It is essential that any examination be conducted in appropriate surroundings and, hopefully, the days of dingy 'examination rooms' in district police stations have been eliminated. Unless the police can provide adequate premises, then the doctor must insist on the examination taking place either in their own health centre or surgery or in hospital.

When a woman or girl of mature enough years to understand the situation presents with an allegation of a sexual offence, the doctor is present primarily as a carer and healer, but may also have a forensic function in obtaining evidence for a subsequent prosecution. It must be made clear at the outset to the victim what is entailed in the examination and the possible consequences, including a court appearance. Only a small proportion of women subjected to a sexual assault ever report to either a doctor or the police and, of these, a considerable number decline to allow the matter to go further. Unfortunately, even with the great improvements of recent years, women can be subjected to a lengthy and harrowing experience of criminal investigation and court appearance, so they must be given the opportunity to decline to co-operate in such a process if they so wish.

This aspect is separate from the medical examination to determine the presence of any injuries that may need treatment and also the possible sequelae of venereal infection, pregnancy, and psychological damage.

Where a woman presents herself to a doctor, either in general practice or hospital, the doctor must assume that she has come for purely medical reasons, but must enquire of her whether she wishes to take the matter further in respect of a criminal investigation and charges against an assailant. If she does not, then the matter proceeds on purely medical lines, but if she does so wish to press charges then the police must be notified immediately so that they can be present or represented from the outset together with the facilities for collecting forensic evidence.

In the other type of instance, a woman or girl will be brought to a doctor (often under standing contractual arrangements with a police surgeon) for examination, in which case the forensic and medical aspects are combined from the outset.

However presenting, after an explanation of the procedure and consequences, the doctor must obtain informed consent from the woman or, in the case of a young girl too immature to provide consent, from the parents or guardians. Such consent should be witnessed by an independent person other than a close relative.

The choice of doctor undertaking the examination may be difficult. In the present climate, there is a strong call for women to have the absolute right to demand examination by a female doctor, although this is not always possible from sheer logistical or geographical reasons. Even in the police surgeon community, there are insufficient women police surgeons who have the necessary technical and court expertise, compared with a larger number of male police surgeons. Wherever possible the woman's wishes must be acknowledged, but cannot always be conceded, especially as time may be of the essence in the examination of a sexual offence. Where a male doctor is the examiner, a chaperone is absolutely essential. The victim often has a relative or friend present, but there should also be an independent chaperone such as a woman police officer or preferably a member of the nursing or surgery staff.

Before the examination commences, it is wise to enquire whether the clothing that the woman is wearing was that worn at the time of the alleged offence. Many women immediately bathe and change clothing after a sexual assault and obviously different clothing is useless for forensic examination, as the original clothing should be sent to the laboratory. If the clothing worn was that in place at the time of the assault, a change of clothing should be obtained from the patient's home, as the original clothing will be retained for forensic examination. Attention to this point can save considerable embarrassment of having a woman left dressed only in an examination room gown whilst more appropriate garments are obtained.

If the examination is to be conducted with police investigation and prosecution in mind, then the police will provide a 'sexual offences kit' for the collection and retention of laboratory specimens. In addition, the usual containers and swabs for clinical investigation should be to hand, for the taking of blood and swabs for possible venereal infection.

Before the examination commences, the doctor should take a full general history. The purpose of this is partly to establish a friendly and sympathetic rapport with the patient and also to assess her emotional state. If the girl is very young, she should not be distressed by long questioning about the circumstances, but these should be obtained from the adult parent or companion present. With a more mature woman, careful questioning should be made to ascertain her version of the events, as well as general details of her health, and menstrual and pregnancy history, etc. Part of the purpose of this is to arrive at an opinion about her probable truthfulness, mental state, and general awareness of sexual matters. This is not 'playing detective', as would be the case in dealing with a homicide, but a legitimate part of the examination. In spite of objections by some women's organizations, an enquiry into the recent sexual history is essential, as otherwise legitimate consenting intercourse in recent days cannot be separated from the effects of a sexual assault. An important part in examination is the detection of semen in the vagina, but unless the examiner knows of legitimate sexual activity in the preceding day or two, no interpretation of this finding can be made, as spermatozoa can be recovered from the vagina from 24 to 72 h after intercourse, and even longer from the cervical canal.

The general demeanour of the complainant, including her appearances, such as dishevelled clothing, soiled skin and clothing, hair, state of agitation or emotion, should be noted. In the case of teenage girls, her apparent age should be compared with her stated age, as well as an opinion as to her maturity, mode of dress, and make-up, compared with her real age. The latter points are of particular legal relevance if a girl is between 13 and 16 years of age. Although the minute scientific details of the examination are the concern of the forensic laboratory, the doctor is the only person with the opportunity to observe the original state of the clothing including disorder of the way it is worn, possibly indicating violent displacement or hurried replacement. The woman should undress on a sheet of brown paper provided in the forensic kit, so that any foreign material such as dirt from the scene of assault, foreign hairs, etc. are collected for laboratory examination. Although this should be done under the direct observation of a female doctor, it is probably better that in the case of a male doctor the policewoman or other female chaperone should supervise this more embarrassing part of procedure. The woman then wears an examination gown for the remainder of the process.

A general clinical examination should then be conducted, starting well away from the perineal area. This is partly for its own value and partly to reassure the victim; an abrupt and immediate genital examination is to be deprecated, especially in an overwrought and possibly hysterical young woman.

The whole body should be examined for injuries, soiling, and blood and seminal stains, particular attention being paid to the back of the upper arms, the shoulder blades and buttocks, as well as the more obvious places such as thigh, neck, face, and breasts. Where the offence has allegedly taken place out of doors, there may be grass, leaves, or mud smears on the buttocks or back.

Teeth marks or suction petechiae from the assailant's mouth may be found on the neck or breasts or abdomen and there may even be a laceration of the nipples by teeth. Bruising of the lips and even tearing of the inner aspect against teeth may be found due to blows or rough kissing. If any bites or mouth marks are suspected, photographs and preferably the attendance of a forensic dentist may be required, as the teeth marks may be matched against a possible assailant. If fresh and unwashed, it is advisable to rub a water-moistened throat swab on the mouth marks to retrieve any dried saliva, which may be matched against the blood group of a secreting assailant.

Any suspicious seminal stains on the thighs or other part of the body should be cut away from hairs if dried or captured by moistened swab if on the skin surface. A similar swab should be taken from the mouth if there is the slightest possibility of oral penetration. The latter may not be mentioned or admitted by the woman, but must always be borne in mind as a possibility.

After complete examination of the rest of the body surface, the genitalia should be examined. A good light is essential and either a left lateral or a lithotomy position used on the examination couch. The use of stirrups is particularly embarrassing and has largely been discontinued. Bruises, scratches, and stains on the thighs and buttocks should be looked for. The pubic hairs should be examined and any matted stains or foreign material cut away and preserved. The pubic hairs should be combed out as non-matching male pubic hair may be present. The police forensic kits contain fine tooth combs for this purpose. A sample of pubic hair should be plucked out at the end of the examination and all samples carefully labelled, packed and retained, although an accompanying police officer is usually responsible for this task.

The vulva should be inspected and palpated for scratches, swelling, bruises, or other traumatic or natural lesions. Vulval, low vaginal and high vaginal swabs should be taken and any visible fluid aspirated with a pipette before any digital examination is made. Smears on microscope slides should not be made unless there is to be a delay of more than a day or so in forwarding the swabs to the forensic laboratory. The state of the hymen and vaginal orifice should be examined. Considerable experience is required to differentiate between the many types of hymen, but any practitioner should be able to recognize a recent tear, with the signs of acute injury, such as tenderness, swelling, and bleeding. It may be difficult or impossible to distinguish lesser degrees of assault from normal intercourse when the only signs are slight reddening of the introitus. The degree of dilatation of the vaginal orifice should be estimated and it should be obvious if the woman or girl has been used to sexual intercourse. Although the state of the hymen is emphasized in most textbooks on the subject, in all but young girls it is frequently of little use in evaluating forceful intercourse unless there are acute traumatic lesions present. The hymen can be examined by inserting a specially designed glass globe on a stem, sometimes with transillumination, which is then partially withdrawn so that the hymen is spread around its circumference.

The use of a speculum is somewhat controversial as some examining doctors consider it not appropriate, especially in children and young girls. However, it undoubtedly gives the best view of the vaginal interior, especially where deep damage is suspected.

Naturally, any serious injuries become a matter for gynaecological treatment, irrespective of any forensic considerations.

It must always be borne in mind, especially in sexually mature women, that forceful sexual intercourse without consent may be perpetrated without any physical signs whatsoever in the genitalia. In such cases, better evidence might be available from more general injuries such as restraint bruising on the arms, abrasions, soiling, and bites, etc.

Other samples are usually taken, including fingernail clippings, in case the woman has managed to scratch the assailant and gather foreign skin or fibres, etc. underneath the nails. Blood samples must be taken both for DNA grouping of the woman, alcohol analysis, and any further samples for clinical requirements. For DNA, two EDTA tubes of 5 to 10 ml volume are required and for alcohol, about 5 ml should be placed in a bottle containing fluoride for preservation. These are usually present in the forensic kit. It is usual to take an anal swab, even if there is no admission of anal penetration, and also a saliva sample for control purposes compared with that of the assailant.

At the conclusion of the examination, a full, comprehensive, and contemporaneous report must be written. Dates and times are essential and also names of those present at the examination.

All samples taken by the doctor should be recorded and there are usually special police labels available for each, which must be signed and dated by the doctor who retrieves the samples.

The final matter is the interpretation of the findings and this may be the most difficult part of the procedure. The following questions need to be addressed:

1. Is there evidence of recent sexual activity?
2. Is there evidence that this was forceful– beyond enthusiastic consenting intercourse?
3. Did ejaculation occur?
4. Are there other injuries present?
5. Are any of these sexual in nature (breasts, pubis, etc.)?
6. Is there evidence of anal or oral intercourse?
7. Is there evidence of restraint or resistance, in the form of bruising or abrasions?

In addition to these forensic matters, the doctor must also be concerned about possible pregnancy and the venereal infection. Consideration must be given to offering the 'morning after pill', such as Eugynon 50, if the intercourse took place within 72 h. An alternative would be the fitting of an intrauterine device within the first 5 days. Later, follow-up for the possibility of venereal infection should be made, initiated by the sending of swabs for microbiological examination at the time of examination. The whole problem of rape counselling must be considered and offered where appropriate.

This account is necessarily a brief abbreviation of an extremely complex and difficult problem and as stated at the outset, wherever possible, is best left to those who habitually deal with sexual offences.

Medical reports

Doctors are frequently asked for reports on their patients, from a whole range of sources. In the medicolegal context, such requests may come from lawyers, police, courts, public prosecutors, coroners, insurance companies, etc. All such requests must be viewed very seriously, as a doctor's pronouncements may have far-reaching effects in both criminal, civil, insurance, and other official proceedings. For a doctor to make a false or reckless statement may be both a criminal offence and one that may involve him or her in disciplinary proceedings, with potential loss of the right to practise medicine.

In general, medical reports are often of poor quality, even those emanating from senior doctors. Certain guidelines can greatly improve the quality of such reports which may be of vital interest to the patient or his dependants.

Before submitting any report on a patient, one over-riding consideration has to be addressed—consent. With very few exceptions, no information may be released to a third party without the informed consent of the patient or, if dead, their next of kin or legal representatives. It can be a matter for professional disciplinary action, as has been taken by the General Medical Council on a number of occasions in the United Kingdom if a doctor releases information without the prior approval of the patient. Even where it might be assumed that there is implied consent, this cannot be taken for granted. For example, although police frequently require statements from doctors concerning criminal injuries after assault these cannot be provided as a matter of course. Although in most cases the injured victim is only too willing to provide information that could lead to the prosecution of their assailant, in family disputes, especially between husband and wife (or partners), there may be no wish to pursue the other party and the doctor cannot therefore assume that they can provide a report without prior reference to the patient.

In general, it is for the party requiring the report to obtain the consent. Where a doctor receives a request from a lawyer requesting a medical report on a patient, the doctor must be scrupulous in determining whether that lawyer acts for the patient or for some other person or organization. Unless the requesting letter specifically states that either the lawyer is representing that patient or that the patient's consent has been obtained, the doctor should abstain from offering any report until the matter is clarified. In hospital situations, junior doctors should never offer reports without reference to either their consultant or to the hospital administration. Patients who are asked for consent for such statements must be made aware of the reason for the request and not be misled by default into thinking that this is related to their clinical management.

Police have no more right to obtain a statement from a doctor than anyone else and, in the United Kingdom a Code of Practice has been drawn up between the Association of Chief Police Officers and the British Medical Association to try to regularize the relationship between police officers and medical staff in the obtaining of statements concerning injured patients.

Once consent has been obtained, the doctor must next look at the reason for which the report has been requested. Many medical reports are of little or no value because the response of the doctor is not appropriate to the requirements of the party requesting the report. This is often the fault of the requestors, including lawyers, for not being sufficiently clear about the nature of the information they need. Where the doctor cannot discern from the instructing letter the nature of the assistance required, they should contact the writer and request more specific instructions. This is particularly so in matters of opinion rather than fact (see below).

Medical witnesses fall into two main groups, the professional and the expert witness. The professional witness is a witness as to fact, as might any citizen be witnessing an assault or road accident, although the facts are medical in nature. Junior doctors, certainly up to the middle training grades in hospital service, are almost inevitably professional witnesses and should not venture into the expert witness field. A professional witness will relate actual facts, such as the condition of a patient on admission, the time and date of admission, the description of injuries or disease processes present, and the chronology and extent of treatment and progress. These are factual matters, which should be given without comment.

The other category is the expert witness, usually of consultant or higher academic status, although doctors in senior training grades may also venture some distance down this path. The vital difference between the professional witness and the expert witness is that the latter gives opinion instead of, or in addition to, factual evidence. For example, a pathologist may give factual evidence about their findings at a post-mortem examination but then go on to express an opinion about how certain injuries may have caused death. A pure expert witness is someone who will give an opinion upon facts generated by others.

The form of the report varies greatly with the nature of the case but in general follows the conventional clinical pattern of history-taking and examination. The time and place of the examination is extremely important, especially if the report is being made for the police or prosecution. A brief history should be offered as given by the patient, because although this may be deemed heresay in some legal proceedings, it is still direct evidence of what the doctor learned during the examination.

Next a full description of physical findings should be made, this varying greatly according to the nature of the examination. If concerned with injuries, there is a need to adhere to conventional descriptions of the lesions. This is something done poorly by many doctors, who confuse abrasions, contusions, and lacerations. An abrasion is a surface injury that does not penetrate the full thickness of the skin, a bruise is extravascular leakage of blood beneath the skin and a laceration is a tear through the full thickness of the skin. Knife wounds are a subclass of lacerations caused by a cutting edge and, where longer than the depth, may be termed slashes; where deeper than the length they may be termed stab wounds.

Unless the report is being generated solely for other doctors, it is essential that medical jargon and obscure medical terminology be avoided. Where reports are intended for lawyers, police, or the courts, etc. commonplace terms should be employed. For example, abrasions may be called 'grazes', contusions called 'bruises', lacerations termed 'tears' and incised wounds 'cuts'.

Whatever the nature of injuries, their size and position should be recorded carefully, another frequent defect in medical reports. The dimensions of a bruise or abrasion should be measured in two axes and a description given of the appearance, such as linear markings in a brush abrasion or the colour changes in a bruise. Slashes or stab wounds should be measured as to length and a description of the wound margins offered. The position of all injuries should be described by reference to nearby anatomical landmarks. For example, the centre of a stab wound on the chest should be measured from the midline and from the clavicle, jugular notch, internipple line, or costal margin, according to the most convenient landmark. Too many medical reports merely record vague descriptions such as 'there was a scratch on the left side of the back'. As many months or even years may elapse between the examination and the matter coming to court or other legal scrutiny, it is essential to have a full and accurate report; memory becomes useless in trying to reconstruct the events at a later date.

For more clinical reports, the report follows the usual style and format of a clinical record in hospital or general practitioner notes. Indications of relevant ancillary investigations should be incorporated. If the report is of the expert variety, then opinions about causation and prognosis may be required. As stated at the outset, it is essential to learn from the person requesting the report what features are actually important, as otherwise a mass of redundant fact and opinion may obscure the essentials, or even replace them.

Confidentiality of such reports must be maintained scrupulously and the report delivered only to the person commissioning it. No copies should be supplied to any other person without the consent of the commissioning authority.

Medical confidentiality and consent

Within the Hippocratic Oath there is a firm commitment of all doctors to maintain strict confidentiality concerning the patient's clinical condition. It is sometimes erroneously called 'medical secrecy', implying some conspiracy on the part of doctors, but it must always be remember that the confidentiality belongs to the patient, not the doctor, who is merely the custodian of the patient's right to confidentiality.

Apart from being an ethical duty, confidentiality is an essential tool in medical practice; without the public awareness of a doctor's dedication to silence, many patients would be reluctant to provide a full history, to the detriment of their diagnosis and treatment. Confidentiality does not cease with death and a doctor must not release any information other than that which is in the public domain, such as information revealed in court proceedings, including an inquest.

Confidentiality may only be broken in one of the following circumstances:

1. With the consent of the patient or his/her legal representative. Indeed, not only may the doctor release information at the patient's request, but he *must* divulge it, as the information is not theirs to either withhold or divulge.

2. There is no automatic right of relatives to be told medical facts about a patient except in the case of children, although the age at which this becomes legitimate is rather hazy in English law and depends more upon the maturity of the child than a chronological age. However, it is obviously perverse for a doctor to refuse to tell a spouse or partner that a person has a certain medical condition, especially when that person is in a caring role. More distant relatives have no right of information and, where the medical condition has certain attributes, usually connected with sexual matters, venereal disease, pregnancy, or abortion, the patient may not wish the doctor to tell even the closest relative. In certain situations, where the relative is the carer, the doctor may have to use their own judgement as to disclosure, if the patient's condition and prognosis may depend upon revelation. However, as always, the doctor may be required to justify their decision not to accede to the patient's insistence on confidentiality.

3. As a statutory duty, many medical conditions have to be notified to some official authority under the law of the land. Examples are births and deaths, various infectious diseases, occupational conditions, drug dependence, termination of pregnancy etc. Here the doctor has no choice, as it would be a statutory offence not to notify such matters and the consent of the patient is not required.

4. All courts of law, whether civil, criminal, or coroners' inquests, have a legal right to demand that the doctor reveals any medical information whatsoever if the doctor is called as a witness under oath. On rare occasions, the doctor may demur on grounds of medical confidentiality, but if the judge or coroner insists, then further reluctance to divulge is at the risk of being in contempt of court, with a fine or even imprisonment as the penalty. No legal action can be taken against the doctor who reveals medical information at the behest of a court, as this is absolutely privileged and carries no risk of a subsequent action for defamation or breach of confidence.

5. In the community interest in some situations, the doctor's ethical duty of confidentiality may conflict with their duty as a citizen. Where the doctor has information about a criminal offence, he or she must decide whether they feel the public good outweighs the need for confidentiality. This would occur occasionally in matters such as theft or fraud, etc., but may be relevant if the doctor knows of serious assaults, rapes, or even homicide, which may be repeated by a person they know to be dangerous, psychopathic, or mentally disordered.

    More often, the danger to the community is less dramatic, but may involve a public transport driver whom the doctor deems unfit to continue that employment. The patient may be reluctant to alter their employment voluntarily or to undergo further examination at the behest of their employer. If the doctor cannot persuade the employee to do this, then in certain situations the doctor should communicate their fears to a person directly involved in the situation, preferably another doctor. An industrial medical officer might be the obvious recipient of such information, but if no such person exists then the managing director of the employing firm should be informed. Where a doctor has a patient who develops epilepsy or fits, there may be the need to communicate with the medical officer of the Driving and Vehicle Licence Centre if the patient cannot be persuaded to voluntarily acknowledge their unfitness to drive.

    Sometimes infectious diseases may require a breach of confidentiality, but most situations such as this are covered by statutory laws, especially where persons involved in food handling are concerned. A more common situation concerns child abuse, and here the over-riding consideration is the safety of the child concerned. In all these cases, the doctor may have to justify their breach of confidentiality to various bodies, including the General Medical Council. When in doubt, he or she is strongly advised to consult colleagues, especially more senior doctors and, in the case of child abuse, specific consultants such as paediatricians. Where any doubt remains, the doctor's own protection or defence society can provide expert advice.

The problem of confidentiality in young persons is extremely difficult and, in the United Kingdom, has been more complicated by the Gillick case, which went to the House of Lords for decision. This concerned a mother who forbad a Health Authority to offer contraceptive advice to her teenage daughters, but opened much wider issues in relation to confidentiality in adolescence and children. Although the age of majority in the United Kingdom is 18, the Family Law Reform Act (1969) allows people of 16 years and over free choice in matters of medical treatment, and thus confidentiality must be maintained between such young persons and the doctor in the usual way. Below 16, the issue is less clear since the Gillick case, but the current advice of the General Medical Council is that where a child below the age of 16 consults a doctor for advice or treatment and is not accompanied by a parent or guardian, the doctor must particularly have in mind the need to foster and maintain parental responsibility and family stability. Before offering advice or treatment the doctor should be satisfied, after careful assessment, that the child has sufficient maturity and understanding to appreciate what is involved. For example, if the request is for treatment for a pregnancy or contraceptive advice, the doctor should be satisfied that the child has sufficient appreciation of what is involved in relation to his/her emotional development, family relationships, problems associated with the impact of pregnancy and/or its termination, and the potential risks to health of sexual intercourse and certain forms of contraception at an early age.

If the doctor is satisfied of the child's maturity and ability to understand, they must none the less seek to persuade the child to involve a parent in the consultation. If the child continues to refuse, the doctor must decide in the patient's best medical interest whether or not to offer advice or treatment. The doctor should, however, respect the rules of professional confidentiality. If the doctor is not so satisfied, they may decide to disclose the information learnt from the consultation: if the doctor choses to do this, the patient should be informed accordingly, and the doctor's judgement concerning disclosure must always reflect both the patient's best medical interest and the trust the patient places in the doctor.

CONSENT

No mentally competent adult (over 16) person need seek or accept medical diagnosis and treatment if they do not wish it. Thus all medical intervention must be preceded by consent, otherwise the actions of the doctor may constitute an assault.

Consent is basically identical in all its forms, but there are several categories, which have differences in practical terms within a doctor's professional activities. Most medical practice is conducted with implied consent, where the very fact of a patient presenting before the doctor implies that he or she is willing to undergo diagnosis and treatment to a certain level. This implied consent covers the usual diagnostic procedures of history-taking, palpation, percussion, auscultation, and general physical examination. Even here, consent is usually taken further by the conventions of polite behaviour, in that the doctor will usually request the patient to remove their shirt or blouse with the explanation that they wish to listen to their chest, etc.

For more invasive techniques of diagnosis or treatment, specific consent has to be obtained for each item of practice. In the taking of a blood sample, for example, the doctor must explain what they wish to do and the reasons for doing it, which the patient is quite entitled to reject. This obtaining of specific consent is known as express consent, and holds good only for one particular action. The old practice of bygone years where a 'blunderbuss' consent was obtained on admission to hospital for all further procedures is now defunct as part of the patronizing attitude of medicine, which by now should be extinct.

Express consent is often obtained in writing, almost always where a general anaesthetic or surgical procedure of any significance is contemplated. Written consent is no better in law than oral consent, but is much easier to validate if a dispute arises. Witnessed oral consent can be difficult to prove later if the witness has vanished and documentary evidence, signed by the patient and witnessed by another party, is at least a permanent record to be kept in the medical notes.

However, consent of any type, whether written or not, is invalid if it is not informed consent. This concept has become much more important in recent years, and has been the subject of many legal actions where the patient claims that they did not give proper consent because they did not understand the implications of the procedure due to a failure of the doctor to sufficiently explain them.

All consent, therefore, must be obtained in the light of a proper explanation given in understandable language, which explains the nature of the procedure proposed and the major risks associated with it. This applies not only to matters such as surgical operations, anaesthetics, or complex invasive diagnostic procedures, but also to the use of certain drug regimes that carry the risk of side-effects.

The degree to which a patient should have a full explanation varies greatly according to the complexity of the proposed procedure, to the doctor's estimation of the ability of the patient to understand the explanation, and to the relative risks involved. Although in North America it is common for virtually every possible risk to be explained, several legal cases in the United Kingdom, such as the Sidaway case, which reached the House of Lords for decision, has settled on major risks as the criterion for explanation. A balance has to be made between the fullness of information and the possibility of frightening off a patient by reciting every risk, including remote risks. For example, every surgical operation carries the risk of a fatal pulmonary embolism, but it would be obviously nonsensical and dangerous to recite this to every patient with acute appendicitis requiring an emergency operation. The legal cases that have established that peer review, i.e. the opinion of practising doctors in the same specialty, should be used to decide what risks should be explained to the patient in relation to any given procedure and, although such opinions vary considerably, the consensus is that exceptional risks need not be explained to the patient. However, every doctor has to make up his or her own mind on each occasion as to the degree of information that must be offered before consent can be considered to be valid.

Consent is obtained in the usual way from conscious, mentally sound persons over 16 years of age without any complications concerning the ability to give valid consent. Where procedures involving marital relations are involved, such as sterilization and termination of pregnancy, the wishes of the spouse are usually sought, although are not legally necessary.

Below the age of 16 years, consent should be sought from the parent or guardian, except in the case of emergencies. However, this does not invalidate consent from some persons below the age of 16 years, if that person is judged by the doctor to have sufficient maturity of mind to appreciate the significance and risks of the proposed procedure. It is always good medical practice for a doctor to make every effort to involve the parents or someone *in loco parentis* in the decision.

Where the parent or guardian of a person below the age of 16 years refuses permission for an urgent or diagnostic therapeutic procedure, the doctor's position is governed partly by personal ethics and partly by a legal mechanism, although in recent years this is usually subservient to the doctor's decision. The situation usually arises from religious objections, notably Jehovah's Witnesses in respect of blood transfusions. Where transfusion is held to be a life-saving matter, the doctor may proceed according to his or her own conscience and trust that the court will uphold his or her view if it should come to litigation. Again the doctor is strongly advised to seek the advice of fellow physicians, especially of more senior level. A formal alternative now rarely used is to seek a court order, even in an emergency situation, to transfer the custody of a child to a fit person under the Children Act (1989), who then authorizes the medical procedure. The Department of Health in the United Kingdom has directed that this procedure be abandoned and, if a doctor acts in good faith in urgent circumstances, they may rest assured that their protection or defence society and employing authority will uphold their decision, even against the parent's objections.

Consent obviously cannot be obtained where a patient is unconscious and, in an emergency situation, the doctor (preferably with the acquiescence of colleagues) should proceed to act in the patient's best interest. However, in such emergency situations only that which is necessary for the preservation of life and health should be undertaken, and no additional non-urgent procedures added on, a principle that applies to all medical practice where the patient has consented only to specific treatment. A surgeon should not be tempted to remove some other minor lesion *en passant*, during an anaesthetic given for the main consented condition.

In the case of mentally impaired persons, if the procedure is not related to the mental defect and the patient is able to understand the nature of the procedure and has given consent, then this is valid. Where the patient is unable to understand the nature of the illness and proposed treatment the legal situation is unclear, as no one, not even the relatives, court or judge can give consent on behalf of mentally disordered patients. What is usually done is that the doctor seeks approval of their actions from the guardian, relative, or responsible medical officer and can even apply to the court for a declaration of approval.

Where the procedure is related to the mental disorder of the patient, then complex rules exist under a variety of legal statutes including the Mental Health Act (1983) and the Mental Health (Hospital Guardianship and Consent to Treatment) Regulations (1983).

REFERENCES

Department of Health (1983). *The removal of cadaveric organs for transplantation – a code of practice including the diagnosis of brain death.* Department of Health, London.

Gee, D.J. and Mason, J.K. (1990). *The courts and the doctor.* Oxford University Press, Oxford.

Knight, B. (1991). *Forensic pathology.* Edward Arnold, London.

Knight, B. (1991). *Simpson's forensic medicine*, 10th edn. Edward Arnold, London.

Knight, B. (1992). *The legal aspects of medical practice*, 5th edn. Churchill Livingstone, Edinburgh.

McLay, W.D.S. (ed) (1990). *Clinical forensic medicine.* Pinter Publishers, London.

Mason, J.K. (1983). *Forensic medicine for lawyers*, 2nd edn. Butterworths, London.

Mason, J.K. and McCall Smith, R.A. (1991). *Law and medical ethics*, 3rd edn. Butterworths, London.

Section 30 *Sports medicine*

30 Sports medicine

A. YOUNG

INTRODUCTION

Man moves by muscular activity. Good clinical practice demands an understanding of exercise physiology. Indeed, the acute and chronic effects of exercise should be an integral part of the syllabus in every medical specialty. It would be both futile and inappropriate to try to cover all the medical aspects of exercise in a single chapter. This one will not deal with the health benefits of physical activity in general, comprehensively reviewed elsewhere. Instead, it will concentrate specifically on aspects of recreational exercise, or sport.

The increasing availability of leisure time and the growth of sports participation mean that sports medicine is now an important part of Western medical practice. It includes topics ranging from the enhancement of elite performance to ensuring safe participation despite the presence of disease or disability. The particular topics to be considered in this chapter are sudden cardiac death, the management of sport-related injuries, and the clinical physiology of endurance sports.

Sudden cardiac death
FREQUENCY

Sudden death during sport tends to attract the attention of the press but is, in fact, very rare. Vigorous exercise carries only a very small absolute risk; a study from Rhode Island gave a figure of approximately 1 death per 7600 middle-aged joggers, half of whom had a premortem diagnosis of ischaemic heart disease. Nevertheless, this was still seven times the death rate during sedentary activities. A Seattle study supported these figures (Table 1) but also put the increased risk during exercise into perspective. Thus, although vigorous physical activity carries a transiently increased risk of sudden cardiac death, this is greatest in those who are habitually least active and is outweighed in those who are habitually most active by a decreased overall risk.

PREVENTION

Exercise electrocardiography has been advocated as a screening procedure for all middle-aged sportsmen. Those who support such a course admit that an appreciable number of those at risk would not be identified but point out that, among asymptomatic men, subsequent overt coronary disease is 10 to 20 times more common in those with an abnormal exercise ECG. The other side of the coin, however, is that, among asymptomatic men, more than 70 per cent of those with an abnormal exercise ECG will have arteriographically normal coronary arteries, normal thallium perfusion scintigraphy, and will not develop overt coronary disease within the next 5 years. To have a chance of postponing the death of one asymptomatic middle-aged jogger per year, one would have to perform at least 15 000 tests, 10 per cent of which would be abnormal. This implies at least 1000 false-positives, an epidemic of iatrogenic cardiac handicap.

Medical evaluation is not a prerequisite for exercise training unless there are symptoms suggestive of myocardial ischaemia, strongly positive risk factors for coronary disease, a family history of premature sudden death or dysrrhythmias, or a personal history of exercise-induced syncope. Instead, anyone unaccustomed to vigorous exercise should be taught that its intensity should at first be modest and should then increase only gradually. The exercising public should also be taught how to recognize symptoms suggestive of underlying cardiac disease and to seek medical advice should they occur.

Sports injuries
DIRECT SOFT-TISSUE TRAUMA

Many sports put the participants at risk of direct trauma to muscle, tendon, ligament, and subcutaneous tissues by contact with the ground, the opponent, a ball or an opponent's bat or stick. Strict enforcement of the rules, a properly prepared playing surface, and tuition in the skills of the sport will prevent some of these injuries but they can never be avoided completely.

Acute treatment

Much of the pain and disability resulting from soft-tissue trauma is due not to the injury itself but to bleeding in and around the damaged tissues. Extravasated blood causes pain and limitation of movement at first by a space-occupying effect, then by causing local inflammation. Later, rehabilitation is hindered by fibrotic adhesions. Acute management concentrates on preventing this sequence of events.

The prevention of bleeding depends on ice, compression, and elevation (mnemonic 'ICE'). The local application of cold for 10 to 20 min will induce vasoconstriction and has the added benefit of relieving pain. Venous hydrostatic pressure at the site of injury is reduced by elevation of the injured limb for 2 to 24 h. Extravasation of blood is limited by a compression bandage applied immediately the ice is removed, and maintained for 2 to 24 h. Consider the contrast with the usual sequence of events after injury. After encouraging further bleeding by attempting to play on, the injured player retires from the game and maintains vasodilation by soaking in a hot bath. This is followed by a couple of hours standing, or at best sitting, enjoying a drink of vasodilating alcohol. Then they wonder why the sprained ankle is swollen, stiff, and painful the next day. Elevation is not only the simplest of the three measures to implement, it is probably also the most important and the most neglected.

Recovery is faster if a non-steroidal anti-inflammatory agent is administered, in full dosage, for the first 3 to 5 days after soft-tissue injury. There may be an advantage in starting treatment with a double strength 'loading' dose but this has not been demonstrated in a trial. A history of dyspepsia is, of course, a relative contraindication to the use of an anti-inflammatory.

Muscle and tendon

Acute management follows the standard general guidelines. Prompt orthopaedic advice should be obtained if there is complete or substantial rupture. A palpable defect is an indication for orthopaedic referral, although not necessarily for surgery.

The patient with a large inter- or intramuscular haematoma should be immobilized for 24 to 48 h, if necessary by admission to hospital. Compression and immobilization of the elevated limb can be achieved by a padded compression bandage or by the evacuation of air from a flexible bag of polystyrene beads fitted snugly around it. On the rare occasions when decompression is required, this can be done with a large bore needle under ultrasonographic guidance.

Table 1 *The relative risk of sudden cardiac death during vigorous physical activity by middle-aged men with no clinically recognized coronary heart disease*

Source	Habitual frequency of high-intensity exercise	Overall (24-h) incidence of sudden cardiac death (per 10^8 person-hours)	Relative risk during high-intensity exercise	
			Mean	95% confidence limits
Thompson *et al.* (1982)	High or very high	Not known	3.5	2–13
Siscovick *et al.* (1984)	Very high	5	5	2–14
	High	6	13	5–32
	Low	14	56	23–131
	Nil	18	–	–

Ligament and joint

The same general guidelines apply. Complete rupture (as indicated by joint instability or subluxation) requires orthopaedic referral. It may be possible to demonstrate instability only by stress radiographs taken under anaesthesia. Orthopaedic advice should also be obtained if there is any block to knee movement, implying the possibility of meniscal injury.

The accumulation of fluid within the first hour after injury implies haemorrhage, most often due, in the knee, to partial or complete tears of the anterior cruciate ligament. Prompt orthopaedic referral is indicated, with a view to early arthroscopy. Remember that a torn joint capsule (e.g. a torn collateral ligament) may accompany the cruciate ligament injury and will allow blood to escape from the knee joint, making the haemarthrosis less obvious.

Rehabilitation

Absolute rest is usually inappropriate after the first 24 h. The indiscriminate use of plaster casts and similar devices is to be deprecated. Rather than immobilization, it is better to think in terms of activity that is selective, graded, and protected. A hinged brace may be helpful, allowing free movement within a predetermined range and plane.

The first aim is to preserve maximal movement and strength without disturbing the soft, new scar forming across the deficit in the torn tissue. As the scar matures, it is necessary to stimulate remodelling of its randomly oriented collagen into the organized orientation that will give maximal mechanical strength in the direction of future imposed stresses. This requires the regular controlled application of gradually increasing tension in the same direction(s). Isometric muscle contractions should be started 24 h after injury, gradually increasing in intensity. Passive movement should begin at the same time, gradually increasing in range and progressing to forceful but controlled stretch.

Before return to competition can be permitted, balance and coordination skills, both conscious and unconscious, must be relearned. This requires the careful introduction of controlled dynamic activity, increasing gradually in both intensity and complexity. Especially in the case of severe ligament injuries, the 'relearning' of skills may depend, in part, on the regeneration of sensory nerve endings.

Joint injury and muscle weakness

Rehabilitation may be complicated by severe weakness of muscles acting across damaged joints. This is due partly to atrophy and partly to reflex inhibition of anterior horn cells by afferent stimuli arising in and around the joint (Fig. 1).

Ultrasound scanning and computerized tomography have shown that thigh muscle atrophy after knee injury is so localized to the quadriceps that its severity cannot be predicted accurately from measurements of thigh circumference. It is not unusual for the quadriceps to shrink by 30 to 50 per cent. There is a widespread belief that vastus medialis is more susceptible to atrophy than the rest of the quadriceps. There is little

evidence for this; the atrophy is merely more obvious. It is also often said that vastus medialis is active only in the last 15 ° of extension. This too is false, although its activity is especially important towards full extension as it maintains patellar alignment. Inability to achieve full voluntary knee extension against gravity reflects quadriceps weakness and a mechanically disadvantageous position, not selective weakness of vastus medialis. Despite its severity, quadriceps wasting may be explained entirely by shrinkage of muscle fibres; simultaneous scans and biopsies suggest that there is no reduction in the number of muscle fibres. Full recovery of muscle mass should, therefore, be possible.

Reflex inhibition of quadriceps may be a very potent phenomenon. Even in the absence of perceived pain, a maximal effort may achieve only 10 per cent of the muscle's normal maximal activation. The experimental infusion of sterile saline into a normal subject's knee has a similar effect. Substantial inhibition may be produced by the infusion of as little as 20 ml, a volume that is barely detectable clinically.

The fact that the quadriceps may be severely inhibited in the absence of any perceived pain has considerable implications for the resumption of full sporting activity. Even an apparently trivial knee effusion may weaken the quadriceps sufficiently to increase greatly its susceptibility to further injury. A similar argument probably applies at other joints.

It is essential to treat the cause of the inhibitory afferent activity. In addition, there is some evidence that the preservation of muscle mass and strength may be enhanced by electrically stimulated muscle contractions; effectiveness may depend on the choice of stimulation frequency.

OVERUSE INJURIES

Growing public enthusiasm for sport, and for distance running in particular, has increased the frequency with which stress fractures and friction syndromes (peritendinitis, tenosynovitis, and periostitis) are

Fig. 1 'Vicious circles', of joint damage and muscle weakness. (Reproduced from Stokes, M. and Young, A. (1984). *Clinical Science*, **67**, 7–14, by permission of The Biochemical Society.)

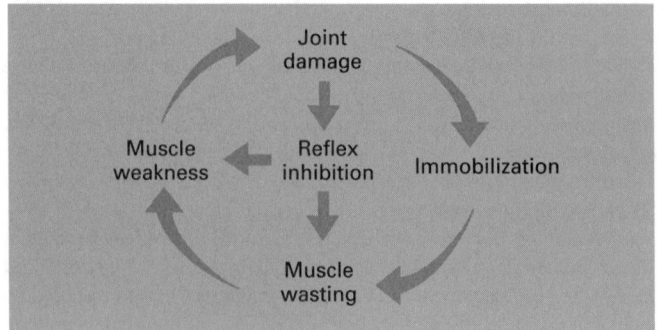

encountered in everyday practice (Fig. 2). To differentiate between them one must establish not only the pain's site, nature, distribution, speed of onset, and persistence after exercise, but also its timing in each stride, the effect of different speeds, terrains, and gradients, and the separate effects of joint angle and weight-bearing.

In the recreational athlete the explanation is usually 'too much too soon'. In the experienced elite performer it is 'too much, too long, and too often'. Other factors may be a change of footwear, terrain, or running speed. Overuse injuries are treated by rest, relief of local inflammation, and the gradual reintroduction of controlled and protected activity. If recurrence is to be prevented, it is important also to ensure that the future training load is controlled more carefully and adjusted more gradually. For example, changes from endurance running to sprinting, or from road to track must be gradual. Shoes should be examined for the adequacy of arch support and heel-cushioning. The squash racket's handle should be thickened to prevent further strains of the common extensor origin. The swimmer's arm action should be analysed to reduce impingement of rotator cuff tendons on the coracoacromial arch. The road runner should be advised to interpose the occasional run on grass.

Stress fracture

The repeated application of stress to a bone may result in a 'fatigue' or 'stress' fracture. The most common sites are the tibia, the distal fibula, and the second and third metatarsals. Femoral stress fractures are also encountered, neck and shaft fractures being about equally common. There is no history of acute trauma, there need not be any pain at rest, and radiographs may at first appear normal. Later, however, the radiographs may show callus formation (Fig. 3). A bone scintigram may be necessary to confirm the diagnosis when the radiograph is negative. A simpler 'bedside' test is the sharp pain produced by insonation of the suspect area of bone with a physiotherapist's ultrasound applicator. This may be particularly useful in order to distinguish between a tibial stress fracture and medial shin soreness. The latter is a common complaint, probably due to periostitis, presenting as localized pain and tenderness on the medial edge of the distal tibial shaft, requiring a shorter period of rest than a stress fracture and responding to oral anti-inflammatories, local steroid injection, and local ultrasound.

The immediate aims of treatment are to avoid complete fracture and to allow the bone to mend. This requires abstinence from running (Table 2). Weight-bearing should be avoided if it is painful. Casting is rarely required. Stress fractures of the femoral neck do not usually require internal fixation but orthopaedic advice should be obtained. Strength and endurance should be maintained by isometric exercises and by a change of activity, for example, to cycling (for metatarsal or fibular fractures) or to swimming.

Friction syndromes

The local inflammatory response to overuse may be evident, with pain, swelling, discoloration, warmth, and palpable (or even audible) crepitation. Sometimes, however, examination may reveal little or nothing. Re-examination immediately after a provocation run may then be helpful.

Fig. 3 (a) A normal radiograph does not exclude the possibility of a stress fracture. (b) A further radiograph 2 weeks later may show evidence of callus formation. (Reproduced from Young, A. and Green, R.W. (1985). *Update* **30**, 1132.)

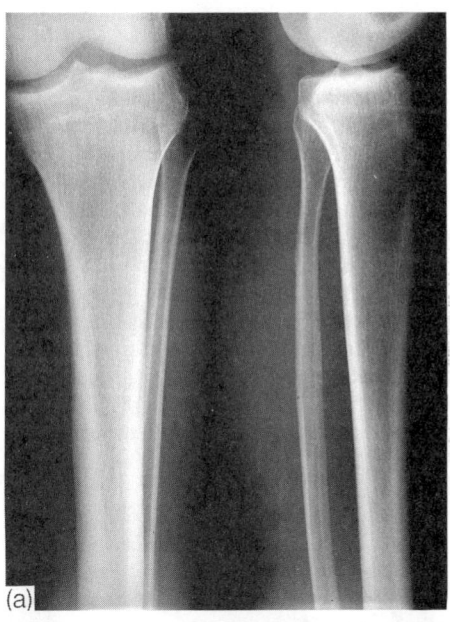
(a)

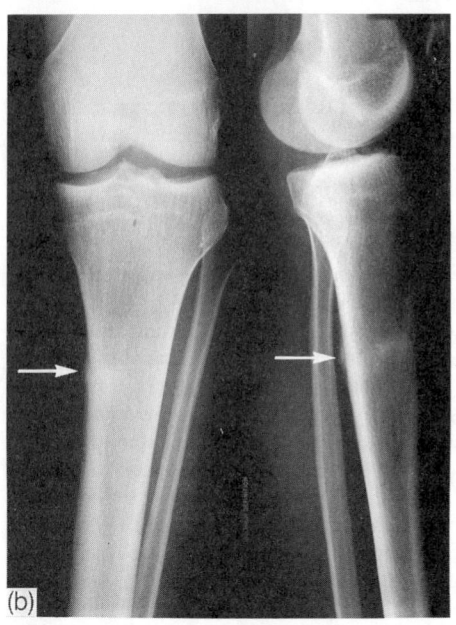
(b)

Fig. 2 Common sites of exercise injuries in joggers and runners. (Reproduced from Young, A. (1983) in *Preventive medicine in general practice* (ed. M. Gray and G. Fowler). Oxford, University Press, p. 160.)

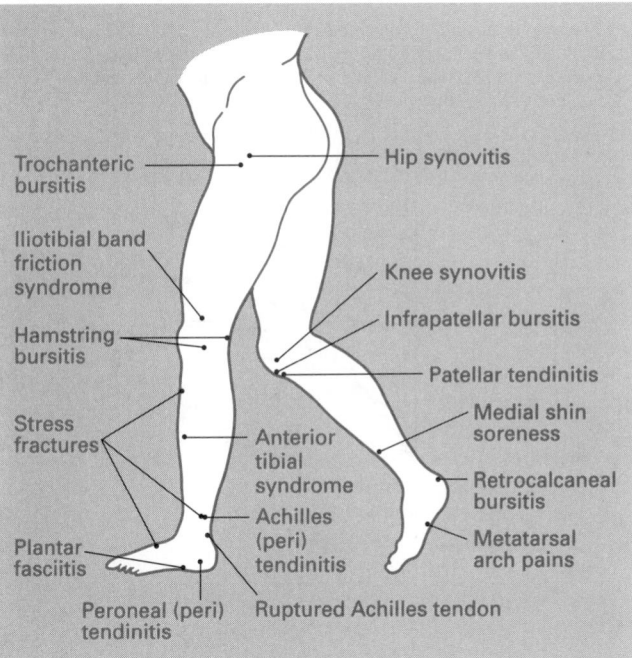

Trochanteric bursitis
Hip synovitis
Iliotibial band friction syndrome
Knee synovitis
Infrapatellar bursitis
Hamstring bursitis
Patellar tendinitis
Medial shin soreness
Stress fractures
Anterior tibial syndrome
Retrocalcaneal bursitis
Achilles (peri) tendinitis
Metatarsal arch pains
Plantar fasciitis
Peroneal (peri) tendinitis
Ruptured Achilles tendon

Table 2 *Stress fracture: recommended periods of abstinence from running*

Metatarsal	2–4 weeks
Fibula	3–4 weeks
Tibial shaft	4–6 weeks
Proximal tibia	8–10 weeks
Femur	3–4 months
Others	Individual

Reproduced from Orava, S. (1980). *British Journal of Sports Medicine* **14**, 40–4, with permission.

There are few patients in whom the problem cannot be resolved by an oral non-steroidal anti-flammatory drug, possibly a local injection of steroid, 1 to 2 weeks relative rest, stretching, isometric strengthening, and the gradual resumption of activity. (Note that injection into the substance of a tendon should usually be avoided lest it predispose to rupture.) Stretching is important to prevent local fibrosis and adhesions, especially within a stenosed tendon sheath. Surgical decompression is occasionally required to relieve achilles peritendinitis, synovitis of the extensor tendons of the oarsman's forearm, or iliotibial band friction.

The iliotibial band friction syndrome seems to cause unnecessary diagnostic difficulty, sometimes even being mistaken for a lesion of the lateral meniscus. Tendoperiostitis develops where the iliotibial band passes over the lateral femoral epicondyle and also has a small insertion into it. The pain usually starts after 1 or 2 miles and becomes steadily worse. It may radiate proximally to the thigh or distally to the tibia. Running downhill in heavy boots, in a tight circle, or with the foot inverted (e.g. to relieve a blister) may all be precipitating factors. Pain usually subsides rapidly after exercise but may still be felt for a day or two when using stairs. The diagnosis is confirmed by passively flexing the knee while maintaining thumb pressure over the lateral femoral epicondyle; tenderness is observed between 30 ° and 60 ° of flexion, as the iliotibial band passes between the bony prominence and the examining thumb.

Enthesitis

Inflammation at a tendon's point of insertion into bone (e.g. tennis elbow) is the result of repeated partial tears and subacute local inflammation. The principles of management include a combination of those for a tendon tear and for an overuse injury.

TRAUMA AND VIRAL INFECTIONS

There is no doubt that infection of the facial skin with herpes simplex virus (HSV) (see Section 7) is easily spread by abrasive contact during sport, especially between wrestlers or between rugby front-row forwards. Because the vesicular eruption is readily traumatized, it may be misdiagnosed. Viral shedding has probably ceased after 4 days but the referee has no independent corroboration of the duration of the eruption. Therefore, any crusted or vesicular eruption of the beard area should debar the player from participation until fully healed.

There is concern that several sports (notably wrestling, judo, rugby, and boxing) offer opportunities for the traumatic application of one player's blood to another player's broken skin, permitting the transfer of blood-borne viruses such as hepatitis B virus (HBV) and human immunodeficiency virus (HIV). No one should be allowed to compete with a freely bleeding injury, an uncovered open wound, or heavily blood-stained clothing. Rugby League and Union have introduced an imaginative rule to reduce the disadvantage caused by adherence to this principle. Although a player must leave the field until the bleeding has been staunched, his team is allowed to field a temporary substitute while he is absent without this counting against their quota of substitutes.

Endurance sports
AEROBIC FITNESS

Aerobic exercise is exercise whose oxygen requirements, after the initial adjustment period, are met in full while it is being performed. It can be continued, therefore, for periods upwards of 5 min. During a bout of aerobic exercise there are increases in pulmonary ventilation, cardiac output, and muscle blood flow so that the transport of oxygen from the atmosphere to the working muscles can be maintained at a level sufficient to meet the muscles' requirements. Repeated bouts of aerobic exercise produce adaptations throughout the oxygen transport system so that the oxygen demands of future exercise can be met with less disturbance of the resting state. This improvement in the homoeostasis of the oxygen transport system is associated with a reduced subjective perception of exertion.

It seems highly likely that regular vigorous aerobic activity can contribute to the prevention of coronary heart disease. There is no doubt that it improves exercise performance and exercise tolerance both in health and even in the presence of angina pectoris, intermittent claudication or chronic airflow obstruction, making the performance of ordinary everyday activities significantly easier. It improves glucose tolerance, contributes to weight control, and may even promote a sense of well-being and 'positive health'. These health benefits depend on the 'training' exercise being repeated regularly and being more vigorous than that encountered in everyday life. To induce a training effect, there must be overload. Hence the medical value of sport.

Measurement

The physiologist's traditional measure of aerobic fitness is the aerobic power or maximal oxygen uptake ($\dot{V}O_2$ max), i.e. the greatest rate at which a person can utilize atmospheric oxygen during continuous exercise. Aerobic training increases $\dot{V}O_2$ max: inactivity, such as bed rest, reduces it. These changes are quite rapid; 10 to 30 per cent changes may occur within a few weeks and, in extreme cases, a 100 per cent change may occur within 2 to 3 months of a major change in habitual physical activity (Fig. 4).

Most current tests of aerobic fitness, whether based on a treadmill, step-test or cycle ergometer, depend on measuring $\dot{V}O_2$ max, or some index from which it can be predicted. Even tests that measure the rate of heart rate recovery after exercise are indirect indicators of $\dot{V}O_2$ max. A typical $\dot{V}O_2$ max for a 20-year-old man might be 45 ml/kg.min. An

Fig. 4 Changes in maximal oxygen uptakes of five subjects before and after bed rest and at various intervals during training. (Reproduced from Saltin *et al.* (1968). *Circulation* **38**, Suppl. VII, by permission of the author and the American Heart Association.)

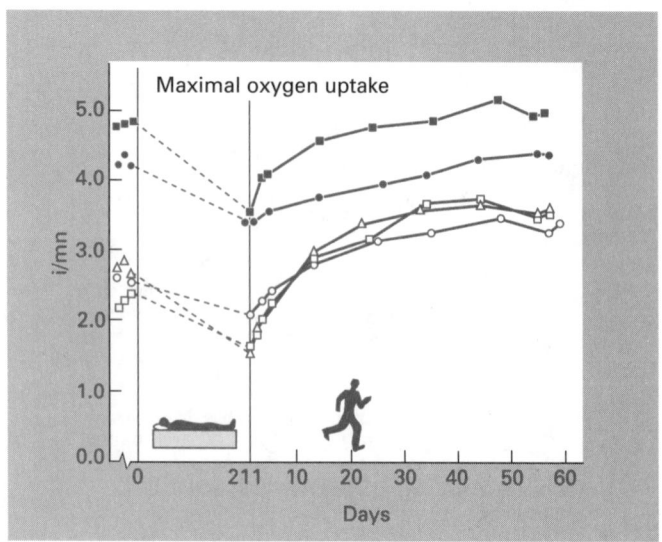

elite endurance athlete might have a value of 70 to 80 ml/kg.min. Less than half of the difference between these values can be ascribed to the effects of training. The rest reflects the elite performer's congenital advantage over the average person.

The ability to sustain exercise at a fixed submaximal proportion of $\dot{V}O_2$ max is probably a more sensitive indicator of an individual's state of training (i.e. the extent to which he or she has realized their personal potential for aerobic fitness). The improvements in performance experienced by the recreational runner or jogger probably owe more to improvement in this 'endurance' aspect of aerobic fitness than to any increase in $\dot{V}O_2$ max. For the elite performer its importance is that they may be able to utilize 75 to 85 per cent of their $\dot{V}O_2$ max throughout most of a marathon, instead of 60 to 70 per cent when only moderately trained. Other than by testing subjects to exhaustion, this aspect of aerobic fitness can be assessed by measuring the percentage of $\dot{V}O_2$ max that can be attained without stimulating anaerobic glycolysis, i.e. without significant accumulation of lactate. For example, a recreational runner's preparation for a marathon produced no change in $\dot{V}O_2$ max but the workrate corresponding to a blood lactate of 2 mmol/l increased from 75 per cent to 82 per cent of his $\dot{V}O_2$ max and the running speed corresponding to 2 mmol/l improved from 8.2 mph (7 min 19 s per mile) to 9.0 mph (6 min 40 s per mile).

Central mechanisms

Maximal oxygen uptake is closely linked with maximal cardiac output. As training produces little change in maximal heart rate (if anything, it reduces it), the increase in $\dot{V}O_2$ max with training is closely related to the increase in stroke volume. Not only does the heart get bigger, ventricular emptying during exercise becomes more complete. The trained person can achieve a greater cardiac output (and therefore a greater oxygen uptake) at any given heart rate.

Peripheral mechanisms

Trained muscles are better able to extract oxygen from their blood supply. The size and number of mitochondria and the density of muscle capillaries are increased, with the result that diffusion distances and capillary flow velocities are reduced. Thus the trained muscle requires a smaller total blood flow to achieve the same rate of oxygen consumption. The larger mitochondrial fraction is associated with a substantially increased muscle content of oxidative enzymes, ensuring that the muscle can utilize the enhanced availability of oxygen. These, incidentally, are the mechanisms behind the improvement in walking distance that the patient with stable intermittent claudication can achieve by training; the total blood supply to the claudicating muscle is not increased, only the muscle's ability to extract oxygen from it.

These changes are strictly local; they are more pronounced in the muscles, and even in the individual muscle fibres, which were used most during the training exercise. After one-legged training an exercise test with the trained leg shows the expected increase in $\dot{V}O_2$ max, in stroke volume, and in power output at a fixed submaximal heart rate. During exercise with the untrained leg, however, these indices remain close to their control values. Similarly, arm training reduces the heart rate response to arm work but not to leg work, whereas leg training reduces the heart rate response to leg work but not to arm work.

It is not long since the pendulum swung from central to peripheral factors as chief determinants of the upper limit to the training-induced improvement in $\dot{V}O_2$ max. The dominance of central factors, however, has been restored by experiments in which maximal exercise was performed by a limited mass of muscle. These have shown that muscle is capable of an oxygen uptake (per unit muscle mass) much greater than that achieved in whole body exercise. The current consensus is that the increase in $\dot{V}O_2$ max with training is limited by the improvement possible in circulatory haemodynamics, that is, by the increase in cardiac output and by its improved distribution. The prime role of the peripheral adaptations is believed to be metabolic. The peripheral adaptations allow greater use of lipid oxidation as a source of energy during prolonged

exercise, sparing the relatively limited glycogen stores and postponing fatigue. The shorter capillary–mitochondrion diffusion distance may facilitate free fatty acid uptake. The enzymes required for translocation of free fatty acids into the mitochondria and for their β-oxidation are increased. The increased capillary density also means that lipoprotein lipase activity is increased, possibly allowing greater utilization of circulating triglycerides during exercise. (Increased lipoprotein lipase activity may also explain the apparently 'cardioprotective' increase in the proportion of high density/low density lipoproteins seen in those undertaking regular vigorous aerobic exercise.)

CARBOHYDRATE METABOLISM
Glycogen loading

Carbohydrate is stored in the body as glycogen, usually about 100 g in the liver and 350 g in muscle. The quadriceps glycogen of trained volunteers is completely depleted after about 90 min of strenuous pedalling. The availability of muscle glycogen becomes limited during the second half of a marathon ('hitting the wall'). The runner then relies more on fat as the fuel and is unable to sustain the same high percentage of $\dot{V}O_2$ max. (In a 24-h run, power output falls to about 50 per cent $\dot{V}O_2$ max.)

It has been known for over 50 years that a low, or high, carbohydrate diet can substantially reduce, or increase, the time for which submaximal exercise (say about 70 per cent $\dot{V}O_2$ max) can be continued. The time to exhaustion when pedalling depends on the initial glycogen content of the quadriceps. Furthermore, if exercise to exhaustion is followed by 2 to 3 days on a diet rich in carbohydrate, the muscle glycogen store is not only restored but shows a 'rebound' effect, reaching double its normal concentration. A classic study used one-legged pedalling to demonstrate that glycogen depletion and rebound super-repletion are both confined to the muscle which has been exercised.

The typical elite marathon runner probably exhausts the muscle glycogen at least twice a week and can start a race with a supranormal muscle glycogen concentration by tapering training for 2 to 4 days before the race and eating a diet rich in carbohydrate (and with a correspondingly reduced protein content). Complex carbohydrate is preferred because slow absorption encourages glycogen storage rather than incorporation into fat.

Additional glucose
Before exercise

There is a strong temptation to consume sugar or glucose just before the start of endurance exercise. This is not a good idea, however, as it suppresses fatty acid mobilization and so hastens exhaustion of muscle glycogen. Fatty acid mobilization depends not only on circulating adrenaline (high levels before and during a race) but also on the progressive suppression of insulin release as the exercise proceeds. The latter mechanism is inhibited by the absorption of a carbohydrate load just before the start of the exercise. Easily digestible carbohydrate should be consumed no later than 3 h before the start.

Pre-exercise caffeine, as strong coffee, may enhance endurance performance by its lipolytic effect, increasing the availability of fatty acids to muscle. For many people, however, any benefit is more than counterbalanced by the disadvantages of its diuretic effect. Laboratory findings cannot always be applied in real life.

During exercise

Endurance is improved by the ingestion of glucose in the later stages of prolonged exercise, for example, after the first hour of a marathon. This does not cause secretion of insulin, perhaps because of the high circulating level of adrenaline. The effectiveness of oral glucose depends also on the rate of gastric emptying and the rate of intestinal absorption. The higher the carbohydrate concentration of the fluid, the slower the stomach empties. To try and give a high concentration of glucose may be counterproductive. During heavy exercise the maximal rate of gastric emptying is about 25 ml/min. Thus, to try and give a large volume of dilute glucose solution may not be effective. It seems best to take small frequent drinks of a solution containing 5 g of glucose/100 ml water, aiming to achieve 1 l/h.

SOME EXERCISE-INDUCED 'ABNORMALITIES'
Amenorrhoea
Oligomenorrhoea and amenorrhoea are more common among distance runners than among non-exercising women. Contributory factors include low body weight, loss of body fat, and perhaps also the emotional stresses associated with a time-consuming training schedule and with competition. It seems clear, however, that exercise itself has an independent effect. Weekly mileage correlates positively with the prevalence of amenorrhoea and negatively with the length of the luteal phase of the menstrual cycle. In some individuals, menstruation may be restored by an injury-induced break from exercise even if weight gain is carefully avoided. The most telling evidence, however, comes from a prospective study in which 28 previously untrained women followed a 2-month programme of progressive training. Alterations of luteal function were as common among those who allowed their weight to fall as among those who deliberately maintained a constant weight, affecting over 60 per cent of both groups of women. Even in the constant weight group, nearly half the women lost the 'surge' of luteinizing hormone (LH). Nevertheless, there is also an interaction with weight loss; both delay of the menses and loss of the LH surge were more common in the weight-loss group.

When consulted by the amenorrhoeic runner, it is as well to remember that runners are susceptible to all the other causes of amenorrhoea, including pregnancy. If pregnancy testing is negative and menstruation does not resume when mileage is temporarily reduced, specialist referral is essential.

A shortened luteal phase is unlikely to be harmful, and is also unlikely to be detected without specific assessment. Should this progress to loss of ovulation but continuing oestrogen production, however, there is a theoretical risk of endometrial hyperplasia and adenocarcinoma by the action of oestrogen on an endometrium unprotected by progesterone. Cyclical treatment with a progesterone analogue might be justifiable, under specialist guidance.

Exercise-induced hypogonadism may be even more pronounced, so that oestrogen levels are suppressed. As the urogenital epithelium is oestrogen dependent, this may increase the likelihood of urethritis and atrophic vaginitis. More important, there is also the possibility of bone atrophy, analogous to the acceleration of calcium loss after the normal menopause. Despite the fact that regular exercise can slow bone loss in elderly women, there is the paradoxical possibility that hypo-oestrogenic amenorrhoea induced by severe exercise may cause bone loss in young women. Cyclical administration of an oestrogen and a progestagen has been advocated but, until the topic is better understood, should not be started without specialist advice.

Finally, it is reassuring to note that exercise-induced amenorrhoea appears to cause no impairment of future fertility.

Anaemia
Iron-deficiency anaemia impairs the aerobic exercise performance of untrained people. In well-trained endurance athletes, although total body haemoglobin is increased, haemoglobin concentration, serum iron, serum ferritin, transferrin saturation, and bone-marrow haemosiderin are all lower than normal. Haematocrit may be 5 to 10 per cent less than in matched controls.

'Sports anaemia' has usually been attributed to iron deficiency, supposedly because of iron losses in sweat or in repeated bouts of haemoglobinuria. This may not be the case. The lower haemoglobin concentration of the endurance athlete may be only a dilutional effect of the increased plasma volume, which results from repeated endurance exercise. It has been suggested that a further factor may be a normal, physiological response to prolonged periods of high intensity exercise with

a high degree of oxygen extraction from haemoglobin. This would increase the concentration of 2,3-diphosphoglycerate in red cells, shifting the oxyhaemoglobin dissociation curve to the right. This in turn may lead to erythropoietin production being reduced, so that the oxygen delivery capacity of arterial blood remains constant. It is also suggested that prolonged running results in a slight increase in intravascular haemolysis. The resulting haemoglobin–haptoglobin complex is taken up by hepatocytes. This shift in red cell catabolism from the reticuloendothelial system to hepatocytes may explain the reduced haemosiderin content of the distance runner's bone-marrow.

On the other hand, 'low-weight' athletic women (such as endurance runners) are at risk of true iron-deficiency due to an inadequate dietary intake. Therefore, although there is no reason to treat 'sports anaemia' with iron, an empirical trial of oral iron may be justified to exclude an element of true iron-deficiency anaemia.

'Treatment' of healthy athletes with recombinant erythropoietin probably enhances endurance performance. Not only is it illegal, it also carries considerable theoretical risks, due to an exaggerated hypertensive response to exercise and to increased blood viscosity (especially in the context of prolonged events normally associated with substantial dehydration). It has been suggested that there might be a link with at least some of a spate of mysterious deaths of up to 19 Dutch and Belgian cyclists between 1987 and 1990.

Rhabdomyolysis (see also Section 25)
'Physiological'
The high levels of creatine kinase (CK) and other muscle proteins in plasma for several days after strenuous exercise, such as marathon running (Fig. 5), are due to leakage of protein from skeletal muscle. They may be associated with microscopic mechanical disruption of muscle cells, especially after downhill running or other exercise involving lengthening of active muscles ('eccentric' contractions). There is no evidence that marathon running damages a healthy, well-perfused myocardium, despite the fact that post-race plasma levels of creatine kinase, myoglobin, aspartate transaminase, lactate dehydrogenase, and tropomyosin normally rise to the same extent as after myocardial infarction. Increased circulating levels of the so-called 'cardiac-specific' isoenzyme CK-MB, of the ratio of CK-MB to total creatine kinase, and of the cardiac-specific lactic dehydrogenase isoenzyme may be adequately explained by the increased proportion of these isoenzymes in endurance-trained muscles.

In the rare instance of a collapsed marathon runner who requires admission to hospital, it may prove difficult to decide whether there is myocardial damage, especially if the normal electrocardiogram shows apparent abnormalities. The acute-phase protein response to marathon running is small but after longer distances it too may resemble the response to a small myocardial infarction. For the future, the radioimmunoassay for cardiac troponin-I may be able to distinguish between 'physiological' rhabdomyolysis and myocardial damage. In the meantime, however, the certain identification of myocardial injury or ischaemia in a marathon runner requires scintigraphic demonstration of technetium pyrophosphate uptake by myocardium or abnormalities of thallium perfusion imaging.

Major
Catastrophic exertional rhabdomyolysis is rare, but may be life-threatening, as the release of large amounts of myoglobin causes acute tubular necrosis. Predisposing factors include dehydration, hyperthermia (see below), and repeated eccentric contractions. The rapid and forceful eccentric quadriceps contractions which provide the decelerating force in squat jumps explain why this exercise has given its name to the potentially lethal exercise-induced rhabdomyolysis sometimes seen in military recruits undergoing their initial training ('squat jump syndrome'). Downhill running produces more muscle damage than uphill running.

An inborn deficiency of carnitine palmityl transferase may result in the very rare syndrome of recurring bouts of severe, exercise-induced rhabdomyolysis.

The patient will be nauseous, vomiting, and ill. The muscles may be swollen, tender, aching, and weak and there may be anuria or the passage of small quantities of 'Coca-cola' urine. Urine will be positive for 'blood' on strip-testing; microscopy will show no red cells but perhaps some pigment casts. Plasma creatine kinase levels will be hugely elevated, perhaps 100 times the upper limit of normal. The damaged muscle tissue takes up calcium and releases phosphate, creatine, and purines. The result is that, for a given degree of renal failure, the plasma calcium is unusually low and plasma levels of potassium, phosphate, creatinine, and urate are unusually high. Hospitalization and cardiac monitoring are mandatory, forced alkaline diuresis may facilitate myoglobin excretion, and the hyperkalaemia must be controlled. In some cases a period of dialysis is required.

POPULAR MARATHONS AND MASS RUNS

'Popular', or non-elite, running events have become very popular, with fields of many hundreds or even thousands participating over courses

Fig. 5 Changes in (a) serum total creatine kinase and (b) plasma myoglobin in young men who had completed a marathon (running times: mean = 194 min, range =163–280 min). (Reproduced from Cummins, P. *et al.* (1987). *European Journal of Clinical Investigation* **17**, 317–24, by permission.)

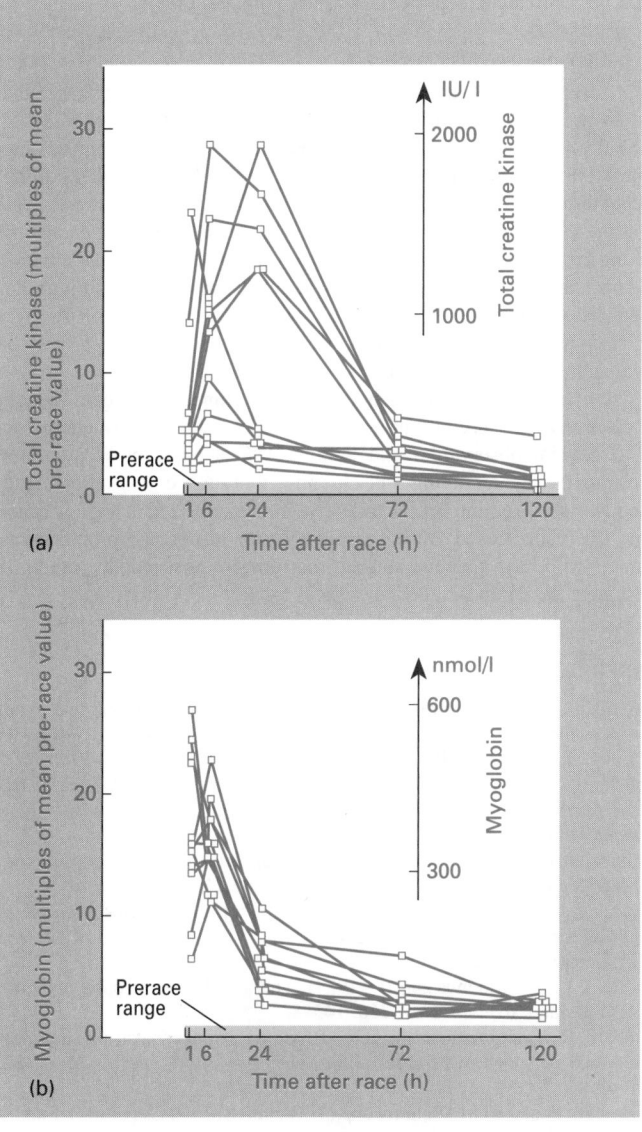

from 10 km up to the full marathon distance of 26 miles 385 yards (42.2 km). Even in marathons, a very high proportion of participants are non-elite, inexperienced, and possibly underprepared. In half-marathons, not only are the numbers even bigger (more than 25 000 in the Great North Run), a higher proportion may be ill-prepared but set to 'have a go'. The experienced runners' training enables them to meet the homoeostatic challenges of prolonged running. They also know how to prevent undue strain or 'decompensation' when doing so, using pace judgement and technical knowledge, and 'listening to their bodies'. This may not be true for the participants in a mass run.

It is essential, therefore, that mass running events should have enough medical and paramedical personnel, trained and equipped to deal with hypovolaemia, hyperthermia, and hypothermia, and (in diabetic runners) hypoglycaemia. Local hospitals are unlikely to have to admit more than one or two runners, but must be party to the overall planning. Their staff must be warned of the biochemical derangements that are 'normal' after prolonged exercise, and should also be reminded of the essentials of management of exertional heat injury and acute rhabdomyolysis.

The positioning of medical facilities requires considerable care and thought. The police and ambulance services must be asked to help plan for the occasional need for rapid evacuation (of a collapsed runner or of a local resident). The size and positioning of first aid posts and medical stations must take account of the stages of the race where most of the problems will arise, of the probable frequency of problems at each stage, and of the sheer numbers involved. Less than 0.1 per cent are likely to need detention in a race medical area but, with a field of 20 000, there may be 20 such 'collapses'. In order to ensure sufficient spare capacity, it is recommended that there should be provision for a 0.75 per cent collapse rate, including one intensive care bed per 10 000 runners.

Treatment for relatively trivial problems (blisters, cramps, chafing) will be required for only about 1 per cent but there should be provision, at the finish area, for a 5 per cent treatment rate plus first aid posts every 2 to 2.5 miles around the course. These posts must also be able to cope with a 5 to 10 per cent (probably 5 per cent) contact rate, for non-medical 'treatments' such as new shoelaces, safety pins, or encouragement/ sympathy.

Medical responsibility for a mass run is not something to be undertaken lightly or at the last minute. The medical director must be involved in every stage of planning. For example, medical advice sheets should be sent to each entrant with the notification that their entry has been accepted. A sample advice sheet and fuller guidance on staffing numbers, preparation, and disposition are available elsewhere.

Hypovolaemia

Trained runners may lose as much as 5 or 6 per cent of body weight in the course of a marathon, representing perhaps 3 to 4 litres of fluid. Under hot conditions, fluid losses may be even greater. Maximal muscle blood flow and adequate cerebral blood flow are maintained, despite the reduction in plasma volume, by cutaneous and splanchnic vasoconstriction. There comes a point, however, when these mechanisms can no longer compensate for the loss of blood volume and may even cease to operate. This is especially likely when venous return is no longer maintained by the pumping action of the leg muscles. Relaxation of compensatory vasoconstriction may occur as much as 20 min after the finish, resulting in collapse if fluid losses have not been adequately restored in the meantime. (There is an analogy with the way that vasoconstriction can maintain blood pressure in the face of severe haemorrhage but may then suddenly fail just when all seems well.) The main medical post should be placed sufficiently beyond the finish line that the incoming tide of runners does not hinder staff carrying a shocked and collapsed runner from the clothing claim area. The organization of the finish area must be adequate for large numbers of athletes finishing together so that they are not required to stand still, queuing to pass the finish marshals or to collect their clothes. (In the Great North Run, the peak period sees 500 runners per minute finishing together.)

Adequate fluid replacement during the run is, of course, the best way to prevent hypovolaemic collapse. The medical director is responsible for ensuring that the organizers provide sufficient drink stations and that the runners are educated in their importance. Runners should be fully hydrated at the start and should take additional fluid early in the race, before they feel thirsty. Water or a dilute glucose solution is recommended.

Hypovolaemia predisposes to hyperthermia (see below). The impaired physical performance of hypovolaemia may predispose to hypothermia (see below). Hypovolaemic collapse may both simulate and accompany either hypothermia or hyperthermia. Every confused or collapsed runner, with or without signs of peripheral circulatory collapse, must have their rectal temperature recorded.

Hypovolaemic collapse usually responds well to rest, leg elevation, and oral rehydration. Intravenous fluid is rarely required but is indicated in the confused or deteriorating patient or if fluid losses continue (by vomiting or diarrhoea, the result perhaps of overintense splanchnic vasoconstriction).

Hyperthermia (see also Section 8)

The rate of heat production while running is high; 75 per cent of the energy expended is converted to heat. When running fast, the rate of heat production may be greater than the body's capacity to dissipate heat. There are numerous, well-documented examples of rectal temperatures of 40 to 42 °C at least 10 min after running, even under rather mild environmental conditions and especially in the shorter events (10 km to half-marathon).

Sweating is the most important avenue of heat dissipation. Anything which impedes sweat loss will increase the risk of hyperthermia, for example, still or humid atmospheric conditions, excess clothing, or dehydration. Other predisposing factors may include a high ambient temperature, lack of fitness, obesity, age extremes, inadequate heat acclimatization, recent illness (e.g. cold or 'flu), previous history of heat stroke, or a susceptibility to malignant hyperthermia.

The prevention of heat injury depends, therefore, on education of participants and organizers and on adequate fluid replacement. The American College of Sports Medicine has provided guidelines, including the recommendation that an event should be cancelled if environmental conditions are such that WGPT > 28 °C. (WGPT = 0.7 wet bulb temperature + 0.2 globe temperature + 0.1 dry bulb.) In the United Kingdom, where summer temperatures are lower than is usual in North America, runners will be less acclimatized and the cancellation threshold should probably be lower.

It is essential to recognize that severe heat injury can also occur under relatively mild environmental conditions. This is especially true for military exercises and training, where the clothing may be physiologically inappropriate. Failure to prepare for and to recognize cases of exercise-related heat exhaustion in such circumstances is inexcusable.

Runners and first aiders alike should be taught to recognize the early warnings of hyperthermia, such as piloerection, chilling, throbbing head, unsteadiness, nausea, and cessation of sweating. These need not be present, however, and the runner may continue to sweat profusely while deteriorating and developing a staggering gait, mental disturbance, and slurred speech. Even the unconscious patient with cold, clammy skin may well be hyperthermic. A rectal temperature is mandatory in any collapsed, confused or fitting runner.

The essentials of treatment are intravenous fluid replacement and heat loss; the number and severity of complications is directly related to the delay in starting them. In order to promote the loss of heat by evaporation, the patient is shaded, stripped, wetted, and fanned. Cold water and cold air should not be used, as they would promote cutaneous vasoconstriction, impeding core-to-surface heat transfer. Both water and air should be applied at room temperature. Immersion in cold water is contraindicated but ice packs may be applied over major vessels in groins and axillae. These measures should be reduced when the rectal temperature is between 38 and 38.5 °C, lest there should be an overshoot into hypothermia.

Serious complications are managed along the lines described elsewhere in this book, e.g. rhabdomyolysis (see above and Section 25), acute tubular necrosis (Section 20), hepatic necrosis (Section 14), disseminated intravascular coagulation (Section 22) or haemorrhage (with hypoprothrombinaemia, hypofibrinogenaemia, or thrombocytopenia) (Section 22).

Sickle cell trait

During basic training, black recruits with sickle cell trait had a 27-fold increased risk of non-traumatic sudden death unexplained by pre-existing disease. These deaths were often associated with some combination of hyperthermia, rhabdomyolysis, and acute renal failure. There are also anecdotal case reports suggesting an association between sickle cell trait and catastrophic thermal injury and rhabdomyolysis. Presumably, loss of renal concentrating ability puts such individuals at an increased risk of hypovolaemia and, therefore, hyperthermia. Moreover, there may be the potential for a moderate degree of exercise-induced, local, muscle damage to develop into a self-perpetuating combination of impaired muscle blood flow, intramuscular hypoxia and sickling, and muscle necrosis. Individuals with sickle cell trait may have a particular need to observe the standard advice about gradual and adequate physical conditioning and about maintenance of hydration during prolonged exertion. It is unlikely, however, that their participation in sporting activities need be restricted except perhaps at very high altitude.

Hypothermia (see also Section 8)

Heat loss may outstrip heat production. Even in the same race, one runner may have a rectal temperature of > 40 °C and another < 36 °C. Factors predisposing to hypothermia include a low ambient temperature, rain, wind, ectomorphy, slow running speed, and inadequate clothing. Hypothermia is most likely to develop in the runners who are slowest over the second half of a marathon. Runners should be educated against setting off too fast; fatigue reduces the rate of metabolic heat production and increases the likelihood of hypothermia, especially if clothing has been discarded earlier in the race. A water- and windproof top layer which is light enough to be carried (e.g. a large polythene bag) may be a valuable preventive measure.

The hypothermic runner may present with impaired speech, thought or co-ordination. Rectal temperature must be measured; values below 36 °C require observation and below 34 °C demand close attention. Treatment is by removing wet clothing, thorough drying, dressing in adequate dry clothing and a reflective foil blanket, and warm drinks. The foil blanket used alone provides totally inadequate protection to runners who have finished and will not prevent post-race hypothermia if runners are denied immediate access to warm, dry clothing.

REFERENCES

American College of Sports Medicine (1987). Position stand on the prevention of thermal injuries during distance running. *Medicine and Science in Sports and Exercise*, **19**, 529–33.

Bouchard, C., Shephard, R.J., and Stephens, T. (eds.) (1994). *Physical activity, fitness, and health; international proceedings and consensus statement*. Human Kinetics, Champaign, Illinois.

Eichner, E.R. (1992). Sports anemia, iron supplements, and blood doping. *Medicine and Science in Sports and Exercise*, **24**, S315–8.

Greig, C. and Young, A. (1992). Aerobic exercise. In *Oxford textbook of geriatric medicine* (ed. J.G. Evans and T.F. Williams), pp. 601–4. Oxford University Press, Oxford.

Hallberg, L. and Magnusson, B. (1984). The aetiology of 'sports anemia'. *Acta Medica Scandinavica*, **216**, 145–8.

Hubbard, R.W. and Armstrong, L.E. (1990). Exertional heatstroke: an international perspective. *Medicine and Science in Sports and Exercise*, **22**, 2–48.

Kark, J.A., Posey, D.M., Schumacher, H.R., and Ruehle, C.J. (1987). Sickle-cell trait as a risk factor for sudden death in physical training. *New England Journal of Medicine*, **317,** 781–7.

Loveday, C. (1990). HIV disease and sport. In *Medicine, Sport and the Law* (ed. S.D.W. Payne), pp. 81–6. Blackwell Scientific Publications, Oxford.

Sawka, M.N. (1992). Current concepts concerning thirst, dehydration, and fluid replacement. *Medicine and Science in Sports and Exercise*, **24,** 643–87.

Siscovick, D.S., Weiss, N.S., Fletcher, R.H., and Lasky, T. (1984). The incidence of primary cardiac arrest during vigorous exercise. *New England Journal of Medicine*, **311,** 874–7.

Sutton, J.R. (1992). $\dot{V}O_2$max – new concepts on an old theme. *Medicine and Science in Sports and Exercise*, **24,** 26–58.

Thompson, P.D. (1982). Cardiovascular hazards of physical activity. In *Exercise and Sport Sciences Reviews*, Vol. 10 (ed. R.L. Terjung), pp. 208–35. Franklin Institute Press, Philadelphia.

Thompson, P.D., Furk, E.J., Carleton, R.A., and Stur, W.Q. (1982). Incidental death during jogging in Rhode Island from 1975 though 1980. *Journal of the American Medical Association*, **247,** 2535–8.

Tunstall-Pedoe, D. (ed) (1984). Popular marathons, half marathons, and other long distance runs: recommendations for medical support. *British Medical Journal*, **288,** 1355–9.

Young, A. (1992). Strength and power. In *Oxford textbook of geriatric medicine* (ed. J.G. Evans and T.F. Williams), pp. 597–601. Oxford University Press, Oxford.

Young, A. (1993). Current issues in arthrogenous inhibition. *Annals of the Rheumatic Diseases*, **52,** 829–34.

Section 31 *Medicine in old age*

31 Medicine in old age

F. I. CAIRD and J. GRIMLEY EVANS

Ageing in the sense of senescence is characterized by a loss of adaptability of an individual organism as time passes. As we grow older our homeostatic mechanisms on average become less sensitive, slower, less accurate, and less well sustained. If we did not undergo senescence we would still ultimately die from accident, disease, predation, or warfare, but the risk of death would remain constant with age or might even fall as natural selection progressively seeded out the less successfully adaptive individuals. With age-associated loss of adaptability, mortality rates rise with age and this is the biological marker of senescence.

Senescence in the human first becomes apparent just before the age of puberty. Mortality rates fall from early infancy through childhood but around the age of 12 or 13 they start to rise again (Fig. 1). Except for perturbations in early adult life due to deaths from accidents and violence, the subsequent rise in age-specific mortality rates is continuous and broadly exponential throughout adult life. There is no discontinuity in later life to provide any biological justification for separating 'the elderly' from the rest of the adult human race.

We age at different rates, and interindividual variation in physiology and functional capability increases with age. Age therefore tells us something about the average performance of groups of individuals but very little about the performance of a single individual. Many people aged 80 function within the 'normal' range for people in early adult life. It is bad science as well as bad medicine to choose what treatment should be offered to elderly individuals solely on the basis of their age. Treatment should be determined on the basis of individual assessments of function and functional reserve and the presence or absence of multiple pathology. Making such assessments is an important part of modern medicine.

The components of age differences

Although widely taught, there is little point in attempting to distinguish between 'normal ageing' and 'disease'. No one has provided an adequate definition of normal ageing, and disease has a range of different definitions. The important questions to be asked of age-associated phenomena is not whether they are normal ageing or disease but how and why they arise and what can be done about them. There are particular dangers in categorizing conditions as 'normal ageing' since this is often taken to imply that doctors have no responsibility for doing anything about them even if they are potentially remediable.

Table 1 summarizes the sources of differences between young and old people. Some are due to true ageing, that is to say changes that have actually occurred to individuals as they have grown older but others, although frequently mistaken for ageing, are due to other factors. Because of selective survival people who reach old age will be different from those who died in middle age. This has been demonstrated for some genetic factors such as those determining lipoprotein patterns or HLA haplotypes associated with susceptibility to particular diseases. Selective survival is also associated with lifestyle and possibly with personality factors.

If ageing is defined in terms of change in adaptability, it can only be assessed by offering identical challenges to individuals of different ages and measuring their responses. Differential challenge refers to the fact that society is organized in such a way that older people tend to be offered more severe challenges than face the young, but their poorer outcome is attributed to age. Hypothermia has been more common among old than young people in Britain partly because of age-associated changes in metabolism, but also because older people tend to live in the worst and coldest houses. Some of the grossest examples of differential challenge are unfortunately in the Health Services, where old people are frequently offered worse treatment, and in wards and departments with lower levels of staffing and equipment, than are the young. One survey found that 40 per cent of coronary care units had an upper age limit for thrombolytic therapy following myocardial infarction, even though, in terms of numbers of lives saved, this treatment is probably more effective among old people than among young. Efforts are now being undertaken to abolish such 'ageism' in health care.

Cohort effects are most prominent in the field of mental functioning in societies which have been changing rapidly over the past century. Intelligence takes different forms in different cultures, and the society for which older people were educated was very different from that in which young people are now being brought up. In longitudinal studies where individuals are tested against their own former selves rather than against other people younger than themselves, it is found that mental function declines much less and much later than appears from cross-sectional studies. Moreover, some age-associated functional changes can be compensated for. As an example, cross-sectional studies show an apparent decline with age in the ability to learn new material. Studies have shown, however, that older people can learn well if taught by methods appropriate to their cultural background and sensitive to the maintenance of motivation and to pace.

True ageing is the consequence of an interaction between extrinsic (environmental and lifestyle) and intrinsic (genetic) factors. Intrinsic

Table 1 *Sources of age differences*

True ageing	Intrinsic (genetic)
	Extrinsic (environment and lifestyle)
Non-ageing	Selective survival
	Differential challenge
	Cohort effects

Fig. 1 Age- and sex-specific mortality rates, England and Wales 1988.

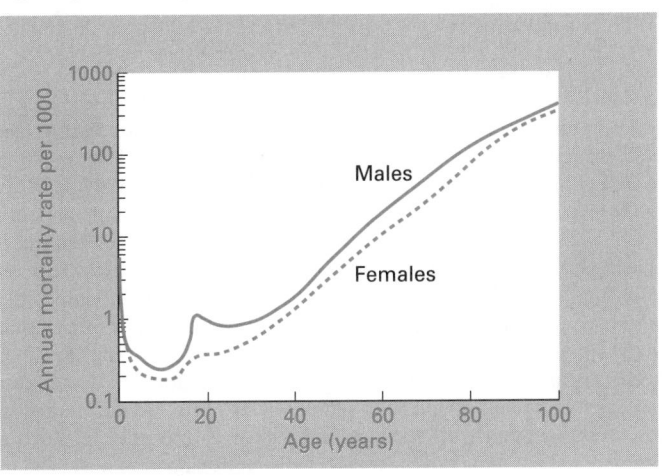

factors in ageing are thought to reflect particularly the accuracy of repair of damage to cells arising from such ubiquitous agencies as heat, radiation, and the free radicals generated during cellular metabolism. In addition, individuals will vary in their susceptibility as well as their exposure to environmental factors affecting metabolism and physiology. In genetically predisposed individuals a high dietary salt intake may cause a rise in blood pressure; some others may be liable to develop diabetes and coronary heart disease in response to a Western-type diet high in calories and animal fat. Cigarette smoke has a variety of effects that accelerate ageing; it impairs lung function, has anti-oestrogenic effects, brings forward the age of the menopause, and reduces bone density. Patterns of physical exercise have an important effect on functional ability in later life.

Ageing and medicine

Table 2 lists some important general characteristics of disease in later life. Multiple pathology is common and because of age-associated loss of adaptability, illness in old age is often characterized by a cryptic and non-specific presentation. For example, reduced ability to metabolize bacterial toxins and slowness in mounting an inflammatory response may cause pneumonia in an old person to present as acute delirium before there are any physical signs in the chest. A myocardial infarction may be painless in later life and present as mental confusion due to reduced cardiac output or as an inexplicable fall. Reduced sensation in the peritoneum may delay the diagnosis of appendicitis or perforated peptic ulcer. The slowness of the aged body in mounting its defences can lead to rapid deterioration unless an accurate diagnosis is made and correct treatment instituted urgently. Because of this urgency, and on account of the cryptic presentation of multiple pathology, older patients require on average more investigations than do younger adults if similar levels of diagnostic accuracy are to be attained.

Reduced adaptability of old age also causes a high incidence of secondary complications both of disease and treatment which calls for careful surveillance by medical and nursing staff. Good-quality medical and nursing care for older people requires scrupulous attention to detail, since even the smallest error of judgement or lack of observation may have serious consequences for the patient.

While younger patients usually have sufficient functional reserve to convalesce spontaneously after an illness, there is a more frequent need for active rehabilitation to help an elderly patient recover fully. Plans for this need to be an early consideration, since rehabilitation is most effective if started as soon as possible after the onset of acute illness. Loss of adaptability leads to an increased importance of environmental factors both in the genesis and in the management of illness in later life. In particular the rehabilitation plan must also take into account the demands that the patient's home environment will dictate. Some modification to the home, or provision of services, may be necessary to close the 'ecological gap' between what the environment demands and what the patient can do. Such 'prosthetic' supports will reduce the patient's independence and autonomy, however, and should not be introduced without the patient being also helped to be as independent as possible by the 'therapeutic' interventions of medicine, nursing, physiotherapy, and occupational and speech therapy, where indicated.

Age-associated physiological changes

Anatomical and physiological changes with ageing are described in almost every body system. They mostly become apparent in early or middle adult life but their magnitude and practical significance vary considerably. Significant and progressive alterations in average body composition appear in the fifth decade of life. There is a decline in lean body mass with a corresponding fall in oxygen consumption, largely attributable to a decline in muscle bulk. However, until extreme old age average body weight remains constant or may increase, owing to an increase in body fat. This change in body composition has important

Table 2 *Characteristics of disease in old age*

Multiple pathology
Non-specific or cryptic presentation
Rapid deterioration if untreated
High incidence of secondary complications
Need for rehabilitation
Importance of environmental factors

Table 3 *Commonly used laboratory data for which reference ranges are essentially unchanged in old age*

Serum sodium
Serum bicarbonate
Serum chloride
Serum magnesium
Serum aspartate transaminase
Serum lactate dehydrogenase
Serum alanine transferase
Serum amylase
Serum 5'-nucleotidase
Serum creatinine kinase
Serum bilirubin
Haemoglobin and red-cell indices
Coagulation tests
Thyroid hormones

From Hodkinson (1992).

effects on pharmacokinetics, but is also the background against which must be set age-associated changes in nutrition, and in cardiovascular, respiratory, and renal function, and the interpretation of their measurement.

The blood volume falls with age, and there is a slight decline in haemoglobin concentration, more evident in women than in men, so that in women aged over 75 a haemoglobin concentration in the range 11.5 to 11.9 g/dl should not necessarily be interpreted as anaemia. The structure and composition of red cells and the dynamics of haematopoiesis remain unaltered. The white cell count falls slightly, the principal decrease being in the lymphoctye count, but the platelet count and platelet function are unaltered.

Normal values for elderly people for some common biochemical measurements are given in Tables 3 and 4. The concentrations of major electrolytes are unaffected by age except for a tendency for the mean serum calcium to decline. Before the menopause, serum calcium concentrations are lower in women than men, and after that event higher; this probably reflects the loss at the menopause of the restraining influence of oestrogens on parathyroid hormone activity. There is a very small reduction in serum albumin concentration in healthy elderly people, which is not clinically significant; the much greater reduction in levels in many elderly people in hospital is due to the effects of disease, reflects its severity and duration, and is a predictor of its outcome.

The principal anatomical alterations in the cardiovascular system include an increase in the amount of fibrous tissue in the skeleton of the heart and in the myocardium and valves, and accumulation of lipofuscin in the myocardial fibres (a change of no evident functional significance). There is a decrease in the elasticity of the aorta and its main branches, accompanied by an increase in their diameter and length. Interpretation of changes in cardiovascular function in old age is made difficult by the very high prevalence of unequivocal heart disease (at least 50 per cent in the United Kingdom). There is no doubt of a minor decline of resting heart rate, and of greater changes in intrinsic heart rate (that is, the heart rate after combined sympathetic and parasympathetic blockade), and in maximum heart rate on exercise; these changes probably relate to a decrease in the number of pacemaker cells in the sinoatrial node, and to

Table 4 *Commonly used laboratory data where reference ranges are altered in older persons*

Test	Reference range in old age	Change in old age
Serum albumin	33–49 g/l	Lowered
Serum globulin	20–41 g/l	Raised
Serum potassium	3.6–5.2 mmol/l	Raised
Blood urea	3.9–9.9 mmol/l	Raised
Serum creatinine	52–159 μmol/l	Raised
Serum uric acid	148–461 μmol/l	Raised
Serum calcium (women)	2.18–2.68 mmol/l	Raised
Serum calcium (men)	2.19–2.59 mmol/l	Unchanged
Serum phosphate(women)	0.94–1.56 mmol/l	Raised
Serum phosphate (men)	0.66–1.27 mmol/l	Lowered
Serum alkaline phosphatase	22–82 Iu/l	Raised
Random blood glucose	3.4–9.3 mmol/l	Raised
Leucocyte count	3100–8900/mm^3	Lowered

From Hodkinson (1992).

alterations in their reactivity to sympathetic and parasympathetic stimuli. Cardiac output at rest has long been thought to fall with age, but this is not so. The mean arteriovenous oxygen difference is unaltered. Pulmonary vascular pressures are unchanged (except for a slight rise on exercise), as is pulmonary blood volume. The mean systemic arterial pressure rises in most, but not all populations; it cannot therefore be an intrinsic age change, but represents the response of susceptible people to environmental factors, probably including excessive salt intake. In those populations in which it does change, the rate of rise with age of systolic arterial pressure is greater than that of diastolic; this increase in pulse pressure is probably an expression of the reduced elasticity of the aortic compression chamber.

Owing to diminished compliance (due to heart wall hypertrophy and probably cross-linking of proteins) the older heart takes longer to fill during diastole than does the young heart. The older patient is therefore less tolerant of tachycardia than the young; this may contribute to the often severe consequences of the onset of atrial fibrillation and to an intolerance of medication that increases heart rate. The older heart is also less able to respond to demand for increase in cardiac output by an increase in rate; it therefore increases output more by the Frank–Starling mechanism.

The interpretation of respiratory function changes with age is complicated by the high prevalence of cigarette smoking in many populations. Total lung volume does not alter, but vital capacity falls and residual volume increases with age, so that over the age of about 60 the critical closing volume exceeds the functional residual volume. Ventilatory capacity falls with age, at a slower rate in non-smokers than smokers. Ventilation–perfusion inequality increases slightly, probably mainly as a result of increasing inequality of ventilation. These changes in lung function reflect especially a decrease in elasticity of the lungs and in respiratory muscular strength, but their overall consequences are minimal in terms of their effects upon the blood gases (Pao$_2$ falls slightly), doubtless because they do not exceed the age-associated reduction in oxygen consumption and carbon dioxide production.

Age changes in renal function are well documented. The glomerular filtration rate falls by approximately 1 per cent per year over the age of 40, as do tubular reabsorptive and secretory capacities. These changes exceed the decline in lean body mass, so that serum urea and creatinine concentrations rise slightly. The response to an acid load is impaired, and the maximum rate of secretion of hydrogen ion falls; changes in blood pH in response to an acid load are thus greater in magnitude and longer in duration than in younger people. The response to antidiuretic hormone is reduced, and water conservation thus less efficient. This is accompanied by a delayed response to fluid deprivation, due at least in part to impaired thirst mechanisms, which result in elderly people being

at increased risk of dehydration. Conversely, some elderly people, typically hypertensive women, show an enhanced thirst response to diuretics (perhaps particularly amiloride) with increased water intake and hyponatraemia.

The mechanism of these alterations is unknown, although loss of nephrons contributes. Their importance lies particularly in the pharmacokinetics of renally excreted drugs.

In the gastrointestinal tract, gastric atrophy becomes increasingly common as age advances, but hydrogen ion secretion is often unaltered. Minor atrophic changes in the mucosa of the small bowel are described, and there is evidence of slight impairment of absorption of some nutrients; this is rarely of clinical significance, but calcium absorption is reduced because of diminished sensitivity to vitamin D. Reduction in the motility of the large bowel is common and may partly reflect diverticular disease or chronic purgative abuse.

There is an age-associated reduction in hepatic mass and blood flow, of approximately 30 per cent, but none in cellular structure or enzyme concentrations or function. Overall changes in hepatic function, as measured by conventional tests such as serum bilirubin and hepatic enzymes are minor. Reduction in the hepatic metabolism of some drugs is, however, well documented.

The major changes with age in the bony skeleton are discussed in Section 19. The most important manifestation of the decline in bone mass is a reduction in the mechanical strength of bone and an increase in the tendency to fracture. Vertebral fractures start to appear at the time of the menopause in women and increase in prevalence thereafter. The great majority of limb bone fractures in old age are caused by simple falls, and there is an exponential increase in risk of falling after the age of 60 or so; women are more likely than men to fall. It is therefore not surprising that there is a similarly exponential increase in risk of proximal femoral fracture, again with a much higher risk in women, over the same age range. However, distal forearm fractures do not increase in incidence through old age. This may indicate that the older one is the less likely one is in a fall to throw out an arm in time as a protective response.

The reasons for the virtually universal occurrence of osteoarthritic changes in many joints are uncertain but may include the mechanical effects of time-related wear and tear, age-associated changes in the metabolism of joint cartilage, or a disease process unrelated to age. The epidemiology of knee osteoarthritis suggests that wear and tear from occupation, injury, and obesity is important. Obesity seems both to predispose to arthritis of the knee and to be a factor in making the arthritis painful. Weight loss is therefore an important therapeutic element. In contrast, osteoarthritis of the hip seems to be a long-term consequence of minor (or major) forms of congenital dysplasia of the hip, and the effects of occupation and obesity are much less clear. There is evidence of a genetic predisposition to the syndrome of generalized osteoarthritis.

In the endocrine system, apart from the obvious changes in ovarian function at the menopause, there are minor declines in circulating thyroid hormone levels, a reduction in the rate of secretion of insulin in response to raised blood sugar levels, and a decline in insulin sensitivity (that is, in glucose disposition per unit of circulating insulin at a given blood glucose). The release of antidiuretic hormone in response to osmotic loads increases, perhaps in association with reduced renal responsiveness and changes in the sensitivity of blood volume receptors. There is little evidence of any abnormality of parathyroid, adrenal, or pituitary function as a universal feature of old age. The response of the adrenals and of adrenocorticotrophic hormone secretion to stress is essentially unaltered.

Age changes in the nervous system are among the most important, because of their great significance in the psychology and psychiatry of ageing, and in the production of disorders of movement. Their anatomical basis is complex and as yet imperfectly understood. The numbers of neurones in some parts of the nervous system (for example, the motor neurones of the spinal cord, the Purkinje cells of the cerebellum, the cells of the substantia nigra and the neocortex—the latter to a variable degree in different cortical areas) fall with age, but there are no changes in other parts (for example, several clearly defined brain-stem nuclei). Anatomical abnormalities of the neurones that remain are also described, including the accumulation of lipofuscin and loss of dendrites and dendritic spines in cortical neurones. The anatomical basis of alterations in cortical function may thus be due both to a reduction in number of neurones, and in connections between them. There is a reduction in peripheral nerve conduction velocities, both motor and sensory, differing in different nerves, and reflecting a fall-out of fibres of all sizes. There is also an increase in the variability of nerve conduction velocities, which probably contributes to the inaccurate transmission of information, and may impair the cognitive function of the brain as a parallel computer.

Central autonomic nuclei (for example the intermediolateral cell column in the spinal cord) and first- and second-order autonomic neurones outside the central nervous system show a fall in cell numbers. Changes in autonomic function include alterations in control of heart rate (see above), and abnormalities of temperature regulation. The threshold for appreciation of skin temperature changes may increase by as much as tenfold. This may be an important reason for old people's inability to recognize temperature change, and thus to respond by appropriate behaviour to falls in environmental temperature. There may also be failure of cutaneous vasoconstriction in response to cold, and of vasodilatation and sweating in response to increasing body temperature, the last partly due to reduction in the number of sweat glands. Failure of vasoconstriction is clearly important in reducing the response to falling core temperature, as is failure of shivering, thus making hypothermia more likely. Coexisting undernutrition, even of brief duration, may also reduce hepatic thermogenesis. The impairment of vasomotor and sudomotor responses to heat will increase the likelihood of heatstroke.

Failure of the blood pressure response to postural change is also important. Baroreceptor responses are blunted, perhaps as a result of sclerotic changes in the carotid sinus, and there may in addition be failure of central and perhaps peripheral vasoconstrictor responses to falling blood pressure.

Age changes in the eye and ear are well documented. Decrease in elasticity of the lens begins very early in life, but only becomes symptomatic in the fifth decade, when presbyopic hypermetropia results from failure of accommodation, which is probably due to changes both in the lens itself and in its capsule and suspensory ligaments. High tone deafness (presbyacusis) has several mechanisms, and is partly an intrinsic true age change, although there is little doubt of the importance of prolonged exposure to industrial and other environmental noise. Impaired vestibular function is also described.

Clinical assessment of the elderly patient

The process of history-taking requires modification for elderly patients. The sensitive clinician talking to someone much older than himself should realize that he may be talking across a cultural divide, and should have the courtesy to reduce the speed of his speech to the polite usage of earlier generations. More time is required to obtain an adequate history from an elderly patient if he or she is deaf, and perhaps suffers from impairment of memory. Questions need to be simple and straightforward. It is sometimes only possible to establish that a symptom exists, while its duration is uncertain, or the converse, that something whose nature is uncertain has been amiss for a definite time. The duration of symptoms and the sequence of their development are often more important than their precise nature. If there is temporary or permanent impairment of memory, it is essential to take a history from some other person—a relative, or someone who has been caring for the patient.

A full assessment involves the co-operation of physician, nurse, physiotherapist, occupational therapist, and social worker, but preliminary enquiry can be undertaken by the physician and nurse. Short standard mental and physical function tests should be part of the routine clinical examination of old people. For patients in hospital the short mental function test shown in Table 5 is widely used. Scores of 7 or less are pathological and imply some form of mental dysfunction such as depression, delirium, dementia, or oligophrenia. The mental function test only detects gross problems and a search for evidence of early or mild mental disability requires a more elaborate test, and the help of a clinical psychologist should be sought. For physical function (so-called activities of daily living assessment) there are many scales available; the Barthel index or one of its modifications (Table 6) is widely used to assess progress in rehabilitation as well as static levels of ability.

Systematic enquiry should follow the usual lines. The past history is more important in elderly patients, because there is more of it; medical records of previous illnesses may constitute vital evidence. An accurate drug history is essential, covering as much of the past as possible, and non-prescribed as well as prescribed drugs. A clear account of the time scale of drug therapy and of the dates of starting and stopping individual drugs will go far to clarify the complexities of symptoms due to drugs, and to their withdrawal—both common in elderly patients. A dietary history is, on occasion, of importance, although it may only be possible to identify the grossest deficiencies. An accurate account of psychiatric symptoms is vital, since deterioration in mental state is the most common factor limiting the possibility of investigation or of rehabilitation in physical disease.

A detailed account of the patient's social circumstances is essential, and of the physical and emotional environment at home. Such knowledge is vital if physical rehabilitation is to be effective in re-establishing the patient at home; this can best be obtained by visiting the house itself. No assessment is complete without information on what relatives the patient has, where they live, and what they are able to contribute to his or her welfare. It is essential to decide what supporting community services the patient requires and is receiving, and to know what are available locally, and how best to obtain them.

Principles of drug therapy in old age

Appropriate drug therapy remains one of the most important aspects of the medicine of old age, since drugs are more often prescribed for elderly people, multiple pathology is a temptation to polypharmacy, and the adverse effects of some drugs may increase with age. Nevertheless, inappropriate prescribing remains the most common simple cause of adverse drug reactions. It has been claimed that at least 10 per cent of admissions of elderly patients to hospital in the United Kingdom are drug-induced, and likely therefore to be iatrogenic.

Understanding of alterations in pharmacokinetics with age is advancing rapidly. Drug absorption in general varies little with age, although

Table 5 *Abbreviated mental test score (MTS)*

Age
(must be correct)

Time
(correct to nearest hour without looking at watch or clock)

42 West Street
(give this or similar address, ask for it to be repeated to ensure
  that it has been heard correctly. Ask for it at the end of the
  test)

Month
(exact)

Year
(exact, except in January or February when previous year is
  acceptable)

Name of place
(if not in hospital ask for type of place or area of town)

Date of birth
(exact)

Start of the Second World War
(exact year)

Name of present monarch

Count backwards from 20 to 1
(prompt if necessary, 20, 19, 18 . . ., but no further prompts.
  Patients can hesitate and self-correct but no other errors
  allowed)

Score 8–10 probably normal
       7 probably abnormal
       0–6 abnormal
Change in score of 3 or more is probably significant

Table 6 *The Barthel index of activities of daily living*

Bowels	
Continent	2
Occasional accidents	1
Incontinent	0
Bladder	
Continent	2
Occasional accidents	1
Incontinent	0
Feeding	
Independent	2
Needs some help	1
Dependent	0
Grooming, face/hair/teeth/shaving	0
Independent	1
Needs help	0
Dressing	
Independent	2
Can do half	1
Dependent	0
Transfer	
Independent	3
Minor help needed	2
Major help (can sit)	1
Unable	0
Toilet use	
Independent	2
Needs some help	1
Dependent	0
Walking	
Independent	3
Walks with one stick	2
Wheelchair independent	1
Unable	0
Stairs	
Independent	2
Needs some help	1
Dependent	0
Bathing	
Independent	1
Dependent	0
Total score	

a substantial increase in the absorption of levodopa, probably due to reduced dopa decarboxylase in the gastric mucosa, is an important exception. The bioavailability of those drugs, such as propranolol, which are extensively degraded in the liver, may be greatly increased by a reduction in their first-pass metabolism. The binding of drugs to serum albumin may be reduced in ill elderly people in whom serum albumin concentrations are frequently low and the ease with which one drug displaces another from albumin may be increased. There is, however, little evidence that these changes are of major practical importance.

The volume of distribution of some drugs is reduced; that of digoxin may be correlated with reduced muscle Na/K ATPase. That of others (for example, diazepam) is increased. The fall in lean body mass and body water might be expected to reduce the volume of distribution of water-soluble drugs, and the increase in body fat to increase that of fat-soluble drugs, but other poorly understood factors may play a greater part. Changes in the volume of distribution make it difficult to interpret changes in plasma half-life as a measure of drug elimination; this is most satisfactorily expressed in terms of clearance. The associations of age with other aspects of drug distribution are poorly understood. Thus the apparent increase in sensitivity of the elderly brain to nitrazepam, which is not explained by any change in its plasma kinetics, may be due to alterations in the blood–brain barrier, or in the kinetics of drugs in the cerebrospinal fluid, or to a pharmacodynamic effect.

Alterations in drug elimination are undoubtedly the most important pharmacokinetic differences so far demonstrated. The age-associated fall in glomerular filtration rate is accompanied by a parallel decrease in the elimination of drugs principally excreted by this route (for example, digoxin), but in this instance and others, additional, disease-related reduction in glomerular filtration is also very important. Drugs princi-

pally eliminated by renal tubular secretion (for example the penicillins and aminoglycosides) share in this reduction in rate of elimination; this may be important when high urinary concentrations of antibiotic are required in the treatment of urinary tract infections, and in the case of the aminoglycosides is responsible for the relation of ototoxicity to age. Toxic serum concentrations may follow the giving of standard adult doses to elderly patients. The situation with regard to drugs eliminated by the liver varies. The elimination rates of some decline with age, but not of others. It is not entirely clear what determines these differences, but delayed elimination, and in certain cases delayed formation of active metabolites, will prolong the duration of action of some drugs.

There are at present few well-documented examples of age-associated differences in pharmacodynamics. The effect of warfarin on the synthesis of clotting factors is increased in elderly subjects. Some of the cardiac effects of sympathomimetic amines and β-blockers are reduced, perhaps because of a reduction in the number and/or sensitivity of β-adrenergic receptors. In practice this may be cancelled out by the increased bioavailability of some β-blockers and consequent higher serum levels. No age effect on α-adrenoceptors has been shown.

Other factors not strictly kinetic or dynamic may alter the response of elderly patients to drugs. The chronic administration of thiazide and related diuretics produces little change in whole-body potassium in the middle-aged, but in elderly patients is a prime cause of potassium depletion. The difference lies in the substantially lower average dietary potassium intake of old people, in whom diuretic-induced urinary potassium loss can easily exceed intake, and so make depletion inevitable. Potassium supplements should therefore always accompany diuretic therapy for elderly people, or potassium-sparing combination drugs may be used as they are more palatable and more effective.

The compliance of elderly patients with prescribed drug therapy is imperfect, although perhaps no more so than that of the young and middle-aged when cognitive function is unimpaired. The most satisfactory way of improving compliance is to reduce to a minimum the demands made on the patient. Complex drug regimens are inappropriate. Simplicity of prescribing (the use, for instance, of once-daily dosage schedules if possible), clear instruction, reinforced by written indications of what is required, and appropriate packaging and labelling (practical matters often thought to be beneath the attention of doctors), can do much to improve compliance. Provided the prescription is correct, these measures ensure the maximum benefit at the minimum risk.

Some common clinical problems

URINARY INCONTINENCE

This is a socially disabling affliction that affects approximately 2 per cent of middle-aged men and 12 per cent of middle-aged women, and increases with age to a prevalence of around 8 per cent in men and 16 per cent in women aged over 75 years. A number of classifications of urinary incontinence have been advanced; Table 7 sets out one common form. The patient with acutely developing incontinence due to illness or injury should be reassured, but every effort should be made to ensure that it does not continue into a chronic form. Many patients with dementia become incontinent, but incontinence should never be attributed solely to dementia unless the latter is severe, and until all treatable causes have been excluded. Functional incontinence due to inability of an old person to reach a toilet in time is unnecessarily prevalent, particularly in hospitals where old people with mobility problems may have their beds too far from a toilet and where nurses cannot (or do not) answer bells promptly. Overflow incontinence when the bladder is only able to overcome an outlet obstruction at high volumes is common in men with prostate difficulties. It is diagnosable by postvoiding ultrasound examination and often requires surgical intervention. Where this is not feasible, medical approaches include α-adrenergic blockers (given with care on account of the risk of hypotension); there may prove to be a place for antiandrogenic therapy to reduce prostatic hypertrophy. Urge incontinence is usually mainly due to instability of the detrusor muscle of the bladder, but may also arise through irritation of the bladder by infected urine; it then responds to appropriate antibiotic therapy. The contractions of an unstable bladder may be inhibited by anticholinergic drugs, but these must be used with care as they may induce glaucoma and constipation, while lipid-soluble anticholinergic drugs may cross the blood–brain barrier and cause delirium. Although newer preparations such as oxybutynin are popular with some, this drug is not conspicuously better than the longer-established propantheline.

The certain diagnosis of unstable bladder and associated urethral dysfunctions requires invasive investigation, including cystometry. In practice most cases or urinary incontinence can be dealt with empirically, and invasive investigation should be reserved for the more intractable cases. It is useful for medical and nursing teams in primary or hospital care to agree on a general plan for approaching problems of incontinence. Figure 2 outlines one example of such an approach. In many instances urinary incontinence may be a problem only at night. If this is not due to nocturnal epilepsy, it often has to be managed in a pragmatic way. A drug with anticholinergic effects, such as imipramine, may be of value. Setting an alarm clock to wake the patient to empty his or her bladder prophylactically may be of benefit. For some patients a small

Table 7 *Forms of urinary incontinence*

Acute	Transitory due to illness, delirium, epilepsy, etc.
Established	Infection—may be the consequence rather than the cause of incontinence. Treatment should not be continued if incontinence persists after the urine is sterile
	Functional—difficulty in getting to a toilet
	Stress—loss of urine on coughing or straining
	Urge—often due to precipitate bladder contractions
	Overflow—secondary to obstruction of bladder outflow. Diagnosis may need postvoiding ultrasound. May be due to constipation.
	Fistulous—for example, fistula between bladder and vagina
	Disinhibitory—occurs in frontal brain damage and dementia
	Behavioural—a form of social manipulation (rare)

dose of a rapidly acting diuretic in the afternoon followed by restriction of fluids until bedtime will enable the cardiovascular system to reabsorb fluid pooled during the day in the lower limbs without an inconvenient increase in urinary output. The use of dDAVP or other analogues of vasopressin at bedtime in order to produce an antidiuresis during the night should be avoided as this may result in fluid overload and hyponatraemia.

FAECAL INCONTINENCE

Faecal incontinence, with or without associated urinary incontinence, affects around 1 per cent of people aged over 65. Faecal and double incontinence are associated with a range of anorectal and neurological disorders, including dementia. In later life the commonest cause is rectal or sigmoid overloading due to constipation (faecal impaction). In middle-aged women a pelvic neuropathy, sometimes possibly a consequence of childbirth, is encountered as a cause of faecal incontinence, which may be improved by surgical intervention. Any form of acute or chronic diarrhoea will also lead to incontinence in a proportion of cases. Faecal impaction most commonly occurs in the rectum and can be readily diagnosed by rectal examination. 'High' impaction can occur at the rectosigmoid junction and above, and may need to be diagnosed by a plain abdominal radiograph. High impaction must always raise the possibility of obstruction by a carcinoma or inflammatory stricture due to diverticulitis. Treatment of impaction requires enemas and suppositories, rarely manual evacuation, and then a regular regime of stool-softening medication such as lactulose.

In some cases where faecal incontinence is an intractable problem it can be ameliorated by giving constipating medication such as codeine phosphate or loperamide with bowel lavage once a week. This is not an easy regimen to establish but can be of help for an old person who wishes to remain in his or her home.

FALLS

Falls are an important cause of morbidity among elderly people. Apart from the immediate hazards of falling, which include contusions, lacerations, fractures, head injury, hypothermia, pneumonia, pressure sores, and rhabdomyolysis, there is considerable long-term morbidity from the induced fear of further falls. This may lead to increasing immobility and possibly to premature institutionalization. In the general population, one-fifth of people aged 65 to 69 fall once or more during a year; this proportion doubles by the age of 80. It is therefore impracticable for every fall to be followed by a full diagnostic evaluation. Old people who fall more than twice in a 1-year period, or whose fall is inexplicable, need further assessment. Some falls are due largely to environmental hazards such as poor lighting or loose stair carpets. These are well worth identifying in individual patients, but this is not an effective means of preventing falls in the community as the great majority of apparent hazards will not, in fact, be responsible for a fall.

Table 8 lists some of the specific medical causes of falls that may need to be considered. If the patient finds himself or herself on the floor and cannot remember actually falling, this suggests either epilepsy or syncope. Full investigation of syncope will include tilt table testing and carotid sinus massage (see Chapter 24.4.2); this can be of benefit as cardio-inhibitory syncope can be effectively treated with a pacemaker. Postural hypotension is a common problem (see below) and is most commonly due to drugs. Postprandial hypotension is also common; if severe, periods of rest after meals may be the only treatment to offer, although caffeine has been shown in some studies to be helpful if given at the right time. The unstable knee is a common problem in old age, particularly if an illness or some other cause of reduced activity allows the strength of the quadriceps to fall below the level critical to maintaining stability of the partially flexed knee. Pain or an effusion in the knee can also reduce quadriceps strength by reflex inhibition. The unstable knee due to inadequate quadriceps strength is a diagnosis well worth making as it can often be effectively treated by exercises directed by a physiotherapist.

Rehabilitation

The principles of geriatric medicine are well illustrated by the approach to rehabilitation. The central concept in rehabilitation is to foster the natural recovery from illness, to avoid adding iatrogenic problems, and to prevent and treat secondary complications of disease and its treatment. For each patient a care plan is defined. This is based on a full diagnosis and knowledge of the likely pattern of recovery from illness, the patient's present level of functioning, and the demands that his or her home environment are likely to make. The care plan defines objectives, what treatment is to be offered to the patient, and what progress is to be expected. At regular intervals the patient's functional state is reviewed by the multidisciplinary team and compared with the original plan. If there is a mismatch, the reason should be sought. Has some new illness intervened? Has a complication of illness (such as reactive depression) arisen? Was the original assessment of probable progress unrealistic? On the basis of this review the plan is updated and revised if necessary. The overall strategy necessitates a realistic view of the patient and his or her psychological state, diseases and disabilities, an organized setting, and a co-ordinated method of management, usually involving a large number of points of detail. Although there may be little scientific evidence that rehabilitation as at present conducted affects eventual outcome (for example in stroke), it is highly unlikely that all its benefits are psychological, while the consequences of a lack of rehabilitation (for example contractures and unnecessary immobility) are obvious.

Effective rehabilitation of the elderly patient requires a team of medical, nursing, and paramedical personnel, each with a role. Responsibility for the co-ordination of the activities of the team usually falls to the doctor, although he or she may well not be the most important member of the team at a particular time during the rehabilitation of a patient. Nurses have a central place, because they spend much the most time with the patient, and are thus the best placed both to gather and to transmit information. The functions of the paramedical members of the team (physiotherapist, occupational therapist, speech therapist, and social worker) are the assessment of the patient's disability in terms of their own discipline, treatment by appropriate techniques, and the counselling of the patient and her relatives. The physiotherapist's principal concern is mobility; the occupational therapist's, activities of daily living, the provision of aids, and the adaptation of the patient's home environment to her disabilities. The speech therapist is concerned with communication disorders and their treatment; his or her function in counselling relatives is especially important. The social worker is concerned with the social and family problems presented by illness and disability. Each patient requires an individual rehabilitation programme, and each member of the team must know what is expected. It is vital to involve carers at every stage. The programme must be flexible, and take into account the unforeseen. No irretrievable action should ever be taken which might prevent the patient from benefiting from unanticipated improvement.

The operation of these principles can be illustrated by three common examples encountered in everyday geriatric hospital practice: rehabilitation in acute physical illness, following stroke, and in Parkinson's disease.

Fig. 2 Illustrative algorithm for management of urinary incontinence in elderly patients. 'Refer' indicates referral to specialist urological or gynaecological service.

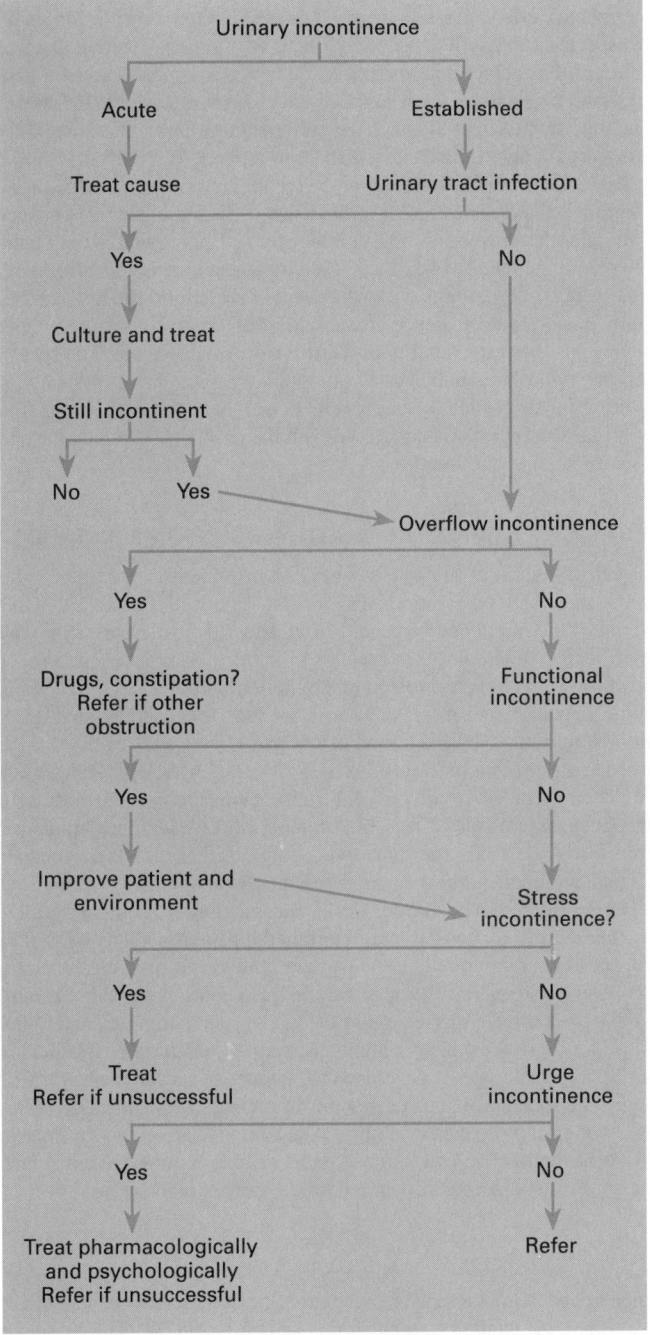

Table 8 *Some medical causes of falls*

Cardiovascular
   Hypotension (postural, exertional, postprandial, drug-
     induced, induced by bed rest)
   Cardiac arrhythmia
   Syncope (micturition, cough, defaecation, carotid sinus
     sensitivity)
Neuromuscular
   Epilepsy
   Transient ischaemic attacks
   Menière's disease
   Parkinsonism and multisystem disorders
   Myopathy
   Neuropathy or myelopathy
   Unstable knee due to quadriceps weakness
   Visual field defect or inattention
   Dementia
   Intermittent delirium (drugs, alcohol, hypoglycaemia)

REHABILITATION IN ACUTE ILLNESS

This should begin immediately on admission to hospital. The patient and his or her relatives should be made aware that discharge is anticipated, and the expectation either of prolonged or even permanent hospitalization must be prevented. When the patient is fit to get out of bed, the natural history of the illness and the time course of recovery require consideration, and the presence of complications should be assessed, including in particular pressure lesions of the skin and postural hypotension. Prevention of the former is an important immediate aspect of rehabilitation, since a full-thickness pressure sore will retard rehabilitation by many weeks; its creation takes a few hours. Postural hypotension may be due to drugs, to biochemical disorders, or to bed rest itself. The patient's mental state requires assessment, with particular attention to intellectual impairment, the presence of depression, and the adequacy of morale. Disability must be assessed in functional terms (for example the ability to feed, dress, maintain continence, and walk; see Table 6), and must be seen against the state preceding the acute illness. A target date for discharge should be set, and arrangements made with relatives and community services to ensure that support is available on the day of discharge and immediately thereafter. When the drug regimen has been reduced to the minimum necessary, it should be explained in detail to the patient, who should be given the responsibility for it, supervised by the nursing staff or ward pharmacist.

REHABILITATION AFTER STROKE

This presents problems of greater complexity. A detailed neurological and functional assessment is the essential starting point, beginning with a determination of mental state, and of problems of communication (deafness and language disorder), with particular attention to receptive dysphasia. In the upper limb, motor function can be most simply assessed from fine finger movements. If these return within 3 weeks, reasonable recovery of upper limb function is likely. Important proprioceptive loss and the phenomena of unilateral sensory inattention imply a poor prognosis for functional recovery, although both tend to improve over a period of 3 or 4 months. In the lower limb, power can be simply tested by asking the patient to lift the leg off the bed. If it can be held for 10 to 15 s, the patient should be able to stand, although disorder of balance or instability of the knee may remain important problems. The prevention of contracture of the knee and ankle and of pressure sores on the heel of the affected leg are essential. Deep venous thrombosis, once common, is now less often seen; prophylactic heparin is rarely used. Sitting and standing balance must be assessed, since it is counterproductive to ask a patient who cannot sit unsupported to stand, or one who cannot stand unsupported to walk.

One of the most common causes of failure to do as well as expected during rehabilitation after stroke is depression. Continuous awareness of its possibility and its rapid recognition are essential. Its treatment is that of depression of any cause.

Epilepsy is a not uncommon associate of cerebrovascular disease, which is its most common cause in later life. Some strokes present as fits or status epilepticus which require pharmacological control. Often in these cases the fits subside after the acute phase and medication can be cautiously withdrawn. A proportion of stroke survivors, perhaps 10 to 15 per cent, develop epilepsy over the 2 years after the stroke, presumably consequent on cerebral scar tissue, and typically in these cases the epilepsy requires lifelong treatment. The epilepsy may present in cryptic form as nocturnal incontinence, pain of sudden onset in the limbs or face, unexplained falls, or episodes of confusion. It may also be mistaken for transient ischaemic attacks if followed by Todd's paresis and an exacerbation of pre-existing neurological signs.

Although thalamic pain is overdiagnosed, pain in hemiplegia is not uncommon and is typically focused on the shoulder of the affected upper limb. Usually there are three elements in the genesis of the pain: first is a peripheral lesion such as a frozen shoulder, a rotator cuff lesion, or an unsuspected subluxation; secondly, there is often an affective element in the form of depression or anxiety; thirdly is a central change in pain threshold, especially if there has been a sensory component to the stroke. It is important to treat the first two factors before resorting to centrally acting drugs such as carbamazepine in an attempt to modify the third.

The functions of the members of the rehabilitation team are essentially as outlined above. The nursing staff are concerned with the maintenance of morale, the prevention of incontinence, and the organization of the patient's immediate environment. The physiotherapist is concerned with balance and with walking, with whatever aid is appropriate. With further improvement, independence in activities of daily living (especially dressing) is the responsibility of the occupational therapist. The speech therapist will play a major part with those with dysphasia, particularly in the serial assessment of improvement of language function. Finally, the social worker will be concerned with the problems of relocation and re-establishment at home.

REHABILITATION OF THOSE WITH PARKINSON'S DISEASE

The rehabilitation of the patient with Parkinson's disease (see Chapter 24.10) illustrates other principles. Mental state is the principal determinant of the likelihood of benefit from drug therapy. Depression may be difficult to diagnose, but responds to antidepressant therapy. Proper use of drugs has a central role in rehabilitation. Initial doses of levodopa should be small, and increase in dose gradual, to a modest final dose; this will minimize the likelihood of adverse effects such as psychiatric disorder, dyskinesia, and postural hypotension. Anticholinergic drugs should rarely be used (the only indication being tremor), because of a high frequency of side-effects, but bromocriptine, selegiline, and newer drugs have essentially the same indications for their use as in younger patients, although starting doses should be lower.

The restoration of mobility is largely a function of proper drug therapy, but the physiotherapist can improve the patient's ability to turn in bed, and encourage confidence in walking, and the proper use of walking aids. The occupational therapist can provide appropriate aids to daily living (for example, for feeding, in the kitchen and bathroom, and in the toilet); a visit to the patient's home is essential to determine which aids will be of benefit. Newly developed techniques of speech therapy are of value. The social problems of families of patients with Parkinson's disease, who face prolonged disability often complicated by the psychiatric effects of the disease and its drug therapy, may require the assistance of a sympathetic social worker and/or voluntary organization.

Psychiatric disorders in old age

Nowhere is the importance of psychiatry in medicine more evident than in old age. A detailed account is given in Section 27. The principal

Table 9 *Some causes of delirium and dementia in old age*

Structural damage to the brain
  For example
    cerebral infarction, Alzheimer's disease, subdural haematoma,
    cerebral tumour (primary or secondary)
Disorders of the cerebral circulation
  For example
    carotid insufficiency, systemic hypotension, congestive cardiac failure
Metabolic brain disorders
  For example
    hypoxia, uraemia, dehydration, electrolyte disorder, thyroid disease, hypoglycaemia, vitamin deficiency (of vitamin B_{12} or folate)
Epilepsy
Drug toxicity
  For example
    poisoning with barbiturates, phenothiazines, alcohol, digitalis, etc.

Table 10 *Simple classification of the severity of dementia*

Mild impairment
  There is definite impairment of memory and calculating ability; such patients are often unable to manage to live alone, and are in need of some degree of supervision
Moderate impairment
  There is in addition disorientation for time, place, or person; such patients can live at home with others, but if their behaviour is disturbed, institutional care may be needed
Severe impairment
  There is in addition difficulty with self-care, in particular initially difficulty with dressing; some have also difficulty in walking, and/or incontinence of urine; such patients need devoted attention to continue to live outside hospital

problems for the physician in geriatric medicine may be summarized as follows.

The recognition of delirium should lead to a vigorous search for causes, with emphasis on the detection of focal neurological signs, cardiac or respiratory failure, a wide range of biochemical disorders, infection in a variety of possible sites, and drug toxicity (see Table 9). The key to the management of delirium is to identify and treat the precipitating cause. As far as possible, sedative drugs should be avoided and the anxiety and disordered behaviour managed by psychological means. Delirious patients have problems with attention, memory, and perception; they are usually also feeling ill and frightened. Good nursing management depends on recognizing the implications of these problems. Patients need to be reassured repeatedly and calmly about where they are and what is happening. The environment should be quiet and free from worrying sounds. A delirious patient may, not altogether unreasonably, interpret a singer of popular music on an unseen ward radio or television as a fellow prisoner being tortured. It is reassuring to delirious old people if doctors are dressed and behave like doctors, and nurses like nurses of more gracious times; being addressed in old age by some overfamiliar ambiguous stranger using one's Christian name can be alarming. It is easier to see what is going on if lighting is adequate for aged eyes. All forms of physical restraint are terrifying; they should not be used.

Assessment of dementia requires detailed enquiry from relatives about how the patient spends his or her time, and about such manifestations as restlessness, wandering, and aggressive behaviour. Observation of the patient's appearance and behaviour during examination provides valuable information; physical examination may show neurological abnormalities depending on the cause. Simple psychometric tests (Table 5) are valuable, and should be a routine part of geriatric clinical examination.

A simple classification of the severity of intellectual impairment is of value, in part because it can provide guidance to the type of care the patient is likely to require. An example is given in Table 10. The management of dementia rests on alteration and simplification of the environment so that the sufferer can cope with it. This implies a need for supervision to maintain socially acceptable behaviour. Drug therapy has little place, but disturbed behaviour by day may need to be treated with small doses of thioridazine, with haloperidol as a valuable alternative in more severe cases.

Some patients with dementia may have been living in such a restricted environment and with so much support from relatives, neighbours, or friends that their cognitive impairment has passed unnoticed. This state may be regarded as a compensated dementia. When removed suddenly to an unfamiliar environment, for example by coming to hospital or being taken on a well-intentioned but ill-advised holiday, they become acutely disoriented and anxious. Unless they are returned rapidly to their familiar environment, this decompensation of dementia may become irreversible.

The recognition and treatment of depression is also essential. To the geriatric physician it most commonly presents as failure to rehabilitate as expected.

A paranoid state may hinder medical treatment if one of the patient's delusions is that he or she is being poisoned by the doctors.

Some old people whose psychiatric state cannot be called normal defy precise categorization. They have shown persistently odd behaviour throughout their lives, have antagonized and driven away all their relatives and friends, and are in consequence solitary, isolated, and difficult. They may live in self-inflicted squalor which brings them to the attention of neighbours and local authority agencies. They may not be intellectually impaired, and are not paranoid, depressed, nor anxious. The term eccentric is as good as any. Recognition is not difficult, but treatment is, since correction of the squalor and disarray in which they live is only of brief benefit.

When to refer a patient to a psychogeriatrician is a further problem. One indication is undoubtedly difficulty in diagnosis, in particular perhaps in distinguishing between dementia and the pseudodementia of depression, or deciding, when both are present, which is the more important. Interpretation of paranoid states may also constitute an indication for referral. A final principal indication is severity of illness. The severely depressed patient should not be denied the undoubted benefits of electroconvulsive therapy when the indications for this exist (for example life-threatening reduction in food or fluid intake). The demented patient whose behaviour is disruptive or aggressive, or is manifest by persistent wandering, is best managed in a psychogeriatric ward by appropriately trained nurses. On occasion the clinical psychologist may assist with behavioural modification.

Cardiovascular disease

The symptoms of heart disease in old age are not infrequently modified. Cardiac pain is often slight; angina may be manifest as a need to stop walking, and the pain of cardiac infarction may be absent, or be overshadowed by other symptoms, such as confusion. As a symptom of heart failure, breathlessness may be replaced by fatigue, which may reflect reduced cardiac output and muscle blood flow, without great increase in pulmonary vascular volumes or pressures; decreased sensory input from the respiratory muscles, heart, and pulmonary vasculature may also be relevant.

Interpretation of cardiovascular signs must also be modified for elderly patients. Reduction in hand blood flow may suppress the signs of increased cardiac output in anaemia or cor pulmonale. Decreased elasticity of the central arterial tree increases pulse pressure, and may mask the peripheral signs of aortic stenosis. The venous pressure is usually more easily visible through the thin skin of an elderly neck, but compression of the left innominate vein between an enlarged aorta and the back of the sternum may result in asymmetrical elevation of the venous pressure, that in the left jugular and subclavian veins being higher than that on the right, a difference abolished by deep inspiration. The true central venous pressure should thus be determined from the right jugular venous system, or after inspiration. The cardiac apex may be difficult to feel, and its site may be displaced by thoracic kyphoscoliosis, but the powerful and prolonged impulse of left ventricular hypertrophy, the diffuse impulse of left ventricular dilatation, and the increased left parasternal pulsation of right ventricular hypertrophy can usually be identified. The elderly heart shows no abnormal auscultatory findings, apart from the frequent presence of a soft ejection systolic murmur. The proper recognition of congestive cardiac failure rests upon the demonstration of breathlessness, elevation of the venous pressure in all phases of respiration, bilateral pulmonary signs (of oedema or effusion), hepatic enlargement (rather than mere downward displacement), and sacral or symmetrical ankle oedema. Basal lung crepitations not cleared by coughing are present in a high proportion of old people without identifiable cause and should not on their own be considered diagnostic of heart failure. A third heart sound is much more suggestive of heart failure than is a fourth sound in later life. The diagnosis of left heart failure is more difficult, but nocturnal or exertional breathlessness or fatigue, Cheyne–Stokes respiration, and evidence of left heart disease should be present. Accurate diagnosis, both of cardiac failure and of its underlying cause, is of great importance, since proper treatment is extremely rewarding, and the drugs used are certainly ineffective, and possibly dangerous, in patients who do not have cardiac failure.

CARDIAC FAILURE

Cardiac failure should initially be treated along the same lines as in the young. The entirely proper enthusiasm for the active and early mobilization of elderly patients has obscured the fact that in cardiac failure physical rest is very important. The patient should initially be nursed in bed or in a chair. Once signs of cardiac failure have disappeared, and weight loss following diuretic therapy has ceased, gradual mobilization may begin, initially with walking to the toilet, and then with longer distances on the flat within the house or ward.

Digitalis therapy is essential in patients with atrial fibrillation and an uncontrolled ventricular response, and may be valuable in those with atrial fibrillation and a slow ventricular rate, and those with sinus rhythm, at least for the first few weeks. Digitalization should be begun with a single oral dose of 0.5 or 0.75 mg of digoxin, followed by a maintenance dose appropriate to the patient's renal function. If this is reasonably normal (serum urea 10 mmol/l or less, and/or serum creatinine 150 µmol/l or less), the maintenance dose should be 0.25 mg/day; if renal function is more impaired, the lower dose of 0.125 mg/day is correct. Digoxin 0.0625 mg/day does not produce therapeutic serum levels unless the glomerular filtration rate is less than 10 ml/min. These simple rules will enable the maximum benefit from digoxin with the minimum risk of toxicity.

Digitalis therapy should be continued indefinitely in patients with atrial fibrillation in whom the ventricular rate rises to above 80 beats/min in the absence of digitalis, but can be discontinued after 3 months in patients in sinus rhythm, particularly when cardiac failure has been precipitated by an event such as myocardial infarction, and there is spontaneous improvement in myocardial function.

Diuretic therapy poses particular problems (see Chapter 15.6.1). Increased urine volumes may result in retention of urine in elderly men, and in incontinence in either sex. Normal bladder function is usually restored when cardiac failure has resolved, and mental state and mobility have improved. Potassium depletion is frequent, and potassium supplements should be given, or potassium-sparing agents used.

The place of angiotensin-converting-enzyme (ACE) inhibitors in the treatment of cardiac failure in elderly patients has been clarified in recent years, and it is now clear that they are of considerable value. They not only improve symptoms, in particular fatigue, but they also reduce mortality from progression of cardiac failure, though not from arrhythmias. Doses should be lower than in younger patients. The usual precautions, in particular for first-dose hypotension, should be taken and contraindications, such as severe renal failure, observed. Routine checking of renal function, say after 1 to 2 weeks of therapy, is essential in all patients.

PAROXYSMAL CARDIAC DYSRHYTHMIAS

These are recognized as causes of syncope and falls. Frequent ventricular ectopic beats or left bundle branch block are common findings in routine ECGs of elderly people and are difficult to interpret in this context. If a dysrhythmia has not been demonstrated at the time of a syncopal episode, 24 h electrocardiogram monitoring is commonly performed, but again the relevance of the commonly found brief episodes of dysrhythmia to a patient's symptoms may be difficult to establish. The combination of syncope and complete heart block, bifascicular block, or the sick sinus syndrome, is an indication for cardiac pacing, perhaps with dual-chamber pacing, whatever the age of the patient, since the quality of life is much improved and its length perhaps increased (Chapter 15.8.2). When the symptoms are those of cardiac failure, a decision is more difficult, but temporary pacing to see if symptoms improve is justifiable. Elderly patients tolerate cardiac pacing extremely well; the expectation of life of octogenarians paced for complete heart block has been shown to be normal.

MYOCARDIAL INFARCTION

In myocardial infarction age is not a contraindication to established regimens of thrombolysis and heparin as used in younger patients. Indeed, the evidence suggests that thrombolytic therapy may save more lives when given to older patients following myocardial infarction than when given to younger patients. The duration of heparin therapy may be extended for patients with large myocardial infarctions or with overt heart failure, or when for any reason bed rest has to be prolonged. Postmyocardial regimens, including aspirin, should normally be used in older patients as in younger. Should overt systemic embolism occur in the context of myocardial infarction, oral anticoagulation will need to be considered, but in the absence of established atrial fibrillation or other reasons for supposing there is a chronic risk of repeated embolism, anticoagulation would not normally be continued beyond 6 weeks.

ATRIAL FIBRILLATION

Large trials have now established that in the absence of contraindications, patients aged 60 and over with atrial fibrillation should have long-term anticoagulation therapy in order to reduce their three- to fivefold increased risk of stroke. Patients with associated valvular disease or dilated left atrium are at even higher risk of stroke. Even in the absence of overt stroke, CT scanning has shown that older patients in atrial fibrillation show a higher prevalence of 'silent' cerebral infarcts; anticoagulation therapy may therefore reduce the subsequent incidence of multi-infarct dementia.

The risks of oral anticoagulant therapy are on average greater for older people than younger. Oral anticoagulants have a more powerful pharmacodynamic affect in later life; older people are more likely to have cryptic peptic ulcer disease and may be more liable to haemorrhagic complications owing to changes in blood vessels and skin elasticity. None the less, there is evidence that this increased risk of haemorrhagic complications from anticoagulant therapy can be overcome by care in prescribing and increased surveillance of therapy. Anticoagulant therapy should only be instituted in patients of any age where good compliance can be expected and adequate surveillance ensured. In atrial fibrillation, anticoagulation need not be of an intense level and an INR of 2 to 2.5 is an appropriate target. It is prudent to reduce pre-existing high blood pressure (see below) before instituting anticoagulant therapy. In young patients, paroxysmal atrial fibrillation does not seem to be associated with an enhanced risk of stroke. The situation is less clear for patients aged over 60 who develop paroxysmal atrial fibrillation without treatable cause, but on the basis of present knowledge they should be anticoagulated because they are likely to move into established fibrillation. Data from the Framingham study suggested that the risk of stroke may be greatest during the 6 months or so before and after an older person becomes established in atrial fibrillation.

DEEP VENOUS THROMBOSIS

Leg vein thrombosis with a clot extending above the popliteal should be treated in elderly patients along conventional lines with short-term heparin followed by oral anticoagulation for 3 months. Continuous anticoagulation will need to be considered in a patient with recurrent thrombosis. Anticoagulant therapy is not normally used for elderly patients with venous thrombosis restricted to veins below the knee, but a proportion of these show later extension which should be watched for and treated appropriately. There is a slight risk of a carcinoma becoming apparent in elderly patients with otherwise unexplained leg vein thrombosis, but the excess risk is less than at younger ages. Apart from care to exclude a pelvic neoplasm, it is rarely profitable to institute a systematic search for occult malignancy in the absence of localizing symptoms or signs.

STROKE

The role of aspirin and heparin in the acute phase following a stroke is undergoing examination in randomized controlled trials. There is a great deal of uncertainty about the indications for anticoagulant therapy following established stroke. Clearly this should only be considered where CT scan has excluded the possibility of the stroke being due to cerebral haemorrhage. For patients who have had a non-haemorrhagic stroke associated with atrial fibrillation, anticoagulant therapy should be considered, but opinions differ as to the appropriate time to start. In the early days following a stroke there is a risk of haemorrhage into a cerebral infarct, but the risk of a further stroke is highest in the early days after an embolus. At present most clinicians would consider starting anticoagulation between 2 and 4 weeks after a non-haemorrhagic stroke in an elderly patient with atrial fibrillation, but more research needs to be done.

In the absence of atrial fibrillation or some other established cardiac source for repeated emboli, it is not usual to use anticoagulant therapy for transient ischaemic attacks. It might, however, be considered for therapeutic trial in a patient with many repeated attacks who has not responded to aspirin therapy. It should not be persisted with, however, if there is not a clear benefit sufficient to outweigh the risk of haemorrhagic complications.

HIGH BLOOD PRESSURE

In Western populations mean systolic blood pressure rises with age until the eighth decade and thereafter shows a fall, due partly to selective survival but partly also to some old people experiencing declines in blood pressure. Average diastolic blood pressure in the population typically peaks in the seventh decade and thereafter declines. It is no longer appropriate to consider the rise of blood pressure with age as 'normal ageing' as it clearly carries with it an increased risk of cardiovascular disease, particularly coronary disease and stroke.

Large trials have now established that treatment of high blood pressure in patients at least up to the age of 80 can reduce the risk of stroke. Treatment of raised blood pressure should now be considered in patients of either sex and any age. Moreover, the benefits have been shown for the treatment of systolic pressure, regardless of whether diastolic pressure is also raised or not. It is best to regard as in need of treatment a sustained systolic pressure of over 160 mmHg, whether or not the diastolic pressure is over 90 mm Hg in a patient under the age of 80. The object of treatment should be to reduce blood pressure to approximately 160/90 mmHg over 2 to 3 months. All effective means of lowering blood pressure carry a significant risk of undesirable side-effects in later life and care needs to be taken in the selection of therapy, and in ensuring reliable compliance and the surveillance of blood pressure levels.

In the absence of contraindications, the first line of treatment in the elderly patient should be a potassium-sparing thiazide diuretic combination such as hydrochlorothiazide 25 mg with triamterene 50 mg once a day. This combination has been shown to be safe and effective; the thiazide diuretic also helps to prevent osteoporosis, a factor of particular significance for women. In young adult patients it is not usually considered necessary to add a potassium-retaining agent or potassium supplements to thiazide therapy for hypertension as dietary intake often matches urinary losses. This may not be true for some older people. If the effect on blood pressure of this or an equivalent dose of thiazide is inadequate, it should not be raised as this would merely increase the risk of side-effects without further benefit to the blood pressure. A second-line drug should be added or substituted. Thiazide diuretics may be contraindicated in diabetics or in patients with a tendency to gout. They also may be associated with impotence in men; the age of a patient should not inhibit the doctor from making a tactful enquiry about the possible importance of this before prescribing.

β-Blockers tend not to be very effective in lowering blood pressure in older people and have a fairly high risk of side-effects. Calcium-channel blockers are effective. For diabetic patients and for those with evidence of heart failure, ACE inhibitors may be the best treatment. These drugs are effective in older patients, but again the risk of side-effects is somewhat greater than in younger patients. Care has to be taken if the patient has been on diuretics, and potassium-retaining drugs such as triamterene or amiloride should be stopped when an ACE inhibitor is started. A base-line estimate of plasma creatinine and urea should be made. In view of the risk of first-dose hypotension, the patient should initially be given a small dose of captopril (2–6.25 mg) and the blood pressure monitored over 3 h. If there is no fall in blood pressure during this period, the likelihood of precipitating hypotension later is low but the patient should be warned of the possibility. The majority of patients who show a significant fall in pressure do so within 1 h of receiving captopril.

It is usual to transfer the older patient from captopril to a drug with single daily dosage in order to improve compliance. Subsequent dosage is tuned by small increments. Plasma creatinine and urea estimation should be repeated a few days and up to 4 weeks after starting ACE inhibitor therapy in view of the risk of renal failure being induced by the drug in those with occult renal artery stenosis. Older patients on antihypertensive treatment should have their lying and standing blood pressure checked at regular intervals of 6 to 8 weeks.

ORTHOSTATIC HYPOTENSION

This is a common phenomenon in elderly people. A drop of 20 mmHg or more in systolic pressure on standing is found in 15 per cent of those aged between 65 and 74, and in 25 per cent over that age. This drop is usually asymptomatic, but if the fall in systolic pressure is substantial, or the standing systolic pressure is 110 mmHg or less, and autoregulation of cerebral blood flow is impaired, then orthostatic syncopal symptoms are likely. The great majority of cases are due to injudicious drug therapy, particularly with thiazides, other hypotensive drugs, tricyclic antidepressants, phenothiazines, benzodiazepines, levodopa, or combinations of drugs. Orthostatic hypotension may develop if bed rest is prolonged, and may obstruct rehabilitation following acute illness. In the small proportion of cases not due to drugs, primary changes in the autonomic nervous system may be responsible; the complete Shy–

Drager syndrome is a distinct rarity. The recognition of orthostatic hypotension depends on a careful history, indicating that the cerebral circulation is impaired immediately after rising from bed or chair. It is confirmed by taking the blood pressure in the standing as well as the lying position; if this is done routinely, many cases of so-called 'vertebrobasilar insufficiency' will be found to have a simple and usually easily remediable cause. Management begins with reduction or discontinuance of the causal drug therapy. Reduction in levodopa dosage will usually lead to a satisfactory compromise between improvement in parkinsonism and incapacitating orthostatic hypotension. When drug therapy is not implicated, or orthostatic hypotension does not disappear when apparently causal drugs are discontinued, raising the head of the bed at night may be of value, but usually treatment with fludrocortisone, 0.1 to 0.3 mg/day, should be combined with tight, full-length elastic stockings, and advice on the gradual achievement of the standing position from lying. Blood pressure falls spontaneously in some older hypertensive patients, sometimes in associated with a reduction in body weight or the onset of debilitating disease, but often for no discernible reason. The first sign of this may be unexplained episodes of postural hypotension in a patient whose antihypertensive therapy has been stable for some time. Symptoms may first appear postprandially. Management is by reduction or withdrawal of antihypertensive treatment.

Bone disease

Osteoporosis and Paget's disease are common in elderly people but are considered in detail elsewhere (see Section 19). Osteomalacia due to inadequate vitamin D activity is well recognized as a problem for women in some Asian immigrant groups to the United Kingdom and is also found in the indigenous elderly population. There is loss of 1α-hydroxylase activity in the ageing kidney which reduces the effective use by the body of endogenous and exogenous vitamin D. In the absence of other specific causative factors such as malabsorption syndromes or anti-epileptic medication, osteomalacia in elderly people largely occurs in the housebound and particular in the north of the United Kingdom. It is now less common than it used to be, probably partly because of reduced levels of industrial and domestic air pollution allowing more ultraviolet light to penetrate to ground level, and partly because of dietary changes. Twenty years ago elderly people tended to eat butter rather than margarine but butter has a variable and low vitamin D content. More recently margarine has become more popular and this is fortified with vitamins A and D. The yet more recent growth in popularity of unfortified low-fat spreads and the likelihood of European Community regulations forbidding the mandatory fortification of margarines may make osteomalacia in the British elderly population once more a health problem.

Frank osteomalacia is associated with the characteristic histological pattern of unossified zones of osteoid visible in bone biopsy. It has also been suggested that minor degrees of vitamin D deficiency may also produce osteoporosis, that is to say reduced bone tissue with normal histology. When vitamin D activity in the body is low and calcium absorption from the gut thereby inadequate, parathyroid secretion is increased so maintaining blood calcium levels at the expense of the bones. This produces the characteristic reduced plasma phosphate (and chloride raised within its normal range) of early (compensated) osteomalacia. Studies among middle-aged women in the United States have shown that in the winter vitamin D levels fall low enough to activate parathyroid hormone leading to loss of bone that may not be fully made up in the following summers. It may emerge that winter supplements of vitamin D will have a place in the prevention of osteoporosis in older people, but on present knowledge this has to be regarded as speculative.

The manifestations of vitamin D deficiency cover a wide spectrum, from asymptomatic biochemical changes to backache and diffuse bone pain; proximal muscle weakness may lead to immobility and falls; mental changes, especially depression, are common; the combination of muscle weakness and osteomalacic changes in bone may cause fractures, particularly of the proximal femur. The diagnosis should always be considered in elderly patients with these features. Radiological evidence in the form of Looser's zones is usually lacking, but isotope bone scanning may reveal areas of increased uptake at the characteristic sites of pseudofractures, such as the medial border of the scapula, the inferior pubic ramus, and the medial femoral neck. Biochemical changes are difficult to interpret because of age-associated changes in serum calcium and alkaline phosphatase (see Table 4). There is also a substantial overlap in serum vitamin D concentrations between undoubted normality and undoubted vitamin D deficiency. The single most satisfactory diagnostic measure is probably a therapeutic trial of vitamin D. Alfacalcidol in a dose of 1 microgram/day should be given, together with calcium supplements. If osteomalacia is the diagnosis, bone pain and other physical and mental symptoms will disappear within a few days, the serum phosphate and calcium will rise within a week or two, and the alkaline phosphatase begin to fall, but much more slowly. The vitamin D supplementation should then be reduced to maintenance levels, and plasma calcium concentrations monitored regularly to prevent hypercalcaemia.

The prevention of osteomalacia in the residents of long-term care institutions should be an important concern of geriatricians and of general practitioners providing medical care to nursing and residential homes for older people. Exposure to small doses of ultraviolet light has been shown to produce substantial effects on serum 25-hydroxyvitamin D levels of institutionalized elderly patients, but there are possible hazards to both patients and staff from overdosage of ultraviolet light. Dietary replacement of butter by margarine fortified with vitamin D, taking every opportunity for controlled exposure to natural sunlight, and consideration of vitamin D supplementation for the particularly vulnerable, at least in winter, are simpler and safer approaches.

Metabolic and endocrine disorders

DIABETES MELLITUS

The definition, and thus the diagnosis, of diabetes becomes more difficult with advancing age. Glucose tolerance, whether tested orally or intravenously, shows a steady decline with age, and the incidence of newly discovered frank diabetes rises. The mean decline in glucose tolerance is such that if the standard diagnostic criteria used in middle age are applied to those over the age of 70, over 50 per cent of elderly people would be 'diabetic'. Severe glucose intolerance accompanied by symptoms of diabetes leaves no doubt that the patient should be treated as diabetic, but asymptomatic mild impairment of glucose tolerance can scarcely be regarded in the same way. Help with resolution of these difficulties is provided by revision of the blood glucose criteria for the diagnosis of diabetes, and the introduction of the concept of impaired glucose tolerance (Table 11), and the measurement of glycosylated haemoglobin in doubtful cases (precise normal values vary somewhat from laboratory to laboratory but seem unaffected by age). If diabetes is diagnosed according to the criteria shown, almost all symptomatic elderly patients will be diagnosed as diabetic. The category of impaired glucose tolerance includes many elderly people, but follow-up of this group suggests neither a much greater excess risk of the development of true diabetes nor of its specific complications, but rather an increased susceptibility to atherosclerotic vascular disease.

The factors influencing the age change in glucose tolerance are poorly understood. Obesity is probably less, and diabetogenic drugs more important than has been thought. Genetic factors are more important than in younger insulin-dependent patients, and the diabetes-promoting influence of multiparity persists in women at least to the age of 80. The probable physiological mechanism involved in the impairment of glucose tolerance with age is a combination of reduction both in the effectiveness of the action of insulin and in insulin secretion in response to hyperglycaemia.

The clinical presentation of diabetes in old age is different from that at younger ages. Many are diagnosed as a result of routine testing during

Table 11 *WHO guidelines for diagnosis of diabetes mellitus and impaired glucose tolerance (stated in terms of venous whole blood, true glucose measurements, following a 75 g oral glucose load where appropriate)*

1. Diabetes mellitus is diagnosed when:
   (1) The fasting blood glucose concentration equals or exceeds 7 mmol/l (126 mg/dl) on more than one occasion
   (2) The blood sugar concentration 2 h after a 75 g oral glucose load equals or exceeds 10 mmol/l (180 mg/dl) irrespective of the fasting concentration

2. Impaired glucose tolerance exists when the 2 h blood glucose concentration falls between 7 and 10 mmol/l. Action with impaired glucose tolerance depends upon individual circumstances

a medical or surgical illness, some because of the development of disorders associated with diabetes (for example peripheral vascular disease, cataract), and relatively fewer because of classical symptoms such as weight loss, polyuria, and pruritus vulvae. A small proportion present with life-threatening metabolic decompensation.

The management of newly discovered diabetes in old age is based on diet, oral hypoglycaemic agents, and insulin. Its most important aspect is the education of the patient and of those caring for him or her in the nature of the condition and the objectives of treatment. Dietary treatment should be advised for every old person in whom a definite diagnosis of diabetes is made. Reduction in carbohydrate intake to 120 to 150 g/day, with maintenance of normal protein intake, is usually all that is needed. Advice should be simple, flexible, and repeated, should allow adequate variety to take account of the individual's own preferences, and should avoid setting inappropriate dietary patterns.

Oral hypoglycaemic agents should be used if dietary therapy does not result in reduction in hyperglycaemia within a few weeks. Tolbutamide, gliclazide, and glibornuride are to be preferred, while longer-acting drugs such as chlorpropamide and glibenclamide should not be used. Limitation of dosage, and prompt discontinuance if food intake falls, are important to prevent hypoglycaemia. The combination of a short-acting sulphonylurea and metformin is often appropriate.

In elderly patients with acutely disordered diabetes, insulin should not be withheld. In the long term, it should be given to those in whom oral therapy fails. There is also a small group of thin, elderly men whose diabetes is insulin-dependent from the first; it should never be thought that such diabetes does not or cannot occur in old age. Single daily injections of insulin are preferable to multiple. Regular blood or urine testing is necessary, and the fact that the renal threshold for glucose rises slightly with age should not deter from this necessary discipline. Many elderly diabetics, especially those on insulin, benefit from the support and advice given by regular attendance at a diabetic clinic.

Approximately one case in six of diabetic ketosis occurs in patients over the age of 60. Ketosis is usually precipitated by infection, but multiple causes are common. The degree of metabolic decompensation is often greater in elderly than in younger patients. Vigorous rehydration and insulin therapy (see Chapter 11.11) are essential, but the mortality remains high. Non-ketotic hyperosmolar coma is virtually confined to elderly patients, but how this state arises is far from clear. It may occur postoperatively even in mild diabetes, and should be watched for in this situation. Treatment with large amounts of intravenous fluid and small doses of insulin produces slower improvement than in ketosis, and the mortality, mostly due to arterial occlusion, is again substantial.

The evidence for the relationship between control of diabetes and the development of complications in old age is not entirely satisfactory. Good control retards the development of the specific complications of diabetes, but cannot be relied upon to prevent progression of established

lesions. In the elderly, glucose intolerance (and presumably therefore poorly controlled diabetes) is more important than, for instance, hypercholesterolaemia as a risk factor for cardiac failure, intermittent claudication, and stroke, but less important than cigarette smoking in respect of intermittent claudication, or than raised blood pressure in respect of cardiac failure or stroke.

The specific complications of diabetes occur more frequently in elderly than in young patients. The majority of patients blind from diabetes are over the age of 60. The prognosis of diabetic retinopathy in old age is less favourable than in middle age, but photocoagulation remains effective treatment for many macular lesions. Cataract extraction is three or four times more common in elderly diabetics than in non-diabetics, although the visual indications for operation are the same. The results of operation are excellent, except when preoperative visual impairment is partly due to pre-existing retinopathy. The neurological complication of diabetes particularly associated with old age is amyotrophy (see Chapter 11.11). Its clinical recognition is important, because of its generally good prognosis, and the need to avoid unnecessary investigation. The principal emphasis in the management of foot lesions is on preventive measures, such as simple foot hygiene, proper footwear, avoidance of damaging extremes of heat and cold, and, if necessary, attendance at a chiropody clinic. It is important to remember that many old people have difficulty in checking their feet.

HYPOTHYROIDISM

Most cases of hypothyroidism in old age are of autoimmune origin, though previous thyroid surgery and radio-iodine therapy account for a considerable proportion. Classical clinical presentations probably only occur in a quarter of patients. Signs and symptoms such as cold intolerance, hair loss, and coarsening of the skin, are less common than an insidious decline in general health and mobility, and psychiatric manifestations, in particular depression. Hypothyroid coma, sometimes associated with severe headache and fits, and hypothermia (sometimes precipitated by phenothiazines) are less common but important presentations. The most useful physical signs are change in voice and delayed relaxation of tendon reflexes.

Cautious initial replacement therapy is advisable, beginning with thyroxine 25 μg/day, particularly if overt heart disease coexists. Adequacy of treatment may be established by an eventual fall in serum thyroid stimulating hormone to normal; doses of 100 to 150 μg/day are usually adequate. Relapse due to discontinuance of treatment is regrettably frequent, and the responsible doctor must ensure that lifelong treatment is in fact lifelong. Poor compliance may necessitate supervision by a relative, neighbour, or visiting nurse. Simplification of treatment by weekly administration of 70 per cent of the total weekly dose of thyroxine or twice-weekly administration of half the dose has its advocates.

HYPERTHYROIDISM

Hyperthyroidism is less common in old age than hypothyroidism, but perhaps even more likely to present in an atypical manner, so that a high index of suspicion is required if this important (because so easily treatable) condition is to be diagnosed. Weight loss, anorexia, gastrointestinal, and cardiovascular symptoms predominate. Cardiac failure, usually with atrial fibrillation resistant to digitalis, is the most important cardiac presentation, and proximal myopathy is not infrequent. The eye signs and goitre are less common in elderly patients, and apathy or depression may be prominent. Untreated hyperthyroidism in old age is a serious threat to life. Treatment is best begun with carbimazole, followed, when thyroid function has returned to normal, by radio-iodine. In mild cases radio-iodine alone will be adequate, but the correct dose is difficult to determine, and the patient may remain undertreated for months. Lifelong follow-up is necessary, because whether or not a dose of radio-iodine sufficient to abolish thyroid function is used, hypothyroidism is a common sequel. An alternative is to use an ablative dose of radio-iodine initially with replacement by thyroxine when thyroid stimulating hormone levels rise.

Disorders of temperature regulation

Elderly people often show evidence of disordered thermoregulation, and they are thus particularly liable to be sensitive to extremes of environmental temperature.

HYPOTHERMIA

Most elderly patients with hypothermia present after a period of 2 or 3 days of relatively cold weather, but it is entirely possible for hypothermia to develop in hospital in midsummer at United Kingdom latitudes, especially if disease or drugs play an important part. The fall in central temperature occurs over 24 to 48 h, and its principal manifestations are progressive ataxia and slowing of cerebration, leading to stupor, and finally coma. On clinical examination, the skin on unexposed surfaces, such as the axilla, chest, and abdomen, feels cold to touch. There may be oedema of the face and eyelids resembling that of myxoedema, but due to redistribution of fluid between the intra- and extracellular compartments, and resolving with correction of the hypothermia. The pulse is slow, unless severe physical illness has raised it towards normal, and the blood pressure is difficult to record or low. Cerebration is slow but may be remarkably accurate even in the presence of considerable reduction in body temperature. Tendon reflexes are normal unless there is associated hypothyroidism. The diagnosis is made by recording the rectal temperature; this should be done without delay on all occasions when the oral temperature is recorded at 35°C or less. The principal investigation that may show characteristic but by no means universal features is the electrocardiogram, with bradycardia and J-waves (Fig. 3). In severe hypothermia there is often atrial fibrillation with a slow ventricular response.

Hypothermia in elderly patients has a high fatality, related to its cause in the individual case (those due to drugs usually recover; those due to severe physical illness usually die), its severity, and its complications (particularly pneumonia and pancreatitis). Its management is difficult. There is no rational basis for the use of steroids, while intravenous fluids are dangerous because they may produce pulmonary oedema; intravenous glucose is not metabolized, since insulin is ineffective in the hypothermic state. A slow rise in body temperature (optimally 0.5°C per hour) should be produced by exposing the patient to a relatively high ambient temperature of 30°C. Improvement is shown by an increase in rectal temperature and pulse rate, a maintained blood pressure, and improvement in conscious level. If hypothyroidism is suspected, liothyronine should be given, but only when the central temperature has risen to normal.

The elderly patient who has recovered from hypothermia should be regarded as at risk from a further episode, and relatives and social agencies should be mobilized to ensure maintenance of an adequate temperature in the home. The long-term prognosis is better in patients who have survived an episode of hypothermia of known cause. Many are alive 3 years later, as against none of those without a clear cause, whose failure of temperature regulation is presumably due to serious abnormality of the relevant physiological mechanisms.

HYPERTHERMIA

Hyperthermia may be an equal hazard. An increase in mortality in continuing care wards and of elderly people at home has been recognized during heat waves. The absence of appropriate behavioural responses is probably as important as impairment of physiological responses. The paramount need is to collect elderly people at risk into environments that can be kept cool. There is little useful guidance about the management of grossly raised body temperatures in elderly patients, except to maintain fluid intake.

Fig. 3 ECG from a hypothermic patient illustrating the Osborne (J wave) seen in V5 and 6. The characteristic is a deflection lying between the QRS complex and the beginning of the ST segment. The pathophysiology of the J wave is uncertain.

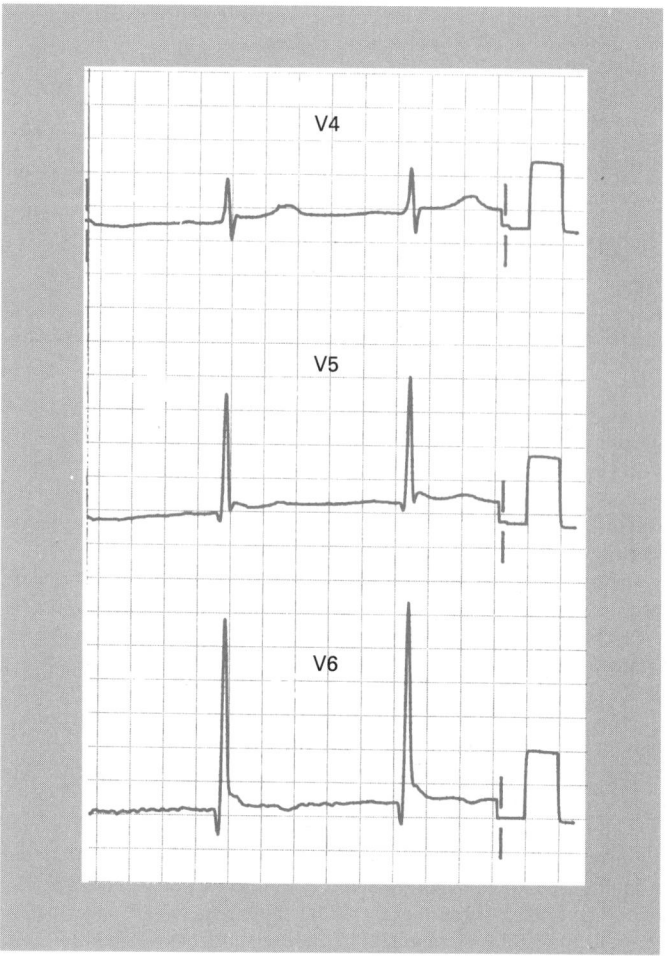

REFERENCES

Andrews, K. (1987). *Rehabilitation of the older adult.* Edward Arnold, London.

Caird, F.I. (1982). *Neurological disorders in the elderly.* Wright, Bristol.

Comfort, A. (1979). *The biology of senescence*, (3rd edn). Churchill Livingstone, Edinburgh.

Finch, C.E. (1990). *Longevity, senescence and the genome.* University of Chicago Press, Chicago.

Grimley Evans, J. and Williams, T.E. (ed.) (1992). *The Oxford textbook of geriatric medicine.* Oxford University Press, Oxford.

Hodkinson, H.M. (1992). Reference values for biological data in older persons. In *The Oxford textbook of geriatric medicine*, (ed. J. Grimley Evans and T.F. Williams), pp. 723–8. Oxford University Press, Oxford.

Kane, R.L., Grimley Evans, J., and Macfadyen, D. (ed.) (1990). *Improving the health of older people. A world view.* Oxford University Press, Oxford.

Lowenthal, D.T. (ed.) (1992). *Geriatric cardiology.* F.A. Davies, Philadelphia.

Marks, R. (1987). *Skin disease in old age.* Martin Dunitz, London.

Nuñez, J.F.M., and Cameron, J.S. (1987). *Renal function and disease in the elderly.* Butterworth, London.

O'Malley, K. (1984). *Clinical pharmacology and drug treatment of the elderly.* Churchill Livingstone, Edinburgh.

Section 32 *Terminal illness*

32 Terminal illness

M.J. BAINES

'I conceive it the office of the physician not only to restore the health but to mitigate pains and dolours; and not only when such mitigation may conduce to recovery but when it may serve to make a fair and easy passage'
FRANCIS BACON (1561–1626)

Modern scientific medicine is involved with the diagnosis and treatment of disease and is aimed at its cure or, at any rate, its remission. Such a view regards death as a disaster, the doctor's ultimate failure. Yet this attitude ignores the physician's responsibility to manage the process of dying by 'mitigating pains and dolours' and by giving appropriate support to the dying patient, the family, and the professional carers.

In the 1960s a number of influential reports drew attention to the suffering of the dying, and during that decade the modern hospice movement was born. Since then there has been a rapidly increasing and worldwide concern for the dying; palliative medicine has been established as a medical discipline, hospices have been founded in every continent, and the World Health Organization has taken a leading role in advocating pain relief and palliative care for all who need them (World Health Organization 1990).

The diagnosis of dying

'There is a general understanding that terminal care refers to the management of patients in whom the advent of death is felt to be certain and not too far off and for whom medical effort has turned away from therapy and become concentrated on the relief of symptoms and the support of both patient and family'
(Holford 1973)

The decision that active treatment, aimed at prolongation of life, is no longer appropriate must always be difficult. Yet such decisions must be made. To continue in an attempt to cure the incurable adds to the patient's distress and makes good symptom control and psychological support much more difficult.

IN CANCER PATIENTS

The decision to abandon active treatment is most commonly made in patients with advanced malignant disease, with the expectation of a steadily deteriorating situation. It is partly for this reason that palliative medicine has concentrated on cancer patients and most writing, including this chapter, is based on experience with this group. However, many cancer patients die with pneumonia, uraemia, or organic brain disease, and it is to be expected that much of the symptom control that has been developed will have wider application.

IN OTHER DISEASES

Over the past few years those working in other branches of medicine have described their criteria for stopping active treatment, or for recognizing that death is inevitable. They may include reference to the particular symptoms that develop during the process of dying and the expected span of life once active treatment is stopped.

In most of the common respiratory or cardiovascular diseases, the diagnosis of dying is made by exclusion, after a failure to respond to standard therapeutic and rehabilitative endeavours. It is often the experienced nurse who will first recognize the situation and this is usually just a few days before death.

In psychogeriatric patients there is often a prolonged period of dying, with a survey showing that 'over two thirds of patients lingered just short of death for many weeks and half of these protracted deaths featured distress, with or without pain'.

The increased use of life-sustaining technology has brought its own problems, with the inevitable ethical issues over whether such treatment is withheld or withdrawn. A survey of patients on long-term renal dialysis showed that 22 per cent of deaths were due to stopping treatment. A large majority of the competent patients made this decision for themselves; with incompetent patients, the doctor usually brought up the subject and discussed it with the family. Patients survived a mean of 8 days after dialysis was stopped.

Decisions to limit treatment are frequently made in a neurosurgical unit when signs of a poor prognosis are noted or there is a failure to respond to treatment. Median survival of 5 days was found after such a treatment-limiting decision.

Further studies are needed to describe how the diagnosis of dying is made in other diseases and how the specific problems that emerge in the last days or weeks of life can be controlled.

Appropriate treatment

A patient needs appropriate treatment at all stages of the illness. However, deciding which treatment is appropriate is often difficult, for it requires an understanding of the active treatment available with its likely response rate and side-effects. It also requires judgement about the patient's general condition, prognosis, psychological state, and wishes for the future. Doctors are not committed to every manoeuvre possible to prolong life but must be equally concerned with the relief of suffering.

Three stages in the treatment of the cancer patient have been described and are shown in Fig. 1.

Curative treatment is attempted for about half of all cancer patients, using one or more of the three treatment modalities: surgery, radiotherapy, and chemotherapy. The aim is survival or a long-term remission, and the toxicity of treatment may be high. However, about 50 per cent of those who have received curative treatment will eventually relapse.

Palliative treatment is appropriate, from the outset, for 50 per cent of cancer patients and for the further 25 per cent who have relapsed. Such

Fig. 1 Stages in cancer treatment.

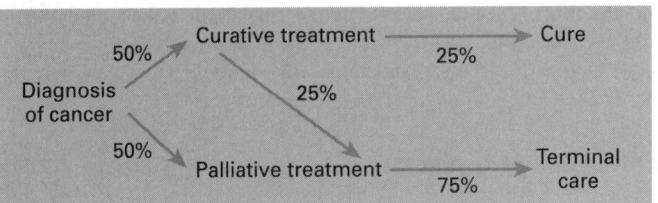

Table 1 *Prevalence of symptoms in terminal illness (percentage of patients)*

	Cancer, hospice[a]	All diseases, hospital[b]	Non-cancer, hospital and home[c]	Motor neurone disease, hospice[d]	AIDS, hospice[e]
Weakness	92	88		90	61
Anorexia	75	92	38		41
Pain	69	69	67	57	60
Dyspnoea	50	69	49	47	11
Nausea/vomiting	49	54	27		21
Constipation	48	54	32	65	18
Cough	47	77	18	53	19
Insomnia	29	88	36	48	
Confusion	27	35	38		29
Bedsores	25	61	14		
Catheter/ incontinence	20	31	33	15	
Slurred or absent speech				80	
Dysphagia	25		17	79	
Dribbling			14	38	

[a]Symptoms of patients with advanced cancer on hospice admission.

[b]Terminally ill patients in a general hospital, 58% cancer, 42% non-cancer (Hockley *et al.* 1988).

[c]Symptoms in the last year of life in non-cancer patients (Searle, 1991).

[d]Patients with motor neurone disease on hospice admission (O'Brien *et al.* 1992).

[e]Patients with AIDS on hospice admission (Moss 1990).

treatment is not aimed at cure. It may prolong life but it is mainly directed at symptom control and maintaining the quality of life. Appropriate palliative treatment may cause mild or short-lived side-effects.

Some 75 per cent of cancer patients in the developed world will eventually require terminal care. The aim of treatment in terminal illness is purely the relief of physical and emotional distress and no side-effects of treatment are acceptable.

In rare situations, appropriate treatment to relieve terminal suffering may shorten life (see below). This is permissible provided the doctor's aim is only the relief of suffering. This reflects the so-called double effect theory and is incorporated into English law in one of the few decided cases in this area (R. v. Bodkin Adams 1957). On the other hand, some patients, thought to be dying, are able to resume active therapy once their symptoms and mental state improve with appropriate treatment.

However, the skills developed in palliative medicine have wide application. The control of pain and vomiting, the breaking of bad news, the support of frightened children, and many other aspects of palliative care are relevant to patients and families facing all types and stages of illness.

Symptom control in terminal illness

The patient who is dying of a chronic illness usually presents a complex clinical picture. The causative illness, whether advanced cancer, chronic respiratory failure, or stroke, often leads to widespread physical changes with reduced resistance to infection, impairment of hepatic or renal function, and marked debility. It is therefore not surprising that dying patients develop a multiplicity of symptoms in their last weeks or months of life. The foundation of good terminal care is meticulous attention to these symptoms, for without this it is difficult, perhaps impossible, to give the necessary emotional support to the patient and family.

Prevalence of symptoms

A number of studies have been undertaken to determine the prevalence of symptoms in different groups of dying patients; those with and with-

out cancer and also those with motor neurone disease and AIDS (Table 1).

Such studies show the considerable level of suffering during the last months of life in those with chronic illness. The prevalence of pain is remarkably similar in all patient groups, between 57 and 69 per cent. Dyspnoea, anorexia, constipation, and insomnia are also common. However, there are some major differences; the elderly (over 75 years) have a higher incidence of confusion (49 per cent) and faecal incontinence (28 per cent). Communication difficulties and a distressing, but nonspecific, agitation are also common in older patients. Patients with motor neurone disease develop major problems with speech and swallowing. Those with advanced AIDS may have severe diarrhoea due to Cryptosporidium and other infections.

Relatives caring for the dying are often equally concerned with psychological symptoms, and report the patient's depression (36 per cent) and bad temper (25 per cent).

Diagnosis of symptoms

Palliative treatment involves making a diagnosis of the cause, or causes, of each symptom. For example, a patient with breast cancer may be nauseated due to liver metastases, hypercalcaemia, or constipation. In the patient who is terminally ill this diagnosis will usually be based on a careful history and physical examination with the minimum of investigations. The diagnosis should include the anatomical site and pathological process involved, any contributing biochemical abnormality and the psychological and social components. The information should be recorded using problem-orientated notes. For example, Mr S.L. (62), squamous carcinoma of left bronchus. Dyspnoea due to tumour and a large left pleural effusion, exacerbated by a chest infection and his increasing anxiety about the future.

Principles of treatment

Although a patient may have an advanced or terminal illness it is often possible to reverse the cause (or one of the causes) of a particular symptom, with resultant improvement. Even if the cause of the symptom proves irreversible, a knowledge of the mechanism involved will point to the correct symptomatic treatment. For example, uraemic vomiting requires different management from the vomiting of malignant gastroduodenal obstruction.

Most symptoms in terminal illness are amenable to treatment with appropriate medication. The symptoms are usually persistent and therefore require regular medication 'by the clock' to maintain control. The dose interval will depend on the plasma half-life of the drug used. For example, both morphine and diazepam are used for malignant dyspnoea. Morphine, in solution, has a plasma half-life of about 3 h and therefore should be given 4 hourly. Diazepam, however, has a plasma half-life of over 30 h and can be given in a single nightly dose.

The oral route is preferred and can often be used until shortly before death. However, if the patient is vomiting, dysphagic, or semiconscious, many drugs can be administered by subcutaneous infusion, using a portable syringe driver, or rectally. Repeated intramuscular injections should be avoided and intravenous infusions are contraindicated (see below).

Psychological factors play a considerable part in exacerbating the physical symptoms of terminal illness. A sympathetic explanation of the disease, its symptoms, treatment, and future course will often allay the fears of a patient and family, help them to talk together, and result in a lessening of tension and pain.

Good symptom control requires regular and frequent review as the situation changes and new symptoms develop.

In the sections that follow, many of the major symptoms caused by terminal illness are discussed, with their common causes and suggested treatment. Although most of the clinical experience and research in this field are based on patients with advanced cancer, it is expected that there is wide application to those dying from other diseases.

Anorexia

A reduced desire for food is common, and indeed, expected, as the patient's health deteriorates. However, appetite and the ability to eat continue to rate highly in quality of life studies, even in very ill patients. A poor appetite seems to cause more family stress than any other symptom, for relatives and carers often equate the giving of food with the maintaining of life and feel that it is their main way to show care.

The treatment options are as follows:

Correction of causative factors

Infections, depression, and hypercalcaemia should be treated appropriately. Pain, nausea, and constipation require symptomatic treatment. Good mouth care is important.

Dietary measures

Hyperalimentation, using enteral or parenteral methods, has not been shown to increase survival in patients with advanced cancer and is not appropriate for the terminally ill. Simple dietary measures are helpful; these include the serving of small portions, the imaginative use of nutritional supplements, and, perhaps, alcohol before a meal.

Appetite stimulants

Corticosteroids in low dosage, prednisolone (15–30 mg daily) or dexamethasone (2–4 mg daily) normally lead to improvement in appetite within a week. Megestrol acetate, in doses from 160 to 800 mg daily, has also been shown to improve appetite and reduce weight loss. However, the additional cost of high-dose progestogens suggest that they should be reserved for patients who fail to respond to corticosteroids or when these are contraindicated.

Cancer pain

Pain is the symptom most expected and most feared by cancer patients and their families. Sadly, this fear has often been justified for, in the past, cancer pain has been poorly understood and inadequately treated. Fortunately the situation is now improving and most patients with cancer in the developed world should be guaranteed good pain relief throughout their illness. In the developing world, where about 80 per cent of patients present with advanced or terminal disease, the situation is gradually improving, mainly due to the initiative of the World Health Organization in promoting the wide availability of oral morphine for cancer patients.

Pain has been described as a somatopsychic experience, with its intensity depending both on the extent of tissue damage and on the patient's psychological state. In patients with advanced cancer the pain will be exacerbated by associated physical symptoms, such as vomiting or dyspnoea, and by the inevitable fear of deterioration, separation, and death.

Diagnosis of cancer pain

It is important to make a diagnosis as to the cause of pain or, more often, pains. Most patients with advanced cancer have more than one pain, some caused directly by the tumour, others resulting from treatment, debility, or concurrent illness. The use of a body chart is recommended, with space for the severity, nature, and time span of pain plus the presumptive diagnosis.

Most chronic cancer pain is nociceptive, in that it is caused by mechanical or chemical stimuli in bone, viscera, etc. and conducted along intact somatosensory pathways. However, a significant proportion of cancer pain is neuropathic, caused by damage in the central or peripheral nervous system.

Fig. 2 Treatment of cancer pain.

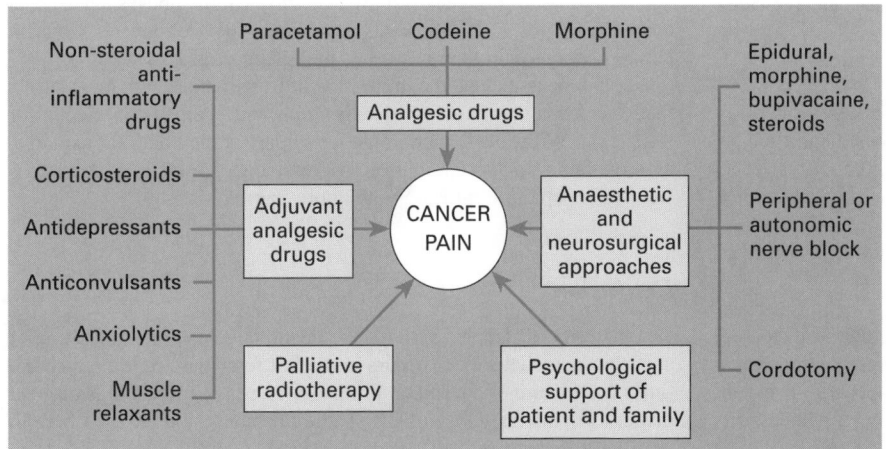

MANAGEMENT OF PAIN

The very complexity of cancer pain with its multiple causes, exacerbating factors, and psychological issues means that a combination of treatments is likely to be needed. This is shown in Fig. 2.

Analgesic drugs

Analgesic drugs are the mainstay of treatment. They should be given as soon as pain develops, regularly and, if possible, by mouth. The dose should be individually determined, being the lowest compatible with pain control. For example, oral morphine may prove effective at 5 to 10 mg 4 hourly but occasionally 1000 mg daily, or even higher, is required.

Paracetamol (1000 mg 4 hourly) is recommended for the treatment of mild pain. If this proves ineffective, the choice is between using a weak opioid, such as codeine or dextropropoxyphene (as in co-proxamol), or a low dose of a strong opioid. With escalating pain or a very sick patient it is advisable to start treatment with morphine or to change to it directly from paracetamol.

Morphine

Morphine is well absorbed when given by mouth, mainly in the proximal small bowel. Buccal and rectal absorption are more variable. Metabolism occurs mainly in the liver, where morphine is broken down into glucuronides, and it is in this form that most renal excretion occurs. The active metabolite, morphine-6-glucuronide passes only slowly into the cerebrospinal fluid and it is this fact that probably accounts for the poor analgesic effect of single oral doses of morphine compared with the good results with repeated administration. The plasma half-life of morphine is about 3 h, so morphine should be given 4 hourly to maintain a satisfactory plasma level (unless a controlled release preparation is used).

Preparations of morphine

1. Morphine sulphate tablet or solution, given 4 hourly.
2. Controlled release morphine sulphate tablet or granules, given 12 hourly.
3. Morphine injections, given 4 hourly. Parenteral to oral potency ratio is about 3:1 in patients receiving regular morphine. Diamorphine is identical in action to morphine; if it is available (as in the United Kingdom), it is preferred for injection because of its greater solubility. Diamorphine, or morphine, is given by injection or subcutaneous infusion only if the patient is unable to take oral drugs; there is little evidence that these routes improve pain control.
4. Epidural morphine is given 12 hourly, or by infusion. The ratio of epidural dose: oral dose is 1:10. The role of epidural morphine remains unclear for there are very few randomized trials comparing it with oral morphine. For the moment it should probably be reserved for patients whose pain has been found to be opioid sensitive (neuropathic pain is only occasionally relieved) but when oral morphine causes unacceptable side-effects.

Problems with morphine

Drowsiness usually wears off after a few days. About 30 per cent of patients feel nauseated on starting morphine so an antiemetic such as metoclopramide should be given to prevent this, it can usually be stopped after a week. Constipation should be avoided by prescribing laxatives routinely. A dry mouth is a common side-effect and requires regular mouth care. Respiratory depression is minimal, if it occurs at all, with regular oral morphine (see below).

Tolerance, although widely feared, is a minor problem. When an increasing dose of morphine is needed this is usually due to increased pain from the advancing malignancy. Addiction, an overpowering drive to take a drug for its psychological effects, does not appear to occur in patients with pain. Physical dependence does develop but if pain lessens

after radiotherapy, a nerve block, or simply a lower level of anxiety, it is possible to reduce the dose of morphine slowly without producing withdrawal symptoms.

Alternatives to morphine

Although morphine is the recommended strong analgesic, there are a few patients who complain of severe nausea or drowsiness which they attribute to the drug, and others who refuse to have it. For such patients it is necessary to have alternatives to oral morphine. These are shown in Table 2, which can also be used in converting to morphine from other drugs.

Adjuvant analgesic drugs

The correct use of adjuvants may mean that morphine is not required, or it may be possible to give it in a lower dose. Response to adjuvant analgesic treatment is variable so it is recommended that, unless delayed response is likely, the drug is discontinued after a week if there is no improvement. The use of adjuvant drugs in various types of cancer pain is summarized in Table 3.

Other treatment

Radiotherapy may be helpful, even during the last weeks of life, provided that it is given without delay and with the minimum number of treatments. Fortunately, 80 per cent of patients with a painful bony metastasis gain relief from a single fraction.

The value of anaesthetic techniques will depend on the availability of an anaesthetist specializing in pain control. Some useful procedures are shown in Table 3. Transcutaneous electrical nerve stimulation (TENS) is occasionally useful for the control of cancer pain; acupuncture has rarely been found to be effective.

Chronic benign pain

Chronic pain of non-malignant origin is very common in the course of terminal illness, being reported by 67 per cent of non-cancer patients in the last year of life. There are many causes, including arthritis, back problems, pressure sores, and the pain of immobility from stroke or severe disability. The management of many of these conditions is covered elsewhere. The principles of treatment for benign pain are the same as those for cancer pain. It is important to make a clear diagnosis, institute specific therapy if possible, use analgesic and adjuvant drugs regularly, and give appropriate psychological support.

Non-opioid analgesics (paracetamol and aspirin), non-steroidal anti-inflammatory drugs, and weak opioids (codeine and co-proxamol) are preferred. But with severe pain, for example, from gangrene, morphine should be given in adequate doses and often combined with an appropriate psychotropic drug to relieve distress.

Tricyclic antidepressants and anticonvulsants are used for neuropathic pain such as post-herpetic and trigeminal neuralgia, diabetic neuropathy, and the thalamic pain caused by stroke. Physical methods, such as local anaesthetic sprays, TENS, and acupuncture seem of greater value in chronic benign pain than in pain of malignant origin.

Nerve blocks include the infiltration of trigger areas with local anaesthetic, epidural steroids for root irritation and sympathetic blocks for ischaemia. With severe pain in the lower part of the body, for example, an inoperable fractured femur or progressive gangrene, it is worth considering an epidural infusion with bupivacaine.

Confusion

The majority of people, as they near death, develop some alteration of consciousness. This often occurs in the last few hours of life but sometimes is a feature of a terminal illness for weeks or more and is of great distress to patients and families. The term 'confusion' is used here to

Table 2 *Alternatives to oral morphine*

Name	Dose interval (hours)	Tablet	Morphine equivalent (as 4 hourly solution)	Comment
Buprenorphine	8	0.2 mg 8 hourly	7 mg	Given sublingually Less physical dependence Probable ceiling dose at 3–5 mg/24 h
Dextromoramide	2	5 mg (and 10 mg)	15 mg (peak effect)	Too short-acting for regular use
Methadone	8–12	5 mg	7.5 mg single dose	Long plasma half-life (2–3 days) Accumulation occurs.
Oxycodone	8	30 mg suppository 8 hourly	15 mg	Preferred analgesic suppository
Pethidine	2–3	50 mg	5 mg	Weak oral analgesic Short-acting
Phenazocine	8	5 mg 8 hourly	20 mg	Useful alternative to morphine Sublingual administration possible.

Table 3 *Adjuvant therapy in cancer pain*

Type of pain	Adjuvant drug	Other treatment
Bone pain	Non-steroidal antiinflammatory drugs (NSAID), e.g. naproxen 500 mg twice a day	Palliative radiotherapy Immobilization, e.g. surgical fixation
Neuropathic (deafferentation) pain	Amitriptyline 25 mg at night with increasing dose Carbamazepine 100 mg three times a day with increasing dose Flecainide 100–200 mg/24 h	Epidural steroids +/− bupivacaine TENS
Pancreatic or liver pain	NSAID	Coeliac plexus block
Intestinal colic (from inoperable obstruction)	Hyoscine butylbromide 60–200 mg 24/h	
Headaches (from raised intracranial pressure)	Dexamethasone 16 mg/24 h, reducing as possible	Cranial irradiation
Chest wall pain	NSAID	Intercostal or thoracic paravertebral block
Lymphoedema		Compression bandaging

describe the symptoms of both the acute confusional state and dementia. It includes memory loss, inappropriate behaviour, aggression, disorientation, and paranoia. Psychiatrists generally use the term 'confusion' in the specific instance of disorientation in time, or for place or person.

CAUSES OF CONFUSION

It is important to seek a diagnosis of the cause (or causes) of confusion. This may indicate some reversible factor but, even if this is not the case, the patient and family will be relieved to know that the altered behaviour is due to physical disease rather than impending insanity.

Potentially reversible causes of confusion which arise in the terminally ill include medication, especially opioids, psychotropic drugs, and corticosteroids (although steroid psychosis is rare). Infections and biochemical changes are often treatable and cerebral oedema associated with tumours can be reduced with dexamethasone. Nocturnal confusion may be due to anoxia and hypercapnia. Some elderly patients become acutely confused on hospital admission but, on enquiry, it emerges that they have a mild degree of dementia and were 'just about' coping at home.

MANAGEMENT OF CONFUSION

Reversible causes should be sought and treated appropriately. Non-drug methods of management are always required. Staff should try to under-

stand what the patient is experiencing while not agreeing with the misconception behind it. A familiar routine is helpful, if possible in home surroundings.

The 'quietly muddled' patient requires no medication, and sedative drugs may worsen things. Psychotropic drugs are used to reduce agitation, hallucinations, or paranoia. Trifluroperazine or haloperidol are usually effective and cause little sedation. Thioridazine or chlorpromazine can be substituted if sedation is required.

Constipation

Constipation is the infrequent, difficult passage of small, hard faeces. In the patient with terminal illness, constipation is rarely caused by a reversible condition such as hypercalcaemia. Much more often the cause is a combination of the following: inactivity, a diet low in roughage, general weakness, confusion, and the constipating effect of drugs such as opioids, phenothiazines, and tricyclic antidepressants.

ASSESSMENT

A careful history will note the patient's previous bowel habit, as well as the recent frequency of defaecation and characteristics of the stool. Abdominal and rectal examinations are important to avoid misdiagnosis.

MANAGEMENT

The advice to increase activity and add fibre to the diet is rarely possible in the very ill patient so, in practice, laxatives and rectal measures are required. Laxatives are often divided into those that primarily stimulate peristalsis and those whose main effect is to soften and bulk the stool. This is not pharmacologically tenable as increased stool size, in itself, causes increased peristalsis, but the division remains useful in the clinical choice of laxatives.

Faecal softeners retain water in the bowel by osmosis or increase water penetration of faeces. They include magnesium sulphate or hydroxide, lactulose, and poloxamer.

Stimulant laxatives increase colonic muscle activity. They include senna, bisacodyl, and danthron.

Constipation, in the terminally ill, is best managed with a combination of both types of laxative. This will avoid either painful colic or a rectum loaded with soft faeces, problems that arise if a stimulant or a softening laxative is given alone. Examples include lactulose and bisacodyl, magnesium hydroxide and liquid paraffin emulsion with senna, and codanthramer (danthron and poloxamer). The dose should be gradually increased until a regular soft bowel action is obtained.

Suppositories, an enema, or manual removal may be needed if the patient presents with a loaded rectum or if the laxative regimen is ineffective. It is a good general rule to perform a rectal examination on the third day if the bowels have not opened, inserting a glycerine or bisacodyl suppository if the rectum is loaded.

Cough

Cough receptors are found at all levels of the respiratory tree and can be stimulated by mechanical or chemical means. Common causes of cough include bacterial or viral infections, primary or secondary tumours involving the respiratory tract, cardiac failure, asthma or chronic obstructive airways disease, and smoking.

Specific treatment aimed at relieving the cause of coughing should be given unless the patient is too ill. Such treatments include antibiotics, diuretics, bronchodilators, corticosteroids, and radiotherapy. If specific treatment is inappropriate or ineffective, symptomatic treatment must be offered. These measures include the following.

Simple linctus

This seems to soothe the pharynx and reduce coughing. Proprietary preparations offer no advantages.

Steam inhalations

Steam inhalations or nebulized saline aid the expectoration of viscid sputum, especially if they are followed by physiotherapy.

Opioids

Opioids such as codeine, morphine, and methadone suppress the cough reflex centrally. They should be reserved for those with a dry cough, those too weak to expectorate, or occasionally at night if the cough disturbs sleep. Codeine, 30 to 60 mg 4 hourly, is often effective, but with an intractable cough, usually caused by lung cancer, morphine is needed. Morphine, 5 mg 4 hourly, is the starting dose; this can be increased until relief is obtained.

Nebulized local anaesthetic

The use of 5 ml of 2 per cent lignocaine 4 hourly has occasionally been of benefit, but many patients find it unacceptable.

Dysphagia

Difficulty in swallowing can be caused by malignant or benign obstructive lesions involving the pharynx or oesophagus. Neurological causes include cerebrovascular disease, cerebral tumours, and motor neurone disease. Dysphagia can be caused, or exacerbated, by pain on swallowing, a dry mouth, and anxiety.

Having diagnosed the cause of dysphagia, specific treatment may be possible. Thrush infections of the mouth or oesophagus should be treated with nystatin or fluconazole. Oesophageal cancer can be treated with radiotherapy, laser therapy, bouginage, or an indwelling flexible oesophageal tube. Radiotherapy should be considered for mediastinal lymphadenopathy but, if the patient is not fit enough, the dysphagia may respond temporarily to corticosteroids (dexamethasone, 8 mg/day) which cause shrinkage of peritumour inflammatory oedema.

If such specific treatment is not possible, then dietary modification is required. In general, patients with obstructive lesions need a nourishing but fluid diet, whereas those with neurological problems prefer semisolid food. Correct positioning and adequate time for feeding is important.

Drugs for symptom relief should be continued but may need to be given by subcutaneous infusion or rectally. The use of a nasogastric tube or gastrostomy for feeding is controversial. They should probably be used for patients with localized head and neck cancer who are in good general condition but avoided in those with widespread metastatic disease. Most patients with severe dysphagia sooner or later develop an aspiration pneumonia, which should usually be treated symptomatically.

Dyspnoea

Dyspnoea is defined as a distressing difficulty in breathing. It is therefore a subjective symptom (like pain) and its severity may be poorly related to tachypnoea or to pulmonary pathology. Breathing is under the control of the respiratory centres, and these are stimulated by chemical changes in the blood ($\uparrow$ $P\text{CO}_2$, $\downarrow$ $P\text{O}_2$, $\uparrow$ H^+), by afferent impulses from the lung, heart, chest wall, diaphragm, and from higher centres.

It is important to seek a diagnosis of the cause (or causes) of breathlessness in the terminally ill patient. Such causes include infection, primary or secondary lung tumour, chronic obstructive airways disease, cardiac failure, pleural effusion, pulmonary embolus, and anxiety. In most patients these should, in the first instance, be treated actively provided that necessary symptomatic measures are used as well. For example, low-dose oral morphine will ease the dyspnoea and pain from a chest infection; it can be withdrawn later if the infection resolves with antibiotics and physiotherapy.

However, as the disease progresses, the place for active treatment becomes less. The patient may not improve following pleural aspiration or a course of antibiotics and it may be decided that the side-effects of a treatment, such as anticoagulation, outweigh its possible benefits.

A significant number of terminally ill patients will express to their families, or to medical and nursing staff their 'readiness to go' or their hope that 'things won't be dragged out'. Such wishes must be respected when a decision about active treatment is made. The patient and family should be reassured that dyspnoea and pain will be relieved even if, for example, antibiotics are not prescribed.

SYMPTOMATIC TREATMENT OF DYSPNOEA

Explanation and adjustment

Severe dyspnoea is frightening and the resultant anxiety exacerbates the symptom. Medical and nursing staff should encourage patients to express their fears, usually of choking or suffocating, and give careful explanation and reassurance. Simple measures such as an open window, a fan, or a backrest in bed may help, as can relaxation techniques and breathing exercises.

Morphine

This is the most effective symptomatic treatment for dyspnoea and has been used in patients with advanced cancer, chronic obstructive airways disease, and motor neurone disease. Its mechanism of action remains unclear; it reduces the sensitivity of the respiratory centre to stimuli, but, when opioids are administered over a period, tolerance to this occurs. Morphine also causes peripheral vasodilation, helpful when there is pulmonary oedema. It appears to reduce the sensation of dyspnoea more than it reduces the level of ventilation.

Clinical experience indicates that regular oral morphine, starting with 2.5 to 5 mg 4 hourly and increasing slowly if needed, to 20 mg 4 hourly is safe and effective. The role; if any, for nebulized morphine remains unclear.

Bronchodilators

These may prove helpful even when there is no obvious wheeze, especially in patients with a history of smoking or chronic bronchitis.

Benzodiazepines

Diazepam, 2 to 10 mg at night, is used for its anxiolytic effect, sometimes in combination with morphine.

Hyoscine (scopolamine) and atropine

These drugs are used, in combination with diamorphine or morphine, to lessen the 'death rattle' which can occur in the last hours of life. The dose is 0.3 mg to 0.6 mg 4 hourly by injection, or up to 2.4 mg over 24 h by subcutaneous infusion.

Oxygen

The use of oxygen in the dyspnoea of terminal illness is controversial, as is the role of hypoxia in causing this symptom. In most patients, dyspnoea can be relieved more easily by morphine. This avoids the use of an oxygen mask or nasal cannulae; barriers between the patient and family.

RESPIRATORY EMERGENCIES

These include a major haemoptysis, pulmonary embolus, or acute tracheal compression. Intravenous midazolam or diazepam, 10 to 20 mg, should be given slowly, or diazepam rectal solution, 10 to 20 mg. An alternative is an injection of diamorphine, 5 mg, with hyoscine, 0.4 mg.

Insomnia

Many patients with terminal illness sleep poorly due to unrelieved physical or mental distress. Before prescribing a hypnotic it is necessary to enquire if sleep is disturbed by pain or discomfort, sweats or cramp, fear of incontinence, or any other physical symptom for which appropriate relief can be given. More often anxiety, depression, or a fear of dying in the night prevent normal sleep. A careful enquiry will usually uncover such factors and they can be helped by counselling, with perhaps, the addition of psychotropic drugs. However, in spite of these measures, many patients request a hypnotic. These include:

1. Temazepam 10 to 30 mg. The most useful hypnotic, a short-acting benzodiazepine with a plasma half-life of 6 to 8 h.
2. Chlormethiazole 1 to 2 caps (192–384 mg). A useful hypnotic for the elderly or confused, it has a plasma half-life of 3 to 4 h.
3. Diazepam 5 to 10 mg. This benzodiazepine has a very long half-life with a risk of accumulation. However, it is of value as a hypnotic where there is associated intractable dyspnoea, or for the short-term management of severe anxiety.
4. Amitriptyline or another sedative tricyclic antidepressant is used when insomnia is associated with clinical depression.

Nausea and vomiting

Vomiting results from impulses reaching the vomiting centre in the medulla which contains both histamine and muscarinic cholinergic receptors. It can be stimulated in the following ways:

(1) from the chemoreceptor trigger zone where dopamine receptors are concentrated;
(2) from vagal afferents from the gastrointestinal tract;
(3) from the vestibular apparatus (this, like the vomiting centre, contains both histamine and muscarinic cholinergic receptors);
(4) directly, from raised intracranial pressure; or
(5) from psychological causes, especially anxiety.

Thus nausea and vomiting have a large range of potential causes originating in many parts of the body.

ASSESSMENT

The causes of vomiting in the patient who is terminally ill can usually be determined from a careful history and clinical examination. Note should also be taken of the volume, content, and timing of vomits. A biochemical profile may be needed, but other investigations are rarely necessary or appropriate.

In many patients, the predominant cause of vomiting can be identified and an antiemetic drug selected that is relatively specific for the mechanism involved. Other patients have vomiting with multifactorial causation and need a combination of antiemetics and other treatment.

ANTIEMETIC DRUGS

A large number of antiemetic drugs has been found useful and research is continuing, with the development of new agents. Table 4 lists recommended antiemetics, with their site of action, dosage, and available routes. Other antiemetics include corticosteroids, which potentiate the effect of antiemetics used in chemotherapy and may reduce peritumour oedema in some cases of obstructive vomiting. Ondansetron blocks serotonin receptors in the gut and chemoreceptor trigger zone. It has proved very effective in the prevention of chemotherapy-induced vomiting, but its role in palliative medicine has not yet been fully evaluated.

MANAGEMENT

Suggested treatment for some causes of vomiting is as follows:

Opioid-induced vomiting

About 30 per cent of patients starting morphine feel nauseated during the first week of treatment. Either metoclopramide or haloperidol should be given prophylactically.

Uraemia

Haloperidol is usually effective but sometimes the sedating phenothiazine, methotrimeprazine, is required.

'Squashed stomach syndrome'

This is caused by external pressure and is treated with metoclopramide or domperidone.

Gastric outlet obstruction

Treatment is started with metoclopramide. If this is ineffective, it is worth trying dexamethasone 8 mg/day by injection. Nasogastric suction is occasionally required.

Inoperable intestinal obstruction

Treatment is started with haloperidol or cyclizine. The antiemetic will usually be given with diamorphine (for pain) and hyoscine butylbromide (for colic). The somatostatin analogue, octreotide 0.3 mg–1.0 mg/24 h, by subcutaneous infusion, reduces gastrointestinal secretions and is used, with benefit, in intractible obstructive vomiting. Methotrimeprazine is sometimes required in the terminal stage of the disease.

Table 4 *Recommended antiemetics*

Name	Main site of action	Neurotransmitter receptors	Dose (mg 24 h)	Routes
Cyclizine	Vomiting centre	Histamine and muscarinic cholinergic	100–200	0,1,SC
Domperidome	Upper gut Chemoreceptor trigger zone	Dopamine	30–180	O,R
Haloperidol	Chemoreceptor trigger zone	Dopamine	1.5–15	0,1,SC
Metoclopramide	Upper gut Chemoreceptor trigger zone	Dopamine	30–100	0,1,SC
Methotrimeprazine	Chemoreceptor trigger zone	Dopamine	50–200	0,1,SC

0, oral; 1, intramuscular; R, rectal; SC, subcutaneous infusion (the preferred route in severe vomiting using a syringe driver)

Raised intracranial pressure

Dexamethasone is the treatment of choice; if contraindicated, cyclizine is usually effective.

Vestibular disturbance

Both cyclizine and hyoscine are effective.

Sore mouth

A dry or painful mouth is common in those with terminal disease. Causes include drugs with anticholinergic effects, dehydration, thrush, and poorly fitting dentures.

Good oral hygiene is most important. Teeth and dentures should be cleaned regularly. Mouthwashes with chlorhexidine 0.2 per cent or povidone-iodine 1 per cent both moisten and cleanse the mouth. Chewing pineapple chunks, which contain the enzyme ananase, will clean a furred tongue.

Thrush infections are common and should be treated with nystatin suspension or with the systemic antifungal drugs, fluconazole or ketoconazole.

Buccal analgesics include benzydamine (Difflam®), an NSAID absorbed through the mucosa, and choline salicylate (Bonjela®), which can be applied to ulcerated areas before meals. Triamcinolone in Orabase® is used for painful aphthous ulcers.

The last days

The correct management of the last few days of life involves the care of both patient and family. The way in which the death is handled will influence the family's grief, bereavement and their ability to cope with the future. Those who visit the bereaved will be only too aware how the last hours become imprinted on the memory, with unanswerable questions 'I wonder if she was trying to say something to me?' 'Do you think he was in pain?'

MEDICAL MANAGEMENT

As death approaches there is usually a gradual increase in drowsiness and weakness, but it is often the experienced nurse who will recognize that this is not a temporary deterioration but represents the imminence of death. This 'diagnosis of dying' needs to be confirmed by the doctor who should then review the medication, stopping all drugs except those for symptom relief. Drugs to withdraw include antibiotics, diuretics, antihypertensives, antidepressants, and laxatives. Corticosteroids and NSAIDs are usually continued until the patient cannot swallow.

Studies have shown that two-thirds of patients continue to take some oral medication until the last day of life, but essential drugs must be charted so that, if swallowing becomes impossible, they can be given regularly by injection or suppository. These essential drugs are as follows:

Morphine or diamorphine

The oral dose should be converted to the dose for injection and given either by subcutaneous infusion or 4 hourly (see above).

Anticonvulsants

These should be replaced by diazepam suppositories, 10 to 20 mg twice a day, or by midazolam by subcutaneous infusion.

Hyoscine hydrobromide

Hyoscine hydrobromide, 0.4 to 0.6 mg 4 hourly, or up to 2.4 mg/24 h by subcutaneous infusion, may be needed to relieve the 'death rattle'.

Psychotropic drugs

While most patients become more drowsy and lapse into coma as death approaches, some become restless and agitated. This may be due to unrelieved pain or a distended bladder or rectum but frequently no cause can be identified. Benzodiazepines (diazepam and midazolam), phenothiazines, and phenobarbitone have proved effective in this situation. Suggested doses are:

Diazepam suppositories
10 to 20 mg 8 hourly.

Midazolam
30 to 100 mg/24 h, by subcutaneous infusion.

Methotrimeprazine
25 to 50 mg 4 to 8 hourly or by subcutaneous infusion.

Chlorpromazine
Up to 300 mg/24 h can be given by intramuscular injection or by suppository. It is too irritant to use subcutaneously.

Phenobarbitone

Phenobarbitone 200–600 mg/24 h by subcutaneous infusion. A separate syringe driver will be needed as it cannot be mixed with other drugs.

Care for the family

It is essential that the close family are informed that death is approaching. They will usually understand that the question 'How long?' cannot be accurately answered and accept 'Just a few hours (or days)'. It is to be hoped that they will have been involved already in discussions about the illness and its outcome, but many will wish to ask specific questions about the process of dying and the continuing need for medication and nursing care at this stage.

Many relatives are distressed when the patient is unable to take food or water and some request that tube feeding is given. Medical and nursing staff need to take time to explain what is happening. 'He won't eat and therefore he will die' needs to be turned to 'He is dying and therefore doesn't need to eat'. Reassurance must be given that a degree of dehydration, at this stage, does not cause symptoms.

The natural urge of families to 'do something' for someone who is dying can be harnessed by skilled nursing staff. Relatives can help with practical things such as mouth care, washing, and turning. They should be reminded that hearing and touch are the last senses to go, so their physical contact and speech can continue to bring comfort.

Staff should help the family to be present at the death, if this is what they want. But many people have not witnessed a death (except on television) and need help about what to expect, for example the changing pattern of breathing.

After death

However much the death has been expected, the actual moment comes as a profound emotional and physical shock. Families therefore need a time of quiet privacy to absorb what has happened and to express their emotions in their own way. After this there is the time for staff to show their sympathy; simple prayers may be welcomed followed by the inevitable, but essential, cup of tea.

Some family members will wish to help with washing and dressing the body; all will value assurance that this will be done with care and respect, taking into account their wishes and their cultural or religious practices.

Psychological aspects of terminal illness

An understanding of the main psychological and social aspects of terminal illness is as essential to the physician as a knowledge of the methods of pain control. Patients and their families place considerable emphasis on their doctor's ability to communicate effectively and to understand their emotions as well as their physical condition. Yet studies have shown that many doctors have received minimal training in this area and lack the necessary skills.

Talking about death

Communication between doctor and patient was no problem in Hippocratic times for the advice to physicians was:

> 'Reveal nothing to the patient of his future or present condition, for this has caused many patients to take a turn for the worse'

Unfortunately, this tradition of silence persisted for centuries and is still followed in many parts of the world. However, Western society in the past 30 years has seen a dramatic change, with the vast majority of cancer patients knowing the diagnosis and being informed about the progress of their illness. This change has come about because of the wishes of patients for information and because it has been shown that anxiety and depression are reduced when open discussion is welcomed.

However, as the disease progresses and death approaches, the problem of communication emerges again, with many doctors and most families finding it extremely difficult to talk about the imminence of death or the process of dying. But the majority of dying patients have been shown to be aware of what is happening, so that communication with them must be a two-way process, listening as well as speaking. This will enable the patient to direct the flow of conversation, at his or her own pace, expressing worries or hopes and receiving information. Most will be relieved when they can, often over a period, come to share their thoughts and fears with their families and with medical and nursing staff.

Although most dying patients come to a stage of understanding and acceptance, there remains a small group who use the psychological defence of denial. This can work effectively, shielding them from the truth that is too painful to bear. Provided such a defence is working, it should be allowed to continue. But if it is creating major problems, such as severe anxiety, then the denial should be gently but firmly challenged.

On occasions, this truthful approach proves unacceptable to family members. They may try to insist that the patient is not told the diagnosis, often saying that their relative will lose hope and stop fighting if he or she realizes that death is inevitable and close. It is always worth exploring this reluctance for the truth to be shared. There may well be the memory of someone who had a similar illness and died in pain. Sometimes members of the family wish to protect themselves and feel that a cheerful facade, pretending that all is well, will make the final weeks easier. But often collusion is an act of love, as both patient and relative genuinely hope to avoid distress for their loved one.

It requires time to talk over these matters, but the doctor's first duty is to the patient who has a right to know the situation, if he asks, even against the wishes of the family. However, such a confrontation is rare and most families will agree that the doctor can, gently, explore what the patient knows and answer questions truthfully. They will be reassured to hear that such an approach actually reduces anxiety, for the most worried patients are those who are isolated with their fears about dying, unable to share them with family or staff.

Fears of dying

The fear of dying is universal; virtually everyone is afraid at some stage in their final illness, for death remains the great unknown. In the past, doctors have tended not to become involved with their patient's fears of dying. They probably felt inadequate in dealing with them and left them, in the hope that they would be dealt with by nurses, social workers, or clergy. However, many of these fears require medical explanation and reassurance and almost all dying patients value the opportunity to share their fears with the doctor they have come to know.

The most common fear of the dying is that of uncontrolled pain. Many patients fear that pain-relieving drugs, especially the opioids, will lose their effect and pain will become unbearable. They need reassurance that this never occurs and that pain control in the last days of life is always possible, although sometimes the necessary drugs may cause drowsiness. Other fears that are often expressed are those of dependence, incontinence, and confusion. It is obviously not honest to deny the possibility of these but patients are helped by explanation of practical steps that could be taken if they arise, for example increased nursing help, a catheter, or an appropriate change of medication.

Many elderly patients dread the prospect of the final stages of life being prolonged 'artificially' and are reassured to know that this will not be done. In younger patients the fear of death is usually associated with anger, the feeling that they have been 'cheated of life' and have much living left to do. Those of all ages fear separation, and worry how the family will cope without them, especially if there are young children, an old or frail spouse, or major financial or emotional problems.

These are only some of the fears of the dying but they illustrate the urgent need for open communication at this time, involving patient, doctor, and family. Some fears are groundless and can be relieved by explanation and reassurance, but all are lessened by being shared.

Anxiety and depression

It is inevitable that everyone facing death should, at times, feel anxious and depressed. Patients may find themselves unable to concentrate, irritable, unable to sleep, and worried about the future. These are normal responses to a crisis and, in most cases, resolve fairly rapidly with help from family and friends.

Some patients, however, continue to have high levels of anxiety and depression (both are usually present, although one may predominate) that persist for weeks or months and impair social activities and relationships. This syndrome is termed an 'adjustment reaction' and occurs in about 30 per cent of cancer patients. Symptoms often fluctuate in severity from day to day and patients can be distracted. This helps to distinguish it from the less common major affective or anxiety disorders. Treatment of an adjustment reaction is with short-term supportive psychological help, giving information, helping the patient to find practical steps to help make the necessary adjustment, and emphasizing past strengths and coping mechanisms. Anxiolytic or antidepressant drugs are sometimes needed in addition to these measures.

The diagnosis of clinical depression in a patient with terminal illness is difficult, and the distinction between profound sadness and depression may be blurred. The normal biological indicators, such as poor appetite, insomnia, and loss of energy are of little value. The diagnosis depends on psychological symptoms especially a sense of worthlessness, guilt, and anhedonia—a lack of pleasure in all, or almost all, activities. About 10 per cent of terminally ill cancer patients become seriously depressed; the prevalence in other life-threatening illnesses is not known.

Depressed patients are treated with a combination of antidepressants and psychological measures. Tricyclic antidepressants are started at a low dose, usually 25 mg at night, and increased until beneficial effect is found. Amitriptyline or dothiepin are used for the patient who is anxious and depressed, imipramine or lofepramine (70 mg twice daily) for the retarded patient. The more recently developed antidepressants, the 5-HT inhibitors, appear equally effective but have fewer side-effects.

Many of the severely anxious patients seen during their terminal illness have a long history of chronic anxiety with exacerbations under stress. These are more difficult to help than those with acute anxiety precipitated by their illness. Anxiety may be expressed as a constant feeling of unease or persistent worrying thoughts. It may cause problems such as palpitations or panic attacks and exacerbate physical symptoms such as pain, vomiting, and dyspnoea.

Most terminally ill, anxious patients require an anxiolytic drug in addition to psychological support and, if possible, relaxation therapy. Diazepam has a very long half-life and can be given in a single dose of 2 to 10 mg at night. A β-blocker, such as propranolol, may help to relieve the physical symptoms of anxiety.

Support for the family

The news that someone is dying has a profound effect on all members of the family and so, in palliative medicine, the focus of care must shift from the patient alone and be concerned with the whole family group. In many hospices a simple genogram or family tree is made when the patient is first seen (Fig. 3). This immediately shows the size of the family and previous losses by death or separation. In addition, as details are given, some of the family's strengths and resources will become apparent. There is no 'normal' family, they come in many shapes and sizes. However, a family which has stayed together has developed a balance, each person filling his or her own role. The diagnosis of terminal illness can destabilize this and, as a result, can cause profound stress as the main roles in the family have to be reassessed and reallocated.

Doctors need to be aware of some of these family stresses and gently encourage an open discussion of these changes. It might be thought that 'planning for the future' means 'giving up the fight' but most can accept that 'we can hope for the best but also plan for the worst'.

Feeling that the spouse will cope and the family stay together undoubtedly helps someone to die peacefully. Many of the bereaved find comfort as they take up new tasks which were discussed and approved by their husband, or wife, or mother before the death occurred.

Children facing bereavement

The urge to protect children from distress is very strong. In the past, when a parent was dying, children were often sent away to grandparents or at any rate shielded, as far as possible, from a knowledge of what was happening, and from the parents' emotions. However, these measures only served to exclude and isolate the child, leaving him or her unsupported and confused, perhaps feeling responsible for the illness or fearing that it was contagious. Information is, of course, picked up by children at all times. They will hear phrases from the doctor's conversation or sense crying in the bedroom and they will observe physical changes in the parent.

Whenever possible, children need preparation before the death; they need to be given information in a form that they can understand and have the chance to ask questions and to express and share their feelings. Parents, not surprisingly, find this task or preparation immensely difficult and they will often appreciate professional help. Doctors must be willing to meet with the whole family, to give explanations of illness and death that can be understood by a 5-year-old, or 10-year-old. A social worker or nurse will usually be present too, but children, especially the older ones, often need to meet the doctor as well.

Children facing the death of a parent need reassurance about their own continuing care; who will look after them or take them to school. These issues are, of course, very painful, and parents need reassurance that showing grief in front of children is appropriate and not harmful. Children should be encouraged to continue visiting. They need the chance to say goodbye and the opportunity to choose whether or not to attend the funeral.

Sadly, much adult suffering has been caused by a badly handled childhood bereavement. However, with appropriate preparation and help, bereaved children can develop into happy and healthy adults.

Spiritual pain

Faced with serious illness or impending death many patients will begin to think more deeply about their life and its meaning. Some will have

Fig. 3 A genogram of the Smith family.

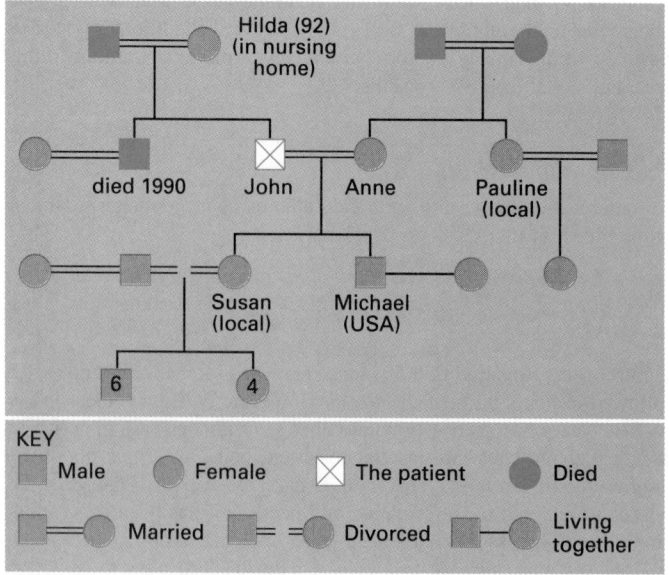

a profound sense of guilt and failure about the past, things left undone or failed relationships. Others feel deeply the meaninglessness of life, that there is no point or purpose in it. A few are troubled by the fear of what happens after death.

These, and other considerations, are aspects of spiritual pain and are very real to many dying patients. Doctors need increasingly to be aware of these issues, to have thought out their own beliefs and to be able, sensitively, to offer spiritual help if this is asked for. They should be aware of the patient's religious beliefs so that the specific practices of the Christian, Jew, Moslem, Hindu, or Buddhist can be adhered to. If the patient has even a vague church connection he or she will probably appreciate an offer to contact the priest or minister.

However, the burning questions that start 'Why me?', 'If only', 'What is the point of it all?' cannot wait until the chaplain is summoned. They may arise during a physical examination or following an enquiry about last night's sleep. Yet the questioners do not expect a solution to the problem of suffering; they are asking for the doctor's response and continuing concern, the willingness to stay with them in their suffering, while often having no answers.

Bereavement

Bereavement is something which all people go through at some time in their lives, but a major bereavement remains a bewildering and frightening experience. The bereaved may be overwhelmed by physical or psychological symptoms which they do not understand and suspect that they are seriously ill or going mad.

Immediately after the death there is usually a period of numbness lasting some days but this is followed by a long period when the bereaved person may feel exhausted, eat and sleep poorly, and often feel depressed, guilty, or angry—even with the dead person. Slowly, over many months, these feelings fade, though the 'pangs of grief' may continue, especially at anniversaries. Doctors need to be familiar with the stages of normal grief and mourning so that they can recognize when grief is delayed, inhibited, or becomes chronic and professional help is needed. Even a single visit after death is of value. It helps the bereaved to ask questions about the illness which may have troubled them, it encourages the expression of feelings, and reassures of continuing help if needed.

Ethical issues in terminal illness

Ethical decisions about treatment are being made all the time in hospitals, hospices, and homes, but it is only recently that the frequency and content of ethical problems have been studied and documented. For example, a significant ethical problem was found in 25 per cent of patients admitted to the medical unit of a general hospital. When terminal illness is present, the frequency of such ethical decisions increases. In a large survey from The Netherlands medical decisions concerning the end of life were taken in 38 per cent of all deaths (54 per cent of all non-acute deaths).

The law and the treatment of the terminally ill

The law, in the United Kingdom, gives some guidelines to doctors as they treat the dying. These can be summarized as follows:

1. A patient who is conscious and lucid and refuses treatment must have his wish respected. If the patient is incompetent, his parent(s) or legal guardian can speak for him, but only if they act in his best interests.
2. When a patient is near death, a doctor is not obliged to embark on, or continue, heroic (or extraordinary) treatment which has no prospect of benefiting the patient. Such treatment includes artificial nutrition and hydration.

3. The doctor has an obligation to relieve pain and make the patient comfortable. If, to ease pain, the doctor must take measures which may hasten death, this is permissible, provided the principal aim is the relief of pain.
4. The doctor may not embark on any conduct with the primary intention of causing the patient's death, nor facilitate suicide.

Types of ethical decisions

The Dutch study highlighted three types of ethical decisions concerning the end of life. In 17 per cent of patients the decision was about the advisability of stopping, or not starting, treatment that was expected to prolong life. Such treatment would include high-technology measures, such as life-support machines or renal dialysis. Decisions would also cover the prescription of antibiotics for a moribund patient with pneumonia, transfusion of a patient whose dying was associated with haematemesis or melaena, and the use of feeding tubes in a patient too weak to swallow.

In a further 17 per cent of patients the ethical decision concerned the advisability of giving drugs for pain, especially the opioids, in dosages that doctors feared might shorten life; in 1.8 per cent of cases the decision was about euthanasia.

Obviously, too many ethical dilemmas arise during the management of a terminal illness for them all to be covered in this chapter, but the problems of shortening life with drugs, hydration in the dying, and euthanasia will be discussed, below.

Do opioids shorten life?

Doctors working in palliative medicine continue to be surprised by articles in the press and from the euthanasia lobby stating that to relieve pain in some patients it is necessary to use such high doses of morphine that life is shortened. Their daily experience in hospices is that the appropriate dose of morphine probably lengthens life. Even if high doses are needed to control severe pain, the pain-free patient often recovers appetite, and resumes activity, and a zest for living.

There are, however, two unusual situations in which medication for symptom control may shorten life. The first is when a patient presents with severe malignant dyspnoea associated with pain and the appropriate treatment is with oral morphine, carefully titrating the dose until relief is obtained. The second dilemma is with a patient in a severe, agitated delirium when benzodiazepines or other psychotropic drugs are needed to relieve intolerable distress. The resultant respiratory depression or sedation is these cases may sometimes shorten life, but the aim of treatment in each situation is to relieve suffering.

NUTRITION AND HYDRATION IN TERMINAL ILLNESS

In the past, malnutrition and dehydration often accompanied deaths resulting from prolonged illness, because sick and dying people could not consume adequate amounts of food and water. However, with the availability of intravenous fluids and tube feeding, these methods have been used for the terminally ill as well as for those with curable disease. The aims of such treatment are to extend life, to relieve the supposed distress of dehydration, and, perhaps, to comply with the request of relatives.

However, over the past few years there has been a reappraisal of the value of continuing hydration for the very ill patient with no prospect of recovery. Recent studies have shown that dehydration, in terminal illness, is not painful and that patients rarely complain of thirst. In fact, continuing hydration may actually increase the distress of dying, leading to problems with pulmonary oedema, incontinence, and the 'death rattle'. Some well-publicized cases in the United States and the United Kingdom have brought into public awareness the issues involved. An increasing proportion of the population have expressed the view that they do not wish their death to be prolonged by artificial means.

For all these reasons, intravenous fluids are only given if the cause of dehydration is reversible, for example, hypercalcaemia. The only distressing symptom of terminal dehydration is a dry mouth, and this can easily be treated with local measures. Staff need time to explain this approach to the family. 'He won't drink and therefore he will die' needs to be turned into 'He is dying and therefore does not need to drink'.

Voluntary euthanasia

There is considerable pressure, at the present time, for a change in the law to allow doctors, under certain strict conditions, to administer a lethal injection at the patient's request. It appears that 1.8 per cent of all deaths in The Netherlands are due to euthanasia.

Doctors working in hospices are united in opposing any change in the law, believing that euthanasia is not the answer to terminal suffering and that there is a better alternative.

There continue to be well-reported cases where terminal pain has not been controlled, even with massive doses of opioids. However, as this chapter details, pain control is more sophisticated than just morphine, and various adjuvant therapies are often needed. Pain, in the dying, can always be relieved, although sometimes at the cost of drowsiness, or, very occasionally, keeping the patient asleep.

The last days of life are often times of personal growth and family unity, strengthening the ties that are so important in bereavement.

Many fear that 'voluntary' euthanasia would not remain voluntary for long. There are major economic forces at work with an ageing population, and unspoken pressures on the elderly and dependent who often feel that they are a burden on their families.

Conclusion

The hospice movement was born through one woman's response to an individual who was dying. The work thus started by Dame Cicely Saunders led to the foundation of a medical speciality, palliative medicine, which, from its inception was committed to 'efficient loving care'. Efficiency must utilize and develop skills based on the most recent scientific work. Loving care depends less on our skills and more on our compassion and humanity, the quality of relationship which develops between ourselves and the patient.

It is, of course, costly for staff to develop such relationships, with the inevitable pain and the bereavement which follow. We need to share this with others in the multidisciplinary team and plan for formal—or more often, informal—ways of supporting each other. This will enable us to remain close to people in their suffering and find, in so doing, a deepening of our own understanding and maturity.

Our greatest support will come from the work itself. Giving effective pain and symptom control is very satisfying and it is rewarding to see an anxious and denying patient come to terms with the illness and, by sharing this, help the family to face the future. The dying have much to teach us all about the meaning of life, for it is at this time that people are at their most mature and their most courageous.

REFERENCES

American Psychiatric Association (1987). *Diagnostic and statistical manual of mental disorders,* (3rd edn, revised). Washington, DC.
Ashby, M. and Stoffell, B. (1991). Therapeutic ratio and defined phases: proposal of ethical framework for palliative care. *British Medical Journal* **302,** 1322–4.
Black, D. and Jolley, D. (1990). Slow euthanasia? The deaths of psychogeriatric patients. *British Medical Journal* **300,** 1321–3.
British Medical Association (1988) *Euthanasia: report of the working party to review the British Medical Association's guidance on euthanasia.* BMA, London.
Du Boulay, S. (1994). *Cicely Saunders.* (revised edn.) Hodder and Stoughton, London.
Hinton, J. (1994). Can home care maintain an acceptable quality of life for patients with terminal cancer and their relatives? *Palliative Medicine,* **8,** 183–96.
Hockley, J.M., Dunlop, R., and Davies, R.J. (1988). Survey of distressing symptoms in dying patients and their families in hospital and the response to a symptom control team. *British Medical Journal* **296,** 1715–17.
Holford, J.M. (1973). *Terminal care. Care of the dying. Proceedings of a National Symposium.* HMSO, London.
Moss, V. (1990). Palliative care in advanced HIV disease: presentation, problems, and palliation. *AIDS* **4,** (Suppl.1), S235–S242.
Neu, S. and Kjellstrand, C.M. (1986). Stopping long term dialysis. *New England Journal of Medicine* **314,** 14–20.
O'Brien, T., Kelly, M., and Saunders, C. (1992). Motor neurone disease: a hospice perspective. *British Medical Journal* **304,** 471–3.
Report of the Select Committee on Medical Ethics. (1994). HMSO, House of Lords, Paper, 21:1.
Searle, C. (1991). Death from cancer and death from other causes: the relevance of the hospice approach. *Palliative Medicine,* **5,** 12–19.
Van Der Maas, P.J., Van Delden, J.J.M., Pijnenborg, L., and Looman, C.W.N. (1991). Euthanasia and other medical decisions concerning the end of life. *Lancet* **338,** 669–74.
World Health Organization (1990). *Cancer pain relief and palliative care.* WHO, Geneva.

FURTHER READING

Palliative Medicine. A quarterly journal, published by Edward Arnold, London.
Doyle, D., Hanks, G., and MacDonald, N. (ed.) (1993). *Oxford textbook of palliative medicine.* Oxford University Press, Oxford.
Saunders, C. and Sykes, N. (1993). *The management of terminal malignant disease,* (3rd ed.). Edward Arnold, London.
Searle, C. and Cartwright, A. (1994). *The year before death.* Avebury, Aldershot.
Stedeford, A. (1984). *Facing death: patients, families and professionals.* Heinemann Medical Books, Oxford.
Wall, P.D. (ed.) (1994). *Textbook of pain,* (3rd edn.). Churchill Livingstone, London.
Worden, W.J. (1991). *Grief counselling and grief therapy,* (2nd ed.). Tavistock/Routledge, London.

Section 33 *Reference intervals for biochemical data*

33 Reference intervals for biochemical data

A. M. GILES and P. HOLLOWAY

Classification of laboratory results

Intervals are presented in the following format; for individual tests see general text

Introduction

The precise quantitation of substance in easily accessible body fluids is an intergral part of clinical assessment of patients. The results are used in screening for disease as well as in diagnosis and for monitoring the response to therapy in established disease. Much diagnostic weight rests on single determinations and patterns of biochemical tests. To this end it is important to consider biological variations between healthy individuals, inherent variations in laboratory methods, and the errors of sampling and hospital practice which can influence every determination. The first (and the last) are the provinces of the physician ordering the test. The second is the concern of the laboratory which provides quality control and the reference ranges for the test.

'Normal range' and 'abnormal' results

Clinical diagnostic decisions may depend equally upon finding a 'normal' result for any test requested. The physician should be clear as to the meaning of these terms. An important task of the clinical biochemist is, therefore, to provide relevant sets of reliable reference data. Whilst for any individual the ideal reference value for an analyte should be that obtained when that individual is healthy, in practice laboratory test results are interpreted by comparision to traditional but often inadequately defined reference intervals (formerly termed 'normal' ranges). The wide belief that biological data assume a gaussian distribution is inappropriate. Most biological data are not symmetrically distributed and require statistical tools which assume other kinds of distribution or are independent of distribution form. Ideally each laboratory should establish sets of reference intervals derived from local reference (a more appropriate term to 'normal') populations.

Reference interval

In the past many texts quoted a 'reference range' defined as the mean ± 2 standard deviations from the mean of results obtained from the reference population. This is, however, not now the commonest method applied to clinical biochemistry tests. Many of the 'intervals' quoted in clinical practice are in fact derived from a skew-distribution calculated from the geometric mean to include 95 per cent of values obtained from what is considered to be a 'healthy' population (95 per cent confidence intervals). The merits of a diagnostic test are determined by the relationship between the data for healthy and unhealthy populations and an example of a relatively poor test is given in Fig. 1. By whatever criteria it is obtained, the reference interval is compounded of both physiological variation and the irreducible error. More elaborate statistical handling of human biochemical data is available for individual tests, but is not generally required in making a diagnosis. By way of warning, however, it will readily be appreciated that if this criterion of health (viz. biochemical results within 95 per cent limits for the given value), is applied to multiple tests in any individual, then with a battery of say 12 tests theoretically only 50 per cent of 'normal' individuals will be found to be 'healthy'. An important example of the limitations of strict referral to the 'reference interval' is highlighted by plasma total cholesterol measurements within certain populations where established reference intervals may be considered to contain a considerable proportion of individuals with 'undesirable' or 'unhealthy' values. In such situations it may be appropriate to define an 'ideal' or 'optimum' range for that parameter.

In conclusion, the use of the following tables of reference intervals for biochemical tests must, therefore, include an appreciation of the limitations in reference intervals of analytical variation and differences between methods of analysis, as well as the differences of sex, age, posture, diet and other biological variables, and sampling that contribute to such an operation. The physician should constantly bear in mind the need to see individual results of laboratory tests in their clinical context and not to hesitate in questioning an unexpected or unlikely result.

The reference intervals given here are established for laboratory investigations available at the John Radcliffe Hospital in Oxford, UK. Throughout the tables intervals are given in SI and conventional units.

Fig. 1 Theoretical distributions of an analyte in healthy (symmetrical) and unhealthy (negatively skewed) populations.

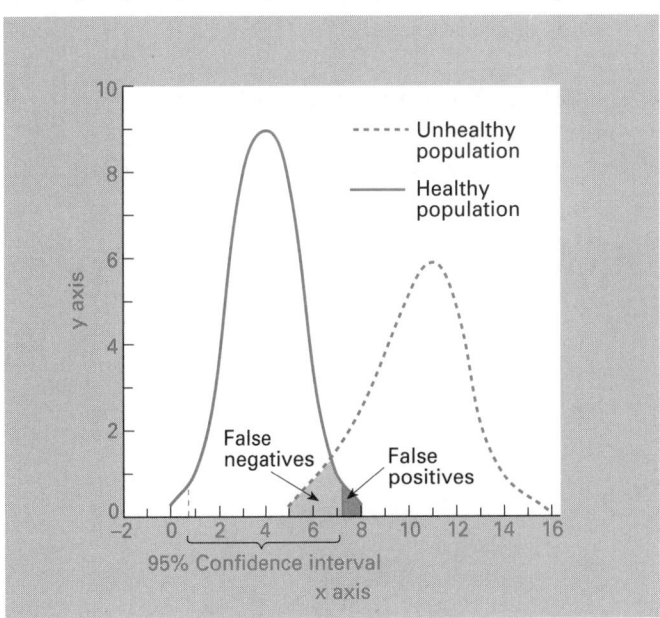

Table 1 *Everyday tests*

Determination	Sample†	SI units	Conventional units
Alcohol	B or P	Legal limit (UK)	
		<17.4 mmol/l	<80 mg/dl
Albumin	P	35–50 g/l	3.5–5.0 g/dl
Albumin—pregnancy	P	25–38 g/l	2.5–3.8 g/dl
Ammonia	P	<40 µmol/l	<68 µg/dl
α-Amylase	P	25–180 somogyi units/dl	46–330 U/l
Anion gap	P		
$(Na^+ + K^+) - (HC)_3^- + Cl^-)$		12–16 mmol/l	12–16 mmol/l
Bilirubin	P	3–17 µmol/l	0.2–1.0 mg/dl
Bicarbonate*	P	22–28 mmol/l	22–28 mEq/l
Calcium (ionized)	P	1.0–1.25 mmol/l	4.0–5.0 mg/dl
Calcium (total)	P	2.12–2.65 mmol/l	8.5–10.6 mg/dl
Calcium (total)—pregnancy	P	1.95–2.35 mmol/l	7.8–9.4 mg/dl
Chloride	P	95–105 mmol/l	95–105 mEq/l
Copper	P	12–26 µmol/l	76–165 mg/dl
Creatinine	P	70–150 µmol/l	0.7–1.7 mg/dl
Creatinine—pregnancy	P	24–68 µmol/l	0.27–0.76 mg/dl
Cholesterol‡	P	3.9–7.8 mmol/l	150–300 mg/dl
Digoxin			
Children	P	2.0–3.0 nmol/l	1.6–2.3 ng/ml
Adults		1.0–2.0 nmol/l	0.8–1.6 ng/ml
Glucose (fasting)	P	4.0–6.0 mmol/l	72–108 mg/dl
Glycated haemoglobin (HbAlC)	B	5–8%	
Iron	S	M 14–31 µmol/l	78–174 µg/dl
		F 11–30 µmol/l	62–168 µg/dl
Total iron-binding capacity (TIBC)	S	45–75 µmol/l	250–420 ug/dl
Lactate			
(venous)	B	0.5–2.2 mmol/l	4.5–19.8 mg/dl
(arterial)		0.5–1.6 mmol/l	4.5–14.4 mg/dl
Lactate	CSF	<2.8 mmol/l	<25.5 mg/dl
Magnesium	P	0.75–1.05 mmol/l	1.5–2.1 mEq/l
Osmolality	P	278–305 mosmol/kg	
Phosphate (inorganic)	P	0.8–1.45 mmol/l	2.48–4.5 mg/dl
Potassium	P	3.5–5.0 mmol/l	3.5–5.0 mEq/l
Protein (total)	P	60–80 g/l	6.0–8.0 g/dl
Sodium	P	135–145 mmol/l	135–145 mEq/l
Urea	P	2.5–6.7 mmol/l	15–40 mg/dl
Urea—pregnancy	P	2.0–4.2 mmol/	12–25 mg/dl
Urea nitrogen	P	1.16–3.12 mmol/l	7.0–18.7 mg/dl
Uric acid*	P	M 210–480 µmol/l	3.5–8.1 mg/dl
	P	F 150–390 µmol/l	2.5–6.5 mg/dl
Uric acid—pregnancy	P	F 100 –270 µmol/l	1.7–4.5 mg/dl
Zinc	P	6–25 µmol/l	39–163 µg/dl

These values are age-dependent.

*See Table 4.

†B = whole blood; S = serum; P = plasma; U = urine.

M = male; F = female.

‡Figures refer to current distribution in the United Kingdom. Desirable upper limit 5.2 mmol/1 (200 mg/100 ml).

Table 2 *Everyday tests for diagnostic enzymes*

Enzyme	Method	Sample[†]	Reference intervals	
Acid phosphatase	Kind King 37°C			
Total		S	1–5	U/L
Prostatic		S	0–1	U/L
Alkaline phosphatase*	Bessey-Lowry 37°C	P	Adult 80–250	U/L
Alanine-transaminase (ALT (SGPT))	Boehringer German OPT 37°C	P	5–35	U/L
Angiotension converting enzyme		S	21–54	U/l
Aspartate-transaminase (AST (SGOT))	Boehringer German OPT 37°C	P	15–42	U/L
α-Amylase	Cassaway 37°C	P	25–180	Somogyi units/dl
Creatine kinase (CK)	Boehringer German NAC activated 37°C	P P	M 24–195 F 24–170	U/L U/L
Creatine kinase MB (CKMB)	Szaszg 37°C		32–184	U/L
Gammaglutamyl transferase (γGT)	Goldbarg *et al.*	P	M 11–51 F 7–35	U/L U/L
Lactate dehydrogenase (total) (LDH)	Scandinavian SCE 37°C	P	110–250	U/L
Pseudocholinesterase		P	2.25–6.9	kU/l

Cholinesterase	Phenotype	Percentage inhibition with	
		Fluoride	Dibucaine
Normal homozygote	$Ch_1{}^UCh_1{}^U$	40–50	82–88
Abnormal homozygote	$Ch_1{}^DCh_1{}^D$	70–81	14–30
	$Ch_1{}^FCh_1{}^F$	30–35	60–73
Abnormal heterozygote	$Ch_1{}^UCh_1{}^D$	44–60	60–68
	$Ch_1{}^UCh_1{}^F$	37–41	70–79
	$Ch_1{}^DCh_1{}^F$	47–52	59–63

Enzyme	Method	Reference intervals	
Urinary *N*-acetyl-β-D-glucosaminidase (NAGase) (in normal urine age 25–35)	Methoxynitrovinylphenol (MNP) release— Cortecs Diagnostics[‡]	M 1.49–4.5 F 2.5–5.4	U/l U/l

These values are age-dependent.

*See Table 4.

[†]S = serum; P = plasma.

M = male; F = female.

[‡] Manley *et al.* (1994). *Diabetic Medicine*, **11**, 534–44.

Table 3 *Blood gases*

		SI units		Conventional units	
Anion $(Na^+ + K^+) - (HCO_3{}^- + Cl^-)$		12–16	mmol/l	12–16	mEq/l
Arterial carbon dioxide	($Pa\text{CO}_2$)	4.7–6.0	kPa	35–45	mmHg
Mixed venous carbon dioxide	($Pv\text{CO}_2$)	5.5–6.8	kPa	41–51	mmHg
Arterial oxygen	($Pa\text{O}_2$)	11.3–12.6	kPa	85–95	mmHg
Mixed venous oxygen	($Pv\text{O}_2$)	4.0—6.0	kPa	30–45	mmHg
Newborn arterial oxygen		5.3–8.0	kPa	40–60	mmHg
H^+ ion activity		36–44	nmol/l	36–44	mEq/l
Arterial pH		7.35–7.45			
Bicarbonate (arterial—whole blood)		19–24	mmol/l	19–24	mmol/l
Bicarbonate (venous—plasma)		22–28	mmol/l	22–28	mmol/l
Bicarbonate (cord blood)		14–22	mmol/l	14–22	mmol/l
Base excess		±2	mmol/l	±2	mEq/l
Carboxyhaemoglobin:					
Non-smoker		<2%			
Smoker		3–15%			
Toxic at		>15%			
Coma at		>50%			

Table 4 *Paediatric reference intervals*

	Sample	SI units		Conventional units	
Alkaline phosphatase (*p*-nitrophenyl phosphate method at 37°C)	P				
<1 year		30–250	IU/l	30–250	IU/l
1–14 years		150–570	IU/l	150–570	IU/l
>14 years		80–250	IU/l	80–250	IU/l
Ammonia	P	<40	μmol/l	<68	mg/dl
Aspartate transaminase	P				
1–3 years		20–60	U/l		
4–6 years		15–50			
Bicarbonate	P				
Infants		18–22	mmol/l	18–22	mEq/l
Older children		20–26	mmol/l	20–26	mEq/l
Bilirubin	P				
First week of life		100–200	μmol/l (total)	6–11.6	mg/dl
After first week of life and		2–14	μmol/l (total)	0.11–0.8	mg/dl
Throughout childhood		0–0.4	μmol/l (direct)	0–0.02	mg/dl
Calcium	P				
1–3 weeks		1.9–2.85	mmol/l	7.6–11.40	mg/dl
3 weeks and above		2.12–2.65	mmol/l	8.5–10.6	mg/dl
β-Carotene	S				
<1 year (upper limit falls with age up to 3½ years)		1.3–6.3	μmol/l	69–338	μg/dl
3½ years onwards		1.9–2.8	μmol/l	102–150	μg/dl
Creatinine*	P				
Cord blood		57–100	μmol/l	0.6–1.13	mg/dl
2 weeks–6 years		33–61	μmol/l	0.37–0.69	mg/dl
6 years–10 years		39–70	μmol/l	0.44–0.80	mg/dl
>12 years		49–81	μmol/l	0.55–0.90	mg/dl
Creatinine clearance 3–13 years	U and P	94–142	ml/min per 1.73 m²		
Creatine kinase (method—CK Boehringer at 37°C)	P				
Neonates		75–400	U/l		
Infants 3–12 months		10–145	U/l		
Children 1–15 years		15–130	U/l		
Glucose (fasting)≠					
Cord	S	2.5–5.3	mmol/l	45–96	mg/dl
premature/low birth weight		1.1–3.3	mmol/l	20–60	mg/dl
Neonate		1.67–3.3	mmol/l	30–60	mg/dl
1 day		2.2–3.3	mmol/l	40–60	mg/dl
1–7 days		2.8–4.6	mmol/l	50–85	mg/dl
>7 days		3.3–5.5	mmol/l	60–100	mg/dl
Immunoreactive trypsin	B	<70	μg/l		
	S	<130	μg/l		
Total protein	P				
First month		51	g/l (mean)		
First year		61	g/l (mean)		
Children					
1–6 years		61–78	g/l		
7–16 years		66–82	g/l		

Immunoglobulins∞	S	IgG (g/l)	IgA (g/l)	IgM (g/l)
Cord		5.2–18.0	0–0.02	0.02–0.2
Weeks				
0–2		5.0–17.0	0.01–0.08	0.05–0.2
2–6		3.9–13.0	0.02–0.15	0.08–0.4
6–12		2.1–7.7	0.05–0.4	0.15–0.7

	Sample	SI units		Conventional units
		IgG (g/l)	IgA (g/l)	IgM (g/l)
Months				
3–6		2.4–8.8	0.1–0.5	0.2–1.0
6–9		3.0–9.0	0.15–0.7	0.4–1.6
9–12		3.0–10.9	0.20–0.7	0.6–2.1
Years				
1–2		3.1–13.8	0.3–1.2	0.5–2.2
2–3		3.7–15.8	0.3–1.3	0.5–2.2
3–6		4.9–16.1	0.4–2.0	0.5–2.0
6–9		5.4–16.1	0.5–2.4	0.5–1.8
9–12		5.4–16.1	0.8–2.8	0.5–1.9
12–15		5.4–16.1	0.8–2.8	0.5–1.9

	Sample	SI units		Conventional	
Lactate	P} venous	0.5–2.2	mmol/l	4.5–19.8	mg/dl
	} arterial	0.5–1.6	mmol/l	4.5–14.4	mg/dl
	B	0.5–1.7	mmol/l	4.5–15.3	mg/dl
	CSF	<2.8	mmol/l	<25.5	mg/dl
Metadrenaline: urine (upper limits of normal in children: total metadrenaline					
0–1 years	U	2.8	mmol/mol creatinine	4.5	μg/mg creatinine
1–2		3.0	mmol/mol creatinine	5.4	μg/mg creatinine
2–5		1.8	mmol/mol creatinine	3.0	μg/mg creatinine
5–10		1.6	mmol/mol creatinine	2.8	μg/mg creatinine
10–15		1.0	mmol/mol creatinine	1.8	μg/mg creatinine
15–18		0.5	mmol/mol creatinine	0.7	μg/mg creatinine
Phosphate (inorganic)·	P				
Newborn		1.20–2.78	mmol/l	3.7–8.6	mg/dl
Young children		1.29–1.78	mmol/l	4.0–5.5	mg/dl
15 years (girls)		0.9–1.38	mmol/l	2.8–4.3	mg/dl
17 years (boys) (over the age of 7 years there is a steady fall to reach adult levels at 15–17 years)		0.83–1.49	mmol/l	2.6–4.6	mg/dl
Potassium	P				
Newborn		up to 6.6	mmol/l		
Older than 1 month–6 years		4.1–5.6	mmol/l		
Boys 7–16 years		3.3–4.7	mmol/l		
Girls 7–16		3.4–4.5	mmol/l		
Uric acid	P				
Childhood (will rise until adulthood—further during puberty in boys but not in girls)		0.06–0.24	mmol/l	1.0–4.0	mg/dl
Boys 16 years		0.23–0.46	mmol/l	3.8–7.7	mg/dl
Girls 16 years		0.19–0.36	mmol/l	3.2–6.0	mg/dl
Thyroid stimulating hormone outside neonatal period	S	0.5–5.0	mU/l	0.5–5.0	μU/ml
Sweat sodium		10–40	mmol/l	10–40	mEq/l
Sweat chloride		0–30	mmol/l	0–30	mEq/l

*Values depend also on gestational age.

⌐Typical definition of hypoglycaemia:
low birth weight	<1.5 mmol/l	<27 mg/dl
normal weight 0–3 days	<1.7 mmol/l	<31 mg/dl
>3 days	<2.2 mmol/l	<40 mg/dl

∞Values taken from Milford Ward, A., Riches, P. G., Fifield, R., and Smith, A.M. (eds.) (1993). *Handbook of Clinical Immunochemistry.* 4th edn. PRU Publications. (ISBN 0-948722-03-7).

·Affected by diet—particularly milk fed.

P = plasma; S = serum; U = urine; B = whole blood; CSF = cerebrospinal fluid.

33 REFERENCE INTERVALS FOR BIOCHEMICAL DATA

Table 5 *Hormones*

	Sample	SI units		Conventional units	
Adrenaline	P	0.03–1.31	mmol/l	6–240	ng/ml
Noradrenaline	P	0.47–4.14	mmol/l	9–760	ng/ml
ACTH	P	3.3–15.4	pmol/l	<10–80	ng/l
Adrenaline	U	<100	nmol/24 h	11–49	µg/24 h
Aldosterone	P	Recumbant 100–450 Midday-twofold increase of recumbant level	pmol/l	3–13	ng/dl
Aldosterone[≠]	U	10–50	nmol/24 h	4–18	mg/24 h
Angiotension II	P	5–35	pmol/l	5.2–36.0	pg/ml
Antidiuretic hormone (ADH)	P	0.9–4.6	pmol/l	1–5	ng/l
Calcitonin	P	<27	pmol/l	<100	ng/l
Catecholamines	U	<2.6	µmol/24 h	<440	µg/24 h
Cortisol	P	00:00 h 80–280	nmol/l	3–10	µg/dl
		09:00 h 280–700	nmol/l	10–25	µg/dl
(free)	U	<280	mmol/24 h	<10	µg/dl
Follicular stimulating hormone	P/S				
Follicular phase		0.5–5.0	U/l	0.5–5.0	mIU/ml
Ovulatory peak		8–15	U/l	8–15	mIU/ml
Luteal phase		2–8	U/l	2–8	mIU/ml
Postmenopause		>30	U/l	>30	mIU/ml
Male		0.5–5.0	U/l	0.5–5.0	mIU/ml
Gastrin	P	<40	pmol/l	<80	ng/l
Glucagon	P	<50	pmol/l	<17.7	ng/dl
Growth hormone	P	<20	mU/l	<20	µU/ml
Human chorionic gonadotrophin	S	<5	U/l	<5	U/ml
Insulin (fasting)	P	<15	mU/l	<15	µU/ml
Insulin C-peptide (fasting)	P	<0.4	nmol/l		
Insulin-like growth factor 1	P	0.52–3.4	kU/l	0.52–3.4	U/ml
Luteinizing hormone	P/S				
Premenopausal		6–13	U/l	6–13	mIU/ml
Follicular phase		3–12	U/l	3–12	mIU/ml
Ovulatory peak		20–80	U/l	20–80	mIU/ml
Luteal phase		3–16	U/l	3–16	mIU/ml
Postmenopause		>30	U/l	>30	mIU/ml
Male		3–8	U/l	3–8	mIU/ml
Normetadrenaline (adults)	U	<3	µmol/24 h		
Metadrenaline (adults)	U	<2	µmol/24 h		
3-Methoxytyramine (adults)	U	<2	µmol/24 h		
Neurotensin	P	<100	pmol/l		
17β-Oestradiol	P				
Follicular phase		75–260	pmol/l	20–70	pg/ml
Mid cycle		370–1470	pmol/l	100–400	pg/ml
Luteal phase		180–1100	pmol/l	50–300	pg/ml
Male		<220	pmol/l	<60	pg/ml
Parathormone (intact)	P	<0.9–5.4	pmol/l	3.6–22	mg/dl
Pancreatic polypeptide (PP)	P	<200	pmol/l	<830	ng/l
Progesterone	P	M <5	nmol/l	<1.6	ng/ml
Post ovulation		F 15–77	nmol/l	4.7–24	ng/ml
Follicular		<3	nmol/l	<1	ng/ml
17-Hydroxyprogesterone	P (newborn)	7–16	nmol/l	230–530	ng/dl
Prolactin	P	M <450	U/l	<450	mIU/ml
		F <600	U/l	<600	mIU/ml
Renin activity	P				
Recumbent		1.1–2.7	pmol/ml/h	4.8–11.9	µg/dl/h
Erect after 30 min		3.0–4.3	pmol/ml/h	13.2–19	µg/dl/h
Depends on diuretics, salt intake, etc.					

	Sample	SI units		Conventional units	
Sex hormone binding protein	S	M 10–62	nmol/l		
		F 40–137	nmol/l		
Somatostatin	P	<100	pmol/l	<16.3	ng/dl
Testosterone	P/S	M 9–42	nmol/l	2.6–12.1	ng/ml
		F 1–2.5	nmol/l	0.3–0.7	ng/ml
Thyroid stimulating hormone	P	0.5–5.5	mU/l	0.5–5.5	mIU/ml
Thyroid binding globulin	P	13–28	mg/l	13–28	mg/l
Tri-iodothyronine (T3)		1.0–3.0	nmol/l	65–195	ng/dl
Free T$_3$ (FT3)		3.3–8.2	pmol/l	214–533	pg/dl
Thyroxine (T4)	P	70–140	nmol/l	5.4–10.7	μg/dl
Free T$_4$ (FT4)	P	9–25	pmol/l	0.7–1.7	ng/dl
Vasoactive intestinal polypeptide (VIP)	P	<30	pmol/l	<100	ng/l

Care should be taken in infants and children in the interpretation of normal ranges.

*Values vary with dietary sodium and plasma renin activity.

P = plasma; U = urine; S = serum.

Table 6 *Tumour markers*

	Sample	Normal range	
Alpha-fetoprotein (AFP)	S	<10	kU/l
Carcinoembryonic antigen (CEA)	S	<10	μg/l
Neurone specific enolase	S	<12	μg/l
Prostatic specific antigen* (PSA)	S	<4	μg/l
Human chorionic gonadotrophin (HCG)	S	<5	IU/l
Ca125	S	<35	U/ml
Ca19–9	S	<33	U/ml

*Hybridtec assay.

S = serum.

Table 7 *Vitamins and related tests*

Vitamins	Sample	SI units		Conventional units	
Vitamin A					
Retinol	S	M 1.06–3.35	μmol/l	30–96	μg/dl
		F 0.84–2.95	μmol/l	24–84	μg/dl
β-Carotene*	S	M 0.01–6.52	μmol/l	0.5–350	μg/dl
		F 0.019–2.93	μmol/l	1.02–158	μg/dl
Thiamine (B$_1$)	P	>40	nmol/l	>1	μg/dl
As red cell thiamine diphosphate	B			320–550	ng/g haemoglobin
As red cell transketolase		<1.3	TPP α effect		
Riboflavine (B$_2$)					
As red cell glutathione reductase	B	<70% activation			
Pyridoxine (B$_6$)					
As red cell aspartate transaminase	B	<150% activation			
Vitamin B$_{12}$	S	150–750	ng/l		
Folate	S	4.8–6.4	nmol/l	2.1–2.8	μg/l
	B (red cell)	0.36–1.44	μmol/l	160–640	g/l
Vitamin D metabolites:					
25-OHD*	S	17–125	nmol/l	7–50	μg/l
1,25 (OH)D$_3$		50–120	pmol/l	20–50	pg/ml
Vitamin E (α-tocopherol)	S	11.5–35	μmol/l	5–15	μg/ml

*See Table 4.

*Upper limit reduced by ~ one-half in winter.

S = serum; P = plasma; B = blood. M = male; F = female.

Table 8 *Intermediary metabolities (after overnight fast)*

	Age 21–40 years		Age 41–60 years		Age 61–75 years	
	Conventional units	SI units	Conventional units	SI units	Conventional units	SI units
Glucose	75.2–98.8 mg/dl	4.18–5.9 mmol/l	71.6–108 mg/dl	3.98–6.02 mmol/l	73–109 mg/dl	4.06–6.07 mmol/l
Lactate	3.56–10.72 mg/dl	0.40–1.19 mmol/l	3.69–10.22 mg/dl	0.41–1.14 mmol/l	4.15–8.73 mg/dl	0.46–0.97 mmol/l
Pyruvate	0.02–0.14 μg/dl	0.03–0.16 mmol/l	0.03–0.13 μg/dl	0.03–0.14 mmol/l	0.03–0.10 μg/dl	0.03–0.12 mmol/l
Alanine	1.63–4.2 mg/dl	0.18–0.48 mmol/l	1.83–4.0 mg/dl	0.21–0.45 mmol/l	1.51–3.42 mg/dl	0.17–0.39 mmol/l
Glycerol	0.25–0.93 mg/dl	0.03–0.10 mmol/l	0.28–0.85 mg/dl	0.03–0.10 mmol/l	0.30–1.28 mg/dl	0.03–0.14 mmol/l
Non-esterified fatty acids	1.59–18.6 mg/dl	0.06–0.7 mmol/l	5.32–19.9 mg/dl	0.20–0.75 mmol/l	3.99–23.6 mg/dl	0.15–0.89 mmol/l
3-Hydroxy-butyrate	0.05–3.48 mg/dl	0.01–0.34 mmol/l	0.10–2.25 mg/dl	0.01–0.22 mmol/l	0.13–6.46 mg/dl	0.01–0.62 mmol/l
Acetoacetate	0.1–1.46 mg/dl	0.01–0.15 mmol/l	0.07–1.60 mg/dl	0.01–0.16 mmol/l	0.09–2.82 mg/dl	0.01–0.28 mmol/l
Total ketone bodies		0.02–0.44 mmol/l		0.02–0.30 mmol/l		0.02–0.84 mmol/l
Triglyceride	27.4–222 mg/dl	0.31–2.51 mmol/l	47.8–195 mg/dl	0.54–2.20 mmol/l	46.9–226 mg/dl	0.53–2.56 mmol/l
Insulin		1.8–15.0 m.i.u./l		2.0–13.2 m.i.u./l		1.9–12.3 m.i.u./l

Values from one Unit (Newcastle/Southampton, UK). Alberti, K. G. (1978). *Clinical Chemistry,* **24,** 1591.

Table 9 *Lipids and lipoproteins*

	Sample	SI units		Conventional units	
Cholesterol*	P	3.9–7.8	mmol/l	150–300	mg/dl
Ideal upper limit		5.2	mmol/l	200	mg/dl
Acceptable upper limit		6.5	mmol/l	250	mg/dl
Triglyceride (fasting)	P	0.55–1.90	mmol/l	48.6–168	mg/dl
Non-esterified (free) fatty acids (NEFA)	S	M 0.19–0.78	mmol/l	5.1–20.9	mg/dl
		F 0.06–0.9	mmol/l	1.6–24	mg/dl
Lipoproteins (as cholesterol)					
LDL	S	1.55–4.4	mmol/l	60–170	mg/dl
Ideal upper limit		3.4	mmol/l	130	mg/dl
Acceptable upper limit		4.2	mmol/l	160	mg/dl
HDL	S	0.8–2.0	mmol/l	30–77	mg/dl
Ideal	S	M >0.9	mmol/l	>35	mg/dl
Ideal		F >1.2	mmol/l	>46	mg/dl

*Values increase with age.

P = plasma; S = serum.

Table 10 *Proteins and immunoproteins*

	Samples	Reference interval	
Albumin	P	35–50	g/l
α_1-Antitrypsin	S	107–209	mg/l
β_1-Transferrin	S	1.2–2.0	g/l
Complement C_3		65–190	mg/dl
C_4		15–50	mg/dl
Caeruloplasmin	S	16–60	mg/dl
C1 esterase inhibitor	S	15–35	mg/dl
C-reactive protein (CRP)	S	<10	mg/l
CSF IgG/albumin ratio		<22	%
Ferritin	S	14–200	µg/l
Fibrinogen	P	2–4	g/l
Fibrinogen degradation products	S	<0.8	µg/l
Haptoglobins	S	0.6–2.6	g/l
Immunoglobulins*			
IgG	S	6.0–13.0	g/l
IgA		0.8–3.0	g/l
IgM		0.4–2.5	g/l
IgE		<120	kU/l
Total protein	P	60–80	g/l
	U	<140	g/l
β_2-Microglobulin	S	<3	mg/l
	U	4–370	µg/l or 30–370 µg/24 h
Thyroid microsomal antibodies	S	M <1/400	
	S	F (<44 years) <1/400	
	S	F (>44 years) <1/6400	
Viscosity	S	1.4–1.9	(ratio to water)

*See Table 4.

P = plasma; S = serum; U = urine.

P

Erratum

These entries are missing from the printed index